Unit VIII Hematologic System

Unit IX Cardiovascular and Lymphatic Systems

Unit X Pulmonary System

Unit XI Renal and Urologic Systems

Unit XII Digestive System

Unit XIII Musculoskeletal System

Unit XIV Integumentary System

Unit XV Multiple Interacting Systems

PATHOPHYSIOLOGY

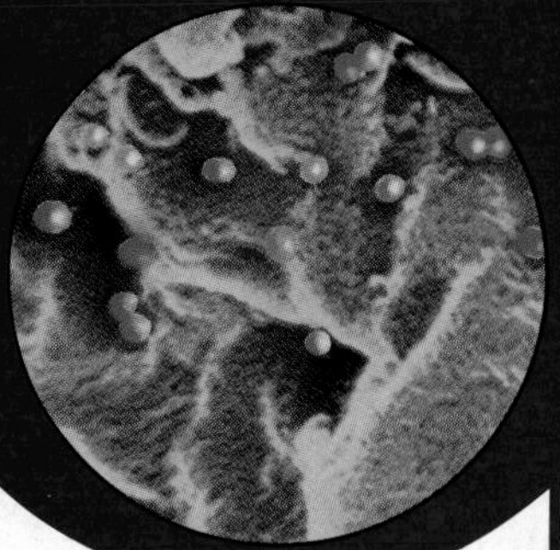

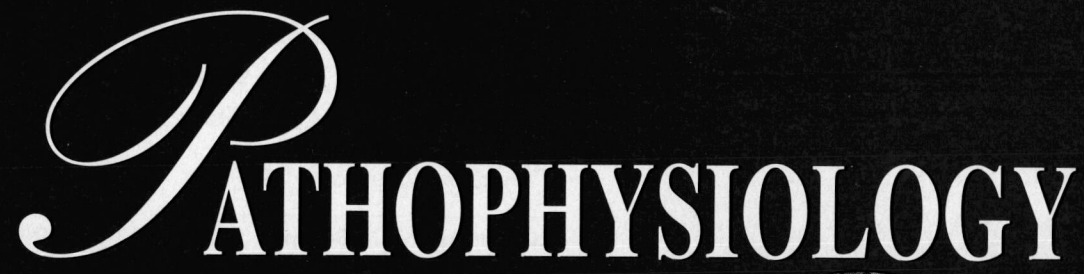

THE BIOLOGIC BASIS FOR DISEASE IN ADULTS & CHILDREN

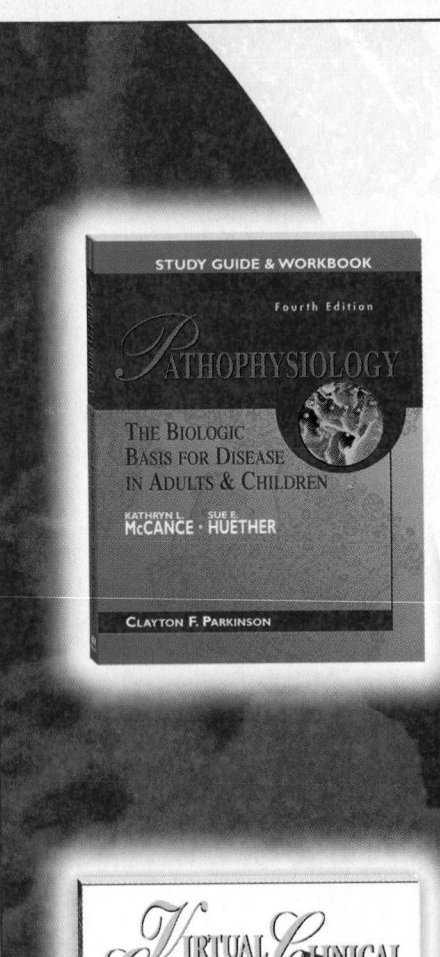

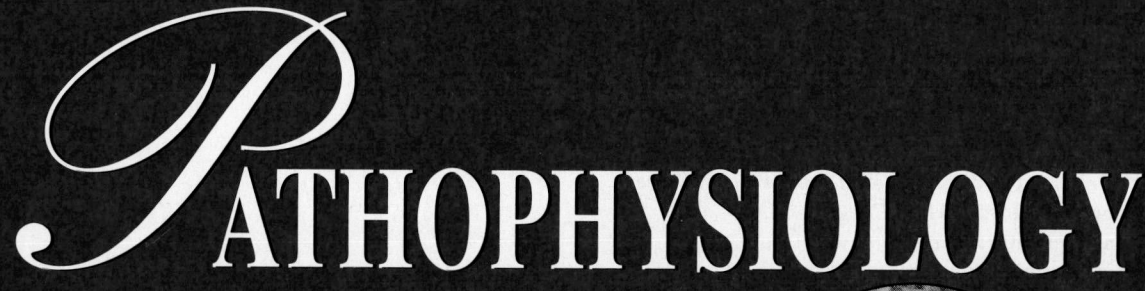

PATHOPHYSIOLOGY

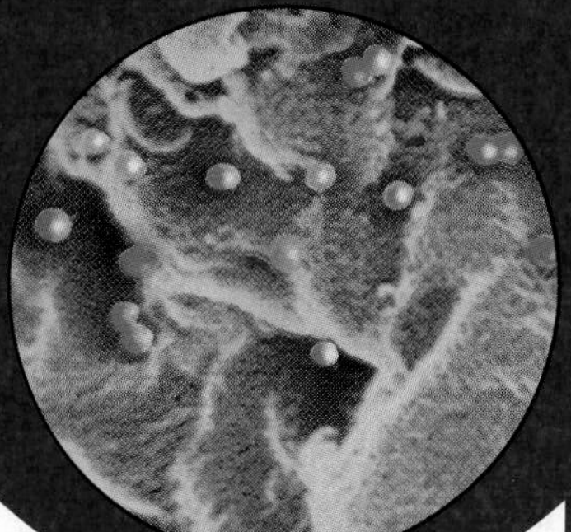

THE BIOLOGIC BASIS FOR DISEASE IN ADULTS & CHILDREN

KATHRYN L. McCANCE, RN, PhD
Professor, College of Nursing
University of Utah
Salt Lake City, Utah

SUE E. HUETHER, RN, PhD
Professor, College of Nursing
University of Utah
Salt Lake City, Utah

Fourth Edition
With 1400 illustrations

Mosby
An Affiliate of Elsevier

Mosby
An Affiliate of Elsevier

Vice President and Publishing Director: *Sally Schrefer*
Executive Editor: *Darlene Como*
Managing Editor: *Brian Dennison*
Project Manager: *Catherine Jackson*
Project Specialist: *Jeff Patterson*
Designer: *Kathi Gosche*

FOURTH EDITION

NOTICE
Pharmacology is an ever-changing field. Standard safety precautions must be followed, but as new research and clinical experience broaden our knowledge, changes in treatment and drug therapy may become necessary or appropriate. Readers are advised to check the most current product information provided by the manufacturer of each drug to be administered to verify the recommended dose, the method and duration of administration, and contraindications. It is the responsibility of the licensed prescriber, relying on experience and knowledge of the patient, to determine dosages and the best treatment for each individual patient. Neither the Publisher nor the editors assume any liability for any injury and/or damage to persons or property arising from this publication.

Mosby, Inc.
11830 Westline Industrial Drive
St. Louis, Missouri 63146

Printed in China

ISBN 0-323-01438-0

05 06 07 08 09 9 8 7 6 5 4

CONTRIBUTORS

Pat Wills Alcoser, MSN, CPNP
Pediatric Nurse Practitioner
Texas Children's Hospital
Houston, Texas

Kathleen M. Baldwin, RN, PhD, CEN, CCRN, ANP, GNP
Associate Professor and Director of Graduate Studies
Harris School of Nursing
Texas Christian University
Fort Worth, Texas

Barbara J. Boss, RN, PhD, CFNP, CANP
Professor of Nursing, School of Nursing
University of Mississippi Medical Center
Jackson, Mississippi

Valentina L. Brashers, MD
Associate Professor of Nursing
Clinical Assistant Professor of Medicine
University of Virginia Health Sciences Center
Charlottesville, Virginia

Kristen Lee Carroll, MD
Assistant Professor, Department of Orthopedics
University of Utah
Salt Lake City, Utah

Jean Anne Connor, RN, MS, CPNP
Pediatric Nurse Practitioner
Stonybrook Division of Pediatric Cardiology
University Hospital and Medical Center
Stonybrook, New York

Christy L. Crowther, RN, BSN, MS, CRNP
Adult Nurse Practitioner
Chesapeake Orthopaedic & Sports Medicine Center
Glen Burnie, Maryland;
Clinical Instructor, Department of Family Medicine
University of Maryland School of Medicine
Baltimore, Maryland

Deborah B. Evers, RN, DNS(c), CPN
Associate Professor, Parent-Child Nursing
Charity School of Nursing
Delgado Community College
New Orleans, Louisiana

Deborah K. Froh, MD
Assistant Professor of Pediatrics
University of Virginia
Charlottesville, Virginia

Todd C. Grey, MD
Chief Medical Examiner, State of Utah;
Associate Clinical Professor, Department of Pathology
University of Utah School of Medicine
Salt Lake City, Utah

Mary Fran Hazinski, RN, MSN, FAAN
Clinical Specialist, Division of Trauma
Departments of Surgery and Pediatrics
Vanderbilt University Medical Center;
Consultant, Pediatric Critical Care
Vanderbilt Children's Hospital
Nashville, Tennessee

Marilyn Jo Hockenberry, RN-CS, PhD, PNP, FAAN
Professor, Baylor College of Medicine;
Director of Nurse Practitioners
Texas Children's Cancer Center
Texas Children's Hospital
Houston, Texas

Carolyn Hollingshead, PhD, RD
Adjunct Instructor (Clinical)
Division of Foods and Nutrition
University of Utah
Salt Lake City, Utah

Marilyn E. Jenkins, RN, MBA, CNA
Director of Nursing
Cincinnati Burns Hospital
Shriners Hospitals for Children
Cincinnati, Ohio

Robert E. Jones, MD
Associate Clinical Professor
Department of Endocrinology
University of Utah School of Medicine
Salt Lake City, Utah

Lynn B. Jorde, PhD
Professor and Associate Chairman
Department of Human Genetics
University of Utah School of Medicine
Salt Lake City, Utah

Elizabeth Kassner, RN, MS, CPNP, CPON
Pediatric Nurse Practitioner
Texas Children's Cancer Center
Texas Children's Hospital
Baylor College of Medicine
Houston, Texas

Nancy E. Kline, RN, PhD, CPNP
Assistant Professor of Pediatrics
Baylor College of Medicine;
Pediatric Nurse Practitioner
Texas Children's Hospital
Houston, Texas

Jonathan Leo, PhD
Associate Professor of Anatomy
Western University of Health Sciences
Pomona, California

Thom J. Mansen, RN, PhD
Associate Professor, College of Nursing
University of Utah
Salt Lake City, Utah

Stephen E. Morris, MD, FACS
Associate Professor of Surgery
Co-Director, Intermountain Burn Center
Salt Lake City, Utah

Leona A. Mourad, RN, MS, ONC
Associate Professor Emeritus
Ohio State University, College of Nursing
Columbus, Ohio;
Nursing Consultant
Mourad Consultant Associates
Santa Barbara, California

Noreen Heer Nicol, RN, MS, FNP
Dermatology Clinical Specialist/Nurse Practitioner
Chief Clinical Officer
National Jewish Medical and Research Center;
Clinical Senior Instructor
University of Colorado School of Nursing
Denver, Colorado

Katherine Padgett, RN, MN
Associate Professor, Charity School of Nursing
Delgado Community College
New Orleans, Louisiana

Marianne R. Piano, RN, PhD
Associate Professor
University of Illinois at Chicago
Chicago, Illinois

Lee K. Roberts, PhD
Senior Vice President of Research and Technical Development
PowderJect Vaccines, Inc.
Madison, Wisconsin

Kristynia M. Robinson, RN, PhD, FNPc
Associate Professor of Nursing;
Director of Grants and Research
Idaho State University
Pocatello, Idaho

Neal S. Rote, PhD
Director of Research
Department of Obstetrics and Gynecology
MetroHealth Medical Center;
Professor of Reproductive Biology and Pathology
Case Western Reserve School of Medicine
Cleveland, Ohio

Jane Shelby, PhD
Associate Professor of Surgery
Department of Surgery
University of Utah
Salt Lake City, Utah

Richard A. Sugerman, PhD
Professor of Anatomy
Western University of Health Sciences
Pomona, California

Lorey Takahashi, PhD
Assistant Professor, Department of Psychology
University of Hawaii
Honolulu, Hawaii

REVIEWERS

Sr. Rose Terese Bahr, RN, PhD, FAAN
Professor of Nursing and Chair
Division of Community Health Nursing
School of Nursing, Catholic University of America
Washington, DC

Jane Ball, RN, DrPH, CPNP
Director, Emergency Medical Services for Children
National Resource Center
Children's National Medical Center
Washington, DC

Beverly Bartlett, RN, PhD
Assistant Professor, College of Nursing
University of Rhode Island
Kingston, Rhode Island

Mary K. Beard, MD, FACOG
Clinical Professor, Department of Obstetrics and Gynecology
University of Utah;
Private Practice, LDS Hospital
Salt Lake City, Utah

Carroll Conner Bouman, RN, PhD
Clinical Nurse Specialist in Cardiopulmonary Nursing;
Faculty Member, School of Nursing
University of Rochester
Rochester, New York

John Carey, MD, MPH
Associate Professor
Chief, Division of Medical Genetics
School of Medicine, University of Utah
Salt Lake City, Utah

Dana H. Clarke, MD
Medical Director, Diabetes Health Center
Salt Lake City, Utah

Miguel da Cunha, PhD
Associate Professor
University of Texas Health Sciences Center at Houston
Houston, Texas

Joyce Dains, RN, DrPH, JD, CS, FNP
Assistant Professor, Baylor College of Medicine
Houston, Texas

Lydia DeCastro-Svetich, RN, MS
Associate Professor, Orvis School of Nursing
University of Nevada, Reno
Reno, Nevada

Carol DeMoss, RN, MS, CS
Clinical Nurse Specialist
Visiting Nurse Association of Allegheny County
Pittsburgh, Pennsylvania

Dennis M. DePace, PhD
Department of Anatomy, Hahnemann University
Philadelphia, Pennsylvania

Dorothy Doughty, RN, MN, CETN
Program Director
Enterostomal Therapy Nursing Education Program
Emory University
Atlanta, Georgia

Harmon J. Eyre, MD
Professor of Medicine, Division of Hematology/Oncology
School of Medicine, University of Utah
Salt Lake City, Utah

Kathy Gardner, MS(c)
Instructor, Pathophysiology
North Dakota State University
Fargo, North Dakota

Nancy Gibson, RN, FNP
Salt Lake City, Utah

Mikel Gray, RN, PhD, CUNP, CCCN, FAAN
Nurse Practitioner and Associate Professor
Department of Urology and School of Nursing
University of Virginia
Charlottesville, Virginia

Judith Hall, RN, PhD
Assistant Professor, School of Nursing
University of Texas at Arlington
Arlington, Texas

Laurel Halloran, RN, PhD
Assistant Professor, Clinical Nurse Specialist
Department of Nursing
Western Connecticut State University
Danbury, Connecticut

K.C. Hayes, DVM, PhD
Director, Foster Biomedical Research Center;
Professor and Chairman, Biology Department
Brandeis University
Waltham, Massachusetts

List includes reviewers of first, second, third, and fourth editions.

Mary Beth Hayward, RN, MSN
Associate Professor, School of Nursing
Medical College of Ohio
Toledo, Ohio

Ruthellyn Hinton, RN, MS, MN
Associate Professor, School of Nursing
Pittsburg State University
Pittsburg, Kansas

Marilyn Humphrey, RN, MA
Coordinator, Nursing Program
Chabot College
Hayward, California

Kirtly Parker Jones, MD
Associate Professor and Vicechair for Academic Affairs
Department of Obstetrics and Gynecology
University of Utah
Salt Lake City, Utah

Linda Jones, RN, MS, CS, OCN
Assistant to the Associate Director for Nursing Oncology
University of Rochester Cancer Center;
Assistant Professor of Clinical Nursing
University of Rochester School of Nursing
Rochester, New York

Norman L. Keltner, RN, EdD, CRNP
Associate Professor
University of Alabama School of Nursing
University of Alabama at Birmingham
Birmingham, Alabama

Sr. Joan Klemballa, RN, MA
Associate Professor, Division of Nursing Education
University of District of Columbia
Washington, DC

Helene J. Krouse, RN, PhD
Assistant Professor, School of Nursing
Boston College
Chestnut Hill, Massachusetts

Michele T. Laraia, RN, PhD
Assistant Professor, College of Medicine
Department of Psychiatry and Behavioral Sciences
Medical University of South Carolina
Charleston, South Carolina

Renee Leasure, RN, PhD, CCRN
Assistant Professor, School of Nursing
University of Oklahoma
Oklahoma City, Oklahoma

Mary Lentz, RN, PhD
Assistant Professor, School of Nursing
University of Pittsburgh
Pittsburgh, Pennsylvania

Stacey Levine, RN, PhD
Associate Professor, University of Alberta
Clinical Sciences Department
Edmonton, Alberta, Canada

Leslie Marshall, RN, PhD
Associate Professor, College of Nursing
University of Iowa
Iowa City, Iowa

Patricia Maybee, RN, MS, CCRN
Department of Instruction, College of Nursing
Clemson University
Clemson, South Carolina

Mary Beth McDowell, RN, MN
Assistant Professor, College of Allied Health and Nursing
Eastern Kentucky University
Richmond, Kentucky

Mary Ellen McMorrow, RN, EdD, CCRN
Professor, Department of Nursing
College of Staten Island, City University of New York
Staten Island, New York

Diane Melancon, RN, MSN
Associate Professor of Nursing Education
San Antonio College
San Antonio, Texas

Christine Miaskowski, RN, PhD, FAAN
Professor and Chair, Department of Physiological Nursing
University of California
San Francisco, California

Kenneth Morgan, PhD
Associate Professor
Department of Epidemiology and Biostatistics
McGill University
Montreal, Canada

Leona A. Mourad, RN, MS, ONC
Associate Professor, Emeritus
The Ohio State University;
Nursing Consultant, Mourad Consultant Associates
Dublin, Ohio

Christine Mudge-Grout, RN, MS
Clinical Nurse Specialist, Nephrology/Transplant
Department of Nursing
University of California at San Francisco
San Francisco, California

Virginia L. Neelon, RN, PhD
Associate Professor, School of Nursing
University of North Carolina at Chapel Hill
Chapel Hill, North Carolina

Mary Ann Nihart, RN, MA, CS
Clinical Nurse Specialist, Turning Point Center
San Francisco, California

Donna Patterson, RN, MSN
Assistant Professor, College of Nursing
Villanova University
Villanova, Pennsylvania

Ann Peterson, RN, BS, BSN
Endocrine Clinical Nurse Specialist
Nursing Department, National Institutes of Health
Bethesda, Maryland

Karen A. Pfeifer, RN, MSN, CNA, ONC
Director of Nursing Resources
Zale Lipshy University Hospital
Dallas, Texas

Nancy Redeker, RN, MSN, PhD
Instructor, College of Nursing
Rutgers University
Newark, New Jersey

Linda L. Robertson, RN, PhD
Assistant Professor, School of Nursing
University of Pittsburgh
Pittsburgh, Pennsylvania

Connie Robinson, RN, MN
Assistant Professor, School of Nursing
University of California at San Francisco
San Francisco, California

David B. Roll, PhD
Professor of Medicinal Chemistry
College of Pharmacy, University of Utah
Salt Lake City, Utah

Amy Perrin Ross, RN, MSN, CNRN
Neuroscience Clinical Nurse Specialist
Loyola University Medical Center
Maywood, Illinois;
Triton College
Continuing Education Center for Health Professionals
River Grove, Illinois

Phyllis Russo, RN, EdD
Chairperson, Undergraduate Nursing
College of Nursing, Seton Hall University
South Orange, New Jersey

Ann Sedore, RN, PhD
Associate Professor, College of Nursing
Syracuse University
Syracuse, New York

Janice Selekman, RN, DNSc
Associate Professor
Generic Baccalaureate Program Director
Department of Nursing, Thomas Jefferson University
Philadelphia, Pennsylvania

Mary Ann Siefert, RN, MS
Primary Childrens Hospital
Salt Lake City, Utah

Barbara Peterson Sinclair, RN, MN
Director, OB/GYN Nurse Practitioner Program
School of Nursing, California State University
Los Angeles, California

Patricia A. Stuckey, RN, MSN, OCN
Assistant Professor, Medical-Surgical Nursing
Virginia Commonwealth University
Medical College of Virginia School of Nursing
Richmond, Virginia

Patricia J. Thompson, RN, PhD
Associate Professor, College of Nursing
University of Arkansas for Medical Sciences
Little Rock, Arkansas

Arthur Vander, PhD
Department of Physiology, University of Michigan
Ann Arbor, Michigan

Filomena Varvaro, RN, PhD
Assistant Professor, School of Nursing
University of Pittsburgh
Pittsburgh, Pennsylvania

Sharon Wahl, RN, MSN, EdD
Professor, Department of Nursing
San Jose State University
San Jose, California

Eleanor A. Walker, BNS, MS
Assistant Professor, School of Nursing
Catholic University of America
Washington, DC

Connie A. Walleck, RN, MS, FCCM
Senior Associate Director of Nursing
University Hospital, SUNY Health Science Center
Syracuse, New York

Lin C. Weeks, RN, MS, CNAA
Administrative Director, Hospital Education
Hermann Hospital
Houston, Texas

Pamela B. Weilitz, RN, MSN
Pulmonary Clinical Nurse Specialist
Barnes Hospital
St. Louis, Missouri

Raymond L. White, PhD
Professor and Co-Chairman, Human Genetics Department
Investigator of Howard Hughes Medical Institute
School of Medicine, University of Utah
Salt Lake City, Utah

Gail M. Wilkes, RN, MS, OCN
Clinical Nurse Specialist in Oncology
Boston City Hospital
Boston, Massachusetts

Elizabeth Hahn Winslow, RN, PhD, FAAN
Associate Professor, School of Nursing
University of Texas at Arlington
Arlington, Texas

PREFACE

The fourth edition of *Pathophysiology: The Biologic Basis for Disease in Adults and Children* is better than ever. Thorough updating of content with state-of-the-art information was our top priority. In addition, the following specific goals were achieved:

- Increased attention to differences in etiology and epidemiology, pathophysiology, clinical manifestations, and treatment according to gender and age
- Linkage of relevant contemporary biology to all disease states
- Increased integration of health promotion and disease prevention with updating of risk factors, the relationship between nutrition and disease, screening recommendations, and other therapeutic approaches
- Scrupulous attention to presentations of emerging new data on controversial topics such as the role of hormones in cancer causation

ORGANIZATION AND CONTENT: WHAT'S NEW IN THE FOURTH EDITION?

The organization of this textbook has been well received and therefore was not changed for this edition. The book is divided into two parts—Part One: "Central Concepts of Pathophysiology: Cells and Tissues," and Part Two: "Pathophysiologic Alterations: Organs and Systems."

Part One: Central Concepts of Pathophysiology: Cells and Tissues

Part One begins with an in-depth study of the cell and progresses to cover the underlying processes of disease. Concepts covered include cell signaling and cell communication processes; cytokines and their biologic activities; genes and common genetic diseases; cell injury; fluid and electrolyte and acid-base balance; immunity, inflammation, and wound healing; stress, coping, and illness; and tumor biology and metastasis. Significant revisions and additions to Part One include the following:

- Newly discovered cellular organelles—for example, vaults and cellular adhesion molecules
- New section on signal transduction
- Major rewrite on chemokines and inflammation
- New content on tissue transplantation and fungal infection, and a partially rewritten discussion of AIDS
- Extensively rewritten content on environmental risk factors and genes implicated in cancer
- New section on detoxification and cancer

Part Two: Pathophysiologic Alterations: Organs and Tissues

Part Two is a systematic survey of diseases within body systems. Each unit focuses on a specific body system and begins with an anatomy and physiology chapter to provide a basis of comparison for understanding the alterations brought about by disease. The discussion of each disease in the alterations chapters is developed in a logical manner that begins with an introductory paragraph on etiology and epidemiology, followed by pathophysiology, clinical manifestations, and evaluation and treatment. Separate chapters are dedicated to pediatric pathophysiology, and sensitivity is paid to gender and age. Significant revisions and additions to Part Two include the following:

- New content on the mechanisms of chronic pain
- Extensive rewrite of Chapter 17, "Neurobiology of Schizophrenia, Mood Disorders, and Anxiety Disorders"
- Rewritten discussion of diabetes mellitus and the cellular action of insulin
- Rewritten content on the biologic effects of the hormones estrogen and progesterone
- Extensive rewrite of Chapter 22, "Alterations of the Reproductive System," including much new information on hormones and cancer
- New section on hematopoiesis and the stem cell system
- Extensively rewritten discussion of anemias, acute blood loss, and polycythemia
- New section on atherosclerosis, minerals and hypertension, hormones and heart disease, acute coronary syndromes, and myocardial infarction
- Rewritten section on asthma and the associated inflammatory process
- New content on obesity
- Extensive rewrite of Chapter 42, "Alterations of Musculoskeletal Function in Children," including a new section on benign tumors and nonaccidental trauma
- New content on proinflammatory and antiinflammatory mediators for both adults and children with septic shock

ART PROGRAM

Extensive work was performed to create an outstanding art program, with meticulous attention directed toward the creation of new art and the revision of existing art. Hundreds of new full-color illustrations and photographs were added to this edition. As a result, the art program is spectacular! Notable is the strategic placement of new figures to illustrate difficult concepts that often challenge understanding. Also included are many new, high-quality, full-color photographs of clinical manifestations, pathologic specimens, and clinical imaging techniques. Additional colors have been added to the algorithms allowing the essential concepts to more easily emerge.

FEATURES TO PROMOTE LEARNING

We added to this edition an "Introduction to Pathophysiology," found after the table of contents, that defines and describes pathophysiology and explains its significance and importance. We also used a special heading to underscore the consistent treatment of each disease—Pathophysiology, Clinical Manifestations, and Evaluation and Treatment. Furthermore, we have added an Index of Special Features to the end of the text to help readers easily locate information of particular interest.

We added two new features to the third edition: *What's New?* and *Nutrition & Disease* (most of which were contributed by Carolyn Hollingshead) boxes. With the contributors we carefully updated these feature boxes and added many more throughout the text. In addition, we maintained our standard aids to maximize learning: chapter outlines with page numbers, introductory paragraphs prefacing each chapter, key terms in boldface type within chapters and end-of-chapter lists of key terms with page numbers, updated and highlighted content on aging, figure titles in boldface type, and summary reviews in an outline format.

ANCILLARIES

The online ***Instructor's Electronic Resource*** is free to instructors who adopt the textbook for course work. This time-saving resource consists of an Instructor's Manual, Test Bank, and Electronic Image Collection. The Instructor's Manual includes learning objectives, lecture outlines, a synopsis of difficult concepts, and critical thinking exercises. The Test Bank offers approximately 2000 true/false, multiple choice, and matching test questions with an answer key. The Electronic Image Collection—new to this edition—provides more than 200 illustrations from the text for use in presentations such as PowerPoint.

MERLIN is **M**osby's **E**lectronic **R**esource **L**inks and **I**nformation **N**etwork, an innovative website that provides WebLinks to numerous Internet resources, content updates, author information, and more. The MERLIN site designed for this text includes hundreds of links to authoritative sites related to pathophysiology, all conveniently organized by the textbook's table of contents. If you have chosen this textbook for a course you are teaching, ask your Mosby sales representative for a passcode to access this resource.

Many students have found the ***Study Guide and Workbook*** to be very helpful to them as they read this textbook and prepare for classroom examinations. The Study Guide includes foundational objectives to help students review the background knowledge necessary for chapter comprehension, a memory bank of key terms, learning objectives with corresponding textbook page numbers, a practice examination for each chapter, and a concise summary of key chapter concepts. Case studies are also included for each of the disease chapters.

Virtual Clinical Excursions is a groundbreaking new workbook and CD-ROM. The CD-ROM provides a simulated hospital setting with five patients with diverse conditions and backgrounds. In this interactive environment, students observe patient interviews and physical examinations, access laboratory and diagnostic test data and medication administration records, monitor vital signs, and evaluate patient progress. Each workbook lesson complements the textbook content and directs students to apply in practice what they are learning from the text.

For instructors seeking more in-depth case studies, particularly for advanced students, ***Clinical Applications of Pathophysiology: Assessment, Diagnostic Reasoning, and Management*** by Valentina L. Brashers is suggested. This unique workbook reviews 27 common health problems and illustrates how pathophysiologic concepts play a role in patient care with clinical link diagrams and case studies for each disorder. Questions are integrated throughout the case studies to promote continual critical thinking and can be used as course assignments. Answers to the case study questions are available free to instructors who adopt the workbook for course use.

For further information about ancillaries for this text and supplemental resources, contact your Mosby sales representative or call Faculty Support at 800-222-9570.

ACKNOWLEDGMENTS

Our contributors are amazing! The updating of this edition was an awesome task. The contributors worked diligently to stay current while keeping the text easy to read with much style. For your continued commitment to excellence, we thank you.

Piecing together of all the changes and additions to the manuscript while continuing to work courteously with an exhausted bunch is not an easy task. Once again this task was done brilliantly by Sue Meeks. She whipped the manuscript—and us—into shape and did it seemingly without us even knowing it. Thank you, Sue. We are deeply grateful for your magic wand.

Managing Editor Brian Dennison was a key player in this revision. Without a doubt, his attention to detail has made this edition better than ever. He was tenacious in his management of the art program. Thank you, Brian. Executive Editor Darlene Como finessed the larger picture. Her oversight and direction of the revision were right on and often saved us much time and energy. Thank you, Darlene, for your wise counsel. We are sincerely grateful to Project Specialist Jeffrey Patterson. Jeffrey was always available, orchestrated the people behind the scenes to produce well-edited text and well-arranged pages, and kept this book on course despite numerous obstacles. Thank you, Jeffrey. Our Book Designer, Kathi Gosche, did a spectacular job! The full-color design is elegant and highly usable. In addition, Kathi had great patience and included us in the decision-making. Thank you, Kathi. To Sally Schrefer, we owe our greatest respect, for without her this book would not exist.

Once again we would like to thank the outstanding medical illustrator, Barbara Cousins. Not only is her work dramatic in both color and content, but her first drafts were remarkably accurate! We are grateful to two outstanding photographers, Dennis Kunkel and Ed Reschke. Both contributed a number of fantastic and unique color micrographs. We thank the Department of Dermatology at the University of Utah School of Medicine, which provided numerous photos of skin lesions.

Thank you to the many colleagues and friends at the University of Utah College of Nursing, School of Medicine, Eccles Medical Library, and College of Pharmacy. In particular we would like to thank Lyn Pearse, Becky Nielson, and Cathy Groos who were all very helpful with many of the administrative details.

Special thanks are given to colleagues and students, particularly nursing, medical, and pharmacy students, for your letters, e-mail messages, and phone calls. It is for all of you that we have become so motivated to do the best job possible. Thank you.

Most importantly, we thank our families, especially John, Mae, Eric, Mark, Greg, Beth, and Anne. Your continued enthusiasm and support make it all possible.

Kathryn L McCance

Sue E Huether

CONTENTS

Unit IV Cellular Proliferation: Cancer

PART TWO Pathophysiologic Alterations: Organs and Systems

Unit V Neurologic System

Introduction to Pathophysiology

The word root "patho-" is derived from the Greek word *pathos*, which means suffering. Thus *pathophysiology* means the study of suffering caused by *pathology* (abnormality or disease) of *physiology* (bodily functions). More simply, it is the science dealing with disease caused by alteration of function. *Pathogenesis* is the origin and development of a disease process.

Pathophysiology is one of the most important bridging sciences between preclinical and clinical courses for students in the health sciences and requires in-depth study at an early stage in the curriculum. The definitions or conceptual models of pathophysiology that we carry in our minds influence what we do with our observations and what rationale we provide for our actions. Therefore the clinician must understand that while pathophysiology is a science, it also designates suffering in people; the clinician should never lose sight of this aspect of its definition.

As students study clinically related sciences, they learn to recognize and categorize disease. From the formulation of a differential diagnosis one understands the different *clinical manifestations*, the signs and symptoms of certain pathologies. These understandings structure further investigations, treatment plans, and evaluation. The interaction of these activities determines clinical outcomes and treatment success. Still, the concept of disease can be inherently ambiguous and elusive; many pathologies remain hidden and resist easy classification. One should appreciate that the naming and diagnosing of diseases involve evaluative judgments as well as scientific fact and that the process is as much a social endeavor as it is a scientific one. Some diseases, such as tuberculosis, identify a highly specific causative or etiologic agent or process. Others, such as Alzheimer disease or arthritis, indicate pathologic changes of unclear cause. In addition, syndromes and functional disorders simply describe multiple symptoms and signs that frequently occur together. Does commonality exist in all of these labels?

The answer is both yes and no and depends on our conception of health and disease. In the strictest sense, objective scientific facts help us know if an individual is healthy or suffering from disease. However, the individual's conception of disease is based on personal beliefs and histories, professional and lay healers who interact with that individual, and society at large. Each idea or construct has the power to influence other ideas and constructs, and each relationship has the ability to shape the way disease is understood and experienced.[1] In short, defining and understanding disease is tremendously ambiguous. Perhaps the most important and desirable trait for the new student of pathophysiology is an open and tolerant mind. To believe that science alone can overcome ignorance and that clinical training and technology can overcome ineptitude only encourages arrogance and undermines the scientific purpose.

Pathophysiology has had great success in explaining the mechanisms and clinical manifestations associated with infectious diseases. Syndromes of unclear etiology such as headache and fibromyalgia have proven to be troublesome. Even more difficult are multifactorial conditions, such as atherosclerosis or type 2 diabetes mellitus, in which several interacting factors contribute to the etiology. Learning how interacting factors relate to one another to increase morbidity or actually cause disease contributes to an appreciation of how emerging concepts revolutionize current understandings. For example, for many years the bacterial forms seen in gastric biopsies were interpreted as contaminants. It took several decades to understand the bacterial origin of gastritis, peptic ulcer disease, and even gastric carcinoma. Such findings are a major revolution in thought, and currently there is reason to believe that atherosclerosis may include infectious and inflammatory mechanisms interacting with key risk factors such as high lipids. The implications of thinking that is open and creative for screening, diagnosing, and treating are monumental! However, several interacting factors can still explain and confirm an individual's subjective feelings of suffering, such as pain or fatigue.

The language that clinicians use to discuss diseases and their manifestations is powerful. Lives are altered by a few words uttered by a clinician in a white coat or uniform. "AIDS," "cancer," and "heart attack" have become culturally ingrained symbols that portend an individual's future. While some futures are determined by scientific evidence, others are determined by subjective experience.[2] For example, a person diagnosed with a familial disease may ask, "Will I suffer like my mother did?" This questioning influences the individuals' suffering.

In conclusion, pathophysiology—the understanding of disease—requires both descriptive evidence and an evaluative component regarding suffering and the language we use to describe it. Combining objective and subjective perspectives requires new conceptual models that take into account the complex interactions among the body, mind, culture, and spirit.

REFERENCES

1. Magid C: Developing tolerance for ambiguity, *JAMA* 285(1):88, 2001.
2. Goldstein J: In the twilight: life in the margins between sick and well, *JAMA* 285(1):92, 2001.

CHAPTER 1

Cellular Biology

KATHRYN L. McCANCE

CHAPTER OUTLINE

An understanding of cellular biology is increasingly necessary for an understanding of disease. An overwhelming amount of information is revealing how cells behave as a multicellular "social" organism. At the heart of cellular biology is cellular communication ("cellular crosstalk")—how messages originate and are transmitted, received, interpreted, and used by the cell. Fossil records suggest that unicellular organisms resembling bacteria were present on earth 3.5 billion years ago, yet it took another 2.5 billion years for the first multicellular organisms to appear. It seems that this delay was slow because multicellularity needed elaborate signaling mechanisms to evolve that would allow cells to crosstalk. Streamlined conversation between, among, and within cells maintains social acceptance. Intercellular signals allow each cell to determine its position and specialized role. Cells must demonstrate a "chemical fondness" for other cells to maintain the integrity of the entire organism. When they no longer tolerate this fondness, the conversation breaks down and cells either adapt (sometimes altering function) or become vulnerable to isolation, injury, or disease.

PROKARYOTES AND EUKARYOTES

Living cells generally are divided into two major classes—eukaryotes and prokaryotes. The cells of higher animals and plants are eukaryotes, as are the single-celled organisms fungi, protozoa, and most algae. Prokaryotes include cyanobacteria (blue-green algae), bacteria, and rickettsiae. Prokaryotes traditionally were studied as core subjects of molecular biology. Current emphasis is on the eukaryotic cell; much of its structure and function has no counterpart in bacterial cells.

Eukaryotes (*eu* = good; *karyon* = nucleus) are larger and have more extensive intracellular anatomy and organization than do prokaryotes. Eukaryotic cells have a characteristic set of membrane-bound intracellular compartments, called *organelles,* that includes a well-defined nucleus. **Prokaryotes** contain no organelles, and their nuclear material is not encased by a nuclear membrane. Prokaryotic cells are characterized by lack of a distinct nucleus.

In addition to having structural differences, prokaryotic and eukaryotic cells differ in chemical composition and biochemical activity. The *nuclei* of prokaryotic cells carry genetic information in a single circular chromosome, and they lack a class of proteins called *histones,* which in eukaryotic cells bind with deoxyribonucleic acid (DNA) and are involved in the supercoiling of DNA (see Fig. 1-2). Eukaryotic cells have several chromosomes. Protein production, or synthesis, in the two classes of cells also differs because of major structural differences in ribonucleic acid (RNA) protein complexes. Other distinctions include differences in mechanisms of transport across the outer cellular membrane and in enzyme content.

CELLULAR FUNCTIONS

Cells become specialized through the process of **differentiation,** or maturation, so that some cells eventually perform one kind of function and other cells perform other functions. Highly developed functions, such as movement, are often associated with the absence of some other property, such as hormone production, which is more highly developed in some other type of specialized cell. The eight chief cellular functions follow:

1. *Movement.* Muscle cells can generate forces that produce motion. Muscles that are attached to bones produce limb movements, whereas those that enclose hollow tubes or cavities move or empty contents when they contract. For example, the contraction of smooth muscle cells surrounding blood vessels changes the diameter of the vessels; the contraction of muscles in walls of the urinary bladder expels urine.
2. *Conductivity.* Conduction as a response to a stimulus is manifested by a wave of excitation, an electrical potential, that passes along the surface of the cell to reach its other parts. Conductivity is the chief function of nerve cells.
3. *Metabolic absorption.* All cells take in and use nutrients and other substances from their surroundings. Cells of the intestine and the kidney are specialized to carry out absorption. Cells of the kidney tubules reabsorb fluids and synthesize proteins. Intestinal epithelial cells reabsorb fluids and synthesize protein enzymes.
4. *Secretion.* Certain cells, such as mucous gland cells, can synthesize new substances from substances they absorb and can secrete the new substances to serve as needed elsewhere. Cells of the adrenal gland, testis, and ovary can secrete hormonal steroids.
5. *Excretion.* All cells can rid themselves of waste products resulting from the metabolic breakdown of nutrients. Membrane-bound sacs (lysosomes) within cells contain enzymes that break down, or digest, large molecules, turning them into waste products that are released from the cell.
6. *Respiration.* Cells absorb oxygen, which is used to transform nutrients into energy in the form of adenosine triphosphate (ATP). Cellular respiration, or oxidation, occurs in organelles called *mitochondria.*
7. *Reproduction.* Tissue growth occurs as cells enlarge and reproduce themselves. Even without growth, tissue maintenance requires that new cells be produced to replace cells that are lost normally through cellular death. Not all cells are capable of continuous division, and some cells, such as nerve cells, cannot reproduce.
8. *Communication.* Communication is critical for all the other functions above that enable the survival of the society of cells. Pancreatic cells, for instance, secrete and release insulin to tell muscle cells to take up sugar from the blood for energy. Constant communication allows the maintenance of a dynamic steady state.

STRUCTURE AND FUNCTION OF CELLULAR COMPONENTS

Fig. 1-1 shows a "typical" eukaryotic cell. It consists of three components: an outer membrane called the *plasma membrane,* or *plasmalemma;* a fluid filling called **cytoplasm;** and the "organs" of the cell-membrane–bound intracellular organelles, among them the nucleus.

Nucleus

The **nucleus,** which is surrounded by the cytoplasm and generally is located in the center of the cell, is the largest membrane-bound organelle. Two membranes compose the **nuclear envelope** (Fig. 1-2, *A*). The outer membrane is continuous with membranes of the endoplasmic reticulum. The nucleus contains the **nucleolus,** most of the cellular DNA, and the DNA-binding proteins, the histones, that regulate its activity. The length of DNA in eukaryotic cells is so great that the risk of breakage is high. Therefore the histones that bind to DNA cause the folding of DNA into chromosomes (Fig. 1-2, *C*). The wrapping of DNA into tight packages of chromosomes is essential for cell division in eukaryotes.

The primary functions of the nucleus are cell division and control of genetic information. Other functions include the replication and repair of DNA and the transcription of the information stored in DNA. Genetic information is transcribed into RNA, which can be processed into messenger, transport, and ribosomal RNA and introduced into the cytoplasm, where it directs cellular activities. Most of the processing of RNA occurs in the nucleolus. (The role of DNA and RNA in protein synthesis is discussed in Chapter 4.)

Cytoplasmic Organelles

Cytoplasm is an aqueous solution **(cytosol)** that fills the **cytoplasmic matrix**—the space between the nuclear envelope and the plasma membrane. The cytosol represents about half the volume of a eukaryotic cell. It contains thousands of enzymes involved in intermediate metabolism and is crowded with ribosomes making proteins. Newly synthesized proteins remain in the cytosol if they lack a signal for transport to a cell organelle.[1] The organelles suspended in the cytoplasm are enclosed in biologic membranes, which enables them simultaneously to carry out functions that require different biochemical

FIG. 1-1 Typical or composite cell. A, Artist's interpretation of cell structure. **B,** Color-enhanced electron micrograph of a cell. Both show the many mitochondria known as the "power plants of the cell." Note, too, the innumerable dots bordering the endoplasmic reticulum. These are ribosomes, the cell's "protein factories." (From Thibodeau GA, Patton KI: *Anatomy and physiology,* ed 4, St Louis, 1999, Mosby.)

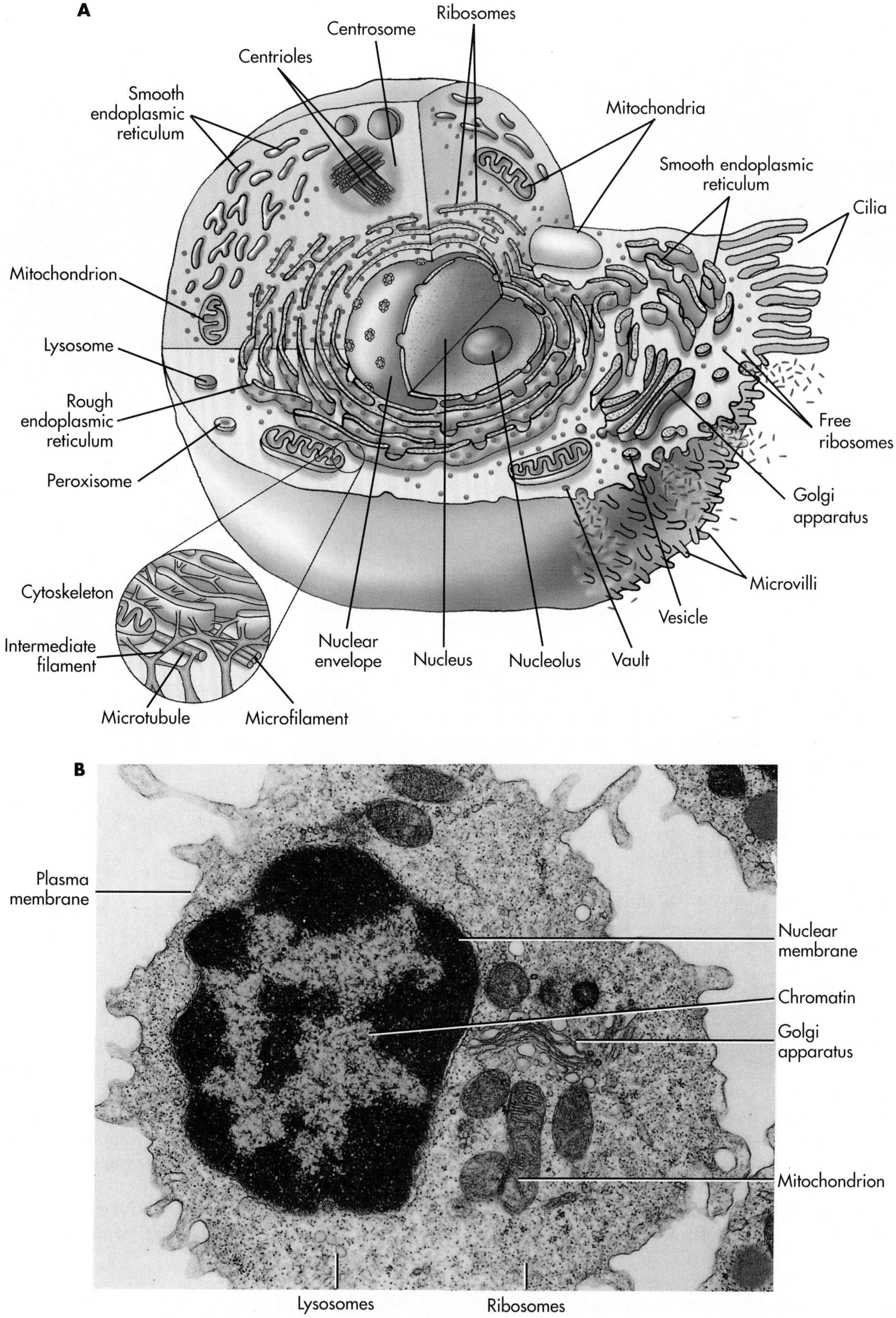
A
Ribosomes
Centrosome
Centrioles
Smooth
endoplasmic
reticulum
Mitochondria
Smooth endoplasmic
reticulum
Cilia
Mitochondrion
Lysosome
Rough
endoplasmic
reticulum
Peroxisome
Free
ribosomes
Golgi
apparatus
Microvilli
Cytoskeleton
Vesicle
Intermediate
filament
Nuclear
envelope
Nucleus
Nucleolus
Vault
Microtubule
Microfilament
B
Plasma
membrane
Nuclear
membrane
Chromatin
Golgi
apparatus
Mitochondrion
Lysosomes
Ribosomes

FIG. 1-1 For legend see opposite page.

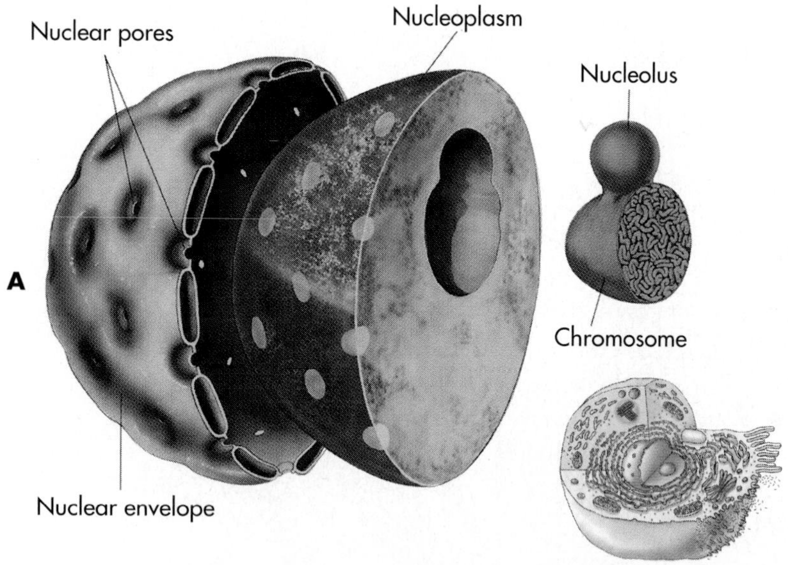

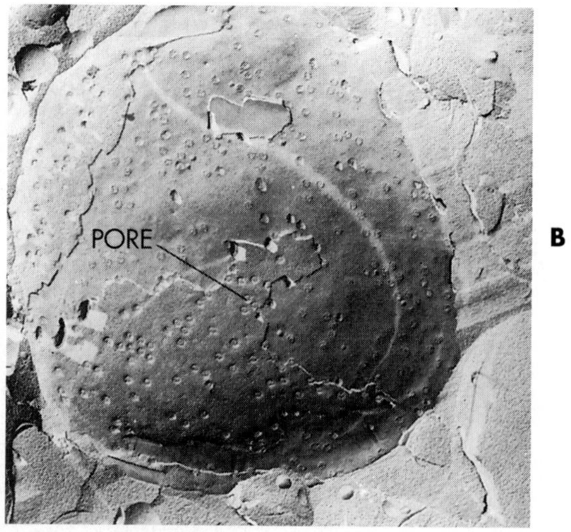

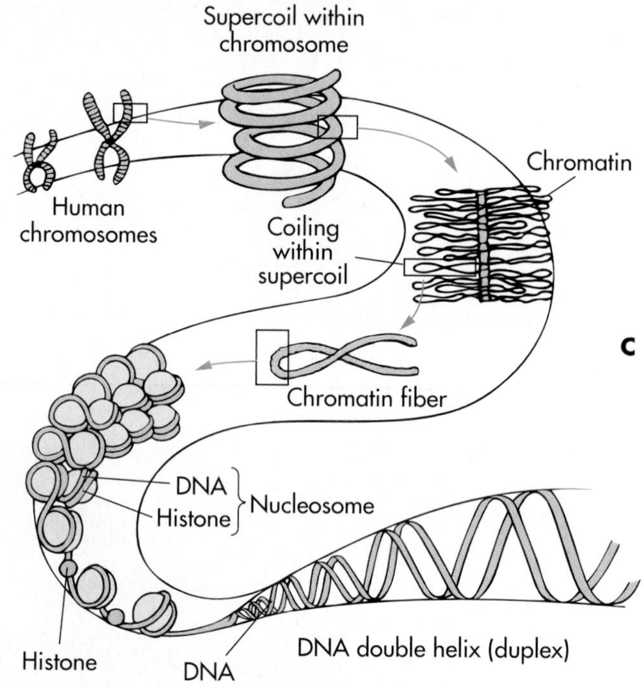

FIG. 1-2 The nucleus. The nucleus is composed of a double membrane, called a *nuclear envelope,* that encloses the fluid-filled interior, called *nucleoplasm.* The chromosomes are suspended in the nucleoplasm (here shown much larger than real size to show the tightly packed DNA strands). **A,** Swelling at one or more points of the chromosome occurs at a nucleolus where genes are being copied into RNA. The nuclear envelope is studded with pores. **B,** The pores are visible as dimples in this freeze etch of a nuclear envelope. **C,** How DNA is coiled within a chromosome. (**B** from Raven PH, Johnson GB: *Biology,* St Louis, 1992, Mosby.)

environments. These functions, many of which are directed by coded messages carried from the nucleus by RNA, include synthesis of proteins and hormones and their transport out of the cell, isolation and elimination of waste products from the cell, metabolic processes, breakdown and disposal of cellular debris and foreign proteins (antigens), and maintenance of cellular structure and motility. Also, the cytosol functions as a storage unit for fat, carbohydrate, and secretory vesicles.

Ribosomes

Ribosomes are RNA-protein complexes (nucleoproteins) that are synthesized in the nucleolus and secreted into the cytoplasm, possibly through pores in the nuclear envelope. These tiny organelles may float free in the cytoplasm or attach themselves to the outer membranes of the endoplasmic reticulum (see Fig. 1-1). Their chief function is to provide sites for cellular protein synthesis.

Endoplasmic Reticulum

The **endoplasmic reticulum** (*endo* = within; *plasma* = cytoplasm; *reticulum* = network) is a membrane factory that specializes in the synthesis and transport of the protein and lipid components of most of the cell's organelles. It consists of a network of tubular or saclike channels (cisternae) that extend throughout the cytoplasm and are continuous with the outer nuclear membrane (Fig. 1-3). The folded membranes that form the cisternae of the endoplasmic reticulum may be *rough* (granular) or *smooth* (agranular). The rough endoplasmic reticulum is rough because ribosomes and ribonucleoprotein particles are attached to it (see Fig. 1-3). Some of the proteins synthesized by these ribosomes remain in the endoplasmic reticulum, and others are used to construct membranes of other organelles (the Golgi complex, lysosomes, peroxisomes, nucleus) and of the cell itself.

Smooth endoplasmic reticulum does not contain ribosomes or ribonucleoprotein particles (see Fig. 1-1). Rather, membranous surfaces of the smooth endoplasmic reticulum contain enzymes involved in the synthesis of steroid hormones and are responsible for a variety of reactions required to remove toxic substances from the cell. The endoplasmic reticulum communicates with the Golgi complex and interacts with other organelles, particularly lysosomes and peroxisomes.

Golgi Complex

The **Golgi complex** (or **Golgi apparatus**) is a network of flattened, smooth membranes and vesicles frequently lo-

A

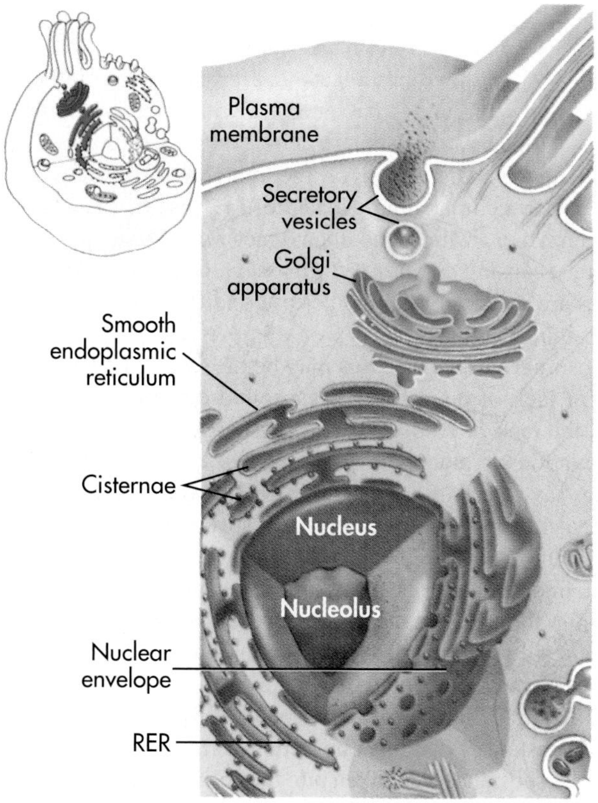

B

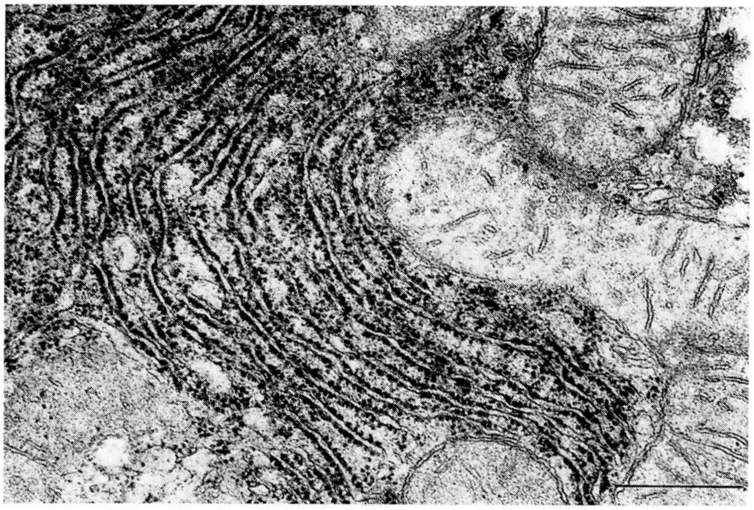

FIG. 1-3 Endoplasmic reticulum (ER). A, The ER consists of rough endoplasmic reticulum (RER) arranged into ribosome-coated cisternae and vesicles of smooth endoplasmic reticulum (SER). **B,** Electron micrograph of rough and smooth ER. (**B** courtesy C. Kelloes and M. Farmer, Center for Advanced Ultrastructural Research, University of Georgia.) (From Lindsay DT: *Functional human anatomy,* St Louis, 1996, Mosby.)

A B

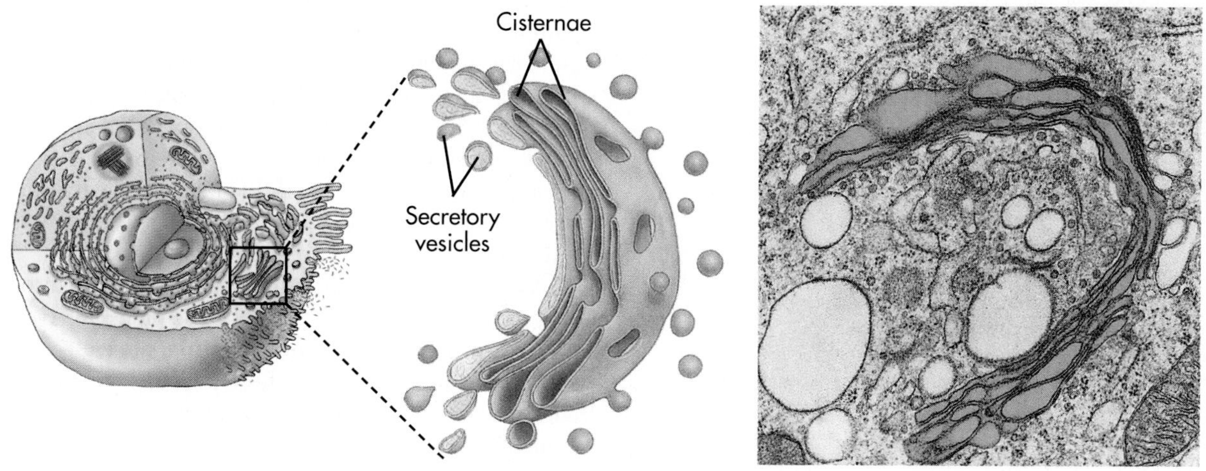

FIG. 1-4 Golgi apparatus. A, Schematic representation of the Golgi apparatus (complex), showing a stack of flattened sacs, or cisternae, and numerous small membranous bubbles, or secretory vesicles. **B,** Transmission electron micrograph showing the Golgi apparatus highlighted with color. (From Thibodeau GA, Patton KI: *Anatomy and physiology,* ed 4, St Louis, 1999, Mosby.)

cated near the nucleus of the cell (Fig. 1-4). Proteins from the endoplasmic reticulum are processed and packaged into small, membrane-bound vesicles called **secretory vesicles,** which collect at the end of the membranous folds of the Golgi bodies—called **cisternae.** The secretory vesicles then break off from the Golgi complex and migrate to a variety of intracellular and extracellular destinations, including the plasma membrane. The vesicles fuse with the plasma membrane, and their contents are released from the cell. The best known vesicles are those that have coats made largely of the protein **clathrin** and are called *clathrin-coated vesicles.* They bud from the Golgi complex on the outward secretory pathway and from the plasma membrane on the inward endocytotic pathway (see p. 22). Many molecules, including lipids, proteins, glycoproteins, and enzymes of lysosomes, pass through the Golgi complex at some stage in their maturation. The Golgi complex is probably the director of macromolecular traffic (e.g., protein, polynucleotide, polysaccharide molecules) in the cell[1] (Fig. 1-5).

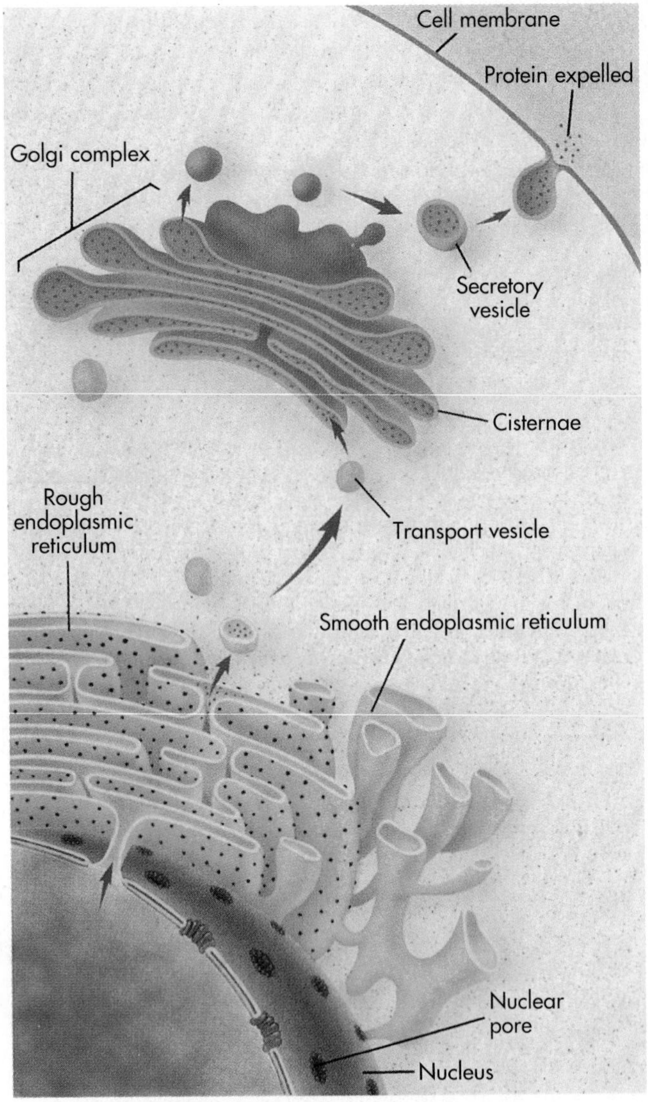

FIG. 1-5 How the internal membrane system of a cell packages a protein for export. The instructions for making a protein that is destined for export from a cell, such as a digestive enzyme made by a pancreas cell, are first transcribed from DNA by RNA in the nucleus. The RNA then leaves the nucleus through a nuclear pore and proceeds to a ribosome located on the rough endoplasmic reticulum (ER). There it provides instructions for the correct sequence of amino acids for synthesizing that particular digestive enzyme. When enzyme synthesis is complete, the enzyme travels through the ER and is then encapsulated in a transport vesicle. The transport vesicle fuses with a Golgi body, releasing the enzyme. In the Golgi complex the enzyme is further modified and is then shunted to the ends of the Golgi complex, or cisternae. There the enzyme waits for a secretory vesicle, which will carry it to the perimeter of the cell, the cell membrane. The secretory vesicle membrane then fuses with the cell membrane, and the enzyme is released outside the cell. (From Raven PH, Johnson GB: *Understanding biology*, ed 3, Dubuque, Iowa, 1995, Brown.)

Lysosomes

Lysosomes (*lyso* = dissolution; *soma* = body) are saclike structures that originate from the Golgi complex (see Fig. 1-1). They contain more than 40 digestive enzymes called *hydrolases,* which catalyze bonds in proteins, lipids, nucleic acids, and carbohydrates. Lysosomes function as the intracellular digestive system (Fig. 1-6). Lysosomal enzymes are capable of digesting most cellular constituents down to their basic forms, such as amino acids, fatty acids, and sugars.

The lysosomal membrane acts as a protective shield between the powerful digestive enzymes within the lysosome and the cytoplasm, preventing their leakage into the cytoplasmic matrix. Disruption of the membrane by various treatments or cellular injury leads to a release of the lysosomal enzymes, which can then react with their specific substrates, causing *cellular self-digestion.* Lysosomal abnormalities are involved in a number of conditions that involve cellular injury and death.

Lysosomal storage diseases may be the result of a genetic defect or lack of one or more lysosomal enzymes. For example, the lack of lysosomal α-1,4-glucosidase leads to an accumulation of glycogen in lysosomes known as *Pompe disease*. Tay-Sachs disease is characterized by an accumulation of GM2 ganglioside (a lipid) in lysosomes as a result of the deficiency or absence of lysosomal hexosaminidase A. In gout, undigested uric acid accumulates within lysosomes, damaging the lysosomal membrane. Subsequent enzyme leakage results in cell death and tissue injury.

Lysosomes are necessary for normal digestion of cellular nutrients, intracellular debris, and potentially harmful extracellular substances that must be removed from the body. Extracellular substances are taken into the cell and encapsulated in a membrane-bound vesicle. Lysosomes merge with the vesicle to form a digestive vacuole. Lysosomes remain fully active by maintaining a low internal pH. They do this by pumping hydrogen ions into their interiors. The hydrolytic enzymes are only maximally active at acid pH values. Lysosomes that are not active do not maintain such an acid internal pH. Lysosomes in this "holding pattern" are called **primary lysosomes.** When a primary lysosome fuses with a vacuole or other organelle, its pH falls and the hydrolytic enzymes become activated. When it becomes active, it is called a **secondary lysosome,** or heterophagosome.

As cells complete their life span and die, lysosomes digest the resultant cellular debris. Lysosomes involved in this process, which is called **autodigestion,** are called **autolysosomes,** or autophagosomes. In living cells, cellular debris is encapsulated within a vesicle that reacts with a lysosome to complete its degradation. This process is called **autophagy.** Autophagy also occurs during starvation, enabling the cell to use a part of its own substance for fuel without doing itself irreparable harm.

Products of autophagy (and of phagocytosis, the ingestion of harmful foreign substances; see Chapter 7) pass out of the lysosome and are reused by the cell. Indigestible material is stored in vesicles called **residual bodies,** whose contents are actively expelled from the cell (see Fig. 1-6). High concentrations of lipids may accumulate within the residual bodies and remain there for a long time. The lipids are eventually oxidized, and a pigmented substance containing polyunsaturated fatty acids and proteins accumulates in the cell. This pigmented substance, termed *lipofuscin,* is often called "age pigment" and is noted in older individuals (see Chapter 2).

WHAT'S NEW? Vaults: A Newly Discovered Organelle

In the 1990s, researchers identified another organelle—**vaults.** Vaults are cytoplasmic ribonucleoproteins, much larger than ribosomes, and shaped like octagonal barrels (see illustration below). Their name comes from their multiple arches, which reminded their discoverers of vaulted or cathedral ceilings. A single cell can contain thousands of vaults. Vaults were identified only recently because of changes in staining techniques. The function of vaults may be related to their octagonal shape. Similarly, the pores in the membrane surrounding the nucleus (see Fig. 1-2, *B*) are also octagonally shaped and the same size as vaults, leading to speculation that vaults may be cellular "trucks." Further, vaults would dock at nuclear pores, pick up molecules synthesized in the nucleus, and deliver their load elsewhere in the cell. Because at any given time about 5% of the vaults are localized near the nuclear pores, it is thought that vaults may be carrying messenger RNA (mRNA) from the nucleus to the ribosomal sites of protein synthesis within the cytoplasm. Recent observations suggest that vaults transport several copies of untranslated RNA and that they are transported along cytoskeletal-based cellular tracks—much like an assembly line.[2] Researchers are investigating the role of vaults in cancer cells' resistance to drug therapy. Perhaps transporting chemotherapy drugs to sites for exocytosis from the cancer cell increases the drugs' elimination. Although the normal cellular function of the vault is as yet undetermined, the structure of the vault is consistent with a role in either subcellular transport or sequestering large nuclear protein assemblies.[3]

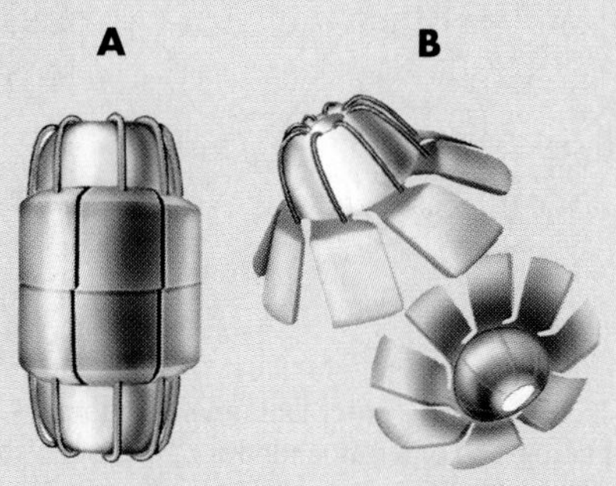

Vaults. A, Schematic three-dimensional representation of a vault, an octagonal barrel-shaped organelle believed to transport messenger RNA from the nucleus to the cytoplasmic ribosomes. **B,** Schematic representation of an opened vault, showing its octagonal structure. (Redrawn from Sherwood L: *Human physiology: from cells to systems*, ed 3, Belmont, Calif, 1997, Wadsworth. Reprinted with permission of Wadsworth, a division of Thomson Learning.)

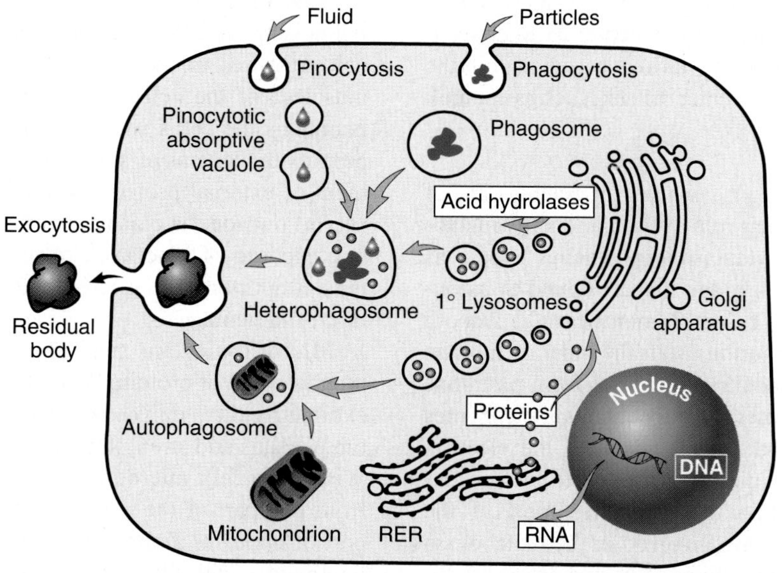

FIG. 1-6 Lysosomes. Primary (1°) lysosomes, which originate from the Golgi apparatus, give rise to heterophagosomes and autophagosomes. Undigested material in phagosomes is extruded from the cell or remains in the cytoplasm as lipofuscin-rich residual bodies. RER, rough endoplasmic reticulum. (From Damjanov I: *Pathology for the health-related professionals*, ed 2, Philadelphia, 2000, W.B. Saunders.)

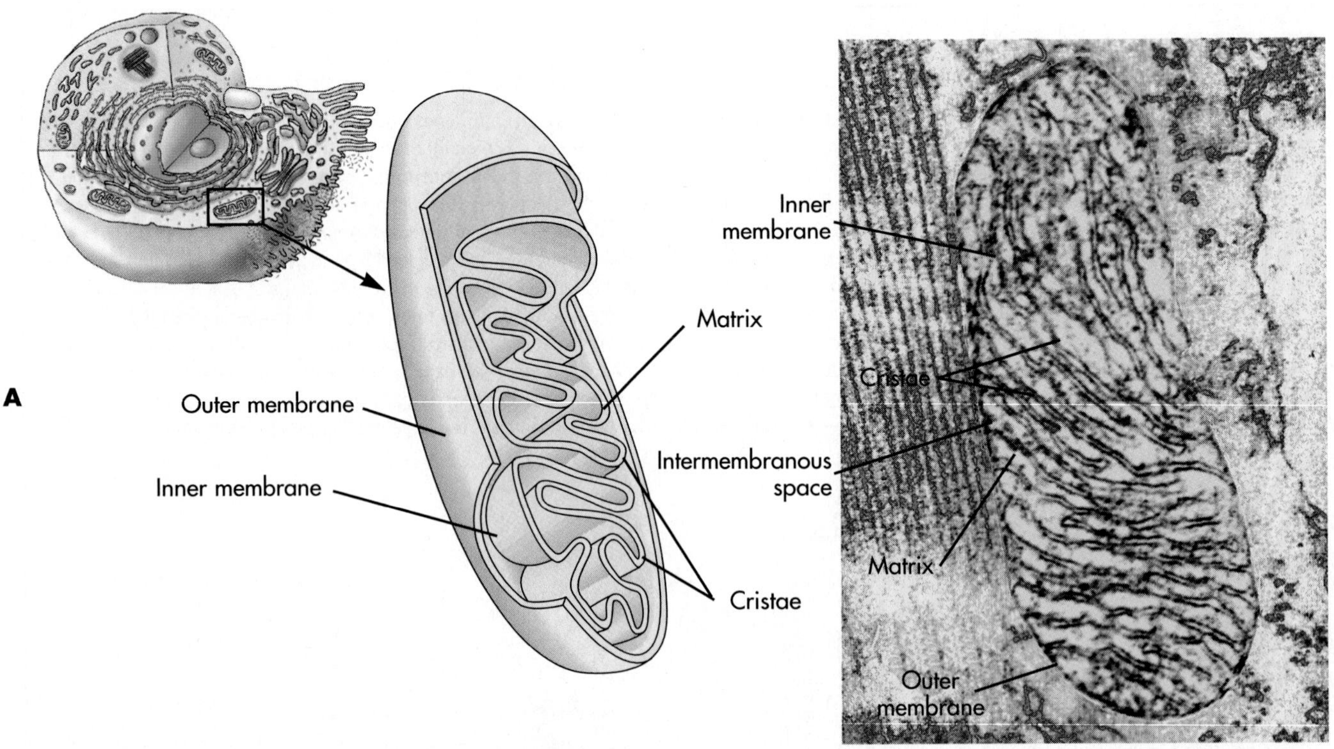

FIG. 1-7 Mitochondrion. A, Cutaway sketch showing outer and inner membranes. Note the many folds (cristae) of the inner membrane. **B,** Transmission electron micrograph of a mitochondrion. Although some mitochondria have the capsule shape shown here, many are round or oval. (From Thibodeau GA, Patton KI: *Anatomy and physiology*, ed 4, St Louis, 1999, Mosby.)

Peroxisomes

Peroxisomes (microbodies) are similar to lysosomes in microscopic appearance, but they are larger and oval or irregular in shape. Apparently derived from the smooth endoplasmic reticulum (ER), peroxisomes contain several oxidative enzymes that either produce or use hydrogen peroxide, for example, the enzyme catalase, which accelerates, or catalyzes, the conversion of two hydrogen peroxides to water and oxygen (see discussion of free radicals in Chapter 2). Such reactions are important in detoxifying various wastes within the cell or foreign components that enter the cell, such as ethanol.

Mitochondria

Mitochondria (*mito* = thread; *chondros* = granule) are of much interest because of their role in cellular energy metabolism (see p. 14). These cytoplasmic organelles appear as spheres, rods, or filamentous bodies that are bound by a double membrane (Fig. 1-7). The **outer membrane** is smooth and surrounds the mitochondrion itself; the inner membrane is convoluted in the mitochondrial matrix to form partitions called **cristae.** The **inner membrane** contains the enzymes of the respiratory chain—the name given to the electron transport chain. These enzymes are essential to the process of oxidative phosphorylation that generates most of the cell's ATP. Metabolic pathways involved in the metabolism of carbohydrates, lipids, and amino acids and special pathways involving urea and heme synthesis are located in the mitochondrial matrix.

The outer membrane is permeable (passable) to many substances, but the inner membrane is highly selective and contains many transmembranous transport systems. The inner membrane contains a transporter to move electrically charged calcium (calcium ions). (Membrane transport is discussed on p. 17.)

Cytoskeleton

All eukaryotic cells contain elaborate and specialized internal structures in the cytosol that provide the "bones and muscles" of the cell—the **cytoskeleton.** The cytoskeleton maintains the cell's shape and internal organization, and it permits movement of substances within the cell and movement of external projections (cilia or microvilli; flagella in sperm) outside the plasma membrane. The internal skeleton is composed of a network of protein filaments; two of the most important are microtubules and actin filaments, or microfilaments.

Microtubules are small, hollow, cylindric, unbranched tubules made of protein. When found together, microtubules exhibit rigidity, unlike the rest of the cytoplasm. Microtubules thus add strength to the cell's structure (Fig. 1-8, *A*). Within the cell, microtubules support and move organelles from one part of the cytoplasm to another, facilitate transport of impulses along nerve cells, and have roles in the inflammatory and immune responses and hormone secretion. Microtubules are also involved in external movement, or motility, of some cells.

A

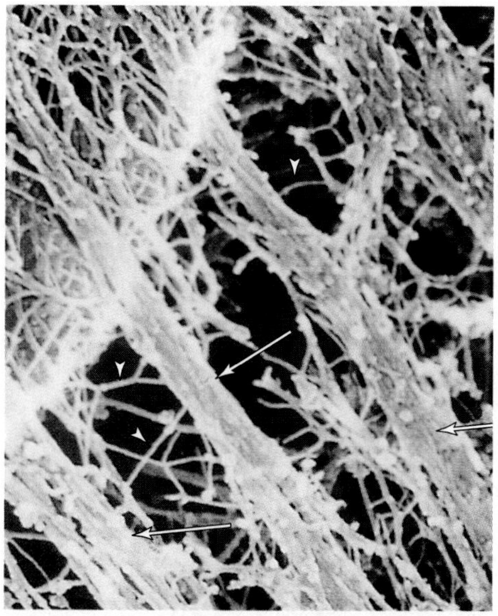

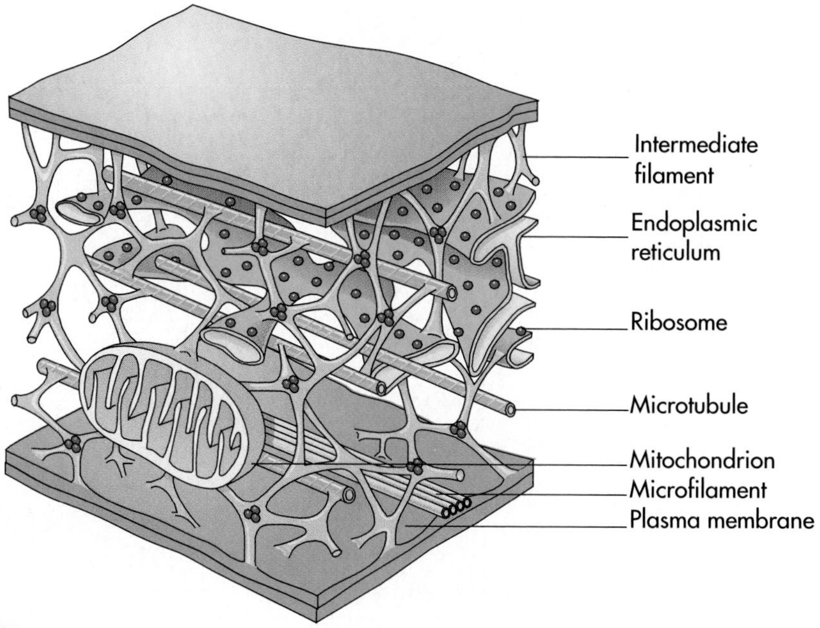

B

C

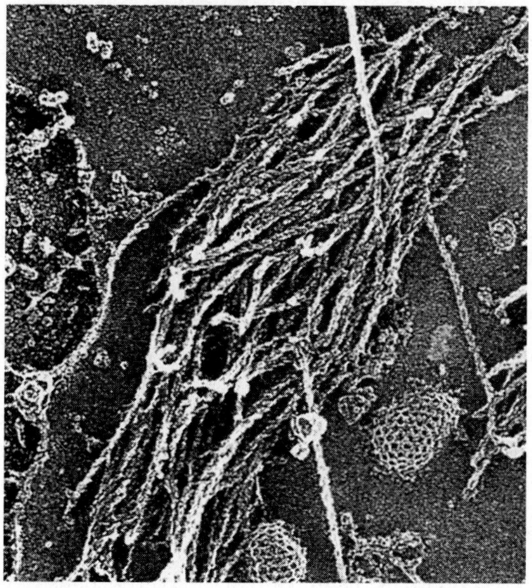

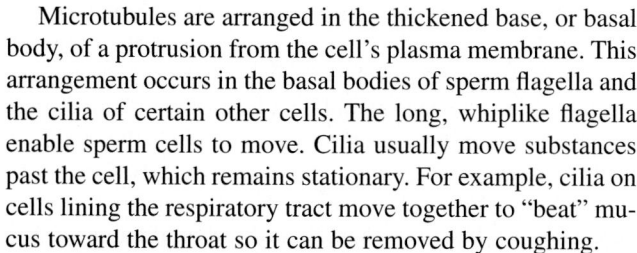

FIG. 1-8 Cytoskeleton. A, Color-enhanced electron micrograph of a portion of the cell's internal framework. The letter N marks the nucleus, the arrowheads mark the intermediate filaments, and the complete arrows mark the microtubules. **B,** Artist's interpretation of the cell's internal framework. Note that the "free" ribosomes and other organelles are not really free at all. **C,** Cytoskeleton showing several actin filaments (352,500). (**A** and **B** from Thibodeau GA, Patton KI: *Anatomy and physiology,* ed 4, St Louis, 1999, Mosby. **C** from Erlandson SL, Magney JE: *Color atlas of histology,* St Louis, 1992, Mosby.)

Microtubules are arranged in the thickened base, or basal body, of a protrusion from the cell's plasma membrane. This arrangement occurs in the basal bodies of sperm flagella and the cilia of certain other cells. The long, whiplike flagella enable sperm cells to move. Cilia usually move substances past the cell, which remains stationary. For example, cilia on cells lining the respiratory tract move together to "beat" mucus toward the throat so it can be removed by coughing.

While the cell is not in the process of division, only a few microtubules are assembled; cellular division (mitosis) or defense (phagocytosis) does, however, induce a cycle of rapid assembly and disassembly. Microtubules involved in cellular division are arranged in a **centriole.** Centrioles always consist of nine bundles containing three microtubules each. During division the pairs of centrioles split and migrate to opposite poles of the cell (see p. 25).

Alterations of microtubular function are implicated in disease processes. For example, alterations in actin microfilament act as a driving force for cell extension during cancer spread.[4]

Actin filaments (microfilaments) are smaller fibrils that generally occur in bundles rather than singly (Fig. 1-8, *C*). Like microtubules, actin filaments are associated with cellular locomotion and maintenance of cell and tissue shape.[4] In addition, microfilaments are necessary for regulating cell growth.[5] Cellular locomotion depends on contractile properties that involve both microtubules and actin filaments. Anesthetic drugs can affect both structures, disrupting intracellular movement and cellular motility.

Plasma Membranes

Whether they surround the cell or enclose an intracellular organelle, membranes are exceedingly important to normal physiologic function because they control the composition of the space, or compartment, they enclose. Membranes can include or exclude various molecules, and because of selective transport systems, they can move molecules into or out of the space (Fig. 1-9). By controlling the movement of substances from one compartment to another, membranes exert a powerful influence on metabolic pathways. In addition to these functions, the plasma membrane has an important role

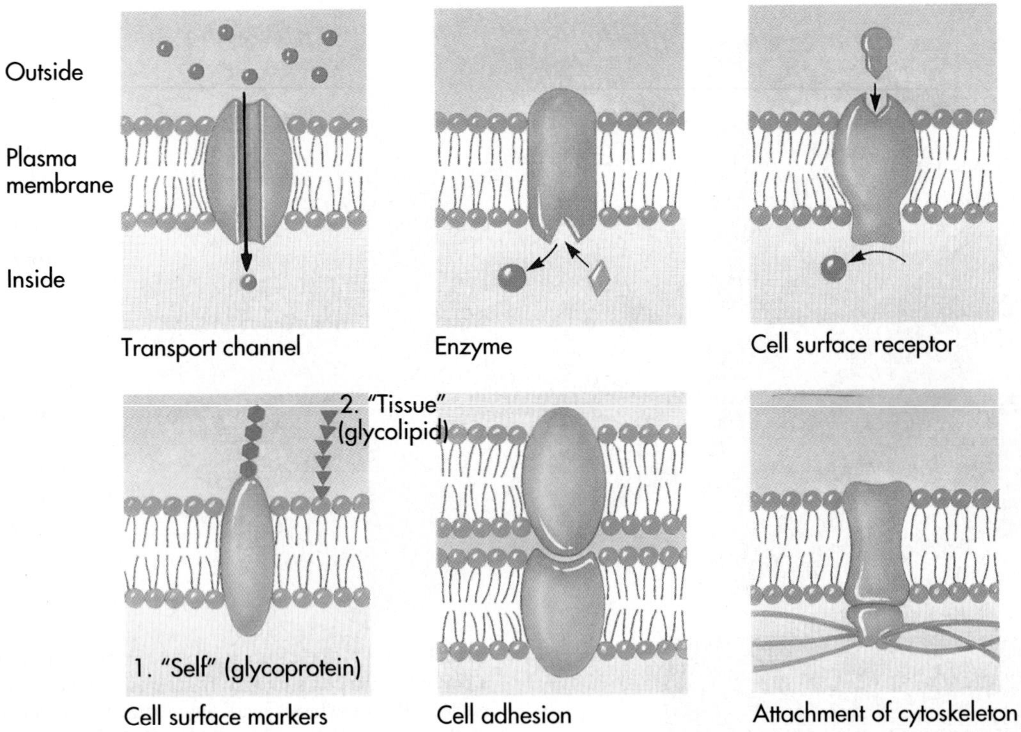

FIG. 1-9 Functions of plasma membrane proteins. The plasma membrane proteins illustrated here show variety of functions performed by the different types of plasma membranes. (From Raven PH, Johnson GB: *Understanding biology,* ed 3, Dubuque, Iowa, 1995, Brown.)

in cell-to-cell recognition. For example, protein receptors for hormones and for other chemical signals are associated with the membrane and act as markers that identify a cell to its neighbors. Other functions of the plasma membrane include cellular mobility and the maintenance of cellular shape (Table 1-1).

Membrane Composition

The outer surface of the plasma membrane is not smooth but dimpled with cavelike indentations known as **caveolae** ("tiny caves"). Caveolae were not thought to be functionally significant until the mid-1990s when evidence suggested that they (1) serve as a repository for some receptors, (2) provide a new route for transport into the cell, and (3) act as the initiator for relaying signals from several extracellular chemical messengers into the cell's interior (see p. 23).[6]

The major chemical components of all membranes are lipids and proteins, but the percentage of each varies among different membranes. Lipid molecules are the most abundant, but the protein molecules are so large that in total mass these two constituents are roughly equal. The structure of a plasma membrane is shown in Fig. 1-10. Intracellular membranes have a higher percentage of proteins than do plasma membranes, presumably because most enzymatic activity occurs within organelles. Carbohydrates are mainly associated with plasma membranes, where they are combined chemically with lipids, forming glycolipids, and with proteins, forming glycoproteins.

Lipids

The basic component of the plasma membrane is a bilayer of lipid molecules—phospholipids, glycolipids, and cholesterol (respective ratios 70:5:25). The lipids are responsible for the structural integrity of the membrane. Each lipid molecule is said to be amphipathic. An **amphipathic molecule** is one in which one part is hydrophobic (uncharged, or "water hating") and another part is hydrophilic (charged, or "water loving") (see Fig. 1-10). The membrane spontaneously organizes itself into a bilayer because of these two incompatible solubilities. The hydrophobic region (hydrophobic tail) of each lipid molecule is protected from water, whereas the hydrophilic region (hydrophilic head) is immersed in it. The bilayer's structure accounts for one of the essential functions of the plasma membrane: it is impermeable to most water-soluble molecules (molecules that dissolve in water) because they are insoluble in the oily core region. The bilayer serves as a barrier to the diffusion of water and hydrophilic substances while allowing lipid-soluble molecules, such as oxygen (O_2) and carbon dioxide (CO_2), to diffuse through it readily. Because the bilayer is fluid at temperatures above freezing, components of the cellular environment move slowly and selectively across the membrane all the time. (Components of the cellular environment are discussed in Chapter 3.)

Proteins

Research suggests two ways to classify membrane proteins. One way is classification as peripheral or integral proteins.

Table 1-1 Plasma Membrane Functions

Cellular Mechanism	Membrane Functions
Structure	Usually thicker than the membranes of intracellular organelles Containment of cellular organelles Maintenance of relationship with cytoskeleton, endoplasmic reticulum, and other organelles Outer surfaces in many cells are not smooth but are studded with cilia or even smaller cylindric projections called microvilli; both are capable of movement; caveolae are also outer indentations Maintenance of fluid and electrolyte balance
Protection	Barrier to toxic molecules and macromolecules (proteins, nucleic acid, polysaccharides) Barrier to foreign organisms and cells
Activation of cell	Hormones (regulation of cellular activity) Mitogens (cellular division, see Chapter 4) Antigens (antibody synthesis, see Chapter 8) Growth factors (proliferation and differentiation, see p. 26 and Chapters 10 and 24)
Transport	Diffusion and exchange diffusion Endocytosis (pinocytosis and phagocytosis); receptor-mediated endocytosis Exocytosis (secretion) Active transport
Cell-to-cell interaction	Communication and attachment at junctional complexes Symbiotic nutritive relationships Release of enzymes and antibodies to extracellular environment Relationships with extracellular matrix

Modified from King DW, Fenoglio CM, Lefkowitch JH: *General pathology: principles and dynamics,* Philadelphia, 1983, Lea & Febiger.

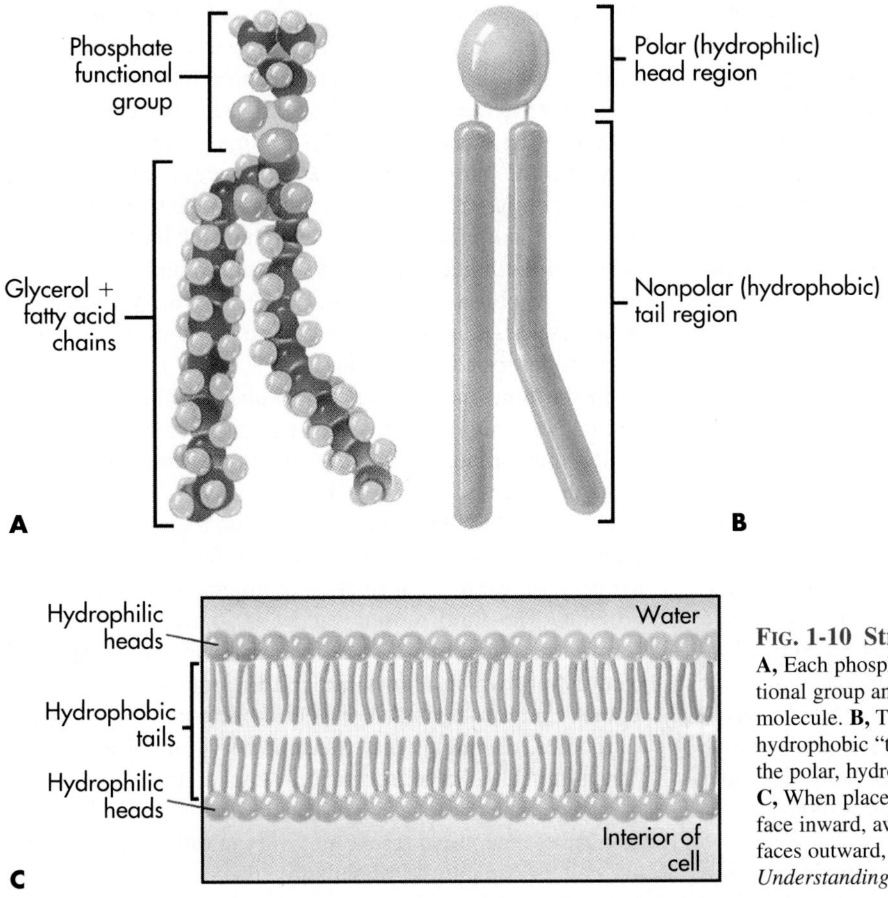

FIG. 1-10 Structure of a phospholipid molecule. **A,** Each phospholipid molecule consists of a phosphate functional group and two fatty acid chains attached to a glycerol molecule. **B,** The fatty acid chains and glycerol form nonpolar, hydrophobic "tails," and the phosphate functional group forms the polar, hydrophilic "head" of the phospholipid molecule. **C,** When placed in water, the hydrophobic tails of the molecule face inward, away from the water, and the hydrophilic head faces outward, toward the water. (From Raven PH, Johnson GB: *Understanding biology*, ed 3, Dubuque, Iowa, 1995, Brown.)

Integral membrane proteins are those embedded in the lipid bilayer linked to either *phosphatidylinositol,* a minor phospholipid, or a fatty acid chain. The integral proteins can be removed from the membrane only by detergents that solubilize (dissolve) the liquid. **Peripheral membrane proteins** are not embedded in the bilayer but reside at one surface or the other, bound to an integral protein.

Although the classification of membrane proteins as peripheral or integral is commonly used, it does not describe how proteins are associated with the bilayer. The second mode of classification does so by taking into account the membrane-spanning, or transmembranous, nature of membrane proteins[1] (see Fig. 1-11). According to this classification, proteins are associated with the lipid bilayer in four ways:

1. Some proteins, called **transmembrane proteins,** extend across the bilayer and are exposed to an aqueous environment on both sides of it.
2. Some intracellular proteins extend their polypeptide chain partially through the bilayer by means of a fatty acid chain.
3. Some cell-surface proteins are attached to the bilayer by a covalent linkage (i.e., a specific oligosaccharide).
4. Some proteins do not extend even partially through the bilayer but are bound to the membrane by noncovalent linkages with other membrane proteins.

Proteins exist in densely folded molecular configurations rather than straight chains, so an excess of hydrophilic units is at the surface of the molecule and an excess of hydrophobic units is inside. Although membrane structure is determined by the lipid bilayer, membrane functions are determined largely by proteins. For example, proteins facilitate transport across membranes by serving as receptors, enzymes, or transporters. Proteins act as (1) recognition and binding units (receptors) for substances moving in and out of the cell; (2) pores or transport channels for various electrically charged particles called *ions* or *electrolytes* and specific carriers for amino acids and monosaccharides; (3) specific enzymes that drive active pumps that promote concentration of certain ions, particularly potassium (K^+), within the cell while keeping concentrations of other ions, for example, sodium (Na^+), below concentrations found in the extracellular environment; (4) cell surface markers, such as **glycoproteins** (proteins attached to carbohydrates) that identify a cell to its neighbor; (5) **cell adhesion molecules (CAMs)** or proteins allowing cells to hook together and as attachments to the cytoskeleton for maintaining cellular shape; and (6) catalysts of chemical reactions, for example, lactose to glucose (see Fig. 1-9). (Membrane transport is discussed on p. 17.)

The interaction of plasma membrane proteins with lipids is complex and is currently the subject of much research. The role of proteins in the onset and progression of disease is important because of their enzymatic, transport, and recognition-receptor functions in cellular physiology.

Carbohydrates

A significant amount of carbohydrate is contained within the plasma membrane in the form of glycoprotein. Intercellular recognition, which is required for tissue formation, is an important function of membrane glycoproteins. Abnormal surface carbohydrate markers have been identified in certain tumor cells, leading investigators to claim that these markers are involved in tissue growth. Cells do not "trespass" their boundaries and overgrow their own territory.

Membrane Fluidity: The Fluid Mosaic Model

In the 1960s GL Nicholson and SJ Singer proposed the popular fluid mosaic model for biologic membranes (Fig. 1-11). The model, which is continually being modified, presents integral proteins as pieces of a mosaic that float singly or as aggregates in the fluid lipid bilayer. The protein molecules serve to (1) transport other molecules into and out of the cell; (2) facilitate (catalyze) membrane reactions; (3) receive messages, thus acting as receptors for extracellular and intracellular signals; and (4) create structural linkages between the external and internal cellular environments. The fluid mosaic model accounts for the flexibility of cellular membranes, their self-sealing properties, and their impermeability to many substances.

New revisions of the model now state that most membrane proteins do not enjoy unrestricted, lateral movement. Instead, multiple modes of diffusion and transport indicate a mix or heterogeneity in the membrane. Thus some proteins may randomly diffuse, others are confined or static, and still others are tethered to the cytoskeleton. The degree of a membrane's fluidity depends on temperature. At lower temperatures the lipids are in a gel crystalline state, and at higher temperatures they become highly fluid. These properties are critical for cellular growth, division, and receptor function. Because *some* proteins are free to move within the plasma membranes (like floating icebergs), certain foreign proteins (antigens) may become buried in the bilayer, emerging at the surface only after injury and then attracting antibodies (proteins produced by the immune system), which attack host cells. Antigens and antibodies, which are the cause and effect of the immune response, are discussed in Chapter 6. The burial and reemergence of antigens may be one cause of autoimmune disease, described in Chapter 8.

In the fluid mosaic model, cellular membranes are dynamic. Not only do some lipids and proteins move laterally on the membrane, but also ions and other molecules move through it. Cells, however, do have ways of immobilizing specific membrane proteins in a specific region of the membrane. Confinement may be necessary for certain functions to occur, for example, formation of intercellular junctions by proteins. The fluid mosaic model is logical in that it describes the membrane as existing in a state of change and modulation, which allows the cell to protect itself actively against injurious agents. Hormones, bacteria, viruses, drugs, antibodies, chemicals that transmit nerve impulses (neurotransmitters), and other substances attach to the plasma membrane by means of receptor molecules on its outer layer. The number of receptors present may vary at different times, and the cell is capable of modulating the effects of injurious agents by altering receptor number and pattern.[7] This aspect

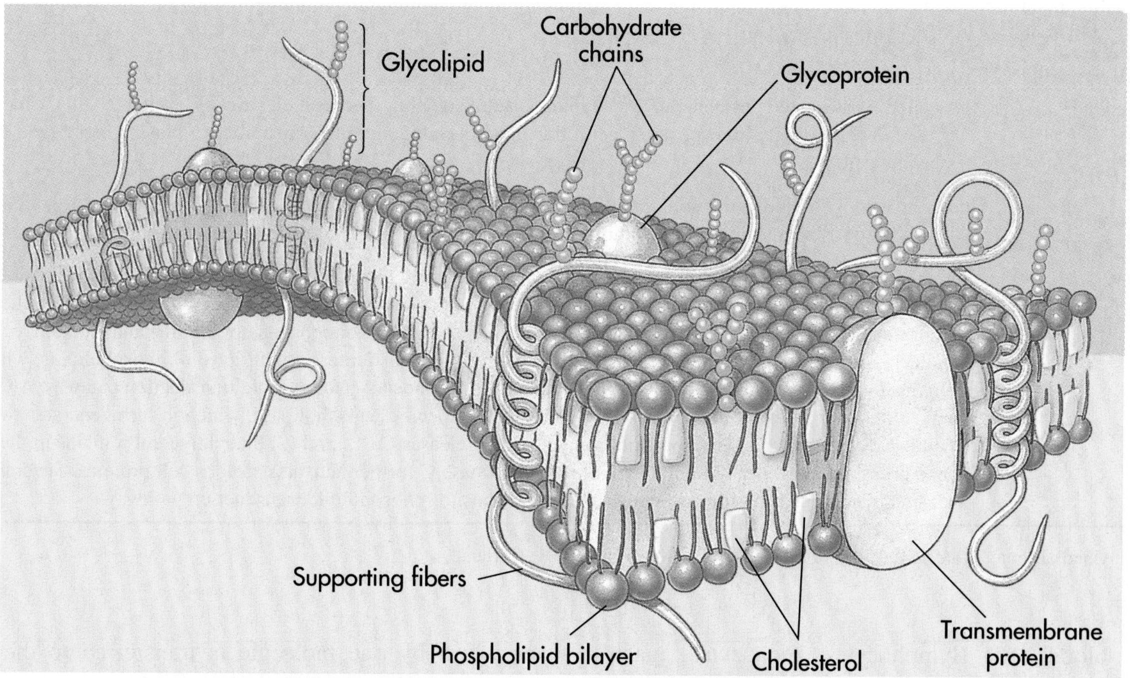

FIG. 1-11 Fluid mosaic model. Schematic, three-dimensional view of the fluid mosaic model of membrane structure. The lipid bilayer provides the basic structure and serves as a relatively impermeable barrier to most water-soluble molecules. (Modified from Thibodeau GA, Patton KI: *Structure and function of the human body,* ed 11, St Louis, 2000, Mosby.)

of the fluid mosaic model has drastically modified previously held concepts concerning the onset of disease.

The concentration of cholesterol in the plasma membrane affects membrane fluidity. Increased concentration results in less fluidity on the membrane's hydrophilic outer surface and more fluidity at its hydrophobic core. Changes in cholesterol content are factors in some diseases. In cirrhosis of the liver, for example, the cholesterol content of the red blood cell's plasma membrane increases. This causes an overall decrease in membrane fluidity that seriously affects the cell's ability to transport oxygen.

Cellular Receptors

Cellular receptors are protein molecules on the plasma membrane, in the cytoplasm, or in the nucleus that are capable of recognizing and binding with specific smaller molecules called **ligands.** Hormones, for example, are ligands. Recognition and binding depend on the chemical configuration of the receptor and its smaller ligand, which must fit together somewhat like pieces of a jigsaw puzzle (see Chapter 19).

Plasma membrane receptors are particularly important for cellular uptake of ligands (Table 1-2). They protrude from or are exposed at the external surface of the membrane, often attached to integral proteins. Some of these recognition units have all the mobile properties related to membrane fluidity. The ligands that bind with membrane receptors include hormones, neurotransmitters, antigens, complement components, lipoproteins, infectious agents, drugs, and metabolites. The past several years have brought many new discoveries concerning the specific interactions of cellular receptors with their respective ligands. In many instances this information has provided a basis for understanding disease.

Although the chemical nature of both ligands and the receptors to which they bind differs, receptors are classified on the basis of their location and function (see Cellular Communication and Signal Transduction). Cellular type determines overall cellular function, but plasma membrane receptors determine which ligands a cell will bind with and how the cell will respond to binding with each. For example, the ability of a hormone or a neurotransmitter to stimulate a cell is regulated by the specificity and number of receptors present on the plasma membrane. Specific processes also control intracellular mechanisms. Hormone binding, for example, depends on special messenger molecules that regulate protein synthesis within the cell (see Chapter 19). Neurotransmitters (discussed in Chapter 13) also operate by causing special messengers to react with specific receptors.

Receptors for different drugs are found on the plasma membrane, in the cytoplasm, and in the nucleus. Membrane receptors have been found for certain anesthetics, opiates, endorphins, enkephalins, antibiotics, cancer chemotherapeutic agents, digitalis, and other drugs. Membrane receptors for endorphins, which are opiate-like peptides isolated from the pituitary gland, are found in large quantities in pain pathways of the nervous system (see Chapters 13 and 14). With binding, the endorphins (or drugs like morphine) change the cell's permeability to ions, increase the concentration of molecules that regulate intracellular protein synthesis, and initiate molecular events that modulate pain perception.

Receptors for infectious microorganisms, or antigen receptors, bind bacteria, viruses, and parasites. Antigen receptors

Table 1-2 Classes of Plasma Membrane Receptors

Type of Receptor	Description
Channel linked	Also called ligand-gated channels; involve rapid synaptic signaling between electrically excitable cells. Channels open and close briefly in response to neurotransmitters changing ion permeability of plasma membrane of post-synaptic cell.
Catalytic	Once activated by ligands, function directly as enzymes. Composed of transmembrane proteins that function intracellularly as tyrosine-specific protein kinases.
G-protein linked	Indirectly activate or inactivate plasma membrane enzyme or ion channel; interaction mediated by guanosine triphosphate (GTP)–binding regulatory protein (G protein). When activated, a chain of reactions occurs that alters concentration of intracellular messengers, such as cyclic adenosine monophosphate (cAMP) and calcium, or signaling molecules. Other target proteins' behavior also altered. May also interact with inositol phospholipids, which are significant in cell signaling, and molecules involved in the inositol-phospholipid transduction pathway. A G protein–linked receptor activates the enzyme phosphoinositide-specific phospholipase, which in turn generates two intracellular messengers: (1) inositol triphosphate ($InsP_3$) releases Ca^{++}, and (2) diacylglycerol remains in the plasma membrane and activates protein kinase C. Protein kinase C further activates various cell proteins. Several different plasma membrane receptors are known to use the inositol-phospholipid transduction pathway.

Data from Alberts B et al: *Molecular biology of the cell,* ed 4, New York, 2001, Garland.

on white blood cells (lymphocytes, monocytes, macrophages, granulocytes) recognize and bind with antigenic microorganisms and activate the immune and inflammatory responses (see Chapters 6 and 7).

CELLULAR METABOLISM

All the chemical tasks of maintaining essential cellular functions are referred to as **cellular metabolism.** The energy-using process of metabolism is called **anabolism** (*ana* = upward), and the energy-releasing process is known as **catabolism** (*cata* = downward). Metabolism provides the cell with the energy it needs to synthesize (produce) cellular structures.

Dietary proteins, fats, and starches are hydrolyzed in the intestinal tract into amino acids, fatty acids, and glucose. These constituents are then absorbed, circulated, and taken up by the cell, where they may be used for various vital cellular processes, including the production of ATP. The process by which ATP is produced is one example of a series of reactions called a **metabolic pathway.** A metabolic pathway involves several intermediate steps whose end products are not always detectable. A key feature of cellular metabolism is the directing of biochemical reactions by protein catalysts, or enzymes. Most biochemical reactions in a pathway are catalyzed by a specific enzyme. Each enzyme has a high affinity for a **substrate**—a specific substance that is converted to a product of the reaction.

Role of Adenosine Triphosphate

For a cell to function, it must be able to extract and use the chemical energy contained within the structure of organic molecules. When 1 mole of glucose is metabolically broken down in the presence of oxygen into carbon dioxide (CO_2) and water (H_2O), 686 kilocalories (kcal) of energy are released. In a test tube this energy is released as heat. Because a cell cannot transform heat into work, chemical energy, rather than heat, is created by metabolism. The chemical energy lost by one molecule is transferred to the chemical structure of another molecule by an energy-carrying or transferring molecule, such as ATP. The energy stored in ATP can be used in a variety of energy-requiring reactions and in the process is generally converted to adenosine diphosphate (ADP) and inorganic phosphate (Pi). The energy available as a result of this reaction is about 7 kcal/mol of ATP. In addition to its use in synthesis (anabolism) of organic molecules, ATP is used by the cell for muscle contraction and active transport of molecules across cellular membranes. The function of ATP is not only to *store* energy but also to *transfer* it from one molecule to another. Energy is stored by molecules of carbohydrate, lipid, and protein, which, when catabolized, transfer energy to ATP.

Food and Production of Cellular Energy

The process of catabolism of the proteins, lipids, and polysaccharides found in food can be divided into three phases (Fig. 1-12). In phase 1, large molecules are broken down into their smaller subunits—proteins into amino acids, polysaccharides into simple sugars, and fats into fatty acids and glycerol. These processes are called **digestion** and occur outside the cell by the action of secreted enzymes.

In phase 2 the small molecules enter cells and are further broken down in the cytoplasm. Most of the sugars are converted into pyruvate. Pyruvate then enters mitochondria and is converted to the acetyl groups of acetyl coenzyme A (acetyl CoA). Acetyl CoA, like ATP, releases energy when it is hydrolyzed. The most important part of phase 2 is the lysis (splitting) of glucose, known as **glycolysis** (Fig. 1-13). Glycolysis produces a net of two molecules of ATP per glucose molecule through the process of **oxidation,** or the removal and transfer of a pair of electrons. This process, often called **oxidative cellular metabolism,** involves 10 biochemical reactions. In reactions 1 through 5, glucose is converted to two, three-carbon aldehyde (glyceraldehyde-3-phosphate [G3P]),

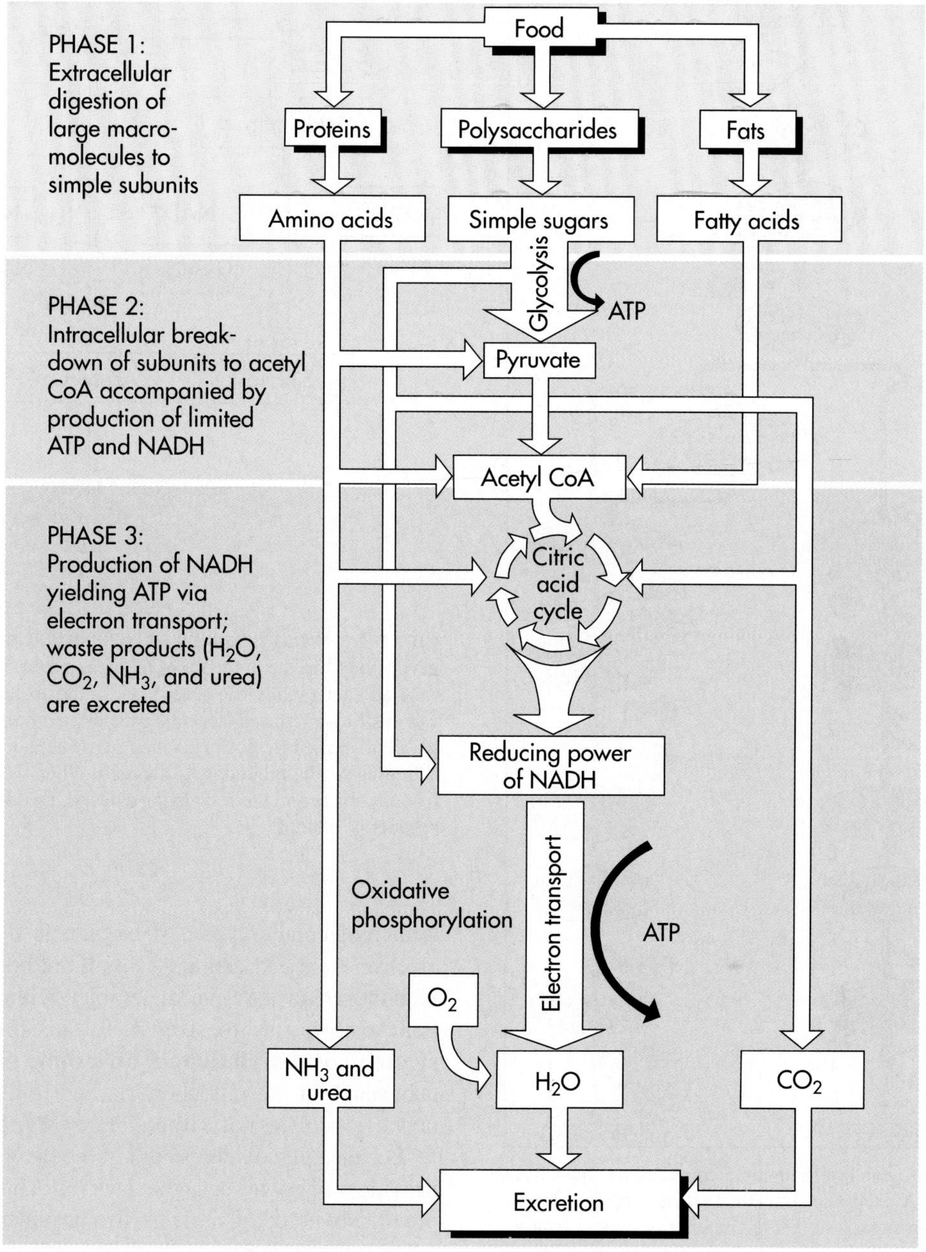

FIG. 1-12 Three phases of catabolism, which leads from food to waste products. These reactions produce ATP, which is used to drive other processes in the cell.

which requires energy in the form of ATP. The next five reactions convert G3P molecules into pyruvate molecules and generate four molecules of ATP for each two molecules of G3P. In addition, two molecules of NADH are further oxidized to produce four more molecules of ATP. After subtracting two molecules of ATP to drive the reactions, the net yield is six ATP molecules for each molecule of glucose.

Phase 3 occurs when the acetyl group of acetyl CoA is completely degraded to CO_2 and H_2O. It is in this final phase that most of the ATP is generated. Phase 3 begins with the **citric acid cycle** (also called the **Krebs cycle** or the **tricarboxylic acid cycle**) and ends with oxidative phosphorylation. The citric acid cycle accounts for approximately two thirds of the total oxidation of carbon compounds in most cells. Its major end products are CO_2 and two dinucleotides, NADH and $FADH_2$. NADH and $FADH_2$ transfer their electrons into the electron-transport chain.

Oxidative Phosphorylation

Oxidative phosphorylation occurs in the mitochondria and is the mechanism by which the energy produced from carbohydrates, fats, and proteins is transferred to ATP. During the breakdown (catabolism) of foods, many of the reactions involve the removal of electrons from various intermediates. These reactions generally require a coenzyme (a nonprotein carrier molecule), such as nicotinamide adenine dinucleotide (NAD), to transfer the electrons and thus are called **transfer reactions.**

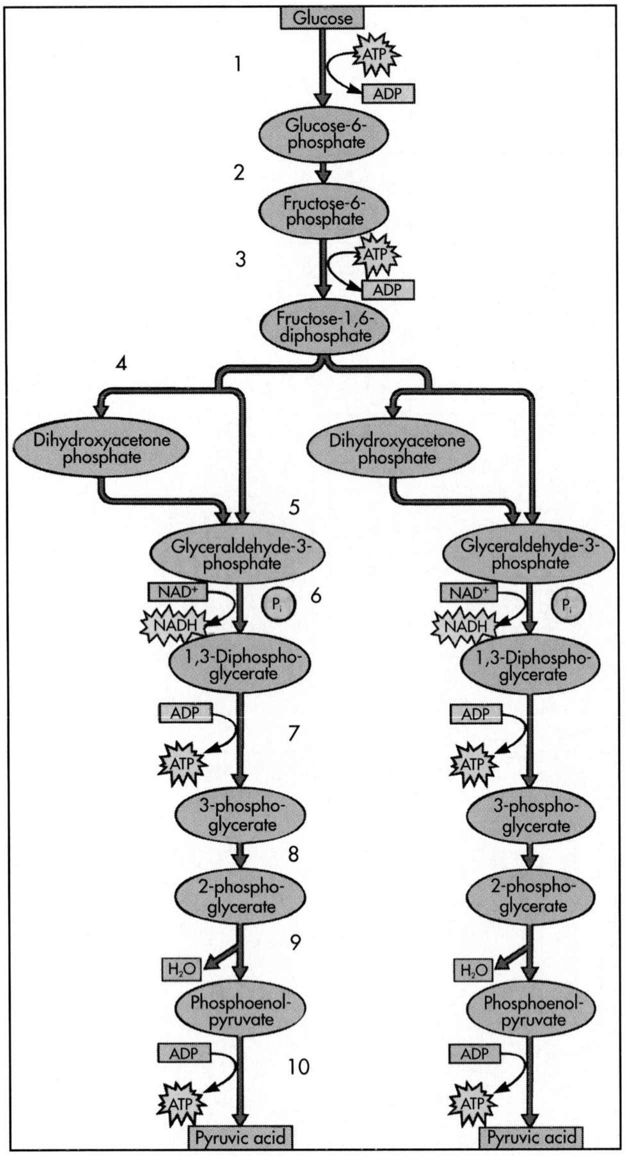

FIG. 1-13 Glycolysis. Each of the numbered reactions is catalyzed by a different enzyme. At step 4, a six-carbon sugar is broken down to give two three-carbon sugars, so that the number of molecules at every step after this is doubled. Reactions 5 and 6 are the reactions responsible for the net synthesis of ATP and NADH molecules. (Modified from Thibodeau GA, Patton KI: *Anatomy and physiology,* ed 4, St Louis, 1999, Mosby.)

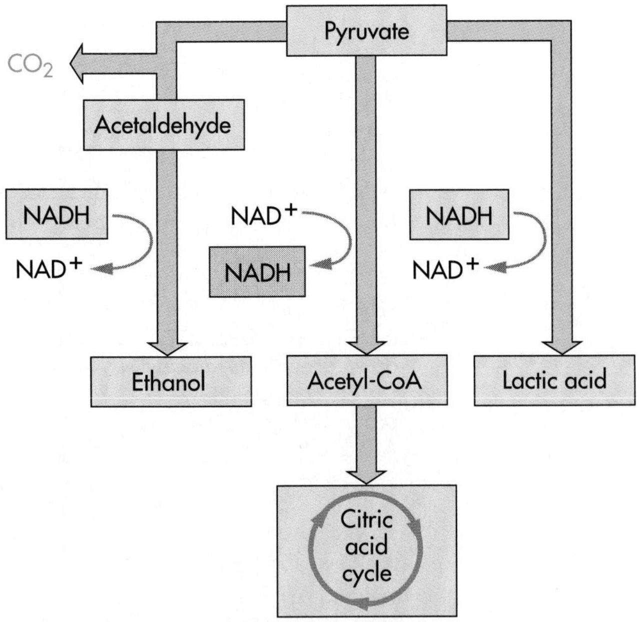

FIG. 1-14 What happens to pyruvate, the product of glycolysis? In the presence of oxygen, pyruvate is oxidized to acetyl CoA and enters thr citric acid cycle. In the absence of oxygen, pyruvate instead is reduced, accepting the electrons extracted during glycolysis and carried by NADH. When pyruvate is reduced directly, as it is in muscle, the product is lactic acid. When CO_2 is first removed from pyruvate and the remainder reduced, as it is in yeasts, the product is ethanol.

In oxidative phosphorylation, molecules of NAD and flavin adenine dinucleotide (FAD) transfer electrons they have gained from the oxidation of substrates to molecular oxygen, O_2. The electrons from reduced NAD and FAD, NADH and $FADH_2$, are transferred to a series of carrier molecules (the **electron-transport chain**) on the inner surfaces of the mitochondria with the release of hydrogen ions. Some of the carrier molecules are a group of brightly colored iron-containing proteins known as **cytochromes** that accept a pair of electrons. After passing through a sequence of different cytochromes, these electrons are eventually combined with molecular oxygen. If oxygen is not available to the electron-transport chain, ATP will not be formed by the mitochondria. Instead, an anaerobic (without oxygen) metabolic pathway synthesizes ATP. This process, called **substrate phosphorylation,** or **anaerobic glycolysis,** does not take place in the mitochondria and is linked to the breakdown (glycolysis) of carbohydrate (Fig. 1-14).

Because glycolysis occurs in the cytoplasm of the cell, it provides energy for cells that lack mitochondria. However, as previously noted, glycolysis also provides energy to the cell when oxygen delivery is insufficient or delayed. The reactions in anaerobic glycolysis involve the conversion of glucose to pyruvic acid (pyruvate) with the simultaneous production of ATP. With the glycolysis of one molecule of glucose, two ATP molecules and two molecules of pyruvate are liberated. If oxygen is present, the two molecules of pyruvate move into the mitochondria, where they enter the citric acid cycle. If oxygen is absent, pyruvate is converted to lactic acid and released into the extracellular fluid (see Fig. 1-14). The conversion of pyruvic acid to lactic acid is reversible; therefore, once oxygen is restored, lactic acid is quickly converted back to either pyruvic acid or glucose. The anaerobic generation of ATP from glucose, through the reactions of glycolysis, is not as efficient as the aerobic generation of ATP. The addition of an oxygen-requiring stage to the catabolic process (stage 3) provides cells with a much more powerful method for extracting energy from food molecules.

MEMBRANE TRANSPORT: CELLULAR INTAKE AND OUTPUT

Cells continually take in nutrients, fluids, and chemical messengers from the extracellular environment and expel metabolites or the products of metabolism and end products of lysosomal digestion. Intake and output, or transport, occurs by different mechanisms, depending on the characteristics of the substance to be transported. Water and small, electrically uncharged molecules move easily through pores in the plasma membrane's lipid bilayer. This process, called **passive transport,** will occur naturally through any semipermeable barrier. It is driven by osmosis, hydrostatic pressure, and diffusion, all of which depend on the laws of physics and do not require life. The process is passive in that it does not require any expenditure of energy by the cell.

Other molecules cannot be driven across the plasma membrane solely by forces of diffusion, hydrostatic pressure, or osmosis because they are too large or are ligands that have bound with receptors on the cell's plasma membrane. Some of these molecules are moved into the cell by mechanisms of **active transport,** which requires life, biologic activity, and the expenditure of metabolic energy by the cell. Unlike passive transport, which can be duplicated across any semipermeable barrier in a laboratory, active transport occurs only across living membranes that (1) use energy generated by cellular metabolism and (2) have receptors that are capable of recognizing and binding with the substance to be transported. Large molecules (macromolecules), along with fluids, are transported by means of endocytosis (taking in) and exocytosis (expelling). Water and electrically charged molecules are transported by protein channels embedded in the plasma membrane. Ligands enter the cell by means of receptor-mediated endocytosis.

Movement of Water and Solutes

Cellular membranes are semipermeable and generally allow passage of water and small particles of dissolved substances called **solutes.** The movement of solute molecules through membranes is related to their size, solubility, electrical properties, and concentration on either side of the membrane. Small, lipid-soluble particles, such as oxygen, carbon dioxide, and urea, can readily pass the lipid bilayers of the plasma membrane. Larger, water-soluble particles may pass through pores in the membranes. Although large protein molecules, such as albumin and globulin, pass through membranes by endocytosis, they influence the movement of water by exerting an osmotic effect (see p. 18).

Body fluids are composed of two types of solutes: **electrolytes,** which are electrically charged and dissociate into constituent **ions** when placed in solution; and nonelectrolytes, such as glucose, urea, and creatinine, which do not dissociate. Electrolytes account for approximately 95% of the solute molecules in body water. Electrolytes exhibit **polarity** by orienting themselves toward the positive or negative pole. Ions with a positive charge are known as **cations** and migrate toward the negative pole, or cathode, if an electrical current is passed through the electrolyte solution. **Anions** carry a negative charge and migrate toward the positive pole, or anode, in the presence of electrical current. Anions and cations are located in both the intracellular fluid (ICF) and extracellular fluid (ECF) compartments, although concentration of particular ions varies depending on their location. (Fluid and electrolyte balance between body compartments is discussed in Chapter 3.) For example, Na^+ is the predominant extracellular cation, and K^+ is the principal intracellular cation. The difference in ICF and ECF concentrations of these ions is important to the transmission of electrical impulses across the plasma membranes of nerve and muscle cells.

Electrolytes are measured in milliequivalents per liter (mEq/L) or milligrams per deciliter (mg/dl). Milliequivalents per liter indicate the number of electrical charges per unit volume of fluid. The term *milliequivalent* thus indicates the chemical-combining activity of an ion, which depends on the electrical charge, or valence, of its ions. In abbreviations, valence is indicated by the number of plus or minus signs. Monovalent ions, or ions with one charge, include sodium (Na^+), chloride (Cl^-), and potassium (K^+). Divalent ions, which have two charges, include calcium (Ca^{++}) and magnesium (Mg^{++}). One milliequivalent of any cation can combine chemically with 1 mEq of any anion: one monovalent anion will combine with one monovalent cation. Divalent ions combine more strongly than monovalent ions. To maintain electrochemical balance, one divalent ion will combine with two monovalent ions (e.g., $Ca^{++} + 2\ Cl^- = CaCl_2$).

Passive Transport

Diffusion

Diffusion is the movement of a solute molecule from an area of greater solute concentration to an area of lesser solute concentration. This difference in concentration is known as a **concentration gradient.** Particles in a solution move randomly in any direction. If the concentration of particles in one part of the solution is greater than in another part, the particles distribute themselves evenly throughout the solution. According to the same principle, if the concentration of particles is greater on one side of a permeable membrane than on the other side, the particles diffuse spontaneously from the area of greater concentration to the area of lesser concentration until equilibrium is reached. The higher the concentration on one side, the greater the diffusion rate. The overall effect of diffusion is the passive movement of particles "down" a concentration gradient, that is, from an area of high concentration to an area of low concentration.

The diffusion rate is influenced by differences of electrical potential across the membrane (see p. 23). Because the pores in the lipid bilayer are often linked with Ca^{++}, other cations (e.g., Na^+ and K^+) diffuse slowly because they are repelled by positive charges in the pores.

The rate of diffusion of a substance depends also on its size (diffusion coefficient) and its lipid solubility (Fig. 1-15). Usually, the smaller the molecule and the more soluble it is

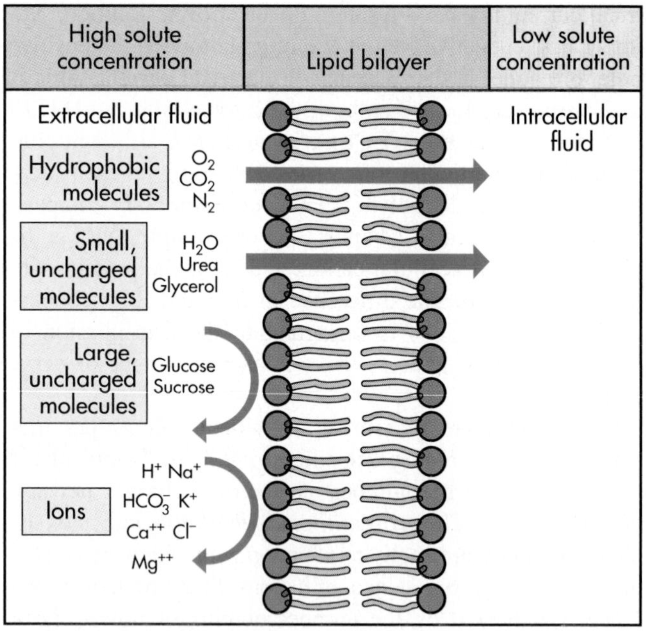

FIG. 1-15 Passive diffusion of solute molecules across plasma membrane. Oxygen, nitrogen, water, urea, glycerol, and carbon dioxide can diffuse readily down the concentration gradient. Macromolecules are too large to diffuse through pores in the plasma membrane. Ions may be repelled if the pores contain substances with identical charges. If the pores are lined with cations, for example, other cations will have difficulty diffusing because the positive charges will repel one another. Diffusion can still occur, but it occurs more slowly.

in oil, the more hydrophobic or nonpolar it is and the more rapidly it will diffuse across the bilayer. Oxygen, carbon dioxide, and the steroid hormones are all examples of nonpolar molecules. Water-soluble substances, such as sugars and inorganic ions, diffuse very slowly, whereas uncharged lipophilic ("lipid-loving") molecules, such as fatty acids and steroids, diffuse rapidly. Ions and other polar molecules generally diffuse across cellular membranes more slowly than lipid-soluble substances.

Water readily diffuses through biologic membranes because water molecules are small and uncharged. Although the mechanism is not known with certainty, the dipolar structure of water allows it to cross rapidly the regions of the bilayer containing the lipid head groups. Lipid head groups constitute the two outer regions of the lipid bilayer.

Hydrostatic Pressure

Hydrostatic pressure is the mechanical force of water pushing against cellular membranes. In the vascular system, hydrostatic pressure is the blood pressure generated in vessels by the contraction of the heart. Blood reaching the capillary bed has a hydrostatic pressure of 25 to 30 mm Hg, which is sufficient force to push water across the thin capillary membranes into the interstitial space, a process known as *filtration*. Hydrostatic pressure is partially balanced by osmotic pressure: there is a net movement of water out of the capillary partially balanced by osmotic forces that tend to pull water into the capillaries. Water that is not osmotically attracted back into the capillaries moves into the lymph system (see discussion of Starling forces in Chapter 3).

Osmosis

Osmosis is the movement of water "down" a concentration gradient, that is, across a semipermeable membrane from a region of higher water concentration to a lower water concentration. For osmosis to occur, the membrane must be more permeable to water than to solutes and the concentration of solutes must be greater so that water moves more easily. Osmosis is directly related to both hydrostatic pressure and solute concentration but *not* to particle size or weight. For example, particles of the plasma protein albumin are small but more concentrated in body fluids than the larger and heavier particles of globulin. Therefore albumin exerts a greater osmotic force than globulin.

Osmolality controls distribution and movement of water between body compartments. The terms *osmolality* and *osmolarity* are often used interchangeably in reference to osmotic activity, but they define different measurements. **Osmolality** is a measure of the number of milliosmoles per kilogram of water, or the concentration of molecules per *weight* of water. **Osmolarity** is a measure of the number of milliosmoles per liter of solution, or the concentration of molecules per *volume* of solution. When solute is added to water, the volume is expanded and includes the original liter of water plus the volume occupied by the solute particles. In measuring osmolarity, the volume of water is therefore reduced by an amount equal to the volume of added solute.

In solutions that contain only dissociable substances, such as Na^+ and Cl^-, the difference between the two measurements is negligible. In considering all the different solutes in plasma (e.g., proteins, glucose, lipids), however, the difference between osmolality and osmolarity becomes more significant. In plasma, less of the plasma weight is water and the overall concentration of particles is therefore greater. The osmolality will be greater than the osmolarity because of the smaller proportion of water. Osmolality is thus the preferred measure of osmotic activity in clinical assessment of individuals.

The normal osmolality of body fluids is 280 to 294 mOsm/kg. The osmolality of intracellular and extracellular fluid tends to equalize and so provides a measure of body fluid concentration and thus the body's hydration status (see Chapter 3). Hydration is also affected by hydrostatic pressure, since the movement of water by osmosis can be opposed by an equal amount of hydrostatic pressure. The amount of hydrostatic pressure required to oppose the osmotic movement of water is called the **osmotic pressure** of the solution. Factors that determine osmotic pressure are the type and thickness of the plasma membrane, the size of the molecules, the concentration of molecules or the concentration gradient, and the solubility of molecules within the membrane. Examples of movement of water in relation to hydrostatic and osmotic forces occur in the glomerulus in the kidney (see Chapter 34) and in the capillaries of the microcirculation (see Chapter 28).

Effective osmolality is sustained osmotic activity and depends on the concentration of solutes remaining on one side of a permeable membrane. If the solutes penetrate the membrane and equilibrate with the solution on the other side of the membrane, the osmotic effect will be diminished or lost. For example, urea is a small solute that readily diffuses across cellular membranes. Solutions containing urea rapidly lose their effective osmolality because they rapidly equilibrate. Solutes too large to pass through the membrane thus sustain an effective osmolality, meaning that they enhance osmotic activity. Plasma proteins are examples of molecules that provide effective osmolality because they normally do not cross cellular membranes.

Plasma proteins also influence osmolality because they have a negative charge. The principle by which the plasma protein charge influences osmolality is known as *Gibbs-Donnan equilibrium,* and it affects the distribution of ions across cellular membranes. Gibbs-Donnan equilibrium occurs when fluid in one compartment contains small diffusible ions such as Na^+ and Cl^-, together with large, nondiffusible charged particles, such as plasma proteins. Because the body tends to maintain an electrical equilibrium, the nondiffusible protein molecules cause asymmetry in the distribution of small ions. Anions such as Cl^- are thus driven out of the cell or plasma, and cations such as Na^+ are attracted. The protein-containing compartment will maintain a state of electroneutrality, but the osmolality will be higher. The overall osmotic effect of colloids, such as plasma proteins, is called the **oncotic pressure,** or **colloid osmotic pressure**.

Tonicity describes the effective osmolality of a solution. (The terms *osmolality* and *tonicity* may be used interchangeably; also see Chapter 3.) Solutions, then, have relative degrees of tonicity. An **isotonic solution** (or isoosmotic solution) has the same osmolality or concentration of particles (285 mOsm/kg) as the ICF or ECF. Examples of isotonic solutions include 5% dextrose in water and normal (0.9%) saline solution. A **hypotonic solution** has a lower concentration and is thus more dilute than body fluids. Water is a hypotonic solution. Consequently, water is osmotically pulled into the cells, causing them to swell or burst. A **hypertonic solution** has a concentration greater than 285 to 294 mOsm/kg. An example of a hypertonic solution is 3% saline solution. Water can be pulled out of the cells by a hypertonic solution, so the cells shrink. The concept of tonicity is important when correcting water and solute imbalances by administering different types of replacement solutions.

Mediated and Active Transport

Mediated Transport

Mediated transport (passive and active) involves integral or transmembrane proteins with receptors having a high degree of specificity for the substance being transported. Inorganic anions and cations (e.g., Na^+, K^+, Ca^{++}, Cl^-, HCO_3^-) and charged and uncharged organic compounds (e.g., amino acids, sugars) require specific transport systems to facilitate movement through different cellular membranes. Rates at which substances are moved by mediated transport mechanisms have often been measured, yet the specific membrane proteins involved have not been identified. Mediated transport is much faster than simple diffusion.

A **transport protein** (carrier protein) is a transmembrane or integral protein that binds with and transfers a specific solute molecule across the lipid bilayer. Each transport protein, or **transporter,** has receptors for a specific solute. When the transporter is saturated—that is, when all receptor sites are occupied by solute molecules—the rate of transport is maximal. Solute binding can be blocked by **competitive inhibitors** that compete for the same receptor site and may or may not be transported by the transport protein. Noncompetitive inhibitors bind elsewhere but can alter the structure of the transporter.

The transporter protein is a multipass, transmembrane protein; that is, its polypeptide chain crosses the lipid bilayer multiple times. This chain forms a continuous pathway enabling solutes to pass across the membrane without coming into direct contact with the hydrophobic interior of the lipid bilayer1 (Fig. 1-16). (Transmembrane proteins are illustrated in Fig. 1-11.)

Another mechanism of mediated transport is the channel protein. The protein transporter creates a water-filled pore or channel across the bilayer through which specific ions can diffuse. These channels are sometimes called *ion channels,* and because they are permeable mainly to K^+, they are also called *K^+ leak channels* (Fig. 1-17). The channel is controlled by a gate mechanism that determines which receptor-bound solutes can move into the channel that is created after receptor-solute contact. Binding stimulates conformational changes in the protein transporter that move the solute through the channel short distances at a time until it reaches the other side of the membrane. Ion channels are responsible for the electrical excitability of nerve and muscle cells and play a critical role in the membrane potential.

Mediated transport systems can move solute molecules singly or two at a time. Two molecules can be moved simultaneously in one direction (a process called **symport**) or in opposite directions (called **antiport**), or a single molecule can be moved in one direction (called **uniport**) (Fig. 1-18).

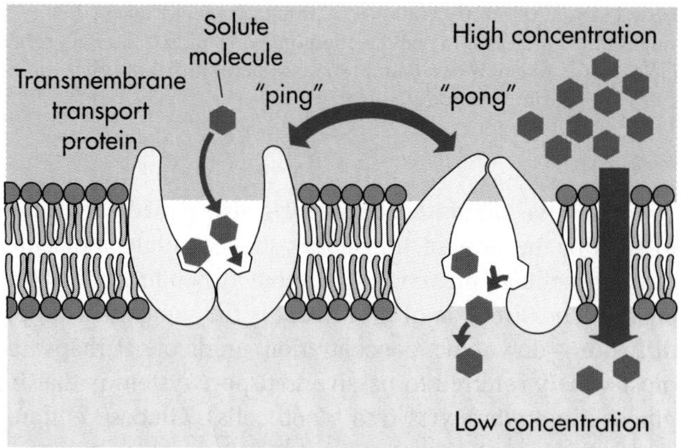

FIG. 1-16 Conformational-change model of mediated transport (facilitated diffusion). The transporter protein has two states, "ping" and "pong." In the ping state, sites for molecules of a specific solute are exposed on the outside of the bilayer. In the pong state, the sites are exposed to the inner side of the bilayer.

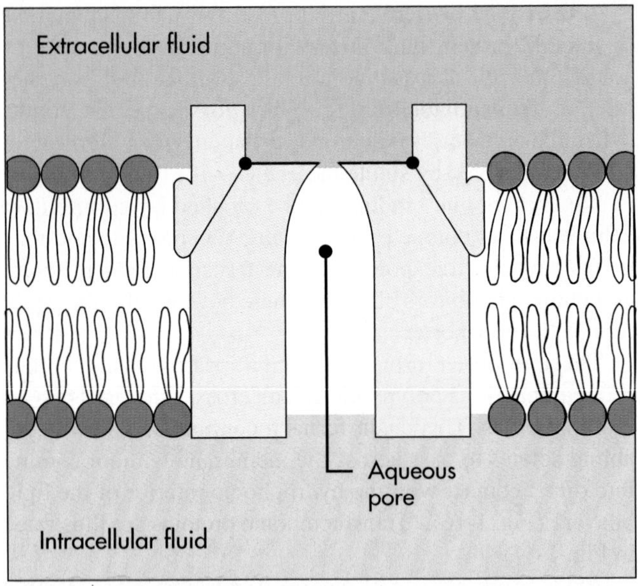

FIG. 1-17 Channel mode of mediated transport (facilitated diffusion). A channel protein forms a water-filled pore across the bilayer through which specific ions can diffuse.

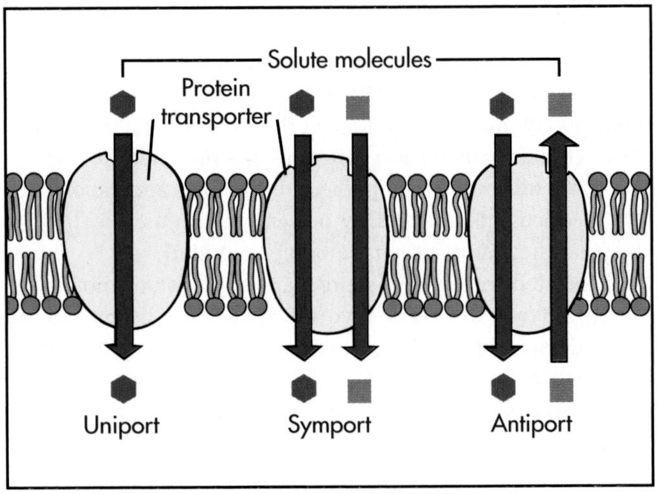

FIG. 1-18 Mediated transport. Simultaneous movement of a single solute molecule in one direction (uniport), of two different solute molecules in one direction (symport), and of two different solute molecules in opposite directions (antiport).

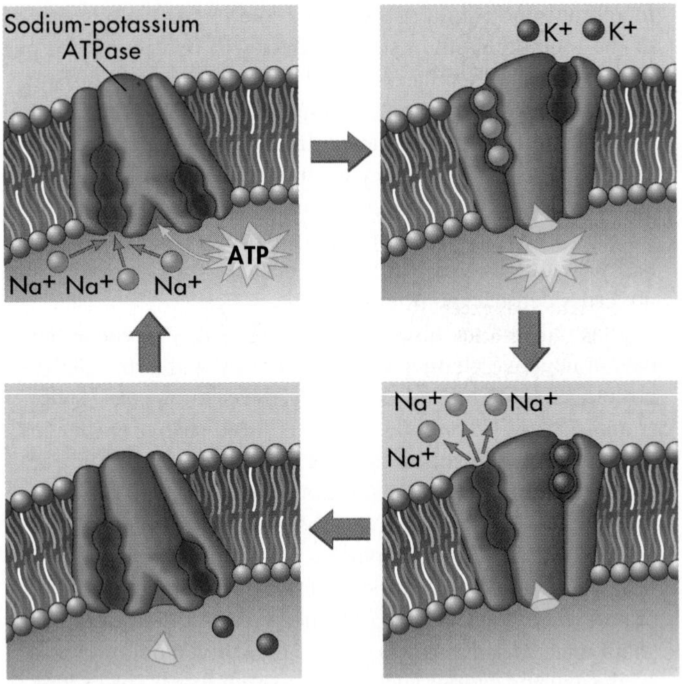

FIG. 1-19 Active transport and the sodium-potassium pump. Three Na^+ ions bind to sodium-binding sites on the carrier's inner face. At the same time an energy-containing ATP molecule produced by the cell's mitochondria binds to the carrier. The ATP breaks apart, transferring its stored energy to the carrier. The carrier then changes shape, releases the three Na^+ ions to the outside of the cell, and attracts two K^+ ions to its potassium-binding sites. The carrier then returns to its original shape, releasing the two K^+ ions and the remnant of the ATP molecule to the inside of the cell. The carrier is now ready for another pumping cycle. (From Thibodeau GA, Patton KI: *Anatomy and physiology,* ed 4, St Louis, 1999, Mosby.)

In **passive mediated transport,** also called **facilitated diffusion,** the protein transporter moves solute molecules through cellular membranes without expending metabolic energy. The direction of movement is the same as in simple diffusion—down the concentration gradient. Perhaps the most widely referred to passive transport system is that for glucose in erythrocytes (red blood cells). Glucose is transported by a uniport mechanism and demonstrates saturation kinetics; that is, the transport system is saturated when all the glucose-specific receptors on the membrane are occupied and operating at their maximal capacity.

The anions Cl^- and HCO_3^- also undergo passive mediated transport in the erythrocyte. This antiport mechanism allows Cl^- movement in one direction and simultaneous HCO_3^- movement in the opposite direction. The directions of movement depend on the concentration gradients of the ions across the membrane.

In **active mediated transport,** also called **active transport,** the protein transporter moves molecules against, or up, the concentration gradient. Unlike passive mediated transport, active mediated transport requires the expenditure of energy. Many active mediated transport systems, or pumps, have ATP as their primary energy source, but not all. Some use the electrochemical gradient of Na^+ across the membrane (Fig. 1-19). Energy in the form of ATP, however, is required for activation of the Na^+ gradient.

A "carrier" mechanism in the plasma membrane mediates the transport of ions, such as Na^+, K^+, H^+, Cl^-, and HCO_3^-, and of nutrients, such as glucose and amino acids. Energy supplied by ATP is required to pump ions against a concentration gradient. The best-known pump is the Na^+-K^+–dependent ATPase pump. It continuously regulates the cells' volume by controlling leaks through pores or protein channels and maintains the ionic concentration gradient necessary for cellular excitation and membrane conductivity (see p. 23). The maintenance of intracellular K^+ concentrations is also required for enzyme activity, including that of enzymes involved in protein synthesis.

Table 1-3 Major Transport Systems in Mammalian Cells

Substance Transported	Mechanism of Transport	Tissues
SUGARS		
Glucose	Passive protein channel	Most tissues
	Active: symport with Na^+	Small intestines and renal tubular cells
Fructose	Passive	Intestines and liver
AMINO ACIDS	Coupled channels	
Amino acid specific transporters	Active: symport with Na^+	Intestines, kidney, and liver
All amino acids except proline	Active: group translocation	Liver
Specific amino acids	Passive	Small intestine
OTHER ORGANIC MOLECULES		
Cholic acid, deoxycholic acid, and taurocholic acid	Active: symport with Na^+	Intestines
Organic anions, e.g., malate, α-ketoglutarate, glutamate	Antiport with counter-organic anion	Mitochondria of liver cells
ATP-ADP	Antiport transport of nucleotides; can be active	Mitochondria of liver cells
INORGANIC IONS		
Na^+	Passive	Distal renal tubular cells
Na^+/H^+	Active antiport, proton pump	Proximal renal tubular cells and small intestines
Na^+/K^+	Active: ATP driven, protein channel	Plasma membrane of most cells
Ca^{++}	Active: ATP driven, antiport with Na^+	All cells, antiporter in red cells
H^+/K^+	Active	Parietal cells of gastric cells secreting H^+
Cl^-/HCO_3^- (perhaps other anions)	Mediated: antiport (anion transporter–band 3 protein)	Erythrocytes and many other cells

Data from Alberts B et al: *Molecular biology of the cell,* ed 4, New York, 2001, Garland; Devlin TM, editor: *Textbook of biochemistry: with clinical correlations,* ed 3, New York, 1992, Wiley; Raven PH, Johnson GB: *Understanding biology,* ed 3, Dubuque, Iowa, 1995, Brown.

NOTE: The known transport systems are listed here; others have been proposed. Most transport systems have been studied in only a few tissues, and their sites of activity may be more limited than indicated.

ATP, Adenosine triphosphate; *ADP,* adenosine diphosphate.

Active Transport of Na^+ and K^+

The active transport system for Na^+ and K^+ is found in virtually all mammalian cells. The Na^+-K^+ antiport system (Na^+ moving out of and K^+ moving into the cell) uses the direct energy of ATP to move these cations. The transporter protein is an enzyme, ATPase. ATPase has a requirement for Na^+, K^+, and Mg^{++} ions. The concentration of ATPase in plasma membranes is directly related to Na^+-K^+ transport activity. Approximately 60% to 70% of the ATP synthesized by cells, especially muscle and nerve cells, is used to maintain the Na^+-K^+ transport system. Excitable tissues (e.g., muscle and nerve tissues) have a high concentration of Na^+-K^+ ATPase, as do other tissues that transport significant amounts of Na^+, for example, kidneys and salivary glands. For every ATP molecule hydrolyzed, three molecules of Na^+ are transported out of the cell, whereas only two molecules of K^+ move into the cell. The process leads to an electrical potential and is called *electrogenic*, with the inside of the cell more negative than the outside. The exact mechanism for transport of Na^+ and K^+ across the membrane is uncertain. One proposal is that ATPase induces the transporter protein to undergo several conformational changes, causing Na^+ and K^+ to move short distances (see Fig. 1-19). The conformational change creates a lowering affinity for Na^+ and K^+ to the ATPase transporter, resulting in the release of the cations after transport.

The sarcoplasmic reticulum of heart muscle and skeletal muscle has an ATP-dependent Ca^{++} active transport system that regulates the Ca^{++} levels in the cell's cytoplasm, which in turn regulates muscle contraction and relaxation cycles (see Chapter 28). The Ca^{++} transport system depends on ATPase activity and is similar to that of Na^+-K^+ ATPase.

The transport of sugars and amino acids across the plasma membrane depends on the simultaneous movement (symport) of Na^+ or Na^+-dependent transport (see Fig. 1-18). Na^+-dependent symport occurs primarily in the plasma membrane of epithelial cells of the kidney tubules and intestines. The transport of glucose is not directly dependent on the hydrolysis of ATP; however, the Na^+ gradient is ATP dependent, and thus ATP is indirectly involved in glucose transport.

The epithelial cells that line the intestines depend on Na^+ to transport various amino acids. Similarly, the uptake of Cl^- by the small intestine depends on Na^+ symport and antiport mechanisms for the secretion of Ca^{++} from the cell.

Table 1-3 summarizes the major mechanisms of transport through pores and protein transporters in the plasma membranes. Many disease states are caused or manifested by loss of these membrane transport systems.

Transport by Vesicle Formation

Endocytosis and Exocytosis

The active transport mechanisms by which the cells move large proteins, polynucleotides, or polysaccharides (macromolecules) across the plasma membrane are very different from those that mediate small solute and ion transport. Transport of macromolecules involves the sequential formation and fusion of membrane-bound vesicles.

In **endocytosis** a section of the plasma membrane enfolds substances from outside the cell, invaginates (folds inward), and separates from the plasma membrane, forming a vesicle that moves into the inside of the cell (Fig. 1-20, *A*). Two types of endocytosis are designated based on the size of the vesicle formed. **Pinocytosis** (cell drinking) involves the ingestion of fluids and solute molecules through formation of small vesicles, and **phagocytosis** (cell eating) involves the ingestion of large particles, such as bacteria, through formation of large vesicles (also called *vacuoles*).

Because most cells continually ingest fluid and solutes by pinocytosis, the terms *pinocytosis* and *endocytosis* are often used interchangeably. In pinocytosis the vesicle containing fluids, solutes, or both fuses with a lysosome, and lysosomal enzymes digest them for use by the cell. In phagocytosis the large molecular substances are engulfed by the plasma membrane and enter the cell so that they can be isolated and destroyed by lysosomal enzymes (see Chapter 7). Substances that are not degraded by lysosomes are isolated in residual bodies and released by the cell by exocytosis. Both pinocytosis and phagocytosis require metabolic energy and often involve binding of the substance with plasma membrane receptors before membrane invagination and fusion with lysosomes in the cell.

In eukaryotic cells, secretion of macromolecules almost always occurs by exocytosis (see Fig. 1-20, *B*). For example, to secrete macromolecules of insulin across plasma membranes, insulin-producing cells store and package insulin molecules in intracellular vesicles, which fuse with the plasma membrane and open to the extracellular space, or matrix, releasing the insulin. Not all secreted substances are secreted into the extracellular matrix. Some adhere to the plasma membrane and are thought to replace segments of the membrane lost through endocytosis or diffuse into the blood to nourish or signal other cells. Recent findings suggest membrane lipids may be a regulator of exocytosis.[8] Exocytosis has two main functions: (1) replacement of portions of the plasma membrane that have been removed by endocytosis and (2) release of molecules synthesized by the cells into the extracellular matrix.

Receptor-Mediated Endocytosis

Ligand binding to *some* plasma membrane receptors leads to clustering, aggregation, and immobilization of the receptors in specialized areas of the membrane called **coated pits** (Fig. 1-21). The pits, which are coated with bristlelike structures (clathrin), deepen and enfold (invaginate), internalizing ligand-receptor complexes and forming a coated vesicle. The clathrin coat or bristles are thought to be responsible for trapping membrane receptors in coated pits. This internal-

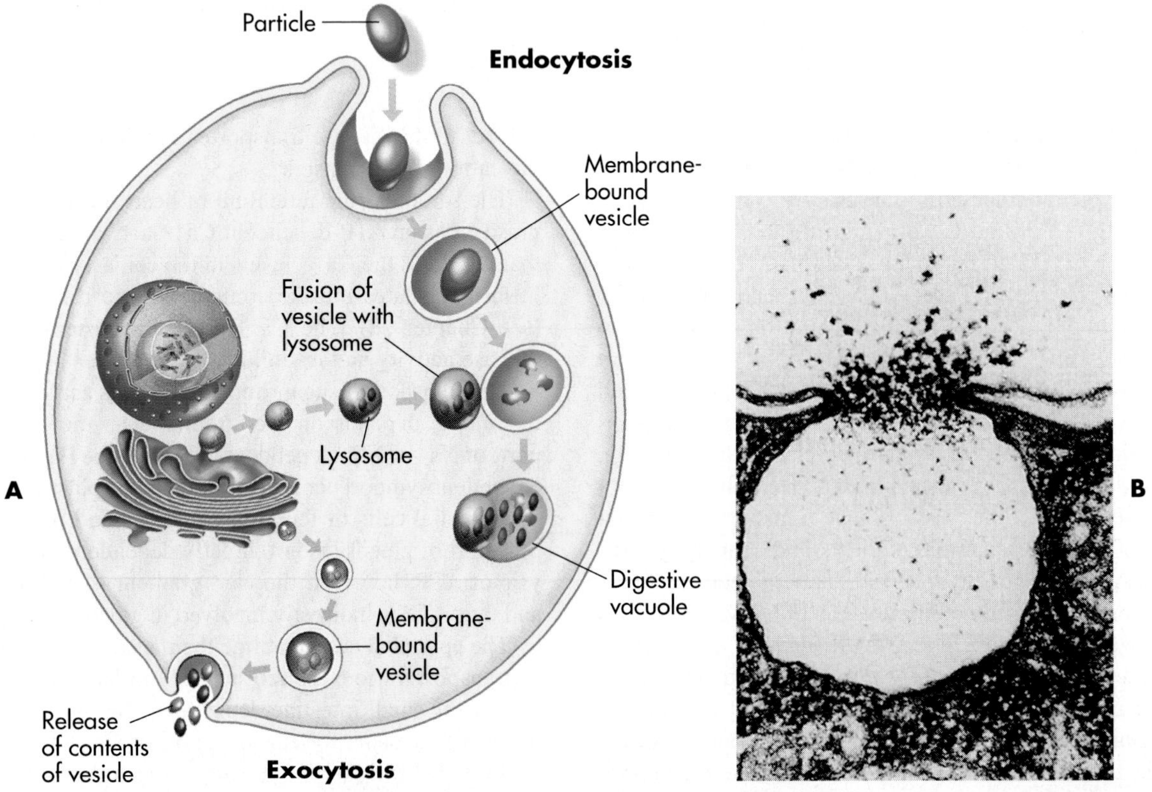

FIG. 1-20 Endocytosis and exocytosis. A, Endocytosis and fusion with lysosome and exocytosis. **B,** Electron micrograph of exocytosis. (**B** from Raven PH, Johnson GB: *Biology,* ed 5, New York, 1999, McGraw-Hill.)

ization process, called **receptor-mediated endocytosis** (**ligand internalization**), is rapid and enables the cell to ingest large amounts of specific ligands without ingesting large volumes of extracellular fluid. Inside the cell, the ingested material is processed by lysosomal enzymes.

The cellular uptake of cholesterol, for example, depends on receptor-mediated endocytosis. Cholesterol (a ligand) is carried primarily in blood plasma attached to an acceptor protein. This cholesterol-protein complex is called low-density lipoprotein (LDL). LDL receptors, which bind LDL to the plasma membrane, control the rate at which cholesterol is transferred into the cell (see Chapter 29).

Caveolae

The outer surface of the plasma membrane is dimpled with tiny flask-shaped pits (cavelike) called *caveolae* (see p. 10). Investigators also label caveolae as specialized membrane **microdomains.** Many proteins, including a variety of receptors, cluster in these tiny chambers. Some of these receptors appear to be important in a new form of cellular uptake of small molecules and ions, for example, the cellular uptake of the B vitamin folic acid. When folic acid binds with its receptors, which are concentrated in the caveolae, the extracellular openings of these tiny caves close off. Closure of the caveolar indentation facilitates the movement of this vitamin across the caveolar membrane into the cytoplasm. Cellular uptake through the opening and closing of caveolae is called **potocytosis.** Potocytosis is thought to be an uptake mechanism for a variety of small molecules and ions, in contrast to receptor-mediated endocytosis, which transports selected large molecules into the cell. In potocytosis the caveolae are thought to *remain* attached to the plasma membrane and not form a membrane-enclosed vesicle such as occurs with endocytosis.

Caveolae not only function as uptake vesicles but also are important sites for signal transduction, a tedious process in which extracellular chemical messages or *signals* are communicated to the cell's interior for execution (see p. 30). Many membrane messengers concentrated in caveolae are important for signal transduction, leading some investigators to call them "signaling organelles."

Movement of Electrical Impulses: Membrane Potentials

All body cells are electrically polarized, with the inside of the cell more negatively charged than the outside. The difference in electrical charge, or voltage, is known as the **resting membrane potential** and is about -70 to -85 millivolts. The difference in voltage across the plasma membrane is a result of the differences in ionic composition of ICF and ECF. Sodium ions have a greater concentration in the ECF, and potassium ions have a greater concentration in the ICF. The concentration difference is maintained by the active transport of Na^+ and K^+ (the sodium-potassium pump), which transports sodium outward and potassium inward (Fig. 1-22). Because the resting plasma membrane is more permeable to K^+ than to Na^+, K^+ can diffuse easily from its area of higher concentration in the ICF to its area of lower concentration in the ECF. Because Na^+ and K^+ are both cations, the net result is an excess of anions inside the cell, resulting in the resting membrane potential.

Nerve and muscle cells are excitable and can change their resting membrane potential in response to electrochemical stimuli. Changes in resting membrane potential

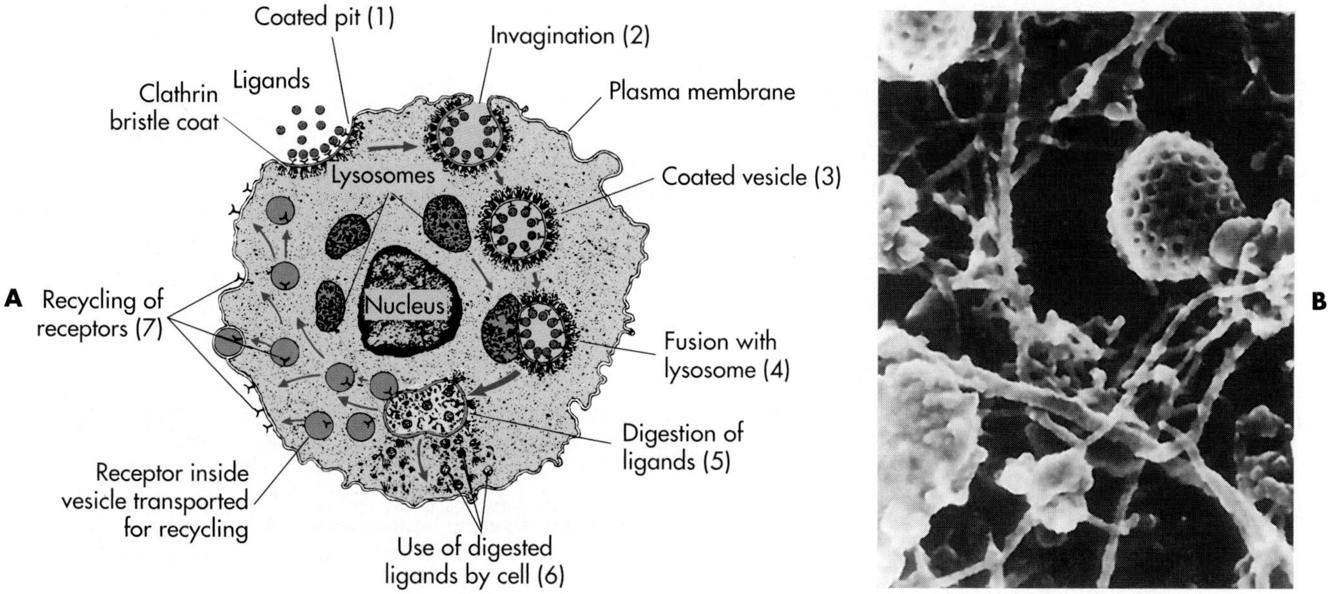

FIG. 1-21 Ligand internalization by means of receptor-mediated endocytosis. A, The ligand attaches to its surface receptor (through the bristle coat or clathrin coat) and, through receptor-mediated endocytosis, enters the cell. The ingested material fuses with a lysosome and is processed by hydrolytic lysosomal enzymes. Processed molecules can then be transferred to other cellular components. **B,** Electron micrograph of a coated pit showing different sizes of filaments of the cytoskeleton (382,000). (Modified from Erlandsen SL, Magney JE: *Color atlas of histology*, St Louis, 1992, Mosby.)

convey messages from cell to cell. When a nerve or muscle cell receives a stimulus that exceeds the membrane threshold value, there is a rapid change in the resting membrane potential known as the **action potential.** The action potential carries signals along the nerve or muscle cell and conveys information from one cell to another. (Nerve impulses are described in Chapter 13.) When a resting cell is stimulated through voltage-regulated channels, the cell membranes become more permeable to sodium. There is a net movement of sodium into the cell, and the membrane potential decreases, or "moves forward," from a negative value (in millivolts) to zero. This decrease is known as **depolarization.** The depolarized cell is more positively charged, and its polarity is neutralized.

To generate an action potential and the resulting depolarization, a critical value known as the **threshold potential** must be reached. Generally this occurs when the cell has depolarized by 15 to 20 millivolts. When the threshold is reached, the cell will continue to depolarize with no further stimulation. The sodium gates open, and sodium rushes into the cell, causing the membrane potential to reduce to zero and then become positive (depolarization). The rapid reversal in polarity results in the action potential.

During **repolarization** the negative polarity of the resting membrane potential is reestablished. As the voltage-gated sodium channels begin to close, voltage-gated potassium channels open. Membrane permeability to sodium decreases, and potassium permeability increases, with an outward movement of potassium ions. The sodium gates close, and with the outward movement of potassium, the membrane potential becomes more negative. The Na^+-K^+ pump then returns the membrane to the resting potential by pumping potassium back into the cell and sodium out of the cell.

During most of the action potential, the plasma membrane cannot respond to an additional stimulus. This time is known as the **absolute refractory period** and is related to changes in permeability to sodium. During the latter phase of the action potential, when permeability to potassium increases, a stronger-than-normal stimulus can evoke an action potential known as the **relative refractory period.**

When the membrane potential is more negative than normal, the cell is in a *hyperpolarized* (less excitable) state. A larger-than-normal stimulus is then required to reach the threshold potential and generate an action potential. When the membrane potential is more positive than normal, the cell is in a *hypopolarized* (more excitable than normal) state, and a smaller-than-normal stimulus is required to reach the threshold potential. Changes in the intracellular and extracellular concentration of ions or a change in membrane permeability can cause these alterations in membrane excitability.

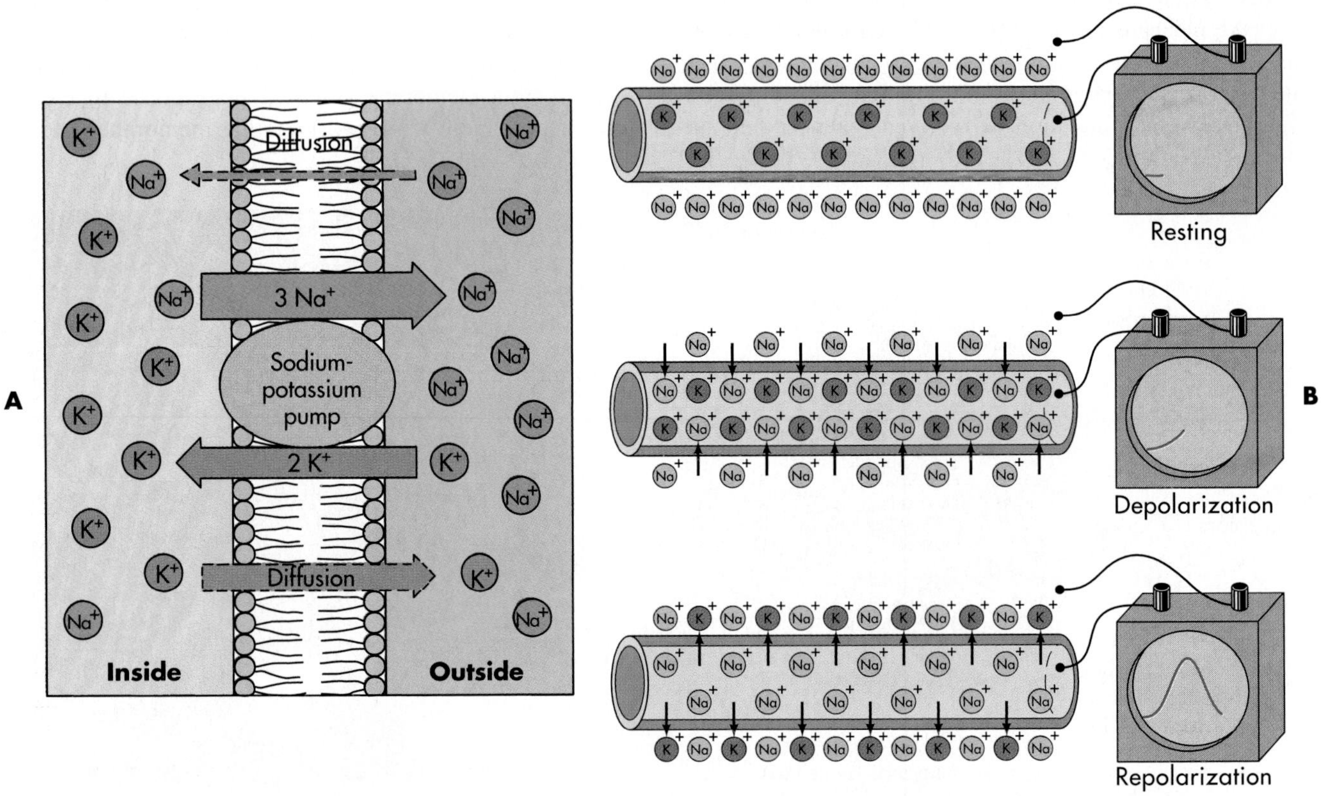

FIG. 1-22 Sodium-potassium pump and propagation of an action potential. A, Concentration difference of Na^+ and K^+ intracellularly and extracellularly. The direction of active transport by the sodium-potassium pump is also shown. **B,** Top diagram represents the polarized state of a neuronal membrane when at rest. The lower diagrams represent changes in sodium and potassium membrane permeabilities with depolarizatrion and repolarization. (From Thibodeau GA, Patton KT: *Anatomy and physiology,* ed 4, St Louis, 1999, Mosby.)

CELLULAR REPRODUCTION: THE CELL CYCLE

Human cells are subject to wear and tear, and most do not last for the lifetime of the individual. In almost all tissues, new cells are created as fast as old ones die. Cellular reproduction is therefore necessary for the maintenance of life. Reproduction of gametes (sperm and egg cells) occurs through a process called *meiosis*, described in Chapter 4. The reproduction, or division, of other body cells (somatic cells) involves two sequential phases: **mitosis,** or nuclear division, and **cytokinesis,** or cytoplasmic division. These two phases occur in close succession, with cytokinesis beginning toward the end of mitosis. Before a cell can divide, however, it must double its mass and duplicate all its contents. Most of the work of preparing for division occurs during the growth phase, called **interphase.** The alternation between mitosis and interphase in all tissues with cellular turnover is known as the **cell cycle.**

Most of the early work on the cell cycle was limited to microscopic observation of mitosis and cytokinesis. Interphase was considered the "resting stage" of the cell. With recent technologic advances a considerable amount has been learned about the interphase part of the cell cycle. During interphase many important processes are taking place as the cell produces DNA, RNA, protein, lipids, and other substances, and each pair of **chromosomes** (paired organelles that carry genetic information) also makes exact copies of itself.

The four designated phases of the cell cycle are (1) the S phase (S = synthesis), in which DNA is synthesized in the cell nucleus; (2) the G_2 phase (G = gap), in which RNA and protein synthesis occurs, the period between the completion of DNA synthesis and the next phase (M); (3) the M phase (M = mitosis), which includes both nuclear and cytoplasmic division; and (4) the G_1 phase, which is the period between the M phase and the start of DNA synthesis (Fig. 1-23).

Phases of Mitosis and Cytokinesis

Interphase (the G_1, S, and G_2 phases) is the longest phase of the cell cycle. During interphase the chromatin consists of very long, slender rods that are jumbled together in the nucleus. Late in interphase, strands of **chromatin** (the substance that gives the nucleus its granular appearance) begin to coil, causing them to shorten and thicken.

The M phase of the cell cycle, mitosis and cytokinesis, begins with **prophase**, the first appearance of chromosomes. As the phase proceeds, each chromosome is seen as two identical halves called **chromatids,** which lie together and are attached at some point by a spindle attachment site called a **centromere**. (The two chromatids of each chromosome, which are genetically identical, are sometimes called *sister chromatids*.) The nuclear membrane, which surrounds the nucleus, disappears. Spindle fibers are microtubules formed in the cytoplasm. **Spindle fibers** radiate from two centrioles located at opposite poles of the cell. The role of the spindle fibers is to pull the chromosomes to opposite sides of the cell.

During **metaphase,** the next phase of mitosis and cytokinesis, the spindle fibers begin to pull the centromeres of the chromosomes. The centromeres become aligned in the middle of the spindle, which is called the **equatorial plate** (or **metaphase plate**) of the cell. This is the stage in which chromosomes are easiest to observe microscopically, since they are highly condensed and arranged in a relatively organized fashion in the two-dimensional equatorial plate.

Anaphase begins when the centromeres split and the sister chromatids are pulled apart. The spindle fibers shorten, causing the sister chromatids to be pulled, centromere first, toward opposite sides of the cell. When the sister chromatids are separated, each is considered to be a chromosome. Thus the cell has 92 chromosomes during this stage. By the end of anaphase, 46 chromosomes are lying at each side of the

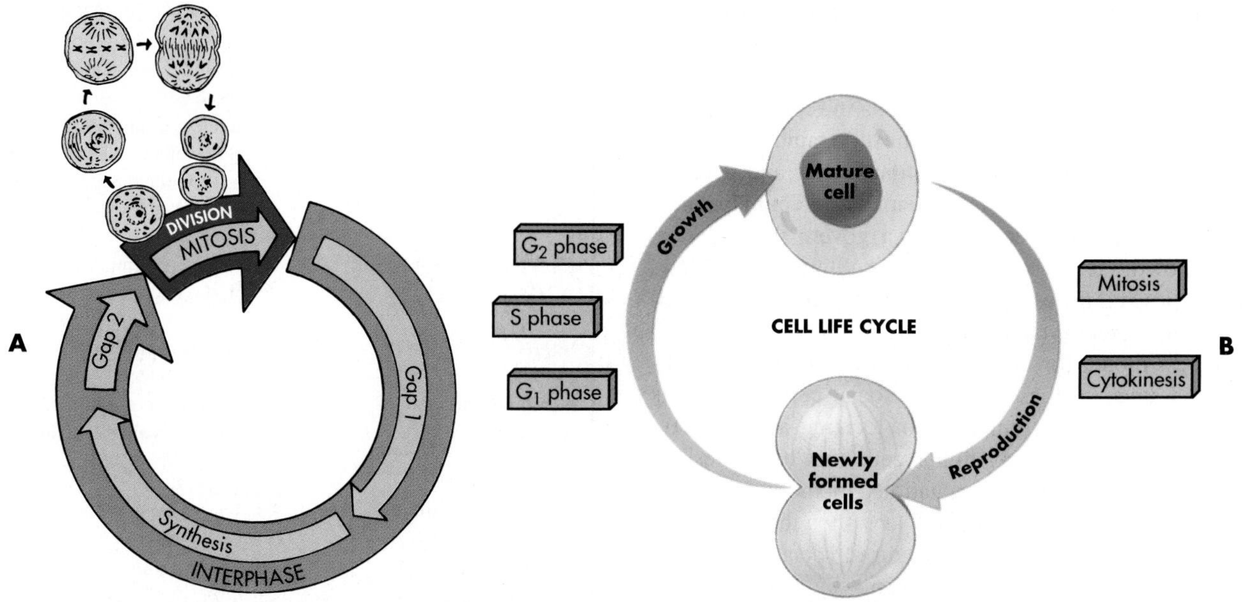

FIG. 1-23 Interphase and the phases of mitosis. (**B** from Thibodeau GA, Patton KT: *Anatomy and physiology,* ed 4, St Louis, 1999, Mosby.)

cell. Barring mitotic errors, each of the two groups of 46 chromosomes is identical to the original 46 chromosomes present at the start of the cell cycle.

During **telophase,** the final stage, a new nuclear membrane is formed around each group of 46 chromosomes, the spindle fibers disappear, and the chromosomes begin to uncoil. Cytokinesis causes the cytoplasm to divide into roughly equal parts during this phase. At the end of telophase, two identical diploid cells, called *daughter cells*, have been formed from the original cell.

Rates of Cellular Division

Although the complete cell cycle lasts 12 to 24 hours, about 1 hour is generally required for the four stages of mitosis and cytokinesis. All types of cells undergo mitosis during formation of the embryo, but many adult cells, such as nerve cells, lens cells of the eye, and muscle cells, lose their ability to replicate and divide. The cells of other tissues, particularly epithelial cells (e.g., of the intestine, lung, skin), divide continuously and rapidly, completing the entire cell cycle in less than 10 hours.

The difference between cells that divide slowly and cells that divide rapidly is the length of time spent in the G_1 phase of the cell cycle. Some cells that divide very slowly remain in the G_1 phase for days or even years. Once the S phase begins, however, progression through mitosis takes a relatively constant amount of time. Once a cell has progressed out of the G_1 phase, there is no turning back; it is committed to completing the S, G_2, and M phases. Times associated with the four successive phases differ.

The mechanisms that control cell division depend on "social control genes" and protein growth factors. Individual cells are members of a complex cellular society in which survival of the *entire organism* is key and not survival or proliferation of just the *individual cells*. To grow and divide, a cell must receive specific positive signals from other cells. Many of these signals *are* protein growth factors that act by overriding intracellular negative controls that block progress of the cell cycle.[1]

When a need arises for new cells, as in repair of injured cells, previously nondividing cells must be rapidly triggered to reenter the cell cycle. With continual wear and tear, the cell birth rate and the cell death rate must be kept in balance. Therefore cell-division controls must govern this balance. Protein growth factors governing the proliferation of different cell types and genes involved in the social control of cell division are currently being identified.[1]

The best model for understanding disruption of cell division and study of these so-called social control genes is tumor biology. Current emphasis in locating and identifying these genes is to study tumor cells that have presumably originated because of mutations to these genes, or proto-oncogenes. Proto-oncogenes are thought to encode key components of the normal system of social controls of cell division[1]; that is, the mechanisms by which signals from a cell's neighbors can impel it to divide, differentiate, or die. Some proto-oncogenes code for growth factors, some for growth factor receptors, some for intracellular regulatory proteins that are involved in cell adhesion, and some for proteins that help relay signals for cell division to the cell nucleus.[1] Although more than 50 proto-oncogenes have been identified, many more are yet to be discovered (see Chapter 10).

Growth Factors

Growth factors, also called *cytokines,* are peptides that transmit signals within and between cells. They have a major role in the regulation of tissue growth and development (Table 1-4). In addition to receiving nutrients, a cell, to proliferate, must receive stimulatory chemical signals (growth factors) from other cells, usually its neighbors. These signals act to overcome intracellular braking mechanisms that tend to restrain cell growth and block progress through the cell cycle.

Different types of cells require different factors; for example, **platelet-derived growth factor (PDGF)** stimulates the production of connective tissue cells. Table 1-4 summarizes the most significant growth factors. Cells that respond to a particular growth factor have specific receptors for the growth factor in their plasma membrane. Recent evidence

Table 1-4 Examples of Growth Factors and Their Actions

Growth Factor	Physiologic Actions
Platelet-derived growth factor (PDGF)	Stimulates proliferation of connective tissue cells and neuroglial cells
Epidermal growth factor (EGF)	Stimulates proliferation of epidermal cells and other cell types
Insulin-like growth factor I (IGF-I)	Collaborates with PDGF and EGF; stimulates proliferation of fat cells and connective tissue cells
Insulin-like growth factor II (IGF-II)	Collaborates with PDGF and EGF; stimulates proliferation of fat cells and connective tissue cells
Transforming growth factor β (TGF-β)	Stimulates or inhibits response of most cells to other growth factors; regulates differentiation of some cell types (e.g., cartilage)
Fibroblast growth factor (FGF)	Stimulates proliferation of fibroblasts, endothelial cells, myoblasts, and other cell types
Interleukin-2 (IL-2)	Stimulates proliferation of T lymphocytes
Nerve growth factor (NGF)	Promotes axon growth and survival of sympathetic and some sensory and CNS neurons
Hemopoietic cell growth factors (IL-3, GM-CSF, M-CSF, G-CSF, erythropoietin)	See Chapter 24

GM, Granulocyte-macrophage; *CSF,* colony-stimulating factor; *M,* macrophage; *G,* granulocyte.

shows that some growth factors are also regulators of other cell processes, such as cellular differentiation. In addition to growth factors that stimulate cellular processes, there are factors that inhibit functions; these factors are not well understood. Cells that are starved of growth factors come to a halt after mitosis and enter the **arrested,** or **G_0, state** of the cell cycle (see p. 25 for cell cycle).[1]

CELL-TO-CELL ADHESIONS

Cells are small and squishy and not like bricks. They are enclosed by a flimsy membrane, yet the cell depends on the integrity of this membrane for its survival. How can cells be formed together strongly, with their membranes intact, to form a muscle that can lift this textbook? Plasma membranes not only serve as the outer boundaries of all cells but also allow groups of cells to be held together robustly, in cell-to-cell adhesions, to form tissues and organs. Once arranged, cells are held together by three different means: the extracellular matrix, cell adhesion molecules in the cell's plasma membrane, and specialized cell junctions.

Extracellular Matrix

Cells can be bound together by attachment to one another or via the **extracellular matrix,** which the cells secrete around themselves. The extracellular matrix is an intricate meshwork of fibrous proteins embedded in a watery, gel-like substance composed of complex carbohydrates (Fig. 1-24). The matrix is like glue; however, it provides a pathway for diffusion of nutrients, wastes, and other water-soluble traffic between the blood and tissue cells. Interwoven within the matrix are three types of protein fibers: collagen, elastin, and fibronectin.

Collagen forms cablelike fibers or sheets that provide tensile strength or resistance to longitudinal stress. Collagen breakdown, such as occurs in osteoarthritis, destroys the fibrils that give cartilage its tensile strength.

Elastin is a rubberlike protein fiber most abundant in tissue that must be capable of stretching and recoiling, like the lungs.

Fibronectin promotes cell adhesion and cell anchorage. Reduced amounts have been found in certain types of cancerous cells allowing cancer cells to travel or metastasize to other parts of the body.

The extracellular matrix is secreted by fibroblasts ("fiber formers"), local cells present in the matrix. The matrix and the cells within it are known collectively as connective tissue because they connect cells together to form tissue and organs. Human connective tissues are enormously varied. They can be hard and dense, like bone; flexible, like tendons or the dermis of the skin; resilient and shock-absorbing, like cartilage; or soft and transparent, like the jelly that fills the eye. In all these examples, the majority of the tissue is occupied by extracellular matrix and the cells that produce the matrix are scattered within it like raisins in a pudding (see Fig. 1-24).[9]

The matrix is not just a passive scaffolding for cellular attachment but also helps regulate the functions of the cells within which it interacts. The matrix helps regulate cell growth and differentiation.

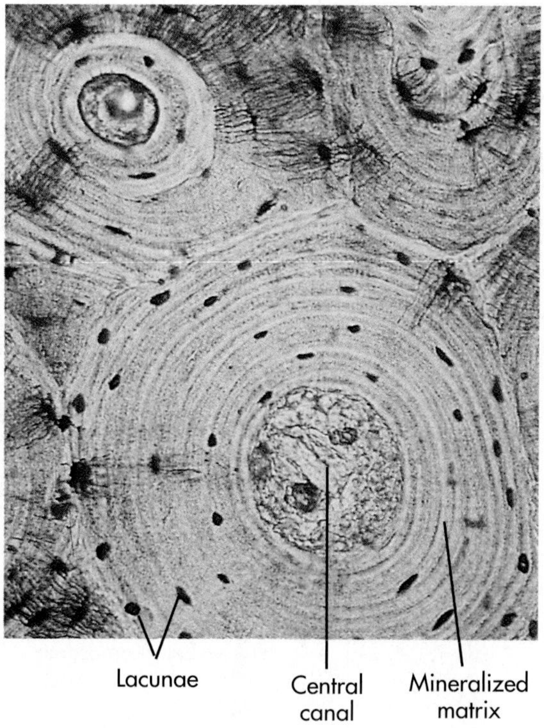

FIG. 1-24 Bone extracellular matrix. The raisin-like dark objects are scattered and embedded in the bone extracellular matrix, which occupies most of the volume of the tissue and provides all of its mechanical strength. (From Thibodeau GA, Patton KT: *Anatomy & physiology*, ed 4, St Louis, 1999, Mosby.)

Specialized Cell Junctions

Cells in direct physical contact with neighboring cells are often linked together at specialized regions of their plasma membranes called **cell junctions.** Cell junctions have two main functions: (1) to hold cells together and (2) to allow small molecules to pass from cell to cell, allowing coordination of the activities of cells that form tissues. The three main types of cell junctions are (1) desmosomes (adhering junctions, or macula adherens), (2) tight junctions (impermeable junctions, or zonula occludens), and (3) gap junctions (communicating junctions) (Fig. 1-25). Together they form the **junctional complex**. **Desmosomes** hold cells together by forming either continuous bands or belts of epithelial sheets or buttonlike points of contact. Desmosomes also act as a system of braces to maintain structural stability. **Tight junctions** serve as a barrier to diffusion, prevent the movement of substances through transport proteins in the plasma membrane, and prevent the leakage of small molecules between the plasma membranes of adjacent cells. **Gap junctions** are clusters of communicating tunnels, **connexons,** that allow small ions and molecules to pass directly from the inside of one cell to the inside of another. Connexons are joining proteins that extend outward from each of the adjacent plasma membranes. Cells connected by gap junctions are considered ionically (electrically) and metabolically coupled. Gap junctions coordinate the activities of adjacent cells. They are important, for example, in synchronizing contractions of heart muscle cells through ionic coupling and in permitting action potentials to spread rapidly from cell to cell

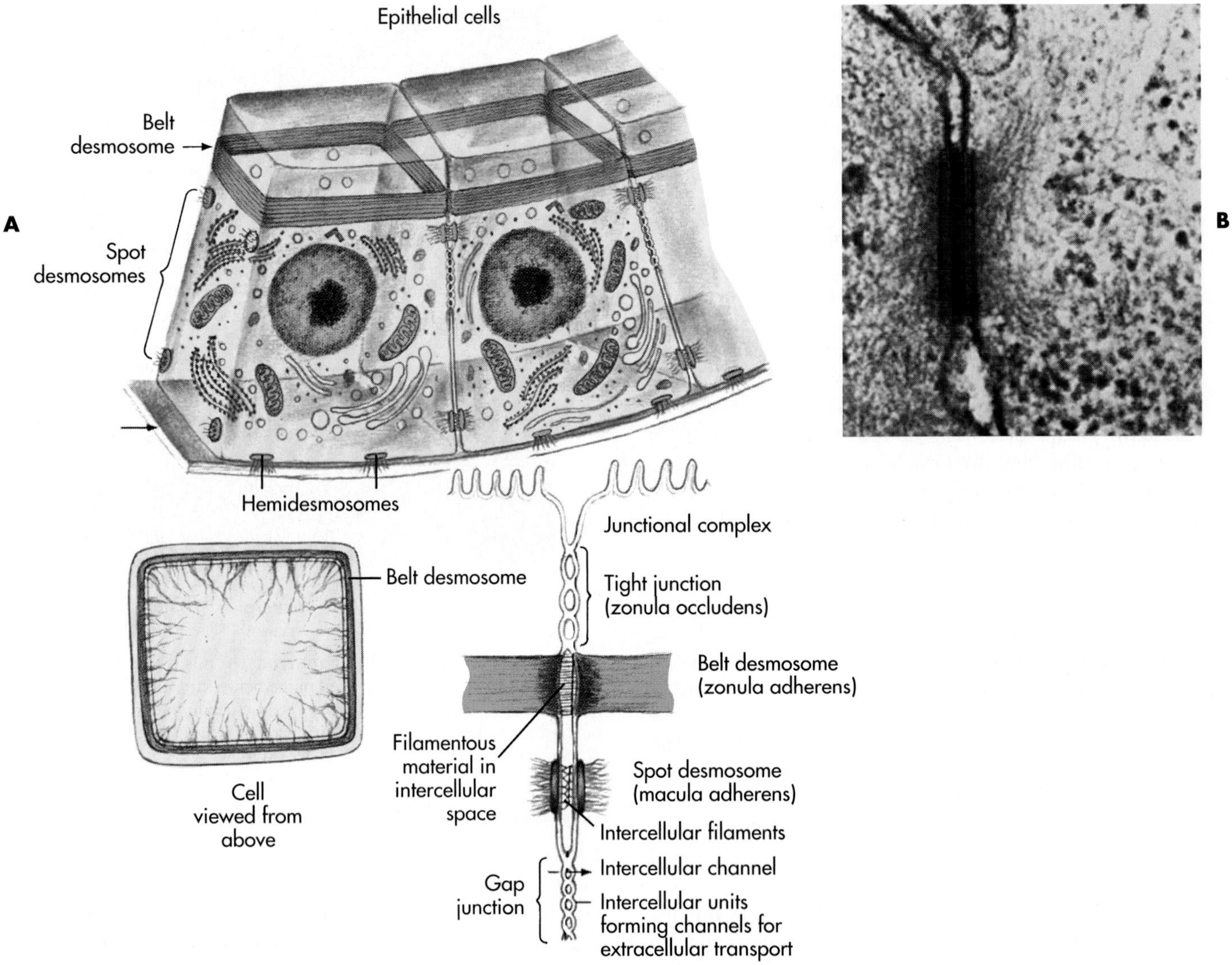

FIG. 1-25 Junctional complex. A, Schematic drawing of a belt demosome between epithelial cells. This junction, also called *zonula adherens,* encircles each interacting cell. The spot desmosomes and hemidesmosomes, like the belt demosomes, are adhering junctions. This tight junction is an impermeable junction that holds cells together but seals them in such a way that molecules cannot leak between them. The gap junction, as a communicating junction, mediates the passage of small molecules from one interacting cell to the other. **B,** Electron micrograph of desmosomes. (From Raven PH, Johnson GB: *Biology,* St Louis, 1992, Mosby.)

in neural tissues. The reason that gap junctions occur in tissues that are not electrically active is unknown. Although most gap junctions are associated with junctional complexes, they sometimes exist as independent structures.

The junctional complex is a highly permeable part of the plasma membrane. Its permeability is controlled by a process called **gating,** which depends on concentrations of calcium ions in the cytoplasm. Increased cytoplasmic calcium causes decreased permeability at the junctional complex. Gating is an important cellular defense mechanism because it enables uninjured cells to seal themselves off from injured neighbors. As damaged cells release calcium, it travels through the junctional complex and increases calcium levels in neighboring cells. (The damaging effects of calcium influx are described in Chapter 2.) This decreases the permeability of the junctional complexes of the neighboring cells, which form a relatively impermeable wall around the injured area.

CELLULAR COMMUNICATION AND SIGNAL TRANSDUCTON

Cells need to communicate with each other to maintain a stable internal environment, or **homeostasis;** to regulate their growth and division and their development and organization into tissues; and to coordinate their functions. Cells communicate in three ways: (1) they form protein channels (gap junctions) that directly coordinate the activities of adjacent cells; (2) they display plasma membrane–bound signaling molecules (receptors) that affect the cell itself and other cells in direct physical contact; and (3) the most common means, they secrete chemicals that signal to cells some distance away (Fig. 1-26). Alterations in cellular communication affect disease onset and progression. In fact, if a cell is unable to perform gap junctional intercellular communication, it is hypothesized that normal growth control and cell differentiation are compromised, favoring cancerous tumor development (see Chapter 10). (Communication through gap junctions is discussed on p. 27, and contact signaling by plasma membrane–bound molecules is discussed on p. 13.) Secreted chemical signals involve communication at a distance. Primary modes of chemical signaling are hormonal, neurohormonal, paracrine, and autocrine (Fig. 1-27).

Hormonal signaling involves specialized endocrine cells that secrete hormone chemicals released by one set of

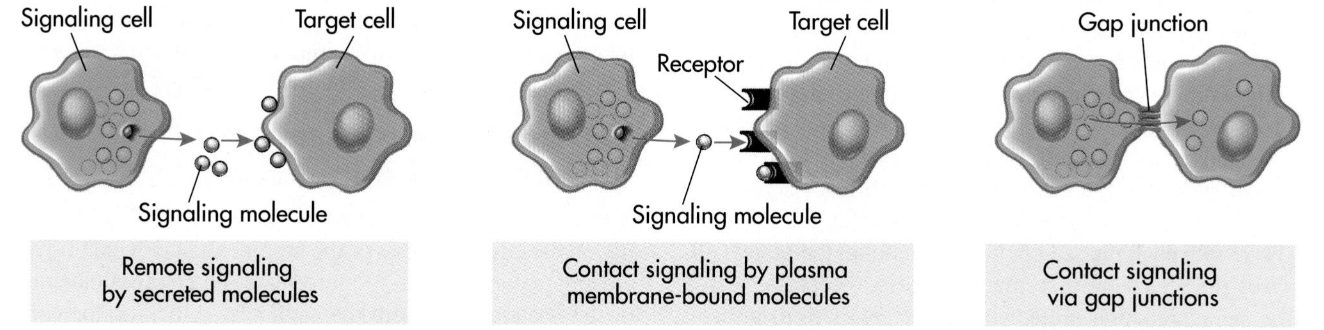

FIG. 1-26 Cellular communication. Three ways in which cells communicate with one another.

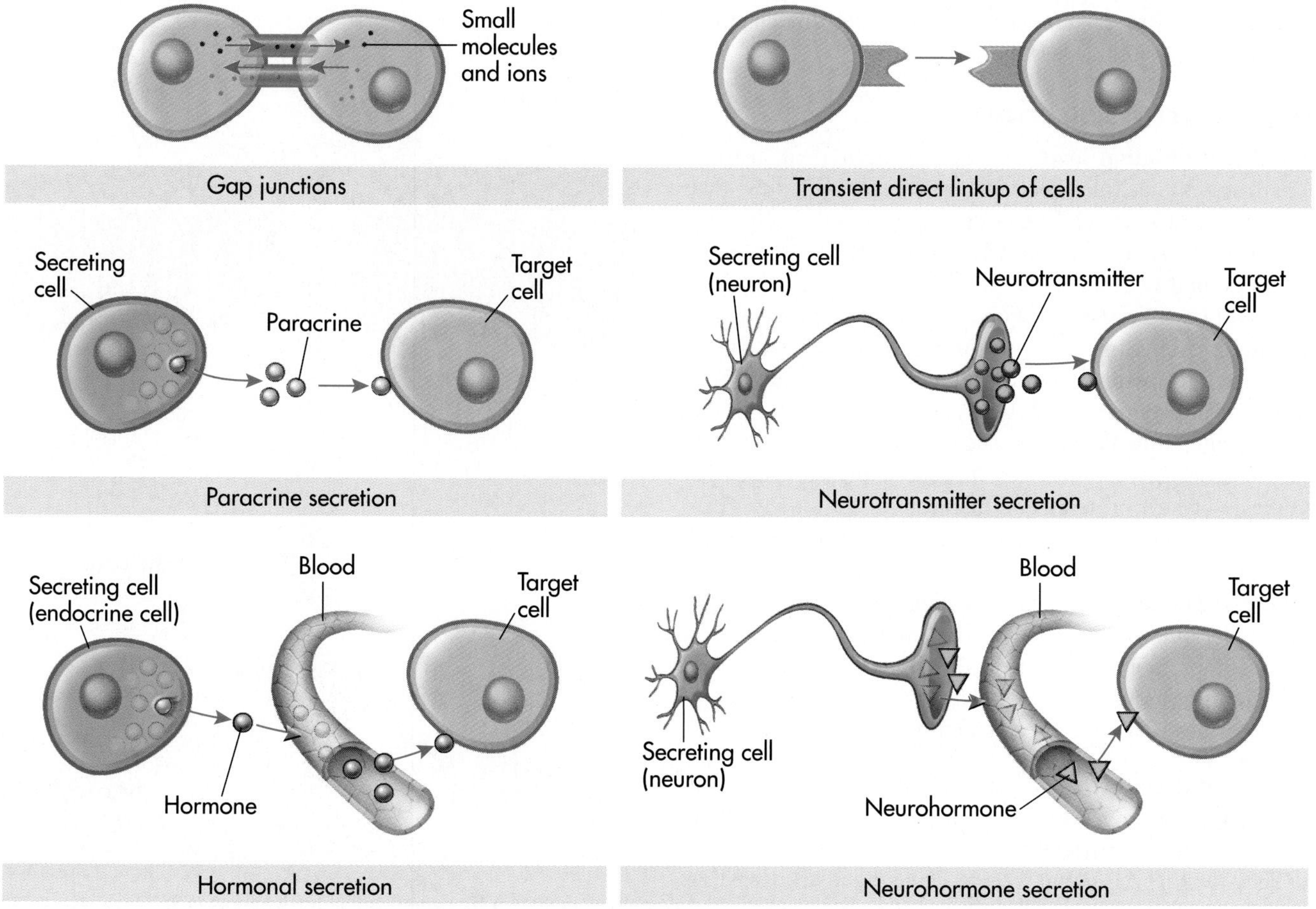

FIG. 1-27 Modes of chemical signaling and cell communication. Paracrines, neurotransmitters, hormones, and neurohormones are all intercellular chemical messengers that accomplish communication between cells. Gap junctions provide the most intimate means of intercellular communication where small molecules and ions are exchanged between interacting cells without even entering the extracellular fluid. Autocrine stimulation (not illustrated) is when the secreting cell targets itself. (Modified from Sherwood L: *Human physiology: from cells to systems*, ed 3, Belmont, Calif, 1997, Wadsworth.)

cells and travel through the tissue and through the bloodstream to produce a response in other sets of cells (see Chapter 19). In **neurohormonal signaling** hormones are released into the blood by neurosecretory neurons. Like endocrine cells, neurosecretory neurons release blood-borne chemical messengers, whereas ordinary neurons secrete short-range neurotransmitters into a small discrete space. In **paracrine signaling,** cells secrete local chemical mediators that are quickly taken up, destroyed, or immobilized. The mediators act only on nearby cells. In **autocrine signaling,** signaling molecules may act back on the cells of *origin* (i.e., *autostimulation*); autocrine circuits function as a component of normal growth-regulatory mechanisms in many adult tissue types.[10,11] Neurons communicate directly with the cells they innervate by releasing neurotransmitters at specialized junctions called *chemical synapses*; the neutrotransmitter diffuses across the synaptic cleft and acts on the postsynaptic target cell (see Fig. 1-28). In each type of chemical signaling, the target cell receives the signal by first attaching to its receptors. Many of the same signaling molecules are receptors used in hormonal, neurohormonal, paracrine, and autocrine signaling. The important differences lie in the speed and selectivity with which the signals are delivered to their targets.[1]

Plasma membrane receptors belong to one of three classes that are defined by the signaling (transduction) mechanism used. Table 1-2 summarizes these receptors.

Signal Transduction

Signal transduction involves incoming signals or instructions from extracellular chemical messengers (ligands) that are conveyed to the cell's interior for execution. Within the outer surface of the plasma membrane specialized protein receptors bind with the selected chemical messengers. This combination of messenger with receptor triggers a cascade of cellular events important to the maintenance of homeostasis, such as membrane transport, cell division and differentiation, movement, secretion, and metabolism. Some types of altered cell behavior, such as increased cell growth and division, involve changes in gene expression and the synthesis of new proteins and therefore occur slowly. Others, such as changes in cell movement, secretion, or metabolism, do not involve the nuclear machinery and therefore occur more rapidly. If deprived of appropriate signals, most cells undergo a form of cell suicide known as programmed cell death, or apoptosis (see p. 74).

Signaling cascades, or relay chains, of intercellular signaling molecules have several important functions (Fig. 1-28):

1. They physically *transfer* the signal from the place at which it is received to some other part of the cell where the response is expected.
2. They *amplify* the signal received, making it stronger; this is caused by a multiplying effect in the pathways; for example, binding of one ligand molecule to a receptor activates a number of adenylyl cyclase molecules.
3. They *distribute* the signal so that it influences several processes in parallel; at any step in the pathway, the signal can *diverge* and be relayed to several different intracellular targets, creating branches in the flow and causing a complex response (see Fig. 1-29).
4. Last, the signal can be *modulated* by other interfering factors prevailing inside or outside the cell.

Two general responses from binding of the extracellular chemical messenger, or **first messenger,** to the membrane receptors occur: (1) opening or closing specific channels in the membrane to regulate the movement of ions into or out of the cell and (2) transferring the signal to an intracellular messenger, or **second messenger,** which in turn triggers a cascade of biochemical events within the cell.

Extracellular Messengers and Channel Regulation

Membrane channels, or "gates," can open and close depending on the circumstances of the first messenger. Opening and closing occur because of conformational changes (shaping) of the proteins that form the channels—blocking the channel (closing) or permitting passage through it (opening). Channel opening and closing can be initiated in one of three ways: (1) by binding of a ligand to a specific membrane re-

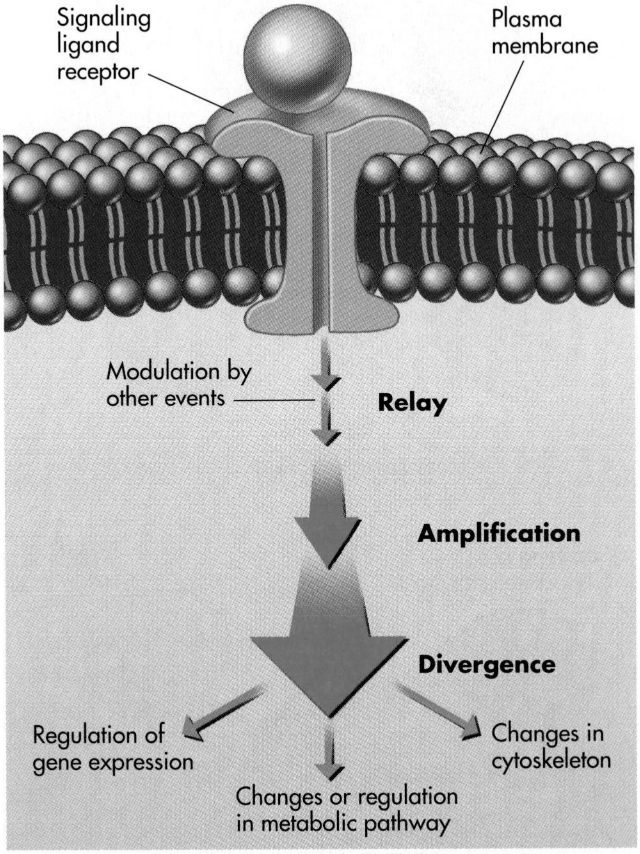

FIG. 1-28 An intracellular signaling cascade. An extracellular chemical messenger (ligand) bonds to a receptor protein located on the plasma membrane where it is transduced into an intracellular signal. This process initiates a signaling cascade that relays the signal into the cell interior, amplifying and distributing it en route. Steps in the cascade can be modulated by other events in the cell.

ceptor that is closely associated with the channel, for example, G proteins; (2) by changes in electric current in the plasma membrane, altering flow of Na^+ and K^+; and (3) by stretching or other chemical deformation of the channel. Fig. 1-29 summarizes ways by which extracellular messengers regulate channel function for the other two methods of controlling channels (see p. 32).

Second Messengers

Many ligands cannot enter their target cells to bring about the desired intracellular response. Instead, the first messengers, or ligands, issue orders by binding with receptors on the surface membrane, triggering a "pass it on" signal. Second messengers are generated in large numbers when the membrane-bound enzyme is activated, and they then rapidly diffuse away

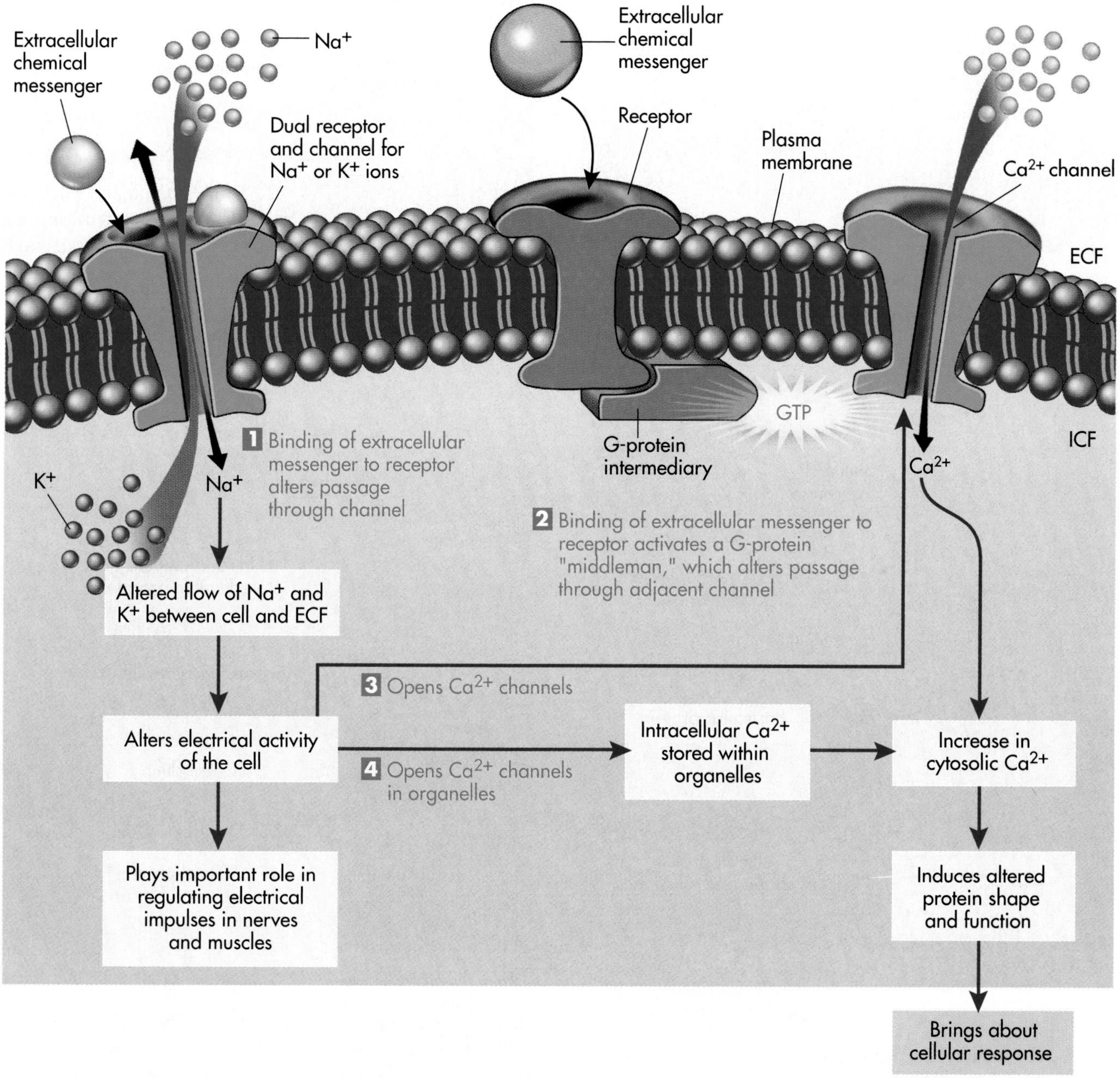

FIG. 1-29 How extracellular messengers regulate channel function. Binding of an extracellular messenger to a dual receptor/channel brings about a quick opening or closing of ion channels, such as Na^+ or K^+ channels, which generates electrical impulses (*1*). A transient opening of membrane Ca^{++} channels occurs when binding of an extracellular messenger to a receptor activates a G-protein intermediary, which alters a nearby ion channel, such as a Ca^{++} channel (*2*). A transient opening of Ca^{++} channels also occurs indirectly in response to electrical impulses produced by extracellular messenger-induced changes in Na^+ and K^+ channels (*3*). Release of Ca^{++} from intracellular stores results when Ca^{++} channels in organelles open in response to electrical impulses (*4*). An increase in cytosolic Ca^{++} arising from pathways 2, 3, or 4 causes changes in the shape and function of specific intracellular proteins to produce the desired cellular response. (Adapted from Sherwood L: *Human physiology: from cells to systems*, ed 3, Belmont, Calif, 1997, Wadsworth.)

from their source, broadcasting the signal throughout the cell (Fig. 1-30). Remember, most cell-surface receptor proteins belong to one of three large classes: ion-channel-linked receptors, G-protein-linked receptors, or enzyme-linked receptors.

The two major second messenger pathways are **cyclic adenosine monophosphate (cyclic AMP, cAMP)** and Ca^{++}. In the cAMP pathway, binding of the ligand to its surface receptor eventually activates the enzyme adenylyl cyclase on the inner surface of the membrane. A membrane-bound "middleman," a **G protein,** acts as an intermediary between

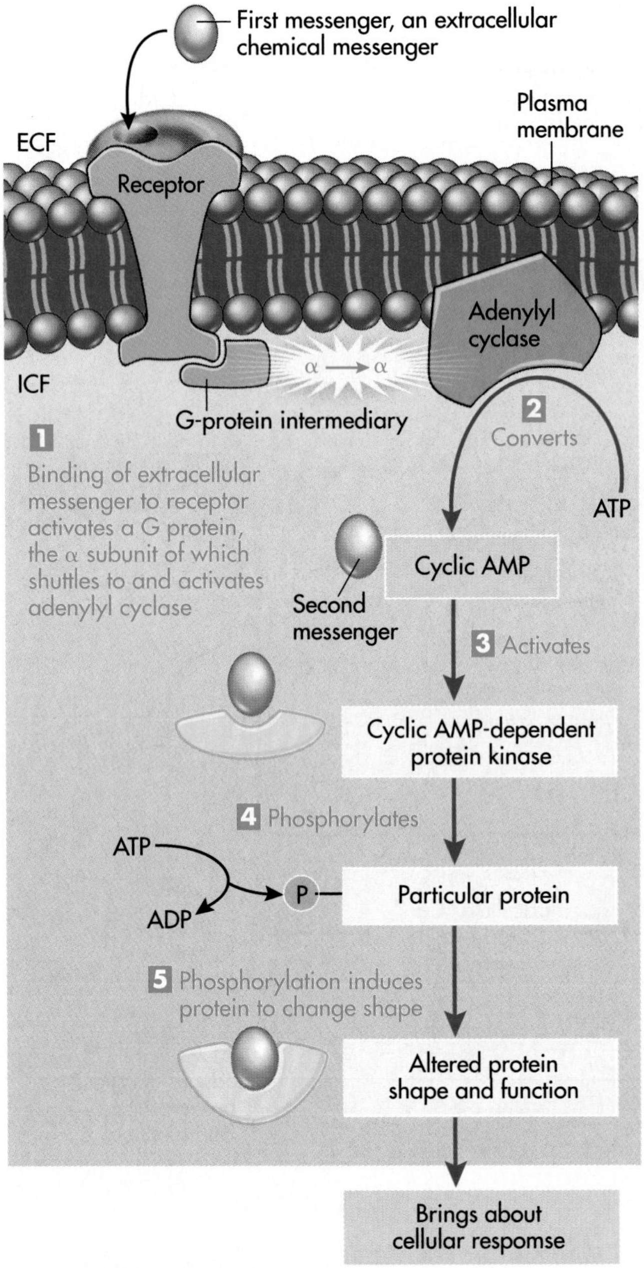

FIG. 1-30 Extracellular messenger and activation of the cAMP second messenger system. The *first messenger*, or binding of an extracellular chemical messenger to a surface membrane receptor, activates the membrane-bound enzyme adenylyl cyclase by means of a G-protein intermediary (*1*), which in turn converts intracellular ATP into cAMP (*2*). cAMP is an intracellular *second messenger*, triggering the cellular response by activating the cAMP-dependent protein kinase (*3*), which in turn phosphorylates (*4*) and therefore modifies (*5*) a specific intracellular protein. The altered protein then directs the cellular response dictated by the extracellular messenger. (Adapted from Sherwood L: *Human physiology: from cells to systems*, ed 3, Belmont, Calif, 1997, Wadsworth.)

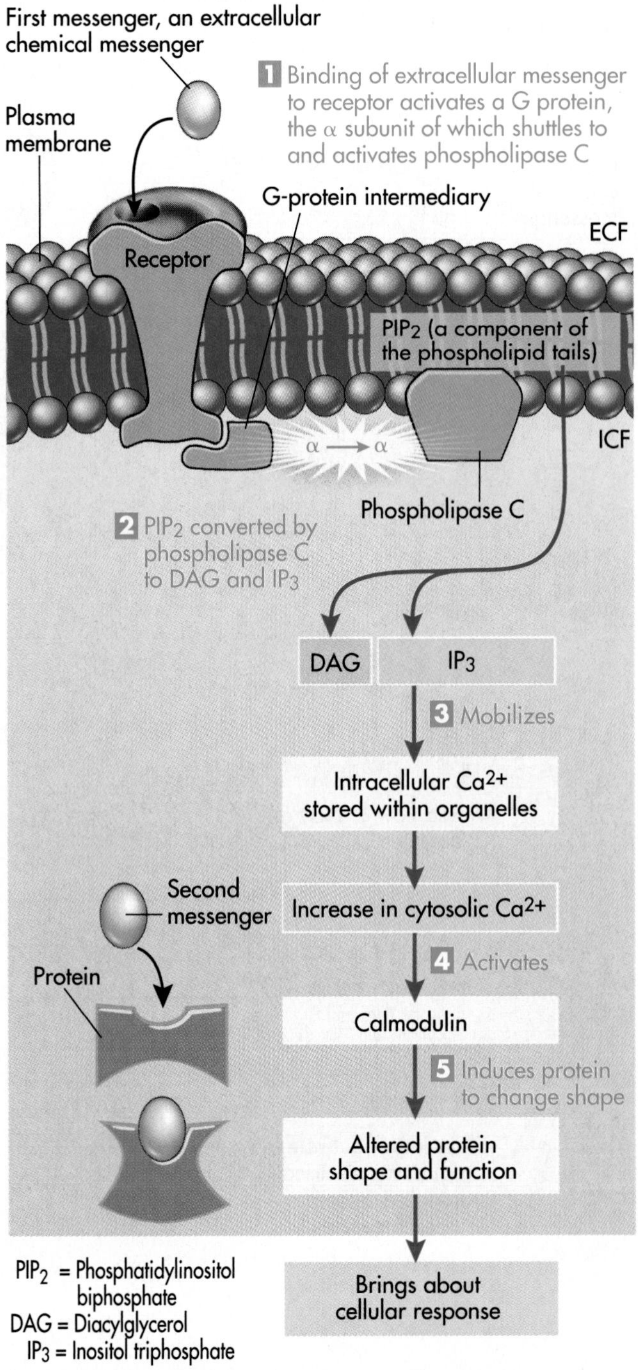

FIG. 1-31 Extracellular messenger and activation of the calcium second messenger system. Binding of an extracellular messenger to a membrane receptor activates the membrane-bound enzyme phospholipase C by means of a G-protein intermediary (*1*). Phospholipase C converts phosphatidylinositol biphosphate (PIP_2) into diacylglycerol (DAG) and inositol triphosphate (IP_3) (*2*). IP_3 then mobilizes Ca^{++} stored within organelles (*3*). Ca^{++}, as a *second messenger*, activates calmodulin (*4*), causing a change in the shape and function of a specific intracellular protein to produce the cellular response (*5*). (Adapted from Sherwood L: *Human physiology: from cells to systems*, ed 3, Belmont, Calif, 1997, Wadsworth.)

the receptor and adenylyl cylcase. G proteins are named because they are bound to guanine nucleotides—**guanosine triphosphate (GTP)** or **guanosine diphosphate (GDP).** An unactivated G protein consists of a complex of alpha (α), beta (β), and gamma (γ) subunits, with a GDP molecule bound to the α subunit. The cAMP pathway with G proteins is summarized in Fig. 1-30.

Instead of cAMP, some cells use Ca^{++} as a second messenger. In this pathway, binding of the first messenger to the surface receptor eventually leads, by means of G proteins, to activation of the enzyme **phospholipase C,** an enzyme **protein effector** (an ion channel for an enzyme) that is bound to the inner side of the membrane. Fig. 1-31 summarizes the Ca^{++} second messenger pathway. The cAMP and Ca^{++} pathways frequently overlap in bringing about a specific cellular response. For example, cAMP and Ca^{++} can influence each other. Calcium-activated calmodulin can regulate adenylyl cyclase and thus influence cAMP; conversely, cAMP-dependent kinase may phosphorylate and thereby change the activity of Ca^{++} channels or carriers. In some instances, both Ca^{++} and cAMP regulate the same intracellular protein. In a few cells, **cyclic guanosine monophosphate (cyclic GMP, cGMP)** serves as a second messenger similar to the cAMP pathway. For example, cGMP is the signal transduction pathway involved in vision. Some cellular responses mediated by cAMP and phospholipase C are summarized in Table 1-5.

A large number of human disorders involve problematic signaling in cells. Cancer, for example, results from genetic mutations leading to the overactivity of proteins in signal-relaying pathways that normally induce the cells to divide. Affected proteins cause cells to behave as if other cells were constantly telling them to reproduce, even when no such orders were sent.[12] Signal blockers are already in use against breast cancer.

TISSUES

The body is made up of four levels of organization: cells, tissues, organs, and systems. Cells of common structure and function are organized into **tissues,** of which there are four primary types: *muscle, neural, epithelial,* and *connective* tissue.

Tissue Formation

To form tissues, cells must exhibit intercellular recognition and adhesion. Specialized cells are thought to form a tissue in one of two ways. First and simplest is mitosis of one or more **founder cells** (the most basic precursor cell). Founder cells are prevented from "wandering away" by macromolecules in the extracellular matrix and by adherence to one another at specialized junctions on their plasma membranes. Mitosis of founder cells forms, for example, epithelial cell sheets (Fig. 1-32).

The second way in which specialized cells form tissues involves their migration to and subsequent assembly at the site of tissue formation. During embryonic development, for example, cells from the neural crest migrate to several different regions, where they differentiate and assemble into a variety of tissues, including those of the peripheral nervous system. Migrant cells are thought to arrive at the site of tissue formation through chemotaxis or contact guidance. **Chemotaxis** is movement along a chemical gradient caused by chemical attraction (see Chapter 7). Cells at the migrant cells' destination secrete a chemical, called *chemotactic factor*, that attracts specific migrant cells. **Contact guidance** is movement along a pathway, or "pavement," in the extracellular matrix.[1]

Tissues are not randomly arranged into organs. No matter how tissue is formed, staying together in groups means that cells must recognize each other and remain distinct from the cells of surrounding tissues. Little is known about the mechanisms involved in these processes.

Types of Tissues

Epithelial Tissue

Epithelial tissue covers most internal and external surfaces of the body. Epithelial cells are closely joined and are attached to a basement membrane or lamina (extracellular matrix), which provides a supporting layer and separates the epithelium from underlying connective tissue (see Fig. 1-32, *A*). Because of its variety of locations, epithelial tissue has several diverse functions, including protection, absorption, secretion, and excretion. For example, the epidermis provides a protective barrier between the host and the outside environment, and the linings of the internal body organs help absorb substances into the body, excrete waste products, and secrete substances into body cavities.

Epithelial cell surfaces differ according to their location and function. Epithelial cells that line body cavities and blood vessels are smooth, whereas other epithelial cells have tiny cytoplasmic projections called **microvilli** on their free

Table 1-5 Hormone-Induced Cell Responses Mediated by cAMP

Signaling Ligands	Target Tissue	Major Response
Epinephrine	Heart	Increase in heart rate and force of contraction
Epinephrine, ACTH	Muscle	Glycogen breakdown
Glucagon	Fat	Fat breakdown
ACTH	Adrenal gland	Cortisol secretion
Antidiuretic hormone	Liver	Glycogen breakdown
Acetylcholine	Pancreas; smooth muscle	Amylase secretion; contraction
Antigen	Mast cells	Histamine secretion
Thrombin	Blood platelets	Serotonin and platelet-derived growth factor secretion; platelet aggregation

cAMP, cyclic adenosine monophosphate; *ACTH,* adrenocorticotropic hormone.

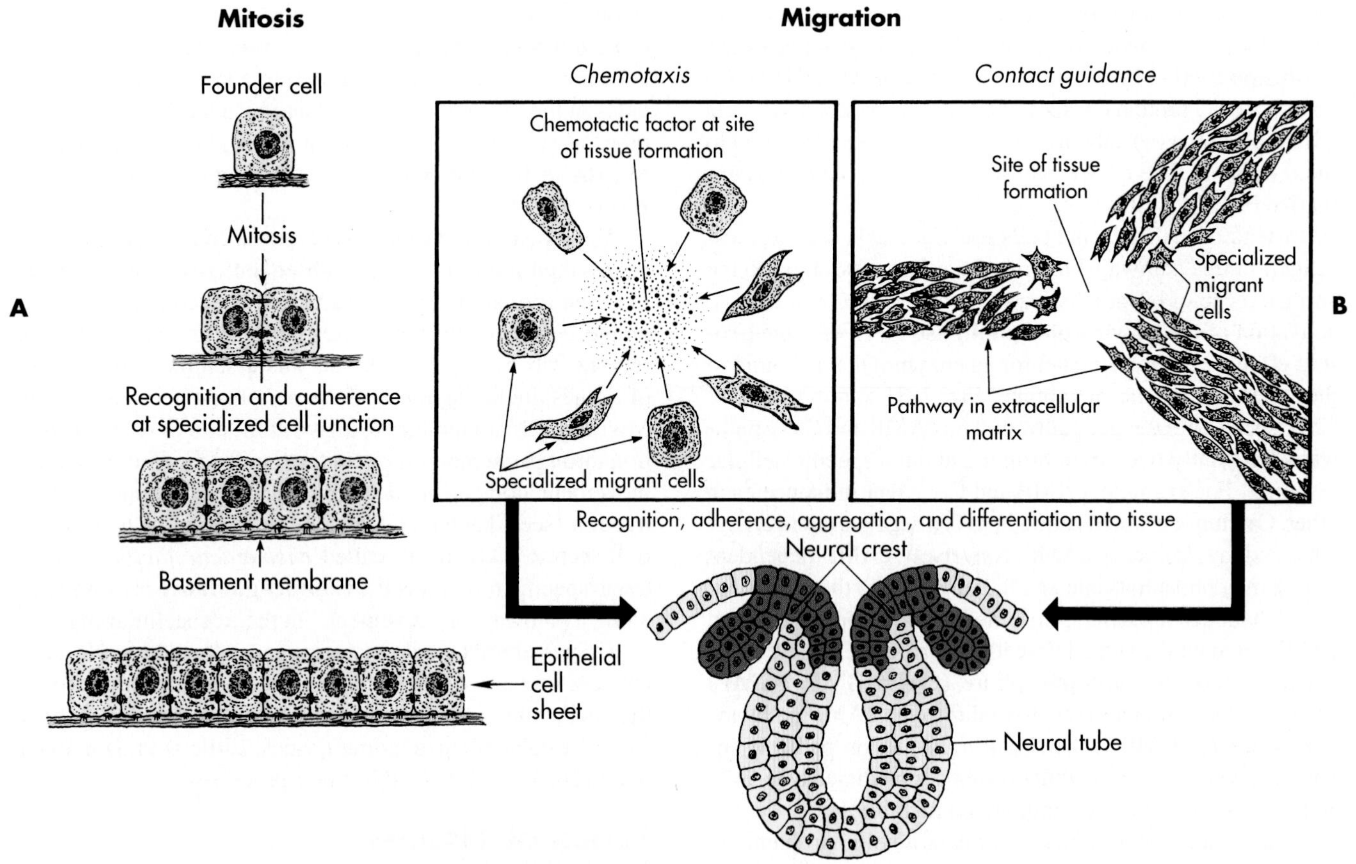

FIG. 1-32 Tissue formation by mitosis and migration. A, Tissue formation by mitosis. Founder cells are kept in place by extracellular matrix and recognition and adherence at cell junctions. **B,** Tissue formation by migration. Specialized cells are attracted to the site of tissue formation by chemotaxis or contact guidance; then they aggregate and differentiate into organized tissue.

surfaces. Microvilli considerably increase the cell's surface area and are found on cells whose main functions are absorption and secretion, such as the epithelial cells lining the digestive tract. **Cilia,** which are hairlike projections that propel mucus, pus, and dust particles out of the body, characterize cells lining the respiratory passages.

Epithelial tissue is classified in two ways: (1) according to the number and arrangement of cell layers and (2) according to cell shape. Epithelium that is formed by a single layer of cells, all of which are in contact with the basement membrane, is called **simple epithelium. Stratified epithelium** has two or more layers of cells, and only the deepest layer is in contact with the basement membrane. Tissue that appears to consist of several cellular layers but is actually a single layer with all cells contacting the basement membrane is called **pseudostratified epithelium.**

Three basic cell shapes are found in epithelium: squamous, cuboidal, and columnar. **Squamous cells** are flat and thin; **cuboidal cells** are as high as they are wide and thus appear square in vertical sections; and **columnar cells** are taller than they are wide and appear rectangular in vertical sections. Overall classifications of epithelial tissue, which take into account both the number of cell layers and cell shape, are summarized in Table 1-6.

Connective Tissue

Connective tissue varies considerably in structure and function but is most common as the framework on which epithelial cells cluster to form organs. Other functions include binding various tissues and organs together, supporting them in their locations, and serving as storage sites for excess nutrients.

In contrast to epithelial tissue, connective tissue is characterized by an abundant extracellular matrix that surrounds few cells. The extracellular matrix is composed of ground substance and fibers. **Ground substance** is a homogeneous mass that varies in consistency from fluid to semisolid gel. Fibers are produced by connective tissue cells (fibroblasts) found within the ground substance. The three types of fibers are collagenous (white), elastic (yellow), and reticular. **Collagenous fibers** are formed of bundles of smaller fibers appearing as wavy bands under the microscope. These fibers are composed of the protein collagen and are strong and inelastic. (Collagen synthesis by fibroblasts is described with respect to tissue repair in Chapter 7.) **Elastic fibers** are long, branching fibers composed of a protein called *elastin* that enables the fibers to return to their original length after stretching. Elastin occurs not only as fibers but also as membranes, particularly the membranes of blood vessels. **Retic-**

Table 1-6 Some Types of Epithelial Tissue With Location and Function

Type of Epithelial Tissue	Location	Function
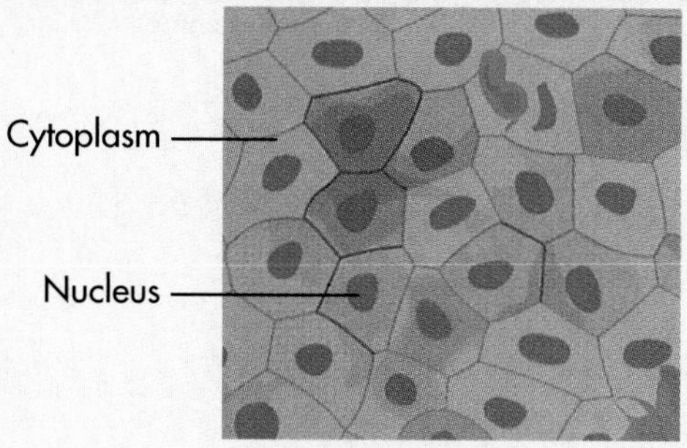 **Simple squamous**	Lines major organs (heart, air sacs of lungs, Bowman capsule of kidney); lines body cavity	Absorption, exchange of materials, filtration, secretion
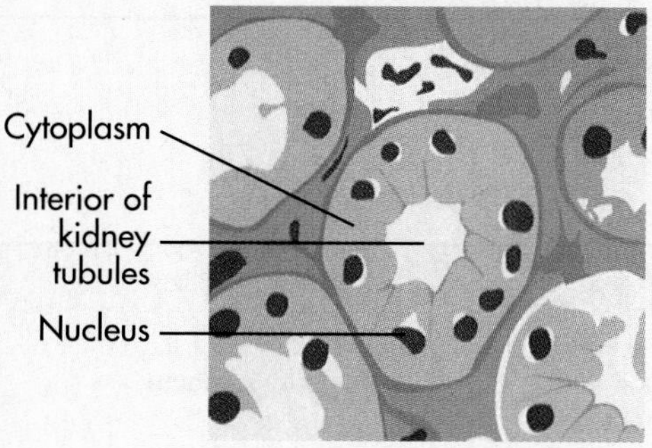 **Simple cuboidal**	Lines tubules and ducts of glands; covers surface of ovary; lines interior of eye	Absorption and secretion
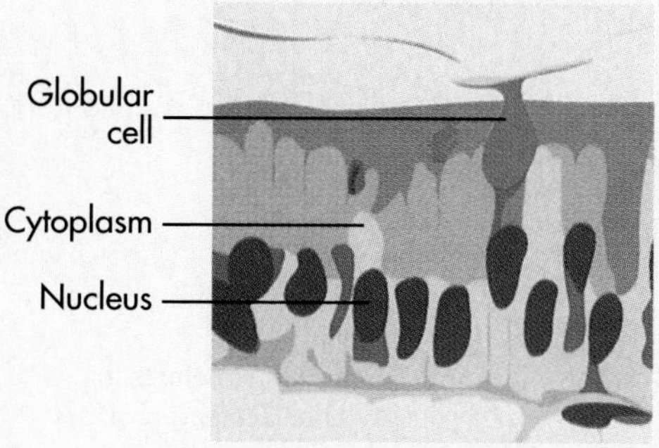 **Simple columnar**	Lines gastrointestinal tract	Secretion from special goblet cells of materials, absorption
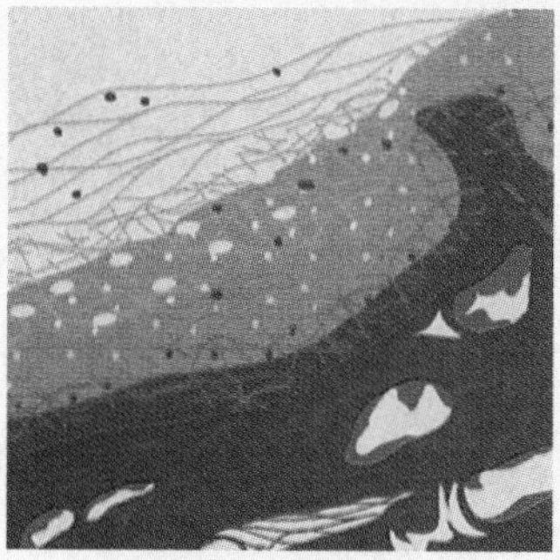 **Stratified squamous**	Lines interior of mouth, tongue, esophagus, vagina	Protection

Continued

ular fibers are thin, short, branching fibers that form an inelastic network made from a collagen-like protein called *reticulum*. Reticular fibers form the internal framework (stroma) to which the epithelial cells of glands are attached. They are found in loose connective tissue, generally in bone marrow and in the **parenchyma** (i.e., the essential substance of an organ rather than its framework) of the liver, spleen, and lymph nodes.

Connective tissues are classified according to the consistency (e.g., loose, dense) of the ground substance and the type and organization of the fibers within it. Table 1-7 summarizes the characteristics of connective tissues.

Table 1-6 Some Types of Epithelial Tissue With Location and Function—cont'd

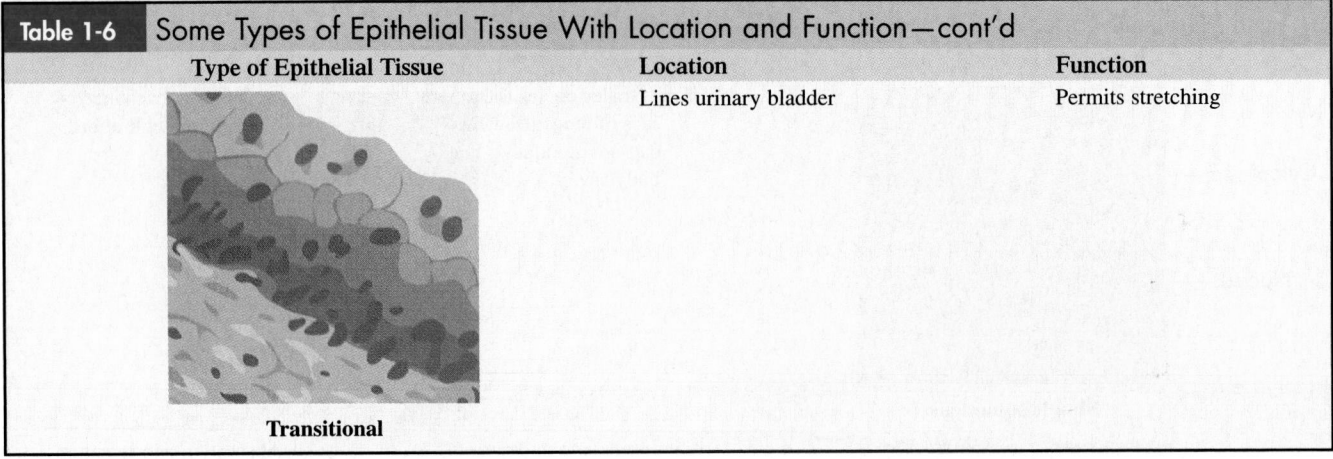

Type of Epithelial Tissue	Location	Function
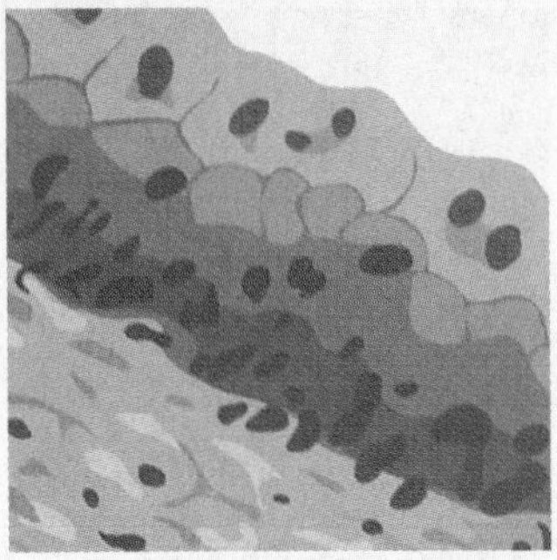 **Transitional**	Lines urinary bladder	Permits stretching

Modified from Raven PH, Johnson GB: *Understanding biology,* ed 3, Dubuque, Iowa, 1995, Brown.

Table 1-7 Types of Connective Tissue With Location and Function

Type of Connective Tissue	Location	Function
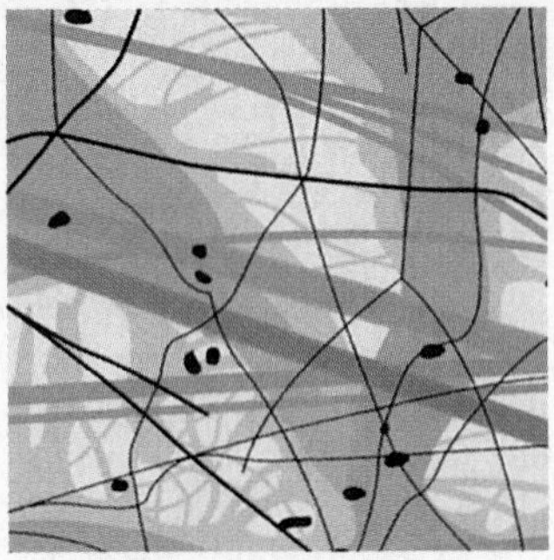 **Loose connective tissue**	Deep layers of skin, blood vessels, nerves, body organs	Support, elasticity
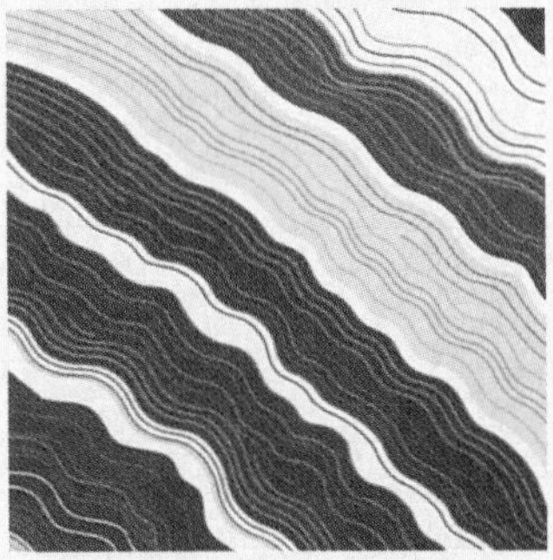 **Dense connective tissue**	Tendons, ligaments	Attaches structures to one another; provides great strength
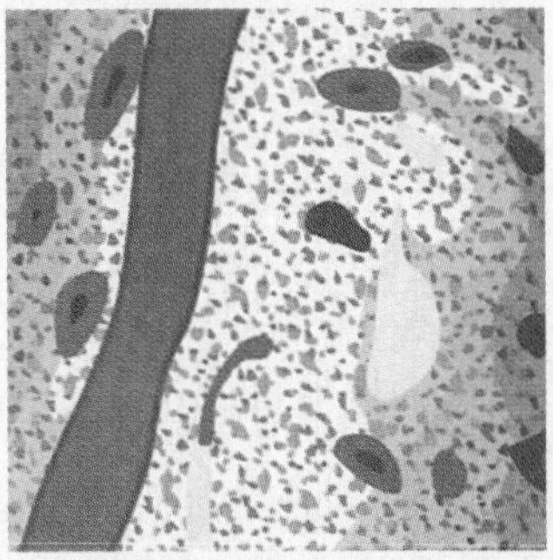 **Elastic connective tissue**	Lungs, arteries, trachea, vocal chords	Provides elasticity

Modified from Raven PH, Johnson GB: *Understanding biology,* ed 3, Dubuque, Iowa, 1995, Brown.

Table 1-7 Types of Connective Tissue With Location and Function—cont'd

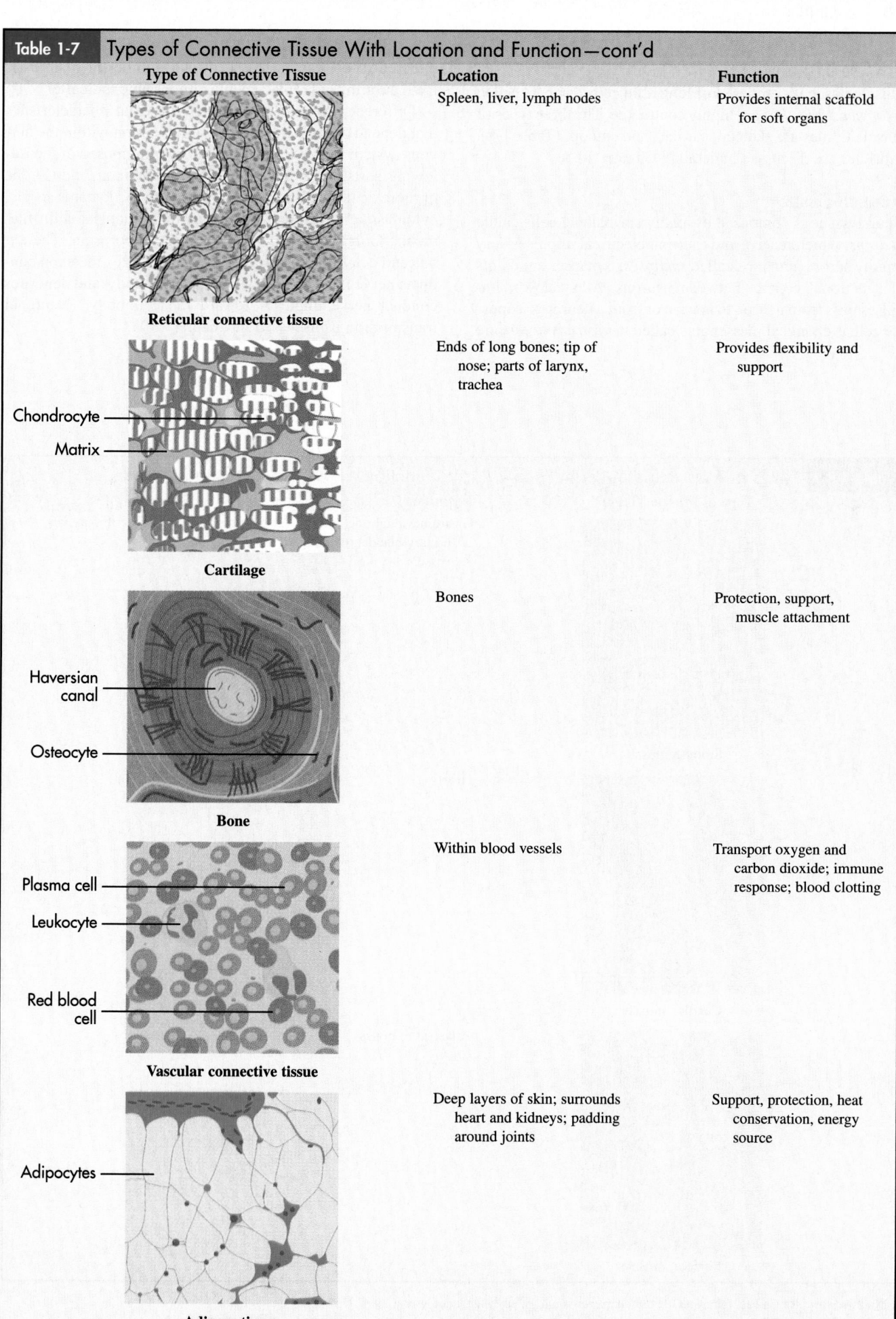

Type of Connective Tissue	Location	Function
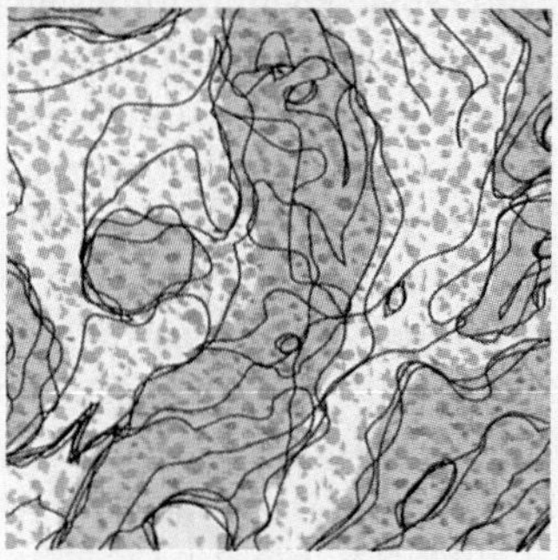 **Reticular connective tissue**	Spleen, liver, lymph nodes	Provides internal scaffold for soft organs
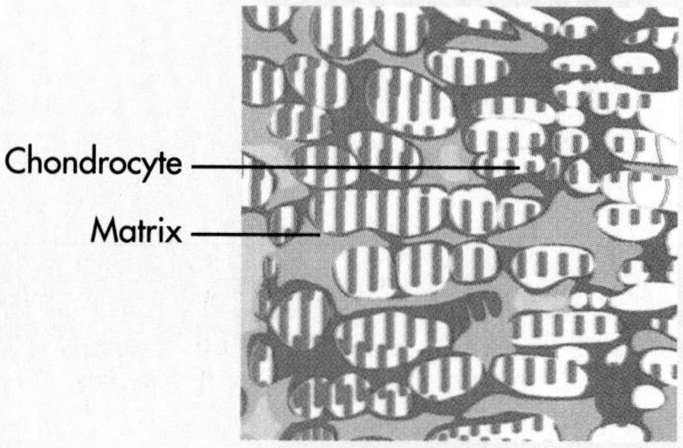 **Cartilage**	Ends of long bones; tip of nose; parts of larynx, trachea	Provides flexibility and support
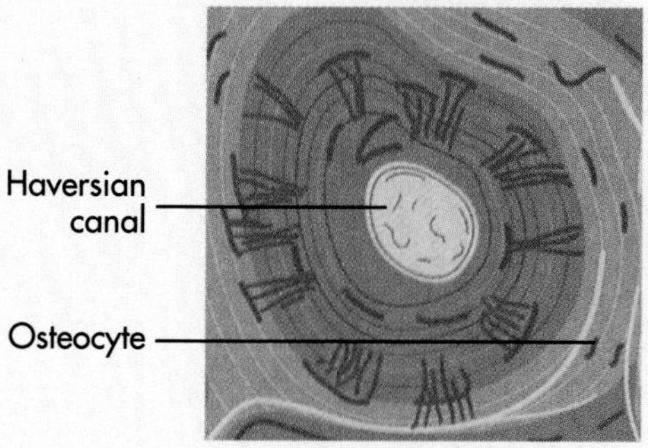 **Bone**	Bones	Protection, support, muscle attachment
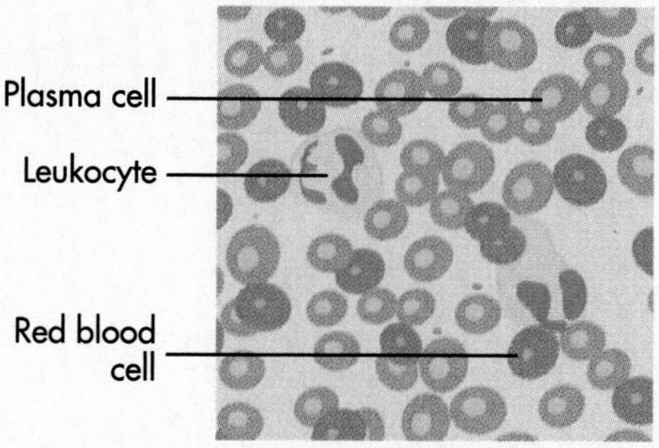 **Vascular connective tissue**	Within blood vessels	Transport oxygen and carbon dioxide; immune response; blood clotting
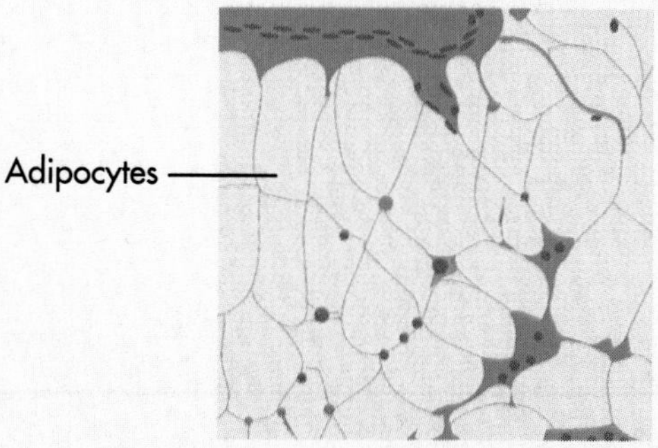 **Adipose tissue**	Deep layers of skin; surrounds heart and kidneys; padding around joints	Support, protection, heat conservation, energy source

Muscle Tissue

Muscle tissue is composed of long, thin cells or fibers called *myocytes*. Myocytes are highly contractile. The three types of muscle tissues are skeletal, cardiac, and smooth (Table 1-8). (Muscles are discussed in detail in Chapter 40.)

Neural Tissue

Neural tissue is composed of highly specialized cells called *neurons*, which receive and transmit electrical impulses very rapidly across junctions called *synapses*. Synapses are points of functional contact between neurons. At synapses, impulses pass from neuron to neuron or from a neuron to a muscle cell as chemical messengers called *neurotransmitters* are released (see Chapter 13). The total number of neurons is fixed at birth, and replacement is impossible thereafter.

Different types of neurons have special characteristics that depend on their distribution and function within the nervous system. All neurons, however, are composed of the following parts: (1) a cell body, (2) a single axon, and (3) one or more dendrites (Fig. 1-33). The cell body contains special cytoplasmic structures, as well as microtubules, actin filaments, Golgi complex, lysosomes, and lipofuscin. The axons and dendrites can be very long. Generally, the axon conducts nerve impulses away from the cell body, and dendrites conduct nerve impulses toward the cell body. (Neuronal transmission is discussed in Chapter 13.)

Table 1-8 Types of Muscle Tissue With Location and Function

Type of Muscle Tissue	Location	Function
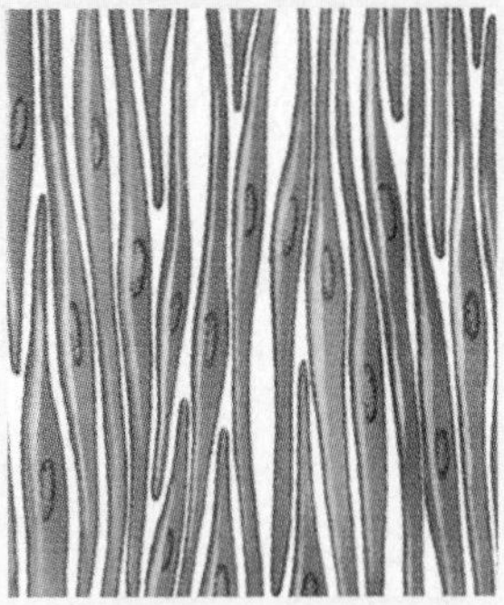 **Smooth muscle**	Gastrointestinal tract, uterus, urinary bladder, blood vessels	Propulsion of materials
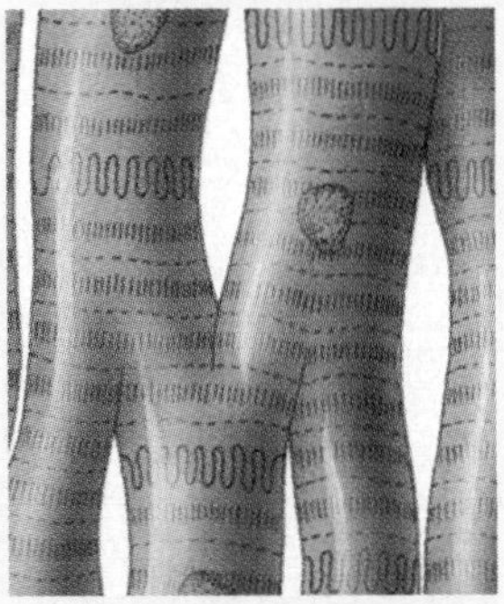 **Cardiac muscle**	Heart	Contraction
 **Skeletal muscle**	Attached to bones	Movement

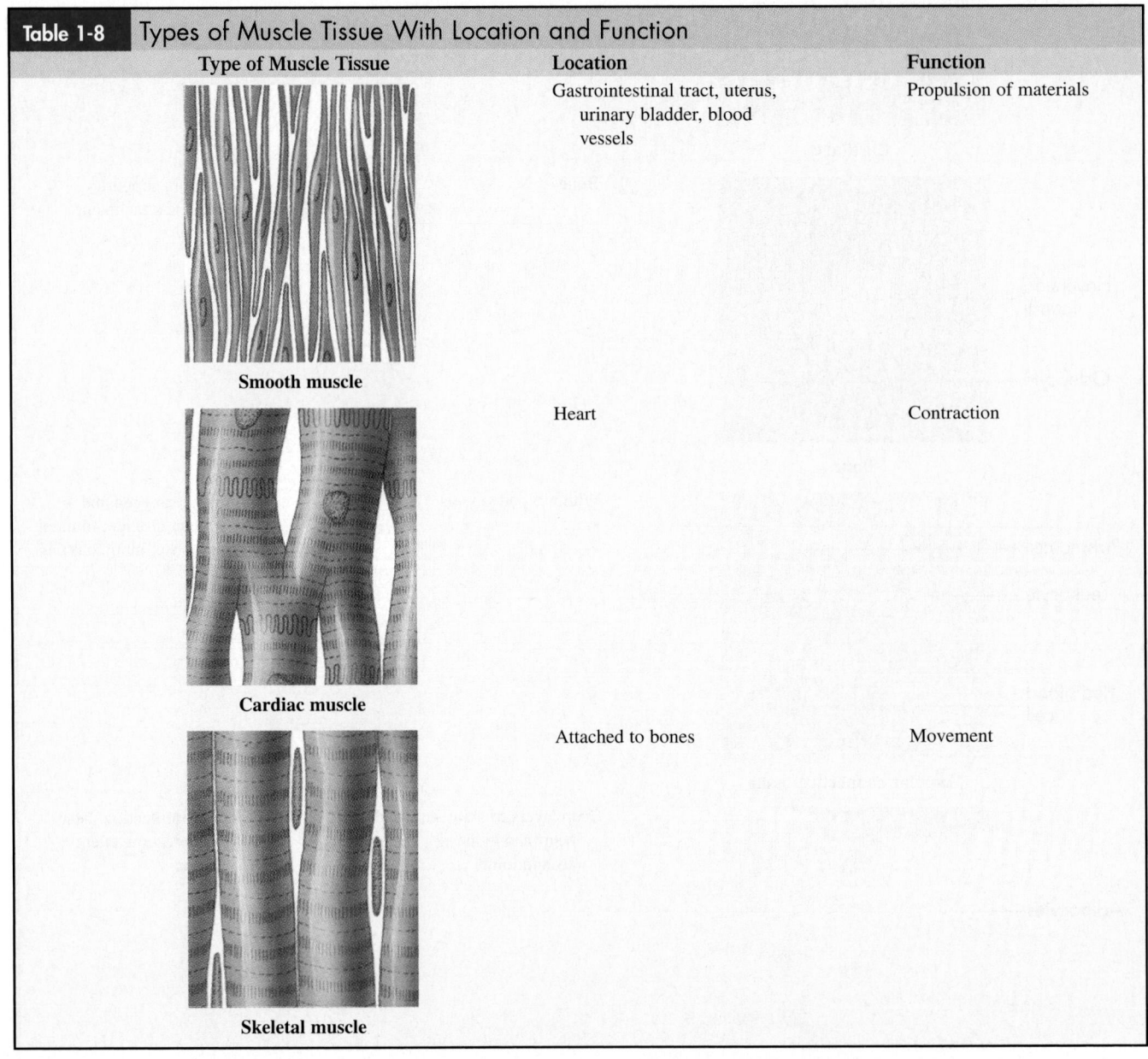

Modified from Raven PH, Johnson GB: *Understanding biology,* ed 3, Dubuque, Iowa, 1995, Brown.

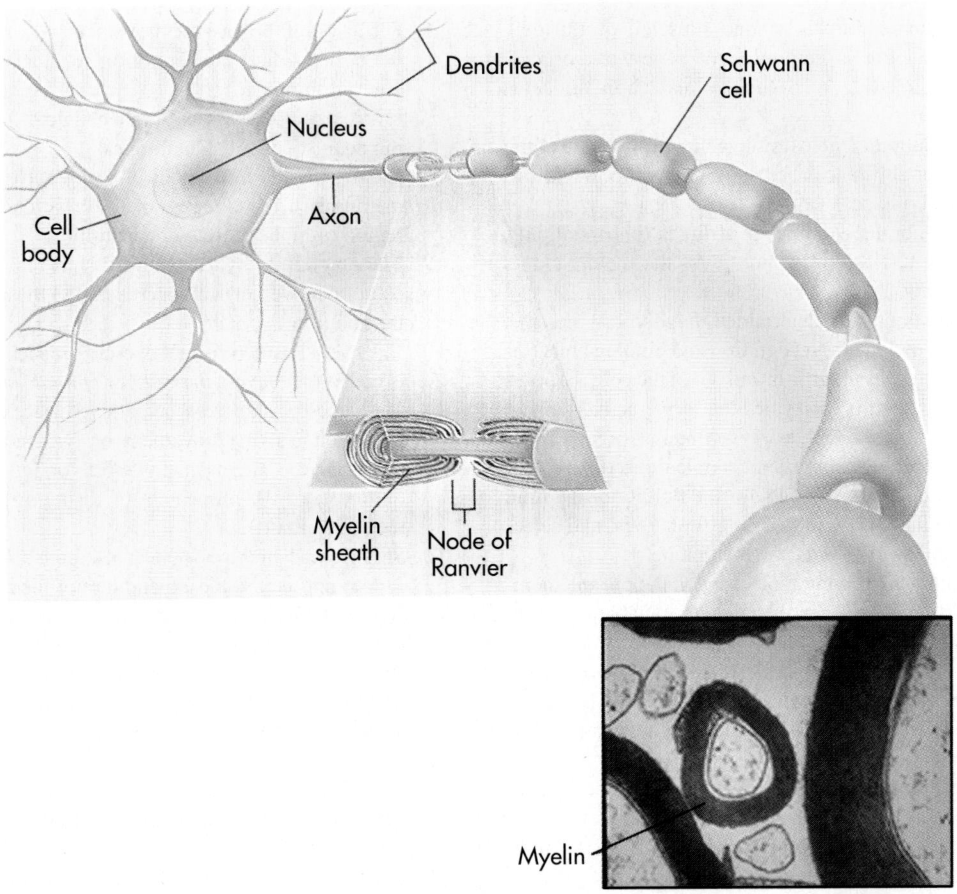

FIG. 1-33 Structure of a typical neuron. Many dendrites carry nerve impulses to the cell body, which then send the nerve impulses along a single, long axon. Long axons are encased at intervals by a myelin sheath. The inset is a micrograph of a myelinated fiber in cross section, showing myelin sheath composed of several layers of myelin, which insulate the axon. (Drawing from Raven PH, Johnson GB: *Understanding biology,* ed 3, Dubuque, Iowa, 1995, Brown; micrograph copyright © Dennis Kunkel, Microscopy, Inc.)

SUMMARY REVIEW

Cellular Functions

1. Cells become specialized through the process of differentiation or maturation.
2. The eight specialized cellular functions are movement, conductivity, metabolic absorption, secretion, excretion, respiration, reproduction, and communication.
3. The eukaryotic cell consists of three general components: the plasma membrane, the cytoplasm, and the intracellular organelles.
4. The nucleus is the largest membrane-bound organelle and is usually found in the cell's center. The chief functions of the nucleus are cell division and control of genetic information.
5. Cytoplasm, or the cytoplasmic matrix, is an aqueous solution (cytosol) that fills the space between the nucleus and the plasma membrane.
6. The organelles are suspended in the cytoplasm and are enclosed in biologic membranes.
7. The endoplasmic reticulum is a network of tubular channels (cisternae) that extend throughout the outer nuclear membrane. It specializes in the synthesis and transport of protein and lipid components of most of the organelles.
8. The Golgi complex is a network of smooth membranes and vesicles located near the nucleus. The Golgi complex is responsible for processing and packaging proteins into secretory vesicles that break away from the Golgi complex and migrate to a variety of intracellular and extracellular destinations, including the plasma membrane.
9. Vaults are newly discovered ribonucleoproteins thought to function as cellular "trucks" carrying mRNA from the nucleus to the ribosomal sites of protein synthesis.
10. Lysosomes are saclike structures that originate from the Golgi complex and contain digestive enzymes. These enzymes are responsible for digesting most cellular substances down to their basic form, such as amino acids, fatty acids, and sugars.
11. Cellular injury leads to a release of the lysosomal enzymes causing cellular self-digestion.
12. Peroxisomes are similar to lysosomes but contain several enzymes that either produce or use hydrogen peroxide.
13. Mitochondria contain the metabolic machinery necessary for cellular energy metabolism. The enzymes of the respiratory chain (electron transport chain), found in the inner membrane of the mitochondria, generate most of the cell's ATP.

Continued

14. The cytoskeleton is the "bone and muscle" of the cell. The internal skeleton is composed of a network of protein filaments including microtubules and actin filaments (microfilaments).
15. The plasma membrane encloses the cell and, by controlling the movement of substances across it, exerts a powerful influence on metabolic pathways.
16. The plasma membrane is a bilayer of lipids (phospholipids, glycolipids) and cholesterol, which gives the membrane its structural integrity.
17. Membrane functions are determined largely by proteins. These functions include (a) recognition and binding units (receptors) for substances moving in and out of the cell; (b) pores or transport channels; (c) enzymes that drive active pumps; (d) cell surface markers, such as glycoproteins; (e) cell adhesion molecules; and (f) catalysts of chemical reactions.
18. The fluid mosaic model accounts for the fluidity of the lipid bilayer and the flexibility, self-sealing properties, and selective impermeability of the plasma membrane.
19. Cellular receptors are protein molecules on the plasma membrane, in the cytoplasm, or in the nucleus, capable of recognizing and binding smaller molecules, called *ligands.*
20. The dynamic nature of the fluid plasma membrane enables it to vary the number of receptors on its surface. The cell is therefore capable of "hiding" from injurious agents by altering receptor number and pattern.
21. The ligand-receptor complex initiates a series of protein interactions, causing adenylyl cyclase to catalyze the transformation of cellular ATP to messenger molecules that stimulate specific responses within the cell.

Cellular Metabolism

1. The chemical tasks of maintaining essential cellular functions are referred to as *cellular metabolism.* Anabolism is the energy-using process of metabolism, whereas catabolism is the energy-releasing process.
2. Adenosine triphosphate (ATP) functions as an energy-transferring molecule. Energy is stored by molecules of carbohydrate, lipid, and protein, which, when catabolized, transfer energy to ATP.
3. Oxidative phosphorylation occurs in the mitochondria and is the mechanism by which the energy produced from carbohydrates, fats, and proteins is transferred to ATP.

Membrane Transport: Cellular Intake and Output

1. Water and small, electrically uncharged molecules move through pores in the plasma membrane's lipid bilayer in the process called *passive transport.*
2. Passive transport does not require the expenditure of energy; rather, it is driven by the physical effects of osmosis, hydrostatic pressure, and diffusion.
3. Larger molecules and molecular complexes (e.g., ligand-receptor complexes) are moved into the cell by active transport, which requires expenditure of energy (by means of ATP) by the cell.
4. The largest molecules (macromolecules) and fluids are transported by the processes of endocytosis (ingestion) and exocytosis (expulsion).
5. Two types of solutes exist in body fluids: electrolytes and nonelectrolytes. Electrolytes are electrically charged and dissociate into constituent ions when placed in solution. Nonelectrolytes do not dissociate when placed in solution.
6. Diffusion is the passive movement of a solute from an area of higher solute concentration to an area of lower solute concentration.
7. Hydrostatic pressure is the mechanical force of water pushing against cellular membranes.
8. Osmosis is the movement of water across a semipermeable membrane from a region of lower solute concentration to a region of higher solute concentration.
9. The amount of hydrostatic pressure required to oppose the osmotic movement of water is called the *osmotic pressure* of the solution.
10. The overall osmotic effect of colloids, such as plasma proteins, is called the *oncotic pressure* or *colloid osmotic pressure.*
11. Mediated transport can be passive or active. Mediated transport includes the movement of two molecules simultaneously in one direction (symport) or in opposite directions (antiport) or the movement of a single molecule in one direction (uniport).
12. Passive mediated transport is also called *facilitated diffusion.* It does not require the expenditure of metabolic energy.
13. Active mediated transport requires metabolic energy (ATP) to move molecules against the concentration gradient.
14. Active transport also occurs by endocytosis, or vesicle formation, in which the substance to be transported is engulfed by a segment of the plasma membrane, forming a vesicle that moves into the cell.
15. Pinocytosis is a type of endocytosis in which fluids and solute molecules are ingested through formation of small vesicles.
16. Phagocytosis is a type of endocytosis in which large particles, such as bacteria, are ingested through formation of large vesicles, called *vacuoles.*
17. In receptor-mediated endocytosis, the plasma membrane receptors are clustered, along with bristlelike structures, in specialized areas called *coated pits.*
18. Endocytosis occurs when coated pits invaginate, internalizing ligand-receptor complexes in coated vesicles.
19. Inside the cell, material ingested by endocytosis is processed and digested by lysosomal enzymes.
20. Caveolae are tiny flask-shaped pits on the outer surface of the plasma membrane. Cellular uptake through the opening and closing of caveolae is called *potocytosis.*
21. All body cells are electrically polarized, with the inside of the cell more negatively charged than the outside. The difference in voltage across the plasma membrane is the resting membrane potential.
22. When an excitable (nerve or muscle) cell receives an electrochemical stimulus, cations enter the cell, causing a rapid change in the resting membrane potential known as the *action potential.* The action potential "moves" along the cell's plasma membrane and is transmitted to an adjacent cell. This is how electrochemical signals convey information from cell to cell.

Cellular Reproduction: The Cell Cycle

1. Cellular reproduction in body tissues involves mitosis (nuclear division) and cytokinesis (cytoplasmic division).
2. Only mature cells are capable of division. Maturation occurs during a stage of cellular life called *interphase* (growth phase).
3. The cell cycle is the reproductive process that begins after interphase in all tissues with cellular turnover. The four phases

of the cell cycle are (a) the S phase, during which DNA synthesis takes place in the cell nucleus; (b) the G_2 phase, the period between the completion of DNA synthesis and the next phase (M); (c) the M phase, which involves both nuclear (mitotic) and cytoplasmic (cytokinetic) division; and (d) the G_1 phase (growth phase, or interphase), after which the cycle begins again.
4. The M phase (mitosis) involves four stages: prophase, metaphase, anaphase, and telophase.
5. The mechanisms that control cell division depend on "social control genes" and protein growth factors.

Cell-to-Cell Adhesions

1. Cell-to-cell adhesions are formed on plasma membranes allowing the formation of tissues and organs. Cells are held together by three different means: (a) the extracellular membrane, (b) cell adhesion molecules in the cell's plasma membrane, and (c) specialized cell junctions.
2. The extracellular matrix includes three types of protein fibers: collagen, elastin, and fibronectin. The matrix helps regulate cell growth and differentiation.
3. The three main types of cell junctions are desmosomes, tight junctions, and gap junctions.

Cellular Communication and Signal Transduction

1. Cells communicate in three ways: (a) they form protein channels (gap junctions); (b) they display receptors that affect intracellular processes or other cells in direct physical contact; and (c) they secrete signals for long-distance communication.
2. Primary modes of chemical signaling include hormonal, neurohormonal, neurotransmitter, paracrine, and autocrine.
3. Signal transduction involves signals or instructions from extracellular chemical messengers that are conveyed to the cell's interior for execution.
4. Signaling cascades, or relay chains, have several important functions, including physically transferring the signal around the cell, amplifying the signal, distributing the signal, and modulating the signal.
5. Two important second messenger pathways are cAMP and Ca^{++}.
6. G protein is an intermediary between the receptor and adenylyl cyclase.
7. Phospholipase C, an enzyme protein effector, is bound to the inner side of the membrane.

Tissues

1. Cells of one or more types are organized into tissues, and different types of tissues compose organs. Organs are organized to function as tracts or systems.
2. Specialized cells are thought to form tissue by mitosis of one or more founder cells or by migration of founder cells and their subsequent assembly at the site of tissue formation.
3. The four basic types of tissues are epithelial, muscle, neural, and connective tissues.
4. Epithelial tissue covers most internal and external surfaces of the body. The functions of epithelial tissue include protection, absorption, secretion, and excretion.
5. Connective tissue binds various tissues and organs together, supporting them in their locations and serving as storage sites for excess nutrients.
6. Muscle tissue is composed of long, thin, highly contractile cells or fibers called *myocytes.* Muscle tissue that is attached to bones enables voluntary movement. Muscle tissues in internal organs enable involuntary movement, such as the heartbeat.
7. Neural tissue is composed of highly specialized cells called *neurons*, which receive and transmit electric impulses very rapidly across junctions called *synapses.*

KEY TERMS

Absolute refractory period, *24*
Actin filament (microfilament), *9*
Action potential, *24*
Active mediated transport, *20*
Active transport, *17*
Amphipathic molecule, *10*
Anabolism, *14*
Anaerobic glycolysis, *16*
Anaphase, *25*
Anion, *17*
Antiport, *19*
Arrested (G_0) state, *27*
Autocrine signaling, *30*
Autodigestion, *6*
Autolysosome, *6*
Autophagy, *6*
Catabolism, *14*
Cation, *17*
Caveolae, *10*
Cell adhesion molecule (CAM), *12*
Cell cycle, *25*
Cell junction, *27*
Cellular metabolism, *14*
Cellular receptor, *13*
Centriole, *9*
Centromere, *25*
Chemotaxis, *33*
Chromatid, *25*
Chromatin, *25*
Chromosome, *25*
Cilium, *34*
Cisterna, *5*
Citric acid cycle (Krebs cycle, tricarboxylic acid cycle), *15*
Clathrin, *5*
Coated pit, *22*
Collagen, *27*
Collagenous fiber, *34*
Columnar cell, *34*
Competitive inhibitor, *19*
Concentration gradient, *17*
Connexon, *27*
Contact guidance, *33*
Crista, *8*
Cuboidal cell, *34*
Cyclic adenosine monophosphate (cyclic AMP, cAMP), *32*
Cyclic guanosine monophosphate (cyclic GMP, cGMP), *33*
Cytochrome, *16*
Cytokinesis, *25*
Cytoplasm, *2*
Cytoplasmic matrix, *2*
Cytoskeleton, *8*
Cytosol, *2*
Depolarization, *24*
Desmosome, *27*
Differentiation, *2*
Diffusion, *17*
Digestion, *14*
Effective osmolality, *18*
Elastic fiber, *34*
Elastin, *27*
Electrolyte, *17*
Electron-transport chain, *16*
Endocytosis, *22*

Continued

KEY TERMS—cont'd

Endoplasmic reticulum, *4*
Equatorial plate (metaphase plate), *25*
Eukaryote, *1*
Extracellular matrix (basement membrane), *27*
Facilitated diffusion, *20*
Fibronectin, *27*
First messenger, *30*
Founder cell, *33*
G protein, *32*
Gap junction, *27*
Gating, *28*
Glycolysis, *14*
Glycoprotein, *12*
Golgi complex (Golgi apparatus), *4*
Ground substance, *34*
Growth factor, *26*
Guanosine diphosphate (GDP), *33*
Guanosine triphosphate (GTP), *33*
Homeostasis, *28*
Hormonal signaling, *29*
Hydrostatic pressure, *18*
Hypertonic solution, *19*
Hypotonic solution, *19*
Inner membrane, *8*
Integral membrane protein, *12*
Interphase, *25*
Ion, *17*
Isotonic solution, *19*
Junctional complex, *27*
Ligand, *13*
Lysosome, *6*
Mediated transport, *19*
Metabolic pathway, *14*
Metaphase, *25*
Microdomain, *23*
Microtubule, *8*
Microvillus, *33*
Mitochondrion, *8*
Mitosis, *25*
Neurohormonal signaling, *30*
Nuclear envelope, *2*
Nucleolus, *2*
Nucleus, *2*
Oncotic pressure (colloid osmotic pressure), *19*
Osmolality, *18*
Osmolarity, *18*
Osmosis, *18*
Osmotic pressure, *18*
Outer membrane, *8*
Oxidation, *14*
Oxidative cellular metabolism (oxidation), *14*
Oxidative phosphorylation, *15*
Paracrine signaling, *30*
Parenchyma, *35*
Passive mediated transport (facilitated diffusion), *20*
Passive transport, *17*
Peripheral membrane protein, *12*
Peroxisome (microbody), *8*
Phagocytosis, *22*
Phospholipase C, *33*
Pinocytosis, *22*
Plasma membrane receptor, ••*13*
Platelet-derived growth factor (PDGF), *26*
Polarity, *17*
Potocytosis, *23*
Primary lysosome, *6*
Prokaryote, *1*
Prophase, *25*
Protein effector, *33*
Pseudostratified epithelium, *34*
Receptor-mediated endocytosis (ligand internalization), *23*
Relative refractory period, *24*
Repolarization, *24*
Residual body, *6*
Resting membrane potential, *23*
Reticular fiber, *34*
Ribosome, *4*
Second messenger, *30*
Secondary lysosome, *6*
Secretory vesicle, *5*
Signal transduction, *30*
Signaling cascade, *30*
Simple epithelium, *34*
Solute, *17*
Spindle fiber, *25*
Squamous cell, *34*
Stratified epithelium, *34*
Substrate, *14*
Substrate phosphorylation, *16*
Symport, *19*
Telophase, *26*
Threshold potential, *24*
Tight junction, *27*
Tissue, *33*
Tonicity, *19*
Transfer reaction, *15*
Transmembrane protein, *12*
Transport protein, *19*
Transporter, *19*
Uniport, *19*
Vaults, *7*

REFERENCES

1. Alberts B et al: *Molecular biology of the cell,* ed 4, New York, 2001, Garland.
2. Hermann C et al: Recombinant major vault protein is targeted to neuritic tips of PC12 cells, *J Cell Biol* 144(6):1163, 1999.
3. Kong LB et al: Structure of the vault, a ubiquitous cellular component, *Structure* 7(4):371, 1999.
4. Mooney DJ, Mikos AG: Growing new organs, *Sci Am* 280(4):60, 1999.
5. Fasshauer M, Iwig M, Glaesser D: Synthesis of proto-oncogene proteins and cyclins depends on intact microfilaments, *Eur J Cell Biol* 77(2):188, 1998.
6. Lofthouse RA et al: Identification of caveolae and detection of caveolin in normal human osteoblasts, *J Bone Joint Surg Br* 83(1):124, 2001.
7. Catt KJ et al: Hormonal regulation of peptide receptors and target cell responses, *Nature* 280:109, 1979.
8. Mizuno-Kamiya M et al: ATP-mediated activation of Ca^{2+}-independent phospholipase A_2 in secretory granular membranes from rat parotid gland, *J Biochem (Tokyo)* 123(2):205, 1998.
9. Alberts B et al: *Essential cell biology,* New York, 1998, Garland.
10. Baserga R, Morrione A: Differentiation and malignant transformation: two roads diverge in the wood, *J Cell Biochem Suppl* 32-33:68, 1999.
11. Gonzalez-Zulueta M et al: Requirement for nitric oxide activation of p21 (ras)/extracellular-regulated kinase in neuronal ischemic preconditioning, *Proc Natl Acad Sci USA* 97(1):436, 2000.
12. Scott JD, Pawson T: Cell communication: the inside story, *Sci Am* 282(6):72, 2000

CHAPTER 2

Altered Cellular and Tissue Biology

KATHRYN L. McCANCE • TODD C. GREY

CHAPTER OUTLINE

Knowledge of the structural and functional reactions of cells and tissues to injurious agents, including genetic defects, is key for the understanding of disease processes. Diseases are now defined and interpreted in molecular terms and not just in general descriptions of altered structure. Altered cellular and tissue biology can be the result of adaptation, injury, neoplasia, aging, or death. (Neoplasia is discussed in Chapters 10 through 12.) Adaptation occurs in response to both normal, or physiologic, conditions and adverse, or pathologic, conditions. For example, the uterus adapts to pregnancy—a normal physiologic state—by enlarging. Enlargement occurs because of an increase in the size and number of uterine cells. In an adverse condition, such as high blood pressure, myocardial cells are stimulated to enlarge by the increased work of pumping. Like most of the body's adaptive mechanisms, however, cellular adaptations to adverse conditions are usually only temporarily successful. Severe or long-term stressors overwhelm adaptive processes, and cellular injury or death ensues.

Cellular injury can be caused by any factor that disrupts cellular structures or deprives the cell of oxygen and nutrients required for survival. Injury may be reversible *(sublethal)* or irreversible *(lethal)* and is classified broadly as chemical, hypoxic (lack of sufficient oxygen), free radical, unintentional or intentional, and immunologic or inflammatory. Cellular injuries from various causes have different clinical and pathophysiologic manifestations.

Cellular death is confirmed by structural changes seen when cells are stained and examined with a microscope. The most important changes are nuclear changes; clearly, without a healthy nucleus, the cell cannot survive.

Cellular aging causes structural and functional changes that eventually lead to cellular death or a decreased capacity to recover from injury. Mechanisms explaining how and why cells age are not known, and distinguishing between pathologic changes and physiologic changes that occur with aging is often difficult. Aging clearly causes alterations in cellular structure and function, yet senescence is both inevitable and normal.

CELLULAR ADAPTATION

Cells adapt to their environment to escape and protect themselves from injury. An adapted cell is neither normal nor injured—its condition lies somewhere between these two states. Cellular adaptations, however, are a common and central part of many disease states. In the early stages of a successful adaptive response, cells may have enhanced function; thus it is hard to know what is a pathologic response vs. an extreme adaptation to an excessive functional demand. The most significant adaptive changes in cells include atrophy (decrease in cell size), hypertrophy (increase in cell size), hyperplasia (increase in cell number), and metaplasia (reversible replacement of one mature cell type by another, less mature cell type). Dysplasia (deranged cellular growth) is not considered a true cellular adaptation but rather an atypical hyperplasia. These changes are shown in Fig. 2-1.

Atrophy

Atrophy is a decrease or shrinkage in cellular size. If atrophy occurs in a sufficient number of an organ's cells, the entire organ shrinks or becomes atrophic. Atrophy can affect any organ, but it is most common in skeletal muscle, the heart, secondary sex organs, and the brain. Atrophy can be classified as *physiologic* or *pathologic*. **Physiologic atrophy** occurs with early development. For example, the thymus gland undergoes physiologic atrophy during childhood. **Pathologic atrophy** occurs as a result of decreases in workload, use, pressure, blood supply, nutrition, hormonal stimulation, and nervous stimulation. Individuals immobilized in bed for a prolonged time exhibit a type of skeletal muscle atrophy called *disuse atrophy*. Aging causes brain cells to become atrophic and endocrine-dependent organs, such as the gonads, to shrink as hormonal stimulation decreases. Whether atrophy is caused by normal physiologic conditions or by pathologic conditions, atrophic cells exhibit the same basic changes.

The atrophic muscle cell contains less endoplasmic reticulum and fewer mitochondria and myofilaments (part of the muscle fiber that controls contraction) than does the normal cell. In muscular atrophy caused by nerve loss, oxygen consumption and amino acid uptake are rapidly reduced. The biochemical changes of atrophy are just beginning to be understood. The mechanisms probably include decreased protein synthesis, increased protein catabolism, or both. The primary pathway of protein catabolism is the **ubiquitin-proteosome** pathway, and signals activating this pathway include metabolic acidosis, glucocorticoids, and thyroid hormone.[1] Proteins degraded in this pathway are first conjugated to ubiquitin (another small protein) and then degraded within a large cytoplasmic proteolytic complex or proteosome.

Atrophy as a result of chronic malnutrition is often accompanied by an increase in the number of **autophagic vacuoles,** which are membrane-bound vesicles within the cell that contain cellular debris—small fragments of mitochondria and endoplasmic reticulum—and hydrolytic enzymes. Atrophic change causes a rapid increase in hydrolytic enzymes, which are isolated in autophagic vacuoles to prevent uncontrolled cellular destruction. Thus the vacuoles proliferate as needed to protect the uninjured organelles from the injured organelles and are eventually taken up and destroyed by lysosomes (a process described in Chapter 1). Certain contents of the autophagic vacuole may resist destruction by lysosomal enzymes and persist in membrane-bound residual bodies. An example of this is granules that contain **lipofuscin,** the yellow-brown age pigment. Lipofuscin accumulates primarily in liver cells, myocardial cells, and atrophic cells.

Hypertrophy

Hypertrophy is an increase in the size of cells and consequently in the size of the affected organ. The cells of the heart and kidneys are particularly responsive to enlargement. The increase in cellular size is associated with an increased accumulation of protein in the cellular components (plasma membrane, endoplasmic reticulum, myofilaments, mitochondria) and *not* with an increase in cellular fluid. Hypertrophy can be *physiologic* or *pathologic* and is caused by specific hormone stimulation or by increased functional demand. For example, physiologic hypertrophy during pregnancy is hormone induced and involves both hypertrophy and hyperplasia. Hypertrophy as an adaptive response—muscular enlargement—occurs in the striated muscle cells of both the heart and skeletal muscles. These cells cannot adapt to increased metabolic demands by mitotic division and production of new cells to share the work. Thus they enlarge and the stimulus appears to be an increased workload. In the heart, pathologic hypertrophy is secondary to hyperten-

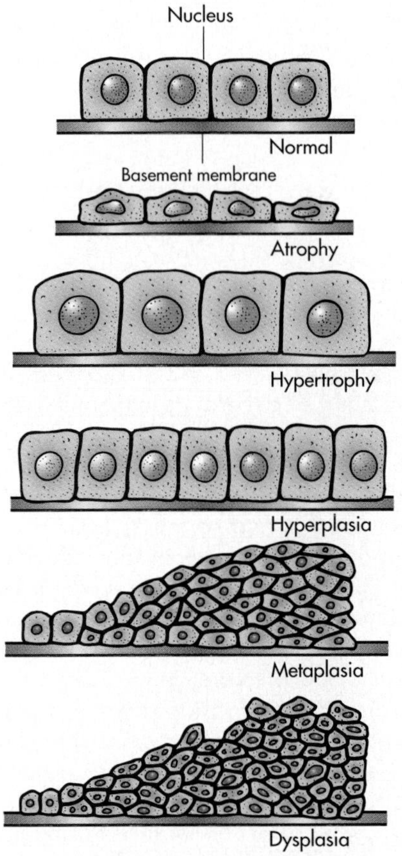

FIG. 2-1 Adaptive alterations in simple cuboidal epithelial cells. (From Lewis SM, Collier JC, Heitkemper MM: *Medical-surgical nursing: assessment and management of clinical problems,* ed 5, St Louis, 2000, Mosby.)

sion or problem valves. In skeletal muscle, physiologic hypertrophy occurs in response to heavy work. Muscular hypertrophy tends to diminish if the excessive workload diminishes.

In myocardial hypertrophy, initial enlargement is caused by dilation of the cardiac chambers, but this is short lived and is followed by increased synthesis of cardiac muscle proteins, allowing muscle fibers to do more work. The nucleus is also hypertrophic with increased synthesis of deoxyribonucleic acid (DNA).[2] Although fully matured (e.g., terminally differentiated) muscle cells are unable to undergo further mitosis, they are capable of increased DNA synthesis. Why cardiac muscle cells are unable to progress through the cell cycle to mitosis is unclear; it may be because of a block that prevents them from entering G_2 of the cell cycle[3] (Fig. 2-2) (see Chapters 1 and 10). Eventually, however, advanced hypertrophy can lead to myocardial failure (Fig. 2-3) (see Chapter 29).

A number of genes are activated during hypertrophy, including the gene for atrial natriuretic factor (ANF). The ANF gene is usually expressed only during early development; however, with cardiac hypertrophy, it is reinduced and the ANF hormone causes salt secretion by the kidney, decreasing blood volume and pressure and reducing hemodynamic load. Other genes activated include regulatory factors (e.g., c-*fos*, c-*jun*), growth factors, vasoactive agents, certain components involved in receptor-mediated signaling pathways, and kinases. The triggers for hypertrophy include two types of signals: mechanical signals, such as stretch, and trophic signals, such as growth factors and vasoactive agents.

After removal of one kidney, the other kidney adapts to an increased demand for work with an increase in both the size and the number of cells. The major contribution to renal enlargement is hypertrophy.

Hyperplasia

Hyperplasia is an increase in the number of cells resulting from an increased rate of cellular division. Hyperplasia as a

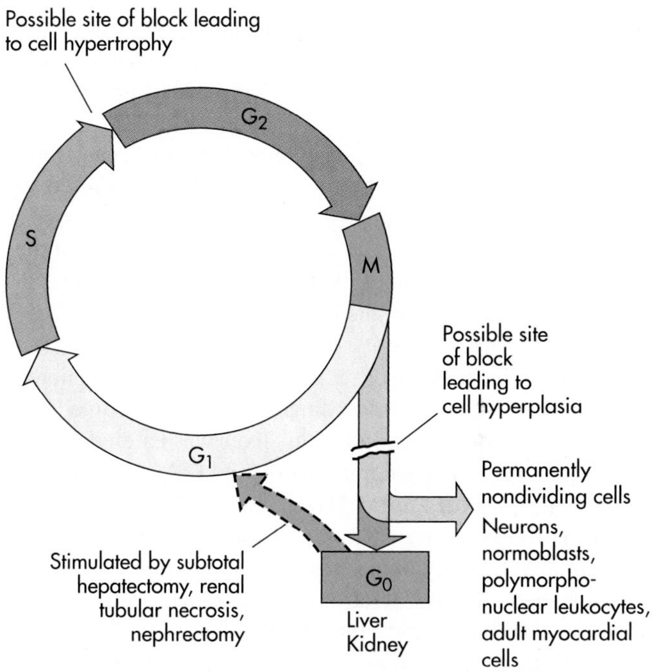

FIG. 2-2 Cell cycle and possible sites of block.

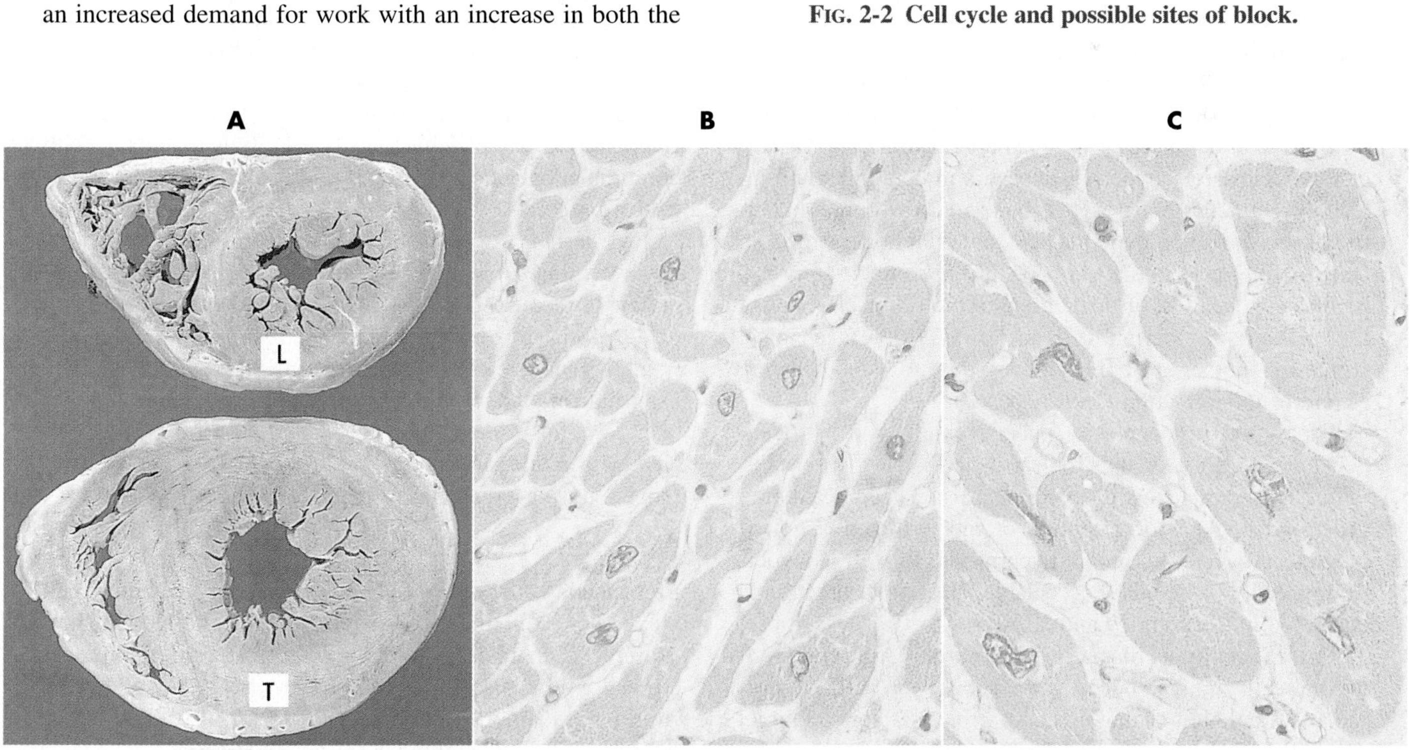

FIG. 2-3 Hypertrophy of cardiac muscle in response to valve disease. A, Transverse slices of a normal heart and a heart with hypertrophy of the left ventricle. (*L,* Normal thickness of left ventricular wall; *T,* thickened wall from heart in which severe narrowing of aortic valve caused resistance to systolic ventricular emptying.) **B,** Histology of cardiac muscle from a normal heart. **C,** Histology of cardiac muscle from a hypertrophied heart. (From Stevens A, Lowe J: *Pathology,* St Louis, 1995, Mosby.)

response to injury occurs when the injury has been severe and prolonged enough to have caused cell death.[2] Loss of epithelial cells and cells of the liver and kidney triggers DNA synthesis and mitotic division. Increased cell growth is a multistep process involving the production of growth factors, which stimulate the remaining cells to synthesize new cell components and, ultimately, to divide. Hyperplasia and hypertrophy often occur together, although the specific mechanism is unknown. Hyperplasia and hypertrophy both take place if the cells are capable of synthesizing DNA; however, in *nondividing cells* (e.g., myocardial fibers) only hypertrophy occurs.

Two types of normal, or physiologic, hyperplasia are compensatory hyperplasia and hormonal hyperplasia. **Compensatory hyperplasia** is an adaptive mechanism that enables certain organs to regenerate. For example, removal of part of the liver leads to hyperplasia of the remaining liver cells (hepatocytes) to compensate for the loss. Even with removal of 70% of the liver, regeneration is complete in about 2 weeks. The remarkable regenerating capacity of the liver was even noted by the ancient Greeks. According to one story, Prometheus was chained to a mountain and his liver was eaten daily by a vulture, only to regenerate every night. A new protein, **hepatocyte growth factor (HGF),** is thought to be a mediator in vitro of liver regeneration.[4] In addition, other in vitro growth factors and cytokines (cell-signaling proteins) that increase hepatic cell regeneration include transforming growth factor–α (TGF-α), epidermal growth factor (EGF), interleukin-6 (IL-6), and tumor necrosis factor–α (TNF-α).

Not all types of mature cells have the same capacity for compensatory hyperplastic growth. Some cells, such as nerve, skeletal muscle, and myocardial cells and the lens cells of the eye, do not regenerate. Skeletal muscle cells, however, can be made by the fusion of myoblasts.[5] Significant compensatory hyperplasia occurs in epidermal and intestinal epithelia, hepatocytes, bone marrow cells, and fibroblasts, and some hyperplasia is noted in bone, cartilage, and smooth muscle cells. An example of compensatory hyperplasia is a callus, or thickening, of the skin as a result of hyperplasia of epidermal cells in response to a mechanical stimulus. Another example is the response to wound healing as part of inflammation (see Chapter 7).

Hormonal hyperplasia occurs chiefly in estrogen-dependent organs, such as the uterus and breast. After ovulation, for example, estrogen stimulates the endometrium to grow and thicken for reception of the fertilized ovum. If pregnancy occurs, hormonal hyperplasia, as well as hypertrophy, enables the uterus to enlarge. (Hormone function is described in Chapters 19 and 20.)

Pathologic hyperplasia is the abnormal proliferation of normal cells and can occur as a response to excessive hormonal stimulation or the effects of growth factors on target cells (Fig. 2-4). Hyperplastic cells are identified by pronounced nuclear enlargement, clumping of chromatin, and one or more enlarged nucleoli. The most common example is pathologic hyperplasia of the endometrium (which is caused by an imbalance between estrogen and progesterone secretion, with oversecretion of estrogen) (see Chapter 22). Pathologic endometrial hyperplasia, which causes excessive menstrual bleeding, is under the influence of regular growth-inhibition controls. If these controls fail, hyperplastic endometrial cells can undergo malignant transformation. (Malignant cell transformation is discussed in Chapter 10.)

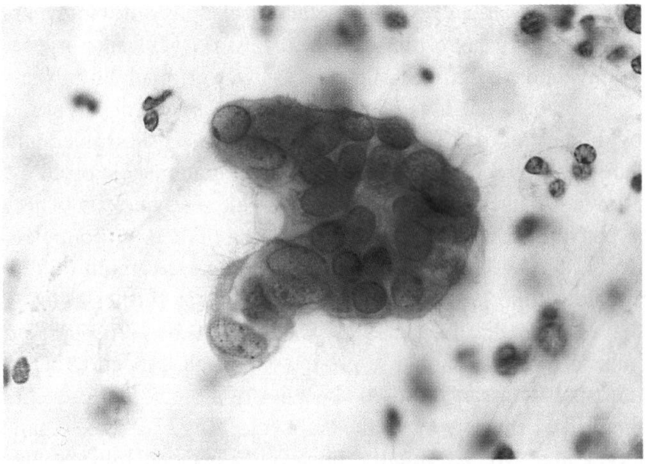

FIG. 2-4 Hyperplasia of bronchial epithelium. (Bronchial brush; Papanicolaou stain.) (From Damjanov I, Linder J: *Anderson's pathology,* ed 10, St Louis, 1996, Mosby.)

Dysplasia: Not a True Adaptive Change

Dysplasia refers to abnormal changes in the size, shape, and organization of mature cells. Dysplasia is not considered a true adaptive process but is related to hyperplasia and is often called **atypical hyperplasia.** Dysplastic changes frequently are encountered in epithelial tissue of the cervix and respiratory tract, where they are strongly associated with common neoplastic growths and often are found adjacent to cancerous cells.

Dysplasia is often classified as mild, moderate, or severe; however, this subjective scheme has prompted recommendations to use either "low grade" or "high grade." Grading of dysplasia, for example, of the female reproductive tract (i.e., Papanicolaou [Pap] smear) is in Chapter 22 (Fig. 2-5). Data indicate that atypical hyperplasia is a strong predictor of breast cancer development.[6] *Neoplasia* is a term associated with malignant tumors. If the inciting stimulus is removed, dysplastic changes often are reversible.

Metaplasia

Metaplasia is the reversible replacement of one mature cell by another, sometimes less differentiated, cell type. The best example of metaplasia is replacement of normal columnar ciliated epithelial cells of the bronchial (airway) lining by stratified squamous epithelial cells (Fig. 2-6). The newly formed squamous epithelial cells do not secrete mucus or have cilia, causing loss of a vital protective mechanism.

Metaplasia is thought to develop from a reprogramming of stem cells existing in most epithelia or of undifferentiated mesenchymal (tissue from embryonic mesoderm) cells pre-

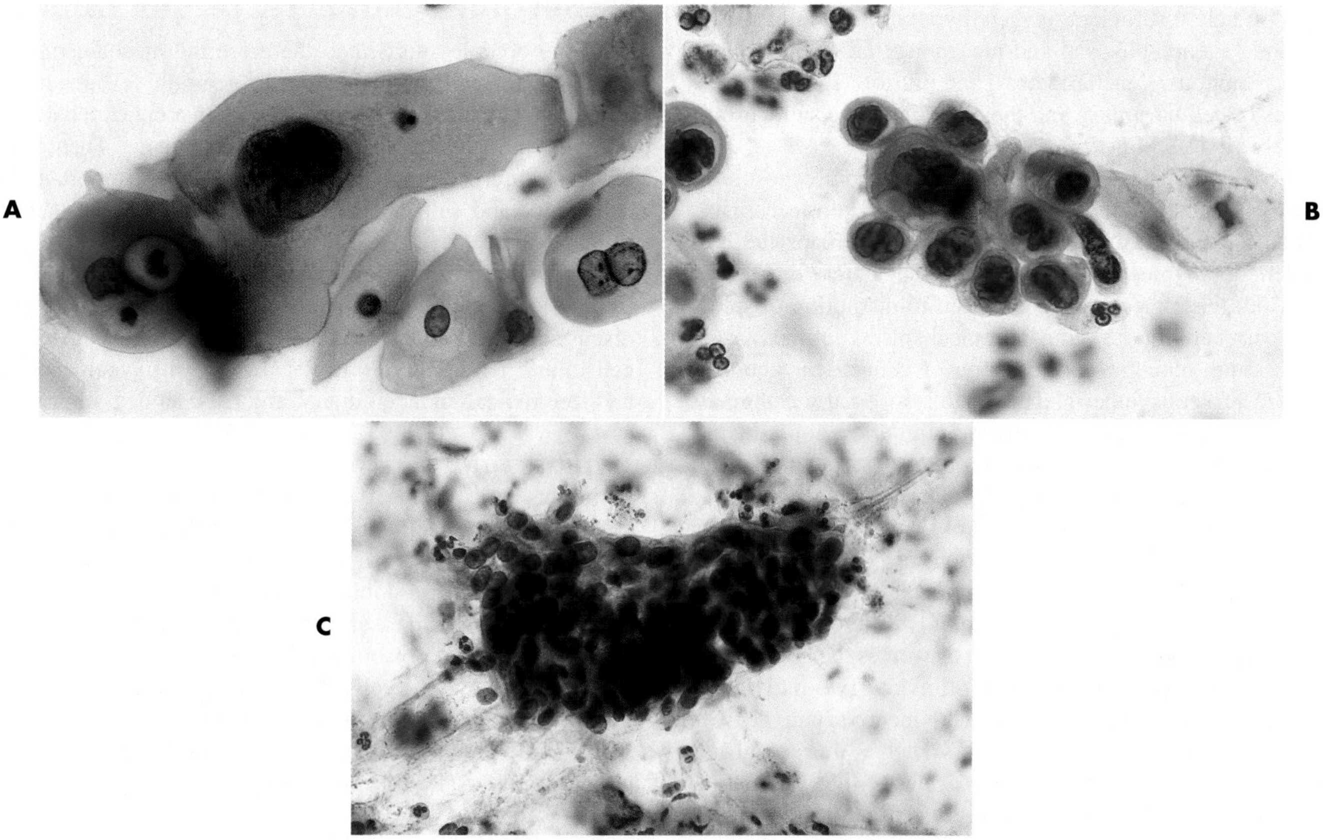

FIG. 2-5 Dysplasia of uterine cervix. A, Mild dysplasia. **B,** Severe dysplasia. **C,** Carcinoma in situ. (From Damjanov I, Linder J: *Anderson's pathology,* ed 10, St Louis, 1996, Mosby.)

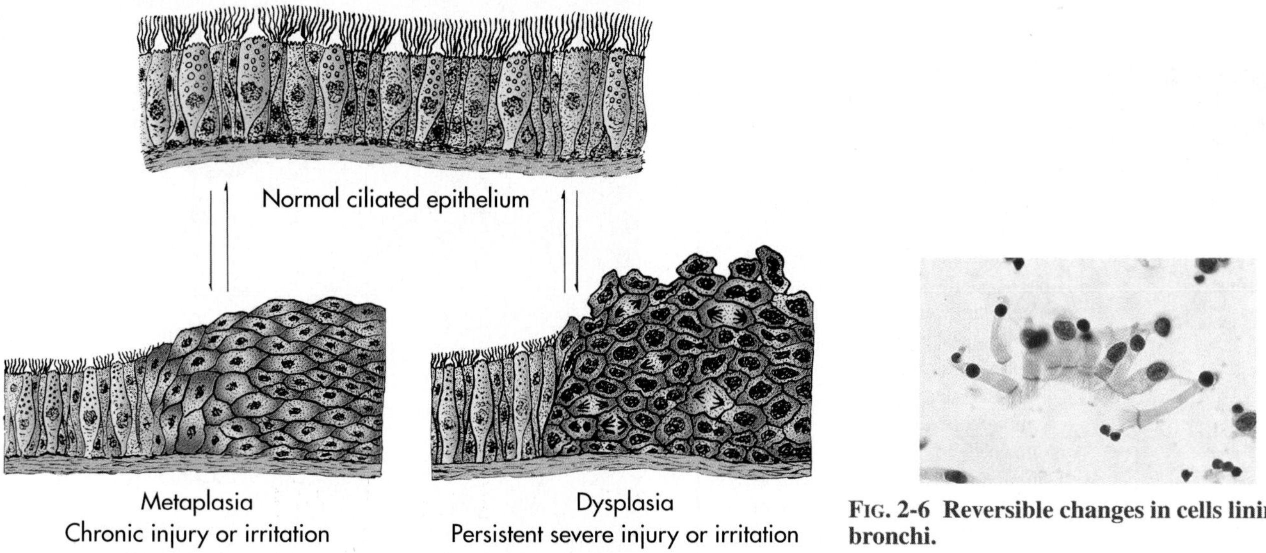

FIG. 2-6 Reversible changes in cells lining the bronchi.

sent in connective tissue. These precursor cells mature along a new pathway because of signals generated by cytokines and growth factors in the cell's environment.

Bronchial metaplasia can be reversed if the inducing stimulus, usually cigarette smoking, is removed. With prolonged exposure to the inducing stimulus, however, cancerous transformation can occur.

CELLULAR INJURY

Most diseases begin with cell injury, and all forms of loss of function derive from cell injury and cell death. Cellular injury occurs if the cell is unable to maintain homeostasis—a normal or adaptive steady state—in the face of injurious stimuli. Injured cells may recover **(reversible injury)** or die **(irreversible injury).** Injurious stimuli include chemical agents, lack of sufficient oxygen (hypoxia), free radicals, infectious agents, physical and mechanical factors, immunologic reactions, genetic factors, and nutritional imbalances. Types of cellular injury and their responses are summarized in Table 2-1 and Fig. 2-7.

Cell injury and cell death often result from exposure to toxic chemicals, infections, and hypoxia. The mechanisms causing chemical and hypoxic injury are perhaps the best understood. (Infections are discussed separately in Chapter 8.) Both these mechanisms can lead to disruption of selective permeability (i.e., transport mechanisms) of the plasma membrane; reduction or cessation of cellular metabolism; lack of protein synthesis; damage to lysosomal membranes, with leakage of destructive enzymes into the cytoplasm; enzymatic destruction of cellular organelles; cellular death (exhibited by nuclear changes); and phagocytosis of the dead cell by cellular components of the acute inflammatory response (see Chapter 7). The extent of cellular injury depends on the type, state (including level of cell differentiation and increased susceptibility to fully differentiated cells), and adaptive processes of the cell, as well as the type, severity, and duration of the injurious stimulus. Two individuals exposed to an identical stimulus may incur varying degrees of cellular injury. Modifying factors, such as nutritional status, can profoundly influence the extent of injury. The precise "point of no return" that leads to cellular death is a biochemical puzzle, and the exact mechanisms responsible for the transition from reversible to irreversible cellular damage are currently debated.

Table 2-1 Progressive Types of Cell Injury and Responses

Type	Responses
Adaptation	Atrophy, hypertrophy, hyperplasia, metaplasia
Active cell injury	Immediate response of "entire" cell
Reversible	Loss of adenosine triphosphate (ATP), cellular swelling, detachment of ribosomes, autophagy of lysosomes
Irreversible	"Point of no return" structurally when severe vacuolization occurs of the mitochondria and Ca^{++} moves into the cell
Necrosis	Common type of cell death with severe cell swelling and breakdown of organelles
Apoptosis, or programmed cell death	Cellular self-destruction for elimination of unwanted cell populations
Chronic cell injury (subcellular alterations)	Persistent stimuli response may involve only specific organelles or cytoskeleton, e.g., phagocytosis of bacteria
Accumulations or infiltrations	Water, pigments, lipids, glycogen, proteins
Pathologic calcification	Dystrophic and metastatic calcification

General Mechanisms of Cell Injury

Cells are complex units, and therefore the mechanisms responsible for cell injury leading to necrotic cell death are numerous and interrelated and depend on a delicate balance between intracellular and extracellular events. There are, however, four common biochemical themes important to cell injury and cell death regardless of the injuring agent (Table 2-2).

Much new information exists on cell injury caused by free radicals, including activated oxygen species. Thus the discussion is expanded to include three common forms of cell injury: (1) hypoxic injury, (2) reactive oxygen species and free radical–induced injury, and (3) chemical injury.

Hypoxic Injury

Hypoxia, or lack of sufficient oxygen, is the single most common cause of cellular injury (Fig. 2-8). Hypoxia can result from a decreased amount of oxygen in the air, loss of hemoglobin or hemoglobin function, decreased production of red blood cells, diseases of the respiratory and cardiovascular systems, and poisoning of the oxidative enzymes (cytochromes) within the cells. The most common cause of hypoxia is **ischemia** (reduced blood supply).

Ischemic injury is often caused by gradual narrowing of arteries (arteriosclerosis) and complete blockage by blood

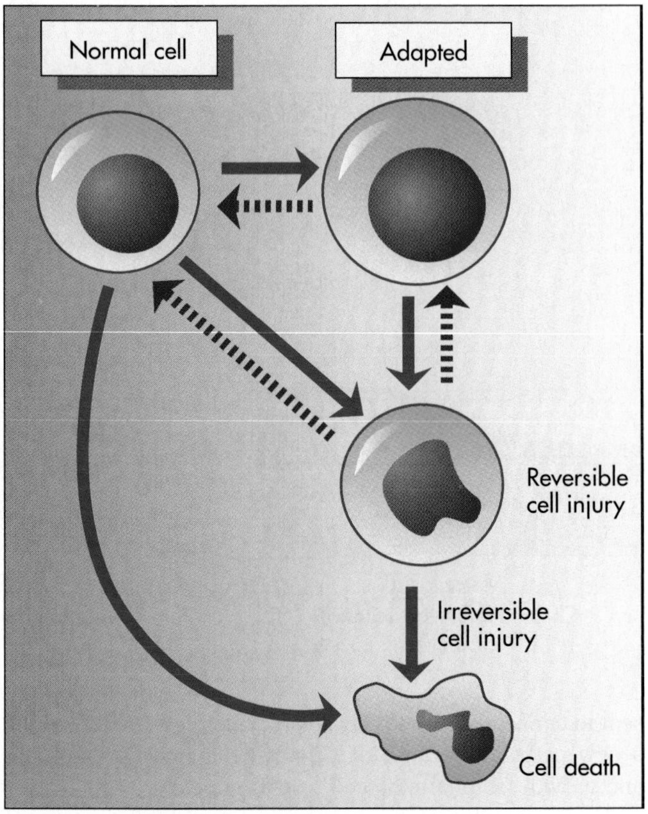

FIG. 2-7 Cellular injury and responses. Relationship among normal, adapted (hypertrophy), and reversibly injured cells and cell death of myocardial cells is depicted here.

clots (thrombosis). Progressive hypoxia caused by gradual arterial obstruction is better tolerated than the sudden acute **anoxia** (total lack of oxygen) caused by a sudden obstruction, such as can occur with an embolus (a blood clot or other plug in the circulation). An acute obstruction in a coronary artery can cause myocardial cell death (infarction) within minutes if the blood supply is not restored, whereas the gradual onset of ischemia usually results in myocardial adaptation. Myocardial infarction and stroke, which are common causes of death in the United States, generally result from atherosclerosis (a type of arteriosclerosis) and consequent ischemic injury. (Vascular obstruction is discussed in Chapter 29.)

Cellular responses to hypoxic injury have been extensively studied in heart muscle. Within 1 minute after blood supply to the myocardium is interrupted, the heart becomes pale and has difficulty contracting normally. Within 3 to 5 minutes, the ischemic portion of the myocardium ceases to

Table 2-2 Common Themes in Cell Injury and Cell Death

Theme	Comments
ATP depletion	Loss of mitochondrial ATP and decreased ATP synthesis; results include cellular swelling, decreased protein synthesis, decreased membrane transport, and lipogenesis, all changes that contribute to loss of integrity of plasma membrane (see text)
Oxygen and oxygen-derived free radicals	Lack of oxygen is key in progression of cell injury in ischemia (reduced blood supply); activated oxygen species (free radicals, $O_2^{\bar{}}$, H_2O_2, OH·) cause destruction of cell membranes and cell structure
Intracellular calcium and loss of calcium steady state	Normally intracellular cytosolic calcium concentrations are very low; ischemia and certain chemicals cause an increase in cytosolic Ca^{++} concentrations; sustained levels of Ca^{++} continue to increase with damage to plasma membrane; Ca^{++} causes intracellular damage by activating a number of enzymes (see text)
Defects in membrane permeability	Early loss of selective membrane permeability found in all forms of cell injury (see text)

ATP, Adenosine triphosphate.

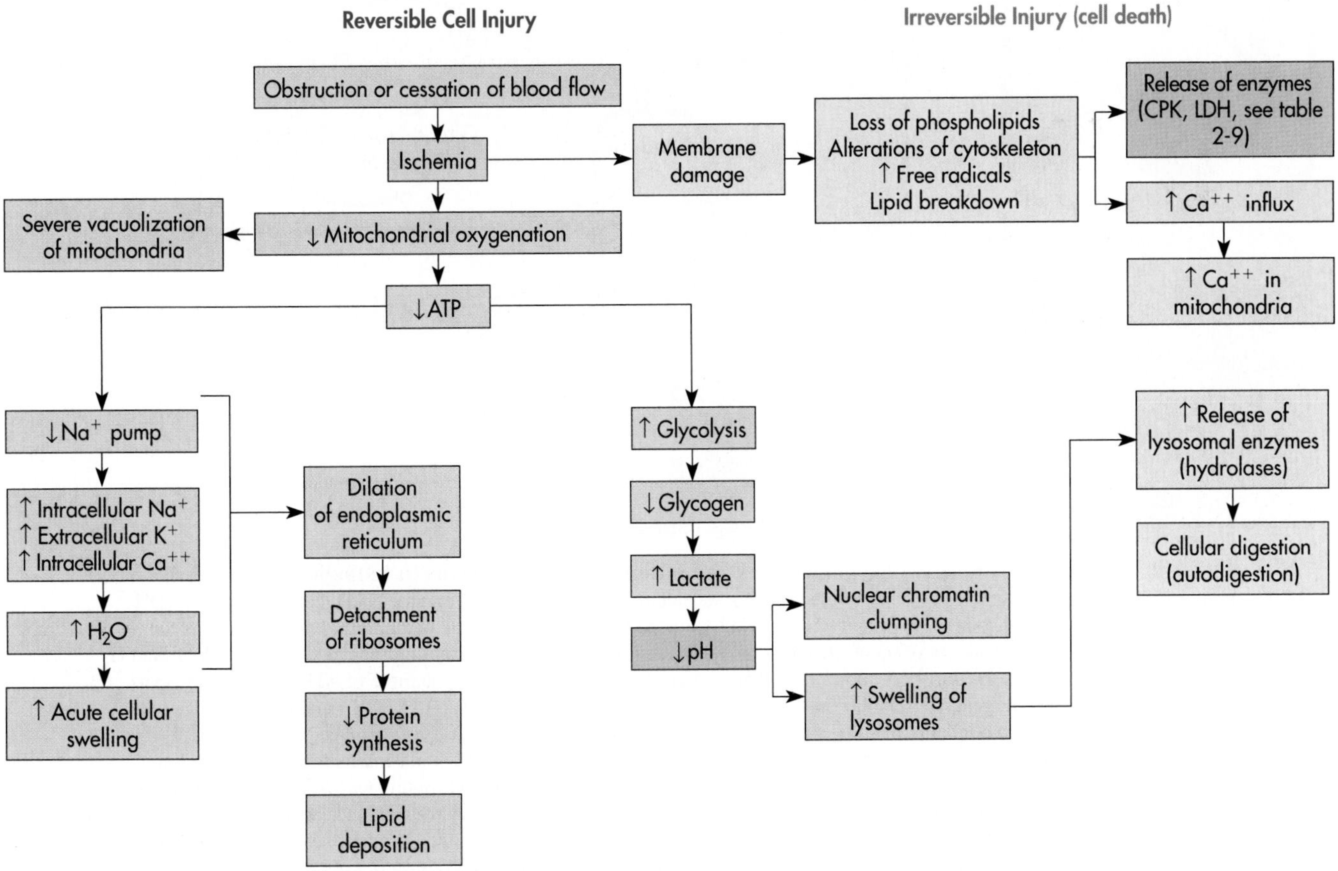

FIG. 2-8 Hypoxic injury induced by ischemia. Purple boxes involve reversible cell injury, and light blue boxes involve irreversible cell death. Green boxes are clinical manifestations.

contract. The abrupt lack of contraction is caused by a rapid decrease in mitochondrial phosphorylation, which results in insufficient adenosine triphosphate (ATP) production. Lack of ATP leads to an increase in anaerobic metabolism, which generates ATP from glycogen when there is insufficient oxygen. When glycogen stores are depleted, even anaerobic metabolism ceases.

A reduction in ATP levels causes the plasma membrane's sodium-potassium pump and sodium-calcium exchange to fail, which leads to an intracellular accumulation of sodium and calcium and diffusion of potassium out of the cell. (The sodium-potassium pump is discussed in Chapter 1.) Sodium and water then can enter the cell freely, and cellular swelling results. The movement of water and ions into the cell causes early dilation of the endoplasmic reticulum. Dilation causes the ribosomes to detach from the rough endoplasmic reticulum, resulting in reduced protein synthesis. With continued hypoxia, the entire cell becomes markedly swollen, with increased concentrations of sodium, water, and chloride and decreased concentrations of potassium. These disruptions are reversible if oxygen is restored. If oxygen is not restored, however, there is vacuolation (formation of vacuoles) within the cytoplasm, swelling of lysosomes, and marked swelling of the mitochondria resulting from mitochondrial membrane damage. Extensive damage also occurs to other cellular membranes. Structurally, this stage is associated with irreversible cell injury. With plasma membrane damage, extracellular calcium moves into the cell and accumulates in the mitochondria. Restoration of oxygen, however, can cause additional injury called **reperfusion injury.** Reperfusion injury results from the generation of high reactive oxygen intermediates, including hydroxyl radical (OH•), superoxide ($O_2^{\bar{\cdot}}$), and hydrogen peroxide (H_2O_2). These radicals can all cause further membrane damage (see p. 51). Antioxidants can decrease the amount of damage, especially superoxide dismutase and vitamin E.[7]

All cells in the body are bathed in a fluid rich in calcium ions. If the plasma membrane's barrier to calcium ions is eliminated or damaged, calcium readily enters and accumulates in the mitochondria, resulting in mitochondrial swelling and rapid death of the cell. Death is caused by calcium accumulation compromising ATP production by the mitochondria. In hypoxic injury caused by atherosclerosis, fail-

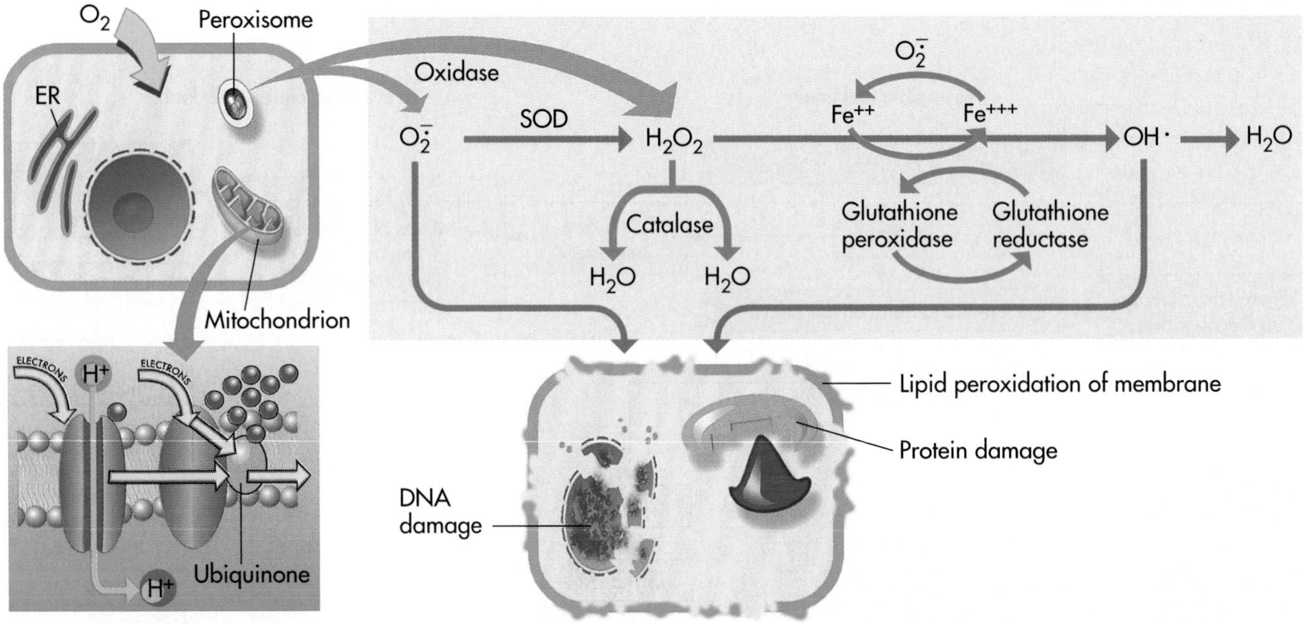

FIG. 2-9 Generation of reactive oxygen species and antioxidant mechanisms in biologic systems. In the mitochondria there are four sites of entry of electrons to the electron transport system: one for NADH and three for $FADH_2$. These pathways meet at the small, lipophilic molecule, ubiquinone (coenzyme Q), at the beginning of the common electron transport pathway. Ubiquinone transfers electrons in the inner membrane, ultimately enabling their interaction with O_2 and H_2 to yield H_2O. In so doing, the transport allows free energy change and the synthesis of one mole of ATP. With the transport of electrons, free radicals are generated within the mitochondria. Reactive oxygen species (H_2O_2, OH•, and $O_2^{\bar{\cdot}}$ and nitric oxide [NO]) act as physiologic modulators of some mitochondrial functions but may also cause cell damage. O_2 is converted to superoxide ($O_2^{\bar{\cdot}}$) by oxidative enxymes in the mitochondria, endoplasmic reticulum (ER), plasma membrane, peroxisomes, and cytosol. O_2 is converted to H_2O_2 by superoxide dismutase (SOD) and further to OH• by the Cu^{++}/Fe^{++} Fenton reaction. Superoxide catalyzes the reduction of Fe^{++} to Fe^{+++}, thus increasing OH• formation by the Fenton reaction. H_2O_2 is also derived from oxidases in peroxisomes. The three reactive oxygen species (H_2O_2, OH•, and $O_2^{\bar{\cdot}}$) cause free radical damage to lipids (peroxidation of the membrane), proteins (ion pump damage), and DNA (impaired protein synthesis). The major antioxidant enzymes include SOD, catalase, and glutathione peroxidase. (Modified from Cotran RS, Kumar V, Collins T: *Robbins pathologic basis of disease,* ed 6, Philadelphia, 1999, W.B. Saunders.)

ure of ATP production further deprives the myocardium of the energy needed for contraction.

Free Radicals and Reactive Oxygen Species

An important mechanism of membrane damage is injury induced by free radicals, especially by activated oxygen species. A **free radical** is an electrically uncharged atom or group of atoms having an unpaired electron. Having one unpaired electron makes the molecule unstable; thus to stabilize it gives up an electron to another molecule or steals one. Therefore it is capable of injurious chemical bond formation with proteins, lipids, carbohydrates—key molecules in membranes and nucleic acids. Free radicals are difficult to control and initiate chain reactions.

Free radicals may be initiated within cells by (1) the absorption of extreme energy sources (e.g., ultraviolet light, x-rays); (2) endogenous, usually oxidative, reactions that occur during normal metabolic processes (Fig. 2-9); or (3) enzymatic metabolism of exogenous chemicals or drugs (e.g., $CCl_3^{\cdot}$, a product of carbon tetrachloride [CCl_4]). Table 2-3 describes the most significant free radicals.

Although wide-ranging effects can occur from these reactive species, three are particularly important for cell injury: (1) lipid peroxidation; (2) alterations of proteins causing fragmentation of polypeptide chains; and (3) alterations of DNA, including breakage of single strands. **Lipid peroxidation** is the destruction of unsaturated fatty acids. Fatty acids of lipids in membranes possess double bonds between some of the carbon atoms. Such bonds are vulnerable to attack by oxygen-derived free radicals, especially $OH^{\cdot}$. The lipid-radical interactions themselves yield peroxides. The peroxides set off a chain reaction resulting in membrane, organelle, and cellular destruction. Because of our understanding of free radicals, a growing number of diseases and disorders have been linked either directly or indirectly to these reactive species (Table 2-4).

It is fortunate that the body can sometimes rid itself of free radicals. Superoxide may spontaneously decay into oxygen and hydrogen peroxide. Table 2-5 and Fig. 2-10 summarize other methods that contribute to inactivation or termination of free radicals. The toxicity of certain drugs and chemicals can be attributed to either conversion of these chemicals to free radicals or the formation of oxygen-derived metabolites.[8] This process is discussed in Chemical Injury.

Chemical Injury

Mechanisms

Chemical injury begins with a biochemical interaction between a toxic substance and the cell's plasma membrane, which is ultimately damaged, leading to increased permeability. Not all the mechanisms causing chemically induced membrane destruction are known; however, the two general mechanisms include (1) direct toxicity by combining with a molecular component of the cell membrane or organelles and (2) reactive free radicals and lipid peroxidation.

Because it has been investigated extensively, carbon tetrachloride (CCl_4) injury is a useful example of chemical injury. Carbon tetrachloride, an agent formerly used in dry cleaning, is injurious to cells because an enzyme system (P-450) in the smooth endoplasmic reticulum of liver cells converts it into $CCl_3^{\cdot}$ (chloromethyl), a highly toxic free radical.

Table 2-3 Biologically Relevant Free Radicals

Free Radical	Comments
Reactive oxygen species (ROS) Superoxide $O_2^{\cdot-}$ $O_2 \xrightarrow{\text{oxidase}} O_2^{\cdot-}$	Generated either (1) directly during autooxidation in mitochondria or (2) enzymatically by enzymes in the cytoplasm, such as xanthine oxidase or cytochrome P-450; once produced, it can be inactivated spontaneously or more rapidly by the enzyme superoxide dismutase (SOD): $O_2^{\cdot-} + O_2^{\cdot-} + 2H^+ \xrightarrow{\text{SOD}} H_2O_2 + O_2$
Hydrogen peroxide (H_2O_2) $O_2^{\cdot-} + O_2^{\cdot-} + 2H \xrightarrow{\text{SOD}} H_2O_2 + O_2$ or oxidases present in peroxisomes O_2 peroxisome $O_2^{\cdot-} \xrightarrow{\text{SOD}} H_2O_2$	Generated by the enzyme superoxide dismutase (SOD) or directly by oxidases in intracellular peroxisomes; NOTE: SOD is considered an antioxidant because it converts superoxide to H_2O_2; catalase (another antioxidant) can then decompose H_2O_2 to $O_2 + H_2O$
Hydroxyl radicals (OH^-) $H_2O \rightarrow H^{\cdot} + OH^{\cdot}$ or $Fe^{++} + H_2O_2 \rightarrow Fe^{+++} + OH^{\cdot} + OH^-$ or $H_2O_2 + O_2^{\cdot-} \rightarrow OH^{\cdot} + OH^- + O_2$	Generated by the hydrolysis of water caused by ionizing radiation or by interaction with metals—especially iron (Fe) and copper (Cu). Iron is important in toxic oxygen injury because it is required for maximal oxidative cell damage
Nitric oxide (NO) $NO^{\cdot} + O_2^{\cdot-} \rightarrow ONOO^- + H^+$ $\uparrow\downarrow$ $OH^{\cdot} + NO_2 \rightleftarrows ONOOH \rightarrow NO_3^-$	NO by itself is an important mediator that can act as a free radical; it can be converted to another radical—peroxnitrite anion ($ONOO^-$), as well as $NO_2^{\cdot}$ and NO_3^-

Data from Cotran RS, Robbins SL, Schoen FJ: *Robbins' pathologic basis of disease,* ed 6, Philadelphia, 1999, Saunders.

Table 2-4 Diseases and Disorders Linked to Oxygen-Derived Free Radicals

Deterioration noted in aging	Iron overload
Atherosclerosis	Lung disorders
Heart disease	Asbestosis
Stroke	Oxygen toxicity
Brain disorders	Emphysema
Ischemic brain injury	Nutritional deficiencies
Aluminum toxicity	Radiation injury
Alzheimer disease	Reperfusion injury
Neurotoxins	Rheumatoid arthritis
Cancer	Skin disorders
Cardiac myopathy	Solar radiation
Chronic granulomatous disease	Burns
Diabetes mellitus	Contact dermatitis
Eye disorders	Bloom syndrome
Macular degeneration	Toxic states
Cataracts	Xenobiotics (CCl_4, paraquat, cigarette smoke, etc.)
Inflammatory disorders	Metal ions (Ni, Cu, Fe, etc.)

Data from Knight JA: Diseases related to oxygen-derived free radicals, *Ann Clin Lab Sci* 25(2):111, 1995; Bergendi L et al: Chemistry, physiology and pathology of free radicals, *Life Sci* 65(18-19)1865, 1999.

Table 2-5 Methods Contributing to Inactivation or Termination of Free Radicals

Method	Process
Antioxidants	Endogenous or exogenous; either blocks synthesis or inactivates (e.g., scavenges) free radicals; includes vitamin E, vitamin C, cysteine, glutathione, albumin, ceruloplasmin, transferrin
Enzymes	Superoxide dismutase,* which converts superoxide to H_2O_2; catalase* (in peroxisomes) decomposes H_2O_2; glutathione peroxidase* decomposes OH· and H_2O_2

*These enzymes are important in modulating the cellular destructive effects of free radicals, also released in inflammation.

In CCl_4 injury, newly formed $CCl_3^\cdot$ rapidly destroys the endoplasmic reticulum of the liver cell by lipid peroxidation breaking down the reticulum's lipid component. The lipid molecules accumulate within the cytoplasm, starting within cisternae of the endoplasmic reticulum (Fig. 2-11). Fatty liver develops because CCl_4 poisoning blocks the synthesis of **lipid-acceptor proteins** (**apoproteins**) that normally bind with triglycerides to form lipoproteins, which are transported out of the cell. Blockage of triglyceride (lipoprotein) secretion begins 10 to 15 minutes after CCl_4 exposure. Fat droplets that accumulate in cisternae of the endoplasmic reticulum combine to form larger droplets and fill vacuoles, which in turn fill the entire cytoplasm. Approximately 10 to 12 hours later, the liver appears grossly enlarged and pale because of the accumulation of fat. (Accumulation of fat is discussed further on p. 68.)

In the meantime, cellular swelling progresses because of alterations in the selective permeability of the plasma membrane. Cellular swelling becomes severe when the plasma membrane loses its ability to prevent the passive inward diffusion of sodium ions, water, and calcium. The most serious consequence of plasma membrane damage is, as in hypoxic injury, to the mitochondria. An influx of calcium ions from the extracellular compartment and their accumulation in the mitochondria cause the mitochondria to swell, an occurrence that is associated with irreversible cellular injury. The injured mitochondria can no longer generate ATP, but they do continue to accumulate calcium ions. The influx of calcium into the mitochondria interferes with oxidative metabolism (by uncoupling oxidative phosphorylation).

Decreasing cellular pH (caused by the loss of oxidative phosphorylation and ATP-stimulating glycolysis), together with fluid and electrolyte imbalances (increased sodium, calcium, and water and decreased potassium), leads to lysosomal membrane injury, causing a leakage of lysosomal enzymes into the cytoplasm. Enzymatic digestion of cellular organelles, including the nucleus and nucleolus, ensues, halting synthesis of DNA and ribonucleic acid (RNA). The leakage of lysosomal enzymes apparently occurs late in chemical injury, well after irreversible lipid accumulation, mitochondrial swelling, and ATP loss.

Chemical Agents

Many chemical agents cause cellular injury. Minute amounts of some, such as arsenic and cyanide, can rapidly destroy enough cells to cause death of the individual. Long-term exposure to air pollutants, insecticides, and herbicides can cause cellular injury. Carbon monoxide, carbon tetrachloride, and social drugs, such as alcohol, can significantly alter cellular function and injure cellular structures. Over-the-counter and prescribed drugs also may cause cellular injury, sometimes leading to death. Accidental or suicidal poisonings by chemical agents cause numerous deaths. The injurious effects of some of these agents—lead, carbon monoxide, and ethyl alcohol—exemplify common cellular injuries.

Lead. Heavy metals, such as **lead,** cause a significant number of childhood poisonings. Lead-based paint, which

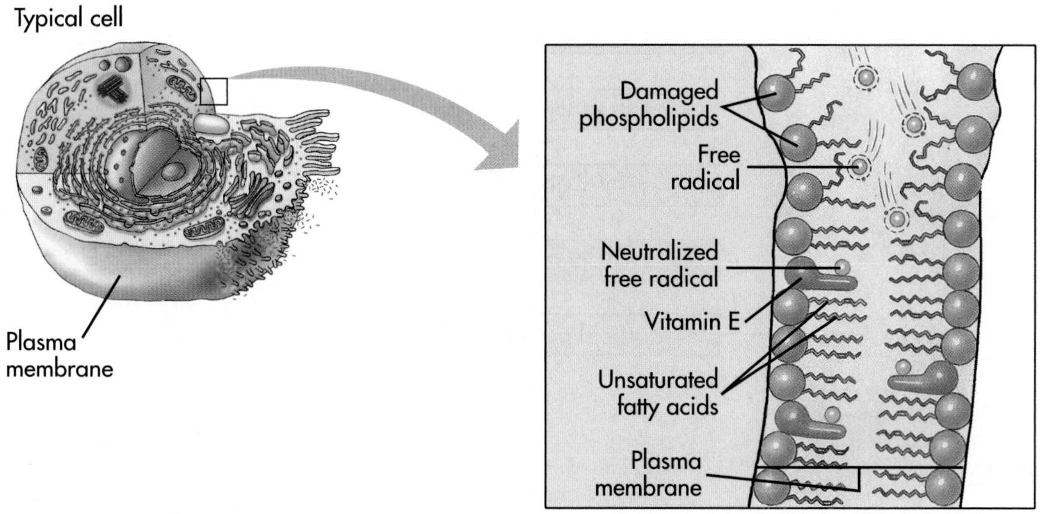

FIG. 2-10 Role of vitamin E. Vitamin E can act as an antioxidant, attracting and neutralizing molecules with unpaired electrons. (From Thibodeau GA, Patton KT: *Anatomy and physiology,* ed. 4, St Louis, 1999, Mosby.)

has a sweet taste, is often ingested by children. Other sources of lead include dust and soil in inner-city urban and, possibly, rural areas, debris from household renovations, formula mixed with lead-contaminated tap water, newsprint, lead water pipes, hair dyes, soldered tin cans, pottery glazes, and contamination from leaded gasoline.[9] Children are particularly vulnerable to lead toxicity because, compared with adults, they absorb lead more readily through the intestines. If nutrition is compromised, especially if dietary intake of iron, calcium, zinc, and vitamin D is insufficient, lead's toxic effects are enhanced.

The organ systems primarily affected by lead include the nervous system, the hematopoietic system (tissues that produce blood cells), and the kidneys. A suggested mechanism by which lead acts on the central nervous system (CNS) is interference with neurotransmitters, which may cause hyperactive behavior and proliferation of capillaries of the white matter and intercerebral arteries.[2] Lead inhibits several enzymes involved in hemoglobin synthesis. A significant manifestation of lead toxicity is anemia caused by lysis of red blood cells (hemolysis). Manifestations of brain involvement include convulsions and delirium and, with peripheral nerve involvement, wrist, finger, and sometimes foot paralysis. Renal lesions can cause tubular dysfunction resulting in glycosuria (glucose in the urine), aminoaciduria (amino acids in the urine), and hyperphosphaturia (excess phosphate in the urine). Gastrointestinal symptoms are less severe and include nausea, loss of appetite, weight loss, and abdominal cramping.

Carbon monoxide. Gaseous substances can be classified according to their ability to asphyxiate (interrupt respiration) or irritate. Toxic asphyxiants, such as carbon monoxide, hydrogen cyanide, and hydrogen sulfide, directly interfere with cellular respiration. **Carbon monoxide** is widely available.

Carbon monoxide is odorless, colorless, and undetectable unless it is mixed with a visible or odorous pollutant. It is produced by the incomplete combustion of such fuels as gasoline. Although carbon monoxide is a chemical agent, the ultimate injury it produces is a hypoxic injury, namely, oxygen deprivation. Normally, oxygen molecules are carried to tissues bound to hemoglobin in red blood cells (see Chapter 28). Because carbon monoxide's affinity for hemoglobin is 300 times greater than that of oxygen, it quickly binds with the hemoglobin, preventing oxygen molecules from doing so. Minute amounts of carbon monoxide can produce significant percentages of **carboxyhemoglobin** (carbon monoxide bound with hemoglobin).

Symptoms related to carbon monoxide poisoning include headache, giddiness, tinnitus (ringing in the ears), nausea, weakness, and vomiting. At risk for carbon monoxide exposure are those who (1) breathe air polluted by gasoline engines or defective furnaces; (2) work in occupations such as coal mining, fire fighting, or engine repair; and (3) smoke cigarettes, cigars, or pipes. The fetus is especially at risk from the effects of carbon monoxide because fetal carboxyhemoglobin levels are likely to be 10% to 15% greater than maternal levels.[10]

Ethanol. Alcohol **(ethanol)** is the number one mood-altering drug in the United States. Because alcohol is not only a psychoactive drug but also a food, it is considered part of the basic food supply in many societies.

A large intake of alcohol has enormous effects on nutritional status. Liver and nutritional disorders are the most serious consequences of alcohol abuse. New understandings of the mechanisms of ethanol-induced liver injury have emerged through the clarification of a new pathway for ethanol oxidation, the microsomal P-450 oxidase pathway.

The major effects of acute alcoholism involve the CNS. After ingestion, alcohol is absorbed, unaltered, in the stomach and small intestine. Fatty foods and milk slow absorption.[11] Alcohol then is distributed to all tissues and fluids of the body in direct proportion to the blood concentration.

Most of the alcohol in the blood is metabolized in the liver through one major and two accessory pathways. The

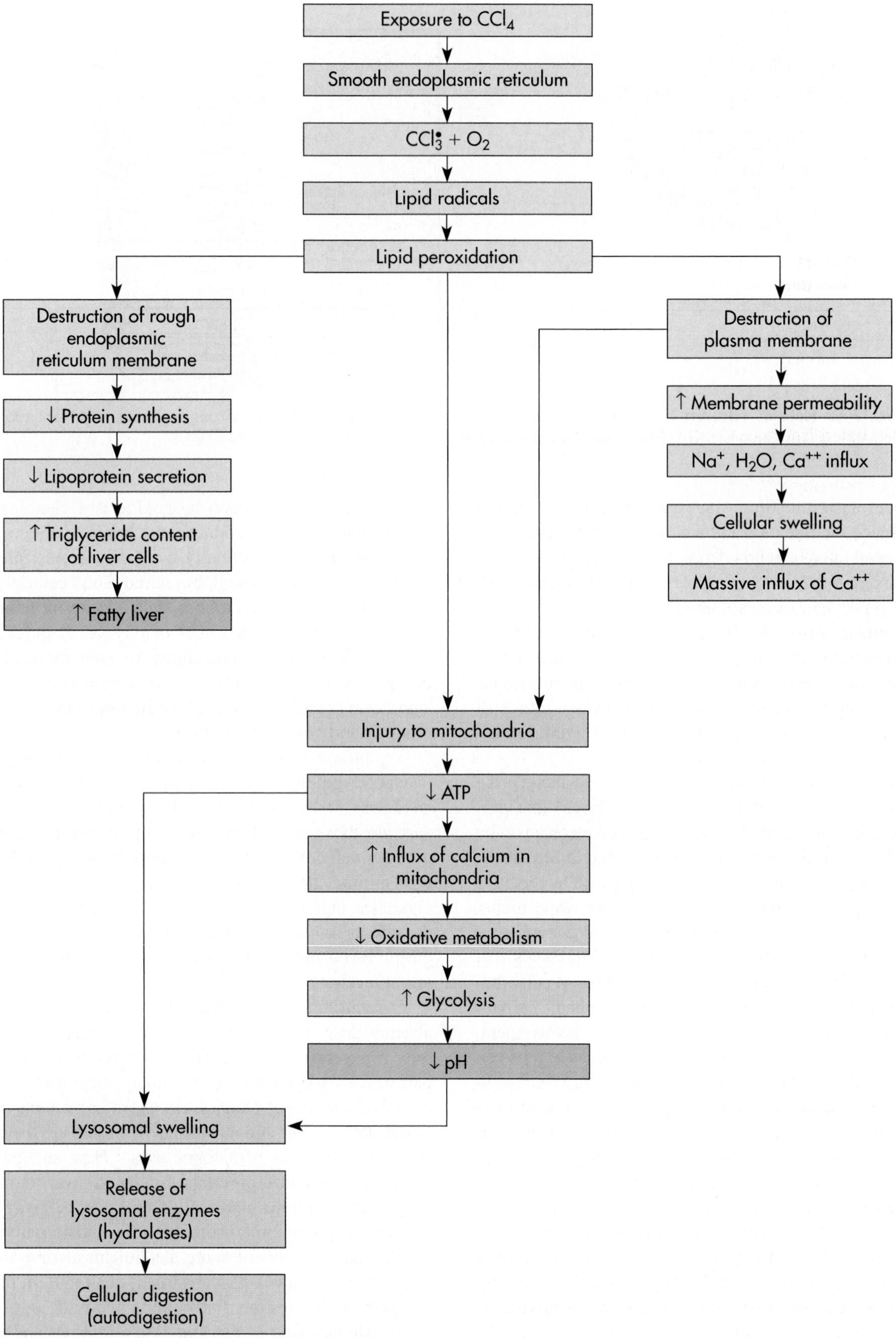

FIG. 2-11 Chemical injury of liver cells induced by carbon tetrachloride (CCl_4) poisoning. Light blue boxes are mechanisms unique to chemical injury; purple boxes involve hypoxic injury. Green boxes are clinical manifestations.

major pathway involves hepatic alcohol dehydrogenase (ADH), an enzyme of the cytosol that catalyzes the conversion of ethanol to acetaldehyde (Fig. 2-12).

The microsomal ethanol oxidizing system (MEOS) depends on cytochrome P-450, an enzyme necessary for cellular oxidation.[12] Activation of MEOS requires a high ethanol concentration and thus is thought to be important in the accelerated ethanol metabolism (i.e., tolerance) noted in people with chronic alcoholism.[12]

Individuals differ in their capability to metabolize alcohol. Genetic differences in metabolism of liver alcohol, including aldehyde dehydrogenases, have been identified.[13] Persons with chronic alcoholism develop certain levels of tolerance because of enzyme induction, leading to an increased rate of metabolism (e.g., P-450).

Acute alcoholism mainly affects the CNS but may induce reversible hepatic and gastric changes. The hepatic changes, initiated from acetaldehyde, include deposition in fat, enlargement of the liver, interruption of microtubular transport of proteins and their secretion, increase in intracellular water, depression of fatty acid oxidation in the mitochondria, increased membrane rigidity, and acute liver cell necrosis (see Chapter 38). In the CNS, alcohol is itself a depressant, initially affecting subcortical structures (probably the brain stem reticular formation).[14] Consequently, motor and intellectual activities become disoriented. Acute alcoholism contributes significantly to more than 50% of motor vehicle fatalities. At higher blood levels, medullary centers become depressed, affecting respiration. Much investigation is underway on the relationship of alcohol and snoring and obstructive sleep apnea (cessation of breathing).[15]

Chronic alcoholism causes structural alterations in practically all organs and tissues in the body, especially the liver and stomach. The precise mechanisms for these widespread effects are controversial, but new evidence supports damage via the generation of free radicals. Acetaldehyde results in the formation of free radicals modulating the activity of the free radical–generating enzyme xanthine oxidase.[16,17] Chronic alcoholism is related to several disorders, including an increased tendency to hypertension, a higher incidence of acute and chronic pancreatitis, and regressive changes in skeletal muscle (see Chapter 38). Ethanol is implicated in the onset of a variety of immune defects, including effects on the production of cytokines involved in inflammatory responses (tumor necrosis factor, interleukin-1, interleukin-6).[18] The deleterious effects of prenatal alcohol exposure (e.g., **fetal alcohol syndrome [FAS]**) have also been noted. FAS can lead to growth retardation, cognitive impairment, facial anomalies, and ocular disturbances.[19,20] Animal studies have shown that ethanol at moderate concentrations inhibits epidermal growth factor–dependent replication of hepatocytes. This finding may account for the growth/development impairment associated with fetal alcohol syndrome and decreased liver regeneration in alcoholic liver disease.[21,22] The wide variety of cellular/biochemical effects of ethanol on fetal tissue is itself a puzzle reflecting a multifactorial prob-

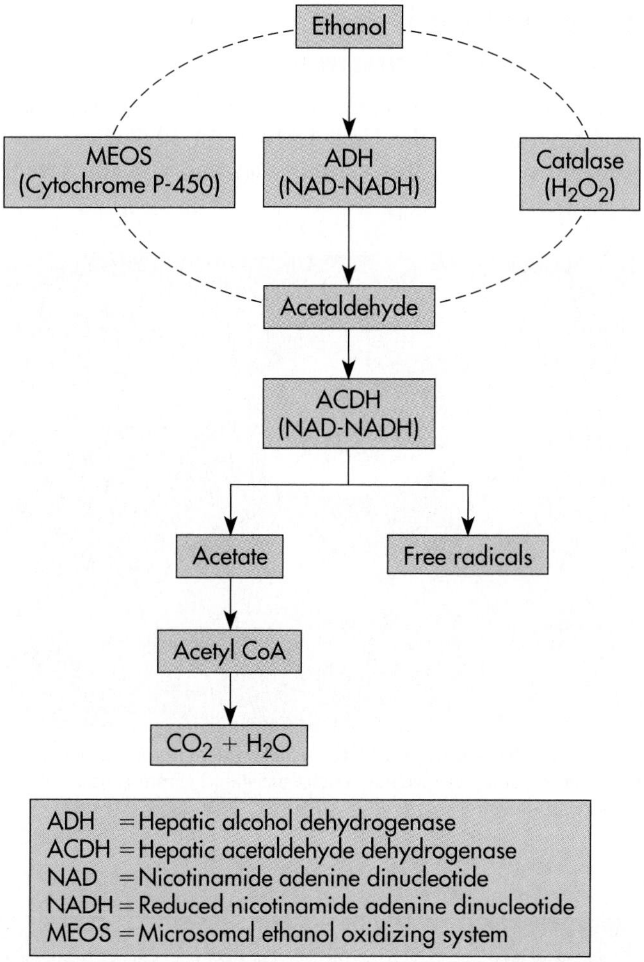

FIG. 2-12 Major pathway of metabolism of alcohol in the liver through ADH.

lem. These effects are conceptually connected to membrane structure and function involving transport systems, membrane fluidity, Na^+-K^+ pump expression, and epidermal growth factor receptor expression.[22] Recent evidence points to oxidative stress as potentially causative of these membrane-related events.[17]

Whatever the cause, people with chronic alcoholism have a significantly shortened life span related mainly to damage to the liver, stomach, brain, and heart. Alcohol is a well-known cause of hepatic injury, terminating in cirrhosis (see Chapter 38) (Fig. 2-13). Although this issue is still controversial, moderate amounts of alcohol may decrease the incidence of coronary heart disease (see Chapter 29).

Social or street drugs. The social or "recreational" use of psychoactive drugs is widespread in many parts of the world. Most popular and dangerous are the drugs marijuana, cocaine, and heroin. The real prevalence of marijuana and heroin use is unknown. Although the prevalence of cocaine use in the general population decreased beginning in 1986, morbidity and mortality related to cocaine increased sharply in the 1990s. Drug trafficking is a prevalent risk behavior among adolescents.[23] Table 2-6 summarizes the effects of these drugs.

Unintentional and Intentional Injuries

Unintentional and intentional injuries are an important health problem in the United States. In 1997 there were 146,400 deaths in this category, an injury death rate of 54.7/100,000.[24] Death is significantly more common for men than women; the overall rate for men is 78.62/100,000 vs. 31.76/100,000 for women. There are also significant racial differences in the death rate, with whites at 53.07/100,000, blacks at 71.43/100,000, and other racial groups at a combined rate of 37.95/100,000. There also is a bimodal age distribution for injury-related deaths, with peaks in the young adult and elderly groups. Unintentional injury is the leading cause of death for people between the ages of 1 and 34 years, with intentional injury (suicide, homicide) ranking between the second and fourth leading cause of death in this age-group. Statistics on nonfatal injuries are harder to document accurately, but they are known to be a significant cause of morbidity and disability and to cost society billions of dollars annually. The more common terms used to describe and classify unintentional and intentional injuries and brief descriptions of important features are discussed here.

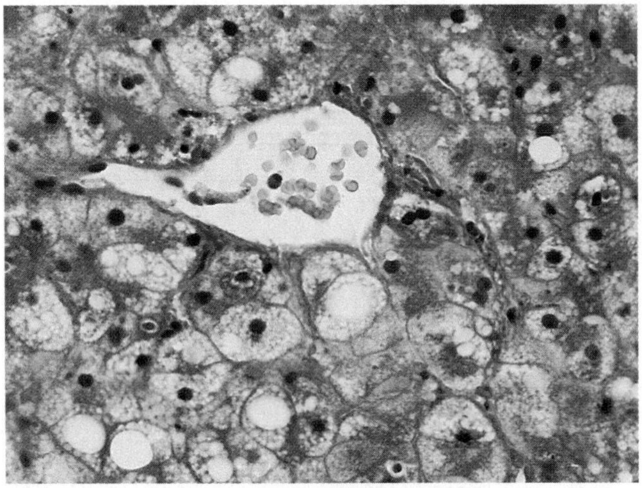

FIG. 2-13 **Alcoholic hepatitis.** Chicken-wire fibrosis extending between hepatocytes. (Mallory trichrome stain.) (From Damjanov I, Linder J: *Anderson's pathology,* ed 10, St Louis, 1996, Mosby.)

Blunt Force Injuries

Blunt force injuries are the result of the application of mechanical energy to the body resulting in the tearing, shearing, or crushing of tissues. They are the most common type of injuries seen in most health care settings. Blunt force injury may be caused by blows (where a moving object strikes the body), impacts (where the moving body strikes a fixed object), or a combination of both. Motor vehicle accidents

Table 2-6 Social or Street Drugs

Type of Drug	Comments
Marijuana	Active substance: delta-9-tetrahydrocannabinol (THC) found in resin of the *Cannabis sativa* plant; with smoking (e.g., "joints"), about 50% is absorbed through the lungs; when ingested only 10% is absorbed; with heavy use the following adverse effects have been reported: alterations of sensory perceptions, cognitive and psychomotor impairment (e.g., inability to judge time, speed, and distance); smoking 3 or 4/day is similar to 20 cigarettes/day with frequency of chronic bronchitis—unknown but may contribute to lung cancer; from animal studies only reproductive changes include reduced fertility, decreased sperm motility, decreased circulatory testosterone; fetal abnormalities include low birth weight and increased frequency of childhood leukemia; increased frequency of infectious illnesses thought to be the result of depressed cell-mediated and humoral immunity.
Cocaine and crack	Extracted from the leaves of the coca plant and sold as a water-soluble powder (cocaine hydrochloride) liberally diluted with talcum powder or other white powders; extraction of pure alkaloid from cocaine hydrochloride is "free-base" called "crack" because it cracks when heated; crack is more potent than cocaine; cocaine is widely used as an anesthetic, usually in procedures of the oral cavity; it is a potent CNS stimulant blocking reuptake of neurotransmitters norepinephrine, dopamine, and serotonin; also increases synthesis of norepinephrine and dopamine; dopamine induces a sense of euphoria, and norepinephrine causes adrenergic potentiation including hypertension, tachycardia, and vasoconstriction; cocaine can therefore cause severe coronary artery narrowing and ischemia; not clear is why cocaine increases thrombus formation; other cardiovascular effects include dysrhythmias, sudden death, dilated cardiomyopathy, rupture of descending aorta (i.e., secondary to hypertension), myocyte apoptosis; effects to the fetus include premature labor, retarded fetal development, stillbirth, hyperirritability.
Heroin	An opiate closely related to morphine, methadone, and codeine; highly addictive, and withdrawal causes intense fear ("I'll die without it"); sold "cut" with similar-looking white powder; dissolved in water it is often highly contaminated; feeling of tranquility and sedation lasts only a few hours and thus encourages repeated intravenous or subcutaneous injections; acts on the receptors enkephalins, endorphins, and dynorphins, which are widely distributed throughout the body with high affinity to the CNS; effects can include infectious complications, especially *Staphylococcus aureus,* granulomas of the lung, septic embolism, and pulmonary edema—in addition, viral infections from casual exchange of needles and HIV; sudden death is related to overdosage secondary to respiratory depression, cardiac output, and severe pulmonary edema.

Data from Cotran RS, Robbins SL, Schoen FJ: *Robbins pathologic basis of disease,* ed 6, Philadelphia, 1999, Saunders; Nahas G, Latour C: *Med J Australia* 156:495, 1992.

and falls are the most common causes, accounting for 43,591 and 12,555 deaths, respectively, in 1997.

Contusion

A **contusion** (bruise) is bleeding into the skin or underlying tissues as a consequence of a blow that squeezes or crushes the soft tissues and ruptures blood vessels without breaking the skin. It may take several hours after injury before any change in skin color is seen. A bruise will be red-purple initially, eventually becoming blue-black, and then gradually changing to yellow-brown or green before fully disappearing (Fig. 2-14). These color changes reflect the progression of tissue damage and healing that develops in the area of underlying injury. The length of time depends on such factors as the extent and location of the injury and the degree of vascularization in the area. Small contusions may resolve in a matter of days, whereas larger ones can take weeks to completely heal. Bruising of soft tissues may sometimes be confined to deeper structures; thus no injury is visible externally. Blood in deeper structures may dissect along fascial planes so discoloration of the skin may be seen in areas not directly injured by the initiating blow or impact, such as bruising of the thigh in a hip or pelvis fracture or "black eyes" in orbital plate fractures. Contusions may also be seen in internal organs in cases of severe injury.

A collection of blood in soft tissues or an enclosed space may also be referred to as a **hematoma** (see Figs. 16-3 and 16-6). A **subdural hematoma** is a collection of blood between the inner surface of the dura mater and the surface of the brain, resulting from the shearing of small veins that bridge the subdural space. Subdural hematomas can result from blows, falls, or sudden acceleration/deceleration of the head, as occurs in *shaken baby syndrome*. An **epidural hematoma** is a collection of blood between the inner surface of the skull and the dura. It is caused by a torn artery and is almost always associated with a skull fracture.

Contusions of the brain may result from (1) a blow or (2) a fall or impact. In blows, when a moving object strikes the stationary head, a cerebral contusion grouped in the portions of the brain underlying the area of scalp and skull injury is known as a *coup* pattern of injury. In falls or impacts, where the moving head strikes a fixed object, a cerebral contusion seen in the area of the brain opposite the external injury is known as a *contrecoup* pattern of injury (see Fig. 16-1). Contrecoup injury results when the head accelerates and the brain lags behind and presses into the areas of the skull directly opposite the direction of motion. When the head suddenly stops, the areas of the brain pressing into the skull are injured. For example, a person who falls directly backward striking the occiput (back of the head) will have cerebral contusions of the frontal and temporal tips (these injuries are discussed further in Chapter 16).

Abrasion

An **abrasion** (scrape) results from removal of the superficial layers of the skin caused by friction between the skin and injuring object. Abrasions vary in size and severity from fine, thin scratches to large denuded areas (road rash). In cases where force is applied in a tangential, nonperpendicular direction to the skin surface, tags of tissue may be heaped up at the trailing or downstream edge of the abrasion. An abrasion will have a pale, moist, yellow-brown appearance at first. The color darkens to brown or even black as the injury dries. The injury may ooze fluid for 1 or 2 days until it is completely covered by a crust, or scab, which eventually flakes off of the underlying regenerated skin.

Abrasions and contusions may have a patterned appearance that mirrors the shape and features of an injuring object (Fig. 2-15). Patterning of injuries can be of crucial important in cases of automobile accidents, assaults, or homicides by

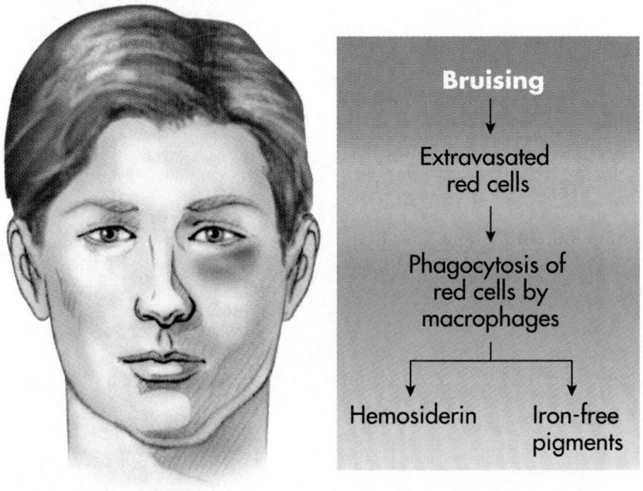

FIG. 2-14 Hemosiderin accumulation is noted as the color changes in a "black eye."

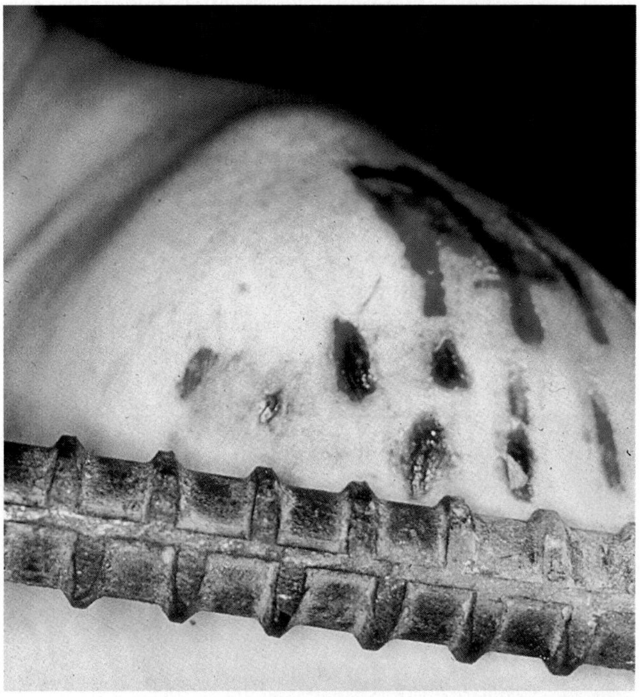

FIG. 2-15 Patterned abrasion caused by a piece of rebar. Note the tissue tags at the inferior margins indicating the downward direction of the blow that caused this injury.

documenting the connection between the victim's injuries and a suspect vehicle or weapon. Bite marks (usually a combination of abrasion and contusion) are another example of a patterned injury that can demonstrate a link between an assailant and victim.

Laceration

A **laceration** is a tear or rip resulting when the tensile strength of the skin or tissue is exceeded. Unlike an incision, where the tissue is cleanly divided by a sharp edge, a laceration is much more jagged and irregular, and the edges will be abraded. The depths of the laceration will be irregular, and there are often tissue "bridges" of small vessels or nerves that have been stretched but not broken, crossing from one side of the wound to the other. If the injuring force is applied perpendicularly to the skin, there will be crushing of the surrounding tissue with associated abrasion and contusion. If force is applied tangentially, there will also be undermining of the wound, with tissues at the trailing edge of the wound lifted away from the underlying structures, creating a pocket in the direction opposite from where the blow came. An extreme example is an **avulsion** (Fig. 2-16), in which a wide area of tissue may be pulled away creating a large flap. Usually, the shallower the angle of incidence of the blow, the more extensive the undermining.

Lacerations of internal organs are not uncommon in blunt impact injuries. Lacerations of the liver, spleen, kidneys, and bowel may occur in cases of blows to the abdomen, often with no visible injury to the abdominal wall seen externally. The thoracic aorta may be lacerated in sudden deceleration accidents. This results from the fact that the arch of the aorta is freely mobile, whereas the descending portion is attached to the spinal column. Rapid deceleration will cause horizontal shearing with either partial or complete transection just below the takeoff of the left subclavian artery. Severe blows or impacts to the chest may also cause rupturing of the heart with lacerations of the atria or ventricles.

Fractures

Blunt force blows or impacts can also cause bone to break or shatter. Fractures are extensively covered in Chapter 41 and are not discussed here.

Sharp Force Injuries

Cutting and piercing injuries accounted for 2864 deaths in 1997. As with all injuries, men have a higher rate (1.59/100,000) than women (0.57/100,000). There are also greater differences among races, with rates in whites 0.79/100,000, blacks 2.93/100,000, and other racial groups 1.0/100,000.

Incised Wounds

An **incised wound** is a cut that is *longer* than it is *deep*. The wound may be straight or jagged, depending on the object used and how the injury occurred, with sharp, distinct edges without abrasion. Because the wound is caused by a sharp edge, the tissues are cleanly divided and there is no tissue bridging or undermining. An incised wound may be thin and narrow or more elliptic and gaping in appearance because of varying lines of tension in the skin, depending on the location and orientation of the wound. Incised wounds tend to produce significant external bleeding with minimal internal hemorrhage. These wounds are often seen in sharp force injury suicides. In most cases, in addition to a deep, lethal cut, there will be multiple superficial incisions grouped in the area known as *hesitation marks* (Fig. 2-17).

Stab Wounds

A **stab wound** is a penetrating sharp force injury that is *deeper* than it is *long*. Because a sharp instrument is used, the depths of the wound are clean and distinct with no underlying or associated crushing injury. The edges are usually clean but may be abraded if the object is inserted deeply with enough force so that a wider, blunter portion of the instrument (e.g., hilt of a knife) impacts the skin. Fig. 2-18 illustrates this type of wound.

A number of features about the blade used may be determined from careful examination of the stab wound. If a *single-edge* blade was used, one margin of the wound will be sharp and the other blunt; if a *double-edge* blade caused

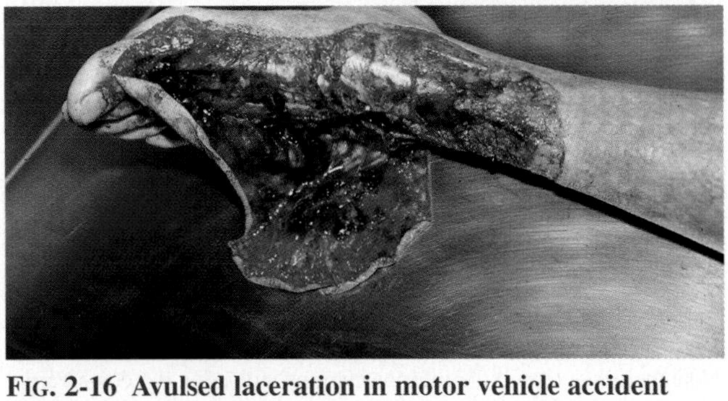

FIG. 2-16 Avulsed laceration in motor vehicle accident victim. The victim was the driver and this injury most likely was caused by the brake pedal.

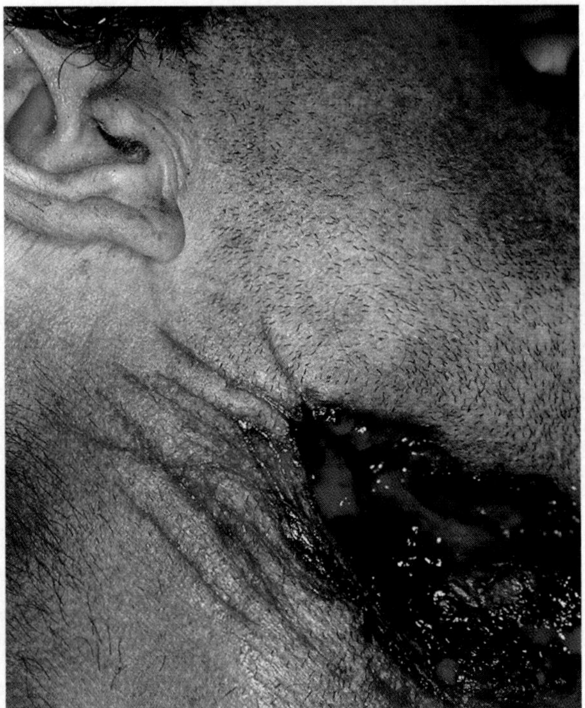

FIG. 2-17 Self-inflicted incised wound of the neck with multiple hesitation marks.

the wound, both margins will have a sharp appearance. Stab wounds produced by a *serrated-edge* blade are often indistinguishable from those made by a *smooth-edge* blade. If there was any hesitation or scraping of the skin edges by the blade, an interrupted pattern of abrasion may be seen but is uncommon. As with incised wounds, skin tension may cause the wound to gape, giving it an elliptic appearance. The edges must be brought into opposition so there is no distortion before trying to determine if the margins are sharp or blunt. The length of the stab wound may or may not correlate with the width of the blade, depending on whether there was any cutting or twisting when the blade was inserted or withdrawn. Once the edges are in opposition, the thickness of the blade may be estimated from the width of the wound. Depth of the wound may not correlate with the length of the blade because the blade was not inserted fully, or, as a consequence of compression of tissues from a forceful thrust, the wound may be deeper than the length of the blade.

Depending on size and location of the stab wound, the amount of external bleeding may be surprisingly small. After an initial spurt, even if a major vessel or the heart is struck, the wound track may be almost completely closed by tissue pressure, allowing only a trickle of visible blood despite copious internal bleeding.

Puncture Wounds

Instruments or objects with sharp points but without sharp edges may produce penetrating **puncture wounds.** A classic example is a wound of the foot caused by stepping on a nail. These injuries often will have abrasion of the edges of the wound, are prone to infection, and can also be quite deep despite a sometimes innocuous external appearance.

Chopping Wounds

Heavy, edged instruments (axes, hatchets, propeller blades) will produce injuries—**chopping wounds**—with a combination of sharp and blunt force characteristics. In addition to cutting, there will usually be associated crushing of the wound edges and underlying tissues.

Gunshot Wounds

Injuries caused by gunfire accounted for 32,436 deaths in the United States in 1997. Of these, 17,566 were suicides, 13,252 homicides, 981 accidents, and 367 classified as undetermined. Men are much more likely to die from gunshot injury than women. The male death rate in 1997 was 21.18/100,000 vs. 3.43/100,000 for women. Black men between the ages of 15 and 24 years have the greatest gunfire injury death rate: 119.89/100,000. To put this statistic into perspective, if this was the rate for the United States as a whole, there would be more than 318,000 gunshot wound deaths per year.

Gunshot wounds may be either penetrating (bullet retained in the body) or perforating (bullet exits). In some cases, the bullet may fragment so pieces of the missile are retained even though there is an exit wound. The most important factors determining the appearance of a gunshot injury are whether it is an entrance or an exit wound and the range of fire.

Entrance Wounds

Although all **entrance wounds** share some common features, the overall appearance is most affected by the range of fire.

Contact range entrance wounds occur when the gun is held so the muzzle rests on or presses into the skin surface, causing a distinctive type of wound. In addition to the hole made by the bullet, there will be searing of the edges of the wound from the flame and hot gases exiting the barrel and soot or smoke deposited on the edges of and in the depths of the wound. In hard contact wounds, where the barrel is firmly pressed into the skin, there may be minimal soot and searing on the outside of the wound but deep penetration of smoke, burning gunpowder fragments, and hot gases into the depths of the injury. In hard contact wounds of the head, where there is only a thin layer of skin and muscle overlying bone, the large amount of gas and explosive energy sent into the wound may cause severe tearing and disruption of the tissues, giving the wound a large, gaping, and jagged appearance—a phenomenon known as **blow back.** In areas of the body with thicker layers of soft tissue, the blow back may not cause tearing but will forcefully drive the skin back onto the end of the barrel, producing a patterned abrasion that mirrors the features of the weapon, known as a **muzzle imprint** (Fig. 2-19).

Intermediate range entrance wounds are surrounded by gunpowder tattooing or stippling (Fig. 2-20). **Tattooing** results from fragments of burning or unburned pieces of gunpowder exiting the barrel and striking the skin surface with enough force to be driven into the epidermis or superficial dermis. **Stippling** results when fragments of powder strike with enough force to abrade the skin but not actually penetrate the surface. This phenomenon can be seen when the muzzle-to-target range of most handguns is less than 48 inches. Beyond this distance, pieces of gunpowder disperse

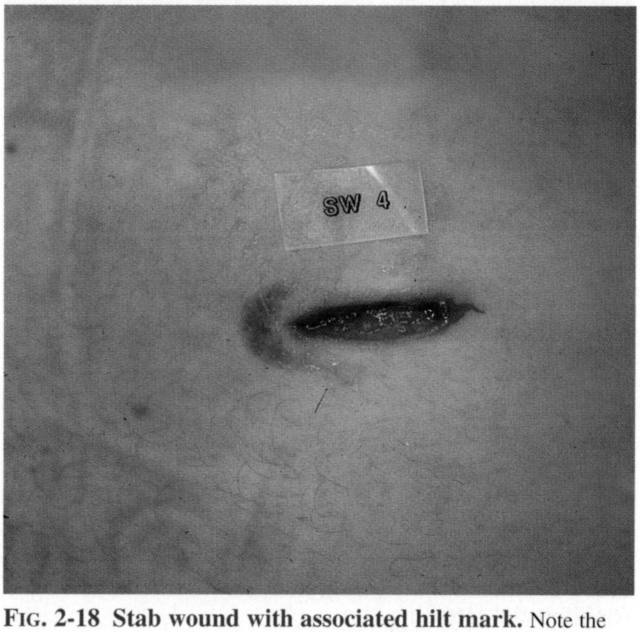

FIG. 2-18 Stab wound with associated hilt mark. Note the sharp margin away from the hilt mark with the blunt margin toward it. This wound was caused by a single-edged knife.

and slow down so much that tattooing or stippling cannot occur. The closer the muzzle is to the skin, the tighter the distribution and greater the density of powder fragments will be around the actual entrance hole. Soot may also be deposited.

An **indeterminate (distant) range entrance wound** occurs when flame, soot, or gunpowder does not reach the skin surface and the only thing striking the body is the bullet. The term *indeterminate* is used rather than *distant* because it does not imply that one can actually determine the range of fire from the appearance of the wound. For example, if an individual is shot through multiple layers of clothing, the entrance wound may have no sooting, searing, or stippling even though the actual range of fire is only a matter of inches; the wound would look the same as if the shot came from a range of 6 meters (20 feet) or more. Indeterminate wounds are characterized by a hole surrounded by a rim of abrasion. The size of the hole can vary according to a number of factors. It is important to remember that one cannot say what caliber of weapon inflicted the wound based solely on the size of the entrance wound. The collar of abrasion results from the fact that the bullet first causes stretching and scraping of the skin before it actually perforates. If the bullet strikes perpendicular to the skin, the margin of abrasion collar is concentrically disturbed about the defect; if it strikes at an angle, the collar is eccentric, with the wider margin pointing in the direction from which the bullet came (Fig. 2-21). If the bullet has struck an intermediary target before hitting the skin, it can be turning and tumbling, producing an irregular abrasion collar.

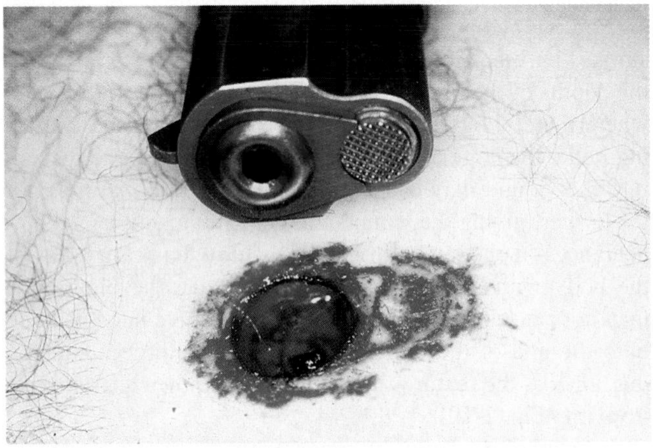

FIG. 2-19 Contact range gunshot wound of the chest with a muzzle abrasion.

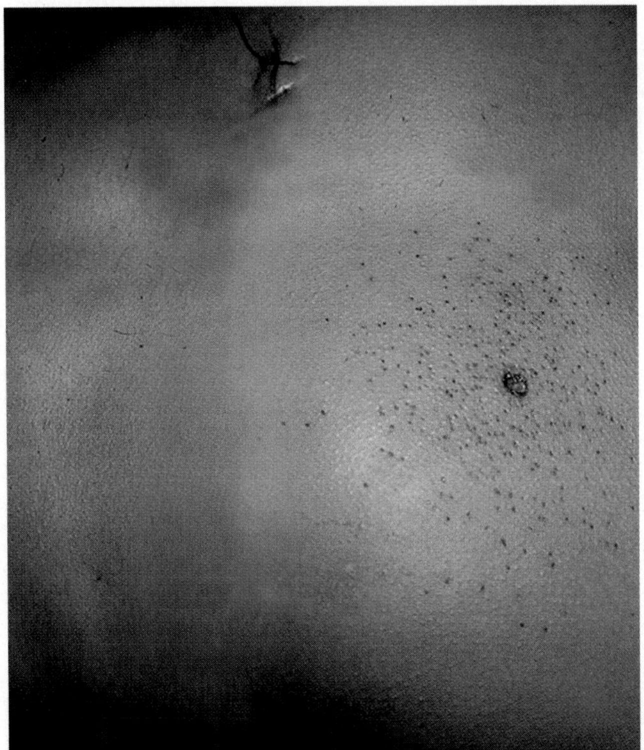

FIG. 2-20 Intermediate range gunshot wound with stippling and tattooing.

Exit Wounds

Exit wounds have the same general appearance no matter what the range of fire. Their shape can vary from round to slitlike to completely irregular. As with entrance wounds, the size does not correlate very well with the caliber of the projectile making the wound. The most important factors affecting exit wounds are the speed of the projectile and the degree of deformation. A smaller, highly deformed bullet exiting at high speed can produce a large, irregular wound, whereas a larger, intact, slower-moving bullet may only make a small hole. Size *cannot* be used to determine if the hole is an exit or entrance wound. In most cases, the margins of an exit wound will *not* have an abrasion collar. An exit wound will have clean edges that can often be reapproximated to cover the defect. The exception is when something is pressing against the skin surface at the exit site, such as tight clothing or the back of a chair. In this situation, the bullet will push the skin against the supporting surface causing rubbing and scraping around the exit defect as it comes out, known as a **shared exit wound.**

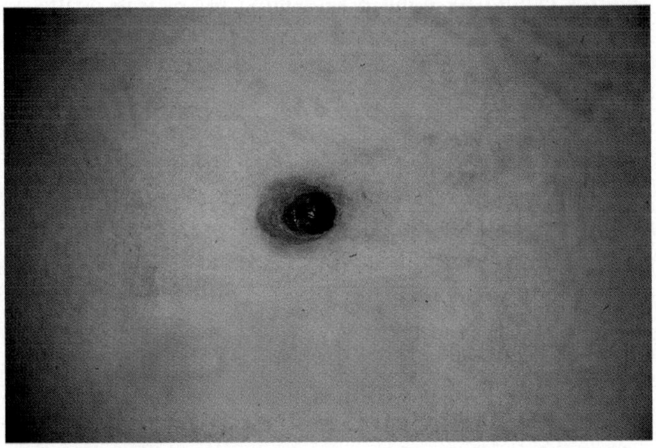

FIG. 2-21 Indeterminate range entrance wound with eccentric collar of abrasion resulting from the bullet striking the skin at an angle.

It is important to remember that because the skin is so elastic and deformable, it is one of the toughest structures for a bullet to go through. It is not uncommon for a bullet to pass entirely through the body and be stopped just beneath the skin. There will often be no visible injury of the overlying skin; however, careful palpation of the area may allow one to locate the bullet.

Wounding Potential of Firearms

The amount of damage done by a bullet is a function of a number of variables. For the most part, the damage caused is a result of the amount of energy transferred to the tissues impacted. The energy a bullet has is determined by the following formula:

$$KE = \frac{1}{2}MV^2$$

where KE is the energy, M is the mass, and V is the speed.

Clearly, increasing the speed of a bullet has a much greater effect on its potential to cause damage than increasing its size. As the bullet passes through tissue and slows down, its energy is dissipated into the surrounding structures. This energy transfer causes tissue destruction in a zone that can be much larger than the actual size of the bullet; the zone of destruction may be several inches in diameter with very high powered bullets. This transfer of energy in head wounds may lead to orbital plate fractures and palpebral ecchymosis (black eyes) or blood draining from the ears even though the path of the bullet does not come near the base of the skull. The amount of damage caused may be exacerbated by the generation of secondary missiles of bone fragments when portions of the skeleton are struck. Some bullets are designed to expand or fragment when they strike an object, thereby increasing the cross-sectional area of the projectile, increasing drag, and enhancing the transfer of energy into the tissues. "Hollow-point" ammunition is an example of this kind of bullet.

Obviously the lethality of a gunshot injury depends on what structures are damaged. Depending on the extent of damage, even gunshot wounds of the brain may not be lethal; however, they are usually immediately incapacitating and lead to significant long-term disability. It is important to remember that a victim with a "lethal" injury (wound of the heart or aorta) may not be immediately incapacitated and may engage in varying degrees of physical activity after being injured. Just because the victim is active or even combative when first evaluated does not mean the individual may *not* have experienced a potentially lethal injury.

Asphyxial Injuries

Asphyxial injuries are caused by a failure of cells to receive or utilize oxygen. Deprivation of oxygen may be partial *(hypoxia)* or total *(anoxia)*. Asphyxial injuries can be grouped into four general categories: suffocation, strangulation, chemical, and drowning.

Suffocation

Suffocation, or oxygen failing to reach the blood, can result from a lack of oxygen in the environment (entrapment in an enclosed space or filling the environment with a suffocating gas) or blockage of the external airways. Classic examples of these types of asphyxial injuries are a child who is trapped in an abandoned refrigerator or a person who commits suicide by putting a plastic bag over the head. A reduction in the ambient oxygen level to 16% (normal is 21%) is immediately dangerous. If the level is below 5%, death can ensue within a matter of minutes. The diagnosis of these types of asphyxial injuries depends on the history of what happened because there will be no specific physical findings.

Diagnosis and treatment in **choking asphyxiation** (obstruction of the internal airways) depend on locating and removing the obstructing material. Injury or disease may also cause swelling of the soft tissues of the airway leading to partial or complete obstruction and subsequent asphyxiation. Suffocation may also result from compression of the chest or abdomen (mechanical or compressional asphyxia) preventing normal respiratory movements. Usual signs and symptoms include florid facial congestion and petechiae (pinpoint hemorrhages) of the eyes and face.

Strangulation

Strangulation is caused by compression and closure of the blood vessels and air passages resulting from external pressure on the neck. This causes cerebral hypoxia or anoxia secondary to the alteration or cessation of blood flow to and from the brain. It is important to remember that the amount of force needed to close the jugular veins (2 kg [4.5 lb]) or carotid arteries (5 kg [11 lb]) is significantly less than that required to crush the trachea (15 kg [33 lb]). It is the alteration of cerebral blood flow in most types of strangulation that causes injury or death—not the lack of air flow. With complete blockage of the carotid arteries, unconsciousness can occur within 10 to 15 seconds.

A noose is placed around the neck, and the weight of the body is used to cause constriction of the noose and compression of the neck in **hanging strangulations.** The body does not need to be completely suspended to produce severe injury or death. Depending on the type of ligature used, there will usually be a distinct mark on the neck, an inverted V with the base of the V pointing toward the point of suspension. Internal injuries of the neck are actually quite rare in hangings, and only in judicial hangings, where the body is weighted and dropped, will significant soft tissue or cervical spinal trauma be seen. Petechiae of the eyes or face may be seen, but they are rare.

In **ligature strangulation,** the mark on the neck is horizontal without the inverted V pattern seen in hangings. Petechiae may be more common because intermittent opening and closure of the blood vessels may occur as a result of the victim's struggles. Internal injuries of the neck are rare.

There will be variable amounts of external trauma on the neck with contusions and abrasions in **manual strangulation** caused either by the assailant or the victim clawing at one's own neck in an attempt to remove the assailant's hands. Internal damage can be quite severe, with bruising of deep structures and even fractures of the hyoid bone and tracheal and cricoid cartilages. Petechiae are common.

Chemical Asphyxiants

Chemical asphyxiants either prevent the delivery of oxygen to the tissues or block its utilization. Carbon monoxide is the most common chemical asphyxiant (see p. 53). **Cyanide** acts as an asphyxiant by combining with the ferric iron atom in cytochrome oxidase, thereby blocking the intracellular utilization of oxygen. A victim of cyanide poisoning will have the same cherry-red appearance as a carbon monoxide intoxication victim because cyanide blocks the utilization of circulating oxyhemoglobin. An odor of bitter almonds may also be detected. (The ability to smell cyanide is a genetic trait that is absent in a significant portion of the general population.) **Hydrogen sulfide (sewer gas)** is a chemical asphyxiant in which victims of hydrogen cyanide poisoning may have brown-tinged blood in addition to the nonspecific signs of asphyxiation.

Drowning

Drowning is an alteration of oxygen delivery to tissues resulting from the breathing in of fluid, usually water. In 1997 there were 4724 drowning deaths in the United States. Although research in the 1940s and 1950s indicated that changes in blood electrolyte levels and volume as a result of absorption of fluid from the lungs may be an important factor in some drownings, the major mechanism of injury is hypoxemia (low blood oxygen levels). Even in freshwater drownings, where large amounts of water can pass through the alveolar-capillary interface, there is no evidence that increases in blood volume cause significant electrolyte disturbances or hemolysis, or that the amount of fluid loading is beyond the compensatory capabilities of the kidneys and heart. Airway obstruction is the more important pathologic abnormality, underscored by that fact that in up to 15% of drownings little or no water enters the lungs because of vagal nerve–mediated laryngospasms. This phenomenon is called *dry-lung drowning*. No matter what mechanism is involved, cerebral hypoxia will lead to unconsciousness in a matter of minutes. Whether this progresses to death depends on a number of factors, including age and health of the individual. One of the most important factors is the temperature of the water. Irreversible injury will develop much more rapidly in warm water than it will in cold water. Submersion times of up to 1 hour with subsequent survival have been reported in children in very cold water. Complete submersion is not necessary for a person to drown. An incapacitated or helpless individual (person with epilepsy or alcoholism, infant) may drown in only a few inches of water.

It is important to remember that there are no specific or diagnostic findings to *prove* that a person recovered from the water is actually a drowning victim. In cases where water has entered the lung, there may be large amounts of foam coming from the nose and mouth, although this can also be seen in certain types of drug overdoses. A body recovered from water with signs of prolonged immersion could just as easily be a victim of some other type of injury who has been put in the water to obscure the actual cause of death. When working with a living victim recovered from water, it is essential to keep in mind that an underlying condition may have led to the person's becoming incapacitated and submersed—a condition that may *also* need to be treated or corrected while correcting hypoxemia and dealing with its sequelae.

Infectious Injury

The pathogenicity (virulence) of microorganisms lies in their ability to survive and proliferate in the human body, where they injure cells and tissues. The disease-producing potential of a microorganism depends on its ability to (1) invade and destroy cells, (2) produce toxins, and (3) produce damaging hypersensitivity reactions (see Chapter 8).

Immunologic and Inflammatory Injury

Cellular membranes are injured by direct contact with cellular and chemical components of the immune and inflammatory responses, such as phagocytic cells (lymphocytes, macrophages) and substances such as histamine, antibodies, lymphokines, complement, and proteases (see Chapter 7). Complement is responsible for many of the membrane alterations that occur during immunologic injury.

Membrane alterations are associated with rapid leakage of K^+ out of the cell and rapid influx of water. Antibodies can interfere with membrane function by binding to and occupying receptor molecules on the plasma membrane. This type of injury is found in certain forms of diabetes mellitus and in myasthenia gravis. Antibodies also can block or destroy cellular junctions, interfering with intercellular communication (see Chapters 6 through 8).

Injurious Genetic Factors

Genetic disorders may be the result of genetic factors that alter the cell's nucleus and the plasma membrane's structure, shape, receptors, or transport mechanisms. For example, enzymatic genetic defects can lead to abnormalities in membrane transport. Genetic disorders that cause structural alterations of the red blood cell include sickle cell anemia, Huntington disease, muscular dystrophy, and abetalipoproteinemia. (Mechanisms causing genetic abnormalities are discussed in Unit II.)

Injurious Nutritional Imbalances

Essential nutrients—proteins, carbohydrates, lipids (fats), vitamins, and minerals—are required for cells to function normally. If these nutrients are not consumed in the diet and transported to the body's cells or if excessive amounts of nutrients are consumed and transported, pathophysiologic cellular effects develop.

Proteins, which consist of chains of amino acids, are the major structural units of the cell and participate in many enzymatic and hormonal functions. Protein deficiency causes a decrease in the intestinal mucosal mass, decreasing the absorptive function. The integrity of the pancreas is also affected, resulting in diminished exocrine secretion. With starvation or malnutrition, the lowered plasma proteins, particularly albumin, cause fluid to move into the interstitium (edema). Protein-calorie malnutrition (PCM) is the predominant worldwide type of malnutrition. Malnourished children are very susceptible to disease and often die of infectious diseases. Even with adequate protein intake, cellular injury can occur if amino acid transport mechanisms fail or are defective. In Fanconi syndrome, for example, renal tubular cells may contain accumulated protein droplets that have been absorbed but cannot be transported.

Glucose is the major carbohydrate obtained from the breakdown of starch (see Chapter 1). **Hyperglycemia** (excessive glucose in the blood) caused by excessive carbohydrate intake may lead to obesity. Deficiencies of glucose result from starvation or from lack of use, as in diabetes. In both conditions the body compensates by metabolizing fat (lipids). (For details on diabetes, see Chapter 20.)

In lipid deficiency, or **hypolipidemia,** the body compensates by mobilizing fatty acids from adipose tissue. This causes an increase in the production and circulation of ketone bodies, which are acidic by-products of lipid metabolism. The excretion of ketone bodies results in loss of water and electrolytes and causes dehydration and thirst. Severe increases in ketone bodies cause ketoacidosis, coma, and death. **Hyperlipidemia,** or an increase in lipoproteins in the blood, results in deposits of fat in the heart, liver, and muscle.

Vitamins are not sources of energy but are necessary for maintaining normal cellular functions. Adequate vitamin intake is necessary because most vitamins are not synthesized by the body. Vitamins are classified as water soluble (thiamine, pyridoxal, cobalamin, ascorbic acid, riboflavin, nicotinic acid, folic acid) or fat soluble (A, D, E, K). They are involved in many reactions, including metabolism of visual pigments (vitamin A), calcium and phosphate metabolism (vitamin D), prothrombin synthesis (vitamin K), and antioxidation reactions (vitamins E and C). Pyridoxal (vitamin B_6) affects amino acid transfer reactions; flavin adenine dinucleotide (FAD), flavin mononucleotide (FMN), and nicotinamide adenine dinucleotide (NAD) help the reaction transfer of electrons (see Chapter 1). Deficiencies in vitamin C result in poor wound healing and scurvy. Vitamin D deficiency causes rickets and problems with healing of fractures. Folate deficiency is associated with plasma and membrane changes of the red blood cell and is particularly a problem in individuals with severe liver dysfunction. Vitamin deficiencies are associated with several other disease states, including cancer (see Chapter 10).

Alterations in plasma membrane functions can be induced by certain nutritional substances. For example, increases in vitamin A consumption can cause lysis of the plasma membrane, releasing hydrolases that damage lysosomal membranes. With insulin deficiency, glucose cannot cross the plasma membrane to enter the cell, causing energy deficits. Nutritional deficiencies also are associated with abnormalities of the chromosomes, nucleus, and DNA synthesis.

Injurious Physical Agents

Injurious physical agents include temperature extremes, changes in atmospheric pressure, radiation, illumination, mechanical factors, noise, and prolonged vibration. Physical injury can result from excessive exposure to many environmental agents, as well as to agents used for the diagnosis and treatment of illness.

Temperature Extremes

Chilling or freezing of cells causes **hypothermic injury** directly by creating high intracellular sodium concentrations, which result from the formation and dissolution of ice crystals. Indirect forms of injury occur because of changes in small blood vessels (the microcirculation). Slow chilling can cause vasoconstriction followed by paralysis of vasomotor control, resulting in vasodilation and increased membrane permeability. This causes cellular and tissue swelling. With an abrupt drop in temperature, vasoconstriction and increased viscosity of the blood cause ischemic injury—infarction and necrosis (cellular death) in affected tissues. With continued exposure to freezing temperatures, vasodilation produces severe swelling that causes degenerative changes in the myelin sheath that surrounds peripheral nerves, resulting in sensory and motor disturbances. Thrombosis also can occur and may lead to gangrene of the affected part. (Gangrene is discussed on p. 73.) These conditions often are called *frostbite*.

Hyperthermic injury (injury caused by excessive heat) varies depending on the nature, intensity, and extent of the injury (Fig. 2-22). A full-thickness burn is an open wound involving skin layers—epidermis, dermis, and subcutaneous layers—and causing extensive loss of fluids and plasma proteins. Cellular regeneration is not possible; therefore skin from a donor or from the host must be grafted to the site. Partial-thickness burns result in reddening of the area as a result of dilation of small blood vessels and increased permeability of cellular membranes, with loss of protein-rich fluid, resulting in the typical "burn blister." In surface epithelial cells, membrane permeability increases, causing both cytoplasmic and nuclear swelling. Temperature-sensitive enzymes with certain cells respond to heat by increasing

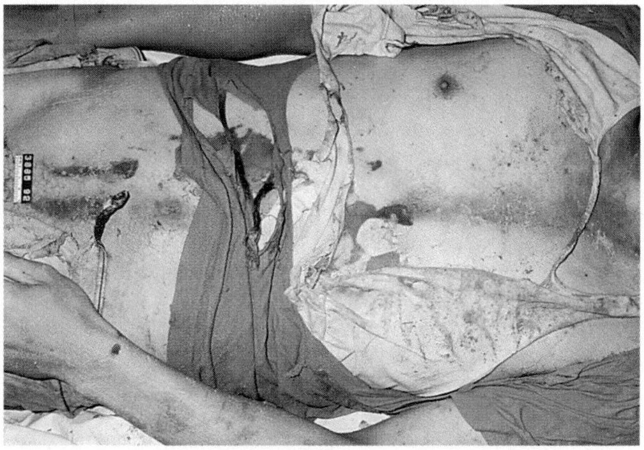

FIG. 2-22 Lightning death with torn and partially burned clothing and cutaneous burn of anterior trunk. (From Damjanov I, Linder J: *Anderson's pathology,* ed 10, St Louis, 1996, Mosby.)

cellular metabolism, with detrimental effects. Intense heat also damages the vascular endothelium and causes coagulation of the blood vessels. (Burns are discussed further in Chapter 45.)

Epidemiologic investigators have reported a relationship between overheating in infants, that is, overdressing infants in the winter, and sudden infant deaths.[25] Studies suggest interactions between body temperature and respiratory responses to hypoxia or increased carbon dioxide (hypercapnia). The hypoxia/*hypo*thermia interaction depresses breathing, reducing the ventilatory response to hypercapnia. The effects of *hyper*thermia seem to be a significant problem only when it accompanies an infection and fever and alters or depresses the breathing responses. (Temperature changes are also discussed in Chapter 14.)

Changes in Atmospheric Pressure

Sudden increases or decreases in atmospheric pressure cause **blast injury,** which can be transmitted by either air (air blast) or water (immersion blast). With sudden increases in pressure, such as in air blast or explosive injuries, tissue injury is caused by compressive waves of air impinging on the body, followed by a sudden wave of decreased pressure. The pressure changes may collapse the thorax, rupture internal solid organs, and cause widespread hemorrhage. In increased pressure caused by immersion blast, water pressure is applied suddenly to all sides of the body, forcing the body up out of water. The positive pressure compresses the abdomen and ruptures hollow internal organs, such as the spleen, kidneys, and liver.

With sudden decreases in pressure, carbon dioxide and nitrogen that are normally dissolved in the blood come out of solution and form tiny bubbles called *gas emboli*. At low atmospheric pressure, such as occurs at altitudes above 15,000 feet, there is a significant decrease in available oxygen. This causes hypoxic injury, and compensatory vasoconstriction shunts blood from the peripheral circulation (in the extremities) to the visceral organs, including the lungs. The combination of increases in pulmonary blood flow and systemic hypoxia causes "high-altitude pulmonary edema"[26] (see Chapter 32).

Deep sea divers and underwater construction workers who return to the surface too quickly develop a form of gas embolism called **decompression sickness** or **caisson disease** ("the bends"). If water pressure is reduced too rapidly, the gases dissolved in blood bubble out of solution, forming emboli. Oxygen is quickly redissolved, but nitrogen bubbles may persist and obstruct blood vessels. Ischemia resulting from gas emboli causes cellular hypoxia, particularly in the muscles, joints, and tendons, which are especially susceptible to changes in oxygen supply. Emboli and interstitial gas accumulate around the joints and skeletal muscles, causing the individual to double up in pain. Tissues of the heart and brain also may be affected by emboli, causing necrosis. The gases can be promptly redissolved in blood by raising the atmospheric pressure. This is accomplished by placing the individual in a decompression chamber. First, pressure is increased until it approximates pressure at the depth to which the diver had descended. This redissolves the gas bubbles in the blood. Then the pressure in the chamber is decreased gradually until it equals pressure at the surface of the water. The slow decrease in pressure slows the gases from bubbling out of solution.

WHAT'S NEW? Roller Coasters and Subdural Hematomas

Japanese researchers reported at least four people developed subdural hematomas after riding high-speed roller coasters. French investigators report six people, after riding roller coasters, developed complications, including arterial dissection, brain stem dysfunction, carotid artery occlusion, and subdural hematomas. In all these individuals, the first symptom experienced was pain. The mechanisms are not understood but probably involve sudden head and neck flexion-extension movements. Signs to watch for are headache, vomiting, or confusion; if they occur, the individual should get to a physician fast.

Data from Fututake T et al: Roller coaster headache and subdural hematoma, *Neurology* 54(1):264, 2000; Kettaneh A, Biousse V, Bousser MG: Neurological complications after roller coaster rides: an emerging new risk? *Presse Med* 29(4):175, 2000.

Ionizing Radiation

Ionizing radiation is any form of radiation capable of removing orbital electrons from atoms. Ionizing radiation is emitted by x-rays, gamma rays, and alpha and beta particles (which are emitted from atomic nuclei in the process of radioactive decay) and from neutrons, deuterons, protons, and pions (all of which are emitted from cobalt or linear accelerators). Occupational exposure to ionizing radiation is mostly limited to alpha- and beta-particle exposure and exposure to x-rays, gamma rays, and neutrons. Radiant energy from sunlight (solar radiation) also can injure cells.

The most abundant source of exposure to ionizing radiation is the environment. This source includes emission from radioactive material inside the body, cosmic rays from outer space, and radiation emitted from such substances as soil and building materials. Environmental radioactivity is emitted primarily by uranium, thorium, and potassium. Other

Table 2-7 Types of Ionizing Radiation and Their Tissue Penetration

Type	Tissue Penetration
X-rays	High
Gamma (γ) rays	High
Beta (β) particles	Low
Alpha (α) particles	Very low
Protons	Intermediate between α and β
Neutrons	High

Data from Damjanov I, Linder J, editors: *Anderson's pathology,* ed 10, St Louis, 1996, Mosby.

sources are x-rays used for medical diagnosis and treatment, uranium and thorium mines, nuclear weapons, and nuclear reactors that generate electricity. Table 2-7 includes types of ionizing radiation and their magnitude of tissue penetration.

The mechanism by which ionizing radiation damages cells is shown in Fig. 2-23. DNA is the most vulnerable target of radiation, particularly the bonds within the DNA molecule. All phases of the cell cycle can be affected by ionizing radiation. Sensitivity of the cell appears to be greatest in G_2, that gap of the cell just before mitosis; irradiation during this phase retards the onset of cell division. Irradiation during mitosis induces chromosomal aberrations. Chromosomal aberrations include breaks, deletions, translocations, and many other structural abnormalities. Membrane molecules and enzymes also are damaged by radiation. The intensity, duration, and cumulative effects of exposure to ionizing radiation determine the extent of injury.

Not all cells and tissues have the same sensitivity to radiation, although all cells can be affected. Radiosensitivity depends on rate of mitosis and cellular maturity. Because fetal cells are both immature and undergoing rapid cycling, the fetus is at great risk for injury caused by ionizing radiation. Particularly vulnerable are embryonic germ cells, which are precursors of ova and sperm. Throughout life, cells of the bone marrow, intestinal mucosa, testicular seminiferous epithelium, and ovarian follicles are susceptible to injury because they are always undergoing mitosis, which ensures the presence of vulnerable, immature daughter cells. A critical target for reactive free radicals, particularly O•, is the DNA.

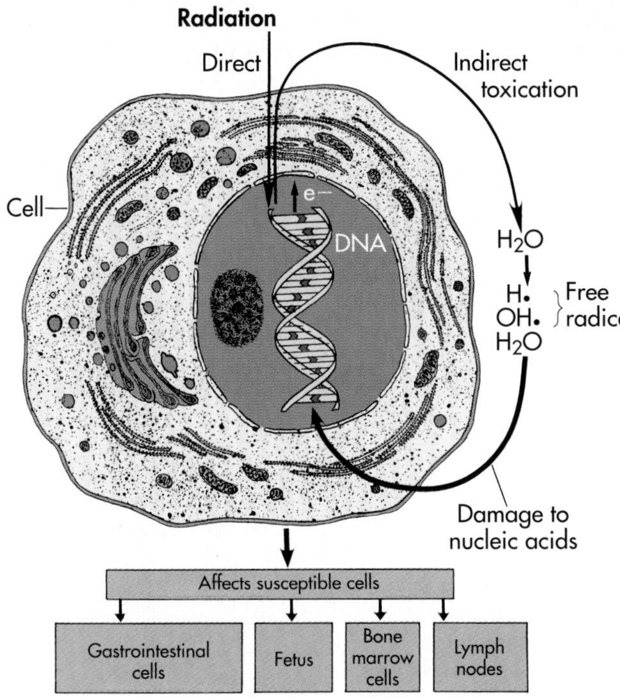

FIG. 2-23 Cellular damage caused by ionizing radiation. Radiation can damage macromolecules in two ways: (1) directly, where the micromolecules are ionized; and (2) indirectly, where water is ionized and produces free radicals that in turn damage macromolecules. Cells that are particularly susceptible to damage are those of the gastrointestinal tract, bone marrow, lymph nodes, fetus, and ovarian follicles.

The effects of ionizing radiation may be acute or delayed. Acute effects of high doses, such as skin redness, skin damage, or chromosomal aberrations, occur within hours, days, or months. The delayed effects of low doses may not be evident for years. Effects are usually (1) somatic, involving the exposed individual's entire body (e.g., leukemia, other cancers); (2) genetic, involving offspring of the exposed individual; or (3) fetal, involving fetuses that are exposed in utero. Data suggest that low-dose exposures may affect apoptosis and epigenetic (a change in gene *expression* and not in the DNA sequence) processes.[27] (The carcinogenic effects of radiation are discussed in Chapter 10, and radiation-induced cancers of the thyroid gland, breast, liver, and bone are discussed in Chapters 20, 22, 38, and 41, respectively.)

Illumination

Illumination has biologic effects that are related to health.[28,29] The harmful effects of fluorescent lighting include eyestrain,

WHAT'S NEW? Cell Phone Effects

Cellular (wireless) phones, which send and receive radio-frequency (RF) radiation signals through their attached antennas, come in digital and analog varieties. The newer digital phones broadcast their communications in discrete bursts of energy, whereas analog phones use continuous signals. The analog phones, being energy hogs, transmit eight times as much energy into the user's head as digital phones. But is this energy a hazard? The epidemiologic evidence for an association between RF radiation and cancer is weak and inconsistent. Recent preliminary data from the Scandinavian countries, worldwide leaders in cell phone use, reported that of 5000 Norwegians, 25% felt warmth on or behind the ear while using their phones and 20% linked frequent headaches and recurring fatigue to cell phone use. The findings were similar in 12,000 Swedes, although the overall rates were lower. Investigators reported that people using analog phones reported more symptoms and more sensations of all kinds; however, the studies were uncontrolled and they did *not* measure RF emissions. As of fall 1999, laboratory studies generally do not suggest that cell phone RF radiation has genotoxic or epigenetic activity; however, more recent studies have noted biologic effects in animals. During the summer of 2000, a 13-country study of brain and other head and neck cancers in cell phone users will begin under the direction of the International Agency for Research on Cancer in Lyon, France. Until we have reliable data, perhaps a prudent approach to cell phones is to discourage use in young, growing children and for adults to use headphones or some other hands-free approach that would remove exposure of the antenna to the head.

Data from Moulder JE et al: Cell phones and cancer: what is the evidence for a connection? *Radiation Res* 151(5):513, 1999; Roti Roti JL et al: Neoplastic transformation in C3H (1/2) calls after exposure to 835.62 MHz FDMA and 847.74 MHz COMA radiation, *Radiat Res* 155(1 Pt 2):239, 2001; Raloff J: Researchers probe cell-phone effects, *Sci News* 157:100, 2000.

obscured vision, and possibly cataract formation. The rapid modulation of light from fluorescent lamps is responsible for eyestrain and headaches.[31] The modulation can be reduced by wearing tinted glasses.[30] The shorter wavelengths in radiant energy in environmental lighting influence the absorption, scattering, and fluorescence, thus obscuring vision.[31]

Studies have demonstrated the in vitro toxicity of halogen lamps.[32] A pilot study of 12 mice illuminated with varying intensities and durations of halogen exposure resulted in benign forms of skin cancer (papillomas) as well as malignant tumor growth. Emission of far-ultraviolet radiation from halogen lamps is thought to be in the range of wavelength responsible for inducing melanoma.[32] Fortunately, prevention is simple if commercial models are available with glass or plastic covers.

Mechanical Stresses

Mechanical injury is caused by physical impact or irritation. Injury may include damage to the nerves surrounding small blood vessels (perivascular) that mediate both vasodilation and vasoconstriction.[33] Recent interest in mechanical injury and blood vessel damage has lead investigators to study balloon catheterization or coronary angioplasty. Coronary angioplasty involves a catheter that is advanced along a blood vessel until it reaches the blocked region of the vessel. The balloon section of the catheter is then inflated, pushing the walls of the blocked vessel outward. Sometimes metal tubes, called *stents,* are inserted to keep the vessel open. Without the stents, however, vessel narrowing, or restenosis, often occurs at the balloon site. The injury causes an adaptive response of hypertrophy of the smooth muscle cells and an increase in macrophage activity. The macrophages release cytokines and growth factors causing intimal cell proliferation and subsequent renarrowing.

The major focus of occupational biomechanics is the response of tissue to mechanical stress, especially the prevention of overexertion disorders of the lower back and upper extremities. Many mechanical stresses can cause *overt* injuries (e.g., a head injury when a worker is struck in the head with a dropped object). Most stresses, however, are subtle and can cause *accumulative* injuries and disorders.[34] Table 2-8 summarizes common types of occupational mechanical stresses and associated types of injury.

Noise

Noise is sound that has the potential for inflicting body harm. The most common pathophysiologic effect of noise is hearing impairment. Noise trauma can be caused by acute loud noise, as well as by the cumulative effects of various intensities, frequencies, and durations of noise.

Two types of hearing loss are associated with noise: (1) acoustic trauma, or instantaneous damage caused by a single sharply rising wave of sound (e.g., gunfire), and (2) noise-induced hearing loss, the more common type, which is the result of prolonged exposure to intense sound (e.g., workplace and leisure-time activities). Hearing loss is a serious complication of critical illness. Individuals in intensive care units can experience hearing loss from mechanical or accidental trauma, ototoxic medications, infections, vascular disorders, autoimmune diseases, and environmental noise.[35] Acoustic trauma can rupture the eardrum, displace the ossicles of the middle ear, and damage the organ of Corti in the inner ear.

If noise has not been too loud or the exposure too long, hearing will return to its original level, a type of hearing loss called a *temporary threshold shift* (TTS). If the noise is louder than a certain value or the exposure time is long, the hearing threshold never returns to its original value, causing a *permanent threshold shift* (PTS). Structural changes associated with TTS, although not fully established, include intracellular changes in the sensory cells (hair cells) and swelling of the auditory nerve endings.[14] With PTS, cochlear blood flow may be impaired and hair cells are damaged with each exposure. Noise-induced hearing loss is gradual and painless. Symptoms of noise-induced hearing loss include loudness recruitment and tinnitus. In loudness recruitment, soft sounds are not heard but loud sounds are heard normally. Tinnitus is a constant, high-pitched ringing that annoys the individual and contributes to loss of sleep.

Table 2-8 Common Types of Occupational Mechanical Stresses and Associated Types of Injury

Mechanical Stresses	Type of Injury
Forceful exertions (e.g., lifting, pushing, pulling of heavy loads)	Low back pain
Awkward trunk postures (e.g., flexion, lateral bending, axial twisting, prolonged sitting)	Low back pain
Whole body vibration (e.g., vibrating seat or platform)	Low back pain; bone deformities; alteration nerve conduction (carpal tunnel syndrome)
Repetitive or prolonged exposure (e.g., to any of the above)	Low back pain; numbness and tingling of wrists and hands
Extreme reaching Low temperatures (e.g., exposure to cold air, tools, materials) Vibration (segmental and whole) Forceful exertions (e.g., friction, balance, posture, pace, use of heavy objects) Ulnar deviation of the wrist	Trauma disorders of upper arms (synovitis, Raynaud phenomenon, bursitis, tendinitis)
Repetitive functions (e.g., walking, climbing stairs, carrying, shoveling, pushing, lifting objects, computer use)	Localized and/or whole body fatigue (shortness of breath, general weakness, hypoxic injury)

MANIFESTATIONS OF CELLULAR INJURY

Cellular Manifestations: Accumulations

Cellular accumulations, also known as **infiltrations,** not only occur when injury is sublethal and sustained in injured cells, but also can occur in normal cells. Common accumulations consist of substances that are normally present, such as fluids and electrolytes, triglycerides (lipids), glycogen, calcium, uric acid, proteins, melanin, and bilirubin. Abnormal accumulations of these substances can occur in the cytoplasm (frequently in the lysosomes) or in the nucleus if (1) the normal, endogenous substance is produced in excess or at an increased rate; (2) an endogenous substance (normal or abnormal) is not effectively catabolized, usually because of lack of a vital lysosomal enzyme; or (3) harmful exogenous materials, such as heavy metals, mineral dusts, or microorganisms, accumulate because of inhalation, ingestion, or infection.

In all storage diseases the cells attempt to digest, or catabolize, the "stored" substances. As a result, excessive amounts of metabolites (products of catabolism) accumulate in the cells and are expelled into the extracellular matrix, where they are taken up by phagocytic cells called *macrophages* (see Chapter 7). Some of these scavenger cells circulate throughout the body, whereas others remain fixed in certain tissues, such as the liver or spleen. As more and more macrophages and other phagocytes migrate to tissues that are producing excessive metabolites, the affected tissues begin to swell. This is the mechanism that causes enlargement of the liver (hepatomegaly) or the spleen (splenomegaly). Enlargement of one of these organs is a clinical manifestation of many of the storage diseases.

Water

Cellular swelling, the most common degenerative change, is caused by the shift of extracellular water into the cells. In hypoxic injury, movement of fluid and ions into the cell is associated with acute failure of metabolism and loss of ATP production. Normally, the pump that transports sodium ions out of the cell is maintained by the presence of ATP and ATPase, the active-transport enzyme. In metabolic failure caused by hypoxia, reduced ATP and ATPase permit sodium to accumulate in the cell, whereas potassium diffuses outward. The increase of intracellular sodium increases osmotic pressure, which draws more water into the cell (transport mechanisms are described in Chapter 1). The cisternae of the endoplasmic reticulum become distended, rupture, and coalesce to form large vacuoles that isolate the water from the cytoplasm, a process called **vacuolation**. Progressive vacuolation results in a more serious condition called **hydropic** or **vacuolar degeneration** (degeneration by water) (Fig. 2-24). If cellular swelling affects all cells in an organ, the organ increases in weight and becomes distended and pale.

Cellular swelling is reversible and is considered to be sublethal. It is, in fact, an early manifestation of almost all types of cellular injury, including severe or lethal cell injury.

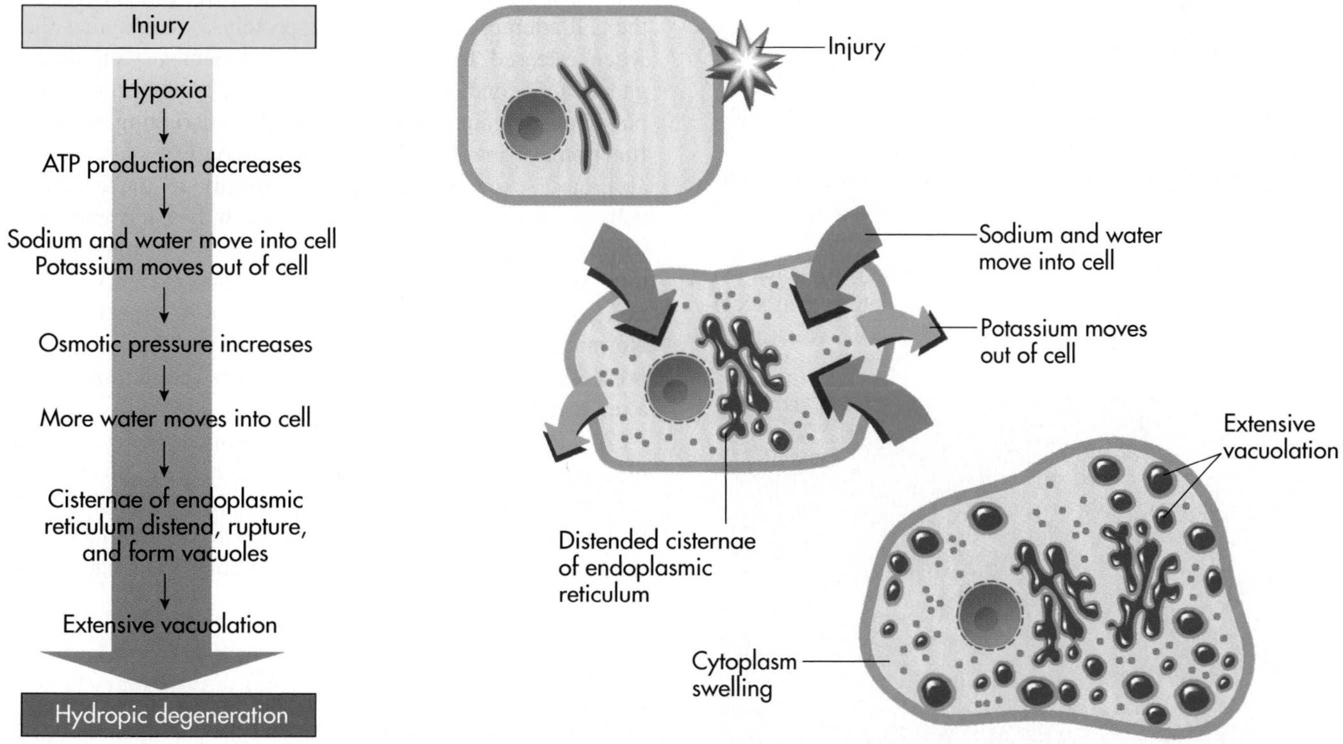

FIG. 2-24 The process of hydropic degeneration. *ATP*, Adenosine triphosphate.

It is also associated with high fever, hypokalemia (abnormally low concentrations of potassium in the blood; see Chapter 3), and certain infections.

Lipids and Carbohydrates

Certain metabolic disorders result in the abnormal intracellular accumulation of carbohydrates and lipids. These substances may accumulate throughout the body but are found primarily in the cells of the spleen, liver, and CNS. Accumulations in cells of the CNS can cause neurologic dysfunction and severe mental retardation. Lipids accumulate in Tay-Sachs, Neimann-Pick, and Gaucher diseases, whereas in the diseases known as mucopolysaccharidoses, carbohydrates are in excess. The mucopolysaccharidoses are progressive disorders that usually involve multiple organs, including liver, spleen, heart, and blood vessels. The accumulated mucopolysaccharides are found in reticuloendothelial cells, endothelial cells, intimal smooth muscle cells, and fibroblasts throughout the body. These carbohydrate accumulations can cause clouding of the cornea, joint stiffness, and mental retardation.[2]

Although lipids sometimes accumulate in heart and kidney cells, the most common site of intracellular lipid accumulation, or **fatty change,** is liver cells. Because hepatic metabolism and secretion of lipids are crucial to proper body function, imbalances and deficiencies in these processes lead to major pathologic changes. Lipid accumulation in liver cells causes an organic condition known as *fatty liver*, or *fatty change* (Fig. 2-25). As lipids fill the cells, vacuolation pushes the nucleus and other organelles aside. Grossly, the liver looks yellowish and greasy.

Lipid accumulation in liver cells occurs after cellular injury sets one or more of the following mechanisms in motion:

1. Increased movement of free fatty acids into the liver (Starvation, for example, increases breakdown of triglycerides in adipose tissue, releasing fatty acids that subsequently enter liver cells.)
2. Failure of the metabolic process that converts fatty acids to phospholipids, resulting in the preferential conversion of the fatty acids to triglycerides
3. Increased synthesis of triglycerides from fatty acids (Increases in an enzyme, α-glycerophosphatase, can accelerate triglyceride synthesis.)

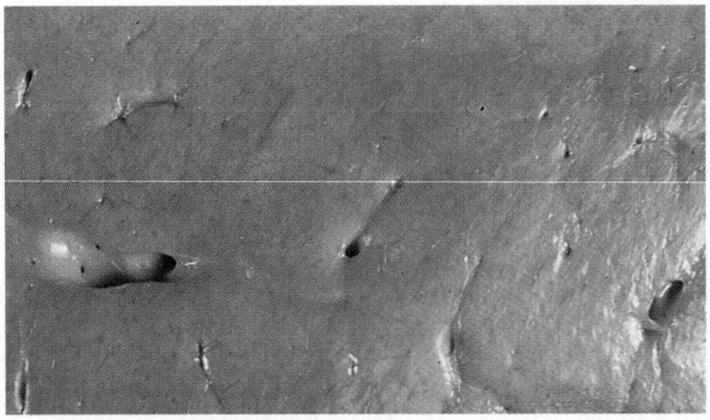

FIG. 2-25 Fatty liver. The liver appears yellow. (From Damjanov I, Linder J: *Pathology: a color atlas,* St Louis, 2000, Mosby.)

4. Decreased synthesis of apoproteins (lipid-acceptor proteins)
5. Failure of lipids to bind with apoproteins and form lipoproteins
6. Failure of mechanisms that transport lipoproteins out of the cell
7. Direct damage to the endoplasmic reticulum by free radicals released by alcohol's toxic effects

Alcohol abuse is one of the most common causes of fatty liver (see Chapter 38). Fatty change caused by alcohol can lead to a form of liver fibrosis called *cirrhosis*. If alcohol intake ceases, the cirrhotic liver can return to a normal size and function. Fatty change from other causes, notably carbon tetrachloride poisoning, is often irreversible.

Glycogen

Intracellular accumulations of glycogen are seen in genetic disorders called *glycogen storage diseases* and in disorders of glucose and glycogen metabolism. Like water and lipid accumulation, glycogen accumulation results in excessive vacuolation of the cytoplasm. The most common cause of glycogen accumulation is diabetes mellitus, a disorder of glucose metabolism (see Chapter 20).

Proteins

Proteins provide cellular structure and constitute most of the cell's dry weight. They are synthesized on ribosomes in the cytoplasm from the essential amino acids lysine, threonine, leucine, isoleucine, methionine, tryptophan, valine, phenylalanine, and histidine. Protein accumulation probably damages cells in two ways. First, metabolites, produced when the cell attempts to digest some proteins, are enzymes that, when released from lysosomes, can damage cellular organelles. Second, excessive amounts of protein in the cytoplasm push against cellular organelles, disrupting organelle function and intracellular communication.

Protein excess accumulates primarily in the epithelial cells of the renal convoluted tubule and in the antibody-forming plasma cells (B lymphocytes) of the immune system. Several types of renal disorders cause excessive excretion of protein molecules in the urine (proteinuria). Normally, little or no protein is present in the urine, and its presence in significant amounts indicates cellular injury and altered cellular function.

Accumulations of protein in B lymphocytes can occur during active synthesis of antibodies during the immune response. The excess aggregates of protein are called *Russell bodies* (see Chapter 6). Russell bodies have been identified in multiple myeloma (plasma cell tumor) (see Chapters 26 and 41).

Pigments

Pigment accumulations may be normal or abnormal, endogenous (produced within the body) or exogenous (produced outside the body). Endogenous pigments are derived, for example, from amino acids (e.g., tyrosine, tryptophan).

They include melanin and the blood proteins—porphyrins, hemoglobin, and hemosiderin (ferritin). Lipid-rich pigments such as lipofuscin (the aging pigment) give a yellow-brown color to cells undergoing slow, regressive, and often atrophic changes. Exogenous pigments include mineral dusts containing silica and iron particles, lead, silver salts, and dyes for tattoos.

Melanin

Melanin accumulates in epithelial cells (keratinocytes) of the skin and retina. It is an extremely important pigment because it protects the skin against long exposure to sunlight and is considered an essential factor in the prevention of skin cancer (see Chapters 11 and 43). Ultraviolet light (e.g., sunlight) stimulates the synthesis of melanin, which probably absorbs ultraviolet rays during subsequent exposure. Melanin also may protect the skin by trapping the injurious free radicals produced by the action of ultraviolet light on skin.

Melanin is a brown-black pigment derived from the amino acid tryptosine. It is synthesized by epidermal cells called *melanocytes* and is stored in membrane-bound cytoplasmic vesicles called *melanosomes.* Melanosomes are particularly abundant in projections of melanocytic cytoplasm, called *dendrites,* from which they are transmitted to neighboring keratinocytes, where melanin accumulation occurs.[8] (Keratinocytes, which constitute 95% of epidermal cells, are discussed with other skin components in Chapter 43.) The dendritic melanocytes form bridges between neighboring keratinocytes and inject melanosomes into the keratinocytes by an unknown mechanism.

Melanin also can accumulate in melanophores (melanin-containing pigment cells), macrophages, or other phagocytic cells in the dermis. Presumably these cells acquire the melanin from nearby melanocytes or from pigment that has been extruded from dying epidermal cells. This is the mechanism that causes freckles.

Although rare, melanin accumulation occurs in the skin of individuals with Addison disease (adrenocortical insufficiency resulting from disorders of the adrenal cortex; see Chapter 20). The increased melaninogenesis (melanin production) seen in Addison disease is caused by the loss of feedback control of adrenocorticotropic hormone (ACTH). Decreased hormonal secretion from the adrenal gland causes increased release of ACTH from the pituitary gland. In Addison disease the increase in melanin occurs presumably because a segment of the ACTH molecule contains the melanin-stimulating hormone (MSH).

An increase in melanin also occurs in the benign form of "pigmented moles" called *nevi* (Fig. 2-26) (see Chapter 43). Malignant melanoma is a cancerous skin tumor that contains melanin and invades normal tissue early and widely and often leads to death.

A decrease in melanin production occurs in the inherited disorder of the melanin metabolism called *albinism.* Albinism is often diffuse, involving all the skin, the eyes, and the hair. Albinism is also related to phenylalanine metabolism. In classic types the person with albinism is unable to convert tyrosine to DOPA (3,4-dihydroxyphenylalanine), an intermediary in melanin biosynthesis. Melanin-producing cells are present in normal numbers, but they are unable to make melanin. Individuals with albinism are very sensitive to sunlight and quickly become sunburned. They are also at high risk for skin cancer.

Hemoproteins

Hemoproteins are among the most essential of the normal endogenous pigments. They include hemoglobin and the oxidative enzymes, the cytochromes. Central to an understanding of disorders involving these pigments is knowledge of iron uptake, metabolism, excretion, and storage (see Chapter 24). Hemoprotein accumulations in cells are caused by excessive storage of iron, which is transferred to the cells from the bloodstream. Iron enters the blood from three primary sources: (1) tissue stores, (2) the intestinal mucosa, and (3) macrophages that remove and destroy dead or defective red blood cells. The amount of iron in blood plasma also depends on the metabolism of the major iron-transport protein, *transferrin.*

Iron is stored in tissue cells in two forms: as ferritin and, when greater levels of iron are present, as hemosiderin. **Hemosiderin** is a yellow-brown pigment derived from hemoglobin. With pathologic states, excesses of iron cause hemosiderin to accumulate within cells. Accumulation of hemosiderin often occurs in areas of bruising and hemorrhage and in the lungs and spleen after congestion caused by heart failure. With a local hemorrhage, the skin first appears red-blue and then lysis of the escaped red blood cell occurs, causing the hemoglobin to be transformed to hemosiderin. The color changes noted in bruising reflect this transformation.

Hemosiderosis is a condition in which excess iron is stored as hemosiderin in the cells of many organs and tissues. This condition is common in individuals who have received repeated blood transfusions or prolonged parenteral administration of iron. Hemosiderosis is also associated with increased absorption of dietary iron, conditions in which iron storage and transport are impaired, and hemolytic anemia.

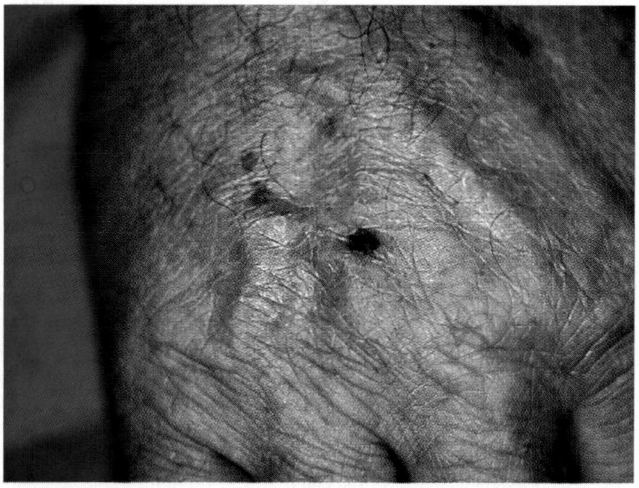

FIG. 2-26 Blue nevus, common type. Nevus is a dark blue-black color and is small and symmetric. (From Damjanov I, Linder J: *Anderson's pathology,* ed 10, St Louis, 1996, Mosby.)

Excessive alcohol ingestion also can lead to hemosiderosis. Normally, absorption of excessive dietary iron is prevented by an iron-absorption process in the intestines. Failure of this process can lead to total-body iron accumulations in the range of 60 to 80 g, compared with normal iron stores of 4.5 to 5 g. Excessive accumulations of iron, such as occur in hemochromatosis (a genetic disorder of iron metabolism and the most severe example of iron overload), are associated with liver and pancreatic cell damage.

It is debatable whether iron accumulation itself causes cellular injury or whether injury is the result of the basic defect that leads to iron storage. The finding that the extent of liver injury (cirrhosis) is related to the extent of iron accumulation[36] suggests that excessive iron accumulation does injure cells.

Bilirubin is a normal, yellow-to-green pigment of bile derived from the porphyrin structure of hemoglobin. Excesses of bilirubin within cells and tissues cause jaundice (icterus), or yellowing of the skin. Jaundice occurs when the bilirubin level exceeds 1.5 to 2 mg/dl of plasma, compared with the normal values of 0.4 to 1 mg/dl. Hyperbilirubinemia occurs with (1) destruction of red blood cells (erythrocytes), such as in hemolytic jaundice; (2) diseases affecting the metabolism and excretion of bilirubin in the liver; and (3) diseases that cause obstruction of the common bile duct, such as gallstones or pancreatic tumors. (For a detailed description of these diseases, see Chapter 38.) Certain drugs, specifically chlorpromazine and other phenothiazine derivatives, estrogenic hormones, and halothane (an anesthetic), can cause the obstruction of normal bile flow through the liver.

Because unconjugated bilirubin is lipid soluble, it can injure the lipid components of the plasma membrane. Albumin, a plasma protein, provides significant protection by binding unconjugated bilirubin in plasma. Unconjugated bilirubin causes two cellular effects: uncoupling of oxidative phosphorylation and a loss of cellular proteins. These two effects could cause structural injury to the various membranes of the cell.

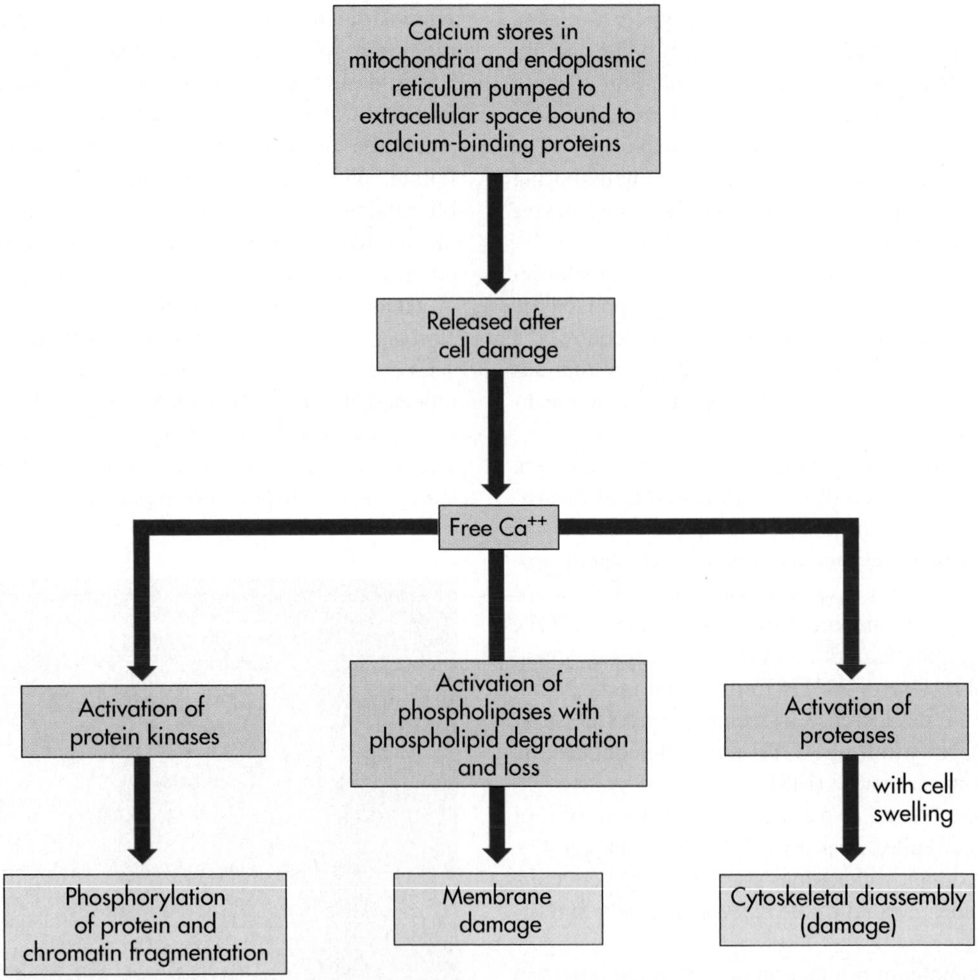

FIG. 2-27 Free cytosolic calcium: a destructive agent. Normally, calcium is removed from the cytosol by ATP-dependent calcium pumps. In normal cells, calcium is bound to buffering proteins, such as calbindin or paralbumin, and is contained in the endoplasmic reticulum and the mitochondria. If there is abnormal permeability of calcium-ion channels, direct damage to membranes, depletion of ATP (i.e., hypoxic injury), calcium increases in the cytosol. If the free calcium cannot be buffered or pumped out of cells, uncontrolled enzyme activation takes place, causing further damage. Uncontrolled entry of calcium into the cytosol is an important final pathway in many causes of cell death.

Calcium

Calcium salts accumulate in both injured and dead tissues (Fig. 2-27). An important mechanism of cellular calcification is the influx of extracellular calcium in injured mitochondria (see pp. 49 and 50). Another mechanism that causes calcium accumulation in alveoli (gas-exchange airways of the lungs), gastric epithelium, and renal tubules is the excretion of acid at these sites, leading to the local production of hydroxyl ions. Hydroxyl ions result in precipitation of calcium hydroxide ($Ca[OH]_2$) and hydroxyapatite ($3Ca_3[PO_4]_2Ca[OH]_2$), a mixed salt. Damage occurs when calcium salts clump and harden, interfering with normal cellular structure and function.

Pathologic calcification can be dystrophic or metastatic. **Dystrophic calcification** is the calcification of dying and dead tissues and occurs in chronic tuberculosis of the lungs and lymph nodes, in arteries with advanced atherosclerosis (narrowing as a result of plaque accumulation), and often in injured heart valves (Fig. 2-28). Calcification of the heart valves interferes with opening and closing of the valves, causing heart murmurs (see Chapter 29). Calcification of the coronary arteries predisposes them to severe narrowing and thrombosis, which can lead to myocardial infarction. Another site of dystrophic calcification is the center of tumors. Over time, the center is deprived of oxygen supply, dies, and becomes calcified. The calcium salts appear as gritty, clumped granules that can become hard as stone. When several layers clump together, they resemble grains of sand and are called **psammoma bodies.**

The exact pathogenic mechanisms responsible for dystrophic calcification are unknown. A popular hypothesis is that with progressive deterioration of dead cells, the exposed denatured (changed) proteins preferentially bind with phosphate ions. The phosphate ions then react with calcium ions to form deposits of phosphate carbonate precipitates and, sometimes, crystalline formations of calcium phosphate. Dystrophic calcification develops slowly and is an explicit marker for the site of dead cells.

Metastatic calcification consists of mineral deposits that occur in undamaged normal tissues as the result of hypercalcemia (excess of calcium in the blood; see Chapter 3). Conditions that cause hypercalcemia include hyperparathyroidism, toxic levels of vitamin D, hyperthyroidism, idiopathic hypercalcemia of infancy, Addison disease (adrenocortical insufficiency), systemic sarcoidosis, milk-alkali syndrome, and the increased bone demineralization that results from bone tumors, leukemia, and disseminated cancers. Hypercalcemia also can occur in some instances of advanced renal failure with phosphate retention, resulting in hyperparathyroidism.[8]

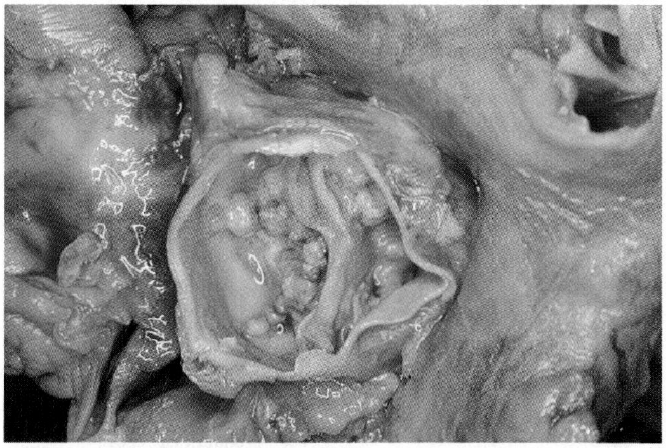

FIG. 2-28 Dystrophic calcification. Calcified aortic valve. (From Damjanov I: *Pathology for the health-related professions,* ed 2, Philadelphia, 2000, W.B. Saunders.)

Urate

In humans, uric acid **(urate)** is the major end product of purine catabolism because of the absence of the enzyme urate oxidase. Serum urate concentration is, in general, stable: approximately 5 mg/dl in postpubertal males and 4.1 mg/dl in postpubertal females. Disturbances in maintaining serum urate levels result in hyperuricemia and deposition of sodium urate crystals in the tissues, leading to painful disorders collectively called *gout.* These disorders include acute arthritis, chronic gouty arthritis, tophus (firm nodular subcutaneous deposits of urate crystals surrounded by fibrosis), and nephritis (inflammation of the nephron).

Chronic hyperuricemia results in the deposition of urate in tissues, cell injury, and inflammation. Because urate crystals are not degraded by lysosomal enzymes, they persist in dead cells.

Systemic Manifestations

Systemic manifestations of cellular injury include a general sense of fatigue and malaise, a loss of well-being, and altered appetite. Fever is frequently present because of biochemicals produced during the inflammatory response (see Chapter 7). Table 2-9 summarizes the most significant systemic manifestations of cellular injury.

CELLULAR DEATH

Necrosis

Cellular death eventually leads to the process of cellular dissolution, or **necrosis.** Necrosis is the sum of cellular changes after local cell death and the process of cellular self-digestion known as autodigestion, or **autolysis** (Fig. 2-29). The structural signs that indicate irreversible injury and progression to necrosis are the dense clumping and progressive disruption of genetic material and disruption of the plasma and organelle membranes. In later stages of necrosis, most organelles are disrupted, and **karyolysis** (nuclear dissolution and lysis of chromatin from the action of hydrolytic enzymes) is underway. In some cells the nucleus shrinks and becomes a small, dense mass of genetic material—a process called nuclear **pyknosis.** The pyknotic nucleus eventually dissolves (by karyolysis) as a result of the action of hydrolytic lysosomal enzymes on DNA. **Karyorrhexis** means fragmentation of the nucleus into smaller particles or "nuclear dust."

Different types of necroses tend to occur in different organs or tissues and sometimes can indicate the mechanism

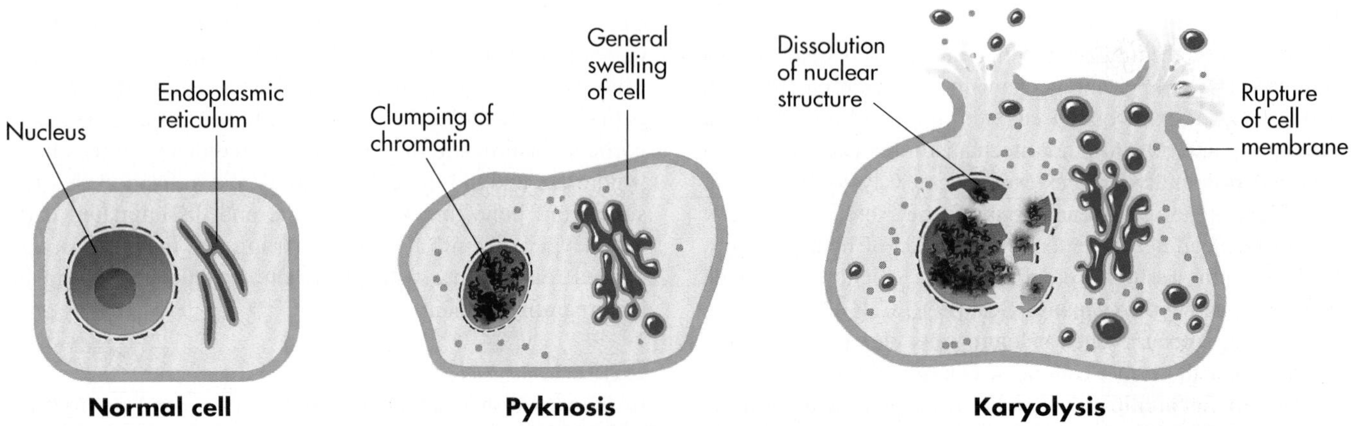

FIG. 2-29 Stages of necrosis.

Table 2-9 Systemic Manifestations of Cellular Injury

Manifestation	Cause
Fever	Release of endogenous pyrogens (interleukin-1, α–tumor necrosis factor, prostaglandins) from bacteria or macrophages; acute inflammatory response
Increased heart rate	Increase in oxidative metabolic processes resulting from fever
Increase in leukocytes (leukocytosis)	Increase in total number of white blood cells because of infection; normal is 5000-9000/mm^3 (increase is directly related to the severity of the infection)
Pain	Various mechanisms, such as release of bradykinins, obstruction, pressure
Presence of cellular enzymes in extracellular fluid	Release of enzymes from cells of tissue*
Lactate dehydrogenase (LDH) (LDH isoenzymes)	Release from red blood cells, liver, kidney, skeletal muscle
Creatine kinase (CK) (CK isoenzymes)	Release from skeletal muscle, brain, heart
Aspartate aminotransferase (AST; SGOT)	Release from heart, liver, skeletal muscle, kidney, pancreas
Alanine aminotransferase (ALT; SGPT)	Release from liver, kidney, heart
Alkaline phosphatase (ALP)	Release from liver, bone
Amylase	Release from pancreas
Aldolase	Release from skeletal muscle, heart

*The rapidity of enzyme transfer is a function of the weight of the enzyme and the concentration gradient across the cellular membrane. The specific metabolic and excretory rates of the enzymes determine how long levels of enzymes remain elevated.

or cause of cellular injury. The four major types of necroses are coagulative, liquefactive, caseous, and fatty. Another type, gangrenous necrosis, is *not* a distinctive type of cell death but refers to larger areas of tissue death.

Coagulative necrosis, which occurs primarily in the kidneys, heart, and adrenal glands, commonly results from hypoxia caused by severe ischemia or hypoxia caused by chemical injury, especially ingestion of mercuric chloride (Fig. 2-30). Coagulation is caused by protein denaturation, which causes the protein albumin to change from a gelatinous, transparent state to a firm, opaque state, similar to that of a cooked egg white. The necrotic tissues appear firm and slightly swollen. Recent evidence indicates that an abnormality in intracellular levels of Ca^{++} (e.g., increased) may be a critical event in coagulation necrosis.[3]

Liquefactive necrosis commonly results from ischemic injury to neurons and glial cells in the brain (Fig. 2-31). Dead brain tissue is readily affected by liquefactive necrosis because brain cells are rich in the digestive hydrolytic enzymes and lipids, and the brain contains little connective tissue. As the cells are digested by their own hydrolases, the tissue becomes soft, liquefies, and is walled off from healthy tissue, forming cysts. (Cyst formation is described in Chapter 7.)

Liquefactive necrosis can result also from bacterial infection, particularly by staphylococci, streptococci, and *Escherichia coli*. In this case the hydrolases are released from the lysosomes of neutrophils, which are phagocytes attracted to the infected area to kill the bacteria. Liquefaction of bacterial cells and neighboring tissue cells by neutrophilic hydrolases results in the accumulation of pus.

Caseous necrosis, which commonly results from tuberculous pulmonary infection, particularly by *Mycobacterium tuberculosis,* is a combination of coagulative and liquefactive necrosis (Fig. 2-32). The dead cells disintegrate, but the debris is not digested completely by hydrolases. Tissues appear soft and granular and resemble clumped cheese, which gives this type of necrosis its name. A granulomatous inflammatory wall encloses areas of caseous necrosis.

Fat necrosis, which occurs in the breast, pancreas, and other abdominal structures, is a specific type of cellular

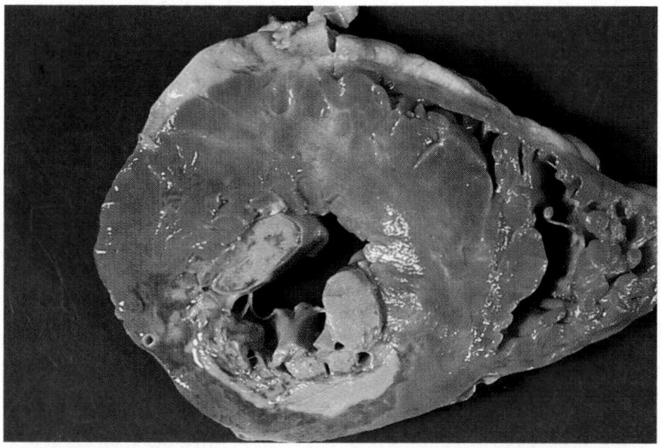

FIG. 2-30 Coagulative necrosis of myocardium of posterior wall of left ventricle of heart. A large anemic (white) infarct is readily apparent; note also the necrosis of papillary muscle. (From Damjanov I, Linder J: *Anderson's pathology,* ed 10, St Louis, 1996, Mosby.)

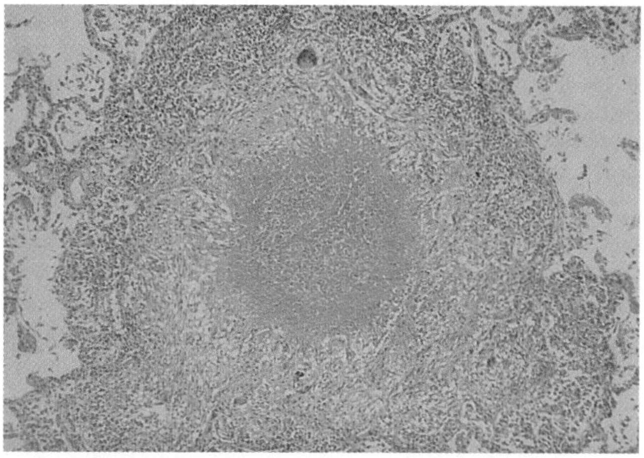

FIG. 2-32 Granuloma with central caseous necrosis typical of pulmonary tuberculosis. (From Damjanov I, Linder J: *Anderson's pathology,* ed 10, St Louis, 1996, Mosby.)

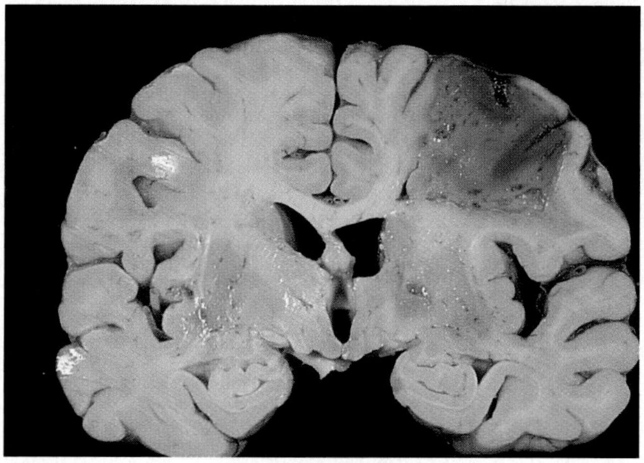

FIG. 2-31 Liquefactive necrosis. Liquefactive necrosis of the brain developed at a large cerebral infarct caused by ischemia. (From Damjanov I, Linder J: *Anderson's pathology,* ed 10, St Louis, 1996, Mosby.)

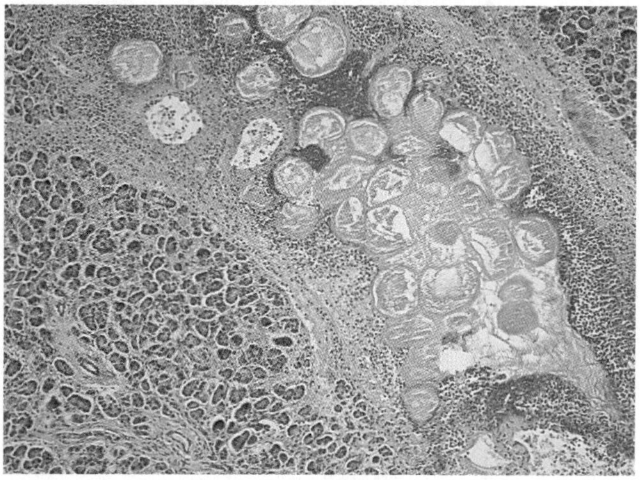

FIG. 2-33 Fat necrosis of pancreas. Interlobular adipocytes are necrotic; these are surrounded by acute inflammatory cells. (From Damjanov I, Linder J: *Anderson's pathology,* ed 10, St Louis, 1996, Mosby.)

dissolution caused by powerful enzymes called *lipases* (Fig. 2-33). Lipases break down triglycerides, releasing free fatty acids, which then combine with calcium, magnesium, and sodium ions, creating soaps (a process known as *saponification*). The necrotic tissue appears opaque and chalk white.

Gangrenous necrosis, a term commonly used in surgical clinical practice, refers to death of tissue and results from severe hypoxic injury, commonly occurring because of arteriosclerosis, or blockage, of major arteries, especially in the lower leg. With hypoxia and subsequent bacterial invasion, the tissues can undergo necrosis. **Dry gangrene** is usually the result of coagulative necrosis. The skin becomes very dry and shrinks, resulting in wrinkles, and its color changes to dark brown or black (Fig. 2-34). **Wet gangrene** develops when neutrophils invade the site, causing liquefactive necro-

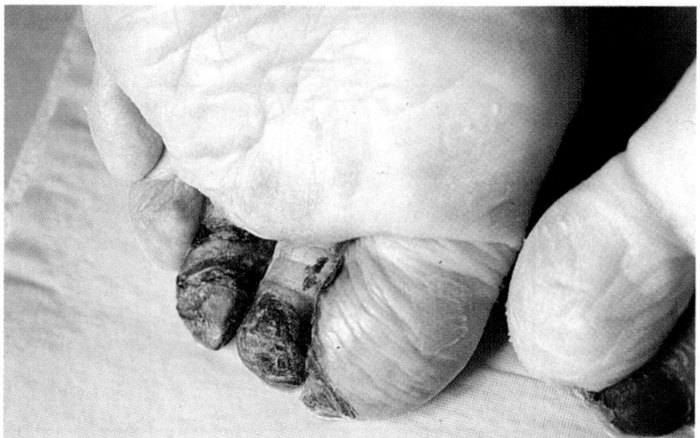

FIG. 2-34 Gangrene of toes. Dry gangrene. (From Damjanov I: *Pathology for the health-related professions,* ed 2, Philadelphia, 2000, W.B. Saunders.)

sis. This usually occurs in internal organs, causing the site to become cold, swollen, and black. A foul odor is present, produced by pus, and if systemic symptoms become severe, death can ensue.

Gas gangrene, a special type of gangrene, is caused by infection of injured tissue by one of many species of *Clostridium.* These anaerobic bacteria produce hydrolytic enzymes and toxins that destroy connective tissue and cellular membranes and cause bubbles of gas to form in muscle cells. Gas gangrene can be fatal if enzymes lyse the membranes of red blood cells, destroying their oxygen-carrying capacity. Death is the result of shock. The condition is treated with antitoxins and supplemental oxygen delivered in a hyperbaric (pressurized) chamber.

Apoptosis

Apoptosis (Greek for "dropping off") is an important, distinct type of cell death[37] that differs from necrosis in several respects (Fig. 2-35). Apoptosis is an active process of cellular self-destruction, called programmed cell death, that is implicated in both normal and pathologic tissue changes.[38] It is responsible for local deletion of cells during normal embryonic development, neurons dying during synaptogenesis, bone cells dying during turnover, lymphocytes dying during

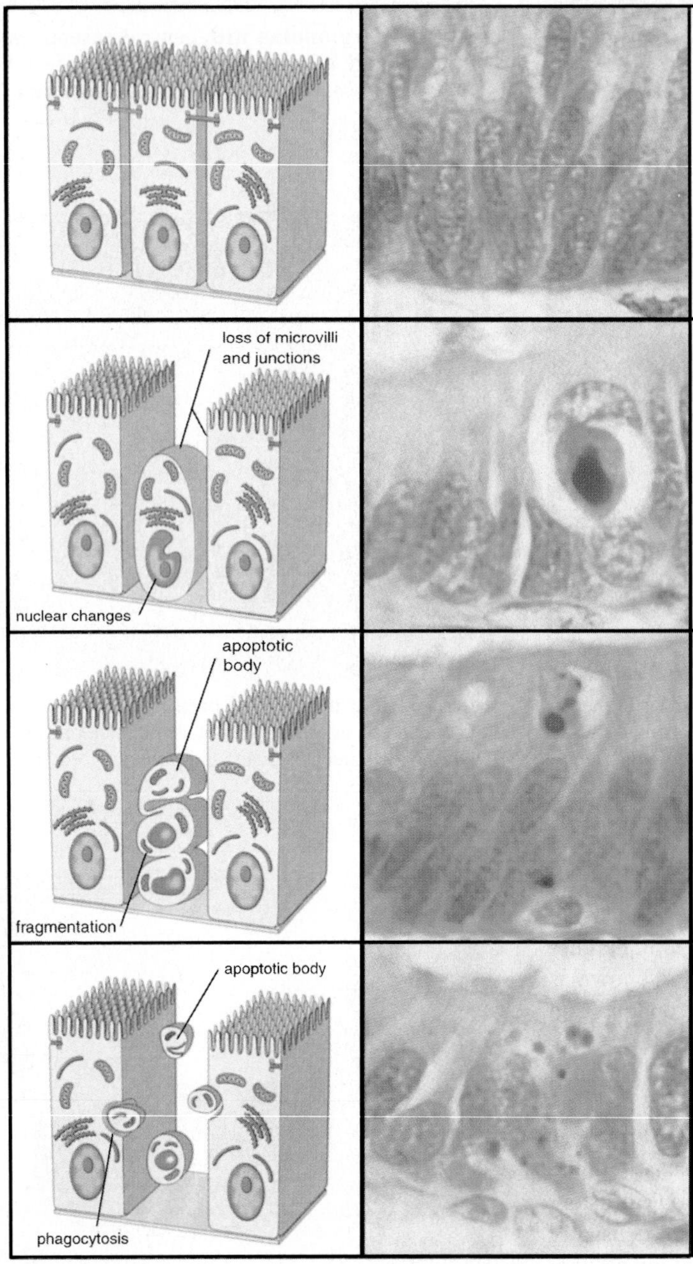

Normal cells are arranged in close contact with each other and are united by cell junctions. Early in the process of apoptosis there is synthesis of enzymes needed to cause cell dissolution, but this is not associated with structural changes. This is termed **priming.** In development many cells are primed for apoptosis and survive only if rescued by a specific trophic factor.

The apoptotic cells lose surface specializations and junctions, shrinking in size. The nuclear chromatin condenses beneath the nuclear membrane. In contrast to necrosis, cell organelles remain normal. Endonuclease enzymes cleave chromosomes into individual nucleosome fragments.

There is splitting of the cell into several fragments known as **apoptotic bodies.** Nuclear fragmentation also occurs. Each fragment contains viable mitochondria and intact organelles. The process takes only a few minutes.

Apoptotic fragments are recognized by adjacent cells, which ingest them by phagocytosis for destruction. Some fragments degenerate extracellularly while others are ingested by local phagocytic cells, not shown on this diagram.

Although apoptosis is a physiologic process, it can also be induced by pathologic conditions.

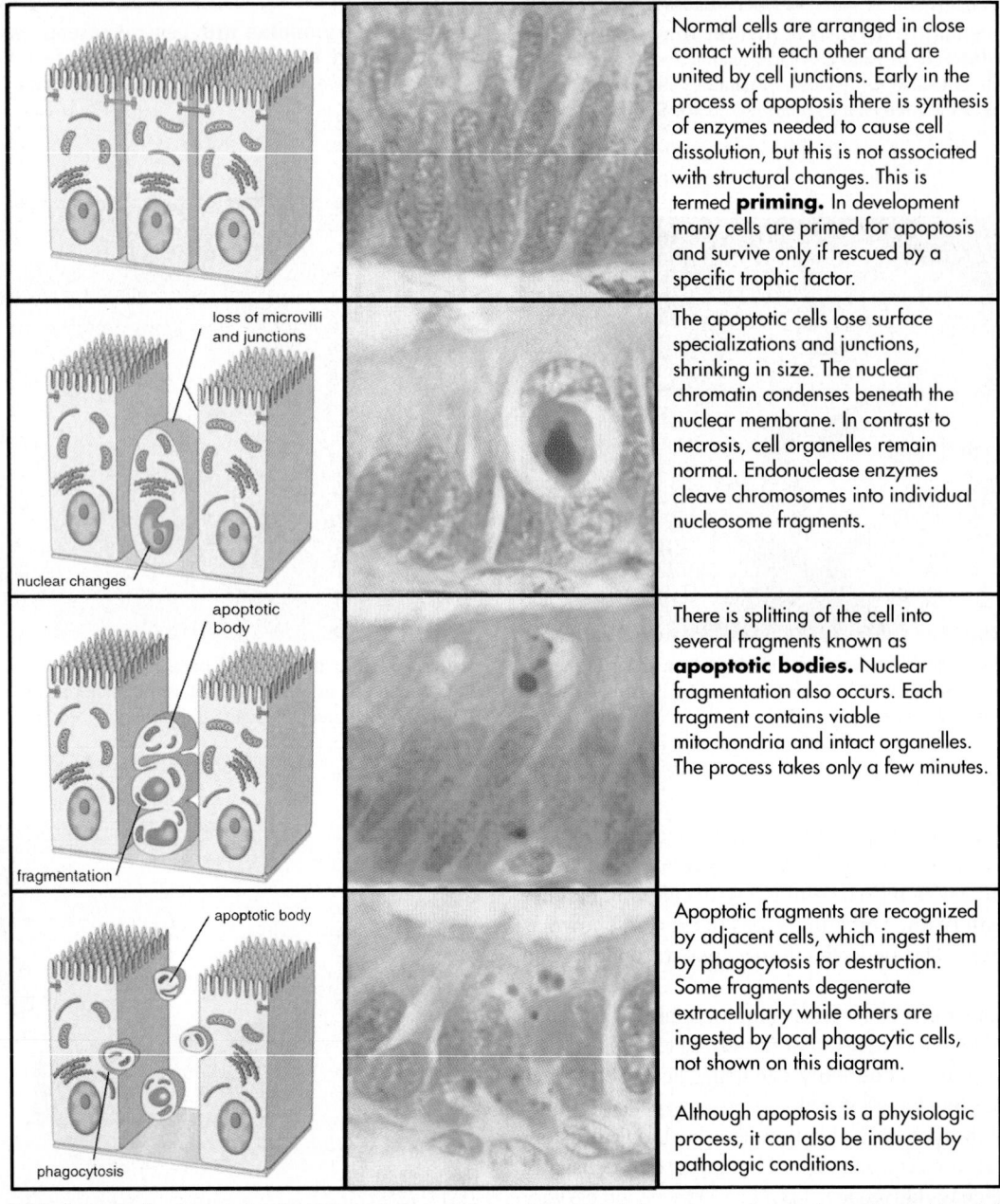

FIG. 2-35 Apoptosis. Apoptosis of cells is a programmed and energy-dependent process designed specifically to switch cells off and eliminate them. This controlled pattern of cell death, termed *programmed cell death,* is very different from that which occurs as a direct result of a severe, damaging stimulus to cells. (From Stevens A, Lowe J: *Pathology,* St Louis, 1995, Mosby.)

receptor repertoire selection, and so on. Apoptosis has been shown to play a major role in endocrine-dependent tissues that are undergoing atrophic change and possibly following axonal injury and in neurodegenerative diseases, such as Alzheimer.[39-41] Apoptosis can occur spontaneously in malignant tumors and in normal, rapidly proliferating cells treated with cancer chemotherapeutic agents and ionizing radiation.[42] Its significance in aging is unknown. Necrosis and apoptosis affect tissues differently. Unlike necrosis, apoptosis affects scattered, single cells. Apoptosis is nuclear and cytoplasmic shrinkage of a cell (i.e., unlike necrosis, in which cells swell and lyse) followed by fragmentation into membrane-bound fragments and subsequent phagocytosis by neighboring, healthy cells.[8] Evidence indicates that apoptosis depends on a tightly regulated cellular program for its initiation and execution.[42] Molecular helpers in this program are present in different subcellular compartments, including the plasma membrane, cytosol, mitochondria, and nucleus. The progression of apoptosis depends on the *interplay* among these compartments and the exchange of specific signaling molecules.[42]

Programmed cell death involves enzymes that cut up other proteins (proteases) that are, themselves, activated by proteolytic activity in response to signals that induce apoptosis.[43] The activated suicide proteases cleave, and thereby activate, other members of the family resulting in an amplifying "suicide" cascade. The activated proteases then cleave other key proteins in the cell, killing it quickly and neatly.[43] With necrosis, cell death is not neat because cells that die as a result of acute injury swell, burst, and spill their contents all over their neighbors causing a likely damaging inflammatory response.[43]

Aging

Aging is usually defined as a normal physiologic process that is universal and inevitable. The basic mechanisms of aging depend on irreversible and universal processes at the cellular and molecular level. To understand aging requires the separation of irreversible processes from potentially reversible mechanisms (i.e., those that result from disease or age-related debilities)—a very difficult task.

Aging traditionally has not been considered a disease because it is "normal"; disease is usually considered "abnormal." Conceptually, this distinction seems clear until the concept of "injury" is introduced; disease has been defined by some pathologists as the result of injury. Aging has been defined as the time-dependent loss of structure and function that proceeds very slowly and in such small increments that it appears to be the result of the accumulation of small, imperceptible injuries—a gradual result of wear and tear.

Injuries may result from unavoidable and universal microinsults caused by continuous bombardment by ultraviolet light, countless mechanical insults, and reactions to metabolites.[44,45] In this context the distinction between aging and disease is unclear. For example, some degree of atrophy of the brain is considered normal in old age until it proceeds far enough to cause clinically significant disability and is called disease. Likewise, most humans have atherosclerosis, and the plaques progress with age, but at what point in this progression is it considered abnormal? These conceptual distinctions have given rise to two general categories of theories of aging. The first category proposes that aging is the result of the accumulation of random injuries and events. The second category proposes that aging is the result of a genetically controlled developmental program, or built-in self-destructive processes. (No matter what conceptual distinction, it seems clear that even in the absence of disease, the individual's frailty increases with age, and death inevitably results!)

Normal Life Span

The **maximal life span** of humans is between 80 and 100 years and does not vary significantly among populations. However, in primitive societies, few individuals reach the maximal life span; most die in infancy and the early years.[46] In societies with improved sanitation, housing, nutrition, and health care, many persons attain the maximal life span. Although the maximal life span has not changed significantly over time, the average life span, or **life expectancy,** has increased. Recently, the death rate for people 65 years of age and older has declined significantly, largely because of decreases in cardiovascular disease.[11] In each successive age-group from 65 years and older, women outnumber men; thus women have a greater life expectancy than men. Increases in life expectancy have resulted in a large elderly population with inherent problems of disability, disease, and socioeconomic hardship.[47]

Life Expectancy and Gender Differences

Life expectancy for females exceeds that for males (the gender gap) except in Bangladesh, Bhutan, India, Nepal, and Pakistan.[48] The female advantage ranges from 4 to 8 years; however, the gender gap is continuing to decrease. International mortality data for 1995 among 15 selected industrialized countries indicate that Iceland had the best recorded age-adjusted rate for men, just ahead of Japan, which has had the lowest mortality rate for more than 20 years.[49] Age-adjusted death rates among U.S. nonwhite men and for men in Scotland were ranked the worst, and among women, the worst mortality rates were in Denmark and Scotland. Although life expectancy values are improving in many countries, U.S. longevity continues to fare poorly in comparison to other developed countries. The U.S. life expectancy for the 1990 to 1995 period for men was ranked thirteenth and for women eleventh. Longevity was the highest for men in Japan and Iceland (76.4 and 76.3 years, respectively) and the lowest for men in Finland (72.0 years). For women, longevity was the best in Japan (82.4 years) and the worst in Denmark (77.8 years). Life expectancies for men during 1995 to 2000 are projected to improve from 1.6 years in New Zealand to 0.4 years in Japan. For women, life expectancy will remain at 80.8 years in Sweden while increasing 0.8 years in the United States, Germany, the United Kingdom, and New Zealand.[49]

Table 2-10 Causes of Current Longevity and Health Differences Between Men and Women

Biologic Hypotheses	Comments
GENETIC	
Female genotype (XX) compared with male genotype (XY)	Little is known about the Y chromosome compared with the X chromosome, especially the significance of the X chromosome to longevity; however, certain genes on the X chromosome are involved in vital functions including blood clotting, muscle function, protection against oxidative damage, DNA synthesis, nucleotide synthesis, and immune response; thus the question raised is, To what extent are these genes critical to longevity?
Increased male mortality during the prenatal period	The incidence in excess male mortality or early die-off during the prenatal period may be attributed to homozygosity of the genes of the X chromosome (one allele instead of two alleles for each gene)
Characteristics of the Y chromosome	The Y chromosome is about one third the size of the X chromosome; few recognized genes are mapped to the Y chromosome
GENETIC AND/OR HORMONAL	
Sex hormones	The levels and balance of the cholesterol-carrying lipoproteins by sex hormones are major factors in the gender gap; sex hormones result in a *healthier* pattern of lipoproteins in women than in men; exogenous estrogens raise protective lipoproteins (high-density lipoproteins [HDL]) and lower nonprotective lipoproteins (low-density lipoproteins [LDL]); male androgens have the opposite effect (see Chapter 29); the pattern in women undergoes a disadvantageous change after menopause; however, the increased death rate for women from cardiovascular disease lags behind that of men by several years. Testosterone decline may be related to increased leptin in men with consequent decrease in body fat; changes in leptin have not been related to changes in estrone in women[50,51]
Neuroendocrine effects, hormones, and the immune system	Sex hormones regulate longevity through their effects on behavior and through the immune system; these effects are interrelated, and the central nervous system is at the center of these relationships; behaviorally, sex hormones affect aggressiveness, territoriality, mate selection, and mating behavior; how these behaviors affect longevity is incompletely understood; reproductive senescence, although life threatening, can contribute to increasing wear and tear and includes cell depletion, cell death, and organ involution; the central nervous system affects the immune system through neuroendocrine mechanisms; sex hormones also affect the immune system; an important question is, How do men and women differ in their perception, handling, and physiologic consequences of stress, and how do these differences relate to the gender gap?
Immune function	The immune system in female mice does appear to be more robust than that in males; it is not clear whether this is related to the antibody genes that map to the X chromosome[52,53]
Cardiovascular effects	Increased myocyte cell loss and myocyte cellular "reactive" hypertrophy is significant in men and women, indicating that gender differences may play a huge role in the detrimental effects of aging on the heart; an increase in mean arterial pressure with age persisted in women beyond 62 yr but not in women younger than 62 yr or in men of any age; endogenous and exogenous androgens are known to decrease HDL cholesterol in men
SOCIAL ROLES	
Multiple roles held by middle-aged women	Differing social roles of men and women are often cited as major causes of the gender gap; the key question is, To what extent do the different roles become sources of stress and thus differentially affect longevity?; data from women 45-55 yr old reveal that the majority of these women are performing multiple roles; although these roles are sources of stress, surprisingly the reported stresses are not translated into negative health outcomes[53,54]; working may play a protective role by alleviating the stress of nurturing roles and thereby prevent morbidity. Over recent decades, time in committed activities shifted in opposite ways for men and women. Men decreased paid work and increased housework, repairs and yard work, and shopping and childcare. Women increased paid work and decreased housework
Occupations and social class	There continues to be an increase in the relative mortality disadvantage of manual relative to nonmanual workers (for many causes of death) for both men and women; as determined by decades of research, the age-adjusted incidence of myocardial infarction declined in both white and blue collar male workers; however, the decline in white collar workers was double that of blue collar workers; no consistent trends in myocardial infarction were observed in women
Risky behavior and social class	Social class differences in smoking behavior (most documented risky behavior) do correspond to observed gender–social class mortality relationships; men with lower levels of education are substantially more likely to smoke than either better educated men or women[12]; however, as the prevalence of smoking among men has declined more rapidly than among women, gender differences in smoking within the blue collar group, although still present, have become less marked

Table 2-10 Causes of Current Longevity and Health Differences Between Men and Women—cont'd

Biologic Hypotheses	Comments
SOCIAL ROLES—cont'd	
Health service use and morbidity differences	Although women report greater use of physical services (particularly preventive services) than men, elderly men have higher hospitalization rates than women; with fewer work obligations, women are more likely to curtail activities and get more bed rest when ill; a more flexible daily schedule made possible by a lower employment rate is a key reason women make more doctor visits for chronic problems[58]; overall, however, women have higher rates of morbidity and therapeutic care than men; women more frequently have short-term illnesses, with higher rates of daily symptoms and higher incidence rates for acute illnesses; thus women have a higher prevalence of many nonfatal chronic conditions, such as arthritis, chronic sinusitis, and digestive conditions; by contrast, men have higher prevalence rates of heart disease, atherosclerosis, emphysema, and other fatal conditions
Other social, psychologic, and emotional issues	Women's excess morbidity in contemporary life is driven by social factors, risks from less satisfying employment, low social support at work, keenly felt stress and unhappiness, stronger feelings of illness vulnerability, fewer formal time constraints, and less physically strenuous leisure activities

Race has a key impact on the gender mortality differences in the United States. Between 1920 and 1970, the gender gap increased among whites by a factor of 6 and by a factor of 8 among blacks. Since 1970, however, the size of the gap has narrowed sharply among whites and has begun to decline among blacks.

Causes of the gender gap have been divided into three very broad areas: biologic (genetic, hormonal), behavioral, and sociocultural (Table 2-10).

Theories and Mechanisms of Aging

Relatively little "indisputable" knowledge exists on the subject of aging. Table 2-11 presents the historical development of aging research. Numerous theories exist about the causes of aging. Many of these theories overlap, interact, and are similar. Some of the theories have focused on a single mechanism—the so-called magic bullet approach to arrest aging. It is doubtful that a single theory will explain all the mechanisms of aging. As stated earlier, there are two general categories of theories of aging: (1) that aging is the result of the accumulation of injurious events, sometimes called *damage-accumulation theories,* or (2) that biologic changes of aging are the result of a genetically controlled developmental program. In the first category, random accumulation of errors in protein structure, mutations in somatic cells, the accumulation of metabolic waste products, and free radical–mediated damage (from highly reactive intermediates produced in the normal course of metabolism, such as hydroperoxides, aldehydes, and ketones) decrease the ability to maintain a physiologic steady state. The accumulation of these injuries increases one's susceptibility to disease. In the developmentally programmed theory of aging, aging is the result of certain genes that program senescence and cell death. Here supporters claim that because maximal life span is genetically determined, the aging process is also.

Evidence exists both for and against any particular theory of aging. However, three major areas of the mechanisms of aging have retained their appeal or have been extensively tested: (1) cellular changes produced by genetic, environmental, and behavioral factors; (2) changes in cellular regulatory, or control, mechanisms, especially in cells of the neuroendocrine, immune, and central nervous systems; and (3) degenerative extracellular and vascular alterations.

Table 2-11 Theories of Aging

Theory	Year	Proponent
Waste product theory	1923	Carrell and Ebeling
Wear-and-tear theory	1924	Pearl
Rate of living theory[a]	1928	Pearl
Neuroendocrine theory (including DHEA and melatonin)	1947	Korenchevsky and Jones
Free-radical theory	1955	Harman
Collagen theory[b]	1957	Verzar
Metabolic theory[a]	1957; 1961	Carlson et al.; Johnson et al.
Somatic mutation theory	1959	Sziliard
Error-catastrophe theory	1963; 1970	Orgel
Cross-linking theory[b]	1968	Bjorksten
Programmed senescence theory	1969	Hayflick
Immunologic theory	1969	Walform
Evolution theory	1977	Kirkwood

Data from Schneider EL: Theories of aging: a perspective. In Warner HR et al, editors: *Modern biological theories of aging,* New York, 1987, Raven; Madison HE:Theories of Aging. In Lueckenotte A: *Gerontologic nursing,* ed 2, St Louis, 2000, Mosby; Hayflick L: *How and why we age,* New York, 1996, Ballantine Books.

NOTE: Theories with the same superscript may represent the same theory.

DHEA, Dehydroepiandosterone.

Genetic and Environmental Factors

Cellular aging results from wear and tear that causes functional changes and eventual cellular death. Cellular damage may occur during replication as a result of factors within the cell, such as DNA and protein mechanisms, or factors outside the cell, such as ionizing radiation. Cells may already be programmed at birth or are injured during life so as to cause errors in mitotic division and in the replication of genetic material, eventually leading to either cellular atrophy or death. Atrophy is common in the thymus, testis, ovary, uterus, and breast of aged individuals, although these organs age differently.

One of the genetic mechanisms of aging is programmed aging. Regardless of damaging environmental factors, some investigators think that each normal cell may have a finite life span during which it can replicate. A classic experiment done by Hayflick[37] demonstrated that fibroblasts are limited to a finite number of generations (40 to 60 doublings). However, proponents do not propose that aging is the result of cells losing their ability to divide. Rather, they believe that an intrinsic program within the human genome progressively slows or shuts down certain physiologic mechanisms, including mitosis.[55]

The **somatic mutation hypothesis** proposes that aging is the result of DNA damage, inefficiency of repair, and loss of integrity of DNA synthesis (i.e., mutations in somatic cells). Somatic mutations increase with age; however, it is not exactly known if this occurs in a linear or exponential fashion, and this increase partly explains the age-related increase in cancer incidence. Somatic mutation of genes that regulate the cell cycle (e.g., *p53,* see Chapter 10) and apoptosis are likely to play a crucial role in cancer initiation.[45] Data suggest that, with aging, life-style factors can contribute to an accumulation of genetic damage.[56] An argument against the somatic mutation theory is that the frequency of mutations in various organs and tissues is thought to be low.[45]

The **catastrophic,** or **error-prone, theory,** initially proposed by Orgel in 1963, stated that the presence of errors in those enzymes involved in transcription and translation, and thus their own synthesis, lead to an increase in errors and eventually to the death of the cell. The theory was later modified by Orgel in 1970, with the possibility that nongrowing cells may not be subject to error catastrophe if the rate of error production did not increase significantly during protein synthesis. Abnormal forms of some, but not all, cellular proteins do appear during senescence but not as a result of errors in protein synthesis as originally predicted.[57] Rather, the abnormal proteins appear to reflect several types of post-translational modifications.[58] The error-catastrophe theory has attracted a great deal of interest. Most of the evidence, however, argues against this theory as originally formulated. The accumulation of altered proteins in aging may result from an increased production or decreased ability of aged cells to degrade their cellular proteins, or both.

Alterations of Cellular Control Mechanisms

The overall effects of aging may be caused by changes in certain cell populations that exert regulatory or control functions, such as cells of the central nervous system, neuroendocrine system, and immune system.[58] The **neuroendocrine theory** of aging purports that a genetic program for aging is encoded in the brain and is controlled and relayed to peripheral tissues through hormonal and neural agents. Possible mechanisms include (1) increased hormonal degradation, (2) decreased rate of hormonal synthesis and secretion, and (3) decreased target-organ sensitivity related to the number of cellular receptors for hormonal ligands, ligand-receptor binding, or ligand internalization (see Chapter 1). (The neuroendocrine theory of aging is discussed further in Chapter 9.)

Proponents of immune theories of aging believe that the immune system is implicated in aging because (1) immune function declines with age; (2) the decline in immune function is related to certain diseases, such as cancer, and to many other secondary effects; and (3) the number of autoantibodies (antibodies that attack body tissues) increases with age. (Changes in the immune system with age are discussed in Chapter 6.)

Degenerative Extracellular Changes

Extracellular factors that affect the aging process include the binding of collagen; the increase in free radicals' effects on cells; the structural alterations of fascia, tendons, ligaments, bones, and joints; and peripheral vascular disease, particularly arteriosclerosis (see Chapter 29).

Aging affects the extracellular matrix with increased cross-linking (e.g., aging collagen becomes more insoluble, chemically stable, but rigid, resulting in a decrease of cell permeability), decreased synthesis, and increased degradation of collagen. These changes, together with the disappearance of elastin and changes in proteoglycans and plasma proteins, cause disorders of the ground substance that result in dehydration and wrinkling of the skin (see Chapter 43). Other age-related defects in the extracellular matrix include skeletal muscle alterations (e.g., atrophy, decreased tone, loss of contractility), cataracts, diverticula, hernias, and rupture of intervertebral disks.

Free radicals of oxygen that result from oxidative cellular metabolism (e.g., respiratory chain, phagocytosis, prostaglandin synthesis) are thought to damage tissues during the aging process (Fig. 2-36). The oxygen radicals produced include superoxide radical, hydroxyl radical, and hydrogen peroxide (see p. 51). These oxygen products are extremely reactive and can damage nucleic acids, destroy polysaccharides, oxidize proteins, peroxidize unsaturated fatty acids, and kill and lyse cells. Oxidant effects on target cells can give rise to malignant transformation through DNA damage. That progressive and cumulative damage from oxygen radicals may lead to harmful alterations in cellular function is consistent with those alterations of aging. This hypothesis is founded on the wear-and-tear theory of aging, which states that damages accumulate with time, decreasing the organism's ability to maintain a steady state. Because these oxygen-reactive species not only can permanently damage cells but also may lead to cell death, there is new support for their role in the aging process.

Of much interest is the relationship between aging and the disappearance or alteration of extracellular substances important for vessel integrity. With aging, lipid, calcium, and plasma proteins are deposited in the walls of vessels. These depositions cause serious basement membrane thickening and alterations in smooth muscle functioning, result-

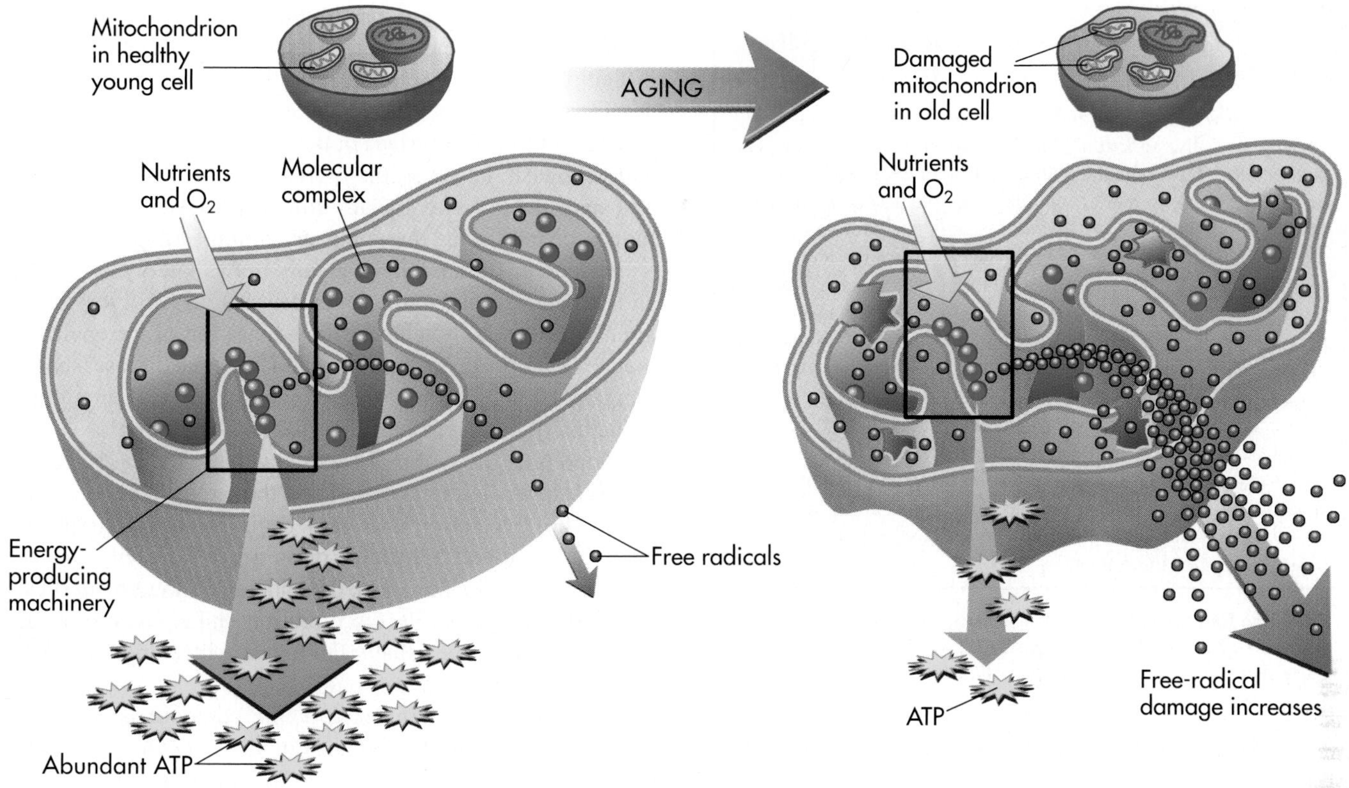

FIG. 2-36 Theory of aging: destructive free radicals.

ing in arteriosclerosis. Arteriosclerosis is a progressive disease that causes serious problems in the aged individual, including stroke, myocardial infarction, renal disease, and peripheral vascular disease.

Cellular Aging

Cellular changes characteristic of aging include atrophy, decreased function, and loss of cells, possibly caused by apoptosis. Loss of cellular function from any of these causes initiates the compensatory mechanisms of hypertrophy and hyperplasia of remaining cells, which can lead to metaplasia, dysplasia, and neoplasia. All these changes can alter receptor placement and function, nutrient pathways, secretion of cellular products, and neuroendocrine control mechanisms. In the aged cell, DNA, RNA, cellular proteins, and membranes are most susceptible to injurious stimuli. DNA is particularly vulnerable to such injuries as breaks, deletions, and additions. Although DNA generally repairs itself with time, the aged cell's capacity for DNA repair is decreased. Lack of DNA repair increases the cell's susceptibility to mutations that may be lethal or may promote the development of neoplasia (see Chapter 10).

Tissue and Systemic Aging

It is probably safe to say that every physiologic process can be shown to function less efficiently with increasing age. The most characteristic tissue change with age is a progressive stiffness or rigidity that affects many systems, including the arterial, pulmonary, and musculoskeletal systems. A consequence of blood vessel and organ stiffness is a progressive increase in peripheral resistance to blood flow. The movement of intracellular and extracellular substances also usually decreases with age as does the diffusion capacity of the lung. Blood flow through organs decreases; for example, renal plasma flow decreases.

Changes in the endocrine and immune systems include thymus atrophy. Although this occurs at puberty, causing a decreased immune response to T-dependent antigens (foreign proteins), increased autoantibodies and immune complexes (antibodies bound to antigen) and an overall decrease in the immunologic tolerance for the host's own cells further diminish the effectiveness of the immune system later in life. The reproductive system loses ova in women, and spermatogenesis in men is decreased. Responsiveness to hormones decreases in the breast and endometrium.

The stomach experiences decreases in the rate of emptying and secretion of hormones and hydrochloric acid. Muscular atrophy diminishes mobility by decreasing motor tone and contractility. **Sarcopenia,** or muscle loss, can occur into old age. The skin of the aged individual is affected by atrophy and wrinkling of the epidermis and alterations in underlying dermis, fat, and muscle.

Total body changes include a decrease in height; a reduction in circumference of the neck, thighs, and arms; widening of the pelvis; and lengthening of the nose and ears. Several of these changes are the result of tissue atrophy and decreased bone mass caused by osteoporosis and osteoarthritis. Body composition changes with age.[59] With middle age there is an increase in body weight (men gain until 50 years of age and women until 70 years) and fat mass followed by a decrease in

WHAT'S NEW? Frailty and Gender: A Biologic Syndrome

Frailty is a wasting syndrome of aging that leaves a person vulnerable to falls, functional decline, disease, and death. The cause of this syndrome is complex but involves a major biologic basis. The biologic model includes sarcopenia, neuroendocrine decline, and immune dysfunction. Several physiologic gender differences may explain different levels of frailty and higher risks for women, including the following: (1) higher baseline levels of muscle mass for men may be protective against frailty; (2) testosterone and growth hormone can provide advantages in muscle mass maintenance; (3) cortisol, which is less dysregulated in older men than women, may also influence muscle mass maintenance; (4) alterations in immune function and immune responsiveness to sex steroids make men more vulnerable to sepsis and infections and women more vulnerable to chronic inflammatory conditions and muscle mass loss; and (5) lower levels of activity and caloric intake may influence greater susceptibility to frailty in women.

Data from Hamerman D: Toward an understanding of frailty, *Ann Intern Med* 130(11):945, 1999; Walston J, Fried LP: Frailty and the older man, *Med Clin North Am* 83(5):1173, 1999.

stature, weight, **fat-free mass (FFM)** (FFM includes all minerals, proteins, and water plus all other constituents except lipids), and body cell mass at older ages. As fat increases, total body water decreases. Increased body fat and centralized fat distribution (abdominal) are associated with non-insulin-dependent diabetes and heart disease. Total body potassium also decreases because of decreased cellular mass. An increased sodium/potassium ratio suggests that the decreased cellular mass is accompanied by an increased extracellular compartment.

Although some of these alterations are probably inherent in aging, others represent consequences of aging. Advanced age increases susceptibility to disease, and death occurs after an injury or insult because of diminished cellular, tissue, and organic function. To determine that an individual "died of old age" would be a monumental if not impossible task.

SOMATIC DEATH

Somatic death is death of the entire person. Unlike the changes that follow cellular death in a live body, **postmortem change** is diffuse and does not involve components of the inflammatory response. Within minutes of death, manifestations of postmortem change appear, eliminating any difficulty in determining that death has occurred. The most notable manifestations are complete cessation of respiration and circulation. The surface of the skin usually becomes pale and yellowish; however, the lifelike color of the cheeks and lips may persist after death from causes such as carbon monoxide poisoning, drowning, and chloroform poisoning.[60]

Body temperature falls gradually immediately after death and then more rapidly (approximately 1.0° to 1.5° F/hr) until, after 24 hours, body temperature equals that of the environment.[61] After death caused by certain infective diseases, body temperature may continue to rise for a short time. Postmortem reduction of body temperature is called **algor mortis.**

Blood pressure within the retinal vessels decreases, causing muscle tension to decrease and the pupils to become dilated. The face, nose, and chin begin to look "sharp" or "peaked" as blood and fluids drain away.[60] Gravity causes blood to settle in the most dependent, or lowest, tissues, which develop a purple discoloration called **livor mortis.** Incisions at this time usually fail to cause bleeding. The skin loses its elasticity and transparency.

Within 6 hours after death, acidic compounds accumulate within the muscles because of the breakdown of carbohydrate and depletion of ATP. This interferes with ATP-dependent detachment of myosin from actin (contractile proteins), and muscle stiffening, or **rigor mortis,** sets in. The smaller muscles are usually affected first, particularly the muscles of the jaw. Within 12 to 14 hours, rigor mortis usually affects the entire body.

Signs of putrefaction are generally obvious about 24 to 48 hours after death. Rigor mortis gradually diminishes, and the body becomes flaccid in 12 to 14 hours. Putrefactive changes vary depending on the temperature of the environment. The most visible is greenish discoloration of the skin, particularly on the abdomen. The discoloration is thought to be related to the diffusion of hemolyzed blood into the tissues and the production of sulfhemoglobin.[56] Slippage or loosening of the skin from underlying tissues occurs at the same time. After this, swelling or bloating of the body and liquefactive changes occur, sometimes causing opening of the body cavities. At a microscopic level, putrefactive changes are associated with the release of enzymes and lytic dissolution called **postmortem autolysis.**

SUMMARY REVIEW

Cellular Adaptation

1. Cellular adaptation is an alteration that enables the cell to maintain a steady state despite adverse conditions.
2. Atrophy is a decrease in cellular size. Amounts of endoplasmic reticulum, mitochondria, and microfilaments are decreased.
3. Physiologic atrophy occurs with early development; for example, the thymus gland involutes and atrophies. Pathologic atrophy occurs as a result of decreases in workload, use, pressure, blood supply, nutrition, hormonal stimulation, and nervous stimulation.
4. Aging causes brain cells and endocrine-dependent organs, such as the gonads, to become atrophic.
5. Hypertrophy is an increase in the size of cells by increased work demands or hormonal stimulation. Hypertrophy can be physiologic or pathologic. Amounts of protein in the plasma membrane, endoplasmic reticulum, microfilaments, and mitochondria are increased.
6. Hyperplasia is an increase in the number of cells caused by an increased rate of cellular division.

7. Compensatory hyperplasia enables certain organs to regenerate. Hormonal hyperplasia is stimulated by hormones to replace lost tissue or support new growth, such as pregnancy.
8. Pathologic hyperplasia is the abnormal proliferation of normal cells in response to excessive hormonal stimulation of growth factors on target cells.
9. Dysplasia, or atypical hyperplasia, is an abnormal change in the size, shape, and organization of mature tissue cells.
10. Metaplasia is the reversible replacement of one mature cell type by another, less mature cell type. Metaplasia is thought to develop from a reprogramming of stem cells existing in most epithelia or of undifferentiated mesenchymal cells in connective tissue.

Cellular Injury

1. Most diseases begin with cell injury. Injured cells may recover (reversible injury) or die (irreversible injury).
2. Cellular injury is caused by a lack of oxygen (hypoxia), free radicals, caustic or toxic chemicals, infectious agents, unintentional and intentional injury, inflammatory and immune responses, genetic factors, insufficient nutrients, or physical trauma from many causes.
3. Cell injury can be acute or chronic, and it can be reversible or irreversible. It can involve necrosis, apoptosis, accumulation, or pathologic calcification.
4. Four biochemical themes are important to cell injury: (a) ATP depletion, (b) oxygen and oxygen-derived free radicals, (c) intracellular calcium and loss of calcium steady state, and (d) defects in membrane permeability.
5. The sequence of events leading to cell death is commonly decreased ATP production, failure of active transport mechanisms (the sodium-potassium pump), cellular swelling, detachment of ribosomes from the endoplasmic reticulum, cessation of protein synthesis, mitochondrial swelling as a result of calcium accumulation, vacuolation, leakage of digestive enzymes from lysosomes, autodigestion of intracellular structures, lysis of the plasma membrane, and death.
6. The initial insult in hypoxic injury is usually ischemia—the cessation of blood flow into vessels that supply the cell with oxygen and nutrients.
7. An important mechanism of membrane damage is injury caused by free radicals. Free radicals are difficult to control and initiate chain reactions.
8. Free radicals can cause (a) lipid peroxidation or the destruction of unsaturated fatty acids, (b) alterations of proteins, and (c) alterations in DNA.
9. The initial insult in chemical injury is damage or destruction of the plasma membrane. Examples of chemical agents that cause cellular injury include carbon tetrachloride, lead, carbon monoxide, and ethyl alcohol.
10. Unintentional and intentional injuries are an important health problem in the United States. Death is more common for men than women and higher among blacks than whites and other racial groups.
11. Injuries by blunt force are the result of the application of mechanical energy to the body resulting in tearing, shearing, or crushing of tissues. The most common types of blunt force injuries include motor vehicle accidents and falls.
12. A contusion is bleeding into the skin or underlying tissues as a consequence of a blow. A collection of blood in soft tissues or an enclosed space may be referred to as a hematoma.
13. An abrasion (scrape) results from removal of the superficial layers of the skin caused by friction between the skin and injuring object. Abrasions and contusions may have a patterned appearance that mirrors the shape and features of an injuring object.
14. A laceration is a tear or rip resulting when the tensile strength of the skin or tissue is exceeded.
15. An incised wound is a cut that is longer than it is deep. A stab wound is a penetrating sharp force injury that is deeper than it is long.
16. Gunshot wounds may be either penetrating (bullet retained in the body) or perforating (bullet exits). The most important factors determining the appearance of a gunshot injury are whether it is an entrance or an exit wound and the range of fire.
17. Asphyxial injuries are caused by a failure of cells to receive or utilize oxygen. These injuries can be grouped into four general categories: suffocation, strangulation, chemical, and drowning.
18. Injury from microorganisms lies in their ability to survive and proliferate in the human body. Injury depends on the microorganisms' ability to invade and destroy cells, produce toxins, and produce damaging hypersensitivity reactions.
19. Activation of inflammation and immunity, which occurs after cellular injury or infection, involves powerful biochemicals and proteins capable of damaging normal (uninjured and uninfected) cells.
20. Genetic disorders injure cells by altering the nucleus and the plasma membrane's structure, shape, receptors, or transport mechanisms.
21. Deprivation of essential nutrients (proteins, carbohydrates, lipids, vitamins) can cause cellular injury by altering cellular structure and function, particularly of transport mechanisms, chromosomes, the nucleus, and DNA.
22. Injurious physical agents include temperature extremes, changes in atmospheric pressure, ionizing radiation, illumination, mechanical stresses (e.g., repetitive body movements), and noise.

Manifestations of Cellular Injury

1. Cellular manifestations of cellular injury include accumulations of water, lipids, carbohydrates, glycogen, proteins, pigments, hemosiderin, bilirubin, calcium, and urate.
2. Accumulations harm cells by "crowding" the organelles and by causing excessive (and sometimes harmful) metabolites to be produced during their catabolism. The metabolites are released into the cytoplasm or expelled into the extracellular matrix.
3. Cellular swelling, the accumulation of excessive water in the cell, is caused by the failure of transport mechanisms and is a sign of many types of cellular injury.
4. Accumulations of organic substances—lipids, carbohydrates, glycogen, proteins, and pigments—are caused by disorders in which (a) cellular uptake of the substance exceeds the cell's capacity to catabolize (digest) or use it or (b) cellular anabolism (synthesis) of the substance exceeds the cell's capacity to use or secrete it.
5. Dystrophic calcification (accumulation of calcium salts) is always a sign of pathologic change because it occurs only in injured or dead cells. Free calcium in the cytosol can cause activation of protein kinases, activation of phospholipases and membrane damage, and damage or disassembly of the cytoskeleton. Metastatic calcification, however, can occur in uninjured cells in individuals with hypercalcemia.
6. Disturbances in urate metabolism can result in hyperuricemia and deposition of sodium urate crystals in tissue, leading to painful disorders called gout.

7. Systemic manifestations of cellular injury include fever, leukocytosis, increased heart rate, pain, and serum elevations of enzymes in the plasma.

Cellular Death

1. Cellular death is manifested as cellular dissolution, or necrosis. Necrosis is the sum of the changes after local cell death and includes the process of autolysis, or cellular self-destruction.
2. The four major types of necrosis are coagulative, liquefactive, caseous, and fat. Different types of necrosis occur in different tissues.
3. Structural signs that indicate irreversible injury and progression to necrosis are the dense clumping and disruption of genetic material and the disruption of the plasma and organelle membranes.
4. Apoptosis, a different type of cellular death, is a process of selective cellular self-destruction that occurs in both normal and pathologic tissue changes.
5. Gangrenous necrosis, or gangrene, is tissue necrosis caused by hypoxia and subsequent bacterial invasion.

Aging

1. It is difficult to determine the physiologic (normal) from the pathologic changes of aging.
2. Humans have an inherent maximal life span (80 to 100 years) that is dictated by currently unknown intrinsic mechanisms.
3. Although the maximal life span has not changed significantly over time, the average life span, or life expectancy, has increased. Life expectancy for females exceeds that for males (gender gap) except in Bangladesh, Bhutan, India, Nepal, and Pakistan.
4. The physiologic mechanisms of aging are apparently associated with (a) cellular changes produced by genetic and environmental factors, (b) changes in cellular regulatory or control mechanisms, and (c) degenerative extracellular and vascular alterations.

Somatic Death

1. Somatic death is death of the entire organism. Postmortem change is diffuse and does not involve the inflammatory response.
2. Manifestations of somatic death include cessation of respiration and circulation, gradual lowering of body temperature, pupil dilation, loss of elasticity and transparency in the skin, muscle stiffening (rigor mortis), and skin discoloration (livor mortis). Signs of putrefaction are obvious about 24 to 48 hours after death.

KEY TERMS

KEY TERMS—cont'd

REFERENCES

1. Kornitzer D, Ciechnover A: Modes of regulation of ubiquitin-mediated protein degradation, *J Cell Phys* 182(1):1, 2000.
2. Kissane JM, editor: *Anderson's pathology,* ed 9, St Louis, 1990, Mosby.
3. Yeldandi AU, Kaufman DE, Reddy JK: Cell injury and cellular adaptations. In Damjanov I, Linder J, editors: *Anderson's pathology,* ed 10, St Louis, 1996, Mosby.
4. Bottaro DP et al: Identification of the hepatocyte growth factor receptor as the c-met proto-oncogene product, *Science* 251(4995):802, 1991.
5. Alberts B et al: *Molecular biology of the cell,* ed 4, New York, 1999, Garland.
6. London SJ et al: A prospective study of benign breast disease and the risk of breast cancer, *JAMA* 267(7):941, 1992.
7. Pryor WA: Vitamin E and heart disease: basic science to clinical intervention trials, *Free Radical Biol Med* 28(1):141, 2000.
8. Bergendi L et al: Chemistry, physiology, and pathology of free radicals, *Life Sci* 65(18-19):1865, 1999.
9. Roberts JW, Dickey P: Exposure of children to pollutants in house dust and indoor air, *Rev Environ Contam Toxicol* 143:59, 1995.
10. Holbrook J: Cigarette smoking. In Rom WH, editor: *Environmental and occupational medicine,* Boston, 1993, Little, Brown.
11. Cassel CK et al, editors: *Geriatric medicine,* ed 2, New York, 1990, Springer-Verlag.
12. Lieber CS: Hepatic, metabolic, and toxic effects of ethanol: 1991 update, *Alcohol Clin Exp Res* 15(4):574, 1991.
13. Noble EP: The gene that rewards alcoholism, *Sci Am Sci Med* 3(2):52, 1996
14. May JJ: Occupational hearing loss, *Am J Ind Med* 37(1):112, 2000.
15. Stradling JR et al: Which aspects of breathing during sleep influence the overnight fall of blood pressure in a community population? *Thorax* 55(5):393, 2000.
16. Lieber CS: Alcohol and the liver: metabolism of alcohol and its role in hepatic and extrahepatic diseases, *Int Sinai J Med* 67(1):84, 2000.
17. Mantle D, Preedy VR: Free radicals as mediators of alcohol toxicity, *Adv Drug React Toxicol Rev* 18(4):235, 1999.
18. Martinez F et al: Interleukin-6 and interleukin-8 production by mononuclear cells of chronic alcoholics during treatment, *Alcohol Clin Exp Res* 28(1):73, 1993.
19. Clark CM et al: Structural and functional brain integrity of fetal alcohol syndrome in nonretarded cases, *Pediatrics* 105(5):1096, 2000.
20. Ikonomidou C et al: Ethanol-induced apoptotic neurodegeneration and fetal alcohol syndrome, *Science* 287(5455):1056, 2000.
21. Boonstra J et al: The epidermal growth factor, *Cell Bio Int* 19(5):413, 1995.
22. Henderson GI et al: Ethanol, oxidative stress, reactive aldehydes, and the fetus, *Front Biosci* 15(4):D541, 1999.
23. Stanton B, Goldbraith J: Drug trafficking among African-American early adolescents: prevalence, consequences, and associated behaviors and beliefs, *Pediatrics* 93(6, pt 2):1039, 1994.
24. Centers for Disease Control: *Injury statistics website,* Washington, DC, 1997, Centers for Disease Control.
25. Wells JC: Can risk factors for over-heating explain epidemiological features of sudden infant death syndrome, *Med Hypotheses* 48(2):103, 1997.
26. Roy SB et al: Haemodynamic studies in high altitude pulmonary edema, *Br Heart J* 31:52, 1969.
27. Trosko JE: Biomarkers for low-level exposure causing epigenetic responses in stem cells, *Stem Cells (Dayt)* 13(suppl 1):231, 1995.
28. Koutz CA et al: Effect of dietary fat on the response of the rat retina to chronic and acute light stress, *Exp Eye Res* 60(3):307, 1995.
29. Weston HC: The effects of age and illumination upon visual performance with clore sights, *Br J Ophthalmol* 32:645, 1948.
30. Wilkins AJ, Wilkinson P: A tint to reduce eye-strain from fluorescent lighting? *Ophthalmic Physiol Opt* 11(2):172, 1991.
31. Ziegman S, Sutliff G, Rounds M: Relationships between human cataracts and environmental radiant energy: cataract formation, light scattering, and fluorescence, *Lens Eye Toxic Res* 8(23):259, 1991.
32. DeFlora S, D'Agostini F: Halogen lamp carcinogenicity, *Nature* 356(6370):569, 1992.
33. Burnstock G, Ralevec V: New insights into the local regulation of blood flow by perivascular nerves and endothelium, *Br J Plast Surg* 47(8):527, 1995.
34. Keyserling WM, Armstrong TJ: Ergonomics. In Last JM, Wallace RB, editors: *Maxey-Roseneau-Last: public health and preventive medicine,* ed 13, Norwalk, Conn, 1992, Appleton & Lange.
35. Halpern NA et al: Hearing loss in critical care: an unappreciated phenomenon, *Crit Care Med* 27(1):211, 1999.
36. Powell LW, Kerr JFR: Pathology of the liver in hemochromatosis, *Pathobiol Ann* 5:317, 1975.
37. Hayflick L: The limited in vitro lifetime of human diploid cell strains, *Exp Cell Res* 37:614, 1965.
38. Kerr JFR, Searle J: Apoptosis: its nature and kinetic role. In Meyn RE, Withers HR, editors: *Radiation biology in cancer research,* New York, 1980, Raven.
39. Lo AC, Houenou LJ, Oppenheim RW: Apoptosis in the nervous system: morphological features, methods, pathology, and prevention, *Arch Histol Cytol* 58(2):139, 1995.
40. Sanders EJ, Wride MA: Programmed cell death in development, *Int Rev Cytol* 163:105, 1995.
41. Robertson JD, Orrenius S, Zhivotovsky B: Review: nuclear events in apoptosis, *J Structural Biol* 129(2/3):346, 2000.
42. Wyllie AH, Kerr JFR, Currie AR: Cell death: the significance of apoptosis, *Int Rev Cytol* 68:251, 1980.
43. Alberts B et al: *Essential cell biology: an introduction to the molecular biology of the cell,* New York, 1998, Garland.
44. Johnson HA, editor: Is aging physiological or pathological? In *Relations between normal aging and disease,* New York, 1985, Raven.
45. Vijg J: Somatic mutations and aging: a re-evaluation, *Mutat Res* 447(1):117, 2000.
46. Poehlman ET et al: Physiological predictors of increasing total and central adiposity in aging men and women, *Arch Intern Med* 155(22): 2433, 1995.
47. Spillman BC, Lubitz J: The effect of longevity on spending for acute and long-term care, *N Engl J Med* 342(19):1409, 2000.

48. Trussel J: Women's longevity, *Science* 270(5237):719, 1995 (letter).
49. Weiss JE, Mushinski M: International mortality rates and life expectancy: selected countries, *Stat Bull Metrop Insurance Co* 80(1):13, 1999.
50. Baumgartner RN et al: Age-related changes in sex hormones affect the sex difference in serum leptin independently of changes in body fat, *Metabolism* 48(3):378, 1999.
51. Ginaldi L et al: Cell proliferation and apoptosis in the immune system in the elderly, *Immunol Res* 21(1):31, 2000.
52. Kahlke V et al: Immune dysfunction following trauma—hemorrhage: influence of gender and age, *Cytokine* 12(1):69, 2000.
53. Ory MG, Warner HR, editors: *Gender, health, and longevity: multidisciplinary perspectives,* New York, 1990, Springer.
54. Verbugge LM, Gruber-Baldini AL, Fozard JL: Age differences and age changes in activities: Baltimore longitudinal study of aging, *J Gerontol Behav Psychol Sci Soc Sci* 51(1):530, 1996.
55. Russell RL: Evidence for and against the theory of developmentally programmed aging. In Warner HR et al, editors: *Modern biological theories of aging,* New York, 1987, Raven.
56. Richter C et al: Oxidants in mitochondria: from physiology to diseases, *Biochem Biophys Acta* 127(1):67, 1995.
57. Cuervo AM, Dice JF: A receptor for the selective uptake and degradation of proteins by lysosomes, *Science* 273(5274):501, 1996.
58. Mera SL: Senescence and pathology of aging, *Med Lab Sci* 49:271, 1992.
59. Baumgartner RN et al: Cross-sectional age differences in body composition in persons 60 years of age, *J Gerontol Med Sci* 50A(6):M307, 1995.
60. Shennan T: *Postmortems and morbid anatomy,* ed 3, Baltimore, 1935, William Wood.
61. Minckler J, Anstall HB, Minckler TM: *Pathobiology: an introduction,* St Louis, 1971, Mosby.

CHAPTER 3

The Cellular Environment: Fluids and Electrolytes, Acids and Bases

SUE E. HUETHER

CHAPTER OUTLINE

The cells of the body live in a fluid environment that requires an electrolyte concentration and pH value (measure of the acidity or alkalinity of a solution) that are regulated within a very narrow range. A balance is maintained by an integration of renal, hormonal, and neural functions. Changes in the composition of electrolytes affect electrical potentials of excitatory cells and cause shifts of fluid from one compartment to another. Alterations in pH disrupt the cellular function of enzyme systems. Fluid fluctuations affect blood volume and cellular function. Disturbances in these functions are common and can be life threatening. Understanding how alterations occur and the body's ability to compensate or correct the disturbance is important to understanding many pathophysiologic conditions.

DISTRIBUTION OF BODY FLUIDS

The fluids of the body are distributed among functional compartments, or spaces, and provide a transport medium for cellular and tissue function. Water moves freely among body compartments and is distributed by osmotic and hydrostatic forces. The **intracellular fluid (ICF)** comprises all the fluid contained within cells. Because the ICF contains twice as many solutes as the ECF, the volume is two times larger than the ECF volume. The **extracellular fluid (ECF)** is all the fluid outside the cells and is divided into smaller compartments. The two main ECF compartments are the **interstitial fluid** and the **intravascular fluid**, which is the blood plasma. Other ECF compartments include the lymph and the transcellular fluids, such as the synovial, intestinal, biliary, hepatic, pancreatic, and cerebrospinal fluid; sweat; urine; and pleural, synovial, peritoneal, pericardial, and intraocular fluids.

The sum of fluids within all compartments constitutes the **total body water (TBW)** (Table 3-1). The volume of TBW is usually expressed as a percentage of body weight in kilograms. The standard value for TBW is 60% of a 70-kg adult male, which is equivalent to 42 L of fluid (Table 3-2). The rest of the body weight is made up of fat and fat-free solids, particularly bone.

Although the amount of fluid within the various compartments is relatively constant, there is exchange of solutes and water between compartments to maintain their unique compositions. The percentage of TBW varies with the amount of body fat and age. Because fat is water repelling (hydrophobic), very little water is contained in adipose cells. Individuals with more body fat have proportionately less TBW and tend to be more susceptible to fluid imbalances that cause dehydration.

Aging and Distribution of Body Fluids

The distribution and amount of TBW change with age (see Table 3-2). In newborn infants, TBW is about 75% to 80% of body weight because infants store less fat. The percentage of TBW decreases to about 67% of body weight during the first year of life. In the immediate postnatal period a physiologic loss of body water occurs amounting to 5% of body weight as the infant adjusts to a new environment. Infants are particularly susceptible to significant changes in TBW because of their high metabolic rate. The turnover of body fluids in infants is caused by their greater body surface area and by their high metabolic rate. The turnover of body fluid therefore is much faster. Loss of fluids from diarrhea can represent a significant proportion of body weight. Renal mechanisms of fluid and electrolyte conservation also may not be mature enough to counter the losses, so dehydration may develop rapidly.

During childhood, TBW slowly decreases to 60% to 65% of body weight. At adolescence the percentage of TBW approaches adult proportions, and gender differences begin to appear. Males eventually have a greater percentage of body water as a function of increasing muscle mass. Females have more body fat and less muscle as a function of estrogens and therefore have less water.

With increasing age the percentage of TBW declines further. The decrease is caused in part by an increased amount of fat and a decreased amount of muscle[1] and by a reduced ability to regulate sodium and water balance. With age the kidney becomes less efficient in producing concentrated urine, and the responses for conserving sodium become sluggish. The normal reduction of TBW in elderly people becomes clinically important with stress, such as fever or dehydration from any cause; loss of body fluids at such times can be severe and life threatening.

Although daily fluid intake may fluctuate widely, the body regulates water volume within a relatively narrow range. The primary sources of body water are drinking, ingestion of water in food, and water derived from oxidative metabolism. Normally, the largest amounts of water are lost through renal excretion. Lesser amounts are eliminated through the stool and through vaporization from the skin and lungs (insensible water loss) (Table 3-3).

Water Movement Between ICF and ECF

The movement of water between ICF and ECF compartments is primarily a function of osmotic forces. (Osmosis and other mechanisms of passive transport are discussed in Chapter 1.) Water moves freely across cell membranes, so the osmolality of TBW is normally at equilibrium. Sodium is the most abundant ECF ion and is responsible for the osmotic balance of the ECF space. Potassium maintains the osmotic balance of the ICF space. The osmotic force of ICF proteins and other nondiffusible substances is balanced by the active transport of ions out of the cell. Normally, the ICF is not subject to rapid changes in osmolality, but when there are changes in ECF osmolality, a net transfer of water from one compartment to another occurs until osmotic equilibrium is reestablished. Fig. 3-1 shows a model of the maintenance of osmotic equilibrium.

Water Movement Between Plasma and Interstitial Fluid

The distribution of water and the movement of nutrients and waste products among the capillary, plasma, and interstitial spaces occur as a result of changes in hydrostatic pressure and osmotic forces at the arterial and venous ends of the capillary. Because water, sodium, and glucose readily move across the capillary membrane, the plasma proteins maintain the effective osmolality by generating plasma oncotic pressure. Osmotic forces within the capillary are balanced by the hydrostatic pressure, which arises from cardiac contraction. The movement of fluid back and forth across the capillary wall is called **net filtration** and is best described by the **Starling hypothesis**:

$$\text{Net filtration} = (\text{Forces favoring filtration}) - (\text{Forces opposing filtration})$$

Table 3-1 Distribution of Body Water

	Percentage of Body Weight	Volume (L)
Intracellular fluid (ICF)	40	28
Extracellular fluid (ECF)	20	14
Interstitial	(15)	(11)
Intravascular	(5)	(3)
Total body water (TBW)	60	42

Table 3-2 Total Body Water in Relation to Body Weight

Body Build	TBW (%) Adult Male	TBW (%) Adult Female	TBW (%) Infant
Normal	60	50	70
Lean	70	60	80
Obese	50	42	60

NOTE: TBW (total body water) is a percentage of body weight.

Table 3-3 Normal Water Gains and Losses (70-kg man)

	Daily Intake (ml)		Daily Output (ml)
Drinking	1400-1800	Urine	1400-1800
Water in food	700-1000	Stool	100
Water of oxidation	300-400	Skin	300-500
		Lungs	600-800
TOTAL	2400-3200		2400-3200

The forces favoring filtration, or movement of water out of the capillary and into the interstitial space, include the capillary hydrostatic pressure and the interstitial oncotic pressure. The forces opposing filtration are the plasma oncotic pressure and the interstitial hydrostatic pressure. Normally, the interstitial forces are negligible because only a very small percentage of plasma proteins crosses the capillary membrane and interstitial fluid moves into cells or is drawn back into the plasma. Thus the major forces for filtration are within the capillary.

As the plasma flows from the arterial to the venous end of the capillary, changes in the force of hydrostatic pressure facilitate the movement of water across the capillary membrane. Oncotic pressure remains fairly constant because plasma proteins normally do not cross the capillary membrane. At the arterial end of the capillary, hydrostatic pressure is greater than capillary oncotic pressure and water filters into the interstitial space. Because of oncotic forces, there is some movement of water back into the capillary, but the net effect is loss of water from the capillary. The movement of water from the plasma causes the hydrostatic pressure within the capillary to decrease. Thus at the venous end of the capillary, oncotic pressure exceeds hydrostatic pressure. Fluids then are attracted back into the circulation, balancing the movement of fluids between the plasma and the interstitial space. The overall effect is filtration at the arterial end and reabsorption at the venous end (Fig. 3-2).

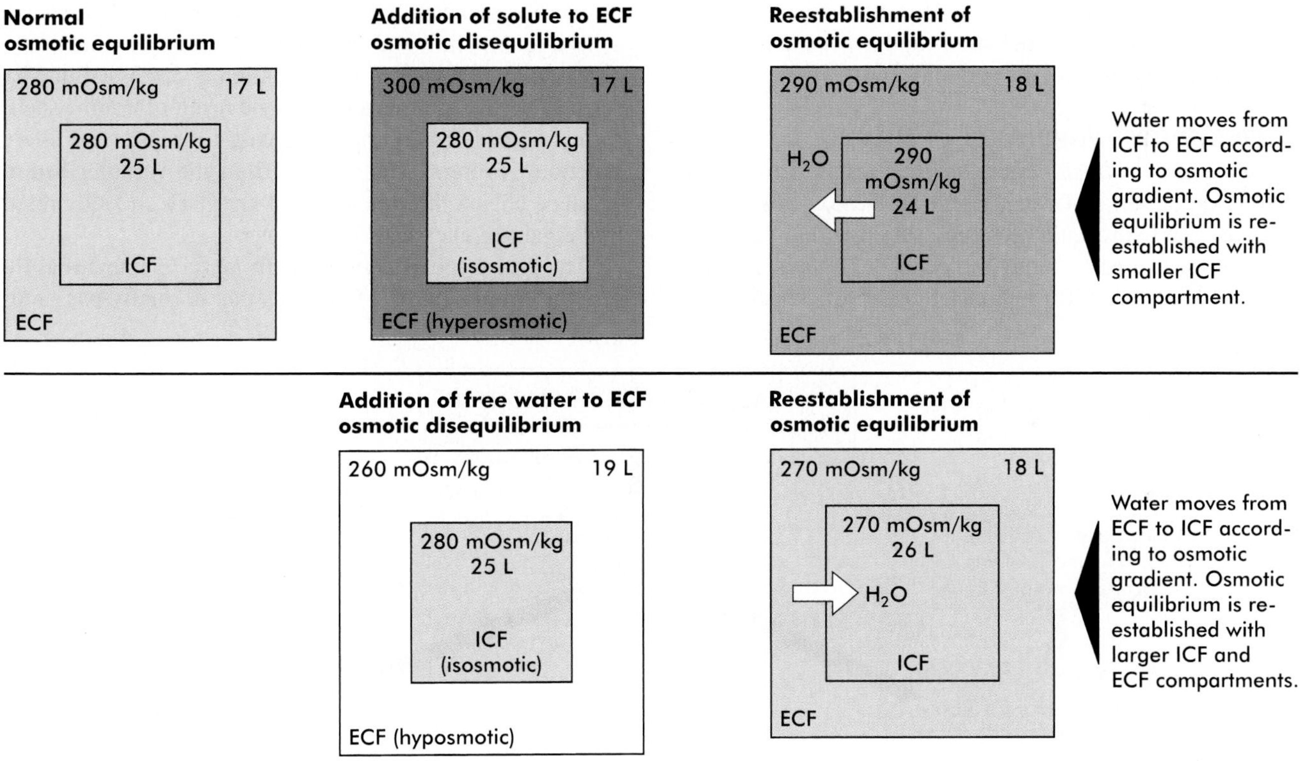

FIG. 3-1 Model of osmotic equilibrium. *ICF*, Intracellular fluid; *ECF*, extracellular fluid.

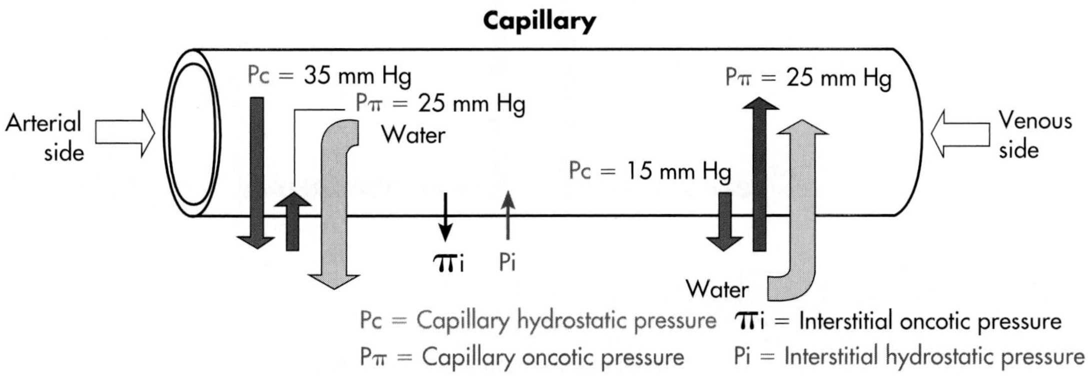

FIG. 3-2 Capillary net filtration forces.

An important factor in capillary filtration of fluid is the integrity of the capillary membrane. Changes in membrane permeability may permit the escape of plasma proteins into the interstitial space. The normal relationship defined by the Starling hypothesis is altered with the osmotic movement of water into the interstitial space, causing tissue edema.

ALTERATIONS IN WATER MOVEMENT

Edema

Edema is the accumulation of fluid within the interstitial spaces. It is a problem of fluid distribution and does not necessarily indicate a fluid excess. In some conditions, sequestered fluids can cause both edema and dehydration. The pathophysiologic process is related to an increase in the forces favoring fluid filtration from the capillaries or lymphatic channels into the tissues. The four most common mechanisms are increased hydrostatic pressure, decreased plasma oncotic pressure, increased capillary membrane permeability, and lymphatic obstruction (Fig. 3-3).

Pathophysiology

An *increase in hydrostatic pressure* can result from venous obstruction or salt and water retention. *Venous obstruction* can cause the hydrostatic pressure of fluid within the capillaries to become great enough to cause fluid to escape into the interstitial spaces. Thrombophlebitis, hepatic obstruction, tight clothing around the extremities, and prolonged standing are common causes of venous obstruction. Congestive heart failure and renal failure are both conditions associated with salt and water retention, which in turn cause volume overload and edema.

Losses or diminished production of plasma albumin contributes to a decrease in plasma oncotic pressure. Decreased oncotic attraction of fluid within the capillary causes fluid to move into the interstitial space. Decreased production of plasma protein may occur with liver disease or protein malnutrition, and losses occur with nephrotic syndrome. The escape of plasma proteins from the serum into the interstitial space also enhances the movement of water from the plasma into the tissues. Losses of plasma proteins occur with glomerular diseases of the kidney, serous drainage from open wounds, hemorrhage, burns, and cirrhosis of the liver.

Increases in capillary permeability are usually associated with inflammation and the immune response. (Immunity is discussed in Chapter 6; inflammation is discussed in Chapter 7.) These responses are often the result of trauma such as burns or crushing injuries, neoplastic disease, and allergic reactions. Proteins then escape from the vascular bed and produce edema through a loss of capillary oncotic pressure and a gain in interstitial fluid proteins.

The lymphatic system normally absorbs interstitial fluid and the small amount of proteins that normally pass across

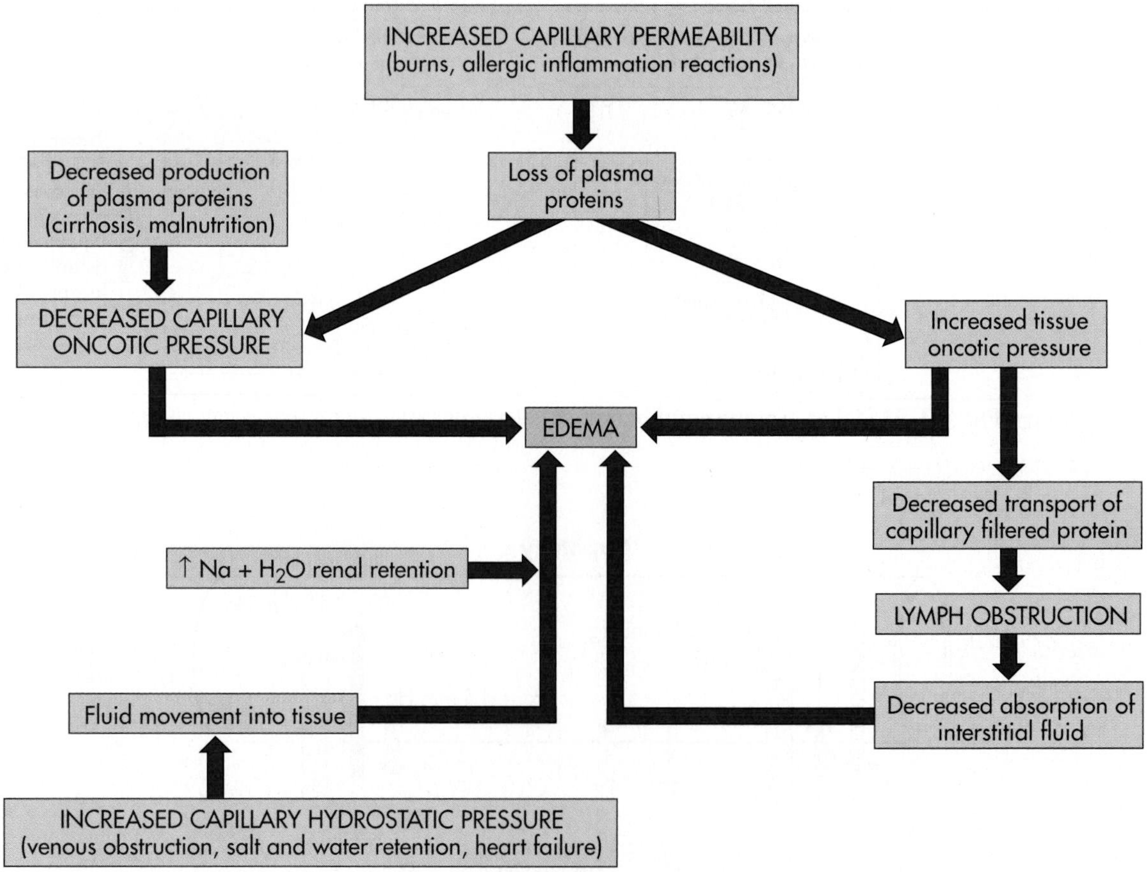

FIG. 3-3 Mechanisms of edema formation.

the capillary membrane. When the lymphatic channels are blocked (because of infection) or are surgically removed, proteins and fluid accumulate in the interstitial space causing **lymphedema.** For example, lymphedema of the arm or leg will occur after surgical removal of axillary and femoral lymph nodes for treatment of carcinoma.[2] Inflammation or tumors may be a cause of lymphatic obstruction leading to edema.

Clinical Manifestations

Edema may be localized or generalized. Some localized edema is limited to the site of trauma, as in a sprained finger or within particular organ systems. This includes cerebral edema, pulmonary edema, pleural effusion, pericardial effusion, and ascites (accumulation of fluid in the peritoneal space). Dependent edema, in which fluid accumulates in gravity-dependent areas of the body, might be a sign of more generalized edema. Dependent edema might appear in the feet and legs when standing and in the sacral area and buttocks when lying down. Dependent edema can be identified by using the fingers to press away edematous fluid in tissues overlying bony prominences. A pit will be left in the skin; hence the term *pitting edema.*

Edema is usually associated with weight gain, swelling and puffiness, tight-fitting clothes and shoes, limited movement of the affected area, and symptoms associated with the underlying pathologic condition. The accumulation of fluid increases the distance required for nutrients, oxygen, and wastes to move between capillaries and tissues. Increased tissue pressure may diminish capillary blood flow. Therefore wounds heal more slowly and the risks of infection and formation of pressure sores increase. Edema of specific organs, such as the brain, lung, or larynx, can be life threatening.

Although the accumulation of fluid is excessive, it is trapped in a "third space" and is not available for metabolic processes. Therefore a state of dehydration can develop as a result of the sequestering of the edematous fluid. An example of such sequestration occurs with severe burns, in which large amounts of vascular fluid are lost to the interstitial spaces, reducing plasma volume and causing shock (see Chapter 45).

Evaluation and Treatment

Specific conditions causing edema require diagnosis. Edema may be treated symptomatically until the underlying disorder is corrected. Supportive measures include elevating edematous limbs, using compression stockings, avoiding prolonged standing, restricting salt intake, and taking diuretics.

SODIUM, CHLORIDE, AND WATER BALANCE

Because water follows the osmotic gradients established by changes in salt concentration, sodium balance and water balance are intimately related. Water balance is primarily regulated by antidiuretic hormone (ADH; also known as *arginine-vasopressin*) from the posterior pituitary. Sodium is regulated by aldosterone from the adrenal cortex.

Water Balance

Secretion of ADH and perception of thirst are primary factors in the regulation of water balance. Thirst is a sensation that stimulates water-drinking behavior. Thirst is experienced when water loss equals 2% of an individual's body weight or when there is an increase in osmolality. Dry mouth, hyperosmolality, and plasma volume depletion activate **osmoreceptors** (neurons located in the hypothalamus that are stimulated by increased osmolality). The action of the osmoreceptors then causes thirst. Drinking water restores plasma volume and dilutes the ECF osmolality.

The secretion of ADH is initiated by an increase in plasma osmolality or a decrease in circulating blood volume and a lowered blood pressure. An increase in plasma osmolality occurs with a deficit of water or an excess of sodium in relation to water. The increased osmolality results in decreased extracellular and interstitial fluid volume and stimulates hypothalamic osmoreceptors. In addition to causing thirst, the stimulated osmoreceptors increase the release of ADH. The action of ADH is to increase the permeability of renal tubular cells to water, and water is then reabsorbed into the plasma from the distal tubules and collecting ducts of the kidney. Urine concentration increases, and the reabsorbed water decreases plasma osmolality, returning it toward normal. Like most hormones, ADH is regulated by a feedback mechanism (Fig. 3-4).

With volume depletion, such as dehydration from vomiting, diarrhea, or excessive sweating, **volume-sensitive**

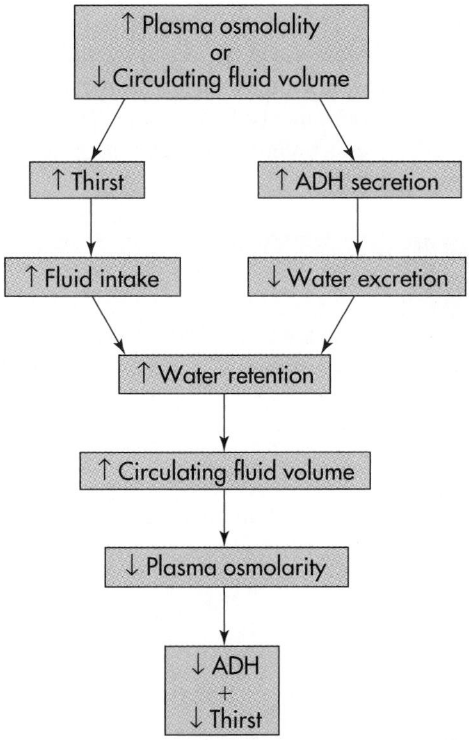

FIG. 3-4 Regulation of thirst and antidiuretic hormone (ADH) secretion.

receptors and **baroreceptors** (nerve endings that are sensitive to changes in volume and pressure) stimulate release of ADH. The volume receptors are located in the right and left atria and thoracic vessels; baroreceptors are in the aorta, pulmonary arteries, and carotid sinus. Secretion of ADH is caused also by a decrease in atrial pressure, as occurs with decreased blood volume. The reabsorption of water mediated by ADH then promotes the restoration of plasma volume.

Sodium and Chloride Balance

Sodium accounts for 90% of the ECF cations (positively charged ions). (The distribution of electrolytes in body compartments is summarized in Table 3-4.) As the most abundant ECF cation, along with its constituent anions (negatively charged ions) chloride and bicarbonate, sodium regulates osmotic forces and therefore regulates water balance. Sodium has many important body functions, including regulation of osmolality (interstitial and intravascular fluid volume), working with potassium and calcium to maintain neuromuscular irritability for conduction of nerve impulses, regulation of acid-base balance (through sodium bicarbonate and sodium phosphate), participation in cellular chemical reactions, and membrane transport.

Chloride is the major anion in the extracellular fluid. It provides electroneutrality, particularly in relation to sodium. The transport of chloride is generally passive and follows the active transport of sodium, so that increases or decreases in chloride are proportional to changes in sodium. Because bicarbonate is the other major anion in the ECF, the concentration of chloride tends to vary inversely with changes in bicarbonate concentration.

The concentration of sodium is maintained within a narrow range (136 to 145 mEq/L), primarily by the kidney in conjunction with neural and hormonal mediators. The average dietary intake of sodium ranges from 5 to 6 g/day; the minimal daily requirement of sodium is 500 mg. Sweating depletes sodium and water volume and increases the body's sodium requirement.

Table 3-4 Distribution of Electrolytes in Body Compartments

	Extracellular Fluid (mEq/L)	Intracellular Fluid (mEq/L)
CATIONS		
Sodium	142	10
Potassium	5	156
Calcium	5	4
Magnesium	2	26
TOTALS	154	196
ANIONS		
Bicarbonate	24	12
Chloride	104	4
Phosphate	2	40-95
Proteins	16	54
Other anions	8	31-86
TOTALS	154	196 (average)

The kidney regulates sodium balance primarily through renal tubular reabsorption. Under normal rates of sodium intake, the tubules of the kidney function to reabsorb sodium. With an excess or deficit of sodium in relation to water, a combination of hormonal, neural, and renal mechanisms acts synergistically to control sodium balance.

The hormonal regulation of sodium balance is mediated by **aldosterone,** a mineralocorticoid synthesized and secreted from the adrenal cortex (see Chapter 19). The secretion of aldosterone is influenced by both circulating blood volume and plasma concentrations of sodium (Na^+) and potassium (K^+) (i.e., aldosterone is secreted when sodium levels are depressed, potassium levels are increased, or renal perfusion is decreased). The action of aldosterone is to increase the reabsorption of sodium and secretion of potassium by the distal tubule of the kidney. As a result, sodium concentration of the ECF is enhanced and potassium is excreted with the urine.

When circulating blood volume is reduced, **renin,** an enzyme secreted by the juxtaglomerular cells of the kidney, is released in response to sympathetic nerve stimulation and decreased perfusion of the renal vasculature. Renin stimulates the formation of **angiotensin I,** an inactive polypeptide, which is then converted into **angiotensin II,** which acts as a hormone. Angiotensin II has two major functions: it stimulates the secretion of aldosterone, and it causes vasoconstriction. The aldosterone then promotes sodium and water reabsorption. The vasoconstriction elevates the systemic blood pressure and restores renal perfusion. The restoration of sodium levels, fluid volume, and renal perfusion then inhibits further release of renin. This sodium and water regulation mechanism is known as the **renin-angiotensin system** (see Chapter 34).

Natriuretic peptides are hormones produced by the heart (atrial natriuretic peptide [ANP]), brain (natriuretic peptide [BNP]), and kidney (urodilatin) and decrease blood pressure and increase sodium and water excretion.[3] ANP is released when there is an increase in transmural atrial pressure (increased volume).[4] Natriuretic hormone is sometimes called a "third factor" in sodium regulation. (Increased glomerular filtration rate is thus the first factor and aldosterone the second factor.)

ALTERATIONS IN SODIUM, CHLORIDE, AND WATER BALANCE

Alterations in sodium and water balance are closely related. Water imbalances may develop because of changes in osmotic gradients caused by gain or loss of salt. Likewise, sodium imbalances occur with alterations in body water volume. Generally, the alterations can be classified as changes in tonicity, or the change in concentration of electrolytes in relation to water (see Chapter 1). Alterations can therefore be classified as isotonic, hypertonic, or hypotonic (Table 3-5).

Isotonic Alterations

Isotonic alterations occur when changes in TBW are accompanied by proportional changes in electrolytes and water. For example, if an individual loses pure plasma or ECF, fluid volume is depleted but the number and type of electrolytes and the osmolality remain in a normal range. Excessive amounts of isotonic body fluids can result from excessive administration of intravenous normal saline or oversecretion of aldosterone with renal retention of both sodium and water. Losses of isotonic body fluids include hemorrhage, severe wound drainage, excessive diaphoresis, intestinal losses, and decreased fluid intake.

Isotonic volume depletion causes contraction of the ECF volume with weight loss, dryness of skin and mucous membranes, decreased urine output, and symptoms of hypovolemia. Indicators of hypovolemia include a rapid heart rate, flattened neck veins, and normal or decreased blood pressure. In severe states, hypovolemic shock can occur (see Chapter 45).

Isotonic volume excesses are most commonly the result of excessive administration of intravenous fluids, hypersecretion of aldosterone, or the effects of drugs such as cortisone. As the plasma volume expands, symptoms of hypervolemia develop. There will be weight gain and a decrease in hematocrit and plasma protein concentration caused by the diluting effect of excess plasma volume. The neck veins may distend, and the blood pressure increases. Increased capillary hydrostatic pressure leads to edema formation. If the plasma volume is great enough, pulmonary edema and heart failure develop.

Table 3-5 Water and Solute Imbalances

Tonicity	Mechanism
Isotonic (isoosmolar) imbalance	Gain or loss of extracellular fluid (ECF) resulting in a concentration equivalent to a 0.9% sodium chloride (salt) solution (normal saline); no shrinking or swelling of cells
Hypertonic (hyperosmolar) imbalance	Imbalances that result in an ECF concentration greater than 0.9% salt solution, i.e., water loss or solute gain; cells shrink in a hypertonic fluid
Hypotonic (hypoosmolar) imbalance	Imbalance that results in an ECF less than 0.9% salt solution, i.e., water gain or solute loss; cells swell in a hypotonic fluid

Hypertonic Alterations

Hypertonic fluid alterations develop when the osmolality of the ECF is elevated above normal. The most common causes are an increased concentration of ECF sodium (hypernatremia) or a deficit of ECF free water. In both instances the hypertonicity of the ECF attracts water from the intracellular space, causing ICF dehydration. A primary increase in ECF sodium causes an osmotic attraction of water and symptoms of hypervolemia. In contrast, a hypertonic state caused primarily by free water loss leads to hypovolemia (Table 3-6).

Hypernatremia

Pathophysiology

Hypernatremia occurs when serum sodium levels exceed 147 mEq/L. Excessive serum sodium may be caused by an

Table 3-6 Causes and Consequences of Hypertonic Imbalances

Causative Factor	Mechanism	ECF Effects	ICF Effects
Increased sodium (hypernatremia)	**Excessive hypertonic salt solutions** Intravenous hypertonic sodium Saline-induced abortions Selected infant formulas **Hyperaldosteronism** **Cushing syndrome**	**Hypervolemia** Weight gain Bounding pulse Increased blood pressure Edema Venous distention **Neuromuscular symptoms** Muscle weakness Seizures	**Intracellular dehydration** Thirst Fever Decreased urine output Shrinkage of brain cells Confusion Coma Cerebral hemorrhage
Water deficit	**Water deprivation** Confusion or coma Inability to communicate Loss of thirst **Water loss** Watery diarrhea Diabetes insipidus Excessive diuresis Excessive diaphoresis	**Hypovolemia** Weight loss Weak pulses Postural hypotension Tachycardia	**Intracellular dehydration** See above
Other factors	Hyperglycemia	Initial dilutional hyponatremia Polyuria Polydipsia Weight loss Hypovolemia Late hypernatremia	**Intracellular dehydration** See above

ECF, Extracellular fluid; *ICF,* intracellular fluid.

acute gain in sodium or a loss of water. Sodium gains cause intracellular dehydration; the movement of water to the ECF may cause hypervolemia. With an accompanying water loss, both ICF dehydration and ECF dehydration occur. Hyperosmolality is a common result of hypernatremia.

High amounts of dietary sodium rarely cause hypernatremia. More commonly, high sodium levels occur because of (1) inadequate free water intake, (2) inappropriate administration of hypertonic saline solution (e.g., as sodium bicarbonate for treatment of acidosis during cardiac arrest), (3) high sodium levels as a result of oversecretion of aldosterone (as in primary hyperaldosteronism), or (4) Cushing syndrome (caused by excess secretion of adrenocorticotropic hormone [ACTH], which also causes increased secretion of aldosterone).[5,6]

Increased sodium in relation to water loss is associated with fever or respiratory infections, which increase the respiratory rate and enhance water loss from the lungs. Diabetes insipidus (excess production of ADH), diabetes mellitus, polyuria, profuse sweating, and diarrhea cause water loss in relation to sodium. Infants with severe diarrhea are particularly vulnerable. Insufficient water intake also can cause hypernatremia, particularly in individuals who are comatose, confused, or immobilized.

Clinical Manifestations

Water is redistributed to the extracellular space, and intracellular dehydration ensues. Convulsions and pulmonary edema are the most serious symptoms. Thirst, fever, dry mucous membranes, hypotension, tachycardia, low jugular venous pressure, and restlessness are associated with hypernatremia as a result of water loss.

Evaluation and Treatment

The serum sodium level is usually more than 147 mEq/L. If there is water loss, urine specific gravity will be greater than 1.030 and hematocrit and plasma proteins will be elevated. The treatment of hypernatremia is to give an isotonic salt-free fluid (5% dextrose in water) until the serum sodium level returns to normal. Hypervolemia and edema require treatment of the underlying clinical condition.

Water Deficit

Pathophysiology

Dehydration is an appropriate term to describe water deficit, but dehydration is also commonly used to indicate both sodium loss and water loss (isotonic or isoosmolar dehydration). Pure **water deficits** (hyperosmolar or hypertonic dehydration) are rare because most people have access to water. Individuals who are comatose or paralyzed will continue insensible water losses through the skin and lungs with a minimal obligatory formation of urine. Hyperventilation caused by fever also may precipitate water deficit. The most frequent cause of water loss is increased renal clearance of free water as a result of impaired tubular function or inability to concentrate the urine, as with diabetes insipidus (see Chapter 20).

Clinical Manifestations

Marked water deficit is manifested by symptoms of dehydration: thirst, dry skin and mucous membranes, elevated temperature, weight loss, and concentrated urine (with the exception of diabetes insipidus). Skin turgor may be normal or decreased. Symptoms of hypovolemia, including tachycardia, weak pulses, and postural hypotension, may be present.

Evaluation and Treatment

An elevated hematocrit and serum sodium concentration are associated with moderate water loss in addition to clinical signs and symptoms.

Treatment is to give water. When intravenous replacement is required, 5% dextrose in water should be used because pure water lyses red blood cells.

Hyperchloremia

Hyperchloremia occurs clinically when there is an excess of sodium or a deficit of bicarbonate. Greater than normal amounts of chloride can be expected with hypernatremia or metabolic acidosis (see p. 106). Ingestion of excessive chloride infrequently accompanies the use of an ammonium chloride diuretic. No specific symptoms are associated with chloride excess.

Alterations in chloride levels are usually secondary to their pathophysiologic processes. Treatment therefore generally is related to management of the underlying disorder.

Hypotonic Alterations

Hypotonic fluid imbalances occur when the osmolality of the ECF is less than normal. The most common causes are sodium deficit **(hyponatremia)** or free water excess. Either of these causes leads to an intracellular overhydration (edema). When there is a sodium deficit, the osmotic pressure of the ECF decreases and water moves into the cell, where the osmotic pressure is greater. The plasma volume then decreases, leading to symptoms of hypovolemia. With free water excess, both the ICF volume and the ECF volume increase, causing symptoms of hypervolemia (Table 3-7) and water intoxication with cerebral and pulmonary edema.[7]

Hyponatremia

Pathophysiology

Hyponatremia develops when the serum sodium concentration decreases to less than 135 mEq/L. Sodium deficits usually cause hypoosmolality with movement of water into cells with cell swelling. Several clinical syndromes may cause hyponatremia. These syndromes may be caused by sodium loss, inadequate sodium intake, or dilution of the body's sodium level.

Pure sodium deficits usually are caused by diuretics[8] and extrarenal losses such as vomiting, diarrhea, gastrointestinal suctioning, or burns. **Inadequate intake** of dietary sodium is rare but can occur in individuals on low-sodium diets, particularly among those taking diuretics. **Dilutional hyponatremias** occur when there is an excess of TBW in re-

Table 3-7 Causes and Consequences of Hypotonic Imbalances

Causative Factor	Mechanism	ECF Effects	ICF Effects
Decreased sodium (hyponatremia)	**Inadequate intake** **Hyperaldosteronism** **Excessive diuretic therapy** Furosemide Ethacrinic acid Thiazides	**Extracellular volume contraction and hypovolemia** (but may not be if there is water excess)	**Increased intracellular water; edema** Brain cell swelling, irritability, depression, confusion Systemic cellular edema, including weakness, anorexia, nausea, and diarrhea
Water excess	**Excessive pure water intake** Excessive administration of hypotonic intravenous solutions Drinking water to replace isotonic fluid losses Tap water enemas Psychogenic polydipsia Renal water retention Syndrome of inappropriate antidiuretic hormone (SIADH)	**Extracellular volume expands with hypervolemia** (but may not be if fluid is trapped in intracellular space)	**Edema** (see above)
Other factors	Isotonic dehydration treated with intravenous D_5W; glucose in D_5W solution is metabolized to water, contributing to hyponatremia Nephrotic syndrome Cirrhosis Cardiac failure	**Hypervolemia** or **hypovolemia**	**Edema** (see above)

ECF, Extracellular fluid; *ICF*, intracellular fluid.

lation to total body sodium or a shift of water from the ICF to ECF space (e.g., administration of mannitol). Replacement of fluid loss with intravenous 5% dextrose in water also can cause a dilutional hyponatremia once the glucose is metabolized, leaving a hypotonic solution with a diluting effect. In addition, excessive sweating may stimulate thirst and intake of large amounts of water, which dilute sodium.

Hyponatremia also may be hypoosmolar or hypertonic. During acute oliguric renal failure, severe congestive heart failure, or cirrhosis, renal excretion of water is impaired. Both TBW and sodium levels are increased, but TBW exceeds the increase in sodium, producing a **hypoosmolar hyponatremia**.

Hypertonic hyponatremia develops with hyperlipidemia, hyperproteinemia, and hyperglycemia. Increases in plasma lipids and proteins displace water volume and decrease sodium concentration. Hyperglycemia increases ECF osmolality and attracts water from the ICF compartment. The osmotic fluid shift to the ECF in turn dilutes the concentration of sodium and other electrolytes.

Clinical Manifestations

Deficits of sodium alter the ability of cells to depolarize and repolarize normally (see Chapter 1). Behavioral and neurologic changes characteristic of hyponatremia include lethargy, headache, confusion, apprehension, seizures, and coma. Pure sodium losses may be accompanied by loss of ECF causing an isotonic **hypovolemia** with symptoms of hypotension, tachycardia, and decreased urine output. Weight gain, edema, ascites, and jugular vein distention are characteristic of dilutional hyponatremias.

Evaluation and Treatment

In hyponatremic states, serum sodium concentration falls to less than 135 mEq/L. With pure sodium deficits, the hematocrit and plasma protein levels may be elevated. Urine specific gravity is less than 1.010 when renal function is normal because sodium is maximally conserved.

Treatment of hyponatremia is related to the contributing disorder. Losses of sodium and water volume are calculated from the clinical evaluation, and appropriate solutions then are selected for replacement. Restriction of water intake is required in most cases of dilutional hyponatremia because body sodium levels may be normal or increased even though serum levels are low. Hypertonic saline solutions are used cautiously with severe symptoms, such as seizures.[9]

Water Excess

Pathophysiology

When the body is functioning normally, it is almost impossible to produce an excess of TBW. Some individuals with psychogenic disorders develop water intoxication from **compulsive water drinking**. Acute renal failure, severe congestive heart failure, and cirrhosis are clinical conditions that can precipitate water excess. **Decreased urine formation** from intrinsic renal disease or decreased renal blood flow contributes to water excess. The overall effect is dilution of the ECF with the movement of water to the intracellular space by osmosis.

Water excess produces a hypotonic or hypoosmolar water imbalance.

The **syndrome of inappropriate secretion of ADH (SIADH)** is another circumstance contributing to excess water.[10] SIADH occurs when factors other than hyperosmolality or hypovolemia stimulate the secretion of or response to ADH. The amount of ADH is inappropriate in relation to sodium levels. Several clinical conditions associated with stress result in SIADH. These include fear, pain, acute infection, brain trauma, surgery, and drugs such as analgesics and anesthetics. The most common cause is cells that secrete ADH in bronchogenic cancer. SIADH is not caused by excess water intake but by decreased renal excretion of water. Therefore the presence of SIADH increases the risk of water excess if intravenous fluids are being administered. Serum sodium and osmolality are reduced. The kidney continues to excrete sodium and urine specific gravity is elevated, but urine volume is decreased or water is reabsorbed.

Clinical Manifestations

The symptoms of water excess are related to the rate at which water loading has occurred. Acute excesses cause confusion and convulsions. Weakness, nausea, muscle twitching, headache, and weight gain are common symptoms of chronic water accumulation.

Evaluation and Treatment

Serum sodium concentration can be decreased, but this also can occur with a pure sodium deficit. Serum osmolality is decreased because water will be in excess of sodium. The hematocrit therefore is reduced from the dilutional effect of water excess.

WHAT'S NEW? Hospital-Acquired Hyponatremia

Severe hyponatremia (serum sodium <120 mmol/L) is the most common electrolyte abnormality among hospitalized individuals. In addition to elderly individuals, children and premenopausal women are at particular risk. Death or brain damage may range from 50% to 83% and is related to cerebral edema, increased intracranial pressure, and cerebral hypoxemia with symptoms of seizure, respiratory arrest, coma, and death. Postoperative hyponatremia is caused by administration of hypotonic fluids and secretion of antidiuretic hormone. Treatment with hypertonic sodium chloride is usually safe with acute hyponatremia. There is the risk of brain myelinolysis if treatment is too rapid. Treatment with urea or mannitol has also been reported. Fluid restriction can be effective in less severe cases. Frequent monitoring with attention to subtle symptoms and early treatment lead to improved outcomes.

Data from Ayus JC, Arieff AI: Chronic hyponatremic encephalopathy in postmenopausal women, association of therapies with morbidity and mortality, *JAMA* 281(24):2299, 1999; Crook MA et al: Review of investigation of management of severe hyponatremia in a hospital population, *Ann Clin Biochem* 36(pt 2):158, 1999; Fraser CL, Arieff AI: Epidemiology, pathophysiology, and management of hyponatremic encephalopathy, *Am J Med* 102(1):67, 1997; Steele A et al: Postoperative hyponatremia despite near-isotonic saline infusion: a phenomenon of desalination, *Ann Intern Med* 126(1):20, 1997.

Withholding fluid for 24 hours is effective treatment if there are no convulsions. Small amounts of intravenous hypertonic sodium chloride can be given when symptoms are severe.

Hypochloremia

Loss of chloride, or **hypochloremia**, is usually the result of hyponatremia, or elevated bicarbonate concentration, as in metabolic alkalosis (see p. 107). Hypochloremia develops with vomiting and loss of hydrochloric acid. Sodium deficit related to restricted intake or use of diuretics is accompanied by chloride deficiency. Cystic fibrosis, for example, is also characterized by hypochloremia. As with hyperchloremia, treatment of the underlying condition is required.

ALTERATIONS IN POTASSIUM, CALCIUM, PHOSPHATE, AND MAGNESIUM BALANCE

Potassium

Potassium is the major intracellular electrolyte and contributes to many important cellular functions. Total body potassium content is about 4000 mEq, with most of it located in the cells. Daily dietary intake of potassium is 40 to 150 mEq/day, with an average of 1.5 mEq/kg body weight. The ICF concentration of K^+ is 150 to 160 mEq/L; the ECF concentration is 3.5 to 4.5 mEq/L. K^+ is found in most body fluids (Table 3-8).

The difference in the concentration is maintained by a sodium-potassium active transport system (Na^+-K^+ ATPase pump). The ratio of ECF K^+ to ICF K^+ is the major determinant of the resting membrane potential, which is necessary for the transmission of nerve impulses. (Membrane transport and membrane potentials are discussed in Chapter 1.) Changes in the ratio of ICF to ECF potassium are responsible for many of the symptoms associated with potassium imbalance.

Potassium is necessary for a variety of metabolic functions. As the predominant ICF ion, it exerts a major influ-

Table 3-8 Approximate Concentration of Electrolytes in Body Fluids

Fluid	Na^+ (mEq/L)	K^+ (mEq/L)	Cl^- (mEq/L)	HCO_3^- (mEq/L)
Saliva	33	20	34	0
Gastric juice*	60	9	84	0
Bile	149	5	101	45
Pancreatic juice	141	5	77	92
Ileal fluid	129	11	116	29
Cecal fluid	80	21	48	22
Cerebrospinal fluid	141	3	127	23
Sweat	45	5	58	0

From Smith LH, Thier SO: *Pathophysiology: the biological principles of disease,* Philadelphia, 1981, Saunders.
Na^+, Sodium; *K^+*, potassium; *Cl^-*, chloride; *HCO_3^-*, bicarbonate; *H^+*, hydrogen.
*The Cl^- concentration exceeds the Na^+, K^+ concentration by 15 mEq/L in gastric juice. This largely represents the secretion of H^+ by the parietal cells.

ence in the regulation of ICF osmolality and provides the balance for intracellular electrical neutrality in relation to hydrogen (H^+) and Na^+. Potassium is required for glycogen deposition in liver and skeletal muscle cells. The significant role of potassium in maintaining the resting membrane potential is reflected in transmission and conduction of nerve impulses, maintenance of normal cardiac rhythms, and skeletal and smooth muscle contraction.

The kidney provides the most efficient regulation of potassium balance. The amount of K^+ excreted varies in proportion to the dietary intake (40 to 120 mEq/day). Potassium is freely filtered by the renal glomerulus, and 90% is reabsorbed by the proximal tubule and loop of Henle. The distal tubule secretes potassium and determines the amount of K^+ excreted from the body. The transport is passive, because K^+ is secreted to the lumen when sodium is reabsorbed. Unlike sodium, however, the renal mechanism for conserving K^+ is weak, even when total body potassium stores are depleted.

Several factors related to passive transport and aldosterone contribute to renal regulation of potassium. These factors include the concentration gradients for potassium at the distal tubule and collecting duct, changes in pH (causing acidosis or alkalosis), changes in electrical potential differences across the distal tubule, and aldosterone levels. (Renal mechanisms are described in more detail in Chapter 34.)

The concentration of potassium in the distal tubular cell is determined primarily by the plasma concentration in the peritubular capillaries. When plasma K^+ concentration increases from increased dietary intake or shifts from the ICF occur, potassium is secreted into the urine by the distal tubules. Decreases in plasma potassium result in decreased distal tubular secretion, although K^+ losses of approximately 5 to 15 mEq/day will continue. Changes in the rate of filtrate flow through the distal tubule also influence the concentration gradient for K^+ secretion. When the flow rate is high, as occurs with the administration of diuretics, the concentration of potassium in the distal tubular urine will be lower, favoring the secretion of potassium.[11]

Changes in pH and thus in hydrogen ion concentration also affect K^+ balance. Hydrogen ions accumulate in the ICF during states of acidosis. During acidosis, potassium shifts out of the cell to the ECF to maintain a balance of cations across the cell membrane. The decreased ICF K^+ results in decreased secretion of K^+ into the urine by the distal tubular cells, contributing to hyperkalemia. In contrast, intracellular fluid levels of hydrogen are diminished during states of alkalosis. Alkalosis causes potassium to shift into the cell, so the distal tubular cells increase their secretion of K^+ into the urine, contributing to hypokalemia.

Besides acting to conserve sodium, *aldosterone is a major factor in potassium regulation.* When potassium concentration is increased, aldosterone is released, stimulating secretion of potassium into the urine by the distal tubules of the kidney. Aldosterone also increases the secretion of K^+ from the sweat glands.

Insulin contributes to the regulation of plasma potassium levels by promoting the movement of potassium into liver and muscle cells. Insulin therefore can be used to treat hyperkalemia, and dangerously low levels of plasma potassium can result from the administration of insulin when potassium levels are depressed. Potassium balance is especially significant in the treatment of conditions requiring insulin administration, such as insulin-dependent diabetes.

Catecholamines also influence K^+ concentration in ECF. β_2 adrenergics stimulate the movement of K^+ into cells, and α adrenergics shift K^+ out of cells.[12]

An interesting aspect of K^+ regulation is the ability of the body to adapt to increased levels of potassium intake over time. A sudden increase in potassium may be fatal, but if the intake of potassium is slowly increased by amounts more than 120 mEq/day, the kidney is able to increase the urinary excretion of potassium and maintain potassium balance. This tolerance to increasing amounts of potassium is known as **potassium adaptation.**

Hypokalemia

Pathophysiology

Potassium deficiency, or **hypokalemia,** develops when the serum potassium concentration decreases to less than 3.5 mEq/L. Because cellular and total body stores of potassium are difficult to measure, changes in potassium balance are described by the plasma concentration, although changes in total body potassium are not always reflected in the plasma potassium concentration. Generally, lowered serum potassium indicates a loss of total body potassium. Because potassium is lost from the ECF, the change in the concentration gradient favors movement of K^+ from the cell to the ECF. The ICF/ECF concentration ratio is maintained, but total body K^+ is depleted.

Extracellular fluid hypokalemia can, however, develop without losses of total body potassium. For example, potassium shifts into the cell during states of respiratory or metabolic alkalosis or after administration of insulin. In the event of alkalosis, K^+ shifts into the cell in exchange for H^+ to maintain plasma acid-base balance. Insulin also promotes cellular uptake of K^+, causing a deficit in ECF potassium.

Plasma K^+ levels may be normal or elevated when total body potassium is depleted. In such instances, potassium shifts from the ICF to the ECF. One of the common causes of this problem is diabetic ketoacidosis, in which the increased hydrogen ion concentration in the ECF causes H^+ to shift into the cell in exchange for potassium. A normal level of potassium is maintained in the plasma, but potassium continues to be lost in the urine, causing a deficit in total body potassium. Severe, even fatal, hypokalemia may occur if insulin is administered without also providing potassium supplements. Thus total body potassium depletion becomes evident when insulin treatment is initiated.

Potassium loss also occurs through normal body functions without causing hypokalemia. Average daily losses of potassium are as follows:

LOCATION	DAILY LOSS (mEq/L)
Stool	5-10
Sweat	0-20
Urine	40-120

Factors contributing to the development of hypokalemia include reduced intake of potassium, increased entry of potassium into cells, and increased losses of body potassium. Dietary deficiency of potassium is a rare cause of hypokalemia. It may occur in elderly individuals with both low protein intake and inadequate intake of fruits and vegetables and in persons with alcoholism or anorexia nervosa. Generally, reduced potassium intake becomes a problem when combined with other causes of potassium depletion.

Shifts of potassium from the extracellular to intracellular space cause apparent deficits in total body potassium. Alkalosis, particularly respiratory alkalosis, is the most common clinical problem. ECF potassium will exchange with ICF hydrogen and correct the alkalosis by increasing the pH of the ECF. Treatment of pernicious anemia with vitamin B_{12} or folate also may precipitate hypokalemia if the formation of new red blood cells causes enough potassium uptake to effect an extracellular decrease in potassium. Catecholamines (β_2 adrenergics) promote intracellular uptake of K^+. Familial hypokalemic periodic paralysis is a rare genetically transmitted disease that also causes potassium to shift into the intracellular space.

Losses of potassium from body stores are most commonly caused by gastrointestinal and renal disorders. Diarrhea (from any cause), intestinal drainage tubes or fistulae, and laxative abuse also may result in hypokalemia. Normally, only 5 to 10 mEq of potassium and 100 to 150 ml of water are excreted in the stool each day. With diarrhea, fluid and electrolyte losses can be voluminous, with several liters of fluid and 100 to 200 mEq of potassium lost per day. Vomiting or continuous nasogastric suction frequently is associated with potassium depletion, partly because of the potassium lost from the gastric fluid but principally because of renal compensation for volume depletion and the metabolic alkalosis (elevated bicarbonate levels) that occurs from sodium, chloride, and hydrogen ion losses. The loss of fluid and sodium stimulates the secretion of aldosterone, which in turn causes renal losses of potassium. The elevated flow of bicarbonate at the distal tubule contributes to renal excretion of potassium because of increased tubular lumen electronegativity.

Renal losses of potassium are related to increased secretion of potassium by the distal tubule. Use of diuretics, excessive aldosterone secretion, increased distal tubular flow rate, and low plasma magnesium concentration all may contribute to urinary losses of potassium. Many diuretics, including thiazides, furosemide, ethacrynic acid, and osmotic diuretics, inhibit the reabsorption of sodium chloride, causing the diuretic effect. The distal tubular flow rate then increases, promoting potassium secretion. If sodium loss is severe, the compensating aldosterone secretion (which causes secondary hyperaldosteronism) may further deplete potassium stores. Primary hyperaldosteronism with excessive secretion of aldosterone from an adrenal adenoma also causes potassium wasting. Many kidney diseases result in a reduced ability to conserve sodium. The disordered sodium reabsorption produces a diuretic effect, and the increased distal tubule flow rate favors the secretion of potassium. Magnesium deficits stimulate renin release and hyperaldosteronism, causing hypokalemia. Several antibiotics, including amphotericin B, gentamicin, and carbenicillin, are known to cause hypokalemia.

◆ *Clinical Manifestations*

A wide range of metabolic dysfunctions may result from potassium deficiency. Carbohydrate metabolism is affected because hypokalemia depresses insulin secretion and alters hepatic and skeletal muscle glycogen synthesis. Renal function is impaired, with a decreased ability to concentrate urine. Polyuria (increased urine) and polydipsia (increased thirst) are associated with decreased responsiveness to ADH. Chronic potassium deficits lasting more than 1 month may damage renal tissue, with interstitial fibrosis and tubular atrophy.

Neuromuscular and cardiac effects of hypokalemia produce the most common symptoms.[13] Neuromuscular excitability is decreased, causing skeletal muscle weakness, smooth muscle atony, and cardiac dysrhythmias. As Chapter 1 describes, the resting membrane potential (E_m) is determined by the *ratio* of extracellular to intracellular potassium ion concentration. Because the concentration of potassium in the ECF is small, only small changes in ECF potassium are required to influence the resting membrane potential and affect neuromuscular excitability. When extracellular potassium levels decrease rapidly and intracellular potassium concentration does not change, the resting membrane potential becomes more negative and the cell membrane is **hyperpolarized.** If the threshold potential (E_t) remains stable, the difference between resting membrane potential and threshold potential increases, requiring a stronger stimulus to initiate an action potential (Fig. 3-5).

Factors such as calcium concentration and pH also contribute to the changes in neuromuscular excitability associated with hypokalemia. Increases in ECF calcium concentration tend to make the threshold potential less negative and decrease membrane excitability, potentiating the neuromuscular effects of hypokalemia.

The onset of symptoms is related to the rate of potassium depletion. Because the body can accommodate slow losses of potassium, the decrease in ECF concentration may be slow enough to allow potassium to shift from the intracellular space. The extracellular to intracellular potassium concentration gradient then is restored toward normal, with less severe neuromuscular changes. With acute losses of potassium, changes in neuromuscular excitability are more profound. Skeletal muscle weakness initially occurs in the larger

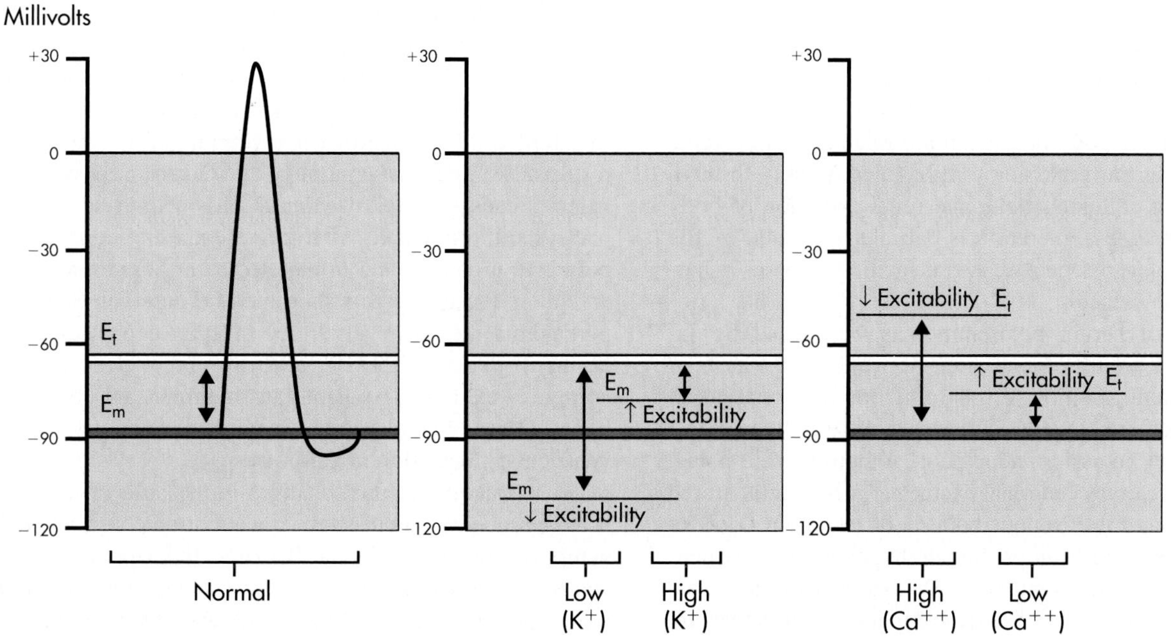

FIG. 3-5 Effects of potassium (K^+) and calcium (Ca^{++}) on membrane excitability. Potassium affects resting membrane potential (E_m), and calcium affects threshold potential (E_t)

muscles of the legs and arms and ultimately affects the diaphragm and depresses ventilation. Paralysis and respiratory arrest then can occur. Loss of smooth muscle tone is manifested by constipation, intestinal distention, anorexia, nausea, vomiting, and paralytic ileus.

The cardiac effects of hypokalemia are related also to changes in membrane excitability (see Fig. 3-5). Because potassium contributes to the repolarization phase of the action potential, hypokalemia delays ventricular repolarization. A variety of dysrhythmias may occur, including sinus bradycardia, atrioventricular block, and paroxysmal atrial tachycardia. The characteristic changes in the electrocardiogram reflect delayed repolarization. For instance, the amplitude of the T wave is decreased; the amplitude of the U wave is increased; and the ST segment is depressed (Fig. 3-6). In severe states of hypokalemia, P waves peak and the QRS complex is prolonged. Hypokalemia also increases the risk of digitalis toxicity.

◆ *Evaluation and Treatment*

The diagnosis of hypokalemia is significantly related to the medical history and the identification of disorders associated with potassium loss. Treatment involves an estimation of total body potassium losses and correction of acid-base imbalances. Further losses of potassium should be prevented, and the individual should be encouraged to eat foods rich in potassium. The maximal rate of oral replacement is 40 to 80 mEq/day if renal function is normal. A maximal safe rate of intravenous replacement is 20 mEq/hr. Because potassium is irritating to blood vessels, a maximal concentration of 40 mEq/L should be used. Serum potassium values can be monitored until normokalemia is achieved.

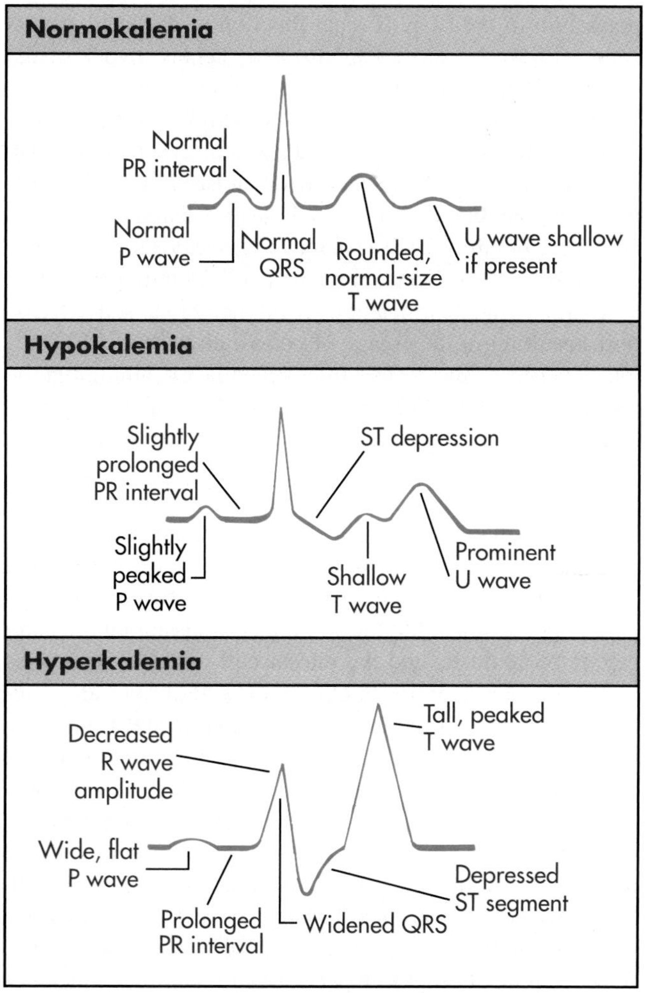

FIG. 3-6 ECG changes with potassium imbalance.

Hyperkalemia

Pathophysiology

An elevation of ECF potassium *above 5.5 mEq/L* constitutes **hyperkalemia**. Because of efficient renal excretion, increases in total body potassium are relatively rare. Acute increases in serum potassium are handled quickly through an increase in cellular uptake and renal excretion of body potassium excesses. Excretion is partially mediated by the secretion of aldosterone, because it facilitates losses of potassium in the urine.

Excesses of serum potassium may be caused by increased intake, a shift of potassium from cells to the ECF, or decreased renal excretion. If renal function is normal, slow, long-term increases in potassium intake are usually well tolerated through potassium adaptation, although acute potassium loading can exceed renal excretion rates. Use of stored whole blood and intravenous boluses of penicillin G or replacement potassium can precipitate hyperkalemia, particularly if renal function is impaired. Dietary excesses of potassium are uncommon, but accidental ingestion of potassium salt substitutes can cause toxicity.

Movement of potassium from the ICF to the ECF occurs with cell trauma or a change in cell membrane permeability, acidosis, insulin deficiency, or cell hypoxia. Burns, massive crushing injuries, and extensive surgeries can cause loss of potassium to the ECF. If renal function is sustained, potassium will be excreted. As cell repair begins, hypokalemia develops without an adequate intake of potassium.

In states of acidosis, hydrogen ions shift into the cells in exchange for ICF potassium and sodium; hyperkalemia and acidosis therefore often occur together. Because insulin promotes cellular entry of potassium, insulin deficits, which occur with conditions such as diabetic ketoacidosis, are accompanied by hyperkalemia. Hypoxia can lead to hyperkalemia by diminishing the efficiency of cell membrane active transport, resulting in the escape of potassium to the ECF. Digitalis overdose may cause hyperkalemia by inhibiting the sodium-potassium ATPase pump, which maintains high intracellular potassium and high extracellular sodium (see Chapter 1).

Decreased renal excretion of potassium commonly is associated with hyperkalemia. Renal failure that results in oliguria (urine output less than 30 ml/hr) is accompanied by elevations of serum potassium. The severity of hyperkalemia is related to the amount of potassium intake, the degree of acidosis, and the rate of cell damage. Decreases in the secretion or renal effects of aldosterone also can cause decreases in the urinary excretion of potassium. For example, Addison disease results in decreased production and secretion of aldosterone and thus contributes to hyperkalemia. Potassium-sparing diuretics (e.g., spironolactone, which inhibits sodium reabsorption and potassium and hydrogen secretion by the distal tubule) also may contribute to hyperkalemia. Frequently, however, these diuretics are used in combination with diuretics that cause potassium wasting in an attempt to balance renal potassium gains and losses.

Clinical Manifestations

Symptoms of hyperkalemia vary, but common characteristics are muscle weakness or paralysis and changes in the electrocardiogram. During mild attacks, increased neuromuscular irritability may be manifested as tingling of lips and fingers, restlessness, intestinal cramping, and diarrhea. Severe hyperkalemia causes muscle weakness, loss of muscle tone, and paralysis. In mild states of hyperkalemia the more rapid repolarization is reflected in the electrocardiogram as narrow and taller T waves with a shortened QT interval. Severe hyperkalemia (serum levels $\geq$ 6.0 mEq/L) depresses the ST segment, prolongs the PR interval, and widens the QRS complex (see Fig. 3-6). Bradydysrhythmias are common in hyperkalemia with alterations in cardiac conduction causing ventricular fibrillation or cardiac arrest.

As with hypokalemia, changes in the ratio of intracellular to extracellular potassium concentration contribute to the symptoms of hyperkalemia. If extracellular potassium concentration increases without a significant change in intracellular potassium, the resting membrane potential becomes more positive and the cell membrane is **hypopolarized** (the inside of the cell becomes less negative or partially depolarized). (Electrical properties of cells are discussed in Chapter 1.) With relatively mild elevations in extracellular potassium, the cell more rapidly repolarizes and becomes more irritable (peaked T waves). An action potential then is initiated more rapidly because the distance between the resting membrane potential and the threshold potential has been shortened. With more severe hyperkalemia, the resting membrane potential approaches or exceeds the threshold potential (wide QRS merging with T wave). In this case the cell is not able to repolarize and therefore does not respond to excitation stimuli. The most serious consequence is cardiac standstill.

Like the effects of hypokalemia, the neuromuscular effects of hyperkalemia are related to the rate of increase in the ECF potassium concentration and the presence of other contributing factors, such as acidosis and calcium balance. Long-term increases in ECF potassium concentration result in shifts of potassium into the cell, because the tendency is to maintain a normal ratio of intracellular/extracellular potassium concentrations. Acute elevations of extracellular potassium affect neuromuscular irritability because this ratio is disrupted.

Because calcium influences the threshold potential, changes in extracellular fluid calcium concentration can augment or override the effects of hyperkalemia. With hypocalcemia the threshold potential becomes more negative, enhancing the neuromuscular effects of hyperkalemia. Hypercalcemia causes the threshold potential to become less negative, counteracting the effects of hyperkalemia on resting membrane potential (see Fig. 3-5).

Evaluation and Treatment

Hyperkalemia should be investigated when there is a history of renal disease, massive trauma, insulin deficiency, Addison disease, use of potassium salt substitutes, or metabolic acidosis. The acuity of the onset of symptoms may be related to the underlying cause.

Management of hyperkalemia is related to treating the contributing causes and correcting the potassium excess. Normalizing the extracellular potassium concentration can be achieved with a variety of methods; the treatment chosen is related to the cause and severity of the problem. Calcium gluconate can be administered to restore normal neuromuscular irritability when serum potassium levels are dangerously high. Administration of insulin and glucose facilitates cellular entry of potassium, and sodium bicarbonate corrects metabolic acidosis and lowers serum potassium. Oral or rectal administration of cation exchange resins, which exchange sodium for potassium in the intestine, can be effective. Dialysis effectively removes potassium when there is renal failure.

Calcium and Phosphate

The total body content of calcium is about 1200 g. Most calcium (99%) is located in bone as hydroxyapatite (an inorganic compound that contributes to bone rigidity), and the remainder is in the plasma and body cells. Of the calcium in the plasma, 50% is bound to plasma proteins (2.5 mEq/L), and about 40% is in the free or ionized form (2.4 mEq/L). The total fraction of calcium circulating in the blood is small (4.5 to 5.5 mEq/L, or 8.6 to 10.5 mg/dl). Ionized calcium has the most important physiologic functions.

Calcium is a necessary ion for many fundamental metabolic processes. It is the major cation for the structure of bones and teeth. It serves as an enzymatic cofactor for blood clotting and is required for hormone secretion and the function of cell receptors. Plasma membrane stability and permeability are directly related to calcium ions, as is the transmission of nerve impulses and the contraction of muscles.

Phosphate is found primarily in bone, with smaller amounts within the intracellular and extracellular spaces. In the serum, phosphate exists in phospholipids and phosphate esters and as inorganic phosphate, which is the ionized form. The normal serum levels of inorganic phosphate range from 2.5 to 4.5 mg/dl and may be as high as 6.0 to 7.0 mg/dl in infants and young children. Intracellular phosphate has many metabolic forms, including the high-energy structures creatine phosphate and adenosine triphosphate (ATP). Phosphate acts as an intracellular and extracellular anion buffer in the regulation of acid-base balance; in the form of ATP it provides energy for muscle contraction.

Calcium and phosphate concentrations are rigidly controlled. They are related by the product of calcium (Ca^{++}) and phosphate ($HPO_4^{=}$), which is a constant ($Ca^{++} \times HPO_4^{=} = K$). Thus, if the concentration of one ion increases, that of the other decreases.

Calcium and phosphate balance is regulated by three hormones: parathyroid hormone (PTH), vitamin D, and calcitonin.[12] Acting together, these substances determine the amount of dietary calcium and phosphate absorbed from the intestine, the deposition and absorption of calcium and phosphate from the bone, and the renal reabsorption and excretion of calcium and phosphate by the kidney.

The parathyroid glands are sensitive to changes in serum calcium concentrations. The parathyroid glands secrete PTH in response to low serum calcium. Calcitonin is stimulated by high serum calcium levels. Parathyroid hormone initiates renal activation of vitamin D. (The specific actions of PTH in relation to calcium and phosphorus are described in Chapter 19.) The renal regulation of calcium and phosphate balance requires PTH. As PTH secretion is stimulated by low levels of serum calcium, there is increased reabsorption of calcium along the distal part of the nephron and inhibition of phosphate resorption by the proximal segment of the nephron. The net result is an increase in serum calcium and urinary excretion of phosphate. Fig. 3-7 summarizes hormonal regulation of calcium.

Another hormone important to calcium and phosphate regulation is vitamin D. Vitamin D (cholecalciferol) is a fat-soluble steroid ingested in food or synthesized in the skin in the presence of ultraviolet light. Several steps of activation are required before vitamin D can act on target tissues. The first step occurs in the liver; final activation is in the kidney. The renal activation of vitamin D begins when the serum calcium level decreases and stimulates secretion of PTH. PTH then acts to increase calcium reabsorption and enhance

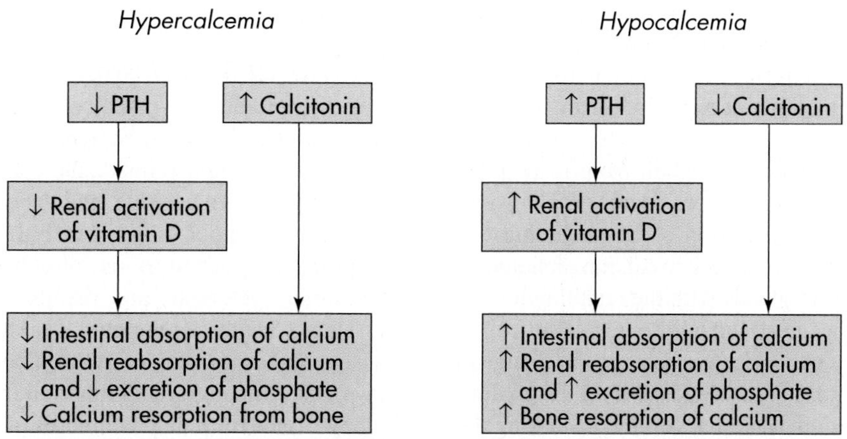

FIG. 3-7 Hormonal regulation of calcium balance. *PTH*, Parathyroid hormone.

renal excretion of phosphate, producing decreased phosphate levels. The combination of low calcium, PTH secretion, and low phosphate thus causes the renal activation of vitamin D. The activated vitamin D then circulates in the plasma and acts to increase absorption of calcium in the small intestine, enhance bone absorption of calcium, and increase renal tubular reabsorption of calcium. When there is renal failure, vitamin D will not be activated; serum calcium levels will decrease; and phosphate levels will increase.

The exchange of calcium and phosphate between serum and bone is regulated also by hormones. When serum calcium levels are low, PTH and vitamin D stimulate the osteoclasts in bone to resorb bone and release calcium and phosphate into the plasma. As calcium levels increase above 12 mg/dl, the thyroid hormone calcitonin opposes the action of PTH and lowers the serum calcium level by stimulating osteoblasts to deposit calcium and form new bone. When calcium levels are low, the secretion of calcitonin is suppressed.

The fractions of serum calcium that are freely ionized or bound to plasma proteins are influenced by pH. In states of acidosis, levels of ionized calcium increase. When alkalosis develops, with an increase in pH, protein-bound calcium increases and the physiologically active, ionized calcium decreases. The decreased concentration of ionized calcium may be great enough to cause symptoms of hypocalcemia, such as tetany.

Hypocalcemia

Pathophysiology

Hypocalcemia occurs when serum calcium concentrations are less than 8.5 mg/dl and ionized levels are less than 4.0 mg/dl. Deficits in calcium are related to inadequate intestinal absorption, deposition of ionized calcium into bone or soft tissue, blood administration, or decreases in PTH and vitamin D.

Nutritional deficiencies of calcium can occur with inadequate sources of dairy products or green, leafy vegetables. Excessive amounts of dietary phosphorus also bind with calcium, so neither mineral is absorbed. Blood transfusions are also a common cause of hypocalcemia because the citrate solution used in storing whole blood binds with calcium. Pancreatitis causes release of lipases into soft tissue spaces, so the free fatty acids that are formed bind calcium, causing a decrease in ionized calcium. Neoplastic bone metastases tend to inhibit bone resorption and increase calcium deposition into bone, thereby decreasing serum calcium levels.

Vitamin D deficiency, which can result from inadequate intake or avoidance of sunlight, causes decreased intestinal absorption of calcium. Malabsorption of fat, including fat-soluble vitamin D, may also contribute to calcium deficiency. Removal of the parathyroid glands with the resulting loss of PTH also causes hypocalcemia. Metabolic or respiratory alkalosis causes symptoms of hypocalcemia because the change in pH enhances protein binding of ionized calcium. Hypoalbuminemia lowers total serum calcium levels by decreasing the amount of bound calcium.

Clinical Manifestations

The clinical manifestations of hypocalcemia are caused primarily by an increase in neuromuscular excitability. Calcium deficits cause partial depolarization of nerves and muscle as the threshold potential approaches the resting membrane potential (see Fig. 3-5). Therefore a smaller stimulus is required for initiating the action potential. The symptoms include confusion, paresthesias around the mouth and in the digits, carpopedal spasm (muscle spasms in the hands and feet), and hyperreflexia.

Two clinical signs are Chvostek sign and Trousseau sign. Chvostek sign is elicited by tapping on the facial nerve just below the temple. A positive sign is a twitch of the nose or lip. Trousseau sign is contraction of the hand and fingers when the arterial blood flow in the arm is occluded for 5 minutes.

Severe symptoms include convulsions and tetany, a continuous severe muscle spasm that can interfere with breathing and cause death. The characteristic electrocardiogram (ECG) change is a prolonged QT interval, indicating prolonged ventricular depolarization and decreased cardiac contractility. Intestinal cramping and hyperactive bowel sounds also may be present because hypocalcemia affects the smooth muscles of the gastrointestinal tract.

Evaluation and Treatment

The health history may signify underlying pathologic conditions that require further evaluation and treatment. Severe symptoms of hypocalcemia require emergency treatment with intravenous 10% calcium gluconate. Oral calcium replacement should be initiated, and serum calcium levels should be monitored. Decreasing phosphate intake facilitates long-term management of hypocalcemia.

Hypercalcemia

Pathophysiology

Hypercalcemia with serum calcium concentrations exceeding 12 mg/dl can be caused by a number of diseases. The most common among these are hyperparathyroidism; bone metastases with calcium resorption from breast, prostate, and cervical cancer; sarcoidosis; and excess vitamin D. Many tumors produce PTH and elevate the serum calcium levels. Sarcoidosis appears to increase vitamin D levels.

Clinical Manifestations

Many symptoms of hypercalcemia are nonspecific. Because serum calcium levels are increased, a greater amount of calcium is also contained inside the cells. The threshold potential becomes more positive, and the cell membrane becomes refractory to depolarization (see Fig. 3-5). Thus many of the symptoms are related to loss of cell membrane excitability. (Membrane potentials and membrane excitability are discussed in Chapter 1.) Fatigue, weakness, lethargy, anorexia, nausea, and constipation are common. Behavioral changes may occur. Impaired renal function frequently develops, and kidney stones form as precipitates of calcium salts. A shortened QT segment and depressed T waves also may be observed on the ECG, with bradycardia and varying degrees of heart block.

Evaluation and Treatment

With elevated serum calcium levels, often a reciprocal decrease in serum phosphate values occurs. Specific diagnostic procedures to identify the contributing pathologic condition are required.

Treatment is related to severity of symptoms and the underlying disease. When renal function is normal, oral phosphate administration is effective. When there is acute illness and high calcium levels, intravenous administration of large amounts of normal saline will enhance renal excretion of calcium. Corticosteroids and the cytotoxic drug mithramycin also are used to treat hypercalcemia. Ultimately, the underlying pathologic condition must be treated.

Hypophosphatemia

Pathophysiology

Hypophosphatemia is a serum phosphate level less than 2.0 mg/dl and is usually an indication of phosphate deficiency. In some conditions, total body phosphate is normal but serum volumes are low. The most common causes are intestinal malabsorption and increased renal excretion of phosphate. Inadequate absorption is associated with vitamin D deficiency, use of magnesium- and aluminum-containing antacids (which bind with phosphorus), long-term alcohol abuse, and malabsorption syndromes. Respiratory alkalosis can cause severe hypophosphatemia because of cellular use of phosphorus for an accelerated glucose metabolism. Increased renal excretion of phosphorus is associated with hyperparathyroidism.

Clinical Manifestations

The consequences of phosphate deficiency are related to reduced capacity for oxygen transport by red blood cells and to disturbed energy metabolism. Transport and release of oxygen are associated with 2,3-diphosphoglycerate (2,3-DPG) and ATP. When phosphate is depleted, 2,3-DPG and ATP levels become low and diminish release of oxygen to the tissues. The oxyhemoglobin curve shifts to the left (see Chapter 31), and hypoxia can occur with bradycardia and varying degrees of heart attack.

Leukocyte and platelet dysfunctions also are associated with hypophosphatemia. There is a greater risk of infection and blood-clotting impairment, with potential for hemorrhage. Nerve and muscle function can be affected with derangement in energy metabolism. Irritability, confusion, numbness, coma, and convulsions develop with severe phosphate losses. Muscle weakness may become serious enough to cause respiratory failure, and cardiomyopathies also can develop. In response to low phosphate levels, bone resorption occurs and may lead to rickets or osteomalacia.

Evaluation and Treatment

To correct the condition, the underlying cause must be identified and treated. Although serum phosphate levels are below normal, the administration of phosphate salts is dangerous, and low phosphate levels are usually not considered life threatening.

Hyperphosphatemia

Pathophysiology

Hyperphosphatemia, or an elevated serum phosphate level of more than 4.5 mg/dl, develops with exogenous or endogenous addition of phosphorus to the ECF or with significant loss of glomerular filtration.[14] Because most phosphate is located in cells, the cell destruction associated with treatment of metastatic tumors with chemotherapy can release large amounts of phosphate into the serum. Long-term use of phosphate-containing enemas or laxatives also may lead to hyperphosphatemia. Hypoparathyroidism can cause elevated phosphate by increasing renal tubular reabsorption of phosphate.

High levels of serum phosphate also lower serum calcium levels, and increased amounts of phosphate and calcium are deposited in bone and soft tissues. Serum calcium levels may become low enough to cause symptoms of hypocalcemia, including tetany.

Clinical Manifestations

Symptoms of hyperphosphatemia are related primarily to low serum calcium levels and thus are comparable to symptoms of hypocalcemia. With prolonged hyperphosphatemia, calcification of soft tissues occurs in the lungs, kidneys, and joints.

Evaluation and Treatment

To correct the condition, the underlying pathologic condition must be identified and treated. Aluminum hydroxide may be administered because it binds phosphate in the gastrointestinal tract and is eliminated. Dialysis is required for management of renal failure.

Magnesium

Magnesium (Mg^{++}) is a major intracellular cation. About 40% to 60% is stored in muscle and bone with 30% in the cells. A small amount (1%) is in the serum. Plasma concentration is 1.8 to 2.4 mEq/L with about one third bound to plasma proteins and the rest in ionized form. Regulation of magnesium metabolism is primarily by the kidney, and low serum levels cause renal conservation of magnesium. Magnesium is a cofactor in intracellular enzymatic reactions and is a cause of neuromuscular excitability. Calcium and magnesium often interact in reactions at the cellular level.

Hypomagnesemia occurs when serum magnesium concentration is less than 1.5 mEq/L and increases in neuromuscular excitability and tetany are present. Malnutrition, malabsorption syndromes, alcoholism, renal tubular dysfunction, metabolic acidosis, and loop and thiazide diuretics can cause magnesium losses. Diabetes mellitus is associated with hypomagnesemia partly as a function of osmotic diuresis.[15] Signs and symptoms of hypomagnesemia are similar to those of hypocalcemia. Depression, confusion, irritability, increased reflexes, muscle weakness, ataxia, nystagmus, tetany, and convulsions may be observed.[15] Treatment is intramuscular or intravenous administration of magnesium sulfate.

Hypermagnesemia, in which magnesium concentration is greater than 2.5 mEq/L, is rare and usually is caused by renal failure. Magnesium-containing antacids (e.g., Gaviscon, Gelusil) can potentiate excess magnesium. Excess magnesium depresses skeletal muscle contraction and nerve function. Signs and symptoms include nausea and vomiting, muscle weakness, hypotension, bradycardia, and respiratory depression.[15] Treatment is avoidance of magnesium-containing substances and removal of magnesium by dialysis.

ACID-BASE BALANCE

Hydrogen ion concentration must be regulated within a narrow range for the body to function normally. Slight changes in amounts of hydrogen can significantly alter biologic processes in cells and tissues. Hydrogen ion is necessary to maintain membrane integrity and the speed of enzymatic reactions. Most pathologic conditions disturb acid-base balance, and the degree of severity may be more harmful than the disease process.

Hydrogen Ion and pH

The hydrogen ion concentration $[H^+]$ is commonly expressed as the pH, the negative logarithm of hydrogen ions in solution. The logarithmic value means that as the pH changes one unit (e.g., 7.0 to 6.0), the $[H^+]$ changes tenfold (i.e., 0.0000001 to 0.000001). The relationship is commonly expressed as follows:

$$pH = \log\frac{1}{[H^+]} \quad \text{or } pH = -\log[H^+]$$

As the $[H^+]$ increases, the pH decreases; likewise, as the $[H^+]$ decreases, the pH increases. The greater the $[H^+]$, the more acidic the solution and the lower the pH. The lower the $[H^+]$, the more basic the solution and the higher the pH. In biologic fluids, a pH of less than 7.4 is defined as acidic and a pH greater than 7.4 is defined as basic.

Different body fluids have different pH values as follows:

BODY FLUID	PH
Gastric juices	1.0-3.0
Urine	5.0-6.0
Arterial blood	7.38-7.42
Venous blood	7.37
Cerebrospinal fluid	7.32
Pancreatic fluid	7.8-8.0

Body acids are formed as end products of cellular metabolism. The average person generates acid in the amount of 50 to 100 mEq/day from the metabolism of protein, carbohydrates, and fats and from loss of base in the stools. To maintain a normal pH, an equal amount of acid therefore must be neutralized or excreted. The lungs, kidneys, and bone are the major organs involved in the regulation of acid-base balance. The systems are interrelated and work together to regulate short- or long-term changes in acid-base status. Body acids exist in two forms: **volatile** (can be eliminated as carbon dioxide [CO_2] gas) and **nonvolatile.** The volatile acid is carbonic acid (H_2CO_3), which is formed from the hydration of carbon dioxide:

Regulated by lung Regulated by kidney

$$CO_2 + H_2O \leftrightarrow H_2CO_3 \leftrightarrow HCO_3^- + H^+$$

Carbonic acid is a weak acid, and, in the presence of carbonic anhydrase, it readily dissociates into carbon dioxide. Approximately 12,000 to 15,000 millimoles of CO_2 is produced per day.[16] The carbon dioxide is then eliminated by pulmonary ventilation. Sulfuric, phosphoric, and other organic acids are nonvolatile strong acids produced from the metabolism of proteins, carbohydrates, and fats. (Strong acids are those that readily give up their hydrogen; weak acids do not.) Nonvolatile acids are eliminated by the renal tubules with the regulation of HCO_3^-. Thus the lungs and kidneys, with the help of body buffer systems, are the prime regulators of acid-base balance.

Buffer Systems

Buffering occurs in response to changes in acid-base status. **Buffers** can absorb excessive H^+ (acid) or OH^- (base) without a significant change in pH. The buffer systems are located in both the ICF and ECF compartments, and they function at different rates. Buffer systems exist as buffer pairs, consisting of a weak acid and its conjugate base (Table 3-9). The most important plasma buffer systems are carbonic acid–bicarbonate and hemoglobin. Phosphate and protein are the most important intracellular buffers.

An important factor for effective buffering is a function known as the *pK value*, which represents the pH at which a buffer pair is half dissociated. Buffer pairs can associate and dissociate (see Table 3-9).

The pK provides a rate constant for the chemical reaction. A buffer system is most effective when the pK for the buffer is close to the pH of the fluid in which the buffer is acting. For the bicarbonate–carbonic acid buffer system, the pK is 6.1. This value is not as high as the pK for other buffer systems (see Table 3-9), but this buffer system is still very effective because carbon dioxide is rapidly removed from the blood by the lungs.

The pK value is also a term in the equation used to determine pH. The relationships among pH, pK, and the ratio of bicarbonate to carbonic acid can be expressed as follows by the *Henderson-Hasselbalch equation:*

$$pH = pK + \log\frac{[HCO_3^-]}{[H_2CO_3]}$$

The pH then can be determined when specific values are included in the equation:

Table 3-9 Buffer Systems

Buffer Pairs	Buffer System	pK Values	Reaction	Rate
HCO_3^-/H_2CO_3	Bicarbonate	6.1	$H^+ + HCO_3^- \rightleftharpoons H_2O + CO_2$	Instantaneous
Hb^-/HHb	Hemoglobin	7.3	$HHb \rightleftharpoons H^+ + Hb^-$	Instantaneous
$HPO_4^=/H_2PO_4^-$	Phosphate	6.8	$H_2PO_4 \rightleftharpoons H^+ + HPO_4^=$	Instantaneous
Pr^-/HPr	Plasma proteins	6.7	$HPr \rightleftharpoons H^+ + Pr^-$	Instantaneous

Organs	Mechanism	Rate
Lungs	Regulates retention or elimination of CO_2 and therefore H_2CO_3 concentration	Minutes-hours
Ionic shifts	Exchange of intracellular potassium and sodium for hydrogen	2-4 hours
Kidneys	Bicarbonate reabsorption and regeneration, ammonia formation, phosphate buffering	Hours-days
Bone	Exchanges of calcium, phosphate, and release of carbonate	Hours-days

HCO_3^-, Bicarbonate; *H_2CO_3*, carbonic acid; *Hb^-*, hemoglobin; *Pr^-*, protein; *$H_2PO_4^-$*, monobasic phosphate; *$HPO_4^=$*, dibasic phosphate; *HPr*, hydrogenated protein; *HHb*, hydrogenated hemoglobin.

$$
\begin{aligned}
pH &= pK + \log \frac{[HCO_3^-]}{[H_2CO_3]} \\
&= 6.1 + \log \frac{24}{1.2} \\
&= 6.1 + \log \frac{20}{1} \\
&= 6.1 + 1.3 \\
&= 7.40
\end{aligned}
$$

Carbonic Acid–Bicarbonate Buffering

The carbonic acid–bicarbonate buffer pair operates in both the lung and the kidney. The greater the carbon dioxide partial pressure (Pco_2), the more carbonic acid is formed. The relationship that exists between carbonic acid (H_2CO_3) and carbon dioxide (Pco_2) can be expressed as follows:

$$H_2CO_3 = 0.03 \times Pco_2 \text{ (mm Hg)}$$

The 0.03 represents the solubility coefficient for carbon dioxide in water. The Pco_2 of arterial blood is normally about 40 mm Hg. Therefore the amount of H_2CO_3 is equal to about 1.2 mmol/L (0.03 × 40). As the amount of carbon dioxide increases or decreases, the amount of H_2CO_3 changes in the same direction.

The relationship between bicarbonate and carbonic acid is usually expressed as a ratio. When the pH is 7.40, this ratio is 20:1 (bicarbonate/carbonic acid). The ratio is defined by the amount of bicarbonate and carbon dioxide (carbonic acid) in the arterial blood. Bicarbonate concentration (HCO_3^-) is normally about 24 mEq/L. Therefore the 20:1 ratio can be developed as follows:

$$\frac{[HCO_3^-] = 24 \text{ mEq/L}}{[H_2CO_3] = (0.03 \times 40 \text{ mm Hg})} = \frac{24}{1.2} = \frac{20}{1}$$

The values for HCO_3^- and Pco_2 (H_2CO_3) can increase or decrease proportionately, but the 20:1 ratio is maintained.

The lungs can decrease the amount of carbonic acid by blowing off CO_2 and leaving water. The kidneys can reabsorb bicarbonate or regenerate new bicarbonate from CO_2 and water. The renal mechanism does not act as rapidly as the lungs, but the two systems are very effective together because acid concentration can be rapidly adjusted by the lungs and bicarbonate is easily reabsorbed or regenerated by the kidneys. The pH equation can be symbolically expressed as follows:

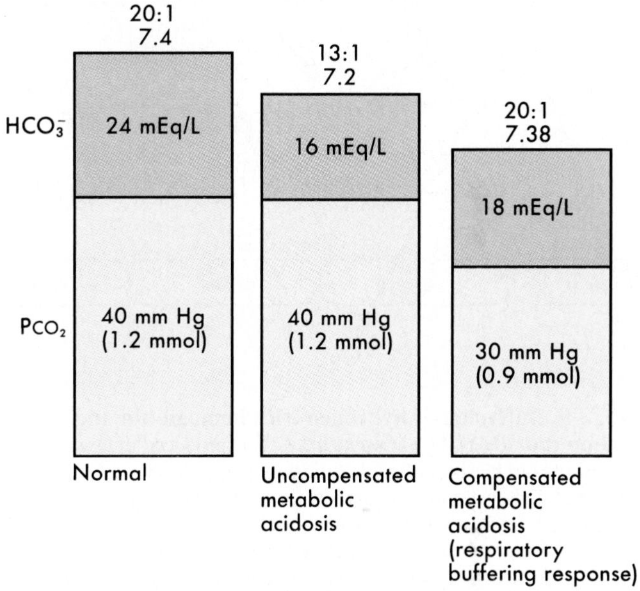

FIG. 3-8 Maintenance of HCO_3^-/Pco_2 (H_2CO_3) ratio in metabolic acidosis.

$$pH = \frac{\text{Base}}{\text{Acid or pH}} = \frac{\text{Renal regulation (slow)}}{\text{Pulmonary regulation (fast)}}$$

or

$$pH = \frac{\text{Metabolic acid-base function}}{\text{Respiratory acid-base function}}$$

Changes in either the numerator or the denominator will change the pH. For example, if the amount of bicarbonate is decreased, the pH also decreases, causing a state of acidosis. The pH can be returned to a normal range if the value of the denominator or the amount of carbonic acid also decreases.

This type of adjustment in pH is known as **compensation.** With compensation, a 20:1 ratio may be achieved, but the actual values for HCO_3^- and H_2CO_3 are not normal. The respiratory system compensates for changes in pH by increasing or decreasing ventilation. The renal system compensates by producing more acidic or more alkaline urine. **Correction** occurs when the values for both components of the buffer pair return to normal (Fig. 3-8).

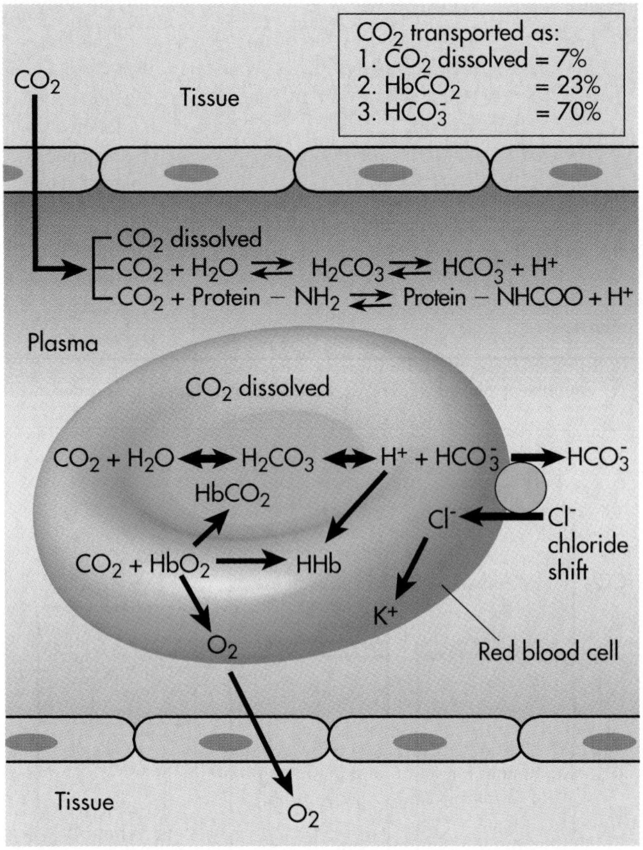

FIG. 3-9 Buffering of hydrogen with hemoglobin and carbon dioxide (CO_2) transport. CO_2 is produced in tissue cells and diffuses to plasma, where it is transported as dissolved CO_2, or it combines with water to form carbonic acid (H_2CO_3), or it combines with protein from which hydrogen has been released. Most of the CO_2 diffuses into the red blood cell and combines with water to form H_2CO_3. The H_2CO_3 dissociates to form hydrogen (H^+) and bicarbonate (HCO_3^-). The HCO_3^- shifts into the plasma and chloride (Cl^-) shifts into the red blood cell to maintain electroneutrality. Hydrogen combines with hemoglobin that has released its oxygen to form HHb, which buffers the hydrogen and makes venous blood slightly more acidic than arterial blood.

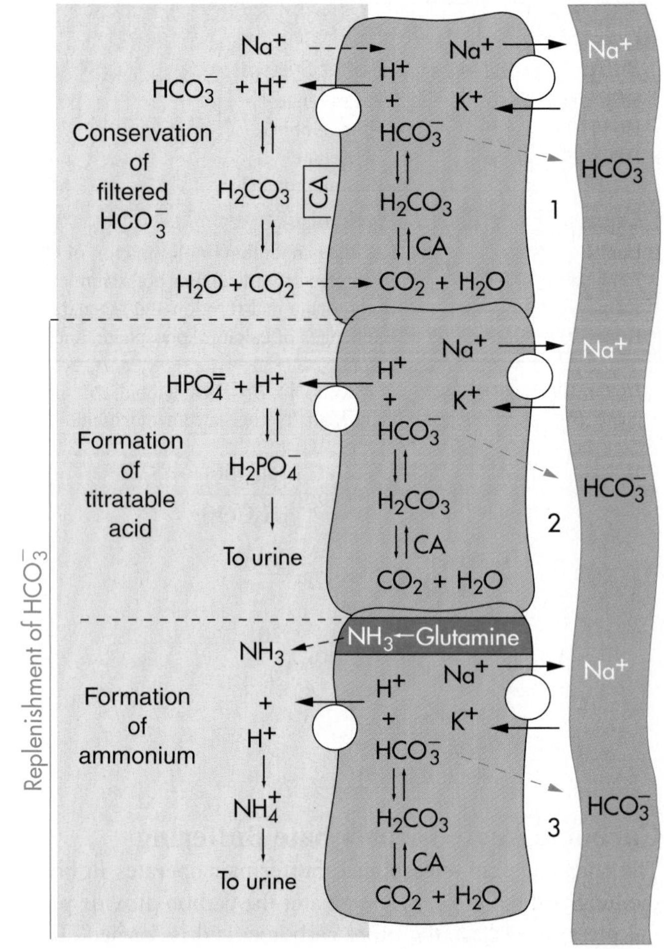

FIG. 3-10 Renal excretion of acid. *1, Conservation of filtered bicarbonate.* Filtered bicarbonate combines with secreted hydrogen in the presence of carbon anhydrase (CA) to form carbonic acid (H_2CO_3), which then dissociates to water (H_2O) and carbon dioxide (CO_2); both diffuse into the epithelial cell. The CO_2 and H_2O combine to form H_2CO_3 in the presence of CA, and the resulting bicarbonate (HCO_3^-) is converted by reabsorption into the capillary. *2, Formation of titratable acid.* Hydrogen ion is secreted and combines with dibasic phosphate ($HPO_4^=$) to form monobasic phosphate ($H_2PO_4^-$). The secreted hydrogen is formed from the dissociation of H_2CO_3, and the remaining HCO_3^- is reabsorbed into the capillary. *3, Formation of ammonium.* Ammonia (NH_3) is produced from glutamine in the epithelial cell and diffused to the tubular lumen, where it combines with H^+ to form ammonium (NH_4^+). Once NH_4^+ has been formed, it cannot return to the epithelial cell (diffusional trapping), and the bicarbonate remaining in the epithelial cell is reabsorbed into the capillary.

Protein Buffering

Both intracellular and extracellular proteins have negative charges and can serve as buffers for H^+, but because most proteins are inside cells, they are primarily an intracellular buffer system. Hemoglobin (Hb) is an excellent intracellular buffer because of its ability to bind with H^+ (forming HHb) and carbon dioxide ($HHbCO_2$). Hemoglobin bound to H^+ becomes a weak acid. Unsaturated hemoglobin (venous blood) is a better buffer than hemoglobin saturated with oxygen (arterial blood). The hemoglobin buffer system is illustrated in Fig. 3-9.

Renal Buffering

The distal tubule of the kidney regulates acid-base balance by secreting hydrogen into the urine and reabsorbing bicarbonate with a maximum acidity of about 4.4 to 4.7. Buffers in the tubular fluid combine with hydrogen ions, allowing more H^+ to be secreted before the limiting pH value is reached. Dibasic phosphate ($HPO_4^=$) and ammonia (NH_3) are two important renal buffers. Dibasic phosphate is filtered at the glomerulus. About 75% is reabsorbed, and the remainder is available for buffering H^+. Secreted H^+ combines with $HPO_4^=$ to form monobasic phosphate ($H_2PO_4^-$). The remaining negative charge on the molecule makes it lipid insoluble, and it cannot diffuse back across the tubular cell and into the blood. Thus it is excreted in the urine (Fig. 3-10).

Ammonia (NH_3) is an important renal buffer. Ammonia is not ionized (does not carry a charge), and therefore it is lipid

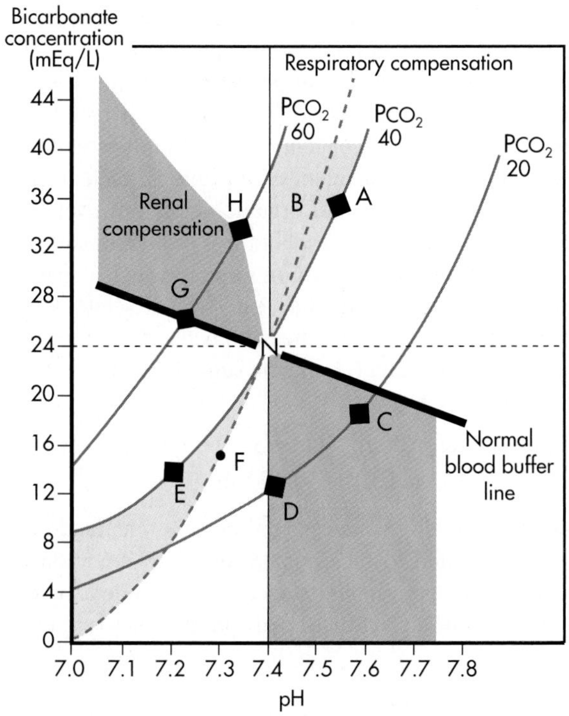

FIG. 3-11 Graph of pH, $P\text{CO}_2$, and bicarbonate relationships. *Solid red lines* represent different carbon dioxide partial pressure ($P\text{CO}_2$) values. *Vertical axis* represents bicarbonate concentration, and *horizontal axis* represents acidity or alkalinity (pH) values. Thus for any indicated $P\text{CO}_2$, there is a corresponding pH and bicarbonate concentration. Any point on the graph predicts the required $P\text{CO}_2$, pH, and bicarbonate values. *Dashed horizontal line* shows behavior of bicarbonate as a pure buffer at 24 mEq/L. The normal blood buffer line represents values that would be obtained if blood were equilibrated at different CO_2 values. Point *N* represents normal values. *Point A* represents metabolic alkalosis, indicated by a normal $P\text{CO}_2$ of 40 and pH greater than 7.4. Respiratory compensation is achieved by hypoventilation, which raises the $P\text{CO}_2$ to *point B* and decreases the pH. Respiratory alkalosis is represented by *point C* and reflects hypocapnia (decreased $P\text{CO}_2$). Renal compensation for respiratory alkalosis is increased renal excretion of bicarbonate to normalize pH at *point D*. Metabolic acidosis at *point E* represents normal $P\text{CO}_2$ and a decrease in bicarbonate and pH. Respiratory compensation by hyperventilation is indicated by *point F*. Respiratory acidosis at *point G* indicates high $P\text{CO}_2$ and low pH values. Renal compensation for chronic high $P\text{CO}_2$ values is indicated by *point H*.

soluble and can cross the cell membrane. The presence of NH_3 in the cell creates a concentration gradient, and it diffuses into the renal tubular fluid where it combines with hydrogen to form ammonium ion (NH_4^+), which is eliminated in the urine (see Fig. 3-10). The renal buffering of hydrogen ions requires the use of CO_2 and H_2O to form H_2CO_3. The enzyme carbonic anhydrase catalyzes the formation of $H^+ + HCO_3^-$. The hydrogen is secreted from the tubular cell and buffered in the lumen by phosphate and ammonia. The bicarbonate is reabsorbed. The end effect is the addition of new bicarbonate, which contributes to the alkalinity of the plasma, because the hydrogen ion is excreted from the body (see Fig. 3-10).

Other Buffers

A cellular ion exchange mechanism is also an important buffering system. The best example is the shift of potassium in exchange for hydrogen during states of acidosis or alkalosis. During acidosis, potassium tends to leave the intracellular space in exchange for hydrogen. The reverse occurs during alkalosis. Although the ionic shifts facilitate buffering, the changes in intracellular or extracellular potassium concentrations may have serious consequences.

Acid-Base Imbalances

Pathophysiologic changes in the concentration of hydrogen ion in the blood lead to acid-base imbalances. **Acidemia** is a state in which the pH of arterial blood is less than 7.35. A systemic increase in hydrogen ion concentration is termed **acidosis. Alkalemia** is a state in which the pH of arterial blood is greater than 7.45. A systemic decrease in hydrogen ion concentration is termed **alkalosis.** Acid-base imbalances may have a metabolic or respiratory etiology or may be mixed. Fig. 3-11 summarizes the relationships among pH, $P\text{CO}_2$, and bicarbonate during different acid-base alterations.

Table 3-10 Primary and Compensatory Acid-Base Changes

	Primary Disturbance			Compensations		
	pH	$P\text{CO}_2$	HCO_3^-	pH	$P\text{CO}_2$	HCO_3^-
Metabolic acidosis	↓	N	↓	↑-N	↓	↓
Metabolic alkalosis	↑	N	↑	↓-N	↑	↑
Respiratory acidosis	↓	↑	N	↑-N	↑	↑
Respiratory alkalosis	↑	↓	N	↓-N	↓	↓

↑-*N,* Increase toward normal; ↓-*N,* decrease toward normal; *pH,* measure of the acidity or alkalinity of a solution; $P\text{CO}_2$, carbon dioxide partial pressure; HCO_3^-, bicarbonate.

Metabolic Acidosis

Pathophysiology

In **metabolic acidosis**, noncarbonic acids increase or bicarbonate is lost from the extracellular fluid (Tables 3-10 and 3-11). This can occur quickly, as in lactic acidosis from poor perfusion, or more slowly, as in renal failure or diabetic ketoacidosis.

The buffer systems compensate for the excess acid and attempt to maintain the arterial pH within a normal range. Buffering by bicarbonate lowers the serum value of this ion. The respiratory system compensates for a metabolic acidosis as the reduced pH stimulates hyperventilation, lowering

Table 3-11 Causes of Metabolic Acidosis

Increased Noncarbonic Acids (Elevated Anion Gap)	Bicarbonate Loss (Normal Anion Gap)
Increased H^+ load	Diarrhea
Ketoacidosis (e.g., diabetes mellitus, starvation)	Ureterosigmoidoscopy
Lactic acidosis (e.g., shock)	Renal failure
Ingestions (e.g., ammonium chloride, ethylene glycol, methanol, salicylates, paraldehyde)	Proximal renal tubule acidosis
Decreased H^+ excretion	
Uremia	
Distal renal tubule acidosis	

the $Paco_2$ and the amount of H_2CO_3 circulating in the blood. The kidneys excrete the excess acid as NH_4^+ and titratable acid ($H_2PO_4^-$). When the acidosis is severe, the buffers are unable to compensate for the increasing H^+ load and the pH continues to decrease. The result is a decrease in the 20:1 ratio of bicarbonate to carbonic acid (Fig. 3-12).

The evaluation of the **anion gap** can be helpful when used cautiously to distinguish different types of metabolic acidosis.[17] Normally, the concentrations of cations and anions in the plasma are equivalent. Some anions, such as protein, sulfates, phosphates, and organic acids, however, are not measured in the common laboratory evaluations of the blood. Therefore the **normal anion gap** represents negative ions not usually measured (sulfate, phosphate, lactate, ketoacids, albumin). A convenient measure is the difference between the sum of Na^+ and K^+ and the sum of HCO_3^- and Cl^-, or about 10 to 12 mEq:

$$\text{Anion gap} = [Na^+ (140) + K^+ (4.0)] - [HCO_3^- (24) + Cl^- (110)] = 10\text{-}12 \text{ mEq/L}$$

In metabolic acidosis a normal anion gap is characteristic of conditions related to bicarbonate loss with retention of chloride to maintain an ionic balance. This is called **hyperchloremic metabolic acidosis.** An elevated anion gap is

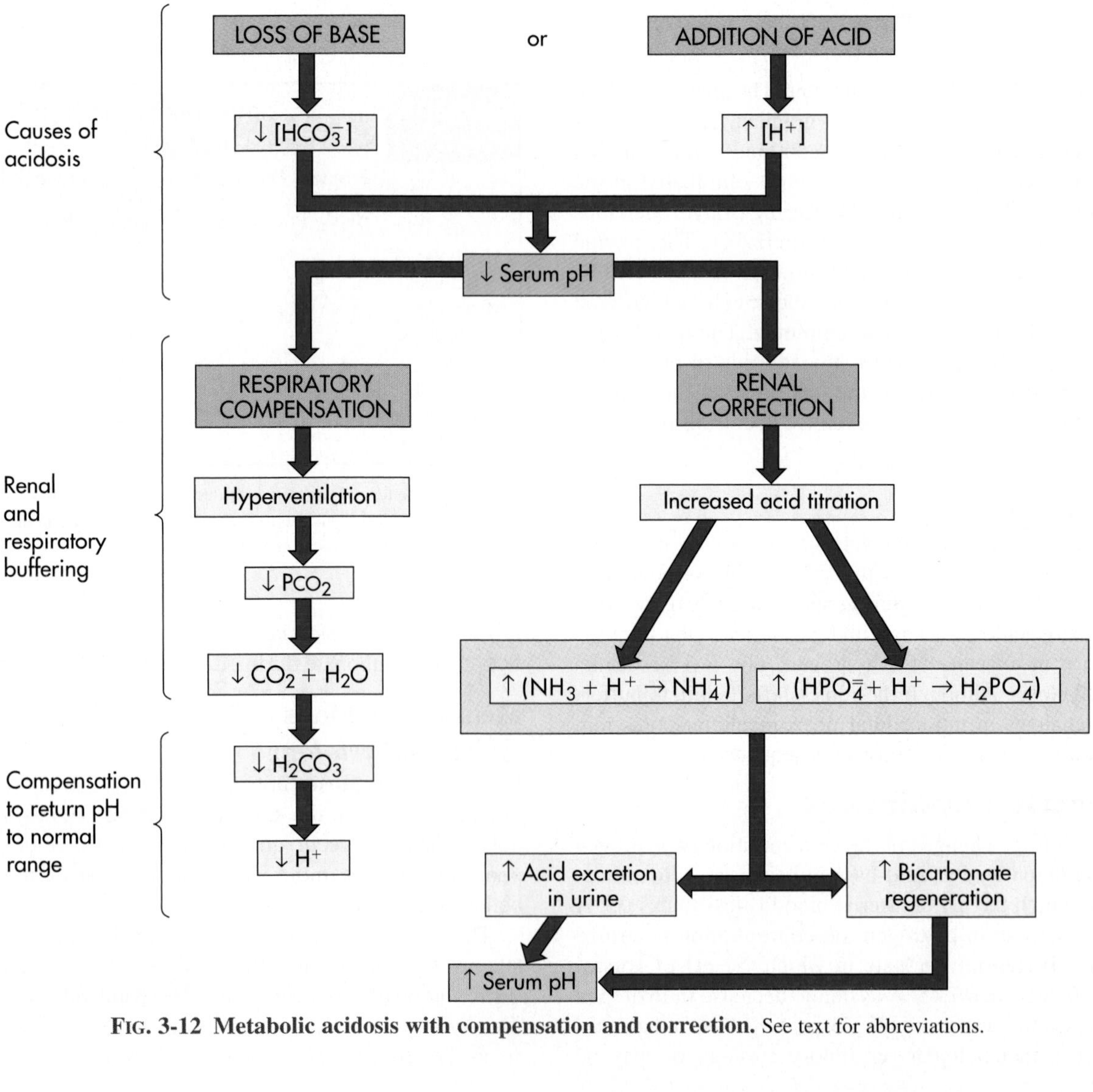

FIG. 3-12 Metabolic acidosis with compensation and correction. See text for abbreviations.

characteristic of acidosis associated with accumulation of anions other than chloride (see Table 3-11).

Clinical Manifestations

Metabolic acidosis is manifested by changes in the neurologic, respiratory, gastrointestinal, and cardiovascular systems. Headache and lethargy are early symptoms, which progress to coma with severe acidosis. Deep, rapid respirations (Kussmaul respirations) are indicative of respiratory compensation. Anorexia, nausea, vomiting, diarrhea, and abdominal discomfort are common. Severe acidosis can compromise ventricular contraction and produce life-threatening dysrhythmias.

Evaluation and Treatment

The diagnosis of metabolic acidosis is established from the health history, clinical symptoms, and laboratory findings. Arterial blood pH is below 7.35, and bicarbonate concentration is less than 24 mEq/L. The underlying condition must be diagnosed to establish effective treatment. During severe acidosis ($pH \leq 7.1$), sodium bicarbonate administration is required to elevate the pH to a safe level, particularly if there is renal failure. Accompanying sodium and water deficits must also be corrected.

Metabolic Alkalosis

Pathophysiology

Metabolic alkalosis is common and occurs when bicarbonate is increased, usually caused by excessive loss of metabolic acids.[18] Among the conditions that can result in metabolic alkalosis are prolonged vomiting, gastrointestinal suctioning, excessive bicarbonate intake, hyperaldosteronism, and diuretic therapy.[19]

When acid loss is caused by vomiting with depletion of ECF and chloride **(hypochloremic metabolic alkalosis),** renal compensation is not very effective because the volume depletion and loss of electrolytes (Na^+, K^+, H^+, Cl^-) stimulate a paradoxic response by the kidneys.[12] The kidneys increase sodium and bicarbonate reabsorption with excretion of hydrogen. Bicarbonate is reabsorbed because the ECF chloride concentration is decreased. When the potassium concentration is depleted, hydrogen moves to the intracellular space and is excreted to maintain an electrochemical balance. The urine is acidic, and the reabsorbed bicarbonate prevents correction of the alkalosis (Fig. 3-13). Correction is achieved when the ECF is expanded with a solution of sodium chloride and potassium. The volume replacement decreases the renal stimulus to reabsorb Na^+, and chloride as an anion is replaced. Bicarbonate then can be lost in the urine, and hydrogen ion excretion decreases, correcting the pH.

With hyperaldosteronism the excess aldosterone causes sodium retention and loss of hydrogen and potassium. Mild volume expansion ensues, and bicarbonate is retained with the sodium, causing alkalosis.

Diuretics, such as thiazides, ethacrynic acid, and furosemide, produce mild alkalosis by enhancing sodium, potassium, and chloride excretion more than bicarbonate excretion.

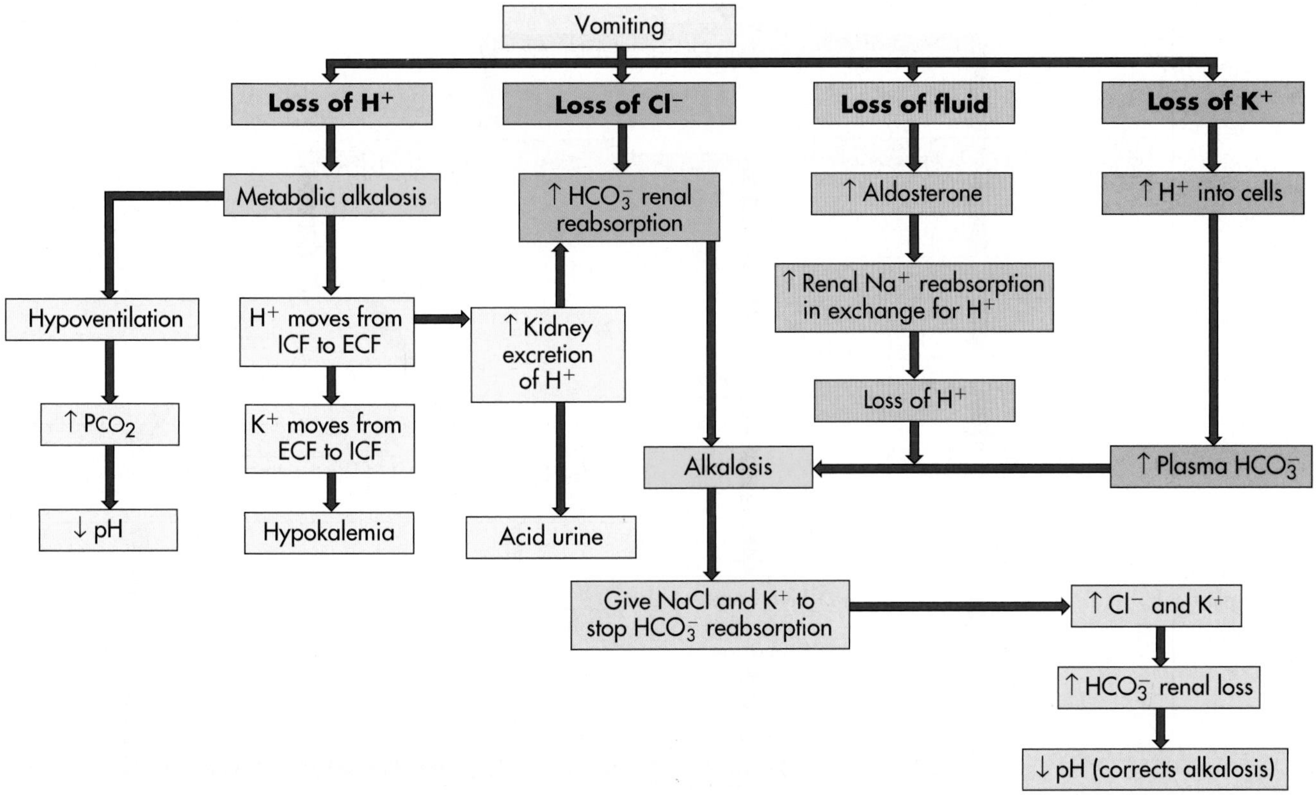

FIG. 3-13 Hypochloremic metabolic alkalosis. See text for abbreviations.

Respiratory compensation for metabolic alkalosis occurs when the elevated pH inhibits the respiratory center. The rate and depth of ventilation are decreased, causing retention of carbon dioxide. The ratio of HCO_3^- to H_2CO_3 is reduced toward normal. Respiratory compensation is not very efficient, however, and chronic or severe metabolic alkalosis requires therapeutic intervention (Fig. 3-14).

Clinical Manifestations

Because of the many causes of metabolic alkalosis, the symptoms vary. Some common symptoms, such as weakness, muscle cramps, and hyperactive reflexes, are related to volume depletion and electrolyte losses. Because alkalosis causes a decrease in ionized calcium, tetany may develop.

Respirations are slow and shallow to increase carbon dioxide content. Confusion and convulsions occur with severe alkalosis. Atrial tachycardia is a potential problem. The oxyhemoglobin curve is shifted to the left (see Chapter 31), decreasing the dissociation of oxyhemoglobin and increasing the risk of dysrhythmias.

Evaluation and Treatment

The health history provides significant clues to the diagnosis of metabolic alkalosis. The arterial pH is above 7.45, and bicarbonate levels exceed 26 mEq/L. With respiratory compensation, the P_{CO_2} rises above 40 mm Hg. With hypochloremic alkalosis, serum chloride values are below normal. Potassium levels are usually depleted because hydrogen is released from the cells in exchange for potassium to help regulate the pH level. The K^+ is then secreted from the distal tubule or kidney cells into the urine.

With hypochloremic alkalosis or contraction alkalosis with volume depletion, a sodium chloride solution is required for correction. The renal stimulus to increase ECF volume by retaining Na^+ is diminished, and HCO_3^- can be excreted as $NaHCO_3$ in the urine. The administration of potassium corrects alkalosis caused by hyperaldosteronism or hypokalemia. The potassium causes hydrogen to move back into the ECF and decreases loss of hydrogen from the distal tubule.

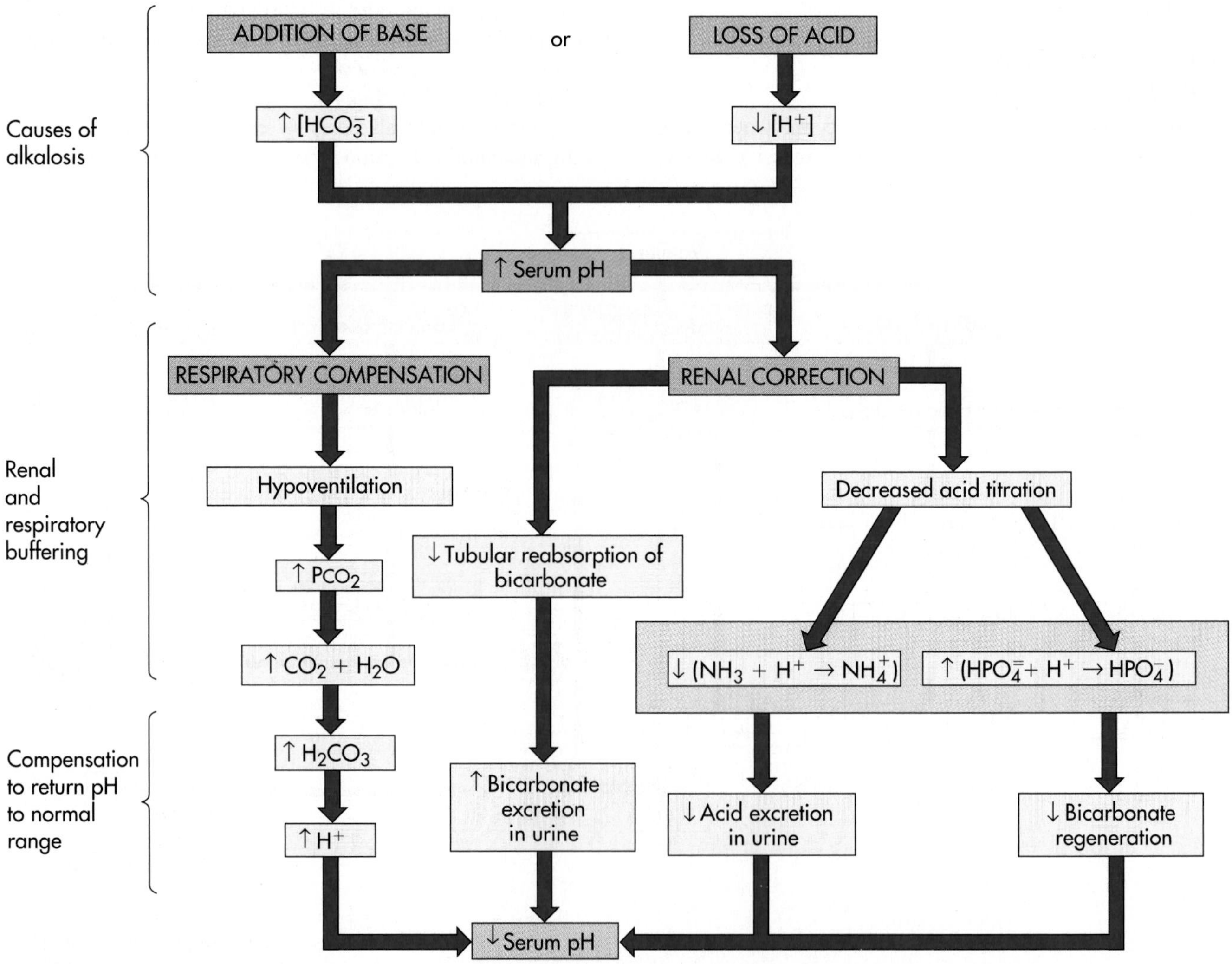

FIG. 3-14 Metabolic alkalosis with compensation and correction. See text for abbreviations.

Respiratory Acidosis

Pathophysiology

Respiratory disorders of acid-base balance are caused by increases or decreases of alveolar ventilation in relation to the metabolic production of carbon dioxide. **Respiratory acidosis** occurs when ventilation is depressed. Carbon dioxide is retained, increasing $[H^+]$ (as H_2CO_3) and producing acidosis. Carbon dioxide excess is called **hypercapnia.** The common causes include depression of the respiratory center (brain stem trauma, oversedation), respiratory muscle paralysis, disorders of the chest wall (kyphoscoliosis, pickwickian syndrome, flail chest), and disorders of the lung parenchyma (pneumonia, pulmonary edema, emphysema, asthma, bronchitis).

Respiratory acidosis may be acute or chronic. Airway obstruction is the most common cause of acute respiratory acidosis. Acute compensation for respiratory acidosis is not effective because the renal buffer mechanism takes time to function. Further, the protein buffers provide marginal compensation, and HCO_3^- is not a good buffer for CO_2. Acute uncompensated respiratory acidosis is characterized by a decreased pH, elevated Pco_2, and normal or slightly increased bicarbonate level.

Chronic respiratory acidosis is commonly associated with chronic obstructive pulmonary disease and deformities of the chest wall. Renal compensation is effective and is established over several days. The acidosis produced from CO_2 retention stimulates the kidney to secrete hydrogen ion and regenerate bicarbonate. Serum bicarbonate and arterial Pco_2 are elevated, and pH will be restored toward normal (Fig. 3-15).

Clinical Manifestations

The symptoms of respiratory acidosis are related to acuity of onset and severity of Pco_2 retention. Initial symptoms include restlessness and apprehension followed by lethargy, muscle twitching, tremors, convulsions, and coma. Neurologic symptoms are caused by a decrease in the pH of cerebrospinal fluid and vasodilation because CO_2 readily crosses the blood-brain barrier. The respiratory rate is rapid at first and gradually becomes depressed because, over time, the respiratory center adapts to increasing levels of CO_2. Cyanosis does not occur unless there is an accompanying hypoxemia, and the skin may instead be pink from vasodilation caused by the acidosis.

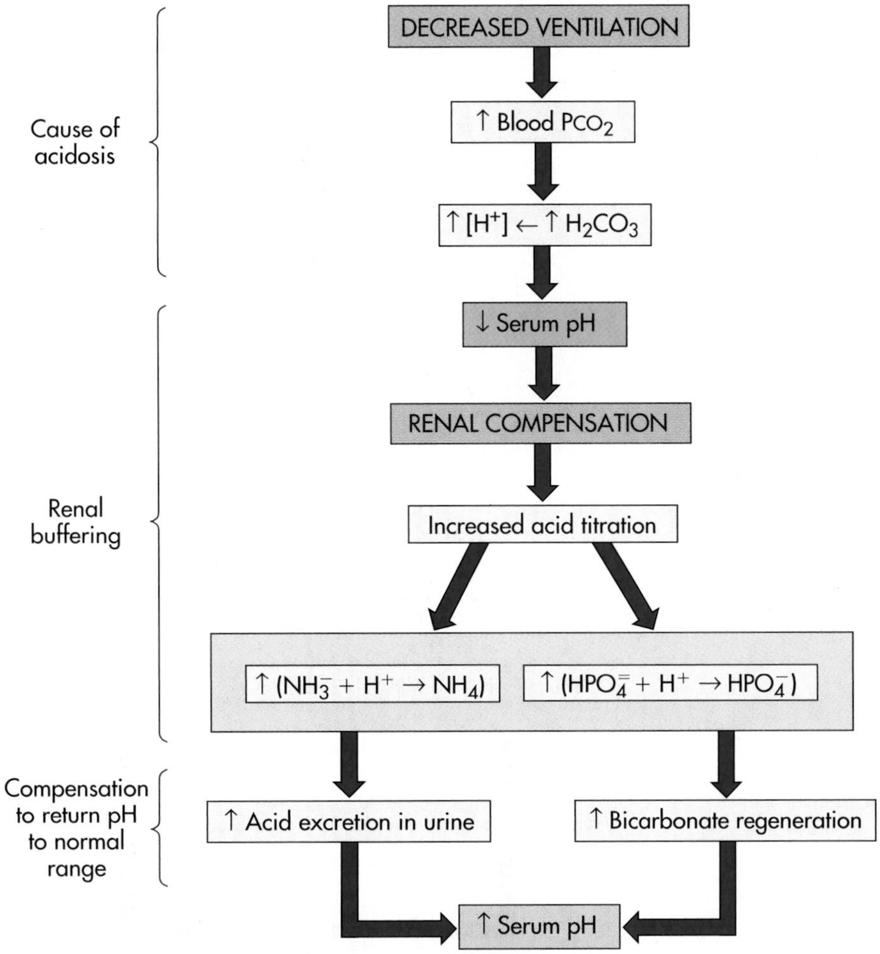

FIG. 3-15 Respiratory acidosis with compensation. See text for abbreviations.

Evaluation and Treatment

The primary diagnostic indicators are an arterial pH less than 7.35 and hypercapnia. Acute respiratory acidosis must be distinguished from chronic acidosis; the health history and clinical laboratory data are therefore helpful. With renal compensation, bicarbonate levels are elevated and the pH is restored toward normal.

The restoration of adequate alveolar ventilation removes excess CO_2. If alveolar ventilation cannot be maintained spontaneously because of drug overdose or neuromuscular disorders, mechanical ventilation is required. The arterial pH, P_{CO_2}, P_{O_2}, and HCO_3^- must be carefully monitored. Rapid reduction of P_{CO_2} can cause respiratory alkalosis with seizures and death.

Renal buffering is usually effective in compensating for uncomplicated chronic respiratory acidosis. The underlying diseases are treated to achieve maximal ventilation. In the presence of hypoxemia and hypercapnia, oxygen can function as a respiratory depressant when the respiratory center is no longer stimulated by the lower pH and elevated P_{CO_2}. Therefore oxygen should be given cautiously.

Respiratory Alkalosis

Pathophysiology

Respiratory alkalosis occurs when there is alveolar hyperventilation and excessive reduction of carbon dioxide (termed **hypocapnia**). Stimulation of ventilation is precipitated by hypoxemia, which may be caused by pulmonary disease, congestive heart failure, or high altitudes; hypermetabolic states such as fever, anemia, and thyrotoxicosis; early salicylate intoxication; hysteria; cirrhosis; and gram-negative sepsis. Improper use of mechanical ventilators can cause iatrogenic respiratory alkalosis. Secondary respiratory alkalosis may develop from hyperventilation stimulated by metabolic or respiratory acidosis.

The onset of respiratory alkalosis occurs within minutes of hyperventilation. Cellular buffers provide immediate compensation with shifts of H^+ from ICF to ECF. The H^+ shifts are not very effective, however, if there is a significant decrease in P_{CO_2}. When there is chronic respiratory alkalosis, renal compensation restores pH toward normal by decreasing H^+ excretion and bicarbonate absorption (Fig. 3-16).

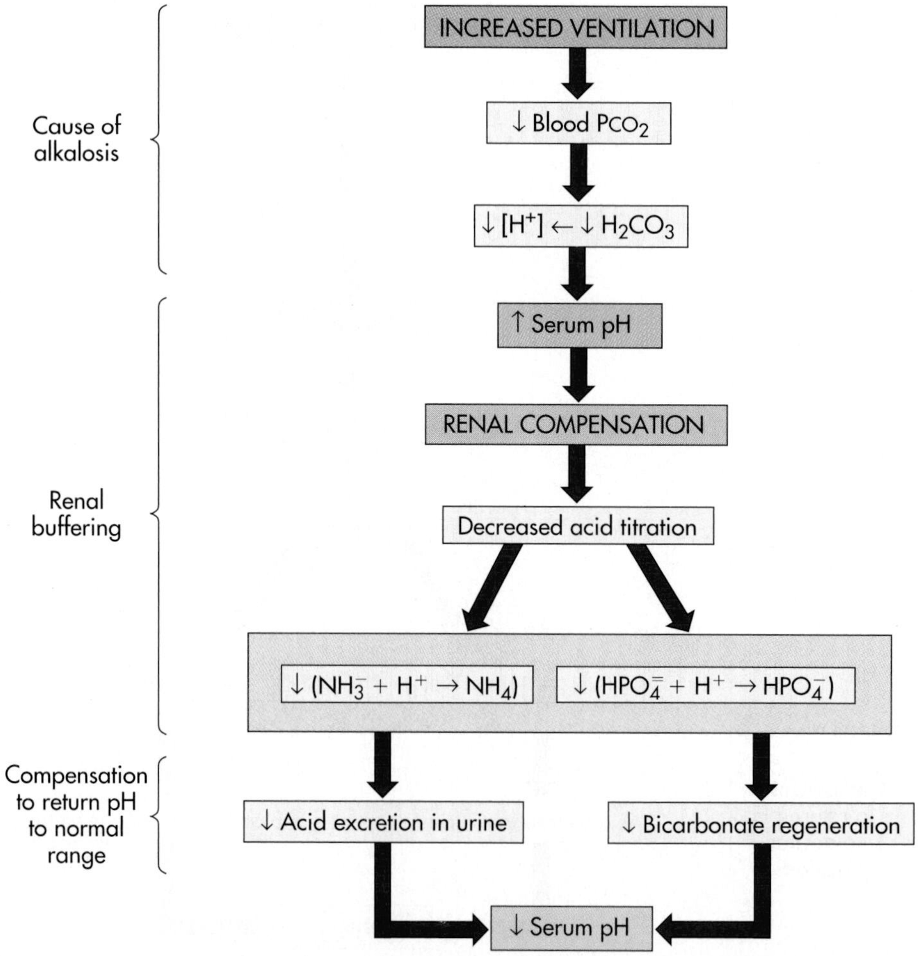

FIG. 3-16 Respiratory alkalosis with compensation. See text for abbreviations.

Clinical Manifestations

Respiratory alkalosis, like metabolic alkalosis, is irritating to the central and peripheral nervous systems. Symptoms include dizziness, confusion, tingling of extremities (paresthesias), convulsions, and coma. Carpopedal spasm and other symptoms of hypocalcemia are similar to those of metabolic alkalosis. Deep and rapid respirations (tachypnea) are primary symptoms that cause respiratory alkalosis.

Evaluation and Treatment

The underlying disturbance must be identified. The arterial pH is above 7.45, and the P_{CO_2} is less than 38 mm Hg. In acute states, bicarbonate levels are normal. With chronic respiratory alkalosis, there is a compensatory decrease in the bicarbonate level and the pH is closer to normal.

Treating the underlying disturbance is the most effective treatment. Hypoxemia must be corrected and hypermetabolic states reversed. Symptoms from hysterical hyperventilation can be corrected by rebreathing from a paper bag, which increases the concentration of inspired carbon dioxide and reverses the respiratory alkalosis.

SUMMARY REVIEW

Distribution of Body Fluids

1. Body fluids are distributed among functional compartments and are classified as intracellular fluid (ICF) or extracellular fluid (ECF).
2. The sum of all fluids is the total body water (TBW), which varies with age and amount of body fat.
3. Water moves between the ICF and ECF compartments principally by osmosis.
4. Water moves between the plasma and interstitial fluid by osmosis and hydrostatic pressure, which occur across the capillary membrane.
5. Movement across the capillary wall is called *net filtration* and is described according to the Starling law.

Alterations in Water Movement

1. Edema is a problem of fluid distribution that results in accumulation of fluid within the interstitial spaces.
2. Edema is caused by arterial dilation, venous or lymphatic obstruction, loss of plasma proteins, increased capillary permeability, and increased vascular volume.
3. The pathophysiologic process that leads to edema is related to an increase in forces favoring fluid filtration from the capillaries or lymphatic channels into the tissues.
4. Edema may be localized or generalized and usually is associated with weight gain, swelling and puffiness, tighter-fitting clothes and shoes, and limited movement of the affected area.

Sodium, Chloride, and Water Balance

1. Sodium and water balance are intimately related; chloride levels are generally proportional to changes in sodium levels.
2. Water balance is regulated by the sensation of thirst and by antidiuretic hormone, which is initiated by an increase in plasma osmolality or a decrease in circulating blood volume.
3. Sodium balance is regulated by aldosterone, which increases reabsorption of sodium by the distal tubule of the kidney.
4. Renin and angiotensin are enzymes that promote or inhibit secretion of aldosterone and thus regulate sodium and water balance.
5. Atrial natriuretic hormone is also involved in decreasing tubular resorption and promoting urinary excretion of sodium.

Alterations in Sodium, Chloride, and Water Balance

1. Alterations in water balance may be classified as isotonic, hypertonic, or hypotonic.
2. Isotonic alterations occur when changes in TBW are accompanied by proportional changes in electrolytes.
3. Hypertonic alterations develop when the osmolality of the ECF is elevated above normal, usually because of an increased concentration of ECF sodium or a deficit of ECF water.
4. Hypernatremia (sodium levels greater than 147 mEq/L) may be caused by an acute increase in sodium or a loss of water.
5. Water deficit, or hypertonic dehydration, is rare but can be caused by lack of access to water, pure water losses, hyperventilation, arid climates, or increased renal clearance.
6. Hyperchloremia is caused by an excess of sodium or a deficit of bicarbonate.
7. Hypotonic alterations occur when the osmolality of the ECF is less than normal.
8. Hyponatremia (serum sodium concentration less than 135 mEq/L) usually causes movement of water into cells.
9. Hyponatremia may be caused by sodium loss, inadequate sodium intake, or dilution of the body's sodium level.
10. Water excess is rare but can be caused by compulsive water drinking, decreased urine formation, or the syndrome of inappropriate secretion of ADH.
11. Hypochloremia is usually the result of hyponatremia or elevated bicarbonate concentrations.

Alterations in Potassium, Calcium, Phosphate, and Magnesium

1. Potassium is the predominant ICF ion; it functions to regulate ICF osmolality, maintain the resting membrane potential, and deposit glycogen in liver and skeletal muscle cells.
2. Potassium balance is regulated by the kidney, by aldosterone and insulin secretion, and by changes in pH.
3. A mechanism known as *potassium adaptation* allows the body to accommodate slowly to increased levels of potassium intake.
4. Hypokalemia (serum potassium concentration less than 3.5 mEq/L) indicates loss of total body potassium, although ECF hypokalemia can develop without losses of total body potassium and plasma K^+ levels may be normal or elevated when total body potassium is depleted.
5. Hypokalemia may be caused by reduced potassium intake, increased ICF-to-ECF potassium concentration, loss of potassium from body stores, increased aldosterone secretion (e.g., caused by hypernatremia), and increased renal excretion.

6. Hyperkalemia (potassium levels greater than 5.5 mEq/L) may be caused by increased potassium intake, a shift from ICF to ECF potassium, or decreased renal excretion.
7. Calcium is a necessary ion in the structure of bones and teeth, in blood clotting, in hormone secretion and the function of cell receptors, and in membrane stability.
8. Phosphate acts as a buffer in acid-base regulation and provides energy for muscle contraction.
9. Calcium and phosphate concentrations are rigidly controlled by parathyroid hormone (PTH), vitamin D, and calcitonin.
10. Hypocalcemia (serum calcium concentration less than 8.5 mg/dl) is related to inadequate intestinal absorption, deposition of ionized calcium into bone or soft tissue, blood administration, or decreased PTH and vitamin D levels.
11. Hypercalcemia (serum calcium concentration greater than 12 mg/dl) can be caused by a number of diseases, including hyperparathyroidism, bone metastases, sarcoidosis, and excess vitamin D.
12. Hypophosphatemia is usually caused by intestinal malabsorption and increased renal excretion of phosphate.
13. Hyperphosphatemia develops with acute or chronic renal failure with significant loss of glomerular filtration.
14. Magnesium is a major intracellular cation and is principally regulated by PTH.
15. Magnesium functions in enzymatic reactions and often interacts with calcium at the cellular level.
16. Hypomagnesemia (serum magnesium concentrations less than 1.5 mEq/L) may be caused by malabsorption syndromes.
17. Hypermagnesemia (serum magnesium concentrations greater than 2.5 mEq/L) is rare and is usually caused by renal failure.

Acid-Base Balance

1. Hydrogen ions, which maintain membrane integrity and the speed of enzymatic reactions, must be concentrated within a narrow range if the body is to function normally.
2. Hydrogen ion concentration is expressed as pH, which represents the negative logarithm of hydrogen ions in solution.
3. Different body fluids have different pH values.
4. The renal and respiratory systems, together with the body's buffer systems, are the principal regulators of acid-base balance.
5. Buffers are substances that can absorb excessive acid or base without a significant change in pH.
6. Buffers exist as acid-base pairs; the principal plasma buffers are carbonic acid–bicarbonate, protein (hemoglobin), and phosphate.
7. Buffer pairs can associate and dissociate; the pK value is the pH at which a buffer pair is half dissociated.
8. The lungs and kidneys act to compensate for changes in pH by increasing or decreasing ventilation and by producing more acidic or more alkaline urine.
9. Correction is a process different from compensation; correction occurs when the values for both components of the buffer pair are returned to normal.
10. Acid-base imbalances are caused by changes in the concentration of H^+ in the blood; an increase causes acidosis, and a decrease causes alkalosis.
11. An abnormal increase or decrease in bicarbonate concentration causes metabolic acidosis or metabolic alkalosis; changes in the rate of alveolar ventilation produce respiratory acidosis or respiratory alkalosis.
12. Metabolic acidosis is caused by an increase in noncarbonic acids or loss of bicarbonate from the extracellular fluid.
13. Metabolic alkalosis occurs with an increase in bicarbonate usually caused by loss of metabolic acids from conditions such as vomiting, gastrointestinal suctioning, excessive bicarbonate intake, hyperaldosteronism, and diuretic therapy.
14. Respiratory acidosis occurs with a decrease of alveolar ventilation and an increase in levels of carbon dioxide, which in turn causes hypercapnia.
15. Respiratory alkalosis occurs with alveolar hyperventilation and excessive reduction of carbon dioxide, or hypocapnia.

KEY TERMS

Acidemia, *105*
Acidosis, *105*
Aldosterone, *90*
Alkalemia, *105*
Alkalosis, *105*
Angiotensin I and II, *90*
Anion gap, *106*
Baroreceptor, *90*
Buffer, *102*
Buffering, *102*
Chloride, *90*
Compensation, *103*
Compulsive water drinking, *93*
Correction, *103*
Decreased urine formation, *93*
Dehydration, *92*
Dilutional hyponatremia, *92*
Edema, *88*
Extracellular fluid (ECF), *85*
Hypercalcemia, *100*
Hypercapnia, *109*
Hyperchloremia, *92*
Hyperchloremic metabolic acidosis, *106*
Hyperkalemia, *98*
Hypermagnesemia, *102*
Hypernatremia, *91*
Hyperphosphatemia, *101*
Hyperpolarized, *96*
Hypertonic hyponatremia, *93*
Hypocalcemia, *100*
Hypocapnia, *110*
Hypochloremia, *94*
Hypochloremic metabolic alkalosis, *107*
Hypokalemia, *95*
Hypomagnesemia, *101*
Hyponatremia, *92*
Hypoosmolar hyponatremia, *93*
Hypophosphatemia, *101*
Hypopolarized, *98*
Hypovolemia, *93*
Inadequate intake, *92*
Interstitial fluid, *85*
Intracellular fluid (ICF), *85*
Intravascular fluid, *85*
Lymphedema, *89*
Metabolic acidosis, *105*
Metabolic alkalosis, *107*
Natriuretic peptide, *90*
Net filtration, *86*
Nonvolatile, *102*
Normal anion gap, *106*
Osmoreceptor, *89*
Potassium adaptation, *95*
Pure sodium deficit, *92*
Renin, *90*
Renin-angiotensin system, *90*
Respiratory acidosis, *109*
Respiratory alkalosis, *110*
Sodium, *90*
Starling hypothesis, *86*
Syndrome of inappropriate secretion of ADH (SIADH), *94*
Total body water (TBW), *85*
Volatile, *102*
Volume-sensitive receptor, *89*
Water deficit, *92*

REFERENCES

1. Chumlea WC et al: Total body water data for adults 18 to 64 years of age: the Fels Longitudinal Study, *Kidney Int* 56(1):244, 1999.
2. Mortimer PS: The pathophysiology of lymphadema, *Cancer* 83(12 suppl, Am):2798, 1998.
3. Ogawa T et al: Characterization of natriuretic peptide production by adult heart atria, *Am J Physiol* 276(6, pt 2):H1977, 1999.
4. Thibault G, Amiri F, Garcia R: Regulation of natriuretic peptide secretion by the heart, *Annu Rev Physiol* 61:193, 1999.
5. Moritz ML, Ayus JC: The changing pattern of hypernatremia in hospitalized children, *Pediatrics* 104(3, pt 1):435, 1999.
6. Polderman KH et al: Hypernatremia in the intensive care unit: an indicator of quality of care? *Crit Care Med* 27(6):1105, 1999.
7. Garigan TP, Ristedt DE: Death from hyponatremia as a result of acute water intoxication in an Army basic trainee, *Mil Med* 164(3):234, 1999.
8. Spital A: Diuretic-induced hyponatremia, *Am J Nephrol* 19(4):447, 1999.
9. Gill G, Leese G: Hyponatremia: biochemical and clinical perspectives, *Postgrad Med J* 74(875):516, 1998.
10. Haycock GB: The syndrome of inappropriate secretion of antidiuretic hormone, *Pediatr Nephrol* 9(3):375, 1995.
11. Ludlow M: Renal handling of potassium, *ANNA J* 20(1):52, 1993.
12. Halperin ML, Goldstein MB: *Fluid, electrolyte, and acid-base physiology*, ed 3, Philadelphia, 1999, W.B. Saunders.
13. Wahr JA et al: Preoperative serum potassium levels and perioperative outcomes in cardiac surgery patients: Multicenter Study of Perioperative Ischemia Research Group, *JAMA* 281(23):2203, 1999.
14. Thatte L et al: Review of literature: severe hyperphosphatemia, *Am J Med Sci* 310(4):167, 1995.
15. Nadler JL, Rude RK: Disorders of magnesium metabolism, *Endocrinol Metab Clin North Am* 24(3):623, 1995.
16. Rose DB, Post T: *Clinical physiology of acid-base and electrolyte disorders*, ed 5, New York, 2000, McGraw-Hill.
17. Oster JR et al: Metabolic acidosis with extreme elevation of anion gap: case report and literature review, *Am J Med Sci* 317(1):38, 1999.
18. Webster NR, Kulkarni V: Metabolic alkalosis in the critically ill, *Crit Rev Clin Lab Sci* 36(5):497, 1999.
19. Galla JH: Metabolic alkalosis, *J Am Soc Nephrol* 11:369, 2000.

CHAPTER 4

Genes and Genetic Diseases

LYNN B. JORDE

CHAPTER OUTLINE

In the nineteenth century, microscopic studies of cells led scientists to suspect that the nucleus of the cell contained the important mechanisms of inheritance. Scientists found that chromatin, the substance that gives the nucleus a granular appearance, is observable in nondividing cells. Just before the cell divides, the chromatin condenses to form discrete, dark-staining organelles, which are called *chromosomes.* (Cell division is discussed in Chapter 1.) With the rediscovery of Gregor Mendel's important breeding experiments at the turn of the twentieth century, it soon became apparent that the chromosomes contained **genes,** the basic units of inheritance. Chromosomes were the subject of much study, but because of poorly developed laboratory techniques, progress was slow. Since the mid-1950s, however, technologic advances have permitted a rapid increase in scientific knowledge of the form, composition, and function of chromosomes.

The primary constituent of the chromatin is **deoxyribonucleic acid (DNA).** Genes are composed of sequences of DNA. By serving as the blueprints of proteins in the body, genes ultimately influence all aspects of body structure and function. **Structural genes** dictate the makeup of proteins. Estimates suggest that there are approximately 50,000 to 100,000 structural genes. An error in one of these genes often leads to a recognizable genetic disease.

To date, more than 11,000 genetic conditions have been identified and cataloged.[1] As infectious diseases come under increasingly effective control, the proportion of beds in pediatric hospitals occupied by children with genetic diseases has risen to one third.[2] In addition, many common diseases that affect primarily adults, such as hypertension, coronary heart disease, diabetes, and cancer, are now known to have important genetic components. (These diseases are also affected by environmental factors. The interaction between genetic and environmental components is discussed in Chapter 5.)

Great progress is being made in the diagnosis of genetic diseases and the understanding of genetic mechanisms underlying them. With the huge strides being made in molecular genetics, gene therapy—the replacement of disease genes with normal ones—has begun. Genetics is now one of the most rapidly advancing fields of medicine.

DNA, RNA, AND PROTEINS: HEREDITY AT THE MOLECULAR LEVEL

DNA

Composition and Structure

Genes are composed of DNA, which has three basic components: the pentose sugar molecule, deoxyribose; a phosphate molecule; and four types of nitrogenous bases. Two of the bases, **cytosine** and **thymine,** are single carbon-nitrogen rings called **pyrimidines.** The other two bases, **adenine** and

guanine, are double carbon-nitrogen rings called **purines.** The four bases are commonly represented by their first letters: A, C, T, and G.

One of Watson and Crick's contributions was to demonstrate how these molecules are physically assembled together as DNA. They proposed the now-famous **double-helix** model, in which DNA can be envisioned as a twisted ladder with chemical bonds as its rungs (Fig. 4-1). The two sides of the ladder are composed of the sugar and phosphate molecules, held together by strong phosphodiester bonds. Projecting from each side of the ladder, at regular intervals, are the nitrogenous bases. The base projecting from one side is bound to the base projecting from the other by a weak hydrogen bond. Therefore the nitrogenous bases form the rungs of the ladder; adenine pairs with thymine, and guanine pairs with cytosine. Each DNA subunit—consisting of one deoxyribose molecule, one phosphate group, and one base—is called a **nucleotide.**

DNA as the Genetic Code

To serve as the basis of genetic inheritance, DNA must be able to direct the synthesis of all the body's proteins. Proteins

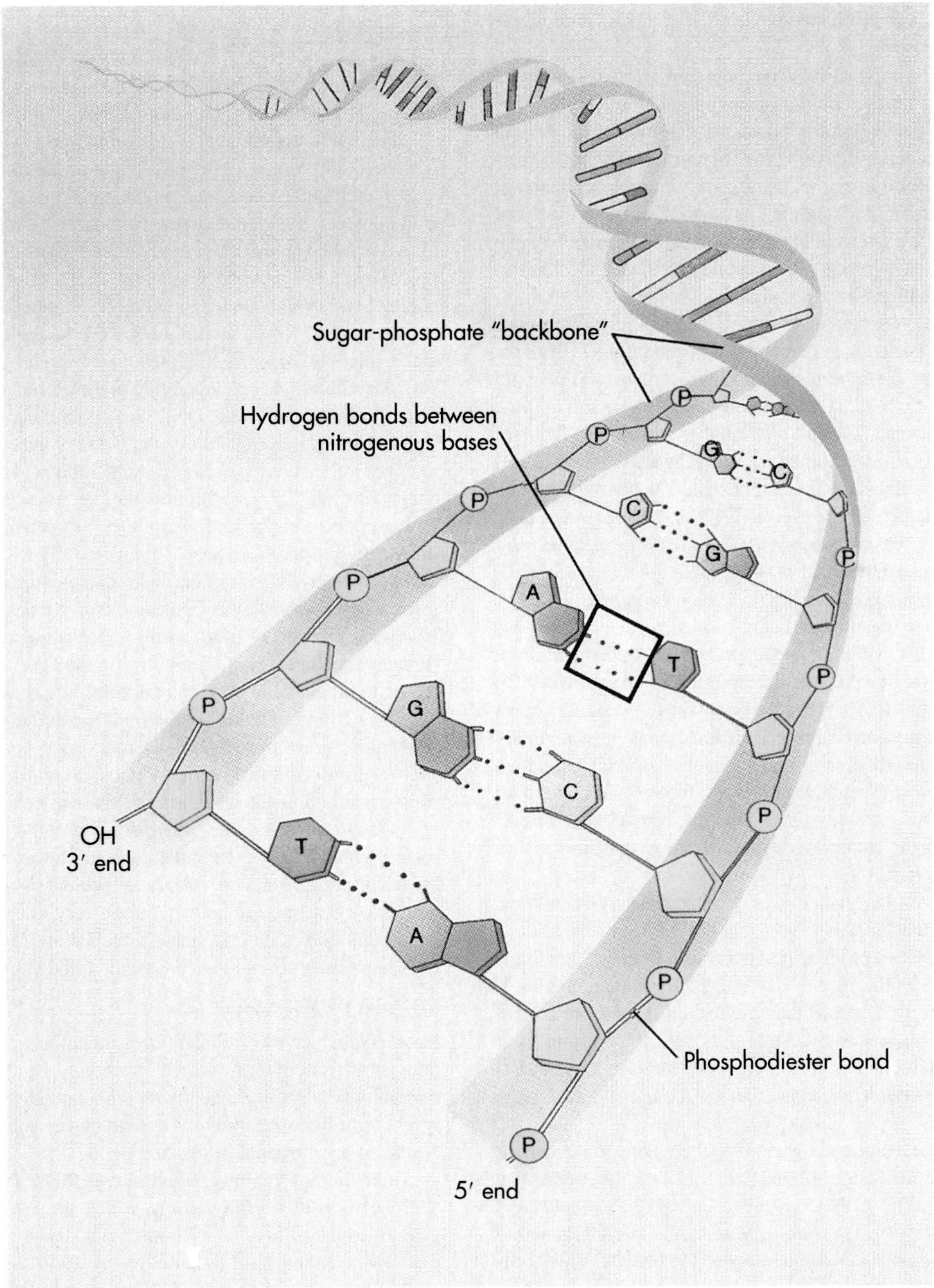

FIG. 4-1 Structure of deoxyribonucleic acid (DNA). In a DNA double helix, only two nitrogenous base pairs are possible: adenine *(A)* with thymine *(T)*; and guanine *(G)* with cytosine *(C)*. The bases are linked in the middle of the molecule by hydrogen bonds. The "backbone" of the DNA molecule is composed of the deoxyribose sugars joined by phosphodiester bonds to phosphate groups *(P)*. (From Raven PH, Johnson GB: *Understanding biology,* ed 3, Dubuque, Iowa, 1995, Brown.)

WHAT'S NEW? Genetic Engineering and Gene Therapy: The "New Genetics"

Terms such as *cloning, genetic engineering,* and *recombinant DNA* have received much exposure in the popular press during the past several years as the news media have recognized the potential importance of these techniques. Indeed they are part of the scientific revolution sometimes known as the *new genetics.*

RECOMBINANT DNA

Genetic engineering refers to laboratory alteration of genes. Most alterations are accomplished by using recombinant DNA techniques, which involve combining the DNA of two or more different organisms. A number of sophisticated methods have been invented to do this; described here is a common approach that is similar in principle to most other approaches.

Among the key components of recombinant DNA research are bacterial plasmids—small, circular pieces of self-replicating DNA that reside in many bacteria but often are not essential to the growth or survival of the bacteria. Plasmids can therefore be extracted from or inserted into bacteria without seriously disrupting bacterial growth or reproduction. Once they are extracted from their bacterial hosts, the plasmids are exposed to restriction endonucleases, which are enzymes that cleave, or cut, the plasmid DNA at a specific nucleotide sequence, called a *restriction site.*

Different restriction endonucleases have different restriction sites. A commonly used restriction endonuclease is called *Eco*RI (from the bacteria that produce it, *Escherichia coli*). *Eco*RI cleaves DNA only when the sequence GAATTC is found on one DNA strand and the complementary sequence is found on the other strand. The DNA of another organism, such as a human, can also be exposed to *Eco*RI and can be cleaved at the same restriction sites. The resulting human restriction fragments, which are pieces of DNA, have exposed ends that have base sequences complementary to those of the cleaved plasmid DNA. The human DNA and plasmid DNA, if mixed together, undergo complementary base pairing (i.e., they recombine).

The result is that the human DNA is incorporated within the plasmid. The plasmids, which now contain human genes in addition to their own, are allowed to reenter bacteria. Selection processes can be applied to pick out the bacteria that contain the desired human genes. These are cultured and allowed to form clones (or genetically identical copies) through normal cell division. Through continued cell division, millions of bacterial clones are formed, all containing the same human gene. Like any other gene, the human gene directs protein synthesis in the bacteria, resulting in the production of human proteins by bacteria.

Because bacteria multiply rapidly, large amounts of a given human protein can be manufactured by using this procedure. It has already been used successfully to produce human insulin in mass quantities. Because the insulin produced this way is actually human insulin, it produces fewer allergic reactions than the insulin taken from animal pancreases. Interferon, a substance that may help the body to fight cancer and viral infections, has also been produced this way, as has human growth hormone, a substance that can be used to cure pituitary dwarfism.

In trying to isolate a particular gene, it is often more convenient to begin work with the messenger ribonucleic acid (mRNA) that codes for the gene product. The mRNA can be purified from body cells, and then an enzyme called *reverse transcriptase* can be used to generate the DNA sequence that is complementary to the mRNA. This complementary DNA (cDNA) can be inserted into plasmids and cloned by using the same recombinant techniques, so that virtually unlimited quantities of the desired gene product can be manufactured.

Recombinant DNA methods have been applied toward the understanding of the single-gene disorder phenylketonuria (PKU), which is the result of a lack of the enzyme phenylalanine hydroxylase. First, mRNA coding for this enzyme was purified from rat liver cells. After attachment of a radioactive "label" to cDNA produced from this mRNA, the cDNA was used as a probe. The probe was exposed to a series of cells that had been manipulated in the laboratory so that each cell line contained only one or a few chromosomes. When the probe hybridized consistently with only the cells containing chromosome 12, it proved that the gene that produces phenylalanine hydroxylase and thus causes PKU is located on this chromosome. Knowing the chromosome location of a gene is a very important step in the diagnosis and understanding of a genetic disease. Ultimately, therapeutic techniques might be developed to correct such disorders by replacing or repairing the abnormal gene.

The use of recombinant DNA techniques to clone DNA sequences has been (and continues to be) of great importance in genetics. However, the cloning process can take a great deal of time, even for well-studied genes. When doing genetic diagnoses, it is often necessary to obtain results very quickly. A newer technique, the polymerase chain reaction (PCR), provides a very rapid means of making millions of copies of a DNA sequence in only a few hours (as opposed to 1 week or more using cloning techniques). PCR basically involves the artificial replication of a DNA sequence, achieved by exposing the DNA strand to alterations in temperature in the presence of free DNA bases. At lower temperatures the DNA undergoes complementary base pairing, and at higher temperatures the DNA strands separate to form new templates for another cycle of replication when the temperature is again lowered. By repeating this temperature cycling over and over, DNA copies can be produced rapidly. This technique is very useful for diagnostic purposes because it requires only a very small sample of blood or other tissue and because a large number of copies can be made in a very short time. In theory, even a single DNA molecule can be copied millions of times using PCR. It is also used extensively in forensic medicine (e.g., in identifying the DNA of criminal suspects by using blood, semen, or hair samples left at the scene of a crime).

The advent of this technology has led to fears that organisms that could pose grave threats to the human species might be created. In 1974 a group of molecular geneticists themselves called a moratorium on recombinant DNA research when its implications began to be realized; however, after much study and the introduction of rules regarding laboratory containment, research was resumed. Because of the elaborate precautions taken to prevent inadvertent creation of harmful organisms and because of the very low probability that such organisms could survive outside the laboratory, the possibility of such an occurrence is now considered to be extremely remote.

GENE THERAPY

An area in which recombinant DNA techniques have generated much interest is gene therapy, which essentially involves the insertion of normal genes. For example, by recombinant DNA methods, a normal gene might be inserted into a human chromosome to counteract the effects of an abnormal or missing gene.

Gene therapy can be applied in two ways. The less controversial approach is somatic cell therapy, which consists of inserting normal genes into the cells of an individual who has a genetic disease. Here a particular tissue, such as bone marrow cells that produce abnormal erythrocytes, would be treated. More controversial is the application of gene therapy very early in embryonic development. By inserting genes into the embryos, all body cells could be altered, including the

WHAT'S NEW? Genetic Engineering and Gene Therapy: The "New Genetics"—cont'd

germ cells. Thus not only would the genetic constitution of the embryo and resulting individual be changed, but also all the descendants of that individual would have altered genetic constitutions. This procedure is sometimes referred to as *germ cell therapy.*

Somatic cell therapy has now been initiated for a number of human diseases, including hemophilia, cystic fibrosis, familial hypercholesterolemia, and several types of cancer.[3,4] The procedure has been quite successful in these individuals, and no serious side effects have been encountered. More than 400 somatic cell gene therapy protocols are now being tested. Because of several important technical and ethical considerations, germline therapy will not be attempted in humans in the foreseeable future.

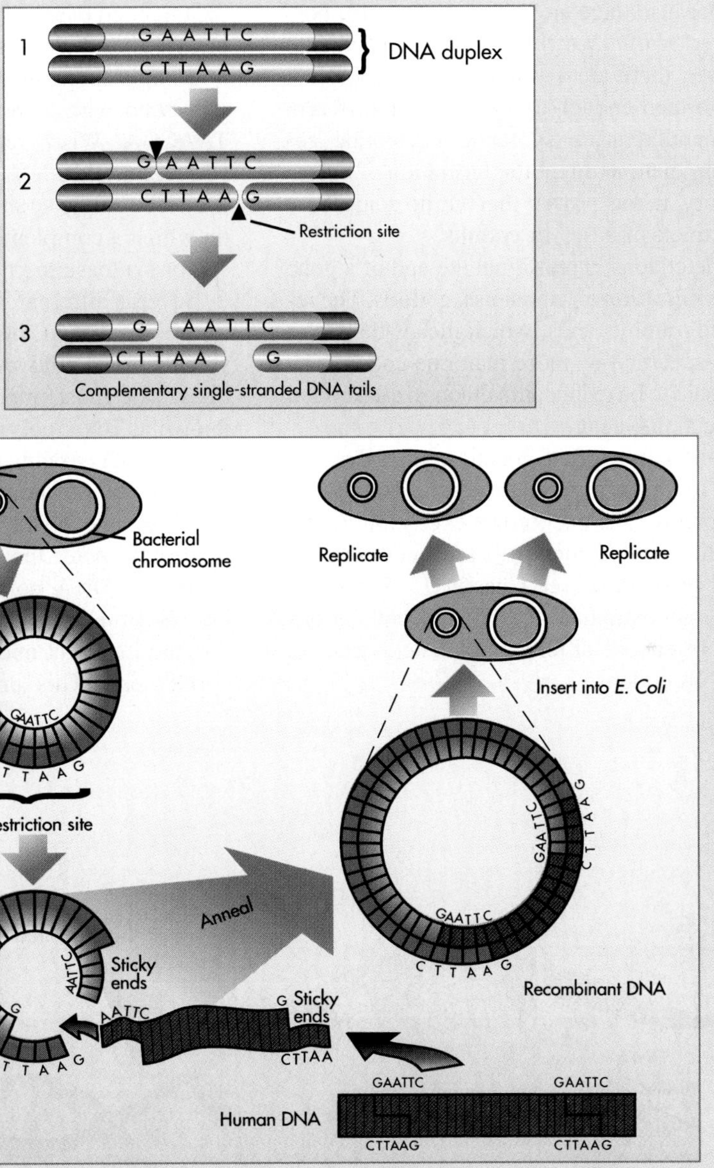

Recombinant DNA technology. Human DNA and circular plasmid DNA are both cleaved by a restriction enzyme, producing sticky ends (*1* to *3*). This allows the human DNA to anneal and recombine with the plasmid DNA. Inserted into the plasmid DNA, the human DNA is now replicated when plasmid is inserted into the bacterium, such as *Escherichia coli (4). G,* Guanine; *A,* adenine; *T,* thymine; *C,* cytosine.

Data and illustration from Jorde LB et al: *Medical genetics,* ed 2, St Louis, 1999, Mosby.

are composed of one or more **polypeptides** (intermediate protein compounds), which are in turn composed of sequences of **amino acids** (organic acids containing NH_2). The body contains 20 different types of amino acids, and the amino acid sequences that make up polypeptides must in some way be specified by the DNA molecule.

Because there are 20 possible amino acids and only four possible bases, each single nucleotide cannot specify an amino acid. Similarly, the amino acids cannot be specified by couplets of bases (e.g., adenine-guanine, thymine-guanine, guanine-cytosine) because there are only 4×4, or 16, possible couplets. If series of three bases are translated into amino acids, however, there are $4 \times 4 \times 4$, or 64, possible combinations—more than enough to specify each different amino acid. By manufacturing synthetic nucleotide sequences and allowing them to direct the formation of amino acids in the laboratory, it was proved that amino acids were specified by these triplets of bases, or **codons.**

Of the 64 possible codons, three signal the end of a gene and are known as **termination,** or **nonsense, codons.** The remaining 61 all specify amino acids, which means that most amino acids can be specified by more than one codon. The genetic code is thus said to be redundant, although each codon can specify only one amino acid.

Another significant feature of the genetic code is that it is universal: all living organisms use precisely the same DNA codes to specify proteins. The one known exception to this rule occurs in mitochondria—cytoplasmic organelles that are the sites of cellular respiration (see Chapter 1). The mitochondria have their own extranuclear DNA. Several codons of mitochondrial DNA encode different amino acids than do the same nuclear DNA codons.

Replication

In addition to having the ability to specify amino acid sequences, DNA must be able to replicate itself accurately during cell division if it is to serve as the basic genetic material. DNA replication consists of the breaking of the weak hydrogen bonds between the bases, leaving a single strand with each base unpaired. The consistent pairing of adenine with thymine and of guanine with cytosine, known as **complementary base pairing,** is the key to accurate replication. The principle of complementary base pairing dictates that the unpaired base will attract a free nucleotide only if the nucleotide has the proper complementary base. Thus a portion of a single strand with a sequence of bases labeled ATTGCT will bond with a series of free nucleotides with the bases TAACGA. When replication is complete, a new double-stranded molecule identical to the original is formed (Fig. 4-2). The single strand is said to be a **template,** or molecule on which a complementary molecule is built, and is the basis for synthesizing the new double strand.

Several different proteins are involved in DNA replication. One protein unwinds the double helix, one holds the strands apart, and others perform different distinct functions. The most important of these proteins is an enzyme known as **DNA polymerase.** This enzyme travels along the single DNA strand, adding the correct nucleotides to the free end of the new strand. Besides adding the new nucleotides, the DNA polymerase performs a proofreading procedure. After the new nucleotide has been added to the chain, the DNA polymerase checks to make sure that its base is actually complementary to the template base. If it is not, the incorrect nucleotide is excised and replaced with a correct one. This procedure, one of the mechanisms of

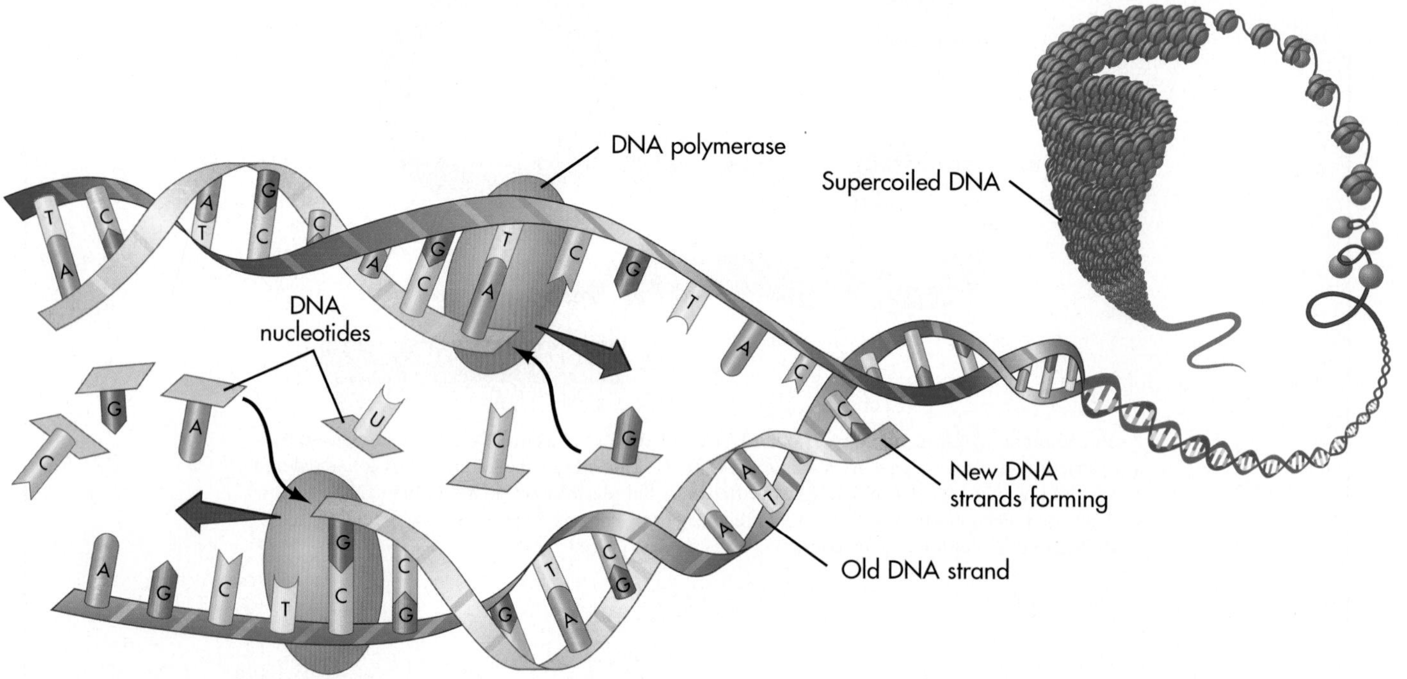

FIG. 4-2 Deoxyribonucleic acid (DNA) replication. *A,* Adenine; *T,* thymine; *G,* guanine; *C,* cytosine. (From Thibodeau GA, Patton KI: *Anatomy & physiology,* ed 4, St Louis, 1999, Mosby.)

DNA repair, substantially enhances the accuracy of DNA replication.

Mutation

A **mutation** is any inherited alteration of genetic material. Chromosome aberrations that cause congenital defects are examples of mutations. Other mutations are subtle and are not observable as chromosome aberrations. One such mutation is the **base pair substitution,** in which one base pair is replaced by another. This substitution sometimes results in a change in amino acid sequence, but because of the redundancy of the genetic code, it may have no consequence. If an amino acid change does not occur, the mutation is termed a **silent substitution.** Profound consequences can result, however, when an amino acid sequence is altered by a base pair substitution. (Many of the serious genetic diseases discussed later are the result of base pair substitutions.)

A second major type of mutation is the **frameshift mutation.** This alteration involves the insertion or deletion of one or more base pairs to the DNA molecule. As Fig. 4-3 shows, these mutations can change the entire "reading frame" of the DNA sequence because codons consist of groups of three base pairs. A frameshift mutation thus can greatly alter the resulting amino acid sequence.

A large number of agents are known to increase the frequency of mutations. These agents are known collectively as **mutagens.** Radiation, such as that produced by x-rays and nuclear fallout, is an important mutagen and is known to cause cell damage (see Chapter 2). Radiation forms electrically charged ions that can produce chemical reactions, which in turn change DNA bases. A variety of chemicals can also induce mutations, often because they are chemically similar to DNA bases. Other chemicals mimic the effects of ionizing radiation, and still others interfere with the process of base pairing. Hundreds of chemicals are now known to be mutagenic in humans or laboratory animals, such as nitrogen mustard, vinyl chloride, alkylating agents, formaldehyde, sodium nitrite, and saccharin. Some of these chemicals, however, are much more potent mutagens than others. Nitrogen mustard, for example, is extremely mutagenic, whereas saccharin is a relatively weak mutagen.

Measurement of the mutation rate in humans is difficult, in part because mutations are very rare events. Current estimates are that the rate of **spontaneous mutation** (a mutation that occurs in the absence of exposure to known mutagens) in humans is about 10^{-4} to 10^{-7} per gene per generation. This rate appears to vary from one gene to another. Certain areas of some chromosomes have particularly high mutation rates and are known as **mutational hot spots.** In particular, sequences consisting of a cytosine base followed by a guanine base (CG) are highly susceptible to mutation and are known to account for a disproportionately large percentage of disease-causing mutations.[5]

From Genes to Proteins

Whereas DNA is formed and replicated in the cell nucleus, protein synthesis takes place in the cytoplasm. The transport of the DNA code from nucleus to cytoplasm and subsequent protein formation involves two basic processes: transcription and translation. Both these processes are mediated by **ribonucleic acid (RNA),** a type of nucleic acid that is chemically very similar to DNA. RNA is also composed of sugar molecules, phosphate groups, and nitrogenous bases. RNA differs from DNA in that the sugar molecule is ribose rather than deoxyribose and in that uracil rather than thymine is one of the four bases. The other bases of RNA, as in DNA, are adenine, cytosine, and guanine. Uracil is structurally very similar to thymine, so it also can pair with adenine. The final difference between RNA and DNA is that, whereas DNA usually occurs as a double strand, RNA usually occurs as a single strand.

Transcription

Transcription is the process by which RNA is synthesized from a DNA template. The result is the formation of **messenger RNA (mRNA)** from the base sequence specified by the DNA molecule. An enzyme called *DNA-dependent RNA polymerase,* or **RNA polymerase,** binds to a **promoter site** on the DNA. A promoter site is a sequence of DNA that specifies the beginning of a gene. The RNA polymerase then pulls a portion of the DNA strands apart from one another, allowing unattached DNA bases to be exposed. One of the DNA strands then provides the template for the sequence of mRNA nucleotides.

The sequence of bases in the mRNA is thus complementary to that of the template strand, and with the exception of the presence of uracil instead of thymine, the mRNA sequence is identical to that of the other DNA strand. Transcription continues until a DNA sequence called a **termination sequence** is reached. Then the RNA polymerase detaches from the DNA, and the transcribed mRNA is freed to move out of the nucleus and into the cytoplasm. Fig. 4-4 summarizes the process of transcription.

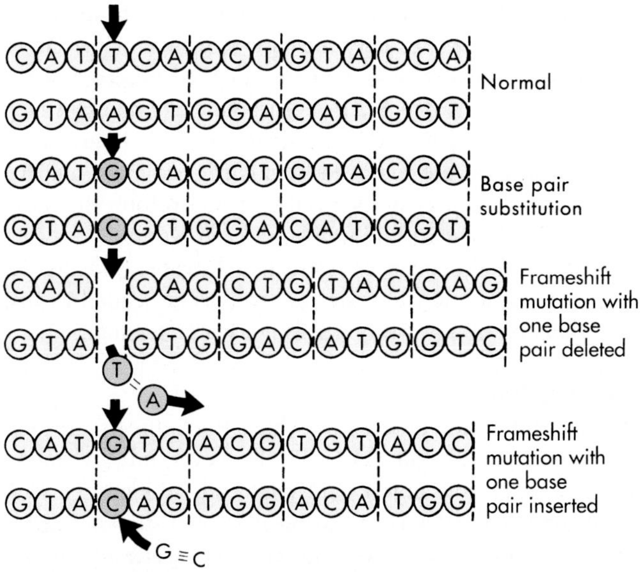

FIG. 4-3 Different kinds of mutations. *A,* Adenine; *T,* thymine; *G,* guanine; *C,* cytosine.

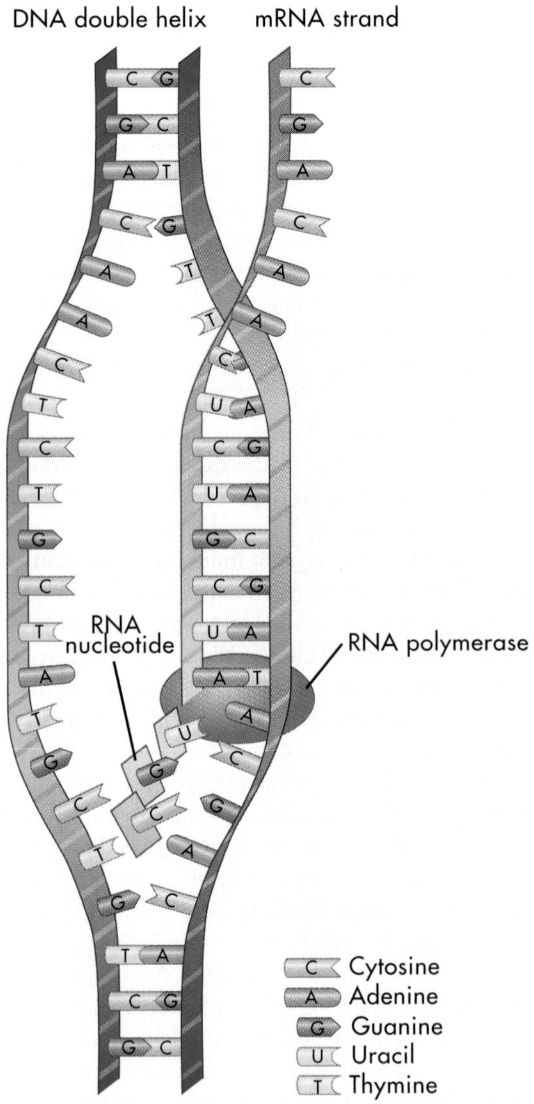

FIG. 4-4 General scheme of ribonucleic acid (RNA) transcription. See text for explanation. (From Thibodeau GA, Patton KI: *Anatomy & physiology,* ed 4, St Louis, 1999, Mosby.)

Gene Splicing

After the mRNA first has been transcribed from the DNA template, it reflects exactly the base sequence of the DNA. The RNA in this state is sometimes called **heterogeneous nuclear RNA (hnRNA).** In eukaryotes an important step takes place before this RNA leaves the nucleus. Many of the RNA sequences are removed by nuclear enzymes, and the remaining sequences are spliced together to form the functional mRNA that will migrate to the cytoplasm.

The excised sequences are called **introns,** and the sequences that are left to code for proteins are called **exons.** The function, if any, of introns is not yet understood.

Translation

Translation is the process by which RNA directs the synthesis of a polypeptide (Fig. 4-5). However, mRNA cannot code directly for amino acids. Instead, it interacts with **transfer RNA (tRNA),** a cloverleaf-shaped strand of about 80 nucleotides. The tRNA molecule has a site for the attachment of an amino acid. At the opposite side of the cloverleaf is a sequence of three nucleotides called the **anticodon.** The anticodon undergoes complementary base pairing with an appropriate codon in the mRNA. The mRNA thus specifies the sequence of amino acids by acting through the tRNA.

The site of actual protein synthesis is the **ribosome,** which consists of roughly equal parts of protein and **ribosomal RNA (rRNA).** During translation (Fig. 4-6) the ribosome first binds to an initiation site on the mRNA sequence. The ribosome then binds the tRNA to its surface so that base pairing can occur between tRNA and mRNA. The ribosome then moves along the mRNA sequence, codon by codon. As each codon is processed, an amino acid is translated by the interaction of mRNA and tRNA.

In this process the ribosome provides an enzyme that catalyzes the formation of covalent peptide bonds between the adjacent amino acids, resulting in a growing polypeptide. When the ribosome arrives at a termination signal on the mRNA sequence, translation and polypeptide formation cease. The mRNA, ribosome, and polypeptide separate from one another, and the polypeptide is released into the cytoplasm to perform its required function.

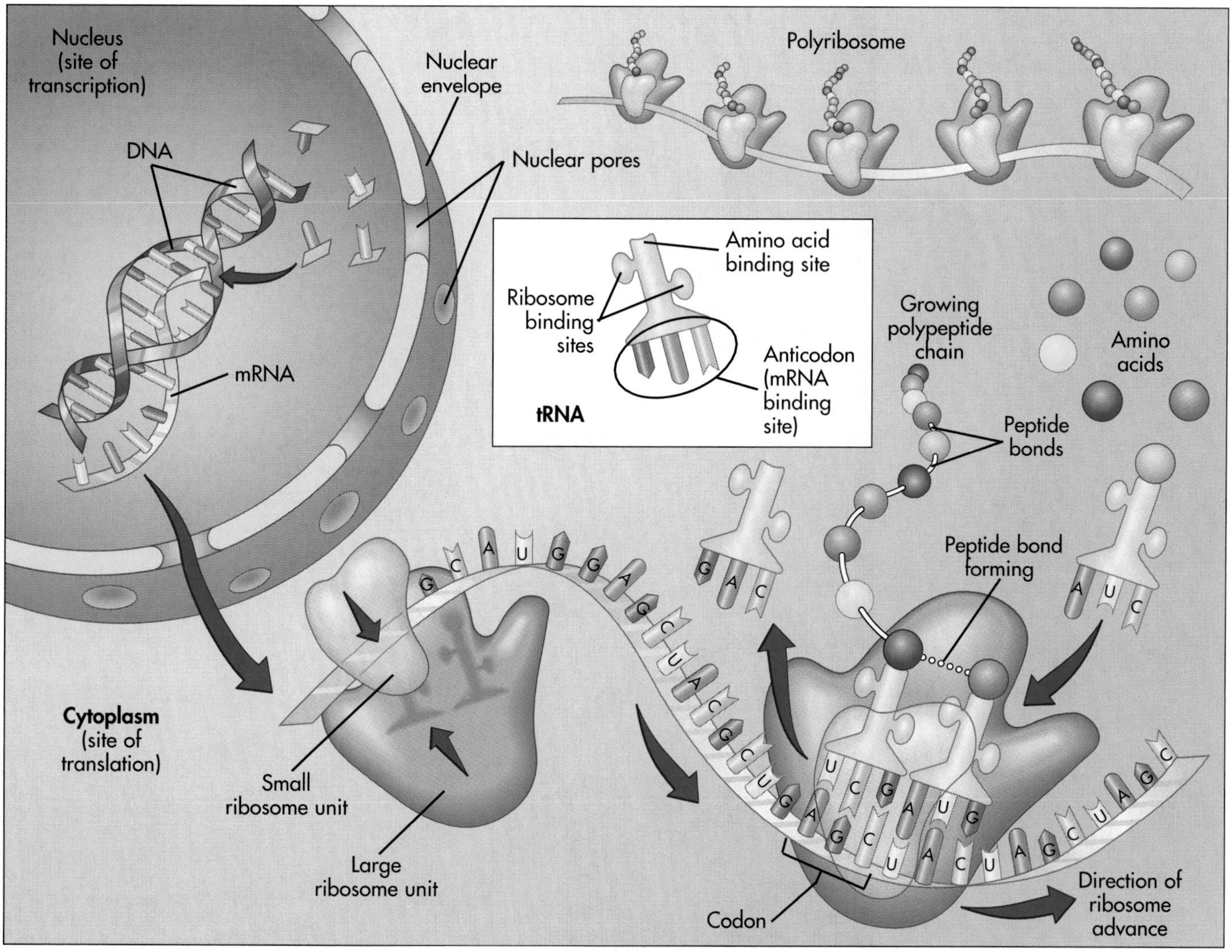

FIG. 4-5 Protein synthesis. Protein synthesis begins with *transcription,* a process in which a messenger ribonucleic acid (mRNA) molecule forms along one gene sequence of a deoxyribonucleic acid (DNA) molecule within the cell's nucleus. As it is formed, the mRNA molecule separates from the DNA molecule and leaves the nucleus through the large nuclear pores. Outside the nucleus, ribosome subunits attach to the beginning of the mRNA molecule and begin the process of *translation.* In translation, transfer RNA (tRNA) molecules bring specific amino acids—encoded by each mRNA codon—into place at the ribosome site. As the amino acids are brought into the proper sequence, they are joined together by peptide bonds to form long strands called *polypeptides.* Several polypeptide chains may be needed to make a complete protein molecule. *A,* Adenine; *C,* cytosine; *G,* guanine; *U,* uracil. (From Thibodeau GA, Patton KI: *Anatomy & Physiology,* ed 4, St Louis, 1999, Mosby.)

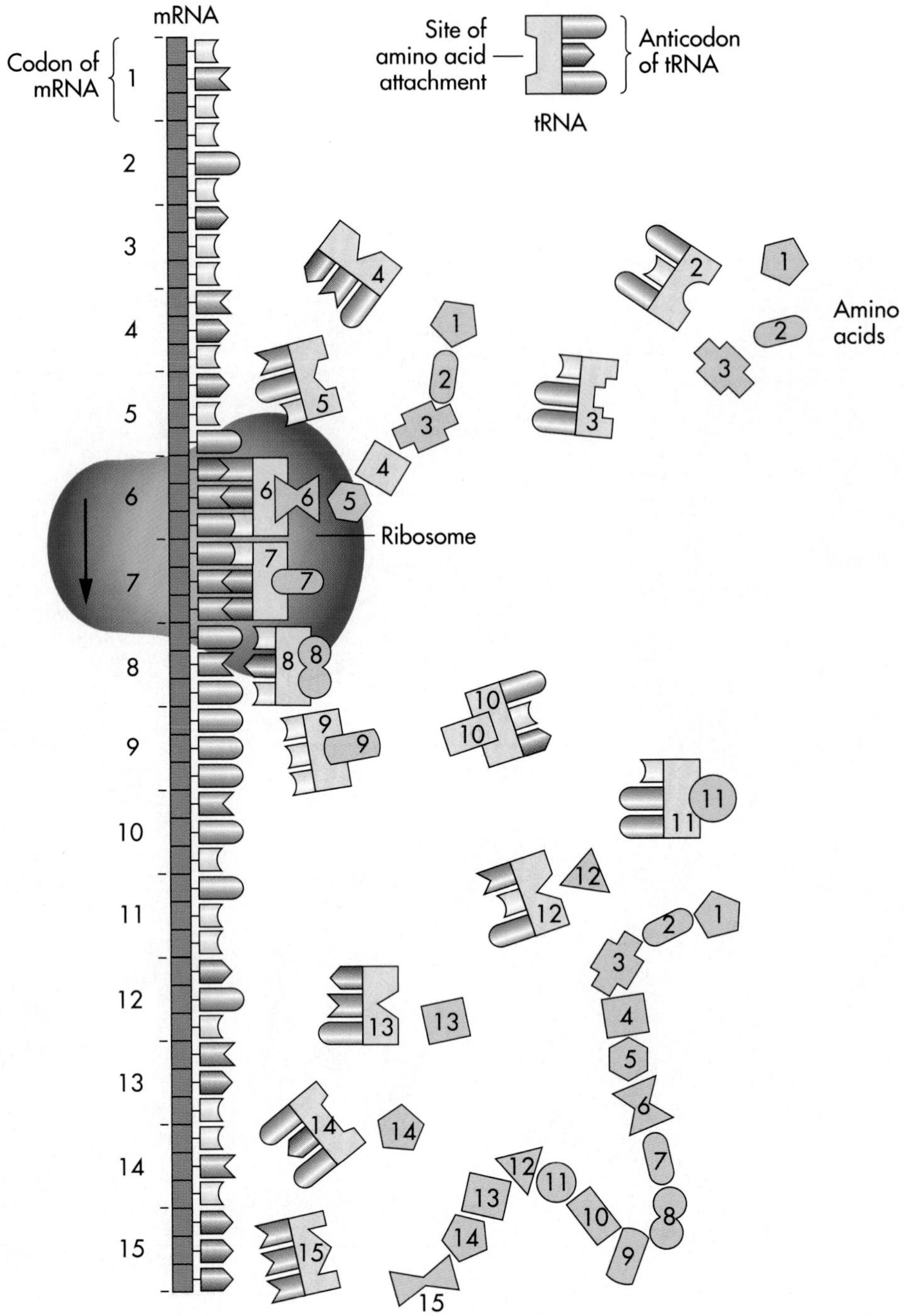

FIG. 4-6 **A ribosome "reading" the code of messenger ribonucleic acid (mRNA) and assembling a polypeptide chain.**

CHROMOSOMES

Human cells can be categorized into two types: the **gametes** (sperm and egg cells) and the **somatic cells,** which include all cells other than gametes. Each somatic cell has 46 chromosomes in its nucleus. These are **diploid cells,** meaning that the chromosomes occur in pairs. Thus each cell actually contains 23 pairs of chromosomes. One member of each pair comes from the individual's mother, and one comes from the father. New somatic cells are formed through mitosis and cytokinesis, through which the cell nucleus and cytoplasm are replicated. (The division process that creates new copies of somatic cells is described in Chapter 1.) Gametes are **haploid cells:** they have only one member of each chromosome pair, giving them a total of 23 chromosomes. The process by which these haploid cells are formed from diploid cells is called **meiosis** (Fig. 4-7).

In 22 of the 23 chromosome pairs, the two members of each pair are virtually identical in microscopic appearance and are thus said to be **homologous** to one another. These 22 chromosome pairs are homologous in both males and females and are termed **autosomes.** The remaining pair of

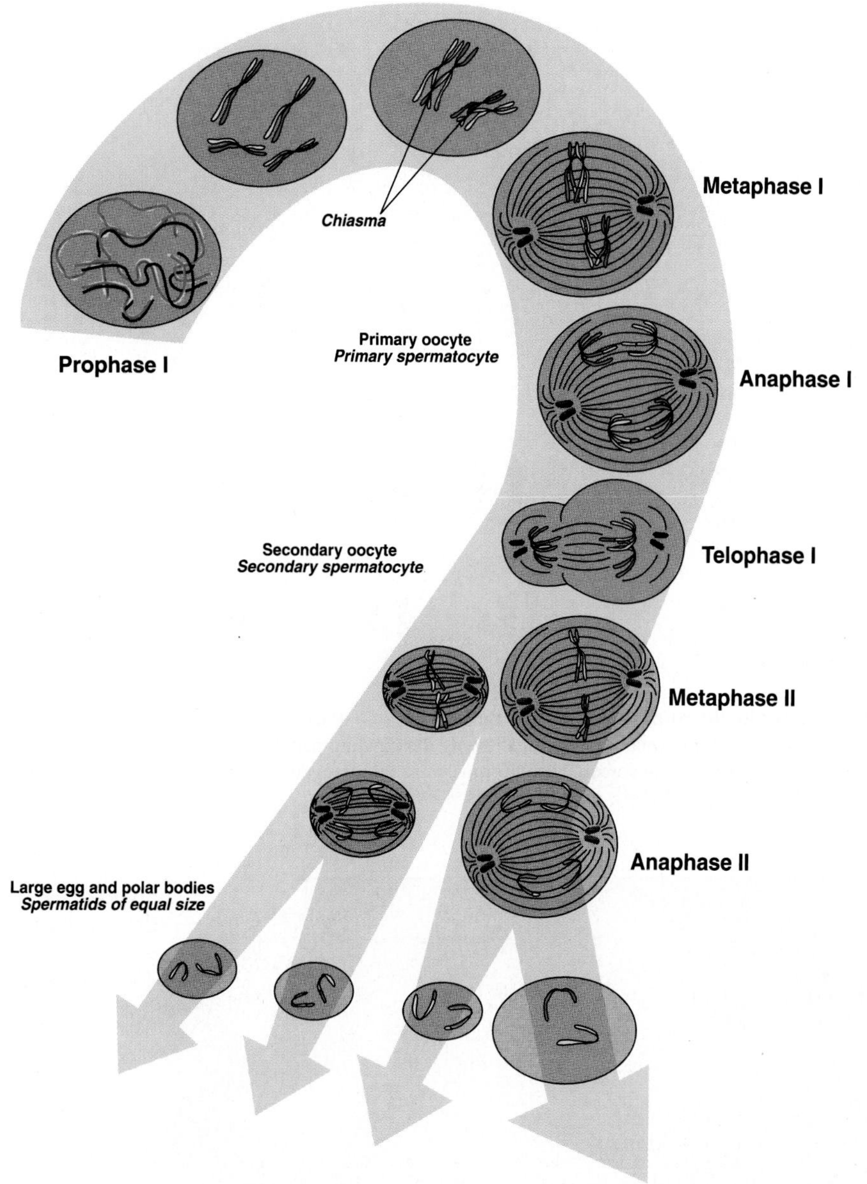

FIG. 4-7 Stages of meiosis. Stages of meiosis, during which haploid gametes are formed from a diploid stem cell. For brevity, prophase II and telophase II are not shown. Note the relationship between meiosis and spermatogenesis and oogenesis. (From Jorde LB et al: *Medical genetics,* ed 2, St Louis, 1999, Mosby.)

chromosomes, the **sex chromosomes,** consists of two homologous X chromosomes in females and a nonhomologous pair, X and Y, in males.

Fig. 4-8, *A,* illustrates a **metaphase spread,** which is a photograph of the chromosomes as they appear in the nucleus of a somatic cell during metaphase. (Chromosomes are easiest to visualize during this stage of mitosis.) A **karyotype** is an ordered display of chromosomes. In Fig. 4-8, *B,* the chromosomes are cut out and arranged according to size, with the **homologous chromosomes** paired together. The 22 autosomes are numbered according to length, with chromosome 1 as the longest and chromosome 22 as the shortest. Some natural variation in relative chromosome length can be expected from person to person, however, so it is not always possible to distinguish each chromosome by its length. Therefore the position of the centromere is also used to classify the chromosomes (Fig. 4-9).

The chromosomes in Fig. 4-8 were stained with a substance that penetrates all areas of the chromosome (a "solid stain"). In the late 1960s and early 1970s, several staining materials were found to bind preferentially to certain areas of chromosomes. The resulting distinctive **chromosome bands** are evident in various patterns in the different chromosomes so that each chromosome can be distinguished easily. One of the most commonly used stains is **Giemsa stain.** By using banding techniques, chromosomes can be unambiguously numbered, and individual variation in chromosome composition can be studied. Missing or duplicated portions of chromosomes, which often result in serious diseases, also can be readily identified.

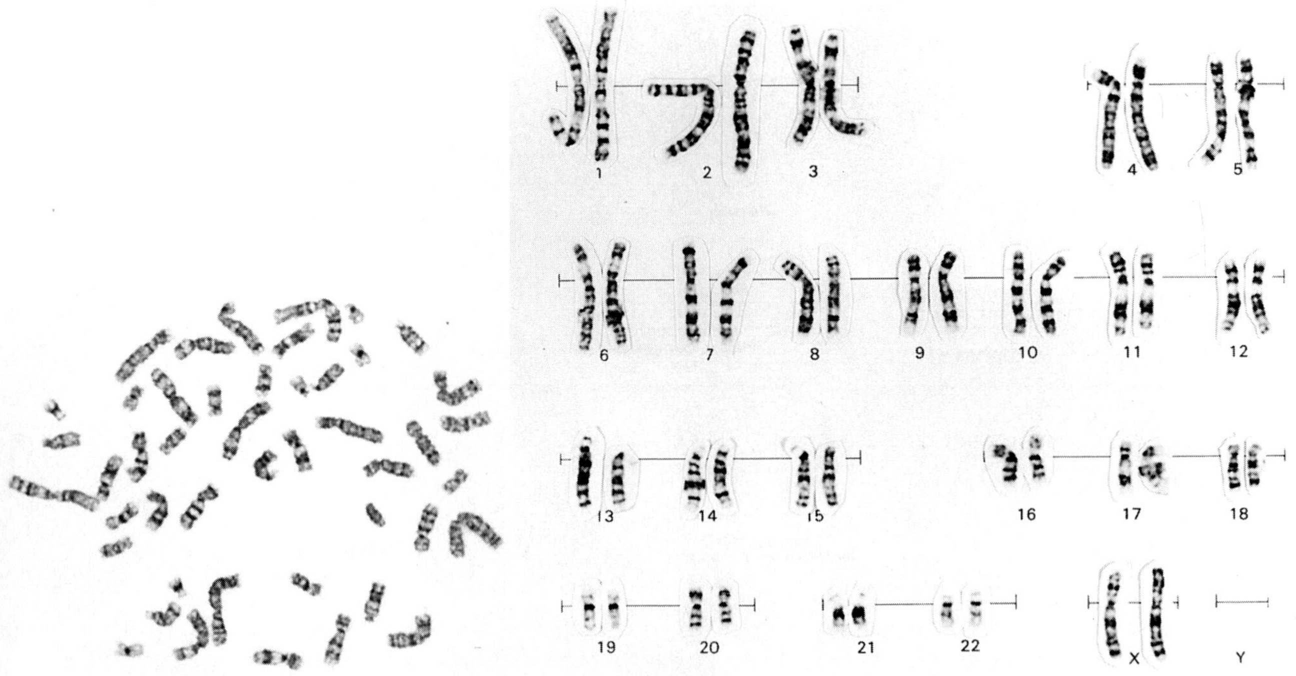

FIG. 4-8 Karyotype of chromosomes. A, G-banded metaphase of a normal cell showing the bands of all normal chromosomes. **B,** G-banded karyotype of a normal female cell showing the banding patterns of the various chromosomes. Identical patterns characterize homologous chromosomes. The chromosomes are arranged from largest to smallest in size. (From Damjanov I, Linder J: *Anderson's pathology,* ed 10, St Louis, 1996, Mosby.)

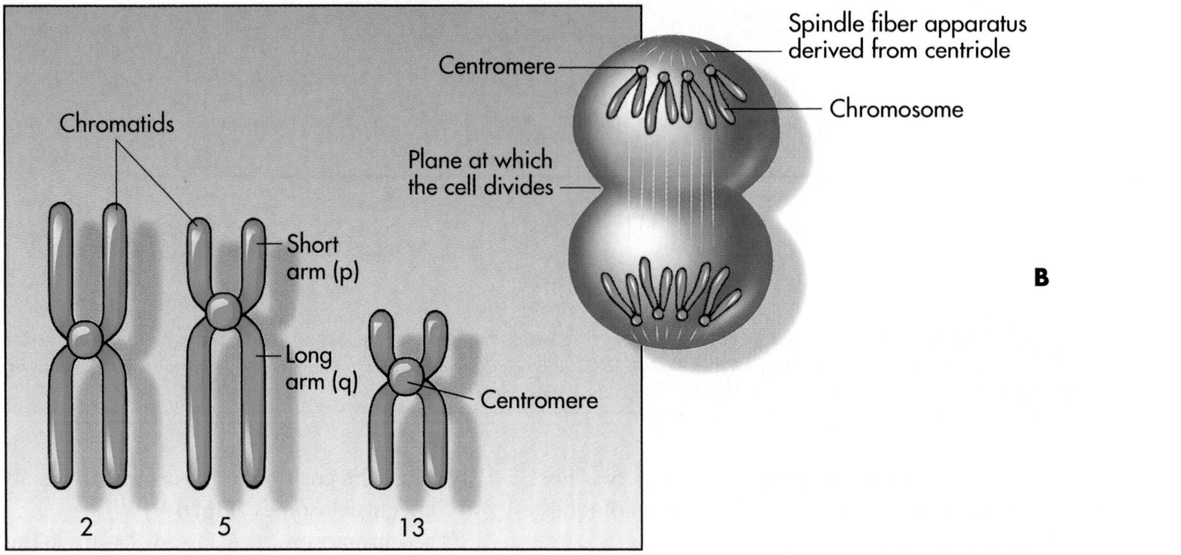

FIG. 4-9 Structure of chromosomes. A, Human chromosomes 1, 5, and 13. Each is replicated and consists of two chromatids. Chromosome 1 is a metacentric chromosome because the centromere is close to middle; chromosome 5 is submetacentric because the centromere is set off from middle; chromosome 13 is acrocentric because the centromere is at or very near the end. **B,** During mitosis, the centromere divides and chromosomes move to opposite poles of cell. At the time of centromere division, the chromatids are designated chromosomes.

Chromosome Aberrations and Associated Diseases

Chromosome abnormalities are the leading known cause of mental retardation and miscarriage. Estimates indicate that a major chromosome aberration occurs in at least 1 in 12 conceptions. Most of these fetuses do not survive to term; in fact, about 50% of all recovered first-trimester spontaneous abortuses have major chromosome aberrations.[6] The number of live births affected by these abnormalities is significant; about 1 in 150 has a major diagnosable chromosome abnormality.[7] See Box 4-1.

Box 4-1

PRENATAL DIAGNOSIS OF CHROMOSOME ABNORMALITIES

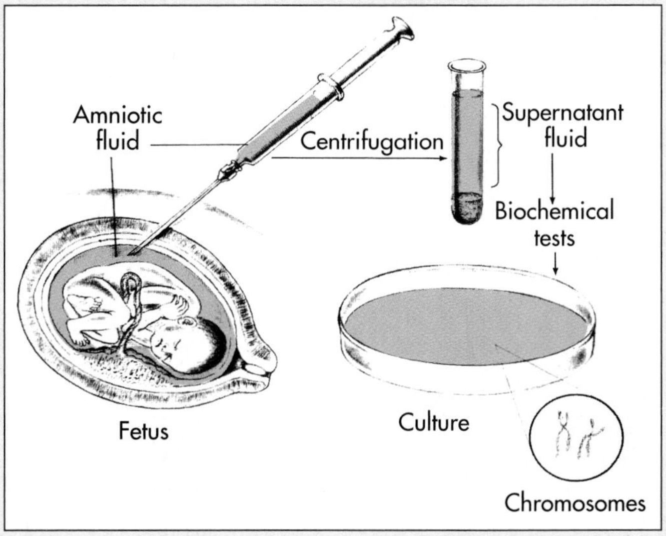

All the chromosome abnormalities discussed here can be detected prenatally, using a procedure called *amniocentesis.* At about the sixteenth week of gestation, a sufficient amount of amniotic fluid is available to enable the withdrawal of a small amount of fluid (2 to 20 ml). This fluid contains live skin cells (fibroblasts) shed by the fetus. These cells can be cultured and karyotyped, and chromosome abnormalities can be detected.

Other disorders can be detected with this procedure. These include most neural tube defects, which cause an elevation of α-fetoprotein in the amniotic fluid, and several hundred diseases caused by mutations of single genes. The procedure involves a risk of losing the fetus, estimated to be about 0.5%. Thus amniocentesis is recommended only for pregnancies known to have an elevated risk for a genetic disease. These include pregnancies of women older than 35 years, in which the risk for Down syndrome and other aneuploidies is elevated, and pregnancies in which parents are known to carry translocations or certain disease genes.

One problem with prenatal diagnosis by amniocentesis is that by the time the sixteenth week of gestation is reached and another 2 or 3 weeks to culture the fibroblasts and test for genetic disease elapse, the mother is near the twentieth week of pregnancy. Pregnancy termination of an affected fetus at this stage can present serious emotional and personal dilemmas as well as some medical risk. For many parents, abortion would be more acceptable for a fetus at an earlier gestational age. A newer technique, *chorionic villus sampling,* consists of extracting a small amount of villous tissue directly from the chorion. This procedure can be performed at 10 weeks' gestation and does not require in vitro culturing of cells because sufficient numbers are directly available in the extracted tissue. Thus the procedure allows prenatal diagnosis at about 2 months' gestation rather than at nearly 5 months' gestation. Chorionic villus sampling involves a slightly higher fetal loss rate than amniocentesis, with most estimates ranging from 1% to 2%.

Data from Wang BT et al: *Am J Med Genet* 53:307, 1994.

Polyploidy

Cells that have a multiple of the normal number of chromosomes are said to be **euploid cells** (Greek *eu* = good or true). Because normal gametes are haploid and most normal somatic cells are diploid, they are both euploid forms. When a euploid cell has more than the diploid number of chromosomes, it is said to be a **polyploid cell.** Several types of body tissues, including some liver, bronchial, and epithelial tissues, are normally polyploid. A zygote having three copies of each chromosome, rather than the usual two, has a form of polyploidy called **triploidy. Tetraploidy,** a condition in which euploid cells have 92 chromosomes, has also been observed. Both these conditions are incompatible with postnatal survival. Nearly all triploid fetuses are spontaneously aborted or stillborn. A few have survived to term but have died shortly after birth. Tetraploidy has been found primarily in early abortuses, although occasionally affected infants have been born alive. Like triploid infants, however, they do not survive. Triploidy and tetraploidy are relatively common conditions, accounting for approximately 10% of all known miscarriages.[6]

Aneuploidy

A somatic cell that does not contain a multiple of 23 chromosomes is an **aneuploid cell.** A cell containing three copies of one chromosome is said to be trisomic (a condition termed **trisomy**) and is aneuploid. **Monosomy,** the presence of only one copy of a given chromosome in a diploid cell, is the other common form of aneuploidy. Among the autosomes, monosomy of any chromosome is lethal, but newborns with trisomy of some chromosomes can survive. This difference illustrates an important principle: in general, loss of chromosome material has more serious consequences than duplication of chromosome material.

Aneuploidy of the sex chromosomes is less serious than that of the autosomes. For the Y chromosome, this is true

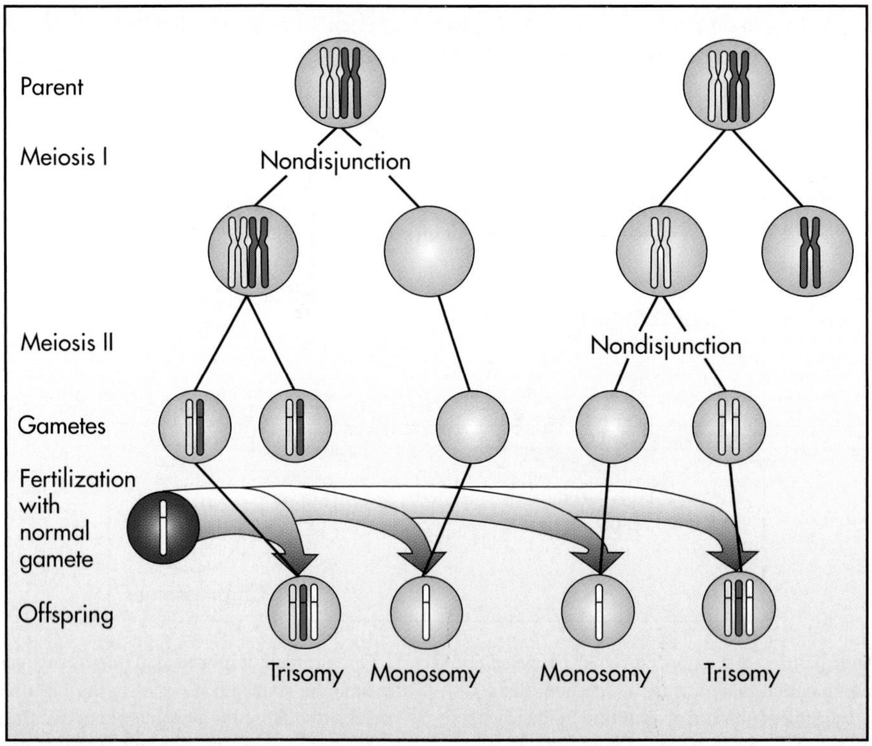

FIG. 4-10 Nondisjunction. Nondisjunction causes aneuploidy when chromosomes or sister chromatids fail to divide properly. (From Jorde LB et al: *Medical genetics,* ed 2, St Louis, 1999, Mosby.)

because very little genetic material is located on this chromosome. For the X chromosome, inactivation of extra chromosomes largely diminishes their effect. A zygote bearing *no* X chromosome, however, will not survive.

Aneuploidy is usually the result of **nondisjunction,** an error in which homologous chromosomes or sister chromatids fail to separate normally during meiosis or mitosis (Fig. 4-10). Nondisjunction during either stage of meiosis produces some gametes that have two copies of a given chromosome and others that have no copies of the chromosome. When such gametes unite with normal haploid gametes, the resulting zygote is monosomic or trisomic for that chromosome. Occasionally, a cell can be monosomic or trisomic for more than one chromosome.

Autosomal Aneuploidy

Trisomy can occur for any chromosome, but the only forms seen with an appreciable frequency in live births are trisomies of the thirteenth, eighteenth, or twenty-first chromosome. Fetuses with most other chromosomal trisomies *do not* survive to term. Trisomy 16, for example, is the most commonly known trisomy among abortuses, but it is not seen in live births.[8]

Partial trisomy, in which only an extra portion of a chromosome is present in each cell, can also occur. The consequences of partial trisomies are not as severe as those of complete trisomies. Trisomies may also occur in only some cells of the body. Individuals thus affected are said to be **chromosomal mosaics,** meaning that the body has two or more different cell lines, each of which has a different karyotype. Mosaics are usually formed by early mitotic nondisjunction occurring in one embryo cell but not in others.

The best-known example of aneuploidy in an autosome is trisomy of the twenty-first chromosome, which causes **Down syndrome** (named after J. Langdon Down, who first described the disease in 1866). Down syndrome was formerly called *mongolism,* but this inappropriate term is no longer used. Down syndrome is seen in 1 in 800 live births.[8] Individuals with this disease are mentally retarded, with intelligence quotients (IQs) usually ranging from 25 to 50. The facial appearance is distinctive (Fig. 4-11), with a low nasal bridge, epicanthal folds (which produce a superficially Asian appearance), protruding tongue, and flat, low-set ears. Poor muscle tone (hypotonia) and short stature are both characteristic. Congenital heart defects affect about one third to one half of live-born children with Down syndrome; a reduced ability to fight respiratory infections and an increased susceptibility to leukemia also contribute to reduced survival rate. By 40 years of age, individuals with Down syndrome virtually always develop symptoms that are nearly identical to those of Alzheimer disease. About three fourths of fetuses known to have Down syndrome are spontaneously aborted or stillborn. About 20% of infants born with Down syndrome die during their first 10 years of life. For those who survive beyond 10 years, average life expectancy is now about 60 years.

About 97% of Down syndrome cases are caused by nondisjunction during the formation of one of the parent's

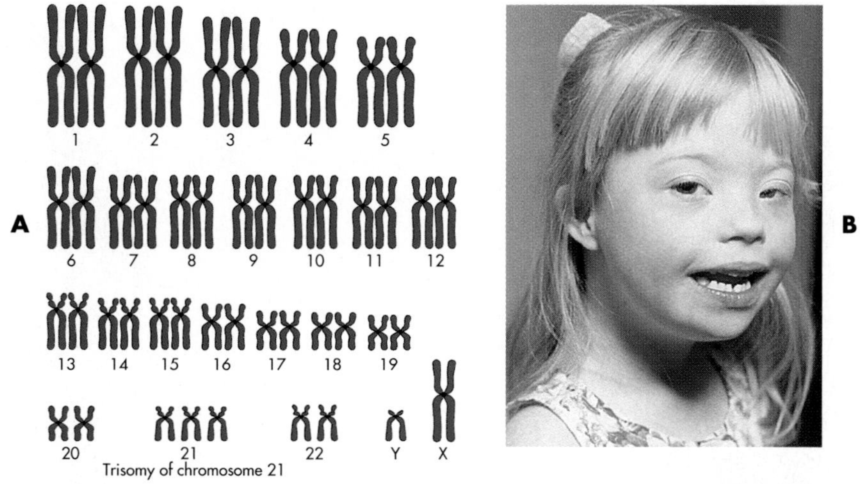

FIG. 4-11 Down syndrome. A, The karyotype of Down syndrome consists of 47 chromosomes and shows trisomy 21. **B,** A child with Down syndrome. (**A** from Damjanov I: *Pathology for the health-related professions,* ed 2, Philadelphia, 2000, W.B. Saunders; **B** courtesy A. Olney and M. MacDonald, University of Nebraska Medical Center, Omaha.)

gametes or during early embryonic development. The remaining 3% result from translocations (discussed later). In approximately 90% to 95% of cases, the nondisjunction occurs in the formation of the mother's egg cell. Paternal nondisjunction is responsible for the remaining cases. Among individuals with Down syndrome, about 1% are known to be mosaics. Because mosaics have a large number of normal cells, the effects of the trisomic cells are attenuated and symptoms are generally less severe.

The risk of having a child with Down syndrome increases greatly with maternal age. As Fig. 4-12 demonstrates, women younger than 30 years have a risk ranging from about 1 in 1000 births to 1 in 2000 births. The risk begins to rise substantially after 35 years, and it reaches 3% to 5% for women older than 45 years. This dramatic increase in risk may be caused by the age of maternal egg cells, which are held in an arrested state of prophase I from the time they are formed in the female embryo until they are shed in ovulation. Thus an egg cell formed by a 45-year-old woman is itself 45 years old. This long suspended state may allow for the accumulation of errors leading to nondisjunction. The risk of Down syndrome, as well as other trisomies, does not appear to increase with paternal age.[9]

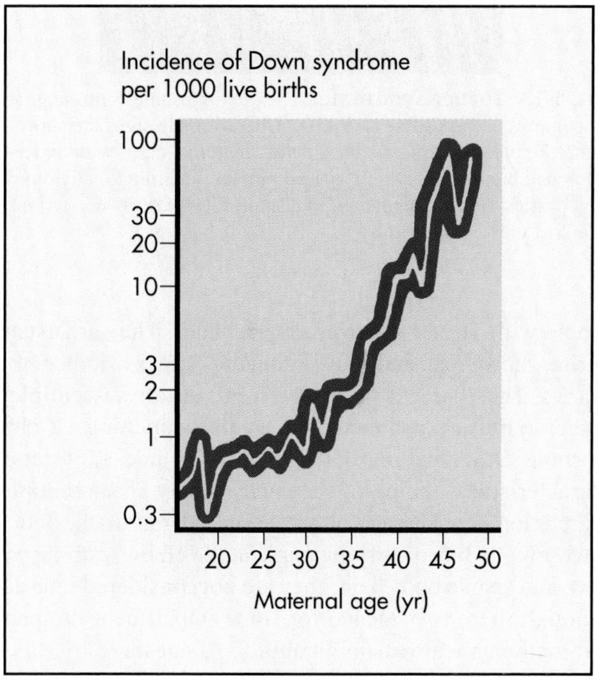

FIG. 4-12 Down syndrome increases with maternal age. Rate is per 1000 live births related to maternal age.

Sex Chromosome Aneuploidy

The incidence of sex chromosome aneuploidies is fairly high. Among live births, about 1 in 400 males and 1 in 650 females have a form of sex chromosome aneuploidy.[10] Because these conditions are generally less severe than autosomal aneuploidies, all forms except complete absence of an X chromosome allow at least some individuals to survive.

One of the most common sex chromosome aneuploidies, affecting about 1 in 1000 newborn females, is trisomy X. Instead of two X chromosomes, these females have three X chromosomes in each cell. Most of them have no overt physical abnormalities, although sterility, menstrual irregularity, or mental retardation is sometimes seen. Some females have four X chromosomes, and they are more often mentally retarded. Those with five or more X chromosomes generally have more severe mental retardation and various physical defects.

A condition that leads to somewhat more serious problems is the presence of a single X chromosome and no homologous X or Y chromosome, so the individual has a total of 45 chromosomes. The karyotype is usually designated 45,X, and it causes a set of symptoms known as **Turner syndrome** (Fig. 4-13). Because they have no Y chromosomes,

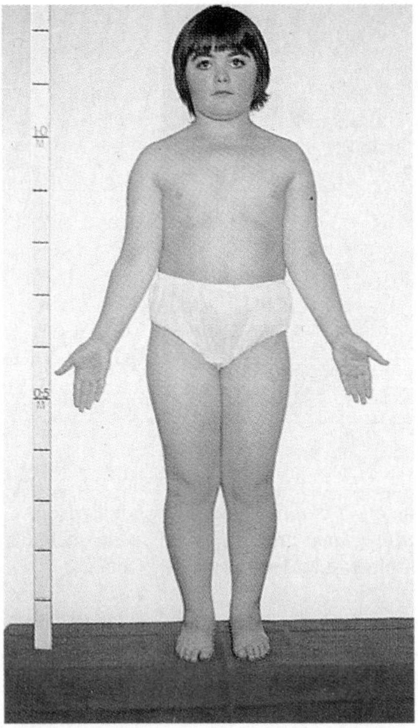

FIG. 4-13 **Turner syndrome.** A sex chromosome is missing, and the person's chromosomes are 45,X. Characteristic signs are short stature, female genitalia, webbed neck, shieldlike chest with underdeveloped breasts and widely spaced nipples, and imperfectly developed ovaries. (From Thibodeau GA, Patton KT: *Anatomy & physiology*, ed 4, St Louis, 1999, Mosby.)

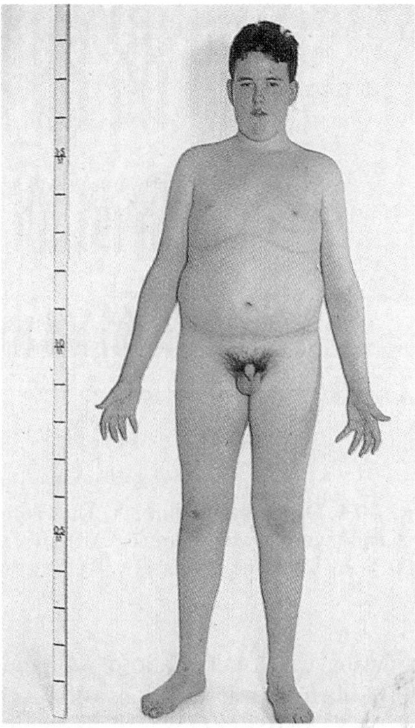

FIG. 4-14 **Klinefelter syndrome.** This young man exhibits many characteristics of Kleinfelter syndrome: small testes, some development of the breasts, sparse body hair, and long limbs. This syndrome results from the presence of two or more X chromosomes with one Y chromosome (genotypes XXY or XXXY, for example). (From Thibodeau GA, Patton KT: *Anatomy & physiology*, ed 4, St Louis, 1999, Mosby.)

people with Turner syndrome are females. They are usually sterile, however, and have gonadal streaks rather than ovaries. These streaks of connective tissue are susceptible to cancer in mosaics who have some cells containing a Y chromosome. Other features of the disorder include short stature, characteristic webbing of the neck, widely spaced nipples, coarctation (narrowing) of the aorta, edema of the feet in newborns, reduced carrying angle at the elbow (cubitus valgus), and sparse body hair. They are not considered retarded, although there is evidence for some impairment of spatial and mathematical reasoning ability. About three fourths of recognized 45,X conceptions inherit their X chromosome from the mother. Thus most cases are caused by a **meiotic error** in the father.

The frequency of Turner syndrome is low compared with that of other sex chromosome aneuploidies: only about 1 in 3000 newborn females is affected.[11] About one half of individuals with Turner syndrome have simple monosomy of the X chromosome; others have one of several more complex X chromosome abnormalities. The 45,X karyotype is extremely common among conceptions, however, and about 15% to 20% of spontaneous abortions with chromosome abnormalities have this karyotype, making it one of the most common single-chromosome aberrations. Thus the condition is highly lethal during gestation: only about 0.5% of 45,X conceptions survive to term. The condition may be relatively benign among live-born females because many or most of these individuals are mosaics. Combinations of 45,X cells with XX, XXX, or XY cells are common among those with Turner syndrome.

Individuals with at least two X chromosomes and a Y chromosome in each cell (47,XXY karyotype) have a disorder known as **Klinefelter syndrome** (Fig. 4-14). Because of the presence of a Y chromosome, these individuals have a male appearance, but they are usually sterile, and about half develop femalelike breasts (a condition called *gynecomastia*). The testes are small, body hair is sparse, the voice is often somewhat high pitched, and a moderate degree of mental impairment may be present. Klinefelter syndrome is found in about 1 in 1000 male births. About two thirds of the cases are caused by nondisjunction of the X chromosomes in the mother, and the frequency of the disorder rises with maternal age. Individuals with the XXXY and XXXXY karyotypes also are considered to have Klinefelter syndrome, and the degree of physical and mental impairment increases with each additional X chromosome. Regardless of the number of X chromosomes, however, these individuals have a male appearance. The presence of a single Y chromosome, which causes the undifferentiated gonads to become testes, always produces a male. As in Turner syndrome, mosaicism is fairly common; the most prevalent combination is XXY and XY cells.

The other sex chromosome aneuploidy that affects males is the 47,XYY karyotype. Individuals with this kary-

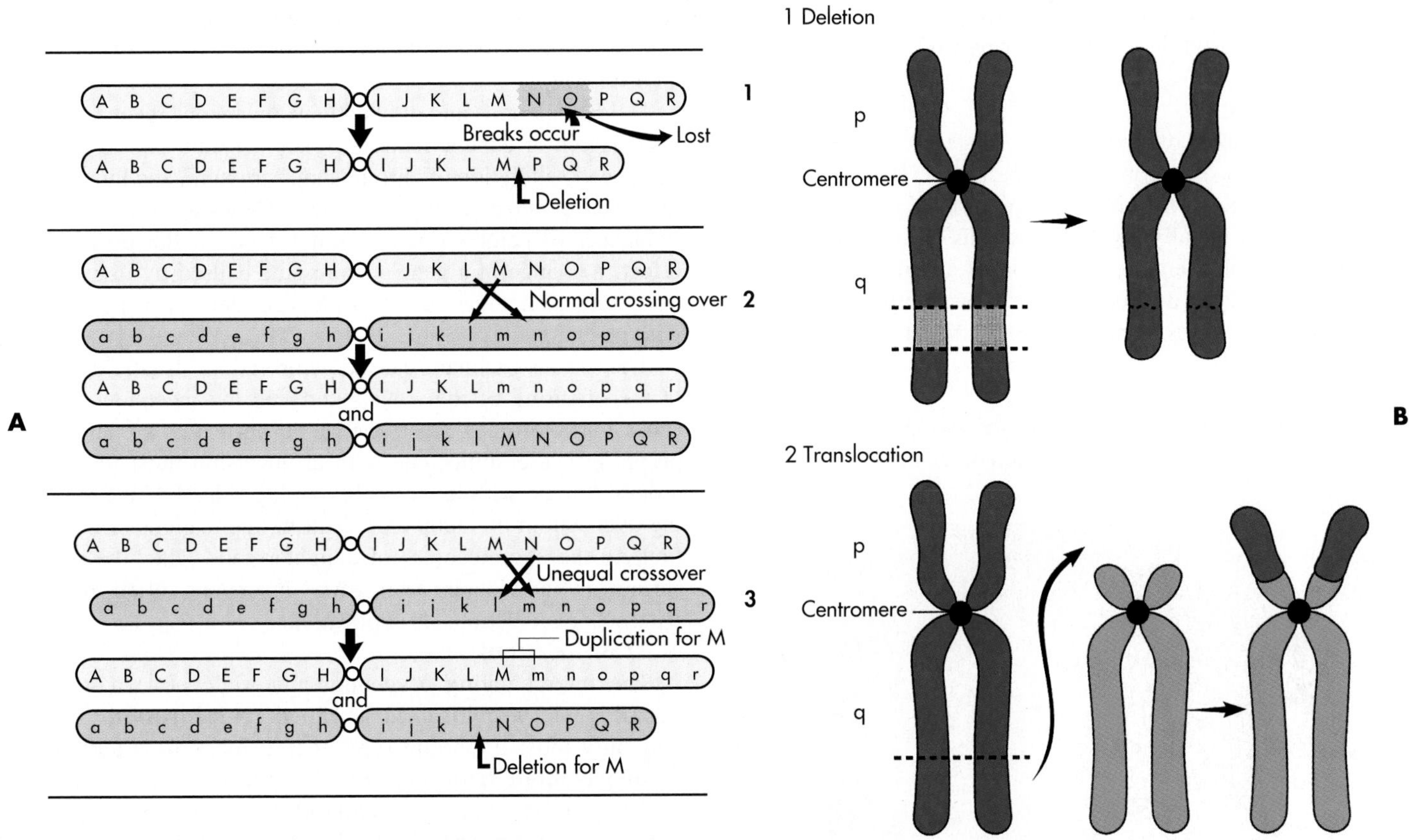

FIG. 4-15 Abnormalities of chromosome structure. A, (*1*) Deletion occurs when a chromosome segment is lost; (*2*) normal crossing over; and (*3*) generation of duplication and deletion through unequal crossing over. **B,** Structural chromosomal abnormalities: (*1*) deletion and (*2*) translocation. (**B** from Damjanov I: *Pathology for the health-related professions,* ed 2, Philadelphia, 2000, W.B. Saunders.)

otype tend to be taller than average, and they have a 10- to 15-point reduction in average IQ. This condition, which causes few serious physical problems, achieved notoriety when it was found that its incidence in prison populations was about 1 in 30 (compared with 1 in 1000 in the general male population). This discovery led to the suggestion that this chromosome might predispose affected individuals to violent, criminal behavior. Several dozen studies have addressed this issue, and they have shown that XYY males are not inclined to commit violent crimes. However, even after adjusting for the effects of decreased IQ, some evidence exists for an increased incidence of behavioral disorders.

Abnormalities of Chromosome Structure

In addition to the loss or gain of whole chromosomes, parts of chromosomes can be lost or duplicated as gametes are formed, and the arrangement of genes on chromosomes can be altered. Unlike aneuploidy and polyploidy, these changes sometimes do not have serious consequences for an individual's health. Some of them can even go entirely unnoticed, especially when very small pieces of chromosomes are involved. Nevertheless, abnormalities of chromosome structure can also produce serious disease in individuals or their offspring.

During meiosis and mitosis, chromosomes usually maintain their structural integrity very well, but **chromosome breakage** occasionally does occur. Mechanisms exist to "heal" these breaks, and generally the break is repaired perfectly with no damage resulting to the daughter cell. Sometimes, however, the breaks remain, or they heal in a fashion that alters the structure of the chromosome. The extent of chromosome breakage is increased in the presence of certain harmful agents, called **clastogens.** Identified clastogens include ionizing radiation, some viral infections, and certain chemicals.

Deletions

Broken chromosomes and loss of DNA cause **deletions** (Fig. 4-15). Usually a gamete with a deletion unites with a normal gamete to form a zygote. The zygote thus has one chromosome with the normal complement of genes and one with some missing genes. Because a fairly large number of genes can be lost in a deletion, serious consequences can result even though one chromosome is normal. The most often cited example of a disease caused by a chromosomal deletion is the **cri du chat syndrome** (Fig. 4-16). The term, which literally means "cry of the cat," describes the characteristic cry of the affected child. Other symptoms include low birth weight, severe mental retardation, microcephaly (smaller than normal head size), heart defects, and the typical facial appearance shown in Fig. 4-16. The disease is caused by a deletion of part of the short arm of chromosome 5.

Duplications

Duplications of chromosome material are, like deletions, a form of chromosome aberration. Because a deficiency of genetic material is more harmful than an excess, duplications usually have less serious consequences than deletions. For example, a deletion of a region of chromosome 5 causes cri du chat syndrome, but a duplication of the same region causes mental retardation but physical traits are nearly normal.

Inversions

An **inversion** is the occurrence of two breaks on a chromosome, followed by the reinsertion of the missing fragment at its original site but in inverted order. Thus a chromosome symbolized as ABCDEFG might become ABEDCFG after an inversion.

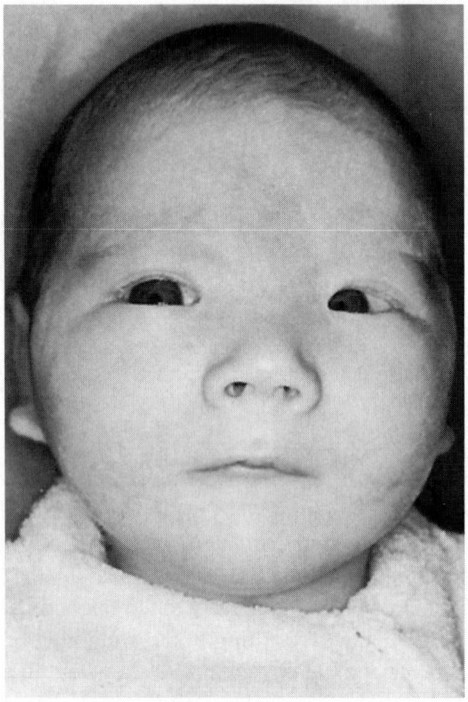

FIG. 4-16 Infant with cri du chat syndrome. Syndrome is caused by deletion of part of the short arm of chromosome 5. (From Thompson MW, McInnes RR, Willard HF: *Genetics in medicine,* ed 5, Philadelphia, 1991, W.B. Saunders.)

Unlike deletions and duplications, inversions result in no loss or gain of genetic material. They are thus said to be a "balanced" alteration of chromosome structure, and they often have no apparent physical effect. Genes are sometimes influenced by neighboring genes, however, and this **position effect,** a change in a gene's expression caused by its position, does sometimes result in physical defects in persons with inversions.

The serious problems caused by inversions usually occur in the offspring of individuals carrying the inversion. Because chromosomes must line up in perfect order during prophase I, a chromosome with an inversion must form a loop to line up with its normal homolog (Fig. 4-17). Crossing over within this loop can result in duplications or deletions in the chromosomes of daughter cells. Thus the offspring of individuals who carry inversions often have chromosome deletions or duplications.

Translocations

The interchanging of genetic material between nonhomologous chromosomes is called **translocation.** The clinically most important type of translocation is termed a **robertsonian translocation.** In this translocation the long arms of two nonhomologous chromosomes fuse at the centromere, forming a single chromosome (Fig. 4-18, *A*). Robertsonian translocations are confined to chromosomes 13 through 15, 21, and 22 since the short arms of these chromosomes are very small and contain no essential genetic material. When a robertsonian translocation takes place, the short arms are usually lost during subsequent cell divisions. Because the carriers of robertsonian translocations lose no important genetic material, they are normal, although they have only 45 chromosomes in each cell. Their offspring, however, may have serious deletions or duplications (Fig. 4-18, *B*). For example, a common robertsonian translocation involves the fusion of the long arms of chromosomes 21 and 14. An offspring who inherits a gamete carrying the fused chromosome receives an extra copy of the long arm of chromosome 21 and thus develops Down syndrome. Robertsonian translocations are

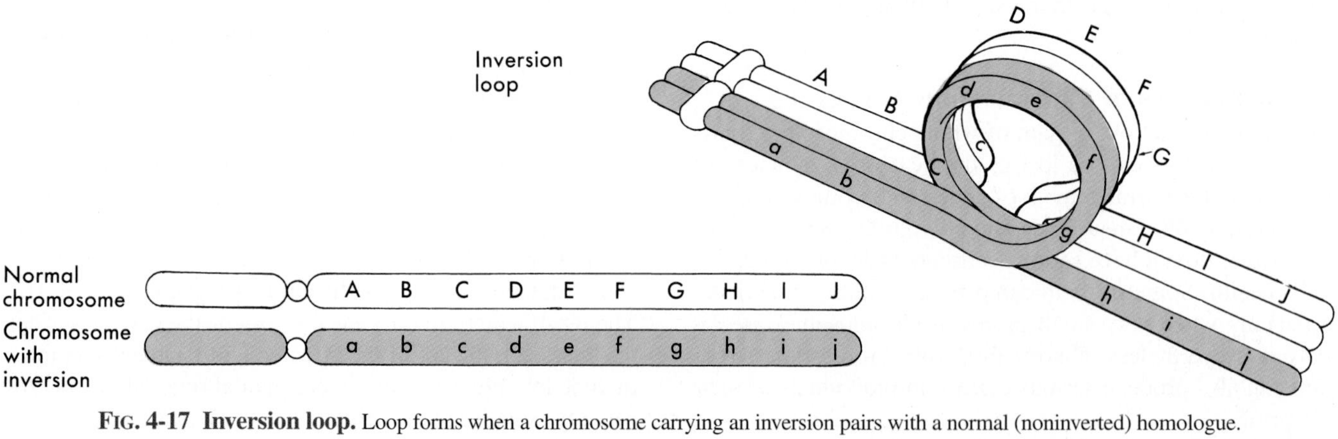

FIG. 4-17 Inversion loop. Loop forms when a chromosome carrying an inversion pairs with a normal (noninverted) homologue.

A

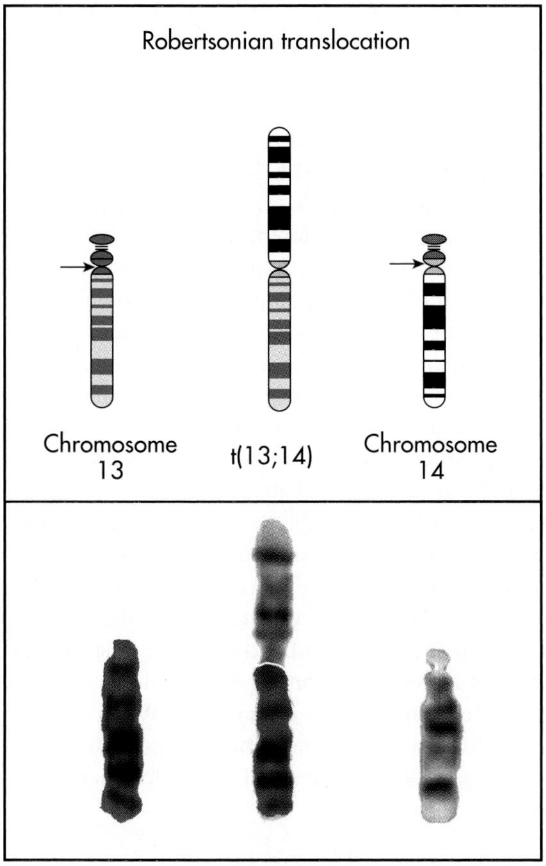

FIG. 4-18 Translocation. A, In a robertsonian translocation, shown here, the long arms of two acrocentric chromosomes (13 and 14) fuse, forming a single chromosome. **B,** The possible segregation patterns for the gametes formed by a carrier of a robertsonian translocation. Alternate segregation (quadrant a alone or quadrant b with quadrant c) produces either a normal chromosome constitution or a translocation carrier with a normal phenotype. Adjacent segregation quadrant a with c or quadrant a with b) produces unbalanced gametes and will result in conceptions with trisomy 14, trisomy 21, monosomy 14, or monosomy 21. (From Jorde LB et al: *Medical genetics,* ed 2, St Louis, 1999, Mosby.)

B

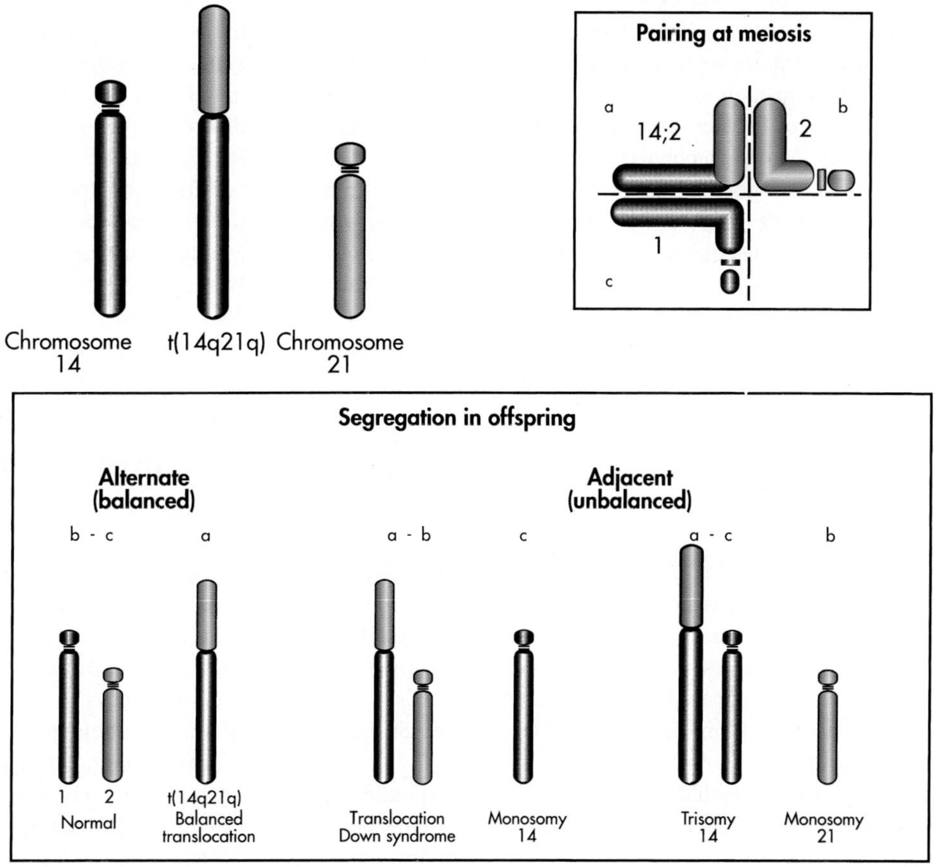

responsible for approximately 3% to 5% of Down syndrome cases. Parents who carry a robertsonian translocation involving chromosome 21 have an increased risk for producing multiple offspring with Down syndrome.

A **reciprocal translocation** occurs when breaks take place in two different chromosomes and the material is exchanged. As with robertsonian translocations, the carrier of a reciprocal translocation is usually normal because the individual has a normal complement of genetic material. However, the carrier's gametes can be normal, can carry the translocation, or can have duplications and deletions.

Fragile Sites

For reasons not yet fully understood, a number of areas on chromosomes develop distinctive breaks and gaps (observable microscopically) when the cells are cultured in a folate-deficient medium. Most of these **fragile sites** have no apparent relationship to disease. However, one particular fragile site, located on the long arm of the X chromosome, is associated with a disorder of considerable importance, both clinically and genetically. This disorder is known as the *fragile X syndrome.* The most important feature of this syndrome is mental retardation. With a relatively high population prevalence (affecting approximately 1 in 2000 to 1 in 4000 individuals), the fragile X syndrome is the second most common genetic cause of mental retardation (after Down syndrome).

Fragile X syndrome involves a puzzling pattern of inheritance. In particular, males who inherit the mutation do not necessarily express the disease condition but they can pass it on to descendants who do express it. Ordinarily, a male who inherits a disease gene on the X chromosome expresses the condition since he has only one X chromosome. Another uncommon feature of this disease is that about one third of carrier females are affected, although less severely than males. Many mechanisms have been proposed to account for the complex mode of inheritance of the fragile X syndrome. Recently it has been shown that unaffected transmitting males have an elevated number (more than about 50) of repeated DNA sequences in the first exon of the fragile X gene. These "repeats" consist of CGG sequences that are duplicated again and again. Affected males have a much larger number of these repeats—200 or more.[12] An increase in the number of these repeated sequences in successive generations can lead to expression of the fragile X syndrome. More than 20 other genetic diseases also are caused by this mechanism.[13,14]

ELEMENTS OF FORMAL GENETICS

The mechanisms by which an individual's set of paired chromosomes produces traits are the principles of genetic inheritance. Mendel's work with garden peas first defined these principles. Later geneticists have refined Mendel's work to explain patterns of inheritance for traits and diseases that appear in families.

Analysis of traits that occur with defined, predictable patterns has helped geneticists link the pieces of the human gene map. Current research focuses on assigning genes to specific locations on chromosomes. Eventually, diseases and defects caused by single genes can be traced and therapies to prevent and treat such diseases can be developed.

Many traits are caused by single genes and are often called *mendelian traits* (after Gregor Mendel). Each gene occupies a position along a chromosome known as a **locus.** The genes at a particular locus can take different forms (i.e., they can be composed of different nucleotide sequences). These different forms are called **alleles.** For example, most people have a type of hemoglobin known as *hemoglobin A,* whose protein sequence is dictated by a single gene. A few individuals have an alternative form of hemoglobin, termed *hemoglobin S,* which differs from hemoglobin A by a single amino acid substitution. The genes coding for hemoglobins A and S are thus two different alleles at a locus. A locus that has two or more alleles that occur with an appreciable frequency in a population is said to be **polymorphic** or a **polymorphism.**

Because humans are diploid organisms, each chromosome is represented twice, with one member of the chromosome pair contributed by the father and one by the mother. At a given locus an individual has one gene whose origin is paternal and one whose origin is maternal. When the two genes are identical, the individual is **homozygous** at that locus. When the genes are not identical, the individual is **heterozygous** at the locus.

Phenotype and Genotype

The composition of genes at a given locus is known as the **genotype.** The outward appearance of an individual, which is the result of both genotype and environment, is the **phenotype.** For example, an infant who is born with an inability to metabolize the amino acid phenylalanine has the single-gene disorder known as *phenylketonuria (PKU)* and thus has the PKU genotype. If the condition is left untreated, abnormal metabolites of phenylalanine will begin to accumulate in the infant's brain and irreversible mental retardation will occur. Mental retardation is thus one aspect of the PKU phenotype. By imposing dietary restrictions to exclude food containing phenylalanine, however, retardation can be prevented. Although the child still has the PKU genotype, a modification of the environment (in this case the child's diet) produces an outwardly normal phenotype.

Dominance and Recessiveness

In many loci the effects of one allele mask those of another when the two are found together in a **heterozygote.** The allele whose effects are observable is said to be **dominant.** The allele whose effects are hidden is said to be **recessive** (from the Latin root for "hiding"). Traditionally, for loci having two alleles, the dominant allele is denoted by an uppercase letter and the recessive allele is denoted by a lowercase letter. When one allele is dominant over another, the heterozygote genotype *Aa* has the same phenotype as the dominant homozygote *AA.* For the recessive allele to be expressed, it must exist in the **homozygote** form, *aa.*

When the heterozygote is distinguishable from both homozygotes, the locus is said to exhibit **codominance.** For example, in the MN blood group, both alleles, *M* and *N,* of the heterozygote are detectable and therefore codominant. Another example is the ABO blood group, in which heterozygotes having the *A* and *B* alleles express both of them as A and B antigens on their red cells (forming blood group AB).

A **carrier** is an individual who has a disease gene but is phenotypically normal. Most genes for recessive diseases occur in heterozygotes who carry one copy of the gene but do not express the disease. Because many recessive genes are lethal in the homozygous state, they are eliminated from the population when they occur in homozygotes. By "hiding" in carriers, however, most recessive genes for diseases survive to be passed on to the next generation.

TRANSMISSION OF GENETIC DISEASES

An important aspect of a genetic disease is the pattern in which it is inherited through the generations of a family, or its **mode of inheritance.** Once the mode of inheritance is known, much can be learned about the disease gene itself and reliable genetic counseling can be given to members of families in which the disease is present (see Chapter 5).

Modes of inheritance were systematically studied by Gregor Mendel, who formulated two basic laws of inheritance. His **principle of segregation** states that homologous genes separate from one another during reproduction and that each reproductive cell carries only one of the homologous genes. Mendel's second law, the **principle of independent assortment,** states that the hereditary transmission of one gene has no effect on the transmission of another. Mendel discovered these laws in the mid-nineteenth century by performing breeding experiments with garden peas. He had no knowledge of chromosomes. Early in the twentieth century geneticists found that the behavior of chromosomes does essentially correspond to Mendel's laws, which now form the basis for the **chromosome theory of inheritance.**

The known single-gene diseases can be classified into four major modes of inheritance: autosomal dominant, autosomal recessive, X-linked dominant, and X-linked recessive. The first two types involve genes known to occur on the 22 pairs of autosomes. The last two types occur on the X chromosome; no good documentation exists of disease genes occurring on the Y chromosome. The number of diseases assigned to each category is growing rapidly. Current catalogs of single-gene traits, which include disease-producing and nonclinical traits (e.g., attached earlobes), list 10,671 known autosomal traits and 624 X-linked traits.[1]

An important tool in the analysis of modes of inheritance is the **pedigree** chart. It summarizes family relationships and shows which members of a family are affected by a genetic disease (Fig. 4-19). Generally, the pedigree begins with one individual in the family, the **proband,** also termed the

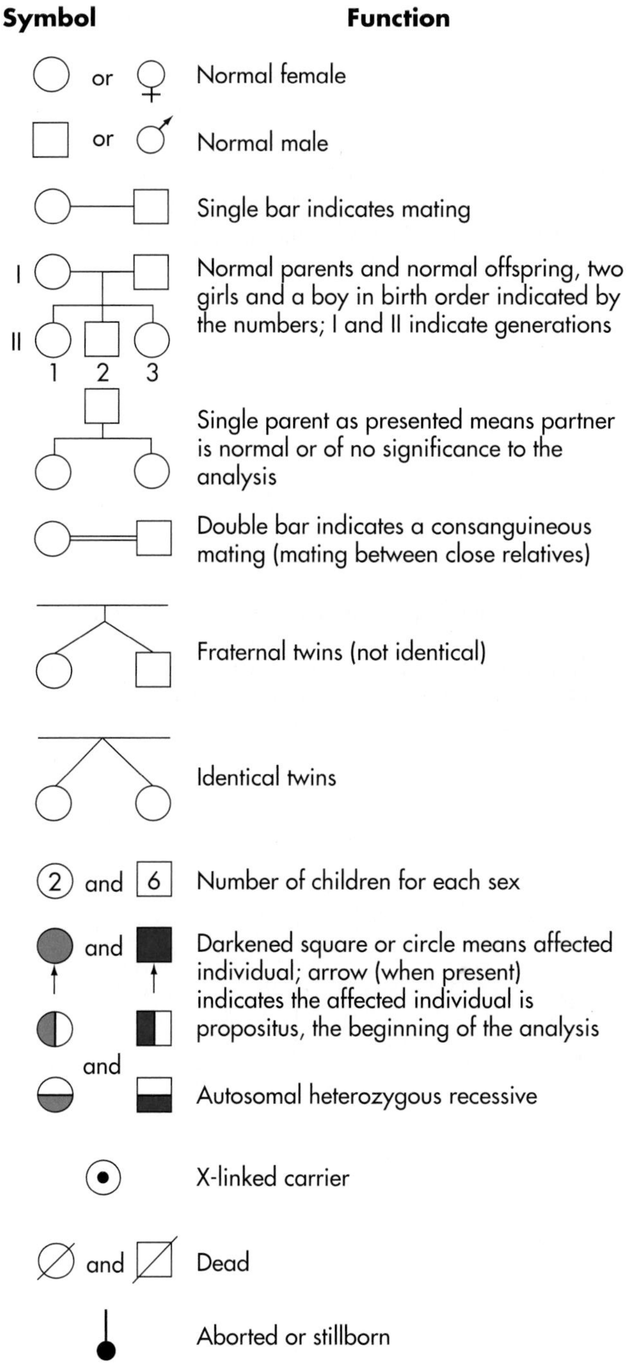

FIG. 4-19 Symbols commonly used in pedigrees.

propositus (male) or **proposita** (female). This individual is usually the first person in the family diagnosed or seen in a clinic.

Autosomal Dominant Inheritance

Characteristics of Pedigrees

Diseases caused by autosomal dominant genes are rare. The most common occur in fewer than 1 in 500 individuals, so it is uncommon for two individuals both affected by the same autosomal dominant disease to produce offspring together. Fig. 4-20, *A,* illustrates this unusual pattern. More often, affected offspring are produced by the union of a normal parent with an affected heterozygous parent. The diagram (Punnett square) in Fig. 4-20 illustrates this mating. The affected parent can pass either a disease gene or a normal gene to his or her children. Each event has a probability of 0.5; thus on the average, half of the children will be heterozygous and will express the disease and half will be normal.

Fig. 4-21, *A,* is a typical pedigree showing the transmission of an autosomal dominant gene. The gene shown here causes achondroplasia (Fig. 4-21, *B*). Several important characteristics of this pedigree support the conclusion that the trait is caused by an autosomal dominant gene:

1. The two sexes exhibit the trait in approximately equal proportions, and males and females are equally likely to transmit the trait to their offspring.

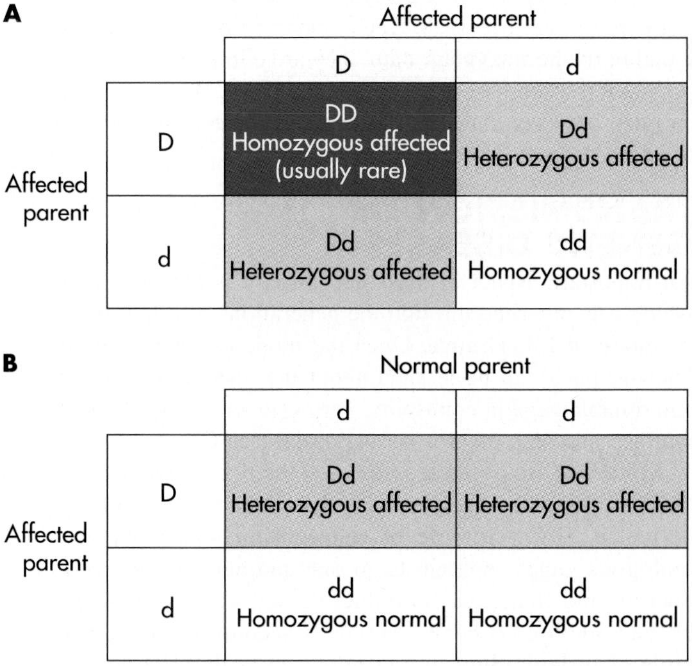

FIG. 4-20 Punnett square and autosomal dominant traits. A, Punnett square for the mating of two individuals with an autosomal dominant gene. Here both parents are affected by the trait. **B,** Punnett square for the mating of a normal individual with a carrier for an autosomal dominant gene.

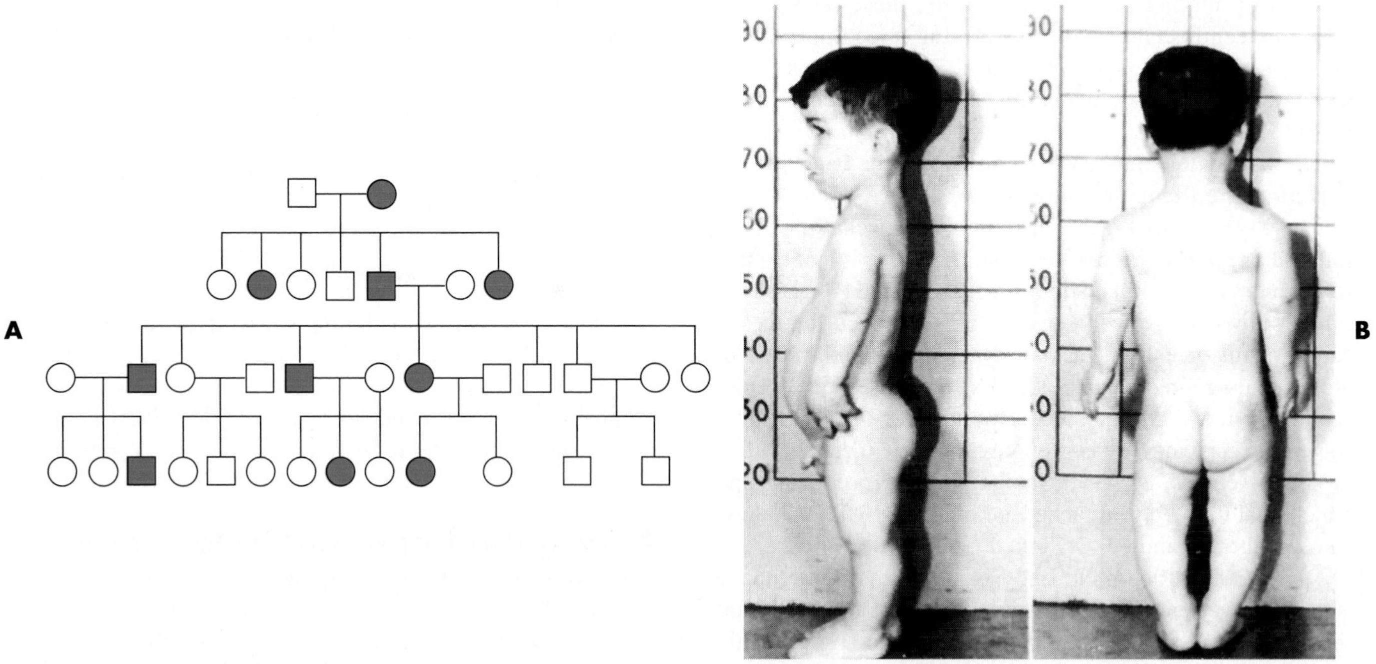

FIG. 4-21 Pedigree for achondroplasia. A, Pedigree showing the transmission of an autosomal dominant disease. **B,** Achondroplasia, an autosomal dominant disorder. (**B** from McKusick VA: *Mendelian inheritance in man,* ed 11, Baltimore, 1994, Johns Hopkins University Press.)

2. There is no skipping of generations. If an individual has achondroplasia, one parent must also have it. If neither parent has the trait, none of the children has it (with the exception of new mutations, as discussed later).
3. Affected heterozygous individuals transmit the trait to approximately half of their children, but because gamete transmission is subject to chance fluctuations, it is possible that all or none of the children of an affected parent may have the trait. When large numbers of matings of this type are studied, however, the proportion of affected children will closely approach one half.

Recurrence Risks

Parents at risk for producing children with a genetic disease nearly always ask the question, "What is the *chance* that our child will have this disease?" When one child has already been born with a genetic disease, the parents can be given a **recurrence risk,** which is the probability that subsequent children also will have the disease. If the parents have not yet had children but are known to be at risk for having children with a genetic disease, an **occurrence risk** (the probability that a child will have a specific disease) can be given. When one parent is affected by an autosomal dominant disease (and is a heterozygote) and the other is normal, the occurrence and recurrence risks for each child are one half.

An important principle is that each birth is an independent event, much like a coin toss. Thus, even though parents may already have had a child with the disease, their recurrence risk remains one half. Even if they have had several children, all affected (or all unaffected) by the disease, the law of independence dictates that the probability that their next child will have the disease is still one half. Parents' misunderstanding of this principle is a common problem encountered in genetic counseling.

If a child has been born with an autosomal dominant disease and there is no history of the disease in the family, the child is probably the product of a new mutation. The gene transmitted by one of the parents has thus undergone a mutation from a normal to a disease-causing allele. The genes at this locus in most of the parent's other germ cells would still be normal. In this situation the recurrence risk for the parent's subsequent offspring is not greater than that of the general population. The offspring of the affected child, however, will have an occurrence risk of one half. Because these diseases often reduce the potential for reproduction, a large proportion of the observed cases of many autosomal dominant diseases are the result of new mutations. For example, approximately seven eighths of all cases of achondroplasia are caused by new mutations.

Occasionally, two or more offspring will present symptoms of an autosomal dominant disease when there is no family history of the disease. Because mutation is a rare event, it is unlikely that this disease would be a result of multiple mutations in the same family. The mechanism most likely to be responsible is termed **germline mosaicism.** During the embryonic development of one of the parents, a mutation occurred that affected all or part of the germline but few or none of the somatic cells of the embryo. Thus the parent carries the mutation in his or her germline but does not actually express the disease. As a result, the unaffected parent can transmit the mutation to multiple offspring. This phenomenon, although relatively rare, can have significant effects on recurrence risks.[15]

Delayed Age of Onset

One of the most well-known autosomal dominant diseases is Huntington disease, a neurologic disorder whose main features are progressive dementia and increasingly uncontrollable movements of the limbs (discussed further in Chapter 16). The latter is known as *chorea* (Greek *khoreia* = dance), and the disease was formerly called Huntington chorea.

One of the key features of this disease is its **delayed age of onset:** symptoms are not usually seen until age 40 years or later. Thus those persons who develop the disease often have had children before they are aware that they have the gene. If the disease were present at birth, nearly all affected persons would die before reaching reproductive age, and the occurrence of the gene in the population would be much lower. From the gene's "point of view," a delayed age of onset is quite advantageous. An individual whose parent has the disease has a 50% chance of developing it during middle age. He or she is thus confronted with a tortuous question: "Should I have children, knowing that there is a 50:50 chance that I may have this disease gene and pass it to half my children?"

Penetrance and Expressivity

Another important variation seen in some autosomal dominant diseases is incomplete penetrance. The **penetrance** of a trait is the percentage of individuals with a specific genotype who also exhibit the expected phenotype. Incomplete penetrance means that individuals who have the gene for a disease may not exhibit the disease phenotype at all, even though the gene and the associated disease may be transmitted to the next generation. A pedigree illustrating the transmission of an autosomal dominant gene with incomplete penetrance is given in Fig. 4-22. Retinoblastoma, the most common malignant eye tumor affecting children, is one disease that typically exhibits incomplete penetrance. About 10% of the individuals who are **obligate carriers** of the gene (i.e., those who have an affected parent and affected children and therefore must themselves carry the gene) do

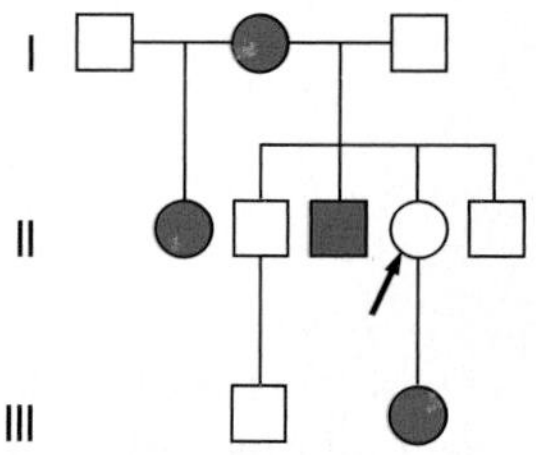

FIG. 4-22 Pedigree for retinoblastoma showing incomplete penetrance. Female with marked arrow in line II must be heterozygous, but she does not express the trait.

not have the disease. The penetrance of the gene is then said to be 90%.

The gene responsible for retinoblastoma has been mapped to the long arm of chromosome 13, and its DNA sequence has been studied extensively. This gene is known as a **tumor-suppressor gene:** the normal function of its protein product is to regulate the cell cycle so that cells do not grow uncontrollably. When a mutation alters the protein, its tumor-suppressing capacity is lost and a tumor can form[16,17] (see Chapters 10 and 18).

A similar complication is variable expressivity. **Expressivity** is the extent of variation in phenotype associated with a particular genotype. If expressivity of a disease is variable, the penetrance may be complete but the severity of the disease can vary greatly. The best-known example of variable expressivity in an autosomal dominant disease is type 1 neurofibromatosis, or von Recklinghausen disease. The gene that causes neurofibromatosis has been mapped to the long arm of chromosome 17, and studies of its DNA sequence indicate that it, like the retinoblastoma gene, is a tumor-suppressor gene.[18] This disease is sometimes called the *elephant man's disease.* However, Joseph Merrick, the man to whom this term was originally applied, probably had a rare disorder called *Proteus syndrome.* The expression of this gene can vary from a few harmless café-au-lait spots ("coffee with milk," describing the light-brown color) on the skin to numerous malignant neurofibromas, scoliosis, seizures, gliomas, neuromas, hypertension, and mental retardation (Fig. 4-23).

A parent with mild expression of the disease—so mild that he or she is not aware of it—can transmit the gene to a child, who can then exhibit severe expression of the disease. As with delayed age of onset and incomplete penetrance, variable expressivity provides a mechanism by which autosomal dominant genes can be maintained at higher prevalence rates in populations.

Several factors can cause variation in expressivity. Genes at other loci can sometimes modify the expression of a disease gene (these are termed *modifier genes*). Environmental factors can also influence the expression of a disease gene. Finally, different types of mutations at a locus can cause variation in severity. For example, a base substitution resulting in a single amino acid change usually produces a mild form of the clotting disorder hemophilia A (Box 4-2). A base substitution resulting in a "stop" codon (and thus premature termination of translation) usually produces a more severe form of hemophilia A.

Genomic Imprinting

Mendel's experimental work with garden peas established that the phenotype is the same whether a given allele is inherited from the mother or the father. Indeed, this principle has been part of the central dogma of genetics. Recently, however, it has become increasingly apparent that this principle does not always hold. A striking example is given by a deletion on the long arm of chromosome 15 (15q11-q13). When the deleted chromosome is inherited from the father, the offspring manifest a disease known as *Prader-Willi syndrome.* This disease phenotype includes short stature, obesity, and hypogonadism. When the deleted chromosome is inherited from the mother, the offspring develop *Angelman syndrome,* which is characterized by mental retardation, seizures, and an ataxic gait. The deletions inherited from the father and the mother are cytogenetically indistinguishable.

A

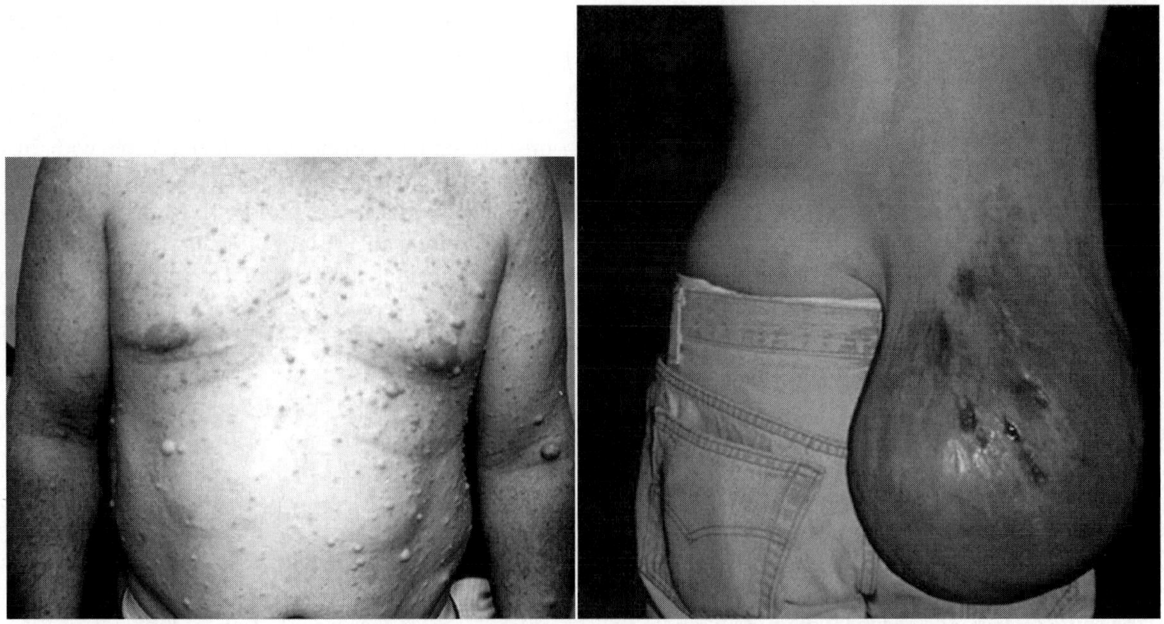

B

FIG. 4-23 Neurofibromatosis. A, Young adult with multiple dermal neurofibromas of the trunk. Note also a *café-au-lait* spot in right upper abdomen. **B,** Individual has a large plexiform neurofibroma hanging from lower right back, causing considerable inconvenience and discomfort (substantially improved by surgical removal of tumor). (From Jorde LB et al: *Medical genetics,* ed 2, St Louis, 1999, Mosby. **B** courtesy Dr. D. Viskochil, University of Utah Health Sciences Center.)

What could cause these differences? It appears that they involve the phenomenon of **genomic imprinting.**[19] The allele inherited from the mother has a different "imprint" from the allele inherited from the father. The imprint alters the activity level of the allele, causing the differences described. The precise way in which genomic imprinting works is not yet understood. However, research with transgenic mice (mice that have had a single foreign gene placed in their genome through recombinant DNA techniques) indicates that the expression level of these transgenes is influenced by the parental origin of the gene (imprinting) *and* that the activity level is associated with the degree of methylation of the gene. Genes that are more highly methylated tend to be transcriptionally less active (i.e., less of the gene is transcribed into messenger RNA). The attachment of methyl groups to DNA may inhibit the binding of proteins that promote transcription. Methylation, which can vary in degree depending on which parent transmits the gene, thus may represent the imprint itself. At this point, however, only an *association* between methylation and imprinting has been

Box 4-2

HEMOPHILIA A AND THE RUSSIAN REVOLUTION

The figure (partial pedigree for descendants of Queen Victoria) is one of the best-known disease pedigrees in existence. It shows the transmission of hemophilia A in the European royal families. This disease, often called a *bleeder syndrome,* is caused by a defect in one of the blood-clotting factors, factor VIII, and can cause severe hemorrhages. In this pedigree Queen Victoria of England was the first known carrier of the disease, and several of her male descendants were affected by it. One of the most historically significant consequences of this pedigree involves the hemophiliac Czarevich Alexis, son of Czar Nicholas II of Russia. Gregori Rasputin, the "mad monk," was reputedly the only person able to prevent the young boy's bleeding episodes and was thus able to gain considerable power over the royal family. Rasputin's destabilizing influence is thought to have hastened the 1917 Bolshevik revolution.

The Russian royal family was again touched by genetics. Modern DNA "fingerprints" and mitochondrial DNA sequence were used to prove that a mass burial near Ekaterinburg, Russia, contained the remains of most of the executed members of the czar's family.

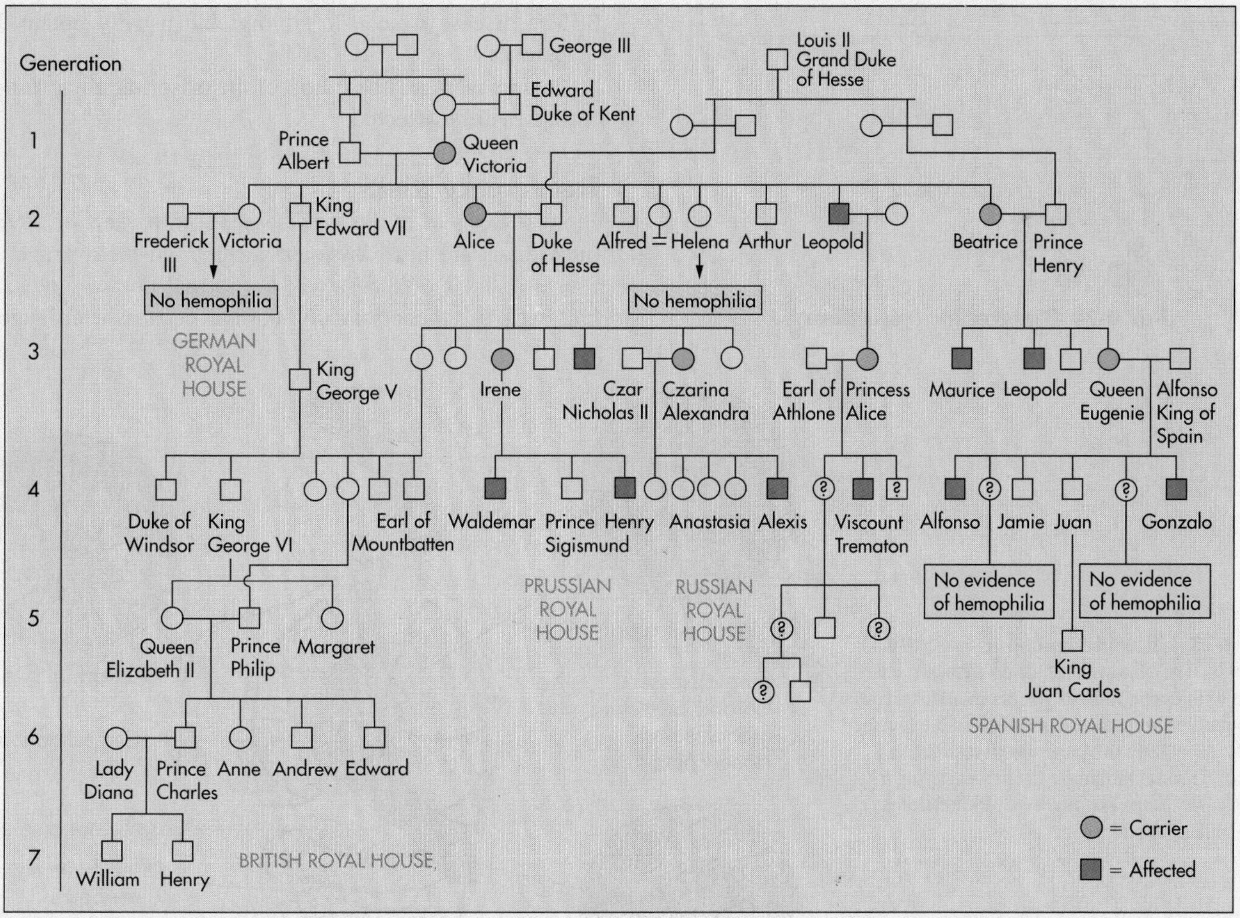

Partial pedigree for descendants of Queen Victoria, showing appearance of hemophilia A in one of her sons and in his descendants and in descendants of her daughters and granddaughters. Royal families of Prussia, Hesse, Battenberg (Mountbatten), Russia, and Spain were thus affected with the disease. The present royal family of England, however, is free of the disease, in spite of inbreeding.

established. It is not at all clear whether methylation is the actual *mechanism* of genomic imprinting.

Autosomal Recessive Inheritance

Characteristics of Pedigrees

Like autosomal dominant diseases, diseases caused by autosomal recessive genes are rare in populations, although the number of carriers for recessive diseases can be high. The most common lethal recessive disease in white children, cystic fibrosis, occurs in about 1 in 2500 births. Approximately 1 in 25 whites carries one copy of the gene for cystic fibrosis (see Chapter 33). Because an individual must be homozygous for a recessive gene to express the disease, the carriers are phenotypically normal. Because most genes for recessive diseases are maintained in normal carriers, they are able to survive in the population from one generation to the next. As with some autosomal dominant diseases, some autosomal recessive diseases are characterized by delayed age of onset, incomplete penetrance, and variable expressivity.

Fig. 4-24 shows a pedigree for cystic fibrosis. The cystic fibrosis gene, which has been mapped to the long arm of chromosome 7, encodes a protein product that forms chloride channels in the membranes of specialized epithelial cells.[20] Defective transport of chloride ions leads to a salt imbalance that results in secretions of abnormally thick, dehydrated mucus (Fig. 4-25). Some of the digestive organs, particularly the pancreas, become obstructed with mucus, causing malnutrition, and the lungs become clogged with mucus, making them highly susceptible to bacterial infections (especially *Pseudomonas*). Death from lung disease or heart failure occurs on average by about 30 years of age. In the pedigree shown here, the two affected individuals are the offspring of the marriage of two first cousins. Marriage between related individuals, termed **consanguinity** (from the Latin root meaning "with blood"), is often a factor in producing children with recessive diseases because related individuals are more likely to share the same recessive genes. Consanguinity is seen most often in rare recessive diseases, since carriers of common recessive diseases have a fairly high probability of encountering one another just by chance.

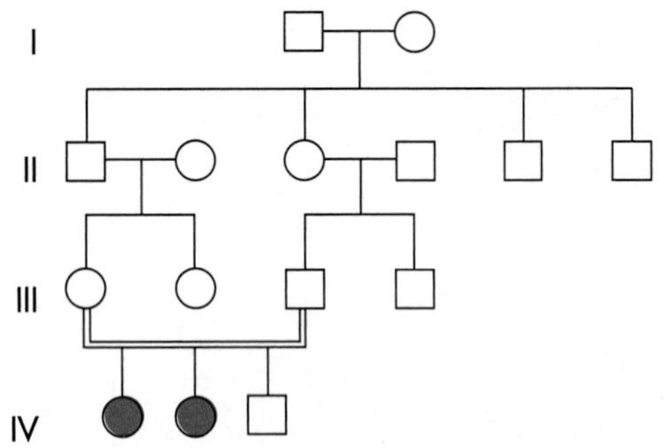

FIG. 4-24 Pedigree for cystic fibrosis.

Important criteria for discerning autosomal recessive inheritance include the following:

1. Males and females are affected in equal proportions.
2. Consanguinity is often present.
3. The disease is seen in siblings but usually not in their parents.
4. On the average, one fourth of the offspring of carrier parents will be affected.

Recurrence Risks

In most cases of recessive disease, both parents of affected individuals are heterozygous carriers. On the average, one fourth of their offspring will be normal homozygotes, one half will be phenotypically normal carrier heterozygotes,

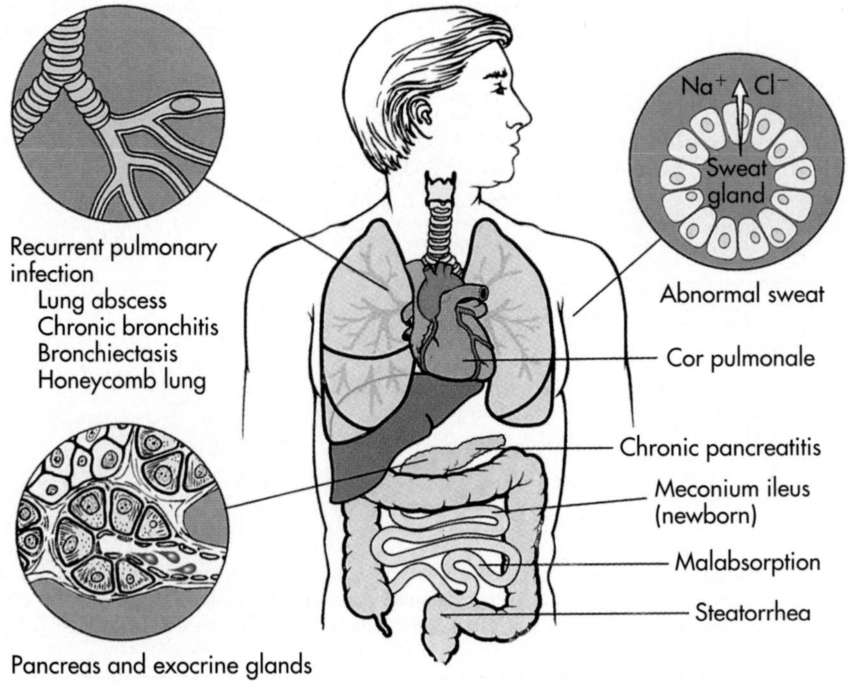

FIG. 4-25 Chloride transport in cystic fibrosis. The abnormal chloride transport associated with cystic fibrosis results in a lack of sodium chloride in the secretions of all exocrine glands, especially the pancreas, intestine, and bronchi. (From Damjanov I: *Pathology for the health-related professions,* ed 2, Philadelphia, 2000, W.B. Saunders.)

and one fourth will be homozygotes with the disease (Fig. 4-26). Thus the recurrence risk for the offspring of carrier parents is 25%. As before, these are the *average* figures. In any given family, there will likely be chance fluctuations, but a study of a large number of families would yield figures close to these proportions.

If two parents have a recessive disease, they each must be homozygous for the disease. Therefore, when two parents are affected by a recessive disease, all their children must also be affected. This observation helps to distinguish recessive from dominant inheritance, because two parents both affected by a dominant gene are nearly always both heterozygotes and thus one fourth of their children will be unaffected.

Because carrier parents usually are unaware that they both carry the same recessive gene, they often produce an affected child before knowing of their condition. Increasingly, **carrier detection tests** that can identify heterozygotes by measuring the reduced amount of a critical enzyme are becoming available. The critical enzyme is totally lacking in a homozygous recessive individual, but an essentially normal phenotype is seen when it is present in a reduced quantity in the carrier. Often carriers can also be detected by direct examination of the disease locus for a mutation. Such testing is especially valuable for siblings of known carriers, who may themselves be carriers. Some recessive diseases for which carrier detection tests are now available are PKU, sickle cell disease, cystic fibrosis, Tay-Sachs disease, hemochromatosis, and galactosemia.

Consanguinity

Consanguinity and **inbreeding** are related concepts. *Consanguinity* refers to the mating of two related individuals, and the offspring of such matings are said to be *inbred.* Consanguinity is often an important characteristic of pedigrees for recessive diseases because relatives share a certain proportion of genes received from a common ancestor. The proportion of shared genes depends on the closeness of their biologic relationship. For example, siblings share one half of their genes on average. With each decreasing degree of relationship, this proportion is reduced by one half. Uncles share one fourth of their genes with nephews and nieces; first cousins share one eighth; first cousins once removed* share one sixteenth; second cousins share one thirty-second; and so on. With consanguineous matings there is a significant increase in recessive disorders. Most empirical studies show that the proportion of offspring of marriages of first cousins who are affected by genetic diseases is approximately double that of the general population.[21] Marriages between first cousins are prohibited in most states of the United States. Marriages between closer relatives (except between double first cousins†) are prohibited throughout the United States.

*First cousins once removed are the offspring of one's own first cousins.
†Double first cousins share both sets of grandparents; ordinary first cousins share just one set of grandparents.

X-Linked Inheritance

Not all genetic diseases are caused by genes located on the 22 autosomes. Some conditions are instead caused by genes located on the sex chromosomes, and that mode of inheritance is **sex-linked.** Because the Y chromosome is not yet known to carry any disease-causing genes, the terms **X-linked** and *sex-linked* are sometimes equated. The former, however, is a more specific term. Only a few diseases are known to be inherited as X-linked dominant traits. Because these diseases are so seldom encountered, only the much more common X-linked recessive diseases are discussed here.

Because females receive two X chromosomes, one from the father and one from the mother, they can be homozygous for a disease allele at a given locus, homozygous for the normal allele at the locus, or heterozygous. Males, having only one X chromosome, are said to be **hemizygous** for genes on this chromosome. A male who inherits a recessive disease gene on the X chromosome will be affected by the disease because the Y chromosome does not carry a normal allele to counteract the effects of the disease gene. Males are always more frequently affected by X-linked recessive diseases, with the difference becoming more pronounced as the disease becomes rarer.

X Inactivation

In the late 1950s Mary Lyon proposed that one X chromosome in the somatic cells of females is permanently inactivated, a process termed *X inactivation.*[22] This proposal, known as the *Lyon hypothesis,* explains why most gene products coded by the X chromosome are present in equal amounts in males and females, even though males have only one X chromosome and females have two X chromosomes. This phenomenon is called **dosage compensation.** The inactivated X chromosomes are observable in many interphase cells as highly condensed intranuclear chromatin bodies, termed **Barr bodies** (after Barr and Bertram, who discovered them in the late 1940s). Normal females have one Barr body in each somatic cell, whereas normal males have no Barr bodies.

The actual process of inactivation occurs very early in embryonic development—approximately 7 to 14 days after fertilization. In each somatic cell one of the two X chromosomes is inactivated. In some cells the X chromosome contributed by the father is inactivated; in others the maternal X

	D	d
D	DD Homozygous normal	Dd Heterozygous carrier
d	Dd Heterozygous carrier	dd Homozygous affected

FIG. 4-26 Punnett square for the mating of heterozygous carriers typical of most cases of recessive disease.

chromosome is inactivated. Because the inactivation process is random, the maternal X chromosome is inactivated in approximately half the cells and the paternal X chromosome is inactivated in approximately half the cells. Once the X chromosome has been inactivated in a cell, all the descendants of that cell have the same chromosome inactivated. Thus inactivation is said to be *random* but *fixed.*

Some individuals do not have the normal number of X chromosomes in their somatic cells. For example, males with Klinefelter syndrome typically have two X chromosomes and one Y chromosome. These males *do* have one Barr body in each cell. Females whose cell nuclei have three X chromosomes have two Barr bodies in each cell, and females whose cell nuclei have four X chromosomes have three Barr bodies in each cell. Females with Turner syndrome have only one X chromosome and no Barr bodies. Thus the number of Barr bodies is always one less than the number of X chromosomes in the cell. All but one X chromosome are always inactivated.

Persons with abnormal numbers of X chromosomes, such as those with Turner syndrome or Klinefelter syndrome, are not physically normal. This situation presents a puzzle because they presumably have only one active X chromosome, just as individuals with normal numbers of chromosomes do. However, the distal part of the short arm of the X chromosome, as well as several other regions on the chromosome arm, is not inactivated. Thus X inactivation is also known to be *incomplete.*

The actual mechanism underlying X inactivation is still not well understood, although the gene responsible for initiating X inactivation has been located.[23] **Methylation** of X chromosome DNA, a process in which DNA is inactivated when cytosine bases are enzymatically converted to 5-methylcytosine, appears to be involved. Inactive X chromosomes can be at least partially reactivated in vitro by administering 5-azacytidine, a demethylating agent.

Sex Determination

The process of sexual differentiation, in which the embryonic gonads become either testes or ovaries, begins during the sixth week of gestation. A key principle of sex determination in the human is that one copy of the Y chromosome is sufficient to initiate the process of gonadal differentiation that produces a male fetus. The number of X chromosomes does not alter this process. For example, an individual with two X chromosomes and one Y chromosome in each cell is still phenotypically a male. Thus it is logical that the Y chromosome must contain a gene that begins the process of male gonadal development.

This gene, termed *SRY* (for "sex-determining region on the Y") has been located on the short arm of the Y chromosome.[24,25] The *SRY* gene lies immediately proximal to the distal tip of the Y chromosome, known as the **pseudoautosomal** region (Fig. 4-27). This portion of the Y chromosome is so named because it pairs with the distal tip of the short arm of the X chromosome during meiosis and exchanges genetic material with it (crossover), just as autosomes do. The DNA sequences of these regions on the X and Y chromosomes are highly similar. The remainder of the X and Y chromosomes, however, do not exchange material and are not similar in DNA sequence. An important piece of evidence that supports *SRY* as the male-determining gene is that female mouse embryos injected with this gene develop as phenotypic males.

Although the *SRY* gene is located on the Y chromosome, the other genes that contribute to male differentiation are located on other chromosomes. Thus *SRY* appears to act as a trigger that initiates the action of genes on other chromosomes (e.g., those that control Sertoli cell differentiation or secretion of müllerian-inhibiting substance). This concept is supported by the fact that the *SRY* gene is similar in sequence to other genes that are known to regulate the transcription of DNA (i.e., they turn other genes on and off).

Occasionally the crossover between X and Y occurs closer to the centromere than it should, placing the *SRY* gene on the X chromosome after crossover. This variation can result in offspring with an apparently normal XX karyotype but a male phenotype. Such XX males are seen in about 1 in 20,000 live births and closely resemble males with Klinefel-

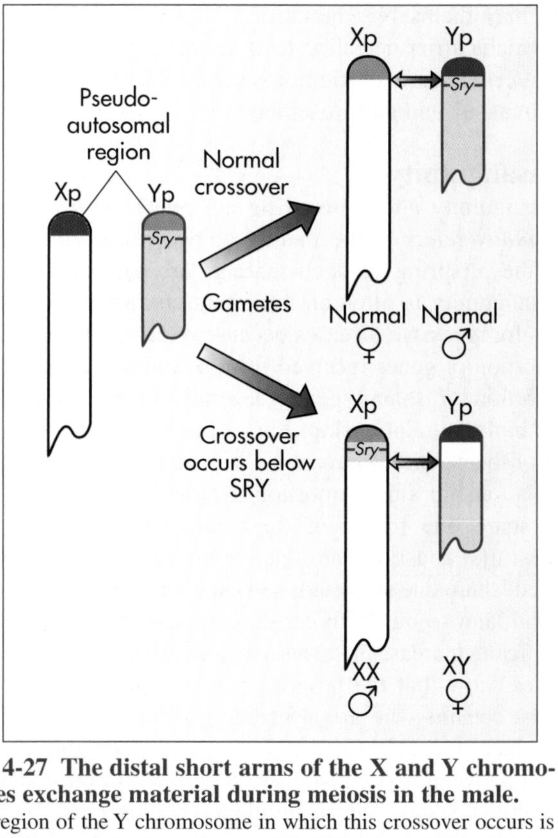

FIG. 4-27 The distal short arms of the X and Y chromosomes exchange material during meiosis in the male. The region of the Y chromosome in which this crossover occurs is called the *pseudoautosomal region.* The *SRY* gene, which triggers the process leading to male gonadal differentiation, is located just outside the pseudoautosomal region. Occasionally, the crossover occurs on the centromeric side of the *SRY* gene, causing it to lie on an X chromosome instead of a Y chromosome. An offspring receiving this X chromosome will be an XX male, and an offspring receiving the Y chromosome will be an XY female. (From Jorde LB et al: *Medical genetics,* ed 2, St Louis, 1999, Mosby.)

ter syndrome. Conversely, it is possible to inherit a Y chromosome that has lost the *SRY* gene (because of either a crossover error or a deletion of the gene). This situation produces an XY female. Such females have gonadal streaks rather than ovaries and have poorly developed secondary sex characteristics.

Characteristics of Pedigrees

X-linked pedigrees show distinctive modes of inheritance. The most striking characteristic is that females are seldom affected. To express an X-linked recessive trait, a female must be homozygous: either both her parents are affected or her father is affected and her mother is a carrier. Such matings are rare.

An important example of an X-linked recessive disease is hemophilia A. The pedigree shown in Box 4-2 demonstrates the following principles of X-linked recessive inheritance:

1. The trait is seen much more frequently in males than in females.
2. Because a father can give a son only a Y chromosome, the trait is never transmitted from father to son.
3. The gene can be transmitted through a series of carrier females, causing the appearance of a "skipped generation."
4. The gene is passed from an affected father to all his daughters, who, as phenotypically normal carriers, transmit it to approximately half their sons, who are affected.

The most common and severe of all X-linked recessive disorders is Duchenne muscular dystrophy (DMD), which affects approximately 1 in 3500 males. As its name suggests, this disorder is characterized by progressive muscle degeneration. Affected individuals are usually unable to walk by 10 to 12 years of age. The disease affects the heart and respiratory muscles, and death caused by respiratory or cardiac failure usually occurs before 20 years. Until recently, the underlying pathologic origin of this disorder was a mystery. However, mapping and cloning of the disease gene (on the short arm of the X chromosome) have greatly increased our understanding of the disorder.[26] The DMD gene is the largest gene ever found in the human, spanning over 2 million DNA bases. It encodes a previously undiscovered muscle protein, termed **dystrophin.** Extensive study of dystrophin indicates that it plays an essential role in maintaining the structural integrity of muscle cells: one end of the protein binds to actin filaments in the cytoplasm of the cell, and the other end binds to a group of membrane-spanning proteins known as the *dystrophin-associated glycoproteins.* When dystrophin is absent, as in individuals with DMD, the cell cannot survive and muscle deterioration ensues.

Most cases of Duchenne muscular dystrophy are caused by deletions of portions of the DMD gene. They generally involve frameshift deletions in which all the amino acids following the deletion are altered. It is interesting that an "in frame" deletion (in which a multiple of three bases is deleted, and the amino acids following the deletion are *not* altered) produces a milder form of muscular dystrophy, the Becker type. These two types of dystrophy are examples of a disease in which different types of mutations at the same locus produce variable expression of the disease.

Recurrence Risks

The most common mating type involving X-linked recessive genes is the combination of a carrier female and a normal male. On the average, the carrier mother will transmit the disease gene to half her sons and half her daughters. As Fig. 4-28, *A,* shows, half the daughters in such a mating will be carriers, whereas half will be normal. Half the sons will be normal, whereas half will have the disease. These are probabilities that indicate what risks can be expected on the *average.* See Box 4-2.

The other common mating type is an affected father and a normal mother (Fig. 4-28, *B*). In this situation all the sons must be normal because the father can transmit only his

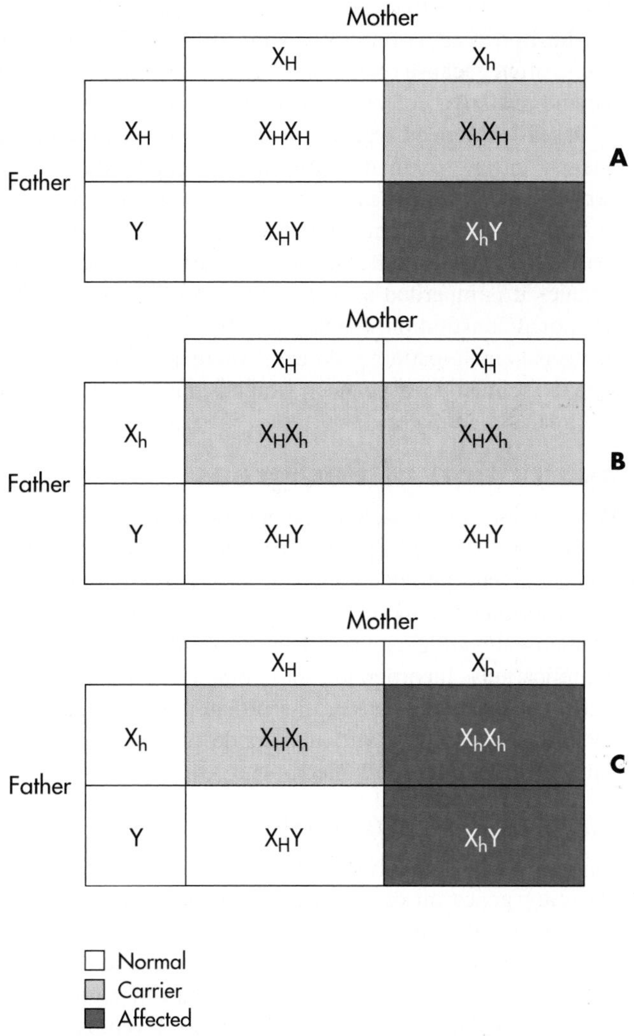

FIG. 4-28 Punnett square and X-linked recessive traits. **A,** Punnett square for the mating of a normal male (X_HY) and a female carrier of an X-linked recessive gene (X_HX_h). **B,** Punnett square for the mating of a normal female (X_HX_H) with a male affected by an X-linked recessive disease (X_hY). **C,** Punnett square for the mating of a female who carries an X-linked recessive gene (X_HX_h) with a male who is affected with the disease caused by the gene (X_hY).

Y chromosome to them. Because all the daughters must receive the father's X chromosome, they will all be heterozygous carriers. Because the sons *must* receive the Y chromosome and the daughters *must* receive the X with the disease gene, these are predictions and not probabilities. None of the children will express the disease.

The final mating pattern, less common than the other two, involves an affected father and a carrier mother (Fig. 4-28, *C*). With this pattern, on average, half the daughters will be heterozygous carriers and half will be homozygous for the disease gene and thus affected. Half the sons will be normal, and half will be affected. Some X-linked recessive diseases, such as DMD, are fatal or incapacitating before the affected individual reaches reproductive age, and therefore affected fathers are rare or nonexistent.

Sex-Limited and Sex-Influenced Traits

Confusion sometimes exists between traits that are sex-linked and those that are sex-limited or sex-influenced. A **sex-limited trait** is one that can occur in only one of the sexes, often because of anatomic differences. Inherited uterine and testicular defects are two obvious examples.

A **sex-influenced trait** is one that occurs much more frequently in one sex than in the other. A good example of a sex-influenced trait is male-pattern baldness, which occurs in both males and females but is much more common in males. In males it is inherited as a dominant trait, whereas in females it is inherited as a recessive trait. Because of their hormonal constitution, females need two copies of the gene to express male-pattern baldness. Another example is autosomal dominant breast cancer, which is much more common in females than males.

Evaluation of Pedigrees

With complications such as incomplete penetrance, variable expressivity, delayed age of onset, and sex-influenced traits, it is not always possible simply to look at a disease pedigree and determine the mode of inheritance. A sophisticated statistical methodologic approach has evolved to deal with such complications. Incorporated into computer programs, these statistical techniques assess the probability of observing a certain pedigree if a particular mode of inheritance (e.g., autosomal dominant with incomplete penetrance) is in effect.

LINKAGE ANALYSIS AND GENE MAPPING

Locating genes on chromosomes and on specific areas of chromosomes is one of the most important endeavors in human genetics. The location of a gene can tell much about the function of the gene, its interaction with other genes, and the likelihood that certain individuals will develop a genetic disease.

Classical Pedigree Analysis

Mendel's second law, the principle of independent assortment, states that an individual's genes will be transmitted to the next generation independently of one another. This law is only partly true, however, because genes located close together on the same chromosome *do* tend to be transmitted together to the offspring. Thus Mendel's principle of independent assortment holds true for most pairs of genes but not those that occupy the same region of a chromosome. Such loci demonstrate **linkage** and are said to be linked.

During the first meiotic stage, the arms of homologous chromosome pairs intertwine and sometimes exchange portions of their DNA (Fig. 4-29) in a process known as **crossing over.** During crossing over, new combinations of alleles can be formed. For example, two loci on a chromosome have alleles *A* and *a* and alleles *B* and *b.* Alleles *A* and *B* are located together on one chromosome arm, and alleles *a* and *b* are located on the other arm. The genotype of this individual is denoted as *AB/ab.*

As Fig. 4-29, *A,* shows, the allele pairs *AB* and *ab* would be transmitted together when no crossing over occurs. However, when crossing over occurs (Fig. 4-29, *B*), all four possible pairs of alleles can be transmitted to the offspring: *AB, aB, Ab,* and *ab.* The process of forming such new arrangements of alleles is called **recombination.** Crossing over does not necessarily lead to recombination, however, because double crossing over between two loci can result in no actual recombination of the alleles at the loci (Fig. 4-29, *C*).

The rate of crossing over can be used to infer the distance between two loci on a chromosome because the probability of crossovers occurring between two loci increases as the loci become more distant. For example, if an individual with genotype *AB/ab* produces recombinant offspring gametes (composition of *Ab* and *aB*) 2% of the time, it is said that the two loci are two map units apart. One **map unit** equals a 1% recombination rate between two loci. When loci on the same chromosome are 50 or more map units apart, they are considered unlinked because their recombination frequency is just as great as it would be if they were on different chromosomes (where the probability of being transmitted together must equal one half). Because they are on the same chromosome, they are said to be unlinked but **syntenic loci.** Recombination frequencies provide a good estimate of actual physical distance between loci at smaller distances, but because of double crossovers, they tend to yield underestimates at larger distances. On average, each map unit is equal to approximately 1 million DNA base pairs.

Pedigrees can be used to determine recombination rates between loci. Fig. 4-30 shows a pedigree in which the rare disease *nail-patella syndrome* (an autosomal dominant disease consisting of malformed patellae and nails) is being transmitted. The individuals in this pedigree have been typed for the ABO blood group, whose locus is also located on chromosome 9. Examination of generations I and II shows that the nail-patella gene must be on the same chromosome arm as the gene for blood type A because the mother, whose blood type was B, was unaffected with the disease. The daughter's genotype would then be *AN/Bn,* where *N* indicates the disease allele and *n* indicates the normal allele. The daughter's husband (individual II-1) must have the genotype *On/On.* If the loci for nail-patella syndrome and the ABO blood group are linked, the children of this union who are affected with nail-patella syndrome should have blood type A; those who are unaffected should have blood type B. In six of seven cases we find this to be true. In one case a recombination occurred (individual III-6), indicating a recombination rate of 1 in 7, or 14%. The two loci are therefore 14 map units apart.

In practice, a much larger sample of families would be used to ensure against statistical artifacts. Also, as with the determination of mode of inheritance, the situation is not always as clear as in Fig. 4-30. Elaborate statistical procedures have been devised to evaluate the probabilities that two loci are linked at a given map distance.

Once a close linkage has been established between a disease locus and a "marker" locus (e.g., a blood group) and once the alleles of the two loci that are inherited together within a family have been determined, reliable predictions of whether a member of a family will develop the disease can be made. If, for example, the recombination rate between a disease locus and a marker locus, such as the ABO blood group, is less than 1%, family members can simply have their ABO blood type assayed to find out, with 99% or greater certainty, whether each member carries the disease gene.

This capability is especially important for diseases with delayed age of onset. Linkage has been established between

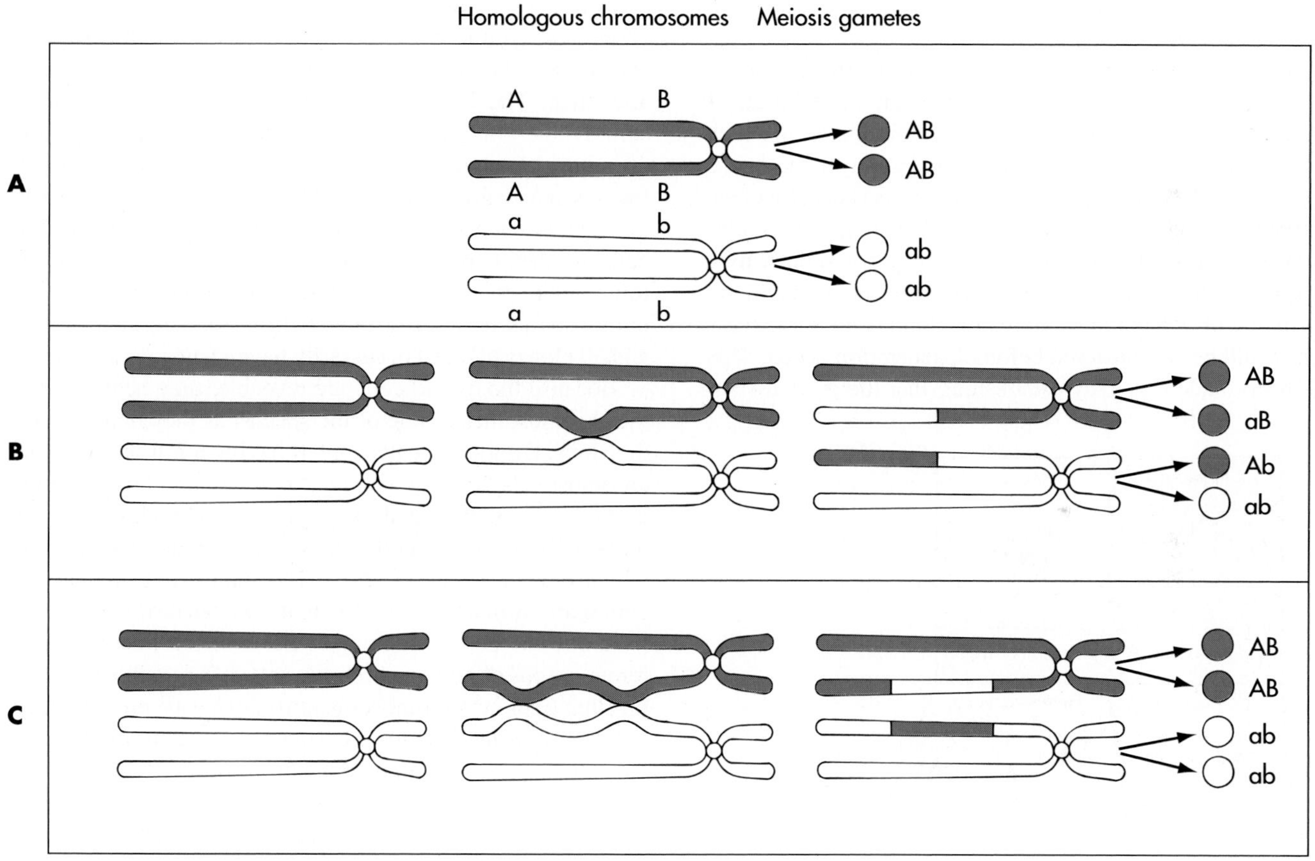

FIG. 4-29 The genetic results of crossing over. A, No crossing over. B, Crossing over with recombination. C, Double crossing over resulting in no recombination.

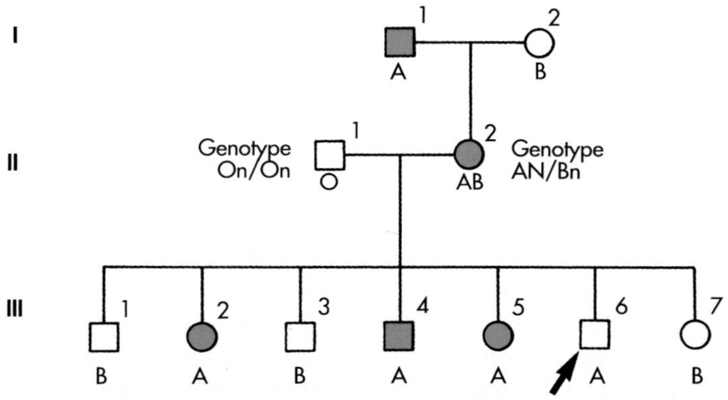

FIG. 4-30 The ABO nail-patella linkage in three generations of a family. Letters below symbols indicate ABO blood groups. Individual III-6 shows recombination.

several DNA polymorphisms and the gene for Huntington disease. Determining this kind of linkage means that it is possible for offspring of an individual with Huntington disease to know whether they also carry the gene and thus could pass it on to their own children. The difficult decision of whether to have children will be made easier for these individuals, although some individuals may prefer to remain uninformed of their genotypes. Other delayed-onset diseases for which linked markers have been found include adult polycystic kidney disease, familial Alzheimer disease, and two forms of autosomal dominant breast cancer (about 5% of breast cancer cases are caused by an autosomal dominant gene). Pinpointing specific mutations in these genes has also made direct genetic diagnosis possible. The advantage of direct diagnosis is that it is more accurate because it tests for the disease-causing mutation itself.

For some genetic diseases, prophylactic treatment is available if the condition can be diagnosed in time. An example of this is hemochromatosis—a recessive genetic disease in which excess iron is retained, causing degeneration of the heart, liver, brain, and other vital organs. Diagnosis is usually made at about 40 years of age in males, after which most individuals survive only a few years. If earlier tests could determine whether an individual had the disease, preventive treatment, consisting of phlebotomies to remove blood and thus excess iron, could be administered before degeneration began. This has been made easier by establishing that the gene for hemochromatosis is closely linked to the human leukocyte antigen (HLA) (see Chapter 6) complex on chromosome 6. Individuals at risk for developing the disease can be determined by assaying their HLA type, and preventive therapy can be given, ensuring an ordinary life span. More recently, the hemochromatosis gene itself has been identified, enabling more precise diagnosis. This example is one instance in which genetics contributes to preventive medicine in its best sense.

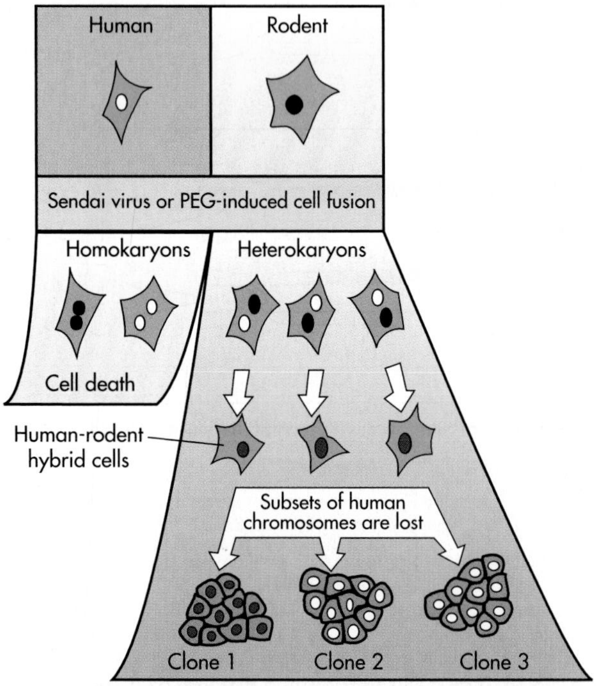

FIG. 4-31 Gene mapping by somatic cell hybridization. Human and rodent cells that fused are selected using a medium such as hypoxanthine, aminopterin, and thymidine (HAT). Hybrid cells preferentially lose human chromosomes, resulting in clones that each have only a few human chromosomes. Each clone is examined to determine whether the gene is present, thus assigning the gene to a specific chromosome. *PEG,* Polyethylene glycol. (From Jorde LB et al: *Medical genetics,* ed 2, St Louis, 1999, Mosby.)

Assigning Loci to Specific Chromosomes

Somatic Cell Hybridization

One of the more surprising biologic discoveries in recent years is that somatic cells from different species, when grown in the same culture, occasionally fuse together to form hybrid cells (Fig. 4-31). This has been done with cells from humans and mice. The resulting hybrid cells contain 86 chromosomes: the 46 human chromosomes together with the 40 mouse chromosomes. The percentage of successful cell fusions can be greatly increased by exposing the cells to certain agents, such as Sendai virus or polyethylene glycol. The cells are then exposed to selective media, such as hypoxanthine, aminopterin, and thymidine (HAT) medium, to weed out those that do not fuse. The hybrid cells are then cloned, and all clones of a cell necessarily have identical karyotypes.

Because the hybrid cells are unstable, they begin to lose the chromosomes of one of the species as they undergo cell divisions. Eventually cells are left having a full set of mouse chromosomes but only one or a few human chromosomes. The cells are karyotyped to determine which chromosomes remain. These sets of cells can then be studied to determine which enzymes they produce. The mouse and human enzymes are sufficiently different that they can be distinguished from one another. By looking at different cell lines with different groups of human chromosomes, it is possible to establish that a certain chromosome must always be present when a certain enzyme is detected. Thus the gene coding for that enzyme must be located on that chromosome.

Sometimes a gene can be assigned to a specific *segment* of a chromosome by using somatic cell hybridization. Translocations in which only part of a single human chromosome is attached to one of the mouse chromosomes occur infrequently. If a human enzyme is still detectable, then the gene coding for this enzyme must be located on the translocated segment of the human chromosome.

In Situ Hybridization

In situ hybridization involves hybridizing a specific piece of radioactively labeled DNA or RNA (a probe) to fixed metaphase chromosomes that have been denatured so that their DNA is single structured. If the radioactive probe matches the DNA of a chromosome segment, it hybridizes and remains at a particular position on the chromosome (hence the term *in situ*). Its position can then be located by autoradiography—a procedure in which the radioactive emissions from the hybridized probe mark its location when exposed to x-ray film.

The procedure is now performed most commonly with nonradioactive fluorescent probes (fluorescent in situ hybridization [FISH]).

In situ hybridization is often combined with somatic cell hybridization to locate genes on chromosomes. Once the cell lines with different combinations of human chromosomes are created by somatic cell hybridization, they can be exposed to radioactively labeled probes. Consistent hybridization of a probe with cell lines containing a certain chromosome demonstrates that the gene corresponding to the probe is located on that chromosome. In some ways, this approach is superior to the enzyme assay technique described previously, since it does not require the in vitro expression of a phenotype (the enzyme).

Complete Human Gene Map: Prospects and Benefits

Rapid progress is currently being made in assigning genes to their chromosomal locations. A number of important genetic diseases have been located on specific areas of individual chromosomes: these include Huntington disease, retinoblastoma, DMD, hemophilia A, cystic fibrosis, PKU, neurofibromatosis, familial breast cancer, and familial Alzheimer disease[27] (Fig. 4-32). Table 4-1 contains a partial list of mapped diseases. The development of thousands of new DNA markers is especially helpful in this effort. A marker map of the human genome has been completed, and the entire sequence of the human genome will be completed by or before 2003 (completion of 90% of the sequence was announced in June 2000). Achievement of this goal serves several purposes:

1. Marker genes will be available to establish close linkages for many genetic diseases. With the establishment of a comprehensive marker map, accurate predictions can be made for the inheritance of most genetic diseases.
2. Knowing the location of genes often yields valuable information about the way genes function and interact with one another. A number of genes with similar functions (e.g., some of the globin genes) are located close to one another on the same chromosome. This characteristic can have important implications for the diseases caused by these genes.
3. Mapping a disease gene is an important step toward isolating and **cloning** the gene (clones are identical copies of genes). Once a gene can be cloned, its DNA sequence can be studied to determine the nature and function of the protein encoded by the gene. Cloning the genes that cause diseases such as cystic fibrosis and DMD has contributed immensely to our understanding of the pathophysiologic aspect of these disorders. In addition, the ability to clone a gene opens up the possibility of gene therapy for the disorder.

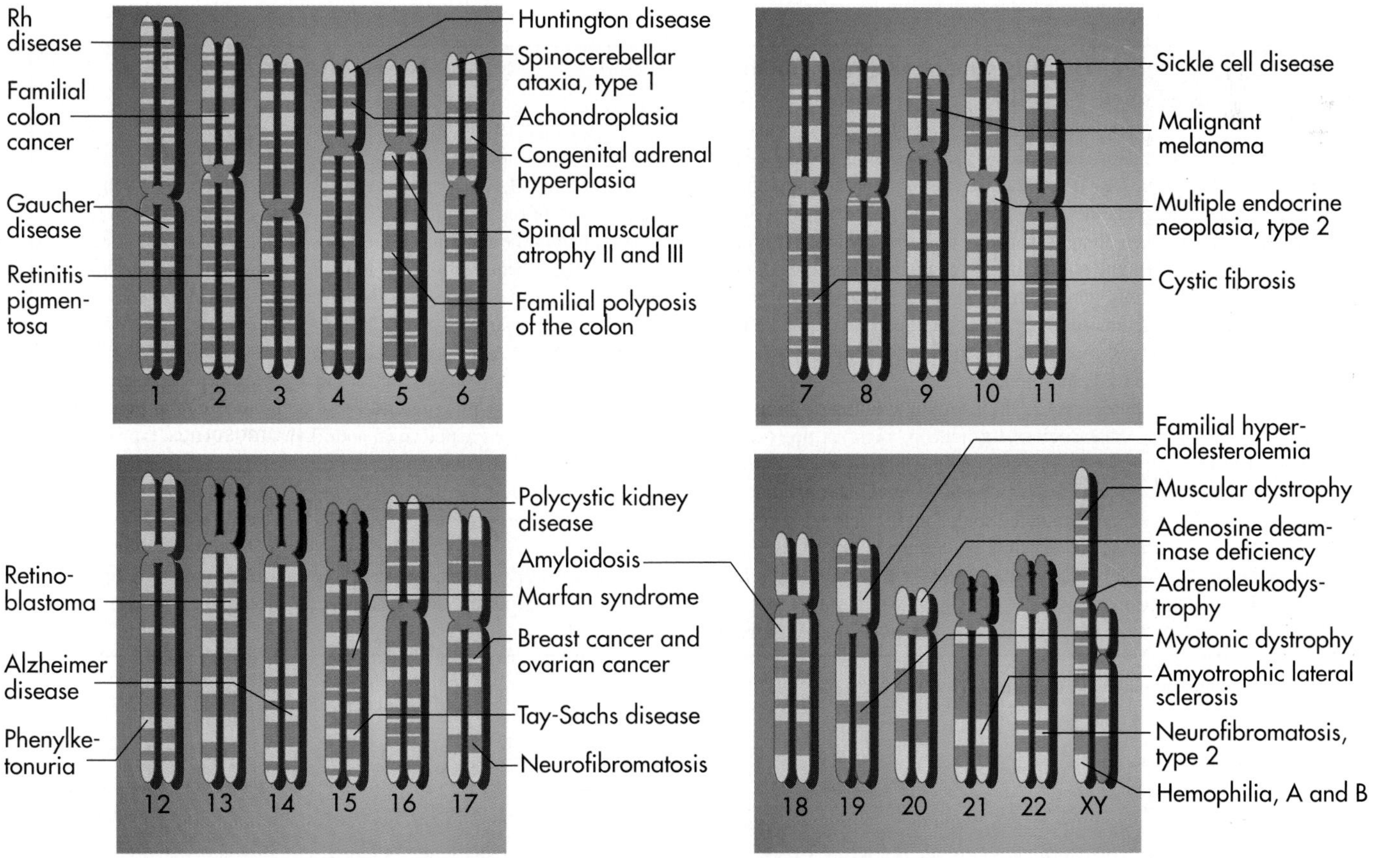

FIG. 4-32 Example of diseases: gene map.

Table 4-1 Important Genetic Diseases Mapped to Specific Chromosome Locations

Disease	Chromosome Location	Gene Cloned*
Huntington disease	4p16	Yes
Cystic fibrosis	7q31	Yes
Hemophilia A	Xq28	Yes
Marfan syndrome	15q15-21	Yes
Sickle cell anemia	11p15	Yes
β-Thalassemia	11p15	Yes
α-Thalassemia	16pter-p12	Yes
Familial breast cancer		
BRCA1	17q21	Yes
BRCA2	13q	Yes
Fragile X syndrome	Xq27	Yes
Phenylketonuria	12q21-qter	Yes
Duchenne muscular dystrophy	Xp21	Yes
Becker muscular dystrophy†	Xp21	Yes
Retinoblastoma	13q14	Yes
Hemochromatosis	6p21	Yes
Familial hypercholesterolemia (LDL receptor defect)	19p13	Yes
Polycystic kidney disease	16p	Yes
α_1-Antitrypsin deficiency	14q31-32	Yes
Familial Alzheimer disease	1q, 14q, 19q, 21q	Yes
Cleft palate	Xq13-21	No
Tay-Sachs disease	15q22-q25	Yes
Neurofibromatosis (classic)	17q11	Yes
Neurofibromatosis (bilateral acoustic form)	22q11-13	Yes
Familial polyposis coli	5q21-22	Yes

*Cloning may be partial or complete.
†Becker muscular dystrophy is an allelic form of Duchenne muscular dystrophy.

WHAT'S NEW? Germline Therapy, Genetic Enhancement, and Human Cloning: Controversial New Issues in Medical Genetics

Although there are many reasonable objections to germline gene therapy, some experts feel it is premature to dismiss it altogether. They point out that germline gene therapy is in many ways technically easier to perform than is somatic cell therapy. In addition, germline therapy offers the possibility of "genetic enhancement," the introduction of favorable genes into the embryo. However, a gene that is favorable in one environment may be quite unfavorable in another (e.g., the sickle cell mutation, which is only advantageous for heterozygotes in a malarial environment).

Another area of controversy is the prospect of cloning humans (McLaren, 2000). Several species (e.g., sheep, pigs, cattle, mice) have been successfully cloned by introducing a diploid nucleus from an adult cell into an egg cell from which the original haploid nucleus was removed. This cell is manipulated so that all the genes can be expressed. There is little doubt that this procedure could be used to clone a human being. Some argue that human cloning offers childless couples the opportunity to produce children to whom they are biologically related or even to "replace" a child who has died. Others respond that this method of creating life is too artificial. In any case, it is important to keep in mind that a clone is only a *genetic* copy. The environment of the individual, which also plays a large role in development, cannot be replicated.

Recently, it became possible to derive embryonic stem cells from early-stage human embryos. These stem cells can potentially be treated to form many types of differentiated cells (e.g., neurons for individuals with Parkinson disease, myocytes for individuals with heart disease). The combination of embryonic stem cell technology and human cloning offers an interesting possibility—a preembryo could, in theory, be created from an individual's own cell, producing embryonic stem cells that would be immunologically a perfect match for the individual.

Although these technologies offer the hope of effective treatment for some recalcitrant diseases, they also present thorny ethical issues. Clearly, decisions regarding their use must be guided by constructive input from scientists, legal scholars, philosophers, and others.

McLaren A: Cloning: pathways to a pluripotent future, *Science* 288:1775, 2000.

SUMMARY REVIEW

DNA, RNA, and Proteins: Heredity at the Molecular Level

1. Genes, the basic units of inheritance, are composed of deoxyribonucleic acid (DNA) and are located on the chromosomes.
2. DNA is composed of deoxyribose, a phosphate molecule, and four types of nitrogenous bases. The physical structure of DNA is a double helix.
3. The DNA bases code for amino acids, which in turn make up proteins. The amino acids are specified by triplet codons of nitrogenous bases.
4. DNA replication is based on complementary base pairing, in which a single strand of DNA serves as the template for attracting bases that form a new strand of DNA.
5. DNA polymerase is the primary enzyme involved in replication. It adds bases to the new DNA strand and performs "proofreading" functions.
6. A mutation is an inherited alteration of genetic material (i.e., DNA).
7. Substances that cause mutations are called *mutagens.*
8. The mutation rate in humans varies from locus to locus and ranges from 10^{-4} to 10^{-7} per gene per generation.
9. Transcription and translation, the two basic processes in which proteins are specified by DNA, both involve ribonucleic acid (RNA). RNA is chemically similar to DNA, but it is single stranded, has a ribose sugar molecule, and has uracil rather than thymine as one of its four nitrogenous bases.
10. Transcription is the process by which DNA specifies a sequence of messenger RNA (mRNA).
11. Much of the RNA sequence is spliced from the mRNA before the mRNA leaves the nucleus. The excised sequences are called *introns,* and those that remain to code for proteins are called *exons.*
12. Translation is the process by which RNA directs the synthesis of polypeptides. This process takes place in the ribosomes, which consist of proteins and ribosomal RNA (rRNA).
13. During translation, mRNA interacts with transfer RNA (tRNA), a molecule that has an attachment site for a specific amino acid.

Chromosomes

1. Human cells consist of diploid somatic cells (body cells) and haploid gametes (sperm and egg cells).
2. Humans have 23 pairs of chromosomes. Twenty-two of these pairs are autosomes. The remaining pair consists of the sex chromosomes. Females have two homologous X chromosomes as their sex chromosomes; males have an X and a Y chromosome.
3. A karyotype is an ordered display of chromosomes arranged according to length and the location of the centromere.
4. Various types of stains can be used to make chromosome bands more visible.
5. About 1 in 150 live births has a major diagnosable chromosome abnormality. Chromosome abnormalities are the leading known cause of mental retardation and miscarriage.
6. Polyploidy is a condition in which a euploid cell has some multiple of the normal number of chromosomes. Humans have been observed to have triploidy (three copies of each chromosome) and tetraploidy (four copies of each chromosome); both conditions are lethal.
7. Somatic cells that do not have a multiple of 23 chromosomes are aneuploid. Aneuploidy is usually the result of nondisjunction.
8. Trisomy is a type of aneuploidy in which one chromosome is present in three copies in somatic cells. A partial trisomy is one in which only part of a chromosome is present in three copies.
9. Monosomy is a type of aneuploidy in which one chromosome is present in only one copy in somatic cells.
10. In general, monosomies cause more severe physical defects than do trisomies, illustrating the principle that the loss of chromosome material has more severe consequences than the duplication of chromosome material.
11. Down syndrome, a trisomy of chromosome 21, is the best-known disease caused by a chromosome aberration. It affects 1 in 800 live births and is much more likely to occur in women over 35 years of age.
12. Most aneuploidies of the sex chromosomes have less severe consequences than those of the autosomes.
13. The most commonly observed sex chromosome aneuploidies are the 47,XXX karyotype, 45,X karyotype (Turner syndrome), 47,XXY karyotype (Klinefelter syndrome), and 47,XYY karyotype.
14. Abnormalities of chromosome structure include deletions, duplications, inversions, and translocations.

Elements of Formal Genetics

1. Mendelian traits are caused by single genes, each of which occupies a position, or locus, on a chromosome.
2. Alleles are different forms of genes located at the same locus on the chromosome.
3. At any given locus in a somatic cell, an individual has two genes, one from each parent. An individual may be homozygous or heterozygous for a locus.
4. An individual's genotype is his or her genetic makeup, and the phenotype reflects the interaction of genotype and environment.
5. At a heterozygous locus, a dominant gene's effects mask those of a recessive gene. The recessive gene is expressed only when it is present in two copies.

Transmission of Genetic Diseases

1. Genetic diseases caused by single genes usually follow autosomal dominant, autosomal recessive, or X-linked recessive modes of inheritance.
2. Pedigree charts are an important tool in the analysis of modes of inheritance.
3. Recurrence risks specify the probability that future offspring will inherit a genetic disease. For single-gene diseases, recurrence risks remain the same for each offspring, regardless of the number of affected or unaffected offspring.
4. The recurrence risk for autosomal dominant diseases is usually 50%.
5. Germline mosaicism can alter recurrence risks for genetic diseases since unaffected parents can produce multiple affected offspring. This situation occurs because the germline of one parent is affected by a mutation but the parent's somatic cells are unaffected.
6. Skipped generations are not seen in classic autosomal dominant pedigrees.

7. Males and females are equally likely to exhibit autosomal dominant diseases and to pass them on to their offspring.
8. Many genetic diseases have a delayed age of onset.
9. A gene that is not always expressed phenotypically is said to have incomplete penetrance.
10. Variable expressivity is a characteristic of many genetic diseases.
11. Genomic imprinting, which may involve methylation, results in differing expressions of a disease gene, depending on which parent transmitted the gene.
12. Most commonly, parents of children with autosomal recessive diseases are both heterozygous carriers of the disease gene.
13. The recurrence risk for autosomal recessive diseases is 25%.
14. Males and females are equally likely to be affected by autosomal recessive diseases.
15. Consanguinity is often present in families with autosomal recessive diseases, and it becomes more prevalent with rarer recessive diseases.
16. Carrier detection tests for an increasing number of autosomal recessive diseases are available.
17. The frequency of genetic diseases approximately doubles in the offspring of first-cousin matings.
18. In each normal female somatic cell, one of the two X chromosomes is inactivated early in embryogenesis.
19. X inactivation is random, fixed, and incomplete (i.e., only part of the chromosome is actually inactivated). It may involve methylation.
20. Gender is determined embryonically by the presence of the *SRY* gene on the Y chromosome. Embryos that have a Y chromosome (and thus the *SRY* gene) become males, whereas those lacking the Y chromosome become females. When the Y chromosome lacks the *SRY* gene, an XY female can be produced. Similarly, an X chromosome that contains the *SRY* gene can produce an XX male.
21. X-linked genes are those that are located on the X chromosome. Nearly all known X-linked diseases are caused by X-linked recessive genes.
22. Males are hemizygous for genes on the X chromosome.
23. X-linked recessive diseases are seen much more frequently in males than in females because males need only one copy of the gene to express the disease.
24. Fathers cannot pass X-linked genes to their sons.
25. Skipped generations are often seen in X-linked recessive disease pedigrees because the gene can be transmitted through carrier females.
26. Recurrence risks for X-linked recessive diseases depend on the carrier and affected status of the mother and father.
27. A sex-limited trait is one that occurs in only one of the sexes.
28. A sex-influenced trait is one that occurs more frequently in one sex than in the other.

Linkage Analysis and Gene Mapping

1. During meiosis I, crossing over occurs and can cause recombinations of alleles located on the same chromosome.
2. The frequency of recombinations can be used to infer the map distance between loci on the same chromosome.
3. Loci that are on the same chromosome are syntenic.
4. A marker locus, when closely linked to a disease-gene locus, can be used to predict whether an individual will develop a genetic disease.
5. A more complete gene map will facilitate marker studies, studies of gene function and interaction, and gene therapy.

KEY TERMS

Adenine, *114*
Allele, *132*
Amino acid, *118*
Aneuploid cell, *125*
Anticodon, *120*
Autosome, *122*
Barr body, *139*
Base pair substitution, *119*
Carrier, *133*
Carrier detection test, *139*
Chromosomal mosaic, *126*
Chromosome band, *123*
Chromosome breakage, *129*
Chromosome theory of inheritance, *133*
Clastogen, *129*
Cloning, *145*
Codominance, *133*
Codons, *118*
Complementary base pairing, *118*
Consanguinity, *138*
Cri du chat syndrome, *129*
Crossing over, *142*
Cytosine, *114*
Delayed age of onset, *135*
Deletion, *129*
Deoxyribonucleic acid (DNA), *114*
Diploid cell, *122*
DNA polymerase, *118*
Dominant, *132*
Dosage compensation, *139*
Double helix, *115*
Down syndrome, *126*
Duplication, *130*
Dystrophin, *141*
Euploid cell, *125*
Exons, *120*
Expressivity, *136*
Fragile site, *132*
Frameshift mutation, *119*
Gamete, *122*
Gene, *114*
Genomic imprinting, *137*
Genotype, *132*
Germline mosaicism, *135*
Giemsa stain, *123*
Guanine, *115*
Haploid cell, *122*
Hemizygous, *139*
Heterogeneous nuclear RNA (hnRNA), *120*
Heterozygote, *132*
Heterozygous, *132*
Homologous, *122*
Homologous chromosome, *123*
Homozygote, *132*
Homozygous, *132*
Inbreeding, *139*
Intron, *120*
Inversion, *130*
Karyotype, *123*
Klinefelter syndrome, *128*
Linkage, *142*
Locus, *132*
Map unit, *142*
Meiosis, *122*
Meiotic error, *128*
Messenger RNA (mRNA), *119*
Metaphase spread, *123*
Methylation, *140*
Mode of inheritance, *133*
Monosomy, *125*
Mutagen, *119*
Mutation, *119*
Mutational hot spot, *119*
Nondisjunction, *126*

KEY TERMS

REFERENCES

1. McKusick VA: *Mendelian inheritance in man,* Baltimore, 1997, Johns Hopkins University Press.
2. Hall JG et al: The frequency and financial burden of genetic disease in a pediatric hospital, *Am J Med Genet* 1:417, 1978.
3. Stephenson J: Gene therapy trials show clinical efficacy, *JAMA* 283:589, 2000.
4. Eck SL: The prospects for gene therapy, *Hosp Pract,* Oct 15, 1999, p 67.
5. Crow JF: Spontaneous mutation in man, *Mutat Res* 437:5, 1999.
6. Hassold TJ: Chromosome abnormalities in human reproductive wastage, *Trends Genet* 2:105, 1986.
7. Tolmie JL: Down syndrome and other autosomal trisomies. In Rimoin DL, Connor JM, Pyeritz RE, editors: *Emery and Rimoin's principles and practice of medical genetics*, vol 1, New York, 1997, Churchill Livingstone.
8. Hassold T, Hunt PA, Sherman S: Trisomy in humans: incidence, origin and etiology, *Curr Opin Genet Dev* 3:398, 1993.
9. Hassold T, Sherman S: Down syndrome: genetic recombination and the origin of the extra chromosome 21, *Clin Genet* 57:95, 2000.
10. Jorde LB et al: *Medical genetics,* ed 2, St Louis, 1999, Mosby.
11. Robinson A, de la Chapelle A: Sex chromosome abnormalities. In Rimoin DL, Connor JM, Pyeritz RE, editors: *Emery and Rimoin's principles and practice of medical genetics*, vol 1, New York, 1997, Churchill Livingstone.
12. Kaufmann WE, Reiss AL: Molecular and cellular genetics of fragile X syndrome, *Am J Med Genet* 88:11, 1999.
13. Margolis RL et al: Trinucleotide repeat expansion and neuropsychiatric disease, *Arch Gen Psychiatry* 56:1019, 1999.
14. Sinden RR: Trinucleotide repeats: biological implications of the DNA structures associated with disease-causing triplet repeats, *Am J Hum Genet* 64:346, 1999.
15. Zlotogora J: Germ line mosaicism, *Hum Genet* 102:381, 1998.
16. Macleod K: Tumor suppressor genes, *Curr Opin Genet Dev* 10:81, 2000.
17. Weinberg RA: How cancer arises, *Sci Am* 275:62, 1996.
18. Gutmann DH et al: The diagnostic evaluation and multidisciplinary management of neurofibromatosis 1 and neurofibromatosis 2, *JAMA* 278:51, 1997.
19. Ben-Porath I, Cedar H: Imprinting: focusing on the center, *Curr Opin Genet Dev* 10:550, 2000.
20. Ziefenski J: Genotype and phenotype in cystic fibrosis, *Respiration* 67:117, 2000.
21. Jorde LB: Inbreeding in human populations. In Dulbecco R, editor: *Encyclopedia of human biology*, vol 5, New York, 1997, Academic Press.
22. Lyon MF: Sex chromatin and gene action in the mammalian X-chromosome, *Am J Hum Genet* 14:135, 1962.
23. Clerc P, Avner P: Genetics: reprogramming X inactivation, *Science* 290:1518, 2000.
24. Swain A, Lovell-Badge R: Mammalian sex determination: a molecular drama, *Genes Dev* 13:755, 1999.
25. Jimenez R, Burgos M: Mammalian sex determination: joining pieces of the genetic puzzle, *Bioessays* 20:696, 1998.
26. Tapscott SJ: Deconstructing myotonic dystrophy, *Science* 289:1701, 2000.
27. Pennisi E: Human genome: finally, the book of life and instructions for navigating it, *Science* 288:2304, 2000.

CHAPTER 5

Genes, Environment, and Common Diseases

LYNN B. JORDE

CHAPTER OUTLINE

Chapter 4 focuses on diseases that are caused by single genes or by abnormalities of single chromosomes. Much progress has been made in identifying specific mutations that cause these diseases, leading to better risk estimates and, in some cases, more effective treatment of the disease. However, these conditions form only a small portion of the total burden of human genetic disease. Most congenital malformations are not caused by single genes or chromosome defects. Many common adult diseases, such as cancer, heart disease, and diabetes, have genetic components, but again they are usually not caused by single genes or by chromosome abnormalities.[1] These diseases, whose treatment collectively occupies the attention of most health care practitioners, are the result of a complex interplay of multiple genetic and environmental factors.

FACTORS INFLUENCING INCIDENCE OF DISEASE IN POPULATIONS

Concepts of Incidence and Prevalence

How common is a given disease, such as diabetes, in a population? Well-established measures are used to answer this question.[2] The **incidence rate** is the number of new cases of a disease reported during a specific period (typically 1 year) divided by the number of individuals in the population. The denominator is often expressed as *person-years.* The incidence rate can be contrasted with the **prevalence rate,** which is the proportion of the population affected by a disease at a specific point in time. Prevalence is thus determined by both the incidence rate and the length of the survival period in affected individuals. For example, the prevalence rate of acquired immunodeficiency syndrome (AIDS) is larger than the yearly incidence rate because most people with AIDS survive for several years after diagnosis.

Many diseases vary in prevalence from one population to another. Cystic fibrosis is relatively common among Europeans, occurring about once in every 2500 births. In contrast, it is quite rare in Asians, occurring only once in every 90,000 births. Similarly, sickle cell disease affects approximately 1 in 600 American blacks,[3] but it is almost never seen in whites. Both these diseases are single-gene disorders, and they vary among populations because disease-causing mutations are more or less common in different populations. (This is in turn the result of differences in the evolutionary history of these populations.) Nongenetic (environmental) factors have little influence on the current prevalence of these diseases.

The picture often becomes more complex with the common diseases of adulthood. Colon cancer, for example, is relatively rare in Japan, but it is the second most common cancer in the United States. Stomach cancer, on the other hand, is common in Japan but relatively rare in the United States. These statistics in themselves cannot distinguish environmental from genetic influences in the two populations. However, because large numbers of Japanese have emigrated, first to Hawaii and then to the U.S. mainland, we can observe what happens to the rates of stomach and colon cancer among the migrants. It is important that the Japanese emigrés have maintained a genetic identity, marrying largely among themselves. In the U.S. population as a whole, the lifetime risk of colon cancer is approximately 5%; in Japan the risk is tenfold lower, only 0.5%. Among the first-generation Japanese in Hawaii, the frequency of colon cancer rises several-fold—not yet as high as in the U.S. mainland but higher than in Japan. Among second-generation Japanese on the U.S. mainland, the colon cancer rates are 5%, equal to the U.S. average. At the same time, stomach cancer has become relatively rare among Japanese-Americans.

These observations strongly indicate an important role for environmental factors in the etiology of cancers of the colon and stomach. In each case, diet is a likely culprit: a high-fat, low-fiber diet in the United States is thought to increase the risk of colon cancer, whereas techniques used to preserve and season the fish commonly eaten in Japan are thought to increase the risk of stomach cancer. This result does not, however, rule out the potential contribution of genetic factors in common cancers. Genes also play a role in the etiology of colon and other cancers.

Analysis of Risk Factors

The comparison just discussed is one example of the analysis of risk factors (in this case, diet) and their influence on the prevalence of disease in populations. A common measure of the effect of a specific risk factor is the **relative risk.** This quantity is expressed as a ratio:

$$\frac{\text{Incidence rate of the disease among individuals exposed to a risk factor}}{\text{Incidence rate of the disease among individuals } \textit{not} \text{ exposed to a risk factor}}$$

A classic example of a relative risk analysis was carried out in a sample of more than 40,000 British physicians to determine the relationship between cigarette smoking and lung cancer. This study compared the incidence of death from lung cancer in physicians who smoked with those who did not. The incidence of death from lung cancer was 1.66 (per 1000 person-years) in heavy smokers (more than 25 cigarettes daily), but it was only 0.07 in the nonsmokers. The ratio of these two incidence rates is 1.66/0.07, which yields a relative risk of 23.7. We can thus conclude that the risk of dying from lung cancer increased by about 24-fold in heavy smokers compared with nonsmokers. Many other studies have obtained similar risk figures.

Although cigarette smoking clearly increases one's risk of developing lung cancer (as well as heart disease, as will be seen below), it is equally clear that *most* smokers do not develop lung cancer. Other life-style factors are likely to contribute to one's risk of developing this disease (e.g., exposure to cancer-causing substances in the air, such as asbestos fibers). In addition, differences in genetic background may be involved. Some studies have shown that mutations in a gene called *FHIT* may make some individuals more sensitive to the carcinogenic effects of tobacco smoke.

Many factors can influence the risk of acquiring a common disease such as cancer, diabetes, or high blood pressure. These include age, gender, diet, exercise, and family history of the disease. Usually, complex interactions occur among these genetic and nongenetic factors. The effects of each factor can be quantified in terms of relative risks. The following discussion demonstrates how genetic and environmental factors contribute to the risk of developing common diseases.

PRINCIPLES OF MULTIFACTORIAL INHERITANCE

Basic Model

Traits in which variation is thought to be caused by the combined effects of multiple genes are **polygenic** ("many genes"). When environmental factors are also believed to cause variation in the trait, which is usually the case, the term **multifactorial trait** is used.[4] Many **quantitative traits** (those, such as blood pressure, that are measured on a continuous numeric scale) are multifactorial. Because they are caused by the additive effects of many genetic and environmental factors, these traits tend to follow a normal, or bell-shaped, distribution in populations.

An example illustrates this concept. To begin with the simplest case, suppose (unrealistically) that height is determined by a single gene with two alleles, *A* and *a*. Allele *A* tends to make people tall, whereas allele *a* tends to make them short. If there is no dominance at this locus, then the three possible genotypes *(AA, Aa, aa)* will produce three phenotypes: tall, intermediate, and short. Assume that the gene frequencies of *A* and *a* are each 0.50. If we look at a population of individuals, we will observe the height distribution depicted in Fig. 5-1, *A*.

Now suppose, a bit more realistically, that height is determined by two loci instead of one. The second locus also has two alleles, *B* (tall) and *b* (short), and they affect height in exactly the same way as alleles *A* and *a*. There are now nine possible genotypes in our population: *aabb, aaBb, aaBB, Aabb, AaBb, AaBB, AAbb, AABb,* and *AABB*. An individual may have zero, one, two, three, or four "tall" alleles, so there are now five distinct phenotypes (Fig. 5-1, *B*). Although the height distribution in our population is not yet normal, it approaches a normal distribution more closely than in the single-gene case just described.

We now extend our example so that *many* genes and environmental factors influence height, each having a small effect. Then there are many possible phenotypes, each differing slightly, and the height distribution approaches the bell-shaped curve shown in Fig. 5-1, *C*.

It should be emphasized that the individual genes underlying a multifactorial trait such as height follow the mendelian principles of segregation and independent assortment, just like any other gene. The only difference is that many of them *act together* to influence the trait.

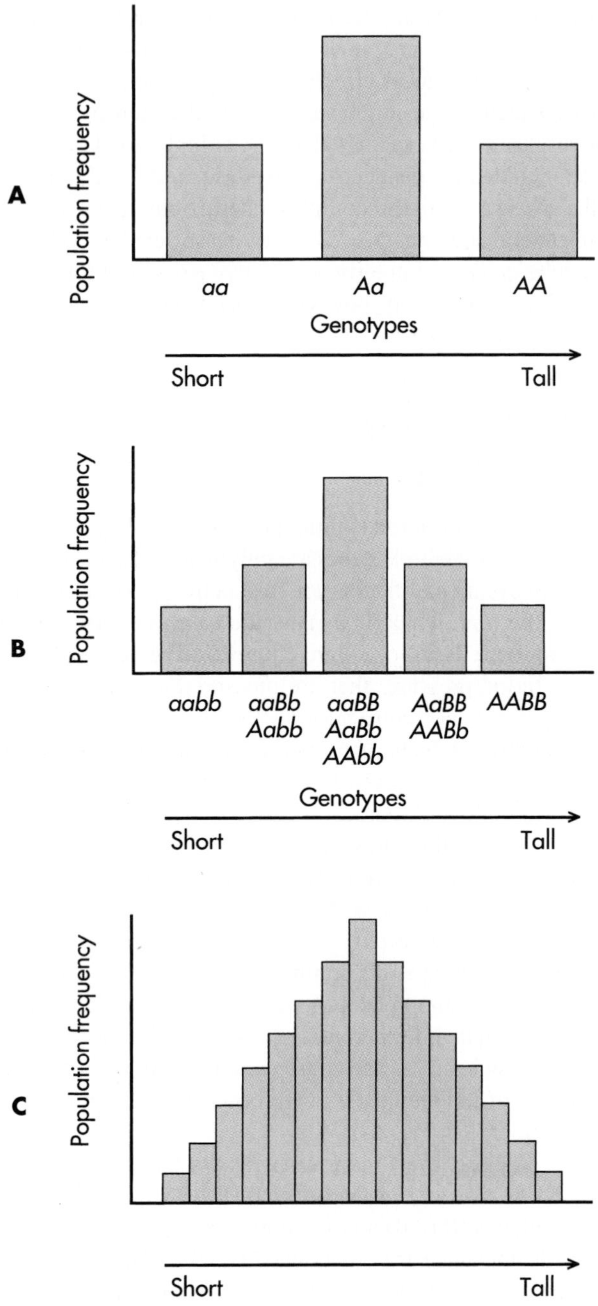

FIG. 5-1 Distribution of height. A, Distribution of height in a population, assuming that height is controlled by a single locus with genotypes *AA, Aa,* and *aa.* **B,** Distribution of height, assuming that height is controlled by two loci. There are now five distinct genotypes instead of three, and the distribution begins to look more like the normal distribution. **C,** Distribution of height, assuming that multiple factors, each with a small effect, contribute to the trait (multifactorial model). (From Jorde LB et al: *Medical genetics,* ed 2, St Louis, 1999, Mosby.)

Blood pressure is another example of a multifactorial trait. A correlation exists between parents' blood pressures (systolic and diastolic) and those of their children. There is good evidence that this correlation is partially caused by genes, but blood pressure is also influenced by environmental factors, such as diet and stress. Two goals of genetic research are the identification and measurement of the relative roles of genes and environment in the causation of multifactorial diseases.

Threshold Model

A number of diseases do not follow the bell-shaped distribution. Instead, they appear to be either present or absent in individuals; yet they do not follow the inheritance patterns expected of single-gene diseases. A commonly used explanation for such diseases is that there is an underlying **liability distribution** for the disease in a population (Fig. 5-2). Those individuals who are on the "low" end of the distribution have little chance of developing the disease in question (i.e., they have few of the alleles or environmental factors that would cause the disease). Individuals who are closer to the "high" end of the distribution have more of the disease-causing genes and environmental factors and are more likely to develop the disease. For diseases that are either present or absent, it is thought that a **threshold of liability** must be crossed before the disease is expressed. Below the threshold, the individual appears normal; above it, he or she is affected by the disease.

A disease that is thought to correspond to this threshold model is *pyloric stenosis,* a disorder that presents shortly after birth and is caused by a narrowing or obstruction of the pylorus, the area between the stomach and intestine. Chronic vomiting, constipation, weight loss, and electrolyte imbalance result from the condition, but it sometimes resolves spontaneously or can be corrected by surgery. The prevalence of pyloric stenosis is about 3 per 1000 live births in whites. It is much more common in males than females, affecting 1 of 200 males and 1 of 1000 females. It is thought that this difference in prevalence reflects *two* thresholds in the liability distribution—a lower one in males and a higher one in females (see Fig. 5-2). A lower male threshold implies that fewer disease-causing factors are required to generate the disorder in males.

The liability threshold concept may explain the pattern of recurrence risks for pyloric stenosis seen in Table 5-1. Note that males, having a lower threshold, always have a higher risk than females. However, the sibling risk also depends on the gender of the proband (i.e., the individual from which the pedigree begins). It is higher when the proband is female than when the proband is male. This reflects the concept that females, having a higher liability threshold, must be exposed to more disease-causing factors than males to develop the disease. Thus a family with an affected female must have more genetic and environmental risk factors, producing a higher recurrence risk for pyloric stenosis in future offspring. It would be expected that the highest risk category would be *male* relatives of *female* probands; Table 5-1 shows that this is the case.

A similar pattern has been observed in a study of *infantile autism,* a behavioral disorder in which the male/female ratio is approximately 4:1. As expected for a multifactorial disorder, the recurrence risks for siblings of male probands (3.5%) is substantially lower than that of siblings of female probands (7%). When the sex ratio for a disease is reversed (i.e.,

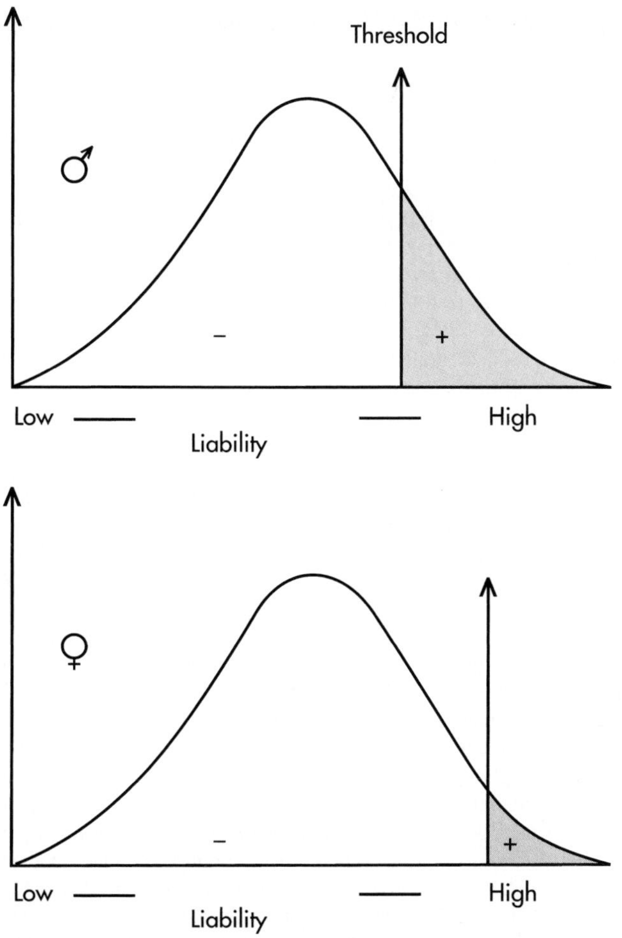

FIG. 5-2 A liability distribution in a population for a multifactorial disease. To be affected with the disease, an individual must exceed the threshold on the liability distribution. This figure shows two thresholds, a lower one for males and a higher one for females (as in pyloric stenosis; see text). (From Jorde LB et al: *Medical genetics,* ed 2, St Louis, 1999, Mosby.)

more affected females than males), one would expect a higher recurrence risk when the proband is male.

A number of other congenital malformations are thought to correspond to this model. They include isolated *cleft lip* and/or *cleft palate (CL/P), neural tube defects (anencephaly, spina bifida), clubfoot (talipes),* and some forms of *congenital heart disease.* In this context, *isolated* means that this is the *only* observed disease feature (i.e., the feature is not part of a larger constellation of findings, as in CL/P secondary to trisomy 13). In addition, many common adult diseases, such as *hypertension, coronary heart disease, stroke, diabetes mellitus* (types I and II), and some *cancers,* are caused by complex genetic and environmental factors and can thus be considered multifactorial diseases.

Recurrence Risks and Transmission Patterns

Whereas recurrence risks can be given with confidence for single-gene diseases (e.g., 50% for typical autosomal dominant diseases, 25% for autosomal recessive diseases), the situation is more complicated for multifactorial diseases.

Table 5-1 Recurrence Risks (%) for Pyloric Stenosis, Subdivided by Genders of Affected Probands and Relatives*

Relatives	Male Probands		Female Probands	
	London	Belfast	London	Belfast
Brothers	3.8	9.6	9.2	12.5
Sisters	2.7	3.0	3.8	3.8

Modified from Carter CO: *Br Med Bull* 32:21, 1976.
*Note that the risks differ somewhat between the two populations.

This is because the number of genes contributing to the disease is usually not known, the precise allelic constitution of the parents is not known, and the extent of environmental effects can vary substantially. For most multifactorial diseases, **empirical risks** (i.e., risks based on direct observation of data) have been derived. To estimate empirical risks, a large series of families is examined in which one child has developed the disease (the proband). Then the siblings of each proband are surveyed to calculate the percentage who have also developed the disease. For example, in the United States about 3% of siblings of individuals with neural tube defects also have neural tube defects (Box 5-1). Thus the recurrence risk for parents who have had one child with a neural tube defect is 3% in the United States. For conditions such as cleft lip/palate that are not lethal or severely debilitating, recurrence risks can also be estimated for the offspring of affected parents. Empirical recurrence risks are, of course, specific for each multifactorial disease.

In contrast to most single-gene diseases, recurrence risks for multifactorial diseases can change substantially from one population to another because gene frequencies as well as environmental factors can differ among populations (note the differences between the London and Belfast populations in Table 5-1).

It is sometimes difficult to distinguish polygenic or multifactorial diseases from single-gene diseases that have reduced penetrance or variable expression. Large data sets and good epidemiologic data are necessary to make the distinction. Several criteria are commonly used to define multifactorial inheritance.

First, *the recurrence risk becomes higher if more than one family member is affected.* For example, the sibling recurrence risk for a *ventricular septal defect* (VSD, a type of congenital heart defect) is 3% if one sibling has had a VSD but increases to approximately 10% if two siblings have had VSDs.[7] In contrast, the recurrence risk for single-gene diseases remains the same regardless of the number of affected siblings. It should be emphasized that this increase does not mean that the family's risk has actually *changed.* Rather, it means that we now have more information about the family's true risk: because they have had two affected children, they are probably located higher on the liability distribution than a family with only one affected child. In other words, they have more risk factors (genetic or environmental) and are more likely to produce an affected child.

Box 5-1

NEURAL TUBE DEFECTS

Neural tube defects (NTDs), which include *anencephaly, spina bifida,* and *encephalocele* (as well as several other less common forms), are one of the most important classes of birth defects, with a birth prevalence of 1 to 3 per 1000.[5] The prevalence of NTDs among different populations varies considerably, with an especially high rate among some northern Chinese populations (as high as 6 or more per 1000 births). In the United States, NTDs are two to three times more common in the eastern than in the western parts of the country. For reasons that are not fully known, the prevalence of NTDs has been decreasing in many parts of the United States and Europe during the past 2½ decades.

Normally the neural tube closes at about the fourth week of gestation. A defect in closure, or a subsequent reopening of the neural tube, results in a neural tube defect. Spina bifida (Fig. 5-3, *A*) is the most commonly observed NTD and consists of a protrusion of spinal tissue through the vertebral column (the tissue usually includes meninges, spinal cord, and nerve roots). About 75% of spina bifida patients have secondary hydrocephalus, which sometimes in turn produces mental retardation. Paralysis or muscle weakness, lack of sphincter control, and clubfeet are often observed. A study conducted in British Columbia showed that survival rates for spina bifida patients have improved dramatically over the past several decades. Fewer than 30% of patients born between 1952 and 1969 survived to 10 years of age, whereas 65% of those born between 1970 and 1986 survived to this age. Anencephaly (Fig. 5-3, *B*) is characterized by partial or complete absence of the cranial vault and calvarium and partial or complete absence of the cerebral hemispheres. At least two thirds of newborns with anencephaly are stillborn; term deliveries do not survive more than a few hours or days.

NTDs are thought to arise from a combination of genetic and environmental factors. In most populations surveyed thus far, empirical recurrence risks for siblings of affected patients range from 2% to 5%. Consistent with a multifactorial model, the recurrence risk increases with additional affected siblings. Studies conducted in Great Britain showed that the sibling recurrence risk was approximately 5% when one sibling was affected and 10% when two were affected. A Hungarian study showed that the overall prevalence of NTDs was 1 in 300 births and that the sibling recurrence risks were 3%, 12%, and 25% after one, two, and three affected offspring, respectively. Recurrence risks tend to be slightly lower in populations with lower NTD prevalence rates, as predicted by the multifactorial model. Recurrence risk data support the idea that the major forms of NTDs are caused by similar factors. An anencephalic conception increases the recurrence risk for subsequent spina bifida conceptions, and vice versa.

NTDs can usually be diagnosed prenatally, sometimes by ultrasound and usually by an elevation in α-fetoprotein (AFP) in the maternal serum or amniotic fluid (see Chapters 10 and 18). A spina bifida lesion can be either open or closed (i.e., covered with a layer of skin). Fetuses with open spina bifida are more likely to be detected by AFP assays.

A major epidemiologic finding is that mothers who supplement their diet with folic acid at the time of conception are less likely to produce children with NTDs. This result has been replicated in several different populations and thus appears to be well confirmed. It has been estimated that as many as 50% to 70% of NTDs can be avoided simply by dietary folic acid supplementation.[6] (Traditional prenatal vitamin supplements have little effect, since administration does not usually begin until well after the time that the neural tube closes.) Because mothers would be likely to ingest similar amounts of folic acid from one pregnancy to the next, folic acid deficiency could well account for at least part of the elevated sibling recurrence risk for NTDs. This is an important example of a *nongenetic* factor that contributes to familial clustering of a disease.

Second, *if the expression of the disease in the proband is more severe, the recurrence risk is higher.* This is again consistent with the liability model, since a more severe expression indicates that the affected individual is at the extreme tail of the liability distribution (see Fig. 5-2). His or her relatives are thus at a higher risk to inherit disease genes. For example, the occurrence of a bilateral (both sides) cleft lip/palate confers a higher recurrence risk on family members than does the occurrence of a unilateral (one side) cleft.

Third, *the recurrence risk is higher if the proband is of the less commonly affected sex* (see the preceding discussion of pyloric stenosis). This is because an affected individual of the less susceptible gender is usually at a more extreme position on the liability distribution.

Fourth, *the recurrence risk for the disease usually decreases rapidly in more remotely related relatives* (Table 5-2). Whereas the recurrence risk for single-gene diseases decreases by 50% with each degree of relationship (e.g., an autosomal dominant disease has a 50% recurrence risk for siblings, 25% for uncle-nephew relationships, 12.5% for first cousins), it decreases much more quickly for multifactorial diseases. This reflects the fact that many genes and environmental factors must combine to produce a trait. All the necessary risk factors are unlikely to be present in less closely related family members.

Table 5-2 Recurrence Risks (%) for First-, Second-, and Third-Degree Relatives

	Risk			
Disease	First Degree	Second Degree	Third Degree	General Population
Cleft lip/palate	4.0	.7	.3	.1
Clubfoot	2.5	.5	.2	.1
Congenital hip dislocation	5.0	.6	.4	.2
Infantile autism	4.5	.1	.05	.04

Finally, *if the prevalence of the disease in a population is* f, *the risk for offspring and siblings of probands is approximately* $\sqrt{f}$. This does not hold true for single-gene traits since their recurrence risks are independent of population prevalence. It is not an absolute rule for multifactorial traits either, but many such diseases tend to conform to this prediction. Examination of the risks given in Table 5-2 shows that the first three diseases follow the prediction fairly well.

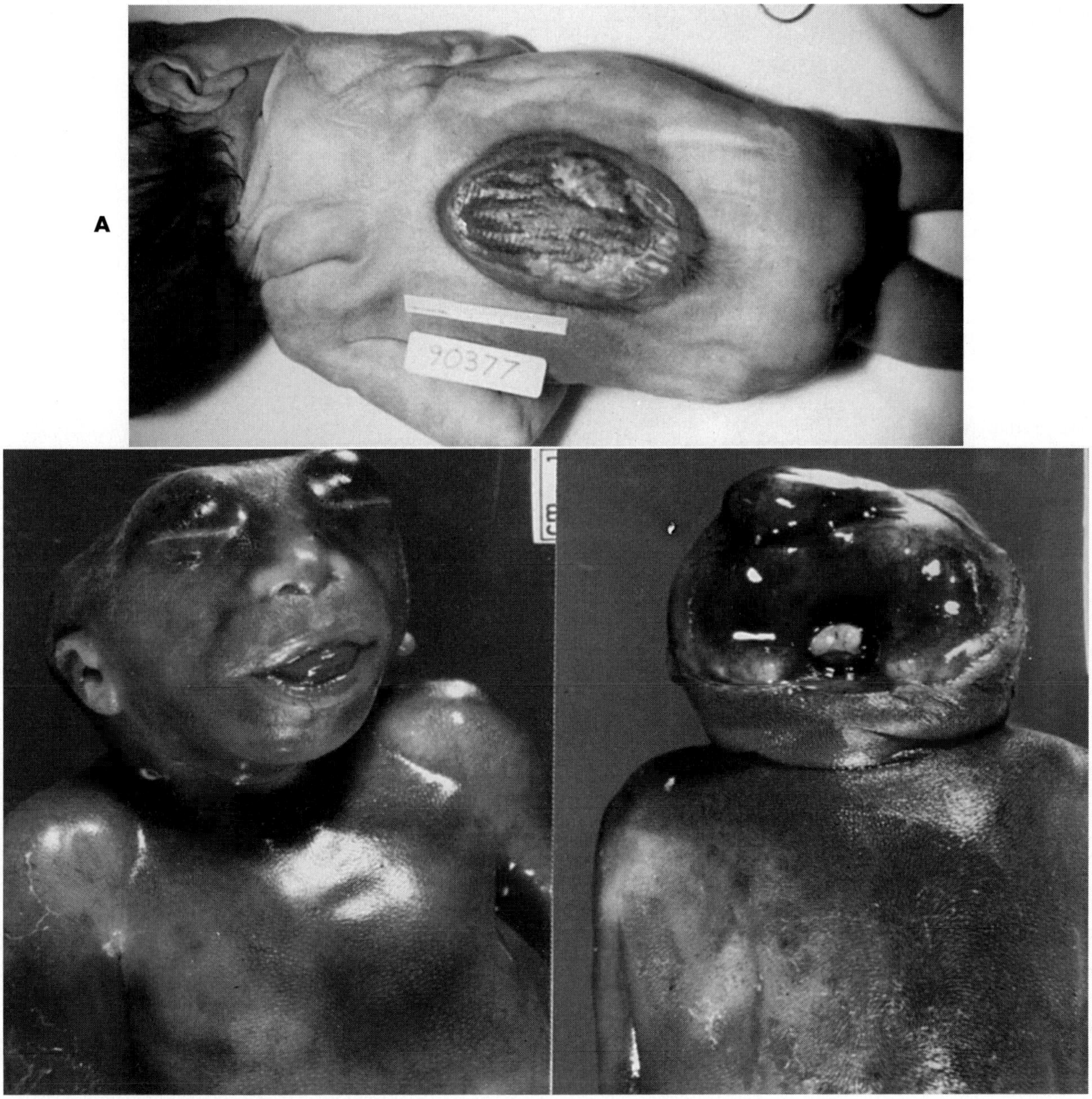

FIG. 5-3 Spina bifida and anencephaly. A, Spina bifida in a newborn. **B,** Anencephaly, showing the absence of the cranial vault. (From Jorde LB et al: *Medical genetics,* ed 2, St Louis, 1999, Mosby.)

However, the observed sibling risk for the fourth disease, infantile autism, is substantially higher than predicted by $\sqrt{f}$.

NATURE AND NURTURE: DISENTANGLING THE EFFECTS OF GENES AND ENVIRONMENT

Family members share genes and a common environment. Family resemblance in traits such as blood pressure reflects both genetic and environmental commonality ("nature" and "nurture," respectively). For centuries people have debated the relative importance of these two types of factors. It is a mistake, of course, to view them as mutually exclusive. Few traits are influenced *only* by genes or *only* by environment. Most are influenced by both. It is useful to try to determine the *relative* influence of genetic and environmental factors. This can lead to a better understanding of disease etiology. It can also help to plan public health strategies. A disease in which the genetic influence is relatively small, such as lung cancer, may be prevented most effectively through emphasis on life-style changes (avoidance of tobacco). When a disease has a relatively larger genetic component, as in breast cancer, examination of family history should be emphasized in addition to life-style modification.

Here, two research strategies are reviewed that are often used to estimate the relative influence of genes and environment: twin studies and adoption studies.

Table 5-3 Concordance Rates in MZ and DZ Twins for Selected Traits and Diseases*

	Concordance Rate		
Trait or Disease	**MZ Twins**	**DZ Twins**	**Heritability**
Affective disorder (bipolar)	.79	.24	>1.00†
Affective disorder (unipolar)	.54	.19	.70
Alcoholism	>.60	<.30	.60
Autism	.92	.00	>1.00
Blood pressure (diastolic)‡	.58	.27	.62
Blood pressure (systolic)‡	.55	.25	.60
Body fat percentage‡	.73	.22	>1.00
Body mass index‡	.95	.53	.84
Cleft lip/palate	.38	.08	.60
Clubfoot	.32	.03	.58
Dermatoglyphics (finger ridge count)‡	.95	.49	.92
Diabetes mellitus	.45-.96	.03-.37	>1.00
Diabetes mellitus (type I)	.55	—	—
Diabetes mellitus (type II)	.90	—	—
Epilepsy (idiopathic)	.69	.14	>1.00
Height‡	.94	.44	1.00
Intelligence quotient (IQ)‡	.76	.51	.50
Measles	.95	.87	.16
Multiple sclerosis	.28	.03	.50
Myocardial infarction (males)	.39	.26	.26
Myocardial infarction (females)	.44	.14	.60
Schizophrenia	.47	.12	.70
Spina bifida	.72	.33	.78

NOTE: Heritability, which is defined as the proportion of the variation in a trait that is due to genetic factors, can be measured as $2(C_{MZ} - C_{DZ})$, where C_{MZ} and C_{DZ} are the concordance rates for MZ twins and DZ twins respectively.
*These figures were compiled from a large variety of sources and represent primarily European and U.S. populations.
†Several heritability estimates exceed 1.0. Because it is impossible for >100% of the variance of a trait to be genetically determined, these values indicate that other factors, such as shared environmental factors, must be operating.
‡Because these are quantitative traits, correlation coefficients are given rather than concordance rates.

Twin Studies

Twins occur with a frequency of about 1 in 100 births in white populations. They are a bit more common in blacks and a bit less common among Asians. **Monozygotic** (MZ, or **"identical") twins** originate when, for unknown reasons, the developing embryo divides to form two separate but identical embryos. Because they are genetically identical, MZ twins are an example of natural clones. **Dizygotic** (DZ, or **"fraternal") twins** are the result of a double ovulation followed by the fertilization of each egg by a different sperm. Thus dizygotic twins are genetically no more similar than siblings. Because two different sperm cells are required to fertilize the two eggs, it is possible for each DZ twin to have a different father. Whereas MZ twinning rates are constant across populations, DZ twinning rates vary somewhat. DZ twinning increases with maternal age until about 40 years, after which it declines.

Because MZ twins are genetically identical, any differences between them should be caused only by environmental effects.[8] MZ twins should thus resemble one another very closely for traits that are strongly influenced by genes. DZ twins provide a convenient comparison, since their environmental differences should be similar to those of MZ twins, but their genetic differences are as great as those between siblings. Twin studies thus usually consist of comparisons between MZ and DZ twins.[9] If both members of a twin pair share a trait (e.g., a cleft lip), it is said to be a **concordant trait.** If they do not share the trait, it is a **discordant trait.** For a trait determined totally by genes, MZ twins should always be concordant, whereas DZ twins should be concordant less often, since they, like siblings, share only 50% of their genes. Concordance rates may differ between opposite-sex DZ twin pairs and same-sex DZ pairs for some traits, such as those that have different frequencies in males and females. For such traits, only same-sex DZ twin pairs should be used when comparing MZ and DZ concordance rates, because MZ twins are necessarily of the same sex.

Table 5-3 gives concordance rates for a number of traits. Note that the concordance rates for contagious diseases such as measles are quite similar in MZ and DZ twins. This is expected, because a contagious disease is unlikely to be influenced markedly by genes. On the other hand, the concordance rates are quite dissimilar for *schizophrenia* and *bipolar affective disorder,* indicating a sizable genetic component for these diseases. The MZ correlations for dermatoglyphics (fingerprints), which are determined almost entirely by genes, are close to 1.0.

At one time, twins were thought to provide a perfect "natural laboratory" in which to determine the relative influences of genetics and environment, but several difficulties

Box 5-2

α_1-ANTITRYPSIN DEFICIENCY: THE INTERACTION OF GENES AND ENVIRONMENT

α_1-Antitrypsin (α_1-AT) deficiency is one of the most common autosomal recessive disorders among whites, affecting approximately 1 in 2500 members of this ethnic group. α_1-AT, synthesized primarily in the liver, is a serine protease inhibitor. It does bind trypsin, as its name suggests. However, α_1-AT binds much more strongly to neutrophil elastase, a protease that is produced by neutrophils (a type of leukocyte) in response to infections and irritants. It carries out its binding and inhibitory role primarily in the lower respiratory tract, where it prevents elastase from digesting the alveolar septi of the lung.

Individuals with less than 10% to 15% of the normal level of α_1-AT activity will experience significant lung damage and typically develop emphysema during their 30s, 40s, or 50s. In addition, at least 10% develop liver cirrhosis as a result of the accumulation of variant α_1-AT molecules in the liver; α_1-AT deficiency accounts for nearly 20% of all nonalcoholic liver cirrhosis in the United States. An important feature of this disease is that cigarette smokers with α_1-AT deficiency develop emphysema much earlier than do nonsmokers. This is because cigarette smoke irritates lung tissue, increasing secretion of neutrophil elastase. At the same time it inactivates α_1-AT, so there is also less inhibition of elastase. One study showed that the median age of survival of nonsmokers with α_1-AT deficiency was 62 years, whereas it was only 40 years for smokers with this disease. Because the combination of cigarette smoking (an environmental factor) and the α_1-AT mutation (a genetic factor) produces more severe disease than either factor alone, it is an example of a gene-environment interaction.

arise. One of the most important is the assumption that the environments of MZ and DZ twins are equally similar. As everyone knows, MZ twins are often treated more similarly than DZ twins. A greater similarity in environment can make MZ twins more concordant for a trait, inflating the apparent influence of genes. In addition, MZ twins may be more likely to seek the same type of environment, further reinforcing environmental similarity. On the other hand, it has been suggested that MZ twins tend to develop personality differences in an attempt to assert their individuality.

Adoption Studies

Studies of adopted children also are used to estimate the genetic contribution to a multifactorial trait. Children born to parents who have a disease but adopted by parents lacking the disease can be studied to find out whether they develop the disease. In some cases such children develop the disease more often than a comparative control population (i.e., adopted children who were born to parents who do *not* have the disease). This provides some evidence that genes may be involved in the causation of the disease, because the adopted children do not share an environment with their affected natural parents. For example, about 8% to 10% of adopted children of a schizophrenic parent develop *schizophrenia,* whereas only 1% of adopted children of normal parents develop schizophrenia.

As with twin studies, several precautions must be exercised in interpreting the results of adoption studies. First, prenatal environmental influences could have long-lasting effects on an adopted child. Second, children are sometimes adopted after they are several years old, ensuring that some environmental influence would have been imparted by the natural parents. Finally, adoption agencies sometimes try to match the adoptive parents with the natural parents in terms of background, socioeconomic status, and so on. All these factors could exaggerate the apparent influence of biologic inheritance.

These reservations, as well as those summarized for twin studies, underscore the need for caution in basing conclusions on twin and adoption studies. These approaches do not provide definitive measures of the role of genes in multifactorial disease nor can they identify specific genes responsible for disease. Instead, they serve a useful purpose in providing a preliminary indication of the extent to which a multifactorial disease may be caused by genetic factors. Currently, sophisticated molecular techniques are being used to identify the specific genes that underlie predisposition to multifactorial diseases.

This discussion should make clear that most common diseases are not the result of either genetics *or* environment. Instead, genetic and nongenetic factors usually interact to influence one's likelihood of developing a common disease. In some cases a genetic predisposition may interact with an environmental factor to increase the risk of disease to a much higher level than would either factor acting alone. A good example of a **gene-environment interaction** is given by α_1-antitrypsin deficiency, a genetic condition that causes pulmonary emphysema and is greatly exacerbated by cigarette smoking (Box 5-2).

GENETICS OF COMMON DISEASES

Some common multifactorial disorders, the congenital malformations, are by definition present at birth. Others, including heart disease, cancer, diabetes, and most psychiatric disorders, are seen primarily in adolescents and adults. Because these disorders are complex, unraveling their genetics is a daunting task. Nonetheless, significant progress is now being made.

Congenital Malformations

Congenital diseases are present at birth. Approximately 2% of newborns present with a congenital malformation; most of these are multifactorial in etiology. Table 5-4 lists some more common congenital malformations. In general, sibling recurrence risks for most of these disorders range from 1% to 5%.

Some congenital malformations, such as cleft lip/palate and pyloric stenosis, are relatively easy to repair and thus are not considered to be serious problems. Others, such as the neural tube defects, usually have more severe consequences. Although some cases of congenital malformations occur in

Table 5-4 Prevalence Rates of Common Congenital Malformations in Whites

Disorder	Prevalence per 1000 Births (Approximate)
Cleft lip/palate	1
Clubfoot	1
Congenital heart defects	4-8
Hydrocephaly	0.5-2.5
Isolated cleft palate	0.4
Neural tube defects	1-3
Pyloric stenosis	3

Table 5-5 Prevalence Figures for Common Adult Diseases

Disease	Number of Affected Americans (Approximate)
Alcoholism	10 million
Alzheimer disease	4 million
Bipolar affective disorder	1 million
Cancer (all types)	6 million
Coronary heart disease	5 million
Diabetes (type I)	1 million
Diabetes (type II)	5-10 million
Epilepsy	2 million
Hypertension	25-30 million
Multiple sclerosis	250,000
Obesity*	50 million
Schizophrenia	2 million

*Defined as 20% or more above ideal body weight.

the absence of any other problems, it is quite common for them to be associated with other disorders. For example, hydrocephaly and clubfoot are often seen secondary to spina bifida, cleft lip/palate is often seen in babies with trisomy 13, and congenital heart defects are seen in many disorders, including Down syndrome.

Environmental factors also cause some congenital malformations. An example is thalidomide, a sedative used during pregnancy in the early 1960s. When ingested during early pregnancy this drug often caused **phocomelia** (severely shortened limbs) in babies. Maternal exposure to retinoic acid, which is used to treat acne, can cause congenital defects of the heart, ear, and central nervous system. Maternal rubella infection can cause congenital heart defects.

Multifactorial Disorders in the Adult Population

Until quite recently, very little was known about specific genes responsible for common adult diseases. With more powerful laboratory and analytic techniques, this situation is changing. This section reviews recent progress in understanding the genetics of the major common adult diseases. Table 5-5 gives approximate prevalence figures for these disorders in the United States.

Coronary Heart Disease

It is well known that coronary heart disease (CHD) is the leading killer of Americans, accounting for approximately 25% of all deaths in the United States. It is caused by *atherosclerosis* (narrowing as a result of the formation of lipid-laden lesions) of the coronary arteries. This narrowing impedes blood flow to the heart and can eventually result in a *myocardial infarction* (destruction of heart tissue caused by an inadequate supply of oxygen). When atherosclerosis occurs in arteries supplying blood to the brain, a *stroke* can result. Many risk factors for heart disease have been identified, including obesity, cigarette smoking, hypertension, elevated cholesterol level, and positive family history (usually defined as having one affected first-degree relative). Many studies have examined the role of family history in CHD, and they show that an individual with a positive family history is two to seven times more likely to have heart disease than is an individual with no family history (this would be the relative risk of heart disease as a result of a positive family history). Generally, these studies also show that the risk increases if (1) there are more affected relatives; (2) the affected relative or relatives are female (the less commonly affected sex) rather than male; and (3) age of onset in the affected relative is early (before 55 years). For example, one study showed that men between the ages of 20 and 39 years had a relative risk of 3.0 for CHD if they had one affected first-degree relative. The relative risk increased to 13 if two first-degree relatives were affected with CHD before 55 years of age.[10]

What part do genes play in the familial clustering of heart disease? Because of the key role of lipids in atherosclerosis, many current studies are focusing on the genetic determination of various lipoproteins.[11] Undoubtedly the most important advance in this area has been the isolation and cloning of the gene for the LDL (low-density lipoprotein) receptor defects that cause *familial hypercholesterolemia* (Box 5-3). Nearly 20 other genes involved in lipid variation, coagulation, and hypertension have been identified, including several genes encoding apolipoproteins (the protein components of lipoproteins) (Table 5-6). Functional analysis of these genes is leading to an increased understanding, and eventually more effective treatment, of CHD.

Environmental factors, many of which are easily modified, are also important causes of CHD. Abundant epidemiologic evidence shows that cigarette smoking and obesity increase the risk of CHD, whereas exercise and a diet low in saturated fats decrease the risk. Indeed, the approximate 50% decline in CHD prevalence in the United States during the past 40 years is usually attributed to a decrease in the proportion of adults who smoke cigarettes, decreased consumption of saturated fats, and an increased emphasis on exercise and a generally healthier life-style.

Hypertension

Systemic hypertension, which is seen in at least 15% of the populations of most developed countries, is a key risk factor

Box 5-3

FAMILIAL HYPERCHOLESTEROLEMIA

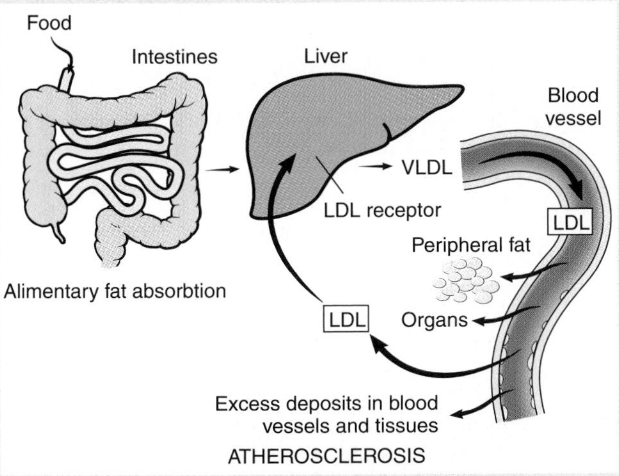

Autosomal dominant familial hypercholesterolemia (FH) is an important cause of heart disease, accounting for approximately 5% of myocardial infarctions in persons under 60 years of age.[12] FH is one of the most common autosomal dominant disorders: in most populations surveyed to date, about 1 in 500 persons is a heterozygote. Plasma cholesterol levels are approximately twice as high as normal (i.e., about 300 to 400 mg/dl), resulting in substantially accelerated atherosclerosis and distinctive cholesterol deposits in skin and tendons (*xanthomas,* Fig. 5-4). Data compiled from five studies showed that approximately 75% of men with FH developed coronary disease and 50% had a fatal myocardial infarction by 60 years. The corresponding percentages for women were lower (45% and 15%) because women generally develop heart disease at a later age than men.

Consistent with Hardy-Weinberg predictions, about 1 in 1 million births is homozygous for the FH gene. Homozygotes are much more severely affected, with cholesterol levels ranging from 600 to 1200 mg/dl. Most experience myocardial infarctions before 20 years of age, and a myocardial infarction at 18 months of age has been reported. If untreated, most FH homozygotes die before 30 years of age.

All cells require cholesterol as a component of their plasma membrane. They can either synthesize their own cholesterol, or, preferably, obtain it from the extracellular environment, where it is carried primarily by low-density lipoprotein (LDL). In a process known as *endocytosis,* LDL-bound cholesterol is taken into the cell via LDL receptors on the cell's surface (Fig. 5-5). FH is caused by a reduction in the number of functional LDL receptors on cell surfaces. Lacking the normal number of LDL receptors, cellular cholesterol uptake is reduced and circulating cholesterol levels increase.

Much of what we know about endocytosis has been learned through the study of LDL receptors. The process of endocytosis and the processing of LDL in the cell are described in detail in Fig. 5-5 (endocytosis is discussed in Chapter 1). These processes result in a fine-tuned regulation of cholesterol levels within cells, and they influence the level of circulating cholesterol as well.

The isolation and cloning of the LDL receptor gene in 1984 were critical steps in understanding exactly how LDL receptor defects cause FH. This gene, located on chromosome 19, is 45 kb in length and consists of 18 exons and 17 introns. It encodes a 5.3-kb messenger ribonucleic acid (mRNA) transcript that ultimately produces a mature protein of 839 amino acids. More than 600 different mutations, including missense and nonsense substitutions as well as insertions and deletions, have been identified in the LDL receptor gene. These can be grouped into five broad classes according to their effects on the activity of the receptor.[13] Class 1 mutations result in no detectable protein product. Thus heterozygotes would produce only half the normal number of LDL receptors. Class 2 mutations in the LDL receptor gene result in production of the LDL receptor, but it is altered such that it cannot leave the endoplasmic reticulum. It is eventually degraded. Class 3 mutations produce an LDL receptor that is capable of migrating to the cell surface but incapable of normal binding to LDL. Class 4 mutations, which are comparatively rare, produce receptors that are normal except that they do not migrate specifically to coated pits and thus cannot carry LDL into the cell. The final group of mutations, class 5, produces an LDL receptor that cannot dissociate from the LDL particle after entry into the cell. The receptor cannot return to the cell surface and is degraded. Each class of mutations reduces the number of effective LDL receptors, resulting in decreased LDL uptake and hence elevated levels of circulating cholesterol. The number of effective receptors is reduced by about half in FH heterozygotes, and homozygotes have virtually no functional LDL receptors.

Understanding the defects that lead to FH has helped to develop effective therapies for the disorder. Dietary reduction of cholesterol (primarily through the reduced intake of saturated fats) has only modest effects on cholesterol levels in FH heterozygotes. Because cholesterol is reabsorbed into the gut and then recycled through the liver (where most cholesterol synthesis takes place), serum cholesterol levels can be reduced by the administration of bile acid–absorbing resins, such as cholestyramine. The absorbed cholesterol is then excreted. It is interesting that reduced recirculation from the gut causes the liver cells to form additional LDL receptors, lowering circulating cholesterol levels. However, the decrease in intracellular cholesterol also stimulates cholesterol synthesis by liver cells, so the overall reduction in plasma LDL is only about 15% to 20%. This treatment is much more effective when combined with agents such as lovastatin that reduce cholesterol synthesis by inhibiting 3-hydroxy-3-methylglutaryl–coenzyme A (HMG-CoA) reductase. Decreased synthesis leads to further production of LDL receptors. When these therapies are used in combination, serum cholesterol levels in FH heterozygotes can be reduced to approximately normal levels.

The picture is less encouraging for FH homozygotes. The therapies just discussed can enhance cholesterol elimination and reduce its synthesis, but they are largely ineffective because homozygotes have few or no LDL receptors. Liver transplants, which provide hepatocytes that have normal LDL receptors, have been successful in some cases, but this option is often limited by a lack of donors. Plasma exchange, carried out every 1 to 2 weeks, in combination with drug therapy, can reduce cholesterol levels by about 50%. However, this therapy is difficult to continue for long periods. Somatic cell gene therapy, in which hepatocytes carrying normal LDL receptor genes are introduced into the portal circulation, is now being tested. It may eventually prove to be an effective treatment for FH homozygotes.

The FH story illustrates how medical research has made important contributions both to our understanding of basic cell biology and to advances in clinical therapy. The process of receptor-mediated endocytosis, elucidated largely by research on the LDL receptor defects, is of fundamental significance for cellular processes throughout the body. Equally important is that this research, by clarifying how cholesterol synthesis and uptake can be modified, has led to significant improvements in therapy for this important cause of heart disease.

Illustration from Damjanov I: *Pathophysiology for the health-related professions,* ed 2, Philadelphia, 2000, W.B. Saunders.

Table 5-6 Single Genes Known to Contribute to Coronary Heart Disease Risk

Gene	Chromosomal Location	Function
Apolipoprotein gene		
Apo *A1*	11q	HDL formation
Apo *A4*	11q	Unknown
Apo *C3*	11q	Unknown
Apo *B*	2p	Chylomicrons; VLDL, IDL, and LDL formation; ligand for LDL receptor
Apo *D*	2p	Unknown
Apo *C1*	19q	LCAT activation
Apo *C2*	19q	Lipoprotein lipase activation
Apo *E*	19q	Ligand for LDL receptor
Apo *A2*	1p	Unknown
Other genes		
Lp(a)	6q	*Lp(a)* particle formation
LDL receptor	19p	Uptake of LDL particles
Lipoprotein lipase	8p	Hydrolysis of lipoprotein lipids
Hepatic triglyceride lipase	15q	Hydrolysis of lipoprotein lipids
LCAT	16q	Cholesterol esterification
Cholesterol ester transfer protein	16q	Facilitates transfer of cholesterol esters and phospholipid lipoproteins

Modified from King RA, Rotter JI, Motulsky AG, editors: *The genetic basis of common diseases,* New York, 1992, Oxford University Press.
HDL, High-density lipoprotein; *VLDL,* very-low-density lipoprotein; *IDL,* intermediate-density lipoprotein; *LDL,* low-density lipoprotein; *LCAT,* lecithin-cholesterol acyltransferase.

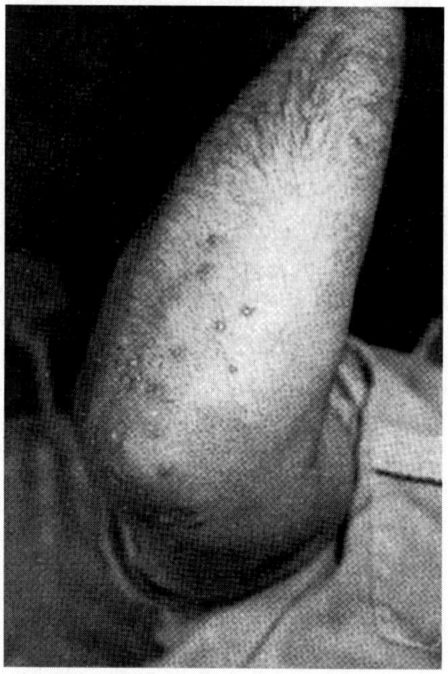

FIG. 5-4 Xanthoma. Xanthomas, or fatty deposits, are clearly visible in an individual familial hypercholesterolemia. (From Jorde LB et al: *Medical genetics,* ed 2, St Louis, 1999, Mosby.)

for heart disease, stroke, and kidney disease. Studies of blood pressure correlations within families indicate that about 20% to 40% of the variation in both systolic and diastolic blood pressure is caused by genetic factors. The fact that this figure is substantially less than 100% indicates that environmental factors also must be important causes of blood pressure variation. The most important environmental risk factors for hypertension are increased sodium intake, decreased physical activity, psychosocial stress, and obesity (but, as discussed below, the latter factor is itself influenced by both genes and environment).

Blood pressure regulation is a highly complex process that is influenced by many physiologic systems, including various aspects of kidney function, cellular ion transport, and heart function. Because of this complexity, it is unlikely that family studies of simple blood pressure will reveal much about genes responsible for hypertension. For this reason most research now focuses on specific components that may influence blood pressure variation, such as angiotensin, angiotensinogen, urinary kallikrein, and sodium-lithium countertransport[14] (Fig. 5-6 and Table 5-7). These factors are more likely to be under the control of smaller numbers of genes. For example, studies have implicated the angiotensinogen gene in the causation of both hypertension and *preeclampsia* (a form of pregnancy-induced hypertension).

Cancer

Cancer is the second leading cause of death in the United States. It is well established that many major types of cancer (e.g., breast, colon, prostate, ovarian) cluster strongly in families. This is caused by both shared genes and shared environmental factors. Although numerous cancer genes are being isolated[15], environmental factors also play an important role in causing cancer. In particular, tobacco use is estimated to account for one third of all cancer cases in the United States, making it the most important known cause of cancer.[16]

Breast Cancer

Breast cancer is the most common cancer among women, affecting approximately 12% of American women who live to 85 years or more. Formerly the leading cause of cancer death among women, it has been surpassed by lung cancer. Breast cancer aggregates strongly in families. If a woman

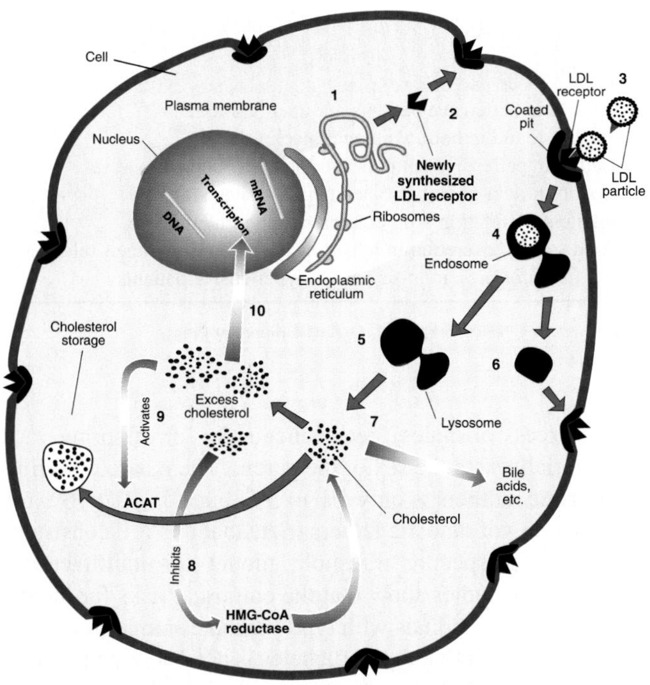

FIG. 5-5 Process of receptor-mediated endocytosis. Numbers in parentheses correspond to numbers shown in the figure. *(1)* The low-density lipoprotein (LDL) receptors, which are glycoproteins, are synthesized in the endoplasmic reticulum of the cell. *(2)* From here, they pass through the Golgi apparatus to the cell surface, where part of the receptor protrudes outside the cell. *(3)* The circulating LDL particle is bound by the LDL receptor and localized in cell-surface depressions called *coated pits* (so named because they are coated with a protein called *clathrin*). *(4)* The coated pit invaginates, bringing the LDL particle inside the cell. *(5)* Once inside the cell, the LDL particle is separated from the receptor, taken into a lysosome, and broken down into its constituents by lysosomal enzymes. *(6)* The LDL receptor is recirculated to the cell surface to bind another LDL particle (each LDL receptor goes through this cycle approximately once every 10 minutes even if it is not occupied by an LDL particle). *(7)* Free cholesterol is released from the lysosome for incorporation into cell membranes or metabolism into bile acids or steroids. Excess cholesterol can be stored in the cell as a cholesterol ester or removed from the cell by associating with high-density lipoprotein (HDL). *(8)* As cholesterol levels in the cell rise, cellular cholesterol synthesis is reduced by inhibition of the rate-limiting enzyme HMG-CoA reductase (3-hydroxy-3-methylglutaryl-coenzyme A reductase). *(9)* Rising cholesterol levels also increase the activity of acyl-CoA:cholesterol acyltransferase (ACAT), an enzyme that modifies cholesterol for storage as cholesterol esters. *(10)* In addition, the number of LDL receptors is decreased by lowering the transcription rate of the LDL receptor gene itself. This decreases cholesterol uptake. (From Jorde LB et al: *Medical genetics,* ed 2, St Louis, 1999, Mosby.)

has one affected first-degree relative, her risk of developing breast cancer doubles. This risk increases if the age of onset in the affected relative is early and if the cancer is bilateral (tumors in both breasts).

An autosomal dominant form of breast cancer accounts for approximately 5% of breast cancer cases in the United States. Genes responsible for this form of breast cancer have been mapped to chromosomes 17 *(BRCA1)* and 13 *(BRCA2)*. Each of these genes has now been cloned.[17] *BRCA1* and *BRCA2* mutations are also associated with an increased risk of ovarian cancer. Cloning of these genes and identification

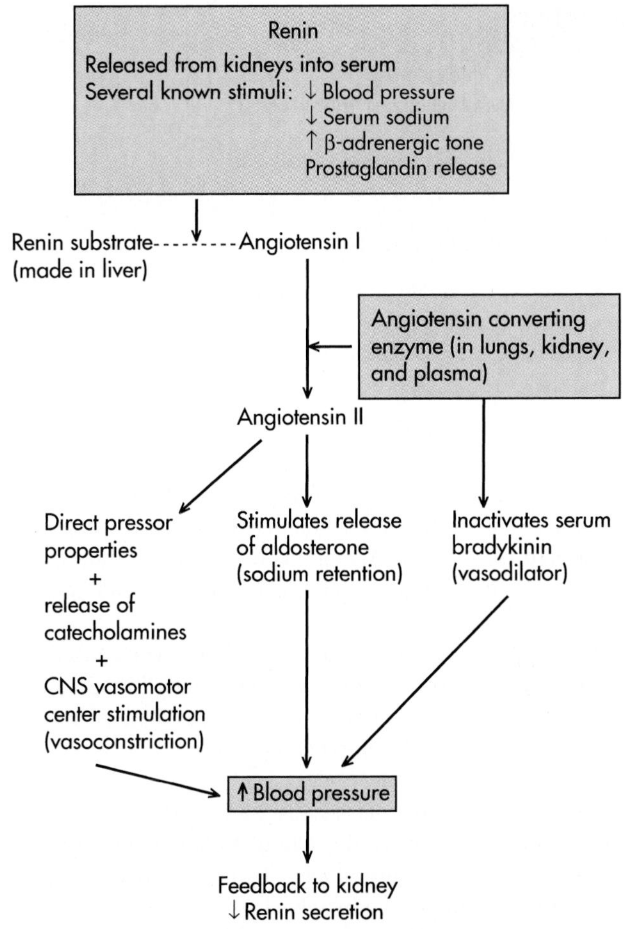

FIG. 5-6 Renin-angiotensin-aldosterone system. *CNS,* Central nervous system. (From Jorde LB et al: *Medical genetics,* ed 2, St Louis, 1999, Mosby.)

of disease-causing mutations may lead to early diagnosis of breast cancer, and the evaluation of these genes' products, which are both involved in deoxyribonucleic acid (DNA) repair, will yield valuable evidence on the etiology of breast cancer in general.

Colorectal Cancer

Colorectal cancer is second only to lung cancer in the number of cases occurring annually in the United States, with 131,200 new cases in 1997.[3] Approximately 1 in 20 Americans will develop colorectal cancer. Like breast cancer, it clusters in families (in fact, familial clustering of this form of cancer was reported in the medical literature as early as 1881). The risk of colorectal cancer in people with one affected first-degree relative is two to three times higher than in the general population.

This familial aggregation is caused in part by subsets of colorectal cancer cases that are inherited as single-gene traits. *Familial adenomatous polyposis* occurs in approximately 1 in 8000 whites. The gene responsible for this disorder was mapped to chromosome 5 several years ago, and the gene itself was subsequently cloned.[18] Cloning of this gene and the study of the probable function of its product have provided important new information on the molecular basis of colorectal cancer.

Table 5-7 Transport Systems Involved in Blood Pressure Regulation

Laboratory Measurement	Positive Findings
Sodium-potassium cotransport (red cells)	Decreased in hypertensive patients and their children Abnormality found in both white and black subjects
Sodium-lithium countertransport (red cells)	Increased in hypertensive patients and their first-degree relatives Abnormality rare or absent in black hypertensive patients No consistent correlation with cotransport abnormalities
Na^+, K^+ ATPase (white cells)	Decreased sodium excretion in hypertensive patients and their relatives Humoral inhibitor present in sera from hypertensive patients

Modified from King RA, Rotter JI, Motulsky AG, editors: *The genetic basis of common diseases,* New York, 1992, Oxford University Press.
Na^+, Sodium; *K^+,* potassium; *ATPase,* adenosinetriphosphatase.

Hereditary nonpolyposis colorectal cancer, which may account for as many as 5% of colorectal cancer cases, is caused by mutations in any of five genes.[19] Cloning of these genes has shown that all of them are involved in the vital process of DNA repair. When this function is compromised, cancer-causing mutations can persist in cells, leading eventually to a tumor.

Other colorectal cancer cases are likely to be caused by a complex interaction of multiple genes. In addition, environmental factors, such as a high-fat, low-fiber diet, are thought to increase the risk of colorectal cancer.

Other Cancers

The genetic basis of various other cancers, including retinoblastoma, has been discussed. Although each of these cancers is relatively rare, study of the causative genes has provided many important insights into the nature of carcinogenesis in general. This will lead to more effective treatment and prevention of all cancers.

Diabetes Mellitus

Like the other disorders discussed in this chapter, the etiology of diabetes mellitus is complex and not fully understood. Nevertheless, progress is being made in understanding the genetic basis of this disorder, which is a leading cause of blindness, heart disease, and kidney failure.[20,21] An important advance has been the recognition that diabetes is actually a heterogeneous group of disorders, all characterized by elevated blood sugar. The focus here is on the two major types of diabetes—type I (insulin-dependent diabetes mellitus [IDDM]) and type II (non-insulin-dependent diabetes mellitus [NIDDM]).

Type I Diabetes

Type I diabetes, which is characterized by T cell infiltration of the pancreas and destruction of the insulin-producing beta cells, usually (but not always) presents before age 40 years. Individuals with type I diabetes must receive exogenous insulin to survive. The pathologic manifestations of the disorder, together with the common finding of antibodies against pancreatic beta cells and a very strong association with several human leukocyte antigen (HLA) class II alleles, suggest that type I diabetes is an autoimmune disorder. Siblings of individuals with type I diabetes face a substantial elevation in risk: approximately 6%, as opposed to a risk of about 0.3% to 0.5% in the general population. Although the sexes are affected in almost equal proportions (there is a slight excess of males), recurrence risks for offspring vary substantially with the sex of the parent. The risk to offspring of diabetic mothers is only 1% to 3%, but it is 4% to 6% for the offspring of diabetic fathers (note that this is inconsistent with the sex-specific threshold model for multifactorial traits). Twin studies show that the empirical risks for identical twins of individuals with type I diabetes range from 30% to 50%. The fact that type I diabetes is not 100% concordant among identical twins indicates that genetic factors are not solely responsible for the disorder. There is good evidence that viral infections, for example, contribute to the causation of type I diabetes in at least some individuals.

The association of specific HLA class II alleles (see Chapter 20) and type I diabetes has been studied intensively. Ninety-five percent of whites with type I diabetes have the HLA DR3 and/or DR4 allele, whereas only about 50% of the general white population has either of these alleles. If an affected proband and a sibling are both heterozygous for the DR3 and DR4 alleles, the sibling's risk of developing type I diabetes is nearly 20% (i.e., about 40 times higher than the risk in the general population). In addition, the presence of aspartic acid at position 57 of the DQβ chain is strongly associated with resistance to type I diabetes. In fact, those who have this amino acid at position 57 are 100 times less likely to develop the disease than are individuals homozygous for other amino acids (alanine, serine, valine). It is probable that this particular amino acid is involved in T cell recognition and that those who lack it are more likely to experience an autoimmune episode.

The insulin gene itself, which is located on chromosome 11p, is another logical candidate for type I diabetes susceptibility. Polymorphisms in and around the insulin gene have been studied extensively, and alleles of some of these polymorphisms are associated with susceptibility to type I diabetes. These associations are not strict: not everybody who carries a given allele will develop type I diabetes. This is expected, given the many other factors, both genetic and nongenetic, that appear to be involved in causing type I diabetes.

Type II Diabetes

Type II diabetes accounts for 80% to 90% of all diabetes cases in the United States. A number of features distinguish it from type I diabetes. Unlike type I diabetes, there is nearly always some endogenous insulin production in persons with type II diabetes and it can often be treated successfully with dietary modification and/or oral drugs. Individuals with type

II diabetes also experience insulin resistance (i.e., their bodies have difficulty using the insulin they produce). This disease typically occurs among people over 40 years of age and, in contrast to type I diabetes, is seen more commonly among obese persons. Neither HLA associations nor autoantibodies are seen commonly in this form of diabetes. Monozygotic twin concordance rates are substantially higher than in type I diabetes, often exceeding 90% (because of age dependence, the concordance rate increases if older subjects are studied). The empirical recurrence risks for first-degree relatives of type II diabetes cases are higher than those for type I, generally ranging from 10% to 15%. The differences between type I and type II diabetes are summarized in Table 5-8.

In spite of the apparently high degree of genetic involvement in type II diabetes, only one specific gene for this disorder has been tentatively identified (a gene-encoding calpain).

The two most important risk factors for type II diabetes are positive family history and obesity (the latter increases insulin resistance). The disease tends to rise in prevalence when populations adopt a more Western diet and exercise pattern. Increases have been seen, for example, among Japanese immigrants to the United States and among some native populations of the South Pacific, Australia, and the Americas. Several studies, conducted on both male and female subjects, have shown that regular exercise can substantially lower one's risk of developing type II diabetes, even among individuals with a family history of the disease. This is partly because exercise reduces obesity. However, even in the absence of weight loss, exercise increases insulin sensitivity and improves glucose tolerance.

A small proportion of type II diabetes cases occurs early in life, typically before 25 years of age. This subset, termed *maturity-onset diabetes of the young* (MODY), can be inherited as an autosomal dominant trait. Studies of MODY pedigrees have shown that about half of cases of the disease are caused by mutations in the glucokinase gene. Glucokinase converts glucose to glucose-6-phosphate in the pancreas. In addition to the glucokinase gene, four other genes, all of which are involved in pancreatic development or insulin regulation, have now been shown to be causes of MODY.

Obesity

Obesity is often defined as a body weight exceeding 20% of the upper limit of the normal range. Using this criterion, approximately 20% of American adults are obese. The body mass index (BMI), defined as weight (in kilograms [kg]) divided by height (in meters [m]) squared, is also used as a measure of obesity. Using the criterion that a BMI above 30 kg/m^2 indicates obesity, 12% of American adults are obese (one of the highest percentages in the world). Although obesity itself is perhaps not a "disease," it is an important risk factor for several common diseases, including heart disease, stroke, and type II diabetes.

As one might expect, a strong correlation exists between obesity in parents and their children. This could easily be ascribed to common environmental effects: parents and children usually share similar dietary and exercise habits. Indeed, it may seem that obesity should be influenced almost exclusively by environmental factors. However, good evidence exists for genetic components as well. Four different adoption studies each showed that the body weights of adopted individuals correlated significantly with their natural parents' body weights but not with those of their adoptive parents. Twin studies also provide evidence for a genetic effect on body weight, with most studies showing significantly higher concordance in MZ twins than in DZ twins. Statistical analyses of family data have shown that major genes, as well as polygenic effects, may be associated with obesity. A gene that encodes leptin, a protein involved in appetite regulation, has been cloned in mice and humans.[22] Leptin injections can reduce obesity in some mice; unfortunately, they do not have a substantial effect in humans.

Table 5-8 Comparison of Major Features of Types I and II Diabetes Mellitus

Feature	Type I Diabetes	Type II Diabetes
Age of onset	Usually <40 yr	Usually >40 yr (except maturity-onset diabetes of the young [MODY])
Insulin production	None	Partial
Insulin resistance	No	Yes
Autoimmunity	Yes	No
Obesity	Not common	Common
Monozygotic (MZ) twin concordance	.55	.90
Sibling recurrence risk	1%-6%	10%-15%

Alzheimer Disease

It is estimated that Alzheimer disease (AD) affects approximately 10% of Americans older than 65 years and as many as half of those older than 85 years. The annual cost of caring for individuals with AD is at least $100 billion. This disorder is characterized by progressive dementia and loss of memory and by the formation of amyloid plaques and neurofibrillary tangles in the brain, particularly in the cerebral cortex and hippocampus. Death usually occurs within 5 to 10 years after the first appearance of symptoms. Individuals with an affected first-degree relative have, on average, a 10% chance of developing the disorder (however, because of the age dependence and heterogeneity of AD, this figure is quite approximate). Although most cases of AD do not appear to be caused by single loci, 5% to 15% follow an autosomal dominant mode of transmission.[23] Early-onset AD (before 65 years of age) accounts for about 25% of AD cases and is much more likely to be inherited in an autosomal dominant fashion.

AD is a genetically heterogeneous disorder. Genes for early-onset AD map to chromosomes 1 and 14, and the two genes encode highly similar protein products that are involved in cleavage of the β-amyloid precursor protein.[24]

Mutations of the β-amyloid precursor protein gene, itself, on chromosome 21, have also been shown to cause early-onset AD in a small minority of individuals. In addition, some cases of the more common late-onset form are associated with an allele of the apolipoprotein E (apo *E*) locus.[23]

A recent compilation of results from many studies showed that, among whites, homozygotes for the apo *E4* allele were 15 times more likely to develop AD than were the rest of the population; heterozygotes having one copy of the allele were approximately three times more likely to develop AD. The risk associated with apo *E4* was even higher for Japanese subjects, but it was somewhat lower for Hispanic and black subjects. The apo *E4* protein product is not involved in cleavage of the amyloid precursor protein but instead appears to be involved in the clearance of amyloid from the brain.

Recently, a genome scan provided evidence for a gene on chromosome 12 that may increase susceptibility to late-onset AD. A gene located within the region implicated by linkage analysis encodes α_2-macroglobulin, a protease inhibitor. Some studies support an association between alleles of this gene and late-onset AD, although the association is not replicated in other studies. It remains to be seen whether this gene plays a significant role in causing AD. Further studies of these various genes will shed light not only on the most common cause of dementia among elderly persons, but also on the aging process in general. Additional studies have implicated a region on chromosome 10 in the causation of AD.

Alcoholism

At some point, alcoholism is diagnosed in approximately 10% of adult males and 3% to 5% of adult females in the United States. The national cost of alcoholism, in terms of lost productivity and direct medical costs, exceeds $165 billion per year. More than 100 studies have shown that this disease clusters in families.[25] The risk of developing alcoholism among individuals with one affected parent is three to five times higher than for those with unaffected parents.

Most twin studies have yielded concordance rates for DZ twins less than 30% and concordance rates for MZ twins in excess of 60%. Adoption studies have shown that the offspring of an alcoholic parent, even when raised by nonalcoholic parents, have a fourfold increased risk of developing the disorder. To control for possible prenatal effects in an alcoholic mother, some studies have included only the offspring of alcoholic fathers. The results have remained the same. One study showed that the offspring of nonalcoholic parents, when reared by alcoholics, did *not* have an increased risk of developing alcoholism. These data argue that there may be genes that predispose some people to alcoholism.

Studies have shown an association between alcoholism and a DNA polymorphism linked to the dopamine D2 receptor gene on chromosome 11q. Because the dopamine receptors are part of the brain's reward pathway, this association has some intuitive appeal. However, many additional studies in other populations have failed to replicate it. It now appears unlikely that this polymorphism contributes importantly to alcoholism susceptibility.[25] Nevertheless, the twin and adoption studies just mentioned are compelling, and it is possible that further studies may reveal genes that do in fact influence susceptibility to this important disease.

It should be underscored that genes may increase one's *susceptibility* to alcoholism. Obviously, this is a disease that requires an environmental component. Regardless of genetic constitution, someone who never consumes alcohol cannot become an alcoholic.

Psychiatric Disorders

The major psychiatric diseases, schizophrenia and affective disorder, have been the subjects of numerous genetic studies.[26] Twin, adoption, and family studies have shown that both disorders aggregate in families.

Schizophrenia

Schizophrenia is a severe emotional disorder characterized by delusions, hallucinations, retreat from reality, and bizarre, withdrawn, or inappropriate behavior. (Contrary to popular belief, schizophrenia is not a "split personality" disorder.) The lifetime recurrence risk for schizophrenia among the offspring of one affected parent is approximately 8% to 10%, which is about 10 times higher than the risk in the general population.[27] As one might expect, the empirical risks increase when more relatives are affected. For example, an individual with an affected sibling and an affected parent has a risk of about 17%, and an individual with two affected parents has a risk of 46%. The risks decrease when the affected family member is a second- or third-degree relative. Details are given in Table 5-9. On inspection of Table 5-9, it may seem puzzling that the proportion of schizophrenic probands who have a schizophrenic parent is only about 5%, which is substantially lower than the risk for other first-degree relatives (e.g., siblings, affected parents, their offspring). This can be explained by the fact that people with schizophrenia are less likely to marry and produce children than are other individuals. There is thus substantial selection against schizophrenia in the population.

Twin and adoption studies also indicate that genetic factors are likely to be involved in schizophrenia. Data pooled from five different twin studies show a 47% concordance rate

Table 5-9 Recurrence Risks for Relatives of Schizophrenic Probands*

Relationship to Proband	Recurrence Risk (%)
Monozygotic twin	44.3
Dizygotic twin	12.1
Offspring	9.4
Sibling	7.3
Niece/nephew	2.7
Grandchild	2.8
First cousin	1.6
Spouse	1.0

Modified from McGue M, Gottesman II, Rao DC: *Behav Genet* 16:75, 1986.

*Figures are based on multiple studies of Western European populations.

for MZ twins, compared with a concordance rate of only 12% for DZ twins. When the offspring of a schizophrenic parent are adopted by normal parents, their risk of developing the disease is about 10%, which is approximately the same as the risk when raised by a schizophrenic biologic parent. Despite numerous studies, no specific gene predisposing to schizophrenia has yet been identified.

Bipolar Affective Disorder

Bipolar affective disorder, also known as *manic-depressive disorder,* is a form of psychosis with extreme mood swings and emotional instability. The incidence of the disorder in the general population is approximately 0.5%, but it rises to 5% to 10% among those with an affected first-degree relative. A study using the Danish twin registry yielded concordance rates of 79% and 24% for MZ and DZ twins, respectively.[28] The corresponding concordance rates for unipolar disorder (major depression) were 54% and 19%. In general, it appears that bipolar disorder is more strongly influenced by genetic factors than is unipolar disorder.

Comments on Psychiatric Disorders

Large-scale linkage studies involving hundreds of polymorphisms throughout the genome have now been carried out for both schizophrenia and bipolar affective disorder. Most of these studies have produced negative results, although a few recent large-scale studies have yielded promising findings. A number of candidate genes have been tested for linkage or association with both diseases. Most of these candidates were chosen on the basis of the known involvement of certain neurotransmitters, receptors, or neurotransmitter-related enzymes in each disease (e.g., schizophrenia can be treated by drugs that block dopamine receptors, and bipolar affective disorder is sometimes treated with lithium). None of the candidate genes tested thus far, including those for sodium-lithium countertransport, various components of the dopaminergic system, and several neurotransmitter-related enzymes (e.g., monoamine oxidase, dopamine-β-hydroxylase, tyrosine hydroxylase), has been shown unequivocally to be linked or associated with either disease.

These results reflect some of the difficulties encountered in doing genetic studies of psychiatric disorders. These disorders are undoubtedly heterogeneous, reflecting the influence of numerous genetic and environmental factors. Also, definition of the phenotype is not always straightforward and it may change through time, significantly complicating genetic analysis.

Some General Principles and Conclusions

Some general principles can be deduced from the results obtained thus far on the genetics of complex disorders. First, the more strongly inherited forms of complex disorders generally have an earlier age of onset (e.g., breast cancer, Alzheimer disease, heart disease). Often these represent subsets of cases in which there is single-gene inheritance. Second, when there is laterality, the bilateral forms are more likely to cluster strongly in families (e.g., breast cancer, cleft lip/palate). Third, although the sex-specific threshold model fits some of the complex disorders (e.g., pyloric stenosis, cleft lip/palate, autism, heart disease), it fails to fit others (e.g., type I diabetes).

A tendency exists, particularly among the lay public, to assume that the presence of a genetic component means that the course of a disease cannot be altered. *This is incorrect.* Most of the diseases discussed in this chapter have both genetic and environmental components. Thus environmental modification (e.g., diet, exercise, stress reduction) can often reduce risk significantly. Such modification may be especially important for individuals with a family history of a disease, since they are likely to develop the disease earlier in life. Those with a family history of heart disease, for example, can often add many years of productive living with relatively minor life-style alterations. By targeting those who can benefit most from intervention, genetics helps to serve the goal of preventive medicine.

In addition, it should be stressed that the identification of a specific genetic lesion can lead to more effective prevention and treatment of the disease. Identification of mutations that cause autosomal dominant breast cancer may enable early screening and prevention of metastasis. Pinpointing a gene responsible for a neurotransmitter defect in a behavioral disorder such as schizophrenia could lead to the development of more effective drug treatments. In some cases, such as familial hypercholesterolemia, gene therapy may be useful. It is important for health care practitioners to help individuals understand these facts.

Although the genetics of common disorders is complex and often confusing, the community health impact of these diseases, together with the evidence for hereditary factors in their etiology, demands that genetic studies be pursued. Substantial progress is already being made. The next decade will undoubtedly witness many further advances in the understanding and treatment of these disorders.

SUMMARY REVIEW

Factors Influencing Incidence of Disease in Populations

1. The incidence rate is the number of new cases of a disease reported during a specific period (typically 1 year) divided by the number of individuals in the population.
2. The prevalence rate is the proportion of the population affected by a disease at a specific point in time.
3. Diseases vary in prevalence from one population to another.
4. Relative risk is a common measure of the effect of a specific risk factor. It is expressed as a ratio of the incidence rate of the disease among individuals exposed to a risk factor divided by the incidence of the disease among individuals *not* exposed to a risk factor.
5. Many factors can influence the risk of acquiring a common disease, such as cancer, diabetes, or hypertension. The factors

can include age, gender, diet, exercise, and family history of the disease.

Principles of Multifactorial Inheritance

1. Traits in which variation is thought to be caused by the combined effects of multiple genes are polygenic.
2. The term *multifactorial* is used when environmental factors also are believed to cause variation in the trait.
3. Many quantitative traits (e.g., blood pressure) are multifactorial.
4. Because traits are caused by the additive effects of many genetic and environmental factors, they tend to follow a normal or bell-shaped distribution in populations.
5. Those diseases, however, that do not follow a bell-shaped distribution appear to be either present or absent in individuals. They do not follow the inheritance patterns of single-gene disease. Instead, such diseases may follow an underlying liability distribution. It is thought that a threshold of liability must be crossed before the disease is expressed.
6. Examples of diseases that correspond to the liability model include pyloric stenosis, infantile autism, neural tube defects, cleft lip/palate, and some forms of congenital heart disease.
7. Many of the common adult diseases, such as hypertension, coronary heart disease, stroke, diabetes mellitus (types I and II), and some cancers, are caused by complex genetic and environmental factors and are thus multifactorial diseases.
8. For most multifactorial diseases, empirical risks, risks based on direct observation of data, have been derived.
9. In contrast to most single-gene diseases, recurrence risks for multifactorial diseases can change significantly from one population to another because gene frequencies, as well as environmental factors, can differ among populations.
10. Several criteria are used to define multifactorial inheritance: (a) the recurrence risk becomes higher if more than one family member is affected; (b) if the expression of the disease in a proband is more severe, the recurrence risk is higher; (c) the recurrence risk is higher if the proband is of the less commonly affected gender; (d) the recurrence risk for the disease usually decreases rapidly in more remotely related relatives; and (e) if the prevalence of the disease in a population is f, the risk for offspring and siblings of probands is approximately $\sqrt{f}$.

Nature and Nurture: Disentangling the Effects of Genes and Environment

1. Family members share genes and a common environment; therefore resemblance in traits, such as blood pressure, reflects both genetic and environmental commonality (nature and nurture, respectively).
2. Few traits are influenced *only* by genes or *only* by environment. Most are influenced by both.
3. When a disease has a relatively larger genetic component, as in breast cancer, examination of family history should be emphasized in addition to life-style modification.
4. Two research strategies often are used to estimate the relative influence of genes and environment: twin studies and adoption studies.
5. Monozygotic twins originate when the developing embryo divides to form two separate but identical embryos.
6. Dizygotic twins are the result of a double ovulation followed by the fertilization of each egg by a different sperm.
7. If both members of a twin pair share a trait, they are said to be *concordant.* If they do not share the same trait, they are *discordant.*
8. Studies of adopted children also are used to estimate the genetic contribution to a multifactorial trait.
9. A genetic predisposition may interact with an environmental factor to increase the risk of disease; this is called a *gene-environment interaction.*

Genetics of Common Diseases

1. Congenital diseases are those present at birth. Most of these diseases are multifactorial in etiology.
2. Multifactorial diseases in adults include coronary heart disease, hypertension, breast cancer, colon cancer, diabetes mellitus, obesity, Alzheimer disease, alcoholism, schizophrenia, and bipolar affective disorder.
3. It is incorrect to assume that the presence of a genetic component means that the course of a disease cannot be altered—most diseases have *both* genetic and environmental aspects.

KEY TERMS

Concordant trait, *156*
Congenital disease, *157*
Discordant trait, *156*
Dizygotic (fraternal) twins, *156*
Empirical risk, *153*
Gene-environment interaction, *157*
Incidence rate, *150*
Liability distribution, *152*
Monozygotic (identical) twins, *156*
Multifactorial trait, *151*
Phocomelia, *158*
Polygenic, *151*
Prevalence rate, *150*
Quantitative trait, *151*
Relative risk, *151*
Threshold of liability, *152*

REFERENCES

1. King RA, Rotter JI, Motulsky AG: *The genetic basis of common diseases,* Oxford, 1992, Oxford University Press.
2. Rothman KJ: *Modern epidemiology,* New York, 1998, Lippincott.
3. American Cancer Society: Cancer statistics, 1997, *CA Cancer J Clin* 47, 1997.
4. Lathrop GM, Terwilliger JD, Weeks DE: Multifactorial inheritance and genetic analysis of multifactorial disease. In Rimoin DL, Connor JM, Pyeritz RE, editors: *Emery and Rimoin's principles and practice of medical genetics*, vol 1, pp 33-46, New York, 1997, Churchill Livingstone.
5. Botto LD et al: Neural-tube defects, *N Engl J Med* 341:1509, 1999.

6. Daly LE et al: Folate levels and neural tube defects: implications for prevention, *JAMA* 274:1698, 1995.
7. Harper PS: *Practical genetic counselling*, ed 5, Oxford, 1998, Butterworth Heineman.
8. Hall JG: Twins and twinning, *Am J Med Genet* 61:202, 1996.
9. Neale MC, Cardon LR: *Methodology for genetic studies of twins and families*, Dordrecht, The Netherlands, 1992, Kluwer Academic Publishers.
10. Hunt SC, Williams RR, Barlow GK: A comparison of positive family history definitions for defining risk of future disease, *J Chron Dis* 39: 809, 1986.
11. Lusis AJ: Athersclerosis, *Nature* 407:233, 2000.
12. Goldstein JL, Brown MS: Familial hypercholesterolemia. In Scriver CR et al, editors: *The metabolic basis of inherited disease,* ed 7, vol 1, New York, 1995, McGraw-Hill.
13. Nicholls P, Young IS, Graham CA: Genotype/phenotype correlations in familial hypercholesterolaemia, *Curr Opin Lipidol* 9(4):313, 1998.
14. Munroe PB, Caulfield MJ: Genetics of hypertension, *Curr Opin Genet Dev* 10:325, 2000.
15. Vogelstein B, Kinzler KW: *The genetic basis of human cancer*, New York, 1998, McGraw-Hill.
16. Trichopoulos D, Li FP, Hunter DJ: What causes cancer? *Sci Am* 275:80, 1996.
17. Bertwistle D, Ashworth A: Functions of the *BRCA1* and *BRCA2* genes, *Curr Opin Genet Dev* 8:14, 1998.
18. Bienz M: APC: the plot thickens, *Curr Opin Genet Dev* 9:595, 1999.
19. Lynch HT, de la Chapelle A: Cancer susceptibility to non-polyposis colorectal cancer, *J Med Genet* 36:801, 1999.
20. Taylor SI: Deconstructing type 2 diabetes, *Cell* 97:9, 1999.
21. Todd JA: From genome to aetiology in a multifactorial disease, type 1 diabetes, *Bioessays* 21:164, 1999.
22. Barsh GS, Farooqi IS, O'Rahilly S: Genetics of body-weight regulation, *Nature* 404:644, 2000.
23. St. George-Hyslop PH: Piecing together Alzheimer's, *Sci Am* 283:76, 2000.
24. Selkoe DJ: Translating cell biology into therapeutic advances in Alzheimer's disease, *Nature* 399:A23, 1999.
25. Reich T et al: Genetic studies of alcoholism and substance dependence, *Am J Hum Genet* 65:599, 1999.
26. Stoltenberg SF, Burmeister M: Recent progress in psychiatric genetics: some hope but no hype, *Hum Mol Genet* 9:927, 2000.
27. Carpenter WT, Buchanan RW: Schizophrenia, *N Engl J Med* 330:681, 1994.
28. Bertelsen A, Harvald B, Hauge M: A Danish twin study of manic-depressive disorders, *Br J Psychiatry* 130:330, 1977.

CHAPTER 6

Immunity

NEAL S. ROTE

CHAPTER OUTLINE

The defense of the human body from infection and injury consists of a complex of interacting and overlapping systems. These systems, innate and immune, complement each other to afford protection from a great variety of injurious environmental agents. Defenses include surface barriers that are normally impenetrable by infectious agents, mechanical and chemical barriers at those surfaces, inflammation, and the immune response.

INNATE DEFENSES

The body's first lines of defense are anatomic barriers: the skin and mucous membranes lining the respiratory, gastrointestinal, and genitourinary tracts. These surfaces are biochemical barriers as well. Sebaceous glands in the skin secrete antibacterial and antifungal fatty acids and lactic acid. Perspiration, tears, and saliva contain an enzyme (lysozyme) that attacks the cell walls of gram-positive bacteria. As a result of these glandular secretions, the surface of the skin is acidic (pH 3 to 5), making it inhospitable to most bacteria.

If an injurious chemical, foreign body, or microorganism penetrates these defenses, the body attempts to eliminate it by mechanical clearance. It may be sloughed off with skin, caught in respiratory mucus and coughed up, vomited from the stomach, or flushed from the urinary tract by urine. Auxiliary defenses are present in the form of the body's normal population of bacteria, or flora, which produce chemicals that inhibit the growth of some invading bacteria. All these defenses are both external and nonspecific; that is, they protect the host as needed against all invaders.

Once external barriers have been compromised, permitting harmful chemicals, foreign bodies, or microorganisms to penetrate cells and tissues, the **inflammatory response,** or **inflammation,** occurs (see Chapter 7). This response, which begins within seconds of injury or invasion, is also nonspecific. It begins with the immediate marshaling of resources by vascular structures at the site of invasion. The affected tissues are soon surrounded by cells and fluids that are equipped to isolate, destroy, and remove the invaders and thereby promote healing.

IMMUNE RESPONSE

The third and last line of defense is the **immune response,** or **immunity.** It occurs much more slowly than the inflammatory response and is specific in that it can confer permanent or long-term protection against specific microorganisms. It can also be induced by vaccination or inoculation. Unlike inflammation, which involves many different plasma systems and cell types, immunity is effected by one type of serum protein (immunoglobulin, or **antibody**) and one type of blood cell (lymphocyte). Table 6-1 summarizes the many defenses against microorganisms.

The inflammatory and immune responses complement one another and interact in complex ways. Because many inflammatory processes are triggered or affected by simultaneous

Table 6-1 Defenses Against Infection

Type of Defense	Specific Mechanism
Surface defenses	Physical barriers: skin, conjunctivae, mucous membranes Mechanical removal: desquamation of skin, tears, mucus, ciliary action, coughing, salivation, swallowing, urination, defecation Normal bacterial flora: antibacterial factors Chemical inhibitors: gastric acid, lactic acid, fatty acids, spermine, lactoperoxidase, bile salts Antimicrobial substances: lysozyme, secretory immunoglobulin A (IgA)
Nonspecific resistance factors	Fever, interferons, complement, lysozyme, C-reactive protein (reacts with bacterial surface polysaccharides and activates complement), lactoferrin (binds and removes iron as a bacterial nutrient), α_1-antitrypsin (inhibits bacterial enzymes)
Inflammation	Soluble factors Clotting system: Hageman factor (factor XII) Complement system: chemotactic factors, anaphylatoxins Kinin system: bradykinin Phagocytes Circulating neutrophils, eosinophils, monocytes/macrophages Fixed macrophages in alveoli, spleen, liver, bone marrow
Immune response	Humoral immune response: B cells, plasma cells, immunoglobulins Cell-mediated immune response: T cells, lymphokines

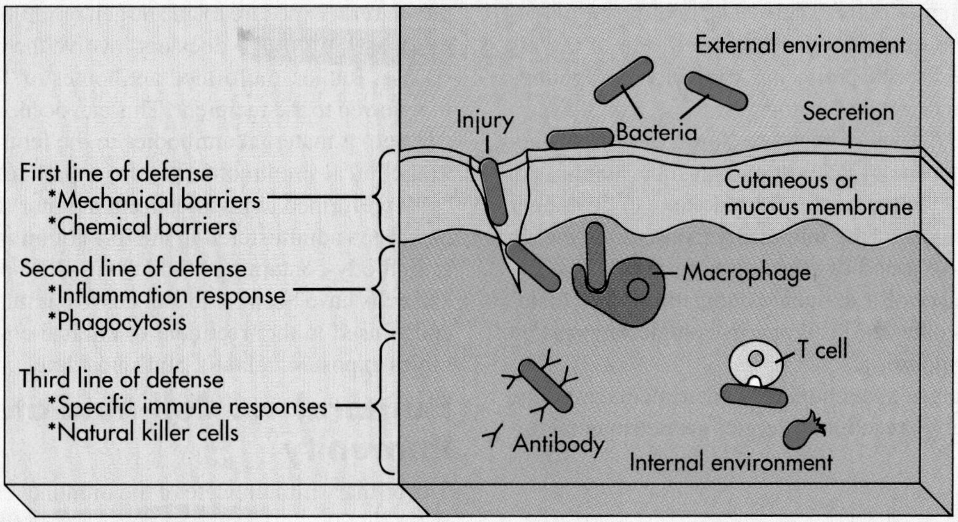

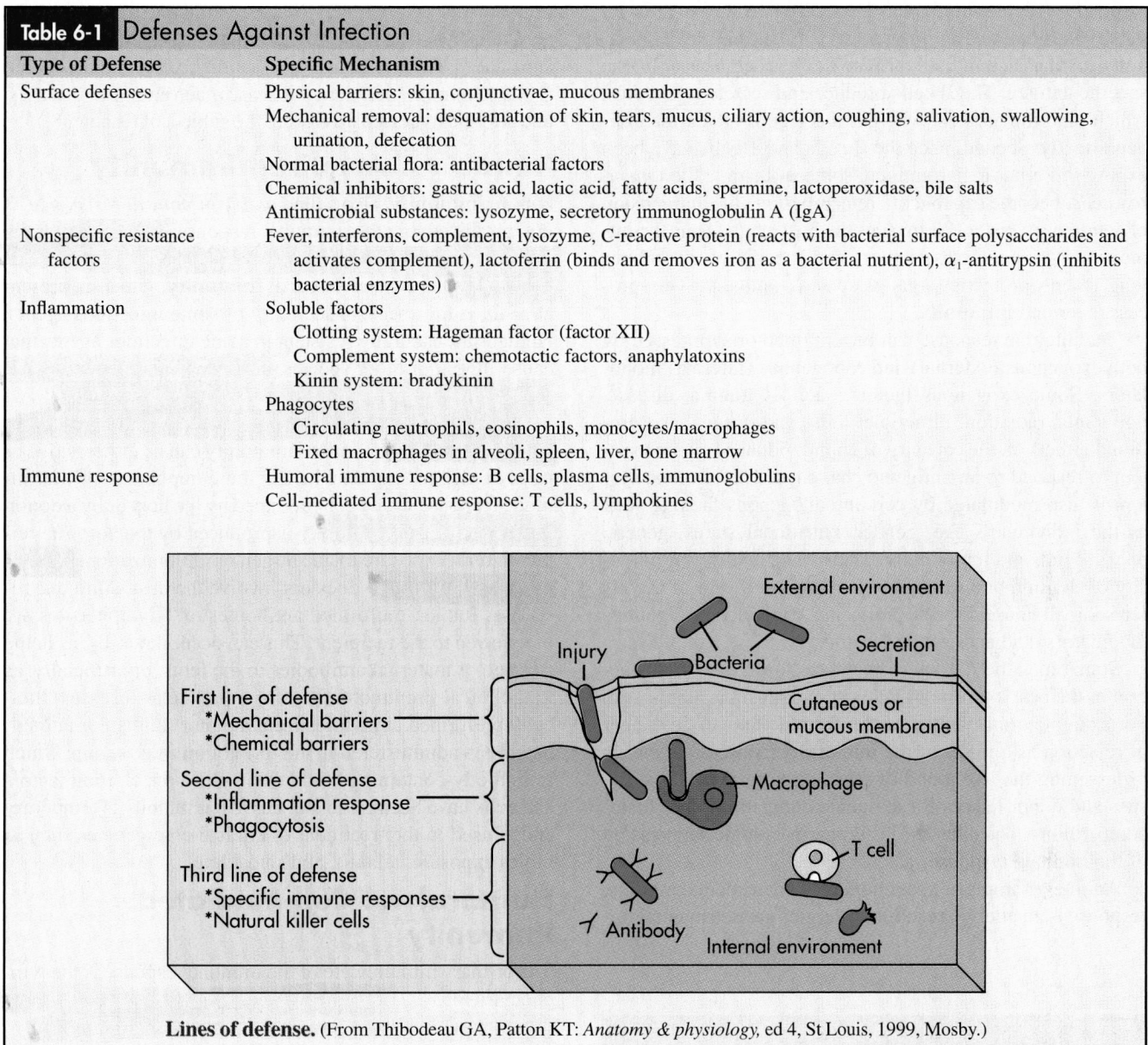

Lines of defense. (From Thibodeau GA, Patton KT: *Anatomy & physiology,* ed 4, St Louis, 1999, Mosby.)

immune processes, an understanding of the immune response is necessary for an understanding of many aspects of inflammation. Therefore the chapters in this unit are presented in the sequence of immunity, inflammation, and diseases of immunity and inflammation. This chapter discusses normal immunity, including the role of antibodies and lymphocytes in protection against infectious organisms. Chapter 7 discusses normal inflammation, including the interactions of the immune and inflammatory responses. Chapter 8 discusses medically relevant aberrations in immunity and inflammation, including allergies, diseases that involve unwanted immunologic destruction of healthy tissue, and diseases that are caused by a deficiency in the normal immune or inflammatory responses. Chapter 9 discusses stress and disease and the relationships among the immune, nervous, and endocrine systems.

CHARACTERISTICS OF IMMUNE RESPONSE

The immune system of the normal adult is continually challenged by a spectrum of chemical substances that it recognizes as foreign, or "nonself." These substances are called *antigens.* Some antigens are on infectious agents, such as viruses, bacteria, fungi, or parasites; some are on noninfectious substances from the environment, such as pollens, foods, and bee venoms; and others are on drugs, vaccines, transfusions, and transplanted tissues.

The body's reaction to antigenic challenges is the immune response, in which physiologic and biochemical interactions cause the maturation and activation of two types of **immunocytes,** or **immunocompetent cells** (Fig. 6-1). The two types of immunocytes, B lymphocytes (B cells) and T lymphocytes (T cells), act in different ways to recognize and respond to specific antigens. They differ from the cells involved in inflammation in two ways. First, they have specificity, so that each individual B or T cell recognizes only one specific antigen. The B cells produce and secrete antibodies, which bind the antigen, whereas the T cells attack the antigen directly. Second, once the B cells and T cells have been exposed to a particular antigen, some of them, called *memory cells,* become capable of "remembering" the antigen and of acting even faster if it invades the host again. Thus the immune system possesses memory and specificity and creates long lasting protection against specific antigens. This process is termed **immunity.**

The immune response can be amplified or suppressed by both exogenous (external) and endogenous (internal) modulators. Some exogenous factors, such as trauma, disease, pollutants, radiation, ultraviolet light, and drugs, have profound effects on the capacity of an individual's immune system to respond to an antigenic challenge. The immune system is also modulated by certain endogenous factors, such as the individual's age, gender, nutritional status, genetic background, and reproductive status. The quality and intensity of the immune response are therefore a sum of the effects of all these factors: antigenic challenge, exogenous modulators, and endogenous factors.

Sometimes the normal immune response does not function in the best interests of the host and must be suppressed. For example, transplanted organs from donors are in danger of rejection as a result of the immune response. One means of lessening the likelihood of rejection is to match host tissues and donor tissues for antigenic compatibility, or histocompatibility. The other means is pharmacologic suppression of the immune response.

Another example of a functioning but detrimental immune response is an allergic reaction. Allergies are detrimental immune responses in which the host's immune system overreacts, or is hypersensitive, to the antigenic properties of certain substances, such as house dust, animal danders, and certain foods. (Immune deficiency diseases, autoimmune diseases, and allergic hypersensitivity are the subject of Chapter 8.)

Innate vs. Acquired Immunity

Innate immunity, also called *native* or *natural resistance,* is not produced by the immune response. Innate immunity consists of all the immune defenses that lack immunologic memory.[1] One type of **natural immunity**, which is present at birth, is the species specificity of some infectious agents. Humans are naturally resistant to some infectious agents that cause illness in other species. For example, humans do not contract canine distemper or serious cases of cowpox.

Acquired immunity is gained after birth as a result of the immune response. Acquired immunity can be either active or passive, depending on whether the components of the immune response have been produced by the host or by a donor. **Active acquired immunity** is produced by the host after either natural exposure to an antigen or immunization. **Passive acquired immunity** does not involve the host's immune response. Rather, preformed antibodies or T lymphocytes are transferred to the recipient. This can occur naturally, as in the passage of maternal antibodies to the fetus, or artificially, as in a clinical immunotherapy for a particular disease. Clinically preformed antibodies from a donor (human or animal) have been administered in the form of immune serum, which is antibody-containing blood from which the clotting factors and cells have been removed. Passive immunity is temporary and is used in the treatment of clinical emergencies such as rabies exposure, tetanus, and snake bite.

Humoral vs. Cell-Mediated Immunity

The primary immunocyte of the immune response is the lymphocyte (Fig. 6-2). The mature **lymphocyte** is a small, round, white blood cell approximately 6 to 10 μm in diameter.

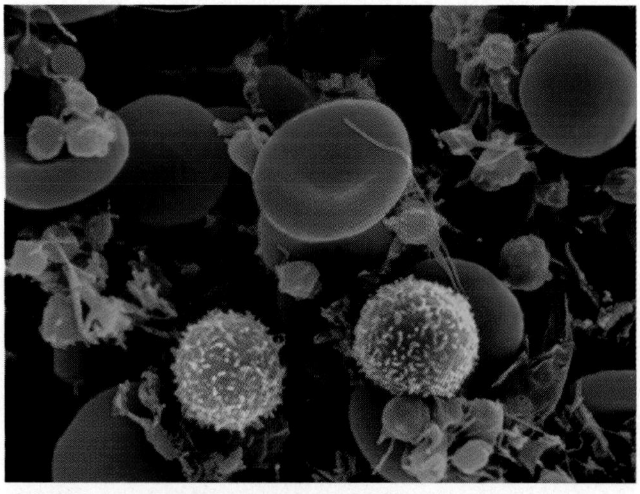

FIG. 6-1 Scanning electron micrograph showing lymphocytes (yellow), red blood cells, and platelets. (Copyright © Dennis Kunkel, Microscopy, Inc.)

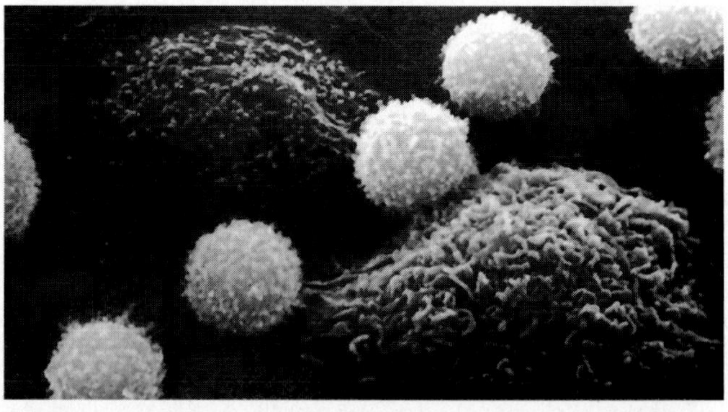

FIG. 6-2 Scanning electron micrograph of lymphocytes and macrophages. The lymphocytes are small and spherical; the macrophages are larger and more irregular in shape. (From Raven PH, Johnson GB: *Biology,* St Louis, 1992, Mosby.)

Lymphocytes originate in the liver and spleen of the fetus and the bone marrow of the child or adult as lymphocyte precursors or stem cells. They are not capable of implementing the immune response. To become immunocompetent, they must migrate through the lymphatics and blood vessels and then through lymphoid tissues in various parts of the body (Fig. 6-3). While passing through these tissues, they mature and undergo changes that commit them to one of two cellular lineages by a process referred to as the **generation of clonal diversity**. The lymphocytes that migrate through one set of lymphoid tissues become **B lymphocytes, or B cells.** When B cells encounter antigens, they are stimulated to mature into plasma cells that produce antibodies by a process referred to as **clonal selection**. B cells are ultimately responsible for **humoral immunity** (see p. 175).

The lymphocytes that migrate through the thymus gland become **T lymphocytes,** or **T cells.** T cells are capable of becoming sensitized to and recognizing specific antigens, which they then attack directly. They are responsible for **cell-mediated immunity** (see p. 184).

WHAT'S NEW? The Interdigitating Dendritic Cell

A key component of innate immunity is one of the most intensely studied components of the past decade—the interdigitating dendritic cell. Cells of this type, principally the Langerhans cells in skin, constantly endocytose extracellular antigens. They become activated and act as antigen-presenting cells when receptors on their surface recognize distinctive pathogen patterns on the surface of microorganisms. Dendritic cells are activated by the release of interferon-α from virally infected cells or an increase in proteins released from the inflammatory process as a result of necrotic cell death. Activated dendritic cells migrate to local lymph nodes, where they present antigen to T cell. Dendritic cells are important in initiating immune responses for which immunologic memory has not been established.

The success of the immune response depends on the interaction between the humoral and cell-mediated responses, which share some components and processes. Differentiation (maturation) of T cells and B cells is shown in Fig. 6-4.

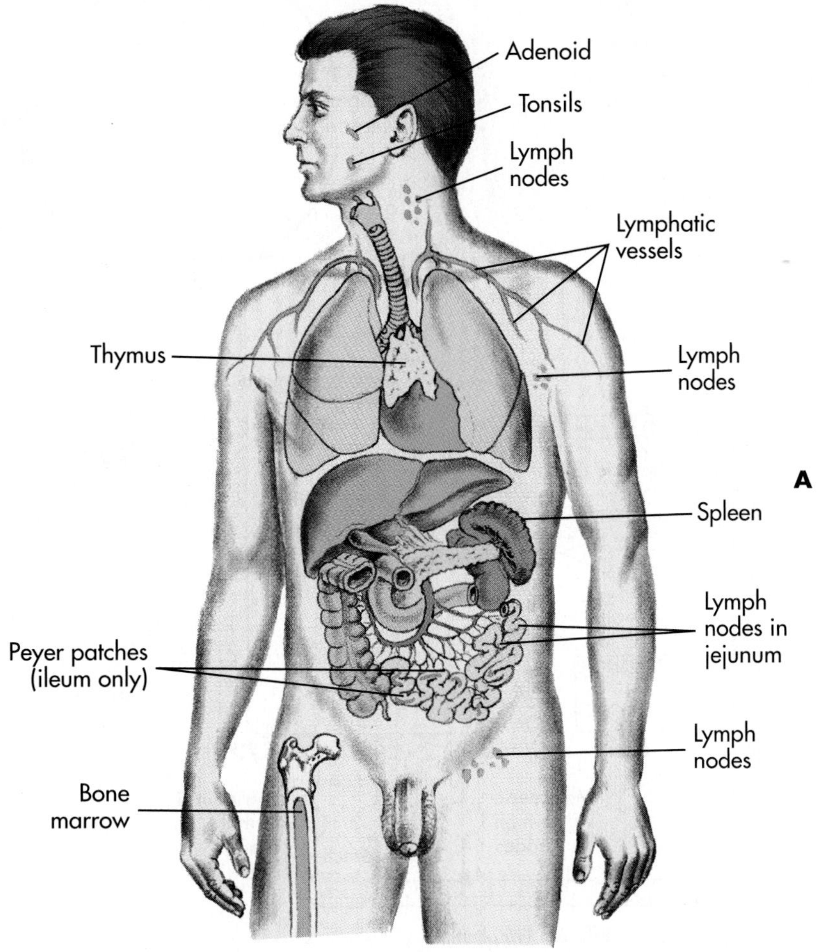

FIG. 6-3 Lymphoid tissues: sites of B cell and T cell differentiation. A, Immature lymphocytes migrate through central (primary) lymphoid tissues: the bone marrow (probable central lymphoid tissue for B lymphocytes) and the thymus (central lymphoid tissue for T lymphocytes). Mature lymphocytes later reside in the T and B lymphocyte-rich areas of the peripheral (secondary) lymphoid tissues.

Continued

B

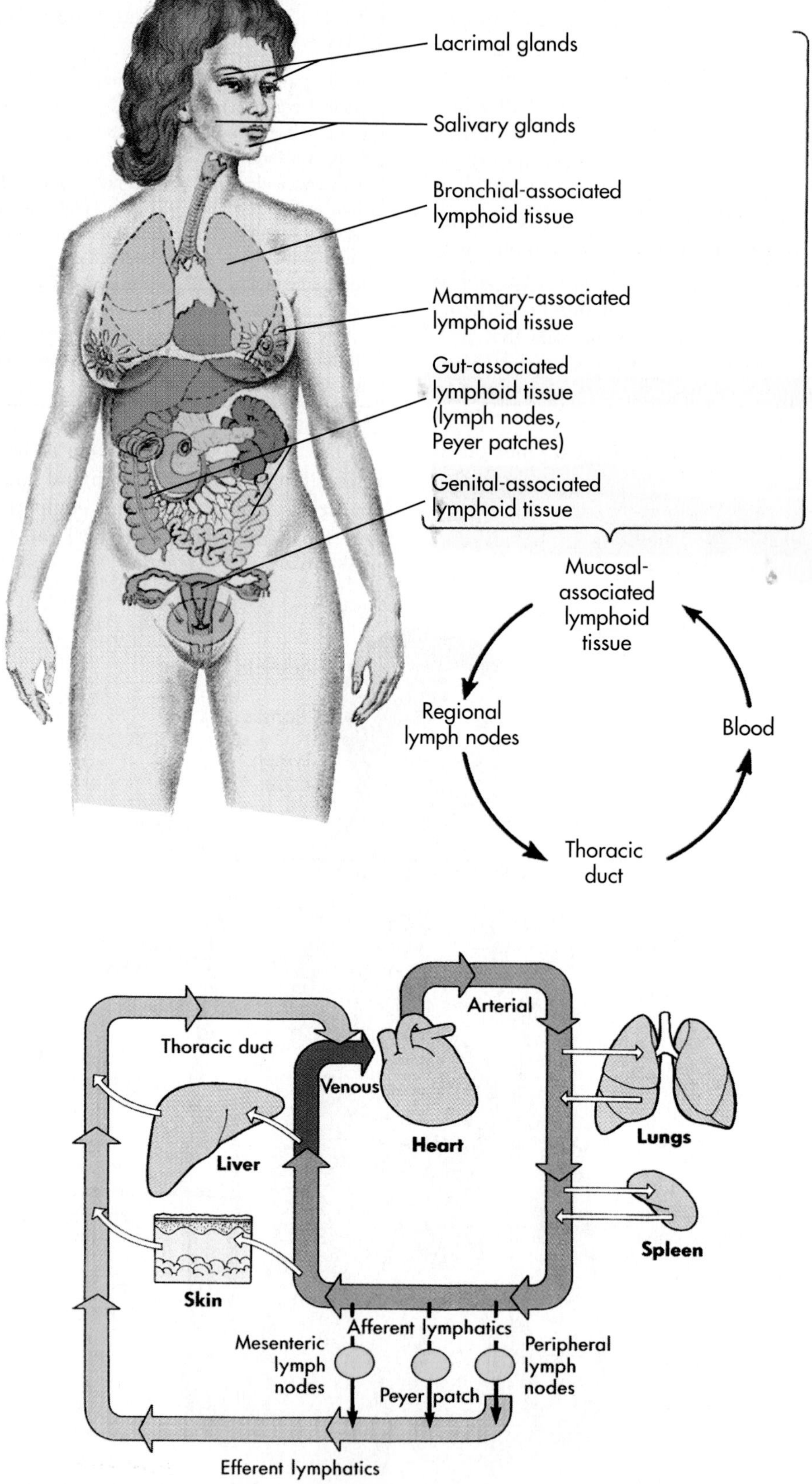

C

FIG. 6-3, cont'd Lymphoid tissues: sites of B cell and T cell differentiation. B, Lymphocytes from the mucosal-associated lymphoid tissues circulate throughout the body in a pattern separate from other lymphocytes. For example, lymphocytes from the gut-associated lymphoid tissue circulate through the regional lymph nodes, the thoracic duct, and the blood and return to other mucosal-associated lymphoid tissues rather than to lymphoid tissue of the systemic immune system. **C,** Pathways of lymphocyte travel. (**C** from Mudge-Grout C: *Immunologic disorders,* St Louis, 1992, Mosby.)

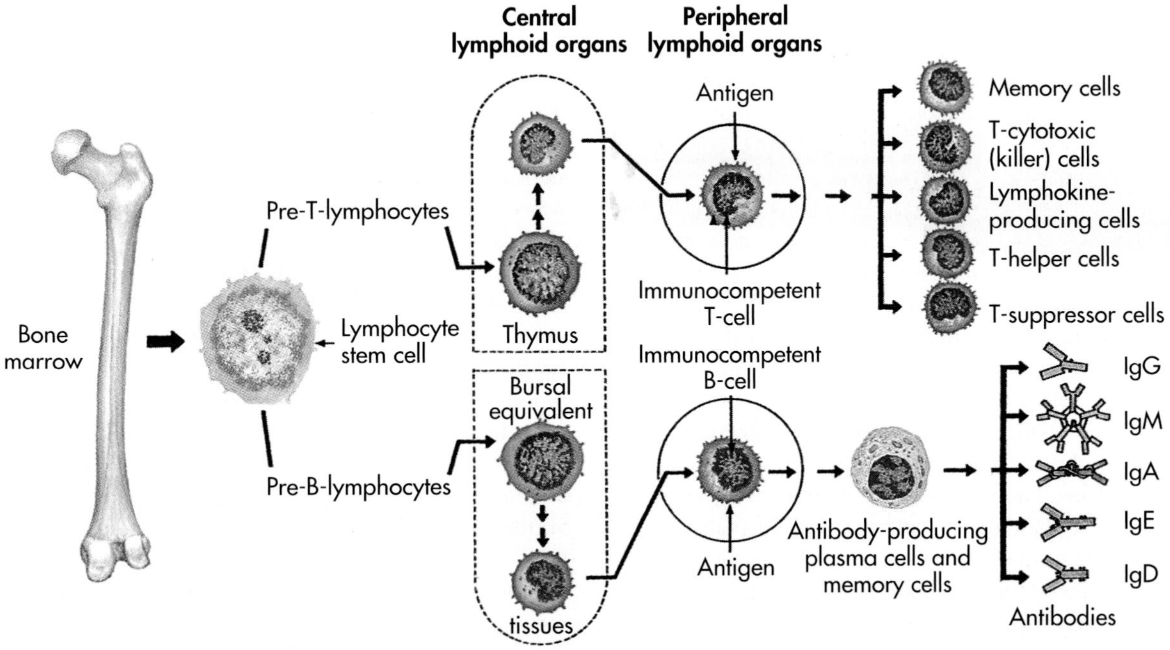

FIG. 6-4 Outcome of T (thymus-derived) and B (bursal-derived) pathways of lymphocyte maturation. Mature cells of the T cell lineage that have different functions usually develop from separate immature T cells. Mature B cells, on the other hand, may directly progress through the production of different classes of antibody against the same antigen.

INDUCTION OF IMMUNE RESPONSE

Antigens and Immunogens

Although the terms *antigen* and *immunogen* commonly are used as synonyms, some technical differences between them are significant. An **antigen** is a molecule or molecular complex that reacts with preformed components of the immune system, such as lymphocytes and antibodies. Antigenicity is the molecule's innate capacity to *react* with those preformed components and is determined by the chemical structure of the antigen molecule. An **immunogen** is an antigen that can also *induce the formation of components of the immune system* (i.e., maturation of T and B lymphocytes, production of antibodies). Therefore a substance may be antigenic—able to react with existing antibodies and mature lymphocytes—yet not immunogenic, that is, not able to induce the immune response.

A molecule is not antigenic unless at least a portion of its chemical structure can be recognized by and bound to specific (matching) receptors on a lymphocyte or antibody molecule. (Receptor function is described in Chapter 1.) The precise portion of the antigen molecule that is configured for recognition and binding is called an **antigenic determinant,** or **epitope.** The matching portion of the receptor on the lymphocyte or antibody is sometimes referred to as an *antigen-binding site, antigen-combining site,* or **paratope.**

Immunogenicity of an antigenic molecule is influenced by (1) foreignness to the host, (2) size, (3) complexity, and (4) quantity. In addition, the antigenic determinant sites must be accessible. Even if an antigen fulfills all these criteria, its ability to act as an immunogen may be affected by its route of entry into the host and by the host's endogenous characteristics, particularly genetic makeup.

Foremost among the criteria for immunogenicity is the antigen's foreignness. The immune system has the exquisite ability to distinguish self **(self-antigens)** from nonself (foreign antigens). Under normal conditions the immune system does not appreciably recognize self-antigens. This is the reason that the immune system is normally tolerant of the host's tissues but is able to reject foreign tissues and destroy infectious agents. **Tolerance,** once thought to be a state of nonresponsiveness in which the immune system passively allowed self-antigens to persist, is now known in some cases to be part of the active immune response. Although some forms of tolerance result from deletion in the central lymphoid organs of B and T cells that react against self-antigens, other forms of tolerance seem to be maintained peripherally. Rather than merely tolerating self-antigens, the immune system prevents their recognition by lymphocytes and antibodies. The response to self-antigens is active suppression of the immune system by specialized T lymphocytes called suppressor T cells, abbreviated Ts (see Fig. 6-4), and by specialized antibody called **antiidiotypic antibody,** abbreviated **anti-ID.** Therefore an antigen that fulfills the criteria of foreignness, size, complexity, and quantity will be immunogenic, whereas a self-antigen that fulfills all the criteria *except* foreignness is a **tolerogenic antigen.**

Molecular size also contributes to an antigen's immunogenicity. In general, large molecules (those bigger than

10,000 daltons), such as proteins, polysaccharides, and nucleic acids, are most immunogenic. Low-molecular-weight molecules, such as amino acids, monosaccharides, fatty acids, and the purine and pyrimidine bases, tend to be unable to induce the immune response. Many molecules in this size range can function as **haptens:** antigens that are too small to be immunogens by themselves but become immunogenic in combination with larger molecules (e.g., penicillin, poison ivy).

The route and vehicle of entry or administration to the host are critical to the immunogenicity of some antigens. This has important clinical implications. The most common routes for clinical administration of antigen are intravenous, intraperitoneal, subcutaneous, intranasal, and oral. Each route preferentially stimulates a different set of lymphocyte-containing (lymphoid) tissues (see Fig. 6-3), inducing different types of cell-mediated or humoral immune responses. Immunogenicity may be altered also by adjuvants (substances that stimulate the immune response) or by other agents that alter the processing of and the response to an antigen.

The genetic makeup of the host plays a critical role in the immune system's ability to respond to many antigens. The genes that affect the immune response are located on chromosome 6, code for HLA antigens, and control the quality and quantity of the host's immune response. (Chromosomes and genetic inheritance are described in Chapter 4.)

Blood Group Antigens

Examples of antigens include those found on the surfaces of erythrocytes, which are known collectively as the **blood group antigens.** More than 80 different red cell antigens are grouped into several dozen blood group systems, each determined by a different locus or set of loci. The most important of these, because they provoke the strongest humoral immune response, are the ABO and Rh systems.

ABO System

Human blood transfusions were carried out as early as 1818, but they were often unsuccessful. Sometimes after a transfusion, the recipient's red blood cells would clump together, thereby blocking the capillaries, and cause death in some instances. In 1901 Karl Landsteiner reported that this reaction was caused by the ABO antigens located on the erythrocyte plasma membranes.

The **ABO blood group** consists of two major carbohydrate antigens, labeled A and B (Fig. 6-5). These are codominant, so individuals can have one of four blood types. Erythrocytes of blood type A carry the A antigen, those of blood type B carry the B antigen, those of blood type AB carry both A and B antigens, and those of blood type O carry neither antigen. A person with type A blood also has anti-B antibodies in the blood. If this person receives blood containing B antigens (i.e., blood from a type AB or B individual), a severe antibody reaction occurs. Similarly, a type B individual (whose blood contains anti-A antibodies) cannot receive blood from a type A or AB donor. Type O individuals, who have neither antigen but have both anti-A and anti-B antibodies, cannot accept blood from any of the other three types. These naturally occurring antibodies, called **isohemagglutinins,** are immunoglobulins of the IgM class and are induced by similar antigens on naturally occurring bacteria in the intestinal tract.

Because individuals with type O blood lack both types of antigens, they are universal donors and anyone can accept small volumes of their blood. Similarly, type AB individuals are universal recipients, because they lack both anti-A and anti-B antibodies. When large volumes of *whole* blood are transfused, however, the donor's antibodies can bind to antigenic determinants on the recipient's erythrocytes. This reaction causes clumping of erythrocytes in the blood. Clump-

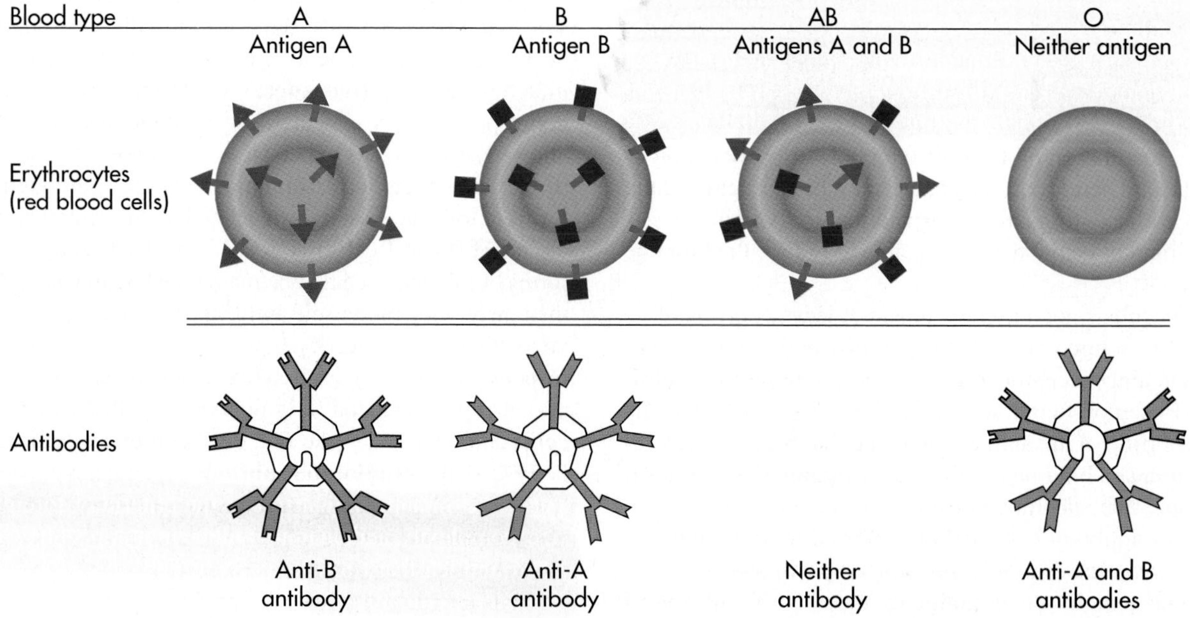

FIG. 6-5 Blood types. The relationship of antigens and antibodies involved in the ABO blood group system.

ing (agglutination) and lysis cause harmful transfusion reactions that can be prevented only by complete and careful ABO matching between donor and recipient.

Rh System

The **Rh blood group** (named after the Rhesus monkey, the animal in which it was first discovered), with its high degree of polymorphism, is a protein antigen system second in complexity only to the HLA system. At least five major antigens and a large number of rare variants have been identified and are expressed only on erythrocytes.[2,3] It appears to consist of three very tightly linked genetic loci, labeled *C, D,* and *E.* Each locus has two alleles labeled *C* and *c, D* and *d,* or *E* and *e.* Distinct antigens are expressed by *C, c, E, e,* and *D,* whereas no distinct antigen has been observed for *d.* Therefore *d* is considered a lack of *D.* The locus of greatest interest is the *D* locus, more commonly expressed as Rh_o (*D*), because it is responsible for Rh maternal-fetal incompatibility and the resulting hemolytic disease of the newborn (see Chapter 27). Persons who have the *DD* or *Dd* genotype have the Rh antigen on their erythrocytes and are called *Rh positive.* The recessive homozygotes, with genotype *dd,* are Rh negative and do not have the Rh antigen. About 85% of North Americans are Rh positive, and about 15% are Rh negative.

HUMORAL IMMUNE RESPONSE

B Lymphocytes

In birds, an organ called the *bursa of Fabricius* is responsible for the maturation of B lymphocytes.[4] Humans have no discrete bursa but do have tissues (probably the bone marrow) that make up the so-called **human bursal equivalent** (see Fig. 6-3). Lymphocytes destined to become B cells circulate through the bursal equivalent, where they undergo hormonally directed proliferation that gives them the capacity to react with antigen and generate diverse antibodies that protect the host against infection (see Fig. 6-4). B cell precursors cannot react with antigen, whereas postbursal B cells produce plasma membrane–bound antibodies of the IgM class, which can bind antigen.

It has been suggested that more than 10^8 different antigenic determinants may be recognized by the mature B cells. Several theories have been generated to explain how such recognition occurs.[5,6] The one most commonly held as correct is that of clonal selection. According to this concept, a large number of B cells with plasma membrane receptors for all potential antigenic determinants are spontaneously generated by genetic rearrangement during fetal life, independent of the presence of antigen (Fig. 6-6). Each B cell, however, responds to only one specific antigen. When the immunocompetent B cells encounter an antigen for the first time, those with specific membrane receptors complementary to that antigen's determinant sites are stimulated to proliferate and differentiate (clonal selection). B cells that have undergone this process are called **plasma cells** and can be found in the blood, secondary lymphoid organs (primarily spleen and lymph nodes), and some inflammatory sites. Thus two proliferative steps take place before antibody production can occur. The first step, the generation of clonal diversity, probably takes place in the bursal-equivalent tissues, is hormonally driven and antigen independent, and results in the generation of immature but immunocompetent B cells with plasma membrane receptors that can recognize virtually any antigenic molecule. The second step, clonal selection, occurs in the peripheral lymphoid organs, is antigen specific and antigen driven, and results in the proliferation and differentiation into antibody-secreting plasma cells. At about the eighth week of gestation in humans, antigen-driven differentiation may begin and proceeds throughout the life of the individual, although generation of clonal diversity primarily occurs in the fetus but probably continues to a low degree in the bone marrow throughout most of adult life.

The clonal selection phase of the immune response is initiated when an antigen binds and interacts with receptors on the surface of the mature B cell, triggering it into a sequence of proliferation and differentiation that results in the production of (1) immunoglobulin-secreting plasma cells and (2) a set of long-lived **memory cells** (see Figs. 6-4 and 6-6). The immunoglobulin-secreting plasma cells are active during the primary immune response. The memory cells are responsible for the secondary response that occurs on future exposure to the antigen (see Fig. 6-13) and for long-term immunity.

Immunoglobulins

Antibodies, or immunoglobulins, are serum glycoproteins produced by plasma cells in response to a challenge by an immunogen. They also serve as receptors on the surface of mature B cells. The term **immunoglobulin** is used to denote all molecules of this type. Antibodies are immunoglobulins known to have specificity for a particular antigen. The five molecular classes of immunoglobulins are IgG, IgA, IgM, IgE, and IgD. These classes are characterized by antigenic, structural, and functional differences (Table 6-2). Within the

Table 6-2 Physicochemical Properties of Immunoglobulins

Class	Subclass	Heavy Chain	Molecular Weight (daltons)	Adult Serum Levels (mg/dl)
IgG	IgG1	(γ_1)	146,000	800-900
	IgG2	(γ_2)	146,000	280-300
	IgG3	(γ_3)	165,000	90-100
	IgG4	(γ_4)	146,000	50
IgM	IgM	(μ)	970,000	120-150
IgA	IgA1	(α_1)	160,000	280-300
	IgA2	(α_2)		50
	sIgA	(α_1, α_2)	385,000	5
IgD	IgD	(δ)	184,000	3
IgE	IgE	(ϵ)	190,000	0.03

Ig, Immunoglobulin; *s,* secretory.

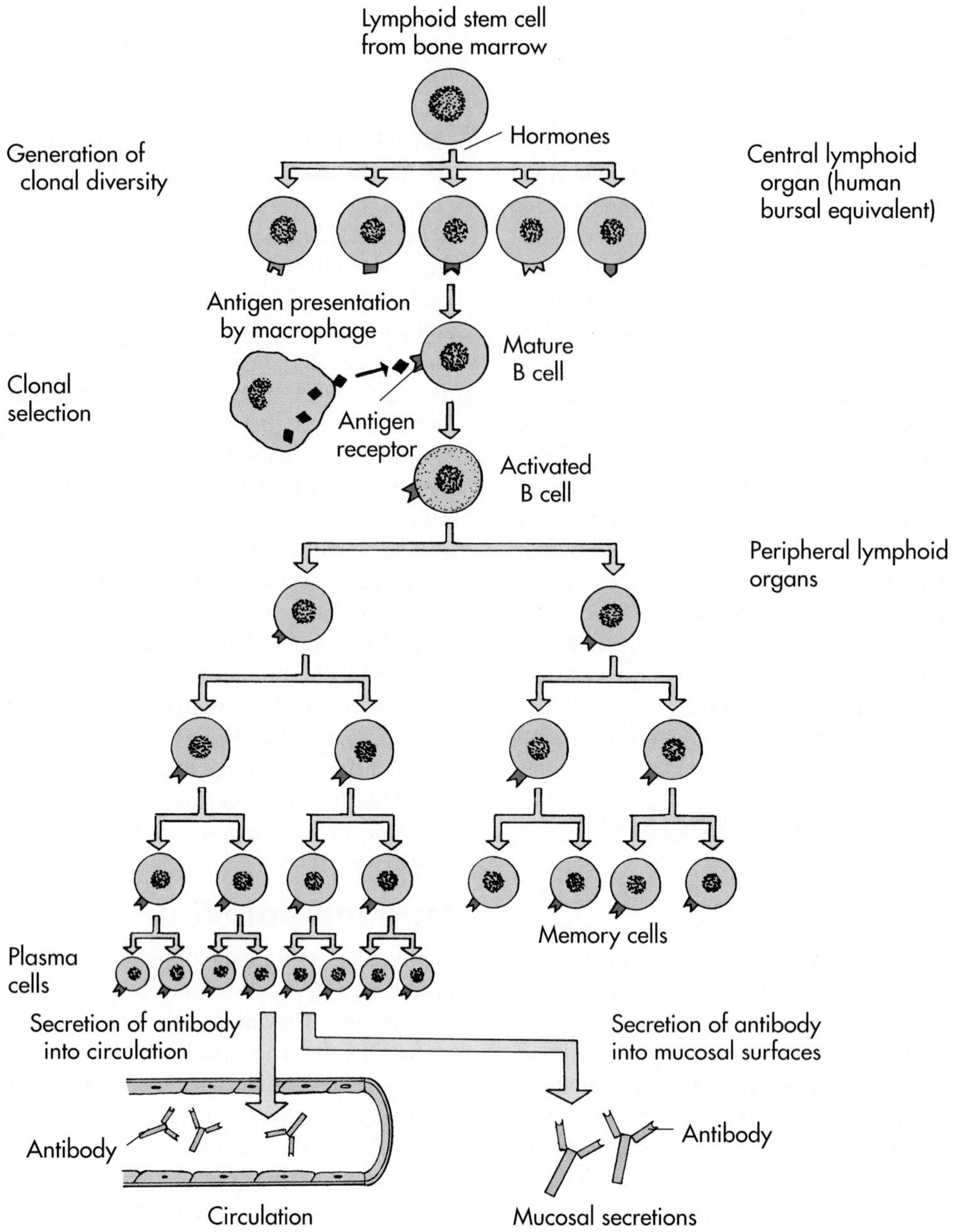

FIG. 6-6 Antibody production: generation of clones of antigen-specific B lymphocytes (B cells). During the generation of clonal diversity, B lymphocyte precursors undergo cellular division in the central lymphoid organs (bursal-equivalent tissues, probably bone marrow) under the control of hormones and without antigen and generate receptors against all possible antigens that may be encountered in the host's adult life. During the clonal selection process, primarily in the peripheral lymphoid organs (spleen and lymph nodes), soluble antigen or antigen presented by macrophages reacts with the clones of B cells having appropriate receptors on their surfaces, causing those cells to proliferate and produce antibody. Clonal selection usually requires the participation of T helper cells.

classes are several distinct subclasses, including four subclasses of IgG and two subclasses of IgA.

Structure of Immunoglobulin Molecules

Structural analysis of the immunoglobulins began with Porter's early studies on the effects of the enzyme papain on IgG.[7] Limited papain digestion cleaved IgG into three fragments, two of which were identical (Fig. 6-7). The two identical fragments were found to retain the antigen-binding activity of the molecule and were termed **antigen-binding fragments (Fab).** The third piece crystallized when separated from the Fab portions and was termed the **crystalline fragment (Fc).**

The Fab portions contain the recognition sites (receptors) for antigenic determinants and confer specificity. The Fc portion is responsible (1) for most of the biologic functions of the molecule, including interactions with the nonspecific effector systems of inflammation, such as the complement cascade (see p. 203), (2) for transport of maternal antibody to the fetus, and (3) for binding to the surface of the effector

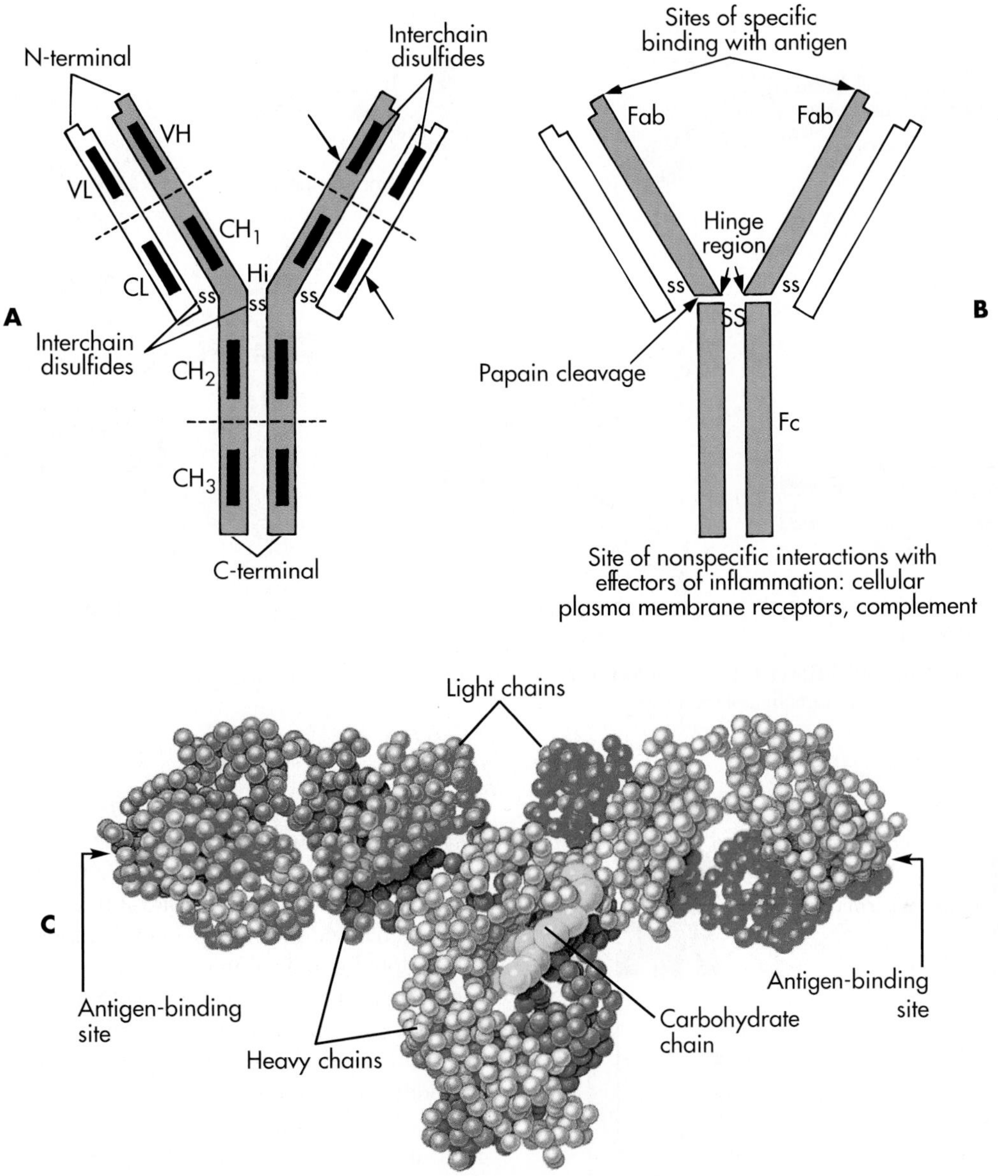

FIG. 6-7 Molecular structure of an antibody. A, The molecule consists of four chains—two light *(L)* and two heavy *(H)*—held together by intrachain and interchain disulfide linkages. The molecule can be divided into regions with variable *(V)* and relatively constant *(C)* amino acid structures (CH_1, CH_2, and CH_3 on the heavy chain). Between the CH_1 and CH_2 regions is the flexible hinge region *(Hi)*. **B,** Experimental fragmentation of IgG into its functional components by limited papain digestion. **C,** In this model of a typical antibody molecule, the light chainsare represented by strands of *red spheres* (each represents an individual amino acid). Heavy chains are represented by strands of *blue spheres*. Note that the heavy chains can complex with a carbohydrate chain. (**C** from Thibodeau GA, Patton KT: *Anatomy and physiology,* ed 4, St. Louis, 1999, Mosby.)

cells of inflammation (polymorphonuclear neutrophils, macrophages, lymphocytes, mast cells, platelets).

The antibody molecule consists of four polypeptide chains—two identical light (L) chains and two identical heavy (H) chains. Both light and heavy chains are divided into variable (V) and constant (C) regions. Among different antibodies the variable region is characterized by a large number of amino acid differences. The light chains of an antibody molecule are of either the kappa or lambda type and also consist of a variable (VL) and a constant (CL) region. Within the same molecule the two heavy chains and two light chains are identical. Each class of antibody has a unique type of heavy chain: gamma (IgG), mu (IgM), alpha (IgA), epsilon (IgE), or delta (IgD) (Fig. 6-8). The light and heavy chains are held together by two major forces: noncovalent bonds and disulfide linkages.

The interaction of the variable region's amino acid sequences on both the heavy and light chains determines the conformation of the antigen-combining site and therefore the antigenic specificity of the immunoglobulin molecule

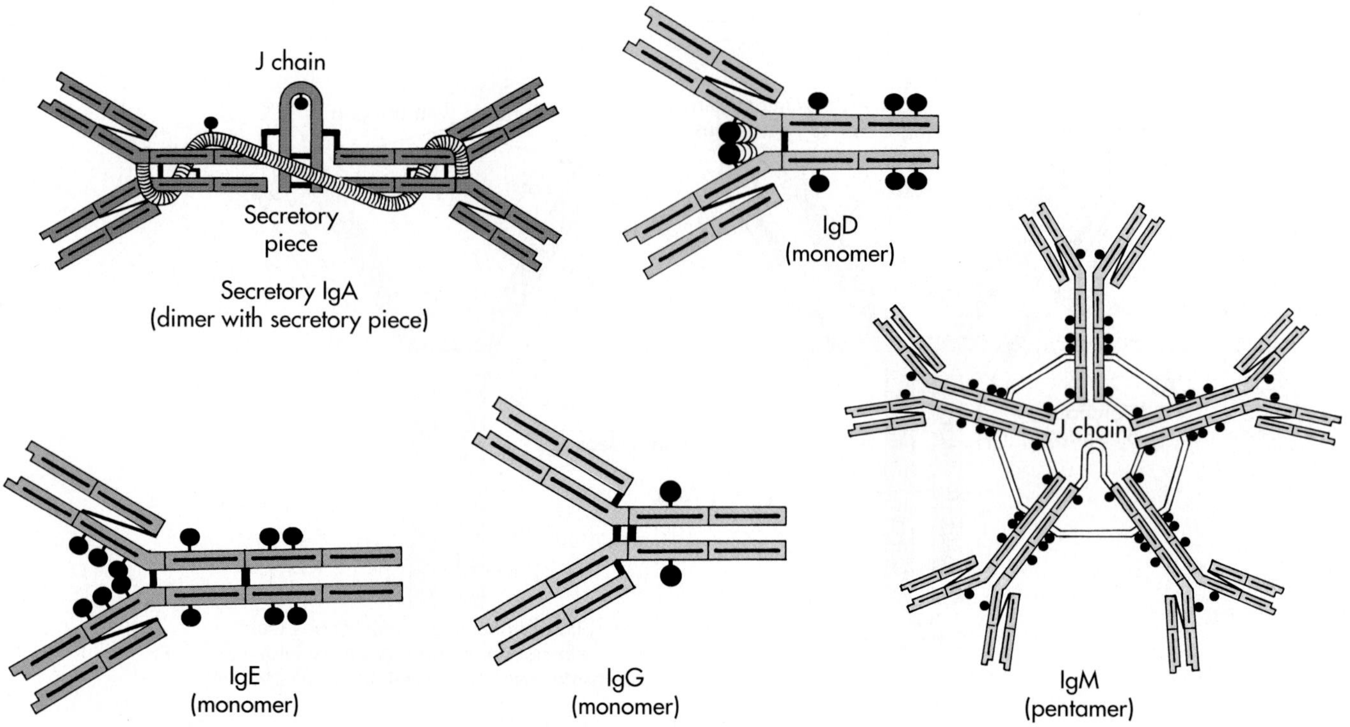

FIG. 6-8 Structure of different immunoglobulins. Secretory IgA, IgD, IgE, IgG, and IgM. The black circles attached to each molecule represent carbohydrate residues.

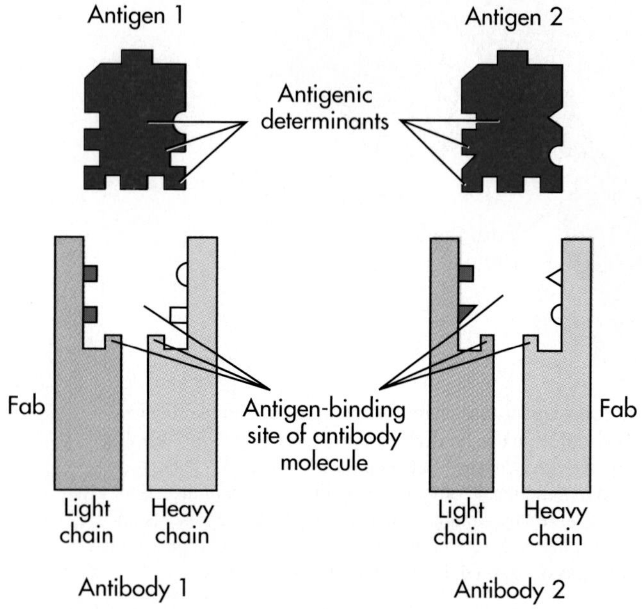

FIG. 6-9 Antigen-antibody binding. The specificity required for antibody binding with an antigen is determined by the shape of the combining site on the antibody. *Fab,* Antigen-binding fragment.

(Fig. 6-9). In some cases the substitution of a single critical amino acid may have a significant effect on the shape of the combining site and specificity of the antibody molecule. The antigen fits into this binding site like a key into a lock and is held there by noncovalent chemical interactions.

Classes of Immunoglobulins

Fig. 6-8 illustrates the structure of the immunoglobulins. IgG constitutes 80% to 85% of the circulating immunoglobulins. The biologic activities attributed to the IgG subclasses are summarized in Table 6-3. IgG is the major class of immunoglobulin in the immune response and is responsible for most of the antibody functions, such as precipitation, agglutination, and complement activation. As a result of selective transport across the placenta, maternal IgG is also the major antibody found in fetal blood.

IgA has two subclasses, IgA1 and IgA2. The predominant antibody in normal body secretions is secretory IgA, which is predominantly IgA2. IgA in the blood is predominantly IgA1. The secretory piece is attached to IgA dimers in the mucosal cells and may protect the molecule against degradative enzymes in secretions. (The biologic role of IgA is discussed on p. 182.)

IgM is the largest immunoglobulin and has 10 theoretic antigenic binding sites, although only 5 are functional. It is the first antibody produced during the initial, or primary, response to antigen (see Fig. 6-13). IgM is synthesized early in neonatal life, and its synthesis may be increased as a response to infection in utero. The trophoblast cells that cover the surface of the placenta lack Fc receptors for IgM; therefore the molecule does not cross the placenta under normal conditions.

Information on the role of IgD is very limited. It is found in very low concentrations in the blood, where it does not appear to have a known function, and is located primarily on

Table 6-3 Biologic Properties of Immunoglobulins

	Complement Activation		Binding to Fc Receptors on						
Subclass	Classic	Alternate	Macrophages	PMNs	Mast Cells	Platelets	Placental Transfer	Presence in Secretions	Induction of Agglutination
IgG1	++	−	+	+	−	+	+++	±	+
IgG2	+	−	−	−	−	+	+	±	+
IgG3	+++	−	+	+	−	+	+++	±	+
IgG4	−	−	−	±	+	+	++	±	+
IgM	++++	−	−	−	−	−	−	+	+++
IgA1	−	+	−	±	−	−	−	+	−
IgA2	−	+	−	±	−	−	−	+	−
sIgA	−	−	−	−	−	−	−	++++	−
IgD	−	±	−	−	−	−	−	−	−
IgE	−	±	?	−	+++	−	−	+	−

Fc, Crystalline fragment; *PMN,* polymorphonuclear neutrophil; *Ig,* immunoglobulin; −, lack of activity; +, relative degree of activity; *sIgA,* secretory immunoglobulin A. (Complement activation and the function of monocytes, PMNs, mast cells, and platelets are described in the section on inflammation, beginning on p. 208.)

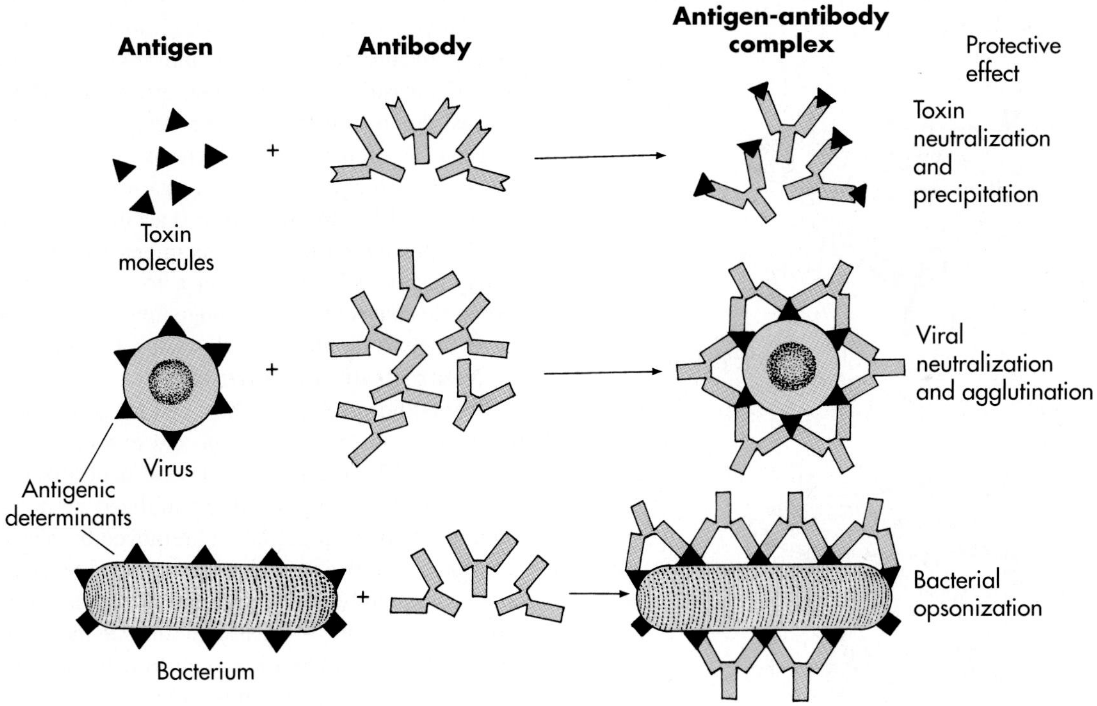

FIG. 6-10 Functions of antibody. Protective activities of antibodies include neutralization of bacterial exotoxins, neutralization of viruses and prevention of their interactions with cellular membranes, and opsonization of bacteria. All of these mechanisms are followed by removal of the antigen by phagocytosis, drainage along with body fluid, or both.

the surfaces of developing B lymphocytes, where it functions as an antigen receptor.

IgE is the least concentrated of any of the immunoglobulins in the circulation (see Table 6-3). It is also the principal antibody in the allergic response (see Chapter 8) and in the prevention of parasitic infections.

Function of Antibodies

The chief functions of antibodies are to protect the host by (1) neutralizing bacterial toxins, (2) neutralizing viruses, (3) opsonizing bacteria (i.e., promoting phagocytosis [see p. 210]), and (4) activating components of the inflammatory response (Fig. 6-10 and Table 6-3).

Normally an antibody circulates in the blood or is suspended in body secretions until it encounters and binds to its appropriate antigen. At that time the antibody may play two roles: (1) it may have a direct effect on the antigen, and (2) it may have an indirect effect on other mechanisms of selfdefense. Directly, the antibody may produce **agglutination** (insoluble antigens clumping together), **precipitation** (soluble antigens falling out of solution), or **neutralization** (inactivation) of the antigen. Which of these occurs is determined by the class of antibody and the characteristics of the antigen. Protection always begins with antigen-antibody binding. The antibody molecule's Fab portions bind with antigenic determinant sites on the antigen. Binding results in **antigen-antibody complexes,** also called **immune complexes.** Antigen-antibody binding may directly affect the antigen by occupying its antigenic determinant sites, rendering them unable to bind with receptors on host cells. For example, viruses that are neutralized in this way are unable to infect cells because the first step in penetrating a host cell is binding with receptors on the cell's plasma membrane.

The indirect effects of antibodies also involve the binding of antigen into antigen-antibody complexes. Once the antigen is bound, however, it is the Fc portion of the antibody molecule that confers indirect protection. Thus antibodies rarely act in isolation (Fig. 6-11).[1,8] Indirect protection consists of (1) enhancement of phagocytosis and (2) activation of plasma proteins that are capable of destroying the antigen. Both these activities involve components of the inflammatory response: phagocytes (see p. 209) and proteins of the complement cascade (see p. 203).

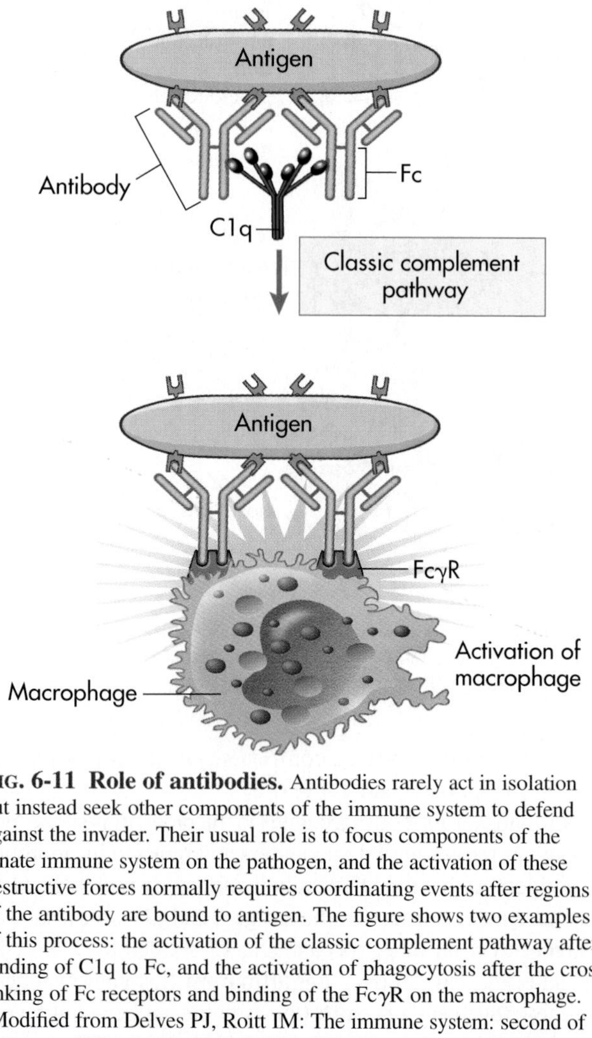

FIG. 6-11 Role of antibodies. Antibodies rarely act in isolation but instead seek other components of the immune system to defend against the invader. Their usual role is to focus components of the innate immune system on the pathogen, and the activation of these destructive forces normally requires coordinating events after regions of the antibody are bound to antigen. The figure shows two examples of this process: the activation of the classic complement pathway after binding of C1q to Fc, and the activation of phagocytosis after the cross-linking of Fc receptors and binding of the FcγR on the macrophage. (Modified from Delves PJ, Roitt IM: The immune system: second of two parts, *N Engl J Med* 343(2):108, 2000. Copyright © 2000 Massachusetts Medical Society. All rights reserved.)

Neutralization of Bacterial Toxins

Many bacteria produce toxins that enhance their pathogenic effects and harm the host in a variety of ways. Fortunately for the host, bacterial toxins are immunogens and are capable of initiating the humoral immune response. One of the principal roles of the antibodies subsequently produced is to function as antitoxins that neutralize bacterial toxins.

The mechanism of neutralization is the formation of antigen-antibody complexes (in this case, toxin-antitoxin complexes), which is the result of antigen-antibody binding (see Figs. 6-9 and 6-10). Simply stated, the antibodies "capture" the toxin molecules by occupying their antigenic determinant sites. This prevents the toxins from binding to tissue cells and exerting their harmful effects. Once the antigen-antibody complexes are formed, they may precipitate out of solution in body fluids or be removed from the body by **phagocytosis** (ingestion by phagocytic cells; see p. 210 for a discussion of phagocytosis).

Detection of the presence of specific antitoxins can aid in the diagnosis of diseases. For example, laboratory tests that detect antistreptolysin O or anti-DNAse (deoxyribonuclease) B measure antibodies that are produced against those toxins; this information can be very useful in the diagnosis of group A streptococcal infections.

Actively induced immunity against many pathogens can be achieved by immunization (vaccination) with their toxins. To prevent harming the recipient, the toxins are chemically inactivated, resulting in a toxoid that has few toxic properties but retains immunogenicity. Vaccines against diseases such as diphtheria and tetanus are toxoids.

Neutralization of Viruses

Antibodies protect the host against some viral infections by preventing the attachment and entrance of viruses into host cells. The mechanism of viral neutralization is shown schematically in Fig. 6-10. Neutralized viral particles may agglutinate or be ingested and removed by phagocytes.

Many viruses (e.g., measles, herpes) are usually inaccessible to antibody after the initial infection because they do not circulate in the bloodstream. Instead they remain in cells and tend to spread by direct cell-to-cell contact. Antibodies against these viruses are most effective in preventing the initial infection but usually play only a minor role in recovery from infection or in preventing recurrent infection. Other viruses, such as polio and influenza, spread from cell to cell through the blood and are more susceptible to the effects of circulating antibodies. These viruses can be controlled by antibodies even after the initial infection.

Protection against many viral infections, such as rubella, can be elicited effectively by vaccination with inactivated viruses. Levels of circulating IgG are usually a good indication of the degree of protection. Because antibody protects against reinfection, some vaccines have been designed to induce antibody production at the site of viral entrance into the body. For example, both oral and injected polio vaccines prevent systemic infection in the recipient, but only the oral preparation readily protects against the carrier state by inducing a secretory IgA response at the usual site of viral entry, which is the gastrointestinal tract.

Opsonization of Bacteria

An **opsonin** is a substance that renders bacteria susceptible to phagocytosis. Antibodies themselves are opsonins; antibodies also induce opsonization by complement component C3b (see p. 203). **Opsonization,** the process of opsonin-enhanced phagocytosis, is necessary because many bacteria have an outer capsule that resists phagocytosis unless antibody is produced against it.

Activation of Inflammatory Processes

One function of an antibody is to act as a bridge that lends specificity to the inflammatory response. One end of the immunoglobulin molecule, Fab, specifically binds to antigens, and the other end, Fc, informs the nonspecific amplifiers of the inflammatory response, both molecular and cellular, that an unwanted substance has invaded the body, either from the outside (e.g., infectious agents) or from within the body (e.g., a malignancy). Antigens are usually complex and bind several antibodies so that when an antigen reacts with the Fab regions of antibody, the Fc portions are held in close proximity to other Fc regions. The clustering of Fc regions results in (1) the binding to and activation of the complement cascade (see p. 203) and (2) the recognition of and binding to receptors (Fc receptors) on the surfaces of inflammatory cells.

Antibodies as Antigens

Because antibodies are proteins, they can serve also as strong antigens and immunogens. For instance, if human IgG is injected into a rabbit, the animal will recognize the human antibody as foreign and begin producing an immune response. That response will be characterized by the production of rabbit antibody that is reactive with the immunogen, the human IgG. Antibody molecules usually contain antigenic determinants that can be classified into one of three groups: isotypic, allotypic, and idiotypic (Fig. 6-12).

Isotypic antigens are species specific, so the antigen differs between species of animals but is the same within the species. These determinants usually are found within the constant regions and are used to differentiate between kappa and lambda light chains and among the different subclasses of heavy chains. For instance, the human gamma heavy chain in IgG1 has an antigenic determinant that is found on IgG1 antibodies in all humans and differs from determinants found on any other class or subclass of human antibody and from those found on IgG1 antibodies from other species of animals. All members of the species will express in their blood a mixture of all isotypes representative of that species. Antibodies against isotypic determinants commonly are used in research and clinical laboratories to differentiate between classes of antibody and between antibodies from different species.

Allotypic antigens are alleles expressed within a species. Antibodies from some members of a species would have a particular antigenic determinant that would differ from the same class and subclass of antibody from another member of the species. Allotypic determinants are also generally found in the constant region of both heavy and light chains, although they differ from the isotypic determinants found in the same general region. Each class or subclass of heavy or light chain has its own set of allotypic determinants. For instance, the gamma heavy chain has a region called *Gm* that is allotypic, of which there are at least 25 known allotypes. Kappa chain has an allotypic region called *Km,* of which there are at least three known allotypes: Km(1), Km(2), and Km(3). Some members of the same species may have kappa chains that bear the Km(1) determinant, and other members of the species will have the Km(2) or Km(3) determinant. If IgG from a Km(1)-bearing individual were injected into a person who possessed only the Km(2) allotype, an antiallotypic antibody against the Km(1) antigenic determinant would be produced.

Idiotypic antigenic determinants are found in the variable regions of heavy and light chains. Commonly an idiotypic determinant will consist of amino acids contributed by each variable region. Because of their location, many idiotypic antigens are found in the combining site on antibody and are characteristic of the antigenic specificity of that molecule. For instance, IgG3 produced against an antigen on the mumps virus will have a characteristic variable region that allows it to bind specifically to that antigen. IgG3 produced in the same individual but against a different antigen, such as tetanus toxoid, will have a different variable region that determines its specificity. Each IgG3 will have a unique set of amino acids in the variable region that will determine the antibody's specificity but will also be recognized as unique idiotypic antigenic determinants. Thus the IgG3 molecules produced in the same individual against mumps and tetanus toxoid will have different idiotypic determinants, although the isotypic and allotypic determinants may be identical. Antibodies produced against idiotypic determinants are called antiidiotypic antibodies and may be normally involved in controlling an individual's immune response against a specific antigen.

Monoclonal Antibodies

Most humoral immune responses are polyclonal; that is, a mixture of antibodies is produced from multiple clones of B

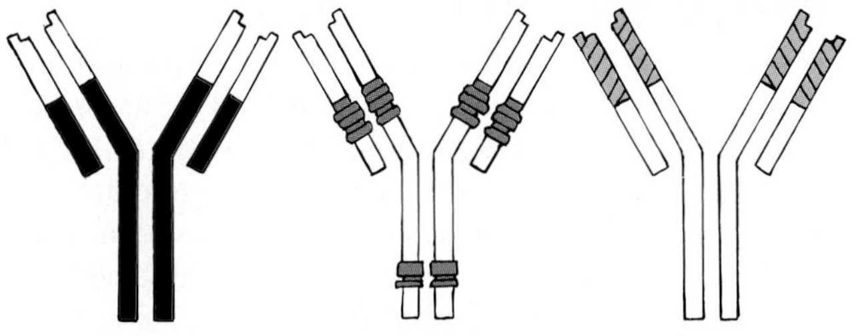

FIG. 6-12 Antibodies as antigens. Antibodies contain three types of antigenic determinants: isotypic, allotypic, and idiotypic.

lymphocytes (see Fig. 6-6). This occurs because most immunogens have multiple antigenic determinants and may stimulate a spectrum of B lymphocytes to proliferate. Each clone secretes antibody that differs slightly from that secreted by other clones, even though all the B cells were stimulated to proliferate by the same immunogen. The antibodies are heterogeneous in immunoglobulin class, amino acid sequence, specificity, and function, and some react more strongly with the antigen than others.

In 1975 César Milstein and Georges Kohler produced an antibody, called a **monoclonal antibody,** that would (1) act against a single specific antigen and (2) be produced by a single clone of B cells that could be maintained indefinitely in the laboratory.[9] Monoclonal antibody was produced by hybridizing B cells from the spleens of mice that had been injected with a specific antigen and "immortal" plasma cells (B cells) from a plasma cell tumor (malignant myeloma). The result was a **hybridoma**, a B cell clone that was both antigen specific and capable of indefinite proliferation. The hybridoma produced monoclonal antibodies. The advantages of monoclonal antibodies over conventional antisera (antibody-containing sera) are that (1) a single antibody of known antigenic specificity is generated rather than a mixture of different antibodies; (2) monoclonal antibodies have a single, constant binding affinity; (3) monoclonal antibodies can be diluted to a constant titer (concentration in fluid) because the actual antibody concentration is known; and (4) the antibody can be easily purified to homogeneity.

The generation of monoclonal antibodies has created new therapeutic and diagnostic possibilities, particularly in the treatment of cancer and early detection of viral infections. Detection of viral infections is generally performed by measuring the specific antibody response against the virus and any antibody that is produced immediately reacts with circulating antigen and therefore cannot be detected by routine serologic tests. Diagnosis is made after viral antigen has been removed from the blood and the patient is recovering. Monoclonal antibody, on the other hand, can be selected against specific antigenic determinants of the virus, produced in large quantities, and used in tests for elevations in circulating viral antigen that appear early in the disease. As a result of hybridoma technology, the clinician can order tests for viral antigens that are specific and diagnostic and detect the disease early in its course.

Secretory Immune System

The immune system within the body is called the **systemic immune system.** A distinct set of lymphoid tissues makes up another, partially independent, immune system at the external surfaces of the body, the **secretory (mucosal) immune system.** Most humoral immune responses occur when antibodies or B cells encounter antigens in the blood, but sometimes this encounter occurs in other body fluids. Some antibodies are present in secretions such as tears, sweat, saliva, mucus, and breast milk, where they can protect the body (or the neonate) against antigens that have not yet penetrated the skin or mucous membranes.

Although antibodies in both blood and secretions are produced by B cells that have matured into plasma cells, antibodies in blood are produced by cells of the systemic immune system, whereas antibodies in secretions are produced by cells of the secretory (mucosal) immune system. The B cells of these two systems follow a different pattern of migration once they leave the bone marrow and enter the lymphatics. Lymphocytes of the systemic immune system travel through the spleen and most lymph nodes (see Fig. 6-3). Lymphocytes of the secretory immune system travel through a different group of lymphoid tissues (see Fig. 6-3): the lacrimal (tear-producing) and salivary glands and lymphoid tissues in the breasts, bronchi, intestines, and genitourinary tract. Immunoglobulins that are secreted at these sites are called *secretory immunoglobulins* (hence secretory IgA) and act locally rather than systemically.

Local protection is necessary to combat antigens (chiefly infectious microorganisms) that are inhaled, are swallowed, or otherwise come in contact with external body surfaces. Once they have taken up residence in the external layers of the body, harmful microorganisms can multiply and the host becomes a carrier. These microorganisms can (1) cause local disease (e.g., cholera), (2) penetrate the skin or mucosa and cause systemic disease (e.g., gram-negative bacterial infection of the blood, or septicemia, if the integrity of the gut is disturbed), (3) not cause disease in the carrier (because of effective systemic immunity) but be spread to other individuals, or (4) pass out of the body without any ill effects (e.g., in feces). The major function of the secretory immune system is to halt viral and bacterial invasion before local or systemic disease develops. When secretory immunoglobulins bind and react with microorganisms, they are unable to attach to and invade mucosal tissue.

IgA is the dominant secretory immunoglobulin, although IgM and IgG also are present in secretions. The primary role of IgA is to prevent the attachment and invasion of pathogens through mucosal membranes, such as those of the gastrointestinal, pulmonary, and genitourinary tracts. To induce protective immunity against some pathogens that enter through these routes, local immunization seems to be preferable to inducing only systemic immunity. The Sabin vaccine against polio is administered orally as an attenuated live virus. This route causes a transient, limited infection and induces effective systemic immunity and secretory immunity, preventing both the disease and the establishment of a carrier state. The Salk vaccine, on the other hand, consists of killed viruses that are administered intradermally. It induces adequate systemic protection but does not generally prevent an intestinal carrier state.

The breast-associated lymphoid tissue is in the trafficking pattern of cells of the secretory immune system, so most antigens to which the mother has been exposed gastrointestinally induce sensitized lymphocytes that migrate to the breast and secrete IgA, IgM, and IgG into the milk. Antibodies against infectious disease agents are found in the milk and may provide protection to the newborn against those pathogens, such as polio, that invade through the gut.

Colostral antibodies do not cross the newborn's gut after the first 24 hours of life and do not have a role in the newborn's systemic immunity.

The mechanisms of antigen-antibody binding are the same in the secretory and systemic immune systems; that is, binding neutralizes or opsonizes the antigen, preventing it from harming the host. The following are major differences between the two systems:

1. Their lymphocytes follow different paths of migration and pass through different lymphoid tissues.
2. The secretory immune response is one of the body's first lines of defense, whereas the systemic response is the body's final defense.
3. The secretory response occurs locally and externally (in body secretions), whereas the systemic response occurs systemically and internally (in blood and tissues).

Primary and Secondary Immune Responses

The immune response to antigenic challenge has classically been divided into two phases—the primary and secondary responses. These phases can be demonstrated by serologic tests that measure plasma concentrations of antibody over time (Fig. 6-13). The initial administration of (or exposure to) most antigens is followed by a latent period, or lag phase, during which mature B cells (called *plasma cells*) produce no detectable antibodies (immunoglobulin [Ig]). After approximately 5 to 7 days, one class of antibody (IgM) can be detected in the circulation. This marks the beginning of the initial response, or **primary immune response,** which is usually dominated by IgM, with lesser amounts of IgG (another class of immunoglobulin). With no further exposure to the antigen, the circulating antibody is catabolized (broken down) and measurable quantities fall. The individual's immune system, however, has been primed. A second challenge by the same antigen results in the **secondary (anamnestic) immune response,** which is characterized by the more rapid production of a larger amount of antibody than the primary response. The rapidity of the secondary immune response is the result of the presence of memory cells. The quantity of IgM produced in the secondary response is about the same as that produced in the primary response. IgG is the predominant antibody class of the secondary response and frequently is present in concentrations several times those of IgM. The greatest differences between the primary and secondary responses are in the amount of IgG that is produced and the rapidity with which antibody appears after antigen challenge.

The primary and secondary responses confer active acquired immunity. When an antigen or vaccine, such as that on rubella virus, enters the host for the first time, the primary immune response is activated. Antibody levels are not high initially, but when the host is exposed to the second rubella vaccination, the secondary response occurs: antibody levels rise immediately and remain elevated for many years. The vaccine does not cause disease because it is made less infectious (attenuated) or otherwise altered before administration so that it is strong enough to elicit the primary immune response but not strong enough to cause illness.

Edward Jenner, an English physician of the late eighteenth century, performed the first well-documented vaccine trial.[10] There are numerous stories about Jenner's experiment, many fanciful. It is known that Jenner recognized that milkmaids were protected from smallpox if they had developed cowpox, a bovine equivalent of smallpox that causes only mild disease in humans. Jenner took material from a

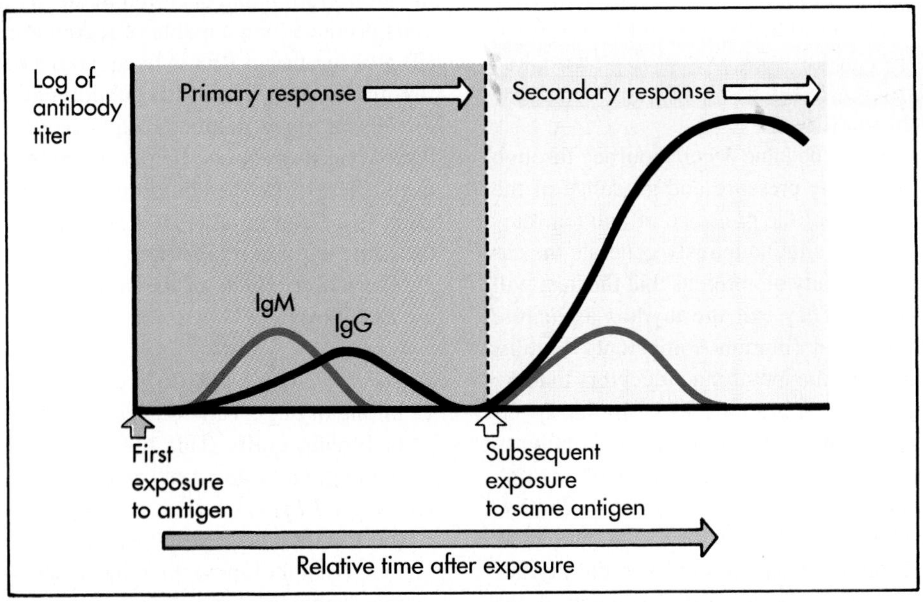

FIG. 6-13 Primary and secondary immune responses. The introduction of antigen induces a response dominated by two classes of immunoglobulins, IgM and IgG. IgM predominates in the primary response, with some IgG appearing later. After the host's immune system is primed, another challenge with the same antigen induces the secondary response, in which some IgM and large amounts of IgG are produced.

cowpox pustule on the hand of an infected milkmaid (reputed to be named Sarah Nelmes in some stories) and injected it into the arm of James Phipps, an 8-year-old boy. After the boy's initial inflammatory reaction to the injection subsided, Jenner injected him with material from a smallpox pustule. Fortunately the experiment was a success, because Jenner is reported to have reinjected smallpox virus into the boy at least 20 times. In 1798 Jenner used the term *vaccination* (*vacca* = cow) to describe his technique.

In Jenner's experiment the antigens on cowpox and smallpox viruses were sufficiently similar that the cowpox antigen functioned as an altered, or attenuated, smallpox antigen. The antibodies and lymphocytes sensitized to recognize and destroy cowpox were able also to recognize the smallpox virus, thereby protecting the immunized child against smallpox.

CELL-MEDIATED IMMUNE RESPONSE

Some lymphocytes are destined to develop into T lymphocytes (T cells), which are responsible for cell-mediated immunity. They are called *T cells* because they are processed through the thymus gland. There are five types of mature T cells, each with a different immune function. Memory cells induce the secondary immune response; **lymphokine-producing cells** transfer delayed hypersensitivity (Td) and secrete proteins (lymphokines) that activate other cells such as **macrophages** (see Chapter 8); **cytotoxic (Tc) cells** attack antigens directly and destroy cells that bear foreign antigens; and **helper T (Th)** and **suppressor T (Ts) cells** control both cell-mediated and humoral processes. (The maturation of T cells is shown in Fig. 6-4.) The Td cell phenotype is probably a subset of Th cells that produces the appropriate lymphokines for activating macrophages but does not provide any other helper function.

The process of T cell proliferation and differentiation shown in Fig. 6-14 is similar to that shown in Fig. 6-6 for B cells. The chief difference is that the generation of clonal diversity takes place in the thymus for T cells and in the human bursal equivalent for B cells.

Lymphocytes destined to become T cells journey through the thymus, where, under the pressure and guidance of the thymic hormones and without the presence of antigen, they are driven to proliferate and simultaneously generate the capacity to recognize the diversity of antigens that the host will encounter throughout life. They exit the thymus as mature and antigenically committed (immunocompetent) T cells. Mature T cells produce plasma membrane receptors that are not antibody but are related molecules with similar specificity for antigens. The **thymus,** which atrophies at puberty and practically disappears in adulthood, consists of a cortex and a medulla interspersed with connective tissue. Prethymic lymphocytes from the fetal liver, spleen, and bone marrow circulate through the bloodstream and seed the thymus during embryonic life. In the postcapillary venules of the thymic medulla, prethymic lymphocytes interact with thymic endothelial cells and enter the body of the thymus. Entrance into the thymus appears to be highly restricted to lymphocytes and also to be unidirectional. The lymphocytes distribute themselves in the thymic meshwork, where they rapidly proliferate in the cortex of the organ and migrate inward to the medulla as they mature into T cells capable of recognizing many different antigens.

During maturation in the thymus, T cells begin producing new proteins that are differentiation related and inserted into the plasma membrane of the cell. These proteins have been identified using monoclonal antibodies and are classified as *cluster of differentiation* (CD) antigens. At least 150 different antigens on a large variety of cells make up the CD system. The functional roles of many of these proteins have been determined, and several important CD antigens participate in the development of the immune response. Because of their association with different immune activities, several CD antigens are markers for particular cells of the immune system. The most important of these are listed in Table 6-4, and their order of appearance in thymocyte development is listed in Table 6-5.

The thymic epithelium produces several hormones involved in the maturation of T cells, including forms of thymosin, thymopoietin, ubiquitin, thymostimulin, and several other hormones. Thymic peptide hormones not only are involved in T cell differentiation within the thymus itself but also may diffuse into the bloodstream and influence uncommitted lymphocytes in the bone marrow and peripheral lymphoid tissues to travel to the thymus. In other words, immature precursor lymphocytes may become irreversibly committed to thymic maturation even before entering the thymus.

Antigenically committed mature T cells exit the thymus through the blood vessels and lymphatics. When mature T cells encounter an antigen they are capable of binding with, they are stimulated to proliferate. This step is different from the proliferation that occurred in the thymus in that (1) all the cells produced are capable of recognizing the same antigen; (2) proliferation is driven by antigen and is not dependent on thymic hormones; and (3) subpopulations of the immature T cells produce mature T cells having different functions (cytotoxicity, memory, helper functions, or suppressor functions). Therefore the end product of antigen-driven proliferation is a large number of T cells capable of acting against the same antigen in a variety of ways.

The major effects of the cell-mediated immune response are as follows:

1. *Cytotoxicity:* Cytotoxic T cells mediate the direct cellular killing of target cells, such as virally infected cells, tumors, or foreign grafts. This function requires cellular contact, binding, and release of toxic substances from the Tc cell.
2. *Delayed hypersensitivity:* The Td cells are involved in the inflammatory response and produce soluble mediators (lymphokines) that influence other cells, such as macrophages.
3. *Memory:* Memory cells are also responsible for the accelerated response to a second antigenic challenge (the secondary immune response).

4. *Control:* Helper T cells facilitate and suppressor T cells inhibit both humoral and cell-mediated immune responses.

Another specialized lymphocyte, the **natural killer (NK) cell,** closely resembles early cells of the T cell lineage. The NK cell expresses only the earliest markers of T cell differentiation, does not bind antigen, and is not induced to proliferate by immunization with antigen. The NK cell can, however, recognize yet undefined chemical changes on the surface of virally infected cells or malignant cells, binding to its target and killing the infected or malignant cell by mechanisms similar to the Tc cell. Targets of NK cells also have generally lost the expression of HLA antigens on their surface. In addition, the NK cell has Fc receptors that can bind to the Fc region of antibody (i.e., IgG) that has coated a target cell. Through these receptors the NK cell can adhere indirectly to and kill an antibody-coated target. This process is called **antibody-dependent cellular cytotoxicity (ADCC),** and when the cell performs this function, it has been referred to as a **killer (K) cell.**

Another system of recognition characteristic of natural killer cells relies on their *killer-activating receptors* and *killer-*

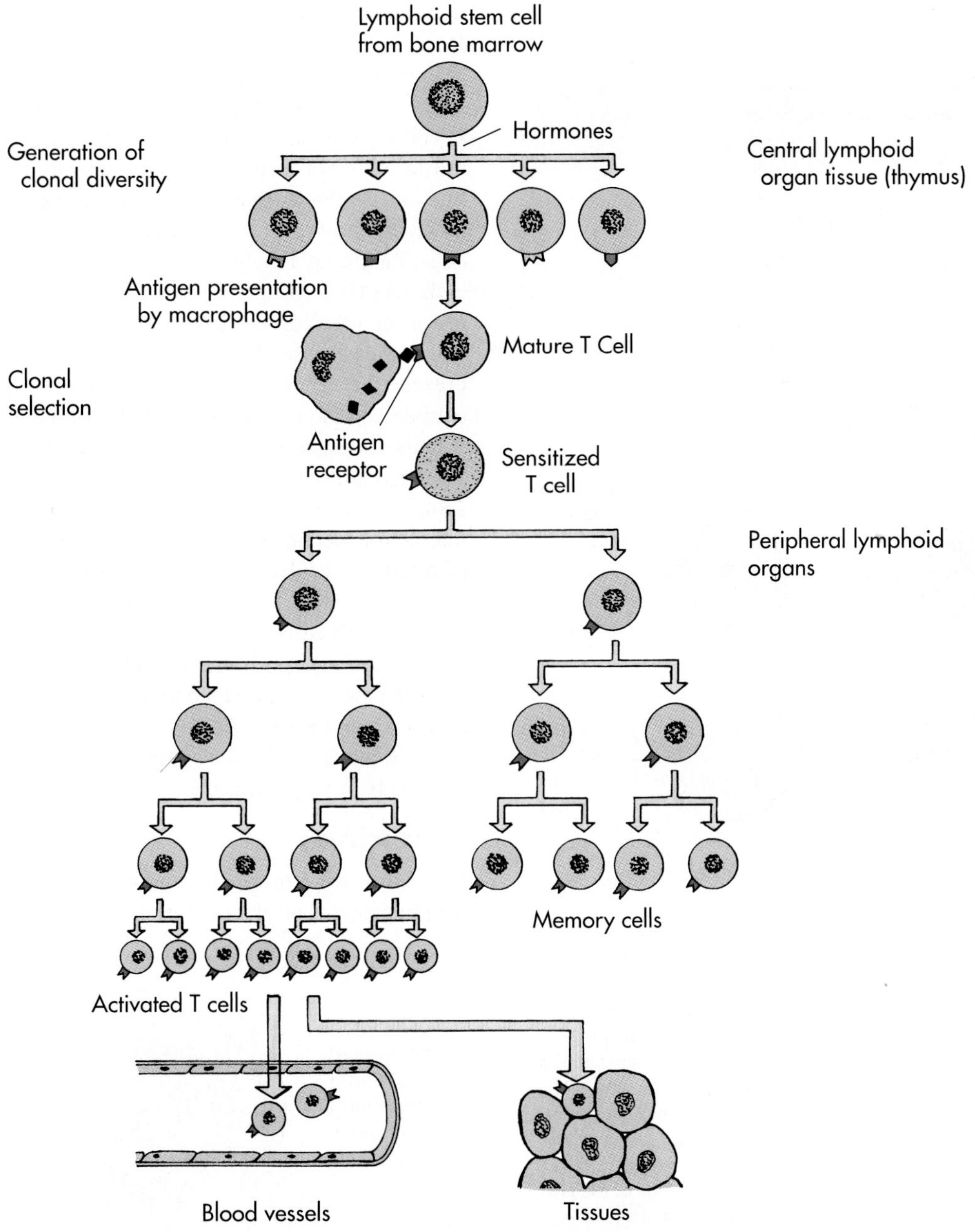

FIG. 6-14 T Cell production: generation of clones of antigen-reactive T lymphocytes. During the generation of clonal diversity, T lymphocyte precursors undergo cellular division in the central lymphoid organ (the thymus) under the control of hormones and without antigen and generate receptors against all possible antigens that may be encountered in the host's adult life. During the clonal selection process, antigen presented by antigen-presenting cells in the peripheral lymphoid organs reacts with the clones of cells expressing appropriate receptors on their surfaces, causing those cells to proliferate and differentiate into functional T lymphocytes.

Table 6-4 CD Antigenic Markers of T Cell Development

CD No.	Cell Type
2	Adhesion molecule with LFA-3, receptor for sheep RBCs
3	Interacts with T cell receptor and CD4 or CD8 to provide signal to nucleus
4	Th cells, adhesion molecule for class II HLA binding and co-receptor
8	Tc and Ts cells, adhesion molecule for class I HLA binding and co-receptor

CD, Cluster of differentiation; *LFA,* leukocyte function–associated antigen; *RBCs,* red blood cells; *Th,* helper T; *HLA,* human leukocyte antigen; *Tc,* cytotoxic T; *Ts,* suppressor T.

Table 6-5 Order of CD Marker Appearance in Thymocyte Development

Earliest thymocyte	CD2+
	CD2,3+
	CD2,3, TCR+
	CD2,3,TCR,4,8+
Most mature thymocyte	CD2,3,TCR,4+ or CD2,3,TCR,8+

CD, Cluster of differentiation.

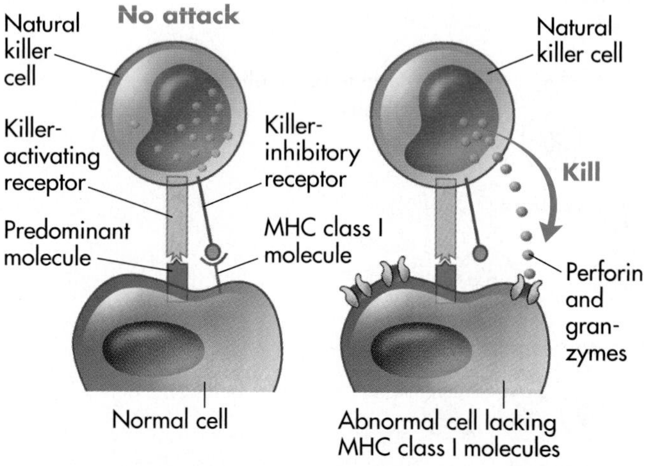

FIG. 6-15 A system used by natural killer cells to recognize normal cells and cells that lack major-histocompatibility-complex class I surface molecules. Killer-activating receptors recognize a number of molecules present on the surface of normal, nucleated cells, and in the absence of inhibitory signal from killer-inhibitory receptors, which recognize major-histocompatibility-complex (MCH) class I molecules, the receptors issue an order to the natural killer cells to attack and kill the other cell. Although all nucleated cells normally express MCH class I molecules on their surface, they can lose this ability. Loss can occur as a result of infection, for example, after herpes virus infection or malignant transformation. The lack of MCH class I molecules means there is no inhibitory signal from the killer-inhibitory receptor and the natural killer cell kills the abnormal target cell by inserting perforin into the members of the target cell and injecting killing enzymes (granzymes). (Modified from Delves PJ, Roitt IM: The immune system: first of two parts, *N Engl J Med* 343(1):37, 2000. Copyright © 2000 Massachusetts Medical Society. All rights reserved.)

inhibitory receptors. The killer-activating receptors recognize a number of different molecules present on the surface of all nucleated cells, whereas the killer-inhibiting receptors recognize major histocompatibility complex (see p. 187) class I molecules, which are also present on all nucleated cells (Fig. 6-15).[1,11,12]

CELLULAR INTERACTIONS IN IMMUNE RESPONSE

Very few antigens can act alone as immunogens. For example, very few can directly induce immature B lymphocytes to become antibody-producing plasma cells. Antigens that do have this capacity are likely to have repeating antigenic determinants (multiple identical antigenic determinant sites). Because these antigens can stimulate B cells without the help of T cells, they are called *T-independent antigens* (Fig. 6-16). The repeating antigenic determinants interact with the B cell's membrane receptors at multiple sites, inducing the cross-linking of receptors and the activation of antibody production. Antigens that cannot induce the immune response independently must first interact with several populations of cells, including T helper (Th) cells and **antigen-presenting cells (APCs).** Antigen-presenting cells are usually macrophage or macrophage-like cells in tissue (i.e., Langerhans cell in the skin; see Figs. 6-6 and 6-14) that process antigen, present the processed antigen to other cells, and produce soluble products (cytokines) that stimulate the other cells. B cells and endothelial cells also have APC activity.

Three cellular interactions occur during an immune response: APC-Th, Th-B, and Th-Tc (Table 6-6). The APC-Th interaction occurs initially, resulting in differentiation and proliferation of the Th cell. After differentiation this Th cell can interact with B cells or Tc cells. As a result of interactions with Th cells, the B cells and Tc cells will undergo differentiation and proliferation. These interactions involve a two-step process: a first signal and a second signal. The first signal is complex and consists of an antigen-specific signal, an adhesion signal, and a cytokine signal. The second signal is provided by cytokines.

Cytokines

Cytokines were originally characterized as low-molecular-weight proteins or glycoproteins (proteins containing carbo-

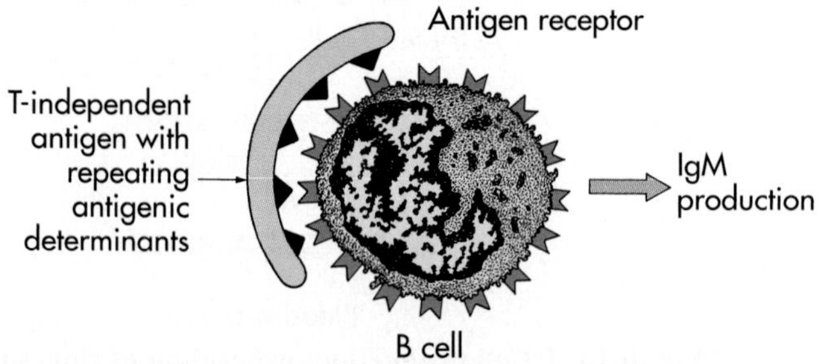

FIG. 6-16 Activation of a B cell by a T cell–independent antigen. Repeating and identical antigenic determinants interact with several receptors on the surface of the B cell and mainly induce the production of IgM.

hydrate) that are secreted by cells participating in the immune response (Table 6-7). They function as messengers of the immune response in that cytokines provide communication among macrophages and various subsets of lymphocytes. During an immune response, one of the participants may release a cytokine, bind to a specific receptor on a neighboring cell, and instruct that target cell to respond in a genetically programmed fashion. Cytokines produced by lymphocytes are referred to as **lymphokines,** and those produced by monocytes and macrophages are called **monokines.** Because of their role in intercellular communication, cytokines have been called *hormones of the immune response.* The effects of these hormones may be on neighboring cells (paracrine), or they may bind to and affect the same cell that produced them (autocrine). (Paracrine and autocrine forms of cellular communication are discussed in Chapters 1 and 10.)

After cytokine stimulation, a target cell may respond in many ways. One of the most common responses is increased production of proteins that are inserted in the plasma membrane and function as receptors. Many of these receptors are specific for various cytokines, but others are necessary for protection against infectious agents, such as receptors for complement component C3b or receptors for the Fc portion of antibody. Most cytokines also will cause the target cell to initiate proliferation and differentiation. Because this effect is common among cytokines, there is a great deal of redundancy in that different cytokines will have similar effects on the same target. The participation of cytokines is essential to the development of an adequate immune response.

Cytokines are produced by a wide variety of cells and guide many other cellular activities beyond the immune response. Many are growth factors that induce the proliferation and differentiation of cells other than lymphocytes, for example, other hemopoietic blood cells (see Chapter 24). In addition, the development and growth of the placenta during pregnancy depend on a variety of cytokines produced by both the mother and the child.

Histocompatibility Antigens

How does the body actually recognize that a substance is foreign? The "code" that brings about this recognition consists of the major **histocompatibility antigens** (also called **HLA antigens**, human leukocyte antigens, or **HLA determinants**), which are proteins found on the surface of nearly every cell in the body. HLA antigens play a role not only in defending the body against infection but also in distinguishing each individual's tissue from the tissues of others.

HLA Complex

The major group of genes producing the HLA antigens is known as the **HLA complex,** or the **major histocompatibility complex (MHC).** This complex consists of four closely linked loci located on the short arm of chromosome 6 (Fig. 6-17). They are labeled A, B, C, and D complex. The antigens produced by the A, B, and C loci (class I antigens) are found on the surfaces of virtually all cells except erythrocytes (red blood cells), and they are involved in the rejection of foreign tissue. The D complex (class II antigens), on the other hand,

Table 6-6 Components of Intercellular Signals During Clonal Selection

	Clonal Selection				
Cellular Interactions	**First Signal**				**Second Signal**
APC-Th	**Antigen:** MHC class II/antigen—CD4/TCR				IL-2
	Adhesion:	*APC*		*Th*	
		B7	—	CD28	
		ICAM1	—	LAF-1	
		LFA-3	—	CD2	
	Cytokine: IL-1				
Th-B	**Antigen:** MHC class II/antigen—CD4/TCR				IL-2, IL-4, IL-5 → IgM
	Adhesion:	*Th*		*B*	IL-2, IL-4, IL-6, IFN-γ → IgG
		CD28	—	B7	IL-5, TGF-β → IgA
		LFA-1	—	ICAM1	IL-4 → IgE
		CD5	—	CD72	
		CD40L	—	CD40	
	Cytokine: IL-2, IL-4, IL-6				
Th-Tc	**Antigen:** MHC class I/antigen—CD8/TCR				IL-2
	Adhesion:	*Th*		*Tc*	
		CD28	—	B7	
		LAF-1	—	ICAM1	
		CD2	—	LFA-3	
	Cytokine: IL-2				

ICAM1, Intercellular adhesion molecule 1; *LAF-1,* leukocyte-activating factor 1; *LAF-3,* leukocyte function-associated antigen 3; see text for other abbreviations.

Table 6-7 Cytokines

Type	Source	Main Functions
INTERLEUKINS (IL)		
IL-1 (α and β)	Predominantly macrophages	↑ Immune response; inflammatory mediator; activates T cells; activates phagocytes; ↑ prostaglandin production; induces a fever
IL-2 (T cell growth factor [TCGF])	Predominantly helper T lymphocytes (Th1); NK cells	↑ T lymphocytes and NK cells; ↑ growth and ↑ T cells
IL-3 (multiple colony-stimulation factor [CSF])	T lymphocytes, mast cells, NK cells	Hematopoietic growth factor for immature hematopoietic precursor cells, ↑ NK cells
IL-4 (B cell growth factor [BCGF])	T (Th2) lymphocytes, helper T cells, mast cells, basophils, eosinophils	Growth factor for T cells, activated B cells, and mast cells; macrophage-activating factor, ↑ IgE reactions
IL-5	T (Th2) lymphocytes, helper T cells, mast cells, eosinophils	↑ Growth and proliferation of activated B cells, ↑ eosinophils, ↑ T cell production
IL-6	Monocytes, T (Th2) and helper T cells, macrophages	B cell stimulatory and differentiation factor; ↑ hematopoiesis, ↑ inflammatory response, fever
IL-7	Bone marrow, thymus	↑ Lymphoid cells
IL-8 (monocyte-derived neutrophil chemotactic factor)	Macrophages, monocytes, T cells	Triggers chemotactic activity of neutrophils and lymphocytes
IL-9	Helper T cells	T cell and mast cell growth factor; maturation of erythroid progenitors
IL-10	Helper T cells	↓ Proliferation of helper T cells; ↑ cytotoxic T cell differentiation; induces MHC antigen expression, ↓ cytokines
IL-11	Bone marrow, stromal cells	↑ Monocyte and B cell function, ↓ some inflammatory cytokines
IL-12	Macrophages, B cells	↑ Helper T cells and production of other lymphocytes and cytokines
IL-13	Activated T cells	↑ Gene expression in nerve and intestinal cells, ↑ osteoclasts, ↑ progenitor cells in bone marrow
IL-14	T cells	B cell growth factor
IL-15	Macrophages	Activity identical to that of IL-2
IL-16	CD8+ T cells	Chemotactic factor and growth factor for CD4+ T cells, chemotactic for eosinophils
IL-17	Helper T cells	↑ IL-6 and IL-8
INTERFERON (IFN)		
IFN-α	Virally infected cells	Provides antiviral protection; ↓ B cell proliferation; ↓ IL-8, (tumor growth, ↑ NK cell
IFN-β	Virally infected cells	Provides antiviral protection; ↑ IL-6, ↓ IL-8
IFN-γ (IL-18)*	T (Th1) lymphocytes, helper T cells, NK cells	Activates macrophages; ↑ B cell differentiation and NK cell activity, ↓ tumor growth
TUMOR NECROSIS FACTOR (TNF)		
TFN-α	Macrophages, T cells, B cells, NK cells, mast cells	↑ Cytokines, ↑ inflammatory and immune responses
TFN-β	T cells	Cytotoxic to tumor cells, ↑ phagocytosis by macrophage and neutrophil, ↑ macrophages, ↑ B cell proliferation
COLONY-STIMULATING FACTORS (CSF)		
G-CSF	Monocytes, fibroblasts	Myeloid growth factor
GM-CSF	T cells, fibroblasts, monocytes, endothelial cells	Myelocytic growth factor
M-CSF	Monocytes, lymphocytes, fibroblasts, endothelial and epithelial cells	Macrophage growth factor
TRANSFORMING GROWTH FACTOR (TGF-β)		
	Lymphocytes, macrophages, platelets, bone	Chemotactic for macrophages, ↑ IL1 production; stimulates fibroblasts for wound healing; inhibits immune response; potentially inhibits mitotic division in other cells

↑, Increased; ↓, decreased; see text for other abbreviations.
*IL-18 is the new designation.

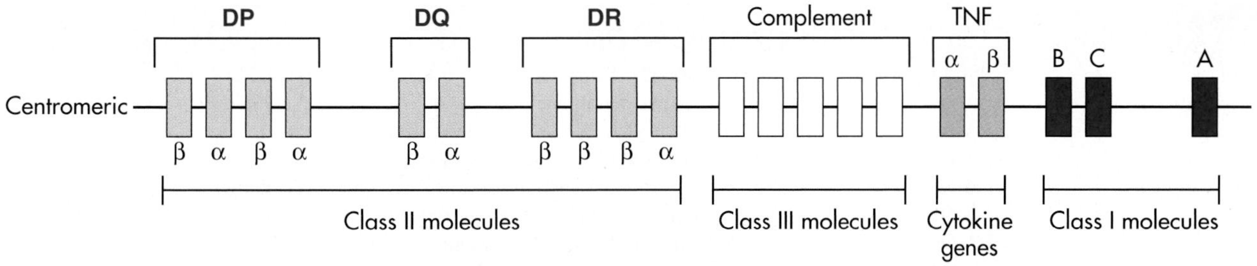

FIG. 6-17 Schematic representations of the HLA complex and its subregions. The relative distances between various genes and regions are not drawn to scale. (From Cotran RS, Kumar V, Collins T: *Robbins pathologic basis for disease*, ed 6, Philadelphia, 1999, W.B. Saunders.)

consists of three separate and independent loci (DR, DP, DQ) that are confined mostly to B lymphocytes, macrophages, some epithelial cells, and transiently to subpopulations of stimulated T lymphocytes.

Each HLA locus has many alleles: at least 21 at A, 42 at B, 10 at C, 17 at DR, 9 at DQ, and 6 at DP. With so many alleles at each HLA locus, many possible allele combinations exist, making it unlikely that two unrelated individuals will have the same HLA composition.

The specific alleles at the six HLA loci on one chromosome are termed the *haplotype.* Each individual has two HLA haplotypes, one for each chromosome. Because the loci are closely linked, the haplotypes are not usually disrupted by recombination and are thus transmitted intact to the offspring. Each parent passes one HLA haplotype to his or her offspring. The offspring then share one haplotype with each parent, and on the average, they share one haplotype with one half of their siblings, both haplotypes with one fourth of their siblings, and no haplotypes with one fourth of their siblings. Monozygotic twins, of course, have identical HLA haplotypes. This coexpression of both maternal and paternal alleles and the tremendous polymorphism make the HLA antigen system useful in determining paternity.

The HLA complex is particularly important in determining the success of tissue grafts and organ transplants. The more similar two individuals are in their HLA makeup, the more likely the success of a transplant from one to the other (they must also have compatible ABO blood types). Even when two people have the same HLA makeup, however, grafts sometimes are rejected because a number of other loci also determine tissue compatibility, although their effects are weaker than those of the HLA system. Thus it is always preferable to obtain a graft or transplant from a closely related individual, such as a sibling, because of a greater chance that a sibling will have the same histocompatibility antigens other than HLA.

Role of HLA Antigens

The function of class I and II antigens is to distinguish self from nonself. Many of the cellular interactions of the immune system require the presentation and recognition of foreign antigens in the context of self-antigens, either class I or II antigenic determinants (Fig. 6-18 and Table 6-8).

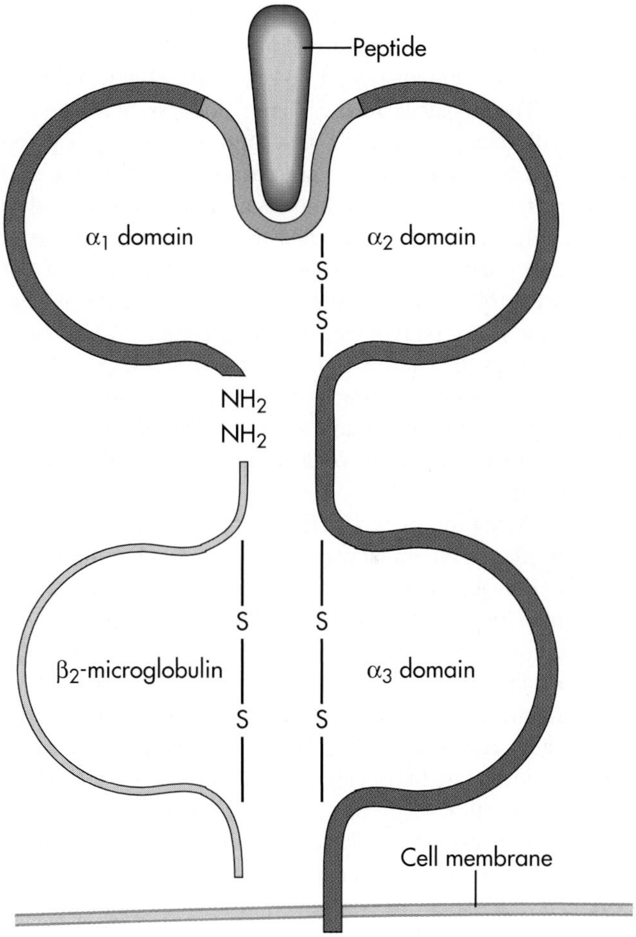

FIG. 6-18 Properties of HLA class I and class II. (From Cotran RS, Kumar V, Collins T: *Robbins pathologic basis for disease*, ed 6, Philadelphia, 1999, W.B. Saunders.)

Genetic loci within the HLA complex also control the quality and quantity of an immune response. These are referred to as **immune response (Ir) genes.**

Antigen Processing, Presentation, and Recognition

When an antigen enters the host, it first equilibrates throughout body fluids. Antigen circulates through the spleen if it enters intraperitoneally or intravenously and to the regional draining lymph nodes if it enters by the subcutaneous or gastrointestinal route. Antigen entering by the bloodstream

Table 6-8 Molecules of Major Histocompatibility Complex

Class	Gene Products	Characteristics
Class I antigens	HLA-A	Single transmembrane polypeptide (alpha chain) complexed with β_2-microglobulin
	HLA-B	Found on all nucleated cells and platelets
	HLA-C	Antigen held by α_1 and α_2 regions
Class II antigens	HLA-DR	Two transmembrane polypeptides (alpha and beta chains)
	HLA-DP	Found on B cells, APCs, and activated T cells
	HLA-DQ	Antigen held by α_1 and β_1 regions

APC, Antigen-presenting cell.

is usually filtered through the red pulp of the spleen, where it encounters splenic lymphocytes. Antigen entering through the interstitial spaces is usually drained by the afferent lymphatics to the regional lymph nodes, where it enters the sinusoids. These spaces in the lymph node architecture are lined with phagocytic cells that ingest antigen. (Lymph nodes and lymphatic vessels are described in Chapter 28.)

At this point a process known as **antigen processing** occurs (Fig. 6-19). After its ingestion by a macrophage in the lymph node, the antigen is degraded. A portion of the degraded antigen is reexposed, or expressed, on the plasma membrane of the phagocyte, which "presents" it to T or B cells (see Figs. 6-6 and 6-14). Antigen processing and presentation are necessary for an immune response to occur. Antigen processing can occur also at many other sites, including other lymphoid organs, the skin, and mucous membranes.

For presentation to occur effectively, the antigen must be in a complex with molecules of class I HLA antigens or class II HLA antigens. The particular HLA class that bears the antigen helps to determine which cell will respond to the presentation of that antigen. For Th cells to respond, the antigen must be presented in a complex with class II HLA antigens, those of the HLA DR,DP,DQ series. For Tc cells and Ts cells to respond, the antigen must be presented in a complex with class I HLA antigens of the HLA-A and HLA-B series. Th cell recognition of antigen therefore is referred to as *class II restricted,* whereas Tc and Ts cell recognition of antigen is referred to as *class I restricted.*

The T cell "sees" the presented antigen through a set of receptors found on the surface of the cell.[13] At least two sets of receptors participate in this interaction; one is antigen specific (the T cell receptor), and the other is independent of the presented antigen (CD4 or CD8). The **T cell receptor (TCR)** is similar to the Fab portion of an antibody in that it consists of two protein chains and contains a combining site that specifically recognizes antigen. The two chains are referred to as *alpha* and *beta chains,* each of which has a variable region and a constant region. The TCR is inserted into the membrane in association with another set of proteins that make up the complex referred to as *CD3.* The combined effects of antigen binding to the TCR and the interaction of CD3 with either CD4 or CD8 at the lymphocyte membrane result in a signal being communicated to the cell as one of the signals for differentiation to begin.

A recently recognized group of antigens has the property of binding simultaneously to certain groups of TCRs at sites away from the normal antigen-specific combining site and to class II antigens (Fig. 6-20). Because the antigen is not limited to reacting with only a few T cells that bear the appropriate antigen-specific TCR, many more T cells will be given an activation signal and initiate differentiation and cytokine production. The resultant increase in the immune response has led to these antigens being referred to as *superantigens.* Several bacteria (e.g., bacteria that cause toxic shock syndrome) secrete superantigens that induce excessive production of cytokines that cause most of the clinical symptoms of the disease.

Before differentiation can proceed, however, a second part of the antigen-specific signal is necessary. That signal is provided through CD4 for Th cells or CD8 for Tc and Ts cells. Neither will recognize the presented antigen directly. Each will bind specifically to regions of the HLA molecule that are away from the site where antigen is being presented. CD4 recognizes a particular amino acid sequence found on class II HLA molecules, and CD8 recognizes a sequence found on class I HLA molecules. The interaction of these molecules with HLA contributes to the physical association of the T cell receptor with antigen and through a cytoplasmic interaction with CD3 provides the signal to initiate T cell differentiation.

In addition to an antigen-specific signal, intercellular communication requires the interaction between complementary sets of adhesion molecules on the surface of each cell. These molecules strengthen the interactions between the cells and provide additional intracellular signals for cellular differentiation and proliferation. Several of these adhesion molecule interactions are listed in Table 6-6.

The macrophage also produces a hormone, **interleukin-1 (IL-1),** that helps the T cell respond. During antigen presentation, IL-1 is released by the macrophage and binds to specific IL-1 receptors on the surface of the Th cell. One of the first steps in Th cell differentiation in response to these multiple signals is the production of another cytokine, IL-2. Without IL-2 production, the Th cell cannot efficiently mature into a functional helper cell. IL-2 has an autocrine effect in that it binds to specific IL-2 receptors on the surface of the same cell that is producing it. The results of the interaction of IL-2 and its receptor are an increased production of both IL-2 and IL-2 receptor, further differentiation of the Th

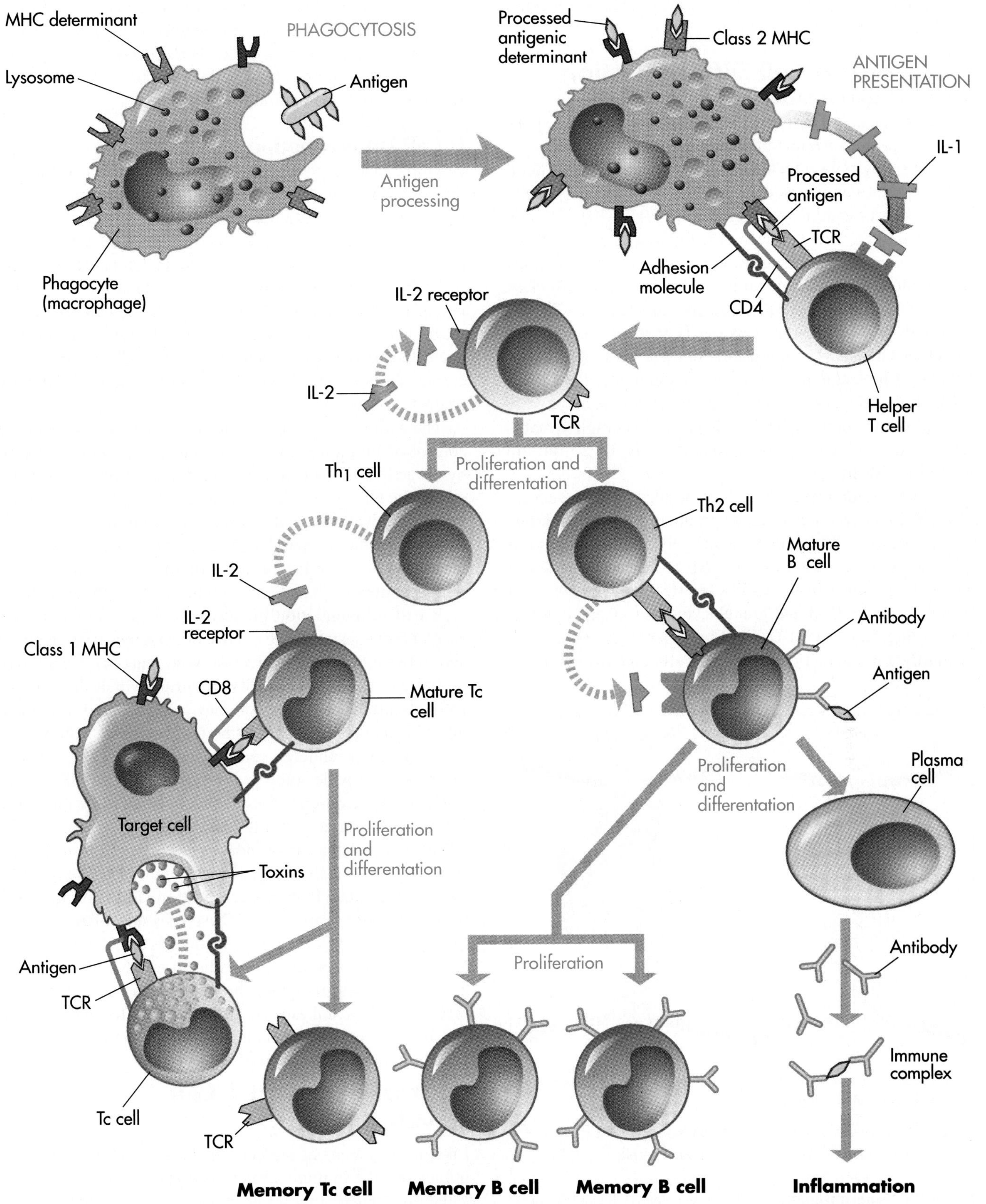

FIG. 6-19 Model of cellular interactions and the immune response. Schematic showing antigen processing, activation, and differentiation of T and B cell immune responses. *Solid arrows* indicate differentiation steps. *Hashed arrows* indicate indirect effects through cytokines (see text).

cell, proliferation of the Th cell, and the production of other cytokines, such as IL-4 and IL-6.

T Cell and B Cell Differentiation

T Cell Differentiation

The development of cytotoxic T cells (Tc), which are responsible for the cell-mediated destruction of such targets as tumor cells or virally infected cells, requires the presentation of foreign antigen in association with class I antigens of the major histocompatibility complex (see Fig. 6-19). Tc cells can see antigen on the surface of antigen-presenting cells or other target cells. For instance, some viruses that infect cells will produce viral-specific antigens that complex with class I HLA antigens on the surface of the infected cell. The Tc cell binds presented antigen with a TCR identical with that found on Th cells. The interaction of CD8 with a portion of the class I molecule provides another differentiation signal. As with Th antigen–presenting cell interactions, a cytokine must also interact with the Tc cell to induce complete maturation and development of cytotoxic activity. IL-2 from the Th cell fulfills this role.

Helper T lymphocytes have been divided into two subsets (Th1, Th2) based on differential production of lymphokines by each subset.[14] Th1 cells more actively produce interferon (IFN-γ), tumor necrosis factor (TNF-β), and IL-2, whereas Th2 cells produce IL-4, IL-5, IL-6, IL-9, and IL-10. Both subsets produce IL-3 and granulocyte/macrophage colony–stimulating factor (GM-CSF). The Th1 cell is responsible primarily for interactions with Tc cells and macrophages (Th1 cells are probably identical with Td cells). The Th2 cell is responsible primarily for interactions with B cells. These two Th cells can suppress each other's function; IFN-γ from the Th1 will suppress Th2 function, and IL-10 from the Th2 will suppress Th1 function.

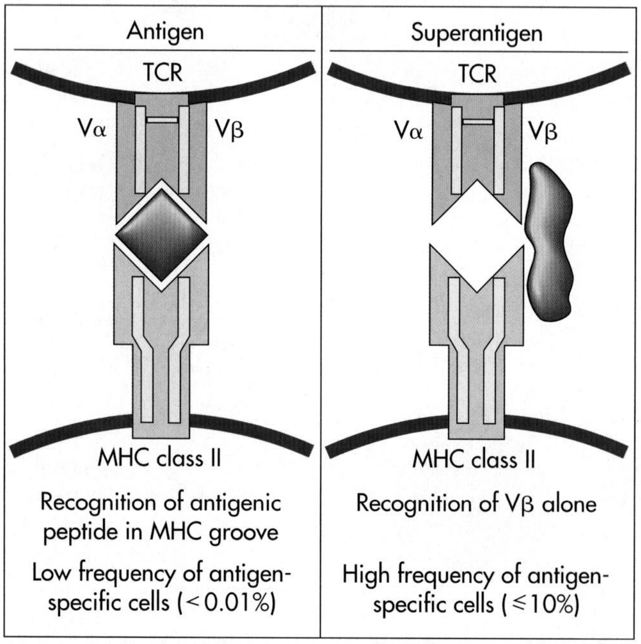

FIG. 6-20 Superantigens. The T cell receptor (TCR) and major histocompatibility complex (MHC) class II molecule are normally held together by processed antigen. Superantigens, such as some bacterial exotoxins, bind directly to the variable region of the TCR-b chain and the MHC class II molecule. Each superantigen activates distinct sets of V b chains independently of the antigen specificity of the TCR.

B Cell Differentiation

B lymphocytes also can recognize antigen, either on the surface of antigen-presenting cells or in soluble form, although the particular antigenic determinant recognized may differ from that recognized by the Th cell. This recognition is apparent from studies using carriers and haptens. Haptens are not normally immunogenic. When haptens are covalently bound to high-molecular-weight proteins (carriers) and injected into an animal, however, the B lymphocytes frequently recognize the hapten and the Th cell recognizes the carrier portion. The result is the production of antibody against the hapten.

The antibody response of the B lymphocytes is under the control of hormones (IL-4 and other interleukins) secreted by the activated Th cell. Some of these hormones probably mimic the effects of antigens with repeating determinants by directly activating the B lymphocytes. Interleukins are not antigen specific, so the Th cell activated by one antigen (i.e., the carrier) can produce a factor that facilitates the production of antibody against another antigen (i.e., the hapten).

B cell differentiation proceeds through multiple stages, each of which is under the control of cytokines (see Fig. 6-19 and Table 6-6). After interaction with antigen, B cells will proliferate, undergo class switch during which the class of antibody produced by the cell may change, and differentiate into plasma cells that are antibody "factories" with no further capacity to undergo cell division. IL-1, IL-2, and IL-4 most likely provide some of the signal to begin differentiation and proliferation. Class switch appears to be under the control of a variety of interleukins and adhesion through CD40. For instance, IL-4 induces class switch to IgG1 and IgE, TGF-β (transforming growth factor-beta) helps class switch to IgA, and IL-6 induces differentiation into IgG- and IgM-secreting plasma cells. The production of pentameric IgM is enhanced by IL-2, which controls J chain expression. Most of these cytokines are produced by Th cells, and each cytokine binds to its target through specific cell membrane receptors. CD40 adhesion is also necessary for class switch, and defects in this molecule will result in defective class switch and overproduction of IgM.

Control of B and T Cell Development

Like most systems of the body that are activated by outside influences, the immune system is conserved by being activated only during time of need and then completely or partially turned off after the threat to the individual has been repelled. Concurrently, the immune system is normally prevented from recognizing and rejecting its own tissue.

Several types of suppressor cells, including Ts cells and some monocytes and macrophages, control both the humoral and cell-mediated activities of the immune system. Suppressor cells appear to vary in specificity, some being antigen specific and others relatively nonspecific for a particular antigen or specific for only one class of antibody or effector cell. Some suppressor cells affect the recognition of antigen, and others suppress the proliferative steps that follow antigen recognition. Tolerance of self-antigens is apparently another suppressor cell function. Although the role of suppressor cells is currently under intense investigation, the degree of their heterogeneity of derivation, function, and specificity is far from determined.

Fetal and Neonatal Immune Function

The normal human infant is immunologically immature at birth. Although cell-mediated immunologic capabilities begin developing early in gestation and probably are completely functional at birth, antibody production, phagocytic activity, and complement activity are clearly deficient. In the last trimester, the fetus appears capable of producing a primary immune response (almost entirely IgM) to antigenic challenge in utero and to infections such as cytomegalovirus, rubella virus, and *Toxoplasma gondii.* The fetus is unable to produce a significant IgG response, however. The capacity to produce IgA is underdeveloped, although some IgA can be detected.

To protect the child against infectious agents in utero and during the first few postnatal months, a system of active transport facilitates the passage of maternal antibodies into the fetal circulation (Fig. 6-21). In the placenta, maternal and fetal blood is separated by a layer of specialized cells termed *trophoblasts.* Immunoglobulins are too large to diffuse across the trophoblastic layer. The trophoblastic cells actively transport immunoglobulins from the maternal to the fetal circulation. Active transport of maternal IgG is mediated by surface receptors that are specific for the Fc portion of free IgG but not for IgM, IgE, or IgA. Active transport sometimes results in higher antibody titers in umbilical cord blood than in maternal blood. (Active transport mechanisms are discussed in Chapter 1.)

At birth, total IgG levels in the umbilical cord are near adult levels. When the source of maternal antibodies is severed at birth, antibody titers in the newborn begin to drop as maternal antibody is catabolized (Fig. 6-22). Thus antibody titers drop rapidly even though the neonate's production of IgG is beginning to rise. This occurs because the rate of catabolism is more rapid than the rate of production. Total immunoglobulin levels reach a minimum at 5 to 6 months in the normal child, occasionally causing transient hypogammaglobulinemia (insufficient quantities of circulating immunoglobulins). Many normal infants experience recurrent mild respiratory tract infections at this time.

Aging and Immune Function

Immune function decreases in old age. T cell function and specific antibody responses to antigenic challenge diminish, yet there is an increase in levels of circulating autoantibodies (antibodies against self-antigens) and immune complexes. In addition, there is an increased incidence of spontaneous monoclonal antibody production without concurrent B cell malignancy (myeloma).

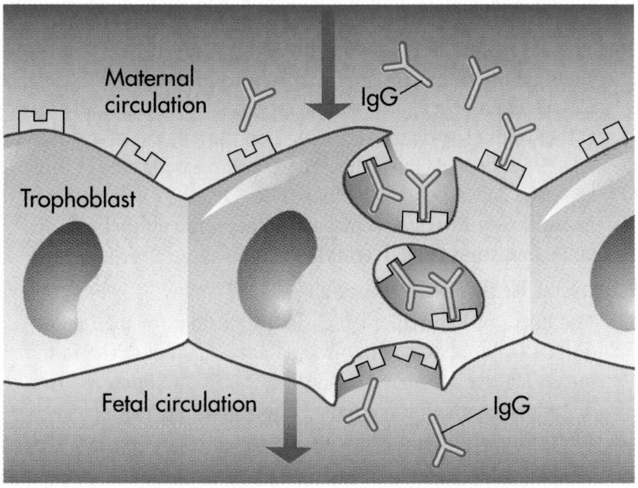

FIG. 6-21 Transport of IgG across the trophoblast. The transport of maternal IgG across the trophoblast and into the fetal circulation is an active process. Maternal IgG binds to crystalline fragment (Fc) receptors on the surface of the trophoblast and is enclosed in vacuoles by the process of endocytosis. Receptors on the trophoblast are specific for the Fc portion of IgG and do not bind other classes of immunoglobulins. The interaction of IgG with the receptors protects the antibody from digestion during transport of the vacuole across the cell. On the fetal side, IgG is released into the fetal circulation by exocytosis (see Chapter 1).

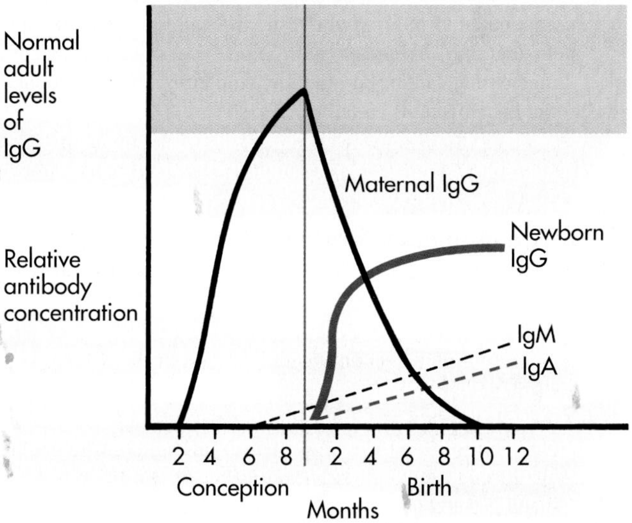

FIG. 6-22 Antibody levels in the umbilical cord blood and neonatal circulation. Early in gestation, maternal IgG crosses the placenta and enters the fetal circulation. At the time of birth, the fetal circulation contains nearly adult levels of IgG, which is almost exclusively maternal, and small amounts of fetal IgM and IgA. After the delivery of the infant, maternal IgG is rapidly catabolized and neonatal IgG production increases.

The central lymphoid organ for T cell development, the thymus, reaches maximum size at sexual maturity and then begins involuting until it is a vestigial remnant by middle age. By 45 to 50 years of age, thymic size is only 15% of its maximum. The level of thymic hormone production and the capacity of the thymus to mediate T cell differentiation decrease with thymic atrophy. Numbers of circulating T cells do not decrease with age, but T cell function may deteriorate. Individuals over 60 years of age generally exhibit decreased delayed hypersensitivity response (as demonstrated by milder positive reactions in tuberculin skin tests), decreased T cell–mediated responses to infections, and decreased T cell activity (as demonstrated by laboratory assays of T cell function).

SUMMARY REVIEW

Innate Defenses

1. The body's first lines of defense are anatomic barriers: the skin and the mucous membrane.
2. If an injurious chemical, foreign body, or microorganism penetrates these defenses, the body attempts to eliminate it by mechanical clearance.
3. Once external barriers have been compromised, the inflammatory response (or second line of defense) occurs.

Immune Response

1. The third line of defense is the immune response, or immunity. Compared with the inflammatory response, the immune response is slower and specific.
2. The inflammatory and immune responses complement one another and interact in complex ways. Because many inflammatory processes are triggered or affected by simultaneous immune processes, an understanding of the immune response is necessary for a complete understanding of inflammation.

Characteristics of Immune Response

1. Immunity is a state of protection, primarily against infectious agents, characterized by memory and specificity.
2. Antigens are chemical substances that react with preformed components of the immune response. Immunogens are antigens that can also induce an immune response. Haptens are antigens that cannot be immunogenic unless they are bound to larger molecules called *carriers.*
3. Self-antigens are antigens on host cells. Self-antigens are normally not recognized as immunogenic by the host's immune system, a condition known as *tolerance.*

Induction of Immune Response

1. The immune response is characterized by the activation of two types of immunocytes: B lymphocytes (B cells) and T lymphocytes (T cells). The activities of B cells compose the humoral immune response, and those of T cells make up the cell-mediated immune response.
2. A B cell develops from a stem cell that matures under hormonal control in bursal-equivalent tissues and develops into a mature plasma cell capable of producing antibody against a specific antigen.
3. Antibodies are plasma glycoproteins that can be classified by chemical structure and biologic activity as IgG, IgM, IgA, IgE, or IgD.
4. Antibodies may protect the host from harmful antigens by recognizing and binding with the antigen's antigenic determinant sites. Occupied antigenic determinants on viruses and bacterial toxins are unable to bind with receptors on host cells and are therefore unable to have injurious effects.
5. The protective effects of antibodies vary with the identity of the antigen. Antibodies opsonize bacteria, neutralize toxins and viruses, and activate inflammatory processes.
6. Antibodies of the systemic immune system function internally—in the bloodstream and tissues. Antibodies of the secretory, or mucosal, immune system function externally—in the secretions of mucous membranes.
7. A T cell develops from a stem cell that matures under hormonal control in the thymus and develops into a cytotoxic T cell, which can kill target cells directly; a delayed hypersensitivity T cell, which produces lymphokines that affect other cells (especially macrophages); a helper T cell, which induces B cells to produce antibody; or a suppressor T cell, which suppresses antibody production and immune function.
8. Antibody production is the final stage of a process requiring the interaction of B cells, helper T cells, and antigen-presenting cells.
9. The body actually recognizes that a substance is foreign through histocompatibility antigens (or human leukocyte antigens). These antigens are proteins found on the surface of nearly every cell in the body. The major group of genes producing the HLA antigens is the HLA complex or the major histocompatibility complex (MHC).
10. The HLA complex consists of four closely linked loci located on the short arm of chromosome 6, known as the A, B, C, and D complex. The antigens produced by the A, B, and C loci (class I antigens) are found on the surface of virtually all cells except erythrocytes. The D complex consists of three separate and independent loci (DR, DP, DQ) that are confined mostly to B cells, macrophages, some epithelial cells, and some stimulated T lymphocytes.

Humoral Immune Response

1. The bursa of Fabricius, which is responsible for the maturation of B lymphocytes in birds, is not a distinct tissue in humans. Humans do have tissues, probably the bone marrow, that make up the human bursal equivalent.
2. According to clonal selection theory, a large number of B cells with plasma membrane receptors for all potential antigenic determinants are spontaneously generated during fetal life.
3. The immune response is initiated when an antigen binds and interacts with receptors on the surface of the immature B cell, triggering it into a sequence of proliferation and differentiation that results in the production of (a) immunoglobulin-secreting plasma cells and (b) a set of long-lived memory cells.

4. Antibodies are immunoglobulins known to have specificity for a particular antigen. The five classes of immunoglobulins are IgG, IgA, IgM, IgE, and IgD.
5. The antigen-binding fragment (Fab) of the antibody contains the receptors for antigenic determinants and confers specificity. The crystalline fragment (Fc) is responsible for most of the biologic functions of the molecule.
6. The chief functions of antibodies are to protect the host by (a) neutralizing bacterial toxins, (b) neutralizing viruses, (c) opsonizing bacteria (promoting phagocytosis), and (d) activating components of the inflammatory response.
7. Most humoral immune responses are polyclonal; however, the generation of monoclonal antibodies—a single antibody of known specificity is generated rather than a mixture of different antibodies—is creating new therapeutic and diagnostic possibilities. A clinician can order tests for viral antigens that are specific and diagnostic and detect the disease early in its course.

Cell-Mediated Immune Response

1. T lymphocytes are responsible for cell-mediated immunity. The five types of mature T cells are memory cells, lymphokine-producing cells, cytotoxic (Tc) cells, helper T (Th) cells, and suppressor (Ts) cells. T cells mature in the thymus and produce plasma membrane receptors specific for antigens.
2. In the thymus, T cells begin producing new proteins that are differentiation related, called cluster of differentiation (CD) proteins (antigens), and that are inserted into the plasma membrane of the cell. Several important CD proteins participate in the development of the immune response.
3. The major effects of the cell-mediated immune response include cytotoxicity, delayed hypersensitivity, memory, and control.
4. The NK cell is a lymphocyte that can recognize chemical changes on the surface of virally infected cells or malignant cells and kill the infected or malignant cells by mechanisms similar to the Tc cell.

Cellular Interactions in Immune Response

1. Antigens that cannot induce the immune response independently must first interact with several populations of cells, including T helper cells, macrophages (as antigen-presenting cells), and cytokines.
2. Cytokines are proteins or glycoproteins secreted by cells participating in the immune response. They function as messengers, enabling communication among macrophages and lymphocytes.
3. When an antigen enters a host, it first equilibrates throughout body fluids. Eventually, antigen encounters macrophages, for example, by circulating through interstitial spaces in the lymph node. At this point, antigen processing occurs.
4. For antigen presentation to lymphocytes to occur, it must be in a complex with molecules of class I HLA antigens or class II HLA antigens. For Th cells to respond, the antigen must be presented in a complex with class II HLA antigens (HLA-DR, -DP, or -DQ). For Tc cells and Ts cells to respond, the antigen must be presented in a complex with class I HLA antigens. During antigen presentation, interleukin-1 (IL-1) is released by the macrophage and binds to receptors of the Th cell. The Th cell then responds by producing IL-2. IL-4 most likely provides a signal to begin differentiation and proliferation of B lymphocytes or antibody production.

Fetal and Neonatal Immune Function

1. Mechanisms of self-defense are naturally somewhat deficient in the fetus and the neonate.
2. The primary immune response is adequate in the fetus and neonate, but the secondary immune response does not develop fully until about 6 months of age. Maternal antibodies protect the neonate for the first 6 months, after which they are catabolized.

Aging and Immune Function

1. T cell function and antibody production in response to a specific antigenic challenge are somewhat deficient in elderly people. Elderly people also tend to have increased levels of circulating autoantibodies (antibodies against self-antigens).

KEY TERMS

KEY TERMS—cont'd

REFERENCES

1. Delves PJ, Roitt IM: The immune system. I, *N Engl J Med* 343(1):37, 2000.
2. Gollin YG: Management of the Rh-sensitized mother, *Clin Perinatol* 22:545, 1995.
3. Rote NS: Pathophysiology of Rh isoimmunization, *Clin Obstet Gynecol* 25:243, 1982.
4. Glick B, Chang TS, Jaap RG: The bursa of Fabricius and antibody production, *Poultry Sci* 35:224, 1956.
5. Burnet FM: *The clonal selection theory of acquired immunity,* London, 1959, Cambridge University Press.
6. Jerne NK: The natural-selection theory of antibody formation, *Proc Natl Acad Sci USA* 41:849, 1955.
7. Porter RR: The hydrolysis of rabbit gammaglobulin and antibodies with crystalline papain, *Biochem J* 73:119, 1959.
8. Delves PJ, Roitt IM: The immune system. II, *N Engl J Med* 343(1):108, 2000.
9. Kohler G, Milstein C: Continuous cultures of fused cells secreting antibody of predefined specificity, *Nature* 256:495, 1975.
10. Jenner E: *An inquiry into the causes and effects of the variolae vaccinae: a disease discovered in some of the western counties of England, particularly Gloucestershire, and known by the name of the cow pox,* London, 1798, Sampson Low.
11. Lanier LL: NK cell receptors, *Annu Rev Immunol* 16:359, 1998.
12. Moretta A et al: Major histocompatibility complex class I-specific receptors on human natural killer and T-lymphocytes, *Immunol Rev* 155:105, 1997.
13. Boniface JJ: T-cell recognition of antigen: a process controlled by transient intermolecular interactions, *Ann NY Acad Sci* 766:62, 1995.
14. Romagnani S et al: TH1 and TH2 cells, *Res Immunol* 149(9):871, 1998.

CHAPTER 7

Inflammation

NEAL S. ROTE

CHAPTER OUTLINE

Inflammation is a biochemical and cellular process that occurs in vascularized tissues. Most of the essential components of the inflammatory process are found in the circulation, and most of the early mediators (facilitators) of inflammation affect the vascular bed so as to increase the movement of plasma and blood cells from the circulation into the tissues surrounding the injury. These substances, known collectively as **exudate,** defend the host against infection and facilitate tissue repair and healing.

As described in antiquity, the superficial hallmarks of inflammation include redness *(rubor),* swelling *(tumor),* heat *(calor),* pain *(dolor),* and loss of function *(functio laesa).* The development of the microscope, however, enabled investigators to detect inflammatory changes at the cellular level. In the nineteenth century, Julius Cohnheim observed three characteristic changes in the microcirculation (arterioles, capillaries, and venules) near the site of an injury. He saw that (1) blood vessels dilated, increasing blood flow to the area; (2) vascular permeability increased, resulting in the outward leakage of plasma, which formed an inflammatory exudate; and (3) white blood cells adhered to the inner walls of vessels and then emigrated through vessel walls to the site of injury.

Inflammation and repair can be divided into several phases (Fig. 7-1). The characteristics of the early inflammatory response differ from those of the later response, and each phase involves different biochemical mediators and cells that function together to (1) destroy injurious agents and remove them from the inflammatory site, (2) wall off and confine these agents so as to limit their effects on the host, (3) stimulate and enhance the immune response, and (4) promote healing.

In contrast to the immune system, which is antigen specific and has memory, the inflammatory response is nonspecific because it takes place in approximately the same way, no matter what the stimulus, and occurs in the same manner, even on second exposure to the same stimulus. The acute response is self-limiting; that is, it continues only until the threat to the host is eliminated. This usually takes 8 to 10 days, from onset to healing. Inflammation is considered chronic if it persists longer than 2 weeks.

ACUTE INFLAMMATORY RESPONSE

The acute inflammatory response begins after lethal or nonlethal cellular injury (Fig. 7-2). Cellular injury may be caused by trauma (mechanical forces), oxygen or nutrient deprivation, genetic or immune defects, chemical agents, microorganisms, temperature extremes, or ionizing radiation. (Mechanisms of cellular injury are described in Chapter 2.)

Unlike the immune response, which takes days to develop, the vascular effects of inflammation are immediate, occurring in seconds. First, arterioles near the site of injury constrict briefly. Vasoconstriction is followed by vasodilation,

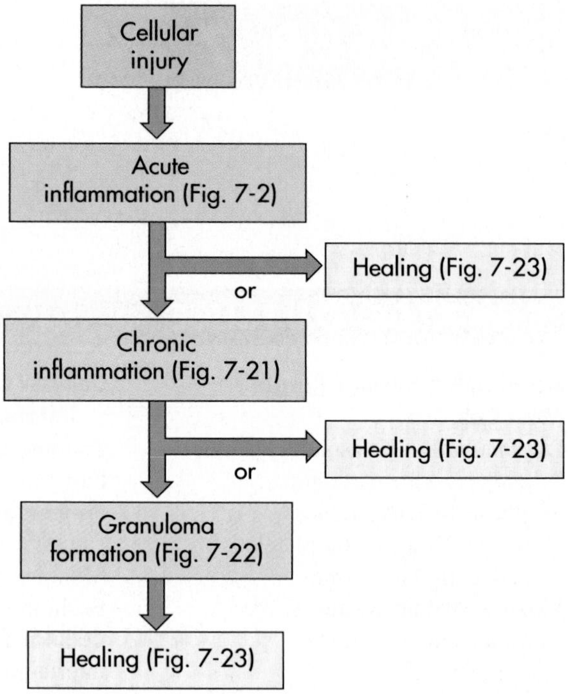

FIG. 7-1 Inflammatory process. Cellular injury leads to acute inflammation, which may result in resolution and healing of the injured site or progress into chronic inflammation. Chronic inflammation in turn may either result in healing or progress into the development of a granuloma. The final step of the process is usually healing and reconstruction of the damaged tissue. The figure numbers refer to those in which more detailed information may be found on that portion of the process.

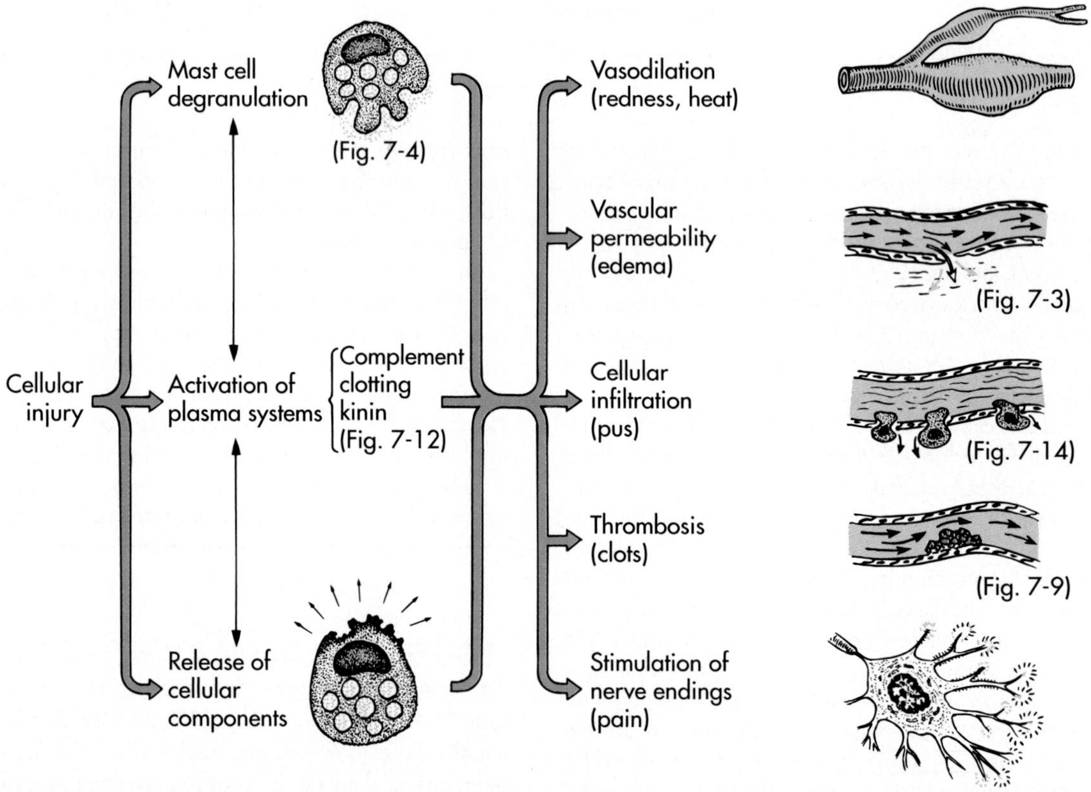

FIG. 7-2 Acute inflammatory response. Inflammation is usually initiated by cellular injury. Mast cell degranulation, the activation of three plasma systems, and the release of subcellular components from the damaged cells occur as a consequence of cellular injury. These systems are interdependent, so that induction of one (e.g., mast cell degranulation) can result in the induction of the other two. The result is the development of microscopic changes in the inflamed site, as well as characteristic clinical manifestations. The figure numbers refer to those in which more detailed information may be found on that portion of the response.

which increases blood flow to the inflamed site. Arteriolar dilation increases pressure in the microcirculation, which may increase the exudation of plasma and blood cells into the tissues. Exudation causes edema and swelling. As plasma moves outward, blood remaining in the microcirculation flows more slowly and becomes more viscous (thick and sticky). Leukocytes (white blood cells) migrate to vessel walls and adhere there. At the same time, biochemical mediators stimulate the **endothelial cells** that line capillaries and venules to retract, creating spaces at junctions between the cells. (Intercellular junctions are described in Chapter 1.) The leukocytes, which otherwise could not penetrate vessel walls, are able to squeeze out through the spaces created by endothelial retraction (Fig. 7-3).

This state of vascular permeability continues throughout acute inflammation, permitting blood cells and plasma proteins to exude continuously into inflamed tissues. Once in the tissues, these cells and proteins act in concert to (1) stimulate and control subsequent inflammatory processes and (2) interact with components of the immune response.

Neutrophils are the first phagocytic leukocytes to arrive at the inflamed site. They phagocytose (ingest) bacteria, dead cells, and cellular debris, and then they die and are removed as pus through the epithelium or the lymphatic system. (The lymphatic system is described in Chapter 28.) The next phagocytes on the scene are monocytes and macrophages, which perform many of the same functions as neutrophils but for a longer time and later in the inflammatory response. Other cells found in inflamed tissues are eosinophils, which help control the inflammatory response and act directly against parasites; basophils, which have a function similar to that of mast cells; and **platelets,** which are cytoplasmic fragments that stop bleeding if vascular injury has occurred (see Chapter 24).

The cells and platelets carry out their roles with the assistance of three major plasma protein systems (the complement, clotting, and kinin systems) and immunoglobulins. The complement system not only activates and assists inflammatory and immune processes but also plays a major role in the direct destruction of cells (especially bacteria). The clotting system traps bacteria in injured tissues and interacts with platelets to prevent hemorrhage. The kinin system helps control vascular permeability. Immunoglobulin is the fourth type of plasma protein that participates in inflammatory processes.

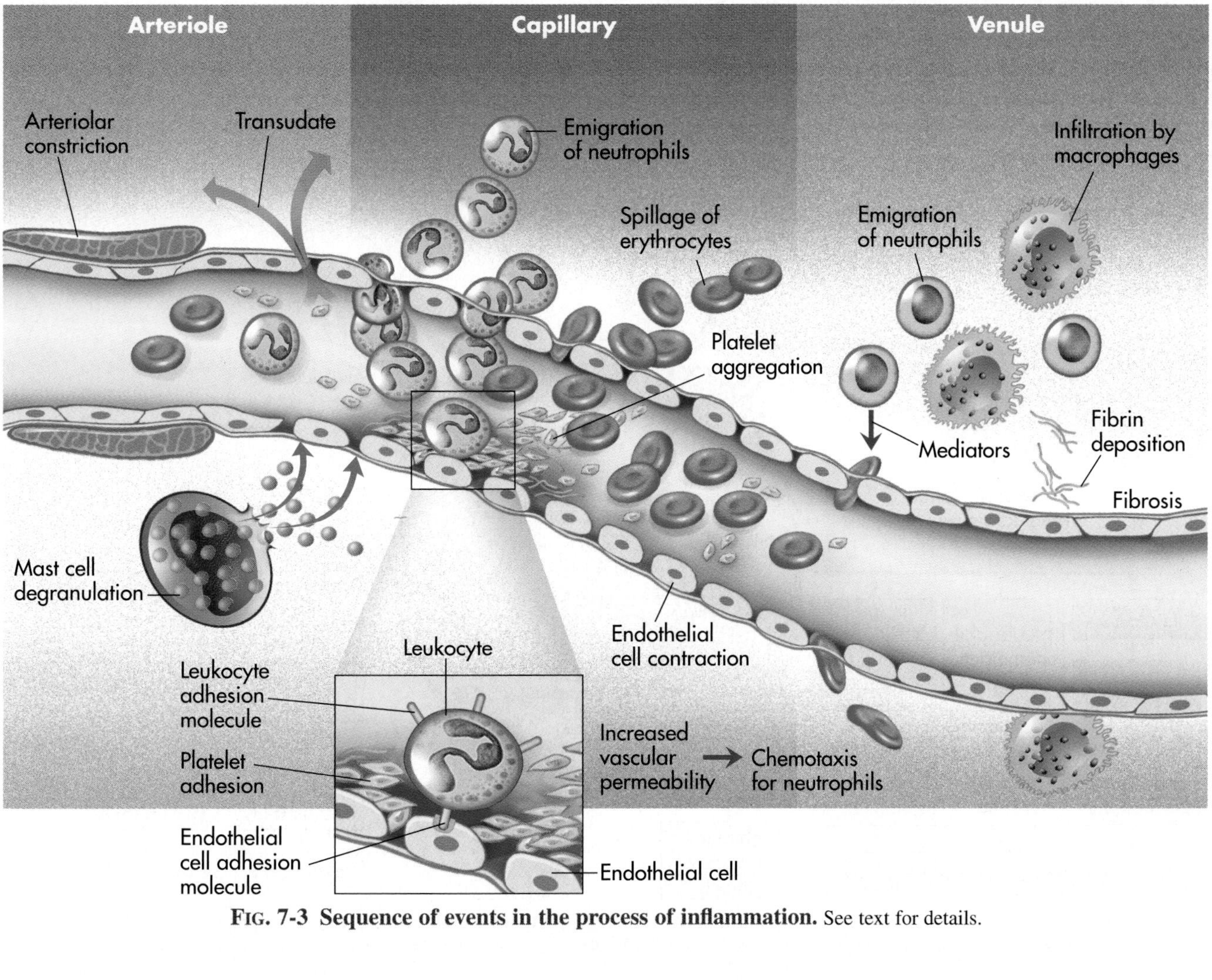

FIG. 7-3 Sequence of events in the process of inflammation. See text for details.

All these cells and protein systems, along with the substances they produce, act at the site of tissue injury to kill microorganisms and remove the debris of "battle," including exudate and dead cells. This prepares the lesion for tissue regeneration or repair, the process known as *resolution.*

Like inappropriate immune processes, inappropriate or exaggerated inflammatory processes have deleterious effects on the host. Even appropriate inflammation can be painful and harm healthy tissues. Further, because inflammation is complex, is nonspecific, and can be triggered and maintained by a great variety of stimuli, it is often difficult to control with drugs.

The function of acute inflammation and the stages by which it proceeds are not difficult to understand. Difficulty occurs when one asks, "How are the various stages initiated, regulated, and ended?" The biochemical mediators and cellular components of the acute inflammatory response form a complex system of interactions that frequently begins with degranulation of mast cells and ends with healing.

MAST CELL

The mast cell is probably the most important activator of the inflammatory response (Fig. 7-4). **Mast cells,** first described by Paul Ehrlich in 1877,[1] are cellular bags of granules located in the loose connective tissues close to blood vessels. **Basophils** are found in the blood and probably function in the same way as tissue mast cells.[2] Mast cells activate the inflammatory response in two ways. The first is **degranulation,** by which they release preformed granular contents into the extracellular matrix. The second is *synthesis* of certain mediators in response to a stimulus.

Degranulation of Vasoactive Amines and Chemotactic Factors

Mast cell degranulation is stimulated by one of the following means:

1. Physical injury, such as heat, mechanical trauma, ultraviolet light, or x-rays
2. Chemical agents, such as toxins, snake and bee venoms, tissue proteases (enzymes), dextran, or a cationic protein released from neutrophils
3. Immunologic means, such as the triggering of IgE-mediated hypersensitivity reactions (see Chapter 8), or direct processes, such as activation of complement components or T lymphocytes (see Fig. 7-5)

Preformed biochemical mediators found in the granules, including histamine, neutrophil chemotactic factor, and eosinophil chemotactic factor of anaphylaxis, are released in seconds and exert their effects immediately. Serotonin, another potent mediator, is released by platelets.

Histamine and serotonin are both vasoactive amines. They cause temporary, rapid constriction of the smooth muscle of large vessel walls; dilation of the postcapillary venules, resulting in increased blood flow into the microcirculation; and increased vascular permeability resulting from retraction of endothelial cells lining the capillaries (see Fig. 7-3).

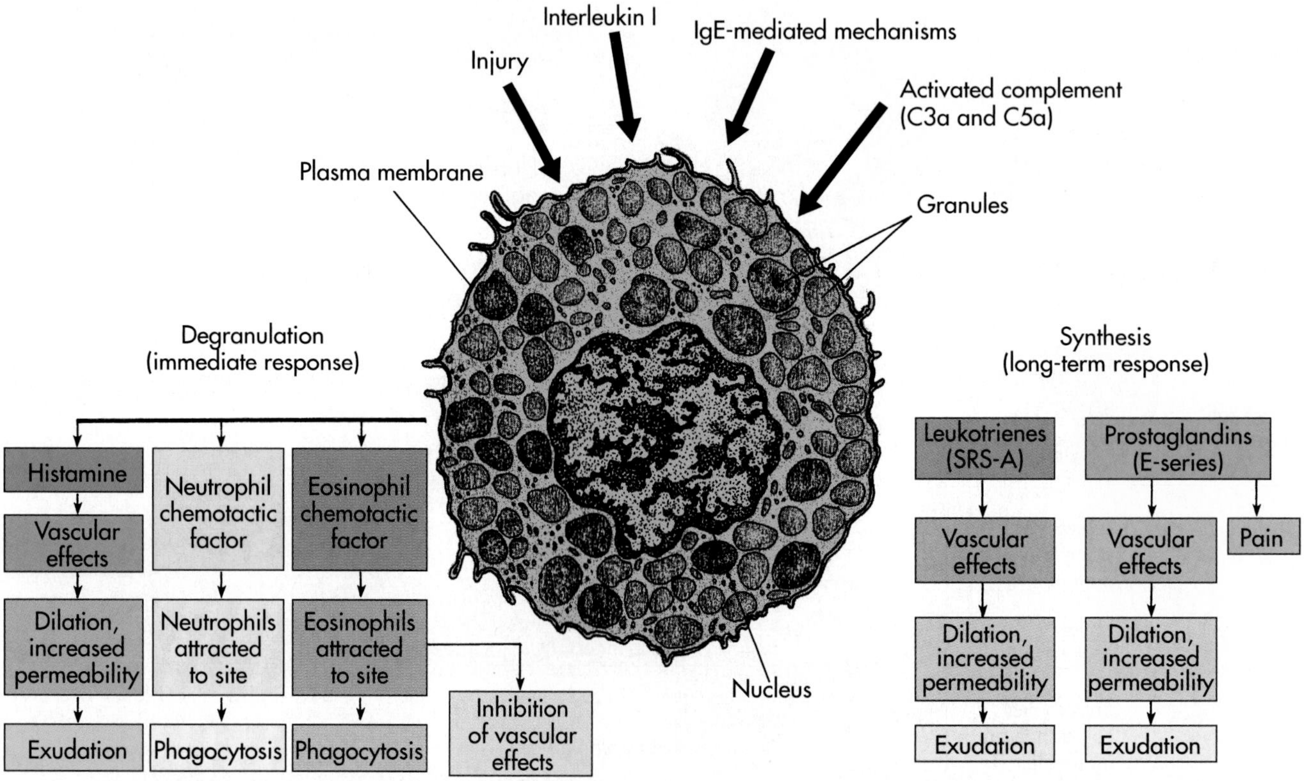

FIG. 7-4 Effects of degranulation *(left)* and synthesis *(right)* by mast cells. The electron micrograph of a tissue mast cell shows darkly stained granules in the cytoplasm (× 9200). *SRS-A,* Slow-reacting substances of anaphylaxis.

Two chemotactic factors, neutrophil chemotactic factor and eosinophil chemotactic factor of anaphylaxis (ECF-A), are also released during mast cell degranulation. A **chemotactic factor** is a biochemical substance that attracts a specific type of leukocyte to the site of inflammation. **Chemotaxis** is directional movement of cells along a chemical gradient formed by a chemotactic factor (Fig. 7-6). Neutrophil chemotactic factor attracts neutrophils to the site of inflammation. Neutrophils are the predominant leukocytes at work during early phases of acute inflammation.

Eosinophil chemotactic factor attracts eosinophils to the inflamed site. Eosinophils are leukocytes that have several functions in the inflammatory response. They are phagocytic and are the body's primary defense against some parasites. Their most important role, however, is to control the mediators of acute inflammation released from mast cells. As with most defense systems of the body, the acute inflammatory response is usually needed only in a circumscribed area and for a limited time. Therefore control mechanisms are necessary to prevent biochemical mediators from evoking more inflammation than is needed. Eosinophils contain several enzymes that degrade the vasoactive amines, thereby controlling the vascular effects of inflammation. These enzymes include histaminase, which mediates the degradation of histamine, and arylsulfatase B, which mediates the degradation of leukotrienes.

Synthesis of Leukotrienes, Prostaglandins, and Platelet-Activating Factor

Leukotrienes, prostaglandins, and platelet-activating factor are mediators synthesized by mast cells (see Fig. 7-4). **Leukotrienes (slow-reacting substances of anaphylaxis [SRS-A])** are acidic, sulfur-containing lipids that produce effects similar to those of histamine, namely, smooth muscle contraction, increased vascular permeability, and perhaps neutrophil and eosinophil chemotaxis. Leukotrienes appear to be important in the later stages of the inflammatory response, because they stimulate slower and more prolonged responses than do histamines. Leukotrienes are produced from a lipid, arachidonic acid, that is released from mast cell

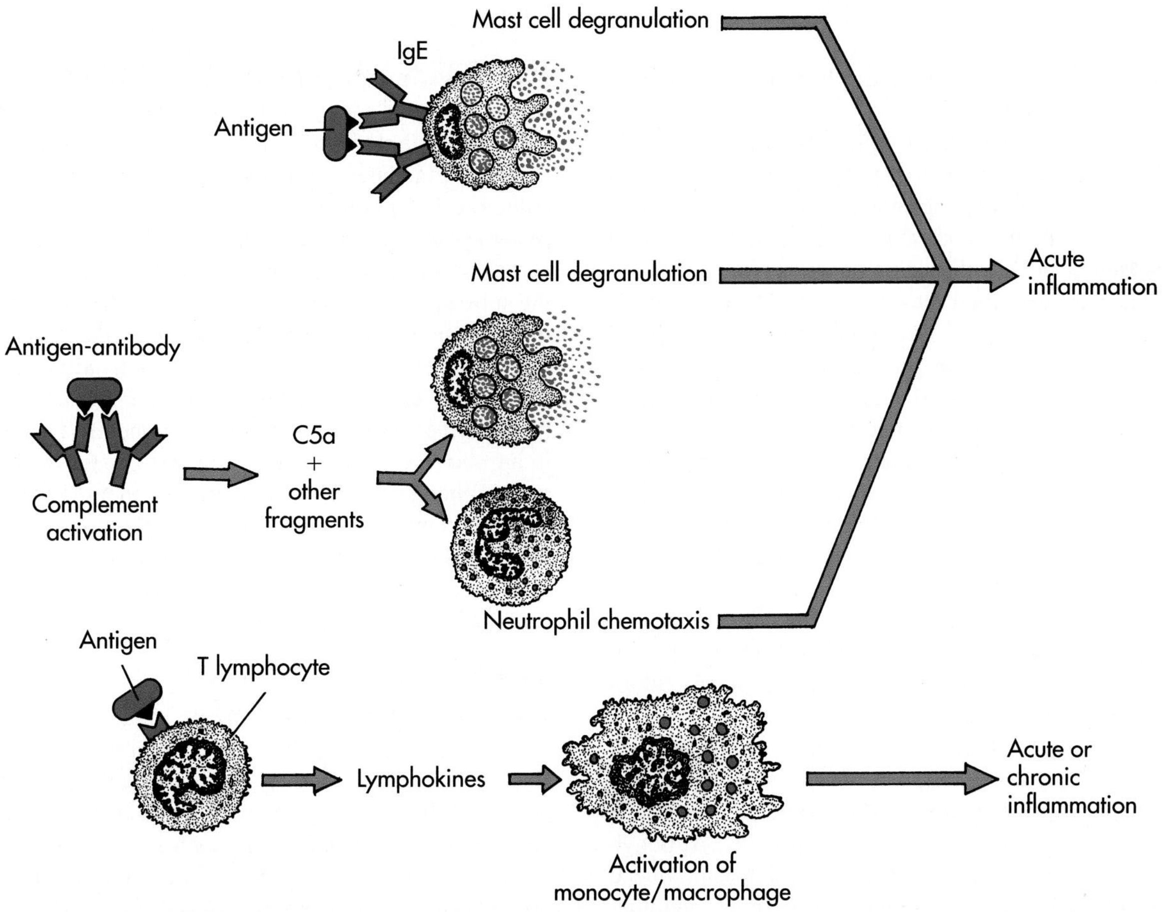

FIG. 7-5 Immunologic mechanisms that activate the inflammatory response. Immunologic factors may affect inflammation through three mechanisms: (1) immunoglobulin E (IgE) can bind to the surface of a mast cell and, after binding antigen, induce the cell's degranulation; (2) antigen and antibody can form immune complexes that activate the complement cascade, releasing small polypeptide fragments, primarily C5a, that have potent biologic activities resulting in mast cell degranulation and neutrophil chemotaxis; and (3) antigen may also react with T lymphocytes, resulting in the production of lymphokines that may contribute to the development of either acute or chronic inflammation.

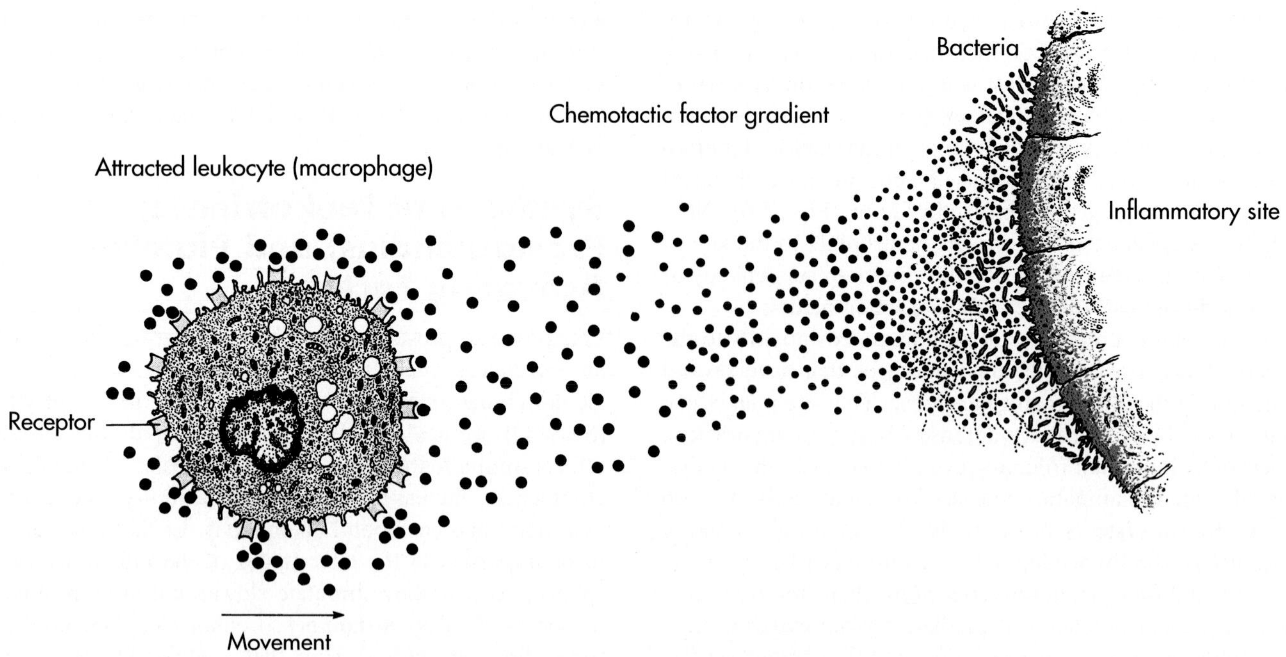

FIG. 7-6 Chemotaxis. Multiple receptors on the leukocyte's plasma membrane sense the area of highest concentration of a chemotactic factor *(dots),* and the leukocyte (usually a phagocyte) moves toward this area.

membranes by an intracellular phospholipase that acts on membrane phospholipids.

The mast cell also synthesizes **prostaglandins,** which, like leukotrienes, cause increased vascular permeability and neutrophil chemotaxis. Prostaglandins also induce pain. Prostaglandins are long-chain, unsaturated fatty acids produced from arachidonic acid by the action of the enzyme cyclooxygenase. They are classified into groups (E, D, A, F, and B) according to their structure. Prostaglandins E_1 and E_2 probably cause increased vascular permeability and smooth muscle contraction; they appear to act directly on postcapillary venules. They also can inhibit some aspects of inflammation by such actions as suppressing both the release of histamine from mast cells and the release of lysosomal enzymes (enzymes responsible for killing and digesting microorganisms) from neutrophils. Enhancement or suppression of the inflammatory response may be related to concentrations of prostaglandins. Aspirin and some other nonsteroidal antiinflammatory agents block the synthesis of prostaglandins of the E series and other arachidonic acid derivatives, thereby inhibiting inflammation.

Platelet-activating factor (PAF) is produced by removal of a fatty acid from the number two position of plasma membrane phosphatidlycholone. The long-chain fatty acid at this position is removed by phospholipase A_2. Although mast cells are a major source of PAF, it can also be produced during inflammation from neutrophils, monocytes, endothelium, and platelets. The biologic activity of PAF is virtually identical with SRS-A, affecting endothelial cells to increase vascular permeability, causing leukocyte adhesion to endothelium, and causing platelet activation.

PLASMA PROTEIN SYSTEMS

Inflammation is mediated by three key plasma protein systems: the complement system, the clotting system, and the kinin system. These systems have several characteristics in common. Each consists of a series of inactive enzymes, or **proenzymes.** When the first proenzyme in the series is converted to an active enzyme, it initiates a cascade in which the substrate of the activated enzyme is the next component of the system. Therefore the entire cascade is activated on activation of the first component. Activation usually involves the enzymatic cleavage of the inactive precursor (proenzyme) into two or more components. The larger one is an active enzyme whose substrate is the next component in the system. The smaller component is usually a potent biochemical mediator of the inflammatory response. Most of these components are short lived because they are inactivated rapidly by other naturally occurring plasma proteins.

Complement System

The complement system consists of at least 10 proteins and makes up 10% of the serum proteins in the circulation (Fig. 7-7). The complement system is perhaps the most important of the plasma protein systems of inflammation because, once activated, its components participate in virtually every inflammatory response.[3,4] In addition, the last few proteins in the complement cascade are capable of killing microorganisms directly.

The complement system can be activated by antigen-antibody complexes, as well as by products released from invading bacteria and by components of the other plasma pro-

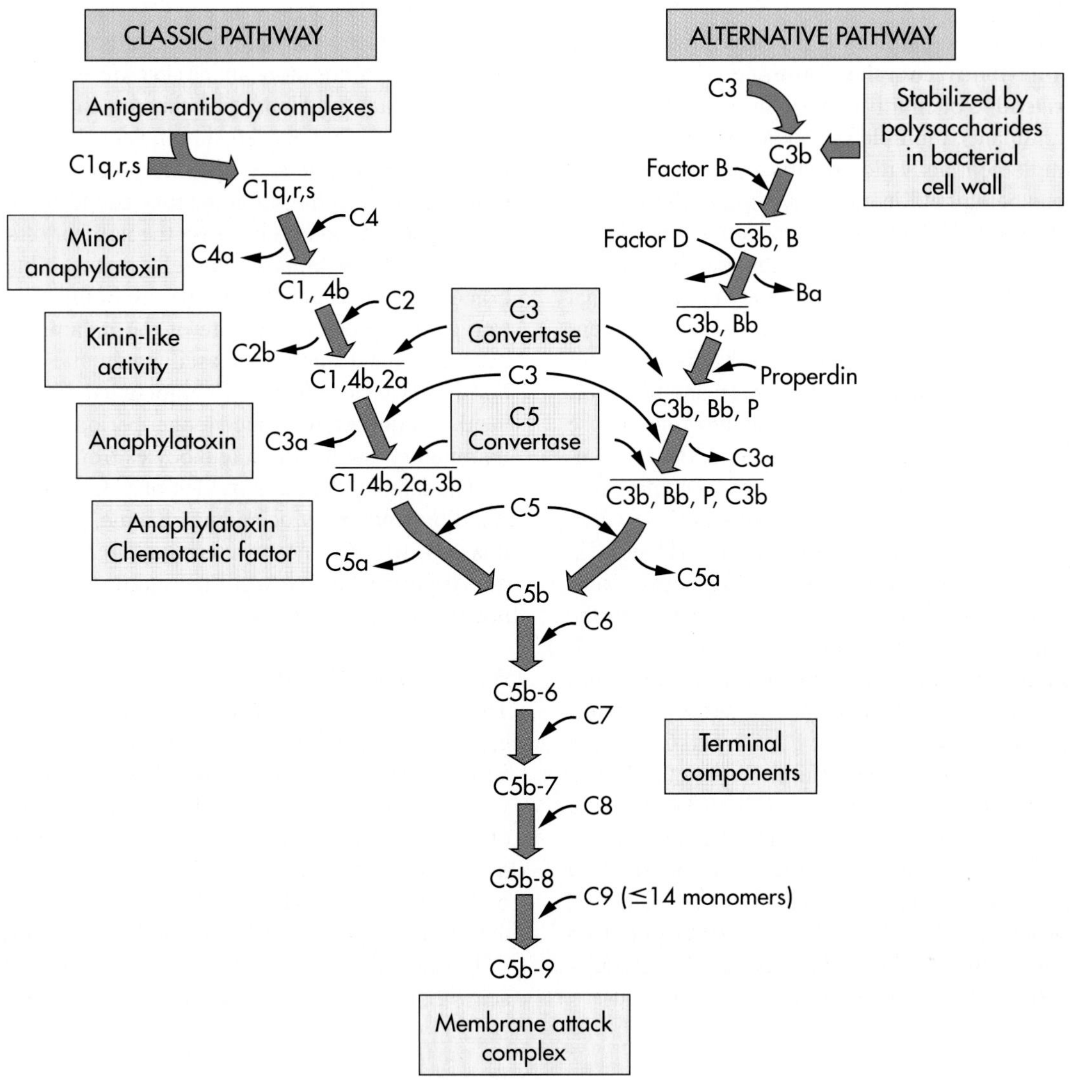

FIG. 7-7 Pathways of activation of the complement cascade. Complement components are cleaved into fragments, or subcomponents (denoted by lowercase letters), during activation. Many of the subcomponents are biochemical mediators of inflammation. The larger activated fragment is usually converted into an active enzyme (indicated by the bar above the fragment) and forms a complex with the preceding components in the cascade. By one nomenclature, the small fragments are the "a" fragments, and the large fragments are the "b" fragments (e.g., C3b is the larger fragment from C3 and Bb is the activated form of factor B), although historically the small C2 fragment has been designated the "b" fragment, as indicated here. The classic pathway is usually activated by antigen-antibody complexes through component C1, whereas the alternative pathway is activated by many agents, such as bacterial polysaccharides, through component C3b. Both pathways produce C3 convertases and C5 convertases, which are enzymatically active complexes that activate C3 and C5, respectively.

tein systems (see Fig. 7-12). The complement system is a nonspecific mechanism of self-defense. Even when it is activated by a specific mechanism, namely, antigen-antibody complexes (the immune system), it mediates inflammation, which is nonspecific. Thus proteins of the complement system (sometimes called *complement components*) are among the body's most potent defenders against bacterial infection.

The two principal routes by which the **complement cascade** is activated are shown in Fig. 7-7. The **classic pathway** is activated when an antigen-antibody complex containing immunoglobulin (IgG or IgM) interacts with the first component of the complement cascade, C1.[5] The **alternative pathway** can be activated by several biologic substances, chiefly bacterial and fungal cell wall polysaccharides (especially endotoxin on gram-negative bacteria). (Bacterial endotoxins are described in Chapter 2.)

Activation of components C1 through C5 produces subunits that enhance inflammation by (1) opsonizing bacteria, (2) attracting leukocytes by chemotaxis, and (3) acting as **anaphylatoxins,** that is, inducing degranulation of mast cells. Components C6 through C9 form complexes capable of creating pores in plasma membranes. The pores permit the influx of water and ions and destruction of the cell. (Cellular injury is discussed in Chapter 2.)

Classic Pathway

Activation of the classic pathway is preceded by formation of an **antigen-antibody complex (immune complex).** Because antigens tend to be multivalent (to have more than one antigenic determinant), multiple antibodies are bound in the complex. Complement activation occurs as a result of antibody Fc regions being held in close proximity. The Fc contains a site that binds C1. The first component of the classic complement cascade, C1, has six sites that can bind to the Fc region and is "fixed" to adjacent antibody molecules that are attached to the antigen. The complex formed by antigen-antibody–complement binding is shown in Fig. 7-8. C1 consists of several subcomponents, including C1q and two molecules each of C1r and C1s. C1r is an enzyme whose substrate is C1s. After binding two Fc regions, the C1q undergoes a conformational change resulting in C1r coming into proximity with C1s. C1r enzymatically activates C1s, which becomes an active enzyme whose substrates are C4 and C2.

Activation of C1 results in the sequential enzymatic activation of all other components of the cascade. Although the cascade continues through the terminal components C6, C7, C8, and C9, the importance of the complement system resides in the activities of the small fragments, or subcomponents, generated during the activation of C4, C2, C3, and C5. C3b, a subcomponent that adheres to the surface of a target cell (e.g., bacterium), is an efficient opsonin. C4a, C2b, C3a, and C5a, which are soluble, low-molecular-weight fragments, are potent activators of the acute inflammatory response. C2b affects smooth muscle, causing vasodilation and increased vascular permeability. C3a, C5a, and to a limited extent C4a are anaphylatoxins; that is, they induce the rapid degranulation of mast cells, with release of histamine (see Fig. 7-4).

The anaphylatoxins C3a and C5a, small polypeptides, are also chemotactic for neutrophils, although C5a is approximately 1000 times more anaphylatoxic and chemotactic than C3a. The dual functions, as a chemotaxic factor and an anaphylatoxin, are not needed simultaneously or to the same degree. Anaphylatoxic activity is necessary early in inflammation and close to the inflammatory site to induce local mast cell degranulation and increase the number of soluble mediators available to enhance vascular permeability. Degranulation of mast cells away from the site of injury would be contrary to the protective nature of the inflammatory response because the substances released would affect healthy neighboring tissues needlessly. Chemotactic activity, on the other hand, is required for a much longer period and distal to the inflammatory site to attract leukocytes from the circulation.

The anaphylatoxic activities of C3a and C5a are inactivated by a naturally occurring enzyme, plasma carboxypeptidase B, which removes a terminal arginine, producing C3a des Arg and C5a des Arg. The removal of the arginine does not affect chemotactic activity.

Alternative Pathway

There is also a nonantibody-mediated (alternative) avenue of entrance into the complement cascade (see Fig. 7-7). The alternative pathway begins with C3b. C3 is spontaneously activated by a number of naturally occurring enzymes. The rate of activation is generally very low, and C3b is usually bound by a complement regulatory protein, factor H, and destroyed by factor I, both of which are found normally in the blood. In the presence of materials such as bacterial polysaccharides, C3b is protected from destruction. The protected C3b can react with another normally occurring component, factor B. The

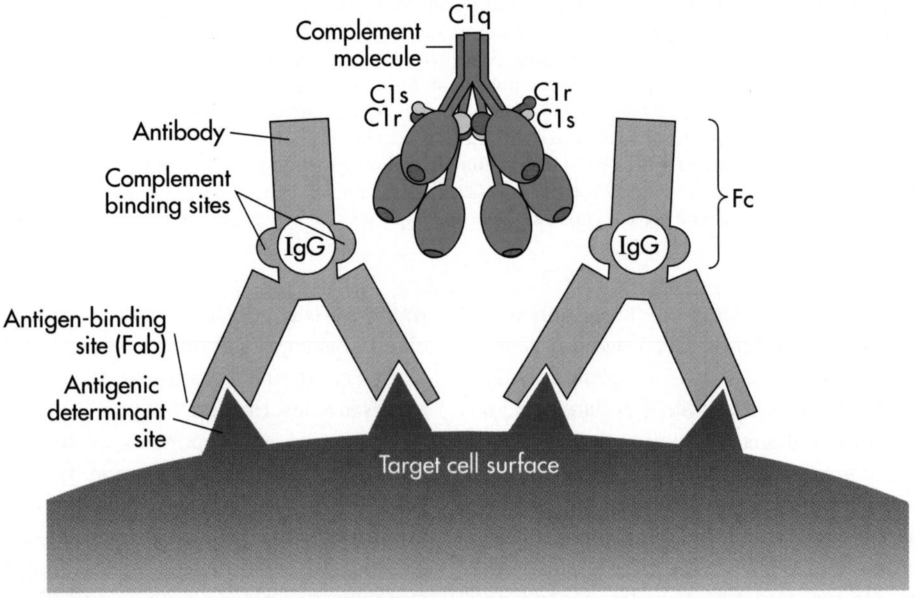

FIG. 7-8 Activation of the first component of complement (C1). It takes two IgG molecules to activate one complement component. Activation of complement cannot occur unless (1) antigen-antibody binding has occurred, placing two Fc regions of the antibody molecule into close proximity; and (2) the complement component can span the gap between two adjacent Fc portions.

complex of C3b and factor B is recognized by an enzyme, factor D, that activates factor B. The resultant C3b,Bb complex is very unstable unless it binds properdin (P). The C3b,Bb,P complex is a C3 convertase (a molecular complex that has C3 as a substrate). The activation of C3 results in a C3b,Bb,P,C3b complex that functions as a C5 convertase. With the activation of C5 the two pathways have joined.

Clotting System

The clotting (coagulation) system is a plasma protein system that forms a fibrinous meshwork at the inflamed site to trap exudates, microorganisms, and foreign bodies. This (1) prevents the spread of infection and inflammation to adjacent tissues, (2) keeps microorganisms and foreign bodies at the site of greatest phagocytic activity, and (3) forms a clot that stops bleeding and provides a framework for future repair and healing. The main substance in this fibrinous mesh is an insoluble protein called *fibrin* that is the end product of the coagulation cascade.

Like the complement cascade, the coagulation cascade can be activated through two different pathways that converge at the point where each pathway produces the same substance (Fig. 7-9). In the complement cascade the classic and alternative pathways converge when each has activated C5 (see Fig. 7-7). In the coagulation cascade the **extrinsic pathway** and the **intrinsic pathway** converge at factor X. From that point the cascade proceeds on a common pathway until fibrin is formed. (The coagulation cascade is discussed further and illustrated in Chapter 24.)

The clotting system can be activated by many substances released during tissue destruction and infection, including collagen, proteases, kallikrein, plasmin, and bacterial endotoxins. In addition, activation of the clotting cascade produces subcomponents that enhance the inflammatory response. The two low-molecular-weight fibrinopeptides released from fibrinogen during fibrin production (especially fibrinopeptide B) are chemotactic for neutrophils and increase vascular permeability by enhancing the effects of bradykinin (formed from the kinin system).

Kinin System

The third plasma protein system with a role in inflammation is the kinin system. The primary kinin is **bradykinin,** which, at low doses, causes dilation of vessels, acts with prostaglandins to induce pain, causes extravascular smooth muscle contraction, increases vascular permeability, and may increase leukocyte chemotaxis. Bradykinin induces smooth muscle contraction more slowly than histamine and may be more important during the prolonged phase of inflammation. Bradykinin, along with prostaglandins of the E series, is probably responsible for endothelial cell retraction and increased vascular permeability in the later phases of inflammation (endothelial cell retraction is shown in Fig. 7-3).

The kinin system is activated by stimulation of the **plasma kinin cascade** (Fig. 7-10). The conversion of plasma prekallikrein to kallikrein is induced by *prekallikrein activator* that is identical with activated of Hageman factor (factor XIIa). Kallikrein then converts kininogen to kinin, the primary kinin being bradykinin. Another source of kinin is the tissue kallikreins in saliva, sweat, tears, urine, and feces. These kallikreins convert serum kininogens to kallidin (Lys-bradykinin), which may be converted to bradykinin by plasma aminopeptidase. Kinins are rapidly degraded and therefore controlled by kininases, which are enzymes present in plasma and tissues.

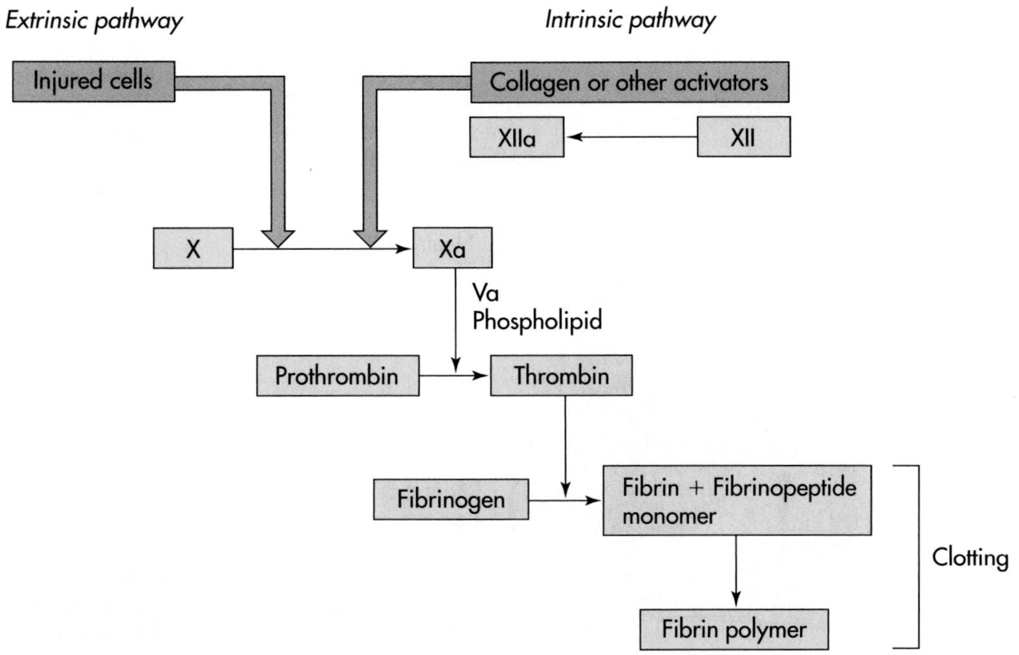

FIG. 7-9 Coagulation cascade. During activation of the coagulation cascade, several components are converted from inactive to active forms. The active components are designated with an "a."

Control and Interaction of Plasma Protein Systems

The activation of the plasma protein systems involved in inflammation produces a large number of very potent, biologically active substances that protect the host from infection. Control of this process is essential for two reasons:

1. The inflammatory process is so important for protection that its activation must be guaranteed; therefore there are multiple means of initiating inflammation.
2. The activities of the biochemical mediators generated during this process are so potent and potentially detrimental to the host that their actions must be confined to injured or infected tissues; therefore multiple mechanisms are available to inactivate or regulate the inflammatory mediators.

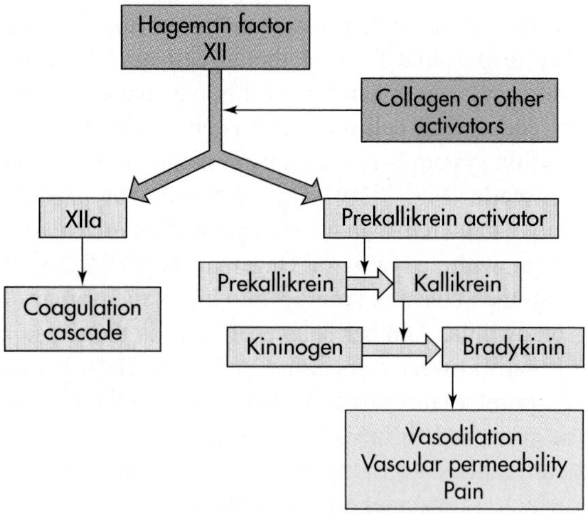

FIG. 7-10 Plasma kinin cascade.

Control is apparent at many levels. Many components of inflammation are rapidly destroyed within seconds by enzymes from the plasma. Two components of the complement cascade, C3a and C5a, are inactivated by the plasma enzyme *carboxypeptidase,* and histamine and leukotrienes are inactivated by the eosinophilic enzymes *histaminase* and *arylsulfatase.* Many other natural inhibitors are present, including antagonists for histamine, kinins, complement components, kallikrein, and plasmin.

Histamine activity is controlled in part by histamine receptors on the host's target cells.[6,7] At least two types of receptors exist for histamine: H1 and H2 receptors (Fig. 7-11). The H1 receptor is responsible for promoting inflammation, whereas inflammation is generally inhibited through the H2 receptor by suppression of leukocytes function and mast cell degranulation. The H1 receptor is present on cells of smooth muscle, especially those of the bronchi, and causes bronchial smooth muscle to contract (bronchoconstriction) when stimulated. The H2 receptor is especially abundant on parietal cells of the stomach mucosa and induces the secretion of gastric acids on stimulation. The distribution of both types of receptors is variable, and frequently they are present on the same cells and may act in an antagonistic fashion. For instance, both receptors are present on neutrophils. Stimulation of H1 receptors results in the augmentation of chemotaxis, whereas H2 stimulation results in its inhibition. The role of H1 and H2 receptors is discussed further in Chapter 8.

Most of the control processes interact, so that the activation or control of one plasma system results in a similar effect on others (Fig. 7-12). Plasmin controls clot formation (by degrading fibrin and fibrinogen) and activates the complement cascade through C1, C3, and C5, as does thrombin.

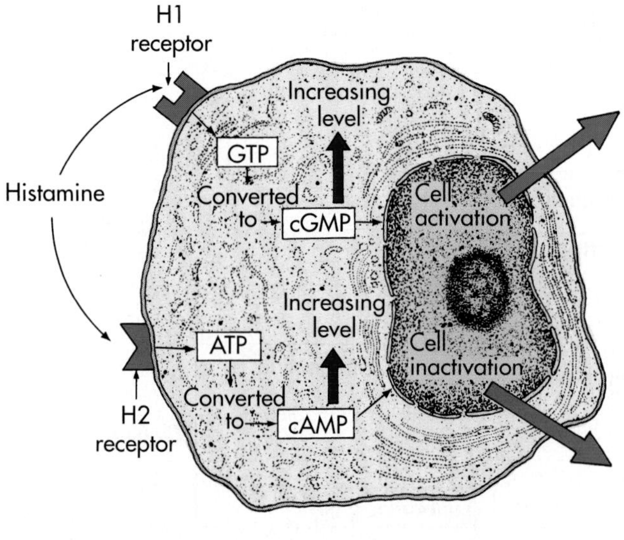

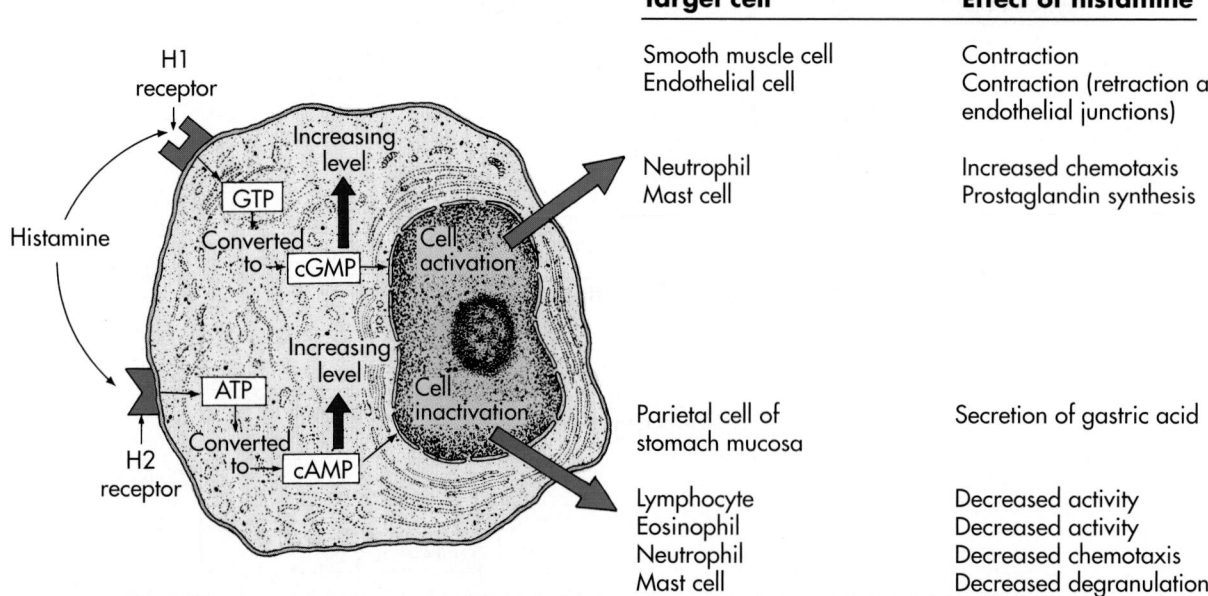

Target cell	Effect of histamine
Smooth muscle cell	Contraction
Endothelial cell	Contraction (retraction at endothelial junctions)
Neutrophil	Increased chemotaxis
Mast cell	Prostaglandin synthesis
Parietal cell of stomach mucosa	Secretion of gastric acid
Lymphocyte	Decreased activity
Eosinophil	Decreased activity
Neutrophil	Decreased chemotaxis
Mast cell	Decreased degranulation

FIG. 7-11 Effects of histamine through H1 and H2 receptors. Effects depend on (1) density and affinity of H1 or H2 receptors on the target cell and (2) the identity of the target cell. *GTP,* Guanosine triphosphate; *cGMP,* cyclic guanosine monophosphate; *ATP,* adenosine triphosphate; *cAMP,* cyclic adenosine monophosphate.

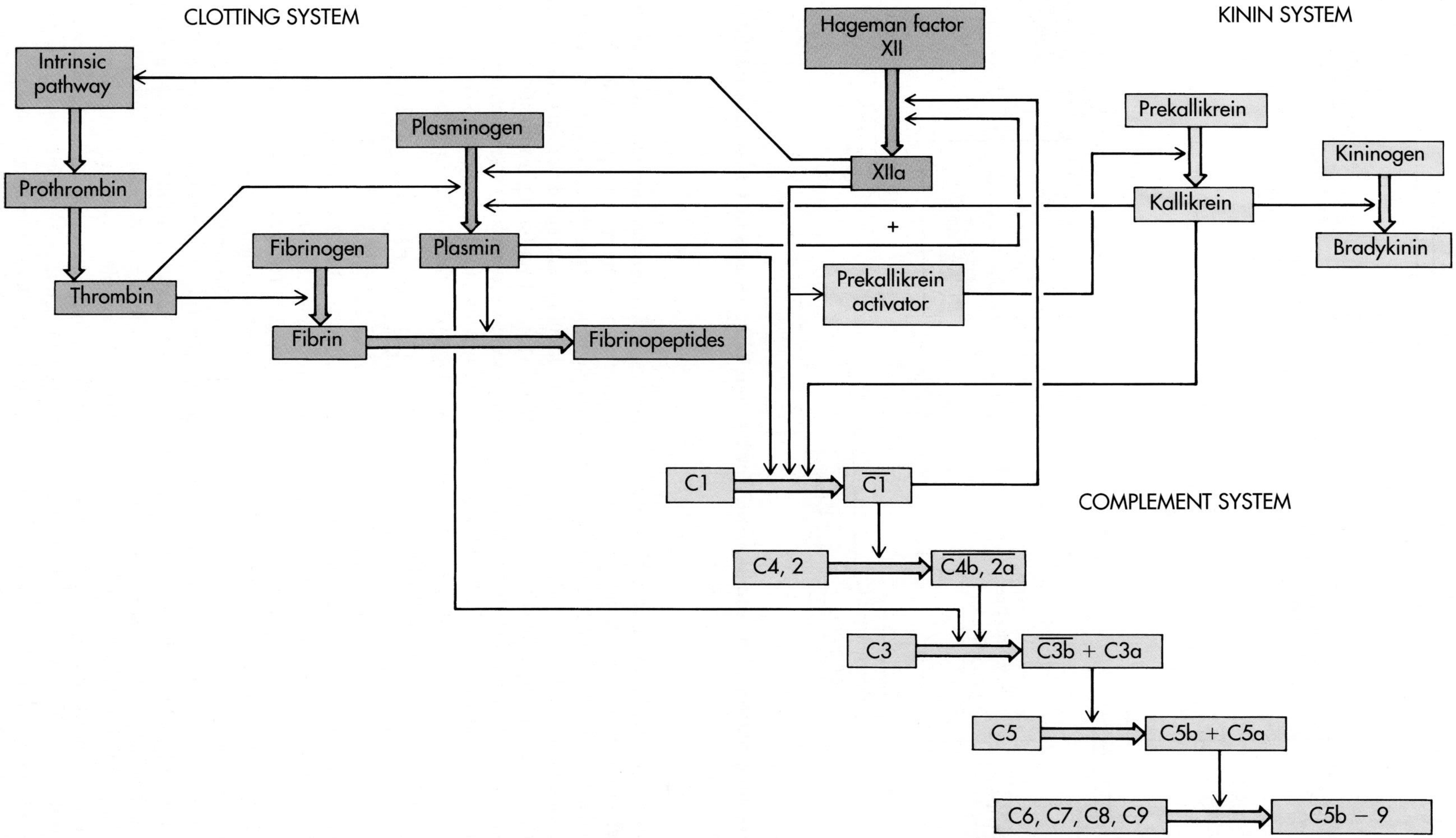

FIG. 7-12 Interaction of the complement, clotting, kinin, and fibrinolytic (plasmin) systems. *Thick arrows* denote the activation of factors within a system. *Thin arrows* denote where a particular factor activates another system.

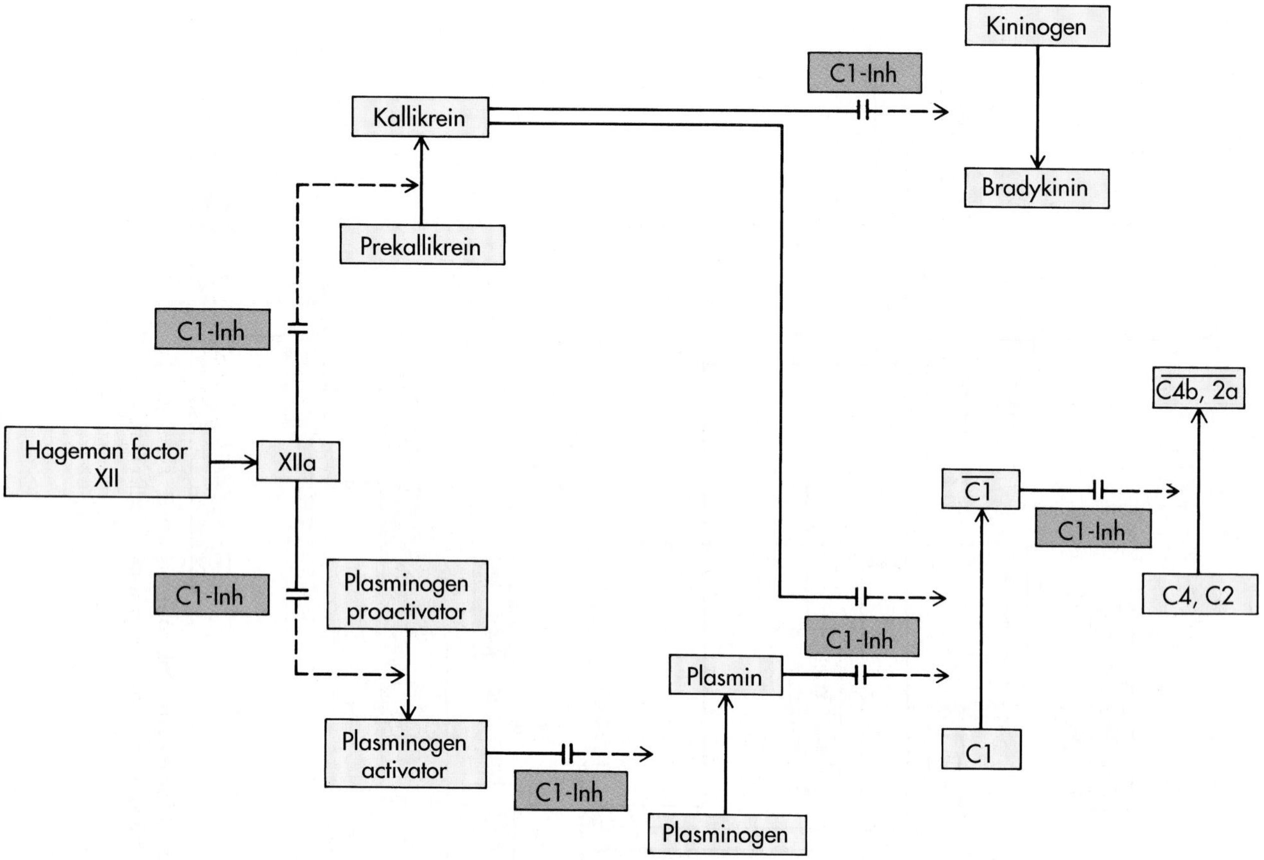

FIG. 7-13 Common control of the complement, clotting, and kinin systems by C1 esterase inhibitor (C1-Inh).

Plasmin also activates the plasma kinin cascade by activating Hageman factor and producing prekallikrein activator. The activation of Hageman factor has four effects: (1) activation of the clotting cascade through factor XI; (2) activation of the fibrinolytic systems through conversion of plasminogen proactivator to plasminogen activator, resulting in the generation of plasmin; (3) activation of the kinin system by a Hageman factor fragment, prekallikrein activator; and (4) activation of C1 in the complement cascade. Plasmin itself exists as a proenzyme, plasminogen, which is activated by several factors, including plasminogen activator generated from the kallikrein system; thrombin generated from the clotting system; bacterial factors, such as streptokinase (produced by hemolytic streptococci); plasminogen activators produced by endothelial cells; and several cellular enzymes released during tissue destruction.

The interaction of control mechanisms is exemplified by the effects of C1 esterase inhibitor.[8] Hereditary angioneurotic edema is an autosomal dominant disease characterized by a deficiency of C1 esterase inhibitor. In individuals with this disease, emotional stress and other stimuli frequently result in recurrent edema in the gastrointestinal tract, respiratory tract, and skin, with death occurring in some cases because of laryngeal swelling. The mechanism appears to be one of episodic, uncontrolled activation of plasmin, resulting in Hageman factor activation, bradykinin production, and C1 activation. C1 esterase inhibitor blocks several steps in the activation of all three cascades, including C1 esterase of the complement system, the effects of activated Hageman factor on the kinin system, and the effects of kallikrein and plasmin (Fig. 7-13). Activation of plasmin may be the most important single cause of hereditary angioneurotic edema, as indicated by the fact that attacks are prevented by ϵ-aminocaproic acid, which prevents the conversion of plasminogen to plasmin.

CELLULAR COMPONENTS OF INFLAMMATION

The two main classes of leukocytes to carry out inflammatory processes are the granulocytes and the monocytes/macrophages. The granulocytes, so-called because of the many enzyme-containing lysosomal granules in their cytoplasm, include the neutrophils, eosinophils, and basophils.[9] Monocytes (the immature forms in the blood) and macrophages (the mature cells in the tissues) have fewer and larger lysosomes in their cytoplasm than do granulocytes. All of these cells are phagocytes (capable of phagocytosis, the ingestion of unwanted matter), but the most important of the phagocytes are the neutrophils and macrophages. Lymphocytes also participate in inflammation, primarily by producing lymphokines.

Another cellular component important to inflammation is the platelet. Platelets are cytoplasmic fragments that circu-

WHAT'S NEW? Adhesion Molecules

Intercellular adhesion molecules (ICAMs) are membrane-bound proteins that allow cellular interaction. Cells can increase or decrease the number of ICAMs on their surface or change their affinity. There are several families of ICAMs, and they are found on vascular endothelium and leukocytes. Integrins are a group of protein adhesion molecules found on many cells and promote adhesion of leukocytes to endothelium and other immune cells. Selectins (types E, P, and L) are expressed on endothelium, platelets, and some leukocytes selectively bind to carbohydrate molecules. During inflammation, ICAMs control binding to leukocytes and platelets and migration of leukocytes in vascular and lymphoid tissue.

Data from Kerr JR: Cell adhesions molecules in the pathogenesis of and host defense against microbial infection, *Mol Pathol* 52(4):220, 1999; Roit I, Male D, Brostoff J: *Immunology,* ed 5, St Louis, 1998, Mosby.

late in the bloodstream until vascular injury occurs. After injury, platelets (1) interact with components of the coagulation cascade to stop bleeding and (2) degranulate, releasing biochemical mediators, such as serotonin, which has vascular effects similar to those of histamine. Their activation is stimulated by many products of inflammation, including collagen, platelet-activating factor (PAF) released from mast cells, and antigen-antibody complexes. (Platelet function is described in detail in Chapter 24.)

Endothelial Cells

Endothelial cell contraction in postcapillary venules and some capillaries leads to increased vascular permeability in inflammation. Histamine, bradykinin, leukotrienes, substance P, and prostaglandins stimulate this process.[10] Endothelial cells also express adhesion molecules (selectins) specific for leukocytes and platelets.[11] **Adhesion molecules** on leukocytes (selectins and integrins; see Chapter 1) promote interaction with the endothelial cells. The adhesion facilitates margination and transmigration of leukocytes across the endothelial cell and basement membrane into the area of inflammation (see Fig. 7-3).

Endothelial cells also release nitric oxide (NO) that causes vasodilation by relaxation of vascular smooth muscle. The response is local and of short duration. NO may also contribute to the regulation of inflammation by suppressing mast cell function and decreasing platelet adhesion and aggregation.[12]

Function of Phagocytes

The neutrophils and macrophages have essentially the same characteristics and functions. Each normally circulates in the bloodstream and is stimulated by inflammation to migrate through vessel walls near an inflammatory lesion. Once in the exudate, each is attracted to the lesion by specific chemotactic factors and kept there by the meshwork formed by fibrinous exudate. Once at the site, each type of cell phagocytoses (ingests) foreign or dead cells until its life span is over. The dead phagocyte then becomes part of the purulent exudate, or *pus,* which leaves the body through the lymphatic system or through the epithelium. Neutrophils and monocytes/macrophages differ chiefly in (1) the speed with which they arrive at the site, with the neutrophils arriving first; (2) the length of time they remain active, with the macrophages being longer lived; (3) the chemotactic factors capable of attracting them; (4) the enzymatic content of their lysosomes, or digestive vacuoles; and (5) their participation in the immune response, with the macrophages being involved in antigen processing and being responsive to lymphokines.

The phagocytes' role begins when the inflammatory response causes them to adhere to capillary and venule walls in a process called **margination,** or **pavementing** (Fig. 7-14). Margination is caused by increased stickiness of the phagocytes and increased adsorption by the endothelial cells lining the vessels as a result of the production of adhesion proteins on the surface of each cell.[13] This is followed by **diapedesis,** or emigration through the retracting endothelial junctions and the basement membrane and out into the surrounding tissues (see Fig. 7-3).

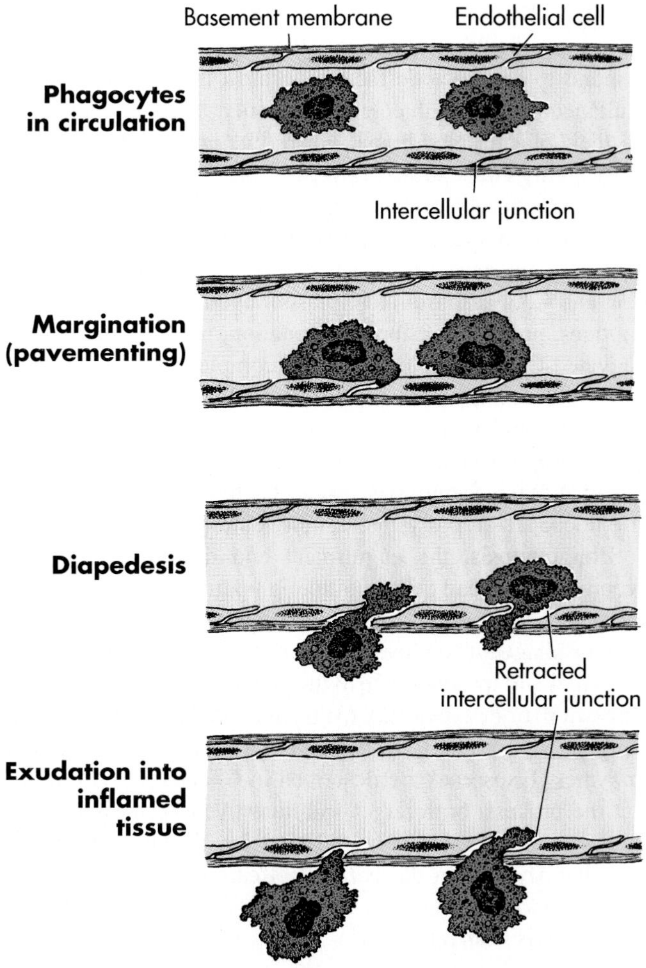

FIG. 7-14 Diapedesis of a phagocyte. Phagocytes are capable of ameboid movement, which allows them to squeeze through intercellular junctions and migrate to inflammatory lesions.

Once phagocytes enter the inflammatory exudate, they are attracted to the inflammatory site by chemotaxis. They respond to chemotactic factors because they can detect simultaneously, through chemoreceptors at multiple locations on their plasma membrane, where chemotactic factors are most highly concentrated (see Fig. 7-6). They then migrate in the direction of highest concentration. The primary chemotactic factors for neutrophils, eosinophils, and monocytes include many bacterial products, complement components C5a and C3a, kallikrein and plasminogen activator, fibrinopeptides, products of fibrin degradation, prostaglandins, the activated C567 complex from the complement system, the eosinophil and neutrophil chemotactic factors released from mast cells, and a monocyte chemotactic factor released from the neutrophil. Histamine, although not chemotactic itself, may facilitate chemotaxis. Some bacterial toxins, such as streptococcal streptolysins, inhibit neutrophil chemotaxis.

Phagocytosis, the engulfment and destruction of microorganisms, dead cells, and foreign particles, begins when the phagocytic cell enters the inflammatory site.[14] The process of phagocytosis involves four steps: (1) recognition of the target and its adherence to the phagocyte, (2) engulfment (ingestion, or endocytosis), (3) fusion with lysosomes within the phagocyte, and (4) destruction of the target by lysosomal enzymes (lysosomes are described in Chapter 1). Throughout the process, both target and digestive enzymes are isolated within membrane-bound vesicles. Isolation protects the phagocyte from the harmful effects of target microorganisms and its own enzymes. Phagocytosis of an opsonized bacterium is illustrated in Fig. 7-15.

Most phagocytes can trap and engulf bacteria that have not been "coated" with an opsonin, but the process is slow and inefficient. Opsonization, usually by antibody or complement component C3b, greatly enhances both recognition and binding (also called *adherence*). Opsonins function as "glue" between the phagocyte and the target cell because receptors on the phagocyte are specific for sites on the opsonin (Fc receptors for antibody, C3b receptors for C3b). This enables the phagocyte to bind opsonized bacteria very tightly to its surface. Although antibody forms a stronger attachment, C3b facilitates phagocytosis to a greater extent.

Engulfment is carried out by small pseudopods that extend from the plasma membrane and surround the adhered microorganism (Fig. 7-16), forming an intracellular phagocytic vacuole, or **phagosome.** The membrane that surrounds the phagosome consists of inverted plasma membrane. After the formation of the phagosome, lysosomes converge, fuse with the phagosome, and discharge their contents, creating a **phagolysosome.** Destruction of the bacterium takes place within the phagolysosome (see Fig. 7-15).

Phagocytosis is accompanied by a burst of metabolic activity in the phagocyte, resulting in the conversion of much of glucose metabolism to the hexose-monophosphate shunt and production of several oxygen-containing molecules that are reactive and highly damaging to cells. This is known as an *oxygen-dependent killing mechanism.* The principal oxygen-dependent mechanism of killing is hydrogen peroxide, especially in conjunction with the lysosomal enzyme *myeloperoxidase* and halide anions (I^-, Cl^-, and Br^-). Myeloperoxidase probably kills by iodination or the formation of toxic chlor-

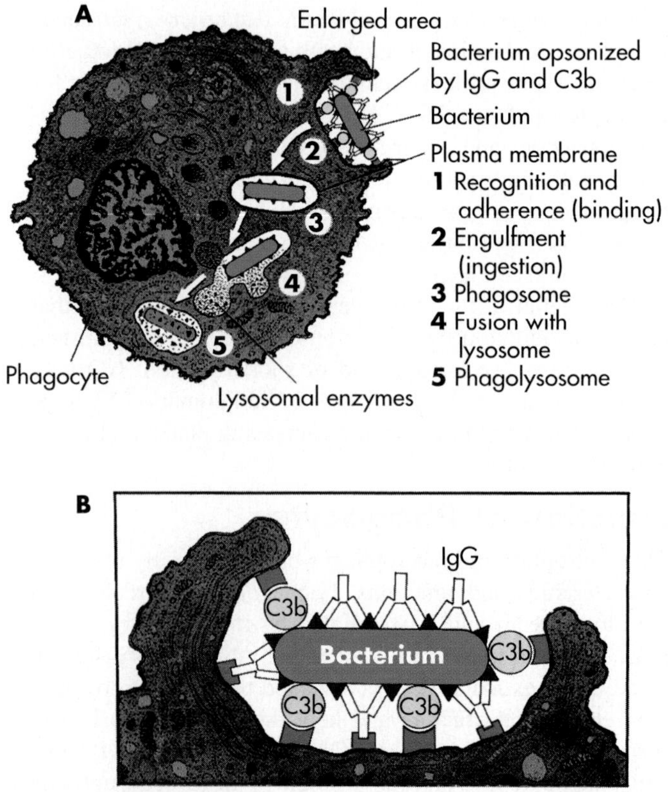

FIG. 7-15 Phases of phagocytosis. A, Opsonized microorganisms bind to the surface of a phagocyte *(1)* and are ingested *(2)* into a phagocytic vacuole, or phagosome *(3)*. Lysosomes fuse with the phagosome *(4),* releasing their digestive enzymes into the vacuole. This results in the formation of a phagolysosome *(5),* within which the microorganism is killed and digested. **B,** Enlargement showing bacterium opsonization. *IgG,* Immunoglobulin G; *C3b,* complement component.

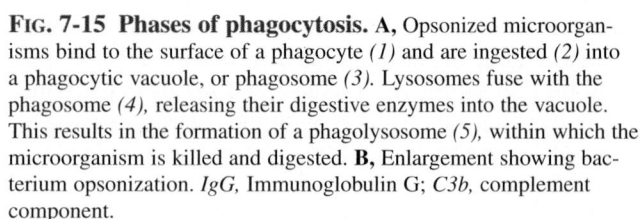

amines and aldehydes on the target cell's surface. The oxygen-independent mechanisms of killing are (1) acid pH (3.5 to 4.0) of the phagolysosome caused by lactic acid production; (2) the cationic proteins, which bind to and damage target cell membranes; (3) lysozyme and elastase, which attack mucopeptides in the target cell wall; and (4) lactoferrin, which inhibits bacterial growth by binding iron.

When the phagocyte dies at the inflammatory site, it lyses (breaks open) and its cytoplasmic contents, including the lysosomal enzymes, are released. Enzymes released from lysosomes can digest the connective tissue matrix, causing much of the tissue destruction associated with inflammation. α_1-Antitrypsin, a plasma protein produced by the liver, inhibits the destructive effects of many enzymes released by dead phagocytes. An inherited deficiency of α_1-antitrypsin often results in chronic lung damage and emphysema as a result of inflammation. (The pulmonary effects of α_1-antitrypsin deficiency are described in Chapter 32.)

Released lysosomal products contribute to other aspects of inflammation. These include increased vascular permeability, chemotaxis for monocytes, breakdown of connective tissues, and activation of the complement and kinin systems.

Polymorphonuclear Neutrophils

The **neutrophil,** or **polymorphonuclear neutrophil (PMN),** is the predominant phagocytic cell in the early inflammatory response, entering the inflammatory site within 6 to 12 hours after the initial injury. Neutrophils arrive first because they are attracted by the immediately generated chemotactic factors, such as complement fragments. Macrophages and lymphocytes, on the other hand, enter the site later, usually after 24 hours, and gradually replace the neutrophils.

Because the neutrophil is a mature cell incapable of division and is sensitive to the acidic environment of inflammatory lesions, it is short lived in the inflammatory site. The primary roles of the neutrophil are removal of debris in sterile lesions, such as burns, and phagocytosis of bacteria in nonsterile lesions.

Monocytes and Macrophages

The **monocyte** is the largest normal blood cell (14 to 20 μm in diameter). Its nucleus is usually indented or horseshoe shaped. It is produced in the bone marrow, enters the circulation, and migrates to the inflammatory site, where it develops into a macrophage. The **macrophage** is generally larger (20 to 40 μm) and is a more active phagocyte than the

A

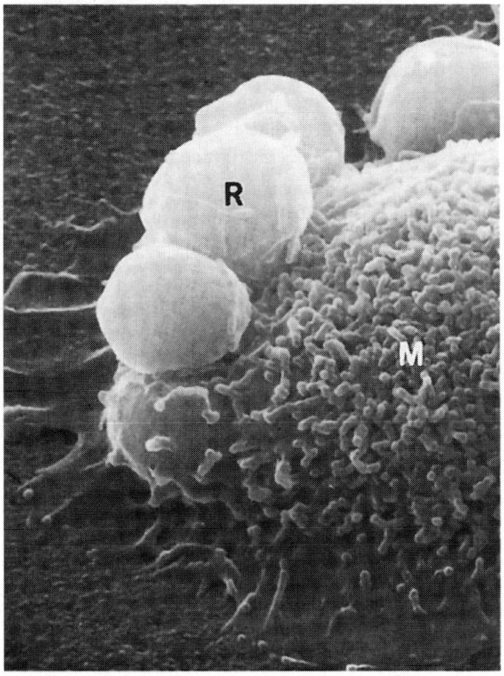

B

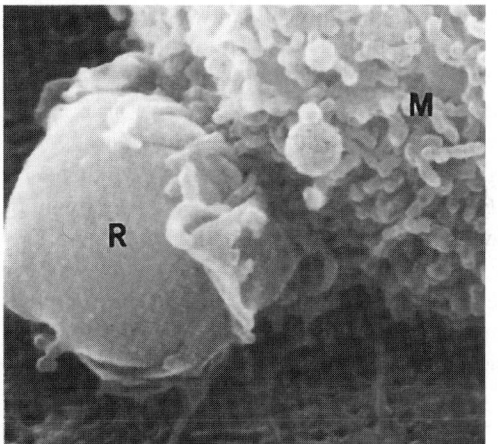

C

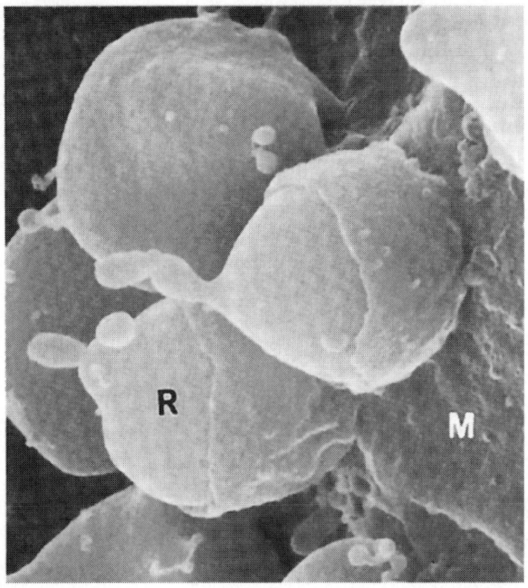

FIG. 7-16 Steps in phagocytosis. This scanning electron micrograph shows the progressive steps in phagocytosis. **A,** Red blood cells *(R)* attach to the surface of a macrophage *(M).* **B,** Part of macrophage *(M)* membrane starts to enclose the red cell *(R).* **C,** The red blood cells are almost totally engulfed by the macrophage. (From King DW, Fenoglio CM, Lefwitch JH: *General pathology: principles and dynamics,* Philadelphia, 1983, Lea & Febiger.)

monocyte (see Fig. 7-16). Monocytes also appear to be the precursors of macrophages that are fixed in tissues (tissue macrophages), including Kupffer cells of the liver and alveolar macrophages of the lungs. (Tissue macrophages are discussed in Chapter 6.)

Macrophage and lymphocyte infiltration characterizes chronic rather than acute inflammation. Macrophages may appear at the inflammatory site soon after the initial neutrophil infiltration (within 24 hours of injury) but usually arrive 3 to 7 days later. They migrate to the site slowly because (1) many of the chemotactic factors that attract them, such as macrophage chemotactic factor, are released by neutrophils and (2) monocytes, the immature macrophages, move somewhat sluggishly.

Macrophages are better suited than neutrophils to long-term defense against infectious agents because macrophages can survive and divide in the acidic inflammatory site, whereas neutrophils cannot. Macrophages also can fuse into larger cells capable of phagocytosing larger targets.

Macrophages have several roles in inflammation and immunity. They are responsive to the soluble products (lymphokines) secreted by T cells, participate in activating the immune response by processing antigen for presentation to lymphocytes (see Fig. 6-19), and are a source of a soluble factor (colony-stimulating factor) that stimulates the growth and differentiation of granulocytes and monocytes in the bone marrow. Macrophages also secrete substances that promote regrowth of tissues during wound healing.

Several bacteria can survive and even thrive inside macrophages. Microorganisms such as *Mycobacterium tuberculosis, Mycobacterium leprae, Salmonella typhi, Brucella abortus,* and *Listeria monocytogenes* can remain dormant or multiply inside the phagolysosomes of macrophages. This occurrence is prevented or ameliorated with the help of the immune system, which is active by the time macrophages have infiltrated the inflammatory site (see Fig. 7-5). Macrophages are further activated, or "turned on," by lymphokines secreted by T cells. Lymphokines increase the killing capacity of the macrophage by increasing its phagocytic activity, size, plasma membrane area, glucose metabolism, and number of lysosomes (Fig. 7-17).

Failure of macrophages to turn on has been traced to defective T cell responses to certain microorganisms. For example, a form of leprosy called *lepromatous leprosy* is characterized by the survival of *M. leprae* that have been phagocytosed by macrophages. In individuals with lepromatous leprosy, T cells fail to secrete the lymphokines needed to transform the macrophages into cells more highly dedicated to killing.

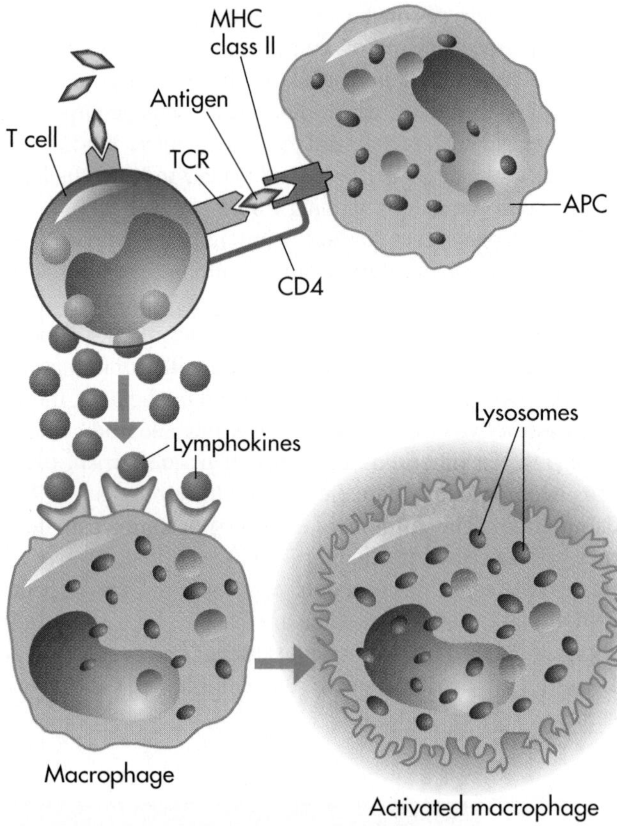

FIG. 7-17 Activation of a macrophage by a lymphokine (macrophage-activating factor [MAF]). Lymphokine is produced by T cells that have been stimulated by an antigen. The ruffled plasma membrane indicates macrophage activation. *APC,* Antigen-presenting cell; *TCR,* T cell receptor.

Eosinophils

Eosinophils are granulocytes that have large numbers of lysosomes containing (1) biochemical mediators that control the vascular effects of serotonin and histamine and (2) a caustic protein that is capable of dissolving the surface membranes of parasites.[15,16] Eosinophils do not phagocytose parasites, many of which are multicellular organisms. Rather, they bind to and degranulate onto the parasite, damaging its surface. This is preceded by the processes shown in Fig. 7-18.

IgE is the chief immunoglobulin involved in allergic hypersensitivity reactions, which are usually detrimental to the host (see Chapter 8). IgE also mediates normal defenses against some pathogenic organisms (see Fig. 7-5). Multicellular parasites, particularly worms, elicit an IgE-mediated allergic response that benefits the host by destroying the parasite. As in allergic reaction, IgE mediates degranulation of mast cells in the presence of soluble antigens. Degranulation releases eosinophil chemotactic factor of anaphylaxis (ECF-A), which attracts eosinophils to the site of parasitic infestation. ECF-A also induces the eosinophil to increase the density of its membrane receptors for opsonins, including complement component C3b and the Fc portions of IgG and IgE. The increased density of receptors for these opsonins enables the eosinophil to bind very tightly to the parasite. The eosinophil is unable to phagocytose the large parasite. Instead of ingesting the organism and enclosing it in a phagolysosome, the eosinophil's lysosomal granules migrate to the surface of the eosinophil and discharge their contents, including highly caustic cationic proteins and major basic protein, onto the parasite's outer membrane. This causes extensive damage to the parasite, and the tight fit between the eosinophil and its target prevents lysosomal contents from damaging neighboring host tissues.

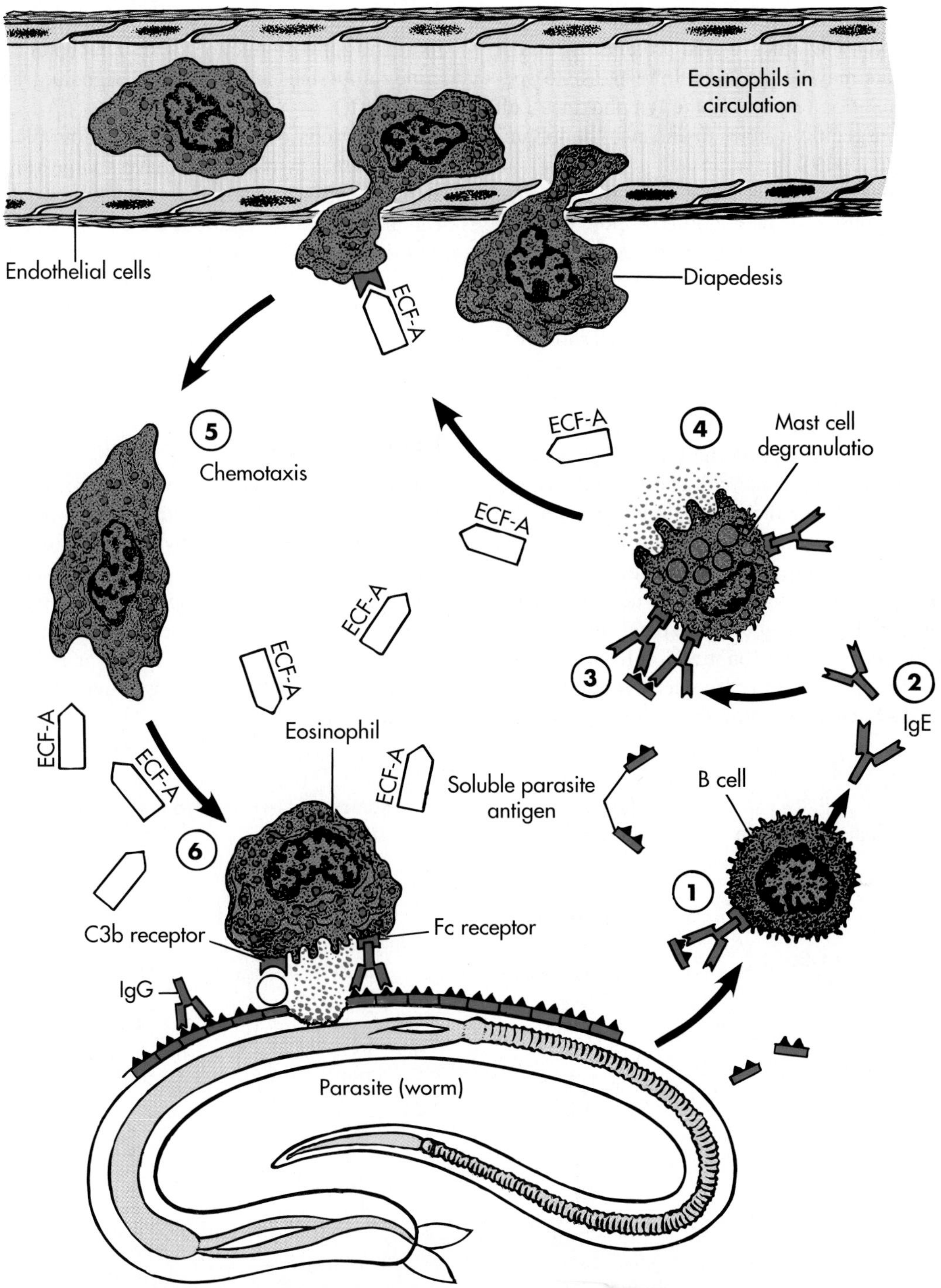

FIG. 7-18 IgE-mediated destruction of a parasite by an eosinophil. Soluble antigen from a parasite binds to an IgE-bearing B cell *(1),* stimulating the B cell to produce IgE *(2),* which binds to Fc receptors on a mast cell. Soluble antigen also binds to IgE on the mast cell *(3),* causing the mast cell to degranulate *(4).* Eosinophil chemotactic factor of anaphylaxis *(ECF-A)* released from the mast cell granules attracts eosinophils out of the circulation and toward the site of inflammation *(5).* IgG and complement component C3b are the opsonins that bind the eosinophil to the parasite. Once bound to the parasite, the eosinophil tries to ingest it and in the process releases its lysosomal enzymes onto the parasite, damaging its outer membrane *(6).*

CELLULAR PRODUCTS

Some host cells produce soluble factors that contribute to nonspecific mechanisms of defense by affecting other, neighboring host cells. In general, these factors are referred to as *cytokines,* but they have been subdivided into *monokines* (produced by macrophages) or *lymphokines* (produced by lymphocytes). (Cytokines are also discussed in Chapter 6.) This division is artificial because most cytokines are also produced by other cells, such as endothelial cells, fibroblasts, and mast cells. The majority of cytokines that are relevant to immunology and inflammation are grouped into interleukins, interferons, and a few other related proteins. Although some of these factors may be produced in response to specific antigenic stimulation (especially the lymphokines), all of them act in a nonspecific manner to enhance the inflammatory response (Fig. 7-19).

Many cells cooperate in producing an effective immune or inflammatory response. The interactions of those cells are governed by cytokines that are produced by cells, secreted from those cells, bind to appropriate target cells, and produce an appropriate response in those stimulated cells. Although most of the effects of cytokines are over short distances (e.g., between cells that are in contact), some effects are mediated over long distances within the body (e.g., the induction of fever by cytokines that are produced at an inflammatory site and act directly on the brain). The specific binding of cytokines to a particular cell is mediated through specific receptors, which are themselves under the regulation of cytokines. For instance, as discussed in Chapter 6, helper T cells (Th) are influenced by interleukin-1 (IL-1) produced by antigen-presenting cells. IL-1 acts in a paracrine manner and mediates neighboring Th cell function by binding to specific IL-1 receptors on the Th cell surface. The Th cell responds by production of another cytokine, interleukin-2 (IL-2). IL-2 acts in an autocrine manner, binding to IL-2 receptors on the same Th cell. The Th cell responds by increasing the production of IL-2 receptor and IL-2. (Paracrine, autocrine, and endocrine signaling are discussed in Chapter 1.)

The actions of cytokines are pleiotropic. This indicates that the same cytokine may have a large variety of different biologic activities depending on the particular target cell to which it binds. In addition, the same cytokine may be produced by a large spectrum of cells, many of which are not part of the immune system. Cytokines may be synergistic (so that their combined activity exceeds the sum of their individual activities) or antagonistic (so that they inhibit each other). A partial list of relevant cytokines is provided in Table 6-7.

Interleukins

The **interleukins (ILs)** are biochemical messengers produced by macrophages or lymphocytes in response to stimulation by an antigen or by products of inflammation.[17,18] Chapter 6 discusses one function of this series of hormones, namely, to enhance the response of lymphocytes and other cells to antigens and other foreign substances. Interleukins, however, are produced by a large variety of cells and have effects on many other cells, frequently independent of antigen stimulation.

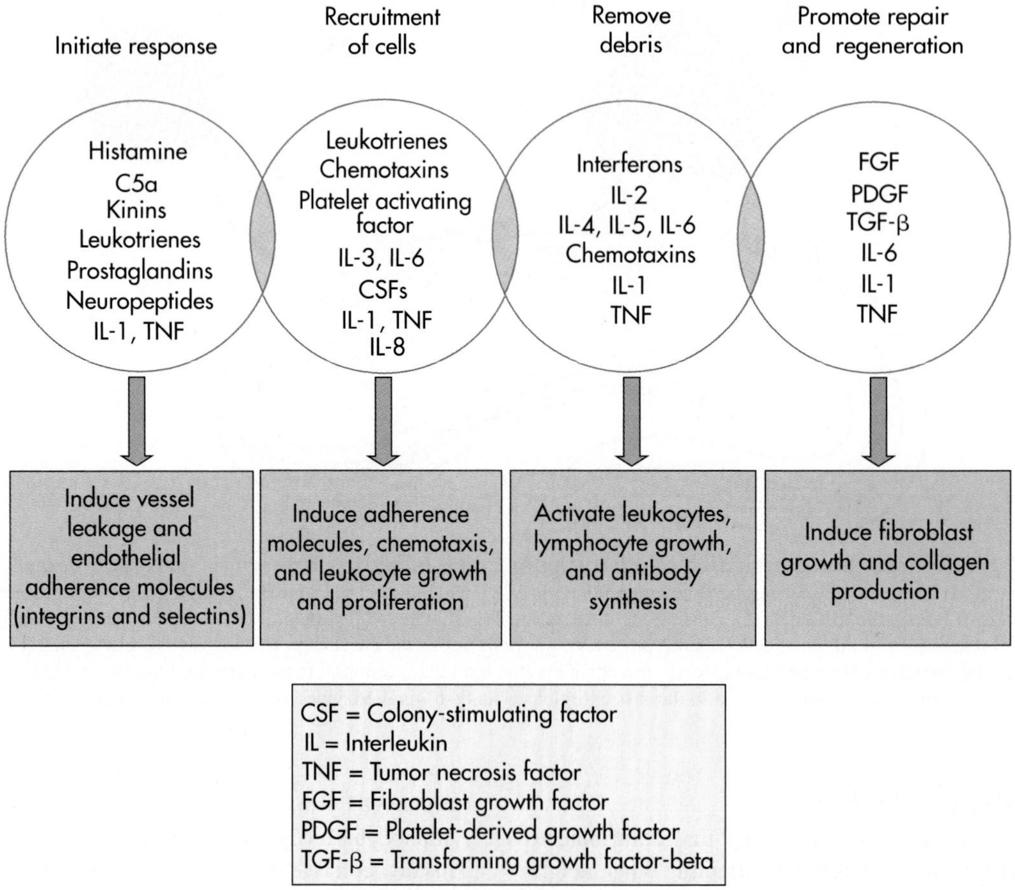

FIG. 7-19 Mediators associated with stages of inflammation. The stages of inflammation overlap and can be concurrent.

IL-1 is produced mostly by macrophages and antigen-presenting cells that have been stimulated by substances associated with tissue injury, including bacteria, endotoxins (bacterial pyrogens), interferon, antigen-antibody complexes, and antigen.[19] IL-1 is a lymphocyte-activating factor that, among other functions, probably augments antibody production by enhancing the production of IL-2 by T helper cells (see Chapter 6). Macrophage-produced IL-1 promotes the growth and function of almost every cell on which it has been tested. It has several effects on neutrophils, including induction of neutrophilia (proliferation that increases the number of circulating neutrophils), chemotaxis, increased hexose-monophosphate shunt activity (i.e., cellular metabolism), and increased lysosomal enzyme activity.

Many other interleukins (see Table 6-7) affect the expression of adhesion molecules by neutrophils and endothelial cells, are chemotactic for phagocytes or lymphocytes, induce the proliferation and release of white blood cells from the bone marrow, and generally enhance inflammation, independent of antigen stimulation.

Lymphokines

Lymphokines, which are produced by T cells in response to antigenic stimulation, are also biochemical mediators that affect other cells of the immune and inflammatory responses (see Fig. 7-5).[20] Although they are produced by cells of the immune system—a specific mechanism of self-defense—lymphokines have nonspecific effects. Many of the lymphokines have been identified as being members of the interleukin or interferon groups.

Different lymphokines have different effects. One lymphokine, called **migration-inhibitory factor (MIF),** is a glycoprotein that inhibits macrophage migration from the inflamed site. Another, **macrophage-activating factor (MAF),** increases the phagocytic activities of macrophages (see Fig. 7-17). MAF activity is most attributable to interferon-gamma (IFN-γ). At least three other lymphokines affect macrophages by causing chemotaxis, promoting maturation of monocytes into macrophages, enhancing macrophage migration along chemotactic gradients, and stimulating macrophages to aggregate or fuse into giant cells. Some lymphokines are chemotactic for the other phagocytes: neutrophils and eosinophils.

Other lymphokines affect lymphocytes, inducing them to produce more lymphokines, proliferate, or diminish their activities. Lymphokines called *lymphotoxins* are nonspecific killers of nonlymphocytes. Tumor necrosis factor–beta (TNF-β) is thought to be the primary constituent of lymphotoxin. A lymphokine called *transfer factor* is a ribonucleoprotein that, when extracted from leukocytes and inoculated into another individual, can transfer immunity from an immunocompetent donor to an immunoincompetent recipient and may be involved in the recruiting of other lymphocytes.

Chemokines

Chemokines are a family of low-molecular-weight (8 to 10 kDa) cytokines or peptides.[21] Most chemokines are either alpha chemokines or beta chemokines depending on their cysteine structure. These molecules are generally proinflammatory and affect a variety of leukocytes, inducing them to move (chemotaxis), grow, become activated, or release stored chemicals from intracellular storage granules (degranulation).[22] Alpha chemokines, such as interleukin 8 (IL-8) and epithelial-dermoid neutrophil attractant (ENA-78), are generally more chemotactic for neutrophils. For example, IL-8 is produced by macrophages, fibroblasts, and endothelial cells and induces migration and activation of neutrophils. Beta chemokines include RANTES, monocyte/macrophage chemotactic proteins (MCP-1, MCP-2, and MCP-3), and macrophage inflammatory proteins (MIP-1α and MIP-1β) and are generally more chemotactic for lymphocytes and monocytes. For instance, RANTES is produced by T cells, endothelial cells, and platelets during chronic inflammation and affects monocytes, natural killer (NK) cells, T cells, basophils, and eosinophils.[23]

Interferon

One of the body's defenses against viral infection is the production of interferon (IFN).[24] (Mechanisms of viral infection are described in Chapter 2.) Interferon does not kill viruses, but it can prevent them from infecting healthy cells. **Interferon** consists of small, low-molecular-weight proteins produced and released by host cells that have been invaded by a virus. Once released, interferon molecules attach themselves to receptors on neighboring host cells. If a neighboring cell is uninfected, the interferon stimulates it to produce an antiviral protein (Fig. 7-20). Interferon has no effect on a cell that is already infected by the virus.

Slightly different kinds of interferon are produced by different types of cells (e.g., neutrophils and macrophages release IFN-α and IFN-β, and T lymphocytes release IFN-γ). All types are host specific but not virus specific; therefore human interferon is effective only in humans, but it is effective against almost all viruses. IFN-α and IFN-β have anti-inflammatory functions, and IFN-γ is proinflammatory and enhances cell-mediated immunity.[25]

LOCAL MANIFESTATIONS OF INFLAMMATION

Because inflammation is a nonspecific defense mechanism, it generally proceeds in the same way, no matter what type of injury has occurred. All the local manifestations of acute inflammation are caused by vascular changes and exudation. Swelling occurs as exudate accumulates. Swelling is usually accompanied by pain caused by pressure exerted by exudate accumulation and the presence of soluble biochemical mediators, such as prostaglandins and bradykinin. Heat and redness are the result of vasodilation and increased perfusion (increased blood flow through the area).

The function of vascular changes and exudation is to deliver leukocytes, plasma proteins, and their biochemical mediators to the site of injury. Exudate and its contents have three functions: (1) to dilute toxins produced by bacteria and toxic products released by dying cells; (2) to carry plasma proteins (including antibody) and leukocytes (both

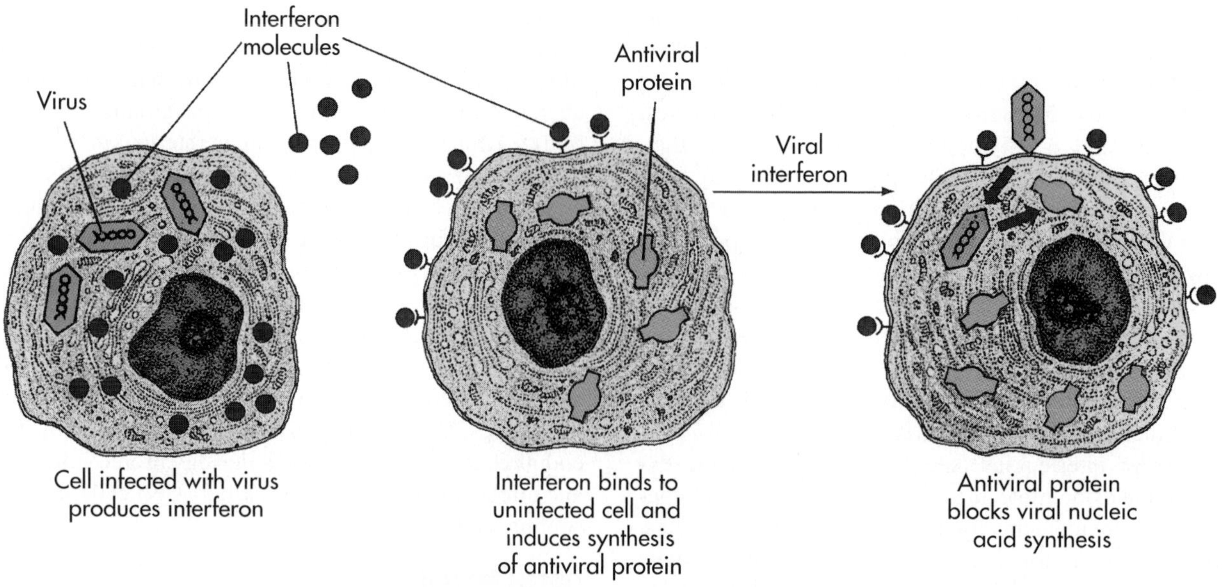

FIG. 7-20 The action of interferon.

phagocytes and lymphocytes) to the site; and (3) to carry away bacterial toxins, dead cells, debris, and other products of inflammation. This third function occurs via channels through the epithelium (sinuses) or through lymphatic vessels. Drainage by lymphatic vessels facilitates the immune response because antigens in lymphatic fluid pass through the lymph nodes, where they stimulate B lymphocytes to become antibody-producing plasma cells or T lymphocytes to become effector T cells. (The lymphatic system is described in Chapter 28.)

Exudate varies in composition, depending on the stage of the inflammatory response and, to some extent, the injurious stimulus. In early or mild inflammation the exudate is watery, or a **serous exudate,** with very few plasma proteins or leukocytes, such as fluid in a blister. In more severe or advanced inflammation the exudate may be thick and clotted, or a **fibrinous exudate,** such as in the lungs of individuals with lobar pneumonia. If a large number of leukocytes accumulate, as in persistent bacterial infections, the exudate consists of pus and is called a **purulent (suppurative) exudate.** Purulent exudate is characteristic of walled-off lesions **(cysts** or **abscesses).** If bleeding occurs, the exudate is filled with erythrocytes and is described as a **hemorrhagic exudate.**

The local manifestations of inflammation can affect all vascularized tissues, but lesions vary, depending on the organ or tissue involved. The lesion resulting from widespread cellular death (necrosis), for example, differs in myocardial (heart muscle), brain, and hepatic (liver) tissue. Cellular death resulting from myocardial infarction (deprivation of oxygen caused by cessation of blood flow) causes a response that proceeds to replacement of the dead tissue with a fibrinous scar. The same injury to brain tissue is more likely to result in the formation of an abscess filled with necrotic tissue (types of necrosis are described in Chapter 2). Destruction of liver tissue stimulates the regrowth, or regeneration, of liver cells.

Because inflammation can occur only in vascularized and perfused tissues, severe tissue damage results in inflammation at the *borders* of the lesion. Examples include perforating injuries, such as wounds or ulcers, and gangrenous lesions, in which an area of a limb or internal organ is killed by bacteria and lack of perfusion.

Local manifestations of inflammation also accompany all types of nonlethal cellular and tissue injury, from fractures or strains of the musculoskeletal system to burn injuries (see Chapter 2). No matter what the cause or where the lesion, inflammation occurs without fail because without it, healing could not occur. Acute inflammation is so closely tied to healing that it is sometimes called the *defense phase of healing.*

SYSTEMIC MANIFESTATIONS OF ACUTE INFLAMMATION

The three primary systemic changes associated with the acute inflammatory response are fever, leukocytosis (a transient increase in circulating leukocytes), and increase in circulating plasma proteins.[26] Fever appears to be induced by mediators (endogenous pyrogens) such as IL-1 that are released from neutrophils and macrophages. Endogenous pyrogen (a fever-causing chemical) acts directly on the hypothalamus, the portion of the brain that controls the body's thermostat. The release of endogenous pyrogen activity occurs after phagocytosis or after exposure of the cell to bacterial endotoxin or to antigen-antibody complexes. (Mechanisms of temperature regulation are discussed in Chapter 14.)

The generation of a febrile response can be beneficial to the defense of the host because the microorganisms that cause some conditions (e.g., syphilis, gonococcal urethritis) are highly sensitive to small increases in body temperature. On the other hand, fever may have some harmful side effects, because it may enhance the host's susceptibility to the effects of endotoxins associated with gram-negative bacterial infections (bacterial toxins are described in Chapter 2).

Table 7-1 Circulating Levels of Acute-Phase Reactants During Inflammation

Function	Increased	Decreased
Coagulation components	Fibrinogen Prothrombin Factor VIII Plasminogen	None
Protease inhibitors	α_1-Antitrypsin α_1-Antichymotrypsin	Inter-α-antitrypsin
Transport proteins	Haptoglobin Hemopexin Ceruloplasmin Ferritin	Transferrin
Complement components	C1s, C2, C3, C4, C5, C9, factor B, C1 inhibitor	Properdin
Miscellaneous proteins	α_1-Acid glycoprotein Fibronectin Serum amyloid A (SAA) C-reactive protein (CRP)	Albumin Prealbumin α_1-Lipoprotein β-Lipoprotein

During many infections, numbers of circulating leukocytes, primarily neutrophils, increase. This increase is usually accompanied by a "left shift" in the ratio of immature to mature neutrophils, so that the more immature forms of neutrophils, such as band cells, metamyelocytes, and occasionally myelocytes, are present in greater than normal proportions. (Chapter 24 discusses the development and maturation of blood cells.) Leukocyte production increases because it is stimulated by several products of inflammation, including complement component C3a. Colony-stimulating factors produced by phagocytes also induce granulopoiesis (formation of granulocytes, namely, neutrophils, eosinophils, and basophils) in the bone marrow, primarily by the proliferation of committed precursors of granulocytes and monocytes (see Chapter 24).

Many plasma proteins, most of which are products of the liver, are increased during inflammation; these are referred to as **acute-phase reactants** (Table 7-1).[27,28] Acute-phase reactants reach maximal circulating levels in 10 to 40 hours. Many are antiinflammatory proteins whose rate of synthesis is increased in the liver (e.g., inhibitors of proteases released during inflammation or proteins that are consumed during inflammation). IL-6, which is induced by IL-1, increases synthesis of acute-phase reactants directly by stimulating liver cells. Administration of IL-1 into animals leads to elevation of most acute-phase reactants, including fibrinogen, C-reactive protein, haptoglobin, amyloid A, α_1-antitrypsin, and ceruloplasmin.[28]

A major systemic complication of infection is *septicemia,* or bacterial infection of the blood. (Septicemia is described briefly in Chapter 2. Its cardiovascular consequences are described in Chapter 29, and anaphylactic shock is described in Chapter 45.)

Acute inflammation can be verified by hematologic tests, which are described in Chapter 24. An increase in blood levels of acute-phase reactants, primarily fibrinogen (see Table 7-1), is usually associated with an increased erythrocyte sedimentation rate. The alteration in plasma proteins probably leads to an enhanced erythrocyte rouleaux formation (stacking of erythrocytes, as in a stack of coins) and increased rates of sedimentation. Although increased erythrocyte sedimentation is a nonspecific reaction, it is considered a good indicator of an acute inflammatory response.

CHRONIC INFLAMMATION

Superficially, the difference between acute and chronic inflammation is purely one of duration, in that chronic inflammation lasts 2 weeks or longer, regardless of cause. Characteristic histologic and mechanistic differences also may be present (Fig. 7-21). Chronic inflammation is sometimes preceded by an unsuccessful acute inflammatory response. For example, if bacterial contamination or foreign objects (e.g., dirt, wood splinter, glass) persist in a traumatic wound, an inflammatory response that is difficult to differentiate from the acute response will continue beyond 2 weeks. Suppuration, pus formation, and incomplete wound healing may characterize this type of chronic inflammation.

Chronic inflammation can occur also as a distinct process without much acute inflammation. Some microorganisms (e.g., mycobacteria that cause tuberculosis) have cell walls with a very high lipid and wax content, making them relatively insensitive to degradation by phagocytes. The persistence of these bacteria continues to stimulate inflammation. Some, such as the microorganisms that cause tuberculosis, leprosy, syphilis, and brucellosis, can survive within the macrophage. In addition, some microorganisms produce toxins that stimulate tissue-damaging reactions even after they are killed. Persistent inflammation can also be the result of prolonged irritation by chemicals, particulate matter, or physical irritants (e.g., inhaled dusts, wood splinters, suture material).

Chronic inflammation is characterized by a dense infiltration of lymphocytes and macrophages. If macrophages are unable to protect the host from tissue damage, the body attempts to wall off and isolate the infected site, thus forming a **granuloma** (Fig. 7-22). Granulomas are formed if neutrophils and macrophages are unable to destroy microorganisms during the acute inflammatory response.[29] Infections

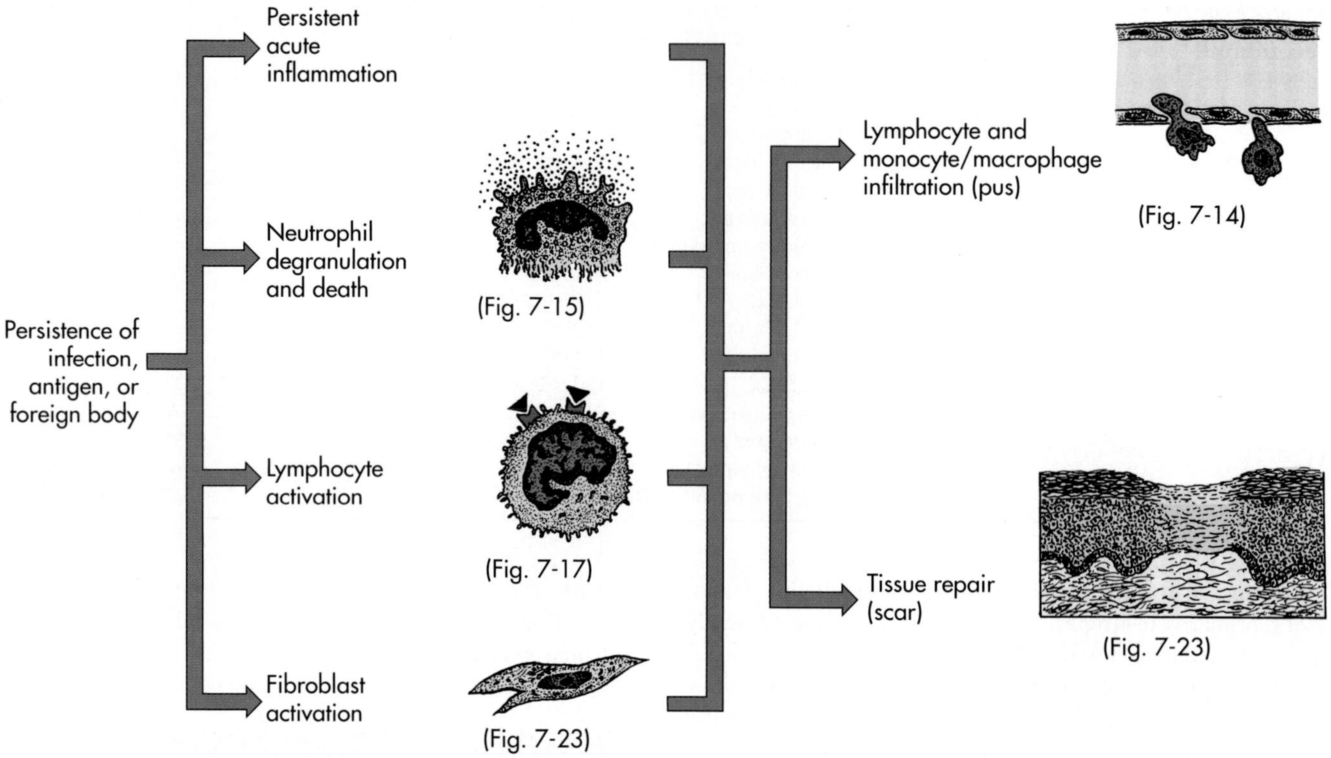

FIG. 7-21 The chronic inflammatory response. Inflammation usually becomes chronic because of the persistence of an infection, an antigen, or a foreign body in the wound. Chronic inflammation is characterized by the persistence of many of the processes of acute inflammation. In addition, large amounts of neutrophil degranulation and death, the activation of lymphocytes, and the concurrent activation of fibroblasts result in the release of mediators that induce the infiltration of more lymphocytes and monocytes/macrophages and the beginning of wound healing and tissue repair. The figure numbers refer to those in which more detailed information may be found on that portion of the response.

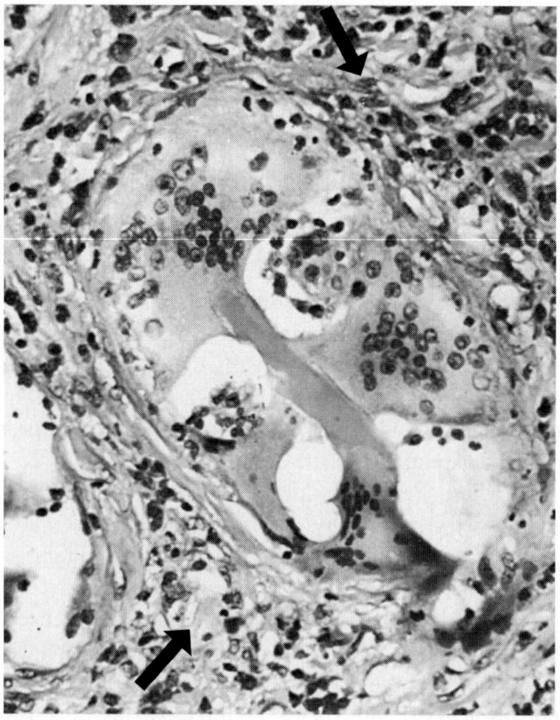

FIG. 7-22 Cross section of a granuloma—granulomatous (de Quervain) thyroiditis. Outside the follicle *(lightly shaded)* are mononuclear inflammatory cells and fibrosis (× 300) *(see arrows).* (From Kissane JM: *Anderson's pathology,* ed 9, St Louis, 1990, Mosby.)

caused by some bacteria (listeriosis, brucellosis), fungi (histoplasmosis, coccidioidomycosis), parasites (leishmaniasis, schistosomiasis, toxoplasmosis), and perhaps large antigen-antibody complexes (rheumatoid arthritis) result in granuloma formation.

Granuloma formation begins when some of the macrophages differentiate into large **epithelioid cells,** cells that are incapable of phagocytosis but capable of taking up debris and other small particles. Other macrophages fuse into multinucleated **giant cells,** which are active phagocytes and can engulf particles too large to be engulfed by single macrophages. The granuloma itself is usually walled off (encapsulated) by fibrous deposits of collagen and may be hyalinized or calcified by deposits of calcium carbonate and calcium phosphate.

The classic granuloma associated with tuberculosis is characterized by a wall of epithelioid cells surrounding a center of dead and decaying tissue (caseous necrosis; see Chapter 2) and mycobacteria. Some of the epithelioid cells fuse into Langhans-type giant cells, with their nuclei distributed in a horseshoe pattern inside the plasma membrane (see Fig. 7-22). The epithelioid cells persist for 3 to 4 weeks, whereas the giant cells live only a few days.

The decay of cells within the granuloma results in the release of acids and the enzymatic contents of dead phagocytes' lysosomes. In this inhospitable environment the cellular debris is broken down into its basic constituents and a clear fluid (liquefaction necrosis; see Chapter 2) remains in the granuloma. Eventually this fluid diffuses out and leaves a hollow, thick-walled structure in the tissue that may remain for the life of the individual.

RESOLUTION AND REPAIR

Destruction of tissue is followed by a period of healing that begins during acute inflammation and may not be complete for as long as 2 years. The most favorable outcome of healing is complete return to normal structure and function. This is possible if damage is minor, no complications occur, or destroyed tissues are capable of **regeneration** (proliferation of remaining cells). Restoration of original structure and physiologic function is called **resolution.**

If extensive damage is present (particularly in tissues incapable of regeneration), if infection results in abscess or granuloma formation, or if fibrin persists in the lesion, resolution is not possible and repair takes place instead. **Repair** is the replacement of destroyed tissue with scar tissue. Scar tissue is composed of **collagen.** It fills in the lesion and restores tensile strength but cannot carry out the physiologic functions of destroyed tissue.

Both regeneration and repair begin during inflammation with phagocytosis of particulate matter in the inflammatory exudate (fibrin from dissolved clots, microorganisms, erythrocytes, and dead tissue cells). This cleanup of the lesion, which also involves dissolution of fibrin clots (or scabs) by fibrinolytic enzymes, is called **débridement.** After débridement, exudate, toxic products, and particulate matter are drained away and vascular dilation and permeability are reversed, preparing the lesion for either regeneration or repair.

Repair, which ends in the formation of scar tissue, always involves processes that (1) fill in the wound, (2) cover or seal the wound, and (3) shrink the wound. These common denominators of wound healing vary in importance and duration among different types of wounds. A clean incision, such as a paper cut or a sutured surgical wound, heals primarily through the process of collagen synthesis. Because sealing of this type of wound has already been facilitated by minimal tissue loss and apposition (joining) of the wound edges, very little sealing (epithelialization) and shrinkage (contraction) are required for healing. Wounds that heal under conditions of minimal tissue loss are said to heal by **primary intention** (Fig. 7-23).

Other wounds do not heal so neatly and easily. Healing of an open wound, such as a stage IV pressure sore (decubitus ulcer), requires a great deal more tissue replacement than healing of a surgical incision. With an open wound, epithelialization, scar formation, and contraction take longer, and healing occurs through **secondary intention** (see Fig. 7-23). Healing by either primary or secondary intention may occur at different rates for different types of tissue and for different types of injury.

Resolution and repair occur in two overlapping phases. The first phase, called the **reconstructive phase,** begins 3 to 4 days after the initial injury and continues for as long as 2 weeks. This phase is also known as the *proliferative, fibroblastic,* or *connective tissue phase.* During the reconstructive phase the lesion is characterized by fibroblast (connective tissue cell) proliferation, which is followed by collagen synthesis by the fibroblasts, epithelialization, and cellular differentiation.

The second phase, the **maturation phase,** begins several weeks after injury and is normally complete within 2 years. The maturation phase is also known as the *differentiation, remodeling,* or *plateau phase.* With maturation there is continuing differentiation of cells, contraction of the wound, scar formation, and remodeling of the scar.

Reconstructive Phase

Because surgical and perforating wounds exhibit all the phases of resolution and repair, they are useful models of both normal and abnormal (dysfunctional) healing. The wound is initially sealed off by a blood clot containing fibrin and trapped cells (erythrocytes and leukocytes). The cross-linked mesh of fibrin is created by activation of the coagulation cascade. The fibrin mesh traps platelets, which further seal damaged vessels by forming a platelet plug (see Chapter 24). Most surgical wounds are completely sealed with fibrin several hours after they have been closed. Sealing creates a barrier to bacterial invasion, although it does not always prevent it. The fibrin seal also helps unite the wound edges. Fibrin provides a framework for the collagen molecules or regenerated tissue cells that ultimately will fill the wound.

For healing to proceed, the fibrin clot must be dissolved and replaced by normal tissue or scar tissue. Enzymatic digestion of the clot usually occurs after activation of the plasma fibrinolytic system (plasmin generation; see Chapter 24) or release of lysosomal enzymes from dead neutrophils. Macrophages invade the dissolving clot and clear away debris and dead cells by phagocytosis. Débridement by macrophages and remaining neutrophils is followed by simple resolution with regeneration of destroyed cells or, if regeneration is not possible, by the process of repair that ends in scar formation (see Fig. 7-23).

Repair begins as **granulation tissue** grows inward from surrounding healthy connective tissue. Granulation tissue is filled with new capillaries that give it a red, granular appearance and is surrounded by fibroblasts and macrophages. First, capillary buds sprout out of vascular endothelial cells around the wound and extend into the débrided areas. Loops form when the young capillaries join *(anastomose).* The loops are more fragile and permeable than mature vessels, resulting in a leakage of erythrocytes and neutrophils. The erythrocytes are phagocytosed by macrophages, and the neutrophils participate in further débridement of the inflammatory lesion. Many of the new capillaries differentiate into arterioles and venules as repair continues. New lymphatic vessels grow into the granulation tissue by a similar process.

The macrophage performs several functions in healing.[30] Besides acting as the primary phagocyte of débridement, it

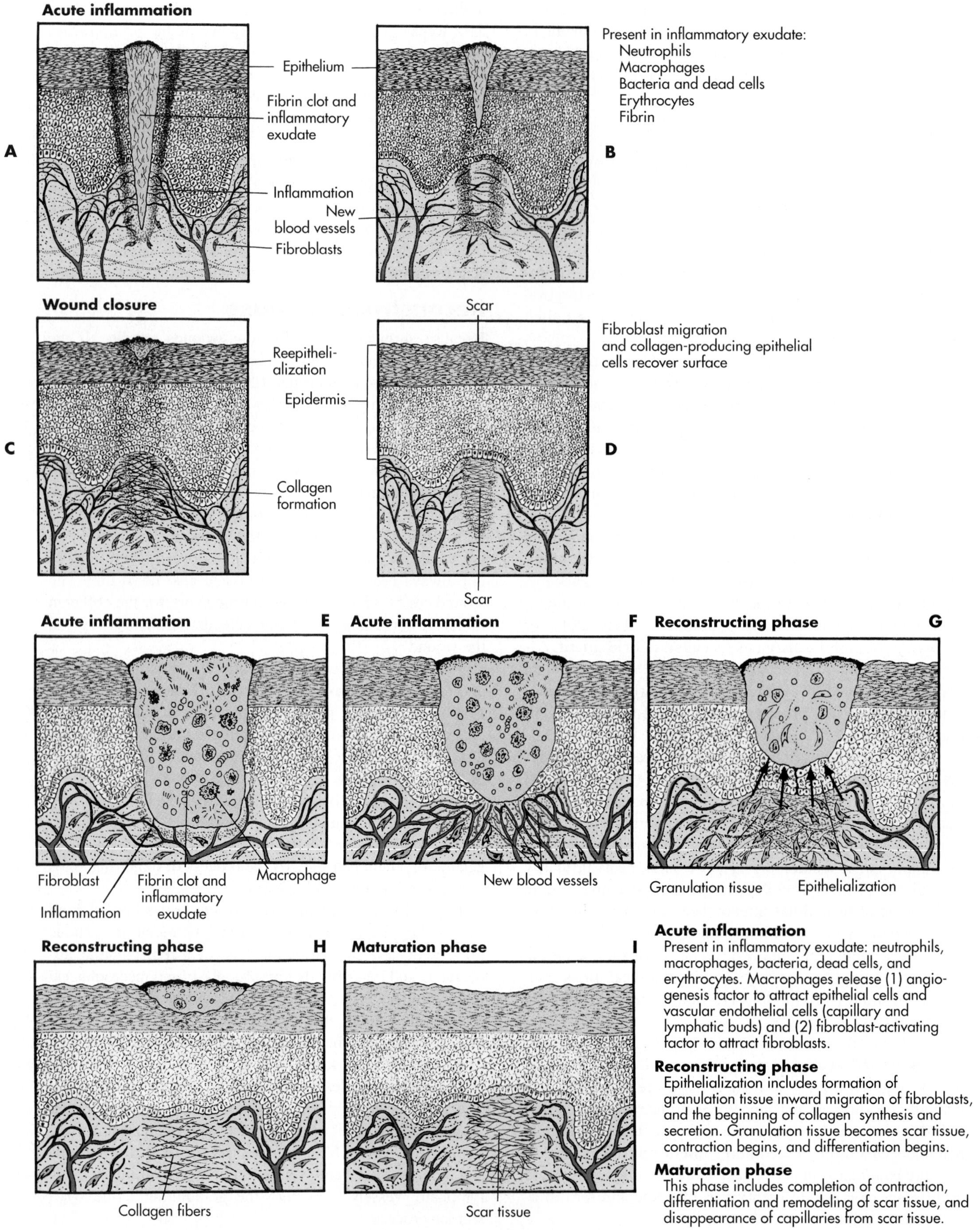
Acute inflammation
A
B
Epithelium
Fibrin clot and inflammatory exudate
Inflammation
New blood vessels
Fibroblasts
Present in inflammatory exudate:
Neutrophils
Macrophages
Bacteria and dead cells
Erythrocytes
Fibrin
Wound closure
C
D
Scar
Reepitheli-alization
Epidermis
Collagen formation
Fibroblast migration and collagen-producing epithelial cells recover surface
Scar
Acute inflammation E
Acute inflammation F
Reconstructing phase G
Fibroblast
Inflammation
Fibrin clot and inflammatory exudate
Macrophage
New blood vessels
Granulation tissue
Epithelialization
Reconstructing phase H
Maturation phase I
Collagen fibers
Scar tissue
Acute inflammation
Present in inflammatory exudate: neutrophils, macrophages, bacteria, dead cells, and erythrocytes. Macrophages release (1) angiogenesis factor to attract epithelial cells and vascular endothelial cells (capillary and lymphatic buds) and (2) fibroblast-activating factor to attract fibroblasts.
Reconstructing phase
Epithelialization includes formation of granulation tissue inward migration of fibroblasts, and the beginning of collagen synthesis and secretion. Granulation tissue becomes scar tissue, contraction begins, and differentiation begins.
Maturation phase
This phase includes completion of contraction, differentiation and remodeling of scar tissue, and disappearance of capillaries from scar tissue.

FIG. 7-23 Wound repair by primary or secondary intention. **A** to **D**, Healing by primary intention. **E** to **I**, Healing by secondary intention.

secretes the following biochemical mediators that promote healing:

- Fibroblast-activating factor, which stimulates fibroblasts to enter the lesion and synthesize and secrete the collagen precursor, procollagen
- Angiogenesis factor, which stimulates vascular endothelial cells to form capillary buds that grow into the lesion
- An unidentified factor that stimulates epithelial cells to grow over and seal the wound's surface

Macrophages also secrete collagenase, which débrides injured collagen fibers in the wound.

As the clot or scab is being dissolved and granulation tissue is being formed, the healing wound must be protected. This is accomplished by **epithelialization,** the process by which epithelial cells grow into the wound from surrounding healthy tissue. Attracted by a factor secreted by macrophages, the epithelial cells migrate under the clot or scab, using proteolytic enzymes to sever the connection between the clot and the wound surface (see Fig. 7-23). Eventually the migrating epithelial cells contact similar cells from all sides of the wound and seal the wound, after which migration and proliferation cease. The epithelial cells remain active, however, undergoing differentiation to give rise to the various epidermal layers (see Chapter 43). Epithelialization of a skin wound can be hastened if the wound is kept moist, preventing the fibrin clot from becoming a scab.

Fibroblasts are the most important cells during the reconstructive phase of wound healing because they synthesize and secrete collagen. Fibroblasts are stimulated by fibroblast-activating factor (from macrophages) to proliferate and enter the lesion. The collagen and connective tissue produced by fibroblasts is laid down in débrided areas about 6 days after the fibroblasts have entered the lesion.[31]

Collagen is the most abundant protein in the body and is the material of tissue repair. It is present in skin, bones, teeth, blood vessels, tendons, cartilage, and connective tissue. Collagen is produced in fibroblasts as a polypeptide of repeating sequences of the amino acids glycine, proline, hydroxyproline, lysine, and hydroxylysine. Proline and lysine are enzymatically hydroxylated after the polypeptide chain is synthesized, and their hydroxylation is absolutely necessary for collagen polymerization and function. Cofactors that are necessary for hydroxylation include iron, ascorbic acid (vitamin C), α-ketoglutarate (from the Krebs cycle), and molecular oxygen (O_2). Absence of these cofactors results in incomplete wound healing.

Immature collagen, termed **procollagen,** is secreted by the fibroblast as a complex of three polypeptide chains cross linked by intermolecular bonds. Procollagen must be activated further by the removal of a small polypeptide sequence by a specific protease. As the scar tissue matures, collagen molecules are cross linked by intramolecular bonds to form collagen fibrils. Cross-linking involves the formation of covalent bonds between lysine residues. At this point the secreted collagen molecules are still of a gel-like consistency in the wound. With further cross-linking the fibrils form fibers. This process takes several months. The collagen initially is deposited randomly, but during remodeling of the scar tissue that has formed, the fibers are dissolved by collagenase and re-formed. During this period the fibers reorient along the lines of mechanical stress and further cross-linking adds strength.

Wound **contraction** is the final process of the reconstructive phase of healing. It is necessary for closure of all wounds, but especially of those that heal by secondary intention. Contraction is noticeable 6 to 12 days after injury. In normal healing, contraction may amount to inward movement of the wound edge by approximately 0.5 mm/day.

The granulation tissue contains **myofibroblasts**—specialized cells that probably cause wound contraction. As the name implies, myofibroblasts have features of both smooth muscle cells and fibroblasts. Microscopically the myofibroblast appears similar to a fibroblast, but it differs in that its cytoplasm contains bundles of parallel fibers similar to those found in smooth muscle cells. These fibers exert a contractile force within the cell. Wound contraction occurs as structures extending from the plasma membrane of the myofibroblast establish connections with neighboring cells. Once connected, myofibroblasts can exert pull on neighboring cells and anchor themselves to the wound bed, promoting contraction.[32]

Maturation Phase

Collagen deposition, tissue regeneration, and wound contraction all begin during the reconstructive phase. When this phase ends, about 2 weeks after injury, these processes are usually not complete. Therefore they continue into the maturation phase, which can continue for years. During the maturation phase, scar tissue is remodeled. Capillaries disappear, leaving an avascular scar. Within 2 to 3 weeks after maturation has begun, the scar tissue has gained about two thirds of its eventual maximum strength.

Epidermal wounds that heal by secondary intention and unsutured internal lesions are seldom completely restored by healing. At best, repaired tissue regains 80% of its original tensile strength. Only epithelial, hepatic (liver), and bone marrow cells are capable of the complete mitotic regeneration known as *compensatory hyperplasia* (hyperplasia is described in Chapter 2). In fibrous connective tissue, such as joints and ligaments, normal healing results in the replacement of the original tissue but the new tissue does not have exactly the same structure or function as the original. Some damaged tissue heals without replacement. For instance, the damage resulting from myocardial infarction heals with a scar composed of fibrous tissue rather than replacing cardiac muscle. Although the composition of healed tissue may differ, the healing process of soft tissues is the same for all wounds.

Dysfunctional Wound Healing

Dysfunctional healing may occur during any phase of the wound-healing process and may involve insufficient repair, excessive repair, or infection. The etiologic cause of dysfunctional healing can be related to a predisposing disorder, such as diabetes mellitus, or to an acquired condition, such as hypoxemia (insufficient oxygen in arterial blood). Numerous drugs and nutrients also can affect wound healing. Wound repair delays healing by reactivating inflammatory processes.

Dysfunction During Inflammatory Response

Healing may be prolonged if bleeding is not stopped during acute inflammation. Hemorrhage in a damaged area delays healing for several reasons. A clot increases the amount of space that granulation tissue has to fill and serves as a mechanical barrier to oxygen diffusion. The accumulation of excess blood cells resulting from hemorrhage prolongs the inflammatory process, because these cells must be cleared before repair. Accumulated blood, which is an excellent culture medium for bacteria, promotes infection and prolongs inflammation by increasing exudation and pus formation. In addition to slowing healing, sepsis can promote excessive scar formation or prevent healing completely.

Excessive amounts of fibrin also are detrimental to healing. The great amount of fibrin that is released in response to injury must eventually be reabsorbed so it will not organize into fibrous adhesions. Adhesions are seldom clinically significant unless they form in the pleural, pericardial, or abdominal cavities. Adhesions in these areas may bind organs together by fibrous bands, the shrinkage of which can distort or strangulate the affected organ.

Many factors may adversely affect the inflammatory process during wound healing. Hypovolemia—decreased blood volume—inhibits inflammation. The physiologic response to hypovolemia is vessel constriction rather than the dilation required to deliver inflammatory cells to the site of injury. Antiinflammatory steroids prevent macrophages from migrating to the site of injury and inhibit their release of collagenase and plasminogen activator.[33] Antiinflammatory steroids also inhibit fibroblast migration into the wound during the reconstructive phase of healing, angiogenesis, wound contraction, and reepithelialization.[34]

Optimal nutrition is important during all phases of healing because metabolic needs are increased. During inflammation the substances most essential for healing are glucose, oxygen, and protein. Because leukocytes need glucose to produce the adenosine triphosphate 59 (ATP) needed for chemotaxis, phagocytosis, and intercellular killing, the wounds of persons with diabetes who receive insufficient insulin heal poorly, mainly because of infection. Persons with diabetes are at risk for ischemic wounds because they are likely to have both small-vessel diseases that impair the microcirculation and altered (glycosylated) hemoglobin, which has an increased affinity for oxygen and thus does not readily release oxygen in tissues. (Hemoglobin's function as the oxygen-carrying component of blood is described in Chapter 24.) Oxygen delivery is compromised also by hypoxemic states. Ischemic tissue is susceptible to infection, which prolongs inflammation. Hypoproteinemia also prolongs inflammation because it impairs fibroblast proliferation.

Wound sepsis is treated in several ways. Most important is the removal or débridement of necrotic tissue and foreign bodies. Débridement is accomplished by surgery or use of absorbent dressings. Wound irrigation and antibiotic therapy also combat infection.

Dysfunction During Reconstructive Phase

Impaired Collagen Synthesis

A number of factors may interfere with the production of collagen in healing tissues. Most of these factors are nutritional. Scurvy, for example, is a condition caused by lack of ascorbic acid. Ascorbic acid is one of the cofactors required for the hydroxylation of the amino acids proline and lysine. Without hydroxylation these amino acids cannot be incorporated into collagen monomers; therefore procollagen is not secreted from the fibroblast. The results of scurvy are poorly formed connective tissue and greatly impaired healing.

Other nutrients play a cofactor role in enzyme systems required for collagen synthesis. These include iron, oxygen, α-ketoglutarate, manganese, copper, and calcium. Usually such minute amounts of these substances are required as cofactors that deficiencies are not clinically significant.

Protein is essential for collagen synthesis. Especially important is the amino acid methionine, which is converted to cystine. The role of cystine in collagen synthesis is twofold: (1) it functions as an important cofactor in enzyme systems required for collagen synthesis; and (2) it contains sulfur, which contributes to the formation of strong disulfide bonds in cross-linked collagen fibrils.

Collagen synthesis may be impaired during the processes of polymerization and cross-linking. After procollagen is secreted from the fibroblast, it must be activated by cleavage of its terminal peptides. Cleavage does not occur, for example, in individuals with Ehlers-Danlos syndrome (type VII). This disease prevents formation of normal connective tissue, causing the skin to be thin and fragile. All forms of Ehlers-Danlos syndrome are characterized by defects in collagen cross-linking. (The role of collagen in bone formation is described in Chapter 40.)

Dysfunctional collagen synthesis also may involve excessive production of collagen. This causes surface overhealing, which is manifested by a keloid or a hypertrophic scar (Fig. 7-24). Both keloid and hypertrophic scars are caused by an imbalance between collagen synthesis and collagen lysis in which synthesis is increased and lysis (degradation) is decreased, but the exact mechanisms are not known.[35,36] A **keloid** is a raised scar that extends beyond the original boundaries of the wound. It invades surrounding tissue and is likely to recur after surgical removal. A familial tendency to keloid formation has been observed, with a greater incidence in blacks than whites. A **hypertrophic scar** is raised but remains within the original boundaries of the wound. Hypertrophic scars tend to regress over time.

Impaired Epithelialization

Epithelialization is suppressed by antiinflammatory steroids, hypoxemia, ionizing radiation, and zinc deficiencies. Wound care technique may greatly influence epithelial cell migration.

External wounds that are draining or healing by secondary intention often are débrided and protected with dressings. The ideal dressing is one that absorbs some drainage without being incorporated into the clot or granulation tissue. Because epithelial cells must migrate across the wound during healing, dressings that débride healthy epithelial cells along with necrotic tissue prolong epithelialization.

Many solutions that traditionally have been used to clean or irrigate wounds are deleterious to the fragile new cells in the wound bed. Normal saline is the most innocuous solution that can be used to cleanse or irrigate a wound that is healing primarily by epithelialization. Solutions such as povidone-iodine and hydrogen peroxide are desiccating (drying) and subsequently inhibit rather than promote epithelial cell migration.

Wound Disruption

A potential complication of wounds that are sutured closed is **dehiscence,** in which the wound pulls apart at the suture line. The greatest incidence of dehiscence occurs 5 to 12 days after suturing. Paradoxically, this is the time when collagen synthesis is at its peak. Approximately 50% of dehiscence occurrences are associated with wound sepsis. Dehiscence also may occur when sutures break because of excessive strain. Obesity increases the risk for dehiscence because adipose tissue is difficult to suture. Wound dehiscence usually is heralded by an increase in serous drainage from the wound. In addition, the individual may report a feeling that "something gave way." Prompt surgical attention is required.

Impaired Contraction

Wound contraction is necessary for healing and is mediated by myofibroblasts.[37] This process may become pathologic when contraction is excessive, resulting in a deformity or **contracture.** Burns are especially susceptible to the development of contractures. Internal contracture may occur in cirrhosis of the liver. Scar tissue that becomes contracted constricts vascular flow, which may contribute to the development of portal hypertension and esophageal varices. Other types of internal contraction deformity include duodenal strictures caused by dysfunctional healing of an ulcer and esophageal strictures caused by lye burns.

Proper positioning and range-of-motion exercises and surgery are among the physical means used to overcome myofibroblast pull and prevent contractures. Biochemical means include control of myofibroblast contraction by the administration of smooth muscle inhibitors (e.g., colchicine) and attempts to inhibit collagen synthesis with drugs that prevent collagen cross-linking or collagenase activity. This treatment is based on the knowledge that collagen can "lock" contracted myofibroblasts into position. Clinical use of pharmacologic methods for control of wound contracture is still largely experimental.

Pediatrics and Mechanisms of Self-Defense

Besides immature or depressed immune function, neonates frequently have transiently depressed inflammatory function. For example, neutrophils and perhaps monocytes may not be capable of chemotaxis. Insufficient response to chemotactic factors appears to be caused by lack of fluidity in the phagocyte's plasma membrane, so that it cannot form pseudopods and migrate. Neonates are prone to infections associated with chemotactic defects, including cutaneous abscesses caused by staphylococci and cutaneous candidiasis. Further, neutrophils in neonates stressed by in utero infection or respiratory insufficiency have diminished oxidative and bacterial responses. (Acquired phagocytic defects, which may be induced by a variety of infections, metabolic disorders, nutrition deficiencies, or drugs, are described in Chapter 8.)

Neonates also are partially deficient in complement, especially components of the alternative pathway. They tend to have a relative deficiency of factor B and to develop severe, overwhelming sepsis and meningitis when infected with bacteria against which there is no transferred maternal antibody.

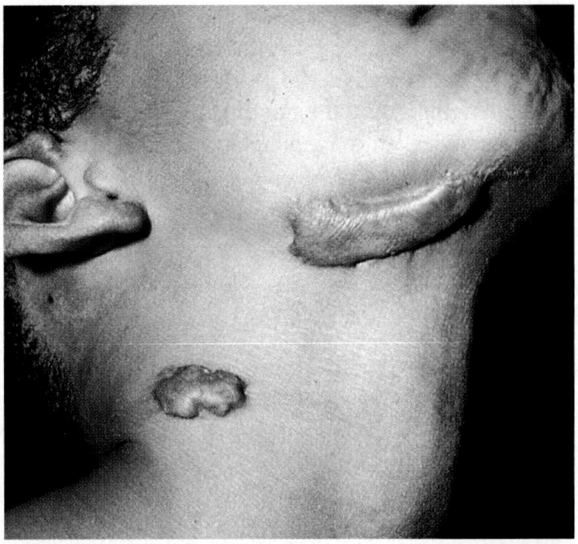

FIG. 7-24 Keloid (scar) formation. Scar caused by excessive synthesis of collagen. Keloid from suture marks in a black individual. (From Damjanov I, Linder J: *Anderson's pathology,* ed 10, St Louis, 1996, Mosby.)

Aging and Mechanisms of Self-Defense

The elderly population is at risk for impaired wound healing. There is no concrete evidence that impaired wound healing is a consequence of normal aging, however. Often impaired healing is associated with chronic illnesses, such as diabetes mellitus or cardiovascular disease. In addition, many elderly persons require medications, such as antiinflammatory steroids, that interfere with healing.

Because of impaired sensation or mobility and physiologic changes in the skin, the elderly are at increased risk for sustaining various wounds. With aging, subcutaneous fat is lost, diminishing a layer of protection. Collagen fibers become thicker and less elastic, thus further contributing to loss of protection.

Diminished immune function may interfere with the elderly person's natural ability to ward off infection in a wound. The regenerative capability of the skin is maintained with aging, but the epidermis undergoes some atrophy that includes atrophy of underlying capillaries. The consequent decrease of perfusion makes the elderly more susceptible than others to the adverse effects of hypoxia (insufficient oxygen) in the wound bed. Aging fibroblasts may have a slower rate of proliferation and attenuate wound healing.[38]

SUMMARY REVIEW

Acute Inflammatory Response

1. Inflammation is a rapid and nonspecific protective response to cellular injury from any cause. It can occur only in vascularized tissue.
2. The macroscopic hallmarks of inflammation are redness, swelling, heat, pain, and loss of function of the inflamed tissues.
3. The microscopic hallmark of inflammation is an accumulation of fluid and cells at the inflammatory site.

Mast Cell

1. The most important activator of the inflammatory response is the mast cell, which initiates inflammation (a) by releasing biochemical mediators (histamine, chemotactic factors) from preformed cytoplasmic granules and (b) by synthesizing other mediators (prostaglandins, leukotrienes) in response to a stimulus.
2. Histamine and serotonin are the major vasoactive amines of inflammation. Both cause constriction of vascular smooth muscles, dilation of capillaries, and retraction of endothelial cells lining the capillaries, which increases vascular permeability.

Plasma Protein Systems

1. Inflammation is mediated by three key plasma protein systems: the complement system, the clotting system, and the kinin system. The components of all three systems are a series of inactive proteins (proenzymes) that are activated in cascade fashion.
2. The complement system can be activated by antigen-antibody reactions (through the classic pathway) or by other products, especially bacterial polysaccharides (through the alternative pathway), resulting in the production of biologically active (anaphylatoxic or chemotactic) fragments and target cell lysis.
3. The clotting system stops bleeding, localizes microorganisms, and provides a meshwork for repair and healing.
4. Bradykinin is the most important kinin protein and causes vascular permeability, smooth muscle contraction, and pain.
5. The inflammatory process is controlled by inhibitory enzymes including histaminase, carboxypeptidase, C1 estrase inhibitor, and α_1-antitrypsin.

Cellular Components of Inflammation

1. The cells involved in the inflammatory process include phagocytic leukocytes (neutrophils, macrophages, and eosinophils), platelets, and lymphocytes.
2. Phagocytic cells engulf and destroy microorganisms by enclosing them in phagocytic vacuoles (phagolysosomes), within which toxic products (especially metabolites of oxygen) and degradative lysosomal enzymes kill and digest the microorganisms.
3. Opsonins, such as antibody and complement component C3b, coat microorganisms and make them more susceptible to phagocytosis by binding them more tightly to the phagocyte.
4. Endothelial cells line the blood vessels and capillaries and retract during inflammation to permit fluids, nutrients, and phagocytic cells into the area of injury.
5. The polymorphonuclear neutrophil (PMN), the predominant phagocytic cell in the early inflammatory response, exits the circulation by diapedesis through the retracted endothelial cell junctions and moves to the inflammatory site by chemotaxis.
6. The macrophage, the predominant phagocytic cell in the late inflammatory response, is highly phagocytic, responsive to lymphokines, and responsible for antigen processing and presentation to lymphocytes.
7. Eosinophils release products that control the inflammatory response and are induced by IgE-mediated mechanisms of hypersensitivity to kill parasitic organisms directly.
8. All of the leukocytes engage in phagocytosis, which is the engulfment and destruction of microorganisms, dead cells, and debris.

Cellular Products

1. The cells involved in immunity and inflammation stimulate other cells by secreting cytokines, especially interferons or interleukins.
2. Lymphokines are cytokines produced by T cells and have their most important effects on macrophages. These effects include chemotaxis, inhibition of migration once the macrophage has entered the inflammatory site, and activation of the macrophage, which makes it a more powerful phagocyte.
3. Interferons are produced by host cells that are already infected by viruses. Once released from infected cells, interferons can stimulate neighboring healthy cells to produce substances that prevent viral penetration.
4. Interleukins are produced by leukocytes that have been stimulated by an antigen. Interleukins stimulate other leukocytes to proliferate or otherwise increase their immune functions. The chief effect of interleukins is to accelerate the immune response.

Local Manifestations of Inflammation

1. Local manifestations of inflammation all involve the same hallmarks of inflammation, but types of exudate and necrosis vary with the injury and the tissue or organ affected.

Systemic Manifestations of Acute Inflammation

1. The systemic effects of inflammation are fever and increases in levels of circulating leukocytes and plasma proteins.

Chronic Inflammation

1. Chronic inflammation lasts 2 weeks or longer. It can occur as a distinct process without much acute inflammation.
2. Chronic inflammation is characterized by a dense infiltration of lymphocytes and macrophages. The body walls off and isolates the host from tissue damage, forming a granuloma.

Resolution and Repair

1. Inflammatory lesions proceed to resolution if little tissue has been lost or injured tissue is capable of regeneration. This is called *healing by primary intention.*
2. Inflammatory lesions that involve extensive damage or tissues incapable of regeneration heal by repair. This process is called *healing by secondary intention.*

Pediatrics and Mechanisms of Self-Defense

1. Neonates frequently have transiently depressed inflammatory function.

Aging and Mechanisms of Self-Defense

1. The elderly person is at risk for impaired wound healing.
2. Diminished immune function may interfere with the elderly person's natural ability to ward off infection in a wound.

KEY TERMS

Abscess, *216*
Acute-phase reactant, *217*
Adhesion molecule, *209*
Alternative pathway, *203*
Anaphylatoxin, *203*
Antigen-antibody complex (immune complex), *204*
Basophil, *200*
Bradykinin, *205*
Chemokines, *215*
Chemotactic factor, *201*
Chemotaxis, *201*
Classic pathway, *203*
Collagen, *219*
Complement cascade, *203*
Contraction, *221*
Contracture, *223*
Cyst, *216*
Débridement, *219*
Degranulation, *200*
Dehiscence, *223*
Diapedesis, *209*
Endothelial cell, *199*
Eosinophil, *212*
Epithelialization, *221*
Epithelioid cell, *218*
Extrinsic pathway, *205*
Exudate, *197*
Fibrinous exudate, *216*
Fibroblast, *221*
Giant cell, *218*
Granulation tissue, *219*
Granuloma, *217*
Hemorrhagic exudate, *216*
Hypertrophic scar, *222*
Interferon, *215*
Interleukin (IL), *214*
Intrinsic pathway, *205*
Keloid, *222*
Leukotriene (slow-reacting substance of anaphylaxis [SRS-A]), *201*
Lymphokine, *215*
Macrophage, *211*
Macrophage-activating factor (MAF), *215*
Margination (pavementing), *209*
Mast cell, *200*
Maturation phase, *219*
Migration-inhibitory factor (MIF), *215*
Monocyte, *211*
Myofibroblast, *221*
Neutrophil, *211*
Phagocytosis, *210*
Phagolysosome, *210*
Phagosome, *210*
Plasma kinin cascade, *205*
Platelet, *199*
Platelet-activating factor (PAF), *202*
Polymorphonuclear neutrophil (PMN), *211*
Primary intention, *219*
Procollagen, *221*
Proenzyme, *202*
Prostaglandin, *202*
Purulent (suppurative) exudate, *216*
Reconstructive phase, *219*
Regeneration, *219*
Repair, *219*
Resolution, *219*
Secondary intention, *219*
Serous exudate, *216*

REFERENCES

1. Ehrlich P: Dietbage zur Kenntnis der Anilinsfarb und Ihrer Verwendung nin ungen der Mikroskopichen technik, *Arch Mikr Anat* 13:263, 1877.
2. Holgate ST: The role of mast cells and basophils in inflammation, *Clin Exp Allergy* 30(Suppl 1):28, 2000.
3. Morgan BP: Physiology and pathophysiology of complement: progress and trends, *Crit Rev Clin Lab Sci* 32L:265, 1995.
4. Czermak BJ, Friedl HP, Ward PA: Complement, cytokines, and adhesion molecule expression in inflammatory reactions, *Proc Assoc Am Physicians* 110(4):306, 1998.
5. Miletic VD, Frank MM: Complement-immunoglobulin interactions, *Curr Opin Immunol* 7:41, 1995.
6. Arrang JM: Molecular and functional diversity of histamine receptor subtypes, *Ann NY Acad Sci* 10:314, 1995.
7. Leurs R, Smit MJ, Timmerman H: Molecular pharmacological aspects of histamine receptors, *Pharmacol Therap* 66:413, 1995.
8. Kwong KY, Maalour N, Jones CA: Uticaria and angiodema: pathophysiology, diagnosis, and treatment, *Pediatr Ann* 27(11):720, 1998.
9. Sampson AP: The role of eosinophils and neutrophils in inflammation, *Clin Exp Allergy* 30(Suppl 1):22, 2000.
10. Vestweber D: Molecular mechanisms that control endothelial cell contacts, *J Pathol* 190(3):281, 2000.
11. Crockett-Torabi E: Selectins and mechanisms of signal transduction, *J Leukoc Biol* 63(1):1, 1998.
12. Pearson JD: Normal endothelial cell function, *Lupus* 9(3):183, 2000.
13. Rep H, Harlan JM: Mechanisms and consequences of phagocyte adhesion to endothelium, *Ann Med* 31(3):256, 1999.
14. Brown EJ: Phagocytosis, *Bioessays* 17:109, 1995.
15. Teixeira MM, Williams TJ, Hellewell PG: Mechanisms and pharmacological manipulation of eosinophil accumulation in vivo, *Trends Pharmacol Sci* 16:418, 1995.
16. Thomas LL: Basophil and eosinophil interactions in health and disease, *Chem Immunol* 61:186, 1995.
17. Lachman LB, Maizel AL: The interleukins: immunoregulatory molecules, *Clin Immunol Newsletter* 4:113, 1983.
18. Milanese C, Richardson NE, Reinherz EL: Identification of a T helper cell–derived lymphokine that activates resting T lymphocytes, *Science* 231(4742):1118, 1986.
19. Saklatvala J: Intracellular signalling mechanisms of interleukin 1 and tumor necrosis factor: possible targets for therapy, *Br Med Bull* 51:402, 1995.
20. Cavaillon JM: Cytokines and macrophages, *Biomed Pharmacother* 48:445, 1994.
21. Murdock C, Finn A: Chemokine receptors and their role in inflammation and infectious disease, *Blood* 95(10):3032, 2000.

22. Gangur BV, Oppenheim JJ: Are chemokines essential or secondary participants in allergic responses? *Ann Allergy Asthma Immunol* 84(6): 569, 2000.
23. Keane MP, Strieter RM: Chemokine signaling in inflammation, *Crit Care Med* 28(4 Suppl):N13, 2000.
24. Kalvakolanu DV: An overview of the interferon system: signal transduction and mechanisms of action, *Cancer Invest* 14:25, 1996.
25. Tilg H, Kaser A: Interferons and inflammation, *Curr Pharm Des* 5(10): 771, 1999.
26. Dinarello CA: Cytokines as endogenous pyrogens, *J Infect Dis* 179(Suppl 2):S294, 1999.
27. Jakab L, Kalabay L: The acute phase reaction syndrome: the acute reactants (a survey), *Acta Microbiol Immunol Hung* 45(3-4):409, 1998.
28. Suffredini AF et al: New insights into the biology of the acute phase response, *J Clin Immunol* 19(4):203, 1999.
29. Munk ME, Emoto M: Functions of T-cell subsets and cytokines in mycobacterial infections, *Eur Respir J* 20:668s, 1995.
30. DiPietro LA: Wound healing: the role of the macrophage and other immune cells, *Shock* 4:233, 1995.
31. Kosir MA et al: Matrix glycosaminoglycans in the growth phase of fibroblasts: more of the story in wound healing, *J Surg Res* 92(1):45, 2000.
32. Nedelec B et al: Control of wound contraction. Basic and clinical features, *Hand Clin* 1(2):289, 2000.
33. Alvarez OM et al: Effect of topically applied steroidal and nonsteroidal anti-inflammatory agents on skin repair and regeneration, *Fed Proc* 43: 2793, 1984.
34. Anstead GM: Steroids, retinoids, and wound healing, *Adv Wound Care* 11(6):277, 1998.
35. Greenhalgh DG: The role of apoptosis in wound healing, *Int J Biochem Cell Biol* 30(9):1019, 1998.
36. Marcus JR et al: Cellular mechanisms for diminished scarring with aging, *Plast Reconstr Surg* 105(5):1591, 2000.
37. Vaughan MB, Howard EW, Tomasek JJ: Transforming growth factor–beta$_1$ promotes the morphological and functional differentiation of the myofibroblast, *Exp Cell Res* 257(1):180, 2000.
38. Khorramizadeh MR et al: Aging differentially modulates the expression of collagen and collagenase in dermal fibroblasts, *Mol Cell Biochem* 194(1-2):99, 1999.

CHAPTER 8

Infection and Alterations in Immunity and Inflammation

NEAL S. ROTE

CHAPTER OUTLINE

The immune system is a finely tuned network that protects the host against foreign antigens, particularly infectious agents. Sometimes this network breaks down, causing the immune system to react inappropriately. Inappropriate immune responses may be (1) exaggerated against environmental antigens (allergy); (2) misdirected against the host's own cells (autoimmunity); (3) directed against beneficial foreign tissues, such as transfusions or transplants (alloimmunity); or (4) insufficient for protection (immune deficiency). All of these can be serious or life threatening. Exaggerated immune responses (allergy) are the most common and usually the least life threatening.

HYPERSENSITIVITY: ALLERGY, AUTOIMMUNITY, AND ALLOIMMUNITY

The inappropriate responses of allergy, autoimmunity, and alloimmunity can be collectively classified as hypersensitivity. **Hypersensitivity** is an altered immunologic reactivity to an antigen that results in a pathologic immune response after reexposure. Allergy, autoimmunity, and alloimmunity (previously termed *isoimmunity*) are differentiated by the source of the antigen against which the hypersensitivity response is directed (Table 8-1). The term **allergy** originally denoted both facets of the immune response: immunity, which is beneficial, and hypersensitivity, which is harmful. Allergy has come to mean the deleterious effects of hypersensitivity to environmental (exogenous) antigens, and immunity means the protective responses to antigens expressed by disease-causing agents.

Autoimmunity is a disturbance in the immunologic tolerance of self-antigens. Many clinical disorders are associated with autoimmunity and are referred to as **autoimmune diseases** (Table 8-2). Autoimmune diseases occur when the immune system reacts against self-antigens and destroys host tissues. Antibodies against self-antigens, termed *autoantibodies,* are produced also by healthy individuals, particularly the elderly. In fact, the aging process may in part represent a deterioration of tolerance to self-antigens. Healthy individuals of all ages may produce autoantibodies, without concurrent overt autoimmune disease, in response to tissue damage. Therefore the presence of low quantities of autoantibodies does not necessarily indicate a disease state.

Table 8-1 Relative Incidences and Examples of Hypersensitivity Reactions*

Target Antigen	Mechanism: Type I (Immunoglobulin E [IgE] Mediated)	Type II (Tissue Specific)	Type III (Immune Complex)	Type IV (Cell Mediated)
ALLERGY	++++	+	+	++
Environmental antigens	Hay fever	Hemolysis in drug allergies	Gluten (wheat) allergy	Poison ivy allergy
AUTOIMMUNITY	±	++	+++	+
Self-antigens	May contribute to some type III reactions	Autoimmune thrombocytopenia	Systemic lupus erythematosus	Hashimoto thyroiditis
ALLOIMMUNITY	±	++	+	++
Other person's antigens	May contribute to some type III reactions	Hemolytic disease of the newborn	Anaphylaxis to IgA in IV γ-globulin	Graft rejection

*The frequency of each reaction is indicated in a range from rare (±) to very common (++++). An example of each reaction is given.

Table 8-2 Disorders Associated with Autoimmunity

System Disease	Organ or Tissue	Probable Self-antigen
ENDOCRINE SYSTEM		
Hyperthyroidism (Graves disease)	Thyroid gland	Receptors for thyroid-stimulating hormone on plasma membrane of thyroid cells
Autoimmune thyroiditis	Thyroid gland	Thyroglobulin; microsomes
Primary myxedema	Thyroid gland	Microsomes
Insulin-dependent diabetes	Pancreas	Islet cells, insulin, insulin receptors on pancreatic cells
Addison disease	Adrenal gland	Surface antigens on steroid-producing cells; microsomes of adrenal cortex
Premature gonadal failure	Ovary	Interstitial cells; corpus luteum
Male infertility	Testis	Surface antigens on spermatozoa
Orchitis	Testis	Germinal epithelium
Female infertility	Ovary	Zona pellucida
Idiopathic hypoparathyroidism	Parathyroid gland	Surface antigens on chief cells (epithelial cells of gland)
Partial pituitary deficiency	Pituitary gland	Prolactin-producing cells; growth hormone–producing cells
SKIN		
Pemphigus vulgaris	Skin	Intercellular substances in stratified squamous epithelium
Bullous pemphigoid	Skin	Basement membrane
Dermatitis herpetiformis	Skin	Basement membrane (immunoglobulin A[IgA])
Vitiligo	Skin	Surface antigens on melanocytes (melanin-producing cells)
NEUROMUSCULAR TISSUE		
Polymyositis (dermatomyositis)	Muscle	Nuclear materials; myosin
Multiple sclerosis	Neural tissue	Unknown
Myasthenia gravis	Neuromuscular junction	Acetylcholine receptors; striations of skeletal and cardiac muscle
Polyneuritis	Nerve cell	Peripheral myelin
Rheumatic fever	Heart	Cardiac tissue (subsarcolemmal membrane); cross reaction with group A streptococcal antigen
Cardiomyopathy	Heart	Cardiac muscle
Postvaccinal or postinfectious encephalitis	Central nervous system	Central nervous system myelin or basic protein
GASTROINTESTINAL SYSTEM		
Celiac disease (gluten-sensitive enteropathy)	Intestine	Gluten
Ulcerative colitis	Colon	Mucosal cells
Crohn disease	Ileum	Unknown
Pernicious anemia	Stomach	Surface antigens of parietal cells; intrinsic factor
Atrophic gastritis	Stomach	Parietal cells
Primary biliary cirrhosis	Liver	Mitochondria; cells of bile duct
Chronic active hepatitis	Liver	Surface antigens, nuclei, microsomes, mitochondria or hepatocytes; smooth muscle

Table 8-2 Disorders Associated with Autoimmunity—cont'd

System Disease	Organ or Tissue	Probable Self-antigen
EYE		
Sjögren syndrome	Lacrimal gland	Antigens of lacrimal gland, salivary gland, thyroid, and nuclei of cells; immunoglobulin G (IgG)
Uveitis	Uveal structures	Antigens of the iris, ciliary body, and choroid
CONNECTIVE TISSUE		
Ankylosing spondylitis	Joints	Sacroiliac and spinal apophyseal joint
Rheumatoid arthritis	Joints	IgG, collagen
Systemic lupus erythematosus	Multiple sites	Numerous antigens in nuclei, organelles, and extracellular matrix
Mixed connective tissue disease	Multiple sites	Ribonucleoprotein and numerous other nucleoproteins
Polyarteritis nodosa (necrotizing vasculitis)	Arterioles (small arteries)	Unknown
Scleroderma (progressive systemic sclerosis)	Multiple organs	Nuclear antigens; IgG
Felty syndrome	Joints	IgG
Antiphospholipid antibody syndrome	Platelets Endothelial cells Trophoblast of placenta	Membrane phospholipids, especially phosphatidylserine
RENAL SYSTEM		
Immune complex glomerulonephritis	Kidney	Numerous immune complexes
Goodpasture disease	Kidney	Glomerular basement membrane
HEMATOLOGIC SYSTEM		
Idiopathic neutropenia	Neutrophil	Surface antigens on polymorphonuclear neutrophils
Idiopathic lymphopenia	Lymphocytes	Surface antigens on lymphocytes
Autoimmune hemolytic anemia	Erythrocytes	Surface antigens on erythrocytes
Autoimmune thrombocytopenic purpura	Platelets	Surface antigens on platelets
RESPIRATORY SYSTEM		
Goodpasture disease	Lung	Septal membrane of alveolus

Alloimmune diseases occur when the immune system of one individual produces an immunologic reaction against tissues of another individual. Alloimmunity can be observed during immunologic reactions against transfusions, grafted tissue, or the fetus during pregnancy.

The mechanism that initiates the onset of hypersensitivity, whether it consists of allergy, autoimmunity, or alloimmunity, is not completely understood. It is generally accepted that genetic, infectious, and possibly environmental factors contribute to hypersensitivity. Most diseases caused by hypersensitivity evolve because of the interactions of at least three variables: (1) an original insult, which alters **immunologic homeostasis** (a steady state of tolerance to self-antigens; more important in autoimmunity than in alloimmunity or allergy); (2) the individual's genetic makeup, which determines susceptibility to the effects of the insult; and (3) an immunologic process that amplifies the insult.

Mechanisms of Hypersensitivity

Diseases caused by hypersensitivity are characterized also by immune mechanisms that initiate inflammation and result in the destruction of healthy tissue (see Table 8-1). These mechanisms are apparent in most hypersensitivity reactions and have been divided into four distinct types: (1) type I (IgE-mediated allergic reactions), (2) type II (tissue-specific reactions), (3) type III (immune complex–mediated reactions), and (4) type IV (cell-mediated reactions)[1] (Table 8-3). This classification is artificial, and seldom is a particular disease associated with a single mechanism only. The four mechanisms are interrelated, and in most hypersensitivity reactions, several mechanisms are at work simultaneously. Some of them are secondary to disease, whereas others are pathognomonic (diagnostic of) and the primary cause of tissue destruction.

Hypersensitivity reactions are immediate or delayed, depending on the time required to elicit the secondary immune response (i.e., for the reaction to appear after reexposure to the antigen). Reactions that occur within minutes are termed **immediate hypersensitivity reactions. Delayed hypersensitivity reactions** may take several hours to appear and are at maximum severity days after reexposure to the antigen.

The most rapid and severe immediate hypersensitivity reaction is **anaphylaxis.** Anaphylaxis occurs within minutes of reexposure to the antigen and can be either systemic (generalized) or cutaneous (localized).[2] Symptoms of systemic anaphylaxis include itching, erythema, vomiting, abdominal cramps, diarrhea, and breathing difficulties. In severe cases, laryngeal edema and vascular collapse may result in respiratory distress, decreased blood pressure, shock, and death. Cutaneous anaphylaxis causes the less severe symptoms of local inflammation.

IgE-Mediated Reactions

Type I reactions are characterized by the production of antigen-specific IgE after exposure to an antigen (Fig. 8-1). Most common allergic reactions are mediated by IgE and therefore are type I reactions. In addition, most type I reactions are against environmental antigens and are therefore allergic. Antigens that cause allergic responses are called **allergens.** It is not known why some antigens are allergens and others are not, but most allergens appear to be proteins that enter the host from the environment.

Role of IgE

In some individuals, exposure to an allergen causes IgE production by selected B cells. Repeated exposure to relatively large doses of allergen usually is required to elicit enough IgE so that the person is "sensitized." IgE binds to Fc receptors on the plasma membranes of mast cells (see Fig. 8-1). The Fc region of IgE and the subclass IgG4 have binding sites specific for receptors on the mast cell. Antibody that binds to mast cells is termed **cytotropic** (able to bind to cell surfaces). **Reagin,** or skin-sensitizing antibody, has been used interchangeably with the term *cytotropic antibody.* The Fc receptors on mast cells bind with IgE that has not previously interacted with antigen.

After the individual is sensitized and with further exposure to the allergen, the allergen's antigenic determinants bind to two molecules of mast cell–bound IgE, cross-linking two IgE-Fc receptor complexes and initiating degranulation of the mast cell and the release of a plethora of mast cell products (see Fig. 8-1, *B,* and Chapter 6). Sometimes the IgE-mediated allergic response is beneficial to the host, as is the case with IgE-mediated destruction of parasites. (This mechanism is described in Chapter 7 and illustrated in Fig. 7-18.)

Mechanisms of IgE-Mediated Hypersensitivity

The products of mast cell degranulation can modulate almost all aspects of an acute inflammatory response. (The effects of biochemical mediators released by mast cells are illustrated in Fig. 7-4). The most potent mediator of IgE-mediated hypersensitivity is histamine, which has effects on key target cells. Acting through certain histamine receptors (H1 receptors) on target cells in the host tissue, histamine contracts bronchial smooth muscles, causing bronchial constriction; increases vascular permeability, causing edema; and causes vasodilation, increasing blood flow into the affected area (see Fig. 7-11). The interaction of histamine with H2 receptors on target cells results in increased gastric secretion and a decrease of histamine released from mast cells and basophils. (Basophils are granulocytes in the blood that are thought to be similar to mast cells.) The action of histamine through H2 receptors suggests an important negative-feedback loop that stops degranulation. That is, the released histamine inhibits release of additional histamine by interacting with H2 receptors on the mast cells. Histamine also may affect control of the immune response through H2 receptors on most cells of the immune system. Another important activity of histamine is its function as a chemotactic factor for eosinophils. In conjunction with eosinophil chemotactic factor of anaphylaxis (ECF-A), histamine enhances attraction of eosinophils into sites of allergic inflammatory reactions and also deactivates and prevents them from migrating out of the inflammatory site. (The role of the eosinophil in inflammation is discussed in Chapter 7.)

Although some control of the allergic response is mediated through histamine receptors, the primary mechanism of control is the autonomic nervous system. The autonomic nervous system includes biochemical mediators (e.g., epinephrine, acetylcholine) that, like the mediators of the inflammatory response, have profound effects on the behavior of target cells in the host tissue. The nervous system mediators bind to appropriate receptors on both mast cells and the target cells of inflammation, thereby controlling (1) release of inflammatory mediators from mast cells and (2) the degree to which target cells respond to inflammatory mediators (see Chapters 1 and 13).

Clinical Manifestations

The clinical manifestations of type I reactions are attributable mostly to the biologic effects of histamine released during mast cell degranulation. The target tissues of the type I response contain large numbers of mast cells and are sen-

Table 8-3 Immunologic Mechanisms of Tissue Destruction

Type	Name	Rate of Development	Class of Antibody Involved	Principal Effector Cells Involved	Complement Participation	Examples of Disorders
I	IgE-mediated reaction	Immediate	IgE	Mast cells	No	Seasonal allergic rhinitis
II	Tissue-specific reaction	Immediate	IgG IgM	Macrophages in tissues	Frequently	Autoimmune thrombocytopenic purpura, Graves disease, autoimmune hemolytic anemia
III	Immune complex–mediated reaction	Immediate	IgG IgM	Neutrophils	Yes	Systemic lupus erythematosus
IV	Cell-mediated reaction	Delayed	None	Lymphocytes Macrophages	No	Contact sensitivity to poison ivy and metals (jewelry)

Ig, Immunoglobulin.

sitive to the effects of histamine released from them. These tissues are found in the gastrointestinal tract, the skin, and the respiratory tract (Fig. 8-2 and Table 8-4).

Gastrointestinal allergy is caused primarily by allergens that enter through the mouth—usually foods. Hypersensitivity frequently is manifested by vomiting, diarrhea, or abdominal pain and may be severe enough to result in malabsorption or protein-losing enteropathy. Foods most frequently implicated in gastrointestinal allergies are milk, chocolate, citrus fruits, eggs, wheat, nuts, peanut butter, and fish. When food is the allergen, the active immunogen may be an unidentifiable product of food breakdown by digestive enzymes. Sometimes the allergen is a drug, an additive, or a preservative in the food. For example, cows treated for mastitis with penicillin yield milk containing trace amounts of this antibiotic. Thus hypersensitivity apparently caused by milk proteins may instead be the result of an allergy to penicillin.

Urticaria, or **hives,** is a dermal (skin) manifestation of allergic reactions. The underlying mechanism is the localized release of histamine and increased vascular permeability,

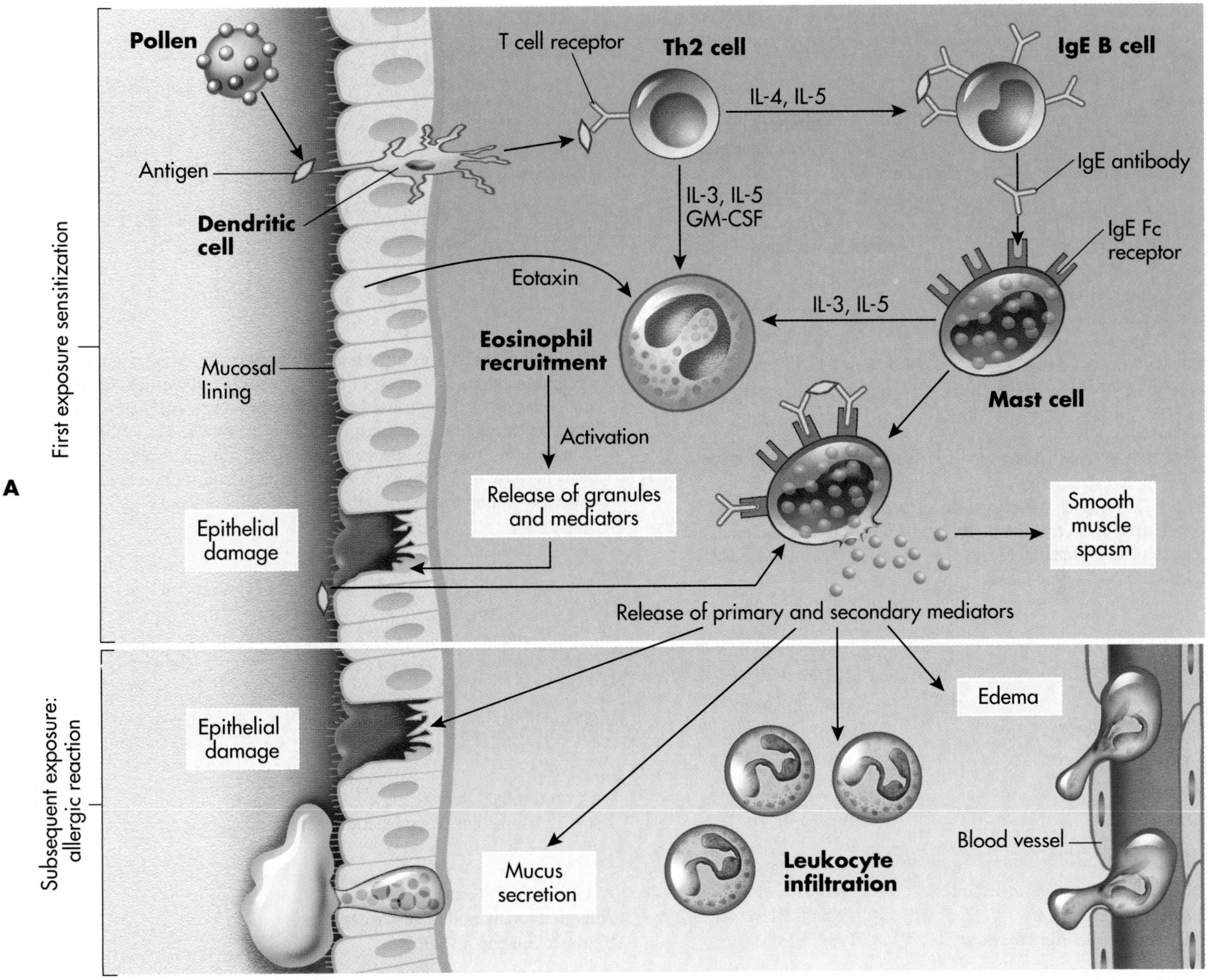

FIG. 8-1 Mechanism of type I IgE–mediated reactions. A, Precursors of Th2 cells by antigen-presenting dendritic cells. The newly made Th2 cells produce cytokines, including IL-3, IL-4, IL-5, and granulocyte-macrophage colony–stimulating factor (GM-CSF). IL-3, IL-5, and GM-CSF promote the survival of eosinophils. IgE-producing B cells increase and secrete IgE. The IgE coats the surface of the mast cell by binding with IgE-specific Fc receptors on the mast cell's plasma membrane. Further exposure to the same allergen crosslinks the surface-bound IgE and activates signals from the cytoplasmic portion of the IgE Fc receptors. These signals initiate two parallel and interdependent processes: one leading to mast cell degranulation and discharge of preformed mediators, and the other newly formed mediators such as arachidonic metabolites. Many local type I hypersensitivity reactions have two well-defined phases. The *initial phase* is characterized by vasodilation, vascular leakage, and, depending on the location, smooth muscle spasm or glandular secretions. These changes usually become evident within 5 to 30 minutes after exposure to the antigen. The *late phase* occurs 2 to 8 hours later without additional exposure to the antigen. The late phase has more intense infiltration of tissues with eosinophils, neutrophils, basophils, monocytes, and T helper cells and tissue destruction in the form of mucosal epithelial cell damage.

Continued

B

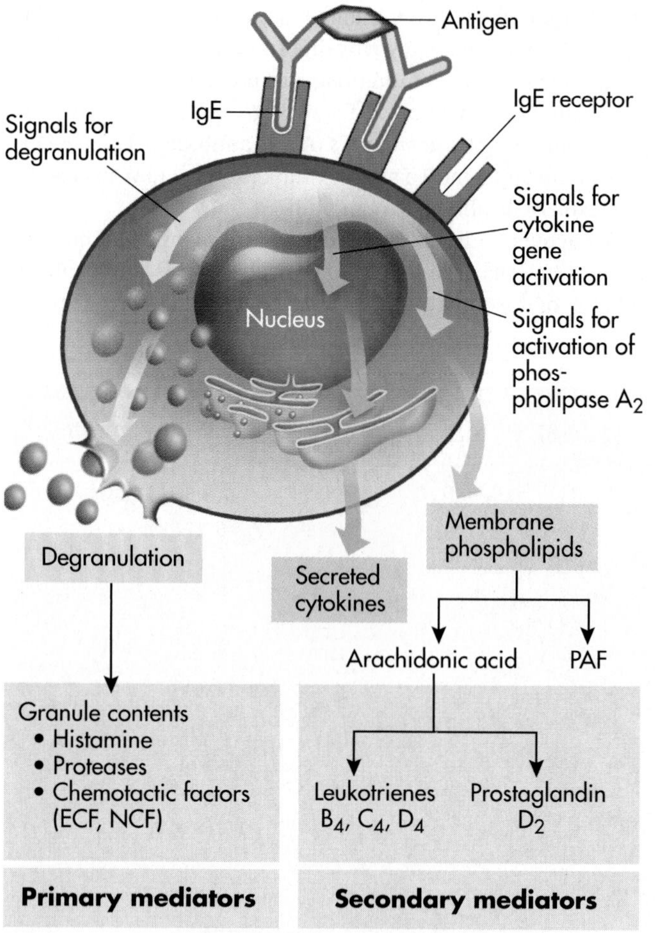

FIG. 8-1, cont'd Mechanism of type I IgE–mediated reactions. B, Activation of mast cells where preformed mediators release primary mediators and newly formed (de novo) mediators release secondary mediators.

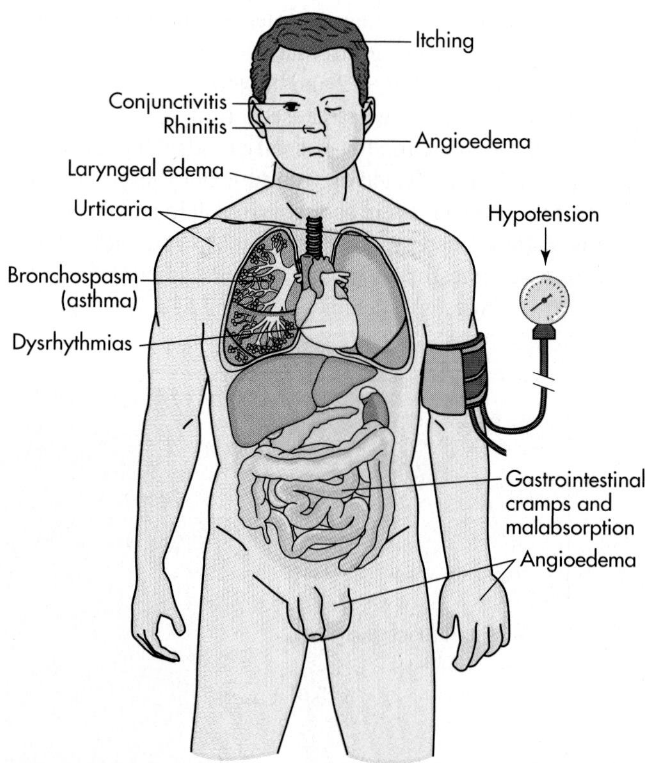

FIG. 8-2 Type I hypersensitivity reactions. Manifestations of allergic reactions as a result of type I hypersensitivity include itching, angioedema (swelling caused by exudation), edema of the larynx, urticaria (hives), bronchospasm (constriction of airways in the lungs), hypotension (low blood pressure) and dysrhythmias (irregular heartbeat) because of anaphylactic shock, and gastrointestinal cramping caused by inflammation of the gastrointestinal mucosa.

Table 8-4 Causes of Clinical Manifestations of Allergy

Typical Allergen	Mechanism of Hypersensitivity	Clinical Manifestation
INGESTANTS		
Foods	Type I	Gastrointestinal allergy
Drugs	Types I, II, III	Urticaria, immediate drug reaction, hemolytic anemia, serum sickness
INHALANTS		
Pollens, dust, molds	Type I	Allergic rhinitis, bronchial asthma
Aspergillus fumigatus	Types I, III	Allergic bronchopulmonary aspergillosis
Thermophilic actinomycetes*	Types III, IV	Extrinsic allergic alveolitis
INJECTANTS		
Drugs	Types I, II, III	Immediate drug reaction, hemolytic anemia, serum sickness
Bee venom	Type I	Anaphylaxis
Vaccines	Type III	Localized Arthus reaction
Serum	Types I, III	Anaphylaxis, serum sickness
CONTACTANTS		
Poison ivy, metals	Type IV	Contact dermatitis

Modified from Bellanti JA: *Immunology III,* Philadelphia, 1985, W.B. Saunders.
*An order of fungi that is stimulated by warmth to grow and proliferate.

resulting in limited areas of edema. Urticaria is characterized by white fluid-filled blisters (wheals) surrounded by areas of redness (flares). The **wheal and flare reaction** is usually accompanied by itching. Not all urticarial symptoms are caused by allergic (immunologic) reactions. Some, termed *nonimmunologic urticaria,* result from exposure to cold temperatures, emotional stress, drugs, systemic diseases, hyperthyroidism, or malignancies (e.g., lymphomas).

Effects of allergens on the mucosa of the eyes, nose, and respiratory tract include conjunctivitis (inflammation of the membranes lining the eyelids), rhinitis (inflammation of the mucous membranes of the nose), and asthma (constriction of the bronchi). Clinical manifestations are caused by vasodilation, hypersecretion of mucus, edema, and swelling of the respiratory mucosa. Because the mucous membranes lining the respiratory tract (accessory sinuses, nasopharynx, and upper and lower respiratory tract) are continuous, they are all adversely affected by the allergic reaction. The degree to which each is affected determines the clinical manifestations of the disease.

The central defect in allergic diseases of the lung, such as asthma, is obstruction of the lumen of the large and small airways (bronchi) of the lower respiratory tract by bronchospasm (constriction of smooth muscle in airway walls), edema, thick secretions, and hyperplasia of smooth muscle and mucus-secreting glands. This leads to ventilatory insufficiency, wheezing, and difficult or labored breathing. Asthma is acute, intermittent, and reversible. Extrinsic asthma is an allergic reaction caused by a known exogenous allergen, whereas intrinsic asthma has no known cause. (Asthma is described further in Chapter 32.)

Genetic Predisposition

Certain individuals who appear to be prone to allergies are referred to as atopic.[3] **Atopic individuals** tend to produce higher concentrations of IgE and to have more Fc receptors on their mast cells. Subtle defects in T lymphocyte function (e.g., a deficiency in IgE-specific suppressor cells) may account for heightened IgE production. The airways and the skin of atopic individuals are also more responsive to a wide variety of both specific and nonspecific stimuli than are the airways and skin of normal individuals. There appears to be a genetic basis for the state; some individuals are genetically predisposed to become sensitized against allergens. In families in which one parent has an allergy, allergies develop in about 40% of the offspring. If both parents have atopic disease, the incidence in offspring is approximately 80%. (Principles of genetic inheritance are discussed in Chapter 4.)

Tests of IgE-Mediated Hypersensitivity

Allergic reactions can be life threatening; therefore it is essential that severely allergic individuals be made aware of the specific allergen against which they are sensitized and instructed to avoid contact with that material. Several tests are available to determine the specific allergen. These tests include skin tests with allergens and laboratory tests for total IgE and allergen-specific IgE.

On injection of an allergen into (intradermal) or onto (epicutaneous or prick test) the skin of a sensitized individual, a local anaphylactic reaction occurs within a few minutes. It consists of a localized swelling and redness, or a wheal and flare reaction. The diameter of the flare reaction is usually indicative of the individual's sensitivity to that allergen. In the most severely allergic individuals, even the extremely small amounts of allergen used for the skin test may evoke a systemic anaphylaxis.

A variety of laboratory tests can detect IgE antibodies. The **radioimmunosorbent test (RIST)** measures circulating levels of total IgE, with atopic individuals usually having elevated levels. The **radioallergosorbent test (RAST)** has been used to measure circulating levels of specific IgE antibodies against many allergens, and the amount of IgE has been found to correlate well with the degree of positive skin test and the severity of clinical symptoms.

Desensitization

Clinical desensitization to allergens can be achieved in some individuals.[4] Minute quantities of the allergen to which the person is sensitive are injected in increasing doses over a prolonged period. This procedure may reduce the severity of the allergic reaction in the treated individual. However, this form of therapy is associated with the risk of systemic anaphylaxis, which, when severe, can be life threatening.[5] Desensitization may work by inducing the production of large amounts of so-called blocking antibodies. A **blocking antibody** presumably competes in the tissues or in the circulation for binding with antigenic determinants on the allergen. Thus neutralized, the antigen is unable to bind with IgE on mast cells. In serum, blocking antibodies are predominantly IgG. The role of blocking antibodies has not been firmly established. Desensitization injections also may stimulate the generation of clones of suppressor T lymphocytes, which inhibit hypersensitivity by suppressing the production of IgE.

Tissue-Specific Reactions

Type II hypersensitivity reactions are generally characterized by the destruction of a target cell through the action of antibody against an antigen on the cell's plasma membrane. In addition to histocompatibility locus antigens (HLAs), most tissues have other antigens. These other antigens are generally called **tissue-specific antigens,** because they are expressed on the plasma membranes of only certain cells. Platelets, for example, have groups of self-antigens that are found on no other cells of the body. Because of limited distribution of tissue-specific antigens, type II diseases are limited to those tissues or organs that express the particular antigen. Environmental antigens (e.g., drugs or their metabolites) also may bind to the plasma membranes of cells (especially erythrocytes and platelets) and function as targets of type II reactions.

There are four general mechanisms by which type II, or tissue-specific, hypersensitivity reactions can destroy or alter cells (Fig. 8-3). All of these mechanisms begin with antibody binding to tissue-specific antigens.

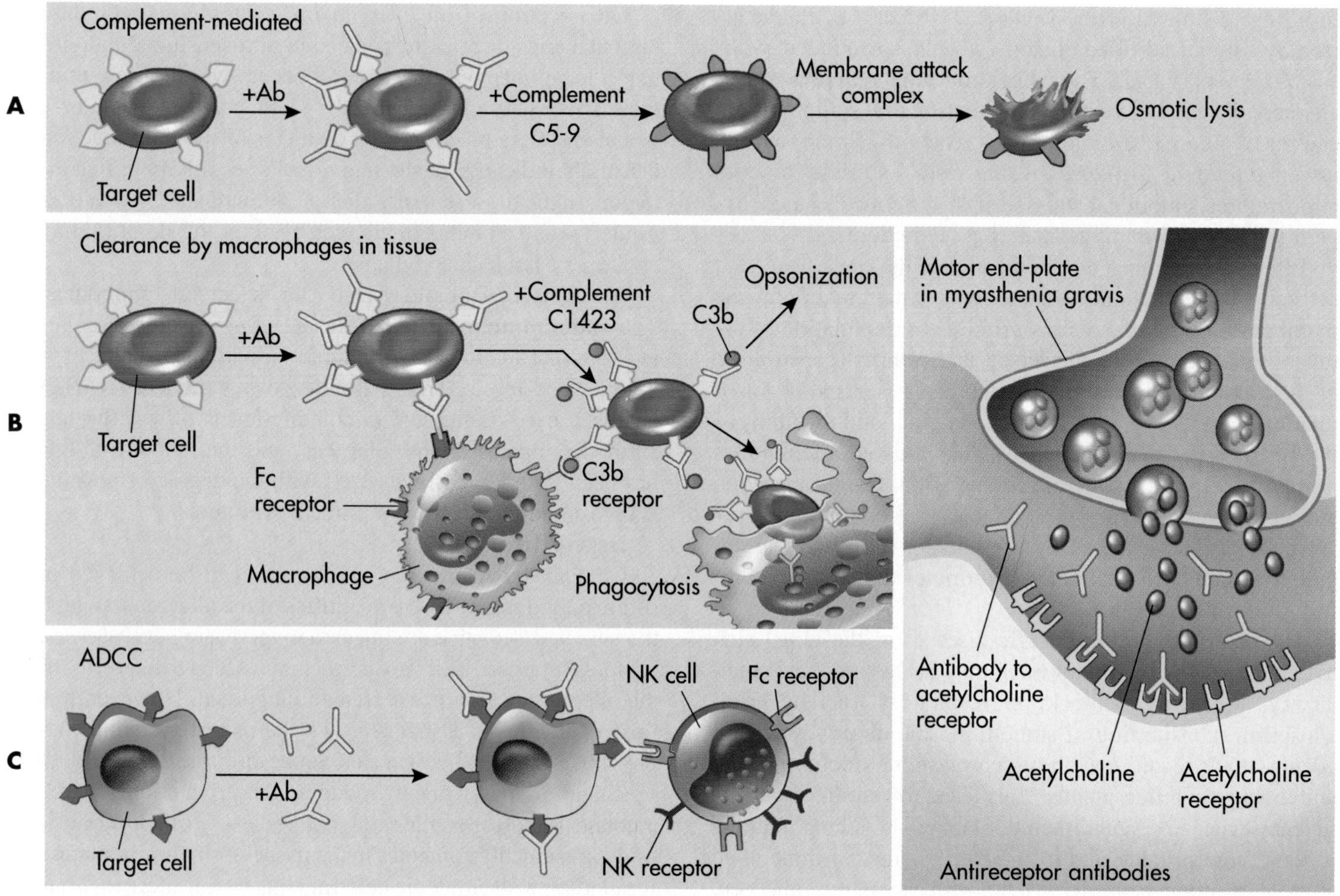

FIG. 8-3 Mechanisms of type II, tissue-specific reactions. Antigens on the target cell bind with antibody and are destroyed or prevented from functioning by **A,** complement-mediated lysis; **B,** clearance by macrophages in tissue; **C,** antibody-dependent cell-mediated cytotoxicity (ADCC). IgG-coated target cells are lysed by cells that have Fc receptors for IgG (e.g., NK cells, macrophages). **D,** Antireceptor antibodies modulate or block the normal function of receptors. This example shows myasthenia gravis where acetylcholine receptor antibodies block acetycholine from attachment to its receptors on the motor end plates of skeletal muscle, impairing neuromuscular transmission and causing muscle weakness.

There are two mechanisms by which antibody and complement may mediate type II hypersensitivity: complement-mediated lysis and opsonization. In the first type, antibody (IgM or IgG) reacts with an antigen present on the surface of the cell, causing activation of the complement system and resulting in the membrane attack complex (C5-9) that lyses the membrane by drilling holes through the bilayer (see Fig. 8-3, *A*). Circulating erythrocytes, for example, are destroyed by complement-mediated lysis in individuals with autoimmune hemolytic anemia (see Chapter 25) or alloimmune reactions to ABO-mismatched transfused blood cells from a donor (Fig. 8-4).

The second mechanism of type II cell destruction is phagocytosis by macrophages of the mononuclear phagocyte system. The Fc receptors on the macrophage recognize and bind the antibody on opsonized (e.g., fixation of antibody or C3b fragment) (see Fig. 8-3, *B*) cells. Phagocytosis of the target cell follows. (Phagocytosis is illustrated in Fig. 7-15.) Antibodies against platelet-specific antigens or against red blood cell antigens of the Rh system will coat those cells at low density, resulting in their preferential removal by phagocytosis in the spleen, rather than by complement-mediated lysis.

The third mechanism of type II host cell destruction is antibody-dependent cell-mediated cytotoxicity (ADCC) (see Fig. 8-3, *C*). This mechanism involves cell destruction by a subpopulation of cytotoxic cells that are not antigen specific (natural killer [NK] cells). Antibody on the target cell is recognized by and bound to Fc receptors on the NK cells, which release toxic substances that destroy the cell.

The fourth mechanism does not destroy the target cell, but rather causes it to malfunction. In this mechanism of type II injury, the damage is done by antibody binding alone (see Fig. 8-3, *D*). The antibody binds to the target cell, occupying and altering receptors that would bind with the various molecules (ligands) required for normal cellular function. For example, in hyperthyroidism (excessive thyroid activity) caused by Graves disease, **autoantibody** activates receptors for thyroid-stimulating hormone (TSH) (a pituitary hormone that controls the production of the hormone

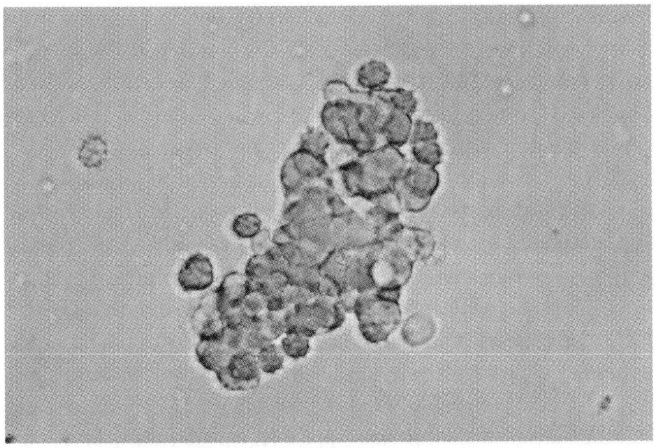

FIG. 8-4 Mismatched transfused blood cells. Agglutination caused by anti-A blood typing system. (Copyright © Ed Reschke.)

thyroxine by the thyroid). The antibody-activated receptors stimulate the thyroid cells to overproduce thyroxine despite decreasing amounts of TSH (see Chapter 20).

Immune Complex–Mediated Injury

Mechanisms

Most type III hypersensitivity diseases are caused by antigen-antibody (immune) complexes that are formed in the circulation and deposited later in vessel walls or extravascular tissues (Fig. 8-5). The primary difference between type II and type III mechanisms is that the antigen in type II hypersensitivity remains at its normal location on the cell surface, whereas the antigen in type III is soluble, having been released into the blood or body fluids. Type III immune complex–mediated reactions therefore are not organ specific, and symptoms have little to do with the antigenic target of the antibody.[6] In some instances, immune complex disease begins with the deposition of antigen in the tissues and is followed by local interactions with antibody and complement. Regardless of whether immune complexes are formed in the circulation or in the tissues, their harmful effects are caused by complement activation, particularly the generation of complement fragments that are chemotactic for neutrophils. The neutrophils attempt to ingest the immune complexes but frequently are unsuccessful because the complexes are bound to the tissues. During the neutrophil's attempts to phagocytose the immune complexes, large quantities of lysosomal enzymes are released into the inflammatory site instead of into phagolysosomes. The attraction of neutrophils and the subsequent release of lysosomal enzymes cause most of the resulting tissue damage.

Fairly large immune complexes are cleared rapidly from the circulation by the tissue macrophages of the mononuclear phagocyte system, whereas very small complexes eventually are filtered from blood through the kidneys, without any pathologic consequences. Intermediate-sized immune complexes (formed at a ratio of antigen to antibody that has a slight excess of antigen) are likely to be deposited in certain target tissues, where they have severe pathologic

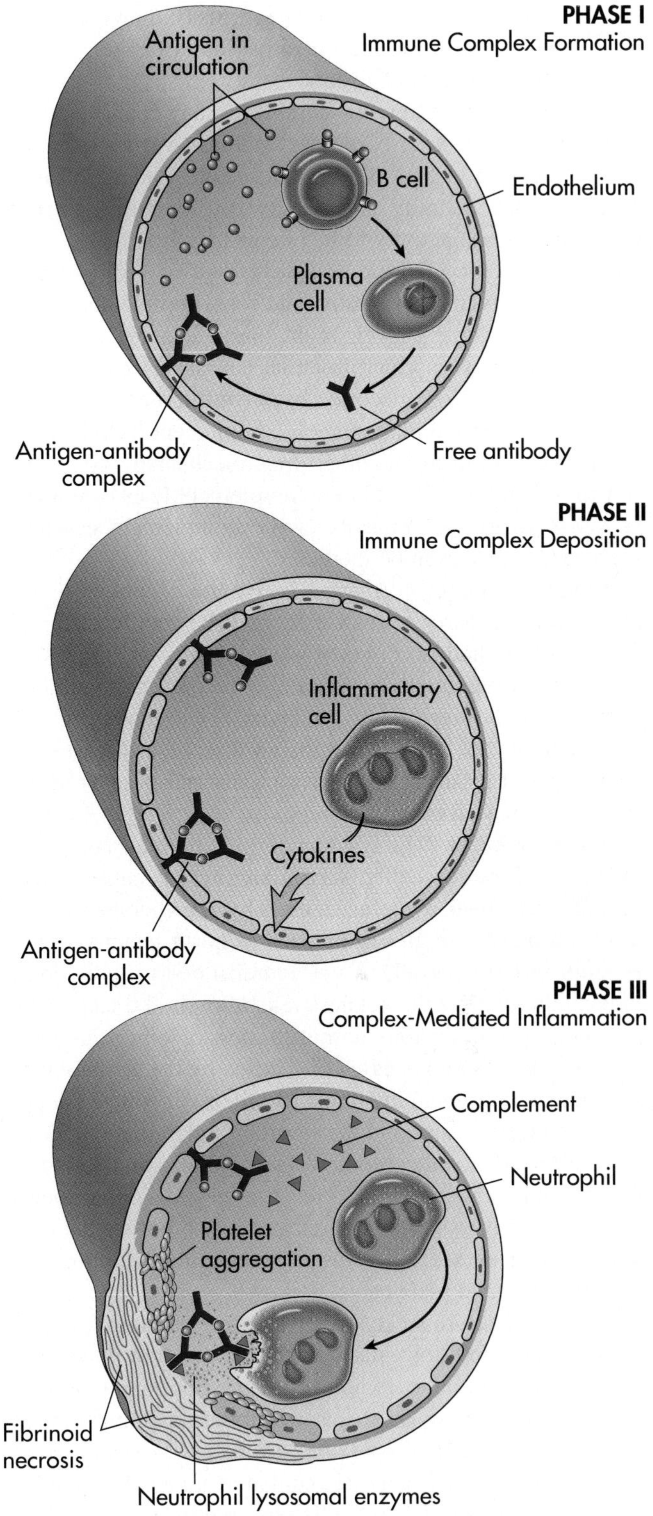

FIG. 8-5 Mechanism of type III, immune complex–mediated reactions. Three sequential phases include phase I with immune complex formation, phase II immune complex deposition, and phase III activation of the complement cascade and generation of complement fragments including C5a. C5a is chemotactic for neutrophils, which migrate into the inflamed area and attach to the IgG and C3b in the immune complexes. The neutrophils degranulate a variety of degradative enzymes that destroy healthy tissues. (From Cotran RS, Kumar V, Collins T: *Robbins pathologic basis of disease,* ed 6, Philadelphia, 1999, W.B. Saunders.)

consequences, such as glomerulonephritis (kidney), vasculitis (vessels), or arthritis (degenerative joint disease).

Immune Complex Disease

The nature of the immune complexes may change and result in changes in severity of the symptoms. Variations in the ratio of antigen to antibody, the class and subclass of antibody, and the quantity and quality of circulating antigen cause the disease activity to be in constant flux.

Because some immune complexes activate complement very effectively and covalently bind some complement components, complement levels in the blood also are in flux. In many conditions in which immune complexes are formed, the individual's blood becomes **hypocomplementemic** (i.e., contains decreased amounts of complement activity). In conditions caused by the other three mechanisms of hypersensitivity (types I, II, and IV), complement levels are unaffected, or some components of the complement cascade, such as C3, may even be increased.

Immune complex formation is dynamic: immune complexes formed early in a disease may be totally different from those formed later in the disease. At any one time, several types of immune complexes may be present simultaneously. With the tremendous potential heterogeneity of immune complexes, it is not surprising that these diseases are characterized by a variety of symptoms and periods of remission or exacerbation of symptoms.

Serum sickness. The systemic form of immune complex–mediated disease is called **serum sickness** because it was initially described as being caused by the therapeutic administration of foreign serum, such as horse tetanus toxin.[7] Foreign serum generally is not administered to individuals today, although serum sickness reactions can be caused by the repeated intravenous administration of other antigens, such as drugs. Serum sickness is caused by the formation of immune complexes in the blood and their generalized deposition in target tissues and the resultant inflammation. Typically affected are the blood vessels, joints, and kidneys. Other manifestations include fever, enlarged lymph nodes, rash, and pain at sites of inflammation. Laboratory findings may include decreased levels of circulating lymphocytes, granulocytes, and platelets.

A form of serum sickness is **Raynaud phenomenon,** an autoimmune condition caused by the temperature-dependent deposition of immune complexes in the peripheral circulation. (Immune complexes that precipitate at temperatures below normal body temperature are called *cryoglobulins.*) The symptoms of Raynaud phenomenon are localized pallor and numbness (usually in the fingers and toes), followed by cyanosis (a bluish tinge resulting from oxygen deprivation) and gangrene or by pain and redness. These signs and symptoms are caused by the temperature-dependent precipitation of immune complexes in the capillary beds of the peripheral circulation and the resulting inflammatory processes.

Arthus reaction. An **Arthus reaction** is an example of a localized immune complex–mediated inflammatory response.[8] It is caused by repeated local exposure to exogenous antigen that reacts with preformed antibody in the walls of blood vessels. Symptoms of an Arthus reaction begin within 1 hour of exposure and peak 6 to 12 hours later. The lesions are characterized by a typical inflammatory reaction, with increased vascular permeability, an accumulation of neutrophils, edema, hemorrhage, clotting, and tissue damage.

Arthus reactions are observed after injection, ingestion, or inhalation of exogenous antigens. Skin reactions can follow subcutaneous or intradermal inoculation with drugs, fungal extracts, or antigens used in skin tests. Gastrointestinal reactions, such as gluten-sensitive enteropathy (celiac disease), follow ingestion of antigen, usually gluten from wheat products (see Chapter 38). Allergic alveolitis (farmer's lung; pigeon breeder's disease) is an Arthus-like acute hemorrhagic inflammation of the air sacs (alveoli) of the lung (see Chapter 32). Allergic alveoliuis is caused by inhalation of fungal antigens, usually particles from moldy hay or pigeon feces.

Cell-Mediated Tissue Destruction

Whereas types I, II, and III hypersensitivity reactions are mediated by antibody, type IV (cell-mediated) reactions are mediated by specifically sensitized T lymphocytes and do not involve antibody (Fig. 8-6). Type IV mechanisms occur as one of two types involving either cytotoxic T lymphocytes (Tc cells) or lymphokine-producing T cells (Td cells). Tc cells can attack and destroy cellular targets directly. Td

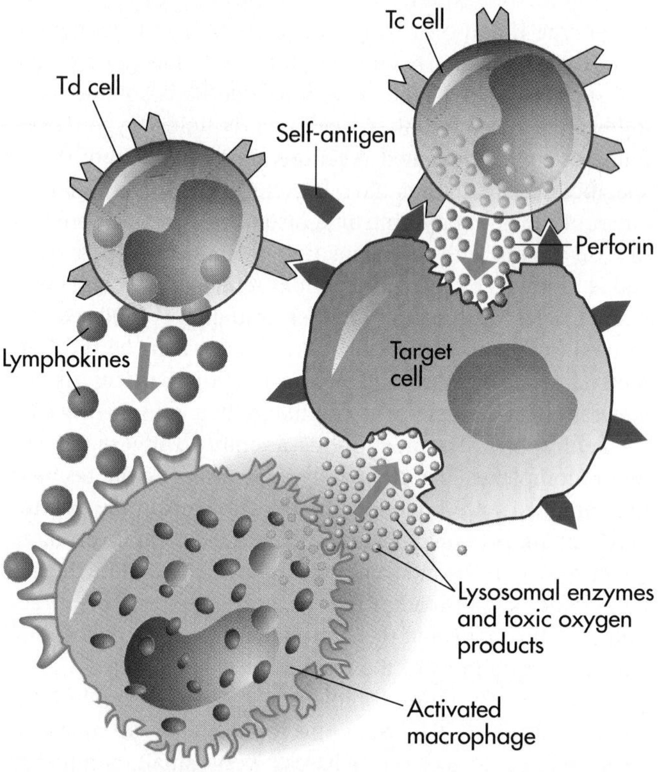

FIG. 8-6 Mechanism of type IV, cell-mediated reactions. Self-antigens from target cells stimulate T cells to differentiate into cytotoxic T cells (Tc), which have direct cytotoxic activity, and T cells involved in delayed hypersensitivity (Td). Td cells, a form of Th cells, produce lymphokines, some of which attract and activate macrophages. The macrophages and enzymes released by them are responsible for most of the tissue destruction.

cells produce lymphokines, which affect various types of cells and can recruit and activate phagocytic cells, especially macrophages, at the inflammatory site. Tissue destruction usually is caused by direct killing by toxins from cytotoxic T cells or the release of soluble factors, such as lysosomal enzymes and toxic oxygen products from macrophages.

Clinical examples of type IV hypersensitivity include graft rejection, tumor rejection, the tuberculin reaction, and allergic reactions resulting from contact with such substances as poison ivy and metals. A type IV component also may be present in many autoimmune diseases such as rheumatoid arthritis, in which the self-antigen is apparently type II collagen (a protein present in joint tissues); autoimmune thyroiditis (Hashimoto disease), in which the self-antigen is a protein on thyroid cells; and insulin-dependent diabetes mellitus, in which the self-antigen is a protein on the beta cell of the pancreas (the cell that normally produces insulin).

A type IV hypersensitivity in the skin was thoroughly described first in 1891 and led to the development of a diagnostic skin test for tuberculosis.[9] The reaction in the skin that follows intradermal injection of antigen into a suitably sensitized individual is called *delayed hypersensitivity* because of its slow onset—24 to 72 hours to reach maximum intensity. The reaction site is also infiltrated with T lymphocytes and macrophages. One of the characteristics of delayed hypersensitivity is that it can be transferred to an unreactive recipient by cells but not by antiserum. This demonstrates that type IV hypersensitivity is mediated by lymphocytes rather than by antibody.

Allergic type IV reactions are elicited by some environmental antigens that are too small to be immunogenic by themselves (haptens).[10] (Immunogenicity is described in Chapter 6.) Antigens with a molecular weight of less than 1000 daltons are not usually immunogenic but become so after binding with a carrier protein in the host. In cases of allergic **contact dermatitis,** the carrier protein is in the skin of the host. The best-known example of allergic contact dermatitis is the delayed reaction caused by contact with poison ivy (Fig. 8-7). The antigen in this instance is a plant catechol, *urushiol,* that reacts with normal skin proteins and evokes a cell-mediated immune response. Skin reactions to industrial chemicals, cosmetics, detergents, clothing, food, metals, and topical medicines (such as penicillin) are elicited by the same mechanism.

Whether a skin reaction is caused by immediate or delayed hypersensitivity may be determined by the distribution of the lesions. The immediate reaction, termed **atopic dermatitis,** is manifested by widely distributed lesions, whereas contact dermatitis consists of lesions only at the site of contact (Fig. 8-8).

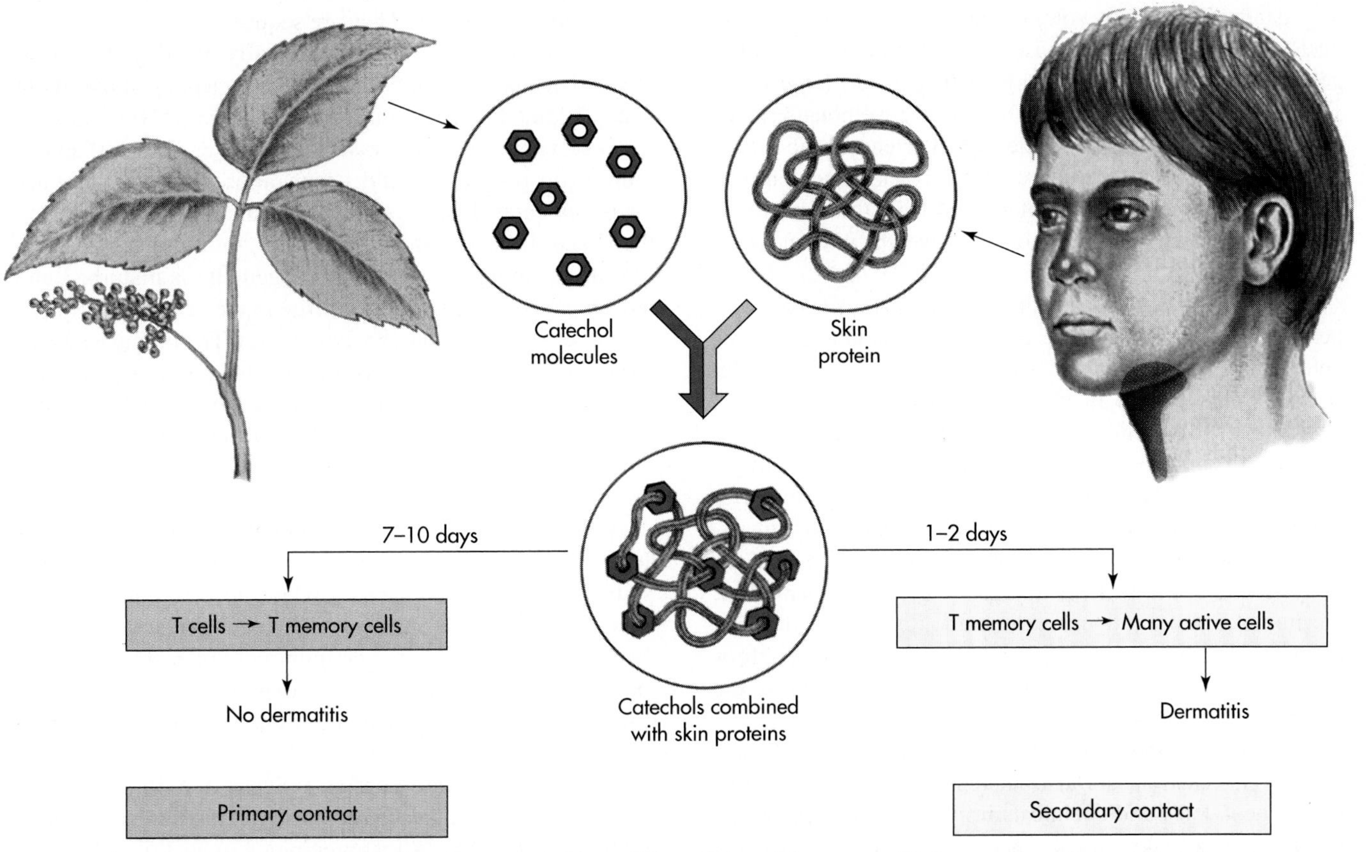

FIG. 8-7 Development of allergic contact dermatitis, a delayed hypersensitivity reaction. Shown here is the development of allergy to catechols from poison ivy. No dermatitis results from the primary contact because the antigens (catechols) are sensitizing the immune response and producing memory T cells. Secondary contact, however, quickly activates a type IV, cell-mediated reaction that causes dermatitis.

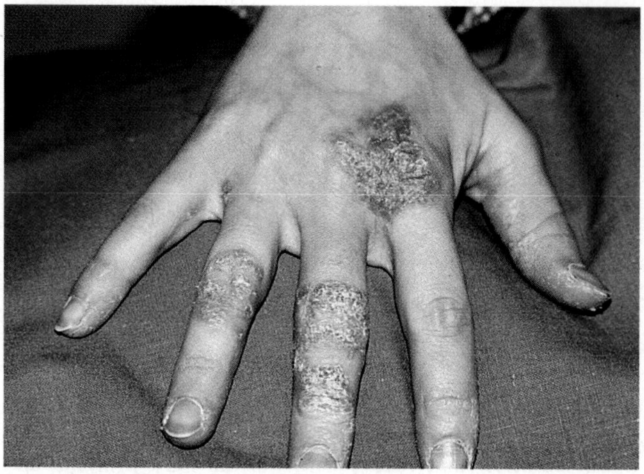

FIG. 8-8 Contact dermatitis. Contact dermatitis caused by a delayed hypersensitivity reaction leading to vesicles and scaling at the sites of contact. (From Damjanov I, Linder J: *Anderson's pathology,* ed 10, St Louis, 1996, Mosby.)

Targets of Hypersensitivity

Allergy

Allergens are environmental antigens that cause atypically exorbitant immunologic responses in genetically predisposed individuals. Typical allergens include pollens (e.g., ragweed, timothy), molds and fungi (e.g., *Penicillium notatum*), foods (e.g., milk, eggs, fish), animals (e.g., cat dander, dog dander), cigarette smoke, and components of house dust (e.g., fecal pellets of house mites). Frequently, the allergen is contained within a particle that is too large to be phagocytosed or is surrounded by a protective nonallergenic coat. The actual allergen is released after enzymatic breakdown (e.g., by lysozyme in secretions) of the larger particle. Most allergens are either haptens that have the capacity to react with proteins or low-molecular-weight immunogenic proteins.

In certain situations an allergen complexes with components of host tissue. The neoantigen, or new antigenic determinant, is recognized as foreign, and the tissue is destroyed. This occurs in allergic reactions to drugs (e.g., penicillin, sulfonamides), in which the drug binds to proteins on the plasma membranes of host cells. The drugs, which are usually haptens, become immunogenic after binding to the host cell's proteins. The immune system attacks the neoantigen on the host cell's membrane and destroys the cell as well. In allergic reactions to penicillin, the immunogenic antigen is a metabolite of penicillin catabolism that binds to the plasma membranes of erythrocytes and induces an antibody response that destroys the cells, causing anemia.

The allergens that induce contact hypersensitivity, a type IV allergic reaction, are also haptens (e.g., metals such as nickel, acetylates and chemicals in rubber, resins in poison ivy and poison oak), which react with normal self-proteins in the skin. When presented in this fashion, these antigens induce a cell-mediated response.

Autoimmunity

Breakdown of Tolerance

Self-antigens usually are tolerated by the host's own immune system. Immunologic tolerance, or immunologic homeostasis, develops in humans during the embryonic period, during which any autoreactive lymphocytes are either eliminated or suppressed. **Autoimmunity** is a breakdown of tolerance in which the body's immune system begins to recognize self-antigens as foreign. The mechanisms of breakdown are many and vary among autoimmune diseases, although in most such diseases the mechanism is unknown. Some of the mechanisms that have been implicated in the development of autoimmunity are (1) exposure within the body of a previously sequestered antigen, (2) the development of a neoantigen, (3) the complications of an infectious disease, (4) the emergence of a previously controlled or "forbidden" clone of lymphocytes with specificity for self-antigens, and (5) an alteration of suppressor T cell or anti–idiotypic antibody function. (Anti–idiotypic antibody is discussed in Chapter 6.)

Sequestered antigen. To be tolerated after birth, a self-antigen must be present in the fetus and exposed to the developing fetal immune system. Some self-antigens are not normally encountered in either fetal or adult life. Certain self-antigens, for example, in the cornea of the eye and in the testicles, are in areas of the body that are not drained by the lymphatics. Therefore these self-antigens never encounter antigen-processing cells in the draining lymph nodes or other lymphoid organs. They are sequestered or hidden from the immune system in **immunologically privileged sites,** so named because foreign tissues can be transplanted into these sites without danger of immunologic rejection. Immunologically privileged sites are vascular, however, so that if an immunologic reaction should occur, antibodies and lymphocytes can enter the site and cause immunologic rejection of the tissue. In some situations, especially trauma, the structure of an immunologically privileged site is disturbed and the previously **sequestered antigens** are released from the damaged tissue and enter the lymphatics. The immune system recognizes these antigens as foreign, and a primary immune response occurs that can inflict extensive immunologic damage to the untraumatized site. An example is sympathetic uveitis, an ocular disease in which physical trauma to one eye results in immunologic injury to the other eye.

Neoantigen. In certain situations a neoantigen that induces an allergic reaction may lead also to autoimmunity. Many **neoantigens** are haptens, which become immunogenic after binding to host proteins. The immune reaction against the neoantigen may lead to an immunologic reaction against the unaltered host protein. Many experimental autoimmune diseases (e.g., experimental autoimmune thyroiditis) can be initiated by this mechanism.

Infectious disease. Foreign antigens from infectious microorganisms can initiate hypersensitivity disease by (1) forming immune complexes that precipitate in host tissues, causing inflammatory disease, or (2) so closely resembling a particular self-antigen (cross reacts with the self-antigen) that they stimulate production of antibodies that also recognize the self-antigen as foreign. Group A streptococci are capable of initiating both these mechanisms, usually as sequelae to streptococcal pharyngitis.

The first mechanism, deposition of immune complexes, is the cause of poststreptococcal glomerulonephritis (inflammation of the kidney). Deposition elicits an inflammatory response that destroys tissues in the glomeruli of the kidney. Because the antigen is foreign, this particular process is allergic. (In Fig. 8-5 this mechanism is illustrated in a blood vessel.) The second mechanism, in which the foreign antigen mimics the molecular structure of a self-antigen, occurs in rheumatic fever and is autoimmune because the target antigen is a self-antigen. In rheumatic fever, streptococcal antigens so closely resemble self-antigens on the heart valve that antibodies produced to incapacitate the streptococci also damage cells of the heart valve.

Forbidden clone. The *clonal deletion theory* on tolerance states that maturing lymphocytes in the central lymphoid organs encounter self-antigen during embryogenesis and, as lymphocytes reactive against self-antigen develop, their clones are prevented, or "forbidden," from maturing. Autoimmunity may result from the survival of a **forbidden clone** and its proliferation later in life. No known autoimmune disease has been shown to be caused by this mechanism, but the pathogenesis of most autoimmune diseases has not yet been discovered. Most likely the only autoreactive clones that are deleted in the central lymphoid organs are those against antigens that are widely distributed in the body, such as self-HLAs or the individual's own blood group A or B antigens.

Suppressor cell dysfunction. Despite the normal development of tolerance, sometimes clones of lymphocytes against self-antigens develop in healthy adults. One of the roles of suppressor T cells may be to suppress the immune responses that these clones activate. Suppressor T cell dysfunction can therefore result in autoimmune disease. If a single antigen-specific population of suppressor cells is affected, a tissue-specific autoimmune disease results. A generalized autoimmune reaction occurs if many suppressor cell populations are dysfunctional. **Systemic lupus erythematosus (SLE),** which is characterized by the production of a large array of autoantibodies, may be caused by a general breakdown in the suppressor cell network.

Original Insult

The cause of some immune diseases is apparent. For example, in drug-induced anemia or thrombocytopenia (decreased numbers of circulating platelets), ample evidence exists that immunologic destruction of erythrocytes or platelets follows the integration of a drug or its metabolite (product of catabolism) into the plasma membranes of the host cells. This causes the immune system to recognize the altered plasma membranes as new and foreign cellular antigens. B cells are stimulated to produce antibody against the drug-cell complex, and immune processes destroy the host cells. Viruses can induce autoimmune reactions by altering the plasma membranes of host cells. In rubella infections, for example, encephalitis can ensue when cells of the nervous system become infected and express virally derived antigens on their plasma membranes. Like the antigenic alterations caused by drug metabolism, virus-induced changes result in the destruction of infected cells by the host's immune system.

The causes of other immune diseases, such as rheumatoid arthritis and SLE, are less clear. Most autoimmune diseases are probably sequelae of preexisting infections that leave no traces to facilitate their identification.

Genetic Factors

Genetic factors that contribute to autoimmunity are easier to identify than pathogenic agents.[11] It is fairly well established that autoimmune diseases can be familial. Affected family members may not all develop the same disease, but several members may have different disorders characterized by hypersensitivity.

The association of diseases with specific HLAs (see Chapter 6) has been recognized only recently and is a relatively nebulous phenomenon. The HLA types of susceptible and resistant individuals have been analyzed for almost every known disease, and, almost universally, individuals with certain diseases are more likely than the general population to have a specific HLA allele or alleles. Some associations are strong; others are more tenuous. The reason some HLA alleles are associated with inappropriate immune function is unclear, but it may directly involve the ability of particular HLA molecules to present antigen or the use of particular HLAs as receptors for disease-causing organisms. These genes may determine an individual's susceptibility to specific infectious agents or the capacity of that individual to mount an immune response against specific antigens. Therefore an individual of a specific HLA type may have inappropriate or exaggerated immune responses against a microorganism, resulting in a hypersensitivity reaction.

Alloimmunity

Alloimmunity occurs when an individual's immune system reacts against antigens on the tissues of other members of the same species. The two clinically relevant examples of this reactivity are (1) transient neonatal diseases (in which the maternal immune system becomes sensitized against antigens expressed by the fetus) and (2) transplant rejection and transfusion reactions (in which the immune system of a recipient of an organ transplant or blood transfusion reacts against antigens on the donor cells).

Because the fetus is a hybrid between the mother and father, it expresses paternal antigens that are not found in the mother. Occasionally, these fetal antigens cross the placenta and elicit an immune response in the mother. Maternal antibody may be transported into the fetal circulation to produce alloimmune disease in the fetus. The mother's immune system produces the antibody, but because her cells do not express the target antigen, she has no manifestations of the disease.

Alloimmune disease may be in conjunction with maternal autoimmune diseases. The mother may be producing an IgG autoantibody specific for maternal self-antigens that are found on fetal cells as well. Therefore symptoms of the same autoimmune disease may affect both mother and child, even though the autoantibody is being produced only by the mother's immune system. This form of disease usually occurs only in association with type II (tissue-specific) reactions. It does not occur in association with IgE-mediated (type I) reactions, immune complex–mediated (type III) reactions, or cell-mediated (type IV) reactions, because the immunologic products of these reactions do not readily cross the placenta and enter the fetal circulation in sufficient quantity.

At birth, the source of the antibody in the fetal circulation is removed. Although symptoms of the alloimmune disease may be manifested in utero or immediately after birth and may be fatal to the fetus or neonate, if symptoms are successfully treated at birth the disease will disappear as the maternal antibody is catabolized.

Examples of immunologic diseases in which the child can be affected include the following antibody-mediated diseases:

1. *Graves disease*—an autoimmune disease in which maternal antibody against the receptor for TSH causes neonatal hyperthyroidism
2. *Myasthenia gravis*—an autoimmune disease in which maternal antibody binds with receptors for neural transmitters on muscle cells (acetylcholine receptor), causing neonatal muscular weakness (see Chapter 16)
3. *Immune thrombocytopenic purpura*—in which maternal antiplatelet antibody destroys platelets in the neonate (see Chapter 27)
4. *Alloimmune neutropenia*—in which maternal antibody against neutrophils destroys neutrophils in the neonate
5. *Systemic lupus erythematosus*—in which diverse maternal autoantibodies induce anomalies (e.g., congenital heart defects) in the fetus
6. *Rh and ABO alloimmunization (e.g., erythroblastosis fetalis)*—in which maternal antibody against erythrocyte antigens induces anemia in the child (see Chapter 27)

Autoimmune and Alloimmune Diseases

Autoimmunity and alloimmunity are exemplified by two disease states, SLE (an autoimmune disease) and transplant rejection (an alloimmune phenomenon). Most of the classic autoimmune diseases, including disorders of the endocrine system (autoimmune thyroiditis and Graves disease), hematologic system (the hemolytic and pernicious anemias), nervous system (myasthenia gravis), and connective tissue in joints (rheumatoid arthritis), are discussed in Unit II of this book.

Systemic Lupus Erythematosus

SLE, which is a chronic, multisystem, inflammatory disease, is one of the most common, complex, and serious of the autoimmune disorders.[12] SLE is characterized by the production of a large variety of autoantibodies against nucleic acids, erythrocytes, coagulation proteins, phospholipids, lymphocytes, platelets, and many other self-components. The most characteristic autoantibodies produced in SLE are against nucleic acids: single-stranded deoxyribonucleic acid (DNA), double-stranded DNA, histones, ribonucleoproteins, and other nuclear materials.

Deposition of circulating immune complexes containing antibody against host DNA produces tissue damage in individuals with SLE. DNA and DNA-containing immune complexes have a high affinity for glomerular basement membranes and therefore may be selectively deposited in the glomerulus. (Kidney structures are described in Chapter 34.) The presence of DNA in the circulation increases from cellular damage in response to trauma, drugs, or infections; it is usually removed in the liver, but removal of circulating DNA is slowed in the presence of immune complexes, thereby increasing the potential for deposition in the kidney. (The liver's role in removing waste products from the blood is discussed in Chapter 37.) Deposition of immune complexes composed of DNA and antibody also causes inflammatory lesions in the renal tubular basement membranes, brain (choroid plexus), heart, spleen, lung, gastrointestinal tract, skin, and peritoneum.

SLE, as with most autoimmune diseases, is seen more frequently in women, especially in the 20- to 40-year-old age-group. Blacks are affected more frequently than whites. A genetic predisposition for the disease has been implicated on the basis of increased incidence in twins and the existence of autoimmune disease in the families of individuals with SLE.

A transient lupus-like syndrome that is indistinguishable both clinically and in the laboratory from spontaneously occurring SLE also can develop from the prolonged use of drugs. The drugs most often implicated are hydralazine (an antihypertensive agent) and procainamide (an antidysrhythmic drug). In genetically susceptible individuals, certain environmental agents, such as ultraviolet light, and several infectious agents may trigger lupus-like immune reactions.

Clinical manifestations of SLE include arthralgias or arthritis (90% of individuals), vasculitis and rash (70% to 80% of individuals), renal disease (40% to 50% of individuals), hematologic abnormalities (50% of individuals, with anemia being the most common complication), and cardiovascular diseases (30% to 50% of individuals). As with most autoimmune diseases, SLE is characterized by frequent remissions and exacerbations. Because the signs and symptoms affect almost every body system and tend to come and go, SLE is extremely difficult to diagnose. This has led to the development of a list of 11 clinical findings. The serial or simultaneous presence of at least four of them indicates that the individual has SLE. The findings are as follows:[13]

1. Facial rash confined to the cheeks (malar rash)
2. Discoid rash (raised patches, scaling)
3. Photosensitivity (skin rash developed as a result of exposure to sunlight)

4. Oral or nasopharyngeal ulcers
5. Nonerosive arthritis of at least two peripheral joints
6. Serositis (pleurisy, pericarditis)
7. Renal disorder (proteinuria of 0.5 g/day or cellular casts)
8. Neurologic disorders (seizures or psychosis)
9. Hematologic disorders (hemolytic anemia, leukopenia, lymphopenia, or thrombocytopenia)
10. Immunologic disorders (positive LE cell preparation, anti–double stranded DNA, anti-Smith [Sm] antigen, false-positive serologic test for syphilis, or antiphospholipid antibodies)
11. Presence of antinuclear antibody (ANA)

Graft Rejection

Transplantation of organs commonly is complicated by an immune response against antigens—primarily HLAs—on the donated tissue. Most of our knowledge on the transplantation of organs is based on renal transplant studies. The primary mechanism of the rejection of transplanted organs is a type IV, cell-mediated reaction. Two randomly chosen individuals are almost certainly antigenically different to some degree. Organ transplants between them could be rejected in approximately 2 weeks without the extensive use of immunosuppressive drugs.

Because HLAs are the principal targets of the rejection reaction, HLA matching of donor and recipient greatly enhances the probability of acceptance of the graft. Matching at each HLA locus is of differential importance; matching at the HLA-DR locus appears to be the most critical for graft acceptance, and matching at HLA-A and HLA-B of slightly lesser importance. (These loci are discussed in Chapter 6.)

Transplant rejection is classified as hyperacute, acute, or chronic, depending on the amount of time that elapses between transplantation and rejection. Hyperacute rejection is immediate and rare. When the circulation is reestablished to the grafted area, the graft may immediately turn white (the so-called *white graft*) instead of a normal pink color. Hyperacute rejection usually occurs in recipients with preexisting antibody to antigens in the graft. As circulation to the graft is established, antibody binds to the grafted tissue and activates the inflammatory response, including the coagulation cascade, which results in stasis of blood flow into the tissue. (Coagulation is described in Chapters 7 and 24.) Biopsies of the graft frequently show deposits of antibody (IgG and IgM), complement, and neutrophils.

Acute rejection is a cell-mediated immune response that occurs approximately 2 weeks after the transplant. This type of rejection occurs when the recipient develops an immune response against unmatched HLAs after transplantation. Immunosuppressive drugs may delay or lessen the intensity of acute rejection. A biopsy of the rejected organ shows an infiltration of lymphocytes and macrophages characteristic of a type IV reaction.

Chronic rejection may occur after a period of months or years of normal function. It is characterized by slow, progressive organ failure. Chronic rejection may be caused by inflammatory damage to endothelial cells lining blood vessels as a result of a weak immunologic reaction against minor histocompatibility antigens on the grafted tissue (see What's New? Emerging Trends in Organ and Tissue Transplantation).

WHAT'S NEW? Emerging Trends in Organ and Tissue Transplantation

Despite great improvements in immunosuppressive therapies to prevent acute rejection, chronic graft rejection remains a significant problem. For example, half of renal allografts (i.e., donor grafts) fail within 10 years of transplantation. Although the mechanisms underlying acute graft rejection are mostly known, chronic rejection is less well understood and probably represents several different immunologic and nonimmunologic processes. Recent advances have suggested that the immune system has more self-regulatory capability than previously appreciated, including so-called *costimulatory receptor signaling.* Optimal T cell responses occur when T cells receive both antigen-specific signals through the T cell receptor and nonantigen-costimulatory signals through accessory cell surface molecules. Costimulatory molecules may have the ability to modulate allograft rejection. Research in T cell costimulation could exploit these regulatory mechanisms to increase graft survival.

From Cecka JM: The UNOS scientific renal transplant registry: ten years of kidney transplants. In Checka JM, Terasaki PI, editors: *Clinical transplants 1997,* Los Angeles, 1998, UCLA Laboratory; Gudmundsdottir H, Turka LA: T cell costimulatory blockage: new therapies for transplant rejection, *J Am Soc Nephrol* 10(6):1356, 1999; Harlan DM, Kirk AD: The failure of organ and tissue transplantation: can T-cell costimulatory pathway modifiers revolutionize the presentation of graft rejection? *JAMA* 282(11):1076, 1999; Nagano H, Tilney NL: Chronic allograft failure: the clinical problem, *Am J Med Sci* 313:305, 1997.

INFECTION

Modern health care has shown great progress in preventing and treating infectious diseases. In developed countries sanitary living conditions, clean water, uncontaminated food, vaccinations, and antimicrobials make death from infectious disease most common among those with debilitating diseases, nutritional deficiencies, or immunosuppression. Infectious disease remains a significant threat to life in many parts of the world, including India, Africa, and Southeast Asia. The recent emergence of new infectious agents and of common agents that have developed resistance to most antimicrobial drugs, however, has greatly increased the risk of severe infection even in developed countries.

Infectious diseases are the number one cause of death worldwide (Table 8-5). Dense populations in developing countries with poor sanitation are victims of plague, cholera, malaria, tuberculosis, leprosy, and schistosomiasis. Only smallpox has been eradicated from the world by vaccination. Vaccination also has eradicated polio from the Western Hemisphere. In the United States, heart disease and malignancies greatly surpass infectious disease as major causes of death (Table 8-6). Although vaccines and antimicrobials have altered the prevalence of infectious disease, mutant strains of bacteria have emerged with resistance to protection previously provided by antimicrobial drug therapy. New diseases, such as legionnaires disease and *Hantavirus,* and the global

Table 8-5 Estimated Annual Number of Deaths by Cause Worldwide (Data from 1999)

Cause of Death	Number	%
Communicable diseases	17,380,000	31.1
Respiratory infections	4,039,000	
HIV/AIDS*	2,673,000	
Perinatal diseases	2,356,000	
Diarrheal diseases	2,213,000	
Tuberculosis	1,669,000	
Childhood diseases	1,554,000	
Malaria	1,086,000	
Maternal diseases	497,000	
Sexually transmitted diseases (excluding AIDS)	178,000	
Meningitis	171,000	
Tropical diseases	171,000	
Hepatitis	124,000	
Noncommunicable diseases	33,484,000	59.8
Cardiovascular diseases	16,970,000	
Malignant neoplasms	7,065,000	
Respiratory diseases	3,575,000	
Digestive system disorders	2,049,000	
Genitourinary disorders	900,000	
Diabetes	777,000	
Nutritional diseases	493,000	
External causes (e.g., accidents, suicide)	5,101,000	9.1

From World Health Organization, Division of Epidemiological Surveillance and Health Situation and Trend Assessment: *Global health situation and projection estimates,* Geneva, 1999, The Organization.
*Global data for acquired immunodeficiency syndrome (AIDS) reported remain highly distorted for three reasons: (1) wide intercountry and interregional differences in the completeness of AIDS case detection and reporting, (2) reporting of AIDS cases to public health authorities and recognition of its importance have occurred in different countries at different times, and (3) pediatric AIDS remains substantially underrecognized and underreported.

spread of acquired immunodeficiency syndrome (AIDS) and drug-resistant tuberculosis are examples of the intense challenge for the prevention and control of infectious disease.

Microorganisms and Humans: A Dynamic Relationship

Many microorganisms find human bodies to be hospitable sites to grow and flourish, provided with nutrients and appropriate conditions of temperature and humidity. In many cases a mutual relationship exists, in which humans and microorganisms benefit (Box 8-1).

For instance, the human gut is colonized by a large variety of microorganisms that make up the normal human flora. These bacteria are provided with nutrients from ingested food and in exchange produce enzymes that facilitate the digestion and utilization of many of the more complex molecules in our diet, produce antibacterial factors (e.g., bacteriocins, colicins) that prevent colonization by pathogenic organisms, and produce usable metabolites (e.g., vitamin K, B vitamins). This homeostasis is normally maintained through the physical integrity of the gut and other mechanisms that guarantee that the immune and inflammatory systems do not attack these symbiotes, and in return they do not attempt to invade and leave the gut. This relationship can be breached as a result of injury releasing intestinal bacteria into the bloodstream, potentially leading to sepsis, shock, and death.

Much of the symbiotic relationship is maintained by the immune and inflammatory systems. If those systems are compromised, many organisms will leave their normal sites and cause infection. Individuals with deficiencies in the immune system easily become infected with *opportunistic organisms,* which are organisms that normally would not cause disease but seize the opportunity provided by the person's decreased immune or inflammatory responses.

True pathogens have devised means to circumvent the normal controls provided by the host's main defensive barriers—the inflammatory system and the immune system. Infection by a pathogen is influenced by several factors:

- *Mechanism of action:* pathogens directly damage cells, interfere with cellular metabolism, and render the cell dysfunctional because of the accumulation of pathogenic substances and toxin production.
- *Infectivity:* ability of the pathogen to invade and multiply in the host; for example, coagulase (an enzyme) that causes coagulation and allows some organisms, such as staphylococci, to clot and form a sticky layer around themselves, protecting themselves against host defenses.
- *Pathogenicity:* the ability of an agent to produce disease depends on its speed of reproduction, extent of tissue damage, and production of toxins.
- *Virulence:* the potency of a pathogen measured in terms of the number of microorganisms or micrograms of toxin required to kill a host—for example, measles is of low virulence; the rabies virus is highly virulent.
- *Immunogenicity:* the ability of pathogens to induce an immune response.
- *Toxigenicity:* a factor important in determining a pathogen's virulence, such as hemolysin, leucocidin, other exotoxins, and endotoxin. Hemolysin destroys erythrocytes, and leucocidin destroys leukocytes; both are products of streptococci and staphylococci.
- *Portal of entry:* the route by which a pathogenic organism infects the host; direct contact, inhalation, ingestion, or bites of an animal or insect. Spread of infection is facilitated by the ability of pathogens to spread through lymph and blood and into tissues and organs, where they multiply and cause disease.

Classes of Infectious Organisms

Infectious disease can be caused by organisms that range in size from 20 nm (poliovirus) to 10 m (tapeworm). Classes of pathogenic organisms and their characteristics are summarized in Table 8-7.

Innate Host Resistance Mechanisms

The first lines of defense against infectious organisms are external barriers, including the skin and mucous mem-

Table 8-6 Death Rates and Percent of Total Deaths for the 15 Leading Causes of Death: United States, 1998

Rank Order*	Cause of Death (Ninth Revision International Classification of Diseases, 1975)	Rate†	Percent of change, 1997 to 1998
1	Diseases of heart	126.6	−3.0
2	Malignant neoplasms, including neoplasms of lymphatic and hematopoietic tissues	123.6	−1.6
3	Cerebrovascular diseases	25.1	−3.0
4	Chronic obstructive pulmonary diseases and allied conditions	21.3	0.9
5	Accidents and adverse effects	30.1	0.0
6	Pneumonia and influenza	13.2	2.3
7	Diabetes mellitus	13.6	0.7
8	Suicide	10.4	−1.9
9	Nephritis, nephrotic syndrome, and nephrosis	4.4	0.0
10	Chronic liver disease and cirrhosis	7.2	−2.7
11	Septicemia	4.4	4.8 (91.3% since 1979)
12	Alzheimer disease	2.6	−3.7
13	Homicide and legal intervention	7.3	−8.8
14	Artherosclerosis	1.9	−9.5
15	Hypertension, with or without renal disease	2.4	4.3

From *National Vital Statistics Report* 48, 2000.
*Rank based on number of deaths.
†Rates per 100,000 population.

Table 8-7 Classes of Human Infectious Organisms

Class	Size	Site of Reproduction	Example
Virus	20-30 nm	Intracellular	Poliomyelitis
Chlamydia	200-1000 nm	Intracellular	Trachoma
Rickettsiae	300-1200 nm	Intracellular	Rocky Mountain spotted fever
Mycoplasma	125-350 nm	Extracellular	Mycoplasma pneumonia
Bacteria	0.8-15 μm	Skin	Staphylococcal wound infection
		Mucous membranes	Cholera
		Intracellular	Streptococcal pneumonia
		Extracellular	Tuberculosis
Fungi	2-200 μm	Skin	Tinea pedis (athlete's foot)
		Mucous membranes	Thrush
		Intracellular	Sporotrichosis
		Extracellular	Histoplasmosis
Protozoa	1-50 mm	Mucosal	Giardiasis
		Extracellular	Sleeping sickness
Helminths	3 mm to 10 m	Intracellular	Trichinosis
		Extracellular	Filariasis

branes. The digestive, respiratory, and genitourinary tracts form a closed barrier between the internal organs and the environment (Fig. 8-9). The second and third lines of defense are the inflammatory response and the immune system.

Once a microorganism penetrates the first lines of defense and invades, the inflammatory response is initiated, especially the phagocytes. The neutrophils actively attack bacteria, engulf them, and destroy the organism (phagocytosis).

The adaptation of the immune system actively neutralizes bacterial defense mechanisms (Fig. 8-10). The complement

Box 8-1

THE MANY RELATIONSHIPS BETWEEN HUMANS AND ORGANISMS

Symbiosis: benefits only the human; no harm to the organism
Mutualism: benefits the human and the organism
Commensalism: benefits only the organism; no harm to the human
Pathogenicity: benefits the organism; harms the human (*opportunism* is a situation in which benign human organisms become pathogenic because of decreased human host resistance)

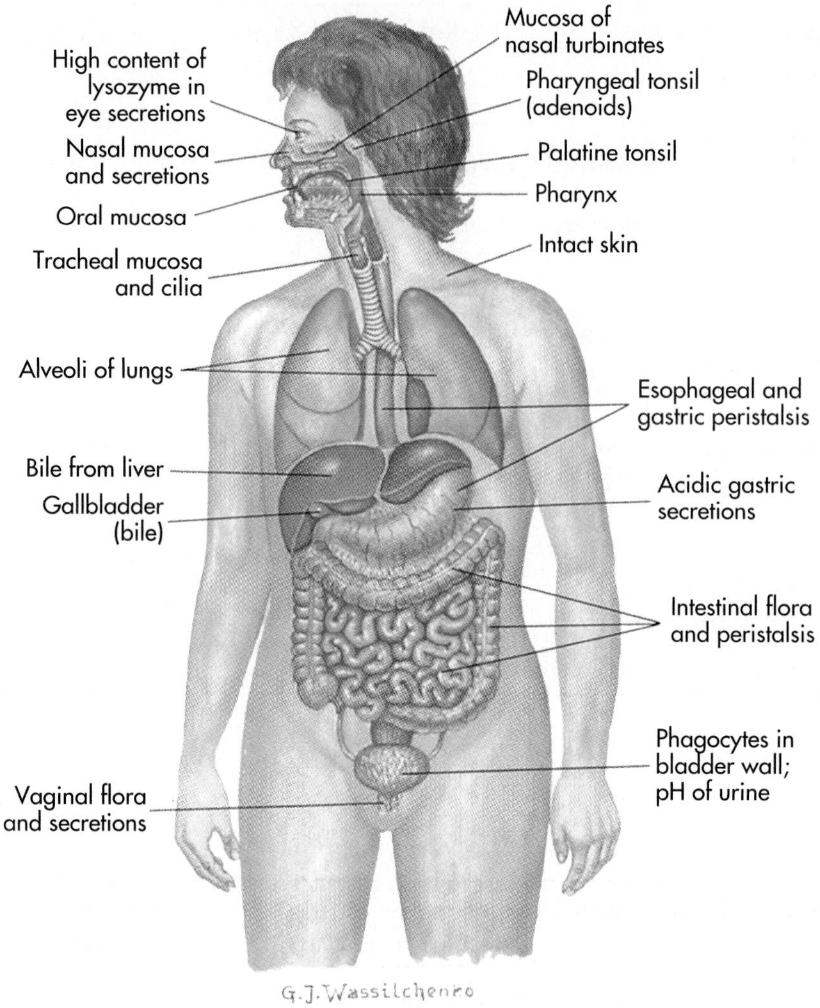

FIG. 8-9 The closed barrier. The digestive, respiratory, and genitourinary tracts form closed barriers between the internal organs and the environment. (From Grimes DE: *Infectious diseases,* St Louis, 1991, Mosby.)

system, through the alternative pathway, produces C3b, which attaches itself to the surface of the bacterium with carbohydrate capsules. C3b functions as a highly effective opsonin that allows adherence between the bacterium and C3b receptors on the phagocyte's surface, thus facilitating phagocytosis. Antibodies also bind to the surface of bacteria, act as opsonins, and can activate complement. Antibodies also are produced against most of the bacterial toxins, neutralizing their effects.

Pathogenic Defense Mechanisms

If the immune system is compromised, infections will not be regulated. As a result, a normally limited and clinically mild viral or bacterial infection will become systemic and potentially fatal to the individual. Some organisms are pathogenic because they have developed mechanisms of modifying the immune response. Table 8-8 contains examples of organisms that fight off or alter the inflammatory or immune systems.

Bacterial Infection and Injury

Bacterial survival and growth depend on the effectiveness of the body's defense mechanisms and on the bacterium's ability to resist these defenses. Many pathogens have devised ways of preventing destruction by the inflammatory and immune systems. For example, some bacteria produce thick capsules of carbohydrate or protein that are antiphagocytic, preventing efficient phagocytosis (Fig. 8-11). Such coatings include the thick polysaccharide covering of the pneumococcus, the waxy capsule surrounding the tubercle bacillus, and the M protein cell wall of the streptococcus.

Because the primary immune response may take 1 week to develop adequately, some pathogens proliferate at rates that surpass the development of a protective response. Cholera causes severe vomiting and watery diarrhea, has a 60% mortality rate, and develops within 2 to 3 days of ingestion. Norwalk virus and rotavirus, which cause severe diarrhea and vomiting, and *Bunyavirus* and *Hantavirus,* which cause hemorrhagic fever, have incubation periods of 24 to 48 hours. Some strains of toxin-producing group A streptococci cause destructive skin infections and pneumonia that may kill an individual within 2 days. Group B streptococci from the maternal vagina may ascend the birth canal, penetrate fetal membranes, and infect the fluid surrounding the fetus. The

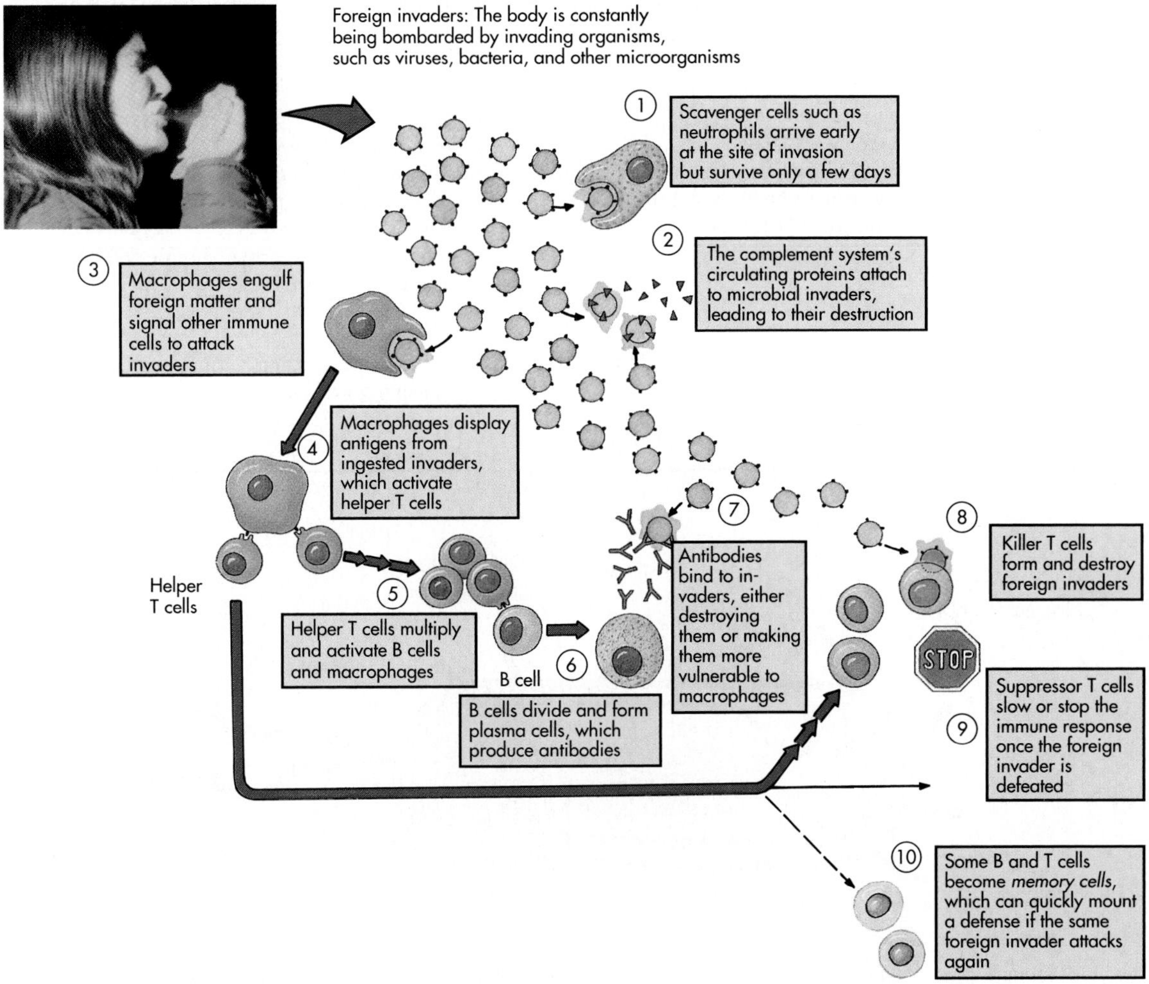

Foreign invaders: The body is constantly being bombarded by invading organisms, such as viruses, bacteria, and other microorganisms
1
Scavenger cells such as neutrophils arrive early at the site of invasion but survive only a few days
2
The complement system's circulating proteins attach to microbial invaders, leading to their destruction
3
Macrophages engulf foreign matter and signal other immune cells to attack invaders
4
Macrophages display antigens from ingested invaders, which activate helper T cells
Helper T cells
5
Helper T cells multiply and activate B cells and macrophages
B cell
6
B cells divide and form plasma cells, which produce antibodies
7
Antibodies bind to invaders, either destroying them or making them more vulnerable to macrophages
8
Killer T cells form and destroy foreign invaders
STOP
9
Suppressor T cells slow or stop the immune response once the foreign invader is defeated
10
Some B and T cells become memory cells, which can quickly mount a defense if the same foreign invader attacks again

FIG. 8-10 Biologic warfare. A brief summary of the immune response. (From Thibodeau GA, Patton KT: *Anatomy and physiology,* ed 4, St Louis, 1999, Mosby.)

Table 8-8 Organisms That Fight Off the Immune System or Cause It to Attack the Host

Organism	Mechanism	Comment
BACTERIA		
Staphylococcus	Produces toxins	Either kills phagocytes or interferes with chemotaxis
Streptococcus		
Mycobacterium tuberculosis	Produces toxins	Prevents infusion of lysosomal granules and formation of phagolysosome
Toxoplasma gondii		
Mycobacteria	Produces enzymes that destroy oxygen metabolites (e.g., catalase, superoxide dismutase)	Prevents killing by O_2-dependent mechanisms
Brucella		
Salmonella typhi		
Neisseria gonorrhoeae	Produces a protease to digest IgA	Infects mucosal surface of urethra
Streptococcus pneumoniae	Produces a protease to digest IgA	Causes pneumonia
Haemophilus influenzae		
Staphylococcus	Produces surface molecules that mimic Fc receptors, which can bind antibody	Protects organism from successful activation of complement cascade and prevents antibody from functioning as an opsonin
Herpes simplex virus		
Group A streptococcus	Contains an antiphagocytic capsular antigen, M protein, that resembles human myocardial antigen	Certain people produce antibody against M protein that also reacts with cardiac tissue, resulting in rheumatic fever (carditis)
Mycoplasma pneumoniae	Expresses antigens similar to those found on human red blood cells	Antibodies can also react with human red blood cells

Continued

Table 8-8 Organisms That Fight Off the Immune System or Cause It to Attack the Host—cont'd

Organism	Mechanism	Comment
VIRUSES		
Influenza	Antigenic mutations ("drift") of antigen on a yearly basis	Immune response developed against previous year's strain is no longer protective
	Severe; virus undergoes antigenic "shift"; genetic recombination between human and avian strains of virus	Because new virus is now very distinct from those found in previous years, no protective immunity preexists, resulting in serious infection
Human immunodeficiency virus (HIV)	Can rapidly mutate its surface antigens	Antibodies produced early in disease will not react with antigens expressed later
PARASITES		
Trypanosoma sp. (sleeping sickness) *Borrelia recurrentis* (relapsing fever)	Activates genes that produce different antigens on their surface	Avoids immune rejection because immune response is unable to identify parasite

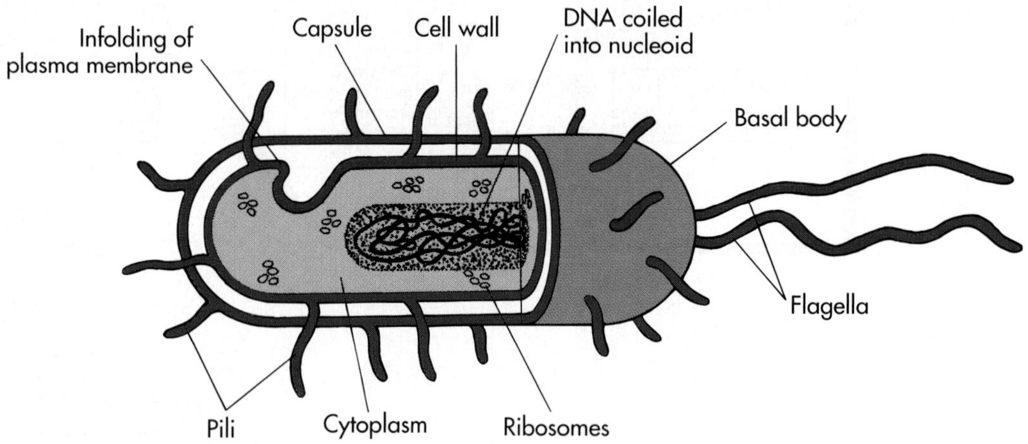

FIG. 8-11 General structure of bacteria. (Redrawn from Mims CA et al: *Medical microbiology,* ed 2, London, 1998, Mosby.)

organism may have already established an active infection of the child's lungs at birth, resulting in a pneumonia that is too advanced to allow successful antibiotic therapy and that has a 50% mortality rate in newborns.

Other bacteria survive and proliferate in the body by producing exotoxins and endotoxins that injure cells and tissues. **Exotoxins** are proteins released during bacterial growth. They are usually enzymes and have highly specific effects. **Endotoxins (lipopolysaccharides [LPS])** are contained in the cell walls of gram-negative bacteria and are released during lysis, or destruction, of the bacteria. Endotoxin may also be released from the membrane of the bacteria, either during bacterial growth or during treatment with antibiotics, which therefore cannot prevent the toxic effects of the endotoxin.[14,15] Bacteria that produce endotoxins are called *pyrogenic bacteria* because they activate the inflammatory process and produce fever. The innermost part of the lipopolysaccharide, *lipid A*, is made of polysaccharides and fatty acids and is responsible for the substance's toxic effects (Fig. 8-12).

Inflammation is the body's initial response to the presence of the bacteria. Vascular permeability is increased, allowing blood-borne substances (i.e., the complement system) involved in bacterial destruction to access the site of infection. Endotoxins increase capillary permeability further by activating the complement cascade. Capillary permeability may increase sufficiently to permit the escape of large quantities of blood, contributing to hypotension and, in severe cases, cardiovascular shock (see Chapter 45). Endotoxin also can activate the coagulation cascade, leading to the syndrome of disseminated (or diffuse) intravascular coagulation.

The ability to produce immunologic hypersensitivity reactions is an important pathogenic mechanism of bacterial toxins. Tissue lesions of many chronic infections are related to the induction of hypersensitivity to the toxin or cell wall component. For example, *M. tuberculosis* causes inflammatory chronic lesions known as *granulomas.*

Some bacteria alter antigens, initiating self-destructive (autoimmune) reactions. Other bacteria produce substances that immunologically "look like" (cross react with) host proteins and cause the body to produce an autoimmune reaction against the cross-reactive antigen in normal tissues.

Bacteremia, or **septicemia,** is the presence of bacteria in the blood and is caused by a failure of the body's defense mechanisms. The usual cause is proliferation of gram-negative bacteria, although a few gram-positive bacteria and

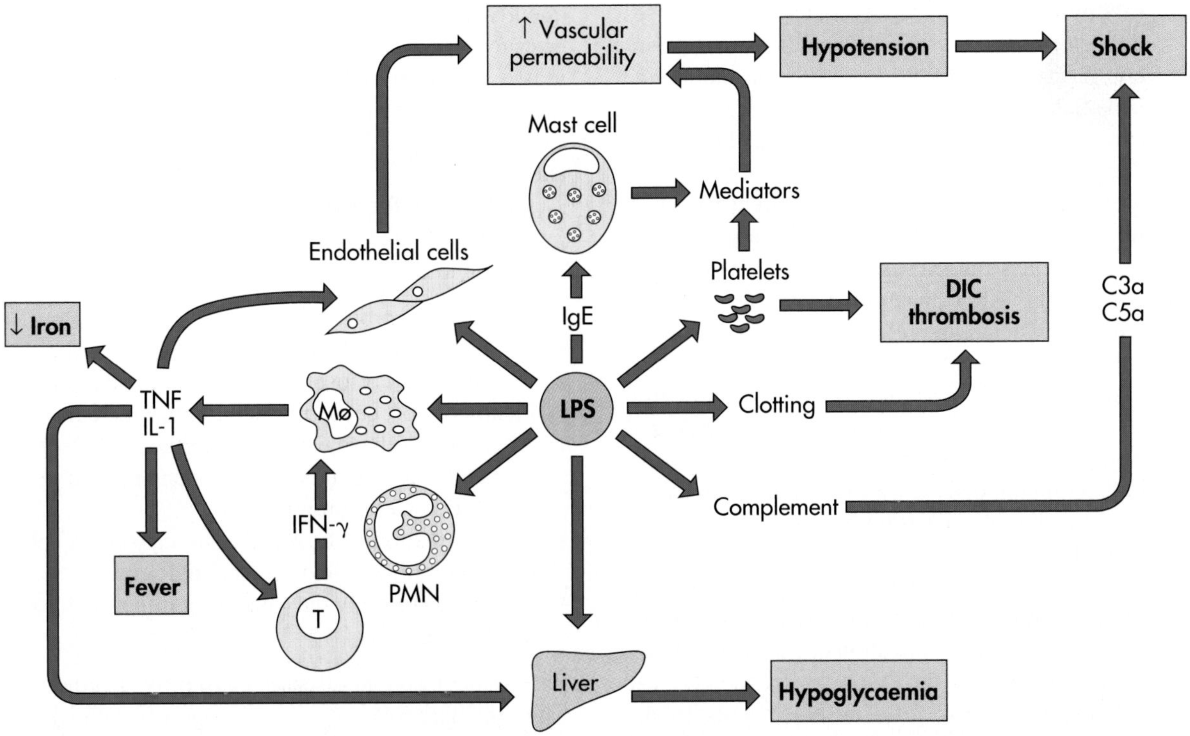

FIG. 8-12 The many activities of lipopolysaccharide (LPS). Bacterial endotoxin (LPS) activates almost every immune mechanism, as well as the clotting pathway, which together make LPS one of the most powerful immune stimuli known. *IgE,* Immunoglobulin E; *DIC,* disseminated intravascular coagulation; *C3a, C5a,* complement components; *TNF,* tumor necrosis factor; *IL-1,* interleukin 1; *Mϕ,* macrophage; *IFN-γ,* interferon-gamma; *PMN,* polymorphonuclear leukocyte; *T,* T cell. (From Mims CA et al: *Medical microbiology,* ed 2, London, 1998, Mosby.)

fungi can cause it. Symptoms of bacteremia are produced by endotoxins. Once in the blood, endotoxins cause the release of vasoactive peptides that affect blood vessels, producing vasodilation, which reduces blood pressure, causes decreased oxygen delivery, and produces subsequent cardiovascular shock (see Chapter 45). Bacteremia is diagnosed from evaluation of blood cultures.

Viral Infection and Injury

Viruses proliferate within cells by taking over the metabolic machinery of host cells and using it for their own survival and replication. Viral diseases are the most common afflictions of humans and include the common cold, the "cold sore" of herpes simplex, and several types of cancer.

Viruses do not produce exotoxins or endotoxins. Viral pathogens bypass many defense mechanisms by developing intracellularly, thus hiding within cells and away from normal inflammatory or immune responses. In many cases, however, because viral agents must spread from cell to cell, the developing immune response eventually cures the infection so the disease is usually self-limiting. Viruses, however, can rapidly produce irreversible and lethal injury in highly susceptible cells in an immunosuppressed host. If a symbiotic relationship is maintained between the host cell and the virus, persistent unapparent infection may result. Cell injury does not occur, and the virus persists until it is activated to replicate (e.g., the cold sores of herpesvirus infection). Immunity may protect the individual from an acute exacerbation only or may be sufficiently strong to prevent disease.

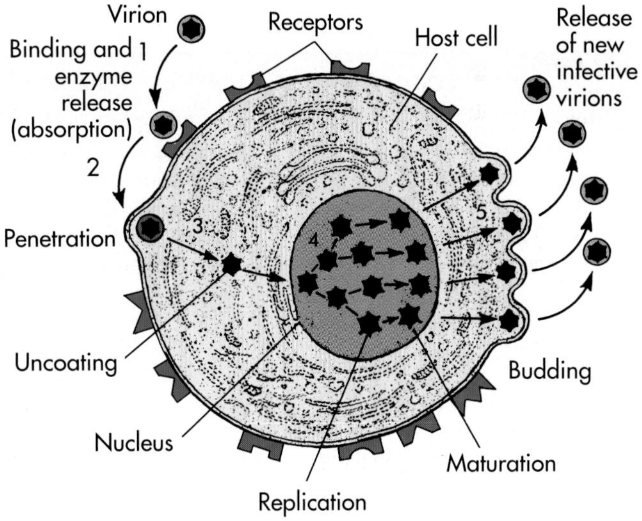

FIG. 8-13 Stages of viral infection of a host cell.

Viral Replication

Virions, or **viral particles,** do not possess any of the metabolic organelles found in prokaryotes (e.g., bacteria) or eukaryotes (e.g., human cells). Unlike bacteria, viruses have no metabolism and are incapable of independent reproduction. Their replication depends totally on their ability to infect a **permissive host cell**—a cell that cannot resist viral invasion and replication. Infection begins when a virion binds to receptors on the plasma membrane of a host cell *(attachment)* (Fig. 8-13). The specificity of the virus for these receptors and the distribution of receptors throughout the host's tissues dictate the range of host cells that a particular virus can infect. Once bound, the virion penetrates the plasma membrane by receptor-mediated endocytosis, by envelope fusion with the plasma membrane, or by directly crossing the plasma membrane.

Viruses contain their genetic information in either DNA or ribonucleic acid (RNA), either of which can be single stranded (ss) or double stranded (ds), and thus are known as DNA or RNA viruses. After penetration, the virus *uncoats* the protective nucleocapsid and releases viral genetic information into the cytoplasm. Most RNA viruses directly produce messenger RNA (mRNA), which is translated into viral proteins, and genomic RNA, which is eventually packaged into new viruses. One particular family of viruses, retroviruses (of which human immunodeficiency virus [HIV] is an example), carries an enzyme (reverse transcriptase) that creates a double-stranded DNA version of the virus. The DNA "provirus" enters the cell's nucleus, where it becomes integrated into the host cell's chromosomal DNA. Most DNA viruses also enter the nucleus, where replication occurs. Some DNA viruses may also integrate into the host's chromosomal DNA.

The translation of viral-specific mRNA results in the production of viral proteins that self-assemble around viral genetic information. New virions then are released from the cell for transmission of the viral infection to other host cells. Enveloped viruses are released through *budding,* in which viral particles are shed enveloped in plasma membrane from the surface of the infected cell. Nonenveloped viruses frequently are released in large numbers concurrent with the destruction of the cell. Viral DNA that has become integrated with host DNA is transmitted to the host's daughter cells during host cell mitosis. By this process, viral genes can become part of the genetic information of the host cell and its progeny.

Cellular Effects of Viruses

Once inside the host cell, virions have many harmful effects, including the following:

- Cessation of protein synthesis
- Disruption of lysosomal membranes, resulting in release of "digestive" lysosomal enzymes that can kill the cell
- Fusion of host cells, producing multinucleated giant cells
- Alteration of the antigenic properties, or "identity," of the host cell, causing the host's immune system to attack the cell as if it were foreign
- Transformation of host cells into cancerous cells, resulting in uninhibited and unregulated growth
- Promotion of secondary bacterial infection by cells damaged by viruses

Examples of human diseases caused by specific viruses are listed in Table 8-9.

Fungal Infection and Injury

Fungi are relatively large organisms with thick walls that grow as either single-celled yeasts (spheres) or multicelled molds (filaments or hyphae) (Fig. 8-14). Some fungi can exist in either form and are called **dimorphic.** The cell walls

Table 8-9 Human Diseases Caused by Specific Viruses

Virus	Pathophysiologic Effects
Papovaviruses (DNA) (papilloma)	Small viruses that induce tumors and cancers in animals, warts (papilloma) in humans
Adenoviruses (DNA)	Medium-sized viruses that cause various respiratory infections in humans; some cause tumors in animals
Herpesviruses (DNA) (herpes simplex, herpes zoster)	Medium-sized viruses that cause various diseases in humans, such as fever blisters, chickenpox, shingles, and infectious mononucleosis; implicated in a type of human cancer called *Burkitt lymphoma*
Poxvirus (DNA) (variola, cowpox, vaccinia)	Very large, complex, brick-shaped viruses that cause diseases such as smallpox (variola), molluscum contagiosum (wartlike skin lesions), cowpox, and vaccinia; vaccinia virus gives immunity to smallpox
Hepatitis B (DNA)	Widespread throughout the world; blood and blood products are the best-documented routes for transmission
Picornaviruses (RNA) (poliovirus, rhinovirus)	Smallest RNA-containing viruses; at least 70 human enteroviruses are known, including the polio virus, coxsackie virus, and echovirus; more than 100 rhinoviruses exist and are the most common cause of colds
Myxoviruses (RNA) (influenza A, B, C)	Medium-sized viruses with a spiked envelope; able to agglutinate red blood cells; cause influenza
Paramyxoviruses (RNA) (measles, mumps)	Structurally similar to myxoviruses but generally larger; cause parainfluenza, measles, mumps
Coronaviruses (RNA)	Associated with upper respiratory tract infections and the common cold
Retroviruses (RNA)	Tumor-associated viruses; cause leukemia and tumors in animals; some members produce "slow" viral infections; cause of AIDS
Arenaviruses (RNA) (lassa)	Possess RNA-containing granules; some members produce "slow" viral infections in humans
Reoviruses (RNA)	Relation to human disease not clear; may be involved in mild respiratory infections and infantile gastroenteritis
Hepatitis A (RNA)	Isolated from chimpanzees; known to be transmitted by humans by close person-to-person contact

Modified from Tortora GJ, Funke BR, Case CL: *Microbiology: an introduction,* ed 3, Menlo Park, Calif, 1989, Benjamin Cummings.
DNA, Deoxyribonucleic acid; *RNA,* ribonucleic acid; *AIDS,* acquired immunodeficiency syndrome.

of fungi are thick and composed of polysaccharides different from the peptidoglycans of bacteria, and they are not motile. The lack of peptidoglycans allows fungi to resist the action of bacterial cell wall inhibitors such as penicillin and cephalosporin. Molds are aerobic, and yeasts are facultative anaerobes. They usually reproduce by simple division or budding.

Diseases caused by fungi are called **mycoses.** Most pathogenic fungi grow as parasites on or near skin or mucous membranes and usually produce mild and superficial disease. Fungi that invade the skin, hair, or nails are known as **dermatophytes.** The diseases they produce are called *tineas* (ringworm), for example, tinea capitis (scalp), tinea pedis (feet), and tinea cruris (groin). Superficial dermatophytes grow in a ringlike, erythematous patch with a raised border. Itching often is intense, and cracking of tissue can occur and lead to secondary bacterial infection. Infections of the scalp are accompanied by scaling and hair loss. (Chapter 43 discusses the various skin disorders caused by fungi.)

Deep infections involving internal organs can be life threatening and are most common in association with other diseases or as an opportunistic infection in immunosuppressed individuals. Fungi causing deep infection enter the body through inhalation or through open wounds. Filamentous forms can multiply extracellularly, but the spherical yeasts multiply within cells, including white blood cells. Some fungi are a part of the normal body flora and become pathologic when immunity is compromised, allowing exaggerated growth and translocation. For example, *Candida albicans* is found in the mouth, gastrointestinal tract, and vagina of many normal individuals. Changes in pH and use of antibiotics that kill bacteria that normally inhibit *Candida* growth permit rapid proliferation, which can lead to superficial or deep infection. Common pathologic fungi are summarized in Table 8-10.

Pathologic fungi release mycotoxins and other enzymes that are damaging to connective tissues, but attachment and invasion by fungi is still not well understood. Phagocytes and T lymphocytes are important in controlling fungi, and low white blood cell counts promote fungal infection.

Fungi are diagnosed by microscopic observation of specimens treated with potassium hydroxide and stained to enhance visualization of spheres and filaments. Specimens also can be cultured. Skin tests are available for species of *Aspergillus.* No vaccines are available to treat fungal disease. Many of the antifungal drugs (e.g., amphotericin B, ketoconazole, fluconazole) used to treat deep or systemic infection are toxic to the host because the fungal cell composition is similar to the host cell. They also can produce significant drug interactions.

Clinical Manifestations of Infectious Disease

The progression from infection to disease follows predictable stages (Fig. 8-15). Clinical manifestations of infectious disease vary, depending on the pathogen and the organ system affected. Manifestations can arise directly from the infecting organism or its products; however, the majority of

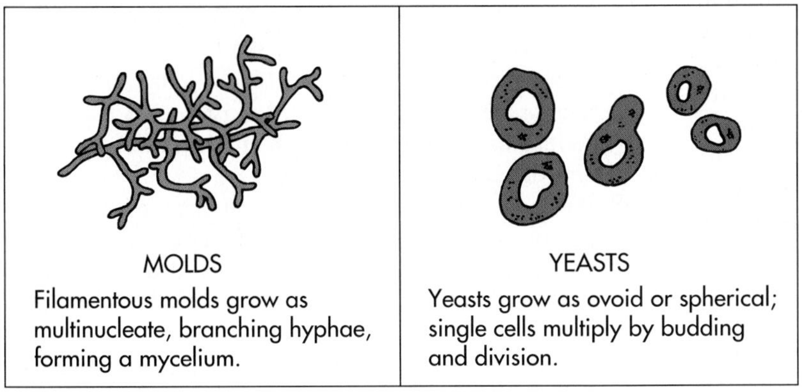

MOLDS
Filamentous molds grow as multinucleate, branching hyphae, forming a mycelium.
YEASTS
Yeasts grow as ovoid or spherical; single cells multiply by budding and division.

FIG. 8-14 Types of fungi. (Redrawn from Mims CA et al: *Medical microbiology,* ed 2, London, 1998, Mosby.)

Table 8-10 Common Pathogenic Fungi

Fungus	Growth Form	Entry	Disease
SUPERFICIAL DERMATOPHYTES			
Microsporum and *Epidermophyton*	Filament	Skin contact	Ringworm, jock itch, athlete's foot
Malassezia furfur	Sphere	Skin contact	Tinea versicolor
DEEP			
Pneumocystis carinii	Sphere	Inhalation	Pneumonia
Histoplasma capsulatum	Sphere	Inhalation	Histoplasmosis
Aspergillus fumigatus	Filament	Inhalation	Aspergillosis and pneumonia
Coccidioides immitis	Unusual form	Inhalation	Coccidioidomycosis
Candida albicans	Sphere	Normal flora of skin, mouth, intestine	Thrush, vaginal yeast infections, systemic infections

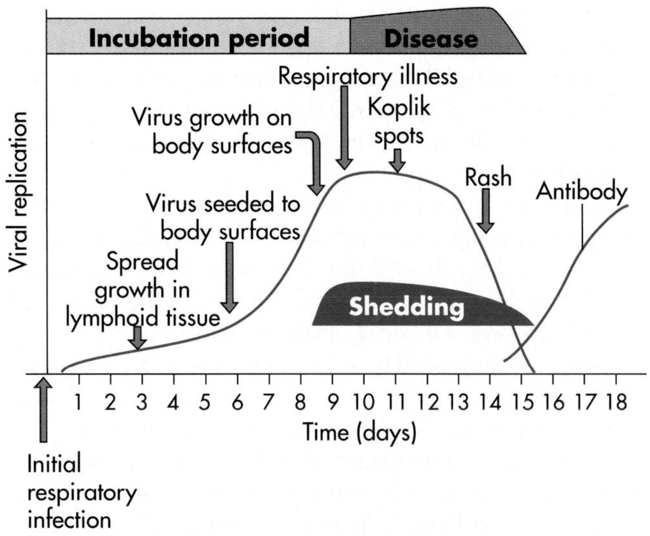

Fig. 8-15 Pathogenesis of measles.

manifestations result from the host's inflammatory and immune responses. Infectious diseases typically begin with the nonspecific or general symptoms of fatigue, malaise, weakness, and loss of concentration. Generalized aching and loss of appetite are common complaints. However, the hallmark of most infectious diseases is fever.

Fever is not failure of the body to regulate temperature; rather, body temperature is regulated at a higher level than normal. Body temperature is regulated by nervous system feedback to the hypothalamus, which functions as a central thermostat. A large number of agents (pyrogens) can produce fever. In current classification, those pyrogens derived from outside the host are termed **exogenous pyrogens** and those produced by the host are termed **endogenous pyrogens.** There is little evidence that exogenous pyrogens cause fever directly. Available data favor an indirect effect of such pyrogens on the hypothalamus that is mediated by endogenous pyrogen (EP) released by cells of the host.[16] A number of hormonelike mediators (cytokines) in cellular and immunologic adaptations have been identified as endogenous pyrogens. They are interleukins 1 and 6 (IL-1 and IL-6), interferon, tumor necrosis factor (TNF), and other cytokines.[16] The mechanism by which these cytokines raise the thermoregulatory set point seems to be through stimulation of prostaglandin synthesis and turnover in both thermoregulatory (brain) and nonthermoregulatory (peripheral) tissue. These mechanisms are discussed in detail in Chapter 13. Although it is generally believed that fever has a beneficial value in infection, the molecular mechanism behind the beneficial effects has not been established. Many investigators, however, consider fever as an adaptive host-defense response.

Recently recognized is the role played by TNF (cachectin) in the pathogenesis of endotoxic shock.[14,15] TNF is a cytokine produced by activated macrophages (e.g., large phagocytic cells) on exposure to endotoxin (see Fig. 8-12). It is sometimes called *cachectin* because of its role in promoting cachexia in individuals with cancer. (Cachexia is discussed in Chapter 10; cytokines are discussed in Chapter 5.)

Countermeasures Against Pathogens: Vaccines and Antimicrobials

The body's innate and innovative responses against microorganisms are numerous and generally involve an interaction between the immune and inflammatory systems. Prophylactic or interventive procedures also have been developed by health care providers to prevent the pathogen from initiating disease (vaccines) or to destroy the pathogen once the disease process has started (antimicrobials).

Vaccines

Many vaccines have been developed to protect against pathogens (Table 8-11). The vaccines and their abbreviations in Table 8-11 are as follows:

1. Hepatitis B virus (Hep B): causes cirrhosis of the liver and liver cancer. The vaccine is a recombinant viral protein.
2. Diphtheria (D): a bacterial infection of the throat; produces a toxin that can lead to heart failure or paralysis. The vaccine is an inactivated form of diphtheria toxin (toxoid).
3. Tetanus (T): a bacterial infection that produces a toxin that attacks the nervous system and may cause death. The vaccine is an inactivated form of the tetanus toxin (toxoid).
4. Pertussis (P) (acellular pertussis [aP]), or whooping cough: a bacterial infection that causes severe coughing in children younger than 5 years. The vaccine may be either a bacterial antigen extract or killed intact bacteria.
5. *Haemophilus influenzae* type b (Hib): a bacterial infection that is commonly contracted by children younger than 5 years and infects the blood, joints, bones, and membrane covering the heart; most common cause of serious bacterial meningitis in children. The vaccine is an extracted bacterial antigen.
6. Polio vaccine (IPV): polio is a viral infection that causes paralysis and death; the vaccine is an attenuated living virus. Recent recommendations are that killed polio vaccine should be used initially, especially for children with suspected immune system defects.
7. Measles and mumps (MM): viruses that cause fever and rash (measles) or inflammation of the salivary glands (mumps); mumps may also cause meningitis. Both vaccines are attenuated living viruses.
8. Rubella (R), or German measles: a viral infection that causes fever and rash; may cause severe birth defects in pregnant women infected in the first trimester.
9. Varicella-zoster (V): a virus that causes chickenpox.
10. Hepatitis A virus (Hep A): recommended in selected areas.

Vaccines induce primary and secondary immune responses under conditions that will not result in disease. Most viral vaccines contain live viruses that are weakened or attenuated so they continue to express appropriate antigens but establish only a limited and easily controlled infection. Most

Table 8-11 Recommended Childhood Immunization Schedule[1]—United States, January–December 2000

Vaccine	Birth	1 mo	2 mo	4 mo	6 mo	12 mo	15 mo	18 mo	24 mo	4-6 yr	11-12 yr	14-16 yr
Hepatitis B[2]	←	Hep B	→									
		←	Hep B	→	←	Hep B	→	→			(Hep B)	
Diphtheria and tetanus toxoids and pertussis[3]			DTaP	DTaP	DTaP		← DTaP	→		DTaP	←	Td
Haemophilus influenzae type b[4]			Hib	Hib	Hib	← Hib	→					
Poliovirus[5]			IPV	IPV	←	IPV	→	→		IPV		
Measles-Mumps-Rubella[6]						← MMR	→			MMR	(MMR)	
Varicella virus[7]						←	Var	→			(Var)	
Hepatitis A[8]									←	Hep A in selected areas	→	

[Open box] Range of recommended ages for vaccination

(Oval) Vaccines to be given if previously recommended doses were missed or were given earlier than the recommended minimum age

[Shaded box] Recommended in selected states and/or regions

From Centers for Disease Control and Prevention: *Recommended childhood immunization schedule—United States, 2000,* 283(7):876, 2000.

On October 22, 1999, the Advisory Committee on Immunization Practices (ACIP) recommended that Rotashield® (rhesus rotavirus vaccine-tetravalent [RRV-TV]), the only U.S.-licensed rotavirus vaccine, no longer be used in the United States (*MMWR* Vol. 48, No. 43, November 5, 1999). Parents should be reassured that children who received rotavirus vaccine before July 1999 are not now at increased risk for intussusception.

[1]This schedule indicates the recommended ages for routine administration of licensed childhood vaccines as of November 1, 1999. Any dose not given at the recommended age should be given as a "catch-up" vaccination at any subsequent visit when indicated and feasible. Additional vaccines may be licensed and recommended during the year. Licensed combination vaccines may be used whenever any components of the combination are indicated and the vaccine's other components are not contraindicated. Providers should consult the manufacturers' package inserts for detailed recommendations.

[2]**Infants born to hepatitis B surface antigen (HBsAg)-negative mothers** should receive the first dose of hepatitis B vaccine (Hep B) by age 2 months. The second dose should be administered at least 1 month after the first dose. The third dose should be administered at least 4 months after the first dose and at least 2 months after the second dose, but not before age 6 months. **Infants born to HBsAg-positive mothers** should receive Hep B and 0.5 mL hepatitis B immune globulin (HBIG) within 12 hours of birth at separate sites. The second dose is recommended at age 1–2 months and the third dose at age 6 months. **Infants born to mothers whose HBsAg status is unknown** should receive Hep B within 12 hours of birth. Maternal blood should be drawn at delivery to determine the mother's HBsAg status; if the HBsAg test is positive, the infant should receive HBIG as soon as possible (no later than age 1 week). **All children and adolescents (through age 18 years)** who have not been vaccinated against hepatitis B may begin the series during any visit. Providers should make special efforts to vaccinate children who were born in or whose parents were born in areas of the world where hepatitis B virus infection is moderately or highly endemic.

[3]The fourth dose of diphtheria and tetanus toxoids and acellular pertussis vaccine **(DTaP)** can be administered as early as age 12 months, provided 6 months have elapsed since the third dose and the child is unlikely to return at age 15–18 months. Tetanus and diphtheria toxoids **(Td)** is recommended at age 11–12 years if at least 5 years have elapsed since the last dose of diphtheria and tetanus toxoids and pertussis vaccine **(DTP),** DTaP, or diphtheria and tetanus toxoids (DT). Subsequent routine Td boosters are recommended every 10 years.

[4]Three *Haemophilus influenzae* type b **(Hib)** conjugate vaccines are licensed for infant use. If Hib conjugate vaccine (PRP-OMP) PedvaxHIB® or ComVax® [Merck]) is administered at ages 2 months and 4 months, a dose at age 6 months is not required. Because clinical studies in infants have demonstrated that using some combination products may induce a lower immune response to the Hib vaccine component, DTaP/Hib combination products should not be used for primary vaccination in infants at ages 2, 4, or 6 months unless approved by the Food and Drug Administration for these ages.

[5]To eliminate the risk for vaccine-associated paralytic poliomyelitis (VAPP), an all-inactivated poliovirus vaccine **(IPV)** schedule is now recommended for routine childhood polio vaccination in the United States. All children should receive four doses of IPV: at age 2 months, age 4 months, between ages 6 and 18 months, and between ages 4 and 6 years. Oral poliovirus vaccine (OPV) (if available) may be used only for the following special circumstances: (1) mass vaccination campaigns to control outbreaks of paralytic polio; (2) unvaccinated children who will be traveling in <4 weeks to areas where polio is endemic or epidemic; and (3) children of parents who do not accept the recommended number of vaccine injections. Children of parents who do not accept the recommended number of vaccine injections may receive OPV only for the third or fourth dose or both; in this situation, health-care providers should administer OPV only after discussing the risk for VAPP with parents or caregivers. During the transition to an all-IPV schedule, recommendations for the use of remaining OPV supplies in physicians' offices and clinics have been issued by the American Academy of Pediatrics (*Pediatrics* Vol. 104, No. 6, December 1999).

[6]The second dose of measles, mumps, and rubella vaccine **(MMR)** is recommended routinely at age 4–6 years but may be administered during any visit, provided at least 4 weeks have elapsed since receipt of the first dose and that both doses are administered beginning at or after age 12 months. Those who previously have not received the second dose should complete the schedule no later than the routine visit to a health-care provider at age 11–12 years.

[7]Varicella (Var) vaccine is recommended at any visit on or after the first birthday for susceptible children, i.e., those whose lack a reliable history of chickenpox (as judged by a health-care provider) and who have not been vaccinated. Susceptible persons aged ≥ 13 years should receive two doses given at least 4 weeks apart.

[8]Hepatitis A vaccine **(Hep A)** is recommended for use in selected states and regions. Information is available from local public health authorities and *MMWR* Vol. 48, No. RR-12, October 1, 1999.

Use of trade names and commercial sources is for identification only and does not constitute or imply endorsement by CDC or the U. S. Department of Health and Human Services. Source: Advisory Committee on Immunization Practices (ACIP), American Academy of Family Physicians (AAFP), and American Academy of Pediatrics (AAP).

bacterial vaccines are killed organisms or extracts of bacterial antigens. Some organisms are not invasive, remaining on the mucosal membranes, but they cause life-threatening disease by the release of powerful toxins that act locally or systemically, including diphtheria, cholera, and tetanus toxins. Vaccination against systemic toxins (e.g., diphtheria, tetanus) has been achieved using **toxoids**—toxins that have been chemically detoxified without loss of immunogenicity. The primary immune response from vaccination is generally short lived; therefore booster injections are used to push the immune response through multiple secondary responses resulting in large numbers of memory cells and long-lasting active immune response with sustained high titers of protective antibody.

Development of a successful vaccine frequently is costly and depends on several factors: identification of the protective immune response; appropriate antigen to induce that response; successful development of that antigen into an effective, cost-efficient, stable, and safe vaccine; and compliance of the susceptible population to achieve a protective level of immunization in the total population. Most vaccine development has focused on preventing the most severe and common infections. With the success of other interventions, such as antibiotic therapy, there has been no perceived need for vaccination against many common and non–life-threatening infections. Even with successful development of a vaccine, a certain percentage of the population will be genetically unresponsive and not produce a protective immune response. Those individuals will be susceptible to the infection and need an effective therapy.

Antimicrobials

Since World War II, antibiotics have had the greatest impact on the success in resisting infection. Antibiotics are natural products of fungi, bacteria, and related organisms and kill or inhibit the growth of other microorganisms. Numerous chemicals or antimicrobials have been identified that either prevent the growth of microorganisms or directly destroy them (Table 8-12). Antibiotics generally act by preventing the function of enzymes or cell structures that are unique to the infecting agent. Because viruses use the enzymes of the host's cells, there has been far less success in developing antiviral antibiotics.

Recent Pathogenic Adaptations

Recently, disease-causing microbial organisms have emerged that have developed mechanisms for circumventing the most modern techniques for destroying or controlling infection, including microorganisms that attack the immune system (HIV) and those that are resistant to multiple antibiotics (e.g., *Mycobacterium tuberculosis*).

HIV is one of the few organisms that directly attacks the central processes involved in the development of an immune response. It infects and destroys the T helper cell, which is necessary to provide help for the maturation of both plasma cells and T cytotoxic cells. Therefore HIV suppresses the immune response against itself and, secondarily, creates a generalized immune deficiency by suppressing the development of immune responses against other pathogens and opportunistic organisms.

The development of vaccines against HIV also has been frustrating because of the large number of changing antigens expressed on the viral surface. HIV can infect also by intercellular fusion between an infected cell in transmitted body fluids and uninfected cells near the mucosal surface. During this mechanism of infection, the virus may remain sequestered in the cell and be resistant to a vaccine-induced immune response.

Since the development of antibiotics, sensitive organisms have mutated and developed resistance to particular antibiotics. Resistance is primarily through inactivation of the drug, alterations of bacterial membrane so that the antibiotic is no longer taken up, or alterations of the target molecule. These changes are generally genetic mutations and can be transmitted directly to neighboring organisms. Penicillin resistance, for example, results from the production of an enzyme (β-lactamase) that breaks down the structure of the antibiotic. Zidovudine (Azidothymidine, AZT) is an antibiotic that suppresses the enzymatic activity of reverse transcriptase, a viral-specific enzyme responsible for the replication of viral RNA and a DNA strand. HIV frequently mutates and produces an AZT-resistant reverse transcriptase.

Table 8-12 Chemicals or Antimicrobials Identified That Prevent Growth of or Destroy Microorganisms

Mechanisms of Action	Agent
Inhibition of synthesis of cell wall	Penicillins
	Cephalosporins
	Monobactams
	Carbapenems
	Vancomycin
	Bacitracin
	Cycloserine
	Fosfomycin
Damage of cytoplasmic membrane	Polymyxins
	Polyene antifungals
	Imidazoles
Metabolism of nucleic acid	Quinolones
	Rifampin
	Nitrofurans
	Nitroimidazoles
Protein synthesis	Aminoglycosides
	Tetracyclines
	Chloramphenicol
	Macrolides
	Clindamycin
	Spectinomycin
	Mupirocin
Modification of energy metabolism	Sulfonamides
	Trimethoprim
	Dapsone
	Isoniazid

Modified from Ellner PD, Neu HCP: *Understanding infectious disease,* St Louis, 1992, Mosby.

The rapid emergence of multiple antibiotic–resistant bacteria has been observed during the past decade. These organisms have developed resistance to almost all currently available antibiotics. For example, *Streptococcus pneumoniae,* which causes pneumonia, meningitis, and acute otitis media (ear infections), was once routinely susceptible to penicillin. Since the 1980s, however, the incidence of penicillin-resistant organisms has risen to 30% in some populations. Many of these are resistant also to multiple antibiotics. In some areas, almost 20% of tuberculosis cases are caused by multiple antibiotic–resistant *M. tuberculosis.* Also, the incidence of drug-resistant gonorrhea, malaria, pneumococcal disease, salmonellosis, shigellosis, and staphylococcal infections has increased dramatically.

Why have multiple antibiotic–resistant organisms appeared? Overuse of antibiotics can lead to the destruction of the normal flora, allowing the selective overgrowth of antibiotic-resistant strains or pathogens that had previously been kept under control. For example, after treatment with the antibiotic clindamycin, the normal intestinal flora can become compromised, allowing the overgrowth of *Clostridium difficile* and the development of pseudomembranous colitis. Also, individuals commonly do not comply with the instructions of health care providers concerning the necessity of completing the therapeutic regimen with antibiotics. This practice allows the selective resurgence of organisms that are more relatively resistant to the antibiotic.

Antibiotic resistance is widespread and spreading. Several studies have confirmed that U.S. rivers are a major reservoir for antibiotic-resistant microbes.[17]

The Future

With the development of multiple antibiotic–resistant strains, creativity to address this new challenge must be rekindled. If currently available antibiotics are no longer effective, alternative forms of therapy must be developed. New antibiotics

WHAT'S NEW? Emerging Infections

In the mid-1970s many microbiologists and physicians believed that infectious disease was on the verge of being controlled as a major cause of death in the United States. That belief was based on the success of public health initiatives, vaccination programs, and the use of antibiotics. Smallpox had been eradicated from the globe (the last reported case was in 1975 in Somalia), measles was almost eradicated in the Western Hemisphere, and many diseases, such as tuberculosis and polio, were on the decline.

Since that time, however, the trend has been reversed completely. Death caused by infection in the United States rose by 58% between 1980 and 1992. Infection is the third leading cause of death in the United States after heart disease and cancer (although many individuals with cancer die of infection) and is the leading cause of death worldwide.

The reversal has occurred because of the emergence of previously unknown infections, the reemergence of old infections that were thought to be under control, and the development of infectious agents that are resistant to multiple antibiotics. The causes for this occurrence are numerous and include the following:

- Vast and rapid urbanization in many areas of the world, resulting in a breakdown in public health programs and a more rapid spread of infection
- Increased travel, allowing more rapid spread of disease from isolated areas to virtually any point around the world in a few hours
- Human encroachment into wilderness areas, resulting in contact with previously sequestered infectious agents
- Antibiotics that are prescribed excessively, that are not taken for a complete course of therapy, or that, even when appropriately used, result in the selection of antibiotic-resistant organisms
- Decreases in federal research budgets to study infectious disease
- Denial by governments, allowing infections to spread in an uncontrolled way
- Increased global warming, allowing insect vectors to spread into and breed in areas that were previously too cool

The emergence of previously unknown infections is not a new event. In the early 1500s syphilis began to spread throughout Europe. It was suggested, probably inaccurately, that Columbus' men brought the disease back from the New World. Although the Italians usually referred to syphilis as the French disease and the French called it the Italian disease, its origins are unclear.

Since 1973, however, more than 30 previously unknown infections have arisen, including Lyme disease (1975), Ebola virus (1976), legionnaires' disease (1978), toxic shock syndrome (1978), AIDS (1981), chronic-fatigue syndrome (1985), hepatitis C virus (1989), hepatitis E virus, (1990), and *Hantavirus* (1993). It is not known how many more infections will be identified.

Concurrently, the incidence and spread of at least 20 well-known infections are increasing. A new strain of cholera that arose in Indonesia in 1961 has spread to Africa and in 1991 to South America. Malaria, dengue fever, and yellow fever are reemerging in areas where they had been eliminated or were unknown. The incidence of tuberculosis is increasing in countries that had reported declines and has risen by almost one third between the mid-1980s and early 1990s. Diphtheria has reemerged as a major health issue in Russia. In 1994 plague was reported in India after being dormant for a generation.

Many common and reemerging infections (e.g., tuberculosis, malaria) have become antibiotic and drug resistant. *Streptococcus pneumoniae,* a common cause of otitis media, pneumonia, and bacteremia, has been treated routinely and successfully with penicillin. Now at least 25% of isolates are penicillin resistant, and some are resistant to multiple antibiotics. Multiple antibiotic–resistant forms of *Staphylococcus aureus,* a primary cause of infections of wounds, surgical incisions, and catheters, are endemic in some hospitals. Some forms of this organism are sensitive to a single antibiotic, vancomycin.

What the future holds is uncertain. Many recent books and movies have been based on the emergence of a new and highly lethal infection from some previously unexplored rain forest. In most cases the dramatized spread and lethality of the infection mimic the possible result of one of many already known infectious agents reaching the general population. To end the drama on a happy note, the heros usually do something that is currently technically impossible, such as clone monkey cells that are producing a protective and curative antibody and produce liters of that antibody within 2 hours (a procedure that would take close to 1 year, if successful at all). The dramas must invent such solutions because, at the moment, no other way of happily concluding such a situation exists.

may solve a portion of the problem or may exacerbate it further. For example, scientists are designing antibiotics that self-destruct, which would decrease contamination in rivers and soil.[18] Other forms of therapy may involve the immune system. If an immune response results in resolution of the infection, use of passive immunotherapy, in which preformed antibodies are given to the individual, may be increased. This form of therapy has been used for decades. Horse serum–containing antibodies were given to treat diphtheria, pneumococcal pneumonia, tetanus, and other diseases in the early twentieth century. Because of foreign proteins in the serum, many individuals developed an immune reaction against the horse proteins and an immune complex–mediated serum sickness. Individuals with an immune deficiency of B cells currently are given intravenous immunoglobulin containing various antibodies against most infectious diseases. Several diseases in persons with intact immune systems have been treated by the administration of human immunoglobulin preparations, including (1) prophylactic administration to prevent hepatitis A in travelers who will enter a region in which the virus is endemic and (2) therapeutic administration to treat hepatitis B and rabies. Recurrent administration of these preparations generally confers passive resistance to most common bacterial and viral infections. More specific therapy with monoclonal antibodies is being evaluated against neonatal infections with the group B streptococci and against gram-negative bacteria that cause septic shock.

Vaccines induce an active immunotherapy in which the individual produces protective antibodies or T cells. The development and widespread use of vaccines against common antibiotic-resistant organisms must now be considered. For example, otitis media, a purulent ear infection, is caused primarily by *Streptococcus, Haemophilus,* and *Staphylococcus.* It routinely has been treated successfully with antibiotics; however, multiple antibiotic–resistant organisms are commonly observed. This may force an evaluation of the use of childhood immunization to prevent this disease. Other vaccines that may be used more widely or may soon be developed include those against cholera, typhoid, malaria, and several other diseases. More novel therapeutic approaches also may require evaluation, such as bacteriophages—viruses that infect bacteria but not humans.

DEFICIENCIES IN IMMUNITY AND INFLAMMATION

Disorders resulting from immune deficiency are the clinical sequelae (results) of impaired function of one or more components of the immune or inflammatory response, including B cells, T cells, phagocytic cells, and complement (Table 8-13 lists defects in phagocytic cells and complement). An **immune deficiency** is the failure of these mechanisms of self-defense to function at their normal capacity. **Congenital (primary) immune deficiency** is caused by a genetic anomaly, whereas **acquired (secondary) immune deficiency** is caused by another illness, such as cancer or viral infection, or by normal physiologic changes, such as aging. Acquired forms of immune deficiency are far more common than the congenital forms.

Whether immune deficiency is congenital or acquired, its chief cause is disruption of lymphocyte function. A stem cell defect may prevent normal lymphocyte development and cause total failure of the immune system; a central lymphoid organ dysfunction may prevent maturation of stem cells into B or T cells; or the final stages of B cell maturation may be disrupted, precluding the production of a specific class of immunoglobulin. Other defects may interfere with intercellular cooperation. For example, helper T cells may be unable to mediate immune interactions. Sometimes enzymatic defects (adenosine deaminase deficiency) in lymphocytes cause a general accumulation of toxic metabolites. Alterations in the inflammatory response, particularly the chemotactic and

Table 8-13 Congenital Defects of Phagocytosis and Complement Function

Type of Defect	Characteristic	Clinical Manifestation
DEFECTS OF PHAGOCYTOSIS		
Quantitative defects	Neutropenia (decreased granulocyte number)	General increase in bacterial infections
Adhesion defects	Decreased neutrophil adhesion to endothelial cells	General increase in bacterial infections
Chemotactic defects	Decreased neutrophil response to chemotactic factors	General increase in bacterial infections
Bacterial killing defects	Decreased bacterial killing because of insufficient H_2O_2 or lysosomal enzymes	Increased bacterial infections—especially with catalase + organisms
COMPLEMENT DEFECTS		
Defects in early classic pathway	Decreased activity of C1, C2, or C4	Mild bacterial infections; systemic lupus erythematosus (SLE)–like syndrome
Defects in alternative pathway	Decreased activity of alternative pathway components—especially factor B	Increased infections with encapsulated bacteria
Defects in C3	Decreased production of C3b	Severe infections, mostly with encapsulated bacteria
Defects in late pathway	Decreased activity of C5, C6, C7, or C8	Recurrent disseminated *Neisseria gonorrhoeae* or *N. meningitidis* infections

phagocytic activities of neutrophils and macrophages or the activity of complement, also can impair host resistance.

The clinical hallmark of immune deficiency is a tendency to develop unusual or recurrent, severe infections. Preschool and school-age children normally have 6 to 12 infections per year, and adults have two to four infections per year. Most of these are not severe and are limited to viral infections of the upper respiratory tract, recurrent streptococcal pharyngitis, or mild otitis media. Potential immune deficiencies are considered if the individual has had severe, documented bouts of pneumonia, otitis media, sinusitis, bronchitis, septicemia, or meningitis or infections with opportunistic microorganisms that normally are not pathogenic (e.g., *Pneumocystis carinii*). Deficiencies in T cell immune responses are suggested when recurrent infections are caused by certain viruses (e.g., varicella, vaccinia, herpes, cytomegalovirus), fungi and yeasts (e.g., *Candida, Histoplasma*), or certain atypical organisms (e.g., *P. carinii*). B cell deficiencies, however, are suggested if the individual has documented, recurrent infections with microorganisms that require opsonization (e.g., encapsulated bacteria) or viruses against which humoral immunity is normally effective (e.g., rubella).

Many immune deficiencies also are associated with other defects; some of these appear to be unrelated to the immune system yet may be life threatening by themselves. Examples include eczema and thrombocytopenia (in Wiskott-Aldrich syndrome); cardiac anomalies, low levels of calcium in the blood, and structural anomalies of the face (in DiGeorge syndrome); and a severe lack of muscular coordination and dilation of the small blood vessels (in ataxia-telangiectasia). The association of these other symptoms sometimes can clarify the pathophysiology of the disease. For instance, in **DiGeorge syndrome** the principal defects are the partial or complete absence of a thymus (resulting in depressed T cell immunity), partial or complete absence of the parathyroid gland (resulting in decreased blood calcium levels), and structural defects in the heart. Each of these anatomic structures originates from the same region in the embryo during the twelfth week of gestation; therefore the defect in DiGeorge syndrome can be traced to an abnormal development at a specific time and in a specific region during embryogenesis (development of the third and fourth pharyngeal pouches).

Routine care of individuals with immune deficiencies must be tempered with the knowledge that the immune system may be totally ineffective. It may be unsafe to administer conventional immunizing agents or blood products to many of these individuals because of the risk that the immunizing agent will cause an uncontrolled infection. Uncontrolled infection is a problem when attenuated vaccines that contain live but weakened microorganisms are used (e.g., live polio vaccine). Although the virus is attenuated enough to be destroyed by a normal immune system, it can survive, multiply, and cause severe disease in an immune-deficient recipient. Further, even simple procedures, such as penetrating the skin for routine blood tests, may lead to fatal septicemia (bacterial infection of the blood) in the immune-deficient person.

Individuals with immune deficiencies are also at risk for **graft-versus-host (GVH) disease.** This occurs if T cells in a graft (e.g., transfused blood) are mature and are therefore capable of the cell-mediated destruction of tissues in the graft recipient. If the recipient's immune system is normal, the grafted T cells are controlled and no tissue destruction occurs. If, however, the recipient's immune system is deficient, the grafted T cells remain unchecked and attack the recipient's tissues.

Congenital Immune Deficiencies

Congenital, or primary, immune deficiency occurs if lymphocyte development is arrested or disrupted in the fetus or embryo[19] (Fig. 8-16). Defects that occur at different stages of stem cell, T cell, or B cell maturation cause different immune-deficiency diseases. Some diseases are caused primarily by a defect in one or the other of the cell lines, although both T and B cell lines may be deficient in some respect. Other congenital immune-deficiency diseases affect stem cells of both cell lines, disrupting both cell-mediated and humoral immune processes. A defect in B cell development results in lower levels of circulating immunoglobulin. The condition in which immunoglobulins are present in insufficient amounts is termed **hypogammaglobulinemia.** The condition in which they are totally or nearly absent is termed **agammaglobulinemia.** (Normal lymphocyte development is discussed in Chapter 6.)

Although most congenital immune-deficiency diseases are rare, much of our current understanding of the development of the immune system and the interactions of the cells in the immune response was developed by studying congenital immune deficiencies or, as they have been called, "experiments of nature." The immune systems of experimental animals have been studied in the laboratory by specifically altering or removing one component of the system and observing the effect of that manipulation on the remainder of the immune response. Studying congenital immune deficiencies allows the opportunity to make similar observations in humans.

The role of bone marrow stem cells in the evolution of the immune system was elucidated by studying children with the most severe deficiencies, **severe combined immune deficiencies (SCIDs).** The most severe form of SCID is **reticular dysgenesis** (failure of blood cells to develop), in which a common stem cell for all white blood cells is absent; therefore T cells, B cells, and phagocytic cells never develop (see Fig. 8-16). Most children with reticular dysgenesis die in utero or very soon after birth.

The common stem cell normally matures into more developed stem cells for individual populations of white blood cells. Most individuals with SCID are deficient only in the maturation of stem cells for lymphocyte development, and therefore they have normal numbers of all other white cells and few, if any, detectable lymphocytes. T and B lymphocytes are few or totally absent in both the circulation and secondary lymphoid organs (spleen, lymph nodes). The thymus is usually hypoplastic (underdeveloped) because of the

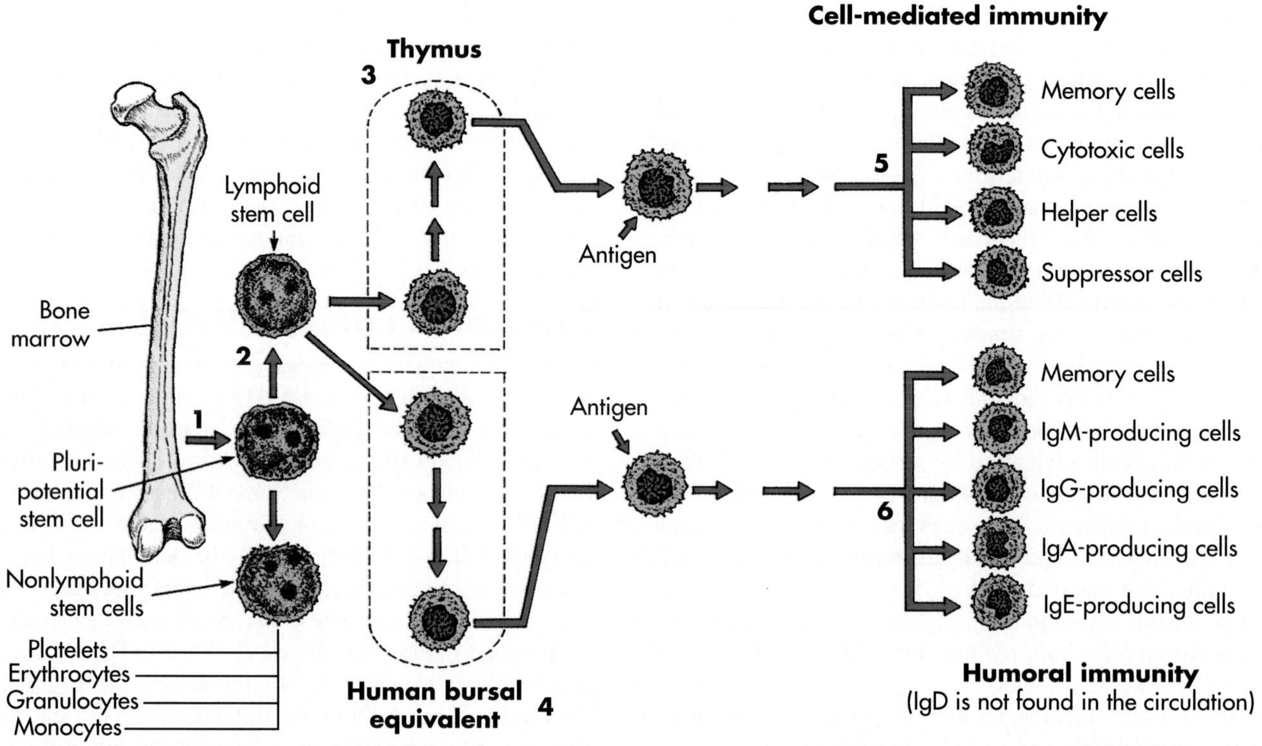

FIG. 8-16 Lymphocyte development defects. Defects in lymphocyte development that may account for congenital immune deficiencies: *(1)* reticular dysgenesis; *(2)* severe combined immune deficiency (SCID); *(3)* DiGeorge syndrome; *(4)* Bruton agammaglobulinemia; *(5)* chronic mucocutaneous candidiasis; and *(6)* selective IgA deficiency. *Ig,* Immunoglobulin.

absence of T cells. Immunoglobulin levels, especially of IgM and IgA, are absent or greatly reduced, although IgG levels may be almost normal in the first months of life because of the presence of maternal antibodies.

Two forms of SCID are caused by autosomal recessive enzymatic defects that result in the accumulation of toxic metabolites to which rapidly dividing cells, such as lymphocytes, are especially sensitive. **Adenosine deaminase (ADA) deficiency** and **purine nucleoside phosphorylase (PNP) deficiency** result in the accumulation of toxic purine metabolism.[20]

Some forms of SCID are X linked and are therefore observed more often in males. One cause has been identified as a mutation in a protein that is part of the receptor for a large number of cytokines, including IL-2 and IL-4. This mutation leads to a shortened (truncated) form of the protein and prevents lymphocytes from responding to several cytokines. Another cause of X-linked SCID is a mutation in one of the proteins of the CD3 complex that is responsible for communication between the T cell receptor (TCR) and the T cell nucleus. This defect prevents a T cell from responding to the interaction of antigen with the TCR.

Stem cells mature in the central or primary lymphoid organs (thymus and bursal-equivalent tissue). The importance of these organs was determined by studying children who failed to develop them during embryogenesis. These children had either a defective thymus (DiGeorge syndrome) or defective bursal-equivalent tissue (Bruton agammaglobulinemia).

DiGeorge syndrome (congenital thymic aplasia or hypoplasia) is caused by the lack, or more commonly partial lack, of the thymus, resulting in lymphopenia with greatly decreased T cell numbers and function[21,22] (see Fig. 8-16).

Bruton agammaglobulinemia is caused by blocked development of B cell precursors into mature B cells because of the lack of normal B cell development in the bursal-equivalent tissue (see Fig. 8-16).[23] The B cells are unable to produce mature B cells because of a mutation in Bruton's tyrosine kinase (Btk), which is required for signal transduction from the IgM antigen receptor, the IL-5 receptor, and the IL-6 receptor. There are few or no circulating mature B cells, although T cell number and function are normal. At 6 months the approximate normal serum concentrations of immunoglobulins are IgG, 400 mg/dl; IgM, 40 mg/dl; and IgA, 30 mg/dl. In 6-month-old children with Bruton agammaglobulinemia, serum IgG levels are well below 100 mg/dl and IgM and IgA are almost absent.

Even if nearly adequate numbers of B and T cells are produced, their cooperation may be defective. The **bare lymphocyte syndrome** is an immune deficiency characterized by an inability of lymphocytes and macrophages to produce class I or class II HLAs. Several forms of this syndrome have been reported: type I, in which class I HLA expression is deficient; type II, in which class II HLA is not expressed; and type III, in which both class I and class II HLA expression is defective. Without HLA expression, antigen presentation and intercellular cooperation cannot occur effectively. Children with this deficiency develop life-threatening infections and usually die before age 5 years.

Some immune deficiencies involve a defect that results in depressed development of a small portion of the immune system and therefore provide information about the function of that portion. For instance, an individual can be unable to produce a certain class of antibody. An example is **Wiskott-Aldrich syndrome** (an X-linked recessive disorder). Here IgM antibody production is greatly depressed because of a mutation in Wiskott-Aldrich syndrome protein (WASp) that is involved in signal transduction. Therefore antibody responses against antigens that elicit primarily an IgM response, such as polysaccharide antigens from bacterial cell walls (e.g., of *P. aeruginosa, S. pneumoniae, H. influenzae,* and other microorganisms with polysaccharide outer capsules), are deficient.[24]

Another defect in which a particular class of antibody is affected is **selective IgA deficiency.** This is the most common type of immune deficiency, having an incidence between 1 in 700 and 1 in 400 individuals. Individuals with selective IgA deficiency are able to produce other classes of immunoglobulins but fail to produce IgA. This suggests a disruption of terminal processes of differentiation, so that immature B cells that are committed to IgA production fail to mature into IgA-producing plasma cells (see Fig. 8-16). Many individuals are asymptomatic, although others manifest a history of severe recurring sinus, lung, and gastrointestinal infections. Individuals with IgA deficiency frequently have chronic intestinal candidiasis (infection with *C. albicans*). (The secretory, or mucosal, immune system is described in Chapter 6.)

Complications of IgA deficiency include severe atopic disease and autoimmune diseases; selective IgA deficiency is two or three times more common in atopic individuals than in others. Secretory IgA normally may prevent the uptake of allergens from the environment. Therefore IgA deficiency may lead to increased allergen uptake and a more intense challenge to the immune system because of prolonged exposure to environmental antigens. One of the most severe complications of IgA deficiency is an anaphylactic reaction that can follow administration of IgA-containing blood products. Serious anaphylactic reactions can occur in individuals totally lacking IgA because the immune system recognizes donor IgA as a foreign antigen. Initial sensitization can occur in fetal life through exposure to maternal IgA or later through the ingestion of maternal IgA in breast milk or bovine IgA in cow's milk. Sensitization also can occur with initial administration of blood products containing IgA. The individual's primed immune system then acts against donor IgA on subsequent exposure.

Other immune deficiencies are characterized by a defect in the capacity to produce an immune response against a particular antigen. In **chronic mucocutaneous candidiasis** the defect is the inability of T lymphocytes to respond against a specific infectious agent, *Candida albicans* (see Fig. 8-16). Individuals with chronic mucocutaneous candidiasis usually have mild to extremely severe recurrent *Candida* infections that involve the mucous membranes and skin. Systemic candidiasis in immunocompetent individuals is extremely rare, although infection of the mucosal lining of the esophagus may develop.

Acquired Deficiencies

Acquired, or secondary, immune and inflammatory deficiency develops after birth and is not related to genetic defects. The following physiologic or pathophysiologic conditions are known to be associated with acquired deficiencies:

- Pregnancy
- Infancy
- Infections, such as rubella (congenital), cytomegalovirus (congenital), measles, leprosy, tuberculosis, or coccidioidomycosis
- Down syndrome
- Malignancies, such as Hodgkin disease, acute or chronic leukemia, nonlymphoid malignancy, or myeloma
- Stress caused by surgery or emotional trauma
- Malnutrition caused by insufficient intake of protein, calories, iron, or zinc
- Aging
- Diabetes
- Alcoholic cirrhosis
- Cell anemia
- Immunosuppressive treatment with corticosteroids, cytotoxic drugs, or ionizing radiation
- Anesthesia

Nutritional Deficiencies

Nutritional status can have a profound effect on immune function. Severe deficits in calorie or protein intake lead to deficiencies in T cell function and numbers. The humoral immune response is less affected by starvation, although complement activity, neutrophil chemotaxis, and bacterial killing within neutrophils frequently are depressed, resulting in infections with organisms that are normally disabled by opsonization and phagocytosis.

Deficient zinc intake can profoundly depress both T and B cell function. Zinc is required as a cofactor for at least 70 different enzymes, some of which are found in lymphocytes and are necessary for their function. Secondary zinc deficiencies may be associated with malabsorption syndrome (failure to absorb zinc), chronic renal disease (loss of zinc in the urine), chronic diarrhea (loss of zinc through the gut), or burns or severe psoriasis (loss of zinc through the skin). Deficiencies of other enzyme cofactors, such as vitamins (pyridoxine, pantothenic acid, folic acid, vitamin A, vitamin E), also may result in severe depressions of both B and T cell function.

Iatrogenic Deficiencies

Iatrogenic disorders are caused by some form of medical treatment (e.g., iatrogenic neutropenia is usually caused by drugs). Some drugs (e.g., cancer chemotherapeutic agents) profoundly suppress blood cell formation in the bone marrow. Other drugs induce immunologic responses that destroy mature granulocytes. The list of drugs having this effect is ever increasing and includes analgesics, antithyroid medications, anticonvulsants, antihistamines, antimicrobial agents, and tranquilizers.

Many drugs also affect B and T cell function, especially against antigens that require the interaction of T helper and B cells for antibody production. These complications have been observed since the advent of potent immunosuppressive (e.g., corticosteroids) and chemotherapeutic drugs as treatment for individuals with transplants, cancer, or autoimmune diseases. Depression of B and T cell formation is manifested as a progressive increase in infections with opportunistic microorganisms (especially *P. carinii*, cytomegalovirus, *C. albicans*, and other fungi), the extent and location of which are unusual.

The immunosuppressive effects of chemotherapeutic drugs are exacerbated by concurrent treatment with ionizing radiation (x-rays). Most cytotoxic drugs and x-rays destroy cells that are proliferating or are in susceptible stages in their cell cycles. Therefore these therapies mainly suppress the primary immune response, which involves proliferation of clones of B and T cells.

Surgery and anesthesia also can suppress both T and B cell function. Transient, severe lymphopenia is a common postoperative condition that can last as long as 1 month. Surgery to remove the spleen (splenectomy) results in a depressed humoral response against encapsulated bacteria (especially *S. pneumoniae, H. influenzae, S. aureus*, the group A streptococci, and *N. meningitidis*), depressed serum IgM levels, and decreased levels of opsonins.

Deficiencies Caused by Trauma

Burn victims are susceptible to severe bacterial infections. Thermal burns appear to be associated with decreased neutrophil function (especially chemotaxis), decreased complement levels, decreased cell-mediated immunity, and decreased primary humoral responses, although secondary humoral responses are normal. The mechanism of this immunosuppression may be twofold. Sera from burned individuals contain nonspecific immunosuppressive factors (will suppress all immune responses, regardless of the antigen involved). In addition, burn victims also have increased suppressor cell function, which may increase antigen-specific suppression.

Deficiencies Caused by Stress

The relationship between emotional stress and depressed immune function recently has become an area of intense research interest. For many decades there were anecdotal reports of increased incidence of infection and malignancy associated with periods of both intense stress (e.g., the loss of a loved one, divorce) and relatively minor stress (e.g., final examination periods at colleges and universities). In addition, early studies showed that immune function, as demonstrated by delayed hypersensitivity skin test results, could be depressed through posthypnotic suggestion.

Only recently has investigation of the mechanisms of this interaction begun.[25] Many lymphoid organs are innervated and can be affected by nerve stimulation. In addition, lymphocytes have receptors for many hormones (e.g., sex hormones, neurotransmitters, and neuropeptides) and can respond to changing levels of these chemicals with increased or decreased function. (Further discussion of the effects of stress on susceptibility to disease is in Chapter 9.)

Acquired Immunodeficiency Syndrome

Acquired immunodeficiency syndrome (AIDS) is currently the best-known example of an acquired dysfunction of the immune system. It is one of the most frightening diseases to appear in modern times. This is because of its extremely high mortality rate, the possibility of transmission by asymptomatic individuals over a period of years, the rapid increase in the number of clinical cases, and the relatively uncontrollable modes of transmission. Approximately 750,000 AIDS cases have been reported in the United States as of this writing (all statistics from Centers for Disease Control and Prevention [CDC]).[26] More than 90% of individuals who develop the most severe form of the disease die within 5 years of diagnosis if untreated, and as of January 1, 2000, approximately 450,000 have died in the United States. It is estimated that in 1991 alone, 55,000 people with AIDS died, the same number of men and women who died during the entire Vietnam War. For several years AIDS was the leading cause of death nationally for people between ages 25 and 44 years. Because of the advent of new therapies, deaths declined by 47% between 1996 and 1997; AIDS dropped to the third leading cause of death in 1996 and to the fifth leading cause of death in 1997. Although deaths have been reduced, approximately 40,000 new cases of HIV infection occur yearly, and half the new cases are in individuals 25 years old or younger. Transmission remains primarily by transplacental or perinatal routes to newborn children, through semen or other body fluids transmitted through homosexual and heterosexual contact, or through blood transmitted during intravenous drug abuse or the medical use of blood products.

AIDS is a worldwide disease. The Joint United Nations Programme on HIV/AIDS estimated that by January 1, 2000, 16.3 million people had died from AIDS (2.6 million in 1999 alone), and 33.4 million were living with HIV/AIDS. Of the 33.4 million HIV-infected people, 22.5 million live in sub-Saharan Africa, 6.7 million in South and Southeast Asia, 1.4 million in Latin America, and 750,000 in the United States.[27,28] The World Health Organization has declared AIDS the most rapidly spreading epidemic in the world.

Epidemiology

The incidence of AIDS in the United States has been decreasing since the early 1990s. Fig. 8-17 illustrates the estimated incidence of AIDS and deaths of adults with AIDS from 1985 to June 1999. The decline in deaths starting in 1996 is due to the success of antiretroviral therapies introduced at that time.[26] The estimated number of persons living with AIDS increased from approximately 174,000 in 1993 to approximately 297,000 in 1998. The proportional distribution by race and ethnicity among people living with AIDS has changed since 1993. In 1998, 39% of persons living with AIDS were white and 40% were black, compared with 46% white and 35% black in 1993. Small changes were seen in proportions of the other racial and ethnic groups.[26] Other important trends are summarized in Figs. 8-18 and 8-19.

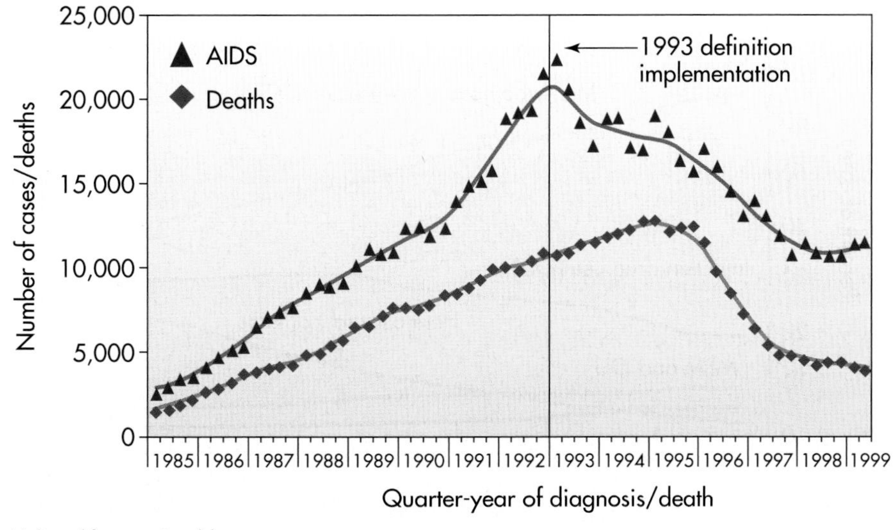

FIG. 8-17 Estimated incidence of AIDS and deaths of adults with AIDS from 1985 to June 1999, United States. Trends in the incidence of AIDS must be viewed in light of change in the history of the epidemic. The expansion of the case definition in 1993 (i.e., including persons at an earlier stage of HIV disease) created a large increase in the number of reported cases. Statistical adjustments are required to properly interpret trends in the AIDS incidence data during the 1990s. However, all AIDS cases and deaths among persons with AIDS, including persons diagnosed under all case definition criteria, are shown here. The *top line* shows the estimated incidence of AIDS from 1985 through June 1999, and the *bottom line* shows estimates of the number of deaths of persons with AIDS. Recent declines in AIDS incidence and deaths are primarily due to the success of antiviral therapies introduced in 1996 that delay disease progression. (From the Centers for Disease Control website, 2000. Available at www.cdc.gov/nchstp/od/nchstp.html.)

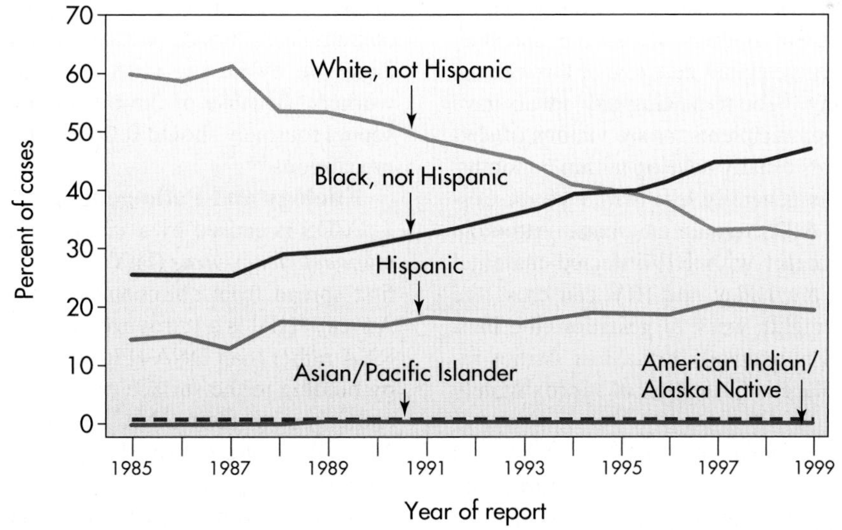

FIG. 8-18 Proportion of AIDS cases by race/ethnicity and year of report from 1985 to 1999, United States. The proportional distribution of AIDS cases among racial/ethnic groups has shifted since the beginning of the epidemic. The proportion of cases among whites has decreased over time, whereas it has increased among blacks and Hispanics. As of 1996, a greater proportion of cases was reported among blacks than whites. The proportion of cases reported among Asians/Pacific Islanders and American Indians/Alaska Natives has remained relatively constant at approximately 1% of all cases. In 1999, 32% of reported AIDS cases were among whites, 47% among blacks, 19% among Hispanics, 1% among Asians/Pacific Islanders, and less than 1% among American Indian/Alaska Natives. The estimated number of persons living with AIDS has increased from approximately 174,000 in 1993 to approximately 297,000 in 1998. The proportional distribution by race/ethnicity among people living with AIDS has changed since 1993. In 1998, 39% of persons living with AIDS were white and 40% were black, compared with 46% white and 35% black in 1993. Small changes were seen in proportions of the other racial/ethnic groups. (From the Centers for Disease Control website, 2000. Available at www.cdc.gov/nchstp/od/nchstp.html.)

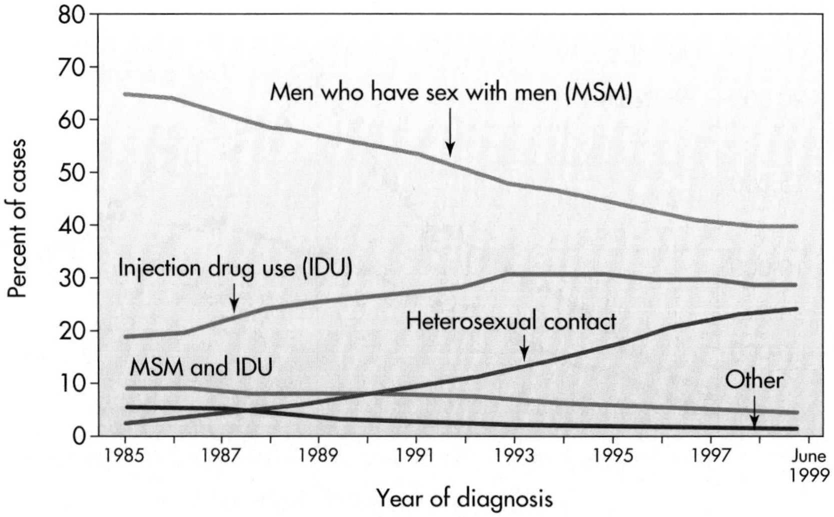

Other includes cases with other or unreported risk exposure. Data adjusted for reporting delays and risk redistribution.

FIG. 8-19 Adult/adolescent AIDS cases by exposure category and year of diagnosis from 1985 to June 1999, United States. The proportion of AIDS cases among men who have sex with men (MSM) has decreased over time from nearly 65% of cases diagnosed in 1985 to approximately 40% of cases diagnosed since 1998. The proportion of AIDS cases among injection drug users increased between 1985 and 1994 and since then has remained stable, accounting for approximately 29% of recently diagnosed cases. Of cases diagnosed in the first half of 1999, nearly 25% were attributed to heterosexual contact; the remaining 2% of cases included those attributed to hemophilia, the receipt of blood or blood products, and those without an identified risk. (From the Centers for Disease Control website, 2000. Available at www.cdc.gov/nchstp/od/nchstp.html.)

More than 8500 cases of AIDS have been reported in children. Most pediatric AIDS cases are newborns who contracted the virus from their mothers across the placenta, from blood exchange during vaginal delivery, or through the milk during breast-feeding.[29] The remaining individuals have hemophilia, are transfusion recipients, or are victims of sexual molestation. Symptoms usually develop within 6 months, and the life expectancy is generally less than 3 years. Certain aspects of pediatric AIDS remain enigmatic. Although the fetus is in direct contact with HIV-infected maternal blood during the entire pregnancy and HIV can cross the placenta as early as the eighth week of gestation, the incidence of pediatric AIDS is relatively low. Most studies report incidences of transplacental infection of approximately 30% or less.

The first reported health care provider to become infected occupationally with HIV was an emergency room nurse who became infected in 1986. The route of infection was probably through cuts in her hand that were exposed to contaminated blood through a gauze pad she was holding on a patient's open wound. More than 40,000 health care workers are infected with HIV. Several thousand health care workers have been exposed to body fluids from HIV-infected individuals, usually through needle sticks or spillage onto unprotected mucous membranes or nonintact skin. At least 56 are documented to have become infected as a result of exposure to body fluids from HIV-infected individuals. These were primarily health care workers who had been stuck accidentally with needles containing virus-contaminated blood or had broken areas of skin exposed to large quantities of contaminated blood. Nurses and clinical laboratory technicians are by far the most commonly infected health care workers. Because of the potential risk, all health care personnel routinely should follow CDC guidelines for universal precautions.[30]

Etiology and Pathogenesis

AIDS is caused by a virus, currently termed *human immunodeficiency virus* (HIV-1) (Fig. 8-20). HIV-1 most likely first spread from chimpanzees to humans in the 1930s in Africa.[31] HIV is a retrovirus carrying genetic information in RNA rather than DNA (Fig. 8-21). Retroviruses infect cells by binding to the surface of a target cell through a receptor and inserting their RNA into the target cell (Fig. 8-22). Through the use of a viral enzyme, reverse transcriptase, the viral RNA is converted to DNA and inserted into the infected cell's genetic material. If the cell is activated, viral proliferation may occur, resulting in production of more infectious virus particles. If, however, the cell remains relatively dormant, the viral genetic material is integrated into the infected cell's DNA, may remain latent for years, and probably is present for the life of the individual.[32]

CD4 is an antigen on the surface of T helper cells that acts as the primary receptor for HIV. The virus infects primarily CD4-positive T helper lymphocytes but also may infect various other cells of the central nervous system that also express the CD4 antigen.[33] Recent studies demonstrate that HIV

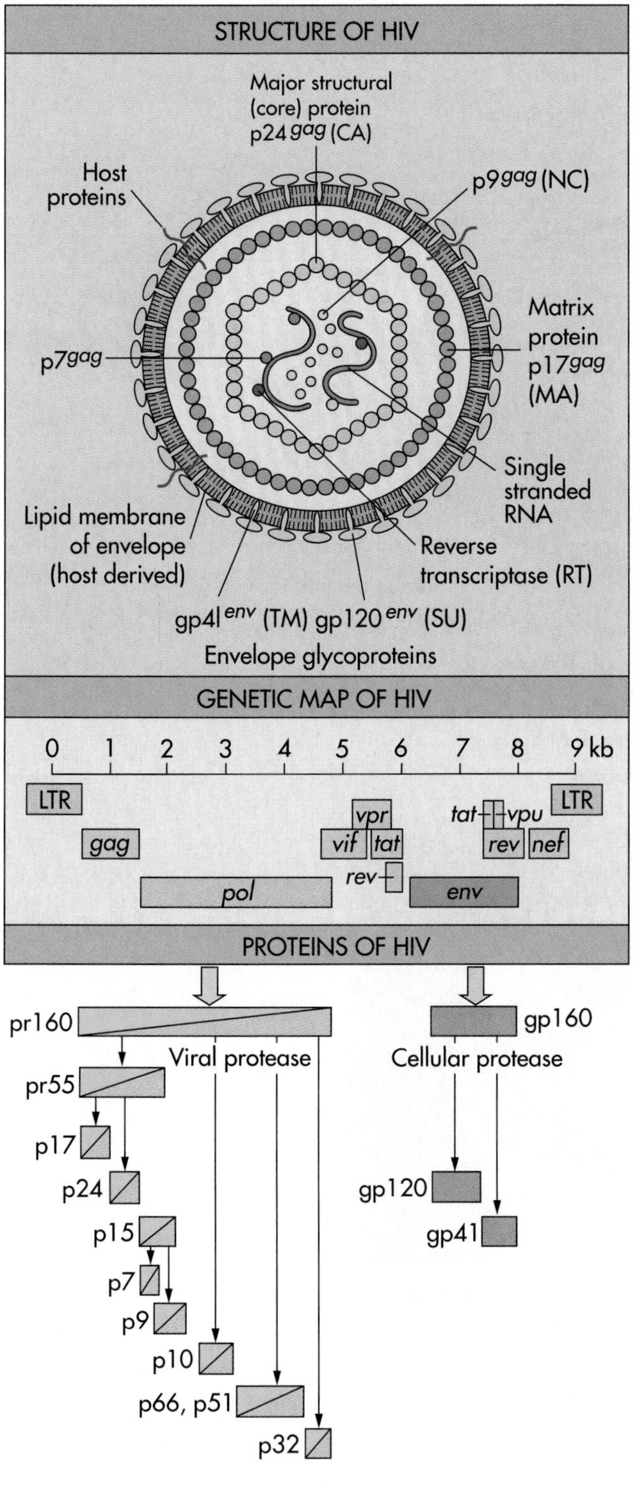

FIG. 8-20 Structure, genetic map, and proteins of human immunodeficiency virus 1 (HIV-1). The HIV-1 virion consists of a core of two identical strands of viral ribonucleic acid (RNA), molecules of reverse transcriptase (RT), nucleic acid binding protein (p9, NC), and a proline-rich protein (p7) encoated in a core capsid structure consisting primarily of the structural protein p24 (CA). The core is encased in a matrix consisting primarily of a protein, p17 (MA). The outer surface is an envelope consisting of the plasma membrane of the cell from which the virus budded and containing normal cellular proteins from the infected cell (host cell) and two viral glycoproteins: a transmembrane gp41 (TM) and a noncovalently attached surface protein, gp120 (SU).

"hitches a ride" on dendritic cells, immune cells that reside in the skin and the mucus-rich lining of the body, which then rushes to activate T cells in the body's lymph nodes.[34] Once activated, the virus causes the destruction of CD4-positive cells, causing a marked decrease in CD4 cells. CD4 cell depletion has a profound effect on the immune system—most notably, a severely diminished response to a wide array of infectious pathogens and malignant tumors (Fig. 8-23). The precise mechanism of the destruction of CD4-positive cells remains unknown, but most of the cells undergoing cellular death do not appear to be infected with HIV.

A second virus, HIV-2, has been identified in West Africa. The first case of HIV-2 in the United States was diagnosed in December 1987 in a recent visitor from West Africa.[35] HIV-2

A

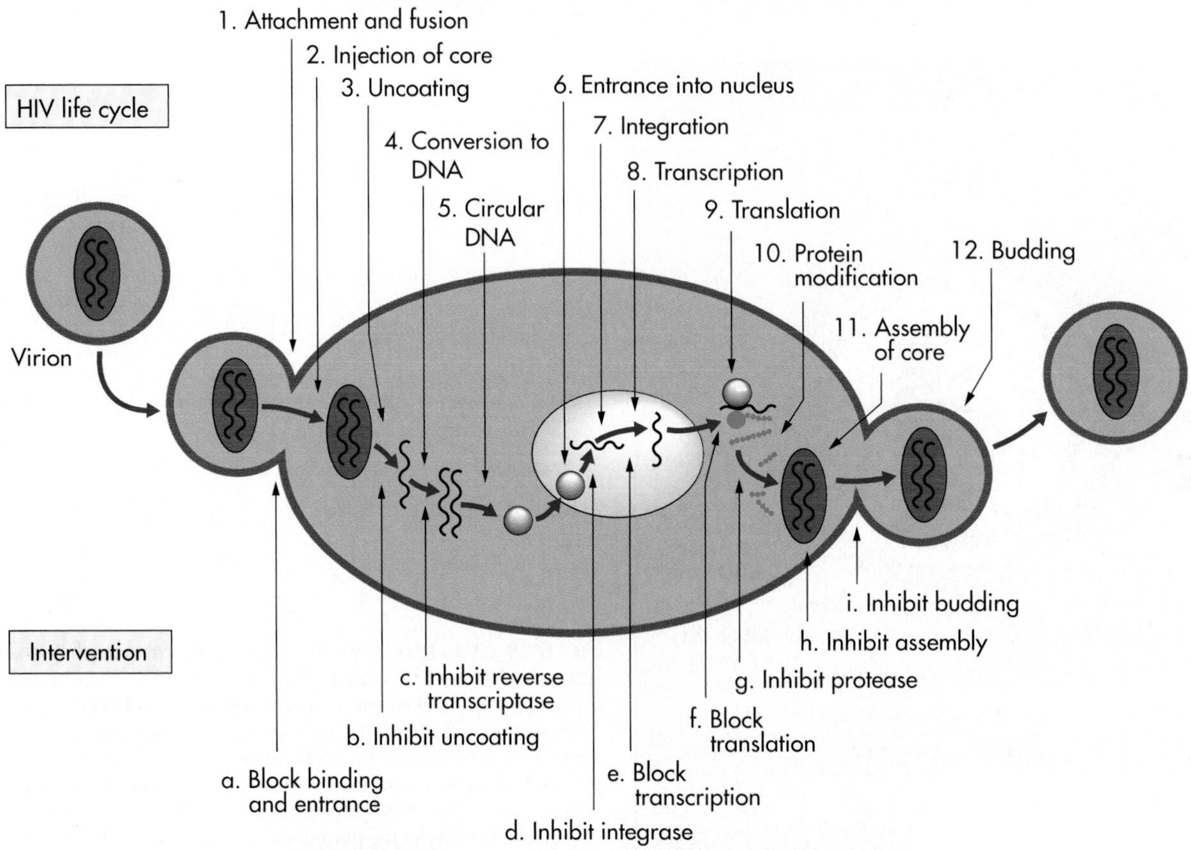

B

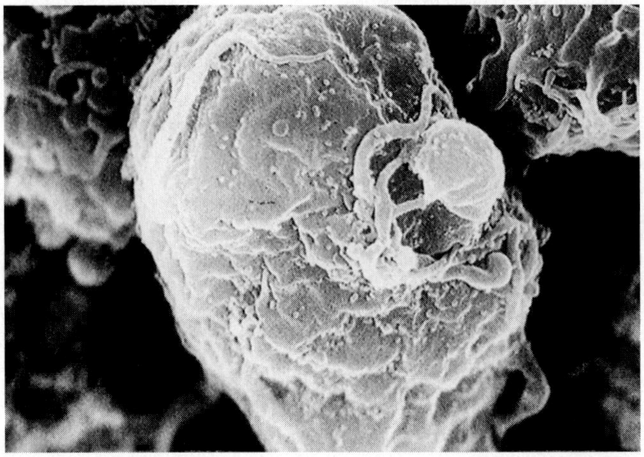

FIG. 8-21 Life cycle and possible sites of therapeutic intervention of human immunodeficiency virus 1 (HIV-1). A, HIV infection begins when a virion, or virus particle *(1)*, binds to specific receptors on the outside of a susceptible cell and the viral envelope and the plasma membrane fuse, and *(2)* the core of the virus is injected into the cytoplasm. Uncoating occurs in the cytoplasm *(3)*, during which the core proteins are removed, and the viral ribonucleic acid (RNA) is released into the infected cell's cytoplasm. *(4)* The single-stranded viral RNA is converted to a double-stranded deoxyribonucleic acid copy (cDNA) by the action of reverse transcriptase. The cDNA becomes circular *(5)* and migrates into the nucleus *(6)*. The cDNA is integrated as a provirus into the cell's own DNA *(7)*. The provirus then either remains latent or *(8)* is transcribed into RNA. Some of the new viral RNA is translated into viral protein precursors at the ribosomes *(9)*. The precursor proteins are modified by viral and cellular proteases into smaller proteins *(10)*. Additional viral RNA and modified viral proteins are assembled into new virions *(11)* that bud from the cell *(12)*. The HIV-1 life cycle is susceptible to blockage at several sites. Some agents (e.g., antibodies against HIV-1 or soluble CD4) could block the binding of the HIV to receptors on the surface of target cells *(a)*. Other agents might keep viral RNA and reverse transcriptase from leaving their protein coat *(b)*. Drugs such as azidothymidine (AZT) and other dideoxynucleosides prevent the reverse transcription of viral RNA into DNA *(c)*. Drugs also may be able to inhibit the viral integrase and prevent insertion of the viral cDNA into the host's chromosomes *(d)*. Antisense oligonucleotides could block the transcription of the provirus *(e)* and translation of mRNA into viral proteins *(f)*. New drugs, protease inhibitors, specifically inhibit the viral protease and prevent the processing of the pr160, which is the precursor of all gag and pol proteins *(g)*. Certain compounds could interfere with viral assembly by modifying such processes *(h)*, and antiviral agents such as interferon could keep the virus from assembling itself and budding out of the cell *(i)*. **B,** Scanning electromicrograph of HIV-infected CD4 lymphocyte showing virus budding from the plasma membrane. (**B,** From Morse SA, Moreland AA, Homes KK, editors: *Atlas of sexually transmitted diseases and AIDS,* London, 1996, Mosby.)

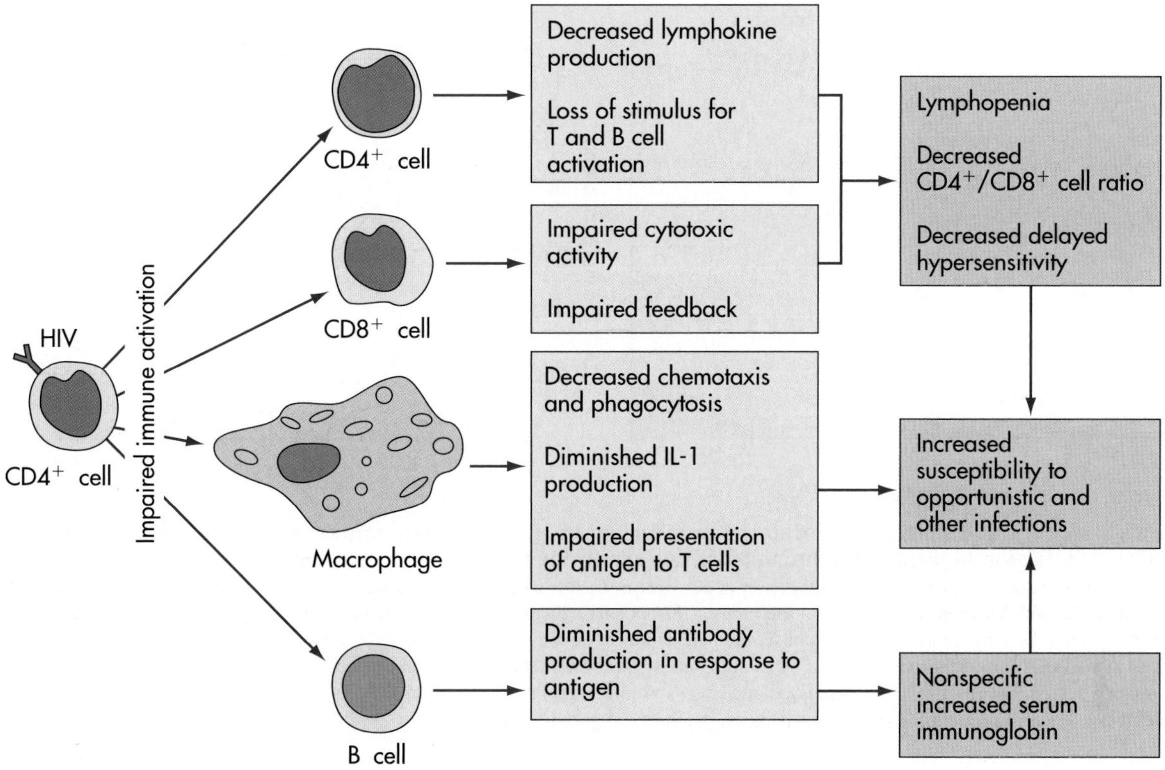

FIG. 8-22 Summary of human immunodeficiency virus (HIV) infection on the immune system. (Redrawn from Morse SA, Moreland AA, Homes KK, editors: *Atlas of sexually transmitted diseases and AIDS,* ed 2, London, 1996, Mosby.)

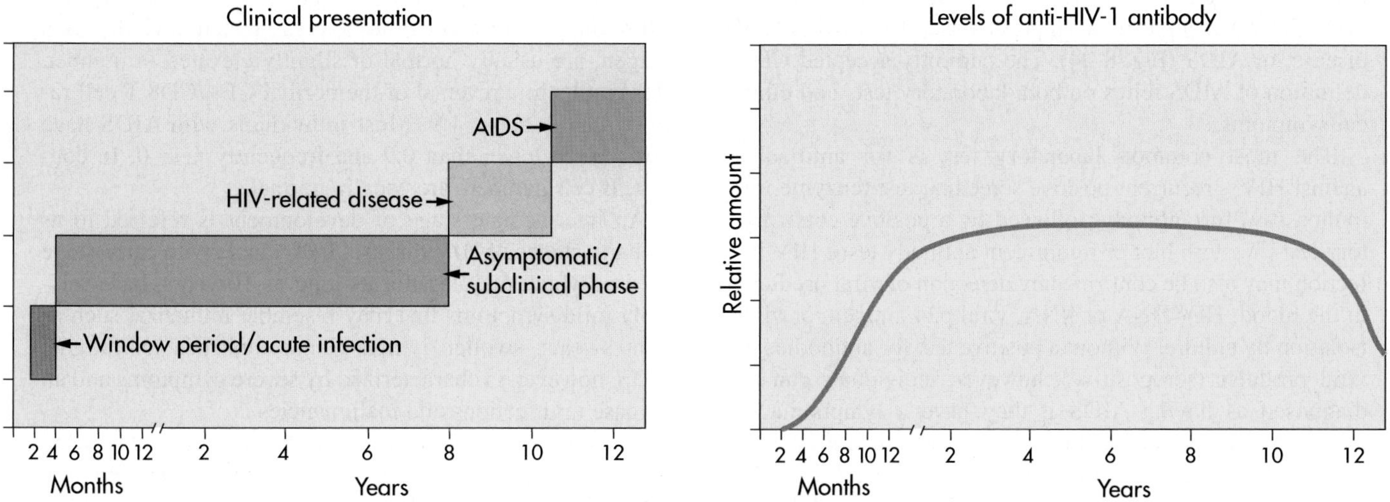

FIG. 8-23 Changes in laboratory levels during progression from human immunodeficiency virus 1 (HIV-1) infection to acquired immunodeficiency syndrome (AIDS). The progression from HIV-1 infection to AIDS is divided generally into four stages, the length of which may vary greatly from patient to patient. During the *initial phase* the patient may experience common and unremarkable symptoms of an acute viral infection. Antibodies against HIV-1 are not yet detectable (window period), but viral products, including p24 antigen, viral RNA, and infectious virus, may be detectable in the blood a few weeks after infection. CD4-positive T cell levels may increase but will remain within normal ranges. During the *second phase* of infection the patient is generally asymptomatic or has slight chronic lymphadenopathy. The virus is replicating in the lymph nodes and other sites, but viral products are being released into the blood sporadically. The patient is seropositive for multiple antibodies against HIV-1, and CD4-positive T cell levels are variable but generally decreasing to below normal ranges.

Continued

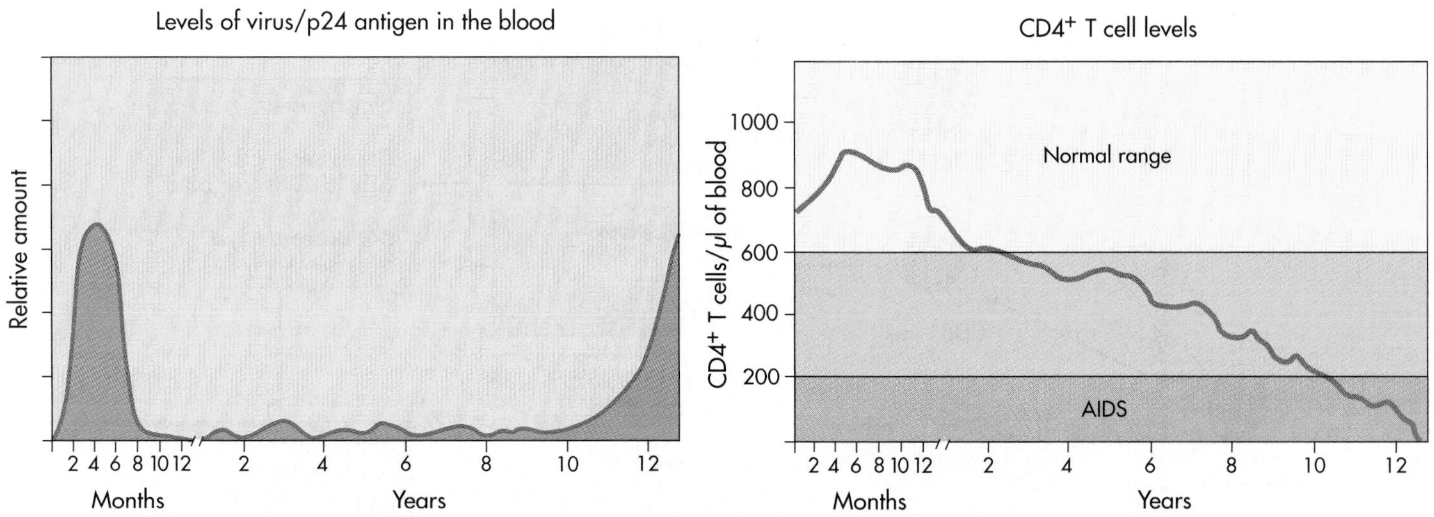

FIG. 8-23, cont'd Changes in laboratory levels during progression from human immunodeficiency virus 1 (HIV-1) infection to acquired immunodeficiency syndrome (AIDS). During the *third phase* the patient develops HIV-related disease—a variety of symptoms of acute viral infection without opportunistic infections or malignancies. Viral products remain detected sporadically in the blood, CD4-positive T cell levels continue to drop, and antibody levels remain high. During the *fourth phase,* the last phase, the patient has been diagnosed with AIDS with a CD4-positive T cell count of less than 200 or opportunistic infections or malignancies. Viral products are released progressively into the blood. As the immune system becomes severely depressed and excess viral antigen is released into the blood, measurable antibody levels decrease. Disease progression usually ends in the death of the patient.

is similar to HIV-1 in route of infection and clinical diagnosis, although it may be less destructive to the immune system and more slowly growing than HIV-1.

Clinical Manifestations

At the time of diagnosis the HIV-infected individual may manifest one of four conditions: serologically negative, serologically positive but asymptomatic, early stages of HIV disease, or AIDS (Fig. 8-24). The currently accepted CDC definition of AIDS relies on both laboratory tests and clinical symptoms.

The most common laboratory test is for antibodies against HIV—recurrent positive screening test (enzyme immunoassay) for antibody, followed by a positive confirmatory test (Western blot or fluorescent antibody test). HIV infection may also be confirmed by detection of viral products in the blood: HIV DNA or RNA, viral p24 antigen, or viral isolation by culture. Without a positive test for antibodies or viral products (seropositive), however, individuals can be diagnosed as having AIDS if they have a lymphoma of the brain and are younger than age 60 years or if they have lymphoid interstitial pneumonitis and are younger than age 13 years. If they are seropositive, the diagnosis of AIDS is made in association with a variety of clinical symptoms involving opportunistic infections (e.g., *Pneumocystis carinii* pneumonia) and other atypical malignancies (e.g., Kaposi sarcoma) (Fig. 8-25 and Table 8-14). Other clinical symptoms of AIDS include persistent lymphadenopathy, weight loss, recurrent fevers, and neurologic abnormalities.

HIV virus also infects the central nervous system, resulting in AIDS dementia complex in the late stages of the disease.[36] Dementia is present in most individuals because of atrophy of cells of the cerebrum and degeneration of the nerve endings. Symptoms include lack of motor coordination and behavioral changes, including psychosis in the most extreme cases.

The major immunologic finding in AIDS is the striking decrease in the number of T helper cells (CD4-positive cells). Suppressor and cytotoxic cells, which have the CD8 antigen, are usually normal or slightly elevated in number. This results in a reversal of the normal CD4/CD8 T cell ratio, which is about 1.9. Most individuals with AIDS have ratios much lower than 0.9 and frequently near 0. In contrast, B cell numbers are usually normal.

An intermediate stage of development is referred to as the early stages of HIV disease. Individuals with early-stage disease, which may last for as long as 10 years, have relatively mild symptoms that may resemble influenza, such as night sweats, swollen lymph glands, diarrhea, or fatigue. AIDS, however, is characterized by severe symptoms and an increase in infections and malignancies.

The presence of circulating antibody against the AIDS virus apparently indicates infection by the virus, although many of these individuals are asymptomatic. Antibody appears rather rapidly after infection through blood products, usually within 4 to 7 weeks. After sexual exposure, however, the individual can be infected yet seronegative for many months. In addition, in the late stages of the disease, some individuals become seronegative because of a deficient immune system. The period between HIV infection and the appearance of antibody is referred to as the **window period.** Although the individual may not have antibody, he or she

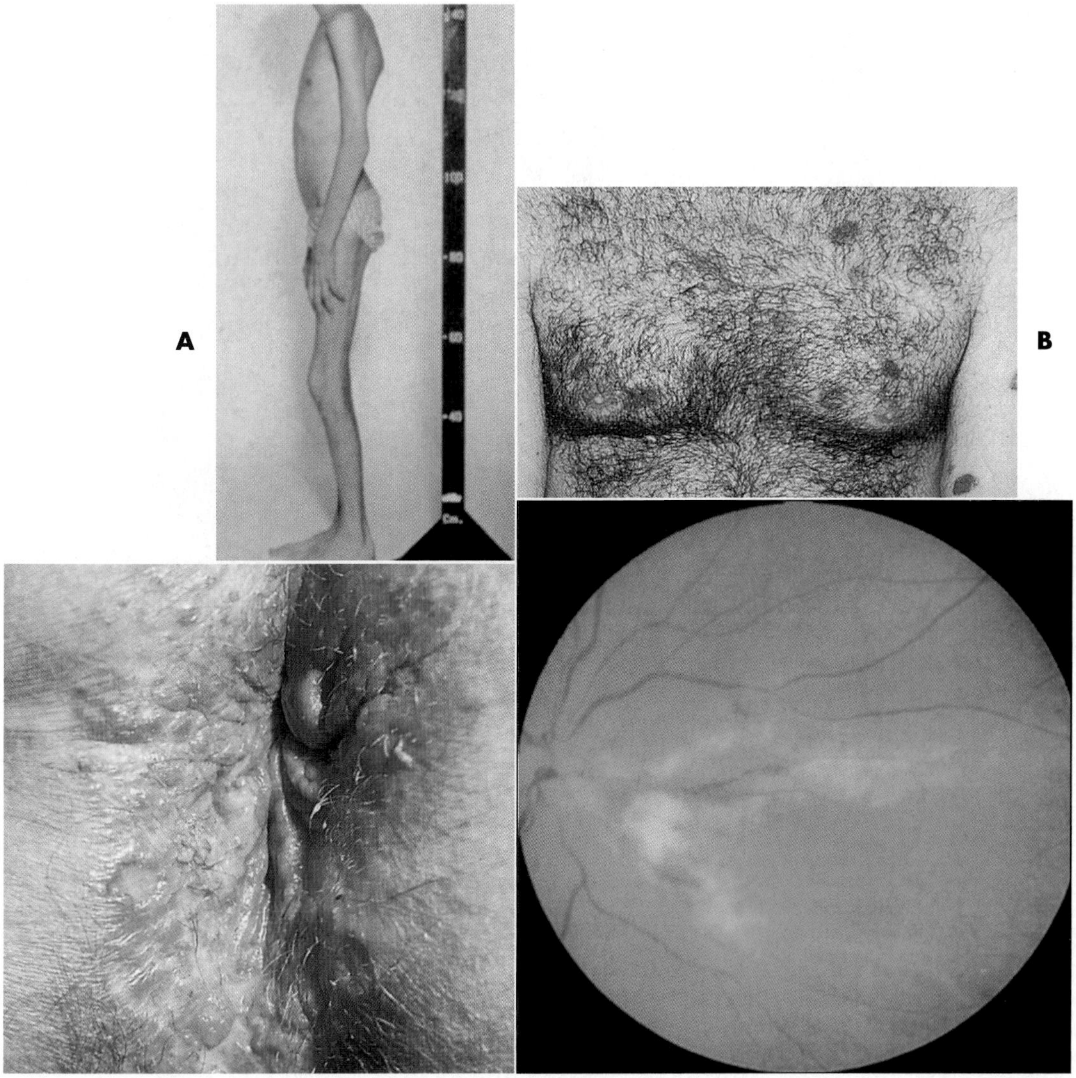

FIG. 8-24 Clinical manifestations of acquired immunodeficiency syndrome (AIDS). A, Severe weight loss from anorexia. **B,** Biopsy-proven Kaposi sarcoma lesions. **C,** Perianal vesicular and ulcerative lesions of herpes simplex infection. **D,** Deterioration of vision from cytomegalovirus retinitis leading to areas of infection; unless treated the progressive impairment will lead to blindness. (**A, D,** From Taylor PK: *Diagnostic picture tests in sexually transmitted disease,* London, 1994, Mosby-Wolfe. **B, C,** From Morse SA, Moreland AA, Holmes KK: *Atlas of sexually transmitted diseases and AIDS,* ed 2, London, 1996, Mosby.)

may have virus growing, be viremic, and be infectious to others within 2 weeks of being infected. Although many individuals are asymptomatic during this initial period, some have clinical indications of an acute retroviral syndrome, including fever, lymphadenopathy, pharyngitis, rash, diarrhea, headaches, and a variety of nonspecfic symptoms.

Estimates are that for every diagnosed case of AIDS, approximately 100 others are HIV infected. It is also estimated that diagnosed cases of AIDS are underestimated by 10% to 15%. The average time from infection to AIDS, without treatment, has been estimated at approximately 10 years. Some estimates are that approximately 99% of HIV-infected individuals would eventually progress to AIDS if they remained untreated.

Treatment and Prevention

Both treatment of ongoing HIV infection and prevention of the initial infection have been difficult to address. HIV has certain characteristics that frustrate attempts to develop effective treatments and vaccines.

Several antibiotics have been tried to prevent viral replication by blocking reverse transcriptase activity (see Fig. 8-21). Reverse transcriptase has a high mutation rate that makes it rapidly become resistant to these antibiotics. The only beneficial use of reverse transcriptase inhibitors alone occurs with treatment of HIV-positive pregnant women in order to affect the risk of infection of their children. Treatment with drugs such as zidovudine decreases perinatal transmission by 66%. Since the introduction of

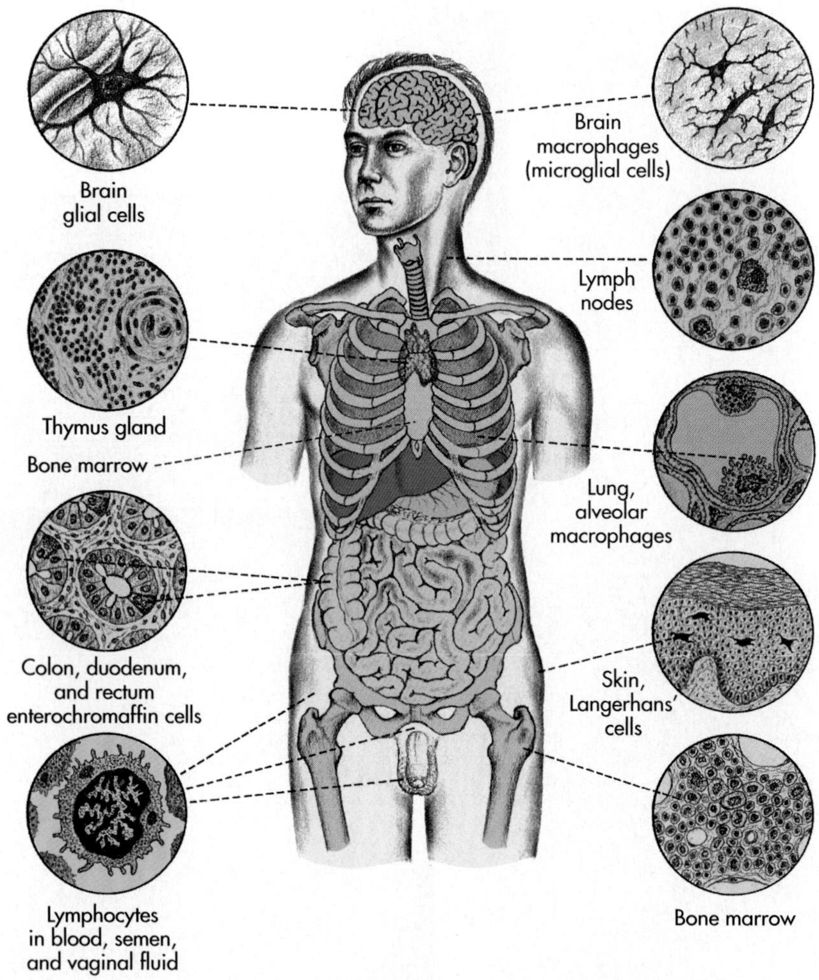

FIG. 8-25 Distribution of tissues that can be infected by human immunodeficiency virus (HIV). Infection is closely linked to the presence of CD4 receptors on host tissue, with the possible exceptions of glial cells in the brain and chromaffin cells in the colon, duodenum, and rectum.

highly active antiretroviral therapy (HAART)—therapy capable of maximally suppressing viral replication—clinical benefits have become profound and durable.[37] HAART consists of a combination of at least three antiretroviral agents. There are currently three classes of antiretrovirals approved by the FDA (Table 8-15).

With the HAART approach, AIDS has become a chronic disease for many patients; CD4 cell counts return to normal, and viral load, measured by HIV RNA in the blood, becomes undetectable. Cessation of treatment, however, frequently results in reexpression of the virus, so that the disease is not cured but only under control.

Recent studies report that a daily regimen of rifampin and pyrazinamide is similar in safety and efficacy to a daily 12-month regimen of isoniazid for prevention of tuberculosis.[38] Isoniazid regimens have problems with adherence, toxicity, and increasing reistance.

A pharmacologic cure for AIDS will be difficult because, like most retroviruses, the AIDS virus incorporates into the genetic material of the host and may never be removed by antibiotic therapy. Therefore drug administration is more often designed to control the virus, rather than eradicate it, and may be necessary for the lifetime of the individual.

The development of an effective AIDS vaccine has been slowed by several major difficulties. First, the AIDS virus is genetically and antigenically variable in a way similar to the influenza virus, so that a vaccine created against one variant may not provide protection against another variant. As many as 30 to 40 different genetic variants have been isolated from the same individual during the progression of the disease. Many of these may coexist in the individual. Second, although AIDS individuals have high levels of circulating antibodies against the virus, these antibodies do not appear to be protective. Therefore, even if an antibody response can be induced by vaccine, that response might not be effective but may even increase infectivity by facilitating viral entrance into cells through opsonization and ingestion of antibody-coated viral particles. It may be more successful to induce Tc cells rather than antibody against HIV antigens. Third, the AIDS virus can be transmitted from cell to cell and initially may enter the body in an infected cell. Microorganisms that spread by cell-to-cell contact are usually not susceptible to circulating antibody. HIV-infected cells also tend

Table 8-14 Laboratory Evaluation of Immune Deficiencies

Function Tested	Laboratory Test	Interpretation of Test
TESTS OF HUMORAL IMMUNE FUNCTION		
Antibody production	Total immunoglobulin levels	Presence of antibody-producing B cells
	Levels of isohemagglutinins	Capacity to produce specific immunoglobulin M (IgM) antibodies
	Levels of antibodies against vaccines—especially diphtheria and tetanus toxoids	Capacity to produce specific immunoglobulin G (IgG) antibodies
	Levels of antibodies against known past infections	Capacity to produce specific IgG or IgM antibodies
B cell numbers	Numbers of lymphocytes with surface immunoglobulin	Presence of circulating B cells
TESTS OF CELLULAR IMMUNE FUNCTION		
Delayed hypersensitivity skin test	Skin test reaction against previously encountered antigens—especially *C. albicans* or tetanus toxoid	Presence of antigen-responsive T cells and cellular interactions (e.g., lymphokine activity and macrophage function)
T cell numbers	Numbers of T cells forming rosettes with sheep erythrocytes or expressing membrane CD3 or CD11 antigen	Presence of circulating T cells
T cell proliferation in vitro	Proliferative response to nonspecific mitogens (e.g., phytohemagglutinin)	Capacity of all T cells to divide in response to nonspecific stimulation (mitogens)
	Proliferative response to antigens (e.g., tetanus toxoid)	Capacity of antigen-reactive T cells to respond to antigen

Table 8-15 Approved Antiretroviral Agents

Type	Generic Name	Action
Nucleoside reverse transcriptase inhibitors	Zidovudine Didanosine Zalcitabine Stavudine Lamivudine Abacavir	After phosphorylation by cellular enzymes, compete with nucleotides for reverse transcriptase binding, incorporate into the growth viral DNA chain, and affect chain termination
Nonnucleoside reverse transcriptase inhibitors	Nevirapine Delavirdine Efavirenz	Interfere with the activity of the reverse transcriptase by disrupting the catalytic site of the enzymes
Protease inhibitors	Saquinavir Ritonavir Indinavir Nelfinavir Amprenavir	Interfere with the cleavage of proteins by the viral protease, causing the production of noninfectious virions
Adjunctive medication	Hydroxyurea	Specific to the S phase of the cell cycle in which it inhibits DNA synthesis

to fuse with other cells, so that infection can spread to uninfected cells without viral particles being produced. It is problematic whether antibodies against HIV prevent intercellular fusion between infected and uninfected cells. Fourth, the only potential experimental animal model for HIV-induced AIDS is the chimpanzee, which is a protected species and relatively unavailable for medical research. This means that the efficacy and toxicity of candidate vaccines may not easily be evaluated.

Clinical Evaluation of Immunity

Individuals with immune deficiencies first go to the health provider with one common symptom: recurrent infections. To delineate the pathophysiology of a particular deficiency, certain observations and tests of the immune system are made. Significant information on the specific immune deficiency can be obtained by noting certain characteristics of the individual, including the presence of any associated anomalies, age, gender, and the types of infections (bacterial, viral, or fungal, and the specific organisms involved). Laboratory evaluation of immune deficiencies is presented in Table 8-14.

Replacement Therapies for Immune Deficiencies

Gamma (γ)–Globulin Therapy

Individuals with B cell deficiencies that cause hypogammaglobulinemia or agammaglobulinemia usually can be treated successfully with administration of γ-globulin. Commercial γ-globulin preparations are usually administered intramuscularly (IM) monthly at dosages determined by body weight (0.2 to 0.6 ml/kg) or by intravenous administration (IVIg). Schedule and dosage are also determined according to titers of circulating immunoglobulins and the incidence of infections in the individual. In a 70-kg adult, a monthly dose can be as high as 42 ml, in which case it may be divided into smaller doses injected IM weekly at different sites to minimize discomfort. Complications of treatment include anaphylactic reactions caused by aggregated immunoglobulins in the preparations (aggregated immunoglobulins, although not immune complexes, can activate inflammation as immune complexes do). Individuals with selective IgA deficiency occasionally develop allergic reactions to IgA in γ-globulin preparations, although commercial γ-globulins usually contain less than 10% of the normal levels of IgM and IgA.

Individuals who need larger amounts of IgM or IgA are given fresh frozen plasma in monthly IV infusions. Dosage is about 10 to 15 ml/kg. Complications associated with plasma therapy include the potential transmission of hepatitis or AIDS. The plasma is irradiated to destroy immunocompetent T cells and avoid GVH disease in individuals with accompanying T cell deficiencies. Administration of fresh frozen plasma is successful in individuals with Wiskott-Aldrich syndrome (IgM deficient), ataxia-telangiectasia (IgA deficient), or complement component deficiencies.

Transplantation and Transfusion

In SCID caused by a lack of stem cells, bone marrow is transplanted from an HLA-matched donor. Other diseases involving depletion of the bone marrow (i.e., aplastic anemia, leukemia requiring eradication of tumor cells in the marrow) also are treated by bone marrow transplantation.[39] At least 75% of bone marrow transplants between individuals who are matched for HLA-A, HLA-B, HLA-C, and HLA-DR are accepted. Most rejections of HLA-matched transplants are because of recognition of minor histocompatibility antigens by individuals who have received multiple transfusions and are, as a result, sensitized against those antigens, which are not evaluated in tissue typing.

GVH disease may develop if the recipient's cells express histocompatibility antigens not found on the donor's cells. GVH disease occurs when immunocompetent T lymphocytes in the grafted material recognize foreign antigens in the recipient, initiating a type IV hypersensitivity reaction against the recipient's tissues. The main target tissues of the reaction are the skin, gastrointestinal mucosa, and liver. Symptoms of a GVH reaction usually appear within 10 to 30 days after the transplant; develop as a skin rash, hepatomegaly, and diarrhea; and may lead to death from infections. GVH disease is not a problem when the recipient is immunocompetent, that is, has an immune system that can control the donor's lymphocytes.

Several attempts have been made to prevent GVH disease by removing mature immunocompetent T lymphocytes from grafts. One procedure is to infuse the graft with monoclonal antibody against plasma membrane antigens found only on mature T cells. Another is to use fetal tissue as the graft. For example, fetal liver, which contains stem cells but not immunocompetent lymphocytes, is sometimes grafted in place of bone marrow if an HLA-matched donor cannot be found.

Reconstitution of thymic function is one therapy for deficiency diseases in which the individual lacks a thymus or thymic function (e.g., DiGeorge syndrome, ataxia-telangiectasia, or chronic mucocutaneous candidiasis). The procedure is to transplant fetal thymus tissue, which lacks immunocompetent T cells, or thymic epithelial cells (the cells that produce the thymic hormones) from which mature T cells have been removed. In some individuals transplantation increases the number of circulating mature T cells, but in most cases improvement is only temporary.

Enzymatic defects that cause SCID (e.g., adenosine deaminase deficiency) have been treated successfully with transfusions of glycerol frozen-packed erythrocytes. The donor erythrocytes contain the needed enzyme and can, at least temporarily, provide sufficient enzyme for normal lymphocyte function.

The administration of soluble materials that affect lymphocyte function can restore T cell function, especially in individuals with Wiskott-Aldrich syndrome or chronic mucocutaneous candidiasis. Transfer factor, a low-molecular-weight nucleoprotein prepared from lymphocyte lysates, can confer specific reactivity against certain antigens and has been used successfully in some individuals. Thymosin, a thymic hormone, also has been used, although with limited success.

Gene Therapy

The first successful therapeutic replacement of defective genes was performed in two girls with SCID caused by an ADA deficiency.[40,41] The normal gene for ADA had been cloned and inserted into a retroviral vector. The gene for ADA had replaced some retroviral genes, resulting in a virus that carried the normal human gene but did not cause disease. The virus was used to infect bone marrow stem cells from these children. The retrovirus inserted the normal ADA gene into the individuals' genetic material. The genetically altered stem cells were infused into the children, resulting in reconstitution of their immune systems.

SUMMARY REVIEW

Hypersensitivity: Allergy, Autoimmunity, and Alloimmunity

1. Hypersensitivity is an inappropriate immune response misdirected against the host's own tissues (autoimmunity); directed against beneficial foreign tissues, such as transfusions or transplants (alloimmunity); or exaggerated responses against environmental antigens (allergy).
2. Mechanisms of hypersensitivity are classified as type I (IgE-mediated) reactions, type II (tissue-specific) reactions, type

III (immune complex–mediated) reactions, and type IV (cell-mediated) reactions.
3. Hypersensitivity reactions can be immediate (developing within an hour) or delayed (developing within hours or days).
4. Anaphylaxis, the most rapid immediate hypersensitivity reaction, is an explosive reaction that occurs within minutes of reexposure to the antigen and can lead to cardiovascular shock.
5. Allergens are antigens that cause allergic responses.
6. Type I (IgE-mediated) reactions are mediated through the binding of IgE to Fc receptors on mast cells and cross-linking of IgE by antigens that bind to the Fab portions of IgE. Cross-linking causes mast cell degranulation and the release of histamine and other inflammatory substances.
7. Type II (tissue-specific) reactions are caused by four possible mechanisms: complement-mediated lysis, opsonization and phagocytosis, antibody-dependent cell-mediated cytotoxicity, and modulation of cellular function.
8. Type III (immune complex–mediated) reactions are caused by the formation of immune complexes that are deposited in target tissues, where they activate the complement cascade, generating chemotactic fragments that attract neutrophils into the inflammatory site.
9. Immune complex disease can be a systemic reaction, such as serum sickness, or localized, such as the Arthus reaction.
10. Type IV (cell-mediated) reactions are caused by specifically sensitized T cells that either kill target cells directly or release lymphokines that activate other cells, such as macrophages.
11. Allergies can be mediated by any of the four mechanisms of hypersensitivity.
12. Clinical manifestations of allergic reactions usually are confined to the areas of initial intake or contact with the allergen. Ingested allergens induce gastrointestinal symptoms, airborne allergens induce respiratory or skin manifestations, and contact allergens induce allergic responses at the site of contact.
13. Atopic individuals are genetically predisposed to the development of allergies.
14. Autoimmunity is a breakdown of immunologic homeostasis, the immune system's tolerance of self-antigens.
15. Autoimmune disease can be caused by the exposure of a previously sequestered antigen, the development of a neoantigen, the complications of infectious disease, the emergence of a forbidden clone of lymphocytes, or an alteration of suppressor T cell function.
16. Alloimmunity is the immune system's reaction against antigens on the tissues of other members of the same species.
17. Alloimmune disorders include transient neonatal disease, in which the maternal immune system becomes sensitized against antigens expressed by the fetus, and transplant rejection and transfusion reactions, in which the immune system of the recipient of an organ transplant or blood transfusion reacts against foreign antigens on the donor's cells.

Infections

1. Infection by a pathogen is influenced by several factors: mechanisms of action, infectivity, pathogeneity, virulence, immunologicity, and toxigenicity.
2. Classes of infectious organisms include viruses, bacteria, chylamydia, rickettsiae, mycoplasma, fungi, protozoa, and helminths.
3. Bacteria injure cells by producing destructive enzymes (exotoxins) or endotoxins. Exotoxins can damage the plasma membranes of host cells or prevent phagocytosis, and endotoxins activate the inflammatory response and produce fever.
4. Bacteremia, or septicemia, is the proliferation of bacteria in the blood. Endotoxins released by blood-borne bacteria cause the release of vasoactive mediators that increase the permeability of blood vessels. Leakage from vessels causes hypotension that can result in septic shock.
5. Viruses enter host cells and use the metabolic processes of host cells to proliferate.
6. Viruses that have invaded host cells decrease protein synthesis, disrupt lysosomal membranes, form inclusion bodies where synthesis of viral nucleic acids is occurring, cause intercellular fusion between host cells to produce giant cells, alter antigenic properties of the host cell, and transform host cells into cancerous cells.
7. Diseases caused by fungi are called mycoses. Most pathogenic fungi grow as parasites on or near skin or mucous membranes and usually produce mild and superficial disease.
8. Fungi that invade the skin, hair, or nails are known as dermatophytes.
9. Most clinical manifestations from infectious disease result from the host's inflammatory and immune responses. The hallmark of most infectious diseases is, however, fever.
10. Many vaccines have been developed to protect against pathogens. Vaccines induce primary and secondary immune responses under conditions that will not cause disease. Most bacterial vaccines are killed organisms or extracts of bacterial antigens. Most viral vaccines contain live viruses that are weakened or attenuated so that they express appropriate antigens but cause only a limited and easily controlled infection.
11. Antibiotic resistance can develop through genetic mutations that inactivate the drug, alter bacterial membranes so that the antibiotic is no longer taken up, or alter the target molecule. Overuse of antibiotics can lead to the destruction of normal flora, allowing the selective overgrowth of antibiotic-resistant strains or pathogens.
12. The development and widespread use of vaccines against common antibiotic-resistant organisms must now be considered.

Deficiencies in Immunity and Inflammation

1. Immune deficiency is the failure of mechanisms of self-defense to function in their normal capacity.
2. Immune deficiencies are either congenital (primary) or acquired (secondary). Congenital immune deficiencies are caused by genetic defects that disrupt lymphocyte development, whereas acquired immune deficiencies are secondary to disease or other physiologic alterations.
3. The clinical hallmark of immune deficiency is a propensity to unusual or recurrent severe infections. The type of infection usually reflects the immune system defect.
4. The most common infections in individuals with defects of cell-mediated immune response are fungal and viral, whereas infections in individuals with defects of the humoral immune response or complement function are primarily bacterial.
5. Severe combined immune deficiency (SCID) is a total lack of T cell function and a severe (either partial or total) lack of B cell function.
6. DiGeorge syndrome (congenital thymic aplasia or hypoplasia) is characterized by complete or partial lack of the thymus (resulting in depressed T cell immunity) and the parathyroid

glands (resulting in hypocalcemia) and the presence of cardiac anomalies.
7. Defects in B cell function are diverse, ranging from a complete lack of the human bursal equivalent function, the lymphoid organs required for B cell maturation (as in Bruton agammaglobulinemia), to deficiencies in a single class of immunoglobulins (e.g., selective IgA deficiency).
8. Defects in phagocyte function, which include insufficient numbers of phagocytes or defects of chemotaxis, phagocytosis, or killing, can result in recurrent, life-threatening infections, such as septicemia and disseminated pyogenic lesions.
9. Acquired immune deficiencies are caused by superimposed conditions, such as malnutrition, medical therapies, physical or psychologic trauma, or infections.
10. AIDS is an acquired dysfunction of the immune system caused by a retrovirus (HIV) that infects and destroys CD4-positive lymphocytes (helper T cells).
11. Immune deficiency syndromes usually are treated by replacement therapy. Deficient antibody production is treated by replacement of missing immunoglobulins with commercial γ-globulin preparations. Lymphocyte deficiencies are treated with the replacement of host lymphocytes with transplants of bone marrow, fetal liver, or fetal thymus from a donor.

KEY TERMS

REFERENCES

1. Gell PGH, Coombs RRA, Lachman PT: *Clinical aspects of immunology,* Oxford, England, 1975, Blackwell Scientific.
2. Portier P, Richet C: De l'action anaphylactique de certains venins, *Comptes Rendus Societie Biologie (Paris)* 54:170, 1902.
3. Marsh DG et al: Genetic basis of IgE responsiveness: relevance to the atopic diseases, *Int Arch Allergy Immunol* 107:25, 1995.
4. Akdis CA, Blaser K: Immunologic mechanisms of specific immunotherapy, *Allergy* 54:31, 1999.
5. Haselden BM et al: Peptide-mediated immune responses in specific immunotherapy, *Int Arch AllergyImmunol* 122(4):229, 2000.
6. Abramson SB, Belmont HM: SLE: mechanisms of vascular injury, *Hosp Pract* 33:107, 1998.
7. Pirquet C, Schick B: *Serum sickness,* Leipzig, Germany, 1905, Franz Denticke.
8. Arthus M, Breton M: Lésions cutanées produites par les injections de sérum, *Comptes Rendus Societe de Biologie* 55:817, 1903.
9. Koch R: Fortsetzung der mitteilungen, ber ein heilmittel gegen tuberkulose, *Deutsche Med Wochenschr* 9:101, 1891.
10. Belsito DV: The diagnostic evaluation, treatment, and prevention of allergic contact dermatitis in the new millennium, *J Allergy Clin Immunol* 105:409, 2000.
11. Theofilopoulos AN, Kono DH: Mechanisms and genetics of autoimmunity, *Ann N Y Acad Sci* 841:225, 1998.
12. Kuper BC, Failla S: Systemic lupus erythematosus: a multisystem autoimmune disorder, *Nurs Clin North Am* 35:253, 2000.
13. Jan EM et al: A critical evaluation of enzyme immunoassays for detection of antinuclear autoantibodies of defined specificities. I. Precision, sensitivity, and specificity, *Arthritis Rheum* 42(3):455, 1999.
14. Calandra T et al: Protection from septic shock by neutralization of macrophage migration inhibitory factor, *Nat Med* 6(2):164, 2000.
15. Baumgartner JD, Calandra T: Treatment of sepsis: past and future avenues, *Drugs* 57(2):127, 2000.
16. Kluger MJ et al: Role of fever in disease, *Ann N Y Acad Sci* 856:224, 1998.
17. Raloff J: Waterways carry antibiotic resistance, *Sci News* 155:356, 1999.
18. Raloff J: Antibiotics may become harder to resist, *Sci News* 157:5, 2000.

19. Conley ME, Notarangelo LD, Etzioni A: Diagnostic criteria for primary immunodeficiencies, *Clin Immunol* 93:190, 1999.
20. Jones AM, Gaspar HB: Immunogenetics: changing the face of immunodeficiency, *J Clin Pathol* 53:60, 2000.
21. Demczuk S, Aurias A: DiGeorge syndrome and related syndromes associated with 22q11.2 deletions, *Annales Genetique* 38:59, 1995.
22. DiGeorge AM: Congenital absence of the thymus and its immunologic consequences. In Bergsma D, McKusick FA, editors: *Immunologic deficiency diseases in man,* National Foundation—March of Dimes Original Article Series, Baltimore, 1968, Williams & Wilkins.
23. Bruton OC: Agammaglobulinemia, *Pediatrics* 9:722, 1952.
24. Thrasher AJ, Kinnon C: The Wiskott-Aldrich syndrome, *Clin Exp Immunol* 120:2, 2000.
25. Masek K et al: Past, present and future of psychoneuroimmunology, *Toxicology* 142:179, 2000.
26. Centers for Disease Control and Prevention: *CDC Web site: www/cdc.gov.*
27. Centers for Disease Control (CDC): HIV/AIDS among racial/ethnic minority men who have sex with men—United States 1998-1998, *MMWR* 49:40, 2000.
28. Satcher D: The global HIV/AIDS epidemic, *JAMA* 281(16):1479, 1999.
29. Castetbon K et al: Letter to editors: risk of HIV transmission through breast feeding, *JAMA* 283(8):999, 2000.
30. Update: Universal precautions for prevention of transmission of human immunodeficiency virus, hepatitis B virus, and other bloodborne pathogens in health-care settings, *MMWR* 37:377, 1988.
31. Cohen J: Searching for the epidemic's origins, *Science* 288(5474): 2164, 2000.
32. Dewhurst SL, da Cruz RL, Whetter L: Pathogenesis and treatment of HIV-1 infection: recent developments, *Front Biosci* 5:D30, 2000.
33. Funke I et al: The cellular receptor (CD4) of the human immunodeficiency virus is expressed on neurons and glial cells in human brain, *J Exp Med* 165:1230, 1987.
34. Raloff J: HIV sexual spread exploits immune sentinals, *Sci News* 157:166, 2000.
35. Update: Acquired immunodeficiency syndrome (AIDS)—worldwide, *MMWR* 37:286, 1988.
36. Pate CA, Mukhtar M, Pomerantz RJ: Human immunodeficiency virus type IVpr induces apoptosis in human neuronal cells, *J Virol* 74(20): 9717, 2000.
37. Gallant JE: Strategies for long-term success in the treatment of HIV infection, *JAMA* 283(10):1329, 2000.
38. Gordin F et al: Rifampin and pyrazinamide vs isoniazid for prevention of tuberculosis in HIV-infected persons: an international randomized trial, *JAMA* 283(11):1445, 2000.
39. Thomas ED: Bone marrow transplantation: a review, *Semin Hematol* 36:95, 1999.
40. Blaese RM: Development of gene therapy for immunodeficiency: adenosine deaminase deficiency, *Pediatr Res* 33:S49, 1993.
41. Onodera M et al: Gene therapy for severe combined immunodeficiency caused by adenosine deaminase deficiency, *Acta Haematol* 101:89, 1999.

CHAPTER 9

Stress and Disease

JANE SHELBY • KATHRYN L. McCANCE

CHAPTER OUTLINE

Modern society is full of stress. As a culture, Americans are champions of the Protestant work ethic, a sixteenth-century philosophy that viewed "idleness as taboo." In *Poor Richard's Almanac,* Ben Franklin counseled new Americans *not to waste time.* Thus driven by this perspective, Americans have devoted time and energy to the invention of time-saving devices. Despite our prosperity, these time-saving inventions have helped create the opposite—the "workaholic" American. Having the capacity to do something often translates into the necessity to do it. For example, computers allow us to endlessly revise documents. Answering machines enable us to return phone calls we would otherwise miss. We have become accustomed to an accelerated way of life, overstimulation, impatience, and suffering from the so-called stress-related disorders.

It is often reported that use of the term **stress** in a biologic sense began with Hans Selye in 1946. In 1914, however, Walter B. Cannon used the term in both a physiologic and a psychologic sense in a paper reporting his psychoendocrine studies.[1] In his report Cannon used such phrases as "great emotional stress" and "times of stress."[1] In 1935 Cannon published another paper, called "Stresses and Strains of Homeostasis." In it he applied the engineering concept of stress and strain in a physiologic context.[2] Cannon thought also that stress involved psychologic factors; his paper stated that physical as well as emotional stimuli can cause stress. The *popularization* of the term, however, began with Hans Selye's work.

The past decade for the first time in history has demonstrated the interactions among social, psychologic, biologic, and behavioral factors in the causes and courses of many diseases. Molecular biologists, immunologists, neurologists, clinicians, and behavioral scientists have begun to explore the role of the neglected half of the mind-body (dualistic) model—the mind. What is emerging is a more holistic and complex model involving biochemical relationships of the central and autonomic nervous systems, the endocrine system, and the immune system and relationships to stress-elicited coping behaviors, such as smoking and poor diet, that can also modify the integrity of the immune system. In addition, stress has been associated with the deterioration of immune-related health outcomes, such as decreased resistance to infection and the onset of worsening of autoimmune diseases. Stress appears to have important implications for the progression of cancer, human immunodeficiency virus (HIV), cardiovascular disease, and other illnesses. Discoveries of these complex links have, in fact, created the field of psychoneuroimmunology.

CONCEPTS OF STRESS

The term *stress* has been used persistently and widely in specialties such as biology, health sciences, and social sciences despite numerous disagreements over its definition. Nevertheless, in recent years stress has been more usefully defined as a *transactional* or *interactional concept.*[3] Transactionally, stress is viewed as the state of affairs arising when a person relates to (i.e., interacts or transacts with) situations in certain ways. People are not disturbed by situations per se but by the ways they appraise and react to situations.[3] In stress a demand *exceeds* a person's coping abilities, resulting in reactions such as disturbances of cognition, emotion, and behavior that can adversely affect a person's well-being.

General Adaptation Syndrome

Selye[4] originally sought to discover a new sex hormone when he discovered the biologic syndrome of stress. In his attempts to discover the new hormone, Selye injected crude ovarian extracts into rats. Repeatedly, he found that the following triad of structural changes occurred: (1) enlargement of the cortex of the adrenal gland, (2) atrophy of the thymus gland and other lymphoid structures, and (3) development of bleeding ulcers of the stomach and duodenal lining. Selye soon discovered that this triad of manifestations was not specific for his ovarian extracts but also occurred after he exposed the rats to other noxious stimuli, such as cold, surgical injury, and restraint. He called these stimuli **stressors.** Selye concluded that this triad or syndrome of manifestations represented a nonspecific response to noxious stimuli. Because many diverse agents caused the same syndrome, Selye suggested that it be called the **general adaptation syndrome (GAS).** In 1959 Selye wrote the following:

> Specific homeostatic mechanisms for the maintenance of body temperature, blood sugar, etc., have been under study since Claude Bernard. The principal contribution of stress research was precisely to show that if we abstract from three specific reactions, there remains a common residual response that is nonspecific in regard to its cause and can be elicited with such diverse agents as cold, heat, x-rays, adrenalin, insulin, tubercle bacilli, or muscular exercise. This is so despite the coexistence of highly specific adaptive reactions to any one of these agents.[5]

Selye later defined three successive stages in development of the GAS: (1) the **alarm stage,** in which the central nervous system (CNS) is aroused and the body's defenses are mobilized (i.e., flight or fight); (2) the **stage of resistance or adaptation,** during which mobilization contributes to flight or fight; and (3) the **stage of exhaustion,** in which continuous stress causes the progressive breakdown of compensatory mechanisms (acquired adaptations) and **homeostasis.** The stage of exhaustion, Selye believed, marked the onset of certain diseases he called **diseases of adaptation.**

The nonspecific physiologic response identified by Selye consists of interaction among the sympathetic branch of the autonomic nervous system (ANS) (see Chapter 13) and two glands—the pituitary gland and the adrenal gland (see Chapter 19). The alarm phase of the GAS begins when a stressor triggers the actions of the pituitary gland and the sympathetic nervous system (SNS) (Fig. 9-1). The resistance or adaptation phase begins with the actions of the adrenal hormones cortisol, norepinephrine, and epinephrine. Exhaustion occurs if stress continues and adaptation is not successful, ultimately causing impairment of the immune response, heart failure, and kidney failure, leading to death.

Selye defined **physiologic stress** as a chemical or physical disturbance in the cells or tissue fluid produced by a change, either in the external environment or within the body itself, that requires a response (i.e., begins the GAS) to counteract the disturbance. Selye identified three components of physiologic stress: (1) the exogenous or endogenous stressor initiating the disturbance, (2) the chemical or physical disturbance produced by the stressor, and (3) the body's counteracting (adaptational) response to the disturbance.[4]

Psychologic Mediators and Specificity

Although Selye's identification of the GAS is regarded as tremendously important and the cornerstone of stress research, the idea that stress is a purely physiologic response is oversimplified. In the mid-1950s, studies showed that activation of the adrenal cortex occurred in humans in response to psychologic stressors;[6] in monkeys with conditioned emotional responses;[7] and in humans subjected to a stressful interview technique.[8] In the early 1960s, researchers found that plasma cortisol levels in groups of subjects increased while they watched war movies and decreased while they viewed Disney nature films.[9,10] Later, Mason[11] demonstrated in a series of experiments that occurrence of the GAS depended on psychologic factors surrounding the stressors. Mason demonstrated that several factors, including degrees of discomfort, unpleasantness, or suddenness of the stress, could account for the presence or absence of the physiologic stress response.

Another challenge to Selye's concept of the GAS focused on his idea that stressors cause a general or nonspecific response.[12] The triad of adrenocortical enlargement, thymus and lymphoid shrinkage, and gastrointestinal ulceration may not be as nonspecific as Selye believed it to be.[13]

Research in the past 25 years has shown the remarkable sensitivity of the pituitary gland and adrenal cortex to emotional, psychologic, and social influences (see What's New? Cancer and Psychologic Stress). Thus it is difficult to know whether it is the way an individual thinks and feels about a physical stressor or the stressor itself that produces the neuroendocrine responses. In experiments in which psychologic reactions were minimized, physical stressors did not appear to stimulate the pituitary or adrenal cortex in a nonspecific way. For example, fasting monkeys who were given nonnutritive placebo food to minimize the discomfort of an empty gastrointestinal tract did not secrete adrenocortical hormones.[11] In another experiment, in which precautions were taken to avoid discomfort, exposure of human subjects to heat actually suppressed adrenocortical hormone levels.[14]

Homeostasis as a Dynamic Steady State

Stressors cause a series of reactions that alter the **dynamic steady state** or the net effect of all the turnover reactions. **Turnover** is the process of synthesis and breakdown of all body substances. These may be short-term or long-term alterations. For example, the normal concentration of glucose in the blood is 80 ± 10 mg/dl. The concentration of glucose increases with acute stress, such as a burn injury, and then slowly returns to normal. If blood glucose remains high in the absence of a known stressor, it is diagnosed as a sign of disease—probably diabetes mellitus. Prolonged, unrelenting stress can cause a chronic elevation of glucose levels that leads to diabetes mellitus.[15]

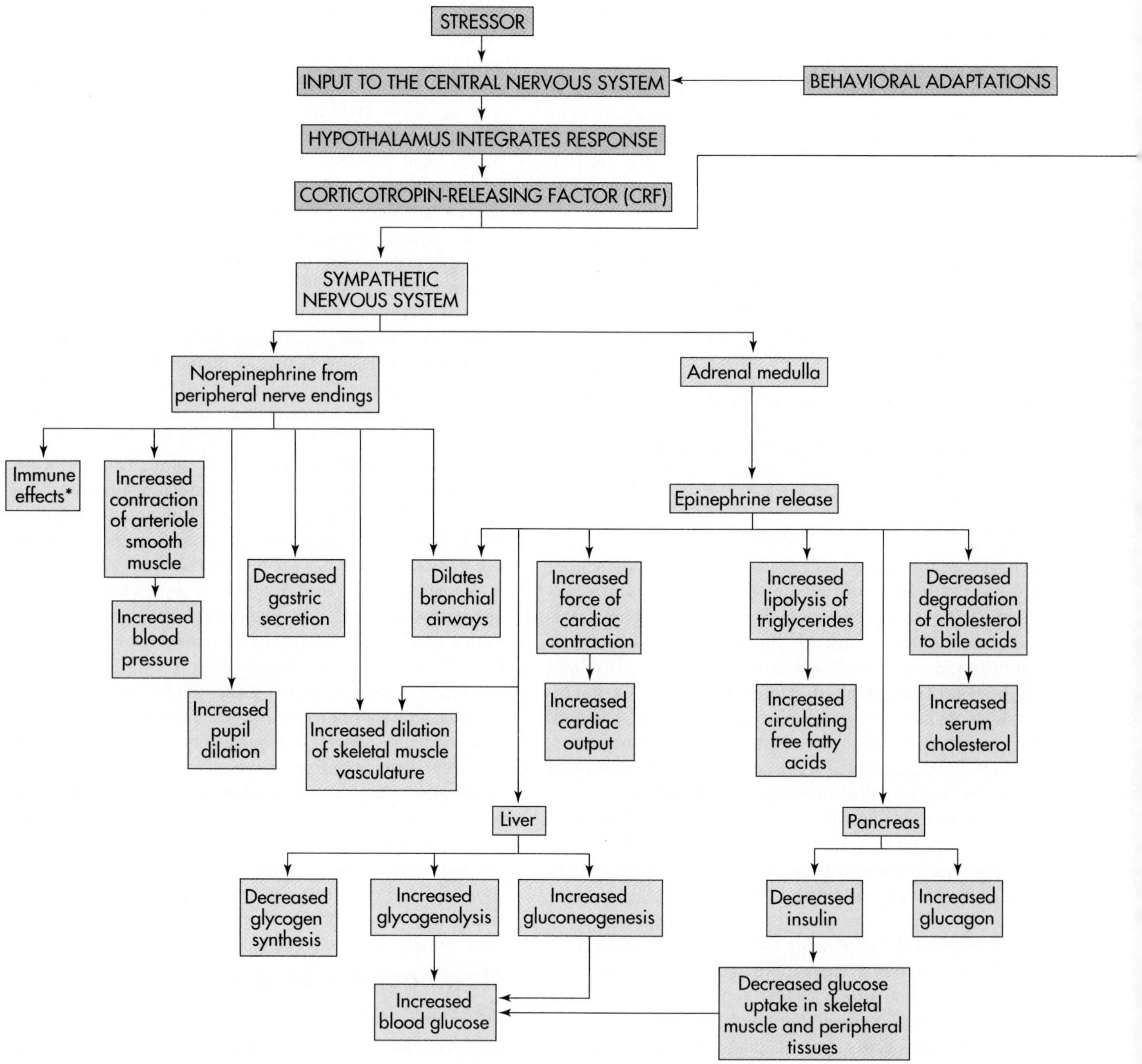

FIG. 9-1 The stress response. *ACTH,* Adrenocorticotropic hormone; *ADH,* antidiuretic hormone; *PMNs,* polymorphonuclear leukocytes; *RNA,* ribonucleic acid. See text for explanation of hormone functions.

*See p. 281 for immune effects.

†Unclear whether endorphins originate from pituitary gland or central nervous system.

‡Explained in text.

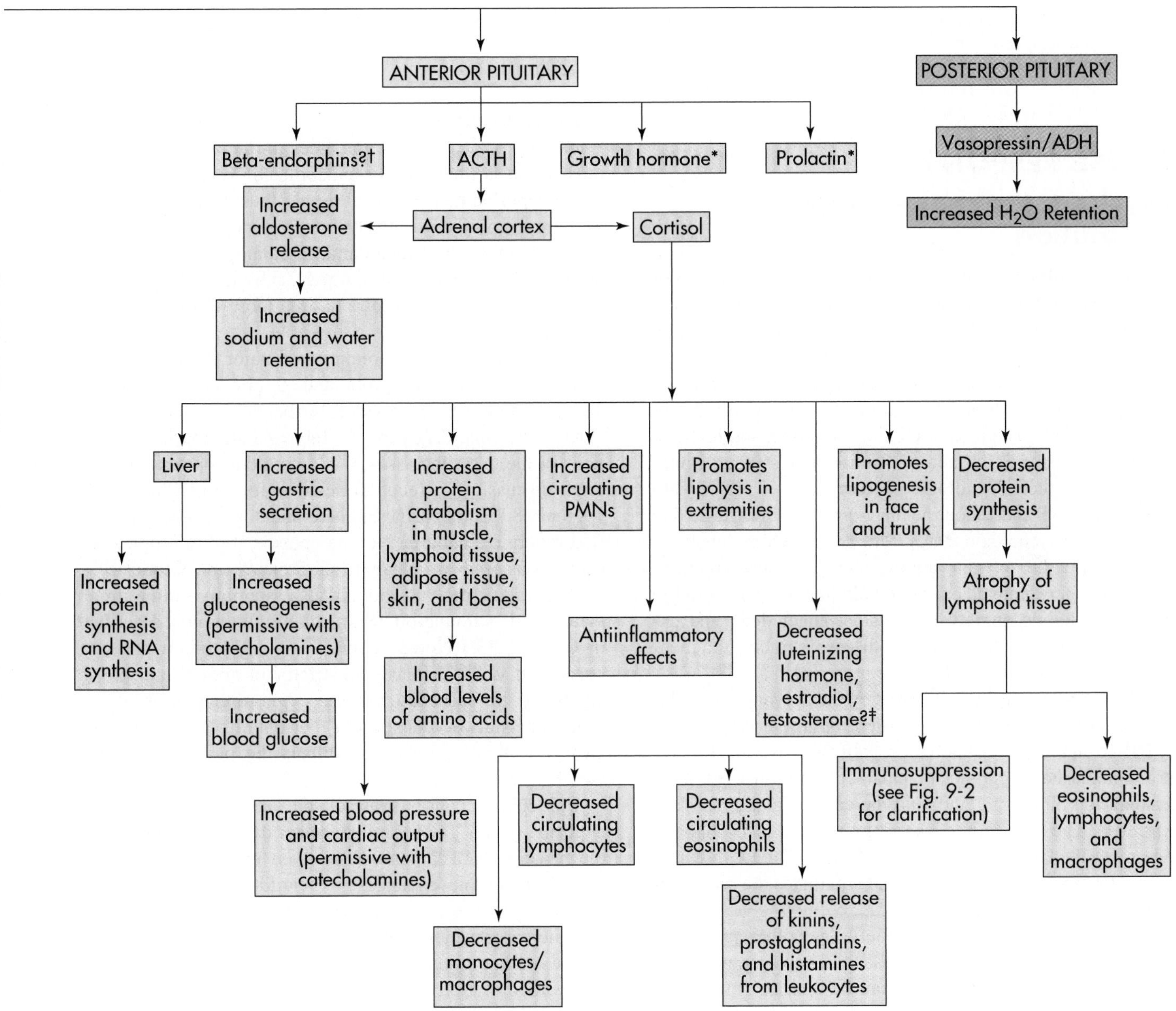

FIG. 9-1, cont'd For legend see opposite page.

WHAT'S NEW? Cancer and Psychologic Stress

There is substantial evidence from both healthy populations and individuals with cancer linking psychologic stress with immune down-regulation. Psychologic stressors are implicated in decreasing natural killer (NK) cells, and distress or depression is correlated with two important processes for carcinogenesis: (1) poorer repair of damaged DNA and (2) alterations in apoptosis. Conversely, the possibility that psychologic interventions may increase immune function and survival among individuals with cancer merits further research, as does the evidence that social support may be a key psychologic mediator.

Data from Kiecolt-Glaser JK, Glaser R: Psychoneuroimmunology and cancer: fact or fiction? *Eur J Cancer* 35(11):1603, 1999.

STRESS RESPONSE

Psychoneuroimmunologic Regulation

Psychoneuroimmunology is the study of the interaction of consciousness *(psycho),* brain and central nervous system *(neuro),* and the body's defense against external infection and abnormal cell division *(immunology).* Psychoneuroimmunology assumes that all immune-related disease is multifactorial, or the result of interrelationships among psychosocial, emotional, genetic, neurologic, endocrine, and immune systems and behavioral factors. The immune system is integrated with other physiologic processes and is sensitive to changes in CNS and endocrine functioning, such as those that accompany psychologic states. Stressors, such as infection, noise, decreased oxygen supply, pain, malnutrition, heat, cold, trauma, prolonged exertion, radiation, responses to life events (including anxiety, depression, anger, fear, and excitement), obesity, old age, drugs, disease, surgery, and medical treatment, can elicit the stress response.

The **stress response** is initiated by the nervous and endocrine systems, specifically corticotropin-releasing factor (CRF) from the hypothalamus, probably the locus coeruleus–norepinephrine/autonomic (sympathetic) nervous (LC-NE) system, the pituitary gland, and the adrenal gland[2,16-18] (see Fig. 9-1). The activation of these systems redirects adaptive energy to the CNS and stressed body sites. The LC-NE system is located in the brain stem and stimulates the release of norepinephrine throughout the brain, promoting arousal, increased vigilance, increased anxiety, and other protective emotional responses. Extensive research, however, must still be done before these pathways can be conclusively implicated as the major stress response pathways.[1] Reproduction, growth, and thyroid hormone are suppressed during stress and may conserve energy during stress. The adrenocortical hormones and the SNS have been postulated as mediators of enhancement or suppression of immune functioning.[19]

Neuroendocrine Regulation

The SNS is aroused during the stress response and causes the medulla of the adrenal gland to release catecholamines (epinephrine, norepinephrine, and dopamine) into the bloodstream. The adrenal medulla is actually an extension of the SNS because preganglionic fibers from the splanchnic nerve terminate in the medulla, where they innervate the chromaffin cells that produce the catecholamine hormones. Simultaneously, hypothalamic CRF stimulates the pituitary gland to release a variety of hormones, including antidiuretic hormone, from the posterior pituitary gland, and prolactin, growth hormone, and adrenocorticotropic hormone (ACTH) from the anterior pituitary gland. ACTH stimulates the cortex of the adrenal gland to release cortisol. (Relationships between the neuroendocrine and immune systems are discussed on p. 281.)

Catecholamines

Epinephrine, a catecholamine, goes to the liver and skeletal muscle but is then rapidly metabolized. Very little adrenal norepinephrine reaches distal tissue; thus the effects caused by norepinephrine during the stress response are primarily from the SNS.[20,21] Catecholamines cannot cross the blood-brain barrier; they are synthesized locally in the brain.[22] Catecholamines circulate in plasma in a loose association with albumin.[22]

The catecholamines stimulate two major classes of receptors: α-adrenergic receptors and β-adrenergic receptors. These two classes are divided further into two subclasses: (1) α_1 and α_2 and (2) β_1 and β_2. Table 9-1 summarizes the actions of the two subclasses of adrenergic receptors. (A thorough discussion of receptors can be found in Chapters 1, 19, and 28.) Epinephrine binds to and activates both α- and β-adrenergic receptors. Norepinephrine at physiologic concentrations binds primarily to α-adrenergic receptors.[22]

The circulating catecholamines essentially mimic direct sympathetic stimulation. (Sympathetic function is described in Chapter 13.) Norepinephrine regulates blood pressure because it is the primary constrictor of smooth muscle in all blood vessels. During stress, norepinephrine raises blood pressure by constricting peripheral vessels, inhibits gastrointestinal activity, and dilates the pupils of the eye (see Fig. 9-1).

Epinephrine causes some of the same effects as norepinephrine, has a greater influence on cardiac action, and is the principal catecholamine involved in metabolic regulation. Epinephrine enhances myocardial contractility (inotropic effect), increases the heart rate (chronotropic effect), and increases venous return to the heart, all of which increase cardiac output and blood pressure. Epinephrine dilates blood vessels of skeletal muscle. Metabolically, epinephrine causes transient hyperglycemia (high blood sugar) by activating enzymes whose actions promote glucose formation (gluconeogenesis and glycogenolysis in the liver) while inhibiting glucose breakdown. Epinephrine decreases glucose uptake in the muscle and other organs and decreases insulin release from the pancreas. The decrease in insulin release prevents glucose from being taken up by peripheral tissue and thus preserves it for the CNS. Epinephrine also mobilizes free fatty acids and cholesterol by stimulating

Table 9-1 Physiologic Actions of α-and β-Adrenergic Receptors

Receptor	Physiologic Actions
$\alpha 1$	Increased glycogenolysis; smooth muscle contraction (blood vessels, genitourinary tract)
$\alpha 2$	Smooth muscle relaxation (gastrointestinal tract); smooth muscle contraction (some vascular beds); inhibition of lipolysis, renin release, platelet aggregation, and insulin secretion
$\beta 1$	Stimulation of lipolysis; myocardial contraction (increased rate, increased force of contraction)
$\beta 2$	Increased hepatic gluconeogenesis; increased hepatic glycogenolysis; increased muscle glycogenolysis; increased release of insulin, glucagon, and renin; smooth muscle relaxation (bronchi, blood vessels, genitourinary tract, gastrointestinal tract)

lipolysis, freeing triglycerides and fatty acids from fat stores, and inhibiting the degradation of circulating cholesterol to bile acids. The metabolic actions of epinephrine aid the metabolic actions of cortisol, which are similar. Table 9-2 summarizes other well-known effects of adrenal catecholamines. All of these effects prepare the body to take physical action: to fight or flee. Stressors commonly associated with catecholamine release by the adrenal medulla include exercise, thermal changes, and acute emotional states.

Catecholamines can modify the numbers of cells of the immune system circulating in the blood.[1] Injection of epinephrine into healthy human subjects is associated with a transient increase of the number of lymphocytes (e.g., T, G, and natural killer cells) in the peripheral blood. Specifically, T cytotoxic and natural killer (NK) cells increase with little change in B lymphocytes. The main change is with NK cells.[1] Qualitatively, lymphocyte responsiveness of T and B lymphocytes is reduced. Similar quantitative and qualitative changes are found 5 to 6 minutes after injection of a psychologic or physical stressor.[23] The effect of catecholamines on the alteration of lymphocyte function is short lived, lasting only about 2 hours.[1] This suggests that for catecholamines to have an effect on immune function that can predispose to illness, their levels must be chronically elevated. This is supported by a study of stress duration and susceptibility to infection.[24] It is unclear whether the increase in lymphocytes is from the bone marrow or peripheral tissues.

Table 9-2 Physiologic Effects of Catecholamines*

Organ	Process or Result
Brain	Increased blood flow Increased glucose metabolism
Cardiovascular system	Increased rate and force of contraction Peripheral vasoconstriction
Pulmonary system	Increased oxygen supply Bronchodilation Increased ventilation
Muscle	Increased glycogenolysis Increased contraction Increased dilation of skeletal muscle vasculature
Liver	Increased glucose production Increased gluconeogenesis Increased glycogenolysis Decreased glycogen synthesis
Adipose tissue	Increased lipolysis Increased fatty acids and glycerol
Skin	Decreased blood flow
Skeleton	Decreased glucose uptake and utilization (decreases insulin release)
Gastrointestinal and genitourinary tracts	Decreased protein synthesis
Lymphoid tissue	Increased protein breakdown (lymphoid tissue shrinks)

Data from Granner DK: Hormones of the adrenal medulla. In Murray RK et al, editors: *Harper's biochemistry,* ed 21, New York, 1993, Lange; Sherwood L: *Human physiology from cells to systems,* ed 3, Belmont, Calif, 1997, Wadsworth.

*Some of these responses require glucocorticoids (e.g., cortisol) for maximal activity (see text for explanation).

Cortisol

The adrenal cortex is activated during stress by ACTH (see Fig. 9-1), increasing adrenocortical secretion of glucocorticoid (steroid) hormones, primarily cortisol. (Cortisol is known also as *hydrocortisone.*) Cortisol circulates in the plasma, both protein bound and free. The main plasma-binding protein is called **transcortin** or **corticosteroid-binding globulin.** The unbound, or free, fraction is approximately 8% of the total plasma cortisol and is the most biologically active fraction of cortisol.[22] Cortisol mobilizes substances needed for cellular metabolism. One of the primary effects of cortisol is the stimulation of gluconeogenesis, or the formation of glycogen from noncarbohydrate sources, such as amino or free fatty acids in the liver. In addition, cortisol enhances the elevation of blood glucose promoted by other hormones, such as epinephrine, glucagon, and somatotropic growth hormone. This action by cortisol is said to be **permissive** for the actions of other hormones. Cortisol also inhibits the uptake and oxidation of glucose by many body cells. The overall action of cortisol on carbohydrate metabolism results in an elevation of blood glucose.

Cortisol also affects protein metabolism. It has an anabolic effect; that is, it increases the rate of synthesis of proteins and ribonucleic acid (RNA) in liver. Cortisol also has catabolic effects in muscle, lymphoid tissue, adipose tissue, skin, and bone.[22] The overall breakdown effect of proteins results in a negative nitrogen balance and an increase in circulating amino acids. Some evidence exists that cortisol depresses transport of amino acids into muscle cells while enhancing their uptake into the liver, where they are converted to glucose. Cortisol also can promote lipolysis in some areas of the body (the extremities) and lipogenesis in others (the face and trunk). The lipid effects of tissue are specific because not all areas show increased fat deposition or lipolysis.[22]

High concentrations of cortisol cause immunosuppression by suppressing protein synthesis, including synthesis of immunoglobulin. Cortisol also alters peripheral blood populations of eosinophils, lymphocytes, and macrophages.[22,25,26] Large doses of cortisol are known to promote atrophy of lymphoid tissue in the thymus, spleen, and lymph nodes.[22] This action of cortisol could account for the lymphoid atrophy observed by Selye. Cortisol may also increase the incidence of lymphocyte *apoptosis* (programmed cell death) during stress.[27,28]

Cortisol directly influences immune responses to antibodies.[29] Physiologically low concentrations of glucocorticoids increase cytokine production by Th2 cells while inhibiting cytokine production by Th1 cells. Decreased Th1 activity would decrease cell-mediated (T cytotoxic response) or delayed-type hypersensitivity reactions.[1,30] High concentrations of glucocorticoids would inhibit both Th1- and Th2-derived cytokines, producing a suppression of all T cell–mediated immune responses (Fig. 9-2).[1]

The ability of therapeutic concentrations of cortisol and other glucocorticoids to suppress the inflammatory response is well documented and provides the basis for the major clinical use of these steroids. Cortisol decreases the number of circulating lymphocytes, monocytes/macrophages, and eosinophils because these cells are shifted from the vascular compartment to other sites, including the bone marrow, lymphoid tissue, and spleen.[23,25] Cortisol enhances the release of polymorphonuclear leukocytes from bone marrow, thus increasing their number in blood, although their effectiveness decreases. Glucocorticoids inhibit the accumulation of leukocytes at the site of inflammation and inhibit the release of substances involved in the inflammatory response (e.g., kinins, plasminogen-activating factor, prostaglandins, and histamine) from the leukocytes.[22] Cortisol inhibits fibroblast proliferation and function at the site of an inflammatory response. This inhibition accounts for the poor wound healing, increased susceptibility to infection, and decreased inflammatory response that often are seen in individuals with chronic glucocorticoid excess. Glucocorticoids are necessary for the maintenance of normal blood pressure and cardiac output. This is another example of how cortisol maximizes the action of the catecholamines (the permissive effect).

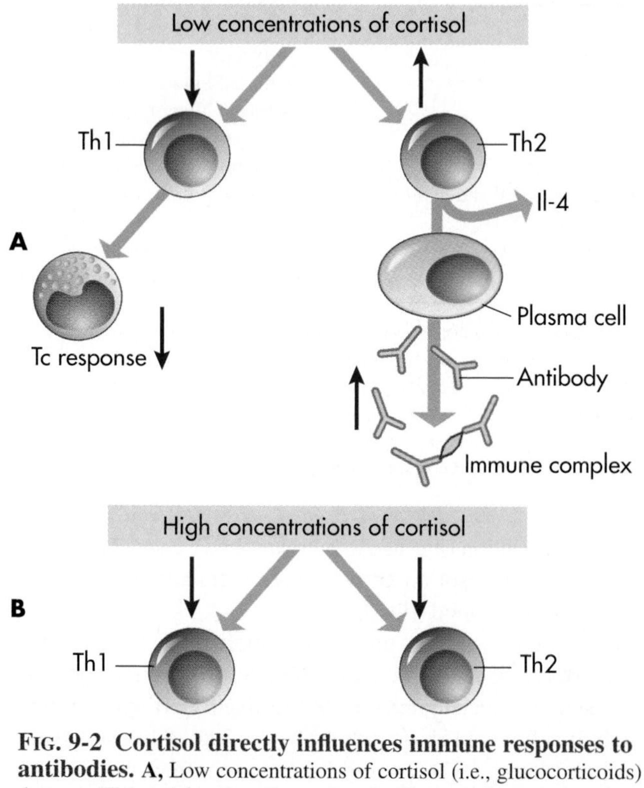

FIG. 9-2 Cortisol directly influences immune responses to antibodies. A, Low concentrations of cortisol (i.e., glucocorticoids) decrease Th1 activity, thus decreasing the T cytotoxic response or delayed-type hypersensitivity. In addition, low concentrations of cortisol increase cytokine production by Th2 cells, increasing the production of antibodies. **B,** High concentrations of cortisol inhibit both Th1- and Th2-derived cytokines, causing a suppression of all T cell–mediated immune responses.

Elevation of glucocorticoid concentration associated with psychologic stress or physical exercise is not as high as that achieved by pharmacologic means.[1] Stress produces an elevation of hormones other than glucocorticoids; the interaction of these various hormones in modifying immune function needs investigation. In the gastrointestinal tract, cortisol promotes gastric secretion. This effect is opposite that of norepinephrine, which reduces gastric secretion. Excessive cortisol may stimulate gastric secretion enough to cause ulceration of the gastric mucosa. This could account for the gastrointestinal ulceration observed by Selye.

Cortisol exerts inhibiting effects by suppressing levels of release of luteinizing hormone, estradiol, and possibly testosterone.[16] The inhibitory effects also render target tissues of sex steroids resistant to these hormones, resulting in hypogonadism.

It is not entirely clear why cortisol secretion during stress is beneficial. It has been suggested that gluconeogenesis promoted by cortisol ensures an adequate source of glucose (energy) for body tissues, and nerve cells in particular. The pooling of amino acids from catabolized proteins may ensure amino acid availability for protein synthesis in certain cells. The redistribution of protein to sites where replacement is critical, such as muscle or cells of damaged tissue, would be beneficial. Short-term, cortisol-induced alterations in immune cell distribution (e.g., traffic) patterns may be adaptive, with a decrease in peripheral blood cell numbers as effector cells locate to sites of injury or inflammation. In addition, decreased immune cell activity by cortisol may be beneficial in some situations because it prevents immune-mediated tissue damage by prolonged cell exposure to high levels of certain cytokines. Whether cortisol-induced effects are adaptive or destructive may depend on the intensity, type, and duration of the stressor, and the subsequent concentration and length of cortisol exposure that target cells of the individual experience. The biologic effects of cortisol are summarized in Table 9-3.

Studies of repeated or chronic stress have revealed variable cortisol responses. In a study using parachute jumping as a stressor, the investigators observed significantly lower cortisol responses than previous jumps in some subjects, whereas other individuals maintained a high level of cortisol.[31] These results suggest that some individuals adapt to stress over time but others remain more susceptible to the effects of stressors.

Other Hormones

Endorphins and Enkephalins

Endorphins and enkephalins (endogenous opiates) are released into the blood as part of the response to stressful stimuli.[32] There are proteins found in the brain with pain relieving capabilities. The secretion of ACTH and β endorphin is stimulated by corticotropin-releasing factor; β endorphins are released from the pituitary gland.[17] There is release of enkephalin from the adrenal medulla. Evidence is accumulating that β endorphins can regulate ACTH secretion and, with ACTH, inhibit hypothalamic CRF secretion, a possible down-regulation pathway of the stress response.[33]

Increased β endorphin levels are associated with a parallel increase in pain threshold (i.e., stress-induced analgesia).[34,35] In a number of conditions or activities in which endogenous opiate activity is increased, subjects not only experience insensitivity to pain but also report increased feelings of excitement, positive well-being, or euphoria.[36] In addition, cells of the immune system synthesize and release opioids when the lymphoid cells are activated.[37] T and B lymphocytes and mononuclear phagocytic cells have receptors for opioids.[1] For example, vigorous running increases β endorphin levels.[38] Endorphins may play a role in the excitement and exhilaration produced by dancing, contact sports, and combat. There is little direct evidence, however, documenting the endorphin system in most of these activities.

Growth Hormone (Somatotropin)

Growth hormone (GH) is synthesized from the anterior pituitary gland and is also produced by lymphocytes and mononuclear phagocytic cells.[39] GH affects protein, lipid, and carbohydrate metabolism. It is involved in tissue repair and may participate in the growth and function of the immune system.[1] Receptors for GH are present on lymphoid cells.[40] This suggests a role for GH in regulating phagocytic function and possibly antigen presentation.[1] GH appears to have enhancing effects on immune function.[1] GH levels increase in the blood after a variety of stressful stimuli, such as cardiac catheterization, electroshock therapy, gastroscopy, surgery, fever, and physical exercise.[29,41] Psychologic stimuli associated with increased levels of GH include examinations, viewing of violent or sexually arousing films, anticipation of exhausting exercise, and certain psychologic performance tests. Prolonged activation of the stress response (chronic stress) leads to suppression of GH and other growth factor effects on target tissues.[42]

Prolactin

Prolactin is released from the anterior pituitary gland and is necessary for lactation and breast development.[43] Prolactin receptors are present in many different tissues, including liver, kidney, intestine, and adrenals. Prolactin is also produced by lymphoid cells.[1,44] Prolactin levels in plasma increase from a variety of stressful stimuli, including gastroscopy, proctoscopy, pelvic examination, and surgery.[45] Prolactin also rises during parachute jumping, during motion sickness, and after examinations.[36] Unlike GH, prolactin levels show little change after exercise. Like GH, however, prolactin appears to require more intense stimuli

Table 9-3 Physiologic Effects of Cortisol

Functions Affected	Physiologic Effects
Carbohydrate and lipid metabolism	Diminishes peripheral uptake and utilization of glucose; promotes gluconeogenesis in liver cells; enhances gluconeogenic response to other hormones; promotes lipolysis in adipose tissue
Protein metabolism	Increases protein synthesis in liver and depresses protein synthesis (including immunoglobulin synthesis) in muscle, lymphoid tissue, adipose tissue, skin, and bone; increases plasma level of amino acids; stimulates deamination in liver
Inflammatory effects	Decreases circulating eosinophils, lymphocytes, and monocytes; increases release of polymorphonuclear leukocytes from bone marrow; decreases accumulation of leukocytes at site of inflammation; delays healing; permissive for vasoconstrictive action of norepinephrine
Lipid metabolism	Lipolysis in extremities and lipogenesis in face and trunk
Immune reserve	Decreases tissue mass of all lymphoid tissues (e.g., decreases protein synthesis); promotes rapid decrease in circulating lymphocytes, eosinophils, basophils, and macrophages; inhibits production of interleukin-1 and interleukin-2; consequently, also blocks cell-mediated immunity and generation of fever
Digestive function	Promotes gastric secretion
Urinary function	Enhances urinary excretion
Connective tissue function	Decreases proliferation of fibroblasts in connective tissue (thus delaying healing)
Muscle function	Maintains normal contractility and maximal work output for skeletal and cardiac muscle
Bone function	Decreases bone formation
Vascular system and myocardial function	Maintains normal blood pressure; permits increased responsiveness of arterioles to constrictive action of adrenergic stimulation; optimizes myocardial performance
Central nervous system function	Somehow modulates perceptual and emotional functioning, essential for normal arousal and initiation of daytime activity; high levels of cortisol associated with decreased recent memory recall*

*Data from Seeman TE et al: Increase in urinary cortisol excretion and memory declines: MacArther studies of successful aging, *J Clin Endocrinol Metab* 82:2458, 1997.

than those leading to increases in catecholamine or cortisol levels. Prolactin levels increase in the plasma after a variety of sexual stimuli, for example, stimulation of the nipple or areola in women. Immune cells also are influenced by prolactin. Prolactin acts as a second messenger for interleukin-2 (IL-2) and is known to have a positive influence on B cell activation and differentiation.[46] Several classes of lymphocytes have receptors for prolactin, suggesting a direct effect of prolactin on immune function. Prolactin secretion is reduced during a stress response, including surgery and trauma, and production of prolactin is reduced in the presence of certain stress-associated cytokines (IL-1 and IL-6).[47]

Testosterone

Testosterone, a hormone secreted by Leydig cells, regulates male secondary sex characteristics and libido. Testosterone levels decrease after stressful stimuli. The decrease in testosterone occurs after stimuli such as ether or anesthesia, surgery, marathon running, and mountain climbing.[48] The mechanism causing decreased levels of testosterone is thought to be exerted by cortisol.

Psychologic stimuli also lead to a decrease in testosterone levels. Men engaged in rigorous combat training and those engaged in the first several weeks of officer candidate school experience significant drops in testosterone levels.[49,50] However, recent data indicate that the psychologic stress associated with some types of competition (pistol shooting) *increases* both testosterone and cortisol, especially in athletes older than 45 years.[51] Individuals with acute illness, such as respiratory failure, burns, and congestive heart failure, show a marked reduction in plasma testosterone.[36]

The direct immunologic effects of sex hormones contribute to the sexual dimorphism seen in the incidence of autoimmune disease[52] and the greater susceptibility to sepsis and mortality in males following injury.[53] Estrogens generally are associated with a depression of T cell–dependent immune function and enhancement of B cell functions, and an-

Table 9-4 Other Hormones That Probably Influence the Stress Response

Hormone	Source	Comments
Melatonin	Produced by pineal gland	Increases during the stress response; release is suppressed by light and increased in the dark; receptors have been identified on lymphoid cells, possibly higher density of receptors on T cells than B cells; suppression of lymphocyte function by trauma was reversed by melatonin (Maestroni, 1999)
Somatostatin (SOM)	Produced by sensory nerve terminals found in and released from lymphoid cells	Natural killer (NK) function and immunoglobulin synthesis is decreased by SOM
Vasoactive intestinal peptide (VIP)	Found in neurons of the central nervous system (CNS) and in peripheral nerves	VIP increases during stress; VIP-containing nerves are located in both primary and secondary lymphoid tissues, around blood vessels, and in the gastrointestinal tract; VIP receptors are on both T and B cells; VIP may influence lymphocyte maturation; cytokine production by T cells is modified by VIP; B cells and antibody production is influenced by VIP
Calcitonon gene–related peptide (CGRP)	Found in spinal cord motor neurons and in sensory neurons near dendritic cells of the skin and in primary and secondary lymphoid tissues	CGRP receptors are present on T and B lymphocytes, thus it is likely that CGRP can modulate immune function; CGRP may enhance the acute inflammatory response because it is a vasodilator; maturation of immune B lymphocytes is inhibited by CGRP; IL-1 is inhibited by CGRP, which is important for the activation of T cells; it has been shown to interfere with lymphocyte activation
Neuropeptide Y (NPY)	Present in the neurons of the CNS and in neurons throughout the body; colocalized in nerve terminals in lymphatic tissues with norepinephrine	Lymphocytes have receptors for NPY and thus may modulate their function (Pettito et al, 1994); Several lines of evidence suggest that NPY is a neurotransmitter and neurohormone involved in the stress response; increased levels of NPY occur in plasma in response to severe or prolonged stress; it may be responsible for stress-induced regional vasoconstriction (splanchnic, coronary, and cerebral); it may also increase platelet aggregation (Rabin, 1999)
Substance P (SP)	Produced by a neuropeptide classified as tachykinin (increases heart rate subsequent to lowering blood pressure) found in the brain, as well as nerves innervating secondary lymphoid tissues	SP increases in responses to stress; receptors for SP are found on the membrane of both T and B cells, mononuclear phagocytic cells, and mast cells; proinflammatory activity induces the release of histamine from mast cells during the stress response; causes smooth muscle contraction, causes macrophages and T cells to release cytokines, and increases antibody production

Data from Maestroni GJ: MLT and the immune-hematopoietic system, *Adv Exp Med Biol* 460:396, 1999; Pettito JM et al: Molecular cloning of NPY-Y1 receptor cDNA from rat splenic lymphocytes: evidence of low levels of expression and NPY binding sites, *J Neuro Immunol* 54:81, 1994; Rabin BS: The nervous system—immune system connection. In *Stress, immune function, and health: the connection,* Wiley-Liss, 1999, New York.

drogens suppress both T and B cell responses.[52] In injury, however, males produce greater amounts of proinflammatory cytokines, a profile that is associated with poor outcome.[54] Additionally, androgens appear to induce a greater degree of immune cell apoptosis following injury, a mechanism that may elicit a greater immunosuppression in injured males versus females.[55] Table 9-4 lists other hormones, including melatonin, substance P, neuropeptide Y, calcitonin gene–related peptide, somatostatin, and vasoactive intestinal peptide.

Role of Immune System

Many immune-related conditions and diseases are associated with stress. The specific stress-induced mechanisms causing these illnesses are not clearly defined. Recent research is focused on the regulatory interactions between the immune system and the nervous and endocrine systems, which may represent mechanistic pathways for stress-associated immune-mediated diseases, including infection, some forms of cancer, allergy, and autoimmunity (Table 9-5).

Table 9-5 Stress-Related Diseases and Conditions

Target Organ or System	Disease or Condition
Cardiovascular system[A-D]	Coronary artery disease
	Hypertension
	Stroke
	Disturbances of heart rhythm
Muscles[E]	Tension headaches
	Muscle contraction backache
Connective tissues[F]	Rheumatoid arthritis (autoimmune disease)
	Related inflammatory diseases of connective tissue
Pulmonary system[G]	Asthma (hypersensitivity reaction)
	Hay fever (hypersensitivity reaction)
Immune system	Immunosuppression or immune deficiency
	Autoimmune diseases
Gastrointestinal system[H]	Ulcer
	Irritable bowel syndrome
	Diarrhea
	Nausea and vomiting
	Ulcerative colitis
Genitourinary system	Diuresis
	Impotence
	Frigidity
Skin[I, J]	Eczema
	Neurodermatitis
	Acne
Endocrine system[K]	Diabetes mellitus
	Amenorrhea
Central nervous system[L-N]	Fatigue and lethargy
	Type A behavior
	Overeating
	Depression
	Insomnia

A. Chemerinski E, Robinson RG: The neuropsychiatry of stroke, *Psychosomatics* 41(1):5, 2000.
B. Hemingway H, Marmot M: Evidence based cardiology: psychosocial factors in the aetiology and prognosis of coronary heart disease, *BMJ* 318(7196):1460, 1999.
C. Pickering T: Cardiovascular pathways: socioeconomic status and stress effects on hypertension and cardiovascular function, *Ann N Y Acad Sci* 896:262, 1999.
D. Williams JE et al: Anger proneness predicts coronary heart disease risk: prospective analysis from the Atherosclerosis Risk in Communities (ARIC) study, *Circulation* 101(17):2034, 2000.
E. Diamond S: Tension-type headache, *Clin Cornerstone* 1(6):33, 1999.
F. Walker JG et al: Stress system response and rheumatoid arthritis: a multilevel approach, *Rheumatology (Oxford)* 38(11):1050, 1999.
G. Gooding V, Kruth M, Jamart J: Joint consultation for high-risk asthmatic children and their families, with pediatrician and child psychiatrist as co-therapists: model and evaluation, *Fam Process* 36(3):265, 1997.
H. Drossman DA: Presidential address: gastrointestinal illness and the biopsychosocial model, *Psychosom Med* 60(3):258, 1998.
I. Howlett S: Emotional dysfunction, child-family relationships and childhood atopic dermatitis, *Br J Dermatol* 140(3):381, 1999.
J. Van Moffaert M: Psychodermatology: an overview, *Psychother Psychosom* 58(3-4):125, 1992.
K. Surwit RS, Williams PG: Animal models provide insight into psychosomatic factors in diabetes, *Psychosom Med* 58(6):582, 1996.
L. Douglas NJ: The psychosocial aspects of narcolepsy, *Neurology* 50(2 suppl 1):S27, 1998.
M. Friedman EM, Irwin MR: A role for CRH and the sympathetic nervous system in stress-induced immunosuppression, *Ann N Y Acad Sci* 771:396, 1995.
N. Johnson SK, DeLuca J, Natelson BH: Chronic fatigue syndrome: reviewing the research findings, *Ann Behav Med* 21(3):258, 1999.

Evidence thus far suggests that the immune, nervous, and endocrine systems communicate through pathways involving hormones, neurotransmitters, neuropeptides, and immune cell products. Various components of immune system responses are potentially affected by all known neuroendocrine-produced factors involved in the stress reaction. Conversely, immune cell–derived cytokines and other products have effects on neurocrine and endocrine cells (see Table 9-4).[56,57] Several pathways appear to regulate communication between these systems with both direct and indirect patterned effects (Fig. 9-3).

Direct influence of the stress response on immune system functioning may occur through hypothalamic and pituitary peptides and by products of the sympathetic branch of the ANS. These factors include CRF, ACTH, endorphins, substance P, epinephrine, norepinephrine, dopamine, serotonin, histamine, GH, vasoactive intestinal polypeptide (VIP), β-endorphin, methionine-enkephalin, leucine-enkephalin, and somatostatin (see Table 9-4).[58-61] Direct suppressive effects of CRF have been reported also on two immune cell types processing CRF receptors—the monocyte-macrophage and CD4 (T helper) lymphocyte.[62] Release of endogenous opiates occurs during stress, and these peptides have been shown to have concentration-dependent, enhancing, and suppressive effects on various immune cells.[58] Immune cells have been shown to have surface β-adrenergic and serotoninergic receptors, as well as receptors for ACTH, CRF, endorphins, GH, prolactin, and steroids.[63-66]

Products of the sympathetic branch of the ANS also influence immune cell behavior. It has been known for some time that there is direct innervation of the thymus, spleen, lymph nodes, and bone marrow.[61] Histochemical studies have verified the presence of cholinergic, adrenergic, and peptinergic nerve terminals in the lymphoid organs and tissues. There is evidence for interaction of norepinephrine released from nerve endings with lymphocytes and macrophages in the spleen, implicating the presence of a route of communication between the ANS and immune system through direct delivery of chemical mediators that alter immune cell behavior in a paracrine (cell to adjacent cell) fashion in the microenvironment of the lymphoid organ.

The pineal gland has a role in regulation of immune response and mediates the apparent effects of circadian rhythm on immunity. Blockage of production of melatonin (by continuous light or by pharmacologic means) results in suppression of immune response, whereas administration of melatonin reverses these effects.[67] This pathway of immunomodulation may be operative in immune changes observed in sleep disturbance and dysregulated circadian rhythm, which is common among elderly and acutely ill and stressed individuals.[68] Melatonin also modulates seasonal changes in immune function and affects tumor development.[69]

Indirect effects of the CNS on immune function involve the hypothalamic-pituitary-adrenal (HPA) axis. This is the most extensively studied pathway, with original interest stemming from early studies showing profound effects of prolonged severe stress on immunologic structures.[70] It was noted that the adrenal gland enlarged with simultaneous involution of the thymus and lymph nodes. Increased levels of circulating glucocorticoids are thought to be an important mechanism, both in the stress-related alterations in immune structures and in suppression of immune response.[70] The increase in glucocorticosteroid (GCS) level is attributable to signaling by pituitary ACTH production. Enhanced production of ACTH by the pituitary is a result of increased hypothalamic CRF. The production of CRF is initiated by a number of stress factors, including high levels of IL-1. Production of IL-1 by activated macrophages and monocytes is inhibited by GCS, suggesting a feedback loop with IL-1, CRF, ACTH, and GCS secretion.[71,72]

The observation that IL-1 can elicit changes in the nervous and endocrine systems by stimulating CRF production in the hypothalamus is part of a growing body of evidence demonstrating immune-induced regulation of the CNS. The release of immune inflammatory mediators IL-6, tumor necrosis factor–beta (TNF-β), and interferon is triggered by bacterial or viral infections, cancer, and tissue injury that in turn initiate a stress response through the HPA pathway described previously. Enhanced systemic production of these cytokines also induces other CNS and behavior changes seen frequently during the acute phase of an infectious episode, acting either directly in a distant systemic "endocrine" way or through the mediation of neuropeptides.[56,73-75] These effects include pyrogenesis (fever), induction of slow wave sleep, and anorexia, all of which are adaptive responses to infection and possibly cancer, with hyperthermia resulting in an inhospitable environment for many microorganisms and tumor cells (by slowing bacterial and tumor growth and viral replication). Slow wave sleep is associated with enhanced release of GH and a reduction in levels of cortisol, which is beneficial for tissue repair and enhanced immune response.[76] Normal and predictive changes in sleep occur in response to infections, and these changes appear to be of important recuperative value to the individual.[77]

Lymphocytes also are known to produce ACTH and endorphins in small amounts, which probably influence immune response in an autocrine or a paracrine manner in the local microenvironment of an ongoing immune response.[66] There is also new evidence that the T cell growth factor (IL-2) can upregulate pituitary ACTH. It appears that the cytokines just mentioned, produced in response to infectious challenge and acting in a distant systemic way, have the greatest influence on neuroendocrine function, with evidence for direct and indirect cytokine effects on nervous and adrenal cell functions. These effects on neuroendocrine function by immune cells indicate an adaptive role for the immune system as a "signal" organ to alert other systems of internal threatening stimuli (e.g., infection, tissue damage, tumor cells) that may upset the dynamic steady state.

The stress-induced alterations in the equilibrium of various neuropeptides and hormones have a significant effect on the immune response. Whether this impact on immune function is suppressive or potentiating depends on the type of immunomodulating factor that is secreted, with some factors

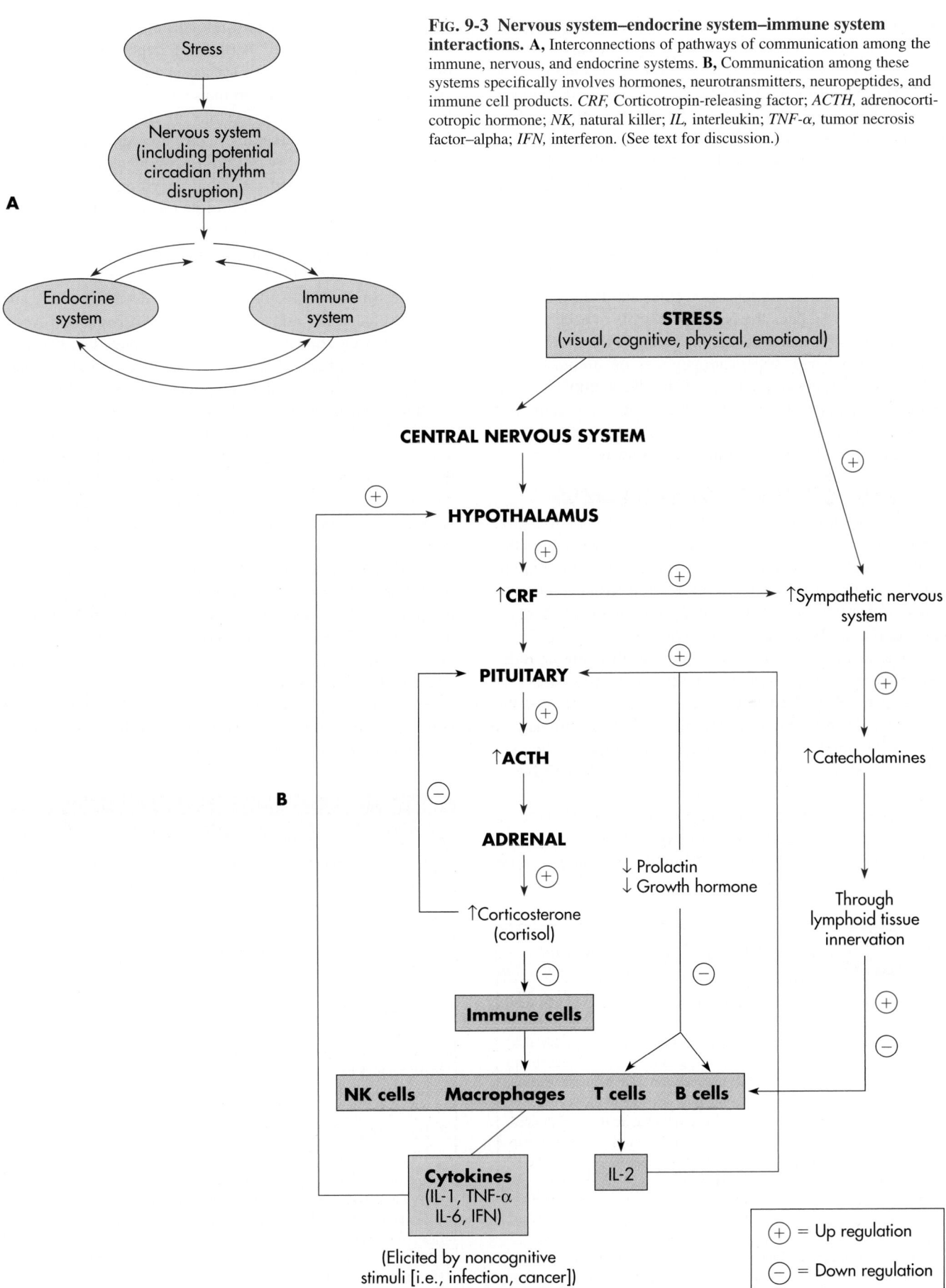

FIG. 9-3 Nervous system–endocrine system–immune system interactions. A, Interconnections of pathways of communication among the immune, nervous, and endocrine systems. **B,** Communication among these systems specifically involves hormones, neurotransmitters, neuropeptides, and immune cell products. *CRF,* Corticotropin-releasing factor; *ACTH,* adrenocorticotropic hormone; *NK,* natural killer; *IL,* interleukin; *TNF-α,* tumor necrosis factor–alpha; *IFN,* interferon. (See text for discussion.)

A

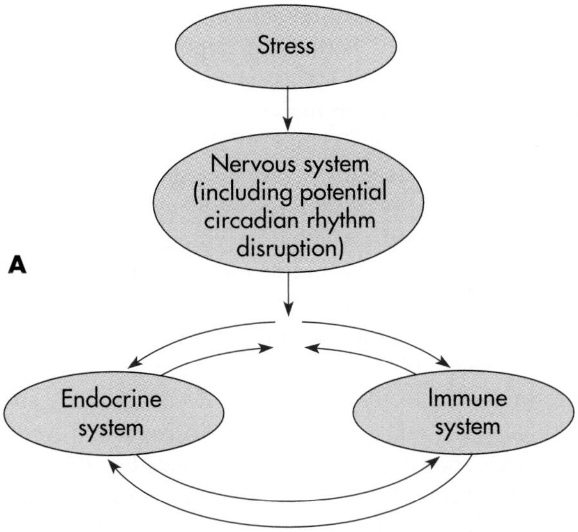

B

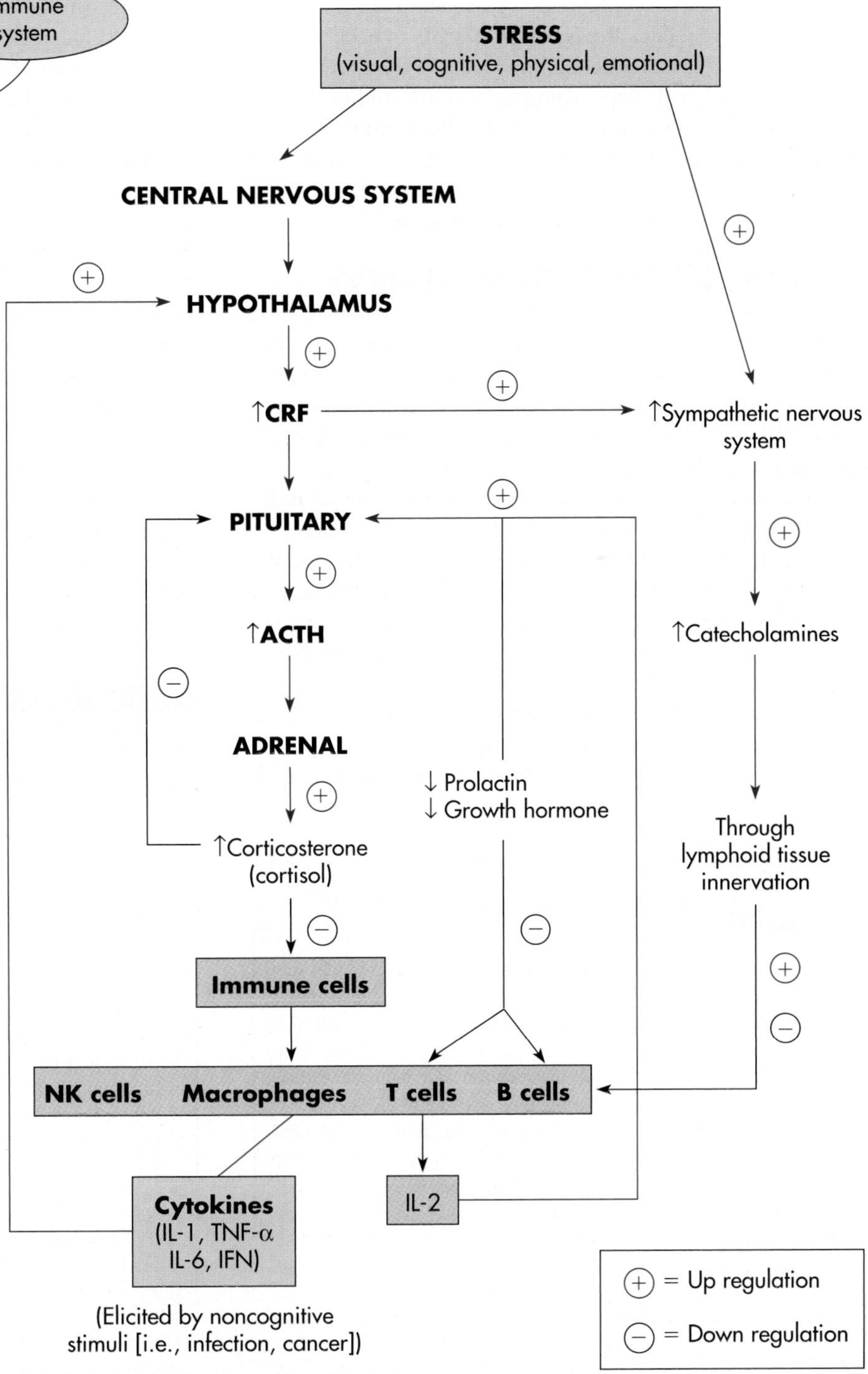

known to have enhancing or suppressing activities, or both, depending on the concentration and length of exposure, the target cell, and the specific immune function studies.[56] The immunomodulatory activity of neuropeptides and neuroendocrine hormones may involve the direct control of biochemical events affecting cell proliferation, differentiation, and function. These factors also may indirectly control immune cell behavior by affecting the production or activity of cytokines.[57]

In summary, a significant body of evidence now supports a link among the nervous, endocrine, and immune systems. The bidirectional communication among these systems involves common use of signal molecules and their receptors, which in turn regulates the behavior of cells in each system. Thus the most recent findings are that (1) there are direct effects of CNS and ANS neuropeptides on immune cells; (2) neurologic-induced endocrine products influence immune cell and neurologic cell function; and (3) immune cell products (cytokines) affect nervous and endocrine cell function through both direct and indirect pathways.

STRESS, COPING, AND ILLNESS

Extreme physiologic stressors, such as severe burn injury, represent a predictable stimulus for the stress responses described previously. A less severe and defined event or situation, however, can be a stressor for one person and not for another. Many stressors, such as fasting or temperature changes, do not necessarily cause a physiologic stress response if psychologic factors are minimized. Stress itself is not an independent entity but a system of interdependent processes that are moderated by the nature, intensity, and duration of the stressor and the perception, appraisal, and coping efficacy of the affected individual, all of which in turn mediate the psychologic and physiologic response to stress (see What's New? Coping Styles and Cancer Progression).

Psychosocial distress may be predictive of psychologic and physical health outcomes. In **psychologic distress** the individual feels a general state of unpleasant arousal after life events, manifest as physiologic, emotional, cognitive, and behavior changes.[78] Periods of depression and emotional upheaval many times are associated with adverse life events and place the affected individual at risk for immunologic deficits, increasing the risk of ill health.[79] A meta-analysis of studies evaluating depression and immunity has revealed a heterogeneity of findings, showing a relationship between depression and reduction in lymphocyte proliferation and NK cell activity.[80] Multiple moderating factors may be important in immune modulation in depressed individuals, including comorbidities such as alcoholism. Psychosocial variables studied have included bereavement, academic pressures (including examinations), life events (positive and negative changes),[79] and aging (Box 9-1). Adverse life events that have been shown to have the most negative effect on immunity have been characterized as uncontrollable, undesirable, and overtaxing the individual's ability to cope.[81,82]

Studies have strengthened the association of stress with potential for illness in humans. One study examined medical students who were immunized with hepatitis B vaccine on the third day of a stressful examination period; the time to seroconversion and level of antibody titer to the vaccine were measured later. The students with the most rapid seroconversion and the highest titers also reported being less stressed and had a good social support system (which may reduce stress).[83] Even more convincing is a study in which the psychologic stress status was determined in healthy individuals after experimentally controlled exposure to respiratory virus by nasal inoculation. Individuals reporting more stress had an increased incidence of clinical cold and respiratory symptoms compared with subjects reporting less stress, and other infections, including HIV, have been shown to be potentially influenced by psychosocial factors.[84-87]

WHAT'S NEW? Coping Styles and Cancer Progression

Although powerful, the biomedical model of disease does not explain all facts about cancer. There is empiric evidence that a hopeless/helpless coping style is associated with unfavorable disease outcome in people with certain cancers. Recent evidence indicates that psychotherapeutic intervention can increase natural killer (NK) cell activity and lymphokine-activated killer cell activity in individuals with malignant melanoma and in those with nonmestastatic breast cancer. These important findings, if confirmed in additional studies, will advance our understanding of mind-body interactions in individuals with cancer.

Data from Ericksen HR et al: The time dimension in stress responses: relevance for survival and health, *Psychiatry Res* 85(1):30, 1999; Garssen G, Goodkin K: On the role of immunological factors as mediators between psychosocial factors and cancer progression, *Psychiatry Res* 85(1):51, 1999; Greer S: Mind body research in psycho-oncology, *Adv Mind Body Med* 15(4):236, 1999.

Box 9-1
AGING AND STRESS: STRESS-AGE SYNDROME

With aging, sometimes a set of neurohormonal and immune alterations, as well as tissue and cellular changes, develops; these changes, which recently have been defined as **stress-age syndrome,** include the following:

- Alterations in the excitability of structures of the limbic system and hypothalamus
- Rise of the blood concentration of catecholamines, antidiuretic hormone (ADH), adrenocorticotropic hormone (ACTH), and cortisol
- Decrease of testosterone, thyroxine, and other hormones
- Alterations of opioid peptides
- Immunodepression
- Alterations in lipoproteins
- Hypercoagulation of the blood
- Free radical damage of cells

Some of the alterations are adaptational, whereas others are potentially damaging. These stress-related alterations of aging can influence the course of developing stress reactions and lower adaptive reserve and coping.

Data from Frolkis VV: *Mech Ageing Dev* 69:93, 1993; Mazzeo RS: Aging, immune function, and exercise: hormonal regulation, *Int J Sports Med* 21(suppl 1):S10, 2000.

Studies have shown adverse changes in immune function following intense exercise, with increased cortisol levels, changes in lymphocyte counts, and alterations in cytokine production.[88] Some of these immune changes could be reduced by administration of carbohydrate beverages to endurance athletes, suggesting that dehydration and decreased tissue perfusion were catalysts for the exercise stress–induced immune changes.

Other clinical situations where the interplay between immunity and psychosocial factors may be evident are cancer and heart disease.[89-91] There is convincing evidence linking cancer with psychologic distress with three possible mechanisms involved. First, NK cell activity, an important first-line immune defense against cancer, is inhibited in stressed or depressed subjects. Stress and depression is also associated with poorer repair of damaged DNA and alterations in the rates of apoptosis of immune and cancer cells. Additional evidence showing a relationship between cancer and psychosocial factors is seen in the enhanced immune function and survival among cancer patients who undergo psychosocial interventions.[89]

New evidence is showing a relationship between immune stimulation, infections, and heart disease.[90] The relationship between stress and cardiovascular health may be mediated by stress-induced changes in immune function, which may potentiate proinflammatory processes and permit infections that lead to heart disease.[91]

In the past decade a significant amount of evidence has accumulated linking severe psychosocial stress resulting from negative life events to a chronic syndrome with mental and physical consequences. Posttraumatic stress syndrome (PTTS) has been described in many populations.[92-94] A cascade model has been proposed to describe the pathogenesis and clinical course of the syndrome that illustrates the clinical, epidemiologic, neurobiologic, and psychosocial components of PTTS.[95] The study of PTTS has contributed to the knowledge of mechanisms involved in the chronic stress and disease relationship, with a recent appreciation of the association of chronic stress with high levels of cortisol production and paradoxic biounavailability of cortisol.[96]

In addition, the interaction with health care providers in a clinical setting, the diagnosis of a major illness, and various medical procedures (e.g., blood draws, injections, examinations, surgical procedures) may represent a significant negative life event to many individuals (Fig. 9-4). These additional stresses may affect the course of illness in these individuals, possibly interfering with the efficacy of the medical intervention. The identification and reduction of stress in the clinical setting therefore is an important area of concern that has particular applicability to clinicians, in both prevention and illness management.

The coping response of individuals may exaggerate or moderate physical consequences of the stress response. The response may be a change in behavior with potentially adverse health effects (e.g., increased smoking, change in eating habits). Serious disturbances of the sleep-wake cycle are observed in many people under stress and in many clinical settings. Recent work has shown that sleep disturbance may exacerbate the pathophysiologic status of certain patient populations.[97-99] Investigators have reported that sleep deprivation and circadian disruption, even in young, otherwise healthy individuals, have detrimental influences on respiratory and immune system function. Even partial sleep deprivation was associated with reduced NK cell activity in healthy

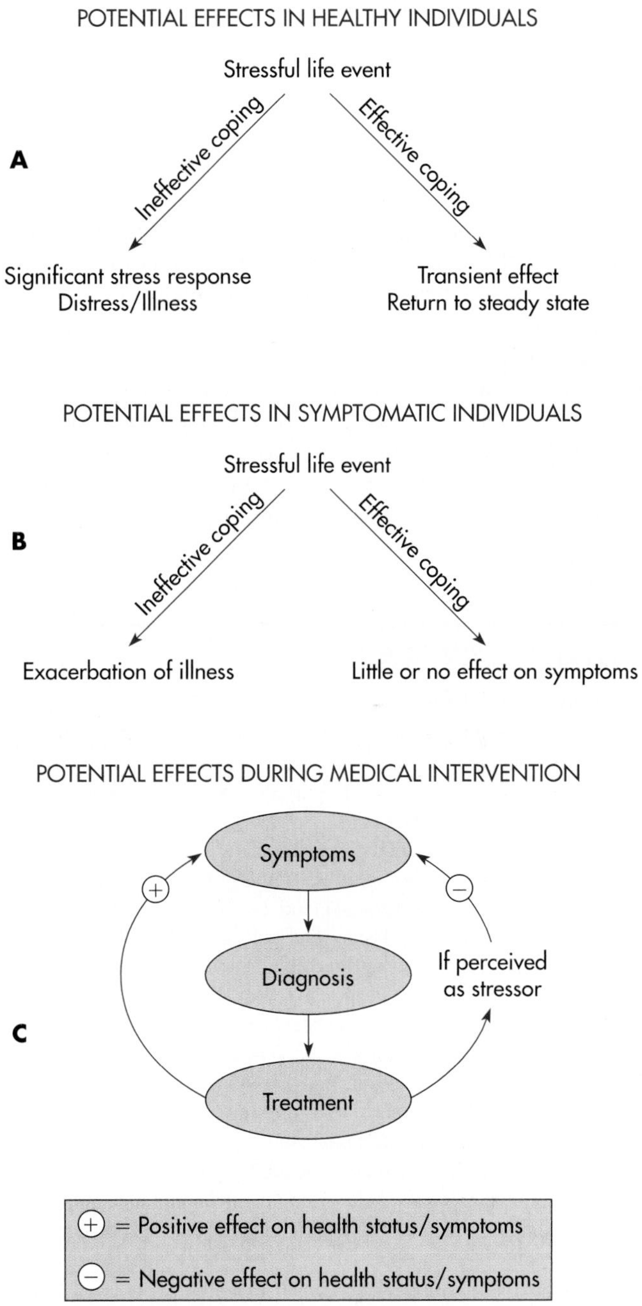

FIG. 9-4 Health outcome determination in stressful life situations is moderated by numerous factors. Whether a life-challenged individual experiences distress or illness depends on the subject's appraisal of the event and the coping strategies used during the stressful period. Models **A** and **B** reflect possible outcomes in stressed healthy and symptomatic individuals. Model **C** illustrates the dynamic clinical setting in which the diagnosis of a serious illness and subsequent medical interventions may be perceived as stressful challenges and have potentially detrimental influences on physical outcome.

subjects, and only recently have seriously ill patients been assessed for adequacy and structure of sleep during recovery.[97]

Adaptive coping strategies, especially those that are problem focused and those that encourage seeking social support,[100,101] are beneficial during stressful experiences. **Coping** is defined as the process of managing stressful demands and challenges that are appraised as taxing or exceeding the resources of the person.[102] The extent to which an individual responds to distress, using effective positive coping strategies, determines the degree of successful moderation of the stress challenge. Conversely, ineffective negative coping attempts may exacerbate the effects of distress on health, thus augmenting the potential for illness.[102] Mediating factors that may influence stress susceptibility or resilience include age, socioeconomic status, gender, social support status, personality, self-esteem, genetics, life events, experiences, and current health status.[103] Although an individual may not be able to avoid stressors and cannot change many of these factors, there is evidence for effective intervention resulting in greater stress resilience and improved psychologic and physiologic outcomes. In a study of nursing home residents randomly assigned to control or social support intervention groups, improved psychologic measures and immune function (NK cell activity) were observed in the experimental group at 6 weeks.[104] In another study, women with recurrent metastatic breast cancer were given either routine follow-up (routine care) or weekly support group sessions. Survival in the support treatment group was an average of 19 months longer than in the routine care group, suggesting a mediating influence of additional support for these women.[26,105]

The importance of social support for seriously ill individuals has focused attention on the health and well-being of family members who function as caregivers. Significant stress manifested as depression, anxiety, and fatigue has been noted in family caregivers of those with cancer, Alzheimer disease, and burn trauma. These studies demonstrated significant suppression of various measures of immune function, with improved function being associated with better perceived social support.[106-108]

Potential interventions for prevention or management of stress-related psychologic or physical problems include both short- and long-term coping strategies. Stress management consists of educational components specific to the individual's problems and relaxation techniques, which may include meditation, imagery, and biofeedback. These approaches may be used on an individual or a support group basis. Incorporation of these approaches into clinical training facilitates the use of stress-reducing methodology in the clinical arena. Future research should focus on the efficacy of such approaches with various populations.

SUMMARY REVIEW

Concepts of Stress

1. *Stress* recently has been defined as the state of affairs arising when a person relates to (i.e., interacts or transacts with) situations in a certain way. Important is how he or she appraises and reacts to situations.
2. Hans Selye identified three structural changes in rats subjected repeatedly to noxious stimuli (stressors): enlargement of the cortex of the adrenal gland, atrophy of the thymus gland and other lymphoid tissues, and gastrointestinal ulceration.
3. Selye believed that the three changes were caused by a nonspecific physiologic response to any long-term stressor. He called this response the *general adaptation syndrome (GAS).*
4. The GAS occurs in three stages: the alarm stage, the stage of resistance or adaptation, and the stage of exhaustion. Diseases of adaptation develop if the stage of resistance or adaptation does not restore homeostasis.
5. Selye identified three components of physiologic stress: the stressor, the physiologic or chemical disturbance produced by the stressor, and the body's adaptational response to the stressor.
6. Other investigators have shown that the physiologic stress response also occurs in response to psychologic or emotional stress.
7. There is disagreement on the nonspecific nature of the stress response because different processes occur in response to specific stimuli, such as exposure to cold or heat.
8. W.B. Cannon defined *homeostasis* as the sum of the processes by which the body maintains itself at a relatively constant composition. This definition has since been modified. *Homeostasis* is now considered to mean the sum of the processes by which the body maintains itself in a dynamic steady state.
9. The function of the physiologic stress response is to maintain the body's dynamic steady state.

Stress Response

1. The stress response involves the nervous system (sympathetic branch of the autonomic nervous system), the endocrine system (pituitary and adrenal glands), and the immune system.
2. The stress response is initiated when a stressor is present in the body or perceived by the mind.
3. The neuroendocrine response to stress consists of sympathetic stimulation of the adrenal medulla to secrete catecholamines (norepinephrine and epinephrine) and stressor-induced stimulation of the pituitary to secrete ACTH, which in turn stimulates the adrenal cortex to secrete steroid hormones, particularly cortisol.
4. In general, the catecholamines prepare the body to act, and cortisol mobilizes energy (glucose) and other substances needed to fuel the action.
5. Epinephrine exerts its chief effects on the cardiovascular system. Epinephrine increases cardiac output and increases blood flow to the heart, brain, and skeletal muscles by dilating vessels that supply these organs. It also dilates the airways, thereby increasing delivery of oxygen to the bloodstream.
6. Norepinephrine's chief effects complement those of epinephrine. Norepinephrine constricts blood vessels of the vis-

cera and skin; this has the effect of shifting blood flow to the vessels dilated by epinephrine. Norepinephrine also increases mental alertness.

7. Cortisol's chief effects involve metabolic processes. By inhibiting the use of metabolic substances while promoting their formation, cortisol mobilizes glucose, amino acids, lipids, and fatty acids and delivers them to the bloodstream. Cortisol also suppresses immune and inflammatory function.
8. The nervous, endocrine, and immune systems communicate through the common use of signal molecules and their receptors, which in turn regulate the behavior of cells in each system during stress challenge.
9. There are direct and indirect pathways of influence among the nervous, endocrine, and immune systems. Neuropeptides have direct effects on immune cells, as well as indirect influences through neuromediated endocrine modulation of immune function. Endocrine products (cortisol) also influence nerve cell behavior. Immune cell products affect both nerve and endocrine cell function, reflecting an adaptive role for the immune system as a "signal" organ to alert other systems of threatening stimuli.
10. Other hormones are affected by the stress response and include increased circulating levels of β endorphins, growth hormone, and prolactin and a decrease in antidiuretic hormone with extreme stress. Testosterone decreases during the stress response.

Stress, Coping, and Illness

1. Stress is a system of interdependent processes that are moderated by the nature, intensity, and duration of the stressor and the coping efficacy of the affected individual, all of which in turn mediate the psychologic and physiologic response to stress.
2. Many studies have linked psychologic distress with altered immune function, and evidence now strengthens the association of stress with potential for illness in humans.

KEY TERMS

Alarm stage, *273*
Coping, *286*
Corticosteroid-binding globulin, *277*
Disease of adaptation, *273*
Dynamic steady state, *273*
General adaptation syndrome (GAS), *273*
Homeostasis, *273*
Permissive, *277*
Physiologic stress, *273*
Psychologic distress, *284*
Psychoneuroimmunology, *276*
Stage of exhaustion, *273*
Stage of resistance or adaptation, *273*
Stress, *272*
Stress-age syndrome, *284*
Stress response, *276*
Stressor, *273*
Transcortin, *277*
Turnover, *273*

REFERENCES

1. Rabin BS: The nervous system—immune system connection. In *Stress, immune function, and health: the connection*. New York, 1999, Wiley-Liss.
2. Kapcala LP et al: The protective role of the hypothalamic-pituitary-adrenal axis against lethality produced by immune, infections, and inflammatory stress, *Annals NY Acad Sci* 77:419, 1995.
3. Ostell A: Coping, problem-solving, and stress: a framework for intervention strategies, *Br J Med Psychol* 64:11, 1991.
4. Selye H: The general adaptation syndrome and the diseases of adaptation, *J Clin Endocrinol* 6:117, 1946.
5. Selye H: *Stress without distress*, Philadelphia, 1974, Lippincott.
6. Hill SR et al: Studies on adrenocortical and psychological responses to stress in man, *Arch Intern Med* 97:269, 1956.
7. Mason JW, Brady JV: Plasma 17-hydroxycortico-steroid changes related to reserpine effects on emotional behaviors, *Science* 124:983, 1956.
8. Hetzel BS et al: Changes in urinary 17-hydroxycorticosteroid excretion during stressful life situations in man, *J Clin Endocrinol* 15:1057, 1955.
9. Handlon JH et al: Psychological factors in 17-hydroxycorticosteroid concentration, *Psychosom Med* 24:535, 1962.
10. Wadeson RW et al: Plasma and urinary 17-OHCS responses to motion pictures, *Arch Gen Psychiatry* 9:146, 1963.
11. Mason JW: Organization of psychoendocrine mechanisms: a review and reconsideration of research. In Greenfield NS, Steinbach RA, editors: *Handbook of psychophysiology,* New York, 1972, Holt, Rinehart, & Winston.
12. Bieliauskas LA: *Stress and its relationship to health and illness,* Boulder, Colo, 1982, Westview Press.
13. Mason JW: A historical view of the stress field, *J Human Stress* 1(1): 6, 1975.
14. Mason JW: Specificity in the organization of neuroendocrine response profiles. In Seeman P, Brown G, editors: *Frontiers in neurology and neuroscience research,* Toronto, 1974, University of Toronto.
15. Surwit RS, Schneider MS: Role of stress in the etiology and treatment of diabetes mellitus, *Psychosom Med* 55:380, 1993.
16. Chrousos GP, Gold PS: The concepts of stress and stress system disorders: overview of physical and behavioral homeostasis, *JAMA* 267(9):1244, 1992.
17. Curtis AL et al: Previous stress alters corticotropin-releasing factor neurotransmission in the locus coeruleus, *Neuroscience* 65:541, 1995.
18. Negrao AB et al: Individual reactivity and physiology of the stress response, *Biomed Pharmacother* 54(3):122, 2000.
19. Ader R, Cohen N: Behaviorally conditioned immunosuppression, *Psychosom Med* 37:333, 1975.
20. Dimsdale JE, Ziegler MH: What do plasma and urinary measures of catecholamines tell us about human response to stressors? *Circulation* 83(suppl II):36, 1991.
21. Herd JA: Cardiovascular response to stress, *Physiol Rev* 71(1):305, 1991.
22. Sapolsky RM, Romero LM, Munck AU: How do glucocorticoids influence stress responses? Integrating permissive, suppressive, stimulatory, and preparative actions, *Endocr Rev* 21(1):55, 2000.
23. Moyna NM et al: The effects of incremental submaximal exercise on circulating leukocytes in physically active and sedentary males and females, *Eur J Appl Phys* 74:211, 1996.
24. Cohen S et al: Types of stressors that increase susceptibility to the common cold in healthy adults, *Health Psychology* 17:214, 1998.

25. Herbert TB, Cohen S: Stress and immunity in humans: a meta-analytic review, *Psychosomatic Med* 55:364, 1993.
26. Spiegel D et al: Effect of psychosocial treatment on survivors of patients with metastatic breast cancer, *Lancet* II:888, 1989.
27. Fukuzuka K et al: Glucocorticoid-induced, caspase-dependent organ apoptosis early after burn injury, *Am J Physiol Regul Integr Comp Physiol* 278(4):R1005, 2000.
28. Hoffman-Goetz L, Zajchowski S: In vitro apoptosis of lymphocytes after exposure to levels of corticosterone observed following submaximal exercise, *J Sports Med Phys Fitness* 39(4):269, 1999.
29. Berne RM, Levy MN, editors: *Principles of physiology,* St Louis, 1990, Mosby.
30. Daynes RA, Aranco BA: Contrasting of glucocorticoids on the capacity of T cells to produce the growth factors interleukin 2 and interleukin 4, *J Immunol* 19:2319, 1989.
31. Deinzer R et al: Adrenocortical responses to repeated parachute jumping and subsequent h-CRH challenge in inexperienced healthy subjects, *Physiol Behav* 61:507, 1997.
32. Guillemin R et al: Beta-endorphin and adrenocorticotropin are secreted concomitantly by the pituitary gland, *Science* 197:1367, 1977.
33. Calogero A et al: Multiple regulatory feedback loops in hypothalamic corticotropin-releasing hormone secretion, *J Clin Invest* 82:767, 1988.
34. Cohen MR et al: Stress-induced plasma beta-endorphin immunoreactivity may predict post-operative morphine usage, *Psychiatr Res* 6:7, 1982.
35. JungKunz G et al: Endogenous opiates increase pain tolerance after stress in humans, *Psychiatr Res* 8:13, 1983.
36. Rose RM: Psychoendocrinology. In Wilson JD, Foster DW, editors: *Williams textbook of endocrinology,* ed 7, Philadelphia, 1985, W.B. Saunders.
37. Cabot PJ et al: Immune cell derived beta-endorphin. Production, release, and control of inflammatory pain in rats, *J Clin Invest* 100:142, 1997.
38. Colt EWD, Wardlaw SL, Franz AG: The effect of running on plasma b-endorphin, *Life Sci* 28:1637, 1981.
39. Weingent DA et al: Characterization of the promoter-directing expression of growth hormone in a monocyte cell line, *Neuroimmunomodulation* 7(3):126, 2000.
40. Kelly PA et al: The prolactin/growth hormone receptor family, *Endocr Rev* 12:235, 1991.
41. Schalach DS: The influence of physical stress and exercise on growth hormone and insulin secretion in man, *J Lab Clin Med* 69:256, 1967.
42. Burguera B et al: Dual and selective actions of glucocorticoid upon basal and stimulated growth hormone release in man, *Neuroendocrinology* 51:51, 1990.
43. Shiu RPC, Friesen HG: Mechanisms of action of prolactin in the control of mammary gland function, *Annu Rev Physiol* 42:83, 1980.
44. Van De Weerdt C et al: Far upstream sequences regulate the human prolactin promoter transcription, *Neuroendocrinology* 71(2):124, 2000.
45. Noel GL et al: Human prolactin and growth hormone release during surgery and other conditions of stress, *J Clin Endocrinol Metab* 35: 840, 1972.
46. Prystowsky MB, Clevenger CV: Prolactin as a second messenger for interleukin 2, *Immunomethods* 5:49, 1994.
47. Jorgensen C, Sany J: Modulation of the immune response by the neuroendocrine axis in rheumatoid arthritis, *Clin Exp Rheumatol* 12:435, 1994.
48. Matsumoto K et al: Plasma testosterone levels following surgical stress in male patients, *Acta Endocrinol* 65:11, 1970.
49. Aakvaag A et al: Testosterone and testosterone-binding globulin (TeBG) in young men during prolonged stress, *Int J Androl* 1:22, 1978.
50. Kreuz LE, Rose RM, Jennings JR: Suppression of plasma testosterone levels and psychological stress: a longitudinal study of young men in officer candidate school, *Arch Gen Psychiatry* 26:479, 1972.
51. Guezennec CY et al: Effect of competition stress on tests used to assess testosterone administration in athletes, *Int J Sports Med* 16(6): 368, 1995.
52. Da Silva JA: Sex hormones and glucocorticoids: interactions with the immune system, *Ann N Y Acad Sci* 876:102, 1999.
53. Offner PJ, Moore EE, Biffl WL: Male gender is a risk factor for major infections after surgery, *Arch Surg* 134(9):935, 1999.
54. Angele MK et al: Sex steroids regulate pro- and anti-inflammatory cytokine release by macrophages after trauma-hemorrhage, *Am J Physiol* 277:C34, 1999.
55. Angele MK et al: Gender dimorphism in trauma-hemorrhage-induced thymocyte apoptosis, *Shock* 12:316, 1999.
56. Aoki N, Ohno Y, Imamura M: Physiological interactions between the immune and endocrine systems: are cytokines hormones? *Med Sci Res* 18:195, 1990.
57. Khansari DN, Murgo AJ, Faith RE: Effects of stress on the immune system, *Immunol Today* 11(5):170, 1990.
58. Dunn AJ: Psychoneuroimmunology for the psychoneuroendocrinologist: a review of animal studies of nervous system-immune system interactions, *Psychoneuroendocrinology* 14:251, 1989.
59. Friedman EM, Irwin MR: A role for CRH and the sympathetic nervous system in stress-induced immunosuppression, *Ann N Y Acad Sci* 771:396, 1995.
60. Jankovic BD: Neuroimmunomodulation: facts and dilemmas, *Immun Letters* 21:101, 1989.
61. Rabin BS et al: Bidirectional interaction between the central nervous system and the immune system, *Clin Rev Immunol* 9(4):279, 1989.
62. Jain R et al: Corticotropin-releasing factor modulating the immune response to stress in the rat, *Endocrinology* 128:1329, 1991.
63. Boranic M et al: Immune response of stressed rats treated with drugs affecting serotoninergic and adrenergic transmission, *Biomed Pharmacother* 44:381, 1990.
64. Borboni P et al: β-Endorphin receptors on cultured and freshly isolated lymphocytes from normal subjects, *Biochem Biophys Res Commun* 163(1):642, 1989.
65. De Souza EB et al: Corticotropin-releasing factor (CRF) and interleukin-1 (IL-1) receptors in the brain-pituitary-immune axis, *Psychopharmacol Bull* 25(3):299, 1989.
66. Weigent DA, Carr DJ, Blalock JE: Bidirectional communication between the neuroendocrine and immune systems: common hormones and hormone receptors, *Ann N Y Acad Sci* 579:17, 1990.
67. Maestroni GJM, Conti A: Anti-stress role of the immuno-opioid network: evidence for a physiological mechanism involving T cell–derived, immunoreactive β-endorphin and metenkephalin binding to thymic opioid receptors, *Int J Neurosci* 61:289, 1991.
68. Schwab RJ: Disturbances of sleep in the intensive care unit, *Crit Care Clin* 10:681, 1994.
69. Nelson RJ, Drazen DL: Melatonin mediates seasonal adjustment in immune function, *Reprod Nutr Dev* 39(3):383, 1999.
70. Ader R, Felten D, Cohen N: Interactions between the brain and the immune system, *Annu Rev Pharmacol Toxicol* 30:561, 1990.
71. Su TP, London ED, Jaffe JH: Steroid binding at sigma receptors suggests a link between endocrine, nervous, and immune systems, *Science* 240:219, 1988.
72. Sundar SK et al: Brain IL-1-induced immunosuppression occurs through activation of both pituitary-adrenal axis and sympathetic nervous system by corticotropin-releasing factor, *J Neurosci* 10:3701, 1990.
73. Busbridge NJ, Grossman AB: Stress and the single cytokine: interleukin modulation of the pituitary-adrenal axis, *Mol Cell Endocrinol* 82:C209, 1991.
74. Hori T et al: Immune cytokines and regulation of body temperature, food intake, and cellular immunity, *Brain Res Bull* 27:309, 1991.
75. Navarra P et al: Interleukins-1 and -6 stimulate the release of corticotropin-releasing hormone-41 from rat hypothalamus in vitro via the eicosanoid cyclooxygenase pathway, *Endocrinology* 128(1):37, 1991.
76. Hall NRS, O'Grady MP: Regulation of pituitary peptides by the immune system, *BioEssays* 11(5):141, 1989.
77. Kreuger JM et al: Sleep, microbes, and cytokines, *Neuroimmunomodulation* 1(2):100, 1994.

78. Thoits PA: Dimensions of life events that influence psychological distress: an evaluation and synthesis of the literature. In Kaplan HB, editor: *Psychosocial stress: trends in theory and research,* Orlando, 1983, Academic Press.
79. Rozlog LA et al: Stress and immunity: implications for viral disease and wound healing, *J Periodontol* 70(7):786, 1999.
80. Irwin M: Immune correlates of depression, *Adv Exp Med Biol* 461:1, 1999.
81. Irwin M et al: Impaired natural killer activity during bereavement, *Brain Behav Immun* 1:98, 1988.
82. Kiecolt-Glaser J et al: Modulation of cellular immunity in medical students, *J Behav Med* 9:5, 1986.
83. Glaser R et al: Stress induced modulation of the immune response to recombinant hepatitis B vaccine, *Psychosom Med* 54:22, 1992.
84. Cohen S: Psychosocial stress and susceptibility to upper respiratory infections, *Am J Respir Crit Care Med* 152:S53, 1995.
85. Evans DL et al: Stress associated reductions of cytotoxic T lymphocytes and natural killer cells in asymptomatic HIV infection, *Am J Psychol* 152:543, 1995.
86. Nott KH, Vedhara K, Spickett GP: Psychology, immunology and HIV, *Psychoneuroendocrinology* 20:451, 1995.
87. Sheridan JF et al: Psychoneuroimmunology: stress effects on pathogenesis and immunity, *Clin Microbiol Rev* 7:200, 1994.
88. Nieman DC: Nutrition, exercise, and immune system function, *Clin Sports Med* 18(3):537, 1999.
89. Kiecolt-Glaser JK, Glaser R: Psychoneuroimmunology and cancer: fact or fiction? *Eur J Cancer* 35(11):1603, 1999.
90. Sharma R, Coats AJ, Anker SD: The role of inflammatory mediators in chronic heart failure: cytokines, nitric oxide, and endothelin-1, *Int J Cardiol* 72(2):175, 2000.
91. Sher L: Effects of psychological factors on the development of cardiovascular pathology: role of the immune system and infection, *Med Hypotheses* 53(2):112, 1999.
92. Bremner JD et al: Neural correlates of memories of childhood sexual abuse in women with and without posttraumatic stress disorder, *Am J Psychiatry* 156(11):1787, 1999.
93. Clohessy S, Ehlers A: PTSD symptoms, response to intrusive memories and coping in ambulance service workers, *Br J Clin Psychol* 38(pt 3):251, 1999.
94. Donnelly CL, Amaya-Jackson L, March JS: Psychopharmacology of pediatric posttraumatic stress disorder, *J Child Adolesc Psychopharmacol* 9(3):203, 1999.
95. Heim C, Ehlert U, Hellhammer DH: The potential role of hypocortisolism in the pathophysiology of stress-related bodily disorders, *Psychoneuroendocrinology* 25(1):1, 2000.
96. Alarcon RD, Glover SG, Deering CG: The cascade model: an alternative to comorbidity in the pathogenesis of posttraumatic stress disorder, *Psychiatry* 62(2):114, 1999.
97. Irwin M et al: Partial sleep deprivation reduces natural killer cell activity in humans, *Psychosom Med* 56:493, 1994.
98. Pollmacher T et al: Influence of host defense activation on sleep in humans, *Adv Neuroimmunol* 5(2):155, 1995.
99. White D et al: Sleep deprivation and the control of ventilation, *Am Rev Respir Dis* 128:984, 1983.
100. Lazarus RS, Folkman S: Coping and adaptation. In Gentry WD, editor: *The handbook of behavioral medicine,* New York, 1987, Guilford.
101. Vitaliano PP et al: Coping as an index of illness behavior in panic disorder, *J Nerv Ment Dis* 175:78, 1987.
102. Folkman S, Lazarus RS: The relationship between coping and emotion: implications for theory and research, *Soc Sci Med* 26:309, 1988.
103. Frolkis VV: Stress-age syndrome, *Mech Ageing Dev* 69:93, 1993.
104. Kiecolt-Glaser J et al: Psychosocial enhancement of immunocompetence in a geriatric population, *Health Psychol* 4:25, 1985.
105. Spiegel D: Psychosocial intervention in cancer, *J Natl Cancer Inst* 85:1198, 1993.
106. Baron RS et al: Social support and immune function among spouses of cancer patients, *J Pers Soc Psychol* 59:344, 1990.
107. Kiecolt-Glaser J et al: Chronic stress and immune function in family caregivers of Alzheimer's disease victims, *Psychosom Med* 45(5):523, 1987.
108. Shelby J et al: Severe burn injury: effects on psychologic and immunologic function in noninjured close relatives, *J Burn Care Rehab* 13(1):58, 1992.

CHAPTER 10

Biology of Cancer

KATHRYN L. McCANCE • LEE K. ROBERTS

CHAPTER OUTLINE

Perhaps no other disease causes more concern, fear, and challenge than cancer. The human responses to cancer are vast and profound, progressing from shock and disbelief to uncertainty and dread of recurrence, to hope and coping, and often to cure. During the next decade, investigators will develop tools for detecting the earliest stages of many cancers—in some cases when the tumor consists of only a few cells—and suppressing them before they have a chance to invade and metastasize. Cancer is in reality a variety of disorders with differing pathophysiologies. Mechanisms of cancer development vary according to the site of the disease and the precipitating cause (Fig. 10-1).

CANCER: A DISEASE OF ABNORMAL GROWTH, DIVISION, AND CELL DIFFERENTIATION

Cells of multicellular organisms are specialized members of a society—a *cellular society.* The goal of this cellular society is survival of the entire organism and not just the individual cell. Therefore some cells must refrain from dividing even when the nutrients are plentiful.[1] Cell division, proliferation, and differentiation are strictly regulated under normal conditions. In this way, organ and tissue mass does not change because a balance is maintained between cell birth rate and cell death rate. When a need arises in an organ or tissue for new cells, however, as in the repair of damage, previously nondividing cells (e.g., resting cells) are rapidly triggered to reenter the division cycle (see Cell Cycle, Chapter 1). Resting cells must be "turned on" for division and proliferation and "turned off" after proliferation has been completed. The cellular control mechanisms that regulate cell birth and cell death are referred to as *social controls* and require *social control genes.* Abnormal cells that disobey the social control mechanisms of normal cell division, proliferation, and differentiation proliferate to form tumors in the body. Virtually every cell in the body, if mutated, has the potential to form tumors.

Social Control Genes and Cellular Division

Genes implicated in cancer broadly include those involved in signal transduction, cell cycle control, DNA repair, cell growth and differentiation (growth factors and growth factor receptors), transcriptional regulation, senescence, and apoptosis (Fig. 10-2; also see Chapter 1).[2] Cell division depends

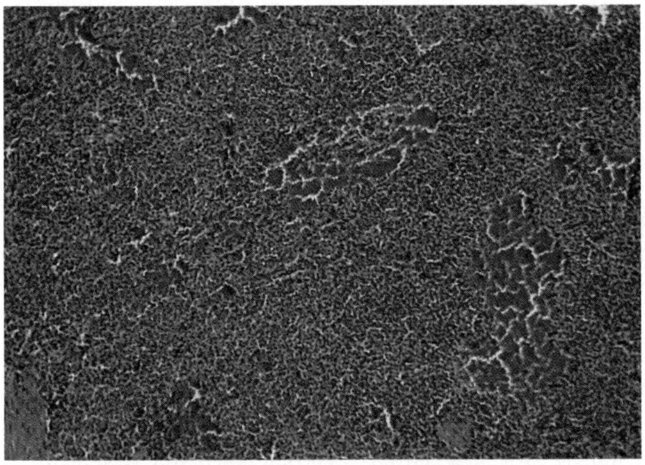

FIG. 10-1 Hairy cell leukemia. The tumor cells diffusely infiltrate the red pulp. Replacement of normal sinus-lining cells by hairy lympocytes leads to pooling of blood and the formation of "blood lakes," which are typical of this disease. (From Damjanov I, Linder J: *Pathology: a color atlas,* St Louis, 2000, Mosby.)

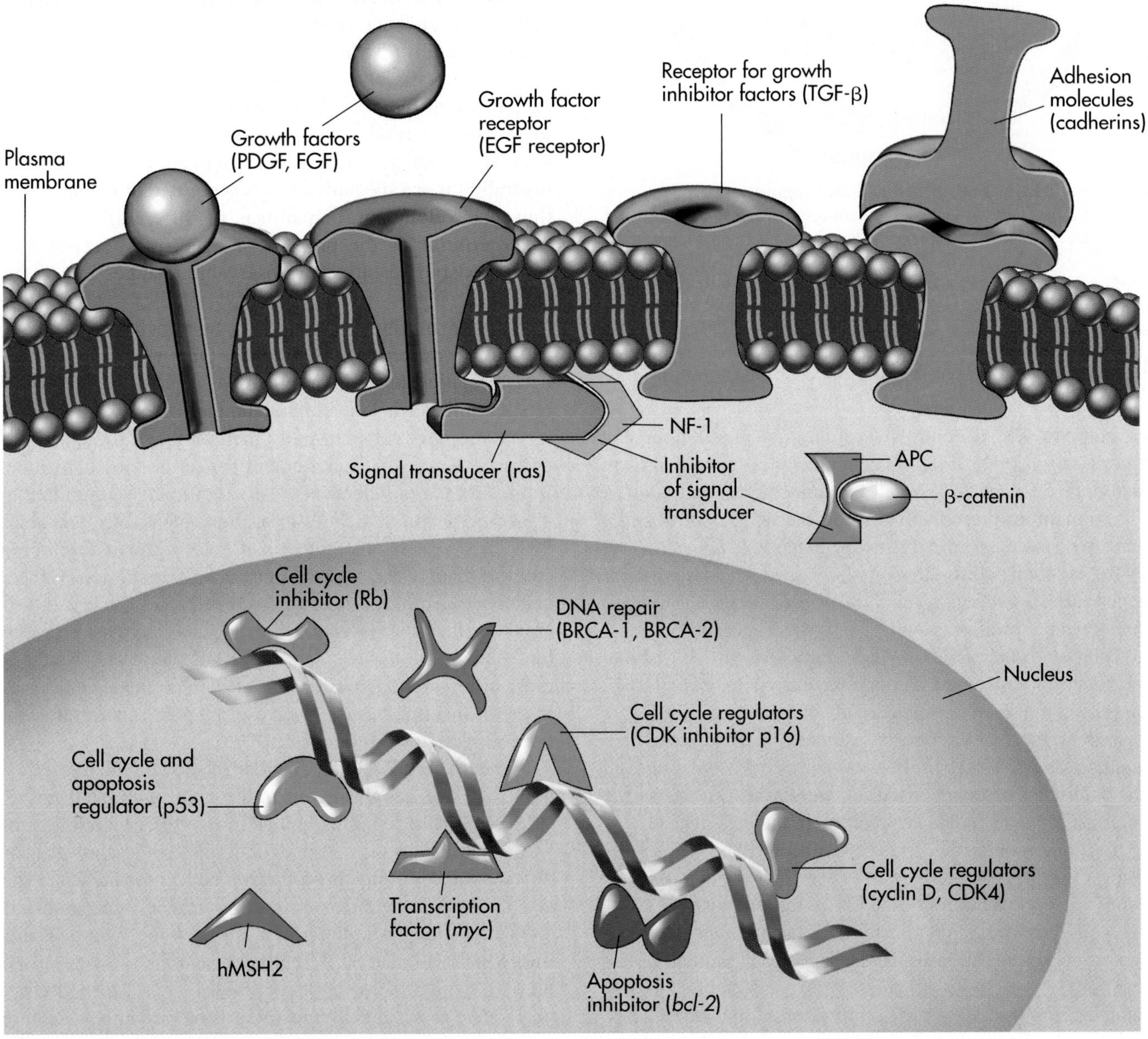

FIG. 10-2 Subcellular localization and functions of major classes of cancer-associated genes. The proto-oncogenes (normal genes that regulate growth and differentiation) are colored *red*, cancer suppressor genes *blue*, DNA repair genes *green*, and genes that regulate apoptosis *purple*. (Redrawn from Cotran RS, Kumar V, Collins T: *Pathologic basis of disease,* Philadelphia, 1999, W.B. Saunders.)

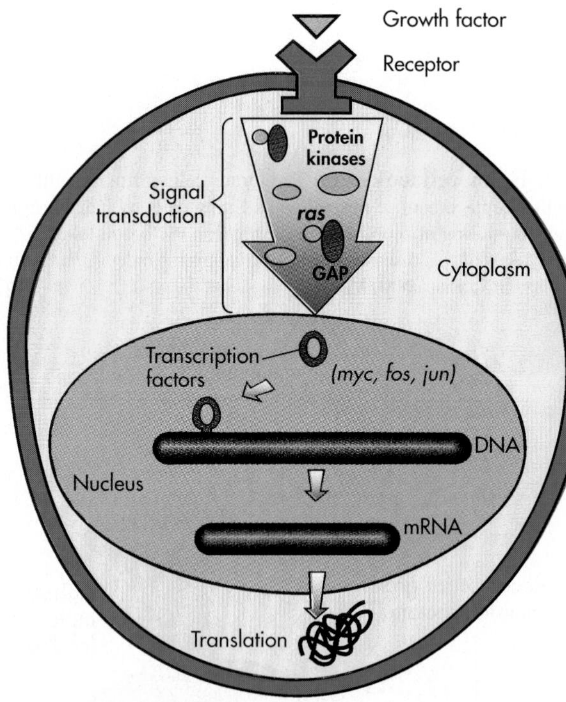

FIG. 10-3 Major features of cellular regulation. External growth factors (proteins and steroid hormones such as epidermal growth factor) bind to membrane-spanning growth factor receptors on the cell surface. These activate signal transduction pathways, in which genes such as *ras* participate. Components of the signal transduction pathway in turn interact with nuclear transcription factors, such as *myc* and *fos,* which can bind with other proteins, such as GTPase-activating protein (GAP), to regulatory regions in DNA. (From Jorde LB, Carey JC, White RL: *Medical genetics,* ed 2, St Louis, 1999, Mosby.)

on complex social controls. Proliferation of different cell types is regulated by different combinations of protein growth factors (see Chapter 1). A cell that undergoes a mutation or set of mutations presumably disrupts the social control genes that give rise to growth factor-regulated cell division (Fig. 10-3). In other words, the protein growth factors of these genes turn on (stimulate) and turn off (inhibit) normal cell division and proliferation (Fig. 10-4). These processes—division and proliferation—are regulated through signal transduction, movement through the cell cycle, DNA repair, transcriptional factors, senescence, and apoptosis. Cancer is caused by the malfunction or mutation of these genes that regulate division and proliferation. The identification and characteristics of many of these *genes* have been one of the great triumphs of molecular biology in the past decade.

Two mutational routes result in uncontrolled cell proliferation that is characteristic of cancer: (1) stimulation of a gene causing *hyperactivity* and (2) inhibition of a gene causing *inactivity.* The stimulation route has a dominant effect, because only one of the cell's two gene copies has mutated. The resulting hyperactivity—that is, overexpression of a growth-related gene product—causes tumor formation. In this case the altered gene is called an **oncogene** (from the Greek *onkos,* a mass or tumor). Conversely, the unaltered normal allele of that gene in a healthy cell is called a **proto-oncogene** (see p. 306). Proto-oncogenes encode products that control cell growth and differentiation. When mutated, they become oncogenes, which can cause cancer. In the inhibitory route the mutation has a recessive effect. In this instance both copies of the cell's particular differentiation gene are inactivated or deleted to free the cell of controlled growth inhibition. The lost gene is called a **tumor suppressor gene** (see p. 308).

In addition to ordinary mutation, another type of genetic change can lead to cancer—change caused by **tumor viruses.** Several types of tumors are associated with viruses. The viruses shed from these tumors can infect normal cells and, as a result of the insertion of the ribonucleic acid (RNA) or deoxyribonucleic acid (DNA) carried by the virus, may transform them into tumor cells (see p. 306).

Cell Differentiation

Cancer cells are defined by two heritable properties—autonomy and anaplasia. **Autonomy** refers to the cancer cell's independence from normal cellular controls. **Anaplasia** (literally, "without form") is the loss of differentiation, the process of developing specialized functions, and organization. In general, the cancer cell has lost its ability to function normally and to control its growth and division. In normal growth and development, cells become irreversibly more specialized or "committed" to a particular line of development, or pathway of differentiation. Thus *differentiation* is the process of acquiring specific new characteristics resulting in observable changes in cellular function.

Transformation is the process by which a normal cell becomes a cancer cell (Fig. 10-5). One mechanism of the transformation process may involve a partial or complete block in the normal developmental pathway toward full differentiation. As cells normally mature, they differentiate to perform the specific functions of the tissue they constitute. In the adult, *undifferentiated cells* (not totally committed to a specific function) are known as pluripotent cells, precursor cells, or *stem cells.* In comparison, cells within a developing embryo display the least amount of differentiation. Cancer cells become more like embryonic cells and are less differentiated (thus the observation that cancerous tissue resembles embryonic tissue) (see Fig. 10-1). As a cell becomes more differentiated, it loses its ability to replicate and ceases to grow. In some tissues, such as the epidermis of the skin, the cell is destined to die (Fig. 10-6).

Cancer is considered a disorder of growth and differentiation because neoplasms resemble undifferentiated tissue. With a partial or complete block in the differentiation pathway, the transformed cell may be trapped in a relatively undifferentiated, highly proliferative cell compartment. The less the tumor resembles normal tissue, the more undifferentiated or anaplastic the tumor is said to be. Tumor **grading,** which estimates differentiation, is thus a gauge of the tumor's degree of malignancy (Table 10-1). As the malignant cells grow and divide, they often lose their mature characteristics and no longer resemble their tissue of origin.

Cancerous growth often depends on derangements of cell differentiation. Differentiation depends on the functioning of the stem cell. Cell populations are renewed by simple duplication by means of **stem cells** (Fig. 10-7, *A*).

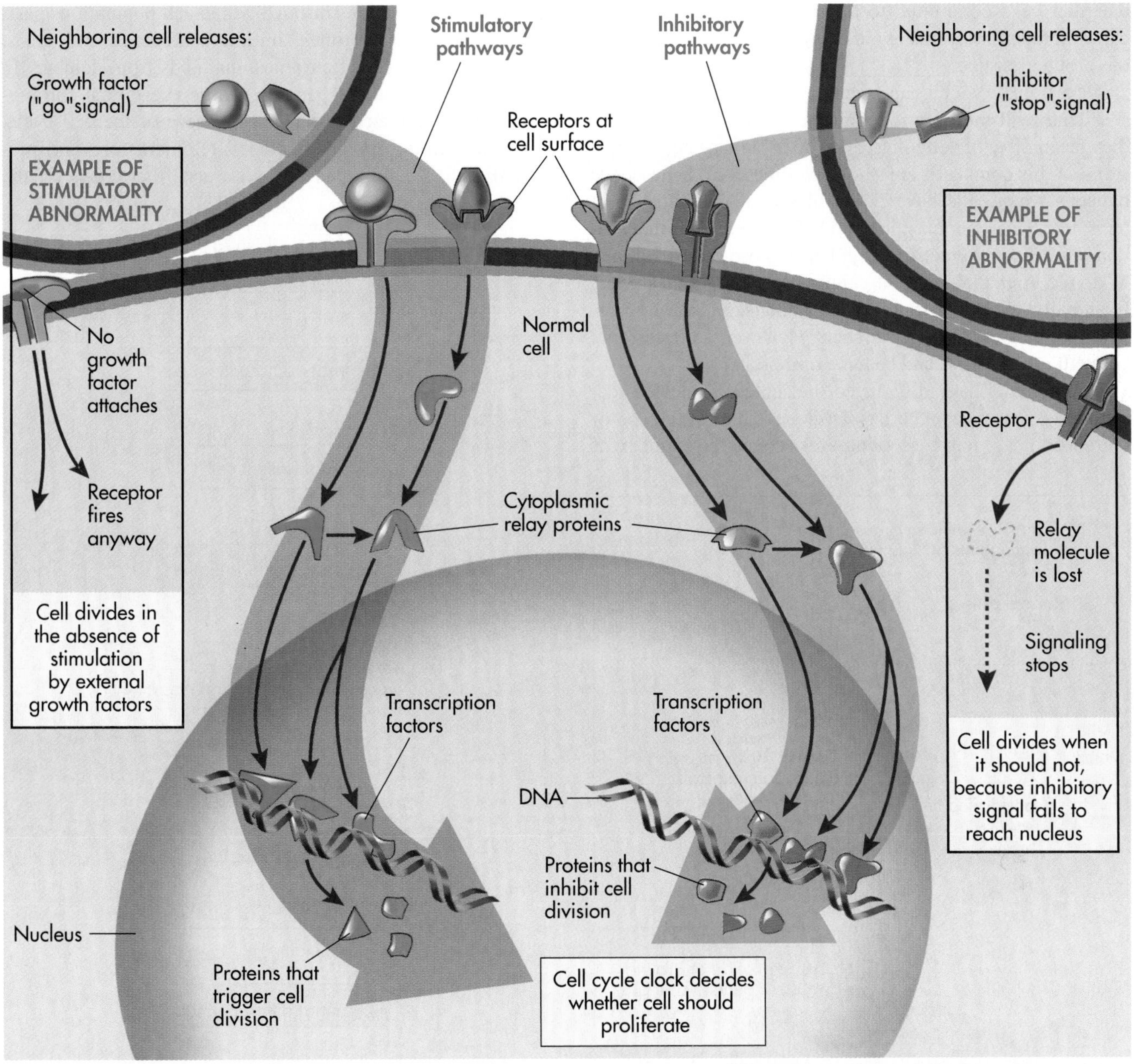

FIG. 10-4 Genetic mutations can cause cancer. Genetic mutations cause stimulatory pathways *(purple)* to issue too many "go signals" or inhibitory pathways *(blue)* can no longer issue "stop signals." A stimulatory pathway will become hyperactive if a mutation (i.e., oncogene) causes any component, such as a growth factor receptor *(box at left)* to issue stimulatory messages autonomously without waiting for signals from upstream. Conversely, inhibitory pathways (e.g., mutations causing tumor-suppressor genes) will be shot down when some constituent, such as a cytoplasmic relay *(box at right)*, is eliminated and thus breaks the signaling chain. (Adpated from Weinberg RA: How cancer arises, *Sci Amer* 275(3):64, 1996.)

The defining properties of a stem cell are these: (1) it is not at the end of the pathway of differentiation; that is, it is not, itself, **terminally differentiated;** (2) it can divide without limit; and (3) when it divides, each daughter cell has a choice—it can remain a stem cell, or it can become irreversibly committed to terminal differentiation (Fig. 10-7, *B*). Normally, each stem cell division generates one daughter stem cell and one cell (although it may be pluripotent—for example, bone marrow stem cells that give rise to several types of blood cells) that is committed to terminal differentiation and a cessation of cell division. If the stem cell divides more rapidly, terminally differentiated cells are produced more rapidly. As already mentioned, regulation of stem cell proliferation with cell growth and terminal differentiation is required to maintain the balance of new cell production and cell destruction within a tissue. To produce a steadily growing tumor, however, a transformed stem cell must cause an imbalance in cell production and cell destruction. An excessive cell division rate for the stem cells will not by itself have this effect.[1] Two derangements in differentiation, however, could presumably cause an imbalance leading to tumor development. First, more than 50% of the daughter cells must remain as stem cells, or second, the process of differentiation must be deranged so that the daughter cells committed to this route retain an ability to carry on indefinitely and avoid being discarded at the end of the production line.[1]

Occasionally a cell can become immortal: it and its descendents will multiply indefinitely. Normally, after a predictable number of doublings, 50 to 60 in human cells, growth stops, at this point cells are said to be **senescent**. Senescence happens when cells have powerful growth-inhibitory proteins, like RB (retinoblastoma) and p53 genes. Cells that sustain in activating mutations in either of these genes continue to divide after their normal counterparts enter senescence. Eventually, the survivors reach a second stage called **crisis**, in which they die in large numbers. However, an occasional cell will escape crisis and become immortal.

Investigators have discovered the molecular device that initiates senescence and crisis. DNA segments at the end of chromosomes, known as **telomeres**, count the number of replicative generations through which cell populations pass, and, at appropriate times, initiate senescence and crisis. Telomere caps protect chromosomal ends from damage. In human cells, telomeres shorten a little every time chromosomes are replicated during the S phase of the cell cycle. Like the plastic tips on shoelaces, telomeres prevent fraying (Fig. 10-8). In a cancer cell, a gene that codes for the

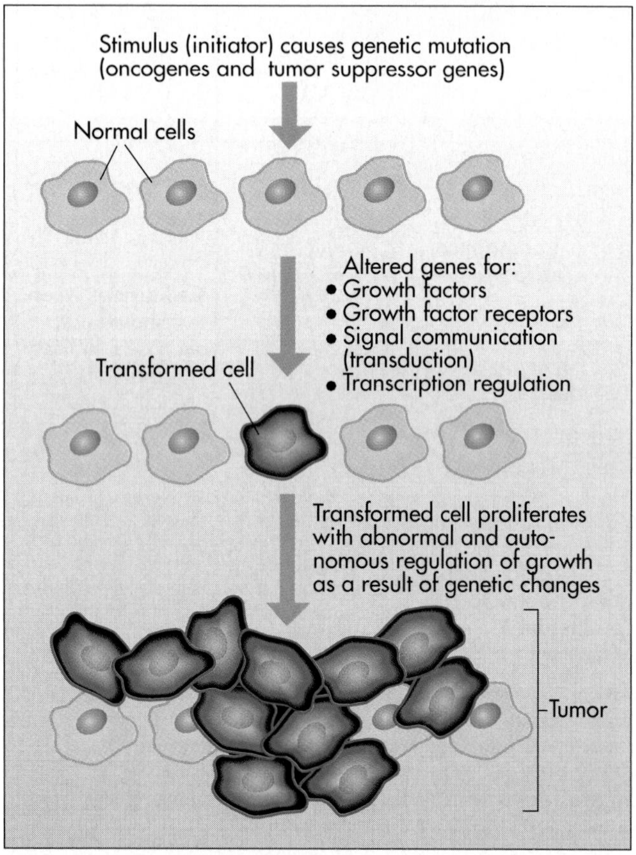

FIG. 10-5 Transformation by altered genetic changes.

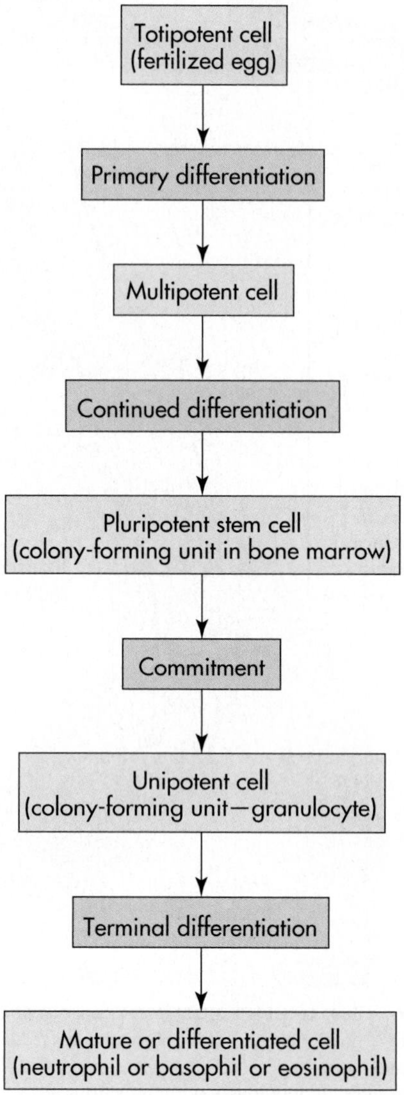

FIG. 10-6 Example of differentiation. Differentiation occurs several times in the lifetime of a granulocyte, with each step further limiting the cell's potential. Eventually the cell terminally differentiates and can no longer divide, and the mature cell dies.

Table 10-1 Tumor Grading: Degrees of Differentiation

Grade	Tumor Characteristics
Grade I: well differentiated	Tumor closely resembles tissue of origin and thus retains some specialized functions
Grade II: moderately differentiated	Tumor has less resemblance to tissue of origin; more variation in size and shape of tumor cells; increased mitoses
Grade III: poorly to very poorly differentiated	Tumor does not closely resemble tissue of origin; much variation in size and shape of tumor cells; greatly increased mitoses
Grade IV: very poorly differentiated	Tumor has no resemblance to tissue of origin; great variation in size and shape of tumor cells

Data from Moosa AR, Robson MC, Schimpff SC, editors: *Comprehensive textbook of oncology,* Baltimore, 1986, Williams & Wilkins.

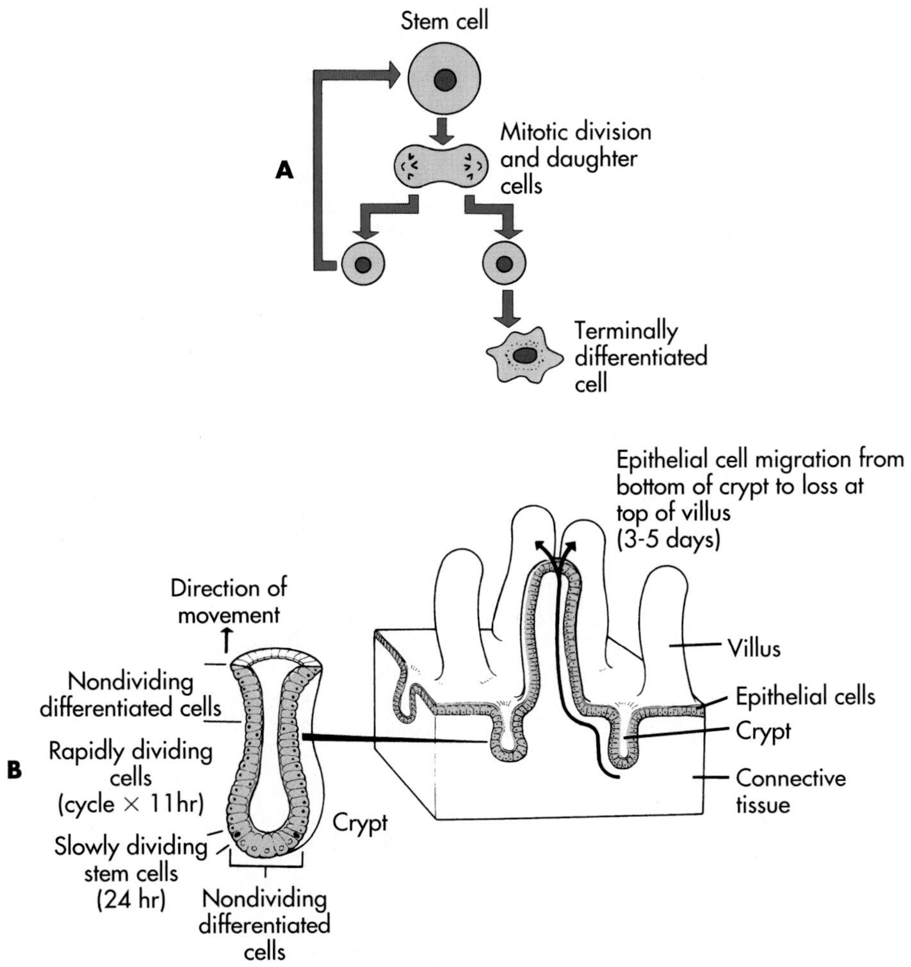

FIG. 10-7 Differentiation of a stem cell. **A,** When a stem cell divides, each daughter cell has a choice: it can either remain a stem cell or go on to become terminally differentiated. **B,** This pattern of cell renewal and proliferation of stem cells in the epithelium forms the lining of the small intestine.

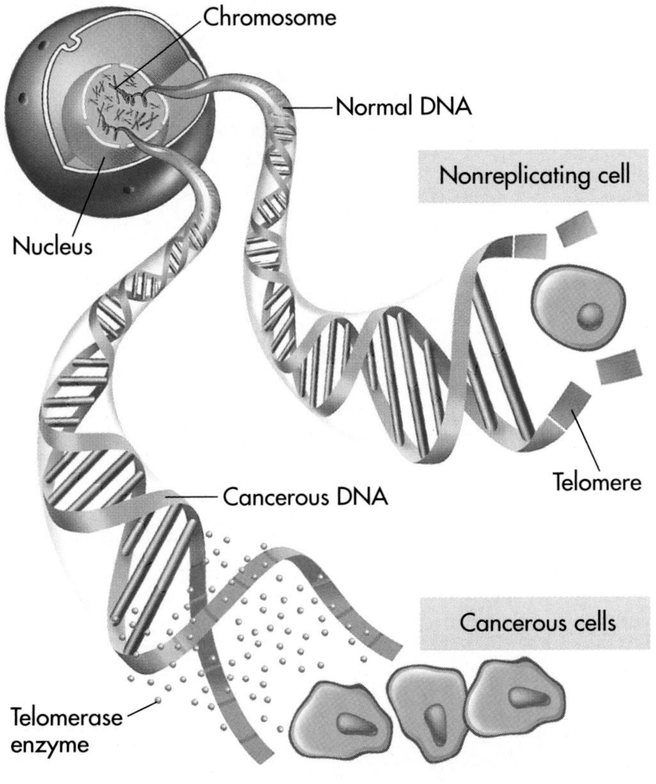

FIG. 10-8 Control of replication. Normal cells cannot divide indefinitely. The end of their chromosomes are controlled by telomeres. Telomeres get shorter with each division until the cells stop dividing. In cancer cells the telomerase gene is "switched on," producing an enzyme that rebuilds the telomeres. Thus the cancer cell continues to divide indefinitely.

Table 10-2 Nomenclature and Classification of Benign and Malignant Tumors*

Cell or Tissue of Origin	Benign Tumor	Malignant Tumor
TUMORS OF EPITHELIAL ORIGIN		
Squamous cells	Squamous cell papilloma	Squamous cell carcinoma
Basal cells	—	Basal cell carcinoma
Glandular or ductal epithelium	Adenoma	Adenocarcinoma
	Cystadenoma	Cystadenocarcinoma
Transitional cells	Transitional cell papilloma	Transitional cell carcinoma
Bile duct	Bile duct adenoma	Bile duct carcinoma (cholangiocarcinoma)
Liver cells	Hepatocellular adenoma	Hepatocellular carcinoma
Melanocytes	Nevus	Malignant melanoma
Renal epithelium	Renal tubular adenoma	Renal cell carcinoma
Skin adnexal glands		
Sweat glands	Sweat gland adenoma	Sweat gland carcinoma
Sebaceous glands	Sebaceous gland adenoma	Sebaceous gland carcinoma
Germ cells (testis and ovary)	—	Seminoma (dysgerminoma)
		Embryonal carcinoma, yolk sac carcinoma
TUMORS OF MESENCHYMAL ORIGIN		
Hematopoietic/lymphoid tissue		
Leukocytes		Leukemias
Granular leukocytes and precursors		Granulocytic leukemia
		Myelocytic leukemias
		Myelogenous leukemias
Plasma cells		Multiple myeloma
Lymphoid		
Nongranular leukocytes and prelymphocytes		Lymphomas
Proliferating lymphocytes and monocytes		Lymphocytic leukemia
Proliferating immature precursor monocytes		Lymphoblastic leukemia
Solid tumors of lymph tissue (thymus, spleen, lymph nodes)		Lymphoma
Neural and retinal tissue		
Nerve sheath	Neurilemoma, neurofibroma	Malignant peripheral nerve sheath tumor
Nerve cells	Ganglioneuroma	Neuroblastoma
Retinal cells (cones)	—	Retinoblastoma
Connective tissue		
Fibrous tissue	Fibromatosis (desmoid)	Fibrosarcoma
Fat	Lipoma	Liposarcoma
Bone	Osteoma	Osteogenic sarcoma
Cartilage	Chondroma	Chondrosarcoma
Muscle		
Smooth muscle	Leiomyoma	Leiomyosarcoma
Striated muscle	Rhabdomyoma	Rhobdomyosarcoma
Endothelial and related tissues		
Blood vessels	Hemangioma	Angiosarcoma
		Kaposi sarcoma
Lymph vessels	Lymphangioma	Lymphangiosarcoma
Synovium	—	Synovial sarcoma
Mesathelium	—	Malignant mesothelioma
Meninges	Meningioma	Malignant meningioma
TUMORS OF UNCERTAIN ORIGIN		
????	—	Ewing tumor

Modified from Murphy GP et al: *American Cancer Society's Textbook of clinical oncology,* ed 3, New York, 2000, American Cancer Society. Reprinted by permission of the American Cancer Society, Inc.

*This list is intended to provide only an introduction to tumor nomenclature.

enzyme telomerase is "turned on" to rebuild the telomere caps, allowing tumor cells to divide endlessly. The result is an immortal cancer cell.

Tumor Classification and Nomenclature

Tumors are classified on the basis of cell type, tissue of origin, whether benign or malignant, degree of differentiation (well, moderately, or poorly), anatomic site, and function. Tumors are named according to the tissues from which they arise, generally with the suffix "oma." Cancers include those of epithelial tissue (**carcinomas**); connective tissue (**sarcomas**); lymphatic tissue (**lymphomas**); glial cells of the central nervous system (**gliomas**); and blood-forming organs, primarily the bone marrow (**leukemias**). The leukemias usually involve an abnormal growth or proliferation of blood-forming cells that infiltrate and replace normal bone marrow and lymphatic tissue. Table 10-2 presents the nomenclature and classification of tumors.

Carcinoma in situ refers to preinvasive epithelial tumors of glandular or squamous cell origin. These tumors have not broken through the basement membrane of their epithelial site. Carcinoma in situ occurs in the cervix, skin, oral cavity, esophagus, and bronchus. In glandular epithelium, in situ lesions occur in the stomach, endometrium, breast, and large bowel. These lesions may erroneously be confused with benign tumors, but both the squamous and glandular cell types show disorganization and atypical changes of epithelium. The time that such lesions remain in situ before becoming invasive is unknown. Some carcinomas of the cervix are known to be preinvasive lesions in situ for several years before they progress to invasive carcinoma or metastatic tumors (see Fig. 10-18, *C*).

CHARACTERISTICS OF CANCER CELLS

Cancer cells differ according to the cell type from which they derive. To apply any definition to *all* cancer cells, however, would be presumptuous. Some tumors retain useful functions and closely mimic normal tissue, whereas others are so disorganized that the tissue of origin is unidentifiable. Cellular characteristics that are standard features of cancerous tissue include local increase in cell number, loss of normal arrangement of cells, variation of cell shape and size, increase in nuclear size and density of staining (reflects an increase in total DNA), increase in mitotic activity, and abnormal mitoses and chromosomes.

Cancer cells are disordered cells with pronounced cellular proliferation and great variation in size and shape. They divide in an uncoordinated fashion, invading and destroying neighboring tissue, a process termed **progression.** Progression is an increase of abnormal biologic properties and not necessarily a progression in tumor size. The biologic worsening is related to the tumor's malignant capabilities or its lack of differentiation. A cancer is therefore a delinquent cell mass. Disorganized cellular relationships are caused by differences between the cell-surface properties of normal and cancerous cells (Fig. 10-9).

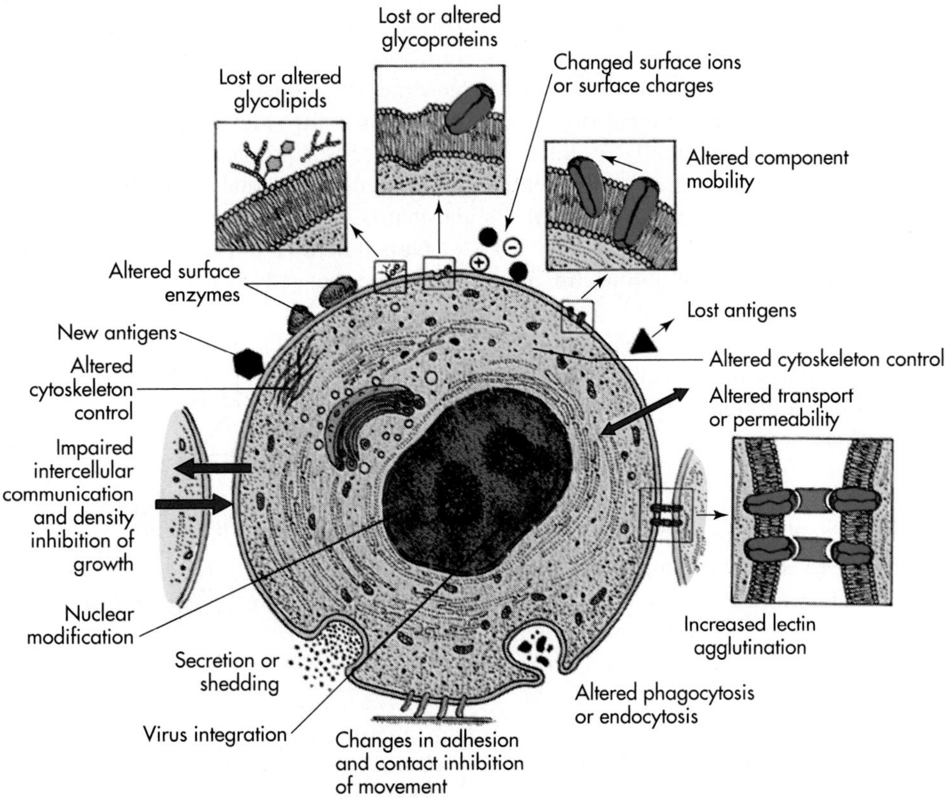

FIG. 10-9 Cell surface changes reported in cancer cells.

Cell-Surface Changes and Their Functional Importance

Glycolipids and Glycoproteins

In cancer cells, cell-surface glycoproteins and glycolipids are lost or modified. Overall, the protein content of the transformed cell is low and the glycolipid content of transformed cell membrane is reduced. Changes in one type of glycolipid, the *glycosphingolipids,* are related to a number of important features of the transformed cell. Glycosphingolipids, by interacting with receptor proteins, may decrease cell responsiveness to growth factors. Decreases or changes in glycosphingolipids may increase the cell's responsiveness to growth factors and promote cellular proliferation.[3]

The effect of glycoprotein and glycolipid changes may be to alter receptor density or configuration of the cell surface, resulting in decreased communication or signaling between cells. These changes may enhance the immune defense against cancer, because altered glycoproteins and glycolipids (as antigens) enable the cancer cells to be recognized by the immune system.[3]

Altered Membrane Transport or Permeability

Cancer cells exhibit a greater metabolic demand for certain substrates, so it seems consistent that they would have enhanced transport for sugars and certain amino acids. Among the most important cell surface changes is the *loss* of large glycoproteins now called **fibronectin,** found in the blood and on normal cell surfaces. Fibronectin is an anchoring molecule. Together with various proteoglycans (a family of protein-carbohydrate complexes), collagen, and elastin, fibronectin holds cells in place in tissue.[3] It is thought to hold receptor molecules in particular arrangements. Fibronectin also contributes to the internal organization of the cell (e.g., cytoskeleton), apparently by interacting with actin filaments and proteins that span the cell membrane. This interaction may contribute to the overall shape of the cell.[4]

Cancer cells may make a defective type of fibronectin, or they may break down fibronectin as they make it.[3] Low levels of fibronectin in cancer cells may cause changes in cellular organization, cell-to-cell adhesion, cellular migration, and cytoskeletal structure. Plasma fibronectin levels rise in the blood of individuals with cancer.

Protease

The sloughing of fibronectin could be caused by an increase in enzymes secreted by cancer cells that break up proteins or protease. Cancer cells secrete plasminogen-activating factor, which activates the inactive protease, plasminogen, into the active form, plasmin. Plasminogen activator may play a role in the degradation of the extracellular matrix during tumor cell invasion. Protease secretion or activation may be needed before the expression or phenotype of the malignant cell can be changed.[4]

Altered Anchoring Junctions and Gap Junctions

Anchoring junctions connect the cytoskeleton of a cell to its neighbor cell or to the extracellular matrix (a loose meshwork of large, extracellular organic molecules that bind cells together) (Fig. 10-10 and see Fig. 1-25). Anchoring junctions are abundant in cardiac muscle, skin epithelium, and the neck of the uterus—tissues that are subjected to severe mechanical stress. Anchoring junctions are classified as two structurally and functionally different types: (1) *adherens junctions* and (2) *desmosomes* and *hemidesmosomes* (see Fig. 1-25). They join the cytoskeleton filaments through intracellular attachment proteins and transmembrane glycoproteins. Normal cells presumably do not divide and proliferate unless they are anchored (see Fig. 10-10).

Cancer cells exhibit **anchorage independence.** Transformed cells have abnormal or decreased cell-cell and cell–extracellular matrix attachments. Without anchorage the transformed cell is allowed to **metastasize,** or grow in new environments. Unlike normal cells, tumor cells continue to divide when they are missing the necessary requirement for anchorage. Anchorage tends to inhibit, rather than to promote, the proliferation of transformed cells.[1] Cell division in normal cells is thought to occur when three things happen: (1) the cell is anchored to the extracellular matrix through anchoring junctions that enable the required cytoskeleton proteins to become organized inside the cell; (2) activation of this organized assembly occurs, typically by one or more growth factors, causing the release of an intracellular signal for cell division; and (3) as a necessary part of the process of releasing the signal, the cell-matrix attachments become partially disassembled.[1] Theoretically, in cancer cells, step 1 (anchorage to the extracellular matrix) is not required to generate the signal to proliferate. A theoretic model comparing anchorage and anchorage independence and proliferation of cells is presented in Fig. 10-11. It is not known why tumor cells fail to make firm attachments to the extracellular matrix.

Gap junctions are actually narrow gaps or channels between adjacent cells, allowing inorganic ions and small water-

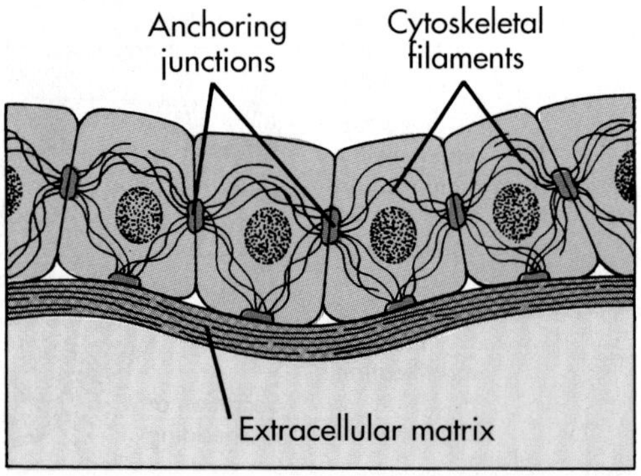

FIG. 10-10 Anchoring junctions. Schematized drawing of anchoring junctions joining cytoskeletal filaments from cell to cell or from cell to extracellular matrix.

soluble molecules to pass directly from the cytoplasm of one cell to the cytoplasm of the other (see Fig. 1-27). Gap junctions are important in regulating metabolic communication and cooperation among cells. Therefore altered gap-junctional intercellular communication (GJIC) may play an essential role in cancer development.[5,6] Evidence for this includes (1) inhibition of GJIC by tumor-causing agents or by activated oncogenes; (2) selective lack of GJIC between transforming and neighboring normal cells; and (3) decrease of GJIC within tumor or transformed cells.[7,8] Investigators have found that many tumor promoters, such as chemicals or growth factors, disrupt or block gap junction function. Further, tumor metastasis has been related to changes in intercellular communication—the more metastatic a tumor becomes, the greater the loss or decrease in intercellular communication.[9]

Tumor Cell Markers

Tumor cell markers are substances produced by cancer cells that are found on tumor plasma membranes or in the blood, spinal fluid, or urine (Table 10-3). Tumor cell markers (also called *biologic markers*) have been associated with cancer for many decades. They include hormones, enzymes, genes, antigens, and antibodies. Tumor cell markers, which vary with the degree of tumor progression, are produced by the cancer cell's genetic material when it is activated during carcinogenesis.

Tumor cell markers can be used in three ways: (1) to screen and identify individuals at high risk for cancer, (2) to help diagnose the specific type of tumor in individuals with clinical manifestations relating to cancer, and (3) to observe the clinical course of cancer. Because tumor markers rarely meet the criteria of specificity, sensitivity, predictability, and feasibility, there are no ideal tumor markers. Therefore tumor markers are known as *borderline* markers and are best used in determining the response to treatment.

A significant problem in diagnosis of cancer from tumor marker assays is that many nonmalignant diseases are associated with tumor markers. The presence of a tumor marker may increase the suggestion of cancer, but it is not used alone as a diagnostic test. The need for the identification of ideal tumor markers remains a high priority because improvement in cancer therapy will depend on earlier detection and tumor identification.

Hormones

Some tumors inappropriately produce hormones, such as adrenocorticotropic hormone (ACTH), insulin, human chorionic gonadotropin (hCG), parathyroid hormones, and erythropoietin. The term **ectopic hormone production** is used to describe the production of hormones by tumors of nonendocrine origin. Detection of certain tumors occurs through abnormally high serum levels of hormones and substrates produced in response to the hormone. hCG, for example, is one of the best clinical detectors or tumor markers. Ectopic ACTH production by certain types of tumors causes the increased adrenal secretion of cortisol.

Enzymes

Cancer causes two types of enzymatic abnormalities: (1) the expression of an immature or fetal form of an enzyme and (2) the ectopic production of enzymes. Of clinical interest

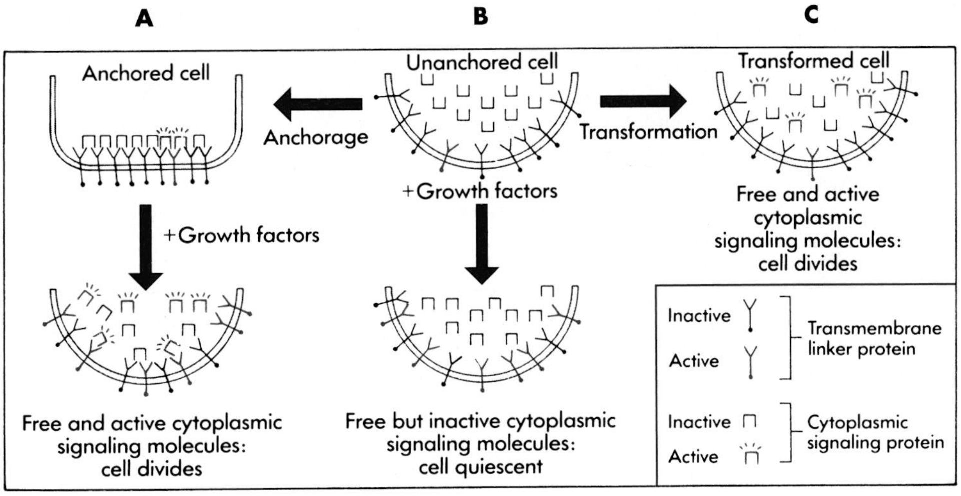

FIG. 10-11 Comparison of normal cell division and proliferation and that of a cancer cell. A hypothetical drawing comparing the normal process of cell division and proliferation (e.g., anchorage, activation of the cell through growth factors to release an intracellular signal for cell division) with that of a cancer cell. **A,** When an anchored cell (normal cell) is stimulated by growth factors, the signaling molecules are "turned on," signaling the cell to divide and weakening the extracellular adhesion so the cell can proliferate. **B,** Normal cells in suspension fail to divide in response to growth factors because very few of the intracellular signaling molecules are bound to the transmembrane protein, allowing them to be turned on. **C,** Cancer cells have reduced adherence and can divide even in suspension because somehow the signaling molecules can turn on the transmembrane proteins.

Table 10-3 Tumor Cell Markers: Selected Examples

Marker	Tumor
Cytology	Aspirates, exudates, urine, brushings (all types)
Antigens	
Carcinoembryonic antigen	Many solid tumors
α-Fetoprotein	Liver, ovary, testis
CA 19-9	Pancreatic or hepatobiliary for staging breast cancer
CA 27-29	
CA 15-3	
Prostate-specific antigen	Prostate
Human chorionic gonadotropin	Ovary
Tumor-specific cell-mediated reactions	
Cytotoxicity tests	Many solid tumors
Delayed hypersensitivity reaction to tumor extracts	Many solid tumors
Ectopic hormones	
Human chorionic gonadotropin	Many tumors
Parathormone	Kidney, lung
Adrenocorticotropic hormone	Lung
Antidiuretic hormone	Lung
Melanin-stimulating hormone	Lung
Thyroid-stimulating hormone	Placenta (choriocarcinoma)
Insulin	Lung
Isoenzymes	
Acid phosphatase	Carcinoma of prostate; breast cancer
Placental alkaline phosphatase	Choriocarcinoma; carcinomas of ovary, pancreas, colon, breast, uterus, bronchus; testicular cancers; reticulum cell sarcoma; Hodgkin disease; multiple myeloma
Nonplacental alkaline phosphatase	Osteogenic sarcoma; parathyroid carcinoma; cancers metastatic to bone from prostate, breast, multiple myeloma, infiltrative cancers of liver, leukemia, reticulum cell sarcoma
Galactosyl transferase	Carcinomas of lung, breast, esophagus, stomach, pancreas, colon, gallbladder; chronic lymphocytic leukemia
Aminopeptidases	Carcinomas of pancreas, liver, stomach lining; carcinoma metastatic to liver
γ-Glutamyl transpeptidase	Carcinomas metastatic to liver
Ribonuclease	Carcinoma of pancreas
Sialyltransferase	Carcinomas of breast, colon, lung, prostate; leiomyosarcoma; leukemia; lymphoma; melanoma
Elevated normal substances	
Immunoglobulins	Multiple myeloma
Insulin	Islet cell tumors
Serotonin	Carcinoid tumors
Parathormone	Parathyroid tumors
Prolactin	Pituitary tumors
Gastrin	Islet cell tumors
Human chorionic gonadotropin	Choriocarcinoma
Calcium	Medullary carcinoma (thyroid), parathyroid tumors
Genes*	Various tumors
Radiographic mammographic density	Breast cancer

Data from King DW, Fenoglio CM, Lefkowitz JH: *General pathology: principles and dynamics,* Philadelphia, 1983, Lea & Febiger; Pagana KD, Pagana TJ: *Mosby's manual of diagnostic and laboratory tests,* St Louis, 1998, Mosby.

*Additional markers include chromosomes and oncogenes (e.g., DNA-binding proteins *c-myc, -myb, -fos*).

are isoenzymes (variable forms of an enzyme). Table 10-3 gives a partial listing of cancer-related isoenzymes.

Extensive research on enzymes and isoenzymes in cancer has clearly shown that cancers do not produce new or unique enzymes. The enzymes or isoenzymes found normally are produced by the noncancerous tissue from which the cancer arises. The tumor may cause the production of enzymes in different or abnormal proportions; however, decreases and increases in enzymes within a given cell type are associated with cancer. These enzyme changes occur mainly within the tumor itself and, unfortunately, are expressed in the circulation only when the tumor is very large or widespread metastases have occurred.[10]

Genes

Technologic advances have enabled researchers to search for tumor markers, such as chromosomes and oncogenes, inside the cell. The Philadelphia chromosome (Ph^1) was the first chromosome marker identified. Because the Ph^1 is present in 95% of individuals with chronic myelocytic leukemia, it is used to establish the diagnosis of the disease.

Oncogene probes and other technologies have enabled researchers to identify more than 20 oncogenes, including the phosphokinases (c-*src, -fps, -yes, -ros*); DNA-binding proteins (c-*myc, -myb, -fos*); and cellular growth factors (e.g., c-*sis*). The search for additional oncogenes is continuing.

Antigens

Cancer cells express "nonself" antigens. Some of these are antigens of tumor-inducing viruses. Others are simply *neo*-antigens *(new)* associated with the cell's transformed state. Although evidence for the existence of unique tumor-*specific* antigens capable of causing tumor rejection in human tumors is weak, human tumors do exhibit tumor-*associated* neoantigens. Many of these antigens normally appear only during embryonic development. In tumors, such antigens are apparently expressed as a result of the reactivation of genes turned off at the end of fetal development. (See p. 323 for a complete discussion of tumor antigens.)

Antibodies

The development of monoclonal antibody (MAb) technology has made antibodies one of the most interesting and potentially rewarding categories of tumor markers. Monoclonal antibody technology produces hybrid cells (i.e., a cancerous cell is fused with an antibody-producing cell to form a hybridoma) that can secrete an antibody to a specific tumor antigen.

Intercellular Changes in Cancer Cells

Cytoskeleton

The "bones and muscles" of the cell constitute the *cytoskeleton.* The cytoskeleton maintains the cell's shape and internal organization, permits the movement of substances within the cell, and permits movement of external projections (cilia or microvilli) from the plasma membrane. The internal skeleton is composed of a network of protein filaments, two of the most important of which are microtubules and actin filaments (microfilaments) (see Fig. 1-9). Microfilaments and microtubules are not well organized in cancer cells or in normal cells during division.

In normal cells, bundles of actin filaments bind to the plasma membrane in a way that allows the filaments to pull on the extracellular matrix—at sites called *focal contacts* or adhesion plaques—or to another cell.[1] Stable arrangements of actin filaments give rise to persistent structures. In cancer cells, focal contacts are disrupted, causing diminished adhesion to extracellular surfaces and forcing the cell to assume a rounded appearance. The cell "rounds up," just as a normal cell does during mitosis.

Microtubules control cell shape, cell locomotion, and cellular division. While the cell is not in the process of division, only a few microtubules are assembled. During cellular division (mitosis) or defense (phagocytosis), microtubules assemble and disassemble rapidly. Antimitotic drugs, such as vinblastine and vincristine, disrupt microtubular function preferentially, killing many rapidly dividing cells. The specific role that microtubules play in cancer cell mobility remains a controversial topic.

Density-Dependent Inhibition of Growth

In the laboratory, when two or more normal cells grown in a single-layer culture come in contact with each other, they tend to stop dividing (proliferating) and form a single layer or sheet of cells called a *confluent monolayer.* The cells do not pile up on one another. This phenomenon is known as **density-dependent inhibition of growth.** Cancer cells, however, usually continue to grow and pile up on top of one another after they have formed a confluent monolayer.

Such phenomena originally were described in terms of "contact inhibition of cell division"; this description is now thought to be misleading. This lack of density-dependent inhibition of growth may be the result of two independent properties: mobility and the amount of growth factors in the medium.[5,11] Thus it is not just the coming in contact with each other that prevents cell proliferation. The old confusing term *contact inhibition of cell division* has now been replaced by *density-dependent inhibition of growth. Contact inhibition of movement,* another confusing term, is an important feature of wound healing in animals. Sheets of epithelial cells at the margin of a wound move rapidly out over the wounded area and cease movement when the cells contact each other across the gap created by the wound.[1]

Transformed cells are more mobile and do not adhere to other cells as well as do normal cells. This property is related to changes in the plasma membrane of the transformed cells, as well as to alteration in the cytoskeleton. Normal cells form tight junctions and other areas of close contact with cells of their own type; transformed cells do not.

Growth Requirements: Inducers of Differentiation

The proliferation of cells is governed by specific combinations of protein growth factors (see Chapter 1). Growth factors act at very low concentrations, most as local chemical mediators—initiators and inhibitors—to help regulate cell population densities. Cancer may result when these factors become unbalanced, when cells cannot respond to growth-suppressor factors, or when cells are chronically stimulated.

Positive and negative regulatory factors that work only in certain types of cells are being identified. Transforming growth factor–β (TGF-β) inhibits the growth of most cells but stimulates fibroblasts, chemotaxis, and the production of collagen and fibronectin by cells. Inhibition occurs because the growth factor "turns off" genes (e.g., that produce platelet-derived growth factor receptors). Other agents known to inhibit growth include interferon-β and tumor necrosis factor. (Cytokines are discussed in Chapter 6). Examples of growth factors and their physiologic actions are presented in Table 1-4 in Chapter 1.

Sachs[12] and others have isolated and characterized both growth inducers and differentiation inducers and have found the following:

1. Growth inducers and differentiation inducers are *different* proteins. Differentiation inducers inhibit growth, and growth inducers cannot cause stem cell progeny to mature.
2. Different growth inducers stimulate cells at different stages of differentiation to produce different inducers of differentiation at different times.

Thus the result is variable numbers of different *types* of differentiated cells derived from the same stem cell type. Because terminally differentiated cells usually no longer divide, differentiation must ultimately neutralize growth inducers. Investigators suggest that whereas normal cells depend on other cells for growth inducer, either cancer cells need little or no growth inducers or they make their own.[13]

Autocrine Stimulation Hypothesis

Transformed cells become independent of growth factors by producing their own growth factors by *autocrine secretion.* (Chemical signaling is discussed in Chapter 1). Malignant and transformed cells have surface receptors for growth factors, as well as the ability to release growth factors. This discovery led to the hypothesis of **autostimulation,** or the **autocrine stimulatory hypothesis,** of cancer. Several mechanisms are proposed by which transformed and malignant cells become *autonomous* with respect to growth factors, including (1) manufacture by transformed cells of their own growth factors; (2) reduction in the amount of growth factor necessary for division; (3) defects of the growth factor receptor on the plasma membrane; and (4) alteration of the receptor signal pathway for second messengers.[13,14] Chapter 1 describes how growth factor binding to membrane receptors initiates a cascade of metabolic events leading to cell division.

All this evidence suggests that the normal processes of cell division and cell differentiation are driven and guided by growth factors and that the cancer cell produces its own growth factor. Growth factors are produced by a highly organized sequence of gene activation and gene suppression. Unraveling these complex genetic sequences may lead to enormous breakthroughs in cancer therapy.

Transformed cells commonly have a complex syndrome of abnormalities. These abnormalities and their functional significance are summarized in Tables 10-4 and 10-5.

Changes in the Nucleus and Cell Protein

The nuclei of malignant cells are often *pleomorphic,* that is, enlarged and variably shaped. Chromatin may clump along the periphery of the nucleus. Alterations include nuclear membrane projections, pockets, blebbing, and fewer nuclear pores, which are associated with DNA replication sites. The rate of mitosis frequently is increased in cancerous tissues. Changes in chromosomes include breaks, deletions, ring forms, and abnormal chromosome karyotypes. For example, frequent changes are reported in chromosomes 1 and 17 in a number of hematologic cancers. A change in chromosome 22 (the Philadelphia chromosome), whereby the long arm is translocated to chromosome 9, is well known in chronic myelocytic leukemia (see Chapter 26).

Other genetic changes are phenotypic, or "translated and transcribed" into protein. Transfer RNA, for example, may have too few or too many methyl groups (CH_3) attached. Proteins that regulate genes and enzymes involved in nucleic acid synthesis may exhibit phenotypic changes, all of which are potential expressions of the malignant state. Although the total significance of phenotypic changes is unknown, pathologists rely on them, along with functional and growth-requirement changes, to identify the transformed state and diagnose cancer. The evidence is strong that phenotypic and other changes result from a defect in the genetic information of the cell.

Table 10-4 Comparison of Normal and Tumor Cells: Cellular Changes Commonly Observed

Growth Characteristics	Normal Cells	Tumor Cells
Density-dependent inhibition of growth	Present	Absent
Growth factor requirements	High	Low
Anchorage dependence	Present	Absent
Proliferative life span	Finite	Indefinite
Adhesiveness	High	Low
Morphology	Flat	Rounded; various shapes; abnormal change
Fibronectin	Present	Reduced
Plasminogen activator	Present	Increased

Table 10-5 Functional Significance of Cellular Changes in Tumor Cells

Change	Functional Significance
Decreased adhesion Disorganized actin filaments (cytoskeleton) Reduced fibronectin Increased production of plasminogen activator	Decreased cell-to-cell adherence, therefore a rounded morphology; increased plasminogen activation, therefore increased extracellular proteolysis
Indefinite proliferative life span Lowered requirement for growth factors Less anchorage dependence Density-dependent inhibition of growth	Abnormalities of growth and mitotic division; increased potential for invasion and metastasis

CAUSES OF CANCER: GENETICS AND CANCER FAMILIES

Is cancer genetic? Does our genetic inheritance *determine* our susceptibility to certain cancers? The answer is yes and no! The genetics of cancer is complex. In attempts to understand the genetics of cancer, researchers study inheritance patterns from one generation to the next (family studies), chromosomes, mutations, and the effects of life-style and environmental agents.

Gene-Environment Interaction

The causes of "common" cancers include environmental factors. Reportedly, environmental agents cause cancer by increasing the frequency of mutations in somatic cells.[15] Most carcinogens are **mutagens,** that is, chemicals that increase the frequency of mutations (see Chapter 4).

Two lines of evidence support the idea that exposure to environmental agents can increase an individual's risk of cancer. The first is based on the identification of environmental agents that have carcinogenic properties.[15] Evidence from both epidemiologic and laboratory studies, for example, shows that cigarette smoke causes lung cancer. Environmental agents, such as chemical carcinogens, x-rays, and ultraviolet radiation, can cause certain types of cancer.

The second line of evidence is based on comparisons of populations with different life-styles. Breast cancer, for example, is prevalent among northern Europeans and Americans but relatively rare among women in Japan. The difficulty lies in determining whether these differences between populations are attributable to life-style factors, to genetics, or to both. The influence of environmental agents was demonstrated in studies of Japanese who emigrated to Hawaii and the U.S. mainland. Researchers studied the changes in incidence of colon and stomach cancer after emigration. In Japan colon cancer is a rare form of cancer. Among the first Japanese emigrants (first generation) in Hawaii, colon cancer incidence rose severalfold but not as high as the overall incidence on the U.S. mainland. Among second-generation Japanese on the U.S. mainland, colon cancer rates rose to the U.S. average. Conversely, stomach cancer is common in Japan but relatively rare in the United States. Japanese on the U.S. mainland have the same low incidence of stomach cancer as the U.S. average. Although these observations implicate environment and life-style in the cause of colon and stomach cancer, they do not rule out genetic factors. The difference in incidence rates could be the result of predisposing genes. One could argue that these genes are less penetrating for colon cancer in Japan because of environmental differences.[15,16]

Inherited Cancer Genes

Most human cancers appear to arise spontaneously, developing without any known prior exposure to a carcinogenic agent. To explain how these neoplasms arise, it was proposed that cancer is caused by genetic factors. It now is known that certain forms of cancer oncogenes (cancer-causing genes) can be introduced into the individual or inherited within some families.

A primary basis of carcinogenesis is damage (mutation) to specific genes. If the genetic events occur in somatic cells, they *are not* inherited by future generations. However, if mutations occur in germline cells, inheritance can occur in cancer-causing genes from one generation to the next (Fig. 10-12). This type of vertical transmission produces families that have a high frequency of specific cancers (Fig. 10-13). In these "cancer families," inheritance of one mutant allele, although rare, seems sufficient to cause a specific form of cancer; almost all individuals who inherit the mutant allele will develop the tumor.[15]

Examples of inherited human cancers include retinoblastoma, a childhood cancer of the eye; Wilms tumor, a childhood cancer of the kidney; neurofibromatosis, fibrosarcomas of nerves; familial breast cancer; and familial polyposis coli, adenomas of the colon. A specific oncogene has been isolated for each of these cancers. Characterization of oncogenes and other genetic risk factors helps to identify individuals who are at risk to develop cancer.[15,17] Early cancer detection and therapy result in better prognoses for at-risk individuals.

Oncogenic Viruses

Viruses were first isolated from certain types of tumors in the early 1900s. These viruses caused cancers when transferred into normal healthy animals. A number of **oncogenic viruses** (cancer-causing viruses) have been isolated, including several associated with human cancers. These oncogenic viruses are true pathogenic agents because they cause a specific type

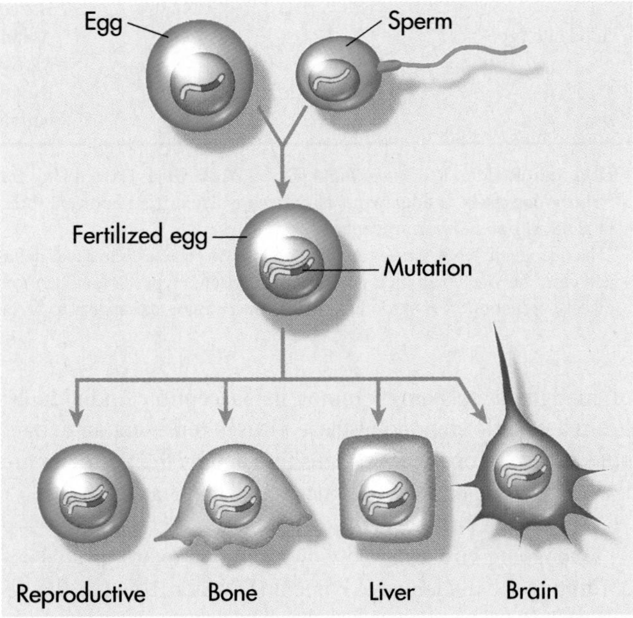

FIG. 10-12 Germline mutation. Inherited mutations are carried in the DNA of reproductive cells. When reproductive cells containing mutations combine to produce offspring, the mutation will be present in *all* the offspring's body cells. (Modified from Lea DH, Jenkins JF, Francomano CA: *Genetics in clinical practice,* Boston, 1998, Bartlett.)

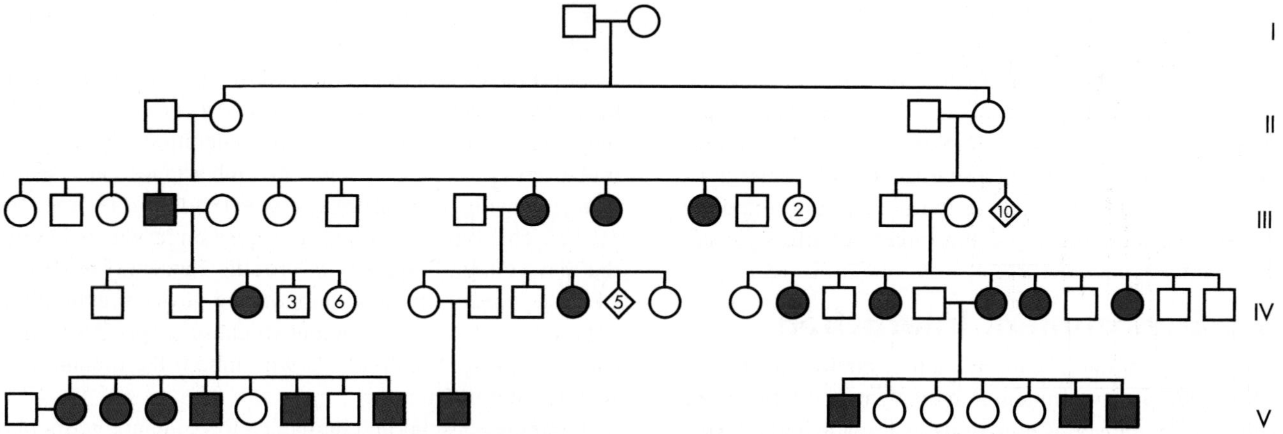

FIG. 10-13 A familial colon cancer pedigree. Darkened symbols represent individuals diagnosed with cancer. (From Jorde LB, Carey JC, White RL: *Medical genetics,* ed 2, St Louis, 1999, Mosby.)

Table 10-6 Classification and Examples of Oncogenic Viruses

Viral Class	Virus	Species of Isolation
ONCOGENIC DNA VIRUSES		
Papovaviruses	Papilloma	Rabbit, human, others
	Polyoma	Mouse
	SV 40	Monkey
Adenoviruses*	Adenovirus 12	Human
Herpesviruses	Epstein-Barr	Human
	Frog herpesvirus	Frog
	Marek disease	Chicken
Hepadenoviruses	Hepatitis B	Human
	Hepatitis C	Human
ONCOGENIC RNA VIRUSES†		
Acute-acting type	Rous sarcoma	Chicken
	Maloney sarcoma	Mouse
	Harvey/Kirsten sarcoma	Rat
Subacute type	Avian leukosis	Chicken
	Mouse mammary tumor	Mouse
	Bovine leukemia	Cow
	Human T leukemia/lymphoma virus	Human

Data from Ruddon R: *Cancer biology,* New York, 1981, Oxford University Press.

*Thirty-one types of adenovirus have been isolated from humans; three of these (types 12, 18, and 31) are highly oncogenic when inoculated into newborn rodents.

†The oncogenic RNA viruses are divided into two classes; the acute-acting types transform cells in vitro, induce rapid disease in vivo, and carry oncogenes in their genome; the subacute types do not cause cell transformation in vitro, have long latency periods for disease induction in vivo, do not possess oncogenes, and appear to be horizontally transmitted.

of malignant or benign tumor in susceptible individuals. From a genetic standpoint these viruses represent an exogenous source of oncogenes. Cells infected by these viruses are transformed when the viral oncogene is activated.

Classification

Oncogenic viruses are divided into two major groups according to the nucleic acid content (DNA or RNA) of the viral particle (Table 10-6). The three main types of oncogenic DNA viruses are papovaviruses, adenoviruses, and herpesviruses. DNA viruses penetrate host cells by the action of their coat proteins. Inside the cell the viral DNA is uncoated and enters the cell's nucleus, where it is inserted (integrated) into the host's DNA. The integrated viral DNA then is transcribed to two "waves" to produce early and late messenger RNAs (mRNAs are described in Chapter 4). Early mRNAs encode for viral proteins that are involved in the replication of the viral DNA. Late mRNAs are transcribed after viral DNA replication and encode for the viral structural proteins. (Viral replication is discussed in Chapter 8, and RNA transcription is discussed in Chapter 4.)

Oncogenic DNA viruses cause tumors in a variety of tissues of different animals. Cancer of the cervix and hepatocellular carcinoma account for about 80% of virus-linked cancer. Hepatitis B virus infection is considered a high-risk factor for hepatocellular carcinoma. In immune-suppressed individuals, Epstein-Barr virus is the causative agent of

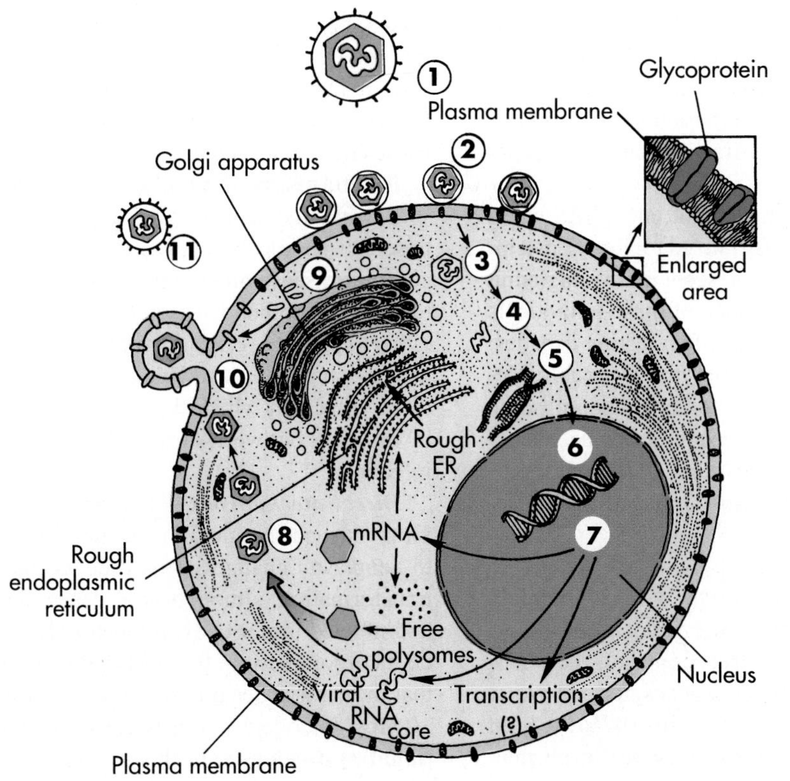

1 Oncogenic retrovirus

2 Absorption—virus binds to cell surface

3 Penetration—virus enters cytoplasm

4 Eclipse—viral RNA freed from core (uncoat)

5 Reverse transcriptase—viral RNA to viral DNA

6 Viral DNA incorporated into host DNA

7 Transcription of host DNA—virus replication
  a. Transcribed v-onc causes transformation
  b. Viral mRNA released to cytoplasm: core protein translated on free polysomes and coat proteins processed on rough endoplasmic reticulum and Golgi apparatus

8 Maturation—core and capsid are assembled in cytoplasm

9 Coat proteins are inserted into plasma membrane

10 Release—virus cores bind to coat proteins and "bud" from cell surface

11 Infectious virus particles

FIG. 10-14 Stages of oncogenic ribonucleic acid (RNA) viral infection. *DNA,* deoxyribonucleic acid; *ER,* endoplasmic reticulum.

Burkitt lymphoma, nasopharyngeal cancer, and B cell lymphoma. Sixty different substrains of human papillomavirus (HPV) have been isolated from benign and malignant human tumors. Certain strains of HPV cause warts, which are benign tumors of the skin, anus, and genitalia. Other strains of HPV cause anogenital carcinoma, oral carcinoma, laryngeal carcinoma, nasal and paranasal carcinomas, as well as conjunctival carcinoma. Except in individuals with the rare disease epidermodysplasia verruciformis, evidence is lacking that HPVs play a role in the induction of either squamous cell carcinoma or melanoma of the skin.[18]

Two other types of viruses have been implicated as causing cancers. These are human immunodeficiency virus (HIV) and the herpes simplex viruses (HSVs). HIV is the causative agent of acquired immunodeficiency syndrome (AIDS), a disease associated with a high incidence of B cell lymphoma and Kaposi sarcoma, a rare form of blood vessel cancer in the skin. HSVs are associated with anogenital and oral cancers. It appears, however, that neither HIV nor HSV is *directly* involved in the development of human cancers.[19]

Retroviruses, a type of RNA virus, contain a unique enzyme, **reverse transcriptase.** This enzyme is required for successful infection by the virus. Before viral replication can occur in the host cell, the viral genome (all the genetic information of the virus) must be transcribed from viral RNA to viral DNA by the reverse transcriptase enzyme (Fig. 10-14). Once the viral genome has been transcribed to viral DNA, it can be integrated into the host's DNA, where it is transcribed and replicated by the host's genetic machinery. Human T cell leukemia-lymphoma virus (HTLV) is an oncogenic retrovirus that is critical for development and progression of adult T cell leukemia-lymphoma (ATLL). HTLV is transmitted both vertically (i.e., inherited by children from infected parents) and horizontally (by breast-feeding, sexual intercourse, blood transfusions, and exposure to infected needles).

Infection by an oncogenic virus is not enough to cause cancer. For example, in some industrialized regions, Epstein-Barr virus can infect 90% of the adolescent and young adult population. Yet only a small percentage of these individuals develop cancer. Long latency periods, often lasting decades; the low number of infected individuals that eventually develop cancer; monoclonality of the tumors; and in some cases exposure to other carcinogenic or promoting agents before the appearance of cancer suggest that additional modifications are required to cause a virally infected cell to develop a malignant phenotype.

Oncogenes

In addition to the genes required by the virus to maintain its integrity as an infectious agent (i.e., virus core proteins, envelope glycoproteins, or reverse transcriptase), the oncogenic virus also possesses specific oncogenes, termed **v-*onc*** (identifying them as viral oncogenes). In 1976 Stehelin showed that cellular oncogenes (termed **c-*onc***) in normal, nontransformed chicken cells and v-*onc* of the avian sarcoma virus had virtually identical nucleic acid sequences. It is now known that cellular oncogenes, c-*onc,* are incorporated into the genomes of various organisms, including humans. Because normal, nontransformed cells carry c-*onc,* a number of conclusions have been drawn concerning the origin and function of these genes.

First, the existence of these c-*onc* throughout evolution in various, unrelated animal species suggests they play an important role in the normal function of the cell. The term *proto-oncogene* sometimes is used to refer collectively to the various c-*onc*. The term *proto-oncogene* also indicates that c-*onc* and v-*onc* genes were probably derived from a common prototype gene. Proto-oncogenes encode for growth factors, growth factor receptors, signal transducers, and nuclear proteins (Table 10-7). Therefore proto-oncogenes both are normal genetic components of the cell and encode for viral products or activities required for cell growth and differentiation. Many viral oncogenes may originate from normal cellular DNA sequences.

Second, some viruses, especially the retroviruses, can incorporate infected host cell genes into their viral genome during their replication process. This explains how oncogenic viruses obtained their proto-oncogenes. Although this suggests the origin of v-*onc,* it does not explain how these viruses transform cells into cancers.

Much research has been directed toward understanding the mechanism or mechanisms by which oncogenic viruses are able to cause cell transformation, leading to the oncogene hypothesis. This hypothesis states that virtually all cells possess oncogenes. Because these c-*onc* are similar to the v-*onc* carried by oncogenic viruses, their activation during viral infections leads to transformation of the cell, which can result in neoplastic cells that are able to form benign or malignant tumors. How oncogenes are activated in normal cells or their role in maintaining the transformed cell phenotype is unknown. Possible mechanisms by which activated oncogenes cause and sustain cell transformation are shown in Fig. 10-15.

Mechanisms of Viral Carcinogenesis

Several mechanisms for viral carcinogenesis are proposed. It should be appreciated, however, that cancer is a complex disease process that can involve a multitude of factors. As with other diseases, the pathogenic agents may have either (1) a direct effect, in which the tumor cells are or were at some stage infected with the oncogenic virus; or (2) an indirect effect, in which the neoplastic cells were not altered by the virus but were stimulated to grow because of the viral infection.

Direct mechanisms. During the infection process the virus may cause mutations in surviving cells that could lead to neoplastic changes. This process may not cause cellular transformation, although viral genes may persist within the noninfected tumor cells. Interestingly, viral genes appear to be incorporated into the host genome randomly, suggesting that the viral genes do not cause transformation directly.

Most oncogenic viruses cause transformation by **insertional mutagenesis.** In this process, the viral genes are incorporated into the host's genome at specific sites. Insertion of the v-*onc* within the host genome can lead to activation of the v-*onc* or c-*onc* genes that are associated with cell transformation. These inserted genes become an inherited trait of all the cancer cells derived from the original transformed cell.

Indirect mechanisms. Because viral infections lead to tissue damage, there is a burst of cell proliferations in the

Table 10-7 Examples of Proto-oncogenes

Oncogene	Chromosome Location	Biologic Function
GROWTH FACTORS		
hst-1	11q13	Heparin-binding growth factor
sis	22q12-q13	Platelet-derived growth factor (PDGF)
GROWTH FACTOR RECEPTORS		
erb A	17q11	Thyroid hormone receptor
src	20q11	Tyrosine protein kinase
raf-1	3p25	Cytoplasmic serine kinase
SIGNAL TRANSDUCTION PROTEINS		
H-*ras*	11p15	Guanosine triphosphate (GTP) binding protein
abl	9q34	Protein kinase
NUCLEAR DNA BINDING PROTEINS		
myb	6q22	Binds DNA
fos	14q24-q31	Interacts with *jun* proto-oncogene to regulate transcription
myc	8q24	Binds DNA

Modified from Jorde LB, Carey JC, White RL: *Medical genetics,* ed 2, St Louis, 1999, Mosby.

damaged tissue after the infection subsides that is associated with the normal repair and healing processes. Actively dividing cells are known to be at higher risk of mutation than resting cells. As a result, these cells are more susceptible to both spontaneous mutagenesis and transformation by a physical or chemical carcinogen. Alternatively, during some viral infections, the host's immune system can become compromised. This reduced immunologic protection can allow neoplastic cells to emerge that would normally be rejected by the host. The role of the immune system in cancer is discussed in

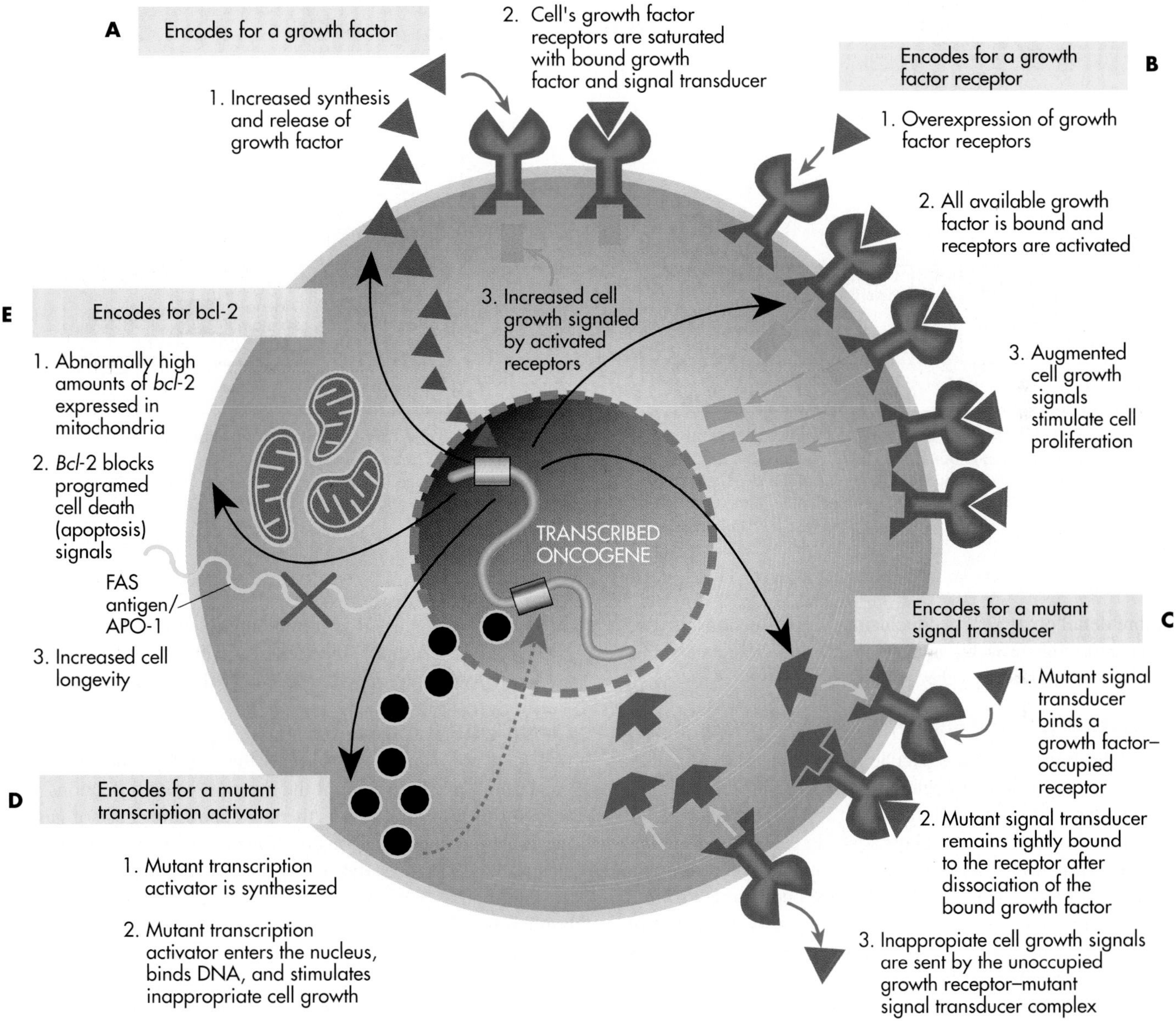
A
Encodes for a growth factor
1. Increased synthesis and release of growth factor
2. Cell's growth factor receptors are saturated with bound growth factor and signal transducer
3. Increased cell growth signaled by activated receptors
B
Encodes for a growth factor receptor
1. Overexpression of growth factor receptors
2. All available growth factor is bound and receptors are activated
3. Augmented cell growth signals stimulate cell proliferation
E
Encodes for bcl-2
1. Abnormally high amounts of bcl-2 expressed in mitochondria
2. Bcl-2 blocks programed cell death (apoptosis) signals
FAS antigen/ APO-1
3. Increased cell longevity
TRANSCRIBED ONCOGENE
C
Encodes for a mutant signal transducer
1. Mutant signal transducer binds a growth factor–occupied receptor
2. Mutant signal transducer remains tightly bound to the receptor after dissociation of the bound growth factor
3. Inappropiate cell growth signals are sent by the unoccupied growth receptor–mutant signal transducer complex
D
Encodes for a mutant transcription activator
1. Mutant transcription activator is synthesized
2. Mutant transcription activator enters the nucleus, binds DNA, and stimulates inappropriate cell growth

FIG. 10-15 Abnormal growth signaling regulated by activated oncogenes underlies neoplastic transformation. Five main oncogene-regulated (either activated c-*onc* or integrated v-*onc*) cell growth–signaling mechanisms induce and sustain the transformed phenotype of neoplastic cells. **A,** The activated oncogene (e.g., *Sis* and *int*-2) encodes for a cell growth factor that is *(1)* synthesized and released in abnormally high amounts. Because of *(2)* excess growth factor availability, the cell's growth factor receptors become saturated with bound growth factor and signal transducer. The growth factor receptors *(3)* remain occupied and activated, sending an augmented signal for stimulated cell growth. **B,** The activated oncogene (e.g., *Erb* a, *erb* b) encodes for a cell growth factor that is *(1)* expressed in abnormally high levels on the cell surface. Because of the high receptor levels *(2)* all available growth factor is bound and the receptor is activated *(3)* sending an augmented cell growth signal. **C,** The activated oncogene (e.g., *Ras*) encodes for *(1)* a mutant signal transducer protein that tightly binds to occupied growth factor receptors. The mutant signal transducer *(2)* remains bound to the receptor even after release of the growth factor from its receptor and *(3)* continues to send a cell growth signal. **D,** The activated oncogene (e.g., *Myc*) encodes for *(1)* a gene transcription activator that *(2)* binds to the DNA promoter region of a gene that stimulates cell growth. **E,** The activated oncogene *(1)* encodes for the *bcl*-2 protein that *(2)* blocks the normal fas antigen/apo-1 mediated signals that induce programmed cell death (apoptosis). Cells that are resistant to normal signals for apoptosis *(3)* have increased longevity and do not respond to the normal signals that drive cell differentiation.

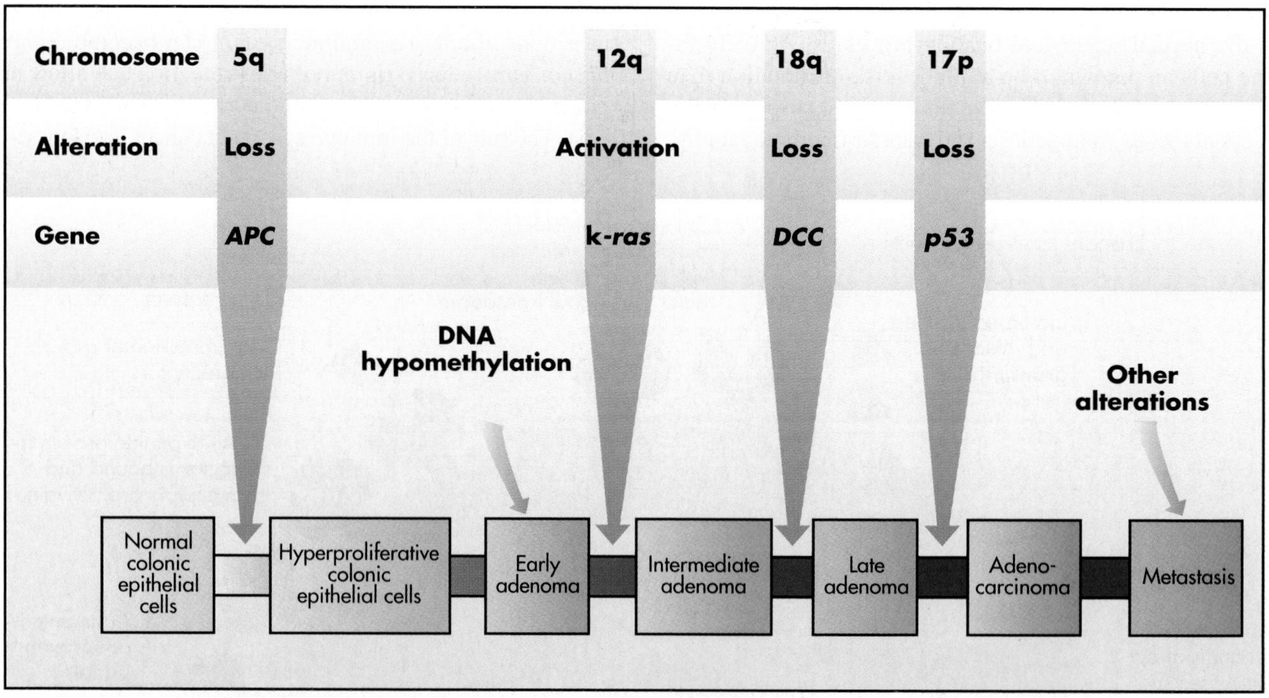

FIG. 10-16 The pathway to colon cancer. Loss of the *apc* (adenomatous polyposis coli) gene transforms normal epithelial tissue lining the gut to hyperproliferating tissue. Hypomethylation of deoxyribonucleic acid (DNA), activation of the k-*ras* proto-oncogene, and loss of the *dcc* (deleted in colon cancer) gene are involved in the progression to a benign adenoma. Loss of the *p53* gene and other alterations are involved in the progression to malignant carcinoma and metastasis. (From Jorde LB, Carey JC, White RL: *Medical genetics,* ed 2, St Louis, 1999, Mosby.)

more detail on p. 322. In conclusion, viral infections may affect carcinogenesis by increasing the individual's risk for neoplasia induced by other means.

Tumor Suppressor Genes

By definition, oncogenes encode for proteins that cause cancer. Because most of the oncogene-derived proteins are cell growth and differentiation factors, it is thought that their unregulated overexpression plays a role in cell transformation. Thus an imbalance in positive growth signals received by the cell causes it to assume the transformed phenotype. Proliferation of normal cells may be regulated by growth-promoting oncogenes counterbalanced by growth-constraining tumor suppressor genes.[20,21]

Tumor suppressor genes encode for proteins that act as negative transducers of growth factor stimulation. The negative growth signals produced by tumor suppressor gene proteins block specific phases of the cell cycle, induce end-stage differentiation, and stimulate cell senescence or death. Carcinogenesis involves *inactivation* of tumor suppressor genes and/or activation of oncogenes (Fig. 10-16, Table 10-8).

Several tumor suppressor genes are involved in inherited human cancers, for example, *rb* in retinoblastoma, *NF1* in neurofibromatosis, *WT1* in Wilms tumor, *BRCA1* in breast cancer. These inherited genes are mutant forms of normal cell growth–regulating genes. The mutation they encode for produces defective regulatory proteins that allow cell transformation. Thus individuals inheriting these genes are prone to develop cancer, having lost normal cell growth and differentiation controls. It is now recognized that the pattern of expression of tumor oncogenes and suppressor genes is associated with tumor induction, growth, and metastasis.[22]

Oncogenic Bacteria

Helicobacter pylori infects more than half of the world's population, making it one of the most prevalent infections.[23] *H. pylori* is now accepted as the most common cause of gastric infection and is responsible for the majority of individuals with peptic ulcer disease, gastric lymphomas, and gastric carcinomas.[23,24,25] The association is stronger with B cell lymphoma of the stomach than with carcinomas. The high prevalence of *H. pylori* infection has been documented most notably in blacks and Hispanics, who also are at high risk for gastric cancer.[24] Treatment of *H. pylori* with antibiotics results in regression of the lymphoma in most cases.[26] The tumors arise in mucosa-associated lymphoid tissue (MALT) and are therefore sometimes called MALTomas. The mechanisms for causing tumor development include (1) dysregulation of the gastric epithelial cells cycle, (2) the formation of DNA adducts (addition of a small chemical group to DNA bases), (3) the generation of free radicals, (4) alterations in growth factor secretion and cytokines, and (5) the effects of decreased gastric secretion. (For further discussion, see Chapter 38.)

Genetic or Epigenetic Changes

The initial problem in understanding tumor development is to discover whether the inheritable aberration is attributable

Table 10-8 Examples of Tumor Suppressor Genes

Gene	Chromosome Location	Proposed Function	Disease Caused by Germline Mutation	Tumors Caused by Somatic Mutation
rb	13q14	Nuclear transcription factor	Retinoblastoma, osteosarcoma	Retinoblastoma, osteosarcoma; breast, lung, prostate, bladder carcinoma
APC	5q12	Possibly involved in cell adhesion	Adenomatous polyposis coli	Colon, pancreatic, stomach carcinoma
NF1	17q11	Guanosine triphosphatase (GTPase) activating protein	Neurofibromatosis type 1	Neuroblastoma, melanoma, colon carcinoma
NF2	22q	Cell membrane–cytoskeletal link	Neurofibromatosis type 2 (bilateral acoustic neuromas)	Central schwannomas and meningiomas
p53	17p13	Transcription/cell cycle regulation	Li-Fraumeni syndrome	Soft tissue sarcoma, breast and colon carcinoma, leukemia and others
VHL	3p25	Possibly in cell adhesion and signal transduction	von Hippel–Lindau disease	Renal cell carcinoma, pheochromocytoma
WT1	11p13	Nuclear transcription factor	Wilms tumor	Nephroblastoma
DCC	18q21	Cell adhesion	Neurofibromatosis type 1 (neural tumors)	Carcinoma of colon and stomach

From Jorde LB, Carey JC, White RL: *Medical genetics,* ed 2, St Louis, 1999, Mosby.

to a genetic change (an alteration in the cell's DNA sequence) or to an **epigenetic change** (a change in the pattern of gene expression without a change in the DNA sequence). The stability of the differentiated state depends on cell memory or heritable epigenetic change. One rare type of tumor, teratocarcinoma—an embryonic tumor containing many varieties of differentiated tissue (e.g., skin, bone, epithelium)—favors an epigenetic origin. Although investigators think cancers are initiated by genetic change, epigenetic change may be important in the future development of the disease. The argument is that most of the agents known to cause cancer cause genetic change or agents that cause genetic change cause cancer. This relationship between carcinogenesis and **mutagenesis** is known for three classes of agents: chemical carcinogens (which cause changes in the nucleotide sequence), ionizing radiation such as x-rays (which typically cause chromosome breaks and translocations), and viruses (which insert foreign DNA into the cell). The role of these agents in cancer is discussed later in this chapter.

CARCINOGENESIS

Understanding of the process of tumor development, **carcinogenesis,** is very limited. Within the past two decades, various theories have greatly influenced views about the carcinogenic process (Box 10-1). These theories or proposed mechanisms of carcinogenesis suggest that the formation of a cancerous tumor is not a "one-hit" event. Instead, *all* of the evidence overwhelmingly supports an evolution of phenotypic and hence presumably genotoxic (DNA toxic) changes from the normal cell to the invasive, metastasizing cell (see Fig. 10-18).

The multistep process of cancer seems to involve loss of the ability of the cell to terminally differentiate (see p. 292), to control growth, to travel to distal tissues, and to invade and colonize these tissues. The tumor, once formed, appears to be derived from a single "outlaw" stem cell.

Box 10-1
THEORIES OR CONCEPTUAL MODELS OF CARCINOGENESIS

Initiation-promotion-progression model
Oncogene and tumor suppressor gene model
Cancer as a disease of differentiation (blocked or partially unblocked ontogeny)
Cancer as a stem cell disease
Cancer as a disease of intercellular communication

Monoclonal Origin

Where evidence is available, it usually confirms that the cancer has a monoclonal origin. For example, the leukemic white blood cells of individuals with chronic myelogenous leukemia are distinguished from the normal cells by a specific chromosomal abnormality (Philadelphia chromosome) (see p. 300). It is doubtful that the genetic mistake responsible for this abnormality would have occurred in several cells at once in the same individual. It is more likely that all the leukemic cells are descendants of the same mutant cell. Other evidence of cancer having a monoclonal origin is from studies of X chromosome inactivation (see Chapter 4). The inactivation of one X chromosome in each cell occurs early in embryonic development and is observable in many interphase cells. Once the X chromosome is inactivated in a cell, all of the descendants of that cell have the same chromosome inactivated. Consequently, X chromosome inactivation can be used as a heritable marker to trace the lineage of cells in the body. In most tumors that have been studied, both benign and malignant, all the tumor cells have been found to have the same X chromosome inactivated. This strongly suggests that the tumor cells originated from a single aberrant cell.[1]

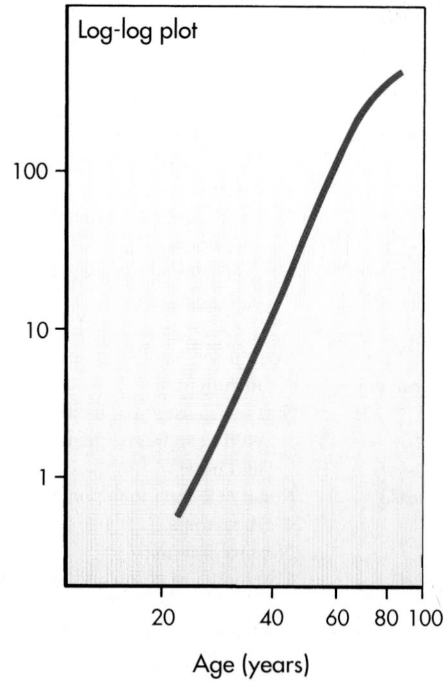

FIG. 10-17 Incidence of cancer rises steeply as a function of age. A cell must accumulate the abnormal effects of several independent accidents before it will give rise to a tumor. (Modified from Alberts B et al: *Molecular biology of the cell,* ed 3, New York, 1994, Garland Press.)

Cell Accidents: A Requisite for Cancer Development

Many lines of evidence indicate that tumor development requires several *independent* rare accidents to occur together in one cell. The evidence involves the relationship of tumor development to age. If a single mutation were responsible, the chance of developing cancer in any given year would be independent of age. For most types of cancer, however, the chance increases at a rapid rate with age (Fig. 10-17). Approximations of three to seven independent random events are typically required to alter a normal cell into a cancer cell; the smaller numbers apply to leukemias, the larger to carcinomas.[1]

The Slow Stages of Cancer Development

Tumor development almost always involves a long delay between the initial causal event and the onset of the disease; for example, the incidence of lung cancer rises steeply after 10 to 20 years of heavy smoking. During this latent period the cancer cells undergo multiple and successive changes. It appears for most cancers that cells of the initial mutant clone undergo further mutation that enables them to divide more rapidly before they terminally differentiate (see Fig. 10-7, *A*). Because of the rapid division and therefore proliferation of cells, the cancer cells begin to outnumber the normal cells as well as those with the primary mutation.

Cancers of the uterine cavity provide a clear example of the early steps in the development of a tumor. These cancers originate from the multilayered cervical epithelium, which is similar to the epidermis of the skin. Normally, proliferation occurs only in the basal layer, and the differentiating cells travel outward from their site of origin. It seems logical that among these basal cells is at least one cell whose line of descendants will not die out in one lifetime—an **immortal stem cell.** Cells moving out toward the surface differentiate into flattened, keratin-rich, nondividing cells as they go and, finally, are sloughed off from the surface (Fig. 10-18, *A*). Examination of Papanicolaou (Pap) specimens from various women shows patches of *dysplasia,* wherein dividing cells are no longer confined to the basal layer and there is disorder in the process of differentiation (Fig. 10-18, *B*). These cells, obtained by a Pap smear, can be viewed under the microscope. If these cells are allowed to progress over a period of years, they give rise to *carcinoma in situ* (Fig. 10-18, *C*). In carcinoma in situ, the cells in all the layers are proliferating and apparently undifferentiated, yet the abnormal cells are still confined to the epithelial side of the basal lamina and are highly variable in size and karyotype. Without treatment the carcinoma in situ cells may still remain harmless or over a period of several years give rise to a malignant clinical carcinoma whose cells cross the basal lamina (see p. 311) and begin to invade the underlying connective tissue (Fig. 10-18, *D*).

Oncogenes and Tumor Suppressor Genes

Proto-oncogenes are known to represent an array of cell growth and differentiation regulatory genes. Oncogenes are generally considered to encode for factors that stimulate cell growth. In contrast, tumor suppressor genes encode for proteins that counteract cell growth signals. (Oncogenes and tumor suppressor genes were introduced earlier on pp. 306-309.) Mutations or gene activation of growth-promoting oncogenes and inactivation of tumor suppressor genes can lead to transformation. Because transformation involves complex processes, it is not surprising that cancers express multiple oncogenes and tumor suppressor genes. Oncogenes involved in human breast carcinoma include growth factors (*int*-2, *hst,* and *bcl*-1); growth factor receptors (*erb*-2, *erb* A, and *erb* B-3); signal transducers *(ras)*; nuclear regulators (*myc, myb,* and *fos*); and suppressors (*rb* and *p53*).[5,15] Further, synergy between specific oncogenes is required for tumor induction. All this suggests that as transformed cells grow and metastasize, various growth and regulatory pathways are activated, as represented by oncogenes and tumor suppressor genes.

Other genetic abnormalities occur in many cancers; these abnormalities include deletions, translocations, and inversions of genes, as well as terminal deletions, monosomy, and trisomy of specific chromosomes (Fig. 10-19). Because these chromosome abnormalities are consistent for certain types of cancer, it is believed they are involved in the carcinogenesis process.[27] Multiple genetic alterations have been well characterized in colorectal carcinoma, including expression of dominant-acting oncogenes *(ras, myc, src)*; inactivation

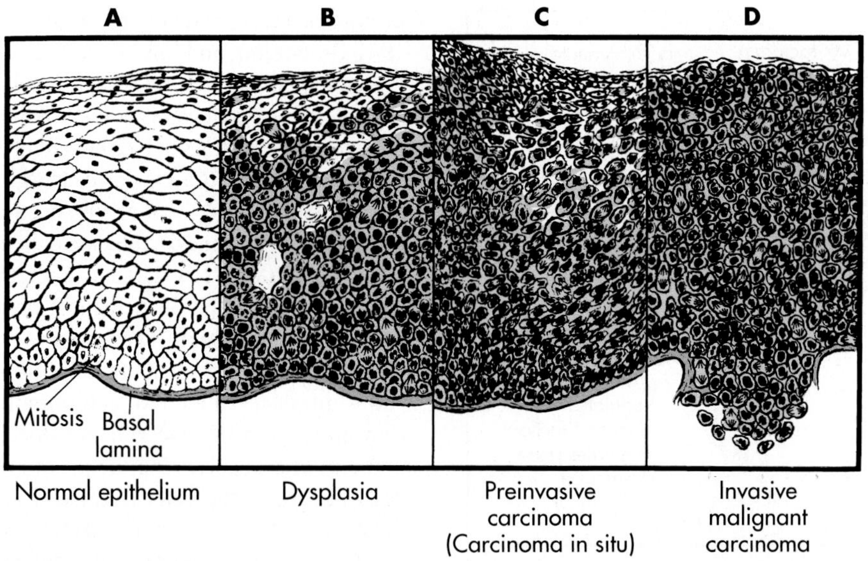

FIG. 10-18 Stages of progression. Stages of progression of development of cancer of the epithelium of the uterine cervix. **A,** Normal. **B,** In dysplasia, the most superficial cells still show signs of differentiation, but this is incomplete and proliferating cells are seen far above the basal layer. **C,** In carcinoma in situ, the cells in all the layers are proliferating and apparently undifferentiated. **D,** Malignancy begins when the cells cross the basal lamina and begin to invade the underlying connective tissue. Several years may elapse from the first signs of dysplasia to the onset of full-blown malignant cancer. (Modified from Alberts B et al: *Molecular biology of the cell,* ed 3, New York, 1994, Garland Press.)

or deletion of suppressor genes *(DCC, p53, APC)*; and deletions from chromosomes 1 and 22 (see Fig. 10-16). This provides further evidence for the role of genetic factors in carcinogenesis.

Stem Cell or Blocked Differentiation

The concept of cancer as a stem cell disease or a disease of differentiation was derived from several observations: (1) the stem cell and the cancer cell both proliferate extensively; (2) cancer cells and stem cells both appear to self-renew or self-generate (see Fig. 10-7); (3) both types of cells act similarly when given radiation therapy; and (4) terminal differentiation can be experimentally (in vitro) induced for both types of cells with natural differentiation factors.

Differentiation depends on the natural functioning of the stem cell progeny (see Fig. 10-7, *B*). A transformed stem cell causes production and cell destruction to be unbalanced in a normal tissue. Two proposed derangements in differentiation, previously discussed, could possibly cause this imbalance and tumor development.

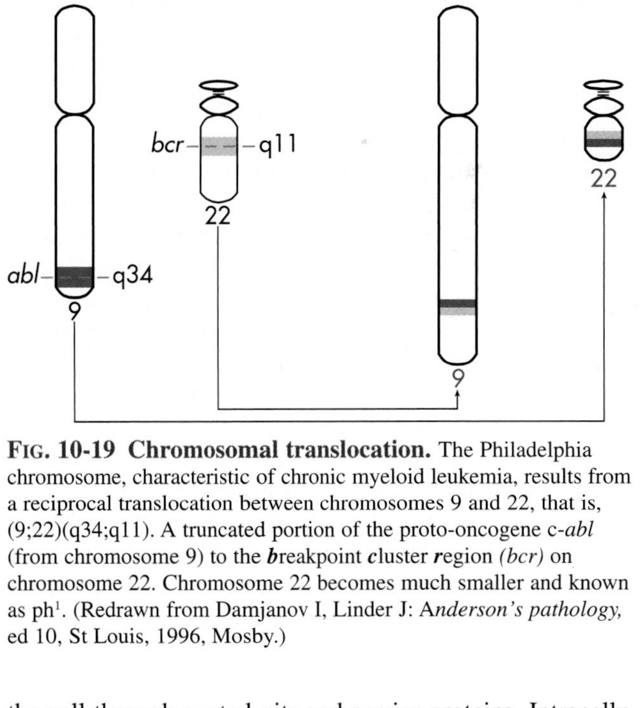

FIG. 10-19 Chromosomal translocation. The Philadelphia chromosome, characteristic of chronic myeloid leukemia, results from a reciprocal translocation between chromosomes 9 and 22, that is, (9;22)(q34;q11). A truncated portion of the proto-oncogene c-*abl* (from chromosome 9) to the ***b***reakpoint ***c***luster ***r***egion *(bcr)* on chromosome 22. Chromosome 22 becomes much smaller and known as ph[1]. (Redrawn from Damjanov I, Linder J: A*nderson's pathology,* ed 10, St Louis, 1996, Mosby.)

Intercellular Communication

All cells that are part of a multicellular organism are able to "talk to" or influence each other (see Chapter 1). Normal tissue growth and differentiation depend on cellular feedback mechanisms that take place through intercellular communication. The delicate integration of the three major types of communication (*intercellular, intracellular,* and *extracellular*) is required (Fig. 10-20). Extracellular communication involves signals from different molecules or ligands, such as neurotransmitters, chemicals, and hormones. These signals are received by specific cell receptors or directly taken into the cell through coated pits and carrier proteins. Intracellular communication occurs when second messengers are activated inside the cell membrane, including cyclic adenosine monophosphate (cAMP), IP^3-diocylglyceride (IP^3-DG), phosphokinase C, Ca^{++} flux, and pH changes. Intercellular communication involves ions and other small molecules that directly communicate with neighboring cells through gap junctions (see Fig. 10-10; also see discussion in Chapter 1 and Fig. 1-28). These three types of cell communication

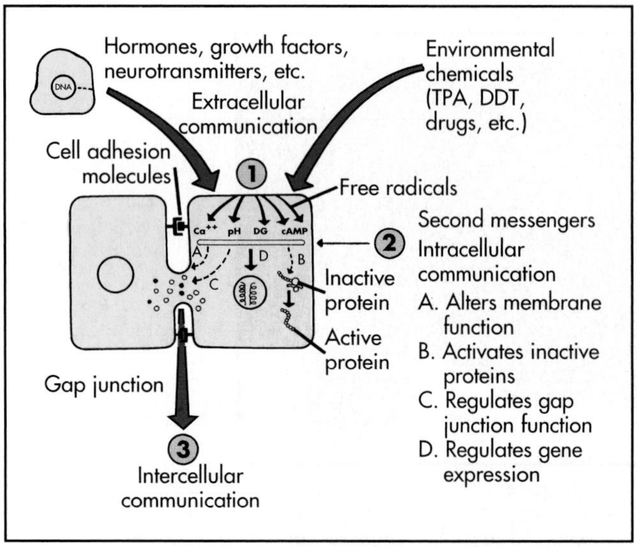

FIG. 10-20 Cellular communication. Proposed link between extracellular and intracellular communication. Schema shows the proposed link between extracellular communication and intercellular communication through various intracellular signaling mechanisms (e.g., transmembrane). It provides a holistic view (mind/body connection) of how the neuroendocrine immune system and other coordinations could occur. Although not shown here, activation or altered expression of various oncogenes and tumor suppressor genes could contribute to the regulation of gap junction function. *TPA,* tissue plasminogen activator; *DDT,* dichlorodiphenyl trichloroethane; *DG,* diocylglyceride; *cAMP,* cyclic adenosine monophosphate.

are closely related and are capable of controlling cellular function.

Investigators propose that gap junction intercellular communication (GJIC) is either blocked or down-regulated in transforming cancer cells, and therefore communication between the transformed cells and normal surrounding cells is lost.[28,29,30] This concept has been incorporated into other theories on carcinogenesis, including the initiation-promotion-progression theory, oncogene theory, and the stem cell theory.

Gap junctions can be down-regulated or blocked by many tumor promoters, such as chemicals or growth hormones. Phorbol esters are known to promote tumors in certain tissues.[31] For example, 12-0 tetradecanoylphorbol-13-acetate (TPA) affects intercellular communication.[31] Investigators demonstrated that TPA decreases communication between transformed and nontransformed cells.[31] Interestingly, communication among transformed cells was less affected by TPA, possibly allowing autonomous growth.

Oncogenes produce abnormal proteins that can take the place of normal hormones, chemicals, or receptors. These oncogene proteins are capable of blocking normal up- and down-regulation of intercellular communication and gap junction function and therefore stimulate tumor cell growth.[6]

Initiation-Promotion-Progression Theory of Carcinogenesis

In 1941 Rous and Kidd hypothesized a two-stage mechanism for the development of cancer involving first an initiation stage (transformation) induced by a mutagen, followed by a promotion stage mediated by another agent[32] (Fig. 10-21). In 1947 Berenblum and Shubik devised a series of experiments that demonstrated the two-stage mechanism for skin cancer. The initiating agent was methylcholanthrene, and the promoting agent was croton oil. Neither agent alone would cause carcinogenesis (i.e., the cancer-causing process required both agents). When two such agents are required to initiate and promote carcinogenesis, they are called **cocarcinogens.**

Initiation or DNA damage (mutation) is the irreversible developmental stage of the cancer precursor cell after exposure to the carcinogen. The initiated cell may not be considered cancerous, however, until a promoting agent acts on that cell to produce an altered, autonomous phenotype. **Promotion** appears to involve cell proliferation and tumor development, thus accelerating the process by which the initiated cells become cancerous. Initiation and promotion mechanisms have not been experimentally shown for all cancers, but the process is most useful when applied to chemical agents, such as benzo[*a*]pyrene found in coal tar or cigarette smoke. Other carcinogens are part of the physical environment (e.g., ionizing and nonionizing radiation) or are biologic agents (e.g., viruses or hormones).

Initiators cause alterations in the DNA. These changes can include one or more complete interruptions of the DNA chain, errors in DNA repair, or an elimination of a base pair (pyrimidine or purine) or sugar. (Normal DNA replication is discussed in Chapter 4.) Promoters may affect cell proliferation by altering cell-to-cell communication or by producing oxygen radicals. Promoters include hormones, drugs, chemicals, plant products, and other environmental factors. These factors induce initiated cells to divide within a tissue. Several agents induce cell division, but only promoters induce tumor development. Promoting agents may interfere with the process of differentiation, usually after division has occurred. In the early stages of epidermal carcinogenesis, the biologic effects of promotion are reversible and are modulated by diet, hormones, and related factors. Table 10-9 compares initiation and promotion substances.

Boutwell[33] suggested that progression of a tumor may be a late phase of promotion. The biologic difference between promotion and progression is unknown, but progression is thought to depend on structural changes in the chromosome and, contrarily, promotion may not cause chromosome abnormalities.

Environmental Risk Factors

Because the exact biochemical cause of cancer is unknown, the traditional emphasis (as part of the initiation-promotion theory) is on those factors with suggested pathogenic mechanisms that increase the incidence of different cancerous tumors. (Methods of risk factor analysis are discussed in Chapter 5.)

Table 10-10 summarizes the estimated new cases and deaths, by gender, for specified sites. Although population trends in incidence rates of cancer are the focus of epidemiologists, laboratory scientists use experimental approaches to determine the effect and nature of environmental factors as initiators or promoters of carcinogenesis. To identify an

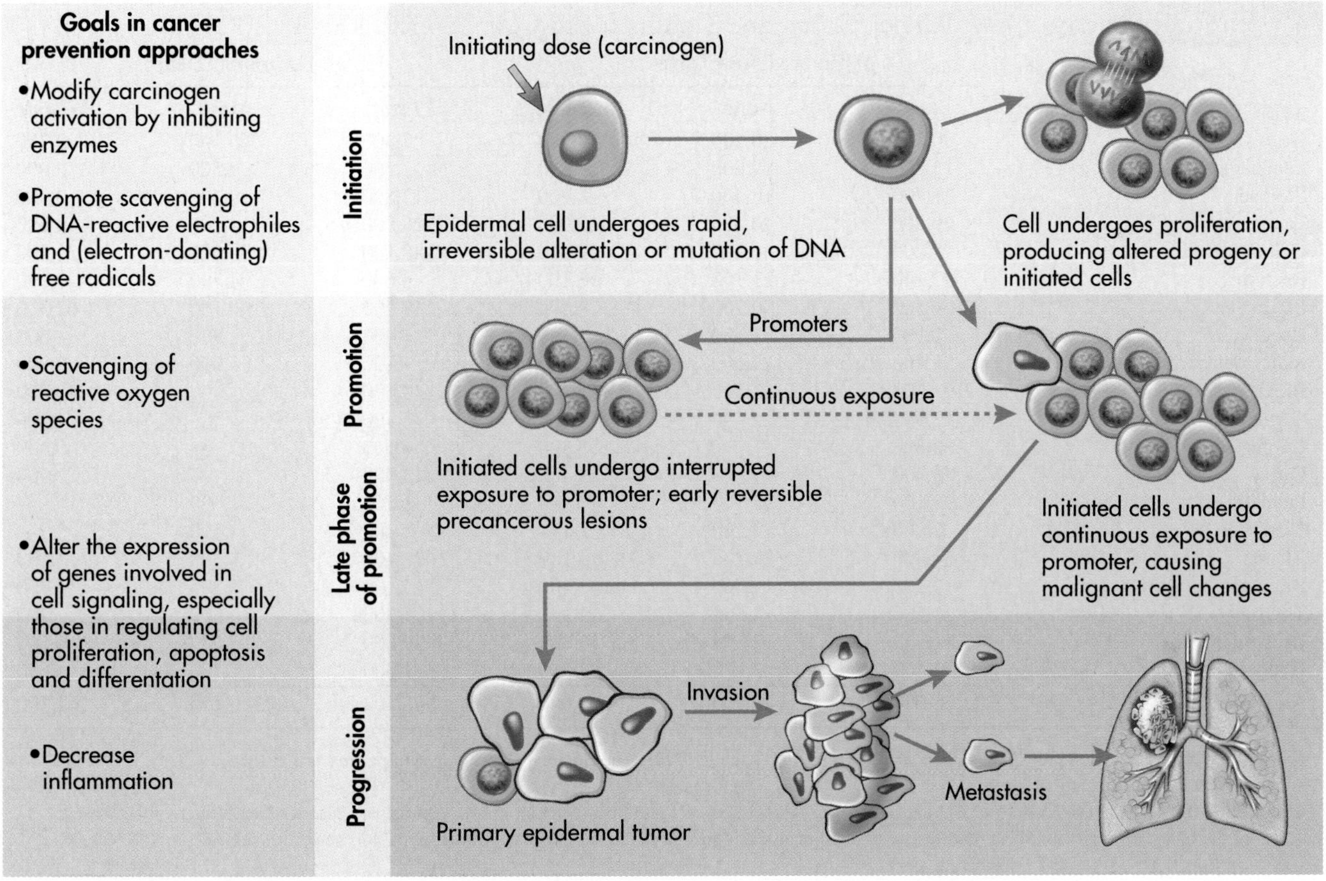
Goals in cancer prevention approaches
•Modify carcinogen activation by inhibiting enzymes
•Promote scavenging of DNA-reactive electrophiles and (electron-donating) free radicals
•Scavenging of reactive oxygen species
•Alter the expression of genes involved in cell signaling, especially those in regulating cell proliferation, apoptosis and differentation
•Decrease inflammation
Initiation
Promotion
Late phase of promotion
Progression
Initiating dose (carcinogen)
Epidermal cell undergoes rapid, irreversible alteration or mutation of DNA
Cell undergoes proliferation, producing altered progeny or initiated cells
Promoters
Continuous exposure
Initiated cells undergo interrupted exposure to promoter; early reversible precancerous lesions
Initiated cells undergo continuous exposure to promoter, causing malignant cell changes
Invasion
Metastasis
Primary epidermal tumor

FIG. 10-21 Multistage theory. Tumor development according to the multistage theory: initiation, promotion, progression. *DNA,* deoxyribonucleic acid

Table 10-9 Initiation and Promotion Substances

Initiators	Promoters
Single exposure to alter cell	Contact after initiator and requires prolonged exposure
Irreversible process	Reversible during early stage
Metabolically converted to reactants that bind covalently to deoxyribonucleic acid (DNA)	Neither metabolic conversion nor covalent binding necessary
High doses carcinogenic	Only weakly carcinogenic without prior treatment of initiator

Data from King DW, Fenoglio CM, Lefkowitz JH: *General pathology: principles and dynamics,* Philadelphia, 1983, Lea & Febiger; Weinstein IB: *Adv Pathobiol* 4:106, 1976.

agent as being an initiator, laboratory scientists must demonstrate that altered DNA changes occur in response to variable doses of that agent—a difficult task at best. Thus the relationship between life-style and carcinogenesis of a given human population can be explored and evaluated from two divergent but equally important approaches: epidemiologic and experimental. Each approach has strengths and weaknesses, and each requires cautionary interpretations. These two perspectives, however, do indicate some agreement about particular agents or conditions that either cause cancer or are associated with an increase in cancer incidence rates.

Personal Behaviors

Tobacco use. Both epidemiologic and experimental data support the conclusion that cigarette smoke is carcinogenic and remains the most important cause of cancer. During the first decades of the twentieth century, lung cancer was rare; however, as cigarette smoking increased, first among men then later among women, the incidence of lung cancer became epidemic.[34] In 1930 the lung cancer death rate for men was 4.9 per 100,000; in 1990 the rate had increased to 75.6 per 100,000.[34] An accomplishment of the second half of the twentieth century has been the reduction of smoking prevalence among persons less than 18 years of age from 42.4% in 1965 to 24.7% in 1997, with the rate for men (27.6%) higher than for women (22.1%). The percentage of adults who never smoked increased from 44% in the mid-1960s to 55% in 1997.[34] The prevalence of smoking was highest among American Indians/Alaskan Natives and second highest among black and Southeast Asian men. The prevalence was lowest among Asian American and Hispanic women.[34] Smoking prevalence among high school seniors has increased to 36.5%. Among high school seniors the prevalence is highest among whites and lowest in blacks.[34] Despite the achievements of the twentieth century, about 48 million U.S. adults smoke cigarettes; half of those who continue to smoke will die from a smoking-related disease. Tobacco use is responsible for one of every five deaths per year.[34] Teen smoking accounts for 85% to 90% of new smokers.[35]

Table 10-10 Estimated New Cancer Cases and Deaths by Sex for Specified Sites, 2001*

	Estimated New Cases			Estimated Deaths		
Types of Cancer	Total	Male	Female	Total	Male	Female
Oral	30,100	20,200	9,900	7,800	5,100	2,700
Esophagus	13,200	9,900	3,300	12,500	9,500	3,000
Stomach	21,700	13,400	8,300	12,800	7,400	5,400
Pancreas	29,200	14,200	15,000	28,900	14,100	14,800
Colon (large intestine)	98,200	46,200	52,000	48,100	23,000	25,100
Rectum	37,200	21,100	16,100	8,600	4,700	3,900
Lung	169,500	90,700	78,800	157,400	90,100	67,300
Bone	2,900	1,600	1,300	1,400	800	600
Skin (melanoma)	51,400	29,000	22,400	7,800	5,000	2,800
Breast	193,700	1,500	192,200	40,600	400	40,200
Cervix	12,900	—	12,900	4,400	—	4,400
Corpus, endometruim	38,300	—	38,300	6,600	—	6,600
Ovary	23,400	—	23,400	13,900	—	13,900
Prostate	198,100	198,100	—	31,500	31,500	—
Testis	7,200	7,200	—	400	400	—
Bladder	54,300	39,200	15,100	12,400	8,300	4,100
Brain and nervous system	17,200	9,800	7,400	13,100	7,200	5,900
Thyroid	19,500	4,600	14,900	1,300	500	800
Leukemias	31,500	17,700	13,800	21,500	12,000	9,500
Hodgkin disease	7,400	3,900	3,500	1,300	700	600
All sites	1,268,000	643,000	625,000	553,400	286,100	267,300

From American Cancer Society: *Cancer facts and figures 2001,* Atlanta, 2001, The Society. Reprinted with permission of the American Cancer Society, Inc.

*Rounded to the nearest 100. Excludes basal and squamous cell skin cancers and in situ carcinomas except urinary bladder. Carcinoma in situ of the breast accounts for about 46,400 new cases annually, and melanoma in situ accounts for about 31,400 new cases annually.

Cigarette smoking increases the incidence of cancer of the bladder, pancreas, and, to a lesser extent, kidney, larynx, oral cavity, and esophagus. These correlations are not surprising, considering the chemical composition of cigarette smoke. These chemicals possess mutagenic capabilities, are absorbed from the lungs into the blood, gain access to distant organs through their distribution by the circulation, and are present in increased concentration in the urine of smokers. Recent studies identify 20 carcinogens in tobacco smoke that cause lung tumors in both laboratory animals and humans.[36] Smoking also increases heart disease, peripheral vascular disease, chronic obstructive pulmonary disease, intrauterine growth retardation, and low birth weight.[34]

The harmful effects of cigarette smoke are worse than those from pipe or cigar smoke. This difference may be attributable to the increased alkalinity of pipe and cigar smoke. Alkaline smoke is more irritating than cigarette smoke and is therefore less readily inhaled into the lungs. The greatest risk among the numerous causes of cancer of the lung is related to the inhalation of tobacco smoke. Low-tar cigarettes do not reduce the risk of lung cancer.

There are hazards for nonsmokers who breathe the smoke of others' cigarettes (passive smoking or environmental tobacco smoke [ETS]). Passive smoking is associated with a modestly increased risk of lung cancers and possibly other cancers and is classified by the Environmental Protection Agency as a known human carcinogen.[37,38] Children are particularly vulnerable to the effects of passive smoke.

Smokeless tobacco (plug, leaf, and snuff) use has changed little since 1970, with a 5% prevalence in 1991 among men, and 2% and 1%, respectively, for women. Smokeless tobacco use is highest among high school white males and lowest among black males.[34] "Dipping snuff," in which a coarse, moist powder is placed between the cheek and gum and nicotine and other carcinogens are directly absorbed through the oral tissue, has caused the greatest concern. Oral cancer occurs more frequently among snuff dippers, as well as pipe and cigar smokers, compared with nontobacco users.[34,39]

Diet. People are constantly exposed to a variety of compounds termed **xenobiotics** (Greek *xenos*, foreign; *bios*, life) that include toxic, mutagenic, and carcinogenic chemicals. Many of these chemicals are found in the human diet. These chemicals can react with cellular macromolecules, such as proteins and DNA, or directly with cell structures to cause cell damage.[40] To counteract these challenges, the body has two defense systems: (1) detoxification enzymes and (2) antioxidant systems (see Chapter 2). The enzymes that activate xenobiotics are called **phase I activation enzymes** and are represented by the multigene cytochrome P450 family, aldehyde oxidase, xanthine oxidases, and peroxidases. **Phase II detoxification enzymes** then further protect against a large array of reactive intermediates and nonactivated xenobiotics.[40] These enzymes are located predominantly in the liver and provide clearance of compounds into the portal circulation, preventing the potential carcinogenic agent(s) from entering the body through the gastroin-

WHAT'S NEW? **How Smokers Get Addicted**

Although smoke delivers a strong hit—about 2 mg of nicotine in each cigarette—and nicotine is considered a powerful addictive drug, there may be others. In a recent report, scientists did positron emission tomography (PET) scans on smokers and abstainers and found that smokers had 40% less of a brain enzyme known as monoamine oxidase B (MAO B). The enzyme breaks down dopamine, a neurotransmitter associated with feelings of pleasure. Because of dopamine's pleasurable effects, it is significant in reinforcing and motivating behavior. Therefore smoking seems to create a self-perpetuating cycle: less MAO B leads to more dopamine, leads to more pleasure, which leads to more smoking, which leads to less MAO B, and so on.

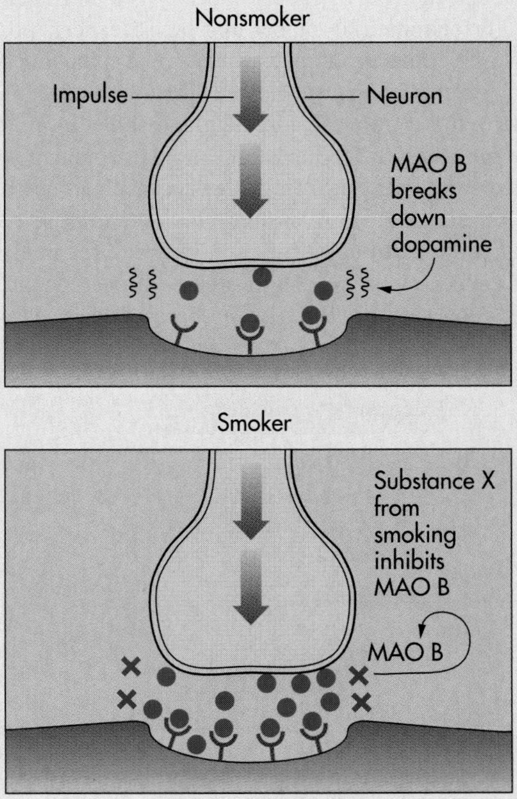

An unknown substance (x) inhibits the activity of the enzyme MAO B, causing an increase in dopamine, increasing the high and therefore the habit.

Data from Fowler JS et al: *Nature* 379:733, 1996.

testinal tract and portal circulation. These enzymes, however, also occur in the barrier skin epithelia and can be induced in other extrahepatic tissue, such as the lung.

Dietary sources of toxic carcinogenic substances include compounds produced in the cooking of fat, meat, or protein, and naturally occurring carcinogens associated with plant food substances, such as alkaloids or mold byproducts.[40] The most studied and most relevant carcinogens produced by cooking are the polycyclic aromatic hydrocarbons benzo-[*a*]pyrene and heterocyclic aromatic amines generated by

NUTRITION & DISEASE

Cancer

General guidelines for cancer protection:

- Low-fat, high-fiber diets
- Increased intake of fruits and vegetables
- Vitamins A, C, E
- Epigallocatechin gallate (found in green tea)
- Phytoestrogens (soy products)
- Decreased use of foods with high amounts of preservatives
- Decreased use of grilled, blackened foods
- Decreased alcohol intake

meat protein. The greatest levels are found in well-done, charbroiled beef. People, likewise, ingest xenobiotics that are environmental or industrial contaminants (e.g., particulate matter of diesel exhaust, contaminating pesticides in food and water supplies) and certain prescribed and over-the-counter medicines.

Nitrates are used as preservatives in fish and meat and may concentrate in the soil and water of some regions. The reaction of nitrites to other nitrosable compounds causes cancer of the glandular stomach in animals. Potentially harmful nitrite reactions can occur when foods are cooked. For example, nitrite-cured bacon, when cooked, yields nitrous acid, which reacts with amines (derivative of ammonia present in many foods) in the meat to form dimethylnitrosamine (DMN). This reaction is favored at an acidic pH and therefore occurs when nitrites and secondary amines are ingested and encounter the acidic gastric juice. Dietary salts also seem to enhance this reaction. The inhabitants of countries with high rates of gastric cancer (e.g., China) ingest large quantities of salted fish and similarly preserved foods.

Certain ingested fats might contribute to the production of carcinogens in the body by increasing the amount of bile acids and cholesterol metabolites in the feces. These metabolites, which include deoxycholic and lithocholic acids, are found in greater quantities in populations who ingest a typical Western fatty diet and in whom colorectal cancer is common.

The most significant dietary factor affecting transport is fiber. Much work has been done to characterize the various components of dietary fiber. (**Fiber** refers to the remnants of the plant cell wall not hydrolyzed by human digestive enzymes.) Although inconclusive, considerable data support the finding that a diet low in fiber is associated with an increased risk of cancer of the colon.[15] High fiber intake is associated with low levels of sex hormones in plasma (e.g., sex hormone–binding globulin, free estradiol, free testosterone), causing a reduction in the bioavailability of the hormones that possibly would reduce the risk of hormone-dependent cancers. It has been suggested recently that because fat intake is related to decreased excretion of biologically active sex hormones and fiber is also related to their levels in plasma, a ratio of fat to total fiber may be a better index of risk than either alone.[1]

Polyunsaturated fatty acids are readily oxidized to yield free radicals and peroxidates that are toxic to cells and related to tumor development. Experiments on animals and humans indicate that polyunsaturated vegetable oils (e.g., omega 6) promote cancer more effectively than do saturated fats, whereas total dietary fat correlates more significantly with cancer incidence and mortality in the epidemiologic data.[41] Omega-3 fatty acids (e.g., fatty fish, cod liver oil), a class of polyunsaturated fats, however, decrease the number and size of tumors and increase the time elapsed before tumors appear.[42,43] The cancer protective effects may be caused by influencing the activity of enzymes and proteins related to intracellular signaling and, ultimately, cell proliferation,[44,45] or by decreasing the blood supply to the tumor by modulating the effects of platelet-activating factor (PAF).[42,46] The destruction of toxic peroxides or radicals may also depend on selenium-containing enzymes. Treatment with selenium has been associated with decreasing mortality from lung, colon, rectal, and prostate cancer.[47] The protective effects were demonstrated with 200 μg per day and its role seems to be one of inhibition of proliferation.[48] Much concern exists, however, over what is a safe range of dietary selenium concentrations that is adequate yet not toxic.

Importantly, many dietary microconstituents from plant sources (e.g., isothiocyanates, dithiolthiones, allyl sulfides, coumarins, and lactones) are correlated with protection against toxicity and cancer.[40] These substances are called **chemoprotectors** (Fig. 10-22). Chemoprotectors protect against both the initiation and promotion phases of cancer, as well as against a broad range of procarcinogens and toxicants. They induce endogenous xenobiotic detoxification enzymes that inactivate carcinogens and toxicants providing protection in a variety of tissues (Fig. 10-23).

Diet seems to function over time to place an individual at risk for cancer. In women, who have a much higher incidence of hormone-dependent cancer than men, diet has been suggested as a main determinant in the cause of some of these cancers.[39,49,50,51,52] Studies have found a consistent relationship between increasing weight in postmenopausal women and the risk of cancer. Obesity is a consistent risk factor for endometrial cancer and breast cancer, possibly because "overnutrition" causes excessive exposure to estrogen. After menopause the only natural estrogens produced are those from the adrenal gland and adipose tissue, so that more adipose tissue causes more estrogen exposure. However, the data regarding breast cancer are inconclusive: international correlational studies and case-control studies show a strong correlation between fat intake and breast cancer rates but cohort studies find no such association.[44] In addition, the rise in obesity correlates with a

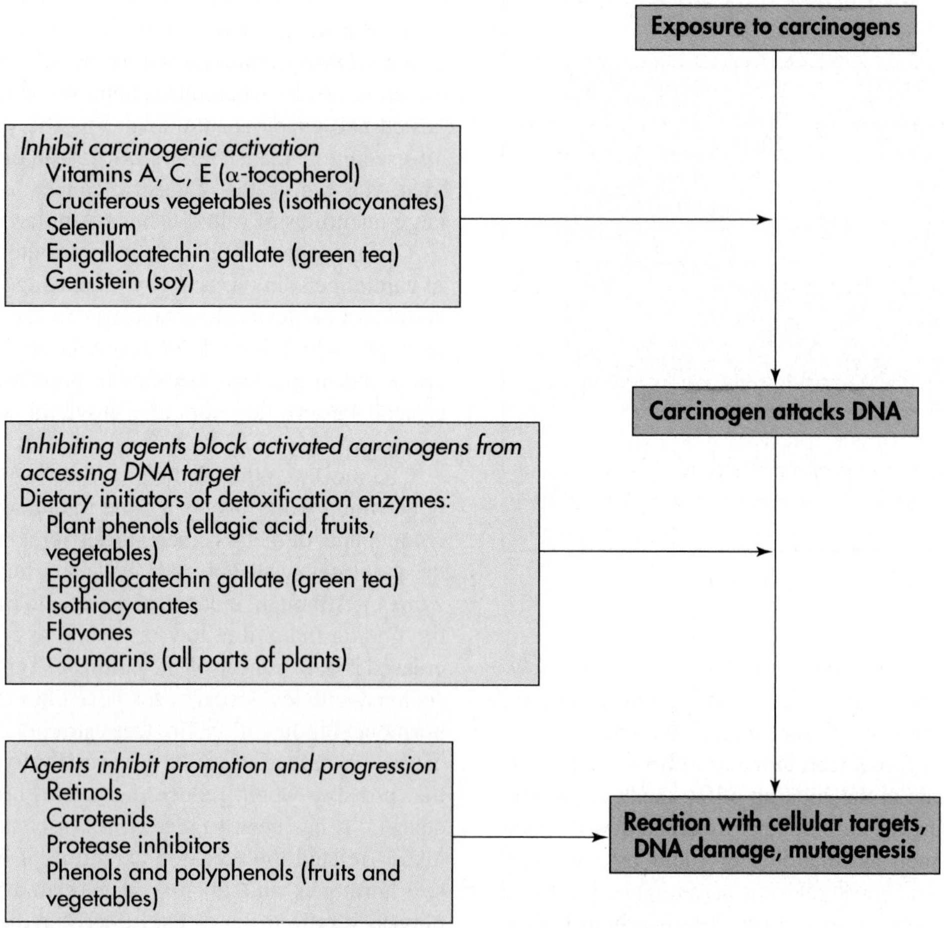

FIG. 10-22 Dietary chemoprotectors.

rise in esophageal cancer in white men. Obesity increases the risk for cancers of the ovary and prostate gland and adenocarinoma of the upper gastrointestinal tract and may also increase the risk of colon cancer and renal cancer (Fig. 10-23).[53,54,55]

Alcohol. Incidence rates for cancer of the mouth, pharynx, larynx, esophagus, and liver are higher in individuals who ingest large quantities of both alcohol and smoke.[11,39,49,56,57] (These cancers are discussed further in Chapter 38.) Wine, beer, and "hard liquor" seem to produce an equivalent effect on cancer risk.[52] Alcohol interacts with smoke, increasing the risk of malignant tumors, possibly by acting as a solvent for the carcinogenic smoke products. Alcohol consumption has been consistently linked to breast cancer and colorectal cancer.[39,52,58,59,60,61,62,63] Mechanisms for increasing the incidence of breast cancer in association with alcohol are unknown and are likely to differ between pre- and postmenopausal women. Mechanisms suggested include the following:

1. The liver's inability to rid the body of carcinogens (including estrogen) with increasing liver damage
2. With increasing liver damage (hyperinsulinemia), progression in precancerous breast lesions stimulated by an insulin increase[64,65]
3. Impairment of the immune system
4. Interference with cell membrane permeability in breast tissue
5. Interactions between estrogen replacement (ERT and HRT) therapy and alcohol as synergistically increasing breast levels of circulating estrogen[66]
6. Activation of insulin-like growth factor 1 receptor in breast tissue by alcohol-related hyperinsulinemia (primarily postmenopausal)[64] (breast cancer is discussed further in Chapter 22)

Alcohol stimulates rectal cell proliferation in the rat, providing a possible mechanism for the observed association with large bowel cancer.[39,49,52]

Sexual and reproductive behavior. The risk of developing cervical cancer is related to the age of first sexual intercourse and to the number of sexual partners.[67] Women who have had one sexual partner are also at risk if that partner has had previous multiple partners. The possible mechanism is a virus transmitted between partners. Studies using molecular analyses reveal that certain types of human papillomavirus (HPV), especially HPV16,[68,69] are causally involved in the development of cancer of the cervix. Although HPV may be a prime determinant worldwide, the importance of cofactors could vary by geographic area. A report by local inhabitants of a town in Utah implicated nearby toxic waste as causing a substantial increase in the incidence of cervical cancer by 150%.[70]

Human papilloma viruses (HPV) types 6 and 11 have been identified as the viruses present in condyloma acuminatum (genital warts). These benign genital lesions replicate in the squamous epithelium. The risk factors associated with the disorder include sexually active young women, multiple sexual partners, and a sexual partner with multiple partners. The most common cause of abnormal Papanicolaou smears is, however, the HPV virus, followed by cervical dysplasia.[68,71,72] Multiple other types of HPV are associated with cancers of the cervix, vulva, penis, and anus.[19]

The incidence of invasive cervical cancer is two and one-half times greater in black women than in white women in the United States.[11] Cervical malignancy also is found more often in women from lower socioeconomic groups.[73,74] Obese women have higher mortality rates for cervical and breast cancer.[75] Cancers of the breast, ovary, and cervix account for 13% of all cancers and 29% of all female cancer deaths in the United States. (These cancers are discussed further in Chapter 22.) Pregnancy and childbearing seem to be protective factors against cancers of the endometrium, ovary, and breast.

Air Pollution

A person inhales about 20,000 L of air in 1 day; thus even modest contamination of the atmosphere can result in inhalation of appreciable doses of pollutants. Concerns are focused on industrial emissions, including arsenicals, benzene, chloroform, vinyl chloride, and acrylonitrile.[76-78] Living close to certain industries is a recognized cancer risk factor, although it is difficult to determine cancer risk from outdoor pollution because of difficulties in estimating long-term exposures and accurately controlling for smoking and radon. One team of investigators estimate that a person must breathe Los Angeles smog for 1 year to inhale the same amount of burnt material that a smoker of two packs per day inhales in 1 day.[79] Other studies that controlled or stratified for smoking demonstrate associations between excess lung cancer rates and heavy metal and aromatic hydrocarbon emissions in polluted air.[77,79]

WHAT'S NEW? Vitamin C May Interfere with Chemotherapy

Recently, investigators reported that because chemotherapy and radiation often destroy cancerous cells through oxidative mechanisms, it is possible that large amounts of antioxidants, such as vitamin C, may actually render cancer treatments less effective. That is, tumor cells compete for the same antioxidants as do normal cells. Studies have shown increased concentrations of vitamin C in certain human tumors as compared with normal tissue. In an animal study designed to determine how human tumor cells take up vitamin C in vivo, investigators reported that tumors (e.g., breast and prostate cancer) rapidly took up vitamin C after the experimental animals had been injected with ascorbic acid. They further determined that the vitamin C was taken up in the form of hydroascorbic acid, which had been *oxidized* from ascorbic acid in the tumor microenvironment. Although it has been established that tumor cells contain high concentrations of vitamin C, it is not known whether vitamin C actually provides malignant cells with a metabolic advantage.

Data from Agus DB, Vera JC, Golde DW: Stromal cell oxidation: a mechanism by which tumors obtain vitamin C, *C Cancer Res* 59:4555, 1999; Stipanuk M: *Biochemical and physiological aspects of nutrition*, Philadelphia, 2000, W.B. Saunders.

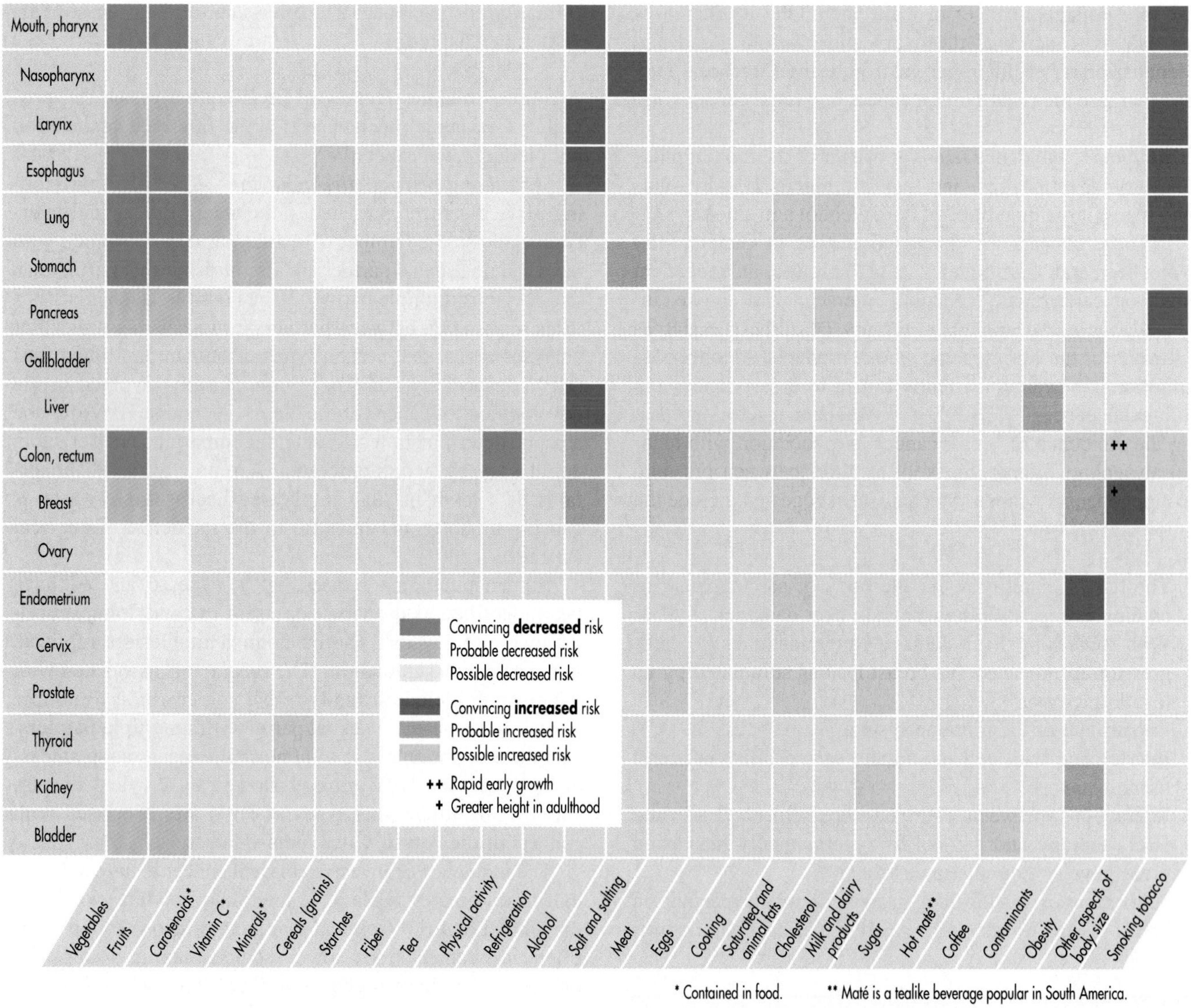

FIG. 10-23 Diet and cancer. (Redrawn from *Nutrition Action Healthletter* [Dec. 1998].)

Indoor pollution generally is considered worse than outdoor pollution, partly because of second-hand smoke or environmental tobacco smoke (ETS). Recently the largest European study done showed a 16% increase in the risk of lung cancer from second-hand smoke in nonsmokers.[80] Another significant indoor air pollutant is radon gas. Radon is a natural radioactive gas that is present in soil, is trapped in houses, and gives rise to radioactive decay products that are known to be carcinogenic to humans.[81,82,83,84,85,86,87] Ten percent of estimated cases of lung cancer are possibly attributable to radon pollution in houses.[76,88] In Sweden the risk for all histologic types of lung cancer, particularly small-cell carcinoma, increased progressively with increasing radon exposure.[87] The most hazardous houses can be identified and modified to prevent radon contamination. Radon increases the risk of lung cancer in smoking and nonsmoking underground miners.[85]

Occupation

Occupational exposures have long been recognized as causes of cancer. Table 10-11 identifies occupational hazards causally associated with cancers in humans.

A substantial percentage of cancers of the upper respiratory passages, lung, bladder, and peritoneum are attributed to occupational factors. Asbestos exposure has accounted for the largest number of occupational cancers but, because of curtailments in exposure, its impact is diminishing. Asbestos exposure and cigarette smoking together act synergistically to produce a 53-fold increase in the risk of lung cancer.[89] Carcinoma of the bladder has been linked to the manufacture of dyes, rubber, paint, and aromatic amines, especially β-napthylamine and benzidine. Benzol inhalation is linked to leukemia in shoemakers and in workers in the rubber cement, explosives, and dyeing industries.

Ultraviolet Radiation

Ultraviolet (UV) sunlight or solar radiation *causes* basal cell carcinoma and squamous cell carcinoma, two common skin cancers found in white individuals. Mutations in two tumor-suppressor genes (TP53 and PTCH) are partially responsible for the nonmelanoma skin cancers.[90] In addition to being a mutagen, sunlight acts as a tumor promoter by favoring the clonal expansion of TP53 mutated cells.[90] Sun-

Table 10-11 Occupational Exposures Related to Cancer

Cancer Site and Casual Agent	Related Occupation
LUNG	
Bischloro-methylether	Ion exchange resin producers
Chromium	Ore and pigment manufacturers
Mustard gas*	Poison gas producers
Radon	Hematite miners and persons exposed to radon
LUNG, PLEURA	
Asbestos	Miners, insulation installers, shipyard workers
LUNG AND SKIN	
Arsenic	Smelter and pesticide workers
Polycyclic hydrocarbons	Workers using mineral oil and tar; coal miners
LUNG AND NASAL	
Nickel	Nickel refiners
Wood dusts†	Nasal sinuses
SKIN	
Ultraviolet (UV) light	Outdoor workers, fishermen
LIVER	
Vinyl chloride	Vinyl chloride workers
Alcohol	Brewery workers
BLADDER	
Aromatic amines	Dye and rubber workers
LEUKEMIA	
Benzene	Workers using glue and varnish
NASAL	
Isopropyl alcohol	Isopropyl alcohol manufacturers
Wood dusts and inorganic-acid mists	Furniture makers
MULTIPLE SITES	
Ionizing radiation	Radium dial painters, uranium miners

*and pharynx
†Not as prevalent in the United States as in Europe

light also has profound effects on the cutaneous immune system, inducing a state of relative immunosuppression that prevents tumor rejection.[91]

Basal cell carcinoma commonly is located on the head and neck. Individuals with these tumors generally have light complexions, light eyes, and fair hair. They tend to sunburn rather than tan and live in areas of high sunlight exposure. These cancers usually arise on areas of the body that receive the greatest sun exposure, although they are not necessarily restricted to these cancer sites. Squamous cell carcinoma is found more commonly in men who work outdoors. These tumors are distributed over the head, neck, and exposed areas of the upper extremities (see Chapter 43).

The incidence of melanoma, a malignant pigmented mole, *correlates* with the amount of exposure to UV light.[8,92] Although the nonmelanoma skin cancers are related to cumulative exposure to UV radiation, melanoma is related to heavy, blistering overdoses at a young age. The relatively recent worldwide increase in melanoma among fair-skinned people is largely attributed to changes in clothing that promote greater exposure. The body areas receiving greater sun exposure vary between the sexes because of clothing differences. Malignant melanomas occur on the upper back and the dorsum of the hands of both sexes and the legs of females. There has been an alarming increase in the incidence of melanoma in the past 4 decades. It has been suggested that changing habits of sun exposure and use of sunscreen lotions may reverse this trend by the year 2020.

Xeroderma pigmentosum is a rare autosomal disease characterized by pigmentation abnormalities and malignancies. Persons with this disease demonstrate excessive skin damage caused by sun exposure at very young ages. People with xeroderma pigmentosum lack enzymes that repair sun-damaged DNA.

Ionizing Radiation

Much of the knowledge of the effects of ionizing radiation on human cancer has stemmed from observations of the Hiroshima and Nagasaki atomic bomb exposures. These unfortunate exposures caused acute leukemias in adults and children and increased frequencies of thyroid and breast carcinomas. Lung, stomach, colon, esophageal, and urinary tract cancers and multiple myeloma lately have been added to the list. At Nagasaki and Hiroshima, leukemia incidence in individuals 15 years or younger reached its peak 6 to 7 years after the explosions and has declined steadily since 1952. Middle-aged people 45 years and older at the time of exposure had a latent period of 20 years before developing acute leukemia. Children conceived after the exposure of their parents to the atomic bombs surprisingly have suffered no increase in any cancer thus far. Human exposure to ionizing radiation includes emissions from x-rays, radioisotopes, and other radioactive sources.

Radiation and carcinogenesis. An important effect of ionizing radiation is thought to be inhibition of cell division. Cells of lymphoid tissue, bone marrow, and intestinal epithelium normally are short-lived, rapidly dividing cells. Symptoms and causes of death from exposure to large doses of whole-body radiation are related to the inability of these cells to divide. For example, the suppression of stem cell (primitive precursor cell) division in the bone marrow can cause the disappearance of granulocytes and cause the remaining stem cells, if there are any, to repopulate the tissues. Depending on how many cells are lost, repopulation may require days, weeks, or longer, which may be too late to reverse the effects.

At low doses of radiation, few dividing cells may be damaged, and in some tissues this may lead to no detectable change in function. Smaller doses, however, can alter the developing fetus.[93] Organ development occurs early and extremely rapidly during pregnancy; exposure of the fetus to radiation can greatly alter cellular integrity and normal development. These effects depend on the number of stem cells available and the stage of fetal development.

Carcinogenesis can occur from mutation or cell transformation caused by radiation (see Chapter 2). Radiation can cause dominant and recessive mutations in the DNA and chromosome aberrations. To produce a carcinogenic effect, these DNA alterations must survive in cells capable of cell division. The DNA-dependent protein kinase (DNA-PK) is a nuclear protein kinase that regulates kinase activity by its association with DNA. Cells deficient in one of the DNA-PK components are hypersensitive to ionizing radiation.[94] Radiation can directly damage macromolecules or carbohydrates, proteins, lipids, and nucleic acids. Indirectly, radiation interacts with substances (generally water) within the cell, producing reactive-free radicals that then interact and damage DNA (see Chapter 2).

Carcinogenesis also can result from gene-environment interactions. Host factors can influence the carcinogenic effects of radiation. For example, although cells can repair some lesions in DNA, some genetic abnormalities alter the repair mechanism, making the individual sensitive to ionizing radiation. Disturbances in the DNA repair mechanism affect the risk of radiation-induced genetic effects and the risk of cancer.

Many other biologic variables affect responses to radiation, including the part and percentage of the body exposed, the individual's age or developmental stage at time of exposure, hormonal balance (e.g., sex hormones regulate cellular growth), genetic integrity, drugs, and other disease processes. Certain drugs can inhibit the immune response by affecting the surveillance role of the lymphoid cells. In the presence of infections, viral nucleoproteins may be introduced into the DNA, rendering the cell susceptible to transformation. Ionizing radiation can cause leukemias and many solid tumors (e.g., thyroid, breast, salivary gland).[93] Compelling data indicate that diagnostic x-rays to the trunk are related to risk of chronic myelogenous leukemia and that the risk increases with increasing x-ray dose to active bone marrow.[93] Solid tumors seldom appear before 10 years after radiation exposure and continue to appear for 30 years or longer after exposure. Leukemia is an exception, appearing within a few years after radiation exposure.

Hormones

The relationship between hormones and human cancer has been studied extensively. Interest began in 1919 when Laek reported that the removal of the ovaries in female mice prevented the development of breast cancer. Four notable types of human cancer—carcinoma of the breast, endometrium, ovary, and prostate—occur in target or hormone-responsive tissues. (These cancers are discussed also in Chapter 22.)

Much current research on hormones and cancer focuses on the direct actions of the sex steroids (estrogens, testosterone, progesterone). Prolactin, a major pituitary hormone, has a direct role in rat mammary cancer growth but its role in human breast cancer is controversial. Studies have found correlations between hyperprolactinemia and metastatic breast cancer.[95,96,97]

Oral Contraceptives

Many epidemiologic studies have found that oral contraceptive (OC) use has no effect on the risk of breast cancer in most women regardless of dose, brand, or type of estrogen or progestin.[58,98,99,100] Some studies, however, have identified subgroups of OC users who have an increased risk of breast cancer. Such subgroups include women with many years of OC use before the age of 25 years, with use before 1971, or with extended use before the first full-term pregnancy; women who use oral contraceptives at 45 years or older; women with a history of biopsy-confirmed benign breast disorders; nulliparous, premenopausal women with an early menarche; women with only one child; and women with a family history of breast cancer.[58,98] Of much interest is OC use in the perimenopausal period, which might increase the risk of breast cancer by prolonging high estrogen and progesterone levels, although the evidence is inconsistent.[101,102]

Ovarian cancer seems to develop from the epithelial cells on the surface of the ovary. The main stimulus for division of these cells is ovulation. After each ovulation, epithelial cells replicate to cover the exposed surface of the ovary. Those factors that *prevent* ovulation help protect against the development of ovarian cancer. Complete and incomplete pregnancies and OC use all reduce the risk of ovarian cancer.[102] In women who have used oral contraceptives for 5 years, endometrial cancer risk is reduced by about 55% relative to that of nonusers. OC use also *may* reduce colorectal cancer.[100]

Male sex hormones—testosterone and its derivative 5-dihydrotestosterone (DHT)—stimulate the growth of target tissues, such as the prostate. Men who take exogenous androgens, however, do not seem to have a higher risk of prostate cancer, whereas women who take estrogens without progestogens after menopause have a higher risk for development of endometrial cancer.

The difficulty in understanding the carcinogenic nature of hormones has been the separation of the hormones as modulators of target tissue growth and function from their potential causative carcinogenic effects. More simply, do hormones cause cancer? do they promote only tumor growth? or do they do both? Most evidence thus far supports their role as promoters of carcinogenesis in target tissues rather than as primary carcinogens; however, estrogen is becoming known as a causative factor, but its exact mechanism is unknown (see WHAT'S NEW? Estrogens and Cancer Update). The sex steroids produce their actions by the receptor mechanism (see Chapters 1 and 21), sensitizing the cell to the carcinogenic insult, promoting the carcinogenic process, and modifying the growth of the established tumor.

Estrogens

Estrogen replacement therapy has been prescribed for women to relieve perimenopausal symptoms (e.g., hot flashes) and to prevent chronic diseases, such as osteoporosis. Long-term use of estrogens by these women has been linked to endometrial cancer and breast cancer.[103,104,105,106,107] The most common type of endometrial carcinoma, endometrioid adenocarcinoma, develops from endometrial hyperplasia coexisting with excess estrogen (estrogen-dominant) exposure. In contrast, serous carcinoma of the endometrium does not seem to be related to estrogenic risk factors (see WHAT'S NEW? Estrogens and Cancer Update).[106]

The synthetic estrogen diethylstilbestrol (DES) also has been linked to cancer. Daughters of women treated with DES to avert habitual abortion have demonstrated a

WHAT'S NEW? Estrogens and Cancer Update

Substantial evidence supports the concept that estrogens can cause breast cancer because they act as regulators of cell proliferation, cell survival, and cell differentiation in animals and in women; the precise mechanism is unknown. The most commonly held theory is that estrogens stimulate proliferation of breast cells and thus statistically increase the chances for genetic mutation that could result in cancer. Another theory is that estrogen metabolism generates oxygen-free radicals and quinones (electron carriers) that produce both stable and unstable DNA metabolites. Both result in genetic mutations that accumulate and could ultimately cause cancer. Estradiol can induce various chromosomal and genetic lesions, including aneuploidy, chromosomal aberrations, gene amplification, and gene mutations, in several cell test systems. It is therefore suggested that estradiol is a carcinogen and capable of inducing genetic lesions in low frequency. In addition, studies strongly support the involvement of increased apoptosis and decreased proliferation after estrogen withdrawal. Further evidence for the role of estrogens in carcinogenesis is related to the enzyme *aromatase* that catalyzes the conversion of androgens to estrogens, which is the major mechanism of estrogen synthesis in the postmenopausal woman. Inhibition of aromatase reduces circulating plasma estrogen; therefore aromatase inhibitors are used in the treatment of breast cancer and are being evaluated for the prevention of breast cancer. Furthermore, antiestrogen drugs (e.g., tamoxifen) have resulted in a 50% reduction in the incidence of contralateral breast cancer.

Data from Brody AM, Njar VC: Aromatase inhibitors and their application in breast cancer treatment, *Steroids* 65(4):171, 2000; Colditz GA: Hormones and breast cancer: evidence of implications for consideration of risks and benefits of hormone replacement therapy, *J Women's Health* 8(3):347, 1999; Dowset HM et al: Clinical studies of apoptosis and proliferation in breast cancer, *Endocr Relat Cancer* 6(1):25, 1999; Goss PE: Risks versus benefits in the clinical application of aromatase inhibitors, *Endocr Relat Cancer* 6(1):325, 1999; Jordan VC: Antiestrogens: clinical applications of pharmacology, *J Soc Gynecol Investig* 7(1 suppl):47, 2000; Liehr JG: 4-hydroxylation of estrogens as a marker for mammary tumors, *Biochem Soc Trans* 27(2):318, 1999; Lin CQ et al: Regulation of mammary epithelial cell phenotypes by the helix-loop-helix protein, Id-1, *Endoc Relat Cancer* 6(1):49, 1999; Santen RH, Harvey HA: Use of aromatase inhibitors in breast carcinoma, *Endocr Relat Cancer* 6(1):75, 1999; Santen RJ et al: The potential of aromatase inhibitors in breast cancer prevention, *Endocr Relat Cancer* 6(2):235, 1999; Yee D, Lee AU: Crosstalk between the insulin-like growth factors and estrogens in breast cancer, *J Mammary Gland Biol Neoplasia* 5(1):107, 2000.

higher than expected percentage of clear cell adenocarcinomas of the vagina.[108] DES and other chemicals (e.g., organochlorines) can mimic a natural estrogen-like response (Fig. 10-24). DES binds to estrogen receptors found inside cells in many parts of the body, including the uterus, breasts, brain, and liver. It can elicit hormone receptors that may be stronger or weaker than those evoked naturally. It manages to sneak through a mechanism that protects the fetus from the development of disruptive effects of excessive estrogen exposure. The use of DES during pregnancy also is associated with an increased risk for breast cancer.[109] Hormone-disrupting chemicals are ubiquitous, and the pathologic conditions they cause may result from even extremely low levels of exposure.

Progestogens and Androgens

Endometrial cells divide in response to estrogen; however, the simultaneous presence of progestogens can decrease or even eliminate such mitotic activity. Progestins are synthetic compounds, such as medroxyprogesterone and acetate, and are *not* the same as natural progesterone—the same is true for estrogen where the majority of studies involve the synthetic estrogen or Premarin. There are over six types of synthetic progestins; thus, it is important to understand what type of progestin is being studied in terms of its biologic effects. Estrogen stimulation "unopposed" by progestogen increases endometrial cancer risk. The impact of combined estrogen (e.g., Premarin) and progestin (i.e., hormone replacement therapy) on risk of breast cancer has been controversial. Although protective effects analagous to those for endometrial cancer have been hypothesized for breast cancer, cyclical use of progestin to stimulate normal menstrual cycles increases mitotic activity in the breast.[45]

Reliable data on the effects of long-term use of combination therapy have only recently become available. These studies provide firm evidence that the addition of progestin to estrogen does not reduce the risk of breast cancer and suggest that risk is actually increased.[45,110,111,112,113] Among current or recent hormone users, the risk of breast cancer was 53% higher for combination therapy and 34% higher for estrogen alone compared with no hormone use.[111] These data were confirmed by the prospective Nurses Health Study and similarly in a Swedish cohort study.[110,112] In the most recent Breast Cancer Detection Demonstration Project, the excess breast cancer risk increased 8% for each year of combined hormone use and by 1% for each year of estrogen-only use.[113] In both the Nurses Health Study and the Breast Cancer Detection Demonstration Project, the majority of women used progestins for 15 or fewer days per month; this pattern appears to increase risk.[45] The biologic mechanisms underlying an effect of exogenous hormones on the breast are complex. The fact that progestins do not down-regulate estrogen and progesterone receptors (at least in 15 or fewer days per month, that is, when it is used cyclically) may contribute to its adverse effects.[114] Moreover, the isozyme of 17B-hydroxysteroid dehydrogenase induced by progestins in the breast predominantly catalyzes the conversion of the less potent estrone to the more potent estradiol.[113,115]

Additional evidence that increased levels of estrogen and progestogens in combination increase breast cancer risk is that early menarche and late menopause with associated increased hormone levels are significant risk factors for this disease (Fig. 10-25). Breast cancer risk is reduced 10% to 20% each year menarche is delayed. In addition, for any given age at menarche, rapid establishment of regular menstrual cycles with the associated increased hormone levels further increases risk.[102] Women who stop menstruating before 45 years old have one half the risk of breast cancer of women who continue to menstruate to 55 years or older.[102]

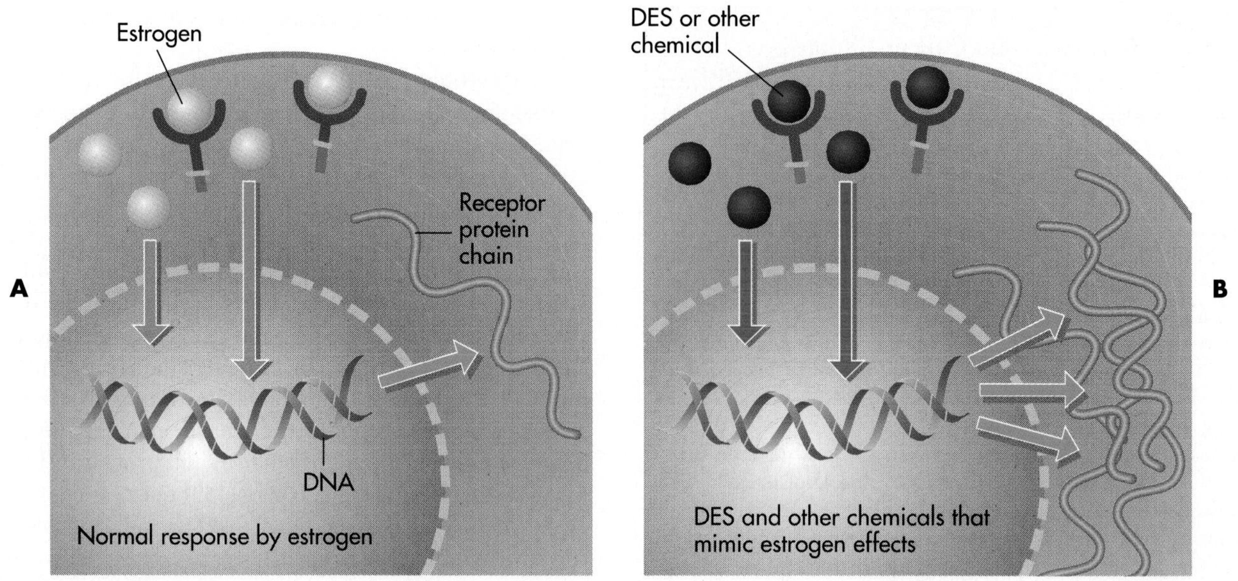

FIG. 10-24 Receptor effects of synthetic chemicals. A, Normal response. A natural estrogen binds to a receptor within the cell and activates the deoxyribonucleic acid (DNA) in the nucleus to produce the appropriate response. **B,** Hormone mimics, diethylstilbestrol (DES), and other synthetic compounds bind to cellular receptors and cause hormonal responses that may be stronger or weaker than those evoked naturally.

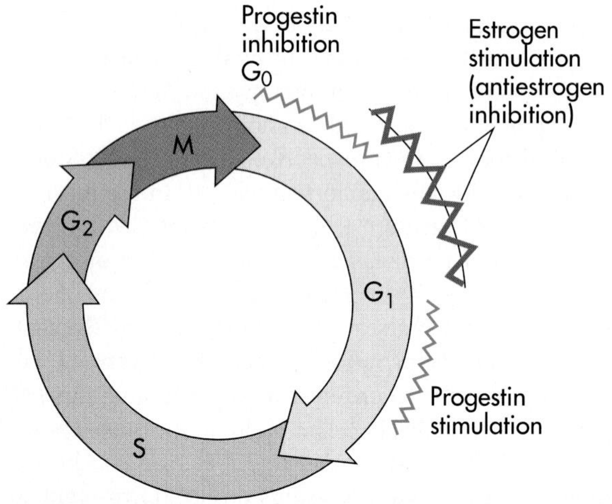

FIG. 10-25 Cell cycle and effects of hormones and hormone antagonists. Blue lines represent times of action of progestins stimulating cells during mid-G_1 period but inhibit progress of cells to reentry into G_1 phase from mitosis (M). Red line represents estrogen stimulating reentry from quiescent G_o state into the cell cycle and also acting during early G_1 phase. Cells are sensitive to growth inhibition by antiestrogen (soon after or until mid-G_1). Cells elsewhere in the cell cycle are essentially insensitive and proceed through S phase and mitosis at the same rate as untreated cells. Thus estrogens and antiestrogens regulate cell proliferation by their actions on a cell cycle control point early to mid-G_1 phase. (The cell cycle is discussed in Chapter 1.)

Breast cancer in men is a rare occurrence, yet the risk factors are similar to those in women and include Western countries, first-degree relatives with breast cancer, increasing age, infertility, obesity, exposure to exogenous estrogens, prior benign breast disease, and exposure to ionizing radiation. A decrease in risk has been related to high fertility, a history of prostate cancer, and exogenous androgens. These observations suggest that risk may be increased by low levels and decreased by high levels of androgens.[116] Although all androgens affect prostatic cells, it is believed that dihydrotesterone (DHT) is the active androgen primarily used by prostatic cancer cells for growth and division.[117,118] Prostate cancer is discussed in detail in Chapter 22.

IMMUNOBIOLOGY OF CANCER

Tumor Immune Surveillance Theory

One conclusion that can be drawn from the viral theory of carcinogenesis is that the induction of altered or abnormal cell products is not necessarily required for cancer cells to develop. The only difference between normal and transformed cells may be the amount, rather than the type, of cellular components (e.g., enzymes, cell surface receptors, plasma membrane–bound proteins) that each possesses. In this regard the overall structural composition of the plasma membranes of normal and transformed cells may be quite similar, if not identical. Thus any differences between normal and cancer cells may be both subtle and possibly imperceptible by the organism.

The immune system of higher organisms, such as humans, has evolved to recognize antigens that are considered to be foreign, or nonself, structures (see Chapter 6). Therefore, if the immune system is capable of recognizing and rejecting tumors, cancer cells must express nonself antigens. The **tumor immune surveillance theory** is based on this assumption.[119]

For some time investigators have been intrigued with the idea that the body could defend itself against the development of cancer. In 1908 a biologist, Dr. Paul Ehrlich, pro-

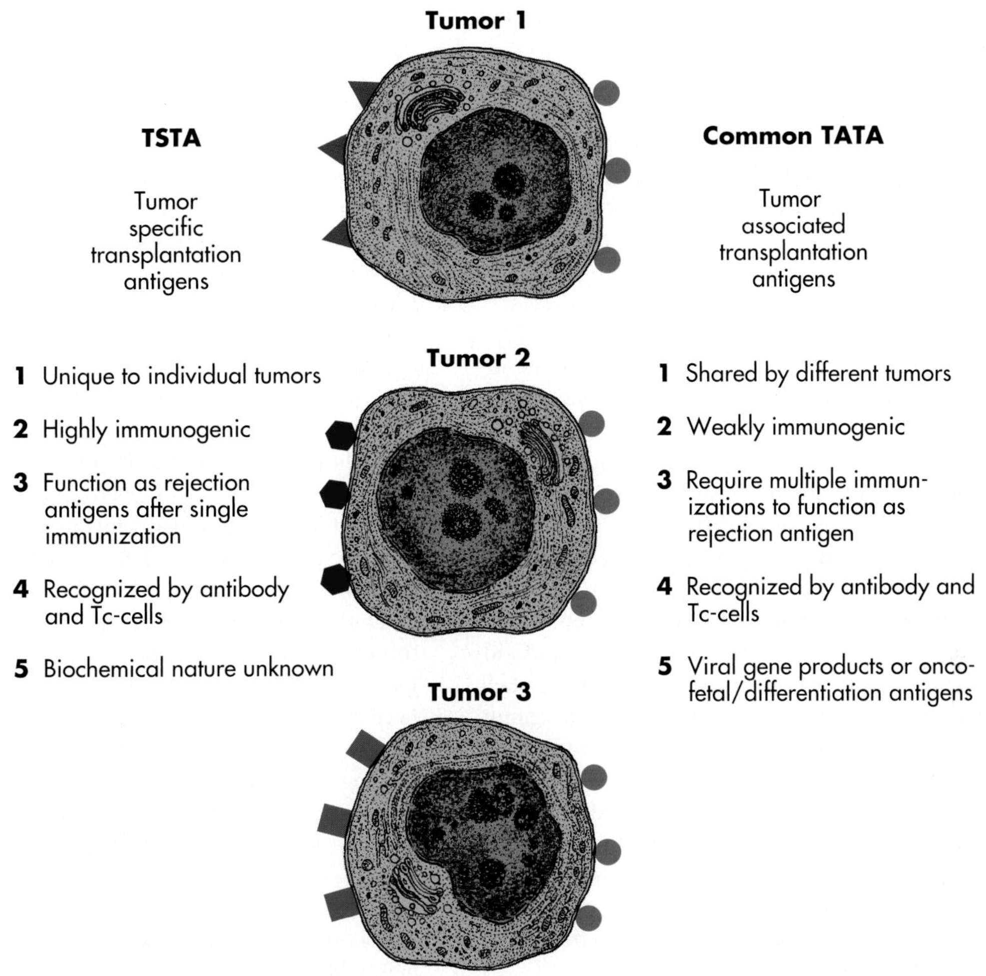
Tumor 1
TSTA
Tumor specific transplantation antigens
Common TATA
Tumor associated transplantation antigens
Tumor 2
1 Unique to individual tumors
2 Highly immunogenic
3 Function as rejection antigens after single immunization
4 Recognized by antibody and Tc-cells
5 Biochemical nature unknown
1 Shared by different tumors
2 Weakly immunogenic
3 Require multiple immunizations to function as rejection antigen
4 Recognized by antibody and Tc-cells
5 Viral gene products or oncofetal/differentiation antigens
Tumor 3

FIG. 10-26 Two general classes of tumor-specific antigens (TSAS).

posed that the transformation process was a common event and that, as a result, cancer cells were constantly arising in normal animals. He proposed that most cancer cells express foreign antigens that make them susceptible to rejection by their host's immune system.

Since that time a number of studies have supported Ehrlich's general concept. Based on this work, Sir Macfarlin Burnet formally proposed the tumor immune surveillance theory in 1970. In short, Burnet proposed that cell-mediated cytotoxicity (i.e., tumor cell killing by immunologic cells such as lymphocytes) evolved because the immune system needed to detect cancer cells. Certain experimental and clinical observations support Burnet's theory, including the identification of tumor antigens, increased risk of certain types of cancers in immune-suppressed individuals, identification of tumor-reactive antibodies in the serum of some individuals with cancer, and demonstration of tumor-specific T cell–mediated cellular immunity (mechanisms of cellular immunity are described in Chapter 6).

Tumor Antigens

Human cancer cells express numerous foreign molecules on their surface that can be recognized by the immune system as **tumor-specific antigens (TSAs).** Several types of molecules have been identified as TSAs. By the strictest definition, TSAs are expressed by tumor cells but not by normal cells. In reality, many of the TSAs expressed by human cancer cells are expressed also by normal cells. This is consistent with the preceding description of cancer. Because cancer is a disease of unregulated cell growth and differentiation, the differences between the molecules expressed on the surfaces of normal and cancer cells are subtle. Thus the recognition of a molecule as a TSA results from a complex interaction between the tumor and its host's immune system.

In the early 1950s Main and Prehn conducted a series of tumor transplantation experiments in mice. These experiments were the first to show that chemically induced mouse skin tumors express transplantation antigens that can immunize their host against the tumor. Further, these antigens were truly TSAs because they were not expressed by normal skin cells. It now is known that TSAs are expressed by most experimentally induced mouse tumors. These mouse tumor transplantation antigens generally are divided into two main groups: (1) tumor-specific transplantation antigens (TSTAs), which are unique for each tumor; and (2) cross-reactive tumor-associated transplantation antigens (TATAs), which are shared by a number of different tumors (Fig. 10-26). The TSTAs are generally the most immunogenic (i.e., they cause the strongest immune response) of the tumor antigens expressed by experimentally induced tumors.

Because transplantation studies cannot be performed with human tumors, much less is known about their ability to elicit a tumor rejection response. Knowledge of human TSAs has come from the study of tumor-reactive antibodies that are obtained from individuals' sera or experimental generation of monoclonal antibodies. Serologically defined human TSAs include viral antigens, oncofetal antigens, oncogene products, and "mutant" proteins and carbohydrates.

Viral Antigens

The **viral antigens** are products expressed by virally transformed cells. Viral antigens are common to all tumors induced by the same virus.

Research suggests that Burkitt lymphoma and nasopharyngeal carcinoma are caused by Epstein-Barr virus (EBV) and produce EBV antigens. Individuals with Burkitt lymphoma have higher antibody titers to EBV antigens than do unaffected individuals of the same age, gender, and geographic location, which is evidence that these tumors express viral antigens. Antibody titers against EBV in individuals with nasopharyngeal carcinoma correlate with the stage of their disease. This suggests that viral antigens are continually expressed by the tumor cells. (Lymphomas are further discussed in Chapter 26.)

Other human cancers that appear to be caused by viruses include T cell leukemias associated with human T cell leukemia virus (HTLV) and cervical carcinomas associated with human papillomaviruses (HPVs).[5,120] It is not known, however, whether these cancers express TSA of viral origin.

Oncofetal Antigens

The **oncofetal antigens** represent molecules that are expressed by cells during certain stages of embryonic development but are absent or expressed at very low concentrations by normal adult cells. The two best characterized antigens in this group are α-fetoprotein and carcinoembryonic antigen.

The **α-fetoprotein (α-FP)** is a serum α-globulin that is secreted by embryonic liver cells. During the first trimester, α-FP constitutes about 90% of the total serum globulins in the blood of human embryos. These levels quickly decline after birth. Individuals with hepatic, pancreatic, and embryonal carcinomas (malignant tumors of epithelial cells) have high levels of α-FP in their serum. Although α-FP appears to be associated specifically with these types of tumors, increased α-FP levels in the blood of individuals with nonneoplastic diseases, such as acute viral hepatitis, also have been observed. It is now known that initial high levels of serum α-FP at the time of liver cancer diagnosis are correlated with a poor prognosis.[121]

The **carcinoembryonic antigen (CEA)** is a glycoprotein that is part of the family of immunoglobulin-related proteins. CEA is associated with the mucous coating of the cells of the fetal gut, pancreas, and liver through the sixth month of gestation. Antibody titers to CEA have been found in the serum of individuals with various types of cancer. For example, 70% of patients with colon cancer, 90% of patients with pancreas cancer, and 35% of patients with breast cancer have detectable CEA antibody titers, compared with normal individuals (about 5% of the normal human population have CEA-reactive antibody titers). As with α-FP, however, serologic titers to CEA have been found in a large percentage of specific groups of normal people (e.g., pregnant women, heavy cigarette smokers) and in individuals with noncancerous diseases.

Malignancies of hematopoietic tissues express a unique form of oncofetal or differentiation antigens.[122] Mature hematopoietic cells arise from a common stem cell population and differentiate through a number of well-defined, lineage-specific stages. For example, the stage of differentiation of T and B lymphocytes can be defined by the cell surface antigens they express. Virtually all cancerous lymphocytes retain and express the antigens from that stage of development in which they were transformed. Pathologists can determine the type and prognosis of the cancer by evaluating the patterns of antigens expressed by these cancers.

One of the best-recognized TSAs expressed by hematopoietic cancers is the common acute lymphoblastic leukemia–associated antigen, referred to as CALLA. It has been shown that **CALLA** is the lymphocyte differentiation antigen CD10. CD10 is expressed by normal bone marrow progenitor cells, bone marrow macrophages and megakaryocytes, germinal center B cells, and mature neutrophils. CD10 also can be detected on a variety of nonhematopoietic cells such as mammary epithelium, fibroblasts, and solid tumors. CD10 expression is a valuable marker of non-B, non-T acute lymphoblastic leukemia (ALL). It has been found that individuals with CD10-positive ALL have a better prognosis than those with B cell, T cell, or CD10-negative non-B, non-T ALL.

Oncogene-Related Antigens

Numerous oncogene-encoded antigens are associated with individual tumors. This finding suggests that complex activation of certain oncogenes is required for transformation of normal cells. A number of oncogene-encoded antigens are expressed by lung cancers.[123] These include *ras, myc,* and *neu.* The oncogene-encoded proteins are associated with cellular growth and differentiation. The antigen *myc* is a nuclear phosphoprotein that binds DNA and regulates transcription. The *neu* protein is similar to epidermal growth factor receptor. Antibodies to the *neu* protein can affect cell proliferation in tumor cells that express this antigen.

A number of mutations are recognized to be associated with certain types of cancers. These mutations are summarized in Table 10-8. For example, 90% of chronic myelogenous leukemias have a translocation of the *bcr* gene (gene for guanosine triphosphate–activating protein) from chromosome 22 to the 59 end of the *abl* proto-oncogene on chromosome 9.

Alternatively, proteins encoded by tumor suppressor genes can be identified as TSAs. For example, retinoblastoma *(rb)* gene, *p53* gene, Wilms tumor gene, and deleted colon cancer *(DCC)* gene products are expressed as tumor antigens. The *rb* and *p53* are nuclear phosphoproteins that can bind several viral oncogene–encoded proteins. Interestingly, both *rb* and *p53* are expressed by lung carcinomas. The deleted colon cancer gene product is a TSA expressed by most colorectal cancers. Another interesting TSA that is a cell growth–regulatory protein is the *MDR1* gene product. Multidrug resistance *(MDR1)* increases the excretion of cancer drugs. Neoplasms that express *MDR1* are usually more resistant to cancer chemotherapy than tumor cells that do not express *MDR1*.

Carbohydrate Tumor Antigens

The tumor-associated carbohydrate antigens arise from alterations in normal glycosylation of proteins or lipids. To some degree, carbohydrate TSAs are oncofetal antigens because many of these antigens are transiently expressed in normal tissues during development and reexpressed by neoplasia.[124] Examples of these types of antigens include the lacto-series of Lewis blood group antigens expressed on glycosphingolipid (GSL) and glycoproteins; the core carbohydrate *o*-linked mucins expressed on glycoproteins; and precursor GSL molecules, such as Gm(3), Gm(2), and 9-*o*-acetyl-GD3, that are expressed by melanoma and other neuroectodermal cancers. Lewis blood group antigens Le^a and Le^b have been detected on gastrointestinal cancers regardless of the Le blood group type of the individual. Le^x and G1 have been found on colorectal and lung cancers.

The expression of the blood group A antigen on lung cancers is associated with a worse prognosis. Most of these antigens are cellular adhesion molecules. These molecules help cells bind with target structures on other cells. Expression of these antigens is thus a prerequisite for metastatic cells to bind vascular endothelium and initiate tissue invasion. Carbohydrate antigen expression has been shown in most cases to correlate with tumor invasiveness and decreased patient survival.

Protein Tumor Antigens

Mouse tumor transplantation experiments conducted in the 1950s suggested that TSAs were new proteins that could be synthesized and expressed only by transformed cells. It is now known that these types of TSA are abnormally expressed proteins with normal function. These TSAs function in proliferation, in enzymatic processes, as receptors, and as cellular structures. These antigens can be located in the nucleus, cytoplasm, plasma membrane, or extracellular compartment. There are numerous examples of these types of TSA.

The major histocompatibility class II antigen, HLA-DR, is not usually expressed by normal epithelial cells. (HLA is discussed in Chapter 6.) However, HLA-DR is expressed, to varying degrees, by melanomas, gastric carcinomas, larynx carcinomas, lung carcinomas, colorectal carcinomas, and breast carcinomas. Except for melanoma, HLA-DR expression is usually observed on tumors with a more favorable prognosis. This may be attributable to the role of class II antigens for stimulating helper T lymphocyte responses (see Chapter 6).

Some protein and glycoprotein TSAs are expressed by tumors and found in the serum of individuals with cancer. The function of these proteins is unknown. Examples include TAG-72, which is expressed by breast, colon, ovary, pancreas, stomach, endometrium, and non–small cell lung carcinomas,[125] and TA-4, an antigen expressed by squamous cell (skin) carcinomas.[126] As mentioned previously, in combination with CEA, TAG-72 expression has diagnostic value for identifying adenocarcinoma. In contrast, TA-4 is elevated in the serum of individuals with squamous cell carcinoma; skin disorders (e.g., psoriasis, atopic dermatitis); and kidney failure. In this regard, TA-4 is of little diagnostic value.

There are several examples of protein TSAs that are enzymes. Prostate-specific antigen (PSA) is expressed by prostate tumors.[127] Increased PSA serum levels are observed in individuals with increased tumor burdens. A strong correlation exists between PSA serum levels and tumor recurrence in individuals undergoing cancer therapy. CO17-1A is a nonsecreted glycoprotein expressed by colorectal carcinomas. It is a cell membrane calcium transporter that is similar in structure to epidermal growth factor and thymosin receptors.[121] Monoclonal antibodies against CO17-1A have tumoricidal properties. These antibodies have been used in immunotherapeutic trials. Metastatic melanomas express a glycoprotein that is melanotransferrin.[128]

A new group of TSA proteins has been identified. These are the stress-induced or heat shock proteins (hsp).[129] A majority of the nonviral TSAs expressed by human cancers are related to hsp.[129] These proteins can bind steroid receptors, immunoglobulin heavy chains, actin, oncogene proteins, and fatty acids.

Concepts about TSA have changed during the past century; that is, the idea that neoantigens are synthesized and expressed by transformed cells is probably incorrect. Based on the current understanding of carcinogenesis and knowledge of the biochemical nature of tumor antigens, clearly "TSA" per se may not exist. Rather, it is more likely that tumor immune surveillance mechanisms respond to tumor-specific epitopes (e.g., antigenic determinants) associated with common cellular molecules. In this regard a variety of modifications in normal molecular expression and association can account for the emergence of tumor-specific epitopes.

Immunologic Defense Against Tumors

When a tumor expresses cell surface TSA, the immune system of an immunologically competent host can reject the tumor. A number of clinical observations strongly support the concept of immunologic involvement in the tumor surveillance process. In the 1700s it was noted that individuals with draining, abscessed tumors lived longer than those whose tumors did not appear to be inflamed. In 1959 Berg reported that women with breast cancer tumors that were infiltrated with lymphocytes had a better prognosis than women whose tumors were free of lymphocytes. For certain types of neoplasia there is an increased risk (2% to 20% increase over the normal population) of developing cancer in individuals who are immunologically suppressed. Such individuals (Table 10-12) include (1) children with immunodeficiency diseases, (2) organ transplant recipients whose immune systems are suppressed with drugs (e.g., cyclosporin A to block graft rejection), (3) individuals with cancer for whom cancer therapy results in the suppression of immune responsiveness (many of the current radiation therapies and chemotherapies that are used to treat various forms of cancer depress the immune system, and these individuals have a high risk of developing secondary tumors), and (4) individuals with AIDS. Immunologic suppression also enhances the growth and recurrence of tumors in individuals with preexisting cancers.[130] These various clinical observations provide strong support for immune surveillance mechanisms and their role in the development of certain types of cancer. By preparing vaccines with cancer antigens, clinicians hope to treat individuals with cancer by stimulating tumor immunity through vaccination.[131]

Table 10-12 Correlation Between Immune Deficiency and Cancer Risk*

Types of Cancer	Increased Risk over Normal Population
Lymphomas	14 times greater
Leukemias	6 times greater
Carcinomas	
Skin (low-sun geographic areas)	4-7 times greater
(high-sun geographic areas)	21 times greater
Uterine cervix	13 times greater
Stomach	11 times greater
Urinary bladder	2 times greater

Data from Penn I: *Clin Exp Immunol* 46:459, 1981; Penn I: *J Pediatr Surg* 29:221, 1994.

*NOTE: There is an increased risk for developing specific types of cancer in individuals with various immune deficiencies versus that of the normal population. The values presented are generalized to include the various immunodeficient conditions. There is no increased risk in immunodeficient individuals for specific cancers not listed.

Immune Mechanisms for Defense Against Cancer

As with other antigens, TSAs can elicit both protective and suppressive immune responses. Certain immune responses are more beneficial than others for protecting the individual against cancer. The cancer defense mechanisms are summarized in Fig. 10-27.

The main involvement of B lymphocytes in a host's defense against cancer is through the production of TSA-reactive antibodies. Many individuals develop antibodies to various TSAs on their tumors. Although antibodies are the basis for identifying and defining tumor antigens expressed by various human cancers, they do not play a major role in protecting the individual against tumor emergence and growth. When effective, antibodies can prevent cancer growth by one of two means. Cytotoxic antibodies can activate complement killing of tumor cells. Alternatively, noncytotoxic antibodies can kill tumors by a mechanism called *antibody-dependent cell-mediated cytotoxicity (ADCC)* (see Chapter 6).

ADCC is a mechanism whereby lymphoid cells capable of killing tumor cells gain the ability to recognize TSA by

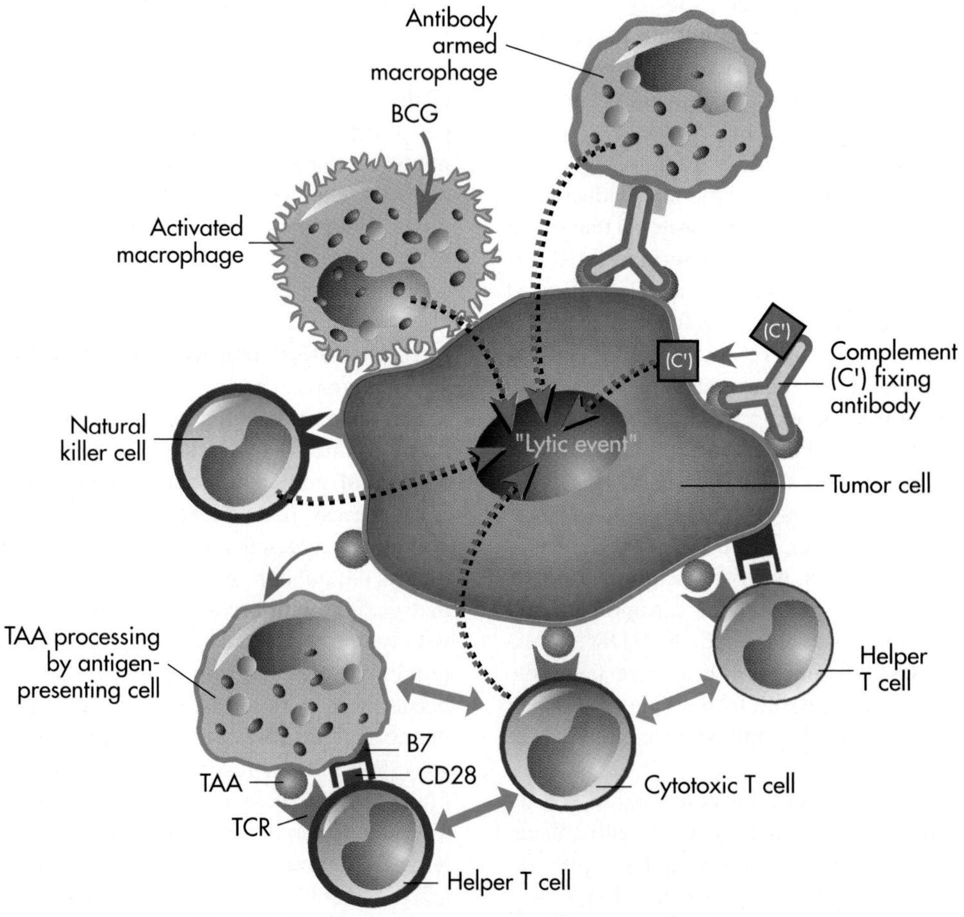

FIG. 10-27 Tumor immune surveillance mechanisms.

binding antibodies to their cell surfaces. The TSA-specific antibodies are bound by the cells' crystallizable fragment (Fc) receptors. The ADCC cells use surface-bound antibody as antigen-specific receptors to bind tumor cells. Once bound to the tumor, ADCC cells deliver a tumor-killing signal (the lytic event). Monocytes; neutrophils; B cells; and certain null cells, called *killer (K)* cells, possess ADCC function. Macrophages with ADCC activity are called *armed macrophages.*

Unlike armed macrophages, nonspecific tumor cell killing can be mediated by activated macrophages. Macrophages can be activated in several ways to lyse tumor cells. One way is by injection of bacterial adjuvants, such as the bacterium *Corynebacterium parvum* and bacille Calmette-Guérin (BCG). Adjuvants have been used in immunotherapy (see Chapter 8). Immune T lymphocytes can release macrophage-activating factors that stimulate macrophages to kill tumor cells. Once activated, macrophages kill tumor cells in a localized, antigen-specific fashion.

Natural killer (NK) and K cells may be the first line of defense against cancer cells. Natural killer cells are present in normal, cancer-free individuals. In mice a transient increase in NK cell activity occurs after TSA and adjuvant stimulation. Mouse strains with high levels of NK cell activity appear to be more resistant to the growth of certain transplantable tumors. Similarly, many individuals with cancer have low levels of NK cell activity. This suggests that NK cells are involved in human tumor immune surveillance.

Cytotoxic T lymphocytes (CTLs) are the most effective mediators of tumor rejection. They are TSA specific and differentiated from resting T cells after antigen presentation by macrophages and activation by helper T lymphocytes. Once activated, CTLs can recognize and kill tumor cells that express the appropriate TSA. Activated CTLs cause tumor rejection by secreting lymphokines (soluble lymphocyte products) that directly lyse tumor cells, inhibit the growth of transformed cells, or stimulate noncommitted cells to join in an antitumor response. These **tumor-infiltrating lymphocytes (TILs)** have been used as a form of cancer immunotherapy. By isolating TILs, expanding them in tissue culture containing the appropriate interleukins, and injecting them back into the individual, oncologists have been successful in treating cancers such as melanoma.

Immune Surveillance Escape Mechanisms

Although the immune system can reject tumors, individuals with normal immunologic function develop cancers. The host-tumor relationship during tumor emergence and progression is thus a complex process. Changes in host immunologic potential (i.e., range of antigenic responses) and characteristics of growing cancer cells (e.g., TAA and TSA expression, growth rate, metabolism) constantly occur. By taking advantage of these changes, many cancers can bypass the host's immune surveillance potential. Ways that tumors escape immunologic rejection include (1) antigenic modulation, (2) secretion of immunosuppressive substances, (3) escape and sneaking through, (4) blocking factor, (5) immunostimulation, and (6) TSA-reactive suppressor T lymphocytes (Ts cells). These escape mechanisms are summarized in Fig. 10-28.

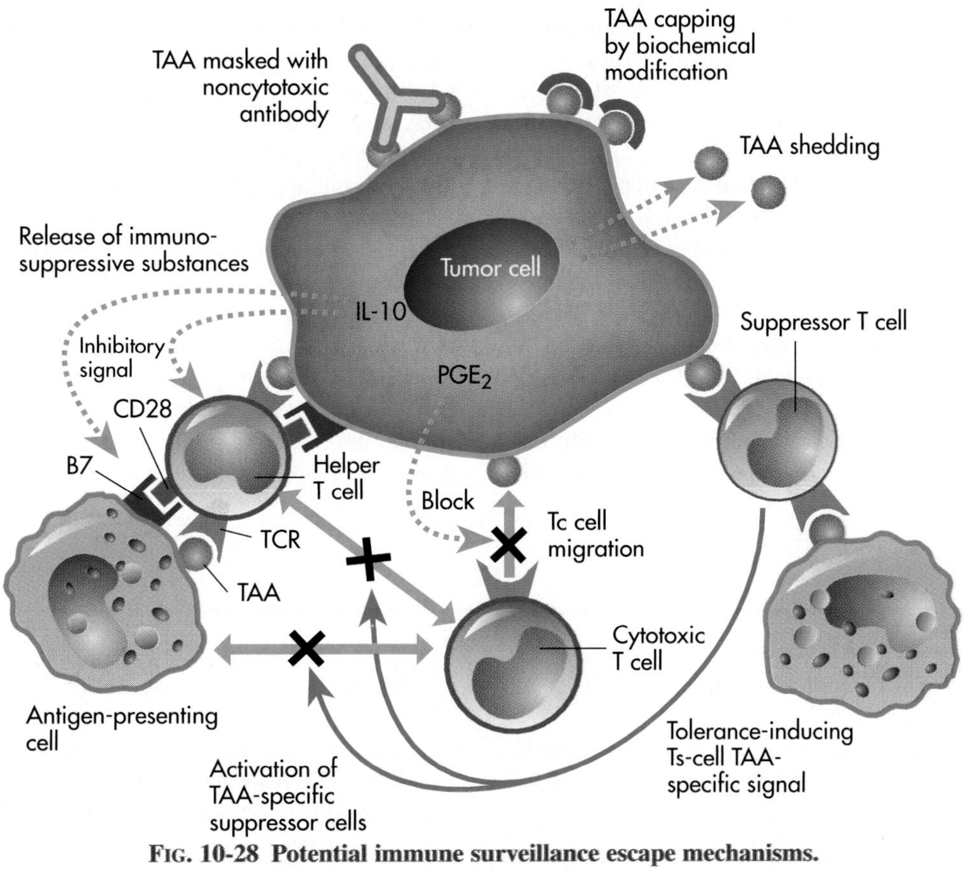

FIG. 10-28 Potential immune surveillance escape mechanisms.

Cancer cells can regulate their expression of cell surface molecules, including TSA. A number of agents, such as cAMP, interferons, interleukins, growth factors, tumor promoters, and retinoic acid, can cause modulation of tumor antigens, such as CEA, TAG-72, and HLA-DR.[125,132] Cancer cells also can mask their TSA by biochemical modifications. Human glioma cells (tumors of the central nervous system) can mask surface antigens with a hyaluronic acid–rich glycosaminoglycan coat. Modulated and masked TSAs are not recognized by the antibodies or cells that mediate effective antitumor immune responses.

Some tumors secrete soluble **immunosuppressive substances**—interleukins and prostaglandins. Prostaglandin E increases cellular cAMP levels in lymphocytes. As a result, lymphocyte proliferation is blocked and clonal expansion of TSA-reactive T lymphocytes cannot occur. This weakens the overall immune response to the tumor.

Tumors arise from a single transformed cell. During progression, cancer cells are actively dividing to increase the tumor mass and changes to the original transformed cell phenotype occur. When a tumor reaches a detectable size, the cells within it are a heterogeneous mixture of subclones. Such a process can facilitate **escape** from host defense mechanisms. This is especially true under conditions in which daughter cells lose or modify their TSA.

Experiments show that some tumors are rejected when a large number of cells are transplanted into a syngeneic host. When fewer cells of the same tumor are transplanted, however, tumors eventually grow in the syngeneic recipients. This observation led to the theory of **sneaking through.** Because tumors originate from a single transformed cell, it is possible that small amounts of TSA are not immunogenic. When a tumor reaches a size at which enough antigen is expressed to stimulate an immune response, it is too large, with too many rapidly growing cells, to be eliminated by the immune system.

Blocking factor, or **blocking antibodies,** can be found in the sera of tumor-bearing animals and in some individuals with cancer. Blocking antibodies bind TSA but do not activate complement or function in ADCC responses. Blocking antibodies inhibit tumor rejection by (1) masking TSA, (2) forming antigen-antibody complexes that cannot be processed by antigen-presenting cells, and (3) inhibiting CTL interaction with the tumor.

Prehn[133] has shown that a "little" **immunologic stimulation** enhances tumor cell growth. When mouse tumor cells were mixed with an optimal number of CTLs and transplanted to syngeneic hosts, the tumors were rejected. In contrast, when tumor cells were mixed with suboptimal numbers of CTL, the tumors grew faster than implants of tumor cells alone. Similar results were obtained when TSA-reactive antibodies were used as the immunologic stimulator. Prehn's studies suggest that in the early phases of an immune response, CTL infiltration into the tumor mass stimulates cancer cell growth. Tumor-infiltrating macrophages appear to have the same growth-enhancing effect.

The various effector functions of the immune system are carefully regulated to avoid potential destruction of normal tissues. One way that the immune system is controlled is by antigen-specific **suppressor T lymphocytes** (Ts cells) (Fig. 10-28). These Ts cells can be elicited by various antigens expressed by progressively growing tumors.[134] Suppressor T-lymphocytes function by (1) blocking other types of immune responses, (2) switching off an ongoing immune response, or (3) modifying the magnitude or type of immune response that is elicited. Increases in the number of circulating Ts cells in the blood of individuals with cancer have been reported.[135]

Active suppression is an effective way for tumors to escape immunologic rejection. Induction of immune suppression by growing tumors may be caused by the immune system's inability to determine whether an actively dividing cell is detrimental (as with transformed cells) or beneficial (as with actively dividing bone marrow cells) to the host. This is a very complex problem because most cell surface molecules (antigens) present on tumor cells are also expressed by their normal cell counterparts.

In addition to antigen-specific Ts cells, **activated macrophages** can exert suppressive activity. Suppression of tumor immune response by macrophages is nonspecific, however, and results in a general depression of the immune system. The mechanism of suppression by macrophages is unknown but appears to be mediated by cytokines.

In conclusion, it appears that tumor growth or rejection depends on complex interactions between cancer cells and the immune system of their host. A range of immunologic protective mechanisms have been identified that cause tumor lysis. Transformation processes, however, can select for cancer cells that escape the host's tumor surveillance system. Further, many carcinogenic agents can cause immune suppression, making individuals more susceptible to the growth of neoplasia.

SUMMARY REVIEW

Cancer: A Disease of Growth, Division, and Cell Differentiation

1. Abnormal cells that disobey the social control mechanisms of normal cell division proliferate to form tumors in the body.
2. Cell division is regulated by different combinations of protein growth factors presumably made by several "social control genes."
3. Two mutational routes result in uncontrolled cell proliferation: (a) stimulation of a gene causing *hyperactivity* and (b) *inhibition* of a gene causing inactivity. Hyperactivity is the

result of a mutation causing overexpression of a growth gene. The gene is called an *oncogene.* Initiation or inactivation of the cell's particular differentiation gene frees the cell of controlled growth. The inactivated or deleted differentiation-promoting gene is called a *tumor suppressor gene.*
4. Another type of genetic change can lead to cancer—those changes caused by tumor viruses.
5. Cancer cells are characterized by anaplasia, or loss of differentiation, and autonomy, or independence from normal cellular controls.
6. In the adult, undifferentiated cells (not totally committed to a specific function) are known as pluripotent cells, precursor cells, or stem cells. Cancer cells become more like embryonic cells and are less differentiated. Cancerous growth depends on derangements of cell differentiation.

Characteristics of Cancer Cells

1. The degree of disorganization varies among tumors, but disordered nuclear and structural components of cells are common.
2. Decreased communication or signaling between cells is the result of alterations in the surface. Because glycolipid and glycoprotein content is reduced, cellular communication is thought to be reduced.
3. Loss of fibronectin contributes to the overall loss in shape, cell-to-cell adhesion, and cellular migration.
4. Cancer cells exhibit anchorage independence with decreased cell-cell and cell–extracellular matrix attachments. Without anchorage, cancerous cells are allowed to metastasize.
5. Tumor metastasis has been related to changes in intercellular communication. Gap junctions are important in regulating communication and are thought to be disrupted or blocked in cancer cells.
6. Tumor cell markers are substances, such as hormones, enzymes, genes, antigens, and antibodies, that denote specific tumors.
7. Several intercellular changes occur in cancer cells, including alterations in the cytoskeleton, density-dependent inhibition of growth, growth requirements, and changes in the nucleus and cell protein.

Genetics of Cancer

1. In rare families, cancer is inherited in an autosomal dominant fashion. The mechanism by which environmental agents cause cancer is reportedly through increasing the frequency of mutation in somatic cells. Most human cancers, however, appear to arise without any known prior exposure to a carcinogenic agent.
2. Usually, mutations in proto-oncogenes accumulate in somatic cells over the years until a cell loses a critical number of growth control mechanisms and initiates a tumor. If damage occurs in cells of the germline, however, an altered form of one of these genes can be transmitted to progeny and predispose them to cancer.
3. Cancer-causing genes, or oncogenes, can be introduced into an individual (e.g., by oncogenic viruses) or inherited within some families.
4. The three main types of oncogenic DNA viruses are papovaviruses, adenoviruses, and herpesviruses. An example of an oncogenic RNA virus is human T cell leukemia-lymphoma virus.
5. Oncogenic viruses possess specific oncogenes called v-*onc.*
6. It is now known that cellular oncogenes, or c-*onc,* are incorporated into the genomes of a variety of different organisms, including humans.
7. The term *proto-oncogene* is used to refer collectively to the various c-*onc.* The term *proto-oncogene* indicates that c-*onc* and v-*onc* genes probably were derived from a common normal prototype gene.
8. Proto-oncogenes encode for growth factors, growth factor receptors, signal transducers, and nuclear proteins.
9. Viruses may cause mutations in surviving (e.g., infected) cells that could lead to neoplastic changes. Most oncogenic viruses cause transformation by a mechanism called *insertional mutagenesis.* Here the viral genes are incorporated into the host's genome at specific sites. The inserted genes are associated with cell transformation.
10. During some viral infections the host's immune system can become compromised, allowing neoplastic cells to emerge that would otherwise be rejected.
11. Tumor suppressor genes encode for proteins that act as inhibitors of growth factor stimulation. Tumor suppressor gene proteins block specific phases of the cell cycle, induce end-stage (e.g., terminal) differentiation, and stimulate cell senescence or death. Carcinogenesis involves inactivation of tumor suppressor genes and activation of oncogenes.
12. Oncogenic bacteria include *Helicobacter pylori. H. pylori* is now accepted as the most common cause of gastric infection and is responsible for the majority of individuals with peptic ulcer disease, gastric lymphomas, and gastric carcinomas.
13. Certain tumors are known to be caused by epigenetic changes, or changes in the pattern of gene expression without changes in the DNA sequence.

Carcinogenesis

1. Carcinogenesis is the process of tumor development.
2. Most evidence confirms that cancer has a monoclonal origin.
3. Because of the complexity of transformation processes, it is not surprising that cancers express multiple oncogenes and tumor suppressor genes.
4. Researchers propose that gap junction intercellular communication is either blocked or down-regulated in transforming cancer cells, and therefore communication between the transformed cancer cells and normal surrounding cells is lost.
5. One theory of carcinogenesis suggests that cancer development occurs in stages: (a) an initiation stage that causes irreversible changes in DNA after exposure to a carcinogen, (b) a promotion stage in which the initiated cells become cancerous, and (c) a progression stage in which the cells become more biologically defective.
6. Initiators and promoters include hormones, drugs, environmental agents, and a variety of personal behaviors. Although the precise biochemical cause of cancer is unknown, these are actually risk factors associated with increased incidence of cancer.
7. Personal behaviors associated with increased cancer risk include smoking and chewing smokeless tobacco, as well as sexual and reproductive behavior.
8. Smoking is associated with cancers of the lung, bladder, larynx, oral cavity, esophagus, and kidney; lung cancer is related to inhalation of tobacco smoke, which contains known carcinogenic compounds.
9. Oral cancer is associated with "dipping snuff."

10. Dietary factors can act as cancer-promoting or cancer-inhibiting agents. People are continually exposed to toxic, mutagenic, and carcinogenic chemicals called xenobiotics.
11. Dietary sources of toxic carcinogenic substances include compounds produced in the cooking of fat, meat, or protein and those associated with plant food substances such as alkaloids or mold byproducts.
12. People ingest xenobiotics that are environmental or industrial contaminants and certain prescribed and over-the-counter medicines.
13. Artificial additives and preservatives in food may include some compounds that are carcinogenic; particularly controversial is the use of nitrites, which react to form direct- or indirect-acting carcinogens when food is cooked.
14. Obesity is associated with endometrial cancer, and high-fat diets, although controversial, are associated with cancers of the breast, endometrium, colon, prostate gland and ovary, and with renal and esophageal cancer in men.
15. Polyunsaturated fatty acids are readily oxidized to yield free radicals and peroxidates that are toxic to cells and related to tumor development.
16. Omega-3 fatty acids (e.g., in fatty fish) decrease the number and size of tumors and increase the time elapsed before tumors appear.
17. Treatment with selenium is associated with decreasing mortality from lung, colon, rectal, and prostate cancer.
18. Incidence rates for cancer of the mouth, pharynx, esophagus, and liver are higher in individuals who ingest large quantities of both alcohol and smoke.
19. Alcohol intake has been consistently linked to breast cancer and colorectal cancer.
20. Age at first sexual intercourse and number of sexual partners are related to development of cervical cancer.
21. Human papillomavirus appears to be the causal agent for cervical cancer.
22. Pregnancy and childbearing seem to be protective factors against cancer of the endometrium, ovary, and breast; other reproductive factors related to decreased risk for breast cancer include late onset of menstruation and early menopause.
23. Air pollution is a concern for causing cancer because of inhalation of emissions, including arsenicals, benzene, chloroform, vinyl chloride, and acrylonitrile. Indoor pollution is considered worse than outdoor pollution because of cigarette smoke and possibly radon gas.
24. Cancers of the upper respiratory tract, lung, bladder, and peritoneum often are attributed to occupational exposures, including asbestos, fossil fuels, dyes, rubber, and paint.
25. Ultraviolet sunlight causes basal cell and squamous cell carcinomas, is associated with malignant melanoma, and is implicated also in increasing the severity of xeroderma pigmentosum.
26. Ultraviolet light damages DNA, inhibits cell division, and can lead to cell death. Damaged DNA can cause cancer by misrepairing itself and creating mutagenic cells that are susceptible to tumor development.
27. Exposure to ionizing radiation is caused by emissions from x-rays, radioisotopes, and other radioactive sources, some of which are industry- or occupation-related exposures.
28. Ionizing radiation inhibits cell division, especially in lymphoid tissue, bone marrow, and intestinal epithelium, which contain normally short-lived, rapidly dividing cells.
29. Carcinogenesis can occur from radiation-induced mutations or cell transformations; mutations may be dominant or recessive and also may cause chromosome aberrations.
30. Genetic factors can alter the repair mechanisms for DNA, so that an individual is particularly sensitive to the carcinogenic effects of ionizing radiation.
31. Biologic variables that affect responses to radiation include the part and percentage of the body exposed, the individual's age or stage of development at the time of exposure, genetic integrity, drugs, and other disease processes.
32. Radiation exposure in the neonate, infant, or child can cause growth retardation; the younger the child, the more vulnerable the child is to the effects of radiation.
33. For cancers that occur in hormone-responsive target tissues, hormones probably act as promoters of carcinogenesis rather than as primary carcinogens; estrogen is becoming known as a causative factor, but its exact mechanism is unknown.

Immunobiology of Cancer

1. Cancer cells express tumor-associated antigens, which are not found on normal, nontransformed cells.
2. Tumor-specific antigens (TSAs) may be caused by synthesis of new molecules, by unmasking of potential tumor-associated antigen, by loss of plasma membrane components, by biochemical modification, or by release of intracellular components.
3. TSAs generally are classified as tumor-specific transplantation antigens (TSTAs) or cross-reactive, tumor-associated transplantation antigens (TATAs).
4. TSTAs are apparently more immunogenic than TATAs and therefore produce a stronger immune response.
5. Tumor antigens include viral antigens, oncofetal antigens (α-fetoprotein and carcinoembryonic antigen), oncogene-related antigens, carbohydrate, and protein tumor antigens.
6. When a developing tumor expresses TSA, an immunologically competent host can recognize these antigens and produce a range of immune responses to reject the tumor.
7. In spite of the immune system's ability to reject cancer cells, some cancer cells are apparently capable of bypassing the host's immune surveillance and, by "escaping," can cause cancer.
8. Proposed immune surveillance escape mechanisms include antigenic modulation, secretion of immunosuppressive substances, escape and sneaking through, selective stimulation of suppressor cells, production of blocking antibodies, and immunostimulation.

KEY TERMS

Activated macrophage, *328*
Anaplasia, *292*
Anchorage independence, *298*
Anchoring junction, *298*
Autocrine stimulatory hypothesis, *302*
Autonomy, *292*
Autostimulation, *302*
Blocking antibody, *328*
Blocking factor, *328*

KEY TERMS—cont'd

CALLA, *324*
Carcinoembryonic antigen (CEA), *324*
Carcinogenesis, *309*
Carcinoma, *297*
Carcinoma in situ, *297*
Chemoprotector, *316*
Cocarcinogen, *312*
c-*onc, 306*
Crisis, *294*
Density-dependent inhibition of growth, *301*
Ectopic hormone production, *299*
Epigenetic change, *309*
Escape, *328*
α-Fetoprotein (α-FP), *324*
Fiber, *315*
Fibronectin, *298*
Gap junction, *298*
Glioma, *297*
Grading, *292*
Immortal stem cell, *310*
Immunologic stimulation, *328*
Immunosuppressive substance, *328*
Initiation, *312*
Insertional mutagenesis, *306*
Leukemia, *297*
Lymphoma, *297*
Metastasize, *298*
Mutagen, *303*
Mutagenesis, *309*
Nitrate, *315*
Oncofetal antigen, *324*
Oncogene, *292*
Oncogenic virus, *303*
Phase I activation enzyme, *314*
Phase II deactivation enzyme, *314*
Progression, *297*
Promotion, *312*
Proto-oncogene, *292*
Retrovirus, *305*
Reverse transcriptase, *305*
Sarcoma, *297*
Senescent, *294*
Sneaking through, *328*
Stem cell, *292*
Suppressor T lymphocyte, *328*
Telomere, *294*
Terminally differentiated, *293*
Transformation, *292*
Tumor cell marker, *299*
Tumor immune surveillance theory, *322*
Tumor-infiltrating lymphocyte (TIL), *327*
Tumor-specific antigen (TSA), *323*
Tumor suppressor gene, *292*
Tumor virus, *292*
Viral antigen, *324*
v-*onc, 306*
Xenobiotic, *314*

REFERENCES

1. Alberts B et al: *Essential cell biology: an introduction to the molecular biology of the cell,* ed 3, New York, 1998, Garland Press.
2. Devereaux TR, Risinger JI, Barrett JC: Mutations and altered expression of the human cancer genes: what they tell us about causes, *IARC Sci Publ* 146:19, 1999.
3. Perillo NL, Marcus ME, Baum LG: Galectins: versatile modulators of cell adhesion, cell proliferation, and cell death, *J Mol Med* 76(6):402, 1998.
4. Blasi F: Molecular mechanisms of protease-mediated tumor invasiveness, *J Surg Oncol* 3:21, 1993.
5. Templeton DJ, Weinberg RA: Principles of cancer biology. In Murphy GP, Lawrence W Jr, Lenhard RE, editors: *ACS textbook of clinical oncology,* ed 2, Atlanta, 1995, American Cancer Society.
6. Trosko JE, Chang CC, Madhuker BV: Symposium: cell communication in normal and uncontrolled growth. Modulation of intercellular communication during radiation and chemical carcinogens, *Radiat Res* 123:241, 1990.
7. Konishi N, Donovan PJ, Waro JM: Differential effects of renal carcinogenesis tumor promoter on growth promotion and inhibition of gap junctional communication, *Carcinogenesis* 11(6):903, 1990.
8. Kricker A, Armstrong BK, Parkin DM: Measurement of skin cancer incidence, *Health Reports* 5:63, 1993.
9. Hamada J et al: Junctional communication of highly and weakly metastatic variant clones from a rat mammary carcinoma in primary and metastatic sites, *Invasion and Metastasis* 11:149, 1991.
10. Moosa AR, Robson MC, Schimpff SC, editors: *Comprehensive textbook of oncology,* Baltimore, 1991, Williams & Wilkins.
11. American Cancer Society: Cancer statistics 1997, *CA Cancer J Clin* 45(1):12, 1997.
12. Sachs L: The molecular control of development in normal and leukemic blood cells, *Int J Dev Biol* 1(suppl):61S, 1996
13. Heldin CH, Westermark B: Mechanism of action and in vivo role of platelet-derived growth factor, *Physiol Rev* 79(4):1283, 1999.
14. Kahn P, Graf T, editors: Malignant transformation as a multistep process. In *Oncogenes and growth control,* New York, 1986, Springer-Verlag.
15. Jorde LB et al: *Medical genetics,* ed 2, St Louis, 1999, Mosby.
16. Cavanee WK, White RL: The genetic basis of cancer, *Sci Am* 272:72, 1995.
17. Kamb A: Role of a cell cycle regulator in hereditary and sporadic cancer, *Cold Spring Harb Symp Quant Biol* 59:39, 1994.
18. zur Hausen H: Papillomaviruses causing cancer: evasion from host-cell control in early events in carcinogenesis, *J Natl Cancer Inst* 92: 690, 2000.
19. Hausen HZ: Viruses in human cancers, *Science* 254:1167, 1991.
20. Weinberg RA: The molecular basis of carcinogenesis: Understanding the cell cycle clock, *Cytokines Molecular Therapy* 2:105, 1995.
21. Weinberg RA: The molecular basis of oncogenes and tumor-suppressor genes, *Ann NY Acad Sci* 758:331, 1995.
22. Yokota J: Tumor progression and metastasis, *Carcinogenesis* 21:497, 2000.
23. Sepulveda AR et al: Molecular identification of main cellular lineages as a tool for the classification of gastric cancer, *Hum Patho* 31(5):566, 2000.
24. Alexander GA, Brawley OW: Association of *Helicobacter pylori* infection with gastric cancer, *Mil Med* 165(1):21, 2000.
25. Smith VC, Genta RM: Role of *Helicobacter pylori* gastritis in gastric atrophy, intestinal metaplasia, and gastric neoplasia [review], *Microse Res Tech* 58(6):313, 2000.
26. Byrd JC et al: Inhibition of gastric mucin synthesis by *Helicobacter pylori, Gastroenterol* 118(6):1072, 2000.
27. Goddard AD, Solomon E: Genetic aspects of cancer, *Adv Hum Genet* 21:321, 1993.
28. Hasler CM, Bennick MR, Trosko JE: Inhibition of gap junction-mediated intercellular communication by alpha-linolenate. *J Physiol* 261:166, 1991.
29. Trosko JE, Chang CC: Stem cell theory of carcinogenesis, *Toxicol Lett* 4(2):283, 1989.
30. Krutovskikh V, Yamasaki H: The role of gap junctional intercellular communication (GJIC) disorders in experimental and human carcinogenesis, *Hilstol-histopathoi* 12(3):761, 1997.
31. Miki H et al: Effect of TPA on intercellular communication in various clones of mouse epidermal cells, *Cancer Res* 50:1324, 1990.
32. Rous P, Kidd JG: Conditional neoplasms and subthreshold neoplastic states, *J Exp Med* 73:365, 1941.
33. Boutwell RK: Some biological aspects of skin carcinogenesis, *Prog Exp Tumor Res* 4:207, 1964.
34. CDC MMWR Weekly Report: Tobacco use—United States 1900-1999, *AMA* 282(23):2202, 1999.

35. Hanson JS: Which straw will break the camel's back, *AJN* 99(11):63, 1999.
36. Hecht SS: Tobacco smoke carcinogens and lung cancer, *J Natl Cancer Inst* 91(14):1194, 1999.
37. Gritz ER, Fiore MC, Henningfield JE: Smoking and cancer. In Murphy GP, Lawrence W, Lenhard RE: *Clinical oncology*, ed 2, New York, 1995, American Cancer Society.
38. Leonard CT, Sachs DP: Environmental tobacco smoke and lung cancer incidence, *Curr Opin Pulm Med* 54(4):189, 1999.
39. Henderson BE, Ross RK, Pike MC: Toward the primary prevention of cancer. *Cancer Sci* 254:1131, 1991.
40. Jones DP, Delong MJ: Detoxification and protective functions of nutrients. In Stipanuk M, ed, *Biochemical and physiological aspects of nutrition*, Philadelphia, 2000, W.B. Saunders.
41. Guthrie N, Carroll KK: Specific versus non-specific effects of dietary fats on carcinogenesis, *Prog Lipid Res* 38:261, 1999.
42. Mukutmoni-Norris M, Hubbard NE, Erickson KL: Modulation of murine mammary tumor vasculature of dietary N-3 fatty acids in fish oil, *Cancer Lett* 150(1):101, 2000.
43. Ogilvie GK et al: Effect of fish oil, arginine, and doxorubicin chemotherapy on remission and survival time for dogs with lymphoma: A double-blind, randomized placebo-controlled study, *Cancer* 88(8): 1916, 2000.
44. Bartsch H, Nair J, Owen RW: Dietary polyunsaturated fatty acids and cancers of the breast and colorectum: emerging evidence for their role as risk modifiers, *Carcinogenesis* 20(12):229, 1999.
45. Willett WC, Colditz G, Stampfer M: Postmenopoausal estrogens—opposed, unopposed, or none of the above [editorial], *JAMA* 283(4): 534, 2000.
46. Martin-Chouly CA et al: Modulation of PAF production by incorporation of arachidonic acid and eicosapentaenoic acid in phospholipids of human leukemic monocyte-like cells THP-1, *Prostaglandins Other Lipid Mediat* 60(4):127, 2000.
47. Vinceti M et al: Mortality in a population with long-term exposure to inorganic selenium via drinking water, *J Clin Epidemiol* 53(10):1062, 2000.
48. Sunde RA: Selenium. In Stipanuk MH, editor, *Biochemical and physiological aspects of human nutrition*, Philadelphia, 2000, W.B. Saunders.
49. *Cover story: Diseases we can't crack. Nutrition Action Health Letter* 26(10):7, 2000.
50. Cotugna N: Dietary factors and cancer risk, *Semin Oncol Nurs* 16:99, 2000
51. Doll R, Peto R: *The causes of cancer,* New York, 1981, Oxford University Press.
52. Henderson BE, Ross RK, Pike MC: Toward the primary prevention of cancer, *Cancer Sci* 254:1131, 1991.
53. Blot WJ, McLaughlin JK: The changing epidemiology of esophageal cancer, *Semin Oncol* 26(5 suppl 15):2, 1999.
54. McLaughlin JK, Lipworth L: Epidemiologic aspects of renal cell cancer, *Semin Oncol* 27(2):115, 2000.
55. Pera M: Epidemiology of esophageal cancer, especially adenocarcinoma of the esophagus and esophagogastric junction, *Recent Results Cancer Res* 155:1, 2000.
56. Franceschi S: Alcohol and cancer, *Adv Exp Med Biol* 472:43, 1999.
57. Trigg DJ, Lait M, Wenig BL: Influence of tobacco and alcohol on the stage of laryngeal cancer diagnosis, *Laryngoscope* 110(3 pt 1):408, 2000.
58. Kelsy J, Gammon MD: The epidemiology of breast cancer, *CA Cancer J Clin* 41:146, 1991.
59. Rohan TE et al: Alcohol consumption and risk of breast cancer: a cohort study, *Cancer Causes Control* 11:239, 2000.
60. Willett WC et al: Fat and the risk of breast cancer, *N Engl J Med* 316(1):22, 1987.
61. Young TB: A case-control study of breast cancer and alcohol consumption habits, *CA Cancer J Clin* 64:552, 1989.
62. Gorins A: Causal interactions of estrogens and alcohol in cancer of the breast, *French Presse Med* 29(12):670, 2000.
63. Wu AH: Diet and breast carcinoma in multiethnic populations, *Cancer* 88(5 suppl):1239, 2000.
64. Stoll BA: Alcohol intake and late-stage promotion of breast cancer, *Eur J Cancer* 35(12):1653, 1999.
65. Yu H, Berkel J: Do insulin-like growth factors mediate the effect of alcohol on breast cancer risk, *Med Hypotheses* 52(6):491, 1999.
66. Ginsberg ES: Estrogen, alcohol and breast cancer risk. *J Steroid Biochem Mol* 69(1):299, 1999.
67. Murthy NS, Mathew A: Risk factors for pre-cancerous lesions of the cervix, *Eur J Cancer Prev* 9(1):5, 2000.
68. Hausen HZ: Papillomaviruses causing cancer: evasion from host-cell control in early events in carcinogenesis, *J Natl Cancer Inst* 92(9): 690, 2000.
69. Southern SA, Herrington CS: Molecular events in uterine cervical cancer, *Sexually Transmitted Infections* 74:101, 1998.
70. Rutter DO: Healing their wounds, *Catalyst* 15(4):12, 1996.
71. Micha JP: Genital warts: treatable warning of cancer, *Female Patient* 9:31, 1984.
72. Goodman A: Role of routine human papillomavirus subtyping in cervical screening, *Curr Opin Obstet Gynecol* 12(1):11, 2000.
73. Devesa SS, Diamond EL: Association of breast cancer and cervical cancer incidences with income and education among whites and blacks, *J Natl Cancer Inst* 65:515, 1980.
74. Kreiger N et al: Social class, race/ethnicity, and incidence of breast cancer, cervix, colon, lung, and prostate cancer among Asian, Black, Hispanic, and White residents of the San Francisco Bay Area, 1988-92 (United States), *Cancer Causes Control* 10(6):525, 1999.
75. Willett WC: Dietary fat and breast cancer, *Toxicol Sci* 52(2 Suppl): 127, 1999.
76. Blair A, Kazerowni N: Reactive chemicals and cancer, *Cancer Causes and Control* 8:473, 1998.
77. Katsouyanni K, Pershagen G: Ambient air pollution exposure and cancer, *Cancer Causes Control* 8(3):284, 1997.
78. Ames BN, Magaw R, Gold LS: Ranking possible carcinogenic hazards, *Science* 236:271, 1987.
79. Epstein SS, Swartz JB: Fallacies of lifestyle cancer theories, *Nature* 289:127, 1981
80. Ong EK, Glantz SA: Tobacco industry efforts subverting International Agency for Research on cancer's second-hand smoke study, *Lancet* 355(9211):1253, 2000.
81. Demers R: Overview of radon, lead, and asbestos exposure, *Am Fam Physician* 44(5 suppl):51S, 1991.
82. Krewski D et al: Characterization of uncertainty and variability in residential radon cancer risks, *Ann N Y Acad Sci* 895:245, 1999.
83. Neuberger T, Allen A: Lung cancer risk form residential radon: Meta-analysis of eight epidemiologic studies, *J Natl Cancer Inst* 89:663, 1997.
84. Polpong E, Borornkitti S: Indoor radon, *J Med Assoc Thailand* 81:47, 1998.
85. Vahakangas KH et al: Mutations of p53 and ras genes in radon-associated lung cancer from uranium miners, *Lancet* 339(8793): 576, 1992.
86. Weisburger JH, Williams GM: Causes of cancer. In Murphy GP, Lawrence W, Lenhard RE: *Clinical oncology,* ed 2, New York, 1995, American Cancer Society.
87. Yngveson A et al: p53 mutations in lung cancer associated with residential radon exposure, *Cancer Epidemio Biomarkers Prev* 8:433, 1999.
88. Krewski D et al: Characterization of uncertainty and variability in residential radon cancer risk, *Ann NY Acad Sci* 895:245, 1999.
89. Humphrey EW, Ward HB, Perri RT: Lung cancer. In Murphy GP, Lawrence W, Lenhard RE: *Clinical oncology,* ed 2, New York, 1995, American Cancer Society.
90. Wilkenkal NM, Brash DE: Ultraviolet radiation induced signature mutations in photocarcinogenesis, *J Ivestig Dermatol Symp Proc* 4(1): 6, 1999.
91. Grossman D, Leffell DJ: The molecular basis of nonmelanoma skin cancer: New understanding, *Arch Dermatology* 133(10):1263, 1997.

92. Bruce AJ, Brodland DG: Overview of skin cancer detection and prevention for the primary care physician, *Mayo Clin Proc* 75(5):491, 2000.
93. Doll R, Wakeford R: Risk of childhood cancer from fetal irradiation, *Brit J Radiol* 70:130,1997.
94. Muller C et al: Regulation of the DNA-dependent protein kinase (DNA-PK) activity in eukaryotic cells, *Biochimie* 81(1):117, 1999.
95. Mandala M et al: Endocrinological study of the dopaminergic regulation of prolactin release in metastatic breast cancer, *Tumori* 85(6):494, 1999.
96. Matera L et al: Prolactin in autoimmunity and antitumor defense, *J Neuroimmunol* 109(1):47, 2000.
97. Wennbo Cohen AD et al: Prolactin serum levels in patients with breast cancer, *Isr Med Assoc* 2(4):287, 2000
98. Gadducci A, Genazzani AR: Steroid hormones in endometrial and breast cancer, *Eur J Gynaecol Oncol* 18:371, 1997.
99. Paul C, Skegg DCG, Spears GFS: Oral contraceptive use and risk of breast cancer in older women, *Cancer Causes Control* 6:485, 1995.
100. Franceschi S, LaVecchia C: Oral contraception and colorectal tumors. A review of epidemiological studies, *Contraception* 58(6):335, 1998.
101. Ostrow RS et al: Detection of papilloma virus DNA in human semen, *Science* 231:731, 1986.
102. Hulka BS: Epidemiologic analysis of breast and gynecologic cancers, *Prog Clin Biol Res* 396:17, 1997.
103. Chiechi LM, Secreto G: Factors of risk for breast cancer influencing postmenopausal long-term hormone replacement therapy, *Tumor* 86(1): 12, 2000.
104. Doren M: Hormonal replacement regimens and bleeding, *Maturitas* 34(suppl 1):517, 2000.
105. Koukoulis GN: Hormone replacement therapy and breast cancer risk, *Ann NY Acad Sci* 900:422, 2000.
106. Sherman ME: Theories of endometrial carcinogenesis: a multidisciplinary approach, *Mod Patho* 13(2):295, 2000.
107. Spady, TH, McComb RD, Shull JD: Estrogen action in the regulation of cell proliferation, cell survival, and tumorigenesis in the rat anterior pituitary gland, *Endocr* 11(3):217, 1999.
108. Herbst AL, Ultelder H, Poskanzer DC: Adenocarcinomas of the vagina: association of maternal stilbestrol therapy with tumor appearance in young females, *N Engl J Med* 284:878, 1971.
109. Kelsey J, Gammon MD: The epidemiology of breast cancer, *CA Cancer J Clin* 41(3):146, 1991.
110. Colditz GA et al: Use of estrogen plus progestin is associated with greater increase in breast cancer risk than estrogen alone, *Am J Epidemiol* 147(suppl):645, 1998.
111. Collaborative Group on Hormonal Factors in Breast Cancer: Breast cancer and hormone replacement therapy: collaborative reanalysis of data from 51 epidemiologic studies of 52,705 women with breast cancer and 108,411 women without breast cancer, *Lancet* 350:1047, 1997.
112. Persson I et al: Risks of breast cancer and endometrial cancer after estrogen and progestin replacement, *Cancer Causes Control* 10:253, 1999.
113. Schairer C et al: Menopausal estrogen and estrogen-progestin replacement therapy and breast cancer risk, *JAMA* 283(4):485, 2000.
114. Hargreaves DF et al: Epithelial proliferation and hormone receptor status in the normal post-menopausal breast and the effects of hormone replacement therapy, *Br J Cancer* 78(7):945, 1998.
115. Peltoketo H et al: Expression and regulation of 17 beta-hydroxysteroid dehydrogenase type 1 [review], *J Endocrinol* 150(suppl):S21, 1996.
116. Alberg AJ, Lam AP, Helzlsouer KJ: Epidemiology, prevention, and early detection of breast cancer, *Curr Opin Oncol* 11(6):435, 1999.
117. Denis LJ, Griffiths K: Endocrine treatment in prostate cancer [review], *Semin Surg Oncol* 18(1):52, 2000.
118. Tsihlias J et al: Involvement of p27Kip1 in G1 arrest by high dose 5 alpha-dihydrotesterone in LNCaP human prostate cancer cells, *Oncogene* 19(5):670, 2000.
119. Stevenson H, Tsang KY: Tumor immunology, *Immunol Series (U.S.)* 58:497, 1993.
120. Hellstrom KE, Hellstrom I: Oncogene associated tumor antigens as targets for immunotherapy, *Fed Am Soc Exp Biol J* 3:1715, 1989.
121. Wahren B, Harmenbert U: Tumour markers in gastrointestinal cancer, *Scand J Clin Lab Invest* 206:21, 1991.
122. Vaickus L, Ball ED, Foon KA: Immune markers in hematologic malignancies, *Crit Rev Oncol Hematol* 11:267, 1991.
123. Souhami RL: The antigens of lung cancer, *Thorax* 47:153, 1992.
124. Spingarn NE, Slocum LA, Weisburger JH: Formation of mutagens in cooked foods. II. Foods with high starch content, *Cancer Lett* 9:7, 1980.
125. Guadagni F et al: Regulation of human tumor antigen expression by biological response modifiers (BMRs), *Annual Ist Super Sanita* 27: 71, 1991.
126. Upham J, Campbell B: Utility of squamous cell carcinoma antigen (SCC Ag) as a tumour marker in pulmonary malignancy, *Respir Med* 86:201, 1992.
127. Cooper EH et al: Tumor markers in prostate cancer, *Cancer* 70:225, 1992.
128. Naftzger C, Houghton AN: Tumor immunology, *Curr Opin Oncol* 3(1):93, 1991.
129. Srivastava PK, Maki RG: Stress-induced proteins in immune response to cancer, *Curr Topics Microbiol Immunol* 167:109, 1991.
130. Penn I: Cancers in renal transplant recipients, *Adv Ren Replace Ther* 7:147, 2000.
131. Dalgleish AG: Cancer vaccines, *Br J Cancer* 82:1619, 2000.
132. McKeever PE, Davenport RD, Shakui P: Patterns of antigenic expression of human glioma cells, *Crit Rev Neurobiol* 6:119, 1991.
133. Prehn RT: Perspectives on oncogenesis: does immunity stimulate or inhibit neoplasia? *J Reticuloendo Soc* 10:1, 1971.
134. Naor D, Duke-Cohan JS: Suppressor cells and malignancy. I. Suppressor macrophages and suppressor T-cells in experimental animals. In Ray PK, editor: *Advances in immunity and cancer therapy,* New York, 1986, Springer-Verlag.
135. Frentz G et al: Increased number of circulating suppressor T-lymphocytes in sun-induced multiple skin cancer, *CA Cancer J Clin* 61:294, 1988.

CHAPTER 11

Tumor Invasion and Metastasis

KATHRYN L. McCANCE • LEE K. ROBERTS

CHAPTER OUTLINE

Tumor development is a multistep process during which genetic and epigenetic events determine the transition from a normal to a malignant metastatic state. In the past 10 years much effort has been made to define the molecular mechanisms underlying progression to the metastatic state and to identify possible molecular targets for therapy. These mechanisms have included control of proliferation; the balance between cell survival and apoptosis; the communication with neighboring cells and the extracellular matrix; the induction of tumor neovascularization (angiogenesis); and, finally, tumor cell migration, invasion, and metastatic dissemination.

The major cause of illness and death as a result of most human malignant diseases is metastasis. Most individuals who have malignant tumors suffer from multiple metastases, too small to be detected, at the time the primary tumor is treated. Consequently, an important goal is to develop new therapies or analytic approaches that can be used for accurate prediction of the metastatic potential of a tumor. The hope is that such therapies will be derived from cell molecular research into the mechanism of invasion and metastases.

HISTORICAL THEORIES OF CANCER INVASION

Critical to understanding current research approaches to invasion and metastasis is knowing, historically, where we have been. Table 11-1 reviews the evolution of research on cancer invasion and metastasis.

TUMOR SPREAD

Tumor spread throughout the body can take several forms: (1) direct invasion of contiguous organs or local spread, (2) metastases to distant organs by lymphatics and veins, and (3) metastases by implantation. Spreading of a tumor depends on its rate of growth, its degree of differentiation, the anatomic presence or absence of barriers, and other unknown biologic factors. The history of progression of most malignant tumors can be divided into four phases: (1) malignant change in the initiating cell called *transformation,* (2) *growth* of the transformed cell, (3) local *invasion,* and (4) distant *metastasis.* The original transformed cell must undergo at least 20 population doublings to produce a tumor weighing about 1 g, which is the smallest clinically detectable tumor (Fig. 11-1).[1]

Local Spread

Invasion, or local spread, is a prerequisite for metastasis and the first step in the metastatic process. The progression of a tumor cell from one of benign proliferation to invasion and metastatic growth is the major cause of poor clinical outcome of individuals with cancer.[2] In its earliest stages, local invasion may occur as a function of direct tumor extension.[2] Eventually, however, cells or clumps of cells become detached from the primary tumor and invade the surrounding interstitial spaces. Possible mechanisms thought to be important in local invasion include (1) cellular multiplication, (2) mechanical pressure, (3) release

Table 11-1 Historical Development of the Cellular Theory of Cancer Invasion and Metastasis

Time Frame	Theory Proposal
Hippocrates (460-370 BC)	First theory on cancer invasion; cancer was a disease of black bile leakage into tissue; black bile diffusion theory (imbalance)
Galen (AD 131-203)	Rejected the notion of an imbalance of black bile; proposed black bile concentrated in areas of invasion (humoral theory)
Paracelsus (1493-1541)	Revised humoral theory that cancer invasion was caused by diffusion of mineral salts
Morgagni (1682-1771)	Performed numerous deposits and described cancer deposits in the liver
Müller (1828)	Established cellular origin of cancer
Recamier (1829)	First to propose that invasion and metastasis were the result of translocation of cells; first to use the term *metastasis*—Recamier was not properly acknowledged for this finding
Virchow (1821-1902)	Was convinced of the cellular nature of tumors but retained the humoral diffusion theory
Thiersch (1822-1895)	Refuted the humoral concept, demonstrated that invasion was a process starting from the primary tumor; reported that cancer cells reached the lymph nodes by cellular embolism (cellular-embolic theory); by the end of the nineteenth century, the cellular theory had become firmly established
Paget (late 1800s)	First to speculate about the factors that promote cellular "seeding" of tumor cells (seed versus soil theory)
Tyzzer (early 1900s)	First scientist to develop an experimental model of metastasis
1900s-1970s	Tumor invasion and metastasis thought to be the result of passive growth pressure and low tumor cell cohesiveness
1960s-1970s	Active mechanisms of tumor growth were investigated (e.g., what mechanisms facilitated the movement of tumor cells through host barriers); possible mechanisms included tumor cell mobility, lytic enzymes, and secretions of other factors
1980s-present	Continuation of mechanisms of tumor growth with a recent emphasis on the *biochemical mechanisms* including angiogenesis, extracellular matrix degradation, host-secreted proteases, tumor cell migration, and tumor cell adhesion.

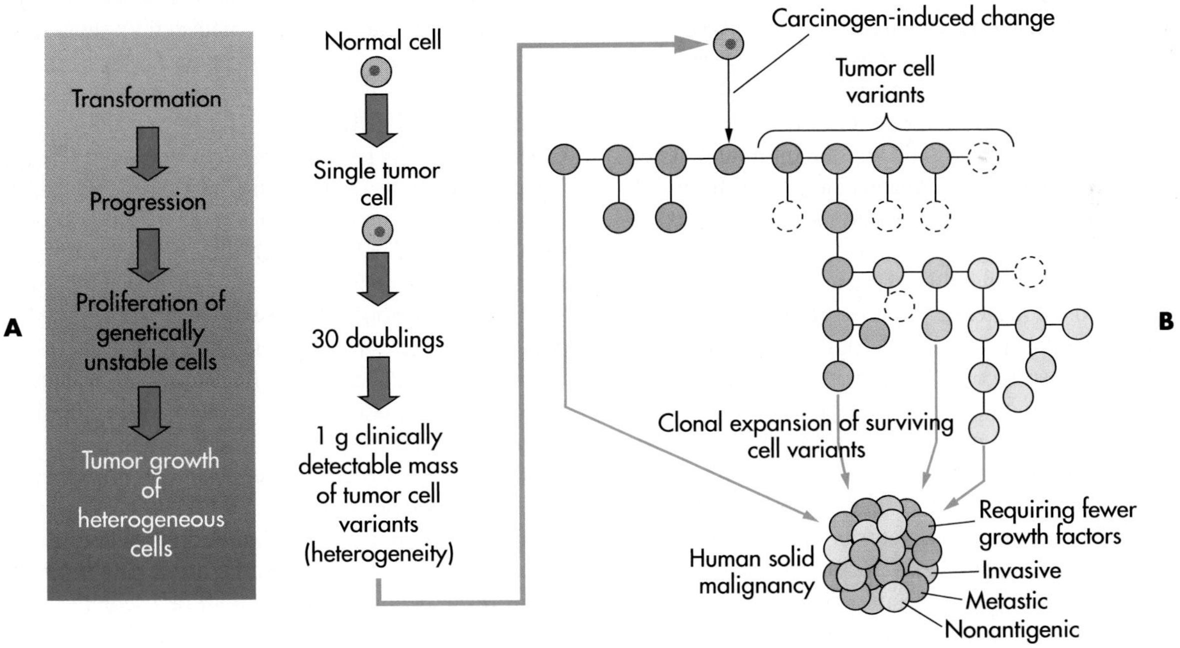

FIG. 11-1 Biology of tumor growth. A, Tumor growth of heterogeneous cells. **B,** Multiple colors represent various cell variants becoming a solid tumor of heterogeneous cells. Heterogeneity therefore causes challenges to treatment.

of lytic enzymes, (4) decreased cell-to-cell adhesion (making cancer cells "slippery"), and (5) increased motility of individual tumor cells.[2]

Cellular Multiplication

The aforementioned mechanisms are not mutually exclusive, and it is likely that in a given tumor any combination of the five may be involved. Invasion depends on the rate of cellular multiplication, which is a function of the cell generation time (through the cell cycle), the number of cells that are dividing (growth fraction), and the cell loss from the tumor. Cells from malignant lesions thus can divide rapidly, but the tumor may not grow because a number of cells are rapidly dying. (The cell cycle is discussed in Chapters 1 and 10.)

Mechanical Invasion

Invasion, in relation to mechanical pressure, is analogous to the way in which plants force their roots through the soil (i.e., by building up pressure that forces sheets, or fingerlike projections, along the lines of least mechanical resistance). Pressure from the growing mass blocks local blood vessels, leading to local tissue death and a reduction in mechanical resistance, which further aids the spread.

Lytic Enzymes

Malignant tumors that invade normal tissues cause significant amounts of degradation to the extracellular matrix (see Chapter 1). Because many animal and human tumors have higher levels of hydrolases (e.g., proteases and collagenases, plasminogen activators, lysosomal enzymes) than do corresponding normal tissues, the concept that malignant tumors produce and secrete lytic enzymes or induce host cells to release proteases (e.g., infiltrating macrophages) that destroy normal tissue has become firmly established.[3,4] Protease activity is regulated by antiproteases. At the invading edge of tumors, the balance between proteases and antiproteases favors proteases. Three classes of proteases have been identified: (1) serine, (2) cysteine, and (3) matrix metalloproteinases (MMPs). MMPs are increased in epithelial cancers and are involved in producing new blood vessels (angiogenesis) that aid in invasion and metastasis.[5] Collagens are the major structural elements of the extracellular matrices where invasion begins (see p. 27). One type of MMP, **type IV collagenase**, cleaves type IV collagen of epithelial and vascular basement membranes. Type IV collagenase is increased in the cells of many highly metastatic tumors. Inhibition of collagenase activity in animal experiments inhibits MMP, greatly reducing metastases.[5] Tumor cells can either release collagenase (e.g., digest collagen) or secrete collagenolytic substances in latent forms that are converted to activate collagenase by lysosomal proteases, such as plasmin.[6]

A number of other proteases that are attached to or released from the cell surface appear to increase tumor invasion through proteolysis, including cysteine proteinases, **cathepsin B and D**, and serine proteases such as **urokinase type plasminogen activator (uPA)**. uPA has been shown to be a prognostic marker in a variety of malignancies, especially breast cancer.[7] Plasminogen activator is increased in tumor cells.[8,9] Plasminogen activator converts the serum proenzyme plasminogen into the protease plasmin, which can degrade a variety of proteins. It is believed that plasminogen activator plays an important role in the degradation of the extracellular matrix during tumor cell invasion. Protease inhibitors can be produced by the host or by the tumor cells themselves. The use of protease inhibitors has been proposed for cancer treatment.[2]

Decreased Cell Adhesion

Cancer cells do not adhere to one another as well as normal cells. This "slippery" trait has been related to fibronectin, which regulates cell attachment, spreading, phagocytosis, cell structure effects, and cell movement; fibronectin also stimulates and generally acts as an anchoring molecule. Cancer cells may make a defective type of fibronectin, or they may break down fibronectin as they make it. Low levels or loss of this anchoring molecule, fibronectin, may help cancer cells "slip" between normal cells in the process of invasion. Similarly, alterations in the cell-to-cell adhesion molecule E-cadherin correlate with the metastatic potential of cancer cells (see Chapter 1 on cell adhesion molecules).

> **NUTRITION & DISEASE**
>
> **Cruciferous Vegetables May Suppress Cancer Invasion**
>
> Indole-3-carbino (I3C) is a compound occurring naturally in cruciferous vegetables (e.g, broccoli, cauliflower). Investigators studied the effects of I3Cs antiinvasion and antimigration activities through estrogen-independent and estrogen-dependent pathways in human breast cancer cell lines. I3C significantly caused a dose-dependent increase in expression of E-cadherin, a cell adhesion molecule. Thus I3C may contribute to suppression of breast cancer invasion and metastasis by increasing E-cadherin and cell attachment.
>
> Data from Meng Q et al: Suppression of breast cancer invasion and migration by indole-3-carbinol: associated with upregulation of BRCA1 and E-cadherin/catenin complexes, *J Mol Med* 78(3):155, 2000.

Increased Motility

Cell movement is key for tumor cells to invade. Stages of invasion include the detachment and subsequent infiltration of cells from the primary tumor into adjacent tissue, as well as the migration of cells through the vascular wall into the circulation (intravasation) and movement out of the vascular wall (extravasation) into a secondary site (Fig. 11-2). Data suggest that tumor cells become mobile to a variety of agents, including extracellular matrix components, some known (e.g., hepatocyte growth factor and epidermal growth factor) and unknown host-derived growth and motility factors, and tumor-secreted or *autocrine motility factors.*[10] This allows a tumor cell to adapt to a variety of tissues. A family of tumor cell–derived (e.g., autocrine) factors or cytokines has now been reported. Thus the **autocrine motility factor hypothesis** specifies that the tumor cell secretes a factor that binds to a specific receptor on the cell surface and stimulates motility (Fig. 11-3). In this way the tumor cell acquires independent and continuous stimulation of its motile behavior, which is necessary for invasion.

Three-Step Theory of Invasion

A three-step theory has been proposed to describe the sequence of biochemical events during tumor cell invasion of the extracellular matrix (Fig. 11-4). These steps occur after tumor cells detach from each other (see Decreased Cell Adhesion). The three steps include tumor cell attachment to the

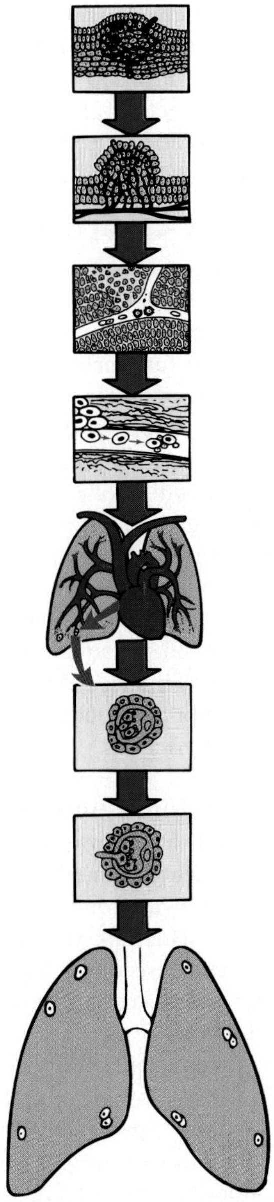

FIG. 11-2 Pathogenesis of metastasis. Initial neoplastic transformation of susceptible cells gives rise to a small population of tumor cells. Vascularization of this initial neoplastic lesion allows further proliferation of tumor cells and enlargement of the primary tumor. Malignant cells within the primary tumor next begin to invade the surrounding host tissue or tissues. Entry of invading tumor cells into lymphatics or blood vessels serves to transport them to distant sites in the body, where they lodge and become arrested in the capillary beds of various organs. The arrested cells then exit from capillaries into the surrounding tissue where, subject to provision of a suitable environment, they proliferate to form metastases. (Redrawn from Poste G, Fidler IJ: The pathogenesis of cancer metastasis, *Nature,* 20:139, 1980.)

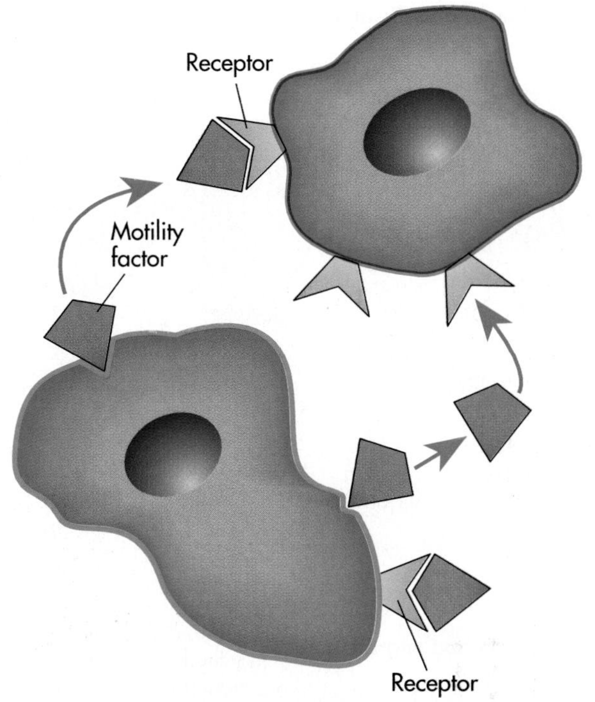

FIG. 11-3 Autocrine motility factor. Certain tumor cells make and secrete a motility factor that can then activate itself or other tumor cells, presumably through a cell surface receptor.

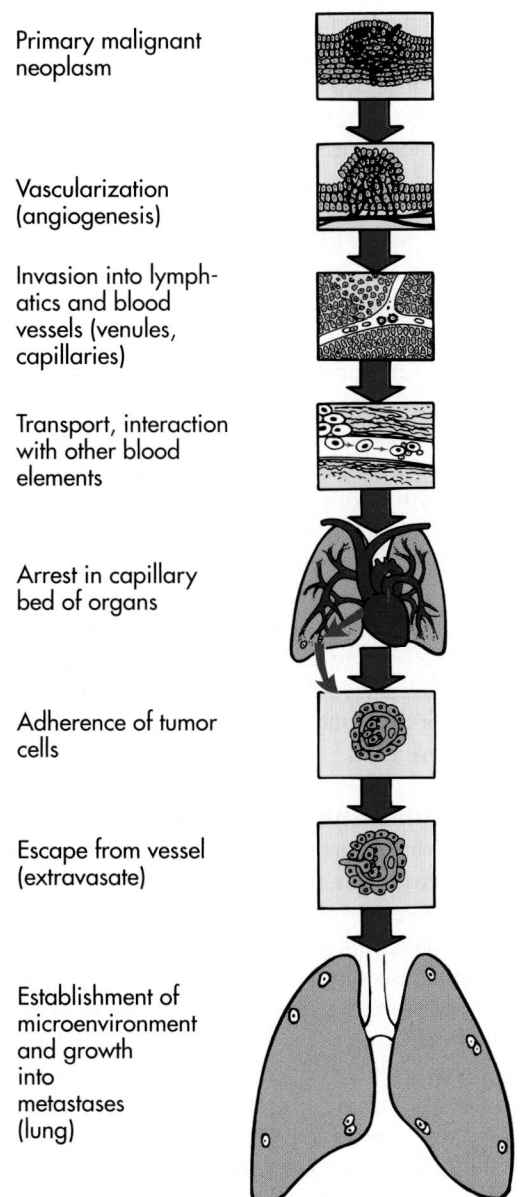

matrix, degradation or dissolution of the matrix, and locomotion into the matrix. The first step, attachment, is mediated by specific attachment factors such as fibronectin and laminin, a complex glycoprotein that is a major constituent of all basement membranes. Tissue compartments are separated from each other by two types of extracellular matrix: (1) basement membranes and (2) interstitial connective tissue. Both types, although organized differently, consist of collagens, glycoproteins, and proteoglycans. Tumor cells interact with the extracellular matrix at several stages in the metastatic process (see Fig. 11-2). A tumor must first navigate the underlying basement membrane and then cross the interstitial connective tissue to eventually get access to the circulation. Membrane vesicles on the cell surface of tumor cells are rich in laminin receptors that enable their attachment to basement membrane.[2] A correlation exists between the invasiveness and the density of laminin receptors to carcinomas of the breast and colon. Laminin forms a bridge between the cell-surface **laminin receptor** and type IV collagen (see Fig. 11-4). In addition to laminin-specific receptors, tumor cells express integrins (adhesion molecules) that can be receptors for many components of the extracellular matrix.[11] Once anchored, the tumor cell in the second step either secretes proteolytic enzymes or induces host cells to produce them, and degradation of the matrix, or step two, begins. Such enzymes may degrade both the attachment proteins and the structural collagenous proteins of the matrix. Type IV collagenase, a powerful proteolytic enzyme, may outnumber the natural protease inhibitors present in the matrix. The third step is tumor cell locomotion into the degraded region of the matrix. Fingerlike projections called *pseudopodia,* which extend from the tumor cell (Fig. 11-5), facilitate movement by attaching to blood vessel walls that

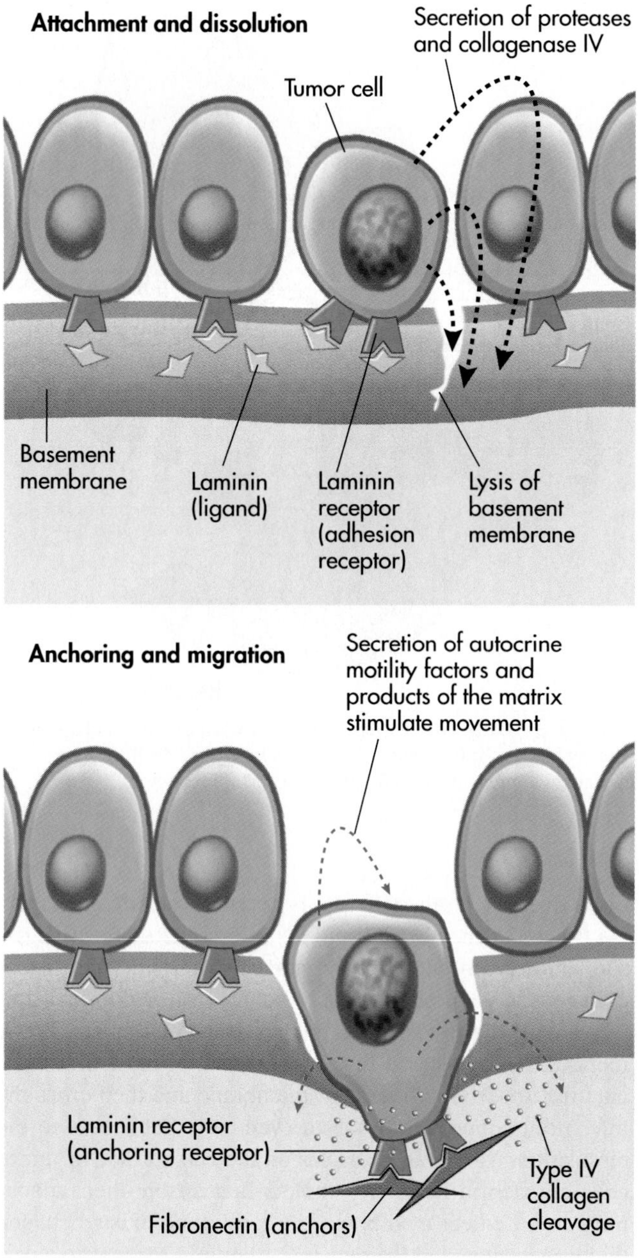

FIG. 11-4 Three-step sequence of tumor invasion: attachment, dissolution, and locomotion. After tumor cells have detached from one another, the first step is tumor cell attachment to the extracellular matrix. Surface receptors on the tumor cell (laminin receptors) bind to parts of the basement membrane (laminin) in the extracellular matrix. Step 2 is degradation of the matrix by tumor cell proteases (collagenase IV and plasminogen activator). The anchored tumor cell either secretes proteolytic enzymes or causes the host cell to secrete the proteolytic enzymes that degrade the matrix in a region very close to the tumor cell surface. Step 3 is the migration (locomotion) of the tumor cell through the degraded basement membrane. During this phase, pseudopodia (fingerlike projections) of the tumor cell cross the basement membrane, enabling the cell to extravasate from the blood vessel into the interstitial tissue.

cross the basement membrane. The tumor cells then extravasate from the vasculature into the interstitial stroma. Theoretically, invasion occurs by cyclic repetition of these steps. The direction of locomotion may be influenced by chemotactic factors (see discussion of autocrine motility factors and Fig. 11-3).

Patterns of Spread: Metastasis

Metastasis, the spread of cancer cells from a primary site of origin to a distant site, is the life-threatening characteristic of malignancy. Local invasion is a condition of metastases. Methods exist for successfully eradicating **primary tumors** (original sites of tumor origin). However, the real challenge for reducing cancer mortality is controlling metastasis, because removal of the primary tumor does not affect the proliferating growth at other sites. Often the primary tumor is not even diagnosed before secondary spread occurs. Three basic mechanisms of metastasis exist: direct or continuous extension, lymphatic spread, and bloodstream dissemination. These mechanisms, however, are not mutually exclusive. Tumor cell spread or dissemination through one mechanism often facilitates metastasis through other mechanisms because tumor cells move through numerous microscopic anatomic connections.

Direct or Continuous Extension

The earliest result of invasion could be called *continuous extension.* Cancerous tumors may extend into several areas without breaking away from the parent tumor, including (1) tissue spaces, (2) lymph vessels, (3) blood vessels, (4) body cavities (serosal seeding), and (5) cerebrospinal spaces.

Direct tumor extension, once thought to result from simple growth pressure only, now is known to be initiated by a complex sequence of events discussed earlier. They are initiated by loss of intracellular adhesion that enables cells to "slip" past one another. Movement of cells through tissue barriers is further influenced by proteases and (autocrine) motility factors (see discussion of local invasion, pp. 336).

Metastasis by Lymphatics and Bloodstream

Metastasis involves a series of sequential steps: (1) extension or local invasion of the surrounding tissue; (2) penetration into blood vessels or lymphatics, or both, and into body cavities; (3) release into the lymph or blood circulation; (4) transport to a secondary site; and (5) arrest, adherence, and proliferation of cells at the secondary site (see Fig. 11-2). Distant cancer spread involves invasion and penetration of tumor cells into blood vessels or lymphatics, or both. Lymphatics and thin-walled venules offer relatively little mechanical resistance to penetration by tumor cells. Blood vessels within tumors offer malignant cells direct access into the circulation. Clusters, single cells, and fragments of tumor cells become separated from the primary tumor site and disseminate by these routes. Clumps of cells have a better chance of successful metastasis than do single cells because clumps involve

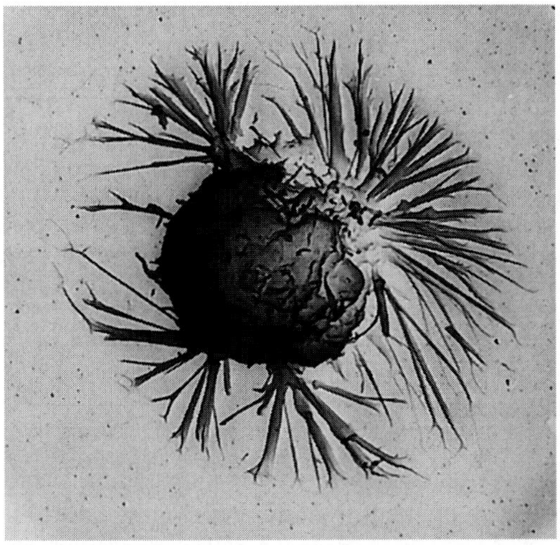

FIG. 11-5 Pseudopodia. Photograph of electron microscopy of a breast cancer cell with fingerlike projections called *pseudopodia.* (Courtesy National Library of Medicine.)

WHAT'S NEW? Adhesion Molecule CD44 and Cancer Metastases

CD44 is an adhesion molecule, a transmembrane protein and member of the cartilage family. It is involved in cell-cell and cell-matrix interactions and signal transduction. CD44 is a major cell surface receptor for hyaluronan, a polysaccharide component of the extracellular matrix. Increased amounts of both CD44 and hyaluronan are reported in solid tumors and tumor-associated fibroblasts. Stimulation of cell migration by hyaluronan has been explained by different mechanisms. Increased interest has been directed at both CD44 and hyaluronan because they are upregulated in neoplasia and CD44, particularly its variants, may be useful as a diagnostic or prognostic marker of malignancy.

Data from Drillenburg P, Pals ST: Cell adhesion receptors in lymphoma dissemination, *Blood* 95(6):1900, 2000; Goodison S, Urquidi V, Tarin D: CD44 cell adhesion molecules, *Mol Pathol* 52(4):189, 1999; Nehls V, Hayen W: Are hyaluronan receptors involved in three-dimensional cell migration? *Histol Histopathol* 25(2):629, 2000; Telen MJ: Red blood cell surface adhesion molecules: their possible roles in normal human physiology and disease, *Semin Hematol* 37(2):130, 2000.

similar (homotypic) adhesions among tumor cells and heterotypic or different adhesions between tumor cells and blood cells, particularly platelets. Platelet tumor clumps appear to enhance tumor cell survival and implantability.[12] Those tumors that arise close to a serous surface can invade through that surface, implant, and become distant metastases. These effusions, also known as *seeding,* occur in the pleural space surrounding the lung and in the peritoneal space surrounding the abdominal cavity.

The most common route for distant metastases is through the lymphatics. Tumors generally lack a well-formed lymphatic network. Lymphatic channels occur at the periphery of the tumor and not within the tumor mass. Tumor cells entering the lymphatic vessels are carried to regional lymph nodes. For many types of cancer, the first evidence of distant spread is a mass in the regional lymph node. An enlarged axillary lymph node, for example, may signal breast cancer; an enlarged inguinal node may indicate a malignant melanoma; an enlarged mesenteric node may be caused by cancer of the gastrointestinal tract. Initially, regional lymph nodes may exert a barrier effect, preventing the further spread of tumor cells into the lymphatic system. Host defenses, such as macrophages and natural killer cells, play an important role in the elimination of circulating tumor cells. Several events can occur in a cancer cell that becomes lodged in lymph nodes, including (1) death as a result of local inflammatory reaction, (2) death because of an incompatible local environment, (3) growth into a discernible lump, (4) sustained dormancy for unknown reasons, or (5) detachment from the nodes and entrance into the efferent lymphatics.

When small lymphatic vessels are penetrated, tumor cell emboli are released into these lymphatic vessels and are responsible for lymphatic metastasis. Shedding of emboli is influenced by changes in vessel pressure, by turbulent alterations in lymphatic flow, and by movements or manipulation of the tumor during diagnostic tests or surgery. Tumor cells eventually move into the regional or systemic venous drainage because of numerous venolymphatic communications.

Hematogenous spread is a complex process that requires tumor cells to penetrate and detach from blood vessels and spread to distant organs, yet it is known that vascularized tumors shed malignant cells constantly as they grow, often releasing millions of cells without producing metastases.[12,13] To establish metastases, tumor cells must "escape" host defenses, survive mechanical trauma in the bloodstream, and lodge in the vascular bed of the target organ. A majority of the tumor cells circulate as single cells and attach directly to the endothelial surface or to preexisting regions of exposed subendothelial basement membrane. Emboli or tumor cells that contain leukocytes, fibrin, or platelets can cause direct embolization in the precapillary venules by mechanical action. The formation of a fibrin-platelet complex is thought to protect tumor cells within the emboli from host defenses and to assist successful attachment to the vascular epithelium. Once arrested in a blood vessel, tumor cells can actively invade the vascular wall and interstitial stroma and invade the parenchyma of the target organ. Arrest and estravasation of tumor emboli at distant sites involve adhesion to the endothelium, followed by emergence through the basement membrane. Involved in these processes are adhesion molecules (e.g., integrins) and proteolytic enzymes (see WHAT'S NEW? Adhesion Molecule CD44 and Cancer Metastases). Growth in the target organ parenchyma requires that a vascular network develop (angiogenesis) and host defenses be ineffective.

Angiogenesis and Angiogenesis Factors

Growth of cancerous colonies depends on an adequate blood supply. Tumor implants cannot grow more than a few

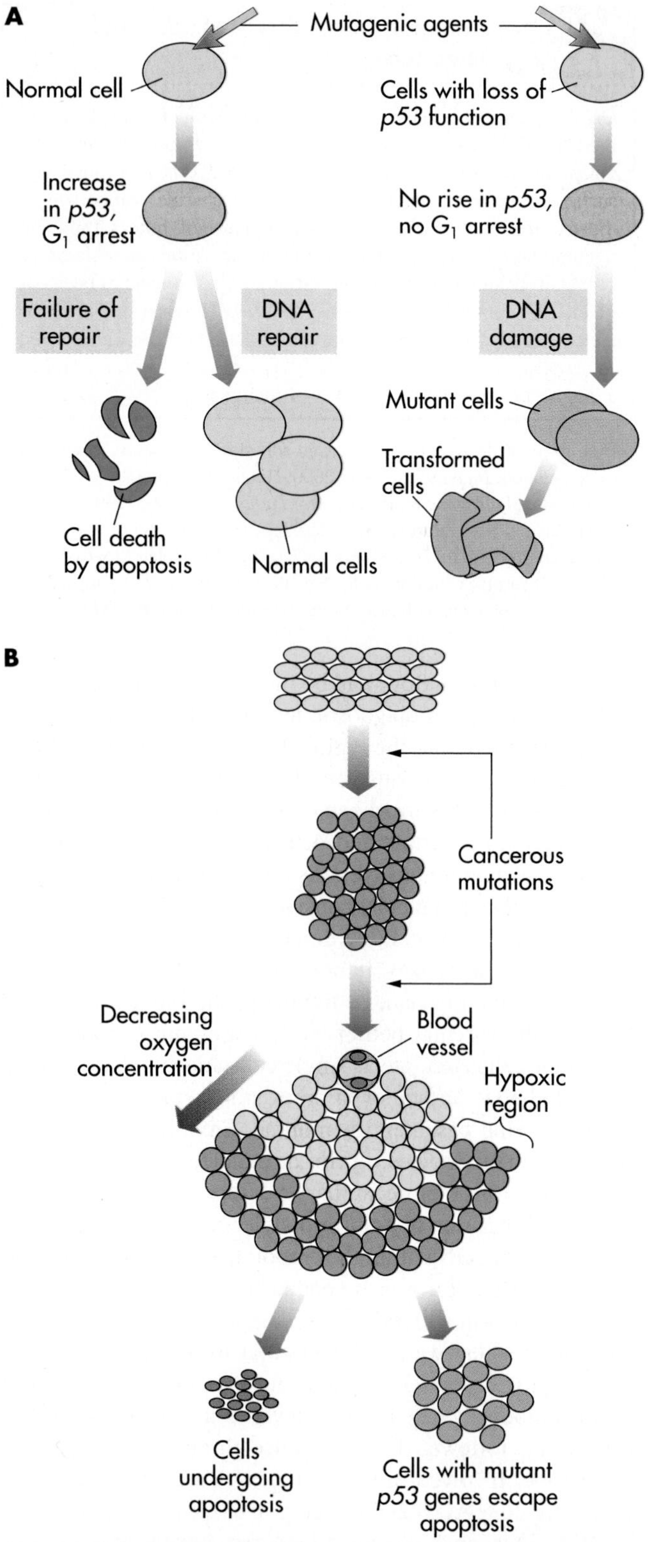

FIG. 11-6 Activation of p53. A, Proposed model for the action of normal and mutant *p53*. **B,** Mutations in normal cells *(left)* result in overgrowth. In response to deoxyribonucleic acid (DNA) damage, the cells produce the protein *p53*. As a tumor increases in size and areas farthest from blood vessels become hypoxic, the cells undergo apoptosis. The only cells to survive and multiply are those with mutations in both copies of the *p53* gene. (*A*, Redrawn from Cotran RS et al: *Robbins pathologic basis of disease*, ed 5, Philadelphia, 1994, W.B. Saunders.)

WHAT'S NEW? Blocking Influx of Ca^{++} Might Inhibit Angiogenesis

Because intracellular calcium is needed to regulate many of the signaling pathways that underlie malignant progression, including angiogenesis, the idea of inhibiting calcium influx is a reasonable new approach. Carboxyamidotriazole (CAI), a synthetic molecule, has been shown to inhibit proliferation, invasion, and metastatic potential of a number of human cancer cell lines in vitro and vivo. CAI inhibits angiogenesis.

Data from Friedrich MJ: Ovarian cancer investigations aim at cell signaling pathways, *JAMA* 281:973, 1999.

millimeters in diameter without developing new blood vessels to "feed" them, a process called **angiogenesis.**[14] Beyond this size, tumors fail to enlarge without vascularization because hypoxia causes apoptosis by activation of p53 (Fig. 11-6 and see p. 341). Perfusion supplies oxygen and nutrients, and newly formed endothelial cells secrete growth factors such as insulin-like growth factor and others that stimulate the growth of nearby tumor cells. It is unclear what triggers blood vessel formation. Several proangiogenic factors have been identified, including vascular endothelial growth factor (VEGF), platelet-derived growth factor (PDGF), transforming growth factor-alpha (TGF-α), basic fibroblast growth factor (bFGF), and angiopoietins.[15,16] Recently, specific inhibitors of angiogenesis have been identified, including platelet factor-4, antiostatin, endostatin, and vasostatin.[16] **Tissue factor (TF)** produced by tumor cells has been implicated in regulation of the "angiogenic switch" that, presumably, regulates the balance of positive and negative angiogenic factors.[17] A major factor may be a sudden drop in the cancer cell's production of thrombospondin—a protein that inhibits the growth of new blood vessels. Normal cells prevent the development of new blood vessels by pumping out thrombospondin.[18,19,20] The development of a new capillary network involves many steps and is similar to the blood coagulation cascade in that one event triggers the next through the action of specific mediators. Therapies aimed at blocking angiogenesis represent a promising therapeutic target. Currently, there are more than 30 angiogenesis inhibitors in clinical trials, and many promising new candidates are under investigation in vitro and in animal models (see "WHAT'S NEW? Therapies in Development," p. 347).[21]

In clinical situations, the rate of spread, as well as the growth of the tumor, is correlated with tumor vascularity. For example, small cell carcinoma of the lung arises in highly vascularized capillary beds and spreads easily and widely to other vascular organs such as the brain.

Growth of Metastases and Metastatic Potential

A metastasis grows and develops when a vascular network is developed, host defenses are evaded, and a compatible environment is available ("the soil"). The metastatic poten-

Table 11-2 Frequent Sites of Distant Metastasis in Some Types of Cancer

Primary Tumor	Major Anatomic Pathways	Frequent Site of Distant Metastasis
Lung	Pulmonary vein, left ventricle	Multiple organs, including brain
Colorectal	Mesenteric lymphatics, portal venous system	Liver
	Inferior vena cava, right ventricle, pulmonary artery	Lungs
Testicular	Lymphatics to the periaortic area to the subclavian veins to the right ventricle	Lungs, liver
Prostate	Batson plexus of paravertebral veins; ilium, lumbar spine	Bones, lung, liver, endocrine glands, central nervous system
Breast	Batson plexus of paravertebral veins, lymph nodes, superior vena cava	Bony skeleton, lungs
Head and neck	Direct extension, Batson plexus	Lymphatics, liver, bone
Ovarian	Direct extension	Peritoneal surfaces, diaphragm
	Omentum and mesenteric veins	Omentum, liver
Sarcoma (extremity)	Inferior vena cava, right ventricle, pulmonary artery	Lungs

tial of many common carcinomas was formerly thought to be related to the size of the primary tumor. New data, however, suggest that the very "stresses" that cancer cells themselves endure, even in very small tumors, may promote the emergence of stronger, more aggressive tumors.[22,23] The microenvironment surrounding the tumor may play a significant role in determining how aggressive the tumor cells become. An environment such as low oxygen (hypoxia) can cause the production of **p53 protein**. Rather than simply arresting cell growth, the p53 protein (also called wild-type p53) activates a cell suicide program called apoptosis (see Chapter 2). In other words, p53 activates the "emergency brake" (see Fig. 11-6, *A*). But if mutations occur in the p53 gene, cells have lost their "emergency brake" against uncontrolled cell growth. These cells do not undergo apoptosis; they survive and may be the strongest, most aggressive cells of the tumor (see Fig. 11-6, *B*). These cells may resurface as stronger renditions of their earlier selves and resist drugs and radiation. More aggressive tumor cells may evolve into larger tumors, or larger tumors may overwhelm host defense mechanisms, thus favoring the survival of malignant cells.

Distribution and Frequent Sites of Distant Metastases

Distant metastasis in many types of cancer appears to take place in the first capillary bed encountered by the circulating cells. Table 11-2 summarizes frequent sites of metastases in various cancers. Patterns of metastasis for certain other tumors, however, are not related to patterns of blood flow or the location of capillary beds. Instead they show preferential growth in certain organs, called **organ tropism**. Ocular melanoma, for example, frequently metastasizes to the liver, and clear cell kidney carcinomas often spread to bone and the thyroid. Organ tropism may be the result of growth factors or hormones present in the target organ, preferential adherence to the surface of certain target organs (sometimes called **tissue-selective homing receptors**), and the presence of chemotactic factors that diffuse from the target organ and cause circulating tumor cells to leave the vessel and gather in the target organs. Organ tropism is determined genetically. Tumor cells contain organ-specific receptors that can discriminate among various vascular beds and preferentially "locate" to certain organs.

Staging

Tumor staging involves the size of the tumor, the degree to which it has locally invaded, and the extent to which it has spread (metastasized). One common scheme for standardizing staging is the *TNM system; T* is for tumor spread, *N* is for node involvement, and *M* is the presence of distant metastasis (Fig. 11-7).

CLINICAL MANIFESTATIONS OF CANCER

Pain

Usually little or no pain is associated with the early stages of malignant disease, but pain occurs in 60% to 80% of individuals who are terminally ill with cancer. Pain is strongly influenced by fear, anxiety, sleep loss, fatigue, and overall physical deterioration. Pain is known to occur through an interaction among psychogenic, cultural, and physiologic components. (The neurophysiology of pain is discussed in Chapter 14.)

General mechanisms that cause pain associated with cancer include pressure, obstruction, invasion of a sensitive structure, stretching of visceral surfaces, tissue destruction, and inflammation. Although the pain may be directly related to the malignancy, it can result from other problems, such as infection. A common cause of pain is bone metastasis, which may be referred away from the involved bone and manifest, for example, as back pain. Bone pain can be caused by periosteal irritation, medullary pressure, or pathologic fractures.

Abdominal pain often is caused by severe stretching from the tumor invasion of the hollow viscus. Tumors that obstruct and distend the bowel cause pain. Small bowel obstructions

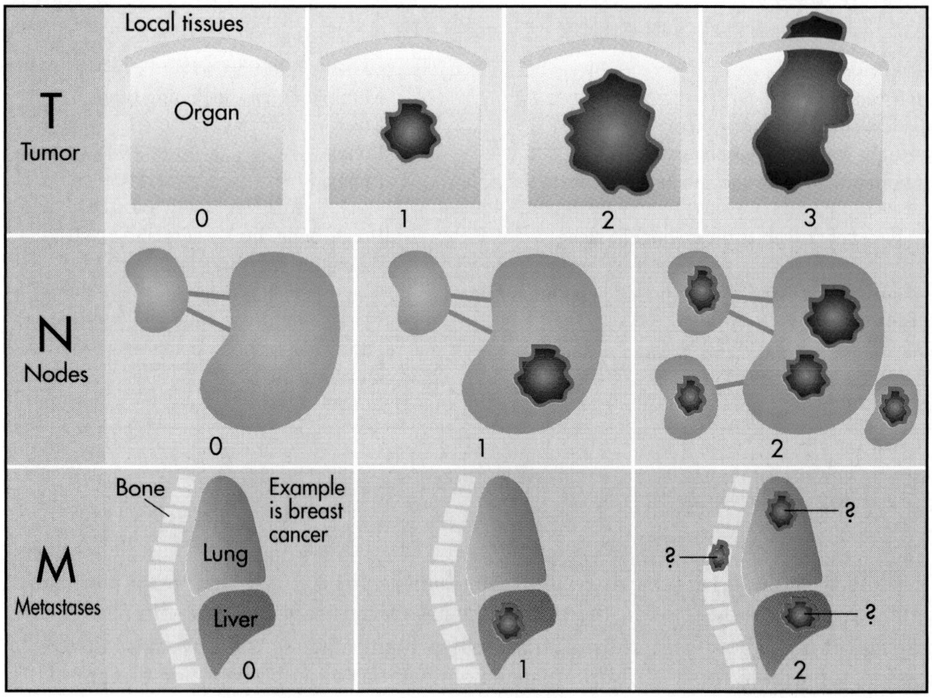

T= Primary tumor; the number equals size of tumor and its local extent. The number can vary according to site.

T0= Breast free of tumor
T1= Lesion <2 cm in size
T2= Lesion 2-5 cm
T3= Skin and/or chest wall involved by invasion

N= Lymph node involvement; a higher number means more nodes are involved.

N0= No axillary nodes involved
N1= Mobile nodes involved
N2= Fixed nodes involved

M= Extent of distant metastases.

M0= No metastases
M1= Demonstrable metastases
M2= Suspected metastases

FIG. 11-7 Tumor staging by the TNM system. (See figure for abbreviations.)

in persons with known malignant disease commonly result from recurrent cancer, surgical adhesions, or new primary tumors. Surgery is often needed to obtain relief. Hepatic malignancies stretch the liver, resulting in a dull pain or a feeling of fullness over the right upper abdominal quadrant.

Tumor compression of nerve endings against a firm surface creates pain. Brain tumors have very little space to grow without compressing blood vessels and nerve endings between the tumor and the cranial vault. Tissue destruction from infection and necrosis can cause pain. The oral area, which frequently has ulcerative lesions, often is infected and painful.

By combining primary treatments, systemic analgesic agents, and other techniques, most individuals with cancer can achieve satisfactory relief of pain. Although cancer pain is a complex problem arising from multiple sources, individuals should be assured that suffering is not inevitable and that relief is attainable.[24]

Fatigue

Fatigue is the most frequently reported symptom of cancer and cancer treatment. The mechanisms that produce fatigue are unknown. Suggested causes include sleep disturbance, various biochemical changes secondary to disease and treatment, numerous psychosocial factors, level of activity, nutritional status, and other environmental and physical factors.[25]

The physiologic understanding of fatigue probably includes mechanisms for decreased muscle contractility. Some individuals with cancer may lose portions of muscle function needed to perform normal physical activities.[25] Other areas of research include muscle function consequences from metabolic products of cancer treatment and associated muscle loss from circulating cytokines (e.g., tumor necrosis factor and interleukin-1 [IL-1]).

Similar to pain, fatigue is a subjective clinical manifestation. Fatigue is described by individuals with cancer as tiredness, weakness, lack of energy, exhaustion, lethargy, inability to concentrate, depression, sleepiness, boredom, lack of motivation, and decreased mental status.[25]

Individuals have reported management of fatigue by changing their expenditure of work, including planning and scheduling activities and work; decreasing nonessential activities; and increasing dependence on others for home management, transportation, and care. Much more research is needed to examine the psychophysiologic mechanisms for fatigue and develop interventions directed at these mechanisms.

Cachexia

The syndrome of **cachexia** includes anorexia; early satiety (filling); weight loss; anemia; asthenia (marked weakness); taste alterations; and altered protein, lipid, and carbohydrate metabolism (Fig. 11-8). Cachexia is the most severe form of malnutrition associated with cancer and results in wasting, emaciation, and decreased quality of life. The anorexia-cachexia syndrome is one of the most common causes of death among individuals with cancer and is present in 80% at death.[26] Anorexia, or loss of appetite, frequently can be attributed to pain, depression, chemotherapy, or radiation therapy. Alterations in taste also can account for the anorexia of cancer. Reductions in sensitivities to sweet, sour, and salty tastes make moderately seasoned foods seem bland. Persons with cancer, especially involving the liver, commonly have an aversion to red meat. Other aversions include coffee and chocolate. Although the process that produces such aversions is unknown, several mechanisms have been suggested, including the following:

1. Poor use of glucose, resulting in an elevation of blood sugar that may depress appetite
2. A decreased supply of insulin, resulting in and causing an elevation of blood sugar, which may depress appetite
3. Increased mobilization of proteins and elevated amino acid level in the blood, which stimulates the satiety center and results in reduced appetite
4. Stimulation of visceral receptors from decreased peristalsis caused by surgery and other treatments, which stimulates the satiety center
5. A reduction in the emotional pleasures of eating or alterations in smell or taste of food, which can depress appetite

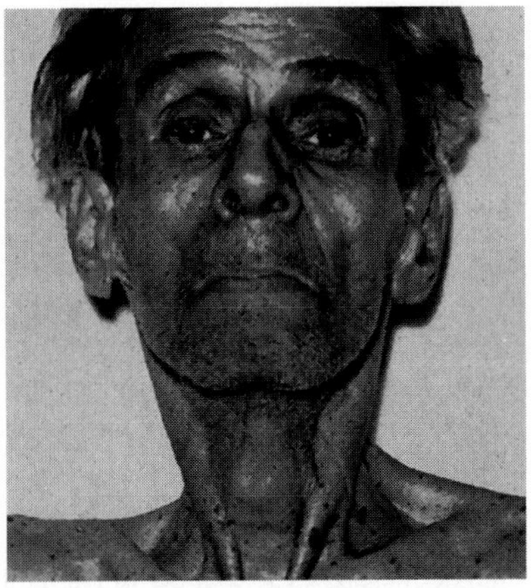

FIG. 11-8 Cachexia. Sunken appearance of the eyes, cheeks, and temporal areas; sharp nose; dry, rough skin. (From Prior JA et al: *Physical diagnosis: the history and examination of the patient,* ed 6, St Louis, 1981, Mosby.)

Anorexia leads to a protein-energy malnutrition (PEM) of three types: (1) malnutrition similar to kwashiorkor, (2) marasmus, and (3) a combination of the two. Kwashiorkor is a form of malnutrition that evolves from a protein-deficient diet, in which calories come primarily from carbohydrates. Because the onset usually is rapid, anthropometric measurements tend to be normal but serum proteins (transferrin, albumin) are decreased. This protein serum decrease (hypoalbuminemia) causes the serum colloid osmotic pressure to decrease, so that fluid escapes to the interstitium and causes edema. Marasmus is a form of malnutrition resulting from a decreased intake of calories and proteins. It is characterized by decreased anthropometric measurements caused by a prolonged and gradual wasting of muscle mass and normal serum albumin. A combination of kwashiorkor and marasmus results in hypoalbuminemia, edema, diminished immunologic competence (which depends on normal protein stores), and an overall physical deterioration. Malnutrition is a major factor contributing to death.[27,28] (Malnutrition is discussed in detail in Chapter 38.)

Progressive weight loss in the person with cancer occurs despite normal or increased food intake. Starvation usually decreases the basal metabolic rate (BMR), but metabolic rates in persons with cancer are high. How increased BMR and weight loss relate to a breakdown of protein and nitrogen loss or negative nitrogen balance is unclear. This increase in BMR may be a result of accelerated metabolic activity of the tumor itself. Malignant cells replicate more rapidly than normal cells and require more food for their growth, but at the expense of the normal tissue. The normal tissue, over time, is sacrificed, and wasting begins to occur. Alterations in protein, lipid, and carbohydrate metabolism undoubtedly play a role.

Carbohydrate metabolism is altered, causing a syndrome that resembles diabetes mellitus. Hyperinsulinemia is present, and many individuals show insulin resistance, hyperglycemia, and an abnormal glucose tolerance test result. These disturbances cause an increased gluconeogenesis, which produces glucose from amino acids. In starvation, protein usually is spared to protect vital structures, but in cancer, protein and fatty acids are used for meeting energy needs. Fatty acids are released from the breakdown of adipose tissue.

An unusual and frustrating component of cancer care is the person's early satiety, or a sense of fullness after only a few mouthfuls of food. The metabolic changes in cancer cachexia appear to be mediated by a complex network of proinflammatory cytokines, especially tumor necrosis factor–α (TNF–α), neuroendocrine hormones, neurotransmitters, eicosanoids, and tumor-derived factors produced by the body in response to the tumor and by the tumor itself. A number of cytokines, including interleukins 1 and 6, interferon, leukemia inhibitory factor, ciliary neurotropic factor, and TNF–α, have been proposed as mediators of the cachetic process.[29]

One of the most significant cytokines is the activated macrophage-produced TNF–α, also called *cachectin* because of its role in the cachexia syndrome. Natural induction of TNF–α is protective; that is, it plays an important role (1) in the defense against viral, bacterial, and parasitic infections; (2) in autoimmune responses; and (3) in the selective destruction of malignant cells.[30] Unregulated TNF is now known to be the basis for development of wasting, cachexia, various inflammatory and/or autoimmune diseases, and septic shock.[30,31,32] (Cytokines are discussed in detail in Chapters 6 and 7.)

Anemia

Anemia is a common disorder associated with malignancy. Most persons with cancer usually have a mild anemia, although 20% may have hemoglobin concentrations below 8 g/dl (normal value, 15 g/dl). Several mechanisms cause anemia in persons with cancer; these include chronic bleed-

WHAT'S NEW? Radiotherapy-Associated Anemia

Only recently has the prevalence of anemia in individuals receiving radiotherapy received much attention. Many people present with anemia before radiotherapy, and even more experience anemia or a worsening of anemia at some point during treatment. The problem of anemia is, however, often ignored because patients may experience only functional anemia, that is, a hemoglobin level less than 12 g/dl. Unless physiologic anemia (hemoglobin = 8 g/dl) is discovered, efforts to correct anemia are often not made. Because hemoglobin levels less than 12 g per dl seem to be associated with tumor hypoxia and poorer outcomes of radiotherapy, ignoring even modest anemia can result in decreased survival and quality of life. Increasing hemoglobin levels 1 to 2 m per dl is usually easily accomplished and there exists the potential for improving outcomes by paying closer attention to this problem.

Data from Harrison LB: Radiotherapy-associated anemia: the scope of the problem, *Oncologist* 5(suppl 2):1, 2000.

ing resulting in iron deficiency, severe malnutrition, medical therapies, or malignancy in blood-forming organs (see WHAT'S NEW? Radiotherapy-Asssociated Anemia). Several of these mechanisms may cause suppression of the action of erythropoietin on the bone marrow, presumably by the release of cytokines.[33] Erythropoietin acts on specific erythroid progenitor cells in the bone marrow to stimulate the release of immature red blood cells (e.g., reticulocytes). Erythropoietin is effective in correcting the anemia associated with cancer. In addition, anemias that occurred after chemotherapy or radiation therapy have also been treated successfully by erythropoietin.[34,35] Chronic bleeding and iron deficiency can accompany colorectal or genitourinary malignancy. Iron also is malabsorbed in persons with gastric, pancreatic, or upper intestinal cancer. In addition, anorexia can cause iron deficiency, although folate deficiency is more common with anorexia.

Anemia can result from chemotherapy, but normochromic (normal hemoglobin concentration) and normocytic (average red cell size) anemias can occur after prolonged administration of alkylating agents or nitrosoureas, both classes of chemotherapeutic agents.[36] Megaloblastic (large red cell) anemias may develop after treatment with methotrexate, which causes abnormal folate metabolism.

Malignancy of the blood-forming organs is associated with a number of hemolytic anemias. An autoimmune hemolytic anemia occasionally develops in persons with chronic lymphocytic leukemia. (Anemia associated with leukemia is discussed in Chapter 25.)

Chemotherapy frequently worsens anemia in individuals with cancer. The administration of recombinant human erythropoietin (r-HuEPO) is safe and can significantly improve the hematocrit and quality of life of anemic individuals receiving myelosuppressive chemotherapy.[35]

Leukopenia and Thrombocytopenia

Direct tumor invasion to the bone marrow causes both leukopenia (a decreased leukocyte count) and thrombocytopenia (a decreased number of platelets). Chemotherapeutic drugs are toxic to the bone marrow, often causing both granulocytopenia and thrombocytopenia. Leukopenia can result from chemotherapy or radiation therapy of areas of the bone marrow. Thrombocytopenia is a major cause of hemorrhage in persons with cancer. It usually results from chemotherapy or bone marrow involvement by the malignancy.

Infection

Infection is the most significant cause of complications and death in persons with malignant disease. When the absolute granulocyte or lymphocyte count falls, the risk of infection increases, and persons with cancer have reduced immunologic functions, debility with advanced disease, and immunosuppression from radiation therapy and chemotherapy. (Factors that predispose persons to infection are summarized in Table 11-3.) Surgery also can lower resistance to infection because removal of large quantities of tissue—together with hemorrhage, dead spaces, and poor tissue perfusion—creates favorable sites for infection. Hospital-related (nosocomial) infections increase because of indwelling medical devices, inadequate wound care, and the introduction of microorganisms from visitors and other patients.

Leukopenia resulting from bone marrow radiation dramatically increases the risk of infection. Mucous membranes and other rapidly dividing cells in the radiation field are prone to irritation and ulceration. Radiation, particularly of the cervix, bladder, and intestinal tract, also can lead to fistula formation or abnormal passages between tissue cavities. Surgery often is required to repair the fistula and eliminate continuous infectious cross-contaminations.

Paraneoplastic Syndromes

Paraneoplastic syndromes are symptom complexes that cannot be explained by the local or distant spread of the tumor or by the effects of hormones released by the tissue from which the tumor arose. About 10% of individuals with malignancy are affected. Although infrequent, paraneoplastic syndromes are significant because (1) they may be the earliest symptom of an unknown cancer, (2) in affected individuals they may represent serious and life-threatening problems, and (3) they may mimic progression and therefore interfere with appropriate treatment. Table 11-4 presents the classifications of paraneoplastic syndromes.

CANCER TREATMENT

Cancer is treated with chemotherapy, radiation therapy, surgery, immunotherapy, and combinations of these modalities (Table 11-5). New proposed therapies are depicted in the figure in WHAT'S NEW? Therapies in Development.

Table 11-3 Factors Predisposing Individuals With Cancer to Infection

Factor	Basis
Age	Many common malignancies occur mostly in older age. Immunologic functions decline with age. General debility reduces immunocompetence. Immobility predisposes to infection. Far-advanced cancer often results in immobility and general debility that worsens with age. Elderly persons are predisposed to nutritional inadequacies. Malnutrition impairs immunocompetence.
Tumor	Nutritional derangements can result. Sites and circumstances favorable to growth of microorganisms (obstruction, serous or blood effusion, ulceration) can be created. Far-advanced disease predisposes patients to debility and immobility. Humoral or cellular immune defects may result. Metastasis to bone marrow may cause leukopenia or other defects in immunity.
Leukemias	Inadequate granulocyte production (impaired phagocytosis) results. Thrombocytopenia (bleeding, breaks in skin integrity) can occur. Late effect: Chronic lung disease from *Pneumocystis carinii* pneumonia can develop during therapy.
Lymphomas and other mononuclear phagocyte malignancies	Humoral and cellular immune defects (anergy, altered immunoglobin production) result. Late effect: Splenectomy in children can cause increased susceptibility to infection.
Treatment: surgery	Invasive procedure interrupts first lines of defense. Radical nature of surgery (removal of large blocks of tissue in lengthy procedures) causes hemorrhage, decreased tissue perfusion, creation of dead spaces, devitalization of tissues. Procedure may be "dirty" surgery (bowel, infected or contaminated areas). Surgery patients are often older and at poor risk. Long preoperative hospitalization often precedes surgery. Patients may have had previous adrenocorticosteroid therapy. Patients may have infections at sites remote from operative area. Nutritional derangements (especially important in head and neck surgery) may result. Lymph node dissection may predispose patient to local infection and impair containment to area. Gynecologic surgery may result in fistulas. Lung surgery may cause bronchopleural fistulas. Debility and immobility may result.

Data from Donovan MI, Girton SF: *Cancer care nursing,* ed 2, New York, 1984, Appleton-Century-Crofts; Murphy GP, Lawrence W, Lenhard RE: *Clinical oncology,* ed 2, New York, 1994, American Cancer Society.

Chemotherapy

Several classes of chemotherapeutic agents are used concurrently to treat different types of cancerous tumors (Table 11-6). The mechanism by which each drug acts to eradicate tumor cells depends largely on its effect on the cell cycle (described in Chapter 1). Malignant tumors have three cellular compartments: (1) cells undergoing mitosis and cytokinesis, (2) cells capable of entering the cell cycle in the G_1 phase (see Fig. 1-23), and (3) cells that do not divide and have irreversibly left the cell cycle (dying malignant cells, differentiated malignant cells, nonmalignant support cells). Cells in compartment 3 will die a natural death without chemotherapy. The specific aim of chemotherapy therefore is to kill cells from compartments 1 and 2—cells that are dividing and cells that are in interphase.

To be curative, chemotherapy must eradicate enough tumor cells so that the body's own defenses can eradicate the remaining cells. Smaller tumors have a faster growth rate and generally are more sensitive to chemotherapy. Few cells in a large tumor are dividing, and as a result, these cells are largely insensitive to chemotherapy.

The development of resistance to one chemotherapeutic agent often results in the coincident development of resistance to other drugs, albeit structurally unrelated. Multidrug resistance is associated with the expression of a cell surface glycoprotein called *P-170.* Cells expressing P-170 have decreased uptake and increased efflux of the drugs to which they are resistant. Multidrug resistance–associated protein gene MRP/MRP1 and its family genes have been isolated and characterized.[37,38,39]

Radiation

The goals of ionizing radiation are (1) to eradicate cancer without producing excessive toxicity during treatment and (2) to avoid damage to normal structures. The application of radiation therefore requires precision and skillful application.

Ionizing radiation leads to damage of important macromolecules, especially deoxyribonucleic acid (DNA). The

Table 11-4 Paraneoplastic Syndromes

Clinical Syndromes	Major Forms of Underlying Cancer	Causal Mechanism
ENDOCRINOPATHIES		
Cushing syndrome	Small cell carcinoma of lung Pancreatic carcinoma Neural tumors	ACTH or ACTH-like substance
Syndrome of inappropriate antidiuretic hormone secretion	Small cell carcinoma of lung; intracranial neoplasms	Antidiuretic hormone or atrial natriuretic hormones
Hypercalcemia	Squamous cell carcinoma of lung Breast carcinoma Renal carcinoma Adult T-cell leukemia/lymphoma Ovarian carcinoma	Parathyroid hormone–related peptide, TGF-α, TNF-α, IL-1
Hypoglycemia	Fibrosarcoma Other mesenchymal sarcomas Hepatocellular carcinoma	Insulin or insulin-like substance
Carcinoid syndrome	Bronchial adenoma (carcinoid) Pancreatic carcinoma Gastric carcinoma	Serotonin, bradykinin, ?histamine
Polycythemia	Renal carcinoma Cerebellar hemangioma Hepatocellular carcinoma	Erythropoietin
NERVE AND MUSCLE SYNDROMES		
Myasthenia	Bronchogenic carcinoma	Immunologic
Disorders of the central and peripheral nervous systems	Breast carcinoma	
DERMATOLOGIC DISORDERS		
Acanthosis nigricans	Gastric carcinoma Lung carcinoma Uterine carcinoma	?Immunologic, ?secretion of epidermal growth factor
Dermatomyositis	Bronchogenic, breast carcinoma	?Immunologic
OSSEOUS, ARTICULAR, AND SOFT TISSUE CHANGES		
Hypertrophic osteoarthropathy and clubbing of the fingers	Bronchogenic carcinoma	Unknown
VASCULAR AND HEMATOLOGIC CHANGES		
Venous thrombosis (Trousseau phenomenon)	Pancreatic carcinoma Bronchogenic carcinoma Other cancers	Tumor products (mucins that activate clotting)
Nonbacterial thrombotic endocarditis	Advanced cancers	Hypercoagulability
Anemia	Thymic neoplasms	Unknown
OTHERS		
Nephrotic syndrome	Various cancers	Tumor antigens, immune complexes

ACTH, adrenocorticotropic hormone; TGF, transforming growth factor, TNF, tumor necrosis factor; IL, interleukin.
From Cotran RS, Kumar V, Collins T: *Robbins Pathologic basis of disease,* ed 6, Philadelphia, 1999, Saunders.

Table 11-5 Examples of Treatment of Site-Specific Cancers

Usual Treatment	Site
Surgery	Colon
	Breast
	Ovary
	Lung
	Thyroid
	Skin
	Uterus
Chemotherapy	Lymphoma
	Leukemia
	Choriocarcinoma
	Ovary
	Breast
Radiation	Breast (all have been combined with surgery)
	Uterus or cervix
	Lymphomas
	Lung
	Combined with surgery in many sites
Hormones	Breast
	Prostate
	Endometrium
Immunotherapy	Melanoma
	Prostate cancer
	Breast cancer?
	Leukemias
	Others?

damage may be (1) lethal, in which the cell is killed; (2) potentially lethal, in which the cell is so severely affected by radiation that modifications in its environment will cause it to die; and (3) sublethal, in which the cell is damaged but subsequently can repair itself. Cellular compartments with rapidly renewing cells are, in general, more radiosensitive. (Cellular effects of ionizing radiation are discussed in Chapter 2.)

Surgery

Surgical therapy is used when the tumor has not yet spread beyond the limits of surgical excision. Surgeons are generally in agreement that if there is any chance of regional lymph node involvement and there is no evidence of distant disease, the lymph nodes also should be removed. **Sentinel nodes** are a limited set of lymph nodes first to receive drainage from any given location. Presumably, cancer metastasizes to these nodes before other nodes. Therefore, new techniques, such as sentinel node localization and biopsy, now allow less invasive tumor staging.[40]

Curative resections are performed if distant metastasis is not evident. The goals of palliative surgery (alleviation without cure) are (1) prevention of symptoms that would have occurred if the individual were not treated and (2) relief of symptoms that are present. Surgery is indicated also for benign tumors that could progress into malignant tumors. Premalignant and in situ tumors of epithelial tissues, such as skin, mouth, and cervix, therefore are removed.

WHAT'S NEW? Therapies in Development—Points of Attack

Cancer develops from a series of mutations. Normally a cell is inhibited from unlimited growth. With cancer the cell can lose its inhibitions to growth and multiply continously.

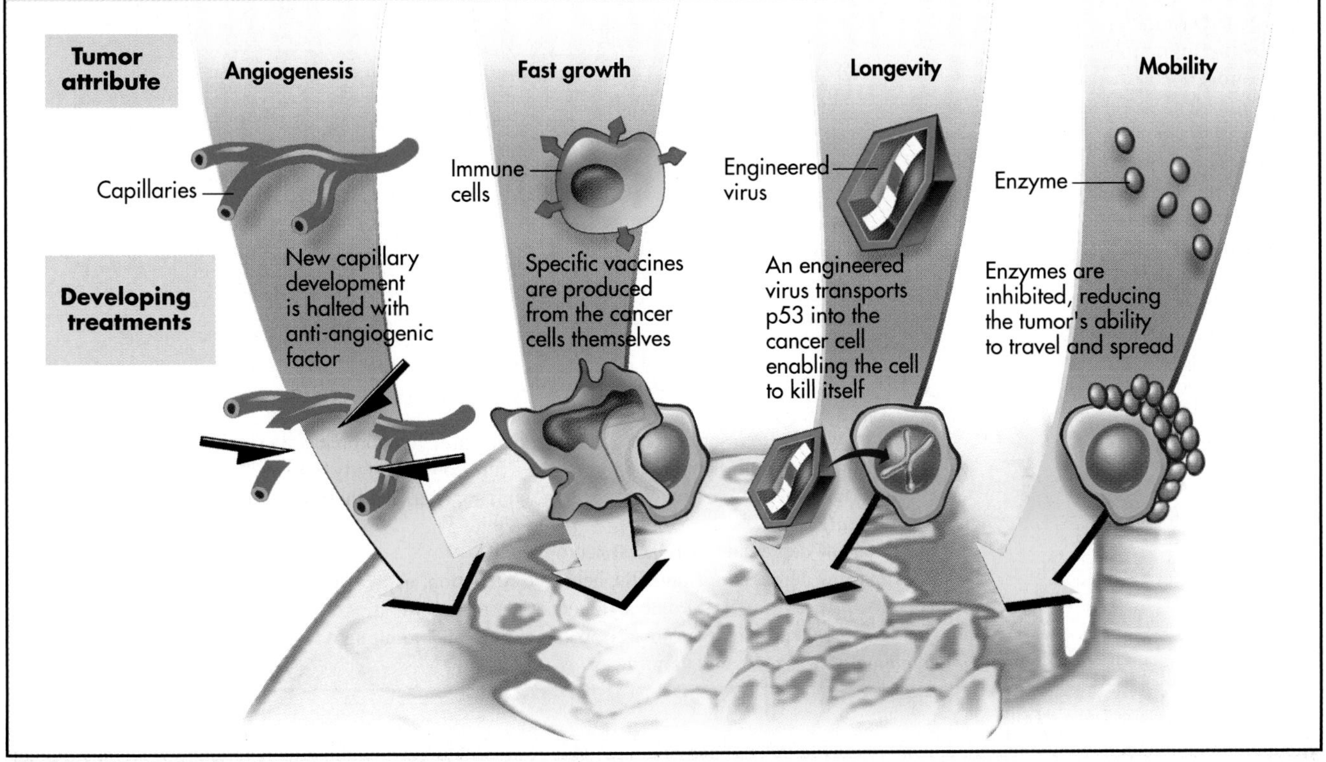

Table 11-6 Examples of Chemotherapeutic Drugs

Drug	Major Toxicity
ALKYLATING AGENTS	
Mechlorethamine Chlorambucil Melphalan Thiotepa Busulfan Cyclophosphamide Ifosfamide	Therapeutic doses: moderate depression of peripheral blood cell count; excessive doses: severe bone marrow depression, leukopenia, thrombocytopenia, and bleeding; maximum toxicity may occur 2-3 wk after last dose; alopecia; nausea and vomiting
ANTIMETABOLITES	
Methotrexate 6-Mercaptopurine 6-Thioquanine 5-Fluorouracil 5-Fluorodeoxyuridine Cytarabine Fludarabine 2-Chlorodeoxyadenosine 2′-Deoxycoformycin Gemcitabine	Oral and digestive tract ulcerations; bone marrow depression with leukopenia, thrombocytopenia, and bleeding; toxicity enhanced by impaired kidney function; alopecia
ANTIBIOTICS	
Doxorubicin Bleomycin Dactinomycin Daunorubicin Plicamycin Mitomycin-C Mitoxantrone	Stomatitis; gastrointestinal injury; bone marrow depression; alopecia; cardiac toxicity at cumulative doses over 500 mg/m^2 (doxorubicin and daunorubicin); pneumonitis and pulmonary fibrosis at cumulative doses over 400 U (bleomycin); hypocalcemia; hepatic toxicity (plicamycin); nausea and vomiting
STEROIDS AND HORMONALLY ACTIVE AGENTS	
Androgen Fluoxymesterone Antiandrogen Flutamide Estrogen Ethinyl estradiol Diethylstilbestrol Antiestrogen Tamoxifen Progestin Megestrol acetate Luteinizing hormone–releasing hormone agonist Leuprolide Aromatase inhibitor Aminoglutethimide Adrenocortical compound Dexamethasone	Fluid retention; masculinization/feminization; hot flashes (sex hormones); hypertension; diabetes; adrenal insufficiency
MISCELLANEOUS DRUGS	
Asparaginase	Anorexia, weight loss, somnolence, lethargy, confusion; hypoproteinemia (including albumin and fibrinogen); hyperlipidemia, abnormal liver function tests, fatty metamorphosis of liver; pancreatitis (rare); azotemia; granulocytopenia, lymphopenia, and thrombocytopenia (usually mild and transient)
Altretamine	Bone marrow depression; peripheral neuropathy
m-AMSA	Bone marrow depression; stomatitis; hepatic dysfunction; nausea and vomiting
Carmustine	Bone marrow depression, thrombocytopenia; nausea and vomiting
Lomustine	Bone marrow depression, thrombocytopenia; nausea and vomiting
Streptozocin	Hypoglycemia; nausea and vomiting

From Krakoff IH: *CA Cancer J Clin* 46:134, 1996.

Table 11-6 Examples of Chemotherapeutic Drugs—cont'd

Drug	Major Toxicity
MISCELLANEOUS DRUGS—cont'd	
Mitotane	Skin eruptions; diarrhea; mental depression; muscle tremors; adrenal insufficiency; nausea and vomiting
Dacarbazine	Bone marrow depression; nausea and vomiting
Hydroxyurea	Bone marrow depression; nausea and vomiting
Etoposide	Alopecia; nausea and vomiting
Cisplatin	Bone marrow depression; renal tubular damage; deafness; nausea and vomiting
Carboplatin	Bone marrow depression; nausea and vomiting
Procarbazine	Bone marrow depression with leukopenia and thrombocytopenia; mental depression; nausea and vomiting
Vinblastine	Alopecia; areflexia; bone marrow depression
Vincristine	Areflexia; muscular weakness; peripheral neuritis; paralytic ileus; mild bone marrow depression
Levamisole	None
Cis-retinoic acid	Cheilitis; stomatitis; conjunctivitis
Paclitaxel	Leukopenia; peripheral neuropathy
Docetaxel	Leukopenia; peripheral neuropathy

Table 11-7 Common Hormonal Agents and Types of Tumors

Agents	Types of Tumors
Corticosteroids	Leukemias
	Hodgkin disease
	Malignant lymphomas
	Breast cancer
	Multiple myeloma
Androgens	Breast cancer
Estrogens	Breast cancer
	Prostate cancer
Antiestrogens	Endometrial cancer
	Breast cancer
Aromatase inhibitors	Adrenal tumors
	Breast cancer
LH-RH analogs	Breast cancer
	Prostate cancer
Antiandrogens	Prostate cancer

LH, Luteinizing hormone; *RH*, releasing hormone.

Hormonal Therapy

Hormonal therapy has been in use for a long time. Table 11-7 lists the commonly used hormonal agents and their primary indications. Their mechanism of action is not known but probably involves receptor manipulations. Presumably by blocking or causing down-regulation of receptors it prevents the cell from receiving normal growth stimulation signals.

Immunotherapy

Chemotherapy and radiation treatments are the most common methods for managing cancer. Although these therapies are effective for certain types of cancer, they have drawbacks. In general, both therapies act by eliminating mitotically or metabolically active cells. Within a tumor mass, however, a significant portion of cells is in a part of the cell cycle that is not affected by either metabolic inhibitors or mitotic poisons. In addition, these therapies have numerous side effects because they affect normal cell populations that, like transformed cells, have high rates of cell division. Cells of the gut epithelium, hair follicles, bone marrow, and gonads are affected by radiation and chemotherapy.

Because cancer is a dynamic disease in which the transformed cells in a tumor mass can adapt to changes in their environment, a single form of cancer therapy that is effective against all types of cancer may not be possible. More specific methods, however, eventually may eliminate transformed cells without damaging normal tissues.

In this regard, immunotherapy (immunologic treatment) holds promise. (The immune system is discussed in detail in Chapter 6.) First, the immune system has specificity for antigen recognition and is highly regulated; thus theoretically antitumor immune rejection responses (described in Chapter 10) can selectively eliminate cancer cells while sparing normal tissues. Second, immune memory cells are long lived and capable of providing extended protection against the emergence of recurrent primary tumor cells and foci of metastatic cancer cells. Third, numerous immunologic mechanisms are able to cause rejection of various types of cancer. Although tumor-immune surveillance provides protection against cancer, certain evasive mechanisms allow tumor cells to escape immune rejection. (Tumor-immune surveillance is described in Chapter 10.) Therefore current research efforts for establishing effective anticancer immunotherapies focus on characterizing the immunogenic properties of various tumor-specific antigens and developing methods to selectively enhance tumor rejection immune responses.

Immunotherapies for the treatment of cancer generally are referred to as **biologic response modifiers (BRMs).** BRMs are mammalian gene products, agents, and clinical protocols that affect biologic responses in host/tumor interactions. BRMs have the following actions:

1. A direct cytotoxic effect on cancer cells
2. The initiation or augmentation of the host's tumor-immune rejection response

Table 11-8 Classification of Biologic Response Modifiers

Major Classification	Specific Examples
Immunomodulating agents	Alkyl lysophospholipids BCG Bestatin *Corynebacterium parvum* Endotoxin Levamisole Muramyldipeptide Picibanil (OK432) Tuftsin
Interferons and interferon inducers	Interferons (alpha, beta, and gamma) Poly IC-LC *Brucella abortus* Viruses
Thymosins	Thymosin α_1 Other thymosin factors Thymosin factor V
Antigens	Tumor-associated antigens Hapten-modified tumor antigens Vaccines
Effector cells	Macrophages Natural killer cells Cytotoxic T cells LAK cells
Lymphokines and cytokines	Colony-stimulating factors Lymphotoxin Interleukins (IL-1, IL-2, IL-3, etc.) Tumor necrosis factor
Colony-stimulating factors	G-CSF, GM-CSF, M-CSF, erythropoietin
Monoclonal antibodies	Cytotoxic antibodies Immunotoxins Phototoxins

BCG, Bacille Calmette-Guérin; *LAK,* lymphokine-activated killer; *G-CSF,* granulocyte colony-stimulating factor; *GM-CSF,* granulocyte-macrophage colony-stimulating factor; *M-CSF,* macrophage colony-stimulating factor.

3. The modification of cancer cell susceptibility to the lytic or tumor-static effects of the immune system

The major classifications of BRMs are presented in Table 11-8. The basis of action and clinical applications of specific BRMs, selected from among the major classifications, are discussed briefly in the remainder of this section.

Immunomodulating Agents

Nonspecific stimulation of the immune system by an adjuvant (a substance that enhances the immune response) has been attempted in individuals with a variety of different cancers (Fig. 11-9). This therapy consists of the administration of an adjuvant (a bacterium), such as *Corynebacterium parvum* or bacille Calmette-Guérin (BCG), an attenuated strain of *Mycobacterium bovis.* Bacterial cell wall extracts, live BCG, or nonviable *C. parvum* is injected at the tumor site. Retardation of tumor growth results through the activation of macrophages, augmentation of natural killer cells, or by some degree of antigenic cross-reactivity between the organism (BCG) and the antigen produced by certain human cancers, such as melanomas.

Some success has been observed in the treatment of genitourinary and lung cancer, usually through combined adjuvant treatments and chemotherapies. The most effective use of this type of immunotherapy, however, has been in the treatment of skin cancers.

Interferons

The interferons are a family of cell-derived proteins that have antiviral and immune modulating activities. The most successful clinical trials have come from the use of interferon-α. Interferon-α is a glycoprotein made by activated leukocytes. In addition to its antiviral activity, interferon-α inhibits tumor growth, enhances natural killer cell activity, and increases cancer cell expression of tumor antigens, thus making them more immunogenic (i.e., eliciting stronger tumor-immune rejection responses). Used either alone or in combination with other treatment modalities, interferon-α has been effective in the treatment of hairy cell leukemia, Kaposi sarcoma (a common cancer of persons with acquired immunodeficiency syndrome [AIDS]), and renal cell carcinoma. Similarly, interferon-α is effective for treating ovarian carcinoma when used after surgical removal of the tumor mass.[41] The use of interferons in cancer therapy is greatly enhanced by the ability to produce these biologic agents by recombinant gene-cloning techniques.

Antigens

Some success in treating skin tumors has been obtained by the application of contact sensitizing agents (materials that cause a hypersensitivity response in the skin), such as dinitrochlorobenzene (DNCB) (Fig. 11-10). With this approach the individual is first sensitized to DNCB through topical application to normal skin, and the tumor is subsequently painted with DNCB.

Tumor regression is thought to occur by inducing a contact hypersensitivity response to the DNCB at the tumor site. (Hypersensitivity reactions are discussed in Chapter 8.) Tumor cells probably are killed because DNCB has become associated with their cell surface and functions as an antigen. This type of therapy, however, is restricted to superficial tumors of the skin.

Research efforts are underway to identify tumor-specific antigens (the various types of antigens are described in Chapter 10) that could be used to develop anticancer vaccines. Ideally, common tumor antigens expressed by a wide range of cancers could be developed as vaccines. These vaccines could be used either as immunotherapies to augment the host's immune response against the tumor or as preventive immunization techniques to inhibit cancer emergence in populations at risk.

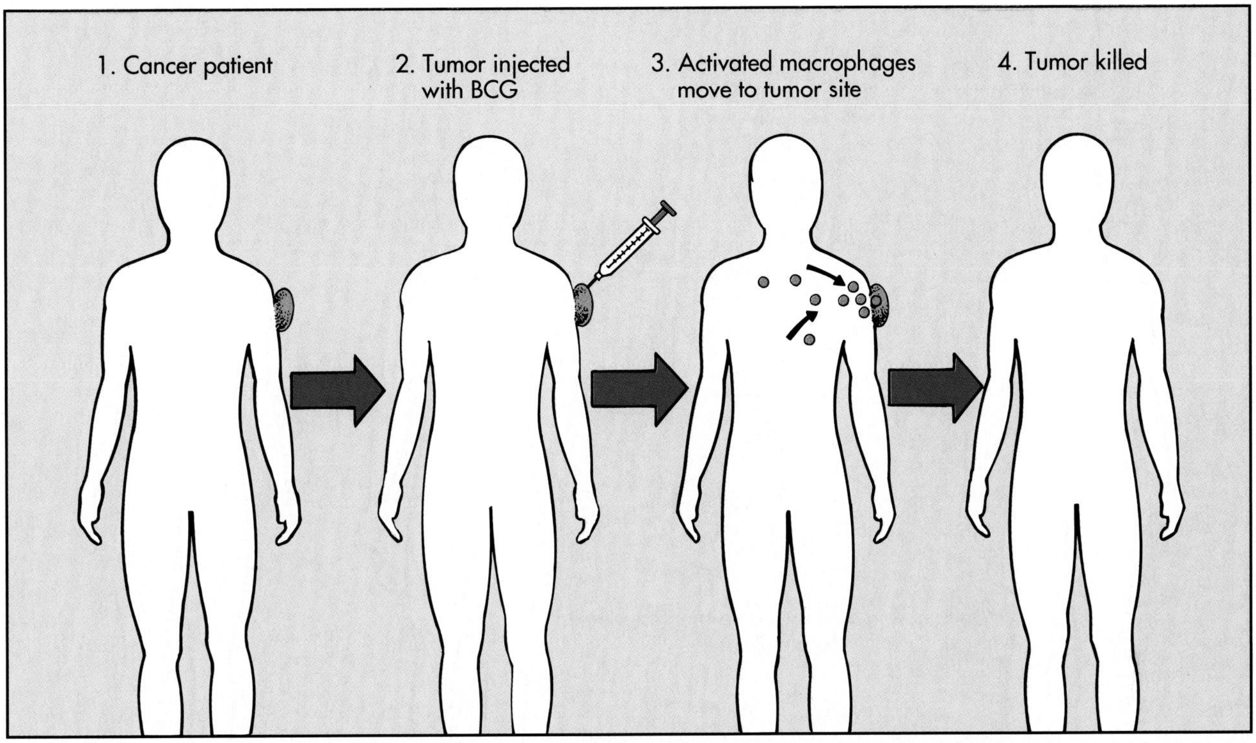

FIG. 11-9 Immunostimulation in cancer therapy. *BCG,* Bacille Calmette-Guérin.

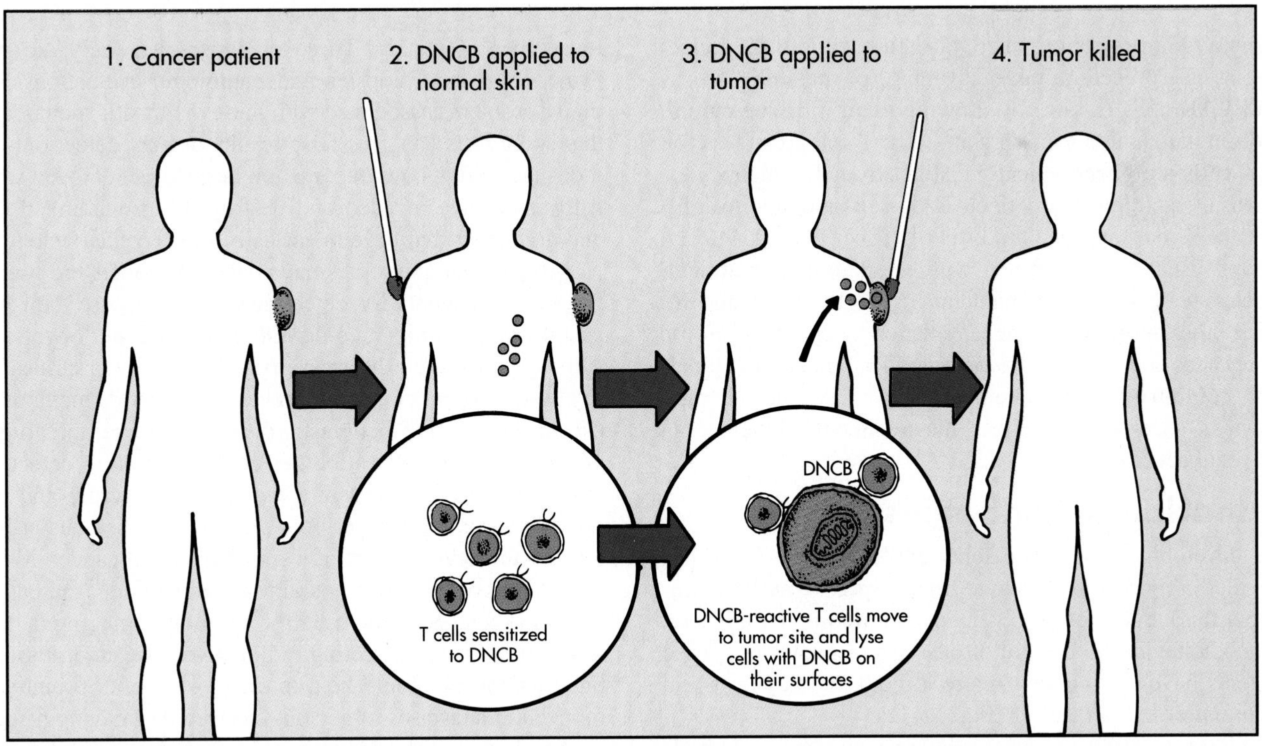

FIG. 11-10 Cancer therapy through antigen modification with dinitrochlorobenzene (DNCB).

Effector Cells and Lymphokines

Theoretically, an effective form of cellular immunotherapy would result from the transfer or augmentation of cytotoxic T cells (Tc cells) that are specific for the antigens expressed by the individual's tumor cells (Fig. 11-11).[42] Because this represents such an attractive form of immunotherapy for cancer, a treatment protocol has been established and is undergoing extensive clinical trials. It is known as *lymphokine-activated killer (LAK) cell therapy.* The idea is to establish tumor-specific cytotoxic cell lines in tissue culture that can

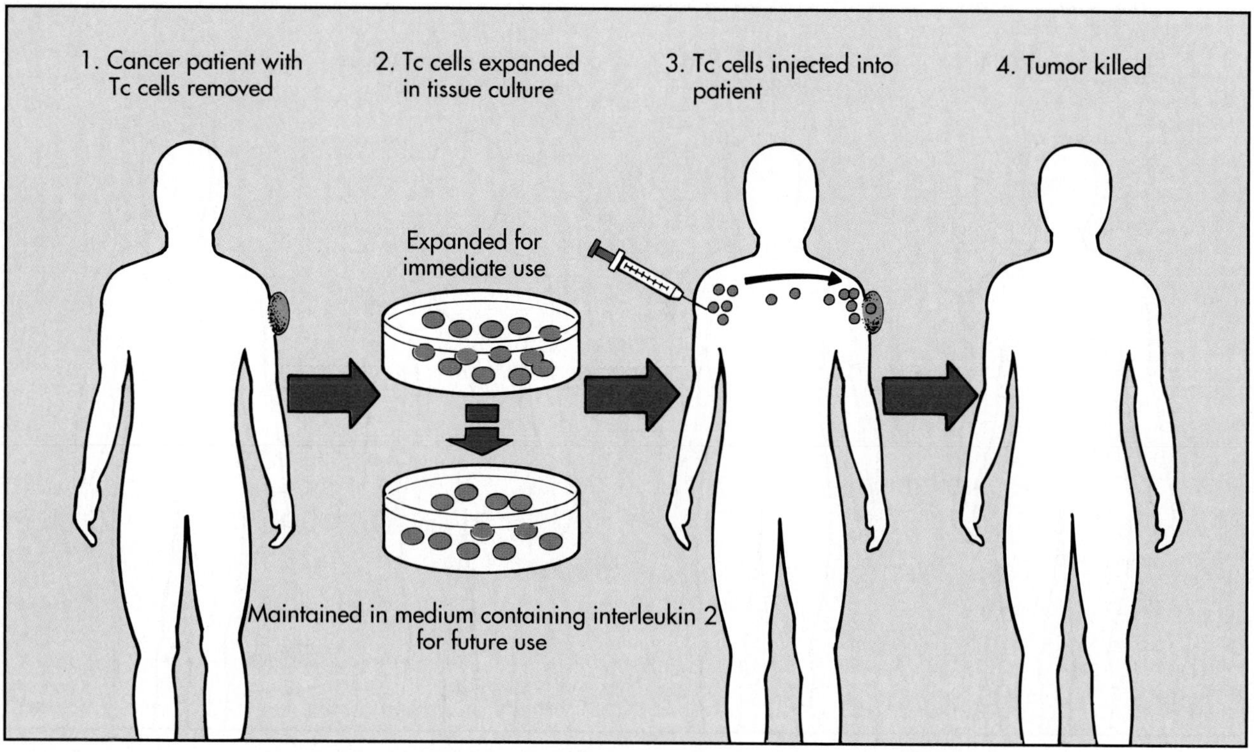
1. Cancer patient with Tc cells removed
2. Tc cells expanded in tissue culture
3. Tc cells injected into patient
4. Tumor killed
Expanded for immediate use
Maintained in medium containing interleukin 2 for future use

FIG. 11-11 Development of cytotoxic T cell (Tc cell) lines for cancer immunotherapy.

mediate tumor rejection when injected back into the cancer patient. The procedure takes advantage of the ability to expand LAK cells in vitro by growing them in tissue culture medium that contains interleukin-2, the T cell growth factor. LAK cells are phenotypically distinct from T lymphocytes. When injected into the patient, LAK cells are able to infiltrate the tumor and mediate lysis of cancer cells. LAK cell therapy usually is combined with interleukin-2 treatment, which is believed to both maintain LAK cell activity and enhance other antitumor immune rejection mechanisms. Some success has been obtained by interleukin-2 treatment alone[43] or in combination with chemotherapy.[44] LAK cell therapy has been used successfully in the treatment of melanoma and renal cell carcinoma.

Monoclonal Antibodies

The development of monoclonal antibody technology has provided a method to generate highly specific antibody reagents that could not be obtained with traditional antisera. (Monoclonal antibodies are discussed in Chapter 6.) These reagents have a promising future in both the diagnosis and treatment of human cancer (Fig. 11-12).

In the past, clinicians have relied on a number of methods to diagnose human cancers. For example, in the case of most skin cancers, the diagnosis can be made by visual examination of the lesion. In contrast, the diagnosis of various soft tissue cancers, such as lung tumors, may require the identification of certain clinical signs (e.g., obstruction, bleeding, pain). Cytologic methods (e.g., Papanicolaou [Pap] smear) or histologic analysis of cells also can be used to diagnose various types of cancer. These diagnoses generally are confirmed by tissue biopsies and pathologic evaluations. The major problems associated with these diagnostic methods are that some tests can give false results or may detect only tumor masses that have become too large to be removed surgically, that have invaded and destroyed surrounding tissues and organs, or that have metastasized to secondary sites.

Monoclonal antibodies have been developed and used as diagnostic reagents for detecting cancer because their high specificity for antigen could reduce the number of false results. Coupled with the appropriate laboratory or clinical assay system, monoclonal antibodies may provide methods for earlier detection of neoplastic disease. For example, highly purified monoclonal antibodies could be used to detect circulating tumor antigens in the individual's serum and thus provide a method for periodic screening of persons at high risk for the development of a specific type of cancer. Monoclonal antibodies, when bound to a radionuclide (radioactive material), also could be used for radiologic imaging (a diagnostic process for detecting radioactive deposits in tissues). Such techniques could help in diagnosing both primary tumors and metastases in persons suspected of having disease.

Another goal is to develop monoclonal antibodies specific for tumor antigens that would mediate tumor rejection without affecting normal tissues. In recent studies, monoclonal antibodies against specific antigens expressed by gastric carcinoma and ricin have been highly effective in causing regression of human tumors grown experimentally in mice.[45,46] The ability to couple cytotoxic substances or cell poisons, such as the alpha chain of ricin (immunotoxins) and

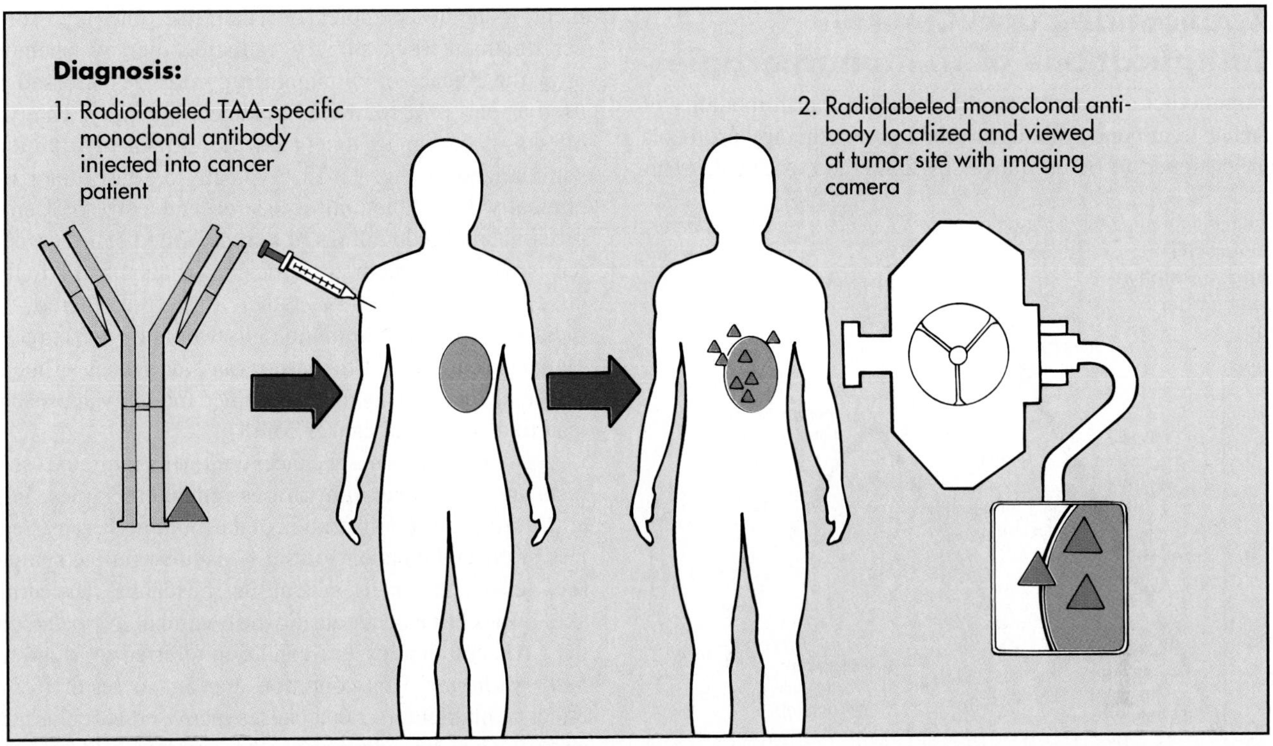

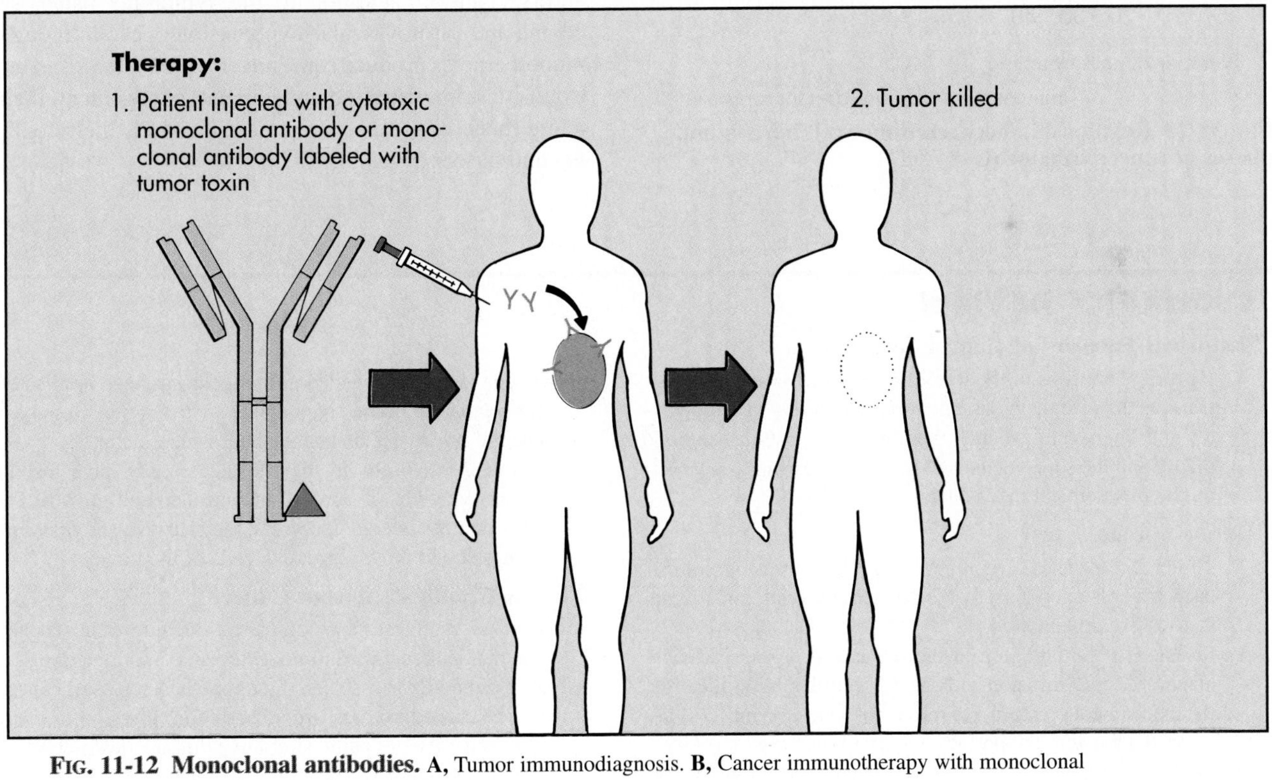

FIG. 11-12 Monoclonal antibodies. A, Tumor immunodiagnosis. **B,** Cancer immunotherapy with monoclonal antibodies. *TAA,* Tumor-associated antigen.

porphyrins (phototoxins), to monoclonal antibodies could greatly enhance the efficacy of these reagents as immunotherapy for cancer. The major problems currently faced in the attempt to use monoclonal antibodies in cancer therapy are (1) developing functional reagents with the appropriate antigen specificities; (2) overcoming clinical complications that are associated with injecting large amounts of foreign antibodies (currently, most monoclonal antibodies can be made only in rodents); and (3) controlling immunoregulatory mechanisms that would eliminate their efficacy. Certainly the potential use of monoclonal antibodies, as well as other forms of immunotherapy, has generated new interest in immune surveillance mechanisms as possible methods for development of immunotherapies for cancer treatment.

Applications and Clinical Complications of Immunotherapies

Immunotherapy represents the so-called fourth modality of cancer treatment. Although some immunotherapy protocols are designed to be used as a single method of cancer treatment, it should be appreciated that, like other types of cancer treatment (i.e., surgery, radiation therapy, chemotherapy), the efficacy of immunotherapy may be increased when used as part of a combined treatment modality. The typical effects of cancer treatment on the growth of a tumor are summarized in Fig. 11-13. Typically a solid tumor is not clinically detectable until it has reached a size of 1 cm, approximately 30 doublings of a transformed cell. Surgery often is used as a method to remove or debulk (partially reduce) the tumor mass. Other forms of therapy (i.e., radiation, chemical, immunologic) would be used to prevent clinical recurrence of the tumor mass or growth of metastatic tumor foci. This type of combined modality approach can lead to a successful cancer cure.

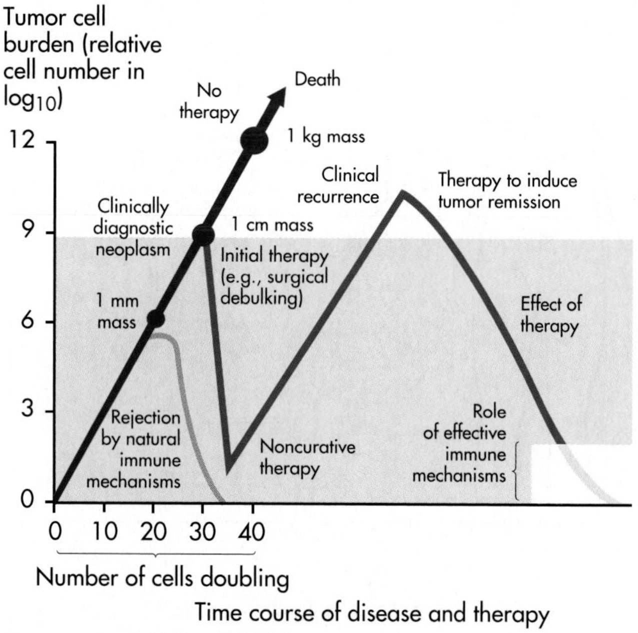

FIG. 11-13 Relationship between tumor cell burden and phases of cancer treatment.

As with other forms of cancer treatment, numerous side effects are associated with various immunotherapies. In general, during the administration of the immunotherapy (regardless of type) the patients usually manifest flulike symptoms (i.e., fever, chills, nausea, vomiting, headache). Urticaria and skin rashes often occur during the treatment. Associated with the LAK cell therapy is a condition referred to as *vascular-leak syndrome*. This condition appears to result from the effect of interleukin-2 that causes increased vascular permeability. Thus, in addition to the symptoms listed, severe edema and cardiovascular hypotension occur. Although immunotherapies produce some adverse side effects and require extensive administration and clinical management, their potential benefit in cancer treatment demands their continued use and further development.

SUMMARY REVIEW

Historical Theories of Cancer Invasion

1. Historical analysis of theories of cancer invasion and metastasis began with the black bile diffusion theory of Hippocrates and later included such theories as the cellular-embolic theory and the seed-versus-soil theory. Today the emphasis is on the biochemical mechanisms of metastasis.

Tumor Spread

1. Tumor spread takes several forms: (a) direct invasion, (b) metastasis of distant organs by lymphatics and veins, and (c) metastasis by implantation.
2. Invasion is the first step in the metastatic process. Mechanisms of local invasion include (a) cellular multiplication, (b) mechanical pressure, (c) release of lytic enzymes, (d) decreased adhesion (slipperiness), and (e) increased motility.
3. The three-step theory of invasion includes (a) tumor cell attachment to the matrix, (b) degradation or dissolution of the matrix, and (c) tumor cell locomotion.
4. Metastasis is the life-threatening characteristic of malignancy. The three mechanisms of metastasis are (a) direct or continuous extension, (b) lymphatic spread, and (c) bloodstream dissemination. These mechanisms are not mutually exclusive.
5. Tumor growth is supported by the development of new blood vessels, a process called *angiogenesis*. Several angiogenic factors have been identified.
6. Tissue factor produced by tumor cells has been implicated in the regulation of the "angiogenic switch" regulating the balance of positive and negative angiogenic factors.
7. If mutations occur in the p53 gene, cells have lost their "emergency brake" against uncontrolled cell growth. These cells do not undergo apoptosis; they survive and may be the strongest and most aggressive cells of the tumor.

Clinical Manifestations of Cancer

1. Clinical manifestations of cancer include pain, cachexia, anemia, leukopenia, thrombocytopenia, and infection.
2. Pain generally is associated with the late stages of cancer. It can be caused by pressure, obstruction, invasion of a structure sensitive to pain, stretching, tissue destruction, and inflammation.
3. Fatigue is the most frequently reported symptom of cancer and cancer treatment.
4. Cachexia (loss of appetite, weakness, inability to maintain weight, taste alterations; altered metabolism) leads to protein-calorie malnutrition and progressive wasting.
5. Anemia associated with cancer usually occurs because of malnutrition, chronic bleeding and resultant iron deficiency, chemotherapy, radiation, and malignancies in the blood-forming organs.

6. Leukopenia is usually a result of chemotherapy (which is toxic to bone marrow) or radiation (which kills circulating leukocytes).
7. Thrombocytopenia is usually the result of chemotherapy or malignancy in the bone marrow.
8. Infection may be caused by leukopenia, immunosuppression, or debility associated with advanced disease.
9. Paraneoplastic syndromes are symptom complexes that cannot be explained by the local or distant spread of the tumor or by hormones released by the tissue from which the tumor arose.

Cancer Treatment

1. Cancer is treated with surgery, radiation therapy, chemotherapy, immunotherapy, and combinations of these modalities.
2. The theoretic basis of chemotherapy is the vulnerability of tumor cells in various stages of the cell cycle. The goal of chemotherapy is to eradicate enough tumor cells so that the body's natural defenses can eradicate remaining cells.
3. Ionizing radiation causes cell damage, so that the goal of radiation therapy is to damage the tumor without causing excessive toxicity or damage to undiseased structures.
4. Surgical therapy is used for nonmetastatic disease, for which cure is possible by removing the tumor, and as a palliative measure to alleviate symptoms.
5. Immunotherapy is appropriate for cancers that cannot be effectively managed by chemotherapy or radiation, usually because enough tumor cells are inactive and invulnerable to these modalities.
6. Forms of immunotherapy known as *biologic response modifiers* include immunomodulating agents, interferons, antigens, effector cells, lymphokines, and monoclonal antibodies.
7. Effector cells and lymphokines provide a form of cellular immunotherapy that involves the transfer of cytotoxic T cells (Tc cells) that are specific for tumor cell antigens.
8. Immunomodulating agents provide nonspecific stimulation of the immune system by means of an adjuvant; they are most effective in treating skin cancers.
9. Antigens cause regression in skin tumors by producing a hypersensitivity response that affects the antigenic properties of the cell surface.
10. Monoclonal antibodies ultimately may be used both as diagnostic reagents for detecting cancer and as a form of cancer therapy in which antibodies specific for tumor antigens would mediate tumor rejection.

KEY TERMS

Angiogenesis, *340*
Autocrine motility factor hypothesis, *336*
Biologic response modifier (BRM), *349*
Cachexia, *342*
Cathepsin B, *336*
Cathepsin D, *336*
Fatigue, *342*
Invasion, *334*
Laminin receptor, *337*
Metastasis, *338*
Organ tropism, *341*
p53 protein, *341*
Paraneoplastic syndrome, *344*
Primary tumor, *338*
Sentinel node, *347*
Tissue factor (TF), *340*
Tissue selective homing receptor, *341*
Type IV collagenase, *336*
Urokinase-type plasminogen activator (uPA), *336*

REFERENCES

1. Cotran RS et al: *Robbins pathologic basis of disease,* ed 6, Philadelphia, 1999, W.B. Saunders.
2. Liotta LA, Clair T: Cancer. Check point for invasion, *Nat* 405(6784):287, 2000.
3. Mandriotta SJ et al: Vascular endothelial growth factor increases urokinase receptor expression in vascular endothelial cells, *J Biol Chem* 270(17):9709, 1995.
4. Mignatti P, Rifkin DB: Biology and biochemistry of proteinases in tumor invasion, *Physiol Rev* 73(1):161, 1993.
5. McCawley LJ, Matrisian LM: Matrix metalloproteinases: multifunctional contributors to tumor progression, *Mol Med Today* 6(6):149, 2000.
6. Hubbard SM, Liotta LA: The biology of metastases. In Baird SB, McCorkle R et al, editors: *Cancer nursing: a comprehensive textbook,* ed 2, Philadelphia, 1996, W.B. Saunders.
7. Duffy MJ et al: Working plasminogen activator: a prognostic marker in multiple types of cancer, *J Surg Oncol* 31(2):130, 2000.
8. Aquirre Ghiso JA et al: Deregulation of the signaling pathways controlling working production. Its relationship with the invasive phenotype, *Eur J Biochem* 263(2):295, 1999.
9. Woodhouse EC et al: General mechanisms of metastasis, *Cancer* 80(8 suppl):1529, 1997.
10. Wells A: Tumor invasion: role of growth factor-induced cell motility, *Adv Cancer Res* 78:31, 2000.
11. Ziober BL et al: Laminin-binding integrins in tumor progression and metastasis, *Semin Cancer Biol* 7:11, 1996.
12. Zhou T, Sargiannidou I, Tuczynski GP: The role of adhesive proteins in the hematogenous spread of cancer, *In Vivo* 14(1):199, 2000.
13. Fidler IJ, Gersten DM, Hart IR: The biology of cancer invasion and metastasis, *Adv Cancer Res* 28:149, 1978.
14. Folkman J et al: Isolating a tumor factor responsible for angiogenesis, *J Exp Med* 133:275, 1971.
15. Anan K et al: Vascular endothelial growth factor and platelet-derived growth factor are potential angiogenic and metastatic factors in human breast cancer, *Surgery* 119(3):333, 1996.
16. Griffioen AW, Molema G: Angiogenesis: potentials for pharmacologic intervention in the treatment of cancer, cardiovascular diseases, and chronic inflammation, *Pharmacol Revl* 52(2):237, 2000.
17. Abdulkadir SA et al: Tissue factor expression and angiogenesis in human prostate carcinoma, *Hum Pathol* 38(4):443, 2000.
18. Lahav J: The functions of thrombospodin and its involvement in physiology and pathophysiology, *Biochem Biophys Acta* 1182(1):1, 1993.
19. Iruela-Arispe ML et al: Antiangiogenic domains shared by thrombospondins and metallospondins, a new family of angiogenic inhibitors, *Ann NY Acad Sci* 886:58, 1999.

20. Maeda K et al: Expression of vascular endothelial growth factor and thrombospondia-1 in colorectal carcinoma, *Int J Mol Med* 5(4):373, 2000.
21. Hagedorn M, Bikfalui A: Target molecules for anti-angiogenic therapy: from basic research to clinical trials, *Crit Rev Oncol Hematol* 34(2):89, 2000.
22. Graeber TG et al: Hypoxia-mediated selection of cells with diminished apoptotic potential in solid tumors, *Nature* 379(6560):88, 1996.
23. Seachrist L: Only the strong survive: the evolution of a tumor favors the meanest, most aggressive cells, *Sci News* 149:216, 1996.
24. Cherny NI: The management of cancer pain, *CA Cancer J Clin* 50(2): 70, 2000.
25. Winningham ML et al: Fatigue and the cancer experience: the state of the knowledge, *Oncol Nurs Forum* 21(1):23, 1994.
26. Nelson KA: The cancer anorexia-cachexia syndrome, *Semin Oncol* 27(1):64, 2000.
27. Davis MP, Dickerson D: Cachexia and anorexia: cancer's covert killer, *Support Care Cancer* 8(3):180, 2000.
28. Wilson RL: Optimizing nutrition for patients with cancer, *Clin J Oncol Nurs* 4(1):23, 2000.
29. Inui A: Cancer anorexia-cachexia syndrome: are neuropeptides the key? *Cancer Res* 59(18):4493, 1999.
30. Habtemariam S: Natural inhibitors of tumor necrosis factor-alpha production, secretion and function, *Planta Med* 66(4):303, 2000.
31. Kapadia SR: Cytokines and heart failure, *Cardiol Rev* 7(4):196, 1999.
32. Yeh SS, Schuster MW: Geriatric cachexia: the role of cytokines, *Am J Clin Nutr* 70(2):183, 1999.
33. Erslev AJ: Erythropoietin and anemia of cancer, *Eur J Haematol* 64(6):353, 2000.
34. Bragga M et al: Erythropoiesis after therapy with recombinant human erythropoietin: a dose-response study in anemic cancer surgery patients, *Vox Sang* 76(1):38, 1999.
35. Gargano G et al: The utility of a growth factor: rHuEPO as a treatment for preoperation autologous blood donation in gynecological tumor surgery, *Int J Oncol* 14(1):157, 1999.
36. Sabatini P: The relationship between anemia and quality of life in cancer patients, *Oncologist* 5(suppl 2):19, 2000.
37. Kumano M et al: Multidrug resistance-associated protein subfamily transporters and drug resistance, *Anticancer Drug Des* 14(2):123, 1999.
38. Roepe PD: What is the precise role of human MDR1 protein in chemotherapeutic drug resistance, *Curr Pharm Des* 6(3):241, 2000.
39. Sikic BI: New approaches in cancer treatment, *Ann Oncol* 6(suppl):149, 1999.
40. Krag D: Sentinel lymph node biopsy for the detection of metastases, *Cancer J Sci Am* 6(suppl 2):S121, 2000.
41. Colombo N et al: Antitumor and immunomodulatory activity of intraperitoneal IFN-gamma in ovarian carcinoma patients with minimal residual tumor after chemotherapy, *Int J Cancer* 51:42, 1992.
42. Appelbaum JW: The role of the immune system in the pathogenesis of cancer, *Semin Oncol Nurs* 8:51, 1992.
43. Melioli G et al: Perilymphatic injections of recombinant interleukin-2 (rIL-2) partially correct the immunologic defects in patients with advanced head and neck squamous cell carcinoma, *Laryngoscope* 102(5): 572, 1992.
44. Mitchell MS: Chemotherapy in combination with biomodulation: a 5-year experience with cyclophosphamide and interleukin-2, *Semin Oncol* 19:80, 1992.
45. Heberman RB: Principles of tumor immunology. In Murphy GP, Lawrence W, Lenhard RE, editors: *Clinical oncology,* ed 2, New York, 1995, American Cancer Society.
46. Pimm MV, Robins RA, Baldwin RW: Capture of recombinant recin A chain by a bispecific anti-RTA:anti-CEA monoclonal antibody pretargeted to a human gastric carcinoma xenograft in nude mice, *J Cancer Res Clin Oncol* 118:367, 1992.

CHAPTER 12

Cancer in Children

ELIZABETH KASSNER • PAT WILLS ALCOSER • MARILYN JO HOCKENBERRY

CHAPTER OUTLINE

Cancer in children is rare, but because so many diseases of childhood have been conquered, cancer is the third leading cause of death in children who have survived their first year.[1] (Trauma remains the leading killer of children and adolescents.) The unique feature of childhood cancer is the short latency time, which contrasts sharply with the long latency period common in adults. In addition, cancers among adults are categorized by the anatomic site of the primary tumor, and cancers in children are categorized by histology.[2] Table 12-1 summarizes the differences between childhood and adult cancers.

INCIDENCE AND TYPES

Both incidence rate and types of cancer that develop vary between children and adults. For example, approximately 9000 children up to 15 years of age are diagnosed with cancer each year, whereas approximately 1,100,000 adults are diagnosed with cancer in the same year.[1] An estimated 12,400 children and young people under the age of 20 will be diagnosed with cancer in the year 2000. In adults, about 1,220,100 new cancer cases are expected to be diagnosed in 2000.[2] Projections reveal that 1 in every 900 persons between the ages of 16 and 44 years will be a survivor of childhood cancer by the year 2000.[3]

Most childhood cancers originate from the **mesodermal germ layer** that gives rise to connective tissue, bone, cartilage, muscle, blood, blood vessels, gonads, kidney, and the lymphatic system. Thus the more common childhood cancers are leukemias, sarcomas, and embryonic tumors. Embryonic tumors originate during intrauterine life. These tumors contain abnormal cells that appear to be immature embryonic tissue unable to mature or differentiate into fully developed functional cells. Embryonic tumors are diagnosed early in life (usually by 5 years of age) and therefore are very rare in adults. **Embryonic tumors** often are named with the term *blast,* which refers to the immature nature of the cells.

Sarcomas and lymphoreticular cancers seen in childhood occur also in adults, but most adult cancers involve epithelial tissue (and are therefore carcinomas). Carcinomas almost never occur in children because these cancers most commonly result from environmental carcinogens and require a long period from exposure to the appearance of the carcinoma. However, epithelial tumors begin to increase between 15 and 19 years of age and become the most common cancer tissue type after adolescence.

By far the most common malignancy in children is leukemia, which accounts for more than one third of childhood cancers (Table 12-2). The second most common group of cancers is tumors of the nervous system, primarily brain tumors. All other pediatric malignancies occur much less frequently. Neuroblastoma and Wilms tumor are both embryonic tumors. Neuroblastoma is a tumor of the sympathetic nervous system. Wilms tumor is a malignancy of the kidney (named after Max Wilms, who identified the tumor); the histologic name is *nephroblastoma.* Rhabdomyosarcoma is a soft tissue sarcoma of striated muscle. Two major bone tumors also occur in children. These are osteosarcoma and Ewing sarcoma (named after James Ewing, who identified this tumor type).

Childhood cancers most often are diagnosed during peak times of physical growth and maturation. In general, they are extremely fast-growing cancers, with 80% having distant spread (metastases) at diagnosis. Many childhood cancers have a peak incidence before the child is 5 years of age. Among these are the leukemias and the embryonic tumors: neuroblastomas, Wilms tumor, and retinoblastoma. Central nervous system tumors are more common from 5 to 10 years of age, and bone tumors, soft tissue sarcomas, and lymphomas are more likely to occur from 10 to 15 years of age.

Overall, cancer is 10% to 25% more common in white than in black children. This is primarily because of the lower incidence of acute lymphocytic leukemia, lymphomas, and Ewing sarcoma in black children. Blacks, however, have a higher incidence of Wilms tumor and osteosarcoma.[2] Some geographic differences also are found. Frequency of cancers by race is illustrated in Table 12-3. In the United States, childhood cancer also is slightly more common in boys than in girls. A newborn male has a 1 in 300 chance of developing cancer by age 20. A newborn female has a 1 in 333 chance of developing cancer by age 20.[4] Some geographic differences are also found. These include increases in Burkitts lymphoma in Africa, osteosarcoma in Spain, retinoblastoma in India, and Hodgkins disease in the United States and Latin America.[3]

ETIOLOGY

Even more so than in adult cancer, the causes of cancer in childhood are largely unknown. Some environmental and host factors are known to predispose a child to cancer, but

Table 12-1 Comparison of Usual Childhood and Adult Cancers

Factor	Childhood Cancers	Adult Cancers
Incidence	Rare, <2% of all cancers	Common, >98% of all cancers
Sites	Involves tissue (e.g., mononuclear phagocyte system, central nervous system [CNS], muscle, bone)	Involves organs (e.g., lung, breast, colon, prostate)
Histology	Most common type—nonepithelial and mesenchymal: sarcomas, embryonic tumors, leukemia, lymphoma	Most common type—epithelial: carcinomas
Latency (from initiation to diagnosis)	Relatively short period	Long period; can be well over 20 yr
Influence of environmental factors in causation	Some environmental factors known, few life-style factors; overall not strong influence shown; more likely an interaction of genetic alterations and environmental factors, called *ecogenetics*	Strong relationship to environmental exposures and life-style factors
Prevention	Minimal strategies known to date	80% estimated to be preventable
Early detection	Generally accidental; small percentage known to be genetically at high risk can be monitored more closely	Possible with adherence to early detection and screening recommendation
State at diagnosis	80% have metastasized	Local or regional
Response to treatment	Very responsive to chemotherapy; tolerate higher doses	Less responsive to chemotherapy
Treatment side effects	Less difficulty with acute toxicity but more significant long-term consequences	More difficulty with acute toxicity but fewer long-term consequences
Prognosis	>65% cure	<60% cure

Data from Fernbach DJ, Vietti T. In Fernbach DJ, Vietti T, editors: *Clinical pediatric oncology,* ed 4, St Louis, 1991, Mosby; Marina NM et al: Pediatric solid tumors. In Murphy GP, Lawrence W, Lenhard RE: *American Cancer Society textbook of clinical oncology,* ed 2, 1995, Atlanta, American Cancer Society; Pizzo PA, Poplack DG, editors: *Principles and practices of pediatric oncology,* ed 3, Philadelphia, 1997, Lippincott-Raven.

Table 12-2 Childhood Cancers by Age SEER 1975–1995

	Percentage of Each Cancer by Age Group		
Site	**<5 yr**	**5-9 yr**	**10-14 yr**
Leukemia	36.1	33.4	21.8
Lymphomas and reticuloendothelial neoplasms	13.9	12.9	20.6
CNS-intracranial and intraspinal neoplasms	16.6	27.7*	19.6
Sympathetic nervous system–neuroblastoma and ganglionneuroblastoma	14.3*	2.7	1.2
Retinoblastoma	6.3*	0.5	0.1
Renal tumors	9.7*	5.4	1.1
Hepatic tumors	2.2*	0.4	0.6
Bone tumors	0.6	4.6	11.3*
Soft tissue sarcomas	5.6	7.5	9.1*
Germ cell tumors	3.3	2.0	5.3*
Carcinomas	0.9	2.5	8.9
Other unspecified	0.5	0.3	0.6
Total	**100**	**100**	**100**

*Peak incidence for disease.

Modified from Ries LA, Percy CL, Bunin GR. In Ries LAG et al, editors: *Cancer Incidence and Survival among children and adolescents: United States SEER Program 1975–1995,* 1999, Bethesda, MD, National Cancer Institute, SEER Program. NIH Pub. No. 99-4649.

causal factors have not been established for most childhood cancers. A number of host factors, many of which are genetic risk factors or congenital conditions, have been implicated in the development of childhood cancer (Table 12-4). The cause of childhood cancer most likely is attributable to the complex interaction of both genetic and environmental factors, now an important area of study called **ecogenetics.**

Most childhood cancers, however, do not lend themselves to early cancer warning signs. Certainly the American Cancer Society's seven warning signs of cancer do not apply because they describe adult, environmentally caused cancers. Although host factors are important in identifying populations of children at risk for cancer, most children who are diagnosed with cancer do not demonstrate any predisposing environmental or host factors.

Table 12-3 Cancers by Race: Incidence per Million Children Younger Than 14 Years of Age, SEER 1974–1991

Cancer Type	White	Black
Leukemia	42.6	26.5
Central nervous system	29.9	25.2
Neuroblastoma	9.7	7.4
Non-Hodgkin lymphoma	9.1	5.4
Hodgkin	7.2	5.0
Wilms tumor	8.1	8.8
Rhabdomyosarcoma	4.7	4.4
Germ cell	3.9	4.2
Retinoblastoma	3.7	4.3
Osteosarcoma	3.3	4.0
Ewing sarcoma	3.2	0.4

Data from Gurney JG et al: Trends in cancer incidence among children in the United States, *Cancer* 78(3):532, 1996.

Genetic Factors

Both oncogenes and tumor-suppressor genes have been associated with the causation of childhood cancers (Table 12-5). Oncogenes are activated through mutation of a proto-oncogene that normally maintains cellular growth and control. Once activated to an oncogene, uncontrolled cell growth—the primary characteristic of cancer cells—results. Oncogenes have been identified in pediatric leukemia, lymphomas, and some solid tumors. Tumor-suppressor genes arise from genes that normally suppress cancer formation but have lost their suppressor function, thus leading to uncontrolled growth. Tumor-suppressor genes have been identified with retinoblastoma and Wilms

Table 12-4 Congenital Factors Associated with Childhood Cancer

Syndrome	Associated Childhood Cancer
CHROMOSOME ALTERATIONS	
Down syndrome	Acute leukemia
13q syndrome	Retinoblastoma
CHROMOSOME INSTABILITY	
Ataxia-telangiectasia	Lymphoma
Bloom syndrome	Acute leukemia, lymphoma, Wilms tumor
Fanconi anemia	Nonlymphocytic leukemia, myelodysplastic syndrome, liver tumor
HEREDITARY SYNDROMES	
Beckwith-Wiedemann syndrome	Wilms tumor, sarcoma, brain tumor, neuroblastoma, hepatoblastoma
Neurofibromatosis	Brain tumor, sarcoma, neuroblastoma, Wilms tumor, nonlymphocytic leukemia
Tuberous sclerosis	Brain tumor
IMMUNE DEFICIENCY DISORDERS	
Congenital	
Agammaglobulinemia	Lymphoma, leukemia, brain tumor
Immunoglobulin A (IgA) deficiency	Lymphoma, leukemia, brain tumor
Wiskott-Aldrich syndrome	Leukemia, lymphoma
Acquired	
Aplastic anemia	Leukemia
Organ transplantation	Leukemia, lymphoma
CONGENITAL MALFORMATION SYNDROMES	
Aniridia, hemihypertrophy, hamartoma, genitourinary anomalies	Wilms tumor
Cryptorchidism	Testicular tumor
Gonadal dysgenesis	Gonadoblastoma
FAMILY SUSCEPTIBILITY	
Twin or sibling with leukemia	Leukemia

Table 12-5 Selected Oncogenes and Tumor-Suppressor Genes Associated With Childhood Cancer

Gene	Associated Pediatric Tumor
ONCOGENES[a]	
abl	Acute lymphoblastoma leukemia
N-*myc*	Neuroblastoma
c-*myb*	Neural tumors, leukemia, lymphomas, rhabdomyosarcoma, Wilms tumor, neuroblastoma
erb B	Glioblastoma
N-*ras*	Neuroblastoma, leukemia
H/K-*ras*	Neuroblastoma, rhabdomyosarcoma, leukemia
TUMOR-SUPPRESSOR GENES[b]	
Rb1	Retinoblastoma, sarcoma
WT1, WT2	Wilms tumor
WT3	Wilms tumor
NF-1	Sarcoma, primitive neuroectodermal tumor, juvenile chronic myelocytic leukemia
NF-2	Brain tumors, melanoma
p16	Brain tumors, leukemia
p53	Sarcoma, leukemia, brain tumors

[a] From Rubnitz JE, Crist WM: Molecular genetics of childhood cancer: implications for pathogenesis, diagnosis, and treatment, *Pediatrics* (100)1:101, 1997.
[b] From Vats TS, Emani A: *Indian J Pediatr* 60:192, 1993.

tumor and are also thought to be associated with rhabdomyosarcoma and neuroblastomas.[5,6,7]

Other genetic factors involve chromosome aberrations or single-gene defects. These chromosome abnormalities include aneuploidy, amplifications, deletions, translocations, and fragility. For example, neuroblastoma is associated with deletion of the short arm of chromosome 1, whereas acute lymphoblastic leukemia commonly demonstrates a fusion of TEL-AML genes and hyperdiploidy.[8]

Some congenital malformations herald the onset of pediatric malignancies. For example, certain syndromes involve easily diagnosed abnormalities, and the children can then be carefully followed and screened for tumor development. One of the more recognized syndromes is the association of trisomy 21 (Down syndrome) with an increased susceptibility to acute leukemia. For children with Down syndrome the risk of developing leukemia is 10 to 18 times greater than in unaffected children. The risk is greatest for children under 5 years of age.[5]

Wilms tumor is particularly recognized for its association with a number of malformations, including genitourinary anomalies—for example, horseshoe kidney, cryptorchidism (undescended testes), and collecting system malformation; aniridia (congenital absence of the iris of the eye); and hemihypertrophy (muscular overgrowth of one half of the body or face). Children diagnosed with Wilms tumor frequently demonstrate one of these congenital abnormalities.[10] Retinoblastoma, a malignant embryonic tumor of the eye, occurs as an inherited defect or as an acquired mutation (see Chapter 18).

Numerous single-gene defects have been associated with the subsequent development of both childhood and adult cancers.[7] For instance, two autosomal recessive diseases involving increased chromosome fragility—Fanconi anemia and Bloom syndrome—are risk factors that evidently predispose the child to acute nonlymphocytic leukemia.[11]

The relative ineffectiveness of the immune surveillance system during intrauterine life may explain the occurrence of embryonic tumors (the immune surveillance system is discussed in Chapter 10). Because this period requires rapid proliferation and differentiation of cells in the developing fetus, cell mutation theoretically could result in embryonic tumors.

Although not determined to be genetically transmitted, a few malignancies seem to demonstrate a familial tendency, suggested by the clustering of specific cancers in a particular family. A child who has a sibling with leukemia has a risk for the development of leukemia that is two to four times greater than for children with healthy siblings.[12] The occurrence of leukemia in monozygous twins is estimated as high as 25%, with an associated degree of risk relative to age.[12] The highest degree of concordance is noted in infant leukemia. Diagnosis after 7 years of age predisposes the unaffected twin to a risk similar to that of the general population.

In families with Li-Fraumeni syndrome (a genetic defect involving the *p53* tumor-suppressor gene), the risk of developing tumors is significantly higher when compared to the unaffected population.[13]

Environmental Factors

Although many adult cancers are associated with environmental agents, few childhood tumors share a strong association. Because of the lengthy latency period required between exposure and development of cancer, early exposure to carcinogens does not result in a tumor until the child is an adult.

Prenatal Exposure

Prenatal exposure to some drugs and to ionizing radiation has been linked to subsequent cancers. Perhaps the most well-known such drug is diethylstilbestrol (DES), a drug taken to avert early abortion. In 1971, DES was identified as a transplacental chemical carcinogen. Adenocarcinomas of the vagina have developed in a small percentage of the daughters of mothers who took DES while pregnant. Other potential transplacental carcinogens have been identified but await further study before any conclusion can be drawn.[14]

Several associations have been found linking parental factors (both nonoccupational and occupational) to the risk of childhood cancer. Exposure to hazardous materials, such

WHAT'S NEW? Parental Smoking Contributes to Childhood Cancer

Parental cigarette smoking accounts for 14% to 15% of all childhood cancers. The exact carcinogenic effect of passive smoke on children is not yet understood. Studies have indicated that maternal smoking is primarily associated with an increased risk of childhood leukemias. The development of leukemia is suspected to occur secondary to transplacental effects on the developing fetus. Paternal cigarette smoking has not been studied as frequently but research has demonstrated a statistically significant correlation with childhood cancers, including leukemia, lymphoma, and CNS tumors. It is hypothesized that cancer results from mutations in the spermatogonia in fathers who smoke. Additional information is needed to determine if the increased incidence is associated with paternal smoking habits or other associated socioeconomic factors, such as maternal education, monthly income, and prenatal care. As the search for the etiology of pediatric cancer continues, paternal smoking warrants further research to determine if these preliminary findings are significant.

Data from Sorahan T et al: Childhood cancer and parental use of tobacco: deaths from 1953-1955, *Br J Cancer* 75:134-8, 1997; Boffetta P, Tredaniel J, Greco A: Risk of childhood cancer and adult lung cancer after childhood exposure to passive smoke: a meta-analysis, *Environ Health Perspect* 108(1):73, 2000; Ji PT et al: Paternal cigarette smoking and the risk of childhood cancer among offspring of nonsmoking mothers, *J NCI* 89:238, 1997; Schuz J et al: Association of childhood cancer with factors related to pregnancy and birth, *Internat J Epidemiol* 28(4):613, 1999.

as petroleum products, solvents, chemicals, and radiation, could lead to genetic changes of the egg or sperm or to transplacental transfer of the carcinogen.[15] Additionally, increased parental age at the time of conception has been linked to a higher incidence of cancer in children.[14,16]

Intrauterine exposure to radiation during pregnancy may be associated with an increased risk for all types of childhood cancer. However, studies of children exposed to atomic fallout in uteri show no increase in childhood cancer.[17,18] Thus it is suggested that women requiring prenatal radiologic studies may have other cancer risks, predisposing the fetus to development of cancer.[15,17,19]

Childhood Exposure

Childhood exposure to drugs, ionizing radiation, or viruses has been implicated as a risk factor that increases susceptibility to specific cancers. In addition to those drug and environmental agents that are known to cause cancer in adults and therefore also are risks for exposure during childhood, a few drugs may particularly increase cancer risk during childhood. These drugs include (1) anabolic androgenic steroids, which are used in the treatment of aplastic anemia or used illegally by teenage athletes for body development and have been associated with subsequent hepatocellular carcinoma; (2) cytotoxic agents used in the treatment of pediatric cancers, which may predispose the child to leukemia in later years; and (3) immunosuppressive agents, particularly those used for transplant surgeries, which have been shown to increase the risk of lymphoma.

Current areas of study focus on the role of childhood environmental exposures to radon gas in the home and electromagnetic fields from residential power lines and the operation of small household appliances. Thus far, results suggest a possible strong association, but further study is needed to determine the significance of any associations.[20,21,22,23]

Although viruses have been implicated in childhood cancers, research has not yet proved a strong association. Viruses have been shown to affect cancer development in some animal models, but causal evidence is only suggestive in humans. (The viral theory of carcinogenesis is discussed in Chapter 10.) In children, the strongest carcinogenic relationship has been shown between the Epstein-Barr virus (EBV) and Burkitt lymphoma. Most African children with Burkitt lymphoma have high titers of antibodies against EBV. Up to 50% of American children with Burkitt lymphoma, however, do not have elevated EBV titers.[24] Therefore, although EBV can induce lymphocyte transformation in laboratory studies, evidence has not yet shown whether the relationship is causal. Investigators are examining the role of viruses in the development of neuroblastomas, Wilms tumor, and osteosarcoma.

PROGNOSIS

Today, childhood cancer is not inevitably fatal. Significant progress has been made in the past 10 years so that approximately 65% of children diagnosed with cancer can now be cured.[3] Overall, children have a more favorable prognosis than do adults.[2] Children appear to be both more responsive to available treatments and better able to tolerate the immediate side effects of therapies. Children with cancer are more likely than adults to be enrolled and treated through clinical trials. Treatment effectiveness is more easily determined, and advances from clinical trials contribute to a higher survival rate in children.[25]

Because childhood cancer should be viewed as a chronic disease instead of a fatal illness, the focus of treatment is on the quality of life. Even those cancers that cannot be cured generally can be treated, resulting in a significant period of quality time. With increasing survival periods, the long-term effects of treatment are under careful investigation. More effective yet less toxic chemotherapy and radiation treatments must be found. Cured children still face residual and late effects of treatment. These late effects are more significant in children than in adults because childhood treatment occurs in a physically immature, growing individual. Potential effects that need further attention include physical impairments, reproductive dysfunction, soft tissue and bone atrophy, learning disabilities, secondary cancers, and psychologic sequelae. More must be learned about the genetic factors associated with childhood malignancies and about the genetic consequences of treatment. Genetic counseling is appropriate for children cured of cancers known to be transmitted genetically (e.g., retinoblastoma).

SUMMARY REVIEW

Incidence and Types

1. Although childhood cancer is rare, it is still the third leading cause of death in children.
2. The unique feature of childhood cancers is the short period of latency, which contrasts sharply with the long latency period common in adults.
3. Common childhood cancers include leukemias, CNS tumors, sarcomas, and embryonic tumors that contain immature fetal tissue that has not differentiated into fully developed cells.
4. Embryonic tumors almost always are diagnosed early and are very rare in adults.

Etiology

1. Because most carcinomas are caused by environmental exposure, these cancers are extremely rare in children, who have not lived long enough to be affected.
2. Host factors are especially important in identifying a child at risk for cancer because environmental risk factors have had less effect on the child's short lifetime.
3. Genetic factors that place a child at risk for cancer include some congenital malformations that are chromosome aberrations or single-gene defects.
4. A familial tendency is evident for a few childhood cancers, including leukemia.
5. Environmental risk factors associated with childhood cancer include prenatal exposure to some drugs and ionizing radiation and postnatal exposure to certain drugs (particularly anabolic steroids and some cytotoxic and immunosuppressive agents), to radiation, and possibly to certain viruses.

Prognosis

1. More than 65% of children diagnosed with cancer are cured.
2. Improved survival for children with cancer has led to investigations for less toxic treatments that minimize residual effects and for more research into the genetic factors associated with cancer in childhood.

KEY TERMS

Ecogenetics, *359* — Embryonic tumor, *357* — Mesodermal germ layer, *357*

REFERENCES

1. Landis SH et al: Cancer statistics, *CA: Cancer J Clinicians* 48(1):6, 1998.
2. American Cancer Society: *Cancer facts & figures 2000,* New York, 2000, The Society.
3. Robinson LL: General principles of the epidemiology of cancer. In Pizzo PA, Poplack DG, editors: *Principles and practices of pediatric oncology*, ed 3, Philadelphia, 1997, Lippincott-Raven.
4. Ries LAG et al, editors: *Cancer incidence and survival among children and adolescents: United States SEER Program 1975–1995*, Bethesda, 1999, National Cancer Institute SEER Program, NIH Pub. No. 99-4649.
5. Marina NM et al: Pediatric solid tumors. In Murphy GP, Lawrence W, Lenhard RE, editors: *American Cancer Society textbook of clinical oncology*, ed 2, Atlanta, 1995, American Cancer Society.
6. Rubnitz JE, Christ WM: Molecular genetics of childhood cancer: Implications for pathogenesis, diagnosis, and treatment, *Peds* 100(1):1, 101, 1997.
7. Ruccione K: Cancer and genetics: What we need to know now, *J Ped Oncol Nurs* 16(3):156, 1999.
8. Wiemels JL et al: Prenatal origin of acute lymphoblastic leukaemia in children, *Lancet* 354(9189):1499, 1999.
9. Hasle H, Clemmensen IH, Mikkelsen M: Risks of leukaemia and solid tumors in individuals with Down's syndrome, *Lancet* 355(9199):165, 2000.
10. Green DM et al, editors: *Principles and practices of pediatric oncology,* ed 3, pp. 733, Philadelphia, 1997, Lippincott-Raven.
11. Clericuzio CL: Recognition and management of childhood cancer syndromes: a systems approach, *Am J Med Genetics* 89(2):81, 1999.
12. Margolin JF, Poplack DG: Acute lymphoblastic leukemia. In Pizzo PA, Poplack DG, editors: *Principles and practices of pediatric oncology*, ed 3, pp. 409, Philadelphia, 1997, Lippincott-Raven.
13. Hisada M et al: Multiple primary cancers in families with Li-Fraumeni syndrome, *J NCI* 90:606, 1998.
14. Schuz J et al: Association of childhood cancer with factors related to pregnancy and birth, *Internat J Epidemiol* 28(4):631, 1999.
15. Smulevich VB, Solionova LG, Belyakova SV: Prenatal occupation and other factors and cancer risk in children: II. Occupational factors, *Internat J Cancer* 83(6):718, 1999.
16. Smulevich VB, Solionova LG, Belyakova SV: Prenatal occupation and other factors and cancer risk in children: I. Study methodology and non-occupational factors, *Internat J Cancer* 83(6):712, 1999.
17. Boice JD, Miller RW: Childhood cancer and adult cancer after intrauterine exposure to ionizing radiation, *Teratology* 59(4):227, 1999.
18. Steiner M et al: Trends in infant leukemia in West Germany in relation to in utero exposure due to Chernobyl accident, *Radiation Environmental Biophysics* 37(2):87, 1998.
19. Meinert R et al: Associations between childhood cancer and ionizing radiation: results of a population-based case-control study in Germany, *Cancer Epidemiol Biomarkers & Preven* 8(9):793, 1999.
20. Feychting M, Floderus B, Ahlbom A: Parental occupational exposure to magnetic fields and childhood cancer (Sweden), *Cancer Causes & Control* 11(2):151, 2000.
21. Kaletsch U et al: Childhood cancer and residential radon exposure—results of a population-based case-control study in Lower Saxony (Germany), *Radiation Environmental Biophysics* 38(3):211, 1999.
22. Sorahan T et al: Maternal occupational exposure to electromagnetic fields before, during, and after pregnancy in relation to risks of childhood cancers: findings from the Oxford survey of childhood cancer, *Amer J Industrial Med* 35(4):348, 1999.
23. UK Childhood Cancer Study Investigators: Exposure to poser-frequency magnetic fields and the risk of childhood cancer, *Lancet* 354(9194): 1925, 1999.
24. Shat A, Magrath I: Malignant non-Hodgkin's lymphomas in children. In Pizzo PA, Poplack DG, editors: *Principles and practices of pediatric oncology*, ed 3, pp. 545, Philadelphia, 1997, Lippincott-Raven.
25. Ungerlieder RS, Ellenberg SS: Clinical trials: design, conduct, analysis, and reporting. In Pizzo PA, Poplack DG, editors: *Principles and practices of pediatric oncology*, ed 3, pp. 385, Philadelphia, 1997, Lippincott-Raven.

CHAPTER 13

Structure and Function of the Neurologic System

RICHARD A. SUGERMAN

CHAPTER OUTLINE

The human nervous system is a remarkable structure responsible for the body's ability to reciprocally interact with the environment and for the regulation of activities involving internal organs. The nervous system literally drives the other systems of the body. It is a network composed of complex structures that transmit electrical and chemical signals between the body's many organs and tissues and the brain.

OVERVIEW AND ORGANIZATION OF THE NERVOUS SYSTEM

Although the nervous system functions as a unified whole, structures and functions have been divided to facilitate understanding. Structurally, the nervous system is divided into the central nervous system and the peripheral nervous system. The **central nervous system (CNS)** consists of the brain and spinal cord, enclosed within the protective cranial vault and vertebrae, respectively. The **peripheral nervous system (PNS)** is composed of the **cranial nerves,** which project from the brain and pass through foramina (openings) in the skull, and the **spinal nerves,** which project from the spinal cord and pass through intervertebral foramina of the vertebrae. Peripheral nerve pathways are differentiated into **afferent pathways (ascending pathways)** that carry sensory impulses toward the CNS and **efferent pathways (descending pathways)** that innervate **effector organs,** such as skeletal, cardiac, and smooth muscle, as well as glands, by transmitting motor impulses away from the CNS. Organs innervated by specific components of the nervous system are called *effector organs.* Cranial nerves are viewed most correctly as modified spinal nerves. Some cranial nerves function similar to spinal nerves, whereas others have specialized sensory tasks, such as smell, taste, sight, and hearing.

Clinically, the PNS can be divided into the somatic nervous system and the autonomic nervous system. The **somatic nervous system** consists of motor and sensory pathways regulating voluntary motor control of skeletal muscle. The **autonomic nervous system (ANS)** also consists of motor and sensory components and is involved with regulation of the body's internal environment (viscera) through involuntary control of organ systems. The ANS is further divided into sympathetic and parasympathetic divisions. Today we understand that some aspects of the ANS can be controlled through mental practice with or without biofeedback techniques.

CELLS OF THE NERVOUS SYSTEM

The two basic types of cells that make up nervous tissue are neurons and supporting cells. The **neuron** is the primary cell of the nervous system. Working in parallel systems, neurons can scan the environment, integrate many systems at higher cognitive levels, and initiate body responses to maintain homeostasis. The supporting cells, such as the **neuroglial cells** of the CNS and the **Schwann cells** of the PNS, provide structural support and nutrition for neurons, increase the speed of nerve impulses, and play a significant role with neurons in processing and storage of information (memory).[1]

Neuron

Neuronal structure varies considerably throughout the CNS. Neurons vary in size from micrometers to several meters and have from one cell process to many cell processes. Even the shapes and complexity of the processes can vary considerably. **Neurons** are specialized cells that share many of the same metabolic activities and constituents as other types of cells. The fuel source for the neuron is predominantly glucose; insulin, however, is not required for cellular glucose uptake in the CNS. Neurons contain many cellular constituents, namely, microtubules, neurofibrils, microfilaments, and Nissl substances. **Microfilaments** and **neurofibrils** are composed of structural proteins and are responsible for structural support within the cell and movement of neuron processes, as seen in amoebas and white blood cells. **Microtubules** also are made of protein and are believed to be involved in the transport of cellular products. **Nissl substances** consist of endoplasmic reticulum and ribosomes and are involved in protein synthesis. The CNS starts out with more neurons than it needs, and those neurons that do not become involved in functional systems die. Some neurons continue to divide for months after birth. Olfactory neurons in the nose continue to divide throughout life.

A neuron (Fig. 13-1) has three components: a cell body (soma) and the thin processes of the cell—the dendrites and axons. Most cell bodies are located within the CNS. Dense, packed cell bodies in the CNS are called **nuclei.** Cell bodies in the PNS are usually found in groups called **ganglia** or **plexuses.** The **dendrites** are extensions that carry nerve impulses toward the cell body. The **dendritic zone** is the receptive portion of a neuron that receives a stimulus and continues further conduction. **Axons** are long, conductive projections from the cell body that carry nerve impulses away from the cell body. The **axon hillock** is the cone-shaped, Nissl-free area where the axon leaves the cell body. The initial segment of the axon has the lowest threshold for stimulation, and, as a result, action potentials begin here.

A typical neuron has only one axon, which may be covered with a segmented layer of lipid material called **myelin,** which acts as an insulating substance. This entire membrane

A

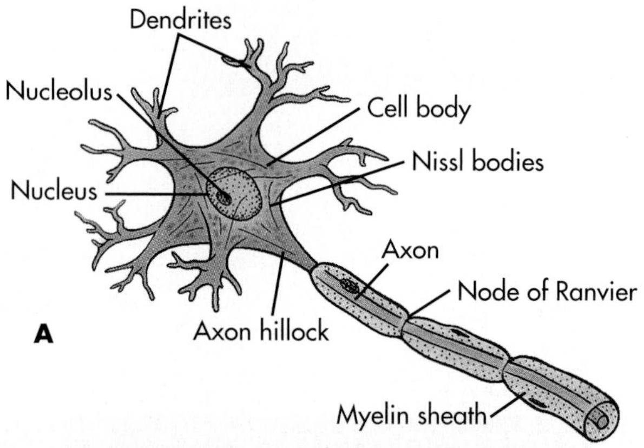

B

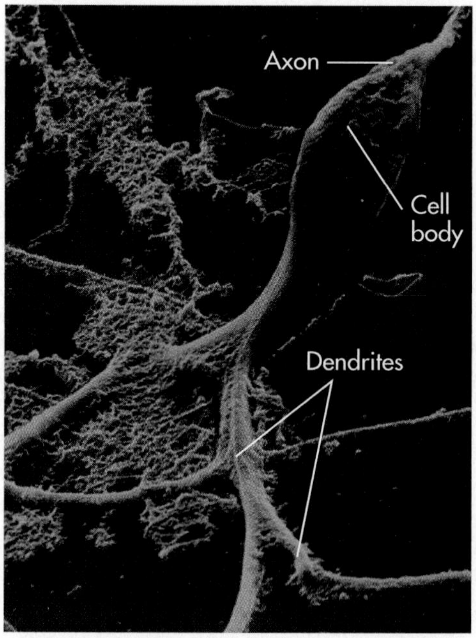

FIG. 13-1 Neuron with composite parts. A, Multipolar neuron: neuron with multiple extensions from the cell body. **B,** Scanning electron micrograph. (**B,** From Thibodeau GA, Patton KI: *Anatomy and physiology,* ed 4, St Louis, 1999, Mosby.)

is referred to as the **myelin sheath;** the thin membrane between the myelin sheath and the **endoneurium,** a delicate connective tissue around each axon in the PNS (see Fig. 13-22, *B*), is the **neurilemma (Schwann sheath).** The neurilemma and the myelin sheath are interrupted at regular intervals by the **nodes of Ranvier.** The **Schwann cell** forms and maintains the myelin sheath, and the nodes of Ranvier form the spaces on either side of the Schwann cell. If the myelin layer is tightly wrapped many times around the axon forming nodes of Ranvier, it increases conduction velocity and the neuron is called *myelinated* (see Fig. 13-1).

Myelin acts as an insulator that allows ions to flow between segments rather than along the entire length of the membrane, resulting in increased velocity. This mechanism is referred to as **saltatory conduction.** If the Schwann cells are loosely wrapped around the axon, it is referred to as *unmyelinated* and conduction velocity is not increased. Axons

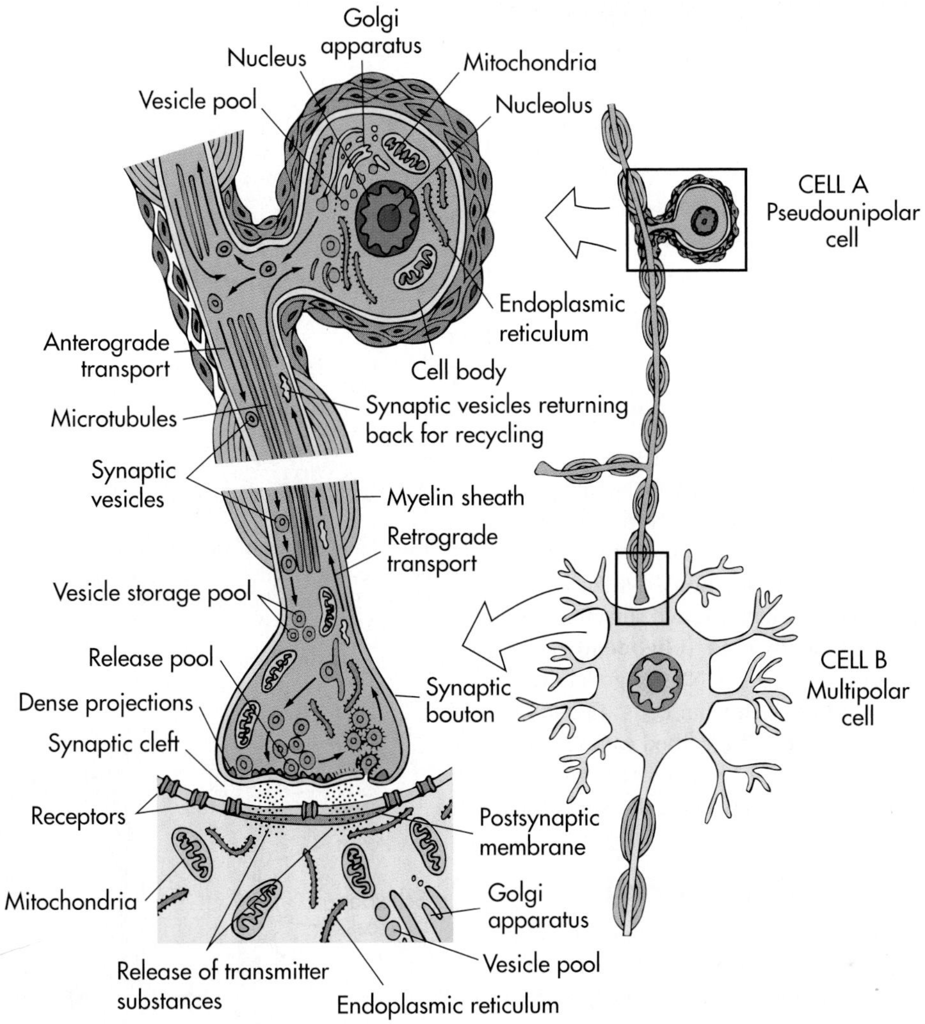

FIG. 13-2 Neuronal transmission and synaptic cleft. Electrical impulse travels along axon of first neuron to synapse. Chemical transmitter is secreted into synaptic space to depolarize membrane (dendrite or cell body) of next neuron in pathway. Cell A represents pseudounipolar cell; cell B represents multipolar cell.

are capable of extensive branching, which occurs at the nodes of Ranvier. Two major principles of information processing in the nervous system are **divergence** and **convergence.** *Divergence* refers to the ability of these branching axons to influence many different neurons. *Convergence* is the term applied to branches of numerous neurons converging on and influencing one or a few neurons. Disorders of the myelin sheath (demyelinating diseases), such as multiple sclerosis and Guillain-Barré syndrome, demonstrate the important role myelin plays in nerve function (see Chapter 15). Besides depending on the myelin coating, conduction velocities also depend on the diameter of the axon. Larger axons transmit impulses at a faster rate.

Neurons are structurally classified on the basis of the number of processes (projections) extending from the cell body. There are four basic types of cell configuration: (1) unipolar, (2) pseudounipolar, (3) bipolar, and (4) multipolar. **Unipolar neurons** have one process that branches shortly after leaving the cell body. One example is found in the retina. **Pseudounipolar neurons** (some authors call them *unipolar*) have one process with its dendritic portion extending away from the CNS and its axon portion projecting into the CNS (Fig. 13-2). The configuration is typical of sensory neurons in both cranial and spinal nerves. **Bipolar neurons** have two distinct processes arising from the cell body. This type of neuron connects to rod and cone cells of the retina. **Multipolar neurons** are the most common and have multiple processes capable of extensive branching. A motor neuron is typically multipolar (see Fig. 13-2).

Functionally, there are three types of neurons (with their direction of transmission and typical configuration noted in parentheses): (1) sensory (afferent, mostly pseudounipolar), (2) associational (interneurons, multipolar), and (3) motor (efferent, multipolar). **Sensory neurons** carry impulses from peripheral sensory receptors to the CNS (Box 13-1). **Associational neurons (interneurons)** transmit impulses from neuron to neuron, that is, from sensory to motor neurons. **Motor neurons** transmit impulses away from the CNS to an effector organ. In skeletal muscle the end processes form a complex neuromuscular (myoneural) junction.

Box 13-1

MAJOR TYPES OF SENSORY RECEPTORS

Nicoceptors (pain)
Mechanoreceptors (touch, pressure, and mechanical deformation or encapsulated endings)
Photochemical (light on the retina)
Chemoreceptors (flavors, odors, oxygen levels, osmolarity of body fluids, and carbon dioxide levels in the blood)
Thermoreceptors (heat and cold)
Proprioception (location of body parts)
Audition and balance (sound and positional movement)

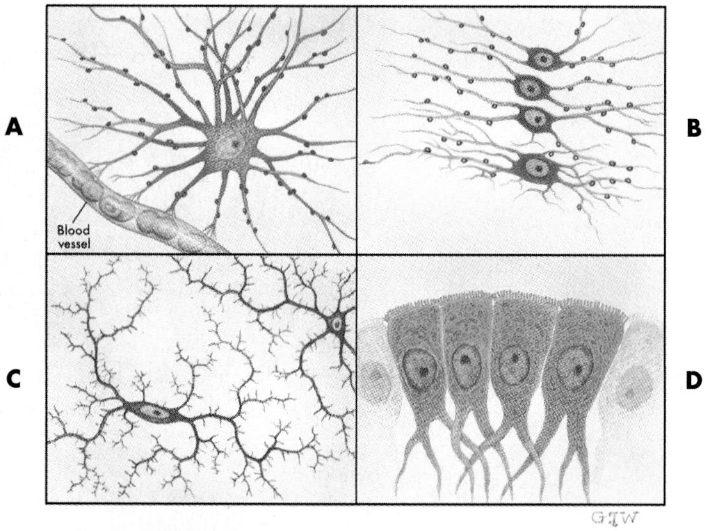

FIG. 13-3 Types of neuroglia cells. A, Fibrous astrocyte; **B,** oligodendrocytes; **C,** microglia cells; **D,** ependymal cells. (Modified from Chipps E, Clanin N, Campbell V: *Neurologic disorders,* St Louis, 1992, Mosby.)

Neuroglia and Schwann Cells

Neuroglia ("nerve glue") are the general classification of cells that support the neurons of the CNS. They make up approximately half of the total brain and spinal cord volume and are five to ten times more numerous than neurons. Different types of neuroglia serve different functions. **Astrocytes,** for example, fill the spaces between neurons and surround blood vessels in the CNS; **oligodendroglia (oligodendrocytes)** function to deposit myelin within the CNS. Oligodendroglia are the CNS counterpart of the Schwann cells. Ependymal cells line the cerebrospinal fluid (CSF)–filled cavities of the CNS. **Microglia** remove debris (phagocytosis) in the CNS. Characteristics of neuroglia and Schwann cells are summarized in Fig. 13-3 and Table 13-1.

Nerve Injury and Regeneration

When an axon is severed, a typical sequence of events, known as *wallerian degeneration,* occurs in the distal axon: (1) a characteristic swelling appears within the portion of the axon distal to the cut, (2) the neurofilaments hypertrophy, (3) the myelin sheath shrinks and disintegrates, and (4) the axon degenerates and disappears. The myelin sheaths re-form into Schwann cells that line up in a column between the cut and the effector organ.

At the proximal end of the injured axon similar changes occur, but only back to the next node of Ranvier. The cell body responds to trauma by swelling and the Nissl substance dispersing (chromatolysis). During the repair process the cell increases in metabolic activity, protein synthesis, and mitochondrial activity. Approximately 7 to 14 days after the injury, new terminal sprouts project from the proximal segment and may enter the remaining Schwann cell pathway. (Fig. 13-4 contains a more detailed representation of these events.) This process, however, is limited to myelinated fibers and generally occurs only in the PNS. The regeneration of axonal constituents in the CNS is limited by an increased incidence of scar formation and the different nature of myelin formation by the oligodendrocyte.

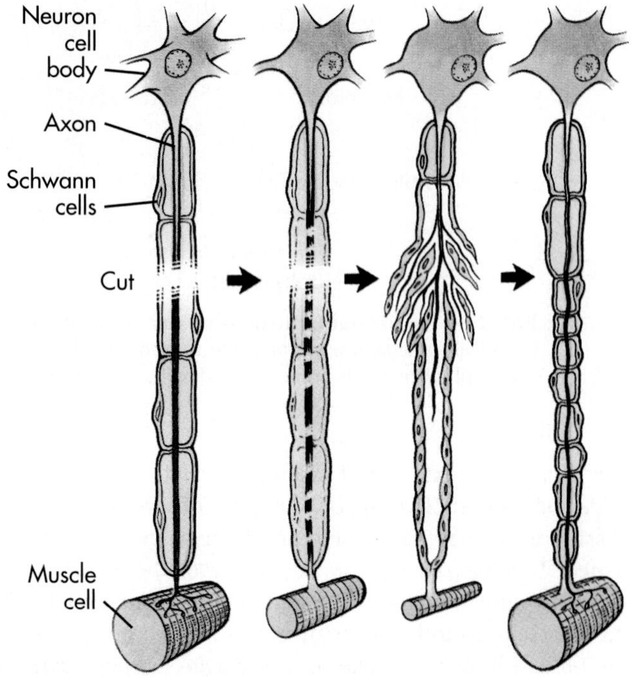

FIG. 13-4 Repair of a peripheral nerve fiber. When cut, a damaged motor axon can regrow to its distal connection only if the neurilemma remains intact (to form a guiding tunnel) and if scar tissue does not block its way.

Nerve regeneration depends on many factors, such as location of the injury, type of injury, the inflammatory responses, and the process of scarring. The closer to the cell body of the nerve, the greater the chances that the nerve cell will die and not regenerate. A crushing injury allows recovery more fully than does a cut injury. Crushed nerves sometimes recover fully, whereas cut nerves often form connective tissue scars that block or slow regenerating axonal branches.

NERVE IMPULSE

Neurons generate and conduct electrical and chemical impulses by selectively changing the electrical portion of their plasma membranes and influencing other nearby neurons by the release of chemicals (neurotransmitters). A neuron in its

Table 13-1 Support Cells of the Nervous System

Cell Type	Primary Functions
Astrocytes	Form specialized contacts between neuronal surfaces and blood vessels Provide rapid transport for nutrients and metabolites Believed to form an essential component of the blood-brain barrier Appear to be the scar-forming cells of CNS, which may be the foci for seizures Appear to work with neurons in processing information and memory storage
Oligodendroglia (oligodendrocytes)	Formation of myelin sheath and neurilemma in CNS
Schwann cells (neurolemmocytes)	Formation of myelin sheath and neurilemma in PNS
Microglia	Responsible for clearing cellular debris (phagocytic properties)
Ependymal cells	Serve as a lining for ventricles and choroid plexuses involved in production of cerebrospinal fluid

CNS, Central nervous system; *PNS,* peripheral nervous system.

unexcited state maintains a resting membrane potential (see Chapter 1). When the membrane potential is raised sufficiently, an action potential is generated (see Fig. 1-24), and the nerve impulse then flows to all parts of the neuron. The action potential response occurs only when the stimulus is strong enough; if it is too weak, the membrane remains unexcited. This property is sometimes termed the *all-or-none response.*

Synapses

Neurons are not physically continuous with one another. The region between adjacent neurons is called a **synapse** (see Fig. 13-2). Impulses are transmitted across the synapse by chemical and electrical conduction (see Figs. 13-2 and 13-13); only chemical conduction is discussed here. The neurons that conduct a nerve impulse are named according to whether they relay impulses *toward* the synapse **(presynaptic neurons)** or *away* from the synapse **(postsynaptic neurons).** Four basic types of connections occur in regions of contact between the presynaptic and postsynaptic neurons. These are between axons (axoaxonic), from axon to cell body (axosomatic), from axon to dendrite (axodendritic), and from dendrite to dendrite (dendrodendritic).

Impulses are transmitted across the synapse by chemical conduction. The conducting substance is called a **neurotransmitter,** and it is often formed in the **synaptic boutons** of the presynaptic neuron's axon and stored in synaptic vesicles within the boutons. Action potentials in the presynaptic neuron cause the synaptic vesicles to release their neurotransmitter or neurotransmitters through the plasma membrane into the **synaptic cleft** (the space between the neurons) and bind to receptor sites on the plasma membrane of the postsynaptic neuron (see Fig. 13-2). Neurons can synthesize more than one neurotransmitter, and postsynaptic membranes can contain more than one type of transmitter-specific receptor.

Neurotransmitters

More than 30 substances are thought to be neurotransmitters, including norepinephrine, acetylcholine, dopamine, histamine, γ-aminobutyric acid (GABA), and serotonin.[2] Many of these transmitters have more than one function. For example, norepinephrine in the brain probably helps regulate mood, functions in dream sleep, and maintains arousal. Several neurotransmitters are amino acids, including GABA, glutamic acid, and aspartic acid. Small chains of amino acids, such as enkephalins and endorphins, also function as neurotransmitters. They (neuropeptides) are involved in the perception and integration of pain, as well as in emotional experiences. Kandel and colleagues[3] define a neurotransmitter as a chemical that "must be synthesized in the neuron, become localized in the presynaptic terminal (synaptic bouton), be released into the synaptic cleft, bind to a receptor site (binding site) on the postsynaptic membrane of another neuron or effector where it affects ion channels and, last, be removed by a specific mechanism from its site of action." Neurotransmitter and neuromodulator substances are listed in Table 13-2.

Because the neurotransmitter is stored on one side of the synaptic cleft and the receptor sites are on the other side, chemical synapses operate in only one direction. Therefore action potentials are transmitted along a multineuronal pathway in only one direction. The binding of the neurotransmitter at the receptor site changes the permeability of the postsynaptic neuron and consequently its membrane potential. Two possible scenarios can then follow: (1) the postsynaptic neuron may be excited (depolarized; **excitatory postsynaptic potentials**

WHAT'S NEW? Brain Synthesis of Neurosteroids

Although the brain is a target site for peripheral steroids, the brain glial cells, cerebellar Purkinje, and other cells also synthesize steroids from cholesterol, such as progesterone, pregnenlone, and dehydroepiandrosterone. These steroids are called neurosteroids and have diverse functions, including modulation of neurotransmitters (e.g., $GABA_A$ and the glutamate and cholinergic systems). Beneficial effects have been shown for memory, learning, stress, depression, regulation of myelination, and neuroprotection and growth of axons and dendrites. Research is advancing potential pharmacologic use of neurosteroids to treat neuropathologies and support normal aging.

Data from Compagnone NA, Mellon SH: Neurosteroids: biosynthesis and function of these novel neuromodulators, *Front Neuroendocrinol* 21(1):1, 2000; Tsutsui D et al: Novel brain function: biosynthesis and actions of neurosteroids in neurons, *Neurosci Res* 36(4):261, 2000.

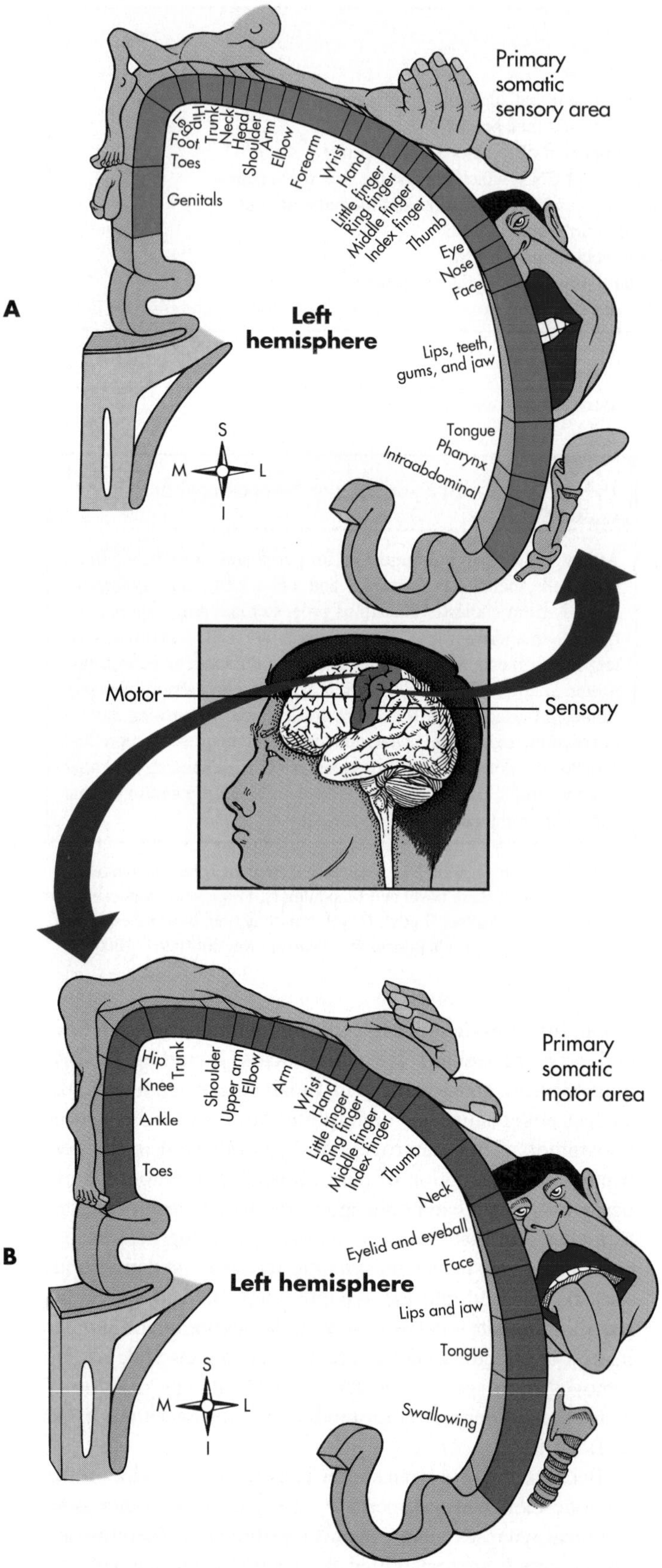

FIG. 13-7 Primary somatic sensory (A) and motor (B) areas of the cortex. (From Thibodeau GA, Patton KI: *Anatomy and physiology,* ed 4, St Louis, 1999, Mosby.)

callosum (commissural fibers). The corpus callosum connects the two cerebral hemispheres and is essential in the coordination of activities between hemispheres, especially specific tasks that may be present in only one hemisphere (see Figs. 13-6, *C,* and 13-14). As a last resort, part or all of the corpus callosum is cut to prevent the spread of epileptic loci (site of seizure activity) through the corpus callosum to the opposite cerebral hemisphere. Epileptic loci often are found in the temporal lobe. This procedure, evolved in the well-known split-brain studies, results initially in temporary aphasia and paralysis.

Inside the cerebrum are numerous tracts (white matter) and nuclei (gray matter). The major **cerebral nuclei** are called *basal ganglia* and include the **corpus striatum** and **amygdala.** The corpus striatum consists of the **lentiform nucleus** (lens shaped), the putamen and globus pallidus, and the ram's horn–shaped caudate nucleus. The **internal capsule** is a thick white matter region in which afferent and efferent pathways, to and from the cerebral cortex, pass through the center of the cerebral hemispheres. The **corpus striatum** appears striped because of the rostral connections between its gray matter and the white matter of the internal capsule.

Functionally, the basal ganglia include, in addition to the corpus striatum, the subthalamic nucleus of the diencephalon and the substantia nigra of the mesencephalon. The basal ganglia plus their interconnections with the thalamus, premotor cortex, red nucleus, reticular formation, and spinal cord are part of the basal ganglia system (extrapyramidal system). The basal ganglia system is believed to exert a fine-tuning effect on motor movements. Parkinson disease and Huntington disease are conditions associated with defects of the basal ganglia (Box 13-2). They are characterized by various involuntary or exaggerated motor movements (see Chapters 15 and 16).

The **limbic system,** first described in 1878 by Broca, is composed of the **Papez circuit** (amygdala, parahippocampal gyrus, **hippocampus,** fornix, mamillary body of hypothala-

Box 13-2

SURGERY FOR PARKINSON DISEASE

Surgical treatment for Parkinson disease can provide gratifying relief from the disabling symptoms of the disease when medical therapies are not effective. The forms of surgery include ablation (thallamotomy, pallidotomy, and subthalamotomy), deep brain stimulation (thalamus, globus pallidus pars internalis, and subthalamic nucleus), and cell graft and gene therapy (mainly of the striatum). Deep brain stimulation is preferred because there is symptom control without tissue destruction. Research is continuing to overcome obstacles associated with cell transplant and gene therapy that boosts dopamine production.

Data from Follett KA: The surgical treatment of Parkinson's disease, *Annu Rev Med* 51:235, 2000; Gross CE et al: From experimentation to the surgical treatment of Parkinson's disease: prelude or suite in basal ganglia research? *Prog Neurobiol* 59(5):509, 1999; Latchman DS, Coffin RS: Viral vectors in the treatment of Parkinson's disease, *Mov Disord* 15(1):9, 2000.

mus, thalamus, and cingulate gyrus), septal area, habenula, other portions of the hypothalamus, and related autonomic nuclei. It is an extension or modification of the olfactory system. Its principal effects are believed to be involved with primitive behavioral responses, visceral reaction to emotion, feeding behaviors, biologic rhythms, and the sense of smell. Expression of affect (emotional and behavioral states) is mediated by extensive connections with the limbic system and prefrontal cortex. Interestingly, the Papez circuit, first postulated in 1937, appears to have as one of its major functions the consolidation of memory through a reverberating circuit.

Diencephalon

The **diencephalon,** surrounded by the cerebrum, is made up of four divisions: **epithalamus, thalamus, hypothalamus,** and **subthalamus** (see Table 13-3 and Fig. 13-6, *B*). The epithalamus (pineal gland) forms the roof of the third ventricle (a brain cavity) and composes the most superior portion of the diencephalon. It has connections and functions closely associated with those of the limbic system. For example, the hormones of the pineal body have been shown to influence reproductive ability, and the secretion of melatonin is associated with circadian rhythms (see Chapter 19).

The largest component of the diencephalon is the thalamus. It is approximately the size and volume of the thumb from the tip to the first joint. It borders and surrounds the third ventricle, and it is a major integrating center for afferent impulses to the cerebral cortex, except olfaction. The perception of various sensations occurs at this level but requires cortical processing for interpretation. The thalamus also serves as a relay center for sensory aspects of motor information from the basal ganglia and cerebellum to appropriate cortical motor areas. Cerebral cortical information also projects to the thalamus, creating reverberating circuits.

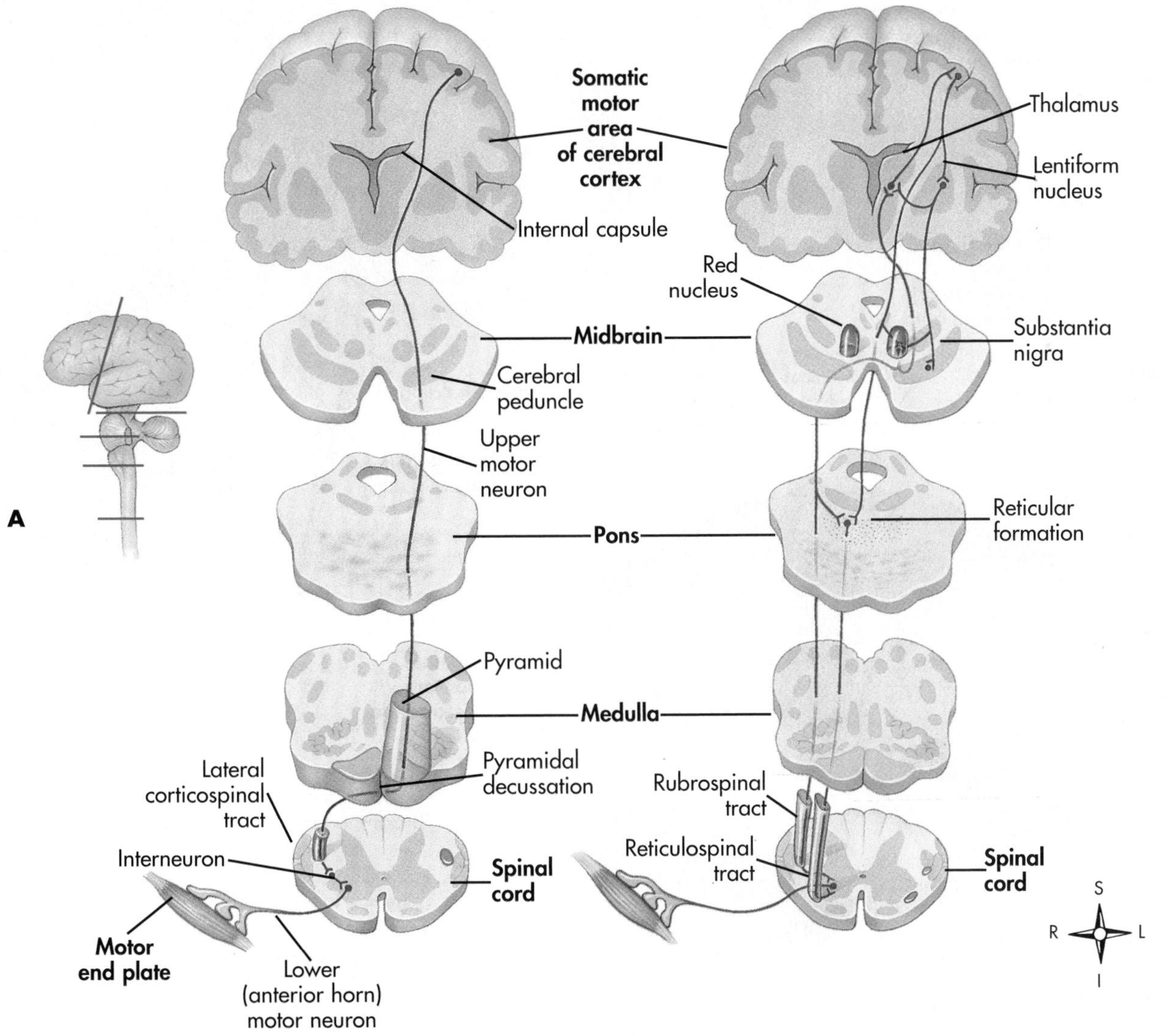

FIG. 13-8 Examples of somatic motor and sensory pathways. A, Motor: the pyramidal pathway through the lateral corticospinal tract and the extrapyramidal pathways through the rubrospinal and reticulospinal tracts. (From Thibodeau GA, Patton KI: *Anatomy and physiology,* ed 4, St Louis, 1999, Mosby.) *Continued*

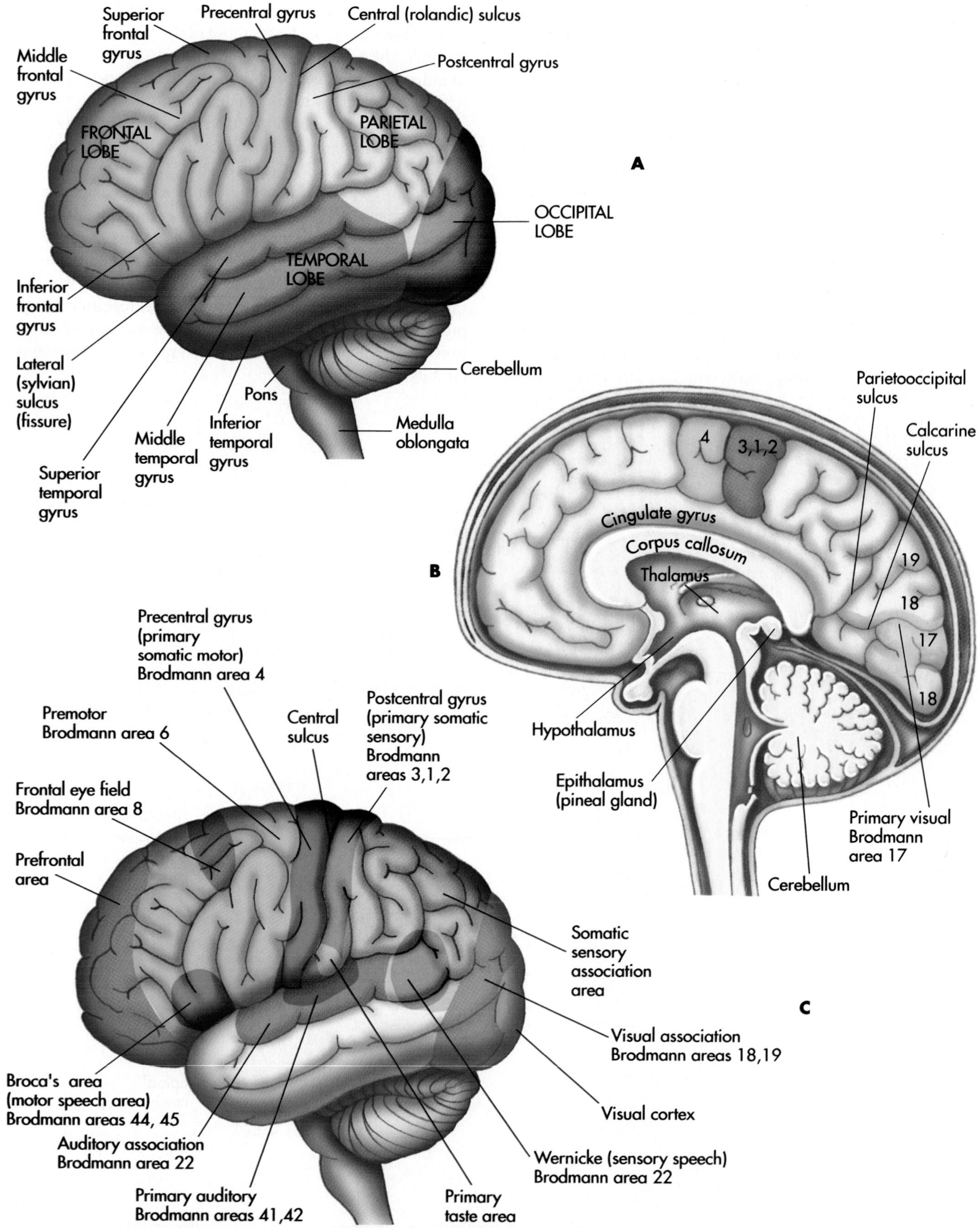

FIG. 13-6 Cerebral hemispheres. A, Left hemisphere of cerebrum, lateral view. **B,** Functional areas of the cerebral cortex, midsagittal view. **C,** Functional areas of the cerebral cortex, lateral view.

and in conjunction with the cerebral cortex is referred to as the **reticular activating system.** Some nuclei within the reticular formation are involved in motor movements.[4]

In general, many major divisions of the brain are associated with different functions, such as the occipital lobe and vision, but attributing specific functions to definite regions of the brain is not entirely accurate. Many activities, such as motor movements and memory, may actually be performed in several regions. Understanding functional specificity is very useful to clinical personnel, especially when attempting to localize pathologic conditions in the nervous system. A neurologist often can localize the site of a tumor, stroke, or bullet wound in an individual just by performing a neurologic examination.

Many attempts have been made to ascribe function to various regions of the cerebral cortex. A German neuropsychiatrist, Brodmann (1868–1918), is credited with postulating various activities to many regions of the cerebral cortex. (Fig. 13-6, *B* and *C*, illustrates these regions and identifies some functional areas.) Another basic CNS principle, **plasticity,** holds that the CNS can change. Children with brain damage may have functional areas "relocate" into other parts of the brain. This propensity for plasticity decreases with age, which explains why older individuals tend not to recover from brain injuries as well as younger individuals. The balance between specificity and plasticity makes understanding brain functions difficult.

Forebrain

Telencephalon

The **telencephalon** consists of the **cerebrum** (the largest portion of the brain), which includes the cerebral cortex and **basal ganglia.** The surface of the cerebrum is characterized by numerous convolutions called *gyri* (see Fig. 13-6, *A*). The gyri greatly increase the cortical surface area. Grooves between adjacent gyri are called **sulci.** Deeper grooves are referred to as **fissures.** The **cerebral cortex** contains the cell bodies and dendrites of neurons, which often are referred to as **gray matter.** Gray matter is organized into columns perpendicular to the surface that receive, integrate, store, and transmit information. **White matter** lies beneath the cerebral cortex and is composed of myelinated nerve fibers.

The two cerebral hemispheres are separated by the longitudinal fissure. The surface of each hemisphere is divided into lobes taking their names from the region of the skull under which each of them lies. The **frontal lobe's** posterior margin is on the **central sulcus (fissure of Rolando,** central fissure), and it borders inferiorly on the **lateral sulcus (sylvian fissure, lateral fissure)** (see Fig. 13-6, *A*). The **prefrontal area** is responsible for goal-oriented behavior (i.e., ability to concentrate), short-term or recall memory, and the elaboration of thought and inhibition on the limbic (emotional) areas of the CNS. The **premotor area** (Brodmann area 6) (see Fig. 13-6, *C*) is involved in programming motor movements. This area contains the cell bodies that form part of the **basal ganglia system** (extrapyramidal system—efferent pathways outside the pyramids of the medulla oblongata). The frontal eye fields (the lower portion of Brodmann area 8), which are involved in controlling eye movements, are located in the middle frontal gyrus.

The **primary motor area** (Brodmann area 4) is located along the **precentral gyrus** forming the **primary voluntary motor area,** which has a somatotopic organization that often is referred to as a *homunculus* (little man) (Fig. 13-7). Electrical stimulation of specific areas of this cortex causes specific muscles of the body to move. The medial part of the longitudinal fissure affects the lower limb and foot, whereas on the lateral surface, the superior third controls the torso and arm, the middle third the hand, and the lowest third the face and mouth/throat. The axons traveling from the cell bodies in and on either side of this gyrus project fibers (axons) that form the **corticospinal tracts** (pyramidal system) that descend into the spinal cord. Cerebral impulses control function in the opposite side of the body, a phenomenon called **contralateral control** (Fig. 13-8, *A*). **Broca speech area** (Brodmann areas 44, 45) is rostral to the inferior edge of the premotor area (Brodmann area 6) on the inferior frontal gyrus. It is usually on the left hemisphere and is responsible for the motor aspects of speech. Damage to this area, commonly as a result of a cerebrovascular accident (stroke), results in the inability to form, or difficulty in forming, words (expressive aphasia or dysphasia) (see Chapter 15).

The **parietal lobe** lies within the borders of the central, parietooccipital, and lateral sulci. This lobe contains the major area for somatic sensory input, located primarily along the **postcentral gyrus** (Brodmann areas 3, 1, 2), which is adjacent to the primary motor area. Communication between the motor and sensory areas (and among other regions in the cortex) is provided by **association fibers.** Much of this region is involved in sensory association (storage, analysis, and interpretation of stimuli). (Fig. 13-7 shows the distribution of functions associated with both the primary motor area and the primary sensory area of the cerebral cortex.)

The **occipital lobe** lies caudal to the parietooccipital sulci and superior to the cerebellum. The primary visual cortex (Brodmann area 17) is located in this region and receives input from the retinas. Much of the remainder of this lobe is involved in visual association (Brodmann areas 18, 19). The **temporal lobe** lies inferior to the lateral sulcus and is composed of the superior, middle, and inferior temporal gyri. The primary auditory cortex (Brodmann area 42) and its related association area (Brodmann area 41) lie deep within the lateral sulcus on the superior temporal gyrus. The **Wernicke area** (posterior portion of Brodmann area 22) is located on the superior temporal gyrus. This area is responsible for reception and interpretation of speech, and dysfunction may result in receptive aphasia or dysphasia. The Wernicke area, along with adjacent portions of the parietal lobe, constitutes a *sensory speech area.* The temporal lobe also is involved as a major area for long-term memory and secondary functions, such as balance, taste, and smell.

Another lobe, the **insula,** lies hidden from view deep in the lateral sulcus. Lying directly beneath the longitudinal fissure is a massive white matter pathway called the **corpus**

[EPSPs]) or (2) the postsynaptic neuron's plasma membrane may be inhibited (hyperpolarized; **inhibitory postsynaptic potentials [IPSPs]**). (Chapter 1 contains a review of electrical impulses and membrane potentials.)

Usually, a single EPSP cannot induce a neuron's action potential and the propagation of the nerve impulse. Whether this occurs depends on the number and frequency of potentials the postsynaptic neuron receives—a concept known as **summation. Temporal summation** (time relationship) refers to the effects of successive impulses received at the same synapse. **Spatial summation** (spacing effect) is the combined effects of impulses a single neuron transmits to different synapses at the same time. **Facilitation** refers to the effect of EPSPs on the plasma membrane potential. The plasma membrane is facilitated when summation brings the membrane closer to the threshold potential and decreases the stimulus required to induce an action potential. The effect that a neurotransmitter has on the plasma membrane potential depends on the balance of these effects. The mechanisms of convergence, divergence, summation, and facilitation allow for the integrative processes of the nervous system.

Table 13-2 Substances That Are Neurotransmitters and/or Neuromodulators

Substance	Location	Effect	Clinical Example
ACETYLCHOLINE			
	Many parts of the brain, spinal cord, neuromuscular junction of skeletal muscle, and many ANS synapses	Excitatory or inhibitory	Alzheimer disease (a type of senile dementia) is associated with a decrease in acetylcholine-secreting neurons; myasthenia gravis (weakness of skeletal muscles) results from a reduction in acetylcholine receptors
MONOAMINES			
Norepinephrine	Many areas of the brain and spinal cord; also in sympathetic ANS synapses	Excitatory or inhibitory	Cocaine and amphetamines,* resulting in overstimulation of postsynaptic neurons
Serotonin	Many areas of the brain and spinal cord	Generally inhibitory	Involved with mood, anxiety, and sleep induction; levels of serotonin elevated in schizophrenia (delusions, hallucinations, and withdrawal)
Dopamine	Some areas of the brain and ANS synapses	Generally excitatory	Parkinson disease (depression of voluntary motor control) results from destruction of dopamine-secreting neurons; drugs used to increase dopamine production induce vomiting and schizophrenia
Histamine		Generally inhibitory	No clear indication of histamine-associated pathologic conditions; histamine apparently is involved with arousal, pituitary hormone secretion, control of cerebral circulation, and thermoregulation
AMINO ACIDS			
γ-Aminobutyric acid (GABA)	Most neurons of the CNS have GABA receptors	Majority of postsynaptic inhibition in the brain	Drugs that increase GABA function have been used to treat epilepsy (excessive discharge of neurons)
Glycine	Spinal cord	Most postsynaptic inhibition in the spinal cord	Glycine receptors inhibited by strychnine
Glutamate and aspartate	Widespread in the brain and spinal cord	Excitatory	Drugs that block glutamate or aspartate are under development; might prevent seizures and neural degeneration from overexcitation
NEUROPEPTIDES			
Endorphins and enkephalins	Widely distributed in the CNS and PNS	Generally inhibitory	The opiates morphine and heroin bind to endorphin and enkephalin receptors on presynaptic neurons and reduce pain by blocking the release of neurotransmitter
Substance P	Spinal cord, brain, and sensory neurons associated with pain, GI tract	Generally excitatory	Substance P is a neurotransmitter in pain transmission pathways; blocking its release by morphine reduces pain

From Seeley R, Stephens TD, Tate P: *Anatomy and physiology,* ed 3, St Louis, 1992, Mosby.
*Increase the release and block the reuptake of norepinephrine.
ANS, Autonomic nervous system; *CNS,* central nervous system; *PNS,* peripheral nervous system; *GI,* gastrointestinal.

Two points could be helpful in understanding the complexity of brain physiology. First, the aforementioned neuromodulators appear to function to raise or lower the membrane potentials of neurons. These chemicals facilitate or inhibit the effect of neurotransmitters. Second, reciprocal synapses between dendrites, that is, one dendrite being able to depolarize or hyperpolarize the membrane potential of another dendrite through the use of neurotransmitters, demonstrate that the interactions between neurons are far more complicated than postulated by simple on-off models of brain function.

CENTRAL NERVOUS SYSTEM

Brain

The human brain enables individuals to reason, function intellectually, express personality and mood, and interact with the environment. The brain is a pinkish gray organ that weighs approximately 3 pounds and has the consistency of tofu or custard. It receives approximately 15% to 20% of the total cardiac output. The three major divisions of the brain, based on embryologic origin, are (1) the forebrain, formed by the two cerebral hemispheres; (2) the midbrain, which includes the corpora quadrigemina, tegmentum, and cerebral peduncles; and (3) the hindbrain, which includes the cerebellum, pons, and medulla (Table 13-3). The midbrain, medulla oblongata, and pons make up the **brain stem,** which connects the hemispheres of the brain, cerebellum, and spinal cord. A collection of nuclei (nerve cell bodies) within the brain stem forms the **reticular formation** (Fig. 13-5). The reticular formation is a large network of connected tissue nuclei that regulate vital reflexes, such as cardiovascular function and respiration. The reticular formation is essential for maintaining wakefulness

Table 13-3 Divisions of the Central Nervous System

Primary Vesicles	Secondary Vesicles	Associated Structures
Forebrain (prosencephalon)	Telencephalon	Cerebral hemispheres
		Cerebral cortex
		Rhinencephalon
		Basal ganglia
	Diencephalon	Epithalamus
		Thalamus
		Hypothalamus
		Subthalamus
Midbrain (mesencephalon)	Mesencephalon	Corpora quadrigemina
		Tegmentum
		Cerebral peduncles
Hindbrain (rhombencephalon)	Metencephalon	Cerebellum
		Pons
	Myelencephalon	Medulla oblongata
Spinal cord	Spinal cord	Spinal cord

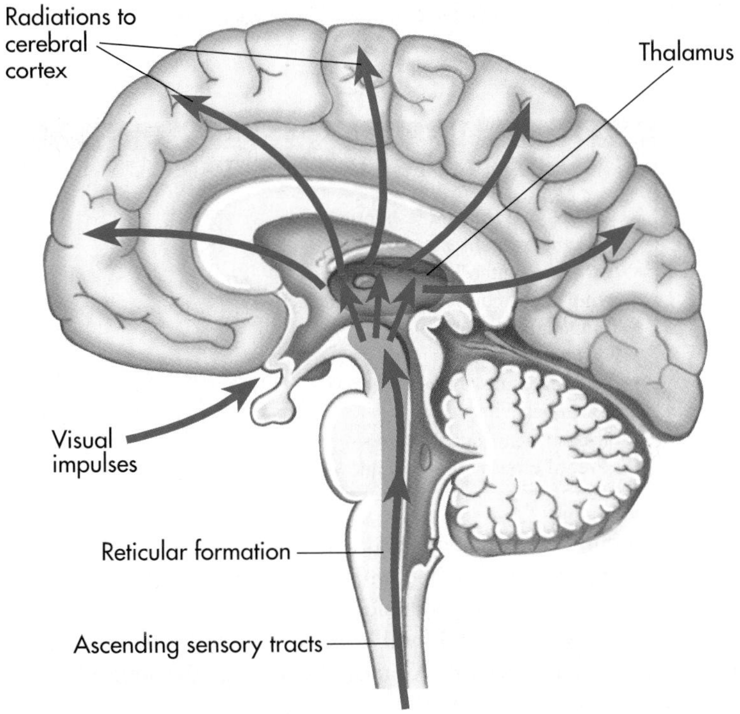

FIG. 13-5 Reticular activating system. System consists of nuclei in the brain stem reticular formation plus fibers that conduct to the nuclei from below and fibers that conduct from the nuclei to widespread areas of the cerebral cortex. Functioning of the reticular activating system is essential for consciousness.

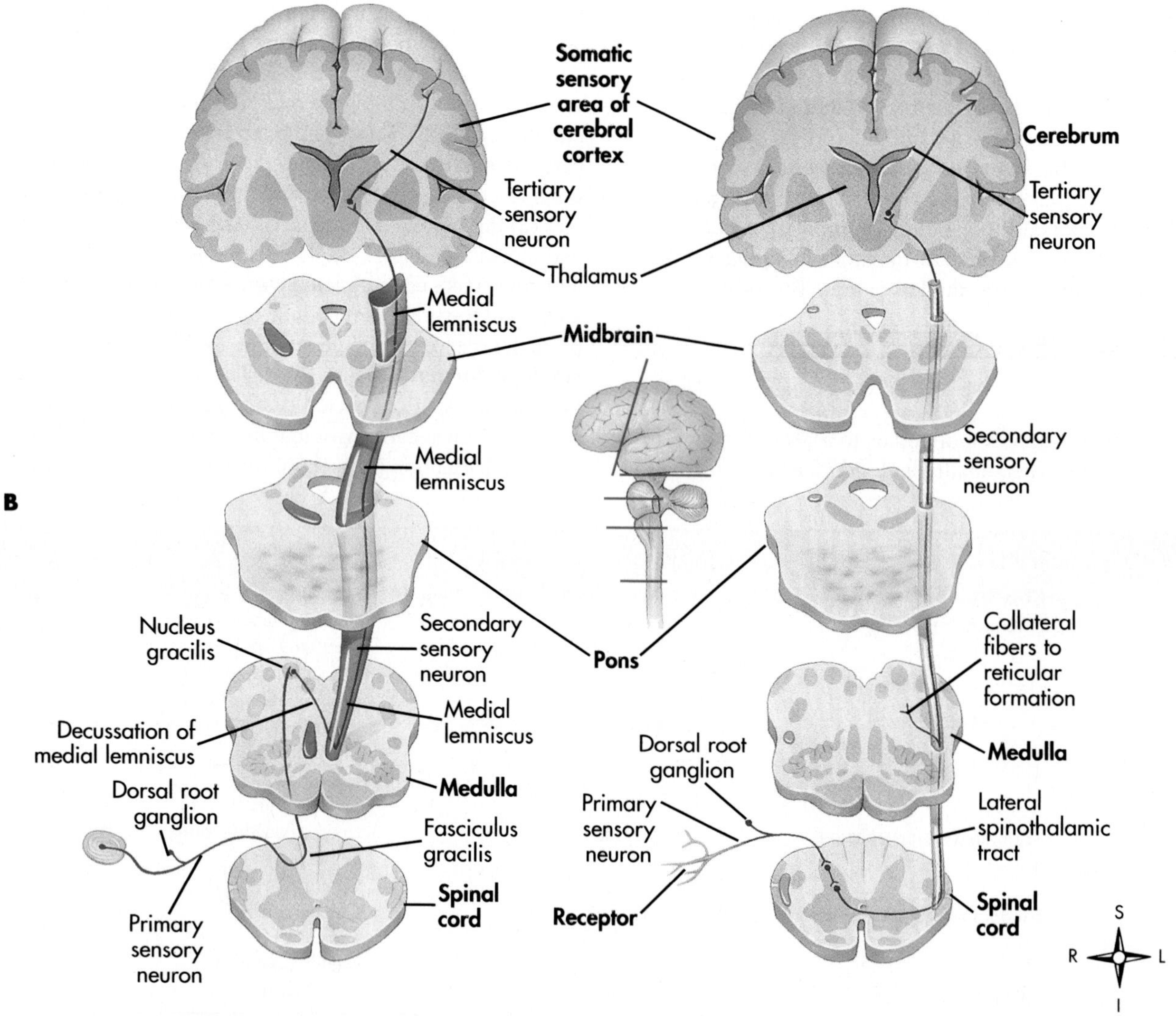

FIG. 13-8, cont'd Examples of somatic motor and sensory pathways. B, Sensory: pathways of the medial lemniscal system that conducts information about discriminating touch and kinesthesis and the spinothalamic pathway that conducts information about pain and temperature. (From Thibodeau GA, Patton KI: *Anatomy and physiology,* ed 4, St Louis, 1999, Mosby.)

The hypothalamus forms the base of the diencephalon. Hypothalamic function falls into two major areas: (1) maintenance of a constant internal environment and (2) implementation of behavioral patterns. Integrative centers control ANS function, regulation of body temperature, endocrine function, and regulation of emotional expression. (Temperature regulation is discussed in Chapter 14.) The hypothalamus exerts its influence through the endocrine system, as well as neural pathways (Box 13-3). (For endocrine functions of the hypothalamus and pituitary, see Chapter 19.)

The subthalamus flanks the hypothalamus laterally. The subthalamus contains the **subthalamic nucleus,** which is part of the basal ganglia system.

Box 13-3

FUNCTIONS OF THE HYPOTHALAMUS

- Visceral and somatic responses
- Affectual responses
- Hormone synthesis
- Sympathetic and parasympathetic activity
- Temperature regulation
- Feeding responses
- Physical expression of emotions
- Sexual behavior
- Pleasure-punishment centers
- Level of arousal or wakefulness

Midbrain

The **midbrain (mesencephalon)** is composed of three structures: the **corpora quadrigemina,** or tectum (composed of the superior and inferior colliculi); the **tegmentum** (containing the red nucleus and substantia nigra); and the basis pedunculi. (The tegmentum and basis pedunculi are collectively the cerebral peduncles.)

The **superior colliculi** are involved with voluntary and involuntary visual motor movements (e.g., the ability of the eyes to *track* moving objects in the visual field). The **inferior colliculi** accomplish similar motor activities but involve movements affecting the auditory system (e.g., positioning the head to improve hearing). The inferior colliculus is also a major relay center along the auditory pathway. The **red nucleus** is a major motor output center that is influenced by the cerebellum. The inferiormost portion of the basal ganglia is the **substantia nigra,** which synthesizes **dopamine,** a neurotransmitter and precursor of norepinephrine. Its dysfunction is associated with Parkinson disease (see Chapter 16). The **basis pedunculi** are made up of efferent fibers of the corticospinal, corticobulbar, and corticopontocerebellar tracts.

Other notable structures of this region are the nuclei and tracts of the third and fourth cranial nerves. The **cerebral aqueduct** (aqueduct of Sylvius), which carries CSF, also traverses this structure. The plugging of this aqueduct is often the cause of hydrocephalus.

Hindbrain

Metencephalon

The major structures of the **metencephalon** are the cerebellum and the pons. The **cerebellum** (see Fig. 13-6, *A* and *B*) is composed of two cerebellar hemispheres covered with small convolutions called *folia.* Each hemisphere is divided by the primary fissure into two lobes (anterior and posterior) that are connected by a midline structure called the **vermis,** meaning worm.

The cerebellum is responsible for both conscious and unconscious muscle synergy and for maintaining balance and posture. This is accomplished through extensive neural connections from the spinal cord and medulla oblongata through the inferior cerebellar peduncle and with the midbrain and higher structures through the superior cerebellar peduncle. The two cerebellar hemispheres receive massive cerebral cortical input through the middle cerebellar pedunculi. These connections allow extensive sampling of visual, vestibular, and proprioceptive data from other regions of the CNS and periphery. Damage to the cerebellum is characterized by ipsilateral (same side) loss of equilibrium, balance, and motor coordination. The cerebellum has ipsilateral control of the body, in contrast to the cerebral cortex, which has contralateral (opposite side) control of the body.

The **pons** (bridge) is easily recognized by its bulging appearance below the midbrain and above the medulla oblongata. Primarily, it transmits information from the cerebellum to the brain stem nuclei and relays motor information from the cerebral cortex to the contralateral cerebellar hemisphere. The pons is an important center for the control of respiration (i.e., rate and relationship of inspiration to expiration). The nuclei of cranial nerves V through VIII are located in this structure.

Myelencephalon

The **medulla oblongata** makes up the **myelencephalon** and is the lowest portion of the brain stem. Reflex activities, such as heart rate, respiration, blood pressure, coughing, sneezing, swallowing, and vomiting, are controlled in this area. The nuclei of cranial nerves IX through XII (see Table 13-6 for discussion) are located in this region. The lowest portion of the reticular formation is found here.

A major portion of the descending motor pathways (i.e., corticospinal tracts) cross to the contralateral side, or decussate, at the inferior medulla oblongata (see Figs. 13-8, *A*). These pathways, together with other areas of decussation in the CNS, are the basis for the phenomenon of contralateral control.

Spinal Cord

The **spinal cord** is the portion of the CNS that lies within the vertebral canal and is surrounded and protected by the **vertebral column.** The spinal cord has many functions, which include a long nerve cable that connects the brain and body, somatic and autonomic reflexes, motor pattern control centers, and sensory and motor modulation. It continues from the medulla oblongata and ends at the level of the first or second lumbar vertebra in adults (Fig. 13-9). The end of the spinal cord, **conus medullaris,** is cone shaped. Spinal nerves continue from the end of the spinal cord and form a nerve bundle called the **cauda equina.** The filament anchor from the conus medullaris to the coccyx is the **filum terminale** (see Fig. 13-9).

Grossly, the spinal cord is divided into sections (8 cervical, 12 thoracic, 5 lumbar, 5 sacral, and 1 coccygeal) that correspond to paired nerves (see Fig. 13-9). A cross section of the spinal cord (Fig. 13-10) is characterized by a butterfly-shaped inner core of gray matter (containing nerve cell bodies). The **central canal** lies in the center of this region and extends through the spinal cord from its origin in the fourth ventricle. The gray matter of the spinal cord is divided into three regions with specific functional characteristics. These regions include the **posterior horn (dorsal horn),** which is composed primarily of interneurons and axons from sensory neurons whose cell bodies lie in the **sensory ganglion (dorsal root ganglion).** At the tip of the posterior horn is the **substantia gelatinosa,** a structure involved in pain transmission (see Chapter 14). The **intermediolateral gray (lateral horn)** contains cell bodies involved with the ANS. The **anterior horn (ventral horn)** contains the nerve cell bodies for efferent pathways leaving the spinal cord by way of spinal nerves. The terms *anterior* and *posterior* are preferred by many authors for describing human spinal cord anatomy, whereas *dorsal* and *ventral* are the common zoologic ("cat and dog") terms.

Surrounding the gray matter is white matter that forms ascending and descending pathways called **spinal tracts** and short ascending and descending integrative pathways. Spinal tracts are named to denote their beginning and ending points. For example, the **spinothalamic tract** carries nerve impulses from the spinal cord to the thalamus in the diencephalon. The white matter is subdivided into columns. These consist of the **anterior column (ventral column), lateral column,** and **posterior column (dorsal column).** (Fig. 13-11 identifies the location and principal activities of the major spinal tracts.)

anteriorly to the base of the brain at the crista galli of the ethmoid bone. The **tentorium cerebelli,** a common landmark, is a membrane that separates the cerebellum below from the cerebral structures above. The tentorium may become involved during periods of increased intracranial pressure caused by an injury to the brain. An injury within the cranial cavity tends to shift intracranial contents, and as structures shift, they tend to be compressed against these rigid membranes, resulting in damage or destruction. A common example is tentorial herniation.

Below the dura mater lies the **arachnoid membrane,** characterized by its filmy, weblike structure. It loosely follows the contours of the cerebral structures but goes over the sulci.

The **subdural space** lies between the dura and arachnoid. Many small bridging veins that have little support traverse the subdural space. Their disruption results in a subdural hematoma (see Chapter 16). The **subarachnoid space,** which contains CSF, lies between the arachnoid and the pia mater (see Fig. 13-14). Damage to intracranial vessels can lead to a condition called *subarachnoid hemorrhage,* which frequently results in signs of meningeal irritation, such as neck stiffness, Kernig sign, and low back pain.

Unlike the dura mater and arachnoid, the delicate **pia mater** (see Fig. 13-14) closely adheres to the surface of the brain and spinal cord and even follows the sulci and fissures. It provides support for blood vessels serving brain tissue. The **choroid plexuses,** structures that produce CSF, arise from the pia mater. The spinal cord is anchored to the vertebrae by extension of the meninges called **denticulate ligaments.** The meninges continue beyond the end of the spinal cord to the lower portion of the sacrum. CSF, contained within the subarachnoid space, also circulates down to the large **lumbar cistern,** which extends from the second lumbar vertebra to the second sacral vertebra. Cisterns are expanded areas of the subarachnoid space. The **cerebellomedullary cistern (cisterna magna)** and the pontine cisterns are two other important cisterns.

The meninges form potential and real spaces important to understanding functional and pathologic mechanisms. For example, between the dura mater and skull lies a potential space termed the **epidural space** (see Fig. 13-14). In the spinal canal there is a real epidural space filled with fatty tissue and a venous plexus. The arterial supply to the meninges consists of blood vessels that lie within grooves in the skull. As a result of trauma, the skull can be fractured and the blood vessels disrupted. The ruptured vessels can lead to an accumulation of blood within the epidural space, called an *epidural hematoma* (see Chapter 16). Persons with alcoholism often fall and injure their head, resulting in an epidural hematoma. An inflammation of the meninges (meningitis) also can have life-threatening implications because of the relative proximity to the brain. (Disorders of the CNS are discussed in Chapter 16.)

Table 13-4 Composition of Cerebrospinal Fluid

Constituent	Normal Value
Na^+	148 mM
K^+	2.9 mM
Cl^-	125 mM
HCO_3^-	22.9 mM
Glucose (fasting)	50-75 mg/dl (60% of serum glucose)
pH	7.3
Protein	15-45 mg/dl
Albumin	80%
Gamma globulin	6%-10%
Cells	
White (lymphocytes)	0-6/mm^3
Red	0/mm^3

Na^+, Sodium; *K^+*, potassium; *Cl^-*, chloride; *HCO_3^-*, bicarbonate.

Cerebrospinal Fluid and the Ventricular System

Cerebrospinal fluid (CSF) is a clear, colorless fluid similar to blood plasma and interstitial fluid. The intracranial and spinal cord structures float in CSF and are protected from jolts and blows. The buoyant properties of the CSF also prevent the brain from tugging on meninges, nerve roots, and blood vessels. (Constituents of CSF are listed in Table 13-4.) Between 125 and 150 ml of CSF, approximately the quantity of a small cup of coffee, is circulating within the **ventricles** (small cavities) and subarachnoid space at any given time. Approximately 600 ml of CSF is produced daily.

The choroid plexuses in the lateral, third, and fourth ventricles produce the major portion of CSF. (Ventricles are illustrated in Fig. 13-14.) These plexuses are characterized by a rich network of blood vessels, supplied by the pia mater, that lie in close contact with the ependymal cells of the ventricles.

The CSF exerts pressure within the brain and spinal cord. When a person is lying down, CSF pressure is approximately 120 to 180 mm of water pressure, or approximately 9 to 14 mm Hg pressure. CSF flow is a result of a pressure gradient between the arterial system and the CSF-filled cavities. Beginning in the lateral ventricles, the CSF flows through the **interventricular foramen (foramen of Monro)** into the third ventricle and then passes through the cerebral aqueduct (aqueduct of Sylvius) into the fourth ventricle. From the fourth ventricle the CSF may pass through either the paired **lateral apertures (foramina of Luschka)** into the pontine cisterns, located along the basal pons, or the midline **median aperture (foramen of Magendie)** into the cerebellomedullary cistern before communicating with the subarachnoid spaces of the brain and spinal cord. The CSF does not, however, accumulate. Instead, it is reabsorbed into the venous circulation through the arachnoid villi, primarily located superior to the falx cerebri in the **superior sagittal sinus.** The **arachnoid villi** protrude from the arachnoid space, through the dura mater, and lie within the blood flow of the venous sinuses. CSF is reabsorbed by means of a pressure gradient between the arachnoid villi and the cerebral venous sinuses. The villi function as one-way valves directing CSF outflow into the blood but preventing blood flow into the subarachnoid space. Thus CSF is derived from the blood, and after circulating throughout the CNS, it returns to the blood.

Samples of CSF are withdrawn for diagnostic purposes either (1) by inserting a needle between the third and fourth lumbar vertebrae into the lumbar cistern (subarachnoid space)—a procedure called **lumbar puncture**—or (2) from an intraventricular catheter. Spinal anesthesias (blocks) are administered in a similar manner.

Vertebral Column

The **vertebral column** (Fig. 13-15) is composed of 33 vertebrae: 7 cervical, 12 thoracic, 5 lumbar, 5 fused sacral, and 4 fused coccygeal. Between each interspace (except the fused sacral and coccygeal vertebrae) is an **intervertebral disk** (Fig. 13-16). At the center of the intervertebral disk is the **nucleus pulposus,** a pulpy mass of elastic fibers. The intervertebral disk functions to absorb shocks, preventing damage to the vertebrae. The intervertebral disk is also a common source of back problems. If too much stress is applied to the vertebral column, the disk contents may rupture and protrude into the spinal canal, causing compression of the spinal cord or nerve roots. The disks can also degenerate.

Blood Supply

Blood Supply to the Brain

The brain receives approximately 20% of the cardiac output, or 800 to 1000 ml of blood flow per minute. Carbon dioxide serves as a primary regulator for blood flow within the CNS. It is a potent vasodilator in the CNS, and its effects ensure an adequate blood supply.

The brain derives its arterial supply from two systems: the **internal carotid arteries** and the **vertebral arteries** (Fig. 13-17). The internal carotid arteries, anteriorly, supply a proportionately greater amount of blood flow. They take their origin from the common carotid arteries, enter the cranium through the base of the skull, and pass through the **cavernous sinus.** After giving off some small branches, they divide into the **anterior** and **middle cerebral arteries.** The vertebral arteries, posteriorly, originate as branches off the subclavian arteries, pass through the transverse foramina of the cervical vertebrae, and enter the cranium through the foramen magnum. They join at the junction of the pons and medulla oblongata to form the **basilar artery.** The basilar artery divides at the level of the midbrain to form paired **posterior cerebral arteries.** Three major paired arteries perfuse the cerebellum and brain stem and have their origins from the posterior arterial supply: the posterior inferior cerebellar artery, off the vertebral artery; and the anterior inferior cerebellar and superior cerebellar arteries, off the basilar artery. The basilar artery also gives rise to small pontine arteries. The large arteries on the surface of the brain and their branches are called **superficial arteries (conducting arteries).** The small branches that project into the brain are termed **projecting arteries (nutrient arteries).** Occluding any of these vessels can cause neurologic signs and symptoms that are often diagnostically unique.

The **arterial circle (circle of Willis)** (Fig. 13-18) is a structure credited with the ability to compensate for reduced blood flow from any one of the major contributors (collateral blood flow). The arterial circle is formed by the posterior cerebral arteries, posterior communicating arteries, internal carotid arteries, anterior cerebral arteries, and anterior communicating artery. The anterior cerebral, middle cerebral, and posterior cerebral arteries leave the arterial circle and extend to various brain structures. (Table 13-5 and Fig. 13-19 illustrate structures served, functional relationships, and pathologic considerations related to occlusion of cerebral arteries.)

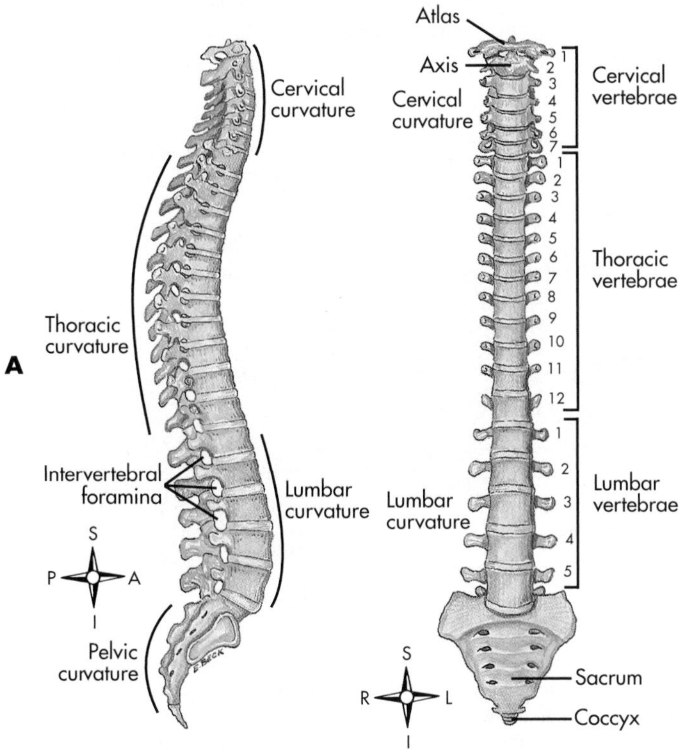

FIG. 13-15 Vertebral column. A, Right lateral view. **B,** Anterior view. (From Thibodeau GA, Patton KI: *Anatomy and physiology,* ed 4, St Louis, 1999, Mosby.)

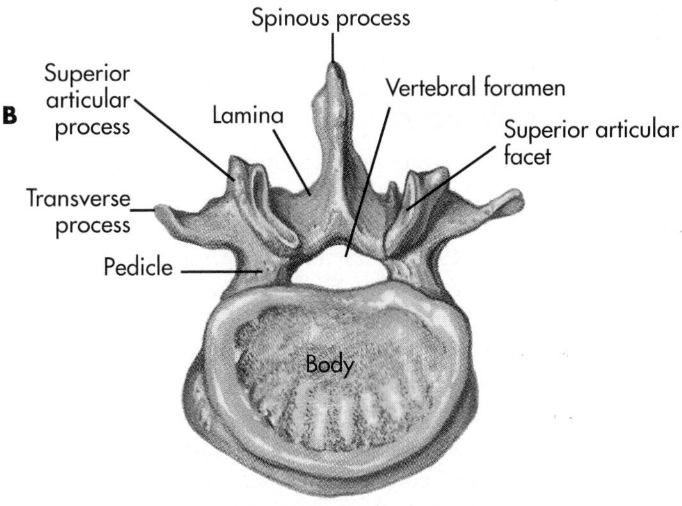

FIG. 13-16 Lumbar vertebra, superior view. (From Thibodeau GA, Patton KI: *Anatomy and physiology,* ed 4, St Louis, 1999, Mosby.)

or association neuron between the afferent and efferent neurons. Transmission time for three-neuron reflexes is slower than in simple reflexes because there are two synaptic delays, rather than one, as well as the delay in crossing the interneuron. The afferent neuron of the reflex arc simultaneously sends sensory information to the effector organ and to higher CNS centers (see Figs. 13-8, *B,* and 14-2). The motor effects from reflex arcs generally occur before perception of the event in the higher centers of the brain. Much of the regulation of the internal environment is mediated by ANS reflexes.

Afferent pathways transmit information from peripheral receptors and eventually terminate in the cerebral or cerebellar cortex or both. Efferent pathways primarily relay information from the cerebrum to the brain stem or spinal cord (see Fig. 13-8, *A*). **Upper motor neurons** (i.e., corticospinal tract) are the classification of motor pathways completely contained within the CNS. Their primary roles include directing, influencing, and modifying reflex arcs, lower-level control centers, and motor (and some sensory) neurons. Generally, upper motor neurons form synapses with interneurons, which then form synapses with lower motor neurons before projecting into the periphery. **Lower motor neurons** (i.e., cranial and spinal efferent neurons) are responsible for direct influence to muscles. Their cell bodies lie in the gray matter of the spinal cord, but their processes extend into the PNS (see Fig. 15-20). Destruction of upper motor neurons usually results in initial paralysis followed within days or weeks by partial recovery, whereas destruction of the lower motor neurons often leads to permanent paralysis. Peripheral nerve damage may be followed by nerve regeneration and recovery. (Injury to motor neurons is discussed in Chapter 15.)

Muscle activity (i.e., stimulation and contraction) is regulated by nerve impulses. Motor neurons innervate one or more muscle cells, forming **motor units** consisting of a neuron and the skeletal muscles it stimulates. The junction between the axon of the motor neuron and the plasma membrane of the muscle cell is called the **neuromuscular (myoneural) junction** (Fig. 13-13). The skeletal muscle neuromuscular junction is more elaborate than the simpler smooth muscle neuromuscular junction.

Motor Pathways

The four clinically relevant motor pathways are the **lateral corticospinal, corticobulbar,** basal ganglia, and **vestibulospinal.** The corticospinal (see Fig. 13-8, *A*) and corticobulbar (see Fig. 15-19) are essentially the same tract and consist of a two-neuron chain. The cell bodies originate in and around the precentral gyrus; pass through the corona radiata of the cerebrum, the internal capsule, middle three fifths of the basis pedunculus, pons, and pyramid; decussate (cross contralaterally) in the medulla oblongata; and form the lateral corticospinal tract of the spinal cord (see Fig. 13-11). The lateral corticospinal tract axons (upper motor neurons) leave the tract to go to specific interneurons or motor neurons in the anterior horn. The lateral corticospinal tract has the same somatotopic organization as the body. These spinal motor neurons project to specific motor units and are lower motor neurons. The corticobulbar (bulbar refers to brain stem) tract can be thought of as the part of the corticospinal tract that innervates the cranial motor nuclei for eye, face, tongue, throat, and neck movement. This tract innervates all the cranial motor nuclei bilaterally except for the facial (spinal), accessory, and hypoglossal nuclei, which receive primarily contralateral innervation. These tracts are involved in precise motor movements. The basal ganglia are part of a system that drives the reticular descending tracts (Fig. 13-11 shows only one of the two reticulospinal tracts). These tracts modulate motor movement by inhibiting and exciting spinal activity. The vestibulospinal tract arises from the lateral vestibular nucleus in the pons and causes the extensor muscles of the body to rapidly contract, most dramatically witnessed when a person starts to fall backward.

Sensory Pathways

The three clinically important spinal afferent pathways are the posterior (dorsal) column, **anterior spinothalamic,** and **lateral spinothalamic** (see Figs. 13-8, *B,* and 13-11). The posterior column has a somatotopic organization with the fasciculus gracilis and fasciculus cuneatus, respectively, carrying lower body and upper body fine touch, two-point discrimination, and proprioceptive information (i.e., **epicritic**). The posterior column is formed by a three-neuron chain. The first neuron of the chain is the primary afferent neuron. It is also the sensory neuron of the reflex arc. After entering the spinal cord it sends its axon ipsilaterally up the spinal cord in a specific part of the posterior funiculus and synapses in one of three posterior column nuclei in the hindbrain. A basketball center has primary afferent neurons that run from the great toe up to the pons, which could be over

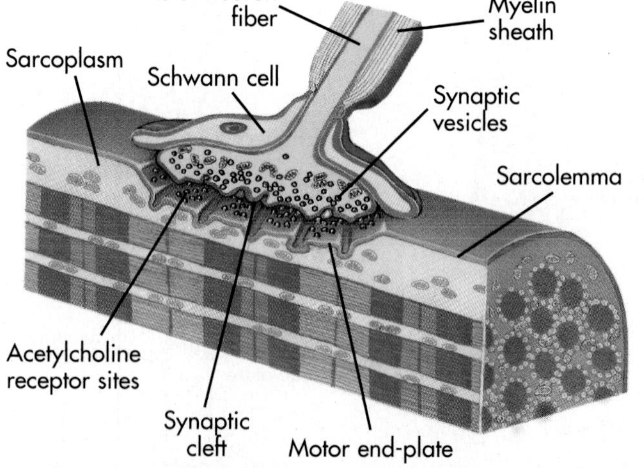

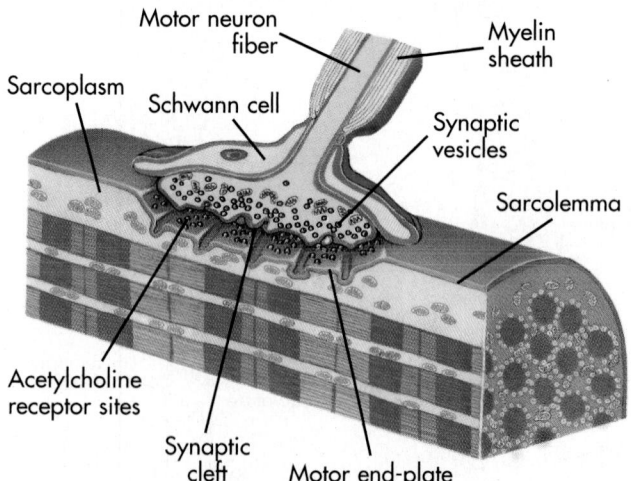

FIG. 13-13 Neuromuscular junction. This figure shows how the distal end of a motor neuron fiber forms a synapse, or "chemical junction," with an adjacent muscle fiber. Neurotransmitters (specifically, acetylcholine) are released from the neuron's synaptic vesicles and diffuse across the synaptic cleft. There they stimulate receptors in the motor end-plate region of the sarcolemma. (From Thibodeau GA, Patton KI: *Anatomy and physiology,* ed 4, St Louis, 1999, Mosby.)

6 feet long. The second-order neuron has its cell body in one of the posterior column nuclei and sends it axon contralaterally and ascends to a specific nucleus of the thalamus and synapses. The third-order neuron, originating in the thalamus, continues the tract into the internal capsule, corona radiata, and postcentral gyrus (Brodmann areas 3, 1, 2) (see Fig. 13-6, *C*). The anterior and lateral spinothalamic tracts are responsible for vague touch and pain and temperature, respectively (see Fig. 13-8, *B*). These modalities are referred to as **protopathic.** Today, the anterior and lateral spinothalamic tracts are combined by many neuroanatomists into the anterolateral system, because these modalities are difficult to localize into finite tracts in the spinal cord. These tracts also form a three-neuron chain. However, the primary afferent neurons synapse in the posterior horn of the spinal cord, not just at the level they enter the intervertebral foramen but in a number of spinal segments above and below their point of entry. This is an example of divergence. The second-order neurons in the posterior horn cross to the contralateral side in the spinal cord and ascend to the same thalamic nucleus as the posterior column pathway and continue on with the posterior column pathway to the postcentral gyrus.

Protective Structures

Cranium

The cranium is composed of eight bones. The cranial vault functions to enclose and protect the brain and its associated structures. The **galea aponeurotica,** which is a thick, fibrous band of tissue overlying the cranium between the frontal and occipital muscles, affords added protection to the bony structure of the skull. The subgaleal space has venous connections with the dural sinuses, and with increased intracranial pressure, blood can be shunted to the space, thus reducing pressure in the intracranial cavity. The subgaleal space is also a common site for wound drains after intracranial surgery.

The floor of the cranial vault is irregular and contains many foramina (openings) for cranial nerves, blood vessels, and the spinal cord to exit. The cranial floor is divided into three fossae (depressions). The frontal lobes lie in the **anterior fossa;** temporal lobes and base of the diencephalon lie in the **middle fossa** (temporal fossa); and the cerebellum lies in the **posterior fossa.** These terms are commonly used anatomic landmarks to describe the location of intracranial lesions.

Meninges

Surrounding the brain and spinal cord are three protective membranes: the dura mater, the arachnoid, and the pia mater. Collectively they are called the **meninges** (Fig. 13-14). The **dura mater** (meaning literally "hard mother") is composed of two layers, with the venous sinuses formed between them. The outermost layer forms the **periosteum (endosteal layer)** of the skull, and the **inner dura or meningeal layer** is responsible for the formation of rigid, double-thickness membranous plates that serve to support and separate various brain structures.

One of these membranous plates (see Fig. 13-14), the **falx cerebri,** dips between the two cerebral hemispheres along the longitudinal fissure. The falx cerebri is anchored

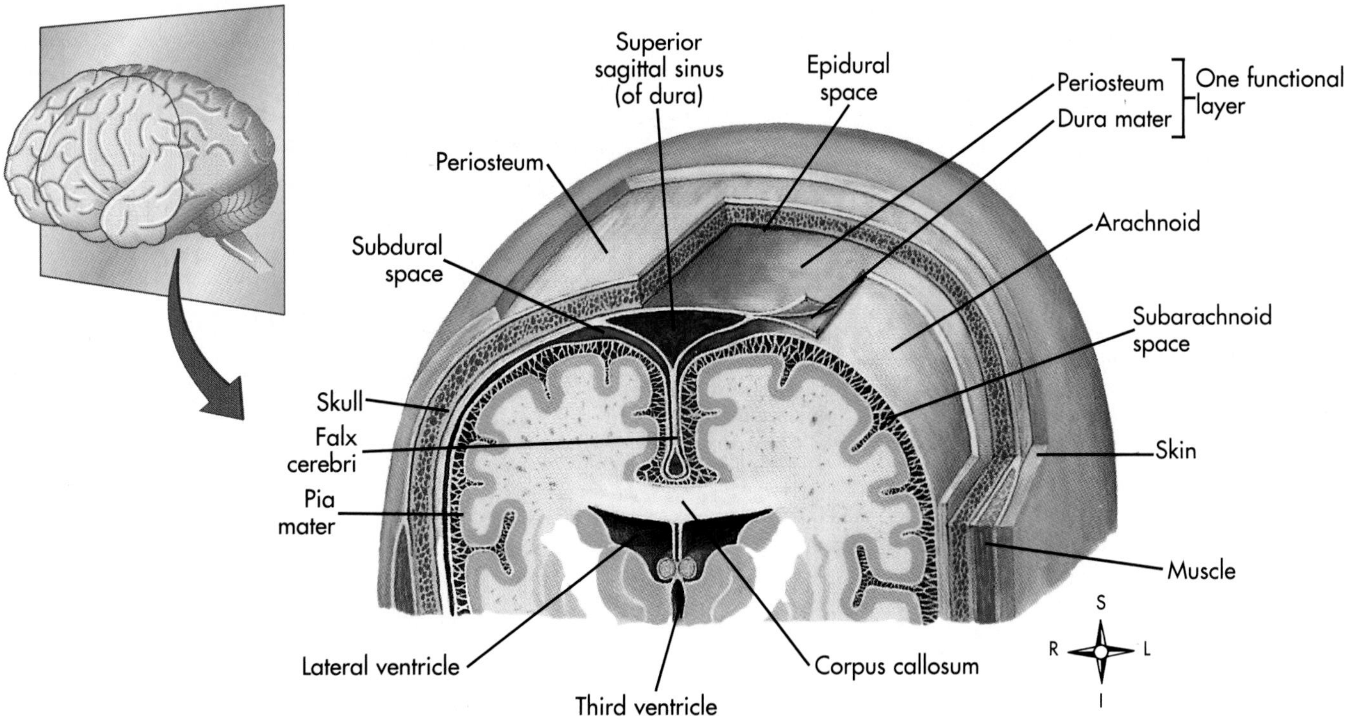

FIG. 13-14 Coverings of the brain. Frontal section of the superior portion of the head, as viewed from the front. Both the bony and the membranous coverings of the brain can be seen. (From Thibodeau GA, Patton KI: *Anatomy and physiology,* ed 4, St Louis, 1999, Mosby.)

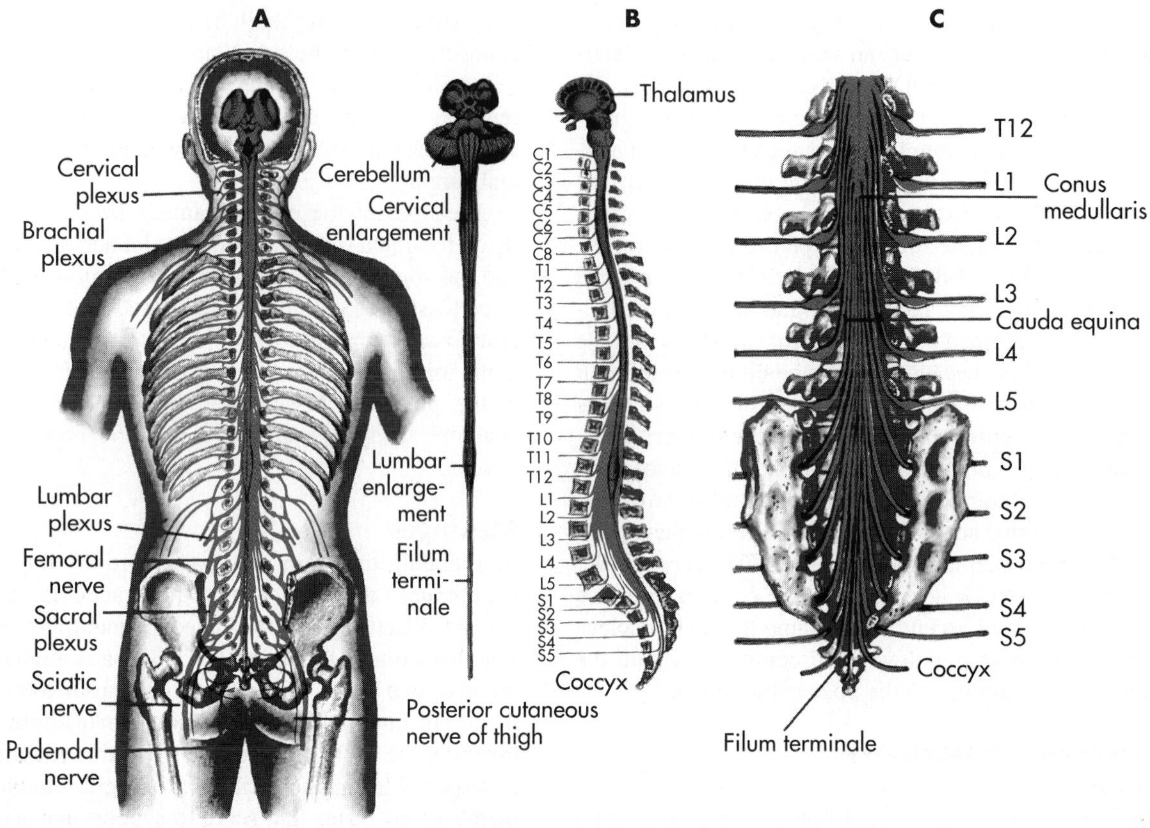

FIG. 13-9 Spinal cord within vertebral canal and exiting spinal nerves. A, Posterior view of brain stem and spinal cord in situ with spinal nerves and plexus. **B,** Anterior view of brain stem and spinal cord. **C,** Enlargement of caudal area showing termination of spinal cord (conus medullaris) and group of nerve fibers constituting the cauda equina. (From Rudy EB, editor: *Advanced neurological and neurosurgical nursing,* St Louis, 1984, Mosby.)

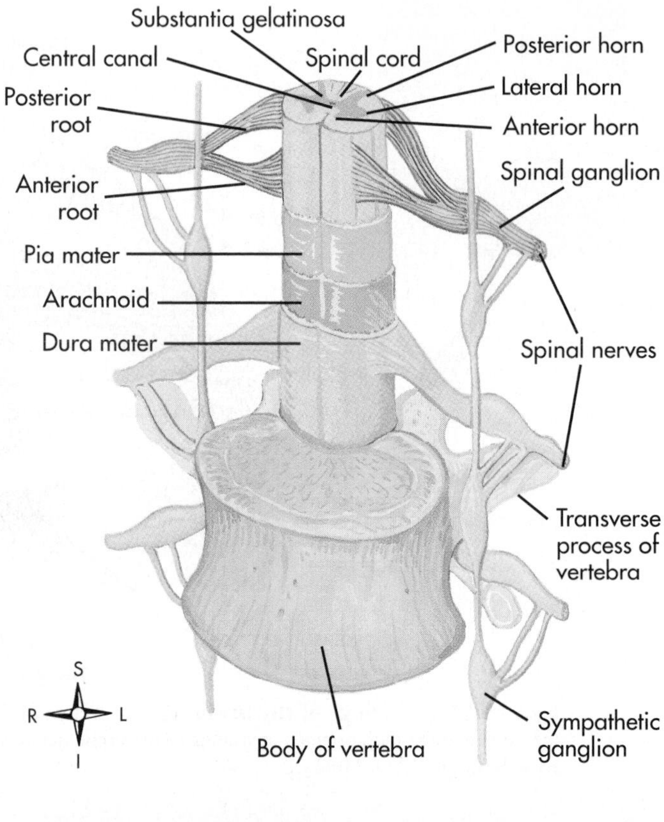

FIG. 13-10 Coverings of the spinal cord. Note how the dura mater extends to cover the spinal nerve roots and nerves. The arachnoid is highlighted in blue and the pia mater in pink. (Modified from Thibodeau GA, Patton KI: *Anatomy and physiology,* ed 3, St Louis, 1996, Mosby.)

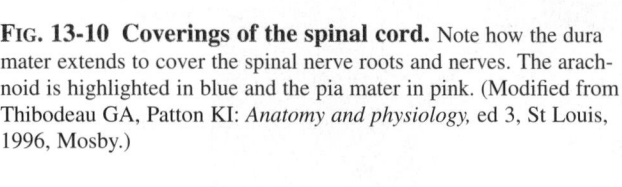

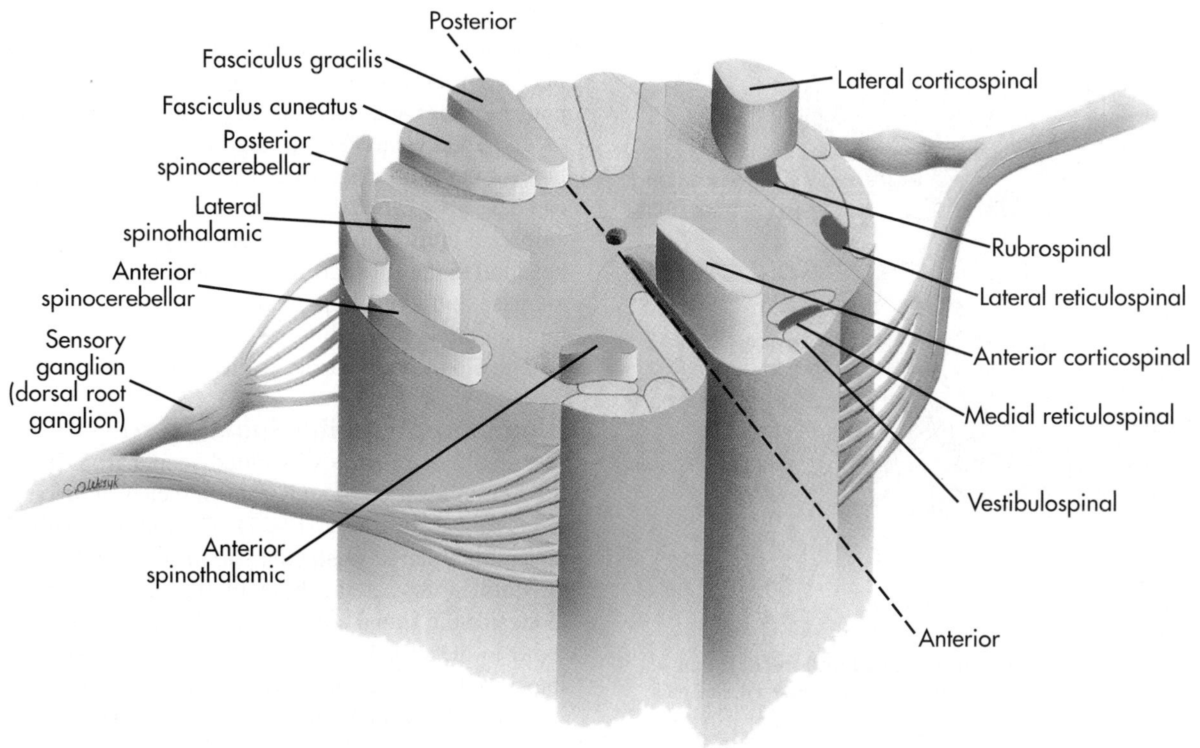

FIG. 13-11 Major tracts of the spinal cord. The major ascending (sensory) tracts, shown only on the left here, are highlighted in blue. The major descending (motor) tracts, shown only on the right, are highlighted in red. The broken line indicates the anteroposterior orientation angle. (From Thibodeau GA, Patton KI: *Anatomy and physiology,* ed 4, St Louis, 1999, Mosby.)

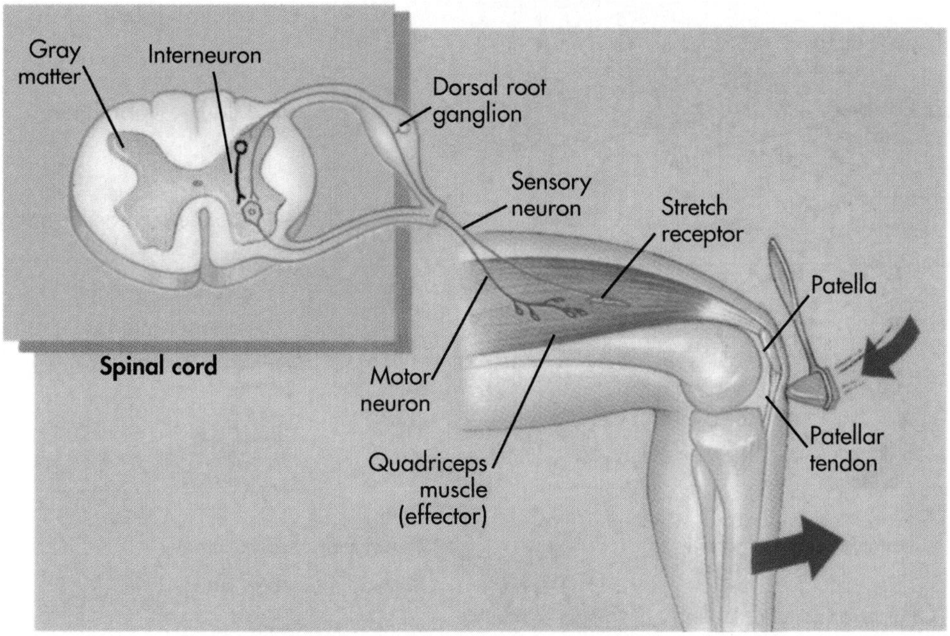

FIG. 13-12 Cross section of spinal cord showing simple reflex arc. (From Thibodeau GA, Patton KI: *Anatomy and physiology,* ed 4, St Louis, 1999, Mosby.)

Neural circuits in the spinal cord, when activated, display specific sets of motor responses. **Reflex arcs** form basic units that respond to stimuli and provide protective circuitry for motor output. Structures mandatory for a reflex arc are a receptor, an **afferent (sensory) neuron,** an **efferent (motor) neuron,** and an effector muscle or gland. The afferent neuron is a pseudounipolar neuron with its cell body in the sensory ganglion. A simple reflex arc may contain only two neurons. (Fig. 13-12 illustrates a simple reflex arc.) Most reflex arcs consist of three neurons that include an interneuron

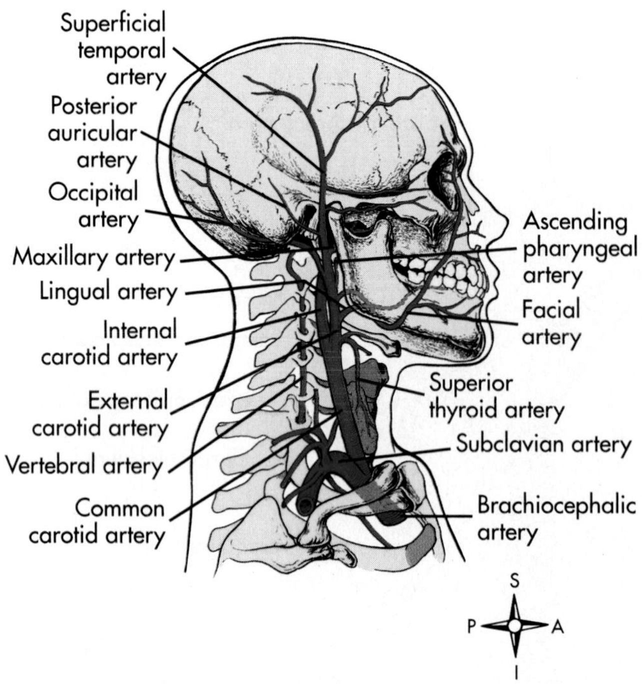

FIG. 13-17 Major arteries of the head and neck. (From Thibodeau GA, Patton KI: *Anatomy and physiology,* ed 4, St Louis, 1999, Mosby.)

Cerebral venous drainage does not parallel (lie side by side) its arterial supply, whereas the venous drainage of the brain stem and cerebellum does parallel the arterial supply of the structures. The cerebral veins are classified as superficial veins and deep cerebral veins. The veins drain into venous plexuses and dural sinuses (formed between the dural layers) and eventually join the internal jugular veins at the base of the skull (Fig. 13-20). Adequacy of venous outflow can have a significant effect on intracranial pressure. For example, in individuals with head injury, turning or letting the head fall to the side partially occludes venous return and can increase intracranial pressure because of decreased flow through the jugular veins.

The blood-brain barrier is discussed in Box 13-4.

Blood Supply to the Spinal Cord

The spinal cord derives its blood supply from branches off the vertebral arteries and from branches from various regions of the aorta (Fig. 13-21). The **anterior spinal arteries** and the paired **posterior spinal arteries** branch off the vertebral artery at the base of the cranium and descend alongside the spinal cord. Arterial branches from vessels exterior to the spinal cord follow the spinal nerve through the intervertebral foramina, pass through the dura, and divide into the anterior and posterior radicular arteries.

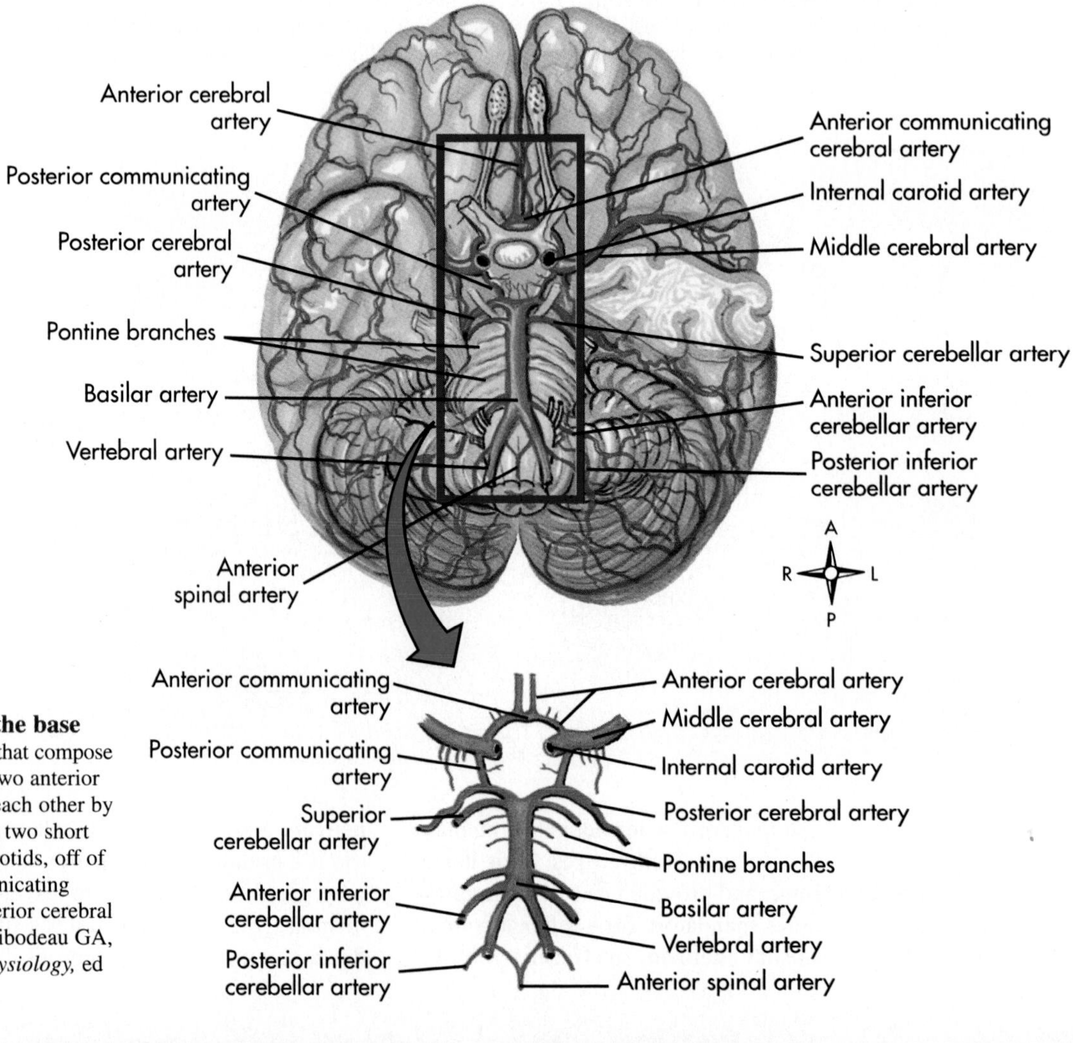

FIG. 13-18 Arteries at the base of the brain. The arteries that compose the circle of Willis are the two anterior cerebral arteries, joined to each other by the anterior communicating two short segments of the internal carotids, off of which the posterior communicating arteries connect to the posterior cerebral arteries. (Modified from Thibodeau GA, Patton KI: *Anatomy and physiology,* ed 4, St Louis, 1999, Mosby.)

Table 13-5 Arterial Systems Supplying the Brain

Arterial Origin	Structures Served	Conditions Caused by Occlusion
Anterior cerebral artery	Basal ganglia; corpus callosum; medial surface of cerebral hemispheres; superior surface of frontal and parietal lobes	Hemiplegia on contralateral side of body, greater in lower than in upper extremities
Middle cerebral artery	Frontal lobe; parietal lobe; temporal lobe (primarily cortical surfaces)	Aphasia in dominant hemisphere and contralateral hemiplegia (see Chapter 15)
Posterior cerebral artery	Part of diencephalon and temporal lobe; occipital lobe	Visual loss; sensory loss; contralateral hemiplegia if cerebral peduncle affected

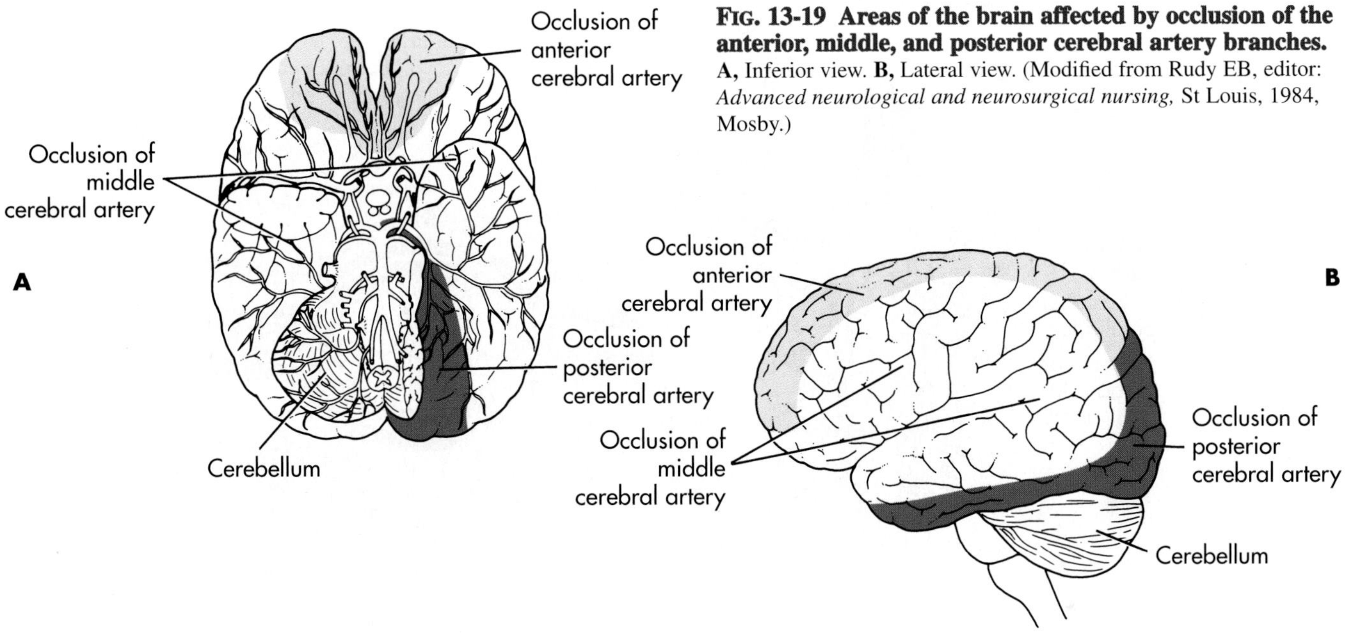

FIG. 13-19 Areas of the brain affected by occlusion of the anterior, middle, and posterior cerebral artery branches. **A,** Inferior view. **B,** Lateral view. (Modified from Rudy EB, editor: *Advanced neurological and neurosurgical nursing,* St Louis, 1984, Mosby.)

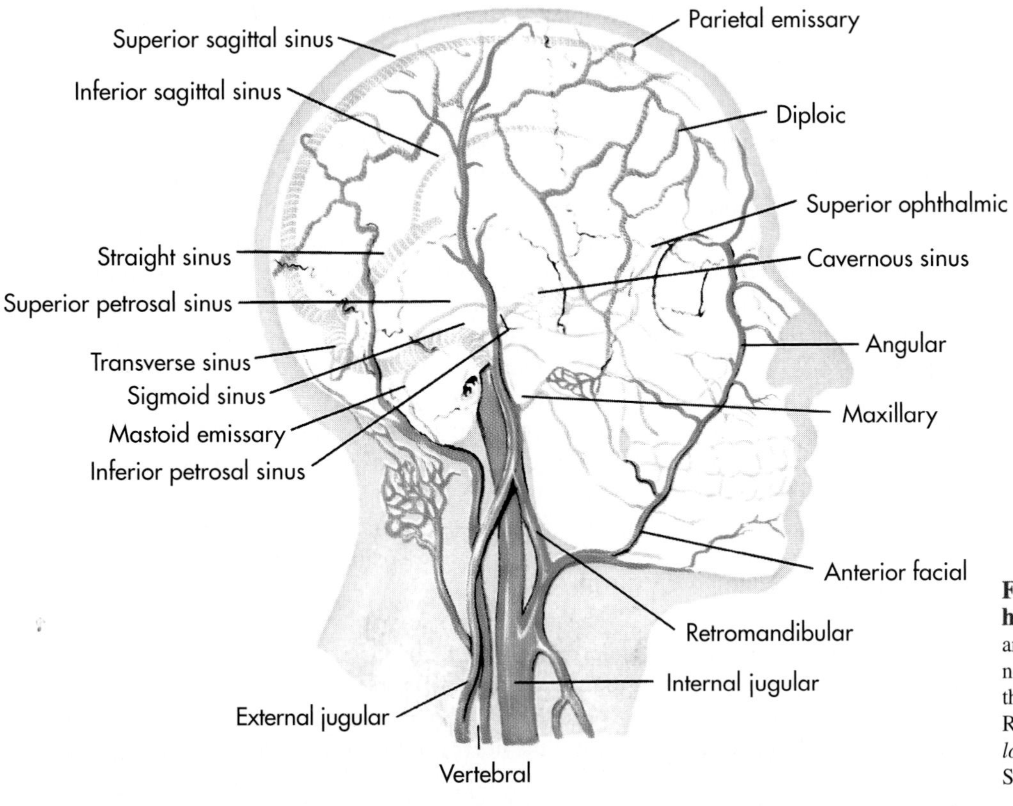

FIG. 13-20 Large veins of the head. Deep veins and dural sinuses are projected on the skull. Note connections (emissary veins) between the superficial and deep veins. (From Rudy EB, editor: *Advanced neurological and neurosurgical nursing,* St Louis, 1984, Mosby.)

Box 13-4

THE BLOOD-BRAIN BARRIER

The **blood-brain barrier** is a term used to describe cellular structures that selectively inhibit certain substances in the blood from entering the interstitial spaces of the brain or CSF. This term emphasizes the impermeability of the nervous system to large and potentially harmful molecules. It is thought that the supporting cells (neuroglia), particularly the astrocytes, and tight junctions between endothelial cells (see Chapter 1) are involved in the formation of the blood-brain barrier. It appears that certain metabolites, electrolytes, and chemicals have differing abilities to cross the brain. This has substantial implications for drug therapy because certain types of antibiotics and chemotherapeutic drugs show a greater propensity than others for crossing the barrier.

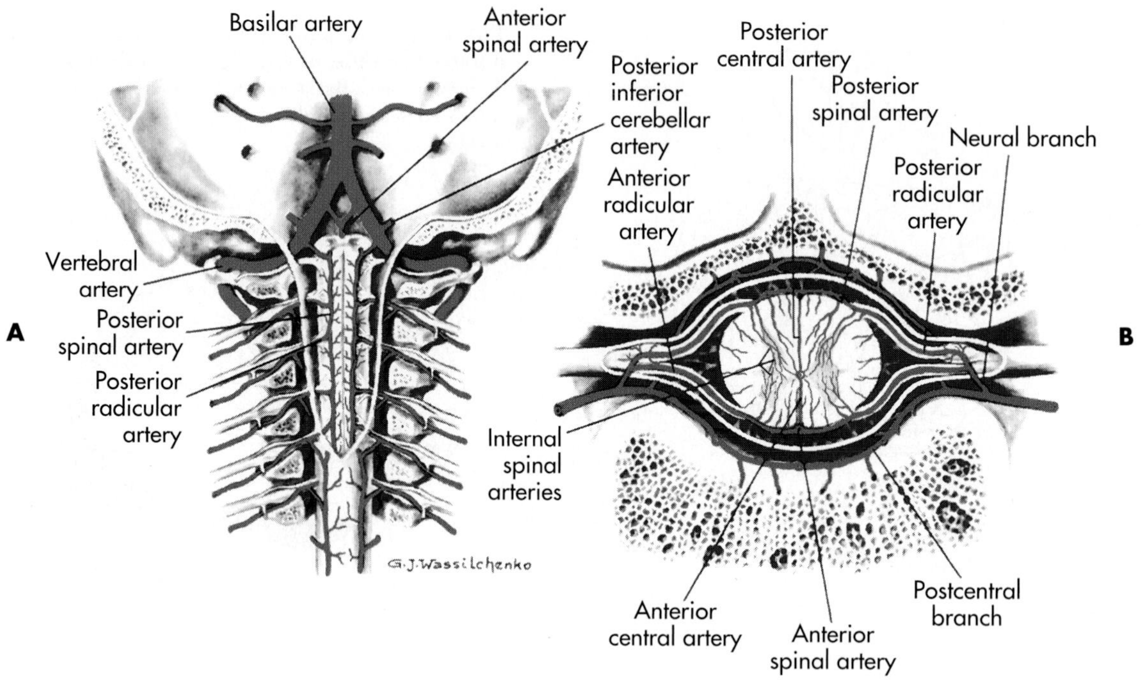

FIG. 13-21 Arteries of the spinal cord. A, Arteries of cervical cord exposed, posterior view. **B,** Arteries of spinal cord diagrammatically shown in horizontal section. (From Rudy EB, editor: *Advanced neurological and neurosurgical nursing,* St Louis, 1984, Mosby.)

The radicular arteries eventually reconnect to the spinal arteries. Branches from the radicular and spinal arteries form plexuses whose branches penetrate the spinal cord, supplying the deeper tissues. Venous drainage parallels the arterial supply closely and drains into venous sinuses located between the dura and periosteum of the vertebrae.

PERIPHERAL NERVOUS SYSTEM

The cranial and spinal nerves, including their branches and ganglia, constitute the PNS. A peripheral nerve (cranial or spinal) is composed of individual axons/dendrites, with most wrapped in a myelin sheath. These individual fibers are arranged in bundles called **fascicles** (Fig. 13-22, *B*). The coverings supply structural support, a blood supply, and interstitial compartments necessary for the supply of essential electrolytes to support nerve impulse conduction.

The 31 pairs of spinal nerves derive their names from the vertebral level from which they exit. There are eight cervical spinal nerves. The first cervical nerve exits above the first cervical vertebra, and the rest of the spinal nerves exit below their corresponding vertebrae. From the thoracic region (and inferiorly) nerves correspond to the vertebral level above their exit.

Spinal nerves contain both sensory and motor neurons and are called **mixed nerves.** They arise as rootlets from the anterior and posterior horn cells of the spinal cord. These two spinal nerve roots converge in the region of the intervertebral foramen to form the spinal nerve (see Fig. 13-10). Shortly after converging, the spinal nerve divides into anterior and posterior rami (branches). The anterior rami (except the thoracic) initially form plexuses (networks of nerve fibers), which then branch into the peripheral nerves. Instead of forming plexuses, the thoracic nerves pass through the intercostal spaces and innervate regions of the thorax.

The main spinal nerve plexuses innervate the skin and the underlying muscles of the limbs. The **brachial plexus,** for example, is formed by the last four cervical nerves (C5 to C8) and the first thoracic nerve (T1). The brachial plexus innervates the nerves of the arm, wrist, and hand. The **lumbar**

A

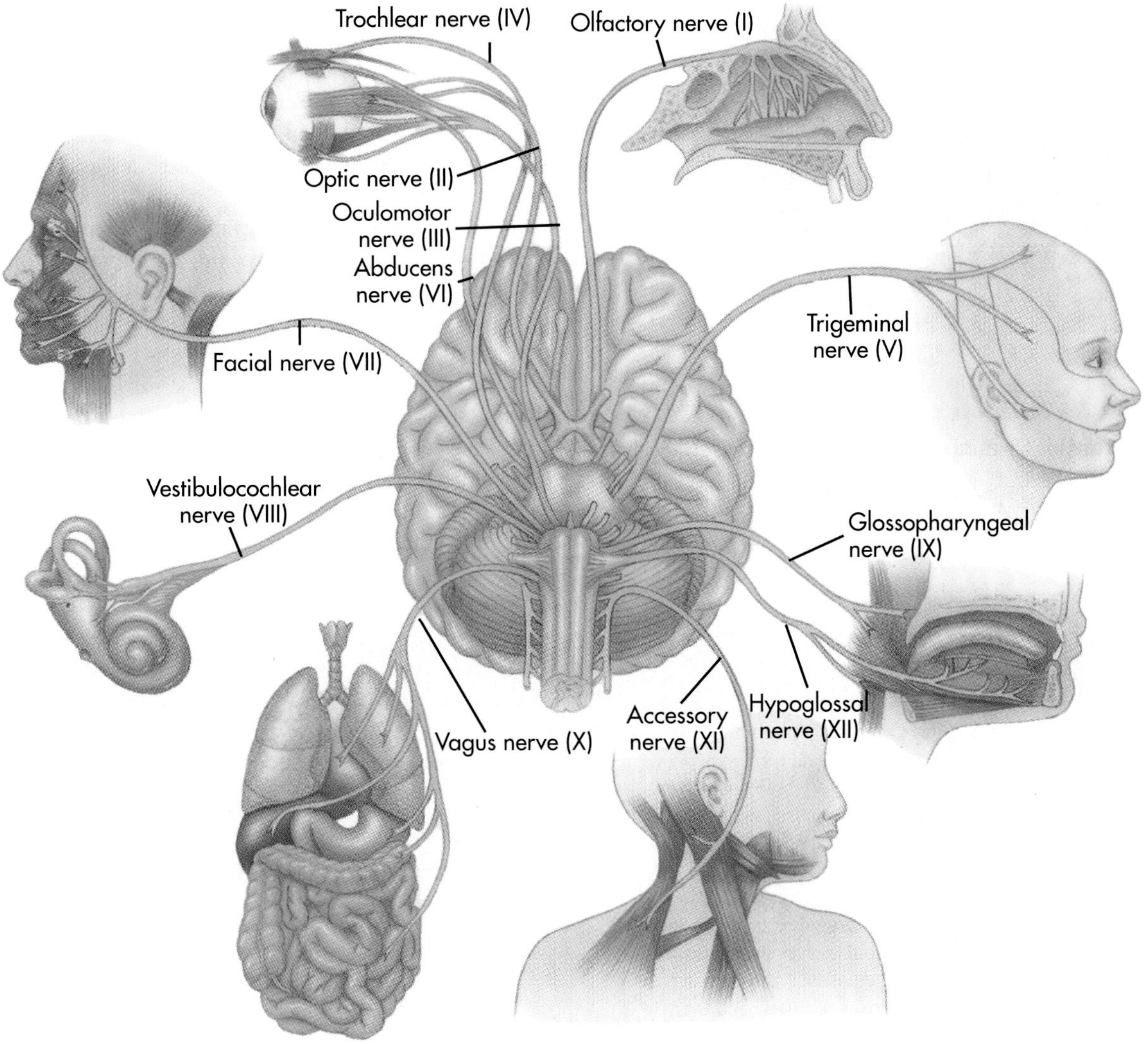

B

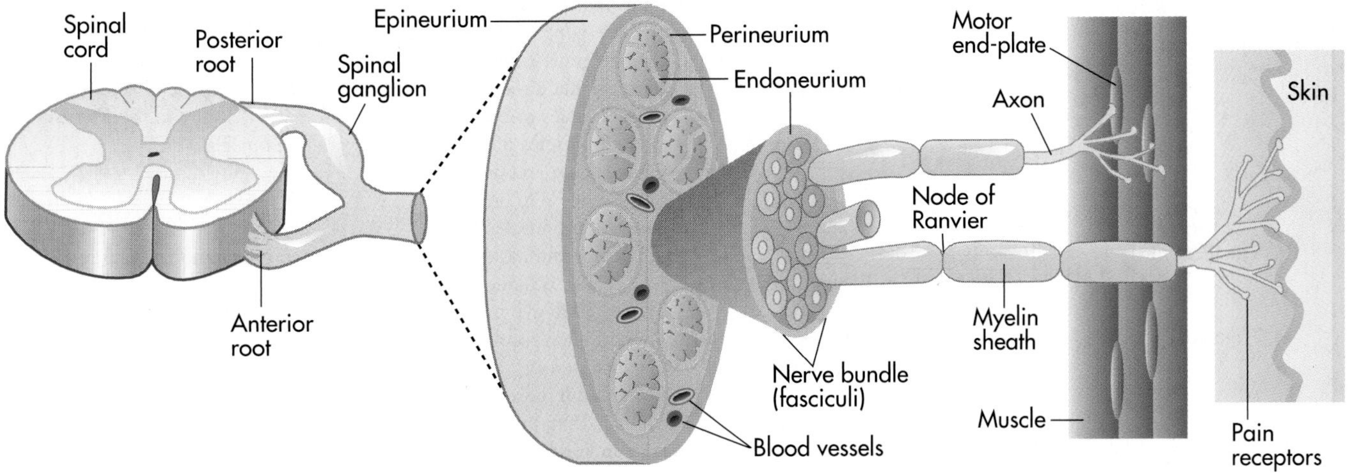

FIG. 13-22 Cranial and peripheral nerves. A, Ventral surface of the brain showing attachment of the cranial nerves. **B,** Peripheral nerve trunk and coverings. (**A, C,** From Thibodeau GA, Patton KI: *Anatomy and physiology,* ed 4, St Louis, 1999, Mosby.)

Continued

C

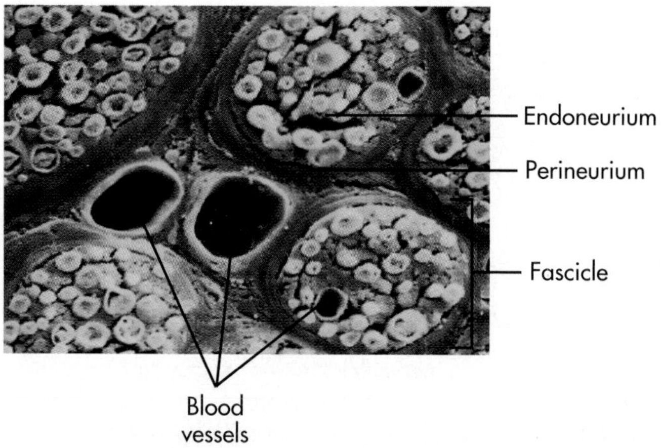

FIG. 13-22, cont'd Cranial and peripheral nerves. C, Scanning electron micrograph of a freeze-fractured preparation of peripheral nerve. (**A, C,** From Thibodeau GA, Patton KI: *Anatomy and physiology,* ed 4, St Louis, 1999, Mosby.)

plexus (L2 to L4) and **sacral plexus** (L5 to S5) contain nerves that innervate the anterior and posterior portions of the lower body, respectively.

The posterior rami of each spinal nerve, with their many processes, are distributed to a specific area in the body. Sensory signals thus arise from specific sites associated with a specific spinal cord segment. Specific areas of cutaneous (skin) innervation at these spinal cord segments are called **dermatomes.** The dermatomes of various spinal nerves are distributed in a fairly regular pattern, although adjacent regions between dermatomes can be innervated by more than one spinal nerve.

Like spinal nerves, cranial nerves are categorized as peripheral nerves. Most of these are mixed nerves (like the spinal nerves), although some are purely sensory or motor. Cranial nerves arise from nuclei in the brain and brain stem. (Fig. 13-22, *A,* illustrates their location, and Table 13-6 describes structural and functional characteristics.)

Table 13-6 The Cranial Nerves

Number and Name	Origin and Course	Function	How Tested
I. Olfactory	Fibers arise from nasal olfactory epithelium and form synapses with olfactory bulbs, which transmit impulses to temporal lobe	Purely sensory; carries impulses for sense of smell	Person is asked to sniff aromatic substances, such as oil of cloves and vanilla, and to identify them
II. Optic	Fibers arise from retina of eye to form optic nerve, which passes through sphenoid bone; two optic nerves then form optic chiasma (with partial crossover of fibers) and eventually end in occipital cortex	Purely sensory; carries impulses for vision	Vision and visual field tested with an eye chart and by testing point at which person first sees an object (finger) moving into visual field; inside of eye is viewed with ophthalmoscope to observe blood vessels of eye interior
III. Oculomotor	Fibers emerge from midbrain and exit from skull to run to eye	Contains motor fibers to inferior oblique, superior, inferior, and medial rectus extraocular muscles that direct eyeball; levator muscles of eyelid; smooth muscles of iris and ciliary body; and proprioception (sensory) to brain from extraocular muscles	Pupils examined for size, shape, and equality; pupillary reflex tested with a pen light (pupils should constrict when illuminated); ability to follow moving objects
IV. Trochlear	Fibers emerge from posterior midbrain and exit from skull and run to eye	Proprioceptor and motor fibers for superior oblique muscle of eye (external eye muscle)	Tested in common with cranial nerve III relative to ability to follow moving objects
V. Trigeminal	Fibers emerge from pons and form three divisions that exit from skull and run to face and cranial dura mater	Both motor and sensory for face; conducts sensory impulses from mouth, nose, surface of eye, and dura mater; also contains motor fibers that stimulate chewing muscles	Sensations of pain, touch, and temperature tested with safety pin and hot and cold objects; corneal reflex tested with a wisp of cotton; motor branch tested by asking subject to clench teeth, open mouth against resistance, and move jaw from side to side
VI. Abducens	Fibers leave inferior pons and exit from skull to run to eye	Contains motor fibers to lateral rectus muscle and proprioceptor fibers from same muscle to brain	Tested in common with cranial nerve III relative to ability to move each eye laterally

AUTONOMIC NERVOUS SYSTEM

Components of the autonomic nervous system (ANS) are located in both the CNS and PNS; however, the ANS is considered part of the efferent division of the PNS, even though visceral afferent neurons are an important part of this system. Many neurons of the ANS travel in spinal nerves and certain cranial nerves. The widespread activity of this system indicates that its components are distributed all over the body. The peripheral autonomic nerves carry mainly efferent fibers. The motor component of the ANS is a two-neuron system consisting of **preganglionic neurons** (myelinated) and **postganglionic neurons** (unmyelinated) (Fig. 13-23). This arrangement contrasts with the somatic nervous system, where a single motor neuron travels from the CNS to the innervated structure. Visceral afferent neurons have their cell bodies in some sensory and cranial ganglia and their fiber processes traveling in peripheral nerves. The CNS has autonomic areas in the intermediolateral horns of the spinal cord, cardiovascular and respiratory centers in the reticular formation, and both sympathetic and parasympathetic areas in the hypothalamus. CNS pathways interconnect all these areas.

The ANS coordinates and maintains a steady state among visceral (internal) organs, such as regulation of cardiac muscle, smooth muscle, and the glands of the body. This system is considered an involuntary system because one *generally* cannot "will" these functions to happen. The ANS is separated both structurally and functionally into two divisions: (1) the **sympathetic nervous system** (Fig. 13-24) and (2) the **parasympathetic nervous system** (Fig. 13-25).

Anatomy of the Sympathetic Nervous System

The sympathetic nervous system functions to mobilize energy stores in times of need (e.g., in the fight-or-flight response) (see Fig. 9-1; see also Chapter 9). The sympathetic division receives its innervation from cell bodies located from the first

Table 13-6 The Cranial Nerves—cont'd

Number and Name	Origin and Course	Function	How Tested
VII. Facial	Fibers leave pons and travel through temporal bone to reach face	Mixed: (1) supplies motor fibers to muscles of facial expression and to lacrimal and salivary glands and (2) carries sensory fibers from taste buds of anterior part of tongue	Anterior two thirds of tongue tested for ability to taste sweet (sugar), salty, sour (vinegar), and bitter (quinine) substances; symmetry of face checked; subject asked to close eyes, smile, whistle, and so on; tearing tested with ammonia fumes
VIII. Vestibulocochlear (acoustic)	Fibers run from inner ear (hearing and equilibrium receptors in temporal bone) to enter brain stem just below pons	Purely sensory; vestibular branch transmits impulses for sense of equilibrium; cochlear branch transmits impulses for sense of hearing	Hearing checked by air and bone conduction by use of a tuning fork; vestibular tests: Bárány and caloric tests
IX. Glossopharyngeal	Fibers emerge from midbrain and leave skull to run to throat	Mixed: (1) motor fibers serve pharynx (throat) and salivary glands, and (2) sensory fibers carry impulses from pharynx, posterior tongue (taste buds), and pressure receptors of carotid artery	Gag and swallowing reflexes checked; subject asked to speak and cough; posterior one third of tongue may be tested for taste
X. Vagus	Fibers emerge from medulla, pass through skull, and descend through neck region into thorax and abdominal region	Fibers carry sensory and motor impulses for pharynx; a large part of this nerve is parasympathetic motor fibers, which supply smooth muscles of abdominal organs; transmits sensory impulses from viscera	Same as for cranial nerve IX (IX and X are tested in common) because they both serve muscles of throat
XI. Spinal accessory	Fibers arise from medulla and superior spinal cord and travel to muscles of neck and back	Provides sensory and motor fibers for sternocleidomastoid and trapezius muscles and muscles of soft palate, pharynx, and larynx	Sternocleidomastoid and trapezius muscles checked for strength by asking subject to rotate head and shrug shoulders against resistance
XII. Hypoglossal	Fibers arise from medulla and exit from skull to travel to tongue	Carries motor fibers to muscles of tongue and sensory impulses from tongue to brain	Subject asked to stick out tongue, and any position abnormalities are noted

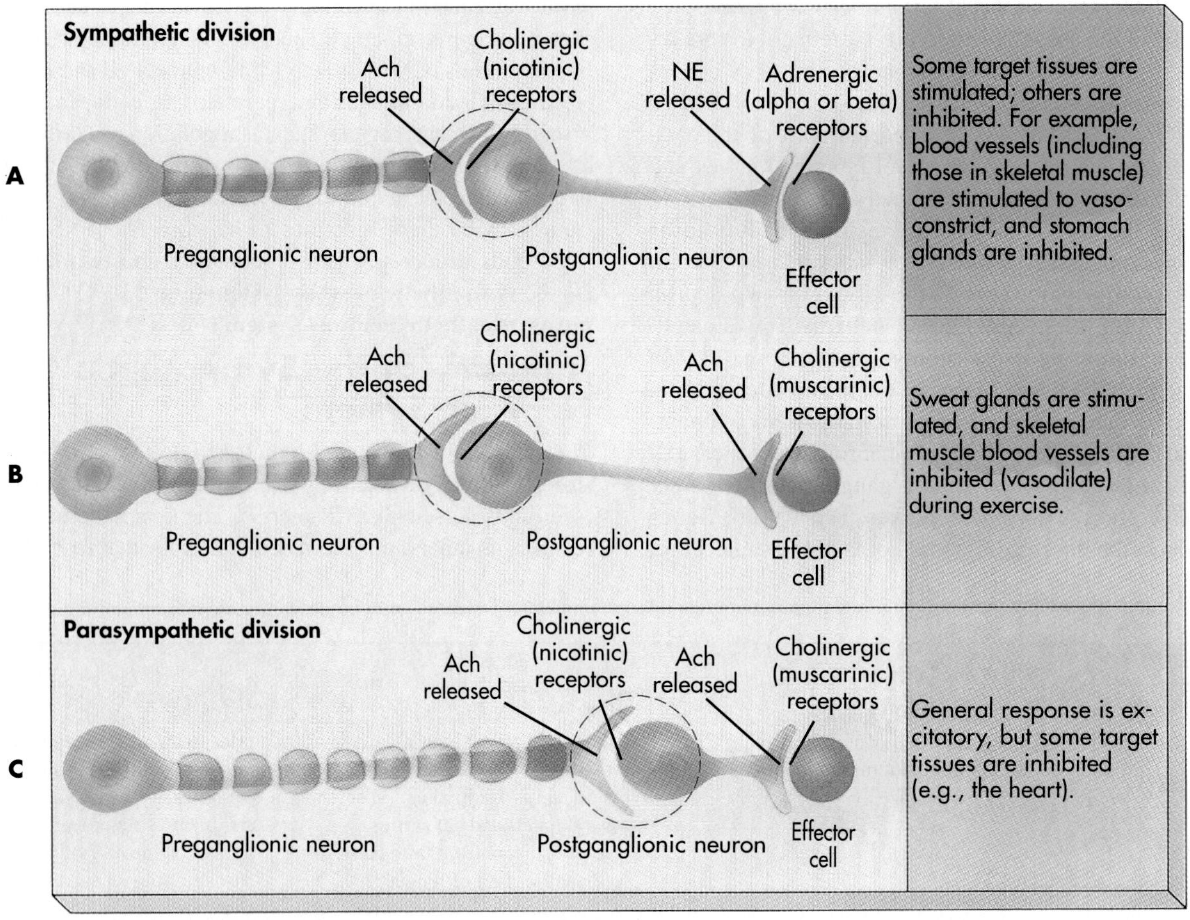

FIG. 13-23 Locations of neurotransmitters and receptors of the autonomic nervous system. In all pathways, preganglionic fibers are cholinergic, secreting acetylcholine *(Ach),* which stimulates nicotinic receptors in the postganglionic neuron. Most sympathetic postganglionic fibers are adrenergic **(A)**, secreting norepinephrine *(NE),* thus stimulating α- or β-adrenergic receptors. A few sympathetic postganglionic fibers are cholinergic, stimulating muscarinic receptors in effector cells **(B)**. All parasympathetic postganglionic fibers are cholinergic **(C)**, stimulating muscarinic receptors in effector cells. (From Thibodeau GA, Patton KI: *Anatomy and physiology,* ed 4, St Louis, 1999, Mosby.)

thoracic (T1) through the second lumbar (L2) regions of the spinal cord and is therefore called the **thoracolumbar division.** The preganglionic axons of the sympathetic division form synapses shortly after leaving the cord in the **sympathetic (paravertebral) ganglia.** At this point the impulse may travel several ways: (1) directly across the same ganglion level and form a synapse with the cell bodies of the postganglionic neuron, (2) up or down the sympathetic chain before forming synapses with a higher or lower postganglionic neuron (divergence), or (3) through the chain ganglion without synapsing (see Fig. 13-24). Some preganglionic axons form pathways called **splanchnic nerves,** which lead to **collateral ganglia** that surround the abdominal aorta. The collateral ganglia are named according to the branches of the aorta nearest them, namely, the **celiac, superior mesenteric,** and **inferior mesenteric.** The preganglionic neurons synapse with postganglionic neurons within the collateral ganglia. These postganglionic neurons leave the collateral ganglia and innervate the viscera below the diaphragm.

Preganglionic sympathetic neurons that innervate the adrenal medulla also travel in the splanchnic nerves and do *not* synapse before reaching the gland. The secretory cells in the adrenal medulla are considered modified postganglionic neurons. Because preganglionic sympathetic fibers are all myelinated, travel to the adrenal medulla is quick, and innervation causes the rapid release of epinephrine and norepinephrine. Epinephrine and norepinephrine are mediators of the fight-or-flight response (see Chapter 9).

Anatomy of the Parasympathetic Nervous System

The parasympathetic nervous system functions to conserve and restore energy. The nerve cell bodies of this division are located in the cranial nerve nuclei and in the sacral region of the spinal cord and therefore constitute the **craniosacral division.** Unlike the sympathetic division, the preganglionic fibers in the parasympathetic division travel to ganglia close to the organs they innervate before forming synapses with the relatively short postganglionic neurons (see Fig. 13-25). Parasympathetic nerves arising from nuclei in the brain stem travel to the viscera of the head, thorax, and abdomen within

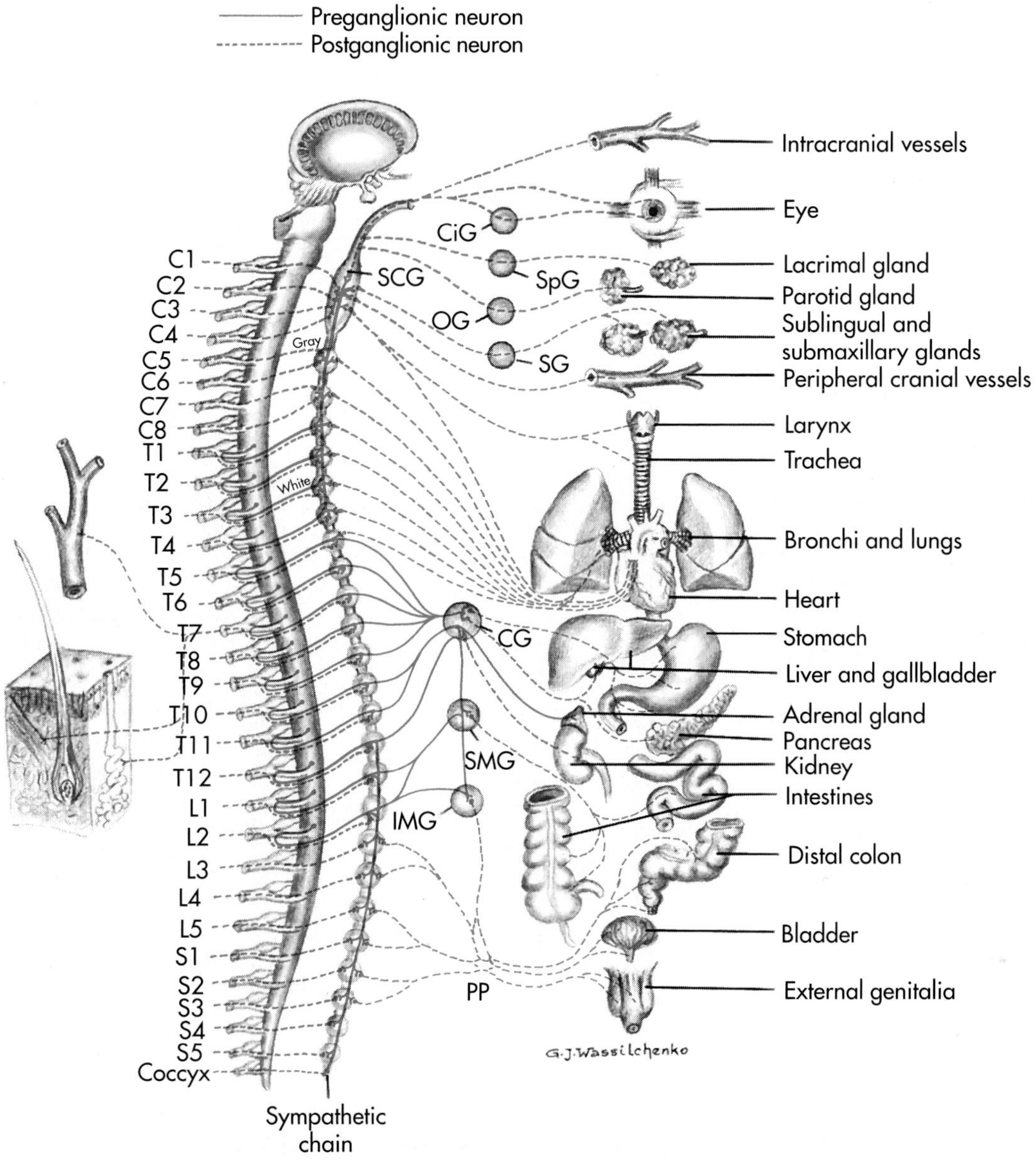

FIG. 13-24 Sympathetic division of the autonomic nervous system. *CiG,* Ciliary ganglion; *SpG,* sphenopalatine ganglion; *SCG,* superior cervical ganglion; *OG,* otic ganglion; *SG,* submandibular ganglion; *CG,* celiac ganglion; *SMG,* superior mesenteric ganglion; *IMG,* inferior mesenteric ganglion; *PP,* pelvic plexus. Fibers of the parasympathetic system pass through the CG and SMG, but these ganglia are not part of the parasympathetic system. (From Rudy EB, editor: *Advanced neurological and neurosurgical nursing,* St Louis, 1984, Mosby.)

cranial nerves—including the oculomotor (III), facial (VII), glossopharyngeal (IX), and vagus (X) nerves.

Preganglionic parasympathetic nerves that originate from the sacral region of the spinal cord run either separately or together with some spinal nerves. The preganglionic axons join together to form the **pelvic nerve,** which innervates the viscera of the pelvic cavity. These preganglionic axons synapse with postganglionic neurons in terminal ganglia located close to the organs they innervate.

Neurotransmitters and Neuroreceptors

Sympathetic preganglionic fibers and parasympathetic preganglionic and postganglionic fibers release **acetylcholine**—the same neurotransmitter released by somatic efferent neurons (Fig. 13-26; also see Fig. 13-23). These fibers are characterized by **cholinergic transmission.** Most postganglionic sympathetic fibers release **norepinephrine** (adrenaline) and thus are considered to function by **adrenergic transmission.** A few postganglionic sympathetic fibers, such as those that innervate the sweat glands, release acetylcholine.

The action of catecholamines (epinephrine, norepinephrine, dopa) varies with the type of neuroreceptor stimulated. It should be remembered that catecholamines also are released by the adrenal medulla gland that physiologically and biochemically resembles the sympathetic nervous system. Two types of adrenergic receptors exist: α- and β-adrenergic receptors. Cells of the effector organs may have only one or

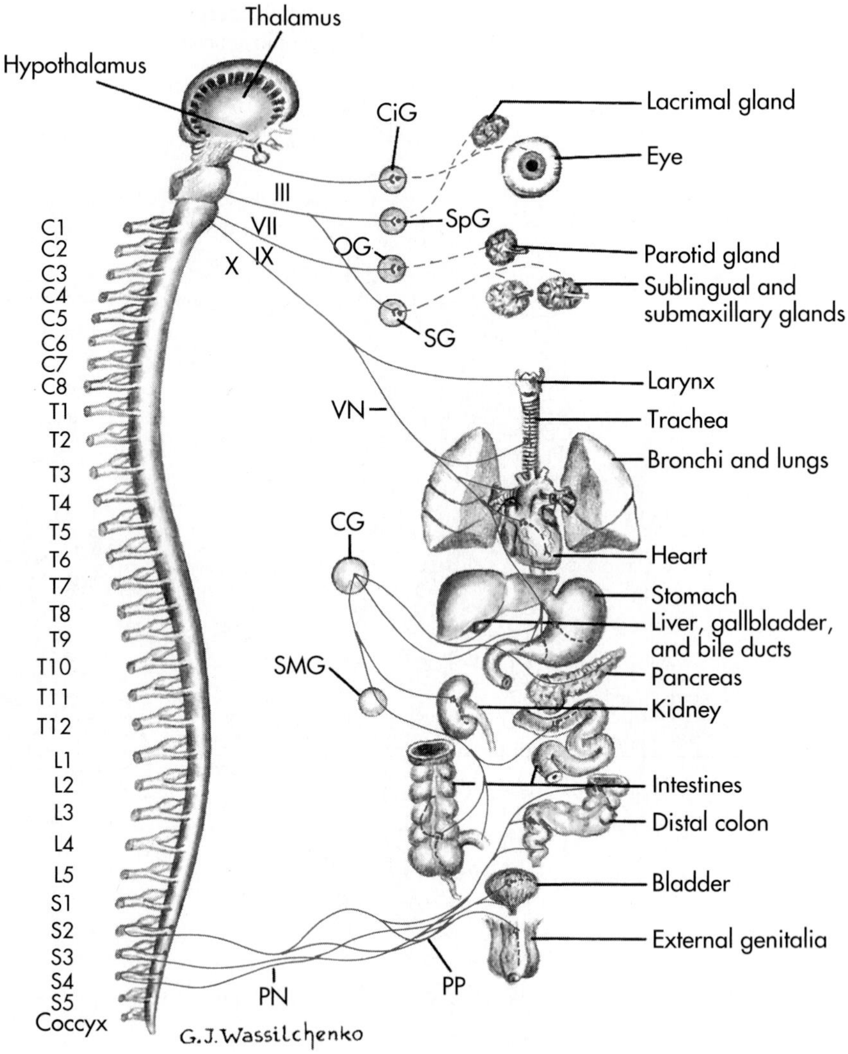

FIG. 13-25 Parasympathetic division of the autonomic nervous system. *CiG,* Ciliary ganglion; *SpG,* sphenopalatine ganglion; *OG,* otic ganglion; *SG,* submandibular ganglion; *VN,* vagus nerve; *CG,* celiac ganglion; *SMG,* superior mesenteric ganglion; *PP,* pelvic plexus; *PN,* pelvic nerve. Fibers of the parasympathetic system pass through the CG and SMG, but these ganglia are not part of the parasympathetic system. (From Rudy EB, editor: *Advanced neurological and neurosurgical nursing,* St Louis, 1984, Mosby.)

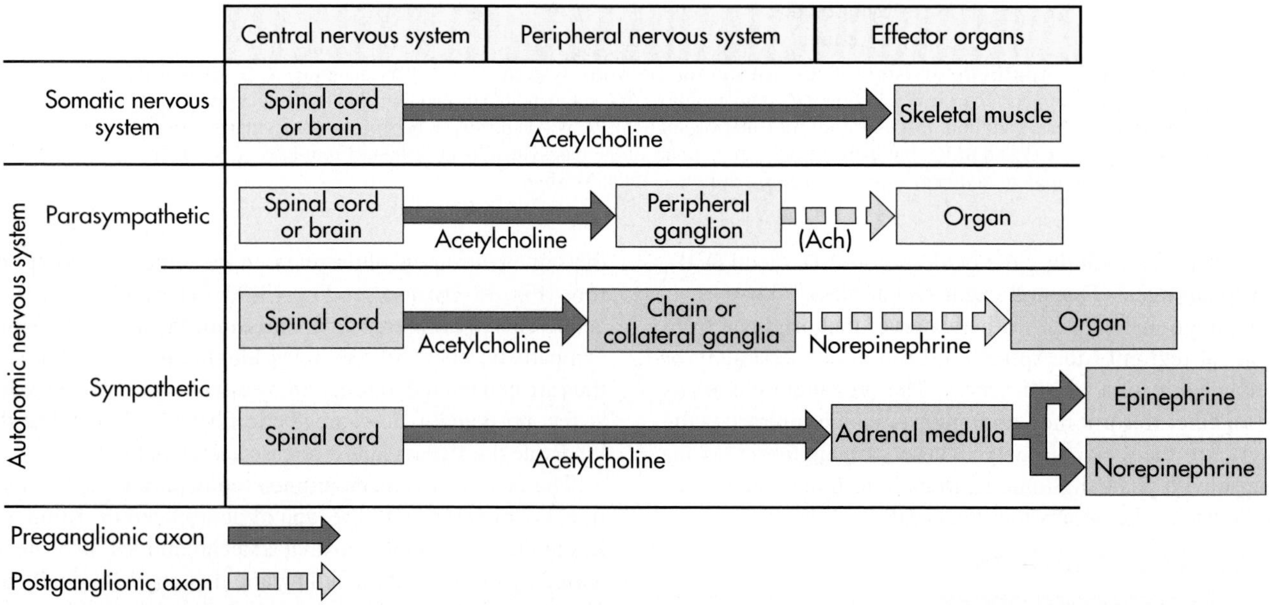

FIG. 13-26 The autonomic nervous system and the type of neurotransmitters secreted by preganglionic and postganglionic fibers. Note that all preganglionic fibers are cholinergic *(Ach).* A somatic nerve is used for comparison.

both types of adrenergic receptors. The **α-adrenergic receptors** have been further subdivided according to the action produced: α_1-adrenergic activity is associated mostly with excitation or stimulation; α_2-adrenergic activity is associated with relaxation or inhibition. Most of the α-adrenergic receptors on effector organs belong to the α_1-adrenergic class. The **β-adrenergic receptors** are classified as β_1-adrenergic receptors (which facilitate increased heart rate and contractility and cause the release of renin from the kidney) and β_2-adrenergic receptors (which facilitate all of the remaining effects attributed to β-adrenergic receptors).[5] Norepinephrine stimulates all α-adrenergic and β_1-adrenergic receptors and only certain β_2-adrenergic receptors. The primary response from norepinephrine, however, is stimulation of the α_1-adrenergic receptors that cause vasoconstriction. Epinephrine strongly stimulates all four types of receptors and induces general vasodilation because of the predominance of β-adrenergic receptors in muscle vasculatures. (Table 13-7 summarizes the effects of neuroreceptors on their effector organs.)

Table 13-7 Actions of Autonomic Nervous System Neuroreceptors

Effector Organ or Tissue	Receptor	Adrenergic Effect	Cholinergic Effect
Eye, iris			
Radial muscle	α_1	Contraction (mydriasis)	—
Sphincter muscle	—	—	Contraction (miosis)
Eye, ciliary muscle	β_2	Relaxation for far vision	Contraction for near vision
Lacrimal glands	—	—	Secretion
Nasopharyngeal glands	—	—	Secretion
Salivary glands	α_1	Secretion of potassium and water	Secretion of potassium and water
	β	Secretion of amylase	—
Heart			
SA node	β_1	Increased heart rate	Decrease heart rate; vagus arrest
Atrial	β_1	Increased contractility and conduction velocity	Decrease contractility; shorten action potential duration
AV junction	β_1	Increased automaticity and propagation velocity	Decrease automaticity and propagation velocity
Purkinje system	β_1	Increased automaticity and propagation velocity	—
Ventricles	β_1	Increased contractility	—
Arterioles			
Coronary	α_1, β_2	Constriction, dilation	Dilation
Skin and mucosa	α_1, α_2	Constriction	Dilation
Skeletal muscle	α, β_2	Constriction, dilation	Dilation
Cerebral	α_1	Constriction (slight)	—
Pulmonary	α_1, β_2	Constriction, dilation	—
Mesenteric	α_1	Constriction	—
Renal	$\alpha_1, \beta_1, \beta_2$, D	Constriction, dilation	—
Salivary glands	α_1, α_2	Constriction	Dilation
Veins, systemic	α_1, β_2	Constriction, dilation	—
Lung			
Bronchial muscle	β_2	Relaxation	Contraction
Bronchial glands	α_1, β_2	Decreased secretion; increased secretion	Stimulation
Stomach			
Motility	α_1, β_2	Decrease (usually)	Increase
Sphincters	α_1	Contraction (usually)	Relaxation (usually)
Secretion	—	Inhibition (?)	Stimulation
Liver	α, β_2	Glycogenolysis and gluconeogenesis	Glycogen synthesis
Gallbladder and ducts	—	Relaxation	Contraction
Pancreas			
Acini	α	Decreased secretion	Secretion
Islet cells	α_2, β_2	Decreased secretion; increased secretion	—
Intestine			
Motility and tone	$\alpha_1, \beta_1, \beta_2$	Decrease	Increase
Sphincters	α_1	Contraction (usually)	Relaxation (usually)
Secretion	α_2	Inhibition (?)	Stimulation
Adrenal medulla	—	—	Secretion of epinephrine and norepinephrine (nicotinic effect)
Kidney			
Renin secretion	α_1, β_1	Decrease; increase	—

Continued

Table 13-7 Actions of Autonomic Nervous System Neuroreceptors—cont'd

Effector Organ or Tissue	Receptor	Adrenergic Effect	Cholinergic Effect
Ureter			
Motility and tone	α_1	Increase	Increase
Urinary bladder			
Detrusor	β_2	Relaxation (usually)	Contraction
Trigone and sphincter	α_1	Contraction	Relaxation
Sex organs, male	α_1	Ejaculation	Erection
Skin			
Pilomotor muscles	α_1	Contraction	—
Sweat glands	α_1	Localized secretion	Generalized secretion
Fat cells	α_2; $\beta_1(\beta_3)$	Inhibition of lipolysis; stimulation of lipolysis	—
Pineal gland	β	Melatonin synthesis	—

Functions

Many body organs are innervated by both the sympathetic and parasympathetic nervous systems. The two divisions frequently cause opposite responses; for example, sympathetic stimulation of the gastrointestinal (GI) tract causes decreased peristalsis, whereas parasympathetic stimulation of the GI tract increases peristalsis. In general, sympathetic stimulation promotes responses that are concerned with the protection of the individual. For example, sympathetic activity increases blood sugar levels and temperature and raises blood pressure. In emergency situations a generalized and widespread discharge of the sympathetic system occurs. This is accomplished by an increased firing frequency of sympathetic fibers and by activation of sympathetic fibers normally silent and at rest (fibers to the sweat glands, pilomotor muscles, and the adrenal medulla, as well as vasodilator fibers to muscle). Regulation of vasomotor tone is considered the single most important function of the sympathetic nervous system. (Fig. 13-27 illustrates some of the most important functions of the sympathetic nervous system; also see Fig. 9-1.)

Increased parasympathetic activity promotes rest and tranquility and is characterized by reduced heart rate and enhanced visceral functions leading to digestion. Stimulation of the vagus nerve in the GI tract increases peristalsis and secretion, as well as relaxation of sphincters. Activation of parasympathetic fibers in the head, provided by cranial nerves III, VII, and IX, causes constriction of the pupil, tear secretion, and increased salivary secretion. Stimulation of the sacral division of the parasympathetic system contracts the urinary bladder and facilitates the process of genital erection.

The parasympathetic system lacks the generalized and widespread response of the sympathetic system. Specific parasympathetic fibers are activated to regulate particular functions. Although the actions of the parasympathetic and sympathetic systems usually are antagonistic, there are exceptions. Changes in the shape of the lens (for near vision) require only oculomotor parasympathetic activity. Most of the blood vessels involved in the control of blood pressure are innervated by sympathetic nerves. Peripheral vascular resistance is increased and decreased by the relative activity of the sympathetic division without a counteracting parasympathetic component. To decrease blood pressure, therefore, it is more important to block or paralyze the continuous (tonic) discharge of the sympathetic system than to promote parasympathetic activity.

Aging and the Nervous System

The CNS mechanisms involved in the aging process are extremely complex, and many questions concerning the neurologic effects of aging have yet to be answered. Some of the identified mechanisms associated with aging are pathologic, but the distinction between these mechanisms and those that are a part of the normal aging process remains somewhat cloudy.

Structural Changes with Aging

The CNS demonstrates many structural changes during the aging process. The primary mechanism responsible for most of these structural changes is a decrease in the number of neurons. Predominant external features of the aging brain include decreased brain weight and size (primarily the frontal hemispheres), increased adherence of the dura mater to the skull, fibrosis and thickening of the meninges, narrowed gyri, and widened sulci with a corresponding increase in the size of the subarachnoid space. The basal ganglia and ventricular system are internal structures that commonly reveal changes with aging. The basal ganglia reveals aberrations in vascular structures, and the ventricles (primarily the lateral and third ventricles) are enlarged, probably because they occupy much of the space left by dead neurons.

Cellular Changes with Aging

Practically every cell type within the CNS reflects specific responses to aging. A decrease in the number of neurons characterizes aging. Although neuronal cell loss is a general feature of aging, the effects are not consistent with deteriorating mental function or age of the individual.[6] Controversy regarding the effects of neuronal cell loss still exists.

Principal cellular changes associated with aging include dendrite structure, lipofuscin deposition, and the presence of

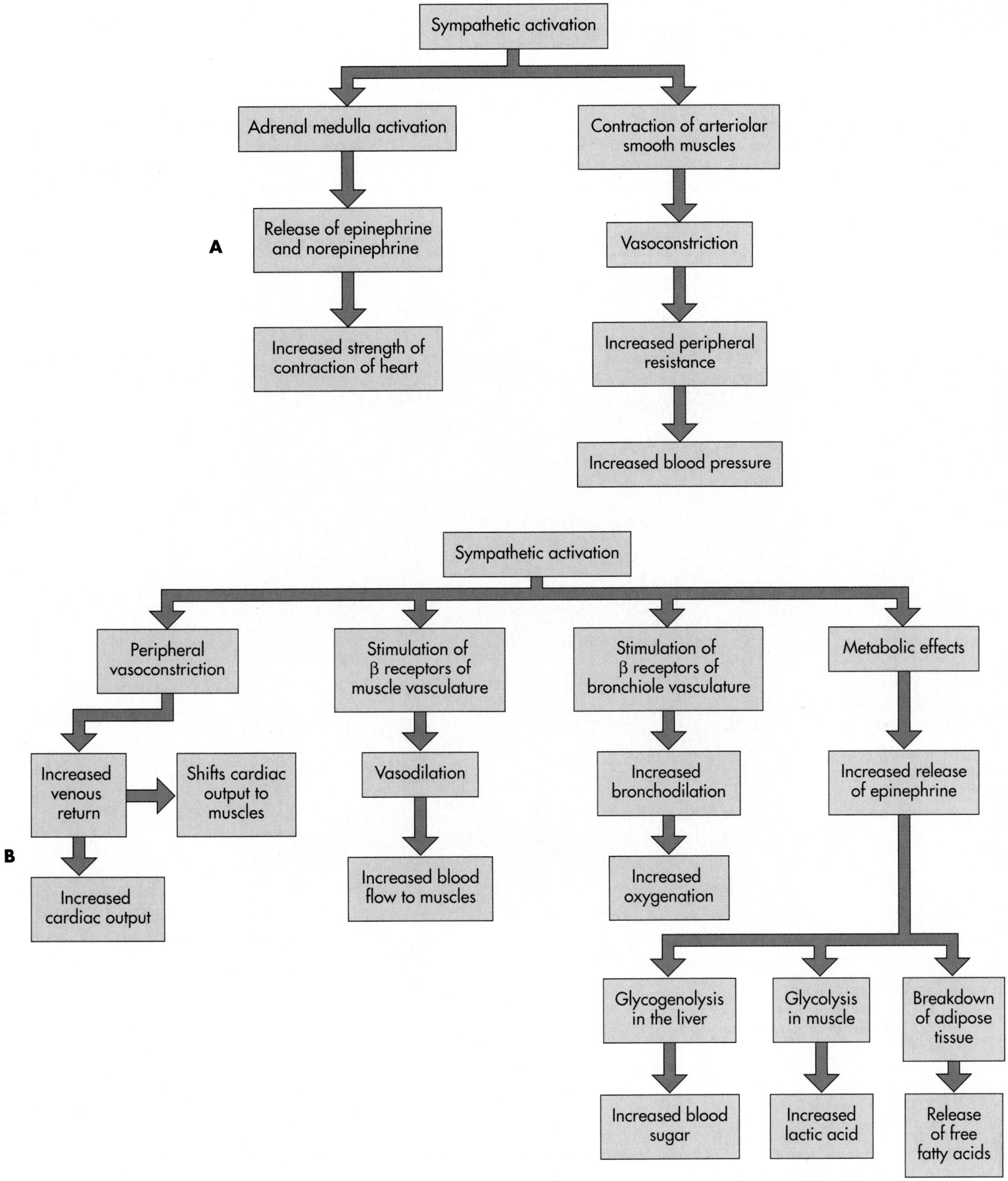

FIG. 13-27 Some important functions of the sympathetic nervous system. A, Regulation of vasomotor tone. **B,** Regulation of strenuous muscular exercise (fight-or-flight response). (See also Chapter 9 and Fig. 9-1 for more detail of the stress response.)

WHAT'S NEW? Reinforcement Center (Nucleus Accumbens)

Recently, a small nucleus (see accompanying figure) in the septal area of the frontal lobe has become a center of intense research. The nucleus accumbens is considered to be the principal site of action for addictive drugs and the anatomic basis of positive reinforcement. The nucleus accumbens has input from the mesencephalon (ventral tegmental area) and many other neural areas. Mesencephalon neurons project dopamine to the nucleus accumbens and can affect its activity. Other neurotransmitters involved in this positive feedback system are GABA, serotonin, and glutamate. Opiates can interfere with this system by allowing too much dopamine to go to the nucleus accumbens. The nucleus accumbens is involved in drug craving and withdrawal symptoms and therefore is clinically important.

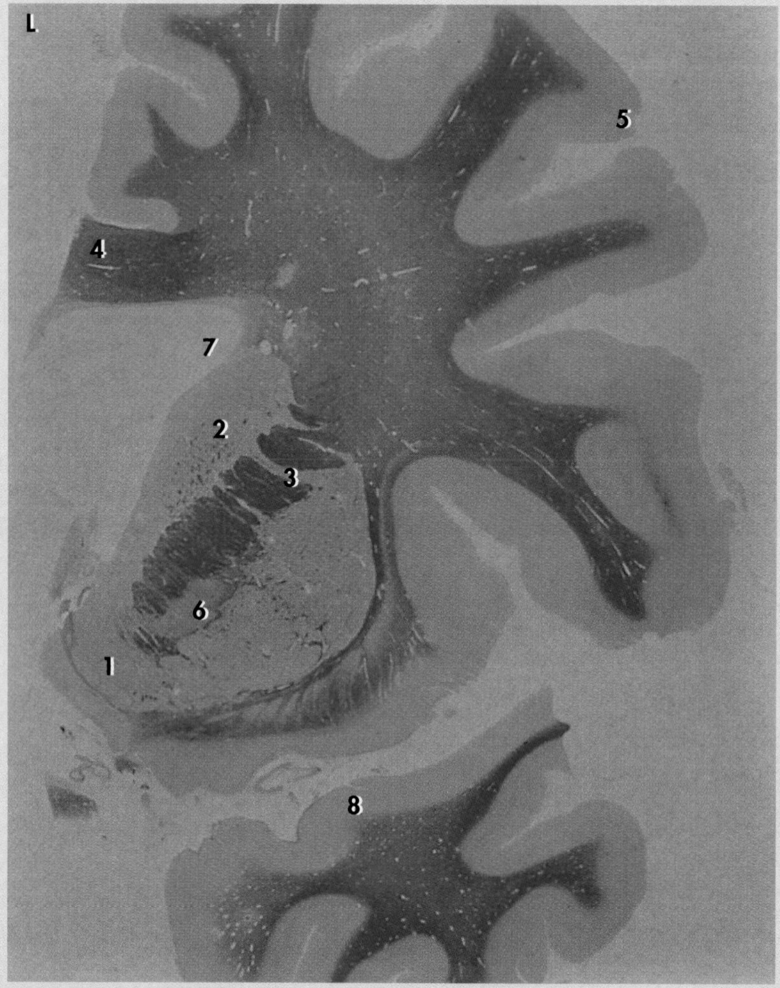

A histologic section through one cerebral hemisphere passing through the paraterminal gyrus to show the underlying nucleus accumbens. Solochrome cyanin and nuclear fast red stain.

1. Nucleus accumbens
2. Caudate nucleus
3. Continuity of caudate nucleus with putamen
4. Corpus callosum
5. Frontal lobe
6. Globus pallidus
7. Lateral ventricle
8. Temporal lobe

(From England MA, Wakely J: *Color atlas of the brain and spinal cord,* St Louis, 1991, Mosby. Copyright © 1991 Marjorie A. England and Jennifer Wakely.)

Data from Brown P, Molliver ME: Dual serotonin (5-HT) projections to the nucleus accumbens core and shell: relation of the 5-HT transporter to amphetamine-induced neurotoxicity, *J Neurosci* 20(5):1952, 2000; Charney DS, Nestler EJ, Bunney BS, editors: *Neurobiology of mental illness,* London, 1999, Oxford University Press.

neurofibrillary tangles, senile plaques, and Lewy bodies. Hirano and Llena[7] described a decreased number of dendritic processes and their multiple synaptic connections. Lipofuscin, a yellow-brown fatty pigment, is found to be deposited intracellularly in increased amounts with age. Controversy still exists concerning whether increasing intracellular quantities of lipofuscin might be associated with disruption of cytoplasmic function, that is, protein synthesis.[8]

Senile plaques (areas of nerve degeneration) are found in the interstitial spaces of the cerebral cortex associated with tissue degeneration. **Neurofibrillary tangles** involve degenerative changes in neural protein fibers. These entities also are common in Alzheimer disease and some other forms of dementia. At present there is growing definitive evidence of a link between quantitative cellular changes and nervous system function in aging individuals.

Closely paralleling cell function is a selective alteration in neurotransmitter function. One potentially fruitful area of research is correlating the effects of acetylcholine (i.e., cholinergic transmission) and defects of memory and cognitive function associated with aging.[8]

Functional Changes with Aging

Because of integrative processes in the CNS, the consequences of aging have widespread implications for critical steady state, psychologic, and social function. Many theories have been proposed to explain the observations of progressive slowing of neurologic responses seen in elderly persons (Table 13-8). Studies of changes in brain electrical activity have been helpful in determining alterations in neural function. Timiras[9] described the relationship between transmission of neural signals and slowing of responses observed in the elderly: "It is evident that the efficacy of the signals may be disturbed not only by irregularities in the action of cells carrying the signals but also by the amount of random background activity." This background activity is termed *neural noise.*

TESTS OF NERVOUS SYSTEM FUNCTION

Skull and Spine Roentgenograms

Roentgenograms (x-ray films) of the skull or spine from multiple angles (views) are used primarily to localize bony defects, bone density, erosion, or calcified structures. The pineal gland in older people becomes calcified and is useful as an internal brain landmark. X-ray films are probably the most commonly used radiologic studies.

Computed Tomography

Computed tomography (CT) creates two-dimensional reconstructions from multiple radiologic images (x-rays) using computer-assisted analysis. It is capable of demonstrating fine distinctions in densities of a variety of tissues. CT imaging is a safe and noninvasive procedure used in evaluating cranial and spinal structures, as well as hemorrhages, tumors, and distortions in the brain because of pressure differences. A variety of contrast media also are commonly used in conjunction with this procedure to aid in enhanced delineation of selected structures.

Magnetic Resonance Imaging

Magnetic resonance imaging (MRI) is now a commonly used testing modality. It uses a static magnetic field, instead of x-rays, to orient physiologic atomic particles. Disruption of this orientation by excitation of the particles using serial radiofrequency pulsations provides the image data. The specific tissue reaction is computer analyzed to give an image

Table 13-8 Common Neurologic Signs in Aging

Neurologic Sign	Examples	Changes in Response
Reflexes	Ankle reflex	Usually the first tendon reflex to be lost in elderly persons
	Superficial reflex	Decreased or absent responsiveness
Primitive reflexes (reflexes seen normally in infancy but that subside with maturity)	Suck and grasp	Reappearance with aging
Sensation	Taste and smell	Progressive deficit
	Pain	Increased pain threshold, although subjective complaints increase
	Vibratory sense	Decreased
	Vision	Decreased visual color sense in a significant percentage of aged persons; pupils commonly smaller; slowing of pupillary relaxation and accommodation
Motor function	Physiologic tremor	Exaggeration of normally unnoticeable resting tremor that is present at all ages
	Neuromuscular control	Decreased, resulting in postural effects
	Posture	Stance commonly shows increased flexion of hips and knees; swaying motion while standing in one position more common
	Gait	Shuffling or shortened stride; loss of arm movement with walking
	Muscular atrophy	Age-associated loss of muscle fibers

of exquisite detail, similar to that provided by CT. The MRI also provides reconstruction of images in three views at right angles (i.e., axial, sagittal, coronal). MRI is reported to have none of the adverse effects associated with radiation examinations.

Magnetic Resonance Angiography

A newer addition to MRI is **magnetic resonance angiography (MRA).** Special imaging techniques allow the visualization of blood vessels in great detail. MRA is likely to become indispensable, alone or in conjunction with cerebral angiography, in detecting and localizing pathologic lesions of the circulatory system of the brain.

Positron Emission Tomography Scan

The **positron emission tomography (PET) scan** uses CT imaging to detect the emission of positive electrons from radioactive substances. These substances are injected into the bloodstream or administered as inhaled gases. As they are distributed in tissues, they display characteristic patterns that indicate physiologic and metabolic processes, for example, glucose and oxygen uptake, cerebral blood flow, neural and neurotransmitter function, and the effects of drugs. As a research tool, PET is being used to visualize the specific brain sites that are involved in the processing of information in the brain.

Brain Scan

The **brain scan** images radionuclide substances (technetium [^{99m}Tc]) that have been introduced into the bloodstream. For example, visualization of tissue uptake of the radioactive agent provides an indication of blood-brain barrier integrity (increased uptake of the agent indicates disruption). This scanning technique also can identify abnormalities in blood flow dynamics and cellular metabolic function. The brain scan is particularly helpful in detecting abnormal vascularity resulting from neoplasms, abscesses, and vascular lesions.

Isotope cisternography is another radionuclide imaging technique that uses brain scan imaging to detect CSF flow, CSF resorption, and integrity of CSF pathways. The radionuclide agent in this case is injected directly into the subarachnoid space. Under normal conditions the agent passes over the cortical surface and is resorbed through the arachnoid villi. Demonstration of the agent in the ventricular system after a specific period of time indicates CSF obstruction; that is, the CSF backflows from the subarachnoid space into the ventricles.

Cerebral Angiography

Angiography is a radiologic technique that demonstrates cerebrovascular blood flow. This technique commonly is performed by the introduction of a small catheter into the femoral artery. The catheter is then passed to the level of the cerebral circulation and through the aorta, and a contrast dye is injected. Serial x-ray films are then taken. These films demonstrate flow of the dye through the cerebral vasculature and provide information on patency, location, size, and flow pattern of the vessels. Another technique used in cerebral angiography is the retrograde (reverse flow) injection of the dye through catheterization of a brachial, axillary, subclavian, or femoral vein.

Myelography

A **myelogram** demonstrates intraspinal anatomy by the introduction of a radiographic dye into the lumbar subarachnoid space or the cerebellomedullary cistern (cisterna magna). The dye is allowed to flow in a cephalic direction, as in the case of a lumbar injection, or inferiorly in a cerebellomedullary cistern puncture. X-ray films are then obtained. The distribution of the dye delineates spinal cord and nerve root structure and integrity.

Echoencephalography (Ultrasound)

Echoencephalography, or **ultrasound,** is a safe, noninvasive procedure using sound waves that are deflected at differing rates, depending on the density of the tissue. Information is processed and displayed on an oscilloscope screen. It is useful primarily in the detection of structural characteristics of intracranial space-occupying mass lesions and the determination of ventricular dimensions, especially in newborns.

Electroencephalography

The **electroencephalograph (EEG)** is a recording of electrical impulses, arising from the cortical surface of the brain, that is detected by scalp electrodes. The recording of brain wave patterns is analyzed for alterations or localization (or both) of specific electrical activity. This test is especially useful in detecting and localizing foci that initiate seizure activity. It is also an important technique in determining, from a person's brain activity, whether the person is legally "brain dead."

Evoked Potentials

Evoked potentials (EPs) are a method of detecting electrical brain activity that results from a stimulus—primarily auditory, visual, or peripheral sensory. Electrical activity is computer formatted to display changes in trends. The primary uses of EPs include perioperative detection of sensory pathway integrity and disease- or drug-related sensory dysfunction.

Cerebrospinal Fluid Analysis

Cerebrospinal fluid (CSF) generally is obtained from the lumbar or cisternal subarachnoid space by means of a hollow needle that allows passive flow. The lumbar puncture is performed most often at the L3–4 interspace (below the level of the spinal cord at L1–2). Cisternal puncture is performed by the insertion of a needle into the cerebellomedullary cistern using an approach from the back of the neck in the region of the foramen magnum. CSF pressure is commonly measured during these procedures. The CSF can be analyzed also for gross characteristics and constituents (color, blood cells, electrolytes, and protein) and cultured for microorganisms (Table 13-9).

Table 13-9 Cerebrospinal Fluid Analysis

Parameters	Normal	Abnormal	Possible Cause
Pressure (initial readings)	120-180 mm H_2O (9-14 mm Hg)	<60 mm H_2O	Faulty needle placement Dehydration Spinal block along subarachnoid space Block of foramen magnum
		>200 mm H_2O	Muscle tension Abdominal compression Brain tumor Subdural hematoma Brain abscess Brain cyst Cerebral edema (any cause) Hydrocephalus
Color	Clear, colorless	Cloudy	Increased cell count Increased microorganisms
		Yellow	Xanthochromic (caused by red blood cell [RBC] pigments) High protein content
		Smoky	Presence of RBCs
Red blood cells	None	Blood-tinged	Traumatic tap
		Grossly bloody	Traumatic tap Subarachnoid hemorrhage
White blood cells	0-6/mm^3	$>10/mm^3$ (Cell counts range from below 100 to many thousands depending on causative factor; all are abnormal findings.)	Occurs in many conditions: Bacterial infections of meninges Viral infections of meninges Neurosyphilis Tuberculous meningitis Metastatic neoplastic lesions Parasitic infections Acute demyelinating diseases Following introduction of air or blood into subarachnoid space
Protein*	15-45 mg/dl (1% of serum protein)	<10 mg/dl	Little clinical significance
		>60 mg/dl	Occurs in many conditions: Complete spinal block Guillain-Barré syndrome Carcinomatosis of meninges Tumors close to pial or ependymal surfaces or in cerebellopontine angle Acute and chronic meningitis Meningeal hemorrhage Demyelinating disorders Degenerative diseases
Glucose	50-75 mg/dl (approximately 60% of blood glucose level)	<40 mg/dl	Acute bacterial meningitis Tuberculous meningitis Meningeal carcinomatosis
		>100 mg/dl	Diabetes
Chloride	700-750 mg/dl; 125 mM	<625 mg/dl	Hypochloremia Tuberculous meningitis
		>800 mg/dl	Not of neurologic significance; correlates with blood levels of chloride

Data From Rudy EB, editor: *Advanced neurological and neurosurgical nursing,* St Louis, 1984, Mosby.
*NOTE: If CSF contains blood, this will raise the protein level.

SUMMARY REVIEW

Overview and Organization of the Nervous System

1. The divisions of the nervous system have been categorized as either structural (central nervous system [CNS] and peripheral nervous system [PNS]) or functional (somatic nervous system and autonomic nervous system [ANS]).
2. The CNS is contained within the brain and spinal cord.

3. The PNS is composed of cranial and spinal nerves, which carry impulses toward the CNS (afferent) and away from the CNS (efferent) to target organs or skeletal muscle.

Cells of the Nervous System

1. The neuron and neuroglial cells make up nervous tissue. The neuron is specialized to transmit and receive electrical and chemical impulses, and the neuroglial cell provides supportive functions. The neuron is further divided into unipolar, pseudounipolar, bipolar, and multipolar categories, according to structure and particular mechanics of impulse transmission.
2. The neuron is composed of a cell body, one or more dendrites, and an axon. A myelin sheath around selected axons forms an insulation that allows quicker nerve impulse conduction.

Nerve Impulse

1. The region between the neurons is the synapse, and the region between the neuron and muscle is the myoneural junction. Neurotransmitters are responsible for chemical conduction across the synapse and myoneural junction. Nerve impulse is predominantly regulated by a balance of inhibitory postsynaptic potentials (IPSPs) and excitatory postsynaptic potentials (EPSPs), temporal and spatial summation, and convergence and divergence.

Central Nervous System

1. The brain is contained within the cranial vault and is divided into three distinct regions: (a) forebrain, (b) hindbrain, and (c) midbrain.
2. The forebrain comprises the two cerebral hemispheres and allows conscious perception of internal and external stimuli, thought and memory processes, and voluntary control of skeletal muscles. The deep portion of the forebrain is termed the *diencephalon* and processes incoming sensory data. The center for voluntary control of skeletal muscle movements is located along the precentral gyrus in the frontal lobe, whereas the center for perception is along the postcentral gyrus in the parietal lobe. The Broca area (rostral to the postcentral gyrus) and the Wernicke area (superoposterior temporal lobe) are major speech centers.
3. The hindbrain allows sampling and comparison of sensory data from the periphery and motor impulses from the cerebral hemispheres for the purpose of coordination and refinement of skeletal muscle movement.
4. The midbrain is primarily a relay center for motor and sensory tracts, as well as a center for auditory and visual reflexes.
5. The spinal cord contains the majority of nerve fibers connecting the brain with the periphery. Reflex arcs are completed in the spinal cord and influenced by the higher centers in the brain.
6. The CNS is protected by the scalp, bony cranium, meninges, vertebral column, and cerebrospinal fluid. Cerebrospinal fluid is formed from blood components in the choroid plexuses of the ventricles and is reabsorbed in the arachnoid villi (located in the dural venous sinuses) after circulating through the brain and spinal cord.
7. The paired carotid and vertebral arteries supply blood to the brain and connect to form the circle of Willis. The major branches projecting from the circle of Willis are the anterior, middle, and posterior cerebral arteries. Drainage of blood from the brain is accomplished through the venous sinuses and jugular veins.
8. Blood supply to the spinal cord originates from the vertebral arteries and branches arising from the aorta.

Peripheral Nervous System

1. The PNS functions to relay information from the CNS to muscle and effector organs through cranial and spinal nerve tracts arranged in fascicles (multiple fascicles bound together form the peripheral nerve).

Autonomic Nervous System

1. The ANS is responsible for the maintenance of a steady state in the internal environment. Two opposing systems make up the ANS: (a) the sympathetic nervous system responds to stress by mobilizing energy stores and prepares the body to defend itself, and (b) the parasympathetic nervous system conserves energy and the body's resources.

Aging and the Nervous System

1. Major structural changes with aging include a decrease in number of neurons and a decrease in brain weight and size.
2. Deposition of lipofuscin and the presence of senile plaques, multiple neurofibrillary tangles, and Lewy bodies are common cellular changes with aging.
3. A progressive slowing of neurologic function occurs with advancing age.

Tests of Nervous System Function

1. Tests of nervous system function include x-ray films, computed tomography, magnetic resonance imaging and angiography, positron emission tomography, brain scan, cerebral angiography, myelography, echoencephalography, electroencephalography, evoked potentials, and analysis of the cerebrospinal fluid.

KEY TERMS

Acetylcholine, *389*
α-Adrenergic receptor, *391*
β-Adrenergic receptor, *391*
Adrenergic transmission, *389*
Afferent pathway (ascending pathway), *363*
Afferent (sensory) neuron, *377*
Amygdala, *372*
Angiography, *396*
Anterior cerebral artery, *381*
Anterior column (ventral column), *375*
Anterior fossa, *379*
Anterior horn (ventral horn), *375*
Anterior spinal artery, *382*
Anterior spinothalamic, *378*
Arachnoid membrane, *380*
Arachnoid villi, *380*
Arterial circle (circle of Willis), *381*
Association fiber, *371*
Associational neuron (interneuron), *365*
Astrocyte, *366*
Autonomic nervous system (ANS), *363*
Axon, *364*
Axon hillock, *364*
Basal ganglia, *371*
Basal ganglia system, *371*
Basilar artery, *381*
Basis pedunculi, *375*
Bipolar neuron, *365*
Blood-brain barrier, *384*
Brachial plexus, *384*
Brain scan, *396*
Brain stem, *369*
Broca speech area, *371*

KEY TERMS—cont'd

Cauda equina, *375*
Cavernous sinus, *381*
Celiac, *388*
Central canal, *375*
Central nervous system (CNS), *363*
Central sulcus (fissure of Rolando), *371*
Cerebellomedullary cistern (cisterna magna), *380*
Cerebellum, *375*
Cerebral aqueduct (aqueduct of Sylvius), *375*
Cerebral cortex, *371*
Cerebral nuclei, *372*
Cerebrospinal fluid (CSF), *380*
Cerebrum, *371*
Cholinergic transmission, *389*
Choroid plexus, *380*
Collateral ganglia, *388*
Computed tomography (CT), *395*
Contralateral control, *371*
Conus medullaris, *375*
Convergence, *365*
Corpora quadrigemina (tectum), *374*
Corpus callosum (commissural fibers), *371*
Corpus striatum, *372*
Corticobulbar, *378*
Corticospinal tract, *371*
Cranial nerve, *363*
Craniosacral division, *388*
Dendrite, *364*
Dendritic zone, *364*
Denticulate ligament, *380*
Dermatome, *386*
Diencephalon, *373*
Divergence, *365*
Dopamine, *375*
Dura mater, *379*
Echoencephalography (ultrasound), *396*
Effector organ, *363*
Efferent (motor) neuron, *377*
Efferent pathway (descending pathway), *363*
Electroencephalograph (EEG), *396*
Endoneurium, *364*
Epicritic, *378*
Epidural space, *380*
Epithalamus, *373*
Evoked potential (EP), *396*
Excitatory postsynaptic potential (EPSP), *367*
Facilitation, *368*
Falx cerebri, *379*
Fascicle, *384*
Filum terminale, *375*
Fissure, *371*
Frontal lobe, *371*
Galea aponeurotica, *379*
Ganglia, *364*
Gray matter, *371*
Hippocampus, *372*
Hypothalamus, *373*
Inferior colliculi, *375*
Inferior mesenteric, *388*
Inhibitory postsynaptic potential (IPSP), *368*
Inner dura or meningeal layer, *379*
Insula, *371*
Intermediolateral gray (lateral horn), *375*
Internal capsule, *372*
Internal carotid artery, *381*
Interventricular foramen (foramen of Monro), *380*
Intervertebral disk, *381*
Lateral aperture (foramen of Luschka), *380*
Lateral column, *375*
Lateral corticospinal, *378*
Lateral spinothalamic, *378*
Lateral sulcus (sylvian fissure, lateral fissure), *371*
Lentiform nucleus, *372*
Limbic system, *372*
Lower motor neuron, *378*
Lumbar cistern, *380*
Lumbar plexus, *384*
Lumbar puncture, *381*
Magnetic resonance angiography (MRA), *396*
Magnetic resonance imaging (MRI), *395*
Median aperture (foramen of Magendie), *380*
Medulla oblongata, *375*
Meninges, *379*
Metencephalon, *375*
Microfilament, *364*
Microglia, *366*
Microtubule, *364*
Midbrain (mesencephalon), *374*
Middle cerebral artery, *381*
Middle fossa (temporal fossa), *379*
Mixed nerve, *384*
Motor neuron, *365*
Motor unit, *378*
Multipolar neuron, *365*
Myelencephalon, *375*
Myelin, *364*
Myelin sheath, *364*
Myelogram, *396*
Neurilemma, *364*
Neurofibril, *364*
Neurofibrillary tangle, *395*
Neuroglia, *366*
Neuroglial cell, *364*
Neuromuscular (myoneural) junction, *378*
Neuron, *364*
Neurotransmitter, *367*
Nissl substance, *364*
Node of Ranvier, *364*
Norepinephrine, *389*
Nucleus, *364*
Nucleus pulposus, *381*
Occipital lobe, *371*
Oligodendrocyte, *366*
Oligodendroglia, *366*
Papez circuit, *372*
Parasympathetic nervous system, *387*
Parietal lobe, *371*
Pelvic nerve, *389*
Periosteum (endosteal layer), *379*
Peripheral nervous system (PNS), *363*
Pia mater, *380*
Plasticity, *371*
Plexus, *364*
Pons, *375*
Positron emission tomography (PET) scan, *396*
Postcentral gyrus, *371*
Posterior cerebral artery, *381*
Posterior column (dorsal column), *375*
Posterior fossa, *379*
Posterior horn (dorsal horn), *375*
Posterior spinal artery, *382*
Postganglionic neuron, *387*
Postsynaptic neuron, *367*
Precentral gyrus, *371*
Prefrontal area, *371*
Preganglionic neuron, *387*
Premotor area, *371*
Presynaptic neuron, *367*
Primary motor area, *371*
Primary voluntary motor area, *371*
Projecting artery (nutrient artery), *381*
Protopathic, *379*
Pseudounipolar neuron, *365*
Red nucleus, *375*
Reflex arc, *377*
Reticular activating system, *371*
Reticular formation, *369*
Roentgenogram (x-ray film), *395*
Sacral plexus, *386*
Saltatory conduction, *364*
Schwann cell, *364*
Schwann sheath, *364*
Senile plaque, *395*
Sensory ganglion (dorsal root ganglion), *375*
Sensory neuron, *365*
Somatic nervous system, *363*
Spatial summation, *368*
Spinal cord, *375*
Spinal nerve, *363*
Spinal tract, *375*
Spinothalamic tract, *375*
Splanchnic nerve, *388*
Subarachnoid space, *380*
Subdural space, *380*
Substantia gelatinosa, *375*
Substantia nigra, *375*
Subthalamic nucleus, *374*
Subthalamus, *373*
Sulci, *371*
Summation, *368*

KEY TERMS—cont'd

REFERENCES

1. Waxman SG: *Correlative neuroanatomy,* ed 24, New York, 2000, Lange Medical Books/McGraw-Hill.
2. Fuller RW: Neural functions of serotonin, *Sci Med* 2(4):48, 1995.
3. Kandel ER, Schwartz JH, Jessell TM, editors: *Principles of neural science,* ed 4, New York, 2000, McGraw-Hill.
4. Pritchard TC, Alloway KD: *Medical neuroscience,* Hershey, PA, 1999, Fence Creek Publications.
5. Benarroch EE et al: *Medical neurosciences,* ed 4, Baltimore, 1999, Lippincott Williams & Wilkins.
6. Scheibel ES, Scheibel BS: Structural changes in the aging brain. In Brody H, Harman D, Ordy JM, editors: *Clinical, morphological, and neurochemical aspects of the aging nervous system,* New York, 1975, Raven.
7. Hirano A, Llena JF: Degenerative diseases of the central nervous system. In Rosenburg RN, editor: *The clinical neurosciences: neuropathology,* vols 1 and 2, New York, 1983, Churchill Livingstone.
8. Wang E, Snyder S, editors: *Handbook of the aging brain,* San Diego, 1998, Academic Press.
9. Timiras PS, editor: *Physiologic basis of aging and geriatrics,* ed 2, Boca Raton, 1994, CRC Press.

CHAPTER 14

Pain, Temperature Regulation, Sleep, and Sensory Function

SUE E. HUETHER • JONATHAN LEO

CHAPTER OUTLINE

Alterations in sensory function may involve dysfunctions of the general or the special senses. Dysfunctions of the general senses include chronic pain, abnormal temperature regulation, tactile dysfunction, and proprioceptive dysfunction. Dysfunctions of the special senses include visual, auditory, vestibular, olfactory, and gustatory (taste) dysfunction.

The special senses of vision, hearing, touch, smell, and taste are the means by which individuals perceive stimuli that are essential in interacting with the environment. Special sensory receptors are connected to specific areas of the cerebral cortex through the afferent pathways of the central nervous system (CNS). Each of the special senses thus involves a connected system of organs and tissues that receives stimuli and portions of the CNS, where sensory stimuli are processed.

All definitions of pain suggest that it is a complex phenomenon composed of sensory experiences that include time, space, intensity, emotion, cognition, and motivation. Pain is an unpleasant phenomenon that is uniquely experienced by each individual; it cannot be adequately defined, identified, or measured by an observer. McCaffery[2] defines pain as "whatever the experiencing person says it is, existing whenever he says it does."

Unlike pain, which is a subjective experience without a precise form of measurement, temperature regulation is measured by clearly defined normal limits. Like pain, however, variations in temperature can signal disease. Fever is a common manifestation of dysfunction and is often the first symptom observed in an infectious or inflammatory condition. If the body's temperature regulatory mechanism is out of balance, the result may be death.

Sleep is a normal, cyclic process that restores the body's energy and maintains normal functioning. Sleep is so essential to both physiologic and psychologic function that sleep deprivation causes a wide range of clinical manifestations. Prolonged deprivation or disruption of sleep ultimately leads to serious dysfunction.

PAIN

The Experience of Pain

Three systems interact to produce pain: (1) the sensory/discriminative system, (2) the motivational/affective system, and (3) the cognitive/evaluative system.[1] The **sensory/discriminative system** processes information about the strength, intensity, and temporal and spatial aspects of pain. These sensations are mediated through afferent nerve fibers, the spinal cord, the brain stem, and the higher brain centers, and they result in prompt withdrawal from the painful stimulus.

The **motivational/affective system** determines the individual's conditioned or learned approach and avoidance behaviors. These behaviors are mediated through the interaction of the reticular formation, limbic system, and brain stem.

The **cognitive/evaluative system** overlies the individual's learned behavior concerning the experience of pain. The individual's interpretation of appropriate pain behavior is learned in several ways; among them are cultural preferences, male and female roles, and experience. The influence of the cognitive/evaluative system may block, modulate, or enhance the perception of pain.

Somatogenic versus Psychogenic Pain

Attempts to categorize pain have suggested two common classes: (1) somatogenic and (2) psychogenic. **Somatogenic pain,** such as the pain of a crushed finger or a heart attack, is pain with a cause. In contrast, **psychogenic pain** is pain for which there is no known physical cause. Psychogenic pain, however, is *not* imaginary pain. It may be just as intense as somatogenic pain and just as distressing. The labels *somatogenic* and *psychogenic* provide some basis for describing pain, but pain is only *primarily* somatogenic or psychogenic; it is rarely, if ever, purely one type or the other.[2]

Acute versus Chronic Pain

The pain experience may be functionally divided into acute and chronic types. **Acute pain** is a protective mechanism that alerts the individual to a condition or experience that is immediately harmful to the body. The onset of acute pain is usually sudden, and the pain is relieved after the chemical mediators that stimulate the nociceptors are removed. Acute anxiety is always associated with acute pain. Anxiety is a response to the threat inherent in the painful experience, including issues surrounding the cause of pain, its treatment, and prognosis. Hope of recovery is also associated with acute pain. Acute pain mobilizes the individual to take prompt action to relieve it.[3]

Chronic pain is persistent—usually defined as lasting at least 6 months. The cause of chronic pain often is unknown, and if the cause is known, the pain does not respond to usual therapy. The onset may be sudden, but chronic pain often develops insidiously so that the individual generally experiences more suffering over time. Individual behavior is adaptive and directed toward modifying the pain. Chronic pain often is associated with a sense of hopelessness and helplessness as the cure becomes more elusive and the time frame protracted. The pain is perceived as meaningless, and depression often results. (Table 14-1 compares the characteristics of chronic and acute pain.)

Pain Threshold and Pain Tolerance

The **pain threshold** is the point at which a stimulus is perceived as pain. The threshold does not vary significantly among people or in the same person over time. Intense pain at one location, however, may cause an increase in the threshold in another location. For example, a person with se-

Table 14-1 Comparison of Acute and Chronic Pain

Characteristic	Acute Pain	Chronic Pain
Experience	An event	A situation, state of existence
Source	External agent or internal disease	Unknown; if known, treatment is prolonged or ineffective
Onset	Usually sudden	May be sudden or develop insidiously
Duration	Transient (up to 6 months)	Prolonged (months to years)
Pain identification	Painful and nonpainful areas generally well identified	Painful and nonpainful areas less easily differentiated; change in sensations becomes more difficult to evaluate
Clinical signs	Typical response pattern with more visible signs	Response patterns vary; fewer overt signs (adaptation)
Significance	Significant (informs person something is wrong)	Person looks for significance
Pattern	Self-limiting or readily corrected	Continuous or intermittent; intensity may vary or remain constant
Course	Suffering usually decreases over time	Suffering usually increases over time
Actions	Leads to actions to relieve pain	Leads to actions to modify pain experience
Prognosis	Likelihood of eventual complete relief	Complete relief usually not possible

Data from Black RG: *Surg Clin North Am* 55(4): 999, 1975.

vere pain in one knee is less likely to experience chronic back pain that is less intense. This phenomenon is called **perceptual dominance.** Because of perceptual dominance, an individual with many painful sites may report only the most painful one. Then, when the dominant pain is diminished, the individual identifies other painful areas.[4]

Pain tolerance is the duration of time or the intensity of pain that an individual will endure before initiating overt pain responses. It is the amount of pain the person will tolerate before outwardly responding to it. Pain tolerance is influenced by the person's cultural perceptions, expectations, role behaviors, and physical and mental health. Pain tolerance generally is decreased with repeated exposure to pain. Tolerance is decreased also by fatigue, anger, boredom, apprehension, and sleep deprivation. Tolerance may be increased by alcohol consumption, medication, hypnosis, warmth, distracting activities, and strong beliefs or faith.[2]

Pain tolerance varies greatly among people and in the same person over time because of the body's ability to respond differently to noxious stimuli. No direct relationship exists between the intensity of painful stimuli and an individual's perception of pain or response to pain.

Children and elderly persons may experience or express pain differently from adults.

Pediatrics and Perception of Pain

Children and infants have anatomic and functional ability to perceive pain. Pain pathways and cortical and subcortical centers for pain perception, as well as neurochemicals associated with pain transmission and modulation, are functional in the preterm and newborn infants.[5] The nociceptor system is functional in fetuses by 24 weeks of gestation.[6] Repetitive, painful experiences and prolonged exposure to analgesic drugs in infants during the neonatal period may permanently alter synaptic and neuronal organization.[7]

Change in facial expression, crying, and body movements are the most consistent expressions of pain in infants. The painful facial expression includes lowered brows drawn together; presence of a vertical bulge and furrows in the forehead between the brows; broadened nasal root; tightly closed, scourged eye fissures; and angular, squarish mouth and chin quiver (Fig. 14-1).[8] Physiologic responses include an increase in heart rate, blood pressure, and respiratory rate. There may be flushing or pallor, sweating, and decreased oxygen saturation. Toddlers also express pain with crying, facial expression, and body language (body tenses, guarding, and hands holding body). Older children, between ages 5 and 18 years, tend to have a lower pain threshold than do adults. Children, like adults, have highly individual responses to pain. The pain must be adequately treated for children of all ages.[9]

Aging and Perception of Pain

Studies on pain perception in the elderly population have yielded conflicting evidence. Some studies show an increase in the pain threshold with aging; others show no change.[10,11] The varied results are probably a function of independent variation in the sensory/discriminative, motivational/affective, and cognitive/evaluative components of the pain experience. In general, studies confirm that an increase in the pain threshold occurs in some elderly people. This change may be caused by peripheral neuropathies and changes in the thickness of the

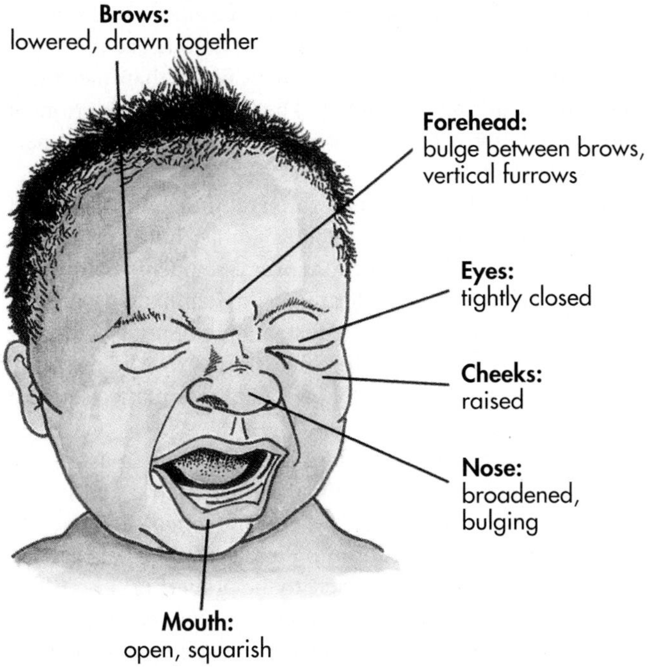

FIG. 14-1 Painful facial expression of infants. (From Wong DL: *Whaley and Wong's essentials of pediatric nursing,* ed 6, St Louis, 2001, Mosby.)

WHAT'S NEW? Pain and Gender

Gender differences in the experience of pain have been documented in both animal and human research. Women report higher pain levels or have less tolerance for pain stimulus intensities, or both. Gender differences exist also in the prevalence of painful diseases; for example, more women are affected by interstitial cystitis, fibromyalgia, and rheumatoid arthritis, and men are more affected by cluster headache. Pain symptoms differ for men and women for diseases such as coronary artery disease, irritable bowel syndrome, and appendicitis. Sex hormones are known to have an effect on the mechanisms and outcomes of opiate analgesia, and in rodents, morphine analgesia is greater in males than in females. A recent human study now suggests that kappa-opioid receptor analgesia is greater in women than in men and may reflect a difference in endogenous pain circuits activated by different opiate receptor subtypes. Continuing research is needed to further understanding of gender differences in the operation of pain mechanisms and the development of more specific pain management strategies.

Data from Fillingim RB, Maixner W: *Pain Forum* 4:209, 1995; Gear RW et al: *Pain* 64:123, 1996; Gear RW et al: *Nat Med* 2(11):1238, 1996; Taenzer AH et al: Gender affects report of pain and function after arthroscopic anterior cruciate ligament reconstruction, *Anesthesiology* 93(3):670, 2000.

skin.[12] (Neuropathies are discussed in Chapter 16.) A decrease in pain tolerance is also evident in older persons, and women appear to be more sensitive to pain than are men.[13]

Neuroanatomy of Pain

The portions of the nervous system responsible for the sensation and perception of pain may be divided into three areas: (1) the afferent pathways, (2) the central nervous system, and (3) the efferent pathways. The afferent portion of the system is composed of **nociceptors** (pain receptors) in the tissues. (As Chapter 13 describes, afferent nerves carry signals to the spinal cord network, which transmits the signal to the brain.) Afferent pathways terminate in the dorsal horn of the spinal cord. Both incoming and descending stimuli modulate pain patterns in the dorsal horn cells. The portions of the CNS involved in the interpretation of pain signals are the limbic system, reticular formation, thalamus, hypothalamus, medulla, and cortex. The ventroposterior and medial thalamic nuclei facilitate discrimination and localization of pain. The limbic and reticular tracts are probably involved in alerting, arousal, and motivational behaviors related to pain. The medulla and hypothalamus activate coping responses, such as "fight or flight," the release of corticosteroids, and cardiovascular responses. The various regions of the brain that modulate spinal pain transmission are complex and integrated. The efferent pathways, composed of the fibers connecting the reticular formation, midbrain, and substantia gelatinosa, are responsible for modulating pain sensation.

Role of Afferent and Efferent Pathways

The nociceptors are at the ends of the small unmyelinated and lightly myelinated afferent neurons. The ends of these neurons respond to chemical, mechanical, and thermal stimuli (Table 14-2). In addition to distal stimulation, nociceptors may be activated more proximally as they pass through areas of entrapment in the spinal column. Heat injury and inflammation associated with rheumatic disease appear initially to lower the threshold and increase the intensity of response to additional painful stimuli. Repeated noxious stimulation to inflamed joints results in an eventual decrease in sensitivity, however.[14] In some instances, physiologic states, such as increased skeletal muscle tone, enhance excitability of nociceptors.[15]

Table 14-2 Stimuli That Activate Nociceptors (Pain Receptors)

Location of Receptor	Provoking Stimuli
Skin	Pricking, cutting, crushing, burning, freezing
Gastrointestinal tract	Engorged or inflamed mucosa, distention or spasm of smooth muscle, traction on mesenteric attachment
Skeletal muscle	Ischemia, injuries of connective tissue sheaths, necrosis, hemorrhage, prolonged contraction, injection of irritating solutions
Joints	Synovial membrane inflammation
Arteries	Piercing, inflammation
Head	Traction, inflammation, or displacement of arteries, meningeal structures, and sinuses; prolonged muscle contraction
Heart	Ischemia and inflammation

Nociceptors are nonencapsulated free nerve endings that can be classified as either *unimodal* or *polymodal*. The unimodal nociceptors respond to only one type of sensory modality (mechanosensitive) and are found in the skin, mucous membranes, and some walls lining body cavities. Polymodal nociceptors, which are the majority of nociceptors, respond to more than one sensory modality (mechanosensitive, thermosensitive, and chemosensitive) and are found widely distributed in deep tissues and skin. Nociceptors are not evenly distributed in the body. For example, the skin has many more nociceptors than the internal structures, and the eye has many more than the arm. This maldistribution of nociceptors affects the relative sensitivity to pain of different areas of the body.

As Fig. 14-2 illustrates, stimulation of nociceptors produces impulses that are transmitted through small Aδ fibers and C fibers to the spinal cord, where they form synapses with neurons in the dorsal horn. From the dorsal horn the nociceptive impulses are transmitted to various parts of the spinal cord and to the rest of the CNS.

The small unmyelinated C polymodal nociceptors are responsible for the transmission of diffuse burning or aching sensations. Because of the size of the fiber and the lack of a myelin sheath, transmission through C fibers is relatively slow. This type of pain is more susceptible to local anesthesia. Transmission through the slightly larger, myelinated A mechanical nociceptors occurs much more quickly. Aδ fibers carry well-localized, sharp pain sensations and are important in initiating rapid reactions to stimuli. The reflex arc to and from the spinal cord is much faster than the transmission of the pain stimulus. Therefore the retraction of the injured body part occurs before the individual perceives the pain.

Most afferent pain fibers terminate in the dorsal horn of the spinal segment that they enter. Some, however, extend toward the head or the foot for several segments before terminating. The Aδ fibers terminate in lamina I (marginal zone) but also in lamina II (substantia gelatinosa) and lamina V of the spinal cord. Most fibers cross over in the cord. Some do not, and this is why pain may return after surgical resection of these fibers.

Secondary neurons transmit the information from the substantia gelatinosa and laminae to the ventral and lateral horn, crossing, in the same or adjacent spinal segments, to the other side of the cord. From there the impulse is carried through the spinothalamic tracts to the brain (Fig. 14-3). The two divisions of the spinothalamic tract that carry pain information to the brain are (1) the neospinothalamic tract (acute pain) and (2) the paleospinothalamic tract (dull and burning pain). The neospinothalamic tract carries information to the midbrain, postcentral gyrus (where pain is perceived), and cortex. The paleospinothalamic tract carries information to the reticular formation, pons, limbic system, and midbrain.

The efferent pathway is responsible for modulation or inhibition of afferent pain signals. Afferent stimulation of the **periaqueductal gray (PAG)** (gray matter surrounding the cerebral aqueduct) in the midbrain stimulates the efferent pathway. Efferent neurons located in the PAG form synapses with structures in the medulla that inhibit pain.[16] From there the impulse is transmitted through the spinal cord to the dorsal horn to impair or block transmission of nociceptive impulses.

Neurophysiology of Pain

Theories of Pain

Theories proposed to describe the mechanisms of pain include the specificity theory, the intensity theory, the pattern theory, and the gate control theory. The **specificity theory** proposes four major categories of cutaneous sensation: (1) touch, (2) warmth, (3) cold, and (4) pain. Each cutaneous sensation is the result of stimulation of specific receptor sites on the skin. Stimulation of the nerve endings of the pain receptors precipitates transmission of the painful stimuli (through Aδ and C fibers) to the spinal cord. The pain neurons form synapses in the substantia gelatinosa and cross to the opposite side of the spinal cord, ascending to the brain through the spinothalamic tract. The perception of pain then occurs in special areas of the thalamus and cerebral cortex.

According to the specificity theory, a direct relationship exists between the stimulus and the perception of pain. Although this theory postulates the existence of specific skin receptors for pain and explains why actual tissue damage causes pain, it fails to account for adaptation to pain and effects of psychosocial factors on pain perception.[17]

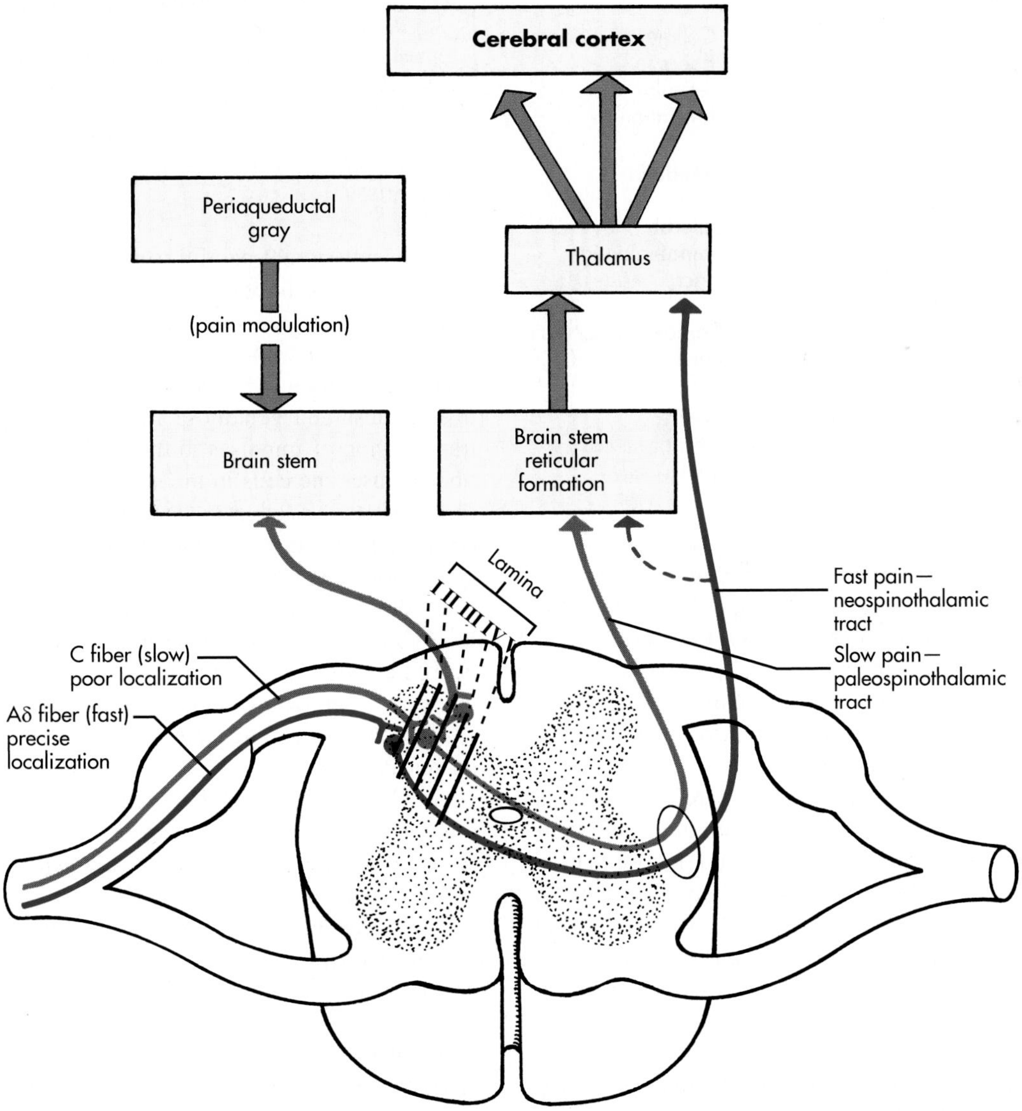

FIG. 14-2 Aδ fibers transmit acute localized pain sensations. The fibers synapse in laminae I and V, cross over, and synapse in the midbrain via the neospinothalamic tract. Neurons in lamina I are excited by thermal and mechanical stimuli and are unaffected by touch or movement of hairs. The small C fibers transmit "slow" or chronic burning sensations. The fibers synapse in laminae II and III, cross over, and synapse in the reticular formations and midbrain via the paleospinothalamic tract.

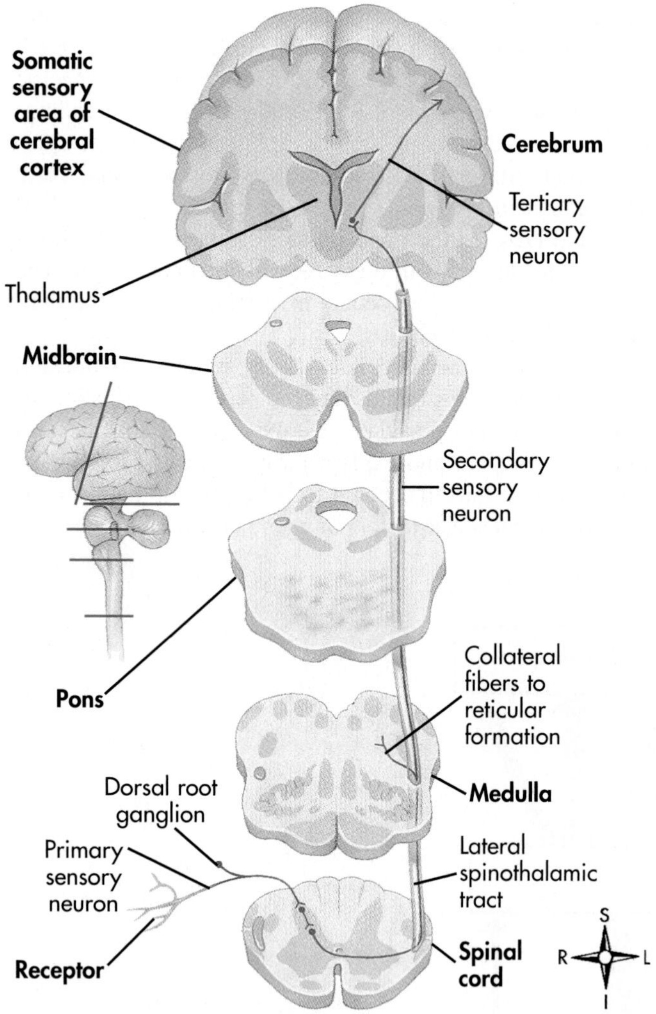

FIG. 14-3 Example of somatic sensory pathway. A spinothalamic pathway that conducts information about pain and temperature. (From Thibodeau GA, Patton KI: *Anatomy and physiology,* ed 4, St Louis, 1999, Mosby.)

The **intensity theory** proposes that pain results from excessive stimulation of sensory receptors. Pain occurs if the stimulus is applied with enough intensity. Excessive stimulation of receptors or a pathologic condition that promotes summation of impulses produced by nonnoxious stimuli can cause pain.[18] The theory does not account for intense stimulation of some sites that produces no pain.

The **pattern theory** suggests that the perception of pain is the result of stimulus intensity (a function of the length of time and the amount of tissue involved) and the summation of the impulses. According to the pattern theory, nonspecific receptors transmit patterns of nerve impulses from the skin to the spinal cord. Certain patterns of impulses then are perceived as pain. Theorists disagree about where the summation occurs. According to some, summation occurs in the spinal cord; according to others, it occurs in the brain. Although the pattern theories do not account for adaptation to pain, they do allow for the many factors that contribute to pain perception.[17]

The **gate control theory** describes how innocuous stimuli transmitted by large myelinated afferent fibers may prevent transmission of painful stimuli.[17] According to this theory, nociceptive impulses are transmitted from specialized skin receptors to the spinal cord through large A and small C fibers (see Fig. 14-2). These fibers terminate in the substantia gelatinosa, in the dorsal horn of the spinal cord. Cells in the substantia gelatinosa function as a gate, regulating transmission of impulses to the CNS. Stimulation of larger fibers causes the cells in the substantia gelatinosa to "close the gate." A closed gate decreases stimulation of trigger cells, decreases transmission impulses, and diminishes pain perception. Persistent stimulation of the large fibers, however, allows adaptation. When adaptation to impulses from large fibers occurs, the result is a relative increase in small neuron activity. Adaptation to larger fibers thus may "open the gate." Scratching and vibration prevent large neuron adaptation and keep the gate closed over prolonged periods, decreasing pain.

Small-fiber input inhibits cells in the substantia gelatinosa and opens the gate. An open gate increases the stimulation of trigger cells, increases transmission of impulses, and enhances pain perception. In addition to gate control through large- and small-fiber stimulation, the CNS, through efferent pathways, may close, partially close, or open the gate (Fig. 14-4).

Cognitive functioning thus may modulate pain perception. Interaction of the cognitive/evaluative, motivational/affective, and sensory/discriminative systems determines the individual's pain response. Although the gate control theory has been extremely influential, it is incorrect with respect to specific details. Namely, the existence of excitatory and inhibitory outputs of C fibers is unlikely.[17,19,20]

WHAT'S NEW? Neuromatrix Theory of Chronic Pain

Melzack has proposed a theory of chronic pain that will provide new directions for pain research. Chronic pain is theorized to be a multidimensional experience produced by patterns of nerve impulses known as "neurosignatures." These nerve impulses are generated in the brain by a widely distributed network known as "the body-self neuromatrix." The "body-self" represents the unique distinction of the self with unity of feeling, experiences, and genetic predisposition. It is multidimensional, including sensory, cognitive, affective, postural, evaluative, and other components. The "neuromatrix" is composed of centers and loops of neurons in the brain whose links and synapses are initially determined genetically but can be changed and modified by sensory inputs. The "neurosignature patterns" may be triggered by sensory inputs from the body or may originate in the brain *independently* of peripheral sensory input. It is the output of the widely distributed "neuromatrix," not input, that generates the "neurosignature pattern" of pain. This explains most types of chronic pain in which there is no discernible cause or correlation between pathology and pain (e.g., phantom limb pain and neuropathies). In summary, neuromatrix theory suggests that the brain can detect and analyze inputs and generate perceptual experience when there is no external input evoked by injury, inflammation, or other pathology. It is representative of the brain's plasticity.

Data from Melzack R: Pain—an overview, *Acta Anaesthesiol Scand* 43:880, 1999.

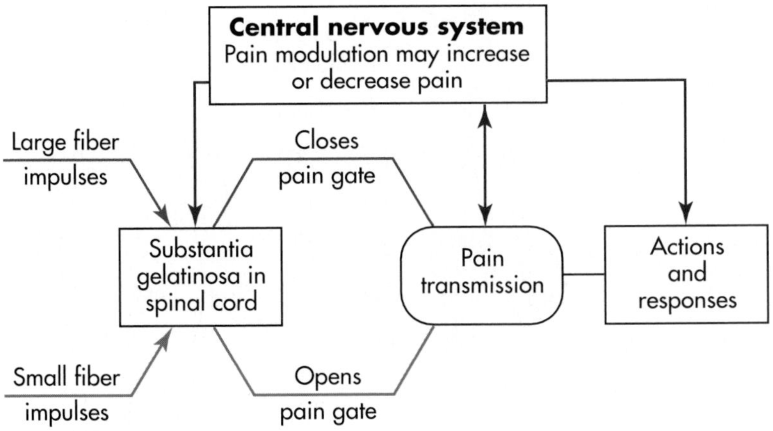

FIG. 14-4 Schematic diagram of the gate control theory of pain mechanism.

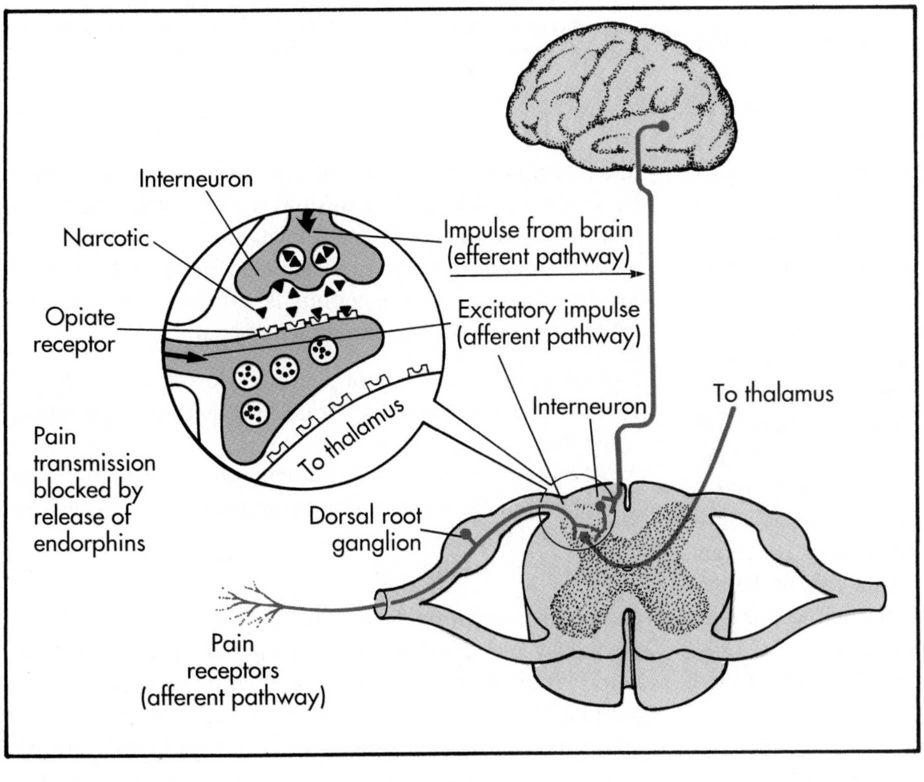

FIG. 14-5 Descending pathway and endorphin response. The biologic receptors of the enkephalins and endorphins are located close to known pain receptors in the periphery and ascending and descending pain pathways.

Neuromodulation

Neuromodulators of pain are found in the pathways that mediate information about painful stimuli, including the periphery, ascending and descending spinal tracts, the cortex, and the gastrointestinal tract.[21] Tissue injury results in the release of prostaglandins (PGs) such as PGE_2 and PGI_2, nitric oxide, bradykinins, and histamine, which depolarize adjacent nociceptors, causing pain. Lymphokines released from lymphocytes in chronic inflammatory lesions may contribute to some types of chronic pain. Substance P, neurokinin A, and calcitonin gene–related peptide are released from peripheral pain receptors and promote the spread of pain locally. Norepinephrine and 5-hydroxytryptamine contribute to pain modulation (inhibition) in the medulla and pons. Substance P and other neurotransmitters contribute to the modulation of pain in both the afferent and efferent fibers of the spinal cord.

Endorphins (endogenous morphines) are a family of neuropeptides that inhibit transmission of pain impulses in the spinal cord and brain.[22] The three classifications of endorphins are (1) β-lipotropin, (2) enkephalin, and (3) dynorphin. **β-Lipotropin** (β-, γ-, and α-endorphin) is a potent endorphin located in the hypothalamus and the pituitary gland. These endorphins may be responsible for general sensations of well-being. **Enkephalin,** found in the neurons of the brain and spinal cord, is a weaker analgesic than other endorphins but is more potent and longer lasting than morphine. **Dynorphin** (a powerful endorphin) is 50 times more potent than β-endorphin. Dynorphin reportedly originates in the neural lobe of the pituitary.[23]

All endorphins act by attaching to **opiate receptors** on the plasma membrane of the afferent neuron (Fig. 14-5). The combination of the opiate receptor and endorphin inhibits the release of excitatory neurotransmitters (i.e., substance P), thus blocking the transmission of the painful stimulus. In much the same way, exogenous opiates relieve pain by attaching to the opiate receptors and augmenting the natural endorphin response.[24] The enkephalin-endorphin receptors also have been identified as specific cellular attachment sites for morphine and other exogenous narcotic molecules.

Stress, excessive physical exertion, acupuncture, intercourse, and other factors increase the levels of circulating endorphins, serotonin, norepinephrine, and other neurotransmitters, raising the pain threshold.[23] Although still controversial, some evidence suggests that high levels of circulating endorphins may play a role in so-called painless myocardial ischemia and infarction.[25]

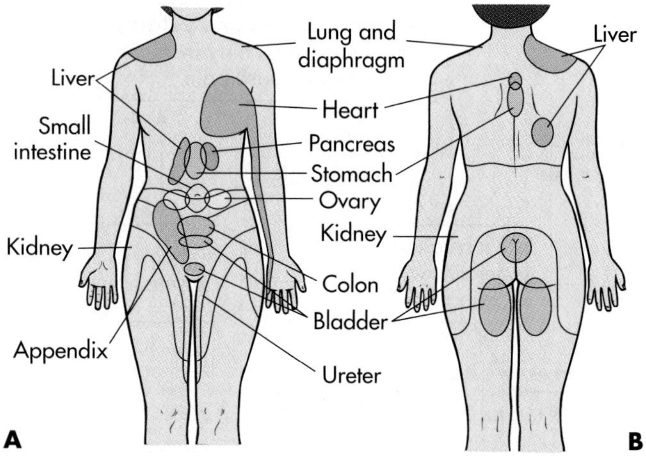

FIG. 14-6 Sites of referred pain. A, Front. **B,** Back. (Redrawn from Phipps WJ, Sands JK, Marck JF: *Medical surgical nursing: concepts and clinical practice,* ed 6, St Louis, 1999, Mosby.)

Clinical Manifestations of Pain

Acute Pain

Acute pain arises from cutaneous, deep somatic, or visceral structures and can be classified as (1) somatic, (2) visceral, and (3) referred. The nervous system is usually intact in acute pain. **Somatic pain** is superficial (coming from the skin or close to the surface of the body) and is either sharp and well localized or dull, aching, poorly localized, and accompanied by nausea and vomiting. **Visceral pain** refers to pain in internal organs, the abdomen, or the skeleton. It is poorly localized because of the lesser number of mechanoreceptors in the visceral structures. It is associated with nausea and vomiting, hypotension, restlessness, and, in some cases, shock. Visceral pain often radiates (spreads away from the actual site of the pain) or is referred. **Referred pain** is pain that is present in an area removed or distant from its point of origin. The area of referred pain is supplied by the same spinal segment as the actual site of pain. Impulses from many cutaneous and visceral neurons converge on the same ascending neuron, and the brain cannot distinguish between the two. Because there are more receptors in the skin, the painful sensation is experienced there.[26] (Common areas of referred pain and their associated sites of origin appear in Fig. 14-6.)

Physiologic Response

Acute pain is a warning of actual or impending tissue injury. Physiologic responses therefore include increased heart rate, increased respiratory rate, elevated blood pressure, pallor or flushing, dilated pupils, and diaphoresis. Blood sugar is elevated, gastric acid secretion and motility decrease, and blood flow to the viscera and skin decrease. Nausea occasionally occurs.

Psychologic and Behavioral Response

Individuals often psychologically respond to acute pain with fear (e.g., fear of diagnosis, fear of continued pain), anxiety, and a general sense of unpleasantness or unease. The stress of fear may in turn contribute to the physiologic signs of pain. Additionally, individuals do not always discuss or report their pain.[27]

Chronic Pain

Chronic pain is prolonged pain (lasts longer than 6 months) that may be persistent (e.g., low back pain) or intermittent (e.g., migraines). Chronic pain may be caused or aggravated by a decreased level of endorphins or a predominance of C-neuron stimulation.[28] Chronic pain is more difficult to manage or control than acute pain (see Table 14-1). The following changes in nerve terminals, afferent fibers, and the CNS may contribute to chronicity of pain:[29]

1. Changes in sensitivity of neurons—lower threshold
2. Spontaneous impulses from regenerating peripheral nerves
3. Alterations in the dorsal root ganglion in response to peripheral nerve injury and neurotransmitters—reorganization of nociceptive neurons
4. Loss of pain inhibition in the spinal cord

Central sensitization is an increase in the excitability of medullary and spinal neurons arising from persistent stimulation from injured peripheral nerves. Prolonged firing of peripheral C-fiber nociceptors causes release of glutamate and aspartate, which act on *N*-methyl-D-aspartate (NMDA) receptors in the spinal cord with release of nitric oxide. This causes the spinal cord neuron to become more sensitive to all of its inputs, including ascending stimuli, resulting in central sensitization.[30]

Central pain is caused by a lesion or dysfunction in the CNS (brain or spinal cord). The lesions of central pain can include infarction, hemorrhage, abscess, degeneration, tumors, or traumatic injury. The pain may represent a large or defined body area. It is usually irritating and constant and can cause considerable suffering. Thalamic pain is a form of central pain involving lesions in the thalamus.

Neuropathic pain is the result of trauma or disease of the peripheral nerves. The pain is often paroxysmal, tingling, burning, or shooting. It can be evoked by movement, and there may be sensitivity in the denervated part of the body. The mechanisms of pain are complex. Injured nerves can become hyperexcitable and generate ectopic discharges with spontaneous firing of some neurons with low thresholds for mechanical, chemical, or thermal stimuli. Accumulation of sodium ion channels at sites of nerve injury and demyelination can promote hyperexcitability. There can also be neuroplastic (the ability of neurons to alter their structure and function) changes at the level of the brain and spinal cord that may modulate pain.[31,32]

Physiologic Response

Physiologic responses to chronic pain depend on whether it is persistent or intermittent. Intermittent pain produces a physiologic response similar to that of acute pain, whereas persistent pain allows for physiologic adaptation. Adaptation produces normal heart and respiratory rates and normal blood pressure. Other physiologic responses to acute pain also become normal, but even though the physiologic responses are normal, the pain is not relieved.

Psychologic and Behavioral Response

Chronic pain produces significant behavioral and psychologic changes.[33] Individuals with chronic pain often are depressed, have difficulty sleeping and eating, and may become preoccupied with the pain. Living with chronic pain requires constant attention to the earliest signs of pain so that the pain-provoking stimuli can be identified and avoided. Persons with chronic pain generally attempt to keep pain-related behavior to a minimum so that they appear as normal as possible. They need to have someone understand that the pain and the need to hide it are usually conflicting drives for those with chronic pain. They tend not to report pain for fear of being labeled complainers. They often deny pain and sometimes engage in activities that provoke pain so that they can keep up with others. Even in learning to pace themselves through the day's activities, they may aggravate the pain.[34]

Chronic Pain Conditions

The most common chronic pain condition is persistent low back pain. This, like many other conditions, is a result of poor muscle tone, inactivity, muscle strain, or sudden vigorous exercise. Other chronic conditions include neuralgias, hyperesthesias, myofascial pain syndrome, and hemiageusias. Chronic pain is associated with cancer in some instances.

Neuralgias are painful conditions that result from an infection or disease that damages a peripheral nerve. Causalgias and reflex sympathetic dystrophies are types of neuralgias. **Causalgia** is a condition causing severe burning pain that may be triggered by normally nonnoxious stimuli such as light touch, sound, or cold. The pain appears 1 to 2 weeks after injury to the brachial plexus, the median nerves, or the sciatic nerves. The severe, diffuse, and persistent pain occurs in the extremity supplied by the injured nerve. Discoloration and changes in the texture of the skin may appear in the affected area. Excessive nail growth may be noted, and swelling and stiffness of proximate joints may occur.

Reflex sympathetic dystrophies occur after peripheral nerve injury and are characterized by continuous, severe, burning pain. The pain often is associated with vasospasm and vasomotor changes. Vasomotor changes usually begin with vasodilation and are followed by vasoconstriction and cool cyanotic and edematous extremities. As muscle wasting occurs, amputation of the involved extremity may be required.

Hyperesthesias are chronic pain conditions characterized by increased sensitivity and decreased pain threshold to tactile and painful stimuli. Stimuli that usually do not produce pain thus become painful. The pain is usually diffuse, modified by fatigue and emotion, and mixed with other sensations. The hyperesthesia may be the result of chronic irritation of the thalamus and other central areas.

Myofascial pain syndromes are the second most common cause of chronic pain. These conditions include myositis, fibrositis, myofibrositis, myalgia, and muscle strain; they involve injury to the muscle and fascia. The pain is a result of muscle spasm, tenderness, and stiffness. These conditions lead to muscle guarding, a behavior that limits muscle motion. In turn, limited motion causes muscle weakness, stiffness, tenderness, and spasm, all of which produce more pain. The pain is described as dull and aching and may be mild to disabling. During the early stages of the disorder, the pain is localized, but as the disorder progresses, the pain becomes more generalized.

Hemiagnosia is a loss of ability to identify the source of pain on one side (the affected side) of the body. Application of painful stimuli to the affected side thus produces discomfort, anxiety, moaning, agitation, and distress but no attempt to withdraw from or push aside the offending stimulus because of an inability to locate the site through normal sensory pathways. Hemiagnosia is associated with stroke that produces paralysis and a hypersensitivity to pain in the affected side.

Phantom limb pain is pain that an individual feels in an amputated limb after the stump has completely healed. It is more likely to appear in individuals who experienced pain in the limb before amputation. If the neuronal pathway from the amputated limb is stimulated at any point along the pathway, action potentials are propagated toward the cortex. CNS integration results in the perception of pain from the receptors in the amputated limb even though it is no longer there. The pain suppression effect of other sensations, such as touch, pressure, and proprioception, from the amputated limb may be a factor in the intensity of phantom limb pain.

Phantom limb pain may be influenced by emotions and sympathetic stimulation and may be associated with trigger points. **Trigger points** are small, hypersensitive regions in the muscle or connective tissue. They may be close to or removed from the area of pain, but stimulation of the trigger point produces pain in a specific area.

Cancer often is associated with chronic pain. Studies done at Memorial Sloan-Kettering Cancer Center indicate three major categories of pain syndromes that result in chronic pain in the individual with cancer.[35] The categories are (1) pain attributed to the advance of the disease, (2) pain associated with treatment of the disease, and (3) pain attributed to coexisting entities (e.g., osteoarthritis) that are unrelated to the disease.

By far the most common cause of chronic pain in the individual with cancer is that attributed to the advance of the disease.[35] Pain can be caused by infection and inflammation, increasing pressure of a growing tumor on nerve endings, stretching of visceral surfaces, or obstruction of ducts and intestine. This pain may be acute, intermittent, or continuous. Therapeutic approaches are partially effective in controlling the pain. Pain from tumor infiltration of nerve tissue; trauma or chemical injury to the nerve; or damage from radiation, chemotherapy, or surgical sectioning of the nerve produces another form of chronic pain referred to as *deafferentation pain.* (Deafferentation refers to a loss of sensory input from a portion of the body.) Deafferentation pain is described as a constant, dull, viselike ache, with paroxysms of burning or electric shock–like sensations. It may lead to hyperactivity of neurons in the spinal cord and thalamus. Deafferentation pain is poorly controlled by peripheral and epidural analgesia.[36,37]

Some individuals experience chronic pain after treatment (see Chapter 10). Chronic postoperative pain occurs in a small percentage of individuals after the following:

1. Thoracotomy, with pain often caused by tumor recurrence or invasion of the chest wall
2. Radical mastectomy, with pain resulting from interruption of the intercostobrachial nerve (which branches from the brachial plexus to the thoracic region)
3. Radical neck dissection, with pain attributable to surgical injury or interruption of the cranial nerves
4. Surgical amputation, which may be followed by phantom limb pain

Chemotherapy, especially treatment with Vinca alkaloids, may be associated with a variety of neuropathies producing painful dysesthesias ("pins and needles" sensations) in the feet and hands. Radiation therapy may result in connective tissue fibrosis and secondary nerve injury that produces pain.[35] Cancer pain is discussed in Box 14-1.

Box 14-1

INADEQUATE CANCER PAIN MANAGEMENT

Cancer pain management remains a formidable problem even though standards and guidelines have been published by the World Health Organization, American Pain Society, and Agency for Health Care Policy and Research. From 45% to 75% of individuals with both early and late stages of cancer experience pain that compromises their daily lives. Barriers to pain control include attitudes and misconceptions about pain management by both clinicians and patients, poor pain assessment, failure of clinicians to obtain adequate pain management consultation, fear of addiction, undermedication, cultural variation in pain responses, restrictive regulations, and inadequate insurance. The sciences and principles of analgesia are well established. New education strategies and accountability procedures are required to achieve optimal pain management for all individuals with cancer.

Data from Cleary JF: Cancer pain management, *Cancer Control* 7(2): 120, 2000; Juarez G, Ferrell B, Borneman T: Cultural considerations in education for cancer pain management, *J Cancer Educ* 14(3):168, 1999; Pargeon KL, Hailey BJ: Barriers to effective cancer pain management: a review of the literature, *J Pain Symptom Manage* 18(5): 358, 1999; Walsh D: Pharmacological management of cancer pain, *Semin Oncol* 27(1):45, 2000.

TEMPERATURE REGULATION

In all homeothermic animals, temperature regulation is achieved through precise balancing of heat production, heat conservation, and heat loss. In humans, body temperature is maintained in a range around 37° C (98.6° F). The normal range is considered to be 36.2° to 37.7° C (97.2° to 99.9° F), but all parts of the body do not have the same temperature. The extremities, for example, are generally cooler than the trunk. The temperature at the core of the body (as measured by rectal temperature) is generally 0.5° C higher than at the surface (as measured by oral temperature). The internal temperature varies normally in response to activity, environmental temperature, and daily fluctuation of **circadian rhythm** (the pattern of each 24-hour day). Oral temperatures generally fluctuate within 0.2° to 0.5° C over a 24-hour period. Women tend to have wider fluctuations that follow the menstrual cycle, with a sharp rise in temperature just before ovulation. In both genders the daily fluctuating temperature peaks around 6 PM and is at its lowest during sleep.[38] Maintenance of body temperature within the normal range is necessary for life.

Hypothalamic Control of Temperature

Temperature regulation is mediated hormonally by the hypothalamus. Peripheral thermoreceptors in the skin and central thermoreceptors in the hypothalamus, spinal cord, abdominal organs, and other central locations provide the hypothalamus with information about skin and core temperatures. If these temperatures are low, the hypothalamus responds by triggering heat production and heat conservation mechanisms.

Increased heat production is initiated by a series of hormonal mechanisms involving the hypothalamus and its connections with the endocrine system (see Chapter 19). The heat-producing mechanism begins with a hypothalamic hormone, thyrotropin-stimulating hormone–releasing hormone (TSH-RH). In turn, TSH-RH stimulates the anterior pituitary to release thyroid-stimulating hormone (TSH), which acts on the thyroid gland, stimulating release of thyroxine (T4), one of the thyroid hormones. This hormone then acts on the adrenal medulla, causing the release of epinephrine (a catecholamine and vasopressive hormone) into the bloodstream (see Chapter 19). Epinephrine causes vasoconstriction, stimulates glycolysis, and increases metabolic rates, thus increasing heat production.

The hypothalamus also triggers heat conservation. The mechanisms of heat conservation involve stimulating the sympathetic nervous system, which is responsible for stimulating the adrenal cortex, increasing skeletal muscle tone, initiating the shivering response, and producing vasoconstriction. The hypothalamus also functions in raising body temperatures by relaying information to the cerebral cortex. Awareness of cold provokes voluntary responses such as increased body movement.

The hypothalamus responds to warmer core and peripheral temperatures by reversing the same mechanisms. The

TSH-RH pathway is shut down. The sympathetic pathway is prompted to produce vasodilation, decreased muscle tone, and increased sweat production. Hypothalamic stimulation of the cerebral cortex provokes voluntary measures to reduce heat production and promote heat loss.

Mechanisms of Heat Production

Body heat is produced by the chemical reactions of metabolism, skeletal muscle tone and contraction, and chemical thermogenesis. Heat is distributed by the circulatory system.

Chemical Reactions of Metabolism

The chemical reactions that occur during the ingestion and metabolism of food and those required to maintain the body at rest (basal metabolism) require energy and give off heat. These processes occur in the body core (liver) and are in part responsible for the maintenance of core temperature.

Skeletal Muscle Contraction

Skeletal muscles produce heat through two mechanisms: (1) gradual increase in muscle tone and (2) rapid muscle oscillations (shivering). Both increasing muscle tone and shivering are controlled by the hypothalamus and occur in response to cold. As peripheral temperature drops, muscle tone increases and shivering begins. Shivering is a fairly effective method for increasing heat production, because no work is performed and all the energy produced is retained as heat.

Chemical Thermogenesis

Chemical thermogenesis, also called *nonshivering thermogenesis,* results from the release of epinephrine. Epinephrine produces a rapid, transient increase in heat production by raising the body's basal metabolic rate. Chemical thermogenesis seems to be different from hormone-triggered increases in the basal metabolic rate. Chemical thermogenesis—through epinephrine—produces a quick, brief rise in basal metabolic rate, whereas the hormone *thyroxine* triggers a slow, prolonged rise.[39] Chemical thermogenesis occurs in brown adipose tissue present mainly in small newborn mammals that have high surface/volume ratios. Brown adipose tissue is rich with mitochondria. Like other small newborn mammals, human infants lose more heat through **conduction** and **convection** than they are capable of generating through normal metabolic mechanisms. Brown adipose tissue therefore plays an important role in maintaining body temperature in the newborn. As with most mammals reared in a temperature-controlled environment, humans gradually lose the capacity for chemical thermogenesis as brown adipose cells dedifferentiate. This can occur as early as 4 weeks after birth.[40] Because of the decrease in brown adipose tissue in the adult, the role of this mechanism of heat production in adults is under investigation.[41]

Mechanisms of Heat Loss

Heat loss is achieved through many mechanisms: (1) radiation, (2) conduction, (3) convection, (4) vasodilation, (5) decreased muscle tone, (6) evaporation, (7) increased respiration, (8) voluntary measures, and (9) adaptation to warmer climates.

Radiation

Radiation refers to heat loss through electromagnetic waves. These waves emanate from surfaces with temperatures higher than the surrounding air. Thus if the temperature of the skin is higher than that of the air, the skin and therefore the body lose heat to the air.

Conduction

Conduction refers to heat loss by direct molecule-to-molecule transfer from one surface to another. Through conduction, the warmer surface loses heat to the cooler surface. Thus the skin loses heat through direct contact with cooler air, water, or another surface. In the same manner, the core of the body loses heat to the cooler body surface.

Convection

Convection is the transfer of heat through currents of gases or liquids. It greatly aids heat loss through conduction by exchanging warmer air at the surface of the body with cooler air in the surrounding space. Convection occurs passively as warmer air at the surface of the body rises away from the body and is replaced by cooler air, but the process may be aided by fans or wind. (The combined effect of conduction and convection by wind is conventionally measured as the *windchill factor.)*

Vasodilation

Peripheral vasodilation increases heat loss by diverting core-warmed blood to the surface of the body. As the core-warmed blood passes through the periphery, heat is transferred by conduction to the skin surface and from the skin to the surrounding environment. Because heat loss through conduction depends on the temperature of the surrounding medium, heat loss through conduction is minimal to nonexistent if the surrounding air is warmer than the body surface.

Vasodilation occurs in response to autonomic stimulation under the control of the hypothalamus. It is useful in instances of moderate temperature elevation. As core temperature increases, vasodilation increases until maximal dilation is achieved. At that point the body must use additional heat loss mechanisms.

Decreased Muscle Tone

To decrease heat production, muscle tone may be moderately reduced and voluntary muscle activity curtailed. These mechanisms explain in part the "washed-out" feeling associated with high temperatures and warm weather. Both decreased muscle tone and reduced activity have a limited effect on decreasing heat production, however, because muscle tone and heat production cannot be reduced below basal body requirements.

Evaporation

Evaporation of body water from the surface of the skin and the linings of the mucous membranes is a major source of heat reduction. Insensible water loss (in the absence of perceptible sweating) accounts for a loss of about 600 ml of water per day. Heat is lost as surface fluid is converted to gas, so that heat loss by evaporation is increased if more fluids are available at the body surface. To speed this process, fluids are actively secreted through the sweat glands. As much as 4 L of fluid per hour may be lost by sweating. Electrolytes are lost with the water. Therefore loss of large volumes through sweating may result in decreased plasma volume, decreased blood pressure, weakness, and fainting. (Alterations in fluid balance are discussed in Chapter 3.)

Like other heat reduction mechanisms, stimulation of sweating occurs in response to sympathetic neural activity and depends on a favorable temperature difference between the body and the environment. In addition, heat loss through evaporation is affected by the relative humidity of the air. If the humidity of the air is low, sweat evaporates quickly, but if the humidity is high, sweat does not evaporate and instead remains on the skin or drips off.

Increased Respiration

Exchanging air with the environment through the normal respiratory process provides some heat loss, although it is minimal. As air is inhaled, the air draws heat from the upper respiratory tract. The air is further warmed in the alveoli by blood in the microcirculation. This warmed air then is exhaled into the environment. This normal process occurs faster at higher body temperatures through an increase in respiratory rates. Thus hyperventilation is associated with hyperthermia. (Normal pulmonary function is discussed in Chapter 31.)

Voluntary Mechanisms

In response to high body temperatures, people typically "stretch out," thereby increasing the body surface area available for heat loss. They also "slow down" or "take it easy," thereby decreasing skeletal muscle work, and they "dress for warm weather." The most efficient dress for warm weather is a light-colored, loose-fitting garment, because light colors reflect heat from the body and loose-fitting garments allow free air movement for convection, conduction, and evaporation to occur.

Adaptation to Warmer Climates

The body of an individual who moves from a cooler to a much warmer climate undergoes a period of adjustment, a process that takes several days to weeks. At first the individual experiences feelings of lassitude, weakness, and faintness with even moderate activity. Body temperatures rise with any work. Within several days, however, the individual experiences an earlier onset of sweating; the volume of sweat is increased; and the sodium content is lowered. Heart rate is decreased and stroke volume increased so that cardiac output remains unchanged. Extracellular fluid volume increases, as does plasma volume. These physiologic adaptations result in improved warm weather functioning and decreased symptoms of heat intolerance. People's work output, endurance, and coordination increase, and their subjective feelings of discomfort decrease.[42]

Mechanisms of Heat Conservation

The body conserves heat and protects core temperature through two important mechanisms: (1) involuntary vasoconstriction and (2) voluntary mechanisms. To preserve core temperature, the skin and periphery are used as an insulating cover.[42]

Vasoconstriction

By constricting peripheral blood vessels, centrally warmed blood is shunted away from the periphery (where radiation, conduction, and convection would allow heat loss) to the core of the body, where heat can be retained. This mechanism takes advantage of the insulating layers of the skin and subcutaneous fat to protect core temperature.

Voluntary Mechanisms

In response to lower body temperatures, individuals typically "bundle up," "keep moving," or "curl up in a ball." Bundling up involves dressing with several layers of clothes that allow air to be trapped between the skin and the clothing, thus providing an additional layer of insulation. Keeping moving, stamping feet, clapping hands, jogging, and other types of physical activity increase skeletal muscle activity and thus promote heat production. Curling up in a ball decreases the amount of skin surface available for heat loss through radiation, convection, and conduction.

Aging and Pediatric Changes in Temperature Regulation

Infants and the elderly require special attention to maintenance of body temperature. Infants produce sufficient body heat but are unable to conserve heat produced. The poor heat conservation is caused by the infant's small body size and greater ratio of body surface to body weight, which give the infant more surface area for heat loss. Infants also have a very thin layer of subcutaneous fat and thus are not as well insulated as adults.[43] Elderly persons have poor responses to environmental temperature extremes as a result of slowed blood circulation, structural and functional changes in the skin, and an overall decrease in heat-producing activities. Other factors affecting thermal regulation in the elderly population include decreased shivering response (delayed onset and decreased effectiveness), slowed metabolic rate, sedentary life-style, decreased vasoconstrictor response, diminished or absent sweating, desynchronization of circadian rhythm, undernutrition, and decreased perception of heat and cold.[44,45]

Both infants and elderly people have difficulty regulating body heat through physiologic mechanisms of heat production and conservation. Health care providers need to be aware of these particular developmental differences, because infants cannot adjust to the environment to compensate for heat loss and elderly people, because of decreased peripheral sensation, may not be alerted to the need to do so.

Pathogenesis of Fever

Fever is a complex, integrated cascade of behavioral, neurologic, and endocrine responses to an immune challenge initiated by endogenous pyrogens.[46] It is a normal adaptive response to cytokines. The thermoregulatory mechanisms of the hypothalamus and brain stem adjust heat production, conservation, and loss to maintain body core temperature at a normal level.[47,48] During fever, this level is raised so that the thermoregulatory centers adjust heat production, conservation, and loss to maintain the core temperature at the new, higher temperature, which functions as a new "set point."[49]

The pathophysiology of fever begins with the introduction of **exogenous pyrogens** (i.e., endotoxins) (Fig. 14-7). The most frequently encountered exogenous pyrogens are the lipopolysaccharide complex in the cell wall of gram-positive bacteria and viruses.[50] **Endogenous pyrogens,** including interleukin-1 (IL-1), interleukin 6 (IL-6), tumor necrosis factor (TNF), and interferon-γ, are produced by phagocytic cells as they destroy microorganisms within the host.[51] The endogenous pyrogens act on brain cells, which release prostaglandin E_2 (PGE_2) and other cytokines.[52] An integrated behavioral, endocrine, and autonomic nervous system response is then initiated. Centers in the hypothalamus and brain stem signal an increase in heat production and heat conservation to raise body temperature to the new level. Peripheral vasoconstriction occurs with shunting of blood from the skin to the body core. Epinephrine release increases metabolic rate, and muscle tone increases. Decreased release of vasopressin reduces the volume of body fluid to be heated. Shivering also may occur. The individual dresses more warmly, decreases body surface area by curling up, and may go to bed in an effort to get warm. Body temperature is maintained at the new level until the fever "breaks."

During fever, arginine vasopressin (AVP), α–melanocyte-stimulating hormone (α-MSH), and corticotropin-releasing factor are released and can act as **endogenous cryogens** to help diminish the febrile response.[53] This antipyretic effect constitutes a negative-feedback loop (see Fig. 14-7).[54] The antipyretic effect may help explain fluctuations in the febrile response. When the fever breaks, the set point is returned to normal. The hypothalamus responds by signaling a decrease in heat production and an increase in heat reduction mechanisms. The result is decreased muscle tone, peripheral vasodilation, flushing of the skin, and sweating. The individual feels very warm, replaces warm clothing with cooler clothes, throws off the covers, and stretches out. Once the body has returned to a normal temperature, the individual feels more comfortable and the hypothalamus adjusts thermoregulatory mechanisms to maintain the new temperature.

Benefits of Fever

Fever production aids responses to infectious processes through several mechanisms.[55] Simple raising of body temperature kills many microorganisms and has adverse effects on the growth and replication of others. Higher body temperatures decrease serum levels of iron, zinc, and copper, all of which are needed for bacterial replication. The body switches from burning glucose to metabolism based on lipolysis and proteolysis, depriving bacteria of a food source. Anorexia and somnolence reduce the demand for muscle glucose.[56] Increased temperature also causes lysosomal breakdown and autodestruction of cells, thus preventing viral replication in infected cells. Acute-phase proteins produced by the liver during inflammation bind cations necessary for bacterial reproduction. Heat increases lymphocytic transformation and motility of polymorphonuclear neutrophils, thus facilitating the immune response. Phagocytosis is enhanced, and production of antiviral interferon may be augmented.[57,58]

Because fever is a beneficial response to infection, suppression of fever by treatment with antipyrogenic medications should be reviewed carefully.[48] Such treatment should be employed only if the fever produces or is high enough to produce serious side effects such as nerve damage or convulsion.

Infection and fever responses in elderly people and in children may vary from those in the normal adult. Older individuals may have decreased or no fever response to infection. The absence of fever responses to infection and therefore the beneficial aspects of fever production may explain the increase in morbidity and mortality rates seen in very elderly persons.[59] In contrast, children develop higher temperatures than adults for relatively minor infections. Febrile seizures may occur with temperatures above 39° C (102.2° F), although most children do not develop febrile seizures until temperatures are much higher. Febrile seizures are more predominant in male children before age 5 years. Febrile seizures are generally brief and self-limiting, lasting less than 5 minutes in 40% of children and less than 20 minutes in 75% of children. Authorities differ over the significance of febrile seizures. Although in most instances there appears to be no long-term effect on the child, a small percentage of children (1% to 2%) may develop epilepsy.[60]

Disorders of Temperature Regulation

Hyperthermia

Hyperthermia (marked warming of core temperature) can produce nerve damage, coagulation of cell proteins, and death. At 41° C (105.8° F), nerve damage produces convulsions in the adult. At 43° C (109.4° F), death results. Hyperthermia is not mediated by pyrogens, and there is no resetting of the hypothalamic set point. Hyperthermia may be accidental or therapeutic. Therapeutic hyperthermia is a form of local or general body-induced hyperthermia. Its purpose is to destroy pathologic microorganisms or tumor cells by facilitating the host's natural immune process through fever production. As a form of treatment, it is generally controversial. The four forms of accidental hyperthermia are (1) heat cramps, (2) heat exhaustion, (3) heat stroke, and (4) malignant hyperthermia.

Heat Cramps

Heat cramps are severe, spasmodic cramps in the abdomen and extremities that follow prolonged sweating and associated sodium loss. Heat cramps usually appear in individuals who are not accustomed to heat or in those who are performing strenuous work in very warm climates. Fever, rapid pulse, and increased blood pressure often accompany the cramps. Treatment involves administration of dilute salt solutions through oral or parenteral routes.

Heat Exhaustion

Heat exhaustion, or collapse, is a result of prolonged high core or environmental temperatures. These high temperatures cause the appropriate hypothalamic response of

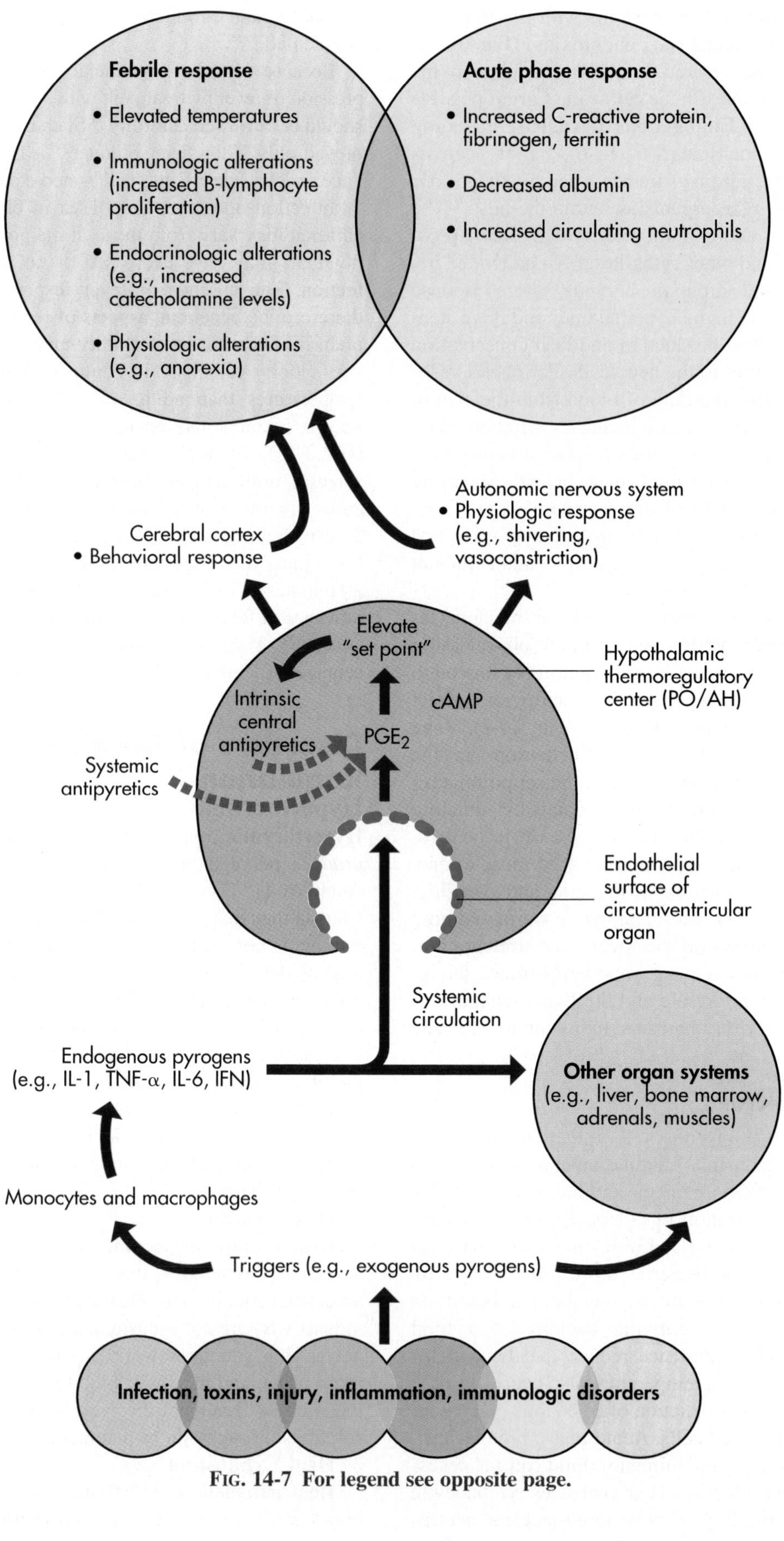

Febrile response
• Elevated temperatures
• Immunologic alterations (increased B-lymphocyte proliferation)
• Endocrinologic alterations (e.g., increased catecholamine levels)
• Physiologic alterations (e.g., anorexia)
Acute phase response
• Increased C-reactive protein, fibrinogen, ferritin
• Decreased albumin
• Increased circulating neutrophils
Autonomic nervous system
• Physiologic response (e.g., shivering, vasoconstriction)
Cerebral cortex
• Behavioral response
Elevate "set point"
Intrinsic central antipyretics
cAMP
PGE2
Hypothalamic thermoregulatory center (PO/AH)
Systemic antipyretics
Endothelial surface of circumventricular organ
Systemic circulation
Endogenous pyrogens (e.g., IL-1, TNF-α, IL-6, IFN)
Other organ systems
(e.g., liver, bone marrow, adrenals, muscles)
Monocytes and macrophages
Triggers (e.g., exogenous pyrogens)
Infection, toxins, injury, inflammation, immunologic disorders

FIG. 14-7 For legend see opposite page.

FIG. 14-7 Pathogenesis of fever and acute-phase response. Certain disease states, through the elaboration of exogenous pyrogens, stimulate monocytes and macrophages to produce endogenous pyrogens such as IL-1, TNF-α, IL-6, and interferon. These pyrogenic cytokines act at the endothelial surface of the circumventricular organ of the preoptic area of the anterior hypothalamus (PO/AH) to induce the production of PGE_2, which elevates the body's thermal set point. Intrinsic central antipyretics and systemic antipyretics exert their effects by decreasing levels of PGE_2. Physiologic and behavioral responses may be invoked to raise body temperature to a new set point. This febrile response must be considered in the context of an overlapping acute-phase response as a global nonspecific response to the original insult. (Modified from Armstrong D, Cohen J: *Infectious diseases,* St Louis, 1999, Mosby.)

profound vasodilation and profuse sweating. Over a prolonged period the hypothalamic responses produce dehydration, decreased plasma volumes, hypotension, decreased cardiac output, and tachycardia. The individual feels weak, dizzy, nauseated, and faint. The symptoms of heat exhaustion cause the individual to stop work, lie down, and rest. Ceasing activity decreases muscle work, causing decreased heat production. Lying down redistributes vascular volume. The individual should be encouraged to drink warm fluids to replace fluid lost through sweating.

Heat Stroke

Heat stroke is a potentially lethal result of a breakdown in control of an overstressed thermoregulatory center. The brain cannot tolerate temperatures over 40.5° C (104.9° F). When core temperature reaches or exceeds 40.5° C (104.9° F), the brain may be preferentially cooled by maximal blood flow through the veins of the head and face, specifically the forehead. Sweat production on the face is maintained even during dehydration. Evaporation of the sweat cools the blood in the veins of the face and forehead; the blood then is returned to the endocranial venous network and sinus cavernosus, cooling the blood in the cerebral arterial vessels that lie in close proximity. Fanning the face enhances this mechanism. In this way the brain can be maintained temporarily at 40° C (104° F), even when core temperatures are higher.[42,61] In instances of very high core temperatures (40° to 43° C [104° to 109.4° F]), the regulatory center may cease to function appropriately. Sweating ceases, and the skin becomes dry and flushed. The individual may be irritable, confused, stuporous, or comatose. Visual disturbances may occur.

As heat loss through the evaporation of sweat ceases, core temperatures increase rapidly. High core temperatures and vascular collapse produce cerebral edema, degeneration of the central nervous system, swollen dendrites, and renal tubular necrosis. Death results unless immediate, effective treatment is initiated.[62]

Treatment includes removing the person from the warm environment, if possible, and using a cooling blanket or cool water bath. Care must be taken to prevent too rapid cooling of the surface, which causes peripheral vasoconstriction and prevents core cooling. Individuals who recover from heat stroke may have permanent damage to the thermoregulatory center and thus may have difficulty tolerating environmental temperature changes.

Children are more susceptible to heat stroke than adults because (1) they produce more metabolic heat when exercising, (2) they have a greater surface area to mass ratio, and (3) their sweating capacity is less than that of adults.[63]

Malignant Hyperthermia

Malignant hyperthermia is a potentially lethal complication of a rare inherited muscle disorder. The condition is precipitated by the administration of volatile anesthetics and neuromuscular blocking agents. About 1 in 200 individuals may be at risk for the muscle disorder. Malignant hyperthermia is caused by either increased calcium release or decreased calcium uptake with muscle contraction. This allows intracellular calcium levels to rise, producing sustained, uncoordinated muscle contractions, which in turn increase muscle work, oxygen consumption, and lactic acid production. As a result of these contractions, acidosis develops and temperature rises (body temperature may rise 1° C [1.8° F] every 5 minutes); approximately 20% of those who develop malignant hyperthermia do not survive. Malignant hyperthermia occurs most often in children and young adults immediately after the induction of anesthesia.

Sympathetic responses and acidosis produce tachycardia and cardiac dysrhythmias, followed by hypotension, decreased cardiac output, and, eventually, cardiac arrest. Increasing temperature, acidosis, hyperkalemia, and hypoxia produce comalike symptoms in the CNS (including unconsciousness, absent reflexes, fixed pupils, apnea, and sometimes a flat electroencephalogram [EEG]). Oliguria and anuria are common, probably resulting from shock, ischemia, and low cardiac output.[64]

Treatment includes withdrawal of the provoking agents and administration of dantrolene sodium (a skeletal relaxant that inhibits calcium release during muscle contraction). Procainamide (Pronestyl) is used to treat cardiac dysrhythmias. Sodium bicarbonate also may be used. Body temperature can be decreased through use of ice bags, a cooling blanket, and iced saline lavage.[64]

Hypothermia

Hypothermia (marked cooling of core temperature) produces vasoconstriction, alterations in microcirculation, coagulation, and ischemic tissue damage. In a controlled situation, such as a surgical procedure, most tissues can tolerate temperatures as low as 7° C. In severe hypothermia (less than 28° C), ice crystals forming on the inside of the cell cause cells to rupture and die. Tissue hypothermia slows the rate of chemical reactions (tissue metabolism), increases the viscosity of the blood, slows blood flow through the microcirculation, facilitates blood coagulation, and stimulates profound vasoconstriction. Hypothermia may be accidental or therapeutic.

Accidental Hypothermia

Accidental hypothermia (temperature below 35° C [95° F]) is generally the result of sudden immersion in cold water or prolonged exposure to cold environments.[65] At particular risk for accidental hypothermia are young persons and elderly persons, because thermoregulatory mechanisms are altered in these two groups.[66] Also at risk are individuals with conditions that diminish the ability to generate heat. Such conditions include hypothyroidism, hypopituitarism, malnutrition, Parkinson disease, and rheumatoid arthritis. Other risk factors include chronic increased vasodilation and decreased thermoregulatory control caused by cerebral injuries, ketoacidosis, uremia, and drug overdoses.[67]

In acute hypothermia, peripheral vasoconstriction shunts blood away from the cooler skin to the core in an effort to decrease heat loss. This peripheral vasoconstriction produces peripheral tissue ischemia. Intermittent reperfusion of the extremities (the Lewis phenomenon) helps preserve peripheral oxygenation. Intermittent peripheral perfusion continues until core temperatures drop dramatically.

The hypothalamic center stimulates shivering in an effort to increase heat production. Severe shivering occurs at core temperatures of 35° C (95° F) and continues until core temperature drops to about 30° to 32° C (86° to 89.6° F). Thinking becomes sluggish and coordination is decreased at 34° C (93.2° F). As hypothermia deepens, paradoxic undressing may occur as hypothalamic control of vasoconstriction is lost and vasodilation occurs with loss of core heat to the periphery. The hypothermic individual therefore feels suddenly warm and begins to remove clothing.[67]

At 30° C (86° F), the individual becomes stuporous; heart rate and respiratory rate decline; and cardiac output is diminished. Cerebral blood flow is decreased. Metabolic rate declines, further decreasing core temperature. Sinus node depression occurs with slowing of conduction through the atrioventricular node. In severe hypothermia (core temperature of 26° to 28° C [78.8° to 82.4° F]), pulse and respirations may be undetectable. Acidosis is moderate to severe. Ventricular fibrillation and asystole are common.[61]

If hypothermia is mild, passive rewarming may be sufficient. Passive rewarming includes provision of warm, dry clothes and warm drinks and performance of isometric exercises to increase heat production and minimize heat loss. Core temperature should be checked as soon as possible.[68]

If core temperature is above 30° C (86° F), active rewarming also may be required. Active rewarming employs warm water baths, warm blankets, heating pads, and warm oral fluids when the individual is fully alert. Active core rewarming is performed when core temperatures have dropped below 30° C (86° F) or when severe cardiovascular abnormalities appear. Core rewarming may be accomplished through administration of warm intravenous solutions, warm gastric lavage, warm peritoneal lavage, inhalation of warmed gases, and, in extreme cases, exchange transfusions, warming blood in a pump oxygenator circuit, and mediastinal lavage.[69]

Rewarming generally should proceed no faster than a few degrees per hour. (Short-term complications of rewarming are listed in Table 14-3.) Long-term complications include congestive heart failure, hepatic and renal failure, abnormal erythropoiesis, myocardial infarction, pancreatitis, and neurologic dysfunctions.

Therapeutic Hypothermia

Therapeutic hypothermia is used to slow metabolism and thus preserve ischemic tissue during surgery or limb reimplantation. The actual mechanism of tissue preservation has been debated.[70] It is possible that the slowed metabolism in hypothermic tissues preserves adenosine triphosphate (ATP).[71] Regardless of the mechanism, however, it is clear that hypothermic ischemic cells remain viable long after normothermic ischemic cells have died. Survival from accidental hypothermia has been reported in individuals with core temperatures at 16° C (60.8° F) and from therapeutic hypothermia with temperatures at 9° C (48.2° F).[61]

The temperature changes of hypothermia place a great deal of stress on the heart. Moderate to severe hypothermia may lead to ventricular fibrillation and cardiac arrest. (This may be the desired outcome in open heart surgery when the heart must be stopped during portions of the surgical procedure.[72]) Prolonged hypothermia may precipitate exhaustion of liver glycogen stores by prolonged shivering. Surface cooling may cause burns, frostbite, and fat necrosis.

Trauma

Major body trauma has varying effects on temperature regulation, depending on the body systems involved. Five types of traumatic injury that usually affect temperature regulation are (1) CNS trauma (discussed in Chapter 16), (2) accidental injury, (3) hemorrhagic shock, (4) major surgery, and (5) thermal burns.

Central Nervous System Trauma

CNS trauma that causes CNS damage, inflammation, increased intracranial pressures, or intracranial bleeding typi-

Table 14-3 Accidental Hypothermia: Complications of Rewarming

Complication	Mechanism
Acidosis	Rewarming stimulates peripheral vasodilation; peripheral blood, returning to the core from the ischemic peripheral tissues, causes a reduction in the pH of core blood
Rewarming shock	As rewarming and vasodilation progress, the body is unable to maintain blood pressure because of reduced fluid volume (from "cold diuresis"), catecholamine depletion (prolonged shivering), and myocardial injury
Deep-ended hypothermia	As colder surface blood is returned to the core, core temperatures may drop; this is also referred to as "after fall" or "after drop"
Dysrhythmia	Rewarming places an additional stress on an already severely stressed myocardium

cally produces a fever greater than 39° C (102.2° F). This temperature, often referred to as a *central fever,* appears with or without relative bradycardia. The temperature is sustained, does not induce sweating, and is highly resistant to antipyretic therapy.

Accidental Injuries

Mild accidental injuries may produce a slight elevation in core temperature. Moderate to severe injuries result in peripheral vasoconstriction with decreased surface and core temperatures. Core temperature is thought to be inversely related to the severity of the injury and may be a result of decreased oxygen transport to the tissues. In severe injuries, shivering is absent and some alteration in thermoregulation is evident.[73]

Hemorrhagic Shock

Loss of blood volume in hemorrhage triggers peripheral vasoconstriction and a slight increase in core temperature. Subsequent decreases in core temperature have been demonstrated in individuals with hemorrhagic shock treated with unwarmed volume-expanding solutions and surgical repair. Volume expansion with warmed solutions is recommended to prevent the deleterious effects of hypothermia on cardiac output, cardiac rhythm, and the immune system.[72]

Major Surgery

Because many victims of trauma undergo major surgical repair, the effect of the surgical procedure on temperature regulation needs to be considered by health care providers. Major surgery often induces significant hypothermia through exposure of body cavities to the relatively cool operating room environment. Other mechanisms that contribute to intraoperative hypothermia include irrigation of body cavities with room temperature solutions, infusion of room temperature intravenous solutions, use of drugs that impair thermoregulatory mechanisms, and inhalation of unwarmed anesthetic agents.[72] Use of warmed irrigating and intravenous solutions may reduce intraoperative hypothermia.

Thermal Burns

Large burn injuries produce significant hypothermia because of the loss of the skin barrier to fluid evaporation and the loss of control of the microcirculation in the skin. Severe burns also compromise the normal insulation of the skin and subcutaneous tissues. (Burns are discussed in Chapter 45.)

SLEEP

Sleep is an active, multiphase process. Although brain activity during sleep varies from wakeful states, an equal amount of energy is consumed during both states.[74] Normal sleep has two phases that can be documented by EEG: rapid eye movement (REM) sleep and non-REM, or slow-wave, sleep.[75,76] Non-REM sleep is divided into four stages based on changes in the EEG pattern (Fig. 14-8):

Stage I—light sleep, with alpha waves interspersed with low-frequency theta waves; slow eye movements
Stage II—further slowing of the EEG with the presence of sleep spindles and slow eye movements
Stage III—low-frequency delta waves with occasional sleep spindles; no slow eye movements
Stage IV—delta waves

The hypothalamus is a major sleep center, and PGD_2 and adenosine may be important endogenous sleep-promoting factors of the basal forebrain.[77,78]

Non–Rapid Eye Movement Sleep

Non-REM (slow-wave) sleep is initiated by the withdrawal of neurotransmitters from the reticular formation and by the inhibition of arousal mechanisms in the cerebral cortex. During non-REM sleep, respiration is controlled by metabolic processes.[79] The basal metabolic rate is decreased by 10% to 15%. Temperature is decreased 0.5° to 1° C (0.9° to 1.8° F). Heart rate decreases by 10 to 30 beats per minute. Respiration, blood pressure, and muscle tone all decrease. Knee-jerk reflexes are absent. Pupils are constricted. During stages I and II, cerebral blood flow to the brain stem and cerebellum is decreased. During stages III and IV, cerebral blood flow to the cortex is decreased.[80] Growth hormone is released during stage IV, and levels of corticosteroids and catecholamines are depressed.

Rapid Eye Movement Sleep

Rapid eye movement (REM) sleep is characterized by desynchronized, low-voltage, fast activity that occurs about every 90 minutes beginning after 1 to 2 hours of non-REM sleep. This sleep is also known as *paradoxic sleep* because the EEG pattern is similar to the normal awake pattern. Alternating periods of REM and non-REM sleep occur throughout the night, with lengthening intervals of REM sleep and

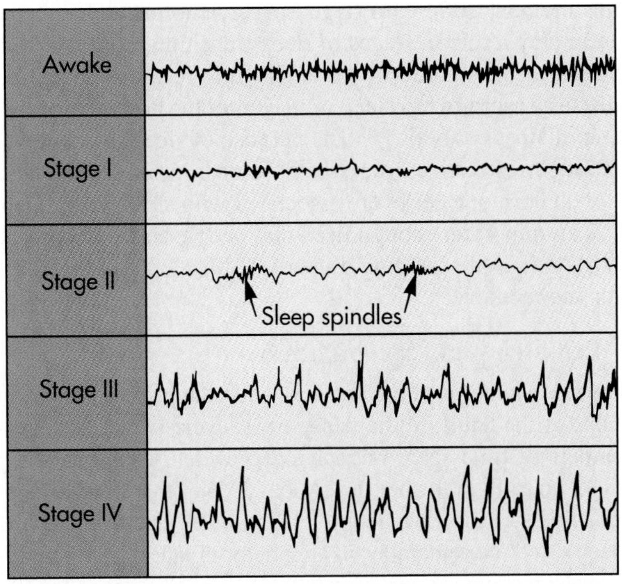

FIG. 14-8 Electroencephalogram (EEG) stages of wakefulness and sleep. *Awake,* Low-voltage fast activity; *stage I,* falling asleep; *stage II,* light sleep with sleep spindles; *stage III,* moderately deep sleep; *stage IV,* deep sleep with slow delta waves. Rapid eye movement (REM) sleep looks similar to awake and stage I.

fewer intervals of deeper stages of non-REM sleep toward morning. REM sleep is characterized by bursts of conjugate rapid eye movement; atonia of antigravity muscles; loss of temperature regulation; alteration in heart rate, blood pressure,[81] and respiration; penile erection in men and clitoral engorgement in women; and a high rate of memorable dreams. Steroids are released in short bursts. During REM sleep, respiratory control is thought to be largely independent of metabolic requirements and oxygen variation. Loss of normal voluntary muscle control in the tongue and upper pharynx may produce some respiratory obstruction. Cerebral blood flow to both hemispheres is increased. About 20% to 25% of sleep time is represented by REM sleep in the adult. REM sleep is controlled by the pontine reticular formation.

Many neurotransmitters are associated with excitatory and inhibitory sleep mechanisms, including catecholamines, acetylcholine, serotonin, histamine, L-tryptophan, prostaglandins, and adenosine.[82] Their mechanism of action is complex and not clearly understood. The reticular formation is primarily responsible for generating REM sleep, and projections from the reticular formation and other areas of the mesencephalon and brain stem produce non-REM sleep.[83] Growth hormone is associated with initiation of sleep, and cortisol rises in the morning.[84]

While asleep, an individual progresses through REM and non-REM sleep in a predictable cycle. Each cycle lasts approximately 90 to 110 minutes, with the individual passing through four to five cycles per night.[85] The first cycle of the night begins with stage I. The individual then progresses through stages II, III, IV, III, II, and REM sleep. A new cycle, beginning with stage II, follows each REM sleep. With each successive cycle, the amount of time spent in stage IV sleep decreases and the amount of time spent in REM sleep increases (Fig. 14-9). The individual who is awakened begins the next cycle with stage I. Acetylcholine and somatostatin play a role in stages of sleep transition. Forced awakenings in the middle of the night may result in increased difficulty returning to sleep or may alter the normal progression of sleep, or both.[86,87] The purpose of sleep is unknown, although restorative processes have been proposed because growth hormone peaks are associated with slow-wave sleep. It is an important enough need that people spend about one third of their life sleeping. Loss of REM sleep impairs learning and memory.[88]

Pediatrics and Sleep Patterns

The sleep patterns of the newborn and young child vary from those of the adult in total sleep time, cycle length, and percentage of time spent in each sleep cycle. Newborns sleep about 16 to 17 hours per day. About 53% of that time is spent in active sleep (REM sleep), 23% in quiet sleep (non-REM sleep), and the remainder in an indeterminate phase. The infant sleep cycle is approximately 50 to 60 minutes in length, with 20 minutes of non-REM sleep and 10 to 45 minutes of REM sleep, in contrast to the adult sleep cycle. Newborns enter REM sleep immediately on falling asleep.[89,90] At about 1 year of age, the infant spends approximately 45% of total sleep time in quiet sleep and 41% in REM sleep. Total sleep time decreases slightly from birth to 1 year. In the American culture, where infants are bottle fed and do not share sleeping space with the mother, infants increase maximum sleep time from 4 to 5 hours to 8 to 10 hours by 4 months of age. They begin to "sleep through the night." In other cultures, where infants are breast fed for up to 2 years and share sleeping space with the mother, they continue to sleep in short bouts and wake frequently to nurse.[91]

In the young child, the sleep cycle length is 45 to 60 minutes, in contrast to 90 to 100 minutes in the adult. The child assumes the adult sleep pattern at some point during the first 2 to 5 years of life.[92]

Aging and Sleep Patterns

The sleep pattern of the older adult differs from that of the younger adult or child. Total sleep time is decreased, and the older individual takes longer to fall asleep. Elderly people awaken earlier in the morning and more frequently during the night. Total REM and stage II time is unchanged, but stage IV sleep decreases by 15% to 30%. On EEG, the spindle indicating stage II sleep is less well formed.[93,94]

These changes in the older adult's sleep pattern may be associated with changes in life-style, physical ailments, lack

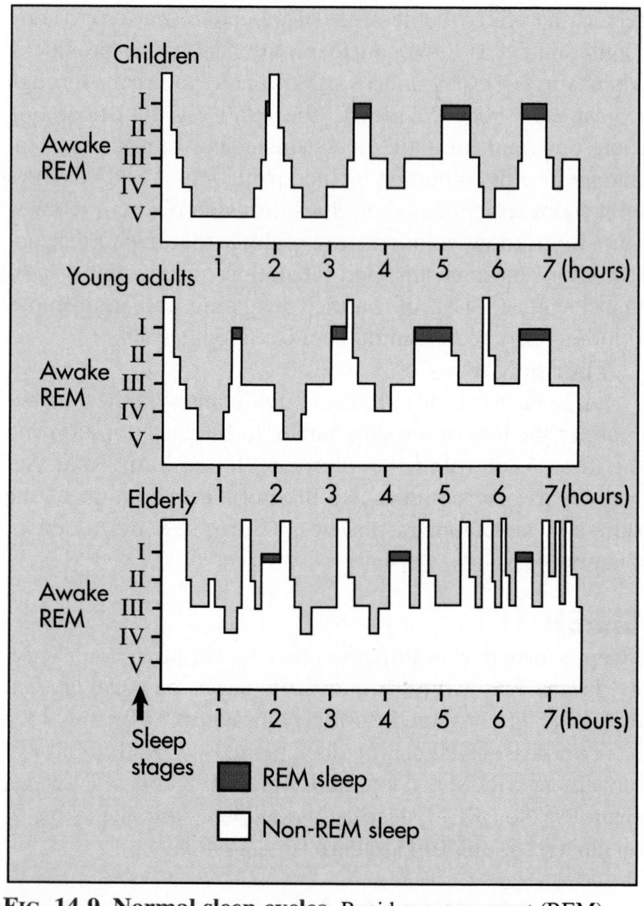

FIG. 14-9 Normal sleep cycles. Rapid eye movement (REM) sleep occurs cyclically throughout the night at intervals of approximately 90 minutes in all age-groups. REM sleep shows little variation in the different age-groups, whereas stage IV sleep decreases with age. In addition, elderly persons awaken frequently and show a marked increase in total time awake.

of daily routine, desynchronization of circadian rhythm, and use of sedatives. Growth hormone and cortisol are diminished in the elderly and may affect sleep patterns.[95] The alteration in sleep pattern typically appears about 10 years later in women than in men. Older adults are less able than younger individuals to tolerate sleep deprivation.[92]

Sleep Disorders

Sleep disorders are classified by their signs and symptoms rather than by their cause. Four classifications of sleep disorders are (1) disorders of initiating sleep; (2) sleep disordered breathing; (3) disorders of the sleep/wake schedule; and (4) dysfunctions of sleep, sleep stages, or partial arousals.

Disorders of Initiating Sleep: Insomnia

Insomnia is defined as the inability to fall or stay asleep. Insomnia may be transient, lasting a few days, and related to travel across time zones, or it may be caused by acute stress. Long-term insomnia is associated with drug or alcohol abuse, chronic pain disorders, or chronic depression. Drugs known to produce insomnia include amphetamines, steroids, central adrenergic blockers, bronchodilating agents, and caffeine.[96]

Sleep Disordered Breathing

The disorders of breathing during sleep are related to airway resistance and exist along a continuum of severity, including upper airway resistance syndrome, obstructive sleep apnea, and obesity hypoventilation syndrome. Sleep disordered breathing affects more men than women.[97] One hypothesis to explain this is that the female hormone progesterone, a respiratory stimulant, may protect premenopausal women from sleep disordered breathing.[98]

Upper airway resistance syndrome is characterized by repetitive increases in resistance to airflow within the upper airway with snoring and brief arousals from sleep and daytime somnolence. The level of negative intrathoracic pressure is the most likely stimulus for arousal, possibly mediated by mechanoreceptors in the upper airway. Hypertension is an important consequence of this disorder, probably resulting from a combination of intermittent hypoxia and hypercapnia, arousals, increased sympathetic tone, altered baroreflex control during sleep, and cardiovascular changes induced by increased negative intrathoracic pressure. Nasal continuous positive airway pressure is the most effective form of therapy.[99,100]

Obstructive sleep apnea (OSA) syndrome affects up to 4% of middle-age adults. Symptoms of OSA include loud snoring, a decrease in oxygen saturation, fragmented sleep, chronic daytime sleepiness, and fatigue. These episodes usually last 10 to 30 seconds and result in the possible development of cardiovascular abnormalities. The obstruction is caused by the soft palate, base of the tongue, or both collapsing against the pharyngeal walls because of decreased muscle tone during sleep. Many individuals are not aware of their heavy snoring and nocturnal arousals and may remain undiagnosed. Potentially fatal systemic illnesses frequently associated with this disorder include hypertension, pulmonary hypertension, heart failure, nocturnal cardiac dysrhythmias, myocardial infarction, and ischemic stroke.[101a]

Treatments include nasal continuous positive airway pressure and dental devices that modify the position of the tongue or jaw. Upper airway and jaw surgical procedures may also be appropriate in selected patients.[101b]

Obesity hypoventilation syndrome is the most severe form of disordered breathing during sleep and is associated with severe morbidity and very high mortality. Most individuals are overweight and have a short, thick neck. Profound obesity is associated with impaired respiratory mechanics and depressed respiratory control, particularly during sleep. Systemic complications include pulmonary hypertension and ischemic heart disease. Daytime sleepiness, fatigue, car accidents, and poor work performance are common.

Continuous positive pressure and airway reconstruction are effective treatments for severe obstructive sleep apnea in the morbidly obese person. Careful selection and identification of potential coexisting obesity hypoventilation syndrome and counseling on weight reduction and avoidance of continual weight gain will improve treatment outcomes.[101c]

Disorders of the Sleep/Wake Schedule

Common disorders of the sleep/wake schedule include rapid time-zone change (jet-lag syndrome), changing sleep schedule with an advance or a delay of 3 hours or more in sleep time, or a change in total sleep time from day to day. These changes in the timing of established sleep schedules have been shown to desynchronize circadian rhythm. Degree of vigilance, performance of psychomotor tasks, and subjective reports of levels of arousal are markedly depressed after alterations in the sleep/wake schedule. Individuals may experience short sleep episodes called *microsleeps* without being aware of decreased vigilance.[102]

It is well established that industrial shift workers exhibit a decrease in accuracy and increased accident proneness.[103] For similar reasons, persons suffering from jet lag require several days to adapt to the new time zone. Travel across time zones requires 2 days to adjust the sleep/wake schedule, 5 days to adjust the body temperature cycle, and 8 days to adjust cortisol secretion. Transmeridian travel requires up to 10 days to adjust the body clock when traveling from east to west. Czeisler's experiments with timed bright-light stimulation have had some success in retiming or resetting the body clock after time-zone shifts.[104]

Parasomnias

Parasomnias are unusual behaviors occurring during sleep, including sleepwalking, night terrors, rearranging furniture, eating food, violent behavior, and enuresis. Three dysfunctions of sleep are common in children: somnambulism (sleepwalking), night terrors (dream anxiety attacks), and enuresis (bedwetting).

Somnambulism

Somnambulism is a disorder primarily of childhood and appears to resolve itself within several years of the onset of the sleepwalking episodes. Sleepwalking occurs in stages III and IV and is therefore not associated with dreaming.

During the sleepwalking episode, the child functions at a very low level of arousal and has no memory of the event on awakening. The greatest concern is for the safety of the child.

Night Terrors

Night terrors are characterized by "sudden apparent arousals in which the child expresses intense fear or emotion."[92] The child, however, is not awake and is very difficult to arouse. Once awakened, the child has no memory of the night terror event. Night terrors occur during stage IV sleep and are not associated with the dreams of REM sleep. Although night terrors occur most often in children, adults may experience them as well. Unlike children, however, adults often display corresponding daytime anxiety.[104]

Enuresis

Enuresis is possibly the most disturbing of the childhood sleep dysfunctions because of the stress society places on nighttime continence and the misconception that children are bedwetting to act out against parents. Bedwetting incidents also are associated incorrectly with dreaming. Laboratory studies of sleep have demonstrated that very few incidents of bedwetting occur when the child is dreaming and that, by far, most incidents occur during non-REM sleep and during the first one third of the night, when the child is most difficult to arouse.[92] Most causes of enuresis are benign and treatable. Evaluations should be completed to detect infections, obstructions, decreased nocturnal secretion of antidiuretic hormone, and neurogenic bladder.[105] Children usually outgrow the enuretic episodes, but management is important to prevent psychologic problems.[106]

Relation between Sleep and Disease

Sleep and disease are interrelated. Some diseases produce alterations in the quantity and quality of sleep or affect sleep stages. These are referred to as **secondary sleep disorders.** In some instances sleep stages produce alterations in certain disease states. These are referred to as **sleep-provoked disorders.** Other entities, such as sudden infant death syndrome (SIDS) and sudden unexplained nocturnal death syndrome (SUNDS), produce unexplained death almost exclusively during sleep.[104]

Secondary Sleep Disorders

The most common causes of secondary sleep disorders are depression, alterations in thyroid hormone secretion (hypothyroidism or hyperthyroidism), pain, and sleep apnea syndromes. Depressed persons have difficulty falling asleep and exhibit less slow-wave sleep, less time spent in REM sleep, early awakening, and less total sleep time. In addition, depressed individuals move through the sleep stages more quickly than do individuals who are not depressed. The same neurotransmitters that may be disturbed in depression also regulate sleep; serotonergic neuron dysfunction also is a possible mechanism.[107] Sleep deprivation paradoxically relieves depression.[104]

Changes in thyroid hormone secretion produce changes in stages III and IV sleep. An increase in thyroid secretion produces an increase in stages III and IV activity, whereas a decrease in thyroid hormone produces a decrease in both stages III and IV sleep.

Chronic pain is a cause of insomnia. Chronic pain inhibits sleep, increases arousals during sleep, and causes prolonged awake intervals during the night. Individuals with chronic pain report not only a decrease in the quantity of sleep but also a decrease in its quality.

Sleep-Provoked Disorders

Some diseases are provoked by certain aspects of sleep. Signs and symptoms of the disease appear during, or are enhanced by, sleep. Diseases that are affected by sleep include coronary artery disease, bronchial asthma, chronic obstructive pulmonary disease (COPD), diabetes, and duodenal ulcers.

Coronary artery disease is most affected during REM sleep. During REM, dreams may provoke nocturnal angina, increased heart rate, and electrocardiogram (ECG) changes. In adults, attacks of bronchial asthma may occur at any time during the night. The attacks cause the individual to spend more of the sleep period awake and thus cause a decrease in stage IV sleep. In children, bronchial asthma attacks are uncommon during the first one third of the night, when stage IV sleep predominates, and occur more frequently during the final two thirds of the night. Stage IV sleep is decreased overall in the child with bronchial asthma. In addition to these changes, asthmatics may experience bronchial spasm during REM sleep.[108]

Persons with COPD experience significantly lowered oxygen tension and increases in carbon dioxide retention during sleep. The lowered oxygen tension is most significant in the tonic phase of REM sleep when voluntary neuromuscular control, including intercostal muscle function, is depressed. Pulmonary spasm and transient pulmonary hypertension result. These changes are particularly evident in the so-called "blue bloater" individual and may contribute to early pulmonary hypertension and cor pulmonale in these persons.[109]

Because blood glucose levels vary during sleep, individuals with uncontrolled diabetes may need careful attention to blood sugar levels during sleep. Studies show that people with duodenal ulcers secrete 3 to 20 times more gastric acid during REM sleep than do people without duodenal ulcers. This increased gastric acid secretion often produces nocturnal epigastric pain.[92]

SIDS affects children primarily in the first 2 years of life and may be related to central sleep apnea episodes. (For further discussion of SIDS, see Chapter 33.)

SPECIAL SENSES

Vision

The eyes are complex sense organs responsible for vision. Within a protective casing, each eye has receptors, a lens system for focusing light on the receptors, and a system of nerves for conducting impulses from the receptors to the brain. Visual dysfunction may be caused by abnormal ocular movements or alterations in visual acuity, refraction, color vision, or accommodation. Visual dysfunction also may be the secondary effect of another neurologic disorder.

External Eye Structures

The external structures protecting the eye include the eyelids (palpebrae), conjunctivae, and lacrimal apparatus (Fig. 14-10). Infection and inflammatory responses are the most common conditions affecting the supporting structures of the eyes. **Blepharitis** is an inflammation of the eyelids caused by staphylococcus or seborrheic dermatitis. Redness, edema, and itching are common symptoms. A **hordeolum (stye)** is an infection of the sebaceous glands of the eyelids, and a **chalazion** is an infection of the meibomian (oil-secreting) gland. These conditions are treated symptomatically.[110]

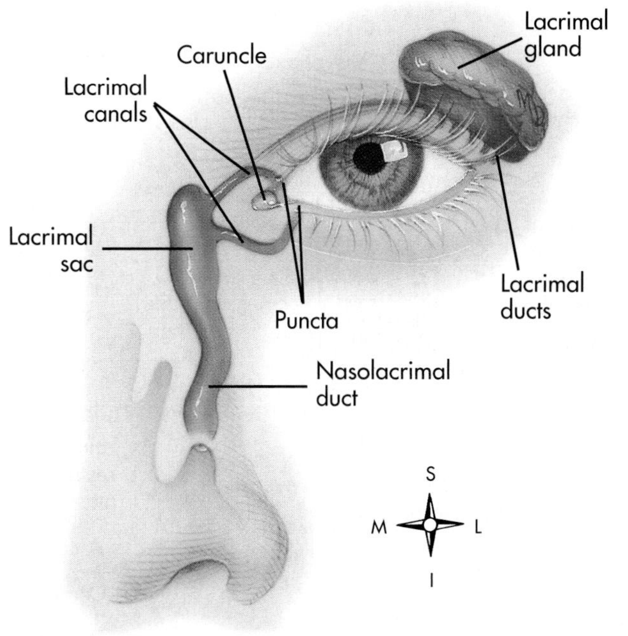

FIG. 14-10 Lacrimal apparatus. Fluid produced by lacrimal glands (tears) streams across the eye surface, enters the canals, and then passes through the nasolacrimal duct to enter the nose. (From Thibodeau GA, Patton KI: *Anatomy and physiology,* ed 4, St Louis, 1999, Mosby.)

Conjunctivitis

Conjunctivitis is an inflammation of the conjunctiva (mucous membrane covering the front part of the eyeball). Conjunctivitis may be caused by bacteria, viruses, allergies, or chemical irritations. The inflammatory response produces redness, edema, pain, and lacrimation. Treatment is related to cause.[111]

Acute bacterial conjunctivitis (pinkeye) is highly contagious and often is caused by gram-positive organisms *(Staphylococcus, Haemophilus, Proteus),* although other bacteria may be involved. The onset is acute, characterized by mucopurulent drainage from one or both eyes. Preventing spread of the organism with meticulous hand washing and use of separate towels is important. The disease frequently is self-limiting and resolves spontaneously in 10 to 14 days. Antibiotic eye drops usually are effective.

Viral conjunctivitis is caused by an adenovirus. Symptoms vary from mild to severe. Some strains of virus cause conjunctivitis and pharyngitis (pharyngoconjunctival fever), and others cause keratoconjunctivitis. Both diseases are contagious, with watering, redness, and photophobia. Treatment is symptomatic.

Allergic conjunctivitis is associated with a variety of antigens, including pollens. There is ocular itching associated with photophobia, burning, and gritty sensations in the eye. Treatment is symptomatic and may include antihistamines, steroids, and vasoconstrictors.

Chronic conjunctivitis is the result of any persistent conjunctivitis. The cause requires identification for effective treatment.

Trachoma (chlamydial conjunctivitis) is caused by *Chlamydia trachomatis.* It often is associated with poor hygiene and is the leading cause of preventable blindness in the world. The severity of the disease varies, but it can involve inflammation and vascularization of the cornea with scarring of the conjunctiva and eyelids, leading to blindness. Chlamydial organisms are sensitive to local or systemic antibiotics.

Keratitis

Keratitis is an infection of the cornea that can be caused by bacteria or viruses. Bacterial infections often cause corneal ulceration and require intensive antibiotic treatment. Type I herpes simplex virus can involve both the cornea and conjunctiva. Common symptoms include photophobia, pain, and lacrimation. Severe ulcerations with residual scarring require corneal transplantation.

The Eye

The wall of the eye is formed of three layers: sclera, choroid, and retina (Fig. 14-11). The **sclera** is the thick, white, outermost layer. It becomes transparent at the **cornea,** the portion of the sclera in the central anterior region that allows light to enter the eye. The **choroid** is the deeply pigmented middle layer that prevents light from scattering inside the eye. The **iris,** part of the choroid, has a round opening, the **pupil,** through which light passes. Smooth muscle fibers control the size of the pupil so that in close vision and bright light the pupil constricts and in distant vision and dim light the pupil dilates.

The innermost layer of the eye, the **retina,** contains millions of rods and cones, special photoreceptors that convert light energy into nerve impulses. In the retina, **rods** mediate peripheral and dim light vision and are densest at the periphery. **Cones,** densest in the center of the retina, are color and detail receptors. The photoreceptive rods and cones are distributed over the entire retina, except where the optic nerve leaves the eyeball. Lack of rods and cones in this area results in the **optic disc,** or blind spot. Lateral to each optic disc is the **fovea centralis,** a tiny area that contains only cones and provides the greatest visual acuity (see Fig. 14-11).

As shown in Fig. 14-12, nerve impulses pass through the optic nerves after leaving the retinas. At the optic chiasm the

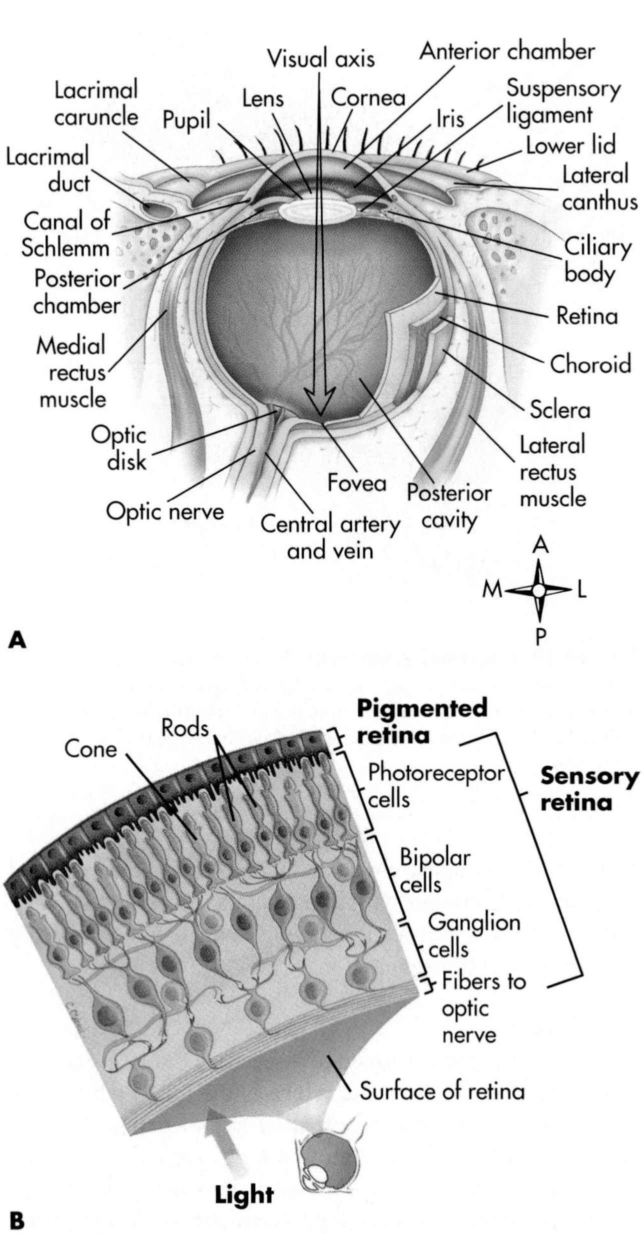

FIG. 14-11 Structure of the eyeball and cell layers of the retina. A, Horizontal section through the left eyeball. The eye is viewed viewed from above. **B,** Pigmented and sensory layers of the retina. (From Thibodeau GA, Patton KT: *Anatomy and physiology,* ed 4, St Louis, 1999, Mosby.)

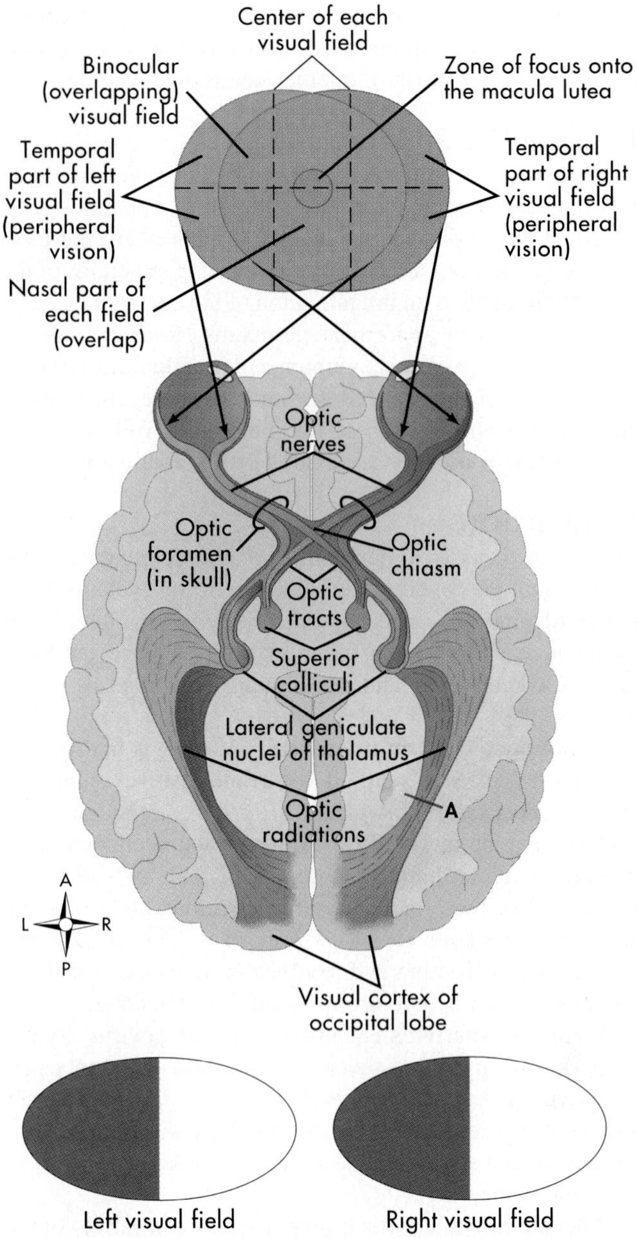

FIG. 14-12 Visual fields and neuronal pathways. Note the structures that make up each pathway: optic nerve, optic chiasm, lateral geniculate body of thalamus, optic radiations, and visual cortex of occipital lobe. Fibers from the nasal portion of each retina cross over to the opposite side at the optic chiasma and terminate in the lateral geniculate nuclei. Location of a lesion in the visual pathway determines the resulting visual defect. Damage at point *A,* for example, would cause blindness in the right nasal and left temporal visual fields, as the ovals beneath indicate. (Trace the visual pathway from point *A* back to the visual field map to see why this is so.) What would be the effect of pressure on the optic chiasm—by a pituitary tumor, for instance? (Answer: It would produce blindness in both temporal visual fields. Why? Because it destroys fibers from the nasal side of both retinas.) (Modified from Thibodeau GA, Patton KI: *Anatomy and physiology,* ed 4, St Louis, 1999, Mosby.)

fibers from the inner (nasal) halves of the retinas cross to the opposite side, where they join fibers from the outer (temporal) halves of the retinas to form the optic tracts. The fibers of the optic tracts synapse in the dorsal lateral geniculate nucleus, and from there the geniculocalcarine fibers pass by way of the optic radiation (or geniculocalcarine tract) to the primary visual cortex in the occipital lobe of the brain.

Light entering the eye is focused on the retina by the **lens**—a flexible, biconvex, crystal-like structure. In youth the lens is transparent and has the consistency of hardened jelly. With age the lens becomes increasingly hard and opaque. The lens divides the anterior chamber into (1) the aqueous chamber and (2) the vitreous chamber. **Aqueous humor,** which fills the aqueous chamber, helps maintain the pressure inside the eye and provides nutrients to the lens and cornea. Aqueous humor is free-flowing fluid, secreted by the ciliary processes and reabsorbed into the canal of Schlemm. If drainage is blocked, pressure within the eye increases (as

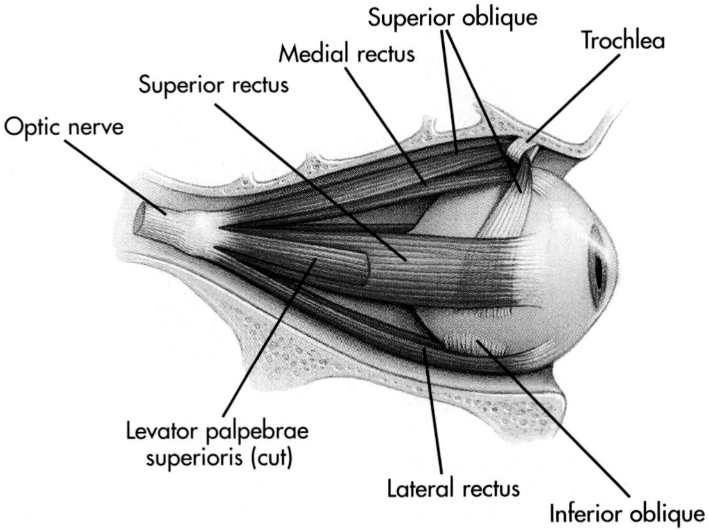

FIG. 14-13 Extrinsic muscles of the right eye. Superior view. (From Thibodeau GA, Patton KI: *Anatomy and physiology*, ed 4, St Louis, 1999, Mosby.)

Table 14-4 Changes in the Eye Caused by Aging

Structure	Change	Consequence
Cornea	Thicker and less curved	Increase in astigmatism
	Formation of a gray ring at the edge of the cornea (arcus senilis)	Not detrimental to vision
Anterior chamber	Decrease in size and volume caused by thickening of lens	Occasionally exerts pressure on Schlemm canal and may lead to increased intraocular pressure and glaucoma
Lens	Increase in opacity	Decrease in refraction with increased light scattering and decreased color vision (green and blue); can lead to cataracts
	Increased firmness, loss of elasticity	Decrease in accommodation for near vision; presbyopia develops by age 50-55 years
Ciliary muscles	Reduction in pupil diameter, atrophy of radial dilation muscles	Persistent constriction (senile miosis); decrease in critical flicker frequency*
Retina	Reduction in number of rods at periphery, loss of rods and associated nerve cells	Increase in the minimum amount of light necessary to see an object

*The rate at which consecutive visual stimuli can be presented and still be perceived as separate.

it does with glaucoma). The vitreous chamber is filled with a gel-like substance called **vitreous humor.** Vitreous humor helps prevent the eyeball from collapsing inward.

The central retinal artery provides blood to the inner retinal surface. Nutrients are supplied to the outer surface of the retina by the choroid. Six extrinsic eye muscles, attached to the outer surface of each eye, allow gross eye movements and permit the eyes to follow a moving object (Fig. 14-13).

Aging and Vision

Changes in the structural components of the eye caused by aging begin at an early age, particularly in the lens of the eye. Changes caused by aging are summarized in Table 14-4. The combined structural changes result in a decline in visual acuity.[112]

Visual Dysfunction

Alterations in Ocular Movements

Abnormal ocular movements occur as a result of oculomotor, trochlear, or abducens cranial nerve dysfunction (see Table 13-6). The three types of eye movement disorders are (1) strabismus, (2) nystagmus, and (3) paralysis of individual extraocular muscles.

Strabismus is the deviation of one eye from the other when the person is looking at an object; it is caused by weak or hypertonic muscle in one of the eyes. The deviation may be upward, downward, inward, or outward. Strabismus in children requires early intervention to prevent the development of **amblyopia** (reduced vision in the affected eye often caused by cerebral blockage of the visual stimuli). The primary symptom of strabismus is **diplopia** (double vision). Strabismus may be caused by a neuromuscular disorder of the eye muscle, diseases involving the cerebral hemispheres, or thyroid disease.

Nystagmus is an involuntary unilateral or bilateral rhythmic movement of the eyes and can occur in infants (congenital) or adults (acquired). It may be present at rest, or it may occur with eye movement. The two major forms of nystagmus are pendular nystagmus and jerk nystagmus. **Pendular nystagmus** is characterized by a regular to-and-fro movement of the eyes in which both phases of the movement are equal in length. In **jerk nystagmus** one phase of the eye movement is faster than the other. Nystagmus may be caused by an imbalance in the normally coordinated reflex activity of the inner ear, vestibular nuclei (connecting the vestibular nerve with vestibulospinal tracts), cerebellum, medial longitudinal fascicle (connecting the mesencephalon with the upper portion of the spinal cord), or nuclei of the oculomotor, trochlear, and abducens cranial nerves (see Table 13-6). Drugs, retinal disease, and diseases involving the cervical cord also may produce nystagmus. Acquired untreated nystagmus can lead to loss of visual acuity.[113]

Paralysis of specific extraocular muscles may cause a variety of abnormalities, including limited abduction, abnormal closure of the eyelid, ptosis (drooping of the eyelid), and diplopia. The abnormalities occur as a result of unopposed muscle activity. Trauma or pressure in the area of the cranial nerves may cause paralysis of specific extraocular muscles. Diseases such as diabetes mellitus and myasthenia gravis also may affect specific extraocular muscles.

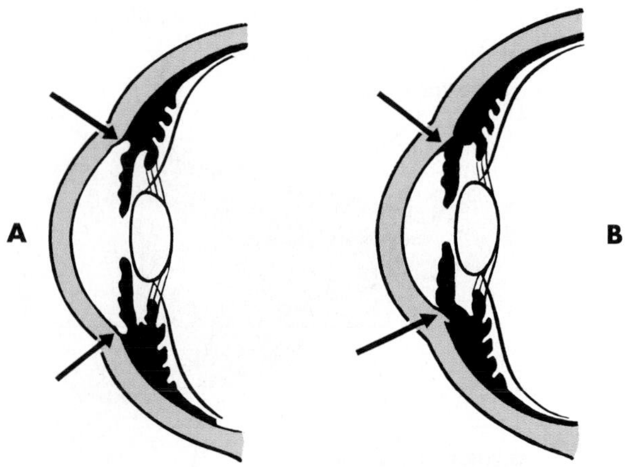

FIG. 14-14 Glaucoma. A, Open-angle glaucoma. The obstruction to aqueous flow lies in the trabecular meshwork. **B,** Closed-angle glaucoma. The trabecular meshwork is covered by the root of the iris. (From Stein HA, Slatt BJ, Stein RM: *The ophthalmic assistant: fundamentals in clinical practice,* St Louis, 1988, Mosby.)

Alterations in Visual Acuity

Visual acuity is the ability to see objects in sharp detail. With advancing age the lens of the eye becomes less flexible and less adjustable. In addition, the sclera changes shape, causing light to fall on the macula (an opaque portion of the cornea). Thus visual acuity declines with age. Visual acuity also may change or diminish for many other reasons. Specific causes of visual acuity changes include (1) amblyopia, (2) scotoma, (3) cataracts, (4) papilledema, (5) dark adaptation, (6) glaucoma, (7) retinal detachment, and (8) macular degeneration.

Amblyopia is a reduction or dimness of vision for unknown reasons. It does not result from a change in refraction (i.e., deviation of light rays) or from any visible changes in the eye. Amblyopia is associated with diseases such as diabetes mellitus, renal failure, and malaria and with toxic substances such as alcohol and tobacco. Amblyopia is the most common cause of vision loss in children.

A **scotoma** is a circumscribed defect of the central field of vision. It is most often a sequel to **retrobulbar neuritis,** an inflammatory lesion of the optic nerve frequently associated with multiple sclerosis (see Chapter 15). Less common causes include the compression of one optic nerve by a retroorbital tumor, neuromyelitis optica (inflammation of the optic nerve), pernicious anemia, and toxic or metabolic causes such as methyl alcohol poisoning and use of tobacco. The precise mechanisms for these conditions causing a scotoma are uncertain, but the result is always a serious impairment in visual acuity.

A **cataract** is a cloudy or opaque area in the ocular lens. The incidence of cataracts increases with age as the lens enlarges. Cataracts develop because of alterations of metabolism and transport of nutrients within the lens. Although the most common form of cataract is degenerative, cataracts also may occur congenitally as a result of infection, radiation, trauma, drugs, or diabetes mellitus. Cataracts cause decreased visual acuity, blurred vision, glare, and decreased color perception. Cataracts are treated by removal of the entire lens and replacement with an artificial lens.

Papilledema is edema and inflammation of the optic nerve at its point of entrance into the eyeball. Generally, papilledema is caused by some obstruction to the venous return from the retina. An early sign is distention of the retinal vein. Obliteration of the physiologic cup (a bright area normally located in the center of the optic disc) follows. Later the optic disc becomes raised above the level of the surrounding retina, and the margins become blurred and indistinct. With severe swelling, hemorrhage and patches of white exudate develop around the disc margins. The three principal causes of papilledema are (1) increased intracranial pressure, (2) retrobulbar neuritis, and (3) changes in the retinal blood vessels. Retinal blood vessel changes are especially prevalent in individuals with diabetes mellitus or hypertension. Such changes account for a large percentage of individuals newly affected with blindness each year. Typically the blood vessels narrow, and hemorrhages and white exudate appear. Ultimately papilledema occurs.

Dark adaptation also affects visual acuity. Low illumination causes impaired visual acuity, particularly in the elderly. The average 80-year-old needs more than twice as much light as a 20-year-old to see equally well. Changes in the quantity and quality of rhodopsin, a substance found in the rods and responsible for low-light vision, are thought to be responsible for reduced dark adaptation in older adults.[114] Vitamin A deficiencies can cause the same phenomenon in individuals of any age.

Glaucoma is characterized by intraocular pressures above the normal pressures of 12 to 20 mm Hg maintained by the aqueous fluid. Genetic causes of glaucoma have recently been reported.[115] The mechanisms of intraocular fluid accumulation are summarized in Fig. 14-14. Chronic increased intraocular pressure first causes loss of peripheral vision, followed by central vision impairment and blindness.[116] Extremely high pressures can cause blindness within days or

Table 14-5 Types of Glaucoma

Type	Mechanism of Increased Pressure
Open-angle glaucoma	Obstruction to outflow of aqueous humor at trabecular meshwork or Schlemm canal; myopia is a risk factor
Narrow-angle glaucoma (angle closure)	Forward displacement of iris toward cornea with narrowing of iridocorneal angle and obstruction to outflow of aqueous humor from anterior chamber
Acute angle closure glaucoma	Acute closure of iridocorneal angle with a sudden rise in intraocular pressure, producing nerve pain and visual disturbances

hours. Loss of visual acuity results from pressure on the optic nerve, which is believed to block the flow of cytoplasm from neuronal bodies in the retina to peripheral optic nerve fibers entering the brain. Lack of nutrients leads to death of the involved neurons. Acute pain may result. The types of glaucoma are summarized in Table 14-5. Glaucoma often is treated with eye drops to reduce secretion or increase absorption of aqueous humor. Surgery may be needed to open the spaces of the trabeculae[117] and reduce intraocular pressure.

Retinal detachment is a common cause of visual impairment and blindness. Risk factors include retinal holes and vitreoretinal traction. Fluid (exudate, hemorrhage, or liquid vitreous) separates the photoreceptors from the retinal pigment epithelium. The separation deprives the outer retina of oxygen and nutrients because the diffusion distance is increased. Communication is also disrupted between the pigment epithelium and photoreceptors. Rhegmatogenous retinal detachment is the most common form of retinal detachment. Causes include intracapsular cataract extraction, severe myopia, lattice degeneration, vitroretinal traction, and trauma. Contraction of fibrous membranes can cause tractional separation of the retinal layers as occurs in proliferative diabetic retinopathy.[118]

Age-related macular degeneration (AMD), loss of central vision, is the major cause of vision loss in individuals over age 60 years. Hypertension, cigarette smoking, and diabetes mellitus are risk factors. There is loss of the outer retina and retinal pigment epithelium of the macula. Loss of the pigment epithelium leads to subretinal neovascularization and degeneration of adjacent photoreceptors. The new vessels leak and bleed, causing retinal detachment and scar formation.[119] Symptoms include blurred vision, difficulty reading, and poor night vision.[120] Progress is being made in new treatments and understanding genetic factors contributing to AMD.[121]

Alterations in Accommodation

Accommodation is the process whereby the thickness of the lens changes. Accommodation is needed for clear vision and is mediated through the oculomotor nerve. Pressure, inflammation, and disease of the oculomotor nerve may alter accommodation. Symptoms include diplopia, blurred vision, and headache. Accommodation is affected also by the decreased flexibility of the lens that occurs with aging. By 60 years of age the lens has become so inelastic that accommodation is not possible.

Loss of accommodation in older adults is termed **presbyopia,** a condition in which the ocular lens becomes larger, firmer, and less elastic. The major symptom is reduced near vision, causing the individual to hold reading material at arm's length. Correction is accomplished through reading glasses or bifocal lenses.

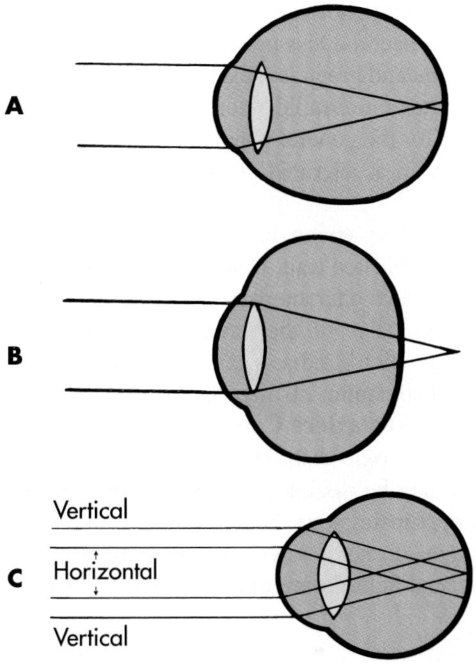

FIG. 14-15 Alterations in refraction. A, Myopic eye. Parallel rays of light are brought to a focus in front of the retina. **B,** Hyperopic eye. Parallel rays of light come to a focus behind the retina in the unaccommodative eye. **C,** Simple myopic astigmatism. The vertical bundle of rays is focused on the retina; the horizontal rays are focused in front of the retina. (From Stein HA, Slatt BJ, Stein RM: *The ophthalmic assistant: fundamentals in clinical practice,* St Louis, 1988, Mosby.)

Alterations in Refraction

Alterations in refraction are the most common visual problem. Errors in refraction are caused by irregularities of the corneal curvature, the focusing power of the lens, and the length of the eye. The major symptoms of refraction alterations are blurred vision and headache. Three types of refraction alterations are myopia, hyperopia, and astigmatism (Fig. 14-15).

In **myopia** (nearsightedness), light rays are focused in front of the retina when the person is looking at a distant object. A concave lens is needed for correction. Myopia requires frequent changes of eyeglasses while the eyeball is lengthening in childhood.

In **hyperopia** (farsightedness), light rays are focused behind the retina when the person is looking at a near object. Hyperopia is corrected with a convex lens. **Astigmatism** is caused by an unequal curvature of the cornea. In astigmatism, light rays are bent unevenly and do not come to a single focus on the retina. Astigmatism may coexist with myopia, hyperopia, or presbyopia. Correction is accomplished with a cylinder lens.

Alterations in Color Vision

Normal sensitivity to color diminishes with age because of the progressive yellowing of the lens that occurs with aging. All colors become less intense, although color discrimination for blue and green is most greatly affected. Color vision deteriorates more rapidly for individuals with diabetes mellitus than for the general population. The deterioration is thought to be an accelerated version of senile color vision deterioration.

Abnormal color vision also may be caused by **color blindness,** an inherited trait. Color blindness is generally an X-linked, recessive characteristic affecting 8% of the male population and 0.5% of the female population. Although many forms of color blindness exist, most commonly the affected individual cannot distinguish red from green.

Neurologic Disorders Causing Visual Dysfunction

Various neurologic disorders may cause visual dysfunction. Vision may be disrupted at many points along the visual pathway, causing a variety of defects in fields of vision. Visual changes do not always cause defects or blindness in the entire visual field; **hemianopia** is the term that describes defective vision in half of a visual field. (Fig. 14-16 illustrates the many areas along the visual pathway that may be damaged and the associated visual changes.)

Because of the anatomy of the optic nerves, injury to the optic nerve causes ipsilateral (same side) blindness but a normal contralateral (opposite side) visual field. Injury to the **optic chiasm** (the X-shaped crossing of the optic nerves), often caused by atherosclerotic ischemia or external compression from trauma or aneurysm, can cause a variety of defects, depending on the location of injury. These defects vary because at the optic chiasm, nerve fibers from the medial half of each retina separate from the lateral half and enter the opposite optic tract.

Because of the normal structure of the visual pathways, destruction of one optic tract causes **homonymous hemianopsia** (complete loss of vision in the inner half of one eye and the outer half of the other). Thus, if an injury to the left optic tract occurs, the individual is blind in the right eye's medial (inner) field and the left eye's lateral (outer) field. If the compression of the optic tract is asymmetric, an incongruous (or uneven) homonymous defect results. Injury to one optic radiation (an ocular pathway in the internal capsule, temporal lobe, or occipital lobe) also causes a homonymous (same field) defect. A major injury in the optic radiation causes homonymous hemianopsia. A lesser injury may cause an upper quadrant homonymous defect. Generally the defects are the same size in both eyes. When the homonymous hemianopsia is caused by an occipital lobe lesion, the area of hemianopsia is split. Although visual acuity may re-

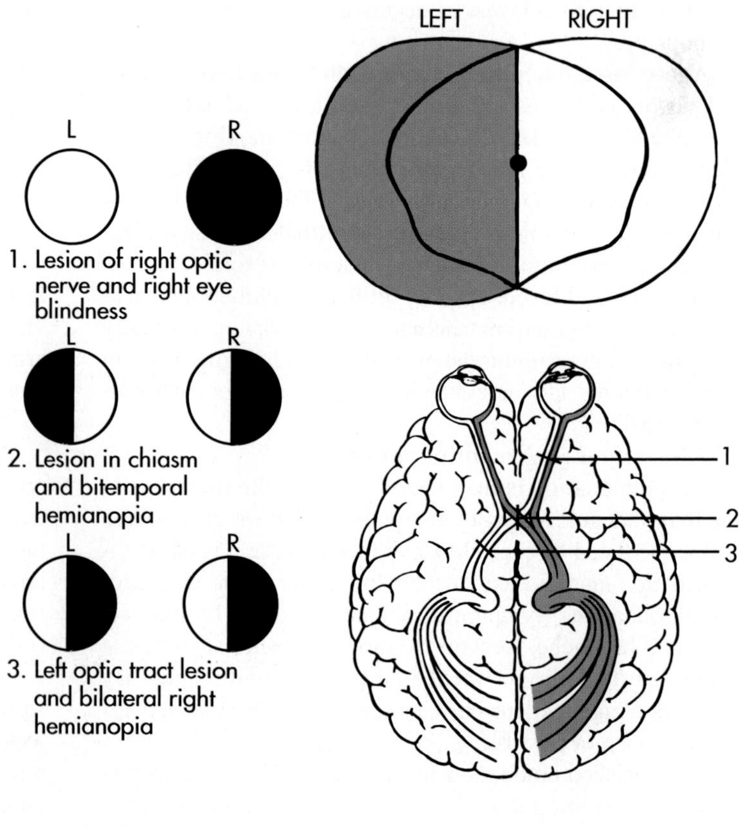

FIG. 14-16 Visual pathway defects. (From Thompson JM et al: *Mosby's clinical nursing,* ed 4, St Louis, 1997, Mosby.)

main unimpaired, reading is difficult because of the inability to group words.

Hearing

The external auditory canal is surrounded by the bones of the cranium. Its opening (meatus) is just above the **mastoid process,** which contains air-filled sinuses called **mastoid air cells.** These promote conductivity between the external and the middle ear.

The Normal Ear

The ear is divided into three areas: (1) the external ear, involved only with hearing; (2) the middle ear, involved only with hearing; and (3) the inner ear, involved with both hearing and equilibrium.

The external ear is composed of the **pinna** (auricle), which is the visible portion of the ear, and the **external auditory canal,** a tube that leads to the middle ear (Fig. 14-17). Sound waves entering the external auditory canal hit the **tympanic membrane** (eardrum) and cause it to vibrate. The tympanic membrane separates the external ear from the middle ear.

The middle ear is composed of the **tympanic cavity,** a small chamber in the temporal bone. Three ossicles (small bones) transmit the vibration of the tympanic membrane to the inner ear. The three ossicles are termed the **malleus (hammer), incus (anvil),** and **stapes (stirrup).** When the tympanic membrane moves, the malleus moves with it and transfers the vibration to the incus, which passes it on to the stapes. The stapes presses against the **oval window,** a small membrane of the inner ear. The movement of the oval window sets the fluids of the inner ear in motion (Fig. 14-18).

The **eustachian (pharyngotympanic) tube** connects the middle ear with the thorax. Normally flat and closed, the eustachian tube opens briefly when a person swallows or yawns, and it equalizes the pressure in the middle ear with atmospheric pressure. Equalized pressure permits the tympanic membrane to vibrate freely. Through the eustachian tube the mucosa of the middle ear is contiguous with the mucosal lining of the throat.

The inner ear is a system of osseous labyrinths (bony, mazelike chambers) filled with a fluid called **perilymph.** The bony labyrinth is divided into the **cochlea,** the **vestibule,** and the **semicircular canals** (see Fig. 14-17). Suspended in the perilymph is a membranous labyrinth that basically follows the shape of the bony labyrinth. The membranous labyrinth is filled with a thicker fluid called **endolymph.**

Within the cochlea is the **organ of Corti,** which contains **hair cells** (hearing receptors). Sound waves that reach the cochlea through vibrations of the tympanic membrane, ossicles, and oval window set the cochlear fluids into motion. Receptor cells on the basilar membrane are stimulated when their hairs are bent or pulled by the movement. Once stimulated, hair cells transmit impulses along the cochlear nerve (a division of the vestibulocochlear nerve) to the auditory cortex of the temporal lobe in the brain (see Fig. 14-18), where interpretation of the sound occurs. Directional hearing is controlled by the angle of the sound source to both ears and axonal delay in conduction in groups of neurons.[122]

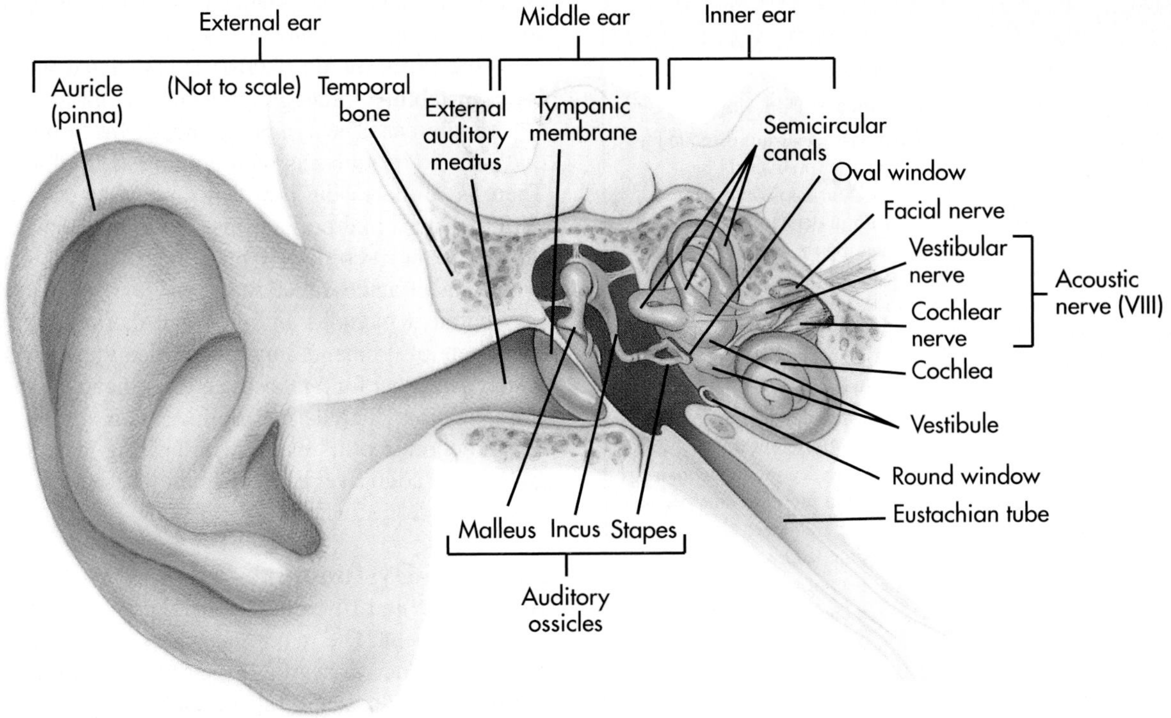

FIG. 14-17 The ear. External, middle, and inner ears. (Anatomic structures are not drawn to scale.) (From Thibodeau GA, Patton KI: *Anatomy and physiology,* ed 4, St Louis, 1999, Mosby.)

The semicircular canals and vestibule of the inner ear contain **equilibrium receptors.** In the semicircular canals the dynamic equilibrium receptors respond to changes in direction of movement. Within each semicircular canal is the **crista ampullaris,** a receptor region composed of a tuft of hair cells covered by a gelatinous cupula. When the head is rotated, the endolymph in the canal lags behind and moves in the direction opposite to the head's movement. The hair cells are stimulated, and impulses are transmitted through the vestibular nerve (a division of the vestibulocochlear nerve) to the cerebellum.

The vestibule in the inner ear contains **maculae,** receptors essential to the body's sense of static equilibrium. As the head moves, **otoliths** (small pieces of calcium salts) move in a gel-like material in response to changes in the pull of gravity. The otoliths pull on the gel, which in turn pulls on the hair cells in the maculae. Nerve impulses in the hair cells are triggered and transmitted to the brain (see Fig. 14-18). Thus the ear not only permits the hearing of a large range of sounds but also assists with maintaining balance through the sensitive equilibrium receptors.

Aging and Hearing

Auditory changes caused by aging are common and incremental. Changes in hearing with aging are summarized in Table 14-6. Approximately one third of people older than 65 years have hearing loss.[123] Changes may occur in both the structural and functional components of the peripheral or central auditory system. Loss of hearing for sounds in the high-frequency range **(presbycusis)** is most common and interferes with understanding speech, particularly high-frequency consonant sounds (e.g., *s, sh, f*). Hearing may be lost in both ears but not at the same time. Elderly individuals from rural areas have less hearing loss than those in noisy cities. The ability to discriminate localization of sound varies with high and low frequencies and diminishes with age.[124] In the low-frequency range, sound localization is a function of the timing of sound arrival between the two ears; localization of high-frequency sounds is a function of sound intensity. Because elderly individuals tend to lose high-frequency hearing first, they may have difficulty localizing high-frequency sounds.

Table 14-6 Changes in Hearing Caused by Aging

Hearing loss affects about one third of older people.[123]

Changes in Structure	Changes in Function
Cochlear hair cell degeneration	Inability to hear high-frequency sounds (prebycusis, sensorineural loss); interferes with understanding speech; hearing may be lost in both ears at different times
Loss of auditory neurons in spiral ganglia of organ of Corti	Inability to hear high-frequency sounds (presbycusis, sensorineural loss); interferes with understanding speech; hearing may be lost in both ears at different times
Degeneration of basilar (cochlear) conductive membrane of cochlea	Inability to hear at all frequencies but more pronounced at higher frequencies (cochlear conductive loss)
Decreased vascularity of cochlea	Equal loss of hearing at all frequencies (strial loss); inability to disseminate localization of sound
Loss of cortical auditory neurons	Equal loss of hearing at all frequencies (strial loss); inability to disseminate localizaton of sound

Ear Infections

Otitis Externa

Otitis externa is the most common infection of the outer ear.[125] The most frequently found microorganisms are *Pseudomonas, Escherichia coli,* and *Staphylococcus aureus.* Infection usually follows prolonged exposure to moisture (swimmer's ear). The earliest symptoms are inflammation with swelling and clear drainage progressing to purulent drainage with obstruction of the canal. Tenderness and pain with earlobe retraction accompany inflammation.

Otitis Media

Otitis media is the most common infection of infants and children. Most children have one episode by 3 years of age. The most common pathogens are *Streptococcus pneumoniae, Haemophilus influenzae*, and *Moraxella catarrhalis.* Respiratory viruses may also have an etiologic role.[126,127] Predisposing factors include allergy, sinusitis, submucous cleft palate, adenoidal hypertrophy, and immune deficiency. Breast-feeding is a protective factor.

Acute otitis media (AOM) is associated with ear pain, fever, irritability, inflamed tympanic membrane, and fluid in the middle ear. The tympanic membrane progresses from erythema to opaqueness with bulging as fluid accumulates. There is an increasing prevalence of AOM caused by penicillin-resistant microorganisms. Otitis media with effusion (OME) is the presence of fluid in the middle ear without symptoms of acute infection.

Treatment includes antimicrobial therapy for AOM and placement of tympanotomy tubes when there is bilateral effusion persistent for 3 months and significant hearing loss.[128] Complications include mastoiditis, brain abscess, meningitis, and chronic otitis media with hearing loss. Speech, language, and cognitive disabilities may be affected by persistent middle ear effusions.

Auditory Dysfunction

Between 5% and 10% of the general population have a hearing impairment. The major categories of auditory dysfunction are conductive hearing loss, sensorineural hearing loss, mixed hearing loss, and functional hearing loss.

Conductive Hearing Loss

A **conductive hearing loss** occurs when a change in the outer or middle ear impairs the sound from being conducted from the outer to the inner ear. Conductive hearing loss occurs when there is interference in air conduction. Conditions that commonly cause a conductive hearing loss include impacted cerumen, foreign bodies lodged in the ear canal, benign tumors of the middle ear, carcinoma of the external auditory canal or middle ear, eustachian tube dysfunction, otitis media, acute viral otitis media, chronic suppurative otitis media, cholesteatoma, and otosclerosis.

Symptoms of conductive hearing loss include diminished hearing and soft speaking voice. The voice is soft because often the individual hears his or her voice, conducted by bone, as loud. In addition, although the cause is unknown, the individual often hears better in a noisy environment than in a quiet one (a condition called *paracusia willisiana*). Treatment of the underlying cause generally improves hearing.[129] A hearing aid is used if the hearing loss is greater than 40 to 50 decibels.

Sensorineural Hearing Loss

A **sensorineural hearing loss** is caused by impairment of the organ of Corti or its central connections. The hearing loss may be gradual or sudden. Conditions that commonly cause sensorineural hearing loss include congenital and hereditary factors, noise exposure, aging, Ménière disease, ototoxicity, and systemic disease (syphilis, Paget disease, collagen diseases, diabetes mellitus). Congenital and neonatal sensorineural hearing loss may be caused by maternal rubella, ototoxic drugs, prematurity, traumatic delivery, erythroblastosis fetalis, and congenital hereditary malfunction. Diagnosis often is made when delayed speech development is noted.

Presbycusis is the most common form of sensorineural hearing loss and is especially common in elderly people. Presbycusis may occur because of atrophy of the basal end of the organ of Corti, a loss in the number of auditory receptors, vascular changes, or stiffening of the basilar membranes. Because of the slow progression of hearing loss, onset of symptoms is gradual. In addition, drug ototoxicities (drugs that cause destruction of auditory function) have been observed after exposure to a variety of chemicals, for example, antibiotics such as streptomycin, neomycin, gentamicin, and vancomycin; diuretics such as ethacrynic acid and furosemide; and chemicals such as salicylate, quinine, carbon monoxide, nitrogen mustard, arsenic, mercury, gold, tobacco, and alcohol. Because of increased concentrations of antibiotics in the endolymph, these drugs generally cause damage to the cells of the cristae and maculae (located in the inner ear) or the cells of the organ of Corti. The increased concentration of drugs in the endolymph is preferentially toxic to the cells.

Diuretics affect hearing primarily by altering the sodium-potassium balance, causing extracellular fluid accumulation and changes in the microstructure of secretory cells. Quinine, mercury, and lead affect the neural pathways of hearing, including the spinal ganglia, the eighth cranial nerve, and the cochlear nucleus. The site of action for the other chemicals, including alcohol and tobacco, has not yet been

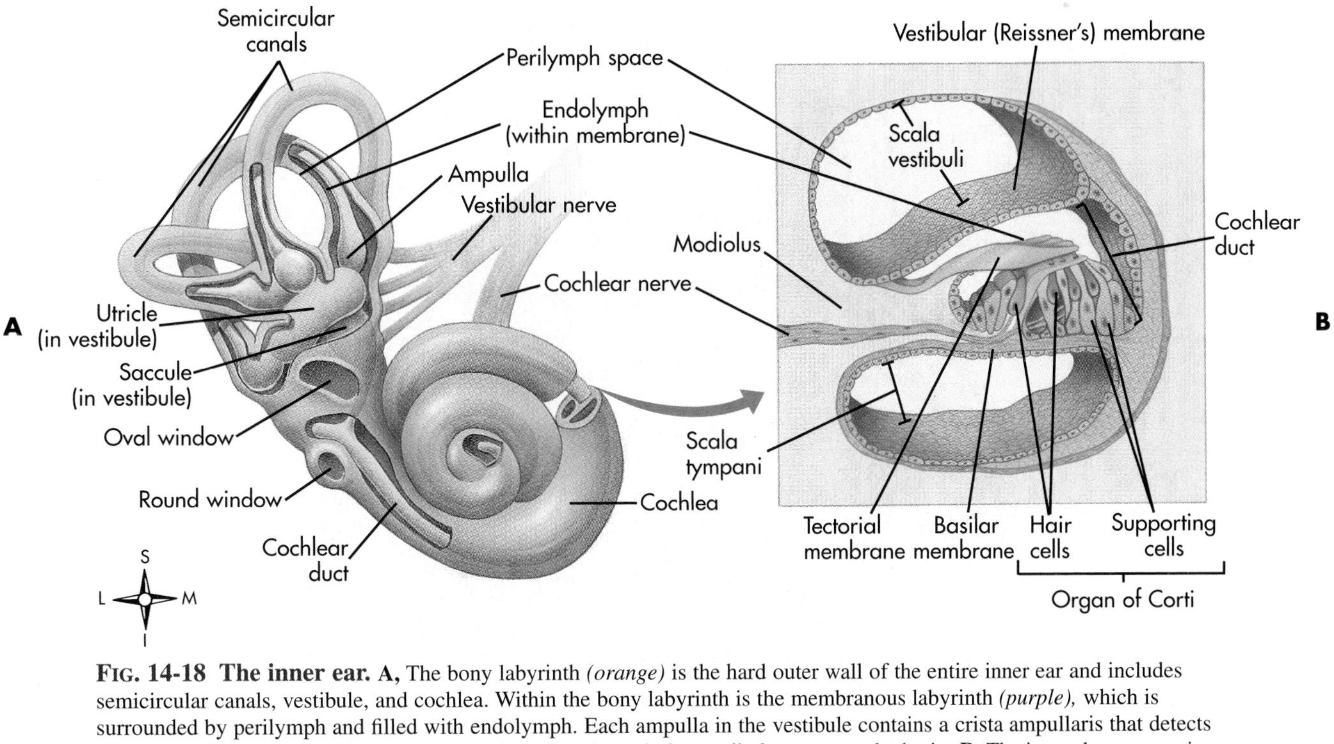

FIG. 14-18 The inner ear. A, The bony labyrinth *(orange)* is the hard outer wall of the entire inner ear and includes semicircular canals, vestibule, and cochlea. Within the bony labyrinth is the membranous labyrinth *(purple),* which is surrounded by perilymph and filled with endolymph. Each ampulla in the vestibule contains a crista ampullaris that detects changes in head position and sends sensory impulses through the vestibular nerve to the brain. **B,** The inset shows a section of the membranous cochlea. Hair cells in the organ of Corti detect sound and send the information through the cochlear nerve. The vestibular and cochlear nerves join to form the eighth cranial nerve. (From Thibodeau GA, Patton KI: *Anatomy and physiology,* ed 4, St Louis, 1999, Mosby.)

determined. In most instances the drugs and chemicals listed previously initially cause **tinnitus** (ringing in the ear), followed by a progressive high-tone sensorineural hearing loss. Care is aimed at prevention of further hearing loss because the loss is usually permanent.

Mixed Hearing Loss

A **mixed hearing loss** is caused by a combination of conductive and sensorineural losses.

Functional Hearing Loss

A **functional hearing loss** occurs for no organic reason. The individual does not respond to voice and appears not to hear. Functional hearing loss is thought to be caused by emotional or psychologic factors. It occurs only rarely.

Olfaction and Taste

Olfaction is a function of cranial nerve I and part of cranial nerve V. Taste is a function of multiple nerves in the tongue, soft palate, uvula, pharynx, and upper esophagus, including cranial nerves VII and IX. Olfaction (smell) dysfunction and taste (gustation) dysfunction may occur separately or jointly. The strong relationship between smell and taste creates the sensation of flavor. If either sensation is impaired, the perception of flavor is altered. (Olfactory structures are illustrated in Fig. 14-19.)

Olfactory cells, which are located in the olfactory epithelium, are the receptor cells for smell. Seven primary classes of olfactory stimulants have been identified: (1) camphoraceous, (2) musky, (3) floral, (4) peppermint, (5) ethereal, (6) pungent, and (7) putrid. The primary sensations of taste are sour, salty, sweet, and bitter. Taste buds sensitive to each of the primary sensations are located in specific areas of the tongue.[130]

Aging and Olfaction and Taste

Olfaction

Sensitivity to odors declines steadily with aging.[131] A study of odor identification indicates an increasing ability from childhood to adolescence and then a decline after 60 years of age. The most significant impairments develop after 80 years.[132] Women generally have better olfactory abilities than men, but the patterns of decline are similar.[133]

The sense of smell begins to degenerate with loss of olfactory sensory neurons and loss of cells from the olfactory bulbs.[134] Loss of olfactory sensitivity and odor identification may diminish appetite and food selection and thus may lead to malnutrition. Safety also may be compromised by an inability to smell toxic or hazardous gases.

Taste

The decline in taste sensation is more gradual than that of smell. Higher concentrations of flavors are required, and elderly persons have difficulty differentiating combinations of flavors.[135] The best-known change with aging is the decline

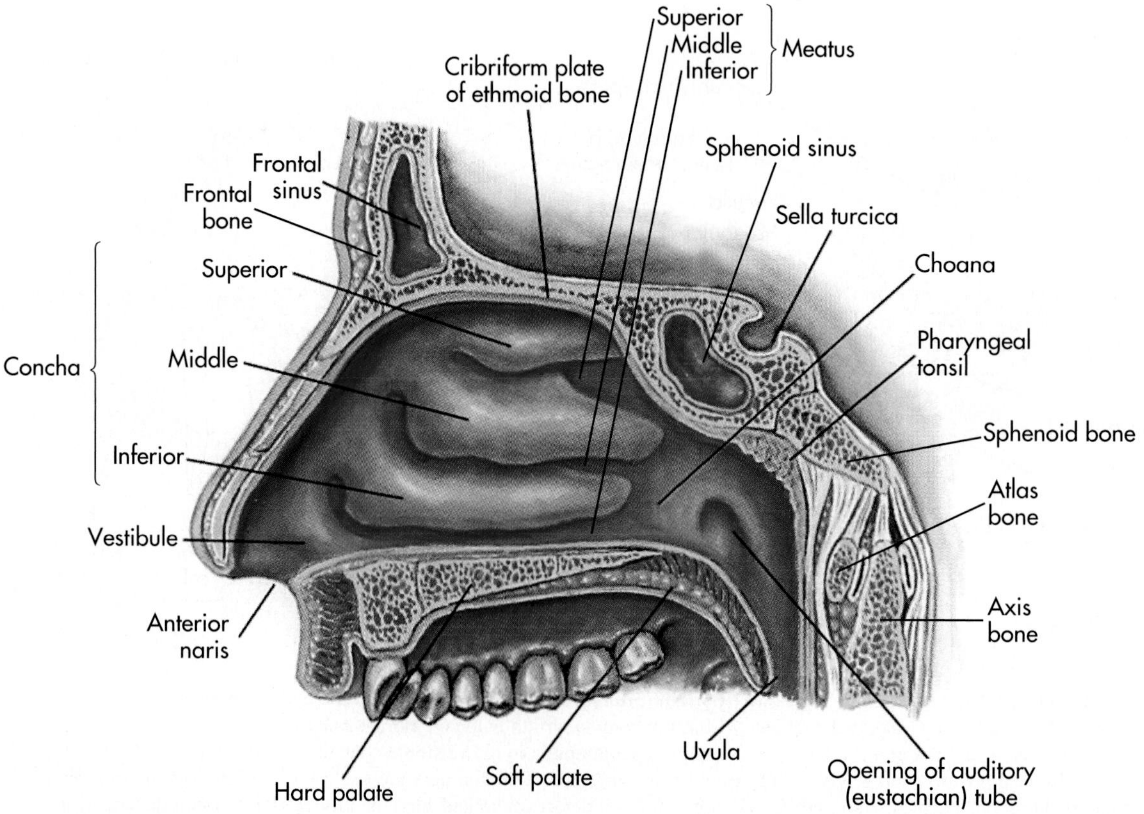

FIG. 14-19 Olfaction. Location of olfactory epithelium, olfactory bulb, and neuronal pathways involved in olfaction. (Modified from Seidel HM et al: *Mosby's guide to physical examination*, ed 4, St Louis, 1999, Mosby.)

in the number of fungiform papillae on the tongue, which decrease by 50% by about 50 years of age.[112] Taste also may be affected by decreased salivary gland secretion. Amylase, contained in saliva, facilitates perception of sweet sensations and also is reduced with aging.

Olfactory Dysfunction

Olfactory dysfunctions include hyposmia, anosmia, hallucinations, and parosmia. **Hyposmia** is the impaired sense of smell, and **anosmia** is the complete loss of smell. When hyposmia or anosmia occurs bilaterally, it is usually the result of rhinitis (inflammation of nasal mucosa), sinusitis, nasal polyps, or excessive smoking.[136] Unilateral hyposmia or anosmia may indicate compression of one olfactory bulb (a bulblike portion of the olfactory nerves) or nerve tract (olfactory nerve pathway), possibly by tumor or head trauma. **Olfactory hallucinations** arise from hyperactivity in cortical neurons and involve smelling odors that are not really present. They are associated with temporal lobe seizures and rarely with schizophrenia. **Parosmia,** an abnormal or perverted sense of smell, may occur with severe depression.[137]

Taste Dysfunction

The sense of taste can be impaired by injury, medications, oral infections, or aging. An alteration in taste also may be attributable to impairment of smell associated with injury near the hippocampus.

Hypogeusia is decrease in taste sensation, and **ageusia** is the absence of taste. Ageusia affecting the entire tongue may follow head injury. Damage to the glossopharyngeal nerve (cranial nerve IX, which innervates the posterior one third of the tongue) causes the loss of the ability to detect bitterness. This loss occurs because the receptors for bitter are located on the base of the tongue. Damage to the facial nerve (cranial nerve VII, which innervates the anterior two thirds of the tongue) causes loss of the ability to detect sour, sweet, and salt tastes. Only bitter tastes can be detected. These losses occur because sour, sweet, and salt receptors are located on the anterior portion of the tongue. **Parageusia** is a perversion of taste in which substances possess an unpleasant flavor. Parageusia occasionally develops for no apparent reason in elderly people and also is common in individuals receiving chemotherapy for cancer. In both cases, parageusia often leads to anorexia and malnutrition.

SOMATOSENSORY FUNCTION

Touch

Touch is not a uniform sensory experience. The sensation of touch involves the fusion of several qualities, including modality, intensity, location, and duration of the sensory stimulus. Receptors sensitive to touch are present in the skin. Meissner and pacinian corpuscles are rapidly adapting receptors, whereas Merkel disks and Ruffini endings are slowly adapting touch receptors. Touch receptors are most numerous in the skin of the fingers and lips and are more scarce in the skin of the trunk. Research suggests that four afferent fiber types mediate tactile sensation.[138] Specific sensory input is carried to the higher levels of the CNS by the dorsal column of the spinal cord and the anterior spinothalamic tract.

Much of the development of the cutaneous senses takes place before birth, but structural growth of the cutaneous senses continues into early adulthood at a reduced rate. Then a gradual decline occurs. Studies have documented loss in tactile sensitivity with advancing age.[139,140] This occurs simultaneously with an increase in the size of pacinian corpuscles and a decrease in the number of corpuscles.

Abnormal tactile perception may be caused by alterations at any level of the nervous system, from the receptor to the cerebral cortex. Any factor that interrupts or impairs reception, transmission, perception, or interpretation of touch also alters tactile sensation. Trauma, tumor, infection, metabolic changes, vascular changes, and degenerative diseases thus may cause tactile dysfunction, which may involve heightened or diminished tactile perceptions.

In addition, most tactile sensations evoke affective responses that determine whether the sensation is unpleasant, pleasant, or neutral. Cerebral and hypothalamic centers influence this response. Sedative drugs and prefrontal injury, which interrupt connections between the prefrontal cortex and subcortical centers, diminish the interpretation of tactile sensations.

Proprioception

Perception and awareness of the position of the body and its parts depend on impulses from the inner ear and from receptors in joints and ligaments. The role of muscle, tendon, and cutaneous receptors is indefinite. Sensory data are transmitted to higher centers, primarily through the dorsal columns and the spinocerebellar tracts, with some data passing through the medial lemnisci and thalamic radiations to the cortex. These stimuli are necessary for the coordination of movements, the grading of muscular contraction, and the maintenance of equilibrium.

A progressive loss of proprioception has been reported in elderly persons.[112] Proprioceptive dysfunction may be caused by alterations at any level of the nervous system. As with tactile dysfunction, any factor that interrupts or impairs the reception, transmission, perception, or interpretation of proprioceptive stimuli also alters proprioception. Two common causes of proprioceptive dysfunction are vestibular dysfunction and neuropathy.

Specific vestibular dysfunctions are vestibular nystagmus and vertigo. **Vestibular nystagmus** is the constant, involuntary movement of the eyeball caused by ear disturbances. This condition occurs when the semicircular canal system is overstimulated. **Vertigo** is the sensation of spinning that occurs with inflammation of the semicircular canals in the ear. The individual may feel either that he or she is moving in space or that the world is revolving. Vertigo often causes loss of balance. Vertigo and nystagmus may occur in a variety of conditions, including labyrinthitis, vestibular neuritis, acute toxic labyrinthitis, and Ménière disease.

Ménière disease is a vestibular disorder that can cause proprioceptive dysfunction. The pathologic basis of Ménière disease is still unclear. The individual with Ménière disease may experience loss of proprioception during an acute attack, so that standing or walking is impossible.

Peripheral neuropathies also can cause proprioceptive dysfunctions. Neuropathies may be caused by a variety of conditions and commonly are associated with renal disease and diabetes mellitus. Although the exact sequence of events is unknown, neuropathies are thought to be caused by a metabolic disturbance of the neuron itself. The result is a diminished or absent sense of body position or position of body parts. Gait changes often occur. (Neuropathies are further discussed in Chapter 15.)

SUMMARY REVIEW

Pain

1. Pain is a complex phenomenon composed of sensory experiences (time, space, intensity) and emotion, cognition, and motivation.
2. Categories of pain include somatogenic pain (with a known physiologic cause), psychogenic pain (without a physiologic cause), acute pain (signal to the person of a harmful stimulus), and chronic pain (persistence of pain of unknown cause or unusual response to therapy).
3. Pain threshold is the point at which pain is perceived. Pain threshold does not vary significantly among people or within the same person over time.
4. Pain tolerance is the duration of time or the intensity of pain that an individual will endure before initiating overt pain response. Tolerance varies widely among individuals and in the same individual over time.
5. Newborns and young children have anatomic and functional ability to perceive pain. Older individuals tend to have a slightly higher pain threshold, probably because of changes in the thickness of the skin and peripheral neuropathies. In all age-groups, women appear to be more sensitive to pain than men.
6. The portions of the nervous system responsible for the sensation and perception of pain may be divided into three areas: (a) the afferent fibers, (b) the central nervous system, and (c) the afferent pathways.
7. The afferent system is composed of nociceptors, Aδ and C fibers, the dorsal horn of the spinal column, and afferent neurons in the spinothalamic tract.
8. Efferent pathways from the periaqueductal gray are responsible for modulation or inhibition of afferent pain signals.
9. The thalamus, cortex, and postcentral gyrus perceive, describe, and localize pain. The reticular formation and limbic system control the emotional and affective response to pain.
10. The specificity theory of pain proposes that pain is caused by stimulation of nerve endings in the skin, transmission of the painful stimuli through A and C fibers to the spinal cord, and ascent of impulses to the brain, causing a direct relationship between the stimulus and the perception of pain.
11. Endorphins inhibit transmission of the pain impulse. They are present in varying concentrations in the neurons in the brain, spinal cord, and gastrointestinal tract.
12. According to the gate control theory, specialized cells within the substantia gelatinosa of the spinal cord act as a gate, opening and closing the afferent pathways to transmission of painful stimuli.
13. The intensity theory proposes that pain results from excessive stimulation of sensory receptors with summation of impulses.
14. According to the pattern theory of pain, pain perception is the result of stimulus intensity and summation of the impulses.
15. Acute pain may be (a) somatic (superficial), (b) visceral (internal), or (c) referred (present in an area distant from its origin). The area of referred pain is supplied by the same spinal segment as the actual site of pain.
16. Physiologic responses to acute pain include increased heart rate, respiratory rate, and blood pressure; pallor or flushing; dilated pupils; and diaphoresis. Blood sugar is elevated; gastric secretion and motility are decreased; and blood flow to the viscera and skin is decreased.
17. Psychologic, behavioral, and physiologic responses to chronic pain include depression, difficulty in sleeping, preoccupation with pain, life-style changes, and physiologic adaptation.
18. Chronic pain may be a result of decreased levels of endorphins, predominance of C neuron stimulation, or leukokinin.
19. Chronic pain conditions include lower back pain, neuralgias, reflex sympathetic dystrophies, hyperesthesias, myofascial pain syndrome, pain hemiagnosia, phantom limb pain, and chronic pain associated with cancer.
20. Pain experienced by infants may have prolonged effect on brain organization and responses to pain.

Temperature Regulation

1. Temperature regulation is achieved through precise balancing of heat production, heat conservation, and heat loss. Body temperature is maintained in a range around 37° C (98.6° F).
2. Temperature regulation is mediated by the hypothalamus. Peripheral thermoreceptors in the skin and central thermoreceptors in the hypothalamus, spinal cord, and abdominal organs provide the hypothalamus with information about skin and core temperatures.
3. Heat is produced through chemical reactions of metabolism, skeletal muscle contraction, and chemical thermogenesis.
4. Heat is lost through radiation, conduction, convection, vasodilation, decreased muscle tone, evaporation of sweat, increased respiration, and voluntary mechanisms.
5. Heat conservation is accomplished through vasoconstriction and voluntary mechanisms.
6. Infants and elderly persons require special attention to maintenance of body temperature. Because of their greater body surface/mass ratio and decreased subcutaneous fat, infants do not conserve heat well. Elderly individuals have poor responses to environmental temperature extremes as a result of slowed blood circulation, structural and functional changes in skin, and an overall decrease in heat-producing activities.

7. Fever is triggered by the release of pyrogens from leukocytes, bacteria, and other cells involved in the immune response. Fever is both a symptom of a disease and a normal immunologic mechanism.
8. Fever involves resetting the hypothalamic thermostat to a higher level. When the fever breaks, the set point is returned to normal.
9. Fever production aids responses to infectious processes. Higher temperatures kill many microorganisms and decrease serum levels of iron, zinc, and copper that are needed for bacterial replication.
10. Hyperthermia (marked warming of core temperature) can produce nerve damage, coagulation of cell proteins, and death. Forms of accidental hyperthermia include heat cramps, heat exhaustion, heat stroke, and malignant hyperthermia. Heat stroke and malignant hyperthermia are potentially lethal developments.
11. Hypothermia (marked cooling of core temperature) slows the rate of chemical reaction (tissue metabolism), increases the viscosity of the blood, slows blood flow through the microcirculation, facilitates blood coagulation, and stimulates profound vasoconstriction. Hypothermia may be accidental or therapeutic.

Sleep

1. Sleep may be divided into rapid eye movement (REM) and non-REM stages, each of which has its own series of stages. While asleep, an individual progresses through REM and non-REM (slow-wave) sleep in a predictable cycle.
2. Sleep is initiated by the withdrawal of neurotransmitters from the afferent formation and by the inhibition of arousal mechanisms in the cerebral cortex. REM sleep is controlled by mechanisms in the pontine reticular formation.
3. The sleep patterns of the newborn and young child vary from those of the adult in total sleep time, cycle length, and percentage of time spent in each sleep cycle. Elderly individuals experience a total decrease in sleep time.
4. During sleep the body is actively engaged in restoring and repairing itself. Sleep deprivation can cause profound changes in personality and functioning.
5. The restorative, reparative, and growth processes occur during slow-wave sleep.
6. Sleep disorders include (a) disorders of initiating sleep (insomnia), (b) sleep disordered breathing, (c) disorders of the sleep/wake schedule (jet lag, shift work), and (d) dysfunctions of sleep, sleep stages, or partial arousals (somnambulism, night terrors, or enuresis).
7. Ingestion of alcohol and some medications can alter or suppress sleep stages, producing sleep disorders.
8. Sleep and disease are interrelated. Some diseases may produce alterations in the quantity and quality of sleep or affect sleep stages. These are referred to as *secondary sleep disorders.* In some instances sleep stages produce alterations in certain disease states. These are referred to as *sleep-provoked disorders.*

The Eye

1. The eyelids, conjunctivae, and lacrimal apparatus protect the eye. Infections are the most common disorders; they include blepharitis, conjunctivitis, chalazion, and hordeolum.
2. Conjunctivitis can be acute or chronic, bacterial, viral, or allergic. Redness, edema, pain, and lacrimation are common symptoms. Chlamydial conjunctivitis is the leading cause of blindness in the world and is associated with poor sanitary conditions.
3. Keratitis is a bacterial or viral infection of the cornea that can lead to corneal ulceration. Photophobia, pain, and tearing are common symptoms.
4. The wall of the eye has three layers: sclera, choroid, and retina. The retina contains millions of photoreceptors known as rods and cones that receive light through the lens and then convey signals to the optic nerve and subsequently to the visual cortex of the brain.
5. The eye is filled with vitreous and aqueous humor, which prevent it from collapsing.
6. Structural eye changes caused by aging result in decreased visual acuity.
7. The major alterations in ocular movement include strabismus, nystagmus, and paralysis of the extraocular muscles.
8. Alterations in visual acuity can be caused by amblyopia, scotoma, cataracts, papilledema, macular degeneration, retinal detachment, and glaucoma.
9. Alterations in accommodation develop with increased intraocular pressure, inflammation, and disease of the oculomotor nerve. Presbyopia is loss of accommodation caused by loss of elasticity of the lens with aging.
10. Alterations in refraction, including myopia, hyperopia, and astigmatism, are the most common visual disorders.
11. Trauma or disease of the optic nerve pathways, or optic radiations, can cause blindness in the visual fields. Homonymous hemianopsia is caused by damage of one optic tract.

The Ear

1. The ear is composed of external, middle, and inner structures. The external structures are the pinna, auditory canal, and tympanic membrane. The tympanic cavity (containing three bones: malleus, incus, and stapes), oval window, eustachian tube, and fluid compose the middle ear and transmit sound vibrations to the inner ear.
2. The inner ear includes the bony and membranous labyrinths that transmit sound waves through the cochlea to the division of the eighth cranial nerve. The semicircular canals and vestibule help maintain balance through the equilibrium receptors.
3. Approximately one third of all people older than 65 years have hearing loss.
4. Otitis extrerna is an infection of the outer ear. Otitis media is an infection of the middle ear common in children.
5. Hearing loss can be classified as conductive, sensorineural, mixed, and functional.
6. Conductive hearing loss occurs when sound waves cannot be conducted through the middle ear.
7. Sensorineural hearing loss develops with impairment of the organ of Corti or its central connections.
8. A combination of conductive and sensorineural loss is a mixed hearing loss.
9. Loss of hearing with no known organic cause is a functional hearing loss.

Taste

1. The perception of flavor is altered if olfaction or taste dysfunctions occur. Sensitivity to odor and taste decreases with aging.
2. Hyposmia is a decrease in the sense of smell, and anosmia is the complete loss of smell. Inflammation of the nasal mucosa and trauma or tumors of the olfactory nerve lead to a diminished sense of smell.

Continued

3. Hypogeusia is a decrease in taste sensation, and ageusia is the absence of taste. Loss of taste buds or trauma to the facial or glossopharyngeal nerves decreases taste sensation.

Touch

1. Touch receptors are located in the skin, and alterations at any level of the nervous system can affect tactile responses.
2. Alterations in touch can result from disruption of skin receptors, sensory transmission, or central nervous system perception.

Somatosensory Function

1. Tactile sensation is a function of receptors present in the skin (pacinian corpuscles), and the sensory response is conducted to the brain through the dorsal column and anterior spinothalamic tract.
2. Alterations in touch can result from disruption of skin receptors, sensory transmission, or central nervous system perception.
3. Proprioception is the position and location of the body and its parts. Proprioceptors are located in the inner ear, joints, and ligaments. Proprioceptive stimuli are necessary for balance, coordinated movement, and grading of muscular contraction.
4. Disorders of proprioception can occur at any level of the nervous system with impaired balance and lack of coordinated movement.

KEY TERMS

Acute bacterial conjunctivitis (pinkeye), *421*
Acute otitis media (AOM), *428*
Acute pain, *402*
Age-related macular degeneration (AMD), *425*
Ageusia, *431*
Allergic conjunctivitis, *421*
Amblyopia, *423*
Anosmia, *431*
Aqueous humor, *422*
Astigmatism, *426*
Blepharitis, *421*
Cataract, *424*
Causalgia, *409*
Chalazion, *421*
Choroid, *421*
Chronic conjunctivitis, *421*
Chronic pain, *402*
Circadian rhythm, *410*
Cochlea, *427*
Cognitive/evaluative system, *402*
Color blindness, *426*
Conduction, *411*
Conductive hearing loss, *428*
Cone, *421*
Convection, *411*
Cornea, *421*
Crista ampullaris, *428*
Dark adaptation, *424*
Diplopia, *423*
Dynorphin, *407*
Endogenous cryogen, *413*
Endogenous pyrogen, *413*
Endolymph, *427*
Enkephalin, *407*
Enuresis, *420*
Equilibrium receptor, *428*
Eustachian (pharyngotympanic) tube, *427*
Exogenous pyrogen, *413*
External auditory canal, *427*
Fovea centralis, *421*
Functional hearing loss, *430*
Gate control theory, *406*
Glaucoma, *424*
Hair cell, *427*
Heat cramp, *413*
Heat exhaustion, *413*
Heat stroke, *415*
Hemiagnosia (to pain), *409*
Hemianopia, *426*
Homonymous hemianopsia, *426*
Hordeolum (stye), *421*
Hyperesthesia, *409*
Hyperopia, *426*
Hyperthermia, *413*
Hypogeusia, *431*
Hyposmia, *431*
Hypothermia, *415*
Incus (anvil), *427*
Insomnia, *419*
Intensity theory, *406*
Iris, *421*
Jerk nystagmus, *424*
Lens, *422*
β-Lipotropin, *407*
Macula, *428*
Malignant hyperthermia, *415*
Malleus (hammer), *427*
Mastoid air cell, *427*
Mastoid process, *427*
Ménière disease, *432*
Mixed hearing loss, *430*
Motivational/affective system, *402*
Myofascial pain syndrome, *409*
Myopia, *425*
Neuralgia, *409*
Night terrors, *420*
Nociceptor, *404*
Non-REM (slow-wave) sleep, *417*
Nystagmus, *423*
Olfactory hallucination, *431*
Opiate receptor, *407*
Optic chiasm, *426*
Optic disc, *421*
Organ of Corti, *427*
Otitis externa, *428*
Otitis media, *428*
Otolith, *428*
Oval window, *427*
Pain threshold, *402*
Pain tolerance, *403*
Papilledema, *424*
Parageusia, *431*
Parasomnia, *419*
Parosmia, *431*
Pattern theory, *406*
Pendular nystagmus, *423*
Perceptual dominance, *403*
Periaqueductal gray (PAG), *405*
Perilymph, *427*
Phantom limb pain, *409*
Pinna, *427*
Presbycusis, *428*
Presbyopia, *425*
Psychogenic pain, *402*
Pupil, *421*
Radiation, *411*
Referred pain, *408*
Reflex sympathetic dystrophy, *409*
Rapid eye movement (REM) sleep, *417*
Retina, *421*
Retinal detachment, *425*
Retrobulbar neuritis, *424*
Rod, *421*
Sclera, *421*
Scotoma, *424*
Secondary sleep disorder, *420*
Semicircular canal, *427*
Sensorineural hearing loss, *429*
Sensory/discriminative system, *402*
Sleep, *417*
Sleep-provoked disorder, *420*

KEY TERMS—cont'd

REFERENCES

1. Sanders SH: Behavioral assessment and treatment of clinical pain: appraisal of current status, *Prog Behav Modif* 8:249, 1979.
2. McCaffery M: Understanding your patient's pain, *Nursing* 80:26, 1980.
3. Melzack R, Wall P: *The challenge of pain,* New York, 1983, Basic Books.
4. Berlin L, Boodell H, Wolff HG: Relation of pain perception and central inhibitory effects of noxious stimulation to phenomenon of excitation of pain, *Arch Neurol* 80:533, 1958.
5. Wolf AR: Pain, nociception and the developing infant, *Paediatr Anaesth* 9(1):7, 2000.
6. Modi N, Glover V: Fetal pain and stress. In Anand KJS, Stevens BJ, McGrath PJ, editors: *Pain research and clinical management,* vol 10, *Pain in neonates,* ed 2, New York, 2000, Elsevier.
7. Anand KJ: Effects of perinatal pain and stress, *Prog Brain Res* 122: 117, 2000.
8. Beyer JE, Wells N: The assessment of pain in children, *Pediatr Clin North Am* 36(4):837, 1989.
9. Golianu B et al: Pediatric acute pain management, *Pediatr Clin North Am* 47(3):559, 2000.
10. Harkins SW, Warner MH: Age and pain, *Behav Soc Sci,* 121, 1977.
11. Zheng Z et al: Age-related differences in the time course of capsaicin-induced hyperalgesia, *Pain* 85(1-2):51, 2000.
12. Kenshalo DR, Hall EC: Thermal thresholds of the rhesus monkey, *J Comp Physiol Psychol* 86:902, 1974.
13. Woodrow KM, Friedman GD, Siegelaub AB: Pain tolerance: differences according to age, sex, and race, *Psychosom Med* 34:548, 1972.
14. Smukler NM: Pain perception, *Bull Rheum Dis* 35(1):1, 1985.
15. Brena SF: Nerve blocks and chronic pain states—an update, *Postgrad Med* 78(4):77, 1985.
16. Urban MO, Gebbhart GF: Supraspinal contributions to hyperalgesia, *Proc Natl Acad Sci USA* 96(4):7684, 1999.
17. Melzack R, Wall P: Pain mechanisms: a new theory, *Science* 150:971, 1965.
18. Bonica JJ: *The management of pain,* vol 1, ed 2, Philadelphia, 1990, Lea & Febiger.
19. Melzack R, Casey KL: Sensory, motivational, and central control determinants of pain: a new conceptual model. In Kenshalto D, editor: *The skin senses,* Springfield, Ill, 1968, Charles C Thomas.
20. Melzack R, Wall P: Psychophysiology of pain, *Int Anesthesiol Clin* 8: 3, 1970.
21. Aimone LD: Neurochemistry and modulation of pain. In Sinatra RS et al, editors: *Acute pain: mechanisms and management,* St Louis, 1992, Mosby.
22. Sorkin LS, Wallace MS: Acute pain mechanisms, *Surg Clin North Am* 79(2):213, 1999.
23. Henry JL: Role of circulating opioids in the modulation of pain, *Ann N Y Acad Sci* 467:169, 1986.
24. West AB: Understanding endorphins: our natural pain relief system, *Nursing* 81:50, 1981.
25. Sheps DS et al: Endorphins are related to pain perception in coronary artery disease, *Am J Cardiol* 59:523, 1987.
26. Seeley RR, Stephens TD, Tate P: *Anatomy and physiology,* ed 2, St Louis, 1992, Mosby.
27. Coward DD, Wilkie DJ: Metastatic bone pain. Meanings associated with self-report and self-management, *Cancer Nurs* 23(2):101, 2000.
28. Almay GL et al: Relationships between CSF levels of endorphins and monoamine metabolites in chronic pain patients, *Psychopharmacology* 67:139, 1980.
29. Whitehead W III, Kuhn WF: Chronic pain: an overview. In Miller TW, editor: *Chronic pain,* vol 1, Madison, Wis, 1990, International Universities Press.
30. Bennett GJ: Update on the neurophysiology of pain transmission and modulation: focus on the NMDA receptor, *J Pain Symptom Manage* 19(1 suppl):S2, 2000.
31. Ossipov MH et al: Spinal and supraspinal mechanisms of neuropathic pain, *Ann N Y Acad Sci* 909:12, 2000.
32. Woolf CJ, Salter MW: Neuronal plasticity: increasing the gain in pain, *Science* 288(5472):1765, 2000.
33. Turk DC: The role of psychological factors in pain management, *Acta Anaesthesiol Scand* 43:885, 1999.
34. Strauss AL, Glasser BG: *Chronic illness and the quality of life,* St Louis, 1975, Mosby.
35. Foley KM: A review of pain syndromes in patients with cancer, *Symp Management Ca Pain* 7, 1984.
36. Foley KM: The treatment of cancer pain, *N Engl J Med* 313:84, 1985.
37. Payne R: Anatomy, physiology, and neuropharmacology of cancer pain, *Med Clin North Am* 71(2):153, 1987.
38. Dinarello CA, Wolff SM: Pathogenesis of fever in man, *N Engl J Med* 298(11):607, March 1978.
39. Himms-Hagen J: Current status of nonshivering thermogenesis. In Ross Laboratories: *Assessment of energy metabolism in health and disease: a report of the first Ross conference in medical research,* Columbus, Ohio, 1980, Ross Laboratories.
40. Benito M: Contribution of brown fat to the neonatal thermogenesis, *Biol Neonate* 48(4):245, 1985.
41. Lowell BB, Spiegelman BM: Towards a molecular understanding of adaptive thermogenesis, *Nature* 404(6778):652, 2000.
42. Yousef MK: Effects of climactic stresses on thermoregulatory processes in man, *Experientia* 43(1):14, 1987.
43. Hammarlund K, Stromberg B, Sedin G: Heat loss from the skin of preterm and full-term newborn infants during the first weeks after birth, *Biol Neonate* 50(1):1, 1986.
44. Collins KJ, Exton-Smith AN: Thermal homeostasis in old age, *J Am Geriatr Soc* 31(9):519, 1983.
45. Fellows IW, MacDonald IA, Bennett T: The effect of undernutrition on thermoregulation in the elderly, *Clin Sci* 69(5):525, 1985.
46. Sarwari AR, Mackowiak PA: Pathogenesis of fever. In Armstrong D, Cohen J, editors: *Infectious diseases,* vol 1, St Louis, 1999, Mosby.
47. Samii A: The neurobiological basis of fever, *Surg Neurol* 45:392, 1966.
48. Saper CB, Breder CD: The neurologic basis of fever, *N Engl J Med* 330(26):1880, 1994.
49. Boulant J: Thermoregulation. In Mackowiak P, editor: *Fever: basic mechanisms and management,* New York, 1991, Raven Press.

50. Cooper KE, Veale WL: Effects of endotoxins on heat tolerance and exercise performance. In Hales JRS, Richards DAB, editors: *Heat stress: physical exertion and environment,* New York, 1987, Elsevier Science Publications.
51. Dinarello CA: Cytokines as endogenous pyrogens, *J Infect Dis* 179(suppl 2):S194, 1999.
52. Coceani F, Akarsu ES: Prostaglandin E_2 in the pathogenesis of fever: an update, *Ann N Y Acad Sci* 856:76, 1998.
53. Mackowiak PA: Concepts of fever, *Arch Intern Med* 158(17):1870, 1998.
54. Armstrong D, Cohen J, editors: *Infectious diseases,* St. Louis, 1999, Mosby.
55. Roberts NJ: The immunological consequences of fever. In Mackowiak P, editor: *Fever: basic mechanisms and management,* New York, 1991, Raven.
56. Luheshi G, Rothwell N: Cytokines and fever, *Int Arch Allergy Immunol* 109(4):301, 1996.
57. Dinarello CA, Wolff SM: Molecular basis of fever in humans, *Am J Med* 72:799, 1982.
58. Kluger MS: The adaptive value of fever. In Mackowiak PA, editor: *Fever: basic mechanisms and management,* New York, 1991, Raven.
59. Yashikawa TT, Norman DC: Approach to fever and infection in the nursing home, *J Am Geriatr Soc* 44(1):74, 1996.
60. Fruthaler GJ: Fever in children: phobia vs. facts, *Hosp Pract* 20(11A):49, 1985.
61. Cabanac M, Brinnel H: The pathology of human temperature regulation: thermiatrics, *Experimentia* 43(1):19, 1987.
62. Clowes GH, O'Donnell TF: Heat stroke, *N Engl J Med* 291:564, 1974.
63. Committee on Sports Medicine: Climatic heat stress and the exercising child, *Pediatrics* 69:808, 1982.
64. Rogers AL, Sturgeon CL: Malignant hyperthermia, *AORN J* 41:369, 1985.
65. Antretter H, Dapunto E, Bonatti J: Management of profound hypothermia, *Br J Hosp Med* 54(5):215, 1995.
66. Reuler R: Hypothermia: pathophysiology, clinical settings, and management, *Ann Intern Med* 89:519, 1978.
67. DeLapp TD: Accidental hypothermia, *Am J Nurs* 83(1):63, 1983.
68. Lee-Chiong TL Jr, Stitt JT: Accidental hypothermia: when thermoregulation is overwhelmed, *Postgrad Med* 99(1):77, 1996.
69. Dean NC: Hypothermia, *Postgrad Med* 82(8):48, 1987.
70. Osterman AL et al: Muscle ischemia and hypothermia: a bioenergetic study using phosphorus nuclear magnetic resonance spectroscopy, *J Trauma* 24(9):811, 1984.
71. Laptook AR et al: Quantitative relationship between brain temperatures and energy utilization rate measured in vivo using 31P and 1H magnetic resonance spectroscope, *Pediatr Res* 38(6):919, 1995.
72. Shaver J et al: Changes in epicardial and core temperatures during resuscitation of hemorrhagic shock, *J Trauma* 24(11):957, 1984.
73. Little RA, Stoner HB: Body temperature after accidental injury, *Br J Surg* 68:221, 1981.
74. Schauf C, Moffet D, Moffett S: *Human physiology,* St Louis, 1990, Mosby.
75. Keenan SA: Normal human sleep, *Respir Care Clin North Am* 5(3):319, 1999.
76. Roth T, Rohers T: Sleep organization and regulation, *Neurology* 54(5 suppl 12):s2, 2000.
77. Hayaishi O: Molecular mechanisms of sleep-wake regulation: a role of prostaglandin D_2, *Philos Trans R Soc Lond B Biol Sci* 29(1394): 275, 2000.
78. Sinton CM, McCarley RW: Neuroanatomical and neurophysiological aspects of sleep: basic science and clinical relevance, *Semin Clin Neuropsychiatry* 5(1):6, 2000.
79. Phillipson EA: State-of-the-art control of breathing during sleep, *Am Rev Respir Dis* 118:909, 1978.
80. Sakai F et al: Normal human sleep: regional cerebral hemodynamics, *Ann Neurol* 7(5):471, 1980.
81. Sei H, Morita Y: Why does arterial blood pressure rise actively during REM sleep? *J Med Invest* 46(1-2):11, 1999.
82. Hayaishi O, Matsumura H: Prostaglandins and sleep, *Adv Neuroimmunol* 5(2):211, 1995.
83. Siegel JM: Mechanisms of sleep control, *J Clin Neurophysiol* 7:49, 1990.
84. Freiss E et al: The hypothalamic-pituitary-adrenocortical system and sleep in man, *Adv Neuroimmunol* 5(2):111, 1995.
85. Kryger MH et al: *Sleep medicine*, Philadelphia, 2000, W.B. Saunders.
86. Campbell SS: Evolution of sleep structure following brief intervals of wakefulness, *Electroencephalography Clin Neurophysiol* 66(2):175, 1987.
87. Kedas A, Lux W, Amodeo S: A critical review of aging and sleep research, *West J Nurs Res* 11(2):196, 1989.
88. Doto L: Sleep stages, memory, and learning, *Can Med Assoc J* 154(18):1193, 1996.
89. Anders TF, Keener M: Developmental course of nighttime sleep-wake patterns in full-term and premature infants during the first year of life, *Sleep* 8(3):173, 1985.
90. Keefe MR: Comparison of neonatal nighttime sleep-wake patterns in nursing versus rooming-in environments, *Nurs Res* 36(3):140, 1987.
91. Elias MF et al: Sleep/wake patterns of breast-fed infants in the first 2 years of life, *Pediatrics* 77(3):322, 1986.
92. Kales A, Kales JD: Evaluation, diagnosis, and treatment of clinical conditions related to sleep, *JAMA* 2229, 1970.
93. Guazzelli M, Feinberg I, Aminoff M: Sleep spindles in the normal elderly: comparison with young adult patterns and relation to nocturnal awakening, cognitive function, and brain atrophy, *Electroencephalography Clin Neurophysiol* 63(6):526, 1986.
94. Mourtazaev MS et al: Age and gender affect different characteristics of slow waves in sleep EEG, *Sleep* 18(7):557, 1995.
95. Kern W et al: Changes in cortisol and growth hormone secretion during nocturnal sleep in the course of aging, *J Gerontol A Biol Sci Med Sci* 51(1):M3, 1996.
96. Kupfer DJ, Reynolds CF: Management of insomnia, *J Engl J Med* 336:341, 1997.
97. Ware JC, McBrayer RH, Scott JA: Influence of sex and age on duration and frequency of sleep apnea events, *Sleep* 23(2):165, 2000.
98. Block AJ: Respiratory disorders during sleep. I, *Heart Lung* 9(6): 1011, 1980.
99. Exar EN, Collop NA: The upper airway resistance syndrome, *Chest* 115(4):1127, 1999.
100. Roux F, D'Ambrosio C, Mohsenin V: Sleep-related breathing disorders and cardiovascular disease, *Am J Med* 108(5):396, 2000.
101a. Friedlander AH et al: Diagnosing and comanaging patients with obstructive sleep apnea syndrome, *J Am Dent Assoc* 131(8):1178, 2000.
101b. Victor LD: Obstructive sleep apnea, *Am Fam Physician* 60(8):2279, 1999.
101c. Li KK et al: Morbidly obese patients with severe obstructive sleep apnea: is airway reconstructive surgery a viable treatment option? *Laryngoscope* 110(6):982, 2000.
102. Monk TH: Shift work. In Kryger MH, Roth T, Dement WC, editors: *Principles and practice of sleep medicine,* ed 3, Philadelphia, 2000, W.B. Saunders.
103. Taub JM, Berger RJ: The effects of changing the phase and duration of sleep, *J Exp Psychol Human Percept Perform* 2(1):30, 1976.
104. Long ME: Sleep, *Natl Geographic* 172(6):786, 1982.
105. Bernard-Bonnin AC: Diurnal enuresis in childhood, *Can Fam Physician* 46:1109, 2000.
106. Harari MD, Moulden A: Nocturnal enuresis: what is happening? *J Paediatr Child Health* 36(1):78, 2000.
107. Thase ME: Treatment issues related to sleep and depression, *J Clin Psychiatry* 61(suppl 11):46, 2000.
108. Lewis DA: Sleep in patients with respiratory disease, *Respir Care Clin North Am* 5(3):447, 1999.
109. McNicholas WT: Impact of sleep on COPD, *Chest* 117(2 suppl):48S, 2000.
110. Carter SR: Eyelid disorders: diagnosis and management, *Am Fam Physician* 57(11):2695, 1998.
111. Morrow FL, Abbott RL: Conunctivitis, *Am Fam Physician* 57(4):735, 1998.

112. Pathy MSJ, editor: *Principles and practices of geriatric medicine,* ed 2, New York, 1991, Wiley.
113. Tusa RJ: Nystagmus: diagnostic and therapeutic strategies, *Semin Opthalmol* 14(2):65, 1999.
114. Jackson RG et al: Aging and dark adaptation, *Vision Res* 39(23):3975, 1999.
115. Damji KF: Advances in molecular genetics of glaucoma: a perspective for the clinician, *Semin Opthalmol* 14(3):171, 1999.
116. Coleman AL: Glaucoma, *Lancet* 354(9192):1803, 1999.
117. Mermoud A, Schnyder CC: Nonpenetrating filtering surgery in glaucoma, *Curr Opin Opthalmol* 11(2):151, 2000.
118. Ross WH, Stockl FA: Visual recovery after retinal detachment, *Curr Opin Opthalmol* 11(3):191, 2000.
119. Bishop PN: Structural macromolecules and supramolecular organization of the vitreous gel, *Prog Retin Eye Res* 19(3):323, 2000.
120. Quillen DA: Common causes of vision loss in elderly patients, *Am Fam Practice* 60(1):99, 1999.
121. Lewis RA, Lupski JR: Macular degeneration: the emerging genetics, *Hosp Pract (Off Ed)* 35(6):41, 2000.
122. Javer AR, Schwartz DW: Plasticity in human directional hearing, *J Otolaryngol* 24(2):111, 1995.
123. Timiras PS: *Physiological basis of aging and geriatrics,* ed 2, Boca Raton, Fla, 1994, CRC Press.
124. Wiley TL et al: Aging and high-frequency hearing sensitivity, *J Speech Lang Hear Res* 41(5):1061, 1998.
125. Brook I: Treatment of otitis externa in children, *Paediatr Drugs* 1(4):283, 1999.
126. Heikkinen T: Role of viruses in the pathogenesis of acute otitis media, *Pediatr Infect Dis J* 19(5 suppl):S17, 2000.
127. Heikkinen T, Chonmaitree T: Increasing importance of viruses in acute otitis media, *Ann Med* 32(3):157, 2000.
128. Klein JO: Management of otitis media: 2000 and beyond, *Pediatr Infect Dis J* 19(4):383, 2000.
129. De la Cruz A et al: Stapedectomy in children, *Otolaryngol Head Neck Surg* 120(4):487, 1999.
130. Scott TR, Giza BK: Issues of gustatory neural coding, *Physiol Behav* 69(1-2):65, 2000.
131. Finkelstein LA, Schiffman SS: Workshop on taste and smell in the elderly: an overview, *Physiol Behav* 66(2):173, 1999.
132. Doty RL: Influence of age and age-related diseases on olfactory function, *Ann N Y Acad Sci* 565:76, 1989.
133. Cain WS, Reid F, Stevens JC: Missing ingredients: aging and the discrimination of flavor, *J Nutr Elderly* 9(3):3, 1990.
134. Bhatnagar KP et al: Number of mitral cells and the bulb volume in the aging human olfactory bulb: a quantitative morphological study, *Anat Rec* 218:73, 1987.
135. Winkler S et al: Depressed taste and smell in geriatric patients, *J Am Dent Assoc* 130(12):1759, 1999.
136. Bromley SM: Smell and taste disorders, *Am Fam Physician* 61(2): 426, 2000.
137. Scott AE: Clinical characteristics of taste and smell disorders, *Ear Nose Throat J* 68(4):297, 1989.
138. Bolanowski SJ et al: Four channels mediate the mechanical aspects of touch, *J Acoust Soc Am* 85(5):1680, 1988.
139. Balin AK, Klingman AM, editors: *Aging and the skin,* New York, 1989, Raven Press.
140. Stevens JC: Age and spatial acuity of touch, *J Gerontol* 47(1):35, 1992.

CHAPTER 15

Concepts of Neurologic Dysfunction

BARBARA J. BOSS

CHAPTER OUTLINE

A person achieves functional adequacy (competence) through complex integrated processes. Three major neural systems account for this functional adequacy: cognitive systems, sensory systems, and motor systems. Alterations in any or all of these affect functional adequacy. Alterations in cognitive and motor systems are discussed in this chapter.

The neural systems basic (core) to the cognitive sphere are (1) attentional systems that provide arousal and maintenance of attention over time; (2) memory and language systems by which information is communicated; and (3) affective, or emotive, systems that mediate feeling tone. These core systems are fundamental to the processes of abstract thinking and reasoning. The products of abstraction and reasoning are organized and made operational through the executive system. The normal functioning of these systems manifests through the motor system in a behavioral array viewed by others as appropriate to human activity and successful living.

ALTERATIONS IN COGNITIVE SYSTEMS

Full consciousness in its broadest sense is both a state of awareness of oneself and the environment and a set of responses to that environment. Full consciousness implies that the individual responds to external stimuli with a wide array of responses. Any decrease in this state of awareness and varied responses is thus a decrease in consciousness.

Consciousness often is viewed as having two distinct components: arousal and content of thought. Arousal, an attentional system, is the state of awakeness that an individual exhibits. Level of arousal is mediated by the reticular activating system, which extends from the medulla to the diencephalon. The reticular activating system provides arousal to the cerebral hemispheres (see Fig. 13-5). Severe alterations in arousal can occur with brain injury both in acute phase and on a long-term basis. Approximately 30% to 40% of survivors of severe brain injury remain in prolonged states of severely reduced consciousness. **Content of thought** (awareness) encompasses all cognitive functions that embody awareness of self, environment, and affective states (i.e., moods). Content of thought is mediated by attentional systems, memory systems, language systems, and executive systems.

Alterations in Arousal (Coma)

Possible causes of an altered level of arousal with acute onset may be separated into three major groups: **structural, metabolic,** and **psychogenic arousal alterations.** Structural causes are divided according to original location of the pathologic condition: supratentorial (above the tentorium cerebelli), infratentorial (subtentorial, below the tentorium cerebelli), subdural (below the dura mater), extracerebral (outside the brain tissue), and intracerebral (within the brain tissue).

Table 15-1 Clinical Manifestations of Metabolic and Structural Causes of Comas

Manifestation	Metabolically Induced Coma	Structurally Induced Coma
Blink to threat (cranial nerves II, VII)	Equal	Asymmetric
Discs (cranial nerve II)	Flat, good pulsation	Papilledema
Extraocular movement (cranial nerves III, IV, VI)	Roving eye movements; normal doll's eyes and calorics	Gaze paresis, nerve III palsy, medial longitudinal fasciculus (MLF) syndrome (internuclear ophthalmoplegia)
Pupils (cranial nerves II, III)	Equal and reactive, may be large (e.g., atropine), pinpoint (e.g., opiates), or midposition and fixed (e.g., glutethimide [Doriden])	Asymmetric and/or nonreactive; may be midposition (midbrain injury), pinpoint (pons injury), large (tectal injury)
Corneal reflex (cranial nerve V, VII)	Symmetric response	Asymmetric response
Grimace to pain (cranial nerve VII)	Symmetric response	Asymmetric response
Motor function movement	Symmetric	Asymmetric
Tone	Symmetric	Paratonic, spastic, flaccid, especially if asymmetric
Posture	Symmetric	Decorticate, especially if symmetric; decerebrate, especially if asymmetric
Deep tendon reflexes	Symmetric	Asymmetric
Babinski sign	Absent or symmetric response	Present
Sensation	Symmetric	Asymmetric

Causes of altered level of arousal also are grouped according to a pathologic process: infectious, vascular, neoplastic, traumatic, congenital (developmental), degenerative, polygenic, and metabolic. Metabolic causes may be further divided into hypoxia, electrolyte disturbances, hypoglycemia, drugs, and toxins (both endogenous and exogenous). All the systemic diseases that eventually produce nervous system dysfunction are part of this metabolic category.

Pathophysiology

Coma is produced by either (1) bilateral hemisphere damage or suppression by hypoxia, hypoglycemia, drugs, or toxins; or (2) a brain stem lesion or metabolic derangement that damages or suppresses the reticular activating system (RAS).[1] Supratentorial processes produce a decreased level of arousal by one of three mechanisms: (1) diffuse bilateral cortical dysfunction, (2) bilateral subcortical dysfunction, or (3) localized hemispheric dysfunction. Disease processes may produce diffuse bilateral cortical dysfunction (e.g., encephalitis) and actually may occur in either the cerebral cortex or the underlying subcortical white matter. Bilateral subcortical dysfunction involves destructive disease that compromises the RAS (e.g., brain stem trauma or cerebrovascular accident) and probably surrounding structures. Localized hemispheric dysfunction generally is caused by masses that directly impinge on deep diencephalic structures or that secondarily compress these structures in the process of herniation. Such localized destructive processes directly impair function of the thalamic or hypothalamic activating systems.

Extracerebral disorders also can produce diffuse bilateral cortical dysfunction. Extracerebral disorders include neoplasms, closed-head trauma with subsequent bleeding, and subdural empyema (accumulation of pus). Intracerebral disorders (those within the brain substance) function primarily as masses. These disorders include bleeding, infarcts and emboli, and tumors.

Infratentorial processes produce a reduction in arousal in one of two ways: (1) there may be direct destruction of the RAS and its pathways, or (2) the brain stem may be destroyed either by direct invasion or by indirect impairment of its blood supply. The most common cause of direct destruction is cerebrovascular disease, but demyelinating diseases, neoplasms, granulomas, abscesses, and head injury also may cause brain stem destruction. In addition, decreased level of consciousness may result from compression of the RAS by a disease process. This compression may occur because of (1) direct pressure on the pons and midbrain, producing ischemia and edema of the neurons of the RAS; (2) upward herniation of the cerebellum through the tentorial notch, thus compressing the upper midbrain and diencephalon; or (3) downward herniation of the cerebellum through the foramen magnum, compressing and displacing the medulla oblongata. Specific causes of compression of the brain stem include hematomas, hemorrhage, and aneurysm; cerebellar hemorrhage, infarcts, abscesses, and neoplasms; and demyelinating disorders.

A wide spectrum of diseases may produce a metabolically induced alteration in arousal. In encephalopathic conditions, widespread direct or indirect interference with neuronal metabolism occurs throughout much of the brain (see Chapter 16). Psychogenic unresponsiveness, although uncommon, may signal general psychiatric disorders. Despite apparent unconsciousness, the person actually is physiologically awake.

Evaluation

Evaluating an altered level of arousal requires distinguishing between organic and functional causes. A further distinction between metabolic and structural causes then is made (Table 15-1). If the cause is structural, the pathologic condition must be localized.

Clinical Manifestations

Patterns of clinical manifestations and their evolution have been identified. The patterns of clinical manifestation are important because they help in determining the extent of brain dysfunction and they serve as indexes for identifying increasing or decreasing central nervous system (CNS) function. The specific clusters of manifestations of abnormal function and their evolution suggest whether the cause of the altered arousal state is supratentorial, infratentorial, metabolic, or psychogenic (Table 15-2). Five categories of neurologic function are critical to the evaluation process: (1) level of consciousness, (2) pattern of breathing, (3) size and reactivity of pupils, (4) eye position and reflexive responses, and (5) skeletal muscle motor responses.

Level of Consciousness

Level of consciousness is the most critical clinical index of nervous system function or dysfunction. An alteration in consciousness indicates either improvement or deterioration of the individual's condition. A person who is alert and oriented to self, others, place, and time is considered to be functioning at the highest level of consciousness, which implies full use of all the person's cognitive capacities.

Because many different terms are used to indicate level of consciousness, definition becomes necessary. The term *unconscious,* for example, has no specific clinical definition and signifies different things to different people. From the normal alert state, levels of consciousness diminish in stages, each of which is clinically defined (Table 15-3).

Pattern of Breathing

Several characteristic respiratory patterns are helpful in evaluating level of brain dysfunction and level of coma. Among these characteristics are rate, rhythm, and pattern of breathing. The breathing patterns can be categorized as hemispheric or brain stem breathing patterns (Table 15-4).

Table 15-2 Differential Characteristics of States Causing Coma

Mechanism	Manifestations
Supratentorial mass lesions compressing or displacing diencephalon or brain stem	Initiating signs usually of focal cerebral dysfunction Signs of dysfunction progress rostral to caudal Neurologic signs at any given time point to one anatomic area (e.g., diencephalon, mesencephalon, medulla) Motor signs often asymmetric
Infratentorial mass of destruction causing coma	History of preceding brain stem dysfunction or sudden onset of coma Localizing brain stem signs precede or accompany onset of coma and always include oculovestibular abnormality Cranial nerve palsies usually manifest "bizarre" respiratory patterns that appear at onset
Metabolic coma	Confusion and stupor commonly precede motor signs Motor signs usually are symmetric Pupillary reactions usually are preserved Asterixis, myoclonus, tremor, and seizures are common Acid-base imbalance with hyperventilation or hypoventilation is common
Psychiatric unresponsiveness	Lids close actively Pupils reactive or dilated (cycloplegics) Oculocephalic reflexes are unpredictable; oculovestibular reflexes are physiologic (nystagmus is present) Motor tone is inconsistent or normal Eupnea or hyperventilation is usual No pathologic reflexes are present Electroencephalogram (EEG) is normal

Table 15-3 Levels of Acute Coma

State	Definition
Confusion	Loss of ability to think rapidly and clearly; impaired judgment and decision making
Disorientation	Beginning loss of consciousness; disorientation to time followed by disorientation to place and impaired memory; lost last is recognition of self
Lethargy	Limited spontaneous movement or speech; easy arousal with normal speech or touch; may not be oriented to time, place, or person
Obtundation	Mild to moderate reduction in arousal (awakeness) with limited response to the environment; falls asleep unless stimulated verbally or tactilely; answers questions with minimum response
Stupor	A condition of deep sleep or unresponsiveness from which the person may be aroused or caused to open eyes only by vigorous and repeated stimulation; response is often withdrawal or grabbing at stimulus
Coma	No verbal response to the external environment or to any stimuli; noxious stimuli such as deep pain or suctioning yield motor movement
Light coma	Associated with purposeful movement on stimulation
Coma	Associated with nonpurposeful movement only on stimulation
Deep coma	Associated with unresponsiveness or no response to any stimulus

With normal breathing, a neural center believed to be located in the forebrain (cerebrum) produces a rhythmic breathing pattern despite lowered arterial carbon dioxide pressure ($PaCO_2$). When neural control at this center is lost as consciousness decreases, the lower brain stem centers regulate the breathing pattern by responding only to changes in $PaCO_2$ levels. The result is the irregular breathing associated with posthyperventilation apnea (PHVA).

The pathophysiology of Cheyne-Stokes respirations (CSR) involves an increased ventilatory response to carbon dioxide stimulation, causing hypercapnia and a diminished ventilatory stimulus. The neural center that causes PHVA thus is related to the CSR, because changes in $PaCO_2$ produce irregular breathing that contributes to overbreathing when stimulated by carbon dioxide. As a result, the $PaCO_2$ level decreases to below normal and, because of the cerebral brain dysfunction, breathing stops until the carbon dioxide reaccumulates to bring the $PaCO_2$ level to normal. In cases of opiate or sedative drug overdose, the respiratory center is depressed and the rate of breathing gradually decreases until respiratory failure occurs.

Certain motor activities related to breathing signify the level of brain dysfunction. Yawning, vomiting, and hiccups are complex reflexlike motor responses that are integrated by neural mechanisms in the lower brain stem. These responses may be produced by compression or diseases that involve tissues in the medulla oblongata. Such disorders include infection, neoplasm, or infarct. Similar responses are produced by dysfunction in the lower brain stem through direct stimulation.

Most CNS disorders produce both nausea and vomiting. Vomiting with no associated nausea indicates direct involvement of the central neural mechanism. Vomiting is associated particularly with CNS injuries that (1) involve the vestibular nuclei (located in the lower pons and medulla oblongata) or their immediate projections, particularly when double vision (diplopia) also is present; (2) impinge directly on the floor of the fourth ventricle; or (3) produce brain stem compression secondary to increased intracranial pressure.

Pupillary Changes

Anatomically, brain stem areas that control arousal are adjacent to areas that control pupils. Pupillary changes thus are a valuable guide to evaluating the presence and level of brain stem dysfunction (Fig. 15-1).

Table 15-4 Patterns of Breathing

Breathing Pattern	Description	Location of Injury
HEMISPHERIC BREATHING PATTERNS		
Normal	After a period of hyperventilation that lowers the arterial carbon dioxide pressure ($PaCO_2$), the individual continues to breathe regularly but with a reduced depth.	Response of the nervous system to an external stressor—not associated with injury to the CNS
Posthyperventilation apnea (PHVA)	Respirations stop after hyperventilation has lowered the PCO_2 level below normal. Rhythmic breathing returns when the PCO_2 level returns to normal.	Associated with diffuse bilateral metabolic or structural disease of the cerebrum
Cheyne-Stokes respirations (CSR)	The breathing pattern has a smooth increase (crescendo) in the rate and depth of breathing (hyperpnea), which peaks and is followed by a gradual smooth decrease (decrescendo) in the rate and depth of breathing to the point of apnea when the cycle repeats itself. The hyperpneic phase lasts longer than the apneic phase.	Bilateral dysfunction of the deep cerebral or diencephalic structures, seen with supratentorial injury and metabolically induced coma states
BRAIN STEM BREATHING PATTERNS		
Central neurogenic hyperventilation (CNH)	A sustained deep rapid, but regular pattern (hyperpnea) occurs, with a decreased $PaCO_2$ and a corresponding increase in pH and increased PO_2.	May result from CNS damage or disease that involves the midbrain and upper pons; seen after increased intracranial pressure and blunt head trauma
Apneusis	A prolonged inspiratory cramp (a pause at full inspiration) occurs. A common variant of this is a brief end-inspiratory pause of 2 or 3 seconds often alternating with an end-expiratory pause.	Indicates damage to the respiratory control mechanism located at the pontine level; most commonly associated with pontine infarction but documented with hypoglycemia, anoxia, and meningitis
Cluster breathing	A cluster of breaths has a disordered sequence with irregular pauses between breaths.	Dysfunction in the lower pontine and high medullary areas
Ataxic breathing	Completely irregular breathing occurs, with random shallow and deep breaths and irregular pauses. Often the rate is slow.	Originates from a primary dysfunction of the medullary neurons controlling breathing
Gasping breathing pattern (agonal gasps)	A pattern of deep "all-or-none" breaths is accompanied by a slow respiratory rate.	Indicative of a failing medullary respiratory center

CNS, Central nervous system.

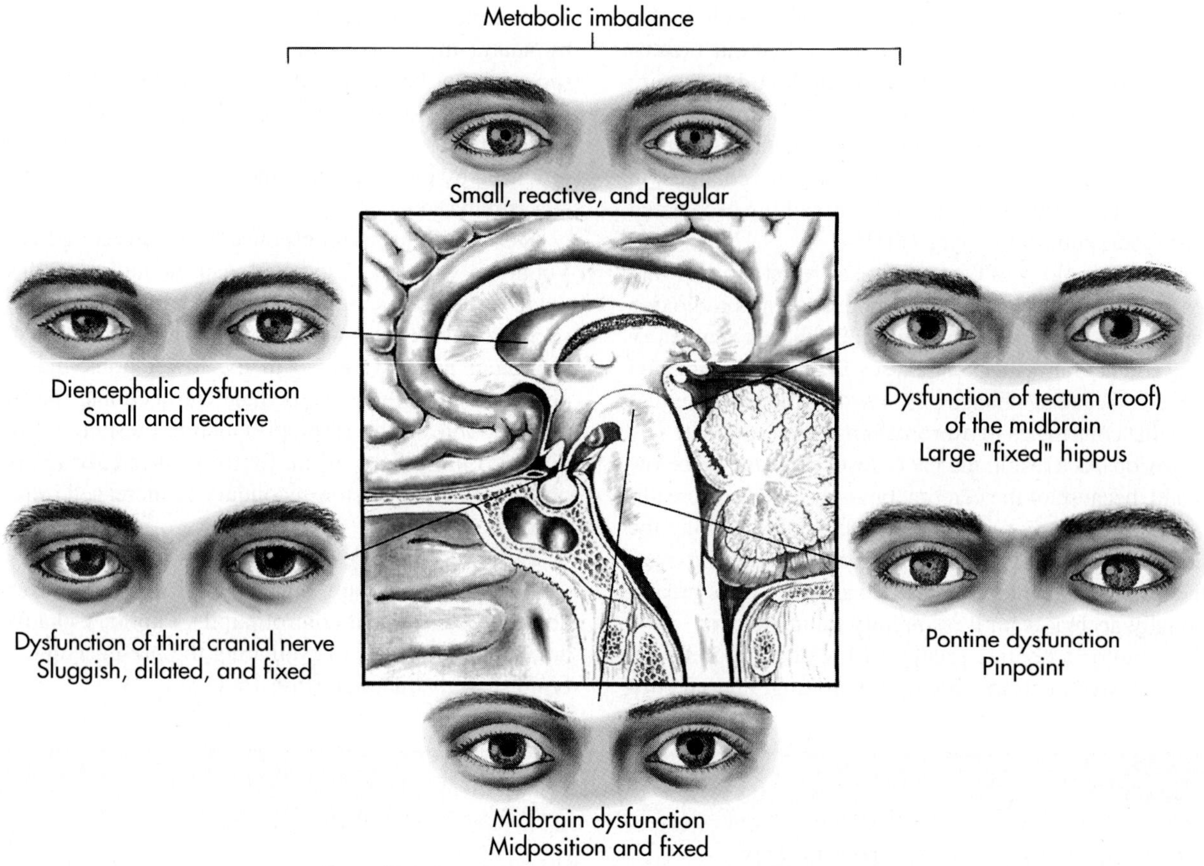

FIG. 15-1 Pupils at different levels of consciousness.

Certain drugs that affect pupils must be considered in the evaluation of pupillary response in comatose states. Atropine, scopolamine, amphetamines, mydriatrics, and cycloplegics in large concentrations fully dilate and fix pupils. Glutethimide in amounts sufficient to produce a coma causes the pupils to become midposition or moderately dilated (4 to 5 mm in diameter), unequal, and frequently fixed to light. Opiates (heroin and morphine) cause pinhole pupils (1.0 mm). Severe barbiturate intoxication may produce fixed pupils.

Severe ischemia and hypoxia produce bilaterally wide (5 mm) and fixed pupils in most instances. Occasionally the pupils remain small (1 to 2.5 mm) or midposition even in the presence of profound hypoxia. Hypothermia also may cause fixed pupils.

Oculomotor Responses

Resting, spontaneous, and reflexive eye movements (oculocephalic [doll's head, doll's eyes] and oculovestibular [caloric] reflexes) undergo change at various levels of brain dysfunction (Table 15-5). Persons with metabolically induced coma, except in cases of barbiturate-hypnotic and phenytoin (Dilantin) poisoning, generally do retain ocular reflexes, however, even when other signs of brain stem damage, such as central neurogenic hyperventilation, are present.

The presence of brisk oculocephalic reflexes and roving eye movements, as well as the failure to elicit nystagmus with instillation of cold or warm water into the external ear canal, indicates a decrease in consciousness (loss of cortical influence) but an intact brain stem (Figs. 15-2 and 15-3).

Destructive or compressive injury to the brain stem causes specific abnormalities of the oculocephalic and oculovestibular reflexes. For example, a skewed deviation, in which one eye diverges downward and the other looks upward, indicates brain stem dysfunction. Destructive or compressive disease processes that involve an oculomotor nucleus or nerve cause the involved eye to deviate outward, producing a resting disconjugate lateral position of the eyes. Unilateral abducens paralysis (paralysis of cranial nerve VI) results in an upward deviation of the ipsilateral eye. With bilateral abducens paralysis, the eyes come together (converge). Reflexive eye movements may be suppressed by drugs, most commonly phenytoin, tricyclics, and barbiturates. Occasionally alcohol, phenothiazines, and diazepam may alter reflex eye movements.

Motor Responses

Motor responses contribute both to evaluating the level of brain dysfunction and to determining the side of the brain that is maximally damaged. The pattern of response is described as (1) purposeful (a defensive or withdrawal movement of limbs to noxious stimuli); (2) inappropriate, or not purposeful (generalized motor movement, posturing, grimacing, or groaning); or (3) not present (unresponsive, no motor response). Purposeful movement requires an intact corticospinal system. Nonpurposeful movement is evidence of severe dysfunction of the corticospinal system.

Table 15-5 Changes in Oculomotor Responses

State	Resting and Spontaneous Eye Movements	Reflexive Eye Movements
Full consciousness	Eyes at rest, still (cortical gaze centers inhibit spontaneous roving eye movements)	Eyes move as the head turns Oculocephalic responses not elicited or inconsistently elicited (frontal gaze centers inhibit brain stem reflexes that fix gaze straight ahead) Oculovestibular (caloric) stimulation produces nystagmus
Cortical dysfunction or disruption of efferent pathways	Conjugate, horizontal, roving eye movements may well be present (cortical gaze centers no longer inhibit these brain stem–generated roving eye movements)	Gaze fixed straight ahead regardless of head position—positive doll's eyes reaction (normal oculocephalic reflexes are no longer inhibited by frontal gaze centers)
Diffuse anoxic damage to cortex	"Ocular dipping"—slow, dysrhythmic downward movement followed by faster, upward movement	Nystagmus is no longer induced by caloric stimulation (normally a cold water stimulus produces deviation of the eyes opposite the irrigated ear; a warm water stimulus deviates the eyes to the same [ipsilateral] side) With an injury that depresses cortical gaze center function, the eyes (and often the entire head) will deviate, or appear to look toward the side of the injured hemisphere With an injury that irritates (stimulates) the neurons of the cortical gaze center, the eyes (and often the entire head) will deviate away from the injured hemisphere (all fibers from the frontal gaze centers decussate and therefore control the function of the contralateral pontine gaze center, which moves the eyes in the ipsilateral direction)
Mesencephalon dysfunction	Roving eye movements cease, and the eyes become immobile and directed ahead (roving eye movements require an intact brain stem) Eyes may turn down and inward	Oculovestibular reflexes become inconsistent and abnormal Loss of Bell phenomenon (upward deviation of eyes on stimulation) (requires intact eye movement pathways from the mesencephalon to pons)
Pontine dysfunction	Loss of spontaneous blinking (requires an intact pons) "Ocular bobbing"—brisk, conjugate, downward movement of eyes with loss of horizontal eye movements	

A

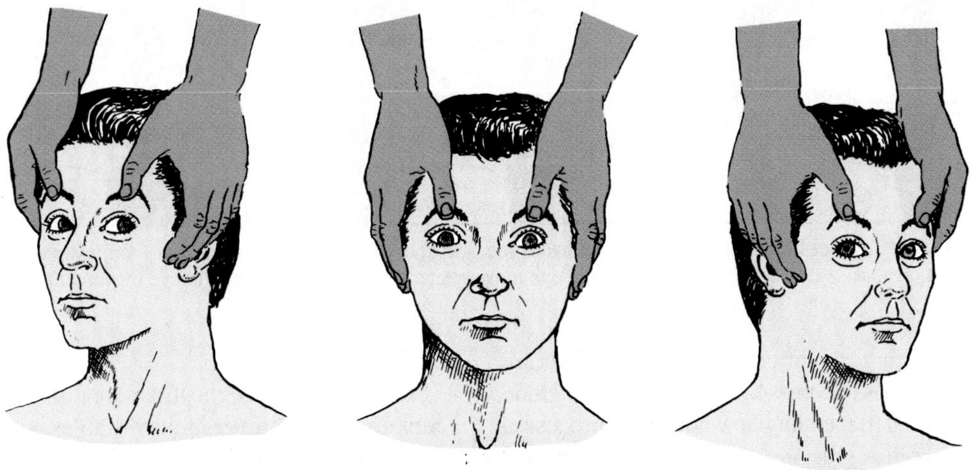

FIG. 15-2 Test for oculocephalic reflex response (doll's eyes phenomenon). A, Normal response—eyes turn together to side opposite from turn of head. (From Rudy EB: *Advanced neurological and neurosurgical nursing,* St. Louis, 1984, Mosby.)

Continued

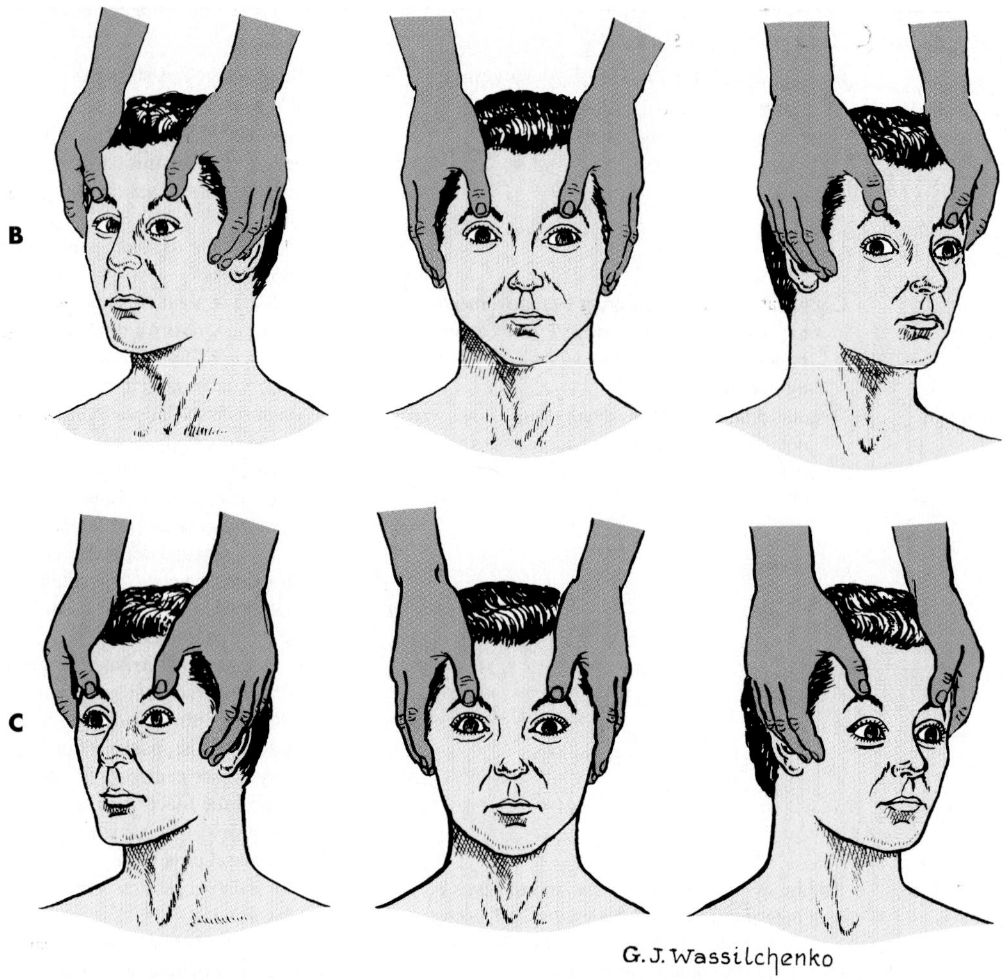

FIG. 15-2, cont'd Test for oculocephalic reflex response (doll's eyes phenomenon). B, Abnormal response—eyes do not turn in conjugate manner. **C,** Absent response—eyes do not turn as head position changes. (From Rudy EB: *Advanced neurological and neurosurgical nursing,* St. Louis, 1984, Mosby.)

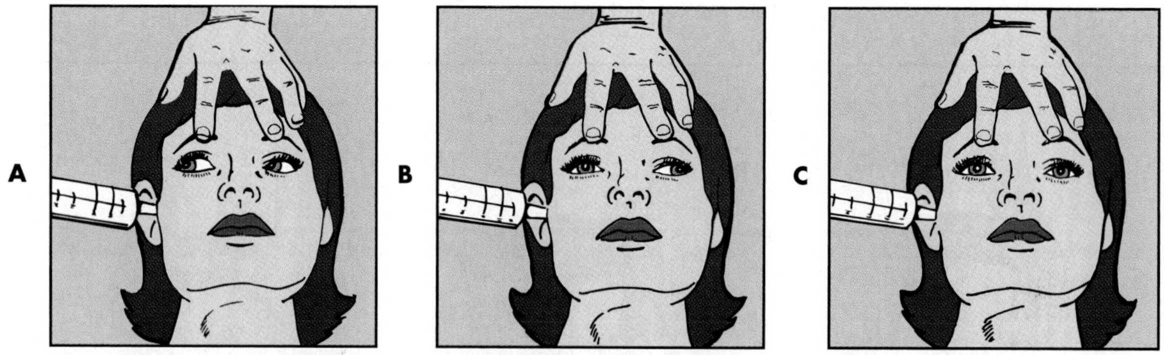

FIG. 15-3 Test for oculovestibular reflex (caloric ice water test). A, Normal response—conjugate eye movements. **B,** Abnormal response—dysconjugate or asymmetric eye movements. **C,** Absent response—no eye movements.

Motor signs indicating loss of cortical inhibition that are commonly associated with decreased consciousness include contralateral or bilateral (depending on whether the process is localized or diffuse) reflex grasping, reflex sucking, snout reflex, palmomental reflex, and rigidity (paratonia) (Fig. 15-4). Abnormal flexor and extensor responses in the upper and lower extremities are defined in Table 15-6 and illustrated in Fig. 15-5.

Outcomes

Categories of prognostic indicators related to outcome of coma include demographic variables, severity indices, neurologic signs, neuroimaging studies, neuromedical markers, psychologic ratings, and outcome scales.[2] Outcome domains fall into two divisions—mortality and extent of disability (morbidity). For coma, the extent of disability division has four domains—recovery of consciousness, residual cognitive

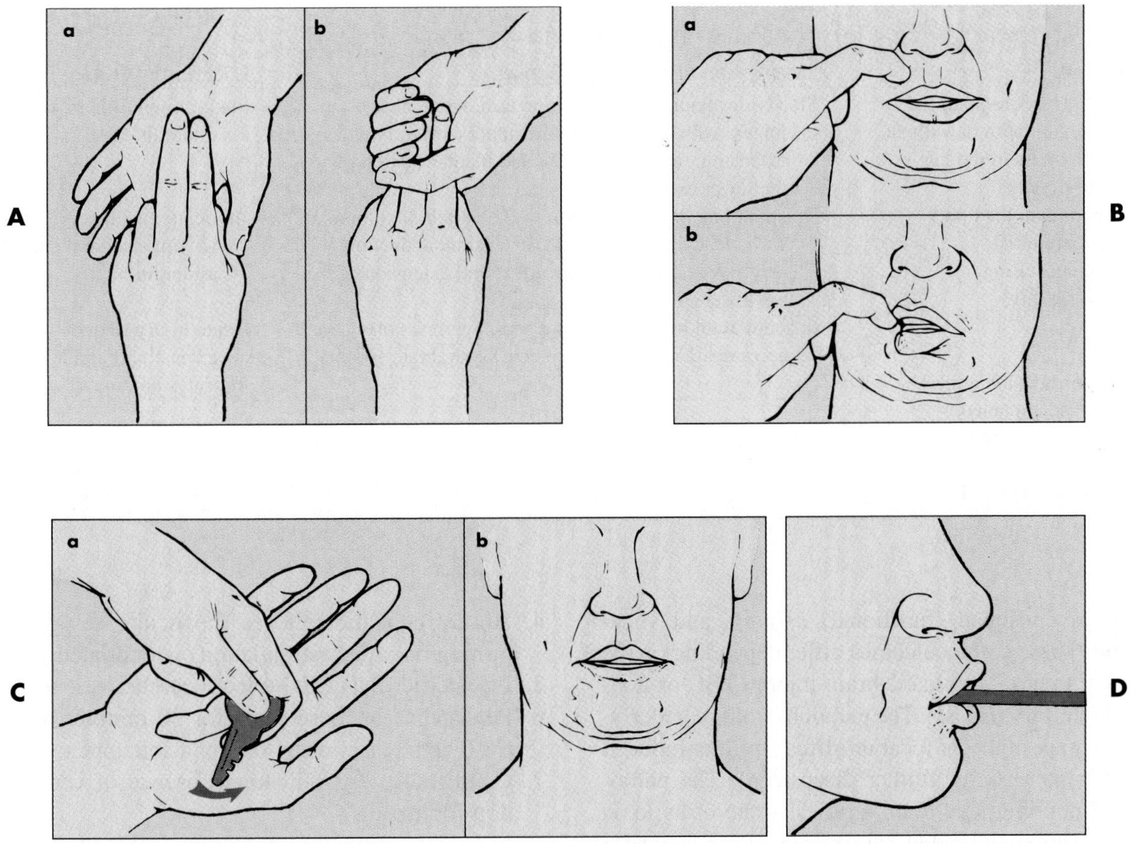

FIG. 15-4 Pathologic reflexes. A, Grasp reflex. **B,** Snout reflex. **C,** Palmomental reflex. **D,** Suck reflex.

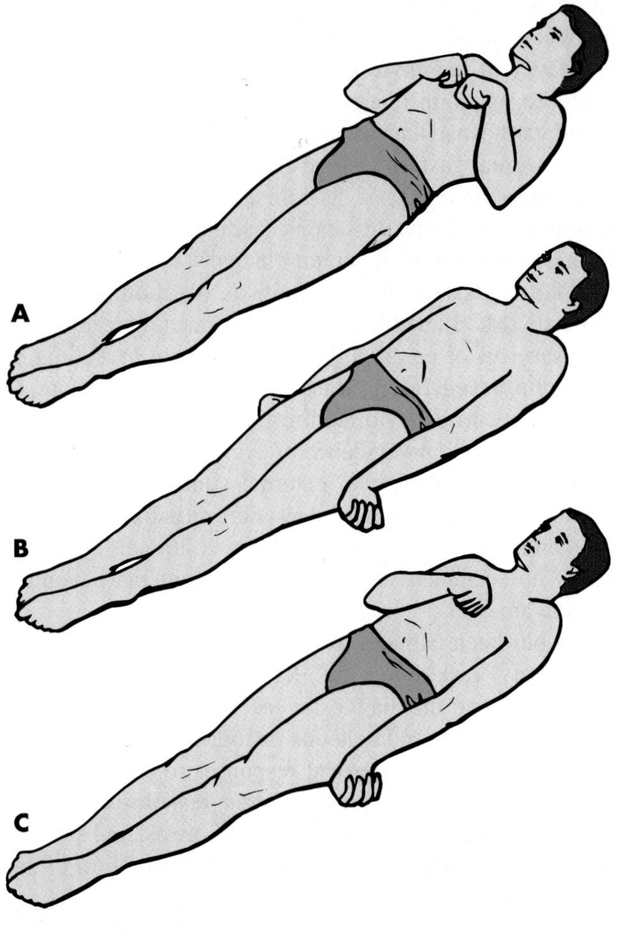

FIG. 15-5 Decorticate and decerebrate responses. A, Decorticate response. Flexion of arms, wrists, and fingers with adduction in upper extremities. Extension, internal rotation, and plantar flexion in lower extremities. **B,** Decerebrate response. All four extremities in rigid extension, with hyperpronation of forearms and plantar extension of feet. **C,** Decorticate response on right side of body and decerebrate response on left side of body. (From Rudy EB: *Advanced neurological and neurosurgical nursing,* St Louis, 1984, Mosby.)

Table 15-6 Abnormal Motor Responses with Decreased Responsiveness

Motor Response	Description of Motor Responses	Location of Injury
Abnormal motor responses, upper extremity flexion with or without extensor responses in the leg (decorticate rigidity)	Slowly developing flexion of the arm, wrist, and fingers with adduction in the upper extremity and extension, internal rotation, and plantar flexion of the lower extremity	Suggest hemispheric damage above midbrain
Extensor responses in the upper and lower extremities (decerebrate posturing, decerebrate rigidity)	Opisthotonos (hyperextension of the vertebral column) with clenching of the teeth; extension, adduction, and hyperpronation of the arms; and extension of the lower extremities	Associated with severe damage involving caudal diencephalon or midbrain
	In acute brain injury, shivering and hyperpnea may accompany unelicited recurrent decerebrate spasms	Acute injury frequently causes limb extension regardless of location
Extensor responses in the upper extremities accompanied by flexion in the lower extremities		Indicates pontine level dysfunction
Flaccid state with little or no motor response to stimuli		Damage to lower pons and upper myelencephalon

dysfunction, psychosocial (functional) domain, and vocational domain. These coma outcomes differ depending on the etiology of the injury—traumatic brain injury (TBI) or nontraumatic brain injury (NTBI). The pathophysiology underlying traumatic brain injury is focal or diffuse trauma-induced injury (see Chapter 16 for further discussion). The pathophysiology of nontraumatic brain injuries is one of hypoxia and ischemia. This may be due, for example, to vascular insult, tumor, hydrocephalus, infection, or anorexia.[2]

Related to mortality, two forms of neurologic death—brain death (brain stem death) and cerebral death—may result from severe TBI and NTBI. **Brain death (brain stem death)** occurs when irreversible brain damage is so extensive that the brain has no potential for recovery and no longer can maintain the body's internal homeostasis. Destruction of the neuronal contents of the intracranial cavity includes the brain stem and cerebellum. On postmortem examination the brain is autolyzing (self-digesting) or already autolyzed.

General agreement holds that brain death has occurred in the absence of discernible evidence of cerebral hemisphere function or function of the brain stem's vital centers for an extended period. In addition, the abnormality of brain function must result from structural or known metabolic disease and *not* be caused by a depressant drug, alcohol poisoning, neuromuscular blockage, or hypothermia. An isoelectric, or flat, electroencephalogram (EEG) (electrocerebral silence) for a period of 6 to 12 hours in a person who is not hypothermic and has not ingested depressant drugs indicates that no mental recovery is possible and usually means that the brain is already dead.

The following clinical criteria determine brain death:[1,3,4]

1. Completion of all appropriate and therapeutic procedures
2. Unresponsive coma (absence of motor and reflex movements)
3. No spontaneous respiration (apnea)—a $PaCO_2$ that rises above 60 mm Hg without breathing efforts, providing evidence of a nonfunctioning respiratory center
4. Absent cephalic reflexes (no ocular responses to head turning or caloric stimulation) with dilated, fixed pupils
5. Isoelectric (flat) EEG (electrocerebral silence)
6. Persistence of these signs for 30 minutes to 1 hour and for 6 hours after onset of coma and apnea
7. Confirming test indicating absence of cerebral circulation (optional)

Cerebral death (irreversible coma) is death of the cerebral hemispheres exclusive of the brain stem and cerebellum. Brain damage is permanent and sufficiently severe that the individual is unable to ever respond behaviorally in any significant way to the environment. The brain, however, may continue to maintain internal homeostasis (normal respiratory and cardiovascular functions, normal temperature control, and normal gastrointestinal function).

Related to the extent of disability, the recovery spectrum of neurobehavioral manifestations (in diagnostic terms, clinical states) after severe brain injury include (1) coma, (2) vegetative state (VS), (3) akinetic mutism, (4) minimally conscious state (MCS), and locked-in syndrome (Table 15-7).[5]

The survivor of cerebral death may remain in a coma or emerge into a **vegetative state (VS).** In **coma,** a state of unarousable neurobehavioral unresponsiveness, the eyes are usually closed with no evidence of eye opening either spontaneously or in response to external stimuli.[6] The person does not follow commands, does not verbalize or mouth words, and has no goal-directed or volitional behavior. There is no sustained visual pursuit movements beyond a 45-degree arc.[7]

A VS has been called a wakeful unconscious state.[5] The Multi-Society Task Force on Persistent Vegetative States (MSTF) identified the diagnostic criteria for VS as (1) periods of eye opening (spontaneous or following stimulation); (2) the potential for subcortical responses to external stimuli, including generalized physiologic responses to pain, such as posturing, tachycardia, and diaphoresis, and subcortical motor responses, such as grasp reflex; (3) return of so-

Table 15-7 Comparison of Clinical Features in Coma, Vegetative State, and Minimally Conscious State

	Clinical Features		
Diagnosis	**Arousal**	**Awareness**	**Communication**
Coma	Eyes do not open spontaneously or in response to stimulation.	No evidence of perception, communication ability, or purposeful motor activity (e.g., command following)	No evidence of yes/no responses, verbalizing, or gesture
Vegetative state	Eyes open spontaneously; sleep-wake cycle resumes; arousal often sluggish, poorly sustained	No evidence of perception communication ability, or purposeful motor activity	No evidence of yes/no responses, verbalization, gesture
Minimally conscious state	Eyes open spontaneously; normal to abnormal sleep-wake cycle; arousal level ranges from obtunded to normal	Reproducible but inconsistent evidence of perception, communication ability, or purposeful motor activity; visual tracking often intact	Ranges from none to unreliable and inconsistent yes/no responses, verbalization, and gesture

From Schacter SC, Saper CB: Vagus nerve stimulation, *Epilepsia* 38(7):677, 1998.

called vegetative (autonomic) functions, including sleep-wake cycles, and normalization of respiratory and digestive system functions; and (4) occasional roving eye movements without concomitant visual tracking ability.[7] The person's eyes open spontaneously or following stimulation, or both. There may be random hand, extremity, or head movements. The individual maintains blood pressure and breathing without support. Brain stem reflexes (pulillary, oculocephalic, chewing, swallowing) are intact. No discrete localizing motor responses are present, and the individual does not speak any comprehensible words or follow commands.

Some survivors of coma progress to a minimally conscious state. The term **minimally conscious state (MCS)** was first used by the International Working Party on Vegetative States[8] and supported by the Brain Injury Interdisciplinary Special Interest Group of the American Congress of Rehabilitation Medicine (ACRM). ACRM defined MCS as a condition of severely altered consciousness in which the person demonstrates minimal but defined behavioral evidence of self or environmental awareness.[9] The clinical features include (1) following simple commands, (2) manipulation of objects, (3) gestural or verbal "yes/no" responses, (4) intelligible verbalization, and (5) stereotypic movements (e.g., blinking, smiling) that occur in a meaningful relationship to the eliciting stimulus and are not attributable to reflexive activity.[6]

Akinetic mutism (AM) is a neurobehavioral state characterized by a severe disturbance in behavioral drive (motivation). Giacino and Zasler[5] describe this state as a subset of the MCS group. Generally, these individuals evidence eye opening with visual tracking and have little or no spontaneous speech or following of commands. Little movement is present. This is not attributable to decreased wakefulness or motor weakness or impairment.

With **locked-in syndrome,** both the content of thought and level of arousal are intact, but the efferent pathways are disrupted. Thus the individual cannot communicate either through speech or through body movement but is fully conscious, with intact cognitive function. The upper cranial nerves (I through IV) often are preserved, however, so that the person possesses vertical eye movement and blinking as a means of communication.

Prognostic indicators for emergence from coma. To date, no indicators except those of brain death predict outcome of coma.[3] Etiology of injury and time since onset of coma are currently the best prognostic indicators of recovery of consciousness or functional outcome. In nontraumatic brain injury, the prognosis can be established earlier than with traumatic brain injury. In traumatic coma, there is a 95% death rate in individuals whose pupillary reflexes or reflective eye movements are absent 6 hours after onset of coma and a 91% death rate if pupils are nonreactive at 24 hours.[3] In nontraumatic coma, absence of any two of the following is an unfavorable sign in the first hours after admission: pupil reflexes, corneal reflexes, or oculovestibular responses. Absence of eye opening and muscle tone in 24 hours predicts death or severe disability.[3]

Recovery of consciousness within 2 weeks is associated with favorable outcomes. Recovery of consciousness after 6 months is correlated with severe disability on the Glasgow Outcome Scale.[6] No recovery without severe disability has ever been documented after 1 year in coma.[6] No emergence from a VS can be expected after 3 months in a VS from hypoxic-ischemic injury and after 1 year from TBI.

Emergence from MCS is confirmed when there is reliable and consistent demonstration of either (1) interactive communication, that is, the ability to answer basic yes/no questions regarding personal or environmental questions, and (2) functional use of objects, that is, the ability to appropriately discriminate among objects.[6] Failure to emerge from MCS within 12 months predicts likelihood of remaining in an MCS.[6]

Seizures

A **seizure** is a sudden, explosive, disorderly discharge of cerebral neurons and is characterized by a sudden, transient alteration in brain function, usually involving motor, sensory, autonomic, or psychic clinical manifestations and an alteration in level of arousal. Seizure disorders, the second most common neurologic disorder, represent a syndrome or symptom, however, and not a specific disease entity. The alteration in level of arousal is temporary.

The term *convulsion,* sometimes applied to seizures, refers to the clonic-tonic (jerky, contract-relax) movement associated with some seizures. The term *epilepsy,* meaning "to be seized by a force from without," generally is applied to conditions in which no underlying correctable cause for the seizures is found so that the seizure activity recurs without treatment. **Epilepsy** therefore is a general term for the primary condition that causes seizures.

Conditions Associated with Seizure Disorders

Any disorder that alters the neuronal environment may cause seizure activity, so that theoretically anyone may experience a seizure. Some persons, however, have a genetic predisposition toward seizure activity; their "seizure threshold" in neuronal tissues apparently is lower. Twenty percent of epilepsies are estimated to have a genetic factor present.[10] The gene responsible for myoclonic epilepsy was isolated to chromosome 21 in 1996.[11]

One third of seizures can be classified as provoked, symptomatic, or secondary, that is, from a known cause or disease. A seizure disorder can be produced by a variety of pathologic processes, including medical diseases, that can extend to involve the nervous system. The onset of a seizure disorder also may indicate the presence of an ongoing primary neurologic disease. Persons with organic brain injury have greater tendencies toward seizure activity than do persons with normal CNS function. Two thirds of seizures are unprovoked, primary, or idiopathic; that is, the etiology or cause is not known. Etiologic factors in seizures generally include (1) cerebral lesions, (2) biochemical disorders, (3) cerebral trauma, and (4) epilepsy, which can result from the following conditions:

Metabolic defects
Congenital malformation
Genetic predisposition
Perinatal injury
Postnatal trauma
Myoclonic syndromes
Infection
Brain tumor
Vascular disease
Drug or alcohol abuse

Causes of recurrent seizures also are age related (Table 15-8). Genetics are probably more of a factor if onset of seizures is before 20 years of age.[10] The incidence of seizures is 20 to 70 per 100,000 persons each year. In persons with seizure disorders, seizure activity may be precipitated by hypoglycemia, fatigue or lack of sleep, emotional or physical stress, febrile illness, large amounts of water ingestion, constipation, use of stimulant drugs, withdrawal from depressant drugs (including alcohol), hyperventilation (respiratory alkalosis), and some environmental stimuli such as blinking lights, a poorly adjusted television screen, loud noises, certain music, certain odors, or merely being startled. Women may have increased seizure activity immediately before or during menses.

Types of Seizure Disorders

Seizures are classified in different ways—by clinical manifestations, site of origin, EEG correlates, or response to therapy. A simplified version of the international classification of epileptic seizures is presented in Table 15-9. **Generalized seizures,** 30% of seizures,[1] involve neurons bilaterally, often do not have a local (focal) onset, and usually originate from a subcortical or deeper brain focus. With a generalized seizure, consciousness always is impaired or lost. **Partial seizures (focal seizures)** involve neurons only unilaterally, often have a local (focal) onset, and usually originate from cortical brain tissue, thereby having a superficial focus. Consciousness may be maintained as long as the seizure activity is limited to one hemisphere in simple partial seizures, but partial seizures may become generalized to involve neurons of the other hemisphere and the deeper brain nuclei. This process is called **secondary generalization.** Con-

Table 15-8 Causes of Recurrent Seizures in Different Age-Groups

Age of Onset	Probable Cause
Neonatal	Congenital maldevelopment, birth injury, metabolic disorders (hypocalcemia, hypoglycemia), vitamin B deficiency, phenylketonuria
Infancy (1-6 mo)	As above; infantile spasms
Early childhood (6 mo–3 yr)	Infantile spasms, febrile convulsions, birth injury and anoxia, infections, trauma
Childhood (3-10 yr)	Perinatal anoxia, injury at birth or later, infections, thrombosis of cerebral arteries or veins, indeterminant cause ("idiopathic" epilepsy)
Adolescence (10-18 yr)	Idiopathic epilepsy, including genetically transmitted types, trauma
Early adulthood (18-35 yr)	Trauma, neoplasm, idiopathic epilepsy, withdrawal from alcohol or other sedative-hypnotic drugs
Middle age (35-60 yr)	Neoplasm, trauma, vascular disease, alcohol or other drug withdrawal
Late life (>60 yr)	Vascular disease, tumor, degenerative disease, trauma

From Adams RD: The convulsive state and idiopathic epilepsy. In Thorn GW et al, editors: *Harrison's principles of internal medicine,* New York, 1985, McGraw-Hill.

sciousness is lost at the point of generalization. In complex partial seizures, consciousness is impaired; that is, the person is unable to respond normally to exogenous stimuli. Sixty percent of seizures are either complex partial seizures or seizures with secondary generalization.

Status epilepticus is the experience of a second seizure, a third seizure, and often subsequent seizures before the person has fully regained consciousness from the preceding seizure or a single seizure lasting more than 30 mintes. The person is still in a **postictal state** (state that follows a seizure) when the next seizure begins. Status epilepticus most frequently results from abrupt discontinuation of antiseizure medications but also may occur in untreated or inadequately treated persons with seizure disorders. The situation is a medical emergency because of the resulting cerebral hypoxia. Mental retardation, dementia, other brain damage, and even death are serious threats. Aspiration also is a great risk. (Terminology associated with seizure activity is defined in Table 15-10.)

Pathophysiology

An **epileptogenic focus** appears to be a group of neurons that evidence a paroxysmal depolarization shift and sudden changes in the usual membrane potential. The plasma membranes of neuronal cells are thought to be more permeable, making them more easily activated by hyperthermia, hypoxia, hypoglycemia, hyponatremia, repeated sensory stimulation, and certain sleep phases. These neurons are hypersensitive and may even remain in a chronic partially depolarized state.

The primary abnormality may be a membrane defect leading to instability in resting potential, abnormalities of potassium conductance or calcium channels, defects of the γ-aminobutyric acid (GABA) inhibitory system, or an abnormality in excitatory transmission enhancement, particularly of the *N*-methyl-D-asparate type.[10] In animal models, a defect in the GABA inhibitory system is the mechanism causing generalized seizures.[10]

The firing of involved epileptogenic neurons becomes increasingly greater in frequency and amplitude. When the

Table 15-9 International Classification of Epileptic Seizures

Traditional Terminology	New Nomenclature
	I. Partial seizures (seizures beginning locally)
Focal motor; jacksonian seizures (occasionally become secondarily generalized)	A. Simple (without impairment of consciousness)
	1. With motor signs
	2. With special sensory or somatosensory symptoms
	3. With autonomic symptoms or signs
	4. With psychic symptoms
Temporal lobe or psychomotor seizures	B. Complex (with impairment of consciousness)
	1. Simple partial onset followed by impaired consciousness
	2. Impaired consciousness at onset—with or without automatisms
	C. Secondarily generalized (partial onset evolving to generalized tonic-clonic seizures)
	II. Generalized seizures (bilaterally symmetric and without local onset)
Limited grand mal	A. Tonic, clonic, or tonic-clonic
Grand mal	B. Absence
Petit mal	1. Simple—loss of consciousness only
	2. Complex—with brief tonic, clonic, or automatic movements
	C. Lennox-Gastaut syndrome
	D. Juvenile myoclonic epilepsy
	E. Infantile spasms (West syndrome)
Drop attacks	F. Atonic (astatic, akinetic) seizures (sometimes with myoclonic jerks)
	III. Specialized epileptic syndromes
Minor motor	A. Myoclonus and myoclonic seizures
	B. Reflex epilepsy
	C. Acquired aphasia with convulsive disorder
	D. Febrile and other seizures of infancy and childhood
	E. Hysterical seizures

Table 15-10 Terminology Applied to a Seizure Disorder

Term	Definition
Aura	A partial seizure experienced as a peculiar sensation preceding the onset of a generalized seizure that may take the form of gustatory, visual, or auditory experience; a feeling of dizziness or numbness; or just "a funny feeling"
Prodroma	Early clinical manifestations, such as malaise, headache, or a sense of depression, that may occur hours to a few days before the onset of a seizure
Tonic phase	A state of muscle contraction in which there is excessive muscle tone
Clonic phase	A state of alternating contraction and relaxation of muscles
Postictal state	The time period immediately following the cessation of seizure activity

intensity of the neuronal discharge reaches a threshold point, the discharge spreads to adjacent normal neurons through corticocortical synapses. If uninhibited at this point, the cortical excitation spreads through interhemispheric tracts to the contralateral cortex and through projection pathways to the subcortical areas of the basal ganglia, thalamus, and brain stem. The excitation spread to the subcortical, thalamic, and brain stem areas corresponds to the **tonic phase** (phase of muscle contraction with increased muscle tone) and is associated with loss of consciousness. Autonomic clinical manifestations also may emerge at this point, and apnea may be present for a few seconds. The excitation is further projected downward to the spinal cord neurons through the corticospinal and reticulospinal pathways.

The **clonic phase** (phase of alternating contraction and relaxation of muscles) begins as inhibitory neurons in the cortex, anterior thalamus, and basal ganglia begin to inhibit the cortical excitation. This inhibition causes an interruption in the seizure discharge, producing an intermittent contract-relax pattern of muscle contractions. The intermittent clonic bursts gradually become more and more infrequent until they finally cease. At this point the epileptogenic neurons are exhausted and the neuronal membranes probably are hyperpolarized.

The maintenance of seizure activity demands a 250% increase in adenosine triphosphate (ATP). Cerebral oxygen consumption is increased by 60%. Although cerebral blood flow also increases approximately 250% during seizure activity, available glucose and oxygen are readily depleted. With a severe seizure the brain tissue may require more ATP than can be produced by the tissues from the available oxygen and glucose. A deficiency of ATP, phosphocreatine, and glucose then occurs, and lactate accumulates in the brain tissues. Severe seizures thus may produce secondary hypoxia, acidosis, and lactate accumulation, all of which are imbalances that may result in progressive brain tissue injury and destruction. Cellular exhaustion and destruction are consequences of these events.

If a seizure focus is active for a prolonged period, a secondary focus, called a **mirror focus,** may develop in normal tissue. This process apparently is caused by the interhemispheric communication, inasmuch as the mirror focus is located in the contralateral cortical area.

◆ *Clinical Manifestations*

The clinical manifestations associated with seizure depend on the type of seizure (Table 15-11). Two types of symptoms often signal an impending generalized tonic-clonic seizure: an **aura,** a partial seizure that immediately precedes the onset of a generalized tonic-clonic seizure, and a **prodroma,** an early manifestation that may occur hours to days before a seizure (see Table 15-10). Both manifestations may become familiar to the person experiencing recurrent generalized seizures and so may help in preventing injuries during the seizure.

◆ *Evaluation and Treatment*

The health history is the most critical aspect in diagnosing a seizure disorder and establishing the cause. The health history is supplemented by the physical examination and laboratory tests of blood and urine (blood glucose, serum calcium, blood urea nitrogen, urine sodium, and creatinine clearance) to identify any systemic diseases known to have seizures as a clinical manifestation. Skull x-ray films, computed tomography (CT) scan, magnetic resonance imaging (MRI), and cerebrospinal fluid (CSF) examination are useful to identify any neurologic diseases associated with seizures. The EEG is useful in assessing the type of seizure and may help determine its focus (Fig. 15-6). Magnetoencephalography is sometimes used for diagnosis (Box 15-1).

Treatment for a seizure disorder is first to correct or control its cause, if possible. If this is not possible, the major means of management is the judicious administration of antiseizure medications. The therapeutic goal is complete suppression of seizure activity without intolerable side effects of the drug. Other medical therapies may include prescription of a ketogenic diet, vagus nerve stimulation,[12,13] and

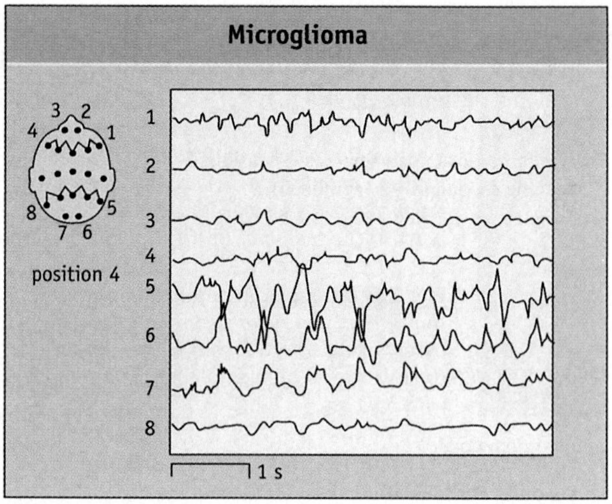

FIG. 15-6 Electroencephalogram showing right posterior temporal sharp activity in individual with a microlioma. (From Perkins GD: *Mosby's color atlas and text of neurology,* London, 1998, Mosby-Wolfe.)

Box 15-1

NOT A SEIZURE

"Storming," also known as autonomic dysfunction syndrome (ADS) or diencephalic seizures, is now thought to consist of proxysmal sympathetic storms. There is activation or disinhibition of the central sympathetic excitatory regions in the brain. The person experiences episodic alterations in body temperature, blood pressure, heart and respiratory rate, size of pupil, and level of consciousness. these signals coincide with hyperhidrosis, vomiting, excessive salivation, and extensor posturing. No evidence of epileptiform activity is found on EEG, nor are antiseizure medications helpful. The condition is best treated with morphine sulfate, bromocriptine, diazepam, clonazepam, or chlorpromazine. "Storming" has been diagnosed in persons with closed-head injury, hydrocephalus, and diencephalic or suprasellar tumors.

Data from Boeve BF et al: Paroxysmal sympathetic storms ("diencephalic seizures") after diffuse axonal head injury, *Mayo Clin Proc* 73:148, 1998.

Table 15-11 Clinical Manifestations Related to Seizure Types

Type	Clinical Manifestations	Site
I. PARTIAL SEIZURES		
A. Simple		
1. With motor symptoms		
a. Without jacksonian march (focal motor seizure—the motor movements do not extend into adjacent areas)	Motor activity is usually clonic. Motor movement elicited by the seizure activity depends on the anatomic-physiologic portion of the irritated cortex, but motor seizures most often begin in the face and hands. Focal seizures begin with slow, repetitive jerking of the body part, which increases in strength and rate over a period of 5 to 15 seconds. The seizure can cease spontaneously, with a gradual decrease in clonic movement.	Primary motor area
b. With jacksonian march (jacksonian seizure—the seizure activity spreads in an orderly fashion of adjacent areas)	Seizure activity spreads to adjacent areas after the initial clonic movement increases; motor movements, for example, would begin in the fingers of one side and spread to the hand, wrist, forearm, arm, face, and finally the lower extremity on the same side of the body. After spreading, the jerking movements in all areas would spontaneously stop.	Primary motor area
c. Adversive seizure	Turning movement of hand and eyes to the side opposite the irritative focus occurs. Often it is associated with contractions of the trunk and extremities. It may remain local or develop into a generalized seizure.	Frontal lobe anterior to the primary motor area
2. With special sensory or somatosensory symptoms (focal sensory seizure); less common than focal motor seizures; any age may be affected	Sensory experience is subjective and confined to the primary sensory modalities (somesthetic, visual, auditory-vestibular, or olfactory). If sensory seizure begins on the hand area of the sensory cortex, the patient experiences numbness, tingling, or "pins and needles" phenomena. Other sensory experiences include burning, a crawling sensation, or a feeling of movement of the body part. Most frequent areas affected include lips, fingers, and toes. May remain local or develop into a generalized seizure.	Sensory cortex Postcentral gyrus (parietal lobe) with involvement of the primary sensory area
B. Complex (temporal lobe or psychomotor seizure)		
1. Simple partial onset followed by impairment of consciousness—common seizures found in both children and adults but in most persons occur before 20 yr old	The person is able to interact with the environment with purposeful, although inappropriate, movements; although the body muscles stiffen, the person does not fall and may even continue the complex activity in which he or she was involved, such as driving (perseverative automatisms); the person may appear "wide eyed." A wide variety of sensory experiences precede the automatism and include illusions; formed hallucinations; primitive visceral, olfactory, and gustatory sensations; and affective and cognitive symptoms. Most characteristic event of a temporal lobe seizure is the automatism; common examples of automatisms are lip smacking, chewing, facial grimacing, swallowing movements, and patting, picking, or rubbing oneself or one's clothing. Temporal lobe seizures generally last 11 sec to 8 min (average 2 min) and are followed by several minutes of postictal confusion.	Temporal lobe and its connections Frontal lobes Other areas
2. Impaired consciousness at onset—with or without automatisms	See above.	
C. Secondarily generalized	Unconsciousness appears. General symptoms are produced.	

Continued

Table 15-11 Clinical Manifestations Related to Seizure Types—cont'd

Type	Clinical Manifestations	Site
II. GENERALIZED SEIZURES		
A. Clonic	Characterized by repetitive clonic jerks of constant amplitude and diminishing frequency.	
B. Tonic (affects infants and children)	Loss of postural tone without evidence of clonicity, with flexion of the upper limbs and extension of the lower limbs.	
	Child assumes an abnormal posture for seconds or minutes without losing consciousness.	
C. Tonic-clonic (grand mal seizure) (affects both children and adults)	A prodromal period of irritability and tension may precede a tonic-clonic seizure by several hours or days; however, in most persons, seizures begin without warning.	Multifocal
	Characteristically tonic-clonic seizures begin with a sudden loss of consciousness and brief flexion; the person falls to the ground and the body stiffens in an opisthotonos position with legs and, usually, arms extended; the jaw snaps shut; a shrill cry may be heard as a result of forceful exhalation of air through the closed vocal cords as the thoracic muscles initially contract; the bladder and, less often, the bowel may evacuate; during the tonic phase, the person is apneic with subsequent cyanosis; pupils are dilated and unresponsive to light.	
	The tonic phase lasts less than 1 min (average 10-15 sec).	
	The clonic phase is characterized by flexion spasm of whole body interrupted by muscular relaxation, muscular contractions accompanied by strenuous hyperventilation; the face is contorted; the eyes roll, and there is excessive salivation with frothing from the mouth; profuse sweating and a rapid pulse are evident. The tongue is often bitten.	
	The clonic jerking subsides in frequency and amplitude over a period of about 30 secs.	
	The tonic-clonic seizure lasts 2-5 min.	
	After the clonic phase, the person is in a stupor or coma for about 5 min; the extremities are limp; breathing is quiet; and the pupils begin to respond to light.	
	When the person awakens, he or she may be confused and disoriented and complains of headache, muscle aching, and fatigue.	
	There is no recollection of the attack.	
	Tonic-clonic seizures may occur at any time of the day or night, whether the person is awake or asleep.	
	The frequency of recurrence may vary from hours to weeks, months, or years.	
D. Absences (petit mal seizures) always occur in children after the age of 4 years and before puberty	Characterized by an abrupt cessation of activity with a momentary arrest of consciousness lasting about 5-10 sec, whereas a few last 30 sec; the eyes become vacant and roll, or the child may stare straight ahead; the lips may droop or twitch.	Multifocal
	The child is responsive if spoken to during the seizure.	
	The child resumes previous activity after a seizure.	
E. Infantile spasms (affects 3-mo to 2 yr age-group)	Characterized by flexor spasms of the extremities and the head (have been described as jackknife seizures).	
	Seizure lasts a few seconds and often appears in clusters with several clusters occurring daily.	
	Infantile spasms associated with metabolic, degenerative, or structural illness in 50% of cases; in other 50% no correlation is noted.	
	Most victims are mentally retarded.	
F. Atonic (drop attack)	Characterized by sudden loss of postural muscle tone. The tone loss may be mild, resulting in a head nod, or more dramatic, including falls.	Multifocal

Table 15-11 Clinical Manifestations Related to Seizure Types—cont'd

Type	Clinical Manifestations	Site
III. SPECIALIZED EPILEPTIC SYNDROMES		
A. Myoclonus and myoclonic seizures	Characterized by sudden, uncontrollable jerking movements of one or more extremities or the entire body. Seizures usually occur in the morning. Consciousness is thought to be preserved. Person often is flung violently to the ground so that injury is a real possibility. Myoclonic seizures can occur in clusters.	Multifocal

WHAT'S NEW? Women with Epilepsy Receive Attention

Lately, women with epilepsy have received attention. There is now a registry for women taking antiseizure drugs at 888-122-1223. Practice guidelines, *Parameters for Management of Women with Epilepsy,* also were published in 1998 by the American Academy of Neurology.

Data from American Academy of Neurology: Parameters for management of women with epilepsy, *Neurology* 51:944, 1998.

surgery. Folic acid supplementation is important. Some antiseizure medications decrease the effectiveness of hormonal contraceptives. In severe cases, psychologic, social, educational, and vocational counseling are often appropriate for the individual and family.

Alterations in Content of Thought (Cognition)

Selective attention (orienting), or a second attentional network, refers to the ability to select from available, competing environmental and internal stimuli specific information to be consciously processed. Certain structures have been demonstrated to contribute to selective attention. The disengagement mechanism is mediated by the right parietal lobe. The move component is mediated by the superior colliculi for visual orienting. The engage component is mediated by the pulvinar of the thalamus. A weak orienting network results in a neglect syndrome.

Sensory inattentiveness is a form of neglect and may be visual, auditory, or tactile. The person with sensory inattentiveness is able to recognize individual sensory input from the dysfunctional side when called on to do so but ignores (i.e., neglects, extinguishes) the sensory input from the dysfunctional side when stimulated from both sides. This phenomenon is called **extinction.** The entire complex of denial of dysfunction, loss of recognition of one's own body parts, and extinction is sometimes referred to as the **neglect syndrome.**

An isolated (pure) **selective attention deficit,** which manifests as a neglect syndrome, rarely, if ever, occurs clinically because typically other deficits also are present. A neglect syndrome may appear temporarily as a result of seizure activity or a postictal state. Temporary or permanent deficits may occur with contusions or subdural hematomas, encephalitis, and ischemic stroke. Progressive neglect deficits may be found with gliomas or metastatic tumor and in Alzheimer and Pick diseases.

Dysmnesia is a disorder of the **recent memory system** defined as the loss of past memories (retrograde amnesia) coupled with an inability to form new memories (anterograde amnesia) despite intact attentional systems. Isolated (pure) dysmnesia is caused by only a limited number of conditions, such as transient global dysmnesia (episodic global dysmnesia), amnestic stroke, and Korsakoff psychosis (amnestic or dysmnestic syndrome), as well as after temporal lobectomy. Many disorders may temporarily or permanently produce dysmnesia that accompanies other deficits of the cognitive systems. A temporary dysmnesia is found during complex partial seizures that persist for a time in the postictal state, in postconcussive states, and in mild posttraumatic brain injury states. A permanent dysmnesia may be seen after subarachnoid hemorrhage or moderate or severe posttraumatic brain injury states; in carbon dioxide poisoning and other hypoxic or anoxic states; in Wernicke encephalopathy, viral encephalitis, and granulomatous meningitides; in tumors; and in Alzheimer and Pick diseases.

Pattern recognition (remote memory, in which permanent memories are stored) is located in the association areas of the temporal, occipital, and parietal lobes. A pure auditory or visual pattern recognition (remote memory) deficit manifests as an isolated agnosia (see p. 457 for etiologic factors). An isolated (pure) **pattern recognition (remote memory) deficit** of tactile sensations rarely occurs clinically because selected attention would likely be affected as well. A temporary auditory, visual, or tactile pattern recognition (remote memory) deficit may appear as a result of seizure activity or a postictal state. A temporary or permanent deficit can occur with temporal, occipital, or parietal lobe contusion; with subdural hematoma or ischemic stroke; and in encephalitis. A progressive pattern recognition (remote memory) deficit may occur in temporal, occipital, or parietal gliomas; in metastatic tumors; and in Alzheimer and Pick diseases.

The prefrontal areas mediate several cognitive functions, called *executive attention functions.* The vigilance system provides the person with the ability to maintain a sustained state of alertness and involves the right frontal areas and the locus ceruleus. Through the neurotransmitter norepinephrine from the locus ceruleus, the speed of the orienting (selective attention) network is increased and the detection function of the anterior cingulate lobe is decreased.

Detection is the recognition of the object's identity and the realization that the object fulfills a sought-after goal (i.e., target selection among competing, complex contingencies). There is conscious execution of an instruction, ensuring that the instructions are followed. The anterior cingulate cortex inhibits automatic responses so that a less routine response can be given. The basal ganglia and cingulate, as well as other frontal areas, function in color, motion, and form detection.

The anterior cingulate plus more lateral sites of the frontal lobes are involved in the representations of information in the absence of a stimulus, such as spatial position of visual events in memory when the event is removed from view. This is called *working memory* (short-term representation memory). Control of activation of these memories is also in these areas. This gives the person control over information processing. These temporary storage areas permit the brain to retrieve instructions and other information needed to guide behavior.

Isolated (pure) **vigilance, detection,** and **working memory deficits** have been discussed in the literature, but their individual occurrence is uncommon because these deficits generally are present simultaneously. Akinetic mutism exemplifies a detection deficit alone. The person orients to external stimuli and can follow with his or her eyes but does not initiate other voluntary activity. There are no goals generated and no plans for carrying out the goals.[14] The combination of vigilance, detection, and working memory deficits, accompanied by other deficits of the cognitive systems, is much more common. Whether the deficits are temporary or permanent depends on the cause and severity of injury. Deficits caused by CNS-depressant drugs, by seizure activity, and, it is hoped, by neurosurgical procedures involving retraction of

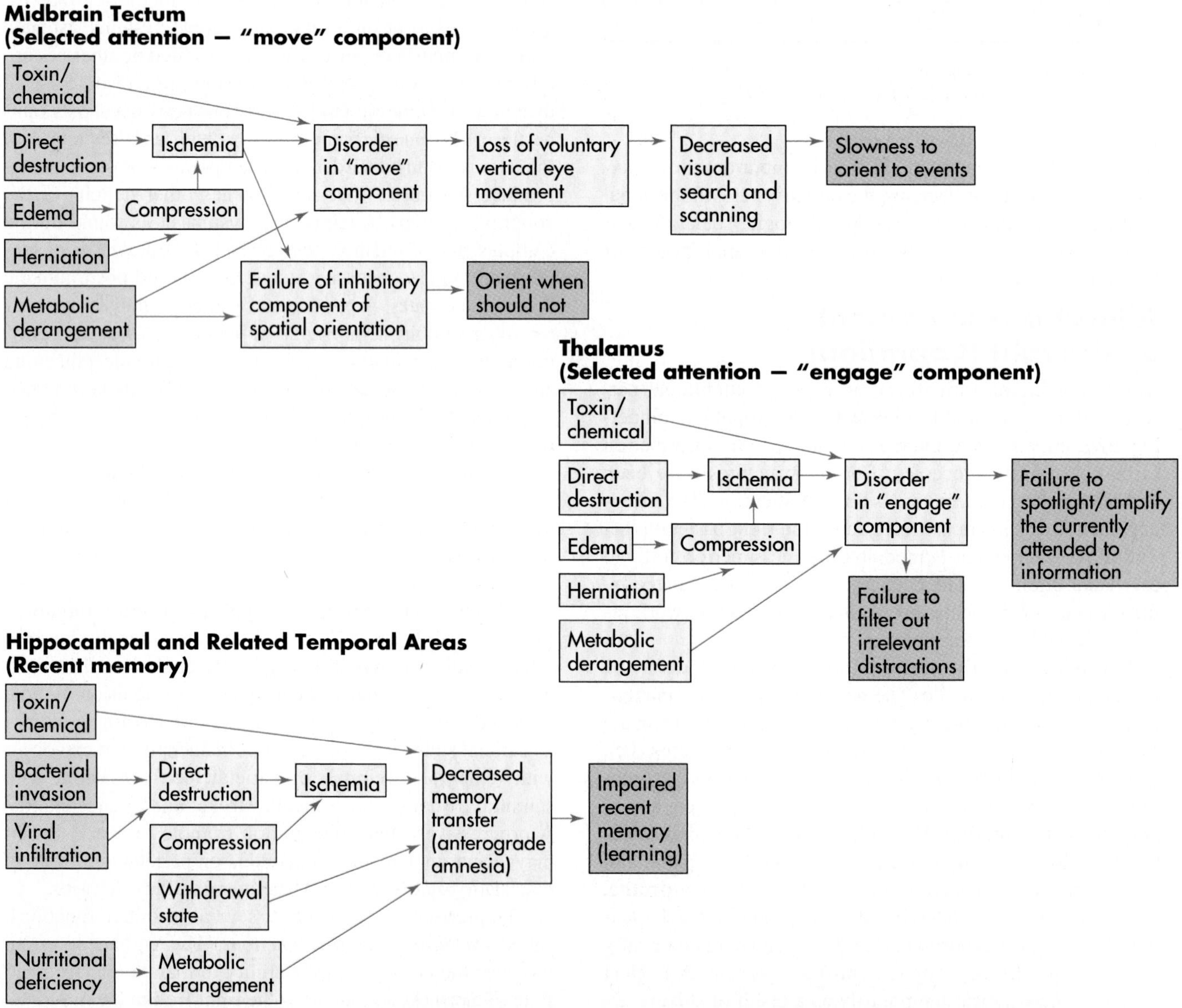

FIG. 15-7 Cognitive network deficits. General pathophysiologic mechanisms underlying cognitive network deficits.

the frontal lobes are temporary. Deficits in postconcussive and mild traumatic brain injury states may prove to be temporary and resolve over time. Permanent deficits are more likely to be found with frontal lobe contusions, moderate or severe posttraumatic brain injury states, ischemic frontal lobe stroke, and neurosurgery that requires frontal lobe resection. Progressive deficits in vigilance, detection, and working memory functions are caused by frontal lobe gliomas, frontal lobe infarcts associated with hypertensive vascular disease, and late Alzheimer and Pick diseases. Persons with schizophrenia have difficulty in clearing working memory of information that is irrelevant to the current task. Additionally, recently encountered visual material that is no longer in plain view cannot be preserved in working memory.

Higher-level thought involves the same neural areas used for sensory-specific computations, but when used voluntarily in thought, these areas are activated from the detection and work memory networks (top-down processing) rather than from bottom-up processing beginning in sensory areas with a specific sensory stimulus. There is a voluntary search for a feature. By reordering component computation, a person produces novel thoughts.[14]

Pathophysiology

Persons with a disease affecting the superior colliculi have a disturbance in the move operation of selective attention, which manifests as a slowness in orienting attention. Persons with parietal lobe disease may experience selective attention deficits related to disengagement from a stimulus. Persons with parietal lobe dysfunction, especially the right parietal lobe, also may experience a unilateral neglect syndrome, the prototype of a selective attention disorder. Persons with a disease affecting the pulvinar of the thalamus have a disturbance in the engage component of selective attention.

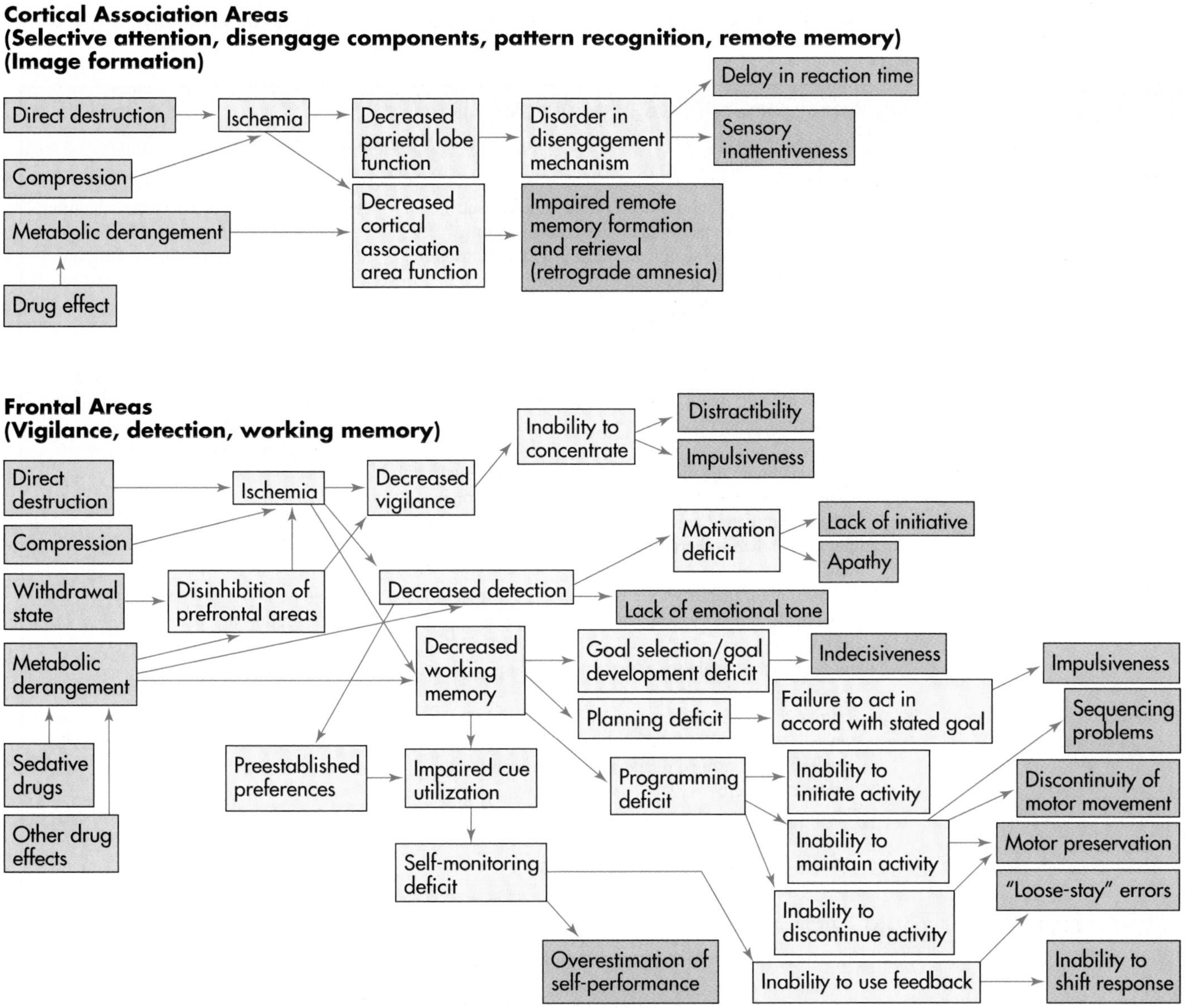

FIG. 15-7, cont'd For legend see opposite page.

A disorder in vigilance may be produced by disease in the right frontal areas. A pathologic condition in the frontal areas also may produce detection and working memory deficits. Impaired higher-level thought may result from a pathologic process in the cortical association areas of the parietal, temporal, and occipital lobes.

The exact pathophysiology of the various disorders of cognitive systems is not fully known. Researchers currently are studying the defects in the elementary operations (components) of each cognitive system. In the past, pathophysiology related to the memory systems was the most studied. Dysmnesia, also known as amnesia, originates from pathologic conditions in the hippocampus and related temporal lobe structures, is the result of a failure to transfer information from working (short-term) to long-term memory, and is a failure to consolidate or retrieve long-term memory stores. Orienting and the executive attentional network are currently receiving intense study.

As a highly general statement, the primary pathophysiologic mechanisms that operate in cognitive systems disorders are (1) direct destruction because of direct ischemia and hypoxia or indirect destruction as a result of compression and (2) the effects of toxins and chemicals. Disinhibition resulting in overactivity, such as seen in some drug withdrawal states, is a pathologic mechanism that can produce detection deficits. The pathophysiologic processes are presented in Fig. 15-7.

Clinical Manifestations

Clinical manifestations of selective attention deficits; pattern recognition deficits; and vigilance, detection, and working memory deficits are presented in Table 15-12.

Evaluation and Treatment

Immediate medical management is directed at diagnosing the cause and treating reversible factors. Rehabilitative measures for cognitive system deficits generally are either compensatory in nature or restorative in nature and have of late been greatly facilitated by computer technology and other electronic-assisted devices. Approaches based on behavioral techniques tend to be compensatory, whereas process-oriented approaches, it is hoped, are restorative.

Table 15-12 Clinical Manifestations of Cognitive Network Deficits

Deficit	Clinical Signs	Symptoms
ATTENTION		
Selective attention (orienting)	Inability to focus attention; decreased eye, head, and body movements associated with focusing on the stimuli; decreased search and scanning; faulty orientation to stimuli causing safety problems	Person reports inability to focus attention, failure to perceive objects and other stimuli (history of injuries, falls, and safety problems)
MEMORY		
Recent (anterograde memory)	*Left hemisphere:* disorientation to time, situation, place, name, person (verbal identification); impaired language memory (e.g., names of objects); impaired semantic memory *Right hemisphere:* disorientation to self, person (visual), place (visual); impaired episodic memory (personal history); impaired emotional memory Either or both hemispheres: confusion; behavioral change	Person reports disorientation, confusion, "not listening," "not remembering"; reports by others of person being disoriented, not able to remember, not able to learn new information
Pattern recognition (remote)	*Left hemisphere:* inability to retrieve personal history, past medical history; unaware of recent current events *Right hemisphere:* inability to recognize persons, places, objects, music, etc., from past	Person reports remote memory problems; others report that person cannot recall formerly known information
Image processing (semantic processing)	Inability to categorize (identify similarities and differences), sort; inability to form concepts; inability to analyze relationships; misinterpretation; inability to interpret proverbs	Reports by others of frequent misinterpretation of data, failure to conceptualize or generalize information
	Inability to perform deductive reasoning (convergent reasoning); inability to perform inductive reasoning (divergent reasoning); inability to abstract; concrete reasoning demonstrated; delusions	Reports by others of predominantly concrete thinking; lack of understanding of everyday situations, health care regimens, and such; delusional thinking
EXECUTIVE ATTENTIONAL NETWORK		
Vigilance	Failure to stay alert and oriented to stimuli	Person reports decreased alertness or ability to orient

Selective attention and executive attentional deficits masquerade as other cognitive deficits. Differential diagnosis of other cognitive deficits is blocked, and learning potential is largely obscured, by the presence of an attention deficit. Therefore diagnosis and treatment of attention deficits are fundamental.

Data Processing Deficits

Agnosia

Agnosia is a defect of pattern recognition—a failure to recognize the form and nature of objects. The disorder involves the loss of recognition through one sense, although the object or person may still be recognized by other senses. Agnosia can be tactile, visual, or auditory. For example, an individual may be unable to identify a safety pin by touching it with a hand but be able to name it when looking at it. Agnosia may be as minimal as a finger agnosia (failure to identify by name the fingers of one's hand) or more extensive, such as a color agnosia.

Agnosia is produced by dysfunction in the primary sensory area or in the interpretive areas of the cerebral cortex (see Fig. 13-6). (The types of agnosia and the associated area that is most commonly involved with each are presented in Table 15-13.) Although agnosia most commonly is associated with cerebrovascular accidents, it may arise from any pathologic process that injures these specific areas of the brain.

Dysphasia

Dysphasia is impairment of comprehension or production of language (semantic processing). With dysphasia, comprehension or use of symbols, in either written or verbal language, is disturbed or lost. **Aphasia** is loss of the comprehension or production of language.

Dysphasias usually are associated with cerebrovascular accident involving the middle cerebral artery or one of its many branches. The language disorders, however, may arise from a variety of injuries and diseases—vascular, neoplastic, traumatic, degenerative, metabolic, or infectious. Dysphasia results from dysfunction in the left cerebral hemisphere, most commonly in the frontotemporal region, particularly around the insula (Fig. 15-8) (see also Fig. 13-6). Most language disorders are caused by acute processes that either resolve or

Table 15-12 Clinical Manifestations of Cognitive Network Deficits—cont'd

Deficit	Clinical Signs	Symptoms
EXECUTIVE ATTENTIONAL NETWORK—cont'd		
Detection	Lack of initiative (anergy); lack of ambition; lack of motivation; flat affect; no awareness of feelings; appears depressed, apathetic, and emotionless; fails to appreciate deficit; disinterested in appearance; lacks concern about childish or crude behavior	Reports by others of laziness or apathy, flat affect or lack of emotional expression, failing to exhibit or be aware of feelings
Mild	Responds to immediate environment but no new ideas; grooming and social graces are lacking	Reports by others of lack of ambition, motivation, or initiative, failure to carry out adult tasks, lack of social graces and new ideas
Severe	Motionless, lack of responding to even internal cues, does not respond to physical needs, does not interact with surroundings	Reports by others of failure to groom or toilet self, unawareness of surroundings and own physical needs
	Inability to use feedback regarding behavior; failure to recognize omissions and errors in self-care, speech, writing, and arithmetic; impaired cue utilization; overestimation of performance	Reports by others of not changing behavior when requested; unawareness of limitations; does not recognize and correct errors in dressing, grooming, toileting, eating, and such; fails to recognize speech and arithmetic errors; careless speech
	Failure to shift response set; failure to change behavior when conditions change; cue utilization may be impaired	Reports by others of failure to use feedback; inability to incorporate feedback (does not correct when feedback is given)
Working memory	Inability to set goals or form goals; indecisiveness	Reports by others of failure to set goals, indecisiveness
	Failure to make plans; inability to produce a complete line of reasoning; inability to make up a story; appears impulsive	Reports by others of failure to plan, impulsiveness, "does not think things through"
	Failure to initiate behavior; failure to maintain behavior; failure to discontinue behavior; slowness to alternate response for the next step; motor perseveration	Reports by others of not knowing where to begin, inability to carry out sequential acts (maintain a behavior), inability to cease a behavior

Table 15-13 Types of Agnosia (Concept Disorders)

Type of Agnosia	Definition	Location of Injury
Tactile agnosia (astereognosis)	Inability to recognize objects by touch	Parietal lobe
Spatial agnosia	Incapacity to find one's way around familiar places; disturbance of perception of space (disorders of [1] topographic [extrapersonal] orientation or [2] topographic and geographic memory [construction])	Parietal lobe
Gertsmann syndrome	Loss of spatial orientation of fingers, body, sides, and numbers	Left angular gyrus (parietal lobe)
Finger agnosia (digital agnosia)	Inability to identify the names of one's fingers	
Right-left confusion	Inability to distinguish right from left	
Agraphia	Inability to write	
Acalculia	Inability to perform mathematic calculations	
Visual agnosia		
Object agnosia	Inability to recognize objects and pictures	Temporooccipital area
Prosopagnosia	Inability to recognize faces	Temporooccipital ventromesial region
Color agnosia	Inability to understand colors as qualities of objects; faulty color concepts and inability to evoke color images in the absence of color blindness; specific types: (1) "hue" problem, (2) color anomia (can not name color)	Inferior occipital cortex in left hemisphere
Body image agnosias (may be spatial)		
Anosognosia	Ignorance or denial of existence of the disease	Right parietal lobe
Autotopagnosia	Loss of ability to identify the body, in whole or in part, or to recognize relationships among various parts	Right parietal lobe
Word blindness (alexia/dyslexia)	Inability to recognize written symbols	Left parietotemporal region
Auditory agnosia (pure word deafness)	Inability to recognize speech sounds	Superior temporal area
Amusia (music deafness)	Loss of capacity to recognize tones and melodies	Right superior temporal area

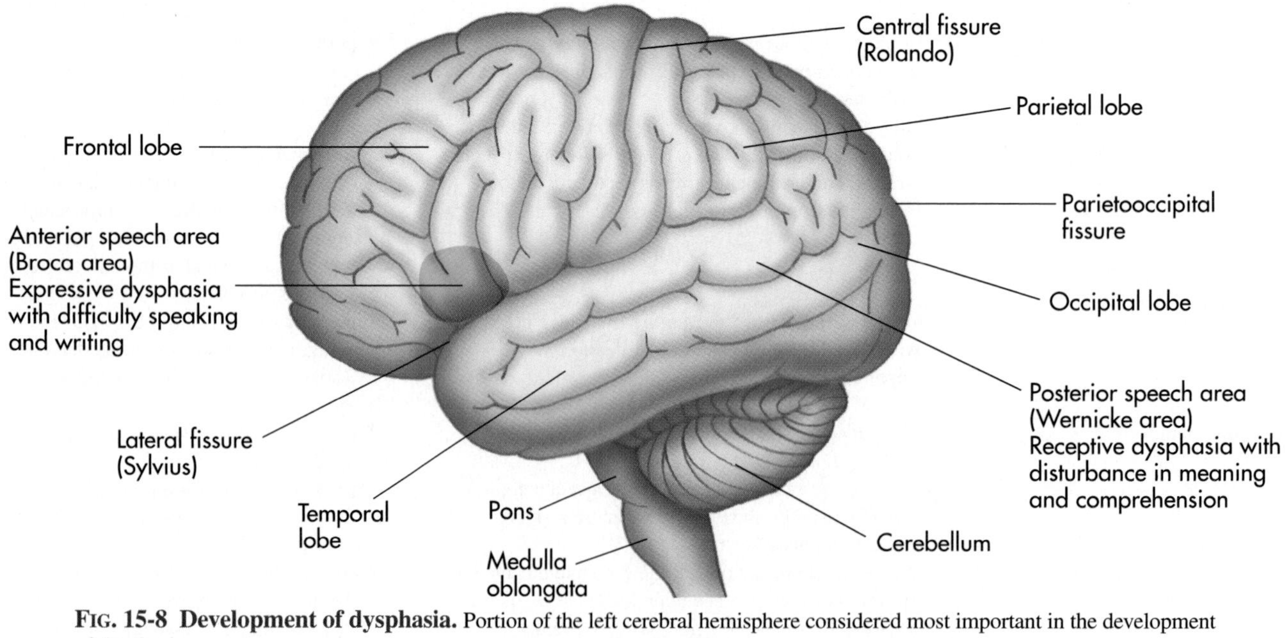

FIG. 15-8 Development of dysphasia. Portion of the left cerebral hemisphere considered most important in the development of dysphasia.

cause a chronic residual deficit. Some language disorders are caused by degenerative disorders that make the dysfunction progressive.

Dysphasias have been classified both anatomically and functionally. Other classifications are linguistic and describe fluency, volume, or quantity of speech. Pure forms of any language dysfunction, however, are rare. **Expressive dysphasias** are characterized primarily by expressive deficits, but a verbal comprehension (auditory-receptive element) deficit may be present. Receptive dysphasias may have expressive deficits. (Table 15-14 compares types of dysphasias; Table 15-15 illustrates some of the language disturbances.)

Dysphasias referred to as **transcortical dysphasias (transcortical sensory dysphasia, mixed transcortical dysphasia, isolated speech center)** involve the ability to repeat (called **echolalia**) and to recite. Speech is fluent but with striking paraphrases. The individual cannot read and write, and comprehension is impaired.

Transcortical dysphasias are caused by hypoxia from prolonged hypotension, carbon monoxide poisoning, or other mechanisms that destroy the border zone (watershed area) of the anterior, middle, and posterior cerebral arteries (see Fig. 13-18). Blood supply is marginal in this region. Hypoxia in this area occasionally may isolate the posterior speech areas or all the speech areas from the remainder of the cortex, although both areas remain intact. The sensory and motor speech areas therefore are functional, but connections with other sensory or motor areas are impaired. Information from the remaining areas of the cortex cannot be transmitted to the Wernicke area to be transformed into language.

Acute Confusional States

Acute confusional states (acute cerebral failure or acute brain failure) result from cerebral dysfunction secondary to such causes as drug intoxication, metabolic disorders, or nervous system disease. A common cause of an acute confusional state is withdrawal from alcohol, barbiturate, or other sedative drug ingestion. Acute confusional states of toxic origin may have either sudden or gradual onset, depending on the amount of exposure to the toxin. These states often occur with febrile illnesses, with systemic diseases such as heart failure, after head injury or anesthesia, postnatally, or with certain focal cerebral lesions.

Pathophysiology

Three pathophysiologic mechanisms probably underlie the development of acute confusional states associated with delirium: (1) injury to nervous tissue, (2) action of toxin or chemical agents on neuronal cells, and (3) disinhibition and overactivity of a previously depressed brain center. Destructive injuries directly affect the nervous tissues and disturb the function of the neurons. In states of intoxication, the direct action of toxins or chemicals on neuronal cells produces dysfunction of the involved cells. In states of withdrawal, the lower brain centers are overactive after the depressant action of the drug wears off, and this overactivity accounts for the development of the acute confusional state.

Clinical Manifestations

The predominant features of an acute confusional state are impaired or lost detection. Because of dysfunction of the anterior cingulate (see Fig. 13-6), the ability to sustain attentional focus is seriously impaired or completely lost. The person is highly distractible and unable to concentrate on incoming sensory information or on any one particular mental or motor task.

The onset of an acute confusional state usually is abrupt rather than insidious. The first clinical manifestations are difficulty in concentration, restlessness, irritability, tremulousness, insomnia, and poor appetite. Later there are top-down processing problems, including misperception, illusion, hallucination, and delirium. Obsessions, compulsive behavior, and rituals may be evident.

In acute confusional states with associated underactivity, the individual exhibits decreases in mental function. Alertness is decreased, as are attention span, accurate perception, and interpretation of the environment. Forgetfulness is prominent. Reactions to the environment are slowed and indecisive. The individual dozes frequently.

Delirium, an acute confusional state associated with overactivity, typically develops over 2 to 3 days. Early clinical manifestations include difficulty in concentrating, restlessness, irritability, insomnia, tremulousness, and poor appetite. Some persons experience seizures. Unpleasant, even terrifying, dreams may occur.

In a fully developed delirium state, the individual is completely inattentive and perceptions are grossly altered. Misperception and misinterpretation are predominant. Hallucinations may be present. The person appears distressed and often very perplexed. Conversation is incoherent. Frank tremor is evident, and a great deal of restless movement is common. Violent behavior may be present. The individual cannot sleep; is flushed; and has dilated pupils, a rapid pulse (tachycardia), temperature elevation, and perfuse sweating (diaphoresis). Delirium typically abates suddenly or gradually in 2 to 3 days, although occasional delirium states persist for several weeks.

Evaluation and Treatment

An acute confusional state is an acute medical problem. The initial goal is to establish that the individual is confused, and the cause must be distinguished as organic or functional (Table 15-16). Next, the goal is to determine whether the confusion is delirium, an acute confusional state with associated underactivity, or an underlying dementia. The precise cause of an acute confusional state is established through the complete history and physical examination. Laboratory tests include an electrocardiogram and blood, urine, CSF, and radiologic studies.

Once the cause is established, treatment is directed at controlling the primary disorder. In an acute confusional state,

Table 15-14 Major Types of Dysphasia

Type	Expression	Verbal Comprehension	Repetition
EXPRESSIVE (BROCA DYSPHASIA, MOTOR)			
	Nonfluent; impairment of ability to find words, difficulty in writing	Relatively intact	Impaired
RECEPTIVE			
Wernicke dysphasia, sensory	Fluent: able to produce verbal language but language is meaningless; words are often inappropriate; words with similar sounds or words with similar meaning are substituted for the correct words; words that are not part of the language may be present; these neologisms may be so extensive as to make the speech entirely incomprehensible; because the person has no means to monitor the language for correctness, errors are not recognized; intonation, accent, cadence, rhythm, and articulation are normal	Impaired (disturbance in understanding all language)	Impaired
Word deafness	Fluent; self-initiated speech is normal	Impaired; hears noise rather than language; language has no meaning and is perceived as foreign	Impaired, cannot repeat
Global (sensory—motor, receptive—expressive)	Nonfluent; produces little speech; at best speaks a few words or phrases	Impaired or completely lost; person understands only the simplest things said	Impaired; not able to repeat
Conduction	Fluent but with paraphrasia in self-initiated speech and writing or reading aloud	Relatively intact	Impaired; not able to repeat
Anomic, nominal (anomia)	Fluent but impaired ability to name objects, persons, qualities, or characteristics; knows what he or she wants to say but cannot find words; may even use desired word in another context but still cannot isolate word when needed	Relatively intact; able to recognize word when it is given	Intact
Transcortical motor	Nonfluent	Relatively intact	Intact
Transcortical sensory	Fluent	Impaired	Intact

all drugs that may be contributing to or causing the condition are discontinued unless the problem is the result of drug withdrawal. Supportive measures are designed to enhance coping skills and to minimize the individual's need for altered cortical functions. Supportive and protective management also involves maintaining the person's intact cortical functions by promoting use of these functions.

Dementing Processes

Dementia is a syndrome that may be caused by a number of different illnesses. Dementia is the progressive failure of many cerebral functions.[15] The dementias are characterized by reduction in cognitive functions (intellectual function). Mental abilities are impaired, with a decrease in orienting, recent memory, remote memory, language, executive attentional functions, and alterations in behavior (Box 15-2).

Dementias can be classified according to etiologic factors (e.g., trauma, tumors, vascular disorders, infections) and according to associated clinical and laboratory signs. Most recently, dementing processes have been grouped as cortical, subcortical, or both (Box 15-3). The culmination of a progressive dementing process is nerve cell degeneration and brain atrophy involving the cerebral cortex, diencephalon, and basal ganglia.

Pathophysiology

Mechanisms in dementing processes include (1) degeneration possibly caused by genetics, inflammation, or biochem-

Name	Reading Comprehension	Writing	Location of Lesion	Cause of Lesion
Impaired	Variable	Impaired	Posteroinferior frontal lobe (Broca area)	
Impaired	Impaired	Impaired	Posterosuperior temporal lobe (Wernicke area)	Occlusion of inferior division of left middle cerebral artery
Impaired	Intact; able to read	Intact; able to write	Pathways connecting the primary auditory cortex and the auditory association areas in the middle third of the left superior temporal gyrus	Small, superficial injury typically associated with occlusion of a branch of the middle cerebral artery
Impaired	Impaired or completely lost	Impaired; produces little written language	Frontotemporal lobe; anterior and posterior speech areas extensively impaired	Occlusion of the left middle cerebral artery of left internal carotid artery; tumors, other mass lesions, and hemorrhage may cause
Impaired	Variable	Impaired	Arcuate fasciculus, supramarginal gyrus, disruption of the large bundle of fibers that arise from the temporal lobe and pass posteriorly around the sylvian fissure and then project anteriorly to the premotor area	Typical cause is embolic occlusion of the ascending parietal or posterior temporal branch of the middle cerebral artery
Impaired	Variable	Variable	Angular gyrus—posterosuperior temporal lobe	
Impaired	Variable	Impaired	Anterior presylvian fissure	
Impaired	Impaired	Impaired	Posterior presylvian fissure	

ical alterations; (2) atherosclerosis, multiple foci of infarction throughout the thalami, basal ganglia, cerebral projection pathways, and associated areas; (3) trauma, lesions in the cerebral convolutions, mainly frontal and temporal, corpus collosum, and mesencephalon; and (4) compression, increased intracranial pressure, and chronic hydrocephalus. For example, persons with Alzheimer disease have a lack of acetylcholine, a neurotransmitter, the first biochemical abnormality that has been demonstrated consistently. Acetylcholine is needed for recent memory at the biochemical level. As the level of acetylcholine is reduced, the individual is able to store less and less information, until all recent memory is lost. The cause for the failure of the enzyme system that produces acetylcholine is not known, but a defect in amyloid metabolism is strongly suspected. Slow-growing viruses probably are associated with some unexplained dementias, such as Creutzfeldt-Jakob disease.

A genetic predisposition probably is a contributing factor to the dementing process. In some instances a familial history of dementia increases by four times the likelihood that dementia will develop. Environmental influences also may play a role in the pathogenesis of dementia. The exact nature of the influence of environmental factors, such as aluminum, is not clearly understood as yet. Causes of dementia are given in Table 15-17.

◆ *Clinical Manifestations*

A summary of the clinical manifestations of the dementias is presented in Table 15-18.

Table 15-15 Examples of Language Disturbances

Disorder		Example
Verbal paraphrasia	Question:	What did the car do?
	Patient:	The car would spit sweetly down the road. (The car sped swiftly down the road.)
Literal paraphrasia	Request:	Say "persistence is essential to success."
	Patient:	Mesastence is instans to success.
Neologism	Question:	What do you call this? (Pointing to a plant.)
	Patient:	It's a logper.
Circumlocution	Question:	What do you call this? (Pointing to a plant.)
	Patient:	Something that grows.
Anomia	Question:	What do you call this? (Pointing to a plant.)
	Patient:	It's . . .
		or
	Question:	What did you do this morning?
	Patient:	Reading.
	Question:	Were you reading a book or a newspaper?
	Patient:	One of those.
Telegraphic style	Question:	Where is your daughter?
	Patient:	New Orleans . . . home . . . Monday.

From Boss BJ: *J Neurosurg Nurs* 16(3):151, 1984.

Table 15-16 Differences between Organic and Functional Confusion

Factor	Organic Confusion	Functional Confusion
Memory impairment	Recent, more impaired than remote	No consistent difference between recent and remote
Disorientation		
Time	Within own lifetime or reasonably near future	May not be related to patient's lifetime
Place	Familiar place or one where patient might easily be	Bizarre or unfamiliar places
Person	Sense of identity usually preserved	Sense of identity diminished
	Misidentification of others as familiar	Misidentification of others based on delusion system
Hallucinations	Visual, vivid	Auditory more frequent
	Animals and insects common	Bizarre and symbolic
Illusions	Common	Not prominent
Delusions	Concern everyday occurrences and people	Bizarre and symbolic
Confusion	Spotty confusion	More consistent
	Clear intervals mixed with confused episodes	No tendency to become worse at night
	Worse at night	

From Morris M, Rhodes M: *Am J Nurs* 72(9):1632, 1972.

Evaluation and Treatment

Establishing the cause for a dementing process may be complicated, but all persons evidencing the clinical manifestations of dementia should be evaluated with laboratory and neuropsychologic testing to identify underlying conditions that may be treatable.

If a specific treatable cause is identified, the appropriate treatment is initiated. For example, an infectious process requires the appropriate antibiotic, and a potentially resectable mass may require neurosurgery. Nutritional deficiencies are corrected. If the cause is metabolic, the imbalance is corrected or the metabolic disorder is treated, or both.

Unfortunately, no specific treatment or cure exists for most progressive dementias. In such instances, therapy is directed at maintaining and maximizing use of the remaining capacities, restoring functions if possible, and accommodating to lost abilities. Assisting the family to understand the dementing process and to learn ways to assist the demented individual is an essential component of supportive management.

Box 15-2

WORLD HEALTH ORGANIZATION DEFINITION OF DEMENTIA

Dementia is a syndrome due to disease of the brain, usually of a chronic or progressive nature, in which there is disturbance of multiple cortical functions, calculation, learning capacity, language, and judgment. Consciousness is not clouded. Impairments of cognitive function are commonly accompanied and occasionally preceded by deterioration in emotional control, social behavior, and motivation.

Alzheimer Disease

Alzheimer disease (dementia of Alzheimer type [DAT], senile disease complex) is a common neurologic disorder.[15]

Box 15-3

CLASSIFICATION OF THE MAJOR CAUSES OF DEMENTIA BASED ON THE OCCURRENCE OF FEATURES OF CORTICAL OR SUBCORTICAL DYSFUNCTION

CORTICAL DEMENTIAS

Alzheimer disease
Pick disease

SUBCORTICAL DEMENTIAS

Extrapyramidal syndromes
- Parkinson disease
- Huntington disease
- Progressive supranuclear palsy
- Wilson disease
- Spinocerebellar degeneration
- Idiopathic basal ganglia calcification

Hydrocephalus
Toxic and metabolic encephalopathies
- Systemic illness
- Endocrinopathies
- Deficiency states
- Drug intoxication
- Heavy metal exposure
- Industrial dementias

Dementia syndrome of depression

DEMENTIAS WITH CORTICAL AND SUBCORTICAL DYSFUNCTION

Multiinfarct dementia
Infectious dementias
- AIDS
- Creutzfeldt-Jakob disease
- Kuru

MISCELLANEOUS DEMENTIA SYNDROMES

Posttraumatic
Postanoxic
Neoplastic

From Cummings JL, Benson DF: *Dementia: a clinical approach,* Stoneham, Mass, 1992, Butterworth.

Table 15-17 Causes of Dementia

Illness	Type of Damage	Treatment Available	Potential Treatment
Dementia of Alzheimer type (DAT)	Plaques, tangles, transmitter defects, abnormal amyloid deposition	+ (?)	Anticholinesterases, nerve growth factor
Vascular dementia	Multiple infarcts, stroke, small vessel disease	+ (?)	Aspirin, lower blood pressure, lower cholesterol
Lewy body dementia	Lewy bodies, transmitter defects	+ (?)	Anticholinesterases
Parkinson disease	Lewy bodies especially in basal ganglia	—	Antiparkinsonian drugs do not help dementia
Frontal lobe dementia	Various, including Pick	—	
Normal-pressure hydrocephalus	Obstructed cerebrospinal fluid flow due to previous damage, e.g., subarachnoid hemorrhage, meningitis	+	Surgery (shunt)
Punch-drunk syndrome	Repeated head injury	+ (?)	Stop the damage
Slow-growing brain tumour	Pressure causes destruction of brain	+	Surgery
Aluminum and other metals	Direct toxic effect	+	Remove the poison
Wilson disease	Toxicity of copper	+	Penicillamine
Alcohol abuse	Toxic effect and thiamine deficiency	+	Abstinence, thiamine treatment
Huntington chorea	Genetic abnormality	—	Screening available
Syphilis (GPI)	Infective	+	Antibiotics
AIDS	Infective, secondary infection	+	Anti-AIDS drugs
CJD	Infection (?)	—	
Vitamin (e.g., B_{12}) deficiencies	Toxic (?)	+	Replacement
Hypothyroidism	Toxic (?)	+	Replacement
Parathyroid disorders	Calcium metabolism altered	+	Medical or surgical

From Jacques A, Jackson GA: *Understanding dementia,* ed 3, London, 2000, Churchill Livingstone.
AIDS, acquired immunodeficiency syndrome; CJD, Creutzfeldt-Jakob disease; GPI, General paralysis of the insane.

Table 15-18 Clinical Manifestations of Dementia

Type	Manifestation
Cortical dementia	Difficulty with naming
	Decreased language comprehension
	Loss of recent memory
	Agnosias
	Apraxia
	Loss of remote memory
	Decreased mathematic skill
	Altered visuospatial relationships
Subcortical dementia	Forgetfulness
	Apathy
	Depression
	Slowed thought processes
	Accident prone
	Personality changes and inappropriate affect
	Loss of motor function: wide shuffling gait with small steps, muscle rigidity, flexion posturing, tendency to fall, abnormal reflexes, bowel and bladder incontinence, immobility

Formerly believed to occur mostly in persons younger than 65 years of age (familial, early-onset dementia), Alzheimer disease (AD) has now been demonstrated to be one of the most common causes of severe cognitive dysfunction in older persons. Its more prevalent forms are late-onset familial Alzheimer dementia (FAD) and nonhereditary, or sporadic, late-onset AD (70% of cases). Both FAD and sporadic, late-onset AD are known as senile dementia of the Alzheimer type (SDAT). AD is also associated with Down syndrome.

◆ *Pathophysiology*

The exact cause of AD is unknown. Several possible theories being investigated include loss of neurotransmitter stimulation by choline acetyltransferase, mutation for encoding amyloid precursor protein, and alteration in apolipoprotein E, which binds beta amyloid.[16] Early-onset FAD includes at least three gene defects on chromosomes 14 (AD3 gene), 19, and 21 (amyloid precursor protein gene) or another gene not yet mapped. Late-onset FAD is linked to a defect in the apolipoprotein E gene on chromosome 19.[17] Each of these mechanisms may be linked to aggregation and precipitation of insoluble amyloid (senile plaques, amyloid plaques) in brain tissue and blood vessels. AD also has been linked to a lysosomal pathway in the breakdown of amyloid precursor protein to yield beta amyloid, a neurotoxic substance coded by chromosome 21. A reduction in protein kinase C and the scavenging of phospholipid from the cell membrane are being studied as the cause for the lysosomal pathway taking precedence. A link between the pathology of AD and aluminum has not been established. Researchers have not yet been able to isolate a virus that causes the disease, but submicroscopic proteinaceous infectious particles (prions) have been isolated. These prions already have been linked to at least one other form of degenerative brain disease. Antibrain

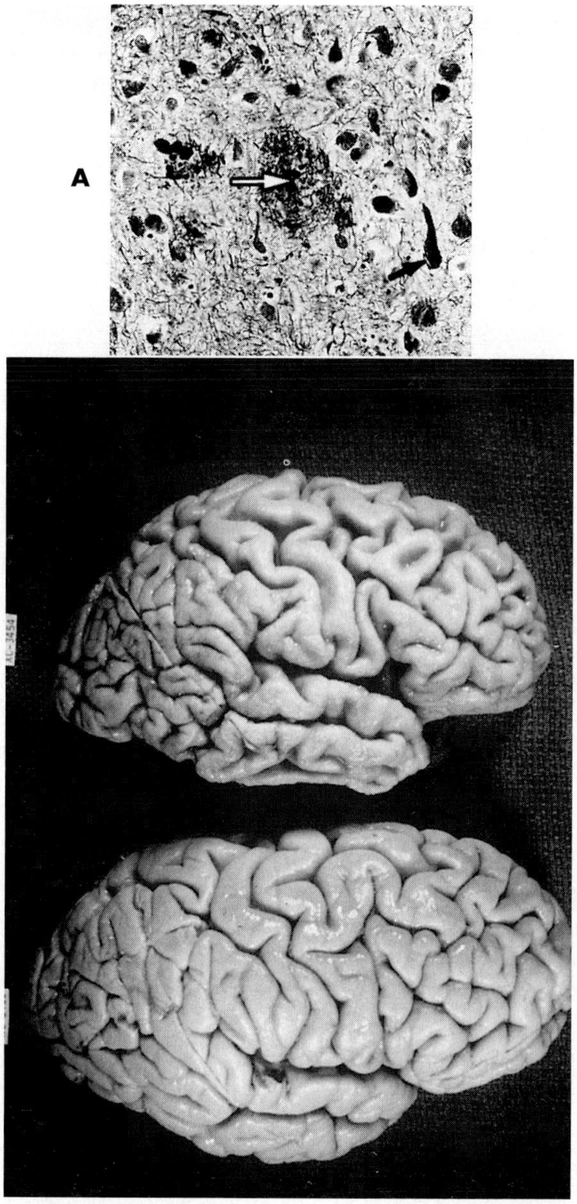

FIG. 15-9 Pathologic changes in Alzheimer disease. **A,** A neuritic (mature) plaque with central amyloid core *(white arrow)* next to a neurofibrillary tangle *(black arrow).* Alzheimer disease **(B)** compared with age-matched and sex-matched control **(C):** reduced size, narrow gyri, and wide sulci, notably in frontal and temporal lobes. (From Damjanov I, Linder J, editors: *Anderson's pathology,* ed 10, St Louis, 1996, Mosby.)

antibodies may account for AD, and an autoimmune cause also is being investigated. One theory is that once plaques form, complement proteins attach to them, attracting microglia (the brain's immune force), which release toxins in an attempt to destroy plaques.[3] Because plaques cannot be destroyed, the assault is endless. In addition, aging and injury also may result in changes that contribute to the development of this disease. Such changes could include decreased oxygen and glucose transport, loss of the blood-brain barrier, and mitochondrial defects that alter cell metabolism and processing of proteins, including amyloid (apo E-IV). Apo E-IV predisposes to late-onset FAD, as well as sporadic late-onset causes. The 3% of persons who are homozygous for apo E-IV have a 90% risk, whereas the 25% who are heterozygous have a 25% risk.[18,19]

Microscopically the protein in the neurons becomes distorted and twisted, forming a tangle called a **neurofibrillary tangle** (Fig. 15-9). Tangles are flame shaped, composed of a microtubule-binding protein called *tau protein.* Cortical nerve cell processes become twisted and dilated because of accumulation of the same filaments that form tangles. Amyloid also is deposited in cerebral arteries, causing an amyloid angiopathy. Groups of nerve cells, especially terminal axons, degenerate and coalesce around an amyloid core. Microscopic examination of these areas of degeneration reveals plaquelike material known as **senile plaques.** These plaques disrupt nerve-impulse transmission. Amyloid and tau proteins have also recently been linked together. Beta amyloid binds to the 7 nicotinic acetylcholine recepor on cholinergic neurons. This binding induces phosphate groups to attach to tau protein.[19] Senile plaques and neurofibrillary tangles are more concentrated in the cerebral cortex and hippocampus. The greater the number of senile plaques and neurofibrillary tangles, the more dysfunction is associated with AD. See Fig. 15-10 for disturbance in blood flow in Alzheimer disease.

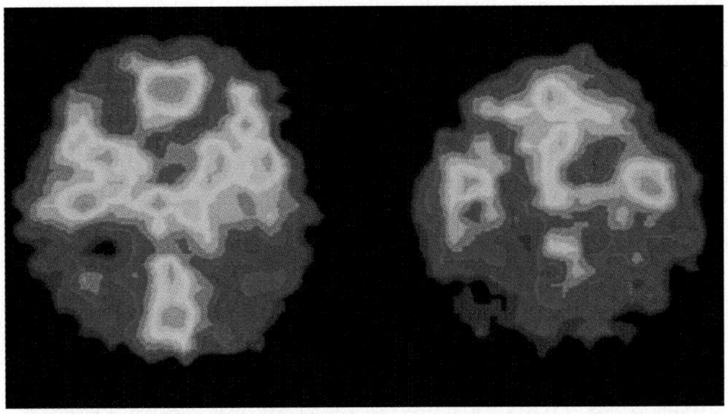

FIG. 15-10 Alzheimer disease. Single photon emission computerized tomography scan showing reduction of temporoparietal blood flow. (From Perkin GD: *Mosby's color atlas and text of neurology,* London, 1998, Mosby-Wolfe.)

Clinical Manifestations

Initial clinical manifestations are insidious and often attributed to forgetfulness, emotional upset, or other illness. The individual becomes progressively more forgetful over time, particularly in relation to recent events. Memory loss increases as the disorder advances, and the person becomes disoriented and confused. The ability to concentrate declines. Abstraction, problem solving, and judgment gradually deteriorate. A failure in mathematic calculation ability, language, and visuospatial orientation occurs. Dyspraxia may appear. The mental status changes induce behavioral changes, including irritability, agitation, and restlessness. Mood changes also result from the deterioration in cognition. The person may become anxious, depressed, hostile, emotionally labile, and prone to mood swings. Motor changes may occur if the posterior frontal lobes are involved. The individual exhibits rigidity (paratonia, gegenhalten), with flexion posturing, propulsion, and retropulsion. Great variability in age of onset, intensity and sequence of symptoms, and location and extent of brain abnormalities occurs among individuals with AD. Box 15-4 presents the clinical findings in each stage of AD.

Box 15-4

CLINICAL FINDINGS IN EACH STAGE OF ALZHEIMER DISEASE

STAGE I (DURATION OF DISEASE: 1 TO 3 YEARS)

Memory—new learning defective, remote recall impaired
Visuospatial skills—topographic disorientation, poor construction
Language—poor word list generation, anomia
Personality—apathy, irritability, depression
Motor system—normal
EEG—normal
CT—normal

STAGE II (DURATION OF DISEASE: 2 TO 10 YEARS)

Memory—recent and remote recall more severely impaired
Visuospatial skills—poor construction, spatial disorientation
Language—fluent aphasia
Calculation—acalculia
Praxis—ideomotor apraxia
Personality—indifference and apathy
EEG—slowing
CT—normal or ventricular dilation and sulcal enlargement

STAGE III (DURATION OF DISEASE: 8 TO 12 YEARS)

Intellectual functions—severely deteriorated
Motor—limb rigidity and flexion posture
Sphincter control—urinary and fecal incontinence
EEG—diffusely slow
CT—ventricular dilation and sulcal enlargement

From Cummings JL, Benson DF: *Dementia: a clinical approach,* Stoneham, Mass, 1992, Butterworth.
EEG, Electroencephalogram; *CT,* computed tomography.

Evaluation and Treatment

The diagnosis of AD is made by ruling out other causes of a dementing process by CT and blood tests. The history, including the mental status examination and the course of the illness, is used for diagnosis. The course of the disorder is highly variable, usually developing over 5 years or more.

Aricept has had a modest effect on cognitive functions in the early stages of AD, but the treatment of AD is directed at decreasing the need for the impaired cognitive function by a compensation technique, such as memory aids, maintaining those cognitive functions that are not impaired, and

NUTRITION & DISEASE

Alzheimer Disease

Weight loss is a major concern for elderly people with Alzheimer disease. The weight loss may be a result of (1) increased incidence of infection, (2) increased energy output because of constant pacing, (3) inadequate food intake, and (4) decreased independence and difficulty in self-feeding. Dementia may lead to memory loss, social isolation, depression, and poor food intake with resultant weight loss. Individuals may forget or refuse to eat, not communicate the need to eat, throw food or hide food, eat spoiled food or nonfood substances, eat favorite foods to the exclusion of eating other foods, take a long time to eat, have difficulty in preparing foods, and be unable to feed themselves. Suggestions for caregivers might include having a service (e.g., Home-Delivered Meals, Meals on Wheels) deliver a daily meal; taking the person to a congregate meal site; offering foods frequently; using finger foods such as Tater Tots, fish sticks, grapes, and crackers; dating refrigerated food and cleaning out the refrigerator on a regular basis; and providing a variety of foods.

Data from Riviere D, Albarede JL, Vellas B: Weight loss in Alzheimer disease, *Am J Clin Nutr* 71(2):S67S, 2000; Riviere S et al: Nutrition and Alzheimer's disease, *Nutr Rev* 57(12):363, 1999.

maintaining or improving the general state of hygiene, nutrition, and health. Environmental management, counseling, education, pharmacotherapy, and health promotion measures provide the foundation on which a comprehensive treatment program is built.

ALTERATIONS IN CEREBRAL HEMODYNAMICS

An injured brain reacts with structural, chemical, and pathophysiologic changes. Critical variables related to cerebral oxygenation include intracranial pressure, blood flow, and oxygen delivery. The pressure and oxygen delivery are critical management issues.

Cerebral Hemodynamics

Increased intracranial pressure (ICP) was the central management issue for many years. It is now recognized that cerebral oxygenation is the critical issue. Several relevant features of cerebral hemodynamics—cerebral blood volume (CBV), cerebral blood flow (CBF), and cerebral perfusion pressure (CPP)—relate to cerebral oxygenation (Box 15-5).

To guide therapeutic management, three critical categories related to cerebral hemodynamics are possible in the injured brain: (1) cerebral oligemia (also called jugular fibrillation), (2) CPP in the normal range (60 to 100 mm Hg) but with an elevated ICP, and (3) cerebral hyperemia. In the treatment algorithms, oxygen saturation measured in the internal jugular vein (SjO_2) is categorized as less than 55%, greater than 55% but less than 70%, or greater than 75%. After SjO_2 is categorized, the ICP must be added to the equation as less than 20 mm Hg or greater than 20 mm Hg. Treatment algorithms are implemented depending on the SjO_2 and ICP that address not only ICP but also CPP.[20,21] The therapeutic goal is to balance ICP and SjO_2.[20,22] Target values for relevant clinical parameters are presented in Table 15-19.

Box 15-5

CEREBRAL HEMODYNAMICS

Cerebral blood volume (CBV) refers to the amount of blood in the intracranial vault at a given time (normally about 10%). Most of this CBV is in the low-pressure venous system. CBV is determined by autoregulation mechanisms that control cerebral blood flow.

Cerebral blood flow (CBF) to the brain is normally maintained at a rate that matches local metabolic needs of the brain and is normally about 750 ml/min (15% to 20% of the cardiac output). CBF is calculated as follows: CBF + CPP/CVR (cardiovascular resistance). Required CBF varies in gray and white matter and is greater in gray matter. CBF is regulated through constriction or dilation of the cerebral vessels predominantly in response to changes in arterial O_2 and CO_2 concentrations. CBF decreases 3% for every 1 mm Hg decrease in CO_2. CBF increases at a PaO_2 of less than 50 mm Hg; CBF is stable (maintained) at a PaO_2 of greater than 80 mm Hg.

Cerebral perfusion pressure (CPP) is the pressure required to perfuse the cells of the brain. The formula to calculate CPP is as follows: CPP = MAP − ICP. Normal CPP is 60 to 100 mg Hg in normal brain tissue. An injured brain requires a CPP of greater than 70 mm Hg. The CPP determines CBF. As CPP decreases to 70 to 80 mm Hg in the injured brain, vasodilation occurs, which increases CBV, also increasing ICP. An increased ICP will decrease CPP.

Oxygen saturation measured in the internal jugular vein ($S\dot{j}O_2$) at the jugular bulb reflects the amount of oxygen still bound as the blood leaves the cranial vault. Cerebral extraction of oxygen (CEO_2) is calculated using the formula $SAO_2 - S\dot{j}O_2/SAO_2 \times 100$.* Normal CEO_2 is 20% to 24%; normal $S\dot{j}O_2$ is 55% to 70%. When oxygen demand exceeds oxygen supply, extraction increases, increasing the $S\dot{j}O_2$. A CEO_2 less than 24% or an $S\dot{j}O_2$ greater than 70% to 75% indicates cerebral hyperemia. Acid-base balance and temperature influence oxyhemoglobin dissociation (see Chapter 31).

*Data from Cruz J: The first decade of continuous monitoring of jugular bulb oxyhemoglobin saturation: strategies and clinical outcomes, *Crit Care Med* 26(2):233, 1998.

Increased Intracranial Pressure

Intracranial pressure normally is 5 to 15 mm Hg, or 60 to 180 cm H_2O. **Increased intracranial pressure** may result from an increase in intracranial content (as occurs with tumor growth), edema, excess cerebrospinal fluid (CSF), or hemorrhage. A rise in intracranial pressure necessitates an equal reduction in volume of the other contents. The most readily displaced content of the cranial vault is CSF. If intracranial pressure remains high after CSF displacement out of the cranial vault, cerebral blood volume is altered, which causes stage 1 of intracranial hypertension. Vasoconstriction and external compression of the venous system occur in an attempt to further decrease the intracranial pressure. Thus, during the first stage of intracranial hypertension, intracranial pressure may not change because of the effective compensatory mechanisms. CSF is reduced through increased

Table 15-19 Therapeutic Management Goals for Patients with Altered Cerebral Hemodynamics

Clinical Parameter	Target Value
Central perfusion pressure	>70 mm Hg
Intracranial pressure	<20 mm Hg
Arterial CO_2 pressure ($Paco_2$)	35 mm Hg
Mean arterial pressure	90 mm Hg
Temperature	34-36°C
Pulmonary capillary wedge pressure	10-15 mm Hg

reabsorption. Blood volume is reduced by compression of intracranial veins. Small increases in volume, however, cause an increase in pressure, and the pressure may take longer to return to baseline. Clinical manifestations at this stage usually are subtle and often transient and include episodes of confusion, drowsiness, and slight pupillary and breathing changes.

If intracranial pressure is still high, a state of intracranial hypertension occurs. With continued expansion of the intracranial content, the resulting increase in intracranial pressure may exceed the brain's compensatory capacity to adjust to the increasing pressure. In this state, the pressure begins to compromise neuronal oxygenation, and systemic arterial vasoconstriction occurs in an attempt to elevate the systemic blood pressure sufficiently to overcome the increased intracranial pressure. This is stage 2 of intracranial hypertension.

As intracranial pressure begins to approach arterial pressure, the brain tissues begin to experience hypoxia and hypercapnia and the individual's condition rapidly deteriorates. Clinical manifestations include decreasing levels of arousal, Cheyne-Stokes respirations or central neurogenic hyperventilation, pupils that become sluggish and dilated, widened pulse pressure, and bradycardia.

Dramatic sustained rises in intracranial pressure are not seen until all the compensatory mechanisms have been exhausted. Once decompensation begins, dramatic rises in intracranial pressure occur over a very short period. **Autoregulation,** the compensatory alteration in the diameter of the intracranial blood vessels designed to maintain a constant blood flow during changes in cerebral perfusion pressure, is lost with progressively increased intracranial pressure. Accumulating carbon dioxide may still cause vasodilation at the local tissue level, but now, without autoregulation, this vasodilation causes the hydrostatic (blood) pressure in the vessels to drop and blood volume to increase. The brain volume is thus further enhanced, and intracranial pressure continues to rise. This is stage 3 of intracranial hypertension. Small increases in volume cause dramatic increases in intracranial pressure, and the pressure takes much longer to return to baseline. As the intracranial pressure begins to approach systemic blood pressure, cerebral perfusion pressure falls and cerebral perfusion slows dramatically. The brain tissues experience severe hypoxia and acidosis.

Increased intracranial pressure in one compartment of the cranial vault is not evenly distributed throughout the other vault compartments. In stage 4, the last stage of intracranial hypertension, brain tissue shifts (herniates) from the compartment of greater pressure to a compartment of lesser pressure (Fig. 15-11). With this shift in brain tissue, the herniating brain tissue's blood supply is compromised, causing further ischemia and hypoxia in the herniating tissues. The herniated brain tissues increase the volume of content within the lower-pressure compartment, exerting pressure on the brain tissue that normally occupies that compartment, thus impairing that tissue's blood supply. Small hemorrhages frequently develop in the involved brain tissue. Obstructive hydrocephalus may develop. The herniation process markedly and rapidly increases intracranial pressure. Mean systolic arterial pressure soon equals intracranial pressure, and cerebral blood flow ceases at this point.

Herniation Syndromes

Supratentorial Herniation

The three types of supratentorial herniation syndromes are (1) uncal (temporal lobe, lateral transtentorial) herniation, (2) central (transtentorial) herniation, and (3) cingulate gyrus herniation. **Uncal herniation** occurs when the uncus or hippocampal gyrus (or both) shifts from the middle fossa through the tentorial notch into the posterior fossa, compressing the ipsilateral third cranial nerve, then the contralateral third cranial nerve, and finally the mesencephalon. Uncal herniation generally is caused by an expanding mass in the lateral region of the middle fossa. The classic manifestations of uncal herniation are a decreasing level of consciousness, pupils that become sluggish before fixing and dilating (first the ipsilateral, then the contralateral pupil), Cheyne-Stokes respirations (which later shift to central neurogenic hyperventilation), and the appearance of decorticate, then later decerebrate, posturing.

Central herniation is the straight downward shift of the diencephalon through the tentorial notch. Causes of central herniation are injuries or masses located around the outer perimeter of the frontal, parietal, or occipital lobes; extracerebral injuries around the central apex (top) of the cranium; bilaterally positioned injuries or masses; and unilateral cingulate gyrus herniation. The individual experiencing transtentorial herniation rapidly passes from a conscious to an unconscious state; from Cheyne-Stokes respirations to apnea; from small, reactive pupils to dilated and fixed pupils; and from decortication to decerebration.

Cingulate gyrus herniation occurs when the cingulate gyrus shifts under the falx cerebri. Little is known about the clinical manifestations of this type of herniation.

Infratentorial Herniation

Two types of infratentorial herniation syndromes may occur. In the most common infratentorial herniation syndrome, a cerebellar tonsil shifts through the foramen magnum because of increased pressure within the posterior fossa. The clinical manifestations of this downward infratentorial

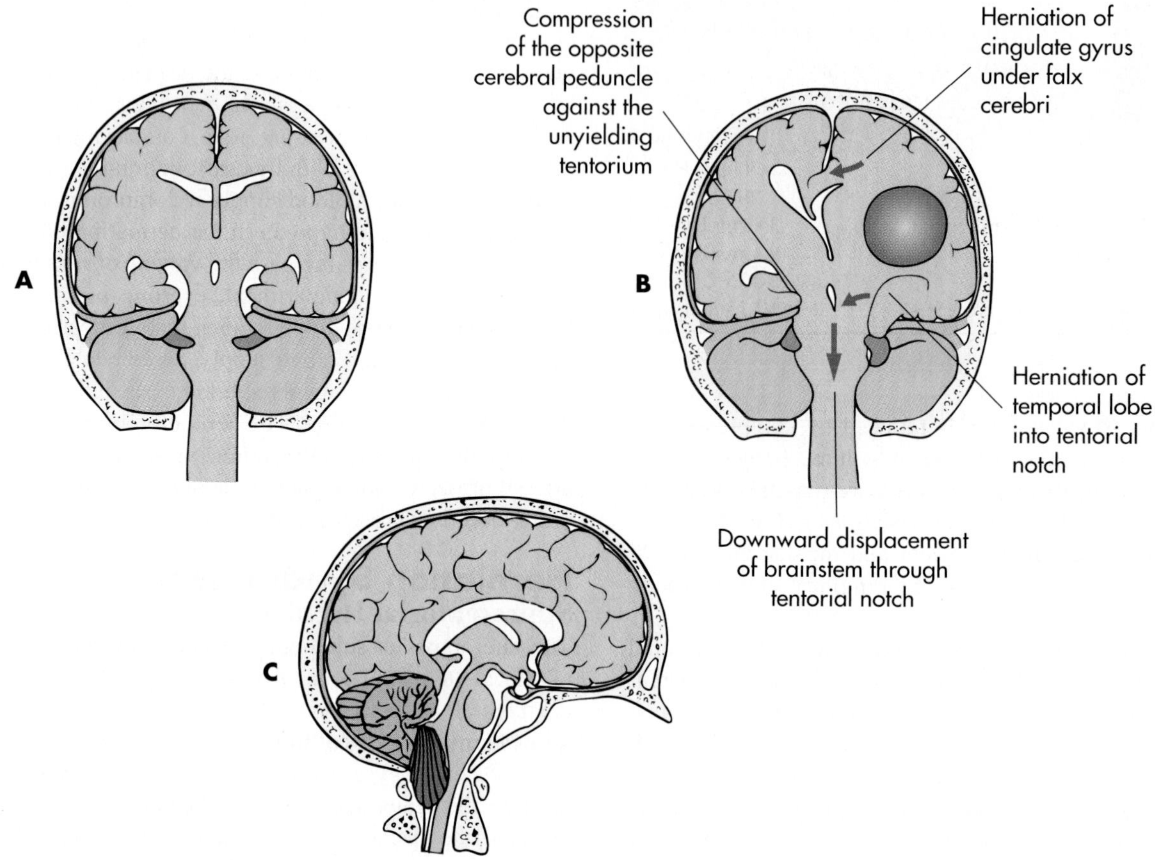

FIG. 15-11 Herniation. A, Normal relationship of intracranial structures. **B,** Shift of intracranial structures. **C,** Downward herniation of the cerebellar tonsils into the foramen magnum.

herniation are an arched, stiff neck; paresthesias in the shoulder area; decreased consciousness; respiratory abnormalities; and pulse rate variations. Occasionally the pressure force is such that an upward transtentorial herniation of a cerebellar tonsil or the lower brain stem results. No specific set of clinical manifestations is associated with this infratentorial herniation syndrome.

Cerebral Edema

Cerebral edema is an increase in the fluid content of brain tissue (Fig. 15-12). Cerebral edema causes an increase in extracellular or intracellular tissue volume after brain insult from trauma, infection, hemorrhage, tumor, ischemia, infarct, or hypoxia. The harmful effects of cerebral edema are caused by the distortion of blood vessels, the displacement of brain tissues, and the eventual herniation of brain tissue from one brain compartment to another.

Four types of cerebral edema are (1) vasogenic edema, (2) cytotoxic (metabolic) edema, (3) ischemic edema, and (4) interstitial edema. **Vasogenic edema** is clinically the most important type. It is caused by the increased permeability of the capillary endothelium of the brain after injury to the vascular structure. The result is a disruption in the blood-brain barrier. Plasma proteins leak into the extracellular spaces, drawing water to them, and the water content of the brain parenchyma increases. Vasogenic edema starts in the area of injury and spreads with preferential accumulation in the white matter of the ipsilateral side because the parallel myelinated fibers separate more easily. Edema then promotes more edema because of ischemia from increasing pressure.

Clinical manifestations of vasogenic edema include focal neurologic deficits, disturbances of consciousness, and a severe increase in intracranial pressure. Vasogenic edema resolves by slow diffusion.

In **cytotoxic (metabolic) edema,** toxic factors directly affect the cellular elements of the brain parenchyma (neuronal, glial, and endothelial cells), causing failure of the active transport systems. The cells lose their potassium and gain larger amounts of sodium. Water follows by osmosis into the cell, so that the cells swell. Cytotoxic edema occurs principally in the gray matter and may increase vasogenic edema.

Ischemic edema follows cerebral infarction. The ischemia has components of both vasogenic and cytotoxic edema. Soon after the onset of ischemia, the initial edema is confined to the intracellular compartment. During the following hours and then over several days, brain cells begin to undergo necrosis and die, releasing lysosomes. In this autodigestive process, the blood-brain barrier's permeability is increased.

Interstitial edema is seen most often with noncommunicating hydrocephalus (see Chapter 16). The edema is caused

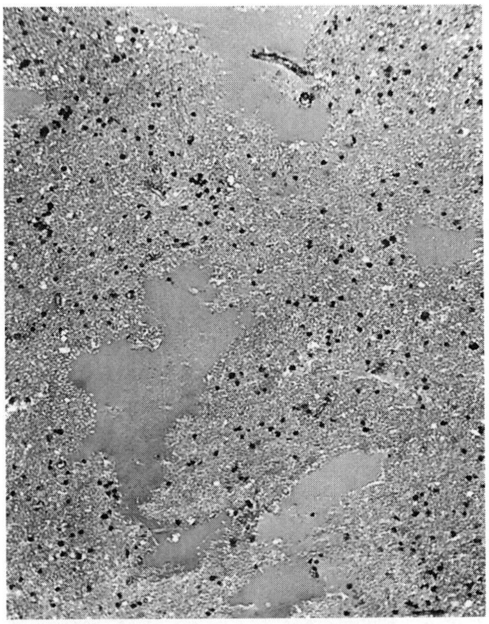

FIG. 15-12 Brain edema. Intercellular lakes of high-protein content fluid. (Hematoxylin-eosin stain; ×90.) (From Kissane JM, editor: *Anderson's pathology,* ed 9, St Louis, 1993, Mosby.)

by transependymal movement of CSF from the ventricles into the extracellular spaces of the brain tissues. The brain fluid volume thus is increased predominantly around the ventricles. The hydrostatic pressure within the white matter increases, and the size of the white matter is reduced because of the rapid disappearance of myelin lipids.

Hydrocephalus

The term **hydrocephalus** refers to a variety of conditions characterized by an excess of fluid within the cranial vault, subarachnoid space, or both. Hydrocephalus occurs because of interference with CSF flow caused by increased fluid production, obstruction within the ventricular system, or defective reabsorption of the fluid. A papilloma (i.e., epithelial tumor) may, in rare instances, cause overproduction of CSF (Fig. 15-13).

Types of Hydrocephalus

Obstruction within the ventricular system, called **noncommunicating hydrocephalus** or *internal (intraventricular) hydrocephalus,* may result from congenital abnormalities in the ventricular system or mass lesions such as a tumor that compresses one of the structures of the ventricular system (see Chapter 18 for additional discussion). Impaired absorption of CSF from the subarachnoid space occurs when an obstructive process disrupts the flow of CSF through the subarachnoid space. The fluid is prevented from reaching the convex portion of the cerebrum, where the arachnoid granulations are located.

Hydrocephalus from impaired absorption may be caused by adhesions from inflammation, as with a meningitis or subarachnoid hemorrhage; compression of the subarachnoid space by a mass, such as a tumor; congenital abnormalities of the subarachnoid space; or high venous pressure within the sagittal sinus. This type of hydrocephalus is termed **communicating (extraventricular) hydrocephalus.** The most common causes of communicating hydrocephalus are subarachnoid hemorrhage, developmental malformation, head injury, and neoplasm.

One form of communicating hydrocephalus is **hydrocephalus ex vacuo,** which arises from cerebral atrophy. CSF fills the unoccupied space. The amount of CSF is increased, but the fluid is not under pressure. Another form of communicating hydrocephalus is **normal-pressure hydrocephalus** (low-pressure, adult, or occult hydrocephalus), which occurs mostly in late middle age. The cause is thought to be arachnoid adhesions that obstruct the subarachnoid space. This form of hydrocephalus is most frequently seen as a complication of head injury and subarachnoid hemorrhage.

Course of the Disease

Hydrocephalus may develop from infancy through adulthood. Congenital hydrocephalus (i.e., ventricular enlargement before birth) is rare. Noncommunicating hydrocephalus is more commonly seen in children. The more frequent type of hydrocephalus in adults is the communicating type. (Hydrocephalus in children is discussed in Chapter 18.)

Most cases of hydrocephalus develop gradually and insidiously over time. **Acute hydrocephalus,** however, may develop in several hours in persons who have sustained head injuries. Acute hydrocephalus contributes significantly to increased intracranial pressure.

Pathophysiology

The obstruction of CSF flow associated with hydrocephalus produces dilation of the ventricles proximal to the obstruction. Obstructed CSF is under pressure, causing atrophy of the cerebral cortex and degeneration of the white matter tracts. There is selective preservation of gray matter. When excess CSF fills a defect caused by atrophy, a degenerative disorder, or a surgical excision, this fluid is not under pressure; therefore atrophy and degenerative changes are not induced.

Clinical Manifestations

The presentation of acute hydrocephalus is one of rapidly developing increased intracranial pressure. The person deteriorates rapidly into a deep coma if not promptly treated. Normal-pressure hydrocephalus has a long-term presentation and develops slowly over time. The individual or family complains of declining memory and cognitive function. An unsteady, broad-based gait with a history of falling is common. Additional clinical manifestations are apathy; inattentiveness; and indifference to self, family, and the environment. Urinary incontinence is present.

Evaluation and Treatment

The diagnosis is made on the basis of physical examination, CT scan, and MRI. A radioisotopic cisternogram may

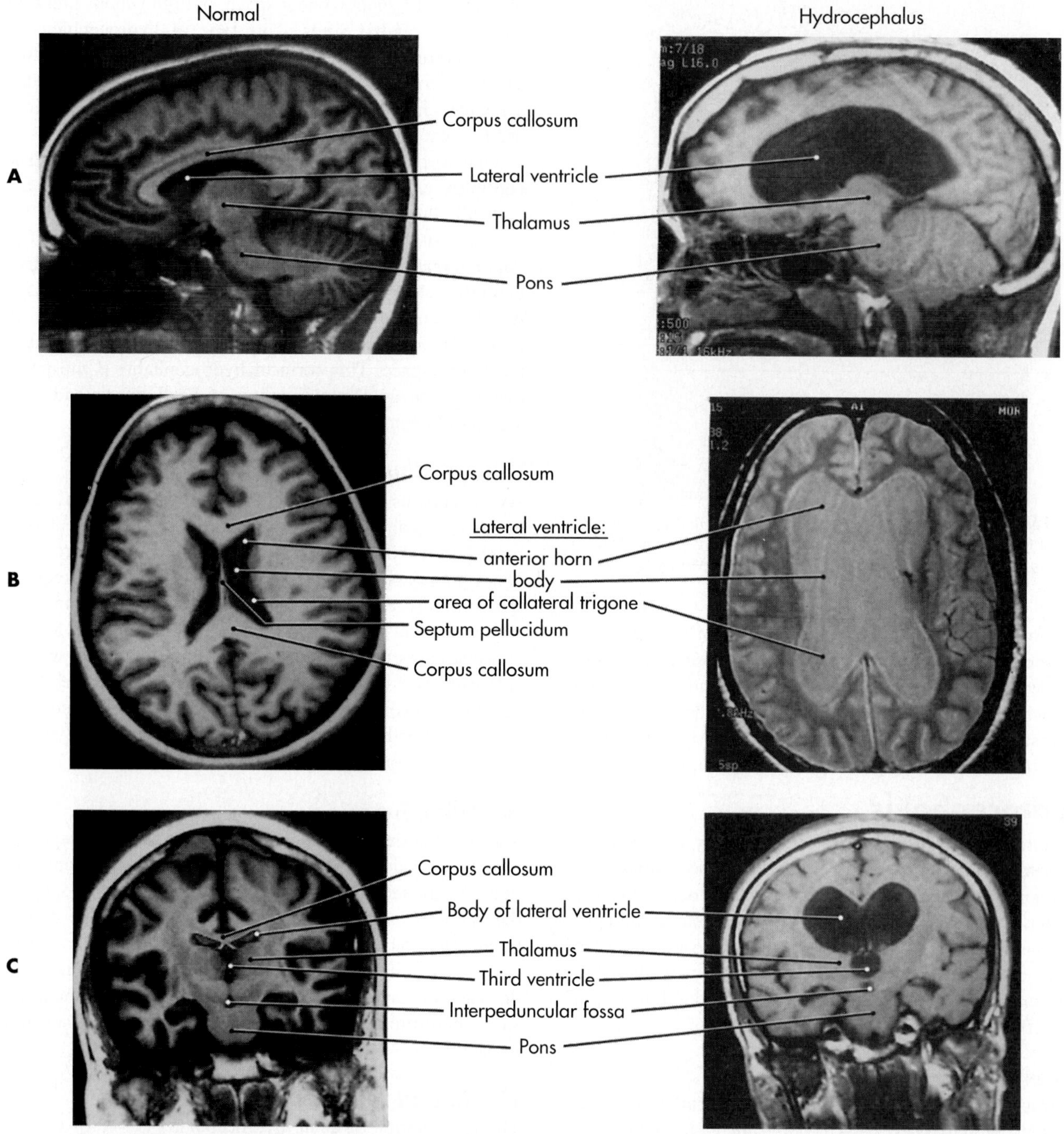

FIG. 15-13 Normal and hydrocephalic brains. Comparison of normal and hydrocephalic brains in sagittal **(A),** axial **(B),** and coronal **(C)** planes as seen in MRI (From Haines DE, editor: *Fundamental neuroscience,* Philadelphia, 1997, Churchill Livingstone.)

be performed to diagnose normal-pressure hydrocephalus. Hydrocephalus can be treated by surgery to resect cysts, neoplasms, or hematomas or by ventricular bypass into the normal intracranial channel or into an extracranial compartment using a shunt. Excision or coagulation of the choroid plexus is needed occasionally when a papilloma is present. In normal-pressure hydrocephalus, reduction in CSF through a diuresis regimen often is used.

ALTERATIONS IN EMOTIONS AND MOOD

Emotions such as anger, hostility, envy, fear, and love all guide behavior and mood and are mediated largely by the limbic system. Alterations in emotions or mood arise from dysfunction in the limbic system; in the hypothalamus, which choreographs the behaviors that accompany emotional and mood states; or in the cerebral cortex, especially the neural tracts of the orbital-frontal cortex that project to the limbic system to exert inhibiting and modulating effects. Changes in the physical, chemical, or electrical status of the frontal lobes, limbic system, or hypothalamus may be associated with significant changes in emotions, mood, and behavior. Changes in emotions, mood, and behavior can result from abscesses, tumors, hemorrhages, metabolic disorders, degenerative disease, and intoxication states.

Pathophysiology

Damage to the frontal lobes and frontolimbic tracts that project inhibitory influences to the limbic system frees the limbic system and leaves it unchecked to generate an array of emotions and mood. Behavior then becomes erratic and unpredictable. Orbitofrontal dysfunction manifests with emotional lability along with disinhibition and impaired social functioning. Pathologic processes within the limbic system itself may produce a deficiency in emotional response, either a lack of impulse (as in the depressive disorder) or excessive impulse, as in certain psychomotor seizures or acute anxiety states. Medial temporal dysfunction involving the limbic system, including the hippocampus and amygdala, manifest with alteration in mood, as well as memory difficulties and disinhibition.

Some recent proposals related to emotions and mood link dysfunction in attentional networks to schizophrenia and depression. Posner and Raichle[14] have proposed that in some forms of schizophrenia an abnormality of the anterior cingulate exists, resulting in an executive attention network deficit. In addition, they have found reduced frontal lobe activity in persons with long-standing schizophrenia, which causes a decrease in working memory functions. Reduced dendrite branching in the frontal lobes has been found in schizophrenia.[23] A gene located on chromosome 13 contributes to at least some cases of schizophrenia, and a sequence on chromosome 8 boosts susceptibility to schizophrenia.[24]

Likewise, increased blood flow to the anterior cingulate and lateral surface of the frontal lobes with a corresponding decrease in blood flow in the posterior brain regions occurs with depression. Posner and Raichle[14] proposed that increased activity in the neural networks involved in internally generated thoughts and information, as well as emotion and mood, may predominate in depression. Overactivity in the amygdala may produce assignment of negative feelings to all thoughts and information.

Hypothalamic dysfunction may excessively arouse the limbic system by supplying too much of a neurotransmitter, resulting in an acute anxiety state or producing associated behaviors without inducing the feelings. For example, tumors that involve the tracts projecting from the hypothalamus are associated with raging behaviors, but the feeling of anger or rage is not present.

Clinical Manifestations

Common among all types of frontal lobe damage is a change in the experience and expression of emotion and mood. The clinical manifestations associated with frontal lobe dysfunction range from excessive, seemingly purposeless activity to spontaneity. Irritability, impulsiveness, mood swings, mood shifts, inability to tolerate frustration, and loss of control occur frequently. Clinical manifestations can include depression, mania, hyperactivity, acute anxiety, acute confusional states, and dementia.

Evaluation and Treatment

Evaluation of alterations in emotion and mood include several strategies: physical and psychologic examinations, CT scans, MRI, EEG, and obtaining appropriate blood chemistry levels. Treatment is directed at preventing injury (including suicide), medically or surgically treating the underlying cause, instituting appropriate drug therapy and psychotherapy, and providing support and guidance to the family. Drugs used to achieve symptomatic control alter the levels of neurotransmitters within the brain tissues. For example, diazepam (Valium) and other drugs compete for the receptors ordinarily occupied by a neurotransmitter so that level of arousal is decreased. Propranolol has been used in panic and anxiety attacks.

ALTERATIONS IN MOTOR FUNCTION

Movements are complex patterns of activity controlled by the CNS. Movements are influenced by the cerebral cortex, the pyramidal system, the extrapyramidal system, and the motor units. Dysfunction in any of these areas can cause motor dysfunction. General motor dysfunctions may produce changes in muscle tone, movement, and complex motor performance.

Alterations in Muscle Tone

Normal muscle tone involves a slight resistance to passive movement. The resistance is smooth, constant, and even throughout the range of motion. Abnormalities of muscle tone are presented in Table 15-20.

Hypotonia

In **hypotonia** (decreased muscle tone), passive movement of a muscle occurs with little or no resistance. Hypotonia is thought to be caused by decreased muscle spindle activity secondary to decreased excitability of neurons. Hypotonia is caused by pure pyramidal tract damage (a rare occurrence) and cerebellar damage. A pure pyramidal tract injury produces hypotonia and weakness. The hypotonia contributes to the ataxia and intention tremor in cerebellar damage and manifests with minimal weakness, with normal or slightly exaggerated reflexes. Hypotonia, often described as flaccidity (a state in which the muscle may be moved rapidly without resistance), occurs when nerve impulses necessary for muscle tone are lost, such as in spinal cord injury or cerebrovascular accident.

Individuals with hypotonia report that they tire easily (asthenia) or are weak, signs that can be observed during their activity attempts. They may have difficulty rising from a sitting position, sitting down without using arm support, and walking up and down stairs, as well as an inability to stand on their toes. Because of their weakness, accident proneness during locomotion and self-care activities is common. Inasmuch as the joints become hyperflexible in hypotonic states, persons with hypotonia may be able to assume positions that require extreme joint mobility. The joints may appear loose, and the knee jerks are pendulous.

The muscle mass atrophies because of decreased input entering the motor unit. Muscle cells gradually are replaced by connective tissue and fat. The muscles are flabby on palpation and are flat in appearance. Fasciculations may be present in some cases.

Hypertonia

In **hypertonia** (increased muscle tone), passive movement of a muscle occurs with resistance. Four types of hypertonia are described: spasticity, gegenhalten (paratonia), dystonia, and rigidity.

Spasticity results from hyperexcitability of the stretch reflexes (overactivation of the alpha motor neurons) and is associated with damage to the motor, premotor, and supplementary motor areas, as well as lateral corticospinal tract damage (Fig. 15-14). Spasticity is accompanied by increased deep tendon reflexes (hyperreflexia) and the spread of reflexes **(clonus).**

Gegenhalten (paratonia) manifests as resistance to passive movement that varies in direct proportion to the force

Table 15-20 Alterations in Muscle Tone

Alterations	Characteristics	Cause
HYPOTONIA	Passive movement of a muscle mass with little or no resistance	Thought to be caused by decreased muscle spindle activity as a result of decreased excitability of neurons
	Difficult to detect; extremity is floppy and allows an excessive movement when displaced	
	Muscles may be rapidly moved without resistance	Occurs typically when nerve impulses necessary for muscle tone are lost
Flaccidity	Associated with limp, atrophied muscles and paralysis	
HYPERTONIA	Increased muscle resistance to passive movement May be associated with paralysis May be accompanied by muscle hypertrophy (see figure 15-17)	Results when the lower motor unit reflex arc continues to function but is not mediated or regulated by higher centers
Spasticity	A gradual increase in tone causing increased resistance until tone suddenly is reduced, which results in clasp-knife phenomenon Velocity dependent (may be absent with slow speed of displacement) Selective distribution (predominates in flexors of the upper extremities and extensors of lower extremities and in pronators compared with supinators)	Exact mechanism unclear; appears to arise from an increased excitability of the alpha motor neurons to any input because of absence of the descending inhibition of the pyramidal systems
Gegenhalten (paratonia)	Resistance to passive movement, which varies in direct proportion to force applied	Exact mechanism unclear: associated with frontal lobe injury
Dystonia	Sustained involuntary twisting movement	Produced by slow muscular contraction
Rigidity	Muscle resistance to passive movement of a rigid limb that is uniform in both flexion and extension throughout the motion Not velocity dependent Activated by contraction of muscles in contralateral extremities Uniform through range in displacement	Occurs as a result of constant, involuntary contraction of muscle
Plastic, or lead-pipe	Increased muscular tone relatively independent of degree of force used in passive movement; does not vary throughout the passive movement	Associated with basal ganglion damage
Cogwheel	The uniform resistance may be interrupted by a series of brief jerks resulting in movements much like a ratchet, "cogwheel" phenomenon	Associated with basal ganglion damage
Gamma	Characterized by extensor posturing (decerebrate rigidity)	Loss of excitation of extensor inhibitory areas by the cerebral cortex decreasing the inhibition of alpha and gamma motor neurons
Alpha		Loss of cerebellum input to lateral vestibular nuclei
MYOTONIA	Impaired relaxation of skeletal muscle after the contraction	

applied and is associated with frontal lobe injury. **Dystonia** manifests as sustained, involuntary twisting movements caused by slow muscle contraction and may be caused by a failure in appropriate reciprocal inhibition of the muscles (Figs. 15-15 and 15-16). Injury to the putamen or its outflow tracts also is associated with hemidystonia.

Rigidity produced by tonic reflex activity mediated by gamma motor neurons may be continuous or intermittent. The involved muscles are firm and tense; the increase in muscle movement is even and uniform throughout the range of passive movement. Four types of rigidity are described: plastic, or lead-pipe, rigidity; cogwheel rigidity; gamma rigidity; and alpha rigidity (see Table 15-20).

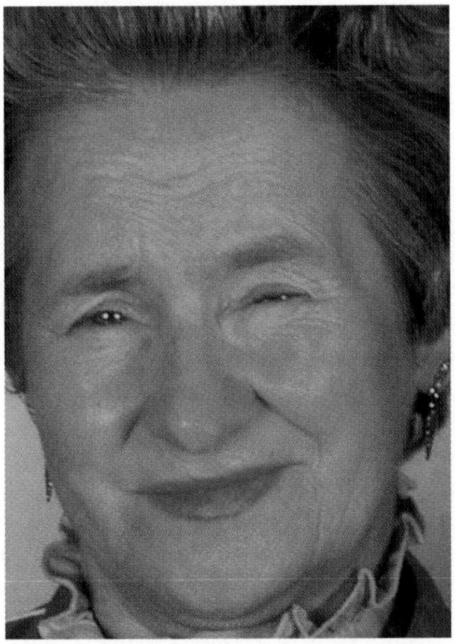

FIG. 15-14 A proxysm of left-sided hemifacial spasm. (From Perkin GD: *Mosby's color atlas and text of neurology,* London, 1998, Mosby-Wolfe.)

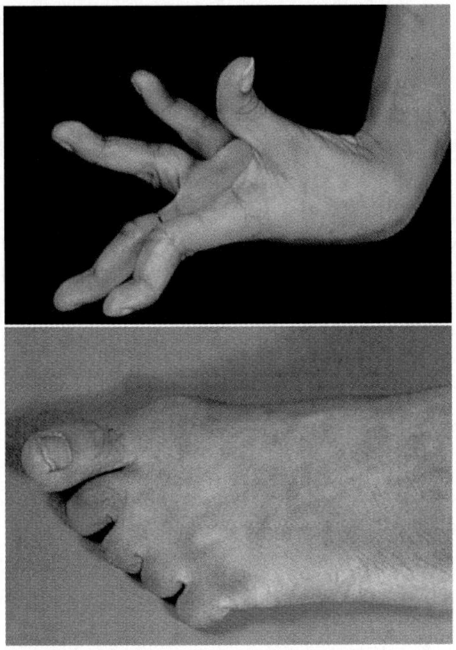

FIG. 15-15 Dystonic posturing of the hand and foot. (From Perkin GD: *Mosby's color atlas and text of neurology,* London, 1998, Mosby-Wolfe.)

Individuals with hypertonia may tire easily (asthenia) or be weak. Passive and active movement is equally affected, except in paratonia, in which more active than passive movement is possible. As a result of hypertonia and weakness, accident proneness during locomotion and self-care activities is common.

The muscles may atrophy because of decreased use of the muscles. However, hypertrophy occasionally may occur in some diseases. Hypertrophy results from overstimulation of muscle fibers. Overstimulation occurs when the motor unit reflex arc remains intact and functioning but is not inhibited by higher centers. The loss of inhibition and the constant state of excitation cause continual muscle contraction, resulting in enlargement of the muscle mass (Fig. 15-17). The muscles are firm on palpation.

Alterations in Movement

Movement requires a change in the contractile state of muscles. Abnormal movements may occur when a variety of CNS dysfunctions alter muscular innervation. Movement disorders are not well understood. Current knowledge has come predominantly from the areas of neuropharmacology and experimental therapeutics. The neurotransmitter *dopamine* has an apparent role in motor function. Some movement disorders (e.g., the akinesias) result from too little dopaminergic activity, whereas others (e.g., chorea, ballism, tardive dyskinesia) result from too much dopaminergic activity. Still others are not related primarily to dopamine function. Movement disorders are not associated necessarily with mass, strength, or tone but are neurologic dysfunctions with either a decreased amount of movement or an excess of movement.

Muscle strength is quantitatively evaluated on a scale of 0 to 4+ or 0 to 5, in which 4+ or 5 is normal and 0 indicates an inability to move against gravity (Table 15-21). Degrees

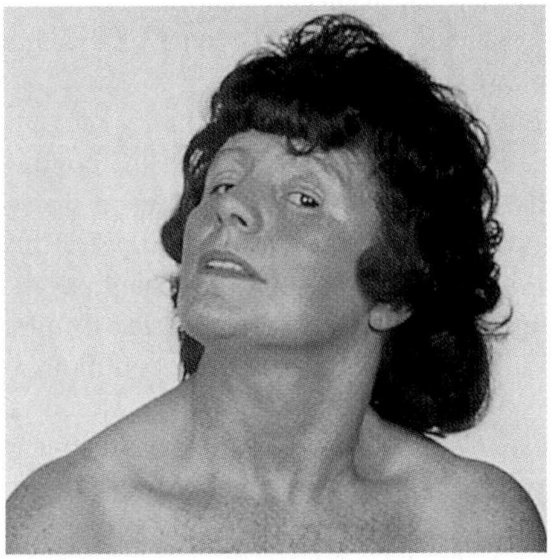

FIG. 15-16 Spasmodic torticollis. A characteristic head posture. (From Perkin GD: *Mosby's color atlas and text of neurology,* London, 1998, Mosby-Wolfe.)

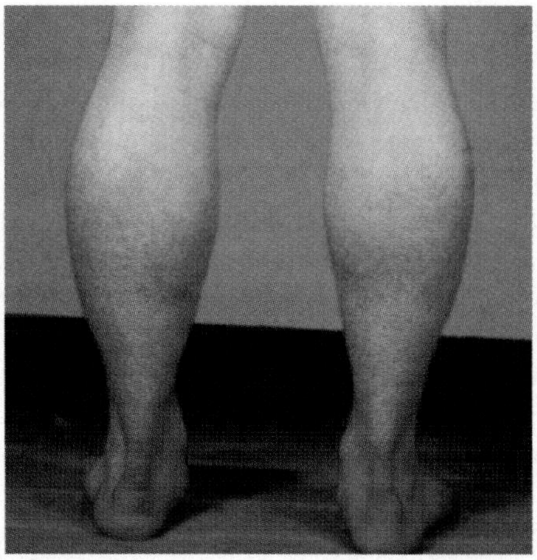

FIG. 15-17 **Pseudohypertrophy of the calf muscles.** (From Perkin GD: *Mosby's color atlas and text of neurology,* London, 1998, Mosby-Wolfe.)

of abnormal muscle strength range from **paresis** (weakness) to **paralysis** (inability of a muscle group to overcome gravity). Sites of paresis and paralysis are named in different ways. **Hemiparesis** refers to weakness on one side of the body; **hemiplegia** indicates paralysis on one side of the body. These conditions result from dysfunction, such as a tumor or cerebrovascular accident, in the brain or brain stem.

Paraplegia refers to paralysis of the lower extremities, whereas **quadriplegia** refers to paralysis of all four extremities. Both paraplegia and quadriplegia may be caused by dysfunction of the spinal cord. Upper cord damage results in quadriplegia, and lower cord damage preserves upper extremity function and causes paraplegia (spinal cord injury is discussed in Chapter 16).

Hyperkinesia

Hyperkinesia (excessive movement) represents the second broad category of abnormal movements. Within this category are a number of specific dysfunctions (Table 15-22). Also included in the general category of hyperkinesias are dyskinesias, that is, abnormal involuntary movements.

Paroxysmal dyskinesias are abnormal, involuntary movements that occur as spasms. The type of dyskinesia varies depending on the specific disorder.

Tardive dyskinesia is the involuntary movement of the face, trunk, and extremities. Although the condition occurs occasionally in individuals with Parkinson disease, it usually occurs as a side effect of prolonged phenothiazine drug therapy or haloperidol (Haldol). The antipsychotic drugs cause denervation hypersensitivity so that it mimics the effect of too much dopamine. The most common symptom of tardive dyskinesia is rapid, repetitive, stereotypic movements. Most characteristic is continual chewing with intermittent protrusions of the tongue, lip smacking, and facial grimacing. Stereotypic movements are believed to be a form of excessive dopaminergic activity.

Other movement disorders under this category are (1) complex repetitive movements, including automatism, stereotype, complex tics, compulsions, perseverations, and mannerisms; (2) positivism (excessive reactions to certain stimuli); and (3) paroxysmal excessive activity, including cataplexy and excessive startle reaction.

Table 15-21 UK Medical Research Council Classification of Muscle Power

Grade	Definition
0	Total paralysis
1	Flicker of contraction
2	Movement with gravity eliminated
3	Movement against gravity
4	Movement against resistance but incomplete
5	Normal power

Hypokinesia

Hypokinesia (decreased movement) is loss of voluntary movement despite preserved consciousness and normal peripheral nerve and muscle function. Types of hypokinesia include paresis and paralysis, akinesia, bradykinesia, and loss of associated movement.

Paresis and Paralysis

Paresis (weakness) is impairment of motor function, that is, partial paralysis with incomplete loss of muscle power. **Paralysis** is loss of motor function, that is, inability of a muscle group to overcome gravity. Two subtypes of paresis and paralysis are described: upper motor neuron paresis and paralysis and lower motor neuron paresis and paralysis (Table 15-23).

Upper motor neuron syndromes. Upper motor neuron paresis and paralysis is known also as spastic paresis and paralysis, and many different terms are used to describe a specific paresis or paralysis. **Hemiparesis** or **hemiplegia** is paresis or paralysis, respectively, of the upper and lower extremities on one side. **Diplegia** is the paralysis of both upper or lower extremities as a result of cerebral hemisphere injuries. **Paraparesis** or **paraplegia** refers to weakness or paralysis, respectively, of the lower extremities. **Quadriparesis** or **quadriplegia** refers to paresis or paralysis of all four extremities. Paraparesis or paraplegia and quadriparesis or quadriplegia may be caused by dysfunction of the spinal cord. Upper cord damage results in quadriparesis or quadriplegia, and lower cord damage preserves upper extremity function and causes paraparesis or paraplegia (spinal cord injury is discussed in Chapter 16).

Upper motor neuron paresis or paralysis is associated with a pyramidal motor syndrome. The **pyramidal motor syndrome** is a series of motor dysfunctions that result from interruption of the pyramidal system (Figs. 15-18 and 15-19). The injury may be in the cerebral cortex, the subcortical white matter, the internal capsule, the brain stem, or the spinal cord. The clinical manifestations of a pure pyramidal injury without other damage are not known, but bilateral interruption of the pyramidal system in monkeys causes hypotonic paralysis, although much control of movement

Table 15-22 Types of Hyperkinesia

Type	Characteristics	Causes
CHOREA*	Nonrepetitive muscular contractions, usually of the extremities of face; random pattern of irregular, involuntary rapid contractions of groups of muscles; disappears with sleep, decreases with resting; increases with emotional stress and attempted voluntary movement	Associated with excess concentration of or a supersensitivity to dopamine within basal ganglia
ATHETOSIS*	Disorder of distal-muscle postural fixation; slow, sinuous, irregular movements most obvious in the distal extremities, more rhythmic than choreiform movements and always much slower; movements accompany characteristic hand posture; slowly fluctuating grimaces	Occurs most commonly as a result of injury to the putamen of the basal ganglion; exact pathophysiologic mechanism is not known
BALLISM	Disorder of proximal-muscle postural fixation with wild flinging movement of the limbs; movement is severe and stereotyped, usually lateral; does not lessen with sleep; ballism is most common on one side of the body, a condition termed *hemiballism*	Results from injury to subthalamus nucleus (one of the nuclei that comprise the basal ganglia); thought to be caused by reduced inhibitory influence in the nucleus, a release phenomenon; hemiballism results from injury to the contralateral subthalamic nucleus
HYPERACTIVITY	State of prolonged, generalized, increased activity that is largely involuntary but may be subject to some voluntary control; not highly stereotyped but rather manifests as continuous changes in total body posture or in excessive performance of some simple activity, such as pacing under inappropriate circumstances	May be caused by frontal and reticular activating system injury
WANDERING	Tendency to wander without regard for environment	"Release" phenomenon; associated with bilateral injury to globus pallidus or putamen
AKATHISIA	Special type of hyperactivity; mild compulsion to move (usually more localized to legs); severe frenzied motion possible; movements are partly voluntary and may be transiently suppressed; carrying out the movement brings a sense of relief; a frequent complication of antipsychotic drugs	Dopaminergic transmission may be involved
TREMOR AT REST	Rhythmic, oscillating movement affecting one or more body parts	Caused by regular contraction of opposing groups of muscles
Parkinsonian tremor	Regular, rhythmic, slow flexion-extension contraction; involves principally the metacarpophalangeal and wrist joints; alternating movements between thumb and index finger described as "pill rolling"; disappears during voluntary movement	Loss of inhibitory influence of dopamine in the basal ganglia, causing instability of basal ganglial feedback circuit within the cerebral cortex
POSTURAL TREMOR		
Asterixis (tremor of hepatic encephalopathy)	Irregular flapping movement of the hands accentuated by outstretching arms	Exact mechanisms responsible unknown; thought to be related to accumulation of products normally detoxified by the liver
Metabolic	Rapid, rhythmic tremor affecting fingers, lips, and tongue; accentuated by extending the body part; enhanced physiologic tremor	Occurs in conditions associated with disturbed metabolism or toxicity, as in thyrotoxicosis (hyperthyroidism), alcoholism, and chronic use of barbiturates, amphetamines, lithium, amitriptyline (Elavil); exact mechanism responsible unknown
Essential (familial)	Tremor of fingers, hands, and feet; absent at rest but accentuated by extension of body part, prolonged muscular activity, and stress	Not associated with any other neurologic abnormalities; cause unknown

*Choreoathetosis involves both chorea and athetosis; precise pathophysiology unknown.

Continued

Table 15-22 Types of Hyperkinesia—cont'd

Type	Characteristics	Causes
INTENTIONAL TREMOR		
Cerebellar	Tremor initiated by movement, maximal toward end of movement	Occurs in disease of the dentate nucleus (one of the deep cerebellar nuclei responsible for efferent output) and the superior cerebellar peduncle (a stalklike structure connected to the pons); caused by errors in feedback from the periphery and errors in preprogramming goal-directed movement
Rubral	Rhythmic tremor of limbs that originates proximally by movement	Results from lesions involving the dentatorubrothalamic tract (a spinothalamic tract connecting the red nucleus in the reticular formation and the dentate nucleus in the cerebellum)
Myoclonus	Series of shocklike, nonpatterned contractions of portion of a muscle, entire muscle, or group of muscles that cause throwing movements of a limb; usually appear at random but frequently triggered by sudden startle; do not disappear during sleep	Associated with an irritable nervous system and spontaneous discharge of neurons; structures associated with myoclonus include the cerebral cortex, cerebellum, reticular formation, and spinal cord

Table 15-23 Upper and Lower Motor Neuron Syndromes

Factor	Upper Motor Neuron Syndromes*	Lower Motor Neuron Syndromes†
Distribution of affected muscles	Muscle groups are affected; when movement is possible, the proper relationship among agonists, antagonists, synergists, and fixators is preserved	Individual muscles may be affected
	Synkinesias (residual movements) are present; attempts to move paralyzed part cause a variety of associated movements; movements of normal limb may cause imitative or mirror movements in the paralyzed limb	Individual muscles may be affected
Muscle tone	Hypertonia, specifically spasticity	Hypotonia, flaccidity
Tendon reflexes	Hyperreflexia with extensor plantar reflex present	Hyporeflexia, no abnormal reflexes present
Atrophy	Slight, caused by disuse	Pronounced atrophy
Fasciculations	Absent	May be present

*Pyramidal motor syndromes.
†All are motor unit syndromes.

eventually returns. In humans, however, injury generally involves more than merely the interruption of the pyramidal system, so that an upper motor neuron paralysis occurs, which indicates involvement of several motor pathways.

The distribution of clinical manifestations varies, depending on the location of the lesion, although certain features are constant. Excessive movements such as clonus and spasms occur regularly, and much variation exists, depending on the suddenness of onset and the age of the individual.

When the pyramidal system is destroyed below the level of the pons, spinal shock occurs. **Spinal shock** is the complete cessation of spinal cord functions below the lesion. It is characterized by complete flaccid paralysis, absence of reflexes, and marked disturbances of bowel and bladder function. The reasons for spinal shock are not fully understood, but a major factor is the sudden destruction of the efferent pathways. If destruction occurs more slowly, spinal shock may not develop (see Chapter 16).

If the pyramidal system is interrupted above the level of the pons, the hand and arm muscles are greatly affected. Paralysis rarely involves all the muscles on one side of the body, however, even when the hemiplegia results from complete damage to the internal capsule. Bilateral movements, such as those of the eye, jaw, and larynx, are affected only slightly, if at all. Predominantly the limbs are affected. Because of their bilateral control, trunk muscles are much less influenced.

Paralysis associated with a pyramidal motor syndrome rarely remains flaccid for a prolonged time. After a few days or weeks, a gradual return of spinal reflexes marks the end of spinal shock. Reflexes then become hyperactive, and muscle tone is increased significantly, particularly in anti-

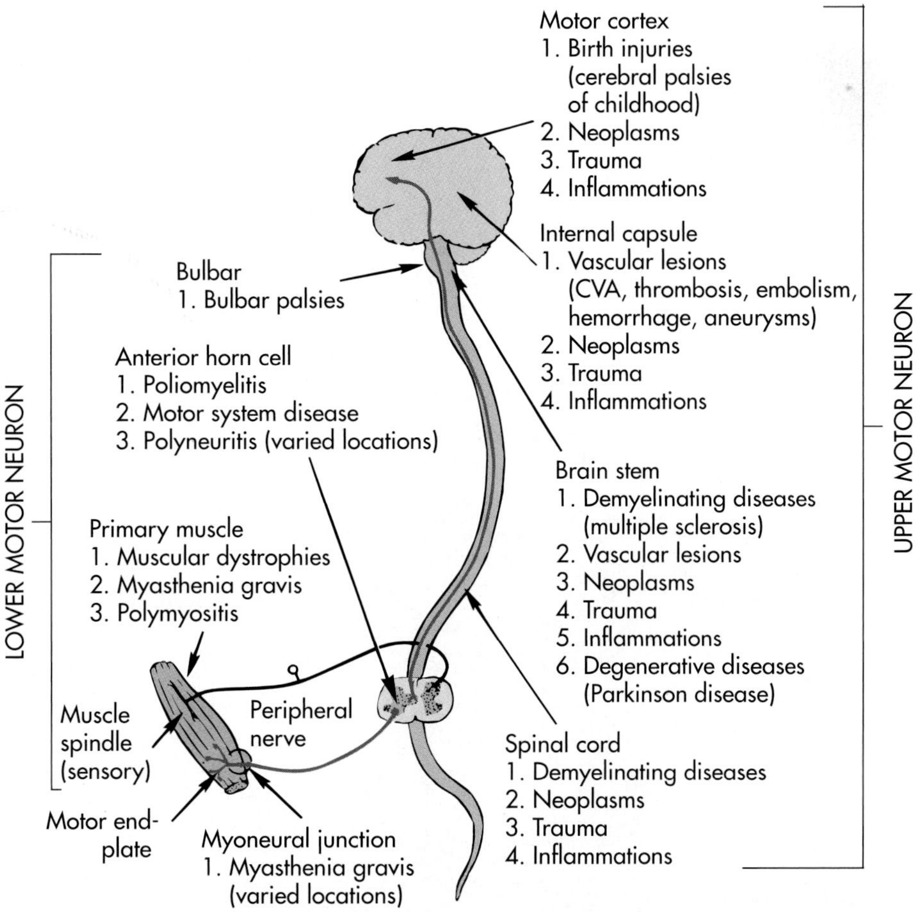

FIG. 15-18 Disturbances in motor function. Disturbances in motor function are classified pathologically along upper and lower motor neuron structures. It should be noted that the second pathologic condition occurs at more than one site in an upper motor neuron, *above right.* A few pathologic conditions involve both upper and lower motor neuron structures. Such as in amyotrophic lateral sclerosis. Other lesion sites include myoneural junction and primary muscle, making it possible to classify conditions as neuromuscular and muscular, respectively.

gravity muscles. Spasticity is common, although rigidity occasionally occurs. Most often, passive range of motion causes the "clasp-knife" phenomenon, probably because of the activation of the two varieties of stretch receptors: (1) the muscle spindles and (2) the Golgi tendon organ. (Muscle function is discussed in Chapter 40.) With pyramidal motor syndrome, predominantly the flexors of the arms and extensors of the legs are affected.

Lower motor neuron syndromes. Lower (primary, alpha) motor neurons are the large motor neurons in the anterior (or ventral) horn of the spinal cord, the motor nuclei of the brain stem, and the axons that originate from these nerve cell bodies (to course in the anterior spinal roots and the spine or in the cranial nerves to reach skeletal muscles) (Fig. 15-20). Dysfunction in this motor system impairs movement, both voluntary and involuntary. The degree of paralysis or paresis is proportional to the number of lower motor neurons affected. If only a portion of the motor units that supply a muscle are affected, only partial paralysis or paresis results. If all the motor units are affected, a complete paralysis results. Other clinical manifestations also are proportional to the degree of dysfunction, but the precise manifestations depend on the location of the dysfunction in the motor unit and in the CNS.

Small motor (gamma) neurons, which function to maintain muscle tone and protect the muscle from injury, also are necessary for normal motor movement. These neurons depend on input from the muscle spindle (arriving through an afferent limb rising to the cord). Dysfunction in this motor system impairs tone and reduces the tendon reflexes, causing hyporeflexia. The muscle is lax and soft, with a decrease in normal tone, or hypotonia, which impairs voluntary and involuntary motor movements. The muscles become susceptible to damage from hyperextensibility because the normal protective mechanisms, which prevent muscle fiber injury, are impaired. The degree of tone loss and the loss of tendon reflexes are proportional to the dysfunction in these reflex motor units.

Generally, in a pathologic process the large and small motor neuron systems are equally affected. Therefore the paresis and paralysis caused by a disorder of the lower motor neurons is called **flaccid paresis** and **flaccid paralysis,**

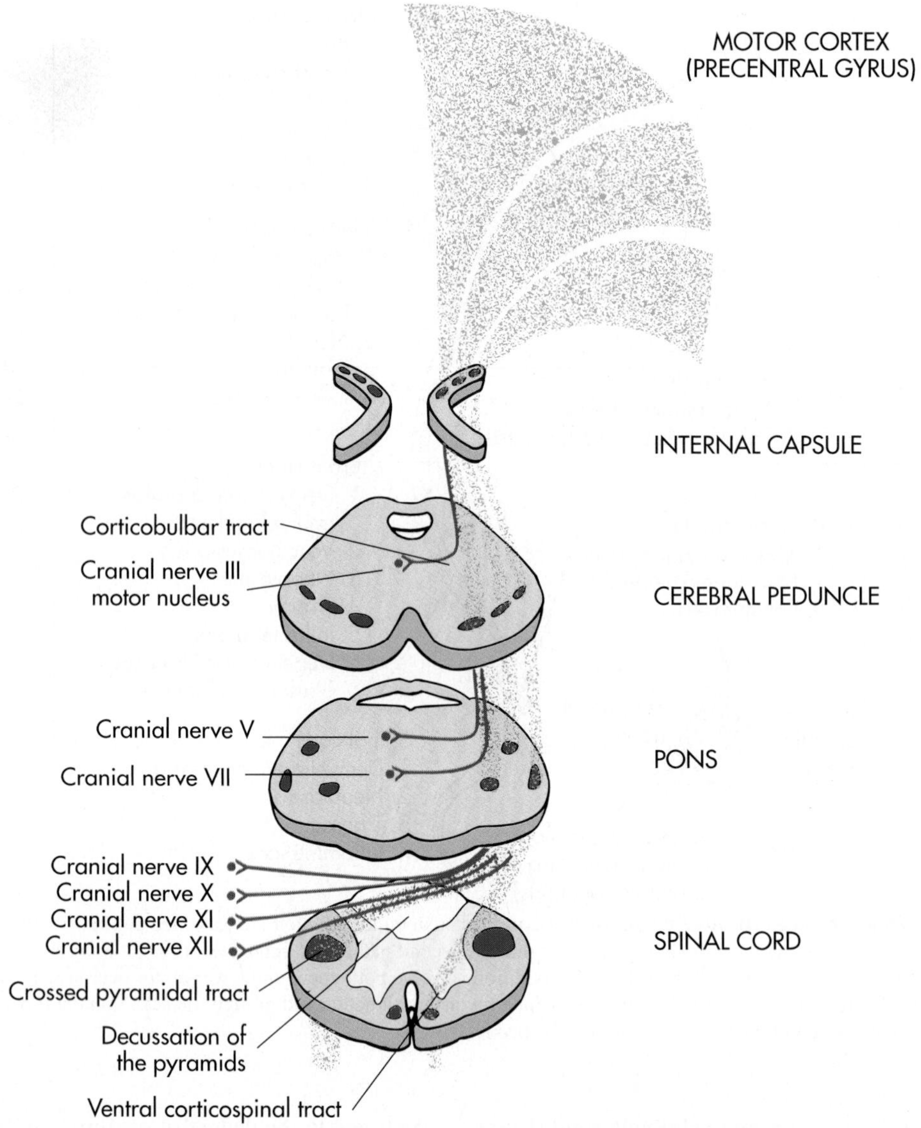

FIG. 15-19 Structures making up the upper motor neuron, or pyramidal, system. Pyramidal system fibers are shown to originate primarily in the cells in the precentral gyrus of the motor cortex; to converge at the internal capsule; to descend to form the central third of the cerebral peduncle; to descend further through the pons, where small fibers are given off to cranial nerve motor nuclei along the way; to form pyramids at the medulla, where most of the fibers decussate; and then to continue to descend in the lateral column of the white matter of the spinal cord. A few fibers descend without crossing at the medulla level.

respectively, because the muscle has reduced or absent tone and is accompanied by hyporeflexia or **areflexia** (loss of tendon reflexes).

A few **gamma neuropathies** (small motor neuron disorders) affect only the gamma motor system. A manifestation of these disorders is a marked reduction in the deep tendon reflexes, which are strikingly out of proportion to the degree of muscle weakness present.

Denervated muscles (i.e., muscles that have lost their nervous system input) undergo atrophy over weeks to months, mostly from disuse. Denervated muscles also demonstrate fasciculations, which are seen as muscle rippling or quivering under the skin. Occasionally, denervated muscles cramp. **Fibrillation** (isolated contraction of a single muscle fiber) also may occur, although this manifestation is not visible clinically.

Amyotrophies. Lower motor neuron syndromes originating in the anterior horn cells or the motor nuclei of the cranial nerves are called **amyotrophies.** Paralytic poliomyelitis is the prototype of these disorders. It involves a severe inflammatory reaction in motor neurons, some of which do not survive, leaving a permanent lower motor neuron syndrome.

Several pathologic processes may give rise to an amyotrophy. A virally induced or postinfectious or postvaccination inflammatory process may injure or destroy anterior horn cells or cranial nerve cell bodies. Most of these inflammatory processes are mild and are followed by rapid cellular recovery.

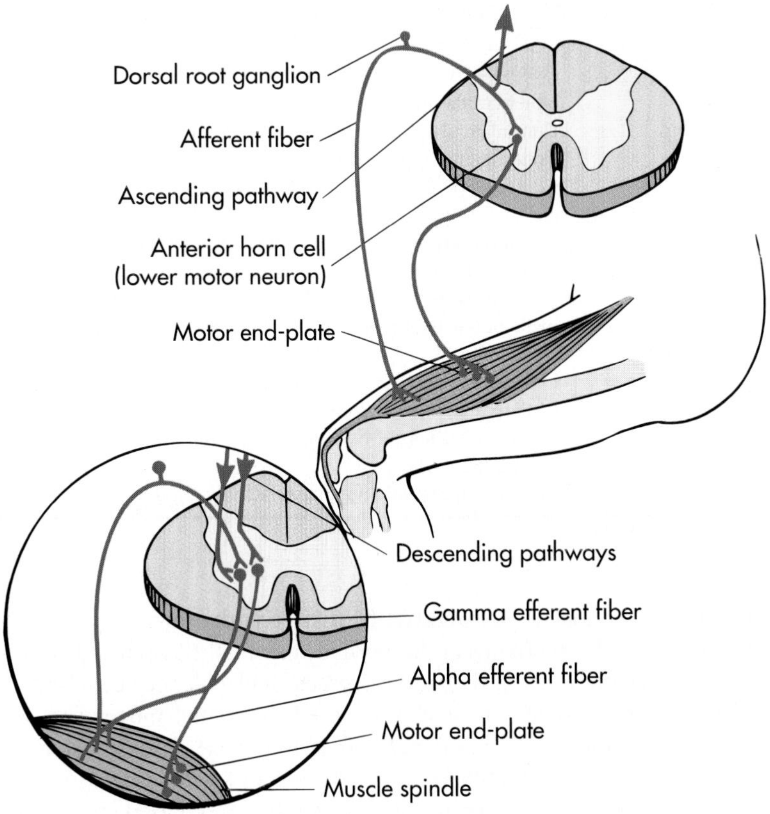

FIG. 15-20 Structures making up a lower motor neuron, including motor (efferent) and sensory (afferent) elements. *Top,* Anterior horn cell (in anterior gray column of spinal cord and its axon), terminating in motor end-plate as it innervates extrafusal muscle fibers in the quadriceps muscle. *Detailed enlargement,* Sensory and motor elements of the gamma loop system. The gamma efferent fiber is shown innervating the polar, or end, region of the muscle spindle (sensory receptor of skeletal muscle). Contraction of muscle spindle fibers stretches the central portion of the spindle and causes the afferent spindle fiber to transmit the impulse centrally to the cord. Muscle spindle afferent fibers in turn synapse on the anterior horn cell and are transmitted by way of gamma-efferent fibers to skeletal (extrafusal) muscle, causing it to contract. Muscle spindle discharge is interrupted by active contraction of extrafusal muscle fibers.

In the amyotrophies, muscle strength, muscle tone, and muscle bulk are affected in the muscles innervated by the involved motor neurons. The paresis and paralysis associated with anterior horn cell injury are segmental, but because each muscle is supplied by two or more roots, the segmental character of the weakness may be difficult to recognize. When cranial nerve motor nuclei are affected (these lack nerve roots and have only small rootlets near the point of exit from the brain stem), the distribution of the motor weakness follows that of the peripheral nerve. The weakness may involve distal muscles, proximal muscles, and the muscles of midline structures. Hypotonia and hyporeflexia or areflexia are present.

The atrophy associated with amyotrophy is segmental when the anterior horn cells of the spinal cord are involved and follows the distribution of the peripheral nerve when the motor nuclei of the cranial nerves are affected. The atrophy may be in distal, proximal, or midline muscles. Fasciculations are particularly associated with primary motor neuron injury, and muscle cramps are common. Mild fatigue is a common complaint. If the pathologic process is limited to the primary motor neuron, no sensory changes are evident.

Because degenerative disorders cause loss of nerve cells in the anterior horn or motor nuclei, the surviving cells are small, shrunken, and filled with lipofuscin. Lost neurons are replaced by astrocytes. The roots or rootlets are thin, and the muscles show denervation and atrophy.

Several brain stem syndromes involve damage to one or more of the cranial nerve nuclei. These are called **nuclear palsies** (Table 15-24) and may be caused by vascular occlusion, tumor, aneurysm, tuberculosis, or hemorrhage.

The anterior horn cells and the motor nuclei of the cranial nerves may be affected secondarily in many severe pathologic processes that primarily involve the peripheral nerves. The condition may extend proximally to affect the nerve roots or rootlets and the motor neurons themselves, a process commonly seen, for example, in Guillain-Barré syndrome. If sufficient numbers of motor neurons are destroyed, permanent loss of motor function results because regeneration of the damaged axons requires a living neuronal cell body.

A group of degenerative disorders principally cause progressive motor cell atrophy. One of these is **progressive spinal muscular atrophy,** in which the anterior horn cells of the spinal cord are the affected motor neurons. This disorder occurs in adults and closely resembles the familial progressive muscular atrophies that occur in infants and children and are considered inherited metabolic disorders (see Chapter 42). If the motor nuclei of the cranial nerves are affected instead of the anterior horn cells, the disorder is labeled **progressive bulbar palsy,** so named because the myelencephalon originally was called the bulb and a degenerative process causes a progressively more serious condition. When any lower motor neuron syndrome involves the cranial nerves that arise from the bulb (i.e., cranial nerves IX, X, and XII), the dysfunction is called a **bulbar palsy.**

The clinical manifestations of bulbar palsy include paresis or paralysis of the jaw, face, pharynx, and tongue

Table 15-24 Examples of Nuclear Palsy Syndromes

Type of Nuclear Palsy	Causes	Associated Clinical Manifestations
Ocular	Upper brain stem tumor Cerebrovascular disease in the vertebro-basilar system Aneurysm Intramedullary bleeding	Other cranial nerve signs Contralateral spastic hemiparesis/hemiplegia Contralateral hyperreflexia Contralateral extensor plantar reflex
Facial	Pontine tumor Cerebrovascular disease in the vertebro-basilar system	Paresis/paralysis of both the upper and lower facial muscles for both voluntary movement and emotionally induced movement
Vagal	Intramedullary tumor Cerebrovascular disease in the vertebro-basilar system	Ipsilateral loss of pain and temperature sensations of the face Contralateral spastic arm and leg paresis/hemiplegia Ipsilateral cerebellar signs
Hypoglossal	Intramedullary tumor Cerebrovascular disease in the vertebro-basilar system	Contralateral loss of position sense and vibration in the arm and leg Contralateral spastic hemiparesis/hemiplegia

musculature. Articulation is affected, especially articulation of the lingual *(r, n, l),* labial *(b, m, p, f),* dental *(d, t),* and palatal *(k, g)* consonants. Modulation is impaired, making the voice rasping or nasal. Pharyngeal reflexes are diminished or lost. Palate and vocal cord movement during phonation is impaired, and chewing and swallowing are affected. The facial muscles are weak, and the face appears to droop. The jaw jerk is decreased. Atrophy eventually becomes apparent, as do fasciculations. All these manifestations become progressively worse, leading to aspiration, malnutrition, possible dehydration, and an inability to communicate verbally.

Akinesia

Akinesia is a decrease in associated and voluntary movements. There is a disturbance in the time it takes to perform a movement. Akinesia is related to dysfunction of the extrapyramidal system, as in parkinsonism. Pathogenesis is related to either a deficiency of dopamine or a defect of the postsynaptic dopamine receptors, which occurs in parkinsonism (see Chapter 16).

Bradykinesia

Bradykinesia is slowness of voluntary movements. There is a disturbance in the time it takes to perform a movement. In bradykinesia all voluntary movements become slow, labored, and deliberate. Bradykinesia consists of (1) difficulty in initiating movements, (2) difficulty in continuing movements smoothly, and (3) difficulty in performing synchronous (at the same time) and consecutive tasks. Difficulty in initiating movements ranges from slight hesitancy to severe **freezing** (transient, helpless immobility). Each intended movement requires effort. Difficulty in continuing motions smoothly causes jerky, irregular, rapid movements, which then decrease in rate and amplitude until they stop. The individual is scarcely aware of the cessation. Difficulty in performing synchronous and consecutive tasks means that each motor act is performed separately. The individual is unable to integrate two acts or to change from one motor pattern to the next with a single smooth motion.

Loss of Associated Neuron Syndromes

In hypokinesia the normal, habitually associated movements that provide skill, grace, and balance to voluntary movements are lost. Decreased associated movements accompanying emotional expression cause an expressionless face, a statuelike posture, absence of speech inflection, and absence of spontaneous gestures. Decreased associated movements accompanying locomotion cause reduction in arm and shoulder movements, in hip swinging, and in rotary motion of the cervical spine.

Alterations in Complex Motor Performance

The alterations in complex motor performance include disorders of posture (stance), disorders of gait, and disorders of expression.

Disorders of Posture (Stance)

An inequality of tone in muscle groups because of a loss of normal postural reflexes results in a posturing of limbs. Many reflex systems govern tone and posture, but the most important factor in posture control is the stretch reflex, in which stretching of extensor (antigravity) muscles causes increased extensor tone and inhibited flexor tone. Four types of disorders of posture are described: (1) dystonic posture, (2) decerebrate posture, (3) basal ganglion posture, and (4) senile posture. Equilibrium and balance are disrupted when postural disorders are present.

Dystonia is the maintenance of an abnormal posture through muscular contractions. When muscular contractions are sustained for several seconds, they are called **dystonic movements,** such as in choreoathetoid movements associated with high levels of L-dopa; when contractions last for longer periods, they are called **dystonic postures,** such as in torticollis. Dystonic postures may last for weeks, causing permanent fixed contractures. Dystonia has been associated with basal ganglia abnormality, but the exact pathophysiologic mechanisms are unknown. One particularly relevant dystonic posture already discussed in this chapter is decorticate (striatal posture or upper motor neuron dysfunction posture), which may be unilateral or bilateral in occurrence. **Decorticate posture** (also referred to as **antigravity posture** or **hemiplegic posture**) is characterized by upper extremities flexed at the elbows and held close to the body and by lower extremities that are externally rotated and extended. Decorticate posture is believed to occur when the brain stem, which facilitates the antigravity position, is not inhibited by the motor function of the cerebral cortex. Upper motor neuron posture is more commonly described as the arm flexed at the elbow, with a wristdrop; the leg inadequately bent at the knee, with the hip excessively circumabducted; and the presence of a footdrop.

Decerebrate posture refers to increased tone in extensor muscles and trunk muscles, with active tonic neck reflexes. When the head is in a neutral position, all four limbs are rigidly extended. The decerebrate posture is caused by severe injury to the brain and brain stem, resulting in overstimulation of the postural righting and vestibular reflexes.

Basal ganglion posture refers to a stooped, hyperflexed posture with a narrow-based, short-stepped gait. This posture abnormality results from the loss of normal postural reflexes and not from defects in proprioceptive, labyrinthine, or visual function. Dysfunctional equilibrium results from the loss of postural stability, and thus the individual is unable to make the appropriate postural adjustment to tilting or loss of balance and falls instead. Dysfunctional righting is the inability to right oneself when changing from a lying or crouching to a standing position or when rolling from the supine to the lateral or prone position. Dysfunctional postural fixation is the involuntary flexion of the head and neck, causing the person difficulty in maintaining an upright trunk position while standing or walking. Basal ganglion dysfunction accounts for this posture.

Senile posture is characterized by an increasingly flexed posture similar to that caused by basal ganglion dysfunction. The posture is associated with frontal lobe dysfunction, but the primary pathophysiology is not well described.

Disorders of Gait

Four predominant types of gait disorder are (1) upper motor neuron dysfunction gait, (2) cerebellar (ataxic) gait, (3) basal ganglion gait, and (4) senile (pseudoparkinsonian) gait. As with posture, equilibrium and balance are affected with gait disturbances.

Several upper motor neuron gaits exist. In the presence of mild upper motor neuron dysfunction, a footdrop may appear only with fatigue. The individual may complain of hip and leg pain. A **spastic gait,** which is associated with unilateral injury, manifests by a shuffling gait with the leg extended and held stiff, causing a scraping over the floor surface. There is an impaired leg swing around the body rather than an appropriate lifting and placing of the leg. The foot may drag on the ground, and the person tends to fall to the affected side. A **scissors gait** is associated with bilateral injury and spasticity. The legs are abducted, causing them to touch each other. As the person walks, the legs are still swung around the body but then cross in front of each other because of adduction. Injury to the pyramidal system accounts for these gaits.

A **cerebellar gait** manifests as a wide-based gait with the feet apart and often turned outward or inward for greater stability. The pelvis is held stiff, and it seems to be independent of the trunk. The individual staggers when walking. Cerebellar dysfunction accounts for this particular gait.

A **basal ganglion gait** and a **senile gait** are both broad-based gaits. The person walks with small steps and a decreased arm swing. The head and body are flexed and the arms semiflexed and abducted while the legs are flexed and rigid in more advanced states. Basal ganglion and frontal lobe dysfunction, respectively, account for these two gaits.

Disorders of Expression

Disorders of expression involve the motor aspects of communication and include (1) hypermimesis, (2) hypomimesis, and (3) dyspraxias and apraxias. Hypermimesis is a disinhibition phenomenon that most commonly manifests as pathologic laughter or crying. Pathologic laughter is associated with right hemisphere injury, and pathologic crying is associated with left hemisphere injury. The exact pathophysiology is not known. Hypomimesis manifests as aprosody, or the loss of emotional language. Receptive aprosody involves an inability to understand emotion in speech and facial expression, whereas expressive aprosody involves the inability to express emotion in speech and facial expression. Aprosody is associated with right hemisphere damage.

Dyspraxia is the partial inability and **apraxia** is the complete inability to perform purposeful or skilled motor acts in the absence of paralysis, sensory loss, abnormal posture and tone, abnormal involuntary movement, incoordination, or inattentiveness. Dyspraxia and apraxia are associated with vascular disorders, trauma, tumor, degenerative disorders, infections, and metabolic disorders. Because the performance of any activity is composed of three parts—(1) the development of the idea, (2) the formulation of the plan of execution, and (3) the motor performance of the activity—three types of dyspraxia have been described (Table 15-25).

True dyspraxias occur when the connecting pathways between the left and right cortical areas are interrupted (Fig. 15-21). Dyspraxias may result from any pathologic process that disrupts the cortical areas necessary for the conceptualization and execution of a complex motor act or the communication pathways within the left hemisphere or between the hemispheres.

Extrapyramidal Motor Syndromes

Because the extrapyramidal system encompasses all the motor pathways except the pyramidal system, two types of motor dysfunction make up the **extrapyramidal motor syndromes:** (1) the basal ganglia motor syndromes and (2) the cerebellar motor syndromes. Unlike pyramidal motor syndromes, both extrapyramidal motor syndromes result in

Table 15-25 Dyspraxias

Types	Description	Location
DYSPRAXIAS DESCRIBING THE COMPONENTS OF A MOTOR ACT		
Ideational	Impairment in ability to comprehend, grasp an idea, or retain the idea of the described act	Diffuse cortical injury, general suppression of cortex
Ideomotor (ideokinetic)	Impairment in ability to formulate an organized idea of action; cannot create mental image (but habitual motor acts may be performed spontaneously or repetitiously)	Associated with left hemisphere dysfunction in the posterosuperior area of temporal lobe and in the inferior areas of parietal and frontal lobes
Motor (limb, kinetic)	Impairment in use of kinesthetic memory patterns (engrams) necessary to perform a motor act; automatic tone and position changes necessary for action do not occur	Associated with premotor area dysfunction, usually limited to contralateral extremity
DYSPRAXIAS RELATED TO SPECIFIC TYPES OF MOTOR ACTIVITY		
Constructional	Impairment in ability to draw or use shapes and designs accurately	May occur with visual association area dysfunction and with posterior parietal lobe injury; more severe when right posterior hemisphere is involved rather than left hemisphere because right parietooccipital area controls visuospatial orientation
Dressing	Impairment in ability to clothe oneself correctly; agnosia and neglect syndrome contribute to dressing dyspraxia and may be entirely responsible for its occurrence	Associated with right parietal injury
Speech	An articulation disorder resulting from impairment of capacity to program positioning of speech musculature and sequencing of muscle movements for volitional production of speech sounds (phonemes); a motor dyspraxia	Associated with dysfunction in Broca area in left hemisphere
	When involvement is more extensive than just muscles used in speech articulation, the dysfunction is called *facial dyspraxia*	Associated with dysfunction in Broca area and premotor areas controlling facial muscles
Gait (frontal lobe ataxia, frontal lobe gait)	Impairment in ability to use extremities effectively and in coordinated manner during ambulation, producing a low, shuffling gait with small, hesitant steps	Associated with loss of integration between cortex and basal ganglion related to stance and locomotion; not a true dyspraxia because dysfunction is not purely cortical
Callosal	An ideomotor dyspraxia in which right arm and leg use is normal but with impairment in ability to perform the same movements with left arm and leg	Associated with anterior corpus callosum injury

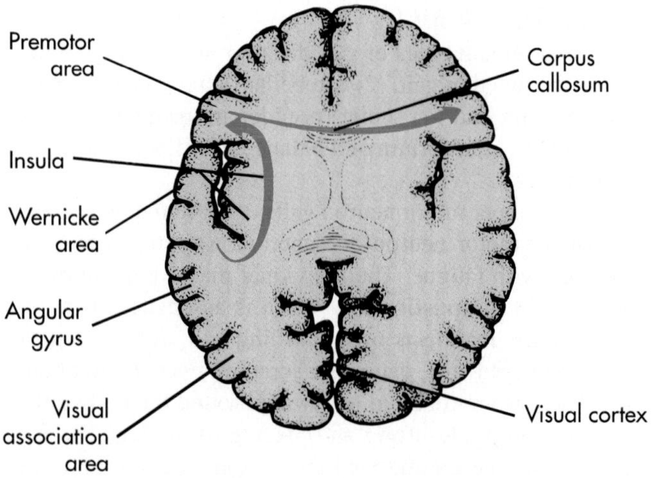

FIG. 15-21 Pathways disrupted in dyspraxias. Formulation of the idea of the motor act is believed to originate in the region of the supramarginal gyrus in the inferior left parietal lobe. This area is connected via associational pathways to the left premotor cortex. The left premotor cortex is connected through the corpus callosum to the right premotor and motor areas. An injury that interrupts the pathways between the left supramarginal gyrus and the premotor region produces a dyspraxia that involves the entire body. An injury that disrupts the callosal pathways produces a dyspraxia of the left side of the body only.

Table 15-26 Pyramidal versus Extrapyramidal Motor Syndrome

Manifestations	Pyramidal Motor Syndrome	Extrapyramidal Motor Syndrome
Unilateral movement	Paralysis of voluntary movement	Little or no paralysis of voluntary movement
Tendon reflexes	Increased tendon reflexes	Normal or slightly increased tendon reflexes
Babinski sign	Present	Absent
Involuntary movements	Absence of involuntary movements	Presence of tremor, chorea, athetosis, or dystonia
Muscle tone	Spasticity in muscles (e.g., clasp-knife phenomenon)	Plastic (equal throughout movement) rigidity or intermittent (cogwheel) rigidity generalized but predominate in flexors of limbs and trunk
	Hypertonia present in flexors of arms and extensors of legs	Hypotonia in cerebellar disease

Table 15-27 Cerebellar Motor Syndromes

Syndrome	Location of Dysfunction	Characteristics
Lateral	Intermediate and lateral corticonuclear zone of anterior and posterior lobes	Muscles of the extremities on the side of the injury become hypotonic with decreased resistance to passive movement Reflexes are hypoactive Ataxia (uncoordination) of extremities is prevalent during voluntary movement, causing some degree of gait disturbance Dysmetria (extremity overshooting its target) occurs Intentional and postural tremors are present
Medial	Medical corticonuclear zone and flocculonodular lobe	Disequilibrium of head and trunk are present during static posture and locomotion Posture and gait are normal Oculomotor disturbances are common Muscle tone is normal Extremities are not ataxic in voluntary movement

movement or posture disturbance without significant paralysis, along with other distinctive symptoms (Table 15-26).

Basal Ganglia Motor Syndromes

Basal ganglia motor syndromes are movement disorders that involve either a paucity or an excess of movements. Stress and nervous tension typically worsen the symptoms, whereas relaxation improves motor performance. Akinesia may occur despite normal strength. Involuntary movements, such as tremor, chorea, ballism, athetosis, and dystonia, also may occur and probably are caused by the loss of the normal modulating effects of the corpus striatum and other parts of the basal ganglia.

Basal ganglia motor syndromes also are characterized by alterations in muscle tone and posture. Rigidity, together with the cogwheel phenomenon, is present in all muscle groups but is most prominent in those that maintain flexed position. Postural abnormalities result from the loss of normal postural reflexes. Dysfunctional equilibrium results from the loss of postural stability.

The symptoms of basal ganglia motor syndromes are explained as an imbalance of dopaminergic and cholinergic activity in the corpus striatum. A relative excess of cholinergic activity produces akinesia and hypertonia. A relative excess of dopaminergic activity produces hyperkinesia and hypotonia. The precise mechanisms by which imbalances of these striatal neurotransmitters cause specific symptoms are unknown.

Cerebellar Motor Syndromes

Cerebellar motor syndromes involve the cerebellum and may result in (1) loss of muscle tone; (2) difficulty with coordination of voluntary movements; (3) minor degrees of muscle weakness, tendency toward fatigue, and impairment of associated movements; and (4) disorders of equilibrium and gait. Cerebellar effects are chiefly ipsilateral (primarily affecting the same side of the body), so damage to the right cerebellum generally causes symptoms on the right side of the body. Predominant symptoms depend on the area of damage within the cerebellum. The two cerebellar syndromes are the lateral syndrome and the medial syndrome (Table 15-27).

Diagnosis of a cerebellar motor syndrome is based on the symptoms, but these may vary because of the individual's attempts at compensation. Further, the nervous system often can operate well despite destruction of parts of the cerebellum, although the mechanisms responsible for this retained function are not fully understood.

SUMMARY REVIEW

Alterations in Cognitive Systems

1. Full consciousness is an awareness of oneself and the environment with an ability to respond to external stimuli with a wide variety of responses.
2. Consciousness has two components: arousal and content of thought.
3. Decreased level of arousal occurs by diffuse bilateral cortical dysfunction, bilateral subcortical (reticular formation, brain stem) dysfunction, and localized hemispheric dysfunction.
4. An alteration in breathing pattern and level of coma reflects the level of brain dysfunction.
5. Pupillary changes reflect changes in level of brain stem function, drug action, and response to hypoxia and ischemia.
6. Abnormal eye movements, including nystagmus and divergent gaze, reflect alterations in brain stem function.
7. Level of brain function manifests by changes in generalized motor responses or no responses.
8. Loss of cortical inhibition associated with decreased consciousness includes abnormal flexor and extensor movements.
9. Cerebral death or irreversible coma represents permanent brain damage, with an ability to maintain cardiac, respiratory, and other vital functions.
10. Brain death results from irreversible brain damage, with an inability to maintain internal homeostasis.
11. Arousal returns in vegetative states and minimally conscious states, but content of thought is absent or markedly reduced, respectively.
12. Seizures represent a sudden, chaotic discharge of cerebral neurons, with transient alterations in brain function. Seizures may be generalized or focal and can result from cerebral lesions, biochemical disorders, trauma, or epilepsy.
13. With a deficit in selective attention, mediated by the brain stem, parietal lobe structures, and the pulvinar, the individual cannot focus on selective stimuli and thus neglects those stimuli.
14. In dysmnesia and amnesia, some past memories are not retrieved and new memories cannot be stored.
15. Frontal areas mediate vigilance, detection, and working memory.
16. With a vigilance deficit, the person cannot maintain alertness.
17. With a detection deficit, the person is unmotivated and unable to use feedback.
18. Some specific disorders of content of thought (cognition) are agnosias, dysphasias, acute confusional states, and dementias, including Alzheimer disease.
19. Agnosias are a defect of recognition and may be tactile, visual, or auditory. They are caused by dysfunction in the primary sensory area or the interpretive areas of the cerebral cortex.
20. Dysphasia is an impairment of comprehension or production of language. Dysphasia may be expressive or sensory.
21. Aphasia is loss of language comprehension or production.
22. Wernicke dysphasia is a disturbance in understanding all language—both verbal and reading comprehension.
23. Conductive dysphasias result from disruption of temporal lobe fibers, with a failure to repeat words but an ability to initiate speech, writing, and reading aloud.
24. Anomic dysphasia is an inability to name objects, persons, or qualities.
25. Transcortical dysphasias involve an inability to repeat and recite.
26. Broca aphasia is an expressive dysphasia of speech and writing but with retention of comprehension.
27. Global aphasia involves both anterior and posterior speech areas, with both expressive and receptive aphasia.
28. Acute confusional states are characterized chiefly by a loss of detection and, in the case of delirium, an intense autonomic nervous system hyperactivity.
29. Alzheimer disease is a chronic, irreversible dementia.

Alterations in Cerebral Hemodynamics

1. Cerebral oxygen is a critical issue.
2. Cerebral perfusion pressure determines cerebral blood flow.
3. An injured brain may experience cerebral oligemia, normal cerebral blood flow but with increased intracranial pressure, or cerebral hyperemia.
4. Increased intracranial pressure may result from edema, excess CSF, hemorrhage, or tumor growth. When intracranial pressure approaches arterial pressure, hypoxia and hypercapnia produce brain damage.
5. Cerebral edema is an increase in the fluid content of the brain resulting from infection, hemorrhage, tumor, ischemia, infarct, or hypoxia.
6. The shifting or herniation of brain tissue from one compartment to another disrupts the blood flow of both compartments and damages brain tissue.
7. Supratentorial herniation involves temporal lobe and hippocampal gyrus shifting from the middle fossa to the posterior fossa; transtentorial herniation with a downward shift of the diencephalon through the tentorial notch; and shifting of the cingulate gyrus herniation under the falx.
8. The most common infratentorial herniation is a shift of the cerebellar tonsils through the foramen magnum.
9. Hydrocephalus comprises a variety of disorders characterized by an excess of fluid within the cranial vault, subarachnoid space, or both. Hydrocephalus occurs because of interference with CSF flow caused by increased fluid production or obstruction within the ventricular system or by defective reabsorption of the fluid.
10. Hydrocephalus can be treated by reducing CSF in the ventricles through the use of shunts and diuretic therapy if resection of the cause is not possible.

Alterations in Emotions and Mood

1. Disorders of the frontal lobes, limbic system, or hypothalamus may be associated with a broad range of changes in emotion and behavior.

Alterations in Motor Function

1. Motor dysfunction may be characterized as alterations of motor tone, movement, and complex motor performance.
2. Hypotonia and hypertonia are the main categories of altered tone.
3. Four types of hypertonia exist: spasticity, gegenhalten, dystonia, and rigidity.
4. Hyperkinesia and hypokinesia are the main categories of altered movement.
5. Included in the category of hyperkinesia are chorea, athetosis, ballism, akathisia, tremor, and myoclonus.

6. Types of hypokinesia include paresis and paralysis, akinesia, bradykinesia, and loss of associated movements.
7. Two subtypes of paresis and paralysis are described: upper motor neuron and lower motor neuron.
8. An upper motor neuron syndrome is characterized by paresis or paralysis, hypertonia, and hyperreflexia.
9. Interruption of the pyramidal tract below the pons results in spinal shock.
10. Lower motor neuron syndromes manifest with impaired voluntary and involuntary movements.
11. Partial paralysis occurs with only partial loss of alpha motor neurons, and total paralysis is complete loss of alpha motor neurons. Loss of gamma motor neurons impairs muscle tone and decreases tendon reflexes.
12. Amyotrophy (e.g., poliomyelitis) is a lower motor neuron syndrome involving the anterior horn cells, with loss of muscle tone and strength resulting in segmental paresis and hyporeflexia.
13. Nuclear palsies involve damage to the cranial nerve nuclei.
14. Bulbar palsies involve cranial nerves IX, X, and XII.
15. Alterations in complex motor performance include disorders of posture (stance), disorders of gait, and disorders of expression.
16. Disorders of posture include dystonic posture, decerebrate posture, basal ganglion posture, and senile posture.
17. Disorders of gait include upper motor neuron gaits, cerebellar gait, basal ganglion gait, and senile gait.
18. Disorders of expression include hypermimesis, hypomimesis, and dyspraxia or apraxia.
19. Dyspraxia is an impairment of the conceptualization or execution of a complex motor act.
20. Extrapyramidal motor syndromes include basal ganglia and cerebellar motor syndromes.
21. Basal ganglia disorders manifest by alterations in muscle tone and posture, including rigidity, involuntary movements, and loss of postural reflexes.
22. Cerebellar motor syndromes result in loss of muscle tone, difficulty with coordination, and disorders of equilibrium and gait.

KEY TERMS

Acute confusional state (acute cerebral failure, acute brain failure), *459*
Acute hydrocephalus, *469*
Agnosia, *457*
Akinesia, *480*
Akinetic mutism (AM), *447*
Alzheimer disease (dementia of Alzheimer type [DAT], senile disease complex), *462*
Amyotrophy, *478*
Aphasia, *457*
Apraxia, *481*
Areflexia, *478*
Aura, *450*
Autoregulation, *467*
Basal ganglia motor syndrome, *483*
Basal ganglion gait, *481*
Basal ganglion posture, *481*
Brain death (brain stem death), *446*
Bulbar palsy, *479*
Central herniation, *467*
Cerebellar gait, *481*
Cerebellar motor syndrome, *483*
Cerebral death, *446*
Cerebral edema, *468*
Cingulate gyrus herniation, *467*
Clonic phase, *450*
Clonus, *472*
Coma, *446*
Communicating (extraventricular) hydrocephalus, *469*
Content of thought, *438*
Cytotoxic (metabolic) edema, *468*
Decerebrate posture, *481*
Decorticate posture (antigravity posture, hemiplegic posture), *481*
Dementia, *460*
Detection deficit, *454*
Diplegia, *474*
Dysmnesia, *453*
Dysphasia, *457*
Dyspraxia, *481*
Dystonia, *480*
Dystonic movement, *480*
Dystonic posture, *480*
Echolalia, *459*
Epilepsy, *448*
Epileptogenic focus, *449*
Expressive dysphasia, *459*
Extinction, *453*
Extrapyramidal motor syndrome, *481*
Fibrillation, *478*
Flaccid paralysis, *477*
Flaccid paresis, *477*
Freezing, *480*
Gamma neuropathy, *478*
Gegenhalten (paratonia), *472*
Generalized seizure, *448*
Hemiparesis, *474*
Hemiplegia, *474*
Hydrocephalus, *469*
Hydrocephalus ex vacuo, *469*
Hyperkinesia, *474*
Hypertonia, *472*
Hypotonia, *471*
Increased intracranial pressure, *466*
Interstitial edema, *468*
Intracranial pressure, *466*
Ischemic edema, *468*
Isolated speech center, *459*
Locked-in syndrome, *447*
Metabolic arousal alteration, *438*
Minimally conscious state (MSC), *447*
Mirror focus, *450*
Mixed transcortical dysphasia, *459*
Neglect syndrome, *453*
Neurofibrillary tangle, *465*
Noncommunicating hydrocephalus, *469*
Normal-pressure hydrocephalus, *469*
Nuclear palsy, *479*
Paralysis, *474*
Paraparesis, *474*
Paraplegia, *474*
Paresis, *474*
Paroxysmal dyskinesia, *474*
Partial seizure (focal seizure), *448*
Pattern recognition (remote memory) deficit, *453*
Postictal state, *449*
Prodroma, *450*
Progressive bulbar palsy, *479*
Progressive spinal muscular atrophy, *479*
Psychogenic arousal alteration, *438*
Pyramidal motor syndrome, *474*
Quadriparesis, *474*
Quadriplegia, *474*
Recent memory system, *453*
Rigidity, *473*
Scissors gait, *481*
Secondary generalization, *448*
Seizure, *447*
Selective attention deficit, *453*
Senile gait, *481*
Senile plaque, *465*
Senile posture, *481*
Sensory inattentiveness, *453*
Spastic gait, *481*
Spasticity, *472*

KEY TERMS—cont'd

Spinal shock, *476*
Status epilepticus, *449*
Structural arousal alteration, *438*
Tardive dyskinesia, *474*
Tonic phase, *450*
Transcortical dysphasia, *459*
Transcortical sensory dysphasia, *459*
Uncal herniation, *467*
Vasogenic edema, *468*
Vegetative state, *446*
Vigilance deficit, *454*
Working memory deficit, *454*

REFERENCES

1. Plum F, Posner JB: *The diagnosis of stupor and coma,* Philadelphia, 1980, FA Davis.
2. Giacino JT, Kalmar K: The vegetative and minimally conscious states: a comparison of clinical features and functional outcome, *J Head Trauma Rehab* 12(4):36, 1997.
3. Ropper AH, Martin JB: Coma and other disorders of consciousness. In Isselbacher KJ et al, editors: *Harrison's principles of internal medicine,* New York, 1994, McGraw-Hill.
4. Walker AE: *Cerebral death,* ed 3, Baltimore, 1985, Urban & Schwarzenberg.
5. Giacino JT, Zasler ND: Outcome after severe traumatic brain injury: coma, the vegetative and minimally responsive state, *J Head Trauma Rehab* 10(1):40, 1995.
6. Giacino JT et al: Development of practice guidelines for assessment and management of the vegetative and minimally conscious states, *J Head Trauma Rehab* 12(4):79, 1997.
7. The Multi-Society Task Force on PVS: Medical aspects of the persistent vegetative state, *N Engl J Med* 330:1572, 1994.
8. Andrews K: International working party on the management of the vegetative state: summary report, *Brain Injury* 10(11):797, 1996.
9. American Congress of Rehabilitation Medicine: Recommendations for the use of uniform nomenclature pertinent to patients with severe alterations in consciousness, *Arch Phys Med Rehabil* 76:205, 1995.
10. Perkin GD: *Mosby's color atlas and text of neurology,* London, 1998, Mosby-Wolfe.
11. Glausiusz J: The genes of 1996, *Discover* 150, 1996.
12. Schacter SC, Saper CB: Vagus nerve stimulation, *Epilepsia* 38(7):677, 1998.
13. Snivelly C, Cownsell C, Lilly D: Vagus nerve stimulator as a treatment for intractable epilepsy, *J Neurosurg Nurs* 30(5):286, 1998.
14. Posner JI, Raichle ME: *Images of mind,* New York, 1994, Scientific American Library.
15. Jacques A, Jackson GA: *Understanding dementia,* ed 3, London, 2000, Churchill Livingstone.
16. Selkoe DJ: The origins of Alzheimer disease: a is for amyoid, *JAMA* 283:1615, 2000.
17. Strittmatter WJ, Roses AD: Apolipoprotein E and Alzheimer's disease, *Annu Rev Neurosci* 19:53, 1996.
18. Nashlund J et al: Correlation between elevated levels of amyloid B peptide in the brain and cognitive decline, *JAMA* 283:1571, 2000.
19. Travis J: New insight into Alzheimer's disease, *Sci News* 156:319, 1999.
20. Bullock R et al: *Guidelines for the management of severe head injury,* Park Ridge, 1995, Brain Trauma Foundation and AANS.
21. Gupta AK, Bullock MR: Monitoring the injured brain in intensive care: present and future, *Hosp Med* 59:704, 1998.
22. Chestnut RN: Treating raised intracranial pressure in head injury. In Naryan RK, Wilberger JE, Povilshock JT, editors: *Neurotrauma,* New York, 1996, McGraw-Hill.
23. Bower B: Dendrite decline in schizophrenia, *Sci News* 157:91, 2000.
24. Bower B: DNA links reported for schizophrenia, *Sci News* 154:151, 1998.

CHAPTER 16

Alterations of Neurologic Function

BARBARA J. BOSS

CHAPTER OUTLINE

Alterations in central nervous system (CNS) function are caused by traumatic injury, vascular disorders, tumor growth, infectious and inflammatory processes, metabolic derangements (including those arising from nutritional deficiencies and drugs/chemicals), and degenerative processes. Alterations in peripheral nervous system function involve the nerve roots (radiculopathies), a nerve plexus, or the nerves themselves (neuropathies). Disorders of the neuromuscular junction also occur.

CENTRAL NERVOUS SYSTEM DISORDERS

Trauma

Brain Trauma

Major head injury or **traumatic brain injury (TBI)** is defined by the National Head Injury Foundation as a traumatic insult to the brain capable of producing physical, intellectual, emotional, social, and vocational changes. Of the 2 million head injuries in the United States each year, 1.6 million are mild injuries not requiring hospitalization. Of the 500,000 TBIs requiring hospitalization, 450,000 persons are admitted to the hospital alive; 80% have mild TBIs, 10% moderate TBIs, and 10% severe TBIs.[1] The Glasgow Coma Scale (GCS) is used to describe injury severity by the international and United States National Traumatic Coma Data Banks. Hallmark of a severe TBI is loss of consciousness for 6 hours or more. TBI classification using the GCS are (1) mild TBI with GCS of 13 to 15, (2) moderate TBI with GCS of 9 to 12, and (3) severe BTI with GCS of 3 to 8.[2] Age and admission GCS are important diagnostic factors in traumatic brain injury.[3,4,5]

Persons at highest risk for TBI are young persons 15 to 30 years of age, infants 6 months to 2 years, young school-age children, and elderly individuals. The male/female ratio for such injury is 3:1. TBI is highest among blacks and in lower-median income families. Persons living in high-crime areas are at greater risk.

Head injuries are broadly categorized into **blunt (closed, nonmissile) trauma** and **open (penetrating, missile) trauma.** Blunt trauma, the more common, involves the head striking a hard surface or a rapidly moving object striking the head. The dura mater remains intact, and brain tissues are not exposed to the environment. Blunt trauma may result in both focal brain injuries and diffuse axonal injuries (Table 16-1). When a break in (penetration of) the dura mater results in exposure of the cranial contents to the environment, open trauma has occurred, which results in focal brain injuries.

The most common types of brain injury are mild concussion and classic cerebral concussion (see p. 493). Of all head injuries, 75% to 90% are not severe (see Table 16-1). Focal brain injury and diffuse axonal injury (DAI) each account for one half of all injuries. Focal brain injury accounts for more than two thirds of head injury deaths; DAI, for fewer than one third. However, DAI accounts for the greatest number of severely disabled survivors, including persons who persist in an unresponsive state or reduced level of consciousness.

In recent years the surviving traumatic brain injury population has changed, mostly because of focus on reducing severity of injury (e.g., passive seat restraints, air bags), reduced transport time, and improved on-the-scene medical management. Improved management of secondary and tertiary injury also is influencing the situation; acute care health professionals are beginning to focus more on morbidity than mortality. As a result, persons with more severe traumatic brain injuries are being admitted to rehabilitation programs.

Cause

Most traumatic brain injuries are caused by motor vehicle accidents (MVAs) (50%) and falls (21%). Sports-related events (10%) and violence (12%) also account for a portion of craniocerebral traumatic brain injuries.[1]

Related to focal brain injuries, objects (e.g., baseball bat, weapon) striking the front of the head usually produce only coup injuries (contusions and fractures) because the inner skull in the occipital area is smooth. Objects striking the back of the head usually result in both **coup** (directly below the point of impact) and **contrecoup** (on the pole opposite the site of impact) **injuries** because of the irregularity of the inner surface of the frontal bones (Fig. 16-1). Objects striking the side of the head may produce coup or contrecoup injuries. The same is true for the head striking an immovable object with little velocity (e.g., a short fall).

Extradural hematomas, a form of secondary injury, are caused most commonly by motor vehicle crashes (MVCs) and occasionally by minor falls and sporting accidents. A temporal fracture causes 90% of temporal lobe extradural hematomas. Direct frontal lobe trauma is associated with frontal extradural hematomas. Posterior extradural hematomas are associated with a fracture across the transverse sinus from an occipital blow.

MVCs are the most common cause of subdural hematomas; 50% of subdural hematomas are associated with skull fractures. Falls, especially in elderly people or in persons with long-term alcohol abuse, are associated with chronic subdural hematomas.

Intracerebral hemorrhage is associated with the presence of contusions. This hemorrhage is caused by forceful impact, usually associated with MVCs and falls from some distance.

Table 16-1 Severity of Trauma Related to Injury, Onset, and Persistence

	Trauma State Induced			
Severity of Trauma	Focal Injury	DAI	Onset of Clinical Manifestations	Persistence of DAI Clinical Manifestations
Mild blunt trauma		Mild concussion	Immediate	Hours to days
Moderate blunt trauma		Classic cerebral concussion	Immediate	Up to 6 mo or longer
	Paraplegia (associated with injury to top of head)		Immediate	
	Blindness (associated with occipital injury)		Immediate	
	Delayed development of unresponsiveness (vasomotor or vasovagal syncopal episode)		Delayed	
Severe blunt trauma		Mild DAI	Immediate	Permanent residual
		Moderate DAI	Immediate	
		Severe DAI	Immediate	
	Acute epidural hemorrhage		Immediate to delayed (2-3 hr)	
	Acute contusional swelling		Delayed onset (few hours after injury)	
	Acute subdural hematoma		Delayed onset (few hours to 1 wk after injury)	
	Subacute subdural hematoma*		Delayed onset (1 to few weeks)	
	Subdural hygroma		Delayed onset	
	Traumatic cerebral hemorrhage*		Delayed onset (as late as 1 wk after injury)	

*May be seen after moderate head injury, especially in elderly persons.
DAI, Diffuse axonal injury.

Compound fractures are caused by objects striking the head with great force or by the head striking an object forcefully. The comments regarding contusion hold true for compound fractures. Temporal blows, related to basilar skull fractures, may produce a fracture involving the middle fossa. An occipital blow may result in a basilar fracture down the occipital bone and across the petrous pyramid. The cervical vertebrae upwardly impacting the base of the skull can produce a posterior fossa **basilar skull fracture.**

Causes of penetrating injuries are missiles (most commonly bullets fired from rifles and handguns) and sharp projectiles (e.g., knives, ice picks, axes, screwdrivers). Most through-and-through injuries are from high-velocity bullets.

Related to DAI, mild concussion and classic cerebral concussion are particularly associated with a moving head striking a hard, unyielding object. A concussion may result from a moving object striking a stationary head, however. Moderate DAI is usually sustained by occupants of vehicles and pedestrians. Sagittal or horizontal (torsional) head motion produces mild or moderate DAI. Severe DAI occurs only in coronal (lateral) head motion and is caused by injuries sustained in MVCs.

Pathophysiology

Damage originates from three mechanisms: primary, secondary, and tertiary injury. Primary injury is caused by the impact and involves neural injury, primary glial injury, and vascular response. In primary glial injury, oligodendroglia is affected by axon injury and by direct mechanical disruption caused by debris and leakage. The vascular response is immediate at the time of injury and involves increased capillary endothelial permeability to solutes. Secondary injury includes cerebral edema, brain swelling, hemorrhage, infection, and increased intracranial pressure. Significant to secondary injury is tissue hypoxia arising from cerebral ischemia (inadequate perfusion and tissue hypoxia). Consequences of ischemia are as follows: (1) ischemic neurons release substances that produce glial permeability to sodium (cytotoxic edema); (2) with energy failure, influxes of calcium through incompetent channels produce electrophysiologic consequences and activation of phospholipases to release free fatty acids with reoxygenation, prostaglandins, and free radicals; and (3) lactic acidosis occurs. Secondary injury occurs from compromise of circulation or brain shift. Tertiary injury is caused by apnea, hypotension, change in pulmonary resistance, and change in electrocardiogram (ECG), specifically ST and T wave changes.

Primary injury. Insight into the nature of the injury and its potential effects can be obtained from information about the causal agent and from the nature, extent, and site of damage. Knowledge of the cellular biology of head injury has progressed dramatically over the past 20 years. Previously, no explanation existed for why persons with similar computed tomography (CT) scans had different clinical pictures or for the electrophysiologic changes in concussion, and outcome was totally unexplained and unpredictable. Technologic advances set the stage for research to uncover different, more satisfactory explanations. Grennarelli and his associates[6] led the way and reconceptualized traumatic brain injury. Their research and that of others have led to the position that two types of injury may occur—focal and diffuse brain injury.

Focal brain injury. **Focal brain injury** is specific, grossly observable brain lesions—cortical contusions, epidural hemorrhage, subdural hematoma, and intracerebral hematoma. The force of impact (translational acceleration) typically produces **contusions** from direct contact (as well as injury to the vault, vessels, and supporting structures) that in turn produce epidural hemorrhage and subdural and intracerebral hematomas. The mechanisms of injury are depicted in Fig. 16-1. Damage results from compression of the

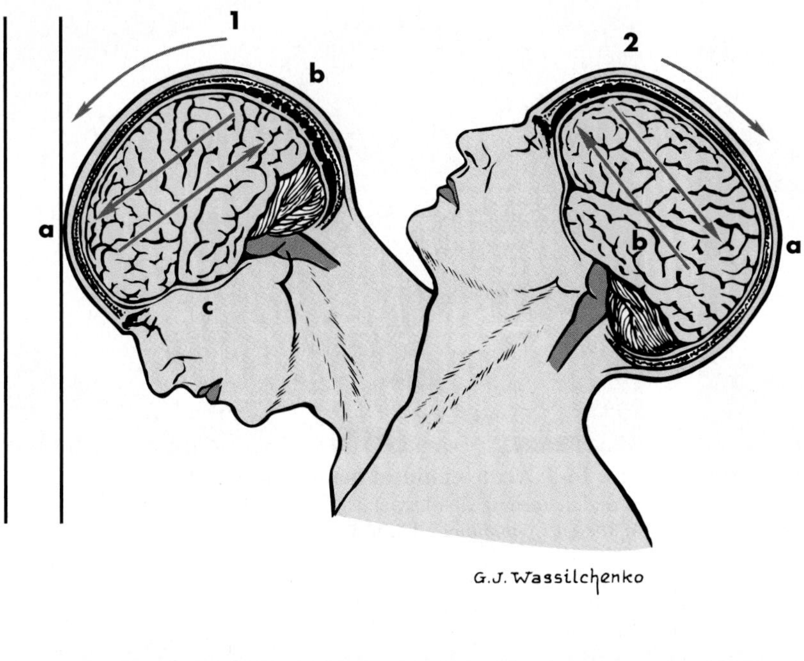

FIG. 16-1 Coup and contrecoup brain injury following blunt trauma. *1,* Coup injury: impact against object; *a,* site of impact and direct trauma to brain; *b,* shearing of subdural veins; *c,* trauma to base of brain. *2,* Contrecoup injury: impact within skull; *a,* site of impact from brain hitting opposite side of skull; *b,* shearing forces through brain. These injuries occur in one continuous motion—the head strikes the wall (coup) and then rebounds (contrecoup). (Modified from Rudy EB: *Advanced neurological and neurosurgical nursing,* St Louis, 1984, Mosby.)

skull at the point of impact and rebound effect. Contusion and bleeding occur because of small tears in blood vessels resulting from these forces. The severity of contusion is associated with the amount of energy transmitted by the skull to underlying brain tissue. In addition, the smaller the area of impact is, the greater the severity of injury, because the force is concentrated into a smaller area. The focal injury may be coup or contrecoup. Brain edema forms around and in damaged neural tissues, contributing to the increasing intracranial pressure (ICP). Within the contused areas are infarction and necrosis, multiple hemorrhages, and edema. The tissue has a pulpy quality. The maximum effects of injury related to contusion, bleeding, and edema peak 18 to 36 hours after severe head injury.

Contusions (Fig. 16-2) are found most commonly in the frontal lobes, particularly at the poles and along the inferior orbital surfaces; in the temporal lobes, especially in the anterior poles and along the inferior surface; and at the frontotemporal junction. They result in changes in attention, memory, executive attentional function (motivation, goal selection or formation, planning, self-monitoring, and use of feedback), affect, emotion, and behavior. Less commonly, contusions occur in the parietal lobes and the occipital lobes. Focal cerebral contusions are superficial, involving just the gyri. Hemorrhagic contusions may coalesce into a large, confluent intracranial hematoma.

Extradural hematomas (epidural hematomas or epidural hemorrhages) represent 1% to 2% of major head injuries and occur in all age-groups, but most commonly in persons 20 to 40 years of age. An artery is the source of bleeding in 85% of extradural hematomas (Fig. 16-3); 15% result from injury to the meningeal vein or dural sinus. Ninety percent of persons also have a skull fracture. The temporal fossa is the most common site of extradural hematoma caused by injury to the middle meningeal artery or vein. The resulting shift of the temporal lobe medially precipitates uncal and hippocampal gyrus herniation through the tentorial notch. Extradural hemorrhages are found occasionally in the subfrontal area (especially in the young and elderly populations), caused by injury to the anterior meningeal artery or a venous sinus, and in the occipital-suboccipital area, which results in herniation of the posterior fossa contents through the foramen magnum. Computed tomography (CT) and magnetic resonance imaging (MRI) show a lens-shaped mass over the surface of the cortex.

Subdural hematomas arise in 10% to 20% of persons with traumatic brain injury. Acute subdural hematomas rapidly develop (within 48 hours) and usually are located at the top of the skull (the cerebral convexities). On CT visualization, they appear as a high-density mass. Bilateral hematomas occur in 15% to 20% of persons. Subacute subdural hematomas develop more slowly, often over 48 hours to 2 weeks. On CT visualization, they appear as a mixed-density mass. Chronic subdural hematomas (commonly found in elderly persons and persons who abuse alcohol who have some degree of brain atrophy with a subsequent increase in the extradural space) develop over weeks to months. Tearing of the bridging veins is the major cause of rapidly developing and subacutely developing subdural hematomas, although torn cortical veins or venous sinuses and contused tissue may be the source. These subdural hematomas act as expanding masses, giving rise to increased intracranial pressure (ICP) that eventually compresses the bleeding vessels (Figs. 16-4 and 16-5). The displacement of brain tissue can result in a herniation syndrome.

The pathogenesis of a chronic subdural hematoma is different. The existing subdural space gradually fills with blood. A vascular membrane forms around the hematoma in ap-

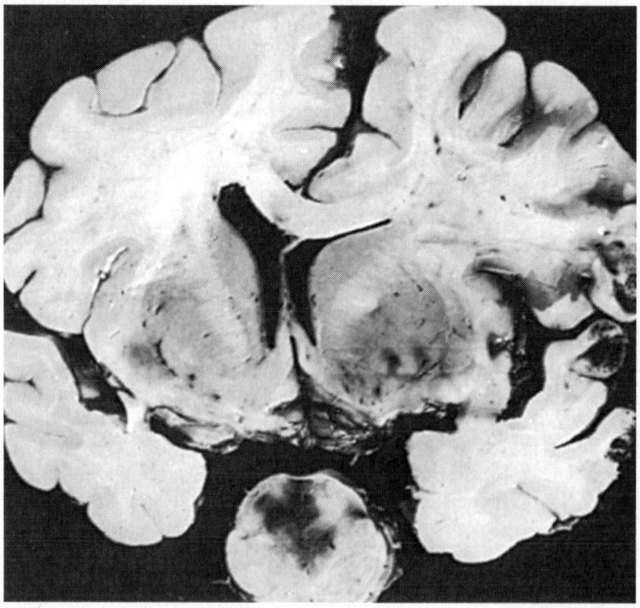

FIG. 16-2 Recent contusions of frontal and temporal lobes. There is displacement of cingulate gyrus and lateral ventricles. Secondary hemorrhages have occurred in lower midbrain and upper pons. (From Kissane JM, editor: *Anderson's pathology,* ed 9, St Louis, 1993, Mosby.)

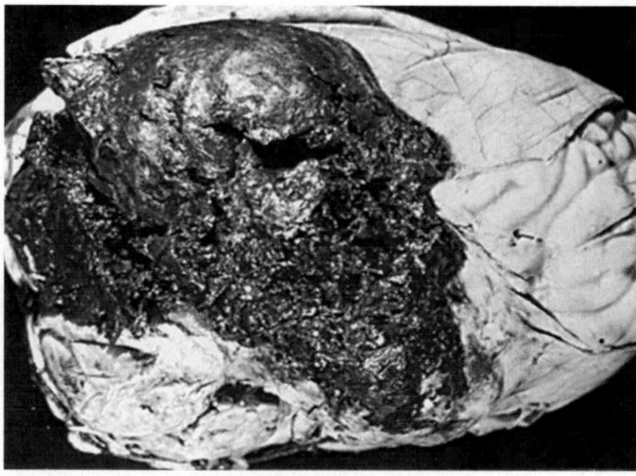

FIG. 16-3 Acute epidural hematoma. Skull fracture with tear of middle meningeal artery and vein. (From Kissane JM, editor: *Anderson's pathology,* ed 9, St Louis, 1993, Mosby.)

proximately 2 weeks. Further enlargement takes place in some persons, but the mechanism of this enlargement is unclear.

Intracerebral hematomas occur in 2% to 3% of persons with head injuries, may be single or multiple, and are associated with contusions. Although most commonly located in the frontal and temporal lobes, intracerebral hematomas may occur in the hemispheric deep white matter. Small blood vessels are traumatized by penetrating injury or shearing forces. The intracerebral hematoma then acts as an expanding mass, resulting in increased ICP and compression of brain tissues with resultant edema (Fig. 16-6). Delayed intracerebral hematomas may appear 3 to 10 days after the head injury.

Open trauma produces discrete (focal) injuries and includes compound fractures and missile injuries. A compound fracture opens a communication between the cranial contents and the environment and should be investigated whenever there are lacerations of the scalp, tympanic membrane, a sinus, an eye, or mucous membranes. Such fractures may involve the cranial vault or the base of the skull (basilar skull fracture). The injury incurred from bone fragments is mainly a tangential injury (injury caused by direct contact) and occasionally a penetrating injury. Bone fragments may lacerate or contuse brain tissues or blood vessels. In addition, cranial nerves may be damaged with a basilar skull fracture.

Missiles include bullets, rocks, shell fragments, knives, and blunt instruments. The mechanisms of injury are crush injury and stretch injury.[6] Crush injury is the laceration and crushing of whatever tissue the missile touches, with the amount of crush related to the degree of fragmentation, deformity, size, and shape. A tangential injury is injury to the coverings of the brain (scalp lacerations), skull fractures, laceration of the meninges, and cerebral lacerations. Projectiles and debris from scalp and skull injury, when driven into the brain substance, produce a penetrating brain injury. Occasionally, projectiles are so forceful that they exit the cranial vault in addition to entering it, producing a through-and-through injury. Primary damage is localized along the path of the penetrating object, and direct tissue disruption along the projectile tract results. A high-velocity bullet produces contusions at the site of entry, caused by bone striking the brain tissue on impact. Bone fragments are driven inward.

Stretch injury involves blood vessels and nerves that are damaged without direct contact due to the amount of tissue stretched secondary to shape, deformation, and striking velocity. Air compressed in front of the bullet exerts an explosive effect on entry, producing extreme distant tissue damage and an immediate primary increase in ICP; a cavity many times greater than the bullet is produced because the brain tissue is propelled away from the tract. The cavity and

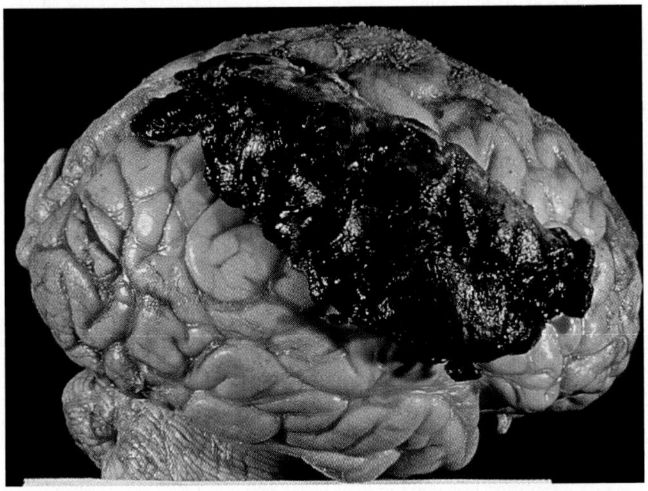

FIG. 16-4 Acute subdural hematoma (dura removed). Leptomeninges are intact. (From Damjanov I, Linder J: *Anderson's pathology,* ed 10, St Louis, 1996, Mosby.)

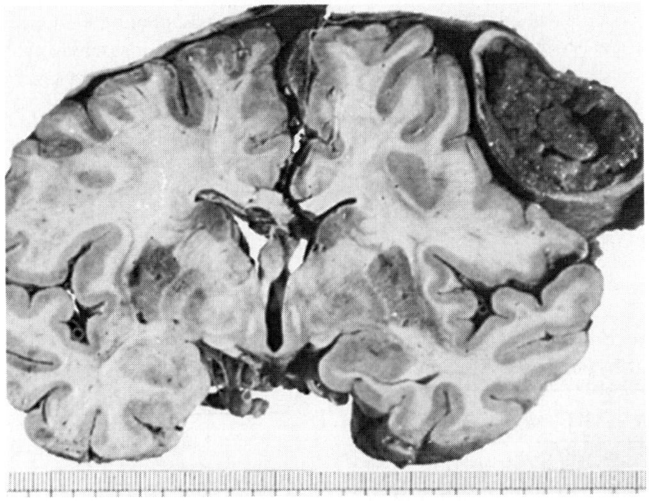

FIG. 16-5 Chronic subdural hematoma. Compression of underlying brain and lateral ventricle. Note bone formation in falx and uncal herniation on side of hematoma. (From Kissane JM, editor: *Anderson's pathology,* ed 9, St Louis, 1993, Mosby.)

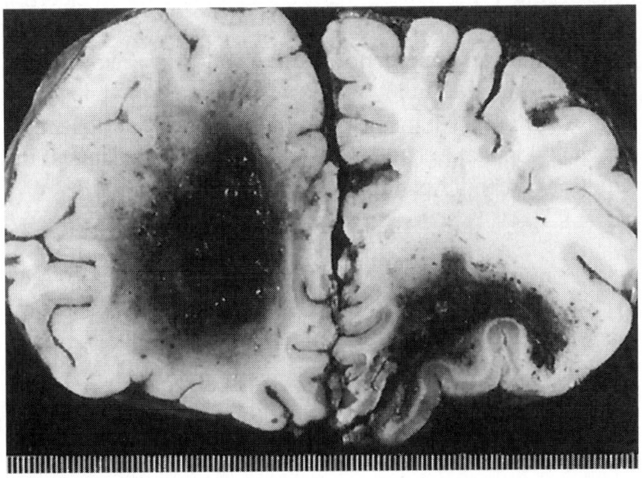

FIG. 16-6 Hematomas. Recent hematomas, resulting from trauma, in frontal lobes. (From Kissane JM: *Anderson's pathology,* ed 8, St Louis, 1985, Mosby.)

pressure produce contrecoup injuries. The intracranial volume is increased directly by the projectile and the debris. The temporary cavity collapses back onto itself, leaving a smaller, permanent cavity. Intracranial bleeding occurs into the permanent cavity and may cause the cavity to expand. Edema in and around the injured brain tissue rapidly develops; edema and bleeding contribute markedly to ICP. This second rise in ICP to 60 to 100 mmHg may last 2 to 5 minutes. Because of acute ischemic damage to the tract, necrosis of tissue begins. Within hours after bullet-induced injury, tissue within 1 cm adjacent to the tract disintegrates. Demyelination of white matter affected by hemorrhage and edema occurs by the second day. Unconsciousness, flaccidity, or decerebrate patients (see Chapter 15) have a 94% mortality.

Diffuse brain injury. **Diffuse brain injury** (diffuse axonal injury, DAI) results from a shaking effect (inertial effects of mechanical input to head associated with high levels of acceleration and deceleration, effects of head motion). Rotational acceleration (twisting movement) is the primary mechanism of injury, producing strains and distortions within the brain (see Fig. 16-1). The brain tissues experience shearing stresses set up by the rotational forces that operate when a freely moving head is struck because of the skull's motion from its attachment to the neck. Shearing, tearing, or stretching of nerve fibers with subsequent axonal damage results. Forces applied axially as a result of centrifugal acceleration of the head establish a gradient of injury severity from the hemispheres to the brain stem.[7] The most severe axonal injuries are located more peripheral to the brain stem, thus accounting for the tremendous cognitive and affective impairments seen in survivors of traumatic brain injury from MVCs. The frontal and temporal axonal tracts are particularly vulnerable. Damage reduces the speed of informational processing and responding and disrupts attention.

The common pathologic substrate in diffuse brain injury is axonal damage (disruption). Pathophysiologically, at the time of injury, the damage can be seen only with an electron microscope and involves either numerous axons alone or axonal injury in conjunction with actual tissue tears. Areas where axons and small blood vessels are torn appear as small hemorrhages, located particularly in the corpus callosum and dorsolateral quadrant of the rostral brain stem at the superior cerebellar peduncle.

Progressively increasing numbers of damaged axons are visible 12 hours to several days after the injury. Chromatolysis of the neurons involving eccentric relocation of the nucleus, swelling of the axon hillock, and redistribution of the rough endoplasmic reticulum in the cell body is evident. During this time the torn axons, which resemble dilated sausage links, also regress into round balls called *retraction balls.* These retraction balls are visible with light microscopy.

The number of retraction balls increases during the first week or two but begins to diminish in 2 to 3 weeks. Clusters of microglia appear in their place. Lastly, astrocytosis (gliosis, equivalent to scarring) occurs at the sites of axonal damage. Demyelination is seen particularly in the long axon tracts of the upper brain stem.

Severity of the diffuse injury correlates with the direction and velocity of rotation, that is, how much shearing force was applied to the brain stem. Fig. 16-7 illustrates the spectrum of the diffuse injury as the magnitude increases. DAI is not associated with intracranial hypertension soon after injury, but acute brain swelling (increased intravascular blood within the brain, vasodilation, and increased cerebral blood volume) frequently is seen.

Several categories of diffuse brain injury exist: mild concussion, classic concussion, mild DAI, moderate DAI, and

NUTRITION & DISEASE

Neurotrauma

Neurotrauma or head injury creates hypermetabolism, hypercatabolism, hyperglycemia, and decreased immune competency. The need for energy and protein increases significantly. Provision of an adequate supply of nutrients results in improved outcomes. One study indicated that initiating nutrition therapy within 72 hours after admission can alter the outcome and survival of the individual. Early small bowel feeding results in a decreased incidence of infection and shorter intensive care unit (ICU) stay. The contribution of specific nutrients is being evaluated. Protein needs are also increased for people with spinal cord injury to a recommended 2 grams protein/kg ideal body weight. The use of indirect calorimetry measurements and calculations of the actual energy expenditure of the individual can prevent overfeeding.

Data from Kirby D: *JPEN* 20:1, 1996; Roberts PR: *New Horiz* 3(3): 506, 1995; Rodriguez DJ, Benzel EC, Clevenger FW: The metabolic response to spinal cord injury, *Spinal Cord* 35:599, 1997.

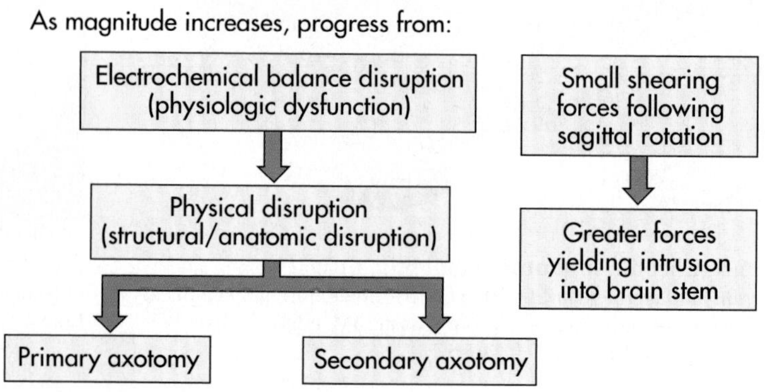

FIG. 16-7 Spectrum of diffuse brain injury.

severe DAI. An organic component is present within each category, in contrast to the previous conceptualization that concussion had no structural injury component.

Mild concussion involves temporary axonal disturbances. Cerebral cortical dysfunction related to attentional and memory systems results, but consciousness is not lost. Three forms have been described:

Grade I Confusion and disorientation accompanied by amnesia (momentary)

Grade II Momentary confusion and retrograde amnesia that develops after 5 to 10 minutes (memory loss involves only events occurring several minutes before injury)

Grade III Confusion and retrograde amnesia present from impact (also anterograde amnesia) (persists for several minutes)

Classic cerebral concussion (*grade IV*) involves diffuse cerebral disconnection from the brain stem reticular activating system and is a phenomenon of physiologic, neurologic dysfunction without substantial anatomic disruption. Evidence of this disconnection is the immediate loss of consciousness, which lasts less than 6 hours. Retrograde and anterograde (posttraumatic) amnesia are present. This type of diffuse injury frequently is associated with focal pathologic findings, especially cerebral contusions that yield focal signs, not loss of consciousness. Two forms of classic cerebral contusion exist: uncomplicated classic cerebral concussion (without focal injury) and complicated classic cerebral concussion (accompanied by focal injury).

Diffuse axonal injury (DAI) produces prolonged traumatic coma lasting more than 6 hours because of axonal disruption. Three forms of DAI exist: mild, moderate, and severe. In **mild DAI,** posttraumatic coma lasts 6 to 24 hours. Death is uncommon, but residual cognitive, psychologic, and sensorimotor deficits may persist. Mild DAI is a relatively uncommon lesion, occurring in 8% of all severe head injuries and 19% of all cases of DAI.

In **moderate DAI,** widespread physiologic impairment exists throughout the cerebral cortex and diencephalon. Actual tearing of some axons in both hemispheres occurs. Basal skull fracture, a focal injury, commonly is associated with moderate DAI. Prolonged coma lasting more than 24 hours is present but prominent brain stem signs do not exist with moderate DAI. Recovery often is incomplete in 93% of those individuals who survive.[3] Moderate DAI is the most common type of DAI and is found in 20% of severe head injuries and 45% of all cases of DAI.

Severe DAI, formerly called *primary brain stem injury* or *brain stem contusion,* involves severe mechanical disruption of many axons in both cerebral hemispheres and those extending to the diencephalon and brain stem. Additional synonyms for severe DAI are listed in Box 16-1. Severe DAI represents 16% of all severe head injuries and 36% of all cases of DAI. Sixty-four percent of persons survive. Thirty percent to 40% stay at low level or reduced states of consciousness for a prolonged period of time.[3,8]

Box 16-1

TERMS DESCRIBING PROLONGED TRAUMATIC COMA

MORE COMMONLY USED TERMS

Brain stem contusion
Cerebral concussion (grade V, prolonged, severe)
Closed head injury
Diffuse degeneration of white matter
Diffuse injury
Edema
Shearing injury

LESS COMMONLY USED TERMS

Central cerebral trauma
Contusion cerebri
Diffuse brain damage of immediate impact type
Diffuse neuronal injury
Diffuse white matter shearing injury
Inner cerebral trauma
Strich injury
Unspecified head injury

Clinical Manifestations, Evaluation, and Treatment

Focal brain injury. The clinical manifestations of a contusion may include immediate loss of consciousness (generally accepted to last no longer than 5 minutes), loss of reflexes with which the individual falls to the ground, transient cessation of respiration, brief period of bradycardia, and decrease in blood pressure (lasting 30 seconds to a few minutes). A momentary increase in cerebrospinal fluid (CSF) pressure and ECG and electroencephalographic (EEG) changes have been demonstrated to occur on impact. Vital signs may stabilize to normal values in a few seconds. Reflexes return next, and the person begins to regain consciousness. Returning to being fully awake and alert takes variable periods, from minutes to days. Regaining a full level of consciousness may be extremely slow, and residual deficits may persist. In some persons, full level of consciousness never returns. Evaluation should include a complete history and physical examination. Skull and spinal radiographs are taken frequently, and a CT scan or MRI may be done. Large contusions and lacerations with hemorrhage may be excised surgically. Otherwise, treatment is directed at controlling ICP and managing symptoms.

Individuals with classic temporal extradural hematomas (i.e., over the temporal lobe) experience a period of loss of consciousness at the time of injury, followed by a lucid period that lasts from a few hours to a few days in one third of persons (if bleeding from a vein). As the hematoma accumulates, a headache of increasing severity, vomiting, drowsiness, confusion, seizure, and hemiparesis may develop. Level of consciousness may dwindle rapidly as the temporal lobe herniation begins. Clinical manifestations of temporal lobe herniation also include ipsilateral pupillary dilation and contralateral hemiparesis.

The diagnosis of an extradural hematoma usually is made with a CT scan or MRI. In some instances, diagnosis is made by history and clinical findings, because time for a CT scan or MRI is not available. The prognosis is usually good if intervention is initiated before bilateral dilation of the pupils. Surgical therapy is evacuation of the hematoma through burr holes, which is followed by ligation of the bleeding vessel or vessels. Extradural hematomas are almost always medical emergencies.

In acute, rapidly developing subdural hematomas, the expanding clots directly compress the brain, giving rise to the clinical manifestations. As the ICP rises, the bleeding veins are compressed and thus bleeding is self-limiting, although cerebral compression and displacement of brain tissue can cause temporal lobe herniation.

An acute subdural hematoma classically begins with headache, drowsiness, restlessness or agitation, slowed cognition, and confusion. These symptoms worsen over time and progress to loss of consciousness, respiratory pattern changes, and pupillary dilation (i.e., the symptoms of temporal lobe herniation). These manifestations are more pronounced than focal manifestations such as dysphasia, dyspraxia, or hemiparesis. Other clinical manifestations may include homonymous hemianopia (defective vision in either the right or the left field), disconjugate gaze, and gaze palsies.

Presenting manifestations of chronic subdural hematomas vary. Of persons affected, 80% have chronic headaches and tenderness over the hematoma on percussion. Most persons appear to have a progressive dementia accompanied by generalized rigidity (paratonia).

Whereas most acute and subacute subdural hematomas are treated with clot evacuation through a burr hole, chronic subdural hematomas (and some that are subacute) require a craniotomy to evacuate the gelatinous blood. The membrane around a chronic subdural hematoma is then dissected away from the dura mater and arachnoid membranes. A technique for percutaneous drainage for chronic subdural hematomas recently has proved successful.

A decreasing level of consciousness is associated with an intracerebral hematoma. Coma or a confusional state from other injuries, however, can make the cause of this increasing unresponsiveness difficult to detect. Contralateral hemiplegia also may occur. As the ICP rises, clinical manifestations of temporal lobe herniation may appear. In delayed intracerebral hematoma, the presentation is similar to that of a hypertensive brain hemorrhage: sudden, rapidly progressive decreased level of consciousness with pupillary dilation, breathing pattern changes, hemiplegia, and bilateral positive Babinski reflexes.

History and physical examination help to establish the diagnosis. CT scan, MRI, and cerebral angiographic visualization confirm the diagnosis. Evacuation of a singular intracerebral hematoma has only occasionally been helpful, mostly for subcortical white matter hematomas. Otherwise, treatment is directed at reducing the ICP and allowing the hematoma to reabsorb slowly.

With open-head injury, most persons lose consciousness. The depth of the coma and the length of the unresponsive state are related to the location of injury, extent of damage, and amount of bleeding. Open-head injury often requires surgery to débride the traumatized tissues to prevent infection and to remove blood clots to help reduce the ICP. ICP also is managed with steroids, dehydrating agents, osmotic diuretics, or a combination of these drugs. Broad-spectrum antibiotics are administered.

The diagnosis of a compound fracture is made through physical examination, skull radiographs, or both. The diagnosis of a basilar skull fracture is made on the basis of clinical findings. Skull radiographs often do not demonstrate the fracture, although intracranial air or air in the sinuses on radiograph, CT scan, or MRI is indirect evidence of a basilar skull fracture.

A compound linear fracture is débrided nonsurgically in cooperative adults and surgically in children and uncooperative adults. Cranioplasty with insertion of bone or an artificial graft may be necessary but often is delayed until antibiotics have been given. Antibiotics are administered after surgery.

Bed rest and close observation for meningitis and other complications are prescribed for a basilar skull fracture. Use of prophylactic antibiotics is controversial because studies have failed to demonstrate that they reduce the rate of infection.

Diffuse brain injury. DAI is associated with physical, cognitive, psychologic/behavioral, and social consequences. Spastic paralysis, peripheral nerve injury, swallowing disorders, dysarthria, visual and hearing impairments, and taste and smell deficits are some of the physical consequences. Common cognitive deficits include disorientation and confusion, short attention span, memory deficits, learning difficulties, dysphasia, poor judgment, and perceptual deficits. Behavioral disorders that emerge include agitation, impulsiveness, blunted affect, social withdrawal, and depression.

Mild concussion is characterized by an immediate onset of clinical manifestations at time of injury and the transitory nature of clinical manifestations. A momentary rise in CSF pressure and changes in ECG and EEG have been demonstrated to occur on impact in the laboratory. No loss of consciousness is experienced. The initial confusional state exists for a moment to several minutes. Amnesia for events preceding the trauma (retrograde amnesia) may be experienced. Anterograde amnesia may exist transiently. Persons may experience head pain and complain of nervousness and "not being oneself" for a short time up to a few days.

In classic cerebral concussion, loss of consciousness lasts as long as 6 hours and reflexes are lost, causing falls. Reflexes are regained as responsiveness returns. Transient cessation of respiration, brief periods of bradycardia, and a decrease in blood pressure lasting 30 seconds or less occur. Vital signs stabilize within a few seconds to within normal limits. Retrograde and anterograde amnesia exist. A confusional state persists for hours to days. The patient experiences head pain, nausea, and fatigue. Attentional and memory system impairments may persist for weeks to months and may include inability to concentrate and forgetfulness. Mood and affect changes may persist for weeks to months and may include nervousness, anxiety reactions, depression, irritability, fatigability, and insomnia.

Some of the effects of a concussion may persist for weeks or months, depending on the severity of the injury. A **postconcussive syndrome** that includes headache, nervousness or anxiety, irritability, insomnia, depression, inability to concentrate, forgetfulness, and fatigability may develop. Treatment entails reassurance and symptomatic relief. Close observation for 24 hours by a reliable individual is indicated so that immediate intervention can be obtained if delayed effects become severe.

In mild DAI, 30% of persons display decerebrate or decorticate posturing; they may experience prolonged periods of stupor or restlessness (see Fig. 15-5).

In moderate DAI, the Glasgow Coma Scale (GCS) score is 4 to 8 initially and 6 to 8 by 24 hours. Thirty-five percent of victims have transitory decerebration or decortication. The person often remains unconscious for days or weeks and on awakening is confused. He or she experiences a long period of posttraumatic anterograde and retrograde amnesia and often has permanent deficits in memory, selective attention, vigilance, detection, working memory, data processing, vision or perception, and language, as well as mood and affect changes ranging from mild to severe.

Severe DAI is associated with brain stem signs that disappear in a few weeks. The person experiences immediate autonomic dysfunction that resolves in a few weeks. Increased ICP appears 4 to 6 days after injury. Pulmonary complications occur frequently, with profound sensorimotor and cognitive system deficits. Severely compromised coordinated movements and verbal and written communication, inability to learn and reason, and inability to modulate behavior also are found.

Diagnosis of focal and diffuse injury is determined by high-resolution CT scan and MRI. Medical management must include management of endocrine and metabolic derangement. Early and late seizures must be prevented and controlled. Storming (diencephalic seizures) must be diagnosed and treated. The role of fluid management has emerged as critically important in the care of individuals with severe brain injuries.

Spinal Cord Trauma

The number of persons with spinal cord injuries (SCIs) is between 32 and 38 million.[9] There are 7800 to 10,000 persons injured each year. Eighty-one percent are men, mostly young adults.[10] The average age is 33.4 years. Fifty percent of the injuries produce paraplegia and 50% produce quadriplegia.[11] MVAs account for 44% of SCIs.[12] Two-thirds of sports-related trauma are diving injuries.[13] Violence accounts for 24% and falls 22% of SCIs.[13] Elderly persons, because of preexisting degenerative vertebral disorders, are particularly at risk for minor trauma resulting in serious spinal cord injury, especially from falls.[14]

Pathophysiology

Spinal cord injuries most commonly occur because of vertebral injuries, which are the result of acceleration, deceleration, or deformation forces most frequently applied at a distance. These forces injure the vertebral or neural tissues by compressing the tissues, pulling or exerting a traction (tension) on the tissues, or shearing tissues so that they slide into one another. These forces may be exerted on the vertebral and neural tissues by hyperextension, hyperflexion, vertical compression, or rotation of the spine (Figs. 16-8 to 16-11). The bones, ligaments, and joints of the vertebral column

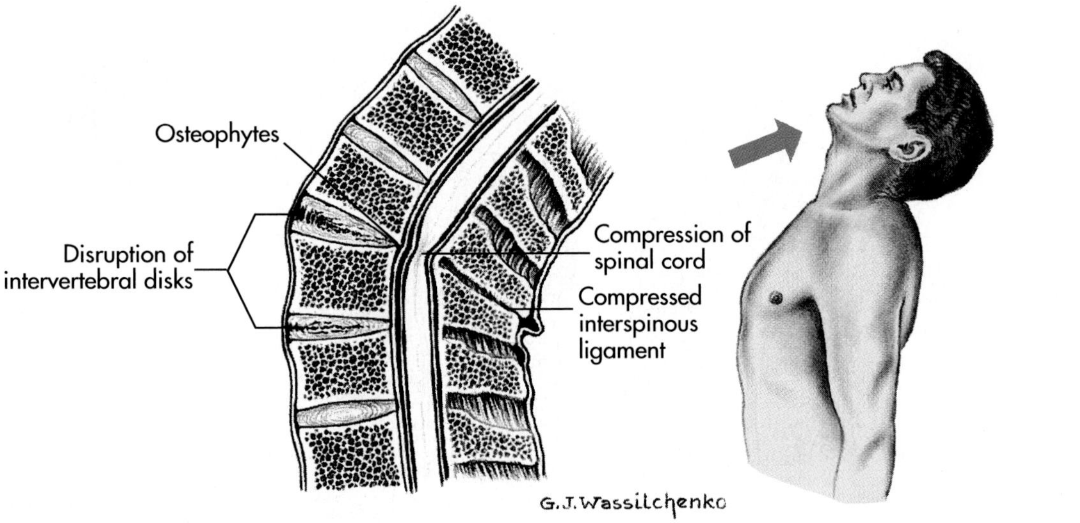

FIG. 16-8 Hyperextension injuries of the spine. Hyperextension can result in fracture or nonfracture injuries with spinal cord damage.

may be damaged. The vertebral column may incur fracture and often compression of one or more elements, dislocation of its elements, or both fracture and dislocation. Vertebral injuries can be classified as (1) simple fracture, a single break usually affecting transverse or spinous processes; (2) compressed (wedged) vertebral fracture, in which a vertebral body is compressed anteriorly; (3) comminuted (burst) fracture, in which a vertebral body is shattered into several fragments; and (4) dislocation.

The vertebrae fracture readily with both direct and indirect trauma. When the supporting ligaments are torn, the vertebrae move out of alignment and dislocations occur. A horizontal

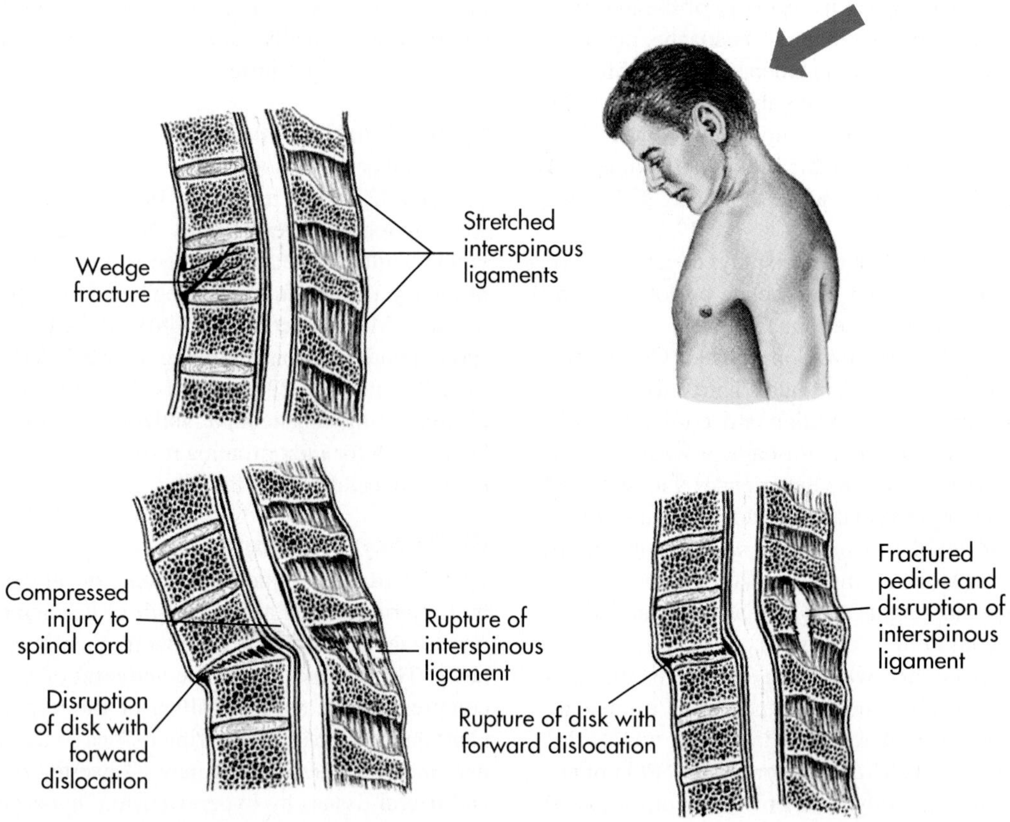

FIG. 16-9 Hyperflexion injury of the spine. Hyperflexion produces translation (subluxation) of vertebrae, which compromises the central canal and compresses spinal cord parenchyma or vascular structures.

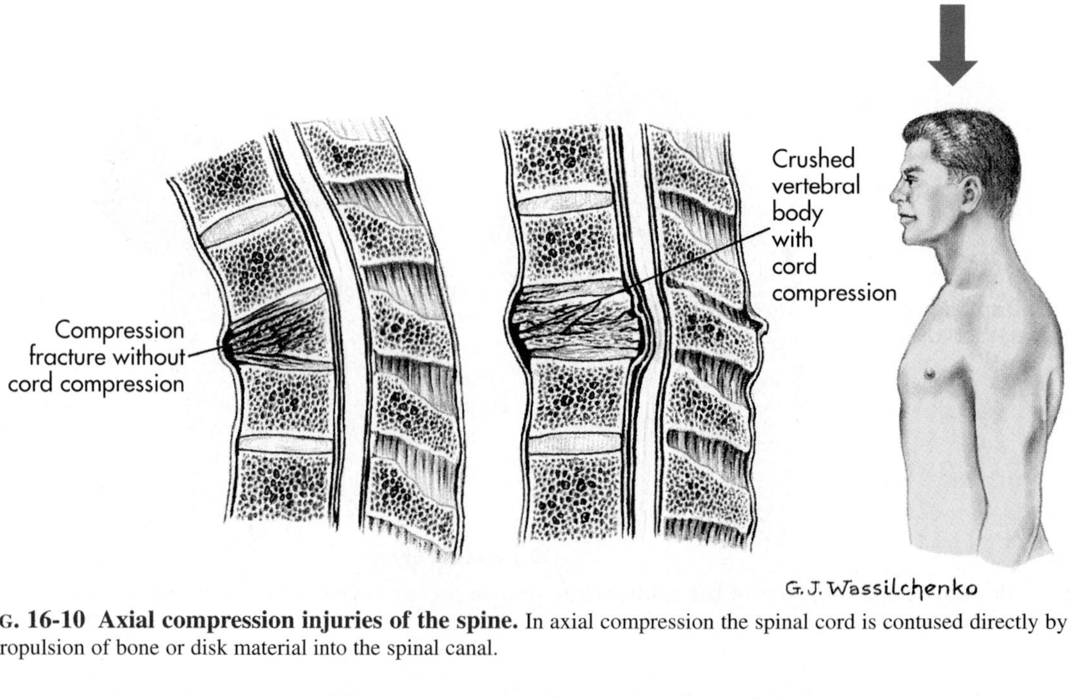

FIG. 16-10 Axial compression injuries of the spine. In axial compression the spinal cord is contused directly by retropulsion of bone or disk material into the spinal canal.

force moves the vertebrae straight forward; if the individual is in a flexed position at the time of injury, the vertebrae are then in an angulated position. Flexion and extension injuries may result in dislocations. (Bone, ligament, and joint injuries are presented in Table 16-2.) Vertebral injuries occur mostly at vertebrae C1 to C2 (cervical), C4 to C7, and T1 (thoracic) to L2 (lumbar) (see Fig. 13-9). These are the most mobile portions of the vertebral column. The cord occupies most of the vertebral canal in the cervical and lumbar regions. The size makes the cord in these areas more easily injured. (Injuries to the cord are summarized in Table 16-3.) Noncontiguous vertebral injuries are not uncommon.[15]

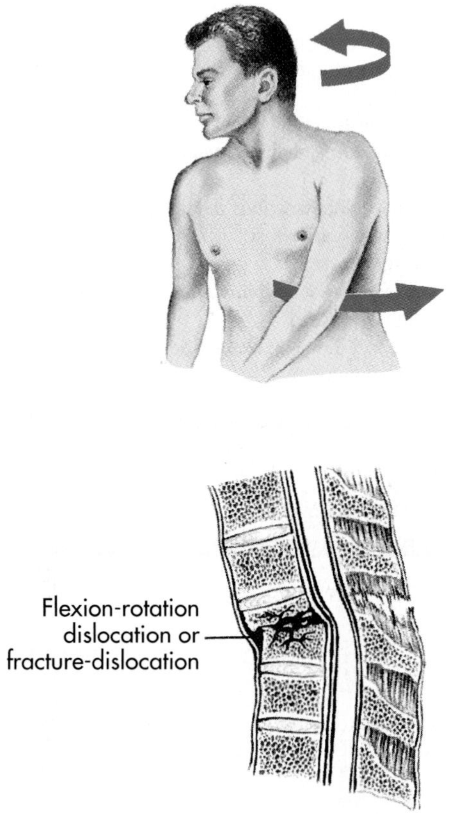

FIG. 16-11 Flexion-rotation injuries of the spine.

Within a few minutes after injury, microscopic hemorrhages appear in the central gray matter and pia arachnoid that increase in size within 2 hours. Edema in the white matter occurs, impairing the microcirculation of the cord. Within 4 hours, numerous swollen axis cylinders develop. Localized hemorrhaging and edema therefore are followed by reduced vascular perfusion and development of ischemic areas. Oxygen tension in the tissue at the injury site is decreased. The microscopic hemorrhages and edema are maximal at the level of injury and for two cord segments above and below it.

Cellular and subcellular alterations and tissue necrosis occur. Electron microscopy has allowed cellular pathogenesis to be described. By 5 minutes after injury, venules of the gray matter are congested and distended by erythrocytes. In 15 to 30 minutes, small hemorrhages occur with extravasation of erythrocytes into perivascular spaces of postcapillary and muscular venules. Within 4 hours there is disruption of myelin, axonal degeneration, and ischemic endothelial injury.

Chemical and metabolic changes in spinal cord tissues include release of toxic excitatory amino acids, accumulation of endogenous opiates, lipid hydrolysis with production of active metabolites, and local free radical release. These changes may produce further ischemia, vascular damage, and necrosis of tissues (autodestruction). Necrosis consumes 40% of cross-sectional cord within 4 hours of trauma and 70% within 24 hours (Fig. 16-12). Cord swelling increases the individual's degree of dysfunction, so that distinguishing the functions to be lost permanently from those that are impaired just temporarily becomes difficult. In the cervical region, cord swelling may be life threatening because of the possibility of resulting impairment of the diaphragm function (phrenic nerves exit C3 to C5) and vegetative functions mediated by the medulla oblongata. Within the first few days of injury, progressive axonal changes occur and necrotic zones develop. Progressive cavitation and coagulation necrosis at the site of injury are termed *posttraumatic infarction.*[15]

Circulation in the white matter tracts of the spinal cord returns to normal in about 24 hours, but gray matter circulation remains altered. Phagocytes appear 36 to 48 hours after injury. There are proliferation of microglia and changes in

Table 16-2 Mechanisms of Vertebral Injury

Mechanisms of Injury	Vertebral Injury	Forces of Injury	Location of Injury
Hyperextension	Fracture and dislocation of posterior elements such as spinous processes, transverse processes, laminae, pedicles, or posterior ligaments	Results from forces of acceleration-deceleration and the sudden reduction in the anteroposterior diameter of the spinal cord	Cervical area
Hyperflexion	Fracture or dislocation of the vertebral bodies, disks, or ligaments	Results from sudden and excessive force that propels the neck forward or causes an exaggerated lateral movement of the neck to one side	Cervical area
Vertical compression (axonal loading)	Shattering fractures	Results from a force applied along an axis from the top of the cranium through the vertebral bodies	T12 to L2
Rotational forces (flexion-rotation)	Ruptures support ligaments in addition to producing fractures	Adds shearing force to acceleration—acceleration forces	Cervical area

astrocytes. Red cells then begin to disintegrate, and resorption of hemorrhages begins. Degenerating axons are engulfed by macrophages in the first 10 days after injury. A cyst with fluid forms.[16] The traumatized cord is replaced by acellular collagenous tissue (a scar), usually in 3 to 4 weeks. Meninges thicken as part of the scarring process.

Clinical Manifestations

Normal activity of the spinal cord cells at and below the level of injury ceases because of loss of the continuous tonic discharge from the brain or brain stem and inhibition of suprasegmental impulses immediately after cord injury, thus causing spinal shock. *Spinal shock* is characterized by a com-

Table 16-3 Spinal Cord Injuries

Injury	Description
Cord concussion	Results in a temporary disruption of cord-mediated functions
Cord contusion	Bruising of the neural tissue causing swelling and temporary loss of cord-mediated functions
Cord compression	Pressure on the cord causing ischemia to tissues; must be relieved (decompressed) to prevent permanent damage to the spinal cord
Laceration	Tearing of the neural tissues of the spinal cord; may be reversible if only slight damage sustained by the neural tissues; may result in permanent loss of cord-mediated functions if spinal tracts are disrupted
Transection	Severing of the spinal cord, causing permanent loss of function
Complete	All tracts in the spinal cord completely disrupted; all cord-mediated functions below the transection are completely and permanently lost
Incomplete	Some tracts in the spinal cord remain intact, together with functions mediated by these tracts; has the potential for recovery although function is temporarily lost
Preserved sensation only	Some demonstrable sensation below the level of injury
Preserved motor nonfunctional	Preserved motor function without useful purpose; sensory function may or may not be preserved
Preserved motor functional	Preserved voluntary motor function that is functionally useful
Hemorrhage	Bleeding into the neural tissue because of blood vessel damage; usually no major loss of function
Damage or obstruction of spinal blood supply	Causes local ischemia

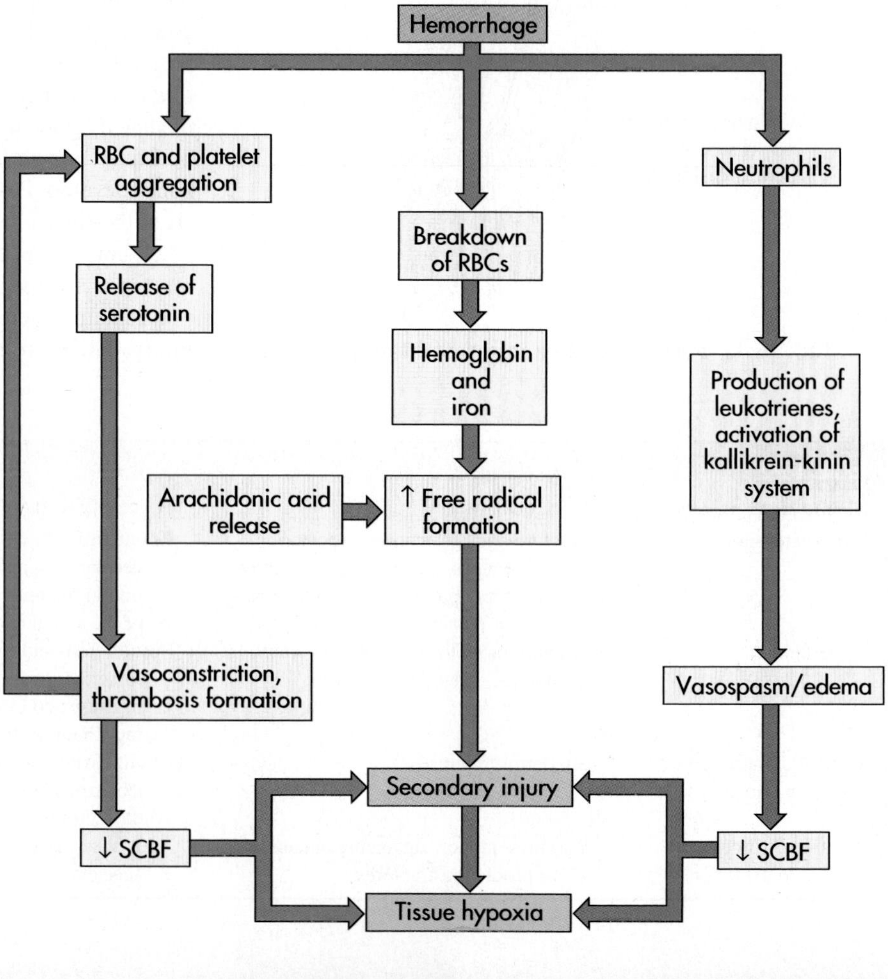

FIG. 16-12 Cascade of metabolic and cellular events that leads to spinal cord ischemia and hypoxia of secondary injury. *RBC,* Red blood cells; *SCBF,* spinal cord blood flow. (Redrawn from Marciano FF et al: *BNI Quarterly* 11(2): 6, 1995.)

plete loss of reflex function in all segments below the level of the lesion. This condition involves all skeletal muscles, bladder, bowel, sexual function, and autonomic control. Severe impairment below the level of the lesion is obvious; it includes paralysis and flaccidity in muscles, absence of sensation, loss of bladder and rectal control, transient drop in blood pressure, and poor venous circulation. The condition also results in disturbed thermal control because the sympathetic nervous system is damaged. This damage causes faulty control of sweating and radiation through capillary dilation. The hypothalamus cannot regulate body heat through vasoconstriction and increased metabolism; therefore the individual assumes the temperature of the air.

Spinal shock may last for 7 to 20 days after onset; it may persist for as short a time as a few days or as long as 3 months. Indications that spinal shock is terminating include the reappearance of reflex activity, hyperreflexia, spasticity, and reflex emptying of the bladder. In persons with cervical or upper thoracic cord injury, a form of distributive shock, called *neurogenic shock,* may be seen in addition to spinal shock, as a result of the loss of sympathetic outflow causing hypotension.

Loss of motor and sensory function depends on the level of injury. All motor, sensory, reflex, and autonomic functions cease below any transected area and also may cease below concussive, contused, compressed, or ischemic areas (Table 16-4). Paralysis of the lower half of the body with both legs involved is termed *paraplegia.* Paralysis involving all four extremities is termed *quadriplegia* (tetraplegia). In complete quadriplegia the level of injury is above C6, and all upper extremity function is lost. In incomplete quadriplegia, function at or above C6 is preserved, leaving the

Table 16-4 Clinical Manifestations of Spinal Cord Injury

Stage	Manifestations
SPINAL SHOCK STAGE	
Complete transection	Loss of motor function 1. Quadriplegia with injuries of cervical spinal cord 2. Paraplegia with injuries of thoracic spinal cord Muscle flaccidity Loss of all reflexes below level of injury Loss of pain, temperature, touch, pressure, and proprioception below level of injury Pain at site of injury caused by a zone of hyperesthesia above the injury Atonic bladder and bowel Paralytic ileus with distention Loss of vasomotor tone in lower body parts; low and unstable blood pressure Loss of perspiration below level of injury Loss or extreme depression of genital reflexes such as penile erection and bulbocavernous reflex Dry and pale skin, possible ulceration over bony prominences Respiratory impairment
Partial spinal cord transection	Asymmetric flaccid motor paralysis below level of injury Asymmetric reflex loss Preservation of some sensation below level of injury Vasomotor instability less severe than with complete cord transection Bowel and bladder impairment less severe than that seen with complete cord transection Preservation of ability to perspire in some portions of the body below level of injury **Brown-Séquard syndrome** (associated with penetrating injuries, arises from a relative hemisection of cord) 1. Ipsilateral paralysis or paresis below level of injury 2. Ipsilateral loss of touch, pressure, vibration, and position sense below level of injury 3. Contralateral loss of pain and temperature sensations below level of injury **Central cord syndrome** (associated with hyperextension or interruption of blood supply) 1. Motor deficit in upper extremities denser than in lower extremities 2. Varying degrees of bladder dysfunction **Anterior cord syndrome** (compromise of anterior spinal artery by occlusion or pressure effect of bone fragments or disk) 1. Loss of motor function below level of injury 2. Loss of pain and temperature sensations below level of injury 3. Touch, pressure, position, and vibration senses intact **Horner syndrome** (injury to preganglionic sympathetic trunk or postganglionic sympathetic neurons of superior cervical ganglion) 1. Ipsilateral pupil smaller than contralateral pupil 2. Sunken ipsilateral eyeball 3. Ptosis of affected eyeball 4. Lack of perspiration on ipsilateral side of face

Data from Boss BJ: The nervous system. In Howe J et al: *The handbook of nursing,* New York, 1984, Wiley & Sons.

Continued

Table 16-4 Clinical Manifestations of Spinal Cord Injury—cont'd

Stage	Manifestations
HEIGHTENED REFLEX ACTIVITY STAGE	Emergence of Babinski reflexes, possibly progressing to a triple reflex; possible development of still later flexor spasms
	Reappearance of ankle and knee reflexes, which become hyperactive
	Contraction of reflex detrusor muscle, leading to urinary incontinence
	Appearance of reflex defecation
	Mass reflex with flexion spasms, profuse sweating, piloerection, and bladder and occasional bowel emptying may be evoked by an autonomic stimulation of skin or from a full bladder
	Episodes of hypertension
	Defective heat-induced sweating
	Eventual development of extensor reflexes, first in muscles of hip and thigh, later in leg
	Possible paresthesias below level of transection: dull, burning pain in lower back, abdomen, buttocks, and perineum

shoulder, upper arm, and some forearm muscle control intact. With acceleration injuries the greatest stress point is C4-5. With a deceleration force the greatest stress point is at C5-6.

Return of spinal neuron excitability occurs slowly. Depending on the degree of damage, either of the following can occur: (1) motor, sensory, reflex, and autonomic functions return to normal; or (2) autonomic neural activity in the isolated segment develops. The sequence of hyperactivity phases, which vary in length, may include (1) minimal reflex activity, (2) flexor spasms, (3) alternation between flexor and extensor spasms, and (4) predominant extensor spasms.

The initial clinical manifestations associated with acute spinal cord injury are rapid loss of (1) voluntary movement in body parts below the level of injury, (2) sensations in the lower extremities and possibly lower trunk (depending on the level of injury), and (3) spinal and autonomic reflexes below the level of injury. The duration of this areflexic state is highly variable. In most persons, reflex activity returns in 1 to 2 weeks.

Gradually reflexes return and become increasingly easier to elicit. A pattern of flexion reflexes emerges, first involving the toes and later the feet and legs. Reflex voiding and bowel elimination appear. Flexor spasms accompanied by profuse sweating, piloerection, and automatic bladder emptying (together called a **mass reflex**) may develop. The ability to sweat when overheated may be disrupted, and extensor spasms may develop, usually after full development of flexor spasms. Sometimes after several months, episodes of autonomic hyperreflexia are elicited.

Autonomic hyperreflexia (dysreflexia) is a syndrome that may occur at any time after spinal shock resolves. The syndrome is associated with a massive, uncompensated cardiovascular response to stimulation of the sympathetic nervous system (Fig. 16-13). The condition is life threatening and requires immediate treatment. Individuals most likely to be affected have lesions at the T6 level or above. Autonomic hyperreflexia is characterized by paroxysmal hypertension (up to 300 mmHg systolic), a pounding headache, blurred vision, sweating above the level of the lesion with flushing of the skin, nasal congestion, nausea, piloerection caused by pilomotor spasm, and bradycardia (30 to 40 beats/min). The symptoms may develop singly or in combination (syndrome) and often are associated with a distended bladder or rectum.

Pathophysiology of hyperreflexia involves the stimulation of sensory receptors below the level of the cord lesion. The intact autonomic nervous system reflexively responds with an arteriolar spasm that increases blood pressure. Baroreceptors in the cerebral vessels, the carotid sinus, and the aorta sense the hypertension and stimulate the parasympathetic system. The heart rate decreases, but the visceral and peripheral vessels do not dilate because efferent impulses cannot pass through the cord.

The most common precipitating cause is a distended bladder or rectum, but any sensory stimulation can elicit autonomic hyperreflexia. Stimulation of the skin or stimulation of the pain receptors may cause autonomic hyperreflexia. Emptying of the bladder or bowel usually relieves the syndrome, and this may be facilitated by drugs, such as phenoxybenzamine.

Evaluation and Treatment

Diagnosis of spinal cord injury is made on the basis of physical, radiologic, and myelographic examination; CT scan; and MRI. For a suspected or confirmed vertebral fracture or dislocation, regardless of the presence or absence of spinal cord injury, the immediate intervention is immobilization of the spine to prevent further injury. Decompression and surgical fixation may be necessary. Corticosteroids are given at the time of injury to decrease secondary cord injury and thereafter for several days. The 21-aminosteroid tirilizad (a lazaroid), an antioxidant and inhibitor of iron-dependent lipid peroxidation, is under study, as are vitamin E and selenium, the opiate antagonist naloxone, calcium channel blockers, glutamate receptor blockers, and growth-promoting and growth-inhibiting factors, including ganglioside GM_1. Nutrition, lung function, skin integrity, and bladder and bowel management must be addressed. Plans for rehabilitation require early consideration.

In cases of autonomic hyperreflexia, intervention must be prompt because cerebrovascular accident (CVA) is possible.

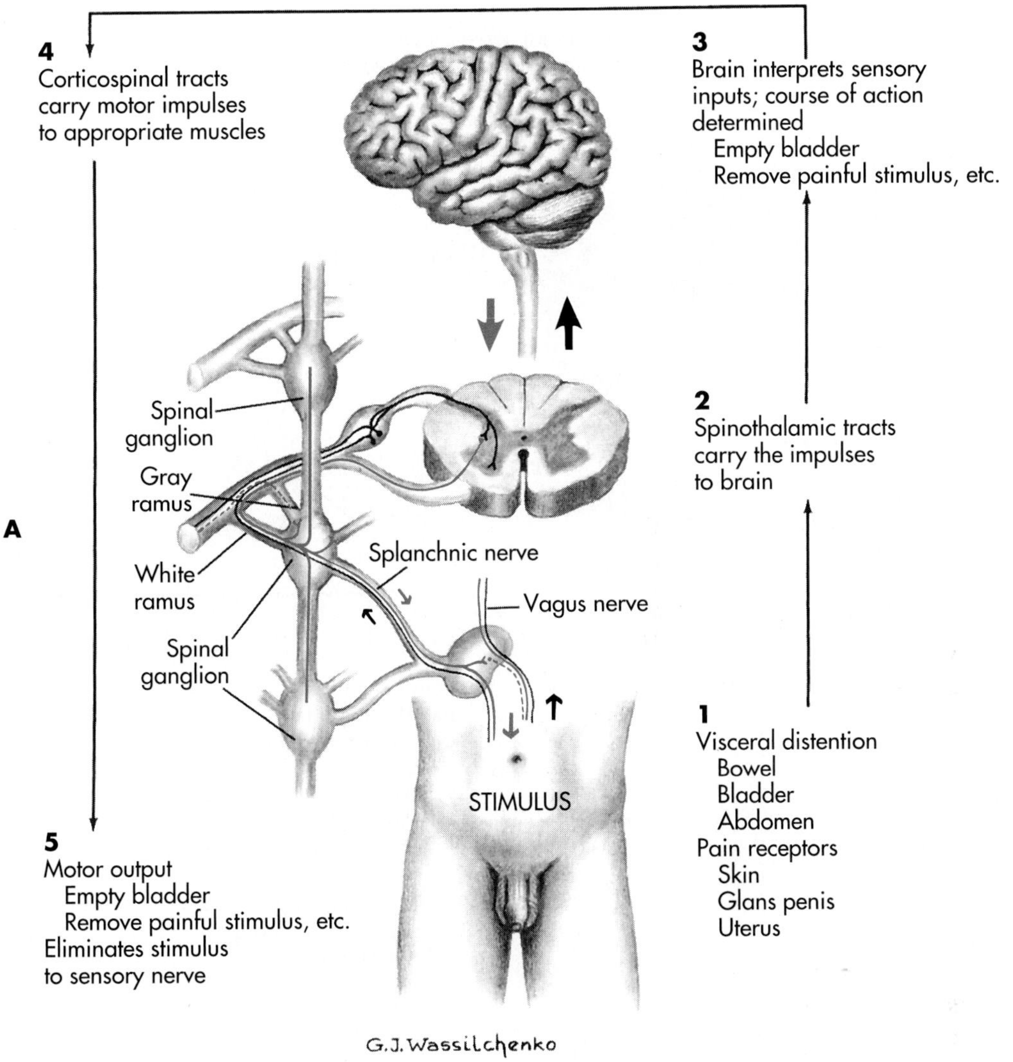

FIG. 16-13 Autonomic hyperreflexia. A, Normal response pathway. (Modified from Rudy EB: *Advanced neurological and neurosurgical nursing,* St Louis, 1984, Mosby.) *Continued*

The head of the bed should be elevated, and the stimulus should be found and removed. Medications may be used if these measures do not effectively reduce blood pressure.

Degenerative Disorders of the Spine

Degenerative changes occur in the vertebral disks. **Degenerative disk disease (DJD)** is a common finding in individuals 30 years of age and older. Only a small percentage of those persons have any functional incapacity because of pain. The causes of DJD include biochemical and biomechanical alterations of the tissue of the intervertebral disk. Fibrocartilage replaces the gelatinous mucoid material of the nucleus pulposus as the disk changes with age. There may be splits in the annulus fibrosis, permitting herniation of elements of nucleus pulposus. There may be shrinkage of the nucleus pulposus that produces prolapse or folding of the annulus with secondary osteophyte formation at the margins of the adjacent vertebral body. The pathologic findings in DJD include disk protrusion, spondylolysis, and/or subluxation and degeneration of vertebrae (spondylolisthesis) and spinal stenosis.

Symptoms result from either (1) disk or annulus protrusion or (2) narrowing of the spinal canal or intervertebral foramen by osteophytes.[17] There may be a congenital narrow canal or congenitally short pedicles.

Posterior disk protrusion in the cervical and thoracic regions lead to cord compression, and cauda equine compression results in the lumbar area. Both situations are called myelopathy. Posterolateral disk protrusions, with or without a contribution from the vertebral body or apophyseal joint osteophytes, lead to nerve root compression (called radiculopathy).

Cervical spondylolysis is a DJD in the cervical spine predominately at C5-C6 and C6-C7. It may present as a cervical radiculopathy or a cervical myelopathy. Clinical manifestations of cervical radiculopathy include[17] neck pain as well as pain in the medial aspects of the scapula, the shoulder, or arm. Sensory symptoms, such as tingling or numbness, follow a dermatomal pattern; weakness follows the pattern of innervation of the affected nerve root and occipital or suboccipital headache (some authorities refute this). Clinical

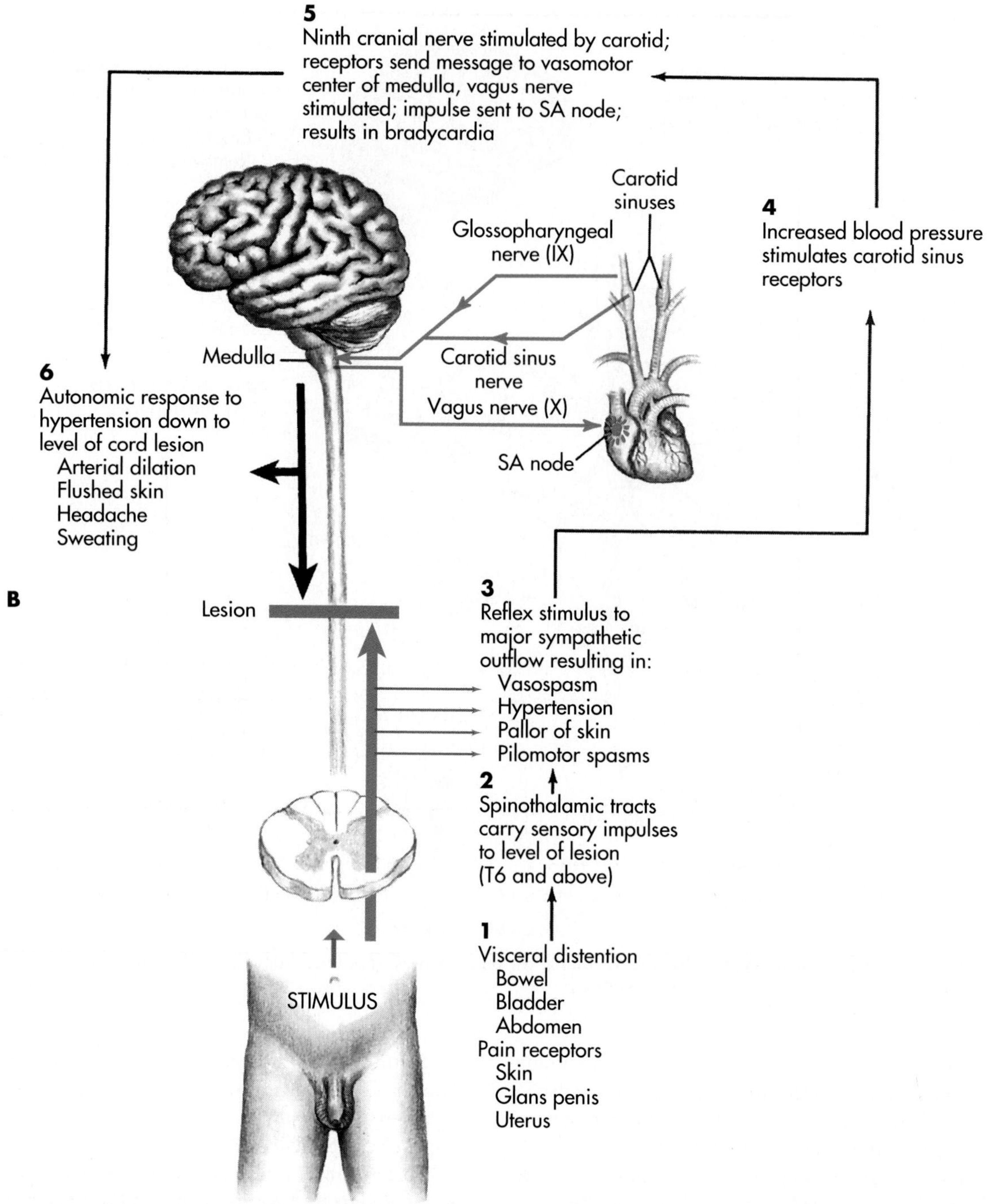
5
Ninth cranial nerve stimulated by carotid; receptors send message to vasomotor center of medulla, vagus nerve stimulated; impulse sent to SA node; results in bradycardia
Carotid sinuses
Glossopharyngeal nerve (IX)
4
Increased blood pressure stimulates carotid sinus receptors
Medulla
Carotid sinus nerve
Vagus nerve (X)
SA node
6
Autonomic response to hypertension down to level of cord lesion
Arterial dilation
Flushed skin
Headache
Sweating
B
Lesion
3
Reflex stimulus to major sympathetic outflow resulting in:
Vasospasm
Hypertension
Pallor of skin
Pilomotor spasms
2
Spinothalamic tracts carry sensory impulses to level of lesion (T6 and above)
1
Visceral distention
Bowel
Bladder
Abdomen
Pain receptors
Skin
Glans penis
Uterus
STIMULUS

FIG. 16-13, cont'd Autonomic hyperreflexia. B, Autonomic dysreflexia pathway. (Modified from Rudy EB: *Advanced neurological and neurosurgical nursing,* St Louis, 1984, Mosby.)

manifestations of cervical myelopathy include[17] difficulty walking, altered sensation in the feet, and sphincter disturbances (occurs late).

Thoracic disk disease is rarely symptomatic, but prolapse is found in one-seventh of scans. Lumbosacral disk disease (lumbar spondylosis) involves the lower two lumbar disks in 90% of persons. There may be (1) lateral disk protrusion (10% of cases) manifesting as pain referred to the anterior thigh and leg; (2) posterolateral disk protrusion; or (3) central disk protrusion manifesting with pain, lower extremity weakness, impaired sphincter function, and saddle anesthesia. Clinical manifestations of posterolateral protrusions (see Fig. 16-14)[17] include pain in back, the sacroiliac joint, and the medial aspect of the buttock and upper thigh; radicular pain exacerbated by movement and straining (medial calf suggests L5, lateral calf suggests S1 root compression); sensory symptoms that are common and segmental in distribution; focal tenderness on palpation of the back; limited range of motion in back and scoliosis secondary to paravertebral spasms; restricted straight leg raising (root at or below L5); positive femoral stretch test (roots of L2, L3, or L4); and focal signs that are determined by root affected.

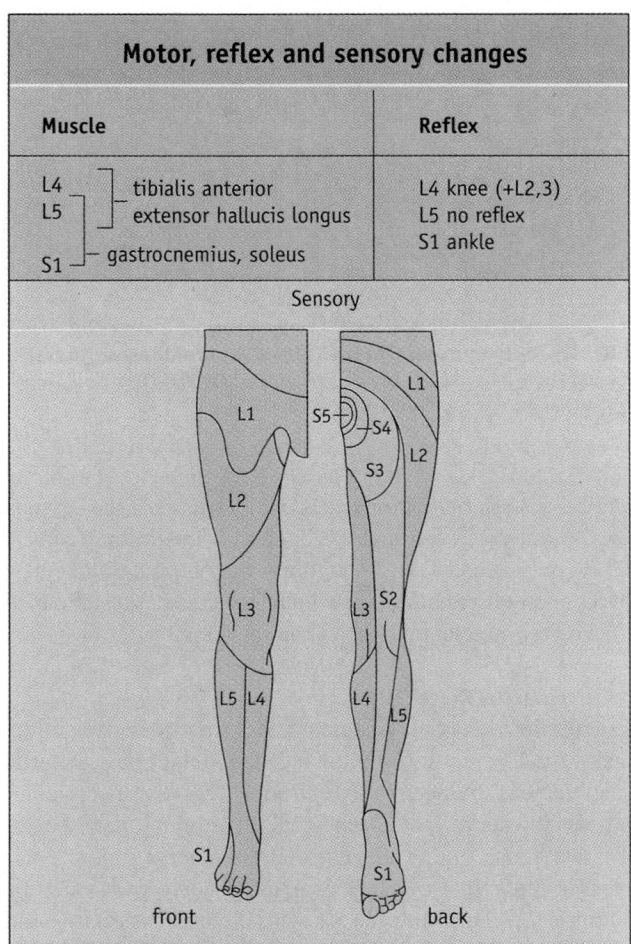

Motor, reflex and sensory changes

Muscle	Reflex
L4, L5 – tibialis anterior, extensor hallucis longus; S1 – gastrocnemius, soleus	L4 knee (+L2,3) L5 no reflex S1 ankle

Sensory

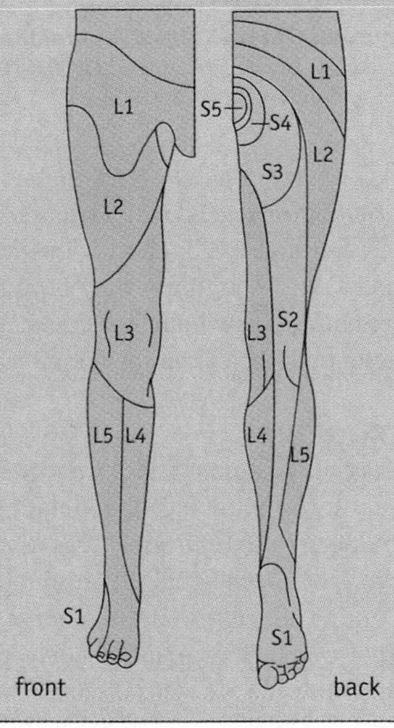

FIG. 16-14 Motor, sensory, and reflex changes in lumbascaral root disorders. (From Perkin DG: *Mosby's color atlas and text of neurology,* London, 1998, Mosby-Wolfe.)

Spondylolysis. **Spondylolysis** is a degenerative process of the vertebral column and associated soft tissue. It is characterized by a structural defect of the spine involving the lamina or neural arch of the vertebra. The most common site affected is the lumbar spine. This defect occurs in the portion of the lamina between the superior and inferior articular facets called the *pars interarticularis.* Mechanical pressure may cause a forward displacement of the deficient vertebra called *spondylolisthesis.*

Heredity plays a significant role, and spondylolysis is associated with an increased incidence of other congenital spinal defects. As a result of torsional and rotational stress, "microfractures" occur at the affected site and eventually cause dissolution of the pars interarticularis.

Spondylolisthesis. **Spondylolisthesis** is a stress factor allowing a vertebra to slide forward in relation to the vertebra below, commonly occurring at L5-S1. Spondylolisthesis is graded from 1 to 4 on the basis of the percentage of slip that has occurred. Individuals with grade 3 or 4 are considered for operative decompression or stabilization or both. Grades 1 and 2 usually are managed symptomatically and with nonsurgical methods.

Box 16-2

STEM CELLS REPAIR RAT SPINAL CORD DAMAGE

Seppa reports that researchers using transplanted fetal mouse stem cells within 9 days of induced spinal cord trauma in rats found that the rats regained their ability to stand on all four legs and to walk.

Data from Seppa A: Stem cells repair rat spinal cord damage, *Sci* 157: 6, 2000.

Spinal stenosis. In **spinal stenosis** the spinal canal may be congenitally narrowed or narrowed by a bulging annulus, a facet hypertrophy, or a thick/ossified posterior longitudinal ligament entrapping a single nerve involving many roots.[17] It is classified as acquired (more common) or developmental (such as occurs in achondroplastic dwarfs). Surgical decompression is recommended for those with long-term symptoms and those who remain unresponsive to medical management.

Low Back Pain

Low back pain affects the area between the lower rib cage and gluteal muscles and often radiates into the thighs. About 1% of individuals with acute low back pain have sciatica, or pain in the distribution of a lumbar nerve root. Sciatica often is accompanied by neurosensory and motor deficits, such as weakness.

The incidence of, or percentage of population affected with, low back pain at some point in life is 60% to 80%, and the annual incidence is 5%.[18] Men and women are affected equally; however, women report low back symptoms more often after the age of 60 years.

Pathogenesis

Most cases of low back pain are idiopathic, and clinicians are unable to provide a precise diagnosis for most individuals with this disorder. The local processes involved in low back pain range from tension caused by tumors or disk prolapse, bursitis, synovitis, rising venous and tissue pressure (found in degenerative joint disease), abnormal bone pressures, problems with spinal mobility, inflammation caused by infection (as in osteomyelitis), bony fractures, or ligamentous sprains to pain referred from viscera or the posterior peritoneum. General processes resulting in low back pain include bone diseases, such as osteoporosis or osteomalacia, and hyperparathyroidism.

Several risk factors have been identified in the pathogenesis of low back pain. They include involvement caused by occupations that require repetitious lifting in the forward bent-and-twisted position, exposure to vibrations caused by vehicles or industrial machinery, and perhaps cigarette smoking.[19] Osteoporosis increases the risk of spinal compression fractures and may be the reason elderly women report more symptoms than men. Genetic predispositions for low back pain include isthmic spondylolisthesis (vertebra slides forward or slips in relation to a vertebra below), spinal osteochondrosis, and spinal stenosis associated with achondroplasia. Variations in posture, such as lordosis and scoliosis of less than 60 degrees, do not appear to increase the risk of low back pain or sciatica. Differences in weight, height, and leg length are controversial as risk factors.

Anatomically, low back pain must come from innervated structures, but deep pain is widely referred and varies from person to person. The nucleus pulposus has no intrinsic innervation; however, when extruded or herniated through a prolapsed disk, it irritates the dural membranes and is responsible for pain referred to the segmental area (see Fig. 16-14). The interspinous bursae can be a source of low back pain between L3, L4, L5, and S1 but also may affect L1, L2, and L3 spinous processes, depending on the closeness of the adjacent pair of spines. The anterior and posterior longitudinal ligaments of the spine and the interspinous and supraspinous ligaments are abundantly supplied with pain receptors, as is the ligamentum flavum. All of these ligaments are vulnerable to traumatic tears (sprains) and fracture. The role of muscle injury in the production of low back pain remains uncertain, even though sprains and strains are the most common diagnoses.[20] The muscle spasms that often are produced during sieges of low back pain are thought to be produced by as yet unknown sensory or motor-reflex pathways.[21] The most commonly encountered causes of low back pain include lumbar disk herniation, degenerative disk disease, spondylolysis, spondylolisthesis, and spinal stenosis. (For a discussion of disk herniation and rupture, see p. 503.)

Evaluation and Treatment

Diagnosis of low back injury is made on the basis of physical, electromyelographic (EMG), epidurographic, diskographic, and MRI examination; CT examination with or without myelography; and nerve conduction studies. Most individuals with acute low back pain benefit from a nonspecific short-term treatment regimen including bed rest, analgesic medications, exercises, physical therapy, and education. Surgical treatments may be indicated if individuals do not respond to medical management. Surgical treatments include diskectomy and spinal fusions. Individuals with chronic low back pain can be treated with antiinflammatory and muscle relaxant medications and exercise programs. Aerobic exercises are a popular treatment and seem to be more effective than traction or low back exercises.[20] Spinal surgery has a limited role in curing chronic low back pain.

Herniated Intervertebral Disk

Herniation of an intervertebral disk is a protrusion of part of the nucleus pulposus (like stepping on an ice cream sandwich) through a tear in the posterior rim of the annulus fibrosus (the fibrous capsule enclosing the gelatinous center of the disk) (Fig. 16-15). Rupture of an intervertebral disk usually is caused by trauma or degenerative disk disease or both. Lifting with the trunk flexed and sudden straining when the back is in an unstable position are the most common causes. Men are more affected than women, with the highest incidence among those 30 to 60 years of age. Most commonly affected are the lumbosacral disks, that is, L5-S1 and L4-5. Disk herniation occasionally occurs in the cervical area, usually at C5-6 and C6-7. Herniations at the thoracic level are extremely rare. The injury may have an immediate onset or an onset within a few hours, or the manifestations of injury may take months to years to develop.

A

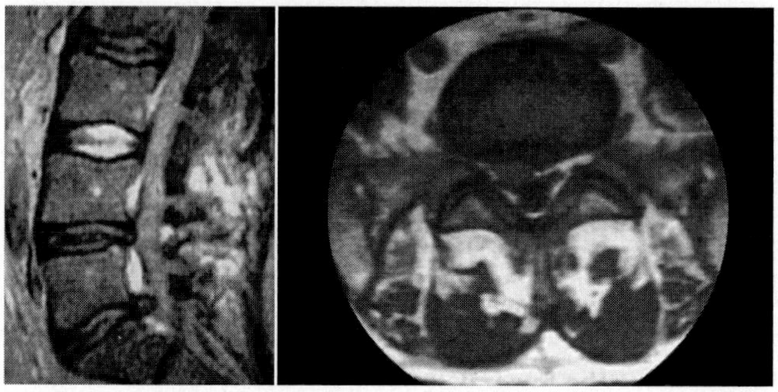

B

FIG. 16-15 Posterolateral disk protrusion. MRI scan, *(a)* sagittal and *(b)* axial sections. (From Perkin DG: *Mosby's color atlas and text of neurology,* London, 1998, Mosby-Wolfe.)

Pathophysiology

In a herniated disk the ligament and posterior capsule of the disk usually are torn, allowing the gelatinous material (the nucleus pulposus) to extrude. This extrusion compresses the nerve root. Occasionally the injury tears the entire disk loose, and it protrudes onto the nerve root or compresses the spinal cord. One or more nerve roots may be compressed. This multiple nerve root compression is found especially at the L5-S1 level, where the cauda equina may be compressed. Large amounts of extruded nucleus pulposus or complete disk herniation (i.e., of both the capsule and the nucleus pulposus) may compress the spinal cord.

Clinical Manifestations

The location and size of the herniation into the spinal canal, together with the amount of space that exists inside the spinal canal, determine the clinical manifestations associated with the injury (see Fig. 16-15). A herniated disk in the lumbosacral area is associated with pain that radiates along the sciatic nerve course over the buttock and into the calf or ankle. The pain occurs with straining, including coughing and sneezing, and usually on straight leg raising. Other clinical manifestations include limited range of motion of the lumbar spine; tenderness on palpation in the sciatic notch and along the sciatic nerve; impaired pain, temperature, and touch sensation in the L5-S1 or L4-5 dermatomes of the leg and foot; decreased or absent ankle jerk; and mild weakness of the foot.

With the herniation of a lower cervical disk, paresthesias and pain are present in the upper arm, forearm, and hand in the affected nerve root distribution. Neck and nerve root pain may be increased by neck motion and straining, including coughing and sneezing. Neck range of motion is diminished. Slight weakness and atrophy of biceps or triceps may occur; the biceps or triceps reflex may decrease. Occasionally signs of corticospinal and sensory tract impairments appear. These include motor weakness of the lower extremities, sensory disturbances in the lower extremities, and presence of a Babinski reflex.

Evaluation and Treatment

Diagnosis of a herniated intervertebral disk is made on the basis of the history; physical, EMG, CT, MRI, myelographic, and diskographic examination; spinal radiographs; and nerve conduction studies. Multiple avenues of therapy are available. The conservative approach comprises traction, bed rest, heat and ice to the affected areas, and an effective analgesic antiinflammatory regimen. The surgical approach is indicated if there is evidence of severe compression (weakness, decreased deep tendon reflexes and bladder/bowel reflexes) or if the conservative approach is unsuccessful.

Cerebrovascular Disorders

Cerebrovascular disease is the most frequently occurring neurologic disorder. More than 50% of persons admitted to general hospitals with neurologic problems have cerebrovascular disease. Any abnormality of the brain caused by a pathologic process in the blood vessels is referred to as a *cerebrovascular disease.* Included in this category are lesions of the vessel wall; occlusion of the vessel lumen by thrombus or embolus; rupture of the vessel; and alteration in vessel permeability, such as increased blood viscosity.

The brain abnormalities induced by cerebrovascular disease are of two types: (1) ischemia with or without infarction (death of brain tissues) and (2) hemorrhage. The common clinical manifestation of cerebrovascular disease is a **cerebrovascular accident (CVA, stroke),** which is a sudden, nonconvulsive focal neurologic deficit.

Cerebrovascular Accidents (Stroke Syndromes)

The incidence of stroke is 600,000 persons per year. Cerebrovascular accidents (CVAs) are the third leading cause of death in the United States, resulting in 160,000 deaths per year. It is the leading cause of disability in the United States.[22] The economic cost is greater than 40 billion dollars per year.[22,23] Five percent to 14% of stroke survivors have a second stroke within 1 year of the first CVA. By 5 years, 24% of females and 42% of males have a second stroke.

The highest incidence of stroke is among people over 65 years of age. Strokes, however, do occur in a 3:10 ratio (28%) in individuals younger than 65 years of age. Stroke tends to run in families and is more common in women. The incidence of stroke is 2.5 times higher in blacks than whites.[17] Blacks suffer greater physical impairments and are nearly 2 times as likely to die from their stroke. Intracranial atherosclerosis is more common in black and Asian populations, whereas extracranial disease is more common in the white population.

The mildest outcome of a CVA is so minimal as to be almost unnoticed. The most severe outcomes are hemiplegia, coma, and death. CVAs (stroke syndromes) are classified according to pathophysiology and thus are ischemic (thrombotic or embolic), global hypoprofusion (as in shock), or hemorrhagic. Risk factors for stroke include the following:

1. Arterial hypertension and both elevated systolic and diastolic blood pressures are independent risk factors.[17]
2. Smoking increases the risk of stroke by 50%.
3. Diabetes increases the risk of ischemic stroke between 2.5 and 3.5 times.
4. Insulin resistance is an independent risk factor for ischemic stroke.[24]
5. Polycythemia and thrombocythemia increase the risk for ischemic stroke.
6. Presence of elevated lipoprotein-a is an independent risk factor for ischemic stroke.
7. Impaired cardiac function increases the risk for ischemic stroke.
8. Hyperhomocysteinemia is a strong and independent risk factor for ischemic stroke.[25]
9. Nonrheumatic atrial fibrillation is associated with a fivefold increase in the incidence of ischemic stroke.[26]
10. Estrogen deficiency is a risk factor in postmenopausal women; however, there are no data on recurrent stroke risk.[27]

Thrombotic Stroke

Thrombotic strokes (cerebral thrombosis) arise from arterial occlusions caused by thrombi formed in the arteries supplying the brain or in the intracranial vessels. The development of a cerebral thrombosis most frequently is attributed to atherosclerosis and inflammatory disease processes (arteritis) that damage arterial walls. Increased coagulation can lead to thrombus formation. Conditions causing inadequate cerebral perfusion (e.g., dehydration, hypotension, prolonged vasoconstriction from malignant hypertension) increase the risk of thrombosis. Over 20 to 30 years, atheromatous plaques (stenotic lesions) tend to form at branchings and curves in the cerebral circulation. The smooth stenotic area can degenerate, forming an ulcerated area of vessel wall. Platelets and fibrin adhere to the damaged wall, and clots form, gradually occluding the artery. The thrombus may enlarge both distally and proximally in the vessel. Portions of the clot break off and travel up the vessel to distant sites where occlusion occurs, producing a stroke syndrome.

Thrombotic strokes may be further subdivided on the basis of clinical manifestations into transient ischemic attacks, strokes-in-evolution, and completed strokes. **Transient ischemic attacks (TIAs)** are experienced by 50,000 Americans per year. They probably represent thrombotic particles causing an intermittent blockage of circulation or spasm. In a true TIA all the neurologic deficits must be completely clear within 24 hours, leaving no residual dysfunction. Recurrence of symptoms is 30% at 3 months, 60% at 6 months, and 80% at 1 year without definitive treatment. Reversible ischemic neurologic defects (RINDs) are signs that persist over 24 hours but eventually disappear completely.

The symptoms of thrombotic strokes occasionally have an abrupt onset but tend to be slowly progressive, evolving in a step-by-step fashion over minutes to hours. The typical development of thrombotic stroke causes the clinical syndrome known as a **stroke-in-evolution (progressive stroke).** An intermittent progression of a neurologic deficit over hours to days is characteristic of thrombotic stroke or slow hemorrhage. The **completed stroke** is a CVA that has reached its maximum destructiveness in producing neurologic deficits, although cerebral edema may not have reached its maximum.

Embolic stroke. An **embolic stroke** involves fragments that break from a thrombus formed outside the brain or in the heart, aorta, common carotid, or thorax. Emboli infrequently arise from the ascending aorta or common carotid artery. The embolus usually involves small vessels and obstructs at a bifurcation or other point of narrowing, thus causing ischemia. An embolus may plug the lumen entirely and remain in place or break into fragments and move up the vessel. Conditions associated with the onset of an embolic stroke include atrial fibrillation; myocardial infarction; endocarditis; rheumatic heart disease; valvular prostheses; atrial-septal defects; and disorders of the aorta, carotids, or vertebral-basilar circulation. Less common contributors to embolic stroke are air, fat, and tumors. Fat emboli sometimes develop with fractures of long bones. Air emboli also can develop after certain types of surgery. In persons who experience an embolic stroke, a second stroke usually follows at some point because the source of emboli continues to exist. Embolization is usually in the distribution of the middle cerebral artery.

Hemorrhagic stroke. **Hemorrhagic stroke (intracranial hemorrhage)** is the third most common cause of CVA (10% of strokes). The most common causes of hemorrhagic stroke are hypertension (56% to 81%), ruptured aneurysms, vascular malformations, bleeding into a tumor, hemorrhage associated with bleeding disorders or anticoagulation, head trauma, and illicit drug use. Risk factors for hemorrhagic stroke include hypertension, previous cerebral infarct, coronary artery disease, and diabetes mellitus.

A hypertensive hemorrhage is associated with a significant increase in systolic and diastolic pressure over several years and usually occurs within the brain tissue. A mass of blood is formed, and its volume increases. Adjacent brain tissue is displaced and compressed. Rupture or seepage into the ventricular system occurs in many cases. Hemorrhages are described as massive, small, slit, or petechial. A massive hemorrhage is several centimeters in diameter; a small hemorrhage is 1 to 2 cm in diameter; a slit hemorrhage lies in the subcortical area; and a petechial hemorrhage is the size of a pinhead bleed. The most common sites for hypertensive hemorrhages are in the putamen of the basal ganglia (a portion of the lentiform nucleus) (55%), the thalamus (10%), the cortex and subcortex (15%), the pons (10%) (Fig. 16-16), and cerebellar hemispheres (10%).

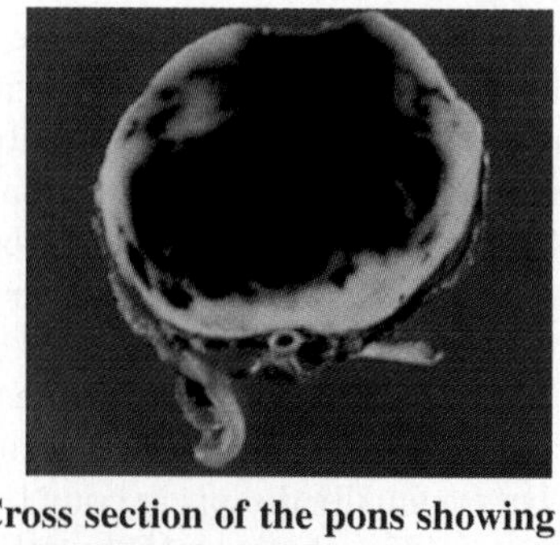

FIG. 16-16 Cross section of the pons showing a hypertensive hemorrhage. (From Perkin DG: *Mosby's color atlas and text of neurology,* London, 1998, Mosby-Wolfe.)

Lacunar stroke. **Lacunar strokes (lacunar infarcts)** are microinfarcts smaller than 1 cm in diameter and involve the small perforating arteries, predominantly in the basal ganglia, internal capsules, and pons. Lacunar infarcts are caused by atherosclerosis and associated with hypertension and diabetes mellitus.[28] Because of the subcortical location and small area of infarction, these strokes may have pure motor and sensory deficits.

Pathophysiology

Cerebral infarction. Cerebral infarction results when an area of the brain loses blood supply because of vascular occlusion. The pathologic manifestation is either (1) a global process that affects neurons most susceptible to ischemia (pyramidal and striatal neurons), Purkinje cells of the cerebral hemispheres, and the border zones at the very end of the arteries of circulation; or (2) a focal process with a central zone of cell loss surrounded by a zone of injured cells (a penumbra) that, if perfused in 1 hour, will survive.[17] Proposed pathogenesis may include (1) abrupt vascular occlusion (e.g., embolus), (2) gradual vessel occlusion (e.g., atheroma), and (3) vessels that are stenosed but not completely occluded. Cerebral thrombi and cerebral emboli are the most common causes of occlusion, but atherosclerosis and hypotension are the dominant underlying processes.

Cerebral infarctions are ischemic or hemorrhagic. In ischemic infarcts (pale infarcts, "white stroke"), cytotoxic ischemic events and interaction between blood elements and blood vessels combine to produce brain injury. The affected area becomes slightly discolored and softens about 6 to 12 hours after the occlusion. Necrosis, swelling around the insult, and mushy disintegration have appeared by 48 to 72 hours after infarction. At a microscopic level, neuronal cell bodies change, myelin sheaths and axis cylinders are interrupted and disintegrate, and there is loss of oligodendrites and astrocytes.

Cellular events involve the following: (1) altered cell membranes in which cell membranes depolarize, allowing calcium influx into the cells, resulting in metabolic effects such as failure of mitochondrial oxidative phosphlylation (responsible for energy production); (2) glutamate release that alters cell membrane permeability to sodium, potassium, and calcium, and thus electrolyte influx pulls water into the cells, resulting in cytotoxic edema; and (3) fall in extra- and intracellular pH due to lactic acid production, resulting in an associated focal vasodilation. Infarcted areas may loose autoregulation.

A syndrome of luxury perfusion in areas adjacent to the infarct develops first from the loss of autoregulation.[17] The vascular bed in this area dilates. Larger, capillary sprouting (neovascularization) supports this luxury perfusion syndrome.

In hemorrhagic infarcts ("red strokes"), bleeding occurs into the infarcted area as a result of restoration of blood flow. Reperfusion occurs when the embolus fragments, or lysis or compressive forces lessen, allowing blood flow to be reestablished into the infarcted area. Most hemorrhagic infarcts are located in the cerebral cortex. Unfortunately, reperfusion has been shown to compromise recovery by accelerating the sequence of metabolically damaging events.[29]

Cerebral hemorrhage. The primary cause of cerebral hemorrhage is hypertension. (Aneurysms and AVMs are discussed on pp. 510 and 511.) The pathogenesis of hypertensive cerebral hemorrhage is not fully understood. Hypertension involves primarily smaller arteries and arterioles, resulting in thickening of the vessel walls, and increased cellularity of the vessels and hyalinization. Necrosis may be present. Microaneurysms in these smaller vessels or arteriolar necrosis precipitates the bleeding.

A mass of blood is formed as bleeding continues into the brain tissue. Adjacent brain tissue is displaced and compressed, producing ischemia and subsequent vasogenic edema. Increased ICP results. Rupture or seepage of blood into the ventricular system occurs in many cases.

The cerebral hemorrhage resolves through reabsorption. Macrophages and astrocytes appear to clear away the blood. A cavity forms, surrounded by a dense gliosis after removal of the blood.

Clinical Manifestations

Because neurons surrounding the ischemic or infarcted areas undergo changes that disrupt plasma membranes, cellular edema results, causing further compression of capillaries. Cerebral edema reaches its maximum in about 72 hours and takes about 2 weeks to subside. Most persons survive an initial hemispheric ischemic stroke unless massive cerebral edema develops. Massive brain stem infarcts, caused by basilar thrombosis or embolism, are almost always fatal, however.

Clinical manifestations of thrombotic stroke vary, depending on the artery obstructed. Different sites of obstruction create different occlusion syndromes (Table 16-5).

With hemorrhagic stroke, clinical manifestations vary according to the location and size of the bleed. Focal neurologic deficits are found in 80% of individuals experiencing hemorrhagic strokes, altered consciousness occurs in 50%,

Table 16-5 Stroke Syndromes Secondary to Occlusion or Stenosis

Location/Vessel	Area of Brain Infarcted	Signs and Symptoms Noted
ANTERIOR AND CENTRAL CIRCULATION	NOTE: The internal carotid enters the circle of Willis and supplies the lateral anterior and central portions of the cerebral hemispheres through the middle cerebral artery and the paramedial frontal lobe superior to the corpus callosum through the anterior cerebral artery; penetrating branches serve the deeper layers of the hemispheres	
Internal carotid	If collateral circulation is intact, there is commonly no infarction; if infarcted, it is in the same area as the middle cerebral artery	• Arterial pressure may be low in the retina • Bruits over the internal carotid artery • Possible retinal emboli • History of transient ischemic attacks (TIAs) • Positive noninvasive studies
Middle cerebral artery (MCA) (most common area); either stem or branches of MCA	Cortical motor area (face, arm, leg) and/or posterior limb, internal capsule, corona radiata	• **Motor:** contralateral hemiparesis or hemiplegia, greater in face and arm than leg
	Cortical sensory area (face, arm, leg) and/or posterior limb of internal capsule	• **Sensation:** contralateral loss in same distribution as motor loss
	Broca area and deep fibers in the dominant hemisphere	• **Speech:** expressive (motor) disorder with anomia (left hemisphere most commonly affected) with nonfluent aphasia and some comprehension defects
	Broca area and deep fibers in the nondominant hemisphere	• **Speech:** dysarthria
	Optic radiations deep in the temporal lobe	• **Vision:** contralateral homonymous hemianopsia or quadranopsia
	Location not known	• **Motor:** mirror movements • **Respirations:** Cheyne-Stokes respirations, contralateral hyperhidrosis, occasional mydriasis
	Posterior limb or internal capsule and adjacent corona radiata	• **Motor:** pure motor hemiplegia
	Penetrating branches of MCA (lenticulostriate branches) into the basal nuclei	• **Motor:** varying degrees of contralateral weakness of face, arm, or leg

Modified from Barker E. *Neuroscience nursing,* St Louis, 1994, Mosby.

Continued

Table 16-5 Stroke Syndromes Secondary to Occlusion or Stenosis—cont'd

Location/Vessel	Area of Brain Infarcted	Signs and Symptoms Noted
ANTERIOR AND CENTRAL CIRCULATION—cont'd		
Middle cerebral artery (MCA) (most common area); either stem or branches of MCA—cont'd		• **Sensory:** little or no loss; if present, contralateral following the motor distribution • **Speech:** transcortical sensory aphasia (communicating pathways are interrupted) • **Perception:** transient visual and sensory neglect on the left if a right lesion
Anterior cerebral artery (ACA) (least common)	Proximal segment: corona radiata (rarely)	• **Motor:** when present, a mild contralateral hemiparesis, greater in leg; with bilateral occlusion of ACA, cerebral paraplegia in both legs can occur
	Main stem (complete occlusion is uncommon, thus areas affected differ and collateral circulation may alleviate signs or symptoms); medial aspect of frontal lobes, caudate nucleus, and corpus callosum are supplied by the ACA	• **Motor:** contralateral paralysis or paresis (greater in foot and thigh); mild upper extremity weakness • **Sensory:** mild contralateral lower extremity deficiency with loss of vibratory and/or position sense, loss of two-point discrimination • **Speech:** may have transcortical motor and sensory aphasia if left hemisphere • Frontal lobe releasing signs • Apraxia
POSTERIOR CIRCULATION	NOTE: The posterior circulation includes the posterior cerebral artery, the vertebral arteries, and the basilar artery; the anatomic territory covered includes the posterior aspects of the hemispheres, the central areas of the thalamus and midbrain, and the brain stem; occlusion of the vessels is most commonly by emboli; effects of infarct in these vessels and their penetrating vessels can be specific or devastatingly global; many complex syndromes have been identified	
Vertebral arteries	Medulla and spinal cord tracts, anterior spinal artery and penetrating branches (medial medullary syndrome)	• **Motor:** contralateral hemiparesis (face spared) and/or impaired contralateral proprioception; flaccid weakness or paralysis of the tongue and/or dysarthria
Basilar artery (three sets of branches)	Midline structures of pons (paramedian branches); three general areas of infarction are common: (1) medial inferior pontine syndrome, (2) medial midpontine syndrome, and (3) medial superior pontine syndrome	• **Motor:** contralateral hemiparesis or hemiplegia, ipsilateral lower motor neuron facial palsy, "locked-in syndrome" • **Sensory:** contralateral loss of vibratory sense, sense of position with dysmetria, loss of two-point discrimination, impaired rapid alternating movements • **Visual:** inferior pontine: diplopia; impaired abduction of ipsilateral eye: internuclear ophthalmoplegia; medial superior; diplopia, internuclear ophthalmoplegia, skewed deviation
	Corticospinal and corticobulbar tracts in pons, sensory tracts of medial and lateral lemnisci, vestibular nuclei, inferior and middle cerebellar peduncles, cranial nerve nuclei and/or fibers, cerebellar connections in tectum, descending sympathetic pathways, central brain stem, pontine tegmentum (vertebral basilar syndrome)	• **Motor:** upper motor neuron type of weakness: paralysis in combinations involving face, tongue, throat, and extremities; dysphagia, facial weakness, dysmetria, ataxia (either trunk or extremities), weak mastication muscles • **Sensation:** combinations of impaired sensation (vibratory, two-point, position sense, pain, temperature), facial hypesthesia, anesthesia of cranial nerve V
Posterior cerebral artery (PCA)	Central territory (thalamic area, dentothalamic tract, cerebral peduncle, red nucleus, subthalamic nucleus, and cranial nerve III)	• **Motor:** contralateral hemiplegia with possible dysmetria, dyskinesia, hemiballism or choreoathetosis, dystaxia, cerebellar ataxia, and tremor; contralateral upper motor neuron palsy; several syndromes are associated: (1) Weber: cranial nerve III palsy and contralateral hemiplegia; (2) thalamoperforate syndrome: superior, crossed cerebellar ataxia or inferior crossed cerebellar ataxia with cranial nerve III palsy (Claude syndrome); (3) decerebrate attacks • **Sensory:** contralateral sensory loss of all modalities without agraphia

Table 16-5 Stroke Syndromes Secondary to Occlusion or Stenosis—cont'd

Location/Vessel	Area of Brain Infarcted	Signs and Symptoms Noted
POSTERIOR CIRCULATION—cont'd		
Posterior cerebral artery (PCA)—cont'd		• **Function:** prosopagnosia (inability to recognize familiar faces), topographic disorientation, memory deficits, alexia, inability to read, color anomia • **Level of consciousness:** in bilateral PCA syndromes, coma with absent doll's eyes or loss of alertness may occur; if tegmentum of midbrain near hypothalamus and third ventricle is damaged, akinetic mutism may occur
SMALL VESSEL DISEASE	Small penetrating vessels in brain parenchyma that supply areas near the basal ganglia are most vulnerable to infarction although any small vessels can occlude deep in the brain and cause injury, producing neurologic signs or symptoms; such infarcts are commonly called *lacunes* (small pit or hollow), a term that is changing in meaning; they can be caused by emboli but are most commonly associated with microatheromas; although they can be found in otherwise healthy people, those with concurrent athersclerosis, **arterial** hypertension, and/or diabetes have a higher incidence of this type of infarct	
	Internal capsule, most commonly	• **Motor:** contralateral hemiparesis on a single side, with equal deficit in face, arm, and leg; often unaccompanied by detectable signs of sensory, visual, and speech loss, depending on location; old term is "pure motor stroke" although evidence suggests that other neurologic signs are present but overlooked because of low intensity
	Thalamus, most commonly	• **Sensory:** complete or partial loss in face, arm, trunk, and leg that appears exactly midline; may be accompanied by pain, hypesthesias, and uncomfortable sensations (hemisensory stroke)
	Pons	• Dysarthria, clumsy hand
	Pons, midbrain, capsule or parietal white matter	• Hemiparesis, ataxia on same side

Once a deep unresponsive state occurs, the person rarely survives. The immediate prognosis is grave. If the person survives, however, recovery of function frequently is possible.

Individuals experiencing intracranial hemorrhage from a ruptured or leaking aneurysm have one of three sets of symptoms: (1) onset of an excruciating generalized headache with an almost immediate lapse into an unresponsive state; (2) headache, but with consciousness maintained; and (3) sudden lapse into unconsciousness. If the hemorrhage is confined to the subarachnoid space, there may be no local signs. If bleeding spreads into the brain tissue, hemiparesis/paralysis, dysphasia, or homonymous hemianopia may be present. Warning signs of an impending aneurysm rupture may include headache, transient unilateral weakness, transient numbness and tingling, and transient speech disturbance. Warning signs, however, often are not present.

Evaluation and Treatment

The newest principle of acute stroke treatment is "time is brain."[29] Time to treatment is often too great considering the time limits for reversibility of brain ischemia. Treatment needs to be initiated within 6 hours of symptom onset.[29] The "future of acute stroke treatment will likely include administration of agents for metabolic intervention by paramedics in the field, followed by perfusion therapy after emergency room evaluation and brain scanning."[29] Drug therapy is designed to prevent further thrombotic events (anticoagulation), augment blood flow (recanalization), reperfuse the tissues (vasodilators, hemodilution, thrombolytics), and protect neurons (metabolic adjustment). To provide anticoagulation and reperfusion, antiplatelets and antithrombotics such as acetylsalicylic acid (ASA), dipyridamine (Persantine), ticlopidine (Ticlid), clopidogrel (Plavix), and combination drugs; heparin; low-molecular-weight heparinoids; and warfarin sodium (Coumadin), as well as thrombolytics such as urokinase/streptokinase, tissue plasminogen (t-PA), ancrod (Arvin), and pentoxifylline may be used.[30] Thrombolytic therapy for acute ischemic stroke, however, has been found to be used in only 2% of persons who were eligible.[31] Metabolic protection is designed to control calcium influx (e.g., calcium channel blockers), excitatory amine activation (e.g., glutamate inhibitors, antagonists), and free radicals (free radical scavenger agents).[32] Cell transplants in stroke are being examined in animal models.

In thrombotic strokes, treatment is directed at supportive management to control cerebral edema and increased ICP. Ancrod (Arvin), a drug, is being tested experimentally to achieve defibrinogenation and thus increase local cerebral blood flow in the ischemic areas. Later surgical intervention to restore blood supply may be indicated. Arresting the disease process by control of risk factors is critical. In embolic strokes, treatment is directed at preventing further embolization by instituting anticoagulation therapy and correcting the primary problem. Rehabilitation is indicated in both thrombotic and embolic stroke. Treatment of an intracranial bleed, regardless of cause, is focused on stopping or reducing the bleeding, controlling the increased ICP, preventing a rebleed, and preventing vasospasm.[33] Occasionally an attempt is made to evacuate or aspirate the blood.

Intracranial Aneurysm

Intracranial aneurysms may result from arteriosclerosis, congenital abnormality, trauma, inflammation, or infection. Cocaine use has been linked to aneurysm formation. The size of the aneurysm may vary from 2 mm to 2 or 3 cm. Most aneurysms are located at bifurcations in or near the circle of Willis, in the vertebrobasilar arteries, or within the carotid system (see Fig. 13-18). Eighty-five percent are in the anterior circulation. Aneurysms may be single, but in 20% to 25% of cases, more than one aneurysm is present. In these instances the aneurysms may be unilateral or bilateral. The incidence of rupture is 11 in 100,000 persons per year. Peak incidence of rupture is among persons from 50 to 60 years of age. Women have a slightly greater incidence of aneurysms.

Pathophysiology

No single pathologic mechanism exists. Aneurysm development is attributed to hemodynamic stress and is believed to be exacerbated by hypertension and certain connective tissue disorders. The smooth muscle coat and elastic lamina of the intracranial artery end at the neck of the aneurysm. The aneurysm wall is composed of fibrous tissue. Aneurysms may be classified on the basis of shape and form (Fig. 16-17).

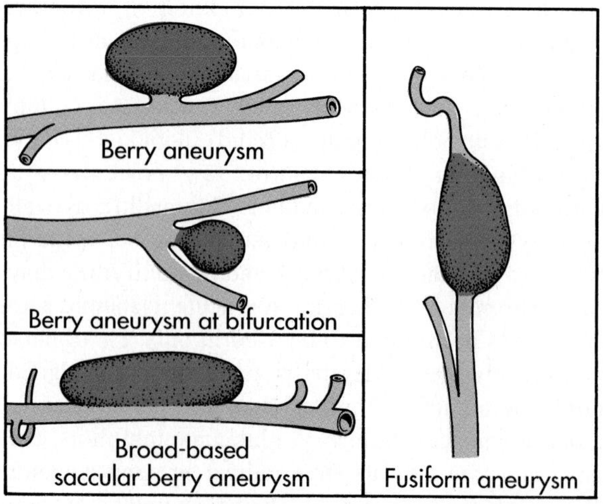

FIG. 16-17 Types of aneurysms.

Saccular aneurysms (berry aneurysms) occur frequently (in approximately 2% of the population) and are probably the result of congenital abnormalities in the media of the arterial wall. The sac gradually grows over time. A saccular aneurysm may be (1) round with a narrow stalk connecting it to the parent artery (Fig. 16-18), (2) broad based without a stalk, or (3) cylindric. Saccular aneurysms are rare in childhood; their highest incidence of rupturing or bleeding is among persons 20 to 50 years of age.

Fusiform aneurysms (giant aneurysms), by definition greater than 25 mm in diameter, make up 5% of all intracra-

A

B

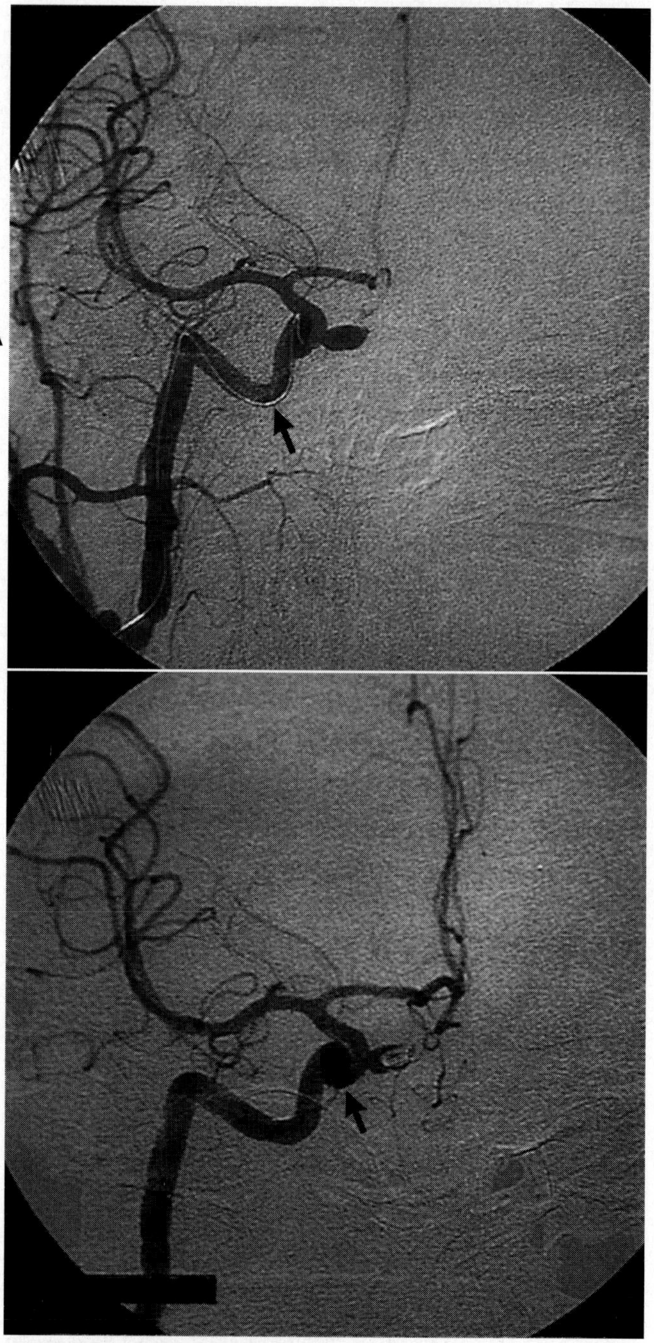

FIG. 16-18 Ophthalmic artery aneyrysm. A, With endovascular coil, **B,** in situ. (From Perkin DG: *Mosby's color atlas and text of neurology,* London, 1998, Mosby-Wolfe.)

nial aneurysms. They occur as a result of diffuse arteriosclerotic changes and are found most commonly in the basilar arteries or terminal portions of the internal carotid arteries. They act as space-occupying lesions. **Mycotic aneurysms** result from arteritis caused by bacterial emboli; these aneurysms are uncommon. **Traumatic aneurysms** are caused by a weakening of the arterial wall by a fracture line, by a penetrating missile, or after neurosurgical or imaging (e.g., angiographic) procedures.

Aneurysms rupture because their walls are thin, causing hemorrhage into the subarachnoid space with rapid spread, producing localized changes in the cerebral cortex and focal irritation of nerves and arteries (see Laplace law, Chapter 28). Because of compression, bleeding ceases with the formation of a fibrin-platelet plug at the point of rupture. Blood undergoes reabsorption through arachnoid villi within 3 weeks.

Clinical Manifestations

Aneurysms are frequently asymptomatic. Of all persons undergoing routine autopsy, 5% are found to have one or more intracranial aneurysms. Clinical manifestations may arise from cranial nerve compression, but the signs vary, depending on the location and size of the aneurysm. Most often, cranial nerves III, IV, V, and VI are affected (see Table 13-6). Unfortunately, the most common first indication of the presence of an aneurysm is an acute subarachnoid hemorrhage, intracerebral hemorrhage, or combined subarachnoid-intracerebral hemorrhage (see p. 512).

Evaluation and Treatment

Diagnosis before a bleeding episode is made using arteriographic examination. After a subarachnoid or an intracerebral hemorrhage, a tentative diagnosis of an aneurysm that has bled is based on clinical manifestations, history, CT scan, and MRI. The treatment of choice for an aneurysm is surgical management. The location and size of the aneurysm and the person's clinical status determine whether invasive therapy is feasible.

Vascular Malformations

Four types of vascular malformation exist: arteriovenous malformation (AVM), cavernous angioma, capillary telangiectasis, and venous angioma.[17] **Cavernous angiomas (malformations)** are sinusoidal collections of blood vessels without interspersed normal brain tissue. They rarely hemorrhage and compose 8% to 15% of all vascular lesions. A **capillary telangiectasis** is dilated capillaries with interspersed normal brain tissue. Hemorrhage is rare and these vascular malformations are associated with Rendu-Oster-Weber disease. **Venous angioma**, the most common vascular malformation found at autopsy (3% of cases), is considered a subset of developmental venous anomalies that occur secondary to arrested development.[8] The result is primitive embryologic veins in a radial pattern feeding a central vein. These rarely hemorrhage.

In an **arteriovenous malformation (AVM),** arteries feed directly into veins through a vascular tangle of malformed vessels (Fig. 16-19). AVMs hemorrhage at a rate of 40% a year. AVMs occur in any part of the brain, and they are usually cone shaped. Their size is highly variable, from malformations of a few millimeters to large ones that extend from the cortex to the ventricle. The large AVMs also may involve the dura mater, including the falx cerebri and the tentorium cerebelli. AVMs occur as frequently in males as in females, and they occasionally occur in families. Although usually present at birth, AVMs exhibit a delayed age of onset and symptoms most commonly occur before 30 years of age.

Pathophysiology

AVMs, which are developmental abnormalities that represent persistence of embryonic patterns of blood vessels, do not have a normal blood vessel structure and are abnormally thin. The involved vessels are thought by some to enlarge over time. The AVM may be fed by one or several arteries. These feeder vessels become tortuous over time and often dilated. With moderate to large AVMs, sufficient blood is shunted into the malformation to deprive surrounding tissue of adequate blood perfusion.

Clinical Manifestations

Clinical manifestations vary. Twenty percent of persons with an AVM have a characteristic chronic nondescript headache,

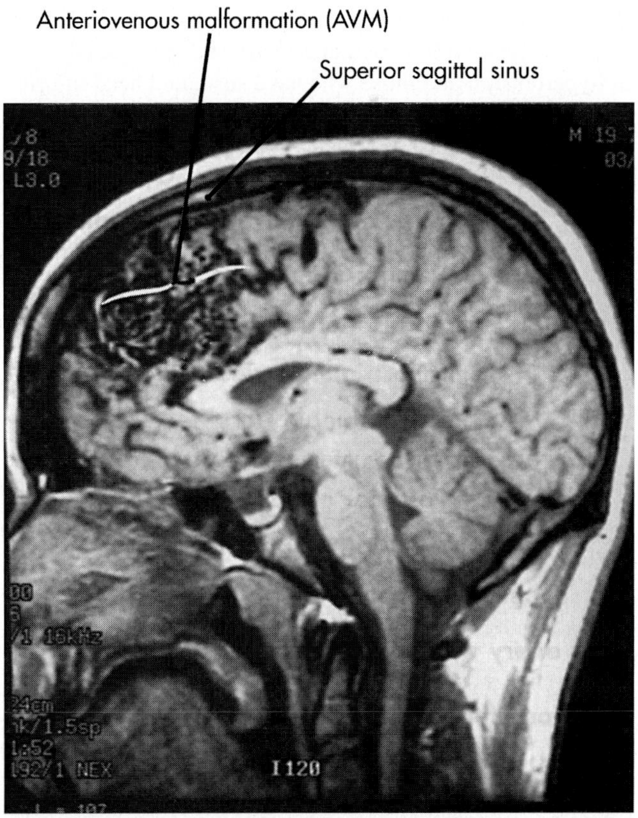

FIG. 16-19 Sagittal magnetic resonance imaging near the midline showing an AVM in the frontal lobe. This lesion includes branches of the anterior cerebral artery and drains into the superior sagittal sinus. (From Haines DE, editor: *Fundamental neuroscience,* Philadelphia, 1997, Churchill Livingstone.)

although some experience migraine. Thirty percent of persons experience seizure disorders caused by compression. Initially, the seizures tend to be focal or jacksonian; generalization often occurs over time. (Seizures are discussed in Chapter 15.) The other 50% suffer an intracerebral, a subarachnoid, or a subdural hemorrhage. Bleeding from an AVM into the subarachnoid space causes clinical manifestations identical to those associated with a ruptured aneurysm. If bleeding is into the brain tissue, focal signs that develop resemble a stroke-in-evolution. Ten percent of persons experience hemiparesis or other focal signs. Hemiparesis usually is caused by compression or rupture. At times, noncommunicating hydrocephalus (see Chapter 15) develops with a large AVM that extends into the ventricle lining.

Evaluation and Treatment

A systolic bruit over the carotid in the neck, the mastoid process, or (in a young person) the eyeball is almost diagnostic of an AVM. CT and MRI examination are used in initial diagnosis, followed by an arteriogram to identify feeding vessels. Treatment options are direct surgical approach, embolization, or radiotherapy. The risk of bleeding is 6% in the first year and 2% to 4% each year thereafter with no intervention.

Subarachnoid Hemorrhage

With a **subarachnoid hemorrhage,** blood escapes from a defective or injured vasculature into the subarachnoid space (Fig. 16-20). Individuals at risk for a subarachnoid hemorrhage are those with intracranial aneurysm, intracranial AVM, or hypertension and those who have sustained head injuries. Subarachnoid hemorrhages often recur, especially from a ruptured intracranial aneurysm.

Pathophysiology

When a vessel is leaking, blood oozes into the subarachnoid space. When a vessel tears, blood under pressure is pumped into the subarachnoid space. The blood is extremely irritating to the meningeal and other neural tissues and so produces an inflammatory reaction in these tissues. Additionally, the blood coats nerve roots, clogs arachnoid granulations (impairing cerebrospinal fluid [CSF] reabsorption), and clogs foramina within the ventricular system (impairing CSF circulation).[34] Intracranial pressure (ICP) immediately increases to almost diastolic levels. ICP returns to near baseline in about 10 minutes. Cerebral blood flow and cerebral perfusion pressure (CPP) decrease. The expanding hematoma acts like a space-occupying lesion, compressing and displacing brain tissue. Granulation tissue is formed, and scarring of the meninges with resulting impairment of CSF reabsorption and secondary hydrocephalus often results. Mortality in subarachnoid hemorrhage at 1 month is 50%.

Clinical Manifestations

Early manifestations associated with leaking vessels are episodic headache, transient changes in mental status or level of consciousness, nausea or vomiting, focal neurologic defects including visual or speech disturbances, cranial nerve palsies, or stiff neck. A ruptured vessel often is accompanied by a sudden throbbing, "explosive" headache. The headache is associated with nausea and vomiting, visual disturbances, motor deficits, and loss of consciousness. These signs all can be related to a dramatic rise in ICP. Meningeal irritation and inflammation often occur, causing neck stiffness (nuchal rigidity), photophobia, blurred vision, irritability, restlessness, and low-grade fever. A positive **Kernig sign** (in which straightening the knee with the hip and knee in a flexed position produces pain in the back and neck regions) and **Brudzinski sign** (in which passive flexion of the neck produces neck pain and increased rigidity) may appear. No localizing signs are present if the bleed is confined completely to the subarachnoid space.

The Hunt and Hess subarachnoid hemorrhage (SAH) grading system is based on description of the clinical manifestations (Table 16-6). Rebleeding is a significant risk with

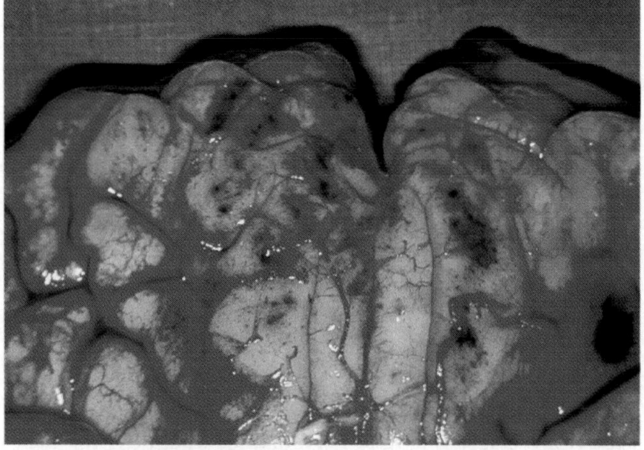

FIG. 16-20 Acute subarachnoid hemorrhage. Acute subarachnoid hemorrhage with focal accentuation over superficial cortical contusions. (From Damjanov I, Linder J, editors: *Anderson's pathology,* ed 10, St Louis, 1996, Mosby.)

Table 16-6 Subarachnoid Hemorrhage Classification Scale

Category	Description
Grade I	Neurologic status intact; mild headache, slight nuchal rigidity
Grade II	Neurologic deficit evidenced by cranial nerve involvement; moderate to severe headache with more pronounced meningeal signs (e.g., photophobia, nuchal rigidity)
Grade III	Drowsiness and confusion with or without focal neurologic deficits; pronounced meningeal signs
Grade IV	Stuporous with pronounced neurologic deficits (e.g., hemiparesis, dysphasia); nuchal rigidity
Grade V	Deep coma state with decerebrate posturing and other brain stem dysfunction

From Cook HA. In Winkleman C, editor: *AACN clinical issues in critical care nursing,* Philadelphia, 1991, Lippincott.

a high mortality (up to 70%). The period of greatest risk is the first month, with the peak incidence of rebleeding during the first 2 weeks after the initial bleed. Rebleeding is manifested by a sudden increase in blood pressure and ICP, along with a deteriorating neurologic status.

Delayed cerebral ischemia, a syndrome of progressive neurologic deterioration, is associated with cerebral artery vasospasm. In persons with a subarachnoid hemorrhage, 40% to 60% experience vasospasms in adjacent and sometimes in nonadjacent vessels. The pathophysiology of vasospasm is unclear. Vasospasm is thought to occur because of the effects of vasoactive substances (e.g., calcium, prostaglandins, serotonin, and catecholamines) on the arteries of the subarachnoid space. Edema, medial necrosis, and proliferation of the intima have been found. Vasospasm causes decreased cerebral blood flow (ischemia) and may produce infarct. The peak time of onset is 3 to 5 days, with maximal narrowing at 5 to 14 days after the initial bleed, but vasospasm may persist for several weeks.

Seizures occur in 25% of persons with an SAH. The incidence of hydrocephalus after a bleed is 20%. Hypothalamic dysfunction, manifested by salt wasting, hyponatremia, and ECG changes, is common.[35]

Evaluation and Treatment

The diagnosis of a subarachnoid hemorrhage is based on the clinical presentation, a noncontrast CT scan, and a lumbar puncture. Arteriographic examination is the definitive diagnostic measure for identifying an aneurysm or AVM. Treatment is directed at control of intracranial pressure, prevention of ischemia and hypoxia of neural tissues, and prevention of rebleeding episodes. Antifibrinolytic drugs may be used to stop rebleeding. Blood pressure is allowed to remain in the high normal range or elevated to that level. Platinum coils and balloon embolization to occlude the aneurysm are used, but microsurgical repair remains the treatment of choice. Calcium channel blockers, such as nimodipine, are used to prevent or reverse vasospasm. Volume expansion or hemodilution through continuous or bolus administration of hetastarch and plasma protein factors to maintain a hematocrit of 33% is used to expand blood volume and augment cerebral perfusion. Thrombolytics, such as ancrod (Arvin) and pentoxifylline, as well as glutamate inhibitors and antagonists and tirilizad (a nonglucocorticoid 21-aminosteroid with antioxidant and iron-chelating action) are being tested. Cerebral angioplasty is being tested for vasospasm. The primary problem must be diagnosed and corrected as well.

Headache

Headache is a common neurologic disorder and is usually a benign symptom. However, it can be associated with serious disease, such as brain tumor, meningitis, and giant cell arteritis. The headache syndromes discussed here are the chronic, recurring type not associated with structural abnormalities or systemic disease and include migraine, cluster, paroxysmal hemicrania, and tension headaches. Characteristics of the major types of headache syndromes are summarized in Table 16-7.

Migraine Headache

Migraine headache affects as many as 11 million people in the United States. The disorder occurs in 15% of women and 6% of men (a 2:1 to 3:1 ratio of female to male), is more common in those 25 to 55 years of age, and can occur in young children. The prevalence in women is highest at 20 to 40 years of age but remains higher than in men into older age. Onset after 50 years of age is rare. Hormonal factors account for most of the gender differences. A positive family history is a common finding, and there is a genetic predisposition to the disorder.[36]

Migraine headache is a benign recurring headache often provoked by a trigger factor and usually accompanied by neurologic dysfunction. Trigger factors may include stress; hunger; weather changes; spring; autumn; sunlight; noise; jet lag; foods, such as red wine, cheese, and chocolate; and menstruation, ovulation, and contraceptives.[37] The International Headache Society[38] has classified the following different clinical subtypes of migraine:

Table 16-7 Characteristics of Common Headaches

	Migraine			
	Without Aura	With Aura	Cluster Headache/ Proximal Hemicrania	Tension Type of Headache
Age of onset	Childhood, adolescence, or young adulthood	Childhood, adolescence, or young adulthood	Young adulthood, middle age	Young adulthood, middle age
Gender	Female	Female	Male	Not gender specific
Family history of headaches	Yes	Yes	No	Yes
Onset and evolution	Slow to rapid	Slow to rapid	Rapid	Slow to rapid
Time course	Episodic	Episodic	Clusters in time	Episodic, may become constant
Quality	Usually throbbing	Usually throbbing	Steady	Steady
Location	Variable, often unilateral	Variable, often unilateral	Orbit, temple, cheek	Variable
Associated features	Prodrome, vomiting	Prodrome, vomiting	Lacrimation, rhinorrhea, Horner syndrome	None

1. Migraine without aura: common migraine
2. Migraine with aura: classic migraine
   a. Migraine with typical aura
   b. Migraine with prolonged aura
   c. Familial hemiplegic migraine
   d. Basilar migraine
   e. Migraine aura without headache
   f. Migraine with acute-onset aura
3. Ophthalmoplegic migraine
4. Retinal migraine

The pathophysiologic basis for migraine is complex and includes neurologic, vascular, and hormonal and neurotransmitter components. Several theories have been proposed to account for the pathogenesis, including the vascular theory, cortical spreading depression, and serotonergic and other neurotransmitter alterations. These theories are summarized in Table 16-8. The phases of a migraine headache are (1) a trigger phase precipitated by external factors; (2) an aura with inhibition of cortical activity and a reduction in blood flow leading to symptoms of scotoma and paresthesias; (3) release of vasoactive neuropeptides, ionic alterations, platelet release of 5-HT, and degranulation of mast cells; and (4) activation of the locus ceruleus and excitation of trigeminal nuclei resulting in vasodilation of dural arteries. The resulting perivascular inflammation leads to the typical headache. Disturbances in the blood-brain barrier in the area postrema cause nausea and vomiting.[39,40]

In migraine with aura, the aura is thought to be caused by a slowly expanding area of reduced cortical activity and reduced blood flow. Reduced blood flow appears to be related to cortical arteriolar vasoconstriction and not vasospasm of larger arteries. Reductions in blood flow are not observed in migraine without aura. The pain of migraine is associated with neurotransmitters and pain fibers from the trigeminal nerve that terminate in the walls of the dural and cortical arteries. The trigeminal nucleus is controlled by the periaqueductal gray matter, which is a central modulator of pain transmission. Projections from the trigeminal nuclei also extend to the cervical spinal cord (C2) and may explain neck pain in addition to headache in migraine.[39]

Migraine headaches without aura, the most common type, last from 4 to 72 hours and are often located on one side. The pain is throbbing, of moderate to severe intensity, and aggravated by physical activity. In migraine with aura, the most common prodromal symptoms are visual (scotomas with luminous angles and scintillating edges, and hemianopsia). Sensory deficits and aphasia may also be present. The aura develops within 5 to 20 minutes and remits within 60 minutes, followed by headache and other symptoms, including nausea, vomiting, photophobia, scalp tenderness; 10% of persons experience diarrhea.

In susceptible women, migraine occurs most frequently before and during menstruation and is decreased during pregnancy and menopause. The cyclic withdrawal of estrogens may trigger attacks of migraine. Cyclic changes in estrogen are absent in pregnancy and after menopause, which could explain the less frequent attacks in some women. Estrogens may act directly on vascular smooth muscle, modulate activity of vasoactive substances at the neurovascular junction, and activate vasoregulatory responses in the hypothalamus.[41] However, no direct evidence has been found to link circulating female sex hormones with the frequency and severity of migraine.[42]

Table 16-8 Pathogenic Theories of Migraine Headache

Theory	Mechanisms
Vascular theory	Abnormalities in cerebral blood flow. Cerebral vasoconstriction during the aura phase and vasodilation during the headache phase; although blood flow is altered it is not adequate to cause ischemia or explain focal symptoms, such as local edema and tenderness; the theory is inadequate to explain the symptoms of migraine.
Cortical spreading depression (CSD)	A reduction in brain and electrical activity. A trigger initiates a reduction in electrical activity and decrease in blood flow that spreads across the cerebral cortex from the occipital region, moving anteriorly at a rate of 2-3 mm/min; flow abnormalities are documented in classic but not common migraine and are probably related to deranged neurologic function; reduced cortical blood flow follows the cortical surface (dural and cortical arterioles) independent of the distribution of the large arteries; reduced cortical blood flow continues after the aura and may be increased or decreased during headache; release of potassium and hydrogen ions during CSD contributes to pain by activating sensory fibers that initiate inflammation and activate trigeminal and brain stem neurons related to pain.
Serotonergic and neurotransmitter alterations	Increased release of serotonin (5-hydroxytryptamine [5-HT]), norepinephrine, substance P, nitric oxide, glutamate, and other sensory substances. Increased release of 5-HT in the dorsal raphe activates neurotransmission to cerebral arteries, altering blood flow, and also affects projections to the visual cortex and visual processing centers; brain increases in glutamate and decreases in magnesium have been documented; afferent and efferent fibers from the trigeminal nerve extend to the wall of cerebral and dural arteries, and the inflammation associated with neurotransmitter release and vascular changes may account for the pain associated with migraine. Activation of N-methyl-D-aspartate receptors by glutamine during cortical spreading depression.

Data from Lauritzen M: *Sci Med* 3(4):32, 1996; Ramadan NM et al: *Headache* 29:590, 1989.

The diagnosis of migraine is made from medical history and physical examination. Clinicians must be skilled in their understanding of different types of headaches, risk factors, family history, and clinical features. Differential diagnosis is confirmed with CT and MRI scans and EEG.[43] A significant number of individuals with migraine have depression as a comorbidity.[44]

The management of migraine includes education that migraine is a chronic physiologic disorder and not psychosomatic. Avoidance of triggers, adequate sleep, regular eating habits, and daily relaxation and meditation can create a headache-protective environment.[45] With the onset of acute migraine, a dark room, ice, and sleep can provide relief. The pharmacologic management of migraine varies with each individual and is related to the severity of the attack. Drug considerations should include antiemetics, nonsteroidal antiinflammatory preparations, ergotamine and dihydroergotamine, and 5-HT antagonists (e.g., sumatriptan). Magnesium administration may help some women with menstrual migraine. Gastric absorption may be decreased during an attack, and routes of administration other than oral (e.g., nasal sprays, intravenous, and rectal) may be used.

The prophylaxis of migraine is considered when attacks cannot be treated effectively. Several drugs may be considered and should *not* be used in combination. Examples include beta-blockers, a calcium antagonist (flunarizine), serotonin antagonists (lisuride, methysergide), nonsteroidal antiinflammatory drugs, dihydroergotamine (DHE), naproxen, valproic acid, and amitriptyline.

Cluster Headache

Cluster headaches occur primarily in men (8:1) between 20 and 50 years of age. Cluster headache has been known also as *histamine cephalalgia, Horton syndrome,* and *erythromelalgia.* These headaches are known as cluster headaches because several attacks can occur during the day for a period of days followed by a long period of spontaneous remission. Cluster headache has an episodic and a chronic form.

The headache attack usually begins without warning and is characterized by severe, unilateral tearing, burning, periorbital, and retrobulbar or temporal pain lasting 30 minutes to 2 hours. One or several attacks may occur in a day, and attacks usually occur at the same time of the day or night. The same side is affected in subsequent episodes. Associated symptoms include lacrimation, reddening of the eye, nasal stuffiness, eyelid ptosis, and nausea. Pain often is referred to the midface and teeth. If the cluster of attacks occurs more frequently without sustained spontaneous remission, they are classified as *chronic cluster headaches* (20% of cases). Alcohol can stimulate an attack during a cluster headache in about 50% to 70% of cases, but it is not a triggering factor during remission.

The etiology and pathophysiology of cluster headache are unknown. There are no consistent changes in cerebral blood flow. Pathogenic mechanisms may include vascular alterations, neurogenic or neuroimmunologic dysregulation of the hypothalamus, dysregulation of the parasympathetic ganglia, sympathetic deficit, and stimulation of the trigeminal nucleus. The rhythmicity of attacks probably is related to disorders of the hypothalamus. There may be altered serotonergic nerve transmission but at different loci than in migraine headache.[46,47]

Prophylactic drugs are used to treat cluster headache. The most effective are prednisone, lithium, methysergide, calcium channel antagonists, and valproate. Acute attacks are managed with oxygen inhalation, sumatriptan, and inhaled ergotamine.

Chronic paroxysmal hemicrania. **Chronic paroxysmal hemicrania (CPH)** is a cluster type of headache that occurs with more daily frequency (4 to 12 times per day) but with shorter duration (20 to 120 minutes). The remission phases are often shorter. The attacks are more common in women, usually after pregnancy. The symptoms are similar to cluster headache. As with cluster headache, there is an episodic and a chronic form. The pathophysiology involves a disorder of sympathetic hyperactivity, but the mechanism is different from cluster headache because there is effective relief of symptoms with indomethacin.

Tension-Type Headache

Tension-type headache is the most common type of headache, occurring in 40% to 60% of the population. The average age of onset is during second decade of life. Female/male ratio is 1:1. It is a mild to moderate bilateral headache with a sensation of a tight band or pressure around the head. The onset of pain is usually gradual. The headache occurs in episodes and may last for several hours or several days. It is not aggravated by physical activity. Chronic tension headache represents headache that occurs at least 15 days per month. Many individuals have both tension-type and migraine headaches.

Both a central mechanism and a peripheral mechanism operate in causing tension headache. The central mechanism probably involves hypersensitivity of pain fibers from the trigeminal nerve. The peripheral mechanism is probably related to contraction of jaw and neck muscles, but the exact mechanisms are unknown. Headache sufferers have more localized pain and tenderness of pericranial muscles.

Mild headaches are treated with ice, and more severe forms are treated with aspirin or nonsteroidal antiinflammatory drugs. Chronic tension headaches are best managed with a tricyclic antidepressant, such as amitriptyline. Naproxen is a second drug of choice. Long-term use of analgesics or other drugs, such as muscle relaxants, antihistamines, tranquilizers, caffeine, and ergot alkaloids, should be avoided.

Tumors of the Central Nervous System

No proven causative agents have been established for tumors of the central nervous system. Carcinogenesis is discussed in Chapter 10.

Cranial Tumors

Tumors within the cranium can be either primary or metastatic. Primary tumors are classified as primary intracerebral tumors or primary extracerebral tumors. Primary intracerebral tumors originate from brain substance, neuroglia, neurons, cells of the blood vessels, and connective tissue. Primary extracerebral tumors originate outside the substance of the brain and include meningiomas, acoustic nerve tumors, and tumors of the pituitary and pineal glands. Metastatic tumors, or secondary tumors, can be found inside or outside the brain substance. Sites of intracranial tumors are illustrated in Fig. 16-21.

CNS tumors include both brain and spinal cord tumors. The incidence is between 3 and 8.4 per 100,000 persons. This incidence seems to increase up to 70 years of age and then decreases. These tumors represent the second most common group of tumors in children. Approximately 70% of all intracranial tumors in children are located infratentorially, and in adults 70% to 75% are located supratentorially.[48] Peripheral nerve tumors are rare in children and common in adults.

Cranial tumors cause local and generalized clinical manifestations. The local effects are caused by the destructive action of the tumor itself on a particular site in the brain and compression causing decreased cerebral blood flow. The effects are varied and include seizures, visual disturbances, unstable gait, and cranial nerve dysfunction. The generalized effects result from increased ICP (Fig. 16-22). Increased ICP may occur because of obstruction of the ventricular system, hemorrhages occurring in and around the tumor, or cerebral edema caused by tumors.

Intracranial brain tumors do not metastasize as readily as tumors in other organs because there are no lymphatic channels within the brain substance. If metastasis does occur, it is usually through seeding of cerebral blood,

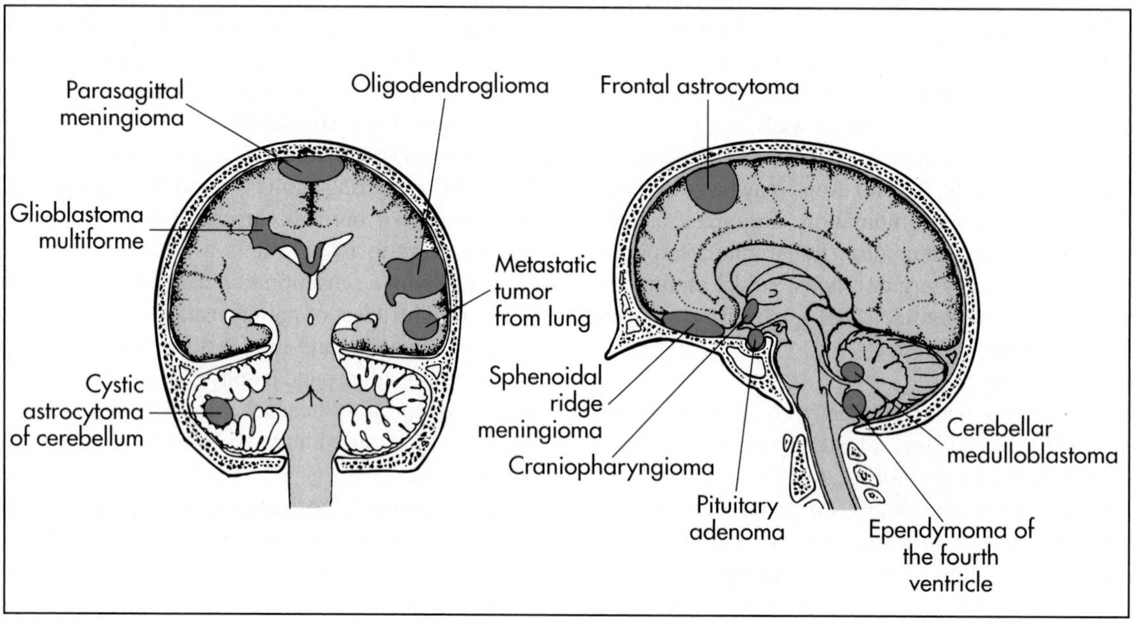

FIG. 16-21 Common sites of intracranial tumors.

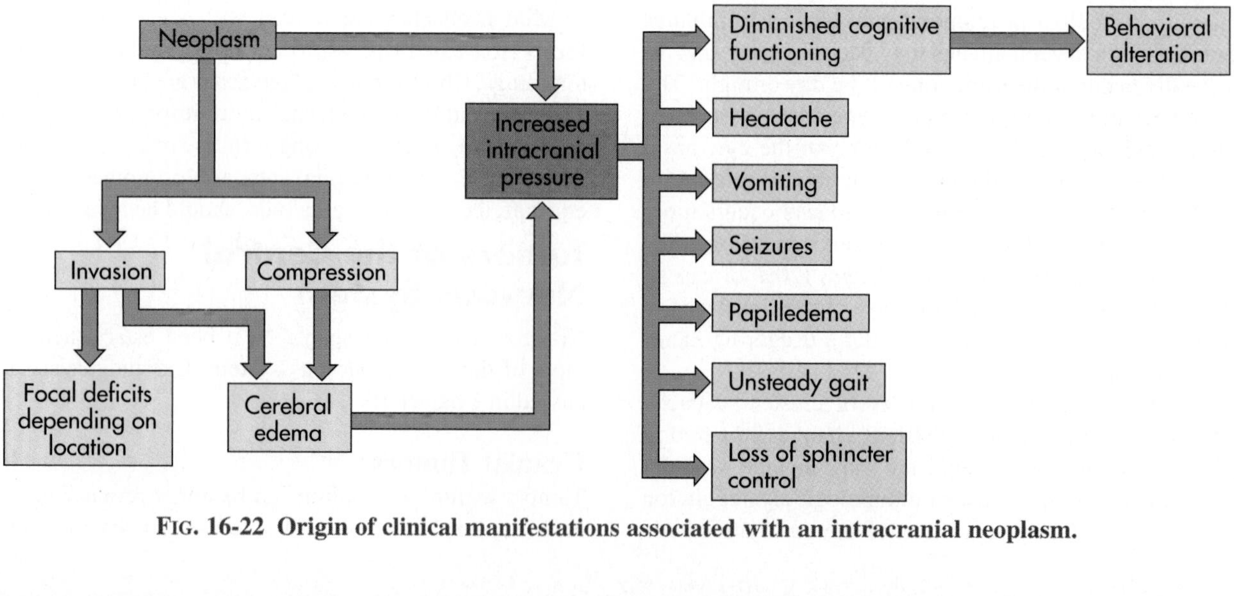

FIG. 16-22 Origin of clinical manifestations associated with an intracranial neoplasm.

through CSF, during cranial surgery, or through artificial shunts.

Primary Intracerebral Tumors

Primary intracerebral tumors, also called **gliomas,** comprise 45% of all adult brain tumors and are both encapsulated and nonencapsulated or invasive tumors[49] (Table 16-9). Typically the invasive tumors invade and destroy adjacent normal CNS tissue, whereas more distal neural and vascular tissues are displaced and compressed, causing ischemia, edema, and increased ICP. Encapsulated tumors generally do not invade adjacent tissues but displace and compress adjacent and distal CNS tissues and vasculature. As with invasive

Table 16-9 Brain and Spinal Cord Tumors

Neoplasm	Location	Characteristics	Cell of origin
GLIOMAS			
Astrocytoma	Anywhere in brain or spinal cord	Slow growing, invasive	Astrocytes
Glioblastoma multiforme	Predominantly in cerebral hemispheres	Highly invasive and malignant	Thought to arise from mature astrocytes
Oligodendrocytoma	Most commonly in frontal lobes deep in white matter; may arise in brain stem, cerebellum, and spinal cord	Relatively avascular, tends to be encapsulated; more malignant form called an oligodendroblastoma	Oligodendrocytes
Ependymoma	Intramedullary: wall of the ventricles, may arise in caudal tail of spinal cord	More common in children, variable growth rates; more malignant, invasive form is called ependymoblastoma; may extend into ventricle or invade brain tissue	Ependymal cells
NEURONAL CELL			
Medulloblastoma	Posterior cerebellar vermis, roof of fourth ventricle	Well demarcated, rapid growing, fills fourth ventricle	Embryonic cells
MESODERMAL TISSUE			
Meningioma	Intradural, extramedullary: sylvian fissure region, superior parasagittal surface of frontal and parietal lobes, olfactory groove, wing of sphenoid bone, superior surface of cerebellum, cerebellopontine angle, spinal cord	Slow growing, circumscribed, encapsulated, sharply demarcated from normal tissues, compressive in nature	Arachnoid cells, may be from fibroblast
CHOROID PLEXUS			
Papillomas	Choroid plexus of ventricular system, lateral ventricle in children, fourth ventricle in adults	Usually benign, slow expansion inducing hemorrhage and hydrocephalus; malignant tumor is rare	Epithelial cells
CRANIAL NERVES AND SPINAL NERVE ROOTS			
Neurilemmoma	Cranial nerves (most commonly vestibular division of cranial nerve VIII)	Slow growing	Schwann cells
Neurofibroma	Extramedullary—spinal cord	Slow growing	Neurilemma, Schwann cells
PITUITARY TUMORS	Pituitary gland; may extend to or invade floor of the third ventricle	Age linked, several types, slow growing, macroadenomas and microadenomas	Pituitary cells, pituitary chromophobes, basophils, eosinophils
GERM CELL TUMORS[70]	Neurohypophysis, hypothalamus, pineal region	Rare, 0.5% of all primary brain tumors; primarily in adolescents; male>female; variable prognosis	Several types: germinoma, embryonal carcinoma, yolk sac tumor, choriocarcinoma, teratoma, mixed germ cell tumor; with different cell origins
BLOOD VESSEL TUMORS			
Angioma	Predominantly in posterior cerebral hemispheres	Slow growing	Arising from congenitally malformed arteriovenous connections
Hemangioblastomas	Predominantly in cerebellum	Slow growing	Embryonic vascular tissue

tumors, encapsulated tumors produce ischemia, edema, and increased pressure. Normal function of the neurons ultimately is impaired by the invasion or compression.

The principal treatment for cerebral tumors is surgical or radiosurgical excision or surgical decompression if total excision is not possible. Chemotherapy, radiation therapy, and hyperthermia also may be used. Supportive treatment is directed at reducing edema. (Cancer treatment is discussed in Chapter 10.)

Astrocytoma. Astrocytomas are the most common primary CNS tumors (50% of all brain and spinal cord tumors). Their etiology remains unknown, but environmental, occupational, and genetic factors are being studied. These tumors are more common in males than females. There are criteria for grading these tumors and two predominant classification systems (Table 16-10). Astrocytomas develop from astrocytes and grow by expansion and infiltration into the normal surrounding brain tissues. These tumor cells are believed to have lost normal growth restraint, and thus they proliferate uncontrollably.

One third of astrocytomas are classified at diagnosis as grade I or grade II astrocytoma. These slow-growing but infiltrative gliomas tend to form cavities (pseudocysts); however, some are firm, noncavitating, avascular, gray-white masses that are difficult to distinguish from normal white matter of the brain. Although these tumors may occur anywhere in the brain or spinal cord, they are located most commonly in the cerebrum, hypothalamus, or pons. Low-grade astrocytomas in adults tend to have a lateral or supratentorial location, and they tend to be midline or near midline in position in children.

Headache may be an early symptom. Approximately half of persons with low-grade astrocytomas experience a focal or generalized seizure. Onset of a focal seizure disorder between the second and sixth decades of life is suggestive of an astrocytoma. Other general or focal neurologic manifestations develop gradually. Increased ICP is usually a late clinical manifestation.

Grade I astrocytomas are treated with surgery and follow-up CT scans. Grade II astrocytomas are treated surgically if they are accessible or by conventional external radiation, local radiation, or stereotactic radiosurgery. Survival time for grade I and II astrocytomas averages 5 to 7 years.

Grades III and IV astrocytomas are found predominantly in the temporal and frontal lobes (Fig. 16-23), as well as in the basal ganglia. These tumors also may be located in the brain stem (Fig. 16-24), cerebellum, and spinal cord. They are found twice as frequently in men as in women, and the 45- to 55-year age-group has the highest incidence. Grades III and IV astrocytomas are often large and well circumscribed with a variegated pattern. The peripheral rim is pinkish gray and solid with a soft, yellow, necrotic center and points of hemorrhage. Microscopically, there is increased cellularity, vascular proliferation, cellular pleomorphism, and necrosis. Necrosis is the principal histologic difference between an anaplastic grade III tumor and a grade IV glioblastoma multiforme.

Grade IV astrocytomas (glioblastoma multiforme) are highly vascular and extensively infiltrative. They may become large enough to extend from the meningeal surface through the ventricular wall. Fifty percent of glioblastomas are bilateral or at least occupy more than one lobe at the time of death.

The typical clinical presentation for a glioblastoma multiforme is that of diffuse, nonspecific clinical manifestations, such as headache, irritability, and personality changes, that progress to more clear-cut manifestations of increased ICP, such as headache on position change; papilledema; or vomiting. Of persons affected, 30% to 40% experience seizure activity. Symptoms may progress to definite focal signs, such as hemiparesis, dysphasia, dyspraxia, cranial nerve palsies, and visual field deficits, in addition to the generalized signs from increased ICP.

Table 16-10 Classification Systems for Astrocytomas

	Kernohan et al. System	Rigertz System	Criteria—Cellular Density, Atypia, Tumor Cell Mitosis
ASTROCYTOMA		Well-differentiated astrocytoma	Increased number of cells
Grade I	Well-differentiated astrocytoma		Least malignant, grow slowly, near normal appearance under microscope
Grade II	More cellular and anaplastic astrocytoma		Abnormal appearance under a microscope, infiltrates, and may recur at a higher grade
GLIOBLASTOMA		Malignant anaplastic astrocytoma	
Grade III	Poorly differentiated astrocytoma		Malignant, many cells undergoing mitosis, infiltrates, and may recur at a higher grade
Grade IV	Poorly differentiated astrocytoma (glioblastoma multiforme)	Glioblastoma multiforme	Increased number of cells undergoing cell division, bizarre appearance under a microscope, widely infiltrates, neovascularization, central necrosis

Diagnosis of high-grade astrocytomas most commonly takes 3 to 6 months from onset of the first clinical manifestations because the person does not recognize the need to consult a health care provider.

Grade III astrocytomas are treated with surgery if they are accessible; radiotherapy; and chemotherapy possibly before, during, and after other therapies. Chemotherapy is given in cycles. With treatment, approximately 55% to 60% of persons with grade III astrocytomas survive 1 year, 30% to 35% survive 2 years, and 10% survive longer than 5 years. Grade IV gliomas are also treated with surgery if accessible, radiotherapy and chemotherapy, or placement of wafers. Nineteen percent of persons with the full treatment regime survive 18 months.

Oligodendroglioma. A far less commonly occurring glioma is **oligodendroglioma,** comprising 5% of all brain tumors and 10% to 15% of all gliomas. Oligodendrogliomas are typically slow-growing, well-differentiated tumors, often with cysts and calcification present. Most are macroscopically indistinguishable from other gliomas. They occur most commonly in persons 40 to 50 years of age and are more common in males than females. Their etiology is unknown. Most oligodendrogliomas are found in the frontal and temporal lobes, often in deep white matter. Twenty percent are in both hemispheres. They may be found also in other parts of the cerebrum, third ventricle, brain stem, cerebellum, and spinal cord. A high incidence of this tumor is found in young adults with a history of temporal lobe epilepsy. Approximately one half of these tumors generally classified as oligodendrogliomas are actually a mixed type of oligodendroglioma and astrocytoma. Malignant degeneration occurs in approximately one third of persons with oligodendrogliomas, and the tumors are then referred to as **oligodendroblastomas.** The tumor rarely becomes a glioblastoma. If there is extension to the pia mater or ependymal wall (see Fig. 13-14), oligodendrogliomas may metastasize to distant CNS sites through the ventriculoarachnoid spaces.

More than 50% of individuals experience a focal or generalized seizure as the first clinical manifestation. Only approximately one half of persons with an oligodendroglioma have experienced increased ICP at the time of diagnosis and surgery, and only one third develop any focal manifestations. The time from first clinical manifestation to surgical intervention often ranges from 2 to 6 years. Treatment options are surgery; radiotherapy (conventional external beam or stereotactic gamma knife and converged beam); and chemotherapy before, during, and after radiation, typically with procarbazine, Lomustine (CCNU), or vincristine (PCV). Eight-five percent of persons survive 5 years if treated with surgery and radiotherapy.

Ependymoma. **Ependymomas** are gliomas that arise from ependymal cells that form the walls of the ventricles and grow either into the ventricle or into adjacent brain tissue; they are not encapsulated (Fig. 16-25 and see Table 16-9). They comprise 6% of all primary brain tumors in adults and 10% in children and adolescents. Among children and adolescents, 60% of those affected are under 5 years of age. Seventy percent of ependymomas occur in the fourth ventricle (i.e., in the posterior fossa) and manifest as difficulty with balance, unsteady gait, uncoordinated muscle movement, and difficulty with fine motor skills. Other common sites for ependymomas are the third ventricle, lateral ventricles, and

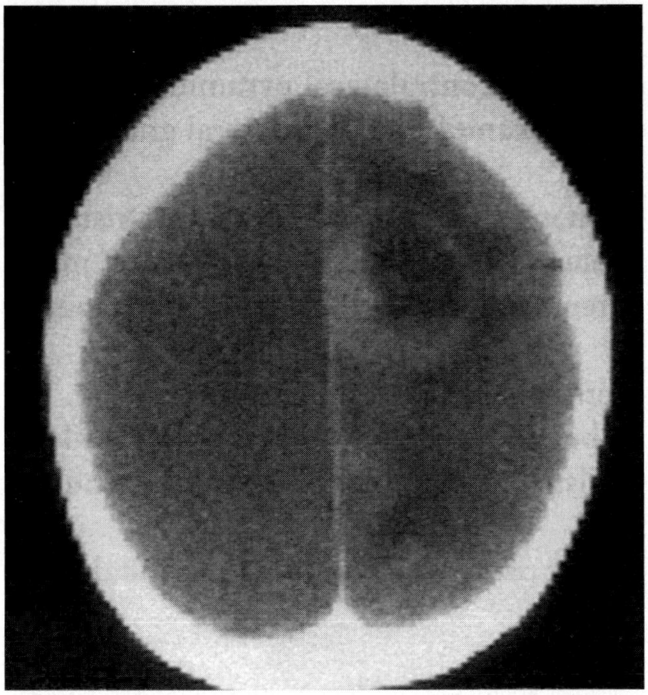

FIG. 16-23 CT showing ring enhancement in a glioma. (From Perkin DG: *Mosby's color atlas and text of neurology,* London, 1998, Mosby-Wolfe.)

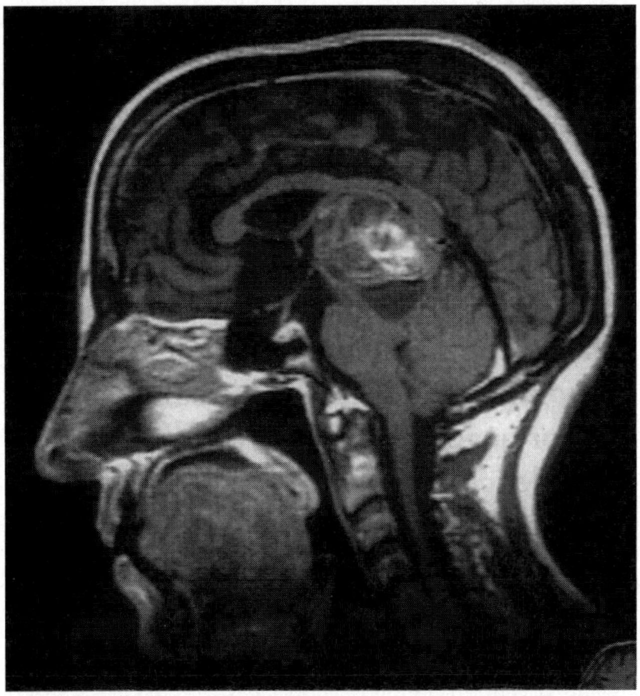

FIG. 16-24 MRI with gadolinium showing a high brain stem glioma. (From Perkin DG: *Mosby's color atlas and text of neurology,* London, 1998, Mosby-Wolfe.)

caudal portion of the spinal cord. The clinical presentation of a lateral and third ventricle ependymoma that involves the cerebral hemispheres is seizures, visual changes, and contralateral weakness of a body part or one side of the body. Approximately 40% of infratentorial ependymomas occur in children younger than 10 years. Occurrence of cerebral (supratentorial) ependymomas is distributed among all ages. Etiology for these tumors is unknown.

Blockage of the CSF pathway by the tumor clinically results in the presence of headache, nausea, and vomiting related to the hydrocephalus produced. Brain stem or upper spinal cord ependymomas may cause neck pain as well.

Clinical manifestations and progression of dysfunction associated with ependymomas may follow a short or long course. The interval between first manifestations and surgery may be as short as 4 weeks with some ependymoblastomas to as long as 7 to 8 years with others.

Ependymomas are treated with radiotherapy of the tumor region and operative site (possibly of the entire brain and spine); stereotactic radiosurgery focused on eradication; and chemotherapy using cisplatin, cyclophephamide, and vincristine. Between 20% and 50% of persons survive 5 years. Some persons benefit from a shunting procedure when the ependymoma has caused a noncommunicating hydrocephalus (see Chapter 15).

Primary Extracerebral Tumors

Meningioma. **Meningioma** constitutes 15% to 20% of all intracranial tumors. The peak incidence is about 45 years of age, with a 2:1 female/male ratio. Meningiomas are considered benign because they are encapsulated and usually do not invade the surrounding brain (Fig. 16-26). These tumors originate from the dura mater or arachnoid membranes. Rarely do meningiomas arise from arachnoid cells of the choroid plexus of the ventricles. Meningiomas most commonly are located in the olfactory grooves, on the wings of the sphenoid bone (at the base of the skull), in the tuberculum sellae (a structure next to the sella turcica), on the superior surface of the cerebellum, and in the cerebellopontine angle and spinal cord. Loss of chromosome 22 has been isolated.

Small meningiomas (less than 2 cm in diameter) often are found on postmortem examination in middle-aged and elderly individuals who had experienced no clinical manifestations and died of totally unrelated causes. The cause of meningiomas is unknown. A meningioma is a sharply circumscribed mass that derives its shape from the space it occupies. A meningioma may extend to the dural surface and erode the cranial bones or produce an osteoblastic reaction. A few meningiomas exhibit malignant, invasive qualities.

Only when meningiomas reach a certain size—at which time they begin to indent the brain parenchyma—do they begin to produce clinical manifestations. Focal seizures are

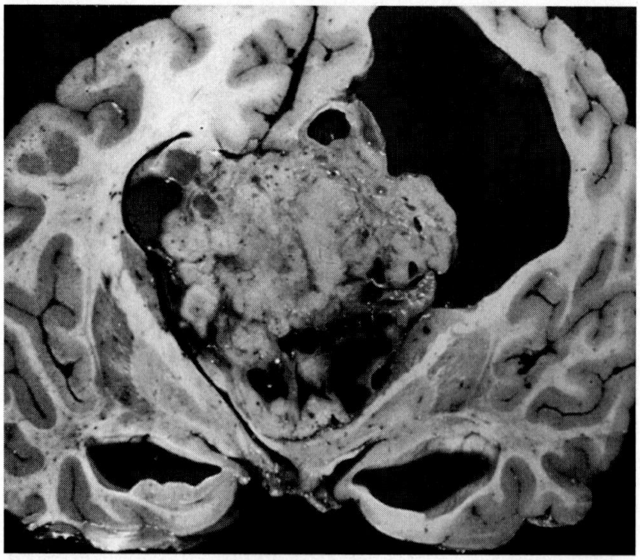

FIG. 16-25 Large septal ependymoma. Note secondary hydrocephalus. (Courtesy Dr. JE Olivera-Rabiela, Mexico City, Mexico. From Rosai J: *Ackerman's surgical pathology,* ed 7, St Louis, 1989, Mosby.)

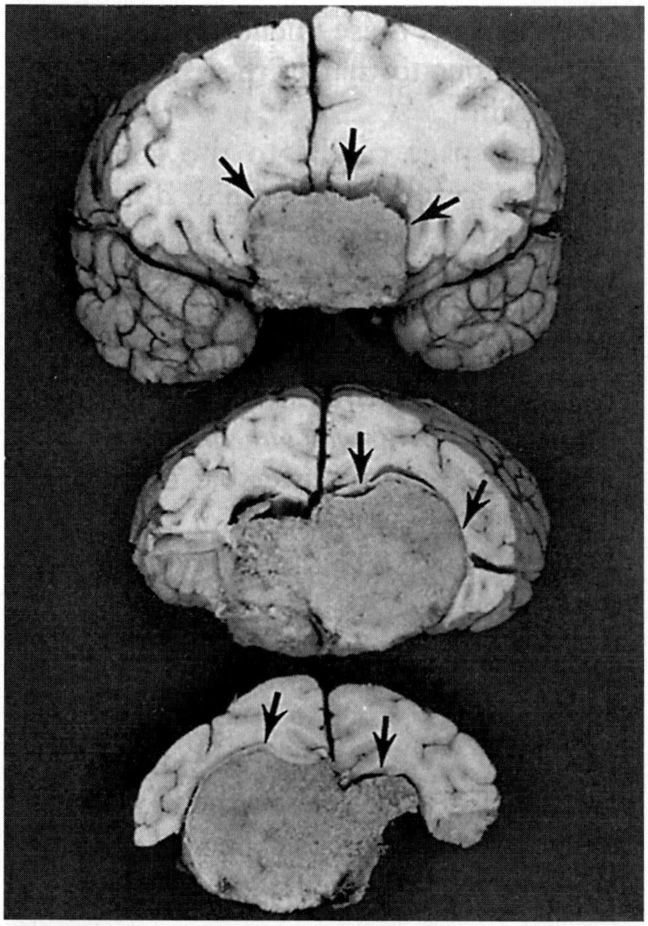

FIG. 16-26 Large olfactory groove meningioma. Note that this tumor has significantly compressed *(arrows)* but not invaded the brain tissue in these sequential slices through the frontal lobe. (Courtesy Dr. Jonathan Fratkin, University of Mississippi Medical Center. From Haines DE, editor: *Fundamental neuroscience,* Philadelphia, 1997, Churchill Livingstone.)

frequently the first manifestation. Other clinical manifestations depend on the tumor's location. Clinical features based on site of origin are as follows:

1. *Sphenoidal wing:* ophthalmoplegia, mild proptosis, and involvement of the ophthalmic division of the trigeminal nerve
2. *Olfactory groove:* anosomia, personality change and visual failure
3. *Parasagittal:* focal seizures of a focal motor or sensory deficit
4. *Parasellar:* evidence of chiasmatic compression

Because of the extremely slow-growing nature of most meningiomas, increased ICP is less common than with gliomas.[17]

With complete surgical excision of the tumor and its meningeal stem, there is still a 20% recurrence rate. Sometimes only partial resection is possible. Radiotherapy is used to slow the tumor growth.

Neurilemmoma. **Neurilemmoma** (neuromas, schwannomas) have now been classified as type 2 neurofibromatosis.[17] Neurofibromatosis is an inherited autosomal disorder. The gene for type 1 is located on chromosome 17 and the gene for type 2 is on chromosome 22. Criteria for the diagnosis of neurofibromatosis types 1 and 2 are presented in Box 16-3.

In type 2 neurofibromatosis the neuroma arises from the sheath of Schwann cells surrounding the axons of the cranial nerves. The tumors most commonly affect persons older than 50 years of age, and women are affected more often than men. The vestibular division of cranial nerve VIII is most commonly affected, although neurilemmomas of the acoustic division of cranial nerve VIII, cranial nerve V, and cranial nerve IX are found (Fig. 16-27).

The tumor originates most commonly just distal to the junction between the nerve root and the brain stem. As the tumor grows, it extends into the posterior fossa to occupy the cerebropontine angle and compress adjacent nerves. Eventually the brain stem is displaced, and the CSF flow is obstructed.

Initial clinical manifestations may include headache, tinnitus, hearing loss, impaired balance, unsteady gait, facial pain, and loss of facial sensations. Later, vertigo with nausea and vomiting, a sense of pressure in the ear, and moderate to severe unsteadiness with rapid position changes may appear. CT scan or MRI can establish the diagnosis. Posterior fossa dye studies may be required. Treatment is by surgical excision of the neurilemmoma. Pituitary tumors are discussed in Chapter 20, and cerebral tumors in children are discussed in Chapter 18.

Metastatic carcinoma. An estimated 25% of persons with cancer develop metastasis to the brain. One third of metastatic brain tumors arise from the lung, approximately one sixth from the breast, and a lesser number from the

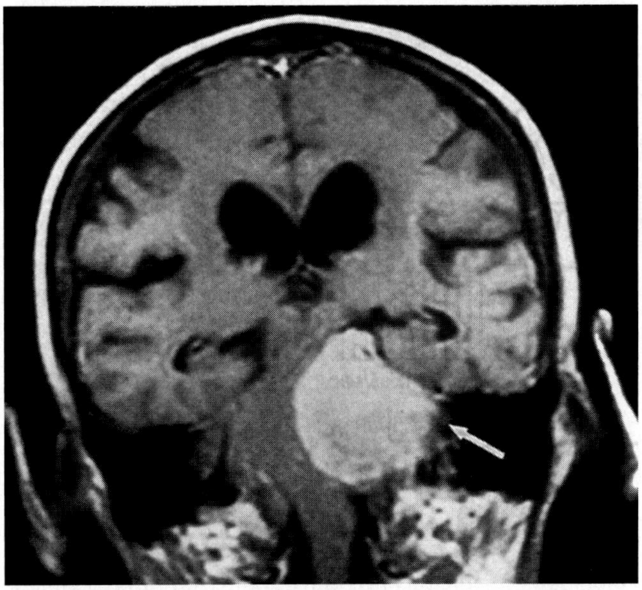

FIG. 16-27 Magnetic resonance imaging (MRI) of an acoustic neuroma (neurilemmoma) of cerebellopontine angle involving the vestibular division of CN VIII. Individual complained of dizziness, nausea, and spatial disorientation. (From Haines DE, editor: *Fundamental neuroscience,* Philadelphia, 1997, Churchill Livingstone.)

Box 16-3

CRITERIA FOR DIAGNOSIS OF NEUROFIBROMATOSIS TYPES 1 AND 2

CRITERIA FOR THE DIAGNOSIS OF NF-1

Two of the following eight criteria
- Six café-au-lait spots over 15 mm in diameter (adults)
- Multiple axillary or inguinal freckles
- One plexiform neurofibroma or two or more neurofibromas of other types
- Optic nerve or chiasmatic glioma
- Lisch iris nodules (two or more)
- Thinning of the cortex of long bones
- Sphenoid dysplasia
- A first degree relative with NF-1

CRITERIA FOR THE DIAGNOSIS OF NF-2

Any one of the three criteria below
- Bilateral VIIIth nerve tumours (as determined by CT or MRI)
- Unilateral VIIIth nerve tumour and first-degree relative with NF-2
- Any two of the following plus first-degree relative with NF-2
  a. plexiform neurofibroma
  b. neurofibroma of another type
  c. meningioma
  d. glioma
  e. schwannoma
  f. presenile posterior cataract

From Perkin GD: *Mosby's color atlas and text of neurology,* 1998, London, Mosby—Wolfe.

gastrointestinal tract and kidney. Melanoma and carcinoma of the gallbladder, liver, thyroid, testes, uterus, ovary, and pancreas also may metastasize to the brain. Other tumors, besides carcinomas, that metastasize only occasionally are rhabdomyosarcomas, Ewing tumors, chorioepithelioma, and lymphoma.

Carcinomas are disseminated to the brain from the circulation. In more than three fourths of persons with metastasis, the metastases are multiple and found in both the cerebrum and cerebellum in a scattered distribution. The metastatic tumors often are located in the meninges and near the brain surface in the gray matter and subcortical white matter. These tumors produce little glial cell reaction in the brain tissue but do cause vasogenic edema in the surrounding brain tissue.

The clinical manifestation of a metastatic brain tumor usually resembles that of a glioblastoma, although several unusual syndromes do exist. Carcinomatous encephalopathy causes headache, nervousness, depressed mood, trembling, confusion, and forgetfulness. In carcinomatosis of the cerebellum, headache, dizziness, and ataxia are found. Carcinomatosis of the craniospinal meninges (carcinomatous meningitis) manifests with headache, confusion, and manifestations of cranial or spinal nerve root dysfunction.

MRI with gadolinum as contrast medium is the most sensitive imaging procedure for metastatic brain tumors. Prognosis is poor. If a solitary tumor is found, surgery or radiation therapy is used, but if multiple tumors exist, symptomatic relief only is pursued.

Spinal Cord Tumors

Spinal cord tumors are relatively rare. The most common primary spinal tumors[50,51] are listed in Box 16-4 and shown in Fig. 16-28. Spinal cord tumors are named to reflect their cell type, growth rate, and structure of origin. Spinal cord tumors are classified as **intramedullary tumors** (originating within the neural tissues) or **extramedullary tumors** (originating from tissues outside the spinal cord). Extramedullary tumors arise from the meninges or roots (forming **intradural tumors**) or from epidural tissue or vertebral structure (forming **extradural tumors**). About 5% of spinal cord tumors seen in general hospital settings are intramedullary, 40% are intradural-extramedullary, and 55% are extradural.

Box 16-4

MOST COMMON PRIMARY SPINAL TUMORS

BENIGN TUMORS

Osteoid osteoma/osteoblastoma
Giant cell tumors
Hemangiomas
Aneurysmal bone cyst

MALIGNANT TUMORS

Chondrosarcoma
Chordoma
Ewing's sarcoma
Osteoarcoma

The axial skeleton is the third most common site for metastasis behind lung and liver metastasis.[50,51] Metastatic spinal cord tumors are three to four times more common than primary spinal cord tumors. They are usually carcinomas from breast, lung, and prostate; lymphomas; or myelomas. Twenty-five percent to 70% involve the vertebral body and are asymptomatic. Metastatic spinal cord tumors are extradural in location. Of extradural tumors, 50% are metastatic and have spread to the spine through direct extension from tumors of the vertebral structures or from extraspinal sources extending through the interventricular foramen or through the bloodstream.

The most common primary extramedullary spinal cord tumors are neurofibromas and meningiomas. These tumors are intradural more often than extradural. Neurofibromas are found most commonly in the thoracic and lumbar regions. Meningiomas are more evenly distributed through the spine. Other extramedullary tumors in order of frequency of occurrence are sarcomas, vascular tumors, chordomas, and epidermoid and similar tumors. Of intradural-extramedullary tumors, 70% are meningiomas, neurofibromas, or sarcomas.

Intramedullary tumors have the same cellular origins as brain tumors. Ependymomas account for 40% of intramedullary spinal cord tumors. Astrocytomas, glioblastomas,

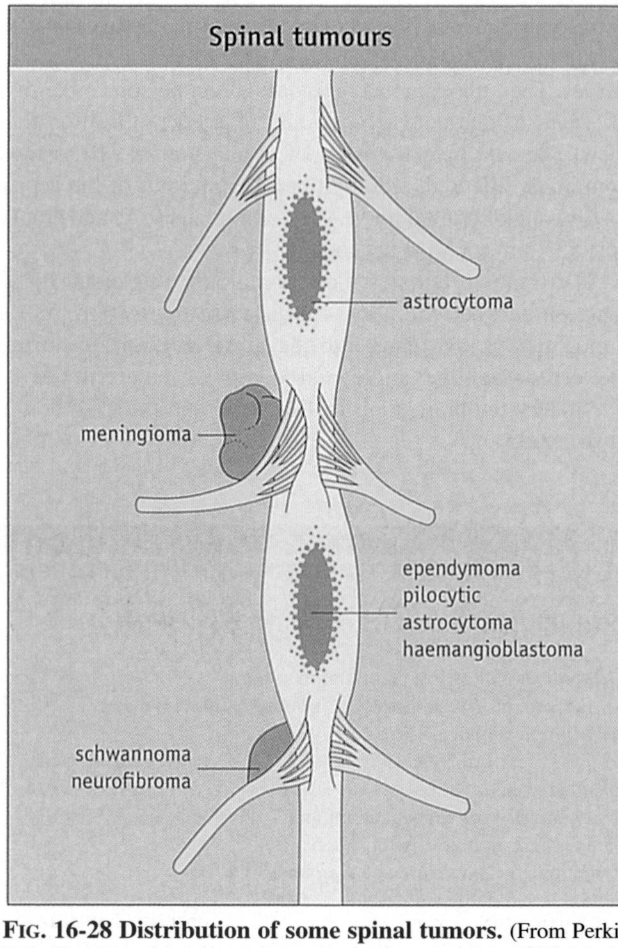

FIG. 16-28 Distribution of some spinal tumors. (From Perkin DG: *Mosby's color atlas and text of neurology,* London, 1998, Mosby-Wolfe.)

oligodendrogliomas, ganglioneuromas, medulloblastomas, hemangiomas, and hemangioblastomas are more or less equally distributed in frequency of occurrence.

Pathophysiology

Extramedullary spinal cord tumors produce dysfunction by compression of adjacent tissue, not by direct invasion. The spinal cord is compressed by the tumor from without, and destruction of the white matter tracts occurs. The spinal canal around the cord becomes filled by tumor.

Intramedullary spinal cord tumors produce dysfunction by both invasion and compression. The cord enlarges from the tumor that is enlarging inside the cord. In addition, distortion of adjacent white matter tracts occurs. Metastases from spinal cord tumors occur from seeding through the CSF; medulloblastomas and ependymomas establish distant implants in this manner.

Clinical Manifestations

The acute onset of clinical manifestations suggests a vascular insult caused by thrombosis of vessels supplying the spinal cord. Clinical manifestations that are gradual and progressive suggest compression. The clinical manifestations associated with spinal cord tumors fall into three major categories: (1) a compressive syndrome (sensorimotor syndrome), (2) an irritative syndrome (radicular syndrome), and rarely (3) a syringomyelic syndrome.

The **compressive syndrome (sensorimotor syndrome)** is associated with compression and is caused less frequently by invasion and destruction of the spinal cord tracts. Symptoms are usually gradual and progressive, and initial manifestations may be asymmetric. With tumors located in the cervical area, the motor dysfunction usually has the following pattern: ipsilateral arm involvement, followed by ipsilateral and contralateral leg involvement, and finally involvement of the opposite arm. With thoracic tumors the pattern of motor involvement is paresis and spasticity of one leg, followed by involvement of the opposite leg. The sensory clinical manifestations of tingling paresthesias have a pattern similar to that of the motor signs. Pain and temperature dysfunctions are found more commonly than touch, vibration, and proprioceptive changes, although posterior column signs also are found frequently. Pain is less well localized than with an irritative syndrome caused by root involvement. Initially the pain and temperature changes are contralateral to the motor deficit (Brown-Séquard syndrome). Bladder and bowel deficits usually appear when paresis develops in the legs.

The **irritative syndrome (radicular syndrome)** combines the clinical manifestations of a cord compression with radicular pain, which is pain in the sensory root distribution and indicates root irritation. The segmental manifestations associated with root irritation include segmental sensory changes that include paresthesias and impaired pain and touch perception; motor disturbances, including cramps, atrophy, fasciculations, and decreased or absent deep tendon reflexes; and ache in the spine. Tenderness of the spinous processes over the tumor is present in about one half of persons with extramedullary tumors. The segmental changes may appear months and sometimes years before the clinical manifestations of compression in benign tumors. The compressive clinical manifestations include an asymmetric spastic paresis of the lower extremities with tumors in the thoracic or lumbar region, paresis of the arms and legs with tumors in the cervical area, decreased or absent pain and temperature perception below the tumor site, posterior column signs, and spastic bladder.

Because they involve the central gray matter of the cord, intramedullary spinal cord tumors (notably ependymomas) may produce **syringomyelic syndrome,** or inflammation of the spinal cord. Inflammation results in the development of tubular (syrinx) cavities in the spinal cord. Occasionally an extramedullary tumor may produce the same effect, although the mechanisms are unknown.

Evaluation and Treatment

The diagnosis of a spinal cord tumor is made through bone scan, needle biopsy guided by CT and positron emission tomography (PET), or open biopsy. Benign or malignant spinal tumor staging may be done (Box 16-5). Involvement of specific cord segments is established.

Treatment varies, depending on the nature of the tumor and the patient's clinical status. Indications for surgery include establishing a tissue diagnosis, neurologic palliation, spinal stabilization, pain relief, and cancer therapy. Surgical resection may involve curretage (piecemeal removal of the tumor) or may be performed en bloc (removal of tumor in one piece). Surgical approaches to the spine include posterior approach (decompression laminectomy), lateral approach, anterior approach (most favored), and combined approaches.[51]

Box 16-5

SPINAL TUMOR STAGING

BENIGN SPINE TUMOR STAGING

S1 Latent, inactive, asymptomatic, are bordered by a true capsule, often confined to vertebra

S2 Active, slowly growing, mildly asymptomatic, has thin capsule and layer of reactive tissue

S3 Aggressive, rapidly growing; often symptomatic; capsule very thin, incomplete, or absent; often invades neighboring compartments

MALIGNANT TUMOR STAGING

Low grade malignant: both 1A and 1B have no true capsule, but a thick pseudocapsule of reactive tissue with islands of tumor

Stage 1A Tumor remains inside of vertebra (intracompartmental)
Stage 1B Tumor outside of vertebra

High grade malignant: rapid growth with continuous seeding nodules

Stage IIA Inside vertebra with skip nodules present
Stage IIB Outside of vertebra
Stage IIIA and IIIB Metastatic high grade intra- and extracompartmental

Posterior and anterior reconstructive surgery may be necessary. Oncologic surgical procedures are classified as intralesional, marginal, wide excision, or radical excision.[50] Indications for external radiation versus surgery are a radiosensitive tumor (e.g., lymphoma), soft tissue compression without instability, a patient who is a poor surgical candidate, paraplegia or advanced paraparesis of greater than 24 hours duration, and an expected survival of less than 3 to 4 months.[50] Chemotherapy, hormonal therapy, and pain management protocols may be appropriate.

Infection and Inflammation of the Central Nervous System

The CNS may be affected directly by bacteria, viruses, fungi, protozoans, and rickettsiae. The resulting infection can be pyogenic, or pus producing. Bacterial toxins also may affect the CNS. The meninges, neural tissues, and vasculature also may be involved in the inflammatory process.

Meningitis

Meningitis (infection of the meninges) may be caused by bacteria, viruses, fungi, parasites, or other toxins. The infections are classified as acute, subacute, or chronic processes, and the pathophysiology, clinical manifestations, and treatment differ for each type of organism.

Bacterial meningitis is primarily an infection of the pia mater and arachnoid, the subarachnoid space, the ventricular system, and the CSF. A systemic or bloodstream infection or a direct extension from an infected area is the access route to the subarachnoid space. The bacterial infection originates in another part of the body. The incidence of bacterial meningitis is 2.5 to 3.5 cases per 100,000 people. The incidence is 20 per 100,000 annually for neonates, and 2 to 9 per 100,000 annually for persons over 60 years of age. The mortality is 25% in adults.[52] Meningococcus *(Neisseria meningitidis)* and pneumococcus *(Streptococcus pneumoniae)* are the common causes of bacterial meningitis in adults. Other common agents are *Streptococcus agalactiae, Haemophilus influenzae*, and enterobacteriaceae.[53] Older patients are more likely to have pneumococcus or Listeria monocytogens.

Meningococcus has been identified worldwide. Meningococcal meningitis occurs predominantly in men and boys and in the fall, winter, and spring of the year. Epidemics of meningococcal meningitis occur in approximately 10-year cycles. Children and adolescents are affected predominantly. With pneumococcal meningitis, young persons and those older than 40 years are mostly affected. Meningitis caused by *Haemophilus influenzae* occurs almost exclusively in children 2 months to 7 years of age. Less common causes are staphylococcus, streptococcus, gonococcus, and gram-negative bacteria.

Aseptic meningitis (viral meningitis, nonpurulent meningitis, lymphocytic meningitis) is an inflammation believed to be limited to the meninges. Young adults are most commonly affected. Clusters of cases tend to occur in the summer and autumn of the year. Aseptic meningitis produces a variety of symptoms and is caused by a variety of infectious agents, most of which are viruses. Enteroviral viruses (echovirus, coxsackievirus, and nonparalytic poliomyelitis), mumps, herpes simplex (type I), adenoviruses, and California virus are the most common causes of aseptic meningitis. Bacterial infections not adequately treated are another cause of aseptic meningitis.

Fungal meningitis is a chronic, much less common condition than bacterial or viral meningitis. The most common fungal infections of the nervous system are histoplasmosis, cryptococcosis, coccidioidomycosis, mucormycosis, candidiasis, and aspergillosis. Fungal meningitis most frequently occurs in persons with impaired immune responses or alterations in normal body flora. Fungal meningitis develops insidiously, usually over days or weeks. Syphilis, tuberculosis, and Lyme disease also are associated with a chronic meningitis.

Tubercular (TB) meningitis, the most common and serious form of CNS tuberculosis, is again on the rise in the United States, especially in persons with acquired immunodeficiency syndrome (AIDS). The tuberculomas erode the pia mater, and the mycobacteria enter the CSF, involving the basal meninges, cerebrum, and spinal nerves. Symptoms include headache, low-grade fever, nausea and vomiting, irritability, difficulty sleeping, and fatigue. These signs and symptoms increase to confusion, stiff neck, significant behavioral changes, and seizures. Hydrocephalus and cranial nerve palsies or cerebral infarcts may occur. Recovery rate is 90% with early diagnosis and treatment with appropriate antituberculosis therapy.

Pathophysiology

The bacteria that commonly cause bacterial meningitis are common inhabitants of the nasopharynx, but a predisposing factor such as a prior upper respiratory infection must be present before the bacteria become blood borne. The method of CNS entry is thought to be through the choroid plexuses. The bacteria or their toxins function as irritants and induce an inflammatory reaction by the meninges (pia mater and arachnoid), the CSF, and the ventricles. The meningeal vessels undergo change, becoming hyperemic and increasingly permeable. Blood cells (neutrophils) migrate into the subarachnoid space, producing an exudate that thickens the CSF and interferes with normal CSF flow around the brain and spinal cord (Fig. 16-29). The exudate has the potential to obstruct arachnoid villi and produce hydrocephalus. The amount of purulent exudate increases rapidly (especially around the base of the brain), causing further inflammation. The exudate extends into the sheaths of the cranial and spinal nerves and into the perivascular spaces of the cortex. Meningeal cells become edematous. The exudate and edematous cells increase ICP. The small and medium-sized subarachnoid arteries, veins, and choroid plexuses undergo inflammatory changes and become engorged, disrupting blood flow and potentially producing thrombosis. Secondary infection of the brain may occur. The cortical neurons also show some changes, including an increase in the number of microglia and astrocytes.

Fungi in the nervous system usually produce a granulomatous reaction with formations of granulomas or gelatinous masses. These usually develop in the meninges at the base of the brain. Fungi also may extend along the perivascular sites in the subarachnoid space and into the brain tissue, producing arteritis with thrombosis, infarction, and communicating hydrocephalus. Meningeal fibrosis develops later in the inflammatory process. Cranial nerve dysfunction, caused by compression, often results from the granulomas and fibrosis.

◆ *Clinical Manifestations*

The clinical manifestations of a bacterial meningitis can be grouped into meningeal signs and neurologic signs.[17] Those clinical manifestations of systemic infection include fever, tachycardia, chills, and petechial rash. The clinical manifestations that arise from the meningeal irritation are a generalized throbbing headache that becomes very severe, photophobia that becomes severe, nuchal rigidity, Kernig sign, and Brudzinski sign. The neurologic signs include a decrease in consciousness, cranial nerve palsies, focal neurologic deficits (such as hemiparesis/hemiplegia and ataxia), and seizures. The irritation and damage to the cranial nerves produced by the inflamed sheaths manifest as follows:

Cranial nerve II: papilledema, blindness
Cranial nerves III, IV, and VI: ptosis, visual field deficits, diplopia
Cranial nerve V: photophobia
Cranial nerve VII: facial paresis
Cranial nerve VIII: deafness, tinnitus, vertigo

Neck stiffness and pain, and possibly head retraction, reflect the irritability of spinal accessory and cervical spinal nerves. Often the vomiting center is irritated, causing projectile vomiting. Confusion and decreasing responsiveness are evidence of cortical involvement. In meningococcal meningitis there is a petechial or purpuric rash involving the skin and mucous membranes. As ICP increases, papilledema may develop and delirium may progress so that the individual reaches an unconscious state.

The clinical manifestations of aseptic meningitis are mild compared with those associated with bacterial meningitis. Mild generalized throbbing headache, mild photophobia, mild neck pain, stiffness, fever, and malaise are all manifestations of aseptic meningitis.

Fungal meningitis develops slowly and insidiously. The first manifestations are often those of dementia or communicating hydrocephalus (see Chapter 15). The individual is characteristically afebrile.

◆ *Evaluation and Treatment*

Diagnosis of bacterial meningitis is based on physical examination, including skin rash, nasopharyngeal smear, and antigen tests. Bacterial meningitis and fungal meningitis are treated with appropriate antibiotic therapy, but resistant strains are becoming an increasing problem. Other supportive measures may be needed. Aseptic meningitis is managed pharmacologically with antiviral drugs and steroids. Vaccinations exist for meningococcal, pneumococcal, and hemophilic meningitis. Chemoprophylaxis for persons exposed to meningococcal meningitis is rifampin.

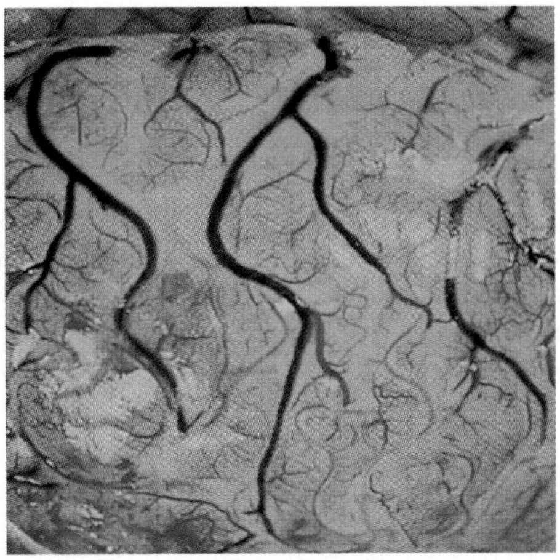

FIG. 16-29 Bacterial meningitis. Lateral surface of the cerebral hemisphere showing a purulent exudate. (From Perkin DG: *Mosby's color atlas and text of neurology,* St Louis, 1998, Mosby-Wolfe.)

Abscess

Abscesses are localized collections of pus within the parenchyma of the brain and spinal cord. The incidence of abscesses is about 1 per 100,000 hospital admissions. Men experience abscesses more frequently than women, with a 2:1 ratio. The median age for abscess formation is 30 to 40 years of age. Abscesses occur (1) after open trauma and during neurosurgery; (2) in association with a contiguous focus of infection, such as the middle ear, mastoid cells, nasal cavity, and nasal sinuses; (3) through metastatic or hematogenous spread from distant foci, such as the heart, lungs, pelvic organs, skin, tonsils, abscessed teeth, osteomyelitis in other than cranial bones, and dirty needles (especially in compromised hosts); and (4) cryptogenically, arising without other associated areas of infections. Streptococci, staphylococci, and bacteroids, often in combination with anaerobes, are the most common bacteria that cause abscesses; however, yeast and fungi also have been found in CNS abscesses. *Toxoplasma gondii* is producing an ever-increasing number of CNS abscesses in persons with AIDS. Eighty percent of abscesses are located in the cerebrum, and 20% are cerebellar. The frontal and temporal lobes are the most common sites. The abscesses are in more than one site in 5% to 20% of cases. Immunosuppressed persons are particularly at risk for abscesses.

Brain abscesses are classified as extradural or intracerebral. **Extradural brain abscesses** are associated with osteomyelitis in a cranial bone. Unlike **intracerebral brain**

abscesses, they rarely arise from a vascular source. **Spinal cord abscesses** are classified as epidural or intramedullary. Individuals with diabetes mellitus show an increased incidence of **spinal epidural abscesses** (which form in the epidural space), whereas debilitated individuals with sepsis more frequently develop **intramedullary spinal cord abscesses** (those within the spinal cord). Epidural spinal abscesses usually originate as osteomyelitis in a vertebra; the infection then spreads into the epidural space. (Osteomyelitis is discussed in Chapter 41.)

Pathophysiology

Organisms gain entrance to the CNS from adjacent sites by direct extension from osteomyelitis or spread along the wall of a vein. Infective emboli carry the organisms from distant sites. Initially, a localized inflammatory process (focal cerebritis) develops, leading to edema, hyperemia, softening, and petechial hemorrhage. There is exudate formation, septic thrombosis of vessels, and aggregates of degenerating leukocytes. The surrounding tissues are edematous. The veins are filled with fibrin and polymorphonuclear leukocytes (white blood cells [WBCs]). After a few days the intense reaction abates, and fibroblasts from capillaries adjacent to the focal cerebritis deposit collagen fibers to contain and encapsulate the purulent focus (Fig. 16-30). The infection becomes delimited with a center of pus and a wall of granular tissue. Encapsulation takes about 2 to 3 weeks. A free (nonencapsulated) abscess is associated with a higher mortality. A mature abscess has three layers: (1) a center of polymorphonuclear leukocytes, (2) a collagenous capsule, and (3) peripheral gliosis. Existing abscesses also tend to spread and form daughter abscesses.

Abscesses arising from the ear frequently are located in the middle or inferior temporal lobe or in the anterolateral cerebellar hemispheres. Abscesses originating from the oral and nasal area most commonly are located in the frontal and temporal lobes. Abscesses from distant foci often occur in multiple numbers in the distal portion of the middle cerebral arteries. In extradural abscesses, pus and granulation tissue accumulate in the extradural space.

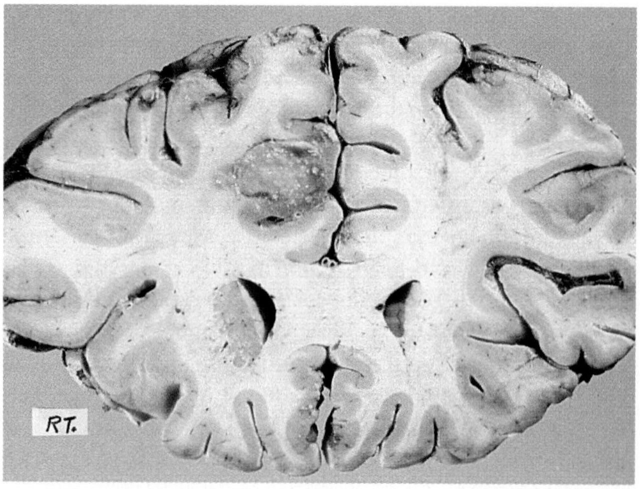

FIG. 16-30 Brain abscess. Early brain abscess appearing as a poorly demarcated area of cerebritis at the gray-white junction. (From Damjanov I, Linder J, editors: *Anderson's pathology,* ed 10, St Louis, 1996, Mosby.)

Clinical Manifestations

Clinical manifestations of brain abscesses are associated with (1) intracranial infection, such as fever and increased sedimentation rate; or (2) an expanding intracranial mass, such as headache, nausea, vomiting, decreasing cognitive abilities, paresis, and seizures. Early clinical manifestations of brain abscesses are low-grade fever, headache, neck pain and stiffness with mild nuchal rigidity, confusion, drowsiness, sensory deficits, and communication deficits. Headache is the most common early symptom. Later clinical manifestations may include inattentiveness (distractibility), memory deficits, decreased visual acuity and narrowed visual fields, papilledema, ocular palsy, ataxia, and dementia. Symptoms depend on the location of the abscess. The development of symptoms may be very insidious, often making an abscess difficult to diagnose. Extradural brain abscesses are associated with localized pain, purulent drainage from the nasal passages or auditory canal, fever, localized tenderness, and neck stiffness; occasionally the individual experiences a focal seizure. Clinical manifestations of spinal cord abscesses have four stages: (1) spinal aching; (2) root pain, which is usually severe, accompanied by spasms of the back muscles and limited vertebral movement because of pain and spasm; (3) weakness caused by progressive cord compression; and (4) paralysis.

Evaluation and Treatment

The diagnosis is suggested on the basis of clinical features and confirmed by CT scan. MRI is helpful when the CT scan does not show an abscess even though it is suggested by clinical features. Surgery is indicated if the diagnosis is in doubt or there are space-occupying problems present. Aspiration through a burr hole or excision through craniotomy with antibiotic therapy may be used. Multiple or surgically inaccessible abscesses are treated with antibiotics, often in conjunction with steroid therapy. In addition, ICP may have to be managed. Because decompression is necessary, spinal cord abscesses are treated with surgical excision or aspiration. Antibiotic and support therapy also is instituted.

Encephalitis

Encephalitis is an acute febrile illness, usually of viral origin, with nervous system involvement. The most common encephalitides are caused by arthropod-borne (mosquito-borne) viruses and herpes simplex, almost exclusively herpes simplex type I (Fig. 16-31). Referred to as *infectious viral encephalitides,* encephalitis also may occur as a complication of systemic viral diseases such as poliomyelitis, rabies, or mononucleosis, or it may arise after recovery from some viral infection such as rubella or rubeola. Encephalitis also may follow vaccination with a live attenuated virus vaccine if the vaccine has an encephalitis component. Such vaccines include measles, mumps, and rubella. Typhus, trichinosis, malaria, and schistosomiasis also are associated with encephalitis. Toxoplasmosis may acutely reactivate in immunosuppressed persons when the once-dormant parasite in cyst form disseminates in brain tissues (see p. 529).

With the exception of the California viral encephalitis, which is endemic, the arthropod-borne encephalitides occur in epidemics, varying in geographic and seasonal incidence (Table 16-11). Eastern equine encephalitis is the most serious but least common of the encephalitides.

Pathophysiology

Evidence of meningeal involvement appears in all encephalitides. The arthropod-borne viral encephalitides cause widespread nerve cell degeneration. Edema and areas of necrosis with or without hemorrhage develop. Increased ICP develops and may progress to herniation. Large degenerative injuries are found in Eastern equine encephalitis,

Table 16-11 Classification and Characteristics of Viruses Causing Encephalitis

Viruses	Incubation Period (days)	Virus	Location	Vector	Season	Affected Population
Eastern equine encephalitis	5-15	*Togaviridae* Alphavirus (formerly group A arbovirus)	Atlantic, Gulf Coast, and Great Lake regions	Mosquito	Midsummer to early fall	Infants, children, and adults >50 yr
Western equine encephalitis	5-10	Same as above	All parts of United States, especially western two thirds of country	Mosquito	Summer to early fall	Infants and young children
Venezuelan encephalitis	2-5	Same as above	Texas, Florida, Mexico; Central and South America	Mosquito	Year round	Infants and young children
St. Louis encephalitis	4-21	*Flaviviridae* Flavivirus group B (formerly group B arbovirus)	United States and Canada, especially Mississippi River, Pacific Coast, Texas, and Florida	Mosquito	Summer and fall	Adults >40 yr; elderly more often affected than younger ages
California encephalitis	5-15	*Bunyaviridae* Bunyavirus (California virus serogroup)	Midwestern United States, eastern seaboard, and Canada	Woodland mosquito	Late summer and early fall	Children <15 yr

From Barker E: *Neuroscience nursing,* St Louis, 1994, Mosby.

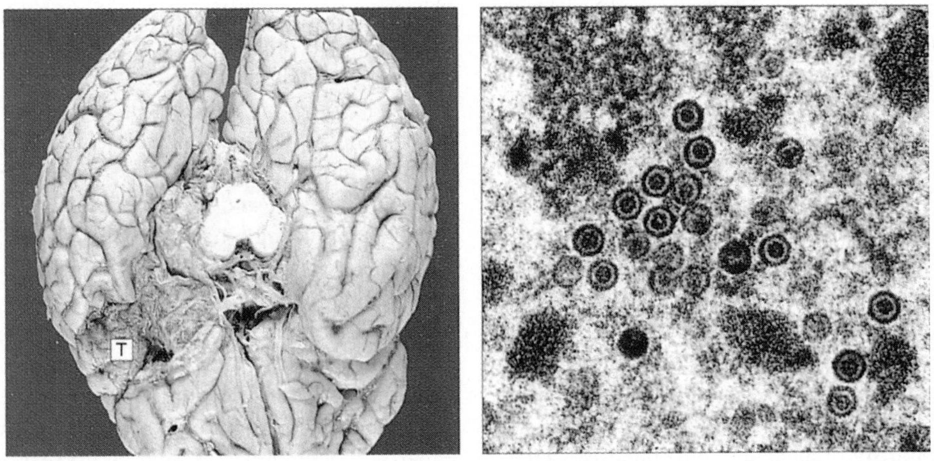

FIG. 16-31 Herpes encephalitis. In herpes simplex encephalitis **(A)** necrosis of the temporal lobes *(T)* is a typical development. Brain biopsy is useful in diagnosis when the virus can be seen by electron microscopy **(B)** as rounded particles with a dense core. Virus can also be identified by immunostaining or culture. In early cases, polymerase chain reaction (PCR) can be used to identify viral deoxyribonucleic acid (DNA) in cerebrospinal fluid samples. (From Stevens A, Lowe J: *Pathology,* St Louis, 1995, Mosby.)

whereas the other arthropod-borne viral encephalitides have microscopic areas of injury and degeneration.

Infectious encephalitis may result from a postinfectious autoimmune response to the virus or from direct invasion of the CNS by the virus. Herpes simplex type I has a tendency to infect the inferomedial surfaces of the temporal and frontal lobes and causes hemorrhagic necrosis.

Clinical Manifestations

Encephalitis may range from a mild infectious disease to a life-threatening disorder. The dramatic clinical manifestations of encephalitis are fever, delirium or confusion progressing to unconsciousness, seizure activity, cranial nerve palsies, paresis and paralysis, involuntary movement, and abnormal reflexes. Signs of marked ICP may be present.

Evaluation and Treatment

Diagnosis is based on medical history and clinical presentation aided by CSF examination and culture, serologic examination, WBC count, CT scan, or MRI. Until very recently, no definitive treatment was available for the viral encephalitides, but herpes encephalitis now is being treated with antiviral agents such as acyclovir and steroids. Supportive therapy is initiated, and measures to control ICP are paramount.

Neurologic Complications of Acquired Immunodeficiency Syndrome

Approximately 40% to 60% of all persons with AIDS have neurologic complications. On postmortem examination, 75% of AIDS victims have nervous system pathologic findings. The CNS pathologic findings in persons with AIDS result from (1) the primary human immunodeficiency virus (HIV) infection, (2) opportunistic infections, (3) neoplasms, and (4) systemic illness. Cerebrovascular complications and complications from the therapeutic drugs used to treat AIDS also may involve the CNS.

A variety of CNS complications of AIDS exist (Box 16-6). Multiple CNS pathologic conditions may be experienced by one person. The most common neurologic disorder is HIV encephalopathy. Other common neurologic disorders are peripheral neuropathies, vacuolar (spongy softening) myelopathy, opportunistic infections of the CNS, and neoplasms.

Although HIV has been isolated in the CSF and brain/spinal cord tissues, the mechanism by which HIV infects the CNS is not known. The virus can be isolated in the CSF at approximately the time of seroconversion. Pathologically, there may be (1) diffuse CNS involvement that produces a variety of clinical manifestations, (2) focal lesions that act as space-occupying lesions, and (3) obstructive hydrocephalus.

Human Immunodeficiency Virus Encephalopathy

HIV encephalopathy (subacute encephalitis, HIV-associated dementia complex, HIV cognitive motor complex, AIDS encephalopathy, AIDS dementia complex, or AIDS-related dementia) may affect both adults and children and is characterized by progressive cognitive dysfunction in conjunction with motor and behavioral alterations. The syndrome typically develops later in the disease but may be an early or a singular manifestation in some persons.

The viral route of entry into the CNS is unclear, but it is believed that HIV encephalopathy is the result of direct brain tissue infection by the virus. HIV is found mostly in white matter subcortical areas affecting macrophages, macrophage-derived multinucleated cells, and microglia, causing an immune-mediated demyelination process in white matter. There is some viral replication in some of the glial cells and, occasionally, within neurons. Multiple small nodules containing inflammatory cells are found scattered throughout the white matter and in subcortical gray matter, such as the basal ganglia and thalami. Multinucleated giant cells are present, as is perivascular inflammation. Focal and diffuse demyelination of white matter and spongy changes of the spinal cord are present. Factors other than direct cell damage are involved, such as released toxins, lymphokines, or other substances. Elevation in CSF levels of quinolinic acid, a neurotoxic metabolite of tryptophan, is correlated with the degree of dementia present. A decreased concentration of adenosine triphosphate (ATP) and inorganic phosphates in the CNS produces a decrease in metabolism.

HIV encephalopathy is insidious in onset and unpredictable in its course. Most persons experience a steady progression characterized by abrupt accelerations of signs over sev-

Box 16-6
NERVOUS SYSTEM COMPLICATIONS OF HIV-1 INFECTIONS

CNS COMPLICATIONS OF HIV-1 INFECTION

Primary HIV-1 encephalopathy
Atypical aseptic meningitis
- Acute: typical meningitis signs
- Chronic: headache syndrome

Spinal vacuolar myelopathy
Opportunistic viral infections
- Progressive multifocal leukoencephalopathy
- Herpesviruses

Nonviral infections
- *Toxoplasma gondii*
- *Cryptococcus neoformans*

Other fungal infections
- Mycobacterial infections
- Bacterial infections

Neoplasms
- Primary CNS neoplasms
- Metastatic neoplasms

Cerebrovascular complications
Complications resulting from systemic AIDS therapy

PERIPHERAL NERVOUS SYSTEM COMPLICATIONS OF HIV-1 INFECTIONS

Distal symmetric peripheral neuropathy
Inflammatory demyelinating polyradiculoneuropathy
Mononeuropathy multiplex
Progressive polyradiculopathy
Other causes of peripheral nervous system dysfunction
- Herpes zoster radiculitis

Cranial neuropathies

eral months to more than 1 year, although some individuals experience an abrupt onset or an accelerated course.

Early clinical manifestations of HIV encephalopathy may be vague. Impaired concentration and short-term memory and retrieval deficits commonly occur. Apathy and lack of motivation may appear; social withdrawal, irritability, and emotional lability appear. Later, difficulties with language, spatial or temporal disorientation, and visual construction appear. Some persons manifest an organic psychosis with agitation, inappropriate behavior, and hallucinosis.

Generalized cognitive system deficits occur later in the course of HIV encephalopathy, often accompanied by psychomotor slowing and decreased speech spontaneity and fluency. Progressive loss of balance, ataxia, spastic paraparesis or paralysis, and generalized hyperreflexia are common motor signs. Decreased writing ability, tremor, myoclonus, and seizure are less commonly seen.

Diagnosis is difficult, especially in early stages. The patient's medical history along with physical examination findings and supporting CSF, CT, and MRI data help to establish the diagnosis. Antiviral agents may be effective, as is dideoxinodine (ddI) along with supportive treatment.

HIV Myelopathy

HIV myeolopathy involving diffuse degeneration of the spinal cord may occur in persons with AIDS and has two forms: vacuolar myelopathy and multinucleated giant cell encephalitis.[17] **Vacuolar myelopathy** is believed to be due to an opportunistic infection, whereas **multinucleated giant cell encephalitis** is believed to be a direct consequence of HIV. The lateral and posterior columns of the lumbar spinal cord are affected in both myelopathies. A progressive spastic paraparesis with ataxia is the predominant clinical manifestation. Leg weakness, upper motor neuron signs, incontinence, and posterior column sensory loss may be present. Diagnosis is made on the basis of history, physical findings, and supporting data from diagnostic procedures. Multinucleated giant cell encephalitis responds to antiviral therapy. Vacuolar myelopathy is treated supportively and does not respond to antivirals.

HIV Neuropathy

HIV neuropathy may have one or a combination of several presentations: a predominantly sensory neuropathy, an autonomic neuropathy, a mononeuritis multiplex, a Guillian-Barré-like syndrome, and a myopathy. The peripheral nervous system may sustain injury in AIDS, manifesting as a peripheral neuropathy or radiculopathy. A progressive radiculopathy of predominantly the dorsal roots of the lumbar and sacral nerves may occur, involving severe myelin and axonal loss. The most common neuropathy is a sensory neuropathy that most commonly occurs later in the disease and is unresponsive to treatment.

HIV has been isolated from peripheral nerves, so it is believed that the virus may directly infect nerves. Patients experience painful, burning dysesthesias and paresthesias, typically in the extremities. Weakness and decreased or absent distal reflexes may be present. Diagnosis is established through history, physical findings, laboratory data, nerve conduction studies, EMG, and possibly biopsy. The most common myopathy is polymyositis; it may be present initially, or it may be a later development. The muscle fiber is infiltrated, initiating inflammation that leads to cellular degeneration and necrosis. The patient experiences muscle weakness of extremities with myalgia and fatigue. Steroids are used therapeutically in polymyositis.

Aseptic Viral Meningitis

Some persons develop an acute aseptic meningitis at approximately the time of seroconversion. This may well represent the initial infection of the nervous system by the HIV. Symptoms include headache, fever, and meningismus. Cranial nerve involvement, especially of nerves V and VII, may appear, but the disease is self-limiting and requires only symptomatic treatment.

Opportunistic Infections

Opportunistic infections may be bacterial, fungal, or viral in origin and produce nervous system disease. Typically, bacterial infections are caused by unusual organisms. Cryptococcal infection is the most common fungal disorder and the third leading cause of neurologic disease in persons with AIDS. In *Cryptococcus neoformans*, small granulomas and cysts are found in the cerebral cortex and later may be present in deep cerebral tissues. The symptoms are vague, such as fever, headache, malaise, and meningismus. Herpes encephalitis and herpes varicella zoster radiculitis may develop. Papovavirus (especially JC virus) in the immunocompromised person with AIDS may produce a demyelinating disorder called progressive multifocal leukoencephalopathy (PML). This virus is found in 90% of healthy persons but is dormant. The virus reactivates to cause PML in 15% of persons with AIDS. Sensory and motor deficits, asphasia, and apraxia are common clinical manifestations. The condition is progressive.

Cytomegalovirus infection. Cytomegalovirus encephalitis is common in persons with AIDS but often not diagnosed while the person is alive. The encephalitis may be present as an acute illness with encephalitis features accompanied by nystagmus and cranial nerve signs. Retinitis is found in 50% of those affected.

Parasitic infection. **Toxoplasmosis** is the most common and occurs in one third of persons with AIDS. CNS toxoplasmosis typically manifests as focal encephalitis. *Toxoplasma gondii,* a protozoan, is thought to reactivate from latent lesions to produce a well-demarcated necrotizing process. Inflammatory infiltrates, thrombotic lesions, and fibrinoid vascular walls are present at the necrotic edge. Marked edema is present adjacent to necrotic areas. Lesions may be multiple and exist throughout the cerebral hemispheres.

Clinical manifestations of CNS toxoplasmosis are focal but highly variable and include clumsiness to hemiplegia, aphasia, seizures, ataxia, cognitive changes, and constitutional symptoms. Fever and headache are common. Toxoplasmosis is difficult to diagnose but is treated effectively with pyrimethamine and sulfadiazine. Allergic response to sulfadiazine can be a problem, and other drugs can be substituted. Persons with AIDS may develop meningitis; encephalitis;

or brain abscesses of fungal, mycobacterial, and bacterial origin.

Central Nervous System Neoplasms

CNS neoplasms associated with AIDS include CNS lymphoma, systemic non-Hodgkin lymphoma, and metastatic Kaposi sarcoma. The precise mechanism of lymphoproliferation is not known. Primary CNS lymphoma is a large-cell lymphoma that presents as rapidly developing and expanding multicentric intracranial mass lesions. There is invasion of the meninges and, possibly, the cranial nerves and spinal cord in systemic non-Hodgkin lymphoma. Metastasis of a Kaposi sarcoma to the CNS is uncommon.

Other Central Nervous System Complications

Persons with AIDS may develop multifocal ischemic infarctions, hemorrhagic infarctions, hemorrhage into tumors, subdural hematomas, and epidural hemorrhage. The precise mechanism of these cardiovascular complications is not yet known. Reported neurologic symptoms produced by AIDS therapeutics include extrapyramidal movements, myoclonus, dysphasia, delirium, and acute myelopathy.

Lyme Disease

Lyme disease, a tick-borne bacterial infection, is now the most common arthropod-borne infection in the United States. It affects all age-groups and involves the peripheral and central nervous systems. Lyme disease is caused by *Borrelia burgdorferi* introduced into the person by tick bite. Infected ticks are endemic in the Midwest, western wooded and coastal areas, and the northeast coast.[54] The microorganism incubates for 3 to 32 days and then migrates to the skin, lymph nodes, and other body systems. The pathologic process progresses through three stages:

Stage I (acute localized). Three weeks after the bite, the disease is characterized by a bull's-eye-like (5 cm in diameter) burning rash, general malaise, flulike symptoms (fever, muscle pain), stiff neck, and headache

Stage II. With acute widespread dissemination of antibodies and immune complexes, cardiac and neurologic involvement predominates. About 10% of persons have cardiac signs and symptoms (palpitations, dizziness, shortness of breath, dysrhythmias, and first-degree heart block). Neurologic signs occur in 10% to 15% of persons and include headache, chronic aseptic (lymphocytic) meningitis, Bell's palsy, encephalitis, and radiculitis. Pathologically, there is a meningeal inflammation, perivascular inflammatory cell formation, and focal demyelination.

Stage III (chronic stage). The third stage may occur up to 2 years after the bite and involves arthritis and involvement of brain parenchyma with encephalitis, chronic neuropathy, and encephalopathy.

Treatment of choice is antibiotic therapy. Minor recurring symptoms are common in 50% of patients.

Degenerative Diseases

Parkinson Disease

Parkinson disease is a commonly occurring degenerative disorder of the basal ganglia (corpus striatum) involving the dopaminergic (dopamine-secreting) nigrostriatal pathway. Nigrostriatal disorders produce a syndrome of abnormal movement called **parkinsonism (Parkinson syndrome, parkinsonian syndrome)** (Fig. 16-32).

Etiologic classification of parkinsonism includes primary (idiopathic) Parkinson disease and secondary parkinsonism (Box 16-7). Primary Parkinson disease involves the loss of pigmented neurons in the substantia nigra, mainly in the ventral and medial portions, associated with reactive gliosis. Secondary parkinsonism is caused by disorders other than Parkinson disease (i.e., trauma, infection, neoplasm, atherosclerosis, toxins, drug intoxication). Drug-induced parkinsonism caused by neuroleptics, antiemetics, and antihypertensives is the most common cause of the secondary form and is usually reversible. Illegal "designer drugs" containing the chemical 1-methyl-4-phenyl-1,2,3,6-tetrahydropyridine (MPTP) have produced a parkinsonian syndrome in users because of severe degeneration of the substantia nigra and locus ceruleus.

The onset of Parkinson disease is after 40 years of age, with mean onset between 58 and 62 years of age.[48] Men are more affected than women. Parkinson disease is one of the most prevalent of the primary CNS disorders and a leading cause of neurologic disability in individuals older than 60 years. The prevalence rate is 30 to 300 per 100,000 persons. An estimated half-million persons in the United States are affected.

Pathophysiology

The pathogenesis of Parkinson disease is unknown. There is an autosomal dominant form but it has atypical features. Epidemiologic data suggest possible genetic, viral, and toxic causes. One hypothesis is that age predisposes the nigrostriatal pathway to damage by environmental toxins. Isolation of the neurotoxic chemical MPTP, demonstration of its ability to produce an irreversible parkinsonian syndrome, and selective destruction of substantia nigra cells have produced a research focus on toxins as causative agents.

Atrophy and neuronal loss are found in the cerebral cortex in more than one half of individuals with Parkinson disease. The principle pathologic feature of Parkinson disease is degeneration of the dopaminergic nigrostriatal pathway, which is composed of neurons of the substantia nigra ("black substance"), with fibers synapsing in the caudate and putamen basal ganglia (Figs. 16-33 and 16-34; see also Fig. 16-32, *A*). In primary (idiopathic) Parkinson disease, Lewy bodies and intracytoplasmic eosinophilic inclusions are found in remaining neurons of the substantia nigra. Similar changes are found in the locus ceruleus and less consistently in the dorsal vagal nucleus and in sympathetic and parasympathetic ganglia.[55] In postencephalitis Parkinson disease, destruction of nigral neurons is widespread and associated with neurofibrillary tangles. Lewy bodies are not present.[55] Signs of inflammation or infection are absent. The severity of Parkinson disease seems to correlate with the degree of neuronal loss in the substantia nigra. Another pathologic feature is significant reduction in certain dopamine receptors (D_1 receptors) in the basal ganglia.

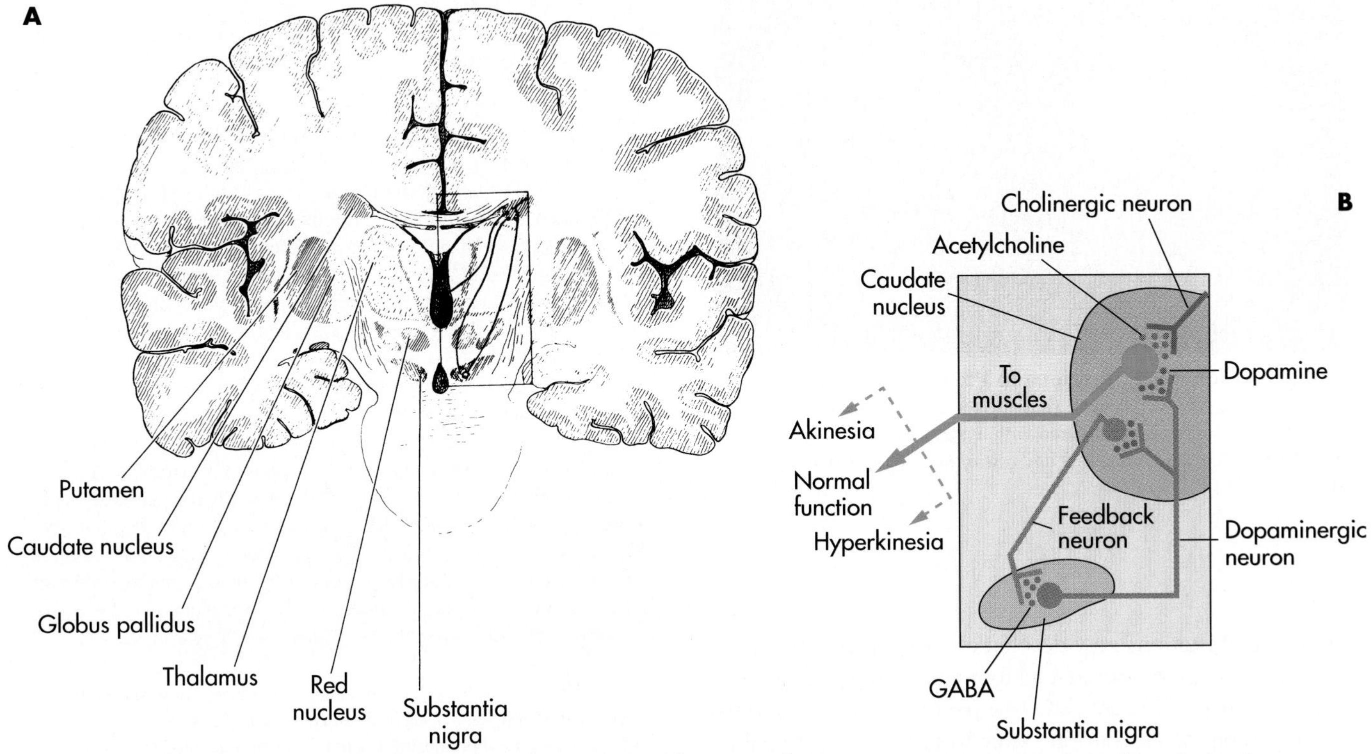

FIG. 16-32 Nigrostriatal disorders produce the Parkinson syndrome. Coronal section of the brain shows the basal ganglia. Pathways controlling normal and abnormal motor function are depicted in a portion of the basal ganglia *(caudate nucleus),* **A,** and shown enlarged in **B.** Dopaminergic synaptic activity is mediated by dopamine. Cholinergic synaptic activity is mediated by acetylcholine. A balance between the two kinds of activity produces normal motor function. A relative excess of cholinergic activity produces akinesia and rigidity. A relative excess of dopaminergic activity produces involuntary movements. Neurons in the caudate nucleus contain gamma-aminobutyric acid *(GABA)* and possibly control dopaminergic neurons in the substantia nigra through a feedback pathway. (**A** from Cutler WP: *Degenerative and hereditary diseases,* ed 7, Washington, DC, 1983, Scientific American Medicine.)

Box 16-7

CLINICAL CLASSIFICATION OF PARKINSONIAN SYNDROMES

1. Idiopathic Parkinson disease
2. Symptomatic parkinsonism
   Postencephalitis
   Drug-induced
   Toxic
   Traumatic
   Atherosclerotic
   Normal pressure hydrocephalus
3. As part of a neuronal degenerate disorder
   Multisystem atrophy
   Progressive supranuclear palsy (PSP)
   Corticobasal degeneration
   Diffuse Lewy body disease

Nigral and basal ganglial depletion of dopamine, an inhibitory neurotransmitter, is the principal biochemical alteration in Parkinson disease (see Fig. 16-32, *B*). Symptom development in basal ganglial disorders is explained as an imbalance of dopaminergic (inhibitory) and cholinergic (excitatory) activity in the caudate nucleus and putamen of the basal ganglia. Dopaminergic-cholinergic balance produces normal motor function. In Parkinson disease, degeneration of

A 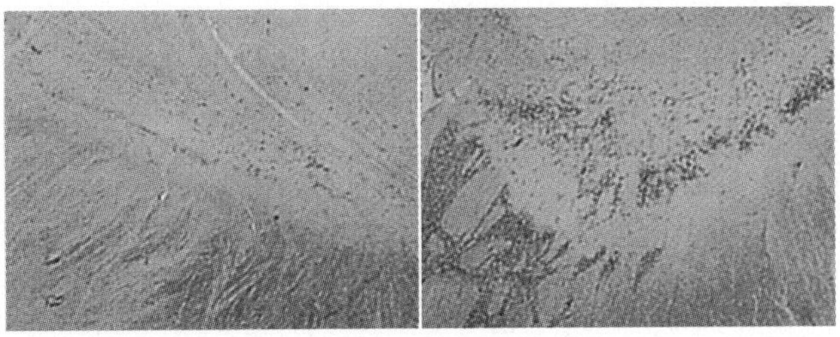 B

FIG. 16-33 Atrophic substantia nigra (A) compared with normal control (B). (From Perkin DG: *Mosby's color atlas and text of neurology,* London, 1998, Mosby-Wolfe.)

the dopaminergic nigrostriatal pathway causes dopamine depletion in the basal ganglia and a relative excess of cholinergic activity in the feedback circuit involving the cerebral cortex, basal ganglia, and thalamus. A relative excess of cholinergic activity in this circuit, as in Parkinson disease, is manifested by hypertonia (tremor and rigidity) and akinesia.

Clinical Manifestations

Symptoms appear after a 60% to 80% loss of pigmented nigral neurons and a loss of 60% to 90% of striatal dopamine occur. The classic manifestations of Parkinson disease are tremor at rest (resting tremor), rigidity (muscle stiffness), akinesia (poverty of movement), and postural abnormalities.

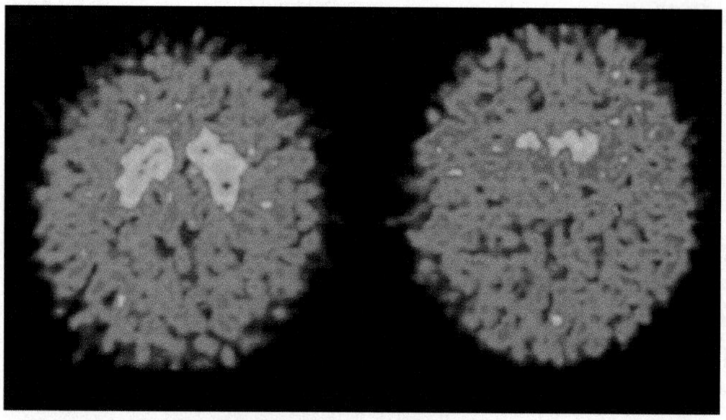

FIG. 16-34 Reduced flurodopa in Parkinson disease. Positron emission tomography scan showing reduced flurodopa uptake in the basal ganglia *(right)* compared with a normal control *(left)*. (From Perkin DG: *Mosby's color atlas and text of neurology,* London, 1998, Mosby-Wolfe.)

NUTRITION & DISEASE

Parkinson Disease

Unintentional weight loss and declining nutritional status occur commonly in individuals with Parkinson disease. Explanations for this weight loss include anorexia, difficulty chewing and swallowing, increased time required to complete a meal, reduced sensitivity to smell and taste, depression, increased energy requirements because of muscular rigidity and increased involuntary movements, side effects of medications, and decreased intestinal absorption of nutrients. Nutritional management might include modifying the textures and consistency of foods if chewing and swallowing are problems, offering food supplements and healthful snacks, providing prosthetic devices, and providing assistance with transportation and procurement of food.

Redistribution of protein may be of benefit, with most of the recommended daily allowance (RDA) for protein provided in the evening and only 10 g of protein in the daytime. Benefits within 1 week were improved daytime mobility at the cost of nighttime rigidity. The other modification is a 5 : 1 ratio of carbohydrate to protein in a meal that stabilizes the plasma levels of large neutral amino acids and allows for titrating levodopa dosages. When this dietary modification is helpful, 70% of the people will follow it for longer than 1 year.

Data from Beyer PL et al: Weight changes and body composition in patients with Parkinson's disease, *J Am Dent Assoc* 95:979, 1995; Davies KN et al: Intestinal permeability and orocaecal transit time in elderly patients with Parkinson's disease, *Postgrad Med J* 72(845):164, 1996; Kempster P, Wahlquist M: Dietary factors in management of Parkinson's disease, *Nutr Rev* 52:51, 1994.

These manifestations may develop alone or in combination, but as the disease progresses, all four are usually present to at least some degree. There is no true paralysis. The symptoms are staged on the Hoehn-Yale scale as follows: *0*, no visible disease; *1*, unilateral involvement; *2*, bilateral involvement; *3*, bilateral involvement with minimal gait difficulty; *4*, bilateral involvement with postural instability; and *5*, bilateral involvement with inability to walk.[55]

Because of the insidious onset, the beginning of symptoms is difficult to document. In early stages of the disease, reflex, sensory, and mental status are usually normal. Autonomic-neuroendocrine symptoms and, in some cases, dementia are also part of the syndrome.

Parkinsonian tremor, rigidity, and bradykinesia. **Parkinsonian tremor,** the most conspicuous and most variable symptom, is usually the first symptom to appear. It is an asymmetric, regular, rhythmic, low-amplitude tremor, with slowly alternating flexion-extension contraction (3 to 4 cycles/sec). Later the tremor becomes symmetric at 7 to 12 cycles per second. It is a tremor at rest, disappearing briefly during the course of a voluntary movement and reappearing when the limb is held in a stationary position. Intensity and amplitude of the tremor vary. The arm is more affected than the leg. The head is involved rarely. Seventy percent of individuals have this tremor, and 20% of persons have a postural (kinesic) tremor or both tremor types. All tremors are increased by stress and anxiety.

Parkinsonian tremor appears to result from instability of feedback from the basal ganglia to the cerebral cortex caused by loss of the inhibitory influence of dopamine in the basal ganglia. Oscillation in the normal feedback cycles of the motor outflow feedback circuit when the muscles are at rest produces the tremor. When the individual performs voluntary movements, the tremor becomes temporarily blocked, presumably because other motor control signals arriving in the thalamus override the abnormal basal ganglial signals. As the disorder worsens, tremor may lessen as rigidity supervenes. The postural tremor is associated with damage to the cerebellodentatofugal pathway to the red nucleus, a pathway that subserves communication from muscle spindles to the thalamus and motor cortex.

Rigidity, a state of involuntary contraction of all skeletal muscles, impedes active and passive movement. The first symptoms of rigidity may be painful muscle cramps in the toes or hands. More commonly the limb feels stiff, heavy, tired, or aching. Rigidity is felt by the examiner as lead-pipe resistance during passive movement that may be interrupted by brief jerks palpable as a cogwheel sensation. The mechanism underlying rigidity is increased resting muscle activity (enhancement of the long-latency stretch reflex).

Akinesia is poverty of associated and voluntary movements. It is the most prevalent and crippling symptom and often is overlooked in the early stages. All striated muscles—extremity, trunk, ocular, facial (Fig. 16-35)—are affected eventually, including muscles of mastication (chewing), deglutition (swallowing), and articulation. The pathophysiology underlying the akinesia is unclear. Micrographia is present. Extreme underactivity in the patient with Parkinson disease makes the person appear stiff, even when resistance to passive movement cannot be felt. Akinesia is a separate phenom-

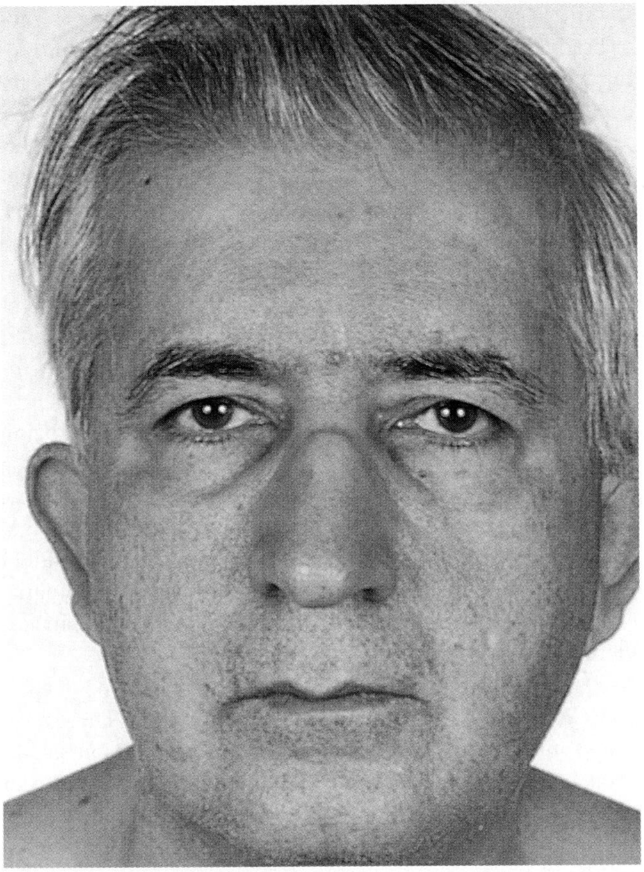

FIG. 16-35 Facial appearance of Parkinson disease. (From Perkin DG: *Mosby's color atlas and text of neurology,* London, 1998, Mosby-Wolfe.)

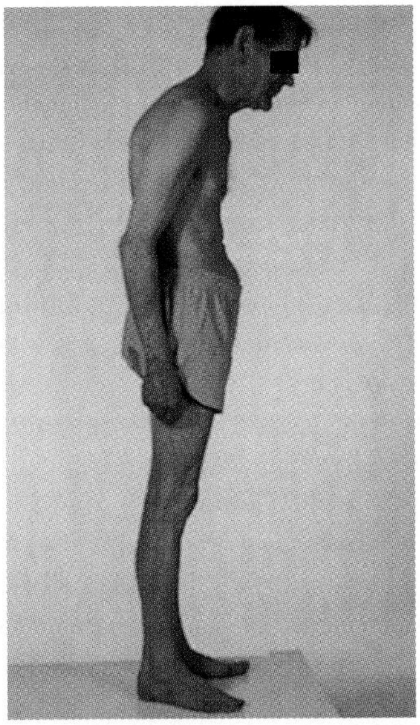

FIG. 16-36 Stooped posture of Parkinson disease. (From Perkin DG: *Mosby's color atlas and text of neurology,* London, 1998, Mosby-Wolfe.)

enon from rigidity and may be severe even in the presence of rigidity. Patients state that they feel "wooden" (as though moving against resistance) and complain of rapid, severe fatigue. Akinesia is attributed to failure of the mechanism programming movement patterns manifested as a defect in the voluntary production of smooth motions at different speeds.

Akinetic symptoms are hypokinesia and bradykinesia. Hypokinesia, or decreased frequency or absence of associated movements, is one of the earliest akinetic symptoms. Individuals with Parkinson disease sit and lie motionless for long periods without the little shifts a normal person makes to prevent discomfort and stiffness. Bradykinesia, or slowness of voluntary movements, is characterized by difficulty initiating, continuing, or synchronizing movements. Both associated and voluntary movements are interspersed by freezing. Freezing may be precipitated by (1) increasing the effort to move, (2) turning, and (3) initiating certain types of tactile and visual contact.

Postural abnormalities. Postural abnormalities are caused by a loss of normal postural reflexes. Three types of postural abnormalities occur in individuals with Parkinson disease: (1) disorders of postural fixation, (2) disorders of equilibrium, and (3) disorders of righting. The disorder of postural fixation associated with Parkinson disease is involuntary flexion of the head and neck. The individual is unable to maintain an upright position of the trunk while standing or walking. The stooped (flexed, forward leaning) posture is characteristic (Fig. 16-36). Postural abnormalities of the hands and feet also occur.

Disorders of equilibrium result from loss of postural stability. The person with Parkinson disease is unable to make the appropriate postural adjustment to tilting or falling and falls like a post when starting to tilt. The festinating gait (short, accelerating steps) of the patient with Parkinson disease is an attempt to maintain an upright position while walking (see Fig. 16-36). Patients also are unable to right themselves when changing from a reclining or crouching position to a standing position and when rolling over from a supine to a lateral or prone position.

Autonomic and neuroendocrine symptoms. Autonomic and neuroendocrine dysfunctions in Parkinson disease produce symptoms that are distressing but not incapacitating. The basal ganglia influence hypothalamic function (autonomic and neuroendocrine) through pathways connecting the hypothalamus with the basal ganglia and cerebral cortex. Common autonomic symptoms in Parkinson disease include inappropriate diaphoresis, orthostatic hypotension, gastric retention, constipation, and urinary retention. A symptom attributed to neuroendocrine dysfunction is seborrhea. Hypothalamic hypersecretion of hormone-releasing factors acting on the anterior pituitary causes hypersecretion of androgenotropic hormones. The androgen excess produces sebum hypersecretion by sebaceous glands. The resulting seborrhea is characterized by oily skin with seborrheic dermatitis along the hairline and in chin-nasal creases.

Cognitive-affective symptoms. Fifty percent of persons with Parkinson disease have a depression that is now believed to be an inherent part of the pathologic state of the disease (an endogenous depression), not a response to the situation. Thirty percent of persons treated on an outpatient basis for Parkinson disease have a dementia, and 80% of persons with Parkinson disease requiring institutional care have dementia as well. Dementia is more common in patients over 70 years of age. Pathologically, in patients with dementia, there are loss of cholinergic cells in the basal nucleus of Meynert; neuronal loss, senile plaques, and neurofibrillary tangles in the neocortex; and amyloid changes in small blood vessels. Lewy bodies are distributed diffusely in many neocortical neurons, making this a Lewy body dementia. The patient evidences disorientation; confusion; memory loss; distractibility; and difficulty with concept formation, abstraction, calculations, thinking, and judgment. Although the symptoms fluctuate, they progressively worsen.

There is also a cognitive disorder unassociated with either a dementia or depression called *bradyphrenia.* This disorder may appear early in the course of the disease and may progress to dementia. Bradyphrenia is caused by disruption of the caudal basal ganglion connections and outflows. The clinical manifestations are slowness of thinking, poverty of thought (diminished imagination and insight), and difficulty formulating thoughts (decreased ability to conceptualize, plan, decide, or improvise). Sleep disturbances also have been documented in persons with Parkinson disease.[56]

Influence of symptoms. Early in the disease, patients often experience a sleep benefit; that is, symptoms decrease with sleep. Also, the symptoms fluctuate in an on-off pattern. Stress influences symptoms adversely, but the underlying mechanism is unclear. The patient's mental status may be further compromised by the side effects of the medication taken to control symptoms.

Late symptoms. The combination of all the parkinsonian symptoms gives the individual a characteristic appearance: a wide-eyed, unblinking, staring expression with the facial muscles smoothed out and almost immobile. Saliva frequently drools from the corners of the slightly open mouth. The skin of the face is frequently greasy. The gait is pathognomonic: the individual walks with slow, short, shuffling steps; the arms are flexed, abducted, and held stiffly at the side; and the trunk is bent slightly forward. The person may break into a run spontaneously or when pushed forward or backward. Because of the disorder of postural fixation, the tendency is to fall to the side.

Evaluation and Treatment

The diagnosis of Parkinson disease is made on the basis of two of the four cardinal symptoms: (1) resting tremor, (2) bradykinesia, (3) cogwheel rigidity, and (4) postural instability. One of the two symptoms must be resting tremor or bradykinesia (criteria from Core Assessment Program for Intracerebral Transplantation [CAPIT]).[18,57] PET shows reduced uptake of 6-[18F]-fluoro-dopa.

The drug therapy includes administration of dopaminergic drugs, such as levodopa (L-dopa), a precursor of dopamine (dopamine does not cross the blood-brain barrier), dopamine agonists, anticholinergic drugs, antihistamines, and amantadine. These drugs are used to decrease akinesia. Because of troublesome side effects and decreased responsiveness to these drugs after 5 years, they are not started until symptoms become incapacitating. Apomorphine is used for the on-off phenomenon and selegiline is used for its neuroprotective properties. Implants of fetal cells are still being studied, as is some ablative surgery (e.g., destruction of a portion of the globus pallidus).[58] Thalmotomy, pallidotomy, and thalamic stimulation are also used at times. Dysphagia and general immobility are special problems of the patient with Parkinson disease, requiring preventive, symptomatic, supportive, and rehabilitative management, such as physiotherapy and speech therapy.[59]

Parkinson disease takes a slowly progressive course for 15 to 20 years before producing total invalidism. The course shows much variation among individuals. The prognosis has been better since the advent of levodopa, but the disorder still shortens life substantially. Pneumonia is the leading cause of death.

Huntington Disease

Huntington disease (HD), also known as chorea, is a relatively rare, hereditary-degenerative disorder diffusely involving the basal ganglia and cerebral cortex. The onset of Huntington disease is usually between 30 and 50 years of age, when the trait may already have been passed to the victim's children. The disorder has a prevalence rate of approximately 5 per 100,000 persons and occurs in all races.

Pathophysiology

Huntington disease is inherited as an autosomal dominant trait with high penetrance. (Mechanisms of genetic inheritance are discussed in Chapter 4.) The genetic defect is on the short arm of chromosome 4, where there is an abnormally long, repeated trinucleotide (CAG)—40 to 70 repeats instead of 9 to 34. Age of onset of symptoms is related to the length of the repeat sequences. Increased length leads to progressively earlier presentations.[60]

The principal pathologic feature of Huntington disease is severe degeneration of the basal ganglia, particularly the caudate and putamen nuclei, and the frontal cerebral cortex (Figs. 16-37 and 16-38). Early in the disease, selective loss of the striatal γ-aminobutyric acid (GABA)/enkephalin pathway to the lateral aspect of the pallidum occurs. The basal ganglia normally contain a preponderance of GABAergic (GABA-secreting) neurons, including the pathway between the basal ganglia and substantia nigra (pallidonigral pathway). Basal ganglia and nigral depletion of GABA, an inhibitory neurotransmitter, is the principal biochemical al-

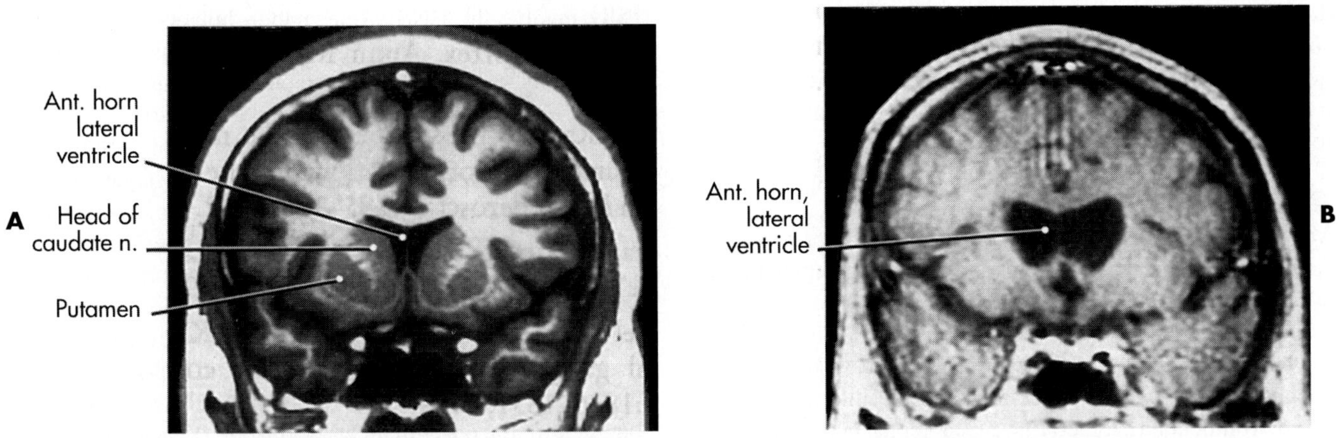

FIG. 16-37 Coronal MRI through frontal lobe and head of the caudate nucleus of a normal individual (A) and an individual with Huntington disease (B). The head of the caudate normally forms a prominent bulge into the anterior horn of the lateral ventricle (**A**, inversion recovery image). Profound cell loss in the neostriatum of Huntington disease greatly diminishes the size of the caudate and renders the lateral wall of the ventricle flat (**B**, T1-weighted image). The slightly wavy appearance of the MRI in *B* is the result of movement (tremor) while the scan was being done. (From Haines DE, editor: *Fundamental neuroscience,* Philadelphia, 1997, Churchill Livingstone.)

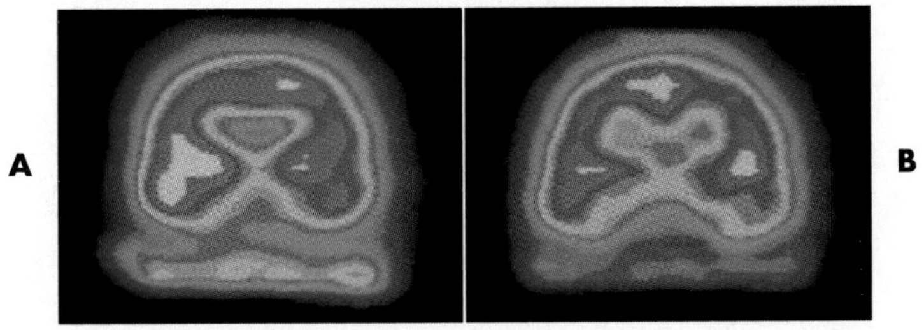

FIG. 16-38 Huntington disease. Single photon emission computerized tomography scan showing reduced caudate blood flow (**A**) compared with normal (**B**). (From Perkin DG: *Mosby's color atlas and text of neurology,* London, 1998, Mosby-Wolfe.)

teration in Huntington disease. Degeneration of the GABAergic pallidonigral pathway causes GABA depletion in the substantia nigra with decreased inhibitory GABA activity on dopaminergic neurons in the substantia nigra and a relative excess of dopaminergic activity in the basal ganglial feedback circuit within the cerebral cortex. A relative excess of dopaminergic activity in this circuit, as in Huntington disease, is manifested by hypotonia and hyperkinesia (involuntary, fragmentary movements such as chorea). Loss of excitatory glutamate may liberate the pathway from the thalamus to the premotor cortex, impairing modulation of movement later in the course of the disease. Within the neurons, producing the fuel for brain activity is difficult, with a resultant buildup of lactic acid.[48]

◆ *Clinical Manifestations*

The classic manifestations of Huntington disease are abnormal movement and progressive dysfunction of intellectual processes (dementia) and thought processes. Any one of these features may mark the onset of the disease. Chorea is the most common type of abnormal movement affecting individuals with Huntington disease. Choreiform movements begin in the face and arms, eventually affecting the entire body. Symptoms of frontal lobe dysfunction include executive attention deficits of short-term memory loss (working memory); reduced capacity to plan, organize, and sequence, as well as bradyphrenia (slow thinking); and apathy. Restlessness, disinhibition, and irritability are common. Affectively, euphoria or depression or both may be present.

◆ *Evaluation and Treatment*

The diagnosis of Huntington disease is based on family history and clinical presentation of the disorder. No known treatment is effective in halting the degeneration or progression of symptoms. The discovery in 1983 of the Huntington disease marker, called *G8,* on chromosome 4 paves the way for presymptomatic diagnosis of the disorder and isolation of the Huntington disease gene. Recombinant genetic techniques may someday prevent or control the disorder.

Multiple Sclerosis

Multiple sclerosis (MS) is a relatively common dysimmune disorder diffusely involving CNS myelin. The peripheral nervous system is not involved. MS is one of many CNS demyelinating disorders. They are acquired conditions and are characterized by degeneration of previously normal myelin with relative preservation of axons. CNS demyelinating disorders are subclassified as primary and secondary. MS and its variants are primary demyelinating disorders. In secondary disorders, CNS demyelination is caused by disorders other than multiple sclerosis.

The onset of MS is usually between 20 and 50 years of age with a peak of age 30. Male/female ratio is about 1:2.[61] MS is the most prevalent CNS demyelinating disorder and a leading cause of neurologic disability in early adulthood. The disease is most prevalent in areas far from the equator. In the United States and Canada the prevalence rate ranges from 30 to 80 per 100,000 persons.[61] MS occurs in all races, but it is chiefly a disorder of whites. Although the disorder does not exhibit a defined inheritance pattern, 15% of persons with MS have an affected relative; Travis[62] believes the gene is the source of the susceptibility. All epidemiologic data point to a relationship between MS and some environmental factor encountered in childhood.

Pathophysiology

MS is currently described as occurring when a previous viral insult to the nervous system has occurred in a genetically susceptible individual with a subsequent abnormal immune response in the central nervous system. T cells become autoreactive to a single myelin protein. Thus the disease is associated with a genetic predisposition and interaction with an environmental risk factor (see Chapter 5). Genetically determined susceptibility is determined by a pattern (haplotype) of histocompatibility antigens (HLA class 1 antigens A3 and B7; and class 2 antigens DRW15, DQW6, and DW2 in whites). Histocompatibility antigen is discussed in Chapter 6. The central components of the pathogenic model are a demyelinating process and nerve fiber loss due to axonal break.[63] Pathologic features of this process are (1) interaction between the systemic immune system and the CNS and (2) demyelinating lesions (plaques and diffuse lesions) in the white matter (Fig. 16-39). (The systemic immune system is discussed in Chapter 6.) In the rat model, immune cells, arriving at the site of myelin sheath damage, discharge glutamate routinely. The glutamate binds to the oligodendrocyte's receptor site and the cell takes it in, accumulating too much glutamate.[64] This in turn causes excessive cell excitation.

Demyelinating lesions (plaques and diffuse lesions) are the second pathologic feature and produce slowing of conduction and finally a conduction block. Plaques characteristically involve the CNS white matter, but occasionally they may extend into the adjacent gray matter. They often coalesce into much larger plaques. In established disease the multifocal, multistaged feature of plaques gives rise to the aphorism that the lesions are "scattered in space and time." Symptoms therefore are multiple and variable. Whether plaques are multiple from the onset of the disease is not known. In many individuals the initial symptoms suggest a single lesion.

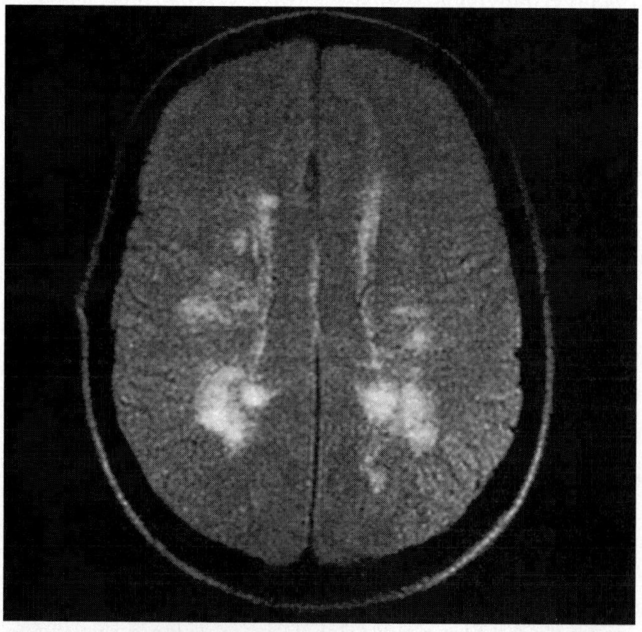

FIG. 16-39 Typical white matter changes on magnetic resonance imaging in multiple sclerosis. (From Perkin DG: *Mosby's color atlas and text of neurology,* London, 1998, Mosby-Wolfe.)

The acute (early) stage of plaque formation is characterized by the process of perivenous demyelination. Most of the neurologic deficits in the acute stage are attributed to inflammatory edema in and around the plaque and to partial demyelination. Symptoms usually remit, partially or completely, weeks after the onset of an early episode.[61] The chronic stage of demyelination and plaque formation is characterized by the process of **gliosis** (glial scarring with late degeneration of axons). Progressive loss of function leads to permanent disability, usually over 20 years.[61]

Although plaques are considered diagnostic of MS, diffuse lesions are common pathologic findings in actively progressive cases. Diffuse lesions are small, widespread areas of perivenular demyelination that do not progress through gliosis. These lesions are sometimes accompanied by edema of surrounding normal brain tissue. The relationship of plaques to diffuse lesions is unknown.

Clinical Manifestations

A variety of events (e.g., infection, trauma, or pregnancy) occurring immediately before the onset or exacerbation of symptoms are regarded as precipitating factors related to MS. Most of the pregnancy-related exacerbations occur 3 months postpartum, suggesting a relation to the stresses of labor and the increased fatigue during the postpartum period rather than to the pregnancy itself.[61]

The major classifications of MS are relapsing-remitting, primary progressive, secondary progressive, and progressive-relapsing (Box 16-8). Initially, 90% of persons present with a relapsing, remitting course. The major manifestations of MS are initial syndromes followed by remissions and established syndromes with no remissions (Box 16-9). Usually persons with late MS have predominantly one of the established syndromes—mixed, spinal, or cerebellar. The initial syndrome depends on the portion of the CNS that is most involved. After years, 50% of individuals appear to have established syndromes of mixed involvement.[61]

Mixed (general) type. Twenty-five percent of persons initially experience retrobulbar or optic neuritis, the manifestations of optic nerve demyelination. The condition usually evolves rapidly over hours to days and is highly suggestive of MS. Involvement may be unilateral or bilateral (although rarely spontaneously). Subjective symptoms are impaired central vision (blurring, fogginess, haziness) and impaired color perception. Signs are decreased central visual acuity; central or paracentral scotoma (area of diminished vision); acquired color vision deficit, especially to red and green; and defective pupillary reaction to light. A variety of field defects may occur. In the acute phase these symptoms may reflect optic papillitis (inflammation and swelling of the optic disc) or retrobulbar neuritis with a normal disc. One third of persons recover completely, and most others improve significantly. Later, pallor of the temporal half of the disc occurs from demyelination of a portion of the optic nerve. (Normal visual function is discussed in Chapter 14.)

The brain stem lesions involve cranial nerves III through XII at the root, nuclear, or corticobulbar (upper motor neuron) level. Internuclear ophthalmoplegia, nystagmus, and dysarthria are the most common brain stem symptoms, followed by deafness, vertigo and vomiting, tinnitus, facial weakness, and facial sensory deficit. Internuclear ophthalmoplegia is lateral gaze paralysis caused by involvement of the medial longitudinal fasciculus, the brain stem pathway that coordinates eye movement. Diplopia and eyeball pain are common complaints. Bilateral internuclear ophthalmoplegia in a young adult is virtually diagnostic of MS.

Cognitive dysfunction recently has been demonstrated to occur early in the disease course. The person experiences decreased short-term memory, recent memory impairment, decreased concentration, word- finding problems, and planning difficulties. Mood alterations are common in MS. Depression is far more common than euphoria.

Spinal type. The spinal type is the second most common type, chiefly involving the spinal tracts and dorsal column. Weakness, numbness, or both in one or more limbs are initial symptoms in 50% of persons with MS. Subjective corticospinal (upper motor neuron) symptoms (stiffness, slowness, weakness) are often unilateral and are a component of fatigability. Spinal signs are usually bilateral (symmetric), with lower limbs more often and more severely affected than upper limbs; spastic paraparesis is probably the most common single neurologic finding in MS.

Bladder and bowel symptoms occur with major spinal cord involvement. Urgency and hesitancy generally precede incontinence. Bladder dysfunction most often involves a small, spastic bladder, although occasionally a large, flaccid bladder may result with retention problems. Neurogenic impotence is often present when sphincter symptoms are present. Bowel incontinence is rare, but constipation is common with severe disease. Subjective dorsal column symptoms are symmetric paresthesias (tingling and numbness) in an unpredictable pattern but with a predilection for lower extremities over upper extremities. Dorsal column signs are vibration, position, and two-point discrimination deficits. Sensory complaints often are not substantiated by objective physical findings but by further diagnostic tests.

Cerebellar type. A nystagmus and ataxia presentation initially is not uncommon and reflects cerebellar and corticospinal involvement. Cerebellar deficits are usually symmetric, with all four limbs involved. With combined corticospinal and cerebellar involvement, the individual has a spastic ataxic gait and ataxia of the arms. Pure cerebellar symptoms are those of motor ataxia, hypotonia, and asthenia (weakness). Manifestations of motor ataxia are decomposition of movement, inability to perform rapid alternating movements (dysdiadochokinesia), and dysmetria. Charcot triad describes a combination of dysarthria, intention tremor, and nystagmus. Hypotonia is manifested by decreased resistance to passive movement, hypoactive deep tendon reflexes, and pendular knee jerk.

Short-lived attacks of neurologic deficits are the temporary appearance or worsening of symptoms. The mechanism of these attacks is complete, reversible conduction block in partially demyelinated axons. Conditions that cause short-lived attacks include (1) minor increases in body temperature or serum Ca^{++} concentration and (2) functional demands exceeding conduction capacity. An increase in body temperature or serum Ca^{++} level increases current leakage

Box 16-8

CLINICAL COURSE OF MS

RELAPSING-REMITTING (RR) MS

Clear relapses (called acute attacks or exacerbations) with either full recovery, or with partial recovery and lasting disability. Between attacks, there is no progression (or worsening) of disease. The most common course of MS.

PRIMARY PROGRESSIVE (PP) MS

Steady progression (or worsening) from onset, with only occasional plateaus or minor recovery. This is a fairly uncommon disease course, and one that may involve different brain and spinal cord damage than do other forms of MS.

SECONDARY PROGRESSIVE (SP) MS

Begins with a pattern of clear-cut relapses and recovery but becomes steadily progressive over time with continued worsening between acute attacks.

PROGRESSIVE-RELAPSING (PR) MS

A rare type that is steadily progressive from onset but also has clear acute attacks.

Box 16-9

ESTABLISHED SYNDROMES OF MULTIPLE SCLEROSIS

MIXED OR GENERALIZED TYPE (50% OF PERSONS)

Optic signs—optic neuritis
Brain stem signs—internuclear ophthalmoplegia, diplopia, vertigo (vomiting), nystagmus, dysarthria
Cerebellar signs—see text

SPINAL TYPE (30% TO 40% OF PERSONS)

Spastic ataxia
Deep sensory changes in the extremities
Bladder and bowel symptoms

CEREBELLAR OR PONTOBULBAR-CEREBRAL TYPE (5% OF PERSONS)

Motor ataxia
Hypotonia
Asthenia

AMAUROTIC FORM (5% OF PERSONS)

Blindness

through demyelinated neurons. Persons with MS may become dramatically worse when body temperature is raised. Hypercalcemia induced by decreased serum pH may aggravate symptoms of MS. Physical and emotional stress impose functional demands that may exceed conduction capacity of affected neurons.

Paroxysmal attacks are sensory or motor symptoms of abrupt onset and short duration (few seconds or minutes). These symptoms include paresthesias, dysarthria and ataxia, and tonic head turning. The mechanism of paroxysmal attacks is nonsynaptic transmission in which nerve impulses are directly transmitted between adjacent demyelinated axons. These impulses arise focally and spuriously in the cervical portion of the spinal cord or in the brain stem. A common paroxysmal symptom, called *Lhermitte sign,* is the momentary paresthesia (shocklike or tingling sensation) that shoots down the trunk or limbs during active or passive flexion of the neck. Bending the neck evokes nonsynaptic impulses in demyelinated axons of the dorsal column in the spinal cord. A person with MS may have many paroxysmal attacks each day. Inciting events include sensory stimulation, voluntary movement, hyperventilation, and emotional stress. Paroxysmal attacks tend to persist for weeks or months and may be followed by progressive symptoms of MS.

Evaluation and Treatment

The diagnosis of MS (definite, probable, or possible) is based on the history and physical examination supported by findings from CSF examination (Table 16-12), evoked response (ER) studies (Fig. 16-40), CT scans of the head, and MRI. Persistently elevated CSF immunoglobulin G (IgG) is found in about two thirds of individuals with MS,[61] and oligoclonal (IgG) bands on electrophoresis are found in more than 90% (Fig. 16-41). ER studies aid diagnosis by detecting decreased conduction velocity in visual, auditory, and somatosensory pathways. MRI is the most sensitive available method of detecting the disease. MRI shows brain stem, optic nerve, and spinal cord lesions not detected by CT. MRI is a good tool with which to monitor progression of the disease.

Treatment has two purposes: (1) acute management of relapses and (2) reducing the frequency of relapses and/or minimizing disease progression ("disease burden").[65,66] Adrenocorticotropic hormone, methylprednisolone, and prednisone are used to shorten the duration of acute relapses. Immunosuppressant therapy may slow progression of the disease. Azathioprine (Imuran) decreases the number of attacks in remitting-relapsing MS. Intravenous cyclophosphamide (Cytoxan) is used in progressive MS. Interferon β-1b (Betaseron, Berlex)[67] and Avonex are choices in relapsing-remitting MS, as well as Copolymer 1 (Copaxone), a synthetic analog of myelin basic protein that acts as a decoy.

Symptom management for fatigue, weakness, vertigo, ataxia, tremor, heat intolerance, spasticity, bladder dysfunction, bowel dysfunction, sexual dysfunction, sensory sensations, pain, cognitive difficulties, depression, and psychosocial issues is essential.[65,66] Supportive and rehabilitative management are directed toward preventing the complications of immobility, especially pressure sores and infections of the pulmonary and genitourinary systems. The average duration of the disease is 30 years.

Table 16-12 Typical Cerebrospinal Fluid Findings in a Multiple Sclerosis Patient

Protein	0.80 g/l
Cell count (all lymphocytes)	15/mm³
Immunoglobulin G/albumin	0.30
Immunoglobulin G index	1.05
Oligoclonal bands	positive

From Perkin GD: *Mosby's color atlas and text of neurology,* 1998, London, Mosby—Wolfe.

Amyotrophic Lateral Sclerosis

Amyotrophic lateral sclerosis (ALS, sporadic motor system disease, sporadic motor neuron disease, motor neuron disease [MND]) is a worldwide degenerative disorder diffusely involving lower and upper motor neurons resulting in progressive muscle weakness leading to respiratory failure and death, usually 2 to 5 years from symptom onset.[68] There are no racial, ethnic, or socioeconomic boundaries.[17] The prevalence rate is 6 to 8 cases per 100,000, with 2 deaths per 100,000. There are 5000 newly diagnosed cases per year in the United States. The term *amyotrophic* (without muscle nutrition or progressive muscle wasting) refers to the predominant lower motor neuron component of the syndrome. Lateral sclerosis, or scarring of the corticospinal tract in the lateral column of the spinal cord, refers to the upper motor neuron component of the syndrome. ALS differs from other motor neuron disorders in that both upper and lower motor neurons are involved.

Classic ALS (Lou Gehrig disease) may begin at any time from the fourth decade of life; its peak occurrence is in the early 50s. Male/female ratio is 3:2, equalizing after menopause. Of persons with ALS, 10% have a familial ALS involving an autosomal dominant pattern with an age-dependent penetrance.[49] ALS was linked to chromosome 21 in 1991. In 1993 a defective superoxide dismutase (SOD) gene was demonstrated to be responsible for 25% of cases of familial ALS.[69]

ALS presentations include crural ALS, proximal or shoulder girdle ALS, and hemiplegic (Mills) ALS. Of persons with ALS, 20% have a benign form of the disease. Subtypes of ALS include primary lateral sclerosis, progressive bulbar palsy, and progressive muscular atrophy.

Pathophysiology

The pathogenesis of ALS is not fully clear. Current data suggest a genetic factor. Persons with familial ALS have a genetic defect on chromosome 21 in the gene that codes for superoxide dismutase, an enzyme that helps destroy free radicals. Abnormal glutamate metabolism and hydrogen peroxide production are also under study as part of the pathogenesis of ALS. RNA strands of echovirus have been isolated in the spinal cord tissue of 15 of 17 persons with ALS who did not have familial ALS.[70]

The principal pathologic feature of ALS is lower and upper motor neuron degeneration, although without inflammation. The number of large motor neurons in the spinal cord, brain stem, and cerebral cortex (premotor and motor areas) is reduced, with ongoing degeneration in the remaining motor neurons. The nuclei of cranial nerves III, IV, and VI are not involved. Death of the motor neuron results in axonal degeneration and secondary demyelination with glial proliferation and sclerosis (scarring) along the corticospinal tract. Inclusion bodies containing the protein *uliquitin* are found in surviving neurons.

Lower motor neuron degeneration denervates motor units. Adjacent, still-viable lower motor neurons attempt to compensate by a process of distal intramuscular sprouting, reinnervation, and enlargement of motor units. The initial symptoms of the disease may be related to lower or upper motor neuron dysfunction or both.

Clinical Manifestations

Weakness may begin in any or all muscles of the body. Muscle weakness in ALS exhibits the following characteristics:

1. Paresis usually begins in a single muscle group.
2. Corresponding muscle groups are asymmetrically affected in a mottled distribution.
3. Gradual involvement occurs in all striated muscles except extraocular muscles and heart and progresses to paralysis with no remissions.
4. Flaccid and spastic paresis may coexist in a single muscle group; flaccid paresis may mask spasticity, which is usually mild.
5. Urethral and anal sphincter weakness is uncommon.
6. No associated mental, sensory, or autonomic symptoms are present. Normal intellectual and sensory functions are sustained until death.

The lower motor neuron syndrome of flaccid paresis consists of weakness of individual muscles, progressing to paralysis, associated with hypotonia and primary muscle atrophy (i.e., atrophy caused by denervation). Hypotonia is manifested by (1) decreased resistance to passive movement, (2) hypoactive or absent deep tendon reflexes, (3) absent abdominal and cremasteric reflexes, and (4) absent Babinski sign. Primary atrophy is manifested by (1) severe, irreversible muscular wasting; (2) fasciculations; (3) metabolically related changes in the skin and appendages; and (4) specific EMG findings. Fasciculations, along with fibrillations, are prominent features of ALS. Metabolic changes include (1) thinning of the skin, (2) thickening of the nails, (3) loss of body hair, and (4) decreased perspiration.

The upper motor neuron syndrome of spastic paresis consists of weakness of movement patterns, progressing to paralysis, associated with spasticity and, in some cases, atrophy secondary to disuse. Spasticity is manifested by (1) clasp-knife phenomenon, evident with passive movement; (2) hyperactive deep tendon reflexes and clonus with severe spasticity; (3) absent abdominal and cremasteric reflexes; and (4) presence of Babinski sign.

Evaluation and Treatment

The diagnosis of the syndrome is based predominantly on medical history and physical examination. EMG and muscle biopsy verify lower motor neuron degeneration and denervation. Muscle biopsy usually is not needed to confirm the diagnosis. Rilutek (Riluzole), an antiglutamate, is the first treatment for ALS.[71] It prolongs life. Treatment is also directed at symptom relief, prevention of complications, maintenance of maximal function, and maintenance of optimal quality of life.[72] Special problems requiring preventive and symptomatic management are communication difficulty caused by dysmasesis and dysphonia, salivation problems with either thick saliva or excessively thin saliva (sialorrhea), and dyspnea caused by diaphragmatic and intercostal

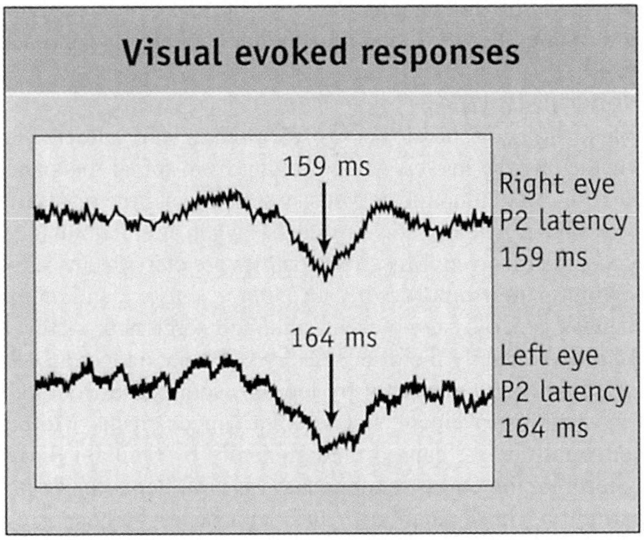

FIG. 16-40 Visual evoked responses showing bilateral delay. (From Perkin DG: *Mosby's color atlas and text of neurology,* London, 1998, Mosby-Wolfe.)

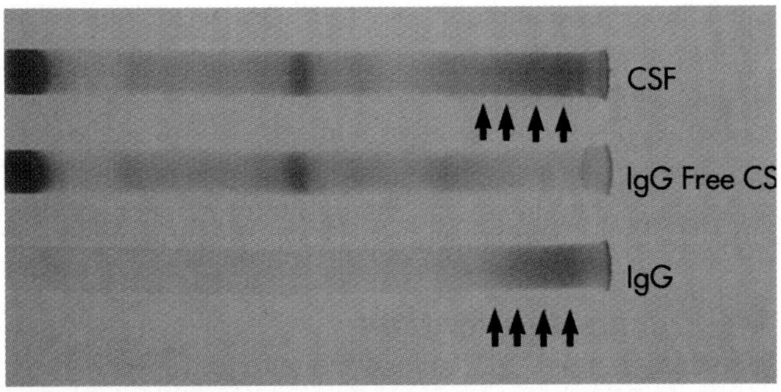

FIG. 16-41 Oligoclonal bands in the cerebrospinal fluid. (From Perkin DG: *Mosby's color atlas and text of neurology,* London, 1998, Mosby-Wolfe.)

weakness. Ventilatory issues become prominent.[73] Supportive and rehabilitation management is directed toward preventing complications of immobility. Psychologic support of the affected individual and the family is extremely important in this disorder. A booket, *Facts about ALS* (1999), is available from the ALS Association in Calabasas Hills, California. An ALS severity scale is also available.[74]

The average duration of life is approximately 2 to 3 years from the appearance of symptoms, but the course of the disease may run from a few months to 15 years. Twenty percent of persons survive 5 years (benign form) and 10% survive 10 years.

PERIPHERAL NERVOUS SYSTEM AND NEUROMUSCULAR JUNCTION DISORDERS

Peripheral Nervous System Disorders

The axons traveling to and from the brain stem and spinal cord neuronal cell bodies may be injured by a multitude of disease processes. Distinct anatomic areas of the axon may be injured, or the spinal nerves may be affected at the spinal roots, at the plexus before peripheral nerve formation, or at the peripheral nerves themselves. The cranial nerves do not have roots or plexuses so are affected only within the nerves themselves. Autonomic nerve fibers may be injured as they travel within certain cranial nerves or emerge through the ventral root and plexuses to travel in the peripheral nerves of the body.

Radiculopathies

As the spinal roots emerge from or enter the vertebral canal, they may be injured or damaged by compression, inflammation, or direct trauma whereby the roots are stretched or torn. **Radiculopathies** are disorders of roots of spinal nerves. **Radiculitis (radiculoneuritis)** refers to an inflammatory disorder of the spinal nerve roots. One or more roots may be affected.

Pathophysiology

Many different pathologic conditions may cause compression, inflammation, or tearing of nerve roots. Roots may be traumatized by a forceful tearing of a nerve, termed *avulsion,* often associated with injuries to the head and shoulders. An acute intervertebral disk prolapse (herniated disk) or a benign tumor may compress nerve roots. Metastatic tumors of the lung, breast, and gastrointestinal tract may produce a carcinomatous meningitis, causing compression and inflammatory changes in nerve roots. Other causes of inflammatory changes in nerve roots are chronic meningitis, neurosyphilis, sarcoidosis, and **inflammatory arachnoiditis** produced by myelography and lumbar punctures.

Clinical Manifestations

The strength, tone, and bulk of the muscles innervated by the involved roots are affected. The pattern and distribution of weakness and atrophy are similar to those of the amyotrophies. Tone and deep tendon reflexes are decreased but rarely absent because the involved muscles are usually innervated by two or more spinal roots. Fasciculations often are present, and mild fatigue may be experienced. Because pathologic processes usually affect both the ventral and dorsal roots, sensory alterations are common.

Diseases that involve spinal roots typically produce local pain; pain on local percussion; pain and paresthesias in the sensory root distribution (called **radicular pain** and **radicular paresthesia**); increased pain with movement, stretching of the root, and maneuvers that transiently increase CSF pressure; sensory loss in a radicular pattern; and spasms of the muscles surrounding the vertebral column (i.e., paravertebral muscle spasms).

Evaluation and Treatment

Diagnostic measures may include spinal films, EMG, lumbar puncture with CSF examination, myelography, and biopsy of tumor masses. Treatment is directed at the cause of the injury and may take the form of surgery, antibiotics, removal of the injurious agent, steroids, and radiation therapy and chemotherapy. Supportive management may include control of the discomfort, protection from further injury, prevention of complications, and rehabilitation where appropriate.

Plexus Injuries

Plexus injuries involve the nerve plexus distal to the spinal roots but proximal to the formation of the peripheral nerves. Such injuries may be caused by trauma, compression, or infiltration, or they may be iatrogenic, caused by positioning during surgery or by an intramuscular injection. Clinical manifestations include motor weakness, muscle atrophy, and sensory loss in affected areas. Paralysis can occur with complete plexus lesions.

The diagnosis is made on the basis of history and clinical manifestations. Therapeutic treatment is directed at removal of the cause, repair and approximation of nervous tissue, prevention of further injury, control of discomfort, prevention of complications, and rehabilitation where appropriate.

Neuropathies

When the peripheral nerves themselves are affected—whether cranial nerves, nerves arising from spinal roots and plexuses, or autonomic nervous system fibers—the resulting syndrome is a neuropathy or **neuritis** when an inflammatory process is involved. Most neuropathies are classified as **sensorimotor neuropathies** because motor, sensory, and reflex changes generally are present, although some neuropathies are predominantly motor or sensory. **Sensory neuropathies** are caused predominantly by leprosy, some industrial solvents, chloramphenicol, and hereditary mechanisms. **Motor neuropathies** are caused predominantly by Guillain-Barré syndrome, infectious mononucleosis, viral hepatitis, acute porphyria, lead, mercury, and triorthocresylphosphates (TCPs). Autonomic fibers may be involved in either a motor or a sensorimotor neuropathy.

Pathophysiology

Although distinct pathophysiologic processes are recognized in a neuropathy, these are not disease specific and may exist simultaneously in any one neuropathy. Wallerian degeneration, in which the axon and myelin distal to the site of axonal interruption degenerate, may be present (see Chapter 13). This type of degeneration is characteristic of a traumatic nerve injury in which the nerve is severed. In some neuropathies the axon may be spared and only the myelin degenerates. Such polyneuropathies are called **segmental demyelinating neuropathies.** This type of degeneration is seen especially in the early phases of many neuropathies. In **axonal degeneration,** distal degeneration of the axon occurs first and is followed by degeneration of the myelin and the axis cylinder. Many pathologic processes may give rise to neuropathy, and one or more nerves may be involved.

Clinical Manifestations

When the axons are affected, muscle strength, muscle tone, and muscle bulk also are affected. Whole muscles or groups of muscles are paretic or paralyzed, and the muscles of the feet and legs often are affected first and more severely. These long, large axons are thought to (1) be more vulnerable to injury because of their size and length, (2) have more Schwann cells available to be injured, and (3) exhibit a "dying back" phenomenon caused by difficulty of the nerve cell body in maintaining the terminal portion of the axon. If unchecked, the pathologic process tends to involve the hands and arms because these have the next longest and largest axons.

Tone and the deep tendon reflexes in the affected muscles generally are decreased in a neuropathy. Atrophy is distributed according to the peripheral nerves involved. The degree and distribution of the atrophy probably depend on the extent of the injury. Fasciculation may be present, especially with associated ventral root or motor neuron changes or both, as in Guillain-Barré syndrome, diabetic neuropathy, and porphyric neuropathy. Mild fatigue may be experienced. A few disorders, notably Guillain-Barré syndrome, produce a pattern of paresis and paralysis that involves all limbs, the trunk, and the neck. Peripheral bifacial and other cranial nerve palsies may be seen with a variety of disorders. Tenderness of the nerve trunks and associated sensory alterations help to distinguish neuropathy from amyotrophy. These include paresthesias and dysesthesias as well as decreased or absent primary sensations (e.g., of temperature, touch, light pain, position, or vibration). Ataxia of gait or limb may arise from the loss of position and vibratory sensations (i.e., proprioceptive sensory loss) and may be enhanced by motor weakness.

Reflexes may be altered. Reflex-mediated autonomic nervous system functions, such as sweating and pupillary size, may be affected. Neuropathies associated with autonomic disturbances include diabetes mellitus, alcoholism and related nutritional neuropathies, amyloidosis, porphyria, Guillain-Barré syndrome, Riley-Day syndrome, and familial sensory neuropathy. In many chronic polyneuropathies the feet, hands, and spine become deformed. Metabolic changes may arise secondary to nerve dysfunction.

Evaluation and Treatment

The diagnostic workup to determine the cause of a neuropathy is often extensive. Early diagnosis and treatment before irreversible neuronal cell damage ensues are of paramount importance. Although axonal regrowth and recovery of function may take months, many neuropathies can be reversed. The therapeutic management is directed first at elimination of the cause, if possible. At least the primary disorder, such as diabetes mellitus, should be controlled. Further damage to the axon must be prevented by avoiding (1) trauma from too-early demand for reuse of the nerve, (2) accidents that cause tissue damage, and (3) hypoxia and ischemia or other deprivation of essential substrates.

Guillain-Barré Syndrome

Guillain-Barré syndrome (Landry-Guillain-Barré syndrome, idiopathic polyneuritis, acute inflammatory demyelinating polyradiculopathy, acute autoimmune neuropathy) is an acquired inflammatory disease that results in demyelination of the peripheral nerves with relative sparing of axons. The disease is characterized by the acute onset of a motor paralysis, usually of an ascending nature. This neurologic disorder occurs throughout the world, affects children and adults of both genders and all age-groups equally, and occurs in all seasons of the year.

The annual incidence rate is 1 to 2 per 100,000 persons with a 4% to 6% mortality rate, and a 5% to 10% morbidity rate (permanent disabling weakness, imbalance, or sensory loss). Precipitating, or at least preceding, events include a mild respiratory or gastrointestinal viral or bacterial infection or other viral illness 1 to 3 weeks or longer before onset of neurologic manifestations, surgical procedures, viral immunizations, and lymphoma or other viral illness. In 60% of patients, *Campylobacter jejuni* is identified as the cause of the preceding infection. Guillilan-Barré syndrome is now classfied into subtypes:[17]

1. Acute inflammatory demyelinating polyradiculoneuropathy
2. Acute axonal motor neuropathy
3. Acute motor and sensory axonal neuropathy
4. Miller-Fisher syndrome
5. Subacute inflammatory demyelinating polyradiculoneuropathy
6. Chronic inflammatory demyelinating polyradiculopathy

Pathophysiology

The neurologic dysfunctions in Guillain-Barré syndrome (GBS) are probably caused by both a humoral- and cell-mediated immunologic reaction directed at peripheral nerve myelin. Lymphocytes infiltrate precedes the influx of macrophages, the cell believed to be responsible for destruction. Macrophages migrate into the areas adjacent to the nerve and attack the myelin surrounding the nerve fibers, causing variable degrees of demyelination of nerve segments. The humoral-mediated component blocks the conduction of nerve impulses to muscles and results in paralysis.[48] Later, there are focal and segmental areas of cellular infiltration by T cell lymphocytes and macrophages in the motor, sensory, autonomic, and cranial nerve pathways. Evidence of reduced suppressor T cell response and abnormal lymphocyte reaction directed against peripheral nervous system myelin has been found. Immunoglobulin M (IgM) antibodies against myelin glycolipid have been found in the serum of GBS patients. Anti-GM1 is more prominent in individuals without sensory symptoms and with prodromal diarrheal illness. Anti-GD1b is more prominent in individuals with prominent sensory symptoms and ataxia. Anti-GQ1b is found in almost all individuals with cranial nerve signs and the Miller-Fisher variant. Antibodies that are cell-mediated responses are thought to be responsible for peripheral nerve demyelination and inflammation. If the process continues, the axons themselves are destroyed by wallerian degeneration. The muscle innervated by the damaged peripheral nerves undergoes denervation and atrophy. If the cell body survives, regeneration of the peripheral nerve takes place and recovery of motor function is likely. If the cell body dies from intense ventral root involvement in the inflammatory-degenerative process, no regeneration is possible. Collateral reinnervation from surviving axons and regenerating axons may take place. In this case, motor recovery is less complete and residual deficits persist.

Clinical Manifestations

Clinical manifestations may vary from paresis of the legs to complete quadriplegia, respiratory insufficiency, and autonomic nervous system instability. Motor signs manifest as an acute or subacute progressive paralysis. Proximal muscles may be involved earlier and more significantly than distal muscles. The paresis/paralysis may be present in an ascending pattern involving limbs, respiratory muscles, and bulbar muscles. Only bulbar muscles may be involved, resulting in dysphagia and dysarthria. Weakness usually plateaus or improves by the fourth week in 90% of persons. After weakness plateaus, strength improves over a period of days to months, with the majority of individuals reaching activity levels similar to their predisease state. Sensory symptoms are common and include paresthesias/dysthesias (tingling, burning, shock-like sensations particularly in the limbs), pain (throbbing, aching particularly in the lower back, buttocks and legs), and numbness. Position and vibratory sensations are more affected than superficial sensation. Deep tendon reflexes are absent or greatly diminished. Respiratory muscle weakness leads to the need for ventilatory support in 10% to 30% of patients. Cranial nerve weakness manifests as facial weakness and bulbar weakness involving chewing, swallowing, and cough. Autonomic dysfunction may manifest as tachycardia or, less frequently, bradycardia; hypotension or hypertension; and loss of or significant increase in sweating in those more severely affected. Patients may undergo a respiratory arrest or cardiovascular collapse. Hyponatremia caused by the syndrome of inappropriate antidiuretic hormone (SAIDH) is common, especially in ventilated individuals.

Evaluation and Treatment

The individual's clinical history helps to diagnose the disorder. Significant signs include paresthesias, paralysis, and CSF findings. The major diagnostic tests are the examination of the CSF, nerve conduction studies, and EMG. The CSF findings include an unusually high protein level (500 mg/dl) without cellular abnormality. Ventilatory support and management of the autonomic nervous system dysfunction are two dominant aspects of the therapeutic management. Plasmapheresis or plasma exchanges within the first two weeks of onset of clinical manifestations are indicated.[75,76] Intravenous immune globulin is used as well as combination therapy.[75,76] After the disorder begins to remit, aggressive rehabilitation should be instituted.

Neuromuscular Junction Disorders

Transmission of the nerve impulse at the neuromuscular junction requires the release of adequate amounts of neurotransmitter from the presynaptic terminals of the axon and effective binding of the released transmitter to the receptors on the membranes of muscle cells (see Fig. 13-13). Nutritional deficits, certain drugs (e.g., reserpine or methyldopa [Aldomet]), and certain disorders that interfere with the synthesis or packaging of the neurotransmitter or its release into the synaptic cleft may result in weakness. Likewise, any pathologic process or drug that interferes with the binding of the neurotransmitter to the receptor may cause weakness.

Marked weakness results from interference with neuromuscular transmission. The distribution of affected muscles is mainly in the bulbar, respiratory, and proximal muscle groups. Botulism toxin has a predilection for the cranial nerves. Eaton-Lambert syndrome affects limb musculature, whereas myasthenia gravis predominantly involves ocular, bulbar, and proximal upper extremity muscles. There is marked fatigability. Muscle tone may be slightly reduced, as may deep tendon reflexes, but the muscle cells are not denervated. Atrophy, if present, is only mild, probably because the small motor system is intact so that tone is maintained to a large degree. Fasciculations or sensory alterations are not present.

The weakness associated with presynaptic dysfunction (as in botulism or Eaton-Lambert syndrome) and that associated with postsynaptic dysfunction (as in myasthenia gravis) are difficult to distinguish clinically, although theoretically some difference should be evident.

Myasthenia Gravis

Myasthenia gravis is a chronic autoimmune disease mediated by antiacetylcholine receptor antibodies that act at the neuromuscular junction; it affects 20,000 to 70,000 persons in the United States. The disease is characterized by exertional fatigue and weakness that worsens with activity, improves with rest, and recurs with resumption of activity. The female/male ratio is 3:2 in younger-aged persons. More males in the older age-group (over 50 years of age) have myasthenia gravis. In 10% to 25% of persons with myasthenia gravis, thymic tumors are found. Of persons with myasthenia gravis, 70% to 80% have pathologic changes in the thymus.[61] Such tumors are more common in males than in females. Myasthenia gravis is an autoimmune disease associated with an increased incidence of other autoimmune diseases, including systemic lupus erythematosus, rheumatoid arthritis, polymyositis, and thyrotoxicosis. (Autoimmune mechanisms are discussed in Chapter 8.) Transitory signs of myasthenia gravis are present in 10% to 15% of infants born to mothers with myasthenia gravis.

Classification of presentations for myasthenia gravis are neonatal myasthenia, congenital myasthenia (neonatal persistent myasthenia), juvenile myasthenia, ocular myasthenia, and generalized autoimmune myasthenia. In **neonatal myasthenia**, onset of signs is 1 to 3 days after birth and the signs persist for a few days to a few weeks. Myasthenia immune globulin is transferred from the mother to the neonate through the placenta. **Congenital myasthenia** presents in infancy and continues into adulthood. The maternal side of the family usually has a positive history for myasthenia gravis. **Juvenile myasthenia** is an autoimmune disorder with a childhood onset usually about 10 years of age. **Ocular myasthenia**, which is more common in males, involves muscle weakness of the eye muscles and eyelids and may include swallowing difficulties and slurred speech as well. **Generalized autoimmune myasthenia** involves the proximal musculature throughout the body and has several courses: (1) a course with periodic remissions, (2) a slowly progressive course, (3) a rapidly progressive course, or (4) a fulminating course.

Pathophysiology

Myasthenia gravis results from a defect in nerve impulse transmission at the neuromuscular junction. The postsynaptic acetylcholine receptors (ACh-R) on the muscle cell's plasma membrane for an unknown reason are no longer recognized as "self" and therefore elicit the generation of antibodies. Acetylcholine receptor antibodies (an IgG antibody) is produced against the acetylcholine receptors. These fix onto the receptor sites and block the binding of acetylcholine. Eventually the antibody action causes the destruction of receptor sites, and the number of receptors on the plasma membrane is reduced. The destruction of receptor sites causes diminished transmission of the nerve impulse across the neuromuscular junction. Muscle depolarization is incomplete or not achieved. The cause of this autosensitization is not known. Evidence supports the autoimmune theory. Clinical and laboratory data show the following:

1. Receptor-binding antibodies are present in 85% to 90% of persons with myasthenia gravis.
2. Passive transfer of myasthenia gravis to animals is possible by injecting serum and IgG from humans with myasthenia gravis.
3. Myasthenia gravis frequently is associated with other autoimmune disorders, such as rheumatoid arthritis, systemic lupus erythematosus, and thyroid disease.
4. Transitory neonatal myasthenia gravis occurs.
5. A strong association between myasthenia gravis and thymus gland hyperplasia exists (0.80).
6. Steroid therapy, antimetabolite drugs, plasma exchange, and thoracic duct drainage all improve the clinical status of the patient with myasthenia gravis.
7. Correlation exists with specific HLA types (HLA-B8).

Clinical Manifestations

Myasthenia gravis typically has an insidious onset. Clinical manifestations may first appear during pregnancy, during the postpartum period, or in conjunction with the administration of certain anesthetic agents. The foremost complaint is muscular fatigue and progressive weakness. The patient often complains of fatigue after exercise and has a recent history of recurring upper respiratory tract infections. The muscles of the eyes, face, mouth, throat, and neck usually are affected first. The extraocular (eye) muscles and the levator muscles are most affected. Manifestations include diplopia, ptosis, and ocular palsies.

The muscles of facial expression, mastication, swallowing, and speech are the next most involved. The results are facial droop and an expressionless face; difficulty chewing and swallowing associated with dietary changes and weight loss; drooling; episodes of choking and aspiration; and a nasal, low-volume but high-pitched monotonous speech pattern.

The muscles of the neck, shoulder girdle, and hip flexors are affected less frequently. When these muscles do become involved, however, the person experiences fatigue requiring periods of rest, weakness of the arms and legs that improves with rest, and difficulty in maintaining head position. The respiratory muscles of the diaphragm and chest wall become weak, and ventilation is impaired. Impairment in deep breathing and coughing predisposes the individual to atelectasis and congestion. In the advanced stage of the disease, all the muscles are weak.

Myasthenic crisis occurs when severe muscle weakness causes extreme quadriparesis or quadriplegia, respiratory insufficiency with shortness of breath and a markedly decreased tidal volume and vital capacity, and extreme difficulty in swallowing. The individual in myasthenic crisis is in danger of respiratory arrest. Myasthenic crisis usually occurs 3 to 4 hours after the patient takes medication.[77]

Cholinergic crisis may arise secondary to drug overdose (anticholinerase drug toxicity). The clinical picture resembles that of myasthenic crisis but the weakness occurs 30 to 60 minutes after taking anticholinergic medication.[77] Other symptoms are also present. Intestinal motility increases and is associated with episodes of diarrhea and complaints of cramping; fasciculation, bradycardia, pupillary constriction,

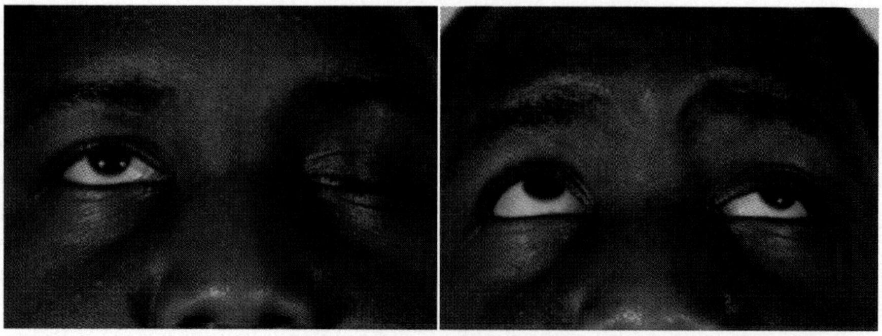

FIG. 16-42 Appearance of the eyes (A) before and (B) after injection of intravenous Tensilon. (From Perkin DG: *Mosby's color atlas and text of neurology,* London, 1998, Mosby-Wolfe.)

increased salivation, and increased sweating are present. These clinical manifestations are caused by the smooth muscle hyperactivity secondary to excessive accumulation of acetylcholine at the neuromuscular junctions and excessive parasympathetic-like activity. As in myasthenic crisis, the individual is in danger of respiratory arrest.

Evaluation and Treatment

The diagnosis of myasthenia gravis is made on the basis of a response to edrophonium chloride (Tensilon), repetitive single-fiber EMG, and antistraited muscle antibodies. The antibodies are found in 80% of persons with generalized autoimmune myasthenia and 55% of persons with occular myasthenia. With intravenous administration of Tensilon, immediate improvement in muscle strength usually persists for 5 to 10 minutes (Fig. 16-42). The EMG is diagnostic in that the muscle fiber weakens readily. Mediastinal CT and MRI are used to determine whether a thymoma is present. Thymus gland abnormalities are seen in 75% of all persons with myasthenia. The progression of myasthenia gravis is highly variable. In some individuals it is mild and spontaneously remits. There is usually a series of relapses, with symptom-free intervals ranging from weeks to months. Over time the disease can progress, leading to death. Ocular myasthenia has a very good prognosis.

Anticholinesterase drugs, steroids, immunosuppressant drugs, cytoxan, and 3,4-DAP are used to treat myasthenia gravis and myasthenic crisis.[78,79] Plasmapheresis may be lifesaving during myasthenic crisis, before and after thymectomy, and at the start of immunosuppressant therapy. For individuals with cholinergic crisis, treatment is to withhold anticholinergic drugs until blood levels fall out of the toxic range, while providing ventilatory support and preventing respiratory complications. Thymectomy is the treatment of choice in individuals with a thymoma.

Myopathies

Myopathy is the term applied to a primary muscle disorder. Many pathologic processes affect muscles and cause loss of functional muscle cells. Within myopathies, muscle strength, tone, and bulk are affected. Primary muscle disease is invariably associated with weakness—usually marked weakness. The distribution of the weakness in myopathy is usually symmetric and proximal, although occasionally the weakness is predominantly distal, such as in myotonic dystrophy. The weakness is associated with mild fatigue. Tone is decreased, as are the tendon reflexes. Atrophy may be present. Some myopathies are associated with muscle hypertrophy as in cretinism and the familial progressive muscular dystrophies of childhood, in which hypertrophied muscles are rubbery and weak. Fasciculations are not present with myopathy because no denervation is present. No sensory changes are found. (Specific myopathies are discussed in Chapter 15.)

SUMMARY REVIEW

Central Nervous System (CNS) Disorders

1. Motor vehicle crashes (MVCs) are the major cause of traumatic CNS injury. Traumatic injuries are classified as closed-head trauma (blunt) or open-head trauma (penetrating). Closed-head trauma is the more common type of trauma.
2. Different types of focal brain injury include contusion (bruising of the brain), laceration (tearing of brain tissue), extradural hematoma (accumulation of blood above the dura mater), subdural hematoma (blood between the dura mater and arachnoid membrane), intracerebral hematoma (bleeding into the brain), and open-head trauma.
3. Open-head trauma involves a skull fracture with exposure of the cranial vault to the environment. The types of open-head trauma (compound fracture, perforated fracture) are linear, comminuted, compound, and basilar skull fracture (in the cranial vault or at the base of the skull).

4. Diffuse axonal injury (DAI) results from the effects of head rotation. The brain experiences shearing stresses resulting in axonal damage ranging from concussion to a severe DAI state.
5. Spinal cord injuries occur most frequently in young men who sustain various kinds of injuries (recreational or travel related) and elderly persons because of preexisting degenerative vertebral disorders.
6. Spinal cord injury involves damage to vertebral or neural tissues by compressing tissue, pulling or exerting tension on tissue, or shearing tissues so that they slide into one another.
7. Spinal cord injury often causes spinal shock with cessation of all motor, sensory, reflex, and autonomic functions below any transected area. Loss of motor and sensory function depends on the level of injury.
8. Paralysis of the lower half of the body with both legs involved is called *paraplegia.* Paralysis involving all four extremities is called *quadriplegia.*
9. Return of spinal neuron excitability occurs slowly. Reflex activity can return in 1 to 2 weeks in most persons with acute spinal cord injury. A pattern of flexion reflexes emerges, involving first the toes and then the feet and the legs. Eventually, reflex voiding and bowel elimination appear and mass reflex (flexor spasms accompanied by profuse sweating, piloerection, and automatic bladder emptying) may develop.
10. Immobilization of the spine is the immediate intervention for a suggested or confirmed vertebral fracture.
11. The pathologic findings in degenerative disk disease (DJD) include disk protrusion, spondylosis, and/or subluxation and degeneration of the vertebrae (spondylolisthesis) and spinal stenosis.
12. Low back pain is pain between the lower rib cage and gluteal muscles and often radiates into the thigh.
13. Low back pain has a high prevalence, affecting 75% to 90% of the population at some time. Sciatica affects about 1% of those with low back pain.
14. Most causes of low back pain are unknown; however, some secondary causes are disk prolapse, tumor, bursitis, synovitis, DJD, osteoporosis, fracture, inflammation, and sprain.
15. Diagnosis of injury to the lower back is made on the basis of physical examination, electromyography (EMG), myelography, computed tomography (CT), and magnetic resonance imaging (MRI).
16. Treatment for low back pain includes bed rest, use of analgesics and antiinflammatory agents, exercise, physical therapy, education, and surgery.
17. Herniation of an intervertebral disk is a protrusion of part of the nucleus pulposus. Herniation most commonly affects the lumbosacral disks (L5-S1 and L4-5). The extruded pulposus compresses the nerve root, causing pain that radiates along the sciatic nerve course.
18. The conservative approach to treatment of an intervertebral rupture is traction and bed rest. Surgery is indicated if there is evidence of severe compression (weakness, chronic pain, decreased deep tendon reflexes, and bladder/bowel reflexes).
19. Cerebrovascular disease is the most frequently occurring neurologic disorder. Any abnormality of the blood vessels of the brain is referred to as a *cerebrovascular disease.*
20. Cerebrovascular disease is associated with two types of brain abnormalities: (a) ischemia with or without infarction and (b) hemorrhage.
21. The most common clinical manifestation of cerebrovascular disease is a cerebrovascular accident (CVA, stroke syndrome).
22. Cerebrovascular accidents are classified according to pathophysiology and include global hypoperfusion and thrombotic (arterial occlusions caused by thrombi), embolic (fragments that break from a thrombus outside the brain), hemorrhagic (intracranial hemorrhage), and lacunar strokes.
23. Treatment for an ischemic CVA includes preventing further thrombotic events, augmenting blood flow, reperfusing tissues, and protecting neurons, as well as supportive management for cerebral edema and increased intracranial pressure. Surgical intervention may be required to restore blood supply.
24. Intracranial aneurysms result from defects in the vascular wall and are classified on the basis of form and shape. They are frequently asymptomatic, but the signs vary according to the location and size of the aneurysm.
25. In cerebral aneurysms, surgical intervention is the treatment of choice before rupture.
26. An arteriovenous malformation (AVM) is a tangled mass of dilated blood vessels. Although sometimes present at birth, AVM exhibits a delayed age of onset.
27. Clinical manifestations of AVM range from headache and dementia to seizures and intracerebral or subarachnoid hemorrhage.
28. A subarachnoid hemorrhage occurs when blood escapes from defective or injured vasculature into the subarachnoid space. When a vessel tears, blood under pressure is pumped into the subarachnoid space. The blood produces an inflammatory reaction in these tissues.
29. Clinical manifestations of a subarachnoid hemorrhage include headache, changes in mental status, transient motor weakness, and numbness and tingling. Vasospasm is a serious complication and may cause ischemia and infarct. Treatment of vasospasm includes use of calcium channel blockers to prevent or reverse vasospasm and augmenting cerebral perfusion by volume expansion and hemodilution.
30. Migraine headache occurs with and without aura and is precipitated by a triggering event. The aura is associated with a spreading wave of cortical depression and decreased blood flow accompanied by scotomas and jagged flashes of light and sensory changes.
31. Etiologic theories of migraine include a central alteration in neurotransmitters, ions, and hormones with altered neural function and blood flow. In women, migraine is associated with the cyclic withdrawal of estrogen.
32. The headache of migraine is throbbing and intense; it may be accompanied by photophobia, nausea, and vomiting.
33. Cluster headaches occur in episodes several times during a day for a period of days at different times of the year. The pain is unilateral, intense, tearing, and burning. Associated symptoms include ptosis, lacrimation, reddening of the eye, and nausea. The etiology is unknown but involves hyperactivity of the sympathetic nervous system. There is an acute and a chronic form.
34. Chronic paroxysmal hemicrania is a cluster headache with more frequent daily attacks; it occurs primarily in women. It responds to treatment with indomethacin.
35. Tension-type headache is the most common type of headache. Both a central mechanism and a peripheral mechanism are associated with the etiology. The headache is bilateral, with the sensation of a tight band around the head.

The pain may last for hours or days. There are acute and chronic forms.

36. Two main types of tumors occur within the cranium: primary and metastatic. Primary tumors are classified as intracerebral or extracerebral. Metastatic tumors can be found inside or outside the brain substance.
37. Central nervous system (CNS) tumors cause local and generalized manifestations. The effects are varied; local manifestations include seizures, visual disturbances, loss of equilibrium, and cranial nerve dysfunction.
38. The principal treatment for brain tumors is surgical or radiosurgical excision or decompression if total excision is not possible. Chemotherapy and radiation therapy also are used.
39. Spinal cord tumors are classified as intramedullary (within the neural tissues) or extramedullary (outside the spinal cord). Metastatic spinal cord tumors are usually carcinomas, lymphomas, or myelomas.
40. Extramedullary spinal cord tumors produce dysfunction by compression of adjacent tissue, not by direct invasion. Intramedullary spinal cord tumors produce dysfunction by both invasion and compression.
41. The onset of clinical manifestations of spinal cord tumors is gradual and progressive, suggesting compression. Specific manifestations depend on the location of the tumor; for example, there may be paresis and spasticity of one leg with thoracic tumors, followed by involvement of the opposite leg.
42. Spinal cord tumors are treated by surgery, radiation therapy, chemotherapy, and hormonal therapy.
43. Infection and inflammation of the CNS can occur by bacteria, viruses, fungi, protozoans, and rickettsiae. The resulting infection of bacterial infections is pus producing, or pyogenic.
44. Meningitis (infection of the meninges) is classified as bacterial, aseptic (nonpurulent), or fungal. Bacterial meningitis is primarily an infection of the pia mater and arachnoid and of the fluid of the subarachnoid space. Aseptic meningitis is believed to be limited to the meninges. Fungal meningitis is a chronic, less common type of meningitis.
45. The meningeal vessels become hyperemic, and neutrophils migrate into the subarachnoid space with bacterial meningitis. An inflammatory reaction occurs, and exudation ensues and increases rapidly.
46. The variety of clinical manifestations depends on the type of meningitis and ranges from throbbing headache to neck stiffness and rigidity and decreasing responsiveness. Specific cranial nerve dysfunction is a common occurrence.
47. Bacterial meningitis and fungal meningitis are treated with appropriate antibiotic therapy; aseptic meningitis is treated with antibiotics, antiviral drugs, and steroids.
48. Brain abscesses often originate from infections outside the CNS. Organisms gain access to the CNS from adjacent sites or spread along the wall of a vein. A localized inflammatory process develops with exudate formation, thrombosis of vessels, and degenerating leukocytes. After a few days the infection becomes delimited, with a center of pus and a wall of granular tissue.
49. Clinical manifestations of brain abscesses include headache, nuchal rigidity, confusion, drowsiness, and sensory and communication deficits. Treatment includes antibiotic therapy and surgical excision or aspiration.
50. Encephalitis is an acute, febrile illness of viral origin with nervous system involvement. The most common encephalitides are caused by arthropod-borne viruses and herpes simplex virus. Meningeal involvement appears in all encephalitides.
51. Clinical manifestations of encephalitis include fever, delirium, confusion, seizures, abnormal and involuntary movement, and increased intracranial pressure.
52. Herpes encephalitis is treated with antiviral agents. No definitive treatment exists for the other encephalitides.
53. The common neurologic complications of acquired immunodeficiency syndrome (AIDS) are human immunodeficiency virus (HIV) encephalopathy, HIV neuropathy, HIV myelopathy, opportunistic infections, cytomegalovirus infection, parasitic infection, and neoplasms. Pathologically, there may be diffuse CNS involvement, focal pathologic findings, and obstructive hydrocephalus.
54. Parkinson disease is a common degenerative disorder of the basal ganglia (corpus striatum) involving degeneration of the dopamine-secreting nigrostriatal pathway. The pathogenesis of Parkinson disease is unknown, but researchers suggest genetic, viral, and environmental toxins as possible causes.
55. Degeneration of the dopaminergic nigrostriatal pathway causes dopamine depletion in the basal ganglia and an excess of cholinergic activity in the cortex, basal ganglia, and thalamus. Tremor and rigidity are caused by the excess cholinergic activity. Progressive dementia may be associated with an advanced stage of the disease.
56. Treatment of Parkinson disease is symptomatic, involving levodopa (L-dopa), a precursor of dopamine. The disease takes a slowly progressive course for 15 to 20 years before producing complete invalidism.
57. Huntington disease (chorea) is a rare hereditary disease involving the basal ganglia and cerebral cortex. It is inherited as an autosomal dominant trait and commonly manifests between 30 and 50 years of age.
58. The major pathologic feature of Huntington disease is severe degeneration of the basal ganglia and the frontal cerebral cortex. The basal ganglia and the substantia nigra exhibit a depletion of neurons that secrete γ-aminobutyric acid (an inhibitory neurotransmitter). This depletion leads to an excess of dopaminergic activity that causes involuntary, fragmentary movements.
59. No known treatment is effective in halting the degenerative process in Huntington disease.
60. Multiple sclerosis (MS) is a relatively common degenerative disorder involving CNS myelin. Although the pathogenesis is unknown, the demyelination is thought to result from an immunogenetic-viral cause. A previous viral insult to the nervous system in a genetically susceptible individual yields a subsequent abnormal immune response in the CNS.
61. The clinical manifestations of MS involve different types: mixed or generalized, spinal, and cerebellar.
62. No treatment is available to cure MS. Steroid and immune therapy is used to acutely manage relapses or reduce frequency of relapses.
63. Amyotrophic lateral sclerosis (ALS) is a degenerative disorder diffusely involving lower and upper motor neurons. The pathogenesis of ALS is not fully known; however, there is lower and upper motor neuron degeneration.
64. Clinical manifestations of ALS may include weakness in all muscles. Flaccid paresis progressing to paralysis is characteristic of the lower motor neuron syndrome. One treatment

is currently available to alter the time course of the ALS syndrome.

Peripheral Nervous System and Neuromuscular Joint Disorders

1. Radiculopathies are disorders of the roots of spinal cord nerves. The roots may be compressed, inflamed, or torn. Clinical manifestations include local pain or paresthesias in the sensory root distribution. Treatment may involve surgery, antibiotics, steroids, radiation therapy, and chemotherapy.
2. Plexus injuries involve the plexus distal to the spinal roots. Paralysis can occur with complete plexus involvement.
3. Neuropathies are the resulting syndrome when the peripheral nerves are affected. Axon and myelin degeneration may be present. Neuropathies are classified as sensorimotor, sensory, or motor. The neuropathies are characterized by varying degrees of paresis and paralysis, and secondary atrophy may be present.
4. Therapy for the neuropathies is directed at the primary cause, such as diabetes mellitus. Axonal regrowth and recovery of function may take months, but many neuropathies can be reversed.
5. Guillain-Barré syndrome is a demyelinating disorder caused by a humoral and cell-mediated immunologic reaction directed at the peripheral nerves. The clinical manifestations may vary from paresis of the legs to complete quadriplegia, respiratory insufficiency, and autonomic nervous system instability. Plasmapheresis or plasma exchange is used in severe disease, followed by aggressive rehabilitation.
6. Myasthenia gravis is a disorder of voluntary muscles characterized by muscle weakness and fatigability. It is considered an autoimmune disease and is associated with an increased incidence of other autoimmune diseases.
7. Myasthenia gravis results from a defect in nerve impulse transmission at the neuromuscular junction. Acetycholine receptor antibody is secreted against the "self" and blocks the binding of acetylcholine. The antibody action destroys the receptor sites, causing decreased transmission of the nerve impulse across the neuromuscular junction.
8. Clinical manifestations of myasthenia gravis include weakness of the muscles of the face and throat and may involve muscles of the diaphragm and chest wall.
9. Treatment of myasthenia gravis involves symptom relief and immunotherapy. The progression of the disease is highly variable; in some individuals it is mild and spontaneously remits.
10. Primary disorders with weakness and atrophy are known as myopathies.

KEY TERMS

KEY TERMS—cont'd

Open (penetrating, missile) trauma, *487*
Parkinson disease, *530*
Parkinsonian tremor, *532*
Parkinsonism (Parkinson syndrome, parkinsonian syndrome), *530*
Plexus injury, *540*
Postconcussive syndrome, *495*
Radicular pain, *540*
Radicular paresthesia, *540*
Radiculitis (radiculoneuritis), *540*
Radiculopathy, *540*
Saccular aneurysm (berry aneurysm), *510*
Segmental demyelinating neuropathy, *541*
Sensorimotor neuropathy, *540*
Sensory neuropathy, *540*
Severe diffuse axonal injury (DAI), *493*
Spinal cord abscess, *526*
Spinal epidural abscess, *526*
Spinal stenosis, *503*
Spondylolisthesis, *503*
Spondylolysis, *503*
Stroke-in-evolution (progressive stroke), *506*
Subarachnoid hemorrhage, *512*
Subdural hematoma, *490*
Syringomyelic syndrome, *523*
Tension-type headache, *515*
Thrombotic stroke (cerebral thrombosis), *505*
Toxoplasmosis, *529*
Transient ischemic attack (TIA), *505*
Traumatic aneurysm, *511*
Traumatic brain injury (TBI), *487*
Tubercular (TB) meningitis, *524*
Vacuolar myelopathy, *529*
Venous angioma, *511*

REFERENCES

1. Marion DW: *Traumatic brain injury*, New York, 1999, Thieme.
2. Bullock R et al: *Guidelines for the management of severe head injury*, New York, 1995, The Brain Trauma Foundation.
3. Giacino JT, Zasler ND: Outcome after severe traumatic brain injury: coma, the vegetative state, and minimally responsive state, *J Head Trauma Rehab* 10(1):40, 1995.
4. Giacino JT et al: Development of practice guidelines for assessment and management of the vegetative and minimally conscious state, *J Head Trauma Rehab* 12(4):79, 1997.
5. van der Naalt J et al: One year outcome in mild to moderate head injury: the predictive value of acute injury characteristics related to complaints and return to work, *J Neurol, Neuros & Psych* 66:207, 1999.
6. Grennarelli TA et al: Influence of the type of intracranial lesion on outcome from severe head injury, *J Neurosurg* 56(1):26, 1982.
7. Simon RH, Sayre JT: *Strategy in head injury management,* Norwalk, Conn, 1987, Appleton & Lange.
8. Kealy KA, Dilger K: Unsuspected venous angioma infarct. a case study. In *AANN 32nd annual meeting program book* (p 136), New Orleans, 2000, AANN.
9. Stewart-Amedei C: Germ cell tumors of the central nervous system. In *AANN 32nd annual meeting program book* (p 212), New Orleans, 2000, AANN.
10. Narayan RK, Wilberger JE Jr, Covlihock ST, editors: *Neurotrauma*, New York, 1996, McGraw-Hill.
11. Sullivan J: Spinal cord injury research: review and synthesis, *Crit Care Nurs Q* 22:80, 1999.
12. Mitcho KJ, Yanko J: Acute care management of spinal cord injury, *Crit Care Nurs Q* 22:60, 1999.
13. DeVivo MJ: Causes and costs of spinal cord injury in the United States, *Spinal Cord* 35(12):809, 1997.
14. Frymoyer J, editor: *The adult spine: principles and practice*, Philadelphia, 1997, Lippincott-Raven.
15. Marciano FF et al: Pharmacologic management of spinal cord injury: review of the literature, *BNI Q* 11(2):209, 1995.
16. Marion DW: Injuries of the spinal cord and spinal column. In Pietzman AB et al, editors: *The trauma manual*, Philadelphia, 1998, Lippincott-Raven.
17. Perkins GD: *Mosby's color atlas and text of neurology*, London, 1998, Mosby-Wolfe.
18. Langston JW et al: Core assessment program for intracerebral transplantation (CAPIT), *Mov Disord* 7(1):2, 1992.
19. Leboeuf Y de C: Does smoking cause low back pain? A review of the epidemiologic literature for causality, *J Manipulative Physiol Ther* 18(4):237, 1995.
20. Mazanec DJ: Back pain: medical evaluation and therapy, *Cleve Clin J Med* 62(3):163, 1995.
21. Weber H: The natural history of disc herniation and the influence of intervention, *Spine* 19(19):2234, 1994.
22. Welch KMA et al, editors: *Primer on cerebrovascular diseases*, San Diego, 1997, Academic Press.
23. Sarasin FP et al: Cost effectiveness of antiplatelet regimens used as secondary prevention of stroke or transient ischemic attack, *Arch Intern Med* 160(18):2773, 2000.
24. Pyorala M et al: Insulin resistance syndrome predicts the risk of coronary heart disease and stroke in healthy middle-aged men: the 22 year follow-up results of the Helsinki Policeman Study, *Arterioscler Thromb Vasc Biol* 20(2):538, 2000.
25. Eikelboom JW: Association between high homocyst(e)ine and ischemic stroke due to large- and small-artery disease but not other etiologic subtypes of ischemic strone, *Stroke* 31(5):1069, 2000.
26. Lestro Henriques I, Bogousslavsky J, van Melle G: Predictors of stroke pattern in hypertensive patients, *J Neurol Sci* 144:142, 1996.
27. Boysen G, Truelsen T: Prevention of recurrent stroke, *Neurolog Sci* 21(2):67, 2000.
28. Bogousslavsky J et al: Stroke subtypes and hypertension. Primary hemorrhage vs infarction, large- vs small-artery disease, *Arch Neurol* 53:265, 1996.
29. Frey JL: The future of acute stroke treatment: lessons from laboratory and clinical research, *BNI Q* 11(3):26, 1995.
30. Osborn TM, LaMonte MR, Gaasch WR: Intravenous thrombolytic therapy for stroke: a review of recent studies and controversies, *An Em Med* 34(2):244, 1999.
31. Kothari R et al: Acute stroke: delays to presentation and emergency department evaluation, *Ann Em Med* 33(1):3, 1999.
32. Hock NH: Neuroprotective and thrombolytic agents: advanced in stroke treatment, *J Neurosi Nurs* 30(3):175, 1998.
33. Broderick J et al: Guidelines for the management of spontaneous intracerebral hemorrhage, *Stroke* 30:905, 1999.
34. Soman P: Severe ventricular dysfunction secondary to subarachnoid hemorrhage, *Clin Cardio* 20(4):402, 1998.
35. DiPasquales G et al: Cardiogenic complications of subarachnoid hemorrhage, *J Neurosurg Sci* 42(suppl 1):33, 1998.
36. Lipton RB, Silberstein SD, Stewart WF: An update on the epidemiology of migraine, *Headache* 36:319, 1996.
37. Robbins L: Precipitating factors in migraine: a retrospective review of 494 patients, *Headache* 34(4):214, 1994.
38. Headache Classification Committee of the International Headache Society: Classification and diagnostic criteria for headache disorders, cranial neuralgias, and facial pain, *Cephalagia* 8(suppl 7):1, 1988.
39. Diener HC, Peatfield RC: Migraine. In Brandt T et al, editors: *Neurological disorders: course and treatment,* San Diego, 1996, Academic Press.
40. Raskin NH: Migraine and other headaches. In *Merritt's textbook of neurology,* ed 9, Baltimore, 1995, Williams & Wilkins.
41. Marcus DA: Interrelationships of neurochemicals, estrogen, and recurring headache, *Pain* 62:(2):129, 1995.
42. Bartelink ML, van Weel C: Migraine in female patients in family practice, *Headache Q Curr Treat Res* 6(3):204, 1995.

43. Kumar KL, Joos SK: Teaching headache management to medicine residents, *Headache* 36(7):446, 1996.
44. Spierlings ELH, van Hoof MJ: Anxiety and depression in chronic headache sufferers, *Headache Q Curr Treat Res* 7(3):235, 1996.
45. Cady RK: Prophylactic therapy of migraine in primary care, *Headache Q Curr Treat Res* (suppl 1):6, 1996.
46. Drummond P: The site of sympathetic deficit in cluster headache, *Headache* 36:3, 1996.
47. Martelletti P, Giacovazzo M: Putative neuroimmunological mechanisms in cluster headache: an integrated hypothesis, *Headache* 36:213, 1996.
48. Barker E: *Neuroscience nursing,* St Louis, 1994, Mosby.
49. American Brain Tumor Association: *A primer of brain tumors*, Des Plaines, 1996, American Brain Tumor Association.
50. Maher de Leon ME, Schell S, Rozental J: Tumors of the spine and spinal cord, *Sem Oncol Nurs* 14:43, 1998.
51. Sundaredon N et al: Tumors of the spine. In Vecht CJ, editor: *Handbook of clinical neurology* (vol 2, p 511), New York, 1997, Elsevier.
52. Phillips FJ, Semor AD: Bacterial meningitis in children and adults: changes in community-acquired disease may affect patient care, *Postgrad Med* 103(b):102, 1998.
53. Pruitt AA: Infections of the nervous system, *Neurol Clin N Am* 16(2):419, 1998.
54. Nadelman RB et al: The clinical spectrum of early Lyme borreliosis in patients with culture-confirmed erythema migrans, *Am J Med* 100(5): 502, 1996.
55. Lieberman A: Hitler, Parkinson's disease and history, *BNI Q* 11(3):4, 1995.
56. Dowling GA: Sleep in older women with Parkinson's disease, *J Neurosci Nurs* 27(6):355, 1995.
57. Defer GL et al: Core assessment program for surgical interventional therapies in Parkinson's disease (CAPSIT-PD), *Mov Disord* 14:572, 1999.
58. Seppa N: The give and take of Parkinson's disease, *Sci News* 156:342, 1999.
59. Yorkston KM, Miller RM, Strand FA: *Management of speech and swallowing disorders in degenerative diseases*, Tucson, 1999, Communication Skill Builders.
60. Stevens A, Lowe J: *Pathology,* London, 1995, Mosby.
61. Adams RD, Victor M, Ropper T: *Principles of neurology,* New York, 1997, McGraw-Hill.
62. Travis J: MS families: it's genes, not a virus, *Sci News* 148(12):180, 1995.
63. Trapp B et al: Axonal transection in the lesion of MS, *NEMJ* (Jan 29):278, 1994.
64. Seppa N: Glutamate glut linked to multiple sclerosis, *Sci News* 157:82, 2000.
65. Halper J, Holland N: New strategies, new hope: meeting the challenge of multiple sclerosis, Part I, *AJN* 98(10):26, 1998.
66. Halper J, Holland N: New strategies, new hope: meeting the challenge of multiple sclerosis, Part II, *AJN* 98(11):39, 1998.
67. Logan-Clubb L, Stacy M: An open-labelled assessment of adverse effects associated with Interferon 1 beta in the treatment of multiple sclerosis, *J Neurosci Nurs* 27(6):344, 1995.
68. Walling AD: Amyotrophic lateral sclerosis: Lou Gehrig's disease, *Am Fam Phys* 59:1489, 1999.
69. Morrison BN, Morrison JH: Amyotrophic lateral sclerosis associated with mutations in superoxide dismutase: a punative mechanism of degeneration, *Brain Res Rev* 29(1):121, 1999.
70. Seppa N: Nerve cells of ALS patients harbor virus, *Sci News* 157:37, 2000.
71. Bromberg MG: Ongoing trials in motor neuron disease, *Expert Opin Invest Drugs* 8(6):884, 1999.
72. Miller RG et al: The ALS practice parameters task force: practice parameters: the care of the patient with amyotrophic lateral sclerosis (an evidence-based review), *Neurol* 52:1311, 1999.
73. Borasio GD, Belinas DF, Yanagisawa N: Mechanical venitlation in amyotrophic lateral sclerosis: a cross-cultural perspective, *J Neurol* 245(suppl 2):S7, 1998.
74. Hillel AD et al: Amyotrophic lateral sclerosis severity scale, *J Neuroepidemiol* 8:142, 1989.
75. Plasma Exchange/Sandoglobulin Guillian-Barré Study Trial Group: Randomised trial of plasma exchange, intravenous immunoglobulin and combined treatment in Guillian-Barré syndrome, *Lancet* 349:225, 1997.
76. Van der Meche FGA, can Doorn PA: Guillian-Barré syndrome and chronic inflammatory demyelinaging polyneuropathy: immune mechanisms and update on current therapies, *Ann Neurol* 30:S14, 1995.
77. Lisak RP, editor: *Handbook of myasthenia gravis,* New York, 1994, Marcel Dekker.
78. Howard JF Jr: Intravenous immunoglobulin for the treatment of acquired myasthenia gravis, *Neurol* 51(6 suppl 5):30, 1998.
79. Keesey J: A treatment algorighm for autoimmune myasthenia in adults, *Ann NY Acad Sci* 841:753, 1998.

CHAPTER 17

Neurobiology of Schizophrenia, Mood Disorders, and Anxiety Disorders

LOREY K. TAKAHASHI

CHAPTER OUTLINE

Mental illnesses are common and have a long history of afflicting humanity. They appear in different cultures and across the socioeconomic spectrum. When mental illnesses are left untreated, the consequences can be devastating. This chapter examines the neurobiology of schizophrenia, mood disorders, and anxiety disorders. The etiology and symptoms underlying these major mental illnesses are diverse and complex. Diagnostic criteria constantly are updated in an attempt to precisely identify and effectively treat the disorders. Even within an illness such as schizophrenia, a number of different symptoms vary in intensity. Some of this variation in symptoms and response to treatment may reflect differences in neural pathologic conditions and function. In schizophrenia, neuroanatomic alterations are found in some individuals. In addition, functional alterations may occur in neurotransmitter systems, such as dopamine. In mood and anxiety disorders, where no clear structural changes are present in the brain, the illness may arise from functional pathologic conditions occurring in specific brain regions. These alterations may stem from a number of differences, including neurochemical secretion and uptake, receptor density, and intracellular functions. Currently, several neurotransmitters and brain regions are identified that may contribute to the disorders.

Knowledge of neurotransmitter systems is critical for the effective treatment of schizophrenia, mood disorders, and anxiety disorders. This information has accumulated rapidly in the latter half of the twentieth century, when it was discovered that certain drugs could mimic or relieve the symptoms of psychopathologic conditions. Today, this information is used to develop new drugs that are more specific in treating illnesses without producing disturbing side effects. Fundamental information on brain function also is expanding rapidly and linking specific brain regions with cognitive and emotional states, as well as suggesting potential targets for therapeutic drugs. Insight into brain function is aided greatly by the advent of powerful neuroimaging techniques that provide a visual evaluation of brain regions associated with mental disorders.

SCHIZOPHRENIA

Schizophrenia is a common and potentially devastating psychiatric illness that strikes 1% of the world's population across all socioeconomic levels. **Schizophrenia** is the term coined originally by Eugene Bleuler in 1911 to describe a collection of illnesses characterized by thought disorders. According to Bleuler, **thought disorders** reflected a break in reality or splitting of the cognitive from the emotional side of one's personality. A schizophrenic individual may exhibit feelings of happiness when recollecting a terrible event or emotional indifference when describing a joyful occasion. Thought disorders are manifested also by incoherent speech, delusions (abnormal beliefs), and hallucinations (imaginary perceptions). These so-called *positive symptoms* (Box 17-1)

Box 17-1

MAJOR SYMPTOMS OF SCHIZOPHRENIA

POSITIVE SYMPTOMS

Hallucinations
- Auditory
- Somatic-tactile
- Visual

Delusions
- Delusions of being controlled
- Delusions of mind reading
- Delusions of reference
- Guilt
- Grandiose
- Persecutory
- Religious
- Somatic
- Thought broadcasting
- Thought insertion
- Thought withdrawal

Positive Formal Thought Disorder
- Circumstantiality
- Derailment
- Distractible speech
- Illogicality
- Incoherence
- Pressure of speech
- Tangentiality

Bizarre Behavior
- Aggressive, agitated
- Clothing, appearance
- Repetitive, stereotyped
- Social, sexual behavior

NEGATIVE SYMPTOMS

Affective Flattening
- Affective nonresponsivity
- Decreased spontaneous movements
- Inappropriate affect
- Lack of vocal inflections
- Paucity of expressive gestures
- Poor eye contact
- Unchanging facial expression

Alogia
- Blocking
- Increase in response latency
- Poverty of speech
- Poverty of speech content

Anhedonia-asociality
- Few recreational interests
- Few social relationships
- Impaired intimacy
- Little sexual interest

Attention
- Social inattentiveness
- Inattentiveness during testing

Avolition-Apathy
- Impaired personal hygiene
- Lack of persistence
- Physical anergia

frequently occur during a **psychotic episode,** when the individual loses touch with reality.

In addition to psychotic episodes, schizophrenic individuals may exhibit blunted affect, apathy, poverty of speech, and lack of social interactions. These characteristics are termed *negative symptoms* (see Box 17-1). Thus schizophrenia is an illness of multiple symptoms often manifested from early adulthood (see Clinical Manifestations). It usually emerges in young adults during their late teens and early twenties, with a slightly earlier onset in males than in females.

Etiology and Pathophysiology

Genetic Predisposition

Genetic epidemiologic studies demonstrate that schizophrenia is a heritable disorder. In monozygotic twins the concordance rate ranges from 30% to 50%. The variable concordance rates may be caused by different diagnostic criteria and methodologic or sampling differences among studies. The concordance rate decreases to 15% in dizygotic twins and siblings. Nevertheless, these rates are considerably higher than the 1% figure found in the general population. Adoption studies further indicate a genetic predisposition to acquire schizophrenia. When adopted into normal families at an early age, children whose biologic parents were schizophrenic are still more likely to acquire the disease than adopted children from normal parents.

Nonetheless, schizophrenia is not a simple genetic disorder. Unlike single-gene Mendelian disorders, where a single locus on the chromosome is clearly linked to the disease, multiple genes located on different chromosomes may be involved in schizophrenia. In addition, as indicated by the 50% concordance rate in monozygotic twins, the genes for schizophrenia have reduced penetrance. That is, an individual may carry the genes for schizophrenia but will not necessarily manifest the illness. Further complicating the search for the genetic bases of schizophrenia is the lack of a consistent set of biologic and phenotypic traits manifested by the illness.

Prenatal and Perinatal Factors

A leading hypothesis for the etiology of schizophrenia suggests that the illness results from neurodevelopmental defects occurring in fetal life. According to this hypothesis, environmental factors interfere with genetically programmed neural development leading to alterations in brain development.[1,2] Several environmental risk factors have been suggested to play a role in the eventual occurrence of schizophrenia. These include exposure to viral infection, prenatal nutritional deficiencies, and perinatal complications.

Viral Infection

The link between a viral infection during pregnancy and the development of schizophrenia was first reported by Mednick and colleagues.[3,4] The results were based on a study of Finnish women exposed to the type A2 influenza virus during the second trimester of pregnancy. Psychiatric diagnosis of their offspring in adulthood indicated a disproportionate increase in schizophrenia. Further, in the Finnish study, women infected with the influenza virus in the first or third trimester produced offspring who were no more likely to be diagnosed with schizophrenia than control subjects. These results support a critical period hypothesis linking viral infection to brain development and schizophrenia. During the second trimester, cortical neurons are developing and rapidly migrating to assume their appropriate position, orientation, and connections. Viral-induced disruption of these neurodevelopmental processes may lead to the structural brain abnormalities observed in schizophrenic individuals.

Subsequent studies examining the prenatal viral hypothesis of schizophrenia have produced a number of inconsistent results.[5] Study differences may stem from unrecognized factors, such as the condition of prenatal nutrition and availability of medication. Conflicting conclusions may arise also from methodologic and statistical differences in the analysis and interpretation of the data.[6]

Nutritional Deficiency

Prenatal nutritional deficiencies increase the risk of neurodevelopmental disorders, such as neural tube defects. In this case, folic acid deficiency during pregnancy is the cause of neural tube defects. The association between prenatal nutritional deficiency and elevated risk of developing schizophrenia was obtained from an examination of records of persons born during the Dutch Hunger Winter of 1944 and 1945.[7] Near the end of World War II, the Nazi blockade of the western Netherlands led to a severe famine that lead to an intake of only 500 and 1000 calories per day. The risk for schizophrenia was determined on the basis of comparing medical records of exposed and unexposed birth cohorts. The study revealed that both males and females conceived at the height of the famine had a twofold increased risk for hospitalized schizophrenia in adulthood. An implication of these results is that appropriate recommendations of specific nutritional supplements during pregnancy may reduce the risk of developing schizophrenia.

Other Developmental Factors

Perinatal complications, such as a difficult delivery at birth and prenatal and perinatal hypoxia, may be associated with increased risk of schizophrenia.[8,9] In the case of hypoxia, some studies point to its effects on altering brain dopamine function. Perinatal complications are associated also with an increased incidence of schizophrenia among individuals born during the winter months. Indeed, one study reported that the risk of schizophrenia was highest during the months of February and March and lowest during August and September.[10]

Neuroanatomic and Functional Abnormalities

Neuroanatomic Alterations

Several structural and functional abnormalities are found in the brain of individuals with schizophrenia.[11,12] Studies using functional brain imaging techniques suggest that no single brain structure is responsible for the pathogenesis of schizophrenia. More likely, dysregulation occurring in a number of different brain regions somehow contributes to the manifestation of the disorder. One prominent brain abnormality is the enlargement of the lateral and third ventricles and widening of fissures and sulci in the frontal cortex (Fig. 17-1). In addition, imaging studies reveal reductions in basal ganglia; thalamus; and temporal lobe, including the amygdala, hippocampus, and parahippocampal gyrus.

Postmortem brain examination of schizophrenic individuals generally supports the brain imaging studies and provides a wealth of evidence consistent with an early neurodevelopmental defect.[1,13] Histologic analyses of the hippocampal formation, which is in the temporal lobe, indicate a marked reduction in dentate granule cell density and a disarray of pyramidal cells in the horn of Ammon. In addition, a significant reduction is found in cell density and volume of the entorhinal cortex, a major subfield of the hippocampal formation receiving diverse cortical information. The reduction in cell size and number probably contributes to the overall decrease in temporal lobe volume. These structural and cellular abnormalities are believed to originate prenatally, most likely during a period of hippocampal cell proliferation and migration. These temporal lobe alterations may be involved in promoting the positive schizophrenic symptoms, such as hallucinations, delusions, thought disorder, and bizarre behavior. Indirect support for this view is based on other work showing that in nonpsychotic individuals, electrical stimulation of the temporal lobe during surgery or temporal lobe epileptic seizures are reported to induce hallucinations and delusions.

Data suggest that the negative symptoms of schizophrenia (i.e., loss of affect, alogia, anhedonia, apathy, cognitive functions) may be the result of pathophysiologic processes occurring in prefrontal cortical regions. This brain area appears to be intricately involved in the initiation and maintenance of goal-directed activities. Individuals with damage to the frontal lobes often exhibit deficits in motivation, emotion,

A

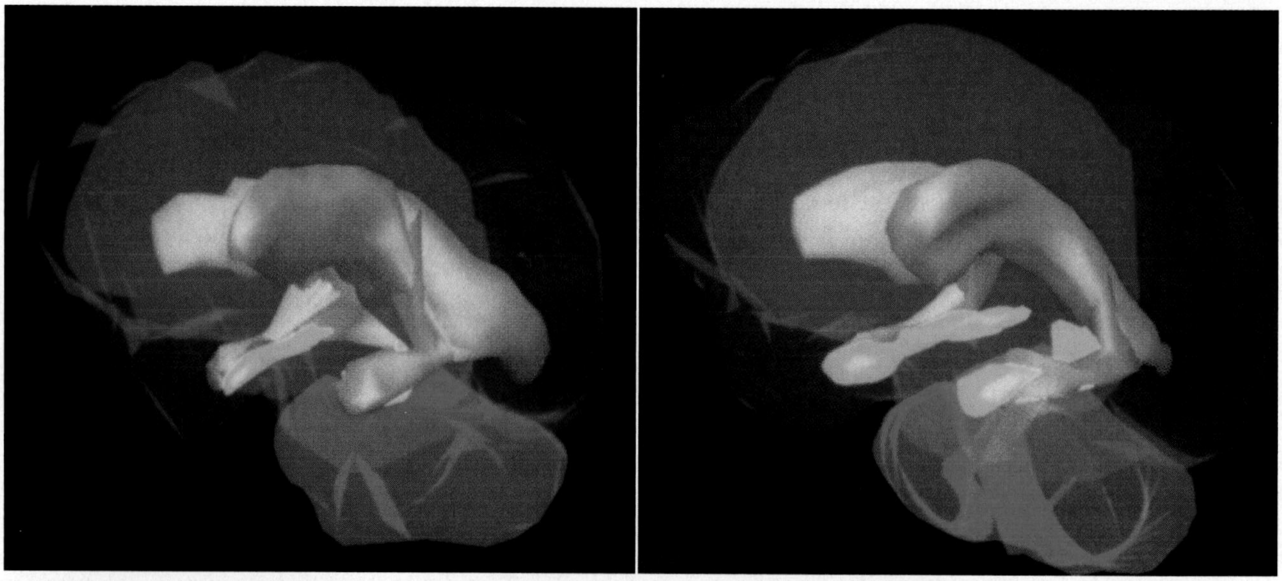

B

FIG. 17-1 Three-dimensional magnetic resonance imaging (MRI) reconstructions showing, A, the cerebroventricles *(gray regions)* and hippocampus *(yellow regions)* of a schizophrenic, and B, a normal individual. Note enlarged cerebroventricles and reduced hippocampal volume of the brain of the schizophrenic individual. (From Gershon ES, Rieder RO: *Sci Am* 267:128, 1992. Original illustrations by Nancy C. Andreason, University of Iowa.)

and organization. One prefrontal region that is extensively studied is the **dorsolateral prefrontal cortex (DLPFC).** This prefrontal region, which corresponds to Brodmann area 9, represents an area actively involved in solving cognitive problems related to **working memory**, which involves the brief storage and use of information. Examples of working memory are mental arithmetic, which involves storing and calculating numbers, as well as solving complex tasks, such as winning a chess match. Working memory is considered to be important also in verbal comprehension and reasoning. During cognitive problem solving, blood flow and metabolism normally increase in the frontal cortex, including the DLPFC. Individuals with schizophrenia, however, often perform poorly on these tests and fail to show an increase in cortical blood flow and metabolism. These studies suggest that the DLPFC is hypoactive in schizophrenia.

Neuropathologic investigations have revealed increased neuronal density in prefrontal area 9 (17%) and occipital cortical area 17 (10%).[14] In addition, cortical thickness is slightly reduced. The lessening in the cortical layer and an increase in neuronal density may be caused by a reduction of neuropil (dendrites and axons). Such a reduction in cortical neuropil could contribute to deficits in cognitive function. Another line of work has shown a reduction in glutamic acid decarboxylase (GAD) messenger ribonucleic acid (mRNA) levels in the DLPFC.[15] GAD is the enzyme responsible for catalyzing the synthesis of **γ-aminobutyric acid (GABA),** the most widespread inhibitory neurotransmitter in the brain. In the DLPFC, approximately 20% to 30% of neurons contain GAD. A reduction in GAD expression may result in reduced GABA production that consequently alters DLPFC cell firing and behavioral patterns.

Neurotransmitter Alterations

Alterations in different neuroanatomic regions may act in concert to compromise neurotransmitter functions, resulting in the onset of schizophrenia. A long-standing neurotransmitter hypothesis of schizophrenia involves dopamine. The **dopamine hypothesis** of schizophrenia suggests that an abnormal elevation in dopaminergic transmission contributes to the onset of schizophrenia. This hypothesis was formulated on the basis of studies indicating that antipsychotic drugs are potent blockers of brain dopamine receptors. A strong positive correlation is found between the clinical potencies of traditional antipsychotic drugs (e.g., chlorpromazine, fluphenazine, and haloperidol) and their affinity for the dopamine D_2 receptor. In addition, drugs that increase dopaminergic transmission— such as levodopa (L-dopa), cocaine, and amphetamine—produce schizophrenic-like psychosis. These drug-induced psychotic states are reversed by dopamine blockers.

Additional evidence revealed that brain concentrations of dopamine or its metabolite, homovanillic acid, were increased in individuals with schizophrenia. Postmortem and neuroimaging studies indicate an increased density of D_2 receptors in brain regions, including the caudate nucleus and nucleus accumbens, especially in individuals manifesting prominent positive symptoms.

The different brain dopamine systems may contribute in various ways to the pathophysiology of schizophrenia (Fig. 17-2). For example, the mesocortical dopamine system plays an essential role in DLPFC functions. Depletion of dopamine in the prefrontal cortex of monkeys produces deficits in cognition and affect. Some investigators report that negative symptoms of schizophrenia may result from decreased dopaminergic transmission in the frontal cortex.[16] This hypodopaminergic transmission in the frontal cortex contrasts with the hypothesized hyperdopaminergic secretion occurring in mesolimbic pathways. The innervation sites of the mesolimbic dopamine system are temporal lobe structures (hippocampal formation and amygdala), as well as the nucleus accumbens and anterior cingulate cortex. Hypersecretion of mesolimbic dopamine pathways may promote the manifestation of positive symptoms.

Although evidence supporting the dopamine hypothesis of schizophrenia is strong, the dysregulation of D_2 receptors cannot account for all aspects of schizophrenia. Whereas the pharmacologic blockade of D_2 receptors occurs rapidly, clinical effects do not appear until after 1 to 2 weeks of treatment. Hence, the antipsychotic effects are not related directly to D_2 blockade or acute suppression of dopamine hypersecretion. D_2-blocking drugs are also clinically ineffective in approximately 20% of persons with schizophrenia. Some of these individuals, however, respond to atypical antipsychotic drugs, such as clozapine, olazapine, and risperidone. These atypical antipsychotic drugs have a higher affinity for the D_4 than the D_2 receptor.[17] In addition, a characteristic of some atypical antipsychotic drugs is their ability to bind to serotonin receptors (5-HT_2).[18] The higher 5-HT_2–D_2 receptor

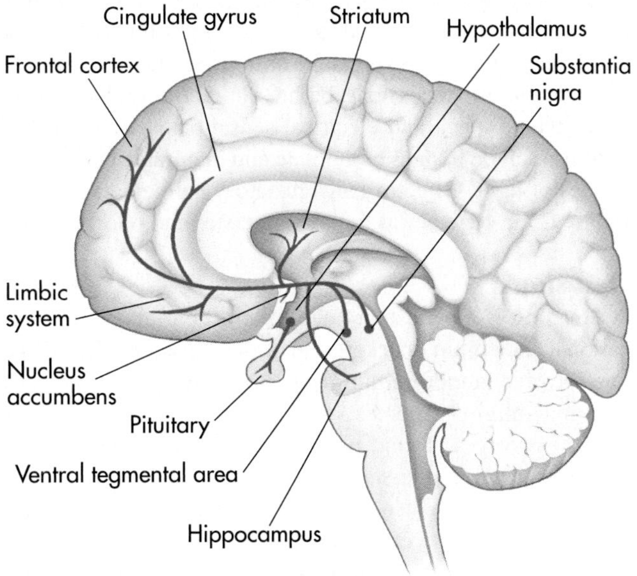

FIG. 17-2 The dopamine system. Dopamine cell bodies are located in the substantia nigra where they project to the stratum (nigrostriatal pathway); and in the ventral tegmental area where they project to the frontal and cingulate cortex (mesocortical pathway), the striatum, the hippocampus and other limbic structures (mesolimbic pathway). Dopamine nuclei are also located in the hypothalamus and project to the pituitary.

binding ratio in comparison with conventional antipsychotic drugs may reflect a normalization of serotonin-dopamine interactions leading to clinical efficacy.

Another neurotransmitter system that may be involved in schizophrenia is glutamate and its actions on the N-methyl-D-aspartate (NMDA) receptor subtype.[16] NMDA antagonists, such as the cyclohexylamine anesthetics phencyclidine (PCP) and ketamine, induce schizophrenic-like symptoms in healthy subjects and exacerbate symptoms in schizophrenic individuals. In schizophrenia, glutamate concentrations in the cerebrospinal fluid (CSF) are reduced along with a reduction in cortical glutamate synthesis. Collectively, these data have led to the hypothesis that NMDA receptor hypofunction occurs in schizophrenia. It should be noted that glutamateric neurotransmission is tightly coupled with GABAergic neurotransmission. As indicated earlier, there is a loss of GABA production in the brain of schizophrenic individuals that could have pathophysiologic consequences for NMDA receptor actions.

Clinical Manifestations

Although there is a tradition to make a distinction between positive and negative symptoms (see Box 17-1) of schizophrenia, current research interests focus on three symptom dimensions. The three core groupings include: (1) psychotic symptoms, such as hallucinations and delusions; (2) disorganized symptoms that include thought disorder and bizarre or inappropriate behavior; and (3) negative symptoms.

Hallucinations

A **hallucination** is a perception experienced without external stimulation of the sense organs. Schizophrenic individuals often experience a variety of sensory hallucinations, including auditory, tactile, visual, gustatory, and olfactory. These hallucinations may appear alone or together. During auditory hallucinations, voices may be heard. Tactile hallucinations may involve touch and electrical sensations. Visual hallucinations include images of animate and inanimate objects and flashes of light. Olfactory and gustatory hallucinations commonly occur together as unpleasant tastes and odors.

Delusions

A **delusion** is a persistent belief that is contrary to the educational and cultural background of the individual. Delusions may involve grandiose, nihilistic, persecutory, somatic, sexual, and religious themes. A common delusion in schizophrenia revolves around paranoid beliefs that may involve spying, conspiracy, persecution, and ridicule. Delusions may also be referential in nature. Referential delusions involve the perception that certain stimuli or events are highly personalized or directed specifically at them. For example, schizophrenic individuals may believe that information provided by a television talk show host is directed at them.

Disorganized Behavior

Disorganized Speech

A common form of disorganized speech is **formal thought disorder,** which involves fluent speech that is difficult to comprehend. The speech is often incoherent as the individual moves from one topic to another unexpectedly (loose associations). Answers to questions are illogical or unrelated, and the person becomes easily distracted when talking.

Another form of disorganized speech is referred to as **poverty of content**. Here the use of vocabularies to convey information is severely retarded despite a fair amount of spoken words. For instance, the same phrases may be used repeatedly throughout a conversation.

Disorganized Behavior

This type of behavior is the conceptual equivalent of disorganized speech. The schizophrenic individual has difficult engaging in goal-directed activities. Behavior may be repetitive (e.g., stereotyped rocking) or aimless in nature and personal hygiene is poorly maintained. Another aspect of disorganized behavior is the manifestation of inappropriate situational affect as exemplified by hostility without provocation or, at the opposite end, childlike silliness in sober situations.

Negative Symptoms

Negative symptoms reflect a diminution or deficit in normal functioning. These symptoms are disabling and include affective flattening, anhedonia, alogia (poverty of speech) and avolition. There is a near absence of emotional or facial expression in **affective flattening**. The same fixed expression is maintained throughout a conversation or in different situations. Individuals with **anhedonia** symptoms are unable to have emotional experiences. They may be unable to experience pleasure or pain and report a sense of detachment from the environment. **Alogia** is the absence of spontaneous speech. Few, if any, words are used to answer questions or to express themselves. Hence, there is an overall reduction in speech production. **Avolition** refers to a deficit in spontaneous or goal-directed activities. An individual may sit tirelessly for prolonged periods of time and must be prodded into completing simple daily tasks.

Treatment

Antipsychotic medications have been used for nearly 50 years to reduce some of the symptoms of schizophrenia. In general, individuals with psychotic symptoms (e.g., hallucinations and delusions) and thought disorder respond to traditional and atypical antipsychotic drugs. However, only 5% to 10% of schizophrenic individuals will be completely relieved of their symptoms. The majority will require long-term maintenance therapy, but the long-term benefits of antipsychotic medication are not always promising. Relapse rates of individuals on maintenance therapy are between 30% and 50%. In addition, side effects that include sedation, weight gain, and extrapyramidal symptoms, such as muscle rigidity, akathesia (motor restlessness), and tremors may complicate long-term maintenance therapy. Tardive dyskinesia, a potentially irreversible movement disorder associated with traditional or convention antipsychotic drugs (e.g., chlorpromazine), is now generally diminished or absent following treatment with new atypical antipsychotics.

Individuals with a high incidence of negative symptoms are likely to have a family history of schizophrenia or neuroanatomic abnormalities, and they may deteriorate progressively. Approximately 10% to 20% of individuals with predominant negative symptoms respond poorly to traditional antipsychotic drugs. These individuals who appear to be refractory to treatment may respond positively to atypical antipsychotic drugs.

In conjunction with pharmacotherapy, psychosocial therapy can facilitate the management of persons with schizophrenia. Psychosocial relationships may assist the individual in developing coping strategies and in identifying stressors and relapse symptoms. In some cases the addition of cognitive behavioral therapy (CBT) may alleviate some of the schizophrenic symptoms that are resistant to medication.[19] One important benefit of psychosocial and family support is the encouragement of compliance with antipsychotic medication, which may require a period of weeks before efficacy occurs.

MOOD DISORDERS: DEPRESSION AND MANIA

Mood refers to a sustained emotional state as opposed to brief emotional feelings, which are termed *affective states.* Normal individuals are capable of experiencing a variety of affective states that include euphoria, joy, surprise, fear, anxiety, sadness, and depression. When emotional states, such as euphoria (mania) and depression, are maintained and become predominant, the individual may be diagnosed with a mood disorder.

Box 17-2 presents the major symptoms of depression and mania. **Major (unipolar) depression** is the most common mood disorder. The lifetime prevalence rate for depression ranges from 8% to 20% of the population. Individuals with major depression experience an unpleasant mood. They are unable to experience pleasure and show a loss of outside interest. When depression becomes too intense and unremitting, individuals may commit suicide. Although depression appears to occur in all age-groups, it may not be diagnosed readily in young children. Females have a twofold greater probability of experiencing a major depression during their lifetime than males.

Approximately 25% of individuals with major depression eventually will experience a manic episode. Individuals experiencing recurrent patterns of depression and mania have a condition called **bipolar disorder** (also known as manic-depression illness) as opposed to *unipolar disorder,* which involves only depression. Bipolar disorder is less common than unipolar depression. It usually emerges in young adulthood and occurs somewhat more frequently in females than in males. In some bipolar individuals, moods alternate rapidly from one to another.

Etiology and Pathophysiology

Genetic Predisposition

A strong genetic basis exists for the development of mood disorders. Monozygotic twin studies reveal concordance rates of 50% to 80% (either bipolar or major depression). Among fraternal twins and first-degree relatives, the rates are approximately 24%. Even among adoptees with a biologic family history of mood disorders, the incidence of having a major depression or bipolar disorder is higher than in control adoptees. The strong tendency for mood disorders to run in families has encouraged a search for the abnormal gene or genes. Some promising molecular genetic findings suggest that regions on chromosomes 18 and 21 may be linked to bipolar disorders.[20]

Nongenetic environmental factors, such as psychosocial stressors, are hypothesized to play an important role in depression. In particular, the first episode of major depression appears to be precipitated by psychosocial stress.[21] The trend toward an earlier onset of depression also is attributed to the greater incidence of stress occurring over the past several decades.

Neurochemical Dysregulation

Individuals with mood disorders respond well to pharmacotherapy. Effective antidepressants, such as monoamine oxidase inhibitors (MAOIs), tricyclic antidepressants (TCAs), and selective serotonin reuptake inhibitors (SSRIs), share the pharmacologic property of increasing the level of **monoamines** (norepinephrine and serotonin), albeit through different mechanisms. In contrast, drugs (e.g., reserpine) that deplete monoamines produce depression. These results are the basis for the monoamine hypothesis, which states that depression occurs following a deficit in brain norepinephrine or serotonin, whereas mania results from elevated concentrations of monoamines (Fig. 17-3).

Further support for the monoamine hypothesis of depression came from an examination of norepinephrine and serotonin metabolites in depressed individuals. The major metabolites of norepinephrine (3-methoxy-4-hydroxyphenylethyleneglycol [MHPG]) and serotonin (5-hydroxyindoleacetic acid [5-HIAA]) were reduced in the cerebrospinal

Box 17-2

MAJOR SYMPTOMS OF DEPRESSION AND MANIA

SYMPTOMS OF DEPRESSION	SYMPTOMS OF MANIA
Depressed mood	Elevated mood
Loss of interests and pleasure	Irritability
Irritability	Inflated self-esteem or grandiosity
Sadness	Decreased need for sleep
Decrease or increase in appetite	Flight of ideas
Insomnia	Excessive talking
Psychomotor agitation or retardation	Pressured speech
Fatigue	Distractibility
Feelings of worthlessness	Increased physical activities
Excessive guilt	Increased pleasurable activities
Poor concentration	Psychomotor agitation
Suicide thoughts	

Data from American Psychiatric Association: *Diagnostic and statistical manual of mental disorders,* ed 4, Washington, DC, 1994, The Association.

fluid of depressed individuals. Other work demonstrated that rapid dietary depletion of tryptophan, the precursor of serotonin synthesis, produced a rapid return to depression in individuals with successful antidepressant treatment.[2] Thus the availability of brain monoamines appears to be considerably reduced in persons with major depression.

The monoamine hypothesis of depression, however, fails to account for the acute biochemical properties of antidepressant drugs and their therapeutic effects. TCAs and SSRIs rapidly block the reuptake, resulting in an immediate elevation in released monoamines. However, the clinical effects of antidepressants do not occur until several weeks of treatment. Further, TCAs and SSRIs vary widely in their ability to block reuptake of monoamines, but they are equally effective over time in the treatment of depression. Increasing knowledge on the diversity of neurotransmitter receptor subtypes, their presynaptic and postsynaptic functions, their responses to antidepressant medications, and their interactions with other neurotransmitter systems should provide future insights into the pathophysiology of depression.

Neuroendocrine Dysregulation

Hypothalamic-pituitary-adrenal (HPA) system abnormalities exist in a large percentage of individuals (30% to 70%) with major depression. HPA system abnormalities are demonstrated in the dexamethasone suppression test. Normally, administration of dexamethasone, a potent synthetic glucocorticoid, suppresses adrenal cortisol secretion because of its negative-feedback effects on the HPA system. However, some individuals with depression exhibit hypersecretion of cortisol and fail to suppress cortisol secretion after dexamethasone administration. In addition, whereas normal individuals typically exhibit a diurnal rise in cortisol secretion at the onset of wakefulness followed by a trough 12 hours later, depressed people continue to exhibit elevated levels of plasma cortisol throughout the evening and early morning hours. It is notable that normalization of the HPA system occurring after antidepressant medication is associated with good treatment response, whereas a persistent dysregulation, such as the failure to suppress plasma cortisol with dexamethasone, is sometimes related to continued depression or relapse.

The search to uncover the basis of this hypercortisolemia in depressed people has led investigators to focus on corticotropin-releasing factor (CRF), a neuropeptide that is released by hypothalamic nerve endings in the median eminence and is the predominant regulator of pituitary adrenocorticotropin (ACTH) secretion (see Chapter 9). Studies indicate that CRF concentrations generally are elevated in

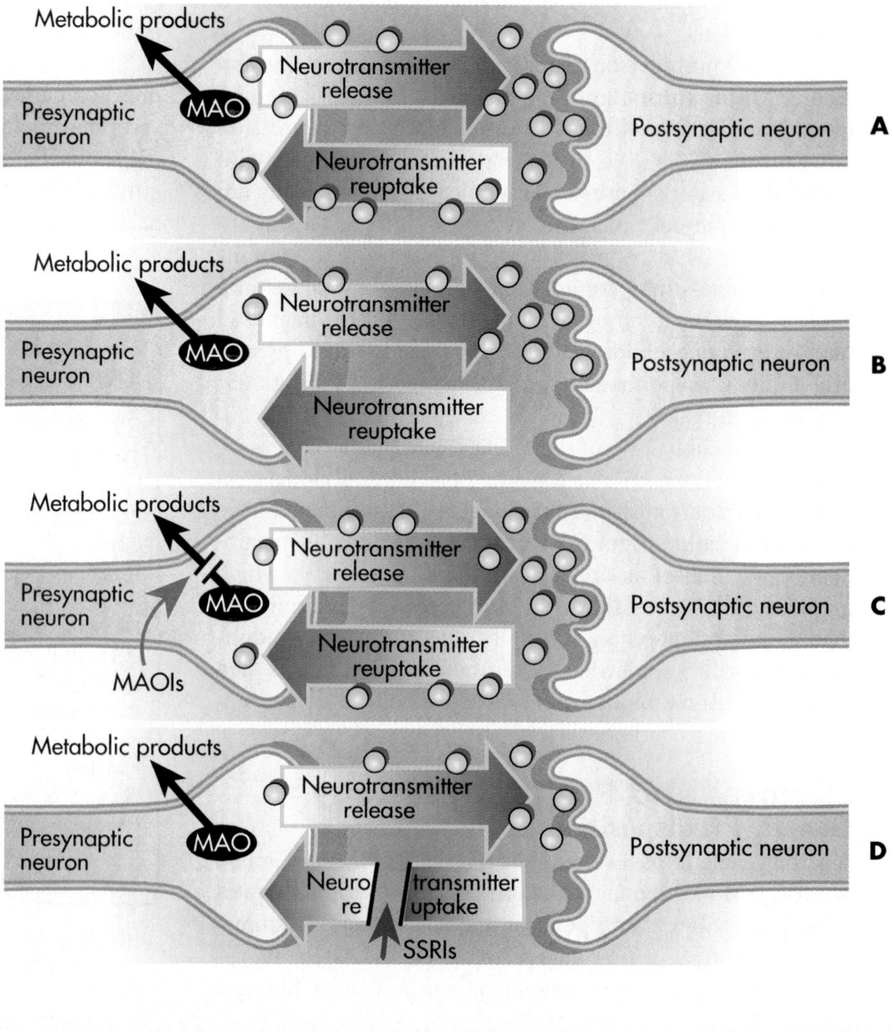

FIG. 17-3 Schematic diagrams showing the sites of actions of antidepressants and their effects on neurotransmitter levels. A, In normal individuals an action potential generated in the presynaptic neuron results in neurotransmitter release into the synapse. Some neurotransmitters bind to receptors on the postsynaptic neuron that leads to activation of second messenger systems (not shown). Neurotransmitters are also removed from the synapse by reuptake into the presynaptic neuron and deanimated by monoamine oxidase (MAO). **B,** In depressed individuals, neurotransmitter levels are hypothesized to be reduced. The mechanisms responsible for this reduction are not understood. **C,** Monoamine oxidase inhibitors (MAOIs) act by preventing the degradation of neurotransmitters, such as norepinephrine and serotonin. As a result, neurotransmitter levels are elevated. MAOIs used in the treatment of depression include phenelzine and tranylcypromine. **D,** The tricyclic antidepressants (TCAs) and selective serotonin reuptake inhibitors (SSRIs) act by reducing the uptake of neurotransmitters from the synapse, leading to increased neurotransmitter levels. Thus TCAs, such as nortriptyline and esipramine, tend to block norepinephrine reuptake, whereas amitriptyline and imipramine also have effects on serotonin reuptake. SSRIs, such as fluoxetine and sertraline, are highly effective in blocking serotonin reuptake.

depression (Fig. 17-4). Further, when some individuals are administered exogenous CRF, they exhibit a decreased ACTH response and decreased CRF receptor concentrations are found in the frontal cortex of depressed suicide individuals. These results suggest that prolonged elevations in CRF secretion, as indicated by elevated CRF levels in the CSF, may downregulate CRF receptors located in both the pituitary and brain. Whether dysregulation of CRF secretion is a primary contributing factor to depression, however, has yet to be determined. CRF activity is neurochemically regulated, and dysfunction of neurotransmitter systems, such as norepinephrine on serotonin, may have a more fundamental role in the pathophysiology of depression.

Individuals with hypothyroidism manifest features that are similar to depression, including depressed mood and cognitive impairments. Furthermore, approximately 20% to 30% of persons with depression have evidence of a dysregulated thyroid system. In addition to some reports of elevated CSF levels in thyrotropin-releasing hormone (TRH), these euthyroid depressed individuals show a blunted thyrotropin (TSH) response to administration of TRH and lack the nocturnal rise in TSH that normally occurs between midnight and the early morning hours.[22] Persistent blunting of the TSH response to TRH is associated with an increased probability of relapse.

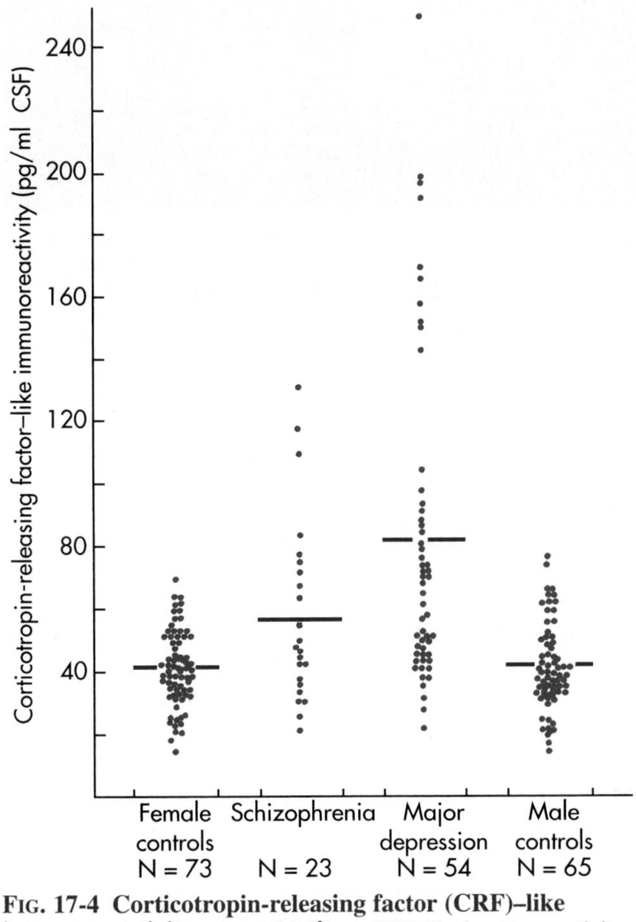

FIG. 17-4 Corticotropin-releasing factor (CRF)–like immunoreactivity concentrations. CRF-like immunoreactivity concentrations in cerebrospinal fluid of female neurologic controls, schizophrenic individuals, depressed individuals, and male neurologic controls. Mean CRF concentrations were elevated significantly in individuals with major depression compared with control and schizophrenic groups. (Redrawn from Banki CM et al: CSF corticotropin-releasing factor-like immunoreactivity in depression ands schizophrenia, *Am J Psychiatry* 144:873, 1987.)

Neuroanatomic and Functional Abnormalities

The dorsal and medial raphe nucleus, located in the central gray of the caudal mesencephalon and rostral pons, contains a large group of serotonin-synthesizing neurons (Fig. 17-5). Postmortem studies of the brain serotonergic system in depressed and suicide victims suggest that cortical serotonin receptor (5-HT_{1A} and 5-HT_{2A}) binding is increased along with possible decreases in serotonin transporter binding. The functional significance of these changes, however, is presently unclear.

Similarly, norepinephrine receptor alterations (β-adrenergic receptor subtypes, α-adrenergic receptors) in the frontal cortex are reported in some suicides with major depression. A particularly interesting preliminary finding is that a reduction in neuron number was found in the rostral locus caeruleus of suicide victims. A reduction in the number of norepinephrine cell bodies has implications for altered functional modulation of all brain regions innervated by locus caeruleus neurons (Fig. 17-6).

In addition to postmortem morphometric studies, modern brain imaging techniques are beginning to reveal a host of structural and functional abnormalities associated with mood disorders. For example, there are reports of reduced frontal lobe volume in depressed individuals and decreased or asymmetric temporal lobe volume in subjects with bipolar illness or depression. In some cases, specific brain abnormalities are

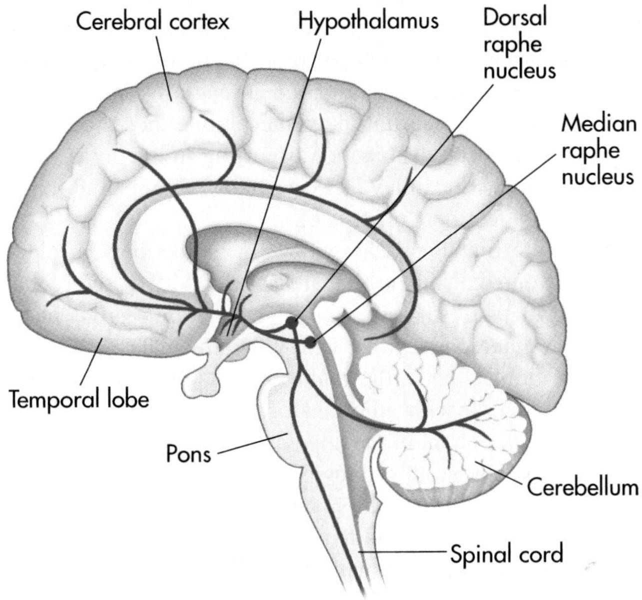

FIG. 17-5 The serotonin system. Serotonin neurons are located in the brain stem raphe nuclei. They project diffusely to all regions of the cortex, temporolimbic regions, the hypothalamus, the basal ganglia, the cerebellum, the brain stem, and the spinal cord.

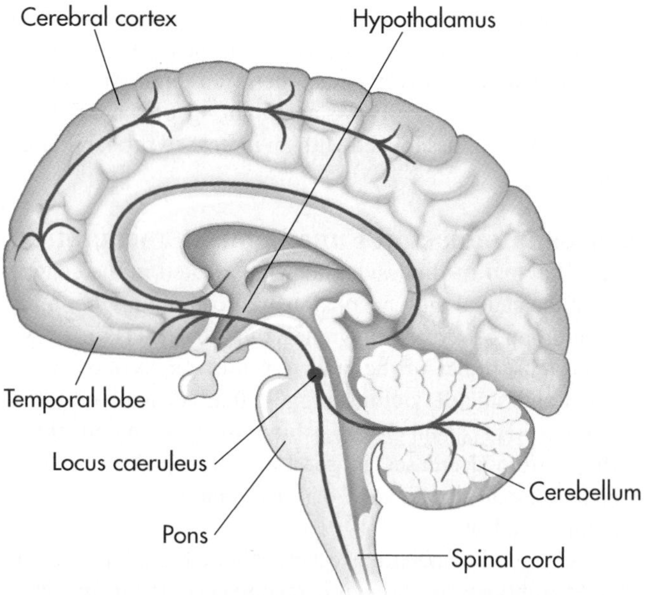

FIG. 17-6 The norepinephrine system. Norepinephrine cell bodies are located in the locus caeruleus, which are situated in the pons. The cell bodies send projections throughout the brain, including the cerebral cortex, temporolimbic regions, the hypothalamus, the midbrain, the cerebellum, the brain stem, and the spinal cord.

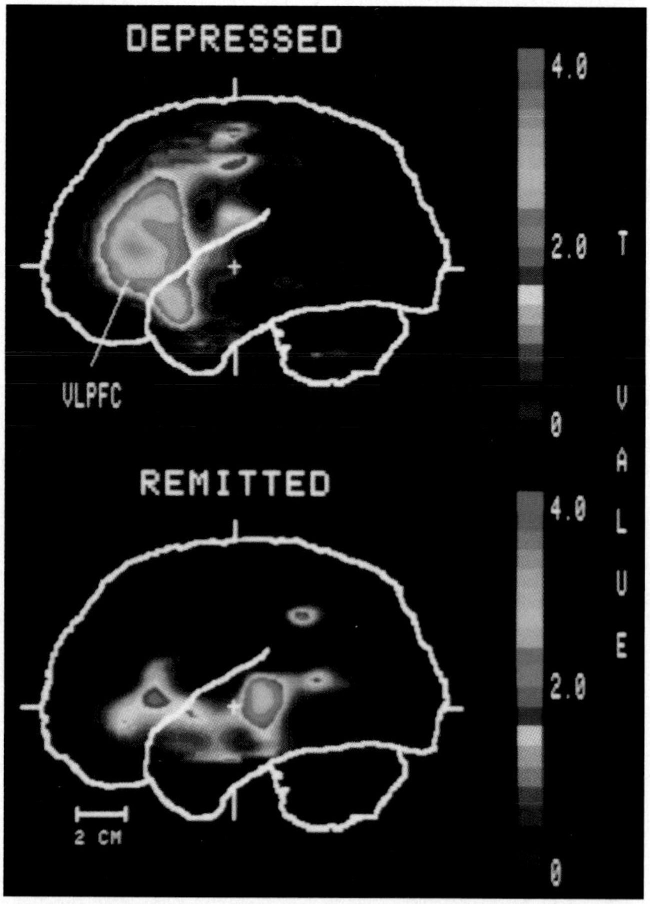

FIG. 17-7 Positron emission tomography (PET) scan showing increased activity in the left prefrontal cortex in a depressed person but not in the remitted person. *VLPFC,* Ventrolateral prefrontal cortex. (From Drevets WC et al: *J Neurosci* 12:3628, 1992. Copyright ©1992 by the Society for Neuroscience.)

associated with a subtype of depressive illness. For instance, there is strong support of enlarged lateral ventricles in late onset or elderly unipolar depression. Similar ventricular enlargements are not present in mid-life depressives, elderly depressives with an early age of illness, or bipolar individuals.

Results of functional imaging studies extend the findings of structural brain abnormalities.[23] In the dorsal lateral and dorsal medial prefrontal cortex, cerebral blood flow and glucose metabolism is reduced in individuals with unipolar and bipolar depression. These abnormalities may be responsible for some of the neuropsychologic impairments occurring during depression. The dorsal lateral abnormalities in depression may be related to retardation in cognitive processing and deficits in speech not altogether unlike those found in schizophrenia. The dysfunction occurring in the dorsal medial prefrontal cortex may be associated with impaired mnemonic and attentional processing.

Other prefrontal cortical regions, including the ventrolateral, ventromedial, and orbital areas, exhibit increased blood flow and metabolism (Fig. 17-7). These brain regions have extensive interconnections with the amygdala, a limbic structure implicated in the evaluation and coupling of sensory information with emotions or affect. Increased blood flow and metabolism in the amygdala of depressed individuals are also observed, and there appears to be a positive relationship between right amygdala metabolic rate and negative affect in depressed individuals.[24] Dysregulation of the amygdala in conjunction with the prefrontal connecting regions may alter the ability of individuals to respond appropriately to stimuli, resulting in a prolonged depressed state. Finally, studies indicate that this increased amygdala activity is reduced along with prefrontal cortical activity to levels that approach normal metabolism and blood flow during antidepressant treatment.

Clinical Manifestations

Depression

Depression is characterized by unremitting feelings of sadness and despair.[25] The **dysphoric** or intensely painful **mood** is accompanied frequently by insomnia, loss of appetite and body weight, and reduced interest in sex. Interest or pleasure in activities decreases dramatically. Sleep disturbances take several forms, including difficulty in initially falling asleep, awakening in the middle of the night and falling asleep after several hours, and early morning wakefulness with an inability to subsequently fall asleep. Individuals also may have reduced motor activity accompanied by marked fatigue. Others may complain of restlessness and agitation. Feelings of worthlessness and guilt are common in depression. The ability to function (e.g., work) and concentrate is greatly diminished. Thoughts of suicide and the risk of suicide are elevated in depressed individuals. Some severely depressed people have psychotic experiences such as hallucinations and delusions. The symptoms of major depression are summarized in Box 17-2. According to DSM-IV,[2] major depression is defined as the occurrence of five or more of these symptoms during a 2-week period in which at least one of the symptoms includes depressed mood or loss of interest or pleasure.

Mania

Manic individuals experience elevated levels of euphoria.[25] Self-esteem is elevated. Feelings of grandiosity are abnormally elevated and may result in psychoses such as delusions and hallucinations. Energy and activity levels are greatly enhanced even after only a few hours of sleep each night. Restlessness and irritability occur frequently in mania. The increased energy, however, does not lead to well-organized plans and thoughts. The individual shows poor judgment in spending money, may become hypersexual, and may make poor business commitments. Other hallmarks of mania are excessive, rapid, loud, and pressured speech. The manic person frequently skips from one topic of conversation to another. In addition, manic individuals are easily distracted both when speaking and when performing tasks. The DSM-VI diagnostic criteria for manic episodes is a period lasting at least 1 week in which the individual experiences an abnormal and persistently elevated, expansive, or irritable mood. During this period, at least three (four if the mood is only irritable) of the manic symptoms listed in Box 17-2 are exhibited.

Treatment

Depression

MAOIs, TCAs, and SSRIs are used in the treatment of depression (see Fig. 17-3). In addition, there are atypical antidepressants, such as nefazodone, trazodone, and mirtazapine, that presumably produce their clinical effects by blocking specific receptors (e.g., $5HT_{2A}$). Initial selection of an antidepressant is based on several considerations, including the person's symptoms, side effects, safety, cost, and convenience. For example, medications that produce sedation may be helpful in treating those with sleep disturbances. Approximately 50% of depressed individuals may not have a favorable response during initial treatment to an antidepressant drug and 10% to 20% of depressed persons may continue to exhibit symptoms after 2 years. Individuals who do not respond to a specific antidepressant within 2 months may be given another antidepressant medication. At present, however, there are no criteria that indicate whether selection of the next antidepressant drug will be efficacious.

A number of side effects are reported with use of antidepressant medications. Commonly reported side effects of MAOIs include sedation or agitation, insomnia, dry mouth, impotence, and weight gain. MAOIs may also induce acute and heightened elevations in blood pressure (e.g., hypertensive crisis) after intake of tyramine-rich foods, such as aged cheeses, sour cream, pods of broad beans, pickled herring, liver, canned figs, raisins, and avocados. In addition, MAOI interactions with TCAs, SSRIs, stimulants, and over-the-counter flu medications are dangerous and should be avoided. Due to these adverse side effect issues, MAOIs are used less frequently that other antidepressant medications.

TCAs may produce sedation, orthostatic hypotension, and weight gain. In addition, some TCAs have moderate anticholinergic side effects, including constipation, urinary hesitancy or retention, dry mouth, blurred vision, and memory impairment. These side effects may be an issue when considering TCA treatment of the elderly. In this case the TCAs desipramine and nortriptyline may be preferred due to their reduced anticholinergic, cardiovascular, and sedative effects.

The most common side effects of SSRIs include sleep disturbances (e.g., insomnia) and nausea. However, agitation, allergic skin reactions, dry mouth, anxiety, altered appetite, and sexual dysfunction have been reported. Unlike MAOIs and TCAs, SSRIs do not appear to have pronounced effects on the cardiovascular or cholinergic systems. A consideration in the selection of SSRIs is whether the individual is taking other psychiatric medications. SSRIs are potent inhibitors of cytochrome P-450 isoenzymes that are involved in drug metabolism. For instance, paroxetine and, to a lesser extent, fluoxetine and norfluoxetine are potent inhibitors of hepatic isozyme CYP2D6, which may then lead to dangerous elevations in blood concentrations of some TCAs and antipsychotic drugs. In addition, SSRIs should not be taken with MAOIs or immediately after discontinuing MAOI treatment. A serotonin syndrome characterized by excitement or autonomic hyperactivity, abdominal pain, rigidity, and hyperthermia may develop that can led to coma or death.

Electroconvulsive therapy (ECT) is used when individuals fail to respond to antidepressants or when they are severely depressed, pregnant, suicidal, or psychotic. ECT is effective in alleviating depressive symptoms in about 50% to 80% of people. Individuals may respond to antidepressant medication after ECT. Although the mechanism of action of ECT is not clear, the procedure is known to produce alterations in monoamine systems.

Recently there has been much interest in using transcranial magnetic stimulation (TMS) of the brain as a treatment for depression.[26,27] TMS is used in neurology for enhancing motor movements by direct magnetic stimulation of the motor cortex. For example, TMS treatment facilitates motor responses and response speed in individuals with Parkinson disease. A few studies have now reported that daily exposure to TMS over the left prefrontal cortex was effective in improving mood in individuals with unipolar and bipolar depression. The basis underlying the improvement in mood is not known but preclinical studies suggest that TMS produces neurochemical changes similar to those of ECT.

Mania

Individuals with bipolar disorder are treated with lithium or other mood stabilizers (e.g., carbamazepine or valproic acid) when the individual does not respond to lithium treatment. The full clinical effects of lithium usually require about 1 week of treatment. As in depression, ECT is administered if individuals with a manic episode do not respond to medication, are pregnant, or have cardiovascular disease.

Frequently reported side effects of lithium treatment include increased thirst, tremors, diarrhea, and weight gain. These side effects diminish over time. One potentially serious side effect of lithium treatment is lithium toxicity. Lithium normally is removed by the kidneys. However, when the body is sodium depleted, the kidneys will reabsorb sodium along with lithium. Individuals receiving lithium treatment are advised to avoid physically demanding exercises that dehydrate the body and to seek medical attention during fever or other conditions that may increase sweating.

Newer treatments for mania include the use of anticonvulsants gabapentin and lamotrigine.[28] Gabapentin is relatively safe, well tolerated, and excreted by the kidneys. Lamotrigine is metabolized by the liver and must be titrated over a period of 2 to 4 weeks because of adverse effects, including dizziness, headaches, somnolence, double vision, and rash.

In addition to pharmacotherapy, psychotherapy may be beneficial to individuals who have difficulty dealing with psychosocial stressors, such as self-esteem, legal problems, fear of recurrence, and interpersonal conflicts affecting the family. Treatment involves a combination of making the individual aware of the bipolar disorder and its treatment, coping with psychosocial stressors, facilitating drug compliance, and monitoring symptom recurrences.

ANXIETY DISORDERS

Fear and anxiety normally arise in threatening or harmful situations. The symptoms may include arousal, tenseness, and increased autonomic activity such as heart rate, blood pressure, and respiration. In addition, individuals tend to engage in protective behavioral responses such as flight and avoidance. These physiologic and behavioral responses are common emotions that reflect individuals' evolutionary heritage. Their expression has allowed humans to adapt and cope under a variety of adverse conditions. However, when these emotions become so intense or are expressed so inappropriately that they undermine the ability to function on a daily basis, anxiety becomes pathologic. Anxiety disorders, which occur in approximately 10% to 30% of the population, can take several forms. This section presents an overview of panic disorder, generalized anxiety disorder, and posttraumatic stress disorder (PTSD).

Panic Disorder

Panic disorder is a well-studied psychiatric condition that consists of multiple disabling panic attacks. Approximately 2% to 3% of women and 0.5% to 1.5% of men have panic disorder. Between panic attacks the individual spends an excessive amount of time worrying about when the next panic attack will occur. These panic attacks are characterized by intense autonomic arousal involving a wide variety of symptoms, including light-headedness, a racing heart, difficult breathing, chest discomfort, generalized sweating, general weakness, trembling, abdominal distress, and chills or hot flashes. In addition, the individual may experience the fear of losing control or dying. The symptoms originally occur spontaneously and vary in length from several minutes to an hour. If they continue for prolonged periods, they can be disabling.

A notable complication in panic disorder is the development of **agoraphobia** or phobic avoidance of places or situations from which escape for help may not be available. For example, the agoraphobic individual will avoid being away from home; standing in line or in a crowd; or riding a train, plane, or automobile. Severe agoraphobia leads to housebound individuals.

Etiology and Pathophysiology

Genetic factors appear to play a large role in panic disorder. The risk of suffering from panic disorder is nearly 20% among relatives of individuals with panic disorder. In contrast, the risk decreases to approximately 2% to 6% among individuals without a family history of panic disorder.

Neuroanatomic and Functional Abnormalities

Although the etiology of panic attacks is not well understood, some factors may be acting on vulnerable brain stem regions to provoke panic attacks. For example, physiologic functions and metabolic demands occurring in the periphery are regulated closely by cells in the brain stem. Information from the cardiovascular and respiratory systems is eventually relayed to the brain stem, resulting in activation of central autonomic pathways. Fearful perceptions and thoughts emanating from the cerebral cortex may contribute by further activating neural circuits in the temporal lobe and brain stem, which may ultimately potentiate the production of panic symptoms. Some individuals are more likely to experience panic attacks after exposure to stress associated with losses (death of loved ones, divorce) or certain situations (near-fatal accidents, trapped in a highly confined place).

Brain regions that may be involved in a panic attack include the locus caeruleus and structures in the temporal lobe (hippocampus and amygdala).[29] The locus caeruleus is located at the pons and contains norepinephrine cell bodies that are responsible for innervating all regions of the forebrain (see Fig. 17-6). Both the hippocampus and the locus caeruleus monitor internal and external signals and show increased activity when aroused. The locus caeruleus is sensitive to changes occurring in the periphery, such as those

WHAT'S NEW? Decreased $GABA_A$–Benzodiazepine Receptor Binding in Panic Disorder

Positron emission tomography (PET), a brain imaging technique, was used to measure $GABA_A$–BZ receptors in the brain of medication-free persons with panic disorder and healthy volunteers. A major reduction in BZ binding was found throughout the brain, especially in the orbitofrontal cortex and insula, which are brain regions associated with anxiety. These results suggest that a reduction in brain $GABA_A$–BZ receptor binding may be an important contributing factor in the pathophysiology of panic disorder.

Data from Malizia AL et al: Decreased brain $GABA_A$–benzodiazepine receptor binding in panic disorder, *Arch Gen Psychiatry* 55:715, 1998.

involving the respiratory and cardiovascular systems. Abnormal hyperactivity of locus caeruleus neurons in response to peripheral autonomic signals may contribute to the onset of panic attacks.

Panic disorder also may involve the brain's GABA–benzodiazepine (BZ) receptor system. BZ receptor sites occur in close proximity to $GABA_A$ receptors. BZ acts by increasing the response in the $GABA_A$ ion channel to GABA, thereby leading to increased chloride ion influx and inhibitory neuronal effects on brain neurotransmitter systems. Of particular relevance to panic disorder, recent brain imaging work revealed a global reduction in brain BZ-binding, which suggests that alterations in inhibitory neuromodulation may contribute to the disorder.[30]

Individuals with panic disorder respond to some pharmacologic agents differently than individuals without panic disorder. That is, administration of panicogenic agents is capable of producing panic attacks only in panic-prone people. In these studies the physical symptoms of panic attacks are reproduced, albeit to only a certain degree, by inhalation of carbon dioxide, yohimbine, caffeine ingestion, sodium lactate, cholecystokinin, and norepinephrine administration. These agents are believed to either directly or indirectly activate the locus caeruleus noradrenergic system,[2] thereby contributing to the production of panic.

Treatment

Panic disorder is highly treatable. Up to 80% of individuals with panic disorder will respond appropriately to cognitive behavioral therapy (CBT) and antidepressant medication, either separately or in combination. During CBT the individual learns that the physical symptoms are not fatal. In addition, he or she learns to control the intensity of anxiety and panic. For example, breathing exercises to control hyperventilation serve to lessen the intense physiologic symptoms of panic, such as elevated heart and respiration rates. Another benefit of CBT is that the individual may become more aware of the benefits and risks of drug medications where the degree of compliance is a critical factor in effective treatment. For some individuals, especially those with no or mild agoraphobia, CBT alone may be effective in the treatment of panic disorder.

Although there are no clinical predicators of drug treatment outcome, antidepressants, such as TCAs and SSRIs, are considered first-line medications for panic disorder with a somewhat superior antipanic efficacy of SSRIs over TCAs. Among the SSRIs, paroxetine and setraline have received FDA indication specifically for panic disorder. Safety and side effect issues of SSRIs and TCAs that apply to mood disorders are also relevant for panic disorders. MAOIs are not used frequently due to their potential adverse effects.

BZs such as alprazolam and clonazepam are another means of treatment for panic disorder; their efficacy may be related in part to their inhibitory effects on locus caeruleus neuronal activity. These drugs are also used as an adjunct or augmentation therapy for individuals that are not fully responsive to SSRIs or TCAs. Short-term side effects of BZ treatment include sedation, ataxia, and cognitive impairment. Some of these side effects, such as sedation, are tolerated with continued use. A potential complication of long-term BZ treatment, however, is physiologic and psychologic dependence. Abrupt BZ withdrawal may produce a withdrawal syndrome, as indicated by symptoms that include heightened reemergence or rebound of anxiety, insomnia, photophobia, and diarrhea. These symptoms may be lessened with gradual tapering off of treatment. Individuals taking BZs may benefit from CBT, which could reduce their reliance on these drugs.

Generalized Anxiety Disorder

Excessive and persistent worries are the hallmarks of **generalized anxiety disorder (GAD).** In the general population the lifetime prevalence rates of GAD range from 4.1% to 6.6%, with somewhat higher rates in women than in men. The individual with GAD worries about life events such as marital relationships, job performance, health, money, or social status. GAD usually emerges in the early 20s, but it can occur in childhood. Symptoms include restlessness, motor tension, irritability, fatigue, difficulty concentrating, and sleep disturbance. Individuals with GAD startle easily and may suffer from depression. The severity of these symptoms fluctuates over time and may be linked to the changing nature of environmental stressors. In general, GAD tends to be a chronic disorder, albeit with age the symptoms may become less severe.

Etiology and Pathophysiology

At present, the etiology and pathophysiology of GAD are poorly understood. However, abnormalities in a few neurotransmitter and receptor systems have been found.[31] Investigators report alterations in the norepinephrine system, with reductions in α_2 receptor binding. In the cerebrospinal fluid of individuals with GAD, one study found a reduction in serotonin levels and another indicated reduced platelet binding of paroxetine, an SSRI.

One of the more prominent alterations of GAD involves the GABA–BZ receptor complex. In GAD individuals, there is a reduction in peripheral BZ receptors, which increase after treatment with BZ drugs (see the following section). Brain imaging work in individuals with GAD appears to further support an alteration in BZ receptors. In comparison to control subjects, GAD subjects show greater homogeneity in cerebral BZ receptor distribution and a significant reduction in the region of the left temporal hemisphere.[32] The therapeutic effects of BZs may lie, in part, in their ability to normalize these BZ receptor alterations.

Treatment

GAD is diagnosed when the individual spends at least 6 months worrying excessively. Treatment of GAD may include behavioral therapy and drug medication. During behavioral therapy the individual learns relaxation techniques to control the anxiety. BZs, such as diazepam, have been traditionally used in the treatment of GAD. Although a majority of individuals with GAD respond to BZ (60%), its use is limited to a short period because of the drug's liability potential (see Treatment section of Panic Disorder, p. 561) and the availability of other medications, including buspirone, TCAs, and atypical antidepresssants.

Buspirone, which has affinity for serotonin receptors ($5\text{-}HT_{1A}$) appears to be as effective as BZs, although the onset of efficacy may take approximately 2 weeks. The advantage of buspirone over BZs is that long-term use does not produce unwanted drug complications, which makes it well suited for certain types of individuals diagnosed with GAD, such as the elderly or those with a history of alcohol abuse. Buspirone's primary side effects, which lessen over time, include dizziness, headaches, nausea, and mild nervousness.

Not all individuals with GAD exhibit a therapeutic response to BZs and buspirone. In addition, many people with GAD are diagnosed with mood and other anxiety disorders. For these individuals, antidepressants (i.e., tricyclics, SSRIs, and atypical antidepressants) may be more efficacious than BZs and buspirone. Results of clinical trials support this treatment alternative as indicated by effective therapeutic responses in people with GAD taking the tricyclic imipramine or the atypical antidepressant trazodone.

Posttraumatic Stress Disorder

Exposure to a terrifying or traumatic event may produce **posttraumatic stress disorder (PTSD).** This disorder was first described in combat situations and called "shell shock" or "war neurosis." Subsequently, exposure to other disasters—including serious accidents, natural disasters such as earthquakes, child abuse, kidnapping, and violent attacks such as rape or mugging—was reported to induce PTSD symptoms. In PTSD the traumatic event is reexperienced persistently by the individual through thoughts or dreams. In some cases, exposure to cues associated with the traumatic event will trigger psychologic distress and intense autonomic arousal. Consequently, the individual attempts to avoid stimuli associated with the trauma. For example, the individual avoids activities that may lead to a recollection of thoughts, feelings, places, or people involved in the trauma. Persistent symptoms of PTSD may include difficulty sleeping, irritability, lack of concentration, hypervigilance, and exaggerated startle response.

Population estimates of PTSD are lower in men (0.5%) than in women (1.2%), and PTSD occurs even in childhood. PTSD in men is usually found among combat veterans, whereas PTSD in women is related to a traumatic event, such as rape or assault. Thus the key etiologic factor leading to PTSD is exposure to a severe stressor, especially those stressors with an emotional impact outside the realm of normal everyday experience. Certain individuals appear to be vulnerable to PTSD. Persons with a history of psychiatric illness (major depression, panic disorder) or those who lack strong social support are more likely to develop PTSD. These individuals may be more sensitive to the effects of the stressor.

The development of PTSD may occur within hours of the traumatic event, or it may be delayed several months or years. A flashback involving images, odors, sounds, and emotions may make the person reenact the event. The duration of the flashback varies from only a few seconds or hours to, in rare cases, several days.

Etiology and Pathophysiology

The primary etiology of PTSD is exposure to a major stressor and may involve several neural structures and neurochemical and hormonal systems.[33] For example, brain imaging studies in combat-related or childhood abuse PTSD victims revealed a reduction in the hippocampal volume. In other studies that measured cerebral activation during exposure to combat-related stimuli, blood flow increased in the amygdala but decreased in the prefrontal cortex of war veterans with PTSD.[34,35] These findings may be particularly relevant for understanding the pathophysiology of PTSD because the hippocampus, the amygdala, and the prefrontal cortex appear to play important roles in the memory of fear responses associated with situational events. At present, however, it is not clear whether these neuroanatomic alterations are risk factors or a consequence of the disorder.

Neurochemical system alterations are reported in individuals with PTSD. In women and sexually abused girls with PTSD, catecholamine and metabolite levels are elevated. Viewing combat films led to elevated levels of epinephrine and norepinephrine in war veterans with PTSD. Furthermore, individuals with combat-related PTSD show a heightened increase in autonomic responses (including heart rate and blood pressure) to yohimbine, an α_2 antagonist, which stimulates central norepinephrine release. These results suggest that norepinephrine hyperactivity may contribute to the symptomatology underlying PTSD.

Alterations in the HPA system are found in individuals with PTSD.[36] The more notable findings are a decrease in cortisol levels and a blunted adrenocorticotropin (ACTH) response to CRF, the neuropeptide that activates pituitary ACTH secretion. It is hypothesized that elevated levels of cortisol at the time of the traumatic event results in enhanced suppression of cortisol feedback that eventually leads to decreased cortisol levels.

Treatment

PTSD usually is diagnosed when symptoms last longer than 1 month. In some cases the symptoms may be short lived and ultimately disappear. In other cases the symptoms may be chronic and last for years. As in GAD, the severity of the symptoms may fluctuate over time. The treatment of chronic PTSD is difficult. Current methods involve psychotherapy and drug treatment. During therapy the individual learns to control the anxiety symptoms. Among war veterans, group or family therapy is supported by the Veterans Administration.

Drug treatment may serve to lessen the recurrent nightmares and flashbacks. Although antidepressants (SSRIs, tricyclics, and MAOIs) are considered first-line medications, individuals with PTSD show only moderate improvement. The tendency to use antidepressants for PTSD is due to the high prevalence of comorbid depression and substance abuse. BZs may be used during the aftermath of a traumatic event to control hyperarousal symptoms such as irritability and muscle tension. However, there is no clear evidence that BZs have clinical efficacy or provide prophylaxis against the development of chronic PTSD. BZs should be used carefully in individuals with chronic PTSD, especially those with a history of drug abuse. Further information on the pathophysiology of PTSDs is needed to determine the effective pharmacologic requirements.

SUMMARY REVIEW

Schizophrenia

1. Schizophrenia is a collection of symptoms characterized by thought disorders. Thought disorders reflect a break between the cognitive and the emotional sides of one's personality.
2. Schizophrenic symptoms appear in early adulthood. Positive symptoms of schizophrenia include hallucinations, delusions, thought disorders, and bizarre behavior. Negative symptoms include flattened affect, alogia, anhedonia, attentional deficits, and apathy.
3. There appears to be a genetic predisposition to acquire schizophrenia.
4. Schizophrenia may result from neurodevelopmental defects occurring in fetal life. Factors that may contribute to neurodevelopmental alterations include early exposure to a viral infection, prenatal nutritional deficiencies, and perinatal complications.
5. Structural and functional brain abnormalities are found in schizophrenia. There is an enlargement of the cerebroventricles and widening of fissures and sulci in the frontal cortex. Histologic analyses reveal a reduction and disarray of cells in the hippocampal formation, a structure in the temporal lobe that plays an important role in cognitive functions.
6. The dorsolateral prefrontal cortex (DLPFC) also plays a role in cognitive functions, and individuals with schizophrenia exhibit decreased blood flow and metabolism in this brain region during cognitive problem-solving tasks. In addition, cortical thickness in the DLPFC is reduced and glutamic acid decarboxylase messenger ribonucleic acid (GAD mRNA) expression is decreased, which may ultimately alter DLPFC cell firing.
7. Alterations in brain dopamine systems accompany schizophrenia. D_2 receptors are elevated in the caudate and nucleus accumbens. In addition, dopamine neurotransmission may be altered in mesocortical and mesolimbic regions of the brain.
8. Positive symptoms, including hallucinations, delusions, and thought disorder, are often acute and manageable with antipsychotic medications that include D_2 receptor–blocking drugs. Individuals who do not respond to D_2 receptor–blocking drugs may respond to atypical antipsychotic drugs that show greater affinity to serotonin receptors. Antipsychotic medication is less effective in treating individuals with schizophrenia who manifest a high incidence of negative symptoms. In addition to pharmacotherapy, psychosocial therapy can assist in the management of schizophrenic individuals by increasing medication compliance and encouraging coping strategies.

Mood Disorders: Depression and Mania

1. Emotional states that are unremitting and disrupt normal functioning of the individual are called *mood disorders.* Major depression and mania are two common mood disorders. The former is characterized by an intense and sustained unpleasant state of sadness and hopelessness, whereas the latter is characterized by extreme levels of energy and euphoria. Individuals with recurrent patterns of depression and mania have a bipolar illness.
2. There is a strong genetic predisposition to develop depression and bipolar illnesses. Psychosocial stressors appear to be important precipitating factors underlying the first episode of major depression.
3. Mood disorders are associated with neurochemical abnormalities. A reduction in brain monoamine neurotransmission is linked to depression, whereas an elevated monoamine level is associated with mania.
4. Individuals with major depression commonly have elevated levels of cortisol. Increased cortisol secretion appears to be a reflection of elevated secretion of corticotropin-releasing factor (CRF), which is also hypothesized to produce some of the symptoms associated with depression. Neuroendocrine abnormalities involving thyroid hormones also are found in depression.
5. Postmortem studies have revealed altered serotonin and norepinephrine receptor binding in the cortex and reduced densities of norepinephrine cell bodies in the locus caeruleus of depressed suicide victims. Functional brain imaging has shown that depressed individuals have alterations in cerebral blood flow to prefrontal and limbic brain regions that include the amygdala, a structure implicated in emotional behavior in depressed individuals. There is a positive relationship between right amygdala metabolic rate and negative affect.
6. Pharmacotherapy is effective in the treatment of mood disorders. Depressed individuals generally respond to MAOIs, TCAs, SSRIs, and atypical antidepressants. Selection of an antidepressant is based on several considerations, including symptomatology, the individual's ability to tolerate the drug's side effects, whether other medications are being taken, cost, and accessibility or convenience. Manic and bipolar individuals are treatable with lithium or mood stabilizers. The clinical effects of the medication usually takes more than a week to develop. Severely depressed and manic people who do not respond to medication are administered ECT and subsequently placed on pharmacotherapy. One potential new treatment for depression is transcranial magnetic stimulation (TMS).

Anxiety Disorders

1. Fear and anxiety are normal emotional states that reflect individuals' evolutionary heritage. However, an anxiety disorder may develop when these states become uncontrollable. Panic disorder, generalized anxiety disorder, and posttraumatic stress disorder (PTSD) are examples of intense fear and anxiety states that require psychiatric treatment.

2. Panic disorder consists of panic attacks characterized by intense autonomic arousal. In addition, heightened fear and anxiety states occur both during and between panic attacks. During a panic attack the individual experiences multiple symptoms, including light-headedness, a pounding heart, and difficulty in breathing. The intense activation of cardiovascular and respiratory systems occurs spontaneously and may last up to 1 hour.
3. Panic disorder may be caused by an oversensitive brain system regulating autonomic functions. Potential brain regions involved in the production of panic attacks are the locus caeruleus, hippocampus, and amygdala. Pathophysiology in the brain $GABA_A$–benzodiazepine receptor system may also contribute to the production of panic attacks. Psychosocial stressors may facilitate the occurrence of panic in vulnerable individuals.
4. Behavioral therapy and antidepressant medication are used to treat panic disorder. In therapy the individual learns to control the intensity of anxiety and panic through breathing exercises and biofeedback techniques. Medication includes the use of monoamine oxidase inhibitors (MAOIs), tricyclic antidepressants, and selective serotonin reuptake inhibitors (SSRIs). Benzodiazepines (BZs) also are prescribed.
5. Generalized anxiety disorder (GAD) is characterized as excessive and persistent worries about life events (e.g., marital relationships, job performance, social status). Individuals with GAD exhibit varying levels of motor disturbances, emotional arousal, and irritability that may be linked to fluctuations in stress. They also may suffer from depression.
6. Although the pathophysiology of GAD is poorly understood, abnormalities in neurotransmitter systems are believed to contribute to the disorder.
7. GAD treatment may include a combination of behavioral therapy (in which the individual learns relaxation techniques) and pharmacotherapy. Although BZs are traditionally used in the treatment of GAD, buspirone and antidepressants are also effective and lack some of the long-term liabilities of BZs.
8. PTSD results from exposure to a life-threatening or traumatic event. Individuals with PTSD have recurring thoughts of the terrifying event. Reenactment of the event varies in duration from a few seconds or hours to several days.
9. Individuals with major depression, with panic disorder, or lacking strong social support are vulnerable to develop PTSD.
10. Reductions in hippocampal volume and altered blood flow in the prefrontal cortex and amygdala are some of the changes found in PTSD. In addition, there are reports of altered norepinephrine and HPA systems in PTSD.
11. Treatment of chronic PTSD is difficult. Current methods involve psychotherapy, which assists the individual to control feelings of anxiety, and pharmacotherapy, which may lessen the recurrent nightmares and flashbacks. Although antidepressasnts and BZs are used, clinical efficacy is modest.

KEY TERMS

γ-Aminobutyric acid (GABA), *553*
Affective flattening, *554*
Agoraphobia, *560*
Alogia, *554*
Anhedonia, *554*
Avolition, *554*
Bipolar disorder, *555*
Delusion, *554*
Depression, *558*
Dopamine hypothesis, *553*
Dorsolateral prefrontal cortex (DLPFC), *553*
Dysphoric mood, *558*
Formal thought disorder, *554*
Generalized anxiety disorder (GAD), *561*
Hallucination, *554*
Major (unipolar) depression, *555*
Manic, *559*
Monoamines, *555*
Mood, *555*
Panic disorder, *560*
Posttraumatic stress disorder (PTSD), *562*
Poverty of content, *554*
Psychotic episode, *551*
Schizophrenia, *550*
Thought disorder, *550*
Working memory, *553*

REFERENCES

1. Bunney BG, Potkin SG, Bunney WE Jr: New morphological and neuropathological findings in schizophrenia: a neurodevelopmental perspective, *Clin Neurosci* 3:81, 1995.
2. Davidson RJ et al: Regional brain function, emotional and disorders of emotion, *Curr Opin Neurobiol* 9:228, 1999.
3. Mednick SA, Huttunen MO, Machon RA: Prenatal influenza infections and adult schizophrenia, *Schizophr Bull* 20:263, 1994.
4. Mednick SA et al: Adult schizophrenia following prenatal exposure to an influenza epidemic, *Arch Gen Psychiatry* 45:189, 1988.
5. Susser E et al: No relation between risk of schizophrenia and prenatal exposure to influenza in Holland, *Am J Psychiatry* 151:922, 1994.
6. Crow TJ: Prenatal exposure to influenza as a cause of schizophrenia, *Br J Psychiatry* 164:588, 1994.
7. Susser E et al: Schizophrenia after prenatal famine, *Arch Gen Psychiatry* 53:25, 1996.
8. Brixey SN et al: Gestational and neonatal factors in the etiology of schizophrenia, *J Clin Psychol* 49:447, 1993.
9. Hollister JM, Laing P, Mednick SA: Rhesus incompatibility as a risk factor for schizophrenia in male adults, *Arch Gen Psychiatry* 53:19, 1996.
10. Mortensen et al: Effects of family history and place of season of birth on the risk of schizophrenia, *N Engl J Med* 340:603, 1999.
11. McCarley RW et al: MRI anatomy of schizophrenia, *Biol Psychiatry* 45:1099, 1999.
12. Schultz SK, Andreasen NC: Schizophrenia, *Lancet* 353:1425, 1999.
13. Falkai P, Bogerts B: The neuropathology of schizophrenia. In Hirsch SR, Weinberger DR, editors: *Schizophrenia*, Cambridge, 1995, Blackwell.
14. Selemon LD, Rajkowska G, Goldman-Rakic PS: Abnormally high neuronal density in the schizophrenic cortex, *Arch Gen Psychiatry* 52:805, 1995.

15. Akbarian S et al: Gene expression for glutamic acid decarboxylase is reduced without loss of neurons in prefrontal cortex of schizophrenics, *Arch Gen Psychiatry* 52:258, 1995.
16. Duncan GE, Sheitman BB, Lieberman JA: An integrated view of pathophysiological models of schizophrenia, *Brain Res Rev* 29:250, 1999.
17. Seeman P, Corbett R, Van Tol HHM: Atypical neuroleptics have low affinity for dopamine D_2 receptors or are selective for D_4 receptors, *Neuropsychopharmacology* 16:93, 1997.
18. Meltzer HY: Clinical studies on the mechanism of action of clozapine: the dopamine-serotonin hypothesis of schizophrenia, *Psychopharmacology* 99:S1827, 1989.
19. Sensky T et al: A randomized control trial of cognitive-behavioral therapy for persistent symptoms in schizophrenia resistant to medication, *Arch Gen Psychiatry* 57:165, 2000.
20. Sanders AR, Detera-Wadleigh SD, Gershon ES: Molecular genetics of mood disorders. In Charney Ds, Nestler EJ, Bunney BS, editors: *Neurobiology of mental illness*, New York, 1999, Oxford.
21. Post RM: Transduction of psychosocial stress into the neurobiology of recurrent affective disorder, *Am J Psychiatry* 149:999, 1992.
22. Barbarino A et al: Nocturnal serum thyrotropin (TSH) surge and the TSH response to TSH-releasing hormone: disassociative behavior in untreated depressive, *J Clin Endocrinol Metab* 71:650, 1990.
23. Delgado PL et al: Serotonin and the neurobiology of depression: effects of tryptophan depletion in drug-free depressed patients, *Arch Gen Psychiatry* 51:865, 1994.
24. Drevets WC: Prefrontal cortical-amygdalar metabolism in major depression, *Ann NY Acad Sci* 877:614, 1999.
25. American Psychiatric Association: *Diagnostic and statistical manual of mental disorders,* ed 4, Washington, DC, 1994, American Psychiatric Association.
26. Belmaker RH, Grisaru N: Magnetic stimulation of the brain in animal depression models responsive to ECS, *J ECT* 14:194, 1998.
27. George MS et al: Low frequency daily left prefrontal rTMS improves mood in bipolar depression: a placebo-controlled case report, *Hum Psychopharmacol* 13:271, 1998.
28. Hilty DM, Brady KT, Hales RE: A review of bipolar disorder among adults, *Psychiat Serv* 50:201, 1999.
29. Goddard AW, Charney DS: Toward an integrated neurobiology of panic disorder, *J Clin Psychiatry* 58(suppl 2):4, 1997.
30. Malizia AL et al: Decreased brain $GABA_A$–benzodiazepine receptor binding in panic disorder, *Arch Gen Psychiatry* 55:715, 1998.
31. Brawman-Mintzer O, Lyudiard RB: Biological basis of generalized anxiety disorder, *J Clin Psychiatry* 58(suppl 3):16, 1997.
32. Tiihonen J et al: Cerebral benzodiazepine receptor binding and distribution in generalized anxiety disorder, *Mol Psychiatry* 2:463, 1997.
33. Charney DS et al: Psychobiologic mechanisms of posttraumatic stress disorder, *Arch Gen Psychiatry* 50:294, 1993.
34. Bremner JD et al: Neural correlates of exposure to traumatic pictures and sound in Vietnam combat veterans with and without posttraumatic stress disorder: a positron emission tomography study, *Biol Psychiatry* 45:806, 1999.
35. Shin LM et al: Visual imagery and perception in posttraumatic stress disorder, *Arch Gen Psychiatry* 54:233, 1997.
36. Kellner M, Yehuda R: Do panic disorders and posttraumatic stress disorder share a common psychoneuroendocrinology? *Psychoneuroendocrinology* 24:485, 1999.

CHAPTER 18

Alterations of Neurologic Function in Children

KATHERINE PADGETT

CHAPTER OUTLINE

Central nervous system (CNS) malformations are responsible for 75% of fetal deaths and 40% of deaths during the first year of life. During the perinatal period, CNS malformations account for 33% of all apparent congenital malformations, and 90% of CNS malformations are defects of neural tube closure. Although embryology is a highly complex and often difficult science, the process of embryonic development explains many of the malformations that occur in children.

Environmental influences also play a significant role in nervous system development. Nutrition, hormones, oxygen levels, and external stimulation all affect normal growth. The proper proportions of essential nutrients are necessary for proliferation of the nervous system tissue. Maternal lifestyle, nutrition, and state of health also have a crucial impact on nervous system development at certain critical periods of maturation.

STRUCTURE AND FUNCTION OF THE NERVOUS SYSTEM IN CHILDREN

The CNS develops from a dorsal thickening of the ectoderm known as the **neural plate.** This plate appears around the middle of the third gestational week and unfolds to form a **neural groove** and **neural folds.** During the fourth gestational week the neural groove deepens; its folds develop laterally; and it closes dorsally to form the **neural tube,** epithelial tissue that ultimately becomes the CNS. The neural tube closes first in the cervical region and then "zippers" in two directions—cranially and caudally (Fig. 18-1).

In the developmental process, some neuroectodermal cells separate from the neural tube but remain between the tube and the surface ectoderm, creating the **neural crest.** This cellular band develops into the cranial and spinal ganglia, more commonly referred to as the peripheral nervous system. Other structures associated with the nervous system arise from mesoderm (**somite**) and include blood vessels, microglial cells, dural and arachnoid layers of the meninges, the capsule of some peripheral sensory nerve endings, and peripheral nerve coverings.

The cranial end of the neural tube forms the brain, and the remainder develops into the spinal cord. The lumen of the neural tube becomes the ventricles of the brain and the central canal of the spinal cord (Fig. 18-2). On either side of the neural tube's inner surface is a longitudinal groove (**sulcus limitans**). Anterior to this region (**basal plate**) the gray matter differentiates into the nuclei of the lower motor neurons. The region posterior to the sulcus (**alar plate**) differentiates into the sensory nuclei of the spinal cord.

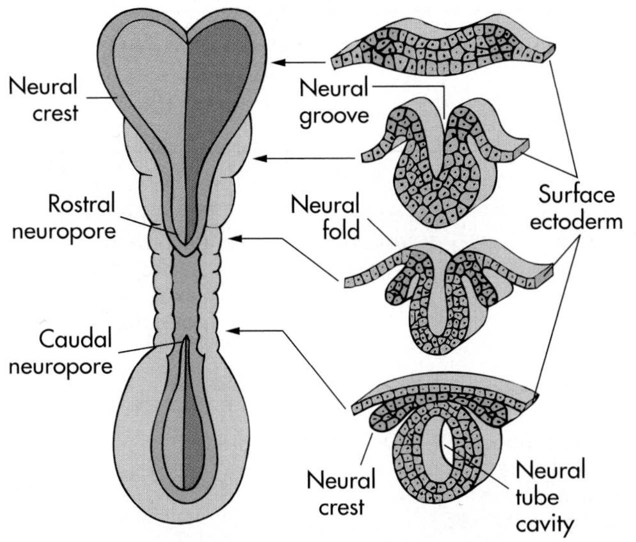

FIG. 18-1 Neural tube at the end of the third week. Neural folds have begun to fuse at the cervical level of the future spinal cord. *Right,* Cross sections of the neural tube at four different levels; at any given level the embryonic central nervous system (CNS) goes through a series of stages resembling these four cross sections. Total length of neural tube at this time is about 2.5 mm.

NUTRITION & DISEASE

Iron and Cognitive Function

Iron deficiency is the single most significant nutrient deficiency, affecting 15% of the world population and causing anemia in 40% to 50% of children. Iron is essential for neurologic activity, including synthesis of dopamine, serotonin, catecholamine, and, possibly, myelin formation. Iron-deficient children have decreased attentiveness, narrow attention span, and perceptual restrictions. In some studies, cognitive deficits in iron can be reversed with iron supplements. Continued research is in progress to determine effects of acute versus chronic iron deficiency and relationships between severity of deficiency and cognitive functioning.

Data from Grantham-MacGregor SM et al: *Proc Nutr Soc* 59(1):47, 2000.

Embryonic development of the nervous system occurs in six stages: (1) dorsal (posterior) induction, (2) ventral (anterior) induction, (3) proliferation, (4) migration, (5) organization, and (6) myelination. (Fig. 18-3 summarizes the embryonic development of the nervous system and identifies disorders associated with interference in any of these stages.) Many different events happen simultaneously, and critical periods must pass uninterrupted if the vulnerable fetus is to develop normally.

In the newborn the bones of the skull are separated, but definite **sutures** (bands of connective tissue) form shortly thereafter. The edges are several millimeters wide to allow for normal growth. At the junctions of the sutures are wider spaces of unossified membranous tissue called **fontanelles.** Sutures and fontanelles close as the skull and brain grow and develop.

On average the posterior fontanelle closes within the first 3 months of life. By 6 months of age, a fibrous union of suture lines occurs and serrated edges interlock. By approximately 20 to 24 months, the anterior fontanelle is closed (Fig. 18-4). At approximately 8 years of age, ossification of the cranial bones is complete; the sutures usually are completely fused and cannot be separated by 12 years of age, even in the presence of increased intracranial pressure (IICP).

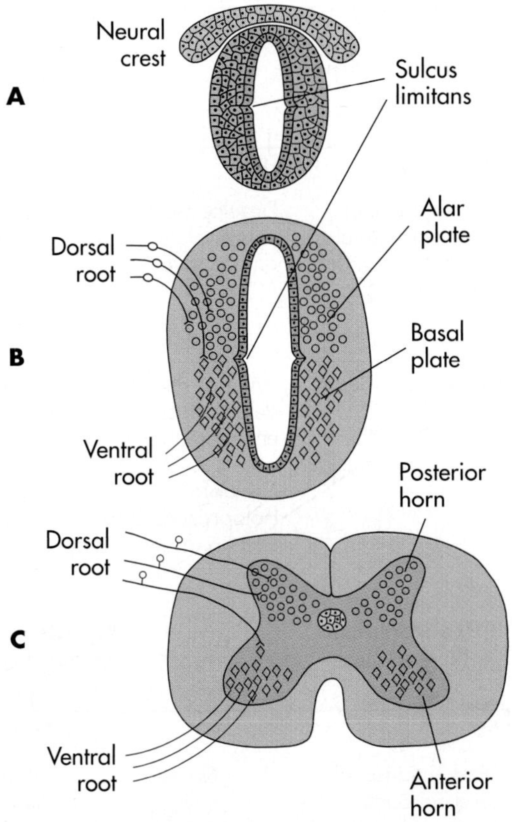

FIG. 18-2 Sulcus limitans and alar and basal plates. A, Neural tube during the fourth week. **B,** Embryonic spinal cord during the sixth week; dorsal root ganglion cells, derived from the neural crest, send their central processes into the spinal cord to terminate mainly in alar plate cells; basal plate cells become motor neurons, whose axons exit in the ventral roots. **C,** Adult spinal cord.

Myelin Sheath

Axons are wrapped in concentric layers of myelin, a lipid-protein sheath (see Chapter 13). Specialized connective tissue cells, which in the peripheral nervous system are called **Schwann cells,** form membranes that wrap around the axon during embryonic development, laying down the lipoprotein lamellae of the myelin sheath. These axons are myelinated, whereas the axons that lack a sheath are thinner, unmyelinated fibers and conduct nerve impulses more slowly. During the first year of life, the presence or absence of various reflexes is indicative of the myelination that has occurred with growth of the infant.

Normal Growth and Development

Human neurologic functioning is primarily at a subcortical level at birth (impulses are handled by the brain stem and spinal cord). Many reflex patterns mediated by brain stem

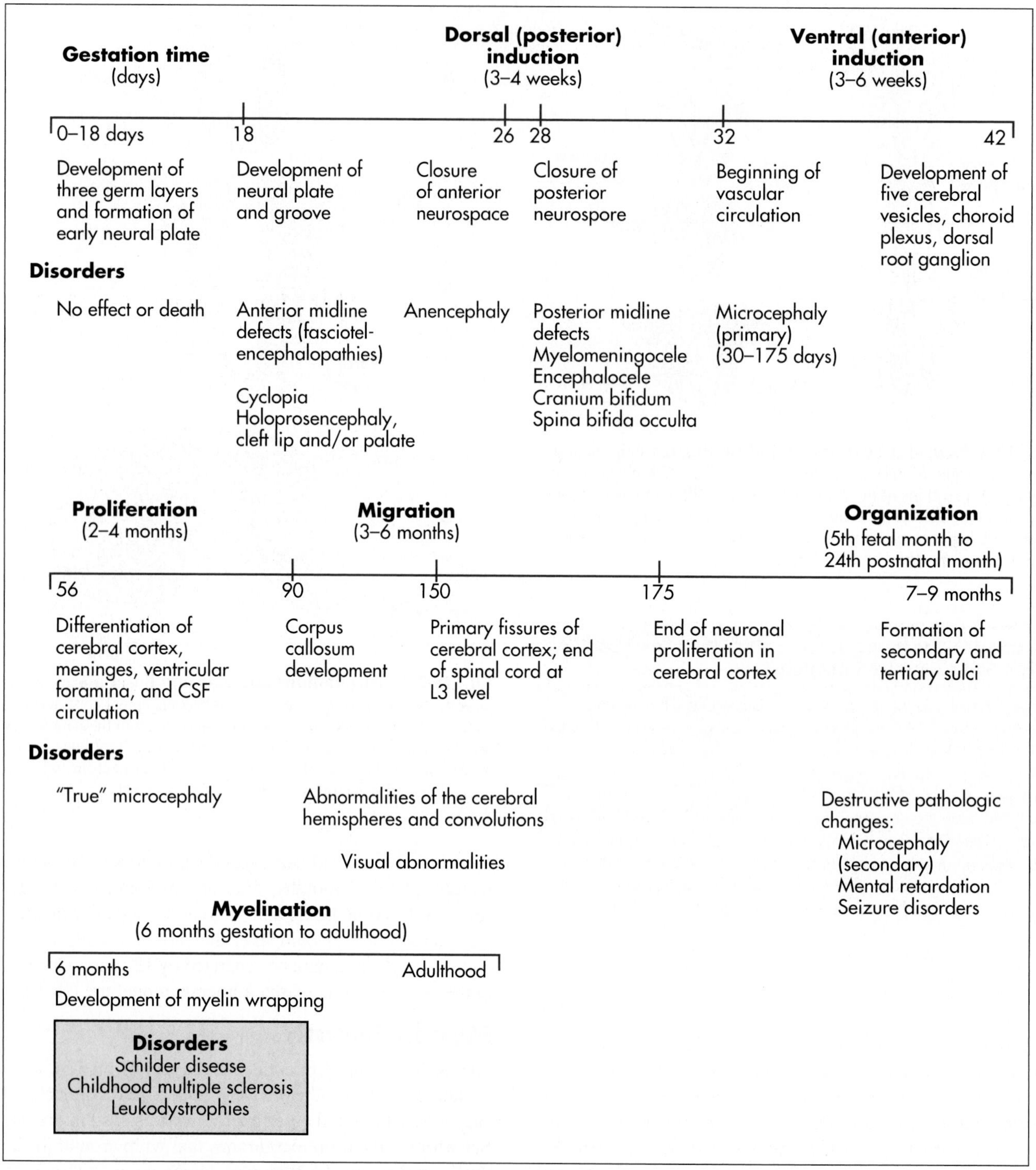

FIG. 18-3 Disorders associated with specific stages of embryonic development.

and spinal cord mechanisms are present at birth and disappear at predictable times during infancy. Table 18-1 summarizes the ages at which reflexes appear and disappear.

Absence of expected reflex responses at the appropriate age indicates general depression of central or peripheral motor functions. Asymmetric responses may indicate lesions in the motor cortex or may occur with fractures of bones after traumatic delivery or postnatal injury. As the infant matures, the neonatal reflexes disappear in a predictable order as voluntary motor functions supersede them. Abnormal persistence of these reflexes is seen in infants with developmental delays or with central motor lesions.

Several differences between adults and children illustrate the pathophysiology of the nervous system in children. First, the head of a normal infant accounts for approximately one fourth of the total height, whereas an adult's head is one eighth of the total body height. Second, the bones of the infant's skull are separated at the suture lines, thus forming two fontanelles or "soft spots": one diamond-shaped anterior fontanelle and one triangular-shaped posterior fontanelle.

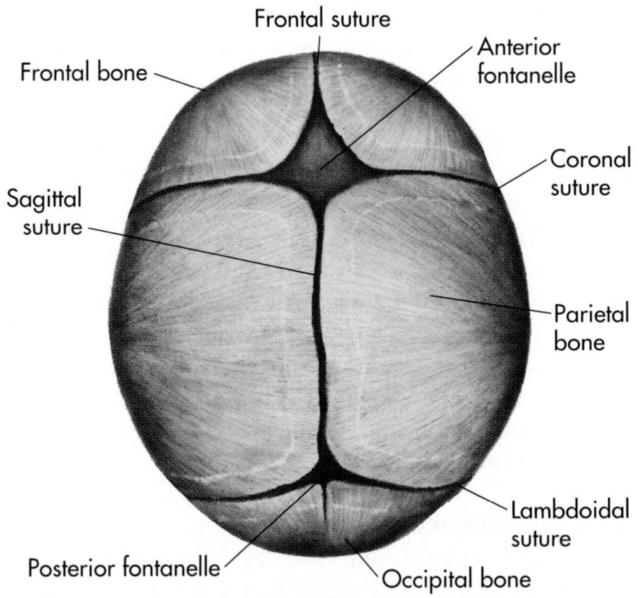

FIG. 18-4 Cranial sutures and fontanelles in infancy. Fibrous union of suture lines and interlocking of serrated edges (occurs by 6 months; solid union requires approximately 12 years). (From Wong DL et al: *Whaley and Wong's nursing care of infants and children,* ed 6, St Louis, 1999, Mosby.)

Table 18-1 Reflexes of Infancy

Reflex	Age at Appearance of Reflex	Age at Which Reflex Should no Longer be Obtainable
Moro	Birth	3 months
Stepping	Birth	6 weeks
Sucking	Birth	4 months awake 7 months asleep
Rooting	Birth	4 months awake 7 months asleep
Palmar grasp	Birth	6 months
Plantar grasp	Birth	10 months
Tonic neck	2 months	5 months
Neck righting	4-6 months	24 months
Landau	3 months	24 months
Parachute reaction	9 months	Persists for life

The posterior fontanelle may be open until 2 to 3 months of age, whereas the anterior fontanelle normally closes by 18 months. Whereas the adult cranium is a closed cavity with sutures firmly holding the cranial bones together, the infant cranium has room for expansion through the fontanelles. An adult's head size will not expand, regardless of intracranial events such as trauma or increased production of cerebrospinal fluid (CSF). The infant's head circumference, on the other hand, increases in size as a result of normal growth up to 5 years of age. The head is the fastest growing body part during infancy. Abnormal intracranial conditions, such as those characterized by IICP, also may result in an increased head circumference in excess of that expected with normal growth. Health care providers carefully monitor head growth during the first 5 years of life by measuring head circumference and comparing the results with a standardized growth chart.

WHAT'S NEW? Reduction of Risks for Neural Tube Defects

Studies indicate that ingestion of multivitamins with folic acid before conception or early in pregnancy may offer protection against the occurrence of neural tube defects. Recent repeated studies demonstrate a 60% to 86% reduction of risks for neural tube defects with periconceptional ingestion of vitamins containing the U.S. recommended daily allowance of 400 mg folic acid.

Data from Abramsky L et al: Has advice on periconceptual folate supplementation reduced neural-tube defects? *Lancet* 354 (9183):998, 1999; Tinkle M, Sterling BS: Neural tube defects: a primary prevention role for nurses, *JOGNN* 26(5):503, 1997; Werler MM et al: Multivitamin supplementation and risk of birth defects, *Am J Epidemiol* 150(7):675, 1999

STRUCTURAL MALFORMATIONS

Defects of Neural Tube Closure

Neural tube defects, which are caused by an arrest of the normal developmental process, have an incidence rate of approximately 0.7 to 1.0 for every 1000 live births in the United States each year. There is a strong association of fetal death with neural tube defects, reducing the actual prevalence of neural defects at birth.[1] Defects of neural tube closure are divided into two categories: posterior defects and anterior midline defects.

Posterior defects are more common. These include **anencephaly** (*an* = without; *enkephalos* = brain) and a group of disorders collectively referred to as the **myelodysplasias** (*dys* = bad; *plassein* = to form). Although myelodysplasia is defined as a defective formation of the spinal cord, the term is used to refer to anomalies of both the vertebral column and the spine.

Anterior midline defects are less common because the inductive processes occur in a relatively short period (2 to 3 days). These developmental defects may cause brain and skull abnormalities. The most extreme form is **cyclopia,** in which the child has a single midline orbit and eye with a protruding noselike appendage above the orbit.

Anencephaly

Anencephaly is an anomaly in which the soft, bony component of the skull and part of the brain are missing. This is a relatively common disorder, with an incidence rate of approximately 0.36 per 1000 total live births in the United States each year.[2] When development is arrested early in anterior closure of the neural tube, the cerebral hemispheres, diencephalon, mesencephalon, cerebellum, brain stem, or spinal cord may be affected. At birth the infant's head, viewed face-on, has a froglike appearance. These infants are stillborn or die within a few days after birth.

Encephalocele

Encephalocele refers to a herniation or protrusion of brain and meninges through a defect in the skull, resulting in a saclike structure. The incidence rate is approximately 1 in 5000 live births in the United States each year.[3] When the defect contains only meninges, it is referred to as a **cranial meningocele.** Most encephaloceles occur in the occipital area, with the remainder found in the frontal, parietal, or nasopharyngeal regions.

Clinical Manifestations

Encephalocele usually is seen at birth as a midline skull defect through which a large mass protrudes (Fig. 18-5). If the defect is located in the nasopharynx, no external anomaly is visible but the child may experience nasal airway obstruction. On examination with a nasal speculum, a smooth, round mass will be visible in the nasal passages. A frontal encephalocele may extend into the orbit of the eye and produce proptosis on the affected side.

Evaluation and Treatment

Diagnosis is based on clinical manifestations and examination of the meningeal sac. With cranial meningocele, surgical repair of the cranial defect affords a good prognosis for most affected infants whose intellectual and motor functioning is normal. An occipital encephalocele may be associated with other findings, such as blindness and cognitive impairment. The size, location, and involvement of the encephalocele help to determine the child's development and intellectual outcome.

Meningocele

A **meningocele,** which is a saclike cyst of meninges filled with spinal fluid, occurs when the neural tube fails to close completely (Fig. 18-6). This cystic dilation of meninges protrudes through the vertebral defect and around the malformed tube. This defect does not involve the spinal cord. Meningoceles occur with equal frequency in the cervical, thoracic, and lumbar spine areas.

Clinical Manifestations

At birth the infant has a protruding sac on the back at the level of the defect. The sac may be covered by a thin layer of muscle and skin and usually appears as raw, fluid-filled tissue. Abnormal neurologic function sometimes is present. Talipes equinovarus (clubfoot), gait disturbance, bladder dysfunction, and upper extremity weakness also have been associated with meningocele. Hydrocephalus commonly is associated with this diagnosis.

Evaluation and Treatment

The diagnosis is made on the basis of clinical manifestations and examination of the meningeal sac. In an effort to preserve neuronal function and minimize potential damage that may occur from infection and manipulation of the fragile sac, surgical closure is optimal during the first 72 hours of life. Functional implications depend on the level and severity of the defect (Table 18-2).

Myelomeningocele

Myelomeningocele (meningomyelocele; spina bifida cystica) is a hernial protrusion of a saclike cyst (containing meninges, spinal fluid, and a portion of the spinal cord with its nerves) through a defect in the posterior arch of a vertebra. Eighty

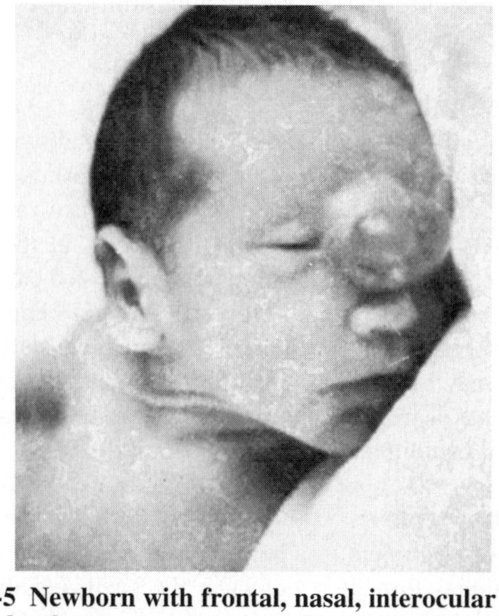

FIG. 18-5 Newborn with frontal, nasal, interocular encephalocele. (Courtesy Dr. Charles Linder, Medical College of Georgia.)

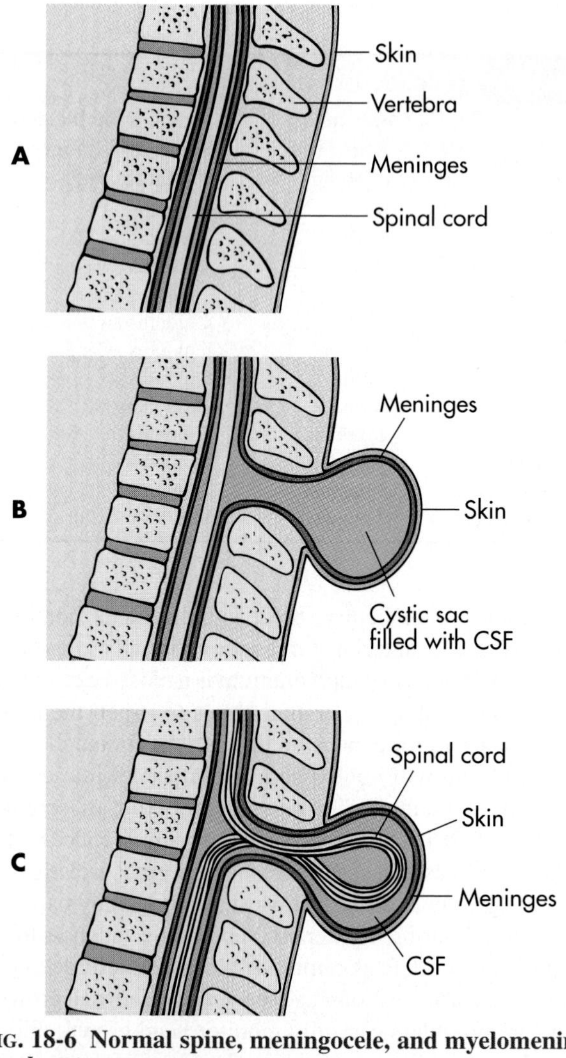

FIG. 18-6 Normal spine, meningocele, and myelomeningocele. Diagram showing section through normal spine **(A)**, meningocele **(B)**, and myelomeningocele **(C)**.

percent of myelomeningoceles are located in the lumbar and lumbosacral regions, the last regions of the neural tube to close. Myelomeningocele has an incidence rate ranging from 0.2 to 0.4 per 1000 live births[4] and thus is one of the most common developmental anomalies of the nervous system.

Pathophysiology

A myelomeningocele is the failure of the neural tube to close, resulting in a cystic dilation of meninges and protuberance of the spinal cord through the vertebral defect. This defect occurs during the first 4 weeks of the gestational period; at the end of this time the neural tube is closed both anteriorly and posteriorly.

Clinical Manifestations

A myelomeningocele is evident at birth as a pronounced skin defect on the infant's back (see Fig. 18-6). The bony prominences of the unfused neural arches can be palpated at the lateral border of the defect. The defect usually is covered by a transparent membrane that may have neural tissue attached to its inner surface. This membrane may be intact at birth or may leak cerebrospinal fluid (CSF), thereby increasing the risks of infection and neuronal damage. Until the defect is closed surgically, CSF may accumulate, resulting in further dilation and enlargement of the sac that may risk further damage to neuronal function.

The actual involvement of the spinal cord has greater implications for the overall function of the infant throughout childhood (see Table 18-2). An absence of neurologic function may occur in some infants with myelomeningocele. Function may be attained if underlying fluid or pus accumulation is prevented from stretching and applying pressure to the neural tissue or if the biochemical alterations do not cause neural tissue to die. Residual neural tissue also may be lost temporarily or permanently at birth because of trauma to the tissue during delivery.

One serious, potentially life-threatening problem associated with myelodysplasia is the **Arnold-Chiari II malformation.** This deformity involves the downward displacement of the cerebellum, cerebral tonsils, brain stem, and fourth ventricle (Fig. 18-7). Arnold-Chiari II malformation compresses and essentially stretches the posterior region of the cerebellum and brain stem downward through the foramen magnum and into the cervical space. The brain stem houses the 12 cranial nerves. Pressure on this region may result in altered function of these nerves or actual palsies.

Table 18-2 Functional Alterations in Myelodysplasia Related to Level of Lesion

Level of Lesion	Functional Implications
Thoracic	Flaccid paralysis of lower extremities; variable weakness in abdominal trunk musculature; high thoracic level may mean respiratory compromise; absence of bowel and bladder control
High lumbar	Voluntary hip flexion and adduction; flaccid paralysis of knees, ankles, and feet; may walk with extensive braces and crutches; absence of bowel and bladder control
Midlumbar	Strong hip flexion and adduction; fair knee extension; flaccid paralysis of ankles and feet; absence of bowel and bladder control
Low lumbar	Strong hip flexion, extension, and adduction and knee extension; weak ankle and toe mobility; may have limited bowel and bladder function
Sacral	Normal function of lower extremities; normal bowel and bladder function

Data from Farley JA, Dunleavy MJ. Myelodysplasia. In Jackson PL, Vessey JA, editors: *Primary care of the child with a chronic condition,* ed 2, St Louis, 2000, Mosby.

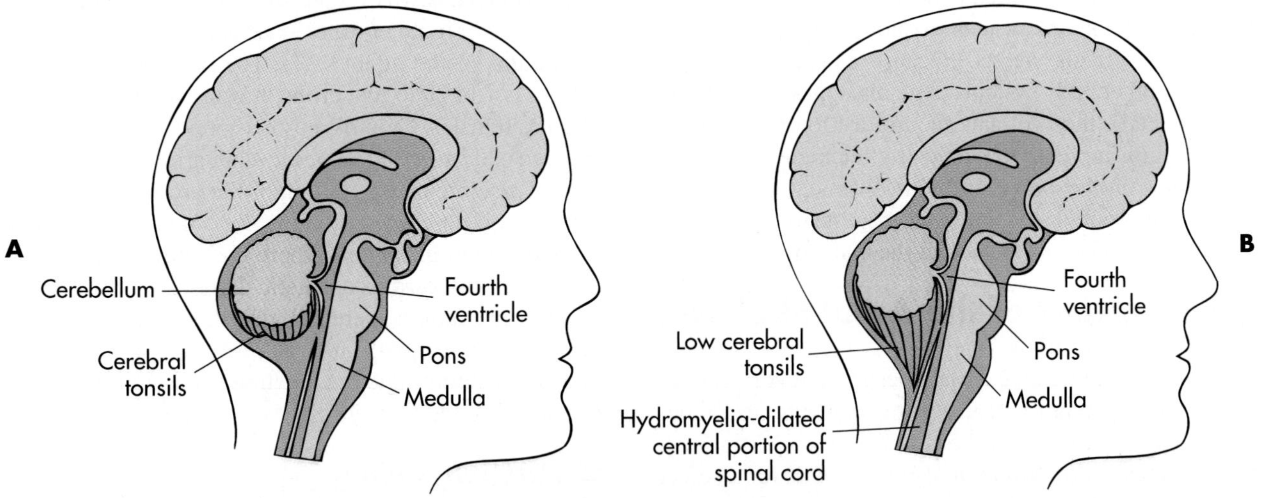

FIG. 18-7 Normal brain and Arnold-Chiari II malformation. Diagram showing normal brain **(A)** and brain with Arnold-Chiari malformation **(B)**.

Dysfunction of the lower cranial nerves is common, and the displacement of this area of the brain results in the compression and elongation of nerves and tissue, which in turn restrict neuronal performance in varying degrees.[5]

Hydrocephalus occurs in 85% of these infants.[6] Seizures also occur in 30% of those with myelodysplasia.[7] Visual and perceptual problems, including ocular palsies, astigmatism, and visuoperceptual deficits, are common.[8] Motor and sensory functions below the level of the lesions are altered. This dysfunction may include degrees of weakness, paralysis, spasticity, and bowel and bladder dysfunction. Often these problems worsen as the child grows and the cord ascends within the vertebral canal, pulling primary scar tissue and tethering the cord.[9] Several musculoskeletal deformities are related to this diagnosis, including clubfoot, dislocation of hip or hips, and poor spinal alignment. Spinal deformities, such as scoliosis and kyphosis, are common.[10]

Tethering of the spinal cord may develop in children with myelodysplasia. The cord becomes caught or tethered from scar tissue as it transcends the vertebral canal with growth. Symptoms related to this problem can include scoliosis, altered gait pattern, changes in muscle strength at or below the lesion, disturbance in urinary and bowel patterns, and back pain.

Evaluation and Treatment

Diagnosis is based on clinical manifestations and examination of the meningeal sac. However, because the pathophysiology of myelodysplasia is determined early in gestation, prenatal diagnosis is possible through ultrasonography. In addition, the presence of a neural tube defect may result in an elevated amniotic fluid α-fetoprotein (AFP) level and subsequent maternal serum AFP levels. Prenatal diagnosis offers the parents the option to terminate the pregnancy or become a candidate for fetal intrauterine repair.[11,12] If they choose to continue the pregnancy, prenatal diagnosis provides the family and the health care team the opportunity to prepare both physically and emotionally for the birth of the child. Cesarean delivery may be recommended to minimize trauma to the open myelomeningocele.[13]

Treatment for the infant with myelomeningocele is early surgical closure of the defect. Because myelodysplasia affects several other body systems (e.g., renal, gastrointestinal, musculoskeletal), these infants require a lifetime, comprehensive, multidisciplinary approach to treatment. The prognosis depends on the extent of the involvement at birth and the success of prophylactic and acute treatment for potential and actual complications that affect the many body systems.

Malformations of the Axial Skeleton

Spina Bifida Occulta

When defects of neural tube closure occur, such as meningocele and myelomeningocele, an accompanying vertebral defect allows the protrusion of the neural tube contents. Such a defect is called **spina bifida.** It also is possible for a defect to occur without any visible exposure of meninges or neural tissue. Because the defect is not apparent to the naked eye (i.e., it is "occult" or hidden), the term **spina bifida occulta** is used. In spina bifida occulta the posterior vertebral laminae have failed to fuse. This extremely common defect occurs to some degree in 10% to 25% of infants. Approximately 80% of these vertebral defects are located in the lumbosacral regions, most commonly in the fifth lumbar vertebra and the first sacral vertebra, and may be detected prenatally with ultrasonic scanning and AFP testing. About 3% of normal adults have spina bifida occulta of the atlas (cervical vertebra 1). The following cutaneous or subcutaneous abnormalities suggest underlying spina bifida:

- Abnormal growth of hair along the spine, which often is either very coarse or very silky
- A midline dimple with or without a sinus tract
- A cutaneous angioma, usually of the "port wine" variety
- A subcutaneous mass, usually representing a lipoma or dermoid cyst

Spina bifida occulta usually causes no serious neurologic dysfunctions.[4] The spinal cord and spinal nerves generally are anatomically and functionally normal. When dysfunctions occur, the common lumbosacral defects cause gait abnormalities, positional deformities of the feet as a result of muscle weakness, or sphincter disturbances of the bladder and bowel. These dysfunctions become evident during periods of rapid growth.

Cranial Deformities

Skull malformations range from minor, insignificant defects to major defects that are incompatible with life.

Acrania

In **acrania** the cranial vault is almost completely absent and an extensive defect of the vertebral column often is present. Acrania associated with anencephaly (absence of brain and spinal column) occurs in approximately 1 per 1000 live births and is incompatible with life. The malformation results from a failure of the cranial end of the neural tube to close during the fourth gestational week. Subsequently, the cranial vault fails to form.

Craniosynostosis

Craniosynostosis (craniostenosis) is the premature closure of one or more of the cranial sutures during the first 18 to 20 months of the infant's life. The incidence of craniosynostosis is 1 in 2000 live births.[14] Males are affected twice as often as females. Craniosynostosis prevents normal skull expansion and causes asymmetric skull growth. Premature closure of a suture causes failure of the growth of the bone located at a right angle to the involved suture. Compensatory growth occurs in regions where the sutures are patent, and this causes the various cosmetic deformities. In the absence of adequate sutures, cerebral growth may exceed the space present. Brain growth may be restricted, and compression may cause neurologic dysfunction from brain damage after 6 months of age (Fig. 18-8).

Pathophysiology

The exact causes of craniosynostosis are unknown, but the condition represents more than a single disorder of embryonic development. One possible explanation is a germ layer disturbance involving the mesenchyma (embryonic connective tissue that gives rise to the connective tissues, blood vessels, and lymphatics). This mesenchymal defect may be caused by a deficiency in enzyme inhibition of ossification. A number of metabolic disorders are accompanied by premature or delayed ossification of cranial bones, suggesting a metabolic mechanism. A genetic defect of hormonal or mineral metabolism may create ossification centers at abnormal sites. Mechanical factors also appear to play a role in craniosynostosis because secondary premature fusion of sutures occurs in microcephaly and after shunting in hydrocephalus.

Clinical Manifestations

Craniosynostosis is classified according to head contour or suture involvement. Final skull contour is determined by the sutures that close, the duration and order of closure, and the ability of other sutures to compensate by expansion. (The frequency and types of craniosynostosis are depicted in Figs. 18-8 and 18-9.)

Premature closure of the sagittal suture, the most common form of craniosynostosis, causes elongation of the skull in the anteroposterior direction. Other anomalies are seen in 25% of these children. When the coronal suture fuses prematurely, the brain expands in a lateral direction. This type of craniosynostosis is associated with a 33% to 66% incidence of associated anomalies. Approximately half of these children are mentally retarded.

Evaluation and Treatment

Diagnosis is made on the basis of physical examination, head circumference measurements, and radiologic examination. Surgical treatment is indicated when closure of multiple sutures causes chronic IICP. Surgery then limits the extent of brain damage. In children with craniosynostosis of one suture, surgery often is performed for cosmetic purposes to limit the appearance of deformity.

Microcephaly

Microcephaly is a defect in brain growth as a whole (see Fig. 18-8). The word *microcephaly* is derived from the

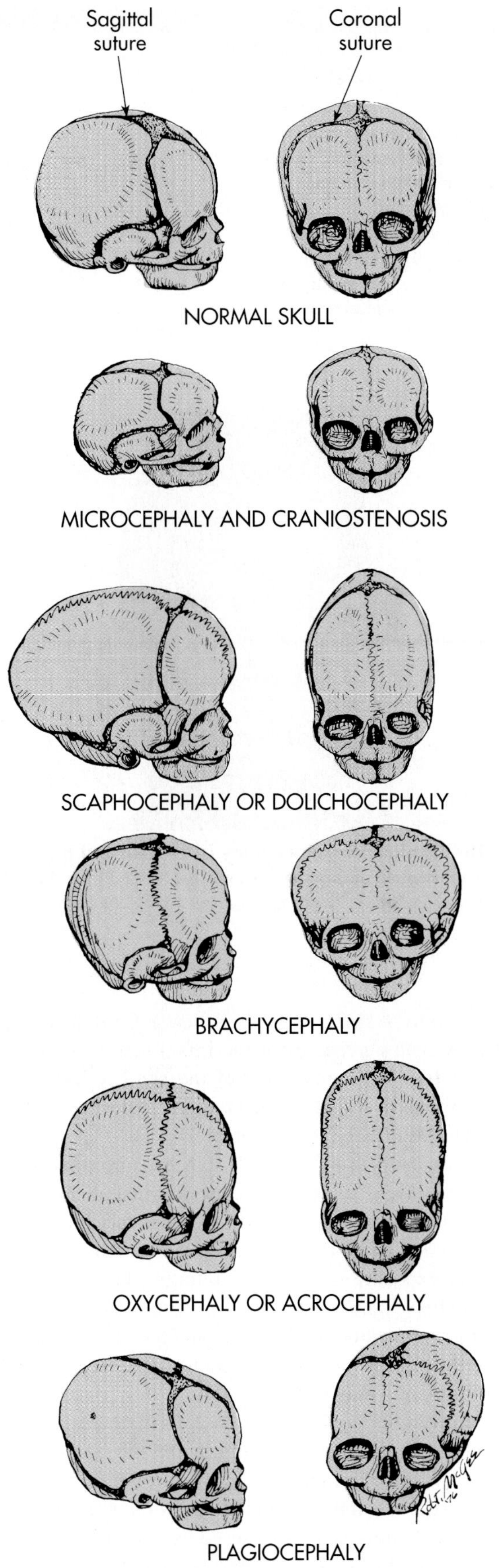

FIG. 18-8 Craniosynostosis. Abnormal head configuration resulting from premature closing of cranial sutures. *Normal skull,* Bones separated by membranous seams until sutures gradually close. *Microcephaly and craniostenosis,* Microcephaly is head circumference more than 2 standard deviations below the mean for age, gender, race, and gestation and reflects a small brain; craniosynostosis is premature closure of sutures. *Scaphocephaly or dolichocephaly* (frequency 56%), Premature closure of sagittal suture, resulting in restricted lateral growth. *Brachycephaly,* Premature closure of coronal suture, resulting in excessive lateral growth. *Oxycephaly or acrocephaly* (frequency 5.8%-12%), Premature closure of all coronal and sagittal sutures, resulting in accelerated upward growth and small head circumference. *Plagiocephaly* (frequency 13%), Unilateral premature closure of coronal suture, resulting in asymmetric growth. (From Wong DL et al: *Whaley and Wong's nursing care of infants and children,* ed 6, St Louis, 1999, Mosby.)

Box 18-1

CAUSES OF MICROENCEPHALY

Defects in Brain Development	Intrauterine Infections	Perinatal and Postnatal Disorders
Hereditary (recessive) microcephaly	Congenital rubella	Intrauterine or neonatal anoxia
Down syndrome and other trisomy syndromes	Cytomegalovirus infection	Severe malnutrition in early infancy
Fetal ionizing radiation exposure	Congenital toxoplasmosis	Neonatal herpesvirus infection
Maternal phenylketonuria	Congenital syphilis	
Seckel syndrome		
Cornelia de Lange syndrome		
Rubinstein-Taybi syndrome		
Smith-Lemli-Opitz syndrome		
Fetal alcohol syndrome		

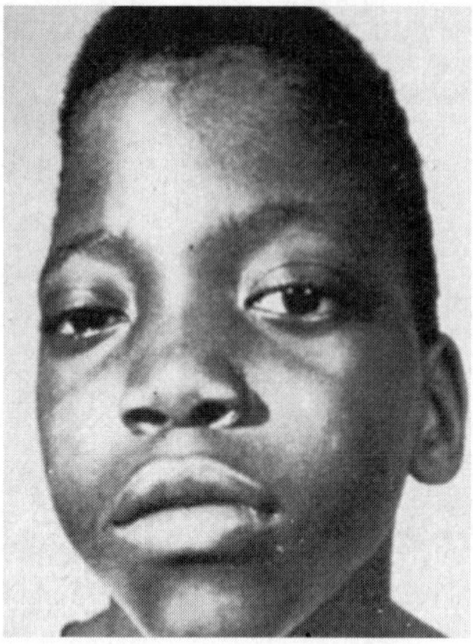

FIG. 18-9 Dolichoscaphocephaly in 14-year-old boy. One of the less threatening of the craniosynostoses. (From Dyken PR, Miller MD: *Facial features of neurologic syndromes,* St Louis, 1980, Mosby.)

Greek (*mikro* = small; *kephale* = head). Cranial size is significantly below average for the infant's age, gender, race, and gestation. The small size of the skull reflects a small brain, except in infants with premature closure of the sutures. The condition is not treatable.

True (primary) microcephaly can be caused by an autosomal recessive disorder, by a chromosomal abnormality, or by toxin exposure during the period of induction and major cell migration (Box 18-1). Radiation, maternal infection, or chemical exposure may be the initiating factor. Secondary microcephaly is associated with a variety of causes. Infection, trauma, metabolic disorders, and anorexia experienced during the third trimester of pregnancy, the perinatal period, or early infancy may be responsible.

Brain weight may be as low as 25% of normal in the microcephalic brain. Both the number and the size of the cortical gyri may be diminished. Growth of the frontal lobes is severely stunted, and the cerebellum often is disproportionately large. In microcephaly caused by perinatal or postnatal disorders, neuronal loss and gliosis may be present in the cerebral cortex. The neurologic manifestations of microcephaly range from decerebrate posture, complete unresponsiveness, and autistic behavior to mild motor impairment, **mental retardation,** and hyperkinesis.

Congenital Hydrocephalus

Congenital hydrocephalus is characterized by an increased volume of CSF. This increase in volume may be caused by a blockage within the ventricular system in which the CSF flows, an imbalance in production of the CSF, or a reduced reabsorption of the CSF that results in ventricular enlargement and IICP. The pressure within the ventricular system pushes and compresses the brain tissue against the skull cavity. When hydrocephalus develops before fusion of the cranial sutures, the skull has the capacity to increase its effort to accommodate this additional space-occupying volume and to preserve neuronal function. The overall incidence of hydrocephalus is approximately 3 per 1000 live births.[9] The incidence of hydrocephalus, excluding the hydrocephalus associated with myelomeningocele, is approximately 0.5 to 1 per 1000 live births, with aqueductal stenosis as the cause for approximately one third of these cases.[2,15] (Types of hydrocephalus are discussed in Chapter 15.)

Pathophysiology

Obstructive hydrocephalus is caused most commonly by congenital aqueduct stenosis. The cerebral aqueduct is narrowed or replaced by multiple channels, or "forks," that end blindly. In a small number of children the stenosis is transmitted as an X-linked recessive trait. The **Dandy-Walker deformity** is a congenital defect of midline cerebellar structures in which hydrocephalus is caused by atresia of the foramina of Luschka or Magendie, leading the ventricular flow of CSF into a "blind pouch." Other causes of obstructions within the ventricular system that can result in hydrocephalus include brain tumors, cysts, trauma, arteriovenous malformations, blood clots, and infections.

CSF travels throughout the ventricular system, surrounds the brain, and is reabsorbed into the venous system by the arachnoid villi. Blockage of the arachnoid villi may occur in conditions such as bacterial or viral meningitis, intraventricular hemorrhage, and subarachnoid hemorrhage, or blockage may result from congenital malformations within this area. In this instance CSF flows or communicates effectively but is unable to be reabsorbed, resulting in hydrocephalus.

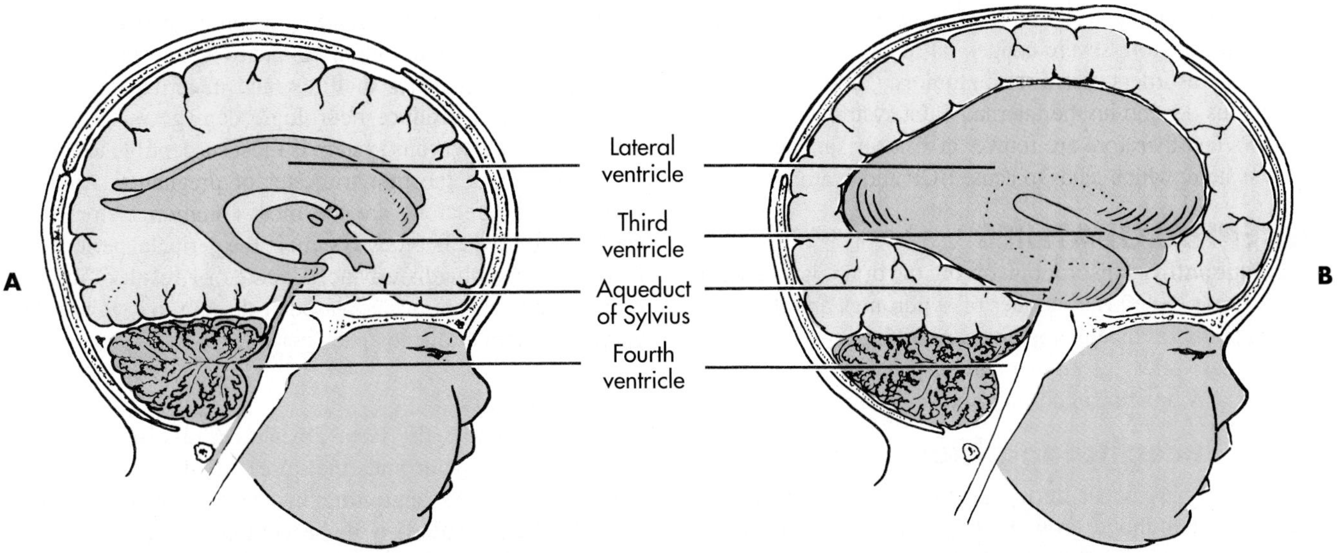

FIG. 18-10 Hydrocephalus. A block in flow of cerebrospinal fluid (CSF). **A,** Patent cerebrospinal fluid circulation. **B,** Enlarged lateral and third ventricles caused by obstruction of circulation—stenosis of aqueduct of Sylvius. (From Wong DL et al: *Whaley and Wong's nursing care of infants and children,* ed 6, St Louis, 1999, Mosby.)

Clinical Manifestations

Congenital hydrocephalus may cause fetal death in utero, or the increased head circumference may require cesarean delivery of the infant. Symptoms of this condition depend directly on the cause and rate of hydrocephalus development. Infants may have no symptoms at birth. During the early weeks of life, the head begins to grow at an abnormal rate. Significant dilation of the ventricles may occur before an abnormal increase in head growth develops. The fontanelles enlarge and become full and bulging (Figs. 18-10 and 18-11). The separation of the cranial sutures leads to a resonant note when the skull is tapped, a manifestation termed **Macewen sign ("cracked-pot" sign).** The eyes may assume a staring expression, with sclera visible above the cornea, called *sunsetting.*

The infant may have difficulty holding the head upright. The scalp skin is thin and shiny, and scalp veins may become prominent. The large cranial vault and the face are disproportionate, and frontal bossing may be present. The infant's cry becomes high pitched as intracranial pressure (ICP) rises; irritability, lethargy, vomiting, and other signs of IICP may develop. Dramatic head growth and enlargement, compression of the optic nerves, and optic chiasm occur in chronic, untreated hydrocephalus. However, because of early surgical intervention, these signs of hydrocephalus rarely are seen. When hydrocephalus develops late in childhood, the head may not have the capacity to enlarge and evidence of IICP is present (see Chapter 15).

The relationship between hydrocephalus and mental retardation has been heavily debated. Correlation between the degree of hydrocephalus and impaired cognitive function often is a result of additional complications, such as severe congenital malformations, acute or chronic infections, or progressive brain tumors. Approximately two thirds of children with uncomplicated congenital hydrocephalus treated successfully with shunting may have normal to borderline intelligence.[15]

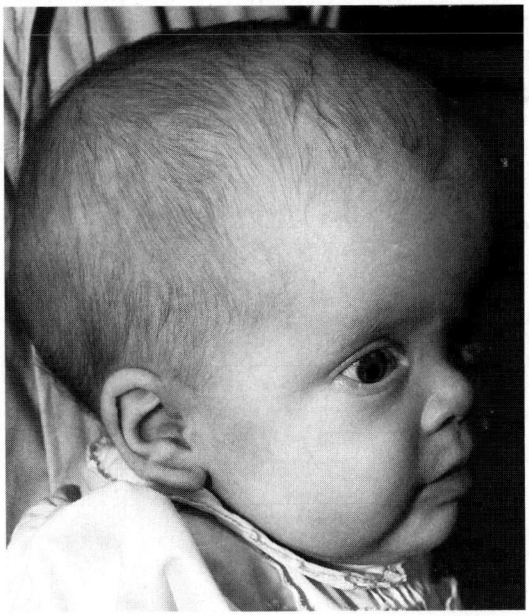

FIG. 18-11 Child with enlarged head caused by hydrocephalus. (From McLaurin DC: *Pediatric neurosurgery,* ed 2, Philadelphia, 1989, W.B. Saunders.)

Evaluation and Treatment

The definitive diagnostic tool for hydrocephalus is computed tomography (CT), and magnetic resonance imaging (MRI) may add information about the specific cause of the hydrocephalus. In infancy, head circumference measurements also are obtained and monitored. The treatment is surgical placement of a shunt to divert the excess CSF from the ventricular cavity to other areas of the body. Several types of shunts are available. The main objective of any shunt system is to decrease ICP and preserve neuronal function. With neurosurgical intervention and follow-up, the 5-year survival usually is greater than 80%. Most deaths that occur within this category result from severe congenital malformations and/or progressive disorders such as brain tumors. Children with hydrocephalus depend on the internal shunt system to maintain safe ICPs and therefore are forever at risk for sudden failure of this system, which leads to acute IICP and death.

ENCEPHALOPATHIES

Encephalopathy, a disorder involving the brain, is a general category that includes a number of syndromes and diseases (see Chapter 15). Encephalopathies in children are associated with a great variety of known and suspected causes. These disorders may be acute or chronic and static or progressive.

Static Encephalopathies

Brain injury may occur during gestation or birth or at any time during childhood growth and development, causing a static, nonprogressive disorder. The clinical manifestations depend on the site and extent of the injury, as well as the age of the child and stage of development at the time of injury. Varying degrees of impairment may result from diffuse or localized injury to the cortex. For example, cerebral palsy results when the motor areas of the brain are injured. Injury to the occipital lobe of the cerebral cortex early in gestation can interfere with normal cerebral maturation and result in future blindness. Cognitive impairment may follow diffuse cerebral injury. Seizures also may develop from cortical injury, particularly if scar tissue remains.

Prenatal factors that affect the developing nervous system may be endogenous or exogenous. The fetus may be affected by impaired embryo implantation, chromosomal abnormalities, infection, trauma, radiation, and toxic substances. Maternal toxemia, diabetes mellitus, and maternal nutritional deficiencies can produce neurologic damage in the fetus. The developing nervous system is most susceptible to injury occurring during the first trimester of pregnancy. Anoxia, trauma, and infections are the most common factors that cause injury to the nervous system in the perinatal period. Infections, metabolic disturbances (acute or a result of inborn errors), trauma, toxins, and vascular disease may injure the nervous system in the postnatal period.

Cerebral Palsy

Cerebral palsy is the term given to a diverse group of nonprogressive syndromes that affect the brain and cause motor dysfunction beginning in early infancy. Cerebral palsy can be classified on the basis of neurologic signs and symptoms. The major types are spasticity, ataxia, dyskinesia, and a mix of one or more of the three. Although cerebral palsy is, by definition, nonprogressive, its clinical manifestations change with growth and maturation of the child.

Cerebral palsy is one of the most common crippling disorders of childhood, affecting nearly 500,000 children in the United States alone. Although the exact incidence is unknown, studies suggest that the incidence is 1 to 2.3 cases of cerebral palsy per 1000 live births.[16] Causes of cerebral palsy are numerous, and both genetic and environmental factors may be responsible. These factors can occur during the prenatal, perinatal, or postnatal period (Table 18-3).

Table 18-3 Cerebral Palsy: Predisposing Factors and Known Causes

Risk Factors	Associated Causes
PRENATAL	
Maternal	Metabolic diseases
	Nutritional deficiencies (e.g., anemia)
	Twin or multiple births
	Bleeding
	Toxemia
	Blood incompatibilities
	Exposure to radiation
	Infection (e.g., rubella, toxoplasmosis, cytomegalic inclusion disease)
	Premature labor
Prematurity	Asphyxia leading to cerebral hemorrhage
Genetic factors	Absence of corpus callosum, aqueductal stenosis, cerebellar hypoplasia
Congenital anomalies of the brain	Unknown causes not evident on clinical examination
PERINATAL	Anesthesia or analgesia during labor and delivery
	Mechanical trauma during delivery
	Immaturity at birth
	Metabolic disorders (e.g., hyperbilirubinemia, hypoglycemia, amino acid disorders, hyperosmolality)
	Electrolyte disturbances (e.g., hypernatremia, hypoglycemia)
POSTNATAL	Head trauma
	Infections (e.g., meningitis, encephalitis)
	Cerebrovascular accidents
	Toxicosis
	Environmental toxins (e.g., lead ingestion, methyl mercury ingestion from contaminated fish)

Pathophysiology

Several factors, alone or in combination, can produce brain damage that leads to cerebral palsy. Prenatal cerebral hypoxia can be responsible for systemic degeneration of immature areas of the brain and can interfere with cell maturation. The severity of the damage depends on the gestational age at the time of the injury and the degree of injury sustained.

Low birth weight and birth asphyxia are commonly identified risk factors for cerebral palsy.[17,18] Hypoxia and asphyxia are known to cause edema in the brain. Lack of oxygen and the incorporation of amino acids during protein synthesis lead to acidosis. Carbon dioxide and lactic acid accumulate with acidosis, causing osmotic pressure changes. This condition contributes to generalized cerebral swelling and CNS damage.

Vascular abnormalities, arterial or venous stasis, and thrombosis can occur as a result of tissue hypoxia or as unrelated structural alterations. These anomalies may result in direct brain trauma that leads to infarction, intraventricular hemorrhage, and subarachnoid hemorrhage. Intraventricular hemorrhage is a common cause of death in newborn infants. Such injuries contribute to CNS damage.

Physical trauma to the central or peripheral nervous system can occur during the birthing process. Linear and depressed fractures are seen in newborn infants when head molding is extreme, with resultant hemorrhages and tears of the tentorium or falx cerebri. Tearing of the superficial cerebral veins is a relatively common occurrence and causes a thin layer of blood over the cerebral convexity. This blood may irritate the brain and result in CNS dysfunction. The infant's position during delivery may cause stretching and damage to nerves. Breech deliveries can cause traumatic injury to the brain stem or spinal cord, resulting in a more localized area of impairment. Malformations of the CNS play an important role in brain injury from perinatal trauma, and they predispose the infant to greater probability of sustained injury to the CNS. Both faulty maturation of the nervous system and a greater vulnerability to perinatal trauma and hypoxia are responsible for a high incidence of neurologic dysfunction in the preterm infant. Genetic, teratogenic, and early pregnancy influences on the development of cerebral palsy are not yet fully understood.[19]

Clinical Manifestations

The syndromes associated with cerebral palsy are classified according to the predominant clinical manifestations. **Spastic cerebral palsy** is associated with increased muscle tone, prolonged primitive reflexes, exaggerated deep tendon reflexes, clonus, rigidity of the extremities, scoliosis, and contractures. This results from motor neuron involvement and injury to the cerebral cortex in either one or both hemispheres and accounts for approximately 65% to 75% of cerebral palsy cases.

Dyskinetic cerebral palsy is associated with extreme difficulty in fine motor coordination and purposeful movements. Movements are jerky, uncontrolled, and abrupt, resulting from injury to the basal ganglia or extrapyramidal tracts. This form of cerebral palsy accounts for approximately 20% to 25% of cases. **Ataxic cerebral palsy** manifests with gait disturbances and instability. The infant with this form of cerebral palsy may have hypotonia at birth, but stiffness of the trunk muscles develops by late infancy. This lack of flexibility exaggerates the infant's inability to balance body position without support. Persistence of this increased tone in truncal muscles affects the child's gait and ability to maintain equilibrium. This form of cerebral palsy accounts for approximately 5% of cases. A child may have symptoms of each of these cerebral palsy types, which leads to a mixed-variety disorder that accounts for approximately 13% of cases.

Children with cerebral palsy often have associated neurologic disorders, such as seizures (35% to 50%), intellectual impairment ranging from mild to severe (50% to 75%), and visual impairment (50%). Because standardized intelligence tests do not allow for the physical handicaps of cerebral palsy, the incidence of associated cognitive impairment is uncertain. Other associated complications include but are not limited to hearing impairment, communication disorders, respiratory problems, bowel and bladder problems, and orthopedic disabilities.[20]

Evaluation and Treatment

Diagnosis of cerebral palsy is made on the basis of neurologic examination and history. The management of children with cerebral palsy varies with age, type and severity of involvement, and associated disorders. Thus the scope of care required by the child and family includes social and educational intervention and a multidisciplinary team approach.

Although the brain injury is static, the clinical picture of cerebral palsy may change with growth and development. Therefore a fundamental component to an effective treatment regimen includes ongoing assessment, evaluation, and revision of the child's overall management plan. The use of intrathecal baclofen pumps and botulinium toxin has shown some improvement in selected children with cerebral palsy.[4,21]

Inherited Metabolic Disorders of the Central Nervous System

A large number of inherited metabolic disorders have been identified. Because these disorders are inherited, their manifestations usually occur in infancy and childhood. Typically these metabolic disorders damage the entire CNS so extensively that these children do not survive to adulthood. The clinical syndromes of the inherited metabolic disorders depend on the nature of the biochemical defect and the stage of nervous system maturation. (Table 18-4 lists some of these inherited metabolic disorders.) Defects in amino acid and lipid metabolism are more common than rarely occurring defects in carbohydrate metabolism.

Defects in Amino Acid Metabolism

Biochemical defects in amino acid metabolism may be classified as (1) those in which the transport of amino acid is impaired, (2) those involving an enzyme or cofactor deficiency, and (3) those grouped around certain chemical

Table 18-4 Inherited Metabolic Disorders of the Central Nervous System

Age of Onset	Disorder
Neonatal period	Pyridoxine dependency, galactosemia, maple syrup urine disease and its variant, phenylketonuria (PKU)
Early infancy	Tay-Sachs disease and its variants, infantile Gaucher disease, infantile Niemann-Pick disease, Krabbe disease (leukodystrophy), Farber lipogranulomatosis, Pelizaeus-Merzbacher disease and other sudanophilic leukodystrophies, spongy degeneration, Alexander disease, Alpers disease, Leigh disease (subacute necrotizing encephalomyelopathy), congenital lactic acidosis, Zellweger encephalopathy, Lowe disease (oculocerebrorenal disease)
Late infancy and early childhood	Disorders of amino acid metabolism, metachromatic leukodystrophy, late infantile GM1 gangliosidosis, late infantile Gaucher and Niemann-Pick diseases, neuroaxonal dystrophy, mucopolysaccharidosis, mucolipidosis, fucosidosis, mannosidosis, aspartylglycosaminuria, amaurotic idiocy (Jansky-Bielschowsky disease, Batten disease, Vogt-Spielmeyer disease, neuronal ceroid lipofuscinosis), Cockayne syndrome
Later childhood and adolescence	Progressive cerebellar ataxias of childhood and adolescence, hepatolenticular degeneration (Wilson disease), Hallervorden-Spatz disease, Lesch-Nyhan syndrome and other uremic states, familial calcification of vessels in basal ganglia and cerebellum, familial polymyoclonus, chronic familial leukodystrophy, homocystinuria, Fabry disease

components, such as sulfur-containing amino acids.[22] Most of the disorders in the literature described to date suggest that the absence of enzymatic activity most often is caused by the genetically determined absence of the enzyme protein.

Diseases caused by an enzymatic deficiency are associated with increased blood concentrations of the amino acid whose degradation pathway is impaired and with the presence of the amino acid in the urine. Because the normal pathway is blocked, small amounts of certain metabolites are found in the blood. Thus in certain diseases, an increase of compromised amino acids and unusual metabolites may appear in blood and urine concentrates.[23]

Phenylketonuria. **Phenylketonuria (PKU)** is an inborn error of metabolism characterized by the inability of the body to convert the essential amino acid phenylalanine to tyrosine (Fig. 18-12). PKU is caused by phenylalanine hydroxylase deficiency and has a prevalence rate of 1 per 10,000 worldwide.[24,25] Because of its genetic component and distribution, this statistical prevalence varies widely on the basis of geographic and ethnic differences.[26] Most natural food proteins contain about 15% phenylalanine, an essential amino acid. Phenylalanine hydroxylase controls the conversion of this essential amino acid to tyrosine in the liver. The body uses tyrosine in the biosynthesis of protein, melanin, thyroxine, and the catecholamines in the brain and adrenal medulla. Phenylalanine hydroxylase deficiency causes an accumulation of phenylalanine in the serum and, subsequently, in the urinary excretion of abnormal metabolites called *phenyl acids.* One of these phenyl acids, phenylpyruvic acid, gives the urine a characteristic musty odor and is responsible for the name given to the disorder. Such high blood levels of phenylalanine prevent sufficient neutral amino acid entry into the brain, which contributes to the neuropathologic process of PKU.[27] Abnormalities occur, such as anomalous development of the CNS, defective myelination, cystic degeneration of the gray and white matter, and disturbances in cortical layers. Unfortunately, brain damage occurs before the metabolites can be detected in the urine, and damage continues as long as phenylalanine levels remain high.

Clinical manifestations related to CNS damage range from mild to severe behavioral disturbances, self-abusive tendencies, and seizures. Because of the lack of tyrosine and its relationship to the biosynthesis of melanin, children with PKU have a characteristic phenotype that includes blond hair, blue eyes, and fair skin. Children with genetically darker complexions may be red haired or brunette.

Less severe variants of this disorder are caused by defects in the phenylalanine hydroxylase *system* rather than the phenylalanine hydroxylase itself. This related disorder, known as **hyperphenylalaninemia (HPA),** occurs when plasma phenylalanine levels rise above normal but do not rise as high as in PKU.[25]

Most children develop normally on a regular diet. Nonselective newborn screening is used to detect PKU and HPA in the United States and in more than 30 countries. Such programs are the greatest source of referrals and allow for accurate interpretation and follow-up of test results, including appropriate genetic and nutrition counseling.[26]

Treatment for PKU involves restriction of phenylalanine in the diet to maintain a nontoxic level. The diet must be supplemented with adequate sources of energy, protein, and nutrients to allow for optimum growth and brain development. Supplementation of tyrosine also may be required if plasma levels are low. The child benefits from ideal management that begins at birth and continues throughout the life span, especially before conception and throughout the mother's pregnancy.[26]

Defects in Lipid Metabolism

Disorders of lipid metabolism are termed **lysosomal storage diseases** because each disorder in this group can be traced to a missing lysosomal enzyme. (Lysosomes, the vesicles within the cell whose primary function is to degrade the breakdown products of cellular metabolism, are dis-

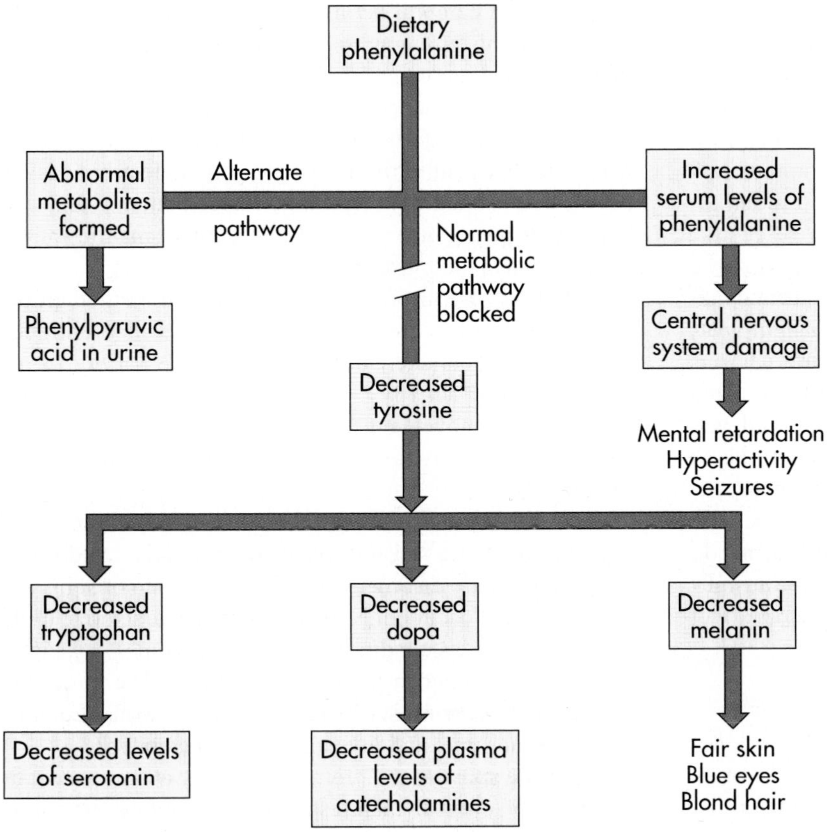

FIG. 18-12 Metabolic errors and consequences in phenylketonuria. (Redrawn from Wong DL et al: *Whaley and Wong's nursing care of infants and children,* ed 6, St Louis, 1999, Mosby.)

cussed in Chapter 1.) An estimated 25 to 30 enzymes within the lysosomes participate in the breakdown of lipids, carbohydrates, proteins, and proteolipids (see Chapter 2). A missing or defective enzyme causes an excessive accumulation of a particular cell function. The enzyme defect may occur in the brain, liver, spleen, bone, or lung, thus involving several organ systems. Therapy has been unsuccessful to date.

Tay-Sachs disease. Perhaps the best known of the lysosomal storage disorders is **Tay-Sachs disease,** an autosomal recessive disorder.[28] Approximately 80% of individuals diagnosed are of Jewish ancestry, although sporadic cases appear in the non-Jewish population.[23]

In Tay-Sachs disease the pathologic changes predominate in the CNS, but neurons throughout the body contain characteristic changes in the cytoplasm. With time, neurons become distorted and balloon, and microglial cells, which also are swollen and filled with large granules, proliferate. Cystic degeneration of the cerebral white matter and atrophy of the cerebellar hemispheres often occur. The number of neurons is diminished. Changes in the spinal cord, particularly in the motor cells of the anterior horn of the cord, also are characteristic. Involvement of this region of the spinal cord results in hypotonia, hyporeflexia, and overall weakness.

Onset of this disease usually occurs when the infant is 3 to 6 months old. A loss of milestones is associated with an excessive startle response. Seizures, muscular rigidity, and blindness become prominent after the first year of life, and head size may increase. Death usually occurs by 2 to 5 years of age. No beneficial therapy has been developed. Genetic counseling programs are available, and some states require screening techniques for couples and those at risk who may be carriers. One in 25 Ashkenazi Jews carry this recessive gene.

Seizure Disorders in Children

Epilepsy

The incidence of epilepsy varies greatly with age. The incidence of epilepsy is estimated to be 0.5% to 1% of children with onset during infancy or childhood.[29] Infants are particularly susceptible during the first 12 months of life. The incidence decreases with age; 75% to 80% of epilepsy cases initially occur before 20 years of age, with 30% of the cases initially occurring within the first 4 years of life. Approximately 181,000 persons in the United States are newly affected each year.[29]

◆ *Pathophysiology*

Seizures are the abnormal discharge of electrical activity within the brain. When a sufficient number of neurons become overexcited, they discharge abnormally, which sometimes results in clinical manifestations. If clinical manifestations do occur, the specific physical activity that occurs may depend on the origin of the electrical activity and its extent within the brain. Repeated recurrence of seizure activity is known as **epilepsy.** Seizures may result from an underlying disorder of the CNS or a disorder that directly or indirectly affects normal CNS function. Certain types of seizures may have a genetic component or familial predisposition, or they can result from maternal diseases or congenital structural anomalies of the CNS. During the newborn period, asphyxia, intracranial hemorrhage, CNS infections, injury, electrolyte imbalances, and inborn errors of metabolism may cause seizures. Etiologic factors of seizures in older infants and children generally are the same as during the first month of life. Often the cause of seizures is unknown.

Seizures and seizure patterns may change as a child grows and develops. The differences between the immature and mature nervous systems may help to explain the changing patterns of clinical seizures with age. The immature nervous system has a reduced capacity for sustaining well-organized seizures. Intracortical connections are poorly developed, and the sending of impulses throughout the cortex is limited. At the cellular level, neurons are less capable of firing in repetitive high-frequency bursts. The excitatory output of a seizure focus is further diminished because the affected neurons do not act synchronously. In addition, changing neurotransmitters, immaturity of cells, and ongoing postnatal factors affect seizure expression in children.

Clinical Manifestations

The clinical manifestations at the time of diagnosis vary depending on the primary cause and the extent and involvement of abnormal electrical discharges within the neuronal tissue. Because of the diversities and complexities that seizure activity invariably displays, an international classification system was adopted. This classification system groups seizures with similar clinical manifestations. Its general purpose is to assist the clinician with the assessment of the clinical course, the identification of the most appropriate treatment, and the evaluation of the individual's response to treatment (see Table 15-8).

The international classification system of epilepsy contains three major groupings: (1) partial seizures, (2) generalized seizures, and (3) unclassified epileptic seizures. Each major grouping is then divided into subsets on the basis of clinical manifestations and electroencephalogram (EEG) findings.

Partial seizures are characterized by seizure activity that begins in and usually is limited to one part of either the left or right hemisphere. A *simple partial seizure* refers to seizure activity that occurs without loss of consciousness. A *complex partial seizure* refers to seizure activity that occurs with impairment of consciousness. The clinical activity displayed by the individual is contingent on the particular part of the cortex from which the seizure is generated. For example, partial seizures may result in abnormal motor activity, such as twitching or loss of tone, or sensory changes, such as tingling or numbness.[30,31]

Simple partial seizures generally are confined to one hemisphere, whereas a complex partial seizure involves both cerebral hemispheres. A simple or complex partial seizure may evolve into a generalized tonic-clonic, tonic, or clonic convulsion.

Generalized seizures are those in which the first clinical manifestations indicate that the seizure activity starts in or involves both cerebral hemispheres. Consciousness may be impaired in this grouping of seizures. The clinical manifestations may include convulsive activity (tonic-tonic, tonic, or clonic activity) or nonconvulsive activity (absence seizures). Absence seizures do not follow a Mendelian pattern of inheritance that results from a single gene defect but, rather, have an autosomal dominant inheritance pattern.[32] Because both hemispheres are involved, the clinical manifestations almost always are bilateral.

Not all seizure disorders fit neatly into a classified grouping. These seizures are referred to as **unclassified epileptic seizures** and characteristically have a wide variety of abnormal clinical activity. Examples of this activity include rhythmic eye movements, chewing, and swimming movements. These activities are commonly seen in neonatal seizures.[33,33a,34]

In addition to the seizures classified by the international system, there are several types of epileptic syndromes. These are seizure disorders that display a group of signs and symptoms that occur collectively and that characterize or indicate a particular condition. Several syndromes associated with epilepsy occur in infants and children. The three syndromes that occur most often are infantile spasms, Lennox-Gastaut syndrome, and juvenile myoclonic epilepsy.

Infantile spasms are a form of epilepsy characterized by a variety of clinical manifestations. The infant may have episodes of sudden flexion or extension movements involving the neck, trunk, and extremities. Clinical manifestations of the resulting spasms may range from subtle head nods to violent body contractions, commonly referred to as *jackknife seizures*. Onset of infantile spasms usually is between 4 and 8 months of age and may be idiopathic or may occur in response to a CNS insult.[35] An EEG will display the classic hypsarrhythmic pattern of epileptic spike and wave discharges on a slow, disorganized background.[36] Infantile spasm manifests a typical clinical course. The "spasms" usually happen in clusters and occur 5 to 150 times per day. They usually are worse when the infant is waking up or falling asleep. Once begun, the seizure activity increases in intensity and severity over time. Invariably a loss of developmental milestones is associated with this syndrome.

Lennox-Gastaut syndrome is an epileptic syndrome characterized by an onset of seizures early in childhood, usually around 1 to 5 years of age. This syndrome includes a variety of generalized seizures—predominantly tonic-clonic, atonic (drop attacks), akinetic, absence, and myoclonic activity. Mental retardation and delayed psychomotor development often are associated with this syndrome.[30,36]

Juvenile myoclonic epilepsy is a primary generalized epilepsy that usually affects adolescents and young adults. Studies have indicated a possible locus on chromosome 6p and 15q14 as a cause for this type of epilepsy.[32] It is a relatively benign form of epilepsy involving myoclonic jerks of the neck, shoulders, and arms. The seizures may occur singularly or repetitively. This form of epilepsy commonly is associated with a normal neurologic examination, normal intelligence, and a positive family history of seizures.[36]

Evaluation and Treatment

Diagnosis of epilepsy and seizure classification are based on history, clinical presentation, physical and developmental examination, and the record of milestone achievements. Evaluation and testing include an EEG to isolate the focus or origin and involvement of seizure activity, CT scan, and/or MRI of the brain to investigate the presence of a lesion or abnormal tissue. A complete metabolic workup must be reviewed to explore the possibility of deficiency or malabsorption.

Specific treatment for epilepsy is directed at the particular clinical manifestations or syndrome of seizure activity and its underlying causes. Treatment usually begins with the use of anticonvulsant medications. Often the epileptic pattern and clinical course require more than one drug to control the abnormal discharges.[34]

Surgery provides treatment for some forms of epilepsy. As with medical interventions, surgical therapy focuses on the particular clinical manifestations of seizure activity. Surgical interventions include resection of brain tissue—that is, partial or complete severing of the corpus callosum. Some seizures are managed through a ketogenic diet. Children with intractable epilepsy have shown some benefit using the vagal nerve stimulator.[37,38]

Prognosis for epilepsy depends greatly on the type and severity of the disorder, the age of onset, coexisting factors, and the type and success of medical, surgical, and nutritional therapy. Several studies have estimated that approximately 40% to 50% of children diagnosed with epilepsy will be seizure free.

Benign Febrile Seizures

Benign febrile seizures occur in 3% to 4% of children younger than 5 years. These seizures usually are brief and self-limited and occur most frequently between the ages of 6 months and 5 years, with peak age at 14 to 18 months.[4,39]

> **NUTRITION & DISEASE**
>
> **Ketogenic Diet in Children with Epilepsy**
>
> The goal of the ketogenic diet in some children with epilepsy is to create and maintain a state of ketosis, which appears to facilitate reduced seizure activity. The diet may be helpful to children who do not respond to conventional therapy or have intolerable side effects. The two basic approaches to the ketogenic diet are (1) a traditional approach with four parts fat to one part carbohydrate/protein in the diet and (2) the medium-chain triglyceride (MCT) approach, in which MCTs make up about 50% to 70% of the diet. Either diet may be unpalatable and difficult to follow, particularly if the child has free access to food. Carbohydrates can be added by 5-g increments after 3-6 months if there has been no seizure activity provided ketosis is maintained. Both dietary approaches include adequate protein for growth. The mechanism is not clearly understood, but it may be caused by a change in neuronal metabolism in which a ketone body behaves as an inhibitory neurotransmitter, producing an anticonvulsant effect on the body. The benefits of the diet usually last less than 2 to 3 years and appear to be less effective with older children.
>
> Data from Katyal NG et al: The ketogenic diet in refractory epilepsy: the experience of Children's Hospital of Pittsburgh, *Clin Pediatr (Phil)* 39(3):153, 2000; Lefevre F, Aronson N: Ketogenic diet for the treatment of refractory epilepsy in children: a systematic review of efficacy, *Pediatrics* 105(4):E46, 2000.

Pathophysiology

The pathogenesis of benign febrile seizures is unknown. A familial incidence of benign febrile seizures indicates a genetic predisposition to the problem. Factors that contribute to susceptibility include age, degree and rate of temperature elevation, and nature of the particular fever-inducing illness. Any disorder producing a high fever may provoke benign febrile seizures in susceptible children.

Clinical Manifestations

Characteristic features distinguish benign febrile seizures from seizures precipitated by fever:

1. Benign febrile seizures are rare before 9 months or after 5 years of age.
2. The convulsion occurs with a rise in temperature greater than 39° C.
3. An acute respiratory or ear infection usually is present, with no evidence of CNS infection or inflammation.
4. Most seizures occur during the first 24 hours of the illness.
5. The convulsion is short (15 minutes or less), generalized, and predominantly tonic.
6. Interictal EEG is normal.
7. The seizure usually does not recur during the same infection.
8. No acute systemic metabolic disorder is present.

Complex febrile seizures have characteristic features similar to these, except that (1) they have a longer duration than do benign febrile seizures, usually longer than 15 minutes; (2) they have focal characteristics; and (3) they usually occur more than once in a 24-hour period. Complex febrile seizures are considered a risk factor for the development of epilepsy.[40]

Evaluation and Treatment

Reduction of elevated body temperature usually controls benign febrile seizures without anticonvulsant medication. In selected individuals, phenobarbital is the most effective medication for preventing recurrence of benign febrile seizures.

Status Epilepticus

Status epilepticus is defined as the state of continuing or recurring seizure activity in which the recovery from seizure activity is incomplete. Seizure activity is unrelenting and usually lasts for 30 minutes or more. Any one of the seizure activities discussed can evolve into status epilepticus. Status epilepticus is a medical emergency that requires immediate intervention.[29]

Acute Encephalopathies

Reye Syndrome

Reye syndrome is characterized by encephalopathy and fatty changes in a variety of organs, especially the liver. The incidence of Reye syndrome has declined sharply over the past 20 years, coinciding with increased public awareness of the association between ingestion of aspirin during illness and subsequent development of Reye syndrome.[41] Although Reye syndrome is becoming increasingly rare in the population, a brief overview of it is important for the following reasons:

1. It may be considered a prototype for acute hepatic encephalopathies.
2. The potential for recurrence is a factor.
3. The use of acetaminophen over aspirin should be considered important and discussed with the parents when obtaining a history.

Pathophysiology

Reye syndrome usually is associated with influenza B or varicella virus infections, although a wide variety of associated viral infections have been reported. A distinct clinical syndrome is apparent. The profound hypoglycemia, hyperammonemia, and an increase in short-chain fatty acids in the serum after liver involvement are responsible for the cerebral manifestations. The liver shows diffuse deposits of lipids and absence of any inflammatory reaction or necrosis. Fatty degeneration of the kidneys leads to azotemia (excess urea in the blood). The brain is extremely edematous.[42,43]

The cause and pathogenesis of Reye syndrome remain unclear. The development of Reye syndrome has been linked to the administration of salicylates (aspirin). The American Association of Pediatrics has recommended not administering aspirin to children who have varicella or flu-like symptoms. A direct relationship clearly exists between this recommendation and the overall decrease in incidence of Reye syndrome. A further reduction may be seen with administration of the varicella vaccine to children between 12 to 18 months of age.[43]

Clinical Manifestations

Typically Reye syndrome develops in a previously healthy child who is recovering from varicella, influenza B, or upper respiratory infection, or gastroenteritis. The various clinical states are as follows:

Stage I Vomiting, lethargy, drowsiness
Stage II Disorientation, delirium, aggressiveness and combativeness, central neurologic hyperventilation, shallow breathing, hyperactive reflexes, stupor
Stage III Obtundation, coma, hyperventilation, decorticate rigidity
Stage IV? Deepening coma, decerebrate rigidity, loss of ocular reflexes, large fixed pupils, divergent eye movements
Stage V? Seizures, loss of deep tendon reflexes, flaccidity, respiratory arrest

Evaluation and Treatment

According to the Centers for Disease Control and Prevention (CDC), the following conditions must be present for diagnosis of Reye syndrome:

1. Acute, noninflammatory encephalopathy documented by (a) alteration in level of consciousness and, if available, (b) a record of CSF containing leukocytes (8/mm^3) and (c) a histologic specimen demonstrating cerebral edema without perivascular or meningeal irritation
2. Hepatomegaly documented by either a liver biopsy or autopsy
3. No more reasonable explanation for cerebral and hepatic abnormalities

The severity of the condition is inversely related to the age of the child at the onset of the illness.

The management of children with Reye syndrome ranges from simple monitoring to extremely complex neurointensive care. Treatment and outcome vary depending on the stage of involvement and the individual child's symptoms.

Intoxications of the Central Nervous System

Drug-induced encephalopathies always must be considered a possibility in the child with unexplained neurologic changes. Such encephalopathies may result from accidental ingestion, therapeutic overdose, intentional overdose, or ingestion of environmental toxins (the most commonly ingested poisons are listed in Box 18-2). About 2 million childhood poisonings that require medical attention occur each year. Approximately 1000 children die each year of poisonings.

High blood levels of lead occur in lead poisoning. If lead poisoning is not treated, lead encephalopathy will result and cause serious and irreversible neurologic damage[44] (Fig. 18-13). Those at greatest risk are children 2 to 3 years of age and those prone to picas. **Pica** is the habitual, purposeful, and compulsive ingestion of nonfood substances such as clay, dirt, and paint chips. Lead intoxication also may occur from long-term exposure to smelters, sniffing of gasoline, and ingestion of airborne lead.

An estimated 225,000 children in the United States and 4% of children 6 months to 5 years of age have excessive amounts of lead in their blood. Black children have a six times greater incidence of symptoms than white children.

Box 18-2
COMMON POISONS

Pharmacologic Agents	Heavy Metals	Miscellaneous Agents
Acetaminophen	Lead	Botulism toxin
Amphetamines	Acute	Alcohols
Anticonvulsants	Chronic	Ethyl, isopropyl, methyl
Antidepressants	Mercury	Pesticides
Antihistamines	Thallium	Organophosphates
Atropine	Arsenic	Chlorinated hydrocarbons
Barbiturates		Mushrooms
Methadone		Venoms
Phencyclidine		Snake bite
Salicylates		Tick paralysis
Tranquilizers		Ethylene glycol

Data from Swaiman KF: *Pediatric neurology: principles and practice,* vol 2, ed 3, St Louis, 1999, Mosby.

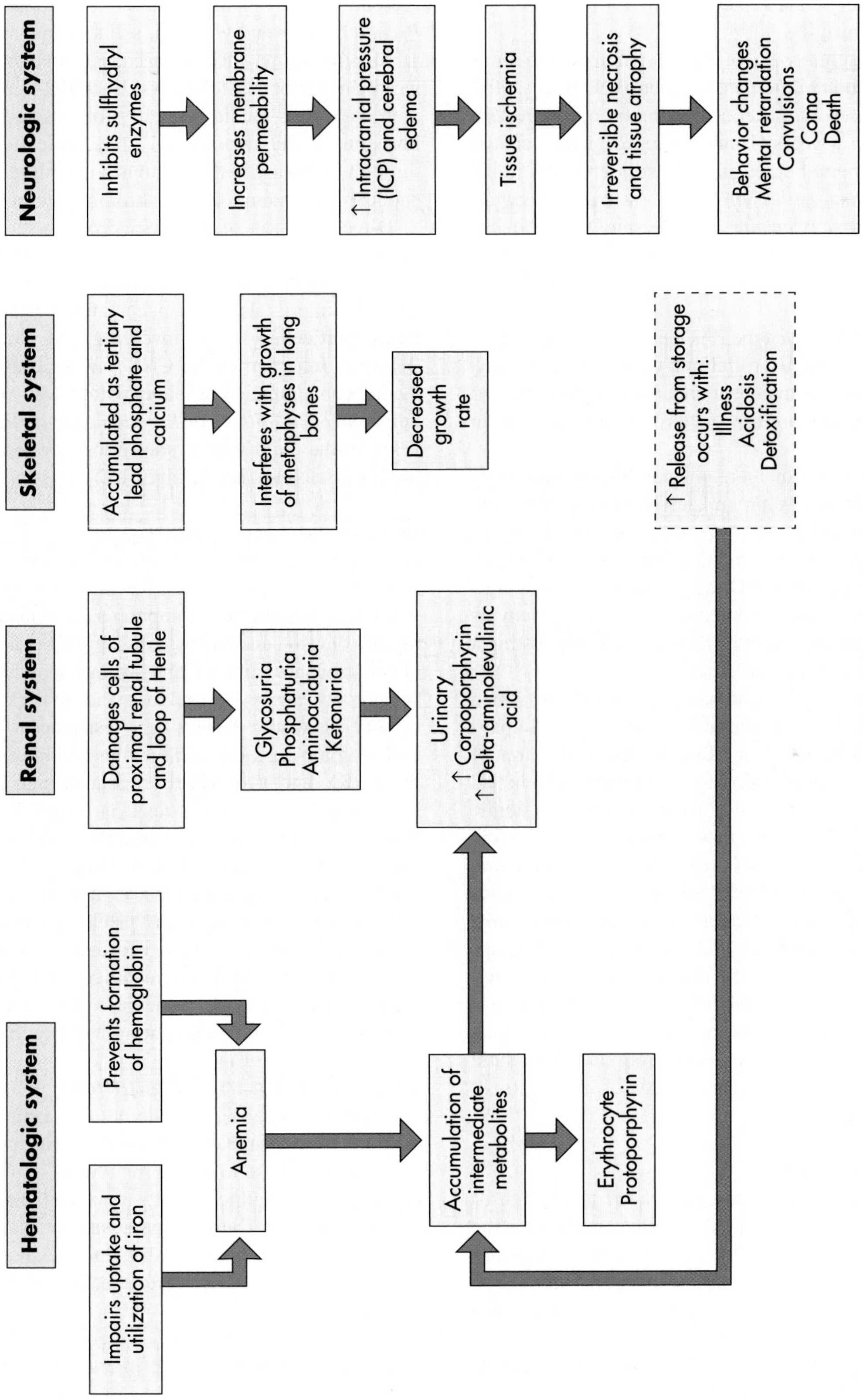

FIG. 18-13 Systemic effects of increased lead absorption in children.

Meningitis

Meningitis refers to inflammation of the meningeal coverings of the brain. The origin of such inflammation and acute encephalopathy can be bacterial or viral.

Bacterial Meningitis

Bacterial meningitis is one of the most serious infections to which infants and children are susceptible.[45] Nearly 90% of all reported cases of bacterial meningitis occur in children younger than 5 years. Three microorganisms account for most of the reported cases of bacterial meningitis in the United States: *Haemophilus influenzae, Neisseria meningitidis,* and *Streptococcus pneumoniae.* Despite the availability of antibiotics capable of killing each of these microorganisms, the general incidence of bacterial meningitis remains unchanged.

Haemophilus influenzae type B is the most common pathogen of bacterial meningitis in children younger than 5 years. Otitis media or sinusitis may be a precursor, because the infections almost always are associated with a bacterium in the blood.

The second most common organism is **Neisseria meningitidis** (meningococcus). Approximately 2% to 5% of healthy children are carriers of *N. meningitidis.* The risk of meningitis in day-care center contacts of children with meningococcal disease is 1 per 1000.[46] During epidemics among military personnel, nasal and oral secretions from as many as 90% of those examined reveal *N. meningitidis,* suggesting a high rate of infectious transmission.

The third organism is **Streptococcus pneumoniae,** which is likely to be found in children older than 4 years. Staphylococcal or streptococcal meningitis can occur in children of any age but shows a predilection for children who have had neurosurgery, skull fracture, or a complication of systemic bacterial infection. Infections that originate in the middle ear, sinuses, or mastoid cells also may lead to *S. pneumoniae* infection in children. In addition, this microorganism tends to occur in children with sickle cell disease or splenectomy. One in every 24 children with sickle cell disease develops pneumococcal meningitis by the age of 4 years. This incidence is 36 times greater than that found in the black population without sickle cell disease and 314 times greater than in white children. *Escherichia coli* and group B β-hemolytic streptococci are the most common causes of meningitis in the newborn period.

Pathophysiology

The cause of bacterial meningitis is related to the age of the child and to a number of factors that predispose the child to bacterial infection or that alter the child's response to an invading microorganism. Any microorganism may be pathogenic under the appropriate circumstances in a given individual.

During the first 2 months of life, the causative organisms are those that reflect the maternal flora or the environment in which the infant has been placed (e.g., gram-negative intestinal bacilli and group B streptococci). Most bacterial meningitis in children 2 months to 12 years of age is caused by *H. influenzae* type B, *S. pneumoniae,* or *N. meningitidis.* In children older than 12 years, meningitis usually is caused by *S. pneumoniae* or *N. meningitidis.* When the child's response has been compromised or when anatomic defects are present, other organisms may be responsible, including *Pseudomonas,* staphylococci, salmonellae, and *Serratia.*

Meningitis may follow bacterial infections of the paranasal sinuses or mastoid cells. Bacterial meningitis in children with otitis media generally follows bacteremia. Direct invasion of the meninges is rare. Infection may spread through the blood to the meninges in children with infective endocarditis, pneumonia, or thrombophlebitis.

Direct invasion of the CNS occurs with fracture of the paranasal sinus, dermoid sinus tracts, or myelomeningoceles if direct communication occurs between the skin and meninges. Meningitis also may occur after neurosurgical procedures, particularly those involving CSF diversion such as shunting. Infection of the CNS may be caused by environmental contamination or manipulation. Meningitis caused by *Staphylococcus aureus* or *Pseudomonas aeruginosa* may develop in the child with cystic fibrosis or severe burns. (For further discussion, see Chapter 16.)

Clinical Manifestations

Acute bacterial meningitis often is preceded by an upper respiratory or a gastrointestinal infection. Fever, headache, vomiting, irritability, photophobia, and nuchal and spinal rigidity develop and can progress rapidly to a decreased level of consciousness and seizures. Irritation of the meninges and spinal roots causes pain and resistance to neck flexion (nuchal rigidity), a positive Kernig sign (resistance to knee extension in the supine position with the hips and knees flexed against the body), and a positive Brudzinski sign (flexion of the knees and hips when the neck is flexed forward rapidly). With severe meningeal irritation the child may demonstrate opisthotonic posturing (rigid arching of the back with the head extended). Meningococcal meningitis can produce a characteristic petechial rash.[47] IICP is caused by cerebral edema and may be increased further by obstruction to the CSF circulation. Thickened meninges and fibrous exudate in the subarachnoid space at the base of the brain obstruct the CSF, resulting in communicating hydrocephalus.

Evaluation and Treatment

A definitive diagnosis is made *only* by examination of CSF obtained from a lumbar puncture. The principles of treatment are similar to those followed for adults (see Chapter 16) and are based on the culture results in which the causative organism is identified. The conjugate vaccine against *H. influenzae* begun during infancy will help prevent nasopharyngeal colonization, thus decreasing the rate and spread of this disease.[46]

The factors that influence outcomes are the age of the child (mortality is highest in infants younger than 1 year), the infective organism (the lowest mortality is in meningococcal meningitis and the highest in meningitis caused by gram-negative enteric organisms), and the duration and extent of inflammation before treatment. Approximately 8% of children with *H. influenzae* meningitis die; 35% of the survivors have serious and permanent sensory or motor dysfunction caused by pressure on the peripheral nerves during the early phases of the illness. Approximately 5% of the children who survive meningitis have hearing deficits; 10% to 15% have cerebral damage, hydrocephalus, motor deficits, or sensory impairments.[48]

Viral Meningitis

The hallmark of viral meningitis, or aseptic meningitis, is a mononuclear response in the CSF and the presence of normal blood glucose level. In some cases the findings with aseptic meningitis are consistent with bacterial meningitis. The clinical manifestations are similar to those in bacterial meningitis, although usually milder. Isolation of the virus is difficult and often impossible. Treatment usually begins with aggressive administration of antibiotics (potential bacterial meningitis) until the diagnosis is confirmed. Treatment may include use of antiviral agents.

HUMAN IMMUNODEFICIENCY VIRUS AND CENTRAL NERVOUS SYSTEM INVOLVEMENT

The human immunodeficiency virus (HIV) subjects the body to multiple, repeated infections. The end stage of this infectious process is called *acquired immunodeficiency syndrome (AIDS).* Through a process of replication, HIV perpetuates and integrates itself into the genetic materials of the organism it infects. The primary pathologic condition of HIV causes specific immunodeficiency that destroys the host's ability to withstand infection. HIV directly invades most major organ systems, including the CNS.[49,50] (HIV and AIDS are discussed in Chapter 8.)

Infants and children have become infected with HIV through a variety of sources. Transmission may occur perinatally through the placenta, by exposure to infected maternal blood and vaginal secretions, and by postpartum ingestion of breast milk. Perinatal transmission accounts for approximately 90% of pediatric AIDS cases in the United States. Infection also can occur from contaminated blood products, although new safeguards with blood products have lessened this risk considerably over the past few years.

The actual incidence of pediatric HIV is not known because no national statistics have been compiled. The CDC estimates that 10,000 to 20,000 infants and children in the United States currently have HIV. This incidence continues to increase rapidly.

Pathophysiology

The HIV infects the T lymphocytes, in particular the CD4 T cells. The virus replicates itself, rendering the CD4 cell nonfunctional. The child is at great risk because the immune system is still developing and therefore has little or no ability to fight this virus (discussed in Chapter 8).

Clinical Manifestations

The clinical diagnosis of HIV in children is very often a difficult task. The CDC revised the classification in 1994 for HIV infection in children younger than 13 years (Box 18-3). The HIV infection may be identified by viral culture of blood or tissue, and the diagnosis is confirmed by the presence of specific antibodies to the virus. However, the presence of passive maternal antibody limits the use of HIV antibody testing in infants in the high-risk category up to 15 months of age. Therefore two definitions of infection in children are necessary: one for prenatally exposed infants up to 15 months of age and one for older children.[51]

HIV affects all body systems. Therefore the clinical manifestations vary greatly from child to child. The initial signs and symptoms may be nonspecific and subtle, and they may progress slowly or rapidly to an acute, life-threatening condition.

A particularly vulnerable site of HIV infection in infants and children is the CNS. HIV encephalopathy is more common in the advanced stages.[52] The revised classification from the CDC requires one of the following progressing findings to be present for at least 2 months,[53] in the absence of a concurrent illness other than HIV that could explain the findings:

1. Failure to attain or loss of developmental milestones, or loss of intellectual ability, verified by standard developmental scale or neuropsychologic tests
2. Impaired brain growth or acquired microcephaly demonstrated by head circumference measurements or brain atrophy demonstrated by CT or MRI with serial imaging required in children less than 2 years of age
3. Acquired symmetric motor deficits manifested by affecting a child 1 month of age or older

The onset of progressive encephalopathy may be a prognostic indicator of a poor outcome.

It may be difficult to completely differentiate the impact of HIV infection on the CNS from the impact of prenatal and perinatal exposure. In addition, other insults may accompany HIV in a young child and affect growth and development, such as drug exposure, prematurity, chronic illness, and a chaotic social atmosphere.[49,51]

Evaluation and Treatment

A definite diagnosis of HIV is made by patient history, viral culture, and clinical manifestations, and a growing number of investigational protocols are available for treatment of children with HIV. In general, treatment is focused on the preservation and maintenance of the immune system, aggressive response to opportunistic infections, and support and relief of symptomatic occurrences (HIV treatment is discussed in Chapter 8).

Acquired immunodeficiency syndrome (AIDS) is the eleventh most common cause of death in children 1 to 4 years of age in 1997.[54] In 1994 the United States Public Health Service (PHS) encouraged the use of Zidovudine to reduce perinatal HIV transmission. The following year (1995), the PHS published guidelines for universal, routine HIV counseling and voluntary HIV testing of pregnant women. This has resulted in a decrease in perinatal HIV transmission.[54] Outcome may depend on the child's age at diagnosis and subsequent onset of symptoms and complications of AIDS.

Box 18-3

PEDIATRIC HUMAN IMMUNODEFICIENCY VIRUS (HIV) CLASSIFICATION

Immunologic Categories	N: No signs/ symptoms	A: Mild signs/ symptoms	B: 1Moderate signs/symptoms	C: 1Severe signs/symptoms
1. No evidence	N1	A1	B1	C1
2. Evidence of moderate suppression	N2	A2	B2	C2
3. Severe suppression	N3	A3	B3	C3

CLINICAL CATEGORIES FOR CHILDREN WITH HIV INFECTION

Category N: Not symptomatic

Children who have no signs or symptoms considered to be the result of HIV infection or who have only one of the conditions listed in Category A

Category A: Mildly symptomatic

Children with two or more of the conditions listed below but none of the conditions listed in Categories B or C:

- Lymphadenopathy
- Hepatomegaly
- Splenomegaly
- Dermatitis
- Parotitis
- Recurrent or persistent upper respiratory infection, sinusitis, or otitis media

Category B: Moderately symptomatic

Children who have symptomatic conditions other than those listed for Category A or C that are attributed to HIV infection; examples of conditions in clinical Category B include but are not limited to:

- Anemia ($\leq$8 gm/dl), neutropenia ($\leq$1000mm^3), or thrombocytopenia ($\leq$100,000mm^3) persisting $\geq$30 days
- Bacterial meningitis, pneumonia, or sepsis (single episode)
- Candidiasis or oropharyngeal (thrush) persisting ($\geq$2 months) in children $\geq$6 months of age
- Cardiomyopathy
- Cytomegalovirus infection with onset before 1 month of age
- Diarrhea, recurrent or chronic
- Hepatitis
- Herpes simplex virus (HSV), somatitis, recurrent (more than 2 episodes within 1 year)
- HSV bronchitis, pneumonitis, or esophagitis with onset before 1 month of age
- Herpes zoster (shingles) involving at least distinct episodes or more than 1 dermatone
- Lieomyosarcoma
- Lymphoid interstitial pneumonia (LIP) or pulmonary lymphoid hyperplasia complex
- Neuropathy
- Nocardiosis
- Persistent fever (lasting $\geq$1 month)
- Toxoplasmosis, onset before 1 month of age
- Varicella, disseminated (complicated chickenpox)

Category C: Severely symptomatic

Children who have any condition listed in the 1987 surveillance case definition of acquired immunodeficiency with the exception of LIP.

Data from Centers for Disease Control and Prevention: 1994 revised classification system for human immunodeficiency virus infection in children less than 13 years of age, *MMWR Morb Mortal Wkly Rep* 43(RR-12):1, 1994.

CEREBROVASCULAR DISEASE IN CHILDREN

Cerebrovascular disease in children differs from that in adults in three ways:

1. An absence of predisposing factors, such as high blood pressure and arteriosclerosis
2. Significant differences in the clinical response related to the developing nervous system and thus a greater capacity for the pediatric brain to recover from vascular insult
3. The anatomic site of the pathologic condition

Cerebrovascular disease can be divided into two categories: occlusive and hemorrhagic.

Occlusive Cerebrovascular Disease

Occlusive disease may result from embolism, thrombosis, or congenital or iatrogenic narrowing of vessels, which leads to a decreased flow of blood and oxygen to areas of the brain. Cardiac anomalies are the most common disorders that lead to complications of cerebral occlusion. Examples include cyanotic and congenital heart disease.

Moyamoya disease is a chronic, progressive vascular disease that results in the progressive stenosis of arterial flow to the brain. Moyamoya, a Japanese term, means "puff of smoke," which describes its appearance on CT examination. The vascularity may be a congenital anomaly, or it can develop as a result of cranial radiation therapy. Treatment is surgical bypass of the occluded region. Regardless of the cause, failure of blood flow to the brain results in an ischemic stroke. Strokes are relatively rare in the pediatric population, with an incidence of approximately 0.63 per 100,000 annually in the United States.

Hemorrhagic Cerebrovascular Disease

Pathophysiology

Congenital arteriovenous malformations are the most common cause of intracranial bleeding and hemorrhagic stroke in children. Hemorrhagic disease may result from vascular anomalies that lead to rupture, such as aneurysm, or from congenital arteriovenous malformation. The rupture and symptomatic development of a cerebral aneurysm are rare in children younger than 19 years. Treatment is surgical repair of the weakened vessel and does not differ from that for the adult population (see Chapter 16).

Clinical Manifestations

The extent of the pathologic condition usually is less extensive in children than in adults. Symptoms may include degrees of hemiplegia (flaccid, spastic), weakness, seizures, high fever, nuchal rigidity, hemianopia, sensory changes, facial palsy, and temporary aphasia.

Evaluation and Treatment

Diagnosis of cerebrovascular disease is made through a series of tests, including CT, MRI, magnetic resonance angiogram (MRA), angiogram, and echocardiogram. History of evolving symptoms and past medical history are of vital importance in accurate diagnosis. Causative factors in the change in vascular flow often are not determined. Malformations vary in size, location, and symptoms, and these factors determine treatment. Options include surgery, radiation therapy, and occlusion of the malformation (see Chapter 16).

Excellent collateral circulation in the child's brain allows for more rapid recovery of motor function. The developing brain, however, may suffer more global, long-term effects, leading to mental retardation, behavior disorders, and seizures.

CHILDHOOD TUMORS

Brain Tumors

Brain tumors are the most common solid tumor and the second most common primary neoplasm in children, second only to leukemia. Overall, brain tumors account for nearly 20% of all childhood cancers, with an annual incidence of 2.4 to 4 per 100,000 in the United States; approximately 2000 cases are diagnosed in each year.[55,56] Brain tumors remain the leading cause of death from disease in children ages 1 to 15 years.[57]

The cause of brain tumors is largely unknown, although genetic, environmental, and immune factors have been implicated in some tumor development. Other considerations and factors that have been investigated in the cause of brain tumors include familial tendencies, radiation, oncologic viruses, and chemical carcinogens. An important area of study has been the relationship of parental occupation to subsequent brain tumors in offspring. Associations have been found with tumors and parental employment, for example, parental exposure to hydrocarbons and employment in the aircraft and paper/pulp industries. Alterations in embryologic development also may play a part in the development of childhood brain tumors. This theory suggests that tumors arise from cells that are "misplaced" during embryonic development, never maturing but later proliferating in this immature form. Chromosomal work has implicated the deletion of chromosome 22 and 17 in some pediatric brain tumors. Further studies are being conducted that may affect the course of treatment for these children.[58] None of these factors, however, has proved significant.

Pathophysiology

Most childhood brain tumors arise from glial tissue, the supportive tissue of the brain. Tumors also may originate in other tissue such as nerve cells, cranial nerves, the pineal and pituitary glands, blood vessels, or neuroepithelium. Brain tumors are classified by the tissue and location from which they arise. Because a uniform pathologic nomenclature has yet to be established, inconsistencies occur when statistical data are compared.

Two thirds of all pediatric brain tumors are found in the posterior fossa region of the brain. This area also may be referred to as *infratentorial* because it is located below the tentorium. The tentorium is the layer of dura mater that separates the cerebellum from the cortex or cerebrum. Thus the area above the tentorium is referred to as the *supratentorial region.* Approximately one third of childhood brain tumors are located in the supratentorial space. On the other hand, in the adult population two thirds of brain tumors are located in the supratentorial region and only one third in the infratentorial region. The types and characteristics of childhood brain tumors are summarized in Table 18-5.

Brain tumors, by virtue of their location, have unique characteristics that distinguish them from tumors found elsewhere in the body. A number of brain tumors in children may be considered histologically benign yet clinically malignant and life threatening because of their location. For example, a tumor located in the brain stem region may appear benign under the microscope, but the clinical presentation threatens and all too often overrides the vital functions of the brain stem.

Types

Medulloblastoma, ependymoma, astrocytoma, brain stem glioma, craniopharyngioma, and optic nerve glioma make up approximately 75% to 80% of all pediatric brain tumors.[59] The location of brain tumors in children is illustrated in Fig. 18-14; specific characteristics, treatment strategies, and prognoses are listed in Tables 18-5 and 18-6.

Table 18-5 Treatment Strategies for Childhood Brain Tumors

Tumor Type	Treatment and Prognosis
Cerebellar astrocytoma	Surgery; possibly curative Radiation and chemotherapy not proved successful but may delay recurrence Survival rate of more than 5 years in 50%-75%; if tumor recurs, it does so very slowly
Medulloblastoma	Surgery, primarily as a partial resection to relieve increased intracranial pressure and "debulk" the tumor Type of treatment is age dependent Radiation as the primary treatment; may include spinal radiation Chemotherapy showing some promise in conjunction with craniospinal radiation 35% 5-year survival rate
Brain stem glioma	Surgery, resection occasionally possible Radiation, primarily palliative treatment Chemotherapy not yet proved beneficial, but new protocols being studied 20% to 40% 5-year survival rate dependent upon total resection
Ependymoma	Tumor possibly indolent for many years Surgery rarely curative; risk of resecting an infratentorial tumor too great Radiation for palliation (current controversy whether local or craniospinal radiation is best) Chemotherapy used for recurrent disease but with disappointing results 20%-80% 5-year survival rate dependent upon total resection
Craniopharyngioma	Surgery possibly successful when a complete resection is performed (partial resection usually requires further treatment) Radiation after partial surgical resection Chemotherapy not commonly used 75% to 85% 5-year survival rate
Optic nerve glioma	Initial treatment controversial Surgery used for diagnosis or relief of hydrocephalus Radiation useful, particularly if the tumor not treated by surgery
Cerebral astrocytoma	Surgery used if resection is possible Radiation useful for all grades of astrocytoma Chemotherapy beneficial in higher-grade tumors, but further study required

Table 18-6 Brain Tumors in Children

Type	Characteristics
Astrocytoma	Arises from astrocytes, often in the cerebellum or lateral hemisphere Slow growing, solid or cystic Often very large before diagnosed Varies in degree of malignancy
Optic nerve glioma	Arises from optic chiasm or optic nerve Slow-growing, low-grade astrocytoma
Medulloblastoma (infiltrating glioma)	Often located in cerebellum, extending into fourth ventricle and spinal fluid pathway Rapidly growing malignant tumor Can extend outside of CNS
Brain stem glioma	Arises from pons or myeloencephalon Numerous cell types Compresses cranial nerves V through X
Ependymoma	Arises from ependymal cells lining ventricles Circumscribed, solid, nodular tumors
Craniopharyngioma	Arises near pituitary gland, optic chiasm, and hypothalamus Cystic and solid tumors that affect vision, pituitary, and hypothalamic functions

Clinical Manifestations

The actual location of the brain tumor dictates the presenting signs and symptoms (discussed in greater detail with each particular brain tumor type). In addition to tumor location and cell type, the rate of growth of the tumor also determines the presenting signs and symptoms. The ability of the brain and intracranial cavity to compensate for tumor growth is directly related to the rate of its growth. This compensatory mechanism allows the components of the intracranial space (blood, brain, and CSF) to adapt temporarily to slow changes in ICP. Therefore slow-growing tumors can grow to enormous size before signs and symptoms are apparent. Conversely, fast-growing tumors allow little time for compensation of the space-occupying lesion, and clinical symptoms occur.

Signs and symptoms of brain tumors in children vary from generalized and vague to those that are localized and

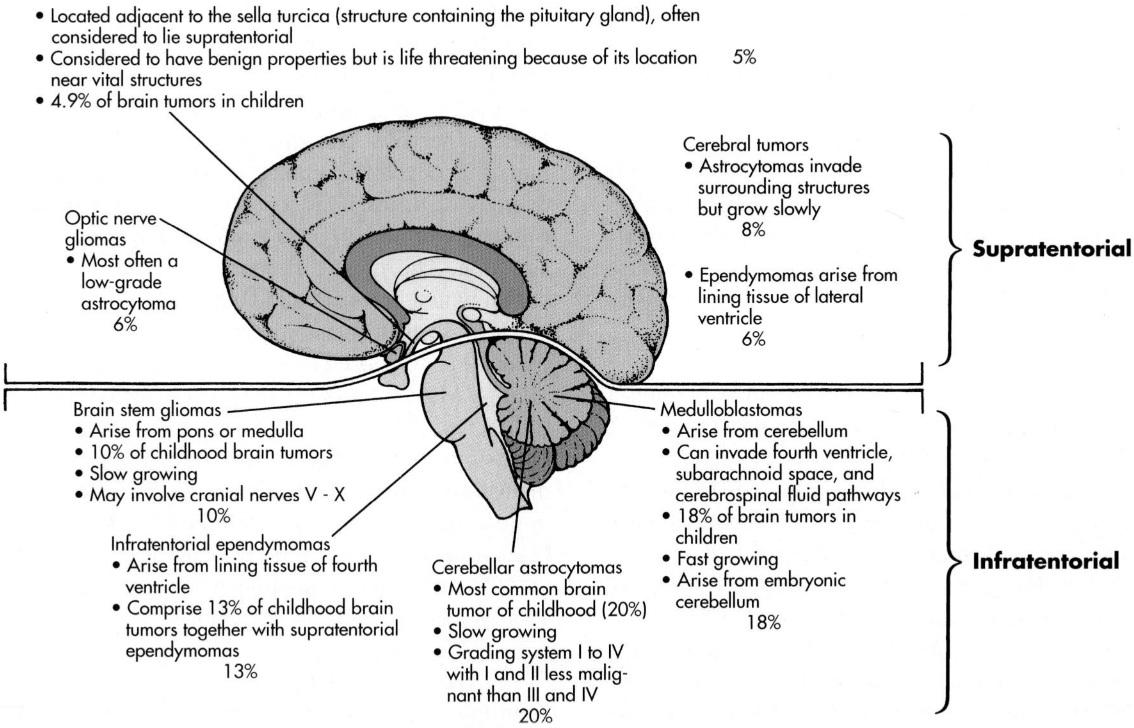
• Located adjacent to the sella turcica (structure containing the pituitary gland), often considered to lie supratentorial
• Considered to have benign properties but is life threatening because of its location near vital structures
5%
• 4.9% of brain tumors in children
Optic nerve gliomas
• Most often a low-grade astrocytoma
6%
Cerebral tumors
• Astrocytomas invade surrounding structures but grow slowly
8%
• Ependymomas arise from lining tissue of lateral ventricle
6%
Supratentorial
Brain stem gliomas
• Arise from pons or medulla
• 10% of childhood brain tumors
• Slow growing
• May involve cranial nerves V - X
10%
Infratentorial ependymomas
• Arise from lining tissue of fourth ventricle
• Comprise 13% of childhood brain tumors together with supratentorial ependymomas
13%
Cerebellar astrocytomas
• Most common brain tumor of childhood (20%)
• Slow growing
• Grading system I to IV with I and II less malignant than III and IV
20%
Medulloblastomas
• Arise from cerebellum
• Can invade fourth ventricle, subarachnoid space, and cerebrospinal fluid pathways
• 18% of brain tumors in children
• Fast growing
• Arise from embryonic cerebellum
18%
Infratentorial

FIG. 18-14 Location of brain tumors in children.

related specifically to the anatomic area. If the tumor is located in the posterior fossa region, the fourth ventricle may become blocked, which leads to hydrocephalus and signs of IICP. IICP also may occur because of the additional mass volume within the fixed container of the skull vault. The symptoms of IICP include headache, vomiting, lethargy, and irritability. If a young child complains of a headache, a thorough investigation should take place because headache is an uncommon complaint in young children. Headache caused by IICP usually is worse in the morning and gradually improves during the day when the child is upright and venous drainage is enhanced. Frequency of headache and other symptoms worsens as the tumor grows. A headache related to IICP generally occurs because of expansion of the lateral ventricle and cerebral hemisphere, which causes a stretching of the pain-sensitive dura mater. Irritability or possible apathy and increased somnolence also may result from IICP. Like headache, vomiting occurs more commonly in the morning. It frequently is not preceded by nausea and may become projectile, differing from a gastrointestinal disturbance in that the child may be ready to eat immediately after vomiting. Other signs and symptoms that can accompany IICP include increased head circumference with bulging fontanelle in children younger than 2 years of age, cranial nerve palsies, and papilledema.

Localized findings relate to the degree of disturbance in physiologic functioning in the area where the tumor is located (see Table 16-9). Infratentorial tumors exhibit localized signs of impaired coordination and balance, including ataxia, gait difficulties, truncal ataxia, and loss of balance. The **medulloblastoma** occurs as an invasive malignant tumor that develops in the vermis of the cerebellum and may extend into the fourth ventricle. The **ependymoma** develops in the fourth ventricle and arises from the ependymal cells that line the ventricular system. The histology of the ependymoma varies, which makes the treatment course and prognosis difficult to establish. Because both tumors are located in the posterior fossa region along the midline, presenting signs and symptoms are similar. In addition to those already described, they may obstruct the fourth ventricle, resulting in hydrocephalus and generalized IICP, headache, nausea and vomiting, and nystagmus (involuntary eye movement).

In contrast, **cerebellar astrocytomas** are located on the surface of the right or left cerebellar hemisphere and cause unilateral symptoms (occurring on the same side of the tumor), such as head tilt, limb ataxia, and nystagmus when the eyes are turned toward the tumor.

Brain stem gliomas often cause a combination of cranial nerve involvement, cerebellar signs of ataxia, and corticospinal tract dysfunction. A common clinical pattern includes unilateral paralysis of cranial nerves with contralateral paralysis of the arm and leg, hyperreflexia, and extensor plantar responses. IICP generally does not occur.

The area of the sella turcica, the structure containing the pituitary gland, is the site of several childhood brain tumors; most common of this group is the **craniopharyngioma.** These tumors may originate from the pituitary gland or the hypothalamus. They are usually slow-growing tumors and may be quite large by the time of diagnosis. Symptoms include headache, seizures, diabetes insipidus, early onset of puberty, and growth delay. Other tumors located in this region of the brain include **optic gliomas.** Tumors that involve the optic tract may cause complete unilateral blindness and hemianopia of the other eye. Optic atrophy is another common finding.

Supratentorial tumors of the cerebral hemispheres in children are not very common. Tumors located in the cortex may cause focal cerebral dysfunction, weakness, hemiparesis, seizures, and visual changes. Involvement of particular lobes may result in more specific localized symptoms. For example, a tumor located in the frontal lobe may cause changes in affect and behavior, and a tumor in the occipital lobe may cause cortical blindness or blindness in one half of the visual field.

Evaluation and Treatment

A child with signs and symptoms of a brain tumor requires a complete workup, including a neurologic, developmental, and ophthalmic examination. CT with contrast enhancement allows direct visualization of the tumor mass. MRI now provides advanced, dramatic examination of the brain and neoplasms. Small, low-grade tumors not seen on CT may be detected by MRI. Although less commonly used, MRA is very helpful in assessing vascularity of the tumor and its relationship to major blood vessels. Myelographic examination may be used to evaluate tumor dissemination along the spinal column. Lumbar puncture to examine CSF for tumor cells also is an option. Tumors more likely to spread throughout the neuraxis include medulloblastomas and ependymomas.

The most useful treatment for brain tumors is surgical resection. Surgery to establish the diagnosis by biopsy or to excise the tumor is part of the initial treatment for most brain tumors. Some brain tumors may be cured with complete resection alone, such as low-grade cerebellar astrocytomas. Contraindications to such interventions are tumors in which surgical resection and biopsy carry a high risk of mortality or serious morbidity (brain stem gliomas). In these instances, diagnosis is made on radiologic evidence and clinical manifestations.

Most brain tumors require additional radiation and chemotherapy. Although these treatments are essential for potential eradication of the brain tumor, radiation to the child's brain is associated with significant morbidity, including both acute and long-term sequelae. Much research and persistence and many investigations are directed at uncovering the secrets to successful treatment of this disease. Prognosis varies according to the type and location of the brain tumor. Historically, survival rates have been low; however, advances have been made with the combination of surgery, radiation therapy, and chemotherapy. Comprehensive care and management of these children and their families are vital. Multidisciplinary teams composed of neurosurgeons, neurologists, neuropathologists, radiation therapists, oncologists, nurses, social workers, physical therapists, and other providers are necessary to provide the continuity and consistency needed to care for these children.

Embryonal Tumors

Neuroblastoma

Neuroblastoma is an embryonal tumor that originates in neural crest cells that normally give rise to the sympathetic ganglia and the adrenal medulla. The primitive neural crest cells (also called *sympathogonia*) are pluripotential (i.e., they give rise to several cell types). They mature into ganglion cells, pheochromocytes (which are found in the sympathetic nervous system), or neurofibrous tissue. Thus tumors that develop from neural crest cells reflect the varying degrees of differentiation of the cells. **Ganglioneuroblastomas** are tumors of an intermediate level of cellular differentiation. The most differentiated tumor is a **ganglioneuroma,** which is considered benign and does not metastasize.

Because neuroblastoma involves a defect of embryonal tissue, it is diagnosed most commonly in young children and infants. Most tumors are diagnosed during the first 2 years of life, and 75% are found before the child is 5 years of age. Occasionally these tumors have been diagnosed at birth with metastasis apparent in the placenta. Neuroblastoma is seen more commonly in white children (9.6 per million) than in black children (7 per million). Although it accounts for 8% to 10% of pediatric malignancies, neuroblastoma causes 15% of cancer deaths in children.[60]

Pathophysiology

Neuroblastoma is the most primitive, or immature, form of the sympathetic nervous system tumors. Areas of necrosis and calcification often are present in the tumor.

Neuroblastoma, more than any other cancer, has been associated with spontaneous remission, commonly in infants who have liver, bone marrow, or skin involvement in addition to the primary site. Remission has been estimated to occur in approximately 7% of cases, but it may occur much more frequently. Neuroblastoma in situ (i.e., noninvasive tumor) has been found during autopsies of infants who died of other causes.

The cause of neuroblastoma is elusive. The tumor has been associated with a number of conditions, including neurofibromatosis and Hirschsprung disease, but most children with neuroblastoma have neither of these conditions. Although familial tendency has been noted in individual cases, a nonfamilial or sporadic pattern occurs in most children with neuroblastoma. Familial cases of neuroblastoma are considered to have an autosomal dominant pattern of inheritance (mechanisms of inheritance are discussed in Chapter 4).

Intense genetic study of neuroblastoma cells has led to some interesting findings. Often these cells show a deletion of the short arm of chromosome 1, which is believed to represent the loss of a tumor response gene. In addition, an oncogene, the N-*myc* oncogene, is present and amplified in neuroblastoma. There is an association between the number of N-*myc* copies present in the neuroblastoma cells and the child's prognosis. The greater the number of copies of the N-*myc* oncogene, the more rapidly progressive and lethal the disease is.[61,62] Further, a gene, the human multidrug-resistant gene *(MDR1),* has been identified and is associated with chemotherapy failure. The *MDR1* gene has been found to be amplified in some neuroblastoma cells after initial treatment with chemotherapy, and the increased presence of *MDR1* is associated with chemotherapy resistance.[63]

Clinical Manifestations

The clinical manifestations of neuroblastoma depend on the location of the tumor. Because neuroblastoma originates where there are elements of sympathetic nervous tissue, the tumor can arise in the sympathetic chain (column of sympathetic ganglia that parallels the spinal column), ganglia of effector organs, peripheral ganglia, adrenal medulla, bladder, and inner genitalia. The most common location is in the retroperitoneal region (65% of cases) and most frequently the adrenal medulla. The tumor is evident as an abdominal mass and may cause anorexia, bowel and bladder alteration, and sometimes spinal cord compression.[60]

The second most common location of neuroblastoma is the mediastinum (area separating the lungs) (15% of cases). There the tumor may cause dyspnea or infection related to airway obstruction. If the tumor is large, compression of the trachea, bronchi, lymphatic vessels, and mediastinal veins often results. Neck and facial edema may then be caused by superior vena cava syndrome. Less commonly, neuroblastoma may arise from the cervical sympathetic ganglion (3% to 4% of cases). Cervical neuroblastoma often causes Horner syndrome, which consists of miosis (pupil contraction), ptosis (drooping eyelid), enophthalmos (backward displacement of the eyeball), and anhidrosis (sweat deficiency).

The initial signs and symptoms of neuroblastoma often are related to metastatic disease. Two thirds of children have metastatic disease at the time of diagnosis. Common sites of metastasis include the skin, with characteristic blue or purple nodules; the liver, causing enlargement; bone, causing pain and pathologic fracture; and bone marrow infiltration, occurring in more than 50% of children. A unique but uncommon site of metastasis is the orbit of the eye, causing an ecchymotic discoloration of the upper and lower eyelids and a "raccoon" eye appearance.

A number of systemic signs and symptoms are characteristic of neuroblastoma, including weight loss, irritability, fatigue, and fever. Intractable diarrhea occurs in 7% to 9% of children and is caused by tumor secretion of a hormone called *vasoactive intestinal polypeptide (VIP).*

More than 90% of children with neuroblastoma have increased amounts of catecholamines and associated metabolites in their urine. High levels of urinary catecholamines and serum ferritin are associated with a poorer prognosis.

Evaluation and Treatment

Initial diagnostic studies are dictated by the location of the primary tumor. Diagnosis begins with a complete physical and neurologic examination. Visualizing examinations, including intravenous pyelogram, CT scan, and MRI of the primary site, provide further information. Investigation of metastatic disease includes skeletal survey, bone scan, liver scan, and bone marrow aspiration and examination. Newer nuclear medicine imaging studies for neuroblastoma, such as ^{131}I-metaiodobenzylguanidine (^{131}I-MIBG) and tumor-specific monoclonal antibody scan, may be helpful. Urinary catecholamine levels are measured by two metabolites, vanillylmandelic acid (VMA) and homovanillic acid (HVA). Measurement of these levels requires a 24-hour urine collection. Other laboratory analyses are likely to include ferritin; serum neuron-specific enolase (NSE), an enzyme produced by neuronal tissues; and gangliosides, lipid molecules that may be shed from the surface of tumor cells.

The diagnosis of neuroblastoma is confirmed by surgical biopsy. Occasionally the biopsy may be avoided if bone marrow aspiration shows tumor infiltration and significant elevation of urinary catecholamines. For many years there was no agreement on a staging system for neuroblastoma. Finally in 1986, an international group proposed a single staging system that was adopted in 1987. A special stage (IV-S) is designated for infants who otherwise would be classified as having early-stage disease but who also have metastatic disease involving the liver, skin, or bone.

Treatment is based on the extent of the disease and prognostic markers, such as age, n-*myc* copy numbers, and high serum ferritin or NSE levels. Early-stage disease is treated by primary excision of the tumor. Because neuroblastoma is a radiosensitive tumor, postoperative radiation therapy may be used for residual disease; however, multiagent chemotherapy is now the predominant treatment modality.[60]. The success of radiation therapy in early-stage disease, however, is controversial.

High-risk neuroblastomas are being treated with high-dose chemotherapy and radiotherapy followed by transplantation of purged autologous bone marrow. Additional treatment may include 13-*cis* retinoic acid. These combined treatments have increased survival rate in some to 3 years.[64]

Stage IV-S disease requires very little treatment, primarily because of the high rate of spontaneous regression. Low-dose radiation treatment or single-course chemotherapy may be used to reduce large tumors.

Retinoblastoma

Retinoblastoma is a rare congenital eye tumor of young children that originates in the retina of one or both eyes (Fig. 18-15). It has been highly studied and is of much interest to geneticists. Retinoblastoma demonstrates both an inherited and an acquired form. Retinoblastoma rarely is diagnosed after the child is 5 years of age. The inherited form of the disease generally is diagnosed during the first year of life and often involves multiple tumors and sometimes both eyes. The acquired disease most commonly is diagnosed in children 2 to 3 years of age and involves unilateral disease.

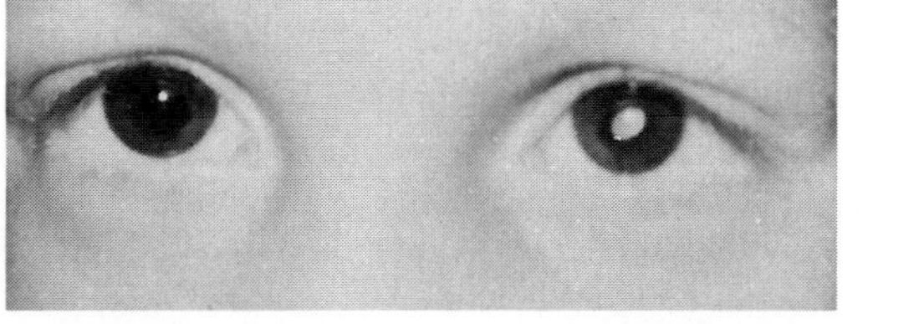

FIG. 18-15 **Retinoblastoma.** Prominent white reflex (caused by retinoblastoma) in dilated pupil of left eye. (From Kissane JM, editor: *Anderson's pathology,* ed 9, St Louis, 1990, Mosby.)

Although retinoblastoma is the most common pediatric intraocular tumor, the prevalence rate is estimated between 1 in 17,000 and 1 in 34,000 live births.[65]

Pathophysiology

Approximately 40% of retinoblastomas are inherited, and the remaining 60% are acquired. In the early 1970s Knudson[66] proposed the "two-hit" hypothesis to explain the occurrence of both hereditary and acquired forms of the disease. This hypothesis predicts that two separate transforming events or "hits" must occur in a normal retinoblast cell to cause the cancer. Further, it proposes that in the inherited form the first "hit" or mutation occurs in the germ cell (inherited from either parent) and the mutation is contained in every cell of the child's body. Only a second, random mutation in a retinoblast cell is necessary to transform that cell into cancer. Multiple tumors are observed in the inherited form because these second mutations are likely to occur in several of the approximately 1 to 2 million retinoblast cells. In contrast, the acquired form of retinoblastoma requires two independent "hits" or mutations to occur in the same somatic cell (after the egg is fertilized) for transformation to cancer. This is much less likely to happen. Fig. 18-16 illustrates the two-mutation model for these two patterns of mutation.

The gene location in which the initial retinoblastoma mutation occurs is on the long arm of chromosome 13, band q14. The gene responsible for retinoblastoma, a tumor suppressor gene, is called the *Rb gene*. The first "hit" inactivates one allele of the *Rb* gene, and the second "hit" inactivates the other allele of the gene. Without the normal functioning of the *Rb* gene, production of protein growth regulators that control retinal cell growth is lacking. Because the gene is inactivated, lack of cell growth control results in unregulated proliferation and tumor development.[67]

The *Rb* gene also has been implicated in other cancers, and survivors of hereditary retinoblastoma may be at increased risk for second cancers, particularly osteosarcoma but also cancer of the lung, breast, prostate, and bladder. Al-

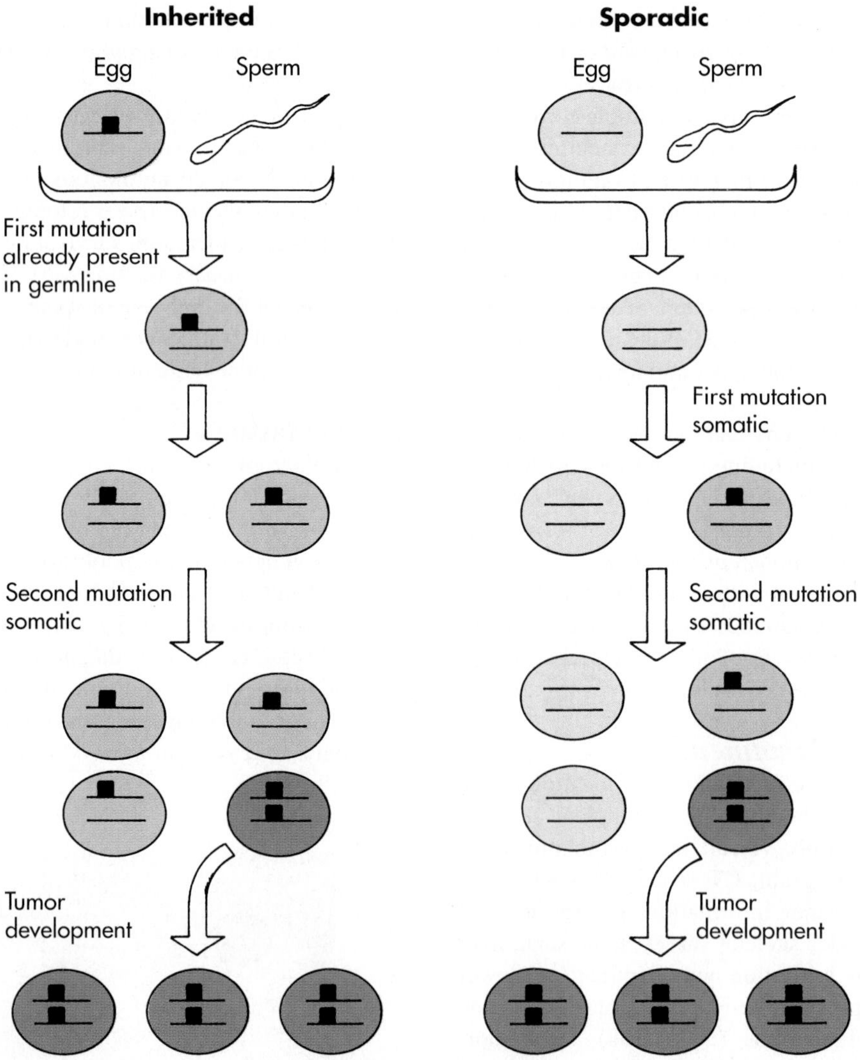

FIG. 18-16 The two-mutation model of retinoblastoma development. In inherited retinoblastoma, the first mutation is transmitted through the germline of an affected parent. The second mutation occurs somatically in a retinal cell, leading to development of the tumor. In sporadic retinoblastoma, development of a tumor requires two somatic mutations.

though retinoblastoma occurs in the very young child, second tumors can develop when survivors are in their 20s and 30s; such tumors generally are resistant to therapy.

Clinical Manifestations

Retinoblastoma grows as one or more tumors in the retina and extends into the vitreous humor. Free-floating, small tumors in the vitreous humor may attach to the surface of the retina in multiple areas and proliferate (Fig. 18-17). The tumor also can invade the optic nerve by infiltrating through the cribriform plate of the ethmoid bone or can spread through the sheath around the nerve. In either case the tumor can gain access to the subarachnoid space and the CNS. The tumor spreads into the choroid in 25% of children with retinoblastoma. Because the choroid is highly vascular, metastasis by means of hematogenous spread is possible. When hematogenous spread occurs, metastatic sites include the bone marrow, long bones, lymph nodes, and liver. Should the tumor invade the orbit, lymphatic spread is possible. Spontaneous regression occurs, although infrequently, and may be caused by the tumor's outgrowing its blood supply.

The primary sign of retinoblastoma is leukokoria, a white pupillary reflex also called *cat's eye reflex,* that is caused by the mass behind the lens (see Fig. 18-15). At this point the tumor is large enough that a light shone into the eye is reflected back by the tumor, making the pupil appear white. Other signs and symptoms include strabismus; a red, painful eye; and limited vision. Any of these signs and symptoms in a child younger than 4 years of age warrants careful ophthalmologic examination of both eyes. Similarly, any newborn with a known genetic risk for retinoblastoma should have routine ophthalmologic examinations.

Evaluation and Treatment

Diagnostic evaluation for retinoblastoma includes documentation of family history; complete ophthalmologic examination; and metastatic studies that include bone marrow aspiration, lumbar puncture for spinal fluid examination, bone scan, and additional radiologic and CT studies of the orbit and brain. Because of the potential hereditary risk to a child's siblings, all siblings younger than 4 years also should receive ophthalmologic evaluations.

Because retinoblastoma is a treatable tumor, dual priorities are saving the child's life and restoring useful vision. Radiation therapy is the primary treatment for small tumors. Photocoagulation therapy that destroys the blood vessels to the tumor may be used after radiation therapy if the tumor has failed to completely regress or recurs. Cryotherapy that destroys the tumor by causing intracellular ice crystal formation and disrupting microcirculation may be used as an alternate approach. Large or multiple tumors, indicating more advanced disease, may require enucleation (removal) of the eye. Every attempt is made to preserve vision in at least one eye without jeopardizing the child's survival.[68]

The prognosis for most children with retinoblastoma is excellent, with a greater than 90% long-term survival, although children with metastatic disease at diagnosis have a poor prognosis. Approximately 75% of children have useful vision in the treated eye.

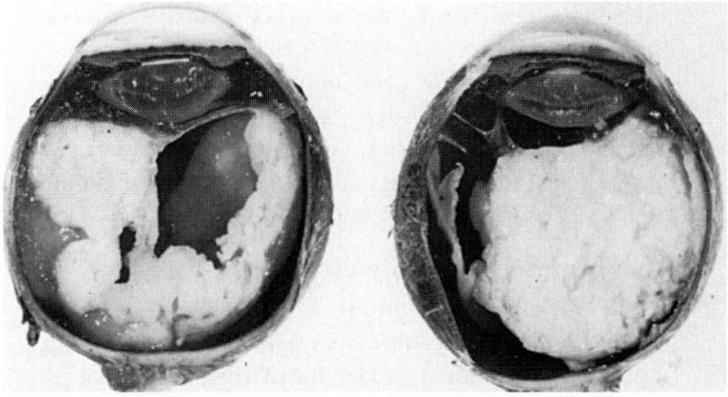

FIG. 18-17 Bilateral retinoblastoma. Presence of white mass consisting of detached retina and neoplastic tissue immediately behind lens in each eye. (From Kissane JM, editor: *Anderson's pathology,* ed 8, St Louis, 1985, Mosby.)

SUMMARY REVIEW

Structure and Function of the Nervous System in Children

1. The central nervous system develops from the neural tube, which is ectodermal in origin. The cranial end of the tube forms the brain, and the spinal cord is formed from the remainder of the tube.
2. The cranial and spinal ganglia form the neural crest.
3. The nervous system develops in six stages, and disruption of any of the stages can lead to malfunction of the nervous system.
4. The bones of the skull are joined by sutures; the wide, membranous junctions of the sutures, known as *fontanelles,* close by 20 months of age.
5. Myelin is a sheath that develops around axons to facilitate speed of nerve impulse conduction. Progressive development of reflexes corresponds to normal maturation of nerve tissue.

Structural Malformations

1. Defects of neural tube closure include anencephaly, encephalocele, meningocele, and myelomeningocele.
2. Failure of the vertebra to close with protrusion of neural tube contents is known as *spina bifida.*
3. Acrania is nearly complete absence of the cranial vault.
4. Premature closure of the cranial sutures causes craniosynostosis and prevents normal skull expansion and compression of growing brain tissue.
5. Microcephaly is lack of brain growth and retarded mental and motor development.
6. Congenital hydrocephalus results from an imbalance between the production and reabsorption of cerebrospinal fluid.

Encephalopathies

1. Static encephalopathies are nonprogressive disorders of the brain that can occur during gestation, birth, or childhood and can be caused by endogenous or exogenous factors.
2. Cerebral palsy can be caused by prenatal cerebral hypoxia or perinatal trauma with symptoms of mental retardation, seizure disorders, or developmental disabilities.
3. Inherited metabolic disorders that damage the nervous system include defects in amino acid metabolism (phenylketonuria) and lipid metabolism (Tay-Sachs disease) and result in abnormal behavior, seizures, and deficient psychomotor development.
4. Seizure disorders are associated with numerous nervous system disorders and more often are a generalized rather than a partial type of seizure.
5. Generalized forms of seizures include tonic-clonic, myoclonic, atonic, akinetic, and infantile spasms.
6. Partial seizures suggest more localized brain dysfunction.
7. Febrile seizures usually are limited to the ages of 9 months to 3 years with a pattern of one seizure per febrile illness.
8. Reye syndrome is associated with influenza B and varicella viruses and symptoms of hypoglycemia, hyperammonemia, and increased serum short-chain fatty acids. Progressive manifestations include lethargy, stupor, rigidity, seizures, and respiratory arrest.
9. Accidental poisonings from a variety of toxins can cause serious neurologic damage.
10. Bacterial meningitis is commonly caused by *Haemophilus influenzae, Neisseria meningitidis,* or *Streptococcus pneumoniae* and may result from respiratory or gastrointestinal infections, with symptoms of fever, headaches, photophobia, seizures, rigidity, and stupor.

Human Immunodeficiency Virus and Central Nervous System Involvement

1. Human immunodeficiency virus (HIV) may be transmitted to infants and children through the placenta, by exposure to infected blood or vaginal secretions, or by ingestion of infected breast milk.
2. The incidence of HIV among children is increasing. The classic symptoms are related to progressive encephalopathy.
3. Acquired immunodeficiency syndrome (AIDS) is the eleventh most common cause of death among children 1 to 4 years of age.

Cerebrovascular Disease in Children

1. Cyanotic and congenital heart disease can be complicated by cerebrovascular occlusion that causes cerebral infarction and brain damage.

Childhood Tumors

1. Brain tumors are the most common tumors of the nervous system and the second most common type of childhood cancer.
2. Tumors in children most frequently are located below the tentorial membrane.
3. Fast-growing tumors produce symptoms early in the disease, whereas slow-growing tumors may become very large before symptoms appear.
4. Symptoms of brain tumors may be generalized or localized. The most common general symptom is increased intracranial pressure (headache, irritability, vomiting, somnolence, and bulging of fontanelles).
5. Localized signs of infratentorial tumors in the cerebellum include impaired coordination and balance. Cranial nerve signs occur with tumors near the brain stem.
6. Supratentorial tumors may be located near the cortex or deep in the brain. Symptoms depend on the specific location of the tumor.
7. Neuroblastoma is an embryonal tumor of the sympathetic nervous system and can be located anywhere there is sympathetic nervous tissue. Symptoms are related to tumor location and size of metastasis.
8. Retinoblastoma is a congenital eye tumor that has both a hereditary and a nonhereditary form.

KEY TERMS

REFERENCES

1. Werler MM: Achieving a public health recommendation for preventing neural tube defects with folic acid, *Am J Public Health* 89(11):1637, 1999.
2. Wiswell TE et al: Major congenital neurologic malformations, *Am J Dis Child* 144:61, 1990.
3. Pollack IF: Management of encephaloceles and craniofacial problems in the neonatal period, *Neurosurg Clin No Amer* 9(1):121, 1998.
4. Behrman RE, Vaughan VC: *Nelson textbook of pediatrics,* ed 16, Philadelphia, 2000, W.B. Saunders.
5. Madsen JR, Scott RM: Chiari malformation, syringomyelia, and intramedullary spinal cord tumors, *Curr Opin Neurol Neurosurg* 6:559, 1993.
6. McLone DG: Care of the neonate with a myelomeningocele, *Neurosurg Clin No Amer* 9(1):111, 1998.
7. Reigel, DH: Infancy through the school years. In Rowley-Kelly F, Reigel DH, editors: *Teaching the student with spina bifida,* Baltimore, 1993, Brookes.
8. Loller DJ: *Learning among children with spina bifida. Spina Bifida Spotlight: 1-6,* Washington, DC, 1993, Spina Bifida Association of America.
9. McGee S, Burkett KW: Identifying common pediatric neurosurgical conditions in the primary care setting, *Neurosurg Clin No Amer* 35(1):61, 2000.
10. Dias M, Veetai L: Pediatric neurosurgical disease, *Pediatr Clin No Amer* 45(6):1529, 1998.
11. Bruner JP et al: Fetal surgery for myelomeningocele and the incidence of shunt-dependent hydrocephalus, *J Am Med Assoc* 282(19):1819, 1999.
12. Simpson JL: Fetal surgery for myelomeingocele: promise, progress and problems, *JAMA* 282(19):1873, 1999.
13. Sutherland RW, Gonzales ET: Current management of the infant with myelomeningocele, *Curr Opin Urology* 9(6):527, 1999.
14. Liptak GS, Serletti JM: Pediatric approach to craniosynostosis, *Peds in Rev* 19(10):352, 1998.
15. Jackson PL: Hydrocephalus. In Jackson PL, Vessey JA, editors: *Primary care of the child with a chronic condition,* ed 3, St Louis, 2000, Mosby.
16. Nelson, KB, Grether JK: Causes of cerebral palsy, *Curr Opin Pediatr* 11(6):487, 1999.
17. Bhushan V, Paneth N, Keily JL: Impact of improved survival of very low birth weight infants on recent secular trends in the prevalence of cerebral palsy, *Pediatrics* 19(6):1094, 1993.
18. Nelson KB et al: Uncertain value of electronic fetal monitoring predicting cerebral palsy, *N Engl J Med* 334(10):613, 1996.
19. Taft TL: Cerebral palsy, *Pediatr Rev* 16(11):411, 1995.
20. Steele S: Cerebral palsy. In Jackson PL, Vessey JA, editors: *Primary care of the child with a chronic condition,* ed 3, St Louis, 2000, Mosby.
21. Awwad Y et al: Intrathecal baclofen therapy for the treatment of cerebral palsy in children, *Annal Neurol* 46(3):466, 1999.
22. Farmer TH, editor: *Pediatric neurology,* ed 3, Hagerstown, Md, 1983, Harper & Row.
23. Swaiman KF, Wright FS: *The practices of pediatric neurology: principles and practice,* St Louis, 1989, Mosby.
24. Guldberg P et al: Phenylalanine hydrolase gene mutations in the United States: report from the maternal PKU collaborative study, *Am J Hum Genet* 59(1):84, 1996.
25. Schmidt K, Kaufman S, Woo SLC: The hyperphenylalaninemias. In Scriver CR et al, editors: *The metabolic basis of inherited disease,* vol 1, ed 6, New York, 1989, McGraw-Hill.
26. Schmidt K: Phenylketonuria. In Jackson PL, Vessey, JA, editors: *Primary care of the child with a chronic condition,* ed 3, St Louis, 2000, Mosby.
27. Kaufman S: An evaluation of the possible neurotoxicity of metabolites of phenylalanine, *J Pediatr* 114:895, 1989.
28. Sermon K et al: Simultaneous amplification of the two most frequent mutations of infant Tay-Sachs disease in single blastomeres, *Hum Reprod* 10(8):2214, 1995.
29. Shafer PO: Epilepsy and seizures advances in seizure assessment, treatment, and self-management, *Neurosurg Clin No Amer* 34(3)743, 1999.
30. Holmes GL: *Diagnosis and management of seizures in children,* Philadelphia, 1987, W.B. Saunders.
31. Penry JK: *Epilepsy: diagnosis, management, quality of life,* ed 2, New York, 1986, Raven.
32. Robinson LL, Gardiner M: Genetics of childhood epilepsy, *Arch Dis Childhood* 82(2):121, 2000.
33. O'Donohoe NV: *Epilepsies of childhood,* ed 3, Oxford, 1994, Butterworth-Weinemann.
33a. Pellock JM: Seizures and epilepsy in infancy and childhood, *Neurol Clin* 11(4):755, 1993.
34. Pellock JM: Managing pediatric epilepsy syndromes with new antiepileptic drugs, *Pediatrics* 104(5 part 1 of 2):1106, 1999.
35. Rantala H et al: Risk factors of infantile spasms compared with other seizures in children under 2 years of age, *Epilepsia* 37(4):362, 1996.
36. Dreifuss FE: Prognosis of childhood seizure disorders: present and future, *Epilepsia* 35(suppl 2):S30, 1994.
37. Camfield PR, Camfield CS: Vagal nerve stimulation for treatment of children with epilepsy, *J Pediatr 134*(5):532, 1999.
38. Murphy JV: Left vagal nerve stimulation in children with medcially refractive epilepsy, *J Pediatr* 134(5):563, 1999.
39. Baumann RJ, Duffner PK: Treatment of children with simple febrile seizures: the AAP practice parameter, *Pediatr Neurol* 23(1):11, 2000.
40. Kudsen FU et al: Long term outcome of prophylaxis for febrile convulsions, *Arch Dis Child* 74(1):13, 1996.
41. Monto AS: The disappearance of Reye's syndrome—a public health triumph, *New Eng J Med* 340(18):1423, 1999.
42. Belay ED et al: Reye's syndrome in the United States from 1981 though 1997, *New Eng J Med* 340(18):1377, 1999.
43. Ward MJ: Reye's syndrome: an update, *Nurs Practitioner* 22(12):45, 1997.
44. Johnston MV, Goldstein GW: Selective vulnerability of the developing brain to lead, *Curr Opin Neurol* 11(6):689, 1998.
45. Pong A, Bradley JS: Bacterial meningitis and the newborn infant, *Infect Dis Clin No Amer* 13(3):711, 1999.
46. Feigin RD, Pearlman E: Bacterial meningitis beyond the neonatal period. In Feigin RD, Cherry JD, editors: *Textbook of pediatric infectious diseases*, ed 4, Philadelphia, 1998, W.B. Saunders.
47. King DS: Central nervous system infections, *Nrsg Clin No Amer* 34(3):761, 1999.
48. Kaplan SL: Clinical presentations, diagnosis, and prognostic factors of bacterial meningitis, *Infect Dis Clin No Amer* 13(3):579, 1999.
49. Fahrner R: Pediatric HIV infections and AIDS. In Jackson PL, Vessey JA, editors: *Primary care of the child with a chronic condition,* ed 3, St Louis, 2000, Mosby.
50. Tardieu M: HIV-1 and the developing central nervous system, *Developmentl Med Child Neurol* 49:843, 1998.
51. Tardieu M et al: HIV-1 related encephalopathy in infants compared with children and adults, *Neurol* 54(5):1089, 2000.
52. Mofenson LM: Viral infections. In Feigin RD, Cherry JD, editors: *Textbook of pediatric infectious diseases*, ed 4, Philadelphia, 1998, W.B. Saunders.
53. Centers for Disease Control and Prevention: 1994 revised classification system for human immunodeficiency virus infection in children less than 13 years of age, *MMWR Morb Mortal Wkly Rep* 43(RR-12):1, 1994.
54. Lindgren ML, Steinberg S, Bayers RH: Epidemiology of HIV/AIDS in children, *Pediatr Clin No Amer* 47(1):1, 2000.
55. Kun LE: Brain tumors challenges and directions, *Pediatr Clin No Amer* 44(4):907, 1997.
56. Packer JR: Brain tumors in children, *Arch Neurol* 56(4):421, 1999.
57. Packer RJ: Brain tumors in children, *Curr Opin Pediatr* 7(1):64, 1995.
58. Biegel JA: Genetics of pediatric central nervous system tumors, *J Pediatr Hemotol & Oncol* 19(6):492, 1997.
59. DiRocco C, Jannell A: Intracranial supratentorial tumors: classification, clinical findings, surgical management, *Rays* 21(1):9, 1996.

60. Castleberry RP: Biology and treatment of neuroblastoma, *Pediatr Clin No Amer* 44(4):919, 1997.
61. Maris JM, Matthay KK: Molecular biology of neuroblastoma, *J Clin Oncol 17*(7):2264, 1999.
62. Schmidt ML et al: Biological factors determine prognosis in infants with stave IV neuroblastoma, *J Clin Oncol 18*(6):1260, 2000.
63. Goldstein LJ et al: Expression of the multidrug resistance, MDR1, gene in neuroblastomas, *J Clin Oncol* 8(1):128, 1990.
64. Matthay KK et al: Treatment of high-risk neuroblastoma with intensive chemotherapy, radiotherapy, autologous bone marrow transplantation, and 13-cis-retinoic acid, *New Eng J Med* 341(16):1165, 1999.
65. Abramson DH et al: Presenting signs of retinoblastoma, *J Pediatr* 132(3):505, 1998.
66. Knudson AG: Mutation and cancer: a statistical study of retinoblastoma, *Proc Natl Acad Sci USA* 68:620, 1971.
67. Rubnitz JE, Crist WM: Molecular genetics of childhood cancer: implications for pathogenesis, diagnosis, and treatment, *Pediatrics* 100(1):101, 1997.
68. Fontanesi J et al: Treatment outcomes and dose response relationships in infants younger than 1 year treated for retinoblastoma with primary irradiation, *Med Pediatr Oncol* 26(50):297, 1996.

CHAPTER 19

Mechanisms of Hormonal Regulation

MARIANN R. PIANO • SUE E. HUETHER

CHAPTER OUTLINE

The endocrine system is composed of various glands located throughout the body (Fig. 19-1). These glands are capable of synthesizing and releasing special chemical messengers called **hormones.** The endocrine system has five general functions:

1. Differentiation of the reproductive and central nervous systems in the developing fetus
2. Stimulation of sequential growth and development during childhood and adolescence
3. Coordination of the male and female reproductive systems, which makes sexual reproduction possible
4. Maintenance of an optimal internal environment throughout the life span.
5. Initiation of corrective and adaptive responses when emergency demands occur

Hormones convey specific regulatory information among cells and organs.

MECHANISMS OF HORMONAL REGULATION

The endocrine glands respond to specific signals by synthesizing and releasing hormones into the circulation. Although a wide variety of hormones function within the body, they share certain general characteristics:

1. Hormones have specific rates and patterns of secretion. Three basic secretion patterns are (a) diurnal patterns, (b) pulsatile and cyclic patterns, and (c) patterns that depend on levels of circulating substrates (e.g., calcium, sodium, potassium, or the hormones themselves).
2. Hormones operate within feedback systems, either positive or negative, to maintain an optimal internal environment.
3. Hormones affect only cells with appropriate receptors and then act on these cells to initiate specific cell functions or activities.
4. The kidneys excrete hormones, whereas the liver metabolizes hormones—inactivating them and rendering the hormone more water soluble for renal excretion.

Hormones may be classified according to their structure, gland of origin, effects, or chemical composition. (Table 19-1 categorizes hormones based on structure.) The secretion and mechanisms of action of hormones represent an extremely complex system of integrated responses. Although much has been learned about these complex systems, many of the specific mechanisms of action are not yet understood. The endocrine and nervous systems work together to regulate responses to the internal and external environments.

Regulation of Hormone Release

The release of hormones occurs either in response to an alteration in the cellular environment or in the process of maintaining a regulated level of certain hormones or certain substances. Hormone release is regulated by chemical factors, endocrine or hormonal factors (a hormone from one endocrine gland controlling another endocrine gland), and neural control. Of these regulatory mechanisms, endocrine regulation by way of feedback circuits (systems) is one of the most important ways in which hormonal secretion is maintained within a physiologic range.

Negative feedback is the most common type of feedback system. In a negative-feedback system, plasma levels of one type of hormone influence the level of other types of hormones. An example of hormone negative feedback is shown in Fig. 19-2, *A*. Increased anterior pituitary release of follicle-stimulating hormone (FSH) and luteinizing hormone (LH) stimulates the maturation and release of the ovum into the oviduct. Mature follicular cells secrete estrogen, and the corpus luteum secretes progesterone. Once *estrogen* levels reach a certain plasma peak, feedback onto the anterior pituitary inhibits further secretion of FSH. Estrogen also inhibits the release of gonadotropin-releasing hormone (GnRH) from the hypothalamus. (GnRH stimulates anterior pituitary release of FSH and LSH.) In this example, regulation of estrogen release is achieved at two levels: at the level of the hypothalamus (long feedback loop) and at the level of the anterior pituitary (short feedback loop).

Negative-feedback systems are important in maintaining hormones within physiologic ranges. The lack of negative-feedback inhibition on hormonal release often results in pathologic conditions. As discussed in Chapter 20, various hormonal imbalances and related conditions are caused by excessive hormone production, which is the result of failure to "turn off" the system. These negative-feedback regulatory systems are diagrammed in Fig. 19-2, *B*.

An example of neural regulation is the release of epinephrine from the adrenal medulla as a result of activation of the sympathetic division of the autonomic nervous system in response to stress. When the stress is removed, the nervous stimulation decreases and less epinephrine is released.

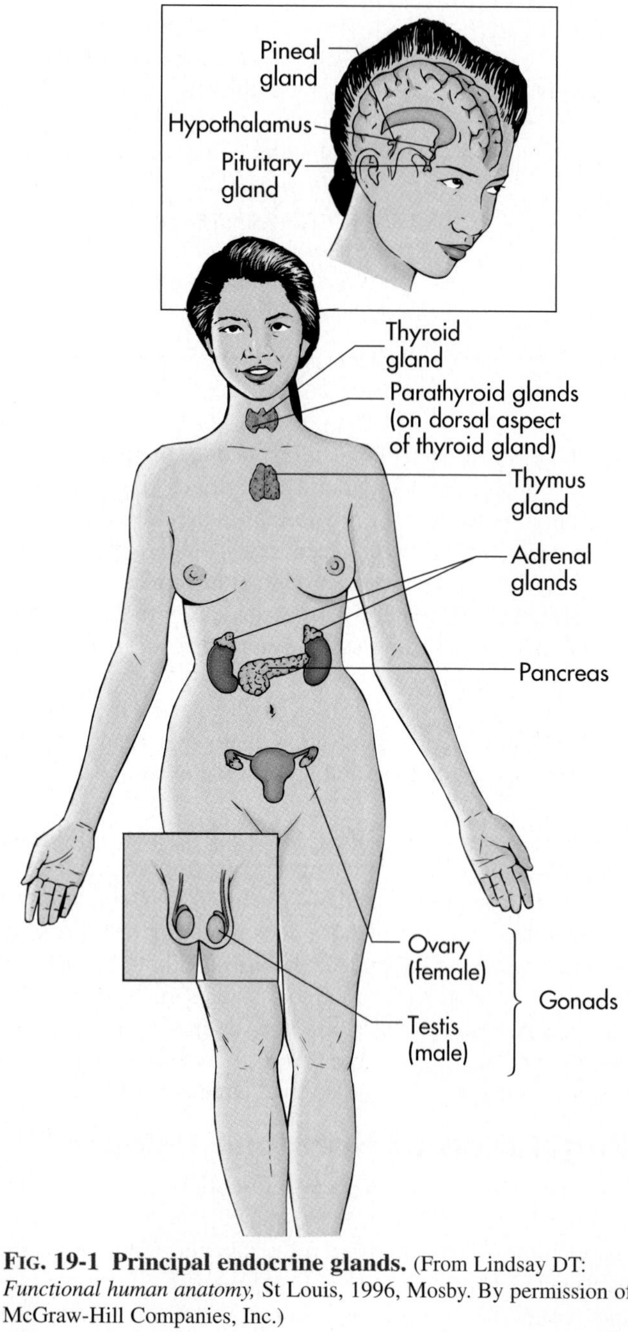

FIG. 19-1 Principal endocrine glands. (From Lindsay DT: *Functional human anatomy,* St Louis, 1996, Mosby. By permission of McGraw-Hill Companies, Inc.)

Table 19-1 Structural Categories of Hormones

Structural Category	Examples
Peptides	Growth hormone
	Insulin
	Parathyroid hormone
	Prolactin
Glycoproteins	Follicle-stimulating hormone
	Luteinizing hormone
	Thyroid-stimulating hormone
Polypeptides	Adrenocorticotropic hormone
	Antidiuretic hormone
	Calcitonin
	Endorphins
	Glucagon
	Hypothalamic hormones
	Lipotropins
	Melanocyte-stimulating hormone
	Oxytocin
	Somatostatin
	Thymosin
	Thyrotropin-releasing hormone
Amines	Epinephrine
	Norepinephrine
	Thyroxine (both thyroxine [T_4] and triiodothyronine [T_3])
Lipids	
Steroids (cholesterol is a precursor for all steroids)	Estrogens
	Glucocorticoids (cortisol)
	Mineralocorticoids (aldosterone)
	Progestins (progesterone)
	Testosterone
Derivatives of arachidonic acid	Leukotrienes
	Prostacyclins
	Prostaglandins
	Thromboxanes

Data from Seeley RR, Stephens TD, Tate P: *Anatomy & physiology,* ed 3, St Louis, 1995, Mosby.

Hormone Transport

Once hormones are released into the circulatory system by the endocrine glands, they are circulated throughout the body. Peptide or protein hormones (insulin, pituitary, hypothalamic, parathyroid) are water soluble and circulate in free (unbound) forms. Water-soluble hormones generally have a short half-life because they are catabolized by circulating enzymes. For example, insulin has a half-life of 3 to 5 minutes and is catabolized by insulinases. Lipid-soluble hormones, such as cortisol and adrenal androgens, are primarily circulated bound to a carrier or binding protein (Table 19-2). A small percentage of the lipid-soluble hormone circulates in a free or active form. For example, approximately 10% of the circulating cortisol is free, whereas 75% is bound

Table 19-2 Binding Proteins, Their Hormones, and Variables That Affect Their Circulating Levels

Binding Protein	Hormone	Factors That Increase Binding Protein Levels	Factors That Decrease Binding Protein
Corticosteroid-binding globulin	Cortisol Progesterone	Estrogen	Liver disease
Sex hormone–binding globulin	Dihydrotestosterone Testosterone Estradiol	—	Androgens Hypothyroidism Liver disease
Thyroid-binding globulin	Thyroxine (T_4) Triiodothyronine (T_3)	Estrogen Hyperthyroidism	Testosterone Glucocorticoids Liver disease
Albumin	All lipid-soluble hormones	Estrogen	Liver disease Malnutrition Renal disease

T_4, Thyroxine; T_3, triiodothyronine.

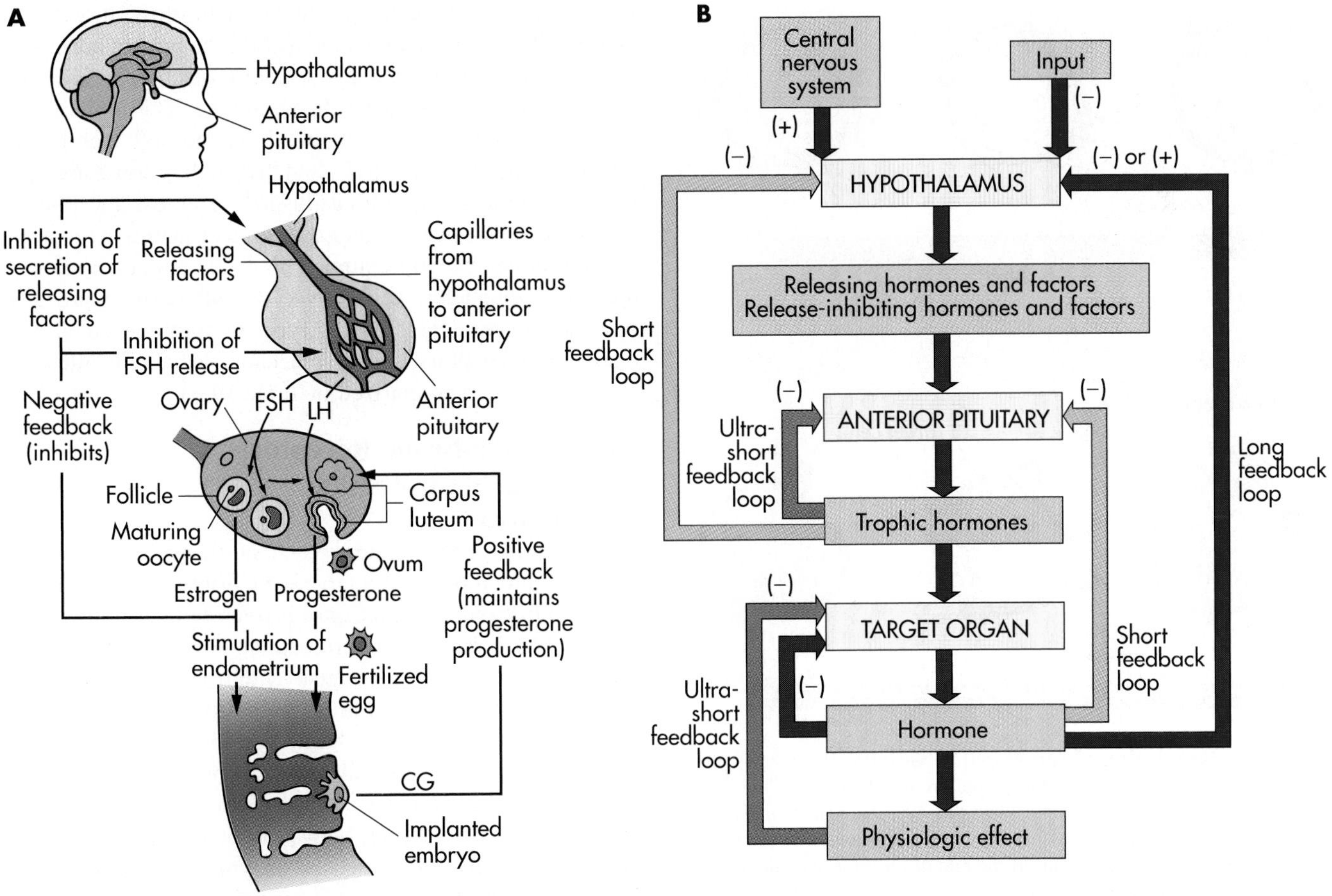

FIG. 19-2 Feedback loops. A, Endocrine feedback loops involving the hypothalamus-pituitary gland and end organs (endocrine regulation). **B,** General model for control and negative feedback to hypothalamic–pituitary target organ systems. Negative-feedback regulation is possible at three levels: target organ (ultrashort feedback), anterior pituitary (short feedback), and hypothalamus (long feedback).

to corticosteroid-binding globulin. A large change in the concentration of binding protein can affect the concentration of free hormone and, therefore, hormone effects (see Table 19-2). As discussed later, water-soluble hormones bind to one of four classes of cell surface receptors, whereas lipid-soluble hormones diffuse through the plasma membrane and bind to cytosolic or nuclear receptors.

Cellular Mechanisms of Hormone Action

When a hormone is released into the circulatory system, it is distributed throughout the body, but only those cells with appropriate receptors for that hormone are affected. The **target cell** hormone receptors have two main functions: (1) to recognize and bind with high affinity to their particular hormones and (2) to initiate a signal to appropriate intracellular effectors.

The sensitivity of the target cell to a particular hormone is related to the total number of receptors per cell. Low concentrations of hormone increase the number of receptors per cell; this is called **up-regulation** (Fig. 19-3, *A*). High concentrations of hormone decrease the number of receptors; this is called **down-regulation** (Fig. 19-3, *B*). Thus the cell can adjust its sensitivity to the concentration of the signaling hormone.

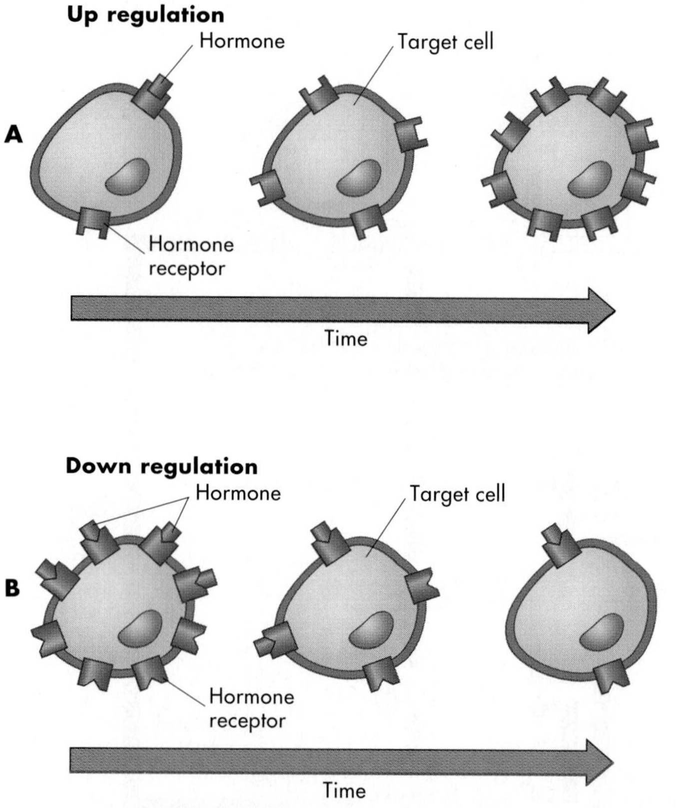

Fig. 19-3 Regulation of target cell sensitivity. If synthesis of new receptors occurs faster than degradation of old receptors, the target cell will have more receptors and thus be more sensitive to the hormone. This phenomenon, **A,** often is called *up-regulation* because the number of receptors goes up. If the rate of receptor degradation exceeds the rate of receptor synthesis, the target cell's number of receptors will decrease, **B.** Because the number of receptors and thus the sensitivity of the target cell go down, this phenomenon often is called *down-regulation.* Shading in box represents hormone concentration. (From Thibodeau GA, Patton K: *Anatomy & physiology,* ed 4, St Louis, 1999, Mosby.)

Hormones have two general types of effects on target cells: direct and permissive. **Direct effects** are the obvious changes in cell function that specifically result from stimulation by a particular hormone. **Permissive effects** are less obvious hormone-induced changes that facilitate the maximal response or functioning of a cell. For example, insulin has a direct effect on skeletal muscle cells with insulin receptors, causing increased glucose transport into these cells. Insulin also has a permissive effect on mammary cells, facilitating the response of these cells to the direct effects of prolactin.

Some hormones have biphasic pharmacologic effects that are dependent on the concentration of the hormone. For example, low or physiologic levels of antidiuretic hormone (ADH) (i.e., levels that are secreted in response to dehydration) stimulate renal tubular reabsorption of sodium and water. However, at supraphysiologic levels (i.e., what can be achieved by exogenous administration), ADH acts as a vasoconstrictor.

Hormone Receptors

Hormone receptors may be located on the plasma membrane or in the intracellular compartment of the target cell. Water-soluble hormones, which include the protein hormones and the catecholamines, have a high molecular weight and cannot diffuse across the cell membrane. They interact or bind with receptors located in or on the cell membrane. Steroid hormones, vitamin D, and thyroid hormones are lipid soluble. These hormones easily diffuse across the plasma membrane and bind to either cytosolic or nuclear receptors. The hormone–receptor complex binds to a specific region in the deoxyribunucleic acid (DNA) and alters the expression of a specific gene (Fig. 19-4). (Types of hormones, their corresponding receptors, and the mechanisms by which they affect the cell are summarized in Table 19-3).

Plasma Membrane Receptors and Signal Transduction

First Messenger

Receptors for most water-soluble hormones are located on the plasma membrane of a target cell. Sometimes a hormone or ligand that binds to a receptor is referred to as a **first messenger.** This is because a hormone binding to its specific receptor represents the first signal within an elaborate signal transduction cascade. **Signal transduction** is the process by which extracellular signals (e.g., hormones) are communicated into a cell. In general, signal transduction involves a series of steps that includes receptor activation or binding of a hormone to its receptor, activation of a G protein (transducer) and membrane-associated enzyme (effector enzyme), and production of a second messenger (Fig. 19-5). The final event is activation of an intracellular enzyme, such as protein kinase A or C.

The signal transduction process begins at the receptor. Receptors on the plasma membrane are continuously synthesized and degraded, so the receptor number can vary from one cell type to another. Various physiochemical conditions can affect both the receptor number and the affinity at which the hormone binds to its receptor. Some of these physiochemical conditions are the fluidity and structure of the plasma membrane, pH, temperature, ion concentration, diet, and the presence of other chemicals (e.g., drugs).

Cell surface receptors usually are classified into four types: (1) G protein–linked receptors, (2) ion-channel receptors, (3) tyrosine-kinase linked receptors (cytokine-receptor superfamily), and (4) receptors with intrinsic enzyme activity (also referred to as receptor tyrosine kinase [RTK] receptors). With the exception of insulin, most water-soluble hormones—such as adrenocorticotropic hormone (ACTH), glucagon, norepinephrine, and epinephrine—activate G protein–linked receptors. Other hormones, such as angiotensin II, activate both G protein–linked and ion-channel receptors. It is thought that insulin activates an RTK receptor, although the signal transduction pathway associated with insulin binding differs from other types of ligands binding to RTK receptors.[1]

Second-Messenger Molecules: cAMP, IP_3 and DAG, Ca^{++}, and cGMP

Cyclic adenosine monophosphate (cAMP). Second-messenger molecules are the initial link between the first signal (hormone) and the inside of the cell (Table 19-4). For example, binding of epinephrine to a β-adrenergic receptor subtype activates (through a stimulatory G protein [G_s] the enzyme adenylyl cyclase. Adenylyl cyclase catalyzes the conversion of adenosine triphosphate (ATP) to the second messenger, 3',5'-cAMP (see Fig. 19-5). Elevation of cAMP activates the enzyme cAMP-dependent protein kinase A. Kinase enzymes, by adding a phosphate moiety to cellular proteins, either activate or deactivate intracellular proteins or enzymes. In cardiac muscle, cAMP-dependent protein kinase phosphorylation of cellular membrane proteins associated with the L-type channel increase the influx of Ca^{++} into the cell. Increased intracellular Ca^{++} levels increase

Table 19-3 Types of Hormones, Their Receptors, and Their Mechanisms of Action

Hormone	Type of Receptor	Mechanism of Action
WATER-SOLUBLE HORMONES		
Glycoproteins, amines, small peptides and proteins (except insulin)	Plasma membrane receptors	Second messengers: cAMP, cGMP, Ca^{++}, IP_3, DAG
Insulin	Plasma membrane receptors	Involves receptor autophosphorylation and activation of the receptor protein tyrosine kinase
LIPID-SOLUBLE HORMONES		
Steroid hormones	Nuclear receptors	Nuclear translocation and altered genome transcription
Thyroid hormones (iodothyronines)	Nuclear receptors Cytosolic receptors	Altered genome transcription

cAMP, Cyclic adenosine monophosphate; *cGMP,* cyclic guanosine monophosphate; *IP_3,* inositol trisphosphate; *DAG,* diacylglycerol.

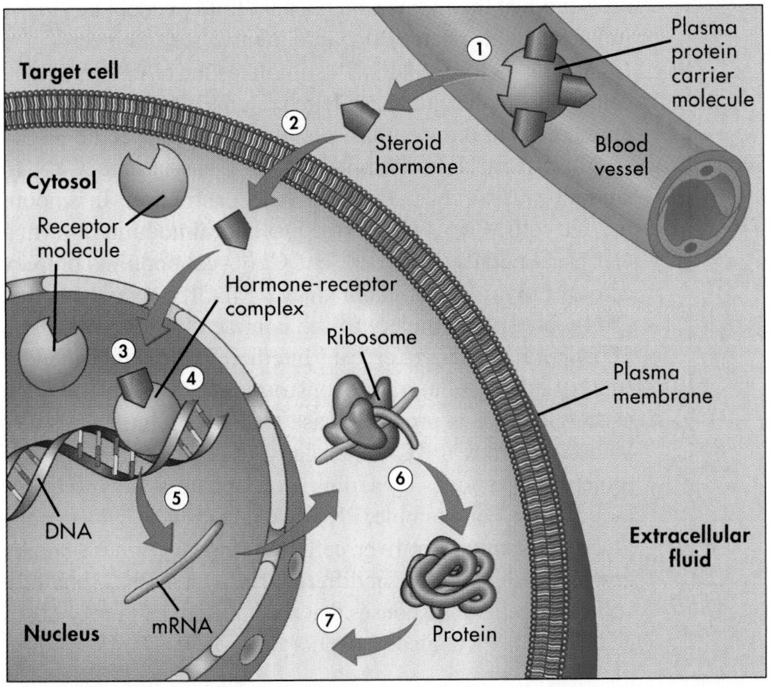

FIG. 19-4 Steroid hormone mechanism. Lipid-soluble steroid hormone molecules detach from the carrier protein *(1)* and pass through the plasma membrane *(2)*. Hormone molecules then diffuse into the nucleus where they bind to a receptor to form a hormone–receptor complex *(3)*. This complex then binds to a specific site on a deoxyribonucleic acid (DNA) molecule *(4)*, triggering transcription of the genetic information encoded there *(5)*. The resulting messenger ribonucleic acid (mRNA) molecule moves to the cytosol, where it associates with a ribosome, initiating synthesis of a new protein *(6)*. This new protein—usually an enzyme or channel protein—produces specific effects on the target cell *(7)*. (Modified from Thibodeau GA, Patton K: *Anatomy & physiology,* ed 4, St Louis, 1999, Mosby.)

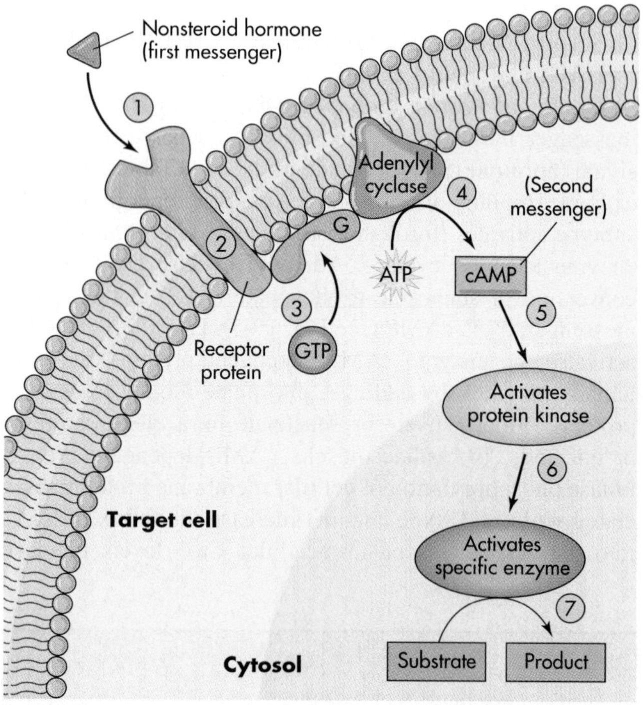

FIG. 19-5 Example of a second-messenger mechanism. A nonsteroid hormone *(first messenger)* binds to a fixed receptor in the plasma membrane of the target cell *(1)*. The hormone–receptor complex activates the G protein *(2)*. The activated G protein reacts with guanosine triphosphate (GTP), which in turn activates the membrane-bound enzyme adenylyl cyclase *(3)*. Adenylyl cyclase catalyzes the conversion of adenosine triphosphate (ATP) to cAMP *(second mesenger) (4)*. cAMP activates protein kinase A *(5)*. Protein kinases activate specific intracellular enzymes *(6)*. These activated enzymes then influence specific cellular reactions, thus producing the target cell's response to the hormone *(7)*. (Redrawn from Thibodeau GA, Patton K: *Anatomy & physiology,* ed 4, St Louis, 1999, Mosby.)

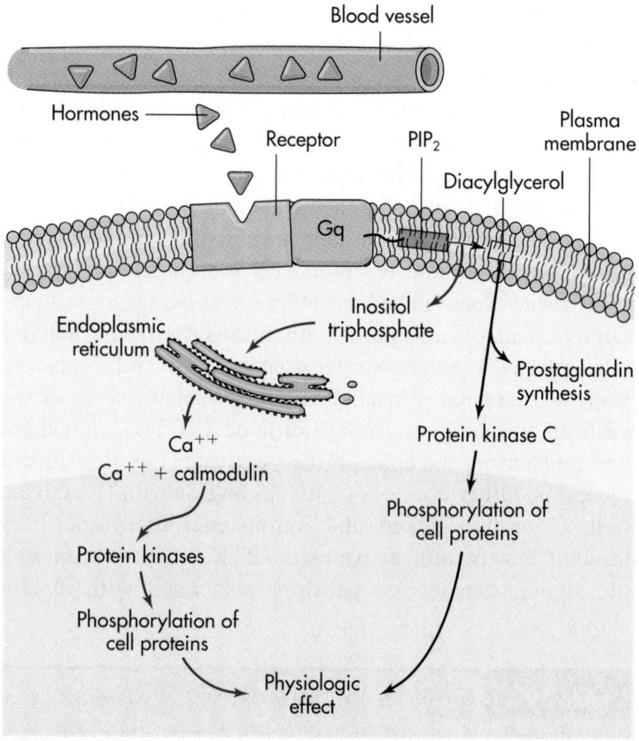

FIG. 19-6 Calcium, inositol triphosphate, and diacylglycerol as second messengers. See text for details.

Table 19-4 Second Messengers Identified for Specific Hormones

Second Messenger	Associated Hormones
Cyclic AMP	Adrenocorticotropic hormone (ACTH)
	Luteinizing hormone (LH)
	Human chorionic gonadotropin (hCG)
	Follicle-stimulating hormone (FSH)
	Thyroid-stimulating hormone (TSH)
	Antidiuretic hormone (ADH)
	Thyrotropin-releasing hormone (TRH)
	Parathyroid hormone (PTH)
	Glucagon
Cyclic GMP	Atrial natriuretic peptide
Calcium	Angiotensin II
	Gonadotropin-releasing hormone (GnRH)
	Antidiuretic hormone (ADH)
IP_3 and DAG	Angiotensin II
	Luteinizing hormone–releasing hormone (LHRH)

AMP, Adenosine monophosphate; *GMP,* guanosine monophosphate; *IP_3,* inositol trisphosphate; *DAG,* diacylglycerol.

myocardial contractility. The actions of cAMP are terminated by the enzyme phosphodiesterase III (PDE), which hydrolyzes cAMP into inactive adenosine monophosphate (AMP) (see Fig. 19-5).

Inositol trisphosphate (IP_3) and diacylglycerol (DAG). The binding of norepinephrine to an α_1-adrenergic receptor or angiotensin II to AT_1 receptors activates the enzyme phospholipase C. A G protein, designated G_q, couples the α_1-adrenergic receptor to phospholipase C. This enzyme breaks down the membrane phospholipid phosphatidylinositol 4,5-bisphosphate (PIP_2) into the two second messengers IP_3 and DAG (Fig. 19-6). IP_3 stimulates the release of stored calcium from the endoplasmic reticulum. In several cell types an increase in intracellular calcium activates specific physiologic effects. For example, an increase in free Ca^{++} in smooth muscle cells results in vasoconstriction. In smooth muscle cells, Ca^{++} binds to the protein calmodulin to form a Ca^{++}–calmodulin complex. The Ca^{++}–calmodulin complex activates myosin light-chain kinase (MLCK), an enzyme that adds a phosphate moiety to the contractile protein myosin. Phosphorylated myosin can interact with actin, thereby causing contraction or vasoconstriction.

DAG activates protein kinase C (PKC). Similar to other kinase enzymes, PKC either activates or deactivates other proteins or enzymes by adding a phosphate moiety to cellular proteins. For example, PKC phosphorylates and activates glycogen synthase in liver cells. Glycogen synthase breaks down stored glycogen. In different cell types, PKC initates a variety of cellular responses that are linked to cell metabolism and growth. PKC also phosphorylates several transcription

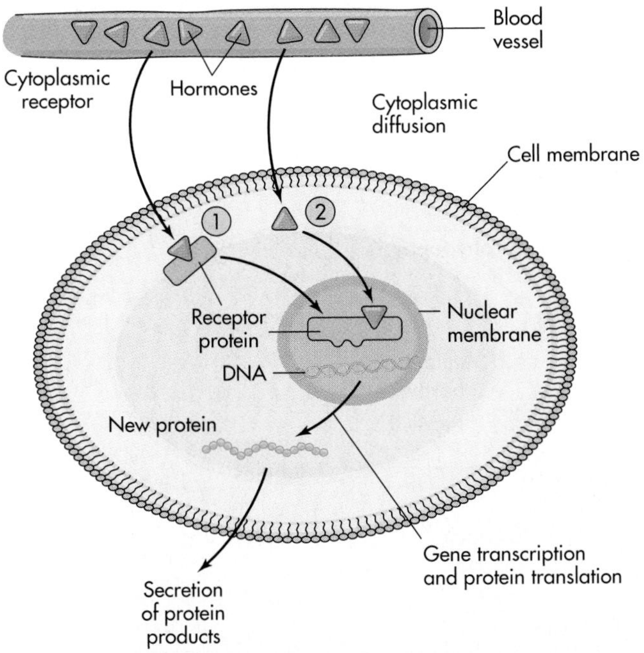

FIG. 19-7 Lipid-soluble hormone signaling process. Free hormones readily diffuse across the cell membrane and either *(1)* attach to a receptor in the cytosol or *(2)* attach to an a receptor molecule in the nucleus.

factors that lead to the induction of new protein synthesis and cell growth. There is evidence that activation of PKC is linked to carcinogenesis and abnormal accelerated growth in some cell types.

Calcium (Ca^{++}). In addition to being an important ion that participates in a multitude of cellular actions, Ca^{++} is also considered an important second messenger. Calcium release from intracellular stores is triggered by IP_3. Ca^{++} release from these intracellular stores activates many cellular responses. For example, vasopressor or ADH stimulation in liver cells leads to the production of IP_3, which in turn leads to an increase in intracellular Ca^{++}. An increase in intracellular Ca^{++} is associated with the enhanced breakdown of glycogen into glucose-1-phosphatase. In most cell types, Ca^{++} binds to the intracellular protein calmodulin and it is the Ca^{++}–calmodulin complex that is responsible for activation of specific proteins. As just noted, the Ca^{++}–calmodulin complex in smooth muscle cells activates MLCK. MLCK phosphorylates myosin; phosphorylated myosin can interact with actin, thereby causing contraction or vasoconstriction.

Cyclic guanosine monophosphate (cGMP). The production of the second messenger 3'-5' cGMP is associated with the activation of the intracellular enzyme guanylyl cyclase. cGMP activates cGMP-dependent kinase, which in turn activates a number of physiologic processes. The effects of various ligands, such as atrial natriuretic factor and nitric oxide (endothelium-derived relaxing factor), are mediated by the second messenger cGMP.

Steroid (Lipid-Soluble) Hormones

The lipid-soluble hormones are classified as steroid hormones and include androgens, estrogens, progestins, glucocorticoids, mineralocorticoids, and thyroid hormones. Steroid hormones are relatively small hydrophobic molecules (synthesized from cholesterol) and therefore cross the plasma membrane by simple diffusion (see Chapter 1). Some steroid hormones bind to receptor molecules in the cytoplasm and then diffuse into the nucleus, whereas others bind to receptors in the nucleus. The resulting hormone–receptor complex binds to a specific site on the promoter region of deoxyribonucleic acid (DNA). This binding activates ribonucleic acid (RNA) polymerase, which stimulates DNA transcription and increased synthesis of specific proteins (increased gene expression) (Fig. 19-7).

STRUCTURE AND FUNCTION OF THE ENDOCRINE GLANDS

Hypothalamic–Pituitary System

The hypothalamic–pituitary axis forms one of the most important and prominent portions of the endocrine system. The hypothalamic–pituitary axis produces a number of releasing/inhibitory hormones and tropic hormones, respectively, that affect a number of diverse body functions (Fig. 19-8). For example, the functions of the thyroid gland, adrenal gland, and male and female reproductive glands, as well as somatic growth and lactation, are regulated by hormones originating from the hypothalamic–pituitary axis.

The hypothalamus is divided into several nuclei and nuclear areas and is located at the base of the brain (Fig. 19-9). The pituitary gland is located at the sella turcica (a saddle-shaped depression on the superior surface of the sphenoid bone). The communication or anatomic connection (blood vessels and neural tract) between the hypothalamus and anterior and posterior pituitary is quite elaborate and well described. However, simply described, the hypothalamus is connected to the anterior pituitary by way of portal hypophysial blood vessels (Fig. 19-10), whereas the hypothalamus is connected to the posterior pituitary by way of a nerve tract referred to as the *hypothalamohypophysial tract* (Fig. 19-11). These connections are vital to the functioning of the hypothalamus–pituitary system. For example, ADH and oxytocin are synthesized in hypothalamic neurons but are stored and secreted by the posterior pituitary. ADH and oxytocin travel to the posterior pituitary by way of the hypothalamohypophysial nerve tract. Second, there are several releasing/inhibitory hormones, such as corticotropin-releasing hormone (CRH), that are synthesized in the hypothalamus and control the release of tropic hormones, such as ACTH, from the anterior pituitary (Table 19-5). These releasing hormones are secreted into the portal hypophysial blood vessels and travel to the anterior pituitary, where they stimulate the secretion of tropic hormones such as ACTH. Other releasing/inhibiting hormones synthesized in the hypothalamus that influence the release of anterior pituitary tropic hormones include thyrotropin-releasing hormone (TRH), growth hormone–releasing factor (GRF), gonadotropin-releasing hormone (GnRH), somatostatin, prolactin-inhibiting factor (PIF), and

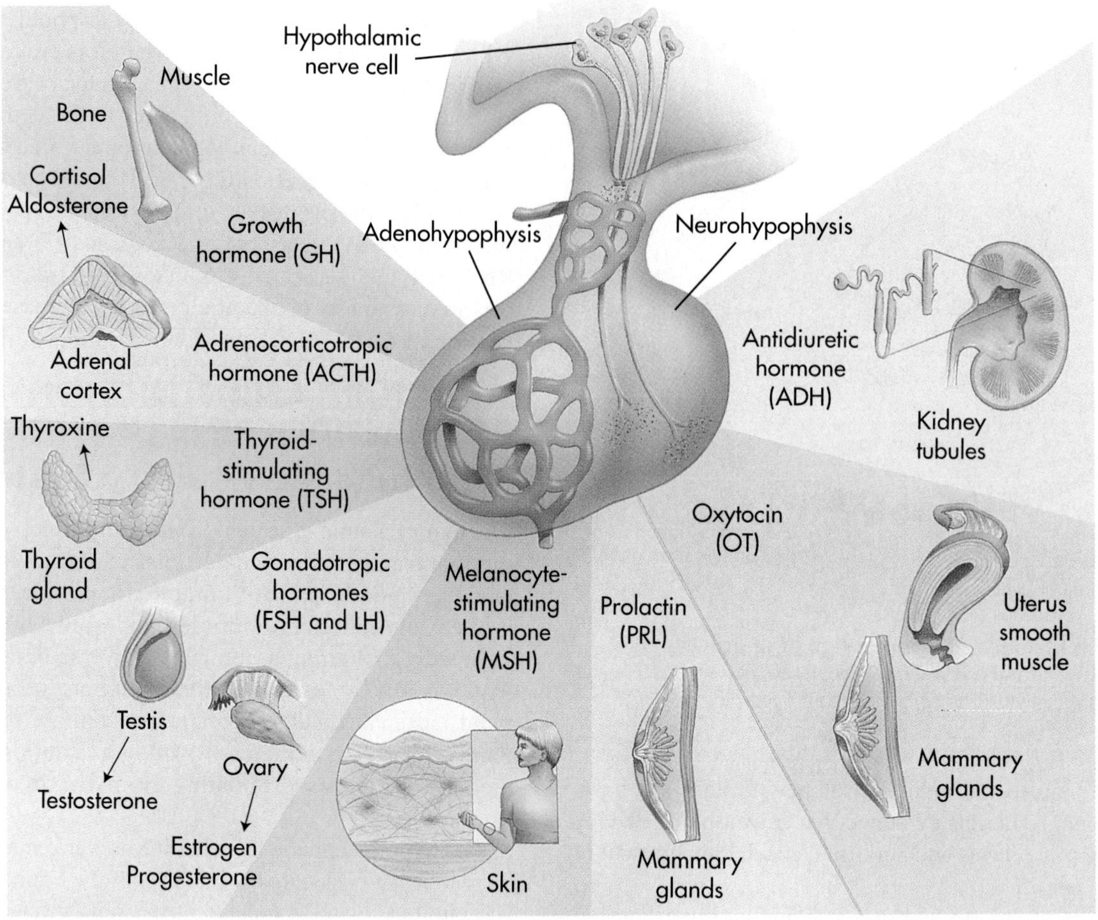

Fig. 19-8 Anterior pituitary hormones and their target organs. Adrenocorticotropic hormone *(ACTH);* thyroid-stimulating hormone *(TSH);* follicle-stimulating hormone *(FSH);* luteinizing hormone *(LH);* male analog of LH *(interstitial cell–stimulating hormone [ICSH]);* melanocyte-stimulating hormone *(MSH);* growth hormone *(GH).* (Modified from Thibodeau GA, Patton K: *Anatomy & physiology,* ed 4, St Louis, 1999, Mosby.)

Table 19-5 Hypothalamic Hormones (Hypophysiotropic Hormones)

Hormone	Target Tissue	Action
Thyrotropin-releasing hormone (TRH)	Anterior pituitary	Stimulates release of thyroid-stimulating hormone (TSH) Modulates prolactin secretion
Gonadotropin-releasing hormone (GnRH)	Anterior pituitary	Stimulates release of follicle-stimulating hormone (FSH) and luteinizing hormone (LH)
Somatostatin	Anterior pituitary Gastrointestinal tract	Inhibits release of growth hormone (GH) Decreases gastric motility, intestinal secretion, and secretion of TSH, parathyroid hormone, renin, glucagon, and insulin
Growth hormone–releasing factor (GRF)	Anterior pituitary	Stimulates release of GH
Corticotropin-releasing hormone (CRH)	Anterior pituitary	Stimulates release of adrenocorticotropic hormone (ACTH) and β-endorphin
Substance P	Anterior pituitary	Inhibits synthesis and release of ACTH Stimulates secretion of GH, FSH, LH, and prolactin
Prolactin-inhibiting factor (PIF; possibly dopamine)	Anterior pituitary	Inhibits secretion of prolactin
Prolactin-releasing hormone (PRH)	Anterior pituitary	Stimulates secretion of prolactin

substance P. These are also referred to as the **hypophysiotropic hormones.**

Some of the aforementioned hypothalamic releasing/inhibiting hormones are referred to as releasing *hormones* rather than releasing *factors.* The primary difference between a releasing factor and a releasing hormone is that the chemical structure (amino acid sequence) has been identified for a releasing hormone, whereas even though there is good evidence for the existence of releasing factors, their amino acid structure has not been identified.

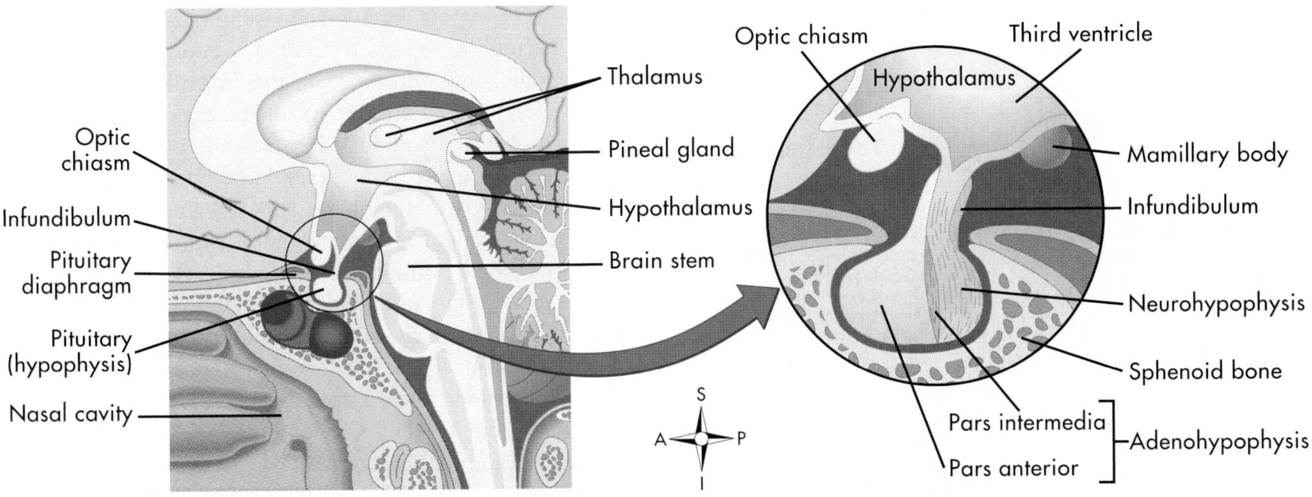

FIG. 19-9 Location and structure of the pituitary gland (hypophysis). The pituitary gland is located within the sella turcica of the skull's sphenoid bone and is connected to the hypothalamus by a stalklike infundibulum. The infundibulum passes through a gap in the portion of the dura mater that covers the pituitary (the pituitary diaphragm). The inset shows that the pituitary is divided into an anterior portion, the adenohypophysis, and a posterior portion, the neurohypophysis. The adenohypophysis is further subdivided into the pars anterior and pars intermedia. The pars intermedia is almost absent in the adult pituitary. (From Thibodeau GA, Patton K: *Anatomy & physiology,* ed 4, St Louis, 1999, Mosby.)

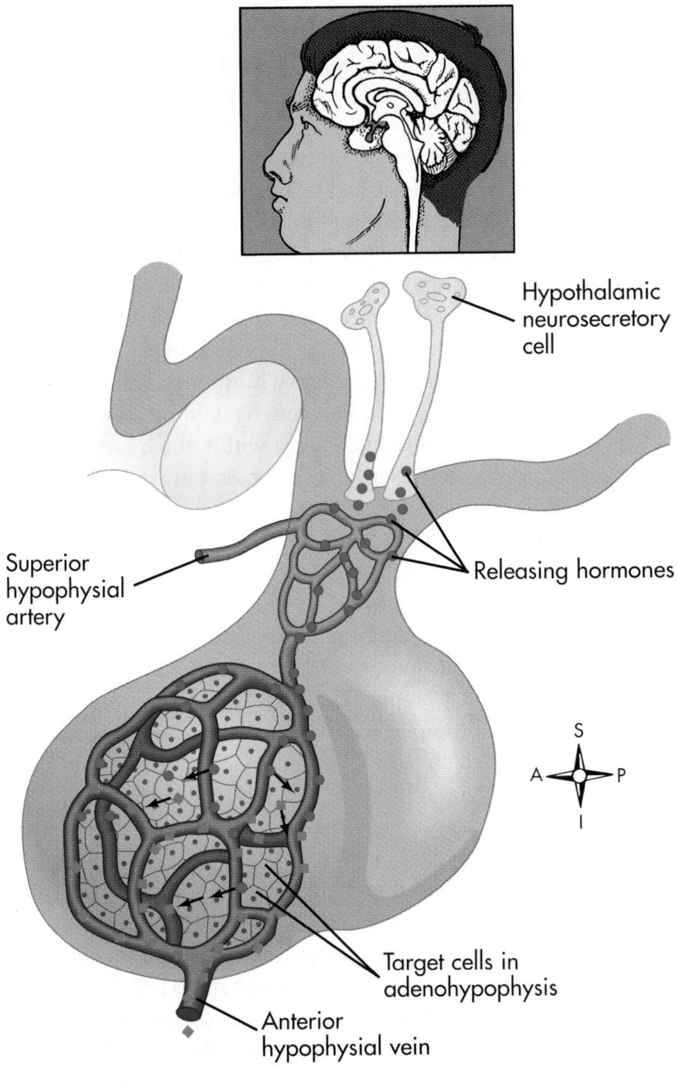

FIG. 19-10 Hypophysial portal system. Neurons in the hypothalamus secrete releasing hormones into veins that carry the releasing hormones directly to the vessels of the adenohypophysis, thus bypassing the normal circulatory route. (From Thibodeau GA, Patton K: *Anatomy & physiology,* ed 4, St Louis, 1999, Mosby.)

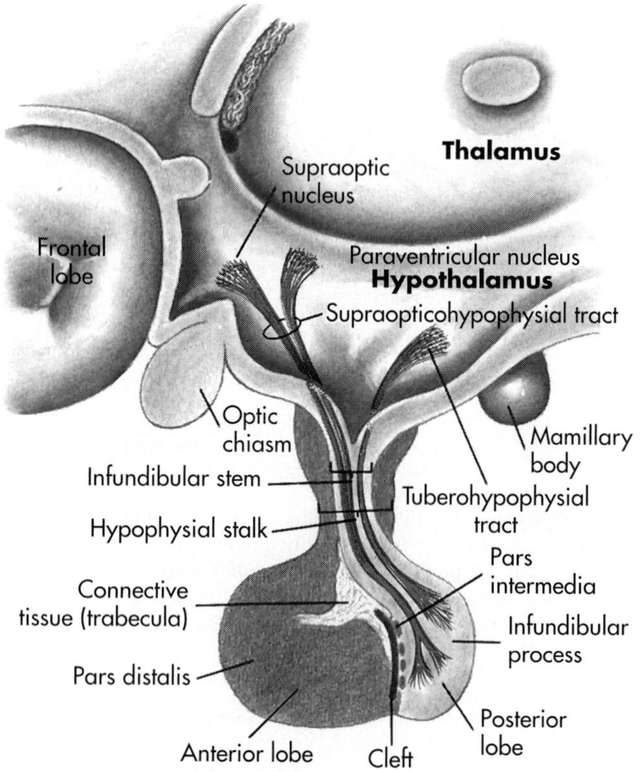

FIG. 19-11 Nerve tracts from hypothalamus to posterior lobe of pituitary gland. (From Thompson JM et al: *Mosby's manual of clinical nursing,* ed 4, St Louis, 1997, Mosby.)

Embryology and Anatomy of the Hypothalamic–Pituitary Axis

The anterior pituitary (adenohypophysis) accounts for 75% of the total weight of the pituitary gland. It is composed of three regions: (1) the pars distalis, (2) the pars tuberalis, and (3) the pars intermedia. The **pars distalis** is the major component of the anterior pituitary and the source of the anterior pituitary hormones. The **pars tuberalis** is a thin layer of cells on the anterior and lateral portions of the infundibular stem. The **pars intermedia** lies between the two lobes of the pituitary gland. In the adult the distinct intermediate lobe disappears and the individual cells are distributed diffusely throughout the pars distalis and pars nervosa (neural lobe).[2]

The posterior pituitary (neurohypophysis) arose embryologically from an outpouching of the floor of the third ventricle within the brain. The posterior hypothalamus consists of three parts: (1) the median eminence located at the base of the hypothalamus, (2) the infundibular stem, and (3) the infundibular process, also known as the *pars nervosa* or *neural lobe.* The **median eminence** is composed largely of the nerve endings of axons that arise primarily in the ventral hypothalamus. The median eminence often is designated as part of the posterior pituitary but contains at least 10 biologically active hypothalamic-releasing hormones, as well as the neurotransmitters dopamine, norepinephrine, serotonin, acetylcholine, and histamine. The median eminence therefore might be more appropriately considered part of the hypothalamus. The infundibular stem contains the axons of neurons that originate in the supraoptic and paraventricular nuclei of the hypothalamus. The infundibular stem thus connects the pituitary gland to the brain. Axons originating in the hypothalamus terminate in the **infundibular process,** which secretes the hormones of the posterior pituitary.

Because of the anatomic location and connection of the pituitary gland to the brain, several neurotransmitters as well as physical and emotional stressors influence the release of specific hypothalamic releasing/inhibitory hormones and their respective tropic hormones. For example, the neurotransmitter norepinephrine stimulates the secretion of CRH, TRH, and GnRH, whereas the neurotransmitter γ-aminobutyric acid (GABA) inhibits CRH, TRH, and GnRH secretion. In terms of tropic hormone release from the anterior pituitary, norepinephrine stimulates the secretion of thyroid-stimulating hormone (TSH), growth hormone (GH), LH, and FSH, whereas the secretion of ACTH is inhibited. Physical (trauma) and emotional (pain) stress, as well as hypoglycemia, can influence the release of stimulating hormones such as CRH, therefore ultimately affecting the amount of ACTH (the tropic hormone) released by the anterior pituitary. This example emphasizes the integrated and coordinated function of the hypothalamic–pituitary axis.

Hormones of the Posterior Pituitary

The posterior pituitary secretes two polypeptide hormones: (1) **antidiuretic hormone (ADH),** also called *vasopressin,* and (2) **oxytocin.** These peptide hormones are similar in structure, differing by only two amino acids. They are synthesized, along with their binding proteins, the neurophysins, in the supraoptic and paraventricular nuclei of the hypothalamus (see Fig. 19-11). Once synthesized, these hormones and their carrier proteins are packaged in secretory vesicles. They are moved down the axons of the infundibular stem to the infundibular process for storage. The posterior pituitary thus can be seen as a storage and releasing site for hormones synthesized in the hypothalamus.

Similar to the anterior pituitary hormones, the release of ADH and oxytocin is influenced by neurotransmitter release. There are well-defined areas within the hypothalamus and other brain stem areas where noradrenergic norepinephrine–containing fibers innervate vasopressin and oxytocin neurons. Stimulation of these areas results in an increase in ADH and oxytocin release.

Antidiuretic Hormone

The major homeostatic function of the posterior pituitary is the control of plasma osmolality as regulated by ADH, or vasopressin (see Chapter 3). At physiologic levels, ADH acts to increase the permeability of the distal renal tubules and collecting ducts (see Chapter 34). This increased permeability leads to an increase in water reabsorption and the production of more concentrated urine. These effects may be inhibited by hypercalcemia, prostaglandin E, and hypokalemia. ADH has no direct effect on electrolyte levels.

ADH originally was named *vasopressin* because in extremely high doses it does cause vasoconstriction and a resulting increase in arterial blood pressure. These levels are not reached physiologically, but this effect may be achieved pharmacologically. For example, high doses of ADH (as the

Table 19-6 Tropic Hormones of the Anterior Pituitary and Their Functions

Hormone	Secretory Cell Type	Target Organs	Functions
Adrenocorticotropic hormone (ACTH)	Corticotropic	Adrenal gland	Increased steroidogenesis Synthesis of adrenal proteins contributing to maintenance of the adrenal gland
Melanocyte-stimulating hormone (MSH)	Melanotropic	Anterior pituitary	Promotes secretion of melanin and lipotropin by anterior pituitary; makes skin darker
Somatotropic hormones Growth hormone (GH)	Somatotropic	Muscle, bone, liver	Regulates metabolic processes related to growth and adaptation to physical and emotional stressors, including skeletal growth, muscle growth, increased protein synthesis, increased liver glycogenolysis, increased fat mobilization
		Liver	Induces formation of somatomedins, or insulin-like growth factors (IGF) that have actions similar to insulin
Prolactin	Lactotropic	Breast	Milk production
Glycoprotein hormones			
Thyroid-stimulating hormone (TSH)	Thyrotropic	Thyroid gland	Increased production and secretion of thyroid hormone Increased iodine uptake
Luteinizing hormone (LH)	Gonadotropic	In women: ovarian follicle	Ovulation, progesterone production
		In men: Leydig cells	Regulates spermatogenesis, testosterone production
Follicle-stimulating hormone (FSH)	Gonadotropic	In women: ovarian follicle	Follicle maturation, estrogen production
		In men: Leydig cells	Spermatogenesis
β-Lipotropin	Corticotropic	Adipose cells	Fat breakdown and release of fatty acids
β-Endorphins	Corticotropic	Adipose cells	Analgesia; may regulate body temperature, food and water intake

drug vasopressin) may be administered to achieve hemostasis during hemorrhage.

The secretion of ADH is regulated primarily by the osmoreceptors of the hypothalamus, located near or in the supraoptic nuclei (osmoreceptors are stimulated by increased osmolality). The plasma osmolality is maintained at the mean set point of approximately 280 mOsm/kg. As plasma osmolality increases, the rate of ADH secretion increases.

Other mechanisms affect ADH secretion. ADH secretion is increased by changes in intravascular volume. Intravascular volume changes are monitored by mechanorecceptors in the left atrium and in the carotid and aortic arches. A volume loss of 7% to 25% acts through these receptors to stimulate ADH secretion. This mechanism for regulating ADH secretion is much less sensitive than that of the osmoreceptors. Stress, trauma, pain, exercise, nausea, nicotine, exposure to heat, and drugs such as chloroform and morphine also increase ADH secretion, apparently by activating cholinergic neurotransmitters in the hypothalamus. ADH secretion decreases with a decrease in plasma osmolality, an increase in intravascular volume, hypertension, and alcohol ingestion.

Oxytocin

Oxytocin is primarily responsible for contraction of the uterus and milk ejection in lactating women and may have a role in sperm motility in men, although this effect has not yet been clearly elucidated. In both genders, oxytocin has an antidiuretic effect similar to that of ADH. The mechanisms by which this effect is achieved appear similar to those of ADH, but the physiologic significance is not clear. (The function of this hormone is discussed in Chapter 21.)

The release of oxytocin has been studied more extensively in women than in men. In the woman, oxytocin is secreted in response to suckling and mechanical distention of the female reproductive tract. Oxytocin is required for the milk "let-down" reflex. Stimulated by sucking, oxytocin binds to its receptors on myoepithelial cells in the mammary tissues and causes contraction of those cells. This results in increased intramammary pressure and milk expression.

Oxytocin also acts on the uterus to stimulate contractions. Its role in initiating labor has been debated because levels of oxytocin do not increase until near the end of labor. It is hypothesized that at this stage oxytocin functions to enhance effectiveness of contractions, to promote delivery of the placenta, and to stimulate postpartum contractions to prevent excessive bleeding.[3]

Hormones of the Anterior Pituitary

The anterior pituitary is composed of two main cell types: (1) the **chromophobes,** which appear to be nonsecretory; and (2) the **chromophils,** which are considered the secretory cells of the adenohypophysis. The chromophils are subdivided into six secretory cell types, and each cell type secretes one or more specific hormones (Table 19-6).

The tropic hormones secreted by the anterior pituitary include ACTH, melanocyte-stimulating hormone (MSH), LH, GH, prolactin, FSH, and TSH. The actions of these anterior pituitary tropic hormones are summarized in Table 19-6. Even though six major stimulatory hormones are released by the anterior pituitary, they can be grouped into three categories: corticotropin-related hormones (ACTH, β-lipoprotein, MSH, and related endorphins), somatomammotropins (GH and prolactin), and glycoproteins (LH, FSH, and TSH). The corticotropin-related hormones are all derived from the precursor pro-opiomelanocortin. Pro-opiomelanocortin is the precursor for ACTH and β-lipoprotein, and within the ACTH amino acid sequence exists MSH. In general, the regulation of the anterior pituitary hormones is achieved by (1) feedback of hypothalamic releasing/inhibitory hormones and factors, (2) feedback from target gland hormones (i.e., cortisol, estrogen), and (3) direct effects of neurotransmitters.

Thyroid and Parathyroid Glands

The thyroid gland, located in the neck just below the larynx, produces hormones that control the rates of metabolic processes throughout the body. The parathyroid glands are located near the thyroid. The four parathyroid glands function to control serum calcium levels.

Thyroid Gland

The **thyroid gland** is composed of two lobes that lie on either side of the trachea, inferior to the thyroid cartilage (Fig. 19-12). The lobes are joined by a small band of tissue, the **isthmus,** which crosses the anterior surface of the trachea and larynx at the cricoid cartilage. The normal thyroid gland is not visible on inspection, but it may be palpated on swallowing, which causes upward displacement of the gland.

The thyroid gland is composed of **follicles.** The follicles are composed of follicular cells that surround a viscous substance called *colloid.* The follicular cells synthesize and secrete some of the thyroid hormones. Neurons terminate on blood vessels within the thyroid gland and on the follicular cells themselves. Acetylcholine, catecholamines, and other peptides directly affect secretory activity of the follicular cells and thyroid blood flow.[4]

Also found in the tissue of the thyroid are parafollicular cells, or **C cells.** The C cells secrete various polypeptides, including calcitonin and somatostatin.[4] **Calcitonin,** also called *thyrocalcitonin,* acts to lower serum calcium levels by direct, rapid, and significant inhibition of bone-resorbing osteoclasts and promotion of osteoblasts that result in bone formation. (Bone resorption is explained in Chapter 41.) The metabolic consequences of calcitonin deficiency or excess, however, have not yet been identified in humans (Table 19-7).

Regulation of Thyroid Hormone Secretion

Thyroid hormone (TH) is regulated through a negative-feedback loop involving the hypothalamus, the anterior pituitary, and the thyroid gland (see Fig. 19-2). (Fig. 19-12 illustrates the thyroid and parathyroid glands.) The initiating hormone is termed **thyrotropin-releasing hormone (TRH),** and it is synthesized and stored within the hypothalamus. TRH is released into the hypothalamic–pituitary portal system and circulates to the anterior pituitary, where it stimulates the release of thyroid-stimulating hormone (TSH). TRH is

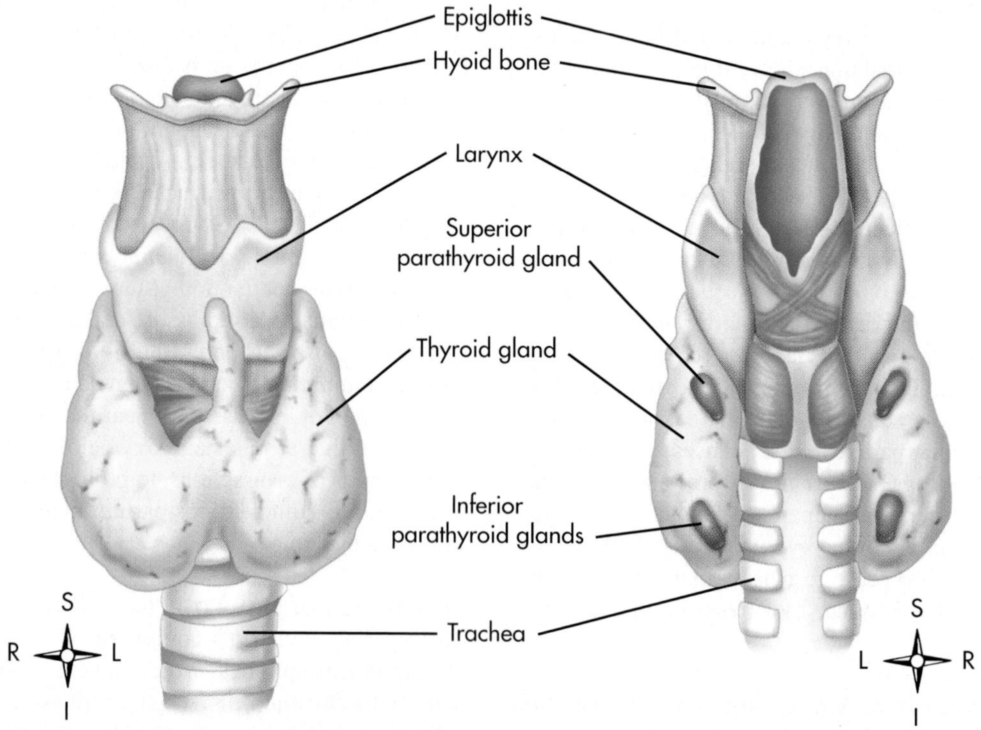

Fig. 19-12 Thyroid and parathyroid glands. Note the relationship of the thyroid and parathyroid glands to each other, to the larynx (voice box), and to the trachea. (From Thibodeau GA, Patton K: *Anatomy & physiology,* ed 4, St Louis, 1999, Mosby.)

increased with exposure to cold, stress, and decreased levels of thyroxine (T_4).

Thyroid-stimulating hormone (TSH) is a glycoprotein hormone synthesized and stored within the anterior pituitary. Once TSH is secreted by the anterior pituitary, it circulates to bind with TSH receptor sites located on the outer side of the thyroid cell's plasma membrane. The effects of TSH on the thyroid include (1) an immediate increase in the release of stored thyroid hormones, (2) an increase in iodine uptake and oxidation, (3) an increase in thyroid hormone synthesis, and (4) an increase in the synthesis and secretion of prostaglandins by the thyroid. Thyroid gland hormones and their regulation and function are summarized in Table 19-7.

When TH is secreted by the thyroid gland, it acts on the thyroid gland, the anterior pituitary, and the median eminence to regulate further TH production. Thyroid hormones have a negative-feedback effect and inhibit TRH and TSH, which decreases TH synthesis and secretion.

Synthesis of Thyroid Hormone

The thyroid gland is stimulated to produce thyroid hormone by TSH, by low serum iodide levels, or by drugs interfering with the thyroid gland's uptake of iodide in the blood. (Iodide is the inorganic or ionic form of iodine and is the form in which iodine enters the thyroid gland.) The first step in the synthesis of TH is to increase the uptake of iodide (an iodine compound) into the thyroid gland. Because there is an iodine concentration gradient of about 30:1 to 40:1 between the thyroid gland and the blood, iodine is moved by active transport from the extracellular fluid to the thyroid follicular cells. (Mechanisms of active transport are discussed in Chapter 1.) Before being used to form TH, however, the iodide must be oxidized to iodine. This reaction is facilitated by the enzyme thyroidal peroxidase inside the follicular cells. The major naturally occurring source of iodine is seafood; in the United States iodine is added to salt and flour. Approximately 25% of ingested iodine is trapped by the thyroid gland.

For the synthesis of TH to occur, another molecule, thyroglobulin, also must be present. **Thyroglobulin** is a large glycoprotein synthesized within the follicular cell. After its synthesis the uniodinated thyroglobulin is released into the colloid. (Colloid is a general term referring to proteins that are stored outside the cell, close to the cell membrane.) Iodine then combines with tyrosine in the thyroglobulin to form iodotyrosines. Two major iodotyrosines are monoiodotyrosine (MIT), with one iodine molecule, and diiodotyrosine (DIT), with two iodine molecules. Several hours after the iodotyrosines are formed, coupling of the iodotyrosines takes place to form iodothyronines, two of which are active thyroid hormones. The exact mechanism for this coupling is not clearly understood. The most commonly held view is that two DIT molecules are coupled to form **thyroxine (T_4)** and one DIT molecule and one MIT molecule are joined to form **triiodothyronine (T_3)**. The thyroid gland normally produces 90% T_4 and 10% T_3. In the body tissues, however, T_4 is converted to T_3, and T_3 probably has the greatest metabolic effects. Once released into the circulation, T_3 and T_4 are transported bound to one of three carrier proteins: thyroxine-binding glubulin, thyroxine-binding prealbumin (transthyretin), or albumin.

Table 19-7 Thyroid Gland Hormones and Their Regulation and Function

Hormone	Regulation	Functions
Thyroxine (T_4) and triiodothyronine (T_3)	T_4 and T_3 levels are controlled by TSH Hormones show diurnal variation with a peak during late evening Influences on amount secreted Gender Pregnancy Gonadal- and adrenal cortical–increased steroids = ↑ levels Exposure to extreme cold = ↑ levels Nutritional state Chemicals GHIH = ↓ levels Dopamine = ↓ levels Catecholamines = ↑ levels	Regulates protein, fat, and carbohydrate catabolism in all cells Regulates metabolic rate of all cells Regulates body heat production Acts as insulin antagonist Maintains growth hormone secretion, skeletal maturation Affects CNS development Necessary for muscle tone and vigor Maintains cardiac rate, force, and output Maintains secretion of GI tract Affects respiratory rate and oxygen utilization Maintains calcium mobilization Affects RBC production Stimulates lipid turnover, free fatty acid release, and cholesterol synthesis
Calcitonin	Elevated serum calcium—major stimulant for calcitonin Other stimulants Gastrin Calcium-rich foods (regardless of serum Ca^{++} levels) Pregnancy Lowered serum calcium—suppresses calcitonin release	Major function: lowers serum calcium by opposing bone-resorbing effects of PTH, prostaglandins, and calciferols by inhibiting osteoclastic activity Also lowers serum phosphate levels May also decrease calcium and phosphorous absorption in GI tract

From Phipps WJ, Sands JK, Marek JF: *Medical-surgical nursing: concepts and clinical practice,* ed 6, St Louis, 1999, Mosby.
CNS, Central nervous system; *GI,* gastrointestinal; *GHIH,* growth hormone–inhibiting hormone; *RBC,* red blood cell; *PTH,* parathyroid hormone.

Thyroid hormones affect many body tissues, primarily by affecting growth and maturation of tissues. Similar to some steroid hormones, thyroid hormones bind to intracellular receptor complexes and then influence the genetic expression of specific proteins. Thyroid hormones also affect cell metabolism by altering protein, fat, and glucose metabolism and, as a result, heat production and oxygen consumption are increased.

It is important to note that thyroid hormones exert a number of permissive effects on many organs, which are rather modest at physiologic thyroid hormone levels. However, these effects can become very pronounced when there is either high or low levels of circulating thyroid hormones. For example, in the heart, T_3 stimulates the synthesis of specific contractile proteins (e.g., α-myosin heavy chain), sarcolemmal ion pumps (Na^+–K^+–ATPase pump, Ca^{++}–ATPase pump) and membrane receptors (β-adrenergic receptors). Therefore in hyperthyroidism, which is associated with elevated levels of thyroid hormones, cardiac effects include increased heart rate and cardiac output, as well as the development of a cardiomyopathy. Thyroid hormones also affect the respiratory center, contributing to the normal hypoxic and hypercapnic drive. In severe hypothyroidism, ventilation can become very depressed. Thyroid hormone also stimulates bone resorption and hyperthyroidism is associated with osteopenia, hypercalcemia and hypercalciuria. Other manifestations of thyroid hormone alteration are explained in Chapter 20.

Parathyroid Glands

Two pairs of parathyroid glands normally are present. They are small and located behind the upper pole of the thyroid gland and behind the lower pole (see Fig. 19-12). The number of parathyroid glands, however, may range from two to six.

The parathyroid glands produce **parathyroid hormone (PTH),** a regulator of serum calcium. PTH is regulated primarily by the level of ionized plasma calcium, although these regulatory mechanisms are not precisely clear. Calcium also increases intraparathyroid destruction of PTH but apparently does not affect the rate of PTH synthesis.

Magnesium and phosphate levels also affect PTH secretion. Hypomagnesemia in persons with normal calcium levels acts as a mild stimulant to PTH secretion. In hypocalcemic persons, hypomagnesemia decreases PTH secretion. Hyperphosphatemia leads to hypocalcemia, probably because of calcium-phosphate precipitation in soft tissue and bone. Alterations in serum phosphate levels therefore may indirectly influence PTH secretion by affecting serum calcium levels (Fig. 19-13). The overall effect of PTH is to decrease serum phosphate concentration.

Once the parathyroid gland is stimulated, PTH is secreted. On release, PTH enters the circulation in unbound form. The hormone attaches to plasma membrane receptors in target tissues, where the biologic effects of PTH are mediated primarily by activation of the adenylyl cyclase system (see Chapter 1).

PTH is the single most important factor in the regulation of serum calcium levels (Fig. 19-14). To achieve regulation of serum calcium, PTH acts directly on bone and on the kidneys. In bone, PTH has at least two effects. The effect of intense acute stimulation involves the breakdown and resorption of bone (see Chapter 41). Chronic stimulation by PTH results in bone remodeling, a process in which bone is broken down and re-formed.

In the kidneys, PTH acts on its plasma membrane receptor in the distal and proximal tubules of the nephron to increase reabsorption of calcium and to decrease reabsorption of phosphorus respectively. PTH also decreases proximal tubule reabsorption of bicarbonate. In the kidney, PTH stimulates the synthesis of a biologically active form of vitamin D (1,25 dihydroxy vitamin D), a potent stimulator of calcium and phosphate transport in the intestine. In this way PTH apparently increases gastrointestinal absorption of calcium.

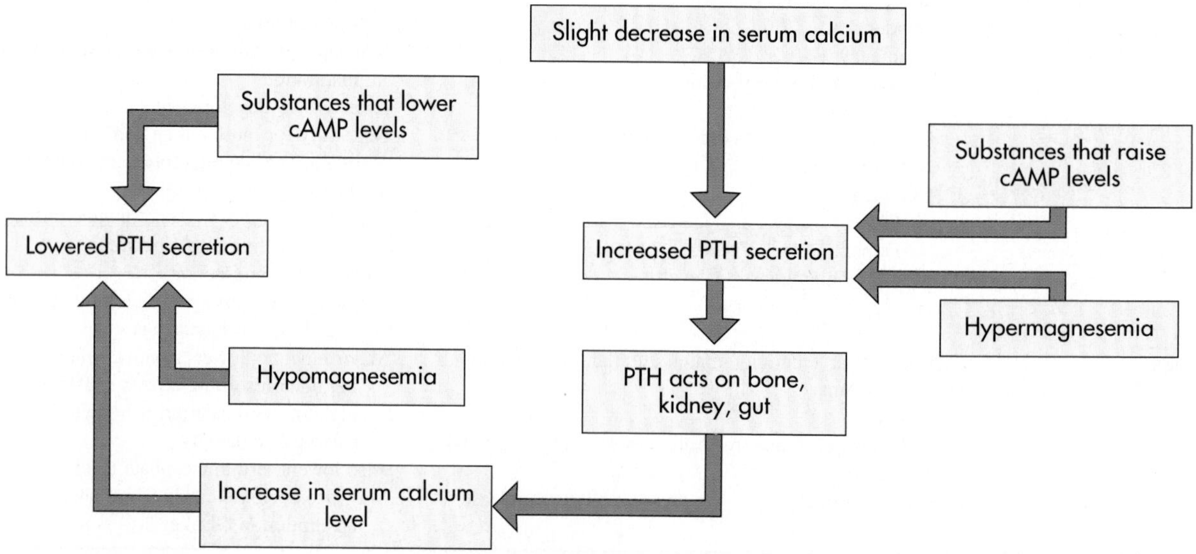

FIG. 19-13 Variables affecting parathyroid hormone (PTH) secretion. *cAMP,* Cyclic adenosine monophosphate.

Endocrine Pancreas

The **pancreas** is both an endocrine gland that produces hormones and an exocrine gland that produces digestive enzymes. (The exocrine pancreas is discussed in Chapter 37.) The pancreas therefore is responsible for much metabolism within the body. A major disorder of the endocrine pancreas is diabetes mellitus.

The pancreas is located behind the stomach, between the spleen and the duodenum. It houses the **islets of Langerhans,** which secrete **glucagon** and **insulin,** hormones that help to regulate much of the carbohydrate, fat, and protein metabolism within the body. The islets of Langerhans have three types of hormone-secreting cells: **A cells,** which secrete glucagon; **B cells,** which secrete insulin; and **D cells,** which secrete gastrin or somatostatin or both. The A cells and D cells are located at the periphery of the islet, and B cells are located in the middle. F cells, a fourth type of pancreatic cell, secrete pancreatic polypeptide. (The pancreas is illustrated in Fig. 19-15). Nerves from both divisions of the autonomic nervous system innervate the pancreatic islets.

Insulin

The B cells of the pancreas synthesize insulin from the precursor, proinsulin. Proinsulin is formed from a larger and earlier precursor molecule, preproinsulin. Proinsulin is composed of an A peptide and a B peptide connected by a C peptide and two disulfide bonds. C peptide is cleaved by proteolytic enzymes, leaving the A and B peptide chain connected by the disulfide bonds. The bonded A and B chains become insulin. Insulin circulates freely in the plasma and is not bound to a carrier.

WHAT'S NEW? Diabetes and Islet Cell Transplant

Clinical trials are currently in progress for transplantation of pancreatic islet cells for the treatment and potential cure of type 1 diabetes mellitus. Islet cell transplant would provide physiologic control of glucose metabolism and prevent the life-threatening complications of diabetes.

The advantages of islet cell transplant over pancreas transplant include the following:

1. It is a safe and simple procedure.
2. It has potential to be an outpatient procedure.
3. It has potential for cell banking by cytopreservation.
4. It has potential for pretransplant genetic immunomodulation.
5. It provides xenogenic (nonhuman) sources of cells.

These advantages and the progress in genetic engineering hold promise for widely available cell therapy for treatment of IDDM.

Data from Inoue K, Mayamoto M: Islet transplantation, *J Hepatobiliary Pancreat Surg* 7(2):163, 2000; Lee MK, Bae YH: Cell transplantation for endocrine disorders, *Adv Drug Deliv Rev* 42(1-2):103, 2000; Soria B et al: Engineering pancreatic islets, *Pflugers Arch* 440(1):1, 2000.

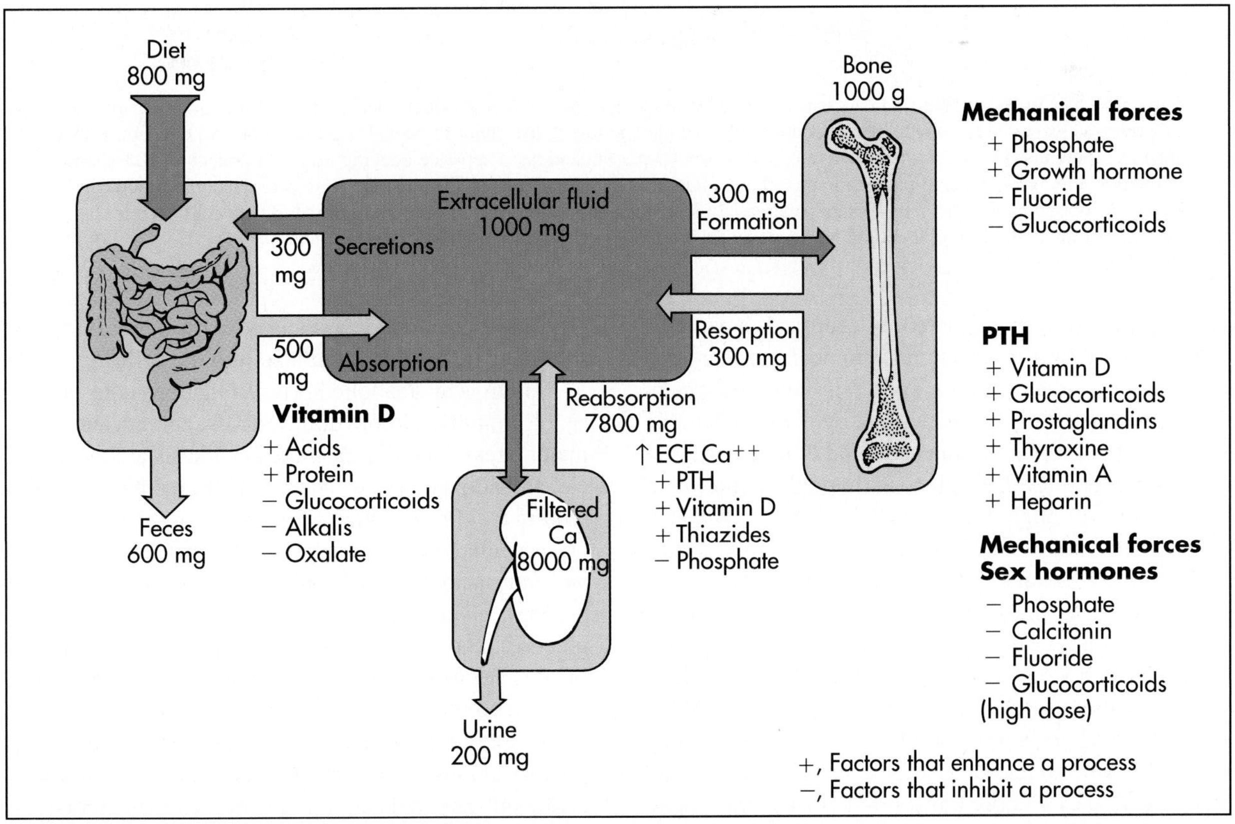

FIG. 19-14 Normal calcium metabolism regulated by parathyroid hormone (PTH). *ECF,* Extracellular fluid; *PTH,* parathyroid hormone; *Mg,* magnesium.

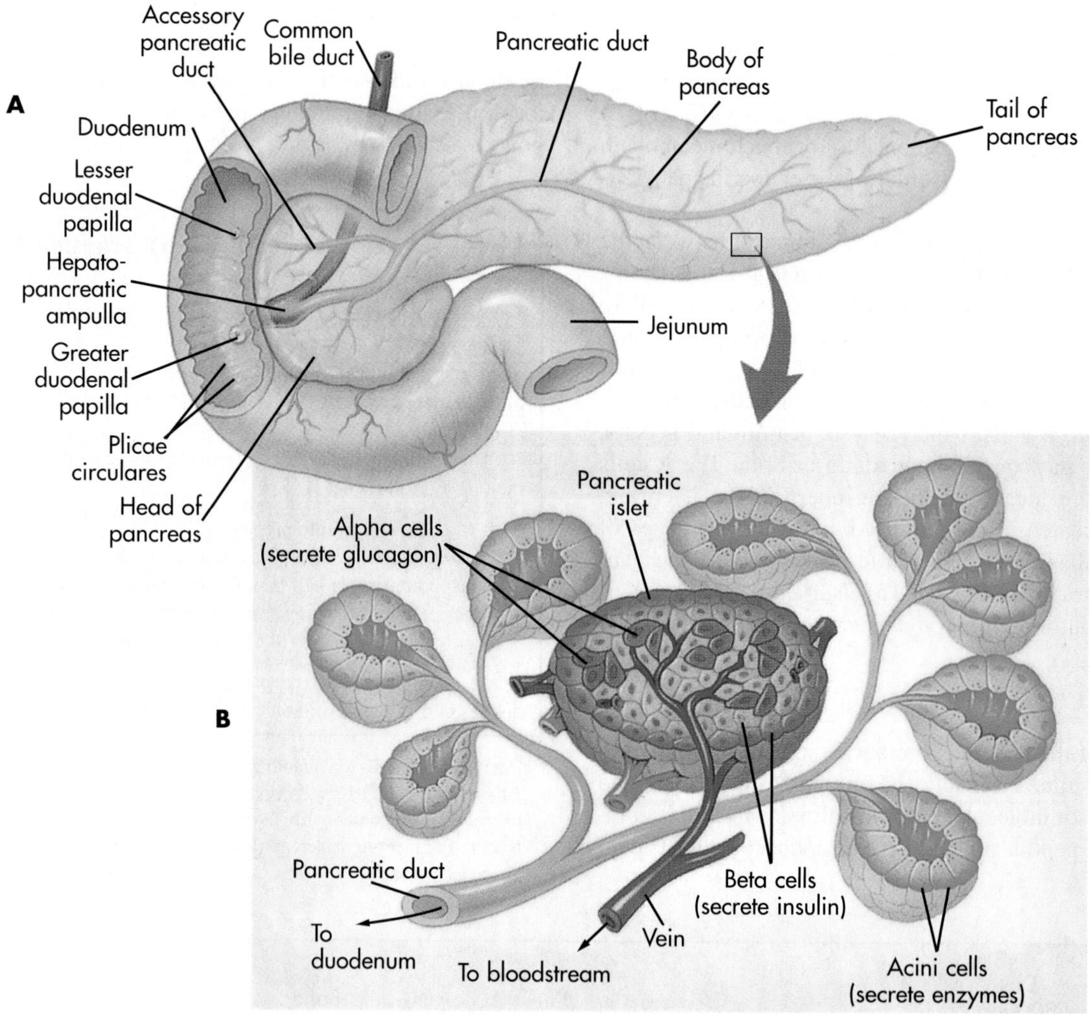

Fig. 19-15 The pancreas. A, Pancreas dissected to show main and accessory ducts. The main duct may join the common bile duct, as shown here, to enter the duodenum by a single opening at the major duodenal papilla, or the two ducts may have separate openings. The accessory pancreatic duct is usually present and has a separate opening into the duodenum. **B,** Exocrine glandular cells (around small pancreatic ducts) and endocrine glandular cells of the pancreatic islets (adjacent to blood capillaries). Exocrine pancreatic cells secrete pancreatic juice, alpha endocrine cells secrete glucagon, and beta cells secrete insulin. (From Thibodeau GA, Patton K: *Anatomy & physiology,* ed 4, St Louis, 1999, Mosby.)

Secretion of insulin is regulated by chemical, hormonal, and neural control. Insulin secretion is promoted by increased blood levels of glucose, amino acids (arginine and glucagon), and gastrointestinal hormones and by parasympathetic stimulation of the B cells. Insulin secretion diminishes in response to low blood levels of glucose (hypoglycemia), high levels of insulin (through negative feedback to the B cells), and sympathetic stimulation of the A cells in the islets. Prostaglandin (PGE2) also inhibits insulin secretion.[5]

Insulin facilitates the rate of glucose uptake into many cells within the body. Binding of insulin to its RTK receptor subtype initiates a series of events that involves autophosphorylation of the insulin receptor substrate (IRS1) and the activation (phosphorylation) of other proteins, including GRB2, a PI-3 kinase, and a tyrosine phosphatase. The net effect is that GLUT4 glucose transporters, which are located below the plasma membrane, are transported (exocytosis) to the outside of the plasma membranes. Translocation of the GLUT4 transporter is associated with a tenfold to twentyfold increase in glucose uptake into the cell (Fig. 19-16).

Insulin is an anabolic hormone that promotes the synthesis of proteins, carbohydrates, lipids, and nucleic acids. The major sites of insulin-promoted synthesis are the liver, muscle, and adipose tissue. The brain and red blood cells do not require insulin for glucose transport. In the liver, insulin increases glucose uptake; stimulates synthesis of glycogen and fatty acids; and inhibits gluconeogenesis (glucose formation), glycogenolysis (the splitting of glycogen to form glucose), and ketogenesis (formation of ketones from fats). In muscle, insulin increases uptake of glucose and amino acids, increases glycogen synthesis, stimulates protein synthesis, and inhibits protein breakdown (proteolysis). In adipose tissue, insulin increases glucose uptake, stimulates fatty acid synthesis, and inhibits fat breakdown (lipolysis). The net effect of insulin in these tissues is to stimulate cellular metabolism. Overall, however, the major consequence of in-

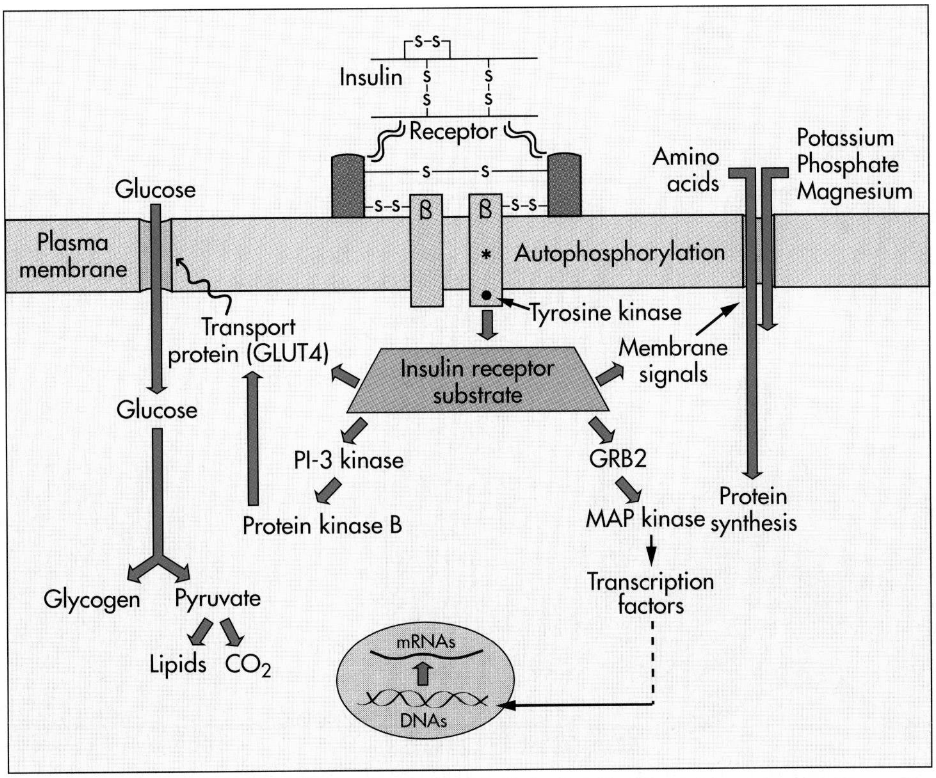

FIG. 19-16 Insulin action on cells. Binding of insulin to its receptor causes autophosphorylation of the receptor, which then itself acts as a tyrosine kinase that phosphorylates insulin receptor substrate (IRS1). Numerous target enzymes, such as protein kinase B and MAP kinase are activated and these enzymes have a multitude of effects on cell function. The glucose transporter, GLUT4, is recruited to the plasma membrane, where it facilitates glucose entry into the cell. The transport of amino acids, potassium, magnesium, and phosphate into the cell is also facilitated. The synthesis of various enzymes is induced or suppressed, and cell growth is regulated by signal molecules that modulate gene expression.

sulin release is to decrease blood glucose. Insulin also facilitates the intracellular transport of potassium.

Insulin is metabolized in the liver and kidney by enzymes that split disulfide bonds. Very little insulin is excreted unchanged in the urine.

Glucagon

Glucagon is produced by the A cells of the pancreas and by a number of cells lining the gastrointestinal tract. High glucose levels cause glucagon release to be inhibited; low glucose levels and sympathetic stimulation promote glucagon release, particularly in the liver. Amino acids, such as alanine, glycine, and asparagine, also stimulate glucagon secretion. A protein-rich meal has the same effect.

Glucagon acts primarily in the liver and increases blood glucose by stimulating glycogenolysis and gluconeogenesis. Glucagon acts as an antagonist to insulin. Much controversy exists regarding the role of glucagon in carbohydrate regulation, both normally and in diabetes mellitus. Glucagon also stimulates lipolysis, which has a ketogenic effect from the metabolism of free fatty acids in the liver.

Somatostatin

The somatostatin produced by D cells is a hormone essential in carbohydrate, fat, and protein metabolism (i.e., homeostasis of ingested nutrients). It differs from hypothalamic somatostatin, which inhibits release of growth hormone. Little is known about pancreatic somatostatin, but it probably is involved in the regulation of A cell and B cell function within the islets. Presumably, somatostatin inhibits both glucagon and insulin secretion, and it may prevent excess secretion of insulin.

Adrenal Glands

The **adrenal glands** are paired, pyramid-shaped organs located behind the peritoneum and close to the upper pole of each kidney. Each gland is surrounded by a capsule, embedded in fat, and well supplied with blood from the phrenic and renal arteries and the aorta. Venous return on the left is to the renal vein and on the right is to the inferior vena cava.

Each adrenal gland consists of two separate portions: an inner medulla and an outer cortex. These two portions have different embryonic origins, different structures, and different hormonal functions. In effect, each adrenal gland functions like two separate glands, although there are interrelationships between functions of each portion (Fig. 19-17).

The **adrenal cortex,** or outer region of the gland, accounts for 80% of the weight of the adult gland. The cortex is histologically subdivided into three zones. The outer layer, the **zona glomerulosa,** constitutes approximately 15% of the

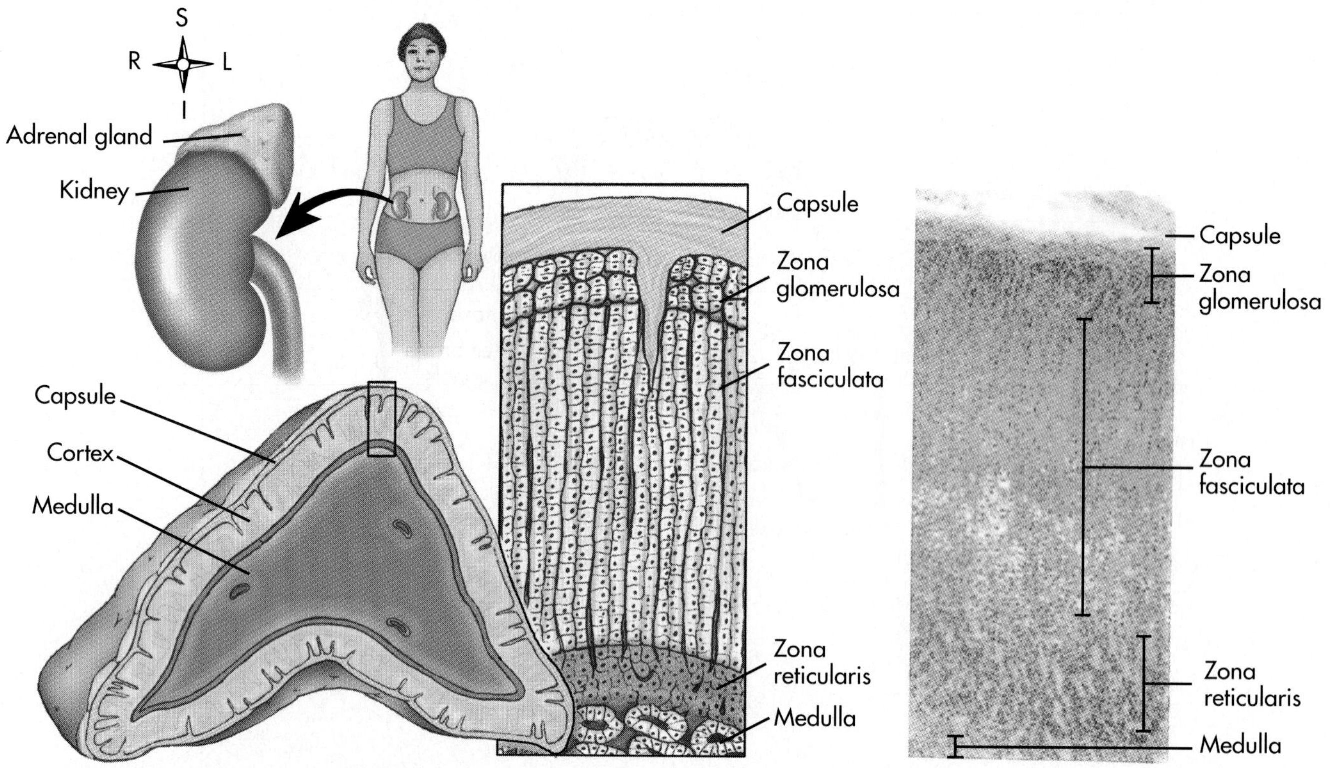

Fig. 19-17 Structure of the adrenal gland showing cell layers (zonae) of the cortex. Zona glomerulosa secretes aldosterone. Zona fasciculata secretes abundant amounts of glucocorticoids, chiefly cortisol. Zona reticularis secretes minute amounts of sex hormones and glucocorticoids. A portion of the medulla is visible at lower right in the photomicrograph (×35) and at the bottom of the drawing. (From Thibodeau GA, Patton K: *Anatomy & physiology,* ed 4, St Louis, 1999, Mosby.)

cortex and primarily produces the mineralocorticoid aldosterone. The middle layer, the **zona fasciculata** (78% of the cortex), and the inner layer, the **zona reticularis** (7% of the cortex), secrete other mineralocorticoids, the adrenal androgens and estrogens, and the glucocorticoids. The **adrenal medulla,** accounting for 20% of the gland's total weight, secretes the catecholamines epinephrine (adrenaline), norepinephrine, and dopamine. Both sympathetic and parasympathetic cholinergic fibers innervate the adrenal medulla; the adrenal cortex does not appear to be directly innervated.

Adrenal Cortex

The adrenal cortex secretes several steroid hormones, including the glucocorticoids, the mineralocorticoids, and the adrenal androgens and estrogens. These hormones are all synthesized from cholesterol. The cells of the adrenal cortex must be stimulated by the hypophysiotropic hormone **adrenocorticotropic hormone (ACTH)** for cholesterol to be used in steroidogenesis. Steroidogenesis is not totally dependent on ACTH,[6] but there appears to be an ACTH-independent baseline glucocorticoid secretion of 3% to 10%.[7] The best-known pathway of steroidogenesis involves the conversion of cholesterol to pregnenolone, which is then converted to the major corticosteroids.

Little storage of the steroid hormones occurs in the adrenal gland. The adrenal cortex also contains a high concentration of ascorbic acid and vitamin A; the functional roles within the adrenal glands are not known at present.

Glucocorticoids

The glucocorticoids have metabolic, antiinflammatory, and growth-suppressing effects. They also influence levels of awareness and sleep patterns.[8,9] The term **glucocorticoid** refers to those steroid hormones that have direct effects on carbohydrate metabolism. These hormones increase blood glucose concentration by promoting gluconeogenesis in the liver and by decreasing uptake of glucose into muscle cells, adipose cells, and lymphatic cells. In extrahepatic tissues the glucocorticoids stimulate protein catabolism and inhibit amino acid uptake and protein synthesis. In hepatic tissue, however, glucocorticoids act primarily to stimulate glucose formation and synthesis of enzymes that mediate glucocorticoid effects. The ultimate effect on the body is protein breakdown (catabolism).

The glucocorticoids act at several sites to inhibit immune and inflammatory reactions (described in Chapter 8). These include depressing proliferation of T lymphocytes, including those that produce the antiviral protein interferon; decreasing natural killer cell activity; reversing macrophage activity; and suppressing the synthesis, secretion, and actions of chemical mediators involved in inflammatory and immune responses. These chemical mediators include interleukins, prostaglandins, leukotrienes, bradykinin, serotonin, and histamine.[10,11]

Other actions of the glucocorticoids include increasing circulating erythrocytes, leading to polycythemia; increasing the appetite; promoting fat deposits in the face and cer-

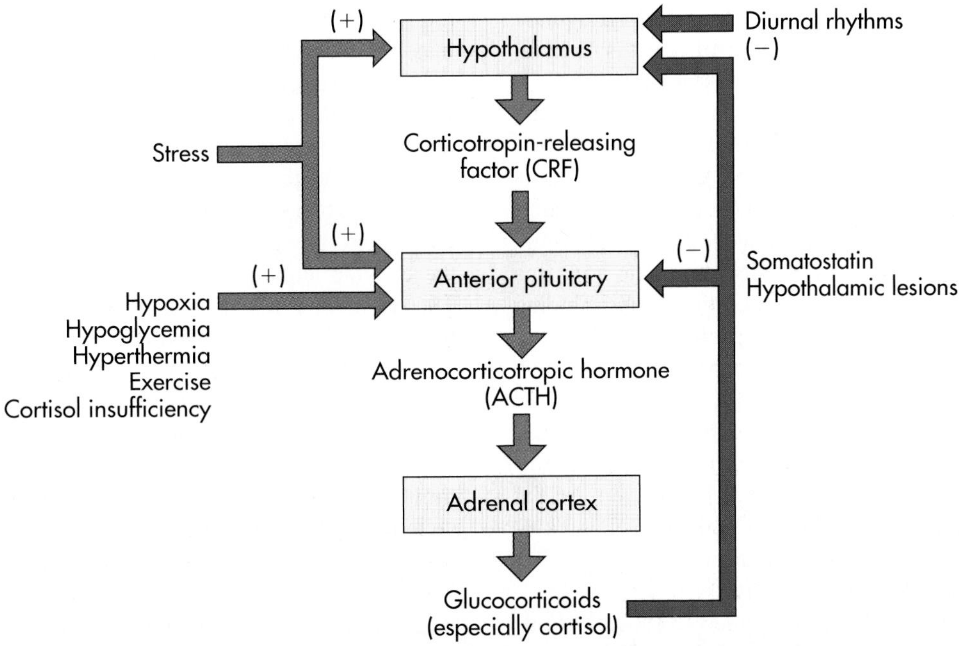

FIG. 19-18 Feedback control of glucocorticoid synthesis and secretion.

vical areas; increasing uric acid excretion; decreasing serum calcium levels, possibly by inhibiting gastrointestinal absorption of calcium; suppressing the secretion and synthesis of ACTH; and suppressing growth hormone (GH) secretion so that somatic growth is inhibited. The glucocorticoids also have important "permissive" effects, sensitizing arterioles to the vasoconstrictive effects of norepinephrine.

Glucocorticoids appear to potentiate the effects of catecholamines, thyroid hormone, and GH on adipose tissue. It also has been speculated that a metabolite of cortisol may act like a barbiturate and depress nerve cell function in the brain. This may account for the noted effects on mood associated with steroid fluctuation in disease or stress.[12]

The most potent of the naturally occurring glucocorticoids is **cortisol.** It is the main secretory product of the adrenal cortex and is necessary for the maintenance of life and for protection from stress (see Chapter 9 and Fig. 9-1). Cortisol has a biologic half-life of approximately 90 minutes, with the liver primarily responsible for its deactivation.

The secretion of cortisol is regulated primarily by the hypothalamus and the anterior pituitary gland (Fig. 19-18). In the hypothalamus, corticotropin-releasing hormone (CRH) is produced in several nuclei and stored in the median eminence. Once released, CRH travels through the portal vessels to stimulate the production of ACTH, β-lipotropin, γ-lipotropin, endorphins, and enkephalins by the anterior pituitary. ACTH is the main regulator of cortisol secretion and adrenocortical growth.

Three factors appear to be primarily involved in regulating the secretion of ACTH: (1) high circulating levels of cortisol and synthetic glucocorticoids suppress both CRH and ACTH, whereas low cortisol levels stimulate their secretion; (2) diurnal rhythms affect ACTH and cortisol levels (in persons with regular sleep/wake patterns, ACTH peaks 3 to 5 hours after sleep begins and declines throughout the day; and cortisol levels follow a similar pattern); and (3) stress has been shown to increase ACTH secretion, leading to increased cortisol levels. (Neurologic mechanisms regulating sleep are discussed in Chapter 14.) A form of ACTH (i.e., ir ACTH) also is produced by the cells of the immune system. It is detectable through laboratory techniques, and physiologically it appears to exert the usual feedback effects (see Chapter 9). This mechanism may account in part for integration of the immune and endocrine systems.

Once ACTH is secreted, it binds to specific plasma membrane receptors on the cells of the adrenal cortex and on other extraadrenal tissues. Because both adrenal and extraadrenal tissues have ACTH receptors, a number of effects result from stimulation by ACTH. (These are summarized in Box 19-1.) Both adrenal and extraadrenal effects appear to

Box 19-1

EFFECTS OF ADRENOCORTICOTROPIC HORMONE

ADRENAL

Maintenance of gland size
Depletion of ascorbic acid
Activation of adenylyl cyclase
Conversion of cholesterol to pregnenolone
Maintenance of enzymes active in converting pregnenolone to other steroids
Accumulation of cholesterol
Secretion of cortisol and adrenal androgens

EXTRAADRENAL

Melanocyte stimulation
Activation of tissue lipase

be mediated through the activation of the adenylyl cyclase system. The most well-known extraadrenal effect is melanocyte stimulation, which causes increased pigmentation.[13]

Once ACTH stimulates the cells of the adrenal cortex, cortisol synthesis and secretion immediately occur. In the normal person the secretory patterns of ACTH and cortisol are nearly identical. After secretion, most cortisol circulates in bound form. Fifteen to thirty percent is bound to albumin, and 55% to 75% is tightly but reversibly bound to a plasma glycoprotein called *transcortin,* or corticosteroid-binding globulin. Transcortin levels are significantly elevated by increased estrogen levels that occur with pregnancy and hormone therapy. Ten to fifteen percent of the cortisol secreted circulates unbound. The unbound portion is free to diffuse into cells, but only those cells with specific intracellular glucocorticoid receptors respond to cortisol stimulation. ACTH is rapidly inactivated in the circulation, and the liver and kidneys remove the deactivated hormone.

Mineralocorticoids: Aldosterone

Mineralocorticoid is the term applied to those steroids that directly affect ion transport by epithelial cells, causing sodium retention and potassium and hydrogen loss. **Aldosterone** is the most potent of the naturally occurring mineralocorticoids. The primary role of aldosterone is to conserve sodium. This is accomplished by increasing the activity of the sodium pump of the epithelial cells. (The sodium pump is described in Chapter 1.)

The initial stages of aldosterone synthesis occur in the zona fasciculata and zona reticularis. The final conversion of corticosterone to aldosterone, however, apparently is confined to the zona glomerulosa. Aldosterone synthesis and secretion are regulated primarily by the renin–angiotensin system (described in Chapter 34), although other factors also may be involved. Sodium and potassium levels may directly affect aldosterone secretion; however, the mechanisms involved are not understood. ACTH may transiently stimulate aldosterone synthesis but does not appear to be a major regulator of aldosterone secretion.

Aldosterone secretion is stimulated by angiotensin II. The conversion of angiotensin I to angiotensin II is stimulated by the enzyme angiotensin I–converting enzyme (Fig. 19-19). The conversion of angiotensinogen to angiotensin I is stimulated by renin (see Fig. 19-19). Renin secretion is stimulated primarily by sodium and water depletion and a diminished effective blood volume. (The postulated relationships among these factors are summarized in Fig. 19-20.)

When sodium and potassium levels are within normal limits, approximately 50 to 250 mg of aldosterone are secreted daily. Fifty to seventy-five percent of the secreted aldosterone binds to plasma proteins, including albumin, transcortin, and an α_1-acid glycoprotein (AAG). The relatively large proportion of unbound aldosterone contributes to its rapid metabolic turnover in the liver, its low plasma concentration, and its short half-life of approximately 15 minutes. The main site of aldosterone degradation is the liver, with the metabolic end products excreted by the kidney.

In the kidney, aldosterone acts on the ascending portion of the loop of Henle; the distal, predominantly convoluted tubule; and the collecting ducts to increase sodium ion reabsorption and increase potassium and hydrogen ion excretion. High levels of aldosterone may result in alkalosis and hypokalemia (see Chapter 3). (Kidney function is discussed in Chapter 34.) This renal effect takes 1 1/2 to 6 hours to occur after stimulation by aldosterone.

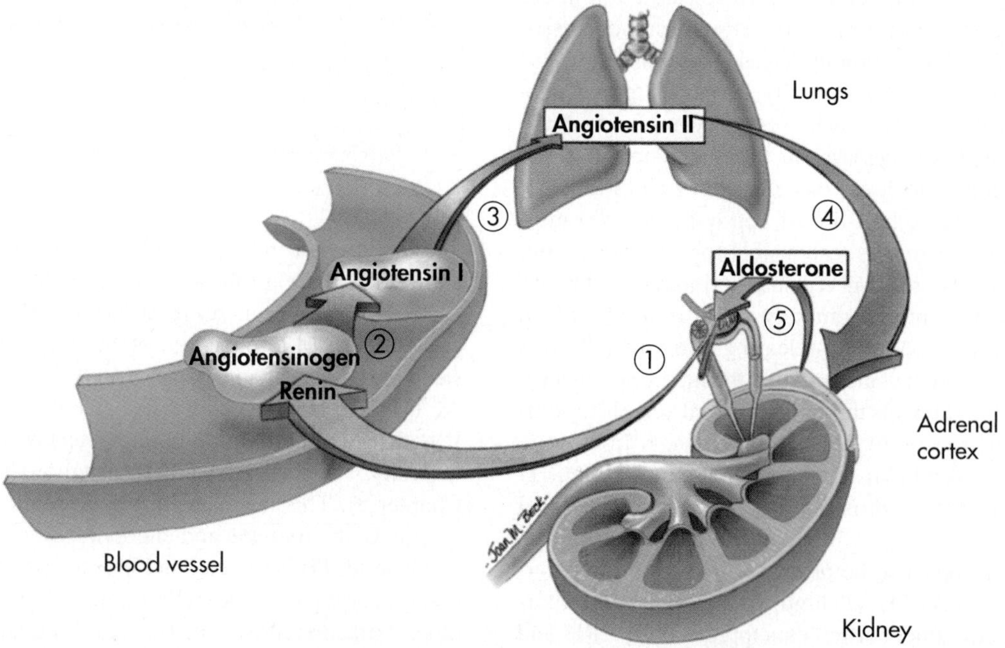

Fig. 19-19 Renin-angiotensin mechanism for regulating aldosterone secretion. (From Thibodeau GA, Patton K: *Anatomy & physiology,* ed 4, St Louis, 1999, Mosby.)

Adrenal Estrogens and Androgens

Estrogen secretion by the normal adrenal cortex is so minimal as to be considered physiologically unimportant. The adrenal cortex also secretes androgens. Some of the weakly androgenic substances secreted by the cortex are then converted by peripheral tissues to stronger androgens, such as testosterone, thus accounting for some androgenic effect initiated by the adrenal cortex. An increased capacity for peripheral conversion of adrenal androgens to estrogens occurs in particular cases, however, including aging, obesity, liver disease, and hyperthyroidism.[14,15] The modulation of adrenal androgen secretion is not well understood. ACTH appears to be the major regulator rather than the gonadotropins. The biologic effects and metabolism of the adrenal sex steroids do not vary from those produced by the gonads (see Chapter 21).

Adrenal Medulla

The adrenal medulla, together with the sympathetic divisions of the autonomic nervous system, is embryonically derived from neural crest cells. The major products secreted by the adrenal medulla are the catecholamines epinephrine (adrenaline) and norepinephrine, although the medulla is only a minor source of norepinephrine.

Catecholamine production in the adrenal medulla consists of approximately 75% to 85% epinephrine and approximately 15% to 25% norepinephrine. Epinephrine is about 10 times more potent than norepinephrine in producing direct metabolic effects. The adrenal medulla synthesizes the catecholamines from the amino acid phenylalanine (Fig. 19-21).

The regulation of adrenal catecholamine release is complex. Secretion is increased by ACTH and the glucocorticoids. The catecholamines apparently exert a direct inhibiting influence on their own secretion by decreasing the formation of the rate-limiting enzyme tyrosine hydroxylase. Other stimuli to adrenal medullary secretion include sympathetic nerve stimulation, hypoglycemia, hypoxia, hypercapnia, acidosis, hemorrhage, glucagon, nicotine, pilocarpine, histamine, and angiotensin II. On stimulation of the adrenal medullary cell, cytoplasmic storage granules that contain the catecholamines

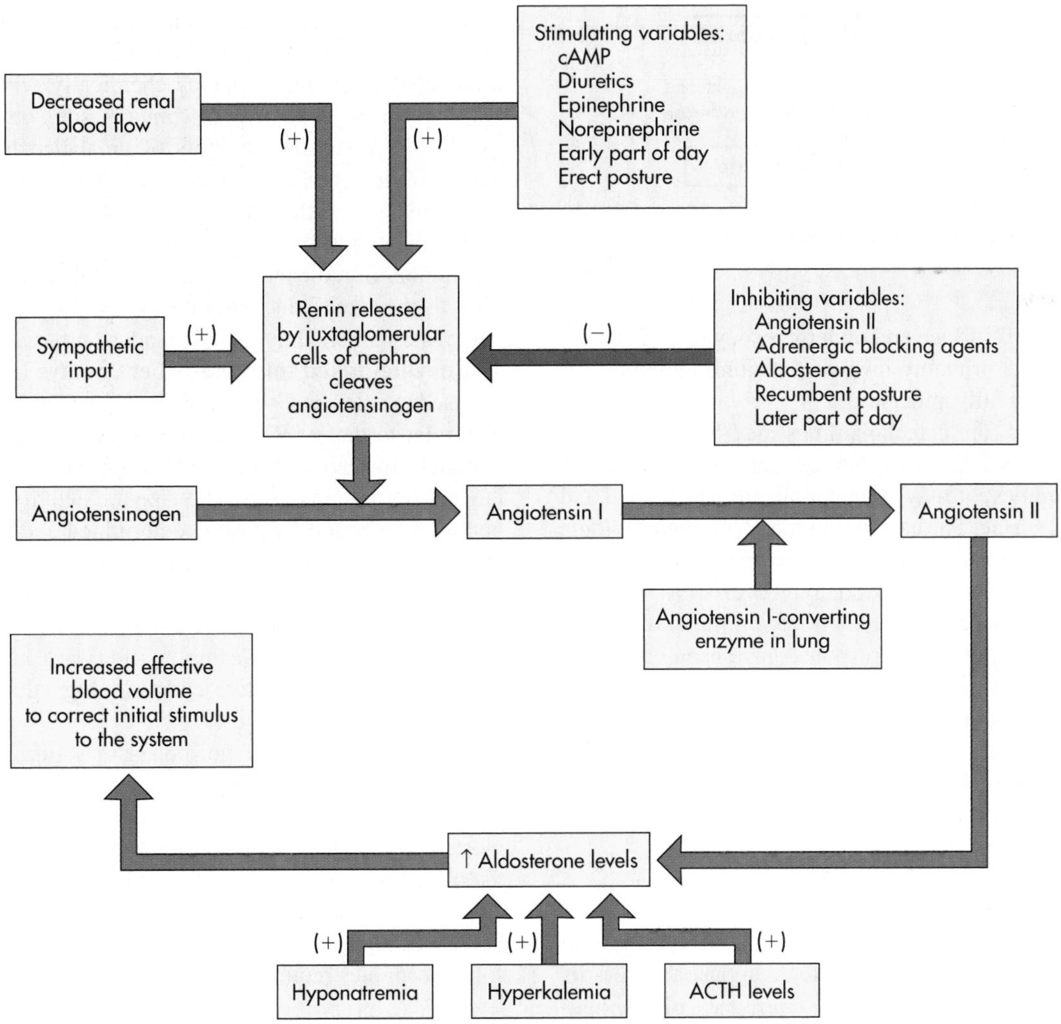

FIG. 19-20 The feedback mechanisms regulating aldosterone secretion. *cAMP,* Cyclic adenosine monophosphate; *ACTH,* adrenocorticotropic hormone.

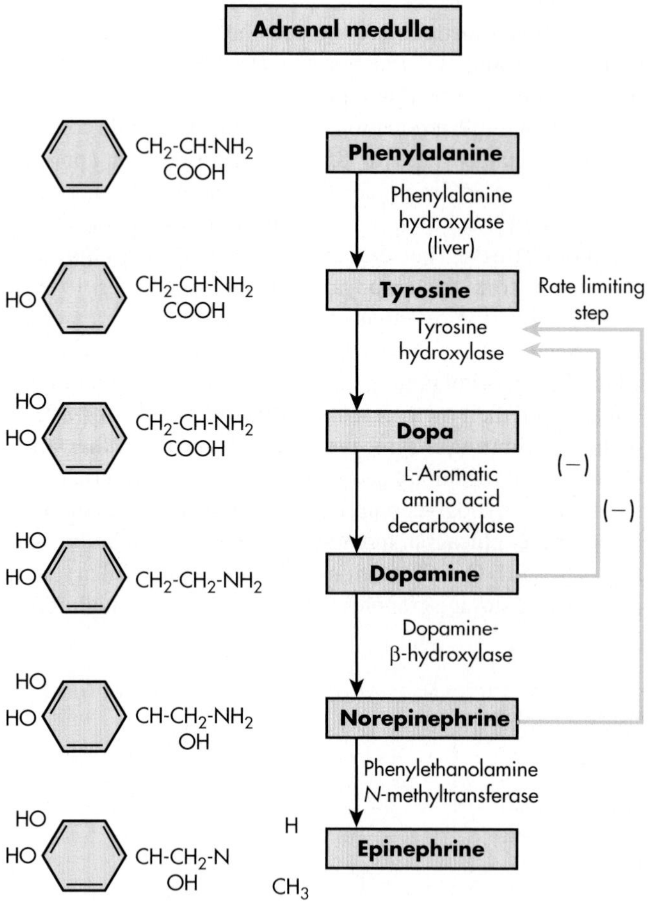

FIG. 19-21 Synthesis of catecholamines.

migrate to the cell surface and undergo exocytosis. The control of exocytosis probably involves calcium, although this mechanism is not fully understood.

Once released, the catecholamines may bind to various target cells, may be taken up by neurons for storage in new cytoplasmic granules, or may be metabolically inactivated and excreted in the urine. The catecholamines exert their biologic effects after binding to a plasma membrane receptor in target cells. This binding activates the adenylyl cyclase system.

Catecholamines have diverse effects on the entire body. Their release and the body's response have been characterized as the "fight or flight" response (see Fig. 9-1 and Table 9-2). In general, the metabolic effects of catecholamines promote hyperglycemia through a variety of mechanisms and through interfering with usual glucose regulatory feedback mechanisms.

Neuroendocrine Response to Stressors

The endocrine system acts together with the nervous system to respond to stressors. The integrated response to stressors also includes the immune system. Hormones of the neuroendocrine system affect components of the immune system, and mediators produced by immune components regulate the neuroendocrine response.

Perception that an event is stressful may be essential to the emotional arousal and initiation of the stress response (discussed in Chapter 9). Some events, such as bacterial invasion, can activate the stress response without emotional arousal. The hypothalamus receives input from a variety of areas within the brain and ultimately directs the neuroendocrine response to stress through the actions of corticotropin-releasing factor (CRF), the locus ceruleus–norepinephrine autonomic (sympathetic) nervous system, and the pituitary–adrenal axis. In addition to the neuroendocrine components of the stress response, the gamma motor neuron system is activated to increase skeletal motor tone. Enhanced availability of vital substrates occurs, and growth and reproduction are inhibited to preserve energy for protective responses.[16] Details of the stress response are presented in Chapter 9.

Tests of Endocrine Function

Tests of the endocrine system involve several general types of clinical evaluation.[17] Measurement of hormone level is accomplished by radioimmunoassay, by enzyme-linked immunosorbent assay, and less commonly by bioassay. **Radioimmunoassay (RIA)** is an immunologic technique in which known amounts of antibody and radiolabeled hormone are placed in an assay tube with the unlabeled hormone. The radiolabeled hormone competes chemically with the nonlabeled hormone molecules for binding sites on the antibodies. When increasing amounts of unlabeled hormones are added to the assay, the limited binding sites of the antibody can bind less of the radiolabeled hormone. Therefore the higher the concentration of unlabeled hormone is, the fewer the number of radioactive "counts," or labeled hormone, that bind to the fixed concentration of antibody. A quantitative value is established by use of standard reference curves.

Enzyme-linked immunosorbent assays (ELISAs) also are used to determine circulating hormone levels. The method is similar to that of RIA but is less expensive and easier to conduct. Instead of radiolabeled hormones, an enzyme-labeled hormone is used. The enzyme activity in either the bound or unbound fraction is determined and related to the concentration of the unlabeled hormone.

A **bioassay** involves the use of graded doses of hormone in a reference preparation and then comparison of the results with an unknown sample. Bioassays are used more commonly in investigative endocrinology than in clinical laboratories.

The concentration of hormones in serum can be measured to assess endocrine function in health and disease. If the serum level is greater or less than the reference values, more definitive tests are required to determine the source of the problem. Measurement of individual hormones does not always permit differentiation between normal and abnormal. For an accurate interpretation, the broad normal range of some hormones requires a knowledge of previous hormonal levels.[18]

The major problems in evaluating the endocrine system include (1) the complexity of the clinical presentation because of multiple organ system involvement, (2) the nonspecific nature of complaints frequently associated with endocrine dysfunction, and (3) the inappropriate use of laboratory test interpretations.

Aging and the Endocrine System

The precise relationship between aging and the endocrine system is not clear. Perhaps most important, the question of whether changes in endocrine function are a consequence or a cause of aging has yet to be resolved. These relationships have been difficult to identify, in part because of a number of age-related variables that may coexist, such as acute and chronic nonendocrine disease; use of medications; alterations in diet, body composition, and weight; and changes in sleep/wake cycles.[8,9]

Theories About the Effects of Aging

Investigation into the role of the endocrine glands and their interactions in the aging process has generated much data, although the evidence is contradictory. Altered biologic activity of hormones, altered circulating levels of hormones, altered secretory response of the endocrine glands, altered metabolism of hormones, and loss of circadian control of hormone secretion are among the findings.[19]

Theories of cellular damage deal with adverse cellular conditions that produce the biologic effects associated with aging. (These theories are discussed in Chapter 2.) The endocrine system has not been specifically implicated in any of these theories, particularly as a causative variable. The cellular changes or consequences described by these theories, however, do affect endocrine glands and might contribute to endocrine gland dysfunction or alterations in responsiveness of target organs. For example, the loss of self-regulatory patterns of the immune system leads to an autoimmune phenomenon characterized by either autoimmunity or immunodeficiencies. These mechanisms may account for the onset of type II diabetes mellitus (see Chapter 20).

Theories of stress and adaptation suggest that body structures wear out from overuse or are no longer able to adapt to the cumulative effects of physiologic stress. One such endocrine function that may be affected is the sympathoadrenal axis. Exhaustion of this axis may be associated with an inability of the body to respond effectively to stressors.

Theories of programmed change are concerned with genetic control of cell function. Certain secretory cells may be programmed genetically to secrete hormones for a prescribed length of time. Changes seen with female reproductive function may represent the phenomenon of programmed change.

All changes in cellular activity—as a result of damage, programmed change, or wear and tear—may affect neuroendocrine regulation. Impaired secretion of hypothalamic regulatory factors and hormones or impaired hypothalamic feedback sensitivity may contribute to impaired control of an optimal internal environment. The dynamic equilibrium of the endocrine system also may be affected by altered secretion of neurotransmitters within certain areas of the brain, affecting hypothalamic and pituitary function. Such alterations may include an excess or deficit in secretion of pituitary hormones and loss of appropriate secretory pattern of those hormones. Loss of endocrine steady states may be associated with or contribute to aging.

Effects of Aging on Specific Glands

Thyroid Gland

Changes in thyroid structure and function occur with aging. Structurally, some glandular atrophy and fibrosis occur with nodularity and increasing inflammatory infiltrates. These infiltrative changes may reflect age-related autoimmune damage.[20]

Changes relative to thyroid hormone and its function are more difficult to assess. One difficulty is finding older adults who are free of all systemic and thyroid-related illness, so that the resulting changes can be attributed to aging. Much of the available data is contradictory. Most evidence, however, supports the following age-related changes:[21,22]

1. T_4 secretion and turnover are decreased.
2. Plasma levels of T_3 decline, especially in men.
3. Hypothyroidism is seen with increasing frequency as age advances.
4. Overall TSH secretion is diminished.
5. Responsiveness of plasma TSH concentration to TRH administration is reduced, especially in men.

In addition, the average dose for TH replacement appears to be lower in elderly persons because the peripheral metabolism of TH decreases with age.[20] TH must be replaced slowly in elderly individuals with coronary artery disease to prevent angina and myocardial infarction.[23] Clinical signs of thyroid disease are more difficult to detect in elderly persons.[24]

Parathyroid Glands

An age-related alteration in PTH secretion has been proposed to explain alterations in calcium homeostasis that have been noted in older adults. Such an alteration, however, has not been documented consistently. Calcium intake, especially in women, tends to decrease with aging. The average daily intake of 450 to 500 mg/day causes a negative calcium balance greater than 40 mg/day and may be related to the absolute bone loss of approximately 1.5% per year. Older adults show decreased intestinal adaptation to variations in calcium intake. Many older adults also have a mild, persistent hypercalciuria, which indicates a defective renal mechanism for responding to decreased calcium intake. Decreased circulating levels of vitamin D also have been documented.

The decrease in calcium intake, an age-related decrease in circulating vitamin D, and a blunted response of older persons to PTH may explain these changes seen in aging.[25] Additional investigation into mechanisms of altered calcium metabolism is required before the age-associated alterations can be explained.

Adrenal Glands

The adrenal cortex loses some weight and has more fibrous tissue after the age of 50 years. Age does not appear to affect the feedback mechanisms involved in maintaining glucocorticoid levels, but the decrease in the metabolic clearance rate of the glucocorticoids is age related.

The metabolic clearance of cortisol decreases with an age-related decline in liver and kidney function. Further, less cortisol appears to be used by the body when aging is accompanied by a loss of lean body mass. Both decreased clearance and reduced use of cortisol contribute to higher circulating cortisol levels, but diurnal variation is maintained.[26] Because feedback mechanisms are intact, the higher cortisol levels cause a decrease in cortisol secretion. Plasma levels of the adrenal androgens, as well as urinary excretion of the metabolic end products, decrease gradually but dramatically with age, to as much as 50% to 70% of the young adult level. This change appears to reflect a decline in the function of the zona reticularis. The effects of decreased secretion are obscured, however, by the effects of aging on gonadal androgen secretion (see Chapter 21). Because cortisol secretion does not vary significantly with aging, the decrease in secretion of adrenal androgens probably is independent of ACTH. Change in both the testis and hypothalamic–pituitary axis may be responsible for decreased testosterone levels.[27] Circadian patterns of ACTH and cortisol secretion change with aging.[28]

Posterior Pituitary

Although hyponatremia is a common finding in older persons,[29] it appears related to changes in renal function rather than to ADH-related mechanisms. Morphologic studies have not shown significant age-related degenerative changes in the neuroendocrine pathways that regulate the synthesis and secretion of ADH. It appears that ADH secretion is augmented when stimulated by changes in osmotic concentration, whereas baroreceptor-mediated ADH secretion is reduced.[8,9]

Anterior Pituitary

The anterior pituitary in older persons is characterized by a number of morphologic changes, including increases in fibrosis, focal necrosis, iron deposits, and microadenoma formation and a moderate decrease in size.[30]

SUMMARY REVIEW

Mechanisms of Hormonal Regulation

1. The endocrine system has diverse functions, including sexual differentiation, growth and development, and continuous maintenance of the body's internal environment.
2. Hormones are chemical messengers synthesized by endocrine glands and released into the circulation.
3. Hormones have specific negative- and positive-feedback mechanisms. Most hormone levels are regulated by negative feedback, in which hormone secretion raises the level of a specific hormone, ultimately causing secretion to subside.
4. Endocrine feedback is described in terms of short, long, and ultrashort feedback loops.
5. Water-soluble hormones circulate throughout the body in unbound form, whereas lipid-soluble hormones (i.e., steroid and thyroid hormones) circulate throughout the body bound to carrier proteins.
6. Hormones affect only target cells with appropriate receptors and then act on these cells to initiate specific cell functions or activities.
7. Hormones have two general types of effects on cells: direct effects, or obvious changes in cell function, and permissive effects, or less obvious changes that facilitate cell function.
8. Receptors for hormones may be located on the plasma membrane or in the cytosol or nucleus of the target cell.
9. Water-soluble hormones act as first messengers, binding to receptors on the cell's plasma membrane. The signals initiated by hormone–receptor binding are then transmitted into the cell by the action of second messengers.
10. Second messengers that have been identified include cyclic adenosine monophosphate (cAMP), cyclic guanosine monophosphate (cGMP), calcium, inositol trisphosphatase (IP_3), and diacylglycerol (DAG).
11. For cells that have cAMP as their second messenger, a series of interactions within the plasma membrane must activate adenylyl cyclase.
12. For cells that have calcium as their second messenger, a rise in intracellular calcium causes calcium to bind with calmodulin, a regulatory protein. This step then initiates other intracellular processes.
13. Lipid-soluble hormones (including steroid and thyroid hormones) may cross the plasma membrane through diffusion. These hormones either bind to cytoplasmic proteins or diffuse directly into the cell nucleus and bind to nuclear receptors.

Structure and Function of the Endocrine Glands

1. The pituitary gland, consisting of anterior and posterior portions, is connected to the central nervous system through the hypothalamus.
2. The hypothalamus regulates anterior pituitary function by secreting releasing hormones and releasing factors into the portal circulation. Releasing hormones have identified chemical structures; releasing factors have hormonal properties but no definitive chemical identification.
3. Hypothalamic hormones include prolactin-inhibiting factor (PIF), which inhibits prolactin secretion; thyrotropin-releasing factor (TRF), which affects release of thyroid hormones; gonadotropin-releasing hormone (GnRH), which facilitates release of adrenocorticotropic hormone (ACTH) and endorphins; and substance P, which inhibits ACTH release and stimulates release of a variety of other hormones.
4. The posterior pituitary secretes antidiuretic hormone (ADH), which also is called *vasopressin,* and *oxytocin.*
5. ADH controls serum osmolality, increases permeability of the renal tubules to water, and causes vasoconstriction when administered pharmacologically in high doses. ADH also may regulate some central nervous system functions.
6. Oxytocin causes uterine contraction and lactation in women and may have a role in sperm motility in men. In both men and women, oxytocin has an antidiuretic effect similar to that of ADH.

7. Hormones of the anterior pituitary are regulated by (a) secretion of hypothalamic-releasing hormones or factors, (b) negative feedback from hormones secreted by target organs, and (c) mediating effects of neurotransmitters.
8. Hormones of the anterior pituitary include ACTH, melanocyte-stimulating hormone (MSH), somatotropic hormones (growth hormone [GH] and prolactin), and glycoprotein hormones (follicle-stimulating hormone [FSH], luteinizing hormone [LH], and thyroid-stimulating hormone [TSH]).
9. The two-lobed thyroid gland contains follicles, which secrete some of the thyroid hormones, and C cells, which secrete calcitonin and somatostatin.
10. Regulation of thyroid hormone (TH) levels is complex and involves the hypothalamus, anterior pituitary, thyroid gland, and numerous biochemical variables.
11. Thyroid hormone (TH) secretion is regulated by thyroid-releasing hormone through a negative-feedback loop that involves the anterior pituitary and hypothalamus.
12. TSH, which is synthesized and stored in the anterior pituitary, stimulates secretion of TH by activating intracellular processes, including uptake of iodine necessary for the synthesis of TH.
13. Once secreted, TH acts on the thyroid gland, the anterior pituitary, and the median eminence to regulate further TH production.
14. Synthesis of TH depends on the glycoprotein thyroglobulin, which contains a precursor of TH, tyrosine. Tyrosine then combines with iodine to form precursor molecules of the thyroid hormones thyroxine (T_4) and triiodothyronine (T_3).
15. When released into the circulation, T_3 and T_4 are bound by carrier proteins in the plasma, which store these hormones and provide a buffer for rapid changes in hormone levels.
16. Thyroid hormones alter protein synthesis and have a wide range of metabolic effects on proteins, carbohydrates, lipids, and vitamins. TH also affects heat production and cardiac function.
17. The paired parathyroid glands normally are located behind the upper and lower poles of the thyroid. These glands secrete parathyroid hormone (PTH), an important regulator of serum calcium levels.
18. PTH secretion is regulated by levels of ionized calcium in the plasma and by cAMP within the cell. Some other substances—hormones, neurotransmitters, and ions—affect PTH secretion by inhibiting cAMP or by changing calcium levels.
19. In bone, PTH causes bone breakdown and resorption. In the kidney, PTH increases reabsorption of calcium and decreases reabsorption of phosphorus and bicarbonate.
20. The endocrine pancreas contains the islets of Langerhans, which secrete hormones responsible for much of the carbohydrate metabolism in the body.
21. The islets of Langerhans consist of A cells, B cells, and D cells.
22. D cells secrete somatostatin, which inhibits glucagon and insulin secretion.
23. B cells secrete preproinsulin, which is ultimately converted to insulin.
24. Insulin is a hormone that regulates blood glucose concentrations and overall body metabolism of fat, protein, and carbohydrates.
25. A cells produce glucagon, which is secreted inversely to blood glucose concentrations.
26. The paired adrenal glands are situated on the kidneys. Each gland consists of an adrenal medulla, which secretes catecholamines, and an adrenal cortex, which secretes steroid hormones.
27. The steroid hormones secreted by the adrenal cortex are all synthesized from cholesterol. These hormones include glucocorticoids, mineralocorticoids, and adrenal androgens and estrogens.
28. Glucocorticoids directly affect carbohydrate metabolism by increasing blood glucose concentration through gluconeogenesis in the liver and by decreasing use of glucose. Glucocorticoids also inhibit immune and inflammatory responses.
29. The most potent naturally occurring glucocorticoid is cortisol, which is necessary for the maintenance of life and for protection from stress. Secretion of cortisol is regulated by the hypothalamus and anterior pituitary.
30. Cortisol secretion is related to secretion of adrenocorticotropic hormone (ACTH), which is stimulated by corticotropin-releasing hormone (CRH). ACTH binds with receptors of the adrenal cortex, which activates intracellular mechanisms (specifically cAMP) and leads to cortisol release.
31. Mineralocorticoids are steroid hormones that directly affect ion transport by epithelial cells, causing sodium retention and potassium and hydrogen loss.
32. Aldosterone is the most potent of the naturally occurring mineralocorticoids. Its primary role is to conserve sodium.
33. Aldosterone secretion is regulated by the renin–angiotensin system.
34. Aldosterone acts by binding to a site on the cell nucleus and altering protein production within the cell. Its principal site of action is the kidney, where it causes sodium reabsorption and potassium and hydrogen excretion.
35. Androgens and estrogens secreted by the adrenal cortex act in the same way as those secreted by the gonads.
36. The adrenal medulla secretes the catecholamines epinephrine and norepinephrine. Catecholamines are synthesized from the amino acid phenylalanine. Their release is stimulated by sympathetic nervous system stimulation, ACTH, and glucocorticoids.
37. Catecholamines bind with various target cells and are taken up by neurons or excreted in the urine. They cause a range of metabolic effects that generally are characterized as the "flight or fight" response.
38. The endocrine system acts together with the nervous system to respond to stressors.
39. The response to stressors involves activation of the sympathetic division of the autonomic nervous system and activation of the endocrine system.
40. The adrenal glands and the sympathetic neurons that innervate these glands form the sympathoadrenal axis.
41. Activation of the sympathetic neurons causes the activation of an enzymatic pathway that increases catecholamine synthesis, leading to manifestations of the "fight or flight" response, hyperglycemia, and immune suppression.
42. Both hyperglycemia and immune suppression appear to be adaptive responses that are essential in the body's ability to react to stressors.
43. Other hormones that are secreted in response to stress include growth hormone, prolactin, testosterone, ADH, and insulin.

Aging and the Endocrine System

1. Endocrine changes that may be associated with aging include altered biologic activity of hormones, altered circulating levels of hormones, altered secretory responses of endocrine glands, altered metabolism of hormones, and loss of circadian control of hormone release.
2. Cellular damage associated with aging, genetically programmed cell change, and chronic wear and tear may contribute to endocrine gland dysfunction or alterations in responsiveness of target organs.
3. Aging apparently causes atrophy of the thyroid gland and is associated with infiltrative glandular changes. Secretion of thyroid hormones may diminish with age.
4. Aging is associated with alterations in calcium steady states, which may be related to alterations in PTH secretion from the parathyroid glands.
5. Age-related changes in adrenal function include decreased clearance of glucocorticoids and a decrease in levels of adrenal androgens. The effects of these changes, however, are offset by feedback mechanisms that maintain glucocorticoid levels and by gonadal secretion of androgens.

KEY TERMS

REFERENCES

1. Lodish H et al: *Molecular cell biology,* ed 4, New York, 2000, WH Freeman and Company.
2. Reichlin S: Neuroendocrinology. In Wilson JD et al, editors: *Williams textbook of endocrinology,* ed 9, Philadelphia, 1998, W.B. Saunders.
3. Kacson B: *Endocrine physiology,* New York, 2000, McGraw-Hill.
4. Braverman LE, Utiger RD: *Werner and Ingbar's The thyroid: a fundamental and clinical text,* ed 8, Philadelphia, 2000, Lippincott Williams & Wilkins.
5. Robertson RP: Dominance of cyclooxygenase-2 in the regulation of pancreatic islet prostaglandin synthesis, *Diabetes* 47(9):1379, 1998.
6. Weber MM et al: Interleukin-3 and interleukin-6 stimulate cortisol secretion from adult human adrenocortical cells, *Endocrinol* 138(5):2207, 1997.
7. Neville AM, O'Hare MJ: *The human adrenal cortex,* New York, 1982, Springer Verlag.
8. Rupprecht R, Holsboer F: Neuroactive steriods: mechanisms of action and neuropsychopharmacological perspectives, *Trends Neurosci* 22(9):410, 1999.
9. Steiger A et al: Effects of hormones on sleep, *Horm Res* 49(3-4):125, 1998.
10. Morand EF, Leech M: Glucocorticoid regulation of inflammation: the plot thickens, *Inflamm Res* 48(11):557, 1999.
11. Rook GA: Glucocorticoids and immune function, *Baillieres Best Pract Res Clin Endocrinol Metab* 13(4):567, 1999.
12. Gard PR, Pelagatti S: *Human endocrinology,* Old Tappan, NJ, 1998, Pearson Education.
13. Abel-Malek Z et al: The melanocortin-1 receptor and human pigmentation, *Ann N Y Acad Sci* 885:117, 1999.
14. Meikle WA, Daynes RA, Araneo BA: Adrenal androgen secretion and biologic effects, *Endocrinol Metab Clin North Am* 20(2):381, 1991.
15. Bulun SE et al: Aromatase in aging women, *Semin Reprod Endocrinol* 17(4):349, 1999.
16. Sapolsky RM, Romero LM, Munck AU: How do glucocorticoids influence stress responses? integrating permissive, suppressive, stimulatory, and preparative actions, *Endocr Rev* 21(1):55, 2000.
17. Hall JE, Nieman J: *Handbook of diagnostic endocrinology*, Totowa, NJ, 2000, Humana Press.
18. Wilson JD et al, editors: *Williams textbook of endocrinology,* ed 9, Philadelphia, 1998, W.B. Saunders.
19. Quau WB, Timiras PA: *Hormones and aging,* Boca Raton, Fla, 1995, CRC Press.

20. Mariotti S et al: Thyroid autoimmunity and aging, *Exp Gerontol* 33(6):535, 1998.
21. Chiovato L et al: Thyroid diseases in the elderly, *Baillieres Clin Endocrinol Metab* 11(2):152, 1997.
22. Samuels MH: Subclinical thyroid disease in the elderly, *Thyroid* 8(9):803, 1998.
23. Urban JR: Neuroendocrinology of aging in the male and female, *Endocrinol Metab Clin North Am* 21(4):921, 1992.
24. Trivalle C et al: Differences in the signs and symptoms of hyperthyroidism in older and younger patients, *J Am Geriatr Soc* 44(1):50, 1994.
25. Haden ST et al: The effects of age and gender on parathyroid hormone dynamics, *Clin Endocrinol* 52(3):329, 2000.
26. Van Cauter E, Leproult R, Kupfer DJ: Effects of gender and age on the levels and circadian rhythmicity of plasma cortisol, *J Clin Endocrinol Metab* 81(7):2468, 1996.
27. Veldhuis JD: Nature of altered pulsatile hormone release and neuroendocrine network signalling in human ageing: clinical studies of the stomatotropic, gonadotropic, corticotropic, and insulin axes, *Novartis Found Symp* 227:163, 2000.
28. Deuschle M et al: With aging in humans the activity of the hypothalamus-pituitary-adrenal system increases and its diurnal amplitude flattens, *Life Sci* 61(22):2239, 1997.
29. Miller M et al: Apparent idiopathic hyponatremia in an ambulatory geriatric population, *J Am Geriatr Soc* 44(4):404, 1996.
30. Lurie SN, Doraiswamy PM, Husain MM: In vivo assessment of pituitary gland volume with magnetic resonance imaging: the effect of age, *J Clin Endocrinol Metab* 71:505, 1990.

CHAPTER 20

Alterations of Hormonal Regulation

ROBERT E. JONES • SUE E. HUETHER

CHAPTER OUTLINE

Function of the endocrine system involves complex interrelationships and interactions that maintain dynamic steady states and provide growth and reproductive capabilities. Dysfunction of the endocrine system initially was described in terms of excessive or insufficient function of the endocrine gland with alterations in hormone levels. Alterations in function were thought to be caused by either hypersecretion or hyposecretion of the various hormones, leading to abnormal hormone concentrations in the blood. Techniques for studying the various components of the endocrine system have improved, and evidence has shown that dysfunction may result from abnormal receptor function or from altered intracellular response to the hormone-receptor complex.

MECHANISMS OF HORMONAL ALTERATIONS

Significantly elevated or depressed hormone levels may result from a variety of causes (Fig. 20-1). Feedback systems that recognize the need for a particular hormone may fail to function properly or may respond to inappropriate signals (see Chapter 19). Dysfunction of an endocrine gland may involve the gland's failure to produce adequate amounts of biologically free or active hormone forms. This failure may occur when the secretory cells are unable to produce or obtain an adequate quantity of required hormone precursors or when they are unable to convert the precursors to the active hormone. A gland also may synthesize or release excessive amounts of hormone. Once hormones are released into the circulation, they may be degraded at an altered rate or they may be inactivated by antibodies before reaching the target cell. Ectopic sources of hormones (hormones produced by nonendocrine tissues) may result also in abnormally elevated hormone levels. This mechanism operates without benefit of the normal feedback system for hormone control. In these cases the ectopic hormone production is said to be *autonomous.*

Recently, research has been directed toward understanding causes for the failure of the target cell to respond to its hormone. The general types of abnormal target cell responses currently recognized are receptor-associated disorders and intracellular disorders. Receptor-associated disorders have

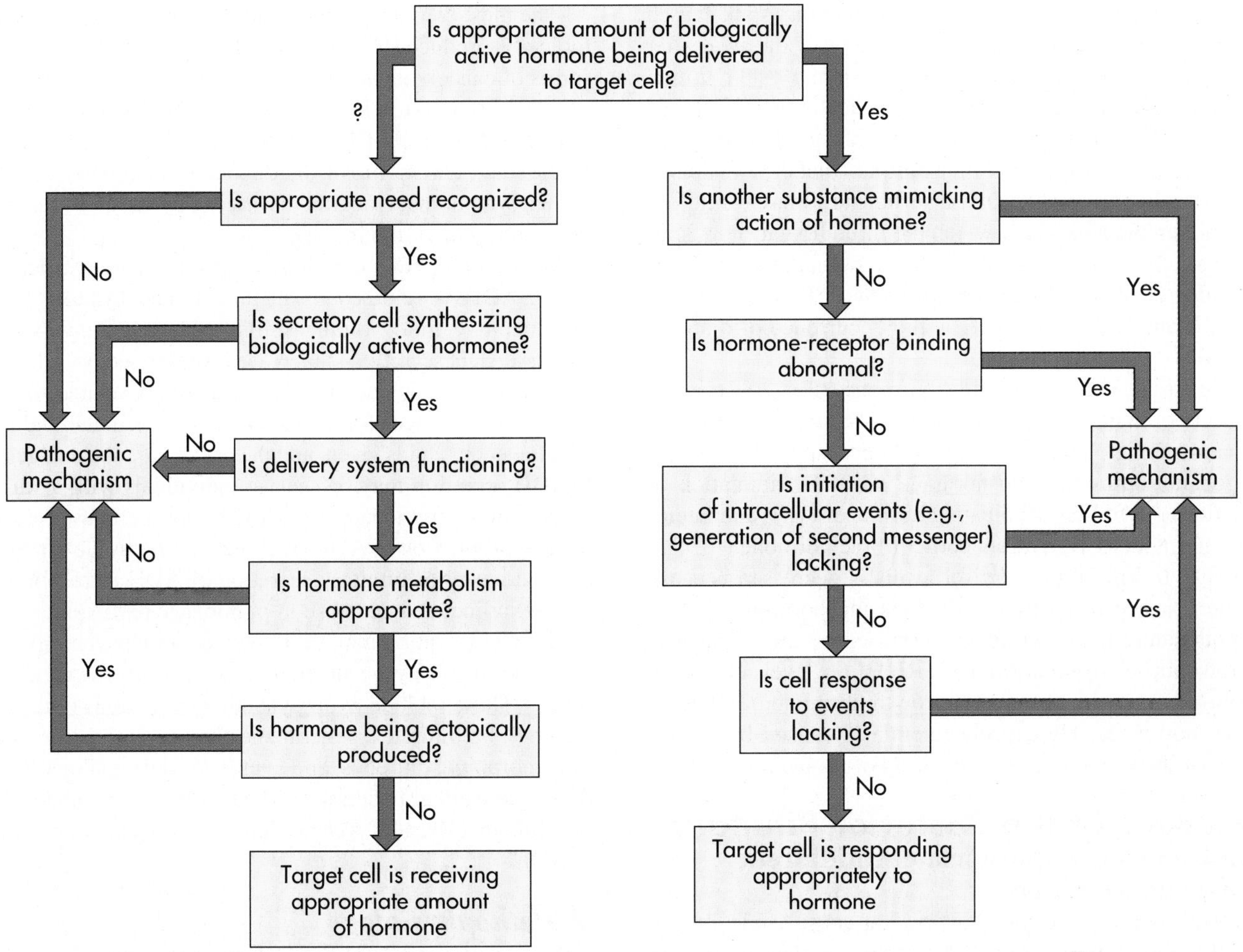

FIG. 20-1 Hormone delivery to cells. Phases at which pathogenic mechanisms may develop in delivering appropriate amounts of hormone to the cells.

been identified primarily in water-soluble hormones, such as insulin.[1] These types of disorders are usually one of the following: (1) a decrease in the number of receptors, leading to decreased or defective hormone-receptor binding; (2) impaired receptor function, resulting in insensitivity to the hormone; (3) presence of antibodies against specific receptors that either reduce available binding sites or mimic hormone action, exaggerating target cell response; or (4) unusual expression of receptor function, as occurs in some tumor cells with abnormal receptor activity.

Intracellular disorders may involve inadequate synthesis of the second messenger, such as cyclic adenosine monophosphate (cAMP), needed to transduce the hormonal signal into intracellular events. The target cell for water-soluble hormones may have a faulty response to hormone-receptor binding and thus fail to generate the required second messenger. The cell also may have an abnormal response to the second messenger if levels of intracellular enzymes or proteins are altered. (Second messengers for various hormones are listed in Table 19-4.) Both of these pathogenic mechanisms result in failure of the target cell to express the usual hormonal effect.

Pathogenic mechanisms affecting target cell response for lipid-soluble hormones, such as thyroid hormone or glucocorticoids, either occur less frequently or are recognized less frequently than those affecting the water-soluble hormones. These hormone-resistant states have been generally linked to mutations in the nuclear receptor for the hormone or, in some instances, to alterations in nuclear coregulators.[2,3] The number of receptors may be decreased, or those receptors may have an altered affinity for hormones. Both mechanisms would affect hormone-receptor binding. Alterations in generation of new messenger ribonucleic acid (mRNA) or absence of substrates for new protein synthesis also may occur, resulting in altered target cell response.

ALTERATIONS OF THE HYPOTHALAMIC–PITUITARY SYSTEM

Documenting abnormal release of hypothalamic-releasing hormones has been difficult because of the relative inaccessibility of the hypothalamic–pituitary unit in the brain and the short half-life and small concentrations of the hypothalamic hormones. The most common hypothalamic diseases probably result from interruption in the pituitary stalk caused by destructive lesions of the stem, rupture of the stem after head injury, surgical transection of the stem, or stem tumor. In these cases, interruption of the physical connections between the hypothalamus and the pituitary gland causes apparent pituitary disease. For example, diabetes insipidus (antidiuretic hormone [ADH] insufficiency) may result, depending on the location at which the infundibular stem is interrupted. If the lesion is close to the hypothalamus, diabetes insipidus is likely; the farther away the lesion is from the hypothalamus, the less likely is the occurrence of diabetes insipidus.

The absence of hypothalamic hormones (Fig. 20-2) causes a variety of manifestations. In women the menses cease, and in men spermatogenesis is impaired because of the absence of gonadotropin-releasing hormone (GnRH) stimulation of gonadotropin follicle-stimulating hormone (FSH) and luteinizing hormone (LH). Adrenocorticotropic hormone (ACTH) response to low serum cortisol levels is decreased because of the absence of corticotropin-releasing hormone (CRH). Hypothalamic hypothyroidism is caused by the absence of thyrotropin-releasing hormone (TRH). Low levels of growth hormone cause the absence of growth hormone (GH) regulatory hormones. Hyperprolactinemia is caused by an absence of the usual inhibitory controls of prolactin secretion.

Diseases of the Posterior Pituitary

Syndrome of Inappropriate Antidiuretic Hormone Secretion

Diseases of the posterior pituitary that cause clinically observable symptoms are rare. If they do occur, they usually are related to abnormal ADH (vasopressin) secretion. **Syndrome of inappropriate ADH (SIADH) secretion** is characterized by high levels of ADH in the absence of normal physiologic stimuli for its release.[4] In order to make the diagnosis of SIADH, the individual should have both normal adrenal and thyroid function because thyroid hormone and glucocorticoids are essential for free water clearance by the kidneys.[5]

The most common cause of elevated levels of ADH is ectopically produced ADH. SIADH is associated with some forms of cancer, apparently because of the ectopic secretion of ADH by tumor cells. Tumors that have been reported in association with SIADH include small cell adenocarcinoma of the lung, carcinoma of the duodenum and pancreas, leukemia, lymphoma, Hodgkin disease, sarcoma, and squamous cell carcinoma of the tongue.

Transient SIADH may follow pituitary surgery, because stored ADH is released in an unregulated fashion. When postoperative fluid volume shifts occur after any type of surgery, ADH secretion is increased for 5 to 7 days. The precise mechanism is uncertain, but it is likely related to fluid and volume changes following surgery, the amount and type of intravenous fluids given, and the use of narcotic analgesics. SIADH secretion may be seen in individuals with a variety of infectious pulmonary diseases. It may be caused by the ectopic production of ADH by infected lung tissue[6] or by increased posterior pituitary secretion of ADH in response to a hypoxia-induced decrease in pulmonary perfusion.[7]

SIADH secretion may be associated with psychiatric disease and also may occur after treatment with a variety of drugs.[8] These include hypoglycemic medications (chlorpropamide), barbiturates, general anesthetics, vincristine, nicotine, morphine, diuretics, and synthetic ADH analogs. These drugs serve either to simulate ADH release or to enhance the physiologic effects of ADH or have a biologic action similar to ADH.

Pathophysiology

The cardinal features of SIADH are symptoms of water intoxication due to enhanced renal water retention or increases in total body water that lead to hyponatremia (low serum sodium), hypoosmolarity, and urine that is inappropriately concentrated with respect to serum osmolarity. These features lead to hyponatremia and hypoosmolality. In SIADH, ADH is released continually. Water retention results from the normal action of ADH on the renal tubules and collect-

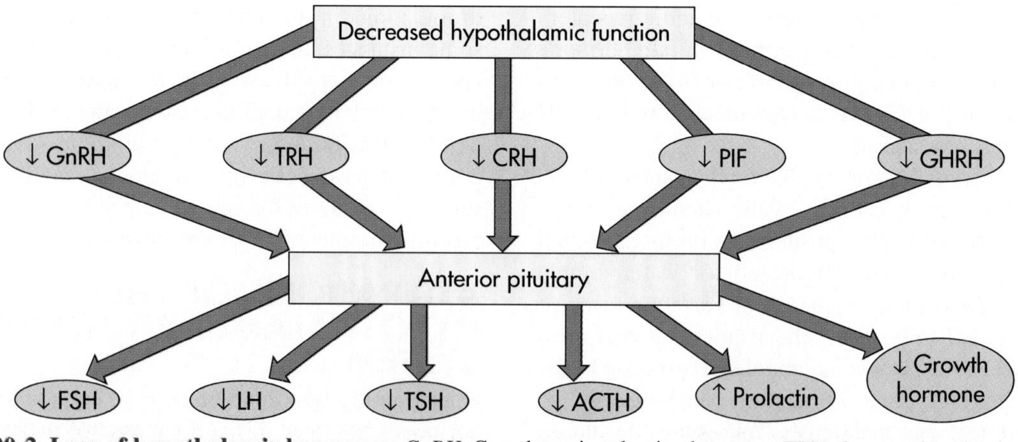

Fig. 20-2 Loss of hypothalamic hormones. *GnRH,* Gonadotropin-releasing hormone; *TRH,* thyrotropin-releasing hormone; *CRH,* corticotropin-releasing hormone; *FSH,* follicle-stimulating hormone; *LH,* luteinizing hormone; *TSH,* thyroid-stimulating hormone; *ACTH,* adrenocorticotropic hormone; *PIF,* prolactin inhibitory factor (probably dopamine); *GHRH,* growth hormone releasing hormone.

ing ducts, increasing their permeability to water and increasing water reabsorption by the kidneys. (Renal function is discussed in Chapter 35.) An expansion of extracellular fluid volume results, and a dilutional hyponatremia develops.

Clinical Manifestations

A diagnosis of SIADH requires the following signs: (1) serum hypoosmolality and hyponatremia, (2) urine hyperosmolarity (i.e., the osmolality of the urine is greater than expected for the concomitant serum osmolality), (3) urine sodium excretion that matches sodium intake, (4) normal adrenal and thyroid function, and (5) absence of conditions that can alter volume status (e.g., congestive heart failure, hypovolemia from any cause, or renal insufficiency).

The symptoms of SIADH are primarily the result of hyponatremia. The severity and the sudden onset of the hyponatremia determine the extent of the symptoms. Even if hyponatremia develops slowly, serum sodium levels below 110 to 115 mEq/L are likely to cause severe and sometimes irreversible neurologic damage. Thirst, impaired taste, anorexia, dyspnea on exertion, fatigue, and dulled sensorium occur when the serum sodium decreases rapidly from 140 to 130 mEq/L. Severe gastrointestinal symptoms, including vomiting and abdominal cramps, occur with a drop in sodium from 130 to 120 mEq/L. With a serum sodium level below 115 mEq/L, confusion, lethargy, muscle twitching, and convulsions may occur. Symptoms usually resolve with correction of hyponatremia.

Evaluation and Treatment

Serum electrolyte levels, serum osmolality and urine volume, urine electrolyte levels, and urine osmolality are adequate measures of the presence of SIADH. The treatment of SIADH involves the correction of the underlying causal problems; emergency correction of severe hyponatremia by administration of hypertonic saline; and, most important, fluid restriction to 600 to 800 ml/day. Careful monitoring is important. If hyponatremia is too rapidly corrected, a severe neurologic syndrome, central pontine myelinolisis, can ensue.[9] Resolution usually occurs within 3 days, with a 2- to 3-kg weight loss due to enhanced free water clearance. No drug therapy is available to suppress ectopically produced ADH; however, demeclocycline, which causes the renal tubules to develop resistance to ADH, may be used to treat resistant or chronic SIADH.

Diabetes Insipidus

Diabetes insipidus is related to an insufficiency of ADH, leading to polyuria and polydipsia. The two types of diabetes insipidus are a neurogenic or central form and a nephrogenic or renal form.[10] Neurogenic diabetes insipidus is the category most frequently encountered in clinical practice. The neurogenic form is caused by insufficient amounts of ADH; the nephrogenic form is caused by an inadequate response to ADH. Psychogenic polydipsia, commonly referred to as compulsive water drinking, may be difficult to differentiate from true diabetes insipidus.

The neurogenic form of diabetes insipidus occurs when any organic lesion of the hypothalamus, pituitary stalk, or posterior pituitary interferes with ADH synthesis, transport, or release. These lesions include primary brain tumors, hypophysectomy, aneurysms, thrombosis, infections, and immunologic disorders. Diabetes insipidus is a well-recognized complication of closed-head trauma.

The nephrogenic form of diabetes insipidus is usually an acquired disorder. An idiopathic form has also been documented and usually occurs in genetically predisposed individuals. Nephrogenic diabetes insipidus is usually associated with end-organ failure, with an insensitivity of the renal tubule to ADH, particularly the collecting tubules. Nephrogenic diabetes insipidus is generally related to disorders and drugs that damage the renal tubules or inhibit the generation of cAMP in the tubules. These disorders include pyelonephritis, amyloidosis, destructive uropathies, polycystic disease, and intrinsic renal disease, all of which lead to irreversible diabetes insipidus. Drugs that may induce a generally reversible form of nephrogenic diabetes insipidus include lithium carbonate, general anesthetics such as methoxyflurane, and demeclocycline.

Pathophysiology

Individuals with diabetes insipidus will have partial or total inability to concentrate urine. In individuals with psychogenic polydipsia, polyuria results from both the volume of fluids ingested plus an effective washout of the renal medullary concentration gradient (see Chapter 35).

Insufficient ADH secretion causes immediate excretion of large volumes of dilute urine, leading to an increase in plasma osmolality. In conscious individuals the thirst mechanism is stimulated and induces polydipsia. For unknown reasons the person usually craves cold drinks. The urine output is varied. In about one half of cases, urine volume is 4 to 8 L/day, whereas in one fourth of the cases it is 8 to 12 L/day. With profound ADH deficiency, output may be greater than 12 L/day. The urine specific gravity is low, from 1.00 to 1.005. If the individual with diabetes insipidus cannot keep up with the urinary loss of water, hypernatremia occurs. Serum electrolytes generally are not affected. Dehydration develops rapidly without ongoing fluid replacement.

In nephrogenic diabetes insipidus, ADH levels are normal or high but the collecting ducts do not increase their permeability to water in response to ADH. There is a familial form of the disorder, or it may be associated with the drugs lithium or demeclocycline or the anesthetic methoxyflurane.

Idiopathic neurogenic diabetes insipidus usually has an abrupt onset, and many individuals can specifically recall the date of onset of their symptoms. Those with posttraumatic or postneurosurgical diabetes insipidus may develop a classic three-phase syndrome. Initially, significant diuresis occurs, apparently as a result of acute damage to the hypothalamic centers involving ADH secretion. The second phase is one of antidiuresis, which may represent necrosis of denervated tissue of the posterior pituitary with release of ADH into the circulation. The final phase is one of polyuria and polydipsia, reflecting a permanent loss of the ability to secrete adequate amounts of ADH. Antidiuretic hormone does not have to be completely absent for polyuria and polydipsia to occur.

Clinical Manifestations

The clinical manifestations of diabetes insipidus are caused by the absence of ADH. These signs and symptoms include polyuria, nocturia, continuous thirst, polydipsia, low urine specific gravity, low urine osmolality,[11] and high-normal plasma osmolality (300 mOsm or more).[7] Plasma osmolality is always higher than urine osmolality in diabetes insipidus after 8 hours of water deprivation. Untreated individuals with long-standing diabetes insipidus may develop a large bladder capacity and hydronephrosis (see Chapter 35).

Evaluation and Treatment

Diabetes insipidus must be distinguished from other polyuric states, including diabetes mellitus, osmotically induced diuresis, and psychogenic polydipsia. Water restriction is a useful test because people without diabetes insipidus respond with a rapid decrease in urine volume (800 mOsm/kg), whereas persons with diabetes insipidus have no decrease in urine volume and maintain a urine osmolarity of approximately 100 mOsm/kg. The diagnosis of diabetes insipidus is generally established through water deprivation testing or by correlating the clinical presentation with serum osmolarity and plasma ADH levels. In individuals with true diabetes insipidus, water deprivation testing can be hazardous. If the individual loses more than 3% of their pretest body weight, circulatory collapse and shock can ensue. The diagnosis of psychogenic polydipsia can be extremely difficult and differentiation from nephrogenic diabetes insipidus (due to the washout of renal concentrating gradient) is based upon plasma ADH levels.[11]

Treatment of neurogenic diabetes insipidus is based on the extent of the ADH deficiency and on individual variables such as age, endocrine and cardiovascular status, and lifestyle. Individuals who have a urine output in excess of 9 L per day and a urine osmolality of less than 100 mOsm/kg after a dehydration or water restriction test generally require ADH replacement.[12]

Replacement therapy for symptomatic central or neurogenic diabetes insipidus includes administration of the synthetic vasopressin analog DDAVP (desmopressin) given intranasally or orally. Drugs that potentiate the action of otherwise insufficient amounts of endogenous ADH, such as chlorpropamide, may be used in individuals with incomplete ADH deficiency. Clofibrate, thiazides, chlorthalidone, and carbamazepine are used in a limited fashion with mildly affected individuals;[13] however, these agents cannot be recommended to treat more symptomatic individuals.

Diseases of the Anterior Pituitary

Disorders of the anterior pituitary may involve either hypofunction or hyperfunction of the gland. **Hypopituitarism** is defined as a range of dysfunction, from the absence of selective pituitary trophic hormones to complete failure of hormonal functions of the anterior pituitary. Pituitary hypofunction may result from intrinsic pituitary process or from a hypothalamic disorder. The most common causes of hypopituitarism lie within the pituitary. Functional hypopituitarism may be seen in systemic illnesses such as anorexia nervosa; starvation; or severe, systemic illness. **Hyperpituitarism** generally is caused by a pituitary adenoma.

Anterior pituitary hypofunction may result from infarction of the gland, removal or destruction of the gland, or space-occupying lesions such as pituitary adenomas or aneurysms that compress otherwise normal secreting pituitary cells and lead to compromised hormonal output. Growth hormone–secreting cells are most sensitive to pressure. Hyperfunction of the anterior pituitary generally implies an adenoma composed of secretory pituitary cells.

Hypopituitarism

In terms of endocrine replacement therapy, it is not important to differentiate the level of functional loss (hypothalamic vs pituitary); it is critical to address the underlying lesion if either neurosurgical intervention or special medical therapy is warranted to treat a neoplastic process.

One cause of hypopituitarism is pituitary infarction. Infarction may be seen in conjunction with Sheehan syndrome (postpartum pituitary necrosis). Pituitary infarction is also seen with shock; pituitary apoplexy; sickle cell disease; and, rarely, during pregnancy in women with diabetes mellitus. Other causes of hypopituitarism are head trauma; infections (e.g., meningitis, syphilis, tuberculosis); vascular malformations; surgical ablation related to tumor removal; and, rarely, granulomatous lesions. The pathogenesis and consequences of Sheehan syndrome illustrate the anatomic relationships and physiologic consequences of panhypopituitarism.

Pathophysiology

The pituitary gland is extremely vascular and is therefore extremely vulnerable to ischemia and infarction. The likelihood of infarction is increased with the increased size and vasculature of the gland, which occurs during pregnancy. In 1961 Sheehan and Stanfield proposed that the primary pathologic mechanism in postpartum pituitary infarction is vasospasm of the artery supplying the anterior pituitary. A frequently identified cause is some event that leads to circulatory collapse and compensatory vasospasm. If vasospasm is sustained for more than several hours, tissue necrosis occurs. The pituitary gland may be particularly susceptible to necrosis because its blood supply, through the hypophysial system, is already partially deoxygenated and, especially in the hyperplastic pituitary of pregnancy, oxygen demands are increased.

After tissue necrosis, edema occurs. Expansion of the pituitary within the fixed compartment of the sella turcica further impedes blood supply to the pituitary. A second mechanism, which may be involved in pituitary infarction in the postpartum woman (Sheehan syndrome), is an increased risk for intravascular coagulation. In such individuals, excessive fibrin is deposited in the pituitary vessels, predisposing the woman to decreased blood supply and infarction of the pituitary.[14]

◆ *Clinical Manifestations*

The signs and symptoms of hypofunction of the anterior pituitary are highly variable and depend on the affected hormones. If all hormones are absent (a condition termed **panhypopituitarism**), the individual experiences cortisol deficiency from lack of ACTH, thyroid deficiency from lack of thyroid-stimulating hormone (TSH), diabetes insipidus from lack of ADH, and gonadal failure and loss of secondary sex characteristics from absence of FSH and LH. GH and, consequently, insulin-like growth factor I levels are low, which results in delayed growth in children and a vague, multisymptom syndrome in adults (Fig. 20-3). In addition, postpartum women are unable to lactate because of the absence of prolactin.

ACTH deficiency is a potentially life-threatening disorder, because cortisol is required for functional maintenance. ACTH deficiency is usually encountered with generalized pituitary hypofunction; it rarely occurs as an isolated event. Within 2 weeks of the complete absence of ACTH, symptoms of cortisol insufficiency develop, including nausea, vomiting, anorexia, fatigue, and weakness. The resulting hypoglycemia is caused by increased insulin sensitivity, decreased glycogen reserves, and decreased gluconeogenesis associated with hypocortisolism. In women, loss of body hair and decreased libido may be caused by decreased adrenal androgen production.

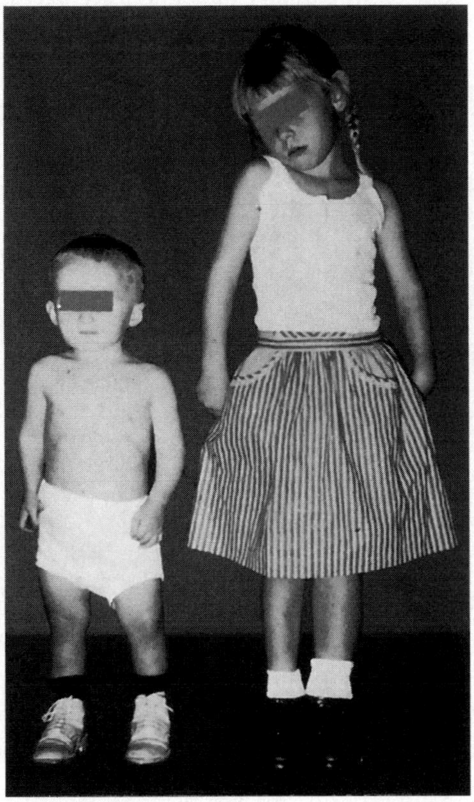

FIG. 20-3 Hypopituitary dwarfism. A 4-year-old boy whose height is 25 inches. Girl is also 4 years old and has a normal height of 39 inches. Dwarf has a normal face, as well as head, trunk, and limbs of approximately normal proportions. (From Brasher HR, Raney RB: *Shand's handbook of orthopaedic surgery*, ed 10, St Louis, 1986, Mosby.)

ACTH deficiency may limit maximum aldosterone secretion, although the renin-angiotensin system is capable of stimulating some aldosterone secretion. Glomerular filtration rate is decreased with ACTH deficiency and may explain the decreased urine output. (Renal function is described in Chapter 34.)

TSH deficiency is rarely seen in isolation but frequently occurs in conjunction with other pituitary hormone deficiencies. The effects of decreased TSH levels may become apparent 4 to 8 weeks after the onset of hypothyrotropinemia. Cold intolerance, dryness of skin, mild myxedema, lethargy, and decreased metabolic rate occur as a result of hypothyroidism induced by decreased TSH levels. The symptoms are usually less severe than those associated with primary hypothyroidism.

The onset of FSH and LH deficiencies in women of reproductive age is associated with amenorrhea and atrophic vagina, uterus, and breasts. In postpubertal males, atrophy of the testes and decreased beard growth occur. Both men and women experience a decrease in body hair and diminished libido. FSH and LH deficiencies frequently occur as a result of pressure on the gonadotropes from other sources, such as tumors. If there is enlargement caused by tumor, symptoms may include headache and visual disturbances with blurring and field defects.

◆ *Evaluation and Treatment*

The diagnostic tests evaluating hypopituitarism are well defined and must be interpreted together with the individual's signs and symptoms. Radioimmunoassay is used to measure hormone levels, and both the trophic pituitary and target hormones must be assessed. Radiographic assessment of the pituitary (MRI or CT scans) may demonstrate enlargement of the pituitary, abnormal areas of enhancement suggestive of an adenoma, deviation of the pituitary stalk, or evidence of a locally aggressive tumor. However, some radiographic findings may be nonspecific and require a clinical correlation to establish a diagnosis. In cases of circulatory collapse, immediate therapy with glucocorticoids and intravenous fluids is critical. Thyroid and cortisol replacement therapy must be maintained. Gender-specific sex steroid replacement therapy is also initiated to improve general well-being and to prevent osteoporosis.

Hyperpituitarism: Primary Adenoma

Pituitary adenomas are usually benign, slow-growing tumors that frequently arise from cells of the anterior pituitary. The incidence of pituitary adenomas may be as high as 22%, but most of these adenomas are microscopic and asymptomatic. Before the widespread use of higher resolution MRI scanning, most of these incidentally discovered lesions (incidentalomas) were found on postmortem examination. The vast majority of pituitary incidentalomas are hormonally silent and do not pose significant hazards to the individual.[15] The cause of pituitary adenomas is not known. The mortality associated with pituitary tumors usually is attributable to alterations in hormone secretion or to invasion or impingement of surrounding structures caused by expanding adenomas.[16]

Pathophysiology

Local expansion of pituitary adenomas causes both neurologic and secretory effects. Neurologically, the tumor may impinge on the optic chiasm if it extends upward from the sella turcica. This causes a variety of visual disturbances, depending on the portion of the nerve that is compressed. If the tumor is locally aggressive, it may invade the cavernous sinus and cause cavernous sinus thrombosis with impairment of the function of the oculomotor, trigeminal (V_1, V_2), trochler, and abducens cranial nerves, evoking symptoms relative to their function. Extension also may involve the hypothalamus, disturbing hypothalamic control of wakefulness, thirst, appetite, and temperature.

The adenomatous tissue secretes the hormone of the cell type from which it arose, without regard to the needs of the body and without benefit of regulatory feedback mechanisms. Because of the pressure exerted by a tumor growing in the unexpandable sella turcica, those secreting cells of the anterior pituitary that are most sensitive to pressure also may be affected (growth hormone–secreting cells, FSH- and LH-secreting cells). The result of such pressure is hyposecretion of these hormones, and surgical debulking of pituitary tumors has been associated with a return of normal anterior pituitary function.[17]

Clinical Manifestations

The clinical manifestations of pituitary adenomas are related to tumor growth and hormone hypersecretion and hyposecretion. Effects from an increase in tumor size include such nonspecific complaints as headache, fatigue, neck pain or stiffness, and seizures. Visual changes produced by pressure on the optic chiasm include visual field impairments (frequently beginning in one eye and progressing to the other) and temporary blindness. If the tumor infiltrates other cranial nerves, neurologic function is affected.

The pressure produced by a pituitary adenoma is also associated with a paradoxical effect on neighboring anterior pituitary cells, which results in hyposecretion of other anterior pituitary hormones. For example, hyposecretion of GH almost always occurs, and in adults the symptoms of growth hormone deficiency are subtle and may include fatigue (altered by composition) or lower psychosocial achievement.[18,19] Gonadotropic hyposecretion frequently results in menstrual irregularity in women, decreased libido, and receding secondary sex characteristics in both men and women. If the tumor exerts sufficient pressure, thyroid and adrenal hypofunction may occur because of lack of TSH and ACTH. These result in the symptoms of hypothyroidism and hypocortisolism.

Evaluation and Treatment

Diagnosis of pituitary adenoma involves physical and laboratory evaluations, including pertinent hormone assays and radiographic examination of the skull. This may be accomplished by computed tomographic (CT) scanning or dynamic magnetic resonance imaging (MRI) used in conjunction with contrast material. Dynamic MRIs provide superior imaging and greater sensitivity in comparison to CT scans.

The goal of treatment is to protect the individual from the effects of tumor growth and to control hormone hypersecretion while minimizing damage to appropriately secreting portions of the pituitary. Individuals can be treated with specific medications (dopaminergic agonists, octreotide, or specific hormone antagonists),[20] neurosurgical adenomectomy, or radiation therapy depending upon the tumor type, extent of tumor growth, and the suitability of the individual for specific types of treatment.

Hypersecretion of Growth Hormone: Acromegaly

Acromegaly occurs in adults who are exposed to continuously excessive levels of GH. In children and adolescents whose epiphyseal plates have not yet closed, the effect of increased GH levels is termed **giantism** (Fig. 20-4).

Acromegaly is a relatively uncommon disease, estimated to occur in about 40 persons per million.[21] Approximately 15% of all pituitary tumors release excessive GH.

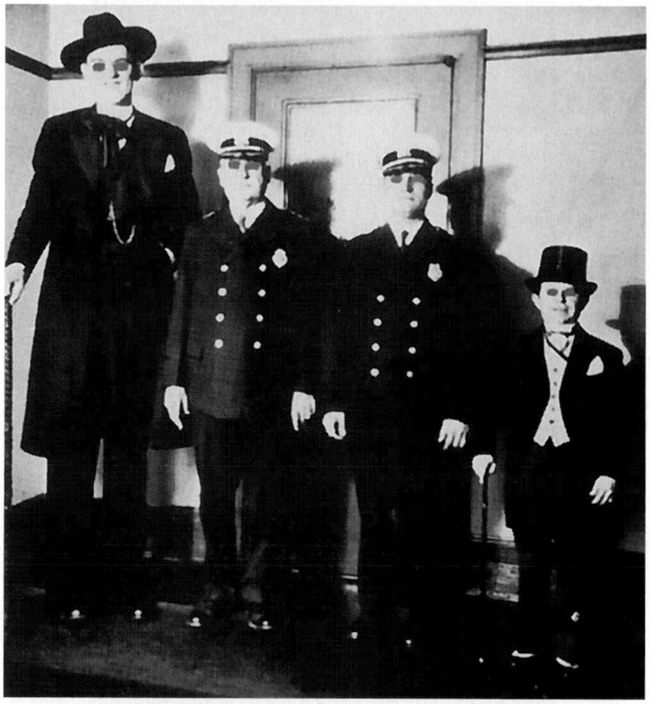

FIG. 20-4 Giantism. A pituitary giant and dwarf contrasted with normal-size men. Excessive secretion of growth hormone by the anterior lobe of the pituitary gland during the early years of life produces giants of this type, whereas deficient secretion of this substance produces well-formed dwarfs. (From Thibodeau GA, Patton K: *Anatomy & physiology*, ed 4, St Louis, 1999, Mosby.)

The most common cause of acromegaly is a primary autonomous GH-secreting pituitary adenoma. Acromegaly occurs more frequently in women than men and is diagnosed most frequently in adults in their 40s and 50s, although the disease is usually present for years preceding the diagnosis.

Acromegaly is a slowly progressive disease that, if untreated, is associated with a decreased life expectancy. The increased number of deaths associated with acromegaly apparently are caused by an increased occurrence of hypertension and diabetes mellitus that leads to coronary artery disease.[22] Malignancies, in particular colon cancer, are also more common in individuals with acromegaly.

Pathophysiology

With a GH-secreting adenoma, the usual GH baseline secretion pattern is lost, as are sleep-related GH peaks. A totally unpredictable secretory pattern ensues. With only slight elevations of GH, insulin-like growth factor 1 levels increase, stimulating growth. In the adult, epiphyseal closure has occurred and increased amounts of GH and insulin-like growth factor 1 cannot stimulate further long bone growth. Instead, these elevations cause connective tissue proliferation and an increase in the cytoplasmic matrix, as well as bony proliferation that results in the characteristic appearance of acromegaly.

GH acts on the renal tubules to increase phosphate reabsorption, leading to mild hyperphosphatemia. The metabolic effects of GH hypersecretion include impaired carbohydrate tolerance and increased metabolic rate. Hyperglycemia may be seen as a result of GH's inhibition of peripheral glucose uptake and increased hepatic glucose production, followed by compensatory hyperinsulinism and, finally, insulin resistance. Diabetes mellitus occurs when the pancreas is unable to secrete enough insulin to offset the effects of GH. Not surprisingly, because of the aforementioned changes in glucose utilization, approximately one third of people with GH abnormalities have glucose intolerance and half of these patients develop diabetes mellitus.[23]

Clinical Manifestations

As a result of connective tissue proliferation, individuals with acromegaly have enlarged tongues, interstitial edema, increase in the size and function of sebaceous and sweat glands (leading to increased body odor), and coarse skin and body hair. The coarse skin condition becomes very apparent when procedures such as inserting an intravenous needle are performed; the skin is very thick and difficult to penetrate (Fig. 20-5). Bony proliferation involves periosteal vertebral growth and enlargement of the facial bones and the bones of the hands and feet (Fig. 20-6). The associated growth results in protrusion of the lower jaw and forehead and a need for increasingly larger sizes of shoes, hats, rings, and gloves.

Because insulin-like growth factor 1 stimulate cartilaginous growth, the increased insulin-like growth factor 1 levels cause elongation of ribs at the bone-cartilage junction, leading to a barrel-chest appearance and increased proliferation of cartilage in joints. This in turn causes backache, arthralgia, and arthritis. These are early manifestations of acromegaly. When shaking hands with an individual with acromegaly, one can palpate the large soft tissues. With bony

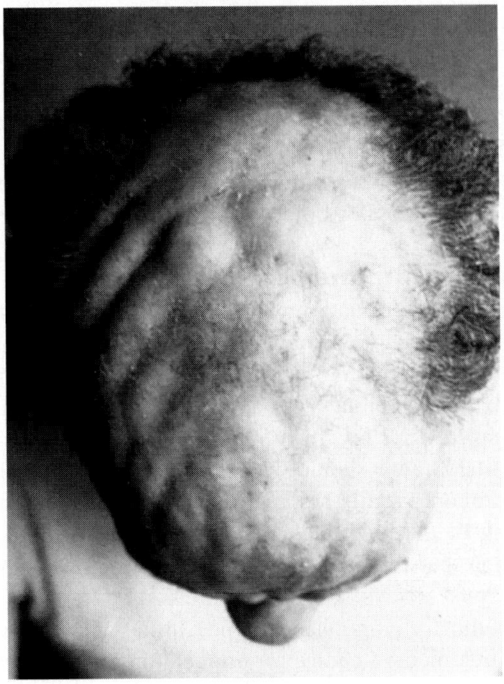

FIG. 20-5 Acromegaly. Note thickening of skin on scalp. (From Thibodeau GA: *Anatomy & physiology*, St Louis, 1987, Mosby.)

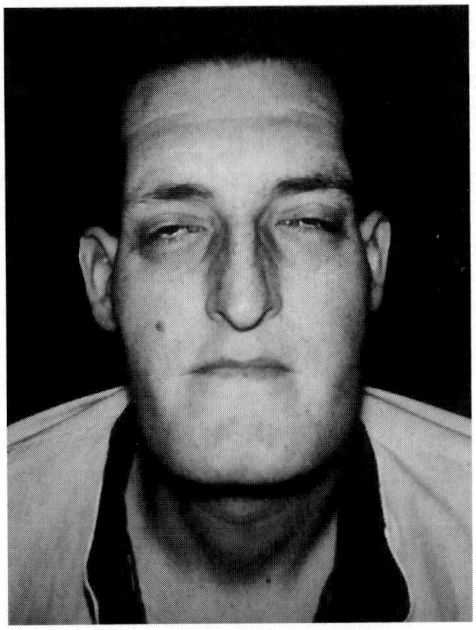

FIG. 20-6 Acromegaly. Note large head, forward projection of jaw, and protrusion of frontal bone. (From Thibodeau GA: *Anatomy & physiology*, St Louis, 1987, Mosby.)

and soft tissue overgrowth, entrapment of nerves may occur, leading to peripheral nerve damage as manifested by weakness, muscular atrophy, footdrop, and sensory changes in the hands.

Although the associated pathophysiology is not understood at present,[24] hypertension and left heart failure are seen in one third to one half of individuals with acromegaly. Headache occurs in 50% to 87% of cases and does not appear related to GH levels, size, or extension of the tumor or presence of hypertension. Because of a space-occupying lesion, central nervous system symptoms of headache, seizure activity, visual disturbances (e.g., bitemporal hemianopia from compression of the optic chiasm), papilledema, and compression hypopituitarism may occur.[25]

If compression hypopituitarism does occur because of a large GH-secreting adenoma, the secretion of the gonadotropins may be affected. This causes amenorrhea in women and loss of libido and erectile dysfunction in men. The secretion of prolactin-inhibiting factor is impaired in 30% to 40% of individuals with acromegaly, which results in hyperprolactinemia.

Evaluation and Treatment

Diagnosis of GH hypersecretion involves measurement of serum GH by radioimmunoassay at basal conditions and in response to glucose administration. The goals of treatment are to normalize or reduce GH secretion, if possible, allowing normal pituitary function and relieving or preventing complications related to tumor expansion. The treatment of choice in acromegaly is surgical removal of the GH-secreting adenoma. Treatment by radiation therapy may be effective when rapid control of GH levels is not essential, when the individual is not a good surgical candidate, or when hyperfunction persists after subtotal resection. Octreotide, a somatostatin analog, has been shown to be extremely effective in lowering elevated growth hormone levels, reversing many of the clinical manifestations of the disease, and causing tumor shrinkage in nearly one half of individuals.[26]

Hypersecretion of Prolactin: Prolactinoma

Pituitary tumors that secrete prolactin, **prolactinomas,** are the most common of hormonally active pituitary tumors encountered in clinical medicine.[27] Prolactin is under tonic inhibitory hypothalamic control through the secretion of dopamine. The physiologic actions of prolactin include breast development during pregnancy, postpartum milk production, and suppression of ovarian function in nursing women. Pathologic elevation of prolactin in women results in amenorrhea, nonpuerperal milk production (galactorrhea), hirsutism, and osteopenia due to estrogen deficiency. Hyperprolactinemia in men causes hypogonadism and erectile dysfunction.[28]

Approximately 30% of pituitary tumors secrete prolactin; however, there are many conditions or medications that can elevate prolactin in the absence of pituitary pathologic condition. For example, renal failure, polycystic ovarian disease, primary hypothyroidism, breast stimulation, or even venipuncture can increase prolactin levels. Medications that can increase prolactin block the effects of dopamine at the pituitary or stimulate proliferation of prolactin-secreting cells (lactotrophes). These include antipsychotics (respiridone, chlorpromazine), metoclorpramide, tricyclic antidepressants, methyldopa, and estrogens. Any process that interferes with the delivery of dopamine from the hypothalamus to the lactotrophes (pituitary stalk tumor, pituitary stalk transection, or compressive pituitary tumor) also results in hyperprolactinemia. Because TRH stimulates prolactin secretion in addition to enhancing TSH release, prolactin may be elevated in patients with primary hypothyroidism.

Pathophysiology

The hallmark of a prolactinoma is sustained increases in serum prolactin. Indeed, tumor size roughly correlates with the degree of prolactin elevation. Hyperprolactinemia has several reproductive consequences. Prolactin suppresses GnRH pulses at the hypothalamus, impairs pulsatile pituitary gonadotropin release, and blunts the gonadal responsiveness to gonadotropins. In estrogen- and progesterone-primed breasts, milk production is stimulated.

Clinical Manifestations

Women with hyperprolactinemia generally present with galactorrhea (nonpuerperal milk production) and menstrual disturbances including amenorrhea. In susceptible women, hirsutism develops due to estrogen deficiency. If detected after many years, estrogen deficiency may also result in osteoporosis. Menstrual abnormalities and galactorrhea are alarming symptoms in women, and, as a result, women generally present earlier in the course of the illness and are found to have microadenomas ($<$1 cm in size) that are less likely to have associated compressive or impingement symptoms. Men, on the other hand, frequently present with headache or visual impairment because they may minimalize or overtly ignore symptoms of hypogonadism (erectile dysfunction or loss of libido).[29]

Evaluation and Treatment

The diagnostic evaluation of hyperprolactinemia starts with a careful history to exclude medications that may cause elevations in prolactin. Symptoms of hypothyroidism should be elicited, and screening with a serum TSH is mandatory. If serum prolactin is less than 50 ng/ml, a careful search for a nonpituitary cause should be pursued. Prolactin levels over 200 ng/ml are usually associated with a prolactinoma. MRI scanning of the pituitary is often helpful in detecting prolactinoma, but the chance of finding an unrelated incidentaloma must always be considered.

Dopaminergic agonists (bromocriptine and cabergoline) are the treatment of choice for prolactinomas,[30] and their use is frequently associated with both a rapid reduction in the size of the tumor and a reversal of the gonadal effects of hyperprolactinemia. Restoration of fertility in previously anovulatory women is common. In individuals resistant or intolerant to these medications, transsphenoidal surgery and radiotherapy are options.

ALTERATIONS OF THYROID FUNCTION

Hyperthyroidism

Thyrotoxicosis

Pathophysiology

Thyrotoxicosis is a condition that results from increased levels of circulating thyroid hormone (TH).[31] Hyperthyroidism is a form of thyrotoxicosis in which excess thyroid hormones are secreted by the thyroid gland. Thyrotoxicosis has a variety of causes. Identifying the cause is important because the treatment and expected outcome vary accordingly. Specific diseases that can cause hyperthyroidism include Graves disease; toxic multinodular goiter; toxic adenoma; and, very rarely, follicular thyroid carcinoma and TSH-secreting pituitary adenomas. Thyrotoxicosis not associated with hyperthyroidism (because thyroid hormone is not being actively synthesized) includes thyroiditis (either subacute or painless) or ingestion of excess TH. Each of these conditions is associated with specific pathophysiology and manifestations. All forms of thyrotoxicosis share some common characteristics.

Clinical Manifestations

The clinical features of thyrotoxicosis are attributable to the metabolic effects of increased circulating levels of thyroid hormones. This usually results in an increased metabolic rate with heat intolerance and an increased tissue sensitivity to stimulation by the sympathetic division of the autonomic nervous system. The major manifestations are summarized in Table 20-1. Goiter is almost always present.

Evaluation and Treatment

The diagnosis of thyrotoxicosis is based upon symptoms of thyroid hormone excess and documentation of increased circulating thyroid hormone levels. Elevated serum free

Table 20-1 Systemic Effects of Hyperthyroidism

System	Clinical Manifestations	Mechanisms Underlying Clinical Manifestations
Endocrine	Enlarged thyroid gland (goiter) (97%-99% of cases); systolic or continuous bruit over thyroid; increased cortisol degradation; hypercalcemia and decreased PTH secretion; diminished sensitivity to exogenous insulin	Hyperactivity of the thyroid gland; excess bone resorption leading to hypercalcemia and a disruption of PTH-regulating mechanisms; increased insulin degradation
Reproductive	Oligomenorrhea or amenorrhea in women, erectile dysfunction and decreased libido in men; increased serum estradiol and estrone but lower than normal levels of free estradiol and estrone	Menstrual cycle alterations that may be related to hypothalamic or pituitary disturbances; increase in sex hormone–binding globulin
Gastrointestinal	Weight loss and an associated increase in appetite; increased peristalsis leading to less formed and more frequent stools; nausea, vomiting, anorexia, abdominal pain; increased use of hepatic glycogen stores and of adipose and protein stores; decrease in serum lipid levels (including triglycerides, phospholipids, and cholesterol); changes in vitamin metabolism leading to decrease in tissue stores of vitamins	Increased catabolism leading to the body's inability to meet its metabolic needs; malabsorption of fat; increased glucose absorption; increase in cholesterol excretion in feces and cholesterol conversion to bile salts; impaired conversion of B vitamins to their coenzymes, causing increased need for water-soluble and fat-soluble vitamins
Integumentary	Excessive sweating, flushing, and warm skin; heat intolerance; hair fine, soft, and straight; temporary hair loss; nails that grow away from nail beds, palmar erythema	Hyperdynamic circulatory state
Sensory (eyes)	Ocular manifestations including elevated upper eyelid leading to decreased blinking and a staring quality; fine tremor of lid; infiltrative ocular changes associated with Graves disease	Overactivity of Müller muscle
Cardiovascular	Increased cardiac output and decreased peripheral resistance; tachycardia at rest; loud heart sounds; supraventricular dysrhythmias, left ventricular dilation and hypertrophy	Hypermetabolism and need to dissipate heat
Nervous	Restlessness; short attention span; compulsive movement; fatigue; tremor; insomnia; emotional lability	Not clearly defined; alterations in cerebral metabolism resulting from excess thyroid hormone
Pulmonary	Dyspnea; reduced vital capacity	Weakness of respiratory muscles

PTH, Parathyroid hormone.

thyroxine (T_4), triiodothyronine (T_3), and radioactive iodine uptake (RAIU) are common in hyperthyroid states.

Treatment is directed at controlling excessive TH production, secretion, or action. The major types of therapy currently used to achieve these goals include drug therapy, radioactive iodine therapy, and surgery.

Graves disease

Graves disease is the most common cause of hyperthyroidism. The cause of Graves disease has been debated for many years, and current research has linked this disorder to autoimmunity (see Chapter 8). Graves disease is a familial disorder,[32] characterized as a multisystem syndrome consisting of one or more of the following: (1) hyperthyroidism, (2) diffuse thyroid enlargement (goiter), (3) ophthalmopathy, and (4) dermopathy. The prevalence is less than 1% in the U.S. population.[33] It occurs more commonly in women.

The pathology of Graves disease indicates that normal regulatory mechanisms are overridden by immunologic mechanisms. Substances termed *thyroid autoantibodies* (or *thyroid-stimulating immunoglobulins*) of the immunoglobulin G (IgG) class are found in more than 95% of subjects with Graves disease.[34] The hyperfunction of the thyroid gland leads to suppression of TSH and TRH, because the immune system is not controlled by feedback from elevated levels of thyroid hormone. The hyperfunction of the thyroid gland is reflected in a dramatically increased iodine uptake and increased rate of thyroid gland metabolism, which may in turn contribute to the hypervascularity and enlargement of the gland. The disproportionate increase in T_3 production reflects long-term hyperstimulation of the thyroid gland. A decrease in the concentration of thyroid-binding globulin, combined with the increased production of thyroid hormone, causes increased circulating levels of thyroid hormone responsible for many of the thyrotoxic symptoms.

A small number of individuals with Graves disease experience **pretibial myxedema (Graves dermopathy)**, characterized by subcutaneous swelling on the anterior portions of the legs and by indurated and erythematous skin. These manifestations occasionally appear on the hands as well.

Many individuals with Graves disease experience ocular manifestations (Fig. 20-7). Two categories of ocular manifestations are associated with Graves disease: (1) functional abnormalities resulting from hyperactivity of the sympathetic division of the autonomic nervous system and (2) infiltrative changes involving the orbital contents with enlargement of the ocular muscles. Functional abnormalities occur in most individuals with Graves disease. These abnormalities include a lag of the globe on upward gaze or a lag of the upper lid on downward gaze. This manifestation does not appear to affect ocular function and appears to resolve with treatment for hyperthyroidism.

Infiltrative ophthalmopathy may occur with Graves disease, although the ophthalmopathy appears to be a separate immune-mediated disorder. Graves ophthalmopathy is also an immune-mediated disease.[35] It appears in 50% to 70% of individuals with Graves disease[36] and is characterized by edema of the orbital contents; protrusion of the globe; paralysis of the extraocular muscles; and damage to the retina and optic nerve, which may lead to blindness. These changes result in exophthalmos, periorbital edema, and extraocular muscle weakness leading to diplopia. The individual may experience irritation, pain, lacrimation, photophobia, and blurred vision. Occasionally, decreased visual acuity, papilledema, visual field impairment, exposure keratosis, and corneal ulceration may occur.

Unfortunately, current treatment for Graves disease does not reverse the infiltrative ophthalmopathy or the pretibial myxedema. Therapy for these problems is palliative, although skin lesions rarely require treatment.

Hyperthryroidism due to Nodular Thyroid Disease

Enlargement of the thyroid gland is referred to as a **goiter.** The thyroid gland normally enlarges in response to an increased secretion of TH that occurs in puberty; pregnancy; iodine deficiency; and immunologic, viral, or genetic disorders. The increased number of follicles is a compensatory mecha-

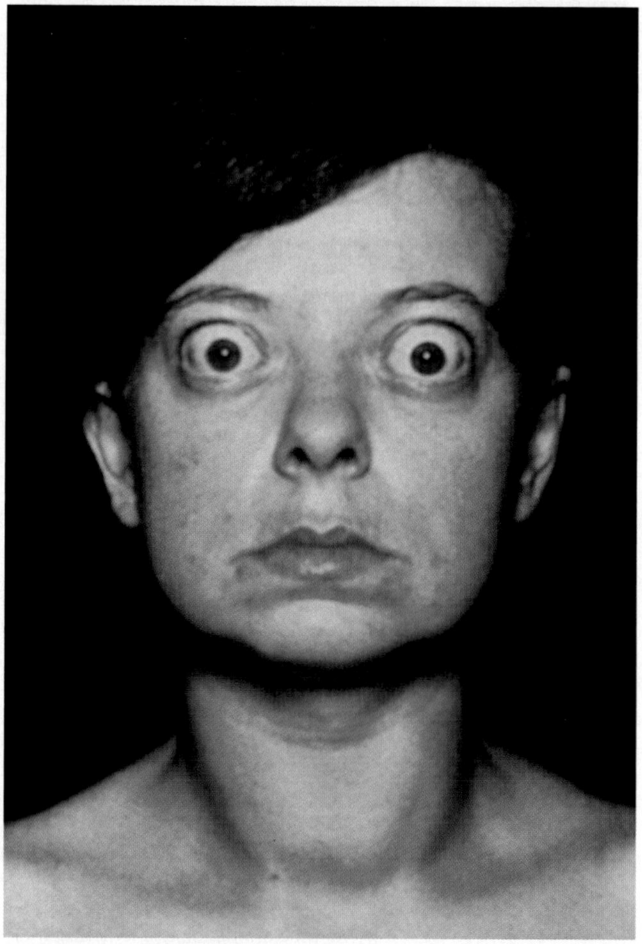

FIG. 20-7 Thyrotoxicosis (Graves disease). Note large and protruding eyeballs in association with a large goiter. (Seidel et al: *Mosby's guide to physical examination*, ed 4, St Louis, 1999; courtesy Paul W Ladenson, MD, The Johns Hopkins University and Hospital, Baltimore.)

nism in response to increased TSH levels. When the condition requiring increased TH resolves, TSH secretion normally subsides and the thyroid gland returns to its original size.

Irreversible changes may have occurred in some follicular cells, however, so that such cells now function autonomously. Hyperthyroidism may result from these irreversible changes. On the other hand, some of these clusters of cells may cease to function, and the remainder of the gland then functions to supply the remainder of the body's need, and a euthyroid state is achieved and maintained. If the autonomously functioning cells produce sufficient or excessive TH for the usual body requirement, the remainder of the gland undergoes involution, becoming normal but inactive tissue. This condition may result in euthyroidism or hyperthyroidism, depending on the amount of TH produced.

Once thyrotoxicosis results, the condition generally is termed **toxic multinodular goiter**; however, only one nodule may become hyperfunctioning. This is termed a **toxic adenoma**. The manifestations of hyperthyroidism resulting from toxic multinodular goiter or a toxic adenoma are similar to those of Graves disease, although infiltrative ophthalmopathy and myxedema do not occur. The symptoms usually develop slowly and appear over time.[37]

Thyrotoxic Crisis

Thyrotoxic crisis (thyroid storm) is a rare but dangerous worsening of the thyrotoxic state, in which death occurs within 48 hours without treatment.[38] The condition may develop spontaneously, but it occurs most frequently in individuals who have undiagnosed or partially treated severe hyperthyroidism and who are subjected to excessive stress from other causes. These causes may include infection, pulmonary or cardiovascular disorders, emotional distress, dialysis, plasmapheresis, or inadequate preparation for thyroid surgery.

The systemic symptoms of thyrotoxic crisis include hyperthermia; tachycardia, especially atrial tachydysrhythmias; high-output heart failure; agitation or delirium; and nausea, vomiting, or diarrhea contributing to fluid volume depletion. The symptoms may be attributed to increased β-adrenergic receptors and catecholamines.[37] The treatment is designed (1) to reduce both circulating TH levels by inducing a block of thyroid hormone synthesis (i.e., propylthiouracil) and thereby reducing their effects to eliminate the precipitating disorder, and (2) to provide symptomatic and supportive care.

Hypothyroidism

Hypothyroidism is the most common disorder of thyroid function. **Hypothyroidism** is caused by a deficient production of TH by the thyroid gland. Hypothyroidism may be primary or secondary. Primary causes include (1) defective hormone synthesis resulting from autoimmune (circulating antithyroid antibodies) thyroiditis, endemic iodine deficiency, or antithyroid drugs (goitrous hypothyroidism); and (2) congenital defects or loss of thyroid tissue after treatment for hyperthyroidism. Causes of secondary hypothyroidism, which are less common, include conditions that cause either pituitary or hypothalamic failure.

Pathophysiology

In primary hypothyroidism the loss of functional thyroid tissue leads to a decreased production of TH. The response is an increased secretion of TSH that may lead to goiter. On the other hand, the cellular infiltration that occurs in autoimmune thyroiditis may also cause thyroid enlargement independently of the trophic actions of TSH. Secondary hypothyroidism is caused most commonly by failure of the pituitary to synthesize adequate amounts of TSH. Pituitary tumors or the results of their treatment are the most common causes of secondary hypothyroidism.

Hypothyroid Conditions

Primary Hypothyroidism

There are several causes of primary hypothyroidism. Some are associated with spontaneous recovery and resultant euthyroidism, whereas others are linked to permanent hypothyroidism. Spontaneous recovery of thyroid function is seen in three conditions—subacute thyroiditis, painless thyroiditis, and postpartum thyroiditis.[39] **Subacute thyroiditis** is a nonbacterial inflammation of the thyroid often preceded by a viral infection. It is accompanied by fever, tenderness, and enlargement of the thyroid. The inflammatory process results initially in elevated levels of thyroid hormone due to release of stored thyroglobulin and later in hypothyroidism before the gland recovers normal activity. Symptoms may last for 2 to 4 months, and nonsteroidal antiinflammatory agents, beta-blockers, and possibly thyroid hormone supplementation may be required during the course of the illness. **Painless thyroiditis** has a course similar to subacute thyroiditis, but it is pathologically identical to Hashimoto disease. **Postpartum thyroiditis** generally occurs within 6 months of delivery, occurs in up to 7% of all women, and has a course similar to painless thyroiditis. Pathologic specimens suggest it is related to Hashimoto disease as well. Spontaneous recovery is seen in over 95% of individuals affected with these forms of thyroiditis. **Autoimmune thyroiditis** (**Hashimoto disease, chronic lymphocytic thyroiditis**) results in destruction of thyroid tissue by circulating thyroid antibodies and infiltration of lymphocytes. Hashimoto disease also has a genetic disposition.[40] Other causes of primary hypothyroidism include radioiodine ablation, thyroidectomy, and medications (lithium and amiodarone). Goiter formation is commonly observed.

Clinical Manifestations

Hypothyroidism generally affects all body systems, with the extent of the symptoms closely related to the degree of TH deficiency. The onset is usually insidious over months or years. The lowered levels of TH result in decreased energy metabolism and heat production. The individual develops a low basal metabolic rate, cold intolerance, lethargy, tiredness, and slightly lowered basal body temperature (Table 20-2). The decrease in TH leads to increases in TSH production and may lead to goiter.

Table 20-2 Systemic Manifestations of Hypothyroidism

System	Clinical Manifestations	Mechanisms Underlying Clinical Manifestations
Neurologic	Confusion, syncope, slowed speech and thinking, memory loss; lethargy, headaches, hearing loss, night blindness; slow, clumsy movements; cerebellar ataxia; slow alpha-wave activity and loss of amplitude in EEG; reduced cAMP response to epinephrine, glucagon, and PTH stimulation	Decreased cerebral blood flow leading to cerebral hypoxia; reduced intracellular processes caused by decreased β-adrenergic activity that may be related to a decrease in the number of β-adrenergic receptor sites
Endocrine	Increased TSH production in primary hypothyroidism; enlarged pituitary thyrotropes, increase in serum prolactin levels with galactorrhea; decreased rate of cortisol turnover but with normal serum cortisol levels	Impaired TH synthesis or defects in iodide trapping leading to compensatory TSH production; chronic overstimulation of thyrotropes by TRH and by TSH synthesis; stimulation of lactotropes by TRH related to increased prolactin levels; decreased deactivation of cortisol
Reproductive	Decreased androgen secretion in men, increased estriol formation in women; low total hormone values but with increased amounts of unbound hormone; anovulation, decreased libido, and a high incidence of spontaneous abortion in women; erectile dysfunction, decreased libido, and oligospermia in men	Altered metabolism of estrogens and androgens; decreased levels of sex hormone–binding globulin
Hematologic	Decrease in red cell mass leading to normocytic, normochromic anemia; macrocytic anemia associated with vitamin B_{12} deficiency and inadequate folate or iron absorption in the gastrointestinal tract	Decreased basal metabolic rate and reduced oxygen requirements, decreased production of erythropoietin, possible relationship between TH and optimal hematologic response to vitamin B_{12}
Cardiovascular	Reduction in stroke volume and heart rate causing lowered cardiac output; increased peripheral vascular resistance to maintain systolic blood pressure; normal response to exercise but with alterations in circulatory system at rest (prolonged circulation time and decreased blood flow to tissues); cool skin and cold tolerance; enlarged heart; decreased intensity of heart sounds and variety of ECG changes (sinus bradycardia, prolonged PR interval, depressed P waves, flattened or inverted T waves, and low-amplitude QRS complexes); cardiac tamponade (although rare)	Decreased metabolic demands and loss of regulatory and rate-setting effects of TH; protein-mucopolysaccharide-rich fluid in the pericardial sac associated with enlarged heart; pericardial effusions associated with heart sounds and ECG changes
Pulmonary	Dyspnea; myxedematous changes in respiratory muscles leading to hypoventilation and carbon dioxide retention, which contribute to myxedema coma	Pleural effusions associated with dyspnea, although effusions may be asymptomatic
Renal	Reduced renal blood flow and glomerular filtration rate leading to decreased renal excretion of water; increase in total body water and dilutional hyponatremia; reduced production of erythropoietin	Hemodynamic alterations associated with reduced blood flow and filtration; increased total body water related to decreased excretion and mucinous deposits in tissue
Gastrointestinal	Decreased appetite; constipation, weight gain, and fluid retention; decreased absorption of most nutrients; decreased protein metabolism leading to retarded skeletal and soft-tissue growth and slightly positive nitrogen balance; edema; decreased glucose absorption and delayed glucose uptake; elevated serum lipid values	Reduced intake and reduced peristaltic activity that may progress to fecal impaction; water absorption related to prolonged transit time; fluid retention associated with myxedematous changes; edema associated with high concentrations of exchangeable albumin in the extravascular space caused by increased capillary permeability to proteins; depressed insulin degradation; depressed lipid synthesis and degradation
Musculoskeletal	Muscle aching and stiffness; slow movement and slow tendon jerk reflexes; decreased bone formation and resorption, increased bone density; aching and stiffness in joints	Decreased rate of muscle contraction and relaxation contributing to slow movement and reflexes
Integumentary	Dry, flaky skin; dry, brittle head and body hair; reduced growth of nails and hair, slow wound healing	Reduced sweat and sebaceous gland secretion
	Myxedema	Accumulation of hyaluronic acid, which binds water and causes a puffy appearance
	Cool skin	Decreased circulation to skin

EEG, Echoencephalogram; *cAMP,* cyclic adenosine monophosphate; *PTH,* parathyroid hormone; *TH,* thyroid hormone; *TSH,* thyroid-stimulating hormone; *TRH,* thyrotropin-releasing hormone; *ECG,* electroencephalogram.

The characteristic sign of severe or long-standing hypothyroidism is **myxedema,** which is histologically similar to the pretibial myxedema deposits that often occur with Graves disease. Myxedema is a result of an alteration in the composition of the dermis and other tissues. The connective fibers are separated by an increased amount of protein and mucopolysaccharides.

This protein-mucopolysaccharide complex binds water, producing nonpitting, boggy edema, especially around the eyes, hands, and feet and in the supraclavicular fossae (Fig. 20-8). Binding with water is also responsible for thickening of the tongue and the laryngeal and pharyngeal mucous membranes. This results in thick, slurred speech and hoarseness, both common in hypothyroidism.

Myxedema coma, a medical emergency, is a diminished level of consciousness associated with severe hypothyroidism. Signs and symptoms include hypothermia without shivering, hypoventilation, hypotension, hypoglycemia, and lactic acidosis. Older patients with severe vascular disease and with moderate or untreated hypothyroidism are particularly at risk for developing myxedema coma. It also may occur after overuse of narcotics or sedatives or after an acute illness in hypothyroid individuals.

Evaluation and Treatment

In addition to the clinical symptoms of hypothyroidism, a decrease in both total and free T_4 is present in myxedema; however, **subclinical hypothyroidism**, defined as an elevation in TSH with normal levels of circulating TH, is more common and also responds to levothyroxine supplementation.[46] TSH concentration increases from loss of negative feedback from thyroid hormone. When hypothyroidism is caused by pituitary deficiencies, serum TSH levels are decreased or are inappropriately normal in the face of low levels of TH. Hormone replacement therapy is the treatment of choice for hypothyroidism. Thyroid hormone is available as a synthetic hormone (levothyroxine) which is preferred over the crude extract from animal thyroid glands (desiccated thyroid).

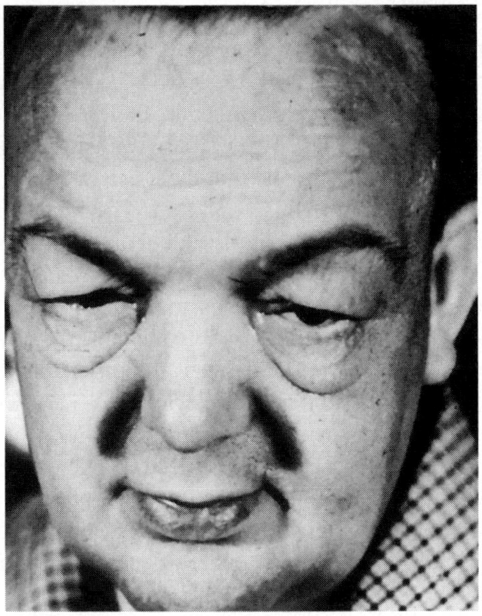

FIG. 20-8 Myxedema. Note edema around eyes and facial puffiness. (From Thibodeau GA: *Anatomy & physiology*, St Louis, 1987, Mosby.)

The restoration of normal TH levels should be timed appropriately; a regimen of hormonal therapy depends on the individual's age; the duration and severity of the hypothyroidism; and the presence of other disorders, particularly cardiovascular disorders. The goal is maximal metabolic restoration consistent with the individual's overall well-being and normalization of TSH levels in individuals with primary hypothyroidism.

Congenital Hypothyroidism

Congenital hypothyroidism, classified as a rare form of primary hypothyroidism, occurs in infants as a result of absent thyroid tissue (thyroid agenesis) and hereditary defects in thyroid hormone synthesis. Thyroid agenesis occurs more frequently in female infants, with permanent abnormalities in 1 of every 4000 live births.[41]

Thyroid hormone is essential for embryonic growth, particularly of brain tissue. The infant will be mentally retarded if there is no thyroxine (T_4) during fetal life, but this can be partially reversed with administration of T_4 immediately after birth.

Clinical manifestations of hypothyroidism may not be evident until after 4 months of age. Signs and symptoms include difficulty eating, hoarse cry, and protruding tongue caused by myxedema of oral tissues and vocal cords; hypotonic muscles of the abdomen with constipation, abdominal protrusion, and umbilical hernia; subnormal temperature; lethargy; excessive sleeping; slow pulse; and cold, mottled skin. Skeletal growth is stunted because of impaired protein synthesis, poor absorption of nutrients, and lack of bone mineralization. The child will be dwarfed, with short limbs, if not treated (cretinism) (Fig. 20-9). Dentition is often delayed. Mental retardation is a function of the severity of hypothyroidism and the delay before initiation of treatment.

Hypothyroidism is difficult to identify at birth, but high birth weight, hypothermia, delay in passing meconium, and

WHAT'S NEW? Maternal Hypothyroidism and Fetal Development

Thyroid hormone is crucial for the normal development of the central nervous system, and it has been observed that maternal thyroid hormone deficiency during pregnancy may adversely affect the child's neuropsychiatric development. A recent study documented that untreated maternal thyroid hormone deficiency during pregnancy was associated with a 7 point lower score on full-scale IQ testing of offspring. Additionally, 19% of the affected children had IQ scores less than 85. Given this profound effect of maternal hypothyroidism on fetal development, aggressive screening and treatment of thyroid disease during pregnancy is warranted.

Data from Haddow JE et al: Maternal thyroid deficiency during pregnancy and subsequent neuropsychological development of the child, *N Engl J Med* 341:549, 1999.

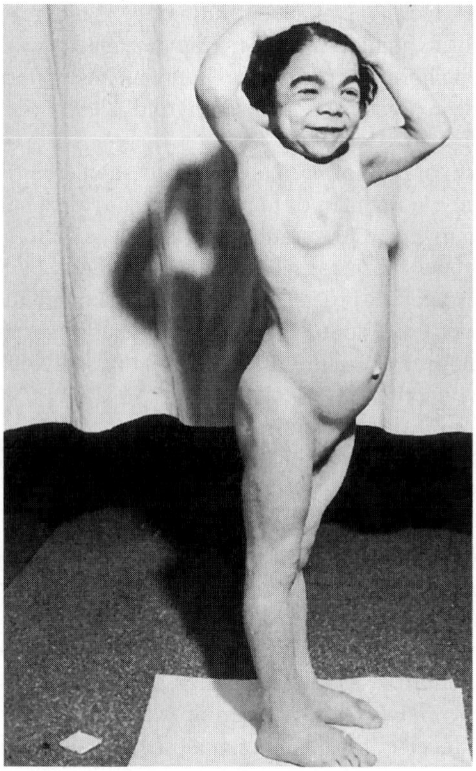

FIG. 20-9 Adult cretin. Note characteristic facial features, dwarfism (44 inches), absent axillary and scant pubic hair, poorly developed breasts, potbelly, and small umbilical hernia. (From Schneeberg NG: *Essentials of clinical endocrinology*, St Louis, 1970, Mosby.)

neonatal jaundice are suggestive signs. Cord blood can be examined in the first days of life for T_4 and TSH levels. Treatment is administration of T_4. There is a high probability of normal growth and intellectual function if treatment is started before the child is 3 or 4 months old.

Thyroid Carcinoma

Thyroid carcinoma is the most common endocrine malignancy but is relatively rare, accounting for 19,500 new cases annually and approximately 0.5% of all cancer deaths per year.[42] The most consistent causal risk factor in the development of thyroid cancer appears to be exposure to ionizing radiation,[43] especially exposure during childhood or puberty. The nuclear reactor accident at Chernobyl in 1986 clearly emphasizes this risk factor.[44]

Most individuals with thyroid carcinoma have normal T_3 and T_4 levels and are therefore euthyroid. Thyroid cancer typically is discovered as a small thyroid nodule or as a metastatic tumor most commonly occurring in the lungs, brain, or bone. Changes in voice and swallowing and difficulty in breathing are related to tumor growth impinging on the trachea or esophagus. The diagnosis of thyroid carcinoma is generally made by fine-needle aspiration of a thyroid nodule. Ultrasonography and radioisotope scanning are rarely helpful in assessing the malignant potential of a thyroid nodule.

Treatment for thyroid carcinoma remains controversial, primarily because of the rarity of the disease, its protracted nature, and the relatively low mortality regardless of the method of treatment. Treatment of well-differentiated tumors includes a near-total or total thyroidectomy, postoperative radioactive iodine, and suppression of TSH with levothyroxine. Anaplastic thyroid carcinoma carries a grave prognosis, and palliation with surgical debulking, external beam radiotherapy, or chemotherapy may be offered.[45]

ALTERATIONS OF PARATHYROID FUNCTION

Hyperparathyroidism

In general, **hyperparathyroidism** is characterized by a greater than normal secretion of parathyroid hormone (PTH). The causes of hyperparathyroidism are classified as either primary or secondary, and their associated pathophysiologic mechanisms are somewhat different.

Pathophysiology

Primary hyperparathyroidism is characterized by greater than normal secretion of PTH by one or more of the parathyroid glands.[47] In primary hyperparathyroidism, normal feedback mechanisms, such as elevated serum levels of ionized calcium, fail to inhibit PTH secretion by the parathyroid gland. **Secondary hyperparathyroidism** is caused by an increase in PTH secondary to a chronic disease state, such as chronic renal failure or malabsorption, which causes a decrease in serum ionized calcium levels (hypocalcemia). The chronic renal failure–induced hypocalcemia serves as the stimulus for increased PTH secretion and renal and gastrointestinal calcium absorption in an attempt to reestablish normal ionized calcium levels. Since vitamin D metabolism is impaired in renal failure, eucalcemia cannot be restored unless vitamin D supplements are administered. Hypercalcemia does not occur in secondary hyperparathyroidism because the parathyroid tissue is not autonomous and is only responding to a physiologic stimulus (hypocalcemia). Hypercalcemia is a hallmark of primary hyperparathyroidism. Many systems are altered in individuals with primary and secondary hyperparathyroidism; the effects of excessive PTH secretion on various organ systems are summarized in Table 20-3.

The cause of primary hyperparathyroidism is unknown; however, recent data suggest that there are two mechanisms for the development of this condition. The first is a clonal proliferation of parathyroid cells with a higher threshold for calcium feedback, and the second is generalized growth of parathyroid tissue. The former is most likely the cause of adenomas, and the latter is probably the cause for hyperplasia. There is also a familial form of the disease that has an autosomal dominant pattern of inheritance.[48] The most common cause of secondary hyperparathyroidism is chronic renal failure. Other causes include dietary deficiency in vitamin D or calcium; decreased intestinal absorption of vitamin D or calcium; and ingestion of drugs, such as phenytoin, phenobarbital, and laxatives, which decrease intestinal absorption of calcium.

Clinical Manifestations

Hypersecretion of PTH causes excessive osteoclastic activity, resulting in bone resorption. (Bone resorption is discussed in

Table 20-3 Manifestations of Primary Hyperparathyroidism

Symptoms	Responsible Derangements	Mechanisms
Renal colic, nephrolithiasis, recurrent urinary tract infections, renal failure	Hypercalcemia, hyperphosphaturia, proximal renal tubular bicarbonate leak, urine pH > 6	Calcium phosphate salts precipitate in alkaline urine, renal pelvis, and collecting ducts; calcium oxalate stones also formed
Abdominal pain, peptic ulcer disease	Hypercalcemia-stimulated hypergastrinemia	Elevated hydrochloric acid secretion
Pancreatitis	Hypercalcemia	Etiology of relationship unknown
Bone disease, osteitis fibrosa and cystica, osteoporosis	PTH-stimulated bone resorption, metabolic acidosis	Osteoporosis now more commonly encountered, but other disorders more specific for hyperparathyroidism
Muscle weakness, myalgia	PTH excess, possible direct effect on striated muscle and on nerves	Characteristic myopathic changes in muscle histology (neuropathy of type I and type II muscle fibers)
Neurologic and psychiatric problems	Hypercalcemia	Neuropathy; electroencephalographic changes present
Polyuria, polydipsia	Hypercalcemia	Direct effect on renal tubule to decrease responsiveness to antidiuretic hormone
Constipation	Hypercalcemia	Decreased peristalsis of gastrointestinal tract
Anorexia, nausea, and vomiting	Hypercalcemia	Central stimulation of vomiting center
Hypertension	Renal disease, direct effect of calcium on arterial smooth muscle, pheochromocytoma	Plasma renin activity elevated or normal
Arthralgia and arthritis	Gout, pseudogout, periarticular classification	Hyperuricemia, chronic renal failure with high calcium × phosphate product

From Rabin D, McKenna TJ: *Clinical endocrinology and metabolism: principles and practice,* New York, 1982, Grune & Stratton.
PTH, Parathyroid hormone.

Chapter 40.) Pathologic bone changes include pathologic fractures, kyphosis of the dorsal spine, and compression fractures of the vertebral bodies. Parathyroid hormone hypersecretion and its resulting hypercalcemia increase the renal filtration load of calcium, leading to hypercalciuria.

Hypercalcemia also affects proximal renal tubular function, causing metabolic acidosis and production of an abnormally alkaline urine. PTH also enhances the renal excretion of phosphate, which results in hypophosphatemia (low serum phosphate) and hyperphosphaturia (increased urine phosphate). The combination of these three variables—hypercalciuria, alkaline urine, and hyperphosphaturia—predisposes the individual to the formation of calcium stones. Kidney stones are frequently formed in the renal pelvis or in the renal collecting ducts and may be associated with infections. Both kidney stones and renal infection may lead to impaired renal function. Hypercalcemia also impairs the concentrating ability of the renal tubule by decreasing its response to ADH.

Chronic hypercalcemia of hyperparathyroidism is associated with mild insulin resistance, necessitating increased insulin secretion to maintain normal glucose levels. Hypercalcemia also affects the muscular, nervous, and gastrointestinal systems. (The clinical symptoms of primary hyperparathyroidism are summarized in Table 20-3.)

Evaluation and Treatment

The diagnosis of hyperparathyroidism is relatively straightforward. The concurrent findings of increased ionized calcium in the face of elevated or inappropriately normal intact PTH (which documents an abnormal feedback mechanism) are suggestive. Hypercalciuria (>4 mg/kg per 24 hours), a benign, inherited condition, familial hypocalciuric hypercalcemia (FHH), is likely to be present. Because FHH is caused by a mutation in the transmembrane calcium receptor and is not associated with the classical complications of hyperparathyroidism, treatment is unnecessary. On the other hand, the definitive treatment of hyperparathyroidsm is surgery.[49] Surgery is generally reserved for individuals with documented complications of hyperparathyroidism (osteoporosis, nephrolithiasis, or gastrointestinal or neuropsychiatric complications) or severely elevated serum calcium levles (>1 mg/dl above the upper limit or normal for the laboratory).

If intact PTH levels are low, the differential diagnosis shifts to hypercalcemia of malignancy, granulomatous diseases (sarcoidosis), excessive calcium ingestion, or to hypervitaminosis A or D. Treatment of these conditions depends upon the underlying cause.

Hypoparathyroidism

Hypoparathyroidism (abnormally low PTH levels) most commonly is caused by damage to the parathyroid glands during thyroid surgery. Postoperatively induced hypoparathyroidism occurs in approximately 1% of all individuals undergoing thyroid surgery, with the incidence increasing to 10% after repeated neck explorations. This is because of the anatomic proximity of the parathyroid gland to the thyroid gland.

Pathophysiology

In hypoparathyroidism a lack of circulating PTH causes a depressed serum calcium level and an increased serum phosphate level. In the absence of PTH the abilities to resorb calcium from bone and to regulate calcium reabsorption from the renal tubules are impaired. The phosphaturic effects of PTH are lost, resulting in hyperphosphatemia.

Hypoparathyroidism can occur also from hypomagnesemia, although the effects of hypomagnesemia on the peripheral metabolism and clearance of PTH are not clearly understood. Once serum magnesium levels return to normal, however, PTH secretion returns to normal, as does peripheral tissues' responsiveness to PTH. Hypomagnesemia may be related to chronic alcoholism, malnutrition, malabsorption, increased renal clearance of magnesium caused by the use of aminoglycoside antibiotics or certain chemotherapeutic agents, or prolonged magnesium-deficient parenteral nutritional therapy.

Clinical Manifestations

Symptoms associated with hypoparathyroidism are related to hypocalcemia. Hypocalcemia causes a lowering of the threshold for nerve and muscle excitation so that a nerve impulse may be initiated by a slight stimulus anywhere along the length of a nerve or muscle fiber. This is manifested as muscle spasms; hyperreflexia; clonic-tonic convulsions; laryngeal spasms; and, in severe cases, death from asphyxiation.

Other symptoms of hypocalcemia are caused by mechanisms that are not yet understood. These symptoms include dry skin; loss of body and scalp hair; hypoplasia of developing teeth; horizontal ridges on the nails; cataracts; basal ganglia calcifications (which may be associated with a parkinsonian syndrome); and bone deformities, including brachydactyly and bowing of the long bones.

Phosphate retention caused by increased renal reabsorption of phosphate is associated also with hypoparathyroidism. Hyperphosphatemia is associated with inhibition of the renal enzyme necessary for the conversion of vitamin D to its most active form. This tends to depress serum calcium levels further by reducing gastrointestinal absorption of calcium.

Evaluation and Treatment

A low serum calcium level and high phosphorus level in the absence of renal failure, intestinal disorders, or nutritional deficiencies are diagnostic of hypoparathyroidism. Intact PTH levels are low in hypoparathyroidism but they are elevated in an inherited condition associated with hypocalcemia and resistance to PTH, pseudohypoparathyroidism.

The treatment of hypoparathyroidism is directed toward the alleviation of hypocalcemia. In acute states this involves parenteral administration of calcium, which allows correction of serum calcium within minutes. Maintenance of serum calcium is achieved with pharmacologic doses of an active form of vitamin D and oral calcium. The recommended daily dose of calcium is 1 to 3 g.

Hypoplastic dentition, cataracts, bone deformities, and basal ganglia calcifications do not respond to the correction of hypocalcemia, but the other symptoms of hypocalcemia are reversible. As serum calcium levels return to normal, phosphaturia usually is stimulated. This leads to a return to normal serum phosphate levels. In some individuals, however, the absence of the phosphaturic effect of PTH causes a persistent hyperphosphatemia.

Significant elevations of phosphorus should be treated with drugs that inhibit gastrointestinal absorption of phosphate and thus prevent ectopic calcifications. Such calcifications are likely to occur if the mathematical product of the serum calcium and serum phosphate levels exceeds 70 (i.e., $Ca^{++} \times PO_4^{-3} > 70$). In such instances, calcifications can be expected.

DYSFUNCTION OF THE ENDOCRINE PANCREAS: DIABETES MELLITUS

Diabetes mellitus is not a single disease but a group of clinically heterogeneous disorders with glucose intolerance in common. It encompasses many causally unrelated diseases and includes many different etiologies of disturbed glucose tolerance.[50] The Greeks initially described diabetes as a condition generally occurring in young, lean people characterized by weight loss, increased appetite, excessive urination, and insatiable thirst (polyphagia, polyuria, and polydipsia). Later, a second type was described in older, obese individuals.

The term *diabetes mellitus* is now used to describe a syndrome characterized by chronic hyperglycemia and other disturbances of carbohydrate, fat, and protein metabolism. In 1979 the National Diabetes Data Group published the first standardized diagnostic criteria and classification scheme for diabetes.[51] Based on an exponential proliferation of knowledge, these diagnostic criteria were revised and the classification was simplified in 1997.[52] Terms from the older classification scheme—insulin-dependent diabetes (IDDM) and noninsulin-dependent diabetes (NIDDM)—have been changed to type 1 diabetes and type 2 diabetes. The classes of gestational diabetes (GDM) and impaired glucose tolerance (IGT) were retained, and a new category, impaired fasting glucose (IFG), was devised. Types 1 and 2 diabetes are the most common and are discussed in greatest detail in this text. Table 20-4 describes the terminology and characteristics of the conditions associated with abnormal glucose metabolism.

The diagnosis of diabetes is based on one of the following:[52]

1. More than one fasting plasma glucose level greater than or equal to 126 mg/dl
2. Plasma glucose value in the 2-hour sample (2hPG) of the standard oral glucose tolerance test (OGTT) greater than or equal to 200 mg/dl, confirmed on subsequent day
3. Casual (any time of day without regard to time since last meal) plasma glucose level greater than 200 mg/dl, combined with classic symptoms of polydipsia, polyphagia, and polyuria

Normal fasting glucose is less than 110 mg/dl in the morning. IFG is defined as a fasting glucose greater than or equal to 110 mg/dl but less than 126 mg/dl. Glucose tolerance is normal if the 2-hour postload glucose level is less than 140 mg/dl. IGT is defined as a 2-hour postload glucose level greater than or equal to 140 but less than 200 mg/dl. Any abnormality of glucose tolerance has potentially serious consequences.

Table 20-4 Classification and Characteristics of Diabetes Mellitus

Name	Previous Synonyms	Characteristics
TYPE 1: PRIMARY B CELL DEFECT OR FAILURE Immune-mediated diabetes common form (~90%)	Juvenile diabetes Juvenile-onset diabetes Ketosis-prone diabetes Brittle diabetes Idiopathic diabetes Insulin-dependent diabetes mellitus (IDDM)	Cellular mediated autoimmune destruction of pancreatic B cells Individual prone to ketoacidosis Little or no insulin secretion Insulin dependent 75% of individuals develop before 30 yr of age, can occur up to the tenth decade Usually not obese
Idiopathic (~10%)	Other types	No defined etiologies; absolute requirement for insulin replacement therapy in affected individuals may come and go
TYPE 2 DIABETES: INSULIN RESISTANCE WITH INADEQUATE INSULIN SECRETION	Adult-onset diabetes Maturity-onset diabetes Stable diabetes Ketosis-resistant diabetes Non-insulin-dependent diabetes mellitus (NIDDM)	Usually not insulin-dependent but may be insulin requiring Individual not ketosis prone (but may form ketones under stress) Obesity common in the abdominal region Generally occurs in those older than 40 yr, but the frequency is rapidly increasing in children Strong genetic predisposition Frequently associated with hypertension and dyslipidemia
OTHER FORMS Genetic defects of the B cell	Secondary diabetes Maturity-onset diabetes of the young (MODY)	Genetic abnormalities such as inability to convert proinsulin to insulin, mutation of insulin molecules or mitochondrial deoxyribonucleic acid (DNA), glucokinase abnormalities
Genetic defects in insulin action		Mutations in the insulin receptor with hyperinsulinism or hyperglycemia or severe diabetes
Pancreatic diseases	Secondary diabetes	Any process that diffusely injures the pancreas
Drug- or chemical-induced B cell dysfunction		Impaired insulin secretion or antagonism of insulin by counter-excess regulatory hormones
Endocrinopathies		Inibition of insulin secretion
Infections		B cell destruction by viruses: *cytomegalovirus, congenital rubella*
Uncommon forms of immune-mediated diabetes mellitus		Few known conditions Anti-insulin receptor antibodies Reported with "stiff man syndrome" and individuals receiving interferon-α
Other genetic syndromes sometimes associated with diabetes mellitus		Down, Klinefelter, Turner and Wolfram syndromes
GESTATIONAL DIABETES MELLITUS	Asymptomatic diabetes Subclinical diabetes Latent diabetes	Glucose intolerance first recognized during pregnancy, most likely in the third trimester Following pregnancy, glucose may normalize, remain impaired, or progress to diabetes mellitus Occurs in 1%-14% of all pregnancies; 40%-60% will develop diabetes mellitus within 15 yr after gestation
Impaired fasting glucose (IFG)		Fasting plasma glucose ≥ 110 and <126 mg/dl
Impaired glucose tolerance (IGT)		Abnormal response to oral glucose tolerance test: 2hPG ≥ 140 and <200 mg/dl 10%-25% will convert to type II diabetes within 10 yr Many with IGT are obese

Data from Gavin J et al: Report of the expert committee on the diagnosis and classification of diabetes mellitus, *Diabetic Care* 20(7): 1183, 1997.

Numerous epidemiologic studies have shown an increased risk of cardivoascular disease and premature death in individuals with glucose intolerance.[53] In addition, individuals with abnormal glucose tolerance have a 3% to 7% yearly risk of developing overt diabetes. In comparison, the individual's *lifetime* risk of acquiring diabetes is around 7% to 10%.

In nonpregnant individuals an OGTT consists of the administration of a 75-g oral glucose load after a 10-hour fast followed by measurement of plasma glucose 2 hours later. It is unnecessary and potentially harmful to perform an OGTT in patients who already meet criteria for diabetes based upon their fasting plasma glucose level. IGT results primarily from reduced suppression of hepatic glucose output caused by abnormal pancreatic islet cell function.[54] Intravenous glucose tolerance tests are rarely used because they are generally less sensitive than OGTTs and may cause painful venous thrombosis. Another mechanism, used primarily to identify the plasma glucose concentration over time, is the measurement of **glycosylated hemoglobin**, but due to the lack of standardization of this measurement, it is not considered a diagnostic test for diabetes. In the normal 120-day life span of the red blood cell, glucose molecules join hemoglobin, forming glycosylated hemoglobin. In individuals with poorly controlled diabetes, increases in the quantities of three glycosylated hemoglobins (A_{1a}, A_{1b}, and A_{1c}) are noted. Once a hemoglobin molecule is glycosylated, it remains that way. A buildup of glycosylated hemoglobin within the red cell reflects the average level of glucose to which the cell has been exposed during its life cycle. Measuring glycosylated hemoglobin assesses the effectiveness of therapy by monitoring long-term serum glucose regulation.[55]

Types of Diabetes Mellitus

Type 1

Although the cause is unknown, **type 1 diabetes mellitus** accounts for approximately 10% of all diabetes mellitus in the Western world. The incidence of the condition is increasing in some areas, with other areas showing no change in incidence.[56] Several studies suggest that the incidence and prevalence are higher for whites than for nonwhites, with the highest rate found in Finland and the lowest rate in Japan. Variations occur, however, even within individual countries. (Table 20-5 summarizes the epidemiology of diabetes mellitus.)

Type 1 diabetes mellitus is thought to be the result of a genetic-environmental interaction. Between 10% and 13% of individuals with newly diagnosed type 1 diabetes have a first-degree relative (parent or sibling) with type 1 diabetes. Diagnosis has a seasonal distribution, with more cases reported during autumn and winter in the northern hemisphere. Diagnosis is rare during the first 9 months of life and peaks at 12 years of age.

Pathophysiology

Two distinct types of type 1 diabetes have been identified: immune and nonimmune. In immune-mediated diabetes mellitus, environmental-genetic factors are thought to result in cell-mediated destruction of B cells. In the common form, markers of immune destruction, including autoantibodies to islet cells and/or to insulin and to glutamic acid decarboxylase (GAD_{65}),[57,58] are found in 85% to 90% of individuals when fasting hyperglycemia is initially detected. Human leukocyte antigen (HLA)–DR4 is strongly associated with this phenomenon. The HLA-DR3 marker is associated with diabetes and other autoimmune disorders, such as Graves, Hashimoto, and Addison diseases.[59] Nonimmune type 1 diabetes occurs secondarily to other diseases such as pancreatitis.

Historically, type 1 diabetes mellitus has been thought to have an abrupt onset. More recently, however, prospective studies show a distinctive natural history involving genetic susceptibility; a long preclinical period; immunologically mediated destruction of B cells, eventually leading to insulin deficiency; and hyperglycemia. Generally, this latent period is longer in older individuals and frequently results in misclassification of an older type 1 individual as having type 2 diabetes.

Genetic Susceptibility

Although the exact nature of genetic susceptibility is not yet understood, research findings support an HLA link. (HLA loci and associated histocompatibility antigens are discussed in Chapter 6.) The strongest association with type 1 diabetes is with alleles HLA-DR4 and HLA-DR3. The risk of developing type 1 diabetes increases five to eight times when one of those specific loci is present. When the individual is heterogenous for HLA-DR3 and HLA-DR4, the risk is 20 to 40 times higher than that of the general population. Specific human antigens also are thought to decrease the risk of developing type 1 diabetes, with HLA-DR2 associated with an unusually low risk. Current theories of causation hold that islet cell destruction occurs predominantly in genetically susceptible people.

Long Preclinical Period

Research has demonstrated the presence of islet cell autoantibodies (ICAs) for years before the occurrence of symptoms. These immune markers precede evidence of B cell deficiency and have been found in 85% to 90% of type 1 diabetes cases at the time of clinical onset.[60] Autoantibodies against insulin (IAAs) also have been noted. Researchers speculate that IAAs may form during the process of active islet cell and B cell destruction. ICAs and IAAs are probably the result of the autoimmune process rather than the cause.[55] They tend to disappear with time. $AntiGAD_{65}$ antibodies are more persistent, which makes them clinically useful in differentiating the etiology of diabetes in a given individual.[57]

Immunologically Mediated Destruction of B Cells

The presence of islet cell antibodies provides strong evidence for an autoimmune origin and pathogenesis of type 1 diabetes. Research suggests that a local or organ-specific suppressor deficit may induce the autoimmune phenomenon.[50] The precise sequence of events that trigger migration or attachment of immune cells to the pancreatic islets has not yet been determined. Environmental mechanisms are thought to play a role in the destruction by direct toxicity, increasing the susceptibility of the B cells to another mechanism or triggering an

Table 20-5 Epidemiology and Etiology of Diabetes Mellitus

	Type 1 Diabetes: Primary B Cell Defect or Failure	Type 2 Diabetes: Insulin Resistance With Inadequate Insulin Secretion
INCIDENCE		
Frequency	One of the most common childhood diseases (10% of all cases of diabetes mellitus) Range from 29.5/100,000 (Finland) to 1.6/100,000 (Japan)	Accounts for most cases (≈90%) Prevalence rate in United States (for age 18 yr and older): 6.6%* Prevalence for Pima Indians (western American Indian group): 39.9%
Change in incidences	Increased incidences in British Isles, Finland, Norway, Denmark, Israel, Germany, and Poland; stable elsewhere	Incidence has risen in United States since 1940
CHARACTERISTICS		
Age at onset	Peak onset at age 11 to 13 yr (slightly earlier for girls than for boys) Rare in children younger than 1 yr and adults older than 30 yr	Risk of developing diabetes increases after age 40 yr; in general, incidence increases with age into the 70s; among Pima Indians, incidence peaks between ages 40 and 50 yr, then falls
Gender	Similar in males and females	In the United States, more females than males
Racial distribution	Rates for whites 1.5-2 times higher than for nonwhites Higher rates for those of Scandinavian descent than for those of central or southern European descent	Certain racial groups may be more likely to develop type 2 diabetes when exposed to a particular environment Common in migrant groups encountering a different environment (e.g., Polynesians moving from traditional to western life-style) In the United States, risk is highest for American Indians; rates are higher for Pacific Islanders, Japanese, Puerto Ricans, Hispanics, and blacks than for whites
Socioeconomic status	Conflicting data	A disease of the affluent in developing nations but more common among those of lower incomes and less education in the United States
Seasonal distribution	More new cases documented during fall and winter in the northern hemisphere	No known association
Childbirth association	No association documented	Effect of parity on subsequent development of type 2 diabetes varies among different populations
Obesity	Generally normal or underweight	Frequent contributing factor to precipitate type 2 diabetes among those susceptible; a major factor in populations recently exposed to westernized environment Increased risk related to duration, degree, and distribution of obesity
ETIOLOGY		
Common theory	*Autoimmune:* genetic and environmental factors, resulting in gradual process of autoimmune destruction in genetically susceptible individuals *Nonautoimmune:* Unknown Strong association with HLA-DR3 and HLA-DR4	Disease results from genetic susceptibility (although the precise gene or genes have not yet been determined) combined with environmental determinants and other risk factors Associated with long-duration obesity
Heredity	Risk to sibling: 5%-10%; risk to offspring: 2%-5%	Risk to first-degree relative (child or sibling): 10%-15%
Presence of antibody	Islet cell autoantibodies (ICA) and/or autoantibodies to insulin, and autoantibodies to glutamic acid decarboxylase (GAD_{65}) are present in 85%-90% of individuals when fasting hyperglycemia is initially detected	Islet cell antibodies not present
Insulin resistance	Insulin resistance rare	Insulin resistance is generally caused by altered cellular metabolism and an intracellular postreceptor defect
Insulin secretion	Severe insulin deficiency or no insulin secretion at all	Typically increased at time of diagnosis, but progressively declines over the course of the illness

Data from Gavin J et al: Report of the expert committee on the diagnosis and classification of diabetes mellitus, *Diabetic Care* 20(7): 1183, 1997.

autoimmune response to B cells. Specific environmental factors linked to type 1 diabetes are presented in Box 20-1.

Hyperglycemia and Other Symptoms

Before hyperglycemia occurs, 80% to 90% of the function of insulin-secreting B cells of the islet of Langerhans must be lost. B cell abnormalities are present long before the acute clinical onset of type 1 diabetes. The initiating events of B cell destruction may differ from the final event that precipitates clinical symptoms.

Regardless of the cause, a disequilibrium of hormones produced by the islets of Langerhans occurs in diabetes mellitus. Considerable evidence suggests that both A cell and B cell functions are abnormal and that both a lack of insulin and a relative excess of glucagon (produced by A cells) exist in type 1 diabetes.

Considerable data has documented that, in the absence of glucagon, the generation of both hyperglycemia and hyperketonemia is considerably delayed compared to conditions where glucagon is present. Thus the full metabolic syndrome is caused by both hormones, a finding that ultimately may provide an entirely new therapeutic approach to the management of diabetes mellitus. Relative hyperglucagonemia occurs in every form of diabetes mellitus. The concentration of glucagon therefore is relatively high in comparison with the relative or absolute deficiency of insulin, and elevated blood glucose levels fail to suppress the production of glucagon. Overproduction of glucose and ketones, as occurs in uncontrolled diabetes mellitus, results from excessive glucagon relative to the amount of effective insulin. The ratio of insulin to glucagon in the portal vein—and not the concentration of each hormone—controls hepatic glucose and fat metabolism.

Box 20-1

SPECIFIC ENVIRONMENTAL FACTORS LINKED TO TYPE 1 DIABETES

DRUGS AND CHEMICALS

Alloxan
Streptozocin
Pentamidine
Vacor (a rodenticide)

NUTRITIONAL INTAKE

Bovine milk
High levels of nitrosamines

VIRUSES

Mumps and coxsackievirus—type 1 diabetes does occur rarely as a complication of viral infections, but no evidence of substantial relationship exists

Rubella—40% of individuals with congenital rubella infection develop type 1 diabetes later

Cytomegalovirus (CMV)—persistent CMV infections appear to be relevant to pathogenesis of some cases of type 1 diabetes

Data from Dahlquist G: *Autoimmunity* 15(1):61, 1993; Karjalainen J et al: *N Engl J Med* 327(5):302, 1992.

Clinical Manifestations

Type 1 diabetes mellitus affects the metabolism of fat, protein, and carbohydrates. Glucose accumulates in the blood and appears in the urine as the renal threshold for glucose is exceeded, producing an osmotic diuresis and symptoms of polyuria and thirst. In addition, protein and fat breakdown occur because of the lack of insulin, resulting in weight loss.

Initial clinical manifestations of type 1 diabetes are generally acute. The individual often has the classic symptoms of polyuria, polydipsia, and polyphagia (Table 20-6). Weight loss and wide fluctuations in blood glucose levels occur.

Ketoacidosis, caused by increased levels of circulating ketones in the absence of the antilipolytic effect of insulin, is also common. Accumulation of ketone bodies causes a drop in pH and triggers the buffering system associated with metabolic acidosis (see Chapter 3). Acetone then is blown off, giving the breath a sweet or fruity odor. Occasionally, diabetic coma caused by ketoacidosis is the initial presenting manifestation of the disease.

Evaluation and Treatment

The diagnosis of diabetes is not difficult when the symptoms of polydipsia, polyuria, polyphagia, weight loss, and hyperglycemia are present in fasting and postprandial states. Under the above circumstances, an OGTT is not needed and its use is contraindicated. In fact, an OGTT is rarely needed to diagnose type 1 diabetes.[61] Age, diet, drugs, activity, and presence of other disease must be considered when performing and interpreting the OGTT.

Table 20-6 Clinical Manifestations and Rationale for Type 1 Diabetes Mellitus

Manifestations	Rationale
Polydipsia	Because of elevated blood sugar levels, water is osmotically attracted from body cells, resulting in intracellular dehydration and stimulation of thirst in the hypothalamus
Polyuria	Hyperglycemia acts as an osmotic diuretic; the amount of glucose filtered by the glomeruli of the kidneys exceeds that which can be reabsorbed by the renal tubules; glycosuria results, accompanied by large amounts of water lost in the urine
Polyphagia	Depletion of cellular stores of carbohydrates, fats, and protein results in cellular starvation and a corresponding increase in hunger
Weight loss	Weight loss occurs because of fluid loss in osmotic diuresis and the loss of body tissue as fats and proteins are used for energy due to the effects of insulin deficiency
Fatigue	Metabolic changes result in poor use of food products, contributing to lethargy and fatigue; sleep loss from severe nocturia also contributes to fatigue

Currently, treatment regimens are designed to avoid high and low levels of glucose. The Diabetes Control and Complications Trial (DCCT) was designed to evaluate the effects of glucose control on the appearance or progression of the early vascular and neurologic complications of type 1 diabetes.[62] In June 1993 the National Institutes of Health announced research results showing a link between glycemic control and development of diabetic complications. The research compared individuals whose blood sugars were tightly controlled (with blood glucose checks four times per day, three or more insulin injections daily or insulin pump, and meal planning) with those who received standard treatment. Intensively treated individuals who achieve similar metabolic control of near-normal glucoses can expect a 50% to 75% reduction in the risk of developing or progression of retinopathy, neuropathy, and nephropathy after 8 to 9 years. These changes begin to appear at 3 to 4 years.[61] Although long-term complications were decreased in the tightly controlled group,[62] achieving near-normal glucose levels was accompanied by risks, such as severe hypoglycemia and weight gain.[62] Management of diabetes mellitus requires individual planning according to type of disease, age, and activity level, but all type 1 individuals require some combination of insulin, meal planning, exercise, and self-monitoring.

Insulin

Insulin administration is used to reduce blood glucose levels and to avoid or lessen the long-term complications of diabetes. Exogenous insulin has been used only since 1922. Before the advent of recombinant deoxyribonucleic acid (DNA) techniques for synthetic insulin production, insulin was extracted primarily from beef or pork pancreata. The structure of human, porcine, and bovine insulins is fairly similar.

Beef insulin is the most immunogenic. Pork insulin more closely resembles human insulin and is therefore less immunogenic. Human insulin has virtually replaced animal-derived insulins, which are only available on a compassionate-use basis. New bioengineered insulins (in which specific amino acid substitutions have been made in the normal human insulin molecule) have provided additional flexibility to the management of people with diabetes.[63] Ultrashort-acting insulins (insulin lispro and aspart) allow better control of postprandial glucose levels,[64] and a long-acting insulin analog, glargine, seems to provide a stable 24-hour basal level of insulin,[65] which is essential in mimicking normal islet cell function. All types of insulin are routinely packaged as 100 units per ml (U100); lesser (U40 or U80) or greater (U500) strengths are available from manufacturers if warranted. Treatment with zinc or protamine concentrations renders the insulin longer lasting.

Insulin is broken down by gastric enzymes and thus may not be given orally. In the management of type 1 diabetes, insulin most commonly is given subcutaneously one to four times daily. Continuous subcutaneous insulin infusion (CSII) is an alternative treatment using a small, battery-powered infusion pump. Glucose and insulin levels may fluctuate widely, and self-monitoring though capillary blood glucose and urine testing is essential.[66] Although insulin is essential in the treatment of type 1 diabetes mellitus, it is associated with a variety of complications, including insulin hypertrophy, antibodies, allergy, resistance, and edema. These complications are distinctly rare in individuals using recombinant human insulin.

Meal Planning

The individual with type 1 diabetes mellitus must consume sufficient calories to achieve and maintain normal weight for height and age. Caloric intake should be regulated with consideration of age, activity, and severity of the diabetes. In general, approximately 55% to 60% of the total calories should be derived from carbohydrates, with less than 30% derived from fats, and 15% to 20% from proteins. The recommended percentage of calories from fat depends on desired glucose, lipid, and weight outcomes.[67] A meal plan based on the individual's usual food intake should be determined and used as a basis for integrating insulin therapy into the usual eating and exercise patterns. Meals and snacks should be planned according to the peak action times of insulin. Intensive insulin therapy, such as multiple injections or CSII, combined with carbohydrate counting, provides a more flexible meal planning option.

Exercise

Exercise by individuals with type 1 diabetes may result in an inability to regulate blood glucose levels.[45] Accommodations must be made for the safe inclusion of exercise, possibly by including adjustments of food and/or insulin doses as guided by frequent self-monitoring of blood glucose (SMBG). Hypoglycemia, hyperglycemia, ketosis, cardiovascular ischemia and dysrhythmia, exacerbation of proliferative retinopathy, and lower-extremity injury are significant potential complications of exercise.[67] Metabolic response to exercise is affected by many variables, such as fitness, duration, and intensity of exercise, and time of exercise related to insulin administration and meals.[68]

Transplantation

Transplantation is designed to establish a normoglycemic, insulin-independent state. Pancreas transplants have been performed since 1966.[69] Research suggests that normal glucose may be maintained for longer than 5 years after pancreatic transplant.[70] Clinical trials on islet transplantation are in progress.[71] As with any transplant, rejection remains a problem, and lifelong immunosuppression is necessary.

Experimental Treatments

New pharmacologic approaches are being tested. The National Institute of Diabetes and Digestive and Kidney Diseases (NIDDK) has initiated a large-scale clinical trial to determine if autoimmune type 1 diabetes mellitus can be prevented with "immunizations" using low doses of insulin or with oral insulin-like agents.[72]

Type 2

Type 2 diabetes mellitus is much more common than type 1. The incidence of the disease has risen in the United States since 1940. Current U.S. disease prevalence in those older than 18 years is 6.6%. In addition, one case is undiagnosed for each known case in the United States. Prevalence varies by ethnic group, with the condition more common in native

Americans, Hispanics, and blacks in the United States. Prevalence also varies by environment. For example, prevalence among Polynesians living traditionally is 2.9% compared with 12% among migrants.[56] A genetic-environmental interaction appears to be responsible for the condition.

Pathophysiology

The cause of the common form of type 2 diabetes mellitus is unknown; the genetics of this form of diabetes are complex and not clearly defined. It affects people primarily after the age of 40 years, many of whom are obese.[73]

Cellular resistance to the effect of insulin is a major factor in the type 2 syndromes. Insulin resistance is defined as a suboptimal response of insulin-sensitive tissues (especially liver, muscle, and adipose tissue) to insulin and has been demonstrated in youthful relatives of people with type 2 diabetes. It is thought that many years of compensatory hyperinsulinemia exist before the clinical appearance of the diabetes. The insulin resistance is heightened by obesity (present in 60% to 80% of type 2 individuals), inactivity, illnesses, medications, and age. Abnormal glucagon secretion also has been demonstrated.[74] A significant body of evidence has accumulated that indicates that defects in insulin secretion can lead to insulin resistance and vice versa. Once type 2 diabetes has become established, it is impossible to determine in any given individual whether the primary defect originated in the B cell or in peripheral or hepatic tissues.[75] Eventually the B cell responsiveness to the glucose stimulus diminishes and hyperglycemia supervenes; yet most type 2 individuals, obese or lean, are still hyperinsulinemic at the time of diagnosis but have a relative deficiency of insulin. The islet dysfunction may be caused by a decrease in B cell mass, abnormal function of the B cells, or some combination.

Pancreatic changes in individuals with type 2 diabetes mellitus are nonspecific and have been observed to a lesser degree in nondiabetic persons. Amyloid of the islets occurs in 10% to 40% of the pancreata from individuals with type 2 diabetes. The extent of amyloid deposits is positively correlated with the age of the individual and the duration and severity of the disease.[76] Amyloid formation is associated with islet cell destruction.[77]

The initial hepatic lesion is fatty infiltration (also called nonalcoholic steatohepatitis or NASH) and has been linked in several epidemiologic studies to risk factors associated with insulin resistance including obesity and elevated serum triglycerides.[78] NASH may progress to varying degrees of cirrhosis resulting in alterations of portal blood flow and diminished intrahepatic concentrations of insulin, which may negatively affect hepatic glucose output.

A decrease in the weight and number of B cells generally occurs in type 2 diabetes, but the cause is unclear. The decrease in B cells is progressive over time. To confuse the issue further, the ratio of A cells to B cells may be completely normal in the individual with type 2 diabetes, and most individuals with type 2 diabetes have plasma and pancreatic insulin levels that are not decreased. This latter finding supports the hypothesis that diabetes is a disorder caused by both insulin and glucagon, so that a deficiency of insulin and an excess of glucagon may be either relative or absolute. An inherited secretory deficiency of the B cells also may play a role.[73]

Type 2 diabetes usually is caused by some combination of genetic-environmental interaction, although the contribution of each component varies under different circumstances. The most powerful risk factor for type 2 diabetes, identified by a World Health Organization study group,[79] is obesity. (Risk factor analysis is discussed in Chapter 5.) Abdominal adiposity, defined as a waist-to-hip ratio greater than 1, and increased visceral adiposity[80] appears to be the greatest risk factor. Excessive caloric intake predisposes an individual to type 2 diabetes by contributing to obesity.

In the obese, insulin has a decreased ability to influence glucose uptake and metabolism in the liver, skeletal muscles, and adipose tissue. Multiple theories have been presented to explain this phenomenon. One theory postulates that a decreased number of insulin receptors in the plasma membrane causes decreased insulin binding. Another theory holds that postreceptor events in insulin-sensitive cells are responsible for the insulin resistance.[81] A third theory states that hyperinsulinemia, which often occurs in the early stages of type 2 diabetes, is a compensatory adaptation to insulin resistance in tissues. This theory suggests that elevated levels of circulating insulin are induced by obesity until the pancreas cannot continue to overproduce insulin. Still another theory holds that overeating leads to hyperinsulinemia, which necessitates the development of peripheral insulin resistance to protect against hypoglycemia.[73] In any event the mechanism responsible for insulin receptor binding or postreceptor activity may be improved through weight loss. Other forms of type 2 diabetes mellitus range from genetic defects in insulin action to association with other genetic syndromes (see Table 20-4). The overwhelming problem associated with all type 2 diabetes is insulin resistance with inadequate insulin secretion.

Clinical Manifestations

Clinical manifestations of type 2 diabetes are often nonspecific. Although younger people may develop the condition, it generally affects those older than 30 years. The individual often is overweight, dyslipidemic, hyperinsulinemic, and hypertensive. A unique manifestation of insulin resistance in women of reproductive age is the polycystic ovary syndrome (POS).[82] Women with POS have a risk seven times the average for developing diabetes later in life. The onset is frequently slow and insidious. Some studies show that the onset of type 2 diabetes occurs at least 7 years before its diagnosis.[83] The individual with type 2 diabetes may show some classic symptoms of diabetes but more often will have nonspecific symptoms such as fatigue, pruritus, recurrent infections, visual changes, or paresthesias (Table 20-7).

Evaluation and Treatment

The diagnosis of type 2 diabetes is similar to that of type 1 (see p. 644). As with type 1 diabetes, the goal of treatment for individuals with type 2 diabetes is the restoration of near-euglycemia (a normal blood glucose level) and correction of related metabolic disorders. Dietary measures, including restriction of the total caloric intake, are of primary importance in the overweight individual. As the obese individual loses weight, the body's resistance to insulin often diminishes so that weight loss results in improved glucose tolerance. Nonobese individuals with type 2 diabetes should consume calories consistent with their ideal weight and pattern of activity. The emphasis for medical nutrition therapy (MNT) in type 2 diabetes should be placed on achieving glucose, lipid, and blood pressure goals.

Although the first approach to treatment of the individual with type 2 diabetes is appropriate meal planning, exercise and medication may be needed for optimal management. Sulfonylurea, biguanide, thiazolidinediones, and α-glucosidase inhibitors are useful in treating some individuals with type 2 diabetes. Use of oral hypoglycemic agents requires a pancreas capable of synthesizing insulin. Sulfonylureas acutely augment B cell insulin secretion. Biguanides (metformin) inhibit hepatic glucose production and increase the sensitivity of peripheral tissue to insulin.[84] α-Glucosidase inhibitors decrease postprandial hyperglycemia through delaying carbohydrate digestion and absorption. The thiazolidinedione class of insulin-sensitizing compounds activate a novel nuclear receptor termed the peroxisome proliferator activator receptors (PPARγ), which in turn regulates cellular carbohydrate and lipid metabolism.[85] Because the pathogenesis of type 2 diabetes involves a combination of insulin resistance and a relative insulin deficiency, it is common to combine therapeutic agents from different classes of oral agents in order to achieve acceptable glycemic control.[86]

Exercise is an important aspect of treatment for the individual with type 2 diabetes. Physical training improves glucose control.[45] Exercise reduces postprandial blood glucose levels, diminishes insulin requirements, lowers triglyceride and cholesterol levels, and increases the level of high-density lipoprotein (HDL) cholesterol. In addition, exercise is a valuable adjunct to weight loss for the overweight individual. Hypoglycemia may result, however, when the exercising individual receives sulfonylurea or insulin therapy. Research suggests that regular, vigorous exercise is associated with a decreased incidence of type 2 diabetes, thus helping prevent the condition.[87]

Acute Complications of Diabetes Mellitus

Hypoglycemia

Hypoglycemia is a lowered plasma glucose level. Its causes may be exogenous, endogenous, or functional (Tables 20-8, 20-9, and 20-10 for a summary of causes). In general, hypoglycemia occurs when blood glucose levels are below 35 mg/dl in newborns for the first 48 hours of life and 45 to 60 mg/dl in children and adults. Evidence also indicates that

Table 20-7 Clinical Manifestations and Rationale for Type 2 Diabetes Mellitus

Manifestations	Rationale
Recurrent infections (e.g., boils and carbuncles; skin infections) and prolonged wound healing	Growth of microorganisms is stimulated by increased glucose levels; impaired blood supply hinders healing
Genital pruritus	Hyperglycemia and glycosuria favor fungal growth; candidal infections, resulting in pruritus, are a common presenting symptom in women
Visual changes	Blurred vision occurs as water balance in the eye fluctuates because of elevated blood glucose levels; diabetic retinopathy is another cause of visual loss
Paresthesias	Paresthesias are common manifestations of diabetic neuropathies
Fatigue	Metabolic changes result in poor use of food products, contributing to lethargy and fatigue

Table 20-8 Exogenous Causes of Hypoglycemia

Exogenous Cause	Predisposing Factor	Occurrence
Insulin	Intentional or accidental overdose; may be combined with inadequate food intake, unusually increased exercise, decrease in insulin requirement, or potentiating medications	Most frequent cause of hypoglycemia
Sulfonylurea agents	Intentional or accidental overdose; may be combined with inadequate food intake, increased exercise, or potentiating medications	Frequent cause of hypoglycemia
Alcohol	Particularly likely in chronically malnourished or acutely food-deprived individuals	Occurs within 6-36 hr of ingesting moderate to large amounts of alcohol
Other agents	Salicylates, hypoglycines, pentamidine	Common in children younger than 2 yr
Exercise	Increased duration and intensity of exercise increase glucose uptake and normally decrease insulin secretion	Occurs with both insulin and sulfonylurea administration and intense exercise but may be unpredictable in onset

Table 20-9 Endogenous Causes of Hypoglycemia

Exogenous Cause	Predisposing Factors	Occurrence
Organic hypoglycemia	Insulinoma	Uncommon neoplasm of B cells of islets of Langerhans
	Nesidioblastosis and B cell hyperplasia	Rare disease causing persistent hypoglycemia of infancy
Extrapancreatic neoplasms	May be mesenchymal tumors, hepatomas, adrenocortical carcinomas, gastrointestinal tumors, lymphomas, or leukemias	Rare; most common in adults 40-70 yr of age
Inborn errors of metabolism	Hereditary fructose intolerance	Rare autosomal recessively inherited inborn error of metabolism
	Fructose-1,6-disphosphatase deficiency	Rare autosomal recessive disease
	Galactosemia	Autosomal recessive disease; hypoglycemia less common than in fructose intolerance
	Phosphoenolpyruvate carboxykinase deficiency	Reported in a few infant cases
	Inborn errors in glycogen metabolism, leucine sensitivity	Reported in von Gierke disease, Hers disease, and type IXb glycogen storage disease

Table 20-10 Functional Causes of Hypoglycemia

Dysfunction	Precipitating Factors	Occurrence
Alimentary hypoglycemia	Rapid dumping of carbohydrates into the upper small intestine	Postgastrectomy
Spontaneous reactive hypoglycemia	Syndrome of unknown cause with symptoms such as diaphoresis, tachycardia, tremulousness, headache, fatigue, drowsiness, and irritability	Rarely diagnosed throughout the world; widely diagnosed in United States, prompting American Diabetes Association and Endocrine Society to issue statement that entity is probably overdiagnosed; it is a benign condition
Alcohol-promoted reactive hypoglycemia	Drinking on an empty stomach	More common with drinks containing both alcohol and glucose or saccharin (e.g., beer, gin and tonic, rum and cola, whisky and ginger ale)
Posthyperalimentation hypoglycemia	Rapid discontinuation of total parenteral alimentation	Easily prevented by gradually reducing parenteral administration (alimentation)
Endocrine-deficiency states	Glucocorticoid deficiency	A danger for any person with adrenal insufficiency
	Growth hormone deficiency	Particularly during a prolonged fast
Severe liver deficiency	Insufficient glucose output by the liver	Fasting hypoglycemia
Lack of body stores for protein, fat, and carbohydrates	Profound malnutrition	Frequent; also found with relative frequency in kwashiorkor
Prolonged muscular exercise	Metabolism of energy-producing substances	Occurs if exercise is too prolonged or severe or if nutritional intake and carbohydrate stores are insufficient
Functional or transient hypoglycemia in infancy	Transient neonatal hypoglycemia	Occurs in 10% of live births, during first 3 days of life
	Maternal diabetes	Caused by beta-cell hyperplasia and possibly relative hypoglucagonemia
	Erythroblastosis fetalis	Frequently associated with erythroblastosis fetalis
	Leucine-induced hypoglycemia	Generally in infants younger than 6 mo of age; severe hypoglycemia attacks may occur postprandially or after short periods of fasting
	Ketotic or ketogenic hypoglycemia	One of the most common forms of hypoglycemia in childhood, occurs after food deprivation in children 1-8 yr old; generally, spontaneous recovery before 10 yr old
	Maple sugar urine disease	Frequent in those with maple sugar urine disease

some individuals may become symptomatic before glucose levels decrease to 60 mg/dl if the decrease is relatively rapid.[88] Hypoglycemia occurs most frequently in individuals with diabetes mellitus treated with insulin (Table 20-11 lists predisposing factors). It occurs in more than 90% of those with type 1 diabetes and limits the management of the disease.[88] Hypoglycemia in diabetes is sometimes called *insulin shock* or *insulin reaction.*

Symptoms result from either activation of the sympathetic nervous system (adrenergic symptoms) or from an abrupt

Table 20-11 Common Acute Complications of Diabetes Mellitus (DM)

Hypoglycemia in Persons with DM	Diabetic Ketoacidosis	Hyperglycemic Nonketotic Syndromes
SYNONYMS		
Insulin shock, insulin reaction	Diabetic coma syndrome	Hyperosmolar hyperglycemia nonketotic coma
PERSONS AT RISK		
Individuals taking insulin Individuals with rapidly fluctuating blood sugar Individuals with type 2 diabetes taking sulfonylurea agents	Individuals with type 1 diabetes Individuals with nondiagnosed diabetes	Elderly or very young individuals with type 2 diabetes, nondiabetics with predisposing factors, persons with renal insufficiency, individuals with undiagnosed diabetes
PREDISPOSING FACTORS		
Excessive insulin or sulfonylurea agent intake, lack of sufficient food intake, excessive physical exercise, abrupt decline in insulin needs (e.g., renal failure, immediately postpartum), simultaneous use of insulin-potentiating agents or beta-blocking agents that mask symptoms	Stressful situation such as infection, accident, trauma, emotional stress; omission of insulin; medications that antagonize insulin	High-carbohydrate diets (e.g., tube feedings, total parenteral nutrition), prolonged mannitol diuresis, peritoneal dialysis or hemodialysis with hyperosmolar dialysate, medications antagonizing insulin
Typical onset		
Rapid	Slow	Slowest
PRESENTING SYMPTOMS		
Adrenergic reaction: pallor, sweating, tachycardia, palpitations, hunger, restlessness, anxiety, tremors Neurogenic reaction: fatigue, irritability, headache, loss of concentration, visual disturbances, dizziness, hunger, confusion, transient sensory or motor defects, convulsions, coma, death	Malaise, dry mouth, headache, polyuria, polydipsia, weight loss, nausea, vomiting, pruritus, abdominal pain, lethargy, shortness of breath, Kussmaul respirations, fruity or acetone odor to breath	Polyuria, polydipsia, hypovolemia, dehydration (parched lips, poor skin turgor), hypotension, tachycardia, hypoperfusion, weight loss, weakness, nausea, vomiting, abdominal pain, hypothermia, stupor, coma, seizures
LABORATORY ANALYSIS		
Serum glucose below 30 mg/dl in newborn (first 2-3 days) and below 55-60 mg/dl in adults	Glucose levels 300-750 mg/dl, reduction in bicarbonate concentration, increased anion gap, increased plasma levels of β-hydroxybutyrate, acetoacetate, and acetone	Glucose levels 600-4800 mg/dl, lack of ketosis, serum osmolarity above 350 mOsm/L, elevated blood urea nitrogen and creatinine

cessation of glucose delivery to the brain (neuroglycopenic symptoms) or borth. Symptoms frequently vary among individuals but tend to be consistent for each person. Adrenergic reactions occur when the decrease in blood glucose is rapid with tachycardia, palpitations, diaphoresis, tremors, pallor, and arousal anxiety. The response is probably generated when the hypothalamus senses decreased glucose levels. The neuron receives inadequate supplies of carbohydrates to metabolize and is thus unable to maintain normal function. Cellular malnutrition (neuroglycopenia) produces further symptoms, including headache, dizziness, irritability, fatigue, poor judgment, confusion, visual changes, hunger, seizures, and coma. Hypoglycemia unawareness is a phenomenon that occurs in individuals without appropriate autonomic warning symptoms before development of neuroglycopenia. These individuals have reduced counterregulatory hormone responses.[89] If an individual is receiving a beta-blocking medication, the autonomic symptoms may be blunted, and recovery from hypoglycemia may be delayed because of impaired glycogenolysis and hampered delivery of gluconeogenic substrates to the liver.

When hypoglycemic symptoms are nonspecific, the safest treatment is to provide some form of glucose, because failure to provide glucose may precipitate convulsions, coma, and death. Prevention of hypoglycemia episodes through alternate therapeutic regimens, individualizing target blood glucose levels, frequent self-monitoring of blood glucose, and proper education should be the goal.

Diabetic Ketoacidosis

Ketoacidosis, a serious complication of diabetes mellitus, is a common cause for hospital admissions, and average mortality rates throughout the United States are 5%. **Diabetic ketoacidosis (DKA)** develops when there is an absolute or

NUTRITION & DISEASE

Reactive Hypoglycemia

Idiopathic reactive hypoglycemia is postprandial hypoglycemia. The probable mechanisms are increased insulin-mediated glucose disposal related to increased nonoxidative glucose metabolism and inadequate counterregulatory glucagon secretion. Symptoms occur 2 to 5 hours after a meal and include weakness, fatigue, rapid heartbeat, sweating, and trembling. Symptoms of reactive hypoglycemia are similar to those of panic attack and are differentiated by measuring blood glucose. Blood glucose levels are measured in symptomatic individuals within a few hours after eating a meal. If the symptoms and low blood sugar (less than 50 mg/dl) occur together and if the symptoms are relieved by eating, a diagnosis can be confirmed. Nutrition therapy is directed to adopting eating habits that keep the blood sugar as stable as possible. Eating five to six small meals rather than three large ones prevents symptoms, with meals and snacks containing carbohydrates, protein, and fat. Restricting or eliminating caffeine and alcohol is also helpful.

Data from *Tufts University Diet Nutr Lett* 13(10):4, 1995; Herbel G, Boyle PJ: Hypoglycemia: pathophysiology and treatment, *Endocrinal Metab Clin North Am* 29(4):725, 2000.

relative deficiency of insulin and an increase in insulin counterregulatory hormones: catecholamines, cortisol, glucagon, and growth hormone. Under these conditions, hepatic glucose production increases, peripheral glucose usage decreases, fat mobilization increases, and ketogenesis is stimulated (Fig. 20-10). The most common precipitating factor is intercurrent illness, such as infection, trauma, surgery, or myocardial infarction. Interruption of insulin administration also may result in DKA. In 20% to 30% of the cases, no precipitating factors are noted. Emotional factors and stress, particularly in children, are thought to contribute to the development of DKA.[90]

Pathophysiology

Catecholamines, cortisol, glucagon, and growth hormone antagonize insulin by increasing glucose production. In addition, catecholamines, cortisol, and growth hormones decrease use of glucose. Insulin deficiency results in decreased glucose uptake, an increased release of fatty acids, and accelerated gluconeogenesis and ketogenesis. Relatively increased glucagon levels are simultaneously responsible for activation of the gluconeogenic (glucose-forming) and ketogenic (ketone-forming) pathways in the liver. Because of the insulin deficiency, hepatic overproduction of β-hydroxybutyrate and acetoacetic acids causes increased ketone concentrations. Ordinarily, ketones used by tissues as an energy source regenerate bicarbonate. This balances the loss of bicarbonate, which occurs when the ketone is formed. Hyperketonemia (increased blood ketone levels) may be a result of impairment in the use of ketones by peripheral tissue, which permits strong organic acids to circulate freely.[90] Bicarbonate buffering then does not occur, and the individual develops a metabolic acidosis.

Clinical Manifestations

The signs and symptoms of DKA are fairly nonspecific, and an individual rarely progresses to complete coma without intervention. Polyuria and dehydration result from the osmotic diuresis associated with hyperglycemia. Here the plasma glucose level is higher than the individual's renal threshold, allowing much glucose to be lost in the urine. Although water deficits may reach 100 ml/kg body weight, they generally are not as severe as those experienced by the individual with hyperosmolar nonacidotic diabetes. Sodium, phosphorus, and magnesium deficits are common. The most important electrolyte disturbance, however, is a marked deficiency in total body potassium. Although the serum potassium may appear normal or elevated because of volume contraction and a shift of potassium from the cell caused by metabolic acidosis, total deficiencies reach 3 to 5 mEq/kg. Symptoms of diabetic ketoacidosis include Kussmaul respirations (hyperventilation in an attempt to compensate for the acidosis), postural dizziness, central nervous system depression, ketonuria, anorexia, nausea, abdominal pain, thirst, and polyuria.

Evaluation and Treatment

The diagnosis of ketoacidosis is suggested when individuals have symptoms of vomiting, abdominal pain, dehydration, and an acetone odor on the breath. Laboratory findings include serum glucose more than 300 mg/dl, reduced serum bicarbonate, increased anion gap, arterial pH less than 7.30, and presence of urine and serum ketones.

Treatment of DKA involves continual administration of low-dose insulin to decrease glucose levels. Fluids are administered to replace lost fluid volume, and electrolytes—particularly sodium, potassium, and phosphorus—are administered as needed. Fluids and electrolytes should be monitored closely. Electrolyte deficits become apparent as fluid volume is replaced. After the administration of insulin, the concentration of β-hydroxybutyrate promptly begins to decrease and after a slight increase, acetoacetate also begins to decrease. A persistent ketonuria may be observed for several days after treatment. Continuous monitoring of the individual is essential to ensure an uncomplicated recovery from DKA. Health teaching emphasizes predisposing factors and strategies for avoiding DKA.

Hyperosmolar Hyperglycemic Nonketotic Syndrome

Hyperosmolar hyperglycemic nonketotic syndrome (HHNKS)[75] was first described in 1886. HHNKS is more commonly seen with type 2 diabetes.

Pathophysiology

HHNKS differs from DKA in the degree of insulin deficiency (which is more profound in DKA) and the degree of fluid deficiency (which is more marked in HHNKS). Levels of free fatty acids in HHNKS are consistently lower than those found in DKA. HHNKS is characterized also by a lack of ketosis. Because the amount of insulin required to inhibit

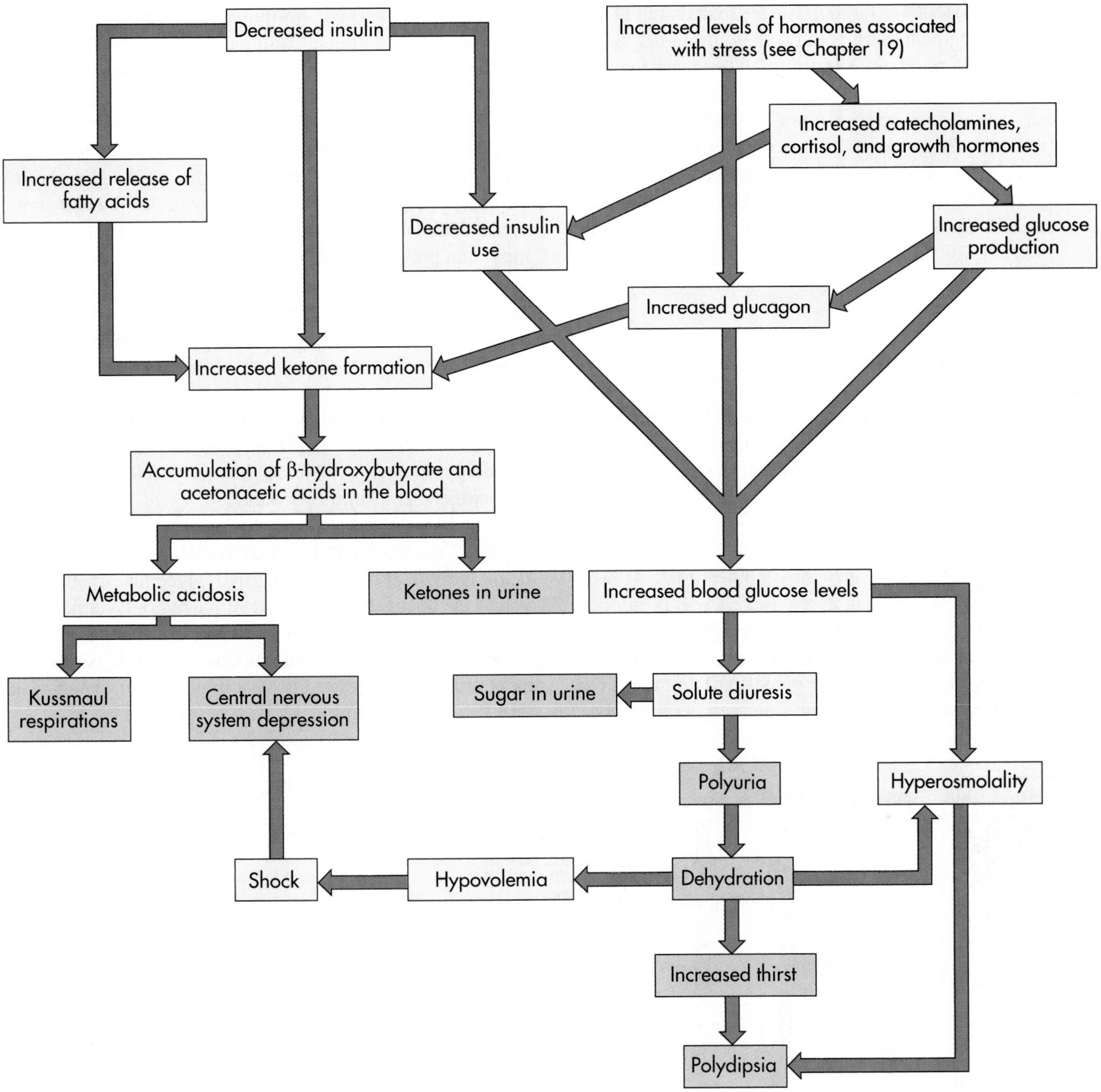

FIG. 20-10 Diabetic ketoacidosis.

fat breakdown is less than that needed for effective glucose transport, insulin levels are sufficient to prevent excessive lipolysis but not to use glucose properly. Glucose levels are considerably higher in HHNKS than in DKA

◆ *Clinical Manifestations*

Glycosuria and polyuria in HHNKS result from the extreme serum glucose elevation. As much as 19 g of glucose per hour may be lost in diuresis, which also causes severe volume depletion and intracellular dehydration. Water losses are generally between 4.8 and 12.6 L, and although some electrolytes are lost with the fluid, the urine is hypotonic. This, along with increased glucose levels, contributes to the increased serum osmolarity. Neurologic changes, such as stupor, correlate with the degree of hyperosmolarity.

◆ *Evaluation and Treatment*

The serum ketone concentration is normal or only mildly elevated in HHNKS. In addition to the depressed mental state, laboratory findings include serum glucose levels higher than 600 mg/dl, serum osmolarity higher than 310 mOsm/L, and blood urea nitrogen (BUN) of 70 to 90 mg/dl. DKA and HHNKS show considerable overlap in symptoms and treatment. An important distinction, however, is that the dehydration in HHNKS is far more severe than that in DKA. Thus fluid replacement, with both crystalloids and colloids, is more rapid. As much as 2000 ml may be given the first hour, together with monitoring of the response to therapy. Potassium deficits may be so extreme in HHNKS that more than 1 week may be needed to correct the total body deficits. Phosphorus and sodium also may be needed. Mortality is also high in HHNKS, currently 14% to 17%, and is related to the age of the individual and comorbid conditions including the severity of the precipitating illness.[91] (Table 20-11 compares the three acute complications described thus far.)

Somogyi Effect

The **Somogyi effect** is a unique combination of hypoglycemia followed by rebound hyperglycemia. The problem is more common in individuals with type 1 diabetes mellitus, particularly in children, and should be investigated whenever fluctuations in blood sugar levels are serious.

Pathophysiology

The Somogyi effect occurs when hypoglycemia stimulates glucose counterregulation, including epinephrine, growth hormone, cortisol, and glucagon release.[88] These hormones serve to increase blood glucose by gluconeogenesis (formation of glucose from nonglucose sources) and glycogenolysis (breakdown of glycogen into glucose). They mobilize fatty acids and proteins while inhibiting peripheral glucose use (Fig. 20-11). These hormones may cause insulin resistance for 12 to 48 hours. Commonly, excessive carbohydrate intake may be a major contributor to rebound hyperglycemia. Also, hypoglycemia generally occurs during the peak of injected insulin; therefore, as counterregulatory hormones are activated and carbohydrate is consumed by the individual, insulin levels are on the decline, which contributes to the subsequent hyperglycemia. The frequency of this phenomenon is debated, and recent studies suggest that it is much less common than previously reported.[61]

Clinical Manifestations

In addition to fluctuating glucose levels, subtle symptoms of hypoglycemia occur. If an individual has nocturnal hypoglycemia, there may be complaints of nightmares and early morning headaches. Both symptoms probably reflect a hypoglycemic state. Ketonuria may occur if the mobilization of energy sources overshoots the body's need for glucose and exogenous insulin is depleted.

Evaluation and Treatment

If the individual has nocturnal hypoglycemia, diagnosis involves the documentation of nighttime hypoglycemia by several plasma glucose analyses at 2 AM, 4 AM, and 7 AM or by using monitors capable of continous glucose sensing. Treatment consists of decreasing insulin dosage or changing the time of administration.

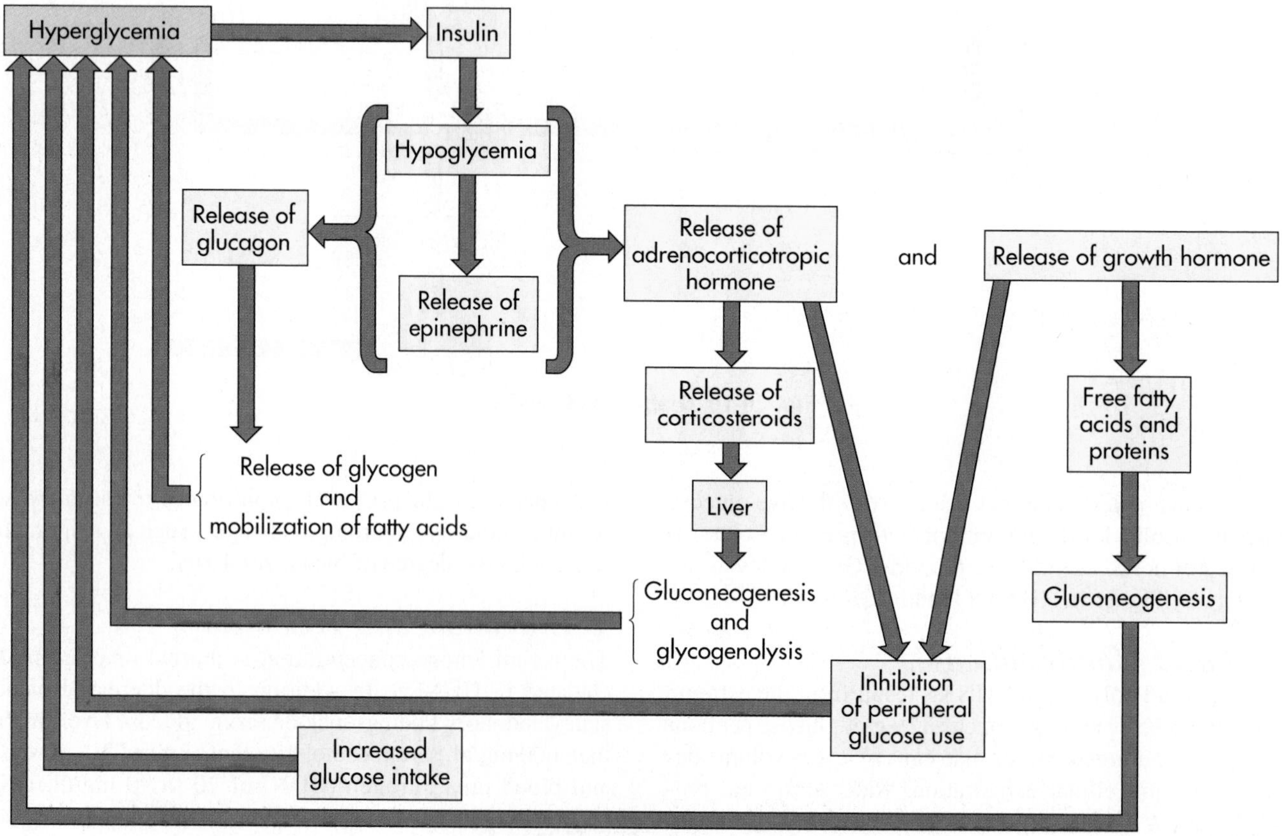

FIG. 20-11 The somogyi effect.

Dawn Phenomenon

The **dawn phenomenon** is an early morning rise in blood glucose concentration with no hypoglycemia during the night. It appears to be related to nocturnal elevations of growth hormone. Growth hormone is a counterregulatory hormone that causes hyperglycemia by decreasing peripheral (other than liver) glucose uptake. Increased clearance of plasma insulin also may be involved. Altering the time and dose of insulin manages the problem. Treating dawn phenomenon may result in the Somogyi effect and vice versa.

Chronic Complications of Diabetes Mellitus

Before the discovery of exogenous insulin, complications in individuals with diabetes had little significance because the survival time was short, especially for individuals with type 1 diabetes. Today, long-term survival is the rule. As a result, the problems of neuropathy, vascular disease, and infection have become important in clinical management. Vascular changes include microvascular disease (e.g., retinopathy and nephropathy) and macrovascular disease (e.g., coronary artery disease, stroke, and peripheral vascular disease).[92] The degree of metabolic control influences the development of complications. Other factors, however, also affect the onset, severity, and progression of complications.[93]

Diabetic Neuropathies

Diabetic neuropathy is the most common cause of neuropathy in the Western world and is probably the most common complication of diabetes. The prevalence is similar for type 1 and type 2,[94] yet the disease remains poorly understood. Neuropathy and other long-term complications are thought to result from the interaction of multiple metabolic, genetic, and environmental factors. The underlying pathologic mechanism may be vascular, metabolic, or a combination of both mechanisms. Neuropathy is classified into two stages: subclinical and clinical. In the subclinical stage, there is evidence that peripheral nerve dysfunctions such as slowed motor and sensory nerve conduction exist without clinical signs. In the clinical stage, symptoms or clinically detectable neurologic deficits are present. Generally, sensory deficits and symptoms are more common than motor involvement.

Diabetic neuropathy is considered to be a form of a "dying back" neuropathy, in which the distal portions of the neurons are initially and eventually more severely affected. The earliest morphologic change in both peripheral nerves and the central nervous system is axonal degeneration that preferentially involves unmyelinated nerve fibers. Schwann cell abnormalities then occur because of changes in the axons they support. Metabolic activity of the Schwann cell is disturbed, causing segmental loss of myelin and the characteristic pattern of demyelination and remyelination observed in long-term diabetic neuropathy. The location of the pathologic condition may include the spinal cord, the posterior root ganglia, or the peripheral nerves. These changes may occur alone or in combination.

Motor nerve conduction velocity, electromyography, and sensory perception have shown abnormalities at the onset of diabetes. Sensory nerve conduction also may be impaired at this stage and is probably the most sensitive index of peripheral neuropathy. These abnormalities may be improved by good glucose control. Although these changes suggest early involvement of the nervous system in individuals with diabetes, they generally are not accompanied by clinical symptomatology.

Various diabetic neuropathies occur, with varying causes, pathogeneses, and clinical backgrounds (Table 20-12). Some of the diabetic neuropathic syndromes are progressive, but many—such as painful peripheral neuropathy, mononeuropathy (wristdrop, footdrop), diabetic amyotrophy, diabetic

Table 20-12 Classification of Diabetic Neuropathies

Location	Characteristics
SOMATIC (PERIPHERAL) NEUROPATHIES	
Lower extremities	Most commonly bilateral, symmetric, and sensory
Asymptomatic	Paresthesias, progressive and irreversible, underlie the development of neuropathic ulcers and Charcot joints
Painful	Pain and paresthesias, particularly nocturnally; anorexia, depression, and irritability; absence of knee and ankle jerk reflexes
Upper extremities	Involves muscle atrophy, asthenia, sensory impairment, and radiculitis
Asymmetric neuropathies	Predominantly motor involvement, absent sensory involvement, sudden onset, severe pain, good prognosis
Diabetic neuropathic cachexia	Profound weight loss with severe pain, spontaneous recovery
VISCERAL NEUROPATHIES (GENERALLY OCCUR WITH PERIPHERAL NEUROPATHIES)	
Cranial nerves	Involves cranial nerve III, leading to pain, diplopia, and ptosis; Involvement of cranial nerve VII leads to Bell palsy
Gastrointestinal tract	Involves decreased esophageal motility, delayed gastric emptying, and diabetic constipation and diarrhea
Genitourinary tract	Insidious and progressive bladder paralysis with urinary retention; sexual dysfunction in males, including retrograde ejaculation and erectile dysfunction
Autonomic nervous system	Includes cardiovascular reflexes, anhidrosis, gustatory sweating, and orthostatic hypotension
Radiculopathy	Spinal cord or root compression, transverse myelitis

neuropathic cachexia, and visceral manifestations associated with autonomic neuropathy (e.g., diabetic diarrhea and orthostatic hypotension)—may spontaneously improve. This suggests that metabolic changes are not completely responsible for the neuropathies. In fact, acute neuropathic syndromes due to nerve infarction may occur during periods of good glucose control. Obviously, much investigation regarding diabetic neuropathies remains to be done. The Diabetes Control and Complications Trial (DCCT) demonstrated a 60% reduction in results related to the appearance of clinical neuropathy and parameters of subclinical nerve dysfunction in the intensive insulin therapy cohort.[62] Similar results are seen in the Kumamoto trial.[95]

Microvascular Disease

Thickening of the capillary basement membrane is characteristic of diabetic microangiopathy and emerges over a period of 1 to 2 years. The thickening eventually results in decreased tissue perfusion. Hyperglycemia is a prerequisite for these microvascular changes and may be related to glycation of structural proteins, which results in the accumulation of advanced glycation end products (AGEs). The frequency of the lesions appears to be proportional to the duration of the disease and blood glucose levels. In the DCCT study, individuals with tightly controlled blood glucose were half as likely to have renal and eye complications as those who received standard treatment.[62] Hypoxia and ischemia of various organs may result from microangiopathy. Two areas often affected are the retina and the kidney.

Retinopathy

The retina is the most metabolically active structure per weight of tissue in the body. Thus the retina is a vulnerable target for microvascular disease in diabetes mellitus. **Diabetic retinopathy** appears to be a response to retinal ischemia resulting from blood vessel changes and red blood cell aggregation. The roles of growth hormone and metabolic control are being explored. The prevalence and severity of the retinopathy are strongly related to the age of the individual and duration of the diabetes and glycemic control. Retinopathy may be present in individuals at the time of diagnosis of type 2 diabetes due to the long preclinical latency of this form of diabetes. The vast majority of individuals with diabetes mellitus have some degree of retinopathy,[96] and retinopathy is closely associated with **diabetic nephropathy,** the so-called renal retinal syndrome.

The three stages of retinopathy are described in Table 20-13. Nonproliferative retinopathy (stage I) is characterized by an increase in retinal capillary permeability, vein dilation, microaneurysm formation, and superficial (flame-shaped) and deep (blot) hemorrhages. Preproliferative retinopathy (stage II) is a progression of retinal ischemia with areas of poor perfusion that culminate in infarcts. Proliferative diabetic retinopathy (stage III) is the result of neovascularization and fibrous tissue formation within the retina or optic disc. Traction of the new vessels on the vitreous humor may cause retinal detachment or hemorrhage into the vitreous humor.

Maculopathy is a progressive process that may accompany the increased retinal capillary permeability, vessel occlusion, and ischemia. If formation of exudates, edema, or ischemia occurs near the fovea, serious loss of vision may result. Laser treatments are used to reduce the rate of vision loss from diabetic macular edema and neovascularization. Vitrectomy is a surgical procedure used to treat an intravitreal hemorrhage secondary to rupture of a neovascular capillary tuft.

Diabetic Nephropathy

Diabetes is the most common cause of end-stage renal disease in the Western world. Approximately 30% of individuals with type 1 and 5% to 10% of those with type 2 diabetes

Table 20-13 Findings in Diabetic Retinopathy

Stages of Retinopathy	Pathologic Findings
NONPROLIFERATIVE RETINOPATHY (STAGE I)	
Venous abnormalities	Increased tortuosity, dilation with irregular constriction; frequency increases with increased severity of retinopathy
Microaneurysms	Mostly thin walled, 15-50 μm in diameter, pathogenesis controversial
Interretinal hemorrhage	Circular and small; may take several months to resorb
Macular edema	Caused by serum leakage through incompetent vessel walls, may resorb in several weeks
Hard exudates	Characteristically "hard" exudates with pattern of exudation irregular in shape and sharply defined may appear and disappear over months to years; common with hypertension; "soft" exudates may appear and disappear more frequently; related to increased retinal capillary permeability
PREPROLIFERATIVE DIABETIC RETINOPATHY (STAGE II)	
Cotton-wool patches	Infarcts of the nerve fiber layer caused by retinal ischemia
Intraretinal microvascular shunts	Tortuous shunts between patent and occluded retinal vessels
PROLIFERATIVE DIABETIC RETINOPATHY (STAGE III)	
Neovascularization	New vessels surrounded by connective tissue; five distinct groups representing different hazards to the eye
Glial proliferation	Often produced to reinforce neovascularization; may occur on optic disc and along vascular arcades
Vitreoretinal traction hemorrhage; retinal detachment	Traction occurring from the vitreous jelly; eventually causes small blood vessels to hemorrhage and retinal detachment to occur

become uremic. The individual typically experiences no clinical signs or symptoms for 10 years in type 1 diabetes or 5 to 8 years in type 2.

The exact process responsible for destruction of kidneys in diabetes is unknown. Mechanisms such as hyperglycemia, hyperfiltration, increased blood viscosity, increased glomerular pressure, albumin, protein kinase C, growth factors, advanced glycation end products, and hypercholesterolemia are being investigated.[97,98,99] The glomeruli are injured by at least two mechanisms: protein denaturation by high glucose levels and adverse effects of intraglomerular hypertension. Renal glomerular changes can occur early in diabetes mellitus and occasionally may precede the overt manifestations of the disease. Glomerular enlargement and glomerular basement membrane thickening, resulting in diffuse intercapillary glomerulosclerosis, develop during the first few years of diabetes. The Kimmelstiel-Wilson nodule, thickening at the center of the glomerular lobules with thickening of the peripheral basement membrane, is distinctive in individuals with diabetes.[100]

Proteinuria, a reliable and consistent sign of renal damage, is the first manifestation of renal dysfunction. Continuous proteinuria generally heralds a life expectancy less than 10 years. The development of more sensitive tests has permitted the detection of small amounts of urinary albumin, microalbuminuria. Earlier intervention with tight glucose control and angiotensin-converting enzyme (ACE) inhibitors or angiotensin II receptor blockers has reduced proteinuria and slowed the progression of nephropathy. Aggressive treatment of hypertension is another therapeutic intervention definitively shown to slow the progression of established renal disease.[101] Scanty information is available to explain the determinants of proteinuria in diabetic nephropathy. Leakage of albumin into glomerular filtrate results from factors other than increased membrane pore size, although these other factors are not yet defined. As renal failure progresses, extensive vascular and extravascular changes occur.

Before the development of proteinuria, no clinical signs or symptoms of progressive glomerulosclerosis are likely to be evident. Later, hypoproteinemia, reduction in plasma oncotic pressure, fluid overload, anasarca (generalized body edema), and hypertension may occur.[102] As renal function continues to deteriorate, individuals with type 1 diabetes may experience hypoglycemia, which necessitates a decrease in insulin therapy. The hypoglycemia occurs because the kidney's ability to metabolize insulin is lost along with other renal functions. As the glomerular filtration rate drops below 10 ml/min, uremic signs such as nausea, lethargy, acidosis, anemia, and uncontrolled hypertension occur (see Chapter 35 for a discussion of renal failure). Impaired kidney function also accelerates retinopathy. Death from renal failure is much more common in individuals with type 1 diabetes mellitus than in those with type 2, because of the association between microalbuminuria and coronary artery disease in individuals with type 2 diabetes.

WHAT'S NEW? Diabetic Complications and Advanced Glycosylation End Products

Persistent exposure to hyperglycemia is an important factor in the development of diabetic microvascular complications. The formation of advanced glycosylation end products (AGE) is the result of accelerated irreversible interaction between glucose and proteins, particularly structural proteins and proteins in the circulation. Receptors for AGEs have been detected on endothelial cells and on monocytes/macrophages. The reaction between AGEs and these receptors leads to cellular damage, including pericyte loss and angiogenesis in retinopathy and mesangial proliferation in nephropathy. There is also an association between AGEs, reactive oxygen species, and cell damage. Pharmacologic prevention of AGE formation is being intensely studied by several groups, but primary prevention through intensive glucose control will provide the same result.

Data from Brownlee M: Negative consequence of glycation, *Metab* 49(2 suppl 1):9, 2000; Yamamoto et al: Roles of the AGE-RAGE system in vascular injury in diabetes, *Ann N Y Acad Sci* 902:163; 2000.

Macrovascular Disease

Macrovascular disease is a major cause of morbidity and mortality among individuals with type 2 diabetes mellitus. The premature atherosclerosis of diabetes has many contributing factors, such as hypertriglyceridemia, low HDL, lipoprotein oxidation, vascular consequences of advanced glycation end products, and altered function. The fibrous plaques of atherosclerosis result from the proliferation of subendothelial smooth muscle in the arterial wall. Other factors in the serum of individuals with diabetes also stimulate this proliferation (Fig. 20-12).

In addition, deposition of lipids in the lesions may be facilitated in individuals with diabetes. Triglyceride elevations with low levels of the protective high-density lipoprotein (HDL) cholesterol are common in individuals with type 2 diabetes mellitus in association with increased quantities of small, dense (very atherogenic) low-density lipoprotein (LDL) cholesterol. Increased levels of the atherogenic oxidized LDL also are seen in hyperglycemic individuals. Further work is needed to clarify the complexities of macrovascular complications.

Coronary Artery Disease

Coronary artery disease (CAD) affects 9.5% to 75% of individuals with diabetes (6% mortality in type 1 patients 45 years of age and younger; 80% mortality in type 2). The risk for those with diabetes is higher than for the general population even when hypertension and hyperlipidemia are taken into account. CAD is the most common cause of death in individuals with type 2 diabetes, but it is also common in those with type 1.[103] Whereas the cardiovascular mortality is increased in all age-groups, mortality is most marked at or before middle age, particularly in women. In general, the prevalence of CAD increases with the duration but not the severity of diabetes.

Myocardial infarction (death of heart muscle as a result of coronary artery occlusion) is the cause of death in 20% of

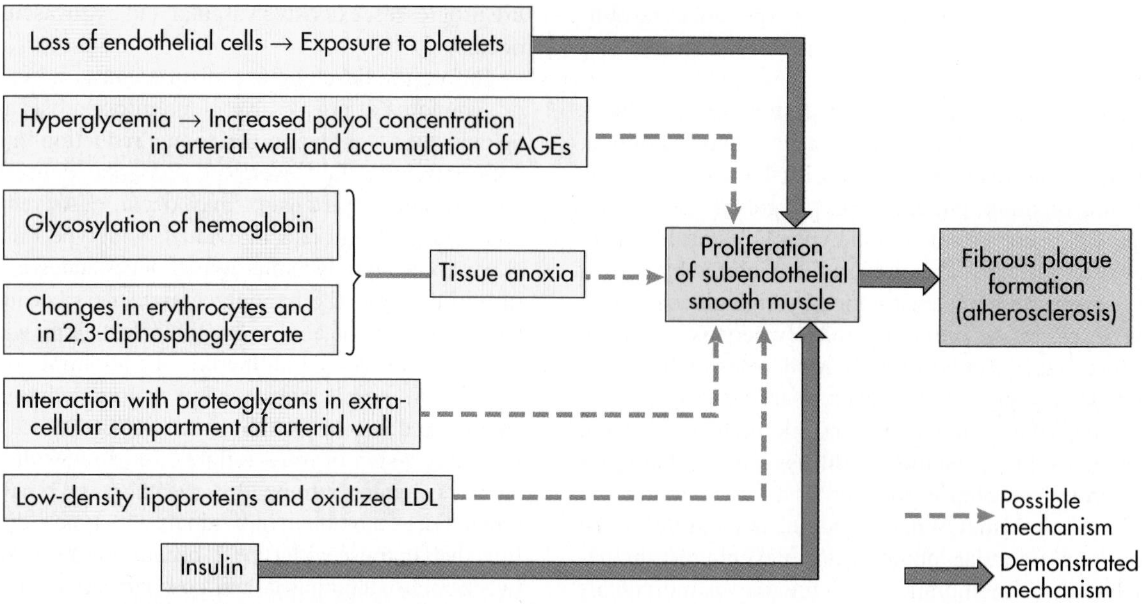

FIG. 20-12 Diabetes mellitus and atherosclerosis. Contributing causes of proliferation of subendothelial smooth muscle in arterial wall, resulting in atherosclerosis.

those with diabetes, and individuals with diabetes mellitus have a higher mortality during the acute phase of myocardial infarctions than do nondiabetic individuals. In addition, the incidence of congestive heart failure is higher in individuals with diabetes, even without myocardial infarction. The reason is unclear but may be related to the presence of increased amounts of collagen in the ventricular wall, which reduces the mechanical compliance of the heart during filling. (Heart disease is described in Chapter 29.)

Stroke

Stroke is twice as common in those with diabetes as in the nondiabetic population.[104] The survival rate for an individual with diabetes after a massive stroke is typically shorter than for a person without diabetes. Hypertension is a definite risk factor (see Chapter 29), and aggressive management of blood pressure in hypertensive individuals with diabetes has been shown to reduce the incidence of stroke.[105] No data are available to evaluate the effects of blood glucose control on the incidence of stroke.

Peripheral Vascular Disease

The increased incidence of peripheral vascular disease (PVD), gangrene, and amputation in diabetic persons has been documented in many studies, particularly in individuals with type 2 diabetes.[92] Fig. 20-13 illustrates how foot lesions of diabetes can lead to amputation. Many individuals with type 2 diabetes have evidence of peripheral vascular disease at the time of their initial diagnosis. The atherosclerotic process in diabetic persons is more common, appears at a younger age, and advances more rapidly than vascular changes in nondiabetic persons. The prevalence of PVD is nearly equal in males and females with diabetes. Age, duration of diabetes, genetics, and additional risk factors influence the development of PVD.

Because of occlusions of the small arteries and arterioles, most of the gangrenous changes of the lower extremities occur in patchy areas of the feet and toes. Smaller vessels often have more advanced disease than larger vessels in the same individuals. Fifty percent of nontraumatic amputations in the United States are performed on individuals with diabetes. Hospital mortality for individuals with diabetes who undergo major amputation is between 10% and 23%. The survival rate after surgery is only 40% at the end of 5 years.[92]

Infection

Increased morbidity and mortality from infectious agents have been documented in those with diabetes.[106] The individual with diabetes is at increased risk for infection throughout the body for at least five reasons. One major reason involves the senses. Impaired vision caused by retinal changes and impaired touch caused by neuropathy diminish the prevention of breaks in the skin by decreasing the early warning systems. Once breaks in skin integrity occur, tissues may have increased susceptibility to infection because of hypoxia, a second reason for susceptibility to infection. Microvascular and macrovascular complications cause decreased oxygen supply to tissues. In addition, the increased content of glycosylated hemoglobin in the red blood cell impedes the release of oxygen to tissues.

The third general reason for infection in individuals with diabetes is that pathogens are able to multiply rapidly once they have gained access to the tissues. Some pathogens proliferate rapidly because the increased glucose in body fluids provides an excellent source of energy. Fourth, the decreased blood supply resulting from vascular changes decreases the supply of white blood cells to the affected area. Fifth, the function of the white cells is impaired. Chemotaxis is abnormal, and phagocytosis is defective. The causes for these mechanisms have not been identified, but the result is an individual at considerable risk for the development of infections. (Factors that promote healing are described in Chap-

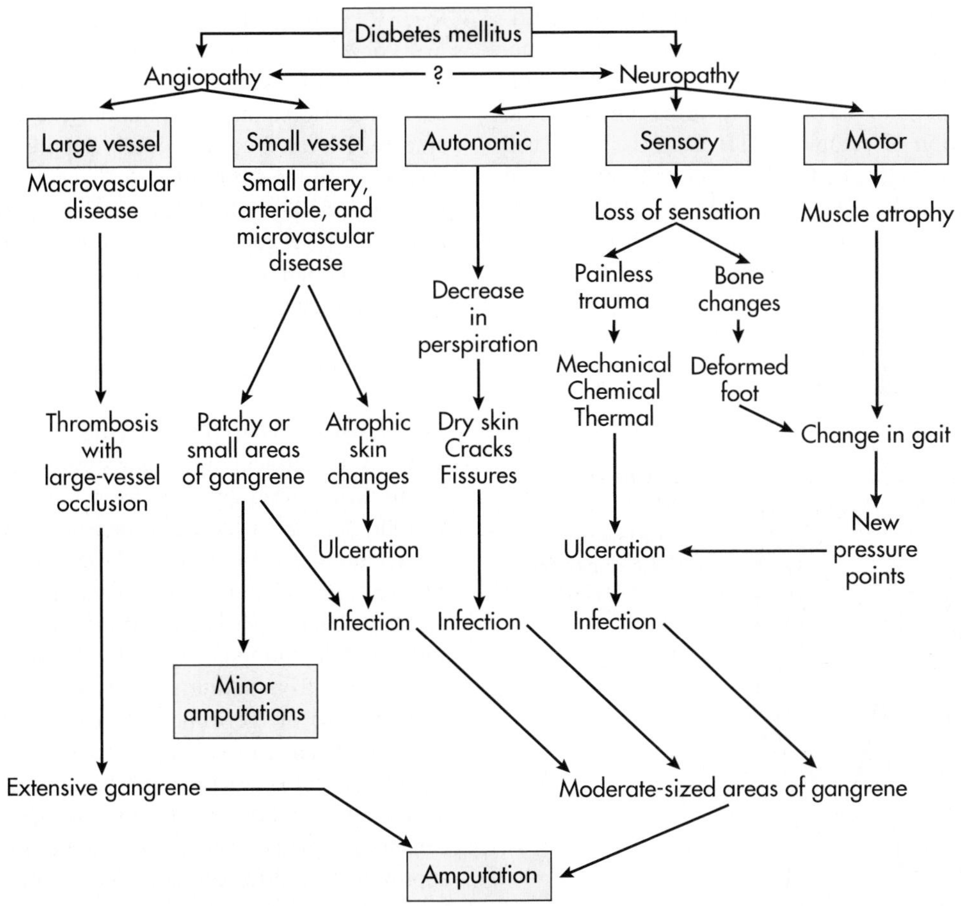

FIG. 20-13 How foot lesions of diabetes can lead to amputation. (From Levin ME, O'Neal LW, Bowker JH: *The diabetic foot*, ed 5, St Louis, 1993, Mosby.)

ter 7.) The risk of infection is especially high for individuals undergoing surgery and for those taking immunosuppressant medications.

ALTERATIONS OF ADRENAL FUNCTION

Disorders of the Adrenal Cortex

Disorders of the adrenal cortex are related to either hyperfunction or hypofunction. Hyperfunction that causes increased levels of circulating cortisol leads to Cushing disease, or Cushing syndrome; hyperfunction that causes increased secretion of adrenal androgens and estrogens leads to virilization or feminization; and hyperfunction that causes increased levels of aldosterone leads to hyperaldosteronism, which may be primary or secondary. Hypofunction of the adrenal cortex leads to Addison disease.

Adrenocortical Hyperfunction: Cushing Syndrome, Cushing Disease

Cushing syndrome refers to chronic **hypercortisolism** (excessive levels of circulating cortisol) caused by hyperfunction of the adrenal cortex. **Cushing disease** is caused by excessive anterior pituitary secretion of ACTH. In addition, a Cushing-like syndrome may develop as a result of the exogenous administration of cortisone.[107]

ACTH-induced Cushing disease is more common in adults and is two to three times more common in women than in men. Cushing syndrome resulting from ectopic ACTH secretion is more common in older adults, particularly men. Adrenal tumors, rather than pituitary tumors, are more common in children, especially girls. Cushing syndrome can occur at any age but usually occurs between 30 and 50 years of age.

Pathophysiology

Hypercortisolism usually is caused by Cushing disease, ectopic ACTH-secreting tumors, or adrenal-secreting tumors. Approximately 75% to 80% of individuals with hypercortisolism have Cushing disease, whereas both ectopic ACTH-secreting tumors and cortisol-secreting adrenal tumors are less often the cause of hypercortisolism.

Although the origin of Cushing disease remains incompletely understood, the vast majority of individuals with Cushing disease have a pituitary microadenoma, which secretes ACTH.[108] In Cushing disease there is a loss of normal feedback inhibition by cortisol because there appears to be a higher set-point for cortisol feedback on CRH and ACTH secretion.

Ectopic ACTH-secreting tumors are nonpituitary tumors that synthesize and hypersecrete ACTH, leading to hypercortisolism. Some tumors also hypersecrete CRH. Tumors associated with episodic secretion of ACTH and hypercortisolism include small cell carcinomas of the lung, thymoma, pancreatic cell tumors, carcinoid tumors, medullary carcinoma of the thyroid, and pheochromocytoma tumors. Even though the secretion of ectopic ACTH from the neoplasm is not under hypothalamic–pituitary control, the normal pituitary release of ACTH is inhibited by the elevated levels of cortisol. However, cortisol fails to inhibit the release of ACTH from the ectopic source.

Autonomous secretion of cortisol can be due to either an adrenal adenoma or, less commonly, to adrenal cortical carcinoma. Elevated cortisol levels suppress CRH and ACTH release secretion from the hypothalamus and anterior pituitary, respectively, which leads to low levels of ACTH. Low levels of ACTH cause atrophy of the remaining normal portions of the adrenal cortex, which over time will alter the cortisol-secreting activity of normal cells. The normal diurnal variation in cortisol secretion is lost in individuals with hypercortisolism regardless of the underlying cause.

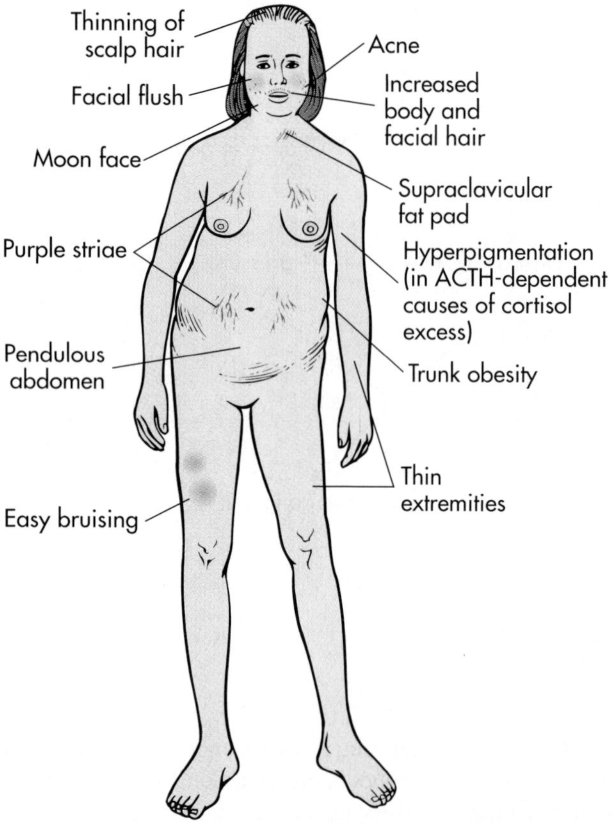

FIG. 20-14 Symptoms of cushing disease.

Clinical Manifestations

Most of the clinical signs and symptoms of Cushing syndrome are caused by hypercortisolism (see Chapter 9). Weight gain is the most common feature and results from the accumulation of adipose tissue in the trunk, facial, and cervical areas. These characteristic patterns of fat deposition have been described as "truncal obesity," "moon face," and "buffalo hump" (Figs. 20-14 and 20-15). Transient weight gain from sodium and water retention may be present because of the mineralocorticoid effects of cortisol, exhibited when cortisol is present in high levels.

Glucose intolerance occurs because of cortisol-induced insulin resistance and increased gluconeogenesis and glycogen storage by the liver. Overt diabetes mellitus develops in approximately 20% of individuals with hypercortisolism. Polyuria, which is sometimes seen in hypercortisolism, is a manifestation of hyperglycemia and resultant glycosuria.

Protein wasting is commonly observed in hypercortisolism and is caused by the catabolic effects of cortisol on peripheral tissues. Muscle wasting, especially obvious in the muscles of the extremities, leads to muscle weakness. In bone, loss of the protein matrix leads to osteoporosis, with pathologic fractures, vertebral compression fractures, bone

A

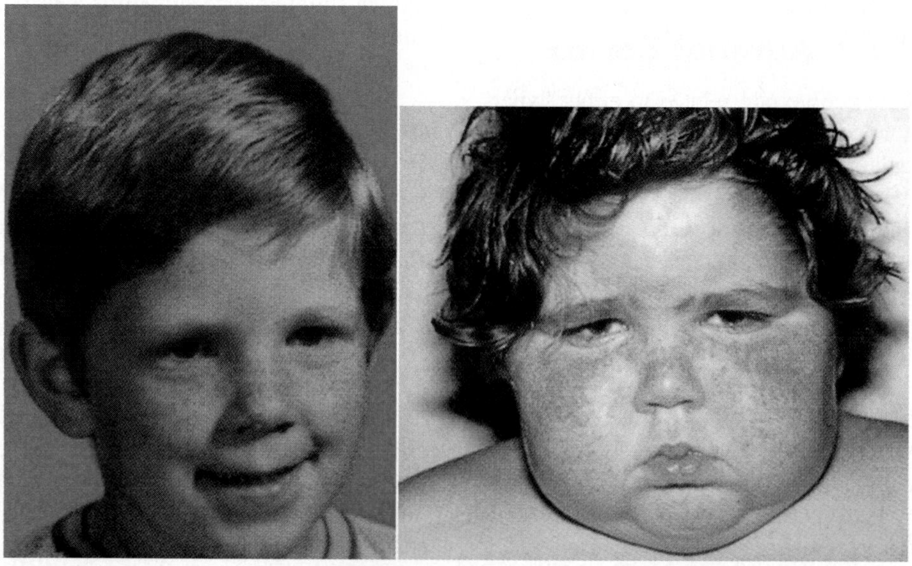

B

FIG. 20-15 Cushing syndrome. A, Patient before onset of Cushing syndrome. **B,** Patient 4 months later. Moon facies is clearly demonstrated. (From Zitelli BJ, Davis HW: *Atlas of pediatric physical diagnosis*, ed 3, London, 1997, Gower.)

and back pain, kyphosis, and reduced height. Bone disease may contribute to hypercalciuria and resulting renal stones, which are experienced by approximately 20% of individuals with disease. Loss of collagen also leads to thin, weakened integumentary tissues through which capillaries are more visible; the tissues are easily stretched by adipose deposits. Together these changes account for the characteristic purple striae most frequently observed in the trunk area. Loss of collagenous support around small vessels makes them susceptible to rupture, leading to easy bruising, even with minor trauma. Thin, atrophied skin is also easily damaged, leading to skin breaks and ulcerations.

Hyperpigmentation in Cushing syndrome is associated with very high serum levels of ACTH. The precise hormonal basis for this hyperpigmentation is still undetermined; however, current speculation focuses on the melanotropic activity of ACTH.[109] The pigmentation involves the mucous membranes, hair, and skin, all of which acquire a characteristic brownish or bronze color.

Cortisol has a permissive effect on the actions of the catecholamines. With elevated cortisol levels, vascular sensitivity to catecholamines is increased significantly, leading to vasoconstriction and hypertension. Elevated blood pressure occurs in most individuals with Cushing syndrome. Chronically elevated cortisol levels also cause suppression of the immune system and increased susceptibility to infections. Consequently, individuals with hypercortisolism experience poor wound healing and are particularly susceptible to superficial fungal infections.

Approximately 50% of individuals with Cushing syndrome experience alterations in their mental status. These may range from irritability and depression to severe psychiatric disturbances such as schizophrenia. The effects of glucocorticoids on mood are complex and are just beginning to be examined.[110]

Females may experience symptoms of increased adrenal androgen levels, increased hair growth (especially facial hair), acne, and oligomenorrhea. Androgen levels rarely become high enough to cause changes of the voice, recession of the hairline, and clitoral hypertrophy unless an adrenal carcinoma is involved. Routine laboratory examinations may reveal hyperglycemia, glycosuria, hypokalemia, and metabolic alkalosis.

Evaluation and Treatment

A variety of laboratory tests must be used to diagnose hypercortosolism and to determine the underlying disorder. These include urinary free cortisol higher than 100 μg per 24 hr, abnormal dexamethasone suppressibility of either urinary or serum cortisol, and simultaneous measurement of ACTH and cortisol. Visualizing procedures, including pituitary MRI or abdominal scanning, are essential in the evaluation. Selective catheterization of the veins draining the pituitary (inferior pertrosal sinus sampling) is very helpful in determining the cause of hypercortisolism and in localizing pituitary tumors.[111] The diagnosis and evaluation of hypercortisolism is one of the most challenging problems in endocrinology.[112]

Without treatment, approximately 50% of individuals with Cushing syndrome die within 5 years of onset. Major causes of death are overwhelming infection, suicide, complications from generalized arteriosclerosis, and hypertensive disease. Treatment is specific for the cause of hypercorticoadrenalism and includes medication, radiation therapy, and surgery. Therefore differentiation among pituitary, adrenal, and ectopic causes of the hypercortisolism is essential for effective treatment.

Hyperaldosteronism

Hyperaldosteronism is characterized by excessive aldosterone secretion by the adrenal cortex. The excessive secretion can result from a primary adrenal disorder, such as an aldosterone-secreting adenoma, or from excessive stimulation of the normal adrenal cortex by substances such as angiotensin II, ACTH, or elevated potassium. Both primary and secondary forms of hyperaldosteronism can occur in individuals. **Primary hyperaldosteronism** refers to an excessive secretion of aldosterone caused by an abnormality of the adrenal cortex. **Secondary hyperaldosteronism** involves excessive aldosterone secretion from an extraadrenal stimulus, most frequently angiotensin II through a renin-dependent mechanism.

Primary hyperaldosteronism (Conn disease, primary aldosteronism) presents a clinical picture of hypertension, hypokalemia, renal potassium wasting, and neuromuscular manifestations. The most common cause of primary aldosteronism is the benign, single adrenal adenoma (80% to 90% of cases), followed by multiple tumors or idiopathic hyperplasia of the adrenals (10% to 15% of cases). Adrenal carcinomas and unknown causes account for the remainder of cases. The incidence of primary hyperaldosteronism is not known, but it is estimated to be the most common cause of secondary hypertension.[113]

Because aldosterone secretion normally is stimulated by the renin-angiotensin system, secondary hyperaldosteronism can be expected to result from sustained elevated renin release and activation of angiotensin II. (Factors that affect renin and aldosterone secretion are summarized in Table 20-14.) Increased renin-angiotensin secretion occurs in a variety of situations. In general, these include decreased circulating blood volume (e.g., in dehydration, shock, or hypoalbuminemia) and decreased delivery of blood to the kidneys (e.g., renal artery stenosis, heart failure, or hepatic cirrhosis). In many of these instances the activation of the renin-angiotensin system and subsequent aldosterone secretion may be seen as compensatory, although in some instances (e.g., congestive heart failure) the increased circulating volume may further worsen the condition.

Increased estrogen levels associated with pregnancy and use of oral contraceptives also increase renin-angiotensin levels, apparently by stimulating renin substrate production by the liver. These pregnancy-induced changes, however, may represent adaptation to pregnancy and are therefore not representative pathophysiologic alterations.

Other causes of secondary hyperaldosteronism are Bartter syndrome, in which the underlying disorder is a

Table 20-14 Physiologic Factors Affecting Renin and Aldosterone Secretion

Factors	Renin Secretion	Aldosterone Secretion
Age	Highest in infants; lowest in the elderly	Highest in infants
Menstrual cycle	Highest in luteal phase (see Chapter 21)	Highest in luteal phase
Sodium intake	Increased by salt restriction Decreased by salt loading	Increased by salt restriction Decreased by salt loading
Potassium status	Increased by K^+ depletion	Decreased by K^+ depletion
Posture	Increased with erect posture	Increased with erect posture
Sympathetic nervous stimulation	Increased by catecholamines	Increased through renin secretion
Time of sampling	Highest before noon; lowest in evening	Diurnal rhythm (as for ACTH)

ACTH, Adrenocorticotropic hormone.

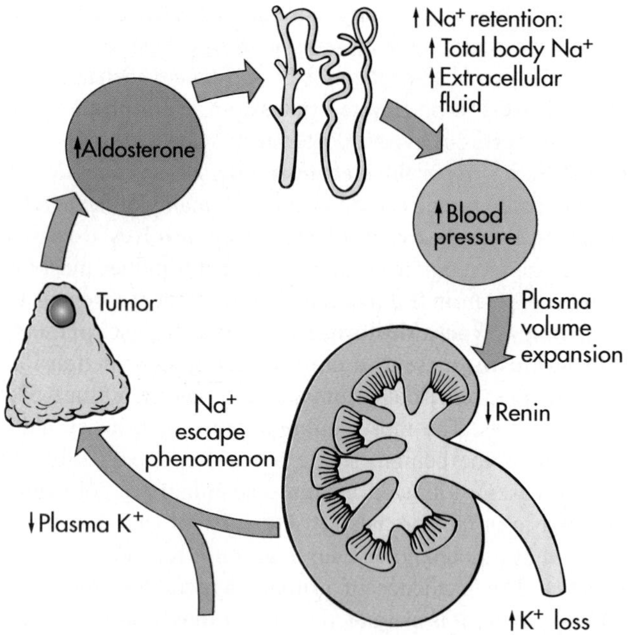

Fig. 20-16 Primary hyperaldosteronism. Pathophysiology of mineralocorticoid excess syndromes in primary hyperaldosteronism.

renal tubular defect leading to hypokalemia, and renin-secreting tumors of the kidney. Such tumors, however, cause secondary hyperaldosteronism. (Renal disorders are discussed in Chapter 35.)

Pathophysiology

In primary hyperaldosteronism, pathophysiologic alterations are caused by excessive aldosterone secretion and the fluid and electrolyte imbalances that ensue. Hyperaldosteronism promotes increased sodium reabsorption with corresponding hypervolemia (see Chapter 3). The extracellular fluid volume overload and suppression of normal feedback mechanisms of renin secretion are characteristic of primary disorders.

Edema usually does not occur with primary aldosteronism, possibly because of the renal tubular "escape" phenomenon that is activated in chronic hyperaldosteronism. The escape phenomenon changes or resets the rate of sodium excretion and prevents more severe sodium retention. The escape phenomenon operates in the proximal tubules and causes additional sodium to pass to the distal tubules, where the sodium is, to some extent, reabsorbed in exchange for potassium. This mechanism, while protecting from excessive sodium reabsorption and edema, increases urinary losses of potassium (Fig. 20-16).

In secondary hyperaldosteronism the effect of increased extracellular volume on renin secretion may vary. If renin secretion is being stimulated by variables other than pressure-initiated cellular changes at the juxtaglomerular apparatus (see Chapter 34), increased circulating blood volume may not decrease renin secretion through feedback mechanisms. This physiologic process is normal in pregnancy and related to increased plasma estrogen.

In Bartter syndrome a state of hypokalemia develops because of defective renal tubular reabsorptive mechanisms. The hypokalemic state may induce the formation of prostaglandins (especially PGE_2) by the renal cells, which stimulates renin and hence aldosterone secretion. The stimulatory effect on aldosterone secretion is offset somewhat by the aldosterone-suppressing effects of hypokalemia.

Potassium secretion also is promoted by aldosterone, so that with excessive circulating levels of aldosterone, hypokalemia occurs (see Chapter 3). In hyperaldosteronism, hypokalemic alkalosis, changes in myocardial conduction, and skeletal muscle alterations may be seen, particularly with severe potassium depletion (i.e., the renal tubules may become insensitive to ADH, thus promoting excessive loss of free water). Rarely, this may result in mild hypernatremia because water is not able to follow the sodium that is reabsorbed.

Clinical Manifestations

Hypertension and hypokalemia are the hallmarks of hyperaldosteronism. Hypertension may result from increased intravascular volume or from a state of aldosterone-mediated vasoconstriction, although the latter mechanism requires very high levels of aldosterone. If hypertension is sustained, the long-term effects of elevated arterial pressure become evident, which include the development of left ventricular dilation and hypertrophy. Because of the increased arterial pressure, renin secretion is typically suppressed, although it is elevated in secondary hyperaldosteronism, which provides a means to clearly differentiate between these conditions.

Aldosterone-stimulated potassium loss can be substantial. Serum potassium levels below 3.0 mEq/L result in the typical manifestations of hypokalemia: hypokalemic alkalosis caused by the movement of potassium from the intercellular to extracellular space in exchange for hydrogen ions as well as renal loss of hydrogen ions to facilitate sodium reabsorption (see Chapter 3). Individuals with hypokalemic alkalosis may experience the following:

1. Tetany and paresthesia caused by an alkalosis-induced lowering of ionized calcium levels
2. Skeletal muscle weakness that can be so severe as to mimic flaccid paralysis
3. Cardiovascular alterations, including depressed T waves and ST segment, appearance of U waves on the electrocardiogram, and ventricular ectopy, which may or may not be associated with syncopy
4. Loss of urine-concentrating mechanisms, leading to polyuria or nocturia

Evaluation and Treatment

A variety of clinical and laboratory measurements are useful in the assessment of hyperaldosteronism.[114] These include blood pressure, serum and urinary electrolyte levels, serum and urinary levels of aldosterone and renin, and aldosterone suppression testing. Blood pressure is elevated; serum sodium may be normal or elevated; and serum potassium is depressed, whereas urinary potassium is elevated (i.e., >30 mmol/day). Serum aldosterone, as measured by radioimmunoassay, usually is greater than 20 ng/dl. Plasma renin activity is generally less than 1 ng/ml/hr for individuals with primary aldosteronism. Serum aldosterone and plasma renin activity both must be measured under controlled situations and after careful dietary regulation of sodium and potassium intake (see Table 20-14). Aldosterone suppression testing commonly is accomplished with fludrocortisone acetate (Florinef) or salt loading. Imaging techniques, such as CT and nuclear magnetic resonance (NMR), may be used to localize an aldosterone-secreting adenoma. Selective venous catheterization of both adrenal veins is also useful.

Treatment includes management of hypertension and hypokalemia, as well as correction of any underlying causal abnormalities. If an aldosterone-secreting adenoma is present, it is generally approached surgically; however, medical management with spironolactone is a viable option in complicated cases.[115]

Hypersecretion of Adrenal Androgens and Estrogens

Hypersecretion of adrenal androgens and estrogens may be caused by adrenal tumors, either adenomas or carcinomas, Cushing syndrome, or defects in steroid synthesis. The clinical syndrome that results depends on the hormone secreted, the gender of the individual, and the ages at which the hypersecretion was initiated. Hypersecretion of estrogens causes **feminization,** the development of female sex characteristics. Hypersecretion of androgens causes **virilization**, the development of male sex characteristics (Fig. 20-17).

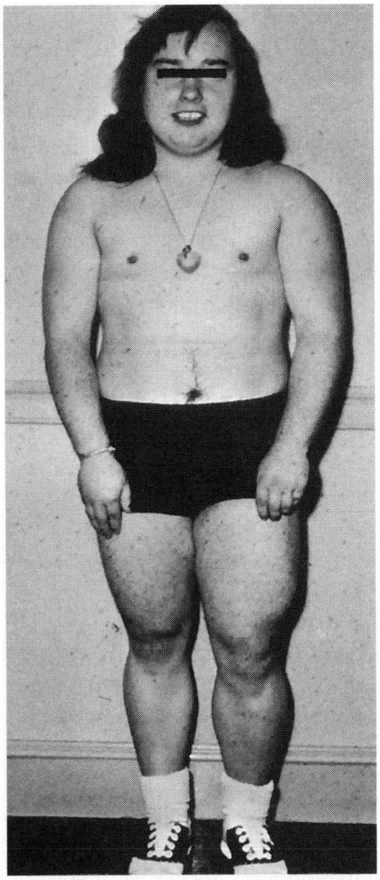

FIG. 20-17 Virilization. Virilization of a young girl by an androgen-secreting tumor of the adrenal cortex. Masculine features include lack of breast development, increased muscle bulk, and hirsutism. (From Thibodeau GA: *Anatomy & physiology*, St Louis, 1987, Mosby.)

The effects of an estrogen-secreting tumor are most evident in males and result in gynecomastia (98% of cases), testicular atrophy, and decreased libido. In female children such tumors may lead to early development of secondary sex characteristics. An androgen-secreting tumor indicates changes more easily observed in females, including excessive facial and body hair growth, hirsutism, clitoral enlargement, deepening of the voice, amenorrhea, acne, and breast atrophy. In children, virilizing tumors promote precocious sexual development and bone aging. Treatment of androgen-secreting tumors usually involves surgical excision.

Adrenocortical Hypofunction

Hypocortisolism (low levels of cortisol secretion) develops because of either inadequate stimulation of the adrenal glands by ACTH or a primary inability of the adrenals to produce and secrete the adrenocortical hormones. In some syndromes, however, there is partial dysfunction of the adrenal cortex so that only synthesis of aldosterone or the adrenal androgens is affected. Hypofunction of the adrenal cortex may affect glucocorticoid or mineralocorticoid secretion or a combination of both.

Primary adrenal insufficiency is termed **Addison disease**. Addison disease is a relatively rare disease, occurring most often in adults 30 to 60 years of age, although it may appear at any time throughout the life span. Addison disease, caused by autoimmune mechanisms, is more common in women.

The most common cause of Addison disease in the United States is autoimmune destruction of the adrenals. Other causes include infections (tuberculosis, fungal, HIV), infiltrative diseases (amyloidosis, metastatic carcinoma), or bilateral adrenal hemorrhage. Adrenoleukodystrophy and adrenomyeloneuropathy are two rare types of X-linked adrenal deficiency that lead to symptoms of hypocortisolism and progressive neurologic symptoms.

Pathophysiology

Addison disease is characterized by elevated serum ACTH levels with inadequate corticosteroid synthesis and output. Before clinical manifestations of hypocortisolism are evident, more than 90% of total adrenocortical tissue must be destroyed.

Idiopathic Addison Disease

Idiopathic Addison disease (organ-specific autoimmune adrenalitis), which causes adrenal atrophy and hypofunction, generally is recognized as an organ-specific autoimmune disease. (Autoimmunity is discussed in Chapter 8.) Autoantibodies are present in 50% to 70% of individuals with idiopathic Addison disease, and this percentage increases in younger persons and in those with other autoimmune diseases. The autoantibodies appear to be specific for the cells of the adrenal cortex. A combination of cell membrane and cytoplasmic antibodies and cell-mediated immune mechanisms contributes to the pathologic findings of the disease. Apparently a genetic defect in immune surveillance mechanisms causes a deficiency of immune-suppressor cells. This deficiency allows the proliferation of immunocytes directed against specific antigens within the adrenocortical cells.[116]

Idiopathic Addison disease frequently is associated with other autoimmune diseases, especially Hashimoto thyroiditis, pernicious anemia, and idiopathic hypoparathyroidism. In these cases, Addison disease may be inherited as an autosomal recessive trait.[117] (Mechanisms of inheritance are described in Chapter 4.)

The adrenal glands in idiopathic Addison disease are smaller than normal and may be misshapen. Microscopically, gland atrophy is evident throughout the cortex, although the medulla appears intact. Extensive diffuse cortical lymphocytic infiltrate supports the immune component of the disease process.

Secondary Hypocortisolism

Secondary hypocortisolism is characterized by low to absent ACTH levels, which cause inadequate adrenal stimulation, adrenal atrophy, and ultimately decreased corticosteroidogenesis. The exogenous administration of glucocorticoids for nonendocrine disease results in this form of hypocortisolism. Successful surgical removal of cortisol-secreting tumors also results in postoperative hypocortisolism. In these cases, increased glucocorticoid levels suppress ACTH production through normal feedback mechanisms. With decreased ACTH levels, corticosteroid synthesis by remaining adrenal tissue is suppressed. Pituitary hypofunction (as occurs in postpartum pituitary infarction [Sheehan syndrome] and panhypopituitarism, hypophysectomy, or isolated ACTH deficiency) causes inadequate ACTH production and secretion and absence of pituitary responsiveness to normal stimulatory mechanisms. In all instances of low ACTH levels, adrenal atrophy occurs, and endogenous adrenal steroidogenesis is depressed.

Clinical manifestations of secondary hypocortisolism are similar to those of Addison disease. One difference is that with the typically low levels of ACTH seen in secondary hypocortisolism, hyperpigmentation does not occur. Second, the renin-angiotensin system is usually normal in these individuals; therefore aldosterone and potassium levels also tend to be normal.

Clinical Manifestations

The symptoms of Addison disease are primarily a result of hypocortisolism and hypoaldosteronism. Decreased adrenal androgen secretion is usually not clinically obvious in males because the adrenals are not a major source of male androgens. Females may experience a loss of some secondary sex characteristics, such as pubic and axillary hair, normally maintained by the adrenal androgens. The symptoms of Addison disease are summarized in Table 20-15.

Evaluation and Treatment

Serum and urine levels of cortisol are depressed with hypocortisolism. In primary adrenal insufficiency (Addision disease), ACTH levels are clearly elevated, and ACTH levels are low in secondary adrenal insufficiency. ACTH levels can only be interpreted in the face of a simultaneous measurement of cortisol. Individuals may develop azotemia due to dehydration, and hyponatremia is common. Hyperkalemia is only seen in Addision disease, but hypoglycemia may be seen in hypocortisolism from any cause. Anemia, eosinophilia, and lymphocytosis are also common. The ACTH stimulation test may be used to evaluate adrenocortical function. This is achieved by administering ACTH and monitoring the serum cortisol levels.

The treatment of Addison disease involves glucocorticoid and possibly mineralocorticoid replacement therapy, together with dietary modifications. All individuals with hypocortisolism require lifetime daily glucocorticoid replacement therapy. In the event of acute stressors, additional cortisol must be administered to approximate the amount of cortisol that might be expected to be secreted if normal adrenal function were present (approximately 100 to 300 mg/day).

The individual's diet should include at least 150 mEq of sodium per day, with sodium intake increased in the event of excessive sweating or diarrhea. Treatment also must include correction of any underlying disorders.

Disorders of the Adrenal Medulla

Adrenal Medulla Hypofunction

No known physiologic alterations are associated with hypofunction of the adrenal medulla. Bilateral adrenalectomy, for example, is followed by a rapid decrease in urinary excretion of epinephrine, but excretion of norepinephrine remains

Table 20-15 Clinical Manifestations and Pathophysiologic Mechanisms of Addison Disease

Clinical Manifestation	Pathophysiologic Mechanism
Weakness and easy fatigability that worsens as the day progresses, seen especially after exposure to stressors	Not known, may be related to hypoglycemia, decreased metabolism of proteins
Gastrointestinal disturbances: anorexia, nausea, vomiting, diarrhea, abdominal pain, weight loss	Not known
Hypoglycemia, manifested by fatigue, mental confusion, apathy, psychosis	Absence of cortisol leads to decreased gluconeogenesis, decreased glycogen storage by liver, decreased metabolism of proteins, increased insulin sensitivity
Hyperpigmentation (only seen in cases of Addison disease with increased ACTH)	Increased secretion of ACTH is accompanied by increased secretion of β-lipotropin and melanocyte-stimulating hormone; both hormones induce pigment changes in epithelial cells
Vitiligo (white patchy areas of depigmented skin)	Autoimmune destruction of melanocytes
Hypotension	Decreased blood volume resulting from hypoaldosteronism causing increased renal sodium losses
Addisonian crisis: severe hypotension and vascular collapse	Combined effects of hypocortisolism, hypoaldosteronism, extracellular volume depletion, and some precipitating stressor (e.g., infection, vomiting, diarrhea); decreased vasomotor tone due to cortisol deficiency

ACTH, Adrenocorticotropic hormone.

relatively stable. Pathophysiologic alterations are instead associated with hyperfunctioning of the adrenal medulla.

Adrenal Medulla Hyperfunction

Adrenomedullary hyperfunction is due to tumors derived from the chromaffin cells of the adrenal medulla. These tumors, **pheochromocytomas**, secrete catecholamines on a continual or episodic basis (Fig. 20-18). Less than 10% of these tumors are malignant; those that are malignant may metastasize to the lungs, liver, bones, or paraaortic lymph nodes. Most pheochromocytomas produce norepinephrine, although large tumors secrete both epinephrine and norepinephrine.

The true incidence of pheochromocytoma in the general population is not known. One tenth of one percent of the hypertensive population have a pheochromocytoma.[118] The tumors are most common in people 40 to 60 years of age, with men and women equally affected.

Pathophysiology

Pheochromocytomas cause excessive production of catecholamines attributable to autonomous functioning of the tumor. Approximately 5% of people with pheochromocytomas have no symptoms because the tumor appears to be nonfunctioning; however, these tumors can release catecholamines in response to stressors, such as abdominal surgery.

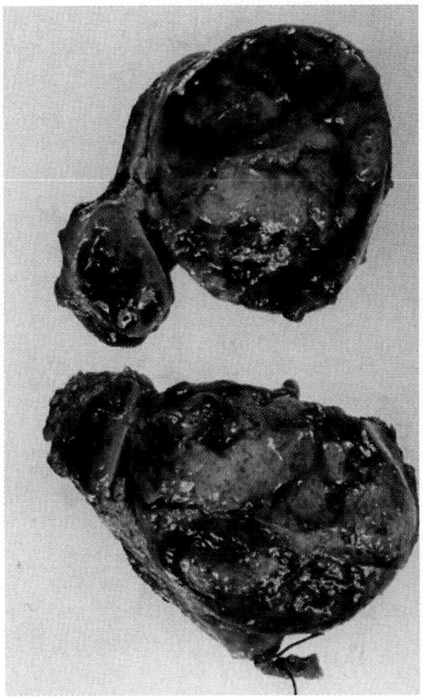

FIG. 20-18 Pheochromocytoma. Gross appearance of adrenal pheochromocytoma. (From Rosai J: *Akerman's surgical pathology*, ed 8, St Louis, 1996, Mosby.)

Clinical Manifestations

The clinical manifestations of a pheochromocytoma are related to the chronic effects of catecholamine secretion and include persistent hypertension associated with diaphoresis, tachycardia, and palpitations. Hypertension is a result of increased peripheral vascular resistance and may be sustained or paroxysmal. Headaches appear because of sudden changes in catecholamine levels in the blood, affecting cerebral blood flow. Hypermetabolism is related to chronic activation of sympathetic receptors in adipocytes, hepatocytes, and other tissues. Glucose intolerance may occur because of catecholamine-induced inhibition of insulin release by the pancreas. Complaints of warmth, heat intolerance, and weight loss are common despite a normal or an increased appetite. Other symptoms of catecholamine excess include excessive sweating, palpitations and tachycardia, and gastrointestinal alterations, especially constipation.

An acute episode of hypertension related to hypersecretion of catecholamines may follow specific events. Exercise, excessive ingestion of tyrosine-containing foods (aged cheese, red wine, beer, yogurt), ingestion of caffeine-containing foods, external pressure on the tumor, and induction of anesthesia all can increase secretion of catecholamines by the tumor.

These tumors tend to be extremely vascular and can rupture. Such an event can cause massive and potentially fatal hemorrhage. Rupture of a pheochromocytoma is characterized by a sudden, unexplained decrease in blood pressure; sudden, severe abdominal pain; and a rigid abdomen.

Evaluation and Treatment

A diagnosis of pheochromocytoma is made when increased catecholamine production is demonstrated in the blood or urine. Individuals with this disorder can have total urine catecholamine levels above 250 mg/day. After elevation of urinary or plasma catecholamines is documented, the site of the tumor is determined using radiographic techniques and surgical exploration of the abdomen. Because of the possibility of metastasis, whole-body scanning may be done.

The usual treatment of pheochromocytoma is surgical excision of the tumor. Medical therapy is used to stabilize blood pressure before surgery. Drugs used include α-adrenergic blocking agents and, possibly later, β-adrenergic blocking agents.[119]

SUMMARY REVIEW

Mechanisms of Hormonal Alterations

1. Abnormalities in endocrine function may be caused by hypersecretion or hyposecretion of hormones, causing alterations in normal hormone levels.
2. Endocrine abnormalities also may be caused by alterations in receptor function through a variety of mechanisms: (a) a decrease in number of receptors, (b) receptor insensitivity to the hormone, (c) antibodies against specific receptors, and (d) defects in second messenger generation or postreceptor defects.
3. Abnormally high levels of circulating hormones sometimes are caused by hormone release from tissues outside the endocrine system (ectopic foci), which may not respond to normal feedback mechanisms, in which case they are said to function autonomously.

Alterations of the Hypothalamic–Pituitary System

1. Dysfunction in the release of hypothalamic hormones probably is related to interruption of the connection between the hypothalamus and pituitary—namely, the pituitary stalk.
2. Disorders of the posterior pituitary include syndrome of inappropriate antidiuretic hormone (SIADH) secretion and diabetes insipidus. SIADH secretion is characterized by abnormally high ADH secretion; diabetes insipidus is characterized by abnormally low ADH secretion.
3. In SIADH, high ADH levels interfere with renal free water clearance, leading to hyponatremia and hypoosmolality. SIADH secretion is associated with certain forms of cancer, apparently because of ectopic secretion of ADH by tumor cells.
4. Diabetes insipidus may be neurogenic, caused by insufficient amounts of ADH, or nephrogenic, caused by an inadequate response to ADH. Its principal clinical features are polyuria and polydipsia.
5. Hypopituitarism is dysfunction of the anterior pituitary that causes failure of hormonal functions. Symptoms may be mild to severe.
6. The most common cause of hypopituitarism is a tumor of the pituitary or subsequent treatment of the tumor (surgical or radiation therapy).
7. Hyperpituitarism is caused by pituitary adenomas. These are usually benign, slow-growing tumors that arise from cells of the anterior pituitary.
8. Expansion of a pituitary adenoma causes both neurologic and secretory effects. Pressure from the expanding tumor causes hyposecretion of cells, dysfunction of the optic chiasm (leading to visual disturbances), and dysfunction of the hypothalamus and some cranial nerves.
9. Hypersecretion of growth hormone (GH) causes acromegaly, in which GH secretion becomes high and unpredictable. Pituitary adenoma is the most common cause of acromegaly.
10. Prolonged, abnormally high levels of GH lead to proliferation of body and connective tissues. Renal, thyroid, and reproductive dysfunction develop slowly, together with a change in bony proportions.

Alterations of Thyroid Function

1. Thyrotoxicosis is a general condition in which thyroid hormone (TH) levels are elevated and produce an exaggerated physiologic response in tissues. The condition can be caused by a variety of specific diseases, each of which has its own pathophysiology and course of treatment.
2. In general, hyperthyroidism has a range of endocrine, reproductive, gastrointestinal, integumentary, and ocular manifestations. These are caused by increased circulating levels of TH and by stimulation of the sympathetic division of the autonomic nervous system.
3. Graves disease, the most common form of hyperthyroidism, is caused by an autoimmune mechanism that overrides normal mechanisms for control of TH secretion.
4. Manifestations of Graves disease can include symptoms of hyperthyroidism, diffuse thyroid enlargement, disorders of the skin, and enlargement of extraoccular muscles.
5. The cutaneous manifestation of Graves disease is pretibial myxedema, a condition characterized by subcutaneous swelling of the legs and, occasionally, the hands.
6. Ocular manifestations of Graves disease are caused by hyperactivity of the sympathetic division of the autonomic nervous system and by immune-induced infiltration of extraoccular muscles.
7. Toxic nodular goiter and toxic multinodular goiter occur when hyperplastic regions of the thyroid become autonomous.
8. Toxic nodular goiters are follicular-cell adenomas that produce symptoms similar to those of Graves disease.
9. Toxic multinodular goiters result from multiple functioning adenomas.
10. Thyrotoxic crisis is a severe form of hyperthyroidism that often is associated with physiologic stress. Without treatment, death occurs quickly.

11. Hypothyroidism is caused by deficient production of TH by the thyroid gland. The condition may be primary or secondary.
12. Primary hypothyroidism transiently occurs in either subacute or painless thyroiditis and spontaneous resolution of hypothyroidism is nearly universal. Chronic lymphocytic thyroiditis, an autoimmune disease, is associated with permanent hypothyroidism.
13. Subacute thyroiditis, a form of hypothyroidism, is a self-limited nonbacterial inflammation of the thyroid gland. The inflammatory process damages follicular cells, causing leakage of triiodothyronine (T_3) and thyroxine (T_4). Hyperthyroidism then is followed by transient hypothyroidism, which is corrected by cellular repair and a return to normal levels in the thyroid.
14. Autoimmune thyroiditis is associated with infiltration or fibrosis of the thyroid, circulating thyroid antibodies, and gradual loss of thyroid function. Autoimmune thyroiditis occurs in those individuals with a genetic susceptibility to an autoimmune mechanism that causes thyroid damage and eventual hypothyroidism.
15. Hypothyroidism also can be caused by hypothalamic–pituitary dysfunction in which TRH and TSH are not produced in sufficient amounts.
16. Thyroid carcinoma is a relatively rare cancer. The most consistent causal risk factor associated with thyroid carcinoma is exposure to ionizing radiation, especially in childhood.
17. Hypothyroidism affects all body systems. Symptoms depend on the degree of TH deficiency. Common manifestations include decreased energy metabolism and heat production.
18. Myxedema is the characteristic sign of hypothyroidism. Myxedema is caused by alterations in connective tissue with water-binding proteins. The excess water leads to edema and thickened mucous membranes.
19. Myxedema coma is a severe form of hypothyroidism, which may be life threatening without emergency medical treatment.

Alterations of Parathyroid Function

1. Hyperparathyroidism may be primary or secondary and is characterized by greater than normal secretion of parathyroid hormone (PTH).
2. Primary hyperparathyroidism is caused by an interruption of the normal mechanisms that regulate calcium and PTH levels. Manifestations include chronic hypercalcemia, increased bone resorption, and hypercalciuria.
3. Secondary hyperparathyroidism is a compensatory response to hypocalcemia and often occurs with chronic renal failure.
4. Hypoparathyroidism, defined by abnormally low PTH levels, is caused by thyroid surgery, autoimmunity, or genetic mechanisms.
5. The lack of circulating PTH in hypoparathyroidism causes depressed serum calcium levels, increased serum phosphate levels, decreased bone resorption, and eventual hypocalciuria.

Dysfunction of the Endocrine Pancreas: Diabetes Mellitus

1. Diabetes mellitus is a complex syndrome that causes a number of physiologic changes, some of which are metabolic processes and others of which are vascular.
2. A diagnosis of diabetes mellitus is based on elevated plasma glucose concentrations. Classic signs and symptoms may be present as well.
3. The two most common types of diabetes mellitus are type 1 and type 2.
4. Type 1 diabetes mellitus is characterized by a lack of insulin and a relative excess of glucagon, which causes improper metabolism of fat, protein, and carbohydrates. There is an immune type and a nonimmune type. The immune type is associated with autoantibodies.
5. Type 1 diabetes mellitus is diagnosed most commonly among whites younger than 30 years of age.
6. In type 1 diabetes mellitus, B cells are destroyed, and islet cell autoantibodies (ICAs and GAD_{65}) appear. The function of these antibodies is unknown, and they tend to disappear with time.
7. Type 1 diabetes mellitus seems to be caused by a gradual process of autoimmune destruction in genetically susceptible individuals.
8. In type 1 diabetes mellitus, lack of insulin and excess glucagon cause hyperglycemia and subsequent loss of glucose in the urine. Polyuria and polydipsia result from osmotic diuresis. Weight loss is a classical symptom of type 1 diabetes.
9. Ketoacidosis is caused by abnormally low levels of insulin and increased levels of glucagon and is associated with increased levels of glucose and ketones.
10. Type 2 diabetes mellitus is caused by genetic susceptibility that is triggered by environmental factors. The most compelling environmental risk factor is obesity.
11. In the obese, insulin has a diminished ability to influence glucose uptake and metabolism.
12. In type 2 diabetes, amyloid deposits in the islets, fatty atrophy of the pancreas and liver, and vascular sclerosis (causing ischemia) generally are present.
13. Some insulin production continues in type 2 diabetes mellitus, but the weight and number of B cells decrease.
14. Because the ratio of A cells to B cells may be normal in the individual with type 2 diabetes, hypotheses suggest that the disease is caused by dysfunctional levels of both insulin and glucagon.
15. Acute complications of diabetes mellitus include hypoglycemia, diabetic ketoacidosis, hyperosmolar hyperglycemic nonketotic syndrome, the Somogyi effect, and the dawn phenomenon.
16. Hypoglycemia is a lowered blood glucose level, which may be related to exogenous, endogenous, or functional causes.
17. Symptoms of hypoglycemia are divided into adrenergic, due to activation of the sympathetic nervous system, and neuroglycopenic, reflecting defective CNS metabolism due to impaired energy generation.
18. Diabetic ketoacidosis develops when there is an absolute or relative deficiency of insulin and an increase in the insulin counterregulatory hormones of catecholamines, cortisol, glucagon, and growth hormone.
19. Hyperosmolar hyperglycemic nonketotic syndrome (HHNKS) is pathophysiologically similar to diabetic ketoacidosis, although levels of free fatty acids are lower in HHNKS and lack of ketosis indicates that some level of insulin is present.
20. The Somogyi effect is a combination of hypoglycemia with rebound hyperglycemia. It is most common in persons with type 1 diabetes mellitus and in children.
21. The dawn phenomenon is an early morning rise in glucose levels caused by nocturnal elevations of growth hormone.

22. Chronic sequelae of diabetes mellitus include diabetic neuropathies, microvascular disease (e.g., retinopathy, nephropathy), macrovascular disease (e.g., coronary artery disease, stroke, peripheral vascular disease), and infection.
23. Diabetic neuropathies may be caused by vascular or metabolic mechanisms or a combination of both.
24. In diabetic neuropathy, axonal and Schwann cell degeneration and metabolic aberrations are related to abnormalities in motor nerve conduction velocity, electromyography, and sensory perception.
25. Microangiopathy is caused by thickening of the capillary basement membrane and eventual decreased tissue perfusion, affecting the microcirculation.
26. Diabetic retinopathy is caused in part by retinal ischemia related to microvascular occlusion associated with diabetes mellitus.
27. Diabetic nephropathy is related to glomerular enlargement and glomerular basement membrane thickening, which in turn cause diffuse intercapillary glomerulosclerosis.
28. Macrovascular disease associated with diabetes mellitus probably is related to the proliferation of fibrous plaques in the arterial wall and to elevated lipid levels.
29. Incidence of coronary heart disease, peripheral vascular disease, and stroke is greater in persons with diabetes than in nondiabetic individuals.
30. Individuals with diabetes are at risk for a variety of infections.
31. Infection may be related to sensory impairment and resulting injury, hypoxia, increased proliferation of pathogens in elevated concentrations of glucose, decreased blood supply associated with vascular damage, and impaired white cell function.

Alterations of Adrenal Function

1. Disorders of the adrenal cortex are related to hyperfunction or hypofunction. No known disorders are associated with hypofunction of the adrenal medulla, but medullary hyperfunction causes clinically defined syndromes.
2. Hypercortisolism is divided into ACTH-dependent (Cushing disease or ectopic ACTH syndrome) and ACTH-independent (adrenal adenoma or adenocarcinoma) mechanisms.
3. Cushing disease is most commonly due to an ACTH-secreting pituitary microadenoma and either ectopic CRH or ACTH production results in a similar clinical syndrome. Cushing syndrome is due to autonomous cortisol production by adrenal tissue.
4. Individuals with Cushing disease lose diurnal and circadian patterns of ACTH and cortisol secretion, and they lack the ability to increase secretion of these hormones in response to a stressor. Individuals experience weight gain, glucose intolerance, protein wasting, bone disease, hyperpigmentation, and immune suppression.
5. Excessive aldosterone secretion causes hyperaldosteronism, which may be primary or secondary. Primary hyperaldosteronism is caused by an abnormality of the adrenal cortex. Secondary hyperaldosteronism involves an extraadrenal stimulus, driven by the renin-angiotensin system.
6. Primary hyperaldosteronism usually is caused by an adrenal adenoma or bilateral nodular hyperplasia. The condition is characterized by hypertension, hypokalemia, renal potassium wasting, and neuromuscular manifestations.
7. Secondary hyperaldosterone secretion is related to a variety of conditions associated with elevated renin release and activation of angiotensin. These include decreased circulating blood volume and decreased renal blood supply, elevated estrogen levels, Bartter syndrome, and renin-secreting tumors.
8. Hyperaldosteronism promotes increased sodium reabsorption, corresponding hypervolemia, increased extracellular volume (which is variable), and hypokalemia related to renal reabsorption of sodium.
9. Adrenal tumors, either adenomas or carcinomas, can autonomously secrete androgens or estrogens.
10. Hypofunction of the adrenal cortex can affect glucocorticoid or mineralocorticoid secretion or both. Hypofunction can be caused by a deficiency of ACTH or by a primary deficiency in the gland itself.
11. Hypocortisolism (low levels of cortisol) is caused by inadequate adrenal stimulation by ACTH or by primary cortisol hyposecretion. Primary adrenal insufficiency is termed Addison disease.
12. Addison disease is characterized by elevated ACTH levels with inadequate corticosteroid synthesis and output.
13. Causes of Addison disease include idiopathic autoimmune disease, tuberculosis of the adrenal gland, familial adrenal insufficiency, amyloidosis, metastatic destruction of the adrenal glands, and adrenal hemorrhage.
14. Secondary hypercortisolism is characterized by low to absent ACTH levels, leading to inadequate adrenal stimulation, adrenal atrophy, and decreased corticosteroidogenesis. The most common cause is withdrawal of exogenous administration of glucocorticoids.
15. Manifestations of Addison disease are related to hypocortisolism and hypoaldosteronism. Symptoms include weakness, fatigability, hypoglycemia and related metabolic problems, lowered response to stressors, vitiligo, hyperpigmentation, and manifestations of hypovolemia and hyperkalemia.
16. Hyperfunction of the adrenal medulla is caused by a pheochromocytoma, which is a catecholamine-producing tumor. Symptoms of catecholamine excess are related to their sympathetic nervous system effects and include hypertension, palpitations, tachycardia, glucose intolerance, excessive sweating, and constipation.

KEY TERMS

Acromegaly, *630*
Addison disease (primary adrenal insufficiency), *661*
Autoimmune thyroiditis (Hashimoto disease, chronic lymphocyte thyroiditis), *635*
Cushing disease, *657*
Cushing syndrome, *657*
Dawn phenomenon, *653*
Diabetes insipidus, *627*
Diabetes mellitus, *640*
Diabetic ketoacidosis (DKA), *649*
Diabetic nephropathy, *653*
Diabetic neuropathy, *653*
Diabetic retinopathy, *654*
Feminization, *661*
Giantism, *630*
Glycosylated hemoglobin, *642*

KEY TERMS—cont'd

REFERENCES

1. Fujimoto WY: The importance of insulin resistance in the pathogenesis of type 2 diabetes, *Am J Med* 108(suppl 16a):9S, 2000.
2. Chrousos GP: A new 'new' syndrome in the world: is multiple postreceptor steroid hormone resistance due to a coregulator defect? *J Clin Endocrinol Metab* 84:4450, 1999.
3. Nagaya T, Seo H: Molecular basis of resistance to thyroid hormone (RTH), *Endocr J* 45:709, 1998.
4. Haycock GB: The syndrome of inappropriate secretion of antidiuretic hormone, *Pediatr Nephrol* 9(3):375, 1995.
5. Keenan AM: Syndrome of inappropriate secretion of antidiuretic hormone in malignancy, *Semin Oncol Nurs* 15:160, 1999.
6. Kovacs L, Lichardus B: *Vasopressin: disturbed secretion and its effects*, Boston, 1989, Dordrecht.
7. Labhart A: *Clinical endocrinology: theory and practice*, Berlin, 1986, Springer-Verlag.
8. Riggs AT et al: A review of disorders of water homeostasis in psychiatric patients, *Psychosomatics* 32(2):133, 1991.
9. Gill G, Leese G: Hyponatremia: biochemical and clinical perspectives, *Postgrad Med J* 74:516, 1998.
10. Blevins LS Jr, Want GS: Diabetes insipidus, *Crit Care Med* 20(1):69, 1992.
11. Goldman L, Bennett JC, editors: *Cecil textbook of medicine*, ed 21, Philadelphia, 2000, W.B. Saunders.
12. Reichlin S, editor: *The neurohypophysis*, New York, 1984, Plenum.
13. Tetiker T, Sert M, Kocak M: Efficiency of indapamide in central diabetes insipidus, *Arch Intern Med* 159(17):2085, 1999.
14. Reid RL, Quigley ME, Yen SSC: Pituitary apoplexy, *Arch Neurol* 42:712, 1985.
15. Aron DC, Howlett TA: Pituitary incidentalomas, *Endocrinol Metab Clin North Am* 29:205, 2000.
16. Aron DC, Tyrrell JB, Wilson CB: Pituitary tumors: current concepts in diagnosis and management, *West J Med* 162(4):340, 1995.
17. Marazuela M et al: Recovery of visual and endocrine function following transsphenoidal surgery of large nonfunctioning pituitary adenomas, *J Endocrinol Invest* 17:703, 1994.
18. Cook DM, Ludlam WH, Cook MB: The adult growth hormone deficiency syndrome, *Ann Int Med* 45:297, 2000.
19. Murray RD et al: Influences on quality of life in GH deficient adults and their effect on response to treatment, *Clin Endocrinol Oxf* 51:565, 1999.
20. Trainer PJ et al: Treatment of acromegaly with the growth hormone-receptor antagonist pegvisomant, *New Eng J Med* 342(16):1171, 2000.
21. Melmed S: Acromegaly, *N Engl J Med* 322:966, 1990.
22. Melmed S et al: Clinical review 75: recent advances in pathogenesis, diagnosis, and management of acromegaly, *J Clin Endocrinol Metab* 80(12):3395, 1995.
23. Ezrin C et al: *Pituitary disease*, Boca Raton, Fla, 1980, CRC Press.
24. Bengtsson BA, Eden S, Ernst I: Epidemiology and long-term survival in acromegaly: a study of 166 cases diagnosed between 1955 and 1984, *Acta Med Scand* 223:327, 1988.
25. Hennessey JV, Jackson IM: Clinical features and differential diagnosis of pituitary tumors with emphasis on acromegaly, *Baillieres Clin Endocrinol Metab* 9(2):271, 1995.
26. Newman CB: Medical therapy for acromegaly, *Endocrinol Metab Clin Clin North Am* 28:171, 1999.
27. Xu RK et al: Pituitary prolactin-secreting tumor formation: recent developments, *Biol Signals Recept* 9(1):1, 2000.
28. Plymate SR, Jones RE: Testicular function in critical illness. In Ober KP, editor: *Contemporary Endocrinology: Endocrinology of Critical Illness,* pp 271, Totowa, NJ, 1997, Humana Press.
29. Luciano AA: Clinical presentation of hyperprolactinemia, *J Reprod Med* 44:1085, 1999.
30. Freda PU et al: Long-term treatment of prolactin-secreting macroadenomas with pergolide, *J Clin Endocrinol Metab* 85:8, 2000.
31. Braverman LE: Evolution of a thyroid status in patients with thyrotoxicosis, *Clin Chem* 42(1):174, 1996.
32. Gough SCL: The genetics of Graves disease, *Endocrinol Metab Clin North Am* 29:225, 2000.
33. McDougall IR: Graves disease, *Med Clin North Am* 75(1):79, 1991.
34. Tonacchera M et al: Patient with monoclonal gammopathy, thyrotoxicosis, pretibial myxedema, and thyroid-associated ophthalmopathy; demonstration of direct binding of autoantibodies in the thyrotropin receptor, *Eur J Endocrinol* 134(1):97, 1996.
35. Bahn RS: Understanding the immunology of Graves ophthalmopathy: is it an autoimmune disease? *Endocrinol Metab Clin North Am* 29:287, 2000.
36. Braverman LE, Utiger RD: *Werner and Ingbar's The thyroid: a fundamental and clinical text*, ed 8, Philadelphia, 2000, Lippincott Williams & Wilkins.
37. Gavin LA: Thyroid crises, *Med Clin North Am* 75(1):179, 1991.
38. Smallridge RC: Metabolic and anatomic thyroid emergencies: a review, *Crit Care Med* 20(2):276, 1992.
39. Schubert MF, Kountz DS: Thyroiditis: a disease of many faces, *Postgrad Med* 98(2):101, 1995.
40. Barbesino G, Chiovato L: The genetics of Hashimoto's disease, *Endocrinol Metab Clin North Am* 29:357, 2000.
41. DeGroot LJ: *Endocrinology*, ed 3, Philadelphia, 1995, W.B. Saunders.

42. American Cancer Society: Estimated new cancer cases by gender, US, 2001, *CA Cancer J Clin* 51:16, 2001.
43. Mizuno T et al: Preferential induction of RET/PTC1 rearrangement by x-ray irradiation, *Oncogene* 19:438, 2000.
44. Farahati T et al: Inverse association between the age at the time of radiation exposure and extent of disease in cases of radiation-induced childhood thyroid carcinoma in Belarus, *Cancer* 88:1470, 2000.
45. Sheaves R et al: *Clinical endocrine oncology*, Oxford, 1997, Blackwell.
46. Ayala AR: When to treat mild hypothyroidism, *Endocrinol Metab Clin North Am* 29:399, 2000.
47. Greenspan FS: *Basic and clinical endocrinology*, Norwalk, Conn, 1991, Appleton & Lange.
48. Dwarakanathan AA et al: Isolated familial hyperparathyroidism with a novel mutation of the MEN1 gene, *Endocr Pract* 6:268, 2000.
49. Walgenbach S, Hommel G, Junginer T: Outcome after surgery for primary hyperparathyroidism: ten year prospective follow-up study, *World J Surg* 24:564, 2000.
50. Palmer JP, Lernmark A: Pathophysiology of type I (insulin-dependent) diabetes. In Porte D, Sherwin RS, editors: *Diabetes mellitus*, ed 5, New York, 1997, Elsevier.
51. National Diabetes Data Group: Classification and diagnosis of diabetes mellitus and other categories of glucose intolerance, *Diabetes* 28:1039, 1979.
52. Gavin J et al: Report of the expert committee on the diagnosis and classification of diabetes mellitus, *Diabetic Care* 20(7):1183, 1997.
53. The DECODE Study Group, European Diabetes Epidemiology Group, Diabetes Epidemiology Collaborative Analysis of Diagnostic Criteria in Europe: Glucose tolerance and mortality: comparison of WHO and American Diabetes Association diagnostic criteria, *Lancet* 354:617, 1999.
54. Mitrakou A et al: Role of reduced suppression of glucose production and diminished early insulin release in impaired glucose tolerance, *N Engl J Med* 326(1):22, 1992.
55. Fajans SS: Classification and diagnosis of diabetes. In Rifkin H, Porte D, editors: *Diabetes mellitus theory and practice*, ed 4, New York, 1990, Elsevier.
56. Bennett PH: Epidemiology of diabetes mellitus. In Porte D, Sherwin RS, editors: *Diabetes mellitus*, ed 5, New York, 1997, Elsevier.
57. Bell DSH: Should anti-glutamic acid decarboxylase antibody levels be determined in new-onset diabetes? *Endocr Prct* 6:214, 2000.
58. Masuda M et al: Autoantibodies to IA-2 in insulin-dependent diabetes mellitus. Measurements with a new immunoprecipitation assay, *Clin Chem Acta* 291:53, 2000.
59. Huang W et al: Although DR3-DQB1*0201 may be associated with multiple component diseases of the autoimmune polyglandular syndromes, the human leukocyte antigen DR4-DQB1*0302 haplotype is implicated only in beta-cell autoimmunity, *J Clin Endocrinol Metab* 81(7):2559, 1996.
60. Roep BO et al: HLA-associated inverse correlation between T cell and antibody responsiveness to islet autoantigen in recent-onset insulin-dependent diabetes mellitus, *Eur J Immunol* 26(6):1285, 1996.
61. Santiago J et al, editors: *Medical management of insulin-dependent (type I) diabetes*, ed 2, Alexandria, Va, 1994, American Diabetes Association.
62. Diabetes Control and Complications Trial Research Group: The effect of intensive treatment of diabetes on the development and progression of long-term complications in insulin-dependent diabetes mellitus, *N Engl J Med* 329:977, 1993.
63. Vajo Z, Duckworth WC: Genetically engineered insulin analogs: diabetes in the new mellenium, *Pharmacol Rev* 52:1, 2000.
64. Gale EA: A randomized, controlled trial comparing insulin lispro with human soluble insulin in patients with type 1 diabetes on intensified insulin therapy. The UK trial group, *Diabet Med* 17:209, 2000.
65. Gillies PS et al: Insulin glargine, *Drugs* 59:253, 2000.
66. American Diabetes Association: Clinical practice recommendations, *Diabetes Care* 19(suppl 1):S1, 1996.
67. American Diabetes Association: Nutritional recommendations and principles for people with diabetes mellitus, *Diabetes Care* 23(suppl 1):S43, 2000.
68. Jones, RE: Management of the exercising diabetic. In Meikle AW, editor: *Contemporary endocrinology: hormone replacement therapy*, p 209, Totowa, NJ, 1999, Humana Press.
69. Sutherland DER et al: Pancreas transplantation. In Porte D, Sherwin RS, editors: *Diabetes mellitus*, ed 5, New York, 1997, Elsevier.
70. Larsen JL, Strata RJ: Consequences of pancreas transplantation, *J Investig Med* 42(4):622, 1995.
71. Shapiro AMJ et al: Islet transplantation in seven patients with type 1 diabetes mellitus using a glucocorticoid-free immunosuppressive regimen, *N Engl J Med* 343:230, 2000.
72. Ingle KL: Calling all physicians for the diabetes prevention trial-type I, *Diabetes Care* 17:1240, 1994.
73. Kahn SE, Porte D: Pathophysiology of type II (noninsulin-dependent) diabetes mellitus: implications for treatment. In Porte D, Sherwin RS, editors: *Diabetes mellitus*, ed 5, New York, 1997, Elsevier.
74. Larsson H, Ahren B: Islet cell dysfunction in insulin resistance involves impaired insulin secretion and increased glucagon secretion in postmenopausal women with impaired glucose tolerance, *Diabetes Care* 23:650, 2000.
75. Raskin P et al, editors: *Medical management of noninsulin-dependent (type II) diabetes*, ed 3, Alexandria, Va, 1994, American Diabetes Association.
76. Westermark P: Pathology of the pancreas in diabetes mellitus. In Porte D, Sherwin RS, editors: *Diabetes mellitus*, ed 5, New York, 1997, Elsevier.
77. Clark A et al: Autoantibodies to islet amyloid polypeptide in diabetes, *Diabetic Med* 8(7):668, 1991.
78. Bellentani S et al: Prevalence of and risk factors for hepatic steatosis in Northern Italy, *Ann Int Med* 132:11207, 2000.
79. World Health Organization (WHO) Study Group: Diabetes mellitus report of a WHO study group, *Tech Rep Series* 727:1, 1985.
80. Cefalu WT: Insulin resistance. In Leahy JL, Clark NG, Cefalu WT, editors: *Medical management of diabetes mellitus,* p 57, New York, 2000, Marcel Dekker.
81. Hsueh WA, Law RE: Insulin signaling in the arterial wall, *Am J Cardiol* 84:21J, 1999.
82. Dunaif A: Insulin action in the polycystic ovary syndrome, *Endocrinol Metab Clin North Am* 28:341, 1999.
83. Harris MI: Epidemiologic studies on the pathogenesis of noninsulin-dependent diabetes mellitus (NIDDM), *Clin Invest Med* 18:231, 1995.
84. DeFronzo RA, Goodman AM, The Multicenter Metformin Study Group: Efficacy of metformin in patients with non-insulin-dependent diabetes mellitus, *N Engl J Med* 333:541, 1995.
85. Komers R, Vrana A: Thiazolidinediones—tools for the research of metabolic syndrome X, *Physiol Res* 47:215, 1998.
86. DeFronzo RA: Pharmacologic therapy for type 2 diabetes mellitus, *Ann Int Med* 131:281, 1999.
87. Manson JE et al: A prospective study of exercise and incidence of diabetes among US male physicians, *JAMA* 268(1):63, 1992.
88. Cryer PE, Gerich JE: Hypoglycemia in insulin-dependent diabetes mellitus: insulin excess and defective glucose counter-regulation. In Porte D, Sherwin RS, editors: *Diabetes mellitus*, ed 5, New York, 1997, Elsevier.
89. Veneman T et al: Induction of hypoglycemia unawareness by asymptomatic nocturnal hypoglycemia, *Diabetes* 42:1233, 1993.
90. Delionback, EE: Diabetic ketoacidosis, In Porte D, Sherwin RS, editors: *Diabetes mellitus*, ed 5, New York, 1997, Elsevier.
91. Matz R: Hyperosmolar nonacidotic diabetes. In Porte D, Sherwin RS, editors: *Diabetes mellitus*, ed 5, New York, 1997, Elsevier.
92. Levin ME, Sicard GA: Peripheral vascular disease in the person with diabetes. In Porte D, Sherwin RS, editors: *Diabetes mellitus*, ed 5, New York, 1997, Elsevier.
93. Skyler JS: Relation of glycemic control of diabetes mellitus to chronic complications. In Porte D, Sherwin RS, editors: *Diabetes mellitus*, ed 5, New York, 1997, Elsevier.
94. Greene DA et al: Diabetic neuropathy. In Porte D, Sherwin RS, editors: *Diabetes mellitus*, ed 5, New York, 1997, Elsevier.
95. Ohkabo Y et al: Intensive insulin therapy prevents the progression of diabetes macrovascular complications in Japanese patients with non-

insulin dependent diabetes mellitus: a randomized, prospective six year study, *Diabetes Res Clin Pract* 28:103, 1995.

96. Nathan DM: Long-term complications of diabetes mellitus, *N Engl J Med* 328(23):1676, 1993.
97. Hsu CY et al: Diabetes, hemoglobin A(1c), cholesterol, and the risk of moderate chronic renal insufficiency in an ambulatory population, *Am J Kidney* 36(2):272, 2000.
98. Odoni G, Ritz E: Diabetic nephropathy—what have we learned in the last three decades? *J Nephrol* 12(suppl 2):S120, 1999.
99. Rossert J, Terraz-Durasnel C, Brideau G: Growth factors, cytokines, and renal fibrosis during the course of diabetic nephropathy, *Diabetes Metab* 26(suppl 4):16, 2000.
100. Harris RD et al: Global glomerular sclerosis and glomerular arteriolar hyalinosis in insulin dependent diabetes, *Kidney Int* 40(1):107, 1991.
101. American Diabetes Association: Consensus statement: treatment of hypertension in diabetes, *Diabetes Care* 16:1394, 1993.
102. Steffes MW, Mauer SM: Diabetic nephropathy: a disease causing and complicated by hypertension, *Clin Chem* 37(10, pt 2):1838, 1991.
103. Fein FS, Scheuer J: Heart disease in diabetes. In Rifkin H, Porte D, editors: *Diabetes mellitus theory and practice*, ed 4, New York, 1990, Elsevier.
104. Bell DSH: Stroke in the diabetic patient, *Diabetes Care* 17(3): 213, 1994.
105. UK Prospective Diabetes Study Group: Tight blood pressure control and risk of macrovascular and microvascular complications in type 2 diabetes (UKPDS 38), *Br Med J* 17:703, 1998.
106. Currie BP, Casey JI: Host defense and infections in diabetes mellitus. In Porte DP, Sherwin RS, editors: *Diabetes mellitus*, ed 5, New York, 1997, Elsevier.
107. McNicol AM: The human adrenal gland: aspects of structure, function, and pathology. In James VH, editor: *The adrenal gland*, ed 2, New York, 1992, Raven.
108. Bardin CW: *Current therapy in endocrinology and metabolism*, ed 6, St Louis, 1997, Mosby.
109. Franco-Saenz R: Diseases of the adrenal cortex. In Mulrow PJ, editor: *The adrenal gland*, New York, 1986, Elsevier.
110. Majewska MD: Steroid hormone metabolites are barbiturate-like modulators of the GABA receptor, *Science* 232:1004, 1986.
111. Wiggam MI et al: Bilateral inferior petrosal sinus sampling in the differential diagnosis of adrenocorticotropin-dependent Cushing's syndrome: a comparison with other diagnostic tests, *J Clin Endocrinol Metab* 85:1525, 2000.
112. Davies JS et al: Diagnostic dilemmas in Cushing's syndrome, *Ann Clin Biochem* 37:85, 2000.
113. Young WF Jr: Primary aldosteronism: a common and curable form of hypertension,*Cardiol Rev* 7(4):207, 1999.
114. Melby JC: Diagnosis of hyperaldosteronism, *Endocrinol Metab Clin North Am 20*(2):247, 1991.
115. Ghose RP, Hall PM, Bravo EL: Medical management of aldosterone-producing adenomas, *Ann Int Med* 131: 105, 1999.
116. Wulffraat NM, Drexhage HA, Bottazzo GF: Autoimmune aspects of Addison's disease. In James VHT, editor: *The adrenal gland*, ed 2, New York, 1992, Raven.
117. McGregor AM: Immunoendocrine interactions and autoimmunity, *N Engl J Med* 322:1739, 1990.
118. Hanna NN, Kenady DE: Hypertension in patients with pheochromocytoma, *Curr Hypertens Rep* 1(6):540, 1999.
119. Cryer PE: Pheochromocytoma, *West J Med* 156:399, 1992.

CHAPTER 21

Structure and Function of the Reproductive Systems

KRISTYNIA M. ROBINSON • SUE E. HUETHER

CHAPTER OUTLINE

The male and female reproductive systems have several anatomic and physiologic features in common. Most obvious is their major function, reproduction, through which a 23-chromosome female gamete, the **ovum,** and a 23-chromosome male gamete, the **spermatozoon (sperm cell),** unite to form a 46-chromosome zygote that is capable of developing into a new individual. The male reproductive system produces sperm and delivers them to the female reproductive tract. The female reproductive system produces the ovum and, if it is fertilized, can nurture and protect it (now called the embryo and developing fetus) and expel it at birth. These functions are determined not only by anatomic structures but also by complex hormonal, neurologic, and psychogenic factors.[1,2]

DEVELOPMENT OF THE REPRODUCTIVE SYSTEMS

The structure and function of both male and female reproductive systems depend on steroid hormones called **sex hormones.** Hormonal effects on the reproductive systems begin well before birth and continue for life.

Sexual Differentiation in Utero

During embryonic development, the initial reproductive structures of male and female embryos are homologous (the same) and consist of one pair of primary sex organs, or **gonads,** and two pairs of ducts, the mesonephric ducts (wolffian ducts) and the paramesonephric ducts (müllerian ducts) (Fig. 21-1). Both pairs of ducts empty into an opening called the *urogenital sinus.*

At about 7 to 8 weeks of gestation, the gonads of genetically male embryos produce testosterone. Under the influence of testosterone, the male gonads develop into two testes, which produce sperm. The paramesonephric ducts degenerate and the mesonephric ducts develop into the vas deferens—the two tubes that carry sperm from the testes to the urethra.

In female embryos the gonads produce the primary female sex hormone, estrogen. In the absence of testosterone the two gonads develop into ovaries, which produce ova. In females the mesonephric ducts deteriorate and the lower ends of the paramesonephric ducts join to become the uterus. The upper portions of the paramesonephric ducts develop into the fallopian (uterine) tubes. These two ducts carry ova from the ovaries to the uterus.

Like the internal reproductive structures, the external structures develop from homologous embryonic tissues. During

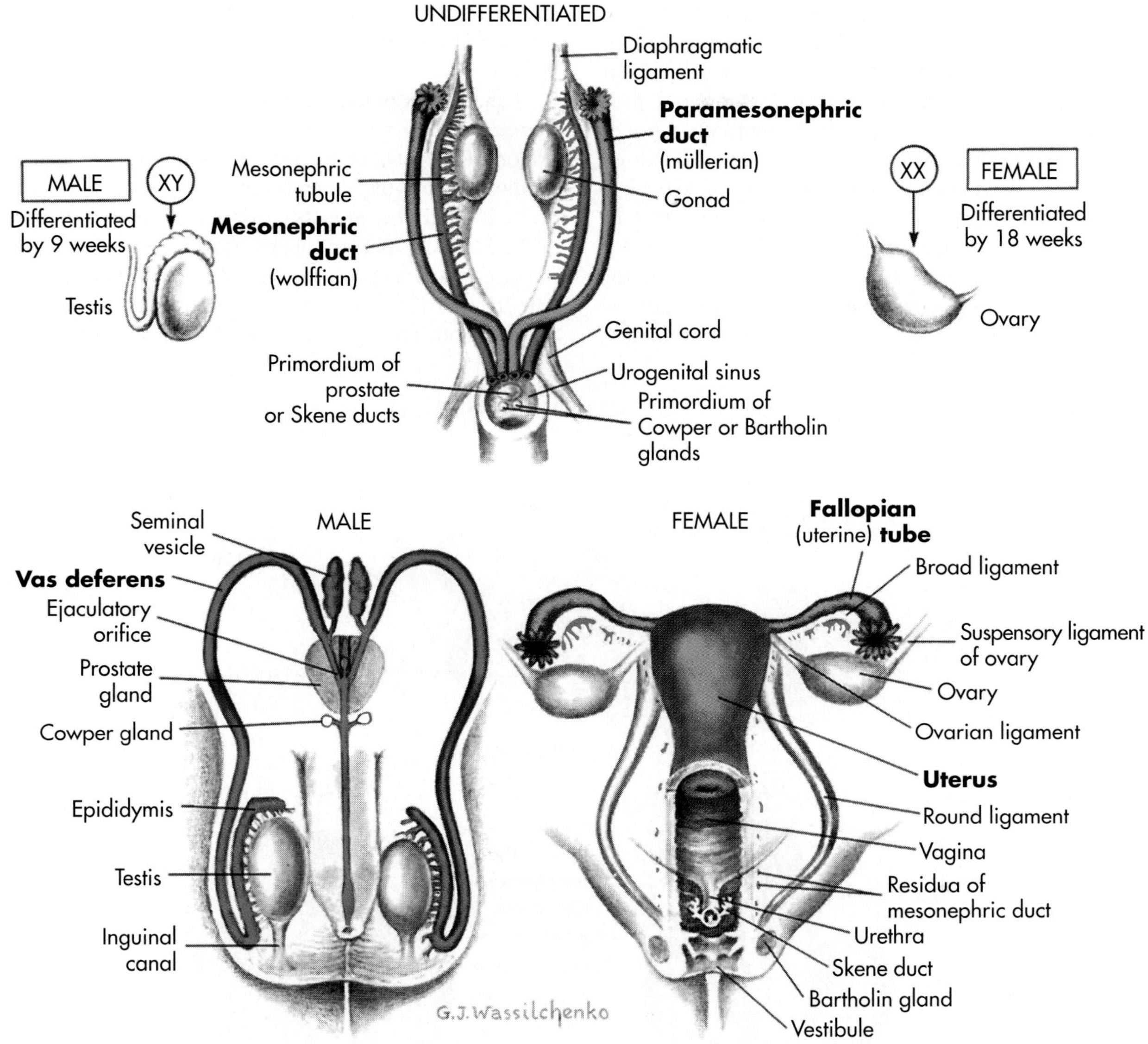

FIG. 21-1 Internal genitalia development. Embryonic and fetal development of the internal genitalia. (Modified from Lowdermilk DL, Perry SE, Bobak IM: *Maternity and women's health care,* ed 6, St Louis, 1997, Mosby.)

the first 7 to 8 weeks of gestation, both male and female embryos develop an elevated structure called the *genital tubercle.* Fig. 21-2 shows how the undifferentiated genital tubercle develops into the external reproductive organs.

Testosterone, which is converted to estrogen in the brain,[2] is necessary for the genital tubercle to differentiate into external male genitalia. By 9 months of gestation the internal and external genital structures are all present and the male gonads (the testes) have descended into the scrotum. Although male differentiation is dependent on testicular hormones and their metabolites, female differentiation occurs in the absence of testosterone; it may even occur in the absence of ovaries,[3] possibly due to the presence of placental estrogens.

Puberty

At term, a sensitive negative-feedback-system, which includes the **gonadostat** (also known as the gonadotropin-releasing hormone pulse generator), is operative in the human fetus. The gonadostat responds to high placental estrogens by releasing low levels of **gonadotropin-releasing hormone (GnRH)**. Soon after birth, sex hormones drop precipitously; negative feedback action of the sex steroids on the hypothalamus and pituitary is removed; and gonadotropins are released. During infancy and early childhood, the gonadostat is remarkably sensitive (6 to 15 times more sensitive than in the adult) to negative feedback,[1] and GnRH secretion is restrained by extraordinarily low levels of estrogen or testosterone. This feedback mechanism is probably an intrinsic neuronal inhibitory system, which suppresses endogenous GnRH secretion and gonadotropin synthesis.[1,2,4] By age 4, low levels of gonadotropins parallel low levels of sex steroids.

Between ages 8 and 12, the gonads begin to produce more sex hormones, initiating sexual maturation, or puberty. In the United States, puberty begins with **thelarche** (breast development) at about 9 years of age in white girls and 8 years of age in African-American girls. In boys it begins later, at approximately 11 years of age. Although the exact trigger for puberty is unknown, it has been linked to obesity and more recently to the presence of **leptin,** a hormone secreted from adipose tissue.[4,5] Leptin, independent of sex hormone production, influences the onset of puberty purportedly through a direct effect on the hypothalamic-pituitary-gonadal axis or indirectly through an unidentified intermediary factor.[5] Leptin levels tend to be higher in African-American girls than in white girls of the same age, which may account for timing of puberty.[6] Puberty usually lasts 2 to 3 years, longer for early developers, and is complete when the individual is capable of reproduction. Puberty is not the same as adolescence. *Puberty* refers solely to sexual maturation; *adolescence* refers to all aspects of development that occur between ages 11 and 19 years.

Puberty is a process that involves a complex series of interrelated physiologic changes leading to reproductive maturation.[4] Reproductive maturation involves the hypothalamic-pituitary axis—the central nervous system, the endocrine system, and the gonads (ovaries or testes) themselves (Fig. 21-3). As puberty approaches, three critical endocrine changes occur: (1) adrenarche, (2) decreased gonadostat sensitivity, and (3) development of a positive feedback system between gonadotropins and GnRH. **Adrenarche** is the in-

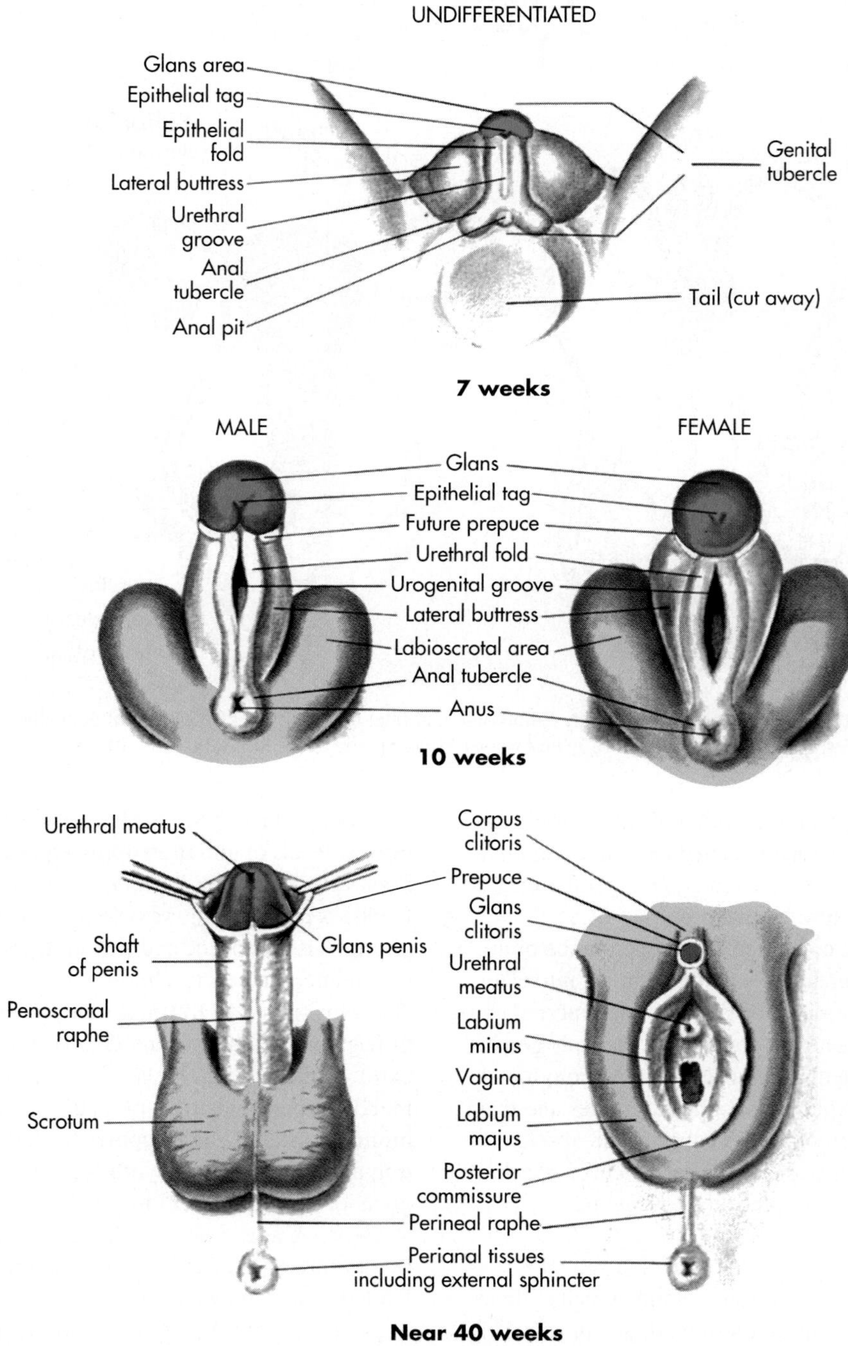

FIG. 21-2 External genitalia development. Embryonic and fetal development of the external genitalia. (Modified from Lowdermilk DL, Perry SE, Bobak IM: *Maternity and women's health care,* ed 6, St Louis, 1997, Mosby.)

creased production of adrenal androgens and occurs in both sexes.[1,2,4] The exact role that adrenarche plays in the initiation of puberty is unclear. Of interest is that adrenarche and **gonadarche** are overlapping but independent developmental processes, that is, adrenarche may occur without gonadarche, and vice versa.[4] Next, through unclear mechanisms, gonadostat sensitivity declines and a pulsatile pattern of GnRH secretion is established. This leads to the third essential endocrine change. GnRH levels increase and stimulate the anterior pituitary to produce gonadotropins: **luteinizing hormone (LH)** and **follicle-stimulating hormone (FSH)**. An increase in nocturnal LH secretion is characteristic of puberty in both boys and girls. A positive feedback loop is created with gonadotropins stimulating the gonads to produce more sex hormones. (The sex hormones are discussed in the sections on the female and male systems.)

Increased sex hormone production causes the genitalia to grow to adult proportions. It also stimulates the development of male and female secondary sex characteristics (increased body hair, voice changes, and breast development). The most important hormonal effects occur in the gonads, however. In

WHAT'S NEW? **Race and Puberty**

Girls in the United States begin puberty at a younger age. White girls enter stage 2 of breast and pubic hair development about 1 year and African-American girls about 2 years earlier than documented standards suggest. Breast development is considered the most reliable sign of pituitary-gonadal axis activation. Pubertal changes do not seem to be related to body weight or adipose tissue, but may be activated by leptin levels. Higher leptin levels are found in African-American girls and may account for earlier onset of puberty in this population. Although breast and pubic hair development may occur at a younger age, average age of menarche remains at 13 years (12.88 years) for white girls and 12 years (12.16 years) for African-American girls. An inverse relationship between the length of the maturation process and onset of puberty seems to exist. Recent studies of young boys between ages 10 and 15 years do not show a significant difference in the timing of puberty based on race.

Data from Kaplowitz PB et al: Reexamination of the age limit for defining when puberty is precocious in girls in the United States: implications for evaluation and treatment, *Pediatrics* 104(4):936, 1999; Wong WW et al: Serum leptin concentrations in Caucasian and African-American girls, *J Clin Endocrinol Metab* 83(10):3574, 1998.

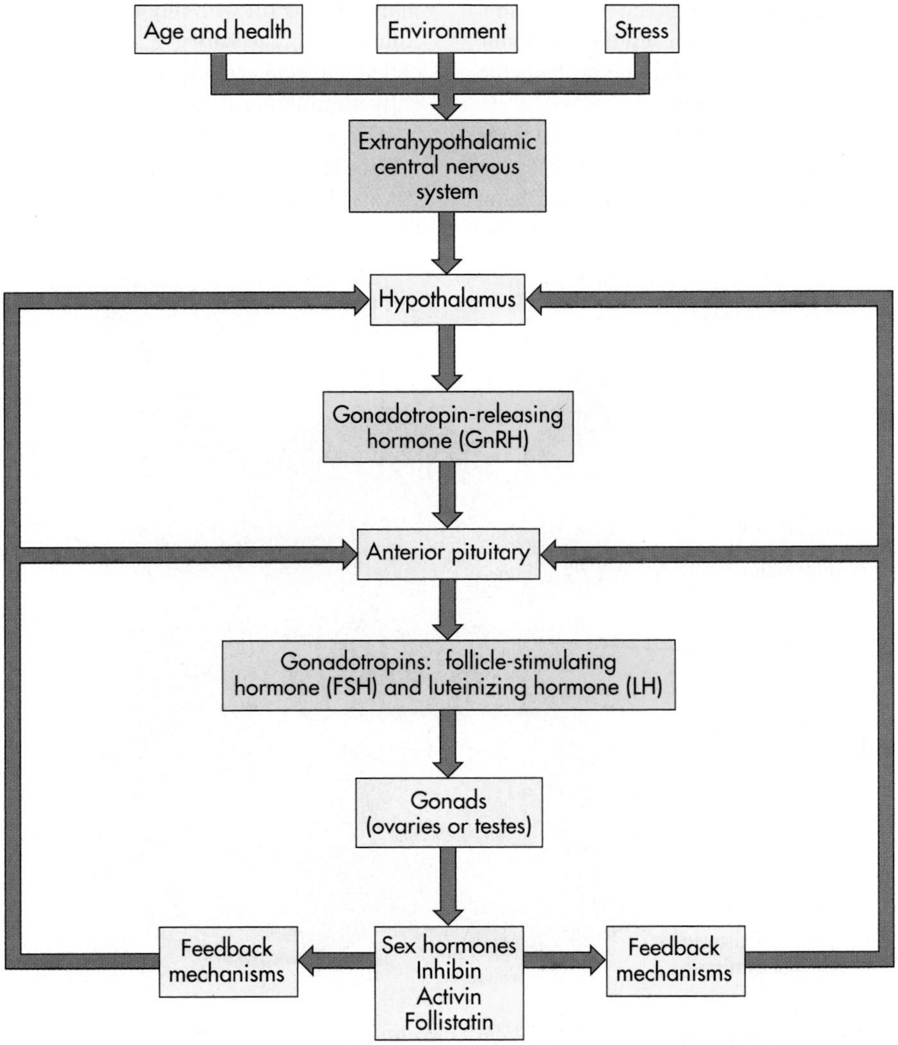

FIG. 21-3 Hormonal stimulation of the gonads. The hypothalamic-pituitary-gonadal axis.

males, the testes begin to produce mature sperm that are capable of fertilizing an ovum. Male puberty is complete with the first ejaculation that contains mature sperm. In females, the ovaries begin to release mature ova. Female puberty is complete at the time of the first ovulatory menstrual period.

THE FEMALE REPRODUCTIVE SYSTEM

The function of the reproductive system is to produce mature ova and, when they are fertilized, to protect and nourish them through embryonic and fetal life and expel them at birth. In females the most important reproductive organs, or genitalia, are internal. They are the ovaries, fallopian tubes, uterus, and vagina. These organs are essential to reproduction. The external genitalia have accessory functions. They protect body openings and play an important role in sexual functioning.

External Genitalia

Fig. 21-4 shows the external female genitalia, which are known collectively as the **vulva,** or pudendum. The **mons pubis** (veneris) is a fatty layer of tissue over the pubic symphysis (joint of the pubic bones). During puberty the mons pubis becomes covered with pubic hair, and its sebaceous and sweat glands become more active. Estrogen causes fat to be deposited under the skin, giving the mons pubis a moundlike shape. This cushion of tissue protects the pubic symphysis during sexual intercourse.

The **labia majora** (singular, **labium majus**) are two folds of skin that arise at the mons pubis and extend back to the fourchette, forming a cleft. Like the mons pubis, the labia majora undergo changes at puberty: the amount of fatty tissue increases, pubic hair grows on the lateral surfaces, and sebaceous glands on the hairless medial surfaces begin to secrete lubricants. Because of an extensive network of nerve endings, the labia majora are highly sensitive to temperature, touch, pressure, and pain and are homologous to the male scrotum (see Fig. 21-2). The principal function of the labia majora is to protect the inner structures of the vulva.

Within the labia majora lie two smaller, thinner folds of skin, the **labia minora** (singular, **labium minus**). Anteriorly, they form the clitoral hood, or prepuce, and frenulum, then split to enclose the vestibule, and converge near the anus, forming the fourchette. The labia minora are hairless, pink, and moist and are well supplied with nerves, blood vessels, and sebaceous glands. These glands secrete a bactericidal fluid that has a distinctive odor and that lubricates and waterproofs the vulvar skin. During sexual arousal the labia minora become swollen with blood.

The **clitoris** is a richly innervated, erectile organ that lies between the labia minora. It is a small, cylindric structure having a glans that is visible and a shaft that lies beneath the skin (see Fig. 21-4). The clitoris is homologous to the male penis. Like the penis, the clitoris is a major site of sexual stimulation and orgasm. With sexual arousal, erectile tissues in the clitoris fill with blood, causing it to enlarge somewhat. Similar to other vulvar glands, the clitoris secretes a fluid, called *smegma,* which has a unique odor and may be erotically stimulating to the male.

The area protected by the labia minora is called the **vestibule.** The vestibule contains the external opening of the vagina, which is called the **introitus,** or vaginal orifice. A thin, perforated membrane called the **hymen** may cover the

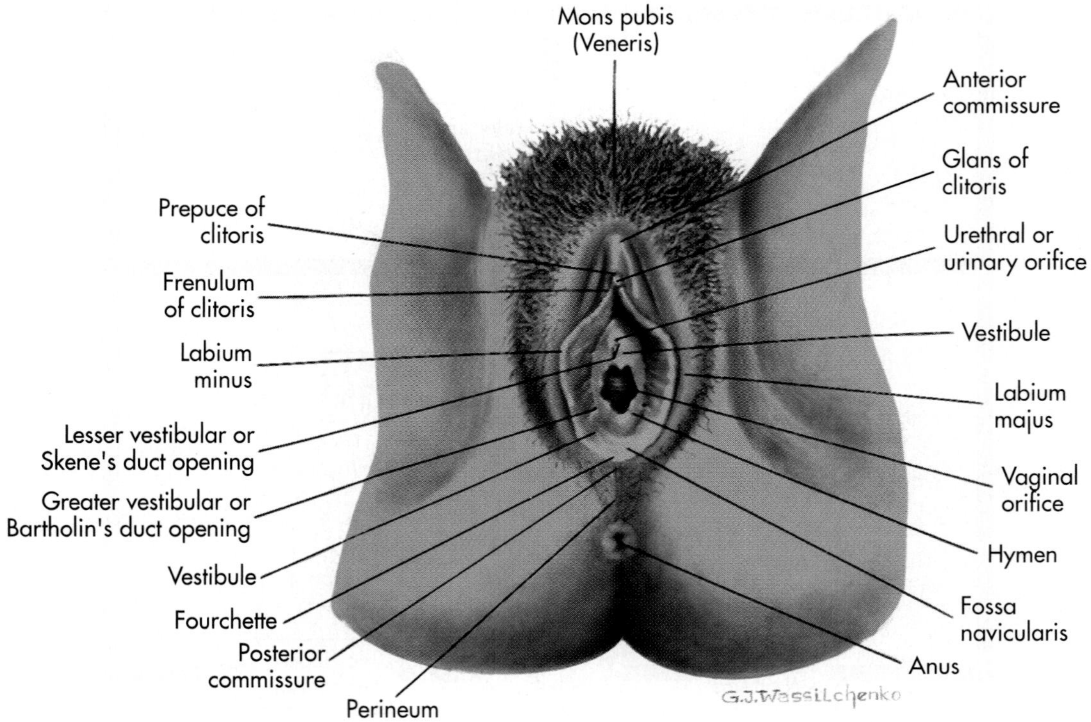

FIG. 21-4 External female genitalia. (Modified from Lowdermilk DL, Perry SE, Bobak IM: *Maternity and women's health care,* ed 7, St Louis, 2000, Mosby.)

introitus. The vestibule also contains the opening of the urethra, or **urinary meatus** (orifice). These structures are lubricated by two pairs of glands: Skene glands and Bartholin glands. The ducts of **Skene glands** (also called the *lesser vestibular* or *paraurethral glands*) open on both sides of the urinary meatus. The ducts of **Bartholin glands (greater vestibular or vulvovaginal glands)** open on either side of the introitus. In response to sexual stimulation, Bartholin glands secrete mucus that lubricates the inner labial surfaces, as well as enhances the viability and motility of sperm. Skene glands help lubricate the urinary meatus and the vestibule. Secretions from both sets of glands facilitate coitus. Also, in response to sexual excitement, the highly vascular tissue just beneath the vestibule fills with blood and becomes engorged.

The less hairy skin and the subcutaneous tissue that lie between the vaginal orifice and the anus are referred to as the **perineum.** Unlike the rest of the vulva, this area has little subcutaneous fat so that the skin is close to the underlying muscles. The perineum covers the muscular **perineal body,** a fibrous structure that comprises elastic fiber, connective tissue, and the common attachment of the bulbocavernosus, the external anal sphincter, and the levator ani muscles (see Fig. 21-4). This area is much larger in the female, and the characteristic median raphe seen in the male generally is absent. The perineum varies in length from 2 to 5 cm or more and stretches remarkably. The length of the perineum and the elasticity of the perineal body influence tissue resistance and injury during childbirth.

Internal Genitalia

Vagina

The **vagina** is an elastic, fibromuscular canal, 9 to 10 cm long, which extends up and back from the introitus to the lower portion of the uterus. As Fig. 21-5 shows, it lies between the urethra (and part of the bladder) and the rectum. Mucosal secretions from the upper genital organs, menstrual fluids, and products of conception leave the body through the vagina, which also receives the penis during coitus. During sexual excitement the vagina lengthens and widens and the anterior third becomes congested with blood.

The vaginal wall is composed of four layers. Its lining is a mucous membrane of squamous epithelial cells. (Types of epithelium are described and illustrated in Chapter 1, Table 1-6.) This layer thickens and thins in response to hormones, particularly estrogen. The squamous epithelial membrane is continuous with the membrane that covers the lower part of the uterus. In women of reproductive age, the mucosal layer is arranged in transverse wrinkles, or folds, called **rugae** (singular, **ruga**). The rugae permit the mucosal layer to stretch during coitus and childbirth. The second layer consists of fibrous connective tissue containing numerous blood and lymphatic vessels. Smooth muscle constitutes the third layer. The outermost layer consists of connective tissue and a rich network of blood vessels.

The upper part of the vagina surrounds the cervix, the lower end of the uterus (see Fig. 21-5). The recessed space around the cervix is called the **fornix** of the vagina. The

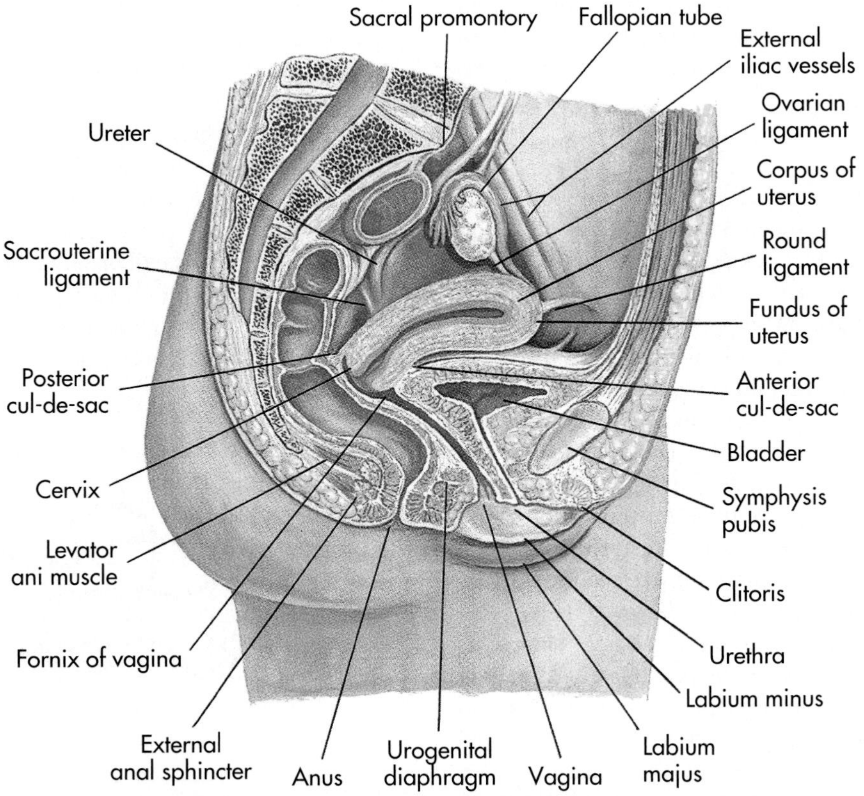

FIG. 21-5 Internal female genitalia and other pelvic organs. Midsagittal view. (Modified from Seidel HM et al: *Mosby's guide to physical examination,* ed 4, St Louis, 1999, Mosby.)

posterior fornix is "deeper" than the anterior fornix because of the angle at which the cervix meets the vaginal canal. In most women this angle is about 90 degrees. A pouch called the **cul-de-sac** separates the posterior fornix and the rectum.

Its elasticity and relatively sparse nerve supply enhance the vagina's function as the birth canal. During sexual arousal the vaginal wall becomes engorged with blood, like the labia minora and clitoris. Engorgement pushes some fluid to the surface of the mucosa, enhancing lubrication. The vaginal wall does not contain mucus-secreting glands; rather, secretions drain into the vagina from the endocervical glands or enter from the vestibule.

Two factors help maintain the self-cleansing action of the vagina and defend it from infection, particularly during the reproductive years: (1) an acid-base balance that discourages the proliferation of most pathogenic bacteria and (2) the thickness of the vaginal epithelium. Before puberty, vaginal pH is about 7.0 (neutral) and the vaginal epithelium is thin. At puberty, the pH becomes more acidic (4.0 to 5.0) and the squamous epithelial lining thickens. These changes are maintained until menopause (cessation of menstruation), at which time the pH rises again to more alkaline levels and the epithelium thins out. Therefore protection from infection is greatest during the years when a woman is most likely to be sexually active. Between puberty and menopause, vulnerability to infection varies somewhat with cyclic changes in pH and epithelial thickness. Both defenses are greatest when estrogen levels are high and the vagina contains a normal population of *Lactobacillus acidophilus,* a harmless resident bacterium that helps maintain pH at acidic levels. Any condition that causes vaginal pH to rise, such as douching or use of vaginal sprays or deodorants, low estrogen levels, or destruction of *L. acidophilus* by antibiotics, lowers vaginal defenses against infection.

Uterus

The **uterus** is a hollow, pear-shaped organ whose lower end opens into the vagina. The functions of the uterus are to anchor and protect a fertilized ovum, provide an optimal environment while it develops, and push the fetus out at birth. In addition, the uterus plays an important role in sexual response and conception. During sexual excitement the opening of the uterus (the cervix) dilates slightly. At the same time, the uterus increases in size and moves upward and backward, creating a tenting effect in the midvagina that results in the cervix "sitting" in a pool of semen. During orgasm, rhythmic contractions facilitate movement of sperm through the cervical os while enhancing physical pleasure.

At puberty the uterus attains its adult size and proportions and descends from the abdomen to the lower pelvis, between the bladder and the rectum (see Fig. 21-5). The uterus of a mature, nonpregnant female is approximately 9 cm long and 6.5 cm wide, with muscular walls 3.5 cm thick. It is held loosely in position by ligaments, peritoneal tissue folds, and pressure of adjacent organs, especially the urinary bladder, sigmoid colon, and rectum. In most women the uterus is anteverted; that is, it is tipped forward so that it rests on the urinary bladder. However, it may be retroverted, or tipped backward. Various degrees of flexion are normal (Fig. 21-6).

Fig. 21-7 shows a cross section of the uterus. The uterus has two major parts: the body, or **corpus,** and the cervix. The top of the corpus, above the insertion of the fallopian tubes, is called the **fundus.** The diameter of the uterine cavity is widest at the fundus and narrowest at the **isthmus,** which is the narrowed part of the corpus just above the cervix. The **cervix,** or "neck of the uterus," extends from the isthmus to the vagina. The passageway between the cervix's upper opening (the internal os) and its lower opening (the external os) is called the **endocervical canal.** The entire uterus, like the upper vagina, is innervated exclusively by motor and sensory fibers of the autonomic nervous system.

The uterine wall is composed of three layers: the perimetrium, the myometrium, and the endometrium (see Fig. 21-7). The **perimetrium (parietal peritoneum)** is the outer serous membrane that covers the uterus. The **myometrium** is the thick, muscular middle layer. The myometrium is thickest at the fundus, apparently to facilitate birth. The **endometrium,** or uterine lining, is composed of a functional layer (superficial compact layer and spongy middle layer) and a basal layer. The functional layer of the endometrium is responsive to sex hormones. Between puberty and menopause this layer proliferates and sloughs off monthly. The basal layer, which is attached to the myometrium, regenerates the functional layer after it sloughs (menstruation).

The endocervical canal does not have an endometrial layer. Rather, it is lined with columnar epithelial cells (see Table 1-6). The endocervical lining is continuous with that of the outer cervix and vagina, but it is not made up of the same type of epithelial cells. The point at which the columnar epithelium of the cervix meets the squamous epithelium of the vagina is called the *transformation zone,* or the **squamous-columnar junction.** The transformation zone is the usual site of cervical dysplasia or carcinoma in situ.

The cervix acts as a mechanical barrier to infectious microorganisms that may be present in the vagina. The external cervical os is a very small opening that contains thick, sticky mucus (the *mucous plug*) during most of the menstrual cycle and all of pregnancy. In addition, the downward flow of cervical secretions moves microorganisms away from the

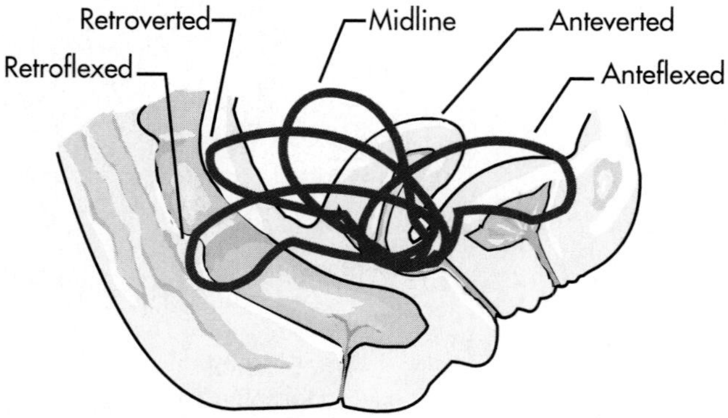

FIG. 21-6 Variations in uterine position.

cervix and uterus. In women of reproductive age, the pH of these secretions is inhospitable to most bacteria. Further, mucosal secretions contain enzymes and antibodies (mostly immunoglobulin A) of the secretory immune system. (The secretory immune system is discussed in Chapter 6.) These defenses do not always prevent infection, even if they are intact. Besides infection, uterine pathophysiology includes displacement of the uterus within the pelvis, benign growths of the uterine wall, and cancer.

Fallopian Tubes

The two **fallopian tubes (oviducts, uterine tubes)** enter the uterus bilaterally just beneath the fundus (see Fig. 21-7). Their function is to conduct the ova from the spaces around the ovaries to the uterus. From the uterus the fallopian tubes curve up and over the two ovaries. Each tube is 8 to 12 cm long and about 1 cm in diameter, except at its ovarian end, which flares out like the bell of a trumpet. This widened end, called the **infundibulum,** is fringed or fimbriated. The **fimbriae** (fringes) move, creating a current that draws the ovum into the infundibulum. Once the ovum has entered the fallopian tube, cilia and peristalsis (muscle contractions) keep it moving toward the uterus.

The ampulla, or distal third, of the fallopian tube is the usual site of fertilization (see Fig. 21-7). Sperm released into the vagina travel upward through the endocervical canal and uterine cavity and enter the fallopian tubes. If an ovum is present in either tube, fertilization can occur. Whether or not the ovum encounters sperm, it continues to travel through the fallopian tube to the uterus. If fertilized, the ovum (now called a *blastocyst*) implants itself in the endometrial layer of the uterine wall. If not fertilized, the ovum breaks down and leaves the uterus with menstrual fluids.

Disorders that affect the fallopian tubes can block the path of both sperm and ovum and cause infertility. Such disorders include congenital malformations, infection, and inflammation.

Ovaries

The **ovaries,** or the female gonads, are the primary female reproductive organs. They have two main functions: secretion of female sex hormones and development and release of female gametes, or ova.

The almond-shaped ovaries are located on both sides of the uterus and are suspended and supported by the mesovarian portions of the broad ligament, ovarian ligaments, and suspensory ligaments (see Fig. 21-7). The ovaries are smaller than their male homologs, the testes. In women of reproductive age, each ovary is 3 to 5 cm long, 2.5 cm wide, and 2 cm thick and weighs 4 to 8 g. Size and weight vary somewhat from phase to phase of the menstrual cycle (see p. 681).

Fig. 21-8 shows a cross section of an ovary. The central part, or medulla, is composed of connective tissue and contains many small arteries, veins, and lymphatics, which enter at the hilum. Surrounding the medulla is the cortex. At birth the cortex of each ovary contains approximately 1 million ova within immature **ovarian follicles.** Follicles grow and undergo atresia continuously and irrevocably during a woman's life. By puberty the number ranges between 200,000 and 400,000 ova. During puberty some of the follicles and the ova within them begin to mature. Between puberty and menopause the ovarian cortex always contains

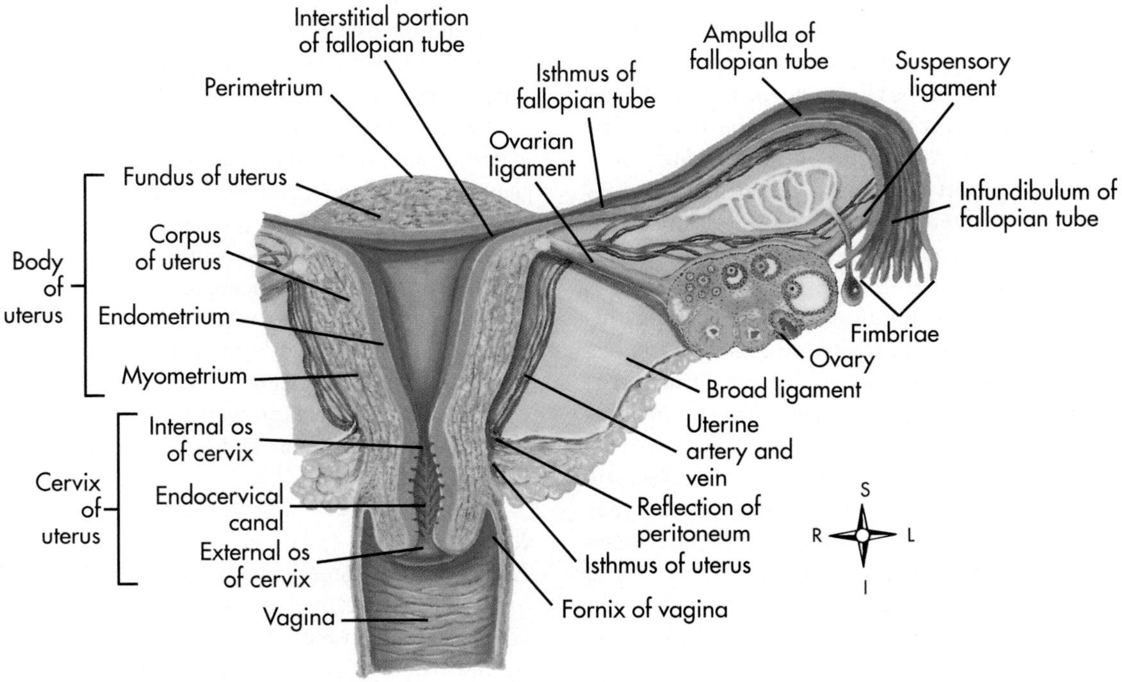

FIG. 21-7 Cross section of uterus, fallopian tube, and ovary. (Modified from Thibodeau GA, Patton KI: *Anatomy and physiology,* ed 4, St Louis, 1999, Mosby.)

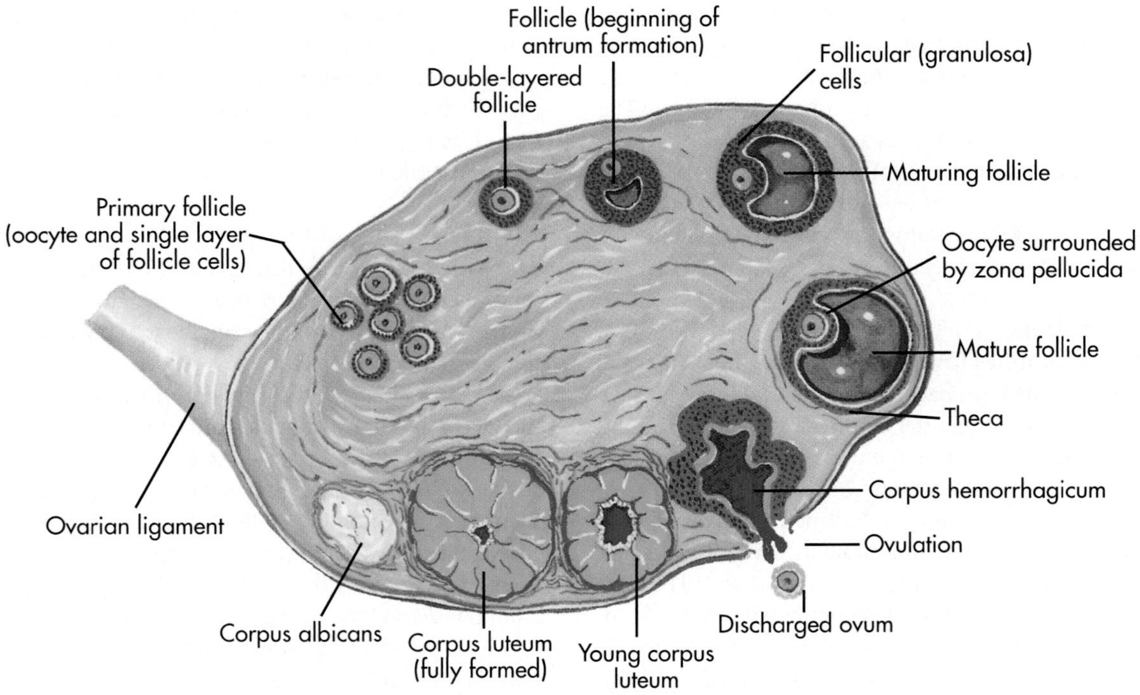

FIG. 21-8 Cross section of ovary during reproductive years. (From Thibodeau GA, Patton KI: *Anatomy and physiology,* ed 4, St Louis, 1999, Mosby.)

follicles and ova in various stages of development. Once every menstrual cycle (about every 28 days), one of the follicles reaches maturation and discharges its ovum through the ovary's outer covering, the germinal epithelium. During the reproductive years, 300 to 500 ovarian follicles mature completely and release an ovum, an event termed **ovulation.** The rest either fail to develop at all or degenerate without maturing completely.[1]

Having ejected a mature ovum, the follicle develops into another structure, the **corpus luteum** (see Fig. 21-8). The immediate fate of the corpus luteum depends on whether the ejected ovum is fertilized. If fertilization occurs, the corpus luteum enlarges and begins to secrete hormones that maintain and support pregnancy. If fertilization does not occur, the corpus luteum secretes these hormones for approximately 14 days and then degenerates, which triggers the maturation of another follicle. The **ovarian cycle**—the process of follicular maturation, ovulation, corpus luteum development, and corpus luteum degeneration—is continuous from puberty to menopause, except during pregnancy. At menopause, this process ceases and the ovaries atrophy.

Four types of cells within the ovarian cortex secrete sex hormones: cells of the stroma, or tissue matrix; two types of cells in the ovarian follicle, **granulosa cells** and **theca cells;** and cells of the corpus luteum (Fig. 21-9). These cells all contain receptors for the gonadotropins (LH and FSH) or for the sex hormones, which are discussed in the next section.

Because hormones regulate ovarian function, any disorder that disrupts hormone secretion or reception by target cells can cause ovarian dysfunction and infertility. Benign or malignant growths, cysts, infection, or inflammation can also cause ovarian pathologic conditions.

Female Sex Hormones

The sex hormones are all steroid hormones, that is, they are synthesized from cholesterol (see Chapter 19). Both male and female sex hormones are present in all adults. However, the female body contains low levels of testosterone and other androgens, and the male body contains low levels of estrogen. Individual effects of sex hormones depend on their amount and concentration in the blood.

The dominant female sex hormones, estrogen and progesterone, are produced by the ovaries. During fetal development, infancy, and childhood, sex hormone production is low. At puberty, hormone production surges, triggering sexual maturation and development of secondary sex characteristics. From puberty to menopause, the sex hormones control the menstrual cycle and are produced cyclically, that is, production surges and diminishes monthly, creating the ovarian and uterine changes associated with the menstrual cycle. Androgens are produced in small amounts by the ovaries and the adrenals and also have important functions in women.

Estrogens

Estrogen is a generic term for three similar hormones: estradiol, estrone, and estriol. **Estradiol (E2)** is the most potent and plentiful of the three and is principally produced by the ovaries (ovarian follicle and corpus luteum). The ovary secretes about 95% of circulating estradiol, with limited amounts secreted by the adrenal cortex. Androgens are converted to estrone in ovarian and peripheral adipose tis-

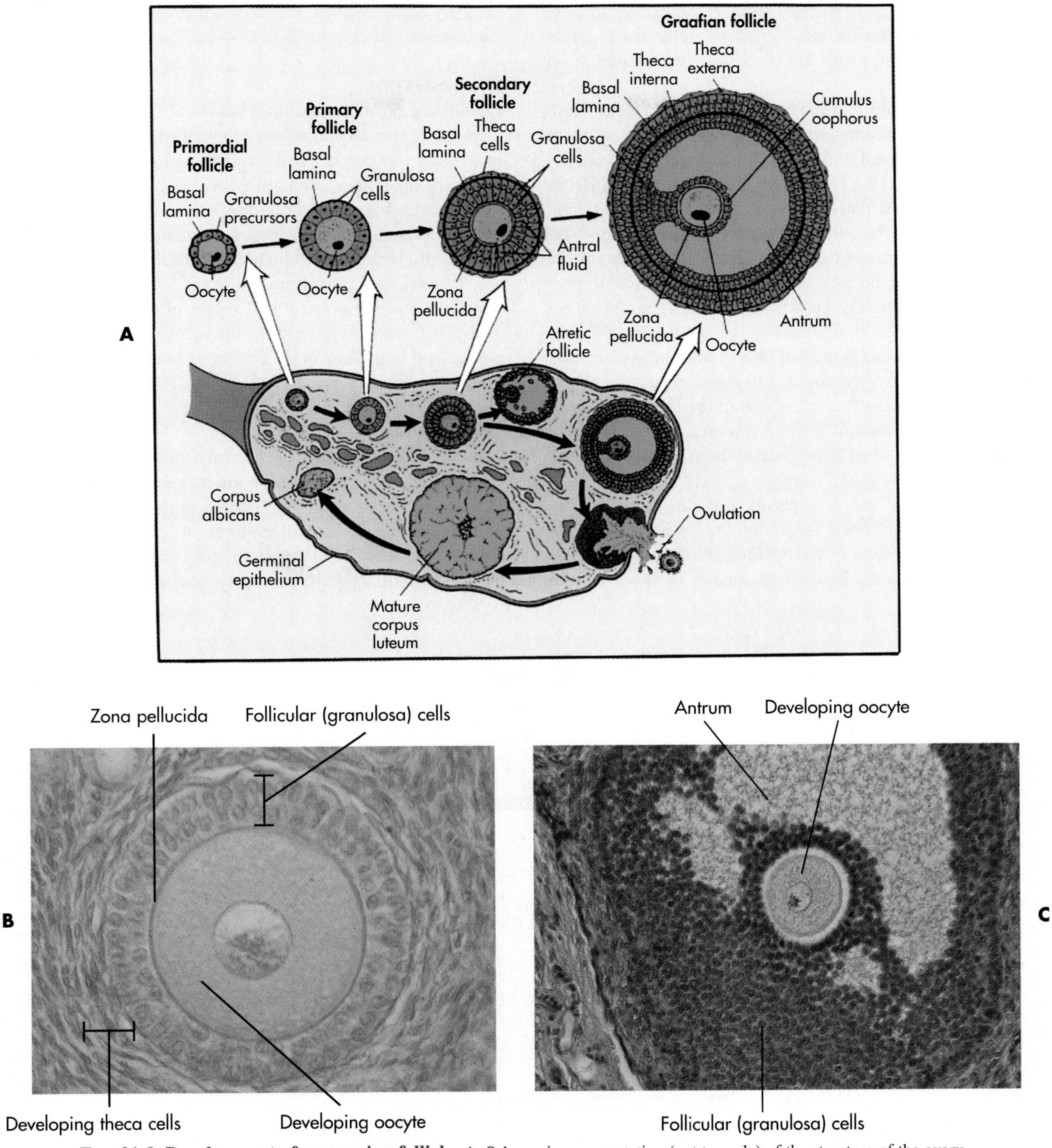

FIG. 21-9 Development of an ovarian follicle. A, Schematic representation (not to scale) of the structure of the ovary, showing the various stages in the development of the follicle and its successor structure, the corpus luteum. **B,** A developing oocyte surrounded by hormone-secreting follicular (granulosa) cells. **C,** More mature ovarian follicle has a fluid-filled cavity called the *antrum.* (**A,** From Berne RM, Levy MN, editors: *Physiology,* ed 4, St Louis, 1999, Mosby. **B, C,** From Thibodeau GA, Patton KI: *Anatomy and physiology,* ed 4, St Louis, 1999, Mosby.)

sue, and estriol is the peripheral metabolite of estrone and estradiol.

Estrogen has numerous biologic effects, many of which involve interactions with other hormones. Estrogen is needed for maturation of reproductive organs, development of secondary sex characteristics, closure of long bones after the pubertal growth spurt, regulation of the menstrual cycle, and endometrial regeneration after menstruation. Estrogen also has metabolic effects on the bones, liver, blood vessels, brain and central nervous system, kidneys, and skin. After menopause, ovarian production of estradiol stops and secretion of estrone is markedly diminished. At this time, the majority of estrogen is derived from extraovarian and extraglandular production of estrones.[7] (Hormone levels during the perimenopause are discussed in the section on menopause, p. 681.)

Like other steroid hormones, estrogens are derived from cholesterol in a complex, enzyme-mediated series of reactions. (Mechanisms of hormone synthesis and action are described in Chapter 19.) The hypothalamus secretes GnRH in a pulsating manner that stimulates gonadotropin (LH and FSH) release from the anterior pituitary. Gonadotropins trigger ovarian production of estrogen. The primary function of LH is to stimulate theca cells of the ovarian follicle to produce androgens, mainly androstenedione. (Androgens are discussed further on p. 689 and in the section on male reproductive function.) Some of these androgens are converted to estrogen by the theca cells themselves, and others diffuse into the granulosa cells. Within the granulosa layer, FSH induces conversion (aromatization) of androgens to estrogens (Fig. 21-10).[4] Estrogens are then released into the bloodstream.

Disturbances of estrogen production can be caused by abnormalities that affect (1) secretion of GnRH by the hypothalamus, (2) secretion of LH or FSH by the anterior pituitary, (3) hormonal feedback mechanisms, or (4) structural integrity of the ovaries. Estrogen's role in the menstrual cycle is described on p. 682.

Progesterone

Luteinizing hormone stimulates the ovary to secrete **progesterone,** the second major female sex hormone. Progesterone is an early product in the enzymatic conversion pathway of estrogen. Small amounts of progesterone are secreted steadily by the adrenal cortex. During the follicular phase, the ovary and the adrenal glands each contribute approximately 50% of total progesterone production. Conversely, large amount are secreted cyclically from the ovary while the corpus luteum is active for about 9 to 13 days after ovulation. With estrogen, progesterone controls the menstrual cycle. The opposing and complementary effects of progesterone and estrogen are listed in Table 21-1.

Androgens

Although **androgens** are primarily male sex hormones, small amounts are produced in the ovary and adrenal cortex in women. Some androgens are precursors of female sex hormones, notably androstenedione. At puberty, androgens contribute to the skeletal growth spurt and cause growth of pubic and axillary hair. The androgens also activate seba-

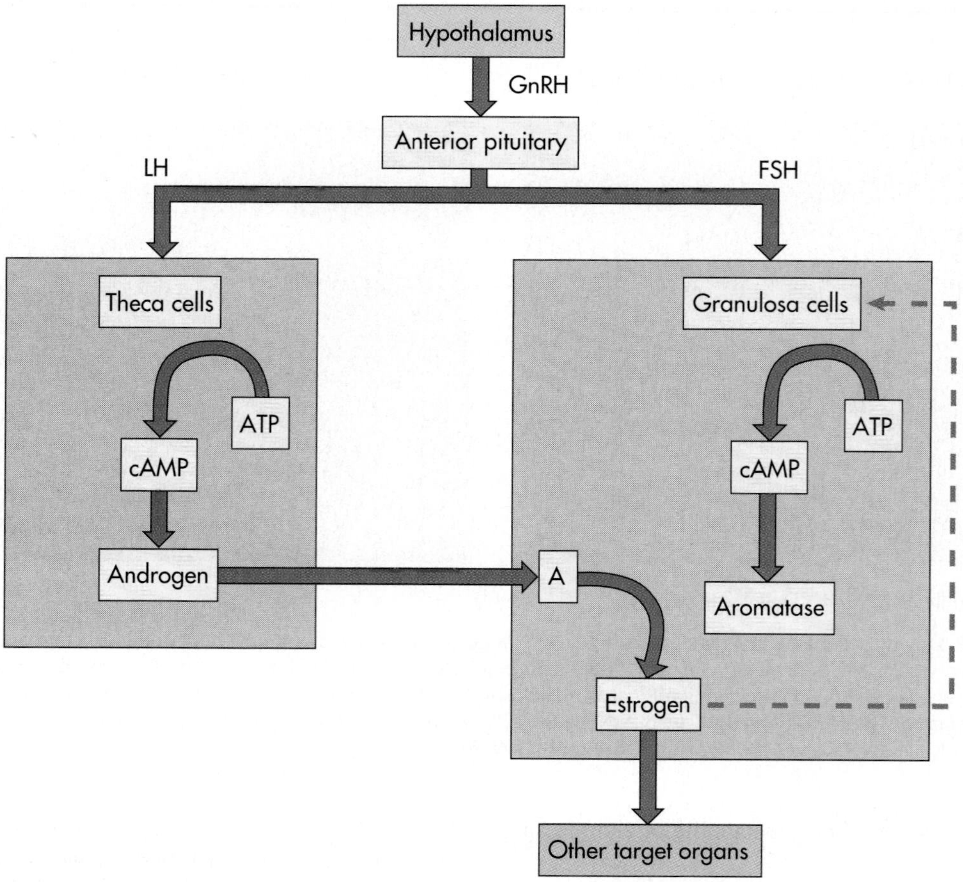

FIG. 21-10 Estrogen. Estrogen production by cells of the ovarian follicle. *GnRH,* Gonadotropin-releasing hormone; *LH,* luteinizing hormone; *FSH,* follicle-stimulating hormone; *ATP,* adenosine triphosphate; *cAMP,* cyclic adenosine monophosphate; *A,* androgen. (Modified from Mishell DR et al: *Comprehensive gynecology,* ed 3, St Louis, 1997, Mosby.)

ceous glands, accounting for some cases of acne during puberty, and play a role in libido.

The Menstrual Cycle

Besides pregnancy, the obvious manifestation of female reproductive functioning is menstrual bleeding (the menses), which starts with **menarche** (first menstruation) and ends with **menopause** (cessation of menstrual flow). In the United States the average age of first menstruation is 12.5 years, with a range from 9 to 17 years. Menarche appears to be related to body weight, especially percentage of body fat (ratio of fat to lean tissue), which theoretically may trigger a change in the metabolic rate and lead to hormonal changes associated with ovulation. The presence of leptin, a hormone secreted from adipose tissue, is thought to inhibit the gonadostat and trigger puberty.[4] At first, cycles are anovulatory and may vary in length from 10 to 60 days or more. As adolescence proceeds, regular patterns of menstruation and ovulation are established at intervals ranging from 30 to 35 days.[8-10] During adulthood, menstruation continues to recur in a recognizable and characteristic pattern, with the length of the menstrual cycle varying considerably among women. If a woman is to experience regular and predictable menstruation, it usually happens by the third decade. Around age 25 in over 40% of cycles, menstrual cycle length is between 25 to 28 days; the percentage increases to 60% between ages 25 and 35 years.[11] The commonly accepted cycle average is 28 (27 to 30) days, with rhythmic intervals of 21 to 35 days considered normal. Approximately 2 to 4 years before menopause (6 to 8 years according to Trealor and colleagues,[9] who studied over 25,000 woman-years in over 2500 women), cycles begin to lengthen again. Menstrual cyclicity and regular ovulation are dependent on (1) the activity of the gonadostat (GnRH pulse generator); (2) the pituitary secretion of gonadotropins; and (3) estrogen (estradiol) positive feedback for the preovulatory LH surge, oocyte maturation, and corpus luteum formation.[4]

Phases

The menstrual cycle consists of three phases of one event, ovulation. During ovulation, an ovum from a mature ovarian follicle is released. The three phases are the follicular/proliferative phase, the luteal/secretory phase, and the ischemic/menstrual phase, known as menstruation (Fig. 21-11).

During **menstruation,** the functional layer of the endometrium disintegrates and is discharged through the vagina. Menstruation is followed by the **follicular/proliferative phase.** This phase is named for two simultaneous processes: maturation of an ovarian follicle and proliferation of the endometrium (see Fig. 21-11). During the follicular/proliferative phase, the anterior pituitary gland secretes FSH, which causes an ovarian follicle to develop. While the follicle is developing, its granulosa cells secrete estrogen and estrogen causes cells of the endometrium to proliferate. By the time the ovarian follicle is mature, the endometrial lining is restored. At this point ovulation occurs.

Ovulation marks the beginning of the **luteal/secretory phase** of the menstrual cycle. The ovarian follicle begins its transformation into a corpus luteum (see Fig. 21-8), hence the name *luteal phase.* LH from the anterior pituitary stimulates the corpus luteum to secrete progesterone, which in turn initiates the secretory phase of endometrial development. Glands and blood vessels in the endometrium branch and curl throughout the functional layer, and the glands begin to secrete a thin, glycogen-containing fluid, hence the name *secretory phase.* If conception occurs, the nutrient-laden endometrium is ready for implantation. If conception and implantation do not occur, the corpus luteum degenerates and ceases its production of progesterone and estrogen. Without progesterone or estrogen to maintain it, the endometrium enters the ischemic (blood-starved) portion of the menstrual phase and disintegrates. Menstruation occurs, marking the beginning of another cycle.

Ovarian cycles appear to have a minimum length of 24 to 26.5 days: the ovarian follicle requires 10 to 12.5 days to develop, and the luteal phase appears relatively fixed at 14 days ($\pm$3 days). Menstrual blood flow usually lasts 3 to 7 days, but it may last as long as 8 days or stop after 1 to 2 days and still be considered within normal limits. Bleeding is consistently scant to heavy and varies from 30 to 80 ml, with most blood loss occurring during the first 3 days of menses. Menstrual discharge consists of blood, mucus, and desquamated

Table 21-1 Complementary and Opposing Effects of Estrogen and Progesterone

Structure	Effect of Estrogen	Effect of Progesterone
Vaginal mucosa	Proliferation of squamous epithelium; increase in glycogen content of cells; layering (cornification) of cells	Thinning of squamous epithelium; decornification
Cervical mucosa	Production of abundant fluid secretions that favor survival and enhance motility of sperm	Production of thick, sticky secretions that tend to "plug" the cervical os
Fallopian tube	Increase of motility and ciliary action	Decrease of motility and ciliary action
Uterine muscle	Increase of blood flow; increase of contractile proteins and uterine muscle and myometrial excitability and action potential; increase of sensitization to oxytocin	Relaxation of myometrium; decrease of sensitization to oxytocin
Endometrium	Stimulation of growth; increase in number of progesterone receptors	Activation of glands and blood vessels; accumulation of glycogen and enzymes; decrease in number of estrogen receptors
Breasts	Growth of ducts; promotion of prolactin effects	Growth of lobules and alveoli; inhibition of prolactin effects

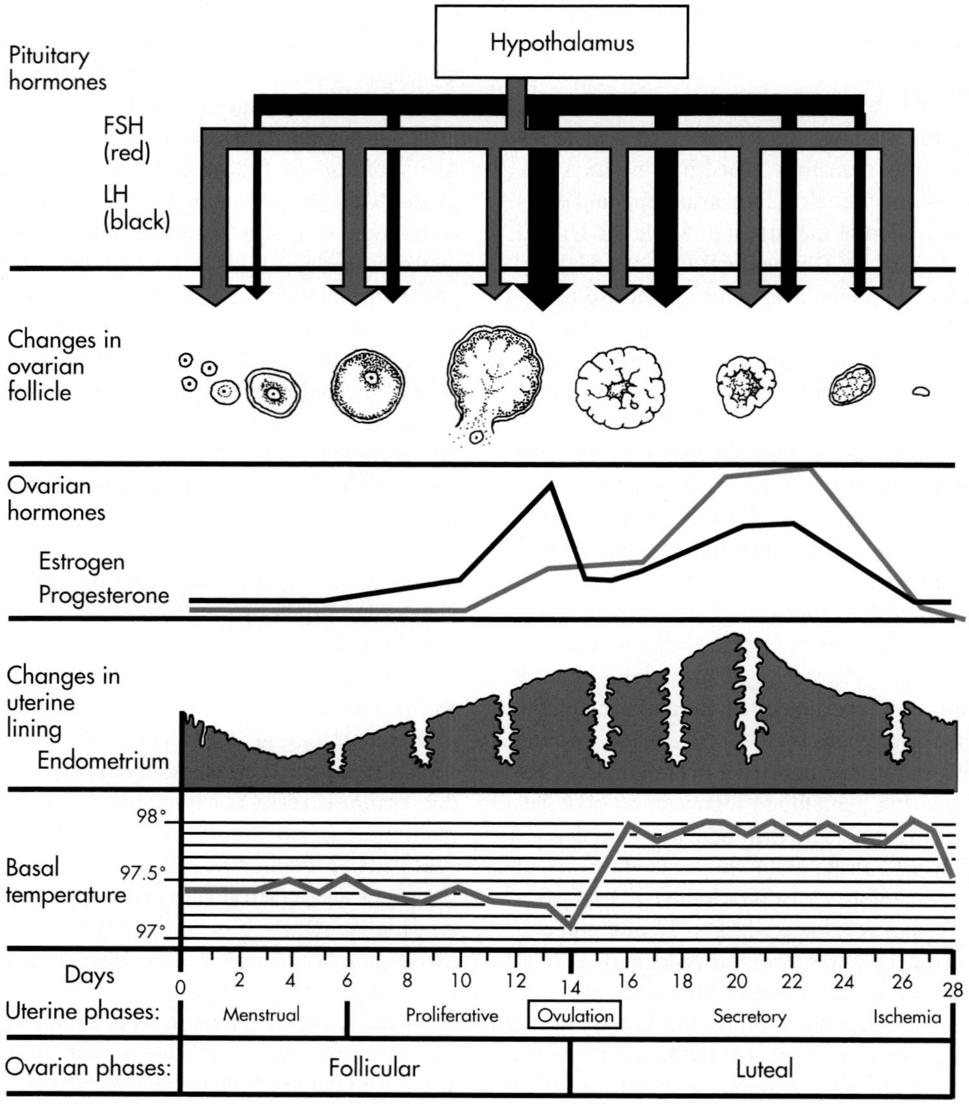

FIG. 21-11 The menstrual cycle. *FSH,* Follicle-stimulating hormone; *LH,* luteinizing hormone. (Modified from Lowdermilk DL, Perry SE, Bobak IM: *Maternity and women's health care,* ed 6, St Louis, 1997, Mosby.)

endometrial tissue and does not clot under normal circumstances. It is usually dark and produces a characteristic musty odor on oxidation. Factors such as severe emotional stress, illness, malnutrition, and seasonal variation may affect the length of the menstrual cycle.[9,12]

Hormonal Controls

Hormonal control of the menstrual cycle depends on complex interactions among the hypothalamus, the anterior pituitary, and the ovaries (or hypothalamic-pituitary-ovarian [H-P-O] axis).[12] GnRH is secreted by the hypothalamus into the hypophyseal portal system and travels to the anterior pituitary, where it stimulates the secretion of LH and FSH. FSH and LH are released from the anterior pituitary in pulses that correspond to the pulsatile secretion of GnRH.

Blood levels of estrogen and progesterone exert a feedback effect on the hypothalamus and the anterior pituitary, thereby determining how much FSH and LH are secreted (Table 21-2). FSH secretion and LH secretion are not completely parallel; that is, FSH and LH are not secreted simultaneously in equal amounts throughout the menstrual cycle. Nonparallel secretion is caused by cyclic changes in feedback mechanisms. During the early follicular phase, low levels of estrogen inhibit the FSH-secreting cells of the anterior pituitary. As the ovarian follicle grows, it produces more and more estrogen. Higher levels of estrogen further suppress FSH release. During the late follicular phase, the preovulatory rise in progesterone facilitates the positive feedback of estrogen; estrogen levels begin to increase, stimulating a surge of FSH and LH secretion from the anterior pituitary. (Progesterone may be necessary also to induce the midcycle FSH peak.) The midcycle surge of LH causes ovulation. Rising estrogen and progesterone levels during the luteal phase may have some inhibitory effect on the anterior pituitary, thereby reducing LH and FSH secretion. Just before the onset of menstruation, FSH and LH levels begin to increase slightly, probably because of declining estrogen and progesterone levels (Fig. 21-12).

Table 21-2 Hormonal Feedback Mechanisms in the Menstrual Cycle

Phase of Cycle and Ovarian Hormone Levels	Feedback to Hypothalamus and Anterior Pituitary	Resultant GnRH, FSH, and LH levels	Ovarian and Menstrual Events
Early follicular phase: estrogen levels low; minute amount of progesterone secreted	Negative and inhibitory	All low	Ovarian follicle develops; endometrium proliferates
Late follicular (preovulatory) phase: estrogen levels high; progesterone increases with small surge before ovulation	Positive and stimulatory	All surge; LH dominates	Process of ovulation begins;endometrial proliferation complete
Ovulatory phase: estrogen levels dip; progesterone levels begin to rise	Negative and inhibitory	All fall sharply	Corpus luteum begins to develop; endometrium enters secretory phase
Early luteal phase: estrogen and progesterone levels high; progesterone dominates	Negative and inhibitory	All continue to decline, but gradually	Corpus luteum fully developed; endometrium ready for implantation
Late luteal phase: estrogen and progesterone levels fall sharply	Negative and inhibitory; feedback lessens slightly	All rise slightly	Corpus luteum regresses; endometrium breaks down; menstruation begins
Menstrual phase: estrogen levels low; minute amount of progesterone secreted	Negative and inhibitory	All low	More ovarian follicles begin to develop; functional layer of endometrium is shed

GnRH, Gonadotropin-releasing hormone; *FSH,* follicle-stimulating hormone; *LH,* luteinizing hormone.

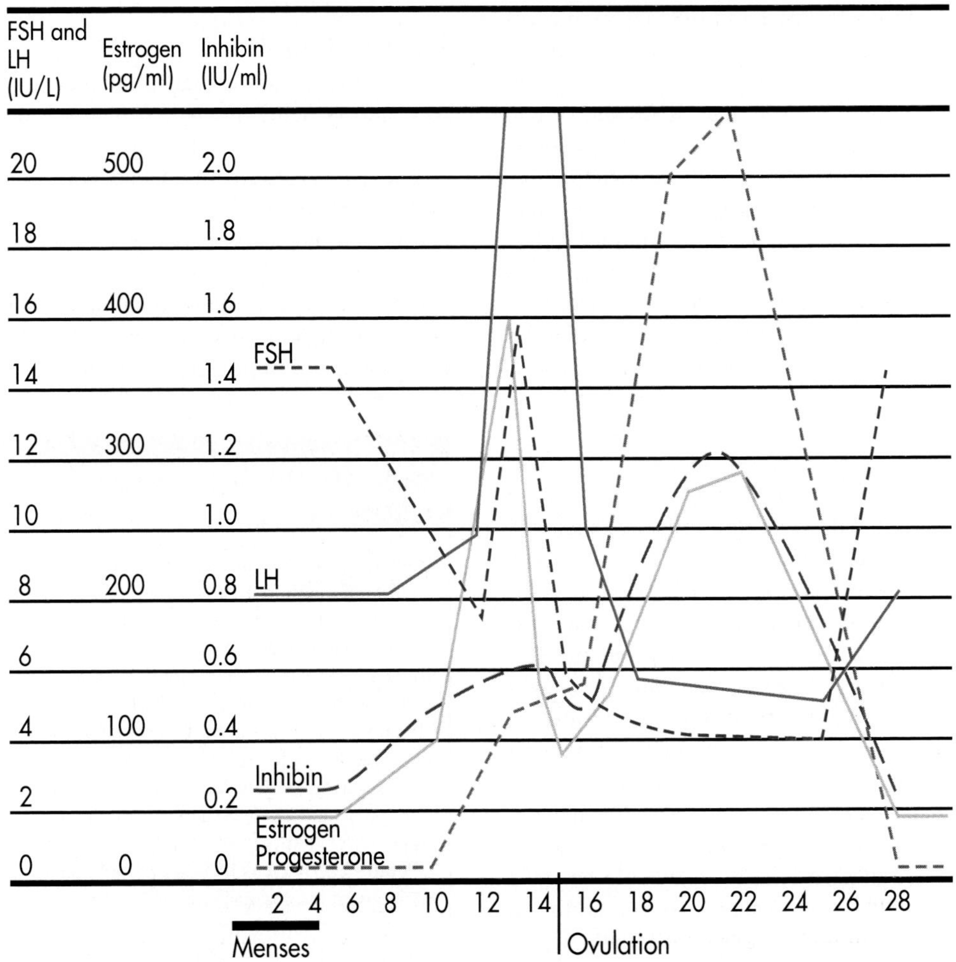

FIG. 21-12 Estrogen, progesterone, gonadotropin, and inhibin fluctuations over the menstrual cycle. Inhibin rises slowly but steadily throughout the follicular phase, peaking at midcycle and again during the midluteal phase. The midcycle peak coincides with surges of luteinizing hormone (LH) and follicle-stimulating hormone (FSH).

A variety of growth factors and autocrine/paracrine peptides influence hormonal control and follicular response.[1,11] During the early follicular stage, FSH stimulates FSH and LH receptors, insulin-like growth factor–I, and production of inhibin and activin; after ovulation, inhibin release comes under the control of LH. **Activin** stimulates FSH release in the pituitary and augments its action in the ovary, possibly by increasing FSH receptors. **Inhibin** inhibits FSH synthesis and secretion, restrains prolactin and growth hormone release, interferes with GnRH receptors, and promotes breakdown of intracellular gonadotropins.[12,13] To a lesser degree, **follistatin,** a polypeptide produced by the pituitary but found primarily in the follicles, suppresses FSH activity, probably by binding to activin. In summary, the balance between activin and inhibin regulates FSH secretion, and follistatin inhibits activin and boosts inhibin activity. Inhibin and activin also regulate LH stimulation of androgen synthesis in theca cells. Fig. 21-12 depicts fluctuating estrogen, progesterone, gonadotropin, and inhibin levels.

Interestingly, inhibins, activins, and follistatins are structurally similar, belonging to the same family of nonsteroidal polypeptides, and are synthesized by granulosa cells in response to FSH. Inhibin is synthesized and secreted from both granulosa and luteal ovarian cells, activin from granulosa cells only, and follistatin from pituitary cells. These peptides are secreted into the follicular fluid and ovarian venous effluent. The expression of these peptides is not liminted to the ovary; they are present in many tissues throughout the body and serve as regulators. Inhibin messenger RNA and activin are also found within the pituitary. Dimers of the β subunits of inhibin (activin) stimulate FSH secretion, whereas α, β-inhibin inhibits FSH.[4,14] Understanding of the function and structural complexity of these polypeptides and their interaction with GnRH, gonadotropins, and sex hormones has increased monumentally over the past decade. New information is gained through research and published on a regular basis.

Ovarian Cycle

By stimulating follicles, gonadotropins initiate their growth and maturation. The most important hormonal event is a rise in FSH. The decline in luteal-phase steroidogenesis and inhibin secretion allows FSH to rise; concurrently there is a slight increase in LH levels (see Fig. 21-12). More specifically, FSH stimulates granulosa cell growth and initiates estrogen production in these cells. At this time a group of ovarian follicles is recruited and begins to mature; the exact number depends on the remaining pool of inactive follicles. As the follicles mature, granulosa cells multiply, increasing estradiol secretion. Within a few days of the cycle, one follicle becomes dominant and the others atrophy. The mechanism for follicular recruitment or dominance is unknown. Once dominance is acquired, it is not transferable but may be related to FSH receptors, blood supply, or the ability to convert androgens to estradiol. The dominant follicle begins to secrete progressively larger amounts of estradiol, which exerts a positive-feedback effect causing the LH surge. (The dynamic process of follicular growth is outlined in Box 21-1.) Ovulation generally occurs 1 to 2 hours before the final progesterone surge, or about 12 to 36 hours after the onset of the LH surge; specific timing may reflect seasonal variations. Progesterone, proteolytic enzymes, and prostaglandins (E and F series) trigger mechanisms controlling follicular rupture and release of the ovum.[1] Possible mechanisms include thinning, stretching, degradation, and digestion of the follicular wall and contraction of smooth muscle cells of the follicle. In studies of human preovulatory follicular cells, as well as luteinized unruptured follicles in women with inflammatory arthritis, the role of prostaglandins "is so well demonstrated that infertility patients should be advised to avoid the use of drugs that inhibit prostaglandin synthesis" (ref. 11, p. 228).

The LH surge also transforms the granulosa cells of the ovulatory follicle into the corpus luteum. The corpus luteum secretes both estrogen and progesterone in amounts that depend, in part, on adequate development of the follicle before ovulation. Progesterone acts both centrally and locally within the ovary to suppress new follicular growth during the early and midluteal phases. If pregnancy does not occur, the corpus luteum persists for 11 to 14 days and then regresses and eventually disappears. An increase in pulse frequency of GnRH from a low level reactivates hormonal control of the menstrual cycle.

Uterine Phases

Uterine phases of the menstrual cycle—proliferative, secretory, and ischemic/menstrual phases—involve cyclic endometrial changes controlled by estrogen and progesterone. Hormonal effects are influenced by the presence of receptors and numerous growth factors, peptides, and enzymes that act as intermediaries between the sex steroids and the endometrium.[4] During the midfollicular phase, increasing levels of estrogen contribute to endometrial repair and proliferation, thus increasing endometrial thickness. Once ovulation occurs and serum progesterone levels increase, the endome-

Box 21-1

DYNAMIC PROCESS OF FOLLICULAR GROWTH

Follicles grow and undergo atresia under all physiologic circumstances. Growth and atresia continue during pregnancy, ovulation, or periods of anovulation and occur at all ages from fetal development to menopause. Maximum number of oocytes (follicles) is found in the fetus at approximately 16 to 20 weeks of gestation. By birth, the number has diminished from 6 to 7 million to 2 million. By puberty, only about 300,000 oocytes remain. During a woman's reproductive years, fewer than 500 oocytes will mature and be released during ovulation. The number of follicles that begin developing during each cycle depends on the residual pool. As a woman ages, fewer numbers of follicles are recruited. Follicular loss accelerates about 10 to 15 years before menopause and seems to coincide with a follicular pool of 25,000.

Data from Kirtley Jones (reproductive endocrinologist): Personal communication, December 2000; Speroff L et al: *Clinical gynecologic endocrinology and fertility,* ed 6, Baltimore, 1999, Lippincott.

trial tissue develops secretory characteristics. If implantation of a fertilized ovum does not take place, endometrial tissue begins to break down approximately 11 days after ovulation. The period of breakdown is sometimes called the *ischemic phase* (see Fig. 21-11). Sloughing of tissue (menstrual bleeding) begins about 14 days after ovulation.

Cervical mucus also undergoes cyclic changes. During the proliferative phase the cervical mucus is thin and watery. Peak estrogen levels occur just before ovulation and maximally stimulate the cervical glands to produce mucus. Cervical mucus becomes thicker and more elastic (spinnbarkeit). In the presence of estrogen, tiny channels develop in the mucus, which allows sperm access to the interior of the uterus. Changes in the consistency of cervical mucus can be used to identify fertile intervals.

Vaginal Response

Vaginal endothelium also responds to cyclic hormonal changes. Under the influence of estrogen, epithelial cells of the vagina grow maximally during the follicular/proliferative phase. After ovulation, layers of keratinized cells overgrow the basal epithelium, a process known as **cornification.** Near the end of the luteal phase, leukocytes invade vaginal epithelium, removing the outer layers in a process termed **decornification.**

Body Temperature

Basal body temperature (BBT) undergoes characteristic biphasic changes during menstrual cycles in which ovulation occurs. During the follicular phase the BBT fluctuates around 98° F (37° C). During the luteal phase, the average temperature increases by 0.4° to 1.0° F (0.2° to 0.5° C). At the end of the luteal phase, 1 to 3 days before the onset of menstruation, BBT declines to follicular-phase levels. The shift in temperature is related to ovulation, corpus luteum formation, and increased serum progesterone levels. Progesterone probably acts on the thermoregulatory center of the hypothalamus to increase body temperature. Changes in BBT are used to document ovulatory cycles but are not useful to predict the exact timing of ovulation.

THE MALE REPRODUCTIVE SYSTEM

In men the external genitalia perform the major functions of reproduction, which are to produce sperm and deliver them to the female reproductive tract.[15] Sperm are produced in the male gonads, the testes, and delivered to the female vagina by the penis. The internal male genitalia have a more accessory function. They consist of conducting tubes and fluid-producing glands, all of which aid in the transport of sperm from the testes to the urethral opening of the penis. The male reproductive and urinary structures are shown in Fig. 21-13.

External Genitalia

Testes

In men the testes are the essential organs of reproduction. Like the ovaries, the testes have two functions: (1) production of gametes (in this case, sperm) and (2) production of sex hormones (in this case, androgens and testosterone). The testes are suspended outside the pelvic cavity because sperm production requires an environment that is 1° or 2° C cooler than body temperature.

During embryonic and fetal life, the testes develop within the abdomen (see Fig. 21-1). Then, about 3 months before birth, the testes start to descend toward the developing scrotum.

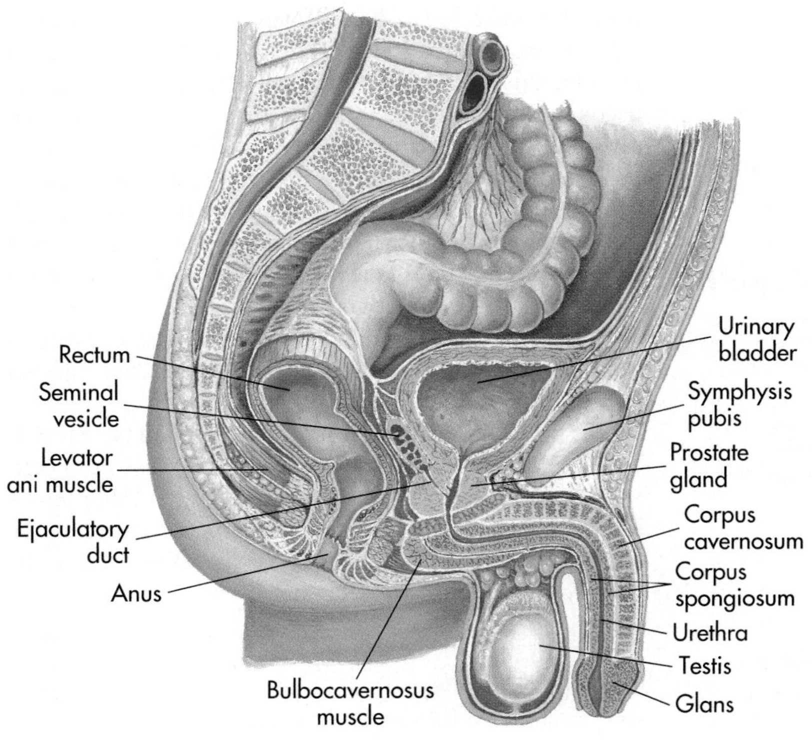

FIG. 21-13 Structure of the male reproductive organs. (Modified from Seidel HM et al: *Mosby's guide to physical examination,* ed 4, St Louis, 1999, Mosby.)

About 1 month before birth, they enter twin passageways called **inguinal canals.** The inguinal canals are vaginal processes created by outpouchings of the peritoneum (lining of the abdominal cavity). The descent of a **testis** is shown in Fig. 21-14. Each testis moves down outside the peritoneum until it is suspended in the scrotal sac by its supply lines: the ducts, blood vessels, lymphatic vessels, and nerves of the **spermatic cord.** When descent is complete, the abdominal end of each vaginal process closes up and the inguinal canal disappears. If peritoneal closure at the site of the inguinal canal is incomplete or weak, an inguinal hernia may occur later in life. The scrotal end of each vaginal process becomes the outer covering of the testis, the **tunica vaginalis.**

Fig. 21-15 shows a sagittal section of a mature testis. The adult testis is ovoid and varies considerably in length (3 to 6 cm), width (2 to 3.5 cm), depth (3 to 4 cm), and weight (10 to 40 g). The testis is almost entirely surrounded by an outer covering, the tunica vaginalis, which separates the testis from the scrotal wall, and an inner covering, the **tunica albuginea.** Inward extensions of the tunica albuginea form septa that separate the testis into about 250 compartments, or lobules, each of which contains several tortuously coiled ducts called **seminiferous tubules.** The seminiferous tubules constitute the bulk (80%) of testicular volume and are the site of sperm production. (Sperm production, termed **spermatogenesis,** is described on p. 689.) Tissue surrounding these ducts contains blood and lymphatic vessels, fibroblastic support cells, macrophages, mast cells, and Leydig cells. **Leydig cells,** which occur in clusters and account for about 1% to 5% of testicular volume, produce androgens, chiefly testosterone.

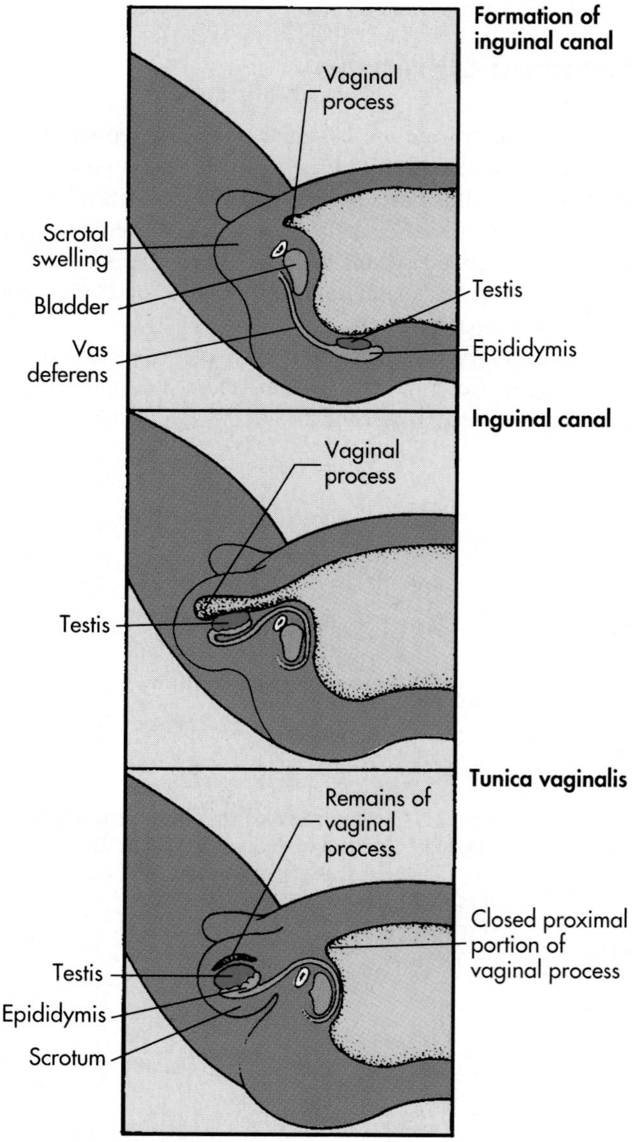

FIG. 21-14 Descent of a testis. The testes descend from the abdominal cavity to the scrotum during the last 3 months of fetal development.

The two ends of each seminiferous tubule join and leave the lobule through a short, straight section called the **tubulus rectus.** Sperm travel from the seminiferous tubules into these straight sections, which lead to the central portion of the testis, the **rete testis.** From the rete testis, sperm move through the **efferent tubules,** or vasa efferentia, to the epididymis, where they mature.

The testes are innervated by adrenergic fibers, whose sole function apparently is to regulate blood flow to the Leydig cells. The testes receive arterial blood from the internal spermatic and differential arteries. Arterial blood flows over the surface of the testes before entering the parenchyma (functional tissues). Surface flow cools the blood to temperatures that promote spermatogenesis, approximately 1.8° to 3.6° F (1° to 2° C) below body core temperature.

Epididymis

The **epididymis** (plural, *epididymides*) is a comma-shaped structure that curves over the posterior portion of each testis (see Fig. 21-15). It consists of a single, highly packed, and markedly coiled (60 to 70 cm when uncoiled) duct measuring 5 cm long, whose structural function is to conduct sperm from the efferent tubules to the vas deferens. The duct can become inflamed from infection by microorganisms that ascend the urethra or from the prostate, causing epididymitis. The epididymis has physiologic functions as well. When sperm enter the head of the epididymis, they are not fully mature or motile, nor are they capable of fertilizing an ovum. During the 12 days (or more) sperm take to travel the length of the epididymis, they receive nutrients and testosterone from the epididymal epithelium, and some biochemical or physiologic mechanism enhances their capacity for fertilization.

The tail of the epididymis is continuous with the **vas deferens,** a duct with muscular layers capable of powerful peristalsis that transports sperm toward the urethra. After traveling the length of the epididymis, sperm are stored in the epididymal tail and vas deferens. The vas deferens enters the pelvic cavity through the spermatic cord.

Scrotum

The testes, epididymides, and spermatic cord are enclosed and protected by the scrotum. The **scrotum** is a skin-covered, fibromuscular sac that is homologous to the female labia majora (see Fig. 21-2). The skin of the scrotum is thin and has rugae (wrinkles or folds), which enable it to enlarge or relax away from the body. At puberty the scrotal skin darkens, develops active sebaceous glands, and becomes sparsely covered with hair. Just under the skin lies a layer of connective tissue (fascia) and smooth muscle, the **tunica dartos** (see Fig. 21-15). The tunica dartos also forms a septum that separates the two testes. Exposure to cold temperatures causes the tunica dartos to contract, pulling the testes close to the warm body. In warm temperatures the tunica dartos relaxes, suspending the testes away from body heat. These mechanisms promote optimal temperatures for spermatogenesis. In addition, scrotal sensitivity to touch, pressure, temperature, and pain protects the testes against potential harm. During sexual excitement, the scrotal skin and tunica thicken, the scrotum tightens and lifts, and the spermatic cords shorten, partially elevating the testes toward the body. As excitement plateaus, the engorged testes increase 50% in size, rotate anteriorly, and flatten against the body, signaling impending ejaculation.

Penis

The **penis** has two main functions: delivery of sperm to the female vagina and elimination of urine. (Urine formation and excretion are the subjects of Chapter 34.) Embryonically, the penis is homologous to the female clitoris (see Fig. 21-2).

Fig. 21-13 shows a sagittal section of the adult penis and its anatomic relation to other urogenital structures. Externally the penis consists of a shaft with a tip, the **glans,** which contains the opening of the urethra. For protection, the skin of the glans folds over the tip of the penis, forming the prepuce, or **foreskin.** At birth, the foreskin is adhered to the glans. Penile erections, which commonly occur, cause the adhesions to break so that by age 3 years the foreskin becomes completely retractable. The skin of the penis is continuous with that of the groin, scrotum, and inner thighs. It is hairless, movable, and darker than surrounding skin.

Internally, the penis consists of the urethra and three compartments: two **corpora cavernosa** and the **corpus spongiosum** (Fig. 21-16). The three compartments are separated by Buck fascia and, like the testes, enclosed by a tunica albuginea. The **urethra** passes through the corpus spongiosum and ends at a sagittal slit in the glans. If the urethra is not completely surrounded by the corpus spongiosum, the meatus may open on the ventral surface of the penile shaft (hypospadias) or on the dorsal surface (epispadias).

Penetration of the female vagina is made possible by the **erectile reflex,** a process in which erectile tissues within the corpora cavernosa and corpus spongiosum become engorged with blood, generally 20 to 50 ml. The erectile tissues consist of vascular spaces, or chambers, which are supplied with blood by arterioles (small arteries). Most of the time the arterioles are constricted, so that not much blood flows through the erectile tissues. Sexual stimulation, however, causes the arterioles to dilate and fill with blood. Their rapid expansion fills the erectile tissues, causing an erection. Erection apparently is maintained by compression or constriction of veins

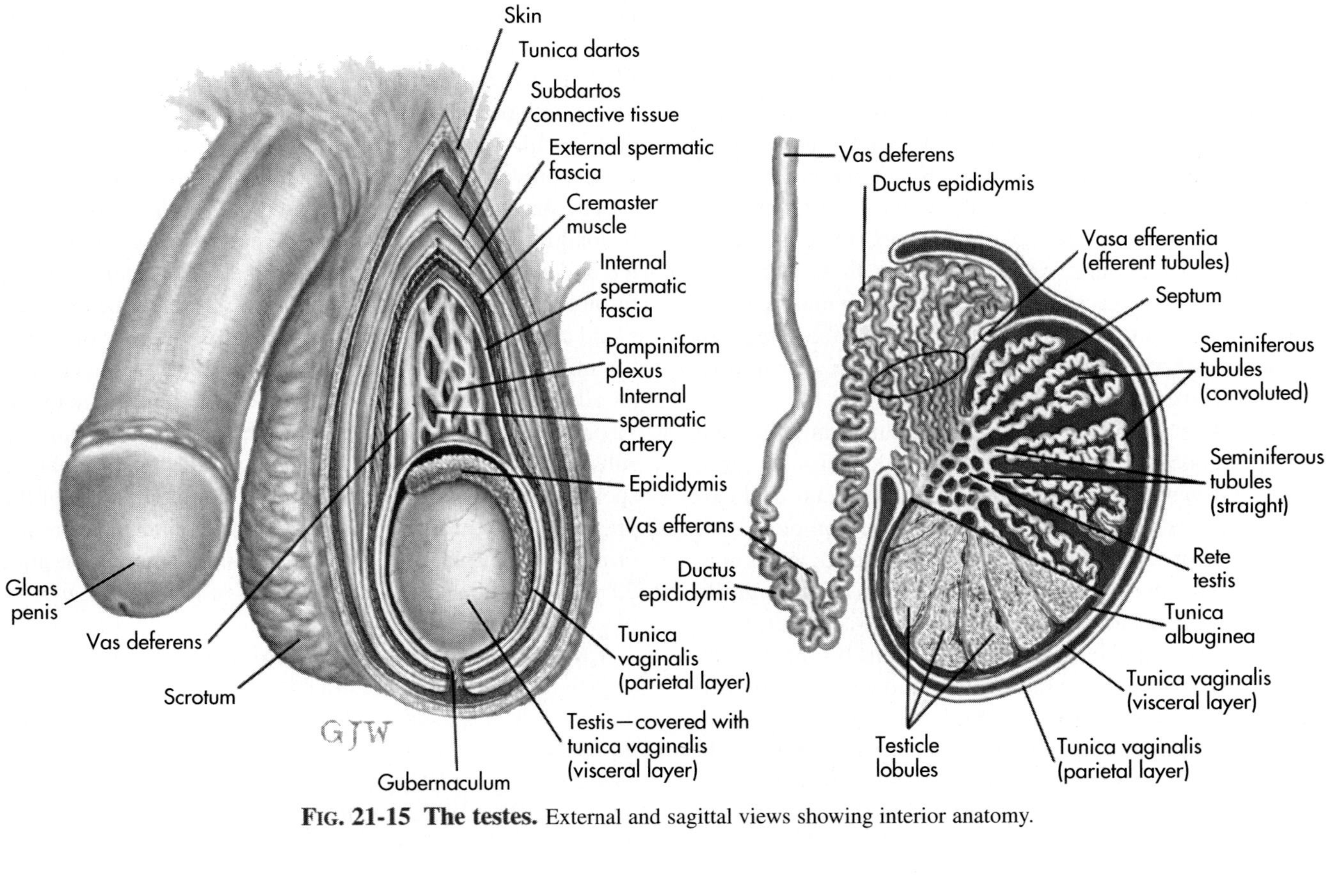

FIG. 21-15 The testes. External and sagittal views showing interior anatomy.

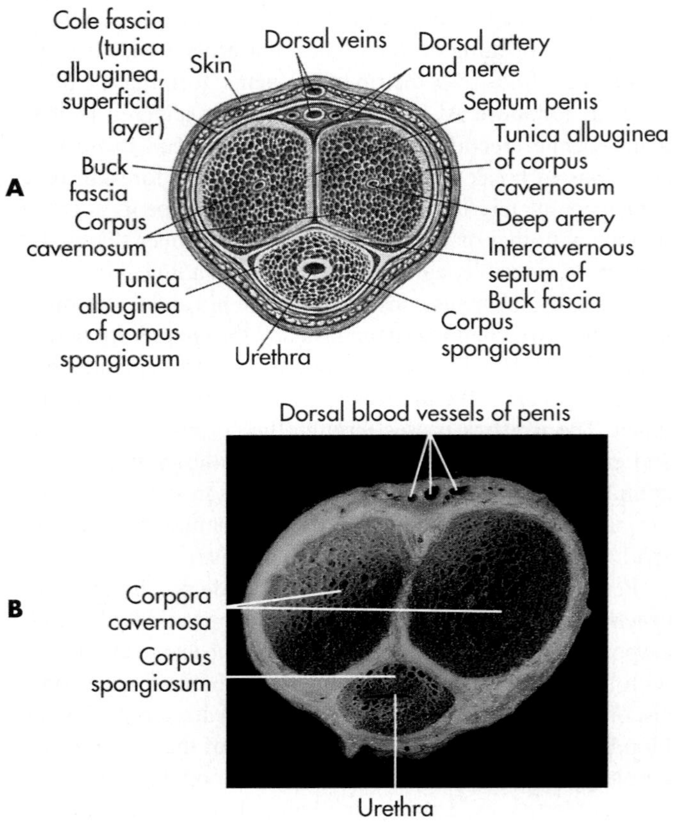

Fig. 21-16 The penis. A, Cross section of the penis. **B,** Cross section of the shaft of the penis showing three columns of erectile, or cavernous, tissue. (**A,** From Thompson JM et al: *Mosby's clinical nursing,* ed 4, St Louis, 1997, Mosby. **B,** From Thibodeau GA, Patton KI: *Anatomy and physiology,* ed 4, St Louis, 1999, Mosby.)

that drain the corpora cavernosa and corpus spongiosum. When sexual stimulation ceases or orgasm and ejaculation occur, these veins open up, blood flows out of the arterioles, and the penis becomes flaccid (soft and pendulous).

Erection is under the control of the autonomic nervous system but can be stimulated or inhibited by central nervous system input. Stimulation of mechanoreceptors of the penis, particularly of the glans, causes parasympathetic nerves of the autonomic nervous system to relax smooth muscle in the walls of penile arterioles. At the same time the effects of sympathetic nerves, which normally cause arteriolar smooth muscle to constrict, are inhibited.

Erections begin in utero and continue throughout life, but ejaculation does not occur until sperm production begins at puberty. Growth of the penis and scrotal contents continues well past puberty, however, and may not be complete until the late teens or early 20s. Penis size, when flaccid, varies considerably; with an erection, differences in penis size diminish. Sexual excitement causes the corpora cavernosa to increase in length and width and become rigid; the penis becomes erect. Stimulation of the glans, which is endowed with copious sensitive nerve endings, provides maximum erotic sensation. With sexual arousal, skin color deepens, the glans doubles in size, and the urethral meatus dilates. Ejaculation occurs with frequent, strong contractions of the vas deferens, epididymis, seminal vesicles, prostate, urethra, and penis.[16]

Internal Genitalia

Fig. 21-13 shows the anatomy of the internal genitalia and their relation to other pelvic organs. The internal genitalia consist of ducts and glands. The ducts—the two vasa deferentia, the ejaculatory duct, and the urethra—conduct sperm and glandular secretions from the testes to the urethral opening of the penis. The glands—the prostate gland, two seminal vesicles, and two Cowper (or bulbourethral) glands—secrete fluids that serve as a vehicle for sperm transport and create an alkaline, nutritious medium that promotes sperm motility and survival. Together, the sperm and the glandular fluids compose **semen.**

Sperm leave the epididymides and travel rapidly through the internal ducts in a process called **emission.** Emission occurs just seconds before ejaculation, at the moment when sexual arousal peaks. Emission always leads to ejaculation.

Emission occurs as smooth muscle in the walls of the epididymides and vasa deferentia begins to contract rhythmically, pushing sperm and epididymal secretions through the vasa deferentia. Each vas deferens is a firm, elastic, fibromuscular tube that begins at the tail of the epididymis, enters the pelvic cavity within the spermatic cord, loops up and over the bladder, and ends in the prostate gland (Fig. 21-17; see also Fig. 21-13). Sperm are moved along by peristaltic contractions of smooth muscle in the walls of the vas deferens.

As sperm leave the ampulla (wide portion) of the vas deferens, the seminal vesicles secrete a nutritive, glucose-rich fluid into the ejaculate (semen). The **seminal vesicles** are a pair of glands, each about 4 to 6 cm long, that lie behind the urinary bladder and in front of the rectum. The ducts of the seminal vesicles join the ampulla of the vas deferens to become the **ejaculatory duct,** which contracts rhythmically during emission and ejaculation. As can be seen in Figs. 21-13 and 21-17, the ejaculatory duct joins the urethra, where both pass through the prostate gland. During emission and ejaculation a sphincter (muscle surrounding a duct) closes, preventing urine from entering the prostatic urethra.

The **prostate gland** is composed of alveoli and ducts embedded in fibromuscular tissue. It measures 4 cm in diameter and weighs approximately 20 g. While semen moves through the prostatic portion of the urethra, the prostate gland contracts rhythmically and secretes prostatic fluid into the mixture. Prostatic fluid is a thin, milky substance with an alkaline pH that helps sperm to survive in the acid environment of the female reproductive tract. In addition, substances in seminal and prostatic fluids help mobilize sperm after ejaculation. Prostatitis is an inflammation of the prostate often caused by infecting microorganisms from the urinary tract. Enlargement of the prostate is common after 50 years of age and is known as *benign prostatic hypertrophy (BPH).*[17]

Cowper glands (bulbourethral glands), whose ducts secrete mucus into the urethra near the base of the penis, are the last pair of glands to add fluid to the ejaculate. Ejaculation occurs as semen reaches the base of the penis and muscles there begin the rhythmic contractions that push semen out. Normally a man ejaculates between 2 and 6 ml of semen, containing 75 million to 400 million sperm. About

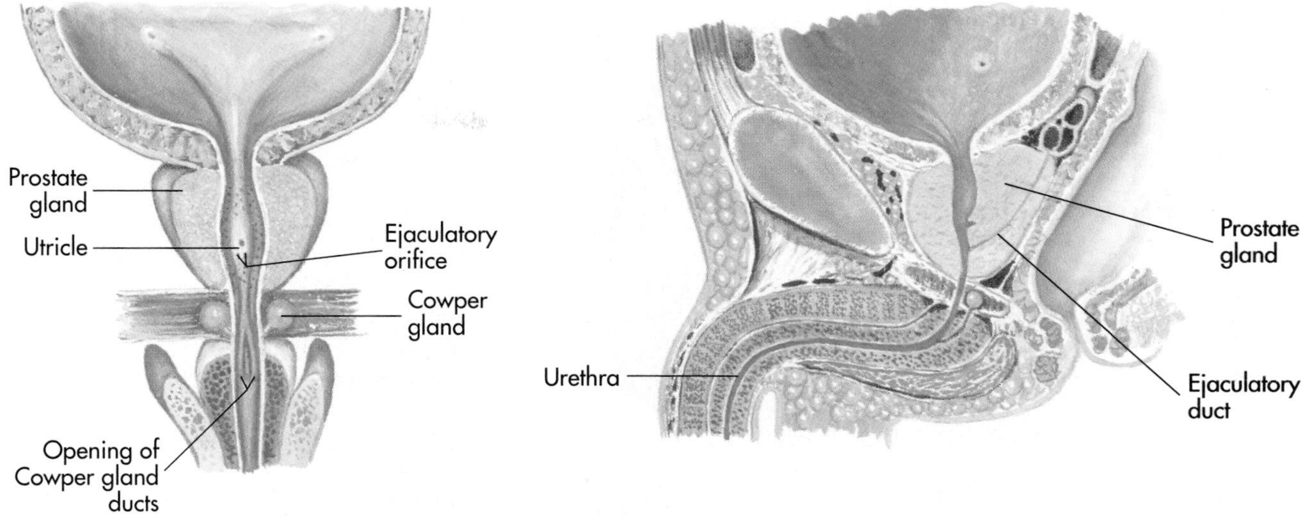

FIG. 21-17 Anatomy of the prostate gland and seminal vesicles. (From Seidel HM et al: *Mosby's guide to physical examination,* ed 4, St Louis, 1999, Mosby.)

98% of the ejaculate consists of glandular fluids; 60% to 70% of volume comes from the seminal vesicles and 20% from the prostate. Therefore the ejaculate of a man who has undergone vasectomy (a surgical procedure that prevents sperm from entering the vas deferens) is not reduced by much: about 2%.

Spermatogenesis

Spermatogenesis begins at puberty and continues for life. In this respect, spermatogenesis differs markedly from oogenesis (production of primordial ova), which occurs during fetal life only.

Spermatogenesis takes place within the seminiferous tubules of the testes (see Fig. 21-15). The basement membrane of each seminiferous tubule is lined with diploid (46-chromosome) germ cells called **spermatogonia** (singular, *spermatogonium*). These cells undergo continuous mitotic division. (Mitotic division, in which a cell divides into two identical cells, is described in Chapter 1.) Some of the spermatogonia move away from the basement membrane and mature, becoming **primary spermatocytes** (Fig. 21-18). The primary spermatocytes undergo meiosis, a type of cell division that results in two haploid (23-chromosome) cells called **secondary spermatocytes.** (Meiosis is described and illustrated in Chapter 4.) The two secondary spermatocytes then undergo meiosis, resulting in four **spermatids.** It is the spermatids that differentiate into spermatozoa, or sperm, each of which contains 23 chromosomes (Fig. 21-19).

The development of spermatids into sperm depends on the presence of **Sertoli cells (nondividing support cells)** within the seminiferous tubules. The spermatids attach themselves to Sertoli cells, from which they receive the nutrients and the hormonal signals they need to develop into sperm.

The process of spermatogenesis, from mitotic division of a spermatogonium to maturation of the spermatids, takes about 70 to 80 days. Mature sperm migrate from the seminiferous tubules to the epididymides, where their capacity for fertilization continues to develop. Although they are completely mature by the time they are ejaculated, the sperm do not become motile (capable of movement) until they are activated by biochemicals in semen and in the female reproductive tract.

Male Sex Hormones

The male sex hormones are androgens. **Testosterone,** the primary male sex hormone, is an androgen. Mainly Leydig cells of the testes and, to a lesser degree, the adrenal glands produce testosterone and other androgens. In men, sex hormone production is relatively constant with some diurnal variation.

The androgens have a number of physiologic actions related to growth and development of male tissues and organs. They are responsible for fetal differentiation and development of the male urogenital system and have some effects on the fetal brain. After birth, the Leydig cells become quiescent until activated by the gonadotropins during puberty. At puberty, androgens cause the sex organs to grow and secondary sex characteristics to develop.

Testosterone affects nervous and skeletal tissues, bone marrow, skin and hair, and sex organs. It has an anabolic effect on skeletal muscle tissue, thereby contributing to the difference in body weight and composition between men and women. Testosterone also stimulates growth of the musculature and cartilage of the larynx, causing a permanent deepening of the voice. Testosterone directly stimulates the bone marrow and indirectly stimulates renal erythropoietin production to achieve increased hemoglobin and hematocrit levels. Because sebaceous gland activity is stimulated by testosterone, acne may develop. In the presence of testosterone, hair becomes coarser in texture and facial hair, axillary hair, and pubic hair grow in male patterns. Later in life, testosterone causes baldness in genetically susceptible individuals. Testosterone is required for spermatogenesis and for secretion of fluid by the prostate gland, seminal vesicles, and Cowper glands. Testosterone is also associated with an increase in libido (sex drive). Other, less-understood, effects

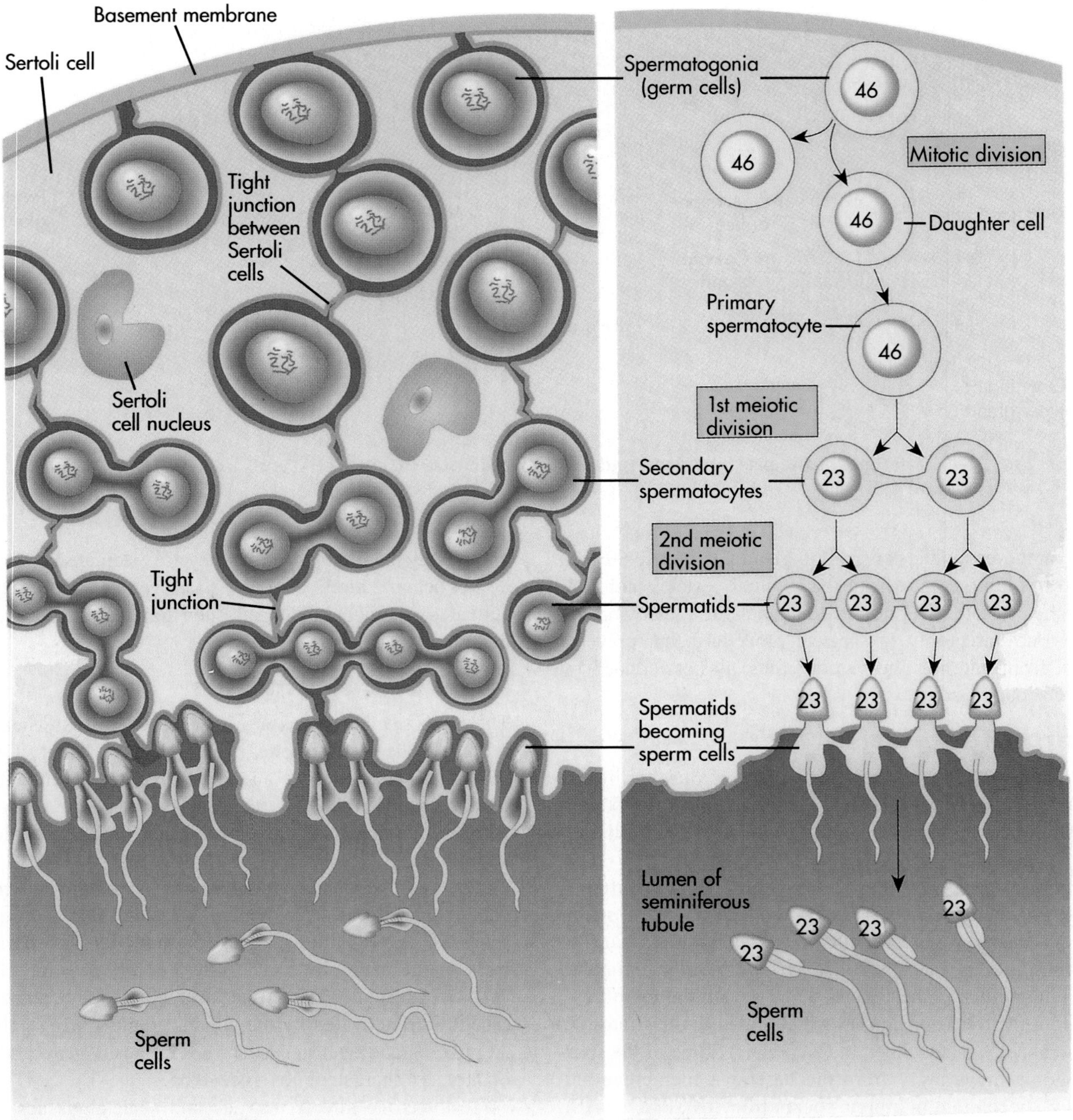

FIG. 21-18 Seminiferous tubule. Section shows process of meiosis and sperm cell formation. (From Thibodeau GA, Patton KI: *Anatomy and physiology,* ed 4, St Louis, 1999, Mosby.)

of testosterone include alterations in fatty acid and cholesterol metabolism.

The regulation of androgen production and spermatogenesis is achieved by a complex feedback system involving the extrahypothalamic central nervous system, the hypothalamus, the anterior pituitary, the testes, and the androgen-sensitive end organs. These relationships, which are essentially the same in women, are summarized in Fig. 21-3. Extrahypothalamic influences include such variables as physiologic and psychologic stress, which may inhibit or augment hypothalamic activity. In the hypothalamus, neurotransmitters regulate GnRH synthesis and pulsatile release into the hypophyseal portal veins. Norepinephrine stimulates GnRH secretion, and serotonin and dopamine inhibit GnRH secretion. GnRH is transported by portal flow to the median eminence of the pituitary gland, where it binds to receptors and stimulates the synthesis and secretion of gonadotropins, LH, and FSH. LH and FSH, which are named for their effects in the female reproductive system, have important effects on the male system as well. LH acts on the Leydig cells to stimulate testosterone secretion, which in turn is enhanced by FSH—FSH binds to Leydig cells and increases the number of LH receptors on the cells. In addition, both FSH and LH are important in the initiation and maintenance of spermatogenesis. LH and FSH secretion are inhibited by testosterone, other androgens, and estradiol. Sim-

A
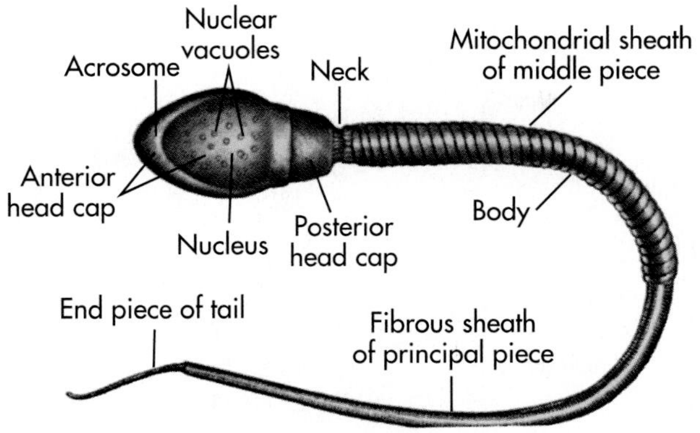

B
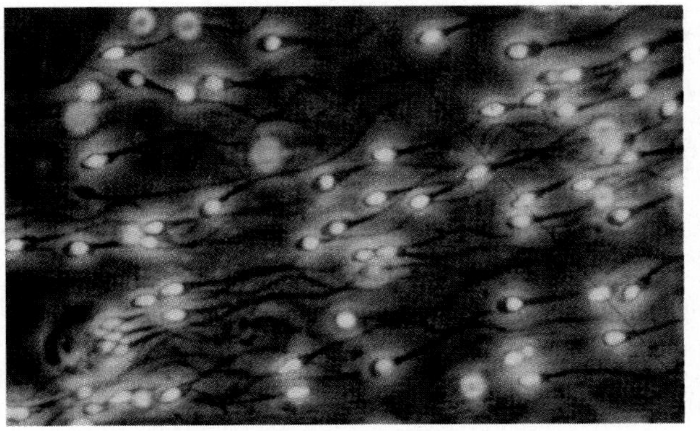

FIG. 21-19 Mature sperm cell (spermatozoon). A, Anatomy of mature sperm cell. **B,** Human sperm with nuclear material glowing with a fluorescent dye. (**A,** From Thompson JM et al: *Mosby's clinical nursing,* ed 4, St Louis, 1997, Mosby. **B,** From Thibodeau GA, Patton KI: *Anatomy and physiology,* ed 4, St Louis, 1999, Mosby.)

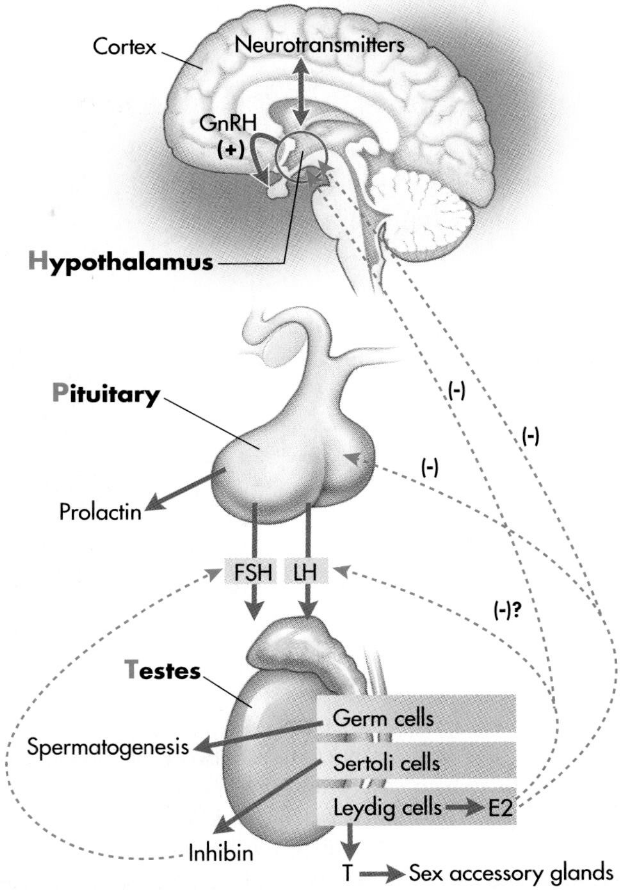

FIG. 21-20 Schematic representation of activity along the H-P-T axis.

ilar to their action in the female gonad, activin and inhibin function as autocrine/paracrine regulators in the male gonad. Activin and inhibin are produced in the Sertoli cells of the testis. Activin stimulates and inhibin inhibits proliferation of spermatogonia by regulating pituitary FSH levels. In addition, activin inhibits and inhibin facilitates LH stimulation of androgen biosynthesis in Leydig cells.

Ninety-eight percent of testosterone, the major steroid hormone produced by the testis, binds to either **sex hormone–binding globulin (SHBG)** or albumin. The remaining 2% remains unbound in the plasma and is free to enter cells and wield its metabolic effects. Changes in the amount of available SHBG affect the amount of testosterone within tissues. The testis secretes only 25% of circulating estrogen (estradiol). The majority is produced by peripheral conversion of testosterone and androstenedione. Estrogens help regulate GnRH and LH secretion. Peripheral conversion of testosterone also produces **dihydrotestosterone (DHT),** another potent androgen. DHT is necessary for external virilization during embryogenesis and androgen activity beginning at puberty and continuing throughout adulthood. **Prolactin,** a polypeptide synthesized and secreted from the pituitary, helps maintain biosynthesis of testosterone. However, elevated prolactin levels suppress biosynthesis.[18]

In summary, hormones secreted at each level of the hypothalamic-pituitary-testicular (H-P-T) axis control and coordinate testicular function (Fig. 21-20) This control is exerted through positive and negative feedback signals by (1) sex steroids that inhibit hypothalamic GnRH secretion and pituitary LH responsiveness to GnRH; and (2) testicular inhibin that inhibits pituitary FSH and, possibly, circulating estrogens (E2). Any disruption along the H-P-T axis may lead to hypogonadism or infertility.

STRUCTURE AND FUNCTION OF THE BREAST

The **breasts** are modified sebaceous glands that lie on the ventral surface of the thorax, within the superficial fascia of the chest wall. They extend vertically from the second rib to the sixth or seventh intercostal space and laterally from the side of the sternum to the midaxillary line. Breast tissue also may extend into the axilla; this tissue is known as the *tail of Spence.*

The Female Breast

The female breast is composed of 15 to 20 pyramid-shaped lobes that are separated and supported by Cooper ligaments (Fig. 21-21). Each lobe contains 20 to 40 lobules (alveoli), which subdivide further into many functional units called **acini** (singular, *acinus*). Each acinus is lined with a layer of epithelial cells capable of secreting milk and a layer of subepithelial cells capable of contracting to squeeze milk from

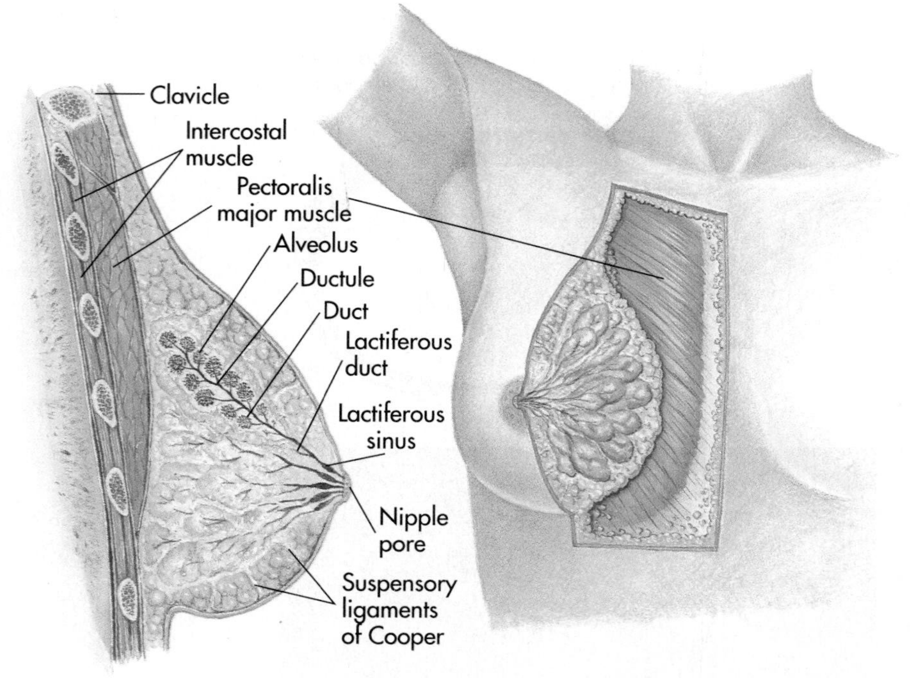

FIG. 21-21 The female breast. (From Seidel HM et al: *Mosby's guide to physical examination,* ed 4, St Louis, 1999, Mosby.)

the acinus. The acini empty into a network of lobular collecting ducts, which empty into interlobular collecting and ejecting ducts. These ducts reach the skin through openings (pores) in the nipple. The lobes and lobules are surrounded and separated by muscle strands and fatty connective tissue. The amount of fatty connective tissue varies from individual to individual, depending on weight and genetic and endocrine factors, and contributes to the diversity of breast size and shape.

An extensive capillary network surrounds the acini and is supplied by the internal and lateral thoracic arteries and the intercostal arteries. Venous return follows arterial supply, with relatively rapid emptying into the superior vena cava. The breasts receive sensory innervation from branches of the second through sixth intercostal nerves and the cervical plexus. This accounts for the fact that breast pain may be referred to the chest, back, scapula, medial arm, and neck. Lymphatic drainage of the breast occurs largely through axillary nodes, but approximately 25% occurs through transpectoral and internal mammary routes (Fig. 21-22).

The **nipple** is a pigmented, cylindric structure that is usually located at the fourth or fifth intercostal space. It measures 0.5 to 1.3 cm in diameter and is approximately 10 to 12 mm in height when erect. On its surface lie multiple openings, one from each lobe. The **areola** is the pigmented, circular area around the nipple. It may be 15 to 60 mm in diameter. A number of sebaceous glands, the **glands of Montgomery,** are located within the areola and aid in lubrication of the nipple during lactation. The nipple and areola contain smooth muscles, which receive motor innervation from the sympathetic nervous system. Sexual stimulation and exposure to cold cause the nipple to become erect.

The fetal and early postnatal development of breast tissue does not depend on hormones, although fetal breast tissue does become progressively responsive to hormonal stimulation. During childhood, breast growth is latent and growth of the nipple and areola keeps pace with body surface growth. (Male breast development normally does not progress any further.) At the onset of puberty in the female, estrogen secretion stimulates mammary growth. Breast development, or thelarche, is usually the first sign of puberty in the female. Full differentiation and maturation of breast tissue occur over approximately 4 years and are mediated by a variety of hormones, including estrogen, progesterone, prolactin, growth hormone, thyroid and parathyroid hormones, insulin, cortisol, and prolactin. Estrogen promotes development of the lobular ducts; progesterone stimulates development of cells lining the acini. Lactation (milk production) occurs after childbirth in response to increased levels of prolactin; prolactin secretion, in turn, is stimulated by breast-feeding. Oxytocin, another hormone released after delivery, controls milk ejection from acini cells. Variations in breast development are listed in Box 21-2.

During the reproductive years, the breast undergoes cyclic changes in response to changes in the levels of estrogen and progesterone associated with the menstrual cycle. During the follicular/proliferative phase of the menstrual cycle, high estradiol levels increase the vascularity of breast tissue and stimulate proliferation of ductal and acinar tissue. This effect is sustained into the luteal/secretory phase of the cycle. During this phase, progesterone levels increase and contribute to the breast changes induced by estradiol. Specific effects of progesterone include dilation of the ducts and conversion of the acinar cells into secretory cells. Most women experience some degree of premenstrual breast full-

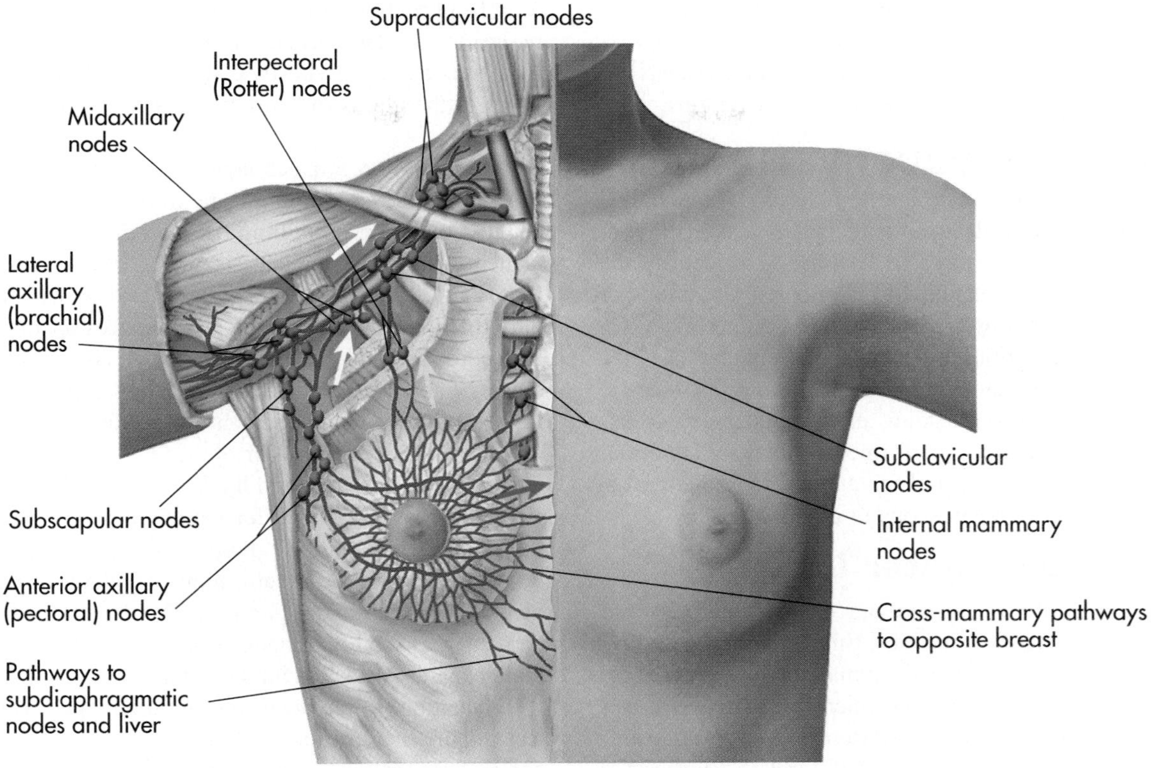

FIG. 21-22 Lymphatic drainage of the female breast. (From Seidel HM et al: *Mosby's guide to physical examination,* ed 4, St Louis, 1999, Mosby.)

Box 21-2

VARIATIONS IN BREAST DEVELOPMENT

- Ectopic breast development may occur in the axilla, abdomen, labia, or back and buttocks (less common) due to development of breast tissue from the milk line, an embryonic mammary ridge of ectoderm.
- Accessory nipples (polythelia) or mammary glands (polymastia) are due to cellular migration along the milk line; polythelia occurs in approximately 1% of the population.
- Failed development of the nipple (athelia) or entire mammary gland (amastia) is rare and may include a complete lack of development, unilateral failure, or extreme asymmetry.
- Symmetric or asymmetric hyperplasia occurs in approximately 1% to 4% of all females.
- In testicular feminization syndrome, the biologic action of testosterone is blocked and full mammary development occurs in a genetic male at puberty.
- In pubescent males, androgens fail to block the development of the mammary bud, which leads to transient unilateral or bilateral gynecomastia.

Data from Runowicz CD: Benign breast disease and screening for malignant tumors. In Copeland LJ, Farrell JF, editors: *Textbook of gynecology,* ed 2, Philadelphia, 2000, W.B. Saunders.

ness, tenderness, and increased nodularity. Breast volume may increase as much as 10 to 30 ml. Because the length of the menstrual cycle does not allow for complete regression of new cell growth, breast growth continues at a slow rate until approximately 35 years of age. Because of the cyclic changes that occur in breast tissue, breast examination should be conducted at the conclusion of or a few days after the menstrual cycle, when hormonal effects are minimal and breasts are at their smallest.

The function of the female breast is primarily to provide a source of nourishment for the newborn. Physiologically, breast milk is the most appropriate nourishment for newborns. Not only does its composition change over time to meet the changing digestive capabilities and nutritional requirements of the infant, but also breast milk contains specific immunoglobulins, especially IgA, and nonspecific antimicrobial factors, such as lysosomes and lactoferrin, which protect the infant against infection. During lactation, high prolactin levels interfere with hypothalamic-pituitary hormones that stimulate ovulation. This mechanism suppresses the menstrual cycle and prevents ovulation. In many parts of the world (so-called underdeveloped or Third World countries), continuous and constant breast-feeding is the major means of contraception. Breasts are also a source of pleasurable sexual sensation and in Western cultures have become a sexual symbol.

The Male Breast

Until puberty, development of the male breast is similar to that of the female breast. In the absence of sufficiently high levels of estrogen and progesterone, the male breast does not develop any further. The normal male breast consists of a small, underdeveloped nipple; some fatty and fibrous tissue; and a few ductlike structures in the subareolar area. The male breast may appear enlarged in obese men because of accumulation of fatty tissue. During puberty some males experience gynecomastia, a condition in which the breasts enlarge temporarily as a result of hormonal fluctuations.

TESTS OF REPRODUCTIVE FUNCTION

Diagnostic tests of the male and female reproductive systems are performed to determine the cause of infertility, to detect the presence of cancerous lesions, or to identify the presence of sexually transmitted infections. (Alterations of the reproductive systems are discussed in Chapter 22; sexually transmitted infections are discussed in Chapter 23.) Procedures include laboratory tests, such as cultures, smears, stains, biopsies, serologic testing, and hormonal assays. Radiographic procedures are performed to identify abnormal growths or structures. Direct observation of reproductive organs is completed by laparoscopy or colposcopy.

Infection and Cancer Tests

Smears, stains, cultures, and serologic testing commonly are used to detect infectious diseases. Smears are prepared by spreading a thick layer of specimen material on a glass slide. The specimen may be evaluated microscopically as a wet mount or dried and stained with different dyes. Gram staining is a technique that allows the differential identification of two categories of bacteria according to the tendency of the microorganism to selectively absorb different components of the stain. Fluorescent antibody testing and deoxyribonucleic acid (DNA) probe testing (nucleic acid hybridization detection method) are fairly quick, inexpensive, and accurate methods that can be used to detect some bacterial and viral infections.

A **culture** is the growth of microorganisms in a nutrient medium selectively prepared to support the growth of particular microorganisms that are obtained from body secretions or tissues. Both bacteria and viruses, such as cytomegalovirus, can be cultured.

Serologic testing identifies whether an antigen-antibody reaction has occurred in response to an infectious microorganism. Several different techniques can be used to identify the formation of antigen-antibody complexes. With immunofluorescent testing, fluorescein-labeled antibodies react with specific antigen, such as the spirochetes of syphilis. The fluorescent pattern of the reaction can be microscopically observed under ultraviolet light. The flocculation (agglutination) test is the precipitation of clumped cells caused by the reaction of antigen with homologous antiserum. The Venereal Disease Research Laboratory (VDRL) test for syphilis is a type of flocculation test. Certain viral diseases can be diagnosed using specific serologic antibody markers, for example, the diagnosis of hepatitis A and hepatitis B viruses. Radioimmunoassay (RIA) and enzyme-linked immunosorbent assay (ELISA) are more specific tests used to document viral infections. Tests used for the diagnosis of sexually transmitted infections are presented in Table 21-3.

Tissue biopsy is the surgical resection of a tissue specimen from a suspected site. The biopsy provides cells and tissues to identify infectious processes and to differentiate benign from malignant conditions and primary from metastatic lesions. In the reproductive tract, tissue may be obtained from the vagina, cervix (by cone or brush biopsy), endometrium of the uterus (by curettage), ovary, testis, prostate, or penis.

Needle biopsy is a technique of aspirating small amounts of tissue by positioning a needle in the tissue and applying negative pressure by pulling back on the plunger of the attached syringe as the needle is moved back and forth at the biopsy site. There is relatively less discomfort with this procedure than with a tissue biopsy that requires opening the surface of the skin to localize the tissue site. Normal findings indicate no abnormal cells or tissues on histologic examination.

The **Papanicolaou smear** is a procedure commonly used for the cytologic examination of the female reproductive tract. Cells from body tissues and fluids (from the vagina or cervix) are stained and examined for the number and types of cells and abnormalities in their morphology. Specimens also may be obtained from the mouth; nipple discharge; or amniotic, pleural, or spinal fluid aspirations. The Papanicolaou smear is particularly useful for diagnosis of premalignant (dysplastic), malignant, atypical, and inflammatory cells.

Evaluations of the breast are commonly performed to detect tumors or to differentiate solid masses from cysts and benign from malignant tumors. Screening or diagnostic mammography, surgical or fine needle biopsy, and ultrasonography are specific examination techniques. Less frequent tests include thermography, which is used for screening; chest x-rays, which are used to detect pulmonary metastases; and computed tomography (CT) scanning, which is used when liver or brain metastases are suspected. **Mammography** is a low-dose radiographic examination used to identify nonpalpable (less than 1 cm) or unrecognized lesions. Breast cancer can be detected by radiography 2 to 3 years before its clinical presentation, providing an excellent prognosis for cure. The American Cancer Society recommends a baseline mammogram of all women at 40 years of age, annual or biannual mammograms between 40 and 49 years of age, and yearly mammograms after 50 years of age.[19]

Ultrasonography is performed chiefly to differentiate cystic from solid lesions; it is not diagnostic of malignancy. **Fine needle aspiration,** an inexpensive and relatively simple procedure, is used to aspirate cysts or to obtain a specimen for **cytologic examination.** The main problem with any needle biopsy or aspiration is sampling error caused by improper positioning of the needle, which creates false-negative test results. The rate of false-positive results with fine needle aspiration is 1% to 2%; the rate of false-negative results is 10%.[20]

Fertility Tests

Tests of reproductive function are performed most commonly when infertility exists. Both the male and female partners are examined, and several diagnostic evaluations may be completed. The types of tests and their normal values are summarized in Tables 21-4 and 21-5. The man is evaluated for number, amount, structure, and motility of sperm and obstruction along the reproductive tract. Tests for women determine whether (1) the reproductive tract

Table 21-3 Diagnosis of Sexually Transmitted Infections

Test	Description	Normal Value
SEROLOGIC TEST FOR SYPHILIS	Detection of antibodies to *Treponema pallidum*	Negative or nonreactive
VDRL	Venereal Disease Research Laboratory (nonspecific)	
RPR	Rapid plasma reagin (more specific)	
FTA	Fluorescent treponemal antibody absorption test (more specific; confirmatory test)	
OTHER TEST FOR SYPHILIS		
Darkfield examination	Direct smear of serous exudate from moist lesions to detect *Treponema pallidum* with corkscrew appearance	Negative
TESTS FOR GONORRHEA		
Culture	Isolation and detection of *Neisseria gonorrhoeae* in urethral, anal, or pharyngeal secretions	No growth
Gram stain	Direct smear and staining of cervical or urethral discharge to identify gram-negative intracellular diplococci with polymorphonuclear (PMN) leukocytes	Negative
DNA probe	Direct detection of DNA (inexpensive and quick)	Negative
TESTS FOR *CHLAMYDIA*		
Tissue culture	Isolation and detection of *Chlamydia trachomatis* from epithelial cells of endocervix and urethra (expensive, time extensive)	No growth
Cervical wet mount	A wet mount preparation of endocervical secretions (EC) can accurately rule out the presence of gonococci and *Chlamydia trachomatis*	EC WBC <5
Antigen detection or DNA probe	Direct immunofluorescent staining of cervical or urethral specimens to detect monoclonal antibodies or genetic probe to detect DNA sequence (both are inexpensive, quick)	Negative
Urine DNA amplification	Universal screening is more effective; future studies are recommended	Negative
TESTS FOR HIV INFECTION		
ELISA (enzyme-linked immunosorbent assay)	Detects the presence of antibodies to human immunodeficiency virus (HIV)	Nonreactive
IFA (indirect fluorescent antibody)	A more specific test for HIV	Nonreactive
WB (Western blot)	A more specific test for HIV	Nonreactive
TESTS FOR VIRAL INFECTIONS		
TORCH test	Detects elevations of IgA or IgM caused by *Toxoplasma,* rubella, cytomegalovirus, syphilis, and herpes simplex in mother and newborn infant; herpes requires more specific testing when result is positive	No elevation in antibodies
Cytomegalovirus (herpes virus 5)	Can be grown in cell culture with samples from urine, cervix, semen, saliva, blood	No growth
HPV testing	Detects human papillomavirus, a primary cause of cervical cancer	Negative

DNA, Deoxyribonucleic acid; *TORCH,* *t*oxoplasmosis, *o*ther, *r*ubella, *c*ytomegalovirus, *h*erpes simplex; *IgA,* immunoglobulin A; *IgM,* immunoglobulin M.

(cervix, uterus, fallopian tubes) is adequately patent to allow for passage of ovum and sperm, (2) ovulation occurs normally, (3) the endometrium is responding normally to hormones, and (4) reproductive tissues are free of tumors or infections. Hormonal assays evaluate the adequacy of pituitary function and target organ response. The position and size of organs or the presence of tumors can be detected by direct observation procedures using a laparoscope or by radiographic studies, such as plain films, computerized scans, or tomography.

Aging and Reproductive Function

Aging and the Female Reproductive System

Menopause is a normal developmental event that is experienced universally by midlife women. In the United States, women reach menopause between ages 48 and 55 years, at a median age of 51.4 years.[7,11] The mean age for smokers is 2 years sooner than nonsmokers (50 versus 52 years).[11,21] Age of menopause tends to be genetically predetermined and

Table 21-4 Tests and Normal Values of Reproductive Function/Fertility

Test	Description	Normal Value
BASIC ASSESSMENT		
Semen analysis (2 samples at least 2 wk apart)	Determines number, motility, and structure of sperm cells	Volume = 2-6 ml Number = >20 million/ml Motility = >50% with forward progression Morphology = >30% normal shape Immunobead test = <20% with adherent particles Sperm Mar test = <10% with adherent particles
	Determines presence of bacteria/leukocytes	$<10^6$ WBC/ml
Antisperm antibody	Detects antibody to sperm	No sperm agglutinins present
INTERMEDIATE ASSESSMENT		
Basal body temperature	Determines whether ovulation has occurred	Decrease in basal body temperature before ovulation followed by a rise in temperature at the time of ovulation
Cervical mucus	Evaluates presence of ovulation from estrogenic effects at ovulation; mucus may also be examined for pH, glucose, or proteins or cultured for presence of infection	Fern pattern appears when cervical mucus dries on a clean slide; mucus is clear, watery, and elastic (spinnbarkeit ≥8-10 cm) with no inflammatory cells
Postcoital cervical mucus (Sims-Huhner test)	Tests ability of sperm to penetrate and maintain motility in cervical mucus 2-4 hr after coitus approximately 1 day before ovulation	≥10 motile sperm in each high-power field; motility in one direction; previous sperm analysis normal
Zona binding test	Nonliving oocytes are surgically removed and bisected; sperm added to the hemioocyte to test fertilizing capability	Bonding <30% predicted failed fertilization 70% of the time Bonding >30% predicted successful fertilization 85% of the time
Ultrasound vaginal scanning	Provides superior quality resolution of the uterine, fallopian, and ovarian structures; also can be used to study folliculogenesis, ovulation, and luteogenesis to detect abnormalities	Normal structures visualized
Falloposcopy	The only method to directly visualize the luminal architecture	Determines if lumen is patent
MORE SPECIALIZED TESTS		
Endometrial biopsy	Determines whether ovulation has occurred by obtaining endometrial tissue on day 26 of 28-day menstrual cycle (or postovulatory day 12)	Finding is "secretory-type" endometrium if ovulation has occurred; read in conjunction with day of cycle and serum progesterone levels
Hysterosalpingogram	Assessment of uterus and fallopian tubes for obstructions using transuterine injection of contrast material and radiography; performed 1-2 days after cessation of menses	No obstruction evident
Uterotubal insufflation (Rubin test)	Assesses patency of fallopian tubes using transuterine tubal insufflation with carbon dioxide and pressure measurement	Pressure <180-200 mm Hg, no obstruction; pressure >200 mm Hg indicates tubal obstruction; repeated studies differentiate obstruction from tubal spasm
Laparoscopy (pelvic endoscopy)	Visualization of reproductive organs using a laparoscope inserted within the pelvic cavity through the abdomen to assess structure or determine presence of adhesions, endometriosis, tumors, or infection	Normal structure and position of organs
Hysteroscopy	Visualization of uterine cavity using modified cystoscope inserted through cervical os; best done during first 14 days of cycle	Absence of intrauterine lesions

WBC, White blood cells.

Table 21-5 Serum Hormone Values

Hormone	Value
Serum progesterone	Normal = >10 ng/dl, presumptive evidence of ovulation; draw level between days 20-25 of 28-day cycle or 6-10 days postovulation <10 ng/ml = inadequate luteal function <3 ng/ml suggests anovulation
Serum testosterone Resulting from diurnal and pulsatile pattern, need serial blood draws	Normal = 300-1200 ng/dl; must be interpreted with serum LH and FSH levels Low values in male hypogonadism
Serum FSH and LH Resulting from diurnal and pulsatile pattern, need serial blood draws	FSH = <22 IU/L LH = 4-24 IU/L High levels in males indicate primary testicular disease; low levels in males indicate hypogonadism caused by hypothalamic-pituitary dysfunction

LH, Luteinizing hormone; *FSH,* follicle-stimulating hormone.

WHAT'S NEW? Perimenopausal Endogenous Ovarian Hyperstimulation Syndrome

Contrary to popular belief, women experience a *hyperestrogenic* state before menopause. In a comprehensive meta-analysis of international research, Dr. Jerilyn Prior concludes that perimenopause (the period from about 5 years before until 1 year after cessation of menstruation) is a time when average estrogen levels are higher than in the fertile stage of a woman's reproductive life. Perimenopausal signs and symptoms, hormone levels, and pathogenesis are similar to the physiologic state experienced by infertile women treated with exogenous ovarian hyperstimulation therapy, hence the name.

It is important to note that there is controversy regarding estrogen levels during perimenopause. Some researchers and clinicians maintain that estrogen levels are slightly elevated during the perimenopause, whereas others continue to espouse the theory of declining estrogen during this time.

Data from Prior JC: Perimenopause: the complex endocrinology of the menopausal transition, *Endocr Rev* 19(4):397, 1998; Speroff L et al: *Clinical gynecologic endocrinology and fertility,* ed 6, Baltimore, 1999, Lippincott.

does not appear to be affected by age at menarche, childbearing or lactation, use of oral contraceptives, socioeconomic class, or race. Besides smoking, younger age at menopause has been associated with abnormal chromosome karyotype (Turner syndrome, gonadal dysgenesis) and undernourishment. Thinner women experience menopause at a slightly younger age, probably related to body fat. Irregular menses in women in their early forties also may be a predictor of an earlier menopause. Alcohol consumption has been associated with later menopause, perhaps due to higher blood and urinary levels of estrogen.[11] Approximately 30% of women experience surgical menopause between ages 22 and 48 years.[7] Peak incidence of hysterectomy, with or without oophorectomy, occurs at age 47 or 48 years, during the perimenopausal transition.[22]

Perimenopause is the transitional period between reproductive and nonreproductive years. The perimenopause usually spans approximately 5 years; 95% of women experience a transition lasting 2 to 8 years.[11,22] Currently there is no universally accepted definition of perimenopause in regard to specific age of onset or duration. Five to 10 years before menopause, approximately 90% of women note mild to extreme variability in frequency and quality of menstrual flow. Perimenopause symptoms depend on the sensitivity of the target tissue receptors. Symptoms usually begin with a shortening of the menstrual cycle, which correlates with shorter follicular phase (FP) lengths, followed by unpredictable or irregular ovulation and a lengthening of the menstrual cycle. Whether early or late, lengthening of cycles uniformly precedes menopause.[11] The perimenopause experience varies between women and from cycle to cycle in the same woman, just as the menstrual experience does in younger, fertile women. It is not uncommon for a woman to experience a short cycle with shortened FP, ovulation, and insufficient luteal phase (LP); followed by a long cycle with extended FP, anovulation, and high E2 levels in the premenstrual phase; followed by a short FP, anovulatory cycle. Variability in cycle length is the norm, and response to the ever-changing hormonal milieu is individual.

Around 37 to 38 years of age, 10 to 15 years before menstruation ceases, women experience accelerated folicular loss that begins when the total number of follicles reaches about 25,000 and ends when the supply of follicles is depleted (see discussion under Hormonal Controls, earlier in this chapter). This loss correlates with a subtle but definite increase in FSH and a decrease in inhibin. Increased FSH stimulation seems to accelerate follicular loss, and declining inhibin production disturbs the negative feedback influence over pituitary secretion of FSH. Perimenopausal cycles are marked by elevated FSH, decreased inhibin, normal LH, and slightly elevated estradiol levels (Fig. 21-23).[11] A hallmark characteristic of impending menopause is the initial "monotropic" FP increase in FSH without corresponding changes in LH levels. Lower inhibin B and increased activin A (a potent stimulator of FSH) levels contribute to this phenomenon.[14]

Increased FSH levels and reduced ovarian secretion of inhibin reflect quality and capability of aging follicles. In a

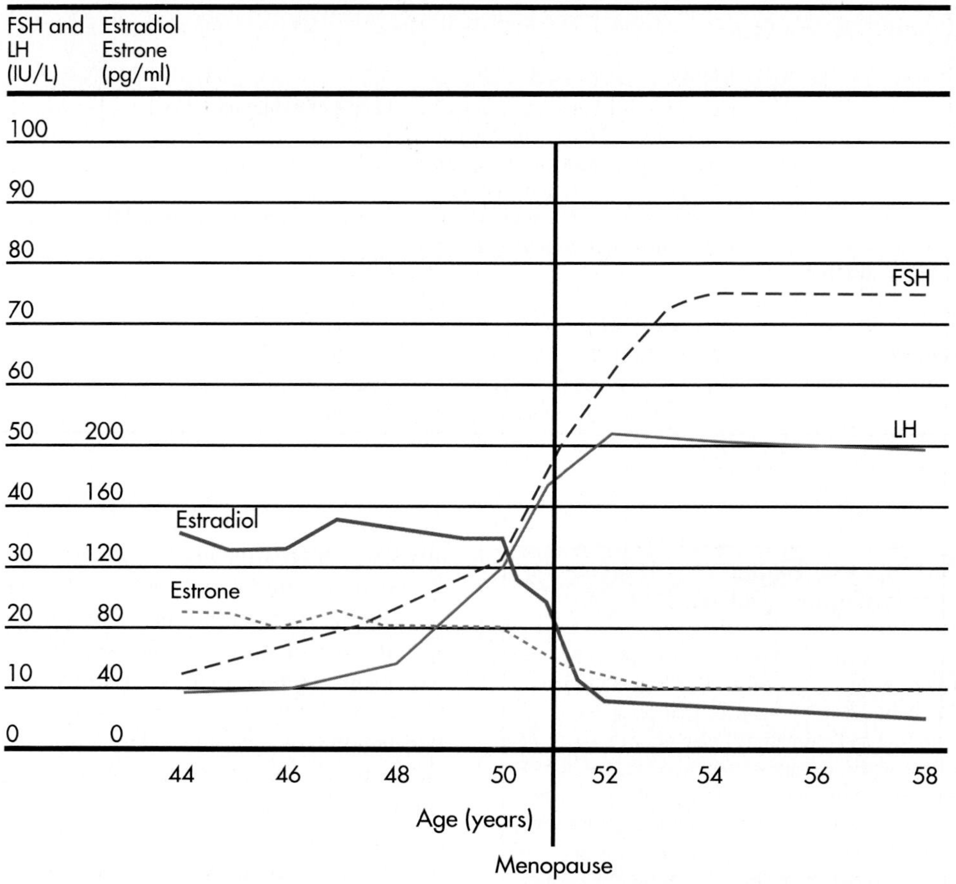

Fig. 21-23 The perimenopausal transition. Mean circulating hormone levels. (From Speroff L et al: *Clinical gynecologic endocrinology and fertility,* ed 6, Baltimore, 1999, Lippincott.)

study of pregnancy rates during in vitro fertilization (IVF), women over 40 years of age had as many oocytes recovered during laparoscopy, equal estrogen and progesterone levels, and similar pregnancy rates when compared with younger women. Yet, despite similar estradiol (E2) levels, inhibin response to exogenous hyperstimulation was significantly lower in the older women. Further, inhibin levels were significantly related to progesterone levels. In this study, 60% of women over 40 years of age who became pregnant through IVF spontaneously aborted, compared with 30% of younger women.[22]

In summary, hormonal findings during the years surrounding menopause indicate that the process of folliculogenesis changes (Box 21-3). Initially, FSH levels are significantly elevated while pulsatile secretion by the pituitary is maintained. Later, LH levels rise. In younger women, FSH stimulates inhibin, which in turn suppresses FSH. However, through an undetermined mechanism, perimenopausal women produce high levels of FSH in early FP and lower FP inhibin levels. The ovary, in response to high FSH, recruits increasing numbers of follicles; these follicles only partially develop, with a net effect of irregular ovulation, lower progesterone levels, and depleted follicle reserve. The increase in developing follicles leads to increased E2 levels. It is believed that lower levels of inhibin and higher levels of activin counteract the usual impact of the negative feedback loop found in younger women.[14,22] Table 21-6 summarizes endocrine events occurring during the perimenopause.

Box 21-3

CHANGES IN OVARIAN FOLLICULOGENESIS DURING THE PERIMENOPAUSE LEADING TO ENDOGENOUS OVERSTIMULATION

↑ FSH → ovarian hyperstimulation → ↑ number of follicles recruited (net effect of follicular depletion) → ↑ estrogen (E2)
↓ Follicular reserve → ↓ inhibin and ↑ activin in FP and LP → ↑ FSH → ↑ number of follicles recruited, partial development, infrequent ovulation → ↑ estrogen (E2) and ↓ progesterone

The majority of health concerns and public health issues focus on menstrual cycle changes, **vasomotor symptoms** or hot flashes/flushes, potential for bone loss (osteoporosis is discussed in Chapter 41), and the emotional symptoms that may accompany the perimenopausal transition.[7,22] Menstrual flooding is one of the most distressing complaints and affects approximately 50% of women. It is also the complaint that in the past put women at high risk for hysterectomy. Flooding is correlated with a change from ovulatory to anovulatory cycles and is associated with unopposed high

Table 21-6 Endocrine Events Associated with Perimenopause

Hormone Changes	Effects
Estradiol (E2) levels	Erratic and intermittent increase
Mean FP level 1 greater than mean FP level in younger women	First in FP (inverse relationship between length of FP and estradiol Level)
FP level may be greater than midcycle peak level in fertile women	Later during premenstrual phase
Ovulatory cycles	Short or insufficient LP (decreased fertility)
Progesterone levels	Decreased in ovulatory cycles; minimal during anovulatory cycles
Anovulatory cycles	Increased to about 50%; perhaps more in later perimenopause
FSH levels	Variable, then increased
LH levels	Normal initially, then increased
Inhibin levels	Correlate with progesterone levels

FP, Follicular phase; *FSH,* follicle-stimulating hormone; *LH,* luteinizing hormone; *LP,* luteal phase.

Table 21-7 Impact of High Estrogen Levels on Menstrual Cycle and Symptomatology

Associated Physiologic Change	Signs/Symptoms
Short follicular phase (FP)	Short cycles
Long FP	Long cycles
Thickened endometrium*	Heavy, long, or unpredictable flow (including clotting and flooding)*
Increase in glandular cells without stromal support produced by progesterone → unstable endometrium	Midcycle spotting
Possible increased production of prostaglandins within endometrial tissue	Flooding (menorrhagia)
	Menometrorrhagia
	Dysmenorrhea
	Breast tenderness, modularity, enlargement
	Water retention
	Emotional stress; new or unpredictable mood swings
	Weight gain
	Vasomotor symptoms
	New onset of migraine headaches; exacerbation of headaches
	Increased premenstrual symptoms

*Symptoms aggravated by anovulatory cycles; leads to dysfunctional uterine bleeding (see Chapter 22).

E2 levels the week before bleeding. Estrogen causes endometrial tissue to thicken. Because women with anovulatory cycles have longer exposure to periods of unopposed estrogen, the mean thickness of their endometrium, as measured by ultrasound, is greater than that of ovulatory women.[7,22] Thicker endometrium without corresponding stromal support from progesterone production leads to heavier periods (with or without flooding and clotting) or midcycle bleeding (Table 21-7).

In the United States, most women and clinicians link hot flashes/flushes, or **vasomotor flush,** with menopause and low estrogen levels. However, a rapid change in estrogen levels (withdrawal or increase), rather than low estrogen levels, induces hot flushes. Vasomotor symptoms are characterized by a rise in skin temperature, dilation of peripheral blood vessels, increased blood flow to the hands, increased skin conductance, and transient increase in heart rate (average of 9 beats per minute and up to 20), followed by a temperature drop and profuse perspiration over the area of flush distribution. Vasomotor flush usually occurs in the face and neck and may radiate into the chest and other parts of the body. Dizziness, nausea, headaches, or palpitations may accompany the flush. Vasomotor symptoms vary in frequency, intensity, and duration, lasting 1 to 5 minutes (mean 2.7 minutes). Anywhere from 11% to 85% of menopausal women experience vasomotor flushes.[7,22] Most (about 60% to 65%) have symptoms for 1 to 5 years, 25% for 6 to 10 years, and 10% to 15% for 10 to 15 years or longer.

Women with higher cyclic E2 levels, that is, premenopausal women with premenstrual vasomotor symptoms and women who report breast, fluid, and premenstrual mood symptoms during the early stages of the perimenopause, are predisposed to withdrawal vasomotor symptoms later in the perimenopausal transition. Anecdotal reports from participants in various research studies suggest that vasomotor symptoms occur just before flow and may be used to predict menstruation.[22] Cyclic vasomotor symptoms, which typically begin early in the perimenopausal transition, differs from noncyclic vasomotor symptoms, which are experienced in late perimenopause. Early vasomotor symptoms typically occur during sleep, often in the early hours of the morning, with few or no daytime vasomotor symptoms; are occasionally preceded by an aura (feelings of anxiety, anger, or panic); and may be associated with nausea, palpitations, dizziness, or faint feelings. Cyclic symptoms tend to occur over several days before and during menses, whereas midcycle vasomotor symptoms are less common and more likely to occur in anovulatory cycles when progesterone does not follow high estrogen midcycle peak. In summary, vasomotor symptoms commonly start when estrogen levels are erratic in the early perimenopause, and they occur in younger women with premenstrual syndrome and high E2 levels. In addition, vasomotor symptoms are highly correlated with a decreased quality of life, especially when sleep is disturbed. Understanding the physiology of vasomotor symptoms and developing a range of nonhormonal and hormonal strategies for control are important priorities in perimenopause research.

Based on the integration of collected data, a temporal chart outlining phases of the perimenopausal transition and associated endocrine changes and symptoms has been developed.[22] Although the transition is divided into five phases, the vast variability in timing and degree of symptoms experienced by individual women may make clear predictions impossible. The information outlined in Table 21-8 provides a template to visualize the complex physiology of the perimenopause and the dynamic changes that occur during this time.

Several other physiologic changes are associated with the postmenopausal period. These changes affect breast tissue, urogenital structures, bone density or risk for osteoporosis, risk for heart disease, possible memory loss or Alzheimer disease, and others. Only changes in the breast and urogenital structures will be addressed here (other topics are addressed in appropriate chapters).

As ovarian function changes, breast tissue involutes. Two phases of involution have been described: the premenopausal phase and the postmenopausal phase. The premenopausal phase occurs between 35 and 45 years of age. During this phase, there is a moderate decrease in mammary tissue. During the postmenopausal phase, glandular breast tissue is significantly reduced and there is some increase of fat deposits and connective tissue. These changes contribute to the reduction in size and firmness of breast tissue.

The urogenital tract undergoes a number of changes. The ovaries begin to decrease in size around age 30 years, and shrinkage accelerates after age 60 years. Gradually, over the years, the uterus atrophies and decreases in size. The vagina shortens, narrows, and loses some of its elasticity. Vaginal walls lose their ability to lubricate quickly. When sexually aroused, postmenopausal women may take 1 to 3 minutes to lubricate, compared with premenopausal women, who take 6 to 30 seconds. Intercourse before adequate lubrication may be painful. The vaginal pH, usually maintained at 4.0 to 6.0 before menopause, increases to between 6.5 and 8.0 and contributes to a higher incidence of vaginitis. The cervix atrophies and the cervical os decreases in size. The vaginal epithelium also atrophies; this atrophy can cause vaginal irritation, burning, itching (pruritus), white discharge (leukorrhea), painful intercourse (dyspareunia), and vaginal bleeding. The labia majora and minora become less prominent, and some pubic hair is lost. Urethral tone declines, as does muscle tone throughout the pelvic area. Urinary frequency, urgency, and incontinence are associated with estrogen deficiency.

Sexually active women have less vaginal atrophy; presumably, sexual activity and stimulation maintains vaginal

Table 21-8 Postulated Perimenopausal Transition Timeline

Phase	Menstrual Physiology	Hormonal Changes	Symptomatology
A	Regular, ovulatory cycles Short cycles, short FP	Intermittent ↑ E2 FSH usually normal Intermittent ↑ FP FSH Low inhibin	Increased breast tenderness, mood swings, fluid retention, premenstrual symptoms Early morning night sweats (vasomotor symptoms) Weight gain, migraine headaches, heavy flow
B	Regular cycles with disturbances in ovulation Short LP Insufficient LP Anovulatory cycles	Intermittent ↑ FP FSH E2 often ↑ Inhibin inappropriately low	Heavy flow ↑ premenstrual symptoms ↑ dysmenorrhea Predictable or ↑ vasomotor symptoms before flow
C	Onset of perimenopause Alternating short, long, or skipped cycles	E2 often quite ↑ E2 normal or low ↑ FSH (slight) ↑ LH Low inhibin	Vasomotor symptoms during waking hours Vasomotor symptoms more persistent, remain cyclic before flow
D	Onset of oligomenorrhea 50% of cycles anovulatory Heavy flow may predict onset of oligomenorrhea	↑ progesterone with ovulation Persistent ↓ FSH ↑ LH Low inhibin	↑ vasomotor symptoms ↑ signs/symptoms of high estrogen after long periods without flow Flow light but unpredictable
E	Final menstrual period plus 1 year	↑ FHS and LH ↓ or normal E2 Consistent low inhibin	↑ intensity and frequency of vasomotor symptoms (although vasomotor symptoms may disappear) ↓ cramps and premenstrual-type symptoms without subsequent flow ↓ breast, mood, and fluid symptoms

E2, Estradiol; *FP,* follicular phase; *FSH,* follicle-stimulating hormone; *LP,* luteal phase.

vasculature and circulation.[11] Regular intercourse (once or twice per week) and masturbation are associated with vaginal pliability, vaginal function, and continued rapid lubrication with arousal.[13]

Aging and the Male Reproductive System

Men maintain reproductive capacity longer than women. There is no known discrete event, comparable to menopause, that characterizes aging of the male reproductive system. Changes do occur, however, in male sexual behavior and in testicular structure and function, including hormonal secretion and spermatogenesis.

Components of male sexual behavior include both sexual drive and erectile and ejaculatory capacity. **Libido,** or sexual drive, is a complex phenomenon that requires a baseline hormonal milieu but is influenced significantly by health status and environmental, social, and psychologic factors. Aging causes specific physical changes that influence erectile and ejaculatory capabilities. Alterations in sexual response include the need for longer stimulation to achieve full erection; slower and less forceful ejaculation, with less pelvic muscle involvement; decreased vasocongestive response; and longer refractory period (time during which erection and ejaculation are not possible), up to 24 hours in some men.

The testes undergo several age-related structural changes, including decreased weight, atrophy, and softening. Degenerative changes in the seminiferous tubules may include thickening of the basement membrane; increase in lumen size; germ cell (spermatogonium) arrest and a decrease in spermatogenic activity; and collapse of tubules, followed by complete obstruction caused by sclerosis and fibrosis. Areas of mild to severe degenerative change may be interspersed with areas having intact tubules. These morphologic changes may result from atherosclerosis (arterial clogging) in the testicular vascular bed.[16] Alterations of the seminiferous tubules do not appear to diminish sperm counts, but they do reduce fertility because a greater percentage of the sperm lack motility or have structural abnormalities.

Aging probably causes changes in the production of male sex hormones and responsiveness of target tissues. Hormone synthesis by the testes, testicular responsiveness to the gonadotropins (FSH and LH), and pituitary secretion of these gonadotropins are altered. Most studies of testosterone levels in aging men show that their serum testosterone levels are lower than levels in younger men.[23-25]

The reduced levels of testosterone may be related to alterations in the Leydig cells, the testosterone producers of the testes. The number of Leydig cells decreases as age increases, perhaps because of atherosclerotic changes in arteries that supply blood to the testes. Even if testosterone levels are not decreased, older men may have less unbound testosterone in their blood, decreasing the amount of unbound hormone available to stimulate target tissues. Decreased testosterone levels have several effects, including functional deterioration of the accessory sex organs (the prostate gland, seminal vesicles, epididymis, and ductus deferens); loss of muscle mass, strength, and endurance; and, in many men, decrease in libido. This last effect may also be caused by alterations in other variables that affect libido.

Serum levels of the gonadotropins, particularly FSH, increase with age. The change in gonadotropin secretion may be similar to that in women and may result from some hypothalamic-pituitary dysregulation of the gonadotropins related to inhibin and activin levels.

SUMMARY REVIEW

Development of the Reproductive Systems

1. Differentiation of female and male genitalia begins around weeks 7 to 8 of embryonic development, when the gonads of genetically male embryos begin to secrete male sex hormones, primarily testosterone. Until that time, the primitive reproductive organs of males and females are homologous (the same).
2. The structure and function of both male and female reproductive systems are controlled by the hypothalamic-pituitary-gonadal [H-P-G] axis, a set of complex neurologic and hormonal interactions that accelerate at puberty and lead to sexual maturation and reproductive capability.
3. Extrahypothalamic factors cause the hypothalamus to secrete gonadotropin-releasing hormone (GnRH), which stimulates the anterior pituitary to secrete gonadotropins—follicle-stimulating hormone (FSH) and luteinizing hormone (LH)—that stimulate the gonads (ovaries or testes) to secrete female or male sex hormones. Paracrine hormones (inhibin, activin, and follistatin) influence the positive and negative feedback loops that occur along the H-P-G axis.
4. Production of primitive female gametes (ova) occurs solely during fetal life. From puberty to menopause, one female gamete matures per menstrual cycle. Production of the male gametes (sperm) begins at puberty; after that, millions are produced daily, usually for life.

The Female Reproductive System

1. The function of the reproductive system is to produce mature ova and, when fertilized, to protect and nourish them through embryonic and fetal life, and expel them at birth.
2. The external female genitalia are the mons pubis, labia majora, labia minora, clitoris, vestibule (urinary and vaginal openings), Bartholin glands, and Skene glands.
3. The internal female genitalia are the vagina, uterus, fallopian tubes, and ovaries.
4. The vagina is a fibromuscular canal that receives the penis during sexual intercourse and is the exit route for menstrual fluids and products of conception. The vagina leads from the introitus (its external opening) to the cervical portion of the uterus.
5. The uterus is the hollow, muscular organ in which a fertilized ovum develops. The uterine walls have three layers: the

endometrium (lining), myometrium (muscular layer), and perimetrium (outer covering, which is continuous with the pelvic peritoneum). The endometrium proliferates (thickens) and sloughs off in response to cyclic hormonal changes. The cervix is the narrow, lower portion of the uterus that opens into the vagina.

6. The two fallopian tubes extend from the uterus to the ovaries. Their function is to conduct ova from the spaces around the ovaries to the uterus. Fertilization normally occurs in the distal third of the fallopian tubes.
7. From puberty to menopause, the ovaries are the site of (1) ovum maturation and release and (2) production of female sex (estrogen and progesterone) and male (androgens) hormones. Female sex hormones predominate and are involved in sexual differentiation and development, the menstrual cycle, pregnancy, and lactation. Androgens in women contribute to prepubertal growth spurt, pubic and axillary hair growth, and activation of sebaceous glands.
8. Developing ovarian follicles (structure that encloses the ovum) produce estrogen (primarily estradiol). The corpus luteum, the structure that develops from the ruptured ovarian follicle after ovulation or ovum release, produces progesterone. Androgens are produced within the ovarian follicle, adrenal glands, and adipose tissue.
9. The average menstrual cycle lasts 27 to 30 days and consists of three phases, which are named for ovarian and endometrial changes: the follicular/proliferative phase, the luteal/secretory phase, and menstruation.
10. Ovarian events of the menstrual cycle are controlled by gonadotropins. High FSH levels stimulate follicle and ovum maturation (follicular phase); then a surge of LH causes ovulation, which is followed by development of the corpus luteum (luteal phase).
11. Ovarian hormones control the uterine (endometrial) events of the menstrual cycle. During the follicular phase of the ovarian cycle, estrogen produced by the follicle causes the endometrium to proliferate (proliferative phase). During the luteal phase, estrogen maintains the thickened endometrium while progesterone causes it to develop blood vessels and secretory glands (secretory phase). As the corpus luteum degenerates, production of both hormones drops sharply, and the "starved" endometrium degenerates and sloughs off, causing menstruation.
12. Cyclic changes in hormone levels also cause thinning and thickening of the vaginal epithelium, thinning and thickening of cervical secretions, and changes in basal body temperature.

The Male Reproductive System

1. The function of the male reproductive system is to produce male gametes (sperm) and deliver them to the female reproductive tract.
2. The external male genitalia are the testes, epididymides, scrotum, and penis. The internal genitalia are the vas deferens, ejaculatory duct, prostatic and membranous sections of the urethra, seminal vesicles, prostate gland, and Cowper glands.
3. The testes (male gonads) are paired glands suspended within the scrotum. The testes have two functions: spermatogenesis (sperm production) and production of male sex hormones (androgens, chiefly testosterone).
4. The epididymis is a long, coiled tube arranged in a comma-shaped compartment that curves over the top and rear of the testis. The epididymis receives sperm from the testis and stores them while they develop further. Sperm travel the length of the epididymis and then are ejaculated into the vas deferens.
5. The scrotum is a skin-covered, fibromuscular sac that encloses the testes and epididymides, which are suspended within the scrotum by the spermatic cord. The scrotum keeps these organs at optimal temperatures for sperm survival (about 1° to 2° C lower than body temperature) by contracting in cold environments and relaxing in warm environments.
6. The penis is a cylindric organ consisting of three longitudinal compartments (two corpora cavernosa and one corpus spongiosum) and the urethra. The urethra runs through the corpus spongiosum. The corpora cavernosa and corpus spongiosum consist of erectile tissue. Externally the penis consists of a shaft and a tip, which is called the *glans*. The glans contains sebaceous glands and the opening of the urethra and is covered by a flap of skin (the foreskin).
7. The penis has two functions: delivery of sperm to the female vagina and elimination of urine. Although semen (sperm and glandular secretions) and urine both exit the penis through the urethra, these two fluids are never in the urethra at the same time.
8. Sexual intercourse is made possible by the erectile reflex, in which tactile or psychogenic stimulation of the parasympathetic nerves causes arterioles in the corpora cavernosa and corpus spongiosum to dilate and fill with blood, causing the penis to enlarge and become firm.
9. Emission, which occurs at the peak of sexual arousal, is the movement of semen from the epididymides to the penis. Ejaculation, which is a continuation of emission, is the pulsatile ejection of semen from the penis. Both emission and ejaculation involve rhythmic contractions of smooth muscle within the internal glands and ducts.
10. Spermatogenesis is a continuous process because spermatogonia, the primitive male gametes, undergo continuous mitosis within the seminiferous tubules of the testes. Some of the spermatogonia develop into primary spermatocytes, which divide meiotically into secondary spermatocytes and then spermatids. The spermatids develop into sperm with the help of nutrients and hormonal signals from Sertoli cells.
11. Production of the male sex hormones is controlled (like production of the female sex hormones) by the hypothalamic-pituitary-gonadal axis and by complex feedback mechanisms. The male hormones are produced steadily, with diurnal variations.

Structure and Function of the Breast

1. Until puberty the female and male breasts are similar, consisting of a small, underdeveloped nipple, some fatty and fibrous tissue, and a few ductlike structures under the areola. At puberty, however, a variety of hormones (estrogen, progesterone, prolactin, growth hormone, insulin, cortisol) cause the female breast to develop into a system of glands and ducts that is capable of producing and ejecting milk.
2. The basic functional unit of the female breast is the lobe, a system of ducts that branches from the nipple to milk-producing units called *lobules*. The lobules contain acini, which are convoluted spaces lined with epithelial cells that

secrete milk and subepithelial cells that contract, moving the milk into the system of ducts that leads to the nipple.
3. Each breast contains 15 to 20 lobes, which are separated and supported by Cooper ligaments.
4. Milk production occurs in response to prolactin, a hormone that is secreted in larger amounts after childbirth. Milk ejection is under the control of oxytocin, another hormone of pregnancy and parturition.
5. During the reproductive years, breast tissue undergoes cyclic changes in response to hormonal changes of the menstrual cycle.

Tests of Reproductive Function

1. Diagnostic tests are performed to evaluate fertility or presence of tumors, infection, or sexually transmitted infections.
2. Smears, stains, cultures, and serologic tests are used to diagnose infections. These tests specifically identify microorganisms or types of infections.
3. Tissue biopsy can be performed by resection or needle aspiration. Specimen analysis permits identification of abnormal cells.
4. The Papanicolaou smear is a cytologic examination of cells taken from body fluids and tissues. Although cells can be obtained from many sites, the smear is most commonly used (with endocervical cells) for diagnosis of cervical carcinoma.
5. Mammography is a low-dose radiographic examination of the breast for cancer detection.
6. Evaluation of fertility includes reproductive hormone assays and assessment of structural alteration or infections and the determination of normal ovulation or adequate sperm motility and count.

Aging and Reproductive Function

1. In women, the transition from fertility to menopause (perimenopause) starts about 5 years before the last menstrual period and ends the following year. During this transition period, the ovaries produce erratic and high levels of estrogen that contribute to such symptoms as hot flush, breast tenderness and nodularity, and migraine headaches. Menstrual cycles shorten and then become irregular as anovulation occurs. Menstruation ceases, and women move into menopause.
2. Menopause begins 1 year after the cessation of menstruation and occurs at the average age of 51.4 years. Levels of sex hormones decrease with the last menstrual cycle.
3. In response to reduced levels of female sex hormones, the reproductive organs atrophy, the vaginal epithelium thins, and glandular secretions diminish and become more alkaline. Continued sexual activity and orgasm reduce vaginal changes.
4. Nonreproductive effects of reduced estrogen levels may include increased risk of osteoporosis and coronary artery disease.
5. Male reproductive function diminishes with age, but it does not cease in healthy men.
6. The testes atrophy and produce less testosterone, and some seminiferous tubules may degenerate and become fibrotic. These changes affect sex drive (libido) and sperm morphology. Although sperm count remains normal, the semen tends to contain more defective and nonmotile sperm.
7. The erectile reflex is somewhat diminished and occurs more slowly as age advances.
8. Reduced testosterone levels cause some loss of function in the internal genitalia and enlargement (hypertrophy) of the prostate gland.

KEY TERMS

KEY TERMS—cont'd

Perimenopause, *697*
Perimetrium (parietal peritoneum), *676*
Perineal body, *675*
Perineum, *675*
Primary spermatocyte, *689*
Progesterone, *680*
Prolactin, *691*
Prostate gland, *688*
Rete testis, *686*
Ruga (rugae, pl.; pertains to vagina and testes), *675*
Scrotum, *686*
Secondary spermatocyte, *689*
Semen, *688*
Seminal vesicle, *688*
Seminiferous tubule, *686*
Serologic testing, *694*
Sertoli cell (nondividing support cell), *689*
Sex hormone, *670*
Sex hormone–binding globulin (SHBG), *691*
Skene gland (lesser vestibular or paraurethral gland), *675*
Spermatic cord, *686*
Spermatid, *689*
Spermatogenesis, *686*
Spermatogonium (spermatogonia, pl.), *689*
Spermatozoon (sperm cell), *670*
Squamous-columnar junction, *676*
Testis, *686*
Testosterone, *689*
Theca cell, *678*
Thelarche, *671*
Tissue biopsy, *694*
Tubulus rectus, *686*
Tunica albuginea, *686*
Tunica dartos, *687*
Tunica vaginalis, *686*
Ultrasonography, *694*
Urethra, *687*
Urinary meatus, *675*
Uterus, *676*
Vagina, *675*
Vas deferens (ductus deferens), *686*
Vasomotor flush, *699*
Vasomotor symptoms, *698*
Vestibule, *674*
Vulva, *674*

REFERENCES

1. Speroff L, Glass RH, Kase NG: *Clinical gynecology, endocrinology, and infertility,* ed 5, Baltimore, 1994, Williams & Wilkins.
2. Roy S: Puberty. In Lobo RA et al, editors: *Infertility, contraception, and reproductive endocrinology,* ed 4, Malden, MA, 1997, Blackwell Science.
3. Persaud TVN: Embryology of the female genital tract and gonads. In Copeland LJ, Farrell JF, editors: *Textbook of gynecology,* ed 2, Philadelphia, 2000, W.B. Saunders.
4. Gordon K, Oehninger S: Reproductive physiology. In Copeland LJ, Farrell JF, editors: *Textbook of gynecology,* ed 2, Philadelphia, 2000, W.B. Saunders.
5. Klein KO et al: Effect of obesity on estradiol level, and its relationship to leptin, bone maturation, and bone mineral density in children, *J Clin Endocrinol Metab* 83(10):3469, 1998.
6. Wong WW et al: Serum leptin concentrations in Caucasian and African-American girls. *J Clin Endocrinol Metab* 83(10):3574, 1998.
7. Dawood MY: Menopause. In Copeland LJ, Farrell JF, editors: *Textbook of gynecology,* ed 2, Philadelphia, 2000, W.B. Saunders.
8. Rics FJ et al: A cross-cultural study of menstrual cycle characteristics of women practicing the sympto-thermal method of natural family planning. In Komenich P et al, editors: *The menstrual cycle,* vol 2, New York, 1981, Springer.
9. Trealor AE et al: Variation of the human menstrual cycle through reproductive life, *Int J Fertil* 12:77, 1967.
10. Vollman RF: The menstrual cycle. In Friedman E, editor: *Major problems in obstetrics and gynecology,* Philadelphia, 1977, W.B. Saunders.
11. Speroff L et al: *Clinical gynecologic endocrinology and fertility*, ed 6, Baltimore, 1999, Lippincott.
12. Golub S: *Periods: from menarche to menopause,* Newbury Park, NJ, 1992, Sage.
13. Shoupe D, Lobo RA: Reproductive neuroendocrinology. In Lobo RA et al, editors: *Infertility, contraception, and reproductive endocrinology,* ed 4, Malden, MA, 1997, Blackwell Science.
14. Reame NE et al: Net increase in stimulatory input resulting from a decrease in inhibin B and an increase in activin A may contribute in part to the rise in follicular phase follicle-stimulating hormone of aging cycling women, *J Clin Endocrinol Metab* 83(10):3302, 1998.
15. Tanango EA, McAninch JW: *Smith's general urology,* ed 16, Norwalk, CT, 1995, Appleton & Lange.
16. Mastroianni L, Coutifaris C: *Reproductive physiology,* vol 1, Carnforth Lanes, UK, Parkridge, NJ, 1990, Parthenon.
17. Lepor H: *Prostatic diseases,* Philadelphia, 2000, W.B. Saunders.
18. Sokol RZ: Male factor in infertility. In Lobo RA et al, editors: *Infertility, contraception, and reproductive endocrinology,* ed 4, Malden, MA, 1997, Blackwell Science.
19. American Cancer Society: *Facts on breast cancer,* New York, 1995, The Society.
20. Guiliano AE: Breast. In Tierney LM, McPhee S, Papadakis MA, editors: *Current medical diagnosis and treatment,* ed 35, Norwalk, CT, 1996, Appleton & Lange.
21. Shoupe D, Brenner PF, Mishell DR: Menopause. In Lobo RA et al, editors: *Infertility, contraception, and reproductive endocrinology,* ed 4, Malden, MA, 1997, Blackwell Science.
22. Prior JC: Perimenopause: the complex endocrinology of the menopausal transition, *Endocr Rev* 19(4):397, 1998.
23. Brenner WJ, Vitiello MV, Primz PN: A loss of circadian rhythmicity in blood testosterone levels with aging in normal men, *J Clin Endocrinol Metab* 56:1278, 1983.
24. Royer GL et al: Relationship between age and levels of total, free, and bound testosterone in healthy subjects, *Curr Therap Res* 35:345, 1984.
25. Vermeulen A, Kaufman JM, Giagulli VA: Influence of some biological indexes on sex hormone–binding globulin and androgen levels in aging or obese males, *J Clin Endocrinol Metab* 81(5):1821, 1996.

CHAPTER 22

Alterations of the Reproductive Systems

KRISTYNIA M. ROBINSON • KATHRYN L. McCANCE

CHAPTER OUTLINE

Alterations of the reproductive system span a wide range of concerns, from delayed sexual development and suboptimal sexual performance to structural and functional difficulties. Many common reproductive disorders carry potentially serious physiologic or psychologic consequences. For example, sexual or reproductive dysfunction, such as impotence or infertility, can dramatically affect self-concept, relationships, and overall quality of life. In terms of serious physiologic consequences, the second leading cause of cancer deaths is prostate cancer in men and breast cancer in women.[1] Conversely, organic and psychosocial problems, such as alcoholism, depression, situational stressors, chronic illness, and medications, can affect ovulation and menstruation, sexual performance, and fertility and may be risk factors for the development of some types of reproductive tract cancers. Often, diagnosis and treatment of reproductive system disorders are complicated because of the stigma and symbolism associated with the reproductive organs and the emotion-laden beliefs and behaviors related to reproductive health. Treatment and diagnosis for any problem may be delayed because of embarrassment, guilt, fear, or denial.

ALTERATIONS OF SEXUAL MATURATION

A variety of congenital and endocrine disorders can disrupt the timing of puberty, or sexual maturation. These disorders may cause puberty to occur too late (delayed puberty) or too early (precocious puberty). Both types of disorders involve the inappropriate onset of sex hormone production by the gonads.

Delayed Puberty

About 3% of children in North America experience delayed development of secondary sex characteristics.[1] The first sign of puberty in girls is thelarche, or breast development. Thelarche should begin by the time a girl is 13 years old. Normally boys tend to mature later than girls, around 14 to 14.5 years of age. In boys the first sign is enlargement of the testes and thinning of the scrotal skin. In **delayed puberty** these secondary sex characteristics show no sign of appearing in a 13-year-old girl or a 14-year-old boy. Clinical diagnosis is made also in the absence of menarche within 5 years of thelarche or by 16 years of age. Boys tend especially to be embarrassed by sexual immaturity;[2] therefore early diagnosis and treatment is recommended, as well as reassurance for both boys and girls.

In 95% of cases, delayed puberty is a constitutional delay; that is, hormonal levels are normal and the hypothalamic-pituitary-ovarian axis is intact, but maturation is happening slowly. Physiologic or constitutional delay tends to be familial and is much more common in boys than in girls (Box 22-1). Constitutional delay is difficult to distinguish from isolated gonadotropin deficiency and can only be diagnosed retrospectively once pubertal progression is complete. For constitutional delay, many clinicians recommend a trial of exogenous sex hormones to reduce embarrassment and enhance self-image and as a diagnostic measure for irreversible hypogonadotropism.[1,2]

The other 5% of cases are caused by some disruption of the hypothalamic-pituitary-gonadal axis (either congenital or acquired) or by a systemic disease. The disruption can consist of deficient secretion of gonadotropin-releasing hormone (GnRH) by the hypothalamus, deficient gonadotropin secretion by the pituitary, or gonadal disorders. A thorough physical examination, including precise body measurements and accurate assessment of sexual maturation, should be done. Careful questioning is imperative to elicit a history of chronic illness, eating disorder, strenuous exercise, drug abuse, anosmia (decreased or absent smell that accompanies Kallman syndrome), signs and symptoms of hypopituitarism, hypothyroidism, Turner syndrome, Klinefelter syndrome, and Tanner staging.[3] Laboratory workup generally consists of x-ray studies for bone age, measurement of thyroid function, serum levels of prolactin and adrenal and gonadal steroids, radioimmunoassay of plasma gonadotropins, and general screening for systemic disorders. Adolescents with high gonadotropin levels require a karyotype, and those with low levels need skull imaging (lateral skull film, computed tomography, or magnetic resonance imaging) to rule out pituitary or other central nervous system infiltrate or tumor.[1] Treatment of pathophysiologic delayed puberty depends on the cause; the goal of treatment is the development of secondary sex characteristics and fertility, when possible.[4,5] Insufficient sex hormone secretion can be corrected by hormone replacement therapy; idiopathic hypogonadotropic hypogonadism and Kallman syndrome,[6] which may be different expressions of the same X-linked chromosomal disorder, are treated with synthetic GnRH. Treatment of Turner syndrome consists of long-term growth hormone therapy with late estrogen therapy.

Box 22-1

CAUSES OF DELAYED PUBERTY

HYPERGONADOTROPIC HYPOGONADISM (INCREASED FOLLICLE-STIMULATING HORMONE [FSH] AND LUTEINIZING HORMONE [LH])

1. Gonadal dysgenesis, most commonly Turner syndrome (45,X/46,XX; structural X or Y abnormalities; or mosaicism)
2. Klinefelter syndrome (47,XXY)
3. Bilateral gonadal failure
   a. Traumatic or infectious
   b. Postsurgical, postirradiation, or postchemotherapy
   c. Autoimmune
   d. Idiopathic empty-scrotum or vanishing-testes syndrome (congenital anorchia) or resistant-ovary syndrome

HYPOGONADOTROPIC HYPOGONADISM (DECREASED LH, DEPRESSED FSH)

1. Reversible
   a. Physiologic delay
   b. Weight loss/anorexia
   c. Strenuous exercise
   d. Severe obesity
   e. Illegal drug use, especially marijuana
   f. Primary hypothyroidism
   g. Congenital adrenal hyperplasia
   h. Cushing syndrome
   i. Prolactinomas
2. Irreversible
   a. Gonadotropin-releasing hormone (GnRH) deficiency (Kallmann syndrome) or idiopathic hypogonad/otropic hypogonadism (IHH)
   b. Hypopituitarism
   c. Congenital central nervous system (CNS) defects
   d. Other pituitary adenomas
   e. Craniopharyngioma
   f. Malignant pituitary tumors

EUGONADISM

1. Congenital anomalies
   a. Müllerian agenesis
   b. Vaginal septum or imperforate hymen
2. Androgen insensitivity syndrome
3. Inappropriate positive feedback

Data from Rudolph AM, Hoffman JIE, Rudolph CD: *Rudolph's pediatrics,* ed 20, Stamford, Conn, 1996, Appleton & Lange; Speroff L, Glass RH, Kase NG: *Clinical gynecologic endocrinology and infertility,* ed 5, Baltimore, 1994, Williams & Wilkins; Saenger P: Growth-promoting strategies in Turner's syndrome, *J Clin Endocrinal Metab* 84(12):4345, 1999.

Precocious Puberty

Precocious puberty is the onset of sexual maturation before age 6 in black girls or age 7 in white girls[7] and age 9 in boys (see Chapter 21 for discussion on puberty). Pre-

WHAT'S NEW? **Lawson Wilkins Pediatric Endocrine Society (LWPES) Proposes New Standards for Defining Precocious Puberty**

According to a 1997 study of more than 17,000 girls ages 3 to 12 years from suburban United States pediatric practices, girls reach thelarche about 1 to 2 years earlier than accepted standards. After an extensive data review, LWPES proposed new guidelines suggesting evaluation of breast or pubic hair development only if one or both occur before age 6 in African-American or age 7 in white girls. Current standards are based on relatively old studies that used small, nondiverse samples, including Marshall and Tanner's study of 192 white orphans from Britain.

Data from Kaplowitz PB et al: Reexamination of the age limit for defining when puberty is precocious in girls in the United States: implications for evaluation and treatment, *Pediatrics* 104(4):936, 1999.

Box 22-2

CAUSES OF ISOSEXUAL PRECOCIOUS PUBERTY

CENTRAL (GONADOTROPIN-RELEASING HORMONE [GnRH] DEPENDENT)

1. Idiopathic, including familial
2. Central nervous system (CNS) abnormalities
   a. Congenital anomalies (hydrocephalus)
   b. Tumors (hypothalamic, pineal, other)
   c. Hypothalamic hamartoma
   d. Postinflammatory/infectious condition
   e. Trauma
   f. Syndromes
      (1) Neurofibromatosis
      (2) Tuberous sclerosis
3. Hypothyroidism (severe)

PSEUDOPRECOCIOUS PUBERTY (GnRH INDEPENDENT)

1. Exogenous sex steroids
2. Gonadal tumors or cysts
3. Adrenal hyperplasia or tumor
4. Ectopic gonadotropin-secreting tumors (chorioepithelioma, hepatoblastoma, teratoma)
5. Familial Leydig cell hyperplasia
6. McCune-Albright syndrome

From Hoekelman RA et al: *Primary pediatric care,* ed 3, St Louis, 1997, Mosby.

cocity is five times more common in girls than boys, with 74% of cases of precocity in girls being idiopathic. Although boys are affected less often, the cause is more likely to be pathologic.

Precocious puberty occurs in three forms: isosexual, heterosexual, and incomplete. **Isosexual precocious puberty** is premature development of appropriate characteristics for the child's sex and may be GnRH dependent or independent.

True isosexual precocious puberty is GnRH dependent and occurs when the hypothalamic-pituitary-gonadal axis is working normally but prematurely. Besides the premature development of secondary sex characteristics, precocity causes premature closure of the epiphysis of long bones, which results in short stature. Idiopathic precocity, or central precocious puberty (CPP), results from failure of central inhibition of the GnRH pulse generator (the gonadostat). The diagnosis of CPP is one of exclusion. When familial, it may be considered constitutional.[1] Because a central nervous system (CNS) lesion may be missed, children with presumed idiopathic precocious puberty require long-term surveillance. More serious causes of central or GnRH-dependent sexual precocity are listed in Box 22-2. Pseudoprecocious puberty, also known as peripheral or GnRH-independent precocious puberty, develops when sex hormones are produced by some mechanism other than stimulation by the gonadotropins. One cause is glandular insufficiency syndromes such as severe hypothyroidism or adrenal insufficiency; others are listed in Box 22-2.

Heterosexual precocious puberty (virilization of a girl or feminization of a boy) causes the child to develop some secondary sex characteristics of the opposite sex. This condition is usually evident at birth and is rare in older children.

Incomplete precocious puberty is the partial development of appropriate secondary sex characteristics. A girl with incomplete precocious puberty might undergo thelarche or adrenarche and, rarely, premature menarche. Premature thelarche is seen in girls between 6 months and 2 years of age. Premature adrenarche tends to occur between ages 5 and 8 years. Premature adrenarche is the consequence of an early increase in the adrenal androgens that leads to early growth of pubic hair and possibly a transient acceleration in growth and bone maturation that has no significant effect on timing of puberty or final height. Sparse hair growth on the genitalia does not represent precocious puberty.

The diagnosis and cause of premature development are often obvious. A thorough history and physical examination are done to determine the velocity of the process and to rule out life-threatening CNS, ovarian, or adrenal neoplasms. Family occurrence helps exclude tumors. The majority of children with precocious puberty are obese.

Treatment for all forms of precocious puberty includes identifying and removing the underlying cause or administering appropriate hormones (Boxes 22-3 and 22-4; see also Box 22-2). In many cases, precocious puberty can be reversed. Management goals include diagnosing and treating intracranial disease; arresting maturation until early teen years; maximizing eventual adult height; reducing emotional problems; and providing contraception, if necessary. The most common form, CPP, is usually treated with potent GnRH agonist analogues, which induce reversible, selective suppression of the pituitary-gonadal axis.[8] Treatment does not seem to affect body composition or increase obesity in children with CPP.[9] Because the majority of these of children are obese and childhood obesity is predictive of obesity and morbidity in adolescence and adulthood, it is important for clinicians to include assessment and management of obesity as part of the treatment for CPP.

Box 22-3

CAUSES OF HETEROSEXUAL PRECOCIOUS PUBERTY

FEMALE

1. Congenital adrenal hyperplasia
2. Androgen-secreting tumors
   a. Adrenal
   b. Ovarian
   c. Teratoma
3. Exogenous androgens

MALE

1. Estrogen-producing tumors
   a. Adrenal
   b. Teratoma
   c. Hepatoma
   d. Testicular
2. Exogenous estrogens
3. Increased peripheral conversion of androgens to estrogens

From Hoekelman RA et al: *Primary pediatric care,* ed 3, St Louis, 1997, Mosby.

Box 22-4

THE THREE FORMS OF PRECOCIOUS PUBERTY

ISOSEXUAL PRECOCIOUS PUBERTY

Premature development of appropriate characteristics for the child's sex

Hypothalamic-pituitary-ovarian axis working normally but prematurely

In about 10% of cases, lethal central nervous system tumor may be the cause[A]

HETEROSEXUAL PRECOCIOUS PUBERTY

Causes the child to develop some secondary sex characteristics of the opposite sex

Common causes: adrenal hyperplasia or androgen-secreting tumors

INCOMPLETE PRECOCIOUS PUBERTY

Partial development of appropriate secondary sex characteristics

Premature thelarche (breast budding) seen in girls between 6 months and 2 years of age

Does not progress to complete puberty (ovulation and menstruation)

Premature adrenarche (growth of axillary and pubic hair) tends to occur between 5 and 8 years of age

Can progress to complete precocious puberty; may be caused by estrogen-secreting neoplasms or may be a variant of normal pubertal development

[A]Kaplowitz PB et al: Reexamination of the age limit for defining when puberty is precocious in girls in the United States: implications for education and treatment, *Pediatrics* 104(4):936, 1999.

DISORDERS OF THE FEMALE REPRODUCTIVE SYSTEM

Hormonal and Menstrual Alterations

Primary Dysmenorrhea

Primary dysmenorrhea is painful menstruation associated with the release of prostaglandins in ovulatory cycles, but not with pelvic disease. The severity of dysmenorrhea is directly related to the duration and amount of menstrual flow. Between 50% and 75% of women ages 15 to 25 years are affected, some (up to 14%) severely enough to miss work or school. Dysmenorrhea usually begins with the onset of ovulatory cycles, around age 15 or 16 years. The incidence steadily rises, peaks in women in their midtwenties, and decreases slowly thereafter.

Pathophysiology

Dysmenorrhea is the result of excessive endometrial prostaglandin production and effect. Women with painful periods produce 10 times as much prostaglandin F ($PGF_{2\alpha}$), a potent myometrial stimulant and vasoconstrictor, as asymptomatic women.[10] Elevated levels of prostaglandins (especially $PGF_{2\alpha}$ and $PGE_{2\alpha}$) are found in endometrial fluid of dysmenorrheic women and correlate positively with pain. Compared with proliferative endometrium, secretory endometrium produces three times the amount of prostaglandins, and the discharged endometrium produces even more.[11] In addition, leukotrienes heighten sensitivity of pain fibers in the uterus and vasopressin contributes to myometrial hypersensitivity, constriction of endometrial blood vessels, and resultant ischemia, endometrial bleeding, and pain caused by prostaglandins.[12] Prostaglandins are primarily released during the first 48 hours of menstruation, when symptoms are the most intense. Women who are anovulatory because they use oral contraceptives do not have primary dysmenorrhea.

Clinical Manifestations

The chief symptom of dysmenorrhea is pelvic pain associated with the onset of menses. The pain frequently radiates into the groin and may be accompanied by backache, anorexia, vomiting, diarrhea, syncope, and headache. The latter symptoms are caused by entry of prostaglandins and prostaglandin metabolites into the systemic circulation. Usually, the discomfort associated with primary dysmenorrhea begins shortly before the onset of menstruation and rarely persists beyond the second day.

Evaluation and Treatment

Primary dysmenorrhea must be differentiated from secondary dysmenorrhea caused by disorders such as endometriosis, pelvic adhesions, inflammatory disease, or uterine fibroid. A thorough medical history and pelvic examination are completed to exclude pelvic pathologic conditions.

In women who desire contraception, primary dysmenorrhea can be relieved with hormonal contraceptives. Hormonal contraception stops ovulation, thereby decreasing prostaglandin synthesis and myometrial contractility. Prostaglandin inhibitors work in 80% of cases and are most effective if started at the first sign of bleeding or cramping. Low-fat diets and regular exercise are thought to prevent or reduce symptoms, and local application of heat, massage, relaxation techniques, and orgasm are common comfort measures.

Primary Amenorrhea

Amenorrhea means lack of menstruation. **Primary amenorrhea** is the failure of menarche and the absence of menstruation by age 14 years without the development of secondary sex characteristics or by age 16 years regardless of the presence of secondary sex characteristics (see p. 706 for discussion of delayed puberty). The causes of primary amenorrhea include a diverse group of abnormalities, such as congenital defects of gonadotropin production (Prader-Willi, Kallmann, and Laurence-Moon-Biedl syndromes); genetic disorders (Turner syndrome); congenital CNS defects, such as hydrocephalus; congenital anatomic malformations of the reproductive system (e.g., absence of vagina or uterus); and acquired CNS lesions, including trauma, infection, and tumors.

Pathophysiology

Pathophysiology can be categorized by compartmentalization. *Compartment IV disorders* include CNS disorders, in particular hypothalamic disorders. In some of the congenital syndromes that cause primary amenorrhea, the hypothalamic-pituitary-ovarian (H-P-O) axis is dysfunctional. The hypothalamus is unable to synthesize GnRH, so the pituitary fails to secrete luteinizing hormone (LH) and follicle-stimulating hormone (FSH). Therefore the ovary does not receive the hormonal signals that normally initiate the ovarian and endometrial changes of the menstrual cycle, and ovulation and menstruation do not occur. Because the ovarian hormones are absent, secondary sex characteristics do not develop.

Compartment III disorders are disorders of the anterior pituitary, including tumors. Some anatomic defects of the CNS, whether congenital or acquired, impinge on the hypothalamic-pituitary unit so as to interfere with or interrupt the secretion of GnRH or FSH and LH. Examples of such defects include hydrocephalus, craniopharyngiomas, and other space-occupying lesions of the CNS (see Box 22-1). Again the target organ, the ovary, does not receive the necessary signals, and ovulation and menstruation do not occur. In some cases these lesions develop between the onset and conclusion of puberty. Therefore skeletal growth may occur and secondary sex characteristics may develop, but sexual maturation is interrupted before menarche, which normally concludes puberty.

Compartment II disorders involve the ovary. Several genetic disorders are associated with primary amenorrhea. These include gonadal dysgenesis (Turner syndrome); testicular feminizing syndrome (male pseudohermaphroditism); and poly-X, or superfemale, syndrome. With the chromosomal abnormalities of Turner syndrome (45,X/46,XX; structural X or Y abnormalities; mosaicism),[5] the ovaries lack gametes and ovarian failure is complete. Without primitive gametes and follicles, follicular development and estrogen secretion cannot occur. Lack of estrogen accounts for failure of secondary sex characteristic development, amenorrhea, and high levels of circulating FSH and LH. In male pseudohermaphroditism the individual is male genetically but female morphologically. The individual does not develop male genitalia because androgen receptors are absent in undifferentiated target organs. The gonads are found either in the abdomen or in the inguinal canal, and they produce both androgens and estrogens. Because target tissues lack androgen receptors but have estrogen receptors, most individuals with male pseudohermaphroditism have female external genitalia and female secondary sex characteristics. With the exception of a small vagina, internal female genitalia are absent, accounting for amenorrhea and infertility.

Compartment I disorders are anatomic defects of the outflow tract associated with primary amenorrhea. They include congenital absence of the vagina and uterus and congenital uterine hypoplasia (infantile uterus). Females without a uterus or vagina usually have normal ovarian function. Therefore skeletal growth occurs and secondary sex characteristics develop in the proper sequence, but menstruation does not occur. In cases of uterine hypoplasia the uterus does not respond to hormonal stimulation during puberty.

Clinical Manifestations

The major clinical manifestation of primary amenorrhea is the absence of the menses. The cause of the amenorrhea determines whether secondary sex characteristics and height are affected.

Evaluation and Treatment

Diagnosis of primary amenorrhea is based on history and physical examination. If ovarian steroid hormone levels are low, the individual has the appearance of an immature female. Physical examination may show structural or physiologic alterations. Laboratory studies may be required to document abnormal levels of gonadotropins and ovarian hormones. Diagnostic imaging is used to document structural abnormalities (Fig. 22-1).

Treatment involves correction of any underlying disorders and hormone replacement therapy to induce the development of secondary sex characteristics (see p. 706 for a discussion of delayed puberty). Surgical alteration of the genitalia may be undertaken to correct structural abnormalities. Hormonal manipulation or embryo transplantation may make pregnancy possible for women with primary amenorrhea.

Secondary Amenorrhea

Secondary amenorrhea is the absence of menstruation for a time equivalent to three or more cycles or 6 months in women who have previously menstruated. A wide variety of disorders and physiologic conditions are associated with secondary amenorrhea. Besides disease, secondary amenorrhea can be triggered by dramatic weight loss, whether the loss results from malnutrition or excessive exercise. Secondary

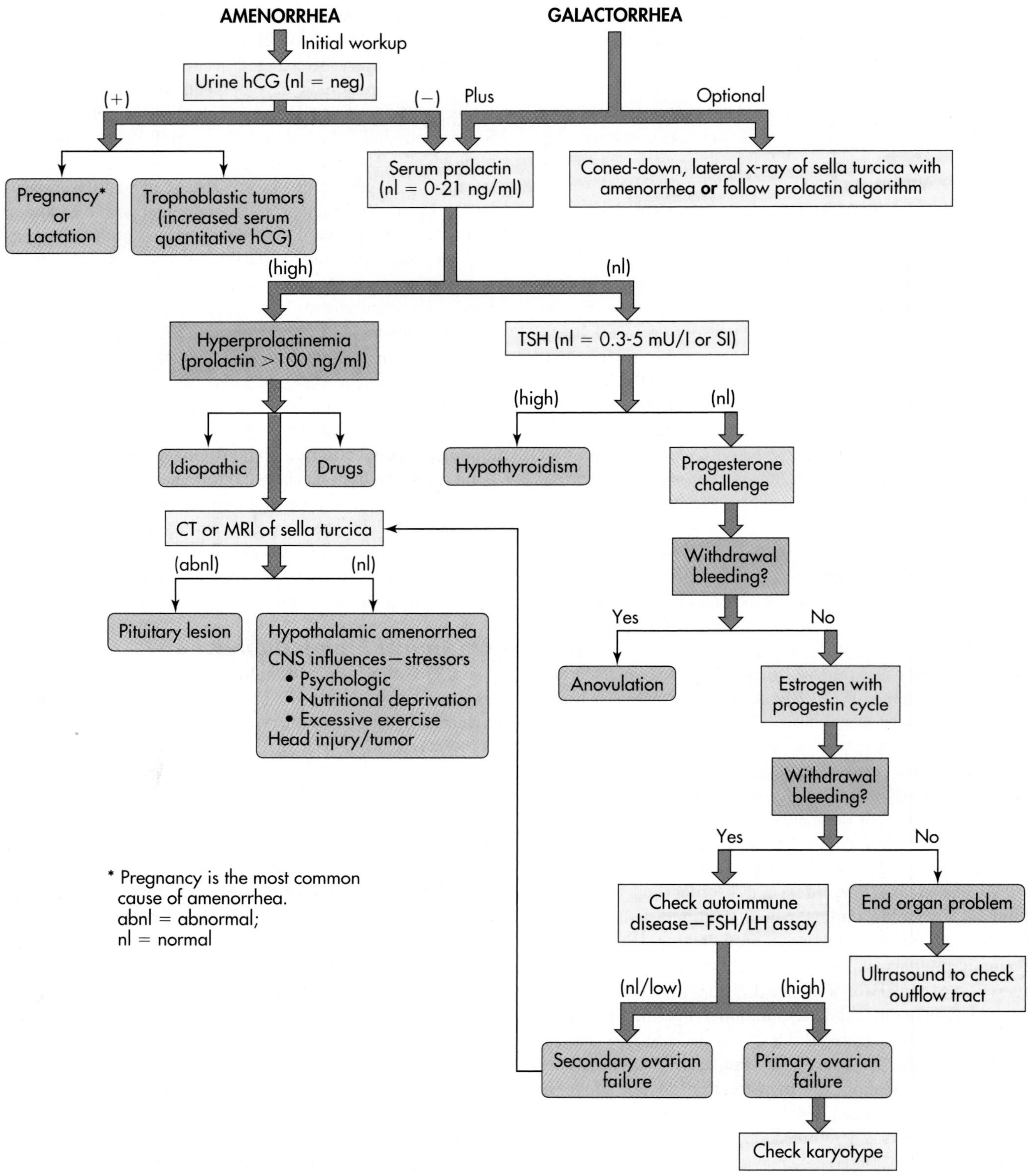

FIG. 22-1 Diagnosis of amenorrhea.

amenorrhea is normal during early adolescence and the perimenopausal period, pregnancy, and lactation.

◆ *Pathophysiology*

The causes of secondary amenorrhea are summarized in Fig. 22-2, and categorization of amenorrhea is discussed on p. 709. In women with normal ovarian steroid hormone levels, secondary amenorrhea is caused by structural abnormalities (müllerian anomalies), Asherman syndrome (removal of the endometrial deciduas basilis), or removal of the uterus (compartment I). In women with elevated ovarian steroid hormone levels, inhibited ovulation leads to amenorrhea (com-

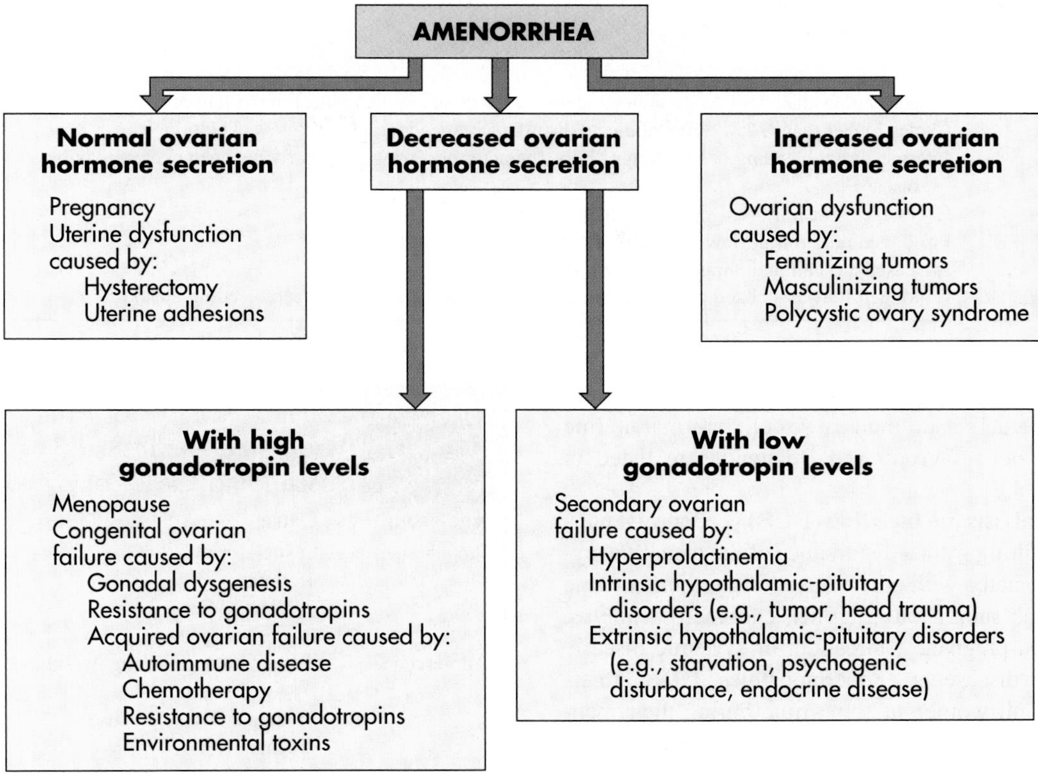

FIG. 22-2 Causes of amenorrhea.

partment II). An excess of ovarian hormones apparently disrupts feedback relationships between the various hormones of the H-P-O axis, preventing ovulation. Specific disorders include premature ovarian failure and consequences of radiation. Depressed ovarian hormone levels, which are associated with a variety of clinical disorders, also cause amenorrhea by preventing ovulation. Lack of ovulation, termed **anovulation,** may result from increased levels of prolactin, decreased levels of gonadotropins, irregular secretion of gonadotropins (compartment III), or abnormally low levels of CNS neurotransmitters (compartment IV). Any of these variables alters the feedback effects that the ovarian hormones have on the hypothalamus and pituitary.

Hyperprolactinemia (overproduction of prolactin by the pituitary) may have short-loop feedback effects that lead to decreased secretion of GnRH by the hypothalamus. The result is a loss of pulsatile LH secretion and an overall reduction in LH levels. Anovulation and secondary amenorrhea may result. In the ovary, elevated prolactin levels appear to inhibit the secretion of progesterone by the granulosa cells of the follicle. This leads to anovulation caused by follicular atresia. These abnormalities may act singly or in combination to cause other alterations in the menstrual cycle.

Clinical Manifestations

The major manifestation of secondary amenorrhea is the absence of menses. Infertility, vasomotor flushes, vaginal atrophy, acne, and **hirsutism** (abnormal hairiness) also may be present, depending on the underlying cause of the amenorrhea.

Evaluation and Treatment

Pregnancy is the most common cause of amenorrhea. Diagnosis of secondary amenorrhea involves the identification of underlying hormonal or anatomic alterations. A woman with secondary amenorrhea and normal secondary sex characteristics should have a complete history and physical examination. Pregnancy is ruled out before any further workup is undertaken. Initial evaluation begins with a measurement of thyroid-stimulating hormone, a prolactin level, and a progesterone challenge to induce withdrawal bleeding. Radioimmunoassay levels of gonadotropins, computed tomography (CT) or magnetic resonance imaging (MRI) imaging of the sella turcica, and ultrasound of the outflow tract may be necessary to determine the cause of amenorrhea (see Fig. 22-1).[13,14] Depending on the cause of the amenorrhea, treatment may involve oral, vaginal, or injectable hormone replacement therapy[11,13,15,16] (e.g., estrogens, thyroid hormone, glucocorticoids, gonadotropins, bromocriptine) or a corrective procedure, such as surgical removal of pituitary tumors. New evidence suggests that insertion of a copper intrauterine device (IUD) may be effective.

Dysfunctional Uterine Bleeding

Menstrual concerns or abnormal bleeding patterns (Table 22-1) are common complaints. Approximately 33% of all gynecologic visits are for irregular genital bleeding. This proportion increases to 69% in the perimenopausal and postmenopausal age-groups.[17] Failure to ovulate as an expression of age, stress, or endocrinopathy is the most common cause of cycle irregularity. Other causes include intrinsic uterine

Table 22-1 Abnormal Menstrual Bleeding

Term	Definition
Polymenorrhea	Cycles shorter than 3 wk; may indicate disturbance in endocrine control of ovulation
Oligomenorrhea	Cycles longer than 6-7 wk; may indicate disturbance in endocrine control of ovulation
Metrorrhagia	Intermenstrual bleeding or bleeding of light character occurring irregularly between cycles; may be a sign of organic disease
Hypermenorrhea	Excessive flow; may be a sign of organic disease
Menorrhea	Prolonged duration of flow
Menorrhagia	Increased amount and duration of flow
Menometrorrhagia	Prolonged flow associated with irregular and intermittent spotting between bleeding episodes

pathologic conditions, pregnancy and its complications, and hematologic disorders. Common causes of abnormal uterine bleeding based on age-group and frequency are listed in Table 22-2.

Dysfunctional uterine bleeding (DUB) is abnormal uterine bleeding resulting from a disturbance of the menstrual cycle. It is not associated with other causes of abnormal uterine bleeding, such as submucous fibroids, endometrial polyps, blood dyscrasias, pregnancy, infection, or systemic disease, such as hepatic disease or endocrinopathies. DUB affects 15% to 20% of all women at some time during their menstrual life and accounts for 25% of gynecologic surgeries.[18]

Table 22-2 Common Causes of Abnormal (Vaginal/Genital) Bleeding in Descending Order of Frequency

Age-group	Cause
Prepubescence	Sexual assault
	Trauma
	Foreign bodies
	Precocious puberty
Adolescence	Anovulation (maturing hypothalamic-pituitary-ovarian axis)
	Trauma and sexual abuse
	Pregnancy
	Pelvic inflammatory disease
	Coagulation disorder
Reproductive years	Pregnancy
	Pelvic inflammatory disease
	Complication of contraceptives
	Endometriosis
	Anovulation
Perimenopause	Anovulation
	Malignancy
	Pregnancy
	Endometriosis
	Benign neoplasms (myomas, adenomyosis)
Postmenopause	Malignancy

Pathophysiology

Greater than 80% of DUB is associated with anovulatory cyles, and the remaining 20% is due to corpus luteum defects or atrophic endometrium.[19] Although DUB may occur at any time during the reproductive years, 20% of cases occur in adolescents and more than 50% of cases occur in perimenopausal women ages 40 to 50 years. Symptoms of hypomenorrhea, followed by missed periods or prolonged intervals between menses, could mark the onset of physiologic perimenopause or may be an early sign of pathologically premature ovulatory failure and secondary amenorrhea. Other conditions associated with chronic anovulation include polycystic ovary syndrome, immaturity of the H-P-O axis, obesity, hyperthyroidism and hypothyroidism, and estrogen-secreting ovarian neoplasms.

DUB secondary to ovarian dysfunction is a result of either progesterone deficiency or relative estrogen excess. In perimenopausal women in their forties and fifties, progesterone secretion is absent or low, yet estrogen (estradiol [E2]) continues to be secreted by the granulosa–theca cell complex, and levels are often erratic and high.[20] (See Chapter 21 for a description of the many hormonal changes associated with the time before and just after menopause.) In the absence of growth-limiting progesterone and periodic desquamation, the endometrium attains an abnormal height with increasing hypervascularity and back-to-back glandularity, but without an intervening stromal support matrix. Menstrual flow may become irregular (metrorrhagia) and excessive (menorrhagia) or both (menometrorrhagia) due to the large quantity of tissue available for bleeding and the random breakdown of tissue that results in exposure of vascular channels. In the absence of adequate progesterone levels, usual endometrial control mechanisms are missing, such as vasoconstrictive rhythmicity, tight coiling of spiral vessels, and orderly collapse, and stasis does not occur. Unopposed estrogen induces a progression of endometrial responses beginning with proliferation, hyperplasia, and adenomatous hyperplasia; over a course of many years, unopposed estrogen may end with atypia and carcinoma.

DUB in ovulatory cycles is less common, and mechanisms underlying the bleeding are associated with organic lesions or corpus luteum defects.[19] Excessive fibrinolytic activity and changes in prostaglandin production may be implicated.

Clinical Manifestations

Ovulatory DUB is cyclic and usually associated with premenstrual symptoms such as breast tenderness, water retention, and cramping. Anovulatory DUB is characterized by unpredictable and variable bleeding in terms of amount and duration. Especially during perimenopause, dysfunctional bleeding also may involve flooding and the passage of large clots, which often indicate excessive blood loss. It is difficult to estimate the severity of blood loss in otherwise healthy women because such women do not become anemic until blood loss exceeds 1.6 L over a short interval.

Evaluation and Treatment

DUB is a diagnosis of exclusion. Treatment goals include preventing or controlling abnormal bleeding, identifying underlying disease, diagnosing any psychosocial pathology that can cause or exacerbate menstrual disorders, and inducing regular menstrual cycles.[21] Usual therapy is hormonal and may consist of intense progestin-estrogen combination therapy, estrogen-only therapy (for acute episodes only), or progesterone-only therapy.[12,15,16,19,20,22] For the woman with idiopathic menorrhagia not associated with anovulatory cycles, prostaglandin synthetase inhibitors may be effective in decreasing blood loss. Desmopressin, a synthetic analog of arginine vasopressin, is used to treat abnormal uterine bleeding in women with coagulation disorders (vonWillebrand disease, which affects about 1% of the population).[19,22] Recalcitrant bleeding may be controlled by suppression of the endometrium followed by ablation. Total or partial ablation of the endometrium has replaced dilation and curettage (D & C) or hysterectomy as the surgical technique of choice for treatment of menorrhagia. Various techniques have been developed, including laser, a resectoscope with a loop or rolling ball electrode, partial rollerball or radiofrequency-induced balloon, and microwave thermal destruction.[19,23-26] The best results are obtained if the endometrium is suppressed for 4 to 6 weeks with either high-dose progestin, GnRH agonist, or danazol. Endometrial ablation is successful in approximately 90% of women; only 50% become amenorrheic. Routine treatment of DUB with D & C or hysterectomy is not recommended. The major indication for a D & C is diagnostic or as a curative procedure in the removal of products of conception, polyps, or focal endometrial hyperplasia.

Polycystic Ovary Syndrome

Polycystic ovary syndrome (PCOS) is the most common endocrine disturbance affecting women, especially young women, and is the leading cause of infertility in the United States.[27-29] Prevalence rates are estimated at between 6% and 10% in the United States, afflicting between 3.2 and 5.4 million young women;[28] similar rates are thought to occur in other countries (Greece and Britain).[27,30] PCOS is familial, and various features of the syndrome may be differentially inherited.[27,31] Confusing the issue is the frequency, expression, and timing of PCOS (polycystic ovaries can be detected in prepubescent children). From 22% to 30% of women have polycystic ovaries on ultrasound, with 80% having one or more symptoms of the syndrome; 80% of women with normal ovaries also experience one or more PCOS symptoms. Signs and symptoms of women with PCOS may change over time. In addition, polycystic ovaries may be associated with Cushing syndrome, congenital adrenal hyperplasia, thyroid disease, androgen-producing adrenal tumors or ovarian tumors (Fig. 22-3), and syndromes with hyperprolactinemia.

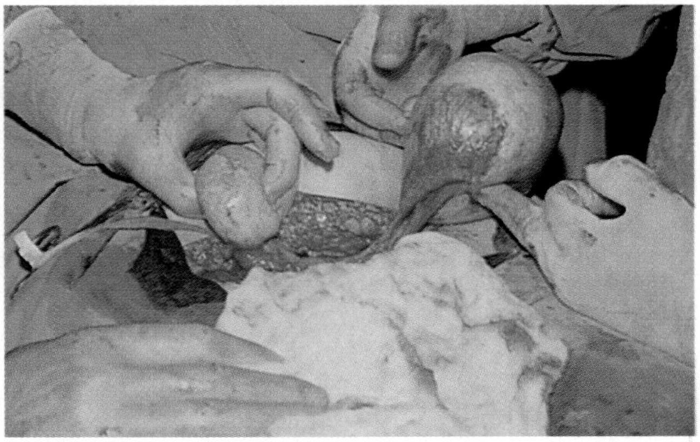

FIG. 22-3 Polycystic ovary. (From Symonds EM, Macpherson MBA: *Diagnosis in color: obstetrics and gynecology,* London, 1997, Mosby-Wolfe.)

WHAT'S NEW? Rethinking the Etiology of Polycystic Ovary Syndrome

"New thinking on polycystic ovary syndrome, an often-overlooked condition that affects millions of women, is paving the way for therapies that address both its short- and long-term consequences" (Nestler, 1999). Polycystic ovary syndrome (PCOS) is now considered a variant of syndrome X, a triadic disease process consisting of hypertension, dyslipidemia, and hyperinsulinemia. Treatment of PCOS with insulin sensitizers seems to increase fertility while decreasing predisposition to type 2 diabetes.

Sources: HealthNews: Polycystic ovary syndrome, 1998. Available at www.onhealth.com/conditions/in-depth/; Amato G et al: Lack of insulin-like growth factor binding protein-3 variation after follicle-stimulating hormone stimulation in women with polycystic ovary syndrome undergoing in vitro fertilization, *Fertil Steril* 72(3):454, 1999; Nestler J: *Insulin resistance and women's health: new insights into polycystic ovary syndrome.* Paper presented at the 14th Annual National Conference of the American Academy of Nurse Practitioners, June 17, 1999.

Pathophysiology

Hyperinsulinemia plays a key role in androgen excess, anovulation, and pathogenesis of PCOS.[27,28,30,32-35] Insulin stimulates androgen secretion by the ovarian stroma and reduces serum sex hormone–binding globulin (SHBG) directly and independently.[28] The net effect is an increase in free testosterone levels. Excessive androgens affect follicular growth, and insulin affects follicular decline by suppressing apoptosis and enabling follicles, which would normally disintegrate, to survive (Fig. 22-4).[27] Further, there seems to be a genetic ovarian defect in PCOS, which makes the ovary either more susceptible to or sensitive to insulin's stimulation of androgen production. Recent research suggests that decreased intraovarian receptors for estrogen receptor–α[31] or insulin-like growth factor–I,[36] increased leptin levels,[37] or direct insulin resistance within selective ovarian cells (fibroblasts)[35] may contribute to this phenomenon.

Several interlinking factors affect the expression of PCOS. Weight gain tends to aggravate symptoms, whereas

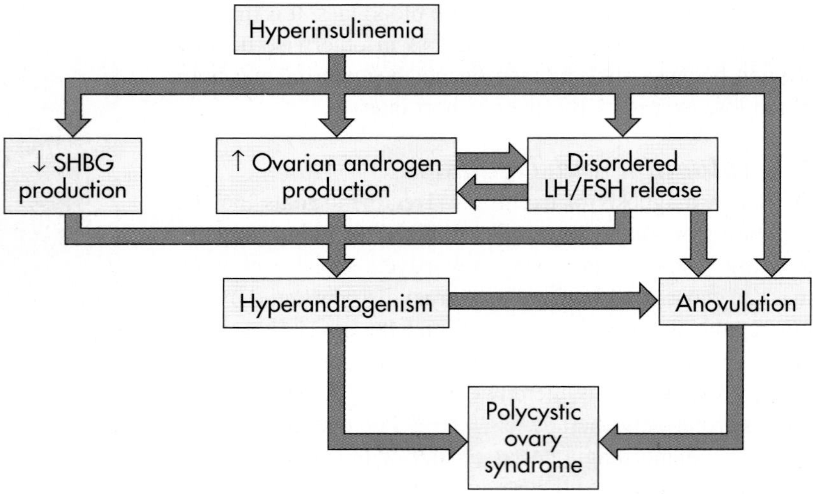

FIG. 22-4 Insulin resistance and hyperinsulinemia in PCOS. See text. *SHBG,* Sex hormone–binding globulin; *LH,* luteinizing hormone; *FSH,* follicle-stimulating hormone.

weight loss may ameliorate some of the endocrine and metabolic events and thus decrease symptoms. Women with PCOS tend to have eating disorders, perhaps due to increased leptin levels (leptin levels are increased in both thin and overweight women). Leptin influences the hypothalamic pulsatility of GnRH and consequent interaction along the entire H-P-O axis. Feedback from the polycystic ovary is disturbed due to changes in ovarian steroid and nonsteroidal (inhibins and related proteins) hormones.

There is dysfunction in folliculogenesis. Inappropriate gonadotropin secretion triggers the beginning of a vicious cycle that perpetuates anovulation. Typically, levels of FSH are low or below normal and LH levels and LH bioactivity are elevated. Persistent LH elevation causes an increase in androgens (dehydroepiandrosterone sulfate [DHEAS] from the adrenal glands and testosterone, androstenedione, and dehydroepiandrosterone [DHEA] from the ovary). Androgens are converted to estrogen in peripheral tissues, and increased testosterone levels cause a significant reduction (approximately 50%) in SHBG, which, in turn, causes increased levels of free estradiol. Elevated estrogen levels trigger a positive-feedback response in LH and a negative-feedback response in FSH. Because FSH levels are not totally depressed, new follicular growth is continuously stimulated, but not to full maturation and ovulation. The accumulation of follicular tissue in various stages of development allows an increased and relatively constant production of steroids in response to gonadotropin stimulation. Thus PCOS is characterized by excessive production of both androgen and estrogen.

Increased androgen secretion by the ovaries contributes to premature follicular atresia and persistent anovulation. In turn, persistent anovulation causes enlarged polycystic ovaries characterized by a smooth, pearly white capsule. This characteristic appearance is caused by a doubling of surface area and increased volume of 2.8 times, doubling of growing and atretic follicles, thickening of the tunica (outermost area) by 50%, increasing cortical stromal thickening by one third and a fivefold increase in subcortical stroma, and escalating hyperplasia.

Clinical Manifestations

PCOS affects females between 15 and 30 years of age. Clinical manifestations of PCOS usually appear at puberty but may appear after a variable period of normal menstrual function and, possibly, pregnancy. The symptoms are related to anovulation and include dysfunctional bleeding or amenorrhea, hirsutism, and infertility. Approximately 38% of women with PCOS are obese.[27,30] Box 22-5 contains a list of signs and symptoms, summary of hormonal disturbances, and complications of PCOS.

Evaluation and Treatment

Diagnosis of PCOS is based on evidence of androgen excess, chronic anovulation, and inappropriate gonadotropin secretion. Tests for impaired glucose tolerance and calculation of glucose-to-insulin ratio and insulin resistance index is recommended. Goals of treatment include reversing signs and symptoms of androgen excess, instituting cyclic menstruation, restoring fertility, and ameliorating any associated metabolic or endocrine, or both, disturbances.[29] Traditionally, treatment of PCOS focused on correcting anovulation and the effects of hyperandrogenism with combined oral contraceptives (COCs), antiandrogens, and fertility agents. With a greater understanding of the role that insulin resistance and hyperinsulinemia play in this disease, insulin sensitizers may be used to decrease insulin, prevent diabetes and heart disease (by reducing microvascular events), and restore fertility. Progesterone therapy is recommended to oppose estrogen's effects on the endometrium and as a means to initiate monthly withdrawal bleeding (at the expense of continued hirsutism). For infertile women, clomiphene citrate, an antiestrogen, is used to facilitate ovulation, although better effects are achieved if therapy is combined with an insulin sensitizer.[28,29,32] Women who are primed with human chorionic gonadotropin (hCG) before in vitro fertilization have greater success in achieving and maintaining pregnancy.[38] For women who do not desire pregnancy, low-dose oral contraceptives may be used to suppress androgen production and hirsutism Approximately 40% of women with

BOX 22-5

CLINICAL MANIFESTATIONS OF POLYCYSTIC OVARY SYNDROME

PRESENTING SIGNS AND SYMPTOMS (% OF WOMEN AFFECTED)

Obesity (38%)
Menstrual disturbance (66%)
Oligomenorrhea (47%)
Amenorrhea (19%)
Regular menstruation (48%)
Hyperandrogenism (48%)
Infertility (73% of anovulatory infertility)
Asymptomatic (20% of those with polycystic ovary syndrome)

HORMONAL DISTURBANCES

Increased insulin (independent of obesity)[A]
Decreased SHBG
Increased androgens (testosterone, androstenedione)
Increased DHEA (occurs in 50% of women)[B]
Increased LH (genetic variant LH-β subunit)[C,D]
Increased prolactin
Increased leptin, especially in obesity (independent of insulin)[C]
Suggested decreased insulin-like growth factor (IGF-I) receptors on theca cells[E]
Possible decreased estrogen receptors (intraovarian and along hypothalamic-pituitary axis)[F]

POSSIBLE LATE SEQUELAE

Dyslipidemia: increased low-density lipoproteins, decreased high-density lipoproteins, increased triglycerides
Diabetes mellitus (30% of women with or without obesity will develop type 2 diabetes mellitus by age 30)[E]
Cardiovascular disease; hypertension
Endometrial carcinoma (anovulatory women are hyperestrogenic)[G,H]

OTHER

Women with PCOS are at increased risk of glucose intolerance and preeclampsia during pregnancy[I]

Adapted from Balen A: Pathogenesis of polycystic ovary syndrome—the enigma unravels? *Lancet* 354:966, 1999.

[A]Diamanti-Kandarakis E et al: A survey of the polycystic ovary syndrome in the Greek island of Lesbos: hormonal and metabolic profile, *J Clin Endocrinol Metab* 84(11):4006, 1999.

[B]Gordon CM: Menstrual disorders in adolescents: excess androgens and the polycystic ovary syndrome, *Pediatr Clin North Am* 46(3):519, 1999.

[C]Orabi HE et al: Serum leptin as an additional possible pathogenic factor in polycystic ovary syndrome, *Clin Biochem* 32(1):71, 1999.

[D]Kurioka H et al: Diagnostic difficulty in polycystic ovary syndrome due to an LH-β-subunit variant, *Eur J Endocrinol* 140:235, 1999.

[E]Couse JF et al: Prevention of the polycystic phenotype and characterization of ovulatory capacity in the estrogen receptor–α knockout mouse, *Endocrinology* 140(12):5855, 1999.

[F]Amato G et al: Lack of insulin-like growth factor binding protein-3 variation after follicle-stimulating hormone stimulation in women with polycystic ovary syndrome undergoing in vitro fertilization, *Fertil Steril* 72(3):454, 1999.

[G]Speroff L, Glass RH, Kase NG: *Clinical gynecologic endocrinology and infertility,* ed 5, Baltimore, 1994, Williams & Wilkins.

[H]Patel SR, Korykowski MT: Treating polycystic ovary syndrome: today's approach, *Womens Health Prim Care* 3(2):109, 2000.

[I]Radon PA, McMahon MJ, Meyer WR: Impaired glucose tolerance in pregnant women with polycystic ovary syndrome, *Obstet Gynecol* 94(2):194, 1999.

PCOS can become pregnant with the proper medical management; this number may increase with current changes in the therapeutic management of PCOS.

Premenstrual Syndrome

Premenstrual syndrome (PMS) is the cyclic recurrence (in the luteal phase of the menstrual cycle) of distressing physical, psychologic, or behavioral changes that impair interpersonal relationships or interfere with usual activities.[39] The prevalence of PMS is difficult to determine. It has been estimated that 5% to 10% of menstruating women have severe to disabling premenstrual symptoms, 3% to 8% have cyclic dysphoria warranting treatment,[40] and 50% or more have mild to moderately distressing symptoms. To confuse matters, it seems that (1) symptoms are experienced to some degree by all adolescent and adult women and are more likely to occur throughout all menstrual phases, (2) the presence and severity of symptoms in any one woman may be inconsistent from month to month, and (3) menstrual phase for peak symptom severity may differ depending on the population studied.[41-43]

Past theories of PMS causes have focused on ovarian, pituitary, and adrenal hormones, as well as insulin, endogenous opioids, prostaglandins, yeast, and bacteria. Support for these varying theories is nonexistent or inconclusive. It is thought that PMS is the result of abnormal tissue response (most likely related to levels of neurotransmitters and neurosteroids)[44] to the normal changes of the menstrual cycle. This biologic response may be triggered by fluctuating estrogen and progesterone levels, which are important but not sufficient to produce PMS. Other mediating factors must exist. The effectiveness of selective serotonin reuptake inhibitors (SSRIs) in relieving premenstrual mood, behavior, or somatic symptoms strongly suggests that PMS is a disorder of decreased synaptic serotonin levels as a mechanism of action. Endorphins and neurosteroids have also been implicated.[40,45,46] A predisposition to PMS runs in families, perhaps because of genetics or environment. A woman's menstrual experience tends to be similar to her mother's or her sister's experience. Although research is limited, further evidence supports a relationship between the severity and frequency of premenstrual symptoms and reports of low general well-being, history of major affective disorder, and personality characteristics, such as perfectionism, increased stress, poor nutrition, lack of exercise, low self-esteem, history of sexual abuse, and family conflict. In turn, when premenstrual symptoms are perceived as distressing, the quality of interpersonal relationships and self-image are negatively affected.

Clinical Manifestations

The pattern of symptom frequency and severity is more important than specific complaints. More than 200 physical, emotional, and behavioral symptoms have been attributed to PMS. Emotional symptoms, particularly depression, anger, irritability, and fatigue, have been reported as the most prominent and the most distressing, whereas physical symptoms seem to be the least prevalent and problematic. Approximately 6% of women have classic PMS, as defined earlier, and 7% report premenstrual magnification of symptoms that occur during the entire cycle. A typical premenstrual symptom pattern may appear after the treatment of a systemic disease. Likewise, underlying physical or psychologic disease may be aggravated premenstrually.

Evaluation and Treatment

Diagnosis of PMS is based on prospective health history and symptoms. Research and diagnostic criteria for premenstrual dysphoric disorder (PMDD) are presented in Boxes 22-6 and 22-7. Because the cause of PMS is complex and cannot be reduced to a single biologic explanation and because the occurrence and severity of PMS are mediated by life-style, social, and psychologic factors, current treatment for PMS is symptomatic. Nonpharmacologic therapies, with or without medication, tend to be more effective in controlling symptoms than medication alone.

Initial treatment focuses on validation of the premenstrual experience, education on PMS and self-help techniques, and elimination of contributing factors or treatment of coexisting disorders. Individual, marriage, or family counseling; anger management and conflict resolution; and stress-reduction techniques, including biofeedback, relaxation and imagery, regular exercise, adequate rest, and time management, are all recommended. Dietary changes, such as eating six small meals each day; increasing intake of complex carbohydrates, fiber, and water; and decreasing caffeine, alcohol, sugar, and animal fat consumption are beneficial.

After a trial of nonpharmacologic therapies, medications may be added to the treatment regimen. Drugs frequently prescribed include vitamin and mineral supplements, SSRIs, antiprostaglandins, and alprazolam. SSRIs relieve symptoms in about 60% of women and may be given continuously or only during the premenstrual period. Long-acting SSRIs, such as fluoxetine, should be tapered to prevent withdrawal symptoms. Progesterone may be used for its muscle relaxant and sedative properties, and its metabolite may work at the γ-aminobutyric acid (GABA) receptor to decrease mood symptoms, even though its efficacy in the treatment of PMS is not documented. Because the edema associated with PMS is a result of local fluid shifts rather than fluid retention, diuretics are not recommended. Women tend to respond immediately to SSRIs whether prescribed intermittently or consistently, suggesting that premenstrual depression is mediated differently than major mood disorders.[44,45]

In severe cases, menses is abolished, which eliminates cyclic ovarian hormones and thus the biologic trigger for

Box 22-6

GENERAL CRITERIA FOR PREMENSTRUAL DYSPHORIC DISORDER

Premenstrual dysphoria is the predominant feature of premenstrual dysphoric disorder (PMDD) and is triggered (not caused) by the endocrine changes that occur in the late luteal phase of the menstrual cycle. Although PMDD is not an accepted diagnostic entity in the *Diagnostic and Statistical Manual of Mental Disorders* (DSM-IV-TR[2000]) text, recognition is given to the severe and incapacitating dysphoria that characterizes the disorder by listing PMDD as an example under "Mood Disorders, Depression, Not Otherwise Specified" in the main text. To encourage further research, PMDD remains in the appendix of DSM-IV. Criteria for PMDD include a rigorous prospective assessment confirming a regular premenstrual pattern of severe depressive symptoms.

Data from American Psychiatric Association: *DSM-IV-TR diagnostic and statistical manual of mental disorders,* ed 4, Washington, DC, 2000, American Psychiatric Association.

Box 22-7

RESEARCH CRITERIA FOR PREMENSTRUAL DYSPHORIC DISORDER

A. In most menstrual cycles during the past year, five (or more) of the following symptoms were present for most of the time during the last week of the luteal phase, began to remit within a few days after the onset of the follicular phase, and were absent in the week postmenses, with at least one of the symptoms being either (1), (2), (3), or (4):
   (1) Markedly depressed mood, feelings of hopelessness, or self-deprecating thoughts
   (2) Marked anxiety, tension, feelings of being "keyed up," or "on edge"
   (3) Marked affective lability (e.g., feeling suddenly sad or tearful or increased sensitivity to rejection)
   (4) Persistent and marked anger or irritability or increased interpersonal conflicts
   (5) Decreased interest in usual activities (e.g., work, school, friends, hobbies)
   (6) Subjective sense of difficulty in concentrating
   (7) Lethargy, easy fatigability, or marked lack of energy
   (8) Marked change in appetite, overeating, or specific food cravings
   (9) Hypersomnia or insomnia
   (10) A subjective sense of being overwhelmed or out of control
   (11) Other physical symptoms, such as breast tenderness or swelling, headaches, joint or muscle pain, a sensation of "bloating," weight gain

   NOTE: In menstruating females, the luteal phase corresponds to the period between ovulation and the onset of menses, and the follicular phase begins with menses. In nonmenstruating females (e.g., those who have had a hysterectomy), the timing of luteal and follicular phases may require measurement of circulating reproductive hormones.
B. The disturbance markedly interferes with work or school or with usual social activities and relationships with others (e.g., avoidance of social activities, decreased productivity and efficiency at work or school).
C. The disturbance is not merely an exacerbation of the symptoms of another disorder, such as Major Depressive Disorder, Panic Disorder, Dysthymic Disorder, or a Personality Disorder (although it may be superimposed on any of these disorders).
D. Criteria A, B, and C must be confirmed by prospective daily ratings during at least two consecutive symptomatic cycles. (The diagnosis may be made provisionally prior to this confirmation.)

Data from American Psychiatric Association: *DSM-IV-TR diagnostic and statistical manual of mental disorders,* ed 4, Washington, DC, 2000, American Psychiatric Association.

PMS. Elimination of menses can be accomplished with the use of oral contraceptives, medroxyprogesterone acetate, or GnRH agonists; emotional symptoms may not be relieved with the latter. In addition, if GnRH analogues are used, then continuous estrogen replacement therapy is needed. Of interest is that women with PMS may experience similar symptoms with synthetic hormones.[45]

Infection and Inflammation

Infections of the genital tract may result from exogenous or endogenous microorganisms. Exogenous pathogens are most frequently sexually transmitted (see Chapter 23). Endogenous causes of infection include microorganisms that are normally present in the vagina, bowel, or vulva. Infection occurs if these microorganisms migrate to a new location or overproliferate or if the immune system and other defense mechanisms are impaired.

A number of skin disorders can affect the vulva. They include reactive dermatitis, contact dermatitis, psoriasis, and impetigo. (For a discussion of skin disorders, see Chapter 43.) Most infectious disorders that affect the vulva and vagina are sexually transmitted, however. These disorders are described in Chapter 23.

NUTRITION & DISEASE

Premenstrual Syndrome

Women who are affected by premenstrual syndrome (PMS) frequently are looking for ways to decrease their symptoms, and dietary interventions are multiple. Dietary changes, such as eating six small meals each day; increasing intake of complex carbohydrates, fiber, and water; and decreasing caffeine, alcohol, refined sugar, and animal fat consumption are beneficial. Recently, a low-fat vegetarian diet was associated with decreased symptoms, possibly because of an increase in serum sex hormone–binding globulin concentration that lowers serum estrogen levels. It also may be helpful to limit sodium intake, and some limited evidence suggests that moderate doses (50 mg/day) of vitamin B_6 may reduce emotional symptoms of depression, irritability, and tiredness. This finding needs to be confirmed. Some researchers have suggested links between serotonin, endorphins, and high sugar intake and PMS risk. One interesting craving is chocolate. Some researchers suggest that a craving for chocolate is an unconscious desire for a compound called phenylethylamine (PEA) in chocolate that stimulates the release of the neurotransmitter dopamine, which regulates mood.

Data from Mahan LK, Escott-Strump S: *Krause's food, nutrition, and diet therapy,* ed 10, Philadelphia, 2000, W.B. Saunders; Barnard ND et al: Diet and sex hormone–binding globulin, dysmenorrhea and premenstrual symptoms, *Obstet Gynecol* 95(2):245, 2000.

Pelvic Inflammatory Disease

Pelvic inflammatory disease (PID) is an acute inflammatory process caused by infection (Fig. 22-5). PID may involve any organ, or combination of organs, of the upper genital tract—the uterus, fallopian tubes, or ovaries—and, in its most severe form, the entire peritoneal cavity. (Infection of the fallopian tubes is termed **salpingitis** [Fig. 22-6]; infection of the ovaries is called **oophoritis.**) Sexually transmitted microorganisms that migrate from the vagina to the uterus, fallopian tubes, and ovaries cause most cases of PID.

Pathophysiology

The development of upper genital tract infections is mediated by a number of defense mechanisms that usually are effective in preventing PID (see Chapter 21). Virulence of the organism, size of the inoculum, and defense status of the individual all determine whether an infectious process results.

PID usually is considered a polymicrobial infection,[47-49] with the majority of cases (up to 84%) caused by mixed nongonococcal/nonchlamydial bacteria, including anaerobes (*Bacteroides* species and peptostreptococci), facultative organisms (*Gardnerella vaginalis, Haemophilus influenzae,* and streptococci), and genital tract mycoplasmas (*Mycoplasma hominis, Mycoplasma genitaliu,* and *Ureaplasma urealyticum*). *Mycoplasma hominis* and *Ureaplasma urealyticum* have been isolated from the endocervic but not the fallopian tubes. *Escherichia coli* has been overemphasized as a causal agent but may contribute to pelvic infections in older women. Recovery of *Neisseria gonorrhoeae* (37% to

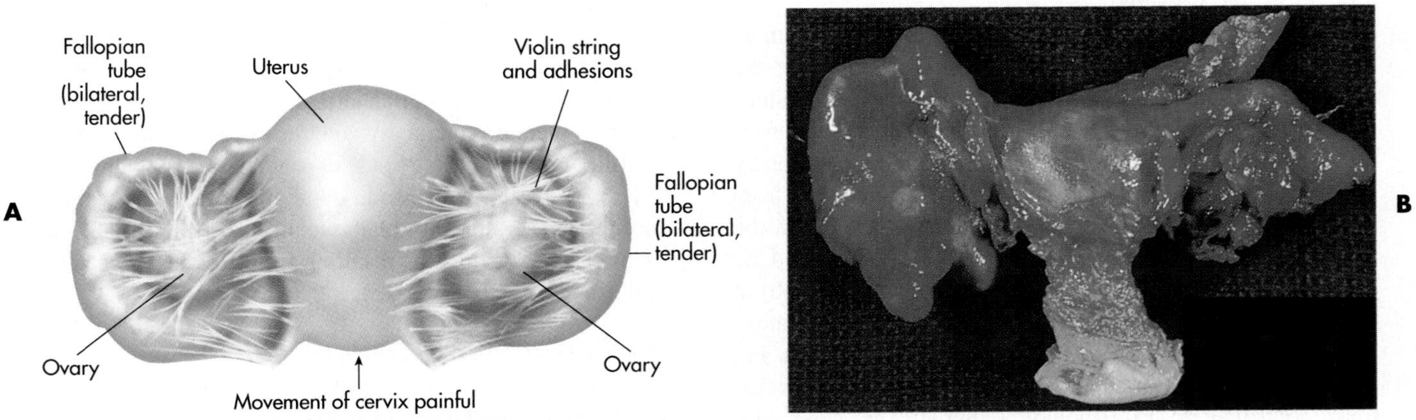

FIG. 22-5 Pelvic inflammatory disease. A, Involvement of both ovaries and fallopian tubes. **B,** Total abdominal hysterectomy and bilateral salpingo-oophorectomy specimen showing unilateral pyosalpinx. (**A,** From Seidel H et al: *Mosby's guide to physical examination,* ed 4, St Louis, 1999, Mosby. **B,** From Morse SA, Moreland AA, Holmes KK: *Atlas of sexually transmitted diseases and AIDS,* ed 2, London, 1996, Mosby-Wolfe.)

A

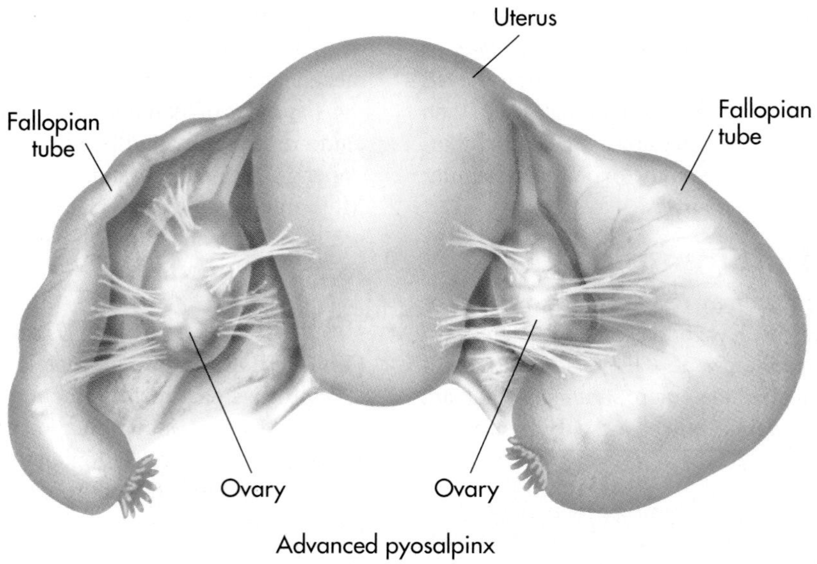

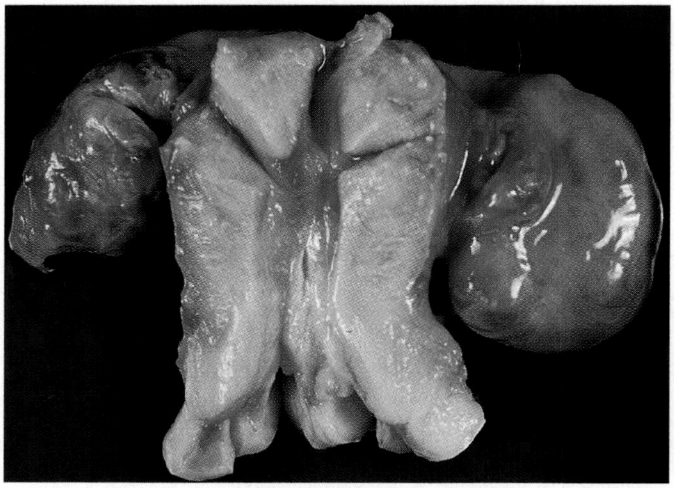

B

FIG. 22-6 Salpingitis. A, Note the swollen fallopian tubes. **B,** Bilateral, retort-shaped, swollen, sealed tubes and adhesions of ovaries are typical of salpingitis. (**A,** From Seidel H et al: *Mosby's guide to physical examination,* ed 4, St Louis, 1999, Mosby. **B,** From Damjanov I, Linder J, editors: *Anderson's pathology,* ed 10, St Louis, 1996, Mosby.)

44%), *Chlamydia trachomatis* (10% to 45%), or both (9% to 12%) is variable; however, facultative or anaerobic bacteria have been insolated in about 50% of women with acute PID. About 25% to 50% of the time, only facultative or anaerobic organisms are recovered.

PID develops when pathogenic microbes ascend from an infected cervix along the endometrial tissue to infect the uterus and adnexae. Gonorrhea or chlamydia may induce changes in the columnar epithelium that lines the upper reproductive tract, causing damage and facilitating invasion by other microorganisms. This observation is supported from the recovery of cytokines, such as interleukin 6, from the cervix and endometrium of women with acute PID,[50] and the presence of antibodies to a chlamydial protein (CHSP60) in animal studies of chronic PID.[51] The resultant inflammatory response leads to tubonecrosis with repeated infections and may predispose a woman to PID.[47,48] Other mechanisms that may contribute to PID include lymphatic drainage with parametrial spread of the infection or the adherance of sexually transmitted bacteria to sperm that travel through the genital tract. Several investigators report that bacterial vaginosis (BV), a bacterial overgrowth of the vagina, has been linked to clinical findings of PID and histologic endometritis. Women with BV are nine times more likely to develop PID.[47,52] (See Chapter 23 for further discussion of BV.) After one episode of pelvic infection, 15% to 25% of women develop long-term sequelae, such as infertility, ectopic pregnancy, chronic pelvic pain, dyspareunia, pelvic adhesions, perihepatitis, and tuboovarian abscess. The incidence of complications increases markedly with repeated infections. Tubal infertility occurs in 8% to 11% of women after one episode, 20% to 30% after two episodes, and 40% to 50% after three episodes.[47] The mortality rate associated with PID is 8% to 9% of cases. Most deaths resulting from PID are caused by septic shock (see Chapter 45).

Clinical Manifestations

The clinical manifestations of PID vary from sudden, severe abdominal pain with fever to no symptoms at all. An asymptomatic cervicitis may be present for some time before PID develops. Of women with salpingitis, 67% to 75% may have a subclinical infection. The first sign of the ascending infec-

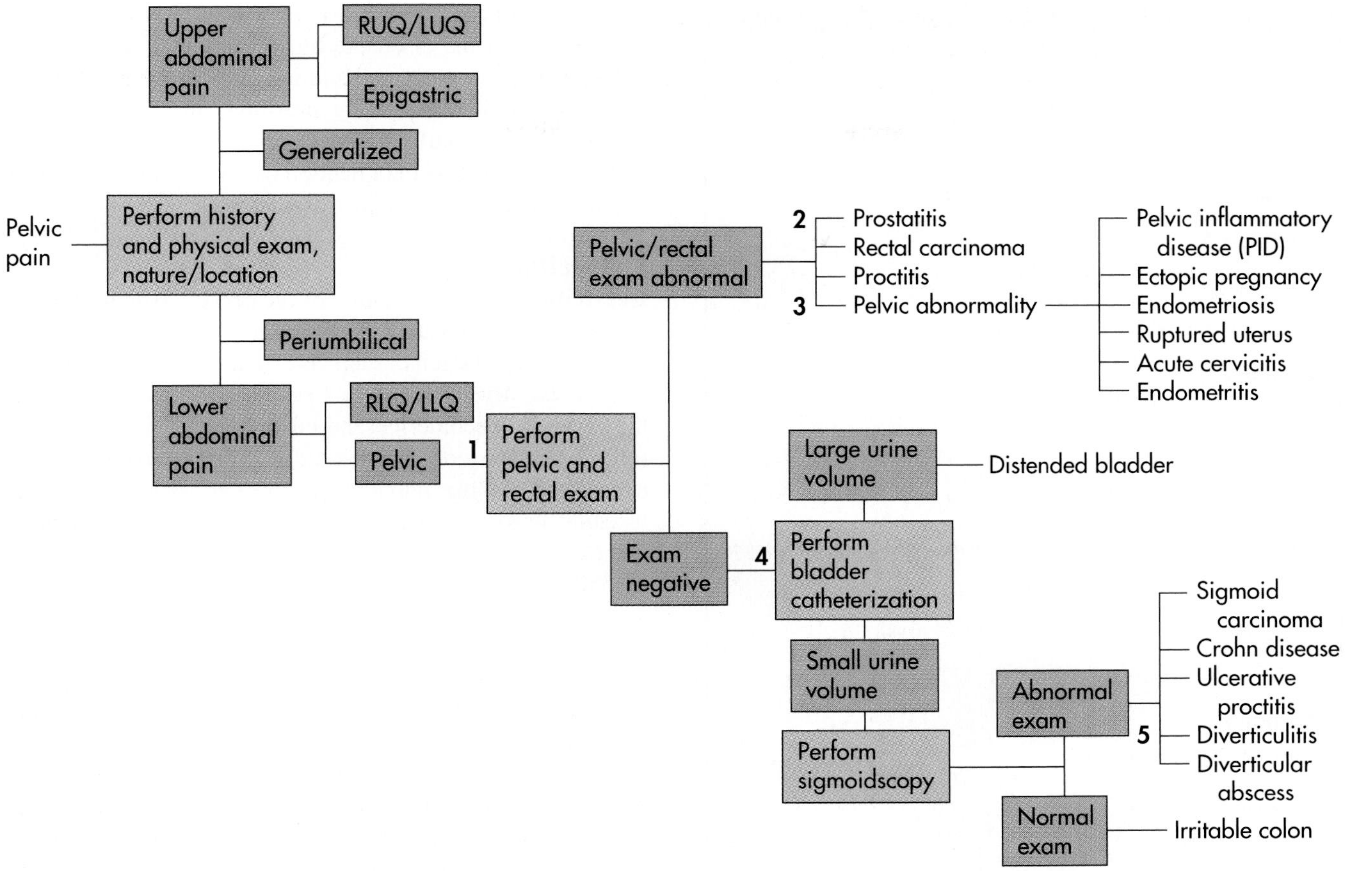

FIG. 22-7 Algorithm or flow chart for pelvic pain. *RUQ,* Right upper quadrant; *LUQ,* left upper quadrant; *RLQ,* right lower quadrant; *LLQ,* left lower quadrant.

tion may be the onset of low bilateral abdominal pain, most often characterized as dull and steady with a gradual onset. Symptoms are more likely to develop during or immediately after menstruation. The pain of PID may worsen with walking, jumping, or intercourse. Other manifestations of PID include dysuria (difficult or painful urination) and irregular bleeding.

Evaluation and Treatment

The diagnosis of PID is based on history, abdominal tenderness with or without rebound, presence of uterine and cervical movement tenderness on bimanual pelvic examination, mucopurulent discharge at the cervical os, white blood cells on Gram stain or wet mount of cervical discharge, leukocytosis, and increased erythrocyte sedimentation rate. To support the diagnosis, a chlamydia smear for fluorescent antibody testing or deoxyribonucleic acid (DNA) testing and a gonorrhea culture or DNA probe are done; sonography, laparoscopy, and culdocentesis are indicated when a woman has recurrent symptoms or symptoms unresponsive to outpatient treatment regimen, fever greater than 38.3° C, or an adnexal mass. Other conditions that cause pelvic pain must be excluded, including ectopic pregnancy, threatened abortion, or appendicitis (Fig. 22-7).

Treatment involves bed rest, avoidance of intercourse, and combined antibiotic therapy (Box 22-8). From 25% to 40% of women require hospitalization for intravenous administration of antibiotics and treatment of peritonitis or a tuboovarian abscess. To prevent recurrence, sexual partners also are treated with antibiotic combinations.[49]

Vaginitis

Vaginitis is infection of the vagina. The major causes of vaginitis are sexually transmitted pathogens (see Chapter 23) and *Candida albicans.* The incidence of sexually transmitted vaginitis remains highest in young women 10 to 24 years of age.[53,54]

The development of vaginitis is related to the overall health of a woman and local defense mechanisms, particularly vaginal pH. The pH of the vagina depends on cervical secretions and the presence of normal flora that help maintain an acidic environment. A neutral or alkaline pH normally occurs before puberty, after menopause, and during pregnancy. The acidic nature of vaginal secretions during the reproductive years provides protection against a variety of sexually transmitted pathogens. Therefore variables that alter the vaginal pH or the bactericidal nature of secretions (see Chapter 21) may predispose a woman to infection. These variables include douching; use of soaps, feminine hygiene sprays, or deodorant menstrual pads or tampons; and conditions associated with increased glycogen content of vaginal secretions, such as pregnancy or diabetes.

Box 22-8

CENTERS FOR DISEASE CONTROL AND PREVENTION RECOMMENDED TREATMENT FOR ACUTE PELVIC INFLAMMATORY DISEASE (1998)

AMBULATORY MANAGEMENT

Regimen A

Ofloxacin, 400 mg PO twice daily for 14 days,
plus
metronidazole, 500 mg PO twice daily for 14 days

Regimen B

Cefoxitin, 2 g IM, plus *probenecid,* 1 g PO in a single dose, concurrently
or
ceftriaxone, 250 mg IM,
or
another parenteral *third-generation cephalosporin* (e.g., *ceftizoxime* or *cefotaxime*).
plus
doxycycline, 100 mg PO twice daily for 14 days

HOSPITAL MANAGEMENT

Regimen A

Cefoxitin, 2 g IV every 6 hr,
or
cefotetan, 2 g IV every 12 hr,
plus
doxycycline, 100 mg IV or PO every 12 hr

Regimen B

Clindamycin, 900 mg IV every 8 hr,
plus
gentamicin loading dose IV or IM (2 mg/kg of body weight) followed by maintenance dose (1.5 mg/kg) every 8 hr (single daily dosing may be substituted)

Data from Centers for Disease Control and Prevention: *1998 Sexually transmitted diseases: treatment guidelines,* 1998, US Dept. of Health and Human Services.

Antibiotics may destroy *Lactobacillus acidophilus,* an anaerobic, gram-positive rod normally found in the vagina that helps maintain an acidic pH. In its absence, alkalinity increases and the vagina is more susceptible to trichomoniasis and bacterial vaginosis; moreover, there may be an overgrowth of *C. albicans,* causing a yeast vaginitis.

Normally, vaginal discharge is a clear, milky, or cloudy secretion with a slippery or clumpy texture. It is nonirritating, has a mild inoffensive odor, and turns yellow after drying. Throughout the menstrual cycle, the amount and texture of a woman's discharge will change in response to hormonal fluctuation. Vaginal secretions increase at the time of ovulation, during pregnancy, and with sexual arousal; just before menstruation, vaginal discharge becomes thick and sticky. Although the amount of vaginal discharge alone is not an indication of infection, any other change in discharge may indicate a problem. Infection is suggested with a marked change in color or if the discharge becomes malodorous or irritating.

Diagnosis is based on history, physical examination, and examination of the discharge by wet mount. Treatment involves developing and maintaining an acidic environment, relieving symptoms (usually pruritus), and administering antimicrobial or antifungal medications to eradicate the infectious organism. If the infection can be sexually transmitted, a woman's partner also will be treated.

Cervicitis

Cervicitis is an inflammation of the cervix. **Mucopurulent cervicitis (MPC)** usually is caused by one or more sexually transmitted pathogens, such as *Trichomonas,* gonorrhea, *Chlamydia, Mycoplasma,* or *Ureaplasma.* Infection causes the cervix to become red and edematous. A mucopurulent (mucus- and pus-containing) exudate drains from the external cervical os, and the individual may report vague pelvic pain, bleeding, or dysuria. The infectious organisms are cultured or identified by immunoassay. Definitive diagnosis is followed by oral antibiotic therapy. Sexual partners are treated.[49]

Vulvitis

Inflammation of the vulva is termed **vulvitis.** Acute vulvitis is an inflammation of the skin (dermatitis) of the vulva and often of the perianal area. Vulvitis can be caused by contact with soaps, detergents, lotions, hygienic sprays, menstrual pads, perfumed toilet paper, or nonabsorbent or tight-fitting clothes. Vulvitis is caused also by vaginal infections (e.g., candidiasis, trichomoniasis) that spread to the labia, where they cause inflammation and edema. Other skin diseases, such as tinea cruris, psoriasis, and inflammation of the apocrine (sweat) glands, can involve the vulva (see Chapter 43).

Avoidance of irritants; wearing loose, cotton clothing; and appropriate antimicrobial or antifungal treatment for recurrent vaginitis are usually effective cures for acute vulvitis. Chronic vulvitis usually is treated with fluorinated hydrocortisone. Biopsy specimens of persistent lesions are examined for the presence of malignancy.

Bartholinitis

Bartholinitis, or **Bartholin cyst,** is an inflammation of one or both of the ducts that lead from the introitus (vaginal opening) to Bartholin glands (Fig. 22-8). The usual causes of bartholinitis are microorganisms that infect the lower female reproductive tract, such as streptococci, staphylococci, and sexually transmitted pathogens. Acute bartholinitis usually is preceded by an infection, such as cervicitis, vaginitis, or urethritis.

Infection or trauma causes inflammatory changes that narrow the distal portion of the duct, leading to obstruction and stasis of glandular secretions. The obstruction, or **cyst,** varies from 1 to 8 cm in diameter and is located in the posterolateral portion of the vulva. The cyst is usually reddened and painful, and pus may be visible at the opening of the duct. The individual may have symptoms of the initiating infection, fever, and malaise.

Most Bartholin cysts are asymptomatic and require no treatment. Chronic bartholinitis is characterized by the presence of a small cyst that is slightly tender but otherwise is

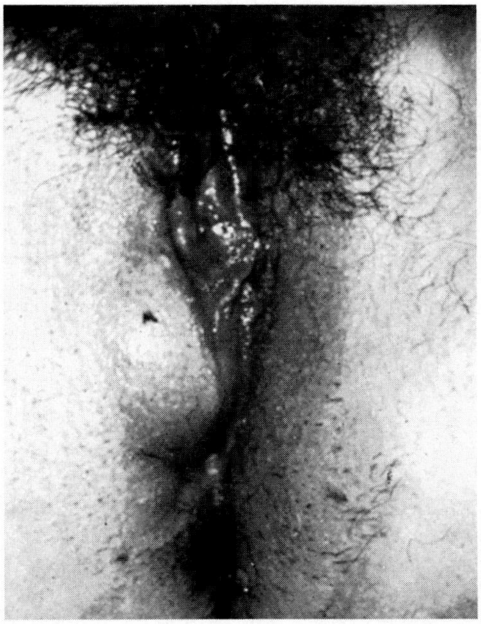

FIG. 22-8 Inflammation of bartholin glands. (From Gardner HL, Kaufman RH: *Benign diseases of the vulva and vagina,* St Louis, 1969, Mosby.)

asymptomatic. Symptoms occur if an exacerbation of infection causes an abscess to form in the gland itself.

Diagnosis of bartholinitis is based on the clinical manifestations and the identification of infectious microorganisms. Antibiotics are given to treat infection, and pain is relieved with analgesics and warm sitz baths. If an abscess forms, it is surgically drained.

Pelvic Relaxation Disorders

The bladder, urethra, and rectum are supported by the endopelvic fascia and the perineal muscles. This muscular and fascial tissue loses tone and strength with aging and may fail to maintain the pelvic organs in the proper position. Progressive relaxation of the pelvic support structures may cause uterine displacement. Uterine displacement can also result if trauma, such as childbirth or pelvic surgery, damages or weakens the supporting structures. Pelvic relaxation is progressive and is related to the inherent strength or weakness of the woman's musculofascial tissue. Malpositioning of the bladder, urethra, or rectum (and hence the uterus) may occur many years after an initial injury to the supporting structure. A strong familial tendency and possibly a multifactorial genetic component place some women at risk for the development of prolapse. Genital prolapse is 80 times more prevalent in whites than in blacks, and, despite grand multiparity, pelvic relaxation is rare in Canadian Indians. Risk factors in nulliparous women, which mimic the impact of childbirth, tend to be occupational activities that require heavy lifting or chronic medical conditions, such as chronic lung disease or refractory constipation. Some women at risk for pelvic organ prolapse have neural abnormalities that interfere with the innervation of the levator ani (see Chapter 21 for a discussion of pelvic support structures).

BOX 22-9

PHYSICAL EXAMINATION TERMS FOR DESCRIPTION OF SUPPORT ABNORMALITIES

Anterior wall support abnormality (further specified as lateral, midline, upper/transverse)
Apical support abnormalities (with or without uterus present)
Posterior wall support abnormality (specify as distal or proximal)

Data from Brubaker L: Abnormalities of pelvic support. In Copeland LJ, Farrell JF, editors: *Textbook of gynecology,* ed 2, Philadelphia, 2000, W.B. Saunders.

BOX 22-10

URINARY, SEXUAL, ANORECTAL (USA) REVIEW OF SYSTEMS FOR PELVIC FLOOR DISORDERS

URINARY

Storage phase: urgency, frequency, nocturia, incontinence (urge, stress, others)
Emptying phase: voiding dysfunction, postural voiding, urinary retention
Sensation: increased (pain, constant urge to urinate), decreased sensation

SEXUAL

Sexual activity: if yes, explore further impact of protrusion; if no, explore reasons
Sexual response: normal/abnormal; same/different
General sensation of protrusion; increased (pain), decreased

ANORECTAL

Storage phase: urgency, frequency, nocturia, incontinence (gas, liquid, solid)
Emptying phase: defecation dysfunction (manually assisted), post-defecation, fullness, constipation
Sensation: increased (pain, constant urge to defecate), decreased (inability to distinguish gas versus stool)

Data from Brubaker L: Abnormalities of pelvic support. In Copeland LJ, Farrell JF, editors: *Textbook of gynecology,* ed 2, Philadelphia, 2000, W.B. Saunders.

Approximately one in nine women in the United States will undergo at least one surgery to treat pelvic organ prolapse or urinary incontinence.[55] At least 30% will have repeat surgical procedures. Because physical examination is an unreliable measure of visceral abnormalities, the trend is to replace urethrocele, cystocele, rectocele, and enterocele with precise terminology that reflects examination findings (Box 22-9). Having a woman stand and strain maximally provides the best information about the degree of pelvic organ relaxation. Physical examination is augmented with imaging by ultrasound, fluoroscope, or magnetic resonance. The urinary, sexual, anorectal (USA) review of systems for pelvic floor disorders provides comprehensive historical data (Box 22-10).

Uterine prolapse is descent of the cervix or entire uterus into the vaginal canal (Fig. 22-9). In severe cases the uterus

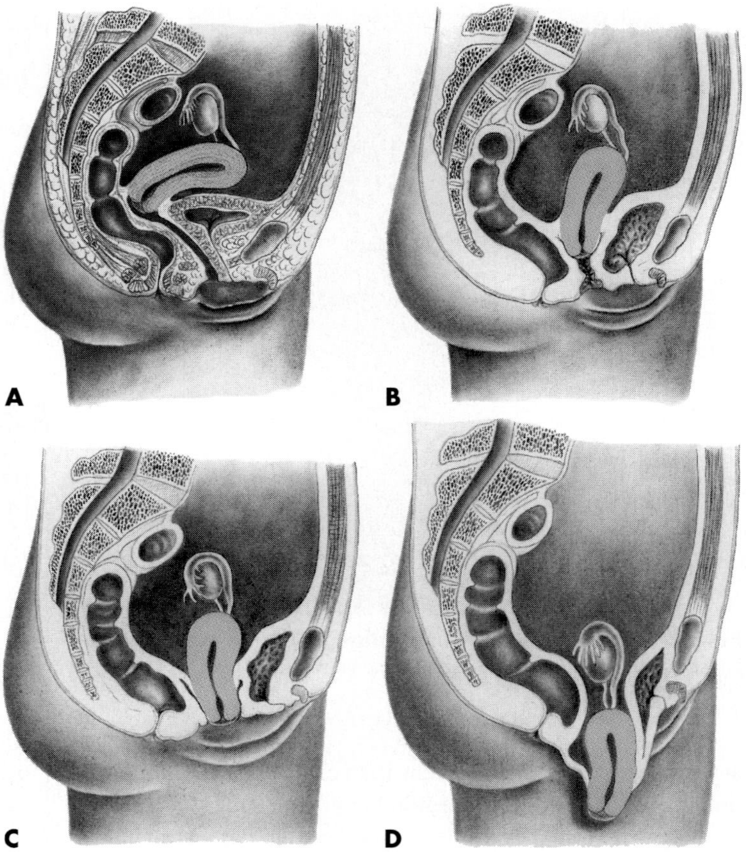

FIG. 22-9 Degrees of uterine prolapse. A, Normal uterus. **B,** First-degree prolapse: descent within the vagina. **C,** Second-degree prolapse: the cervix protrudes through the introitus. **D,** Third-degree prolapse: the vagina is completely everted. (From Seidel H et al: *Mosby's guide to physical examination,* ed 4, St Louis, 1999, Mosby.)

falls completely through the vagina and protrudes from the introitus. First-degree uterine prolapse is not treated unless it causes discomfort. Second- and third-degree prolapse cause feelings of fullness, heaviness, and collapse through the vagina. Symptoms of other pelvic relaxation disorders also may be present. Treatment in these cases is the insertion of a **pessary,** which is a removable mechanical device that holds the uterus in position. The pelvic fascia may be strengthened through Kegel exercises (repetitive, isometric tightening and relaxing of the pubococcygeal muscles) or by a course of estrogen therapy in menopausal women. Surgical repair is the treatment of last resort.

Fig. 22-10 shows vaginal prolapse caused by cystocele and rectocele. **Cystocele** is descent of a portion of the posterior bladder wall and trigone into the vaginal canal and usually is caused by the trauma of childbirth. In severe cases the bladder and anterior vaginal wall bulge outside the introitus. Usually symptoms are insignificant; increased bulging and descent of the anterior vaginal wall and urethra can be aggravated by vigorous activity, prolonged standing, sneezing, coughing, or straining and can be relieved by rest or assumption of a recumbent or prone position. If the cystocele is large, women may complain of vaginal pressure or the feeling of "sitting on a ball." Vaginal pressure may be interpreted as incomplete bladder emptying, which can be controlled by a second voiding a few minutes after the first void or by manually reducing the cystocele before voiding. Occasionally a cystocele causes significant residual urine and bladder infection.

Although commonly associated with urinary stress incontinence, cystocele does not cause it. Dorr[56] states that "stress incontinence is the result of relaxation of the musculofascial supporting tissues of the urethra. Unless special attention is directed to the urethral supports, operative correction of a large cystocele may cause rather than correct stress incontinence."

Medical management includes vaginal pessary; Kegel exercises (prophylactic use produces best outcome); estrogen therapy for postmenopausal women; and, most important, reassurance that pressure symptoms are not the result of a serious condition. Surgical correction is used for severe anatomic injury unresponsive to medical treatment, and its success depends on treatment of generalized urogenital musculofascial supporting tissue relaxation, correction of underlying paravaginal defects, and elimination or prevention of contributing factors that increase intraabdominal pressure, such as pregnancy, constipation, obesity, large pelvic tumors, bronchitis, and heavy manual labor.[56]

Urethrocele, or sagging of the urethra, is commonly associated with cystocele, especially in women with urinary stress incontinence. Like cystocele, urethrocele does not cause urinary incontinence. Urethrocele usually is caused by the shearing effect of the fetal head on the urethra during childbirth. **Cystourethrocele** may occur in nulliparous women and is

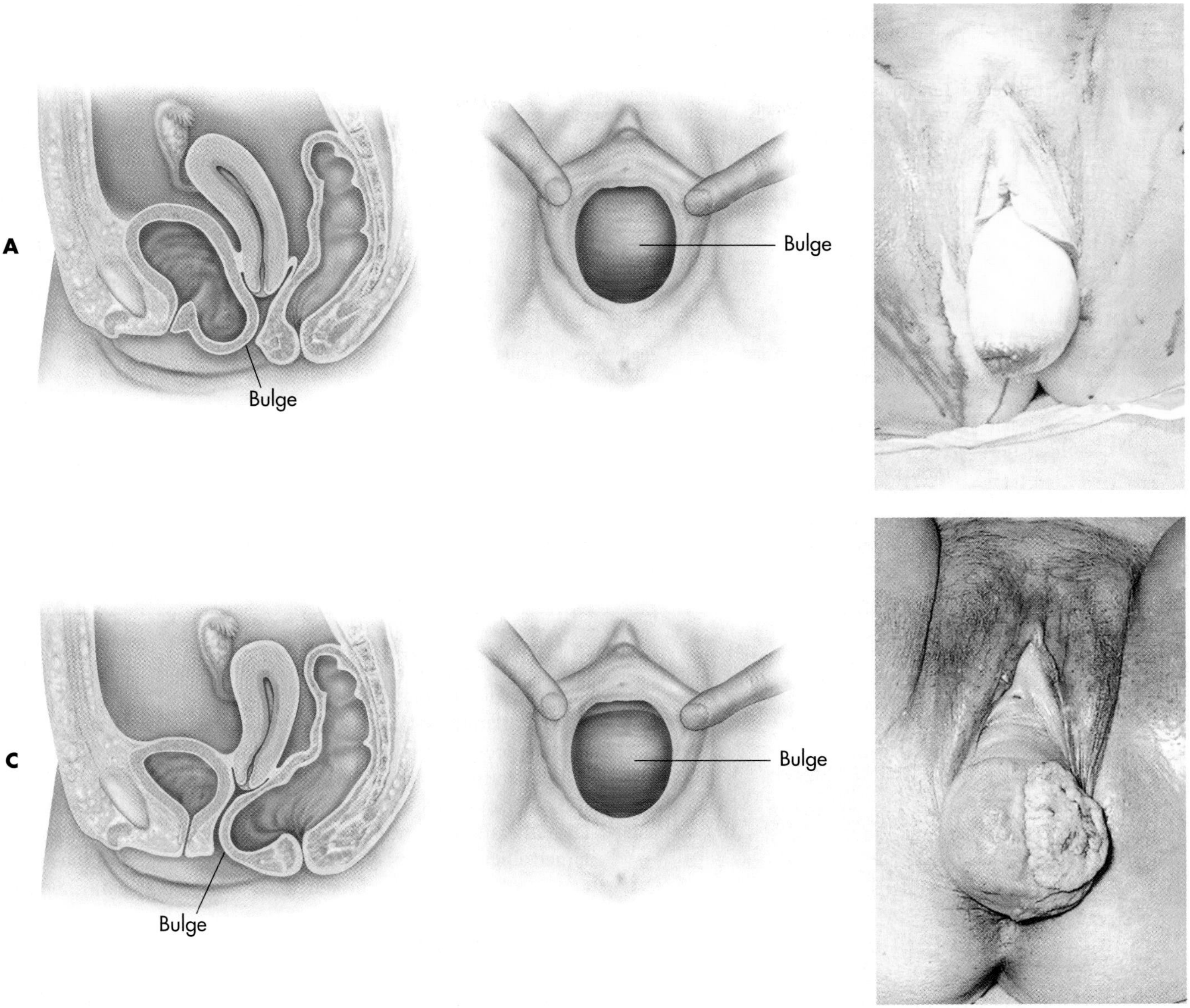

FIG. 22-10 Cystocele and rectocele. **A,** Cystocele. **B,** Large cystocele. **C,** Rectocele. **D,** Rectocele associated with ulceration of vaginal wall. (**A, C,** From Seidel H et al: *Mosby's guide to physical examination,* ed 4, St Louis, 1999, Mosby. **B, D,** From Symonds EM, Macpherson MBA: *Color atlas of obstetrics and gynecology,* London, 1994, Mosby-Wolfe.)

most likely caused by congenital weakness and relaxation of the musculature of the pelvic floor or the endopelvic connective tissues or fascia. Treatment may be necessary after menopause.

A **rectocele** is the bulging of the rectum and posterior vaginal wall into the vaginal canal. During childbirth, all women sustain damage that can lead to a rectocele, but symptoms do not occur until several years after menopause.[56] Familial and genetic predisposition and bowel habits contribute to rectocele development. Lifelong chronic constipation and straining may produce or aggravate a rectocele. Although most rectoceles are asymptomatic, larger ones with extensive relaxation cause vaginal pressure, rectal fullness, and incomplete bowel evacuation. If rectoceles are severe, defecation is difficult and can be accomplished only by applying manual pressure to the posterior vaginal wall. Medical treatment focuses on the management and prevention of constipation and, if needed, the use of a pessary. Rectocele alone (without associated enterocele, uterine prolapse, and cystocele) seldom requires surgery.

An **enterocele** is herniation of the rectouterine pouch into the rectovaginal septum (between the rectum and posterior vaginal wall). It can be congenital or acquired. Congenital enterocele rarely causes symptoms or progresses in size; the acquired form usually is associated with other pelvic relaxation disorders such as uterine prolapse, cystocele, and rectocele. Most large enteroceles are found in grossly obese and elderly persons and can be complicated by rupture or

Table 22-3 Cystocele, Urethrocele, and Rectocele

Condition	Etiology	Symptoms	Treatment
Cystocele	Laceration, stretching, or weakening of supporting fascial tissue; usually caused by prolonged labor, multiple births, or birth of a large baby Paravaginal defects	Usually insignificant Sensation of incomplete emptying of bladder Vaginal pressure or feeling of "sitting on a ball"	Reassurance Depending on age of woman and severity of the condition, includes: Isometric exercise to strengthen the pubococcygeal muscle Estrogen to improve tone and vascularity of fascial support Pessary (a removable device) to hold bladder in position Surgical correction (rarely indicated)
Urethrocele	Pressure of fetal head on urethra and attachments beneath symphysis pubis Familial or genetic predispositions Commonly associated with cystocele in women with stress incontinence	Usually asymptomatic	Isometric exercises (see Cystocele)
Rectocele	Trauma to fascia and levator muscles; usually caused by childbirth Familial or genetic predisposition Lifelong chronic constipation	Constipation or feeling of rectal fullness Difficult defecation Pressure and sensation of fullness in vagina	Isometric exercises and prevention of constipation Surgery (rarely indicated)

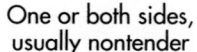

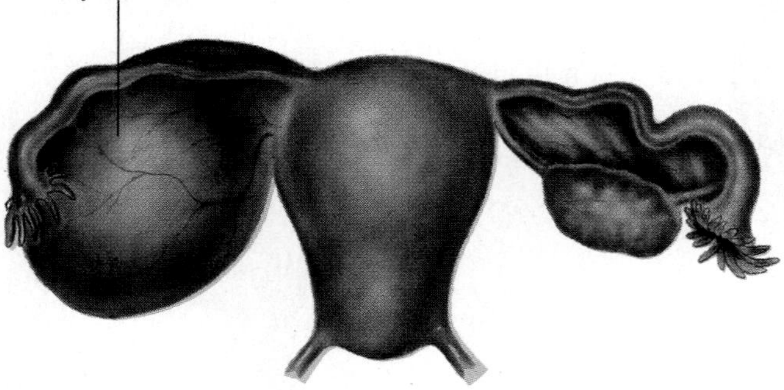

FIG. 22-11 Ovarian cyst. (From Seidel H et al: *Mosby's guide to physical examination,* ed 4, St Louis, 1999, Mosby.)

complete eversion of the vagina with trophic ulceration, edema, and fibrosis. Treatment is surgical. Table 22-3 summarizes the causes, symptoms, and treatment of cystocele, urethrocele, and rectocele.

Benign Growths and Proliferative Conditions

Benign Ovarian Cysts

Benign cysts of the ovary may occur at any time during the life span but are most common between puberty and menopause (Fig. 22-11). Two common causes of benign ovarian enlargement in ovulating women are follicular cysts and corpus luteum cysts. These cysts are called *functional cysts* because they are caused by variations of normal physiologic events. Follicular and corpus luteum cysts are unilateral. They are typically 5 to 6 cm in diameter but can grow as large as 8 to 10 cm.

A **follicular cyst** develops from a dominant ovarian follicle that does not release its ovum but remains active or from a degenerating follicle whose fluid is not reabsorbed. Most follicular cysts are not symptomatic, require no treatment, and either regress or rupture spontaneously within 60 days. A large follicular cyst may cause low back pain, painful intercourse (dyspareunia), chronic lower abdominal pain, and menstrual irregularities.

A **corpus luteum cyst** results from intracystic hemorrhage, occurring during the vascularization stage, about 2 to 4 days after ovulation. It consists of blood, which is replaced by clear fluid that accumulates in the cavity of the corpus luteum. Corpus luteum cysts are less common than follicular cysts, but luteal cysts typically cause more symptoms, particularly if they rupture. Manifestations include dull pelvic pain and amenorrhea or delayed menstruation, followed by irregular or heavier than normal bleeding. Rupture occurs during days 20 to 26 of the menstrual cycle and usually with sexual intercourse. At the time of treatment, most women have acute pain of less than 24 hours' duration, although pain may persist for 1 to 7 days in about 23% of women. A negative β-hCG test rules out ectopic pregnancy. Untrasound confirms presence of a cyst and intraperitoneal fluid, and culdocentesis reveals nonclotting blood. Watching and waiting is warranted if the hematocrit of the fluid is 15% or less. With massive or vigorous bleeding, a laparotomy may be necessary.[57]

Endometrial Polyps

An **endometrial polyp** is a benign mass of endometrial tissue and contains a variable amount of glands, stoma, and

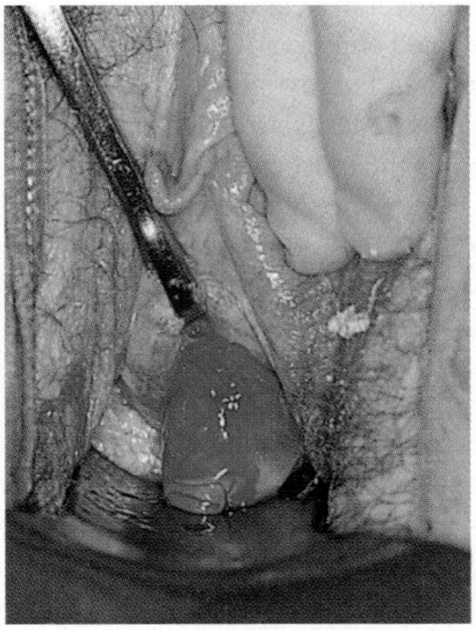

FIG. 22-12 Endometrial polyp. It is protruding through the cervical os. (From Symonds EM, Macpherson MBA: *Color atlas of obstetrics and gynecology,* London, 1994, Mosby-Wolfe.)

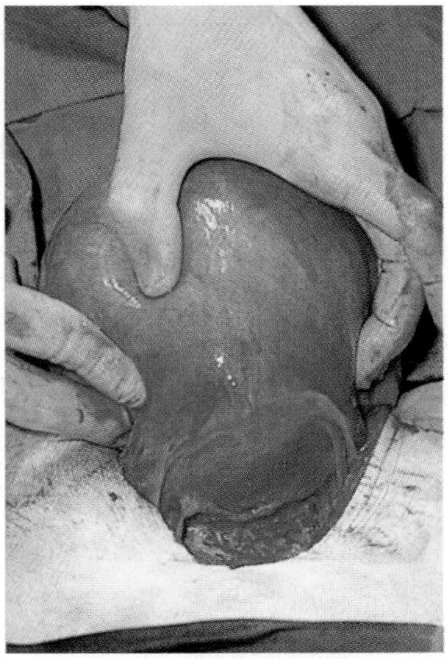

FIG. 22-13 Uterine fibroid. The uterus is irregular because it contains multiple fibroids. (From Symonds EM, Macpherson MBA: *Color atlas of obstetrics and gynecology,* London, 1994, Mosby-Wolfe.)

blood vessels. Endometrial polyps are usually solitary and originate at the fundus but may also be multiple (20% of the time) or originate from the lower uterine segment or upper endocervix and contain mixed epithelium. Polyps are morphologically diverse and are usually classified as hyperplastic, atrophic (or inactive), or functional. In the latter case, the surface epithelium may be "out of phase" with other endometrial tissue. Hyperplastic polyps are often pedunculated and may be mistaken for endometrial hyperplasia or, if large, adenosarcoma (Fig. 22-12). Although polyps most often develop in women between ages 40 and 60 years, they can occur at all ages.[57]

Endometrial polyps are a frequent cause of intermenstrual or excessive menstrual bleeding. Diagnosis is made by hysteroscopy or direct examination of tissue obtained by curettage. The lesions are removed with small, curved forceps. Malignancy is extremely rare, and coexistence of a separate endometrial atypical hyperplasia or adenocarcinoma is common.

Leiomyomas

Leiomyomas, commonly called **uterine fibroids,** are benign tumors that develop from smooth muscle cells in the myometrium (Fig. 22-13). Leiomyomas are the most common benign tumors of the uterus, and most remain small and asymptomatic. Prevalence increases in women ages 30 to 50 years but decreases with menopause. In the United States it is estimated that myomas develop in 30% of white and 50% of black women by age 50 years. The incidence of leiomyomas in black and Asian women is two to five times higher than that in white women.[57]

The cause of uterine leiomyomas is unknown, although their size appears to be related to hormonal fluctuations (particularly estrogen). Uterine leiomyomas are not seen before menarche, and those that develop during the reproductive years generally decrease in size after menopause. Tumors in pregnant women enlarge rapidly but often decrease in size after termination of the pregnancy.

Pathophysiology

Most leiomyomas occur in multiples in the fundus of the uterus, although they may occur singly and throughout the uterus. Leiomyomas are classified as subserous, submucous, or intramural according to their location within the various layers of the uterine wall (Fig. 22-14). Uterine leiomyomas are usually firm and surrounded by a pseudocapsule composed of compressed but otherwise normal uterine myometrium. Degenerative changes, such as ulceration and necrosis, may occur when the leiomyoma outgrows its blood supply and therefore are more common in larger tumors.

Clinical Manifestations

The major clinical manifestations of leiomyomas are abnormal uterine bleeding, pain, and symptoms related to pressure on nearby structures. The leiomyoma tends to make the uterine cavity larger, thereby increasing the endometrial surface area. This increase may account for the increased menstrual bleeding that is associated with leiomyomas. Pain is not an early symptom but tends to occur with the devascularization of larger leiomyomas. It is also associated with blood vessel compression that limits blood supply to adjacent structures. Symptoms of abdominal pressure are slow to develop, apparently because the tumor is relatively slow growing, enabling adjacent structures to adapt to pressure. Pressure on the bladder may contribute to urinary frequency, urgency, and dysuria. Pressure on the ureter may cause it to become distended "upstream" from the pressure point; rectosigmoid pressure may lead to constipation. A sensation

A

B

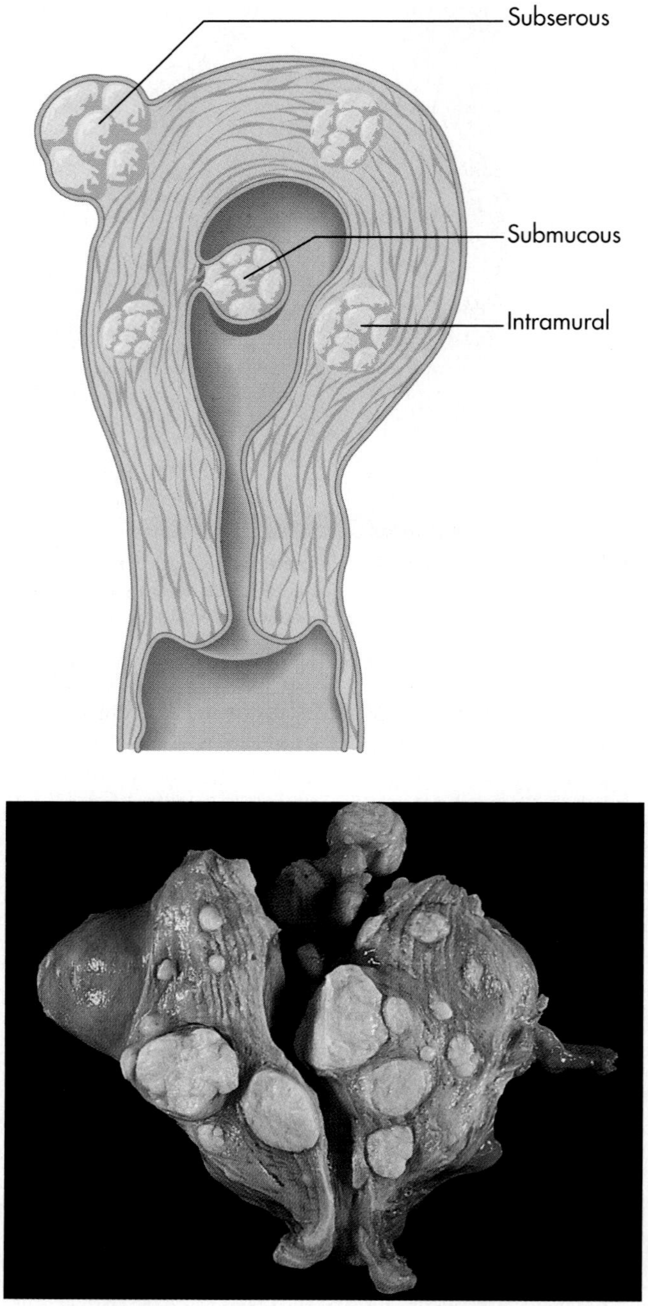

FIG. 22-14 Leiomyomas. A, Uterine section showing whorl-like appearance and locations of leiomyomas, which are also called *uterine fibroids.* **B,** Multiple leiomyomas in sagittal section. Typical, well-circumscribed, solid, light gray nodules distort uterus. (**A,** Redrawn from Novak ER, Woodruff JD, editors: *Novak's gynecologic and obstetric pathology,* ed 6, Philadelphia, 1967, W.B. Saunders. **B,** From Damjanov I, Linder J: *Pathology: a color atlas,* St Louis, 2000, Mosby.)

of abdominal or genital heaviness may be felt with larger tumors.

Evaluation and Treatment

Uterine leiomyomas are suspected when the bimanual examination discloses irregular, nontender nodularity of the uterus. Pelvic sonography or MRI confirms diagnosis.[58] Treatment depends on the symptoms, tumor size, age, reproductive status, and overall health of the individual. Most myomas can be treated conservatively. Conservative treatment is aimed at shrinking the myoma. Use of the antiprogesterone RU486 markedly reduces size. Treatment with GnRH agonists (GnRHa) is the most current therapy. GnRHa produces a hypoestrogenic state that results in diminished arterial uterine blood flow and 30% to 60% reduction in size. Side effects are related to a hypoestrogenic state and include hot flushes, vaginal dryness, decreased libido, memory loss, and osteoporosis. In a small study, these symptoms were minimized with concurrent use of tibolone, a synthetic compound structurally related to noretinodrel.[59] Myomectomy may be undertaken and is the surgical treatment of choice. GnRHa may be used to shrink tumors before surgery, thereby increasing success of myomectomy.[57]

Adenomyosis

Adenomyosis is the presence of islands of endometrial glands surrounded by benign endometrial stroma within the uterine myometrium. It commonly develops during the late reproductive years, with the highest incidence among women in their forties and women on tamoxifen. Adenomyosis has been found in 18% of hysterectomy specimens and 53% of specimens from women taking tamoxifen. Adenomyosis may be asymptomatic or may be associated with abnormal menstrual bleeding, dysmenorrhea, uterine enlargement, and uterine tenderness during menstruation. Secondary dysmenorrhea becomes increasingly severe as disease progresses. On bimanual examination, the uterus is diffusely enlarged, globular, and most tender just before or after menstruation. Diagnosis is confirmed with ultrasonography or MRI.[60] Treatment is symptomatic and, when necessary, is surgical and includes resection of localized areas of adenomyosis or, if severe, hysterectomy. Adenomyosis is unresponsive to hormone treatment, yet three cases of severe adenomyosis treated successfully with GnRHa have been reported.[57]

Endometriosis

Endometriosis is the presence of functioning endometrial tissue or implants outside the uterus. Like normal endometrial tissue, the ectopic (out of place) endometrium responds to the hormonal fluctuations of the menstrual cycle.

The incidence of endometriosis is difficult to determine, particularly in asymptomatic adolescent and fertile women. It is estimated that 10% to 15% of reproductive-age women and 2% to 4% of menopausal women have endometriosis. In addition, as many as 50% of women evaluated for pelvic pain, infertility, or a pelvic mass are diagnosed as having endometriosis. Conversely, endometriosis is found in as many as 31% of fertile asymptomatic women undergoing laparoscopy and 11.3% having hysterectomies.[61] Moreover, the frequency and severity of symptoms do not correlate with the extent or site of lesions.[62] A large study has found that endometriosis outside the ovary, pelvis, or uterus causes an increased risk for endocrine cancers (breast, ovarian, and non-Hodgkin lymphoma).[63]

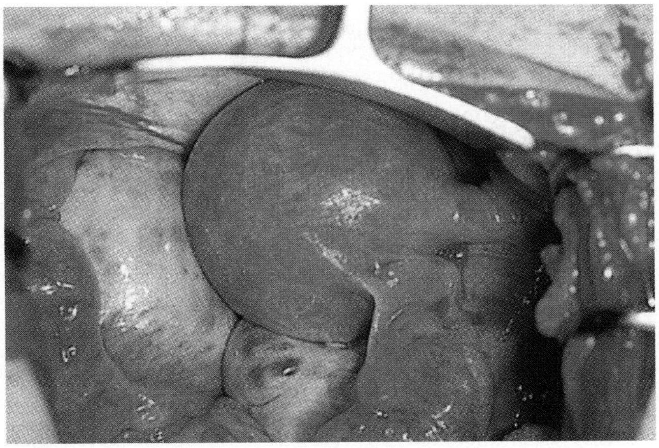

FIG. 22-15 Endometriosis. The uterus is distended, and retrograde spill of menstrual loss has led to the development of endometriosis *(dark purple patches).* (From Symonds EM, Macpherson MBA: *Color atlas of obstetrics and gynecology,* London, 1994, Mosby-Wolfe.)

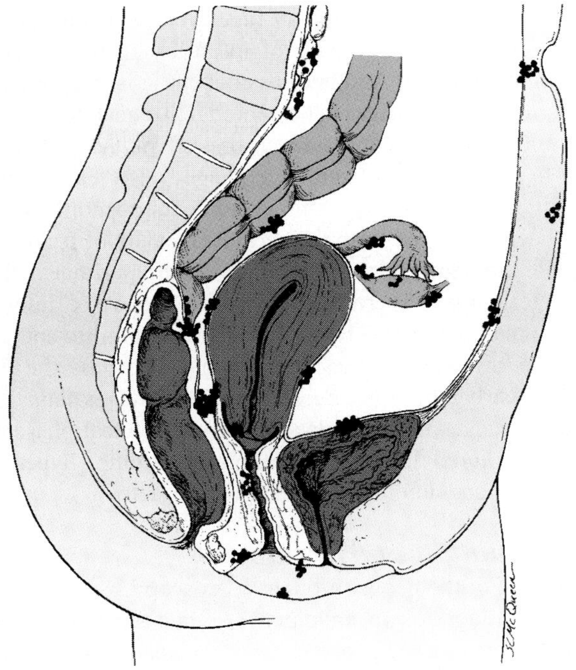

FIG. 22-16 Pelvic sites of endometrial implantation. Endometrial cells may enter the pelvic cavity during retrograde menstruation. (From Herbst AL et al: *Comprehensive gynecology,* ed 2, St Louis, 1992, Mosby.)

The cause of endometriosis is not known, but several theories have been proposed. In 1927 Sampson[64] proposed that endometriosis is caused by the implantation of endometrial cells during **retrograde menstruation,** in which menstrual fluids move through the fallopian tubes and empty into the pelvic cavity (Fig. 22-15). It is now known that retrograde menstruation occurs in almost all women; however, not all women develop endometriosis.

Another theory is that women with endometriosis have a slightly depressed cytotoxic T cell response to endometrial cells or some other defect of the immune response. These alterations may cause the body to tolerate ectopic implantation of endometrial cells. Researchers also have proposed that endometrial cells spread through the lymphatic system or that multipotential cells in the epithelial coverings of reproductive organs are somehow stimulated to develop into endometrial cells. A genetic predisposition to endometriosis has been documented. Studies show that incidence and severity of disease are greatest among women with female relatives who also have endometriosis.[61]

Pathophysiology

Endometrial implants can occur throughout the body. The most common sites of implantation are the ovaries, uterine ligaments, rectovaginal septum, and pelvic peritoneum (Fig. 22-16). Other sites of implantation are the sigmoid colon, small intestine, rectum, appendix, bladder, uterus, vulva, vagina, cervix, lymph nodes, extremities, pleural cavity, lungs, laparotomy scars, and hernial sacs.

Cyclic changes depend on the blood supply of the implants and the presence of both glandular and stromal cells. Given that blood supply is sufficient, the ectopic endometrium proliferates, breaks down, and bleeds in conjunction with the normal menstrual cycle. The bleeding causes inflammation, triggering a cascade of cellular inflammatory mediators, including cytokines, chemokines, growth factors, and protective factors such as secretory leukocyte protease inhibitor[65] and superoxide dismutase.[66] Pain occurs in surrounding tissues. The inflammation may lead to fibrosis, scarring, and adhesions.

Clinical Manifestations

The clinical manifestations of endometriosis are variable in frequency and severity and include primarily infertility and pain,[61] dysmenorrhea, dyschezia (pain on defecation), dyspareunia (pain on intercourse), and, less commonly, constipation, abnormal vaginal bleeding, and, if implants are located within the pelvis, an asymptomatic pelvic mass having irregular, movable nodules and a fixed, retroverted uterus. Most symptoms of endometriosis can be explained by the proliferation, breakdown, and bleeding of the ectopic endometrial tissue with subsequent formation of adhesions. In many instances, however, the degree of endometriosis is not related to the frequency or severity of symptoms. Dysmenorrhea, for example, does not appear to be related to the degree of endometriosis. With involvement of the rectovaginal septum or the uterosacral ligaments, dyspareunia develops. Dyschezia, a hallmark symptom of endometriosis, occurs with bleeding of ectopic endometrium in the rectosigmoid musculature and subsequent fibrosis.

Up to one third of women with infertility have endometriosis.[11,61] The link between endometriosis and infertility is strong, yet the degree of disease and infertililty are not as closely associated. That is, women with untreated minimal to mild disease may have high pregnancy rates or may experience infertility. The exact mechanism for infertility in women with endometriosis is unknown. Infertility may result from mechanical interference with ovulation or ovum transport through the fallopian tube, yet mechanical interference is an unlikely cause of infertility in women with mild endometriosis. Another possible cause is phagocytosis of sperm by macrophages in the reproductive tract. It is known that endometriosis causes macrophages in the peritoneal fluid to become more aggressive phagocytes ("eater cells"; see Chapter 7). However, similar numbers of motile sperm have been recovered from the peritoneal cavity of fertile and infertile women. Elevated cytokines in the peritoneal fluid and interleukin-1 secreted from macrophages of infertile women may play a role by affecting sperm motility and survival, sperm-oocyte interactions, ovum pickup by the fimbriae, or early embryonic development.[61] Other explanations include changes in prostaglandin secretion, luteal phase defect, unruptured luteinizing follicle syndrome, hyperprolactinemia, and autoimmune and genetic factors.

Evaluation and Treatment

Evaluation of the pelvis through laparoscopy is required for definitive diagnosis of endometriosis and should be completed before therapy is begun. Because treatment and prognosis are based on the extent and severity of the disease, a uniform classification system that includes both extent and severity is desirable. However, currently there is no satisfactory classification system for endometriosis.[61,67] Treatment is aimed at preventing or decreasing progression and spread, alleviating pain, and restoring fertility. Current therapies include suppression of ovulation with noncyclic estrogen-progestin COCs, danazol (which diminishes midcycle LH and FSH surge), GnRH agonists/analogues (to create a medical oophorectomy), gestrinone (a 19-nortestosterone derivative and antiprogestational steroid), mifepristone (RU 486) (an antiprogestational and antiflucocorticoid agent that can inhibit ovulation and disrupt endometrial integrity), and atrophy of endometrium with progestogens. A newer therapy is injectable GnRH antagonist, which produces immediate inhibition of gonadotropin release. GnRH antagonists are shorter acting than GnRHa but release histamine at the site of injection. Conservative surgical treatment includes laparoscopic removal of endometrial implants with conventional or laser techniques and presacral neurectomy for severe dysmenorrhea. Effectiveness of therapy can be monitored by CA-125 (carcinoembryonic antigens shed into blood; see p. 296) and may be increased when medical regimens are combined with surgical techniques. All treatments have risks or side effects, and recurrent symptoms develop in as many as 45% of women within 5 years.[61,62]

Cancer

Malignant tumors of the female reproductive system are common. Endometrial carcinoma accounts for approximately 6% of all cancers in women, 4.2% of ovarian tumors, 2.3% of cervical tumors, and less than 1% of other malignant tumors.[68] Malignant neoplasms of the female reproductive tract account for about 1 of 8 (12.5%) diagnosed cancers and 1 of 13 (7.7%) cancer deaths in women in the United States.[68]

Cervical Cancer

Invasive cancer of the cervix accounts for approximately 18% of all gynecologic cancers and 2.3% of all cancers in women in the United States.[68] Mortality rates caused by cervical cancer have declined more than 45% since the early 1970s and an average of 2.1% per year during the years 1992 to 1996. During this same time period, the incidence rate in black women (11.2 per 100,000) exceeded the rate in white women (7.3 per 100,000). In 2001 the American Cancer Society estimated 12,900 new cases of cervical invasive cancer and 4400 cervical cancer deaths.[69]

Because of increased prevalence of Papanicolaou (cytologic) screening, rates of invasive cancer have declined steadily over the past 30 years (greater than 55% since the early 1970s). Although mortality for blacks declined more rapidly than for whites, mortality risks for black women continue to be more than two times those of white women.[68]

Precancerous dysplasia, also called *cervical intraepithelial carcinoma [CIN]* or *cervical carcinoma in situ,* is more frequent than invasive cancer and occurs more often in younger women.[68] An estimated one in eight young women will have cervical dysplasia by age 20, most likely caused by human papillomavirus (HPV) infection.[70] In a large case-control study of 1000 women in 1993, HPV infection accounted for 75% of cases of CIN.[71] According to the Centers for Disease Control and Prevention (CDC),[72] HPV caused 80% of cervical cancers in 1997 and is implicated in almost all cases of CIN (see Chapter 23). However, recent data from an epidemiologic longitudinal study show a strong association between *Chlamydia trachomatis* and cervical squamous cell carcinoma.[73] Mechanisms studied include release of nitric oxide by *C. trachomatis* during infection and inhibition of host cell apoptosis. With chronic chlamydial infections, these mechanisms could initiate carcinogenesis.[73]

Cervical cancer is considered a sexually transmitted disease. Infection of the cervix with HPV, intercourse before 16 years of age, and multiple sexual partners or a male partner with multiple partners places a woman at risk. Smoking is considered a cofactor. Poor nutrition also increases risks, perhaps by depressing the immune system. Likewise, human immunodeficiency virus (HIV)–positive women are at greater risk for developing cervical cancer.[74,75] Specific CDC guidelines for screening and follow-up of abnormal Papanicolaou smears for HIV-positive women are available.[76]

Pathogenesis

Cervical cancer is a progressive disease that is staged according to histology (Table 22-4). Premalignant lesions usually occur 10 to 12 years before the development of invasive carcinoma.

The progressive changes of cervical cells are classified on a continuum from cervical intraepithelial neoplasia, to cervical carcinoma in situ, to invasive carcinoma. **Cervical intraepithelial neoplasia (CIN),** commonly called **cervical dysplasia,** is replacement of some epithelial cells by atypical,

Table 22-4 Clinical Staging for Cancer of the Cervix

Stage	Characteristics
0	Cancer in situ, intraepithelial carcinoma; earliest stage of cancer; cancer confined to its original site
I	Carcinoma confined to cervix (extension to corpus disregarded)
IA	Earliest form of stage I; there is very small amount of cancer, which is visible only under a microscope
IA1	Area of invasion is <3 mm (about 1/8 inch) deep and <7 mm (about 1/3 inch) wide
IA2	Area of invasion is between 3 mm and 5 mm (about 1/5 inch) deep, and <7 mm (about 1/3 inch) wide
IB	Includes cancers that can be seen without a microscope; also includes cancers seen only with a microscope that have spread deeper than 5 mm (about 1/5 inch) into connective tissue of the cervix or are wider than 7 mm
IB1	A IB cancer that is no larger than 4 cm (about 1 3/5 inches)
IB2	A IB cancer that is > 4 cm
II	Cancer has spread beyond the cervix to the upper part of the vagina; cancer does not involve the lower third of the vagina
IIA	Cancer has spread beyond the cervix to the upper part of the vagina; cancer does not involve the lower third of the vagina
IIB	Cancer has spread to the tissue next to the cervix, called the *parametrial tissue*
III	Cancer has spread to the lower part of the vagina or the pelvic wall; cancer may be blocking the ureters (tubes that carry urine from the kidneys to the bladder)
IIIA	Cancer has spread to the lower third of the vagina but not to the pelvic wall
IIIB	Cancer extends to the pelvic wall, blocks urine flow to the bladder, or both
IV	Most advanced stage of cervical cancer; cancer has spread to other parts of the body
IVA	Cancer has spread to the bladder or rectum, which are organs close to the cervix
IVB	Cancer has spread to distant organs beyond the pelvic area, such as the lungs

Reprinted from the American Cancer Society's Cancer Information Database with permission.

neoplastic cells. CIN is graded as mild dysplasia (CIN 1), moderate dysplasia (CIN 2), or severe dysplasia and carcinoma in situ (CIN 3), depending on the depth of epithelial involvement (Fig. 22-17).

In **cervical carcinoma in situ,** all or most of the cervical epithelium shows cellular features of carcinoma, but underlying tissue is not affected. Risk of progression to invasive carcinoma rises steadily with the severity of dysplasia. Women with CIN 1 have a 15% chance of developing malignant lesions. This rate increases to 75% in women with CIN 3.

Carcinoma in situ is most likely to develop in the squamous-columnar junction—the so-called transformation zone—where the columnar epithelium of the cervical lining meets the squamous epithelium of the outer cervix and vagina (Fig. 22-18). In this zone, columnar epithelium is constantly being replaced by squamous epithelium in a process known as *metaplasia.* Metaplasia is thought to be affected by hormonal levels; change in cervical epithelium is not understood as well as endometrial tissue change in response to fluctuating hormones. Because metaplastic cells are at increased risk of incorporating foreign or abnormal genetic material, neoplastic changes are most common in the transformation zone.

The spontaneous regression of carcinoma in situ is extremely rare. Carcinoma in situ is generally a precursor of invasive carcinoma of the cervix. A number of factors, including tumor type, contribute to the rate at which carcinoma in situ becomes invasive. **Invasive carcinoma of the cervix** consists of direct invasion into adjacent tissues and metastasis (spread of cancer cells) through the lymphatics. Adjacent tissues most often involved are the ureters and structures of the lateral pelvic wall, the vaginal stroma and epithelium, and the lower uterine segment and myometrium. The internal, external, and common iliac lymph nodes and the obturator nodes are common sites of lymphatic involvement. A staging system for carcinoma of the cervix is shown in Table 22-4.

Clinical Manifestations

Because cervical neoplasms are asymptomatic, regular cytologic screening (Papanicolaou [Pap] smear) is necessary. About 90% of cervical cancer cases can be detected early through the use of Pap smears.[77] Vaginal bleeding and discharge are common symptoms. Bleeding is variable and may occur after intercourse or between menstrual periods. At times, women will complain of abnormal menses or postmenopausal bleeding. Vaginal discharge is a less common presenting symptom and may be serosanguineous or yellowish in color. A new or foul odor also may be present. Bleeding and discharge are subtle and are likely to be disregarded by premenopausal women, who mistake these signs for variations of normal processes. Postmenopausal women are more likely to seek medical attention if these signs appear. With severe bleeding, symptoms of anemia may occur. Pelvic or epigastric pain is experienced only with large lesions. Advanced disease may cause urinary or rectal symptoms.

Evaluation and Treatment

Cervical cytology is most accurate if cells obtained by endocervical swabbing and ectocervical scraping are examined. When dysplasia is detected, cervical biopsy and curettage are required. Colposcopy is used to identify suggestive sites for biopsy. The transformation zone moves higher into the cervix as age increases, making biopsy more difficult. If invasive carcinoma is found, lymphangiography, CT scan, ultrasonography, or radioimmunodetection methods are used to assess lymphatic involvement. Cystoscopy and proctoscopy also may be performed.

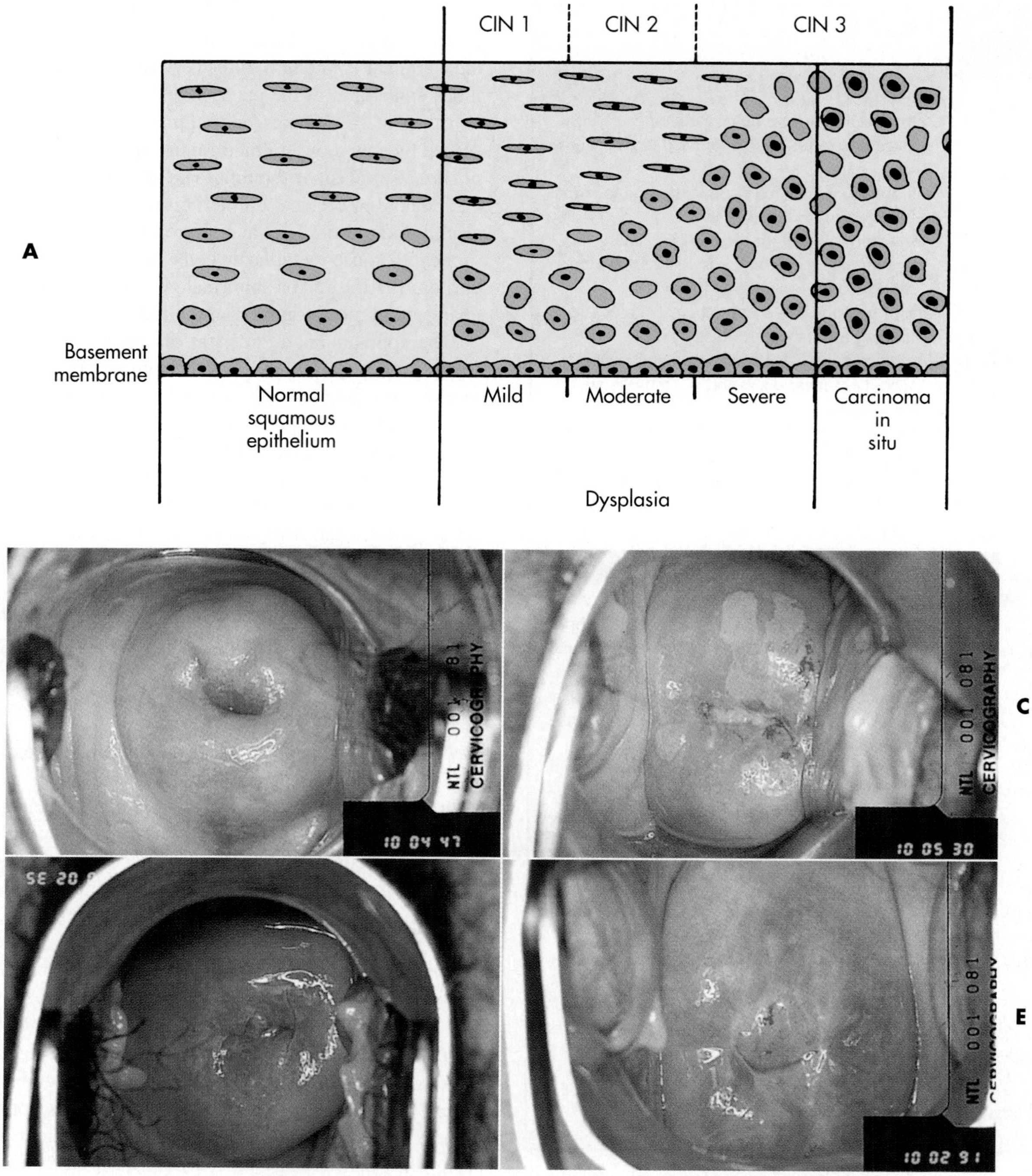

FIG. 22-17 Cervical intraepithelial neoplasia (CIN). A, Diagram of cervical endothelium showing progressive degrees of CIN. **B,** Normal multiparous cervix. **C,** CIN stage 1. Note the white appearance of part of the anterior lip of the cervix associated with neoplastic changes. **D,** CIN stage 2. Lesions reflected in distant capillaries. **E,** CIN stage 3. Lesion predominantly around the external os. (**A,** From Herbst AL et al: *Comprehensive gynecology,* ed 2, St Louis, 1992, Mosby. **B–E,** From Symonds EM, Macpherson MBA: *Color atlas of obstetrics and gynecology,* London, 1994, Mosby-Wolfe.)

The treatment depends on the degree of neoplastic change, the size and location of the lesion, and the extent of metastatic spread. For premalignant change or early cancer (stage 0), cryosurgery or carbon dioxide laser therapy is commonly used; laser treatment may produce better results in the multiparous cervix. Loop diathermy conization and the loop electrosurgical excision procedure (LEEP) are alternative treatments. In LEEP, a small, looped wire with electric current generates heat and burns off cancer cells. Conization is removal of a cone-shaped section of tissue that includes the cancer; high-frequency current is used with cold-knife conization. The amount of tissue removed depends on the location of the lesion. None of these measures affects fertility or childbearing.

For invasive cervical carcinoma, treatment depends on the stage of the tumor (Table 22-5). Surgical intervention may in-

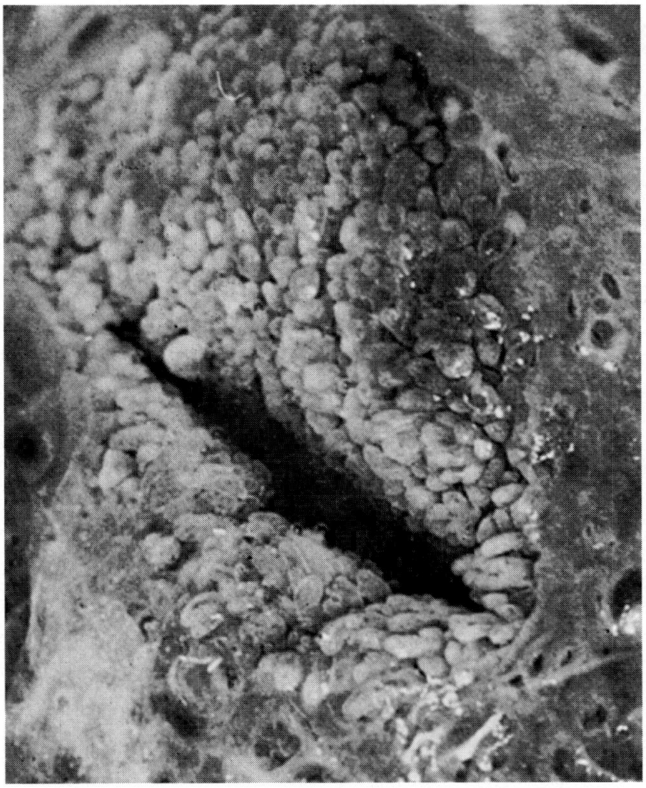

FIG. 22-18 Cervical carcinoma in situ. Typical transformation zone, where the columnar (grapelike) epithelium is replaced by metaplastic epithelium. At its outer edge, the metaplastic epithelium adjoins the squamous epithelium, which extends into the vagina. (From Coppleson M, Pixley E, Reid B: *Colposcopy: a scientific approach to the cervix in health and disease,* Springfield, Ill, 1971, Charles C Thomas.)

Table 22-5 Cervical Cancer Treatment Options

Stage	Treatment
0	Cryosurgery, laser surgery, loop diathermy conization, or loop electrosurgical excision procedure (LEEP)
IA	Surgery (total abdominal hysterectomy, may include oophorectomy), radiation therapy
IB	Surgery (radical hysterectomy with lymph node dissection), internal and external radiation therapy combined
IIA	Surgery (radical hysterectomy with lymph node dissection), internal and external radiation therapy combined
IIB	Internal and external radiation therapy combined
III	Internal and external radiation therapy combined
IVA	Internal and external radiation therapy combined; surgery (exenteration) for removal of uterus, vagina, cervix; could include bladder, colon, or rectum depending on the area of malignant spread
IVB	Radiation therapy for pain symptoms

From American Cancer Society. In *Cancer response system document #10024,* New York, 1995, The Society.

clude a hysterectomy, pelvic lymphadenectomy, and pelvic exenteration. Radiation therapy is used most frequently in cases of small cell cancer with lymphatic involvement. External radiation usually is combined with one or two intracavity implants. Multidrug chemotherapy regimens also have been used. Recent phase 3 trials suggest significant improvement in survival with combined chemotherapy and radiation therapy.[78] Smokers tend to have a higher stage of disease at diagnosis, and their cancer is more resistant to radiation treatment.

With early detection and treatment, prognosis is excellent. Overall, the 5-year survival rate is 70% and increases to 92% with early diagnosis. A cure rate of 100% is possible for women with dysplasia or carcinoma in situ.[69]

Vaginal Cancer

Cancer of the vagina is the rarest of the female genital cancers and accounts for 0.2% of gynecologic cancers.[68] About 75% to 85% are squamous cell–type cancers; the remaining tumors, in descending order of frequency, are adenocarcinomas (15% to 20%), sarcomas (rare), and melanomas (rare). (Types of tumors are described in Chapter 10.) Women with either an in situ or an invasive cervical or vulvar squamous cell cancer are at increased risk for squamous cell abnormality of the vagina.[77] The mean age of women with invasive cancer of the vagina is 55 years; carcinoma in situ occurs about 10 years earlier. Invasive squamous cell cancer affects postmenopausal women, usually in the sixth or seventh decade. Vaginal sarcomas develop in children younger than 5 years and in women in the fifth to sixth decades. Clear-cell carcinomas, the most common form of adenocarcinomas, occur in conjunction with vaginal adenosis in young women with a history of in utero diethystilbesterol (DES) exposure. Metastatic adenocarcinomas arise from the urethra, Bartholin gland, rectum, bladder, endometrium endocervix, ovary, or a distant organ.[77]

Vaginal and cervical cancers are thought to have similar epidemiology. Both start as intraepithelial lesions, occur in sexually active women, and are associated with HPV infection.[74] As mentioned previously, prior carcinoma of the cervix places a woman at higher risk for developing vaginal cancer. In utero exposure to nonsteroidal estrogens also has been considered a risk factor. It has been estimated that 100,000 to 160,000 women were exposed in utero to such nonsteroidal estrogens as DES, dienestrol, or hexestrol from 1960 to 1970. Apparently, exposure to such hormones during the first 3 months of gestation inhibits the normal replacement of columnar epithelium by squamous epithelium in the vagina of the fetus. The columnar epithelium, which is not normally found in the vagina, then may undergo malignant transformation. Not all women exposed to DES in utero develop neoplastic changes in the vagina, however. Between 0.14 and 1.4 cases of vaginal cancer develop per 1000 women at risk. Nineteen years is the average age at which clear-cell carcinoma develops as a result of DES exposure.

Like cervical neoplasms, vaginal cancers are classified as intraepithelial neoplasia (dysplasia), carcinoma in situ, or invasive carcinoma and are staged based on extension into local tissues and metastasis to distant organs. Vaginal cancer is generally asymptomatic, discovered by vaginal cytologic examination, and confirmed by colposcopy and biopsy. The major symptom of invasive cancer, independent of type, is vaginal bleeding (bloody discharge). Advanced disease causes vaginal discharge, vulvar pruritus, rectal or bladder symptoms, and pain or leg edema.

Biopsy techniques confirm the tumor type and determine its size, location, and extent. Treatment depends on these findings and the age of the individual. Vaginal dysplasia or carcinoma in situ is excised with upper vaginectomy, laser ablation or loop electrosurgical excision, cryotherapy, or laser surgery.[77] Topical 5-fluorouracil (5-FU) also may be used. If the lesion is invasive, surgery may include hysterectomy and pelvic bilateral inguinal lymphadenectomy. Radiation and chemotherapy may follow surgery. Approximately 40% of individuals with invasive vaginal cancer develop recurrent cancer, which usually is confined to the pelvic area. The 5-year survival rate is 70% to 75% for early disease, 30% to 40% for stage III, and rare for stage IV.

Vulvar Cancer

Cancer of the vulva is responsible for approximately 0.4% of gynecologic cancers; an estimated 3200 new cases occurred in 1998.[68] The majority (90%) are squamous cell carcinomas, although melanoma (5%), Bartholin gland carcinoma (2%), sarcoma (2%), and adenosquamous carcinoma (1%) may occur.[79] A history of HPV infection or squamous dysplasia of the vagina or cervix is a major risk factor;[74] smoking and coffee use also are considered risk factors.[79] Although it usually affects postmenopausal women (median age of presentation is women in their sixties), vulvar cancer has been diagnosed in women between ages 30 and 90 years. Although leukoplakia and lichen scleroses were believed to be precursors, no prospective studies have been able to confirm such a relationship. Usually, women have a long history of vulvar irritation and pruritus (70%); urinary symptoms and discharge are less common. In addition, women may have a hard ulcerated area of the vulva, large cauliflower lesions, or lesions similar to those of chronic dermatitis. Biopsy confirms the diagnosis. Treatment options include surgery primarily and sometimes radiation with or without chemotherapy.[79] Prognosis depends on lesion size and location, histology, and lymph involvement; risk of metastasis increases with tumor size. The 5-year survival rate is 85% to 90% for stage I and decreases to 20% for stage IV cancer.[79]

Endometrial Cancer and Uterine Sarcoma

Endometrial carcinomas arise within the glandular epithelium of the uterine lining. Cancer of the endometrium is the most common cancer of the pelvic region in women and accounts for 6% of all cancers in women.[68] Estimates include 38,300 new cases in 2001, with approximately 6600 deaths.[69] Although incidence rates are higher in white than in black women, mortality rates in black women are nearly twice as high. Most cases occur in postmenopausal women (Fig. 22-19), with peak incidence occurring in the late fifties to early sixties.[80] The primary risk factor is unopposed estrogen exposure with resultant hyperplasia.[80] The World Health Organization has divided endometrial hyperplasia into two major categories according to whether cytologic atypia is present; only atypical hyperplasia has a significant risk of progressing to well-differentiated endometrial carcinoma.[81] Estrogen-related exposures include estrogen replacement therapy, tamoxifen, early menarche, late menopause, never having children, and a failure to ovulate. Other risk factors include infertility, diabetes, gallbladder disease, hypertension, and obesity. Hereditary nonpolyposis colon cancer, a genetic syndrome, also has been associated with endometrial and ovarian cancer.[82]

Pregnancy and the use of COCs containing synthetic estrogen and progestin have a protective effect.[80] After 12 months of COC use, the risk of endometrial cancer is half that among women who have never used COCs; this effect seems to persist for at least 10 years after birth control pills are discontinued.[48] In addition, controlling obesity, hypertension, and diabetes may reduce an individual's risk of endometrial cancer.

About 75% of endometrial cancers are adenocarcinomas. Abnormal vaginal bleeding is the most common clinical manifestation of endometrial cancer. The bleeding is caused by disruption of the endometrial surface by neoplastic processes. Pain and weight loss are symptoms of late disease.[83]

Screening methods for early detection of endometrial cancer are as effective as those for cervical cancer. Pap smears, which are highly effective in detecting cervical dysplasia, are ineffective in detecting early endometrial cancer.[82] Endometrial biopsies, which allow for direct cytologic sampling of the endometrium, are required for diagnosis and are recommended to screen high-risk women at menopause and periodically. Transvaginal ultrasound (TVUS) is used to measure endometrial thickness and also may be used to screen postmenopausal and high-risk premenopausal women. An endometrial depth of less than 5 mm is suggestive of atrophic endometrium.[20,84] Although serum CA-125 is not a useful screen for endometrial cancer, it may predict the presence of extrauterine disease in women with endometrial cancer.[84] Once cancer is confirmed by biopsy, a laparoscopy may be per-

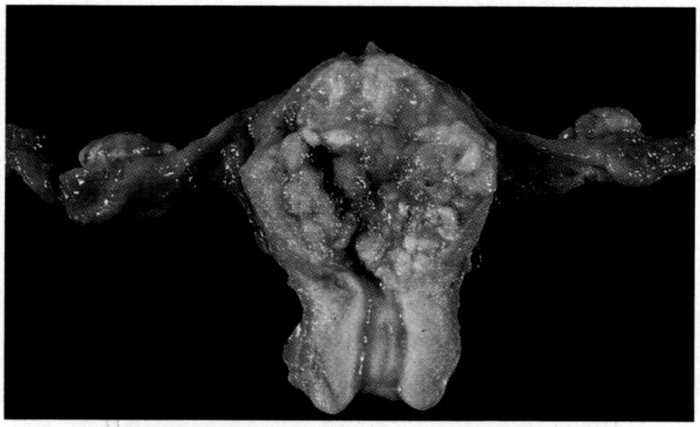

FIG. 22-19 Endometrial cancer. Tumor fills the endometrial cavity. Obvious myometrial invasion is seen. (From Damjanov I, Linder J, editors: *Anderson's pathology*, ed 10, St Louis, 2000, Mosby.)

formed to determine stage of disease. Evaluation for metastasis includes routine blood work, metabolic studies, chest x-ray films, intravenous pyelography (IVP), barium enema, ultrasonography, lymphangiography, CT, MRI, and bone scans.

Treatment is based on the extent of the disease and includes surgical removal of the obvious tumor and radiation for control of residual microscopic disease. Surgical interventions include curettage for carcinoma in situ, total abdominal hysterectomy with bilateral salpingo-oophorectomy, and lymphadenectomy. Chemotherapy or hormone therapy with progesterone may be used. Treatment options for recurrent cancer include radiation and hormone therapy with progestins. Progesterone may benefit individuals with advanced or recurrent disease. The 1-year relative survival rate for endometrial cancer is 93%; the 5-year relative survival rate is 95% with early diagnosis and 64% if diagnosis occurred in the late stage. Relative survival rates for white women exceed those for black women by at least 18% at every stage.

Uterine sarcomas are rare neoplasms that arise from myometrial smooth muscle, endometrial stroma, or more rarely ubiquitous connective tissue elements. Uterine sarcomas constitute 2% to 6% of all uterine malignancies. The average age at diagnosis is the early fifties. There is no epidemiologic association with parity, systemic disease, or prior radiation exposure. However, there is a difference in race-specific incidence; the relative risk for black women compared with white women is 1.6. Symptoms include abnormal uterine bleeding, awareness of a mass, and pelvic pressure or pain. Vaginal discharge is rare. Most commonly, serendipitous diagnosis occurs at the time of surgery for leiomyomas. Treatment consists of total hysterectomy with bilateral salpingo-oophorectomy and selective lymphadenectomy followed by radiation therapy. Five-year survival rates range from 50% in early disease to 5% in advanced disease. Like most cancers, stage is the most important determinant of prognosis. The survival rate at 5 years for stage I disease is 50%. Few women survive advanced-stage disease.[85]

Ovarian Cancer

Cancer of the ovaries is the sixth most frequent cancer in women, other than skin cancer, and ranks fifth as the cause of cancer death in women (Fig. 22-20).[86] In 1998 ovarian cancer accounted for 5.4% of all female cancer deaths[68] and caused more deaths than any female reproductive cancer.[68,86] Incidence rates increase with age and peak between ages 40 and 80 years, with half of all cases in women older than 65 years.[86]

◆ *Pathogenesis*

The cause of ovarian cancer is unknown at present. The risk of the disease is greatest for women with one or more first-degree relatives affected by ovarian cancer. Other risk factors include a personal history of breast cancer and nulliparity. About 90% of families with dominant inheritance of both breast and ovarian cancer have breast cancer susceptibility gene *(BRCA1)* germline mutations.[87,88] Research has found a positive association between family history of uterine, pancreatic, and breast cancer and risk of ovarian cancer. Although previous reports have linked increased parity with reduced risk of ovarian cancer, this may not hold for women with genetic predisposition for ovarian cancer.[87,89] Other potential risk factors include prior use of fertility drugs or hormone replacement therapy (HRT) and diet low in fruits and vegetables and high in fats or whole milk.[86,87] Oral contraceptive use provides the same protection from ovarian cancer as it does from endometrial cancer (see p. 732).[87]

The two major types of ovarian cancer are epithelial ovarian neoplasms and germ-cell neoplasms. Most ovarian malignancies are epithelial ovarian neoplasms, which usually develop from the surface epithelium of the ovary. Epithelial ovarian tumors may be serous, mucinous, endometrioid, or undifferentiated. These tumors are classified as (1) benign, (2) borderline malignant, or (3) frankly malignant. The malignant forms are collectively classed as ovarian adenocarcinomas and account for 90% of all ovarian malignancies. Of the ovarian adenocarcinomas, 40% to 50% are serous epithelial malignancies, which usually involve both ovaries and tend to be bulky. Serous tumors generally affect women from 50 to 55 years of age and are extremely rare in prepubertal girls. The 5-year survival rate is 95% if treated in stage I; however, only 25% of ovarian cancers are diagnosed this early. Five-year survival rates decline with stage of disease: 40% to 60% of women with stage II disease survive 5 years, 15% to 20% with stage III disease survive 5 years, and less than 5% with stage IV disease survive 5 years.[87]

Germ-cell tumors are derived from the primitive germ cells (gametes) of the embryonic gonad and may be either malignant or benign. The benign cystic teratoma accounts for approximately 10% of all ovarian tumors. If the germ-cell tumor is malignant, it tends to be a highly aggressive and rapidly growing tumor with a poor prognosis. Germ-cell tumors almost always occur in children or adolescents.

◆ *Clinical Manifestations*

The intrapelvic location of the ovaries and the range of tumor activity (from slow to rapid and relentless growth) cause

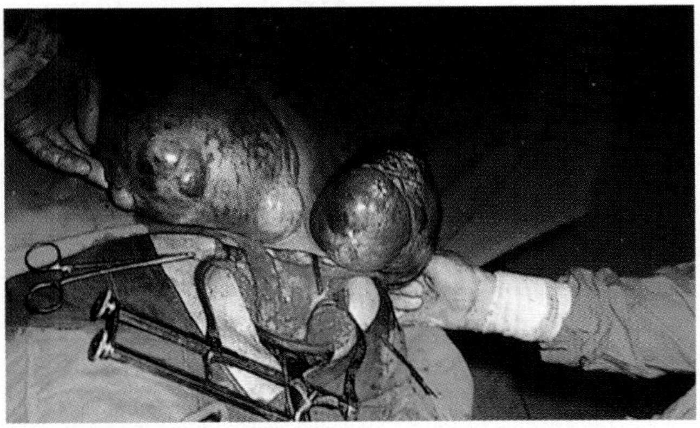

FIG. 22-20 Ovarian tumors. Bilateral multicystic ovarian tumors. (From Symonds EM, Macpherson MBA: *Color atlas of obstetrics and gynecology,* London, 1994, Mosby-Wolfe.)

diverse signs and symptoms. Ovarian cancer generally is considered a silent disease, meaning that by the time the individual experiences symptoms and seeks treatment, the disease has spread beyond the primary site.

The most obvious symptoms are pain and abdominal swelling that arise from the primary ovarian mass or ascites and abdominal distention (Fig. 22-21). Gastrointestinal manifestations may include dyspepsia, vomiting, and alterations in bowel habits caused by mechanical obstruction. Abnormal vaginal bleeding may occur if the postmenopausal endometrium is stimulated by a hormone-secreting tumor. The tumor also may cause ulcerations through the vaginal wall that result in bleeding. There also can be a feeling of pressure in the pelvis and leg pain.[86]

Systemic manifestations of nonmetastatic malignant disease include connective tissue inflammation (dermatomyositis), abnormal pigmentation (acanthosis nigricans), and subacute cerebellar degeneration. Tumor obstruction of vascular channels can cause venous and, occasionally, arterial thrombosis. Alterations in coagulability also occur, contributing to clot formation. Metastasis frequently causes pleural effusion.

A

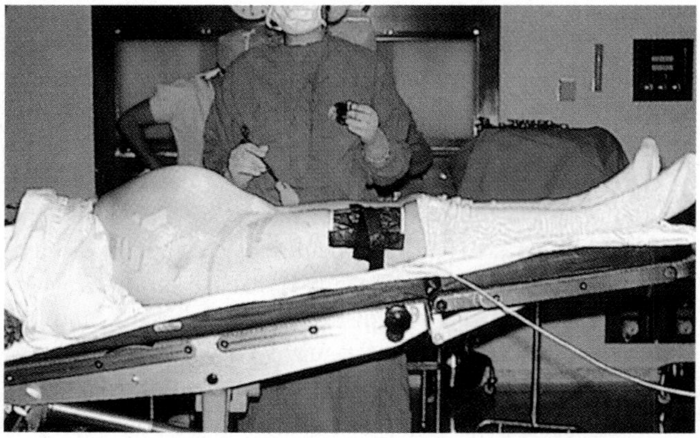

B

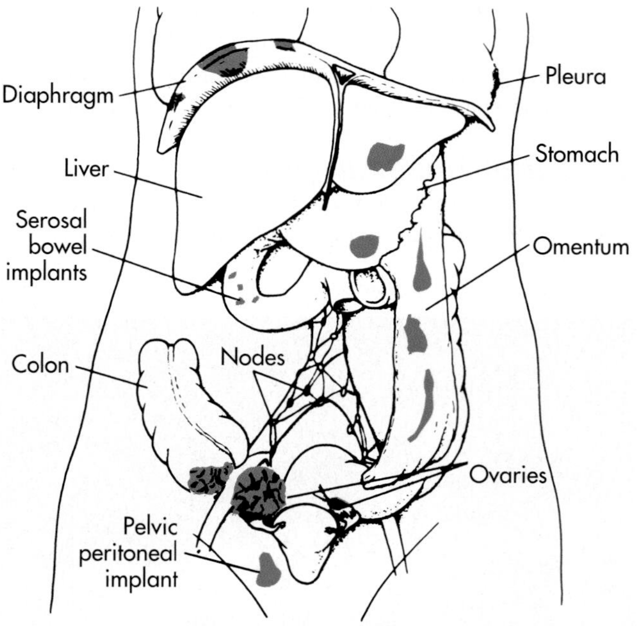

FIG. 22-21 Large malignant ovarian tumor and metastasis of ovarian cancer. **A,** Tumor has caused massive abdominal distention. **B,** Pattern of spread for epithelial cancer of the ovary. (**A,** From Symonds EM, Macpherson MBA: *Color atlas of obstetrics and gynecology,* London, 1994, Mosby-Wolfe, **B,** From DiSaia PJ, Creasman WT: *Clinical gynecologic oncology,* ed 4, St Louis, 1993, Mosby.)

Evaluation and Treatment

Because ovarian cancer has no early symptoms and no effective screening techniques can detect it, disease usually is advanced by the time treatment is sought. Diagnosis is confirmed by biopsy, and extent of the disease is determined by ultrasound, CT, MRI, or other imaging techniques that enable clinicians to localize the tumor mass. Women undergoing surgery for early-stage ovarian cancer need thorough checking for spread to the abdomen and lymph nodes. Staging of disease requires exploratory surgery. The International Federation of Gynecologists and Obstetricians (FIGO) staging system is described in Table 22-6. Other preoperative studies may be used to determine the extent of metastasis. These include an upper gastrointestinal series, barium enema, IVP, mammography, and lymphography.

The search for a tumor marker that could be used as a screen for ovarian cancer is ongoing. Some types of germ cells and, rarely, adenocarcinoma may be associated with increased levels of α-fetoprotein (AFP), hCG, or carcinoembryonic antigen (CA-125). Increased CA-125 levels are found in about 78% to 80% of nonmucinous ovarian cancers; however, elevated levels are produced in 29% of nongynecologic tumors and in a variety of noncancerous conditions, for example, endometriosis, PID, benign ovarian cysts, myomas, and pregnancy. Carcinoembryonic antigen is a nonspecific, nonsensitive test for ovarian cancer; when combined with TVUS it is more sensitive and accurate than is pelvic examination alone. Using a panel of markers may be more sensitive and specific. Further research is needed.[87]

The initial approach to treatment is surgery, which is performed to determine the stage of disease and remove as much of the tumor as possible. Radiation therapy may follow if the tumor is smaller than 2 cm in size and is confined to the abdominopelvic area without involvement of the kidneys or liver. Radiation therapy may be administered externally, intraperitoneally, or in both ways. The success of chemotherapy depends on whether the tumor is a discrete mass, the extent of disease, and whether there has been prior exposure to chemotherapeutic agents. Alkylating agents are given alone or in combination with antimetabolites. At this time, chemotherapy can reduce tumor size, but it does not reduce mortality. In 1991 the U.S. Food and Drug Administration (FDA) approved altretamine as a single agent to treat persistent or recurrent ovarian cancer. Altretamine is used after an initial combination regimen containing an alkylating agent or cisplatin and seems to have the potential to decrease morbidity and possibly mortality. Although CA-125 level does not correlate with tumor staging, changes with chemotherapy can be used to measure tumor response to therapy.[87]

Sexual Dysfunction

Increased awareness of female sexual dysfunction is relatively new, and most of what is known comes from clinical observations and anecdotal reports from women. Adequate research is needed. Both organic and psychosocial disorders can be implicated in sexual dysfunction. Organic problems may be the underlying cause in 10% to 20% of cases and can contribute to another 15%. The exact cause may not always be identified.

As in men, chronic illness can affect sexual functioning and response in women. For example, neuropathy in the pelvic region may increase the threshold for orgasm in diabetic women. Diminished intensity and gradual decline in orgasm may be analogous to the development of impotence in diabetic men. For women with heart disease, problems in sexual functioning more often are related to drug therapy than the disease itself. Table 22-7 outlines possible effects of specified chronic diseases on female sexual functioning.

Sexual anorexia (inhibited sexual desire, decreased libido) may be a biologic manifestation of depression, alcohol or other substance abuse, prolactin-secreting pituitary tumors, or testosterone deficiency. β-Adrenergic blockers used for heart disease also may inhibit sexual desire.

Table 22-6 FIGO* Staging of Carcinoma of the Ovary

Stage	Characteristics
I	Growth limited to the ovaries
IA	Growth limited to one ovary; no ascites
i	No tumor on the external surface; capsule intact (90% 5-year survival with treatment)
ii	Tumor present on the external surface, or capsule(s) ruptured, or both
IB	Growth limited to both ovaries; no ascites
i	No tumor on the external surface; capsule intact
ii	Tumor present on the external surface, or capsule(s) ruptured, or both
IC	Tumor either stage IA or stage IB, with ascites present or with positive peritoneal washings
II	Growth involving one or both ovaries with pelvic extension
IIA	Extension and/or metastases to the uterus and/or tubes
IIB	Extension to other pelvic tissues
IIC	Tumor either stage IIA or stage IIB but with ascites present or with positive peritoneal washings
III	Growth involving one or both ovaries with intraperitoneal metastases outside the pelvis, or positive retroperitoneal nodes, or both; tumor limited to the true pelvis with histologically proven malignant extension to small bowel or omentum
IV	Growth involving one or both ovaries with distant metastases; if pleural effusion is present, there must be positive cytology to allot a case to stage IV; parenchymal liver metastases indicate stage IV
Special category	Unexplored cases that are thought to be ovarian carcinoma

From American Cancer Society: Facts on breast cancer. In *Cancer response document #10020,* New York, 1995, The Society.
*The International Federation of Gynecologists and Obstetricians.

Table 22-7 Possible Effects of Chronic Disease on Sexual Functioning in Women

Disease	Sexual Function
Cerebral palsy	Intact genital sensations, decreased lubrication; difficulty with sexual activity/positioning because of muscle spasticity, rigidity, and/or weakness; pain with positioning caused by contracture of knees and hips or because of increased spasms with arousal
Cerebrovascular accident (CVA)	Difficulties in sexual positioning and sensitivity because of impaired motor strength, coordination or paralysis; decreased sex drive with stroke on the dominant side of the brain
Diabetes	Diminished intensity of orgasm and gradual decline in ability to achieve orgasm; decreased lubrication and/or recurrent vaginal infections with resultant dyspareunia
Chronic renal failure	Decreased arousal; increasingly rare and less intense orgasms; decreased lubrication
Rheumatoid arthritis (RA)	Painful sexual activity/positions because of swollen, painful joints, muscular atrophy and joint contracture; decreased sex drive because of pain, fatigue, and/or medication; genital sensations remain intact
Systemic lupus erythematosus (SLE)	Similar to RA; decreased lubrication and vaginal lesions result in painful penetration
Myocardial infarction (MI)	Most literature male oriented; problems related to medications
Multiple sclerosis (MS)	Diminished genital sensitivity; decreased lubrication; declining orgasmic ability; difficulty with sexual activity because of muscle weakness, pain, or incontinence
Spinal cord injury	Reflex sexual response with injury above sacral area; disrupted response with lesion at or below sacrum; loss of sensation, decreased lubrication; spasticity, incontinence, or pain with arousal; continued orgasmic sensations or sensations diffused in general or to specific body parts, such as breast or lips

Vaginismus is an involuntary muscle spasm in response to attempted penetration. Common causes include prior sexual trauma or fear of sex; organic causes are less common and are similar to those that cause dyspareunia. Even after the underlying organic problem is detected and successfully treated, vaginismus may persist.

Anorgasmia or **orgasmic dysfunction** is the inability of the woman to reach or achieve orgasm. Dysfunction follows a continuum from difficulty in arousal to lack of orgasm. Any chronic illness may affect arousal. Orgasmic dysfunction is linked to organic causes in less than 5% of cases. Diabetes, alcoholism, neurologic disturbances, hormonal deficiencies, and pelvic disorders, such as infections, trauma, and surgical scarring, are specific disorders that may block orgasm. Drugs, such as narcotics, tranquilizers, antidepressants, and antihypertensive medications, also can inhibit orgasm.

Rapid orgasm is a relatively new diagnosis and seems to be rare. In this instance, once orgasm occurs there is little interest in further sexual activity. Rapid orgasm has no known organic cause.

Dyspareunia (painful intercourse) is common. Women may experience pain during arousal, at the time of orgasm, at the initiation of intercourse, midway during intercourse, or after intercourse. The pain may have a burning, sharp, searing, or cramping quality and may be described as external, vaginal, deep abdominal, or pelvic. A variety of psychosocial and organic causes have been identified. Inadequate lubrication may make penetration or intercourse difficult or painful. Drugs with a drying effect, such as antihistamines, certain tranquilizers, and marijuana, and disorders such as diabetes, vaginal infections, and estrogen deficiency can decrease lubrication. Other causes of dyspareunia include skin problems around the introitus or affecting the vulva; irritation or infection of the clitoris; disorders of the vaginal opening, such as scarring from episiotomy, intact hymen, or chronically infected hymenal remnants; bartholinitis; disorders of the urethra or anus; disorders of the vagina, such as infections, thinning of the walls caused by aging or decreased estrogen, or irritation caused by spermicides or douches; and pelvic disorders, such as infection, tumors, cervical or uterine abnormalities, and torn uterine ligaments.

Sexual dysfunction may develop as a coping mechanism. Women with a history of sexual trauma—rape, incest, or molestation—frequently have problems of desire, arousal, or orgasm or experience pain with sexual activity. In extreme cases, total sexual aversion may develop. At other times, sexual dysfunction may be a symptom of marital or relationship problems. Unresolved anger may manifest as inhibited desire or diminished arousal.

Impaired Fertility

Infertility affects approximately 15% of all couples and is defined as the inability to conceive after 1 year of unprotected intercourse. Fertility can be impaired by factors in the man or the woman or both partners. Male factors include diminished quality and production of sperm; important causes of infertility in the female are associated with malfunctions of the fallopian tubes, ovaries, or reproductive hormones. Adhesions from pelvic infection may cause blockage of one or both fallopian tubes, preventing access of the sperm to the ovum. Hormonal or local factors may disrupt ovulation or prevent a fertilized egg from implantation. For unclear reasons, endometriosis also may contribute to infertility. These factors have been discussed previously. A number of diagnostic procedures are required in the routine investigation of the infertile couple (see Table 21-4). In many instances no cause may be identified.

Treatment of infertility is aimed toward correcting problems identified during the diagnostic workup. The best treatment for infertility is prevention, specifically prevention of sexually transmitted infection that can result in scarring and adhesion formation in the reproductive tract of either the man or the woman.

Fertility Tests

Tests of reproductive function are performed most commonly when infertility exists. Both the male and female partners are examined, and several diagnostic evaluations may be completed. The types of tests and their normal values are summarized in Tables 21-4 and 21-5. The man is evaluated for number, amount, structure, and motility of sperm and obstruction along the reproductive tract. Tests for women determine whether (1) the reproductive tract (cervix, uterus, fallopian tubes) is adequately patent to allow for passage of ovum and sperm, (2) ovulation occurs normally, (3) the endometrium is responding normally to hormones, and (4) reproductive tissues are free of tumors or infections. Hormonal assays evaluate the adequacy of pituitary function and target organ response. The position and size of organs or the presence of tumors can be detected by direct observation procedures using a laparoscope or by radiographic studies, such as plain films, computerized scans, or tomography. Before testing and treatment, assessing knowledge of fertility with timing of sexual intercourse is essential. A mature ovum remains viable for 12 to 24 hours, and sperm retain their fertility for up to 5 days and may remain alive in the woman's reproductive tract for up to 9 days. A prospective study showed that almost all pregnancies resulted from sexual intercourse during a 6-day period ending on the day of ovulation.[90]

WHAT'S NEW? UCSF Study Finds Clues to Male Infertility

Flaws in the body's system for repairing DNA, the same problems associated with certain cancers, might explain a significant portion of infertility problems in men. Preliminary findings raise ethical issues regarding the use of high technology to treat infertile men. Infertile men, by technologic means, could unwittingly pass on DNA-repairing flaws to their offspring, predisposing them to infertility and cancer. Scientific findings are reported in the June 2000 issue of the *British Journal of Human Reproduction.*

Data from *Science Report,* Chronical News Services, September 4, 2000.

DISORDERS OF THE MALE REPRODUCTIVE SYSTEM

Disorders of the Urethra

Urethritis and urethral strictures are common disorders of the male urethra. Urethral carcinoma occurs in men older than 60 years, but it is an extremely rare form of cancer.

Urethritis

Urethritis is an inflammatory process of the urethra without concurrent bladder infection that is usually, but not always, caused by a sexually transmitted microorganism. Biologic agents associated with infectious urethritis in males include *Neisseria gonorrhoeae* and *Chlamydia trachomatis, Ureaplasma urealyticum,* and other, less common, mycobacteria; parasites (e.g., *Trichomonas vaginalis*); and viruses (herpes simplex virus, HPV).[91] Infectious urethritis caused by *N. gonorrhoeae* often is called gonococcal urethritis (GU); infection caused by other microorganisms is called nongonococcal urethritis (NGU).[49] (Sexually transmitted urethritis is described in Chapter 23.) Nonsexual origins of urethritis include inflammation or infection as a result of urologic procedures, insertion of foreign bodies into the urethra, anatomic abnormalities, or trauma.

Noninfectious urethritis is rare and is associated with the ingestion of wood alcohol, ethyl alcohol, or turpentine. It is seen also with Reiter syndrome, which involves a number of mucocutaneous lesions.

Symptoms of urethritis include urethral tingling, itching, or burning sensation on urination (dysuria), frequency, and urgency. The individual may note a purulent or clear mucus-like discharge from the urethra. Nucleic acid detection amplification tests allow easy detection of *N. gonorrhoeae* and *C. trachomatis* in first-void urine.[49] Treatment consists of appropriate antibiotic therapy for infectious urethritis and avoidance of future chemical or mechanical irritation.

Urethral Strictures

A **urethral stricture** is a fibrotic narrowing of the urethra caused by scarring. The scars may be congenital but are more likely to result from trauma or untreated or severe urethral infections, most often from long-term use of indwelling urinary catheters. Large catheters and instruments cause internal trauma and ischemia, whereas external trauma, such as pelvic fracture, can partially or completely sever the urethra and cause severe and complex strictures.[92] Urethral carcinoma is a less common cause of urethral stricture. Prostatitis and infection secondary to urinary stasis are common complications. Severe and prolonged obstruction can result in hydronephrosis and renal failure. In addition, chronic, severe strictures may lead to urethral fistulas and periurethral abscesses.[92]

The clinical manifestations of urethral stricture are caused by bladder outlet obstruction. The primary symptom is diminished force and caliber of the urinary stream; other symptoms include urinary frequency and hesitancy, mild dysuria, double urine stream or spraying, and postvoiding dribbling. Symptoms of acute urinary retention may occur in the presence of infection or urinary obstruction. Induration at the stricture site may be palpable. Tender, enlarged masses along the urethra usually indicate periurethral abscesses.

Urethral stricture is diagnosed on the basis of history, physical examination, urinary flow rates, voiding cystourethrogram, and urethroscopy; biopsy confirms carcinoma. Treatment is usually surgical and may involve urethral dilation, urethrotomy, or a variety of open surgical techniques. The choice of surgical intervention depends on the age of the individual and the severity of the problem. Strictures may recur up to 1 year after treatment. Follow-up is necessary during this time; urinary flow measurements and urethrogram help determine extent of residual obstruction.

Disorders of the Penis

Phimosis and Paraphimosis

Phimosis and paraphimosis are both disorders in which the foreskin (prepuce) is "too tight" to be moved easily over the glans penis. **Phimosis** is a condition in which the foreskin cannot be retracted back over the glans, whereas **paraphimosis** is the opposite: the foreskin is retracted and cannot be moved forward (reduced) to cover the glans (Fig. 22-22). Both conditions can cause penile pathologic conditions.

The inability to retract the foreskin is normal in infancy and is caused by congenital adhesions. During the first 3 years of life, these adhesions separate naturally with penile erections and are not an indication for circumcision. Although most cases occur in uncircumcised males, stenosis and resultant phimosis can occur in males with excessive skin remaining after circumcision.[92] Phimosis can occur at any age and is caused most commonly by poor hygiene and chronic infection. Chronic balanoposthitis (inflammation of the glans and prepuce) predisposes older diabetic men to phimosis. It rarely occurs with normal foreskin.

Edema, erythema, and tenderness of the prepuce and purulent discharge are usually the reasons for seeking treatment; inability to retract the foreskin is a less common complaint. Circumcision, if needed, is performed after infection has been eradicated. Complications of phimosis include inflammation of the glans (balanitis) or prepuce (posthitis) and paraphimosis. There is a higher incidence of penile carcinoma in uncircumcised males, but chronic infection, most likely with HPV, is usually the underlying factor in such cases.[93]

Paraphimosis, in which the foreskin is retracted, can constrict the penis, causing edema of the glans. If edema is such that the foreskin cannot be reduced manually, surgery must be performed to prevent necrosis of the glans caused by constricted blood vessels. Severe paraphimosis is a surgical emergency.

Peyronie Disease

Peyronie disease (bent nail syndrome) is a fibrotic condition that causes lateral curvature of the penis during erection (Fig. 22-23). Peyronie disease develops slowly and is characterized by tough, fibrous thickening of the fascia in the

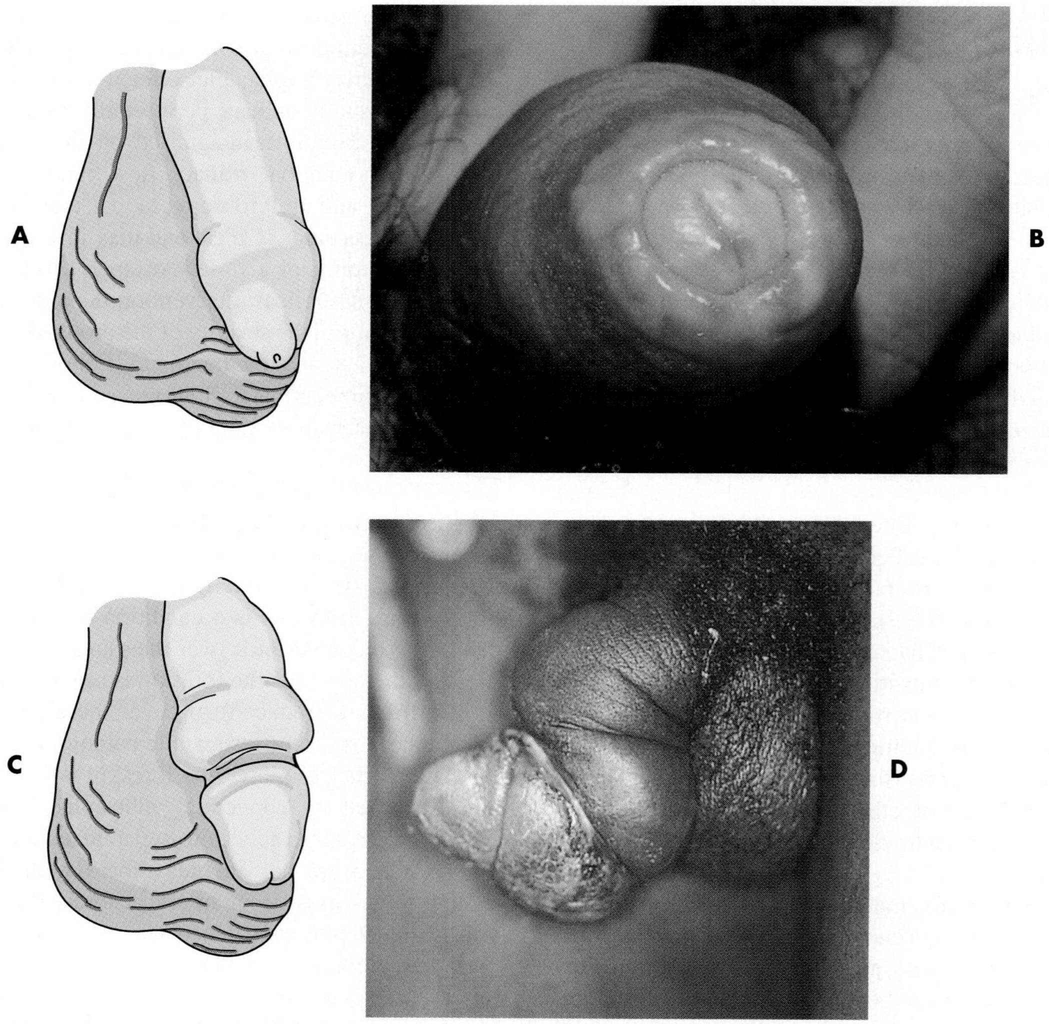

Fig. 22-22 Phimosis and paraphimosis. A, Phimosis: the foreskin has a narrow opening that is not large enough to permit retraction over the glans. **B,** Lesions on the prepuce secondary to infection cause swelling, and retraction of foreskin may be impossible. **C,** Paraphimosis: the foreskin is retracted over the glans but cannot be reduced to its normal position. Here it has formed a constricting band around the penis. **D,** Ulcer on the retracted prepuce with edema. (**A, C,** From Phipps WP, Sand JK, Marek JF: *Medical-surgical nursing: concepts and clinical practice,* ed 6, St Louis, 1999, Mosby. **B,** From Taylor PK: *Diagnostic picture tests in sexually transmitted diseases,* London, 1995, Mosby. **D,** From Morse SA, Moreland AA, Holmes KK: *Atlas of sexually transmitted diseases and AIDS,* ed 2, London, 1996, Mosby-Wolfe.)

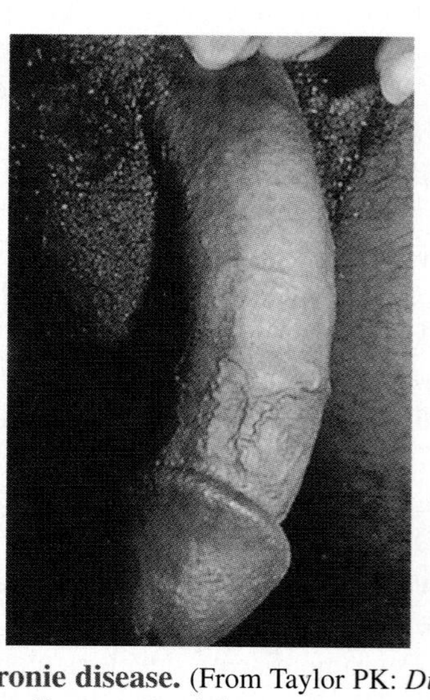

Fig. 22-23 Peyronie disease. (From Taylor PK: *Diagnostic picture tests in sexually transmitted diseases,* London, 1995, Mosby-Wolfe.)

erectile tissue of the corpora cavernosa. A dense, fibrous plaque is usually palpable on the dorsum of the penile shaft. The problem usually affects middle-age men and is associated with painful erection, painful intercourse (for both partners), and poor erection distal to the involved area. In some cases, impotence or unsatisfactory penetration occurs. There is no pain when the penis is flaccid.

Although the exact cause is unknown, a local vasculitis-like inflammatory reaction occurs and decreased tissue oxygenation results in fibrosis and calcification. Peyronie disease is associated with Dupuytren contracture (a flexion deformity of the fingers or toes caused by shortening or fibrosis of the palmar or plantar fascia), diabetes, and the tendency to develop keloids.

There is no definitive treatment for Peyronie disease. Spontaneous remissions occur in as many as 50% of the cases. Pharmacologic therapies that increase oxygenation, such as vitamin E and aminobenzoate potassium (Potaba), may hasten self-resolution if used several times daily for prolonged periods. Plication, as well as surgical resection of the fibrous plaque followed by grafting, has been successful.[92]

Priapism

Priapism is an uncommon condition of prolonged penile erection. It is usually painful and is not associated with sexual arousal (Fig. 22-24). Priapism is idiopathic in 60% of cases; the remaining 40% of cases are associated with spinal cord trauma, sickle cell disease, leukemia, pelvic tumors or infections, or penile trauma. Priapism also has been associated with cocaine use.[94] Currently, intracavernous injection therapy for impotence seems to be the most common cause. Prolonged sexual stimulation often is associated with initial development of the idiopathic type.[92] The two corpora cavernosa within the erect penis are filled with blood and tender to palpation; neither the corpus spongiosum nor the glans is engorged. The vascular congestion is thought to be associated with venous obstruction. If the erection remains over a period of days, edema and fibrosis develop, leading to erectile dysfunction (impotence).

Priapism is a urologic emergency. Treatment within hours is effective and prevents impotence. Conservative approaches include iced saline enemas, ketamine administration, and spinal anesthesia. Needle aspiration of blood from the corpus through the dorsal glans is often effective and is followed by catheterization and pressure dressings to maintain decompression. More aggressive surgical treatments include the creation of vascular shunts to maintain blood flow.[93] Erectile dysfunction results in up to 50% of prolonged cases.

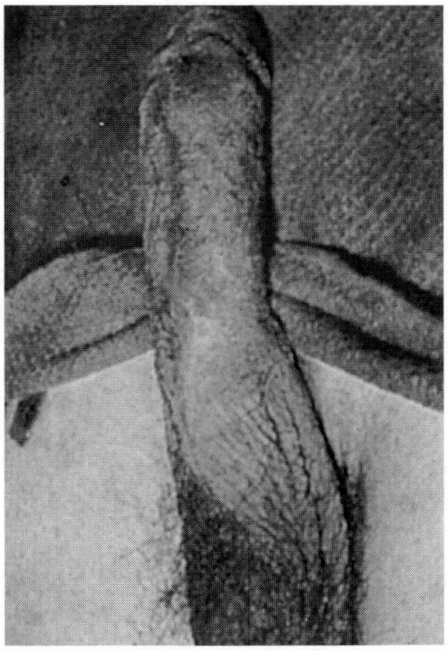

FIG. 22-24 Priapism. (From Lloyd-Davies RW et al: *Color atlas of urology,* ed 2, London, 1994, Mosby-Wolfe.)

Balanitis

Balanitis is an inflammation of the glans penis (Fig. 22-25) and usually occurs in conjunction with posthitis, an inflammation of the prepuce. (Inflammation of the glans and the prepuce is called *balanoposthitis.*) It is associated with poor hygiene and phimosis. The accumulation under the foreskin of glandular secretions (smegma), sloughed epithelial cells, and *Mycobacterium smegmatis* can irritate the glans directly or lead to infection. Skin disorders (e.g., psoriasis, lichen planus, eczema) and candidiasis must be differentiated from inflammation resulting from poor hygienic practices. Balanitis is seen most commonly in men with poorly controlled diabetes mellitus and candidiasis. Antimicrobials are used to treat infection. Circumcision can prevent recurrences and can be considered after the inflammation has subsided.

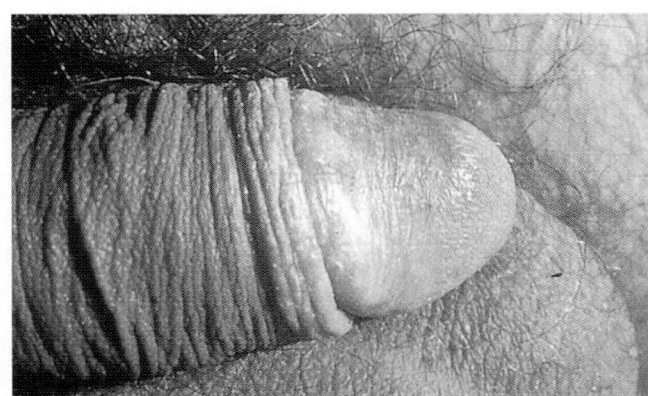

FIG. 22-25 Balanitis. Itchy, red rash on glans of penis secondary to *Candida albicans.* (From Taylor PK: *Diagnostic picture tests in sexually transmitted diseases,* London, 1995, Mosby-Wolfe.)

Penile Cancer

In the United States, carcinoma of the penis is rare and affects about 1 in 100,000 men (Fig. 22-26). Estimates reported by the American Cancer Society indicated that approximately 300 men would die of penile cancer and 1100 new cases would be diagnosed in the year 2000.[93] Although rare in North America and Europe, where it accounts for about 0.2% of cancers and 0.1% of cancer deaths in men, penile cancer may account for up to 10% of cancers in African and South American men.

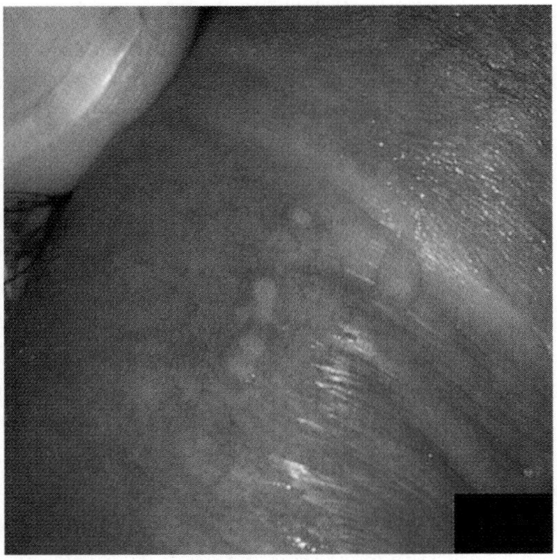

FIG. 22-26 Carcinoma in situ of penis. Flat papules turn white after diagnostic treatment with acetic acid. (From Morse SA, Moreland AA, Holmes KK: *Atlas of sexually transmitted diseases and AIDS,* ed 2, London, 1996, Mosby-Wolfe.)

In the United States, it is twice as common in black men compared with white men[93] and men over age 50.[95] Major risk factors include infection with HPV (mainly serotypes 16, 18, 33, 35, and 45), smoking, and psoriasis treated with combination involving psoralen and ultraviolet light. Although it is considered a disease of the elderly, 20% of men with penile cancer are younger than 40 years.[93]

Before the development of penile cancer, signs of premalignant cancer or epidermal cancer in situ are present.[93,95,96] These include thick, white plaque of leukoplakia that typically involves the meatus; red, inflamed areas of Paget disease; red, velvety, ulcerative lesions of erythroplasia of Queyrat that usually involve the glans; large, invasive, scaly growths of Buschke-Löwenstein tumor; red plaque with encrustations of Bowen disease; and in situ carcinoma that generally affects the penile shaft. Men with leukoplakia or erythroplasia of Queyrat may have concurrent invasive penile carcinoma.[93,97] Pain and bleeding are late signs of penile cancer. Condylomata (genital warts) caused by the HPV may be involved in the development of precancerous lesions (see Chapter 23 for a discussion of HPV). At times the penis might be the site of metastatic spread of solid tumors from the bladder, prostate, rectum, or kidney. Early squamous cell carcinoma and premalignant epidermal lesions are easily treated but are often ignored. Delays in seeking treatment are attributed to denial, embarrassment, failure to detect lesions under a phimotic foreskin, fear, guilt, and ignorance.

Penile cancer is mostly squamous cell carcinoma. Squamous cell carcinoma usually begins as a small, fat, ulcerative or papillary lesion on the glans or foreskin that grows to involve the entire penile shaft. Extensive lesions are associated with metastases and a poor prognosis. These lesions are not as painful as the amount of tissue involvement would seem to indicate. The regional femoral and iliac nodes are common metastatic sites. Rarely, the urethra and bladder are involved. Weight loss, fatigue, and malaise accompany chronic suppurative lesions. Untreated, progressive disease causes death within 2 years.

The specific diagnosis is made by biopsy after examination to document the location, size, and fixation of the lesion. After a positive biopsy, the extent of cancer spread is determine by imaging tests such as ultrasound, CT, or MRI. Fine-needle aspiration of lymph tissue confirms absence or presence of regional adenopathy.[93] About 30% of penile cancers spread to lymph nodes before diagnosis.[95] Distant metastases occur in fewer than 10% of cases and may involve lung, liver, bone, or brain.[97] Staging of penile cancer uses a system created by the American Joint Committee on Cancer (AJCC) and the International Union Against Cancer (UICC). The AJCC/UICC staging system is also known as the tumor, node, metastasis (TNM) system (see Chapter 10).[93] Although this system initially seems cumbersome, it is a simple and easy method of communicating degree of cancer (Box 22-11).

For invasive penile carcinoma, complete excision leaving adequate tumor-free margins is the goal. A simple circumcision may be sufficient for localized lesions of the prepuce. If the primary site is glans and distal shaft, the penis is amputated, leaving a 2-cm margin proximal to the tumor. Inguinal lymph nodes also are removed if metastasis to these structures is known or suspected. Palliative treatment with radiation or chemotherapy may be used when the disease is inoperable and bulky inguinal metastases have occurred. Options for individuals with carcinoma in situ include local excision, radiation, laser surgery, cryosurgery, chemosurgery, or chemotherapy with topical (5%) 5-FU. Differentiation, tumor stage, and age influence prognosis.[98] The 5-year survival rate for stage I disease is greater than 80%;[95] average 5-year survival rate for all stages is 50%.[93]

BOX 22-11

TUMOR, NODE, METASTASIS (TNM)* STAGING FOR PENILE CANCER

STAGE 0

T_{is}, N_0, M_0
T_a, N_0, M_0

STAGE I

T_1, N_0, M_0

STAGE II

T_1, N_1, M_0
T_2, N_0, M_0
T_2, N_1, M_0

STAGE III

T_1, N_2, M_0
T_2, N_2, M_0
T_3, N_0, M_0
T_3, N_1, M_0
T_3, N_2, M_0
T_2, N_1, M_0

STAGE IV

T_4, any N, M_0
Any T, N_3, M_0
Any T, any N, M_1

RECURRENT

Any local or distant penile cancer that returns after treatment

*See Fig. 11-7 on p. 342 for T, N, and M definitions.

Disorders of the Scrotum, Testis, and Epididymis

Disorders of the Scrotum

Men may seek treatment for painful or painless scrotal masses. Masses may be serious (cancer or torsion) or benign (hydrocele or cyst); they may require immediate surgical intervention or allow for careful observation. A flow diagram for diagnosing scrotal masses is provided in Fig. 22-27.[99]

Varicocele, hydrocele, and spermatocele are common intrascrotal disorders.[100-102] A **varicocele** is an abnormal dilation of a vein within the spermatic cord and is classically described as a "bag of worms" (Fig. 22-28). Most (95%) occur on the left side and may be painful or tender. Varicocele occurs in 10% of males and is seen most frequently after puberty. Sudden development of a varicocele in an older man is a late sign of renal tumor.[101] Unilateral right-sided varicoceles are rare and result from compression or obstruction of the inferior vena cava by a tumor or thrombus. Color Doppler ultrasonography is used to confirm the diagnosis.[99]

The cause of varicocele is incompetent or congenitally absent valves in the spermatic veins. The valves that normally prevent backflow are absent or do not close adequately, permitting blood to pool in the veins rather than flow into the venous system. Varicocele decreases blood flow through the

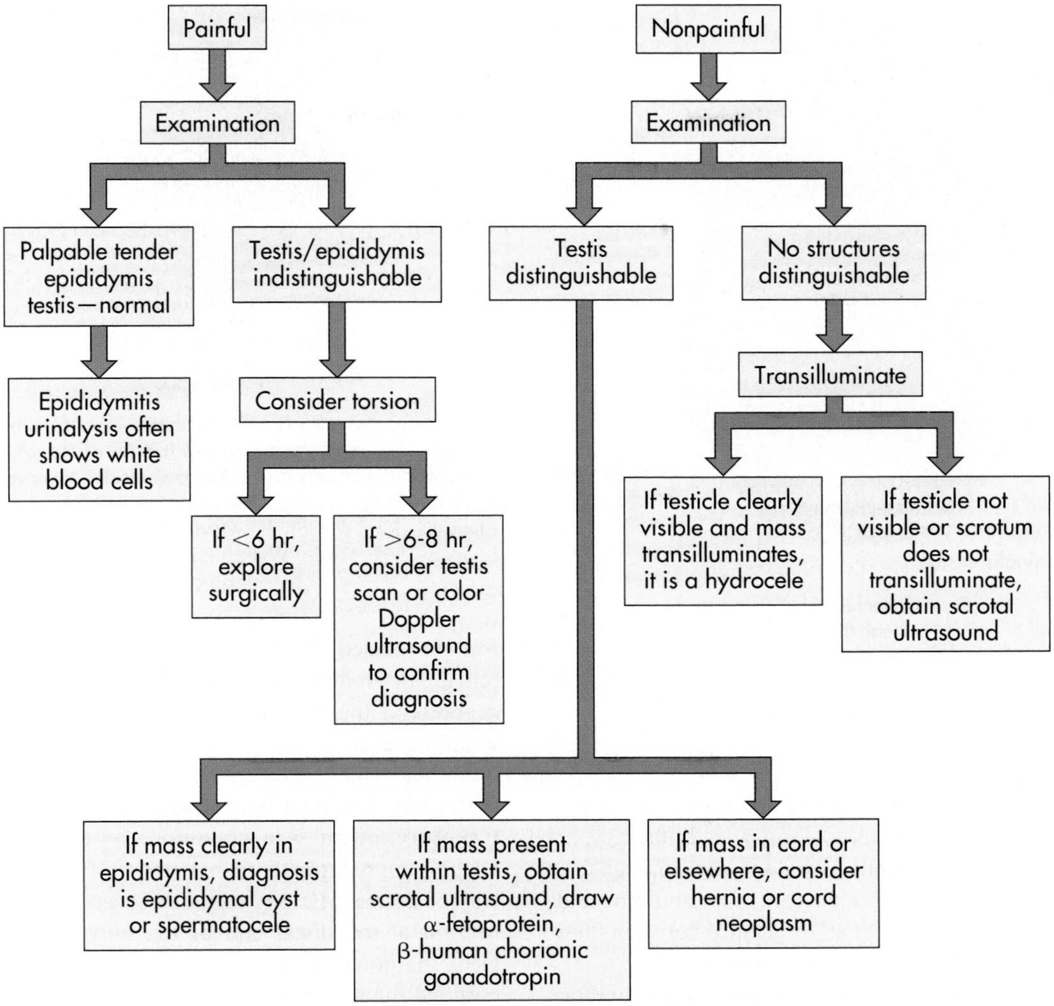

FIG. 22-27 Algorithm of diagnosis of a scrotal mass.

testis. This interferes with spermatogenesis and is a cause of infertility.[100,101] If infertility is a problem, treatment consists of ligation of the spermatic vein or occlusion of the vein by percutaneous methods, such as balloon catheter and sclerosing fluids.[101,103] If varicocele is mild and fertility is not an issue, a scrotal support usually is sufficient to relieve symptoms of scrotal heaviness or "dragging."

A **hydrocele** is a collection of fluid within the tunica vaginalis (Fig. 22-29).[99-101] It is the most common cause of scrotal swelling. Hydroceles occur in 6% of male newborns and are congenital malformations (patent processes vaginalis) that frequently resolve spontaneously in the first year of life. Surgical ligation is recommended if hydrocele persists after age 1 year.[102] Hydroceles in adults may be caused by an imbalance between the secreting and absorptive capacities of scrotal tissues. Hydroceles range in size from slightly larger than the testes to the size of a grapefruit or larger and may be flaccid or tense. Compression of testicular blood supply may lead to atrophy.

The exact mechanism of idiopathic hydrocele is unknown. Secondary hydrocele may result from trauma or infection of

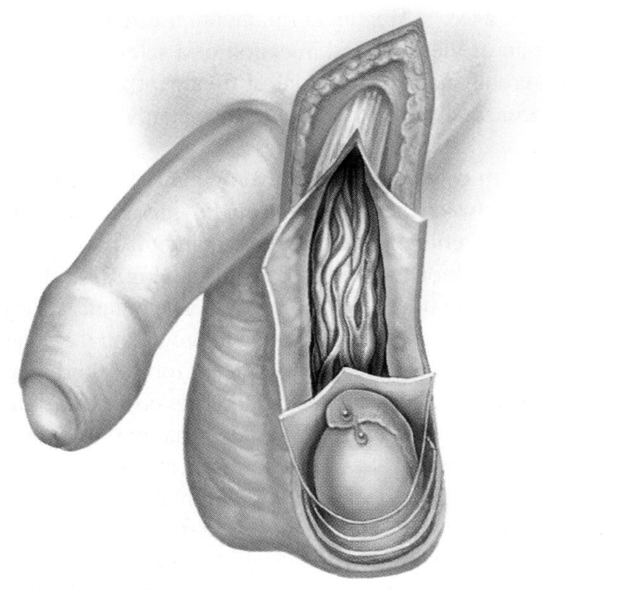

FIG. 22-28 Varicocele. Dilation of veins within the spermatic cord. (From Seidel H et al: *Mosby's guide to physical examination,* ed 4, St Louis, 1999, Mosby.)

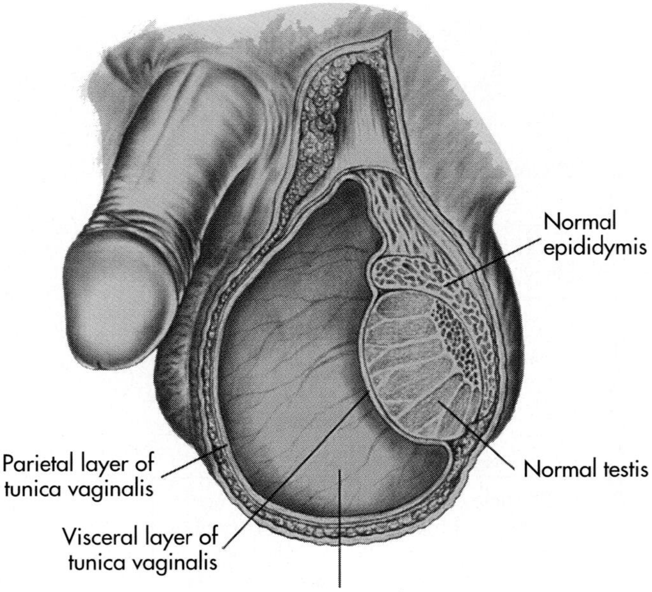

FIG. 22-29 Hydrocele. Accumulation of clear fluid between the visceral and parietal layers of the tunica vaginalis.

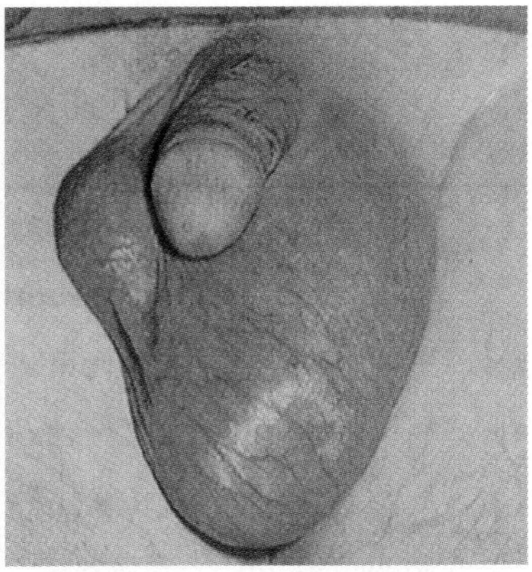

FIG. 22-30 Spermatocele. Retention cyst of the head of the epididymis or of an aberrant tubule or tubules of the rete testis. The spermatocele lies outside the tunica vaginalis; therefore on palpation it can be readily distinguished and separated from the testis. (From Lloyd-Davies RW, Gow JG, Davies DR: *Color atlas of urology,* ed 2, London, 1994, Mosby-Wolfe.)

the testis or epididymis or from a testicular tumor. Rapid accumulation of fluid occurs after local injury, radiotherapy, or infection (epididymitis or orchitis), or it may accompany testicular neoplasm. Chronic hydroceles are more common and occur in men over 40 because of an imbalance between fluid secretion and reabsorption in the tunica vaginalis. A painless, extratesticular mass that easily transilluminates is found on physical examination. Ultrasonography of a large hydrocele, which may conceal a testicular tumor, is recommended. Treatment is usually not required unless a large, bulky hydrocele causes considerable physical discomfort or undesirable cosmetic appearance.[100] Treatment for uncomplicated hydrocele is aspiration of the fluid and injection of a sclerosing agent into the scrotal sac.[99,104] The goal of treatment is to remove the hydrocele and prevent recurrence by sclerosing or excising the tunica vaginalis.

A **spermatocele** is a painless diverticulum of the epididymis located between the head of the epididymis and the testis. In other words, efferent ducts of the epididymis have potential for cystic dilation to form a spermatocele (Fig. 22-30).[99,101] Spermatoceles are filled with milky fluid that contains sperm. Spermatocele is differentiated from a hydrocele in that aspiration of the hydrocele recovers a clear, yellow fluid, and, unlike a hydrocele, a spermatocele does not cover the entire anterior surface of the testis. An epididymal cyst is similar to a spermatocele but does not communicate with the epididymis. Both spermatoceles and epididymal cysts manifest as discrete, firm, freely mobile masses distinct from the testis that may be transilluminated. Epididymal cysts do not require treatment.[99] A spermatic cord tumor may feel like a tense spermatocele but does not contain fluid and will not transilluminate.[101] Spermatoceles that cause pain or discomfort are excised. Usually, however, spermatoceles are asymptomatic or produce mild discomfort that is relieved by scrotal support. Neither hydroceles nor spermatoceles are associated with infertility.

Cryptorchidism and Ectopy

Cryptorchidism is a condition of testicular maldescent, whereas an **ectopic testis** has strayed from the normal pathway of descent. Ectopy may be caused by an abnormal connection at the distal end of the gubernaculum testis that leads the gonad to an abnormal position, usually at the superficial inguinal site. In cryptorchidism the descent of one or both testes is arrested, with unilateral arrest occurring more often than bilateral arrest.[101] The testes may remain in the abdomen, or testicular descent may be arrested in the inguinal canal or the puboscrotal junction. About 3% to 6% of full-term and 20% to 30% of premature male infants have undescended testes at birth;[102] half of such testes descend in the first month of life and a few more at puberty. The incidence of cryptorchidism in adults is 0.7% to 0.8%.[101] Cryptorchidism is commonly associated with vasal or epididymal abnormalities. These congenital anomalies affect about one third to two thirds of newborns with cryptorchidism. Other structural anomalies include posterior urethral valves (less than 5%), upper tract abnormalities (less than 5%), and hypsopadias. The presence of both hypsopadias and cryptorchidism raises the suspicion of mixed gonodal dysgenesis (intersex infant). It has been hypothesized that cryptorchidism may result from an absence or abnormality of the gubernaculum, a cordlike structure that extends from the lower pole of the testis to the scrotum; a congenital gonadal or dysgenetic defect that makes the testis insensitive to gonadotropins (a likely explanation for unilateral cryptorchidism); or lack of maternal gonadotropins (a likely explanation for bilateral cryptorchidism of prematurity).[101] Mechanical possibilities include a short spermatic cord, fibrous bands or adhesions in the normal path of the testes, or a narrowed inguinal canal.

Table 22-8 Diagnosis of Selected Conditions Responsible for the Acute Scrotum

Condition	Onset of Symptoms	Age	Tenderness	Urinalysis	Cremasteric Reflex	Treatment
Testicular torsion	Acute	Early puberty	Diffuse	Negative	Negative	Surgical exploration
Appendiceal torsion	Subacute	Prepubertal	Localized to upper pole	Negative	Positive	Bed rest and scrotal elevation
Epididymitis	Insidious	Adolescence	Epididymal	Positive or negative	Positive	Antibiotics

Chromosomal studies do not support a genetic component. Physiologic cryptorchidism, also called *retractile* or *migratory testis,* is an involuntary retraction of the testes out of the scrotum that occurs with excitement, physical activity, or exposure to cold and is caused by the small mass of prepubertal testis and the strength of the cremaster muscle. This is a common phenomenon that is self-limiting (descent occurs at puberty).

Physical examination discloses the absence of one or both testes in the scrotum and an atrophic scrotum on the affected side. If the undescended testis is in a vulnerable position, for example over the pubic bone, an individual may complain of severe pain secondary to trauma. The adult male with bilateral cryptorchidism may be infertile. Ultrasonography, CT, or MRI can be used to locate an intraabdominal or nonpalpable testis.

Undescended testes are susceptible to neoplastic processes: the risk of testicular cancer is 35 to 50 times greater for men with cryptorchidism or a history of cryptorchidism than for the general male population. Because definite histologic change (decreased Leydig cells, loss of germ cells, and peritubular fibrosis) occurs in the cryptorchid testis by 1 year of age, surgical correction is recommended around that age.[101,105] Treatment often begins with administration of GnRH or hCG, hormones that may initiate descent, making surgery unnecessary. GnRH is given as a nasal spray in Europe and may enhance germ-cell counts even when the testis does not descend.[105] If hormonal therapy is not successful, the testis is located and moved surgically (orchiopexy) in young children or removed (orchiectomy) in adults and children over 10 years of age.[101,105] The testis that is properly placed in the scrotum provides adequate hormonal function and gives the scrotum a normal appearance. A successful operation does not ensure fertility if the testis is congenitally defective. Approximately 20% of males with unilateral undescended testis remain infertile even though orchiopexy is performed by age 1 year; most individuals with treated or untreated bilateral testicular maldescent have poor fertility. In addition, placement of the cryptorchid testis into the scrotal sac does not decrease the potential for malignancy; it does facilitate examination and tumor detection.

Torsion of the Testis

Torsion of the testis is one of several conditions that cause an acute scrotum, which is testicular pain and swelling. Differentiation between testicular torsion and two other common causes of an acute scrotum is based on physical examination and history (Table 22-8).[99,102] More specifically, testicular torsion is a condition in which the testis rotates on its vascular pedicle, interrupting its blood supply (Fig. 22-31) and is responsible for 16% to 42% of cases of boys with an acute scrotum.[102] This event is most common among neonates and pubertal adolescents, but it can occur in males at any age.[99,102] Onset may be spontaneous or follow physical exertion or trauma. Torsion twists the arteries and veins in the spermatic cord, reducing or stopping circulation to the testis. Vascular engorgement and ischemia develop, causing scrotal swelling and pain. These manifestations are not relieved by scrotal elevation (Prehn sign), rest, or scrotal support. On physical examination, men have a tender, high-riding testis, a thickened spermatic cord, and an absent cremasteric reflect. Unlike epididymitis, the epididymis cannot be differentiated from the testis.[102] Diagnostic testing includes urinalysis (to rule out infection) and color Doppler ultrasonography.[90,101,102] Torsion

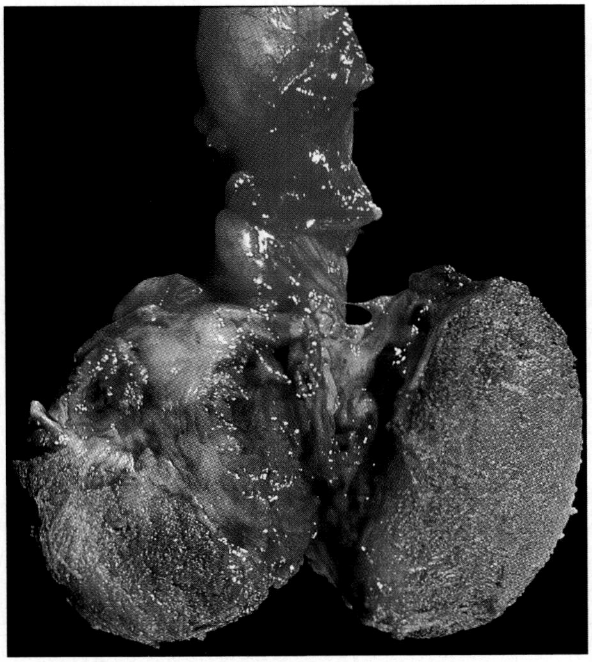

FIG. 22-31 Torsion of the testes. The testes appear dark red and partially necrotic owing to hemorrhagic infarction. (From Damjanov I, Linder J, editors: *Anderson's pathology,* ed 10, St Louis, 1996, Mosby.)

of the testis is a surgical emergency. If the torsion cannot be reduced manually, surgery must be performed within 6 hours after the onset of symptoms to preserve normal testicular function. Surgery includes untwisting the spermatic cord and anchoring both testes in correct position within the scrotum to prevent recurrences. With successful manual detorsion, surgical fixation should be done within a few days.

Orchitis

Orchitis is an acute inflammation of the testes (Fig. 22-32) and is uncommon except as a complication of systemic infection or as an extension of an associated epididymitis (see p. 745).[91] Infectious microorganisms may reach the testes through the blood or the lymphatics or, most commonly, by ascent through the urethra, vas deferens, and epididymis. Most cases of orchitis are actually cases of epididymo-orchitis. Occasionally, in middle-age men, a nonspecific, apparently noninfectious, inflammatory process (called *granulomatis orchitis*) can occur. It seems to be an autoimmune disease that triggers a granulomatous response to spermatozoa.

Mumps is the most common infectious cause of orchitis and usually affects postpubertal males. The onset is sudden, occurring 3 to 4 days after the onset of parotitis. Signs and symptoms include high fever, reaching 40° C (104° F), marked prostration, bilateral or unilateral erythema, edema and tenderness of the scrotum, and leukocytosis. An acute hydrocele may develop. Urinary signs and symptoms, which accompany epididymitis, are absent. Atrophy with irreversible damage to spermatogenesis may result in 30% of affected testes. Bilateral orchitis does not affect androgenic function but may cause permanent sterility.

Treatment is supportive and includes bed rest, scrotal support, elevation of the scrotum, hot or cold compresses, and analgesic agents for relief of pain. If an acute hydrocele develops, it is aspirated. Testicular abscess usually requires orchiectomy (removal of the testis). Appropriate antimicrobial drugs should be used for bacterial orchitis, and corticosteroids are indicated in proved cases of nonspecific granulomatous orchitis.

Cancer of the Testis

Testicular cancer is among the most curable of cancers; for nearly all common types, cure rates are more than 95%. Overall, testicular cancers are rare, accounting for only 1% of cancers and 0.24% of cancers deaths[68] in men, yet they are the most common form of cancer in young men between ages 15 and 35. Approximately 7400 cases and 350 deaths were predicted for 1999,[93] and an estimated 350 men died of testicular cancer in 1997. In the United States, the lifetime probability of developing testicular cancer is 0.2% for white men, an incidence that is four times higher than for blacks. Testicular tumors are slightly more common on the right side than on the left, a pattern that parallels the occurrence of cryptorchidism; about 1% to 2% of primary testicular cancers are bilateral (Fig. 22-33), and 50% of these tumors arise from treated or untreated cryptorchid testes.

Pathogenesis

Ninety percent of testicular cancers are germ-cell tumors, tumors that arise from the male gametes. Germ-cell tumors constitute 90% of testicular cancers and can be broadly classified into two types: seminomas and nonseminomas. Seminomas are the most common, are the least aggressive, and make up about 30% to 35% of testicular cancers. Nonseminomas include embryonal carcinomas, teratomas, and choriocarcinomas, the most aggressive but rare (less than 1%) form of testicular cancer. Testicular cancers can include a mix of types.[106] In addition, testicular tumors can arise from spe-

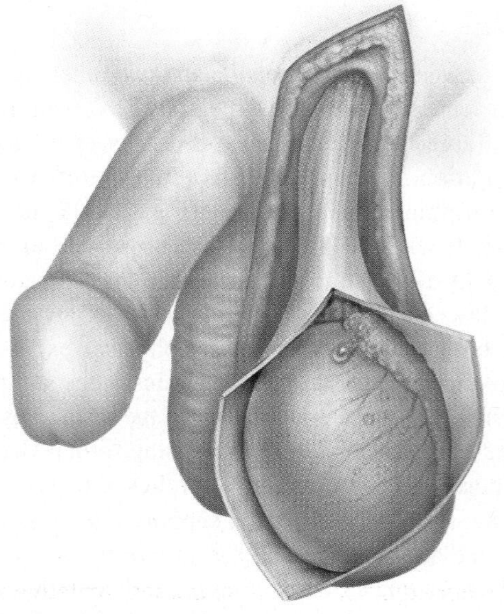

FIG. 22-32 Orchitis. (From Seidel H et al: *Mosby's guide to physical examination,* ed 4, St Louis, 1999, Mosby.)

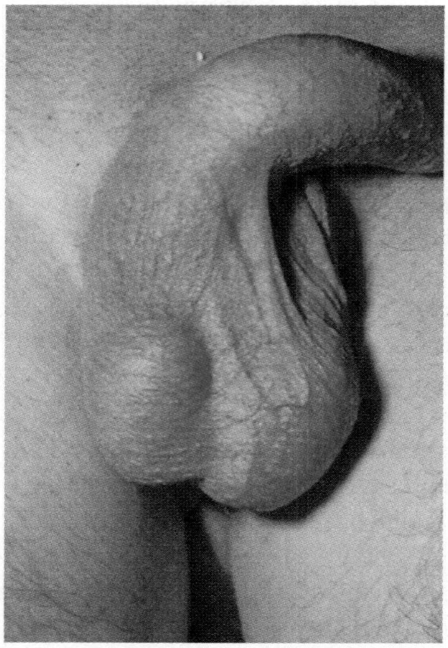

FIG. 22-33 Testicular tumor. (From *400 self-assessment picture tests in clinical medicine,* London, 1984, Wolfe medical publications.)

cialized cells of the gonadal stroma. These tumors, which are named for their cellular origins, are Leydig cell, Sertoli cell, granulosa cell, and theca cell tumors and constitute less than 10% of all testicular cancers.[107]

The cause of testicular neoplasms is unknown. A genetic predisposition is suggested by the fact that the incidence is higher among brothers, identical twins, and other close male relatives. Genetic predisposition is supported further by statistics showing that the disease is relatively rare among black Africans, black Americans, Asians, and native New Zealanders. Risk factors include history of cryptorchidism, abnormal testicular development, Klinefelter syndrome, and history of testicular cancer.[106]

Clinical Manifestations

Painless testicular enlargement commonly is the first sign of testicular cancer. Enlargement is usually gradual and may be accompanied by a sensation of testicular heaviness or dull ache in the lower abdomen.[106,107] Occasionally, acute pain occurs because of rapid growth, resulting in hemorrhage and necrosis. Ten percent of affected men have epididymitis, 10% have hydroceles,[107] and 5% have gynecomastia or hydrocele. Incidence of gynecomastia increases considerably (30% to 45%) in men with Sertoli or Leydig tumors. Approximately 10% of individuals already have symptoms related to metastases at the time of initial diagnosis, which correlates with the typical delay of 3 to 6 months from initial recognition to definitive treatment. Lumbar pain may be present and usually is caused by retroperitoneal node metastasis. Signs of metastasis to the lungs include cough, dyspnea, and bloody sputum (hemoptysis). Supraclavicular node involvement may cause difficulty swallowing (dysphagia) and neck swelling. Alterations in vision or mental status, papilledema, and seizures may be experienced with metastasis to the CNS. Approximately 10% of affected individuals are asymptomatic; the tumor may be detected by the man's sexual partner or incidentally following trauma.

Evaluation and Treatment

An incorrect diagnosis at the initial examination occurs in as many as 25% of men with testicular cancer. Epididymitis and epididymo-orchitis are the most common misdiagnoses; others include hydrocele and spermatocele. Evaluation begins with careful physical examination, including palpation of the scrotal contents with the individual in the erect and supine positions. The abdomen and lymph nodes are palpated to rule out metastases. Signs of testicular cancer include abnormal consistency, induration, nodularity, or irregularity of the testis. A firm, nontender testicular mass or diffuse enlargement is found in the majority of cases. Primary testicular cancer can be assessed rapidly and accurately by scrotal ultrasonography. Tumor markers are higher than normal in the presence of a tumor and may help detect a tumor that is too small to be palpated during physical examination or seen on imaging.[106] Tumor type is identified after inguinal biopsy or orchiectomy. Scrotal incisions may cause dissemination of the tumor and increase the risk of local recurrence and therefore are avoided. Chest x-ray, lymphangiogram, IVP, abdominal ultrasound, and CT are used in clinical staging of disease. Treatment is based on type of tumor, stage of disease, general health, and age. Besides surgery, treatment involves radiation and chemotherapy singly or in combination. A number of factors influence the prognosis (Table 22-9). They include histology of the tumor, stage of the disease, and selection of appropriate treatment. Serum markers, such as AFP, hCG-β, and lactate dehydrogenase, are useful for detecting metastases and assessing responses to therapy. Most individuals treated for cancer of the testis can expect a normal life span, although some have persistent paresthesias, Raynaud phenomenon, or infertility. Almost 90% of disease-related deaths occur in the first 2 years after cessation of therapy; disease-free survival of 3 years is considered a cure. Approximately 10% of men treated for testicular cancer will experience a relapse; if the relapse is discovered early and treated, 99% can be cured. Orchiectomy does not affect sexual function, but infertility can result from chemotherapy or surgical removal of affected abdominal lymph nodes if nerves necessary for ejaculation are severed. After orchiectomy, testicular silicone implants may be used to restore "normal" scrotal appearance.

Epididymitis

Epididymitis, or inflammation of the epididymis, generally occurs in sexually active young males (younger than 35 years) and is rare before puberty (Fig. 22-34). In young men the usual cause is a sexually transmitted microorganism, such as *N. gonorrhoeae* or *C. trachomatis.* Men who practice unprotected anal intercourse may acquire sexually transmitted epididymitis because of *E. coli, H. influenzae,* tuberculosis (especially in regions where incidence of pulmonary tuberculosis is high), *Cryptococcus,* or *Brucella.*[108] In men older than 35 years, Enterobacteriaceae (intestinal bacteria) and *Pseudomonas aeruginosa* associated with urinary tract infections and prostatitis also may cause epididymitis. Besides an infectious etiology, epididymitis may result from a chemical inflammation caused by the reflux of sterile urine into the ejaculatory ducts.[108,109] It is associated with urethral strictures, congenital posterior valves, and excessive physical straining in which increased abdominal pressure is transmitted to the bladder. Chemical epididymitis is usually self-limiting and does not require evaluation or intervention unless it persists.

Pathophysiology

The pathogenic microorganism usually reaches the epididymis by ascending the vasa deferentia from an already infected urethra or bladder. The presence of bacteria initiates the inflammatory response, causing symptoms of bacterial epididymitis. Epididymitis caused by heavy lifting or straining results from reflux of urine from the bladder into the vas deferens and epididymis. Urine is extremely irritating to the epididymis and initiates an inflammatory response called *chemical epididymitis.*

Table 22-9 Testicular Tumors of Germ-cell Origin

Cell Types	Occurrence	Metastatic Pattern	Prognosis/Remission Rate
A. Seminoma (germinoma)	30%-35% of all testicular tumors	Rarely to retroperitoneal lymph nodes	Excellent; tumor usually remains localized and is responsive to radiation; cure rate stages I and II >95%; stages III and IV >80%
B. Nonseminomatous tumors	60% of all testicular tumors		
1. Single cell			
a. Embryonal carcinoma	20%-25% of all testicular tumors; most common testicular tumor in infants and children	Earlier to regional lymphatics, also lung, liver, bone	Good; complete remission rate stages I and II >95%; stages III and IV >70%-80%
b. Teratoma	5%-10% of all testicular tumors (occurs in children and adults)	Through lymphatics and bloodstream; affects same organ systems as embryonal type	Fair
c. Choriocarcinoma	<1% of all testicular tumors	Earliest and widest, initially through bloodstream	Poor; early metastasis
2. Mixed tumors	30%-40% of all testicular tumors		
a. Teratocarcinoma	20%-25% of all testicular tumors	Mixed pattern; depends on cell types	Variable; prognosis becomes that of the most malignant element
b. Other	10%-15% of all testicular tumors	Mixed pattern; depends on cell types	Variable; prognosis becomes that of the most malignant element
i. Teratocarcinoma with seminoma			
ii. Embryonal cancer with seminoma			
iii. Teratoma with seminoma			
iv. Any combination with choriocarcinoma			
3. Non–germ-cell tumors (Leydig cell, Sertoli cell, granulosa cell, and theca cell tumors)	<10%		

Data from American Cancer Society. In *Cancer response system document #10029,* New York, 1995, The Society; Fresti et al with Lanum DL: Carcinoma of the genitourinary system. In Nseys UO, Weinman E, Lamm DL, editors: *Urology for primary care physicians,* Philadelphia, 1999, WB Saunders; Cancer Net: *Cancer facts: questions and answers about testicular cancer,* National Cancer Institute, 2000. Available at www.cancernet.nci.nih.gov/.

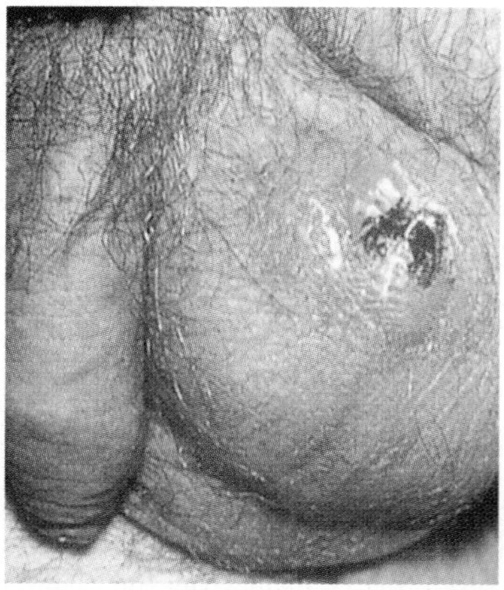

FIG. 22-34 Epididymitis secondary to gonorrhea or nongonococcal urethritis. Secondary to gonorrhea or nongonococcal urethritis, this infection spread to the testes, and rupture through the scrotal wall is threatened. (From Taylor PK: *Diagnostic picture tests in sexually transmitted diseases,* London, 1995, Mosby-Wolfe.)

Clinical Manifestations

Pain is the main symptom of epididymitis. Scrotal or inguinal pain is caused by inflammation of the epididymis and surrounding tissues. The pain is usually acute and severe. Flank pain may occur if, as the urethra passes over the spermatic cord, edematous swelling of the cord obstructs the urethra. The individual may have pyuria and bacteriuria and a history of urinary symptoms, including urethral discharge. The scrotum on the involved side is red and edematous as a result of inflammatory changes. The tail of the epididymis near the lower pole of the testis usually swells first; then swelling ascends to the head of the epididymis. The spermatic cord also may be swollen and tender.

Complications of epididymitis include abscess formation, infarction of the testis, recurrent infection, and infertility. Infarction probably is caused by thrombosis (obstruction by blood clots) of the prostatic vessels secondary to severe inflammation. Recurrent epididymitis may result from inadequate initial treatment or failure to identify or treat predisposing factors. Chronic epididymitis can cause scarring of the epididymal endothelium. Once scarring has occurred, treatment with antibiotics is ineffective because adequate antibiotic levels cannot be achieved within the epididymis.[108,109]

Evaluation and Treatment

A history of recent urinary tract infection or urethral discharge suggests the diagnosis of epididymitis. The relief of pain when the inflamed testis and epididymis are elevated (Phren sign) is also diagnostic. Definitive diagnosis is based on culture or Gram stain of a urethral swab. Epididymal aspiration may be necessary to obtain a specimen, especially if the individual has been taking antibiotics and has sterile urine.

Treatment includes antibiotic therapy for the infection itself (see Chapter 23) and various measures to provide symptomatic relief. Bed rest and scrotal elevation are recommended until the scrotum is no longer tender. Scrotal elevation facilitates maximal lymphatic and venous drainage. Abscess formation is rare with antibiotic therapy. If an abscess occurs and persists, it is drained surgically and an orchiectomy may be indicated. Complete resolution of swelling and pain may take several weeks to months. The individual's sexual partner should be treated with antibiotics if the causative microorganism is a sexually transmitted pathogen.

Disorders of the Prostate Gland

Benign Prostatic Hyperplasia

Benign prostatic hyperplasia (BPH), also called **benign prostatic hypertrophy,** is the enlargement of the prostate gland (Fig. 22-35). (Because the major prostatic changes are caused by hyperplasia, not hypertrophy, benign prostatic hyperplasia is the preferred term.) This condition becomes problematic as prostatic tissue compresses the urethra, where it passes through the prostate. Approximately 80% of men will have prostatic enlargement before age 80 years, and there is a 25% to 30% lifetime chance of needing prostatectomy for BPH once a man reaches 50 years of age.[110] Although BPH is common, its cause remains obscure. Its relationship to aging is well documented, however. At birth the prostate is pea sized, and growth of the gland is gradual until puberty. A period of rapid development continues until the third decade of life, when the prostate reaches adult size (see Chapter 21). Around 40 to 45 years of age, benign hyperplasia begins and continues slowly until death. Although dihydrotestosterone (DHT) is necessary for normal prostatic development, its role in BPH remains unclear. Among all androgen-metabolizing enzymes within the human prostate, 5α-reductase is the most powerful. This reductase corresponds to an age-dependent DHT level. Therefore, although 5α-reductase and DHT decrease with age in the epithelium, they remain relatively constant in the stroma of the prostate gland. Current causative theories of BPH focus on levels and ratios of endocrine factors such as androgens, estrogens, gonadotropins, and prolactin and changes in the balance between autocrine/paracrine growth-stimulatory and growth-inhibitory factors.

A

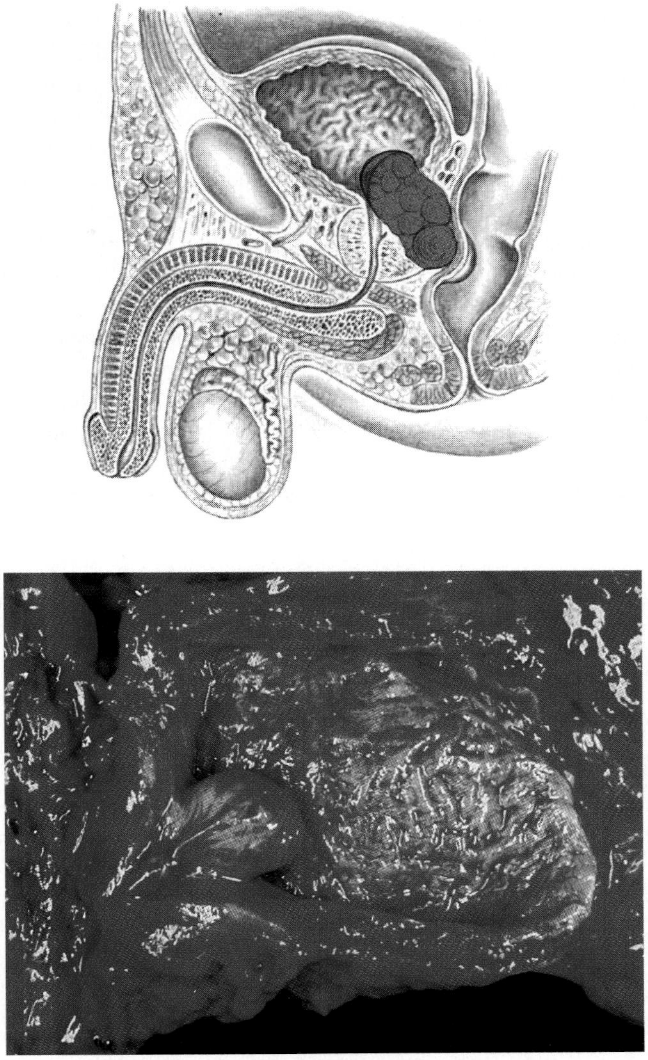

B

FIG. 22-35 Benign prostatic hyperplasia. A, Condition becomes a problem as prostatic tissue compresses the urethra. **B,** Gross appearance of BPH showing transition zone resulting from bulging nodules of varying size. (**A,** From Seidel H et al: *Mosby's guide to physical examination,* ed 4, St Louis, 1999, Mosby. **B,** From Damjanov I, Linder J, editors: *Anderson's pathology,* ed 10, St Louis, 1996, Mosby.)

These factors include insulin-like growth factors (IGFs), epidermal growth factor, nerve growth factor, IGF binding proteins, and transforming growth factor–beta.[111] Other relationships being explored include the interrelationship of the prostatic capsule with α-adrenergic innervation of the prostate and bladder detrusor function.[110]

BPH begins in the periurethral glands, which are the inner glands or layers of the prostate. The prostate enlarges as nodules form and grow (nodular hyperplasia) and glandular cells enlarge (hypertrophy). The development of BPH occurs over a prolonged period, and changes within the urinary tract are slow and insidious. Pathophysiologic effects are a result of complex interactions involving prostatic urethral resistance to the mechanical and spastic effects of BPH, intravesical pressure during voiding, detrusor muscle strength, neurologic functioning, and general physical health.

During the early stages of urethral obstruction, the detrusor muscle hypertrophies to help the bladder force urine out against increasing resistance. Symptoms (Fig. 22-36) are considered obstructive (weak urinary stream, prolonged voiding, abdominal straining, hesitancy, intermittency, incomplete bladder emptying, postmicturitional dribble) or irritative (frequency and repeated urination, nocturia, urgency, incontinence, and bladder pain and dysuria)[112] and may wax and wane.[113] As obstruction progresses, often over a period of several years, the detrusor muscle decompensates and the bladder is unable to empty all of the urine. Increasing volumes of urine are retained until urine retention is chronic. The volume of urine retained may be great enough to produce uncontrolled "overflow incontinence" with any increase in intraabdominal pressure. At this stage the force of the urinary stream is reduced significantly and much more time is required to initiate and complete voiding.

Progressive bladder distention causes sacculations or diverticular outpouchings of the bladder wall, and some neural degeneration of smooth muscle cells occurs. The ureters may be obstructed where they pass through the hypertrophied detrusor muscle. Hematuria, bladder or kidney infection, bladder calculi, acute urinary retention hydroureter, hydronephrosis, and renal insufficiency are common complications.[112] Some men initially have signs of uremia and renal failure. On digital rectal examination (DRE) the hyperplastic prostate is a soft or firm enlargement with smooth mucosal surface and no discernible distinction between lobes; asymmetry is common. The palpated prostate does not always reflect the degree of BPH because a substantial portion of the enlargement is intravesicular.[114]

Patient Information

Name: ______________________

Age: ______________________

Date Completed: ______________________

	Not at all	Less than 1 time in 5	Less than half the time	About half the time	More than half the time	Almost always
1. Over the past month, how often have you had a sensation of not emptying your bladder completely after you have finished urinating?	0	1	2	3	4	5
2. Over the past month, how often have you had to urinate again less than two hours after you finished urinating?	0	1	2	3	4	5
3. Over the past month, how often have you found you stopped and started again several times when you urinated?	0	1	2	3	4	5
4. Over the past month, how often have you found it difficult to postpone urination?	0	1	2	3	4	5
5. Over the past month, how often have you had a weak urinary stream?	0	1	2	3	4	5
6. Over the past month, how often have you had to push or strain to begin urination?	0	1	2	3	4	5
	None	1 Time	2 Times	3 Times	4 Times	5 Times
7. Over the past month, how many times did you most typically get up to urinate from the time you went to bed at night until the time you got up in the morning?	0	1	2	3	4	5

Total I-PSS Score:

	Delighted	Pleased	Mostly Satisfied	Mixed	Mostly Dissatisfied	Unhappy	Terrible
8. If you were to spend the rest of your life with your urinary condition just the way it is now, how would you feel about it?	0	1	2	3	4	5	6

FIG. 22-36 International prostate symptom score (I-PSS). Questionnaires such as the I-PSS allow practitioners to quantitate an individual's BPH symtpoms.

There is no way to reverse progressive BPH, but the hyperplasia is not always progressive. For these reasons, timing of intervention is variable and depends on severity of symptoms and the presence of complications. Annual DREs are used to screen men over 40 years of age for BPH. If marked enlargement, moderate to severe symptoms, or complications are present, transrectal ultrasonography (TRUS) is used to determine bladder and prostate volume and residual urine. Urinalysis, serum creatinine and blood urea nitrogen, uroflowmetry, postvoid residual urine, pressure-flow study, cystometry, and cystourethroscopy are used to determine kidney and bladder function.[112] Physical examination with DRE and prostate-specific antigen (PSA) is conducted to determine hyperplasia.[115] When necessary, the hyperplastic tissue may be removed surgically to prevent the serious consequences of urethral obstruction. Glands under 60 g are treated by transurethral resection, laser therapy, or microwave thermotherapy,[116] whereas larger glands are removed surgically (prostatectomy). A decision diagram is contained in Fig. 22-37. A permanent indwelling catheter is inserted if the individual cannot tolerate surgery. Recently, BPH has been treated successfully with drugs. α-Adrenergic blockers (prazosin and terazosin) are used to relax the smooth muscle of the bladder and prostate. Antiandrogen agents, such as finasteride (Proscar), selectively block androgens at the prostate cellular level and cause the prostate gland to shrink.[47] These drugs offer an alternative to surgery for as many as 75% of men with mild prostate enlargement.[16] Neither the α-adrenergic blockers nor finasteride seems to affect sexual desire or potency; finasteride may cause bone loss and lower levels of PSA. Because of the effect of finasteride on PSA levels, new recommendations for men on finasteride for 6 months or longer state that the serum PSA level should be multiplied by 2 and compared with either age-independent or age-specific upper limits of normal for serum PSA in untreated men with BPH.[25] PSA is used as a screen for prostate cancer. (See Chapter 10 for a discussion of antigens as tumor markers.)

The standard nonsurgical approach to the management of prostatic neoplasm is to decrease androgen (testosterone and its active metabolite DHEA) levels and trigger involution of the gland. Although men with BPH respond favorably to this approach, androgen ablation in men with prostatic cancer is less effective than surgery. One explanation is that local and independent growth factors fully or partially replace the androgen-driven growth signal. Prostatic fibromuscular stroma is a rich source of IGF-II and possesses an abundance of IGF receptors. Recent research supports inhibition of normal IGF-I functions as an alternative or supplement to standard steroid-based therapies for BPH.

Prostatitis

Prostatitis is an inflammation of the prostate. Some degree of prostatic inflammation is present in 4% to 36% of the male population. This percentage increases to 50% in older men. Inflammation is usually limited to a few of the gland's excretory ducts (Fig. 22-38).

Prostatitis is characterized as (1) acute bacterial prostatitis, (2) chronic bacterial prostatitis, or (3) nonbacterial prostatitis. **Prostatodynia** (pain in the prostate) is sometimes considered a form of nonbacterial prostatitis. Men with prostatodynia have the same clinical manifestations as those with nonbacterial prostatitis, but physical and laboratory examinations do not show prostatic pathology. Prostatodynia may not be caused by a pathologic condition of the prostate but rather by spasms in the genitourinary tract or tension in the muscles of the pelvic floor.

A number of defense mechanisms normally protect the lower urogenital tract from infection. Mechanical defenses include urethral length, micturition (urination), and ejaculation. Structural malformations and instrumentation of the genitourinary tract may weaken these defense mechanisms. Chemical defenses include antimicrobial substances in the prostatic fluid. The most important of these is a zinc-containing polypeptide known as *prostatic antibacterial factor.* Coliform bacteria, particularly *Enterobacter, E. coli, Enterococcus, Klebsiella,* and *Pseudomonas,* are common pathogens of bacterial prostatitis. *Ureaplasma* and *C. trachomatis* may also be causative agents of infectious prostatitis.[109]

Bacterial Prostatitis

Acute bacterial prostatitis is an ascending infection of the urinary tract that tends to occur in men between ages 30 and 50 years but is also associated with BPH in older men. Infection stimulates an inflammatory response in which the prostate becomes enlarged, tender, and firm or boggy. The onset of prostatitis may be acute and unrelated to previous illnesses, or it may follow catheterization or cystoscopy.

Clinical manifestations of acute bacterial prostatitis are those of acute cystitis or pyelonephritis. Sudden onset of malaise, low back and perineal pain, high fever (up to 40° C [104° F]), and chills is common, as are dysuria, inability to empty the bladder, nocturia, and urinary retention. Myalgia and arthralgia also may occur. The individual also may have symptoms of lower urinary tract obstruction, such as a slow, small, "narrowed" urinary stream, which may be a medical emergency. Men are acutely ill and may look toxic. Prostatic pain may occur, especially when the individual is in an upright position, because the pelvic floor muscles tighten with standing and compression of the prostate gland occurs. Some individuals experience low back pain, painful ejaculation, and rectal or perineal pain. Palpation discloses an extremely tender, swollen prostate with normal to "boggy" consistency that may be warm to the touch.

Because acute bacterial prostatitis usually is associated with a bladder infection caused by the same microorganism, urine cultures disclose its identity. Prostatic massage may express enough secretions from the urethra for direct bacterial examination, but massage may be painful and increases the risk that the infection will ascend to adjacent structures or enter the bloodstream and cause septicemia. For these

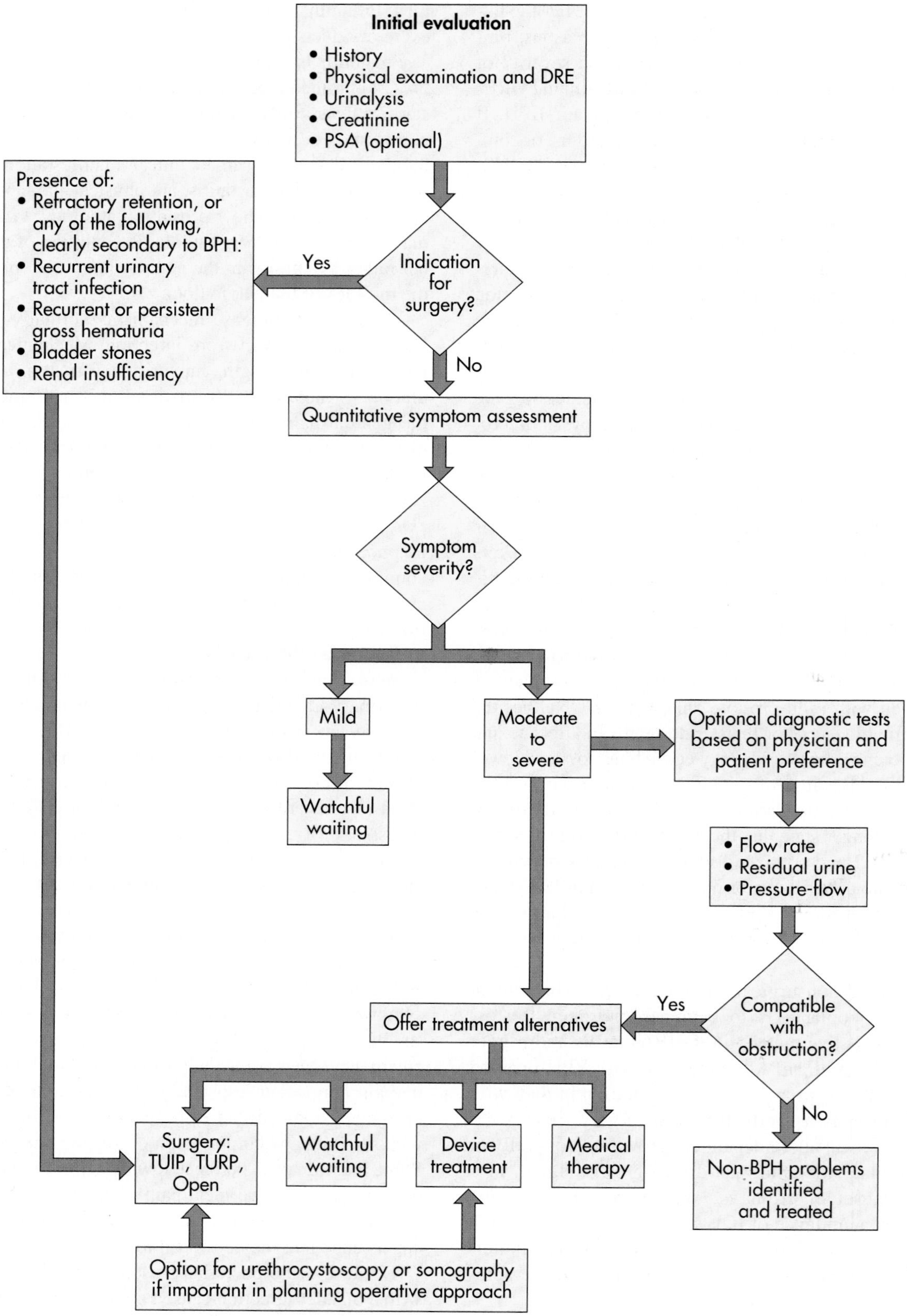

FIG. 22-37 Decision diagram for the diagnosis and treatment of benign prostatic hyperplasia. *DRE,* Digital rectal examination; *PSA,* prostate-specific antigen; *TUIP,* transurethral incision of the prostate; *TURP,* transurethral resection of the prostate. (Adapted from McConnell JD et al: *Benign prostatic hyperplasia: diagnosis and treatment.* Clinical practice guideline no 8, Rockville, Md, 1994, Agency for Health Care Policy and Research, Public Health Services, US Department of Health and Human Services.)

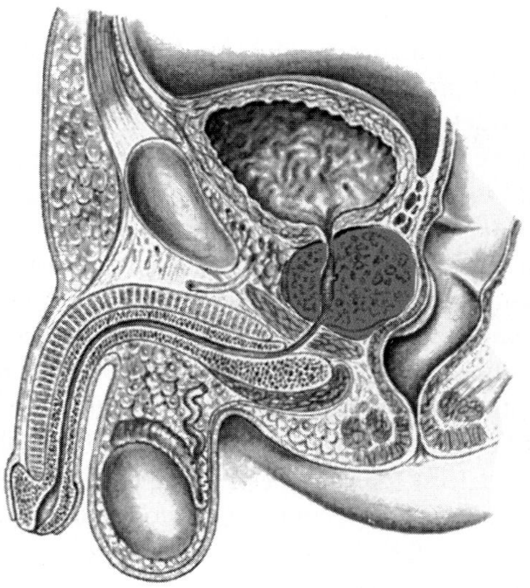

FIG. 22-38 Prostatitis. (From Seidel H et al: *Mosby's guide to physical examination,* ed 4, St Louis, 1999, Mosby.

reasons, prostatic massage generally is contraindicated; transurethral instrumentation also is contraindicated.

Long-term, broad-spectrum antibiotic therapy with fluoroquinolone agents or trimethoprim-sulfamethoxazole for at least 30 to 42 days is recommended to resolve the infection and control its spread. In severe cases the individual is hospitalized and treated with combination intravenous antibiotics, usually an aminoglycoside (gentamicin sulfate, kanamycin sulfate, or tobramycin) and ampicillin for 1 week followed by 4 to 6 weeks of oral antibiotics. Pain relievers, antipyretics, bed rest, and adequate hydration are also therapeutic. Complications include urinary retention that resolves with antibiotic therapy; prostatic abscess that may rupture into the urethra, rectum, or perineum; epididymitis; bacteremia; and septic shock. Urinary retention requiring drainage is best managed with a suprapubic catheter; Foley catheterization is contraindicated during acute infection.

Chronic bacterial prostatitis is characterized by recurrent urinary symptoms and persistence of pathogenic bacteria (usually gram negative) in urine or prostatic fluid.[109] This form of prostatitis is the most common recurrent urinary tract infection in men. Symptoms are variable and may be similar to those of an acute bladder infection: frequency, urgency, dysuria, perineal discomfort, low back pain, and sexual dysfunction. The prostate may be only slightly enlarged or boggy, but fibrosis caused by repeated infections can cause it to be firm and irregular in shape.

When the initial urine sample is bacteria free, prostatic massage is used to express secretions. Subsequently, the first 10 ml of voided urine is collected and examined microscopically. Prostatic secretions showing more than 10 white blood cells per high-power field and macrophages containing fat indicate bacterial infection; diagnosis is confirmed by culture. Prostatic calculi may be seen on pelvic x-ray or TRUS.

Treatment of chronic bacterial prostatitis is difficult because it is often caused by prostatic calculi. Calculi are silent and are found in up to 50% of men with prostatitis, and infected calculi can serve as a source of bacterial persistence and relapsing urinary tract infections.[109] Calculi harbor pathogens within the stone, and consequently pathogens cannot be eradicated from the urinary tract. Permanent cure is achieved by surgical removal of the stones through transurethral prostatectomy, which may not be a viable option for young men. More common symptoms are tempered with chronic suppressive therapy. Quinolones, because of their bioavailability and penetration into prostatic tissue, are the treatment of choice; drug therapy lasts for a minimum of 3 to 4 weeks. If symptoms do not subside, other infectious microorganisms are considered and treated accordingly.[109] Comfort measures include nonsteroidal antiinflammatory drug therapy and liberal use of sitz baths.

Nonbacterial Prostatitis

Nonbacterial prostatitis is the most common prostatitis syndrome and consists of prostatic inflammation without evidence of bacterial infection. Symptoms tend to be milder but are persistent and annoying. Presumably, noninfectious prostatitis or prostadynia is caused by reflux of sterile urine into the ejaculatory ducts as a result of high-pressure voiding.[109] Reflux may be triggered by spasms of the external or internal sphincters. Some men may actually have interstitial cystitis and should be treated accordingly.

Men with nonbacterial prostatitis may complain of pain or a dull ache that is continuous or spasmodic in the suprapubic, infrapubic, scrotal, penile, or inguinal area. Other symptoms are pain on ejaculation and urinary symptoms, such as frequency of urination. The prostate gland generally feels normal on palpation.

Digital examination of the prostate, bacterial cultures of the urogenital tract, microscopic examination of expressed prostatic fluid, urethroscopy, and urodynamic studies are used to verify the diagnosis of nonbacterial prostatitis. Nonbacterial prostatitis is a diagnosis by exclusion.

Therapy is individualized and aimed at decreasing symptoms. α-Adrenergic blockers (e.g., terazosin, doxazonsin, and tamsulosin) may be helpful in decreasing spasms of the prostate muscle. Other treatments include skeletal muscle relaxants, pelvic floor relaxation using biofeedback, and prostatic thermotherapy.[109] Other treatments may include hot sitz baths, bed rest, anticholinergics, and antiinflammatory drugs.

Cancer of the Prostate

In the United States, prostatic cancer is the most commonly diagnosed malignancy and the second leading cause of cancer death in men.[68] In 1998 prostate cancer accounted for about 29.4% of all cancer in men and approximately 13.3% of all cancer deaths; only lung cancer causes more deaths in men.[68,117] An estimated 198,100 new diagnosed cases and 31,500 deaths caused by prostate cancer are expected in 2001.[69] Between 1989 and 1992, incidence rates increased dramatically. This increase was largely due to detection in asymptomatic men using improved screening methods (PSA testing coupled with DRE). Prostate cancer incidence rates are now declining; rates peaked in 1992 among white men and in 1993 for black men. In addition, prostate mortality rates declined significantly between 1992 and 1996.[69]

Overall lifetime incidence is 1 in 10 for all men, with rates in blacks increasing to 1 in 8.[118] By age 85 years, 1 in 6 men will develop prostate cancer. Prostatic cancer tends to be a disease of North American and northwestern European men; it is rare in the Near East, Africa, Central America, and South America. Although the incidence is low in black African men, black African-Americans have the highest rate of prostate cancer in the world and in the United States; incidence rates are more than twice as high in blacks (African-Americans) than whites.

The cause of prostatic cancer is poorly understood. Prostatic cancer is a disease of aging; more than 80% of all prostate cancers are diagnosed in men older than 65 years;[117] prostatic cancer rarely occurs in men younger than 40 years; and incidence increases with advancing age. Most of the androgen-metabolizing enzymes undergo a significant age-dependent alteration.

Dietary Factors

The worldwide distribution of prostate cancer suggests that diet may play a role in the development of this disease, especially if the diet affects hormone levels. Consistency across studies indicates that a high intake of fat (total and especially saturated fat) is a risk factor for prostate cancer, but the strength of the associations is modest and may be greater for African-Americans than for European-Americans.[119-121] Several hypotheses exist concerning the enhancing effect of fat on prostate carcinogenesis, including hormonal mediation and the generation of free radicals. In addition, a low intake of dietary fiber and complex carbohydrates and a high intake of protein are associated with an increased risk of prostate cancer.[121] Controversial is whether obesity or an increased body mass index is a risk factor for prostate cancer.

Individual nutrients or foods and their associations with prostate cancer risk are not strong, yet migration from low-risk areas, such as Japan, to high-risk countries, such as the United States, increases risk considerably.[119] These changes in risk probably reflect differences in life-style and dietary habits. Geographically, individuals who reside in regions with less sunlight have a higher risk of prostate cancer. The highest rates of mortality from prostate cancer in the world are in Scandinavian countries, where exposure to ultraviolet light is low; the link is vitamin D. The Cure of Cancer of the Prostate (CaP CURE) Report states that, of all the risk factors for prostate cancer, only nutrition seems to explain the differences in global distribution of prostate cancer.[122] Diet is especially significant because it affects hormone levels.

Animal studies suggest a protective effect of retinoids (vitamin A) and prostate carcinogenesis; however, consistency is lacking among epidemiologic studies. Vegetarian men have a lower incidence of prostate cancer than omnivorous males.[123] Low levels of dietary selenium are associated with increased prostate cancer risk.[124] Vitamin D (1,25-[OH]2D3) inhibited the growth of certain human prostate cancer cell lines by an androgen-dependent mechanism.[125] Lycopene, a carotenoid found in large amounts in tomatoes that gives them their red color, has been associated with a lower risk of prostate cancer.[126,127]

Hormones

Prostate cancer develops in an androgen-dependent epithelium and is usually androgen sensitive. In addition, a few case reports exist of prostate cancer in men who used androgenic steroids as anabolic agents or for medical purposes, suggestive of a causal relationship.[119,128-130] Population studies have not, however, provided clear and convincing patterns about associations between circulating hormone concentrations and prostate cancer risk.[119] Only a few associations with prostate cancer risk have been observed consistently (in at least three studies), and their associations are weak: (1) slightly higher circulating testosterone and estrogen levels and lower DHEA (sulfate) levels in high-risk African-American men as compared with lower-risk European-American men; and (2) a cytosine-adenine-guanine (CAG) repeat-length polymorphism in the androgen-receptor gene associated with increased risk and increased receptor activity (androgen receptor). Evidence for involvement of activity of the enzyme 5α-reductase, which is critical in androgen activity in the prostate, is contradictory and inconsistent.[119] In men younger than 50 years, circulating levels of androgens and estrogens appear to be higher in men of African descent than in European-American men.

Investigations directed at understanding the hormonal basis of prostate (as well as breast) carcinogenesis have numerous problems. The complexities of interacting hormones and separating out the effects of a single hormone are profound. In addition, only single blood samples are generally available and within-subject variations over time and differences in circadian rhythms cannot be adequately measured.

NUTRITION & DISEASE

Nutrition and Risk Reduction for Prostate Cancer

- Avoid saturated fat
- Avoid specific polyunsaturated fats, including ω-6 fat, linoleic acid (found in safflower and soybean oil), and ω-3 fat α-linolenic acid (found in red meat, mayonnaise, soybean oil, rapeseed oil, and margarine)
- Avoid foods with hydrogenated or partially hydrogenated oil
- Substitute oils with olive oils (use sparingly)
- Decrease total energy intake from calories; avoid refined sugars
- Increase antioxidants, vitamin E (400 IU/day), selenium (from grains, garlic, supplements), green tea, cruficerous vegetables, and fruits
- Increase lycopene (reddest tomatoes available, tomato juice, soup, salads)
- Increase soy (genistein)
- Increase sunshine exposure for daily requirement of vitamin D (200 to 400 IU/day)
- Maintain calcium intake at 1000 mg (19 to 50 years old), 1200 mg (51 and older); switch from cow's milk to soy milk
- Increase fiber (whole grains, beans, cereals)

For documented studies see Arnot R: *The prostate cancer protection plan: the foods, supplements and drugs that could save your life,* Boston, 2000, Little, Brown.

The results of several animal studies do support elevation of bioavailable and bioactive androgens in the circulation and in target tissue as an important risk factor. In fact, some observations indicate that substantial increase in prostate carcinogenesis can be produced by very small elevations of circulating testosterone. Animal studies also indicate that increased biologic activity of the androgen receptor may be associated with prostate cancer.

Vasectomy

Vasectomy has been identified as a possible risk factor for prostate cancer in both case-controlled studies and cohort studies.[131,132] Three mechanisms by which vasectomy could increase risk are (1) elevation of circulating androgens; (2) immunologic mechanisms involving antisperm antibodies; and (3) reduction of seminal fluid levels of 5α-dihydrotesterone, the active metabolite of testosterone in the prostate, in vasectomized men. Other investigators reported a decrease in sex hormone–binding globulin (SHBG) and an increase in the ratio of testosterone to SHBG.[133] These results suggest an elevation of circulating free testosterone following vasectomy.[119]

Familial Factors

Other possible causes are genetic predisposition (familial and hereditary forms). Recent genetic studies suggest that strong familial predisposition may be responsible for 5% to 10% of prostate cancers.[117] Hereditary cancer is an autosomal dominant disease caused by a rare but highly penetrant gene; that is, 88% of gene carriers develop prostate cancer by age 85 years. Hereditary cancer differs from the familial form, which occurs in individuals with a positive family history but who do not exhibit early age of onset.[134] The hereditary form constitutes about 9% of all prostate cancers and approximately 43% of cancers in men less than 55 years of age.[114] There is no clear evidence of a causal link between BPH and prostate cancer even though they may frequently occur together. Recent data substantiate that tobacco use has a significant impact on the occurrence of fatal prostate cancer.[135]

Pathogenesis

More than 95% of prostatic neoplasms are adenocarcinomas,[136] and most occur in the periphery of the prostate. Several histologic grading systems have been developed on the basis of the glandular pattern, the degree of differentiation (anaplasia) of the cancer cells, or both. The biologic aggressiveness of the neoplasm appears to be related to the degree of differentiation rather than the size of the tumor.

Although steroid hormonal factors are strongly implicated in prostate carcinogenesis, little is known about their involvement. Just as the testicles are the male equivalent of the female ovaries, the prostate is the male equivalent of the female uterus; in both situations they originate from the same embryonic cells. This may be important in understanding the role of the associated hormones testosterone, dihydrotestosterone, and estradiol in prostate carcinogenesis.

Testosterone is the major androgen from the interstitial cells of the testis (Lydig cells). Its production in men is almost 5 mg/day. The adrenal cortex contributes the far less potent androstenedione as its major androgen, at about 3 mg/day. In the target tissues and, to a lesser extent, in the testes themselves, testosterone is converted to dihydrotestosterone (DHT) by the enzyme 5α-reductase (Fig. 22-39).

Normally, a small amount of estrogen is produced per day—65 μg of estrone and 45 μg of estradiol—by the aromatization of androstenedione and testosterone, respectively. This reaction is catalyzed by the enzyme system aromatase. A very small quantity of estradiol is released by the testes (see Fig. 22-39); the rest of the estrogens in males are produced by adipose tissue, liver, skin, brain, and other nonendocrine tissue. Thus testosterone is a precursor of the two hormones, DHT and estradiol.

The adult prostate is under control of multiple steroid hormones and paracrine peptide factors (such as insulin-like growth factor [IGF-I]). Most of the androgen-metabolizing enzymes undergo a significant age-dependent alteration. In epithelium, both the 5α-reductase activity and the DHT level decrease with age; whereas in stroma (prostate), not only is the 5α-reductase activity rather constant over the whole age range, but the DHT level is constant as well. In contrast to the relatively unaltered DHT level, the estrogen content follows an age-dependent increase. Thus the age-dependent decrease of the DHT accumulation in epithelium and the concomitant increase of the estrogen accumulation in stroma lead to a tremendous increase with age of the estrogen/androgen ratio in the human prostate.

In addition, there are changes in the balance between autocrine/paracrine growth-stimulatory and growth-inhibitory factors, such as IGFs, epidermal growth factor (EGF), nerve growth factor (NGF), IGF-binding proteins, and transforming growth factor–beta (TGF-β). In animal studies, chronic exposure to testosterone plus estradiol is strongly carcinogenic, whereas testosterone alone is weakly carcinogenic.[119] The mechanism is not clearly understood but appears to involve estrogen-generated oxidative stress and DNA toxicity, and it requires androgen and estrogen receptor–mediated processes, such as changes in sex steroid metabolism and receptor status.[119]

From all of these observations, the following multifactorial general hypothesis of prostate carcinogenesis emerges: (1) androgens act as strong tumor promoters through androgen receptor–mediated mechanisms to (2) enhance the carcinogenic activity of strong endogenous DNA toxic carcinogens, including reactive estrogen metabolites and estrogen—and prostatic-generated reactive oxygen species—and (3) possibly

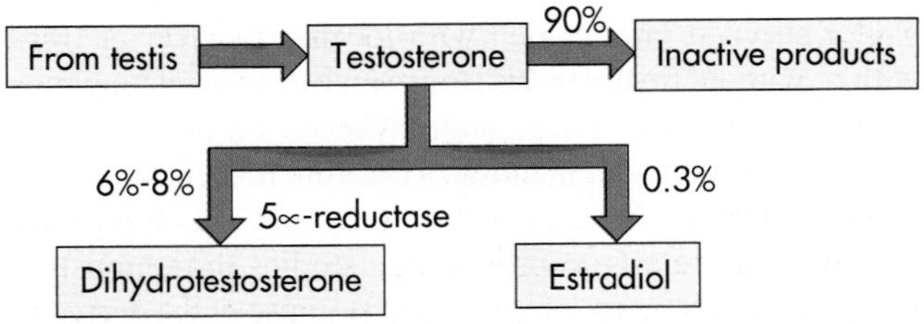

FIG. 22-39 Testosterone and conversion to DHT.

unknown environmental carcinogens. All of these factors are modulated by diet and genetic determinants, such as hereditary susceptibility genes and polymorphic genes, that encode receptors and enzymes involved in the metabolism and action of steroid hormones.[119]

Prostatic cancer is thought to metastasize by local extension and through lymphatic and blood vessels. The most frequent sites of distant metastasis are the lymph nodes, bones, lungs, liver, and adrenals. The pelvis, lumbar spine, femur, thoracic spine, and ribs are the most common sites of bone metastasis. Local extension is usually posterior, although late in the disease the tumor may invade the rectum or encroach on the prostatic urethra and cause bladder outlet obstruction (Fig. 22-40). The spread through blood vessels is illustrated in Fig. 22-41.

Clinical Manifestations

Prostatic cancer often causes no symptoms until it is far advanced. The first manifestations of disease are those of bladder outlet obstruction: slow urinary stream, hesitancy, incomplete emptying, frequency, nocturia, and dysuria. Unlike the symptoms of obstruction caused by BPH, the symptoms of obstruction caused by prostatic cancer are progressive and do not remit. Local extension of prostatic cancer can obstruct the upper urinary tract ureters as well. If rectal obstruction occurs, the individual may experience a large bowel obstruction or difficulty in defecation. Symptoms of late disease include bone pain at sites of bone metastasis, edema of the lower extremities, enlargement of lymph nodes, liver enlargement, pathologic bone fractures, and mental confusion associated with brain metastases.

Evaluation and Treatment

Screening for prostatic cancer includes DRE, PSA blood tests, and TRUS. The American Cancer Society recommends annual DREs for men older than 40 years and an annual DRE and PSA blood test for men older than 50 years (with at least a 10-year life expectancy).[117] Earlier screening with the PSA test is recommended for men at high risk for prostate cancer, such as blacks or relatives of men who have had prostate cancer.[114,117,134,137] It is important to note that PSA levels tend to be higher in blacks at baseline and all stages of cancer.[138] When TRUS is added to the annual DRE and PSA testing, the ability to predict cancer rises significantly, from 41% to greater than 78%. Cancer diagnosis is confirmed through tissue biopsy and microscopic examination of tissue. Lymph node biopsy, bone scans, MRI, and CT may be used to determine metastasis to lymph, bone, or other adjacent tissue.

Recently, controversy over screening has occurred. The 5-year survival rate of men with localized cancer is 100% with or without treatment.[117] However, before screening most men with prostate cancer had advanced disease and died within a few years of diagnosis. Therefore it is unclear which men will benefit from early screening and which will not. Currently, there are no prospective studies to demonstrate benefit or disadvantage of screening. Because of the decreased mortality rate and incidence of advanced disease, some authorities continue to recommend regular screening.[117,137] If a mass is found on DRE or if PSA is greater than 10, TRUS is recommended to confirm presence of mass and to assist with biopsy.[136] PSA is an excellent marker to indicate speed of tumor growth or success of treatment and is routinely used for these reasons.

Treatment of prostatic cancer depends on the stage of the neoplasm (Box 22-12); the anticipated effects of treatment; and the age, general health, and life expectancy of the individ-

A

B

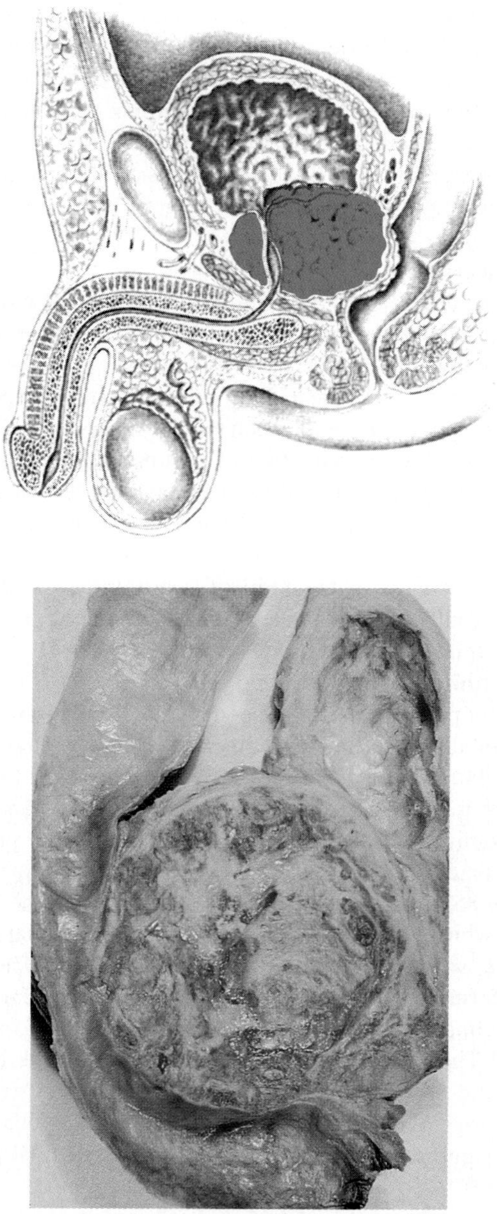

FIG. 22-40 Carcinoma of prostate. A, Frequent sites of distant metastasis are the lymph nodes, bones, lungs, liver, and adrenals. **B,** Carcinoma of the prostate extending into the rectum and urinary bladder. (**A,** From Seidel H et al: *Mosby's guide to physical examination,* ed 4, St Louis, 1999, Mosby. **B,** From Damjanov I, Linder J, editors: *Pathology: a color atlas,* St Louis, 2000, Mosby.)

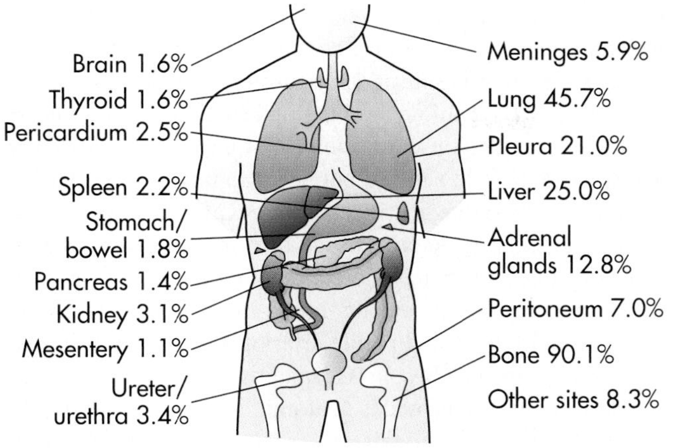

FIG. 22-41 Distribution of hematogeneous metastases in prostate cancer. Study of 556 patients with metastatic prostate cancer. (Adapted from Budendorf L et al: Metastatic patterns of prostate cancer: an autopsy study of 1,589 patients, *Hum Pathol* 31:578, 2000.)

BOX 22-12

STAGING OF PROSTATE CANCER

Treatment and prognosis of prostate cancer depend on the grading or extent of the disease. Newly diagnosed cases can be staged in the following manner:

Stage A (very early)—cancer is confined to the prostate gland, cannot be felt during a rectal examination, and can be seen only with a microscope; local excision at time of biopsy and regular follow-up may be all the treatment required.

Stage B (localized)—cancer is palpable and remains confined to the prostate gland; men are asymptomatic but prostate-specific antigen (PSA) levels will be elevated for those with a mass palpated on digital rectal examination (DRE).

Stage C (regionalized)—tumor has spread to adjacent tissues.

Stage D (advanced)—cancer has recurred in prostate or other parts of body after treatment.

Data from American Cancer Society. *In Cancer response system document #10028,* New York, 1995, The Society; Cancer Net: Prostate cancer, National Cancer Institute, 1998. Available at www.cancernet.nci.nih.goc/wyntle_pubs/prostate.

ual. More recently, the tumor, node, metastasis (TNM) method of staging has been used to determine extent of disease (see Chapter 11, p. 342). Options include no treatment; surgical treatments such as total prostatectomy, transurethral resection of the prostate (TURP), or cryotherapy; nonsurgical treatments such as radiation therapy, hormone therapy, or chemotherapy; watchful waiting; and any combination of these.[117] In addition, new approaches are using immunotherapy.[139] Palliative treatment is aimed at relieving urinary, bladder outlet, or colon obstruction; spinal cord compression; and pain. Treatments at an early stage can cure the disease in most, if not all, men, and treatment for advanced stage can extend life and reduce tumor size, thus preventing or relieving pain. Prognosis and survival rates have improved steadily over the past 50 years. Currently, the overall 5-year survival rate of all stages of prostate cancer is up to 92%; survival rates decline at 10 years (67%) and 15 years (52%).[117]

Treatment for prostate cancer may lead to loss of urinary control, which frequently returns to normal after several weeks or months. Mild stress incontinence can occur after surgery and mild urge incontinence after radiation therapy. Prostate cancer and its treatment can affect sexual functioning. Most men will need assistance (medication) with obtaining an erection for 3 to 12 months after surgery. Sensation of orgasm is not usually affected, but smaller amounts of ejaculate will be produced or men may experience a "dry" ejaculate because of retrograde ejaculation.

Sexual Dysfunction

In males the normal sexual response involves three processes: erection, emission, and ejaculation. **Sexual dysfunction** is the impairment of any or all of these processes. Impairment can be caused by a number of physiologic, psychologic, and emotional factors.

Until the late 1970s, most cases of male sexual dysfunction were thought to be psychogenic. Recent studies of this problem indicate that, in men older than 40 years, organic factors are involved in more than 50% of cases. The causes of organic sexual dysfunction include (1) vascular, endocrine, and neurologic disorders; (2) chronic disease, including renal failure and diabetes mellitus; (3) penile diseases and penile trauma; and (4) iatrogenic factors, such as surgery and pharmacologic therapies. Most of these disorders cause erectile dysfunction.

Pathophysiology

Vascular disorders can prevent erection. Some arterial diseases diminish or interrupt circulation to the penis. This prevents engorgement of erectile tissues in the corpora cavernosa and corpus spongiosum. Rarely, excessive venous drainage of the corpora cavernosa prevents erection.

Endocrine disorders that reduce testosterone production affect sexual function and libido. The reduction may be caused by inadequate secretion of the gonadotropins caused by pituitary dysfunction or hyperprolactinemia. Feminizing tumors and estrogen therapy reduce relative levels of testosterone. Testicular atrophy from any cause also decreases testosterone levels and contributes to sexual dysfunction.

Neurologic disorders can interfere with the important sympathetic, parasympathetic, and CNS mechanisms required for erection, emission, and ejaculation. They include spinal cord injury or tumor, multiple sclerosis, and disorders that cause peripheral neuropathies, such as diabetes mellitus and chronic renal failure. Spinal cord injuries or tumors can alter one or more components of the sexual response, depending on the location of the lesion. For example, in most men with upper motor neuron lesions, reflexogenic erection is possible but emission and ejaculation (i.e., orgasm) are not possible. Lesions affecting the lower motor neurons usually prevent erection. In approximately 40% of such cases, emission and ejaculation are prevented.

Many chronic diseases are associated with sexual dysfunction. In some conditions the sexual dysfunction has a specific physiologic cause. Diabetes mellitus, for example, causes both peripheral vascular and neurologic pathology that can lead to erectile dysfunction. Impotence occurs in about 50% of men undergoing dialysis. Multiple factors are involved, including decreased testosterone levels, autonomic neuropathy, accelerated vascular disease, multiple medications, worsening of primary disease, and psychologic stress. Potency may be restored by successful renal transplantation, except in bilateral transplantation if arterial flow is diminished or interrupted. Cirrhosis of the liver, scleroderma, chronic debilitation, and cachexia also are known to cause impotence. Emotional and psychologic response to chronic illness, such as anxiety, depression, and loss of self-esteem, can affect sexual functioning. In other chronic conditions, sexual dysfunction is associated with low energy levels and loss of libido. The pathophysiologic mechanisms responsible for such changes are not known.

Priapism causes fibrosis of trabeculae (erectile tissues) within the corpora cavernosa, making erection difficult. The penile curvature caused by Peyronie disease does not make erection impossible but may make it extremely painful and intercourse impossible. Penile trauma can damage the erectile tissue, disrupt the posterior urethra, and disrupt the pudendal arteries or nerves.

Iatrogenic factors, including drugs and surgery, have a significant impact on erectile function. The following surgical procedures all carry the risk of erectile dysfunction: radical pelvic surgery; radical prostatectomy; transurethral, suprapubic, or simple retropubic prostatectomy; and aortoiliac surgery. Erectile dysfunction is caused by the severing of small nerve branches that are essential for erection. Aortoiliac surgery, retroperitoneal lymphadenectomy, and sympathectomy cause the loss of ejaculation capacity in some individuals.

A few pharmacologic agents enhance the sexual response, but most have the opposite effect. Men who are taking antihypertensives, antidepressants, antihistamines, antispasmodics, sedatives or tranquilizers, barbiturates, diuretics, sex hormone preparations, narcotics, or psychoactive drugs may experience some degree of sexual dysfunction. Drug-induced sexual dysfunction consists of decreased desire, decreased erectile ability, or decreased ejaculatory ability. Ethyl alcohol may induce alcoholic neuropathy or increased estrogens because of hepatic dysfunction; marijuana depresses testosterone levels; and cigarette smoking contributes to vasoconstriction and venous leakage. A number of pharmacologic agents also diminish the quality or quantity of sperm. A few may cause priapism. Drugs can assist in maintaining an erection.

Evaluation and Treatment

Evaluation of sexual dysfunction includes a physical examination, with particular attention to the genitalia, prostate, and nervous system, and basic laboratory tests to identify the presence of endocrinopathies or other underlying disorders that can cause the dysfunction. If no physiologic cause is found and the condition does not improve with psychotherapy, the man is referred for further investigation of organic causes. Psychologic evaluation is indicated for younger men with a sudden onset of sexual dysfunction or men of any age who are able to achieve but not maintain an erection.

Sophisticated diagnostic techniques can be used to assess penile blood flow, erectile tissue anatomy, nervous system function, and occurrence of erection or emission during sleep (nocturnal emission). Penile blood flow is measured by Doppler techniques and penile arteriography. Corpus cavernosography, in which contrast material is injected into the corpora cavernosa, provides anatomic information about the erectile tissue of the penis. Neuropathic causes of sexual dysfunction are evaluated by measuring the speed of the bulbocavernous reflex. Nocturnal penile tumescence monitoring measures the frequency of nocturnal erections. Depending on the equipment used, this information may be correlated to rapid eye movement (REM) or non-REM sleep.

Treatments for organic sexual dysfunction include both medical and surgical interventions. Nonsurgical interventions include correction of underlying disorders, particularly drug-induced dysfunction and endocrinopathy-related (e.g., reduced testosterone associated with chronic renal failure) dysfunction. Vasodilators and cessation of smoking can benefit individuals with vasculogenic erectile dysfunction. Surgical interventions include penile implants, penile revascularization, and correction of other anatomic defects contributing to sexual dysfunction.

Impairment of Sperm Production and Quality

Spermatogenesis requires adequate secretion of FSH and LH by the pituitary; sufficient secretion of testosterone by the Leydig cells; sufficient function of the Sertoli cells, including secretion of androgen-binding protein, growth factors, inhibin B, and a number of other important (but poorly understood) peptides; and adequate spermatogonia.[140,141] The Leydig cells are located in the testicular interstitum *between* the tubules, and the Sertoli cells and spermatogonia are located *within* the seminiferous tubules. The Sertoli cells extend from the basement membrane to the lumen, display tight junctions between adjacent cells, and form the blood-testis barrier. Inadequate secretion of gonadotropins may be caused by hypothyroidism, hyperadrenocortisolism, hyperprolactinemia, or hypogonadotropic hypogonadism. In these situations, gonadotropin levels are low because of feedback inhibition or idiopathic hyposecretion. In the absence of adequate gonadotropin levels, the Leydig cells are not stimulated to secrete testosterone and sperm maturation is not promoted in the Sertoli cells. Spermatogenesis depends not only on appropriate stimulation by the gonadotropins but also on an appropriate response by the testes. Defects in testicular response to the gonadotropins result in decreased secretion of testosterone and inhibin B and, as a result of normal feedback mechanisms, high levels of circulating gonadotropins. In the absence of adequate testosterone levels, spermatoge-

Table 22-10 Volume and Characteristics of Semen

Characteristic	Normal Semen Quality	Marginal Semen Quality	Abnormal Semen Quality
Semen volume (ml)	2-5	1.5-1.9	<2 or >5
Sperm concentration (× 10^6 ml [million/ml])	≥50	20-49.9	<20
Sperm motility (% motility)	≥50 with forward progression; ≥25 with rapid linear progression within 60 min after collection	40-40.9	<40
Morphology (% with normal morphology)	≥30 oval head forms		<30

Data from McClure RD. In Tanagho EA, McAninch JW, editors: *Smith's general urology,* ed 14, Norwalk, Conn, 1995, Appleton & Lange.

nesis is impaired. Newer research demonstrates the significance of inhibin B as an important marker of the competence of Sertoli cells and spermatogenesis. Inhibin B is strongly correlated with severity of spermatogenic effects. A positive correlation exists between serum inhibin B levels and sperm concentration and testicular volume, and lower levels have been associated with azoospermia, testicular disorders, and infertility.[141]

Impaired spermatogenesis also can be caused by genetic disorders (such as Klinefelter syndrome), myotonic dystrophy, or testicular trauma. Other conditions associated with impaired spermatogenesis include systemic illness, such as renal failure, hepatic disease, or sickle cell disease; exposure to gonadotoxins, such as chemotherapy or radiation; varicocele; and cryptorchidism.

Fertility is adversely affected if spermatogenesis is normal but the sperm are chromosomally or morphologically abnormal or are produced in insufficient quantities. Chromosomal abnormalities are caused by genetic factors and by external variables, such as exposure to radiation or toxic substances. A sperm count of 20 million sperm per milliliter of semen has been suggested as the minimum concentration required for fertility. Average fertile men have 50 to 100 million sperm per milliliter.[103,140]

Sperm motility is another important variable affecting fertility. Motility appears to be affected by the sperm's chemical environment, that is, the characteristics of semen (Table 22-10). Prostatic dysfunction, excessive semen viscosity, presence of drugs or toxins in the semen, and presence of antisperm antibodies are associated with impaired sperm motility. Approximately 3% to 7% of infertile males have antisperm antibodies in their semen. Antisperm antibodies may develop as a result of epididymitis or other inflammation of the genitourinary tract, testicular injury or torsion, a previous vasectomy or biopsy, and cryptorchidism. Antisperm antibodies may be (1) cytotoxic antibodies, which attack sperm and reduce their number in the semen; or (2) sperm-immobilizing antibodies, which impair sperm motility and reduce their ability to traverse the endocervical canal. Intrinsic, biologic factors leading to the production of antisperm antibodies seem to play a greater role than extrinsic factors. The exact mechanism remains unclear.[140]

BOX 22-13

EVALUATION OF MALE PARTNER OF INFERTILE COUPLES*

Thorough history and physical, including imaging for varicocele
Two semen analyses and quantification of serum FSH, LH, testosterone levels, and prolactin if indicated
Semen and urethral cultures
Serum assays or monoclonal antibody testing for white blood cells
Immunobead monoclonal antibody test
Postcoital testing of semen activity and function
Sperm penetration assay
Inhibin B assays or testicular biopsy
Vasogram, TRUS, or other imaging studies

For an in-depth discussion see Kim ED, Lipshultz ED: Male infertility. In Copeland LJ, Farrell JF, editors: *Textbook of gynecology,* ed 2, Philadelphia, 2000, W.B. Saunders.

A male factor contributes to the cause of up to 50% of cases of infertility. As understanding of the male factor in infertility increases, evaluation becomes more complex and essential to appropriate treatment (Box 22-13). Treatment for impaired spermatogenesis involves correction of any underlying disorders and avoidance of radiation or toxins. Androgens, human gonadotropins, and antiestrogens (e.g., clomiphene citrate, tamoxifen citrate) may enhance spermatogenesis. Semen can be modified to improve sperm motility. If conception is desired, the semen is obtained by masturbation (or mechanical device),[140] after which it can be diluted, concentrated, or washed to remove antisperm antibodies. These alterations are followed by artificial insemination.

DISORDERS OF THE BREAST

Disorders of the Female Breast

Galactorrhea

Galactorrhea (inappropriate lactation) is the persistent and sometimes excessive secretion of a milky fluid from the breasts of a woman who is not pregnant or nursing an infant. Galactorrhea, which also can occur in men, may involve one or both breasts and is not associated with breast cancer.

The incidence of galactorrhea is difficult to estimate because of differences among definitions of the condition, examination techniques, and populations of women who have been studied. Prevalence has been documented as 0.1% to 32% of all women.

Pathophysiology

Galactorrhea is not a breast disorder per se. Rather, it is a manifestation of pathophysiologic processes elsewhere in the body. These processes are chiefly hormone imbalances caused by hypothalamic-pituitary disturbances, pituitary tumors, or neurologic damage. Exogenous causes include drugs, estrogen, and manipulation of the nipples. Inappropriate lactation caused by hyperprolactinemia is manifested by the spontaneous appearance of a milky secretion from multiple duct openings, usually from both breasts. Galactorrhea caused by oral contraceptives (OCs) is more likely to occur with high-dose OC use; is characterized by clear, serous, or milky discharge from multiple ducts; and is noticeable during the drug-free interval between OC packets. In premenopausal women, unilateral or bilateral spontaneous multiple duct discharge that increases before menstruation often is caused by fibrocystic change. Unilateral, spontaneous, serous or serosanguineous discharge from a single duct usually is caused by an intraductal papilloma; bloody discharge suggests cancer; bilateral, sticky, multicolored discharge from multiple ducts is often caused by duct ectasia; and purulent discharge indicates a subareolar abscess.[142]

The most common cause of galactorrhea is **nonpuerperal hyperprolactinemia,** or excessive amounts of prolactin in the blood not related to pregnancy or childbirth. Prolactin is a pituitary hormone that stimulates milk production. Nonpuerperal hyperprolactinemia can be caused by any factor that (1) stimulates or overstimulates the prolactin-secreting units of the pituitary gland; (2) interferes with production of **prolactin-inhibiting factor (PIF),** a neurotransmitter (probably dopamine) that inhibits prolactin secretion; or (3) interferes with pituitary receptors for PIF. A variety of exogenous agents and disorders can trigger one of these three mechanisms, thereby causing hyperprolactinemia (Box 22-14).

Several drugs can cause nonpuerperal hyperprolactinemia. They include phenothiazines, reserpine, methyldopa, exogenous estrogens (particularly in high-dose OCs), narcotics, and tricyclic antidepressants.

Hypothyroidism causes increased secretion of hypothalamic thyroid-releasing hormone (TRH), which stimulates prolactin release from the pituitary. Hypothyroidism also is associated with reduced metabolic clearance of prolactin, which prolongs its effects.

Many types of pituitary tumors cause hyperprolactinemia. Prolactinomas cause hyperprolactinemia by secreting prolactin, decreasing production of PIF, or putting pressure on the pituitary stalk such that delivery of PIF to the anterior pituitary is prevented. Growth hormone–secreting pituitary tumors may cause galactorrhea through the intrinsic lactogenic effect that growth hormone appears to have on mammary tissue. Prolactin-secreting lung and kidney tumors also cause hyperprolactinemia.

Chronic stress may cause hyperprolactinemia by inhibiting PIF release. Cervical spinal injuries, head trauma, encephalitis, meningitis, herpes zoster, or thoracotomy scars may stimulate the afferent portion of the suckling reflex arc, which is carried in the second to sixth thoracic nerves. The suckling reflex increases prolactin secretion.

Galactorrhea can be induced by persistent and repeated sucking or squeezing of the nipples and has been documented in women who manipulate their breasts and nipples daily.[143] Monthly examination of the breasts for nipple discharge usually is not associated with the development of galactorrhea.

BOX 22-14

COMMON CAUSES OF HYPERPROLACTINEMIA

PHYSIOLOGIC CAUSES

Exercise
Idiopathic
Pregnancy and postpartum period
Sleep (rapid eye movement [REM] phase)
Stress (trauma, surgery)
Suckling

DRUG CAUSES

Amoxapine
Amphetamines
Anesthetic agents
Butyrophenones
Cimetidine
Estrogens
Hydroxyzine
Methyldopa
Metoclopramide
Narcotics
Phenothiazines
Progestins
Reserpine
Tricyclic antidepressants
Verapamil

PATHOPHYSIOLOGIC CAUSES

Acromegaly
Chronic chest wall stimulation (e.g., postthoracotomy, postmastectomy, herpes zoster)
Cirrhosis
Hypothalamic disease
Hypothyroidism
Pressure on pituitary stalk
Prolactin-secreting tumors
Pseudocyesis (false pregnancy)
Renal failure (especially with zinc deficiency)
Spinal cord lesions

Clinical Manifestations

A small amount of breast milk expressed from the nipple of parous women usually is not a concern, and normal breast milk can be colors other than white. Inappropriate lactation is manifested by the appearance of a milky breast secretion in nonpregnant, nonlactating women from one or both breasts. Most women with galactorrhea experience menstrual abnormality. If a pituitary process is involved, the woman usually experiences hirsutism and infertility; if a hypothalamic lesion is present, she may report such CNS symptoms as intractable headache, visual field disturbances, sleep disturbances, and abnormal temperature, thirst, or appetite.[144]

Evaluation and Treatment

Galactorrhea requires evaluation (1) when it occurs in nulliparous women or in parous women who have not been pregnant or have not breast-fed for 12 months or (2) when it is associated with amenorrhea, headache, visual field abnormalities, or other symptoms implying systemic illness. The evaluation of galactorrhea includes a variety of diagnostic tests. When amenorrhea accompanies galactorrhea, the assessment is the same as for amenorrhea (see Fig. 22-1). Breast secretions are examined for fat globules and neoplastic cells to verify their source. Serum prolactin levels are measured. Because such variables as eating, sleeping, stress, and breast examinations all increase prolactin levels, at least two positive results are needed for a diagnosis of hyperprolactinemia. Prolactin levels greater than 25 to 30 ng/ml (by radioimmunoassay) are considered elevated. Those in the range of 75 to 100 ng/ml are considered to be caused by a pituitary tumor until proved otherwise. Serum thyroxine and thyroid-stimulating hormone levels are measured to rule out hypothyroidism, and LH and FSH levels are obtained if the individual is amenorrheic. CT, MRI, and carotid angiography may assist in the localization of adenomas.

Treatment for galactorrhea consists of identification and treatment of the cause. Medical and surgical therapies may be involved. If a pituitary microadenoma is found, it may be surgically removed, particularly if there has been progressive tumor growth, loss of visual field or acuity, cranial nerve dysfunction, increased intracranial pressure, cerebrospinal fluid leak or obstruction, or infertility. A microadenoma may be treated medically with bromocriptine (Parlodel). This drug controls the tumor but does not cure it, and it must be taken indefinitely. A pituitary macroadenoma usually is treated medically because surgical and radiologic therapies seldom succeed.

Benign Breast Conditions (Fibrocystic Changes)

Fibrocystic changes (FCC) is the most widely accepted term for physiologic nodularity and breast tenderness that waxes and wanes with the menstrual cycle.[145-147] It has become increasingly clear that FCC is a heterogeneous group of lesions that should be diagnosed separately. Microscopic findings of fibrocystic breasts generally include fibrosis, epithelial proliferation, and cyst formation. An estimated 50% to 80% of women normally experience some of these changes. The prevalence of fibrocystic lesions is probably related to hormonal changes, which in turn are affected by genetic background, age, parity, history of lactation, caffeine, and use of exogenous hormones.[145] Although FCC has been considered a risk for breast cancer, only types with epithelial proliferation (e.g., atypical hyperplasia) represent a true risk. For this reason, some authors omit atypical lobular hyperplasia and atypical ductal hyperplasia from their discussion of FCC because they may be considered precursor lesions of breast cancer.

BOX 22-15

CLASSIFICATION OF BREAST BIOPSY TISSUE ACCORDING TO RISK FOR BREAST CANCER

NO INCREASED RISK

Adenosis (sclerosing or florid)
- Apocrine metaplasia
- Macrocysts or microcysts
- Fibroadenoma
- Fibrosis

Mild hyperplasia (3-4 cells deep)
- Mastitis or periductal mastitis
- Squamous metaplasia

SLIGHTLY INCREASED RISK (1.5 TO 2.0 TIMES)

Moderate or florid hyperplasia
- Papilloma

MODERATELY INCREASED RISK (3 TO 5 TIMES)

Atypical hyperplasia (ductal or lobular)

In a review of more than 10,000 breast biopsies, 70% of the women did not have a lesion associated with an increased risk for cancer.[148] Only a small percentage (about 4%) had microscopic changes consistent with an increased risk of cancer. The most important variable on biopsies seemed to be the degree and character of epithelial proliferation. Women with atypical hyperplasia had a relative risk of 5.3, whereas women with atypia and a family history of breast cancer had a relative risk of 11. These findings are supported by those of the Nurses' Health Study. In this study, women whose biopsies showed proliferative disease and atypical hyperplasia had relative risks of 1.6 and 3.7, respectively.[149,150] The College of American Pathologists has classified biopsy tissue according to breast cancer risk. These classifications are listed in Box 22-15. In addition to FCC, many women experience benign breast tumors; these are outlined in Table 22-11 and illustrated in Fig. 22-42. In general, the frequency of chromosome abnormalities is lower in benign lesions than in breast cancer. Genetic aberrations are more common in proliferative than in nonproliferative lesions.[151]

Pathophysiology

Fibrocystic breast changes are of three major types: cystic, fibrous, and epithelial proliferative. **Cysts**, fluid-filled sacs, are the most common feature and are easily treated (Fig. 22-43). Cystic change can be induced in experimental animals by altering ratios of estrogens and progesterones. It is assumed therefore that breast cysts are the result of ovarian alterations, but the exact mechanism is unknown. A variety of substances are secreted into cyst fluid, including polypeptide hormones and both male and female sex steroid hormones. Cystic changes by themselves do not appear to be premalignant alterations; however, with gross cystic breast disease certain proteins in fluid are being used as markers of breast cancer.[152,153] **Gross cystic breast disease (GCBD)** is common in women, especially in the age range between 35 and the menopausal years.[154] Gross cystic disease fluid protein–15 (GCDFP-15), a protein in some breast cysts, and another

Table 22-11 Benign Breast Tumors

Benign Breast Tumor	Risk Factors	Pathophysiology	Clinical Manifestations	Treatment
Fibroadenoma	Puberty, early adulthood; occurs earlier and more frequently in young black women	Slow-growing lesion composed of variable proportions of epithelial and connective tissue; thought to be under influence of estrogen	Painless, firm, elastic, solitary, well-circumscribed mass ~ 1-5 cm in diameter	Excision with a person under local anesthesia; or careful observation
Phyllodes tumor	Middle age	Fibroepithelial tumor characterized by marked proliferation of connective tissue stroma and great size; initially slow growing; 10%-25% may be malignant	Spheric, firm, usually well-circumscribed, multinodular tumor with a diameter of 2-20 cm; trophic cutaneous ulceration is a late manifestation	Local excision of benign or small tumor; simple mastectomy if voluminous or malignant tumor
Intraductal papilloma	Ages 30-50 yr; relatively uncommon	Subareolar tumor consists of epithelial vegetation with central connective tissue axis; found in lactiferous duct	Spontaneous or induced watery, serous, or bloody nipple discharge; small soft, friable, yellow or red, ~ 5-mm, papillomatous growth attached to duct wall by short, thin stalk; rare nipple retraction	Excision of involved duct
Mammary duct ectasia	After menopause or during pregnancy and lactation	Principal lactiferous ducts become dilated and filled with cellular debris; secondary inflammatory reaction; possible rupture of ducts	Subareolar induration or nipple retraction; spontaneous, bloody, sticky, thick, multiple duct discharge; burning pain and swelling of areolar area; palpable mass after rupture	Antibiotic and antiinflammatory therapy
Fat necrosis	Ages 14-80 yr; average age 50 yr; increased in women with fatty, voluminous breasts; trauma	50% are posttraumatic; necrosis secondary to inflammation is more rare	Poorly circumscribed indurated area with yellow or gray necrotic foci	Local excision

protein (GCDFP-24) have recently been used as definitive markers for low-grade breast cancer.[154] Cysts develop more commonly in terminal ducts and lobules.

Fibrous tissue increases progressively until menopause and regresses thereafter. Cysts frequently rupture with release of secretory material into the adjacent tissue. The resulting chronic inflammation and scarring fibrosis contribute to the palpable firmness of the breast.[155] The fibrosis that occurs with cysts and epithelial proliferative lesions therefore is probably a normal process. In younger women it is the sole abnormality in approximately 5% of benign breast biopsy specimens.[156]

Included in the category of **epithelial proliferative disease** are a number of structurally diverse lesions, such as sclerosing adenosis, radial scar, and the lobular and ductal hyperplasias. These changes have the most epidemiologic similarity to breast cancer of all the changes in FCC and primarily carry the most risk for development of a carcinoma.[153]

Sclerosing adenosis is enlargement of one or more lobular units because of an increase in the number of alveolar ducts and an increase in the density of intralobular fibrous tissue. Occasionally, a mass is produced by aggregation of adjacent lobules or uncommonly by excessive enlargement of one lobule.[153] The lumen may contain microcalcifications. Although the differential diagnosis can be difficult from core-needle biopsies and frozen sections, the experienced pathologist using low-power microscopy will rarely confuse it with well-differentiated carcinoma. Calcifications are commonly found in cysts and adenosis and often form suspicious lesions on a mammogram.

Ductal hyperplasia is increased numbers of cells predominantly within the lumen of the terminal ducts and lobular units. It includes a continuum of changes ranging from an insignificant increase in cellularity to features characteristic of **ductal carcinoma in situ (DCIS),** in the latter case constituting a diagnosis of atypical ductal hyperplasia. Con-

A

B

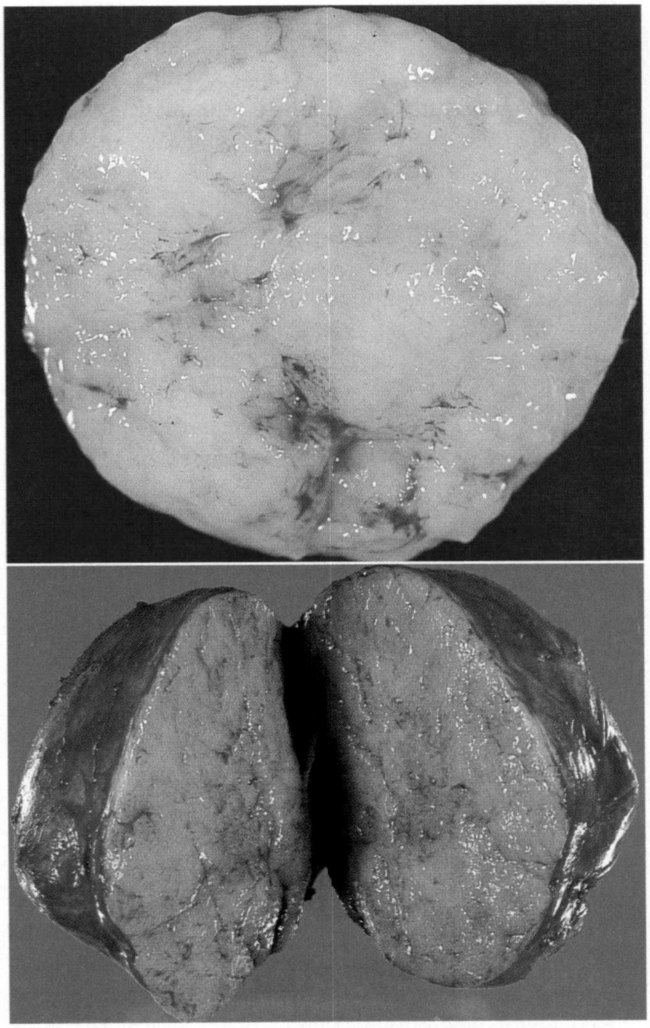

FIG. 22-42 Fibroadenoma. A, Myxoid type of fibroadenoma, showing pale, lobulated, translucent tissue. **B,** Juvenile fibroadenoma showing well-circumscribed mass of tan, fleshy, lobulated tissue. (From Damjanov I, Linder J, editors: *Anderson's pathology,* ed 10, St Louis, 1996, Mosby.)

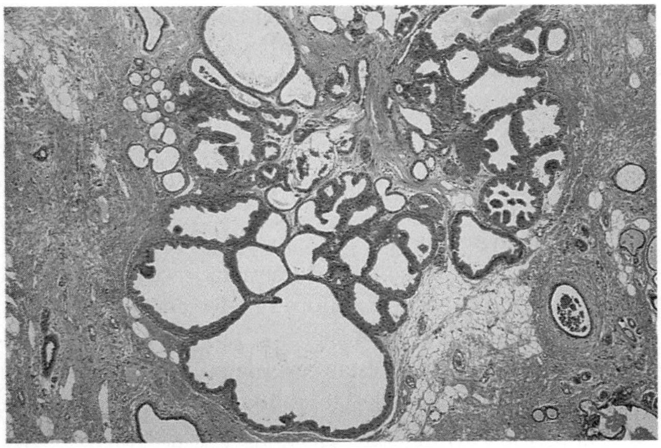

FIG. 22-43 Fibrocystic change. Dilated terminal duct and lobules are lined by epithelium that is either flattened or shows metaplasia. (From Damjanov I, Linder J: *Pathology,* St Louis, 2000, Mosby.)

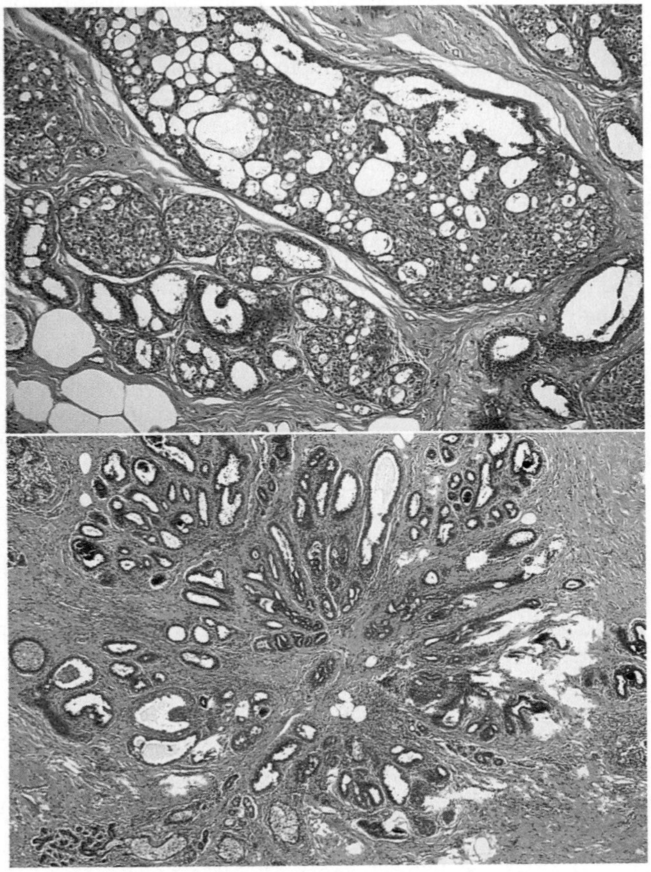

A

B

FIG. 22-44 Hyperplasia. A, Florid duct hyperplasia. The epithelial nests inside the ducts are partially solid and partially cystic. **B,** Radial scar. Central fibrosis is surrounded in a radiating manner by ductlike structures. (From Damjanov I, Linder J: *Pathology: a color atlas,* St Louis, 2000, Mosby.)

troversial is whether DCIS is really a cancer.[157] Experts do not agree because of recent findings that the mortality rate among women diagnosed with DCIS (1978 through 1983 and 1984 through 1989) was only 0.7% after 5 years and 1.9% after ten years.[158] These data indicate that the risk of death from breast cancer in women with DCIS is considerably lower than that of other forms of breast cancer. Thus some experts are of the opinion that about 80% or more of DCIS diagnoses, if left untreated (i.e., lumpectomy, mastectomy, radiation, chemotherapy, tamoxifen) will never proceed to cause death from cancer. The problem is the heterogeneity among types of DCIS, and therefore benign DCIS must be differentiated from problematic DCIS.[159]

Mild hyperplasia exists when there are one or two extra but often incomplete layers of epithelial cells and little or no dilation of the lumen. Moderate hyperplasia and **florid hyperplasia** describe increasing degrees of epithelial proliferation with dilation and filling of the structures (Fig. 22-44, *A*).

Radial scar refers to an irregular, radial proliferation of ductlike mammary epithelial structures with dense central fibrosis (Fig. 22-44, *B*). Radial scar has also been called *radial sclerosing lesions* and *sclerosing papillary proliferation.* Among women with atypical hyperplasia, as compared to women with nonproliferative disease, the relative risk of breast cancer was 5.8 for those with radial scars and 3.8 for those without radial scars. Radial scars are now considered an independent histologic risk factor for breast cancer.[160] The appearance in mammograms, as well as the gross and microscopic appearance, can cause it to be confused with infiltrating ductal carcinoma.[153]

Lobular hyperplasia refers to proliferation of small, uniform cells in the lumen of lobular units. Usually all structures within the lumen are uniformly affected. *Atypical* lobular hyperplasia is when the degree of proliferation and dilation approaches that of **lobular carcinoma in situ (LCIS)**.[153] LCIS has been associated with a moderately increased risk of invasive carcinoma.

Clinical Manifestations

Bilateral pain or tenderness is the most common complaint associated with fibrocystic changes. Discomfort and size of lesions increase as menstruation approaches. Multiple or bilateral masses with a history of transient breast lumps or cyclic pain are common. Symptoms are most common in women ages 30 to 50 years.

Evaluation and Treatment

Breast biopsy is used to make a definitive diagnosis and assess an individual's risk for the development of breast cancer. Mammography may be helpful, but the dense breast tissue frequently seen in young women can make interpretation extremely difficult. Sonography can be used to differentiate a solid mass from a cystic (fluid-filled) mass.

Treatment consists largely of relieving symptoms. The individual can minimize breast pain by wearing a brassiere that provides good support. Cystic pain is reduced by draining the cysts with the person under local anesthesia; however, given time the cysts may disappear without treatment. Many women find that the elimination or reduction of caffeine in their diet reduces both the pain and the nodularity. Women with breast pain also may benefit from a diet low in fat and high in complex carbohydrates.

Danazol, a synthetic androgen, has been used to treat individuals with severe pain caused by proliferative breast disease. Danazol is thought to minimize the hormonal fluctuations to which breast tissue is exposed. Avoidance of high levels of estrogen unopposed by low levels of progesterone may also decrease mutagenesis and proliferation. Depending on the type of progestin/progesterone used and the dose and duration of its application, progesterone may have a predominantly antiproliferative effect.[161-163] The antiproliferative effects are likely to be prerequisites of their function in promoting differentiation (i.e., instead of potential mutagenesis and proliferation).[164]

WHAT'S NEW? Mammographic Densities, Benign Breast Disease, and Breast Cancer Risk

Connective and epithelial tissues are radiologically dense and appear light, an appearance termed *mammographic density*. Mammographic dense tissue appears to indicate proliferation of breast epithelium, stroma, or both.

A large amount of evidence indicates that women with extensive areas of mammographic density are four to six times more likely to develop breast cancer than those with little or no mammographic density. To understand biologically why, investigators estimate the incidence of various histologic types of benign breast disease in relation to mammographic density. Mammographic density in more than 75% of the breast area was associated with an increased risk of incidence of hyperplasia without atypia and of atypical hyperplasia or carcinoma in situ. The relative risk of incident lesions for women with density in more than 75% of the breast was 13.85 for hyperplasia and 9.23 for atypical hyperplasia or carcinoma in situ. Therefore the association between mammographic density and breast cancer risk may be attributable, at least in part, to biologic processes inherent to these histologic features.

Data from Boyd N et al: Mammographic densities and the prevalence and incidence of histological types of benign breast disease. Reference Pathologists of the Canadian National Breast Screening Study, *Eur J Cancer Prev* 9(1):15, 2000.

Cancer

Breast cancer, the most common cancer in American women, is the leading cause of death in women ages 40 to 44 years and the second most common killer after lung cancer of women of all ages. The incidence of breast cancer has risen steadily since 1980 and is leveling off at about 110 cases per 100,000 women (30% of new cancers) (Fig. 22-45). Increased incidence is attributed to growing utilization of screening and diagnostic mammography and to earlier detection.[165] Lifetime risk of breast cancer is 1 in 8 (Table 22-12), with deaths remaining steady at 27.4 per 100,000 women.[165] These mortality rates are seen in white women and are lower in blacks.

Risk factors and possible causes of breast cancer can be classified as reproductive, hormonal, environmental, and familial (Box 22-16 and Table 22-13). Although high-risk populations can be identified, the majority (75%) of breast cancers occur in women whose only risk factors are gender and age.[16,166]

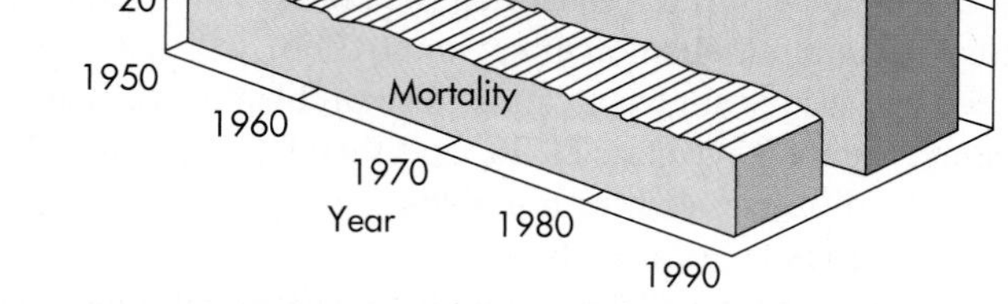

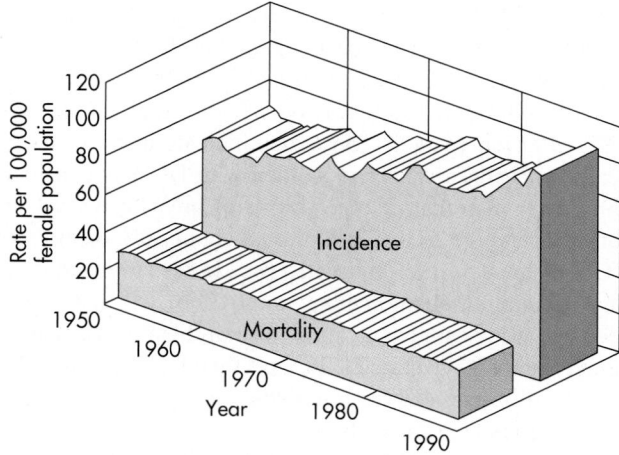

FIG. 22-45 Incidence and mortality rate of breast cancer. Increased incidence of breast cancer but stable mortality rate over the past 40 years. (Modified from Damjanov I, Linder J, editors: *Anderson's pathology,* ed 10, St Louis, 1996, Mosby.)

Reproductive Factors

A woman's age when her first child is born affects her risk for developing breast cancer—the younger she is, the lower the risk.[167] Pregnancies that do not proceed to term apparently have no protective effect. Women who have never given birth are at greater risk than those who have. The duration of a woman's reproductive life also affects her risk of developing breast cancer. Late menarche and early menopause (i.e., a short reproductive life) reduce risk (see Pathogenesis).

Hormonal Factors

The link between breast cancer and hormones is based on five factors that affect risk: (1) the protective effect of an early (i.e., in the twenties) first pregnancy; (2) the protective effect of removal of the ovaries and pituitary gland; (3) the increased risk associated with early menarche, late menopause, and nulliparity; (4) the relationship between types of fat, free estrogen levels, and oxidative changes in estrogen metabolism; and (5) the hormone-dependent development and differentiation of mammary gland structures (see Pathogenesis). The positive relation between endogenous hormone levels and risk of breast cancer supports a biologic mechanism for this relationship.[168] Oral contraceptive use and estrogen replacement therapy may be risk factors for breast cancer. The Collaborative Group on Hormone Replacement Therapy found that the risk of breast cancer increases with longer duration of unopposed estrogen use.[169] Controversial is the risk of breast cancer with hormone replacement therapy (i.e., combined estrogen and progesterone). The combination of continuous estrogen with interrupted or cyclic progestin (synthetic) increases sensitivity to both estrogen and progestin receptors in breast tissue.[170] A recent study found that the combined estrogen-progestin regimen (in which pro-

Table 22-12 Risk of Developing Breast Cancer

By Age (years)	By Ratio
25	1 in 19,608
30	1 in 2525
40	1 in 217
50	1 in 50
60	1 in 26
70	1 in 14
80	1 in 15
Ever*	1 in 8

Data from American Cancer Society. In *Cancer response system document #407002-407038,* New York, 1995, The Society.
*Lifetime risk.

BOX 22-16

SUMMARY: HEREDITARY BREAST CANCER

PREVALENCE: Approximately 12.5% of women will develop breast cancer during their lifetime. About 7% of these women have the hereditary form of breast cancer discussed here (i.e., about 1/150 to 1/200 women in the general population).

SURVIVAL: For all cases of breast cancer diagnosed in the United States from 1986 to 1992, the 5-year survival rates are 85% (whites) and 70% (blacks).

PRESENTATION: The hereditary form of breast cancer is more often bilateral and early onset (premenopausal) than nonhereditary breast cancer.

GENETICS: The mode of inheritance is autosomal dominant. Penetrance for females is 70% to 90% by age 70 years. Males also can be affected, but the penetrance is much lower. Several genes may cause hereditary breast cancer. The most important of these are the breast cancer susceptibility genes *BRCA1* and *BRCA2*. *BRCA1* has been cloned and is located on chromosome 17. Presence of this gene also increases the risk of ovarian cancer. *BRCA2* has been mapped to chromosome 13.

OTHER: *In general,* having one first-degree female relative (i.e., mother or a sister) affected with breast cancer *doubles* a female's risk of developing a breast tumor. If two first-degree relatives develop breast tumors before age 55 years, the risk increases to 54%.

Data from American Cancer Society: *Cancer facts and figures—1995,* Atlanta, 1995, The Society; Lindblom A: *Breast Cancer Res Treat* 34(2):171, 1995; Speroff L, Glass RH, Kase NG: *Clinical gynecologic endocrinology and infertility,* ed 5, Baltimore, 1994, Williams & Wilkins.

Table 22-13 Factors Associated With Increased Risk of Breast Cancer*

Category	Risk Factor	Relative Risk†
Race	Blacks have higher incidence up to age 40 yr; whites have higher incidence over age 40 yr	1.1-1.9
Family history	Breast cancer in first-degree relative before age 60 yr	2.0-3.0
	Premenopausal or bilateral breast cancer	> 4.0
	Breast cancer in two first-degree relatives	4.0-6.0
Previous medical history	Moderate or florid mammary hyperplasia	1.5-2.0
	Mammary papilloma	1.5-2.0
	Atypical mammary hyperplasia	4.0-5.0
Estrogen exposure	Early menarche (before age 12 yr)	1.1-1.9
	Late menopause (after age 55 yr)	1.1-1.9
	Postmenopausal estrogen therapy	1.4
	Oral contraceptive use	1.5
Pregnancy	Nulliparous or late first pregnancy (after age 35 yr)	1.1-1.9
Radiation exposure	Atomic bomb	3.0
	Repeated fluoroscopy	1.5-2.0
Obesity	Fat distribution	1.2
	Hormone levels	
Alcohol abuse	See text for explanation	1.4-2.0

*Normal lifetime risk in white women: 1 in 8.
†Relative risk is defined and discussed in Chapter 5.

gestin was used cyclically fewer than 15 days in the month) was associated with greater increases in breast cancer risk than estrogen alone.[171] Investigators hypothesize that cyclic use of progestins may increase the risk greater than continuous use because it increases sensitivity to both estrogen and progesterone receptors.

Insulin-like growth factors (IGFs) regulate cellular functions involving cell proliferation, differentiation, and apoptosis. Emerging evidence indicates that members of the IGF family, including IGF-I, IGF-II, the IGF-I receptor (IGF-IR), and IGF-binding proteins, play important roles in the development and progression of cancer. IGF-IR, overexpressed in cancer cells, mediates the effects of IGFs and plays a role in cell transformation.[172] IGFs are potent mitogens for estrogen receptor–positive breast cell lines. Interruption of IGF action can inhibit estrogenic stimulation of breast cancer cells. Thus there is cellular crosstalk between the insulin growth factors and estrogen receptors.[173] Interestingly, recent studies have found no evidence that lower intake of total fat decreased risk of breast cancer, but women with breast cancer eating more protein (but not red meat) increased survival.[174,175] This may have some relationship to changes in insulin-like growth factors. Hormones are discussed further in the pathogenesis section.

Environmental Factors and Diet

The environmental causes of breast cancer probably affect the glandular epithelial cells of the breast during the early differential stages from undifferentiated cells to alveolar buds and lobules (see Pathogenesis). During these early phases, mitotic activity and cell division are greater than later in life.[78] High doses of ionizing radiation are associated with an increased risk of breast cancer, especially if exposure occurs during adolescence or pregnancy. These are periods when breast cells are proliferating rapidly.

Conflicting data exist regarding a high-fat diet and breast cancer. Studies in animal models and recent observations in humans, however, have provided evidence that a high intake of ω-polyunsaturated fatty acids (ω-6 PUFAs) stimulates several stages in the development of mammary and colon cancer (and possibly prostate cancer), from an increase in oxidative DNA damage to effects on cell proliferation to free estrogen levels to hormonal catabolic products.[176-179] Conversely, fish oil–derived ω-3 fatty acids seem to *prevent* cancer by influencing the activity of enzymes and proteins related to intracellular signaling and, eventually, cell proliferation.[176] The incidence of breast cancer is significantly higher in populations with high fat intake than in those with low fat intake. Breast cancer is rare in Japan, but not in Japanese immigrants in the United States who adopt Western eating habits.

Investigators have identified potential carcinogens in breast fluid in normal women, especially cholesterol derivatives.[180] Breast fluid is the result of secretions from the cells lining the breast ducts. Breast ductal cells are where the majority of breast cancers develop.[181] These breast secretions have been related to the fat content of the diet. The levels of estrogens are also substantially higher in breast secretions than in blood.[181] Thus fat tissue in the breast may be a source of high concentrations of fat-soluble chemicals (including estrogens), some of which may be carcinogens.[181]

Prospective studies, however, have failed to demonstrate an association between dietary fat and breast cancer risk. Moreover, there is limited evidence that modest reductions in fat intake (less than 30% of caloric intake) reduce breast cancer risk.[182] Further studies are needed to evaluate the benefits of substantially lowering fat intake (20% or less of total calories) and the roles of micronutrient imbalances and childhood nutrition in the development of breast cancer. The role of obesity in breast cancer is complex and seems to be related

NUTRITION & DISEASE

Tumor-Protective Effects of ω-3 Polyunsaturated Fatty Acids and Monounsaturated ω-9 (Oleic Acid)

Dietary fats, specifically ω-6 polyunsaturated fatty acids (PUFAs) and ω-3 PUFAs, affect a variety of steps in the mutistage carcinogenesis process. The effects may be direct or indirect and include (1) peroxidation of double bonds in PUFAs, leading to oxidative stress (for example, oxygen free radicals) and reactive lipid peroxidation products that can cause DNA damage; (2) conversion of essential fatty acids to eicosanoids (prostaglandins, thromboxanes, leukotrienes, hydroxyl and hydroxyperoxy fatty acids), short-lived hormone-like lipids from primarily dietary linoleic acid (ω-6 found in vegetable seeds and oils such as safflower, sunflower, soybean, and corn) (see Fig. 22-49); (3) interaction of fatty acids with signal transduction pathways leading to altered gene expression; (4) with breast cancer, effects on unbound estrogenic metabolism; (5) effects on membrane-bound (lipid-bound) enzymes such as cytochrome P450 that regulate xenobiotic (for example toxic, mutagenic, and carcinogenic chemicals) (see Chapter 10) and estrogen metabolism; and (6) structural and functional changes in cell membranes resulting in alterations in hormone and growth factor receptors.

A reduction in total fat consumption has been shown to reduce circulating estradiol levels by 7% in premenopausal women and 23% in postmenopausal women in Western populations. Important may be the dietary balance between ω-3 and ω-6 fatty acids, especially in women. A diet high in ω-6 PUFAs was widely recommended until recently; its excess intake of ω-6 PUFAs (safflower, corn, soybean, peanut, cottonseed, borage, primrose, and sesame oils and mayonnaise and margarine) may have long-term effects, including neoplastic development, hyperinsulinemia, and atherosclerosis. The Mediterranean diet, higher in ω-3 PUFAs (such as fish oils) and monounsaturated fatty acid (oleic acid, an ω-9 highest in rapeseed and olive oil) are associated with lower rates of breast and colon cancer.

Data from Assmann G et al: International consensus statement on olive oil and the Mediterranean diet: implications for health in Europe, *Eur J Cancer Prev* 6:418, 1997; Bartsch H et al: Dietary polyunsaturated fatty acids and cancer of the breast and colorectum: emerging evidence for their role as risk modifiers, *Carcinogenesis* 20(12):2209, 1999; Latham P et al: Dietary ω-3 PUFA increases the apoptotic response to 1,2-dimethylhydrazine, reduces mitosis and suppresses the induction of carcinogenesis in the rat colon, *Carcinogenesis* 20:645, 1999; Schloss I et al: Dietary factors asssociated with a low risk of colon cancer in coloured West Coast fishermen, *S Afr Med J* 87:152, 1997; Wu AH et al: Meta-analysis: dietary fat intake, serum estrogen levels, and the risk of breast cancer, *J Natl Cancer Inst* 91:529, 1999; Yam D et al: Diet and disease—the Israeli paradox: possible dangers of high omega-6 polyunsaturated fatty acid diet, *Israel J Med Sci* 32:1134, 1996.

to fat distribution, type of fatty acids consumed, and sex hormone levels.[183]

Obesity has been associated with a *reduced* risk of *premenopausal* breast cancer. One mechanism suggested is the direct relationship between irregular menstrual cycling, especially anovulatory cycling and obesity. The anovulatory cycling would result in a decrease in both estrogens and progesterone and therefore a decreased risk of breast cancer. Some obese women have polycystic ovaries. With this condition they may have anovulatory cycling, abnormal menstrual periods, elevated androgens, hyperinsulinemia, and alterations in gonadotropic secretions. It is possible that higher insulin levels increase the enzymatic conversion of testosterone to dihydrotestosterone, rather than estradiol, lowering their estrogen levels.[181]

Obesity, however, is a factor for increasing the risk of breast cancer in *postmenopausal* women. In these women, levels of estrone are directly related to the degree of obesity. Weight gain from perimenopause to postmenopause is also associated with higher estradiol and estrone levels.[181] Estrogen is fat soluble, and therefore a greater degree of fatness that would occur with obesity and aging would also result in a greater storage of estrogens in fat tissue, including fat tissue in the breast.[181] The primary source of estrogen in postmenopausal women is the metabolism of androstenedione (e.g., to estrone), primarily in fat tissue. Another factor relevant to obesity and breast cancer is obesity during childhood or adolescence, which results in a younger age of menarche and, if a later age of menopause (e.g., 55 years), a longer tissue exposure to hormones.

Chemicals in the environment that have a hormone-like effect may increase the risk of breast cancer and other hormone-related cancers.[181] The most significant chemicals may be polychlorinated hydrogens, such as dichlorodiphenyltrichloroethane (DDT). Such chemicals are fat soluble, and the estrogenic effect would require that they bind to the nuclear estrogen receptor and then cause cell division or gene transcription. Because the amount of these environmental estrogens is minute, their effect must be secondary to an abnormal (e.g., mutagenic) response of the estrogen receptor and DNA. Studies have not found an increased risk of breast cancer with exposure to chemicals.[184,185] Because fat-soluble chemicals are transported with lipoproteins (e.g., high-density lipoproteins [HDLs]) in blood and will be higher in women with high lipoprotein levels, as well as obese women, investigators *must* include their measures in studies. So far, these studies have not included lipoprotein levels or the degree of body fat. Further, a long-term follow-up (30 years) of women who were exposed to DES shows a minute increased risk of breast cancer (relative risk 1.35) and no increasing risk over time.[181]

Several studies have shown some correlation between breast cancer and alcohol ingestion. In a large population-based case-control study that included Maine, Massachusetts, New Hampshire, and Wisconsin, recent alcohol consumption and lifetime alcohol consumption were associated with breast cancer risk.[186] The relative risk of developing breast cancer ranged from 1.29 for one alcoholic drink per day to 2.3 for about two drinks per day. The relationship between alcohol and breast cancer risk appears to be present in several forms of alcoholic beverages, but their effects are primarily among premenopausal women.[181] A recent study, however, found that consumption of red wine that is rich in polyphenols could have an antiproliferative effect on breast cancer cell growth.[187] Differences in alcohol intake, however, explain only a small fraction of breast cancer rates.[181,188] A recent, large epidemiologic study found that alcoholic women had a small (15%) increase in breast cancer incidence compared with the general female population.[189]

The mechanisms by which alcohol increases the risk of breast cancer are unknown. Alcohol may hinder the liver's ability to rid the body of cancer-causing agents, impair the body's immune system, or make breast tissue more susceptible to cancer cells. Alcohol stimulates liver enzyme activity, and greater sulfation of estrone thus increases estrones' availability and possibly breast exposure to greater levels of estrone/estradiol.[181] Growth factor systems (ligands and receptors) may be targets of ethanol toxicity.[190] Alcohol combined with estrogen replacement therapy may synergistically enhance the risk. Alcohol can downregulate the expression of *BRCA1* (i.e., the unmutated tumor-suppressor gene), a potent inhibitor of estrogen receptor–α activity, thus increasing estrogen responsiveness.[191] Another mechanism is the possibility that increasing levels of alcohol decrease melatonin levels at night, which might increase circulating estrogen (as well as decrease sleep).[192] It is not known whether decreasing or stopping alcohol consumption in midlife decreases the risk of breast cancer. A recent prospective study found that the excess risk of breast cancer associated with alcohol consumption may be reduced by adequate folate intake. In this study, the risk of breast cancer associated with alcohol was strongest among women with a folate intake less than 300 μg/day.[193]

Familial Factors and Tumor-Related Genes

A history of breast cancer in first-degree relatives (mother or sister) increases a woman's risk two to three times. Risk increases even more if two first-degree relatives are involved, especially if the disease occurred before menopause and was bilateral. In some families, breast cancer occurs at an earlier age and the frequency of bilateral tumors is greater. The presence of breast cancer susceptibility genes is responsible for 5% to 10% of all breast cancer. This figure translates into an estimated prevalence of 200,000 to 600,000 women in the United States.[194] Hereditary breast cancer is transmitted in an autosomal dominant manner (Fig. 22-46). Investigators estimate that 45% of families with apparent autosomal dominant transmission of breast cancer susceptibility and about 90% of families with dominant inheritance of both breast and ovarian cancer harbor *BRCA1* germline mutations.[195] If the median age of onset of breast cancer in families is less than 45 years, the percentage of breast cancer–only families (i.e., do not include ovarian cancer) that are attributed to *BRCA1* mutations rises to almost 70%.[195]

Genes important to the development of cancer regulate diverse cellular pathways, including the progression of cells

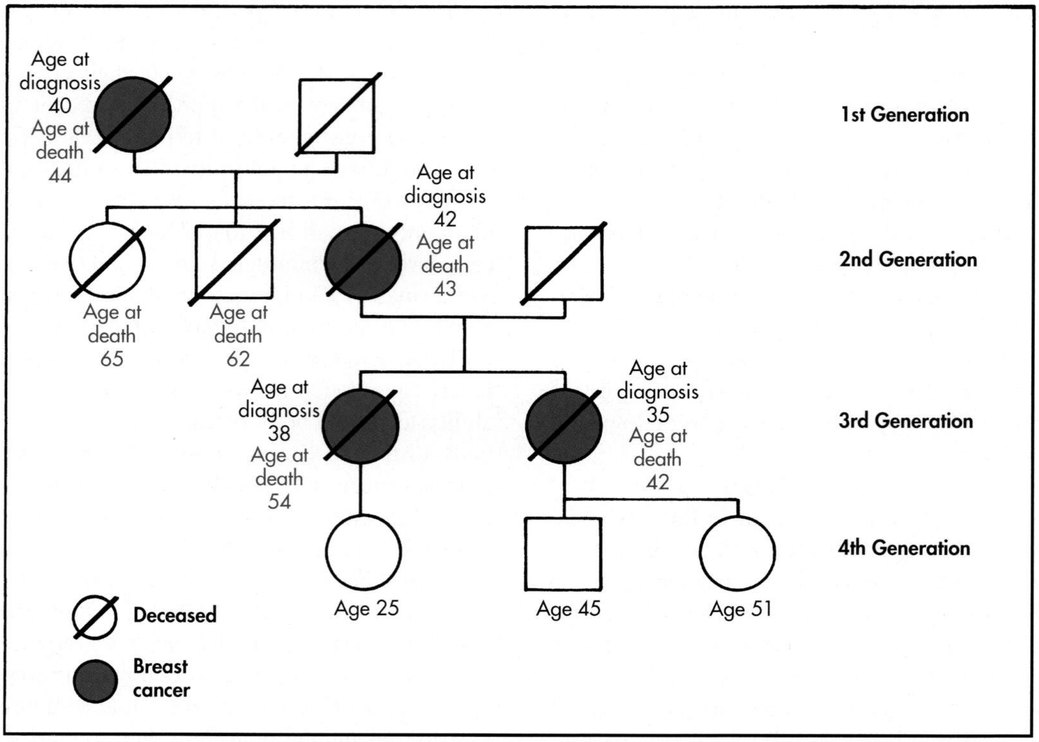

FIG. 22-46 Example of family pedigree for breast cancer. Family pedigree showing cases of breast cancer associated with typical dominant transmission of breast cancer. Other possible genetic alterations related to risk of breast cancer include changes in *p53* and alterations in the estrogen receptor. Numerous somatic mutations in the expression of oncogenes in breast cancer cells have been reported.

through the cell cycle, resistance to apoptosis, and the response to signals that direct cellular differentiation.[196] The inactivation of genes (e.g., tumor-suppressor genes) that contribute to the stability of the genome, itself, can favor errors in other genes that regulate proliferation. The importance of this latter pathway is exemplified by two recent studies linking the function of the *BRCA1* gene with that of the gene for ataxia-telangiectasia mutation (ATM) (Fig. 22-47). A possible new breast cancer susceptibility gene is now being validated on chromosome 13.[197]

Other tumor-related genes include *p53, Bcl-2, HER2,* and *c-myc.* Cells with functional *p53* die by apoptosis, whereas cells lacking *p53* continue to proliferate (see Fig. 11-6). About 40% of breast carcinomas reveal high levels of stabilized, often mutant *p53* protein in their cells; *p53*-related defects in tumor cells correlate with a poor prognosis.

Bcl-2 is a proto-oncogene. *Bcl-2* production decreases or inhibits apoptosis and thereby promotes breast and other cancers. However, the College of American Pathologists has classified it as belonging to category III, meaning insufficient evidence supports it as a prognostic factor.[198]

HER2 protein is overproduced in 25% to 30% of breast cancer cells. It transmits a growth signal to the nucleus. Trastuzumab (Herceptin) blocks the signal, thereby decreasing the growth of the tumor.

C-myc is a proto-oncogene expressed in eukaryotic cells and belongs to the immediate, early growth response genes that are rapidly induced when quiet cells receive a signal to divide. Mutation of *c-myc* is amplified in breast, colon, lung, and many other cancers.

Pathogenesis

Breast cancer is as diverse as the breast itself. Table 22-14 lists the different types of breast carcinomas and summarizes their major characteristics. Most breast cancers arise from the ductal epithelium. Tumors of the infiltrating ductal type do not grow to a large size, but they metastasize early. This type accounts for 70% of breast cancers.

Breast cancer is a disease of the glandular epithelium, and pathogenesis probably involves two or three steps. First, modifications of the DNA of the breast epithelial ductal cells are caused by either genetic alterations, environmental agents, or their interactions. The initiated changes in DNA may occur early in a woman's life—before full differentiation of the breast tissue.[181] Second, growth factors increase the rate of growth of premalignant to malignant cells—the most important of which are estrogen and possibly progesterone. Breast cells produce other growth factors, including IGF, TGF-α, EGF, platelet-derived growth factor, and TGF-β (Fig. 22-48). The production of these factors is to some degree regulated by estrogen.[181] Third, specific oncogenes are progressively modified or specific suppressor genes are lost, leading to advanced metastatic disease.

Unlike most human organs, which are differentiated by the end of fetal life, development and differentiation of the mammary gland occur after puberty. The mammary gland at

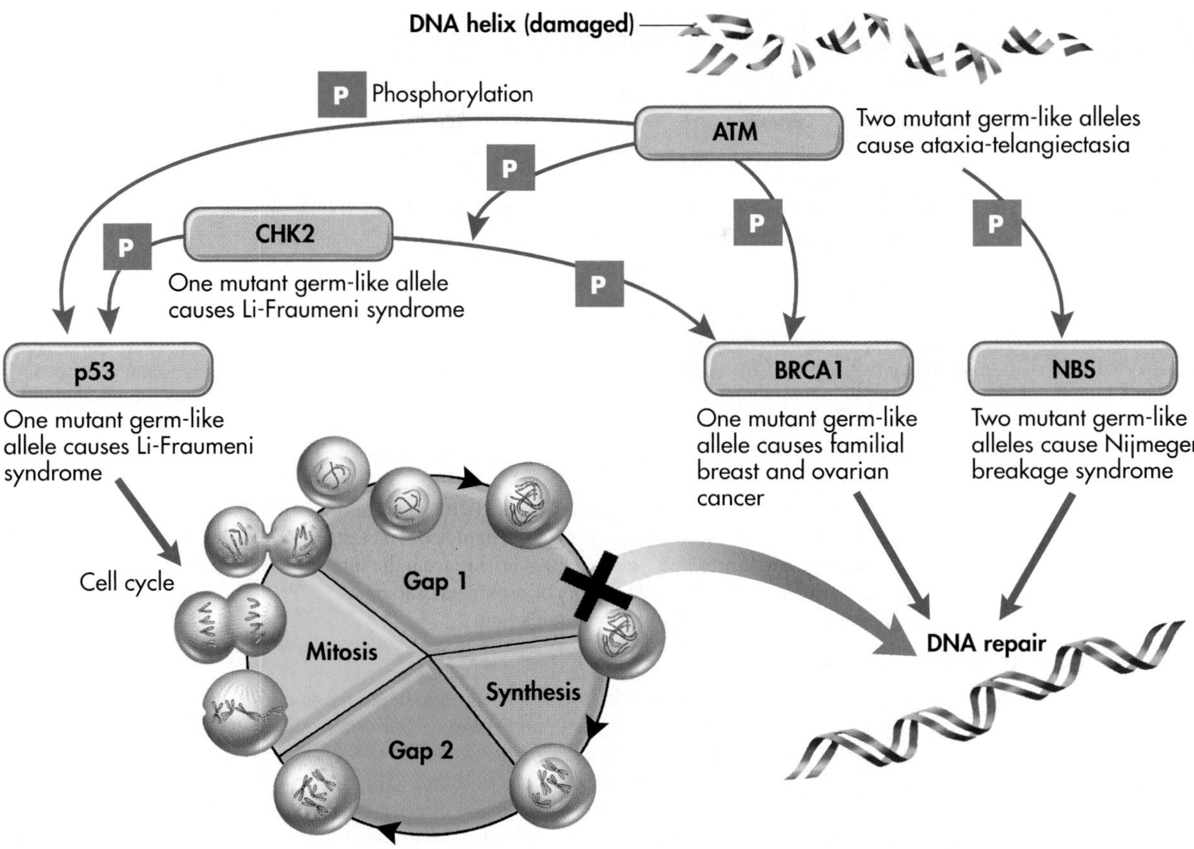

FIG. 22-47 Mutations in genes that regulate cellular proliferation and repair of DNA and lead to breast carcinogenesis. The ataxia-telangiectasia mutated (ATM) gene encodes a protein kinase that activtes (through phosphorylation) the tumor-suppressor *p53* protein either directly or indirectly by activating *CHK2* (a gene that encodes a protein kinase that activates *p53* by adding a phosphate group to it) in response to damage to DNA. The *p53* protein then triggers the arrest of the cell cycle, increasing time for DNA to be repaired. More simply, the ATM gene is necessary to accomplish DNA repair. The *BRCA1* and Nijmegan breakage syndrome (NBS) proteins are also activated by the ATM gene and are thought to be directly involved in the repair of damaged DNA. The inactivating mutations in the genes that encode these proteins increase the risk of breast cancer. (Adpated from Haber D: Roads leading to breast cancer, *N Engl J Med* 343(21):1566, 2000. Copyright © 2000 Massachusetts Medical Society. All rights reserved.)

birth is formed by primary mammary ducts that branch during childhood. At premenarche the duct epithelium proliferates. At menarche, under the influence of progesterone and presumably estrogen, terminal duct tubular units (acini) are formed. Acini are the dynamic structure of the mammary gland (see Fig. 21-20). The number of these acini increases at each menstruation with new budding of structures until approximately 35 years of age.[199,200]

With pregnancy there is an increase in the number of acini, resulting in full differentiation of their structure and function. When pregnancy does not happen, full differentiation of the breast may never be attained. Recently, investigators treated young, virgin rats with hCG, which increases during pregnancy. The treatment induced profuse lobular development of the mammary gland, reduced proliferative activity, and induced the synthesis of inhibin, a secreted protein with tumor-suppressor activity.[201] Thus hCG may induce early DNA changes that control the progression of the differentiation pathway and decrease the risk of breast cancer. At menopause, acini, as well as interlobular fibrous tissues, undergo atrophy, but the large and intermediate duct system persists.[199] Involution of the glandular epithelium continues, and the breast becomes composed mainly of large ducts, increased connective tissue, and fat.

Mammary epithelial cells achieve rapid renewal by a small number of mitotic divisions of immortal stem cells. (Cell renewal is discussed in Chapters 1 and 10.) Because the number of mutations is proportional to the rate and number of stem cell divisions, factors that accelerate cell division can have a carcinogenic effect. Hormones may act as accelerators and influence the susceptibility of the breast epithelium either endogenously or to environmental carcinogens, because hormones control the differentiation of the mammary gland epithelium and thereby regulate the rate of stem cell division. Current knowledge of the mechanisms of differentiation of the mammary gland suggests that especially estrogens and possibly progesterone may be involved in breast carcinogenesis. This hypothesis is supported by two facts: (1) the increased incidence of breast cancer in women (e.g., 100 times more frequent in women than in men) and (2) the association of breast cancer with the events of reproductive life.

Table 22-14 Types of Breast Carcinomas and Major Distinguishing Features

Histologic Type	Distinguishing Features
CARCINOMA OF MAMMARY DUCTS	
Papillary	Well-delineated cystic masses in multiple areas; hemorrhage often present; majority appear in 40- to 60-yr age-group; often involves skin
Intraductal (comedo)	Often accompanied by evidence of infection; well-circumscribed tumors within the duct; well-differentiated tumor cells; rarely ulcerates the skin
Infiltrating Carcinoma	
Ductal	Fibrous, firm, glistening, gray-tan mass with chalky streaks, mixture of patterns; causes discharge from the nipple; represents about 70% of all breast cancer
Mucinous	Usually large (>3 cm in diameter), circumscribed, and encapsulated, glistening appearance, varies in color; two types: pure and mixed; pure tumor is surrounded by mucin; infrequent; found in the lateral half of the breast; tends to occur in women after age 70 yr
Medullary	Encapsulated and grows to be very large (7-8 cm in diameter); commonly infiltrates lymphoid tissue; occurs after age 50 yr
Tubular	Well differentiated with orderly tubules in center (stroma) of mass; associated with noninfiltrating ductal carcinoma; occurs in women about 50 yr of age; nodal metastasis infrequent; occurrence rare
Adenoid cystic	Very rare; well-circumscribed, painless mass arising from the nipple and areola
Metaplastic	Involves cartilage or bone; mixed tumors or osteogenic sarcomas
Squamous cell	Frequent in blacks; originates in ductal epithelium
CARCINOMA OF MAMMARY LOBULES	
Lobular carcinoma in situ	Found in individuals with fibrocystic disease; localized to upper breast quadrants; risk of 10%-35% becoming invasive; occurs frequently in mid-40s; infiltrating variety occurs in early 50s
Infiltrating lobular	Infiltrates from duct; firm mass with chalky streaks
Paget disease	Eczema of the nipple that extends to the areola; cancer usually found underneath the nipple; poorly circumscribed; large Paget cells arise from the duct and directly invade nipple; history of scaly, red rash spreading from the nipple; lesion palpable beneath the nipple, often bilateral; occurs in middle age
Inflammatory carcinomas	Not a histologic type; fairly diffuse within the breast tissue, diffuse edema of the overlying skin; extremely undifferentiated, very rare, most metastasize to axilla
Sarcoma of the Breast	
Cytosarcoma phyllodes	Usually large (>17 cm in diameter); mostly localized but can rupture through the skin; rarely metastasizes to lymph nodes; history of painless nodule present for years before it forms a large mass; ulceration and bleeding of skin often present; occurs in wide age range (ages 13-77 yr)
Fibrosarcoma	Well circumscribed, firm, and usually does not involve the skin or nipple; well differentiated to extremely undifferentiated; arises from connective tissue; extremely rare (e.g., liposarcoma, angiosarcoma)

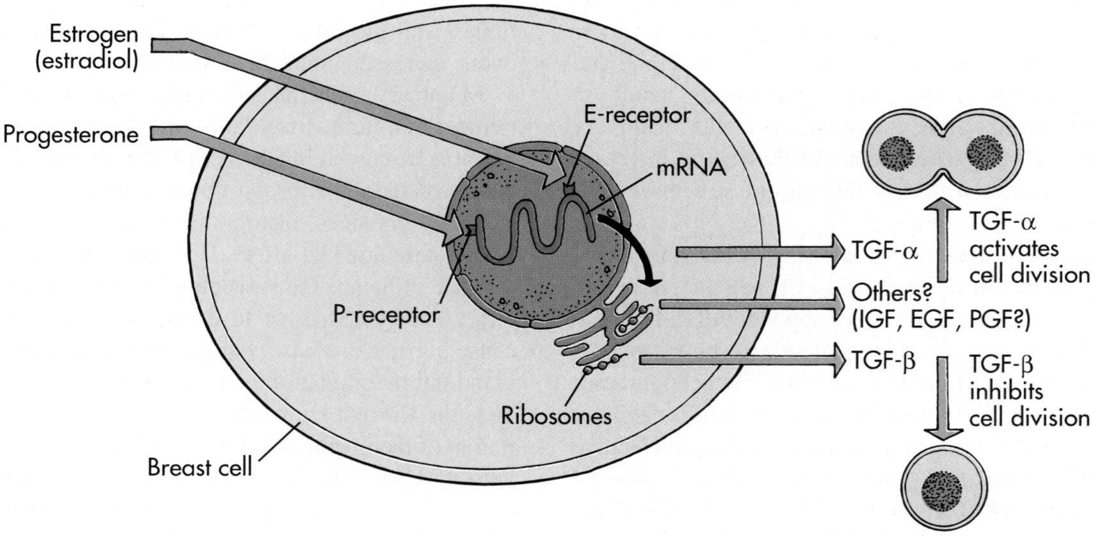

FIG. 22-48 Control of breast cell growth. Two levels of control of breast cell growth: (1) paracrine signaling by estrogen *(E-receptor)* and progesterone *(P-receptor)* steroids and (2) autocrine signaling by locally secreted growth factors, such as transforming growth factor (*TGF-α* and *TGF-β*) and others, including insulin-like growth factor *(IGF)*, epidermal growth factor *(EGF)*, and platelet-derived growth factor *(PGF)*. *mRNA*, Messenger ribonucleic acid.

WHAT'S NEW? Estradiol-Mediated Alterations of Immune Responses

Estrogens can modulate immune responses and immune-mediated diseases, which can predispose to cancer and the development of autoimmune disorders. The mechanisms include pro-oxidant conditions occurring in the course of inflammatory processes. At physiologic doses estradiol (E2) potently induces interleukin-1α (IL-1α), a cytokine that can initiate a cascade of other cytokines, chemotactic factors, and growth factors. Chemotactic factors cause infiltration of phagocytes, which can activate many other cytokines, reactive oxygen species, and reactive nitrogen species. Conversely, E2 inhibits IL-1α–induced IL-6 production. Hence, by suppressing IL-6 formation, E2 increases human epithelial cell proliferation while it also inhibits the activity of natural killer cells, thus enabling tumor growth. E2 mediates macrophage proliferation and decreases cell differentiation. Each of these processes can encourage tumor cell development.

From Cavalieri E et al: Chapter 4: estrogens as endogenous genotoxic agents—DNA adducts and mutations, *J Natl Cancer Institute Monogr* 27:75, 2000; Cutolo M et al: Estrogens, the immune response and autoimmunity, *Clin Exp Rheumatol* 13:217, 1995; Griffiths HR, Lunec J: Molecular aspects of free radical damage in inflammatory autoimmune pathology. In Aruoma OI, Halliwell B, editors: *Molecular biology of free radicals in human disease,* London, 1998, OICA International; Mor G et al: Macrophages, estrogen, and the microenvironment of breast cancer, *J Steroid Biochem Mol Biol* 67:403, 1998; Stadnyk K: AW cytokine production by epithelial cells, *FASEBJ* 8:1041, 1994.

The period of highest proliferative activity of mammary epithelium stem cells is during each ovulatory cycle between puberty and either the first full-term pregnancy or menopause among nulliparous women. The greatest increase in mitotic activity in the breast is during the luteal phase. During the estrogen follicular phase, terminal ductules are few and there is no mitotic activity. During the luteal phase, because of the increased progesterone levels, perhaps on the background of estrogen priming (i.e., cyclic progesterone increases sensitivity of estrogen receptors) or as a result of cooperation between the two hormones, there is increased mitotic activity.[181,197,202] A large body of evidence is accumulating that estrogens induce various types of DNA damage in vitro and in vivo (see What's New? Estradiol-Mediated Alterations in Immune Responses). Although estrogen-induced cell proliferation undoubtedly has an important role in estrogen carcinogenesis, other pathways involving indirect or direct DNA toxicity (i.e., genotoxicity) originate from estrogen metabolites (Box 22-17). Among the metabolites formed during the process of estrogen metabolism and elimination, some are estrogenic (i.e., 4-hydroxycatechol) and some may be protective (i.e., 2-methoxyestrones) through their antioxidant properties or growth and angiogenesis inhibitory activities and promotion of apoptosis.[203] Conversely, the more reactive quinone metabolites are able to form direct adducts (i.e., when carcinogen binds to the DNA) with DNA and may cause oxidative damage to lipids and DNA through redox cycling processes producing reactive oxygen species

BOX 22-17
ESTROGEN CARCINOGENESIS

STANDARD THEORY

Estrogen and perhaps progesterone affect the rate of cell division and thus affect the risk of breast cancer by causing proliferation of breast epithelial cells. Proliferating cells are susceptible to genetic errors during DNA replication; if uncorrected, these errors can ultimately lead to a malignant phenotype.

UPDATED THEORY

Although estrogen-induced proliferation undoubtedly has an important role in the carcinogenic process, mounting evidence supports a complementary pathway involving direct and indirect genotoxicity originating from estrogen metabolites (for example, 4-hydroxy catechol):

- *Indirect:* Oxidative DNA damage through redox cycling leads to reactive oxygen species
- *Direct:* Estrogen-quinone DNA adducts (see Fig. 22-47)

Protective effects: perhaps through 2-methoxy catechol estrogen-mediated growth inhibition, apoptosis, and antiangiogenesis

Data from Feigelson HS, Henderson BE: Estrogens and breast cancer, *Carcinogenesis* 17:2279, 1996.

(Fig. 22-49).[203-205] Estrogen-dependent breast cancer growth may be regulated by positive growth stimulators, such as TGF-α, and negative (inhibiting) growth stimulators, such as TGF-β.[198,206] (The role of other growth factors and hormones on breast mitotic activity may also be important.)

Thus it can be suggested that the risk of carcinogenic mutations is proportional to the *time* required for all stem cells to undergo differentiation. The risk then would be proportional to the duration of the interval separating menarche from the first full-term birth and to the number of ovulatory cycles during this period of time.[199] In human studies an increased risk of breast cancer is associated with young age at menarche, later age at menopause, or longer duration of ovulatory activity. Likewise, a protective effect or decreased risk of breast cancer is associated with young age at first live birth; full-term birth shifts the mammary gland from a proliferative state with high susceptibility to carcinogens to a low-proliferative, low-risk state.[176,199]

Approximately 50% of carcinomas of the breast occur in the upper outer quadrant because most of the glandular tissue of the breast is there (Fig. 22-50). The lymphatic spread of cancer to the opposite breast, to lymph nodes in the base of the neck, and to the abdominal cavity is caused by obstruction of the normal lymphatic pathways or destruction of lymphatic vessels by surgery or radiation. The less common inner-quadrant tumors may spread to mediastinal nodes or Rotter nodes, which are located between the pectoral muscles. Internal mammary chain nodes are frequent sites of metastasis.

Metastases from the vertebral veins can involve the vertebrae, pelvic bones, ribs, and skull. The lungs, kidneys, liver, adrenal glands, ovaries, and pituitary gland are also sites of metastasis.

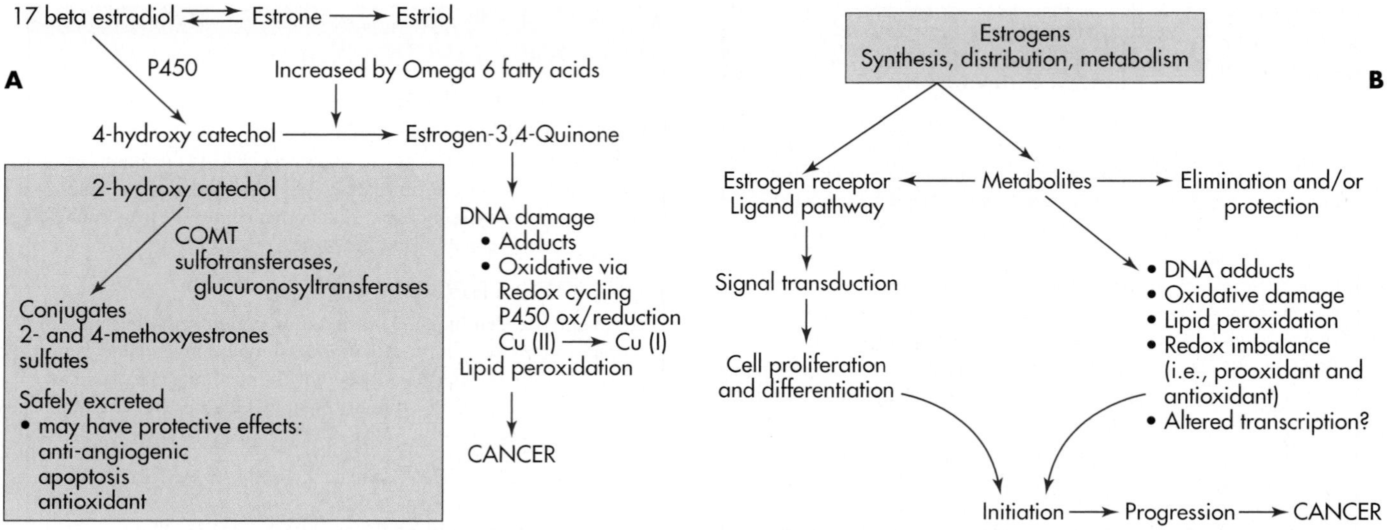

Fig. 22-49 Metabolites of estrogen and their associated carcinogenic effects. A, Metabolites of estrogen and carcinogenic pathway. Genotoxicity can be produced by the 4-hydroxy catechol metabolite. Unstable polyunsaturated fats (ω-6) can increase the production of quinones. Unstable ω-6 fatty acids can be transformed by the effects of oxygen and heat into carriers of free radicals. 2-hydroxy catechol, when methylated, may have protective effects against tumor development. Several enzymes are involved with the metabolism of estrogen, including specific cytochrome P450 isoforms, sulfotransferases, and catechol-*O*-methyltransferase (COMT). These enzymes may be influenced by environmental factors, including fats, alcohol, and xenobiotic exposures. These enzymes also are polymorphic and their distributions may differ among different ethnic populations. **B,** Estrogen receptor and estrogen metabolites on cancer initiation and progression. (**B,** Adapted from Yager JD: Endogenous estrogens as carcinogens through metabolic activation, *J Natl Cancer Institute Monogr* 27:67, 2000.)

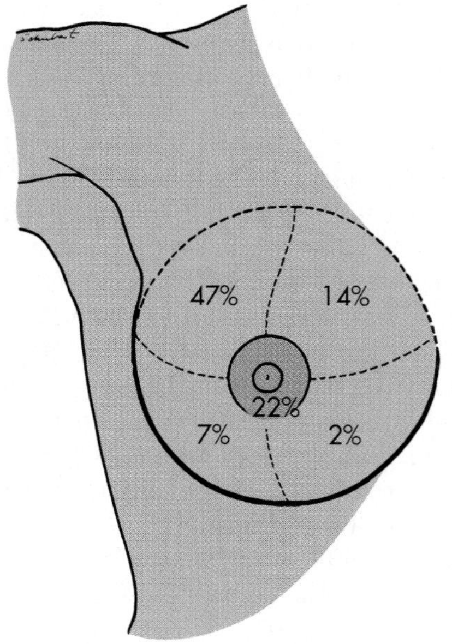

Fig. 22-50 Distribution of carcinomas in different areas of the breast. (From del Regato JA, Spjut HJ, Cox JD: *Ackerman and del Regato's cancer: diagnosis, treatment, and prognosis,* ed 6, St Louis, 1985, Mosby.)

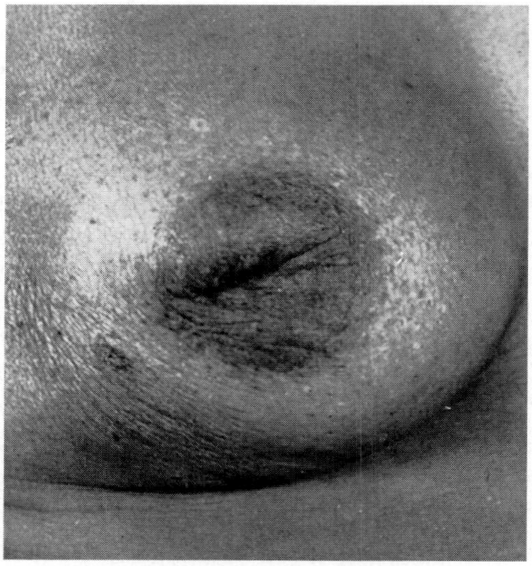

Fig. 22-51 Retraction of nipple caused by carcinoma. (From del Regato JA, Spjut HJ, Cox JD: *Ackerman and del Regato's cancer: diagnosis, treatment, and prognosis,* ed 6, St Louis, 1985, Mosby.)

Clinical Manifestations

The first sign of breast cancer is usually a painless lump. Lumps caused by breast tumors do not have any classic characteristics. Other signs include palpable nodes in the axilla, retraction of tissue (dimpling) (Fig. 22-51), or bone pain caused by metastasis to the vertebrae. Table 22-15 summarizes the clinical manifestations of breast cancers. Manifestations vary according to the type of tumor and stage of disease.

Evaluation and Treatment

Mammography, percutaneous needle aspiration, biopsy or minimally invasive biopsy called **mammotome**, palpation,

Table 22-15 Clinical Manifestations of Breast Cancer

Clinical Manifestation	Pathophysiology
Chest pain	Metastasis to the lung
Dilated blood vessels	Obstruction of venous return by a fast-growing tumor; obstruction dilates superficial veins
Dimpling of the skin	Can occur with invasion of the dermal lymphatics because of retraction of Cooper ligament or involvement of the pectoralis fascia
Edema	Local inflammation or lymphatic obstruction
Edema of the arm	Obstruction of lymphatic drainage in the axilla
Hemorrhage	Erosion of blood vessels
Local pain	Local obstruction caused by the tumor
Nipple/areolar eczema	Paget disease
Nipple discharge in a nonlactating woman	Spontaneous and intermittent discharge caused by tumor obstruction
Nipple retraction	Shortening of the mammary ducts
Pitting of the skin (similar to the surface of an orange *[peau d'orange]*)	Obstruction of the subcutaneous lymphatics, resulting in the accumulation of fluid
Reddened skin, local tenderness, and warmth	Inflammation
Skin retraction	Involvement of the suspensory ligaments
Ulceration	Tumor necrosis

Data from Griffiths MJ, Murray KH, Russo PC: *Oncology nursing: pathophysiology, assessment, and intervention,* New York, 1984, Macmillan.

ultrasonography, and hormone receptor assays are generally used in evaluating breast cancer (Fig. 22-52). Mammography has low specificity in distinguishing between malignant and benign lesions.[207] Responding to the need for earlier, more accurate, and cost-effective methods for cancer detection, investigators are studying alternative methods, including digital mammography, MRI, and ultrasound.[208] The benefits of mammography are unknown in women over 70 years of age and are still debated in those between 40 and 49 years of age. Biopsy is the definitive diagnostic test.

Treatment is based on the extent or stage of the cancer (Box 22-18). The extent of the tumor at the primary site, the presence and extent of lymph node metastasis, and the presence of distant metastases are all evaluated to determine the stage of disease. A new, gentler drug, Herceptin, is available in those women who produce the protein *HER2* (see p. 766). Herceptin blocks the growth-promoting signal produced by *HER2.*

Little is known regarding how dietary factors affect the survival of women with breast cancer. As previously discussed, an increased ratio of ω-3 to ω-6 fatty acids can decrease growth of breast cancer. It is postulated that to minimize oxidative radicals, further dietary supplementation with vitamin E and a retinoid is likely to increase the effectiveness of such a diet.[209] In addition, a recent study found that women eating more protein (but not red meat) increased their survival.[175] Avoidance of hyperinsulinemia, insulin resistance, and the production of insulin-like growth factors may also provide new approaches to cancer prevention.[172]

Surgery, radiation, chemotherapy, hormone therapy, biologic therapy, and bone marrow transplantation may be used to treat breast cancer. The extent of the surgery depends on the tumor's histology, predictability, and stage and the individual's age and medical and psychologic history. Beginning with the most conservative, the surgical procedures commonly used are as follows:

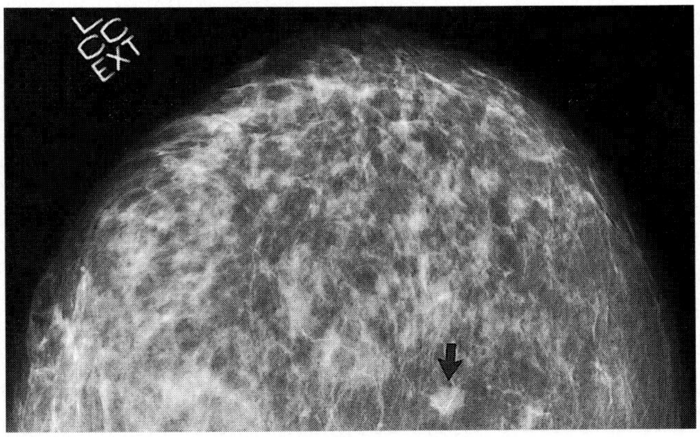

FIG. 22-52 Infiltrating ductal carcinoma. Presurgical mammogram. The ductal carcinoma (nonpalpable, 0.8 cm) was treated by needle-directed excision. (From Damjanov I, Linder J, editors: *Anderson's pathology,* ed 10, St Louis, 1996, Mosby.)

1. Tylectomy or lumpectomy, in which the tumor and a small amount of surrounding tissue are removed
2. Quadrant excision, in which a quadrant of the breast is removed
3. Partial mastectomy or segmental mastectomy, in which a larger amount of tissue is removed
4. Total or simple mastectomy, in which the tumor and all breast tissue are removed (the nipple may or may not be removed)
5. Modified radical mastectomy, in which the breast, pectoralis minor, and axillary contents are removed

Box 22-18

STAGING OF BREAST CANCER

T—PRIMARY TUMOR SIZE

T_X Primary tumor cannot be assessed

T_0 No evidence of primary tumor

T_{is} Carcinoma in situ: intraductal carcinoma, lobular carcinoma in situ, or Paget disease of the nipple with node

T_1 Tumor 2 cm or less in greatest dimension

T_2 Tumor more than 2 cm but not more than 5 cm in greatest dimension

T_3 Tumor more than 5 cm in greatest dimension

T_4 Tumor of any size with direct extension to chest wall or skin

NOTE: Paget disease associated with a tumor is classified according to the size of the tumor

N—REGIONAL LYMPH NODES

N_X Regional lymph nodes cannot be assessed (e.g., previously removed)

N_0 No regional lymph node metastasis

N_1 Metastasis to movable ipsilateral axillary lymph node or nodes

N_2 Metastasis to ipsilateral axillary lymph node(s) fixed to one another or to other structures

N_3 Metastasis to ipsilateral internal mammary lymph node or nodes

M—DISTANT METASTASIS

M_X Presence of distant metastasis cannot be assessed

M_0 No distant metastasis

M_1 Distant metastasis (includes metastasis to ipsilateral supraclavicular lymph node or nodes)

STAGE GROUPING

Stage 0	T_{is}	N_0	M_0
Stage 1	T_1	N_0	M_0
Stage IIa	T_0	N_0	M_0
	T_1	N_1	M_0
	T_2	N_0	M_0
Stage IIB	T_2	N_1	M_0
	T_3	N_0	M_0
Stage IIIA	T_0	N_2	M_0
	T_1	N_2	M_0
	T_2	N_2	M_0
	T_3	N_1	M_0
	T_3	N_2	M_0
Stage IIIB	T_4	Any N	M_0
	Any T	N_3	M_0
Stage IV	Any T	Any N	M_1

Data from Beahrs OH, Hutter RV, Kennedy BJ, editors: *Breast manual for staging of cancer,* ed 45, Philadelphia, 1992, Lippincott.

6. Radical mastectomy, in which the breast, axillary contents, and pectoralis major and minor are removed

Radiation therapy is infrequently used except to prevent metastasis of a small tumor (0.2 cm) that has been surgically excised. Chemotherapy and hormone therapy are most successful as an adjunct to surgery in premenopausal women with hormone-dependent tumors. They are also used in individuals with advanced disease. Endocrine therapy (androgens, estrogens, progesterones, and steroids) may be used to prolong survival time and is thought to be most effective in women with estrogen receptor– and progesterone receptor–positive tumors. Estrogen receptor– and progesterone receptor–negative tumors are unlikely to respond to hormonal therapy. Long-term antiestrogen therapy, such as tamoxifen, has proven efficacy to enhance the survival of individuals with breast cancer. Although tamoxifen maintains bone density and reduces the risk of fatal myocardial infarction, it can have estrogenic effects in the uterus, may cause endometrial cancer, and increases hot flashes. It is not recommended for women intending to become pregnant. In addition, in postmenopausal women, tamoxifen increases the risk of cataracts and blood clots in leg veins. Currently, tamoxifen is not recommended as an agent for prevention of breast cancer in those without breast cancer. Thus new strategies are being studied that have high affinity for breast estrogen receptors but weak affinity for receptors in the uterus. Such a drug, raloxifene, is currently under investigation. Results from the Multiple Outcomes of Raloxifene Evaluation (MORE), a randomized study, found that among postmenopausal women with osteoporosis the risk of invasive breast cancer was decreased by 76%.[210] Newer treatments that include biologic response modifiers (see Chapter 11) and bone marrow transplantation are being used in clinical research trials.

Disorders of the Male Breast

Gynecomastia

Gynecomastia is the overdevelopment of breast tissue in a male. Gynecomastia accounts for approximately 85% of all masses that develop in the male breast and affects 32% to 40% of the male population. If only one breast is involved, it is typically the left. Incidence is greatest among adolescents and men older than 50 years.

Gynecomastia results from hormonal alterations, which may be idiopathic or caused by systemic disorders, drugs, or neoplasms. Gynecomastia usually involves an imbalance of the estrogen/testosterone ratio. The normal estrogen/testosterone ratio can be altered in one of two ways. First, estrogen levels may be excessively high, although testosterone levels are normal. This is the case in drug-induced and tumor-induced cases of hyperestrogenism. Second, testosterone levels may be extremely low although estrogen levels are normal, as is the case in hypergonadism. Gynecomastia also can be caused by alterations in breast-tissue responsiveness to hormonal stimulation. Breast tissue may have increased responsiveness to estrogen or decreased responsiveness to androgen. Alterations of responsiveness may cause many cases of idiopathic gynecomastia.

Besides puberty and aging, estrogen/testosterone imbalances are associated with hypogonadism, Klinefelter syndrome, and testicular neoplasms. Hormone-induced gynecomastia is usually bilateral. Pubertal gynecomastia is a self-limiting phenomenon that usually disappears within 4 to 6 months. Senescent gynecomastia usually regresses spontaneously within 6 to 12 months.

Systemic disorders associated with gynecomastia include cirrhosis of the liver, infectious hepatitis, chronic renal failure, chronic obstructive lung disease, hyperthyroidism, tuberculosis, and chronic malnutrition. It may be that these disorders ultimately alter the estrogen/testosterone ratio, initiating the gynecomastia.

Gynecomastia is frequently seen in males receiving estrogen therapy, either in preparation for a sex-change operation or for prostatic carcinoma. Other drugs that can cause gynecomastia include digitalis, cimetidine, spironolactone, reserpine, thiazide, isoniazid, ergotamine, tricyclic antidepressants, amphetamines, vincristine, and busulfan. Gynecomastia is usually unilateral in these instances.

Malignancies of the testes, adrenals, or liver can cause gynecomastia if they alter the estrogen/testosterone ratio. Pituitary adenomas and lung cancer also are associated with gynecomastia.

Pathophysiology

The enlargement consists of hyperplastic stroma and ductal tissue. Hyperplasia results in a firm, palpable mass, at least 2 cm in diameter and located beneath the areola.

Evaluation and Treatment

The diagnosis of gynecomastia is based on physical examination. Identification and treatment of the cause are likely to be followed by resolution of the gynecomastia. The man should be taught to perform breast self-examination and is examined at 6- and 12-month intervals if the gynecomastia persists. All unilateral breast enlargement in men warrants an evaluation for malignancy; workup includes fine-needle aspiration, cytology, mammography, ultrasound, and biopsy.

Cancer

Male breast cancer (MBC) accounts for 1% of all male cancers and less than 1% of all breast cancers. Breast cancer in men is seen most commonly after age 60 years, with the peak incidence between 60 and 69 years. It has, however, been reported in males as young as 6 years and in adolescents. Possible risk factors include gynecomastia, radiation of the chest wall, and family history of breast cancer, especially in those with germline mutation in *BRCA1* or *BRCA2*. Obesity increases the risk of MBC.[211] The relationship between these factors and risk of disease is not clearly defined.

Male breast tumors frequently resemble carcinoma of the breast in women (see p. 762). The majority of MBCs express estrogen and progesterone receptors.[212] The malignant male breast lesion is usually a unilateral solid mass located near the nipple. Because the nipple is commonly involved, crusting and nipple discharge are typical clinical manifestations. Other findings include skin retraction, ulceration of the skin over the tumor, and axillary node involvement. Patterns of metastasis are similar to those in females.

The diagnosis of cancer is confirmed by biopsy. Because of delays in seeking treatment, male breast cancer tends to be advanced at the time of diagnosis and therefore tends to have a poor prognosis. Treatment protocols are similar to those for female breast cancer, but endocrine therapy is used more frequently for males because a higher percentage of male tumors are hormone dependent. The mainstay of treatment is modified mastectomy with axillary node dissection to assess stage and prognosis.[213] Orchiectomy is performed to treat metastatic disease.

SUMMARY REVIEW

Alterations of Sexual Maturation

1. Sexual maturation, or puberty, should begin in girls between ages 8 and 13 years and in boys between ages 9 and 14 years. Delayed puberty is the onset of sexual maturation after these ages; precocious puberty is onset before these ages.
2. Alterations of sexual maturation can be idiopathic or caused by a disease or congenital anomaly. In most cases of delayed puberty, the hypothalamic-pituitary-gonadal axis is intact but the surge of activity that stimulates puberty is delayed. This situation is common in boys. Precocious puberty, more common in girls, can also be caused by mistiming of the stimulatory surge in a child whose hypothalamic-pituitary-ovarian system is otherwise normal.
3. Precocious puberty can be isosexual (sex appropriate), heterosexual (not sex appropriate), or incomplete (development of one secondary sex characteristic only). Causes of delayed or incomplete puberty can be divided into categories based on gonadotropic secretion: hypergonadotropism (increased levels of follicle-stimulating hormone [FSH] and luteinizing hormone [LH]), hypogonadotropism (decreased LH and FSH levels), and eugonadism.

Disorders of the Female Reproductive System

1. The female reproductive system can be altered by hormonal imbalances, infectious microorganisms, inflammation, structural abnormalities, and benign or malignant proliferative conditions.
2. Menstrual disorders usually involve some disruption of the hypothalamic-pituitary-ovarian axis and subsequent alteration of hormone production, reception by target organs, or feedback mechanisms.
3. Primary dysmenorrhea is painful menstruation not associated with pelvic disease. It results from excessive synthesis of prostaglandins, which cause the myometrium to contract and constrict blood vessels, resulting in ischemic pain.
4. Primary amenorrhea is the continued absence of menarche and menstrual function by 14 years of age without the development of secondary sex characteristics or by age 16 years if these changes have occurred.
5. Secondary amenorrhea is the absence of menstruation for a time equivalent to more than three cycles or 6 months in women who have previously menstruated. Secondary amenorrhea is associated with anovulation.
6. Categorization of amenorrhea as primary or secondary has no clinical significance. Instead, amenorrhea is divided into compartments that reflect the underlying disorder: compartment I, disorders of the outflow tract or uterine target organ; compartment II, disorders of the ovary; compartment III, disorders of the anterior pituitary; and compartment IV,

disorders of the central nervous system (CNS) or hypothalamic factors.

7. Dysfunctional uterine bleeding (DUB) is heavy or irregular bleeding caused by a disturbance of the menstrual cycle.
8. Polycystic ovary syndrome (PCOS) is a problem of persistent anovulation and is thought to be related to syndrome X (hypertension, hyperinsulinemia, and dyslipidemia). Prolonged anovulation leads to infertility, menstrual bleeding disorders, hirsutism, acne, endometrial hyperplasia, cardiovascular disease, and diabetes mellitus in women with hyperinsulinemia. PCOS affects females between 15 and 30 years of age.
9. Premenstrual syndrome (PMS) is the cyclic recurrence of physical, psychologic, or behavioral changes distressing enough to disrupt normal activities or interpersonal relationships. More than 200 emotional, physical, and behavioral symptoms have been attributed to PMS. Emotional symptoms, particularly depression, anger, irritability, and fatigue, are reported as the most distressing symptoms; physical symptoms tend to be less problematic. Treatment is symptomatic and includes self-help techniques, life-style changes, counseling, and selective serotonin reuptake inhibitors (SSRIs).
10. Infection and inflammation of the female genitalia can result from microorganisms from the environment or overproliferation of microorganisms that normally populate the genital tract.
11. Pelvic inflammatory disease (PID) is an acute ascending polymicrobial infection of the upper genital tract and is sexually transmitted.
12. Vaginitis, or vaginal infection, is usually caused by sexually transmitted pathogens or *Candida albicans,* which causes candidiasis. Development is related to the overall health of a woman and local defense mechanisms, particularly vaginal pH. Variables, such as antibiotics, douching, soaps, feminine hygiene sprays, and pregnancy, alter vaginal pH or the bactericidal nature of secretions and predispose a woman to infection.
13. Cervicitis, which is infection of the cervix, can be acute (mucopurulent cervicitis) or chronic. Its most common cause is a sexually transmitted pathogen.
14. Vulvitis is an inflammation of the skin of the vulva. It can be caused by chemical and mechanical irritants, allergens, skin disorders, or spread of vaginal infections, such as candidiasis.
15. Bartholinitis, also called *Bartholin cyst,* is an inflammation of the ducts that lead from the Bartholin glands to the surface of the vulva. Inflammation blocks the glands, preventing the outflow of glandular secretions, and is caused by trauma or infection.
16. The pelvic relaxation disorders—uterine prolapse, cystocele, rectocele, and urethrocele—are caused by the relaxation of muscles and fascial supports, usually with age or after childbirth or other trauma, and are more likely to occur in women with a familial or genetic predisposition.
17. Benign growths and proliferative conditions of the female reproductive tract tend to affect the ovaries (benign ovarian cysts) or uterine tissues (endometrial polyps, leiomyomas, and endometriosis).
18. Benign ovarian cysts develop from mature ovarian follicles that do not release their ova (follicular cysts) or from a corpus luteum that persists abnormally instead of degenerating (corpus luteum cyst). Cysts usually regress spontaneously.
19. Endometrial polyps consist of overgrowths of endometrial tissue and frequently cause abnormal bleeding in the premenopausal woman.
20. Leiomyomas, also called *uterine fibroids,* are tumors arising from the muscle layer of the uterus, the myometrium. Incidence increases in women between ages 30 and 50 years; most myomas remain small and asymptomatic. Adenomyosis is the presence of endometrial glands and stroma within the uterine myometrium.
21. Endometriosis is the presence of functional endometrial tissue (i.e., tissue that responds to hormonal stimulation) at sites outside the uterus. Endometriosis causes an inflammatory reaction at the site of implantation and is a cause of infertility.
22. Most cancers of the female genitalia involve the uterus (particularly the cervix) and the ovaries. Cancer of the vagina is rare.
23. Risk factors for cervical cancer are young age at first coitus, multiple sexual partners, exposure to sexually transmitted infections, and exposure to cigarette smoke.
24. Cervical cancer arises from the cervical epithelium and is considered a sexually transmitted disease. The progressively serious neoplastic alterations are (a) cervical intraepithelial neoplasia (cervical dysplasia), (b) cervical carcinoma in situ, and (c) invasive cervical carcinoma. Smoking is a cofactor.
25. Risk factors for cancer of the vagina are in utero diethylstilbestrol (DES) exposure and prior or concurrent cervical cancer. Like cervical cancers, vaginal cancers arise from the epithelium and are identified as intraepithelial neoplasia (dysplasia), carcinoma in situ, or invasive carcinoma. Most vaginal cancers are secondary in nature. Mean age is 55 years for invasive cancer and 45 years for precursor lesions.
26. The major risk for vulvar cancer is a history of human papillomavirus (HPV) infection or squamous dysplasia of the vagina or cervix. Symptoms include chronic vulvar irritation, pruritus, bloody discharge, and a hard, ulcerated area of the vulva or large cauliflower lesions. Peak incidence is in postmenopausal women, but women age 40 years or younger can be affected.
27. Risk factors for endometrial cancer include obesity, infertility, failure to ovulate, early menarche or late menopause, and tamoxifen or unopposed estrogen therapy. Oral contraceptive use protects against endometrial and ovarian cancers. Peak incidence occurs at 58 to 60 years of age, approximately 10 years later than peak incidence of precursor lesions.
28. Risk factors for ovarian cancer include familial predisposition and personal history of breast cancer. Ovarian cancer causes more deaths than any other genital cancer in women.
29. Awareness of sexual dysfunction is relatively new. Chronic illness, medications, infection, sexual trauma, and a variety of psychosocial concerns have been implicated as causes.
30. Infertility, or the inability to conceive after 1 year of unprotected intercourse, affects approximately 15% of all couples. Fertility can be impaired by factors in the male, female, or both partners.

Disorders of the Male Reproductive System

1. Disorders of the urethra include urethritis (inflammation of the urethra) and urethral strictures (narrowing or obstruction of the urethral lumen caused by scarring).

2. Although noninfectious urethritis can occur, most cases of urethritis result from sexually transmitted pathogens. Symptoms of urethritis include dysuria, frequency, urgency, urethral tingling or itching, and clear or purulent discharge. Treatment consists of appropriate antibiotic therapy and avoidance of future chemical or mechanical irritation.
3. Acquired or congenital scarring that causes urethral stricture can be caused by trauma or by severe or untreated urethral infection. The primary symptom is diminished force and caliber of the urinary stream; other symptoms include urinary frequency and hesitancy, mild dysuria, double urine stream or spraying, and postvoiding dribbling. Treatment is usually surgical.
4. Phimosis and paraphimosis are penile disorders involving the foreskin (prepuce). In phimosis the foreskin cannot be retracted over the glans. In paraphimosis the foreskin is retracted and cannot be reduced (returned to its normal anatomic position over the glans). Phimosis is caused by poor hygiene and chronic infection and can lead to paraphimosis. Paraphimosis can constrict the penile blood vessels, preventing circulation to the glans.
5. Peyronie disease consists of fibrosis, affecting the corpora cavernosa, which causes penile curvature during erection. Fibrosis prevents engorgement on the affected side, causing a lateral curvature that can prevent intercourse.
6. Priapism, a prolonged painful erection not stimulated by sexual arousal, is a urologic emergency. The corpora cavernosa (but not the corpus spongiosum) fill with blood that does not drain out, probably because of venous obstruction. Priapism is associated with spinal cord trauma, sickle cell disease, leukemia, and pelvic tumors. It can also be idiopathic.
7. Balanitis is an inflammation of the glans penis and usually occurs in conjunction with posthitis. It is associated with phimosis, inadequate cleansing under the foreskin, skin disorders, and infections.
8. Cancer of the penis is rare and tends to occur in uncircumcised men with phimosis. Penile carcinoma in situ tends to involve the glans; invasive carcinoma of the penis involves the shaft as well.
9. A varicocele is an abnormal dilation of the veins within the spermatic cord caused by either congenital absence of valves in the internal spermatic vein or acquired valvular incompetence.
10. A hydrocele is a collection of fluid between the testicular and scrotal layers of the tunica vaginalis. Hydroceles can be idiopathic or caused by trauma or infection of the testes.
11. A spermatocele is a cyst located between the testis and epididymis that is filled with fluid and sperm.
12. Cryptorchidism is a congenital condition in which one or both testes fail to descend into the scrotum. Treated or untreated cryptorchidism is associated with infertility and a significantly increased risk of testicular cancer.
13. Testicular torsion is the rotation of a testis, which twists blood vessels in the spermatic cord. This interrupts blood supply to the testis, resulting in edema and, if not corrected within 4 to 6 hours, necrosis and atrophy of testicular tissues.
14. Orchitis is an acute infection of the testes. Pathogenic organisms may reach the testes through the blood or the lymphatics; most commonly, they reach the testes by ascending through the vas deferens and epididymis. Complications of orchitis include hydrocele and atrophy. Granulomatis orchitis, an autoimmune disease, is a nonspecific, noninfectious, inflammatory process that occurs in middle-age men.
15. Testicular cancer is the most common malignancy in males ages 15 to 35 years. Although its cause is unknown, high androgen levels, genetic predisposition, and a history of cryptorchidism, trauma, or infection may contribute to tumorigenesis. Most testicular neoplasms are germ-cell tumors.
16. Spermatogenesis (sperm production by the testes) can be impaired by disruptions of the hypothalamic-pituitary-testicular axis that reduce testosterone secretion and by testicular trauma or atrophy from any cause. Sperm production is also impaired by neoplastic disease, cryptorchidism, or any factor that causes testicular temperature to rise.
17. Sperm quality is impaired by chromosomal abnormalities resulting from genetic factors, irradiation, or toxins. Sperm motility can be impaired by unfavorable constituents or characteristics of semen.
18. Epididymitis, an inflammation of the epididymis, is usually caused by a sexually transmitted pathogen that ascends through the vasa deferentia from an already infected urethra or bladder.
19. Benign prostatic hyperplasia (BPH) is an enlargement of the prostate gland. Symptoms are obstructive or irritative in nature and include urge to urinate frequently, delay in starting urination, and decreased force of stream. BPH can be treated surgically or with medications.
20. Prostatitis can be bacterial or nonbacterial and chronic or acute. Bacterial prostatitis is an infection of the prostate. Acute bacterial prostatitis causes an inflammatory response in which the prostate becomes enlarged, tender, and firm. Chronic bacterial prostatitis is recurrent prostatic infection that eventually causes fibrosis. Nonbacterial prostatitis is prostatic inflammation without evidence of bacterial infection.
21. Prostate cancer is the second leading cause of cancer deaths in men (after lung cancer). Possible causes involve genetic predisposition, dietary factors, and age. Incidence is greatest among northwestern European and North American men (particularly blacks) older than 65 years.
22. Most cancers of the prostate are adenocarcinomas that develop at the periphery of the gland. Because there are no early symptoms, disease is often advanced at the time of diagnosis.
23. Sexual dysfunction in males can be caused by any physical or psychologic factor that impairs erection, emission, or ejaculation. Impairment can be caused by a number of physiologic, psychologic, and emotional factors.

Disorders of the Breast

1. Most disorders of the breast are disorders of the mammary gland, that is, the female breast.
2. Galactorrhea, or inappropriate lactation, is the persistent secretion of a milky substance by one or both breasts in nonpregnant, nonlactating women. Its most common cause is nonpuerperal hyperprolactinemia, a rise in serum prolactin levels that is not associated with pregnancy and childbirth. Hyperprolactinemia can be caused by medications, pituitary tumors, hypothyroidism, chronic stress, or persistent and repeated suckling.
3. *Fibrocystic changes (FCC)* is the most widely accepted term for physiologic nodularity and breast tenderness that waxes and wanes with the menstrual cycle. Microscopic findings of fibrocystic breasts include microcysts, macrocysts, papillomatosis,

adenosis, fibrosis, and ductal epithelial hyperplasia. Although FCC has been considered a risk for breast cancer, only variants with epithelial proliferation represent a true risk. Symptoms of FCC affect women ages 30 to 50 years and include cyclic bilateral breast tenderness and transient breast lumps.

4. Other benign breast conditions include fibroadenomas, mammary duct ectasia (an inflammatory condition), intraductal papillomas, and fat necrosis.
5. Breast cancer is the most common form of cancer in women and second to lung cancer as the most frequent cause of cancer death. The major risk factors for breast cancer are environmental factors, such as a diet high in ω-6 fatty acids; reproductive factors, such as nulliparity; and familial factors, such as a family history of breast cancer. New data on estrogen, estrogen metabolites, and estrogen-dependent growth factors are also implicated.
6. Most breast cancers arise from the ductal epithelium and then may metastasize to the lymphatics, opposite breast, abdominal cavity, lungs, bones, kidneys, liver, adrenal glands, ovaries, and pituitary glands.
7. The first clinical manifestation of breast cancer is usually a small, painless lump in the breast. Other manifestations include palpable lymph nodes in the axilla, dimpling of the skin, nipple and skin retraction, nipple discharge, ulcerations, reddened skin, and bone pain associated with bony metastases.
8. Approximately one third of breast cancers are hormone dependent, or progesterone or estrogen receptor positive. Treatment protocols are often based on whether the tumor is receptor positive or negative.
9. Gynecomastia is the overdevelopment (hyperplasia) of breast tissue in a male. It is first seen as a firm, palpable mass at least 2 cm in diameter located in the subareolar area. Gynecomastia affects 32% to 40% of the male population. Incidence is greatest among adolescents and men older than 50 years.
10. Gynecomastia is caused by hormonal or breast tissue alterations that cause estrogen to dominate. These alterations can result from systemic disorders, drugs, neoplasms, or idiopathic causes.
11. Although breast cancer is relatively uncommon in males, it has a poor prognosis because men tend to delay seeking treatment. Most breast cancers in men are estrogen receptor positive. Incidence is greatest in men in their sixties.

KEY TERMS

Acute bacterial prostatitis, *749*
Adenomyosis, *726*
Amenorrhea, *709*
Anorgasmia (orgasmic dysfunction), *736*
Anovulation, *711*
Balanitis, *739*
Bartholinitis (Bartholin cyst), *720*
Benign prostatic hyperplasia (BPH) (benign prostatic hypertrophy), *747*
Cervical carcinoma in situ, *729*
Cervical intraepithelial neoplasm (CIN) (cervical dysplasia), *728*
Cervicitis, *720*
Chronic bacterial prostatitis, *751*
Corpus luteum cyst, *724*
Cryptorchidism, *742*
Cyst, *720*
Cystocele, *722*
Cystourethrocele, *722*
Delayed puberty, *706*
Ductal carcinoma in situ (DCIS), *760*
Ductal hyperplasia, *760*
Dysfunctional uterine bleeding (DUB), *712*
Dyspareunia (painful intercourse), *736*
Ectopic testis, *742*
Endometrial polyp, *724*
Endometriosis, *726*
Enterocele, *723*
Epididymitis, *745*
Epithelial proliferative disease, *760*
Fibrocystic changes (FCC), *759*
Fibrous tissue, *760*
Florid hyperplasia, *761*
Follicular cyst, *724*
Galactorrhea (inappropriate lactation), *757*
Gross cystic breast disease (GCBD), *759*
Gynecomastia, *772*
Heterosexual precocious puberty, *707*
Hirsutism, *711*
Hydrocele, *741*
Hyperprolactinemia, *711*
Incomplete precocious puberty, *707*
Infertility, *736*
Invasive carcinoma of the cervix, *729*
Isosexual precocious puberty, *707*
Leiomyoma (uterine fibroid), *725*
Lobular carcinoma in situ (LCIS), *762*
Lobular hyperplasia, *762*
Mammotome, *770*
Mild hyperplasia, *761*
Mucopurulent cervicitis (MPC), *720*
Nonbacterial prostatitis, *751*
Nonpuerperal hyperprolactinemia, *758*
Oophoritis, *717*
Orchitis, *744*
Paraphimosis, *737*
Pelvic inflammatory disease (PID), *717*
Pessary, *722*
Peyronie disease (bent nail syndrome), *737*
Phimosis, *737*
Polycystic ovary syndrome (PCOS), *713*
Precocious puberty, *706*
Premenstrual syndrome (PMS), *715*
Priapism, *739*
Primary amenorrhea, *709*
Primary dysmenorrhea, *708*
Prolactin-inhibiting factor (PIF), *758*
Prostatitis, *749*
Prostatodynia, *749*
Radial scar, *761*
Rapid orgasm, *736*
Rectocele, *723*
Retrograde menstruation, *727*
Salpingitis, *717*
Sclerosing adenosis, *760*
Secondary amenorrhea, *709*
Sexual anorexia (inhibited sexual desire, decreased libido), *735*
Sexual dysfunction, *755*
Spermatocele, *742*
Torsion of the testis, *743*
Urethral stricture, *737*
Urethritis, *737*
Urethrocele, *722*
Uterine prolapse, *721*
Uterine sarcoma, *733*
Vaginismus, *736*
Vaginitis, *719*
Varicocele, *740*
Vulvitis, *720*

REFERENCES

1. Reid RL: Amenorrhea. In LJ Copeland, JF Farrell, editors: *Textbook of gynecology,* ed 2, Philadelphia, 2000, W.B. Saunders.
2. Healtheon/WebMD: Hypothalamic disorders. In *Scientific American Medicine,* 1999. Available at www.samed.com/sam/forms/index.htm.
3. Rudolph AM, Hoffman JIE, Rudolph CD: *Rudolph's pediatrics,* ed 20, Stamford CT, 1996, Appleton & Lange.
4. Cacciari E, Mazanti L, Italian Study Group for Turner Syndrome: Final height of patients with Turner's syndrome treated with growth hormone (GH): indications for GH therapy alone at high doses and late estrogen therapy, *J Clin Endocrinol Metab* 84(12):4510, 1999.
5. Saenger P: Growth-promoting strategies in Turner's syndrome, *J Clin Endocrinol Metab* 84(12):4345, 1999.
6. Seminara SB, Hayes FJ, Crowley WF: Gonadotropin-releasing hormone deficiency in the human (idiopathic hypogonadotropic hypogonadism and Kallman's syndrome): pathophysiological and genetic considerations, *Endocr Rev* 19(5):521, 1998.
7. Kaplowitz PB et al: Reexamination of the age limit for defining when puberty is precocious in girls in the United States: implications for evaluation and treatment, *Pediatrics* 104(4):936, 1999.
8. Massachusetts General Hospital Pediatric Endocrine Research Unit. Available at http://mghra-partners.org/narratives/BoepplePA2.html.
9. Palmert MR et al: Is obesity an outcome of gonadotropin-releasing hormone agonist administration? *J Clin Endocrinol Metab* 84(12): 4480, 1999.
10. Pickles VR, Hall WS, Best FA: Prostaglandins in endometrium and menstrual fluid from normal and dysmenorrheic subjects, *Br J Obstet Gynaecol* 72:185, 1965.
11. Speroff L, Glass RH, Kase NG: *Clinical gynecologic endocrinology and infertility,* ed 5, Baltimore, 1994, Williams & Wilkins.
12. Wolf LL, Schumann L: Dysmenorrhea, *J Am Acad Nurse Pract* 11(3): 125, 1999.
13. Reid RL: Amenorrhea. In Copeland LJ, Farrell JF, editors: *Textbook of gynecology,* ed 2, Philadelphia, 2000, W.B. Saunders.
14. Healey PM, Jacobson EJ: *Common medical diagnoses: an algorithmic approach,* ed 3, Philadelphia, 2000, W.B. Saunders.
15. Wetzel W: Micronized progesterone: a new option for women's health care, *Nurse Pract* 24(5):62, 1999.
16. Warren MP, Biller MK, Shangold MD: A new clinical option for hormone replacement therapy in women with secondary amenorrhea: effects of cyclic administration of progesterone from the sustained-release vaginal gel Crinone (45 and 8%) on endometrial morphologic features and withdrawal bleeding, *Am J Obstet Gynecol* 180(1):42, 1999.
17. Mencaglia L, Perino A, Hamou J: Hysteroscopy in perimenopausal and postmenopausal women with abnormal uterine bleeding, *J Reprod Med* 32(8):577, 1987.
18. Weingold AB: Abnormal bleeding. In Kase N, Weingold AB, Gershenson DM, editors: *Principles and practice of clinical gynecology,* New York, 1990, Churchill Livingstone.
19. Kim MH: Dysfunctional uterine bleeding. In Copeland LJ, Farrell JF, editors: *Textbook of gynecology,* ed 2, Philadelphia, 2000, W.B. Saunders.
20. Prior JC: Perimenopause: the complex endocrinology of the menopausal transition, *Endocr Rev* 19(4):397, 1998.
21. Dealy MF: Dysfunctional uterine bleeding in adolescents, *Nurse Pract* 23(5):12, 1998.
22. Oriel KA, Schager S: Abnormal uterine bleeding, *Am Fam Physician* 60(5):1371, 1999.
23. Hodgson DA et al: Microwave endometrial ablation: development, clinical trials, and outcomes at three years, *Br J Obstet Gynaecol* 106: 684, 1999.
24. Aberdeen Endometrial Ablation Trials Group: A randomised trial of endometrial ablation versus hysterectomy for the treatment of dysfunctional uterine bleeding: outcome at four years, *Br J Obstet Gynaecol* 106:360, 1999.
25. Hawe JA et al: Cavaterm thermal balloon ablation for the treatment of menorrhagia, *Br J Obstet Gynaecol* 106:1143, 1999.
26. McCausland AM, McCausland VM: Partial rollerball endometrial ablation: a modification of total ablation to treat menorrhagia without causing complications from intrauterine adhesions, *Am J Obstet Gynecol* 180(6):1512, 1999.
27. Balen A: Pathogenesis of polycystic ovary syndrome—the enigma unravels? *Lancet* 354:966, 1999.
28. Nestler J: *Insulin resistance and women's health: new insights into polycystic ovary syndrome.* Paper presented at the 14th Annual National Conference of the American Academy of Nurse Practitioners, June 17, 1999.
29. Patel SR, Korykowski MT: Treating polycystic ovary syndrome: today's approach, *Womens Health Prim Care* 3(2):109, 2000.
30. Diamanti-Kandarakis E et al: A survey of the polycystic ovary syndrome in the Greek island of Lesbos: hormonal and metabolic profile, *J Clin Endocrinol Metab* 84(11):4006, 1999.
31. Couse JF et al: Prevention of the polycystic phenotype and characterization of ovulatory capacity in the estrogen receptor–α knockout mouse, *Endocrinology* 140(12):5855, 1999.
32. Pugeat M, Ducluzeau PH: Insulin resistance, polycystic ovary syndrome and metformin, *Drugs* 58(suppl 1):41, 1999.
33. Gordon CM: Menstrual disorders in adolescents: excess androgens and the polycystic ovary syndrome, *Pediatr Clin North Am* 46(3):519, 1999.
34. Radon PA, McMahon MJ, Meyer WR: Impaired glucose tolerance in pregnant women with polycystic ovary syndrome, *Obstet Gynecol* 94(2):194, 1999.
35. Book CB, Dunaif A: Selective insulin resistance in the polycystic ovary syndrome, *J Clin Endocrinol Metab* 84(9):3110, 1999.
36. Amato G et al: Lack of insulin-like growth factor binding protein-3 variation after follicle-stimulating hormone stimulation in women with polycystic ovary syndrome undergoing in vitro fertilization, *Fertil Steril* 72(3):454, 1999.
37. Orabi HE et al: Serum leptin as an additional possible pathogenic factor in polycystic ovary syndrome, *Clin Biochem* 32(1):71, 1999.
38. Chian RC et al: Pregnancies from in vitro matured oocytes retrieved from patients with polycystic ovary syndrome after priming with human chorionic gonadotropin, *Fertil Steril* 72(4):639, 1999.
39. Reid R: *Premenstrual syndrome: current problems in obstetrics, gynecology, and fertility,* St Louis, 1985, Mosby.
40. Zerbe KJ: *Women's mental health in primary care,* Philadelphia, 1999, W.B. Saunders.
41. Woods NF et al: *Prevalence of perimenstrual symptoms: final report,* Seattle, 1989, University of Washington.
42. York R et al: Characteristics of premenstrual syndrome, *Obstet Gynecol* 73(4):601, 1989.
43. Roca C, Schmidt PJ, Rubinow DR: A follow-up study of premenstrual syndrome, *J Clin Psychiatry* 60(11):763, 1999.
44. Rosenberg R: *Course and treatment of depression during pregnancy and the postpartum period.* Paper presented at the 8th International Nurse Practitioner Conference, San Diego, September 30, 2000.
45. Rapkin AJ: *Update on the treatments for PMS/PMDD.* Paper presented at the 8th International Nurse Practitioner Conference, San Diego, September 30, 2000.
46. Freeman EW et al: Differential response to antidepressants in women with premenstrual syndrome/premenstrual dysphoric disorder: a randomized controlled trial, *Arch Gen Psychiatry* 56:932, 1999.
47. Lawson MA, Blythe MJ: Pelvic inflammatory disease in adolescents, *Pediatr Clin North Am* 46(4):767, 1999.
48. Hatcher RA et al: *Contraceptive technology,* New York, 1998, Ardent Media.
49. Centers for Disease Control and Prevention: *Sexually transmitted diseases: treatment guidelines, 1998,* Washington, DC, 1998, DHHS.
50. Richter HE et al: The association of interleukin-6 with clinical and laboratory parameters of acute pelvic inflammatory disease, *Am J Obstet Gynecol* 181(4):940, 1999.

51. Peeling RW et al: Antibody response to the chlamydial heat-shock protein 60 in an experimental model of chronic pelvic inflammatory disease in monkeys, *J Infect Dis* 80:774, 1999.
52. Hillier SL et al: Role of bacterial vaginosis-associated microorganisms in endometritis, *Am J Obstet Gynecol* 175:435, 1996.
53. Division of STD Prevention, US Department of Health and Human Services: *Sexually transmitted disease surveillance, 1998,* Atlanta, 1998, Centers for Disease Control and Prevention.
54. Division of STD Prevention, US Department of Health and Human Services: *Sexually transmitted disease surveillance, 1995,* Atlanta, 1996, Centers for Disease Control and Prevention.
55. Brubaker L: Abnormalities of pelvic support. In Copeland LJ, Farrell JF, editors: *Textbook of gynecology,* ed 2, Philadelphia, 2000, W.B. Saunders.
56. Dorr CH: Relaxation of pelvic supports. In DeCherney AH, Pernoll ML, editors: *Current obstetric and gynecologic diagnosis and treatment,* ed 8, Norwalk, Conn, 1994, Appleton & Lange.
57. Adelson MD, Adelson KL: Miscellaneous benign disorders of the upper genital tract. In Copeland LJ, Farrell JF, editors: *Textbook of gynecology,* ed 2, Philadelphia, 2000, W.B. Saunders.
58. Ueda H et al: Unusual appearances of uterine leiomyomas: MR imaging findings and their histopathologic backgrounds, *Radiographics* 19:s131, 1999.
59. Plomaba S et al: Long-term administration of tibolone plus gonadotropin-releasing hormone agonist for the treatment of uterine leiomyonas: effectiveness and effects on vasomotor symptoms, bone mass, and lipid profiles, *Fertil Steril* 72(5):889, 1999.
60. Reinhold C et al: Uterine adenomyosis: endovaginal US and MR imaging features with histopathologic correlation, *Radiographics* 19: s147, 1999.
61. Guarnaccia MM, Silverberg K, Olive DL: Endometriosis and adenomyosis. In Copeland LJ, Farrell JF, editors: *Textbook of gynecology,* ed 2, Philadelphia, 2000, W.B. Saunders.
62. Wardle PG, Hull MG: Is endometriosis a disease? *Baillieres Clin Obstet Gynaecol* 7(4):673, 1993.
63. Brinton LA et al: Cancer risks after a hospital discharge diagnosis of endometriosis, *Am J Obstet Gynecol* 176:572, 1997.
64. Sampson JA: Peritoneal endometriosis due to the menstrual dissemination of endometrial tissue into the peritoneal cavity, *Am J Obstet Gynecol* 14:422, 1927.
65. Suzumori N et al: Expression of secretory leukocyte protease inhibitor in women with endometriosis, *Fertil Steril* 72(5):889, 1999.
66. Ota H et al: Immunohistochemical assessment of superoxide dismutase expression in the endometrium in endometriosis and adenomyosis, *Fertil Steril* 72(1):129, 1999.
67. Canis M et al: Classification of endometriosis, *Baillieres Clin Obstet Gynaecol* 7(4):759, 1994.
68. American Cancer Society: *Cancer facts and figures—1998,* Atlanta, 1998, American Cancer Society.
69. American Cancer Society: *Cancer facts and figures 2001,* Atlanta, 2001, American Cancer Society.
70. Kjaer SK et al: Human papillomavirus—the most significant risk determinant of cervical intraepithelial neoplasia, *Int J Cancer* 65:601, 1996.
71. Schiffman M et al: Epidemiologic evidence showing that human papillomavirus infection causes most cervical intraepithelial neoplasia, *J Natl Cancer Inst* 85(12):958, 1993.
72. Center for Disease Control and Prevention*: Tracking hidden epidemics: trends in the STD epidemics in the United States*, Atlanta, 2000, Centers for Disease Control and Prevention. Available at www.cdc.gov/nchstp/od/.
73. Anttila T et al: Serotypes of *Chlamydia trachomatis* and risk for development of cervical squamous cell carcinoma, *JAMA* 285(1):47, 2001.
74. Center for Disease Prevention and Epidemiology: Anogenital papillomavirus infections, *CD Summary* 47(2), 1998.
75. Klaus BD, Grodesky MJ: Cervical dysplasia in women with HIV, *Nurse Pract* 24(8):79, 1999.
76. Centers for Disease Control and Prevention: USPHS/IDSA guidelines for prevention of opportunistic infections in persons infected with human immunodeficiency virus, *MMWR* 46(RR-12):25, 1997.
77. Hopkins MP: Vaginal neoplasms. In Copeland LH, Farrell JF, editors: *Textbook of gynecology,* ed 2, Philadelphia, 2000, W.B. Saunders.
78. Research report: combination therapy for cervical cancer, *Womens Health Prim Care* 2(60):479, 1999.
79. Gordon AN: Vulvar neoplasms. In Copeland LJ, Farrell JF, editors: *Textbook of gynecology,* ed 2, Philadelphia, 2000, W.B. Saunders.
80. Burke TW, Morris M: Adenocarcinoma of the endometrium. In Copeland LJ, Farrell JF, editors: *Textbook of gynecology,* ed 2, Philadelphia, 2000, W.B. Saunders.
81. Ronnett BM, Kurman, RJ: Endometrial hyperplasia. In Copeland LJ, Farrell JF, editors: *Textbook of gynecology,* ed 2, Philadelphia, 2000, W.B. Saunders.
82. American Cancer Society: *ACS endometrial cancer resource center*, 1999. Available at www3.cancer.org/cancerinfo.
83. American Cancer Society: Endometrial cancer. In *Cancer response system document #10020,* New York, 1995, The Society.
84. Steren AJ: Improved ways of screening for gynecologic cancers, *Contemp Ob Gyn* 75:42, 1995.
85. Nickline JL, Copeland LJ: Uterine sarcomas. In Copeland LJ, Farrell JF, editors: *Textbook of gynecology,* ed 2, Philadelphia, 2000, W.B. Saunders.
86. American Cancer Society: *ACS ovary cancer resource center*, 1999. Available at www3.cancer.org/cancerinfo.
87. Gershenon D: Epithelial ovarian cancer. In Copeland LJ, Farrell JF, editors: *Textbook of gynecology,* ed 2, Philadelphia, 2000, W.B. Saunders.
88. Weber B: Genetic testing for breast cancer, *Sci Am Sci Med* 3(1):12, 1996.
89. Kerber RA, Slattery ML: The impact of family history on ovarian cancer risk: the Utah population database, *Arch Intern Med* 155:905, 1995.
90. Wilcox AJ, Weinberg CR, Baird DD: Timing of sexual intercourse in relation to ovulation, *N Engl J Med* 33(23):1517, 1995.
91. LaRock DR, Sant GR: Lower urinary tract infections in men. In Nseyo UO, Weinman E, Lamm DL, editors: *Urology for primary care physicians*, Philadelphia, 1999, W.B. Saunders.
92. McAninch JW: Disorders of the penis and male urethra. In Tanagho EA, McAninch JW, editors: *Smith's general urology,* ed 14, Norwalk, Conn, 1995, Appleton & Lange.
93. American Cancer Society: *Penile cancer resource center*, 1999. Available at www3.cancer.org/cancerinfo.
94. Altma AL et al: Cocaine associated priapism, *J Urol* 161:1817, 1999.
95. American Cancer Society: Penile cancer. In *Cancer response system document #10005,* New York, 1995, The Society.
96. Nasca MR, Innocenzi D, Micali G: Penile cancer among patients with genital lichen sclerous, *J Am Acad Dermatol* 41:911, 1999.
97. Presti JC, Herr HW: Genital tumors. In Tanagho EA, McAninch JW, editors: *Smith's general urology,* ed 14, Norwalk, Conn, 1995, Appleton & Lange.
98. Lindegarrds JC et al: A retrospective analysis of 82 cases of cancer of the penis, *Br J Urol* 77(6):883, 1996.
99. Kolon TF, Albertsen PC: Diagnosis and treatment of scrotal abnormalities, *Clin Advisor* 47, 2000.
100. Franklin G, Nseyo UO: Anatomic basis of common urologic diseases. In Nseyo UO, Weinman E, Lamm DL, editors: *Urology for primary care physicians,* Philadelphia, 1999, W.B. Saunders.
101. McAninch JW: Disorders of the testis, scrotum, and spermatic cord. In Tanagho EA, McAninch JW, editors: *Smith's general urology,* ed 14, Norwalk, Conn, 1995, Appleton & Lange.
102. Galejs LE, Usaf M: Diagnosis and treatment of the acute scrotum, *Am Fam Physician* 59(4):817, 1999.
103. Del Pizzo JJ, Jarow JP: Management of male infertility. In Nseyo UO, Weinman E, Lamm DL, editors: *Urology for primary care physicians*, Philadelphia, 1999, W.B. Saunders.
104. Rosenthal MS: *The fertility sourcebook,* Los Angeles, 1998, Lowell House.

105. Schenkman EM, Tarry WT: Congenital anomalies. In Nseyo UO, Weinman E, Lamm DL, editors: *Urology for primary care physicians,* Philadelphia, 1999, W.B. Saunders.
106. CancerNet: *Cancer facts: questions and answers about testicular cancer,* National Cancer Institute, 2000. Available at www.cancernet.nci.nih.gov/.
107. Lanum DL: Carcinoma of the genitourinary system. In Nseyo UO, Weinman E, Lamm DL, editors: *Urology for primary care physicians,* Philadelphia, 1999, W.B. Saunders.
108. Gebrosky NP, Nseyo UO: Sexually transmitted diseases. In Nseyo UO, Weinman E, Lamm DL, editors: *Urology for primary care physicians*, Philadelphia, 1999, W.B. Saunders.
109. LaRock DR, Sant GR: Lower urinary tract infections. In Nseyo UO, Weinman E, Lamm DL, editors: *Urology for primary care physicians*, Philadelphia, 1999, W.B. Saunders.
110. Partin AW: Benign prostratic hyperplasia. In Lepor H, editor: *Prostatic diseases,* Philadelphia, 2000, W.B. Saunders.
111. Untergasser G et al: Proliferative disorders of the aging human prostate: involvement of protein hormones and their receptors, *Exp Gerontol* 34(2):275, 1999.
112. Jepson JV, Bruskewitz RC: Clinical manifestations and indications for treatment. In Lepor H, editor: *Prostatic diseases,* Philadelphia, 2000, W.B. Saunders.
113. Barry MJ, Meigs JB: Benign prostatic hyperplasia. In Lepor H, editor: *Prostatic diseases,* Philadelphia, 2000, W.B. Saunders.
114. Narayan P: Neoplasms of the prostate gland. In Tanagho EA, McAninch JW, editors: *Smith's general urology,* ed 14, Norwalk, Conn, 1995, Appleton & Lange.
115. Roehrborn CG: In Lepor H, editor: *Prostatic diseases,* Philadelphia, 2000, W.B. Saunders.
116. Foratos DL, de La Rosette JJ: Heat treatment for the prostate: where do we stand in 2000? *Curr Opin Urol* 11(1):35, 2000.
117. American Cancer Society: Prostate cancer resource center, 1999. Available at www3.cancer.org/cancerinfo.
118. American Cancer Society: Cancer statistics 1997, *CA Cancer J Clin* 47(1):8, 1997.
119. Bosland MC: The role of steroid hormones in prostate carcinogenesis, *J Natl Cancer Inst Monogr* 27:39, 2000.
120. Hayes RB et al: Dietary factors and risks for prostate cancer among blacks and whites in the United States, *Cancer Epidemiol Biomarkers Prev* 8(1):25, 1999.
121. Kolonel LN, Nomura AM, Cooney RV: Dietary fat and prostate cancer: current status, *J Natl Cancer Inst* 91(5):414, 1999.
122. CaP CURE Nutrition Project: *Nutrition and prostate cancer: a monograph from the CaP CURE Nutrition Project,* ed 3, p 4, Jan 1999.
123. Denis L et al: Diet and its preventive role in prostatic disease, *Eur Urol* 35(5-6):377, 1999.
124. Yang M, Sytkowski AJ: Differential expression and androgen regulation of the human selenium-binding protein gene hSP56 in prostate cancer cells, *Cancer Res* 58(14):3150, 1998.
125. Zhao XY et al: 1-Alpha,25-dihydroxyvitamin D3 inhibits prostate cancer cell growth by androgen-dependent and androgen-independent mechanisms, *Endocrinology* 141(7):2548, 2000.
126. Arnot R: *The prostate cancer protection plan: the powerful foods, supplements, and drugs that could save your life,* Boston, 2000, Little, Brown.
127. Giovannucci E et al: Intake of carotenoids and retinol in relation to risk of prostate cancer, *J Natl Cancer Inst* 87(23):1767, 1995.
128. Ebling DW et al: Development of prostate cancer after pituitary dysfunction: a report of 8 patients, *Urology* 49(4):564, 1998.
129. Oosthuzien JM et al: Melatonin and steroid-dependent carcinomas, *Andrologia* 21(5):429, 1989.
130. Roberts JT, Essehigh DM: Adenocarcinoma of prostate in 40-year-old body builders, *Lancet* 2(8509):742, 1986.
131. Giovannucci E et al: A prospective cohort study of vasectomy and prostate cancer in US men, *JAMA* 269(7):873, 1993.
132. Peterson RE et al: Vasectomy and the risk of prostate cancer, *Am J Epidemiol* 135(3):324, 1992.
133. Honda GD et al: Vasectomy, cigarette smoking, and age at first sexual intercourse as risk factors for prostate cancer in middle-aged men, *Br J Cancer* 57(3):326, 1988.
134. Klein EA: An update on prostate cancer, *Cleve Clin J Med* 62(5):325, 1995.
135. Giovannucci E et al: Smoking and risk of total fatal prostate cancer in United States health professionals, *Cancer Epidemiol Biomarkers Prev* 8(4 pt 1):277, 1999.
136. Brown SL, Resnick MI: Transrectal ultrasound and the prostate biopsy: clinical and pathologic issues. In Lepor H, editor: *Prostatic diseases,* Philadelphia, 2000, W.B. Saunders.
137. Tanejo SS: The rationale for early detection of prostate cancer. In Lepor H, editor: *Prostatic diseases,* Philadelphia, 2000, W.B. Saunders.
138. Moule JW et al: Prostate-specific antigen values at the time of prostate cancer diagnosis in African-American men, *JAMA* 274(16):1277, 1995.
139. Salgaller ML: Prostate cancer immunotherapy at the dawn of the new millennium, *Expert Opin Investig Drugs* 9(6):1217, 2000.
140. Kim ED, Lipshultz ED: Male infertility. In Copeland LJ, Farrell JF, editors: *Textbook of gynecology,* ed 2, Philadelphia, 2000, W.B. Saunders.
141. Pierik FH et al: Serum inhibin B as a marker of spermatogenesis, *J Clin Endocrinol Metab* 83(9):3110, 1998.
142. Harney KA, Smith LF: The breast. In DeCherney AH, Pernoll ML, editors: *Current obstetric and gynecologic diagnosis and treatment,* ed 8, Norwalk, Conn, 1994, Appleton & Lange.
143. Haagensen CD: *Diseases of the breast,* Philadelphia, 1986, W.B. Saunders.
144. Kase N, Weingold AB, Gershenon DM, editors: *Principles and practice of clinical gynecology,* ed 2, New York, 1990, Churchill Livingstone.
145. Friedenreich C et al: Risk factors for benign proliferative breast disease, *Int J Epidemiol* 29(4):634, 2000.
146. Minami et al: Risk factors for benign breast disease according to histopathological type: comparison with risk factors for breast cancer, *Jpn J Cancer Res* 89(2):116, 1998.
147. Shirley SE: Beyond fibrocystic disease: the evolving concept of premalignant breast disease, *West Indian Med J* 48(4):173, 1999.
148. Dupont W, Page D: Risk factors for breast cancer in women with proliferative breast disease, *N Engl J Med* 312(2):146, 1985.
159. London SJ et al: A prospective study of benign breast disease and the risk of breast cancer, *JAMA* 267:941, 1992.
150. Marshall LM et al: Risk of breast cancer associated with atypical hyperplasia of lobular and ductal types, *Cancer Epidemiol Biomarkers Prev* 6(5):297, 1997.
151. Lundin C, Mertens F: Cytogenetics of benign breast lesions, *Breast Cancer Res Treat* 51(1):1, 1998.
152. Satoh F et al: Immunohistochemical analysis of GCDFP-15 and GCDFP-24 in mammary and non-mammary tissue, *Breast Cancer* 7(1):49, 2000.
153. Sharkey FE, Allred DC, Valente PT: Breast. In Damjanov I, Linder J, editors: *Anderson's pathology,* ed 10, St Louis, 1996, Mosby.
154. Enrioria PJ et al: Effect of natural "micronized" progesterone on the chorionic gonadotropin concentrations in cyst fluids of women with gross cystic breast disease cancer, *J Steroid Biochem Mol Biol* 73 (1-2):67, 2000.
155. Cotran RS et al: *Robbin's pathologic basis of disease,* ed 6, Philadelphia, 1999, W.B. Saunders.
156. Rivera-Pomar JM et al: Focal fibrous disease of breast: a common entity in younger women, *Virchow's Arch [A] Pathol Anat Histol* 386:59, 1980.
157. Welch HG, Black WC: Using autopsy series to estimate the disease "reservoir" for ductal carcinoma in situ of the breast: how much more breast cancer can we find? *Ann Intern Med* 127(11):1023, 1997.
158. Ernster VL et al: Mortality among women with ductal carcinoma in situ of the breast in the population-based surveillance, epidemiology and end results program, *Arch Intern Med* 160(7):953, 2000.
159. Lishman SC, Lakhani SR: Atypical lobular hyperplasia and lobular carcinoma in situ: surgical and molecular pathology, *Histopathology* 35:195, 1999.

160. Jacobs TW: Radial scars in benign breast-biopsy specimens and the risk of breast cancer, *N Engl J Med* 340(6):430, 1999.
161. Moutsatsou P, Sekeris CE: Estrogen and progesterone receptors in the endometrium, *Ann N Y Acad Sci* 816:99, 1997.
162. Pasqualini JR, Chetrite GS: Estrogen sulfatase versus estrone sulfotransferase in human breast cancer: potential clinical applications, *J Steroid Biochem Mol Biol* 69(1-6):287, 1999.
163. Sitruk-Ware R: Progestins in the menopause, *J Steroid Biochem Mol Biol* 69(1-6):185, 1999.
164. Sutherland RL et al: Estrogen and progestin regulation of cell cycle progression, *J Mammary Gland Biol Neoplasia* 3(1):63, 1998.
165. American Cancer Society: Cancer statistics 1997, *CA Cancer J Clin* 47(1):8, 1997.
166. Guiliano AE: Breast. In Tierney LM, McPhee SH, Papadakis MA, editors: *Current medical diagnosis and treatment,* ed 35, Norwalk, Conn, 1996, Appleton & Lange.
167. American Cancer Society: Facts on breast cancer. In *Cancer response system document #407002-407038,* New York, 1995, The Society.
168. Colditz GA: Hormones and breast cancer: evidence and implications for consideration of risks and benefits of hormone replacement therapy, *J Womens Health* 8(3):347, 1999.
169. Collaborative Group on Hormonal Factors in Breast Cancer: Breast cancer and hormone replacement therapy: collaborative reanalysis of data from 51 epidemiological studies of 52,705 women with breast cancer and 108,411 women without breast cancer, *Lancet* 350(9084):1047, 1997.
170. Casper RF: Estrogen with interrupted progestin HRG: a review of experimental and clinical studies, *Maturitas* 34(2):97, 2000.
171. Schairer C et al: Estrogen-progestin replacement and risk of breast cancer, *JAMA* 284(6):691, 2000.
172. Yu H, Berkel H: Insulin-like growth factors and cancer, *J La State Med Assoc* 151(4):218, 1999.
173. Yee D, Lee AV: Crosstalk between the insulin-like growth factors and estrogens in breast cancer, *J Mammary Gland Biol Neoplasia* 5(1):107, 2000.
174. Holmes MD et al: Association of dietary intake of fat and fatty acids with risk of breast cancer, *JAMA* 281(10):914, 1999.
175. Holmes MD et al: Dietary factors and the survival of women with breast carcinoma, *Cancer* 86(5):826, 1999.
176. Bartsch H et al: Dietary polyunsaturated fatty acids and cancer of the breast and colorectum: emerging evidence for their role as risk modifiers, *Carcinogenesis* 20(12):2209, 1999.
177. Cognault S et al: Effect of an alpha-linolenic acid–rich diet on rat mammary tumor growth depends on the dietary oxidative status, *Nutr Cancer* 36(1):33, 2000.
178. Nakagawa H et al: Effects of genstein and synergistic action in combination with eicosapentaenoic acid on the growth of breast cancer cell lines, *J Cancer Res Clin Oncol* 126(8):448, 2000.
179. Thoennes SR et al: Differential transcriptional activation of peroxisome proliferator-activated receptor gamma by omega-3 and omega-6 fatty acids in MCF-7 cells, *Mol Cell Endocrinol* 160(1-2):67, 2000.
180. Petrakis NL: Nipple aspirate fluid in epidemiologic studies of breast disease, *Epidemiol Rev* 15:188, 1993.
181. Kuller LH: The etiology of breast cancer—from epidemiology to prevention, *Public Health Rev* 23:157, 1995.
182. Byers T: Nutritional risk factors for breast cancer, *CA Cancer J Clin* 74(suppl 1):288, 1994.
183. Deslypere JP: Obesity and cancer, *Metabolism* 44(suppl 9):14, 1995.
184. Kreiger N et al: Breast cancer and serum organochlorines: a prospective study among white, black, and Asian women, *J Natl Cancer Inst* 86:589, 1994.
185. Wolff MS et al: Blood levels of organochlorine residues and risk of breast cancer, *J Natl Cancer Inst* 85:648, 1993.
186. Longnecker MP et al: Risk of breast cancer in relation to lifetime alcohol consumption, *J Natl Cancer Inst* 87(21):923, 1995.
187. Damianaki A et al: Potent inhibitory action of red wine polyphenols on human breast cancer cells, *J Cell Biochem* 78(3):429, 2000.
188. Stampfer MJ, Bechtel SD, Hunter D: Fat, alcohol, selenium, and breast cancer risk, *Contemp Ob Gyn* 37:42, 1992.
189. Kuper H et al: Alcohol and breast cancer risk: the alcoholism paradox, *Br J Cancer* 83(7):949, 2000.
190. Lou J, Miller MW: Ethanol enhances erb B–mediated migration of human breast cancer cells in culture, *Breast Cancer Res Treat* 63(1):61, 2000.
191. Fan S et al: Alcohol stimulates estrogen receptor signaling in human breast cancer cell lines, *Cancer Res* 60(20):5635, 2000.
192. Stevens RG et al: Alcohol consumption and urinary concentration of 6-sulfatoxymelatonin in healthy women, *Epidemiology* 11(6):660, 2000.
193. Zhang S et al: A prospective study of folate intake and the risk of breast cancer, *JAMA* 281(17):1632, 1999.
194. King MC, Rowell S, Love SM: Inherited breast and ovarian cancer—what are the risks? What are the choices? *JAMA* 269:1975, 1993.
195. Weber B: Genetic testing for breast cancer, *Sci Am Sci Med* 3(1):12, 1996.
196. Haber D: Roads leading to breast cancer, *N Engl J Med* 343(21):1566, 2000.
197. Kainu T et al: Somatic deletions in hereditary breast cancers implicate 13q21 as a putative novel breast cancer susceptibility locus, *Proc Natl Acad Sci USA* 15:9603, 2000.
198. Waxman J: A new understanding of the hormonal regulation of endocrine dependent cancer, *Br Med Bull* 47(1):197, 1991.
199. Morabia A, Wynder EL: Epidemiology and natural history of breast cancer, *Surg Clin North Am* 70(4):739, 1990.
200. Russo J, Russo IH: Development of the human mammary gland. In Neville MC, Daniel CW, editors: *The mammary gland: development, regulation, and function,* New York, 1987, Plenum Press.
201. Russo IH, Russo J: Hormonal approach to breast cancer prevention, *J Cell Biochem Suppl* 34:1, 2000.
202. Russo IH, Calaf G, Russo J: Hormones and proliferative activity in breast tissue. In Stoll BA, editor: *Approaches to breast cancer prevention,* Dordrecht, Netherlands, 1991, Kluwer Academic Publishers.
203. Zhu BT, Conney AH: Is 2-methoxyestradiol an endogenous estrogen metabolite that inhibits mammary carcinogenesis? *Cancer Res* 58:2269, 1998.
204. Cavalieri E et al: Chapter 4: estrogens as endogenous genotoxic agents—DNA adducts and mutations, *J Natl Cancer Institute Monogr* 27:75, 2000.
205. Yager JD: Chapter 3: endogenous estrogens as carcinogens through metabolic activation, *J Natl Cancer Institute Monogr* 27:67, 2000.
206. Knabbe C et al: Evidence that transforming growth factor–B is a hormonally regulated negative growth factor in human breast cancer cells, *Cell* 48:417, 1987.
207. Antman K, Shea S: Screening mammography under age 50, *JAMA* 281(16):1470, 1999.
208. Conant EF, Maidment ADA: Breast cancer imaging, *Sci Am Sci Med* 3(1):22, 1996.
209. Stoll BA: Breast cancer and the western diet: role of fatty acids and antioxidant vitamins, *Eur J Cancer* 34(12):1852, 1998.
210. Cummings SR: The effect of raloxifene on risk of breast cancer in postmenopausal women: results from the MORE randomized trial, *JAMA* 281(23):2189, 1999.
211. Hsing AW et al: Risk factors for male breast cancer, *Cancer Causes Control* 9(3):269, 1998.
212. Clark JL et al: Prognostic variables in male breast cancer, *Am Surg* 66(5):501, 2000.
213. Jepson AS, Fentiman IS: Male breast cancer, *Int J Clin Pract* 52(8):571, 1998.

CHAPTER 23

Sexually Transmitted Infections

KRISTYNIA M. ROBINSON

CHAPTER OUTLINE

Throughout recorded history, infectious diseases have threatened humans. Even into the twentieth century, epidemics of diphtheria, typhoid, tuberculosis, cholera, and other catastrophic infections have decimated entire communities almost overnight. Despite medical advances, improved living standards, and better nutrition, new epidemics arise as major public health problems, and some pose lethal threats to individuals and communities. Some of these epidemics are caused by sexually transmitted infections (STIs). At this time, many people consider the number of acquired immunodeficiency syndrome (AIDS) cases and human immunodeficiency virus (HIV) and human papillomavirus (HPV) infections to be at epidemic levels.

Sexually contracted infections affect over 15 million Americans per year, 3 million of whom are teenagers,[1] and account for about one third of the reproductive mortality in the United States. Complications of STIs include pelvic inflammatory disease, infertility, ectopic pregnancy, chronic pelvic pain, neonatal morbidity and mortality, genital cancer, and epidemiologic synergy with HIV transmission. Long-term sequelae of untreated or undertreated STIs may be disastrous and can affect a person's physical, emotional, and financial well-being.

In the past an infection transmitted through sexual intercourse was called a *venereal disease.* Because of its limited scope, the term venereal disease has been replaced with *sexually transmitted infection* (STI). STIs are infections contracted by intimate, as well as sexual, contact and include systemic infections, such as tuberculosis and hepatitis, that can be spread to a sexual partner. Etiology of an STI may be bacterial, viral, protozoan, parasitic, or fungal (Table 23-1). Although the majority of STIs can be treated, viral-induced STIs are considered incurable. The current increase in severity and incidence of STIs can be attributed to demographic, life-style, and behavioral factors. First, many infected individuals do not seek treatment because symptoms are absent, minor, or transient or because health services are inaccessible. Second, increased numbers of single individuals, bisexuality, and premarital or extramarital sexual affairs contribute to rising numbers of lifetime sexual partners and exposure to STIs. Last, indulgence in high-risk sexual behaviors and poor health habits, such as failure to use a condom in nonmonogamous or new relationships, drug use, and douching, increases an individual's risk of exposure or the severity of infection if exposed. Perhaps partly because of risk-taking behavior (unprotected intercourse or selection of high-risk partners), adolescents have the greatest risk for STI exposure and infection. In addition, adolescent women may have a physiologically increased susceptibility to infection because of increased cervical ectopy and lack of immunity. Rates of gonorrhea, chlamydia, vaginitis, cervical condyloma, genital warts, and pelvic inflammatory disease (PID) are all highest in adolescents and decline exponentially with increasing age.

STIs are stereotyped as occurring only among urban poor and minority populations. Because the Centers for Disease Control and Prevention (CDC) does not require that all STIs be reported, private physicians may not report them. Thus reported STIs often come from public health clinics, giving the impression that a greater number of the urban poor and minority populations are inflicted with STIs. In fact, STIs are prevalent among all individuals in all socioeconomic groups.

Table 23-1 Currently Recognized Sexually Transmitted Infections

Causal Microorganism	Infection
BACTERIA	
Campylobacter	Campylobacter enteritis
Calymmatobacterium granulomatis	Granuloma inguinale
Chlamydia trachomatis	Urogenital infections; lymphogranuloma venereum
Polymicrobial	
Gardnerella vaginalis interaction with anaerobes (*Bacteroides* and *Mobiluncus* species) and genital mycoplasmas	Bacterial vaginosis
Haemophilus ducreyi	Chancroid
Mycoplasma	Mycoplasmosis
Neisseria gonorrhoeae	Gonorrhea
Shigella	Shigellosis
Treponema pallidum	Syphilis
VIRUSES	
Cytomegalovirus	Cytomegalic inclusion disease
Hepatitis B virus (HBV)	Hepatitis
Hepatitis C (HCV)	Hepatitis
Herpes simplex virus (HSV)	Genital herpes
Human immunodeficiency virus (HIV)	Acquired immunodeficiency syndrome (AIDS)
Human papillomavirus	Condylomata acuminata
Molluscum contagiosum virus	Molluscum contagiosum
PROTOZOA	
Entamoeba histolytica	Amebiasis; amebic dysentery
Giardia lamblia	Giardiasis
Trichomonas vaginalis	Trichomoniasis
ECTOPARASITES	
Phthirus pubis	Pediculosis pubis
Sarcoptes scabiei	Scabies
FUNGUS	
Candida albicans	Candidiasis

WHAT'S NEW? Sexually Transmitted Infection (STI) Statistical Summary from 1998 CDC Report

Each year in the United States:
- 15 million individuals contract an STI from infected partners
- Two-third of those infected are younger than 25 years

In 1998 there were:
- An estimated 4 million new cases of chlamydia, but only 477,638 new cases were reported
- 650,000 new cases of gonorrhea (more than 500,000 cases were reported in 1993)

8,551 new case of primary and second syphilis (more than 34,000 were reported in 1993)

Untreated or undertreated chlamydia infections are the primary case of *preventable* infertility and ectopic pregnancy.

Viral STIs currently affect more than 56 million people in the United States:
- 1 million with human immunodeficiency virus (HIV)
- 20 million with the human papillomavirus (genital warts)
- 45 million with genital herpes

For more information, call the STD hotline at 1-800-277-8922 or the CDC information line at 1-404-639-1819 or register for electronic reporting through CDC Wonder at 1-404-332-4569.

Data from Division of STD Prevention, Department of Health and Human Services: *Sexually transmitted disease surveillance 1998*, Atlanta, 2000, Centers for Disease Control and Prevention.

SEXUALLY TRANSMITTED UROGENITAL INFECTIONS

Bacterial Infections

Gonorrhea

Gonorrhea is caused by **gonococci** (singular, *gonococcus*), which are microorganisms of the species *Neisseria gonorrhoeae.* Neisser first identified gonococci in stained smears of vaginal, urethral, and conjunctival exudate in 1879. Until 1994 gonorrhea was the most commonly reported communicable infection in the United States. Numbers of reported cases have declined from 620,478 cases in 1991 to 355,642 in 1998,[2] but, when unreported infections are included, the annual number of cases is estimated to be about twice as high.

Although the incidence of gonorrhea has dropped remarkably since the peak of the gonorrhea epidemic in the mid-1970s, the infection rate remains problematic in select groups. In 1998 overall rates of gonorrhea were highest in young adults ages 20 to 24 years.[2] Although the number of reported cases declined in all racial and ethnic groups, the gonorrhea rate remains about 30 times greater for blacks than for non-Hispanic whites. Other demographic and life-style risk factors may include transient or urban residence, early onset of sexual activity, multiple serial or consecutive sex partners, drug use, prostitution, and previous gonorrheal or concurrent STI.[3] The overall rate of gonorrhea has declined 72% since 1975. However, between 1997 and 1998 the rate increased by 8.9%.[2] The risk of developing gonorrhea from intercourse with an infected male partner is 50% to 80% for females, and with an infected female partner it is 20% to 30% for males. The risk increases threefold to fourfold for males after four exposures to an infected partner.

Transmission of gonococcal infection generally requires contact of epithelial (mucosal) surfaces, such as occurs during sexual, oral, or anal intercourse. A pregnant woman can also transmit gonorrhea to her fetus. The infection passes from mother to child across the amniotic membranes, by direct inoculation with a fetal scalp electrode during labor monitoring, or during passage through the birth canal. **Fomites** (contaminated objects) are rarely involved in the transmission of *N. gonorrhoeae,* primarily because the gonococcus requires a rich medium (e.g., body fluids) and an environment high in carbon dioxide (5% to 10%) for growth.

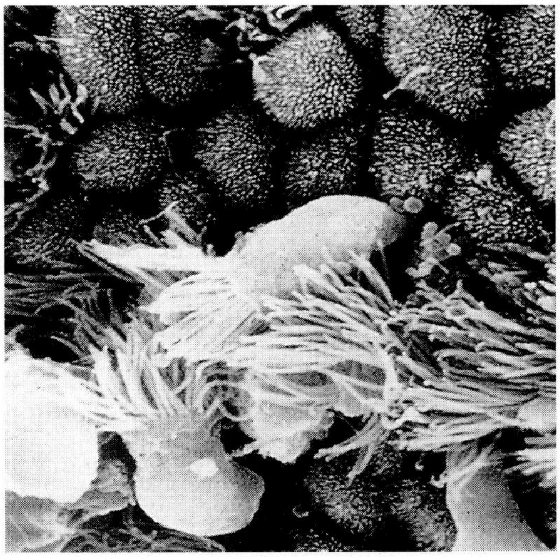

FIG. 23-1 Gonococci. Scanning electron microscopy showing gonococci attached to nonciliated cells from human fallopian tube mucosa. (From Morse SA, Moreland AA, Holmes KK, editors: *Atlas of sexually transmitted diseases and AIDS,* ed 2, London, 1996, Mosby-Wolfe.)

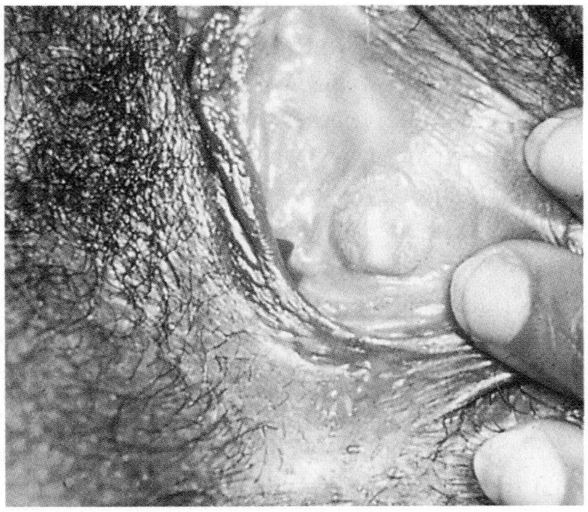

FIG. 23-2 Gonorrhea in a woman. Purulent discharge is visible, with involvement of Bartholin gland. (Examiner would be gloved.) (From Morse SA, Moreland AA, Holmes KK, editors: *Atlas of sexually transmitted diseases and AIDS,* ed 2, London, 1996, Mosby-Wolfe.)

Pathophysiology

Humans are the only natural hosts for *N. gonorrhoeae,* which is an aerobic, non-spore-forming, oxidase-positive, gram-negative coccal (round) microorganism that usually appears in pairs (diplococci), with the adjacent sides slightly flattened. Hairlike filaments, called *pili,* appear to help the microorganisms attach themselves to host cells: the epithelial cells of mucous membranes (Fig. 23-1). Columnar, transitional, and stratified squamous epithelial cells are infected most frequently. First the microorganisms become attached to the plasma membranes (cell walls) of these cells, and then they invade the cells and begin to damage the mucosa. Generally a quick leukocytic (inflammatory) response and exudation at the site of infection occur.

In females the endocervical canal (inner portion of the cervix) is the usual site of original gonococcal infection, although urethral colonization and infection of Skene or Bartholin glands also are common. Several factors can facilitate ascent of gonococci into the uterus and the fallopian tubes, where they cause pelvic inflammatory disease (PID). Among these factors are (1) disintegration of the cervical mucus plug and a rise in vaginal pH above 4.5 during menstruation; (2) uterine cramping that may cause retrograde menstruation, particularly in the presence of an intrauterine contraceptive device; and (3) various microbes that possess virulent potentiating factors for chlamydia or gonococcal PID. Bacteria *(N. gonorrhoeae, Chlamydia trachomatis)* also may adhere to sperm and be transported to the fallopian tubes In the fallopian tubes, progressive mucosal and submucosal invasion and sloughing of normal, ciliated tubal epithelium are accompanied by marked inflammatory response, causing the fallopian tubes to fill with exudate. In males the gonococci typically infect the urethra. Untreated urethral infection causes epididymitis in 1% to 2% of men and, rarely, urethral stricture and sterility. Frequently, concurrent oropharyngeal and anorectal infection can be found in infected men and women.[4,5,6]

Clinical Manifestations

The clinical manifestations of gonorrhea can be categorized as local or systemic and uncomplicated or complicated. Uncomplicated local infections are seen as urethral infections in males and urogenital infections in females. In males the incubation period for urethritis is 3 to 10 days with a range of 12 hours to 3 months.[7] Without treatment, urethritis persists for 3 to 7 weeks, with 95% of men becoming asymptomatic after 3 months. Approximately 60% of those infected suddenly experience marked dysuria (painful or difficult urination) and spontaneous, profuse, mucopurulent discharge from the urethra. However, some individuals have little discharge or urethral itching only, and 5% to 10% never have signs or symptoms. Most cases of untreated gonococcal urethritis resolve spontaneously after several weeks, and more than 95% of individuals are asymptomatic by 6 months after infection.

In females the incubation period varies, but those who develop symptoms do so within 10 days of exposure or within 1 to 2 days after the next menstrual period. The clinical manifestations of uncomplicated gonorrhea in women may be absent (50% of women have asymptomatic infection) or severe; they can include dysuria, increased vaginal discharge, abnormal menses (increased flow or dysmenorrhea), or dyspareunia. Physical examination may disclose cervical friability and erythema (redness) and purulent or mucopurulent discharge from the cervical os. There may be a discharge from the Skene or Bartholin glands if these sites are involved (Fig. 23-2).

Anal and rectal gonococcal infection is found in 30% to 50% of women diagnosed with urogenital gonorrhea. In women, anorectal infection is usually asymptomatic and not necessarily related to anal intercourse. Anorectal gonorrhea most commonly occurs in homosexual men with a history of receptive anorectal intercourse. About 50% of these infected men have symptoms.[7,8]

Symptoms of anorectal gonorrhea range from mild anal pruritus (itching), mucopurulent rectal discharge, and slight rectal bleeding to severe rectal pain, tenesmus (painful and ineffectual straining at stool), and constipation. Physical examination may disclose anal erythema and discharge and evidence of mucosal damage to the anus and rectum, such as friability, edema, and purulent exudate.

Gonococcal pharyngitis occurs primarily in homosexual or bisexual men or heterosexual women after fellatio (oral sexual contact) with an infected partner. Symptomatic pharyngitis is indistinguishable from any other bacterial pharyngitis and can include fever, lymphadenopathy, and tonsillitis. Approximately 60% of these infections are asymptomatic.

Other sites of uncomplicated local infections include the eye, leading to conjunctivitis; however, this is rare in adults. Primary cutaneous infection has also been reported and is usually manifested as a localized ulcer of the genitalia, perineum, proximal lower extremities, or fingers. It is important to determine if such infections are the result of *N. gonorrhoeae* or secondary colonization by a preexisting lesion.

Localized gonococcal infections can be complicated by prostatitis, epididymitis, lymphangitis, and urethral stricture in men and salpingitis, PID, and bartholinitis in women. Chronic salpingitis or perididymitis can cause scarring and tubal adhesions that lead to sterility. Anyone who is infected and remains untreated is at risk for disseminated gonococcal infection.[4,5,6]

Before the advent of antimicrobial therapy, approximately 20% of infected males developed acute epididymitis. Men with this condition report unilateral testicular pain and swelling and commonly have overt urethritis at the same time. Penile lymphangitis is a rare complication with an unclear pathogenesis.[4] Before modern antibiotics, individuals with this condition were at risk for developing urethral strictures; however, this complication is now uncommon if treatment is sought and therapy instituted properly.

Acute salpingitis, or PID, is the most common local complication in females. Approximately 40% of women with untreated cervical gonorrhea develop this condition. Salpingitis is significant in its development because of the potential long-term sequelae associated with it, namely, infertility and ectopic pregnancy.

The onset of symptoms may be rapid and usually occurs during menses. Women may experience chills, fever, nausea, vomiting, and lower abdominal pain that worsen with coughing, sneezing, or intercourse. Abdominal palpation often discloses bilateral lower quadrant tenderness and rebound tenderness resulting from peritoneal irritation caused by tubal exudate. Marked tenderness of the internal genitalia is frequently noted during pelvic examination. Enlargement or masses also may be palpable in the upper genital tract. Abscess of Bartholin gland is also a local complication associated with gonococcal infection in females. Apart from PID, abscess formation of Bartholin gland is the most common complication of gonorrhea in females.

Disseminated gonococcal infection (DGI) is a rare systemic complication brought about by the spread of infection through the bloodstream. Approximately 0.5% of individuals with untreated gonococcal infection develop this complication.[8] Symptoms include fever, rash, and joint swelling or pain.

Spread of *N. gonorrhoeae* to the liver causes a condition known as **perihepatitis** or Fitz-Hugh-Curtis syndrome. *C. trachomatis* also has been identified as a causative agent. Inflammation of the capsule of the liver is the primary pathologic manifestation and produces sudden and intense right upper quadrant pain.[9]

Newborns are at risk most commonly for gonococcal eye infection **(ophthalmia neonatorum)** but also may acquire rhinitis, anorectal infection, or an abscess at the site of electrode placement for fetal monitoring. Onset of symptoms generally occurs 1 to 12 days after birth, with a mean of 4 to 6 days. Affected newborns usually are born to mothers who have had prolonged ruptured membranes. In these cases, immediate treatment with a topical antibiotic is not effective, because the infection is already established. Established infection causes bilateral corneal ulceration, with a profuse yellow or gray purulent exudate and is followed by necrosis, scarring, and compromised vision. Signs of systemic disease are seldom apparent.

Evaluation and Treatment

Clinical signs and symptoms are not sufficient for the differential diagnosis of gonococcal infections. Microscopic evaluation of gram-stained slides of clinical specimens is deemed positive for *N. gonorrhoeae* if gram-negative diplococci with typical "kidney bean" morphology are seen inside polymorphonuclear leukocytes. Such a finding is considered adequate for the diagnosis of gonococcal urethritis in a symptomatic male. Because of the large percentage of infected women without symptoms, routine screening is recommended. For screening purposes or diagnosis of pharyngeal or anorectal gonorrhea, cultures or deoxyribonucleic acid (DNA) genetic probe testing is recommended. For females the Gram stain technique is less accurate and reliable and is replaced with a single culture of endocervical secretions. Because the pharynx or anus and rectum are rarely the only sites of infection for females, routine cultures of these sites are optional.

The many different strains of *N. gonorrhoeae* vary with respect to pathogenicity, virulence, and susceptibility to antibiotics. Two types of plasmid-resistant strains have been identified; they are penicillinase-producing *N. gonorrhoeae* (PPNG), which is resistant to penicillin, and tetracycline-resistant *N. gonorrhoeae* (TRNG). Of all the isolates collected in 1998 by the Gonococcal Isolate Surveillance Project (GISP), 29.4% (a 2% decline since 1995)[10] were resistant to penicillin, tetracycline, or both.[3] In the United States the overall percentage of PPNG isolates has declined from 11.0% in 1991 to 3.0% in 1998,[4] yet the PPNG isolates in some urban areas may be as high as 60% to 75%. TRNG strains have been concentrated along the East Coast of the United States, where they have accounted for about 15% of gonococci. High-level multi-drug–resistant strains are formed when PPNG continues with TRNG. Chromosomally mediated resistant gonococci (CMRNG) are resistant to both penicillin and tetracycline. The prevalence of CRMNG increased from 3.0% in 1989 to 7.2% in 1998.[11] In addition, the number of GISP isolates demonstrating susceptibility to ciprofloxacin, one of the currently recommended treatments for gonorrhea, has decreased from a high of 1.3% in 1994 to 0.5% in 1996. By 1998, the number had increased to 0.9%.[3]

Another major concern is the coexistence of chlamydial infection with gonorrhea.[12] (Chlamydial infections are discussed on pp. 793.) Approximately 20% to 30% of males and a higher proportion of females have coexistent chlamydia infections. Symptoms of chlamydia often go undetected until complications such as PID or urethritis manifest themselves.

Treatment for gonorrhea is influenced by three factors: (1) the spread of infection caused by PPNG and TRNG, (2) the high frequency of chlamydia infection accompanying gonorrhea, and (3) recognition of the serious complications of chlamydia and gonorrhea infections. Beginning in 1989 the CDC[13] recommended that all gonococcal infections be treated as if the organisms were antibiotic resistant and a chlamydia infection coexisted. Current CDC treatment guidelines for uncomplicated gonorrheal infections are listed in Box 23-1; complicated infections require intravenous antibiotic therapy and possible hospitalization.

Sexual partners also are assessed and treated according to these protocols, and sexual contact is avoided until treatment is completed. Condoms are strongly recommended to prevent future infection.

Box 23-1

OUTPATIENT TREATMENT FOR UNCOMPLICATED GONORRHEA INFECTION

One of the following:

Ceftriaxone, 125 mg IM,
or
Ciprofloxacin, 500 mg,
or
Spectinomycin, 2 g IM, (if allergic to penicillin)
or
Cefiximine, 400 mg PO,
or
Ofoxacin, 400 mg PO

Followed by one of these regimens for presumptive coexistent chlamydia:

Azithromycin, 1 g PO (as single dose),
or
Doxycycline, 100 mg PO bid × 7 days,
or
Erythromycin, 500 mg PO qid × 7 days

Syphilis

Syphilis, a disease with local and systemic manifestations, has been well known throughout history. Many famous figures from biblical and Roman times and from the royal families of the Old World were thought or known to have had syphilis.[14] In the early half of the 1900s, an estimated 1 in 4 to 1 in 20 Americans were infected.[15] With the advent of antibiotics and intensive public health efforts during and after World War II, the prevalence of syphilis declined sharply to less than 3 in 1000 Americans in 1985. Between 1986 and 1990, incidence rose to its highest level in 40 years. Recently, the annual reported new cases of primary and secondary syphilis has declined from 50,223 in 1990 to 6,993 in 1998, the lowest number since 1958.[2] Although the incidence in the United States has diminished significantly in the past 3 decades, syphilis remains a problem in certain geographic regions, particularly among blacks. Syphilis facilitates the transmission of HIV infection and seems to contribute to HIV transmission in those parts of the United States, such as the South, where rates of both infections are high.[16] In 1998 the rate of infection was 34 times higher for non-Hispanic blacks than for non-Hispanic whites.[2] During pregnancy, untreated early syphilis results in perinatal death in as many as 40% of cases and, if acquired in the previous 4 years, may lead to fetal infection in more than 70% of cases.[17]

Syphilis occurs primarily in low-income, minority, heterosexual couples who live in the South. Although the rate of primary and secondary syphilis has declined for all racial and ethnic groups since 1990[18] (90% in Hispanics, 85% in non-Hispanic blacks, and 81% in non-Hispanic whites), it is still highest among non-Hispanic black males between the ages of 35 and 39 years.[3] In addition, gonorrhea rates in black adolescents ages 15 to 19 years are more than 28 times higher than rates in white adolescents. Race and ethnicity alone do not alter STI risk but rather act as risk markers that correlate with other more fundamental determinants of health status, such as poverty, access to quality care, and health-seeking behavior. Higher infection rates have been associated with urban areas and with the exchange of sex for drugs, especially crack cocaine.[19] A growing concern is the rapid rise of syphilis infections in the transient and homeless populations.

The current rate of **congenital syphilis (CS)** has paralleled the rates of primary and secondary syphilis diagnosed in minority women over the past 10 years. CS increased 21% between 1986 and 1987[17] and then began to decline. Between 1993 and 1998, the overall rate decreased from 80.7 to 20.6 cases per 100,000 live births.[3] In 1994, 92% of the 1934 infants reported to have CS were born to black or Hispanic women. Although the overall incidence of CS is declining, an increase occurred from 1997 to 1998 in 6 of the 21 states that reported more than five cases in 1998 (Arizona, Missouri, New Jersey, North Carolina, Oklahoma, and South Carolina). In addition, three states (Arkansas, Maryland, and New Jersey) and Puerto Rico had congenital syphilis rates that exceeded the nation's objective for the year 2000, which is 40 cases per 100,000 live births (see *Healthy People 2000: National Health Promotion and Disease Prevention Objectives*).[3] The *Healthy People 2000* objective is many times greater than the rate of CS of most industrialized countries, where syphilis and CS have been nearly eradicated.

Pathophysiology

Treponema pallidum, the cause of syphilis, is an anaerobic bacterium that cannot be cultured in vitro. The treponema (individual microorganism) looks like a corkscrew, with regular, tight spirals and a rotary motion; it can infect any body organ or tissue. Because the bacterium is present in exudate from moist mucosal or cutaneous lesions, the spirochete is transmitted during the first few years of infection. Transmission generally occurs through minor abrasions during sexual intercourse but can occur extragenitally as well. Approximately 30% to 50% of partners who have sexual intercourse with an individual in early-stage syphilis develop the disease.[18]

Syphilis becomes a systemic disease shortly after infection and can be transmitted from a pregnant woman to her fetus as early as the ninth week of gestation. The risk of transmission to the fetus gradually declines with each subsequent pregnancy; therefore a mother who has had several children with severe congenital syphilis may go on to bear a healthy child. After about 8 years, even without treatment, the mother's infection is not transmitted to her fetus.[15]

The course of untreated syphilis consists of four stages: primary, secondary, latent, and tertiary (Box 23-2). **Primary syphilis** begins at the site of bacterial invasion (Fig. 23-3). There *T. pallidum* multiplies in the epithelium, producing a granulomatous tissue reaction called a **chancre.** Some microorganisms drain with lymph into adjacent lymph nodes. Within the nodes and at the site of the chancre, the cell-mediated and humoral immune responses are stimulated.

Secondary syphilis is systemic. During this stage, blood-borne bacteria spread to all major organ systems. The secondary stage is followed by a period during which the immune system is able to suppress the infection. Even without treatment, spontaneous resolution of the skin lesions occurs and the individual enters the latent stage of infection. **Latent**

Box 23-2

PROGRESSION OF UNTREATED SYPHILIS

Stage I, primary syphilis—local invasion: *T. pallidum* multiplies in epithelium, producing granulomatous tissue reaction (chancre); lymph-containing microorganisms drain into adjacent lymph nodes and stimulate immune responses

Stage II, secondary syphilis—systemic disease: blood-borne bacteria spread to all major organ systems; immune system suppresses infection and symptoms regress spontaneously

Stage III, latent syphilis—silent infection: transmission of infection possible even though there are no clinical signs of infection

Stage IV, tertiary syphilis—noninfectious disease: significant morbidity and mortality occur; destructive skin, bone, and soft tissue lesions, or gummas, result from severe hypersensitivity; cardiovascular complications (aneurysms, heart valve insufficiency, heart failure) and neurosyphilis develop

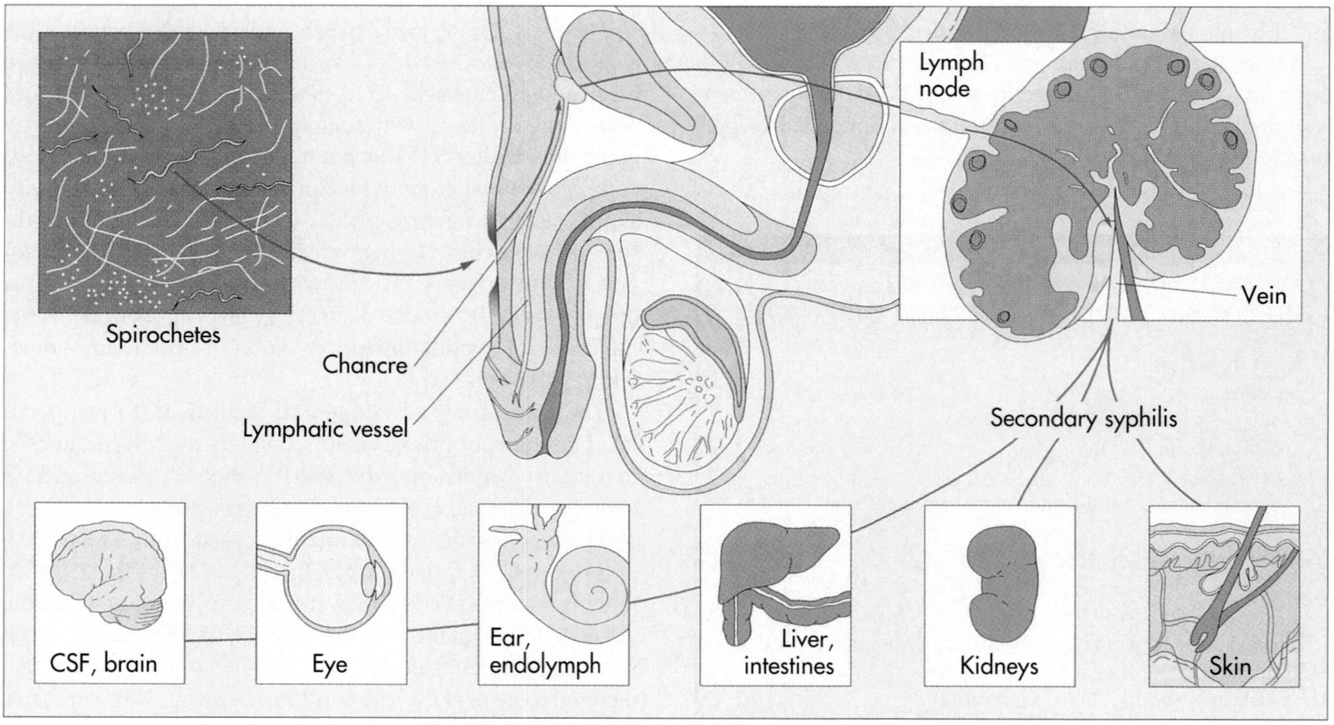

Fig. 23-3 Spirochetes (syphilis) and the progression of disease. Spirochetes enter regional lymph nodes from a skin chancre and then enter the bloodstream. Secondary syphilis is the involvement of systemic organ systems. *CSF,* Cerebrospinal fluid. (From Morse SA, Moreland AA, Holmes KK, editors: *Atlas of sexually transmitted diseases and AIDS,* ed 2, London, 1996, Mosby-Wolfe.)

syphilis may be subdivided into early and late stages; however, no specific criteria delineate one from the other.[19] Medical history and serologic studies show that syphilis is present, but the individual has no clinical manifestations. Transmission is possible during the late and early latent stages.

Tertiary syphilis is the most severe stage, involving significant morbidity and mortality. The pathogenesis of syphilitic manifestations at this stage remains unclear. The destructive skin, bone, and soft tissue lesions (called **gummas**) of tertiary syphilis probably are caused by a severe hypersensitivity reaction to the microorganism. Within the cardiovascular system, infection with *T. pallidum* may cause aneurysms, heart valve insufficiencies, and heart failure. Within the central nervous system (CNS), the presence of *T. pallidum* in cerebrospinal fluid may cause the manifestations of **neurosyphilis.**[15]

The risk of acquiring CS is estimated at 50% in primary and secondary syphilis, 40% in early latent syphilis, and 10% in late latent syphilis.[20] Intrauterine infection causes fetal or perinatal death in 40% of affected infants.[17,21]

Clinical Manifestations

Primary stage. In adults the incubation period of syphilis ranges from 12 days to 12 weeks after exposure and averages 3 weeks. At the site of treponemal entry a sore, or *hard chancre,* develops. Typically the chancre is an eroded, painless, firm, and indurated (hard) ulcer that may be a few millimeters to 2 cm in diameter. Firm, enlarged, and nontender regional lymph nodes accompany chancres. Fig. 23-4 shows typical chancres of the penis and vulva. Syphilitic chancres are not always typical, however. Secondary infection can cause chancres to become necrotic and painful, and lesions on the fingers may be dry, scaly, and papular or moist and vegetative. If left untreated, the chancre of primary syphilis heals in 2 to 8 weeks and then spontaneously disappears, usually without leaving a scar.

Secondary stage. Clinical manifestations of secondary syphilis usually develop 6 weeks after the first appearance of the chancre but may overlap with those of the primary stage. Typically this stage presents with variable systemic symptoms, including low-grade fever, malaise, sore throat, hoarseness, anorexia, generalized adenopathy, headache, joint pain, and skin or mucous membrane lesions or rashes. Cutaneous (skin) rashes are generally papulosquamous (raised and scaly), but any variation or combination of macular (flat), papular (raised), and pustular (pus-filled) lesions may be seen. Often lesions are widespread and bilateral and appear on the palms and soles (Fig. 23-5). Some lesions become hypertrophied, flat, moist, and wartlike or vegetative (e.g., cauliflower-like). These lesions, called **condylomata lata,** are highly contagious and develop on the perineum, vulva, and groin of women (Fig. 23-6) and around the inner thigh and the anal area in both men and women. Besides skin sores, oral mucous membrane lesions (known as mucous patches), lymphadenopathy, pruritus, and alopecia are common. Some individuals develop anemia, leukocytosis, increased sedimentation rate, hepatitis, transitory proteinuria, arthritis, electrocardiographic abnormalities, and CNS symptoms. Regardless of whether treatment is given, the cutaneous lesions generally heal in 2 to 10 weeks, but relapses may occur for several years.[20]

Latent and tertiary stages. The asymptomatic, latent stage of syphilis may be as short as 1 year or as long as a lifetime. After the latent stage, tertiary syphilis may present with gummas, cardiovascular lesions, and neurosyphilis. These manifestations of tertiary syphilis are quite rare because antibiotics can cure syphilis.

Congenital syphilis. CS is characterized by vasculitis, necrosis, fibrosis, and distribution of *T. pallidum* throughout the tissues; it is divided into early and late stages. Signs and symptoms of early CS manifest in the first 2 years of life, and clinical manifestations of the late stage often occur near

A

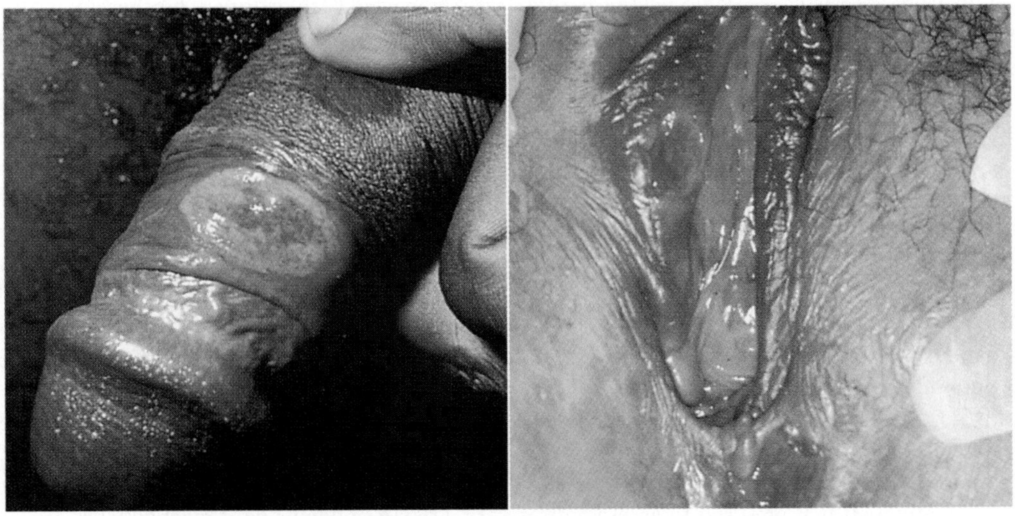

B

FIG. 23-4 Primary syphilis. A, Chancre of the penile shaft. **B,** Multiple primary syphilitic chancres. Labia and the perineum easily show induration and edema of chancres. (Examiner would be gloved.) (From Morse SA, Moreland AA, Holmes KK, editors: *Atlas of sexually transmitted diseases and AIDS,* ed 2, London, 1996, Mosby-Wolfe.)

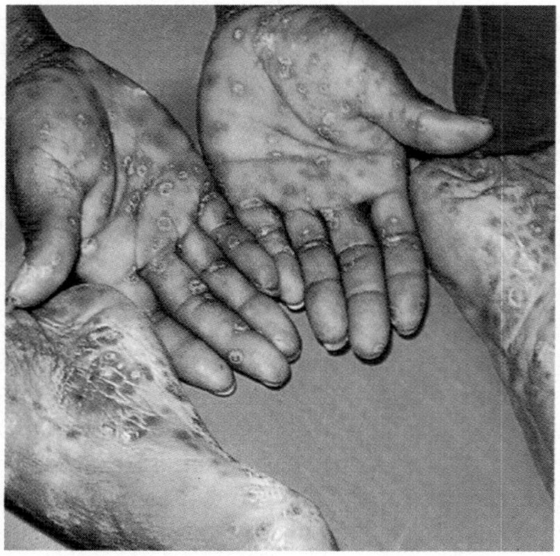

FIG. 23-5 Secondary syphilis. Secondary syphilis to the palms and plantar surfaces. (From Morse SA, Moreland AA, Holmes KK, editors: *Atlas of sexually transmitted diseases and AIDS,* ed 2, London, 1996, Mosby-Wolfe.)

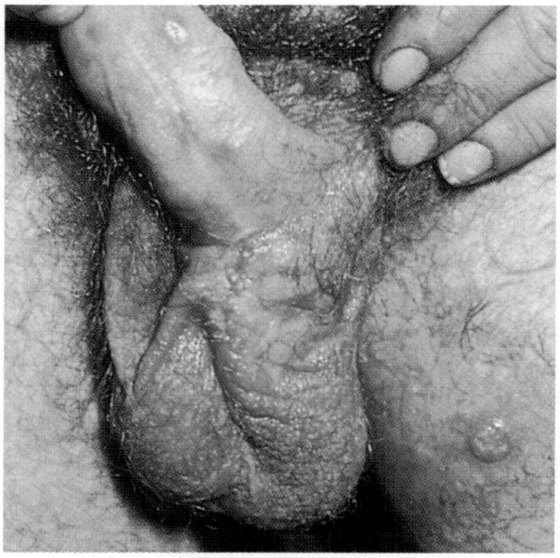

FIG. 23-6 Condylomata lata. Broad-based, moist, darkfield-positive condylomata lata on the thigh. Note the other erosive lesions of secondary syphilis on the penile shaft. (Examiner would be gloved.) (From Morse SA, Moreland AA, Holmes KK, editors: *Atlas of sexually transmitted diseases and AIDS,* ed 2, London, 1996, Mosby-Wolfe.)

puberty. Affected newborns often are premature and show evidence of intrauterine growth retardation, hepatosplenomegaly, bone marrow depression, destructive bone and skin lesions (see Fig. 23-5), retinal inflammation, glaucoma, blood dyscrasia, nephrotic syndrome, and varying degrees of CNS involvement.[15] Late manifestations of classic congenital syphilis correspond to those of tertiary syphilis in the adult and are rare.

Evaluation and Treatment

Because *T. pallidum* cannot be cultured in vitro, early definitive diagnosis of primary or secondary syphilis depends on dark-field microscopy of a specimen taken from a chancre, regional lymph node, or other lesion. If the initial result is negative, the dark-field examination is repeated on two successive days. When suspicion of syphilis—based on history and physical examination—persists, serologic testing is required. An algorithmic approach to the diagnosis of genital ulcers is presented in Fig. 23-7.

Two categories of serologic testing exist: nontreponemal antigen tests and treponemal antibody tests.[22] Nontreponemal antigen tests, which demonstrate the presence of *reagin* (a group of antibodies present in syphilis) in serum, provide indirect evidence of infection. Examples of nontreponemal analysis are the Venereal Disease Research Laboratory (VDRL) antigen and the rapid plasma reagin (RPR) tests (Box 23-3). These tests yield a positive result (presence of reagin) in more than 50% of individuals with primary syphilis and 100% of individuals with secondary disease. When the serologic test is negative and another stage of syphilis is suspected, the test is repeated. If latent or tertiary syphilis is suspected, a treponemal serologic test is done. Treponemal tests are serologic-specific tests that are used to assess antibody response to *T. pallidum* and include the fluorescent treponemal antibody absorption (FTA-ABS) test and the microhemagglutination (MHA-TP) test.

Numerous dermatologic disorders can mimic the skin lesions of secondary syphilis, making differential diagnosis difficult. Again, laboratory confirmation is important; dark-field microscopy of scrapings from the condylomata lata or other skin lesions discloses the treponemata. Serologic tests are almost always strongly positive in this stage.

During the latent stage, individuals continue to have serologic evidence of untreated disease, but confirmation through dark-field microscopy is difficult. Examination of cerebrospinal fluid may confirm that the treponemata are present and the insidious onset of neurosyphilis has begun.

Treatment for all stages of syphilis is parenteral injection of benzathine penicillin G. If the individual has had signs of the disease for less than 1 year, a single dose is appropriate. If signs have been present for more than 1 year, the treatment is three weekly injections. This therapy is also appropriate in pregnancy. There is no evidence to date that *T. pallidum* has developed resistance to penicillin.[3] Individuals who are allergic to penicillin receive oral doxycycline, 100 mg twice daily; or, if the individual is pregnant, she receives oral erythromycin, 500 mg four times daily. Duration of therapy depends on estimated length of infection. Treatment for 14 days is recommended if the individual is infected less than 1 year; treatment is for 28 days if the individual has been infected for longer than 1 year. Because treatment failures do occur, all individuals should have follow-up evaluation. Sexual partners also are examined and treated, and the use of condoms is recommended.

Definitive diagnosis of CS is made by microscopic identification of *T. pallidum* in material from skin lesions or nasal discharge. Probable diagnosis is assumed on the basis of a rising or persistently reactive FTA-ABS value and clinical manifestations. In all cases of maternal syphilis, the goal is to treat the mother to prevent CS. Maternal treatment with penicillin before delivery usually prevents CS. If the infant

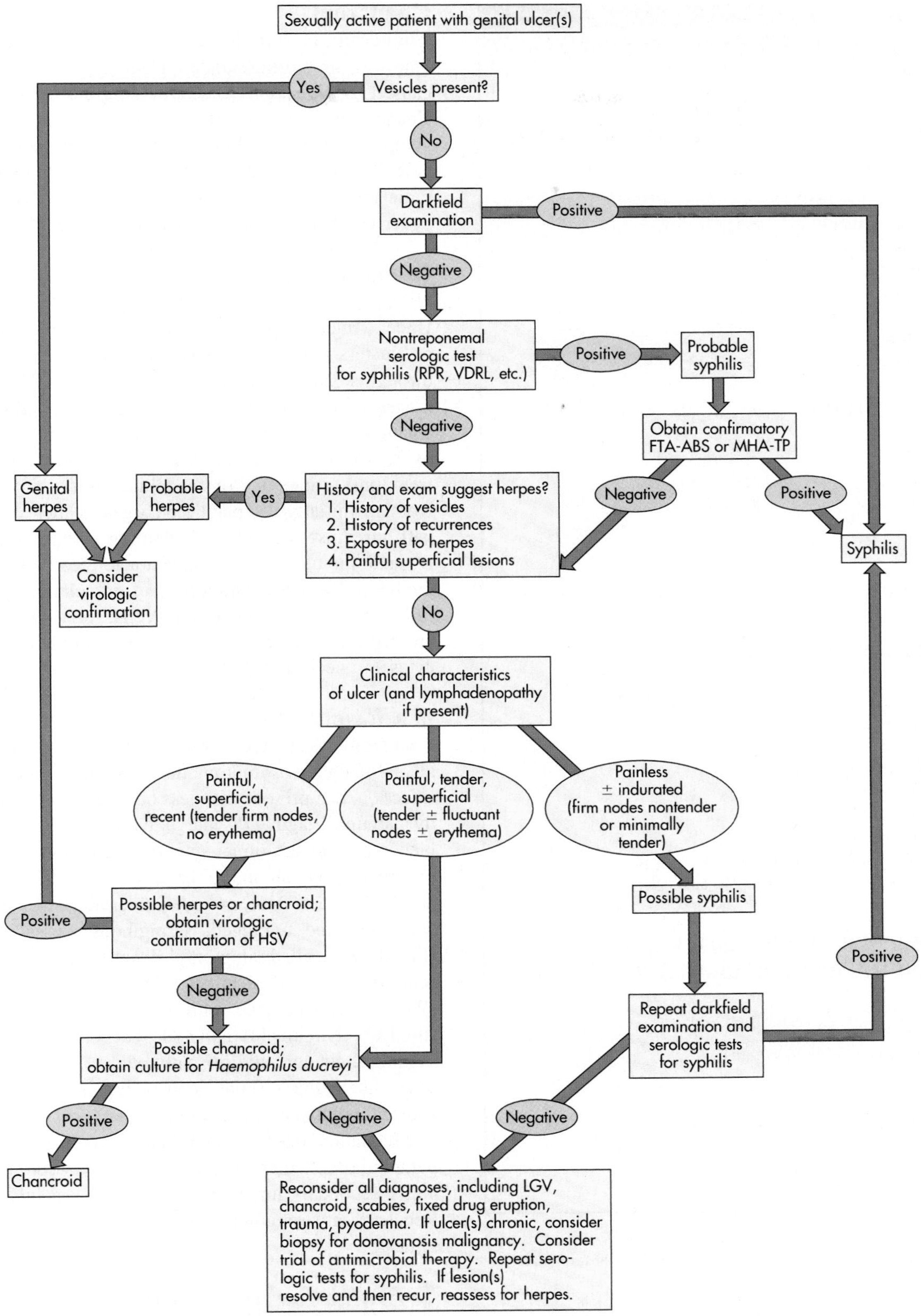

FIG. 23-7 Genital ulceration. Algorithm outlining an approach to the diagnosis of an individual who presents with a genital ulceration. *RPR,* Rapid plasma reagin test; *VDRL,* Venereal Disease Research Laboratory test; *FTA-ABS,* fluorescent treponemal antibody absorption test; *MHA-TP,* microhemagglutination test; *HSV,* herpes simplex virus; *LGV,* lymphogranuloma venereum. (Redrawn from Pitot P, Plummer FA. In Holmes KK et al, editors: *Sexually transmitted diseases,* ed 2, New York, 1990, McGraw-Hill.)

Box 23-3

FALSE-POSITIVE SEROLOGIC TESTS FOR SYPHILIS

REASONS FOR FALSE-POSITIVE, NONTREPONEMAL REACTIONS (VDRL, RPR)

Transient reactions (<6 mos)

Technical error (low titer)
Smallpox vaccination
Mycoplasma pneumonia
Enterovirus infections
Infectious mononucleosis
Pregnancy
Narcotic abuse
Advanced tuberculosis
Scarlet fever
Viral and atypical pneumonia
Brucellosis
Rat-bite fever
Leptospirosis
Measles
Mumps
Lymphogranuloma venereum
Malaria
Trypanosomiasis
Varicella

Chronic reactions (>6 mos)

Malaria
Leprosy
Systemic lupus erythematosus
Narcotic abuse
Other connective tissue diseases
Elderly population
Hashimoto thyroiditis
Rheumatoid arthritis
Reticuloendothelial malignancy
Familial false-positive reaction
Idiopathic

REASONS FOR FALSE-POSITIVE, TREPONEMA-SPECIFIC REACTIONS (FTA-ABS)

Technical error
Inefficient sorbents
Healthy individuals without syphilis
Genital herpes simplex
Pregnancy
Lupus erythematosus (skin only or systemic)
Alcoholic cirrhosis
Scleroderma
Mixed connective tissue disease

VDRL, Veneral Disease Research Laboratory test; *RPR,* rapid plasma reagin test; *FTA-ABS,* fluorescent treponemal antibody absorption test.

requires treatment, penicillin is the drug of choice, because allergy does not pose a problem in the neonatal period. Such infants are then given serologic tests for syphilis at 3, 6, and 12 months. Nearly all tests become nonreactive (negative) by the time the infant is 6 months of age.[17]

Chancroid

Chancroid, or soft chancre, is an acute infectious disease that was first differentiated from syphilis in 1852. It is caused by *Haemophilus ducreyi,* a gram-negative bacillus. Chancroid occurs most frequently in underdeveloped or developing countries. Although incidence in the United States is low, 243 cases were reported to the CDC in 1997[1]; sporadic outbreaks can occur and tend to be associated with poverty, urban prostitution, and illicit drug use.[23]

Pathophysiology

H. ducreyi is a gram-negative bacillus with rounded ends. Under a microscope it is commonly observed in small chains or clusters along mucous strands. Transmission can occur through sexual contact and autoinoculation. There is no evidence of maternal-fetal transfer before or after delivery. Chancroid lesions usually are found on the internal surface of the foreskin or its point of attachment to the penis (the frenulum) in men and on the labia, clitoris, or fourchette in women. Initially the papule enlarges; it then erodes into a soft, circumscribed ulcer containing a superficial exudate. Beneath the ulcer is a lesion characterized by edema, endothelial proliferation, and a base of granulation tissue that is full of lymphocytes and plasma cells. Adjacent lymph nodes are acutely inflamed and full of polymorphonuclear leukocytes and necrotic cells.[24]

Clinical Manifestations

Chancroid has an incubation period of 3 to 10 days.[23] Generally, women are asymptomatic, but depending on the site of infection, can present with less obvious symptoms (dysuria, dyspareunia, vaginal discharge, pain on defecation, or rectal bleeding). Constitutional symptoms are unusual. At the site of inoculation, an initial vesicopustule lesion forms and erodes into a soft ulcer with a necrotic base; surrounding erythema; and a ragged, serpiginous (spreading) border (Fig. 23-8). Unilateral, painful, local lymphadenopathy presents in about half of infected individuals—primarily men. (Women tend to have multiple lesions.) Inguinal **buboes** (fluid-filled inguinal lymph nodes) develop 7 to 10 days after the initial chancre and fill with exudate. In 25% to 60% of cases, the buboes spontaneously rupture. Multiple lesions spread through autoinoculation.

Frequently ulcers on the prepuce may lead to phimosis or paraphimosis. Other complications of chancroid include balanitis, secondary infections, necrosis, and fistula formation. Recalcitrant, serpiginous lesions may take months or years to heal.

Evaluation and Treatment

Chancroid is easily confused with other types of genital ulcers, particularly those of syphilis, genital herpes, and granuloma inguinale (see Fig. 23-8). Unlike the syphilitic ulcer, chancroidal ulcer is painful, tender, and nonindurated. Microscopic analysis of a gram-stained smear from the chancroid helps to identify the microorganism. Definitive diag-

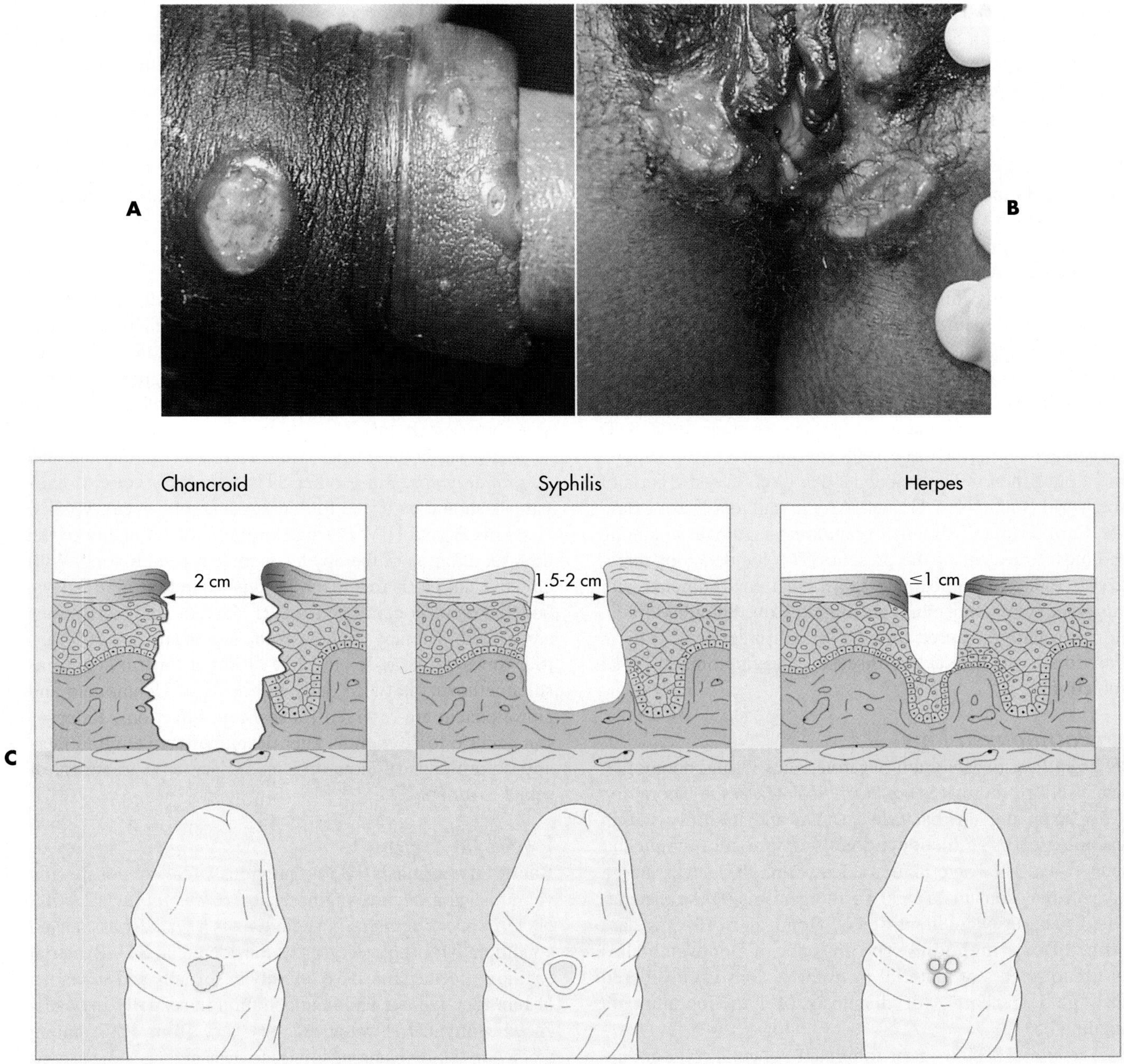

FIG. 23-8 **Chancroid.** **A,** Ulcers on the penile shaft. **B,** Multiple vulvar lesions. **C,** Differences in clinical appearance among chancroid, syphilis, and genital herpes. (From Morse SA, Moreland AA, Holmes KK, editors: *Atlas of sexually transmitted diseases and AIDS,* ed 2, London, 1996, Mosby-Wolfe.)

nosis depends on recovery of *H. ducreyi* from cultured specimens (although special culture medium and conditions are required). Fluorescent monoclonal antibody stains and polymerase chain reaction provide more specific diagnosis but are not routinely available. Because 10% of infected individuals are coinfected with syphilis or herpes simplex virus (HSV), testing includes serologic examination for syphilis and viral culture for HSV. In addition, HIV testing is recommended: chancroid is a cofactor for transmission of HIV.

Resistance to recommended antibiotics has emerged in isolated instances worldwide. Recent treatment recommendations include a single intramuscular injection of ceftriaxone (250 mg) or a single dose of oral azithromycin (1 g). Effective oral multiple-dose regimens include amoxicillin (500 mg) and potassium clavulanate (125 mg) three times daily for 7 days; erythromycin, 500 mg four times daily for 7 days; or ciprofloxacin, 500 mg twice daily for 3 days.[3] Persons infected with HIV have higher rates of treatment failure with single-dose therapy and may require a longer treatment regimen. As a palliative measure, buboes can be aspirated through adjacent, healthy skin. In approximately 5% of cases, relapses at the site of original ulcer have occurred.[23,25] Simultaneous treatment of sexual partners and condom use are recommended to prevent reinfection.

Granuloma Inguinale

Granuloma inguinale (donovanosis) is a chronic, progressively destructive bacterial infection caused by *Calymmatobacterium granulomatis,* which is related to *Klebsiella pneumoniae.* Although sexually transmissible, granuloma inguinale is only mildly contagious and repeated exposure is necessary to cause disease. Often, individuals are coinfected with syphilis.[26]

Indigenous granuloma inguinale no longer occurs in the United States (cases that occur are imported).[23] Of interest, the CDC deleted granuloma inguinale in their 1998 STD surveillance report and the 1998 surveillance report supplement published in November 1999.[2,11] Yet, in some parts of the world (India, New Guinea, Africa, and to a lesser extent the Caribbean and Brazil),[3] granuloma inguinale is among the most prevalent of the present STIs. Incidence of infection is found in tropical and subtropical environments with sustained high temperature and high relative humidity. Infection is usually acquired through sexual intercourse with an individual who has active disease or asymptomatic rectal infection.

Pathophysiology

C. granulomatis is a gram-negative, nonsporing, nonmotile, encapsulated rod that is not easily isolated in the laboratory. After exposure the bacteria survive and multiply within vacuoles of large histiocytic cells or polymorphonuclear leukocytes. The bacteria reproduce within these cells until a vacuole may contain 20 to 30 microorganisms. These bacteria-filled vacuoles were identified by Donovan in 1905 and are termed **Donovan bodies.** The presence of Donovan bodies in tissue smears of material from the lesions is considered the "gold standard" for diagnosis of lymphogranuloma inguinale.[26,27]

The initial lesion is an indurated subcutaneous nodule that is often preceded and accompanied by itching. The primary sites for development of the lesions are the distal penis in males and the introitus in females. Single lesions often coalesce with nearby lesions or form new lesions by autoinoculation of nearby skin surfaces. Progression from the initial nodule to a large, granuloma-heaped ulcer occurs slowly. Secondary infection may occur, increasing tissue damage and residual scarring. The disease may spread to the bones, joints, and liver.

Clinical Manifestations

The incubation period of granuloma inguinale is 8 to 80 days. The initial lesion is an indurated, sharply defined, painless, subcutaneous nodule that is often preceded and accompanied by itching. Nodules bleed easily and contain abundant red, beefy-looking granulation tissue. Progression to a large, granuloma-heaped ulcer occurs slowly; single lesions coalesce or form new lesions by autoinoculation of nearby skin surfaces. Secondary infection may occur, increasing tissue damage and residual scarring. Although systemic symptoms are rare, the disease may spread to the bones, joints, and liver. In some cases, infection spreads to the inguinale area and produces **pseudobuboes.** In these instances, the affected lymph nodes are not directly affected, but the surrounding area may be infected and abscessed.

Evaluation and Treatment

Although the clinical manifestations of this disease are important for diagnosis, confirmation involves microscopic examination in which Donovan bodies are found in a smear or biopsy specimen. Cultures for granuloma inguinale are not available; polymerase chain reaction and serology are available for research only.[23]

Many antibiotics have been used successfully against *C. granulomatis.* Since other STIs frequently coexist, individuals should be tested for chlamydia, gonorrhea, syphilis, Hepatitis B, and HIV. Because of the indolent nature of the disease, duration of therapy tends to be relatively long. With effective antibiotic treatment, lesions begin to heal in 7 days, but treatment is continued for 21 days or until all lesions are healed. Therapy includes oral erythromycin (500 mg) four times daily, or doxycycline (100 mg) or trimethoprim-sulfamethoxazole twice daily for 21 days. Gentamicin and ciprofloxacin are reserved for resistant infections. Relapses can occur 6 to 18 months later despite effective initial therapy, so prolonged follow-up is necessary, as is treatment of sexual partners.[3,23]

Bacterial Vaginosis

Bacterial vaginosis (BV)—previously called nonspecific vaginitis; nonspecific vaginosis; or *Haemophilus, Corynebacterium,* or *Gardnerella* vaginitis—is a sexually associated condition, but is not necessarily considered an STI. Bacterial vaginosis occurs almost exclusively in sexually active women of reproductive age and is uncommon in sexually inexperienced women.[23] Prevalence rates vary from 17% among women in family planning clinics to 37% among some groups of pregnant women.[1] Fifty percent of women with signs of BV are asymptomatic. Lower socioeconomic status, intrauterine device (IUD) usage, multiple or uncircumcised sexual partners, smoking, and increasing parity are associated risk factors.[28,29]

Pathophysiology

The exact etiology of BV is unknown. *Gardnerella vaginalis* and various anaerobes, including *Mycoplasma hominis, Bacteroides,* and *Mobiluncus,* interact and proliferate when lactobacilli (the normal predominant vaginal flora) are decreased or absent. Bacteria adhere to vaginal epithelium, and massive overgrowth occurs and causes a noninflammatory response. Catabolic enzymes degrade proteins to amines. In turn, amines elevate vaginal pH and produce the characteristic fishy odor associated with BV. BV has been implicated

WHAT'S NEW? **Substantial Benefits Derived from Treating Bacterial Vaginosis in Pregnant Women**

A multicenter study of pregnant women recently evaluated the connection between bacterial vaginosis (BV) during pregnancy and preterm, low-birth-weight (LBW) infants. Women were enrolled during routine prenatal visits at 23 to 26 weeks' gestation. At that time they received a complete history and a vaginal examination and vaginal and cervical specimens were collected. BV was determined by vaginal pH >4.5 and wet mount presentation of floral overgrowth and decreased lactobacilli. Of the 10,397 women enrolled, 16% had BV and approximately 5% (504 women) delivered premature, underweight infants (<37 weeks' gestation and <2500 g). At all study centers, increased preterm delivery and LBW were associated with BV.

Logistic regression indicated that a previous preterm LBW infant, prior pregnancy loss, and BV were significant and independent risk factors for the delivery of a preterm underweight infant. Other risks included primigravidity (odds ratio 1.6), smoking (odds ratio 1.4), and black race (odds ratio 1.4). *Gardnerella vaginalis,* bacterioses, and *Mycoplasma hominis* were most strongly tied to BV. Women diagnosed with BV who had both bacterioses and *Mycoplasma hominis* organisms had the highest risk (odds ratio 2.1) of a preterm delivery of an underweight infant; only a history of a preterm delivery of an LBW infant (odds ratio 6.2) was higher. In the United States, LBW infants are more likely to die or to have significant morbidity. At this time, pregnant women are not screened or treated routinely for asymptomatic BV.

Data from Hillier SL et al: *N Engl J Med* 333(26):1737, 1995.

in PID, chorioamnionitis, preterm labor, and postpartum endometritis. Sexual intercourse is believed to be the primary method of transmitting BV, but definitive proof is lacking and the syndrome has been identified in virgins.[23,30]

Clinical Manifestations

BV is characterized by a thin, gray, homogenous, and malodorous discharge that adheres to the vaginal walls but is often copious enough to drain into the vulva. Occasionally the discharge is bubbly or frothy. Usually the vaginal pH is 5.0 to 5.5 and there are no signs of vaginal or cervical inflammation. Individuals often complain of a strong, foul, fishy vaginal odor, particularly after intercourse and during menses. Odor is caused by contact with alkaline secretions, including semen and menstrual discharge. Male partners of infected females may harbor the organisms that are responsible for BV but have no signs or symptoms of active disease.

Evaluation and Treatment

Diagnosis is made by microscopic analysis of a wet mount (a specimen of vaginal secretions placed on a slide and mixed with normal saline). The wet mount shows clue cells, which are considered pathognomonic for BV; absence of lactobacilli; and few or no leukocytes. Clue cells are vaginal epithelial cells that are covered with bacteria and look as if pepper has been sprinkled on them. When a drop of potassium hydroxide (KOH) solution is added to the slide, a characteristic amine odor is released immediately. Cultures are neither useful nor recommended.

The most effective and commonly used treatment for *Gardnerella*-associated BV is a course of oral metronidazole (Flagyl), 500 mg twice daily for 7 days, or 0.75% vaginal gel twice daily for 5 days. Alternative regimens include oral clindamycin, 300 mg twice daily for 7 days, or 2% vaginal cream once daily for 7 days.[3] Clindamycin vaginal suppositories have been newly approved for use as a 3-day treatment regiment in nonpregnant women. Clindamycin cream is oil based, and for up to 72 hours after completing therapy, it may weaken latex condoms. For high-risk pregnant women, metronidazole, 750 mg divided in 3 doses daily for 7 days, is the preferred treatment. BV treatment in women infected with HIV is the same for HIV-negative patients. It is especially important in women who are pregnant, since BV and chorioamnionitis may increase the risk of perinatal transmission of HIV.[23] Some clinicians routinely treat sexual partners; others treat partners only if infection recurs after treatment. Condoms help to prevent future infections.

Chlamydial Infections

Urogenital Infections

Chlamydia is the common name for infections caused by *Chlamydia trachomatis* (CT). *C. trachomatis* is responsible for a variety of syndromes, including acute urethral syndrome, nongonococcal urethritis (NGU), mucopurulent cervicitis, and pelvic inflammatory disease (PID). Chlamydia, the most common bacterial STI in the United States, affects about 3 million individuals annually[31] and is the leading cause of preventable infertility and ectopic pregnancy. In 1998, 49 states reported 607,602 cases of chlamydial infections. Beginning in 1996, all states were expected to report CT infections.[3] Approximately 75% of women with CT infection are asymptomatic.[31] In addition, *C. trachomatis* can be recovered from the urethra in 25% to 60% of men with NGU, in 4% to 35% of men with gonorrhea, in 28% of asymptomatic men whose partners have chlamydial cervicitis, and in 0% to 7% of men without urethritis who are seen in STI clinics.

Evidence of CT infection is rare in sexually inexperienced persons. It is most common among young (less than 20 years old) heterosexuals who have new or multiple partners or who have been diagnosed with gonorrhea. The incidence of CT infection in pregnancy has been estimated between 2% and 30%. Age younger than 25 years (with highest rates in women younger than 20 years), a new sexual partner, and first pregnancy were strongly and independently associated with infection in a recent study of over 7000 pregnant women who were screened for CT at their first prenatal visit. Like gonorrhea, *Chlamydia* infection is transmitted from mother to infant through the infected birth canal (Fig. 23-9). Estimated rate of transmission ranges from 60% to 70%.[32]

Pathophysiology

C. trachomatis is an obligate, gram-negative, intracellular bacterium that lacks the ability to reproduce independently. Like viruses, *Chlamydia* can reproduce only within host cells

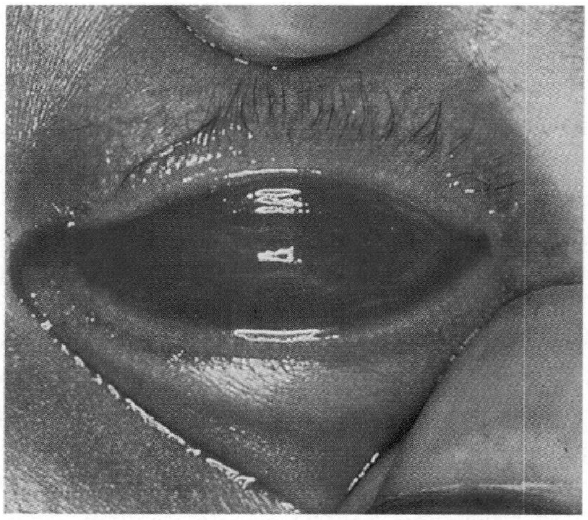

FIG. 23-9 Chlamydial ophthalmia. Reddened conjunctiva seen in this infant. (Examiner would be gloved.) (From Morse SA, Moreland AA, Holmes KK, editors: *Atlas of sexually transmitted diseases and AIDS,* ed 2, London, 1996, Mosby-Wolfe.)

(Fig. 23-10). It is differentiated from other bacteria by its unique two-part growth cycle. The first part consists of an elementary body that is small, resilient, metabolically inert, and able to survive extracellularly. Once this elementary body attaches itself to a receptor host cell, it is able to enter by endocytosis. Once inside the cell, the second part begins and becomes a metabolically active parasite, reproducing within the cell until the cell is destroyed and ruptures, disseminating up to 1000 new elementary bodies. Rarely does this cause a secondary infection. Infection with *C. trachomatis* produces a mononuclear inflammatory reaction rather than a polymorphonuclear inflammatory reaction. The former reaction produces permanent scarring of tissues.[33]

Chlamydia organisms are always pathogens; they are not part of the normal flora of the urogenital tract, despite the fact that infection is often asymptomatic. There are numerous serotypes, or strains, of *C. trachomatis.* Some cause urogenital infection; some, ocular trachoma; and others, lym-

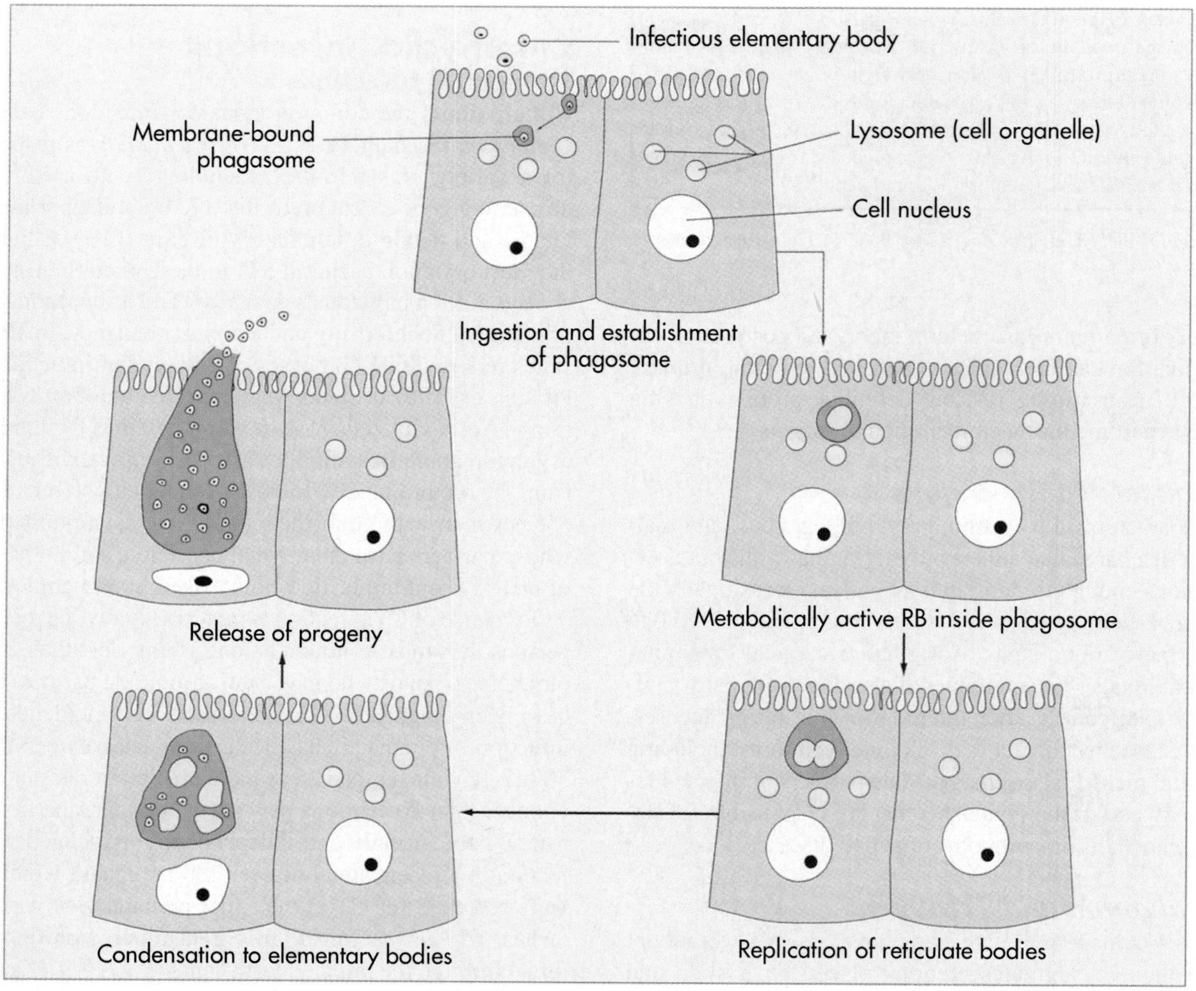

FIG. 23-10 Chlamydial development cycle. The infectious elementary body (EB) attaches to the host cell and is ingested. The EB resides within a membrane-bound endosome (phagosome). Transformation to the metabolically active reticulate body (RB) begins. Next is synthesis of chlamydial constituents and replication of the RBs through fission. A chlamydial inclusion body containing numerous replicative forms can be seen 24 to 28 hours after infection. At 48 to 72 hours after infection, RBs condense to the sporelike EBs. The inclusion body contains several hundred infectious particles at the peak of its maturation. The infectious progeny EBs are released from the infected host cell by extrusion of the inclusion body or by lysis of the host cell. (From Morse SA, Moreland AA, Holmes KK, editors: *Atlas of sexually transmitted diseases and AIDS,* ed 2, London, 1996, Mosby-Wolfe.)

phogranuloma venereum, which is discussed in the next section.

The strains of *C. trachomatis* that cause urogenital infection apparently require squamous-columnar and columnar epithelial cells as hosts. *C. trachomatis* infects and disrupts epithelial tissues but does not seem to invade or destroy deeper tissues or organs. Urogenital chlamydial infections may have a fairly self-limited acute course followed by a chronic, low-grade, persistent infection that lasts for years.[33]

In newborns, several sites may be inoculated with *Chlamydia* during passage through the infected maternal cervix. These include the eye, nasopharynx, rectum, and vagina. The infant also may aspirate infected secretions with its first breaths, resulting in chlamydial pneumonitis and substantial newborn morbidity.

Clinical Manifestations

Asymptomatic chlamydial infection is common. Urogenital infections caused by *Chlamydia* closely parallel those caused by gonorrhea. Both microorganisms infect superficial genital tract tissues, such as mucosa of the urethra and cervix, and both can invade the epididymides, fallopian tubes, and hepatic capsule. Table 23-2 lists the pathophysiologic similarities of chlamydial and gonococcal infections.

Chlamydial infection accounts for 50% to 60% of cases of NGU in men. Clinically, urethritis caused by gonorrhea and chlamydia cannot be differentiated: both have a 7- to 21-day incubation period and cause dysuria. Although urethral discharge in men may be similar in the two infections, chlamydial discharge tends to be more clear and gonococcal discharge more purulent. Men might note a clear, mucous discharge on rising in the morning; dry, clear discharge on their underwear; or mild burning with urination. Chlamydial urethritis is generally milder than gonorrheal urethritis and more likely to be asymptomatic. Symptoms may be intermittent or unnoticeable. Gram-stained smears of the urethral discharge show numerous polymorphonuclear leukocytes, which indicates ongoing inflammation. Screening men without symptoms is not cost effective at this time.

Chlamydial epididymitis can accompany chlamydial urethritis and is characterized by fever and a unilaterally painful, swollen scrotum. Chlamydial infection also causes proctitis (rectal inflammation) in homosexual men and occasionally in heterosexual women and is linked to the practice of receptive anal intercourse. Chlamydial proctitis is generally mild, although it may, like gonorrheal proctitis, cause rectal bleeding, mucous discharge, and diarrhea. Reiter syndrome (urethritis, conjunctivitis, arthritis, and characteristic mucocutaneous lesions) is also associated with untreated chlamydial infections of the urogenital tract.

In young, sexually active women, *C. trachomatis* is a cause of **acute urethral syndrome** (dysuria, urinary frequency, and presence of sterile pus in the urine). *C. trachomatis* also causes asymptomatic urethral infection in women. Chlamydial infection of Bartholin glands can cause purulent discharge and formation of a Bartholin cyst. Women with chlamydial cervicitis may be asymptomatic or may have a yellow mucopurulent discharge from the cervical os and a hypertrophic, edematous, and friable area of cervical ectopy. The woman also may report intermenstrual or postcoital spotting. Although ectopy alone does not indicate a pathologic condition, a raised, erythematous, raw, and friable ectopy is abnormal and strongly suggestive of chlamydial cervicitis (Fig. 23-11). Chlamydial cervicitis is also a leading cause of PID.

Table 23-2 Similarity of Clinical Syndromes Caused by *Chlamydia trachomatis* and *Neisseria gonorrhoeae*

	Clinical Syndrome	
Site of Infection	**N. gonorrhoeae**	**C. trachomatis**
MEN		
Urethra	Urethritis	Nongonococcal urethritis; postgonococcal urethritis
Epididymis	Epididymitis	Epididymitis
Rectum	Proctitis	Proctitis
Conjunctiva	Conjunctivitis	Conjunctivitis
Systemic	Disseminated gonococcal infection	Reiter syndrome
WOMEN		
Urethra	Acute urethral syndrome	Acute urethral syndrome
Bartholin gland	Bartholinitis	Bartholinitis
Cervix	Cervicitis	Cervicitis; cervical atypia
Fallopian tube	Salpingitis	Salpingitis
Conjunctiva	Conjunctivitis	Conjunctivitis
Liver capsule	Perihepatitis	Perihepatitis
Systemic	Disseminated gonococcal infection	Arthritis-dermatitis syndrome

Data from Stamm WE, Holmes KK. In Holmes KK et al, editors: *Sexually transmitted diseases,* ed 2, New York, 1990, McGraw-Hill.

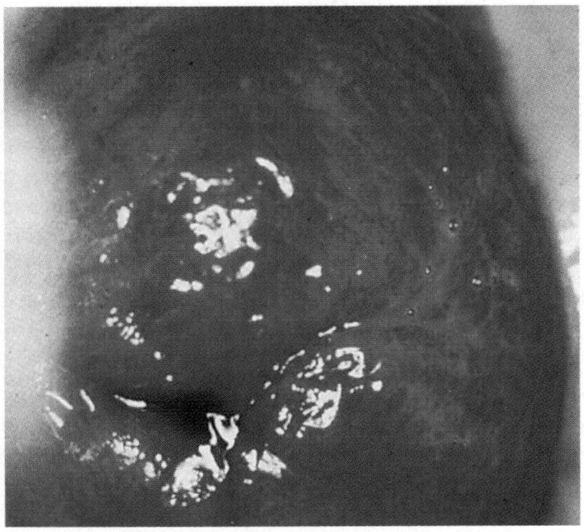

FIG. 23-11 Chlamydial infection. Beefy red mucosa of columnar epithelium. (From Morse SA, Moreland AA, Holmes KK, editors: *Atlas of sexually transmitted diseases and AIDS,* ed 2, London, 1996, Mosby-Wolfe.)

The most common clinical manifestations of chlamydial infections in the newborn are conjunctivitis and pneumonia. Like gonococcal infection, prophylactic treatment with antibiotic eye ointment at birth does not provide complete protection against neonatal conjunctivitis and does not protect against neonatal pneumonia. Chlamydial conjunctivitis begins between 5 and 14 days after delivery, when the infant's eyes begin to water. This discharge may become purulent, and both eyes may become red and swollen. Scarring of the conjunctivae may result, but this infection does not cause blindness, as does the ophthalmia neonatorum caused by *N. gonorrhoeae. C trachomatis* accounts for 20% to 60% of all cases of pneumonia in infants up to 6 months of age.[34] The pneumonia is mild or severe and may accompany the conjunctivitis. Infants with chlamydial pneumonia are seen at 3 to 11 weeks of age with staccato coughing spells, nasal congestion, dyspnea, and minimal fever. Other signs include otitis media, tachypnea, wheezing, bronchospasm, crepitant inspiratory rales, and apneic spells.

Evaluation and Treatment

Methods for diagnosing chlamydial infections include tissue culture techniques, direct chlamydia enzyme immunoassay, fluorescein-labeled monoclonal antibody tests, and DNA probe testing. Currently, DNA screening of urethral or cervical secretions is the most sensitive, specific, and cost-effective diagnostic methods available. Concurrent DNA testing for gonorrhea can be done using the same swab.

C. trachomatis is susceptible to inexpensive, readily accessible antibiotics. Treatment includes antibiotic therapy for infected individuals and all sexual contacts; abstinence or use of condoms during treatment is recommended. A 7-day course of oral doxycycline, 100 mg twice daily; or oral erythromycin or tetracycline, 500 mg four times daily, is effective.[23,35] Erythromycin is the drug of choice in pregnancy. A single 1-g dose of azithromycin taken orally is effective for uncomplicated urethritis and cervicitis and has the advantage of improved compliance and minimal toxicity.[35] Because of the asymptomatic nature of *Chlamydia* and the potential sequelae of untreated infection, extensive widespread screening is warranted.

WHAT'S NEW? Nonculture Techniques Are Inappropriate for Chlamydia Testing in Children

Despite CDC recommendations that cultures are the only appropriate chlamydia test in children, many clinicians tend to use nonculture techniques. Chlamydia causes vaginitis/proctitis in children and culture is necessary to isolate the microorganism. False-positive results occur with enzyme immunoassays due to cross-reaction with microorganisms such as *E. coli*, *S. aureas*, and streptococci. Both false-positive and false-negative reports result from vaginal/rectal testing using nucleic acid amplification tests (polymerase or ligase chain reactions). False-negative findings can be attributed to polymerase inhibitors present in vaginal specimens, whereas false-positives may be caused by amplicon contamination. Using nonculture techniques creates avoidable social, legal, and health problems.

Data from Davis AJ: Nonculture techniques use inappropriate for chlamydia testing in girls, *J Watch: Women's Hlth* 5(2):1, 2000; Hammerschlag MR, Laraque D: Inappropriate use of nonculture tests for the detection of chlamydia trachomatis in suspected victims of child sexual abuse: a continuing problem, *Pediatrics* 104(5):1137, 1999.

Lymphogranuloma Venereum

C. trachomatis (invasive serovars L1, L2, or L3) can cause a chronic STI known as **lymphogranuloma venereum (LGV),** which may be confused with syphilis, herpes, or chancroid. Although LGV is rare in the United States, it has been endemic in Asia and Africa. The infection is acquired during sexual intercourse or through contact with contaminated exudate from active lesions. Inapparent infections and latent disease are rare.[36]

Pathophysiology

The strain of *C. trachomatis* that causes LGV probably penetrates skin and mucous membranes through tiny abrasions. LGV begins as a skin lesion and spreads to genital and rectal lymphatic tissue, where it causes marked inflammation, necrosis, buboes, abscesses of inguinal lymph nodes, and infection of surrounding tissues. Healing occurs by fibrosis after several weeks or months and results in scarring, which damages the lymph nodes and disrupts nodal function. Affected nodes become chronically swollen, hardened, and enlarged. *C. trachomatis* also spreads systematically through the bloodstream and can enter the CNS.[37]

Clinical Manifestations

The primary lesion of LGV appears after an incubation period of 5 to 21 days. The lesion is most commonly a herpetiform (multivesicular) ulcer, but it can take various forms. The ulcer generally is asymptomatic and inconspicuous and heals rapidly, leaving no scar. In men the lesion is found most commonly on the penis or scrotum; in women it is found on the vaginal wall, cervix, or labia. Other signs of primary LGV include a large, tender lymphatic nodule or bubo, urethritis, and cervicitis.

The secondary stage of untreated LGV in men is characterized by inflammation and swelling of the lymph nodes. At first the inguinal bubo is a firm, somewhat painful mass. As the bubo gradually enlarges, it becomes very painful, thereby restricting mobility, and takes on a deep blue color. This color change signals impending rupture of the bubo through the skin. Thick yellow pus may drain from the site for weeks or months. Healing is slow and results in scar formation. Systemic manifestations of secondary LGV include meningitis, pneumonitis, and other major infections. In some cases the bubo does not rupture but rather involutes and becomes firm. Bubo formation is most common in men. In women the inguinal lymph nodes are involved in fewer than one third of cases.

Anorectal LGV may be caused by direct inoculation during anal intercourse, or it may be a chronic or late manifestation of lymphatic spread from the inguinal area. Most individuals with anorectal LGV are women and homosexual men. Clinical symptoms include multiple ulcerations of the rectal mucosa, chronic inflammation, mucopurulent rectal discharge, and rectovaginal fistulas in women. Individuals may have fever, rectal pain, and tenesmus. Rectal strictures, perirectal abscesses, and anal fissures may develop and are the cause of most of the severe morbidity associated with LGV.

Evaluation and Treatment

Clinical manifestations and laboratory tests are used to diagnose LGV. Tests include the LGV complement-fixation tests, isolation of the microorganism in tissue culture, and monoclonal antibody tests. The diagnosis usually is made serologically and by excluding other causes of genital ulcers or inguinal lymphadenopathy. LGV is treated with oral doxycycline, 100 mg twice daily for 21 days. A 21-day course of erythromycin is also effective. Sex partners also should be treated.[3]

Nongonococcal or Nonspecific Urethritis

Nongonococcal urethritis (NGU), also known as *nonspecific urethritis,* is a nonreportable STI. In student health centers and STI clinics, more than 50% of individuals with urethritis have NGU. The morbidity is equal to or greater than that associated with gonorrhea. Approximately 2 million men are affected each year. Most commonly, it affects heterosexual men and men of higher socioeconomic status. NGU may be complicated by epididymitis in heterosexual men under age 35 years, proctitis in homosexual men, and Reiter syndrome.

Pathophysiology

Nongonococcal urethritis is a syndrome caused by a variety of microbes, including *C. trachomatis* and *Ureaplasma urealyticum.* Postgonococcal urethritis occurs in 15% to 35% of men diagnosed with gonorrhea. These men usually have coexistent gonorrheal and chlamydial infection and develop biphasic illness because of the longer incubation period of CT. Chlamydial infections are discussed earlier in this chapter (see p. 793).

C trachomatis is the most frequent cause of NGU (23% to 55%). *Trichomonas vaginalis* and HSV sometimes cause NGU. However, *Ureaplasma, U. urealyticum,* and possibly *Mycoplasma* are implicated in as many as one third of the cases of NGU.[2] Genital colonization with *U. urealyticum* occurs with increasing number of sexual partners. That is, urethral cultures of men with a history of three to five lifetime sexual partners yield *U. urealyticum* whether men have urethritis or not. The difference in symptomatology may be the result of infection by different serotypes. Some of the 14 different serotypes of *U. urealyticum* may be more pathogenic than others. Twenty to thirty percent of men with acute urethritis are negative for *N. gonorrhoeae, C. trachomatis,* and *U. urealyticum.* Some of these men respond to antibiotic treatment; others experience persistent and recurrent infection. There is no clear association between NGU and infection caused by herpes simplex virus, trichomonads, cytomegalovirus, and other organisms.

Clinical Manifestations

Clinically, NGU infection caused by CT cannot be differentiated from NGU caused by another microbe. In both cases, men present after a 7- to 21-day incubation period with complaints of dysuria and mild to moderate white or clear urethral discharge. Discharge may be absent, and urethral itching may be the only symptom. Asymptomatic infection is common.

Evaluation and Treatment

NGU is a diagnosis of exclusion. Urethral exudate is gram stained, and an endourethral swab is taken for DNA probe testing or culture. All patients who have urethritis should be evaluated for the presence of gonococcal and chlamydial infection. A treatment of a single 1g oral dose of azithromycin should be initiated as soon as possible after diagnosis. Doxycycline, 100 mg orally twice a day for 7 days, is also effective. Single-dose regimens have the advantage of improved compliance and of directly observed therapy.[2]

Viral Infections

Genital Herpes

Genital herpes, which causes blisters (cold sores), is the most common infectious genital ulceration in the United States. In fact, genital infection with the herpes simplex virus (HSV) is an epidemic in the United States. Genital herpes can be caused by either of the two serotypes of HSV-type 1 (HSV-1) or type 2 (HSV-2). Although infections caused by the serotypes are clinically indistinguishable, serologic studies show that more than 80% of initial and 98% of recurrent genital HSV infections are caused by HSV-2.

Herpes simplex virus is not a reportable disease, and any reporting that is done is nonstandardized, so national statistics are not available. However, primary HSV infections are estimated to affect 1 million individuals each year. Recurrent infections are mostly asymptomatic (50% to 70%) and affect an estimated 45 million Americans annually.[2] The seroprevalence of HSV-2 is estimated to range from 16% to 20% of the total adult population to 35% to 60% for subgroups, for example, STI clinic patients and black women. The incidence of HSV infection tends to be highest in the teen to young adult age-group (12 to 29 years) and in nonwhite lower socioeconomic groups.[2] Infection with HSV is not commonly associated with other STIs, for example, gonorrhea.[17]

Herpes simplex virus infection is transmitted through intimate contact with a person who is shedding the virus in a secretion or from a peripheral lesion or mucosal surface. Persons without symptoms probably transmit most infections. Transmission rates are not well identified; however, it is estimated that a woman has an 80% to 90% risk of developing genital herpes after being exposed to an infected male. In 1992 Mertz and colleagues[38] studied monogamous heterosexual couples in which one partner had HSV-2 infection.

The noninfected partner seroconverted in 10% of couples over a 1-year period. As many as 70% of such infections seem to be acquired during periods of asymptomatic shedding. Uninfected female partners were at greater risk than males, especially if they were seronegative for HSV-1 antibodies as well. The likelihood of nonsexual transmission of genital herpes, through aerosolized secretions of other fomites, is quite rare and unlikely.[5,33]

Neonatal infections can occur in utero or, more commonly, during the intrapartum or postpartum period. The incidence of neonatal infections has been estimated to be 1 in 2500 to 1 in 20,000 births.[39] Perinatal transmission can cause extensive morbidity and mortality.

Intrauterine transmission can occur through transplacental or ascending infection and can cause spontaneous abortion or premature delivery.[17] Most infections are transmitted intrapartally. Infants are at greatest risk if the mother has a primary infection acquired near the time of delivery (30%-50%) rather than a recurrent infection or an infection acquired during the first half of pregnancy (3%). Ruptured membranes have a role in the development of HSV. Membranes that have been ruptured for more than 6 hours increase the risk for contracting HSV. Fetal monitoring devices also increase the risk of the infant contracting HSV.[40]

Pathophysiology

After initial exposure and entry of the virus at mucocutaneous sites or abraded skin, the virus undergoes replication locally in the dermis and epidermis. This leads to cell destruction, transudation, and vesicle formation. There is spread of the virus to contiguous cells and eventually into sensory nerves. Eventually the virus is transported intraaxonally to the dorsal root, where it remains in a latent stage until it becomes reactivated. During the latent period the genome for the virus is maintained in the host cell nucleus without causing the death of the cell. After oral infection the latent virus resides in the trigeminal ganglion; after genital infection it resides in the dorsal sacral nerve roots.

Latent infections can become reactivated and cause a recurrent infection with similar manifestations. Reactivation of the HSV-2 infection is twice as common as HSV-1 infections, and the likelihood of HSV-2 recurrent infections is 8 to 10 times. Reactivation of HSV is not well understood but may be attributable to physical, hormonal, and immunologic stimuli. Other triggering events may be menstruation, stress, and sun exposure.[32] During reactivation the viral genomes are transported through the peripheral sensory nerves back to the dermal surface.

Clinical Manifestations

Three distinct syndromes associated with HSV infection are first-episode primary genital infection, first-episode nonprimary HSV, and recurrent infections. The manifestations of each one depend on the individual's previous immune state. First-episode primary genital infection occurs when an individual has no antibodies to HSV-1 or HSV-2. The individual has small (1 to 2 mm), multiple, vesicular lesions, which are generally located on the labia minora, fourchette, or penis (Fig. 23-12). They also may appear on the cervix, buttocks, and thighs and are often painful and pruritic. These lesions usually last about 10 to 20 days. The lesions of HSV-1 and HSV-2 are indistinguishable to the naked eye. These wet lesions actively shed virus for about 10 to 14 days, after which they heal by reepithelialization. Small lesions may coalesce into larger ulcers and become secondarily infected.

Systemic manifestations often accompany primary HSV infection, and an individual may experience fever, malaise, myalgias, lymphadenopathy, and urinary retention. Pharyngitis, aseptic meningitis, and hepatitis also may accompany

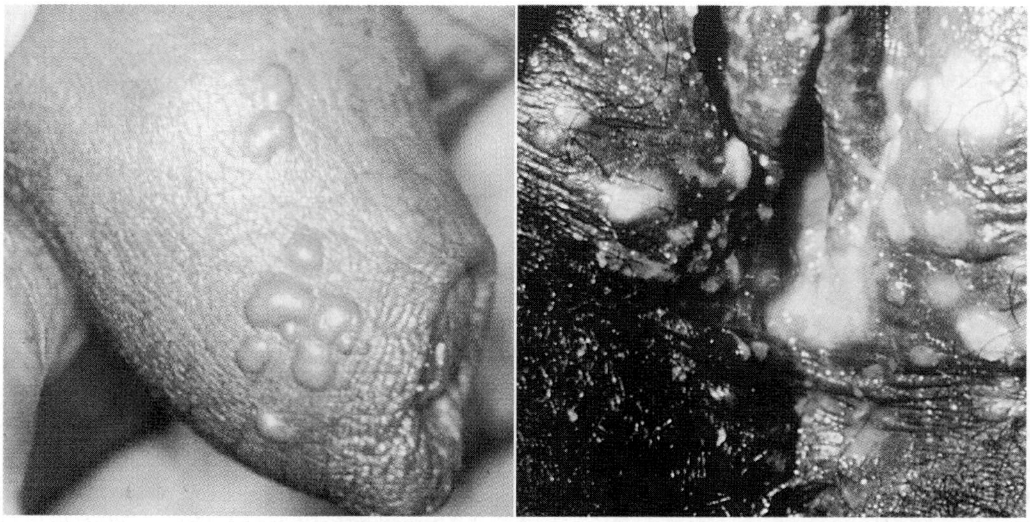

A B

FIG. 23-12 Herpes lesions. A, Early lesions of primary genital herpes. Clear grouped vesicles that frequently result in a scalloped border. **B,** Vulval herpes of several days' duration. Several stages are shown, including clear vesicles, pustules, and grayish exudate. (From Morse SA, Moreland AA, Holmes KK, editors: *Atlas of sexually transmitted diseases and AIDS,* ed 2, London, 1996, Mosby-Wolfe.)

primary HSV infection. Fig. 23-13 illustrates the clinical course of primary genital HSV.

First-episode nonprimary HSV occurs in individuals who have preexisting antibodies. In some individuals the primary infection may not have had any clinical manifestations. The HSV becomes latent within the nerve root and is reactivated at a later date. Compared with primary infection, the first episode of nonprimary HSV is often milder with fewer lesions that are less painful and heal faster. There are also fewer systemic manifestations, and viral shedding is of shorter duration.

Recurrent infections produce mild local symptoms. The number of lesions is greatly reduced, and the lesions are less painful. Lesions are often unilateral, with crusting within 4 to 5 days. Recovery and healing are usually complete within 10 days.

Individuals affected with HSV-2 are more likely to experience recurrent infections. Recurrent infections occur an average of five to eight times per year but may be as frequent as every month or as rare as every few to many years. Individuals may experience prodromal symptoms (e.g., pruritus, tingling, dysesthesias) a few hours to 2 days before the eruption of lesions. Women may experience a vaginal discharge and dysuria, and 44% of men have dysuria. Symptomatic HSV infection of the newborn may occur any time in the first month of life. Manifestations range from a local infection of the eyes, skin, or mucous membranes to a severe, disseminated infection with CNS involvement. About 70% of affected infants present with skin lesions. CNS involvement includes seizures and is associated with a mortality of more than 50% and extensive neurologic sequelae in survivors.

Evaluation and Treatment

Genital HSV infection is suggested if typical genital lesions are present. A presumptive diagnosis of HSV-associated infection is supported by the identification in a Papanicolaou smear of multinucleated giant cells with intranuclear inclusions. Definitive diagnosis is made after viral tissue culture. HSV-1 and HSV-2 are distinguished by fluorescent antibody, neutralization, or other serologic techniques.

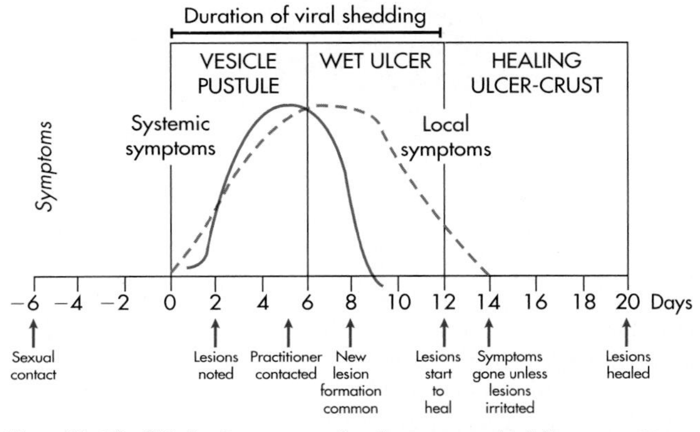

FIG. 23-13 Clinical course of primary genital herpes. (From Corey L: Genital herpes. In Holmes KK et al, editors: *Sexually transmitted diseases,* ed 2, New York, 1990, Mcgraw-Hill.)

There is currently no curative treatment for HSV infection. Oral acyclovir, valaciclovir, peniciclovir, and famciclovir are used for primary and periodic outbreaks and to prevent recurrences. Neither valaciclovir famiciclovir is approved by the U.S. Food and Drug Administration for use in children.[4] Intravenous acyclovir is reserved for severely immunocompromised individuals.[41] Acyclovir-resistant strains of HSV have been identified periodically; no specific definitive resistant strains are known to exist. Although condoms offer some protection, individuals with HSV should refrain from all genital contact when symptomatic and understand that an undetermined risk of transmission exists even during asymptomatic periods.

Condylomata Acuminata

Condylomata acuminata, also called *condyloma* or *genital warts,* is the most common symptomatic viral STI in the United States. Although over 5.5 million cases are diagnosed yearly, incidence is considered underestimated because human papillomavirus (HPV) infection is often subclinical. More sensitive measures of HPV indicate that 28% to 46% of all sexually active young women are infected with the virus. Currently the incidence of condyloma is at epidemic proportions; an estimated 75% of the reproductive-age population has been infected with HPV.[1]

Condylomata acuminata is caused by the human papillomavirus (HPV), of which there are about 70 serotypes. Of these, over 20 infect mucosal surfaces, with 18 to 20 HPV subtypes found in the anogenital area and 2 in the oral cavity.[19,28] The seriousness of genital infection seems to be related to the type of HPV causing the infection. Serotypes 6 and 11 are identified with benign condylomata, and serotypes 16, 18, 31, and 33 have been associated with genital dysplasia; 95% of invasive cervical cancers contain these types. HPV infection is closely associated with multiple sexual partners and early onset of sexual activity and is most common in teens and young adults, 16 to 25 years of age. A growing body of knowledge links HPV infection with cervical and vulvar cancer in females and anorectal and squamous cell carcinoma of the penis in males. Specifically, HPV types 16, 18, 31, 33, and 35 have been associated with squamous intraepithelial neoplasia of the external genitalia (i.e., squamous cell carcinoma in situ, bowenoid papulosis, erythroplasia of Queyrat, or Bowne disease of the genitalia). These HPV types also have been associated with vaginal, anal, and cervical intraepithelial dysplasia and squamous cell carcinoma.[1,2] The association between HPV and cervical cancer depends on HPV type and smoking, parity, immunity, hormonal levels, and nutritional status.[42]

Genital warts are quite contagious, with transmission rates between individuals estimated to be between 38% and 95%. Such a wide range is attributable to the subclinical nature of some infections and various influencing factors that include number of exposures, HPV type, location of lesions, and cellular immunity response. Infants and children also have been identified as being infected with HPV. Infants can be infected in utero and by passage through an infected birth canal. HPV infection in children has been traced to child sexual abuse; however, reports vary in making this connection.[4,43]

Pathophysiology

HPV is a nonenveloped, circular, double-stranded DNA virus that belongs to the Papovaviridae family.[44] Information about HPV was not readily available until the late 1970s, when it became possible to clone the viral genomes directly from infected tissues by recombinant DNA technology.[45]

Transmission of the virus is believed to occur through sexual contact; however, the exact transmissibility of the virus is unknown. HPV is transmissible by fomites and may account for nonsexually transmitted genital warts.[36] The initial infection follows trauma to the epithelium that allows the virus to reach and infect the basal cells of the epithelium, which appear to be supportive of viral propagation. Such minor trauma may occur during sexual intercourse. Epithelial cells that are infected with HPV undergo transformation, proliferate, and form a warty growth. HPV manifestations appear in about 2 to 3 months.

Clinical Manifestations

Condylomata acuminata are soft, skin-colored, whitish pink to reddish brown, discrete growths. They may occur singly or in clusters and may be broad based or pedunculated and feathery or smooth (Fig. 23-14). Sometimes the warts enlarge to form cauliflower-like masses on the male frenulum, glans, foreskin, urinary meatus, shaft, scrotum, or anus and on the female labia, clitoris, perineum, vagina, or anus (Fig. 23-15). Although the lesions are usually not painful, they may cause dyspareunia (painful intercourse) and may be friable and bleed easily. Some individuals complain of pruritus. Cervical lesions are generally flattened and may not be seen easily without colposcopy.[14] Urethral condylomata may occur in men, are always preceded by skin lesions, and can become cancerous.[46] Ninety percent of lesions are found in the distal urethra.

Laryngeal papillomas can occur in infants whose mothers had genital warts at the time of delivery. Clinical manifestations of laryngeal warts include stridor, hoarseness, abnormal cry, cough, and respiratory distress.[39]

Evaluation and Treatment

Generally, diagnosis of condylomata acuminata is made on the basis of clinical manifestations. Koilocytosis (typical cellular changes of HPV infection) seen on the Papanicolaou smear aid in the diagnosis of cervical HPV infection. Pointy, fleshy pink lesions caused by HPV must be differentiated from condylomata lata (the whitish gray, flat lesions) of secondary syphilis. Because HPV infection often accompanies other STIs, gonorrhea culture, chlamydia culture, serologic test for syphilis, and wet mount for other vaginal microorganisms also should be performed. HPV infection also is associated with the development of squamous cell carcinoma; therefore all atypical or persistent lesions should have a biopsy examination. Some clinicians recommend that Papanicolaou smears be repeated every 6 months for women with a history of HPV infection.

Treatments for external genital warts are considered cosmetic—not curative—and include patient-applied therapies (podofilox and imiquimod) and provider-administered therapies (cryotherapy, podophyllin resin, trichloroacetic acid [TCA], bichloroacetic acid [BCA], interferon, and surgery).[3] Cervical and extensive vaginal lesions may be treated with 5-fluorouracil cream or surgical excision with CO_2 laser surgery, cryosurgery, or electrosurgery. Interferons that have general antiviral, antiproliferative, and immunomodulating

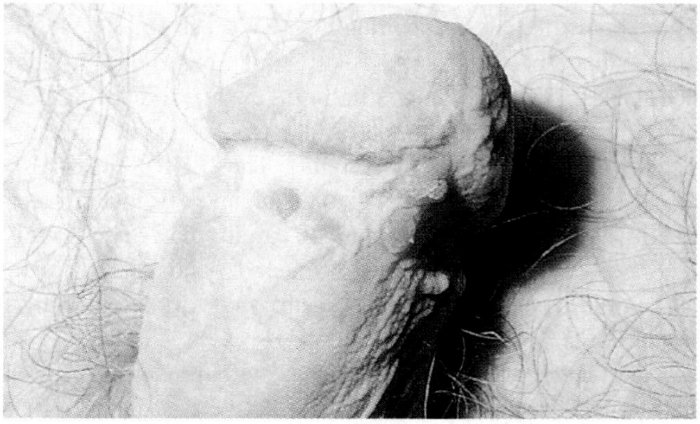

FIG. 23-14 Condylomata acuminata—penile. Asymptomatic, flesh-colored papules are present on the shaft of the penis. (From Morse SA, Moreland AA, Holmes KK, editors: *Atlas of sexually transmitted diseases and AIDS,* ed 2, London, 1996, Mosby-Wolfe.)

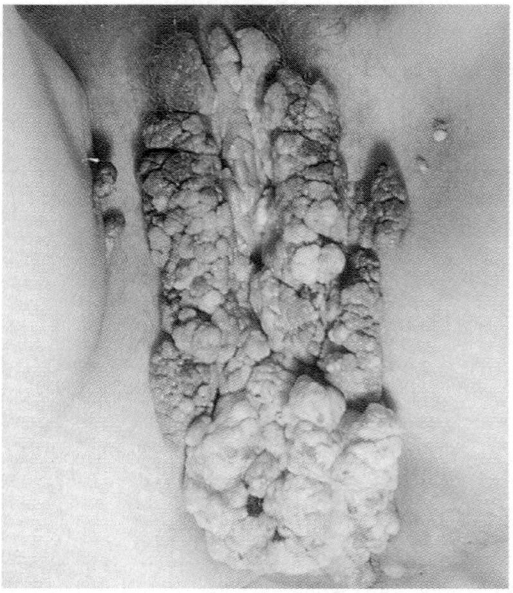

FIG. 23-15 Condylomata acuminata—vulva and perineum. The clinical diagnosis was giant condylomata of Buschke and Löwenstein. Such large and confluent lesions should be carefully examined and multiple biopsies obtained to rule out underlying malignancy. (From Morse SA, Moreland AA, Holmes KK, editors: *Atlas of sexually transmitted diseases and AIDS,* ed 2, London, 1996, Mosby-Wolfe.)

effects have been used successfully in treating stubborn genital warts. Success of treatment depends on response of the immune system. Approximately one third of individuals experience a cure, and another one third experience a decrease in wart size.[17] Surgical excision is the treatment for laryngeal warts in infants.

Molluscum Contagiosum

Molluscum contagiosum is a benign viral infection of the skin in children and adults. Primarily the face, hands, lower abdomen, and genitalia are affected; papules found on other parts of the skin or widely distributed are not uncommon. Individuals with AIDS may develop extensive lesions over the face, neck, and genital region.

Molluscum contagiosum occurs throughout the world and has been a common childhood disease in Papua New Guinea and Fiji. It is much less common in the United States, where incidence is highest among young adults. The childhood disease is transmitted by skin-to-skin contact and fomites (swimming pools, towels, gymnasium equipment) and affects the face, trunk, and limbs. Adult disease is more commonly sexually transmitted and affects the lower abdomen, genitalia, and perianal area.[47] Molluscum contagiosum is most common in males 20 to 29 years of age and in those with multiple sexual partners. The molluscum contagiosum virus is taken into epithelial cells by phagocytosis and replicates within the cytoplasm, where it produces cytoplasmic inclusions **(molluscous bodies)** and cellular hyperplasia. The underlying skin usually is not affected.[48]

After an incubation period of 2 to 7 weeks, white or flesh-colored, round or oval, dome-shaped papules appear. The lesions are relatively small (3 to 5 mm) but occasionally may coalesce to form larger lesions up to 15 mm. The surface has a characteristic central umbilication, from which a thick, creamy core material can be expressed (Fig. 23-16). Generally the lesions are not painful or pruritic unless secondarily infected. The papules may last several months or several years and spread by autoinoculation.

WHAT'S NEW? Self-Collected HPV DNA Samples As an Alternative to Cervical Cytology

Researchers compared self-collected and clinician-collected HPV DNA samples with pap smears for sensitivity in detecting cervical cancer in over 1400 South African women. Abnormal results were confirmed by colposcopy and biopsy. Sensitivity to identify HSIL (high-grade squamous intraepithelial lesions) or cervical cancer was highest in clinician-collected HPV DNA samples (83.9%); there was no significant difference in sensitivity between self-collected cervical samples (66.1%) and pap smears (67.9%). Both clinician- and self-collected cervical samples for HPV had higher false-positive rates (15.1% and 17.1%, respectively) than cytology (3.2% to 12.3%).

Data from Wright TC et al: HPV DNA testing of self-collected vaginal samples compared with cytologic screening to detect cervical cancer, *JAMA* 283(1):81, 2000.

The appearance of the lesions is generally all that is needed to make the diagnosis, although direct microscopic examination of stained material from the core of the papule discloses molluscous bodies within the swollen and rounded epithelial cells. The lesions often heal spontaneously after several months. Other effective means of removing the lesions include curettage and application of liquid nitrogen (cryotherapy) or silver nitrate. Topical acids have been used also but cause scarring. Individuals tend to have lifetime immunity once lesions are healed completely.

Parasitic Infections

Trichomoniasis

Originally discovered in 1836, *Trichomonas vaginalis* was at first thought to be a harmless commensal microorganism. *T. vaginalis* is now known to be one of the most common causes of sexually transmitted lower genital tract infection and urethritis.

Because **trichomoniasis** (infection by *T. vaginalis*) is not a reportable disease, its prevalence can only be estimated. The latest estimates suggest that as many as 5 million cases of trichomoniasis occur each year in the United States,[1] and that *T. vaginalis* accounts for one of four cases of infectious vaginitis.[28] Trichomoniasis is usually found in both sexual partners and often coexists with gonorrhea. Although sexual transmission is clearly the most common means of disease spread, transmission through fomites is theoretically possible. To cause infection, the fomite would have to introduce an inoculum of about 10,000 microorganisms directly into the vagina.[49]

Pathophysiology

T. vaginalis is an anaerobic, unicellular, flagellated, parasitic protozoan that adheres to and damages squamous epithelial

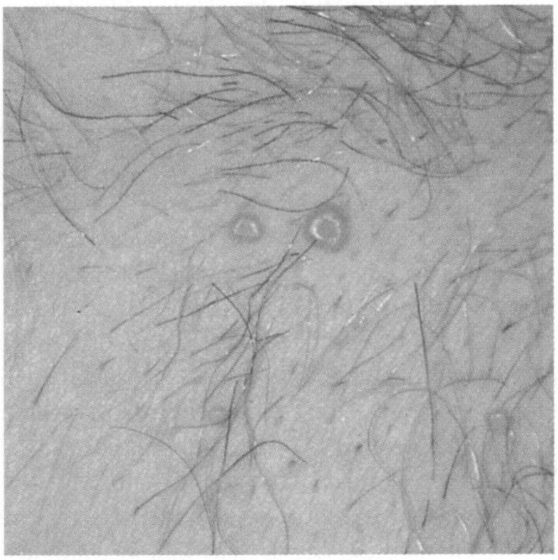

FIG. 23-16 Molluscum contagiosum. Flesh-colored papules of molluscum may be distinguished by their umbilicated centers. The papules contain a white, cheesy substance, which may be stained for the presence of viral inclusion bodies. (From Morse SA, Moreland AA, Holmes KK, editors: *Atlas of sexually transmitted diseases and AIDS,* ed 2, London, 1996, Mosby-Wolfe.)

cells. Because this protozoan selectively affects squamous epithelia, vaginal and urethral tissue is often infected, as are Skene and Bartholin glands. The endocervical canal is not affected because it is lined with columnar epithelium. In men the urethra is the most common site of infection, although the protozoa, called **trichomonads,** also can infect the epididymis and (rarely) the prostate. Zinc, which has potent antibacterial properties, is found in high concentrations in the prostate. Hence many trichomonads are cleared from the male urethra during ejaculation. This action makes urethral trichomoniasis a fairly self-limiting infection in men. Most infections of the male urethra clear up within 2 weeks.

Trichomoniasis is most common in men and women of reproductive age, and it is primarily an infection of the vagina. *T. vaginalis* can induce a marked inflammatory response in the vagina, causing a copious discharge that contains large numbers of polymorphonuclear neutrophils. Trichomonads adhere to but do not invade the squamous epithelial cells.

Clinical Manifestations

Manifestations of vaginal trichomoniasis range from none to severe, with some women reporting an increase in distressing symptoms immediately after menses. Vaginal discharge and internal pruritus are the most common complaints. Dyspareunia and dysuria are also fairly common. Secretions are usually copious, frothy, malodorous, and yellow-green to a gray-green. The vaginal walls may appear erythematous and sore. Rarely, small, punctate red marks, sometimes called *strawberry spots,* are visible. Vaginal pH is usually more than 4.2.

Most men with trichomoniasis remain asymptomatic. Possible clinical manifestations include scant intermittent discharge, slight pruritus, and mild dysuria.

Evaluation and Treatment

History and symptoms are inadequate for diagnosis of trichomoniasis. Fresh secretions have a pH higher than 4.7 and a positive amine odor when mixed with 10% KOH (positive "whiff test").

Microscopic confirmation of the presence of the trichomonads in vaginal secretions or urine provides a definitive diagnosis. In a fresh wet mount preparation that has been warmed slightly, the epithelial cells have relatively clean and sharp edges, the ratio of polymorphonuclear leukocytes to epithelial cells exceeds 1:1, and the trichomonads are visible. The ovoid microorganism is slightly larger than a polymorphonuclear leukocyte and has one rounded, flagellated end and one slightly pointed, flagellated end. The flagella give the trichomonads their characteristic twisting motility. In an acidic environment, such as urine, the trichomonads assume a "balled-up" or spherical shape and become less motile.

The treatment of choice for trichomoniasis is a single dose of metronidazole (Flagyl). The single-dose therapy is effective, has few side effects, and obviates the need for individual compliance with longer regimens. Sexual partners, even if asymptomatic, also are treated and examined for coexisting STIs. The 2-g single dose of metronidazole can be used to treat pregnant women.[3] However, lactating women should suspend breast-feeding for 24 hours after single-dose therapy.[50]

Scabies

Scabies is a rather benign, common parasitic infection that can be spread by skin-to-skin and sexual contact. Discovered by Bonomo in 1687, it is considered to be the first human disease with a known cause.[51]

Scabies has a worldwide distribution, but actual prevalence is unknown.[22] Traditionally the disease was attributed to conditions of poverty, overcrowding, uncleanliness, and sexual promiscuity. Today it is recognized that scabies occurs in individuals with good personal hygiene and is not limited to any social class. Outbreaks of scabies occur every 30 years or so and last about 15 years. The most recent outbreak in the United States began in 1971 and subsided in the 1980s.

Transmission of scabies requires prolonged close skin-to-skin contact, which typically occurs within families or between sexual partners. Nonsexual transmission from patient to nurse has been reported in hospitals during sponge baths and lotion application, and mites have been transferred through infested bedding, clothes, and other fomites.[5]

Pathophysiology

The adult female itch mite, *Sarcoptes scabiei,* is 0.3 to 0.4 mm long and has a life span of about 30 days. Once deposited on human skin, it burrows through the horny layer of the stratum granulosum (Fig. 23-17). Within hours of burrowing, the female begins laying two or three large eggs per day, each of which progresses through larval and nymphal stages to become an adult itch mite in about 10 days. The most common places for scabies to burrow are on the hands (between the fingers) and on the flexor surfaces of the wrists and the extensor surfaces of the elbows. Characteristic lesions may occur on the nipples of women and as pruritic papules on the penile shaft and glans and on the scrotum.[47,52] Pruritic papules may be seen on the buttocks also.[52] Fig. 23-18 shows the typical sites of scabies burrows.

Clinical Manifestations

The classic symptom of scabies is intense pruritus, which may be pronounced at night. The typical burrow of the *S. scabiei* is a short, linear, curved, or S-shaped line (Fig. 23-19). There may be small, erythematous, excoriated larval papules near the burrows. Secondary infections are common and are caused by scratching. In some individuals a hypersensitivity reaction occurs a month or more after the infestation and causes multiple, reddish brown, pruritic nodules to develop on the covered portions of the body—most commonly, the upper thighs, buttocks, male genitalia, and axillary regions. These nodules may persist for more than 1 year despite treatment with a scabicide.

Evaluation and Treatment

Although the diagnosis is often made on clinical grounds, microscopic identification of the mite or its eggs, larvae, or feces is recommended because the symptoms of scabies can

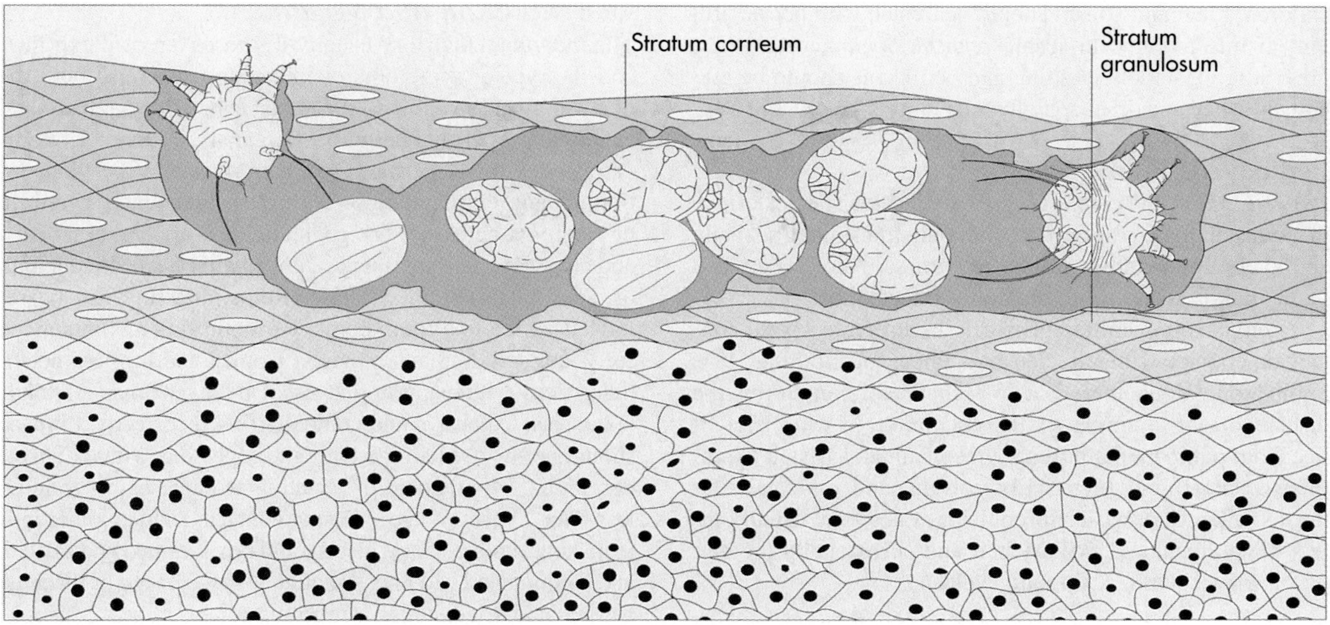

FIG. 23-17 The burrow of *Sarcoptes scabiei*. As the female mite moves through the stratum corneum, she leaves a trail of eggs and scybala behind. When the eggs hatch, the larval forms emerge onto the skin surface. (From Morse SA, Moreland AA, Holmes KK, editors: *Atlas of sexually transmitted diseases and AIDS,* ed 2, London, 1996, Mosby-Wolfe.)

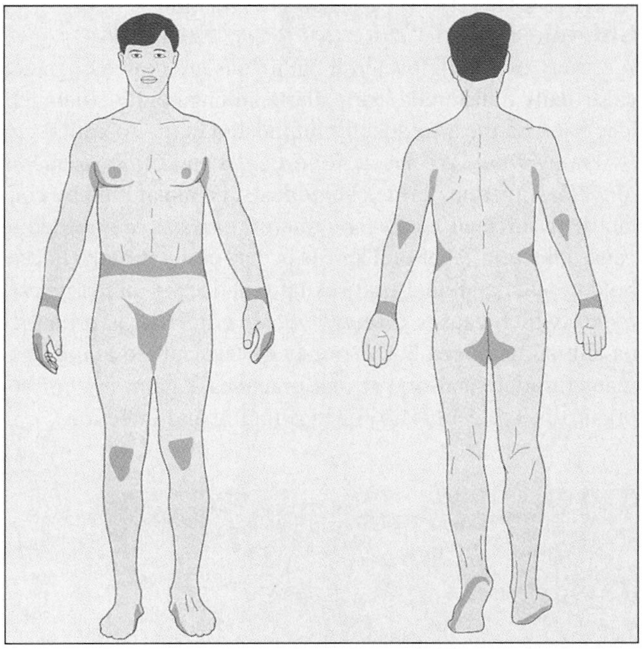

FIG. 23-18 Distribution of skin lesions of *Sarcoptes scabiei* infestation. Unshaded areas are rarely affected in healthy adults. (From Morse SA, Moreland AA, Holmes KK, editors: *Atlas of sexually transmitted diseases and AIDS,* ed 2, London, 1996, Mosby-Wolfe.)

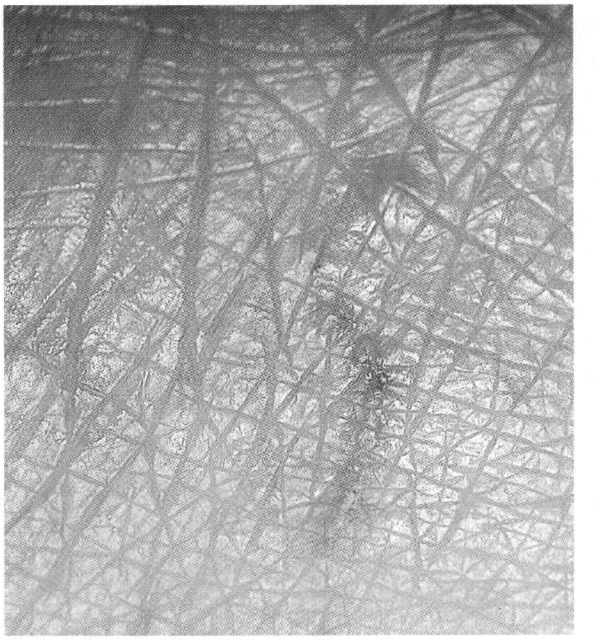

FIG. 23-19 Scabies burrow. An S-shaped burrow with a tiny vesicle at one end. (From Habif TP et al: *Skin disease: diagnosis and treatment,* St Louis, 2001, Mosby.)

imitate those of many other dermatologic conditions. Superficial scrapings from a recently developed, unexcoriated papule or burrow can be observed easily under the microscope; the addition of potassium hydroxide allows easier visualization of the mite.

Preferred treatment is topical application of 5% permethrin massaged and left for 8 to 14 hours. Lindane (1%) lotion or cream applied thinly to all areas of the body below the neck and washed thoroughly at 8 hours and 10% crotamiton applied to the body below the neck nightly for 2 nights and washed thoroughly 24 hours after the second application are effective also.[50,52] Close household and sexual contacts should be treated also. Permethrin has been used safely in infants as young as 2 months and is the treatment of choice for children. Pregnant women should be treated with permethrin only if infestation with scabies can be documented.[50,52] To prevent reinfestation, clothing and bed linens should be machine washed and dried at high temperatures, or dry-cleaned.[3]

Pediculosis Pubis

Phthirus pubis, the crab louse, is one of three species of lice that infest humans. *P. pubis* is commonly transmitted sexually and causes **pediculosis pubis,** or "crabs." Adolescents and young children are most commonly infected.

P. pubis is transmitted primarily by intimate sexual contact or contact with infected bed linens or clothing. It is highly contagious; there is a 95% chance of contracting the disease during a single sexual encounter. The transfer of lice from pubic hair is probably mechanical, assisted by animated scratching; fingernails; towels; and other, similar means rather than by self-propulsion. Pubic lice usually infect the perineal and axillary hair and occasionally the hair of the trunk, beard, scalp, and eyelashes.

Pathophysiology

The crab louse has a 25- to 30-day life cycle from egg to egg that consists of five stages: an egg (or nit) stage, three nymphal stages, and an adult stage, all of which occur in the host. The nits of crab lice are found "glued" to hairs; they are oval, 0.8 by 0.3 mm, and whitish, and they hatch in 5 to 10 days (Fig. 23-20). In the adult stage, pubic lice are grayish, are approximately 1 mm in length, and have a segmented body and claws particularly designed for clinging to pubic hairs. Because lice depend on blood for nutrition, they bite into the skin to obtain food.

Clinical Manifestations

Symptoms range from mild pruritus to severe, intolerable itching, depending on the individual's sensitivity to louse bites. Allergic sensitization occurs in about 5 days, when itching, erythema, and inflammation may worsen. Excessive scratching may lead to secondary infection.

Evaluation and Treatment

The individual's history usually discloses a recent exposure and the typical symptoms of infestation. Because both the lice and nits are visible to the naked eye, a thorough clinical examination permits definitive diagnosis. Pediculosis pubis is treated with 1% permethrin cream rinse or 1% lindane lotion, cream, or shampoo or with over-the-counter pyrethrin or piperonyl butoxide. The pediculicide is applied to infested and adjacent hairy areas and removed after a specified length of time by thorough washing. Remaining nits can be removed with a fine-tooth comb. Permethrin is recommended for young children and pregnant women and has less potential toxicity with inappropriate use. On the other hand, lindane is the least expensive and nontoxic if used correctly. Lindane should not be used after a bath, or by persons with extensive dermatitis, by pregnant or lactating women, or by children less than 2 years of age.[50] Sexual contacts and any other intimate household contacts also should be examined and treated, and clothing and bed linens should be dry-cleaned or machine washed and dried at high temperatures.[3]

SEXUALLY TRANSMITTED INFECTIONS OF OTHER BODY SYSTEMS

Gastrointestinal Infections

Shigellosis and *Campylobacter* Enteritis

A variety of enteric bacterial pathogens are now recognized as sexually transmitted, particularly among homosexual men. The bacteria most frequently implicated in the so-called *gay bowel syndrome* are species of *Shigella* and *Campylobacter. Shigella* infection, termed **shigellosis,** is transmitted by contact with infected feces. Few microorganisms are needed to cause infection. Anal-oral spread occurs easily through household contact and anal-oral sexual practices. *Campylobacter jejuni,* which causes ***Campylobacter* enteritis,** is primarily an animal pathogen but also may be transmitted among humans through anal-oral sexual practices. Again, few microorganisms are necessary for inoculation and infection.

A 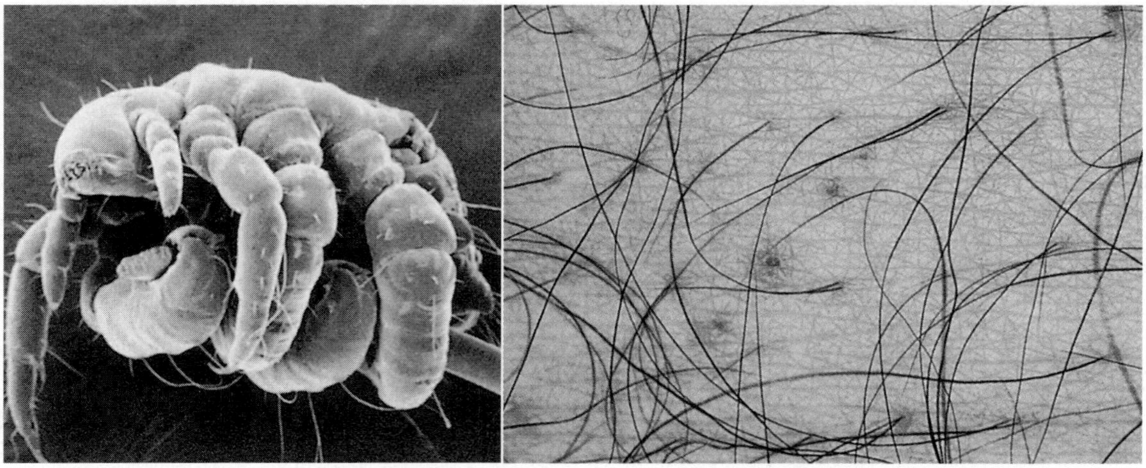 B

FIG. 23-20 Pubic louse and crab louse. A, Pubic louse *(Phthirus pubis)* encircling a pubic hair; the clawlike legs produce a firm grip. **B,** Crab louse bites *(Phthirus pubis).* (From Morse SA, Moreland AA, Holmes KK, editors: *Atlas of sexually transmitted diseases and AIDS,* ed 2, London, 1996, Mosby-Wolfe.)

Pathophysiology

Shigella organisms are nonmotile, gram-negative rods that are related to *Escherichia coli.* They invade and kill intestinal epithelial cells, thereby inducing a marked inflammatory response and diarrhea. *Campylobacter* organisms are highly motile, curved, gram-negative rods that also invade and kill intestinal cells and cause bloody, inflammatory exudate and diarrhea.

Clinical Manifestations

Either microorganism may cause a mild, self-limited gastroenteritis or severe dysentery. After a 24- to 48-hour incubation period, shigellosis begins with fever, abdominal distress, and diarrhea. It may resolve completely or progress to dysentery with severe cramping, abdominal pain, tenesmus, and bloody mucoid discharge from the rectum. *Campylobacter* enteritis typically begins, after a 1- to 7-day incubation period, with sudden fever and abdominal pain followed by diarrhea. Malaise, anorexia, headache, arthralgia, and myalgia are common.[53]

Evaluation and Treatment

Clinical manifestations and cultures of fresh stool samples are used to diagnose shigellosis. Culturing *Campylobacter* is expensive; therefore microscopic analysis of a gram-stained smear of rectal exudate may be used as a diagnostic aid.

Treatment for mild illness includes correction of fluid and electrolyte imbalance. Antidiarrheals are avoided because they may delay clearance of the microorganism. Because both *Shigella* and *Campylobacter* are highly contagious, antibiotic treatment may be advisable even for mild cases. The preferred treatment for shigellosis is oral ciprofloxacin, 500 mg, or norfloxacin, 400 mg, twice daily for 3 days. Oral ciprofloxacin, 500 mg twice daily for 3 to 5 days, or erythromycin, 500 mg four times daily for 5 days, is effective against *Campylobacter* enteritis.[50] Sexual partners are examined and treated, and individuals are instructed to avoid oral-anal contact until the infection is cured.

Giardiasis and Amebiasis

Two enteric protozoa that are sexually transmitted, primarily among homosexual men, are *Giardia lamblia,* the cause of **giardiasis,** and *Entamoeba histolytica,* the cause of **amebiasis.** The incidence of these infections in the male homosexual population has decreased over the past years, presumably because of safer sex practices.[54] Although the principal route of transmission is contaminated drinking water, giardiasis and amebiasis are transmitted also by anal-oral or genital-anal contact.

Pathophysiology

G. lamblia and *E. histolytica* are both parasites having two forms, cysts and **trophozoites** (uncysted protozoa). The cysts are the infective form because they can survive in moist environments outside the host. Giardiasis commonly begins with ingestion of a small number of *G. lamblia* cysts. Once in the upper small bowel, each cyst becomes a trophozoite, which multiplies and attaches to the bowel mucosa. Enzyme deficiencies, inflammation, and immunologic damage then apparently occur, resulting in intestinal malabsorption. Amebiasis begins similarly: the ingested cysts pass to the small or large bowel, where each returns to the trophozoite state, multiplies quickly, and begins to invade the mucosa through cytotoxic activity. Mucosal invasion results in the development of ulcers and an inflammatory response. Individuals infected with *E. histolytica* may excrete up to 45 million cysts per day.

Clinical Manifestations

Giardiasis begins with sudden, explosive diarrhea, distention, and flatulence. Upper gastrointestinal symptoms are also prominent and may include epigastric pain; vomiting; foul, sulfuric burping; and nausea. After the acute illness, which usually lasts several days, milder symptoms may persist for months, with evidence of malabsorption and weight loss. Amebiasis is often asymptomatic. Symptoms that do occur range from mild diarrhea to severe dysentery. Amebiasis may spread from the intestine to other organs, such as the liver.

Evaluation and Treatment

Diagnosis of both entities usually is made by history and microscopic examination of fresh stool specimens for either trophozoites or cysts. Small bowel biopsy may aid in the diagnosis of giardiasis; rectal biopsy may aid in the diagnosis of amebiasis. Serologic testing is useful in the differential diagnosis of symptomatic individuals with amebiasis. Metronidazole is effective against both conditions, but the preferred treatment for giardiasis is oral quinacrine, 100 mg three times daily for 7 to 10 days. The dosage of metronidazole for amebiasis depends on the severity of the infection.[50]

Hepatitis B

Hepatitis is a liver infection that can be caused by six types of viruses: hepatitis A, hepatitis B, hepatitis C, hepatitis D, hepatitis E, and hepatitis G. Each virus causes a syndrome of acute, icteric (jaundice-producing) liver inflammation. Of the three types, the **hepatitis B virus (HBV)** is known to be sexually transmitted. (Hepatitis A, like most other predominantly enteric infections, may be considered an STI because of oral-anal transmission.) Although hepatitis C (HCV) is not currently recognized as an STI, the CDC has listed sexual exposure as an HCV risk factor (Fig. 23-21). Data indicate sexual transmission of HCV appears to occur, but the virus is inefficiently spread through this manner.[35] Additional information about hepatitis is found in Chapter 38.

The prevalence of HBV infection varies dramatically worldwide. In Southeast Asia and Africa, 60% to 80% of the population may harbor serologic evidence of past or current infection. In the United States, approximately 5% to 20% of the general population have evidence of HBV infection. Seropositivity generally increases with age. Serologic tests of STI clinic patients show evidence of past infection in 28%

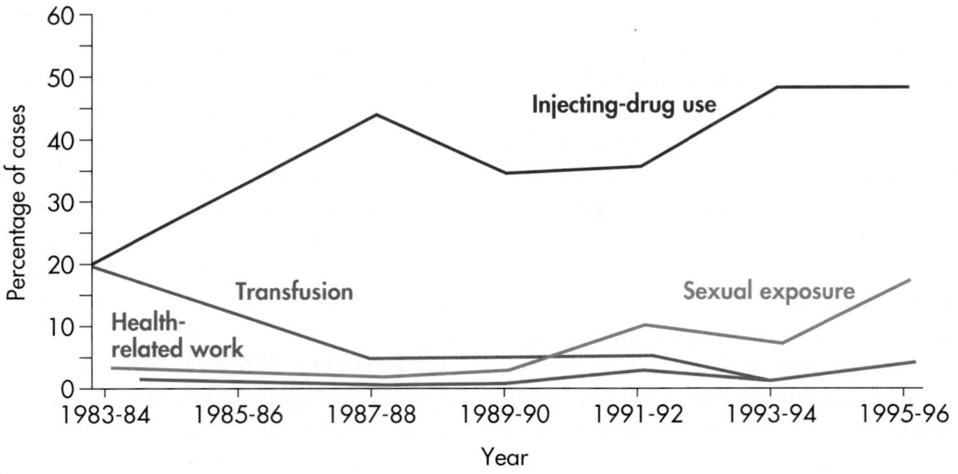

FIG. 23-21 Risk for hepatitis C exposure. Comparison of injecting drug use *(green)*, transfusions *(red)*, health-related work *(blue)*, and sexual exposure *(gold)*. Note the rise in sexually transmitted incidences of hepatitis C over the past 13 years. (From Hepatitis C: What clinicians and other health professionals need to know, 2000. Available at www.cdc.gov/ncidod/diseases/hepatitis/c/edu/default_r.htm.

of individuals ages 25 years and older and 7% in those younger than 25 years.[50] At risk for HBV infection are those with low socioeconomic status, blacks, Indochinese refugees, health care workers, and male homosexuals. In groups of male homosexuals, the seropositivity rates may be as high as 80%. Other groups at risk are intravenous drug users, institutionalized mentally retarded persons, hemodialysis patients, and heterosexual partners of HBV carriers.[55]

Transmission of HBV can occur through needle puncture, blood transfusion, cuts or abrasions in the skin, and absorption by mucosal surfaces. Direct contact with infected body fluids, such as tears, cerebrospinal fluid, synovial fluid, gastric juices, pleural fluid, semen, and urine, may pass the infection. Fomites also can transmit hepatitis: HBV can survive on inanimate objects for up to 1 week.[56]

Perinatal transmission of HBV is relatively common. Neonates whose mothers are infectious have a 70% to 90% chance of becoming infected with HBV during labor or delivery and a 90% chance of becoming chronic carriers.[26] Hepatitis B virus can be found in maternal vaginal secretions, blood, amniotic fluid, saliva, and breast milk.[56]

Hepatitis delta agent is a defective virus that is similar to HBV antigen but cannot cause hepatitis B by itself, requiring the presence of HBV to cause hepatitis. Hepatitis delta infection is rare in the United States, but cases have been documented in intravenous drug users and their sexual contacts and also in recipients of contaminated blood. It commonly is found in homosexuals, persons requiring kidney dialysis, and health care workers.

Pathophysiology

After exposure, HBV passes through the bloodstream to the liver, where it infects liver cells and multiplies. The infection is usually self-limiting, with most patients mounting an effective immune response. Approximately 6% to 10% of infected individuals cannot eradicate the virus and become chronic carriers of HBV.

Clinical Manifestations

Most HBV infections are clinically inapparent and result in solid and permanent immunity. Symptoms of hepatitis usually develop only after a certain HBV antigen has been circulating in the blood for 3 to 6 weeks. Approximately 15% to 20% of individuals develop a prodromal syndrome that is similar to serum sickness. This syndrome is characterized by an erythematous rash, urticaria, polyarthralgias, and arthritis. Symptoms of infection also may include lassitude, anorexia, nausea, vomiting, headache, fever, dark urine, jaundice, and moderate liver enlargement with tenderness. Long-term sequelae include chronic persistent and chronic active hepatitis, cirrhosis, hepatocellular carcinoma, hepatic failure, and death. In neonates who contract HBV, the disease may be manifested in many ways, from mild illness to a severe, fulminant infection with a mortality of 75%.

Evaluation and Treatment

Hepatitis B virus infection is clinically indistinguishable from other types of hepatitis. Diagnosis can be made only through serologic testing.

No specific therapy exists for HBV infection in adults. Treatment consists of supportive care and relief of symptoms. HBV vaccination is recommended for (1) sexually active homosexual and bisexual men, (2) men and women diagnosed with another STI, and (3) persons with more than one sexual partner in the last 6 months.[50]

The infant who is born to a mother with infectious HBV is given HBV immune globulin and Hepatavax-B vaccine within 12 hours of birth. The HBV vaccine is administered again at 1 and 6 months if serologic tests show that a chronic carrier state has not developed.

Systemic Diseases

Epstein-Barr Virus

Recent investigations have indicated that the **Epstein-Barr virus (EBV),** which is transmitted orally, is also capable of being harbored within the male and female genital tracts and transmitted sexually. Further research is needed to specifically identify the role that EBV plays in STIs; however, the significance of EBV infection of the genital tract relates to its ability to transform cells and potentially contribute to the development of cancers in the genital tract.[57]

Acquired Immunodeficiency Syndrome

Epidemiology, modes of transmission, pathophysiology, clinical manifestations, and evaluation and treatment of AIDS are discussed in detail in Chapter 8.

> **WHAT'S NEW? Antiviral Agents and HBV**
>
> During the past decade, numerous antiviral agents have been investigated for treating chronic HBV infection. Interferon alfa-2b has been 40% effective in eliminating chronic HBV infection; persons who become infected during adulthood were most likely to respond to this treatment. Antiretroviral agents (e.g., lamivudine) also have been effective in eliminating HBV infection. Other compounds are still being evaluated. The goal of antiviral treatment is to stop HBV replication. Response to treatment can be demonstrated by normalization of liver function tests, improvement in liver histology, and serorevision from HbeAg-positive to HbeAg-negative. Long-term follow-up of treated individuals suggests that the remission of chronic hepatitis induced by interferon alfa-2b is of long duration.

Cytomegalovirus Infection

Cytomegalovirus (CMV) is a sexually transmissible herpesvirus. It is associated with a number of clinical syndromes in newborns, otherwise healthy adults, and immunosuppressed individuals.

CMV infection causes no specific genital disease, but its incidence is high in individuals being treated for other STIs. CMV infection is prevalent worldwide, especially in developing countries and lower socioeconomic groups. The virus is found in semen, cervical secretions, urine, blood, saliva, breast milk, and stool, and transmission is associated with close (although not always genital) interpersonal contact or direct transfer of cells or body fluids. It is more common in homosexual men and in young women with multiple sexual partners. Intrauterine CMV infection is the most common congenital infection and occurs in 0.5% to 3% of all live births. Like HSV, primary maternal infection carries the greatest risk of transmission and severe consequences. Infected infants can be asymptomatic or may experience varying degrees of sensorineural hearing loss or severe cognitive and psychomotor developmental deficits.[2,58] Perinatal transmission of CMV may occur across the placenta, by contamination with infected secretions during passage through the birth canal, or during breast-feeding.

Pathophysiology

After CMV infects a human cell, it may replicate and destroy the infected cell or become incorporated into the host cell's DNA. Local CMV infections can persist despite the presence of large quantities of systemic antibody to CMV. Cell-mediated immunity seems to have a particular role in protecting against CMV infections. Depression of CMV-specific cell-mediated immunity has been noted in otherwise normal hosts with CMV infection. This may be caused by injury of T cells or macrophages by the cytomegalovirus.[59]

Clinical Manifestations

In healthy individuals, CMV infection can cause a number of mild subclinical or nonspecific illnesses, including mononucleosis, pneumonitis, hemolytic anemia, and thrombocytopenia purpura. In contrast, a CMV infection in an immunocompromised individual, such as a transplant recipient or an individual with AIDS, can cause a devastating, life-threatening illness.

Congenital CMV infection is the most common serious viral infection among infants. Approximately 1% of all infants (40,000) are born with congenital CMV. Of these, 10% (4000) demonstrate typical manifestations of the infection, such as hepatosplenomegaly, intracranial calcifications, microcephaly, smallness for gestational age, and hearing impairments. An additional 10% to 15% of these are asymptomatic at birth; however, they begin to develop manifestations of the infection within the first few months of life. Recent evidence suggests that symptomatic infection of infants is caused by a primary infection of the mother during her pregnancy and not necessarily by reinfection or reactivation of a prior infection.

Evaluation and Treatment

The most definitive diagnostic test for CMV is isolation of the virus, usually through growth in human fibroblast cell culture. Several methods for measuring antibodies to CMV are available, including complement-fixation (CF) tests and indirect immunofluorescent antibody (IFA) tests. These methods frequently are used in clinical situations.

With the increased incidence of CMV infection among immunocompromised individuals (persons with AIDS or transplants), various treatment modalities have been investigated. Ganciclovir is similar to acyclovir and inhibits viral DNA polymerase (see Chapter 4). Relapses of CMV infection are frequent after therapy ceases; thus lifelong therapy is particularly indicated in individuals with AIDS.[45] Acyclovir has been used, but optimum therapeutic benefits have not been established. Future therapies still under investigation include ganciclovir plus CMV immune globulin and vaccine.

Experimental antiviral drugs may prove helpful in the treatment of severe CMV infection, and preliminary studies to develop a vaccine appear promising. No treatment is indicated, however, in most cases of CMV infection.

SUMMARY REVIEW

Sexually Transmitted Urogenital Infections

1. Gonorrhea is a sexually transmitted communicable disease that can be local or systemic. Complications include pelvic inflammatory disease (PID); sterility; and disseminated infection, which is spread through the bloodstream to the skin, joints, and heart.
2. Gonorrhea passed to the fetus from the mother typically manifests as an eye infection and develops 1 to 12 days after birth. Usually ophthalmic antibiotic prophylaxis is not sufficient to prevent infection.
3. Antibiotic coverage for penicillin-resistant strains and chlamydial coinfection is recommended for all individuals diagnosed with gonorrhea and their partners.
4. Syphilis is a sexually transmitted infection (STI) that becomes systemic shortly after infection. The four stages of the disease are (a) primary syphilis with a chancre at the site of infection; (b) secondary syphilis with systemic spread to all body systems; (c) latent syphilis with minimal symptoms or the development of skin lesions; and (d) tertiary syphilis, the most severe stage, with destruction of bone, skin, and soft and neurologic tissues.
5. Congenital syphilis contributes to prematurity of the newborn with bone marrow depression, central nervous system (CNS) involvement, renal failure, and intrauterine growth retardation. Late clinical manifestations are those of tertiary syphilis and are rare.
6. Syphilis is diagnosed by serologic testing and treated with injectable penicillin. Sexual partners are treated also.
7. With chancroid infection, women are generally asymptomatic and men may develop inflamed, painful genital ulcers and inguinal buboes. Incubation period is 1 to 14 days. Single-dose therapy with injectable ceftriaxone or oral azithromycin for both partners is recommended. Persons with human immunodeficiency virus (HIV) may require a longer treatment regimen.
8. Granuloma inguinale (donovanosis) is rare in the United States. The bacteria are gram-negative and survive within macrophages. Localized nodules coalesce to form granulomas and ulcers on the penis in men and labia in women. Antibiotics provide effective treatment. Although rare and mildly infectious, granuloma inguinale is a chronic, progressively destructive bacterial infection. Often individuals diagnosed with granuloma inguinale are coinfected with syphilis.
9. Bacterial vaginosis (BV) is a sexually associated condition caused by an overgrowth of anaerobic bacteria that produce aromatic amines and raise the pH of the vagina, promoting further bacterial growth (without an inflammatory response) and a fishy-smelling odor. "Clue cells" are found on the wet mount. Metronidazole (Flagyl) provides effective treatment. BV has been associated with PID, chorioamnionitis, preterm labor, and postpartum endometritis. Treatment of sexual partners is controversial.
10. Chlamydia is the most common bacterial STI in the United States and the leading preventable cause of infertility and ectopic pregnancy. The causative organism, *C. trachomatis,* localizes to epithelial tissue and can spread throughout the urogenital tract or pass from infected mother to the eyes and respiratory tract of newborn infants during birth. As with gonorrhea, prophylactic eye antibiotic treatment is insufficient to prevent infection. *C. trachomatis* is susceptible to inexpensive, readily accessible antibiotics. Oral doxycycline is the drug of choice in men and nonpregnant women; erythromycin is used for young children and pregnant women. Antibiotic therapy for infected individuals and all sexual contacts is recommended. Because of the asymptomatic nature of chlamydia and the potential sequelae of untreated infection, extensive and widespread screening is warranted.
11. Lymphogranuloma venereum is a chronic STI that is uncommon in the United States. The lesion begins as a skin infection and spreads to the lymph tissue, causing inflammation, necrosis, buboes, and abscesses of the inguinal lymph nodes. Primary lesions appear on the penis and scrotum in men and on the cervix, vaginal wall, and labia in women. Secondary lesions involve inflammation and swelling of the lymph nodes with formation of large blue buboes that rupture and form draining ulcerative lesions. A 21-day course of oral doxycycline or erythromycin is effective. Treatment of sexual partners is recommended.
12. Genital herpes is the most common genital ulceration in the United States and is caused by either type 1 (HSV-1) or type 2 (HSV-2) herpesvirus. Lesions initially appear as groups of vesicles that progress to ulceration with pain, lymphadenopathy, and fever. Herpes simplex virus passes from mother to fetus and can cause spontaneous abortion or prematurity. Acyclovir reduces symptoms but does not cure the disease.
13. Three distinct syndromes are associated with HSV infection: (a) first-episode primary infections, (b) first-episode nonprimary infections, and (c) recurrent infections. Recurrent infections are most often attributable to HSV-2 and are generally milder and of shorter duration.
14. Condylomata acuminata (genital warts) are associated with multiple sexual partners and are highly contagious. The velvety, cauliflower-like lesions occur in the genital and anal areas, vagina, and cervix and are painless. They can be transmitted to the infant at birth. Surgical excision with laser or cryosurgery is most effective.
15. Molluscum contagiosum is a benign viral infection of the skin. It is transmitted by skin-to-skin contact in children and adults. In adults it tends to occur on the genitalia and to be transmitted by sexual contact.
16. Trichomoniasis *(T. vaginalis)* is a common cause of genital infection, vaginitis in women, and urethritis. Both partners usually are infected. Women usually have a copious, malodorous, gray-green discharge with pruritus. Men usually are asymptomatic. Metronidazole is the treatment for both partners.
17. Scabies is a common parasitic infection that can be spread by skin-to-skin contact and sexual contact. The scabies mite burrows through the skin, depositing two or three large eggs per day. Intense pruritus, especially at night, is the most pronounced clinical manifestation. Treatment consists of topical application of a pediculicide.
18. Pediculosis pubis (crabs) is commonly transmitted sexually and is caused by the crab louse, *Phthirus pubis.* The lice bite into the skin for nutrition. Symptoms include mild and severe pruritus. Topical application of prescription or over-the-counter pediculicides is effective treatment.

Sexually Transmitted Infections of Other Body Systems

1. Various enteric bacterial pathogens are now recognized as sexually transmitted, particularly among homosexual men. The infections include shigellosis, *Campylobacter* enteritis, giardiasis, amebiasis, and hepatitis B.
2. Shigellosis is transmitted by contact with infected feces. *Campylobacter* enteritis can be transmitted through anal-oral sexual practices.
3. Giardiasis and amebiasis are transmitted primarily through contaminated drinking water, but they can be transmitted by anal-oral and genital-anal contact.
4. Transmission of hepatitis B virus (HBV) can occur through needle puncture, blood transfusion, cuts in the skin, and contact with infected body fluids.
5. Perinatal transmission of HBV is relatively common.
6. Systemic diseases known to be sexually transmitted include acquired immunodeficiency syndrome (AIDS) (see Chapter 8), cytomegalovirus infection, and Epstein-Barr virus.
7. Epstein-Barr virus may be harbored in the genital tract and passed on through sexual encounters.
8. Cytomegalovirus (CMV) is a sexually transmissible herpesvirus. The infection causes no specific genital disease, but its incidence is high in individuals being treated for other sexually transmitted infections (STIs). The virus is found in semen, cervical secretions, urine, blood, saliva, breast milk, and stool.
9. CMV infection is more common in homosexual men and in young women with multiple sexual partners. It is the most common congenital infection.
10. CMV infection can cause mononucleosis, pneumonitis, hemolytic anemia, and thrombocytopenia purpura. A CMV infection in an immunosuppressed individual can cause a life-threatening illness. No treatment is indicated in most cases of CMV infection.

KEY TERMS

Acute urethral syndrome, *795*
Amebiasis, *805*
Bacterial vaginosis (BV), *792*
Bubo, *790*
Campylobacter enteritis, *804*
Chancre, *786*
Chancroid, *790*
Chlamydia, *793*
Condylomata acuminata, *799*
Condylomata lata, *787*
Congenital syphilis (CS), *785*
Cytomegalovirus (CMV), *807*
Disseminated gonococcal infection (DGI), *784*
Donovan body, *792*
Epstein-Barr virus (EBV), *807*
Fomite, *782*
Genital herpes, *797*
Giardiasis, *805*
Gonococcus, *782*
Gonorrhea, *782*
Granuloma inguinale, *792*
Gumma, *787*
Hepatitis B virus (HBV), *805*
Hepatitis delta agent, *806*
Latent syphilis, *786*
Lymphogranuloma venereum (LGV), *796*
Molluscous body, *801*
Molluscum contagiosum, *801*
Neurosyphilis, *787*
Nongonococcal urethritis (NGU), *797*
Ophthalmia neonatorum, *784*
Pediculosis pubis, *804*
Perihepatitis, *784*
Primary syphilis, *786*
Pseudobubo, *792*
Scabies, *802*
Secondary syphilis, *786*
Shigellosis, *804*
Syphilis, *785*
Tertiary syphilis, *787*
Trichomonad, *802*
Trichomoniasis, *801*
Trophozoite, *805*

REFERENCES

1. National Center for HIV, STD, and TB Prevention: *Tracking the Hidden Epidemics: Trends in the STD epidemics in the United States,* Atlanta, 2000, Centers for Disease Control and Prevention. Available at www.cdc.gov/nchstp/dstd/STD_Index.htm.
2. Division of STD Prevention, Department of Health and Human Services: *Sexually transmitted disease surveillance 1998,* Atlanta, 2000, Centers for Disease Control and Prevention. Available at www.cdc.gov/nchstp/dstd/Stats_Trends.
3. Division of STD Prevention, Department of Health and Human Services: *1998 Guidelines for Treatment of Sexually Transmitted Diseases,* Atlanta, 1998, Centers for Disease Control and Prevention. Available at www.cdc.gov/epo/mmwr/preview/mmwrhtml/00050909.htm.
4. Hook EW III, Handsfield HH: Gonococcal infections in the adult. In Holmes KK et al, editors: *Sexually transmitted diseases,* ed 2, New York, 1990, McGraw-Hill.
5. Pelouze PS: *Gonorrhea in the male and female,* Philadelphia, 1941, W.B. Saunders.
6. Whittington W et al: Gonorrhea. In Morse SA, Moreland AA, Holmes KK, editors: *Atlas of sexually transmitted diseases and AIDS,* ed 2, London, 1996, Mosby-Wolfe.
7. Berger TG, Rothman I: Sexually transmitted diseases in men. In Tanagho EA, McAninch JW, editors: *Smith's general urology,* Norwalk, Conn, 1995, Appleton & Lange.
8. Zenilman JM: Gonorrhea: clinical and public health issues, *Hosp Pract* 28(2a):29, 1993.
9. Sperling RS: Infection protocols: perihepatitis, *Contemp OB/GYN* 37(6): 51, 1992.
10. Division of STD Prevention, Department of Health and Human Services: *Sexually transmitted disease surveillance 1995,* Atlanta, 1996, Centers for Disease Control and Prevention.
11. Division of STD Prevention, Department of Health and Human Services: *Sexually transmitted disease surveillance 1998 supplement,* Atlanta, 2000, Centers for Disease Control and Prevention. Available at www.cdc.gov/nchstp/dstd/Stats_Trends.
12. Leu RH: Complications of coexisting chlamydial and gonococcal infections, *Postgrad Med* 89:56, 1991.
13. Centers for Disease Control: 1989 sexually transmitted diseases treatment guidelines, *MMWR Morb Mortal Wkly Rep* 38:1, 1989.
14. Brandt AM: *No magic bullet: a social history of venereal disease in the United States since 1880,* expanded edition, New York, 1987, Oxford University Press.

15. Sparling PF: Natural history of syphilis. In Holmes KK et al, editors: *Sexually transmitted diseases,* ed 2, New York, 1990, McGraw-Hill.
16. Thompson S, Larsen S, Moreland A: Syphilis. In Morse SA, Moreland AA, Holmes KK, editors: *Atlas of sexually transmitted diseases and AIDS,* ed 2, London, 1996, Mosby-Wolfe.
17. Schultz KF et al: Congenital syphilis. In Holmes KK et al, editors: *Sexually transmitted diseases,* ed 2, New York, 1990, McGraw-Hill
18. Thin RN: Early syphilis in the adult. In Holmes KK et al, editors: *Sexually transmitted diseases,* ed 2, New York, 1990, McGraw-Hill.
19. Hook EW, Marra CM: Medical progress: acquired syphilis in adults, *N Engl J Med* 326(16):1060, 1992.
20. Wooldridge WE: Syphilis: a new visit from an old enemy, *Postgrad Med* 89:193, 1991.
21. Tillman J: Syphilis an old disease, a contemporary problem, *J Obstet Gynecol Neonat Nurs* 21(3):209, 1992.
22. Jacobs RA: Infectious diseases: spirochetal. In McTierney LM, McPhee SJ, Papadakis MS, editors: *Current medical diagnosis & treatment,* ed 35, Norwalk, Conn, 1996, Appleton & Lange.
23. Committee on Infectious Disease: *Red Book 2000.* Elk Grove Village, Ill, 2000, American Academy of Pediatrics.
24. Para MF, Baird IM: Genital ulcer syndromes. In Spagna VA, Prior RB, editors: *Sexually transmitted diseases: a clinical syndrome approach,* New York, 1985, Marcel Dekker.
25. Ronald AR, Albritton W: Chancroid and *Haemophilus ducreyi.* In Holmes KK et al, editors: *Sexually transmitted diseases,* ed 2, New York, 1990, McGraw-Hill.
26. Richens J: The diagnosis of treatment of donovanosis (granuloma inguinale), *Genitourin Med* 67:441, 1991.
27. Hart G: Donovanosis. In Holmes KK et al, editors: *Sexually transmitted diseases,* ed 2, New York, 1990, McGraw-Hill.
28. Hiller S, Holmes KK: Bacterial vaginitis. In Holmes KK et al, editors: *Sexually transmitted diseases,* ed 2, New York, 1990, McGraw-Hill.
29. *Vaginitis.* Washington, DC, 1996, American College of Obstetrics and Gynecology [Technical Bulletin 226:1].
30. Hillier SL et al: Association between bacterial vaginosis and preterm delivery of a low birth-weight infant, *N Engl J Med* 333(26):1737, 1995.
31. Wallin KL et al: Type-specific persistence of human papillomavirus DNA before the development of invasive cervical cancer, *N Engl J Med* 341(22):1633, 1999
32. Sargent SJ: The "other" sexually transmitted diseases: chlamydial, herpes simplex virus, and human papillomavirus infections, *Postgrad Med* 9:359, 1992.
33. Schachter J, Barnes R: Infections caused by *Chlamydia trachomatis.* In Morse SA, Moreland AA, Holmes KK, editors: *Atlas of sexually transmitted diseases and AIDS,* ed 2, London, 1996, Mosby-Wolfe.
34. Peterson IM, Rao R: Genital warts: newly discovered consequences of an ancient disease, *Postgrad Med* 86:197, 1989.
35. Hepatitis C: What clinicians and other health professionals need to know, 2000. Available at www.cdc.gov/ncidod/diseases/hepatitis/c/edu/default_r.htm.
36. Chambers HF: Infectious diseases: bacterial and chlamydial. In McTierney LM, McPhee SJ, Papadakis MA, editors: *Current medical diagnosis and treatment,* ed 35, Norwalk, Conn, 1996, Appleton & Lange.
37. Perine PI, Osoba AO: Lymphogranuloma venereum. In Holmes KK et al, editors: *Sexually transmitted diseases,* ed 2, New York, 1990, McGraw-Hill.
38. Mertz GJ et al: Risk factors for the sexual transmission of genital herpes, *Ann Intern Med* 116(3):197, 1992.
39. Camisa C: Condyloma acuminatum and other human papillomavirus-induced diseases. In Spagna VA, Prior RB, editors: *Sexually transmitted disease: a clinical syndrome approach,* New York, 1985, Marcel Dekker.
40. Stagno S, Whitley RJ: Herpesvirus infection in the neonate and children. In Holmes KK et al, editors: *Sexually transmitted diseases,* ed 2, New York, 1990, McGraw-Hill.
41. Rose FB, Camp CJ: Genital herpes: how to relieve patients' physical and psychological symptoms, *Postgrad Med* 84:81, 1988.
42. Cothran MM, White JE: Update on human papillomavirus, *J Am Acad Nurse Practitioners* 7(12):583, 1995.
43. Derksen DJ: Children with condylomata acuminata, *J Fam Pract* 34: 419, 1992.
44. Alary M et al: Strategy for screening pregnant women for chlamydial infection in a low-prevalence area, *Obstet Gynecol* 82(3):399, 1993.
45. Shah KV: Biology of genital tract human papillomaviruses, *Urol Clin North Am* 19:63, 1992.
46. McAninch JW: Disorders of the penis and male urethra. In Tanagho EA, McAninch JW, editors: *Smith's general urology,* Norwalk, Conn, 1995, Appleton & Lange.
47. Berger TG: Skin diseases of the external genitalia. In Tanagho EA, McAninch JW, editors: *Smith's general urology,* Norwalk, Conn, 1995, Appleton & Lange.
48. Lambert DR, Yoder FW: Ectoparasites and molluscum contagiosum. In Spagna VA, Prior RB, editors: *Sexually transmitted diseases: a clinical syndrome approach,* New York, 1985, Marcel Dekker.
49. Rein MR, Holmes KK: Nonspecific vaginitis, vulvovaginal candidiasis, and trichomoniasis: clinical features, diagnosis, and management. In Remington J, Schwartz MN, editors: *Current clinical topics in infectious diseases,* New York, 1983, McGraw-Hill.
50. Bartlett JG: *Pocket book of infectious disease therapy,* Baltimore, 1995, Williams & Wilkins.
51. Orkin M, Maibach HI: Scabies. In Holmes KK et al, editors: *Sexually transmitted diseases,* ed 2, New York, 1990, McGraw-Hill.
52. Hammerschlag MR, Laraque D. Inappropriate use of nonculture tests for the detection of chlamydia trachomatis in suspected victims of child sexual abuse: a continuing problem. *Pediatrics* 104(5): 1137, 1999.
53. Caldwell JH: The "gay bowel" syndrome. In Spagna VA, Prior RB, editors: *Sexually transmitted disease: a clinical syndrome approach,* New York, 1985, Marcel Dekker.
54. Quinn TC, Stamm WE: Proctocolitis, enteritis, and esophagitis in homosexual men. In Holmes KK et al, editors: *Sexually transmitted diseases,* ed 2, New York, 1990, McGraw-Hill.
55. Lemon SM, Newbold JE: Viral hepatitis. In Holmes KK et al, editors: *Sexually transmitted diseases,* ed 2, New York, 1990, McGraw-Hill.
56. Klein MB: Hepatitis B virus: perinatal management, *J Perinat Neonat Nurs* 1(4):12, 1988.
57. Naher H et al: Subclinical Epstein-Barr virus infection of both the male and female genital tract: indication for sexual transmission, *J Invest Dermatol* 98:791, 1992.
58. Baker ER, Shephard B: Neonatal resuscitation and care of the newborn at risk. In DeCherney AH, Pernoll ML, editors: *Current obstetric and gynecologic diagnosis and treatment,* ed 8, Norwalk, Conn, 1994, Appleton & Lange.
59. Wilson CB: The cellular immune system and its role in host defense. In Mandell G, Douglas RG, Bennett JE, editors: *Principles and practice of infectious diseases,* ed 3, New York, 1990, Churchill Livingstone.

CHAPTER 24

Structure and Function of the Hematologic System

KATHRYN L. McCANCE

CHAPTER OUTLINE

Blood cells travel long distances and thus must be flexible or blood would hardly flow at all. Blood cells act as vehicles—cells and chemicals—that travel along the tens of thousands of miles of blood vessels packed into the human body. Most cells are red blood cells that, like tanker trucks, function as carriers; yet red blood cells maneuver more like sports cars, flexing and deforming to squeeze through capillaries smaller than their own diameters. White blood cells are larger than red blood cells and less flexible. Spherical and stiffer, white cells create more resistance and are much more likely to create "traffic jams." White blood cells travel the main highways, avoiding the small capillaries that red blood cells so expertly squeeze through, but disease can make the white cells "sticky," create traffic jams, and cause the red cells to lose their cargo. These alterations can lead to difficulties in oxygenation, acid-base balance, and immune function and, like a major thoroughfare at rush hour, may alter streamline flow.

COMPONENTS OF THE HEMATOLOGIC SYSTEM

Composition of the Blood

Blood consists of a variety of formed elements (cells and proteins) that circulate in the cardiovascular system suspended in plasma, which is approximately 90% water and 10% dissolved substances (solutes). All of these elements constitute blood volume, which in adults amounts to about 6 quarts (5.5 L). Approximately 45% to 50% of blood volume consists of formed elements, and the remainder is plasma. The continuous movement of blood keeps the formed elements dispersed throughout the plasma, where they are available to carry out their chief functions: (1) delivery of substances needed for cellular metabolism in the tissues, (2) defense against invading microorganisms and injury, and (3) acid-base balance.

Plasma and Plasma Proteins

In adults, plasma accounts for 55% to 60% of blood volume. **Plasma** is a complex aqueous liquid containing a number of organic and inorganic elements (Table 24-1). The concentration of these elements varies depending on diet, metabolic demand, hormones, and vitamins. Plasma differs from serum in that **serum** is plasma that has been altered in the laboratory to remove fibrinogen (a clotting factor) or some other element that is unwanted or unneeded in the sample.

In circulating plasma the dominant elements by weight are the **plasma proteins**, which constitute about 7% of the total plasma weight. The plasma proteins vary in structure and function but can be classified into three major groups:

the **albumins,** globulins, and **clotting factors**. The albumins are the most numerous, followed by the various globulins (immune globulins or γ-globulins) and the clotting factors, chiefly fibrinogen. The plasma proteins are synthesized in the liver, with the exception of the immune globulins, which are synthesized by lymphocytes in the lymph nodes and other lymphoid tissues (see Chapter 6 and p. 817).

Albumin is present at a concentration of about 4 g/dl and is essential for regulating the passage of water and solutes through the capillaries. Because albumin molecules are large and do not diffuse freely through the vascular endothelium, they provide the critical colloid osmotic or oncotic pressure that regulates the passage of water and solutes through the microcirculation (arterioles, capillaries, and venules) (see Chapters 1 and 3). Water and solute particles diffuse out of the arterial portions of the capillaries because blood pressure is greater in arterial than in venous blood vessels (see Chapter 31). Water and solutes move from tissue cells into the venous portions of the capillaries, where the pressures are reversed, with oncotic pressure being greater than intravascular pressure. Albumin also serves as a carrier molecule for both normal components of blood and exogenous agents, such as drugs.

The immune globulins, or antibodies, are synthesized by mature lymphocytes called *plasma cells* in the lymphoid organs, chiefly lymph nodes. The immune globulins include IgA, IgG, IgM, IgD, and IgE. Most of them are critical for defense against infectious microorganisms. (Lymphocyte and antibody function is described in Chapter 6.)

The third important class of plasma proteins is the clotting factors, which promote coagulation and stop bleeding from damaged blood vessels. Fibrinogen is the most plenti-

Table 24-1 Organic and Inorganic Components of Arterial Plasma

Constituent	Amount/Concentration	Major Functions
Water	93% of plasma weight	Medium for carrying all other constituents
Electrolytes	Total < 1% of plasma weight	Maintain H_2O in extracellular compartment; act as buffers; function in membrane excitability
Na^+	142 mEq/L (142 mM)	
K^+	4 mEq/L (4 mM)	
Ca^{++}	5 mEq/L (2.5 mM)	
Mg^{++}	3 mEq/L (1.5 mM)	
Cl^-	103 mEq/L (103 mM)	
HCO_3^-	27 mEq/L (27 mM)	
Phosphate (mostly HPO_4^{--})	2 mEq/L (1 mM)	
$SO4_4^{--}$	1 mEq/L (0.5 mM)	
Proteins	7.3 g/dl (2.5 mM)	Provide colloid osmotic pressure of plasma; act as buffers; bind other plasma constituents (lipids, hormones, vitamins, minerals, etc.); clotting factors; enzymes; enzyme precursors; antibodies (immune globulins); hormones; transporters
Albumins	4.5 g/dl	
Globulins	2.5 g/dl	
Fibrinogen	0.3 g/dl	
Transferrin	250 mg/dl	
Ferritin	15-300 μg/L	
Gases		
CO_2 content	22-20 mmol/L plasma	By-product of oxygenation, most CO_2 content is from HCO_3 and acts as a buffer
O_2	Pao_2 80 torr or greater (arterial); Pvo_2 30-40 torr (venous)	Oxygenation
N_2	0.9 ml/dl	By-product of protein catabolism
Nutrients		Provide nutrition and substances for tissue repair
Glucose and other carbohydrates	100 mg/dl (5.6 mM)	
Total amino acids	40 mg/dl (2 mM)	
Total lipids	500 mg/dl (7.5 mM)	
Cholesterol	150-250 mg/dl (4-7 mM)	
Individual vitamins	0.0001-2.5 mg/dl	
Individual trace elements	0.001-0.3 mg/dl	
Iron	50-150 μg/dl	
Waste products		
Urea (blood urea nitrogen [BUN])	7-18 mg/dl (5.7 mM)	End product of protein catabolism
Creatinine (from creatine)	1 mg/dl (0.09 mM)	End product from energy metabolism
Uric acid (from nucleic acids)	5 mg/dl (0.3 mM)	End product from protein metabolism
Bilirubin (from heme)	0.2-1.2 mg/dl (0.003-0.018 mM)	End product of red blood cell destruction
Individual hormones	0.000001-0.05 mg/dl	Functions specific to target tissue

Data from Vander AJ, Sherman JH, Luchiano DS: *Human physiology: the mechanisms of body function,* ed 2, New York, 1994, McGraw-Hill.

ful of the clotting factors and is the precursor of the fibrin clot (see p. 830). Other plasma proteins include complement proteins, a group of proteins involved in the immune response, a variety of enzymes and their inhibitors, and specific carriers of such elements as iron and copper. The plasma lipids, triglycerides, phospholipids, cholesterol, and fatty acids are carried through the blood as complexes with plasma proteins; they are known as **lipoproteins** (see Chapters 1 and 29).

The electrolytes (electrically charged solutes) of the plasma maintain the osmolarity and pH of blood within a physiologic range (see Table 24-1). (Electrolytes are described in Chapters 1 and 3.)

Cellular Components of the Blood

The cellular elements of the blood are broadly classified as **erythrocytes (red blood cells [RBCs]), leukocytes (white blood cells),** and **platelets (thrombocytes).** The components of the blood are listed in Table 24-2.

Erythrocytes

In 1628 Robert Burton described blood as a "hot, temperate red humor whose office is to nourish the whole body, to give it strength and color being dispersed by the veins through every part of it."[1] A few years later, with the invention of the microscope, researchers learned that erythrocytes give blood its red color.

Erythrocytes are the most abundant cells of the blood, occupying approximately 48% of the blood volume in men and about 42% in women. Erythrocytes are responsible primarily for tissue oxygenation. Their shape, size, and structure reflect their unique function as deliverers of gases throughout the body. The erythrocyte's cytoplasm consists of a solution containing protein (mostly **hemoglobin [Hb],** which carries the gases) and electrolytes, which regulate diffusion through the cell's plasma membrane. The mature erythrocyte lacks the cytoplasmic organelles—a nucleus, mitochondria, and ribosomes—that would enable it to divide or carry out metabolic functions. Therefore it cannot synthesize protein or carry out oxidative reactions. Because it cannot undergo mitotic division, it lives out its life span (approximately 120 days) in the circulation, dies, and is replaced by a new erythrocyte.

The erythrocyte's size and shape are ideally suited to its function as a gas carrier. It is a small disk with two unique properties: (1) **biconcavity** and (2) **reversible deformability** (Fig. 24-1). The flattened, biconcave shape provides a surface area–to–volume ratio that is optimal for gas diffusion into and out of the cell. Reversible deformity enables the erythrocyte to alter its shape to squeeze through the microcirculation and then return to normal. During its 120-day life span, where most of its time is spent within the capillary channels, the erythrocyte, which is 8 μm in diameter, must

Table 24-2 Cellular Components of the Blood

Cell	Structural Characteristics	Normal Amounts of Circulating Blood	Function	Life Span
Erythrocyte (red blood cell) 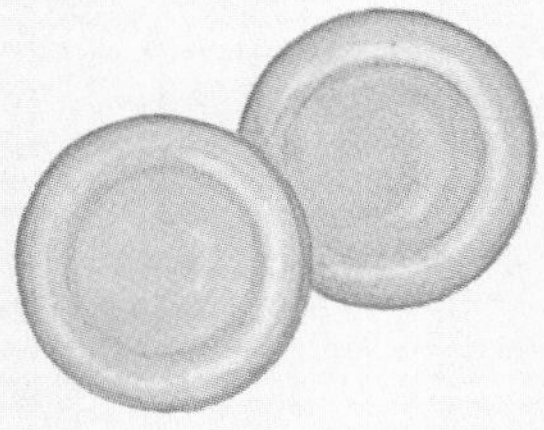	Nonnucleated cytoplasmic disk containing hemoglobin	4.2-6.2 million/mm^3	Gas transport to and from tissue cells and lungs	80-120 days
Leukocyte (white blood cell) 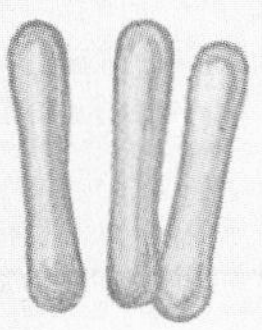	Nucleated cell	5000-10,000/mm^3	Body defense mechanisms	See below
Lymphocyte 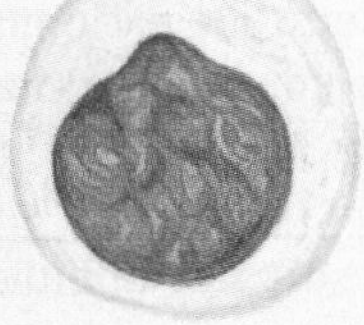	Mononuclear immunocyte	25%-33% of leukocyte count (leukocyte differential)	Humoral and cell-mediated immunity (see Chapter 6)	Days or years depending on type

Continued

Table 24-2 Cellular Components of the Blood—cont'd

Cell	Structural Characteristics	Normal Amounts of Circulating Blood	Function	Life Span
Monocyte and macrophage 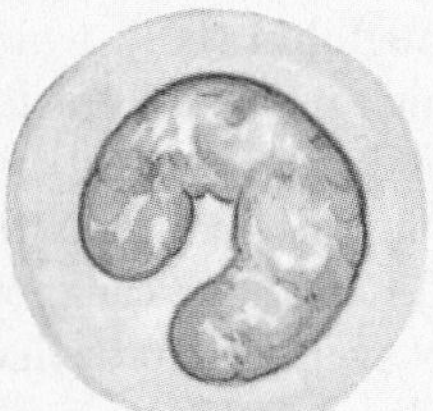	Large mononuclear phagocyte	3%-7% of leukocyte differential	Phagocytosis; mononuclear phagocyte system	Months or years
Eosinophil 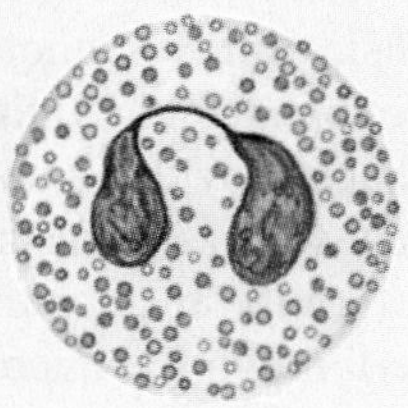	Segmented polymorphonuclear granulocyte	1%-4% of leukocyte differential	Phagocytosis, antibody-mediated defense against parasites, allergic reactions, associated with Hodgkin disease, recovery phase of infection	Unknown
Neutrophil 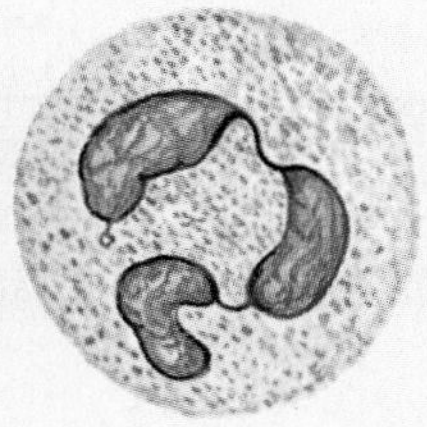	Segmented polymorphonuclear granulocyte	57%-67% of leukocyte differential	Phagocytosis, particularly during early phase of inflammation	4 days
Basophil 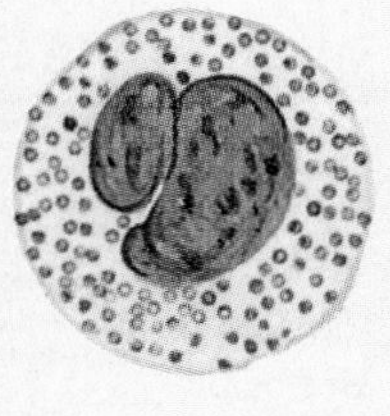	Segmented polymorphonuclear granulocyte	0%-0.75% of leukocyte differential	Secrete chemicals chemotactic for neutrophils*, but associated with allergic reactions and mechanical irritation	Unknown
Platelet 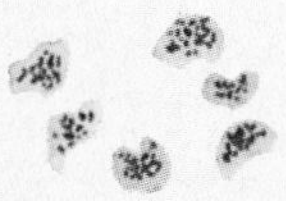	Irregularly shaped cytoplasmic fragment (not a cell)	140,000-340,000/mm^3	Hemostasis following vascular injury; normal coagulation and clot formation/retraction	8-11 days

*Recent data.

repeatedly circulate through splenic sinusoids and capillaries that are only 2 μm in diameter. To do this, the erythrocyte assumes a torpedo-like conformation. The physical arrangement of membrane proteins is responsible for the biconcave shape of the resting cell.

Leukocytes

Leukocytes are white blood cells that defend the body against organisms that cause infection and remove debris, including dead or injured host cells of all kinds (Fig. 24-2). The leukocytes act primarily in the tissues but are transported in the circulation. They are fewer in number than erythrocytes; the average adult has approximately 5000 to 10,000 leukocytes per mm^3 of blood.

Leukocytes are classified according to structure as either granulocytes or agranulocytes and according to function as either **phagocytes** or **immunocytes**. The granulocytes, which

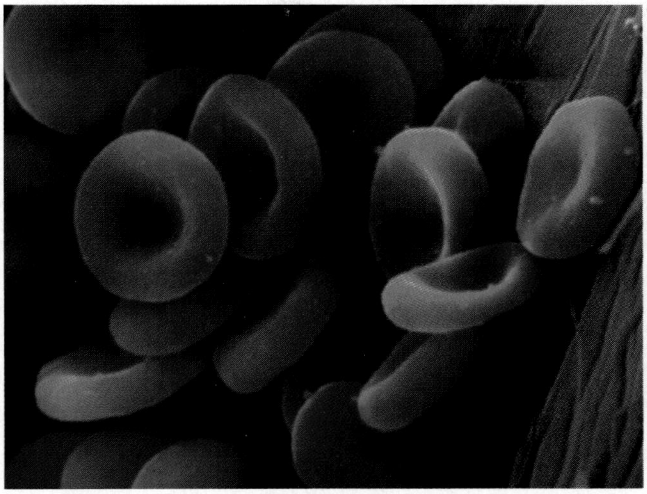

FIG. 24-1 Mature erythrocytes. Scanning electron micrograph of mature erythrocytes on cell wall. (Copyright © Dennis Kunkel Microscopy, Inc.)

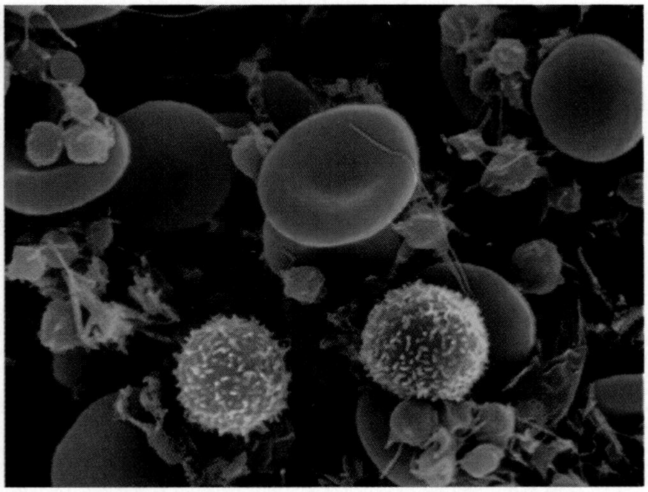

FIG. 24-2 Blood cells. Leukocytes are spherical and have irregular surfaces with numerous extending pili (appears as yellow). Erythrocytes are flattened spheres with a depressed center. Activated platelets are green. (Copyright © Dennis Kunkel Microscopy, Inc.)

include neutrophils, basophils, and eosinophils, are all phagocytes. Of the agranulocytes, the monocytes and macrophages are phagocytes, whereas the lymphocytes are immunocytes (cells that create immunity; see Chapter 6).

Granulocytes. The **granulocytes** are so called because of the many membrane-bound granules in their cytoplasm. The granules contain enzymes capable of killing microorganisms and catabolizing debris ingested by the process of phagocytosis. The granules also contain powerful biochemical mediators with a variety of inflammatory and immune functions. These mediators, along with the digestive enzymes, are released from some granulocytes in response to specific stimuli and from all granulocytes as they reach the end of their natural life span and die. The biochemical mediators have various vascular and intercellular effects, and the enzymes participate in the breakdown of free-floating debris from sites of infection or injury.

Granulocytes are capable of ameboid movement, by which they migrate through vessel walls and then to sites where their action is needed. Migration through vessel walls, called diapedesis, and movement through the tissues, which occurs in response to chemotactic factors, are described and illustrated in Chapter 7.

The **neutrophil (polymorphonuclear neutrophil,** or **PMN**) is the most numerous and best understood of the granulocytes (Fig. 24-3, *A*). Neutrophils constitute about 55% of the total leukocyte count in adults. The cytoplasm of neutrophils contains small lysosomal granules and a central nucleus with two to five distinct lobes. Immature neutrophils are called bands or stabs. Mature neutrophils are called *segmented neutrophils* because of the characteristic appearance of their nucleus.

Neutrophils are the chief phagocytes of early inflammation. Soon after bacterial invasion or tissue injury, neutrophils migrate out of the capillaries and into the inflamed site, where they ingest and destroy microorganisms and debris and then die in 1 or 2 days. The dissolution of dead neutrophils releases digestive enzymes from their cytoplasmic granules. These enzymes dissolve cellular debris and prepare the site for healing. (This final function, called *débridement*, is described in Chapter 7.)

Eosinophils, which have large, coarse granules, constitute only 1% to 4% of the normal leukocyte count in adults (see Fig. 24-3, *B*). Like neutrophils, eosinophils are capable of ameboid movement and phagocytosis. Unlike neutrophils, which ingest cellular debris, eosinophils ingest antigen-antibody complexes and are induced by IgE-mediated hypersensitivity reactions to attack parasites. Eosinophils also help to control inflammatory processes. (Their function in inflammation and defense against parasites is described in Chapter 7.) High eosinophil counts in atopic (allergy-prone) individuals experiencing type I allergic reactions, such as asthma or allergic rhinitis, have led researchers to think that eosinophils participate in hypersensitivity reactions to allergens besides parasites (see Chapter 8).

A complete discussion of **mast cells** is contained in Chapter 7 (see also What's New? box on p. 816).

Basophils, which make up less than 1% of the leukocytes, are structurally similar to the mast cells found throughout extravascular tissue (see Fig. 24-3, *C*). Like the mast cells, whose role in stimulating the inflammatory response is described in Chapter 7, the basophils have cytoplasmic granules that contain vasoactive amines (histamine, bradykinin, serotonin) and an anticoagulant (heparin). The precise function of basophils is poorly understood.

Agranulocytes. The **agranulocytes**—monocytes, macrophages, and lymphocytes—differ from the granulocytes in that they do not contain lysosomal granules in their cytoplasm. The lymphocytes do not contain *any* enzyme-filled digestive vacuoles, and the digestive vacuoles of the monocytes and macrophages are larger and fewer than those of the granulocytes.

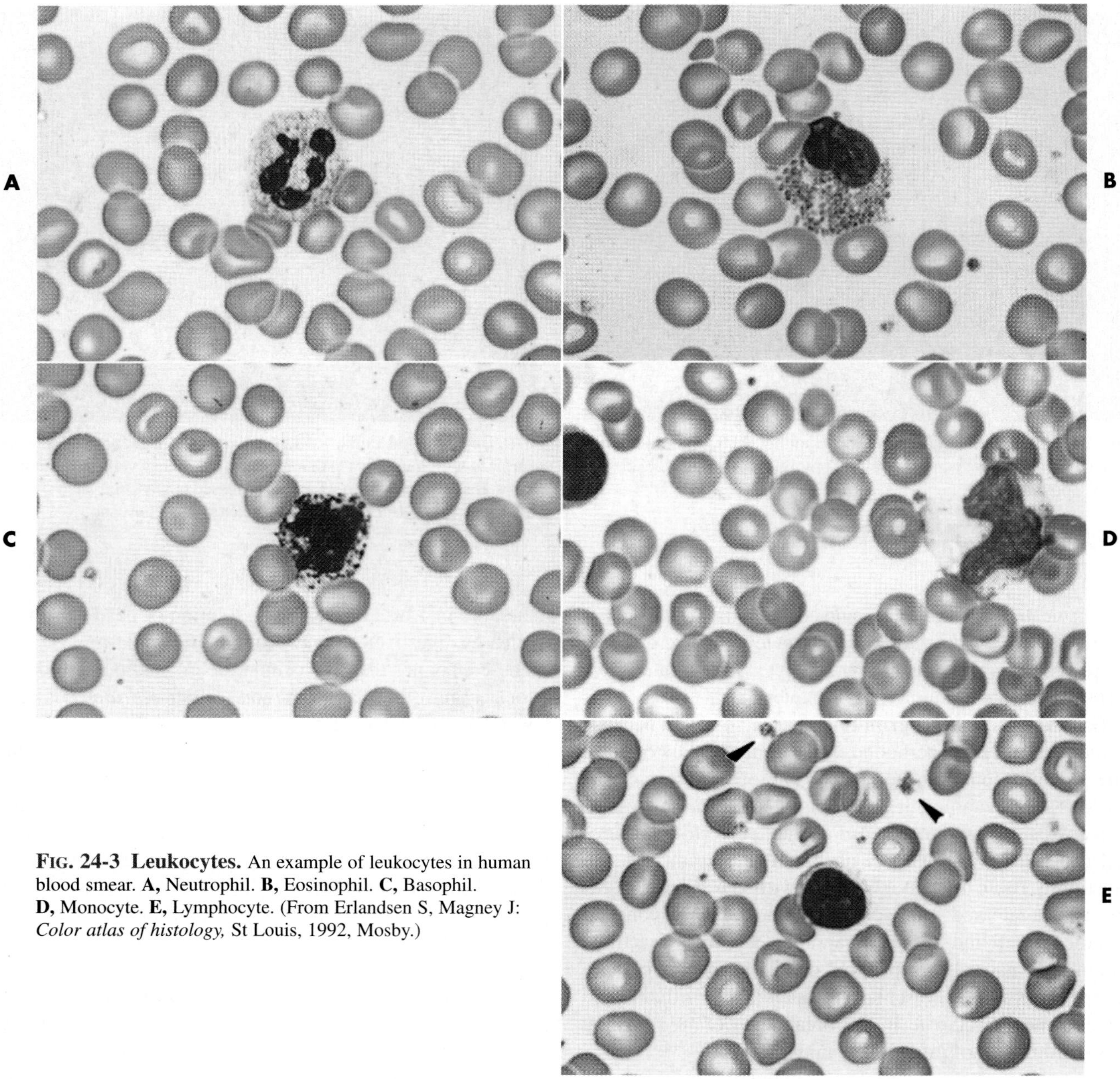

FIG. 24-3 Leukocytes. An example of leukocytes in human blood smear. **A,** Neutrophil. **B,** Eosinophil. **C,** Basophil. **D,** Monocyte. **E,** Lymphocyte. (From Erlandsen S, Magney J: *Color atlas of histology,* St Louis, 1992, Mosby.)

WHAT'S NEW? Mast Cells and Bacteria

Mast cells have had a bad reputation. Through the release of such chemicals as histamine, mast cells can trigger the miseries of allergies. Yet investigators are beginning to report that their role in allergies is an accident. In their recent work, Abraham and colleagues found that mast cells have a surface protein (CD48) that recognizes disease-causing bacteria. Mast cells directly bind to FimH, a protein on a hairlike extension that covers some dangerous bacteria. Thus, mast cells can directly recognize bacteria—but it is unproven whether this function is critical to fighting infection. If it is, it may be possible to activate mast cells at times of infection.

Data from Abraham SN, Malaviga R: Mast cell modulation of the innate immune response to enterobacterial infection, *Adv Exp Med Biol* 279:91, 2000; Travis J: Giving mast cells their proper respect, *Sci News* 165:39, 2000.

The **monocytes** and **macrophages** make up the **mononuclear phagocyte system (MPS),** formerly called the *reticuloendothelial system (RES).* (The MPS is described on p. 818.) Both monocytes and macrophages participate in the immune and inflammatory response because they are powerful phagocytes. They also ingest dead or defective host cells, particularly blood cells.

Monocytes are immature macrophages (see Fig. 24-3, *D*). After monocytes are formed and released by the bone marrow, they enter the bloodstream and circulate for about 36 hours while maturing into macrophages. Some of the circulating macrophages migrate out of the vessels in response to infection or inflammation anywhere in the body. Other macrophages migrate to fixed sites in lymphoid tissues of the liver, spleen, lymph nodes, peritoneum, or gastrointestinal tract, where they are active for months or years. Monocytes participate in immune responses. They ingest and "process" antigens so that the antigens are recognized by T and B lymphocytes (described in Chapter 6). Monocytes have many other biologic properties, including the release of tissue thromboplastin, activators of plasminogen, proteolytic enzymes, and other active agents.

Lymphocytes, which constitute approximately 36% of the total leukocyte count, are the primary cells of the immune response (see Fig. 24-3, *E*). Most lymphocytes are located in lymphoid tissues; only a small percentage circulate in the blood. There are many types of lymphocytes, the most important of which are T cells, B cells, and mature B cells (plasma cells). The life span of the lymphocyte can be days, months, or years, depending on its type and subtype. (Lymphocyte function and dysfunction are described in detail in Unit III.)

Natural killer (NK) cells, which resemble lymphocytes, kill some types of tumor cells and some virus-infected cells without prior exposure. Hence they are named natural killer cells. These large granular lymphocytes account for 5% to 10% of the circulating lymphoid pool and are found mainly in the peripheral blood and spleen. Recent evidence, however, has shown that in the absence of a thymus, fetal thymocytes develop into NK cells instead of T-helper or T-suppressor cells. The same cells maintained in the thymus develop into mature T cells, also called *NKT cells*. Therefore, it is believed that immature thymocytes give rise to T cells or NK cells, depending on the microenvironment. Recently identified and cloned are three distinct NK-specific molecules termed *natural cytotoxicity receptors (NCR)*. They mediate NK cell activation in the interaction and lysis of most tumor cells.[2] These cells are discussed in Chapters 6, 10, and 11.

Platelets

Platelets are not cells, but disk-shaped cytoplasmic fragments. They are formed by fragmentation of very large (40 to 100 μm) cells known as **megakaryocytes** (Fig. 24-4). Platelets are essential for blood coagulation and control of bleeding. **Thrombopoietin (TPO)**, a hormone growth factor, is the main regulator of the circulating platelet mass.[3,4] Presumably, thrombopoietin is activated when the platelet mass is low, causing an increase in serum TPO.[3] They lack a nucleus; therefore they have no deoxyribonucleic acid (DNA) and are incapable of mitotic division. They do, however, contain cytoplasmic granules capable of releasing biochemical mediators when stimulated to do so by injury to a blood vessel.

There are approximately 140,000 to 340,000 platelets per mm^3 of circulating blood. An additional one third of the body's available platelets are in a reserve pool in the spleen. A platelet lives approximately 10 days, after which it dies and is removed by macrophages of the MPS, mostly in the spleen.

Lymphoid Organs

The lymphoid organs, some of which are merely aggregations of lymphoid tissue, are classified as primary or secondary. The **primary lymphoid organs** are the thymus and the bone marrow. The **secondary lymphoid organs** consist of the spleen, lymph nodes, tonsils, and Peyer patches of the small intestine (see Fig. 6-3). All of the lymphoid organs link the hematologic and immune systems in that they are sites of residence, proliferation, differentiation, or function of lymphocytes and mononuclear phagocytes (monocytes and macrophages). (The liver, which also has hematologic functions, is primarily a digestive organ and is described in Chapter 37.)

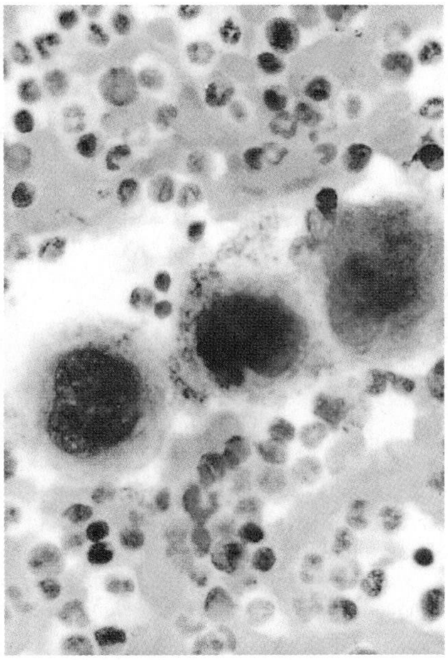

FIG. 24-4 Megakaryocyte and platelets. Note the large number of platelets (purple) surrounding the large megakaryocytes in the center. (Courtesy Miale JB, from *Laboratory medicine: hematology*, ed 6, St Louis, 1982, Mosby.)

Spleen

The **spleen** is the largest of the secondary lymphoid organs. It is a site of fetal hematopoiesis; its mononuclear phagocytes filter and cleanse the blood; its lymphocytes mount an immune response to blood-borne microorganisms; and it serves as a blood reservoir (see Chapter 26).

The spleen is a concave, encapsulated organ that weighs about 150 g and is about the size of a fist (see Fig. 6-3). It is located in the left upper abdominal cavity, curved around a portion of the stomach. Strands of connective tissue (trabeculae) extend throughout the spleen from the splenic capsule, dividing the spleen into compartments. The compartments contain masses of lymphoid tissue called *splenic pulp*. The spleen is interlaced with many blood vessels, some of which are capable of distending to store blood.

Blood that circulates through the spleen comes from the splenic artery, which branches from the descending aorta and reenters the circulatory system through the splenic vein, which feeds into the portal vein. The portion of arterial blood that enters the spleen first encounters the white splenic pulp, which consists of masses of lymphoid tissue containing lymphocytes and macrophages. The white pulp forms clumps around the splenic arterioles and is the chief site of immune

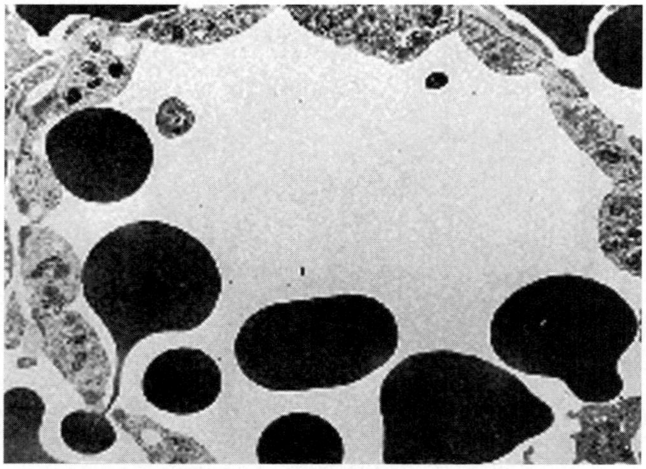

FIG. 24-5 Red cells in the spleen. Transmission electron micrograph of a normal red blood cell traversing the sinus wall in a human spleen. Note how it must deform to reenter the sinus. (From Damjanov I, Linder J, editors: *Anderson's pathology*, ed 10, St Louis, 1996, Mosby.)

and phagocytic function within the spleen. Here blood-borne antigens encounter lymphocytes, initiating the immune response (see Chapter 6).

Some of the blood that enters the terminal capillaries of the spleen continues through the microcirculation and enters highly distensible storage areas called *venous sinuses*. Most of the blood, however, oozes through the extremely permeable capillary walls into the principal site of splenic filtration, the red pulp (Fig. 24-5). Here the resident macrophages of the MPS phagocytose old, damaged, or dead blood cells of all kinds (but chiefly erythrocytes); microorganisms; and particles of debris. Hemoglobin from phagocytosed erythrocytes is catabolized, and heme (iron) is stored in the cytoplasm of the macrophages or released back into the blood plasma (see p. 816 and Fig. 24-13). The macrophages also can remove certain particulate inclusions from erythrocytes without harming the cells themselves. Blood that filters through the red pulp also finds its way into the venous sinuses and hence into the portal circulation.

The venous sinuses (and the red pulp) are capable of storing more than 300 ml of blood. Passive dilation of the venous sinuses enables the spleen to increase its storage capacity as needed by the body. Sudden reductions in blood pressure cause the sympathetic nervous system to stimulate constriction of the sinuses. Constriction, which can expel as much as 200 ml of blood into the venous circulation, helps restore blood volume and increases the hematocrit.

The spleen is not necessary for life or for adequate hematologic function. However, splenic absence from any cause (atrophy, traumatic injury, or removal because of disease) has several effects that indicate its function. For example, leukocytosis (high levels of circulating leukocytes) often occurs after splenectomy. This suggests that the spleen exerts some control over the rate of proliferation of leukocyte stem cells in the bone marrow or their release into the bloodstream. Splenic absence is associated also with decreased levels of iron in the circulation, reflecting the spleen's role in the iron cycle (see p. 827). Immune function decreases in the absence of the spleen. Antibody production in response to small doses of soluble (i.e., blood-borne) antigen diminishes. Finally, the splenic function of removing old and defective blood cells seems to be confirmed by the fact that the blood of individuals lacking spleens contains more morphologically defective blood cells than normal.

Lymph Nodes

Structurally, **lymph nodes** are part of the lymphatic system. Thousands of them are clustered around the lymphatic veins, the vessels that collect interstitial fluid from the tissues and transport it, as lymph, back into the circulatory system near the heart. Functionally, however, lymph nodes are part of the hematologic and immune systems because they are the site of development or activity of large numbers of lymphocytes, monocytes, and macrophages. As the lymph filters through the bean-shaped lymph nodes clustered in the inguinal, axillary, and cervical regions of the body, it is cleansed of foreign particles and microorganisms by the monocytes and macrophages. The microorganisms in lymph stimulate the resident lymphocytes to develop into antibody-producing plasma cells (see Chapter 6). Lymphocytes, monocytes, and macrophages proliferate in the lymph nodes and are released into the lymphatic stream. During an infection the rate of proliferation of macrophages within the nodes is so great that the nodes enlarge and become tender.

Each lymph node is enclosed in a fibrous capsule (Fig. 24-6). Strands of connective tissue (trabeculae) extend inward from the capsule, dividing the node into several compartments. Reticular fibers that extend between the trabeculae divide the compartments into smaller sections. The reticular fibers trap and store large numbers of lymphocytes, monocytes, and macrophages. The node is composed of an outer cortex area and an inner medullary area. Within the cortex of each node are germinal centers, or separate masses of lymphoid tissue. Lymph enters the node through several afferent lymphatic vessels, filters through the sinuses in the node, and leaves by way of efferent lymphatic vessels. Lymph flows slowly through the nodes, which facilitates the phagocytosis of foreign substances within the node and prevents them from reentering the bloodstream.

The Mononuclear Phagocyte System (MPS)

The MPS consists of a line of cells that originate in the bone marrow; are transported by the bloodstream; and, after differentiation to blood monocytes, finally settle in the tissues as mature macrophages. It is composed of monoblasts, promonocytes, and monocytes in bone marrow, monocytes in peripheral blood, and macrophages in tissue. Table 24-3 lists the various names given to macrophages localized in specific tissues.

The cells of the MPS ingest and destroy (by phagocytosis) unwanted materials in the blood and in organs. During

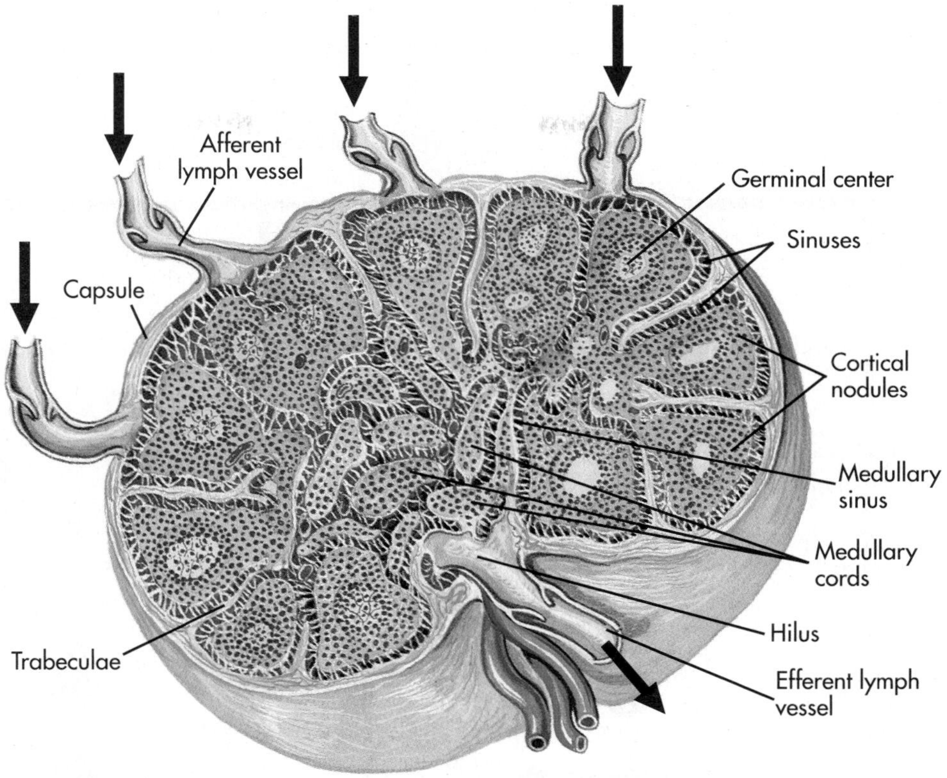

FIG. 24-6 Structure of a lymph node. Several afferent valved lymphatics bring lymph to the node. A single efferent lymphatic leaves the node at the hilus. Note that the artery and vein also enter and leave at the hilus. Arrows show direction of lymph. (From Thibodeau GA, Patton K: *Anatomy & physiology*, ed 4, St Louis, 1999, Mosby.)

inflammation they engulf and digest foreign protein particles, microorganisms, debris from dead or injured cells, defective or injured erythrocytes, and dead neutrophils (see Fig. 7-15). The MPS (mostly in the liver and spleen) also is the main line of defense against bacteria in the bloodstream. In addition, the MPS cleanses the blood by removing old, injured, or dead erythrocytes, leukocytes, platelets, coagulation products, antigen-antibody complexes, and macromolecules (such as lipids and carbohydrates synthesized by the body as the result of faulty metabolism, as in storage diseases). Macrophages also play a role in blood coagulation, wound healing, tissue remodeling, and the control of blood production.

Multiple cell types, including endothelial cells, fibroblasts, and lymphocytes, produce substances called **colony-stimulating factors (CSFs)** which are soluble mediators secreted by cells for the purpose of cell-to-cell communication. CSFs control the production, maturation, and function of granulocytes and monocyte-macrophages (Fig. 24-7, *B*) and the development of blood cells.

The origin and turnover of all the tissue macrophages named in Table 24-3 are not precisely known. It seems clear that once monocytes leave the circulation, they do not return. In the tissues, monocytes differentiate into macrophages without dividing. They can survive many months or even years. Monocytes migrating into inflamed tissues give rise to most of the *reactive* macrophage population. Under

Table 24-3 Mononuclear Phagocyte System*

Name of Cell	Location
COMMITTED STEM CELLS†	Bone marrow
Monoblasts	Bone marrow
Promonoblasts	Bone marrow
Monocytes	Bone marrow and peripheral blood
MACROPHAGES	Tissue
Kupffer cells (inflammatory macrophages)	Liver
Alveolar macrophages	Lung
Histiocytes	Connective tissue
Macrophages	Bone marrow
Fixed and free macrophages	Spleen and lymph nodes
Pleural and peritoneal macrophages	Serous cavities
Microglial cells	Nervous system
Mesangial cells	Kidney
Osteoclasts	Bone
Langerhan cells	Skin
Dendritic cells	Lymphoid tissue

Data from Cotran RS, Kumar V, Collins T: *Robbins pathologic basis of disease,* ed 6, Philadelphia, 1999, W.B. Saunders; Halma C, Daha MR, van-Es-La: *Clin Exp Immunol* 89(10):1, 1992.
*Formerly called the reticuloendothelial system.
†Development of blood cells from stem cells in the marrow is described on this page and illustrated in Fig. 24-7, *A*.

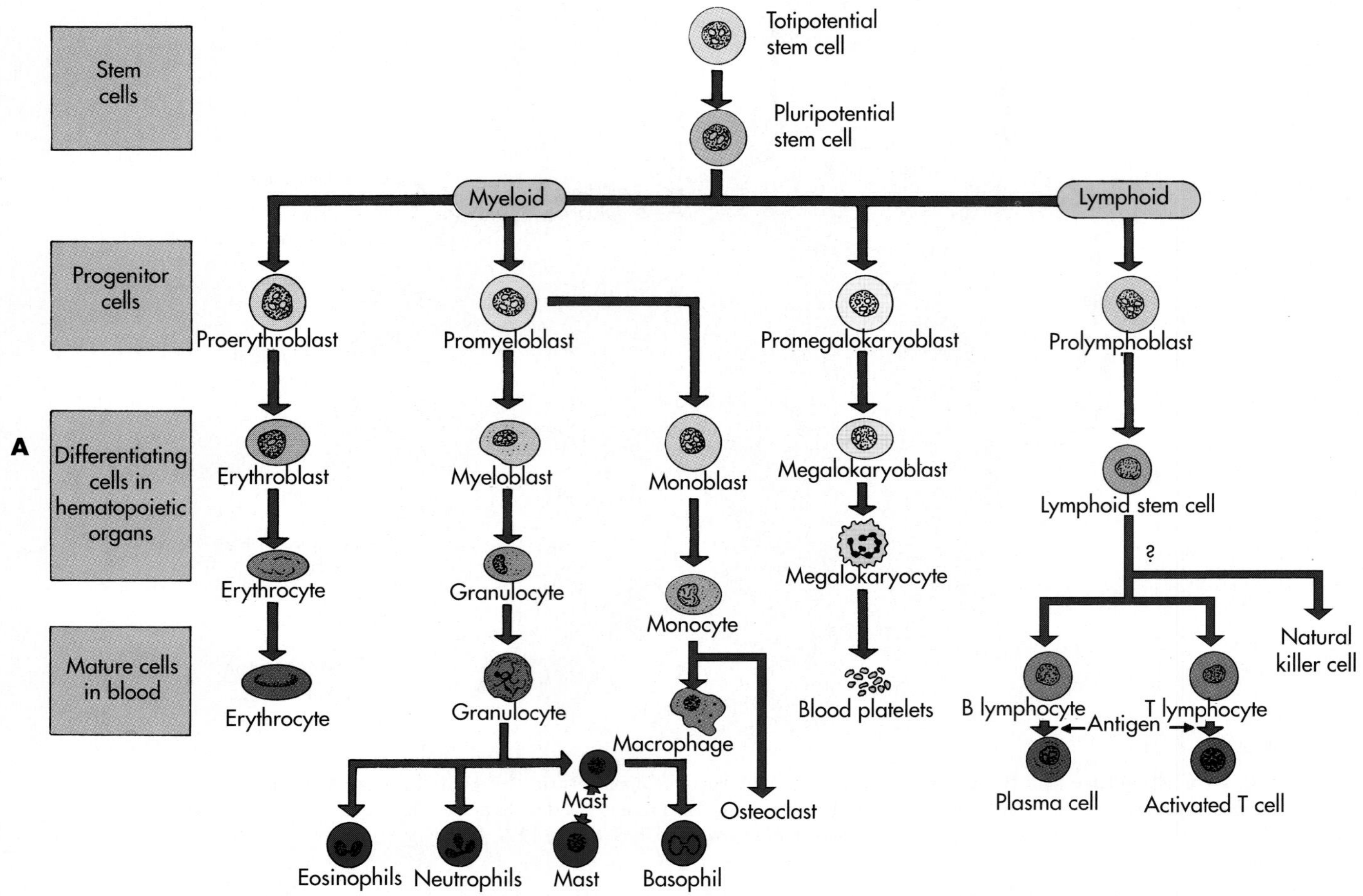

FIG. 24-7 Production, maturation, and function of granulocytes and monocyte-macrophages. A, Bone marrow and stem cell systems. Probable pathways of differentiation, from the totipotential stem cell to mature blood cells. Note the osteoclasts originate from the monocyte lineage. Unknown is the pathway that natural killer cells develop.

normal circumstances, macrophages show little evidence of mitotic division, probably because the levels of CSF production normally are low, but production can be rapidly elevated in response to need, such as an infection.

DEVELOPMENT OF BLOOD CELLS

Hematopoiesis

Blood cell production, termed **hematopoiesis**, occurs in the liver and spleen of the fetus, but after birth it normally occurs only in bone marrow and is known as *medullary hematopoiesis* (see Chapter 27). It is still a mystery why hematopoiesis is restricted to bone marrow after birth.

Hematopoiesis is a two-stage process that involves **mitotic division** (or **proliferation**) and **maturation** (or **differentiation**). Each type of blood cell has parent cells, called **stem cells**, that undergo mitosis when they receive specific biochemical signals indicating that populations of circulating blood cells have diminished to a certain point. The stem cells continue to proliferate until the requisite number of mature daughter cells has entered the circulation. The stem cells of lymphocytes and possibly monocytes are stimulated to proliferate and differentiate by other mechanisms, particularly activation of the immune response, but they too originate in bone marrow.

Hematopoiesis can be divided by activity in the bone marrow by two separate pools: the stem cell pool and the bone marrow pool, with eventual release of mature cells into the peripheral circulation (Fig. 24-8). Investigators propose that in the bone marrow microenvironment a stem cell pool exists where structurally unidentifiable multipotential stem cells and unipotential committed colony-forming units (CFUs) reside. In addition, there is a bone marrow pool that can be divided into two cell pools: cells that are proliferating and maturing and cells that are stored and later released into the peripheral blood. In the peripheral blood, two pools of cells are also categorized: those circulating and those in storage.[5] Those cells stored around the walls of the blood vessels are often called the **marginating storage pool** (see Fig. 24-8).

Certain blood cells proliferate and differentiate simultaneously for a period. Proliferation usually ceases after a number of doubling divisions, but differentiation continues. Recent research provides evidence that separate signaling pathways for proliferation and differentiation exist in erythroid cells.[6,7] Erythrocytes and neutrophils usually are mature before entering the blood. Monocytes and other leukocytes are not. They enter the bloodstream and continue to mature as they travel to the spleen, peritoneal cavity, and lung.

Hematopoiesis continues throughout life to replace blood cells that grow old and die, are killed by disease, or are lost

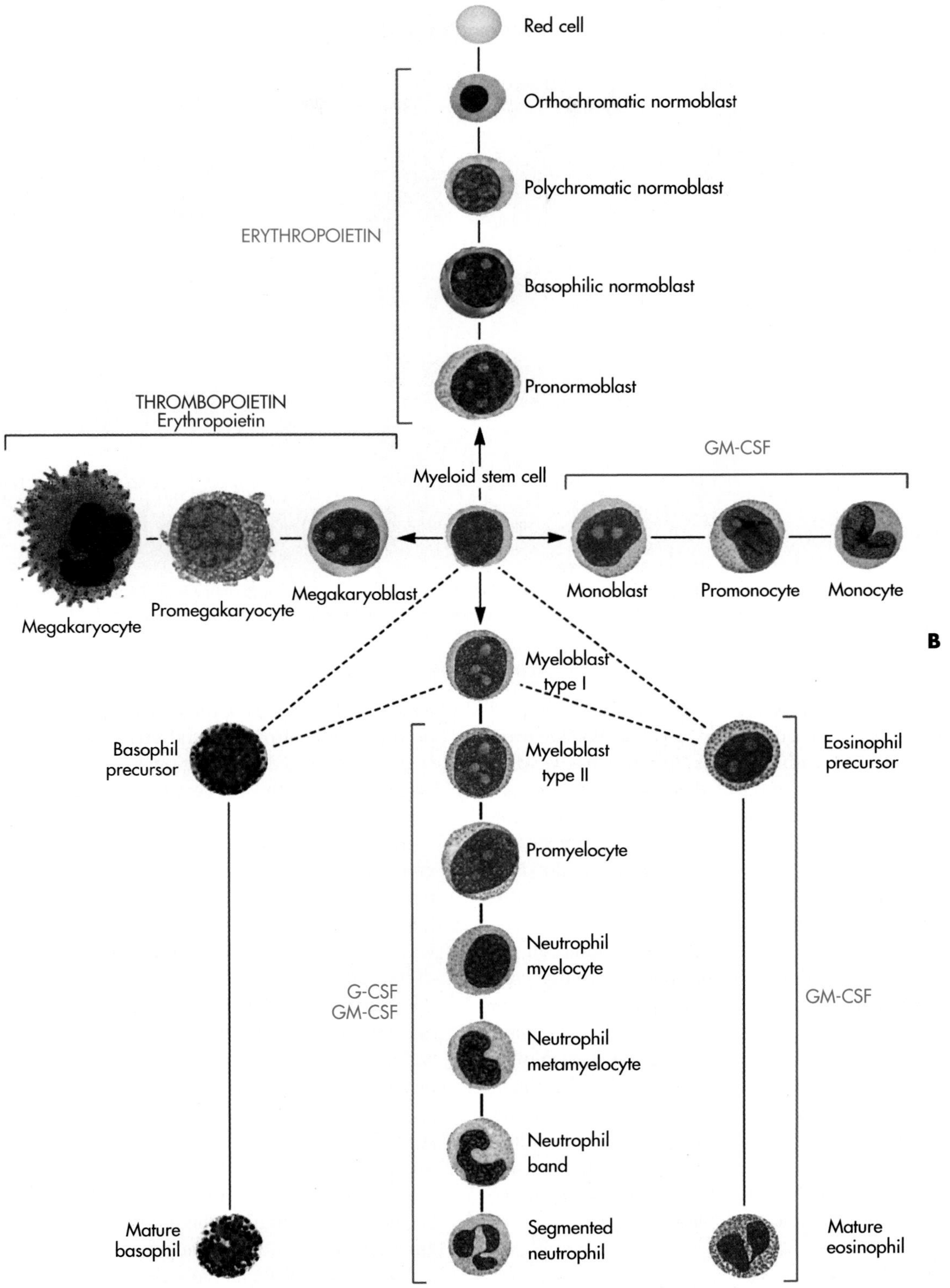

FIG. 24-7, cont'd Production, maturation, and function of granulocytes and monocyte-macrophages. **B,** Schematic representation of myeloid hematopoiesis and major growth factor specificities. *GM-CSF,* Granulocyte-macrophage colony-stimulating factor; *G-CSF,* granulocyte colony-stimulating factor. (B from Damjanov I, Linder J, editors: *Anderson's pathology,* ed 10, St Louis, 1996, Mosby.)

through bleeding. Medullary hematopoiesis increases in response to proliferative disease, hemorrhage, hemolytic anemia (in which erythrocytes are destroyed), chronic infection, idiopathic thrombocytopenic purpura (bleeding caused by platelet insufficiency; see Chapter 26), and other disorders that deplete blood cells. In general, long-term stimuli, such as chronic diseases, cause a greater increase in hematopoiesis than acute conditions, such as hemorrhage. Abnormal proliferation of erythrocytes occurs in polycythemia vera, a myeloproliferative disease.

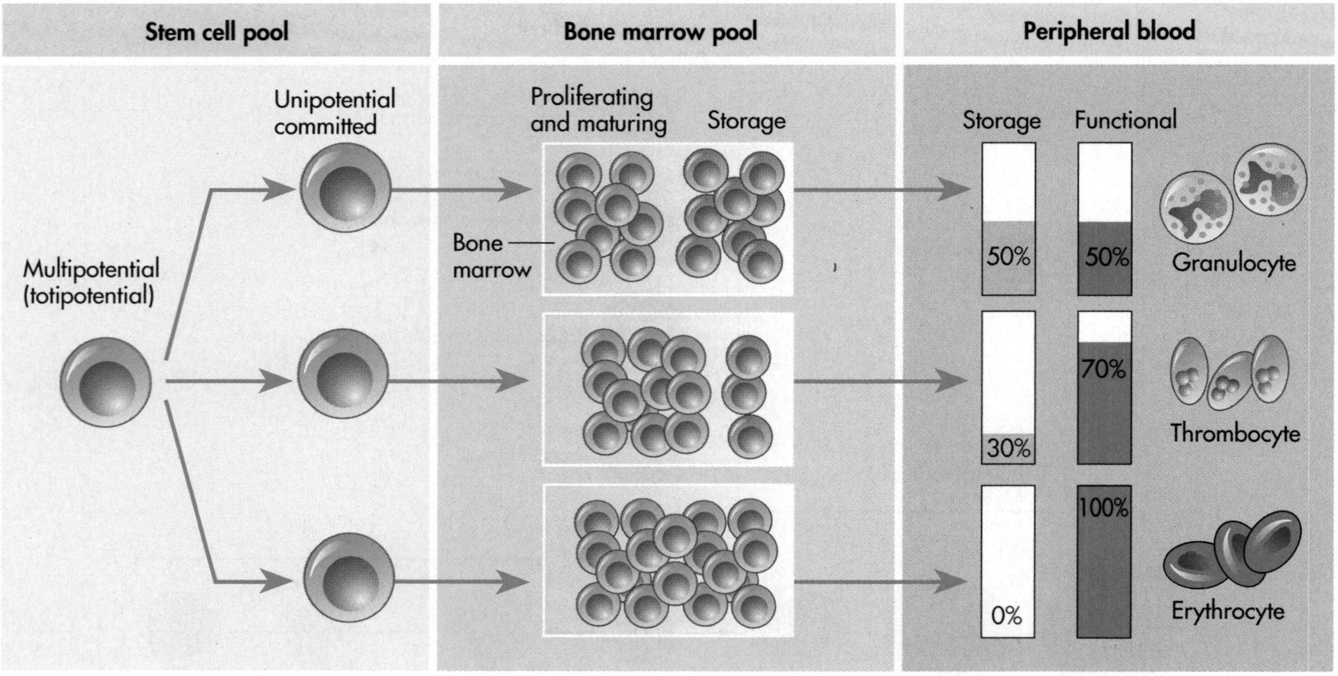

FIG. 24-8 Hematopoiesis. Hematopoiesis from the stem cell pool; activity mainly in the bone marrow and in the peripheral blood. (Modified from Harmening DM, editor: *Clinical hematology and fundamentals of hemostasis,* ed 3, Philadelphia: 1997 F. A. Davis.)

Medullary hematopoiesis can be accelerated by any or all of three mechanisms: (1) conversion of yellow bone marrow, which does not produce blood cells, to red marrow, which does; (2) faster differentiation of daughter cells; and presumably (3) faster proliferation of stem cells. Marrow conversion is stimulated by erythropoietin, the hormone that stimulates erythrocyte production. An increase in blood cell production occurs in response to emergencies, such as infection (see the next section).

In adults, extramedullary hematopoiesis—blood cell production in tissues other than bone marrow—is usually a sign of disease. Extramedullary production of one or more types occurs in disease states that affect erythrocytes (e.g., pernicious anemia, sickle cell anemia, thalassemia, hemolytic disease of the newborn [erythroblastosis fetalis], hereditary spherocytosis) and leukocytes (certain leukemias). Extramedullary hematopoiesis of apparently normal blood cells has been reported also to occur in the spleen and liver and, less frequently, in lymph nodes, adrenal glands, cartilage, adipose tissue, intrathoracic areas, and kidneys.

Stem Cell System

The processes by which blood cells develop from a common ancestor, or stem cell, are known collectively as the **stem cell system**. This system is a hierarchy in which the earliest, most primitive ancestor is the **totipotential hematopoietic stem cell (THSC)** (see Fig. 24-7, *A*). Because these cells have the potential to develop into many types of blood cells, they also are called *multipotential stem cells*. One pathway of development leads to various lymphoid tissues, where T and B lymphocytes mature. The other pathway leads to **myeloid tissue**—the bone marrow. The stem cell of the myeloid pathway is called the *pluripotential myeloid stem cell (PMSC),* or simply the **pluripotential stem cell**. The pluripotential stem cell triggers differentiation of (1) neutrophils and monocytes, (2) eosinophils, (3) erythrocytes, and (4) platelets (see Fig. 24-7, *A*).

Blood cell production in any one pathway requires numerous amplifying cell divisions coupled with complex maturation changes to produce the mature cells that are released into the blood. Regulation of hematopoiesis occurs in two ways: (1) by stromal cells in the marrow that control some of the cellular events by "cell contact processes" and (2) by the interaction of cytokines or regulatory molecules. Stromal cells apparently express **steel factor** (a stem cell factor), which activates stem cells to develop (see What's New? boxes on p. 823). In vitro, hematopoietic cells will survive, proliferate, and differentiate only if they are provided with specific growth factors. These factors are glycoproteins usually called **hematopoietic growth factors** or colony-stimulating factors (CSFs). These factors (cytokines) act as hormones and stimulate the proliferation of progenitor cells and their progeny and initiate the maturation events necessary to produce fully mature cells (i.e., activating specialized functions). Specific CSFs are necessary for the adequate growth of myeloid, erythroid, lymphoid, and megakaryocytic pathways and are required to keep cells alive. CSFs are thought to play a role in preventing programmed cell death (apoptosis) (Table 24-4 and Fig. 24-9).[8,9]

Clinical Uses of Colony-Stimulating Factors

Blood granulocyte numbers (e.g., eosinophils, neutrophils, basophils/mast cells) are normally in the range of 4000 to 6000 cells per microliter, and susceptibility to infection de-

WHAT'S NEW? Bone Marrow Stromal Cells—One Cell with Many Different Faces

Stromal cells (covering or supportive tissue) of the bone marrow exhibit multiple traits of a stem cell population. Recently, they have been shown to differentiate into myocytes, muscle cells, hepatocytes, and glial cells. Human bone marrow stromal cells can be induced to differentiate into neural cells under experimental cell culture conditions. Thus, new is the understanding of bone marrow versatility. If the biologic mechanisms underlying each of the different types of cells become understood, the implications are astonishing. For example, bone marrow might become the reservoir for nerve cells to help with the treatments of spinal cord injuries.

Data from Marshall E: The business of stem cells, *Sci* 287(5457): 1419, 2000; Sanchez-Ramos J et al: Adult bone marrow stromal cells differentiate into neural cells in vitro, *Exp Neurol* 164(2):247, 2000; Seppa N: Do liver stem cells come from bone marrow, *Sci News* 158: 7, 2000; van der Kooy D, Weis S: Why stem cells, *Sci* 287(5457): 1439, 2000; Woodbury D et al: Adult rat and human bone marrow stromal cells differentiate into neurons, *J Neurosci Res* 61(4):364, 2000.

WHAT'S NEW? Embryonic Stem Cells

Investigators recently removed embryonic stem cells from the blastocyst—a group of cells from the egg's protective shell—a few days after fertilization. It is extraordinary that embryonic stem cells have the capacity to grow into any sort of tissue the body will need—blood, nerves, heart, bone, and so forth. The stem cells, in theory, could be used for a vast array of lifesaving therapies—for example, for repairing damaged heart muscle, replacing cells destroyed by Alzheimer disease, and providing new pancreatic cells to produce insulin for diabetics. The key for researchers involves figuring out how to guide stem cells into specific paths of development. Answering all the necessary questions will likely keep scores of investigators busy for years.

Data from Thomson JA et al: Embryonic stem cell lines derived from human blastocysts, *Sci* 282(5391):1145, 1998; Thomson JA, Odorico JS: Human embryonic stem cell and embryonic germ cell lines, *Trends Biotechnol* 18(2):53, 2000.

velops below 1000 cells per microliter. During a natural response to a bacterial infection, granulocytes usually rise to 10,000 to 20,000 cells per microliter. The CSFs can raise white cell numbers even higher. No advantage, however, is gained from extreme numbers because of the formation of toxic products and tissue damage.[8,10] CSFs have been studied in individuals with subnormal hematopoiesis either as a result of diseases such as acquired immunodeficiency syndrome (AIDS), aplastic anemia, or congenital neutropenia or as a consequence of cytotoxic therapy for cancer, including lymphoma and leukemia. The CSFs can stimulate increases in granulocyte-macrocyte populations in such individuals, but responses are quantitatively restricted if the available numbers of stem and progenitor cells have been drastically depleted by chemotherapy or disease. Responses to CSF treatment are evident from the correction of a preexisting disorder, such as in congenital neutropenia or hematopoietic response after cytotoxic therapy (e.g., after bone marrow

Table 24-4 Human Colony-Stimulating Factors (CSFs)

CSF	Cell Origin	Cell Stimulated
M-CSF	Macrophage, fibroblast, endothelial cell	Macrophage
GM-CSF	T cell, macrophage, fibroblast	Neutrophil, macrophage, eosinophil
G-CSF	Macrophage, fibroblast	Neutrophil, eosinophil, basophil
IL-3	T cell, epidermal cell	Neutrophil, macrophage
Erythropoietin	Kupffer and peritubular kidney cells	Erythrocyte
Steel factor (stem cell factor)	Stromal cells in bone marrow and many other cells	Stem cell

Data from Metcalf D: *Science* 254(5031):529, 1991; Rowe JM, Rappaport AP: *J Clin Pharmacol* 32:486, 1992.
M-CSF, macrophage; *GM-CSF,* granulocyte-macrophage; *G-CSF,* granulocyte; *IL-3,* interleukin-3.

transplantation). CSF treatment can result in shorter periods of intensive nursing and hospitalization.[10] Currently, three CSFs are mass-produced in recombinant form and are used to stimulate hematopoiesis, including G-CSF, GM-CSF, and erythropoietin.[11,12]

Bone Marrow

Bone marrow, also called *myeloid tissue* (*myelos* = marrow), is confined to the cavities of bone. Bone marrow consists of blood vessels, nerves, mononuclear phagocytes, stem cells, blood cells in various stages of differentiation, and fatty tissue. Adults have two kinds of bone marrow: red (or active [hematopoietic]) marrow and yellow (or inactive) marrow. The large quantities of fat in inactive marrow make it yellow. Not all bones contain active marrow. In adults, active marrow is in the pelvic bones (34%), vertebrae (28%), cranium and mandible (13%), sternum and ribs (10%), and extreme proximal portions of the humerus and femur (4% to 8%).[11] Inactive marrow predominates in cavities of other bones. (Bones are discussed further in Chapter 40.)

Stem cells in hematopoietic marrow receive the oxygen and nutrients they need for mitosis and maturation from the primary or nutrient arteries of the bones. Branches of these arteries terminate in a capillary network that coalesces into large venous sinuses, which eventually drain into a central vein. Hematopoietic marrow and fat fill the spaces surrounding the network of venous sinuses. Some mechanism of transport enables the newly produced blood cells to traverse narrow openings in venous sinus walls and thus enter the circulation. It is not known whether the movement of the new blood cells forces an opening or whether certain sites open in response to the presence of the newly formed cells. Normally, cells do not enter the circulation until they have differentiated to a certain extent, but premature release is known to occur in certain diseases.

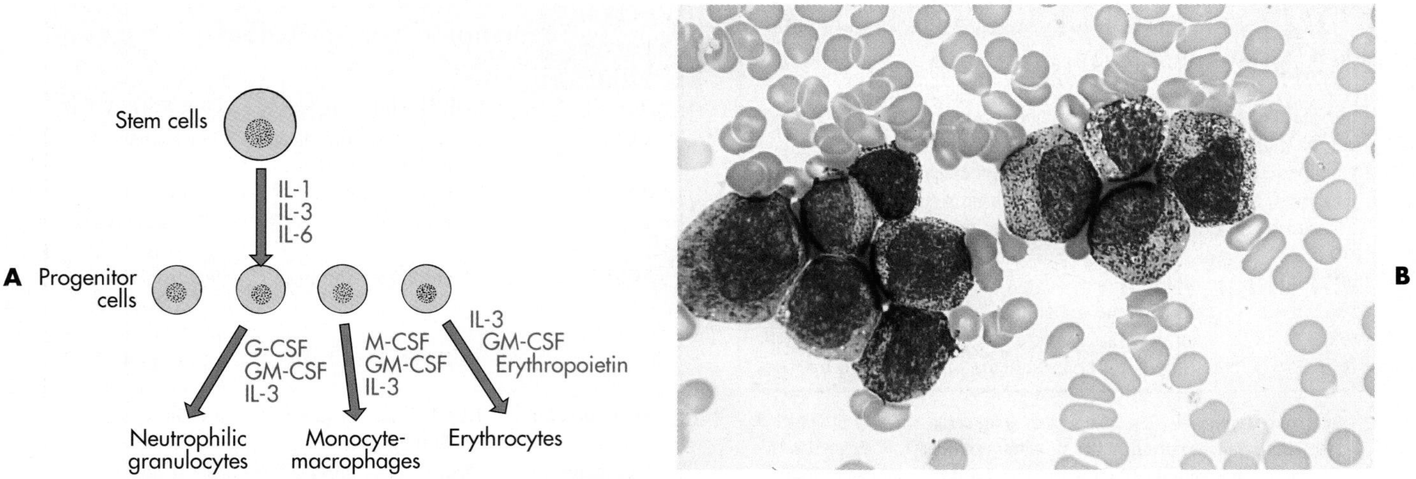

FIG. 24-9 Colony-stimulating factor (CSF) effects. A, Physiologic effects of some CSFs. **B,** Morphologic effects of growth factor. Marrow aspirate from a patient receiving G-CSF showing an early neutrophil response. There is a marked shift toward immaturity in the neutrophils with the majority at the promyelocyte and early myelocyte stages of maturation (Wright-Giemsa stain). *IL,* Interleukin; *G-CSF,* granulocyte colony-stimulating factor; *M-CSF,* macrophage colony-stimulating factor; *GM-CSF,* granulocyte-macrophage colony-stimulating factor. (B from Damjanov I, Linder J, editors: *Anderson's pathology,* ed 10, St Louis, 1996, Mosby.)

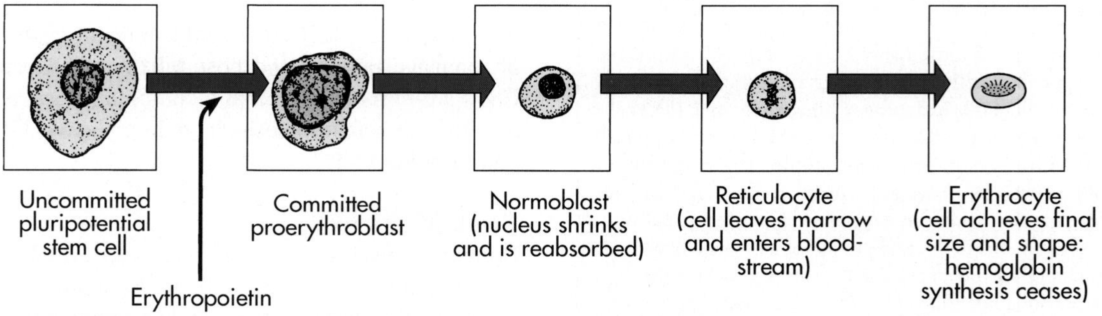

FIG. 24-10 Erythrocyte differentiation. Erythrocyte differentiation from large, nucleated stem cell to small, nonnucleated erythrocyte.

Development of Erythrocytes

For almost 100 years it was believed that erythrocytes developed from lymphocytes that were transformed in the spleen. It was not until the 1850s that the bone marrow was accepted as the site of **erythropoiesis**. It is now known that erythrocytes are derived from precursor cells called **erythroblasts** (Fig. 24-10). Normal erythroblasts are also called **normoblasts**, whereas abnormal ones are called **megaloblasts**.

Erythrocyte development is shown in detail in Fig. 24-10. The proerythroblast (pronormoblast) possesses a huge nucleus, is rich in ribosomes, and can synthesize protein. The signal that causes an increase in circulating erythrocytes is the glycoprotein **erythropoietin**. Erythropoietin stimulates uncommitted stem cells to differentiate into proerythroblasts. Whether hemoglobin has been synthesized at this stage is controversial. Hemoglobin is, however, readily apparent and increases in quantity as nuclear size shrinks throughout the basophilic and polychromatophilic stages. The orthochromatic erythroblast (normoblast) is the smallest of the nucleated erythrocyte precursors. Once the nucleus is lost, the cell that remains is called a **reticulocyte**. Although it lacks a nucleus, the reticulocyte contains polyribosomes (for globin synthesis) and mitochondria (for oxidative metabolism and heme synthesis). The reticulocyte matures to an erythrocyte within 24 to 48 hours. During this period, mitochondria and ribosomes disappear and the cell becomes smaller and more disklike. With these final changes, the erythrocyte loses its capacity for hemoglobin synthesis and oxidative metabolism.

Reticulocytes remain in the marrow approximately 1 day and then are released into the venous sinuses before maturation is complete. Reticulocytes continue to mature in the bloodstream and may travel to the spleen for several days of additional maturation. The normal reticulocyte count is 1% of the total red blood cell count. Approximately 1% of the body's circulating erythrocyte mass normally is generated every 24 hours. Therefore the reticulocyte count is a useful clinical index of erythropoietic activity and indicates whether new red cells are being produced. The concept of "**erythron**" has been used to describe all the tissues that produce

Table 24-5 Structure of Normal Hemoglobin Molecules

Type of Hemoglobin (Hb)	Identity of Polypeptide Chain	Significance
Hb A	$\alpha_2\beta_2$	92% of adult Hb
Hb A_{1c}	α_2(β-NH-glucose)	5% of adult Hb; increased in diabetes (see Chapter 20)
Hb A_2	$\alpha_2\delta_2$	2% of adult Hb; increased in β-thalassemia (see Chapter 25)
Hb F	$\alpha_2\gamma_2$	Major fetal Hb from the third through ninth month of gestation; promotes oxygen transfer across platelets; increase in β-thalassemia
Hb Gower I	ϵ_4 or $\zeta_2\epsilon_2$	Present in early embryo; function unknown
Hb Gower II	$\alpha_2\epsilon_2$	Present in early embryo; function unknown
Hb Portland	$\zeta_2\gamma_2$	Present in early embryo; function unknown

erythrocytes and their precursors. Thus included in this term are stem cells, all stages of developing erythrocytes, and mature red blood cells.

One of the most significant advances in the hematopoietic growth factors has been the development of erythropoietin for use in individuals with chronic renal failure. In 1986 large amounts of recombinant human erythropoietin (r-HuEPO) became widely available for clinical research. Erythropoietin has been used to correct the anemia of chronic renal failure. Several researchers are evaluating the use of r-HuEPO in individuals with AIDS and cancer, as well as enhancing the ability of individuals to donate blood for blood transfusions.[12,13,14] The most significant side effect associated with r-HuEPO is increased blood pressure.[15] Other features that can affect the response to r-HuEPO include blood loss (occult); infection; inflammation; hyperparathyroidism with marrow fibrosis; aluminum toxicity; vitamin B_{12}/folate deficiency; hemolysis; bone marrow disorders; underdialysis; and, possibly, angiotensin-converting enzyme inhibitors.[13]

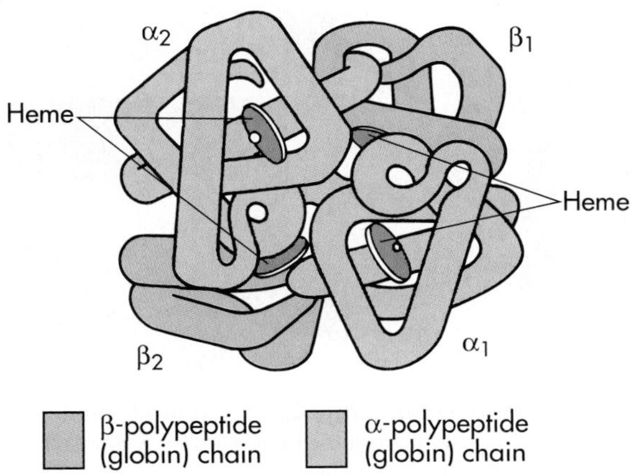

FIG. 24-11 Molecular structure of hemoglobin. Molecule is a spherical tetramer weighing approximately 64,500 daltons. It contains a pair of α-polypeptide and a pair of β-polypeptide chains and several heme groups.

Hemoglobin Synthesis

Hemoglobin, the oxygen-carrying protein of the erythrocyte, constitutes approximately 90% of the cell's dry weight. The cytoplasm of a single erythrocyte can contain as many as 300 hemoglobin molecules. Hemoglobin enables the blood to transport 100 times more oxygen than could be transported dissolved in plasma alone. Hemoglobin is not one molecule but a family of molecules whose members differ slightly in primary structure. Nonetheless, each member is composed of two pairs of polypeptide chains (the **globins**) and four colorful complexes of iron plus protoporphyrin (the **hemes**) (Fig. 24-11).

Hemoglobin synthesis is precisely coordinated by mechanisms not completely understood. Three requisites for hemoglobin synthesis are (1) formation of protoporphyrin, (2) availability of iron (heme), and (3) generation of the proteinaceous globin. Several genes dictate the synthesis of globin in maturing human erythroblasts, each gene resulting in the formation of a structurally different polypeptide chain (alpha, beta, gamma, delta, epsilon, or zeta). Each polypeptide chain contains approximately 150 amino acids and is arranged in the knotted-sausage configuration shown in Fig. 24-11. The chains assemble to form a tetrahedron containing two pairs of identical chains. Hemoglobin A, the most common type of hemoglobin in adults, is composed of two α-polypeptide and two β-polypeptide chains. Seven different types of hemoglobin have been identified in healthy human blood at all stages, from fetal life to adulthood—testimony to the heterogeneity of the molecule (Table 24-5). The timing of synthesis and the relative amount of each type of hemoglobin are determined by complex developmental processes.

Heme is a large, flat, iron-protoporphyrin disk that is capable of carrying one molecule of oxygen (O_2). Recall that hemoglobin contains four heme groups; thus it is capable of carrying four oxygen molecules. Through a series of complex biochemical reactions, **protoporphyrin**, a complex four-ringed molecule, is produced and abounds with ferrous iron. The biochemical reactions of heme synthesis include condensation, oxidation, and reduction, all of which are powered by catalytic enzymes. It is crucial that the iron be correctly charged. Presence of the reduced ferrous iron (Fe^{++}) allows the formation of normal hemoglobin, which is capable of binding oxygen where it is plentiful (in the lungs) and releasing it where it is less plentiful (in the tissues).

Oxidized ferric iron (Fe^{+++}) carries an extra positive charge and results in the formation of **methemoglobin**, an unstable type of hemoglobin that is not capable of binding oxygen. An excess of ferric iron occurs in the presence of certain drugs and chemicals, such as nitrates and sulfonamides.

Hemoglobin that is carrying oxygen is called **oxyhemoglobin**. If all four oxygen-binding sites on the oxyhemoglobin's hemes are occupied by oxygen, the molecule is said to be saturated. Oxyhemoglobin that has released its oxygen or is not bound to oxygen for some other reason is called *reduced hemoglobin*, or **deoxyhemoglobin**. As hemoglobin transfers its oxygen to tissue, it also sheds small amounts of nitric oxide, which dilates the blood vessels and helps to get oxygen into tissues (Fig. 24-12).[16]

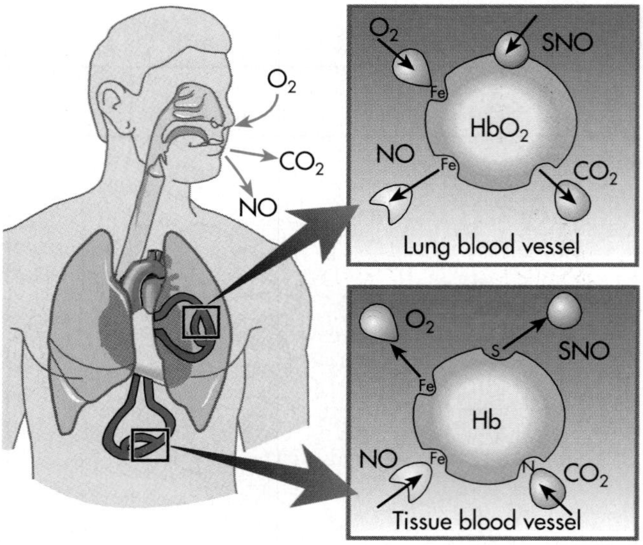

FIG. 24-12 Hemoglobin (Hb) binding to nitric oxide. In the lungs, hemoglobin (Hb) binds nitric oxide (NO) as S-nitrosothiol (SNO). In tissue this SNO is released, and free, circulating NO is bound to a different site for exhalation.

Nutritional Requirements for Erythropoiesis

Normal development of erythrocytes and synthesis of hemoglobin depend on an optimal biochemical milieu and adequate supplies of the necessary building blocks, including protein, vitamins, and minerals (Table 24-6). If these components are lacking, it is usually the result of a nutritional deficiency or a metabolic imbalance in which other organs or tissues use up a disproportionate share of these nutrients or are unable to absorb the needed nutrients. If abnormal distribution of nutrients is prolonged, erythrocyte production slows and anemia (insufficient numbers of functional erythrocytes) may result (see Chapter 25).

Protein is an important structural component of the erythrocyte's plasma membrane, contributing to its strength, flexibility, and elasticity. Amino acid chains form hemoglobin. Without proteins and amino acids, erythrocyte production decreases and the life span of cells that are produced may be shortened because of structural defects. One of the most important proteins is **intrinsic factor (IF),** a glycoprotein necessary for gastrointestinal absorption of vitamin B_{12}. Lack of vitamin B_{12} causes pernicious anemia. IF is secreted by the parietal cells in the gastric mucosa and facilitates vitamin B_{12} uptake at its absorptive site, the ileum.

Table 24-6 Nutritional Requirements for Erythropoiesis

Nutrient	Role in Erythropoiesis	Consequence of Deficiency
Protein (amino acids)	Structural component of plasma membrane	Decreased strength, elasticity, and flexibility of membrane; hemolytic anemia
	Synthesis of hemoglobin	Decreased erythropoiesis and life span of erythrocytes
Cobalamin (vitamin B_{12})	Synthesis of DNA, maturation of erythrocytes, facilitator of folate metabolism	Macrocytic (megaloblastic) anemia
Folate (folic acid)	Synthesis of DNA and RNA, maturation of erythrocytes	Macrocytic (megaloblastic) anemia
Vitamin B_6 (pyridoxine)	Heme synthesis	Hypochromic-microcytic anemia
Vitamin B_2 (riboflavin)	Oxidative reactions	Normochromic-normocytic anemia
Vitamin C (ascorbic acid)	Iron metabolism, acts as a reducing agent to maintain iron in its ferrous (Fe^{++}) form	Normochromic-normocytic anemia
Pantothenic acid	Heme synthesis	Unknown in humans*
Niacin	None, but needed for respiration in mature erythrocytes	Unknown in humans
Vitamin E	Heme synthesis (?); protection against oxidative damage in mature erythrocytes	Hemolytic anemia with increased cell membrane fragility; shortens life span of erythrocytes in individuals with cystic fibrosis
Iron	Hemoglobin synthesis	Iron deficiency anemia
Copper	Required for optimal mobilization of iron from tissues to plasma	Hypochromic-microcytic anemia

Data from Strine-Martin EA, Lotspeich-Steininger CA, Koepke JA: *Clinical hematology: principles, procedures, correlations,* ed 2, Philadelphia, 1998, Lippincott.

DNA, Deoxyribonucleic acid; *RNA,* ribonucleic acid.

*Although pantothenic acid is important for optimal synthesis of heme, experimentally induced deficiency *failed* to produce anemia or other hematopoietic disturbances.

Erythropoiesis cannot proceed in the absence of vitamins, especially B_{12}, folate (folic acid), B_6, riboflavin, pantothenic acid, niacin, ascorbic acid, and vitamin E. Vitamin B_{12} is a large molecule; therefore it requires assistance from IF to penetrate the gastrointestinal mucosa. Once absorbed, vitamin B_{12} is stored in the liver and used as needed in erythropoiesis.

Folate is the second most important vitamin for erythrocyte production and maturation. Folate is necessary for DNA synthesis, being a component of three of the four DNA bases (thymine, adenine, and guanine). Folate also is needed for ribonucleic acid (RNA) synthesis. IF is not required for folate absorption, which occurs principally in the upper small intestine. Folate is stored in and circulates through the liver. Folate deficiency is more common than vitamin B_{12} deficiency and occurs more rapidly. Folate stores can be depleted within a few months, whereas vitamin B_{12} depletion can take years. Folate supplements are prescribed for pregnant women because pregnancy increases the demand for folate and deficiency can cause anemia.

Iron Cycle

Approximately 67% of total body iron is bound to heme in erythrocytes and muscle cells, and approximately 30% is stored bound to ferritin or hemosiderin mononuclear phagocytes (i.e., macrophages) and hepatic parenchymal cells. The remaining 3% (less than 1 mg) is lost daily in urine, sweat, bile, and epithelial cells shed from the gut. Iron not lost is continuously recycled (Fig. 24-13). Recycling is made possible by **transferrin**, a glycoprotein synthesized primarily by the liver but also by tissue macrophages, submaxillary and mammary glands, and ovaries or testes.

Dietary iron is absorbed primarily in the duodenum and proximal jejunum. Some of it passes into the bloodstream, and the rest is sequestered in intestinal epithelial cells as ferritin. This iron is lost when epithelial cells are sloughed off in the intestinal lumen. Iron that is released to the bloodstream is picked up by transferrin, which is the body's major iron-transport molecule. Iron for hemoglobin production is delivered to erythroblasts in erythropoietic bone marrow. Under normal conditions, only one third of the iron-binding sites on transferrin molecules are occupied. It is postulated that iron is transferred from transferrin to erythroblasts in the marrow as follows:

1. The transferrin-iron complex binds to a receptor on the erythroblast's plasma membrane.

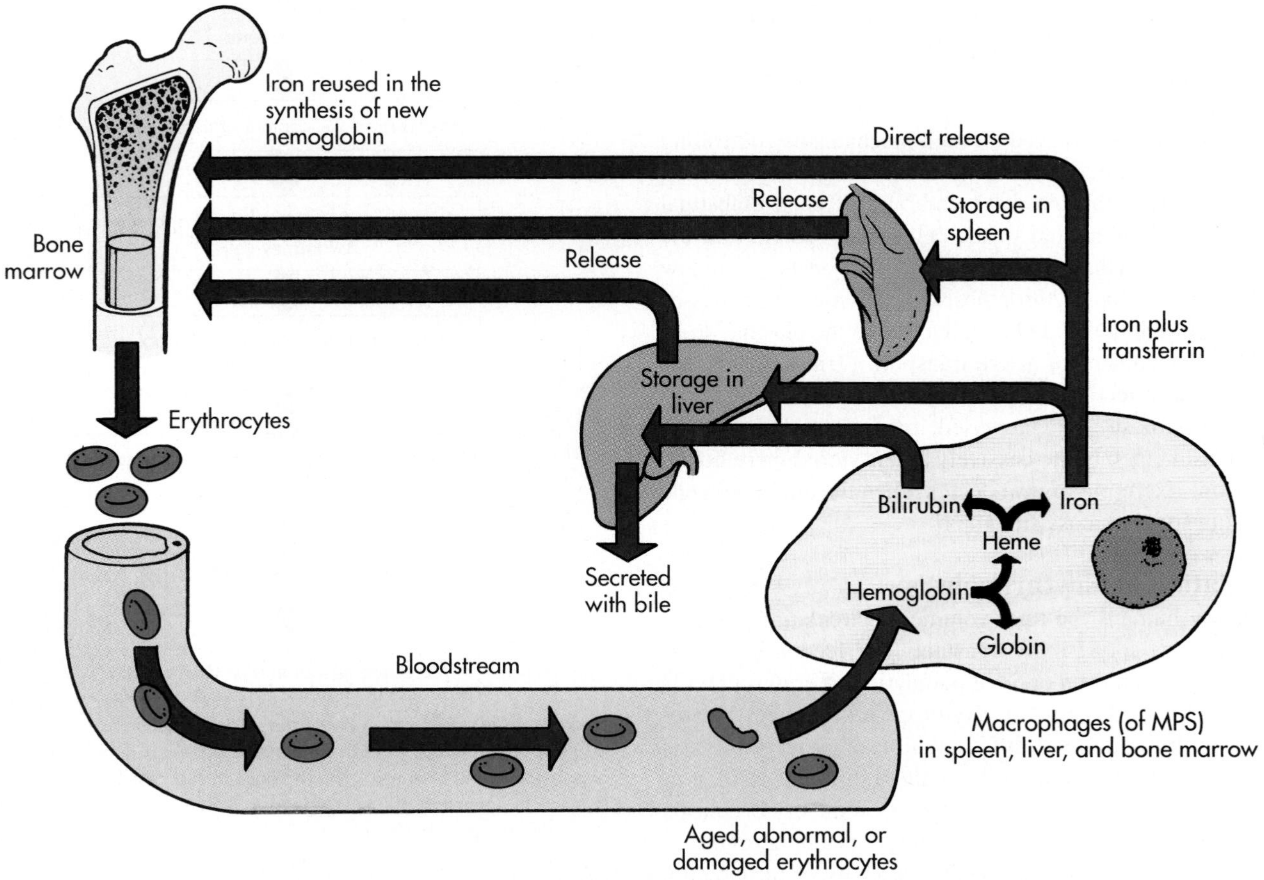

FIG. 24-13 Iron cycle. Iron (Fe) released from gastrointestinal epithelial cells circulates in bloodstream associated with its plasma carrier, transferrin. It is delivered to erythroblasts in bone marrow, where most of it is incorporated into hemoglobin. Mature erythrocytes circulate for approximately 120 days, after which they become senescent and are removed by the mononuclear phagocyte system (MPS). Macrophages of MPS (mostly in spleen) break down ingested erythrocytes and return iron to bloodstream directly or after storing it as ferritin or hemosiderin.

2. The complex moves into the cell, possibly by active transport.
3. Iron is released (dissociated) from transferrin.
4. The dissociated transferrin is returned to the bloodstream (see Fig. 24-13).

Another source of iron for erythropoiesis is the iron stored by ferritin and hemosiderin in the cytoplasm of mononuclear phagocytes (macrophages) resident in the marrow. Once the iron is released into the marrow and incorporated into the erythroblast's mitochondria, the enzyme heme synthetase inserts ferrous iron into protoporphyrin to form heme. Heme then is bound to globin to form hemoglobin. Iron not used in erythropoiesis is stored temporarily as ferritin or hemosiderin and later excreted.

After mature erythrocytes have circulated for 120 days, they are removed from the bloodstream by macrophages of the MPS—chiefly in the spleen. Within the phagolysosomes (digestive vacuole) of the macrophage, the erythrocyte is catabolized and the iron in hemoglobin is oxidized, forming Fe^{+++} (methemoglobin). The heme and globin of methemoglobin dissociate easily, and globin may be reduced to its component amino acids. The iron released by methemoglobin dissociation is stored in the macrophage's cytoplasm as ferritin or hemosiderin or released into the bloodstream, where it is free to bind again to transferrin (see Fig. 24-13). A minute amount of iron is stored in muscle cells by the heme-containing protein **myoglobin**. Unavailable stores of iron are present in cytochromes, catalases, and peroxidase enzymes.

Iron balance is achieved through mechanisms controlling its absorption rather than its excretion. Regulation of iron transport across the plasma membrane of gastrointestinal epithelial cells is related to the cell's iron content and the overall rate of erythropoiesis. If the body's iron stores are low or the demand for erythropoiesis is increased, iron passes rapidly through the epithelial cell and into the plasma, probably by mechanisms of active transport. (Transport mechanisms are described in Chapter 1.) If the body stores are high and erythropoiesis is not increased, iron crosses the epithelial cell's plasma membrane passively and is stored there bound to ferritin. Excretion of iron occurs when the epithelial cells of the intestinal mucosa slough off.

Regulation of Erythropoiesis

In healthy humans the total volume of circulating erythrocytes remains surprisingly constant. The feedback mechanism that maintains an optimal population of erythrocytes is mediated by erythropoietin. Erythropoietin induces the selective proliferation and differentiation of proerythroblasts (see Fig. 24-10). Its earliest effects are to stimulate RNA synthesis, after either binding to receptors on the erythroblast's plasma membrane or entrance into the cell. Hemoglobin synthesis begins hours after initial stimulation by erythropoietin.

Erythropoietin is secreted by the kidney in response to tissue hypoxia (Fig. 24-14). Erythropoietin causes a compensatory increase in erythrocyte production if the oxygen content of blood decreases because of anemia, high altitude, or pulmonary disease. The normal steady-state rate of production of approximately 2.5 million erythrocytes per second in humans can increase up to about 17 million per second under anemic or low-oxygen states.[17] The receptors that detect hypoxia are within the kidney because production of erythropoietin is known to increase after renal artery constriction, which reduces oxygen supply to renal cells.[18] Unlike the peripheral chemoreceptors of the carotid body and aortic arch that send messengers to the brain to increase respiration in individuals with hypoxia, receptors in the kidney are on cells that synthesize and secrete erythropoietin. Thus the body responds to reduced oxygenation of blood in two ways: by increasing intake of oxygen through increased respiration and by increasing the oxygen-carrying capacity of the blood through increased erythropoiesis. Erythropoietin not only stimulates proliferation of committed stem cells in the marrow but also accelerates maturation of existing erythroblasts. (Erythropoiesis also is discussed in the hematopoiesis section.)

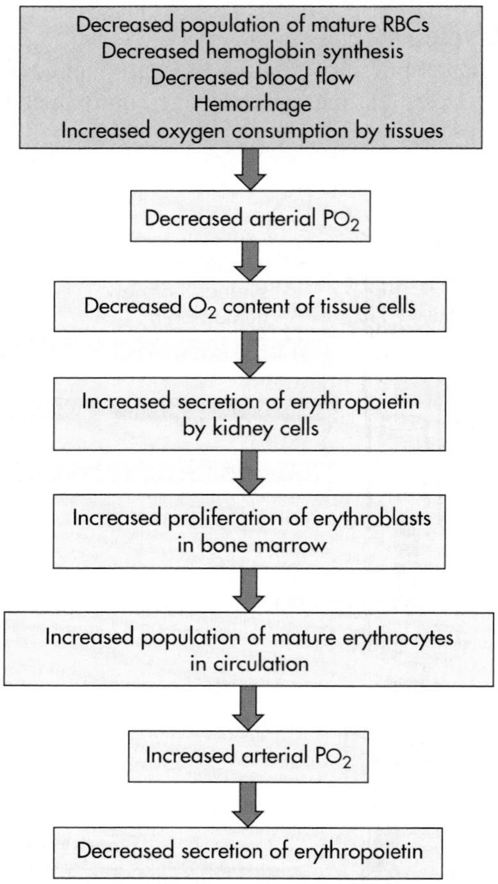

Decreased arterial oxygen levels stimulate production of erythropoietin, which in turn stimulates red cell production and expansion of the erythron. The increase in red cells frequently corrects the problem of low oxygen levels (hypoxia). This restoration to normal oxygen levels alerts the kidney to stop producing erythropoietin (negative feedback). Further erythrocyte production is not needed.

FIG. 24-14 Role of erythropoietin in regulation of erythropoiesis. *RBCs,* Red blood cells; *Po_2,* partial pressure of oxygen in the blood (see Chapter 31).

Normal Destruction of Senescent Erythrocytes

Although mature erythrocytes lack nuclei, mitochondria, and endoplasmic reticulum, they do have cytoplasmic enzymes capable of glycolysis (anaerobic glucose metabolism) and production of small quantities of adenosine triphosphate (ATP). The ATP provides the energy necessary to keep the cell alive and its plasma membrane pliable (see Fig. 24-1). Metabolic processes diminish as the erythrocyte ages. Consequently, less ATP is available to maintain the functions essential for life. The senescent red cell becomes increasingly fragile and loses its property of reversible deformability. Its membrane therefore is susceptible to rupture during passage through narrowed regions of the microcirculation.

Aged red cells are selectively sequestered and destroyed by macrophages of the MPS, primarily in the spleen. If the spleen is dysfunctional or absent, macrophages in the liver (Kupffer cells) take over. The signal that identifies an erythrocyte as senescent and ready for disposal by the MPS is not known. Alterations in the erythrocyte's plasma membrane, including altered ionic and osmotic gradients across it and a decrease in its electrical charge, and an increase in methemoglobin within the erythrocyte all accompany cellular aging. These factors may contribute to sluggish erythrocyte movement through the spleen and other lymphoid tissues, increasing opportunities for phagocytosis by resident macrophages.

Phagocytosis of the erythrocyte is followed by its digestion by proteolytic and lipolytic enzymes within the phagolysosome of the macrophage. Globin is broken down into amino acids, and iron is recycled (see Fig. 24-13). Porphyrin is reduced to bilirubin, which is transported to the liver, conjugated, and finally excreted in the bile as glucuronide (Fig. 24-15). Approximately 6 g of hemoglobin is catabolized daily, producing 200 mg of bilirubin. (Liver function is described in Chapter 37.) Bacteria in the intestinal lumen transform conjugated bilirubin into urobilinogen. A small portion of this urobilinogen is reabsorbed, to be either metabolized further by the liver or excreted by the kidney into the urine. Most of the urobilinogen is excreted in feces.

Conditions causing accelerated erythrocyte destruction increase the load of bilirubin for hepatic clearance, leading to increased serum levels of unconjugated bilirubin and increased urinary excretion of urobilinogen. Gallstones (cholelithiasis) can result from a chronically elevated rate of bilirubin excretion.

Development of Leukocytes

All of the leukocytes arise from stem cells in the bone marrow (their pathways of differentiation are shown in Fig. 24-7, *A*). The granulocytes (neutrophils, eosinophils, and basophils/mast cells) normally mature fully in the marrow and then are

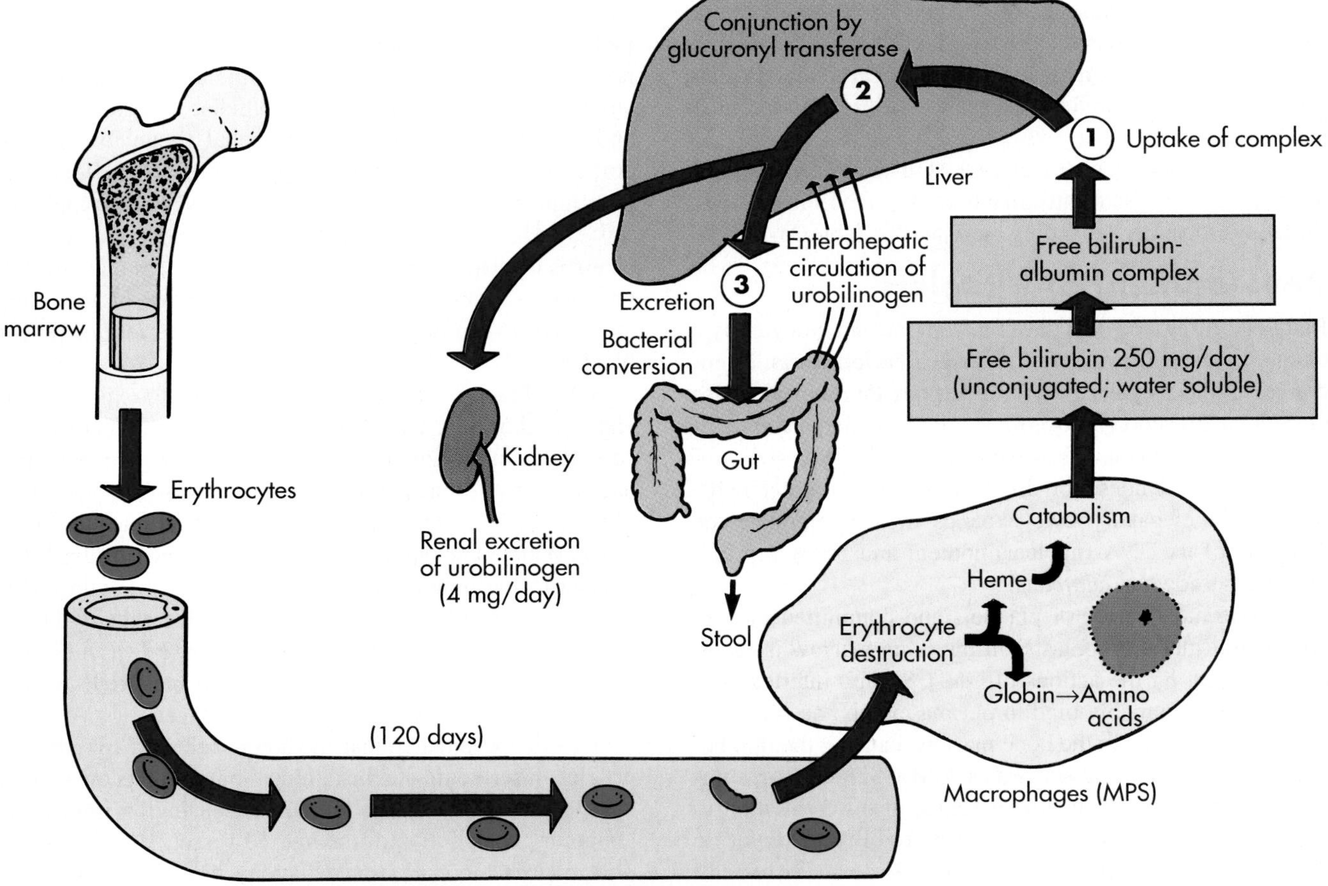

FIG. 24-15 Metabolism of bilirubin released by heme breakdown.

released into the bloodstream. The agranulocytes (monocytes and lymphocytes), however, are released into the bloodstream before they undergo their final phase of maturation. The monocytes mature into macrophages within 1 or 2 days of release, and the lymphocytes travel to lymphoid tissues, where they are stimulated to differentiate into T cells or B cells (see Chapter 6).

The bone marrow exhibits selective retention of immature granulocytes. Hematopoietic growth factors, granulocyte-macrophage colony-stimulating factor (GM-CSF), and granulocyte colony-stimulating factor (G-CSF) are required for granulocyte growth and differentiation. Because elevated blood levels of G-CSF, but not GM-CSF, are seen with infections, G-CSF may be more important as a signal for neutrophils. (Recall that neutrophils are always increased with infection.)

Maintenance of optimal levels of granulocytes and monocytes in the blood depends on the availability of pluripotential stem cells in the marrow, induction of these into committed stem cells, and timely release of new cells from the marrow. The marrow contains a reserve pool that can be rapidly mobilized in response to the body's needs. Once cells are released from the marrow, they join the marginating pool or the circulating pool. The cells in the marginating pool lie along the capillary walls and can move into tissues and mucous membranes. Cells from the circulating pool join the marginating pool to replace the cells that have migrated out of the capillaries. Leukocyte production increases in response to infection, to the presence of steroids, and to reduction or depletion of reserves in the marrow. It is also associated with strenuous exercise, convulsive seizures, heat, intense radiation, paroxysmal tachycardias, pain, nausea and vomiting, and anxiety.

Normally, some leukocytes are lost in saliva, urine, lungs, liver, spleen, and gastrointestinal tract. Most exist in the body from days to years, depending on type (see Table 24-2).

Development of Platelets

Platelets (thrombocytes) develop from megakaryocytes by a unique process of proliferation termed **endomitosis**. In endomitosis the megakaryocyte undergoes the nuclear phase of cellular division (mitosis) but fails to undergo the cytoplasmic phase (cytokinesis) (see Chapter 1). Without cytokinesis the cell does not divide into two daughter cells. Rather, the megakaryocyte expands to accommodate the doubling of its DNA (nuclear) content and breaks up into fragments known as *platelets*.

An optimal number of platelets and committed platelet precursors (megakaryoblasts) in the bone marrow is maintained in part by the actions of GM-CSF and interleukin-3 (IL-3) that presumably bind to plasma membranes of pluripotential stem cells in the bone marrow, causing them to become committed megakaryoblasts. GM-CSF and IL-3 stimulate committed cells at further stages of differentiation to differentiate faster. Rates of the processes of megakaryocyte development, endomitosis, and platelet release are increased.[8]

Platelets, once released, circulate for 10 days before they begin to lose their capacity to carry out biochemical reactions. The initial alteration of function is possibly attributable to proteolytic enzymes present at sites of chronic vascular inflammation. (See Chapter 7 for a discussion of biochemicals involved in inflammation.) Senescent platelets are phagocytosed by neutrophils and monocytes if they are circulating freely or by neutrophils and macrophages if they are part of a clot, or thrombus. Senescent platelets may be removed also by tissue macrophages of the MPS in the liver or spleen.

MECHANISMS OF HEMOSTASIS

Hemostasis means arrest of bleeding. Mechanisms of hemostasis maintain a relatively steady state of blood volume, pressure, and flow through injured blood vessels after vascular damage and bleeding. Three equally important anatomic compartments of hemostasis are platelets, blood proteins (clotting factors), and the vasculature (Fig. 24-16). Hemostasis involves a complex sequence of events: (1) vasoconstriction (vasospasm), (2) formation of a platelet plug, (3) activation of the coagulation (or clotting) cascade, (4) formation of a blood clot, and (5) clot retraction and clot dissolution (fibrinolysis). All of these events involve platelets, clotting, and the blood vessels (vasculature).

Function of Platelets

In hemostasis, platelets adhere to injured vessel walls, undergo granule discharge, and aggregate into clumps or plugs (see Fig. 24-16), releasing biochemical mediators. Normally, platelets circulate freely, suspended in plasma, and do not adhere to endothelial cells that line the vessels. When a vessel is damaged, however, endothelial sloughing occurs and collagen-containing subendothelial tissue is exposed, attracting platelets out of the plasma within 15 to 20 seconds after injury (see Fig. 24-16). The platelets adhere rapidly to this "foreign" surface, after which they undergo dynamic changes in shape from smooth to spiny spheres that develop protrusions (pseudopods), exposing receptors on their surfaces. They then degranulate, releasing a variety of potent biochemicals (see Fig. 24-16, *A*).

Several factors affect platelet adherence to exposed subendothelial tissues. The platelets must contain sufficient concentrations of calcium to change shape, aggregate, degranulate, and activate arachidonic pathways. Adhesion to the vessel subendothelial layer occurs when the platelet receptor binds to von Willebrand factor (e.g., a plasma protein), bridging the platelet to the injury site (see Fig. 24-16, *A*). Erythrocytes apparently increase the rate of platelet adherence by facilitating migration of circulating platelets toward vascular surfaces and by liberating adenosine diphosphate (ADP), which enables platelets to stick to exposed collagen.

Two of the biochemical mediators released by adhered platelets—serotonin and histamine—have effects on smooth muscle in the vascular endothelium, causing an immediate temporary constriction of the injured vessel.[19] Vasoconstriction reduces blood flow and thereby diminishes bleeding.

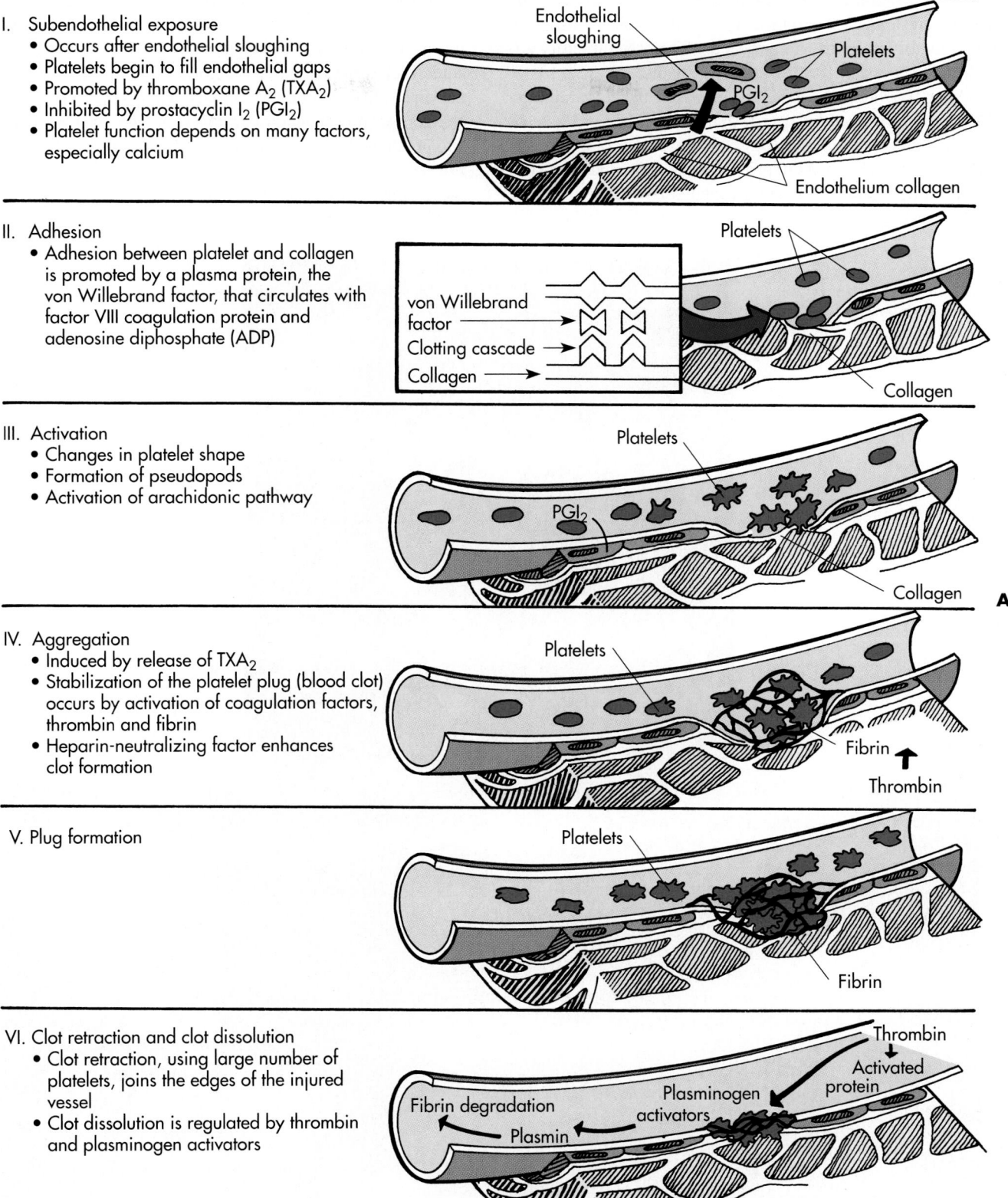

I. Subendothelial exposure
- Occurs after endothelial sloughing
- Platelets begin to fill endothelial gaps
- Promoted by thromboxane A_2 (TXA_2)
- Inhibited by prostacyclin I_2 (PGI_2)
- Platelet function depends on many factors, especially calcium

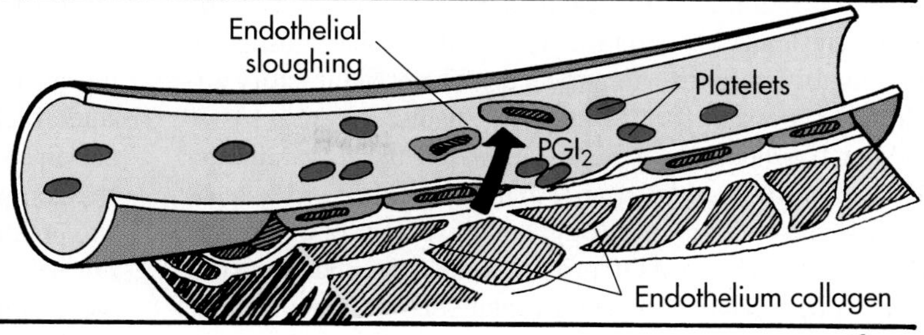

II. Adhesion
- Adhesion between platelet and collagen is promoted by a plasma protein, the von Willebrand factor, that circulates with factor VIII coagulation protein and adenosine diphosphate (ADP)

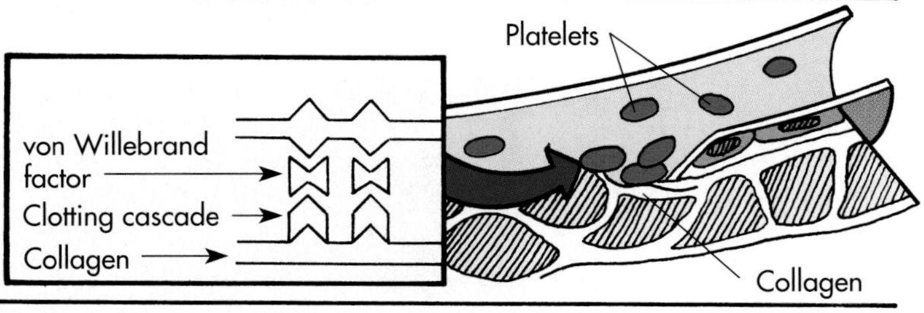

III. Activation
- Changes in platelet shape
- Formation of pseudopods
- Activation of arachidonic pathway

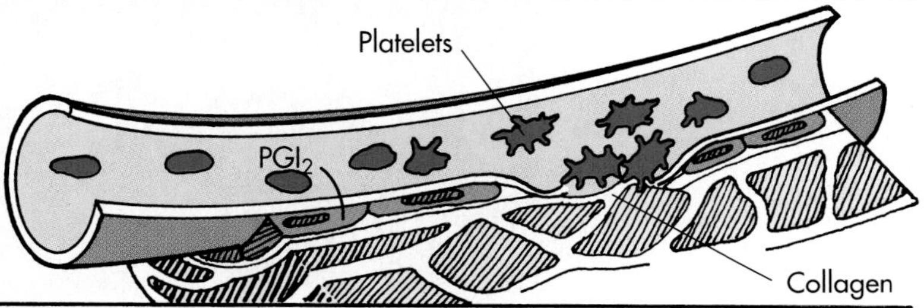

A

IV. Aggregation
- Induced by release of TXA_2
- Stabilization of the platelet plug (blood clot) occurs by activation of coagulation factors, thrombin and fibrin
- Heparin-neutralizing factor enhances clot formation

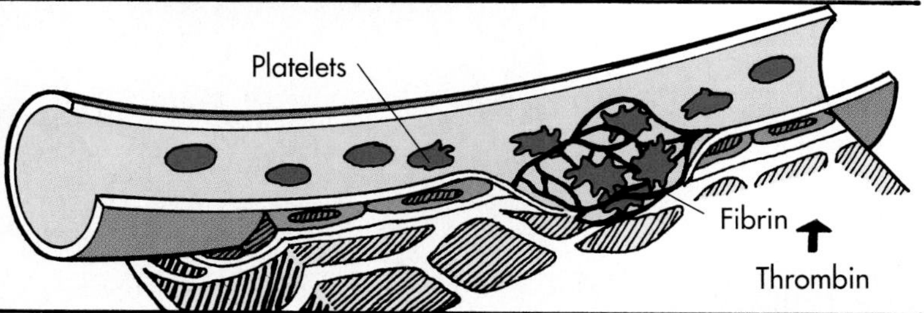

V. Plug formation

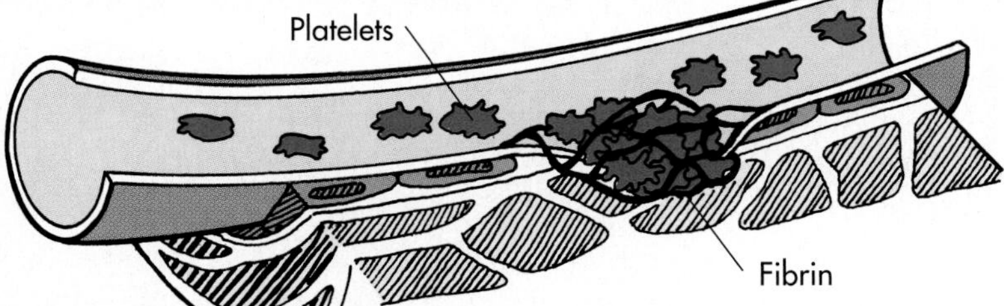

VI. Clot retraction and clot dissolution
- Clot retraction, using large number of platelets, joins the edges of the injured vessel
- Clot dissolution is regulated by thrombin and plasminogen activators

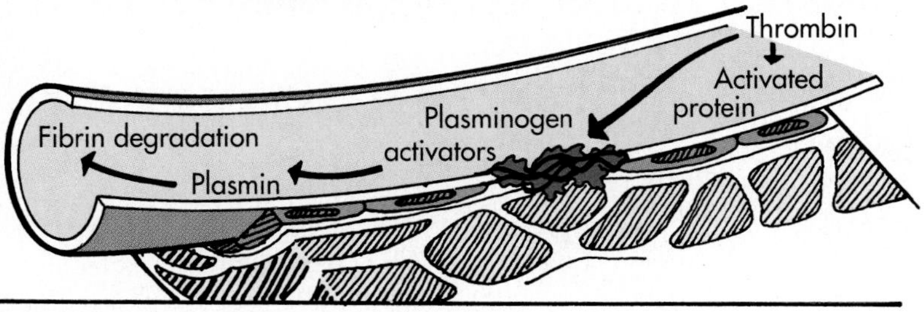

FIG. 24-16 Platelet degranulation. A, Plug formation and clot dissolution.

Continued

(Vasoconstriction also is produced by local reflexes of the nervous system.) Vasodilation soon follows, permitting the inflammatory response to proceed. (The inflammatory response is necessary for healing; see Chapter 7.)

Other biochemical mediators released by degranulation (also called the *platelet-release reaction*) either promote or inhibit platelet activity and the eventual process of clot formation (see Fig. 24-16). ADP promotes the adherence and subsequent degranulation of nearby platelets by causing their plasma membranes to become ruffly and sticky (Fig. 24-17). The new activated platelets cause a platelet plug to seal the injured endothelium. If the effects of ADP were not counteracted and laminar flow were not sufficient, platelet aggregation could continue indefinitely. This is prevented by two antagonistic prostaglandin derivatives, thromboxane A_2 (TXA_2) and prostacyclin I_2 (PGI_2), produced by endothelial cells (see Fig. 24-16, *A*). TXA_2 causes vasoconstriction and promotes the degranulation of other platelets, which then release more

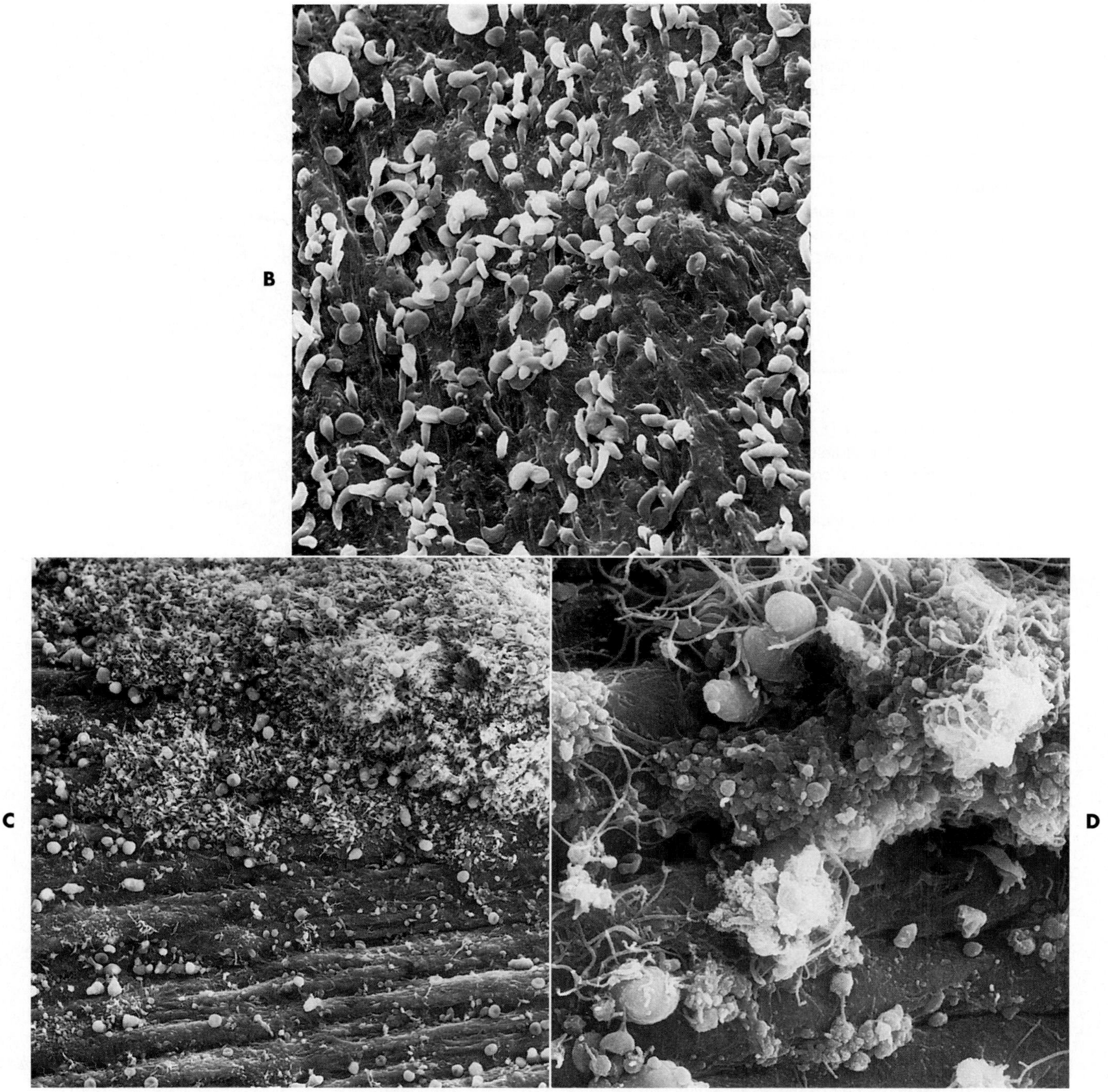

FIG. 24-16, cont'd Platelet degranulation. B, After simple endothelial denudation, platelets adhere to the subendothelium in a monolayer fashion. **C,** Platelet-fibrin thrombus formation. **D,** Higher magnification of the thrombus shows a mixture of red cells and platelets incorporated into the fibrin meshwork. (B to D from Damjanov I, Linder J, editors: *Anderson's pathology*, ed 10, St Louis, 1996, Mosby.)

ADP. PGI_2 inhibits the effects of TXA_2 by promoting vasodilation and inhibiting platelet degranulation. The net effect of TXA_2 and PGI_2 is to permit platelet aggregation to proceed at the site of injury while preventing adherence to normal vascular endothelium. Heparin-neutralizing factor released by platelets (platelet factor 4) enhances clot formation at the site of injury.

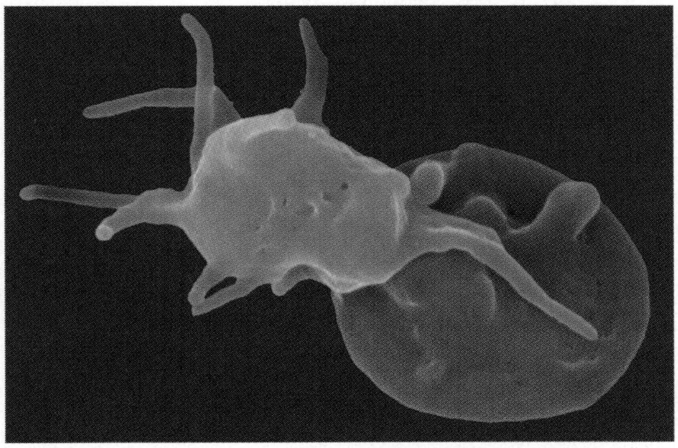

FIG. 24-17 Scanning electron micrograph of moderately active platelet. (Copyright © Dennis Kunkel Microscopy, Inc.)

If blood vessel injury is minor, hemostasis is achieved temporarily by the platelet plug, which usually forms within 3 to 5 minutes of injury. Platelet plugs seal the many minute ruptures that occur daily in the microcirculation, particularly in capillaries. With too few platelets, numerous small hemorrhagic areas called purpuras develop under the skin and throughout the tissues (see Chapter 26).

Function of Clotting Factors

A **blood clot** is a meshwork of protein strands that stabilizes the platelet plug and traps other cells, such as erythrocytes, phagocytes, and microorganisms (Fig 24-18, see also Fig. 24-16, *C* and *D*). The strands are made of fibrin, which normally is not present in the circulation but rather is the end product of the **coagulation cascade,** a series of enzymatic reactions among the clotting factors (Fig. 24-19). According to the cascade theory of coagulation, each coagulation factors is converted to its active form by the preceding factor until fibrin is produced. (Synonyms for the clotting factors

A

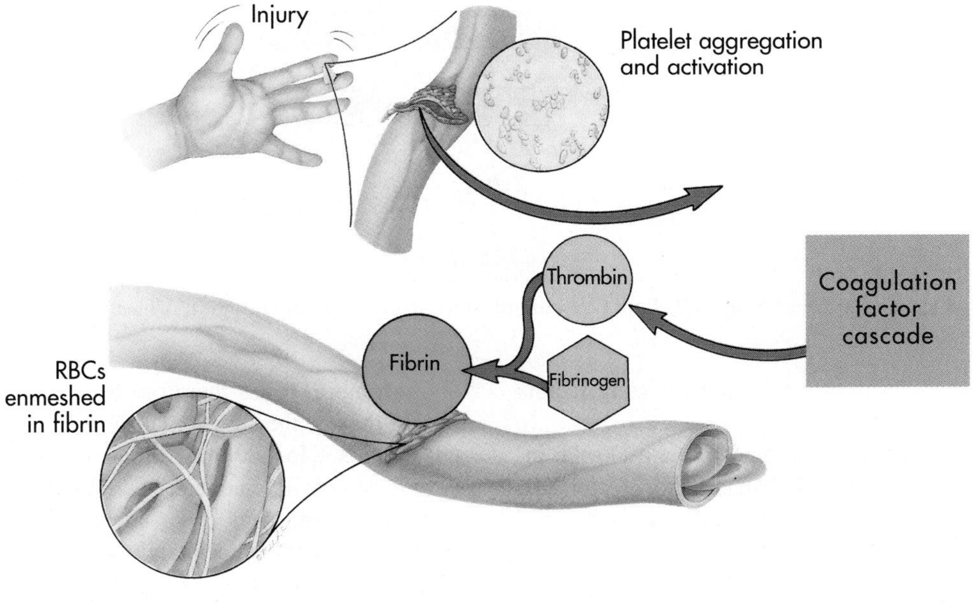

B

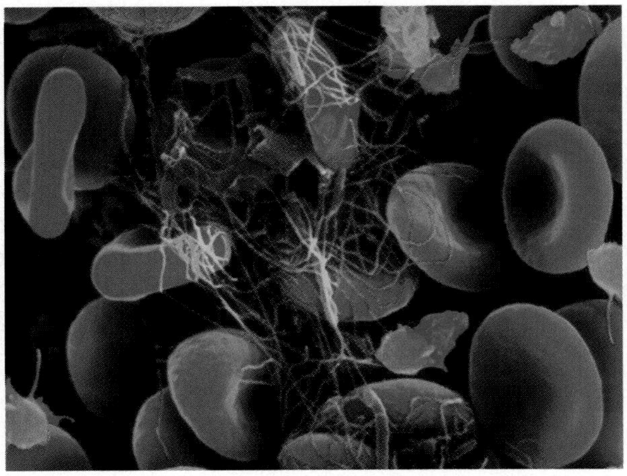

FIG. 24-18 Blood clotting mechanism. A, The clotting mechanism involves release of platelet factors at the injury site, formation of thrombin and trapping of red blood cells (RBCs) in fibrin to form a clot. **B,** An electron micrograph showing entrapped RBCs in a fibrin clot. (A from Thibodeau GA, Patton KT: *Anatomy & physiology*, ed 4, St. Louis, 1999, Mosby. B, copyright © Dennis Kunkel Microscopy, Inc.)

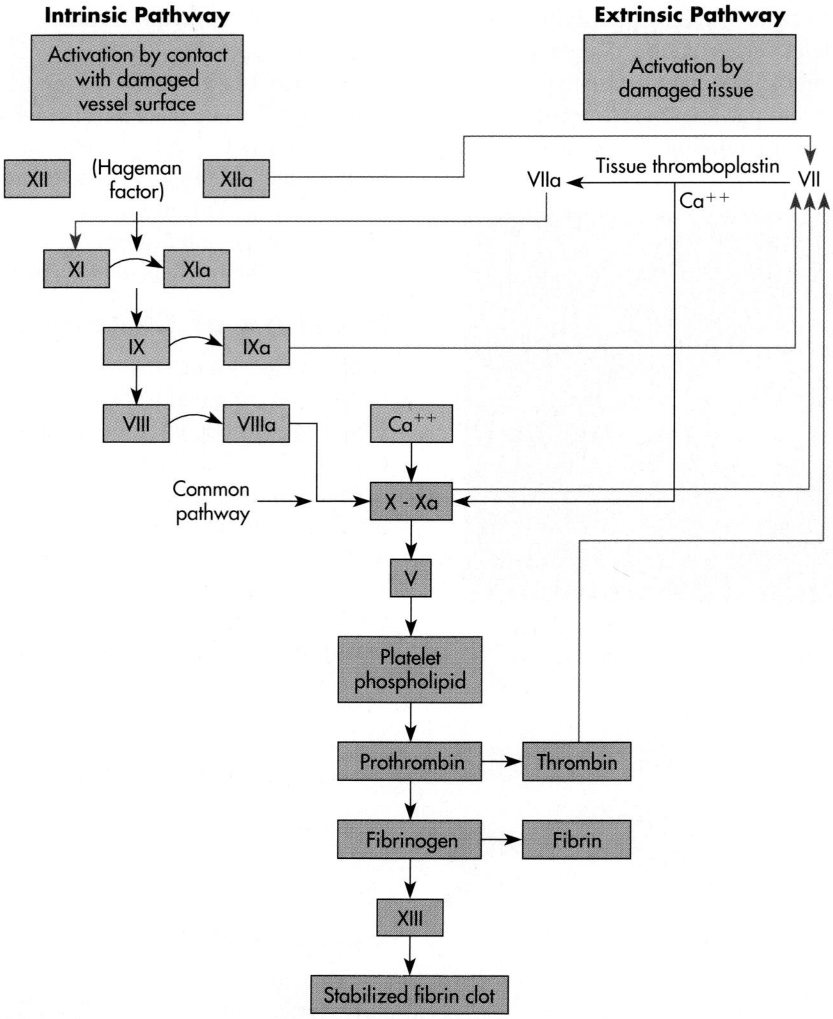

FIG. 24-19 The "cascade" theory of coagulation. Recent changes are shown in blue (see text).

are listed in Table 24-7.) In effect, soluble clotting factors become insoluble fibrin.

The coagulation cascade is initiated through (1) the intrinsic pathway, activated when Hageman factor (factor XII) in plasma contacts with subendothelial substances exposed by vascular injury; and (2) the extrinsic pathway, activated when tissue thromboplastin, a substance released by damaged endothelial cells, contacts with one of the clotting factors, serum prothrombin conversion factor (factor VII). Both pathways lead to a final common pathway when each has activated factor X (Stuart-Prower factor), and this proceeds to clot formation.

Newer Concepts of the Coagulation System

Division of the coagulation process into strictly defined extrinsic and intrinsic pathways has been abandoned because the cascade theory has been modified. Newer concepts are denoted by the blue lines in Fig. 24-19. These changes include (1) that factor VIIa of the extrinsic pathway can directly activate factor IX of the intrinsic pathway; and (2) that factor VII can be activated by factors XIIa, IXa, Xa, and thrombin. It has therefore been hypothesized that factor VII may be the key regulatory protein that initiates blood coagulation.[5] In addition, tissue factor pathway inhibitor (TFPI) is a newly characterized protein involved in the regulation of hemostasis.[20] For simplicity of presentation, the reader should still understand the classic cascade presentation with an awareness of the additional changes. As more information becomes available, the cascade will undoubtedly change.

Control of Hemostatic Mechanisms

The major regulatory events in the clotting processes, including the activation of the clotting factors, the inhibition of these active clotting factors, and the production of circulating anticoagulant proteins, take place on membrane surfaces. The endothelium is a major site of hemostasis. Despite the continual presence of clotting factors and platelets in the circulation, blood normally remains fluid. Two properties of normal vascular endothelium prevent clotting: (1) the smooth texture of the endothelial lining, which prevents adherence of platelets; and (2) the negative charge of protein in the en-

Table 24-7 Coagulation Factors and Synonyms

Factor	Synonym
I	Fibrinogen
II	Prothrombin
V	AC-Globulin
VII	Prothrombin conversion accelerator
VIII:C	Antihemophilic factor
IX	Christmas factor (PTC)
X	Stuart-Prower factor
XI	Thromboplastin antecedent (PTA)
XII	Hageman (contact) factor
XIII	Profibrinoligase
Fletcher factor	Prekallikrein
Fitzgerald factor	High-molecular-weight kininogen
Protein C	Xa inhibitor
Protein S	None

From Bick RL et al, editors: *Hematology: clinical and laboratory practice,* vol II, St Louis, 1993, Mosby.

WHAT'S NEW? Factor XI Increases Clot Risk

People who have a major blood clot in a vein (deep venous thrombosis) are possibly twice as likely as healthy people to have high concentrations of factor XI. The recent finding that factor XI can be activated by thrombin led to a revised model of coagulation (see p. 834). In this model the primary thrombin generation that results in fibrin formation takes place through the extrinsic pathway. Additional thrombin generation takes place inside the fibrin clot through the intrinsic pathway after the activation of factor XI by thrombin. High concentrations of thrombin are formed that are necessary for the activation of *thrombin activatable fibrinolysis inhibitor* (TAFI) Activated TAFI protects the fibrin clot against lysis. The role of factor XI in hemostasis is therefore both procoagulant and antifibrinolytic. The new knowledge of the role of factor XI in coagulation and fibrinolysis may lead to new strategies for the treatment of thrombic disorders.

Data from Bouman BN, Meijers JC: Role of blood coagulation factor XI in downregulation of fibrinolysis, *Curr Opin Hematol* 7(5):266, 2000; Meijers JC et al: High levels of coagulation factor XI as a risk factor for venous thrombosis, *N Engl J Med 342*(10):696, 2000.

dothelial cells, which repels some negatively charged platelets and clotting factors. Damage to the vascular endothelium destroys both of these properties, enabling platelets to adhere and initiating the intrinsic pathway of coagulation.

Once activated, the processes of coagulation are controlled by anticoagulants, some of which are products of the coagulation cascade itself. For example, once a clot has formed, its fibrin strands absorb 85% to 90% of the thrombin subsequently produced at the site. The remaining thrombin is inactivated rapidly by antithrombin III, another plasma protein. Other anticoagulants, most notably heparin, are produced and secreted locally by tissue mast cells and basophils that have been activated by the injury (see Chapter 7). Heparin not only halts the coagulation cascade but also enhances thrombin absorption by fibrin in the clot.

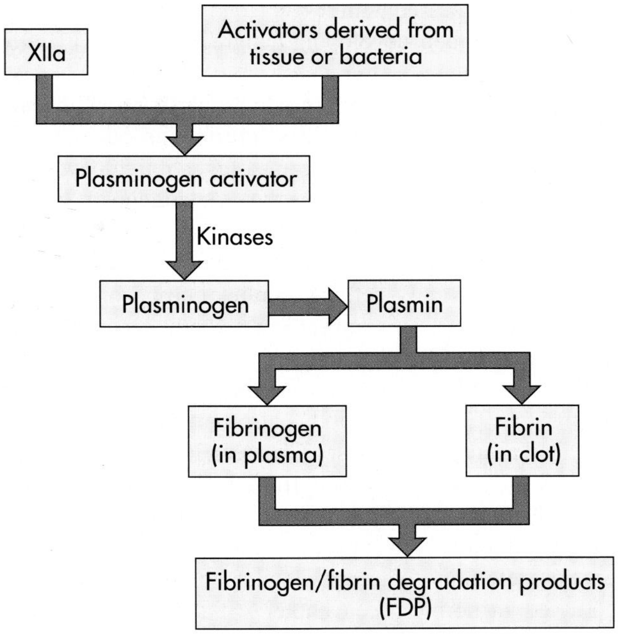

FIG. 24-20 The fibrinolytic system.

Retraction and Lysis of Blood Clots

After a clot is formed, it retracts, or "solidifies." Clot retraction is the final stage of hemostasis. Fibrin strands shorten, becoming denser and stronger, which approximates the edges of the injured vessel wall and seals the site of injury. Retraction is facilitated by the large numbers of platelets trapped within the fibrin meshwork. The platelets, which contain actinomycin-like contractile protein, contract and "pull" the fibrin threads closer together while releasing a factor that stabilizes the fibrin. Contraction expels protein-free serum from the fibrin meshwork. This process usually begins within a few minutes after a clot has formed, and most of the serum is expressed within 1 hour.

Lysis (breakdown) of blood clots is carried out by the **fibrinolytic system** (Fig. 24-20). Lysis is mediated by plasmin (fibrinolysin), a proteolytic enzyme that is activated by substances present during coagulation and inflammation, such as factor XII, thrombin, and lysosomal enzymes. Plasmin splits fibrin and fibrinogen into **fibrin degradation products (FDPs),** which dissolve the clot. The fibrinolytic system removes clotted blood from tissues and dissolves small clots (thrombi) in blood vessels. A balance between amounts of thrombin and plasmin in the circulation maintains normal coagulation and lysis.

CLINICAL EVALUATION OF THE HEMATOLOGIC SYSTEM

Tests of Bone Marrow Function

In tests of marrow function, or hematopoiesis, small amounts of myeloid tissue are removed from the bone cavity and examined under a microscope. Cells contained in the marrow specimen are assessed with respect to (1) relative numbers of stem cells and their developing daughter cells and (2) morphologic structure.

Bone marrow aspiration, in which marrow is withdrawn using a hollow needle, provides information on gross cellular structure; estimation of iron stores in reticulocytes; determination of the ratio of erythrocyte precursor cells to myeloid cells (the normal ratio is 1:3); and the presence or absence of abnormal cells, such as tumor cells. A marrow aspirate that is richly cellular implies normal or increased hematopoiesis but does not indicate whether marrow activity is effective.

Bone aspiration is an important diagnostic test for several anemias (see Chapter 25) and is also performed to diagnose suggested acute leukemia (see Chapters 26 and 27). (Chronic leukemias can be diagnosed from blood samples alone.) Other disorders requiring marrow aspiration for diagnosis or monitoring of disease progression include platelet disorders (to determine whether platelet counts are increased, decreased, or normal; see Chapter 26) and immunoglobulin disorders (to gauge populations of plasma cells and lymphocytes; see Chapter 8).

Bone marrow biopsy, a surgical procedure in which a "slice" of marrow is removed, is performed if (1) aspiration is not diagnostic, (2) tumors are suggested (tumors are more easily detected in biopsy sections), (3) marrow is fibrotic, or (4) populations of more than one type of blood cell are reduced. Because marrow aspiration disturbs marrow structure, only general cellularity (numbers of constituent cells) of the marrow can be gauged. Biopsy specimens provide the most reliable and specific information about marrow cellularity. Marrow biopsy is, however, usually more painful and expensive than marrow aspiration. Therefore biopsy is not performed unless insufficient information is obtained from aspiration.

A direct measure of iron stores can be obtained only from liver or marrow biopsy specimens. The bone marrow technique is preferred, not only because it is safer than liver biopsy but also because the red cell is the immediate source of plasma iron destined for erythrocyte production.

Examination of biopsy specimens and aspirate routinely includes a differential cell count (Table 24-8). The differential cell count involves examining approximately 400 nucleated cells under oil-immersion magnification and counting populations of different stem cells. The relative number of each type of stem cell is expressed as a fraction of 400.

Blood Tests

Blood tests provide information about the absolute and relative numbers of blood cells in a specimen of blood, as well as various structural and functional characteristics of the cells. Deviations from normal can reflect disease, physiologic states (e.g., pregnancy, infancy, old age), injury, or dysfunction in almost any part of the body. Blood tests that reflect chiefly hematologic disorders are listed in Table 24-9.

Table 24-8 Differential Cell Counts in Bone Marrow with Age

Developing Cells in Marrow	Birth	1 mo–1 yr	1-4 yr	4-12 yr	Adult
Erythrocytic series	14	8	19	21	20
Lymphocytic series	14	47	22	18	17
Eosinophilic series	3	3	6	3	3
Neutrophilic series	60	33	50	52	57
Myeloid/erythroid ratio	4:3	4:0	1:3	2:5	1:3

NOTE: Values are percentages of cell types counted during examination of a marrow specimen containing approximately 400 nucleated cells.

Pediatrics and the Hematologic System

Blood cell counts tend to rise above adult levels at birth and then decline gradually throughout childhood. Table 24-10 lists normal ranges during infancy and childhood. The immediate rise in values is the result of accelerated hematopoiesis during fetal life, increased numbers of cells that result from the trauma of birth, and cutting of the umbilical cord.

Average blood volume in the full-term neonate is 85 ml per kilogram of body weight. The premature infant has a slightly larger blood volume of 90 ml per kilogram of body weight, with the mean increasing to 150 mg/kg during the first few days after birth. In both full-term and premature infants, blood volume decreases during the first few months. Thereafter the average blood volume is 75 to 77 ml/kg, which is similar to that of older children and adults.

The hypoxic intrauterine environment stimulates erythropoietin production in the fetus and accelerates fetal erythropoiesis, producing polycythemia (excessive proliferation of erythrocyte precursors) of the newborn. After birth the oxygen from the lungs saturates arterial blood, and more oxygen is delivered to the tissues. In response to the change from a placental to a pulmonary oxygen supply during the first few days of life, levels of erythropoietin and the rate of blood cell formation decrease. The very active rate of fetal erythropoiesis is reflected by the large numbers of immature erythrocytes (reticulocytes) in the peripheral blood of full-term neonates. After birth the number of reticulocytes decreases about 50% every 12 hours so that it is rare to find an elevated reticulocyte count after the first week of life. During this period of rapid growth, the rate of erythrocyte destruction is greater than that in later childhood and adulthood. In full-term infants, normal erythrocyte life span is 60 to 80 days; in premature infants it may be as short as 20 to 30 days; and in children and adolescents it is the same as that in adults—120 days.

In premature infants the postnatal fall in hemoglobin and hematocrit values is more marked than in the full-term

Table 24-9 Blood Tests for Hematologic Disorders

Cell Type and Test	Properly Evaluated by Test	Possible Hematologic Cause of Abnormal Findings
ERYTHROCYTE		
Red cell count	Number (in millions) of erythrocytes/μl of blood	Altered erythropoiesis, anemias, hemorrhage, Hodgkin disease, leukemia
Mean corpuscular volume	Size of erythrocytes	Anemias, thalassemias
Mean corpuscular hemoglobin (MCH)	Amount of hemoglobin in each erythrocyte (by weight)	Anemias, hemoglobinopathy
Mean corpuscular hemoglobin concentration (MCHC)	Concentration of hemoglobin in each erythrocyte (percentage of erythrocyte occupied by hemoglobin)	Anemias, hereditary spherocytosis
Hemoglobin determination	Amount of hemoglobin (by weight)/dl of blood	Anemias
Hematocrit determination	Percentage of a given volume of blood that is occupied by erythrocytes	Hemorrhage, polycythemia, erythrocytosis, anemias, leukemia
Reticulocyte count	Number of reticulocytes/μl of blood (also expressed as percentage of reticulocytes in total red cell count)	Hyperactive or hypoactive bone marrow function
Erythrocyte osmotic fragility test	Cellular shape (biconcavity), structure of plasma membrane	Anemias, hemolytic disease caused by ABO or Rh incompatibility, Hodgkin disease, polycythemia vera, thalassemia major
Hemoglobin electrophoresis	Relative percentage of different types of hemoglobin in erythrocytes	Sickle cell disease, sickle cell trait, hemoglobin C disease, hemoglobin C trait, thalassemias
Sickle cell test	Presence of hemoglobin S in erythrocytes	Sickle cell trait, sickle cell anemia
Glucose-6-phosphate dehydrogenase (G6PD) deficiency test	Deficiency of G6PD in erythrocytes	Hemolytic anemia
HEMOGLOBIN METABOLISM		
Serum ferritin determination	Depletion of body iron (potential deficiency of heme synthesis)	Iron deficiency anemias
Total iron-binding capacity (TIBC)	Amount of iron in serum plus amount of transferrin available in serum (μg/dl)	Hemorrhage, iron deficiency anemia, hemochromatosis, hemosiderosis, iron overload, anemias, thalassemia
Transferrin saturation	Percentage of transferrin that is saturated with iron	Acute hemorrhage, hemochromatosis, hemosiderosis, sideroblastic anemia, iron deficiency anemia, iron overload, thalassemia
Porphyrin analysis (protoporphyrin analysis)	Concentration of protoporphyrin in erythrocytes (μg/dl); an indicator of iron-deficient erythropoiesis	Megaloblastic anemia, congenital erythropoietic porphyria
Direct antiglobulin test (DAT)	Antibody binding to erythrocytes	Hemolytic disease of the newborn, autoimmune hemolytic anemia, drug-induced hemolytic anemia, transfusion reaction
Antibody screen (indirect Coombs test)	Detection of antibodies to erythrocyte antigens (other than the ABO antigens)	Same as for DAT
LEUKOCYTES: DIFFERENTIAL WHITE CELL COUNT (ABSOLUTE NUMBER OF A TYPE OF LEUKOCYTE/μL OF BLOOD)	See below	See below
Neutrophil count	Neutrophils/μl	Myeloproliferative disorders, hematopoietic disorders, hemolysis, infection

Data from Byrne CJ et al: *Laboratory tests: implications for nursing care,* Menlo Park, Calif, 1986, Addison-Wesley; Bick RL et al: *Hematology: clinical and laboratory practice,* St Louis, 1993, Mosby.

NOTE: See Fig. 24-19 and Table 24-7 for information about clotting factors and their sequence of activation in the coagulation cascade.

Continued

Table 24-9 Blood Tests for Hematologic Disorders—cont'd

Cell Type and Test	Properly Evaluated by Test	Possible Hematologic Cause of Abnormal Findings
LEUKOCYTES: DIFFERENTIAL WHITE CELL COUNT (ABSOLUTE NUMBER OF A TYPE OF LEUKOCYTE/μL OF BLOOD)—cont'd		
Lymphocyte count	Lymphocytes/μl	Infectious lymphocytosis, infectious mononucleosis, hematopoietic disorders, anemias, leukemia, lymphosarcoma, Hodgkin disease
Plasma cell count	Plasma cells/μl	Infectious mononucleosis, lymphocytosis, plasma cell leukemia
Monocyte count	Monocytes/μl	Hodgkin disease, infectious mononucleosis, monocytic leukemia, non-Hodgkin lymphoma, polycythemia vera
Eosinophil count	Eosinophils/μl	Hematopoietic disorders
Basophil count	Basophils/μl	Chronic myelogenous leukemia, hemolytic anemias, Hodgkin disease, polycythemia vera
PLATELETS AND CLOTTING FACTORS		
Platelet count	Number of circulating platelets (in thousands)/μl of blood	Anemias, multiple myeloma, myelofibrosis, polycythemia vera, leukemia, disseminated intravascular coagulation (DIC), hemolytic disease of the newborn, idiopathic thrombocytopenic purpura, transfusion reaction, lymphoproliferative disorders
Bleeding time	Duration of bleeding following a standardized superficial puncture wound of the skin, integrity of the platelet plug, measured in minutes following puncture	Leukemia, anemias, DIC, fibrinolytic activity, purpuras, hemorrhagic disease of the newborn, infectious mononucleosis, multiple myeloma, clotting factor deficiencies, thrombasthenia, thrombocytopenia, von Willebrand disease
Clot retraction test	Platelet number and function, fibrinogen quantity and use, measured in hours required for expression of serum from a clot incubated in a test tube	Acute leukemia, aplastic anemia, factor XIII deficiency, increased fibrinolytic activity, Hodgkin disease, hyperfibrinogenemia or hypofibrinogenemia, idiopathic thrombocytopenic purpura, multiple myeloma, polycythemia vera, secondary thrombocytopenia, thrombasthenia
Platelet adhesion studies	Ability of platelets to adhere to foreign surfaces	Anemia, macroglobulinemia, Bernard-Soulier syndrome, multiple myeloma, myeloid metaplasia, plasma cell dyscrasias, thrombasthenia, thrombocytopathy, von Willebrand disease
Platelet aggregation tests	Ability of platelets to adhere to one another	Afibrinogenemia, Bernard-Soulier syndrome, thrombasthenia, hemorrhagic thrombocythemia, myeloid metaplasia, plasma cell dyscrasias, platelet release defects, polycythemia vera, preleukemia, sideroblastic anemia, von Willebrand disease, Waldenström macroglobulinemia, hypercoagulability

Table 24-9 Blood Tests for Hematologic Disorders—cont'd

Cell Type and Test	Properly Evaluated by Test	Possible Hematologic Cause of Abnormal Findings
PLATELETS AND CLOTTING FACTORS—cont'd		
Whole blood clotting time (Lee-White coagulation time)	Overall ability of blood to clot, as measured in minutes in a test tube	Afibrinogenemia, clotting factor deficiencies, excessive fibrinolysis, hemorrhagic disease of the newborn, hypofibrinogenemia, hypoprothrombinemia, leukemia
Circulating anticoagulants (immune globulin G [IgG] antibodies that inhibit coagulation)	Presence of antibodies that neutralize clotting factors and inhibit coagulation, as indicated by prolonged clotting time, prothrombin time, or partial thromboplastin time	Afibrinogenemia, presence of fibrin-fibrinogen degradation products, macroglobulinemia, multiple myeloma, DIC, plasma cell dyscrasias
Partial thromboplastin time (PTT)	Effectiveness of clotting factors (except factors VII and VIII), effectiveness of intrinsic pathway of coagulation cascade, as measured by a test tube (in seconds)	Presence of circulating anticoagulants, DIC, clotting factor deficiencies, excessive fibrinolysis, hemorrhagic disease of the newborn, hypofibrinogenemia and afibrinogenemia, prothrombin deficiency, von Willebrand disease, acute hemorrhage
Prothrombin time	Effectiveness of activity of prothrombin, fibrinogen, and factors V, VII, and X; effectiveness of vitamin K–dependent coagulation factors of the extrinsic and common pathways of the coagulation cascade as measured in a test tube (in seconds)	Hypofibrinogenemia, dysfibrinogenemia, and afibrinogenemia; presence of circulating anticoagulants; DIC; deficiency of factors V, VII, or X; presence of fibrin degradation products, increased fibrinolytic activity, hemolytic jaundice, hemorrhagic disease of the newborn; acute leukemia, polycythemia vera, prothrombin deficiency, multiple myeloma
Thrombin time	Quantity and activity of fibrinogen as measured in a test tube (in seconds)	Hypofibrinogenemia, dysfibrinogenemia, and afibrinogenemia; presence of circulating anticoagulants; hemorrhagic disease of the newborn, polycythemia vera; increase in fibrinogen-fibrin degradation products; increased fibrinolytic activity
Fibrinogen assay	Amount of fibrinogen available for fibrin formation	Acute leukemia, congenital hypofibrinogenemia or afibrinogenemia, DIC, increased fibrinolytic activity, severe hemorrhage
Fibrin-fibrinogen degradation products (fibrin-fibrinogen split products)	Fibrinogenic activity as measured by levels of fibrin-fibrinogen degradation products (in μg/ml of blood)	Transfusion reactions, DIC, internal hemorrhage in the newborn, deep vein thrombosis, pulmonary embolism

Table 24-10 Hematologic Values During Infancy and Childhood

					Differential Counts				
Age	Hemoglobin (g/dl):Mean	Hematocrit (%):Mean	Reticulocytes (%):Mean	Leukocytes (WBC/mm^3): Mean	Neutrophils (%):Mean	Lymphocytes (%):Mean	Eosinophils (%):Mean	Monocytes (%):Mean	Platelets (10^3/mm^3)
Cord blood	16.8	55	5.0	18,000	61	31	2	6	290
2 wk	16.5	50	1.0	12,000	40	48	3	9	252
3 mo	12.0	36	1.0	12,000	30	63	2	5	140-340
6 mo–6 yr	12.0	37	1.0	10,000	45	48	2	5	140-340
7-12 yr	13.0	38	1.0	8,000	55	38	2	5	140-340
Adult	13.0	40	1.0	8,000	55	35	2	5	140-340
Female	14	41	0.8-4.1	7,400	54-62	25-33	1-4	3-7	140-340
Male	16	47	0.8-2.5	7,400	54-62	25-33	1-4	3-7	140-340

infant. In the preschool and school-age child, hemoglobin, hematocrit, and red blood cell counts gradually rise. Metabolic processes within the erythrocytes of neonates differ significantly from those of erythrocytes in the normal adult. The relatively young population of erythrocytes in the newborn consumes greater quantities of glucose than do erythrocytes in adults.

The lymphocytes of children tend to have more cytoplasm and less compact nuclear chromatin than do the lymphocytes of adults. A possible explanation is that children tend to have more frequent viral infections, which are associated with atypical lymphocytes. Even minor infections, in which the child fails to exhibit clinical manifestations of illness, and administration of immunizations may result in lymphocyte changes.[21]

The lymphocyte count is high at birth, continues to rise during the first year of life, and then steadily declines until lower adult values are reached. It is unknown whether these developmental variations are physiologic or a pathologic response to frequent viral infections and immunizations in children.

At birth the neutrophil count is very high and rises during the early days of life.[22] After 2 weeks, neutrophil counts fall to within or below normal adult ranges. By approximately 4 years of age, the neutrophil count is the same as that of an adult.

Eosinophil count is high in the first year of life and is higher in children than in teenagers or adults.[23] Monocyte counts are high in the first year of life and then decrease to adult levels. Platelet counts in full-term neonates are comparable to platelet counts in adults and remain so throughout infancy and childhood.[24]

Aging and the Hematologic System

Blood composition changes little with age. Erythrocyte life span is normal, although erythrocytes are replenished more slowly after bleeding, probably because of iron depletion. Total serum iron, total iron-binding capacity, and intestinal iron absorption are all decreased in the elderly.[25] Iron deficiency is often responsible for the low hemoglobin levels noted in elderly people. The plasma membranes of erythrocytes become increasingly fragile, with portions lost, presumably because of physical trauma inflicted during circulation.

Lymphocyte function decreases with age (see Chapters 6 and 7), causing changes in cellular immunity with some decline in T cell function. The humoral immune system is less able to respond to antigenic challenge.

No changes in platelet numbers or structure have been observed in elderly persons, yet evidence shows that platelet adhesiveness probably increases.[26] Although fibrinogen levels and factors V, VII, and IX tend to be increased in the elderly population, evidence about hypercoagulability is inconclusive.

SUMMARY REVIEW

Components of the Hematologic System

1. Blood consists of a variety of formed elements: about 90% water and 10% solutes. In adults the total blood volume is approximately 5.5 L.
2. Plasma, a complex aqueous liquid, contains three major groups of plasma proteins: albumins, globulins, and clotting factors.
3. The cellular elements of blood are the erythrocytes, leukocytes, lymphocytes, and platelets.
4. Erythrocytes are the most abundant cells of the blood, occupying approximately 48% of the blood volume in men and approximately 42% in women. Erythrocytes are responsible for tissue oxygenation.
5. Leukocytes are fewer in number than erythrocytes and constitute approximately 5000 to 10,000 cells per mm^3 of blood. Leukocytes defend the body against infection and remove dead or injured host cells.
6. Leukocytes are classified as either granulocytes (neutrophils, basophils, eosinophils) or agranulocytes (monocytes, macrophages).
7. Platelets are not cells, but disk-shaped cytoplasmic fragments. Platelets are essential for blood coagulation and control of bleeding.
8. The lymphoid organs are classified as primary (thymus and bone marrow) or secondary (spleen, lymph nodes, tonsils, and Peyer patches of the small intestine).
9. The lymphoid organs are sites of residence, proliferation, differentiation, or function of lymphocytes and mononuclear phagocytes.
10. The spleen is the largest of the secondary lymphoid organs and functions as the site of fetal hematopoiesis, filters and cleanses the blood, and is a reservoir for lymphocytes and other blood cells.
11. The lymph nodes are the site of development or activity of large numbers of lymphocytes, monocytes, and macrophages.
12. The mononuclear phagocyte system (MPS), previously called the *reticuloendothelial system (RES),* is composed of monoblasts, promonocytes, and monocytes in bone marrow, monocytes in peripheral blood, and macrophages in tissue.
13. The MPS is the main line of defense against bacteria in the bloodstream and cleanses the blood by removing old, injured, or dead blood cells; antigen-antibody complexes; and macromolecules.

Development of Blood Cells

1. Hematopoiesis, or blood cell production, occurs in the liver and spleen of the fetus and in the bone marrow after birth.
2. Hematopoiesis involves two stages: (a) proliferation and (b) differentiation, or maturation. Each type of blood cell has parent cells called *stem cells.*
3. Hematopoiesis continues throughout life to replace blood cells that grow old and die, are killed by disease, or are lost through bleeding.
4. Bone marrow consists of blood vessels, nerves, mononuclear phagocytes, stem cells, blood cells in various stages of differentiation, and fatty tissue.
5. Hemoglobin, the oxygen-carrying protein of the erythrocyte, enables the blood to transport 100 times more oxygen than could be transported dissolved in plasma alone.

6. Erythropoiesis depends on the presence of vitamins (especially vitamin B_{12}, folate, B_6, riboflavin, pantothenic acid, niacin, ascorbic acid, and vitamin E).
7. Regulation of erythropoiesis is mediated by erythropoietin. Erythropoietin is secreted by the kidneys in response to tissue hypoxia and causes a compensatory increase in erythrocyte production if the oxygen content of the blood decreases because of anemia, high altitude, or pulmonary disease.
8. Maintenance of optimal levels of granulocytes and monocytes in the blood depends on the availability of pluripotential stem cells in the marrow, induction of these into committed stem cells, and timely release of new cells from the marrow.
9. Specific humoral colony-stimulating factors (CSFs) are necessary for the adequate growth of myeloid, erythroid, lymphoid, and megakaryocytic lineages.
10. Platelets develop from megakaryocytes by a process called *endomitosis*. In endomitosis the megakaryocytes undergo mitosis but not cytokinesis; thus the cell does not divide into two daughter cells.

Mechanisms of Hemostasis

1. Hemostasis, or arrest of bleeding, involves (a) vasoconstriction (vasospasm), (b) formation of a platelet plug, (c) activation of the clotting cascade, (d) formation of a blood clot, and (e) clot retraction and clot dissolution.
2. Two properties of normal vascular endothelium prevent clotting: (a) the smooth texture of the endothelial lining that prevents adherence of platelets and (b) the negative charge of protein in the endothelial cells that repels some negatively charged platelets and clotting factors.
3. Lysis of blood clots is the function of the fibrinolytic system. Plasmin, a proteolytic enzyme, splits fibrin and fibrinogen into fibrin degradation products that dissolve the clot.

Clinical Evaluation of the Hematologic System

1. Tests of bone marrow function include bone marrow aspiration and bone marrow biopsy.

Pediatrics and the Hematologic System

1. Blood cell counts rise above adult levels at birth and then gradually decline throughout childhood.
2. The average blood volume of an infant is 75 to 77 ml/kg, which is similar to that of older children and adults.
3. In response to the change from a placental to a pulmonary oxygen supply during the first few days of life, levels of erythropoietin and the rate of blood cell formation decrease.
4. During the first week of life with rapid growth, the rate of erythrocyte destruction is greater than later in childhood and adulthood.
5. The normal erythrocyte life span is 60 to 80 days in full-term infants, 20 to 30 days in premature infants, and 120 days in children, adolescents, and adults.
6. The lymphocyte count is high at birth, rises during the first year of life, and steadily declines until lower adult volumes are reached.
7. The neutrophil count is very high at birth, falls to adult ranges after 2 weeks, and is the same as for adults by 4 years of age.
8. The eosinophil count is high in the first year of life and is higher in children than in adolescents and adults. Monocyte counts are high in the first year of life and decrease to adult levels.
9. Platelet counts in full-term infants are comparable with those in adults and remain so throughout childhood.

Aging and the Hematologic System

1. Blood composition changes little with age. A delay in erythrocyte replenishment may occur after bleeding, presumably because of iron deficiency.
2. Lymphocyte function appears to decrease with age. Particularly affected is a decrease in cellular immunity.
3. Platelet adhesiveness probably increases with age.

KEY TERMS

Agranulocyte, *815*
Albumin, *812*
Basophil, *815*
Biconcavity, *813*
Blood clot, *833*
Bone marrow (myeloid tissue), *823*
Clotting factor, *812*
Coagulation cascade, *833*
Colony-stimulating factor (CSF), *819*
Deoxyhemoglobin (reduced hemoglobin), *826*
Endomitosis, *830*
Eosinophil, *815*
Erythroblast, *824*
Erythrocyte (red blood cell [RBC]), *813*
Erythron, *824*
Erythropoiesis, *824*
Erythropoietin, *824*
Fibrin degradation product (FDP), *835*
Fibrinolytic system, *835*
Globin, *825*
Granulocyte, *815*
Hematopoiesis, *820*
Hematopoietic growth factor, *822*
Heme, *825*
Hemoglobin (Hb), *813*
Hemostasis, *830*
Immunocyte, *814*
Intrinsic factor (IF), *826*
Leukocyte (white blood cell), *813*
Lipoprotein, *813*
Lymph node, *818*
Lymphocyte, *817*
Macrophage, *816*
Marginating storage pool, *820*
Mast cell, *815*
Maturation (differentiation), *820*
Megakaryocyte, *817*
Megaloblast, *824*
Methemoglobin, *825*
Mitotic division (proliferation), *820*
Monocyte, *816*
Myeloid tissue, *822*
Myoglobin, *828*
Mononuclear phagocyte system (MPS) (reticuloendothelial system [RES]), *816*
Natural killer (NK) cell, *817*
Neutrophil (polymorphonuclear neutrophil [PMN]), *815*
Normoblast, *824*
Oxyhemoglobin, *826*
Phagocyte, *814*
Plasma, *811*
Plasma protein, *811*
Platelet (thrombocyte), *813*
Pluripotential stem cell (pluripotential myeloid stem cell [PMSC]), *822*

KEY TERMS—cont'd

REFERENCES

1. Babior BM, Stossel TP: *Hematology: a pathophysiological approach,* New York, 1984, Churchill Livingstone.
2. Moretta A et al: Surface receptors delivery opposite signals regulate the function of human NK cells, *Semin Immunol* 12(2):129, 2000.
3. Hobisch-Hagen P et al: Low platelet count and elevated serum thrombopoietin after severe trauma, *Eur J Haematol* 64(3):157, 2000.
4. Wang Q et al: Interferon-alpha directly represses megakaryopoiesis by inhibiting thrombopoietin-induced signaling through induction of SOCS-1, *Blood* 96(6):2093, 2000.
5. Harmening DM, editor: *Clinical hematology and fundamentals of hemostasis,* ed 3, Philadelphia: 1997, F.A. Davis.
6. Burke LJ, Baniahmad A: Co-repressors 2000, *FASEB J* 13:1876, 2000.
7. Grandori C et al: The MYC/MAXIMAD network and the transcriptional control of cell behavior, *Annu Rev Cell Div Biol* 16:653, 2000.
8 Alberts B et al: *Molecular biology of the cell,* ed 4, New York, 1999, Garland.
9. Ogilvy S et al: Constitutive Bcl-2 expression throughout the hematopoietic compartment affects multiple lineages and enhances progenitor cell survival, *Proc Natl Acad Sci* 96(26):14943, 1999;
10. Metcalf D: Cellular hemoatopoiesis in the twentieth century, *Semin Hematol* 36(4 suppl 7):5, 1999.
11. Russell WJ et al: Active bone marrow distribution in the adult, *Br J Radiol* 39:735, 1966.
12. Stilgenbauer F et al: Recombinant human erythropoietin in the treatment of cancer, *Antibiot Chemother* 50:106, 2000.
13. Macdougall IC: Meeting the challenges of a new millennium: optimizing the use of recombinant human erythropoietin, *Nephrol Dial Transplant* 13(suppl 23):23, 1998.
14. Moore RD: Human immunodeficiency virus infection, anemia, and survival: *Clin Infect Dis* 29(1):44, 1999.
15. Winearls GC: Recombinant human erythropoietin: 10 years of clinical experience, *Nephrol Dial Transplant* 13(suppl 2):3, 1998.
16. McMahon TJ et al: Functional coupling of oxygen binding and vasoactivity in S-nitrosohemoglobin, *J Biol Chem* 275(22):16738, 2000.
17. Jai L, Bonaventura J, Stamler JS: S-nitrosohaemoglobin: a dynamic activity of blood involved in vascular control, *Nature* 380(6571):221, 1996.
18. Goldwasser E: Erythropoietin: a somewhat personal history, *Perspect Biol Med* 40(1):18, 1996.
19. Fishbach D, Fogdall R: *Coagulation: the essentials,* Baltimore, 1981, Williams & Wilkins.
20. Rosenson RS, Lowe GD: Effects of lipids and lipoproteins on thrombosis and rheology, *Atherosclerosis* 140(2):271, 1998.
21. Mauer AM: *Pediatric hematology,* New York, 1969, McGraw-Hill.
22. Manroe BL et al: The neonatal blood count in health and disease: reference values for neutrophilic cells, *J Pediatr* 95:89, 1979.
23. de Sauvage FJ et al: Stimulation of megakaryocytopoiesis and thrombopoiesis by the c-mpl ligand, *Nature* 369(6481):533, 1994.
24. Albin AR et al: Platelet enumeration in the neonatal period, *Pediatrics,* 28:822, 1961.
25. Garry PJ et al: Effects of iron intake on iron stores in elderly men and women: longitudinal and cross-sectional results, *J Am Coll Nutr* 19(2):262, 2000.
26. McBane RD et al: Fibrinogen, fibrin, and crosslinking in aging arterial thrombi, *Thromb Haemost* 84(1):83, 2000.

CHAPTER 25

Alterations of Erythrocyte Function

THOM J. MANSEN • KATHRYN L. McCANCE

CHAPTER OUTLINE

Alterations of erythrocyte function involve either insufficient or excessive numbers of erythrocytes in the circulation or normal numbers of cells with abnormal components. Anemias are conditions in which there are too few erythrocytes or an insufficient volume of erythrocytes in the blood. Polycythemias are conditions in which erythrocyte numbers or volume is excessive. Each of these two conditions has many causes, and in turn each is known by many names. Anemia and polycythemia are not diseases per se but rather are pathophysiologic manifestations of a variety of disease states.

ANEMIA

Strictly speaking, **anemia** is a reduction in the total number of erythrocytes in the circulating blood or a decrease in the quality or quantity of hemoglobin. Anemias commonly result from (1) impaired erythrocyte production, (2) blood loss (acute or chronic), (3) increased erythrocyte destruction, or (4) a combination of these three.

Classification

Anemias are classified in two ways, according to their etiology or by their morphology (Box 25-1). Morphologic classification is based on two cellular characteristics: size and hemoglobin content. All anemias may be described by these two cellular attributes, making morphologic classification the most common method used (Table 25-1). Cellular size is identified by terms that end in "cytic," whereas hemoglobin content is identified by terms that end in "chromic" (Table 25-2). Additional descriptions of erythrocytes associated with some anemias include **anisocytosis** (assuming various sizes) or **poikilocytosis** (assuming various shapes) (Fig. 25-1).

Clinical Manifestations

The major physiologic manifestation of anemia is a reduced oxygen-carrying capacity of the blood, producing tissue hypoxia. Symptoms of anemia vary in severity and number depending upon the body's ability to compensate for this reduced capacity. If the reduction in red cells is moderate with a gradual onset, compensation may be so successful that the individual is asymptomatic except during periods of physical exertion. As the reduction in red cells continues, symptoms become more evident and alterations of specific organs and compensation effects become more apparent. Compensation occurs by the cardiovascular, respiratory, and hematologic systems. Hematologic findings in various anemias are listed in Table 25-3 on p. 847, and progression and manifestations of anemias are in Fig. 25-2 on p. 848.

A reduction in the number of red blood cells, as seen after hemorrhage, causes a reduction in blood volume. Compensation for a reduced blood volume causes fluids to move from the interstitium into the intravascular space, expanding plasma volume. Although this compensatory mechanism maintains adequate blood volume, the viscosity (thickness) decreases, causing the blood to become "diluted." The diluted blood flows faster and more turbulently than normal blood.

Over time, increased blood flow within the heart chambers causes ventricular dysfunction, cardiac dilation, and heart valve insufficiency. Hypoxia further contributes to anemic cardiovascular alterations by causing the arterioles, venules, and capillaries to dilate, which further increases the flow of blood. Augmented intracardiac blood flow promotes the blood return to the heart, causing it to increase its contractions and rate (cardiac output). These actions meet the increased metabolic demands for oxygen and prevent cardiac congestion. Cardiovascular compensatory mechanisms

Box 25-1

ETIOLOGIC (PATHOPHYSIOLOGIC) CLASSIFICATION OF ANEMIAS

DECREASED OR DEFECTIVE PRODUCTION OF ERYTHROCYTES

Altered hemoglobin synthesis
- Iron deficiency
- Thalassemia
- Anemia of chronic inflammation

Altered deoxyribonucleic acid (DNA) synthesis resulting from deficient nutrients
- Pernicious anemia (decreased B_{12}, folate)

Stem cell dysfunction
- Aplastic anemia
- Myeloproliferative leukemia

Bone marrow infiltration
- Carcinoma
- Lymphoma

Pure red cell aplasia

INCREASED ERYTHROCYTE DESTRUCTION

Blood loss
- Acute—hemorrhage, trauma
- Chronic—gastrointestinal bleeding, menorrhagia

Hemolysis (intracorpuscular defect)
- Membrane—hereditary spherocytosis
- Hemoglobin—sickle cell trait or disease
- Glycolysis—pyruvate kinase
- Oxidation—glucose-6-phosphate dehydrogenase (G6PD) deficiency

Hemolysis (extracorpuscular defect)
- Immune mechanisms—warm antibody/cold antibody
- Infection—clostridial, malarial
- Trauma to erythrocyte—hemolytic uremic syndrome
- Splenic sequestration—hypersplenism

may contribute to the development of congestive heart failure. (Mechanisms of congestive heart failure are described in Chapter 29.)

Tissue hypoxia creates further demands and effects on the pulmonary and hematologic systems. The rate and depth of breathing is increased in an attempt to make more oxygen available to the remaining erythrocytes. Hemoglobin in the erythrocytes releases its oxygen at the tissue level more readily than usual because of an increase in diphosphatidylglycerol (DPG) in the erythrocytes. (Mechanisms of oxygen transport and release by hemoglobin are described in Chapter 31.) When, in the course of the anemia, compensatory mechanisms fail, the individual experiences shortness of breath (dyspnea), a rapid, pounding heartbeat (palpitations), dizzyness, and fatigue even at rest. Decreased blood supply to skeletal and cardiac muscle may also result in muscle pain or claudication and cardiac angina.

When the anemia is severe or rapid in onset, peripheral blood vessels constrict to redirect available blood flow to vital organs. Renal blood flow is decreased and the kidneys, sensing the decreased blood flow, activate the renal renin-angiotensin response. This life-saving maneuver increases salt and water retention to increase blood volume and improve kidney perfusion.

Other manifestations of anemia occur in various organ systems. The skin, mucous membranes, lips, nail beds, and conjunctivae become pale because of reduced hemoglobin concentration. The skin may also become yellowish due to accumulation in the skin of the products of red cell destruction or hemolysis. The skin also suffers from impaired healing and loss of elasticity as well as thinning and early graying of the hair.

If the anemia is caused by a vitamin B_{12} deficiency, the nervous system is affected. Myelin degeneration may occur with loss of fibers in the spinal core. Paresthesias (numbness), gait disturbances, extreme weakness, spasticity, and reflex abnormalities may result. Decreased oxygen supply to the gastrointestinal (GI) tract often produces abdominal pain, nausea, vomiting, and anorexia. A low-grade fever (less than 101° F) occurs in some anemic individuals and may be the result of leukocyte pyrogens being released from ischemic tissues.

Therapeutic intervention for any anemic condition calls for treatment of the underlying disorder and palliation of symptoms. Therapies for anemia include transfusions, dietary correction, and administration of supplemental vitamins or iron.

Macrocytic-Normochromic Anemias

The **macrocytic anemias,** also termed *megaloblastic anemias*, are characterized by defective DNA synthesis that results in ineffecitve erythropoiesis, manifested by unusually large stem cells (megaloblasts) in the marrow that mature into unusually large stem cells (macrocytes) in the circulation. In addition to an increase in size (diameter), the thickness and volume of the cell also increase.[1] Defective DNA synthesis is caused by deficiencies of vitamin B_{12} (cobalamin) or folate, coenzymes that are required for nuclear maturation and the DNA synthetic pathway.

In spite of defective DNA synthesis in megaloblasts, ribonucleic acid (RNA)-controlled processes (RNA replication and hemoglobin synthesis) proceed at a normal rate, causing the cytoplasm and nucleus to grow and develop at unequal rates. Asynchronous cytoplasmic and nuclear development produces megaloblastic stem cells that are larger at all maturational stages than normal stem cells (normoblasts) with a nucleus that is immature and disproportionately small relative to the size of the red cell. With each cell division the disproportion between RNA and DNA becomes more obvious.

As the megaloblastic cell matures and begins to synthesize hemoglobin, chromatin in the nucleus fails to clump normally, resulting in finely distributed chromatin throughout the nucleus. The altered pattern of chromatin deposition also may be used to differentiate normoblasts from megaloblasts. Hemoglobin increases in proportion to the size of the cell; thus the MCHC remains normal and the megaloblastic anemias, in the absence of complications, are normochromic.[1]

Ineffective erythropoiesis also may result in premature cell death within the bone marrow, further reducing the number of erythrocytes and exacerbating the existing anemic condition. Destruction of these red cells produces an increase in serum bilirubin and lactate dehydrogenase.[2]

Table 25-1 Morphologic Classification of Anemias

Morphology and Cause of Reduced Oxygen-Carrying Capacity of the Blood	Name and Mechanism of Anemic Condition	Primary Cause of Associated Disorder
Macrocytic-normochromic anemia: large, abnormally shaped erythrocytes but normal hemoglobin concentrations	Pernicious anemia: lack of vitamin B_{12} (cobalamin) for erythropoiesis; abnormal deoxyribonucleic acid (DNA) and ribonucleic acid (RNA) synthesis in the erythroblast; premature cell death	Congenital or acquired deficiency of intrinsic factor (IF); genetic disorder of DNA synthesis
	Folate deficiency anemia: lack of folate for erythropoiesis; premature cell death	Dietary folate deficiency
Microcytic-hypochromic anemia: small, abnormally shaped erythrocytes and reduced hemoglobin concentration	Iron deficiency anemia: lack of iron for hemoglobin production; insufficient hemoglobin	Chronic blood loss; dietary iron deficiency, disruption of iron metabolism or iron cycle (see Chapter 24)
	Sideroblastic anemia: dysfunctional iron uptake by erythroblasts and defective porphyrin and heme synthesis	Congenital dysfunction of iron metabolism in erythroblasts, acquired dysfunction of iron metabolism as a result of drugs or toxins
	Thalassemia: impaired synthesis of alpha or beta chain of hemoglobin A; phagocytosis of abnormal erythroblasts in the marrow	Congenital genetic defect of globin synthesis
Normocytic-normochromic anemia: destruction or depletion of normal erythroblasts or mature erythrocytes	Aplastic anemia: insufficient erythropoiesis	Depressed stem cell proliferation resulting in bone marrow aplasia
	Posthemorrhagic anemia: blood loss	Acute or chronic hemorrhage that stimulates increased erythropoiesis, which eventually depletes body iron
	Hemolytic anemia: premature destruction (lysis) of mature erythrocytes in the circulation	Any condition that increases fragility of erythrocytes
	Sickle cell anemia: abnormal hemoglobin synthesis, abnormal cell shape with susceptibility to damage, lysis, and phagocytosis	Congenital dysfunction of hemoglobin synthesis
	Anemia of chronic disease: abnormally increased demand for new erythrocytes	Chronic infection or inflammation; malignancy

Table 25-2 Terms Used in Assessment of Erythrocytes

	Erythrocyte Volume	Hemoglobin Content
Normal	Normocytic	Normochromic
Increased	Macrocytic (higher mean corpuscular volume [MCV])	Hyperchromic (higher mean corpuscular hemoglobin concentration MCHC])
Decreased	Microcytic (lower MCV)	Hypochromic (lower MCHC)

In addition to the red cells being affected by defective DNA synthesis, the white cells (neutrophils) also may demonstrate marked enlargement (giant metamyelocytes). Further, other cells throughout the body, particularly those with high turnover rates (intestinal mucosa and other epithelia), may demonstrate enlargement and nuclear abnormalities.[2]

Pernicious Anemia

Pernicious anemia (PA), the most common type of megaloblastic anemia, is caused by vitamin B_{12} deficiency and is associated with the end stage of type A chronic atrophic (autoimmune) gastritis[3] (Figs. 25-1, *C*, and 25-3). *Pernicious* means highly injurious or destructive and reflects the fact that this condition was once fatal. Although rare in individuals less than 30 years of age, it is more common in those of Northern European descent as well as blacks and Hispanics. Females, because of their longer life span[4] are more prone to develop PA, with black females more prone to an earlier onset.[3]

Pathophysiology

The underlying disorder in PA is an absence of intrinsic factor (IF), an enzyme required for absorption of dietary vitamin B_{12}. IF, along with hydrochloric acid, is secreted by gastric parietal cells. Causes of PA include a congenital deficiency in secretion of IF or secretion of a defective IF, partial or complete removal of the stomach (gastrectomy), and gastric atrophy of the parietal cells associated with type A chronic gastritis. Autoimmunity plays a significant role in the development of the condition, characterized by the presence of autoantibodies to gastric parietal cells in the serum and gastric juice. Other characteristics associated with chronic gastric atrophy include achlorhydria, low serum levels of pepsinogen I, hypergastrinemia, and gastric carcinoids.

The early manifestation of the gastric lesion of PA is characterized by chronic infiltration of the gastric submucosa with inflammatory cells; eventuallly extending into the lam-

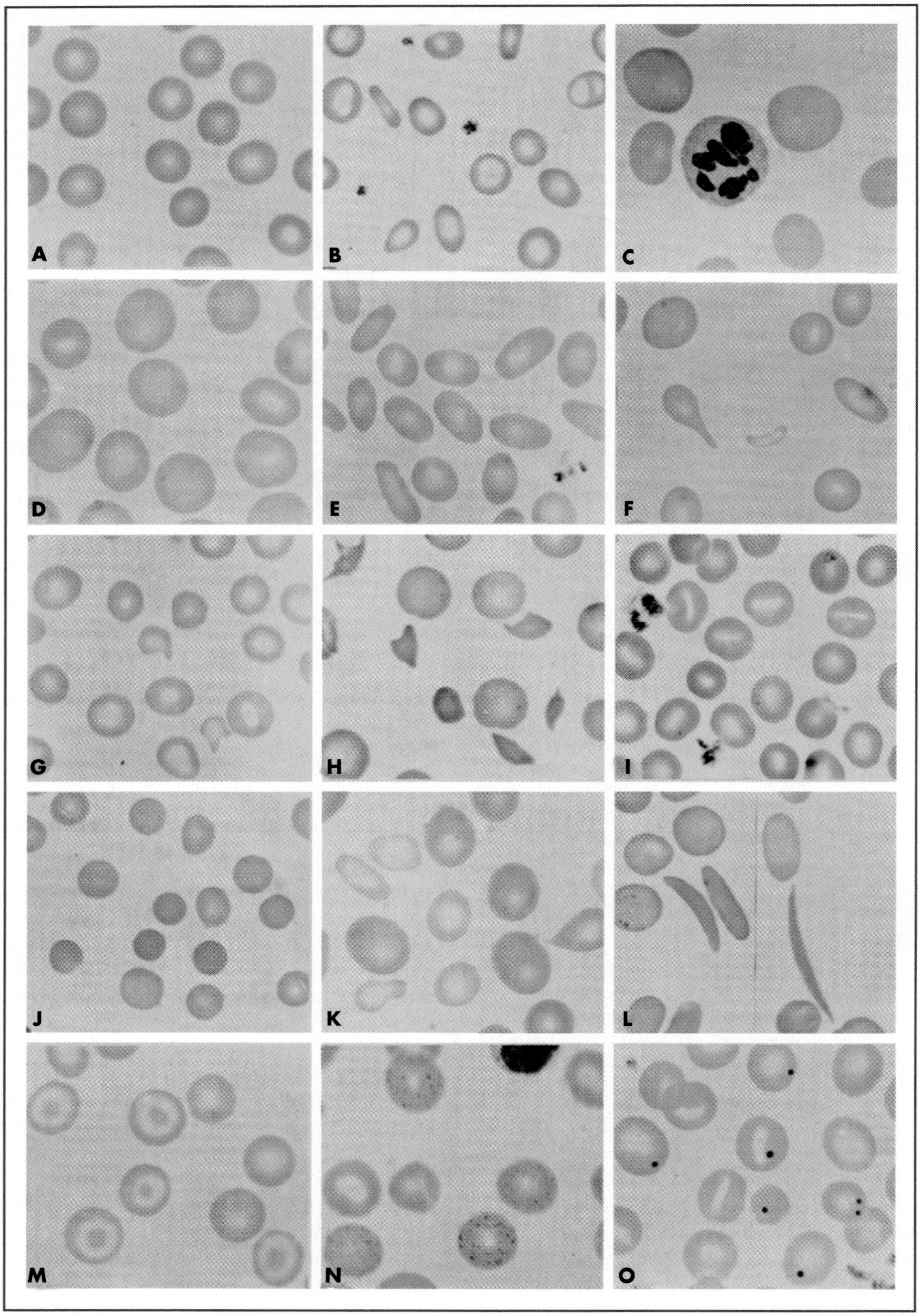

FIG. 25-1 Appearance of red blood cells in various disorders. **A,** Normal blood smear. **B,** Hypochromic microcytic anemia (iron deficiency). **C,** Macrocytic anemia (pernicious anemia). **D,** Macrocytic anemia in pregnancy. **E,** Hereditary elliptocytosis. **F,** Myelofibrosis (teardrop). **G,** Hemolytic anemia associated with prosthetic heart valve. **H,** Microangiopathic anemia. **I,** Stomatocytes. **J,** Spherocytes (hereditary spherocytosis). **K,** Sideroblastic anemia; note the double population of red blood cells. **L,** Sickle cell anemia. **M,** Target cells (after splenectomy). **N,** Basophil stippling in case of unexplained anemia. **O,** Howell-Jolly bodies (after splenectomy). (From Wintrobe MM et al: *Clinical hematology*, ed 8, Philadelphia, 1981, Lea & Febiger.)

Table 25-3 Laboratory Findings for Various Anemias

Test	Pernicious Anemia	Folate Deficiency Anemia	Iron Deficiency Anemia	Sideroblastic Anemia	Aplastic Anemia	Posthemorrhagic Anemia	Hemolytic Anemia	Anemia of Chronic Inflammation
Hemoglobin	Low	Low	Low	Low	Low or normal	Normal or low	Low	Low
Hematocrit	Low	Low	Low	Low	Low or normal	Normal or low	Low	Low
Reticulocyte count	Low	Low	Normal or slightly high or low	Normal or slightly high	Low	Increased	High	Normal
Mean corpuscular volume	High	High	Low	Low	Normal or slightly high	Slightly low	Normal or high	Normal or low
Plasma iron	High	High	Low	High	High	Normal	Normal or high	Low
Total iron-binding capacity	Normal	Normal	High	Normal	Normal	Normal	Normal	Low
Ferritin	High	High	Low	High	Normal	Normal	Normal	Normal
Serum B_{12}	Low	Normal	Normal	Normal	Normal	Normal	Normal	Normal
Folate	Normal	Low	Normal	Normal	Normal	Normal	Normal	Normal
Bilirubin	Slightly high	Slightly high	Normal	High	Normal	Normal	Slightly high	Normal
Free erythrocyte protoporphyrin	Normal	Normal	High	Increased or normal	High	Normal	Normal	Normal or slightly high
Transferrin	Slightly high	Slightly high	Low	High	Normal	Normal	Normal	Slightly low

ina propria and causing degeneration of the parietal and zymogenic cells. Late in the process, the parietal and zymogenic cells are lost and replaced by mucus-containing cells (intestinal metaplasia). The antigen recognized by autoantibodies associated with chronic gastritis has been identified as H^+/K^+ ATPase. This enzyme is responsible for secretion of hydrogen ions by parietal cells in exchange for potassium ions.[3]

Loss of parietal cells leads to the loss of IF, which is the major factor in the development of vitamin B_{12} deficiency and PA. A direct correlation exists between the severity of the gastric lesion and the degree of malabsorption of vitamin B_{12}. Additionally, the autoantibodies present in gastric juice bind with vitamin B_{12} at the IF binding site, preventing the formation of the B_{12}-IF complex.

Genetic factors play a significant role in the development of chronic gastritis and PA as evidenced by the presence of autoantibodies and by the clustering of the disease within families. It is estimated that 20% to 30% of relatives of individuals with PA also have PA. These relatives also demonstrate a higher frequency of the presence of gastric autoantibodies, particularly first-degree female relatives.

Pernicious anemia can be associated with other autoimmune conditions, particularly those that affect the endocrine system, including chronic autoimmunne thyroiditis (Hashimoto thyroiditis), type 1 diabetes mellitus, Addison disease, primary hypoparathyroidism, Graves disease, and myasthenia gravis.[3]

Chronic gastritis may also be secondary to excessive alcohol ingestion, hot tea, and smoking. Individuals with PA are at risk for the development of gastric carcinoma due to intestinal metaplasia. The incidence of carcinoma in individuals with PA is 2% to 3 %.

Clinical Manifestations

Pernicious anemia develops slowly; it may take from 20 to 30 years, with 60 years of age the median age of diagnosis. Because symptoms develop slowly, it is usually severe by the time the individual seeks treatment. Vague early symptoms—including infections; mood swings; and gastrointestinal, cardiac, or kidney ailments—often are ignored. When the hemoglobin has decreased significantly (7 to 8 g/dl), the individual experiences the classic symptoms of anemia: weakness, fatigue, parasthesias of the feet and fingers, and difficulty in walking.

Neurologic manifestations are the result of nerve demyelination and may result in neuronal death. The posterior and lateral columns of the spinal cord also may be affected, causing the individual to experience loss of position and vibration sense, ataxia, and spasticity. These complications pose a serious threat because they are not reversible, even with appropriate treatment. The cerebrum may also be involved with manifestations ranging from mild personality defects and memory loss to obvious psychosis.[3]

Additionally, the individual may experience a loss of appetite, abdominal pain, and a beefy red tongue due to atrophic glossitis. The skin may become "lemon yellow" (sallow) caused by a combination of pallor and icterus. The liver may be enlarged, especially in the elderly, indicating

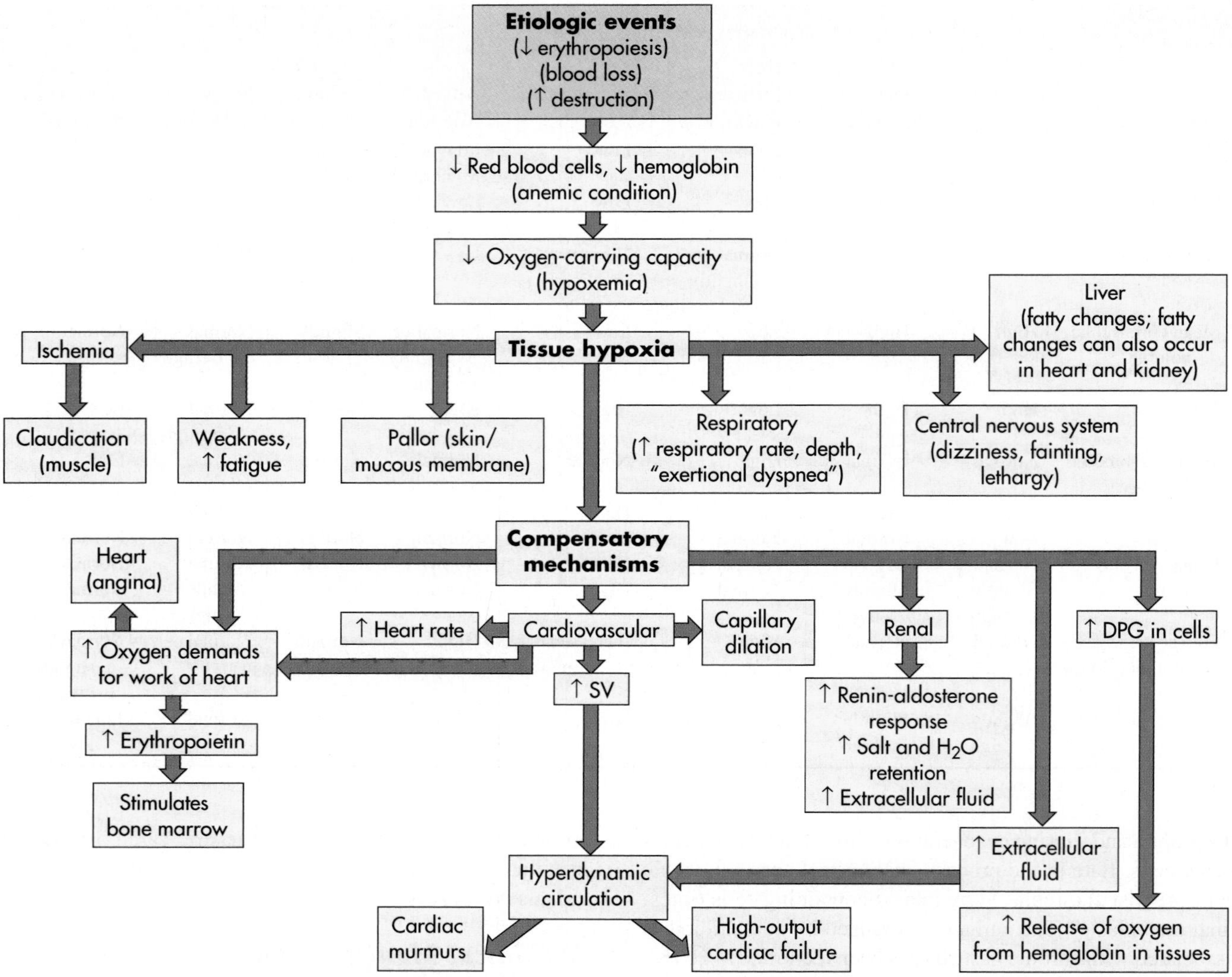

FIG. 25-2 Progression and manifestations of anemia. *SV*, Stroke volume; *DPG*, diphosphatidylglycerol.

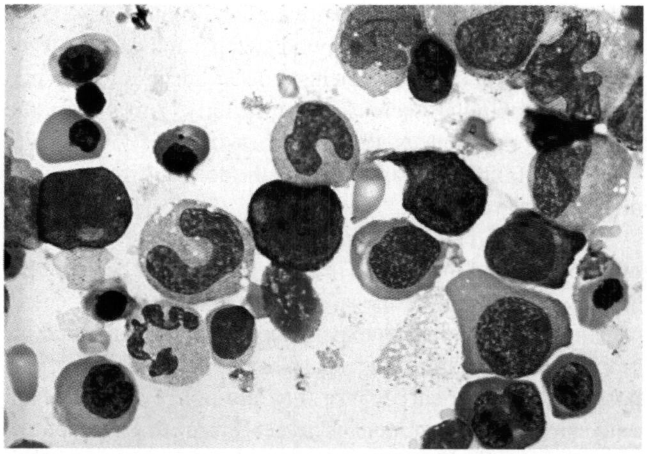

FIG. 25-3 Bone marrow aspirate from individual with pernicious anemia. Bone marrow aspirate smear from an individual with megaloblastic red cell precursors and giant metamyelocytes. The chromatin in the red blood cell nuclei is more dispersed than in normal red cell precursors at comparable stages of maturation; the giant metamyelocytes have dispersed nuclear chromatin in contrast to a normal metamyelocyte, which has condensed chromatin (Wright-Giemsa stain). (From Damjanov I, Linder J, editors: *Anderson's pathology*, ed 10, St Louis, 1996, Mosby.)

right-sided heart failure. The spleen also may be enlarged but nonpalpable.

Evaluation and Treatment

Diagnosis of PA is based on a variety of tests (see Table 25-3), which include blood tests, bone marrow aspiration, serologic studies, gastric biopsy, clinical manifestations, and the Schilling test. In the Schilling test, vitamin B_{12} absorption is measured indirectly by administering radioactive vitamin B_{12} and measuring its excretion in the urine. Low urinary excretion of radioactive vitamin B_{12} is significant for PA. A second test is frequently done to confirm the diagnosis. In the second test, IF may be administered to see if urinary excretion increases. If urinary excretion does not increase, other causes must be considered.[5]

Serologic studies reveal the presence of antibodies, which may also be present in gastric juices. Gastric biopsy reveals total achlorhydria, which is diagnostic for PA, because it is the only gastric lesion causing this condition.

Untreated PA is fatal, usually due to heart failure. Death occurs after a course of remissions and exacerbations lasting from 1 to 3 years. Since 1926, when replacement therapy began, mortality has been reduced significantly. Today, death from PA is rare and any relapses that occur are usually the result of noncompliance with therapy.

Treatment is replacement of vitamin B_{12} (cobalamin). Cyanocobalamin or hydroxocobalamin (1000 micrograms) is administered parenterally on a monthly basis. Initial injections are administered weekly until the deficiency is corrected. Conventional wisdom and practice determined that oral preparations were ineffective because there was no IF to facilitate absorption. However, recent practice has shown that oral administration is beneficial in dosages higher than parenteral dosages.[6,7] There appears to be an alternative mechanism for B_{12} absorption from the stomach that does not depend upon IF.

The effectiveness of cobalamin replacement therapy is manifested by a rising reticulocyte count. Within 5 to 6 weeks, blood counts return to normal. PA cannot be cured, so maintenance therapy must continue for life. Blood transfusions are given if the individual shows signs of circulatory collapse, heart failure, or severe angina pectoris.

Folate Deficiency Anemia

Folate (folic acid) is an essential vitamin that is required for erythrocyte production and maturation. Humans totally depend on dietary intake of folate and require 50 to 200 μg/day, with pregnant and lactating females requiring increased amounts. Folate synthesis takes place in the human intestine, but not in quantities sufficient to make any significant contribution.[8]

The primary biochemical function of folate coenzymes involves the synthesis of purines and prymidines (thyamine, adenine, and guanine) of the four DNA bases and RNA. Folate coenzymes are also involved in the synthesis of thymidylate, which is also an essential precursor of DNA. The clinical manifestations of folate deficiency are apparent when the synthesis of thymidylate is critically impaired.[8]

Absorption of folate occurs primarily in the upper small intestine and is not dependent upon the presence of any other facilitating factor. From the small intestine it is circulated to and through the liver, where it is stored. Folate deficiency is more common that cobalamin deficiency and is frequently associated with alcoholic and other chronically malnourished individuals. Fad diets and diets that are low in vegetables are also identified as causes of folate deficiency. It is argued that the established minimum daily requirement is too low and that at least 10% of persons in North America are folate deficient.[4] Inadequate dietary intake of folate results in the development of a megaloblastic anemia.

The mechanisms that cause the impaired DNA synthesis and destruction of hematopoietic cells in the presence of folate deficiency are not well understood. Apoptosis of erythroblasts in the late stages of differentiation is thought to occur in the presence of folate deficiency.[9,10] Along with anemia, folate deficiency is associated with neural tube defects of the fetus and heart disease, and is also implicated in the development of cancers, specifically colorectal cancers.[11]

Clinical manifestations of folate deficiency anemia are similar to the cachectic, malnourished appearance characteristic of PA. Accompanying the wasted appearance is severe cheilosis, stomatitis, and painful ulcerations of the buccal mucosa and tongue. Gastrointestinal symptoms may be present and include dysphagia (difficulty swallowing), flatulence, and watery diarrhea. In addition, there may be histologic changes and roentgenographic presentations of the GI tract suggestive of sprue.

Neurologic manifestations, such as those seen in PA, are generally not seen in folate deficiency anemia. If they are present, another vitamin deficiency (e.g., thiamine deficiency, which frequently accompanies folate deficiency) is probably the cause.

Treatment for folate deficiency anemia requires daily oral administration of folate preparations. One milligram per day is sufficient for most individuals, although persons with alcoholism may require 5 mg. Alcohol interferes with folate metabolism in the liver and results in profound depletion of folate stores.[12] Prophylactic dosages of 0.1 to 0.4 mg/day are sometimes given during pregnancy. Parenteral administration of folic acid (citrovorum factor or leucovorin) generally is not used except when an overdose of folate antagonists has been administered.[4] After administration of folate, the manifestations of anemia disappear within 1 to 2 weeks.

After the deficiency of folate has been corrected, long-term treatment with folate is not necessary if the individual makes the necessary dietary adjustments to maintain adequate intake. Increased amount of folate (400 μg/day) is recommended as a measure to prevent heart disease because of its ability to reduce homocysteine, which is recognized as a risk factor for the development of atherosclerosis (see Chapter 29).

Microcytic-Hypochromic Anemias

The **microcytic-hypochromic anemias** are characterized by erythrocytes that are abnormally small and contain abnormally reduced amounts of hemoglobin (see Fig. 25-1, *B*). Hypochromia occurs even in cells of normal size.

Microcytic-hypochromic anemia results from various conditions that are caused by (1) disorders of iron metabolism, (2) disorders of porphyrin and heme synthesis, or (3) disorders of globin synthesis. Specific disorders include iron deficiency anemia, sideroblastic anemia, and thalassemia.

WHAT'S NEW? *Helicobacter Pylori* and Iron Deficiency Anemia

H. pylori infection appears to be an additional stressor on women's iron status. Women who are infected with *H. pylori* bacteria were found to have a lower mean level plasma ferritin concentration than noninfected women. Daily intake of iron was the same for both groups. The exact mechanisms causing the reduction are unknown and require further investigation. *H. pylori* in the presence of IDA has also been found to be associated with delayed prepubertal growth in children.

Data from Choe YH et al: *Helicobacter pylori* infection with iron deficiency anaemia and subnormal growth at puberty, *Arch Dis Childhood* 82(2):136, 2000; Peach HG et al: *Helicobacter pylori*: an added stressor in iron status of women in the community, *Med J Australia* 169(41):188, 1998.

Iron Deficiency Anemia

Iron deficiency anemia (IDA) is the most common type of anemia worldwide. It is seen in both developing and developed countries. The overall incidence of IDA is difficult to establish because of the lack of standardized methods and techniques to determine hypoferremia and IDA.[12] Certain populations are known to be at risk for developing hypoferremia and IDA and include those living in chronic poverty, women of childbearing age, and children. In the United States, females demonstrate a higher incidence of hypoferremia (13.9%) than do males (8.3%). The incidence of IDA is also higher in females (4% to 6%) than in males (4%). The incidence peaks in females during their reproductive years and decreases after menopause. Those at highest risk are black females who live in urban poverty.[13] Males demonstrate a higher incidence during childhood and adolescence, with a decrease occurring during young adulthood and an upswing during late adulthood.[12] Children under 2 years are often affected due to the increasing requirement for iron associated with growth.

In well-developed countries the most common cause of IDA is pregnancy and chronic blood loss associated with gastric or duodenal ulcers and neoplasms. Other predisposing conditions include blood loss related to hiatal hernia, cirrhosis, hemorrhoids, and ulcerative colitis. Blood loss of 2 to 4 ml/day (1 to 2 mg of iron) is sufficient to cause hypoferremia and IDA.

Menorrhagia (excessive bleeding during menstruation) is a common cause of primary IDA in females. Related causes of this type of anemia are associated with (1) medications that cause gastrointestinal bleeding (aspirin, nonsteroidal anti-inflammatory drugs [NSAIDs]); (2) surgical procedures that decrease stomach acidity, intestinal transit time, and absorption; (3) insufficient dietary intake of iron; and (4) eating disorders, such as pica or the craving and eating of nonnutritional substances.

Iron is the essential component of hemoglobin and is in constant demand for use in normal erythropoiesis. Iron can be recycled; therefore the body maintains a balance between iron that is in use as hemoglobin and iron that is in storage and available for future hemoglobin synthesis. Blood that is lost from the body reduces the amount of iron that can be recycled from red cells, thus reducing available iron stores (see p. 827).

Iron plays an important role in the body's defense system. Pathogen survival is dependent on iron, and hypoferremia has been hypothesized as an adaptive response to reduce infectious diseases. Current studies indicate that our understanding of the relationship between iron and infection is incomplete.[14]

◆ *Pathophysiology*

Iron deficiency anemia develops slowly through three overlapping states. In stage I, the body's iron stores for erythropoiesis are depleted. Erythropoiesis proceeds normally with the hemoglobin content of red cells remaining normal also. In stage II, iron transportation to bone marrow is diminished and iron-deficient erythropoiesis takes place. Stage III begins when the small hemoglobin-deficient cells enter the circulation in sufficient numbers and replace normal erythrocytes that have reached maturity and have been removed from the circulation. Stage III is associated with IDA and characterized by depletion of iron stores and diminished hemoglobin production.

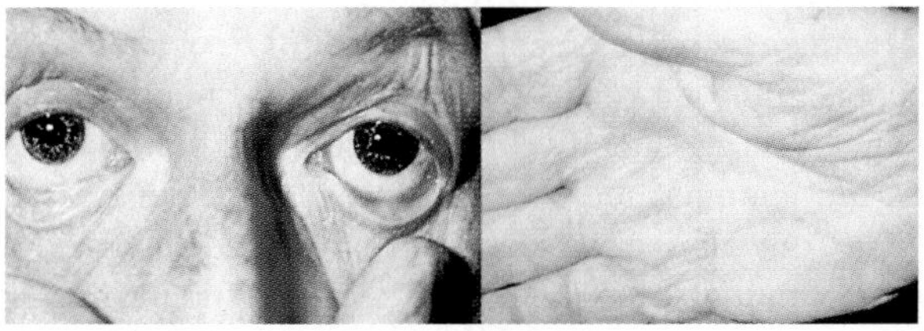

FIG. 25-4 Pallor and iron deficiency. Pallor of the skin, mucous membranes, and palmar creases in an individual with hemoglobin of 9 g/dl. Palmar creases become as pale as the surrounding skin when the hemoglobin level approaches 7 g/dl. (Courtesy Hoffbrand AV, Pettit JE, editors: *Sandoz atlas of clinical hematology*, London, 1988, Gower Medical.)

◆ *Clinical Manifestations*

Symptoms begin gradually and individuals often do not seek medical attention until hemoglobin decreases to a certain level (about 7 to 8 g/dl). Early symptoms include fatigue, weakness, and shortness of breath. Pale earlobes, palms, and conjunctivae (Fig. 25-4) are also common signs.

As the condition progresses and becomes more severe, structural and functional changes in epithelial tissue become apparent (Fig. 25-4). The nails become brittle, thin, coarsely ridged, and spoon-shaped or concave (koilonychia) as a result of impaired capillary circulation (Fig. 25-5). The tongue becomes red, sore, and painful, which is caused by atrophy of the papillae (glossitis) (Fig. 25-6). The degree of pain experienced is directly associated with the amount of iron deficiency.[15] Individuals also experience dryness and soreness in the epithelium at the corners of the mouth, known as *angular stomatitis*. Difficulty in swallowing is associated with a "web" of mucus and inflammatory cells at the juncture between the hypopharynx and esophagus. Dysphagia is also exacerbated by hyposalivation. These IDA epithelial lesions have the potential to become malignant. Recent studies have also documented that IDA is associated with malignancies, particularly of the GI tract.[16]

Because iron is a component of compounds other than hemoglobin (cytochromes, myoglobin, catalase), deficiencies probably alter several tissue enzymes. Deficient iron enzymes may cause many of the clinical manifestations. Individuals with IDA also exhibit gastritis, neuromuscular alterations, irritibility, headache, numbness, tingling, and vasomotor disturbances. The pathogenesis of neurologic symptoms is unknown but may be caused by hypoxia in already compromised cerebral vessels. Gait disturbances are rare. Mental confusion, memory loss, and disorientation frequently are as-

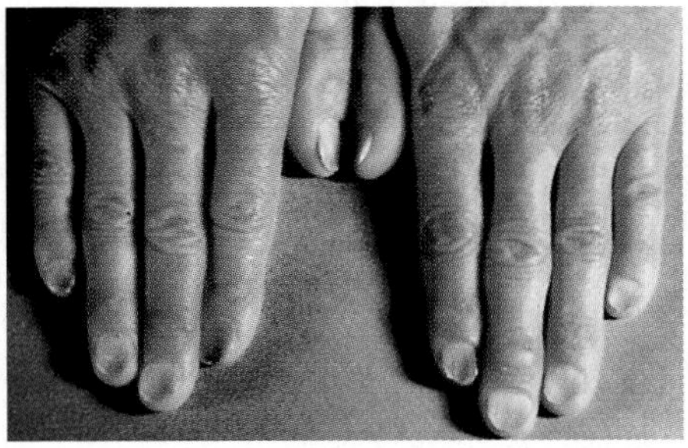

FIG. 25-5 Koilonychia. The nails are concave, ridged, and brittle. (Courtesy Hoffbrand AV, Pettit JE, editors: *Sandoz atlas of clinical hematology*, London, 1988, Gower Medical.)

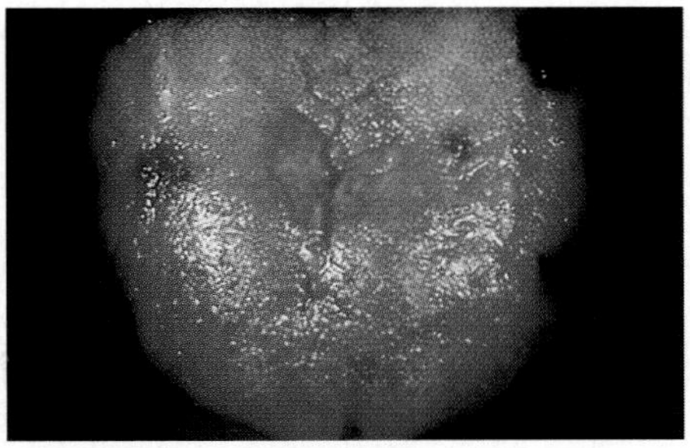

FIG. 25-6 Glossitis. Tongue of individual with iron deficiency anemia has bald, fissured appearance caused by loss of papillae and flattening. (Courtesy Hoffbrand AV, Pettit JE, editors: *Sandoz atlas of clinical hematology*, London, 1988, Gower Medical.)

sociated with anemia in the elderly population and may be wrongly perceived as normal events related to aging.

Evaluation and Treatment

Evaluation is based on clinical manifestations and laboratory tests (see Table 25-3). Iron stores are measured directly by bone marrow biopsy or indirectly by tests that measure serum ferritin, transferrin saturation, or total iron-binding capacity. A sensitive indicator of heme synthesis is the amount of free erythrocyte protoporphyrin (FEP) within erythrocytes. An important new hematologic parameter for detection of IDA is the concentration of the soluble fragment of transferrin receptor. Evaluation of the receptor allows for the differentiation of IDA as a primary condition from IDA that occurs in the presence of anemia of chronic disease.[17]

The first step in treatment of IDA is to identify and eliminate (i.e., rule out) sources of blood loss. Without this strategy, any pharmacologic therapy is ineffective. Iron replacement therapy is very effective in the treatment of IDA. In fact, the most conclusive evidence for the diagnosis of IDA is an increase in hemoglobin of 1 to 2 g/dl after iron therapy is initiated. Iron preparations are administered orally, intramuscularly, or intravenously. Iron preparations are available in ferrous or ferric forms; however, the ferrous form is preferable because it is more readily absorbed. The ferrous form is available as sulfate, gluconate, or fumarate. The sulfate form is the cheapest and most commonly used.[18]

Recommended dosage for initial iron replacement therapy is 150 to 200 mg/day; however, recent studies have found that dosages as low as 60 mg/day are effective in certain individuals.[18] Once therapy has begun, individuals demonstrate a rapid decrease in fatigue, lethargy, and other associated symptoms. Hematocrit levels should improve within 1 to 2 months of therapy; however, the serum ferritin level is a more precise measurement of improvement and total body stores of iron. Once the serum ferritin level reaches 50 μg/L, adequate replacement of iron has occurred.[18] Replacement therapy is usually continued for 6 to 12 months after bleeding has been contained; however, therapy may continue for as long as 24 months. Daily therapy (325 mg/day) for menstruating females may be required until menopause.

Sideroblastic Anemia

Sideroblastic anemias (SAs) are a heterogenous group of disorders characterized by anemia of varying severity due to inefficient iron uptake resulting in dysfunctional hemoglobin synthesis. Ringed sideroblasts within the bone marrow are diagnostic of SA. Ringed sideroblasts are erythroblasts that contain iron granules that are not synthesized into hemoglobin, but instead are distributed in a perinuclear collar arrangement around one third or more of the nucleus (see Fig. 25-1, *K*). Individuals with SA also have increased tissue levels of iron.

Pathophysiology

SAs have various causes; however, they share the commonality of altered heme synthesis in the erythroid cells in bone marrow. SAs are either hereditary or acquired, with acquired SAs being the most common. Acquired SAs occur as a primary disorder with no known cause (idiopathic) or associated with other myeloproliferative or myelodysplastic conditions. Reversible SAs result from various conditions, such as alcoholism, reactions to certain drugs, copper deficiency, and hypothermia.[19]

Hereditary SAs occur almost exclusively in males, supporting a recessive X-linked transmission; however, autosomal transmission affecting females has been documented.[4] SAs have also been associated with autosomal recessive transmission, genetic and mitochondrial mutations, and deficiencies of ferrochelatase.[19] The anemia in all conditions is usually present in infancy or childhood, but it is not uncommon for it to remain undetected until midlife. In some instances, other symptoms, such as diabetes or cardiac failure resulting from tissue iron overload, may be the first manifestation of SA. Differentiation of SA from idiopathic hemachromotosis needs to be confirmed because both are characterized by tissue iron deposition.

The severity of the anemia is quite variable; even when there is little to no anemia present, qualitative alterations of the erythrocytes (e.g., decreased MCV and increased red cell volume distribution width) may be evident.[20] **Dimorphism,** in which both normocytic and normochromic cells are seen concomitantly with microcytic-hypochromic cells, may be present and is seen more commonly in individuals with mild anemia, female carriers, or those who are being treated with pyridoxine. Anisocytosis and poikilocytosis also are seen on examination of the blood smear.

Hereditary SA (XLSA) has been shown to be caused by missense mutations in the erythroid-specific ALA synthetase gene ALAS2.[21] ALAS2 is the first enzyme used in the heme biosynthetic pathway, using pyridoxal phosphates as cofactors for the synthesis of protoporphyrin IX. Protoporphyrin IX is normally combined with iron to produce heme. Reduction in the synthesis of protoporphyrin IX results in the accumulation of iron in the erythrocyte.

Acquired idiopathic sideroblastic anemia (AISA) manifests no similar defect in protoporphyrin IX levels; in fact, the levels are increased rather than decreased.[22] The mechanism for the development of AISA is that iron is not converted (reduced) from the ferric form (Fe^{+3}) to the ferrous form (Fe^{+2}). Iron is stored as the ferric form but requires conversion to the ferrous form for use in heme synthesis. The electrons for this conversion are provided by the mitochondrial electron chain located on the mitochondrial DNA (mtDNA), which is located near the inner mitochodrial membrane, making it vulnerable to damage by oxygen free radicals generated by the respiratory chain. The proposed hypothesis for the development of AISA is that damage to mtDNA causes a respiratory chain defect that interferes with the reduction of iron, allowing accumulation of ferric iron within the mitochondrial matrix.[22]

SA associated with alcoholism is related to nutritional deficiencies, particularly folate. Alcohol impairs the synthesis of heme by reducing the activity of specific enzymes along the heme biosynthetic pathway and also by the direct effects of alcohol and/or acetaldehyde on the heme biosynthetic steps or mitochondrial metabolism.[19]

Specific drugs are also causes of reversible SA and include antituberculous agents (INH, pyrazinamide, and cycloserine) and chloramphenicol. Antituberculous agents interfere with vitamin B_6 metabolism, which reduces ALA synthesis, thus decreasing heme generation. Chloramphenicol produces SA by direct mitochondrial injury, which impairs heme synthesis, as well as erythroid differentiation and proliferation.[19]

Reversible SA from copper deficiency in humans is extremely rare and has been associated with individuals who have had a gastrectomy or prolonged parenteral nutrition without the addition of copper supplements. Copper deficiency is reported to interfere with conversion of ferric iron to ferrous iron. Hypothermia as a contributing factor has also been described and is thought to be a consequence of diminished heme synthesis and iron incorporation into hemoglobin that occurs at reduced body temperatures.

Clinical manifestations

In addition to the cardiovascular and respiration manifestation common to all anemias, individuals with SA demonstrate signs of iron overload, identified as **erythropoietic hemochromatosis**.[19] Mild to moderate enlargement of the spleen (splenomegaly) and liver (hepatomegaly) occur; however, liver function remains normal or only slightly impaired. The occurrence of abnormal skin pigmentation (bronze colored) is occasionally seen. Neurologic and epithelial alterations associated with anemias are absent. Disturbances in heart rhythm, along with congestive heart failure, are major life-threatening complications associated with cardiac iron overload. These manifestations are, fortunately, rare and occur late in the progression of the disease. Young children and infants who are severely affected may demonstrate growth and developmental impairment.

Evaluation and Treatment

Initially, SA may be mistaken for deficiency of stem cells in the marrow (**hypoplastic anemia**) or iron deficiency anemia. (Laboratory findings are listed in Table 25-3). Bone marrow examination establishes the diagnosis. The marrow is packed with erythrocyte stem cells, and mononuclear phagocytes in the marrow are loaded with iron in the form of hemosiderin. Platelet and leukocyte values are generally normal; however, they may be reduced if splenomegaly is present. The presence of sideroblasts confirms the diagnosis of SA.

Individuals with hereditary SA are initially treated with pyridoxine therapy in doses of 50 to 200 mg per day. Approximately one third of individuals with hereditary SA respond to this therapy; however, the response to this treatment is variable. An optimal response manifests as reticulocytosis, with blood hemoglobin levels returning to normal within 1 to 2 months and low FEP levels returning to normal. Morphologic abnormalities of cells, however, do not disappear, even in the presence of normal ALA synthetase activity and hemoglobin. A less than optimal response is noted when hemoglobin levels are elevated but stabilize at less than normal levels. When a response to pyridoxine therapy is observed, lifelong maintenance therapy at a lowered dosage is instituted. Discontinuing therapy will initiate a relapse. For individuals who do not respond to pryidoxine, blood transfusions are necessary to relieve symptoms and permit growth and development.

Individuals who demonstrate evidence of iron overload need to undergo iron depletion therapy to prevent or minimize organ damage. Phlebotomies are generally well tolerated and preferable for individuals who have a mild to moderate anemia without other complications, such as heart disease. Once all the stored iron is removed, maintenance phlebotomies are performed on a continuing basis. Individuals who have severe anemia and/or depend on transfusions become extremely overloaded with iron. In such instances, deferoxamine, an iron-chelating agent, is administered to eliminate stored iron.

Individuals with acquired SA infrequently respond to pyridoxine. Fortunately, these affected individuals are rarely incapacitated by SA. In the absence of abnormalities of other blood cells and without iron overload, progression takes place over many years. Transfusion therapy and iron overload therapy is the same as for hereditary SA when indicated.

Death from SA is relatively rare and often secondary to complications such as infection, bone marrow failure, liver failure, or cardiac failure and/or arrythmias. Idiopathic SA has the potential to convert to **myelodysplastic syndrome,** with the possibility of the affected individual developing acute myeloblastic leukemia.

Normocytic-Normochromic Anemias

Normocytic-normochromic anemias are characterized by erythrocytes that are relatively normal in size and hemoglobin content but insufficient in number. These anemias have no common etiology, pathologic mechanisms, or morphologic characteristics. They are less common than the macrocytic-normochromic and microcytic-hypochromic anemias. Five distinct anemia conditions—aplastic anemia, posthemorrhagic anemia (acute blood loss), hemolytic anemia, anemia of chronic inflammation, and sickle cell anemia—exemplify the diversity of the normocytic-normochromic classification. (Sickle cell anemia is discussed in Chapter 27).

Aplastic Anemia

Aplastic anemia (AA) is a condition characterized by **pancytopenia**, which is a reduction or absence of all three types of blood cells. Pancytopenia results from failure or suppression of bone marrow to produce adequate amounts of blood cells (Fig. 25-7). The pathologic lesion identified with aplastic anemia is a hypoplastic bone marrow, which is replacement of the normal cellular bone marrow with fat.[23] The rate or decline in the quantity of blood cells is related to their life span; thus red cells are last to demonstrate a reduction in numbers. The rate of decline is often chronic, allowing the individual to adapt to the reduction and maintain a new level of hematologic function. This condition may be referred to as *hypoplastic anemia* rather than aplastic. In approximately 50% of people, the anemia progresses rapidly, leading to death from overwhelming infection or bleeding.

The incidence of AA is relatively rare, with an annual incidence rate of 2 new cases per million reported in Europe and Israel.[24] The incidence in developing countries is somewhat higher, presumably because of unregulated use of and exposure to certain chemicals known to cause AA.

Aplastic anemias are acquired or hereditary, with acquired anemias classified further as primary or secondary. **Fanconi anemia** is a rare genetic anemia characterized by pancytopenia because of defects in DNA repair. This anemia develops early in life and is accompanied by multiple congenital anomalies.

Idiopathic AA (primary acquired) accounts for approximately 50% of all confirmed cases, with about 80% occurring after 50 years of age. In instances where AA develops in individuals younger than 30 years of age, secondary causes should be investigated.

Secondary AA is caused by a variety of known chemical agents and ionizing radiation. Chemical agents include benzene; arsenic; and various drugs, such as chloramphenicol and alkylating and antimetabolite chemotherapeutic drugs (6-mercaptopurine, vincristine, and busulfan). Other drugs known to cause AA are identified in Table 25-4. The development of AA with these agents is generally dose related, and the effect can be controlled with appropriate dosages. In other instances, AA might develop after the use of small amounts of these drugs (idiosyncratic), with the anemia following a severe, rapid, irreversible progression.

Total body irradiation also causes AA and, in certain instances, may be used therapeutically for this effect. Infections are also known to cause AA, with viruses being the most common agent. Viral infections that have been identified as causing AA include the human immunodeficiency virus (HIV) infections and hepatitis (non-A, non-B, non-C, and non-G virus). The Epstein-Barr virus has been implicated as well. Human parvovirus B19 infection has also been identified as a cause of AA when the individual has an underlying hematologic or immunologic disorder.[25] The severity of the anemia does not appear to be related to the severity of the infection.

Another condition associated with AA is **pure red cell aplasia (PRCA)**, in which only the red cells are affected. PRCA is a rare disorder and has been associated with autoimmune, viral, and neoplastic (leukemias) disorders; infiltrative disorders of the bone marrow (myelofibrosis); renal failure; hepatitis; mononucleosis; and systemic lupus erythematosus. A thymoma often is found in association with PRCA and is also present in **Diamond-Blackfan syndrome,** a congenital disorder.

A

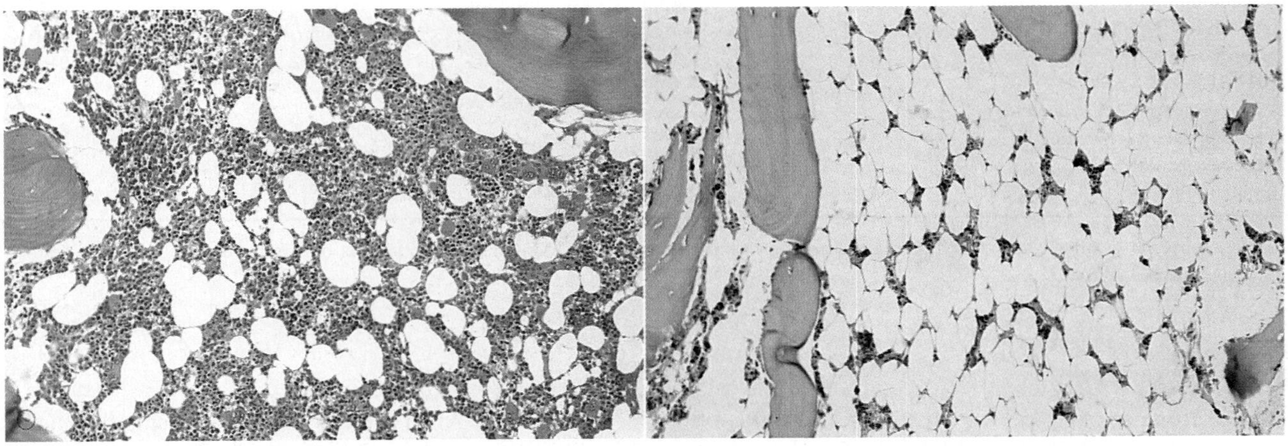

B

FIG. 25-7 Aplastic anemia. A, Normal bone marrow of an adult. Hematopoietic cells account for approximately 40% of marrow's cellularity. **B,** There is a marked reduction in hematopoietic cells with expansion of fat cells. (From Damjanov I, Linder J: *Pathology: a color atlas,* St Louis, 2000, Mosby.)

Table 25-4 Anemias Secondary to Drug Effects

Drug	Hemolytic	Megaloblastic	Sideroblastic	Aplastic
ANTIBIOTICS				
Amphotericin B				X
Trimethoprim-sulfamethoxazole (Bactrim)		X		
Chloramphenicol (Chloromycetin)			XX	XXXX
Erythromycin	X			X
Sulfisoxazole (Gantrisin)				X
Penicillin	XXX			X
Sulfanilamide/sulfonamides	XX			X,X*
Streptomycin	X			X
ANTICONVULSANTS				
Phenytoin (Dilantin)		XXX		XXX,X*
Mephenytoin		XXX		XXX
Primidone (Mysoline)		XX		
Phenobarbital		XX		
Trimethadione (Tridione)				XXX
ANTIINFLAMMATORIES				
ASA (aspirin)				X*
Colchicine		X?		
Gold compounds				XX
Ibuprofen (Motrin)	X			X
Indomethacin (Indocin)				X
Phenacetin	XXX			
Phenylbutazone				XX,X*
ANTIHYPERTENSIVE/DIURETICS				
Methyldopa (Aldomet)	XXX			
Acetazolamide (Diamox)				X
Thiazides	X			
TRANQUILIZERS				
Chlordiazepoxide (Librium)				X
Chlorpromazine (Thorazine)	XX			X
Meprobamate				X
ORAL HYPOGLYCEMICS				
Chlorpropamide (Diabinese)	X			
Tolbutamide (Orinase)				X,X*
IMMUNOSUPPRESSANTS				
Azathioprine (Imuran)			X	X*
Cyclosporine	X			
MISCELLANEOUS AGENTS				
Benzene	XX			XX
Cimetidine (Tagamet)				X
Heparin				X*
INH (isoniazid) } Anti-TB agents	XX			
PASA (paraaminosalicylic acid) } Anti-TB agents	XX	X		
Pyridium (phenazopyridine HCl)				XX
Potassium perchlorate				XX
Quinine/quinidine	XX			

X, Rare number of reported cases; *XXXX*, substantial number of reported cases; *XX, XXX*, intermediate number of reported cases; *X**, "pure red cell" aplasia.

Pathophysiology

Although it is generally known what causes AA, the exact mechanism by which the anemia develops and progresses remains unknown. Recent evidence includes an autoimmune process mediated by interferon-γ (IFN-γ), a product of lymphocytes and killer T cells capable of inhibiting hematopoiesis. Other factors produced by the T cells include tumor necrosis factor (TNF), which also has an inhibitory effect on hematopoiesis.

The actual process of suppression by lymphokines IFN-γ and TNF is thought to occur during early and late hematopoiesis of progenitor and stem cells.[23] The crucial feature of suppression is cell killing by cell-programmed death. Both lymphokines have demonstrated triggering of the Fas receptor on CD34 progenitor cells, which initiates apoptosis.[24] IFN-γ and TNF also induce the production of nitric oxide synthetase and nitric oxide by marrow cells, which also contributes to immune-mediated cytotoxicity and removal of hematopoietic cells.[23] The process by which autoimmunity is initiated is unknown.

Clinical Manifestations

The onset of symptoms is insidious and related to the rapidity with which the bone marrow is destroyed and replaced. Initial symptoms depend on which cell line is affected. When the onset is rapid, symptoms associated with hypoxemia, pallor, and weakness along with fever and dyspnea may be the first manifestations related to decreased red cell population. A slower onset is manifested by progressive weakness and fatigability advancing toward infection and hemorrhaging when the white cell and platelet population is affected. Common sites for hemorrhaging include the nose, mouth, or GI tract. Menorrhagia and purpura may also be evident; however, purpura is not necessarily a classic indication of AA and may not be representative of the degree of thrombocytopenia.

A waxy pallor of the skin is generally demonstrated by the time the condition has been diagnosed. The skin may also demonstrate a brownish pigmentation. Late manifestations of the condition include ulcerations of the mouth and pharynx or a low-grade cellulitis in the neck. Splenomegaly is extremely rare; if it is present, other conditions that may imitate AA should be ruled out. Neurologic changes are only evident when hemorrhages have occurred within the system; however, some individuals have complained of parasthesias.

Commonly, the red cells appear normal in spite of the severity of the anemia. Occasionally, the red cells are macrocytic, with anisocytosis and poikilocytosis, and also may appear immature. Initially, the individual's hemoglobin concentration may be as low as 7 g/dl, with the volume of packed red cells at 0.20 L/L or lower.[26] Concomitantly, the white cells and platelets are markedly reduced.

Evaluation and Treatment

Bone marrow biopsy is necessary to examine fat content and stromal elements and to determine whether the anemia involves bone marrow. Marrow biopsied from individuals with typical AA contains yellowish white material consisting mainly of fat, fibrous tissue, and lymphocytes.[26] Bone marrow characteristics may vary widely; for example, the bone marrow may be aplastic, hypoplastic, normal, or hyperplastic.[26]

Up until the last 20 years, treatment involved the search for the cause, removal of exposure to the potential causative agent, treatment of the anemia by transfusion, and prevention and treatment of infection and hemorrhage. Stimulation of blood cell production was also used and in some instances splenectomy was recommended. The prognosis with these forms of treatment was extremely poor. In acute cases, 25% of individuals succumbed within 4 months, demonstrating a rapid and fatal progression. Approximately 70% died within 5 years and only about 10% experienced complete recovery. Newer forms of treatment, such as bone marrow transplant, immunotherapy, and identification of high-risk individuals, has decreased mortality significantly.[27]

Allogenic bone marrow transplant (BMT) remains the preferred and most successful method for treatment of AA.[28,29] For those individuals unable to undergo such treatment or who lack a suitable sibling donor, immunosuppression remains the treatment of choice. Current therapies with immunosuppression include antithymocyte globulin (ATG), antithoracic duct lymphocyte globulin (ALG), cyclophosamide, and cyclosporine A either alone or in combination. Immunosuppression therapy may be combined with hematopoietic growth factor.[30] Survival rates of 80% have been reported for both types of treatment.[28]

Both forms of treatment are associated with specific problems. The major complication of BMT is graft-versus-host disease (GVHD) and the lethal complications that accompany it (see Chapter 8). Immunosuppression therapy has the risk of developing treatment failure and/or late myeloproliferative or malignant conditions. These late conditions include paroxysmal nocturnal hemoglobinuria (PNH), myelodysplastic syndrome (MDS), acute leukemia, or solid tumor.[31]

Posthemorrhagic Anemia (Acute Blood Loss)

Posthemorrhagic anemia is a normocytic-normochromic anemia caused by acute blood loss from the vascular space. Initial manifestations of this event depend on the severity of blood loss. If the blood loss is severe, the manifestations are related to loss of blood volume rather than loss of hemoglobin. The immediate effects of volume depletion are more significant than loss of circulating blood cells because volume loss reduces mean systemic filling pressure, resulting in a decreased venous return.

A normal, healthy young adult can tolerate a blood loss of 500 to 1000 ml (10% to 20%) without experiencing any symptoms. The same individual with rapid blood loss of 1500 to 2000 ml (30% to 40%) will be asymptomatic in the recumbent position but will experience lightheadedness and dizziness when upright.[32] Clinical manifestations are discussed in Table 25-5.

Within 24 hours of blood loss, lost plasma is replaced by mobilizing water and electrolytes from tissues and interstitial spaces into the vascular system. The hemodilution that results lowers the hematocrit; concurrently, there is often a rapid elevation of circulating neutrophils and platelets. Neutrophils can rise to levels between 10,000 to 30,000 per microliter within a few hours as a result of a shift of marginated leukocytes into the circulation and a release of leukocytes from the bone marrow.[33] The platelet count can rise to levels of about 1,000,000 per microliter. In severe hemorrhage, more immature cells—metamyelocytes, myelocytes, and nucleated red blood cells—may enter the circulation. Tissue oxygenation reduction stimulates the production of erythropoietin, and bone marrow responds by increasing production of RBCs (reticulocytes). Iron recovery from destroyed red blood

Table 25-5 Clinical Manifestations of Acute Blood Loss of Increasing Severity

Volume Lost		
% TBV	ml	Clinical Manifestations
10	500	None; rarely notice vasovagal syncope in blood donors
20	1000	Person at rest difficult, if not impossible, to detect volume loss; tachycardia is common with exercise and a slight drop in blood pressure with postural change
30	1500	Neck veins are flat in supine position; exercise tachycardia and postural hypotension are usually present; resting supine blood pressure and pulse can still be normal
40	2000	Central venous pressure, cardiac output, and arterial blood pressure are below normal even at rest and supine position; individual commonly has air hunger; a rapid, thready pulse; and cold, clammy skin
50	2500	Severe shock, lactic acidosis, death

TBV = total blood volume.
Data based on a 70-kg person with a total blood volume of 5000 ml.
Adapted from Hillman RS: Acute blood loss anemia. In Beutler E et al, editors: *William's hematology,* ed 5, New York, 1995, McGraw-Hill.

cells may occur if the acute blood loss is internal; however, if blood is lost externally, iron stores may be depleted and erythropoiesis impeded. Hemorrhage that is chronic (occult [i.e., bleeding] ulcer or neoplasm) produces adaptations that are less prominent, and the individual experiences an iron deficiency anemia when iron reserves become depleted.

Initial treatment for acute blood loss is restoration of blood volume by intravenous administration of saline, dextran, albumin, or plasma. Large volume losses may require transfusion of fresh whole blood; however, allergenic substances within the plasma or cells can interfere with volume expansion and even produce volume contraction.[33] The actual anemia may not require treatment unless it is associated with iron, folate, or cobalamin deficiency. Evidence of a return to normal is provided when the erythrocytes regain their normal size and shape. However, as the bone marrow begins to produce more erythrocytes, there is an increase (10% to 15% after 7 days) in reticulocytes. Changes in the appearance of red blood cells (polychromatophilia and macrocytosis) associated with reticulocytosis may give the impression that an underlying hemolytic process is occurring. A normal erythrocyte count is usually noted in 4 to 6 weeks, but hemoglobin restoration may take 6 to 8 weeks.

Hemolytic Anemia

Premature, accelerated destruction of erythrocytes, either episodically or continuous, is a clinical manifestation of many disease states and is the predominant event in **hemolytic anemias**. The bone marrow adapts to red cell destruction by accelerating erythropoiesis, and can do so to eight times normal levels. If this increased production can accommodate red cell destruction, the condition is identified as a hemolytic disorder. When erythropoiesis is incapable of keeping up with destruction, a true hemolytic anemia develops.[34]

Pathophysiology

Classification of hemolytiac anemias is somewhat problematic because there is not one system that is entirely satisfactory. Most commonly, hemolytic anemias are classified as acquired or inherited.[34] Hereditary anemias are caused by intrinsic (cellular) abnormalities, typically of the erythrocyte's plasma membrane or cytoplasmic contents (enzymes of hemoglobin). Acquired hemolytic anemias are caused by extrinsic (extracellular) defects such as infection, chemical agents (drugs, toxins, and venom), trauma, physical agents, and abnormal immune responses. Causes of acquired and hereditary hemolytic anemias are listed in Table 25-6.

Hemolysis occurs within blood vessels (intravascular) or lymphoid tissues (extravascular) that filter blood—that is, spleen and liver. Intravascular hemolysis is the least common and is related to physical destruction of red cells or complement-mediated lysis facilitated by antibodies that act as a lysin, opsonin, or agglutinin.

Extravascular hemolysis, occurring within lymphoid tissue, is most common and is caused by macrophage destruction and/or digestion of the mononuclear phagocyte system (MPS). Erythrocytes that have become more rigid are slowed down in their passage through the spleen and are thus more vulnerable to phagocytosis. Erythrocytes coated with immunoglobulin G (IgG) are particularly vulnerable.[35]

Immunohemolytic anemias, previously identified as **autoimmune hemolytic anemias (AHAs)**, are caused by extravascular hemolysis and are associated with autoimmune mechanisms, although in some instances they are mediated by drugs. Hemolytic anemias due to antibodies that coat erythrocytes but do not directly react as hemolysins have been identified as the most common form of autoimmune anemia.[36]

Classification of immunohemolytic anemias depends on the antibody involved. The types of antibodies involved include warm antibody, cold agglutinin, and cold hemolysis. **Warm antibody hemolytic anemia**, the most common form, primarily affects females over the age of 40. The mediating antibody is immunoglobulin G (IgG) that is specific for erythrocyte antigens and has a maximum binding capacity to the surface of the erythrocyte at body temperature (37° C). In approximately half of individuals affected, the condition is idiopathic and primary; in the other half there is some underlying, predisposing condition such as lymphomas, leukemias (CLL), other neoplastic disorders, systemic lupus erythematosus, or exposure to one or more

Table 25-6 Causes of Hemolytic Anemias

Type of Hemolytic Disorder	Primary Cause or Associated Disorder	Mechanisms of Erythrocyte Destruction
ACQUIRED FORMS		
Immune system–mediated hemolysis	Transfusion reaction Hemolytic disease of the newborn (see Chapter 27) Autoimmune hemolytic anemia (see text)	Antibody-mediated erythrocytes by enzymes of the complement system (see Chapter 7)
Traumatic hemolysis	Presence of prosthetic heart valves Structural abnormalities of the heart Hemolytic uremic syndrome Disseminated intravascular coagulation Hemodialysis	Physical destruction of erythrocytes by "mechanical" means (trauma)
Infectious hemolysis	Bacterial infection (clostridia, cholera, typhoid fever) Protozoal infection (malaria, toxoplasmosis)	Infection of erythrocytes
Toxic (chemical) hemolysis	Exposure to toxic chemical agents Hemodialysis or uremia Venoms	Chemical injury of erythrocytes (see Chapter 2)
Physical hemolysis	Burns Radiation	Heat or radiation injury (see Chapter 2)
Hypophosphatemic hemolysis	Hypophosphatemia (phosphate deficiency in plasma; see Chapter 3)	Diminished cellular production of substances required for erythrocyte life and function
HEREDITARY FORMS		
Structural defects	Plasma membrane defects	Fragility of the erythrocyte
Enzyme deficiencies	Deficiency of glycolytic enzymes Deficiency of metabolic enzymes (i.e., glucose-6-phosphate dehydrogenase deficiency)	Diminished cellular function
Defects of globin synthesis or structure	Sickle cell anemia	Increased membrane fragility and deformation during sickle crises
	Thalassemia	Defective hemoglobin structure and function
	Miscellaneous hemoglobin defects	Defective hemoglobin structure and function

From Lee GR et al: *Wintrobe's clinical hematology,* ed 9, Philadelphia, 1993, Lea & Febiger.

drugs that produce a secondary form of the anemia. Red cell destruction results not from intravascular hemolysis but rather from extravascular processes. IgG-coated red cells bind to the Fc receptors on monocytes and splenic macrophages, causing erythrocytes to undergo spheroidal transformation. Transformation is the result of partial loss of the cell membrane from attempted phagocytosis of the IgG-coated cell. The red cells are then sequestered in the spleen and removed from circulation.

The actual mechanisms of autoantibody formation remain largely unknown; however, two models have been developed of **drug-induced hemolysis** (Fig. 25-8). These are the hapten model and the autoantibody model. The **hapten model**, which is based upon penicillin and cephalosporins, proposes that these drugs act as a hapten and combine with the red cell membrane to induce antibody formation directed against the cell-bound drug. Red cell destruction proceeds as previously described. This form of anemia usually follows a large intravenous infusion of the antibiotic and occurs 1 to 2 weeks following the initiation of therapy. Drug-induced anemias may precipitate intravascular hemolysis as a result of complement fixation or extravascular hemolysis in the mononuclear phagocytic system.

The **autoantibody model** is based upon the drug α-methyldopa, which somehow initiates production of antibodies that become directed against intrinsic red cell antigens, particularly Rh blood group antigens. It is estimated that 10% of individuals taking the antihypertensive drug α-methyldopa develop detectable antibodies but that only 1% actually develop clinically significant hemolysis.[37]

Cold agglutinin immune hemolytic anemia is mediated by IgM and occurs less frequently than warm antibody hemolysis, affecting mostly older females. Cold antibodies have a red cell binding capacity that occurs at colder temperatures—lower than 31° C—with maximal binding capacity at 0° C to 4° C. Cold agglutinin anemia causes red cells to clump together, causing manifestations of ischemia. This is a characteristic manifestation of Raynaud phenomenon, in which an individual's fingers and toes experience blanching and numbness followed by cyanosis, redness, throbbing pain, and paresthesias upon exposure to cold temperatures. Ischemia is caused by clumping of red cells in the capillaries as a result of agglutination and fixation of complement or hyperviscosity related to high levels of IgM.[2] The ischemic manifestations generally disappear upon exposure to warmer temperatures. Once warming occurs, the antibody may dis-

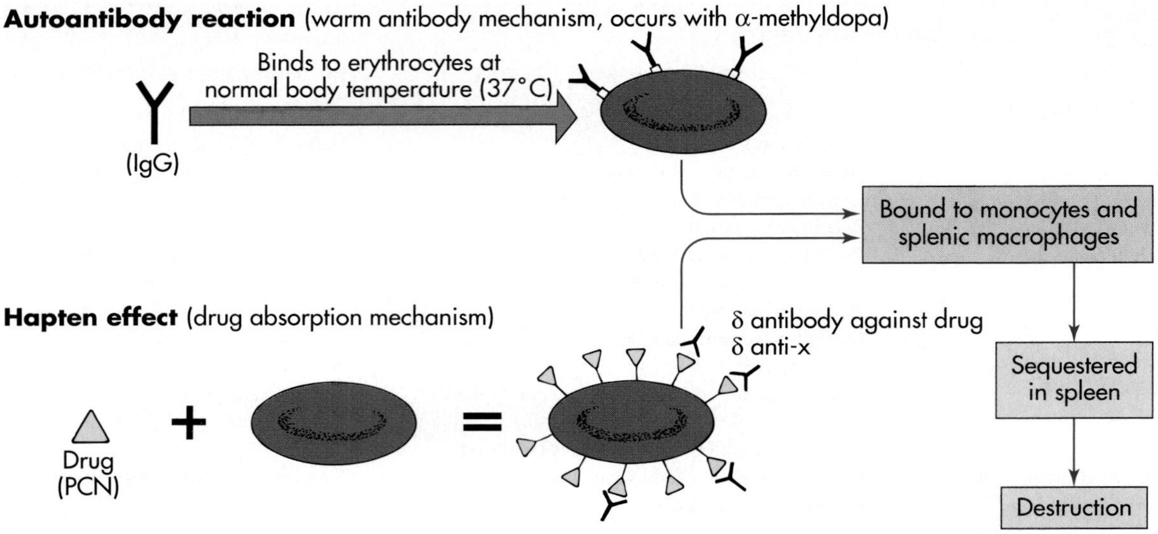

FIG. 25-8 Drug-induced hemolysis.

sociate itself from the erythrocyte; however, if it does not, hemolysis may occur. Cold agglutinin anemia is more a condition related to vascular obstruction rather than hemolysis. Conditions that are associated with cold agglutinin anemia are infectious mononucleosis, mycoplasmal pneumonia, and lymphoid malignancies. It also has been identified with the Epstein-Barr virus, cytomegalovirus infection, mumps, and legionnaires disease.

Cold hemolysis hemolytic anemia is a rare disorder associated with autoantibodies characteristic of the condition paroxysmal cold hemoglobinuria, which is distinguished by acute intermittent massive hemolysis following exposure to cold temperatures. Complement fixation is the identified cause of hemolysis. The autoantibodies, which are IgG in nature and directed against the P blood group antigen, attach to red cells upon exposure to cold temperature and fix complement. Interestingly, it is not until the temperature becomes elevated that hemolysis occurs and is mediated by the lytic complement cascade. This condition is associated with various infections, such as mycoplasmal pneumonia, measles, mumps, and nonspecific viral and "flu" syndromes. A chronic form is related to syphilis. The actual mechanisms by which autoantibodies are produced remain unknown.

Clinical Manifestations

The presence and severity of signs and symptoms of hemolytic anemia depend on the degree of anemia and hemolysis and the success of compensatory erythropoiesis. The severity of anemia varies widely from individual to individual, even in individuals who have the same illness. Severe disease is commonly diagnosed shortly after birth or within the first year of life. Mild to moderate anemia is more common because the shortened erythrocyte survival time is offset by increased erythropoiesis. Some individuals have no symptoms of anemia and it remains undetected unless some other complication develops during the course of the disease.

Jaundice (icterus) is present if heme destruction exceeds the liver's ability to conjugate and excrete bilirubin. Jaundice is first noticed in the neonatal period. Children and adults with congenital hemolytic anemia may not have icterus, or it may be mild enough that it goes unnoticed. Faint scleral icterus may be the only indication of hemolytic disease in many individuals.

Acute conditions that disrupt the delicate equilibrium of accelerated erythropoiesis and red cell destruction may precipitate a crisis. The most common type of crisis is aplastic and results from failure of bone marrow red cell production. The most common cause of aplastic crisis is human parvovirus B19 infection.[34]

Frequently, individuals with congenital hemolytic disorders demonstrate splenomegaly, which is often only mild in nature. In some cases the spleen may become quite enlarged and may be the cause of discovery of the underlying hemolytic disorder. Another underlying condition that may be the cause of determining the presence of the anemic disorder is the development of gallstones.

Children who have hemolytic anemia often demonstrate skeletal abnormalities due to expansion of erythroid bone marrow during the active phase of growth and development. These alterations are more pronounced in the bony structures of the face and skull (see Chapter 27). In some instances, pathologic fractures may also result. Cardiovascular and respiratory manifestations vary with the degree of anemia.

Evaluation and Treatment

Evaluation is based on clinical manifestations, bone marrow studies, and blood tests (see Table 25-3). Abnormally increased numbers of erythrocyte stem cells are found in the marrow, a finding termed *erythroid hyperplasia*. Accelerated erythropoiesis causes large numbers of fragile and immature erythrocytes (stem cells and reticulocytes) to be released prematurely into the circulation. These cells are observed in blood smears.

Acquired hemolytic anemias are treated by removing the cause or treating the underlying disorder. Acute fulminating hemolytic anemia (hemolytic crisis) is treated with fluid and electrolyte replacement to prevent shock and renal damage, which may be caused by red cell debris clogging the kidney tubules. Transfusions of blood products sometimes are given. Splenectomy is performed if the spleen is the major site of hemolysis and splenomegaly is significant.

Steroids are beneficial in treating some forms of immunohemolytic anemia. Folate is also used in treating chronic hemolytic disease to prevent megaloblastic crisis because long-term erythrocyte turnover increases folate requirements.

Anemia of Chronic Disease

Anemia of chronic disease (ACD) is a mild to moderate anemia associated with chronic conditions, including acquired immunodeficiency disease (AIDS); chronic inflammatory disorders, including RA, SLE, acute and chronic hepatitis, and inflammatory bowel conditions; chronic renal failure; and malignancies. The anemia develops after 1 to 2 months of active disease. The severity of the anemia is related to that of the underlying disorder and may by asymptomatic or a coincidental clinical finding. Morphologically, ACD is usually normocytic-normochromic, but it may also be hypochromic and microcytic. The exact incidence of ACD is unknown. Because it is associated with so many pathologic conditions, it is probably second only to iron deficiency in overall incidence.

Pathophysiology

Three pathologic mechanisms cause ACD: (1) decreased erythrocyte life span, (2) ineffective bone marrow response, and (3) altered iron metabolism. Overall, the manifestations of ACD appear to be mediated by activation of the cellular immune response that causes release of specific cytokines. Initiation of this response appears to be the common factor among the various conditions that are associated with ACD. Activation of macrophages is the beginning step, after which cytokines are released that act on other cells, such as lymphocytes, endothelial cells, and fibroblasts, to cause erythropoietic suppression or act directly on effector cells.[38] Specific cytokines that have been implied in ACD include tumor necrosis factor–α (TNF-α), interferon-γ (IFN-γ), interleukin-1β (IL-1β), and interleukin-6 (IL-6).[39,40]

The decreased erythrocyte life span appears to be attributable to red cell destruction mediated by some extrinsic factor that renders the erythrocyte more vulnerable to phagocytosis. Activated macrophages and hemolysis caused by bacterial toxins or tumor secretions have been suggested as factors that contribute to red cell destruction.[41] Individuals with RA who have ACD demonstrate increased levels of IL-1, suggesting that red cell destruction is facilitated by this factor. The precise mechanism by which red cell destruction is mediated remains unclear.[38]

Failure to increase erythropoiesis in response to decreased numbers of red cells is the erythropoietic defect in ACD. Instead of accelerating production of erythrocytes, red cell production continues at a normal rate. Erythropoietic failure results from suppression of erythroid progenitor cells by cytokines released from activated macrophages and lymphocytes, such as TNF-α and IFN-γ. The suppression of erythropoiesis appears to be related to failure of the bone marrow to respond to erythropoietin.[39] Concomitant with suppression of bone marrow function, there is a reduced amount of iron in the blood, impairing the ability of bone marrow to synthesize hemoglobin.

Impaired iron metabolism is the third contributing factor to the pathogenesis of ACD (Fig. 25-9). **Lactoferrin** is hypothesized to be the cause of this dysfunction. Lactoferrin, a protein in the plasma, closely resembles transferrin, the protein that normally binds with plasma iron and transports it to the bone marrow for hemoglobin synthesis. Under normal conditions lactoferrin is present in the blood in only small amounts. During periods of inflammation and infection, however, neutrophils release lactoferrin, making it more available to compete with transferrin. The affinity of iron for lactoferrin is 260 times greater than for transferrin. Lactoferrin-bound iron is removed by the MPS and converted into ferritin, the storage form of iron.

Another protein, **apoferritin**, is implicated in altered iron metabolism. Apoferritin is produced in greater amounts in inflammatory and malignant conditions and also has a greater affinity for iron than transferrin. Apoferritin-bound iron is converted to storage, thus also contributing to a reduction of iron available for hemoglobin synthesis.

Clinical Manifestations

Anemia of chronic disease has fewer and milder manifestations than most other anemias. Manifestations depend on the degree of anemia. As a rule, disability caused by chronic disease limits physical activity; consequently, hemoglobin levels are adequate to accommodate an affected individual's activities. If hemoglobin levels drop significantly, however, clinical manifestations of iron deficiency anemia appear.

Evaluation and Treatment

The significant finding in ACD is iron deficiency in the marrow despite normal or increased iron stores elsewhere in the body. (Blood test findings are listed in Table 25-3). Individuals with ACD but demonstrating no evidence of inflammatory or infectious conditions are screened for the presence of malignancies.

Anemia of chronic disease does not respond to iron replacement therapy because iron is prevented from being transported to the bone marrow. Use of erythropoietin in treatment of ACD associated with arthritis, malignancies, and AIDS has met with limited success.[42] The principle treatment is alleviation of the underlying disorder unless the individual develops symptoms related to the anemia, which then necessitates further treatment.

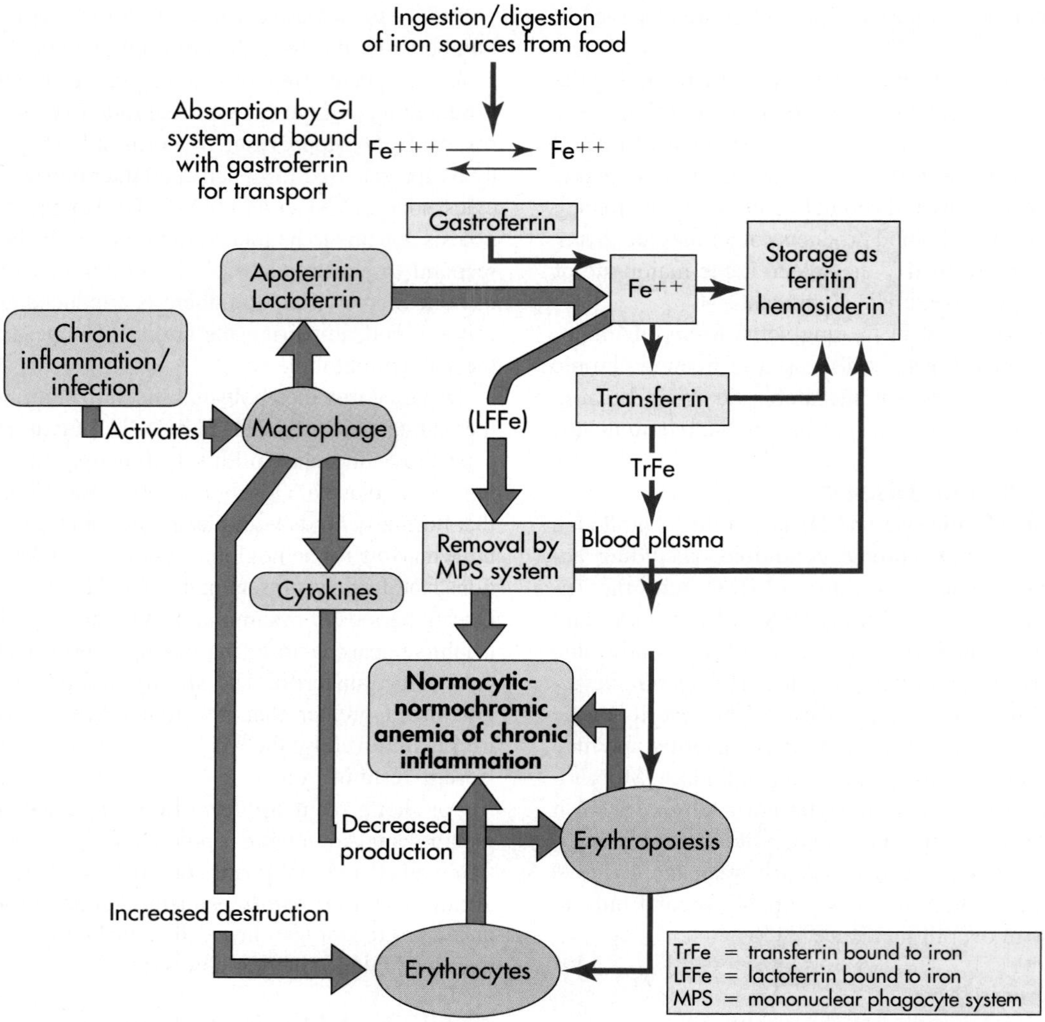

FIG. 25-9 Pathophysiology of anemia of chronic disease. Normal iron metabolism is indicated by the narrow arrows. Abnormal mechanisms that are instrumental in the development of anemia of chronic inflammation are indicated by thick arrows. (See discussion in text.)

MYELOPROLIFERATIVE RED CELL DISORDERS (POLYCYTHEMIA)

Hematologic dysfunction results from an overproduction of red cells as well as a deficiency. One or more marrow elements may be produced in excess as a response to exogenous (radiation, drugs) or endogenous (physiologic compensatory response, immune disorder) signals. Overproduction of white cells results in leukemia (see Chapters 26 and 27). An excess of red cells produces a group of disorders classified as **polycythemia** (Table 25-7).

Polycythemia exists in two forms: relative and absolute. **Relative polycythemia** is a condition in which there is hemoconcentration of the blood that may accompany alterations associated with dehydration. Its development is of minor consequence and resolves with appropriate fluid administration or treatment of the underlying condition.

Absolute polycythemia consists of two forms: primary and secondary. Secondary polycythemia is the most common and is essentially a physiologic response to hypoxia caused by appropriate secretion of erythropoietin. Individuals who live at higher altitudes (i.e., above 10,000 ft), smokers (who have increased levels of CO in their blood), individuals with COPD, and those with congestive heart failure develop secondary polycythemia. Secondary polycythemia also develops in individuals who have abnormal hemoglobin (e.g., $Hb_{San\ Diego}$ or $Hb_{Chesapeake}$), which has an increased affinity for oxygen.[2] Absolute secondary polycythemia may be caused by inappropriate secretion of erythropoietin by tumors associated with renal cell carcinoma, hepatoma, and cerebellar hemangioblastomas.[37] The absolute primary form of polycythemia is known as polycythemia vera.

Polycythemia vera (PV), also called polycythemia rubra vera, is a chronic, clonal alteration characterized by an increase in red cells as well as increased white cells and platelets and splenomegaly. Hypercellularity of the bone marrow is another distinguishing feature and is characterized by hyperplasia of myeloid, erythroid, and megakaryocyte precursors. PV was first described in 1892 by M.H.

Table 25-7 Types of Polycythemia

Type of Polycythemia	Mechanism of Increased Erythropoiesis	Cause or Associated Disorder
Absolute primary polycythemia (polycythemia vera)	Excessive proliferation of erythroid precursors in marrow; increased sensitivity of pluripotential stem cell to erythropoietin	Unknown
Absolute secondary polycythemia	Physiologic increase in erythropoietin secretion by the kidneys in response to underlying systemic disorder (appropriate)	Tissue hypoxia caused by cardiopulmonary disorders (chronic obstruction pulmonary disease, congestive heart failure), decreased barometric pressure, cardiovascular malformations causing mixing of arterial and venous blood, methemoglobinemia, carboxyhemoglobinemia, smoking, obesity, abnormal hemoglobin with increased oxygen affinity
	Nonphysiologic* increase in erythropoietin secretion (inappropriate)	Renal disorders, cerebellar hemangioblastomas, hepatoma (liver tumor), ovarian carcinoma, uterine leiomyoma, pheochromocytoma, adrenocortical hypersecretion
Familial polycythemia	Genetically induced increase in erythroid precursors of the marrow Decreased 2,3-diphosphoglycerate (2,3-DPG) Increased sensitivity of stem cells to erythropoietin Increased erythropoietin secretion	Genetic defect
Relative polycythemia	Reduced plasma volume (hemoconcentration)	Dehydration

*Nonphysiologic means that there is no obvious physiologic explanation for hypersecretion of erythropoietin.

Vasques, a French physician, and was studied extensively by William Osler in the early 1900s. Not until the 1960s was more learned about the condition, at which time a link between polycythemias and all kinds of neoplasias affecting stem cells was investigated.

Polycythemia vera is relatively rare and is considered a condition of older individuals, with a peak incidence occurring between 60 and 80 years of age and a median of 55 to 60 years of age; however, it has been observed in individuals under 40 years of age.[43,44] PV appears to be more common in males; however, the difference between genders is not overwhelmingly significant. It also is more common in whites (particularly those of Northern European Jewish ancestry) than in blacks. Polycythemia is rarely found in children or in multiple members of a single family; however, an autosomal dominant form exists that is characterized by increased production of erythropoietin.

Pathophysiology

PV is a neoplastic, nonmalignant condition characterized by an insidious, abnormal proliferation of bone marrow stem cells dominated by senseless, self-destructive expansion of red cells despite normal to below normal erythropoietin levels.

The underlying cause of PV remains unknown. The most likely cause of PV is acquired genetic alterations in the stem cell leading to a disturbance of normal cellular growth pattern.[44] Laboratory studies have found that red cell precursors are able to grow independent of erythropoietin and become more sensitive to other growth factors. Because all three cell lines may be affected, clinical manifestations of the disorder overlap; however, in each condition, one cell lineage predominates. Specific mechanisms for preferential involvement have been suggested. One possible mechanism is that the abnormal clone of the progenitor cell responds differently to hematopoietic growth factors, including erythropoietin. A second possible mechanism proposes that two lesions are involved—one on the pluripotential stem cell and a second on the committed progenitor cell compartment. A third hypothesis suggests that hematopoietic differentiation is a random development not controlled by hematopoietic growth factors; thus a mutation that occurs in a cell that randomly develops erythroid potential will result in PV.[45,46]

Individuals with PV develop endogenous erythroid colonies, the hallmark of PV, which give rise to progenitor cells and ultimately mature blood cells. These colonies develop in the absence of erythropoietin. Recent evidence suggests that cellular proliferation appears to be facilitated by protein phosphorylation.[44] Various substances have also been identified which may facilitate cellular proliferation. The tumor suppression gene SHP-1 appears to be one responsible agent by interacting with several growth factor receptors, including the erythropoietin receptor.[44] Other substances that have been investigated include interlukin-3 (IL-3), granulocyte-macrophage growth factor (GM-CSF), and stem cell factor (SCF). Another agent may be insulin-like growth factor I (IGF-I).[45]

Clinical Manifestations

Clinical manifestations of absolute PV result from marrow erythropoiesis with increased cellularity of the blood that increases blood volume and viscosity. The major complication of PV is an increased development of thrombi and occlusion of major and minor blood vessels, which may lead to tissue and/or organ ischemia or infarction (tissue injury and/or death). Thrombosis and occlusion of vessels occur in approximately 40% of individuals with PV and are directly correlated with hematocrit levels. Increases in thrombocytes as well as dysfunctional platelets also contribute to this hypercoagulable state.

Circulatory alterations prevalent in PV, caused by the sticky, thick blood and sluggish blood, give rise to specific manifestations, such as plethora (ruddy, red color of the face, hands, feet, ears, and mucous membranes) and engorgement of the retinal and cerebral vessels. Individuals also experience headache, drowsiness, delirium, mania, psychotic depression, chorea, and visual disturbances. Death from cerebral thrombosis is approximately five times greater in individuals with PV.

Cardiovascular alterations are also observed in individuals with PV. Cardiac function, in spite of the previously identified vascular alterations, remains quite normal. Cardiac workload and output remain essentially unchanged; however, increased blood volume may lead to elevated blood pressure. Coronary blood flow may be affected and lead to the onset of angina; however, actual myocardial infarctions caused by PV are relatively rare. Other evidence of cardiovascular involvement is the development of Raynaud phenomenon and thromboanginitis obliterans.

Additionally, gastrointestinal involvement may occur, indicated by the development of gastric and duodenal thrombosis with resultant hemorrhaging. The development of mesenteric thrombosis requires immediate medical intervention. Splenomegaly and hepatomegaly are common due to pooling of blood in these organs; consequently; individuals may develop portal hypertension. The respiratory system, generally not affected by PV, becomes involved if thrombosis and embolization occur.

A unique feature of PV (and one potentially instrumental in diagnosis) is extreme, painful itching. The pruritis appears to be exacerbated by heat or exposure to water (aquagenic pruritis), may be painful, and may be associated with swelling.[43] The itching may be so problematic that individuals avoid exposure to water (hot/warm baths/showers). Cool water does not appear to cause as severe a reaction. The intensity of the itching appears to be directly related to the concentration of mast cells in the skin; however, relief is not obtained by use of antihistamines or topical lotions.[4]

Evaluation and Treatment

Diagnosis of PV is made from blood and laboratory findings. Blood manifestations include an absolute increase in red blood cells, with hematocrits ranging from 18 to 24 g/dl and red cell counts of 7 to 10 $\times$ 10^{12}. Absolute total blood volume is also increased and moderate increases of white blood cells and platelets may also be observed. Erythrocytes appear normal; however, anisocytosis may occasionally be seen. Bone marrow examination may be done, but its use is controversial and there is no definitive criteria that are used to establish the diagnosis. Typically the marrow is hypercellular but not in such a manner as to differentiate it from other myeloproliferative disorders.

Treatment of PV consists of reducing erythrocytosis and blood volume, controlling symptoms, and preventing thrombosis. Erythrocytosis and increased blood volume are reduced by phlobotomy. Three hundred to 500 milliliters are removed two or three times per week until hematocrit levels drop sufficiently. Subsequent phlobotomies may be done every 3 to 4 months to maintain appropriate hematocrit levels (less than 45). Frequent phlobotomies also reduce the amount of iron available so that the individual may become iron deficient, a condition that impedes erythropoiesis, thus reducing the need for frequent phlobotomies. Phlebotomy is also somewhat controversial because it may also contribute to the development of thrombosis; thus its use needs to be individualized. Smokers should quit and individuals with congestive heart failure and/or chronic obstructive pulmonary disease require appropriate medical intervention.

Radioactive phosphorus (^{32}P) is another agent used to treat PV. Its main effect is to suppress erythropoiesis; it is considered an effective and easily tolerated therapy. Radioactive phosphorus is generally effective for an extended period, and as many as 18 months may elapse between treatments. Side effects of ^{32}P treatment include suppression of hematopoiesis resulting in anemia, leukopenia, or thrombocytopenia. Development of acute leukemia is also a major side effect of ^{32}P, generally after 7 or more years of treatment, which makes this therapy more useful in elderly individuals. Two other chemotherapeutic agents that have been used as myelosuppressive agents in treatment of PV—chlorambucil and busulfan—have been discontinued because of the increased incidence of associated leukemia. Hydroxyurea, a nonalkylating myelosuppressive drug, is now the most widely used agent. The incidence of thrombosis and leukemia is greatly reduced; however, this needs to be monitored further.[43] IFN-α is gaining in popularity and efficacy in treatment of PV. Interferon inhibits the growth of the abnormal clone, which leads to the reduction of the clinical and laboratory signs of myeloproliferation.[47] Use of interferon for PV is a relatively new treatment; it is unknown whether there might be long-term effects associated with its use.

Without proper treatment, 50% of individuals with PV die within 19 months of the onset of initial symptoms. Death is caused by thrombosis or hemorrhage. Conversion to acute myeloid leukemia (AML) occurs in 10% of individuals, which is a significant potential adverse outcome of PV and is generally refractory to conventional interventions. Conversion to AML is thought to be directly related to treatment associated with specific cytotoxic agents.

Although PV is a chronic disorder, with appropriate therapy, remissions occur and prevention of significant morbidity and mortality is possible. Survival for 10 to 15 years is common.

SUMMARY REVIEW

Anemia

1. Anemia is defined as a reduction in the number or volume of circulating red cells or an alteration in hemoglobin.
2. Anemias can be classified according to (a) erythrocyte size or concentration of hemoglobin, (b) cause of low blood count, or (c) the kinetics of why constant and adequate numbers of mature erythrocytes are not maintained in the circulation.
3. Clinical manifestations of anemia may be demonstrated in all organs and tissues throughout the body. Decreased oxygen delivery to tissues causes fatigue, dyspnea, syncope, angina, compensatory tachycardia, and organ dysfunction.
4. Macrocytic-megaloblastic anemias, characterized by larger than normal red cells with smaller than normal nuclei, most commonly are caused by deficiency of vitamin B_{12} (due to a lack of IF) or folate. Pernicious anemia can be fatal unless vitamin B_{12} is replaced; replacement is generally by injection, but larger than normal doses given orally may be just as effective.
5. Microcytic-hypochromic anemias are characterized by abnormally small red cells with insufficient hemoglobin content. The most common cause is iron deficiency.
6. Iron deficiency anemia usually develops slowly, with gradual insidious onset of symptoms. Fatigue, weakness, dyspnea, alteration of various epithelial tissues, and vague neuromuscular complaints result.
7. Iron deficiency anemia is usually a result of blood loss or poor nutritional intake. Once the source of blood loss is identified and corrected, oral iron replacement therapy can be initiated. Elevated reticulocyte count is a good index of response to iron therapy.
8. Sideroblastic anemia (SA) results from impaired iron metabolism, which leads to dysfunctional hemoglobin synthesis and in turn produces abnormal cellular sequestration of iron. SAs may be hereditary or acquired, and treatment varies depending on the cause.
9. Normocytic-normochromic anemias are characterized by insufficient numbers of normal erythrocytes. Included in this category are aplastic, posthemorrhagic, and hemolytic anemias and anemia of chronic disease.
10. In aplastic anemia, erythrocyte stem cells are underdeveloped, defective, or absent. Unless the cause is determined, bone marrow aplasia results in death.
11. Sudden blood loss from hemorrhage results in a normocytic-normochromic anemia. Restoration of blood volume by plasma expanders or transfusions may diminish subjective symptoms of anemia. Hemoglobin restoration may take 6 to 8 weeks.
12. Premature destruction of erythrocytes (hemolytic anemia) may be acquired or hereditary. Of the acquired forms, autoimmune reaction and drug-induced hemolysis are the most common.
13. Failure of erythropoiesis in anemia of chronic disease may result in release of cytokines and lactoferrin by phagocytic cells. Lactoferrin has been shown to cause abrupt decreases in plasma iron levels by interfering with the normal iron cycle.

Myeloproliferative Red Cell Disorders (Polycythemia)

1. Polycythemia vera is characterized by excessive proliferation of erythrocyte precursors in the bone marrow. Signs and symptoms result directly from increased blood volume and viscosity. Therapeutic phlebotomy to remove excessive blood volume and use of radioactive phosphorus have been helpful in decreasing the excessive red cell pool.

KEY TERMS

Absolute polycythemia, *860*
Anemia, *843*
Anemia of chronic disease (ACD), *859*
Anisocytosis, *843*
Aplastic anemia (AA), *853*
Apoferritin, *859*
Autoantibody model, *857*
Autoimmune hemolytic anemia (AHA), *856*
Cold agglutinin immune hemolytic anemia, *857*
Cold hemolysis hemolytic anemia, *858*
Diamond-Blackfan syndrome, *853*
Dimorphism, *851*
Drug-induced hemolysis, *857*
Erythropoietic hemochromatosis, *852*
Fanconi anemia, *853*
Hapten model, *857*
Hemolytic anemia, *856*
Hypoplastic anemia, *852*
Immunohemolytic anemia, *856*
Iron deficiency anemia (IDA), *850*
Lactoferrin, *859*
Macrocytic anemia (megaloblastic anemia), *844*
Microcytic-hypochromic anemia, *849*
Myelodysplastic syndrome, *852*
Normocytic-normochromic anemia, *853*
Pancytopenia, *853*
Pernicious anemia (PA), *845*
Poikilocytosis, *843*
Polycythemia, *860*
Polycythemia vera (PV), *860*
Posthemorrhagic anemia, *855*
Pure red cell aplasia (PRCA), *853*
Relative polycythemia, *860*
Sideroblastic anemia (SA), *851*
Warm antibody hemolytic anemia, *856*

REFERENCES

1. Lee GR: Anemia: a diagnostic strategy. In Lee GR et al, editors: *Wintrobe's clinical hematology,* p 908, Baltimore, 1999, Williams & Wilkins.
2. Chandrosoma P, Taylor CR: *Concise pathology,* ed 2, Norwalk, Conn, 1995, Lange.
3. Toh B et al: Pernicious anemia, *New Eng J Med* 337(20):1441, 1997.
4. Jandl JH: *Blood: textbook of hematology,* Boston, 1996, Little, Brown & Co.
5. Brigden SA: Shilling test still useful in pernicious anemia? *Postgrad Med* 106(5):37, 1999.
6. Lederle FA: Oral cobalamin for pernicious anemia: back from the verge of extinction, *J Am Geriatric Soc* 46:1125, 1998.

7. Paauw DS: Did we learn evidence based medicine in medical school? Some common medical mythology, *J Am Board Fam Practice* 12(2): 143, 1999.
8. McNulty H: Folate requirements for health in different population groups, *Br J Biomed Sci* 52:110, 1995.
9. Huang RF et al: Folate deficiency induces a cell cycle-specific apoptosis in HepG2 cells, *J Nut* 129(1):25, 1999.
10. Koury MJ, Horne DW: Apoptosis mediates and thymidine prevents erythroblast destruction in folate deficiency anemia, *Proc Nat Acad Sci USA* 91(9):4067, 1994.
11. Duthie SJ: Folic acid deficiency and cancer: mechanisms of DNA instability, *Br Med* Bull 55(3):578, 1999.
12. Lee GR: Iron deficiency and iron deficiency anemia. In Lee GR et al, editors: *Wintrobe's clinical hematology,* p 979, Baltimore, 1999, Williams & Wilkins.
13. Hord J: Anemia and coagulation disorders in adolescents, *Adol Med* 10(3):359, 1999.
14. Fishbane S: Review of issues relating to iron and infection, *Am J Kidney Dis* 34(4 suppl 2):S47, 1999.
15. Osaki TE et al: The pathophysiology of glossal pain in patients with iron deficiency anemia, *Am J Med Sci* 318(5):324, 1999.
16. Lindsay JO et al: The investigation of iron deficiency anemia—a hospital based audit, *Hepatogastronenterol* 46(29):2887, 1999.
17. Cook JD: The measurement of serum transferrin receptor, *Am J Med Sci* 318(4):269, 1999.
18. Little DR: Ambulatory management of common forms of anemia, *Am Fam Physician* 59(6):1598, 1999.
19. Bottomley SS: Sideroblastic anemias. In Lee GR et al, editors: *Wintrobe's clinical hematology,* p 1022, Philadelphia, 1999, Febiger.
20. Wiley JS: Sideroblastic anemias. In Hoffman R et al, editors: *Hematology: basic principles and practice,* ed 2, New York, 1996, Churchill Livingstone.
21. May A, Bishop DF: The molecular biology and pyridoxine responsiveness of x-linked sideroblastic anemia, *Haematologica* 83:56, 1998.
22. Gatterman N: From sideroblastic anemia to the role of mitochondrial DNA mutations in myelodysplastic syndrome, *Leukemia Res* 24(2): 141, 2000.
23. Young NS: Hematopoietic cell destruction by immune mechanisms in acquired aplastic anemia, *Sem Hematol* 37(1):3, 2000.
24. Young NS: Acquired aplastic anemia, *J Am Med Assoc* 282(3):271, 1999.
25. Sabella C, Goldfarb J: Parvovirus B19 infections, *Am Fam Physician* 60(5):1455, 1999.
26. Williams DM: Pancytopenia, aplastic anemia, and pure red cell aplasia, In Lee GR et al, editors: *Wintrobe's clinical hematology,* p 1449, Baltimore, 1999, Williams & Wilkins.
27. Frickhofen N, Rosenfeld SJ: Immunosuppressive treatment of aplastic anemia with antithymocyte globulin and cyclosporine, *Sem Hematol* 37(1):56, 2000.
28. Bacigalupo A et al: Treatment of acquired severe aplastic anemia: bone marrow transplantation compared with immunosuppressive therapy—the European group for blood and marrow transplantation experience, *Sem Hematol* 37(1):69, 2000.
29. Tisdale JF et al: Cyclophosphamide and other new agents for the treatment of severe aplastic anemia, *Sem Hematol* 37(1):102, 2000.
30. Marsh JCW: Hematopoietic growth factors in the pathogenesis and for the treatment of aplastic anemia, *Sem Hematol* 37(1):81, 2000.
31. Socie G et al: Late clonal diseases of treated aplastic anemia. *Sem Hematol* 37(1):91, 2000.
32. Lee GR: Acute posthemorrhagic anemia. In Lee GR et al, editors: *Wintrobe's clinical hematology,* p 1485, Baltimore, 1999, Williams & Wilkins.
33. Hillman RS: Acute blood loss. In Beutler E et al, editors: *William's hematology,* ed 5, New York, 1995, McGraw-Hill.
34. Lee GR: Hemolytic disorders: general considerations. Megaloblastic and nonmegaloblastic macrobytic anemias. In Lee GR et al, editors: *Wintrobe's clinical hematology,* p 1109, Baltimore, 1999, Williams & Wilkins.
35. Delmaire M et al: Is there a mechanical factor of haemolysis in patients with positive IgG type direct antiglobulin test? *Br J Haematol* 80:91, 1992.
36. Beutler E, Luzzatto L: Hemolytic anemia, *Sem Hematol* 36(4 suppl 7): 38, 1999.
37. Cotran RS et al: *Robbin's pathologic basis of disease,* ed 6, Philadelphia, 1999, W.B. Saunders.
38. Means JRT: The anemia of chronic disorders. In Lee GR et al, editors: *Wintrobe's clinical hematology,* p 1011, Baltimore, 1999, Williams & Wilkins.
39. Allen DA et al: Inhibition of CFU-E colony formation in uremic patients with inflammatory disease: role of IFN-gamma and IFN-alpha, *J Invest Med* 47(5):204, 1999.
40. Voulgari PV et al: Role of cytokines in the pathogenesis of anemia of chronic disease in rheumatoid arthritis, *Clin Immunol* 92(2):153, 1999.
41. Richer S: A practical guide for differentiating between iron deficiency anemia and anemia of chronic disease in children and adults, *Nurs Practitioner,* 22(1):82, 1997.
42. Drueke TB: Modulating factors in the hematopoietic response to erythropoietin, *Am J Kidney Dis* 18:87, 1991.
43. Means JRT: Polycythemia vera. In Lee GR et al, editors: *Wintrobe's clinical hematology,* p 2374 Baltimore, 1999, Williams & Wilkins.
44. Provan D, Weatherall D: Red cells II: acquired anaemias and polycythemia, *Lancet* 355(9211):1260, 2000.
45. Fernandes-Luna JL et al: Pathogenesis of polycythemia vera, *Haematologica* 83:150, 1998.
46. Weinberg RS: In vitro erythropoiesis in polycythemia vera and other myeloproliferative disorders, *Sem Hematol* 34(1):64, 1997.
47. Lengfelder E et al: Interferon alpha in the treatment of polycythemia vera, *Annals Hematol* 79:103, 2000.

CHAPTER 26

Alterations of Leukocyte, Lymphoid, and Hemostatic Function

THOM J. MANSEN • KATHRYN L. McCANCE

CHAPTER OUTLINE

The many disorders involving leukocytes range from purely reactive alterations, such as leukocytosis, to proliferative disorders, such as leukemia. An event of importance to hematology has been its increasing relationship with oncology. Many hematologic disorders are malignancies, and many nonhematologic malignancies metastasize to bone marrow. Thus a large portion of this chapter is devoted to malignant disease.

Because the only role of clotting (hemostasis) is to stop bleeding, this interesting self-regulatory system is obviously essential to survival. It is remarkable that blood clots when shed and normally does not clot within blood vessels. Platelets—through a renaissance of research interest—are known to have roles in clotting, wound healing, inflammation, and phagocytosis of foreign matter. They also play deleterious roles, however, in the pathogenesis of many diseases. This chapter also covers various clotting factors and their control systems.

ALTERATIONS OF LEUKOCYTE FUNCTION

Leukocyte function is affected if too many or too few cells are present in the blood or if the cells that are present are structurally or functionally defective. The presence of too many or too few cells, the so-called **quantitative disorders,** can be the result of bone marrow dysfunction or premature destruction of cells in the circulation. Many quantitative alterations, however, originate in the circulation or lymphoid organs in response to invasion by infectious microorganisms.

The **qualitative disorders** consist of disruptions of leukocyte function in mechanisms of self-defense. Phagocytic cells (granulocytes, monocytes, macrophages) may lose their capacity to function as effective phagocytes; lymphocytes may lose their capacity to respond to antigens. (Qualitative disruptions of inflammatory and immune processes caused by leukocyte disorders are described in Chapter 8.) Other leukocyte alterations are not primarily immune or inflammatory defects but rather are hematologic defects. These disorders include infectious mononucleosis and cancers of the blood—leukemia and multiple myeloma.

Quantitative Alterations of Leukocytes

Quantitative alterations are increases and decreases in numbers of leukocytes in the blood. **Leukocytosis** is present when the leukocyte count is higher than normal; **leukopenia** is present when the count is lower than normal. Leukocytosis or leukopenia may affect a specific type of leukocyte.

Leukocytosis and leukopenia can result from a variety of physiologic conditions and alterations. Leukocytosis is a normal protective response to physiologic stressors, such as invading microorganisms, strenuous exercise, emotional changes, temperature changes, anesthesia, surgery, pregnancy, and some drugs, hormones, and toxins. It is also caused by pathologic conditions, such as malignancies and hematologic

Table 26-1 Other Conditions Associated with Neutrophils, Eosinophils, Basophils, Monocytes, and Lymphocytes

Condition	Cause	Example
NEUTROPHIL		
Neutrophilia	Inflammation or tissue necrosis	Surgery, burns, MI, pneumonitis, rheumatic fever, RA
	Infection	Gram-positive (staphylococci, streptococci, pneumococci), gram-negative (*Escherichia coli, Pseudomonas* species)
	Physiologic	Exercise, extreme heat or cold, third-trimester pregnancy, emotional distress
	Hematologic	Acute hemorrhage, hemolysis, myeloproliferative disorder, CGL
	Drugs or chemicals	Epinephrine, steroids, heparin, histamine, endotoxin
	Metabolic	Diabetes (acidosis), eclampsia, gout, thyroid storm
	Neoplasms	Liver, GI tract, bone marrow
Neutropenia	Decreased marrow production	Radiation, chemotherapy, leukemia, aplastic anemia, abnormal granulopoiesis (megaloblastic anemia)
	Increased destruction	Splenomegaly, hemodialysis, immune reaction
	Infection	Gram-negative (typhoid), viral (influenza, hepatitis B, measles, mumps, rubella), severe infections, protozoal infections (malaria)
EOSINOPHIL		
Eosinophilia	Allergy (type I)	Asthma, hay fever, drug sensitivity
	Infection	Parasites (trichinosis, hookworm), chronic (fungal, leprosy, TB)
	Malignancies	CML, lung, stomach, ovary, Hodgkin disease
	Dermatoses	Pemphigus, exfoliative dermatitis (drug induced)
	Drugs	Digitalis, heparin, streptomycin, tryptophan (eosinophilia-myalgia syndrome), penicillins, propranolol
Eosinopenia	Stress response	Trauma, shock, burns, surgery, mental distress
	Drugs	Steroids (Cushing syndrome)
BASOPHIL		
Basophilia	Inflammation	Infection (measles, chickenpox), hypersensitivity reaction (immediate)
	Hematologic	Myeloproliferative disorders (CGL, polycythemia vera, Hodgkin disease, hemolytic anemia)
	Endocrine	Myxedema, antithyroid therapy
Basopenia	Physiologic	Pregnancy, ovulation, stress
	Endocrine	Graves disease
MONOCYTE		
Monocytosis	Infection	Bacterial: SBE, TB, recovery phase of infection Rickettsiae: Rocky Mountain spotted fever, typhoid fever Protozoa: malaria
	Hematologic	Monocytic leukemia, myeloproliferative disorders, Hodgkin disease, agranulocytosis
	Physiologic	Normal newborn
Monocytopenia	Rare	Chronic diseases: ulcerative colitis, Crohn disease, RA, SLE
LYMPHOCYTE		
Lymphocytosis	Physiologic	4 months to 4 years
	Acute infections	Infectious mononucleosis, CMV infection, pertussis, hepatitis, mycoplasma pneumonia, typhoid
	Chronic infections	Congenital syphilis, tertiary syphilis
	Endocrine	Thyrotoxicosis, adrenal insufficiency
	Malignancies	ALL, CLL, lymphosarcoma cell leukemia
Lymphocytopenia	Immune deficiency syndromes	AIDS, agammaglobulinemia
	Lymphocyte destruction	Steroids (Cushing syndrome), radiation, chemotherapy
	Malignancies	Hodgkin disease
	Debilitating illness	CHF, renal failure, TB, SLE, aplastic anemia

MI, Myocardial infarction; *RA,* rheumatoid arthritis; *CGL,* chronic granulocytic leukemia; *GI,* gastrointestinal; *TB,* tuberculosis; *SBE,* subacute bacterial endocarditis; *SLE,* systemic lupus erythematosus; *CMV,* cytomegalovirus; *ALL,* acute lymphocytic leukemia; *CLL,* chronic lymphocytic leukemia; *AIDS,* acquired immunodeficiency syndrome; *CHF,* congestive heart failure.

disorders. Unlike leukocytosis, leukopenia is never normal or beneficial. When the leukocyte count decreases to below $1000/mm^3$, the individual is at risk for infection. With counts below $500/mm^3$, serious life-threatening infections may occur. Leukopenia can be caused by radiation, anaphylactic shock, systemic lupus erythematosus, and certain chemotherapeutic agents.

Granulocytes and Monocytes

Increased numbers of circulating granulocytes (neutrophils, eosinophils, basophils) and monocytes are primarily a response to microbial invasion. Increased numbers occur also as a result of myeloproliferative disorders (polycythemia vera, chronic myelocytic leukemia) that increase stem cell proliferation in bone marrow.

Decreased numbers occur when infectious processes exhaust the supply of circulating granulocytes and monocytes, drawing them out of the circulation and into infected tissues faster than they can be replaced. Decreases also can be caused by disorders that suppress marrow function.

Granulocytosis begins with the release of white cells that have been stored in the venous sinuses of the marrow. Because the neutrophil is the most numerous of the granulocytes, the term *granulocytosis* often is used to describe **neutrophilia** (Table 26-1). Neutrophilia is present in the early stages of infection or inflammation and is confirmed when the absolute neutrophil count exceeds $7500/\mu l$.[1] Stored neutrophils are approximately 20 to 40 times greater in number than circulating neutrophils. When the neutrophil count increases greatly—more than $100,000/\mu l$ (usually seen only in myelocytic leukemia)—the blood viscosity may greatly increase so that thrombosis or occlusion of blood vessels occurs. Emptying of the venous sinuses stimulates granulopoiesis to replenish neutrophil stores in the marrow. Specific conditions associated with neutrophilia are identified in Table 26-1.

When the demand for circulating neutrophils exceeds the supply, the marrow begins to release immature neutrophils (and other leukocytes) into the blood. Premature release of the immature white cells is responsible for the phenomenon identified as a **shift-to-the-left.** The shift-to-the-left refers to the microscopic detection of disproportionate numbers of immature leukocytes in peripheral blood smears. The phenomenon can be understood if one visualizes cellular differentiation and maturation to progress from left to right, as shown in Fig. 24-7, *A.* (The shift-to-the-left is sometimes called a **leukemoid reaction** because it is similar to morphologic findings in blood smears of individuals with leukemia.) As infection or inflammation diminishes and granulopoiesis replenishes circulating granulocytes, a **shift-to-the-right,** or return to normal, occurs.

Neutropenia is the condition associated with a reduction in circulating neutrophils. Clinically, neutropenia exists when the neutrophil count is less than $2000/\mu l$. A reduction in neutrophils occurs in severe prolonged infections when production of granulocytes cannot keep up with demand.

WHAT'S NEW? WHIM Syndrome

The acronym WHIM stands for warts, hypogammaglobulinemia, infections, and myelokathexis. *Myelokathexis* refers to the retention of white cells in the marrow, which becomes hypercellular. The first identification of this syndrome was in 1964. Myelokathexis is also associated with a chronic, noncyclic neutropenia and a release of defective marrow cells into the circulation. The hypermature neutrophils are bizarre in form with condensed nuclei connected by long, stringy filaments and vacuolated cytoplasm that suggests apoptosis. Stress and fever increase the release of neutrophils. Hypogammaglobulinemia is also marked and associated with recurrent upper respiratory infections. Individuals also have numerous warts in various locations of the body that result in premalignant cervical and vulval dysplasia. Females are more likely to be affected than males, and research to find evidence for genetic transmission is continuing.

Data from Gorlin RJ et al: WHIM syndrome, an autosomal dominant disorder: clinical, hematological and molecular studies, *Am J Med Genet* 91:368, 2000.

Other causes of neutropenia in the absence of overwhelming infection may be (1) decreased neutrophil production or ineffective granulopoiesis, (2) reduced neutrophil survival, and (3) abnormal neutrophil distribution and sequestration.[2] Ineffective or defective neutrophil production may be caused by hematologic disorders, for example, hypoplastic anemia or aplastic anemia, leukemia, or drug- or toxin-induced neutropenia. The megaloblastic anemias (vitamin B_{12} and folate deficiency) are also known to cause neutropenia.[3] Starvation and anorexia nervosa also cause neutropenia because of an inadequate supply of protein building blocks.[4] Reduced neutrophil survival is seen in autoimmune disorders, particularly systemic lupus erythematosus and rheumatoid arthritis. Abnormal neutrophil distribution and sequestration are associated with hypersplenism and pseudoneutropenia. These two manifestations in the presence of rheumatoid arthritis make up what is known as Felty syndrome.[3]

If neutrophils are drastically reduced (less than $500/\mu l$) and the entire granulocyte count is extremely low, a serious condition called **granulocytopenia** or **agranulocytosis** results. The usual cause is interference with hematopoiesis in the bone marrow or increased cell destruction in the circulation. Chemotherapeutic agents commonly used in treating hematologic and other malignancies cause bone marrow suppression. Multiple drugs are known to cause agranulocytosis (Table 26-2). Clinical manifestations of agranulocytosis include infection (particularly of the respiratory system), general malaise, septicemia, fever, tachycardia, and ulcers in the mouth and colon. If untreated, sepsis caused by agranulocytosis results in death within 3 to 6 days. Other conditions associated with neutropenia are identified in Table 26-1.

Eosinophilia, an absolute increase (greater than $450/\mu l$) in the total numbers of circulating eosinophils, has a variety of causes. Allergic disorders (type I) associated with asthma,

Table 26-2 Drugs Associated with Neutropenia and Agranulocytosis

Drug Group	Neutropenia	Agranulocytosis
Analgesics, sedatives, antiinflammatory agents	Gold compounds; phenylbutazone; indomethacin	Phenacetin; barbiturates; aminopyrine; dipyrone
Antibiotics	Cephalosporins; semisynthetic penicillins	Sulfonamides; chloramphenicol; methicillin
Antithyroid agents	Methimazole	Propylthiouracil
Psychotropic agents	Tricyclic antidepressants	Phenothiazines
Anticonvulsant agents	Trimethadione	Phenytoin
Antiarrhythmic agents	Procainamide; quinidine	

hay fever, and drug reactions are frequently cited as causes. Hypersensitivity reactions trigger the release of eosinophilic chemotaxic factor of anaphylaxis (CTF-A) and histamine from mast cells, attracting eosinophils to the area. Areas abundant in mast cells, such as the respiratory and gastrointestinal tracts, are particularly common sites for eosinophil invasion. Other causes of eosinophilia are associated with dermatologic disorders, such as atopic dermatitis, eczema, and pemphigus. Various types of eosinophilic scleroderma-like diseases have also been reported to occur in association with hemato-oncogenic disorders (i.e., eosinophilic cellulitis [Well syndrome] and eosinophilic fasciitis).[5] Most recently, increased numbers of eosinophils have been identified with eosinophilia-myalgia syndrome (EMS), which is associated with ingestion of tryptophan, and a relationship between EMS and fibromyalgia syndrome (FMS) has been suggested.[6]

Parasitic invasion also is associated with eosinophilia, particularly metazoan parasites. Eosinophils are attracted out of the circulation to the site of infestation, where they degranulate powerful enzymes onto the parasites. (This process is described and illustrated in Chapter 7.) Other conditions that cause eosinophilia are detailed in Table 26-1.

Eosinopenia, a decrease in circulating numbers of eosinophils, generally is caused by migration of eosinophils into inflammatory sites. It also may be seen in Cushing syndrome and as a result of stress caused by surgery, shock, trauma, burns, or mental distress. Other conditions causing eosinopenia are detailed in Table 26-1.

Basophilia is rare and when present generally is seen as a response to inflammation and hypersensitivity reactions of the immediate type. Basophils contain histamine that is released during an allergic reaction. An increase in basophils is seen also in myeloproliferative disorders, such as chronic myeloid leukemia and myeloid metaplasia. Other conditions associated with basophilia are listed in Table 26-1.

Basopenia is seen in hyperthyroidism, acute infection, and long-term therapy with steroids. A decrease in basophils is seen also during ovulation and pregnancy. Other conditions associated with basopenia are listed in Table 26-1.

Monocytosis, an increase in numbers of circulating monocytes, is often transient and correlates poorly with disease states. When present, it most commonly occurs with neutropenia associated with bacterial infections, particularly in the late stages or recovery stage, when monocytes are needed to phagocytize surviving microorganisms and debris. Increased numbers of monocytes also may indicate marrow recovery from agranulocytosis. Monocytosis often is seen in chronic infections such as tuberculosis (TB) and subacute bacterial endocarditis (SBE). Recently, peripheral monocytosis has been found to correlate with the extent of myocardial damage following myocardial infarction.[7] Other conditions associated with monocytosis are identified in Table 26-1.

Monocytopenia, a decrease in numbers of circulating monocytes, is rare, and not much is known about this condition because of the small numbers of monocytes generally present in the blood. Monocytopenia, however, has been identified with hairy cell leukemia and prednisone therapy.

Lymphocytes

Quantitative alteration of lymphocytes occurs when lymphocytes are activated by antigenic stimuli, usually microorganisms (see Chapter 6). A **lymphocytosis** is rare in acute bacterial infections and occurs most commonly in acute viral infections, particularly those caused by the Epstein-Barr virus (a causative agent in infectious mononucleosis). Other specific disorders associated with lymphocytosis are listed in Table 26-1.

Lymphocytopenia may be attributable to abnormalities of lymphocyte production associated with neoplasias and immune deficiencies, as well as destruction by drugs, viruses, or radiation. It also is known to occur in individuals for no apparent reason. Other conditions associated with lymphocytopenia are identified in Table 26-1. It has been hypothesized that the lymphocytopenia associated with heart failure and other acute illnesses may be caused by elevated levels of cortisol. The mechanisms in other disease states are not well understood.[8]

The most recent condition in which lymphocytopenia is a major problem is acquired immunodeficiency syndrome (AIDS). The lymphocytopenia associated with this condition is caused by the human immunodeficiency virus (HIV), which is cytopathic for T-helper lymphocytes. (For a more detailed discussion of AIDS, see Chapter 8.)

Infectious Mononucleosis

Infectious mononucleosis (IM) is an acute, self-limiting, neoplastic lymphoproliferative clinical syndrome characterized by acute infection of B lymphocytes (B cells). The most common etiologic agent is the Epstein-Barr virus (EBV), a ubiquitous, lymphotrophic, gamma-group herpesvirus,[9] which was first recognized as the causative agent in IM in the late 1960s.[10] EBV accounts for approximately 85% of all IM cases.[11] Other etiologic agents that may cause symptoms resembling IM are viruses (cytomegalovirus [CMV], adenovirus, HIV, hepatitis A, influenza A and B, and rubella), as well as the bacteria *Toxoplasma gondii, Corynebacterium diphtheriae,* and *Coxiella burnetti.*[12] IM caused by CMV is generally noted in older individuals, with fever and malaise the major complaints; the major manifestations of EBV-induced IM are pharyngitis and lymphadenopathy.[10]

IM usually affects young adults between ages 15 and 35 years, with the peak incidences occurring between 15 and 19 years; males have a later peak (18 to 23 years) than females (15 to 16 years). Children from low socioeconomic environments are particularly susceptible to infections with EBV. It is estimated that 50% to 85% of these children acquire EBV infection by the time they are 4 years of age.[9] Infection with EBV at this early stage is usually asymptomatic and provides the individual with immunity to later infections.[13] The incidence of IM is estimated to be 45 per 10,000 individuals. IM is uncommon in individuals over age 40 years.

The primary route of transmission of EBV is through saliva from close personal contact (i.e., kissing, hence the term "kissing disease"). However, the virus may be present in other mucosal secretions of the genital, rectal, and respiratory tract, as well as blood. No evidence of aerosol transmission has been documented.[9] The course of the infection begins with widespread invasion of B lymphocytes, all of which possess an EBV receptor site. Initially, the sites of invasion are the oropharynx, nasopharynx, and salivary epithelial cells with simultaneous spread to the lymphoid tissue and B cells.[12] Infection of B cells permits the virus to enter the bloodstream, which systematically spreads the infection.[14]

In the immunocompetent individual, EBV invasion triggers an *immunopathologic* response. Unaffected B cells are transformed into immortal plasmacytoid cells that produce antibodies (immunoglobulins A, M, and G [IgA, IgM, and IgG]) against the virus. Concomitantly, there is a massive activation and proliferation of cytotoxic T cells (CD8) to assist the B cell response of attacking the virus directly (see Chapter 6). The proliferation of clones of B and T cells and removal of dead and damaged leukocytes are largely responsible for the swelling of lymphoid tissues (lymph nodes, spleen, tonsils, and occasionally liver). Sore throat and fever, two of the earliest manifestations of IM, are caused by inflammation at the site of viral entry (and initial infection), namely, the mouth and throat. The proliferation of B and T cells is also responsible for the rise in absolute lymphocyte count and the presence of atypical lymphocytes (Downy cells), which are actually CD8 cytotoxic T cells.[14]

The incubation period of IM is approximately 30 to 50 days. Initial symptoms (including headache, malaise, fatigue, arthralgia, fever, chills, dysphagia, and anorexia) may appear during the first 3 to 5 days after introduction of EBV. These symptoms may vary in severity for the next 7 to 20 days. At the time of diagnosis the individual usually has the classic triad of symptoms: fever, pharyngitis, and lymphadenopathy of the cervical lymph nodes. The pharyngitis is usually diffuse and often accompanied by a whitish or grayish green, thick exudate. Enlargement of the spleen and liver also may occur.[15] Splenomegaly has been estimated to occur in approximately 41% to 100% of affected individuals.[12]

Approximately 3% to 10% of adults over age 40 have never been infected with EBV and are susceptible to IM later in life.[16] In individuals over age 40, these classic symptoms generally are not present and it is more difficult to diagnose IM. If an individual has an elevated temperature that cannot be explained and persists for longer than 2 weeks, EBV infection should be suspected, particularly in the presence of abnormal liver function tests with hepatomegaly and jaundice. Other neurologic manifestations that may be present in the older individual include peripheral neuropathy and Guillain-Barré syndrome.[17]

On rare occasions, individuals with IM may have other organ systems affected by EBV. These include neurologic alterations, such as meningitis, encephalitis, Guillain-Barré syndrome, Bell palsy, optic neuritis, mental impairment, transverse myelitis, cerebellar ataxia, and demyelinating diseases. Ocular manifestations also may develop, including eyelid and periorbital edema, dry eyes, keratitis, uveitis, conjunctivitis, retinitis, oculoglandular syndrome, choroiditis, papillitis, and ophthalmoplegia.[17] In children, Reye syndrome has also been associated with EBV infection.

Pulmonary manifestations may develop; however, these are rare. When present, they may include hilar and mediastinal lymphadenopathy, interstitial pneumonitis, and pleural effusion. Incidences of pneumonia and respiratory failure have been documented; however, they are more likely to develop in immunocompromised individuals.

IM is usually self-limiting, and recovery occurs in a few weeks. Severe clinical courses with complications are rare, occurring in only 5% of cases. Fatalities associated with IM involve fulminant hepatitis, hemophagocytic syndrome, and splenic rupture.[18] Splenic rupture is the most common cause of death and appears to be the only gender-related factor associated with IM, with 90% of cases occurring in males.[14] Rupture of the spleen may occur spontaneously without evidence of trauma and most often occurs between 4 and 21 days after onset of symptoms.[12] Airway obstruction from massive edema of the Waldeyer ring is another complication associated with IM,[14] as is autoimmune hemolytic anemia, which occurs in approximately 3% to 5% of cases.[19]

Treatment of IM is supportive and includes rest and alleviation of symptoms with analgesics and antipyretics. Ibuprofen and acetaminophen, not aspirin, are used with children and adolescents because of the reported incidence of Reye syndrome with EBV infection. Pharyngitis of streptococcal origin, which occurs in 20% to 30% of cases, is treated with penicillin or erythromycin. Ampicillin is contraindicated because it causes a rash in most individuals with IM.[10]

Bed rest and avoidance of strenuous activity should be included in the therapy. Steroids may be used, but only in the presence of severe complications (e.g., impending airway obstruction)[15] or other organ system involvement (e.g., nervous system manifestations, thrombocytopenic purpura, myocarditis, pericarditis).[17] Acyclovir has been used with immunosuppressed individuals; however, clinical improvement has been minimal and therefore it is not recommended for standard treatment. IM and EBV infection were thought to be associated with chronic fatigue syndrome in the past, but that relationship is no longer reported to exist.[9]

Serologic tests to determine a heterophile antibody response are necessary to diagnose EBV infection. **Heterophilic antibodies** are a heterogeneous group of IgM antibodies that are agglutinins against nonhuman red blood cells (e.g., sheep, horse). These antibodies may be detected by either qualitative methods (monospot) or qualitative methods (heterophile antobody test).

The monospot test is limited because other infections (e.g., CMV, adenovirus) and toxoplasmosis also produce heterophilic antibodies. The percentage of individuals with IM who have heterophilic antibodies in their blood increases relative to the time of onset of symptoms. Some individuals do not produce heterophilic antibodies, and children under age 4 years also do not produce heterophilic antibodies. For these reasons, 5% to 15% of monospot tests yield a false-positive result.[17] Specificity for EBV infection may be increased with newer viral-specific serology tests that identify EBV-specific antibodies (e.g., viral capsid antigen, IgG and IgM, and EBV antigen). These tests are more expensive and labor intensive and thus should be used in instances where the monospot test is not appropriate.

Leukemias

Leukemia is a clonal malignant disorder of the blood and blood-forming organs causing an accumulation of dysfunctional cells and a loss of cell division regulation. The common pathologic feature of all forms of leukemia is an uncontrolled proliferation of leukocytes. The excessive proliferation of the leukemia cells results in an overcrowding of bone marrow, which causes a decreased production and function of normal hematopoietic cells.

The first description of a "leukemic" individual was by Velpeau in 1827.[20] His patient, a 63-year-old florist and seller of lemonade "who had abandoned himself to the abuse of spiritus liquor and of women, without, however, becoming syphilitic," became ill in 1825. This patient had great swelling of the abdomen, fever, weakness, and symptoms related to urinary stones. On autopsy he was found to have a very large liver and spleen and blood and pus resembling the color of yeast and red wine.[20] Not until 1945, however, did the physiologist Bennet and the pathologist Virchow separately describe leukemia. Virchow coined the term *white blood (weissus blut)* and later the term *leukemia.* He is largely credited with discoveries that have led to current knowledge of the pathology of leukemia.

Since Virchow's time the classification of leukemia has become increasingly complex. Leukemias are classified as either chronic or acute and as either myeloid or lymphoid. The classification system for leukemia is based on the type of cell that predominates; the type of leukemia is named according to the point at which cell maturation is arrested (Fig. 26-1). In 1976 the French-American-British Cooperative Group developed criteria for the classification of acute leukemias. This classification system is based on structure, number of cells, genetics, identification of surface markers, and histochemical staining. These findings produce important therapeutic and prognostic information.

The two major forms of leukemia, acute and chronic, are classified by predominant cell type and the rate at which the affected individual develops clinical symptoms. **Acute leukemia** is characterized by undifferentiated or immature cells, usually a blast cell. The onset of disease is abrupt and rapid. Disease progression results in a short survival time. In **chronic leukemia** the predominant cell is mature in appearance but does not function normally. The onset of disease is gradual, and the prolonged clinical course results in a relatively longer survival time. The past two decades have shown advances in remission induction rates, as well as survival. Thus progress has occurred as a result of more effective chemotherapeutic agents, improved blood product and antimicrobial support, and specialized nursing care.[21] Chemotherapy and bone marrow transplants have significantly increased the survival time for individuals with acute leukemia.

Leukemias occur with varying frequencies at different ages and are more common in adults (approximately 28,200 cases per year) than children (approximately 2600 cases per year).[22] Acute lymphoblastic leukemia is the most common type in children and accounts for more than two thirds of all cases (see Chapter 27). Acute nonlymphoblastic leukemia (approximately 9000 cases per year) and chronic lymphocytic leukemia (approximately 8100 cases per year) are the most common types in adults.[22] The sites of highest overall incidence are the United States, Canada, Sweden, and New Zealand.

Pathogenesis

Leukemias are considered clonal disorders in that a single progenitor cell undergoes transformation. An interesting paradox is that leukemic cells apparently divide more *slowly* and take longer to synthesize deoxyribonucleic acid (DNA) than other blood precursors. Acute leukemia therefore is not caused by rapid cellular proliferation but is instead caused by the blocking of differentiation. Leukemic cells do accumulate relentlessly in most affected individuals, and they compete with normal cellular proliferation. Thus acute leukemia has been termed an *accumulation* disorder, as well as a *proliferation* disorder.

Although the exact cause of leukemia is unknown, it is clear that causal risk factors acting together with a genetic predisposition can alter nuclear DNA. The leukemic cell is then unable to mature and respond to normal regulatory mechanisms. Abnormal chromosomes are reported in 40% to 50% of patients with acute leukemia, and certain chromosomes are repeatedly more involved than others. It thus appears that a mutation in a single cell gives rise to some leukemias.

Although the genetic mechanism remains unknown, studies indicate a statistically significant tendency for leu-

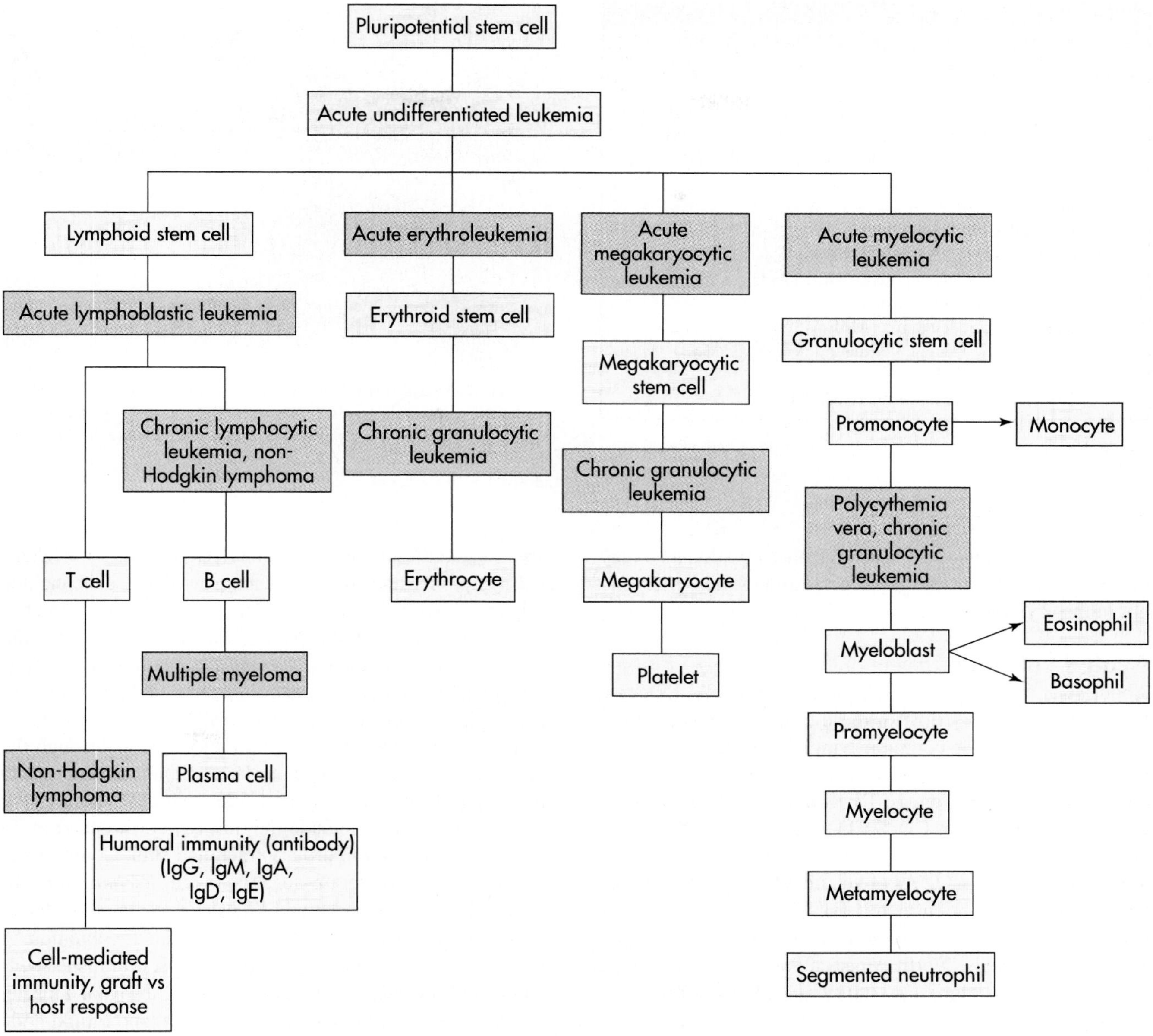

FIG. 26-1 Cell-specific leukemias. Differentiation pathways of blood-forming cells and reported sites of block resulting in cell-specific leukemias. *Ig,* immunoglobulin.

kemia to recur in families. This tendency to cluster is seen among twins and siblings in certain families. Hereditary abnormalities are also associated with an increased incidence of leukemia, Down syndrome, Fanconi aplastic anemia, Bloom syndrome, ataxia-telangiectasia, trisomy 13 (Patau syndrome), Wiskott-Aldrich syndrome, and congenital X-linked agammaglobulinemia.

Acquired disorders that progress to acute leukemia include chronic myelocytic leukemia (CML), polycythemia vera, myelofibrosis, Hodgkin disease, multiple myeloma, ovarian cancer, chronic lymphocytic leukemia (CLL), and sideroblastic anemia. Large doses of ionizing radiation are associated with an increased incidence of myelogenous leukemia. Viruses are known to cause leukemia in certain animals, but they have not yet been proved to cause leukemia in humans. Drugs that cause bone marrow depression (e.g., chloramphenicol, phenylbutazone, and certain alkylating agents, such as cytoxan) also can predispose an individual to leukemia. Acute myelogenous leukemia (AML) is the most frequently reported secondary cancer after high doses of chemotherapy for Hodgkin disease, multiple myeloma, ovarian cancer, non-Hodgkin lymphoma, and breast cancer (Box 26-1).

In some cases the development of leukemia occurs in the most primitive blood precursors—pluripotential stem cells—which give rise to all other blood cells (see Fig. 26-1). The leukemia blasts, or precursor cells, literally "crowd out" the marrow and cause cellular proliferation of the other cell lines to cease (Fig. 26-2). Normal granulocytic-monocytic, lymphocytic, erythrocytic, and megakaryocytic stem cells cease to function, causing **pancytopenia** (a reduction in all

Box 26-1

CLASSIFICATION OF ACUTE MYELOID LEUKEMIAS

Acute myeloblastic leukemia, minimally differentiated (AML-M0)
Acute myeloblastic leukemia without maturation (AML-M1)
Acute myeloblastic leukemia with maturation (AML-M2)
Acute promyelocytic leukemia (AML-M3)
- Hypergranular type
- Microgranular variant

Acute myelomonocytic leukemia (AML-M4)
- Increased marrow eosinophils (AML-M4-EO)

Acute monocytic leukemia (AML)
- Acute monoblastic leukemia (AML-M5A)
- Acute monocytic leukemia, differentiated (AML-M5B)

Erythroleukemia (AML-M6)
Acute megakaryoblastic leukemia (AML-M7)

From Damjanov I, Linder J: *Pathology: a color atlas,* St Louis, 2000, Mosby.

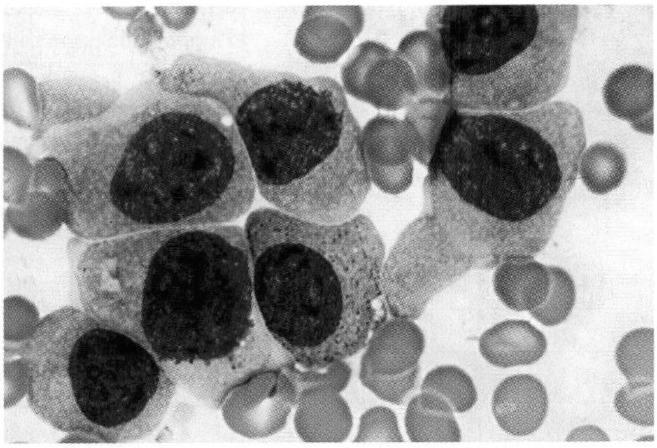

FIG. 26-2 Acute monoblastic leukemia (M5A). The bone marrow contains monoblasts, which are larger than normal myeloblasts and usually have abundant cytoplasm, frequently with scattered granules. (From Damjanov I, Linder J: *Pathology: a color atlas,* St Louis, 2000, Mosby.)

cellular components of the blood). Transformation also may occur specifically in the granulocyte-monocyte series and not in the erythrocyte series.

Acute Leukemias

About 80% of acute lymphoblastic leukemias (ALLs) arise from the B cell line. Most of these cases express the common ALL antigen or common lymphocytic leukemia antigen (CALLA), designated CD-10.[23] About 15% to 20% of all ALL cases arise from the T cell lineage. These cells express the T cell antigens CD-5, CD-7, or CD-10. A very small percentage of ALL cases lack either B or T cell origin and are termed *null cell ALL.* As of yet, no AML-specific surface antigens have been identified.[23] For all types of acute leukemia the mortality rate for the United States is about 7 per 100,000 individuals. North America and the Scandinavian countries have the highest mortality rates; Eastern European countries, Asia (except Japan), and Central America have the lowest mortality rates. The higher mortality rate in Japan is the result of the atomic bombs. Black Americans consistently have shown a lower mortality rate than whites.

Leukemia strikes both genders and all ages. Incidence rises steeply, however, beyond 50 years of age. The 5-year survival rate for individuals with leukemia is 43%, partly because of very poor survival rates of individuals with some types of leukemia, such as acute myelocytic. Over the past 30 years, however, there has been a dramatic improvement in survival of individuals with ALL: from a 5-year survival rate of 4% for those diagnosed in the 1960s, to 38% in the early 1970s, to 59% in the mid-1990s. In children the improvement has been from 4% to 81% (see Chapter 27).[22] The decrease in mortality rate for ALL appears to be the result of chemotherapy.

Clinical Manifestations

The clinical manifestations of all the varieties of acute leukemia are generally similar. (Mechanisms associated with common manifestations are summarized in Table 26-3.) Signs and symptoms related to bone marrow depression include fatigue caused by anemia, bleeding resulting from thrombocytopenia (reduced numbers of circulating platelets), and fever caused by infection. Bleeding can occur in skin, gums, mucous membranes, and gastrointestinal and genitourinary tracts. Signs of bleeding include petechiae and ecchymosis visible in dependent areas, discoloration visible through the skin, gingival bleeding, hematuria, and midcycle menstrual bleeding or heavy bleeding associated with menstruation.

Sites of infection include the oral cavity, throat, respiratory tract, lower colon, urinary tract, and skin. Common organisms include the gram-negative bacilli *Escherichia coli, Pseudomonas aeruginosa,* and *Klebsiella pneumoniae*. Fever is an early sign. Chills and tissue infiltration are common.

Anorexia is associated with weight loss, diminished sensitivity to sour and sweet tastes, wasting away of muscle, and difficulty in swallowing. Liver, spleen, and lymph node enlargement are more common in ALL than in acute nonlymphocytic leukemia (ANLL). Splenomegaly and hepatomegaly usually occur together. The leukemic individual often experiences abdominal pain and tenderness and breast tenderness.

Neurologic manifestations are frequent and may be caused by either leukemic infiltration or cerebral bleeding. Headache, vomiting, papilledema, facial palsy, blurred vision, auditory disturbances, and meningeal irritation can occur if leukemic cells infiltrate the cerebral or spinal meninges. Because chemotherapeutic agents do not pass the blood-brain barrier, leukemia cells can grow easily.

Evaluation and Treatment

Because leukemia frequently is confused with other conditions, early detection is difficult. Persistent symptoms indicate the need for intensive medical investigation. The diagnosis is made through blood tests and examination of bone marrow (Fig. 26-3).

Table 26-3 Clinical Manifestations and Related Pathophysiology in Leukemia

Clinical Manifestations	Laboratory Abnormalities	Cause	Comments
Anemia	Either a decrease or normal number of erythroblasts; key is the relative *proportion* of erythroblasts to total count; decreased iron in mature RBC	Decreased RBC production may be caused by decreased stem cell input or ineffective erythropoiesis or both; proposed reasons are: 1. Replacement of ESCs by leukemic clone 2. Inhibition of ESCs by leukemic cells 3. Inhibition of pluripotent stem cell 4. Decreased erythropoietin responsiveness from impaired interaction of ESCs with T lymphocytes (in leukemia there is an increase in T lymphocytes) 5. Hemorrhage 6. Splenic pooling of RBC 7. Drug therapy	In acute leukemia, anemia is usually present from beginning, often the first symptom noticed, and severe; mild form without symptoms is common in CML and CLL; hemorrhage is common in acute forms, occasional in CML, but rare in CLL
Bleeding, purpura, petechiae, ecchymosis, thrombosis, or hemorrhage	Decreased and possibly abnormal platelets; abnormal clotting	Reduction in megakaryocytes leading to thrombocytopenia	Bleeding occurs more commonly in acute than in chronic leukemia
DIC	Abnormal promyelocytes; hypofibrinogenemia; prolonged prothrombin, thrombin, and reptilase times; elevated fibrin degranulation products; and decreased levels of factor V, fibrinogen, and platelets	Proliferation of promyelocytic granulocytes with an excessive release of procoagulants from granules within the leukemic promyelocyte	Correction of coagulopathy in DIC is dependent on the successful treatment of leukemia
Infection	Infection is likely with an AGC below 500/mm³ (AGC is the proportion of neutrophils and bands to the total white blood cell count)	Infections are caused by organisms endogenous to the host or present in the environment; granulocytopenic persons have an impaired inflammatory response; immune deficiency resulting from chemotherapy, corticosteroids, and the disease process contributes to the infection	Major sites of infection are the alimentary tract sinuses, lungs, and skin; prevention of infection focuses on the restoration of host defenses, decreasing invasive procedures, and reducing colonization of organisms
Weight loss	Decreased 24-hr urinary creatinine excretion; hypoalbuminemia	Condition can be attributed to pain, depression, chemotherapy, radiation therapy, some unknown circulating inhibitor, and alterations in taste	Causes of weight loss are poorly understood; severe alterations in taste; highly seasoned foods seem bland, aggravate condition; patients with liver involvement often detest red meat; some patients have good appetites in the morning but become satiated later; increased metabolism also aggravates the condition
Bone pain	Frequently no radiographic evidence of bone problems	Result of bone infiltration by leukemic cells or intramedullary infarction	If combination drug regimens are ineffective, radiation therapy is used
Elevated uric acid	Normal excretion of uric acid is 300-500 mg/day; the leukemic patient can excrete 50 times more; uric acid precipitates (urates) are commonly found in the proximal collecting tubules and pelvises of the kidney; oliguria and concentrated urine are sometimes found	Uric acid is a normal by-product of protein catabolism; nucleic acid catabolism is accelerated in the leukemic patient; uric acid precipitation occurs at an acidic, or low, pH; urate precipitation in the leukemic patient is increased from dehydration caused by anorexia or fever and drug therapy	Hyperuricemia is present in both acute leukemia and CML; kidney pathologic manifestations can be prevented by ensuring increased urine flow, increasing urine pH by administering sodium bicarbonate, or decreasing acid production through allopurinol, which inhibits the enzyme xanthine oxidase

RBC, Red blood cell; *ESC,* erythropoietic stem cell; *CML,* chronic myelocytic leukemia; *CLL,* chronic lymphocytic leukemia; *DIC,* disseminated intravascular coagulation; *AGC,* absolute granulocyte count.

Continued

Table 26-3 Clinical Manifestations and Related Pathophysiology in Leukemia—cont'd

Clinical Manifestations	Laboratory Abnormalities	Cause	Comments
Liver, spleen, and lymph node enlargement	Biopsy is abnormal for liver and spleen	Leukemic cell infiltration causes splenic, hepatic, and lymph node enlargement; lymph nodes also undergo leukemic proliferation as in CLL	

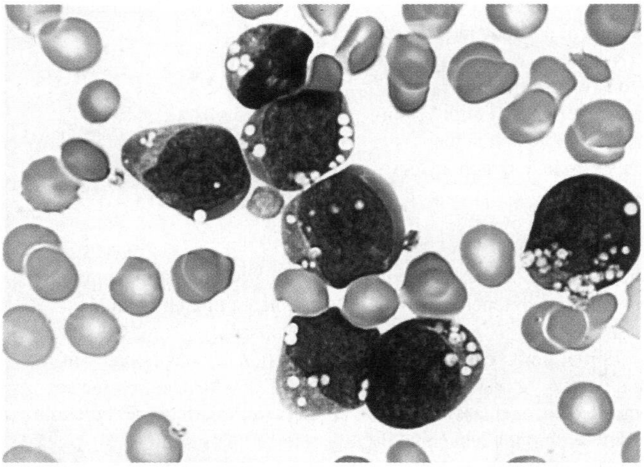

FIG. 26-3 Acute lymphoblastic leukemia. L3 lymphoblasts in a marrow aspirate. The cytoplasm contains sharply outlined cytoplasmic vacuoles (Wright-Giemsa stain). (From Damjanov I, Linder J, editors: *Anderson's pathology,* ed 10, St Louis, 1996, Mosby.)

Chemotherapy is the treatment of choice for leukemia. Two controversial treatments are immunotherapy agents that induce differentiation of immature granulocytes (i.e., *cis*-retinoic acid) and marrow transplants. Drugs are used in various combinations. Supportive measures include blood transfusions, antibiotics, antifungals, and antivirals. Allopurinol is used for preventing production of uric acid (which is elevated from cellular death because of treatment). Bone marrow transplantation as a treatment has been increasing during the past two decades. Improvements in histocompatibility testing, transfusion support, conditioning regimens, and antibiotics have increased survival after transplantation.[24,25] Although there has not been a marked improvement in response or survival of ANLL, dramatic improvements in survival and response of people with ALL have occurred. Future studies will define the role of biotherapy in the treatment of leukemia and perhaps improve survival rates.

Improved survival rates in individuals with acute leukemia have occurred in the past three decades. Factors influencing increased survival rate include the use of combined and multimodality treatment regimens, improved supportive services such as blood banking and nutritional support, and microbial treatment.

Chronic Leukemias

The two main types of chronic leukemias are myelocytic (CML) and lymphocytic (CLL). These two disorders have distinct clinical and morphologic features. CMLs represent clonal, neoplastic expansion of the multipotent myeloid stem cell, whereas CLLs involve neoplastic transformation of lymphoid cells, mainly of the B cell lineage. Unlike cells in acute leukemia, chronic leukemic cells are well differentiated and can be readily identified. Individuals with chronic leukemia have a longer life expectancy, usually several years from the time of diagnosis.

Pathophysiology and Clinical Manifestations

The chronic leukemias have a presentation and progression different from the acute leukemias. Chronic leukemia advances slowly and surreptitiously, without warning. Symptoms—when they do appear—include splenomegaly, extreme fatigue, weight loss, night sweats, and low-grade fever.

The incidence of CML is approximately 1 per 100,000 people. CML is a myeloproliferative disorder, as are polycythemia vera, primary thrombocytosis, and idiopathic myelofibrosis (invasion of bone marrow by fibrous tissue).

The Philadelphia chromosome is a diagnostic marker of CML (Fig. 26-4, *A*). The Philadelphia chromosome results from a reciprocal translocation between the long arms of chromosomes 9 and 22 and is demonstrable in all blood cell precursors, meaning that the disease originates in a progenitor stem cell (see Chapter 4). The median age for persons with Philadelphia chromosome–positive CML is 40 to 45 years. Identifying the Philadelphia chromosome allows the clinician to follow the transformation process. Transformation is identified in erythroid, megakaryocytic, and macrophage cell lines. With such strong evidence that CML begins in a stem cell, however, it is *not* clear why myeloid cells predominate (i.e., in the chronic phase). The chromosome appears not to be genetically transmitted but to occur because of mitotic error. Evidence thus indicates that CML has a clonal origin. The malignant transformation arises from pluripotential stem cells or lymphoid stem cells (see Fig. 26-1). Structural cellular abnormalities are not readily identified in CML. Absent or low levels of the enzyme neutrophil alkaline phosphatase, with subsequent decreased phagocytic capabilities, do, however, indicate that cells fail to differentiate normally.

Although the Philadelphia chromosome is present in erythrocytes, monocytes, and megakaryocytes, erythrocytes and platelets are produced and function relatively normally. The acute effects of CML resemble those of acute leukemia but with more prominent and painful splenomegaly. Liver function rarely is altered despite enlargement, and lympha-

A

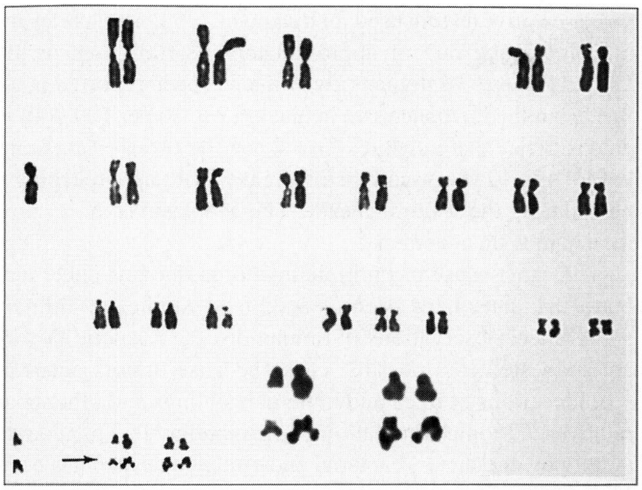

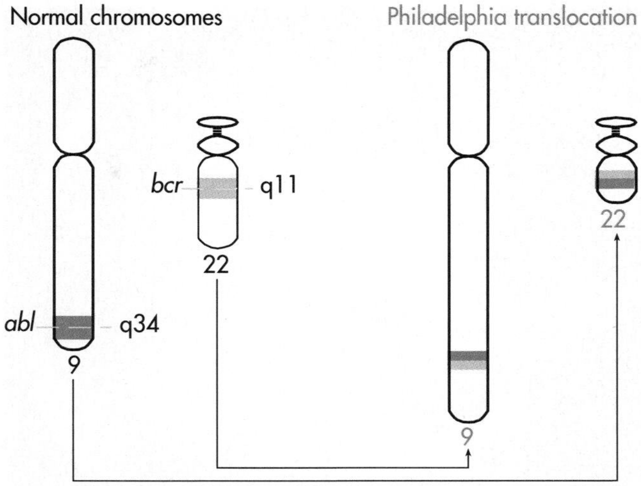

B

C

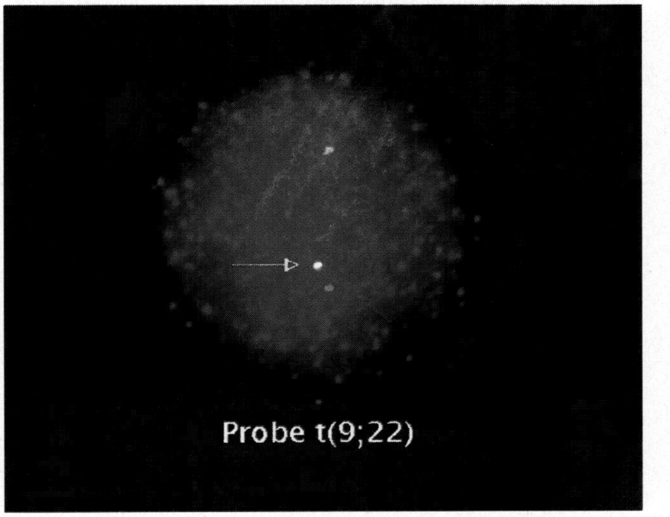

FIG. 26-4 Philadelphia chromosome. A, Metaphase spread of marrow cell in chronic myelocytic leukemia. Ph1 chromosome (*arrow* and enlarged inset) is recognized by partial deletion of long arm. **B,** Schema of the Philadelphia (Ph) translocation (1) seen in chronic myelocytic leukemia. The Ph1 chromosome results from an exchange of materials between chromosomes 9 and 22, that is, t(9;22)(q34;q11). Because chromosome 22 gives up much more of its long arm than that translocated to it from chromosome 9, chromosome 22 becomes much abbreviated and known as Ph1. **C,** Chronic myelogenous leukemia (CML) is characterized by a reciprocal exchange of chromosomal material (translocation) between chromosomes 9 and 22. Probes specific for the involved regions, that is, abl gene (chromosome 9) and bcr (breakpoint cluster region on chromosome 22), are labeled with a green- and red-emitting signal, respectively (made by ONCOR, Gaithersburg, Md). If a translocation is present (bringing abl and bcr into proximity), a yellow-white signal is seen, as in this cell from an individual with CML. (**A,** Courtesy Dr. A.K. Sinha, Houston, Texas. From del Regato JA, Spjut HJ, Cox JD: *Ackerman and del Regato's cancer,* ed 2, St Louis, 1985, Mosby. **B, C,** From Damjanov I, Linder J, editors: *Anderson's pathology,* ed 10, St Louis, 1996, Mosby.)

denopathy generally is found only in the acute phase of the disease. Hyperuricemia invariably is present and produces gouty arthritis. Infections, fever, and weight loss are common findings in patients with CML.

CLL involves malignant transformation predominantly of B cells, although T cell CLL occurs less commonly (Fig. 26-5). The major pathophysiologic deficit in CLL of B cells is their failure to mature into plasma cells that synthesize immunoglobulin (antibody; see Chapter 6). A possible mechanism responsible for CLL of B cells is a deficiency of normal helper T cells with an increase in suppressor T cells. Together, the T cell abnormalities might account for the impaired differentiation of B cells in CLL.

Suppression of humoral immunity caused by reduction in normally functioning B cells is the most significant effect of CLL. Individuals are at risk both for infections commonly combated by B cell–produced immunoglobulins and for the development of autoimmune diseases that result in secondary cancers. Anemia, thrombocytopenia, and neutropenia are typically present with overt CLL (see Table 26-3). Invasion of most organs is uncommon, but infiltration does oc-

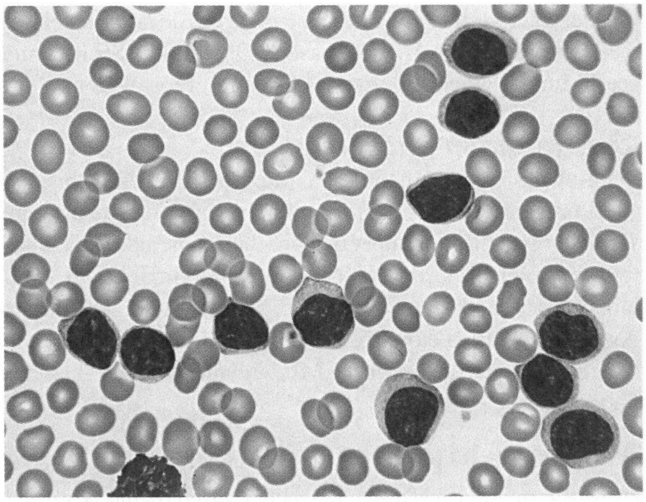

FIG. 26-5 Blood smear from an individual with B cell chronic lymphocytic leukemia and autoimmune hemolytic anemia. There are numerous well-differentiated lymphocytes with a high nuclear/cytoplasmic ratio and condensed nuclear chromatin (Wright-Giemsa stain). (From Damjanov I, Linder J, editors: *Anderson's pathology,* ed 10, St Louis, 1996, Mosby.)

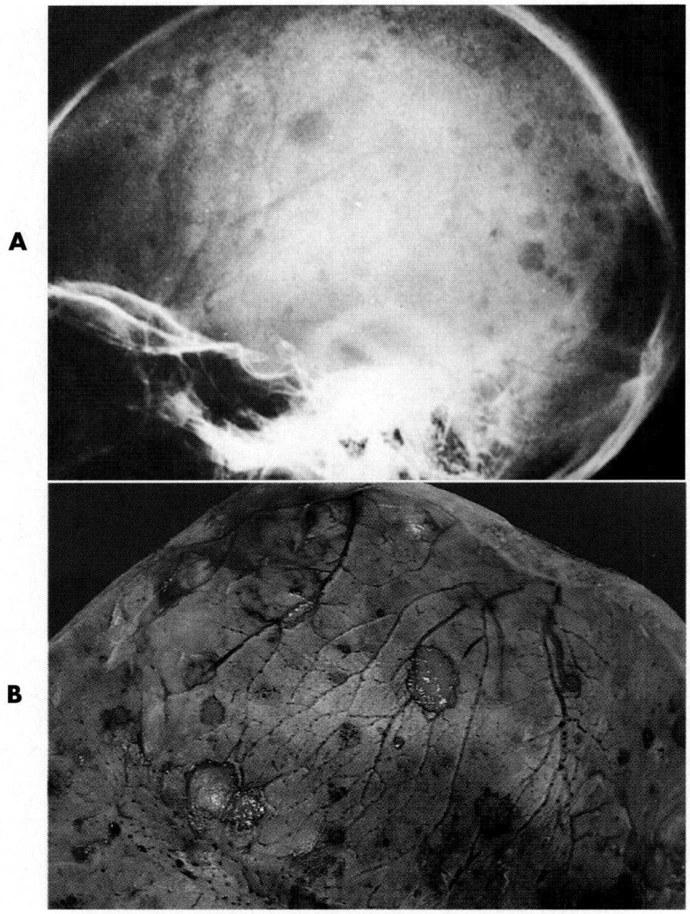

FIG. 26-6 Multiple myeloma. A, The radiograph shows lytic lesions. **B,** The skull contains lytic (punched-out) lesions. (From Damjanov I, Linder J: *Pathology: a color atlas,* St Louis, 2000, Mosby.)

cur in lymph nodes, liver, spleen, and salivary glands. Central nervous system involvement is rare. Elevated levels of the enzyme lactic dehydrogenase (LDH) and hyperuricemia are common, whereas hypercalcemia rarely is evident.

Evaluation and Treatment

State-of-the-art treatment for CML does not cure the disease, prevent blastic transformation, or prolong the average survival time. New therapeutic approaches include bone marrow transplantation, biologic response modifiers, and combination chemotherapy (see Chapter 11). When appropriate donors are available, marrow transplantation should be considered for individuals with CML who are younger than age 50 years.

Multiple Myeloma

Multiple myeloma is a B cell cancer caused by the proliferation of malignant plasma cells. Multiple myeloma is characterized by multiple malignant tumor masses of plasma cells scattered throughout the skeletal system and sometimes in soft tissue (Fig. 26-6). The reported incidence of multiple myeloma has doubled in the past two decades, possibly because of more sensitive testing used for diagnosis.[22,26] It now has an annual incidence rate of approximately 48,100 cases in the United States.[22] Malignant myeloma has been reported in all races, but the incidence rate in blacks (7 to 10 per 100,000) is at least twice that in whites (3 to 4 per 100,000).[22,26] It is rare before age 40 years, and then increases with age, reaching a peak during the seventh decade. The neoplasm is more common in men than women.

The exact cause of multiple myeloma remains uncertain, but a few clues have been gleaned from studies of animals and clinical observations of human disease. Genetic factors are suggested as a possible cause because tumors occur in specific strains of mice and in human siblings and other near relatives. Chronic stimulation of the mononuclear phagocyte system by chemicals, bacteria, and viral agents also has been suggested as a possible cause. Excessive production of an antibody protein by abnormal plasma cells, called *monoclonal gammopathy of undetermined significance* (MGUS), is related to the development of myeloma in 20% of those affected.[22]

Pathophysiology

Malignant plasma cells arise from one clone of B cells that produce abnormally large amounts of one class of immunoglobulin (usually IgG, occasionally IgA, and rarely IgM, IgD, or IgE). Recent studies support involvement of early B lymphocytes, such as hematopoietic stem cells, as the origin of myeloma. These data suggest that myeloma originates in the bone marrow and moves through the circulation to and from extramedullary sites, probably lymph nodes, which are required for their development. Subsequently, the myeloma cells return to the bone marrow or soft-tissue sites, using adhesion molecules (see Chapter 10) for "homing" to sites that can provide the environment for expansion and maturation. Development of myeloma is governed by cytokines, whereby interleukin-6 (IL-6) has an essential role.[27] (Lymphocytes and cytokines are described in Chapter 6.) The abnormal immunoglobulin produced by the malignant transformed plasma cell is called the **M protein.** The M protein is responsible for many of the clinical manifestations of the disease. M protein that is produced in excessive amounts results in ineffective antibody production. **Bence Jones proteins,** the light chains of immunoglobulin molecules, are present in the urine. These proteins may result in damage to renal tubular cells.

Multiple myeloma becomes evident as diffuse destructive bone lesions (Fig. 26-7). The bones most commonly affected are the vertebrae (66%), ribs (44%), skull (41%), pelvis (28%), femur (24%), clavicle (10%), and scapula (10%).[28] The lesions progressively destroy the cortical bone. (Bone structures are described in Chapter 40.) Myeloma cells produce matrix-metalloproteinase-9 (MMP-9) and MMP-2. MMPs probably have major roles in (1) the infiltration of bone and other tissues by the myeloma cells, (2) the osteolytic bone destruction caused by overactive osteoclasts, (3) extracellular matrix remodeling by bone marrow stromal

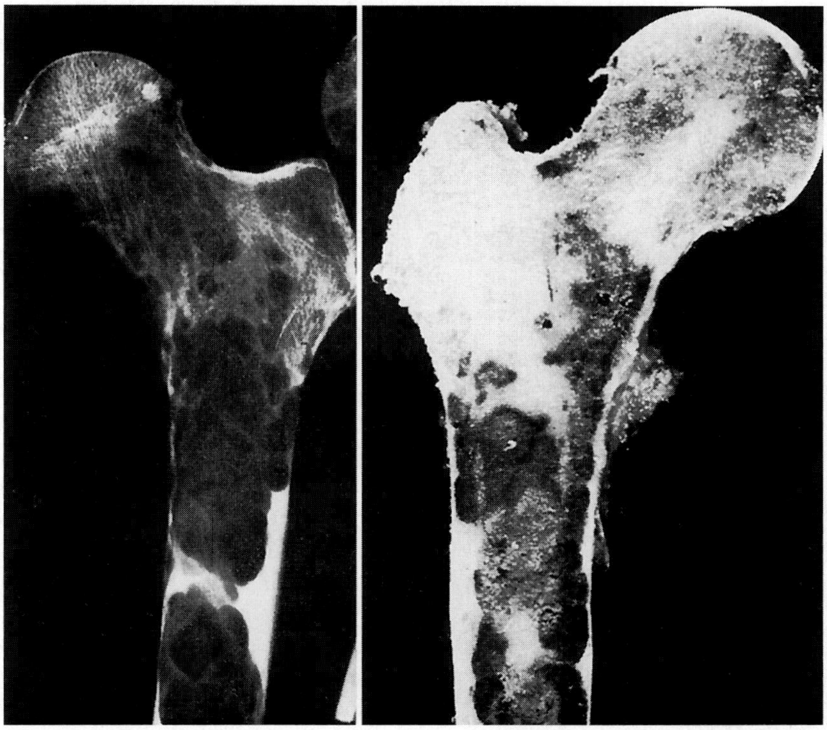

FIG. 26-7 Multiple (plasma cell) myeloma. A, Roentgenogram of femur showing extensive bone destruction caused by tumor. Note absence of reactive bone formation. **B,** Gross specimen from same individual; myelomatous sections appear as dark granular sections. (From Kissane JM, editor: *Anderson's pathology,* ed 9, St Louis, 1990, Mosby.)

cells, (4) promoting the invasion of the endothelial cells that form new blood vessels and sustain tumor cells, and (5) promoting the growth of myeloma cells.[29]

Clinical Manifestations

Clinical manifestations are the result of (1) infiltration and destruction of organs, particularly bone, by the neoplastic plasma cells and (2) an M protein consisting of an excess of immunoglobulins with altered physiologic properties and immune function. Infiltration of bones by malignant plasma cells causes pain and pathologic fractures. Because of an excessive accumulation of neoplastic plasma cells, the most common presenting symptom is bone pain. The production of osteoclast activating factors by the myeloma cells results in extensive osteolysis (breakdown of bone), bone pain, and pathologic fractures. Hypercalcemia resulting from bone resorption can cause neurologic disturbances, such as confusion, lethargy, and weakness, and can contribute to renal disease.

A major clinical manifestation is recurrent infections resulting from suppression of the humoral (antibody-mediated) immune response. Cell-mediated immune function (i.e., T cell function) is relatively normal.[30] Humoral immune function is thought to be suppressed by unknown factors secreted from malignant plasma cells. These factors activate macrophages that inhibit maturation of B cells into plasma cells that would be capable of producing immunoglobulins normally.[31,32] Renal disease, a complication of multiple myeloma, is thought to be the result of Bence Jones proteinuria. The excreted Bence Jones proteins may be toxic to the tubular epithelial cells of the kidney.[33]

Evaluation and Treatment

Diagnosis of multiple myeloma is made by radiographic and laboratory studies and biopsy of a lesion. Chemotherapy, radiation therapy, plasmapheresis (exchange), and marrow transplant have been used for treatment. Individuals with multiple bony lesions, if untreated, rarely survive longer than 6 to 12 months. Recent safe synthetic inhibitors of MMPs are available and may prove useful in limiting the growth and spread of myeloma cells.[29] The median survival for all stages of multiple myeloma is 3 years.[34]

ALTERATIONS OF LYMPHOID FUNCTION

Lymphadenopathy

Normally, lymph nodes are not palpable or only barely palpable. Nodes are generally classified as tender or nontender, and movable or fixed. **Lymphadenopathy** is characterized by enlarged lymph nodes (Fig. 26-8). Localized lymphadenopathy usually indicates drainage of an inflammatory lesion. Generalized lymphadenopathy occurs less frequently as a result of infection and therefore usually is associated with a malignant or nonmalignant disease. Lymphadenopathy reflects significant diseases more often in adults than in children.

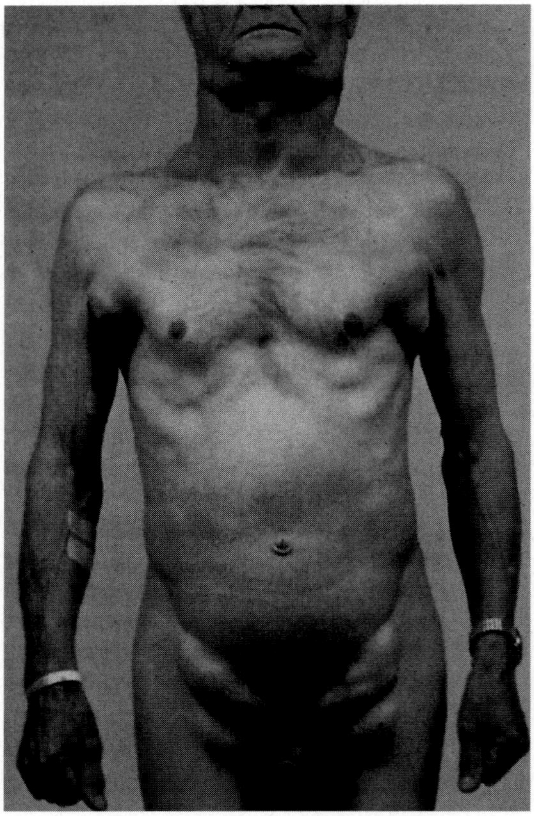

FIG. 26-8 Lymphadenopathy. Individual with lymphocyte leukemia with extreme but symmetric lymphadenopathy. (Courtesy Dr. A.R. Kagan, Los Angeles. From del Regato JA, Spjut HJ, Cox JD: *Ackerman and del Regato's cancer,* ed 2, St Louis, 1985, Mosby.)

Enlargement of the lymph node often is caused by an increase in size and number of the germinal centers within the node caused by proliferation of lymphocytes or monocytes (immature macrophages). Enlargement also may be caused by invasion of the node by malignant cells or cells not normally present within the node. Palpable nodes, however, do not always indicate serious disease and may only indicate a reaction to minor trauma or infection of a specific structure. The location and size of the enlarged node are important factors in diagnosing the cause of the lymphadenopathy, as are the individual's age, gender, and geographic location. Generalized lymphadenopathy occurs with non-Hodgkin lymphomas, CLL, histiocytoses, and disorders that produce lymphocytosis. In general, lymphadenopathy results from four types of conditions: (1) neoplastic diseases, (2) immunologic or inflammatory conditions, (3) endocrine disorders, or (4) lipid storage diseases. Diseases of unknown cause, including autoimmune diseases and reactions to drugs, also may lead to generalized lymphadenopathy.

Malignant Lymphomas

The most significant advances in cancer treatment have been in the management of lymphomas. Lymphomas involve the proliferation of lymphocytes, histiocytes and their precursors, and derivatives in lymphoid tissues. Lymphomas display a wide spectrum of clinical and histologic patterns. There are three major categories of lymphoid malignancies based on morphologic appearance and the cell of origin: B cell, T cell (non-Hodgkin lymphomas), and Hodgkin disease. Hodgkin lymphoma, non-Hodgkin lymphomas, and lymphoid leukemias are included because these disease entities have both solid and blood-circulating phases, making the distinction between them artificial. Subtypes within each disease category may be further categorized into prognostic groups indicating the range of clinical aggressiveness or behavior of the tumor (Table 26-4). Histopathologic parameters in Hodgkin disease do not predict or have prognostic value.

The classification of neoplastic lymphoid disorders has undergone significant changes in the past 10 years that reflect advances in understanding of the functional and genetic heterogeneity of the immune system. Information about lymphoid neoplasms and their tumors has resulted in recognition of new lymphoid neoplasms and the refinement of previously recognized disease categories. In the 1950s Rappaport developed a classification system based on growth patterns (diffuse or nodular) and cytology of lymphocytes (undifferentiated, well differentiated, poorly differentiated, histiocytic). This classification system was further refined in the early 1970s by Lukes and Collins in the United States and Lennert at the University of Kiel, Germany, based on morphology related to lymphocyte lineage. Both classification systems recognized the significance of follicular nodulation as a significant marker in B cell differentiation.

More recently, the *Working Formulation of Clinical Usage* has been the most widely used method for lymphoma diagnosis in the United States and is the basis for most American lymphoma clinical trials. Since 1982 the *Working Formulation* has provided a morphologic classification scheme with prognostic relevance. However, the *Working Formulation* does not include new syndromes identified based on the advanced immunologic and genetic techniques used to evaluate malignant lymphoid tumors. In addition, despite understanding about the relationship between Hodgkin disease and non-Hodgkin lymphoma, Hodgkin disease remains separated from the lymphoma classification. At this time a proposal for a new classification system is being deliberated (Table 26-5), based on morphology and when necessary on immunology, cytogenetics, and molecular biology.[35]

Malignant lymphomas are the fifth most common cause of death from cancer in the United States. Incidence rates differ with respect to age, gender, geographic location, and socioeconomic class. New estimates for 2001 are 62,300 new cases, including 7400 cases of Hodgkin disease and 54,900 cases of non-Hodgkin lymphoma. Since the 1970s, incidence rates for non-Hodgkin lymphoma have increased more than 65%. A large portion of this increase has been attributed to lymphomas developing in association with AIDS.[36] Incidence of Hodgkin disease has declined over the same period, especially among elderly persons.

Table 26-4 Classification of Lymphoid Neoplasms

Lymphoid Neoplasms	Prognostic Group
B CELL NEOPLASMS	
1. Precursor B cell neoplasm	
a. Precursor B lymphoblastic leukemia	Highly aggressive
b. Precursor B lymphoblastic lymphoma	Highly aggressive
2. Peripheral B cell neoplasms	
a. B cell chronic lymphocytic leukemia (CLL),	Indolent
prolymphocytic leukemia (PLL),	Moderately aggressive
small lymphocytic lymphoma (SLL)	Indolent
b. Lymphoplasmacytoid lymphoma/immunocytoma	Indolent
c. Mantle cell lymphoma	Moderately aggressive
d. Follicle center lymphoma, follicular	
(1) Grade I or II	Indolent
(2) Grade III	Moderately aggressive
e. Marginal zone B cell lymphoma	Indolent
Extranodal (MALT type +/− monocytoid B cells)	
f. Hairy cell leukemia	Indolent
g. Plasmacytoma/plasma cell lymphoma	Indolent
h. Diffuse large cell lymphoma*	Aggressive
i. Burkitt lymphoma	Highly aggressive
T CELL AND PUTATIVE NATURAL KILLER (NK) CELL NEOPLASMS	
1. Precursor T cell neoplasms	
a. Precursor T lymphoblastic lymphoma	Highly aggressive
b. Precursor T lymphoblastic leukemia	Highly aggressive
2. Peripheral T cell and NK cell neoplasms	
a. T cell chronic lymphocytic leukemia/promyelocytic leukemia	Moderately aggressive
b. Large granular lymphocytic leukemia (LGL)	
(1) T cell type	Indolent
(2) NK cell type	Aggressive
c. Mycosis fungoides/Sezary syndrome	Indolent
d. Peripheral T cell lymphomas, unspecified*	Aggressive
e. Angioimmunoblastic T cell lymphoma (AILD)	Moderately aggressive
f. Angiocentric lymphoma	Moderately aggressive or aggressive
g. Intestinal T cell lymphoma (+/− enteropathy associated)	Aggressive
h. Adult T cell lymphoma/leukemia (ATL/L)	
(1) Smoldering	Indolent
(2) Chronic	Moderately aggressive
i. Anaplastic large cell lymphoma (ALCL), CD30+, T cell and null cell types	Aggressive
HODGKIN DISEASE (HD)	
1. Lymphocyte predominance	
2. Nodular sclerosis	
3. Mixed cellularity	
4. Lymphocyte depletion	

*This subtype is more likely to include more than one disease entity.

Hodgkin Disease

Pathogenesis

Hodgkin disease is a malignant lymphoma first characterized by Thomas Hodgkin in 1832. Hodgkin disease can be distinguished from other lymphomas by the presence of Reed-Sternberg cells surrounded by a background of benign-appearing host inflammatory cells (Fig. 26-9). It is widely accepted that the Reed-Sternberg cells or their variant represents the malignant transformation of cells.[37] The identity of the normal counterpart of the Reed-Sternberg cells and the molecular events resulting in its malignant transformation remain controversial. Although the Reed-Sternberg cell is necessary for diagnosis, it is not specific to Hodgkin disease, and in rare instances cells resembling Reed-Sternberg cells can be found in benign illness as well as other forms of neoplasia, including non-Hodgkin lymphoma and carcinoma. Hodgkin disease arises in a single node or chain of nodes and spreads characteristically to anatomically contiguous nodes.

Attempts to understand the development of the neoplastic cell of Hodgkin disease have remained inconclusive. The origin of the Reed-Sternberg cell may differ for various subtypes of disease, such as activated lymphoid cells with features of B cell, T cell, or monocytic cell lines. Epstein-Barr virus has also been linked to Hodgkin disease.[38]

Table 26-5 A Comparison of the Working Formulation Classification and the Proposed Revised European-American Classification

	Revised European-American Classification	
Working Formulation	**B Cell Neoplasms**	**T Cell Neoplasms**
1. Small lymphocyte consistent with CLL	**B cell CLL/PLL/SLL**	**T cell CLL/PLL**
	Marginal zone/MALT	LGL
	Mantle cell	ATL/L (chronic and smoldering types)
Plasmacytoid	**Lymphoplasmacytoid marginal zone/MALT**	
	B cell CLL/PLL, SLL	
2. Follicular, predominantly small cleaved cell	**Follicular center, follicular grade II**	
	Marginal zone/MALT	
3. Follicular, mixed small cleaved and large cell	**Follicle center, follicular grade II**	
	Marginal zone/MALT	
4. Follicular, large cell	Follicle center, follicular grade III	
5. Diffuse, small cleaved cell	**Mantle zone**	**T cell CLL/PLL**
	Follicle center, diffuse small cell	LGL
	Marginal zone/MALT	ATL/L
		Angioimmunoblastic
		Angiocentric
6. Diffuse, mixed small and large cell	**Large B cell lymphoma (rich in T cells)**	**Peripheral T cell, unspecified**
	Follicle center, diffuse small cell	ATL/L
	Lymphoplasmacytoid	Angioimmunocentric
	Marginal zone/MALT	Angiocentric
	Mantle cell	Intestinal T cell lymphoma
7. Diffuse, large cell	Diffuse large B cell lymphoma	**Peripheral T cell, unspecified**
		ATL/L
		Angioimmunoblastic
		Angiocentric
		Intestinal T cell lymphoma
8. Large cell immunoblastic	Diffuse large B cell lymphoma	**Peripheral T cell, unspecified**
		ATL/L
		Angioimmunoblastic
		Angiocentric
		Intestinal T cell
		Anaplastic large cell
9. Lymphoblastic	Precursor B lymphoblastic	Precursor T lymphoblastic
10. Small noncleaved cell	Burkitt	Peripheral T cell, unspecified
Burkitt	High-grade B cell, Burkitt-like	
Non-Burkitt	Diffuse large B cell	

From Harris NL: A practical approach to the pathology of lymphoid neoplasms: a revised European-American Classification from the International Lymphoma Study Group. In DeVita VT, Hellman S, Rosenberg SA, editors: *Important advances in oncology 1995,* Philadelphia, 1995, Lippincott.

There is evidence of proto-oncogene involvement in the transformation of Hodgkin disease cells. The transformed cells release cytokines (IL-1, IL-2, IL-5, IL-6; tumor necrosis factor–alpha and tumor necrosis factor–beta; interferon-gamma; granulocyte-macrophage colony–stimulating factor [GM-CSF]; granulocyte colony–stimulating factor [G-CSF]; tumor growth factor–beta) that result in local and systemic reactions.[39] The four histologic subtypes of Hodgkin disease (Table 26-6) are based on the nonmalignant background of the involved node rather than the appearance of the malignant cell.

The incidence of Hodgkin disease is approximately 2.6 per 100,000 men and 2.2 per 100,000 women.[22] Incidence rates for Hodgkin disease have declined, especially among the elderly population.[22] The decrease in incidence in the older population is attributed to improved diagnostic accuracy. The incidence is higher in whites than blacks. There is a bimodal incidence pattern for Hodgkin disease in economically advantaged countries: the Netherlands, Denmark, and the United States have the highest incidence of Hodgkin disease, and Japan and Australia have the lowest. The overall incidence is lower in economically underdeveloped countries, with proportionately more cases occurring at older ages. Hodgkin disease peaks at two different ages: early in life in the second and third decades, and later in life during the sixth and seventh decades.

Clinical Manifestations

Many of the characteristic clinical features (Box 26-2) of Hodgkin disease can be explained by the expression of cytokines and hematopoietic growth factors by the malignant cells. These factors may act in a complex autocrine and paracrine

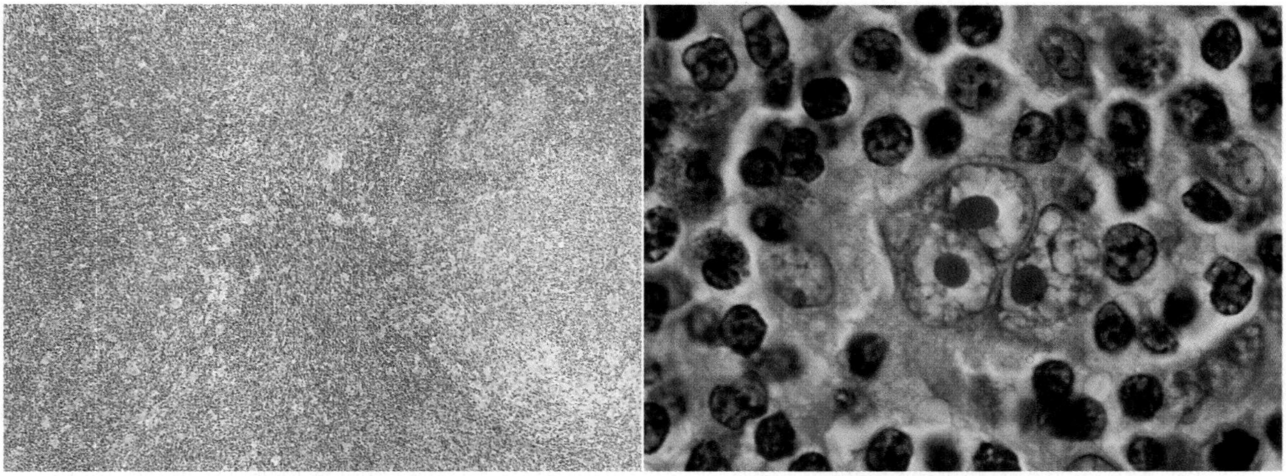

FIG. 26-9 Lymph nodes. A, Lymphocytes and histiocytes Hodgkin disease (L&H HD), nodular type. Large nodules with small, round lymphocytes, histiocytes, and scattered L&H cells. **B,** Diagnostic Reed-Sternberg cell. A large multinucleated or multilobed cell with inclusion body–like nucleoli surrounded by a halo of clear nucleoplasm. (From Damjanov I, Linder J, editors: *Anderson's pathology,* ed 10, St Louis, 1996, Mosby.)

Table 26-6 Subtypes of Hodgkin Disease

Subtype	Incidence	Clinical Presentation
Lymphocyte predominance	Found in all ages, but more common in adults than in children Incidence in males exceeds that in females	Peripheral node involvement Spares the mediastinum Usually localized at diagnosis Survival is long with or without treatment Late relapses common
Nodular sclerosing	Found in all ages, but most common in adolescents and young adults Incidence in females equals or exceeds that in males	Mediastinal involvement Stage and bulk of disease have prognostic significance
Mixed cellularity	Common in adults Incidence in males exceeds that in females	Stage more advanced than in nodular sclerosis and lymphocyte predominance subtypes Involves lymph nodes, spleen, liver, or marrow
Lymphocyte depletion	Least common variant Most common type in elderly persons, human immunodeficiency virus (HIV)–positive individuals, and persons in nonindustrialized countries	Abdominal lymphadenopathy; spleen, liver, and bone marrow involvement, without peripheral lymphadenopathy Stage is more advanced at diagnosis

loop, stimulating both the malignant and nonmalignant stromal cells to proliferate and secrete other growth factors.

An enlarged painless mass, found most commonly in the neck, is frequently an initial sign of Hodgkin disease (Fig. 26-10). Pain may accompany the enlarged node associated with Hodgkin disease. Rarely, pain may be brought on or exacerbated with the ingestion of alcohol. The discovery of an asymptomatic mediastinal mass on routine chest x-ray is not unusual. The cervical, axillary, inguinal, and retroperitoneal lymph nodes are most commonly affected in Hodgkin disease (Fig. 26-11). Local symptoms caused by pressure and obstruction are produced by lymphadenopathy. Intermittent fever, without other symptoms of infection, and drenching night sweats are relatively common clinical presentations of Hodgkin disease. These constitutional symptoms and weight loss have been associated with poor diagnosis. The Cotswold Staging Classification System is used for Hodgkin disease (Table 26-7). The staging system is based on medical history and physical examination to identify the presence of symptoms, palpable lymphadenopathy, and other findings on

Box 26-2

CLINICAL MANIFESTATIONS OF HODGKIN DISEASE

PHYSICAL FINDINGS

Adenopathy
Mediastinal mass
Splenomegaly
Abdominal mass

SYMPTOMS

Fever, weight loss, night sweats
Pruritus

LABORATORY FINDINGS

Thrombocytosis
Leukocytosis
Eosinophilia
Elevated erythrocyte sedimentation rate (ESR)
Elevated alkaline phosphatase

PARANEOPLASTIC SYNDROMES

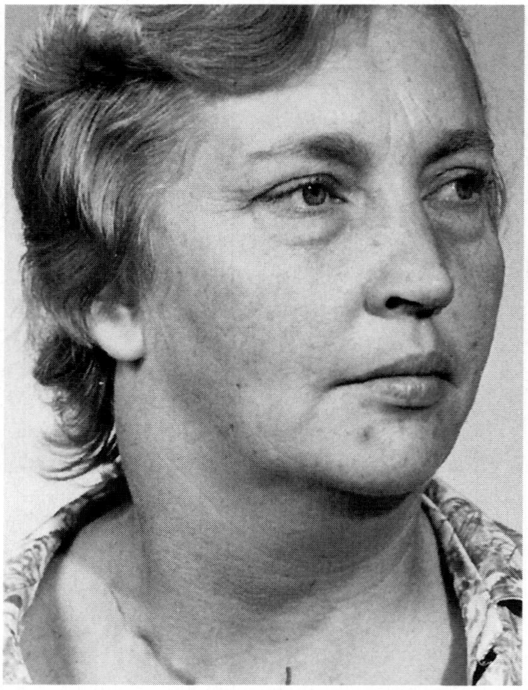

Fig. 26-10 Hodgkin disease and enlarged cervical lymph node. Typical enlarged cervical lymph node in the neck of a 35-year-old woman with Hodgkin disease. (From del Regato JA, Spjut HJ, Cox JD: *Ackerman and del Regato's cancer,* ed 2, St Louis, 1985, Mosby.)

Table 26-7 Cotswold Staging Classification System

Stage	Criteria
I	Involvement of a single lymph node region or lymphoid structure (i.e., spleen, thymus, Waldeyer ring)
II	Involvement of two or more lymph node regions on the same side of the diaphragm (the mediastinum is a single site, hilar lymph nodes are lateralized); the number of anatomic sites should be indicated by a suffix (i.e., II_3)
III	Involvement of lymph node regions or structures on both sides of the diaphragm Stage III_1: with or without splenic hilar, celiac, or portal nodes Stage III_2: with paraaortic, iliac, mesenteric nodes
IV	Involvement of extranodal site(s) beyond that designated "E" Modifying characteristics A: no symptoms B: fever, drenching sweats, weight loss X: bulky disease >1/3 widening of mediastinum >10-cm maximum dimension of nodal mass E: involvement of a single extranodal site contiguous or proximal to known nodal site CS: clinical stage PS: pathologic stage

Data from Lister TA, Crowther D: Staging for Hodgkin's disease, *Semin Oncol* 17:696, 1990.

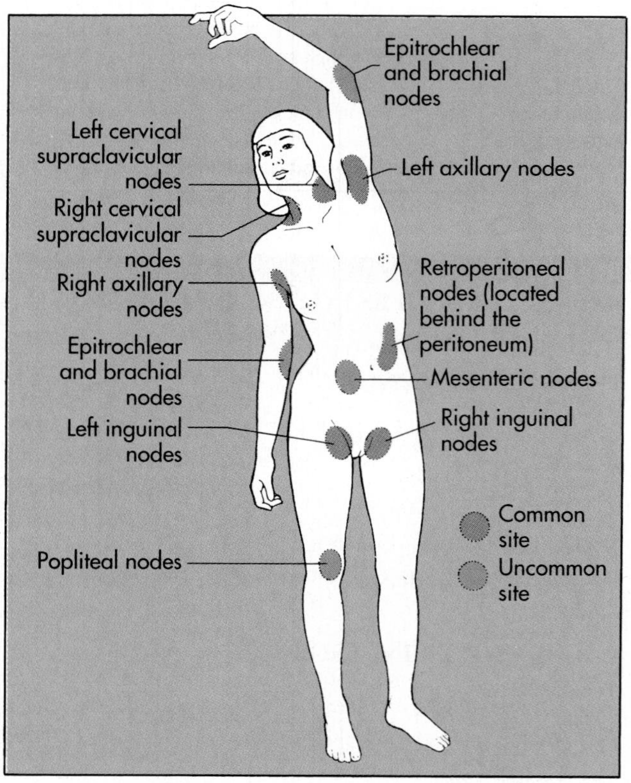

Fig. 26-11 Common and uncommon involved lymph node sites for Hodgkin disease.

radiographic and hematologic studies. The staging system has been able to establish a correlation between anatomic extent of the disease and prognosis. Prognostic factors include clinical stage, histologic type, tumor cell concentration and tumor burden, constitutional symptoms, and age.

Although Hodgkin disease rarely arises in the lung, mediastinal and hilar node adenopathy can cause secondary involvement of the trachea, bronchi, pleura, or lungs. Retroperitoneal nodes can involve vertebral bodies and nerves, causing displacement of ureters. Spinal cord involvement is more common in the dorsal and lumbar regions than in the cervical region. Although uncommon, skin manifestations include psoriasis and eczematoid lesions, causing itching and scratching.

As a result of direct invasion from mediastinal lymph nodes, pericardial involvement can cause pericardial friction rub, pericardial effusion, and engorgement of the neck veins. The gastrointestinal tract and urinary tract rarely are involved. Anemia frequently is found in individuals with low serum iron and iron-binding capacity. Other laboratory findings include elevated sedimentation rate, leukocytosis, and eosinophilia. With advanced stages of Hodgkin disease, leukopenia occurs.

Splenic involvement of Hodgkin disease depends on histopathologic type. The spleen is involved in 60% of cases of mixed cellularity and lymphocyte depletion types. With lymphocyte predominance and nodular sclerosis types, only 34% of cases reveal splenic involvement.

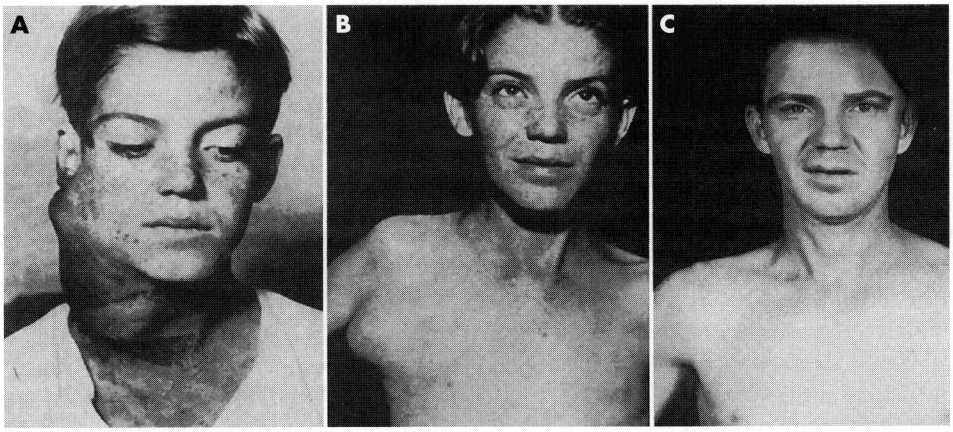

FIG. 26-12 Cervical Hodgkin disease. A, Young boy with extensive cervical Hodgkin disease. **B,** Appearance several years later, when axillary manifestations developed. **C,** Appearance 23 years after initial treatment with radiation. (From del Regato JA, Spjut HJ, Cox JD: *Ackerman and del Regato's cancer,* ed 2, St Louis, 1985, Mosby.)

Evaluation and Treatment

Because of the variability in symptoms, early definitive detection may be difficult. Asymptomatic lymphadenopathy can progress undetected for several years. Careful evaluation, including chest x-ray films, lymphangiography, and biopsy, should be carried out for individuals with fever of unknown origin and peripheral lymphadenopathy. About three of every four individuals diagnosed with Hodgkin disease are cured. Irradiation and chemotherapy have been responsible for the successful treatment of Hodgkin disease (Fig. 26-12). The 5-year survival rate is 82%.[22]

Non-Hodgkin Lymphoma

Pathophysiology

Non-Hodgkin lymphoma is the generic term for a diverse group of disorders characterized by the malignant transformation of the lymphoid system not microscopically characterized by the Reed-Sternberg cells and cellular changes seen in Hodgkin disease (see Table 26-4). The molecular rearrangements of specific oncogenes and immunoglobin genes are important to understanding the development of non-Hodgkin lymphoma.

In addition, environmental agents and inherited genetic abnormalities may participate in the development of irreversible chromosomal changes. Chromosomal mutations result in the transformation or loss of critical oncogenes and tumor-suppressor genes. Non-Hodgkin lymphoma appears to be multicentric in origin with an early tendency to spread widely.

The incidence rate of non-Hodgkin lymphoma is approximately 8.1 per 100,000 men and 5.7 per 100,000 women.[22] Non-Hodgkin lymphoma is a disease of the middle years, usually found in persons older than age 50 years.

As is the case in Hodgkin disease, the etiology of most non-Hodgkin lymphomas is unknown. Several factors suggest possible causal relations: altered immunologic states, such as organ transplant related to immunosuppression and AIDS; Epstein-Barr virus and human T cell lymphotropic virus type 1 (HTLV-I); and exposure to irradiation and chemical substances.

Table 26-8 Clinical Differences Between Non-Hodgkin Disease and Hodgkin Disease

Characteristic	Non-Hodgkin Disease	Hodgkin Disease
Nodal involvement	Multiple peripheral nodes	Localized to single axial group of nodes (i.e., cervical, mediastinal, para-aortic)
	Mesenteric nodes and Waldeyer ring commonly involved	Mesenteric nodes and Waldeyer ring rarely involved
Spread	Noncontiguous	Orderly spread by contiguity
B* symptoms	Uncommon	Common
Extranodal involvement	Common	Rare
Extent of disease	Rarely localized	Often localized

*Fever, weight loss, night sweats.

Clinical Manifestations

The clinical manifestations of individuals with non-Hodgkin lymphoma are similar to those of Hodgkin disease. Differences in clinical features are noted in Table 26-8. Non-Hodgkin lymphoma usually manifests as localized or generalized lymphadenopathy. The cervical, axillary, inguinal, and femoral chains are the most frequent sites of lymph node enlargement. Generally, the swelling is painless and the nodes have enlarged and transformed over a period of months or years. Extranodal sites of involvement are the nasopharynx, gastrointestinal tract, bone, thyroid, testes, and soft tissue. Some individuals have retroperitoneal and abdominal masses with symptoms of abdominal fullness, back pain, ascites, and leg swelling.

Evaluation and Treatment

Individuals with non-Hodgkin lymphoma can survive for long periods. Survival with nodular lymphoma ranges up to 15 years. Individuals with diffuse disease generally do not survive as long. Many investigators believe that more aggressive treatment increases the cure rate. Autologous stem cell transplantation recently has been proposed for recurrent disease when no curative regimen exists and for persons with poor-risk lymphomas. High-grade non-Hodgkin lymphoma is seen with increasing frequency in persons with AIDS and has an extremely poor prognosis.

Burkitt Lymphoma

Burkitt lymphoma is a tumor with unique clinical and epidemiologic features. It occurs in children from east-central Africa and New Guinea and involves primarily the jaw and facial bones (Fig. 26-13). EBV is associated with Burkitt lymphoma in African children. The virus is found in nasopharyngeal secretions.[40]

The American type of Burkitt lymphoma usually involves the abdomen and is characterized by extensive marrow replacement. The cancerous cell is a B cell that undergoes cancerous transformation and progression. The African variety has been treated successfully with radiation therapy and cyclophosphamide. The American type is more resistant to treatment.

Conditions That Mimic Lymphomas

Certain other clinical conditions mimic the malignant lymphomas. These conditions include TB, syphilis, systemic lupus erythematosus, lung cancer, and bone cancer. An important distinction between lymphomas and other conditions is that lymphomas usually involve localized lymphadenopathy. Infectious precursors of malignant lymphomas are characterized by more generalized lymphadenopathy with systemic signs and symptoms.

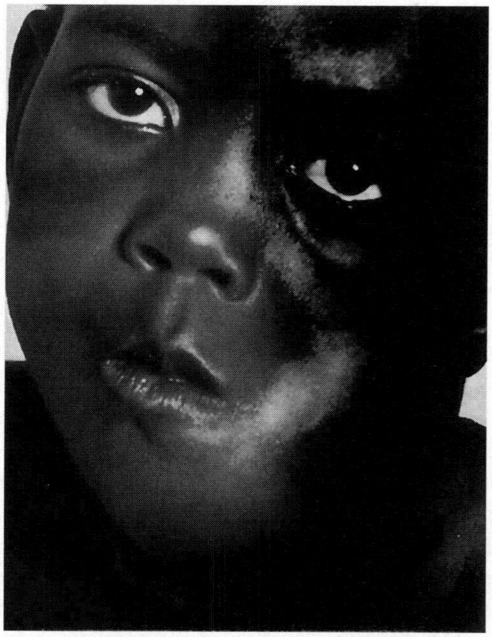

FIG. 26-13 Burkitt lymphoma. Burkitt lymphoma involving the jaw in young African boy. (Courtesy Dr. J.N.P. Davies, Albany, NY. From del Regato JA, Spjut HJ, Cox JD: *Ackerman and del Regato's cancer,* ed 2, St Louis, 1985, Mosby.

ALTERATIONS OF SPLENIC FUNCTION

The spleen has been an organ of mystery and perplexity since ancient times. Its relationship to other organs and disease processes, particularly the immune and hematologic systems, was not identified until the eighteenth century. The complexities of splenic function are still not totally understood, and its mysteries are still under investigation. The spleen is a useful organ, but its functions overlap those of other organs so that one is capable of living a normal, healthy life without the spleen.[41]

In the past, enlargement of the spleen **(splenomegaly)** was identified with various disease states. It is now recognized that splenomegaly is not necessarily pathologic because some individuals may have an enlarged spleen without any evidence of disease. However, it may be one of the first physical signs of underlying conditions and its presence should not be ignored.[8] In conditions where splenomegaly is present, the normal functions of the spleen may become overactive and produce a condition known as **hypersplenism.**

The concept of an overactive spleen dates to 1866; however, the term *overactive spleen* was not uniformly applied to specific conditions and confusion existed over the clinical use and meaning of the term. Current criteria for overactive spleen include (1) anemia, leukopenia, thrombocytopenia, or combinations of these; (2) cellular bone marrow; (3) splenomegaly; and (4) improvement after splenectomy.[42] It is recognized that individuals may seek treatment for problems without having met all these clinical criteria; therefore there is still uncertainty as to the relevance and clarity of this condition. Hypersplenism may be further categorized as *primary,* when no etiologic factor for its presence is identified, and *secondary,* when splenomegaly is the result of some other identified condition.[42]

Overactivity of the spleen results in hematologic alterations that affect all blood components. Sequestering of red cells, granulocytes, and platelets results in a reduction of all circulating blood cells. The spleen may sequester up to 50% of the red cell population, thereby upsetting the normal physiologic concentration of red cells in the circulating blood.[43] The rate of splenic pooling is directly related to spleen size and the degree of increased blood flow through it. In addition to this pooling, the sequestered red cells also are exposed to splenic conditions that accelerate destruction, further contributing to the decreased red cell concentration. These combined activities result in anemia.

Anemia is further potentiated by an increase in blood volume, which produces a dilutional effect on the already reduced concentration of red cells. Anemia has been identified as the result of sequestering. The dilutional effect, as well as the removal and destruction of red cells, depends primarily on the degree of splenomegaly.

White cells and platelets also are affected by sequestering, although not to the same degree as the red cell. Again, the size of the spleen is the determining factor in the number of cells sequestered.

Specific conditions that cause secondary splenomegaly and the resulting hypersplenism are myriad and are related to all other categories of disease that affect individuals, such as infectious, metabolic, circulatory, endocrinologic, and neoplastic, as well as purely mechanical alterations.[8] Specific diseases related to the various classifications of splenomegaly are detailed in Box 26-3. Different pathologic processes produce splenomegaly and are briefly described.

Acute inflammatory or infectious processes cause splenomegaly because of an increased demand for defensive activities. Acutely enlarged spleens secondary to infection may become so filled with erythrocytes that their natural rubbery resilience is lost and they become fragile and vulnerable to blunt trauma.[43] Traumatic rupture of the spleen is a complication in individuals with infectious mononucleosis; rupture occurs mostly in males between the fourth and twenty-first day of acute illness.[9]

Congestive splenomegaly is accompanied by ascites, portal hypertension, and esophageal varices and is seen most commonly in hepatic cirrhosis. Splenic hyperplasia develops in any disorder in which splenic workload is increased and is associated most commonly with various types of anemia (hemolytic) and chronic myeloproliferative disorders (i.e., polycythemia vera).

Infiltrative splenomegaly is caused by engorgement of the macrophages with indigestible materials associated with various "storage diseases." Tumors and cysts are neoplastic disorders that cause actual growth of the spleen. Metastatic tumors of the spleen are rare and may result from skin, lung, breast, and cervical primary sites.[8]

Treatment for hypersplenism is splenectomy; however, it is not always the treatment of choice. It is generally beneficial to perform a splenectomy when the spleen is exerting destructive effects on the red cells, and splenectomy is not performed when the spleen is exerting favorable effects, such as antibody production and hematopoiesis. Splenectomy should be performed for clinical indicators and not necessarily for specific conditions.[41] Splenectomy for splenic rupture no longer is considered mandatory in light of the possibility of overwhelming sepsis after removal. Repair and preservation of the ruptured spleen is now considered before the decision to remove the spleen is made.

Individuals are able to lead normal lives after splenectomy, but hematologic abnormalities persist after removal of the spleen. The red cells become thinner, broader, and wrinkled as a result of increases in surface area and membrane lipids.[43] The white cell count increases dramatically 1 week after removal and then levels off to approximately 40% above normal. Platelets also rise immediately after surgery and then level off to above-normal levels for the duration of the individual's life. Increased platelet levels have been implicated in ischemic heart disease in males because of increased thrombocytosis and hypercoagulability.[43]

Box 26-3

DISEASES RELATED TO CLASSIFICATION OF SPLENOMEGALY

INFLAMMATION OR INFECTIONS

1. Acute
   a. Viral (hepatitis, infectious mononucleosis, cytomegalovirus)
   b. Bacterial (salmonella, gram negative)
   c. Parasite (typhoid)
2. Subacute or chronic
   a. Bacterial (subacute bacterial endocarditis, tuberculosis)
   b. Parasite (malaria)
   c. Fungal (histoplasmosis)
   d. Felty syndrome
   e. Systemic lupus erythematosus
   f. Rheumatoid arthritis

CONGESTIVE

1. Cirrhosis
2. Heart failure
3. Portal vein obstruction (portal hypertension)
4. Splenic vein obstruction

INFILTRATIVE

1. Gaucher disease
2. Amyloidosis
3. Diabetic lipemia

TUMORS OR CYSTS

1. Malignant
   a. Polycythemia rubra vera
   b. Thrombocytopenia
   c. Chronic leukemia (chronic myelocytic leukemia, chronic lymphocytic leukemia)
   d. Hodgkin disease
   e. Acute leukemia
   f. Metastatic solid tumors
2. Nonmalignant: hamartoma
3. Cysts
   a. True: lymphangiomas, hemangiomas, epithelial, endothelial
   b. False: hemorrhagic, serous, inflammatory

ALTERATIONS OF PLATELETS AND COAGULATION

Alterations of platelets and coagulation affect hemostasis, either by preventing hemostasis or by causing it to occur when it is not needed. (Hemostasis is described in Chapter 24.) Platelet and coagulation disorders can prevent hemostasis to varying degrees, causing (or failing to cause) internal or external hemorrhage. Diffuse hemorrhage into skin tissues that is visible through the skin causes a red-purplish discoloration identified as a **purpura.** Purpuric disorders occur when there are not enough normal platelets to plug damaged vessels or prevent leakage from the many minute tears that occur daily in normal capillaries. Coagulation disorders tend to result in more serious internal bleeding and usually are caused by a deficiency of one or several clotting factors.

Disorders in which coagulation proceeds needlessly tend to result from vascular abnormalities that stimulate clotting. These disorders are known collectively as **thromboembolic disease.**

Disorders of Platelets

Quantitative or qualitative abnormalities of platelets can interrupt normal blood coagulation and prevent hemostasis. The quantitative abnormalities are thrombocytopenia, a decrease in the number of circulating platelets, and **thrombocythemia,** an increase in the number of platelets. Qualitative disorders affect the structure or function of individual platelets and can coexist with the quantitative disorders. Qualitative disorders usually prevent platelet adherence and aggregation, preventing formation of a platelet plug.

Thrombocytopenia

Thrombocytopenia is defined as a platelet count below 100,000 platelets/mm^3 of blood. A count of 50,000/mm^3 or less increases the potential for hemorrhage associated with minor trauma. Spontaneous bleeding can occur with counts between 10,000/mm^3 and 15,000/mm^3, resulting in petechiae, ecchymoses, larger purpuric spots, or frank bleeding from mucous membranes.[44] Severe bleeding results if the count is below 10,000/mm^3 and can be fatal if it occurs in the gastrointestinal tract, respiratory system, or central nervous system.

Before the diagnosis of thrombocytopenia is made, it is important to determine if a **pseudothrombocytopenia** is present. This phenomenon occurs in approximately 1 in 1000 to 1 in 10,000 situations and is an in vitro artifact that occurs when platelets counted in a blood smear by automatic cell counting are agglutinated by IgG, IgM, or IgA in the presence of ethylenediaminetetraacetic acid (EDTA).[44,45] The agglutinated platelets are not counted, and it appears that the individual may have thrombocytopenia when in fact it is a false representation of the total platelet count.

Another situation that mimics thrombocytopenia is a dilutional effect observed after massive transfusion of packed cells, which are generally platelet poor. This occurs when an individual has received more than 10 units of blood within a 24-hour period. The hemorrhage that necessitated the transfusion accelerates a loss of platelets, which further contributes to the thrombocytopenic state.

Thrombocytopenia is also the result of increased sequestering of platelets by the spleen secondary to hypersplenism (congestive) (hypersplenism is discussed on p. 884). Hypothermia has also been identified as a cause of thrombocytopenia. Temperatures below 25° C appear to be necessary for this condition to be present. After rewarming, levels of platelets return to normal, suggesting that the platelets are sequestered and later released.[44]

Thrombocytopenia is often secondary to other acquired or congenital conditions that may cause decreased production of platelets or decreased platelet survival. Congenital conditions are rare and include thrombocytopenia with absent radii (TAR) syndrome, Wiskott-Aldrich syndrome, May-Hegglin syndrome, and autosomal recessive thrombocytopenia. The acquired states are more common and include such conditions as viral infections (e.g., EBV, rubella, CMV, and HIV). Thrombocytopenia also may accompany nutritional deficiency states associated with vitamin B_{12}, folic acid, and iron. Bone marrow replacement and bone marrow hypoplasia (aplastic anemia) also may precipitate thrombocytopenia. Drugs (e.g., thiazides, estrogens, quinine-containing medications) and chemotherapy and toxins (e.g., ethanol, cocaine-specific toxins) are also implicated as causing thrombocytopenia.

Heparin is identified as the most common cause of drug-induced thrombocytopenia. Approximately 5% to 15% of individuals treated with heparin develop heparin-induced thrombocytopenia (HIT).[46] HIT is an immune-mediated, adverse drug reaction caused by IgG antibodies that recognize complexes of heparin and platelet factor 4, leading to platelet activation through platelet Fc γIIa receptors.[47] The hallmark of HIT is a decrease in platelets beginning 5 to 10 days after administration of heparin.[47] If HIT is not recognized and treated, intravascular aggregation of platelets causes rapid development of arterial and venous thrombosis. Venous thrombosis is most common and results in deep venous thrombosis and pulmonary emboli. A majority of arterial thromboses affect the large arteries of the lower extremities, causing acute limb ischemia. In addition, arterial thrombosis leads to cerebrovascular accidents and myocardial infarctions. Other major arteries (renal, mesenteric, upper limb) may also be affected.[47]

Thrombocytopenia also is caused by increased platelet destruction. The major cause of platelet destruction is **immune thrombocytopenic purpura (ITP).** The incidence of ITP is estimated to be 1:10,000 in the general public, but precise statistics are not available.[48] This condition was formerly known as *idiopathic thrombocytopenic purpura;* however, recent studies have confirmed an autoimmune process in the destruction of platelets, hence the change from idiopathic to immune. Ninety-five percent of the time, IgG is the antibody that adheres to the platelet and initiates its destruction. Platelet surface membrane proteins become antigenic, stimulating the immune system to produce autoantibody. The antigenic response probably begins in the spleen, prompting autoantibody production. Other antibody-producing tissues, particularly bone marrow, also begin to produce autoantibody. The autoantibodies produced target either platelet glycoprotein (GP)IIb/IIIa or GPIb/IX.[49] It is estimated that about 75% of individuals with ITP produce these autoantibodies.

Other immunoglobulins (IgM and IgA) also have been identified as initiating destruction of platelets.[50] The majority of the destruction of platelets takes place in the spleen when the antibody-bound platelet comes in contact with the mononuclear phagocyte cells. The liver is the major organ involved when IgM is the antibody.

ITP is a common disease in adults and is frequently a chronic condition more prevalent in females. The incidence is highest in the young adult group (20 to 40 years old), but ITP is found in all age categories. The acute form is more prevalent in children and frequently follows a viral illness. In children, the disease typically lasts from 1 to 2 months but may last as long as 6 months followed by a complete remission. However, approximately 7% to 28% of children may develop the chronic form.[48]

Initial manifestations include minor problems, such as development of petechiae and purpura over the course of several days, that progress to major hemorrhage from mucosal sites, epistaxis, hematuria, menorrhagia, and bleeding gums. Rarely will an individual present with intracranial bleeding or other sites of internal bleeding.

No specific guidelines existed for the diagnosis and treatment of ITP until recently. Since 1994, guidelines established by a panel of the American Hematological Society have been used for diagnosis and treatment of ITP in children and adults.[51] Diagnosis of ITP is based on a history of bleeding and associated symptoms, such as weight loss, fever, and headache. Risk factors are also identified, such as HIV infection, and medications are screened as a potential cause of ITP, as well as any family history of bleeding. Physical examination signs are also evaluated for types of bleeding, location, and severity. Evidence of other infections (bacterial, HIV) and thrombosis are also assessed. Other diagnostic tests include complete blood count (CBC) and peripheral blood smear.

Treatment of ITP is palliative and not curative, focusing on inactivation or removal of the site of platelet destruction and antiplatelet antibody production, specifically the spleen.[48] Treatment is initiated when platelet counts are less than 20,000 to 30,000 or less than 50,000 with evidence of bleeding from mucous membranes or at high risk to develop bleeding.[52]

Initial therapy for ITP is infusion of glucocorticoids (prednisone), which prevents sequestering and further destruction of platelets. If platelet counts do not increase appropriately, splenectomy is considered. Splenectomy, however, is not without risk, and approximately 10% to 20% of individuals who undergo splenectomy suffer a relapse and require further treatment.[45] In these relapsed individuals, it is thought that other reticuloendothelial organs, particularly the liver, have emerged as a reservoir for platelets.[48]

Further treatment for ITP includes intravenous immunoglobulin (IVIg), anti–(Rh) D, danazol, and vinca alkaloids (chemotherapeutic agents). Anti–(Rh) D is used as an alternative to splenectomy or to delay the need for one. It is also hoped that its use may induce a remission of ITP.[53] Immunosuppressives (azathioprine and cyclophosphamide) also are used, but only for individuals who are intolerant of other therapies.[45]

Thrombocytopenia is also a manifestation of **thrombotic thrombocytopenic purpura (TTP),** a thrombotic microangiopathy in which platelets aggregate and cause occlusion of arterioles and capillaries within the microcirculation. This is a relatively uncommon syndrome occurring in about 1:1,000,000 individuals with a preference for females in their thirties.[54] TTP is rarely observed in infants and the elderly. TTP is increasing in incidence, and this appears to be a true increase rather than a result of improved recognition.[55]

Platelet aggregation is the key pathologic feature, but the etiology remains unknown. Several hypotheses have been postulated, including abnormal interaction between damaged vascular endothelium and platelets precipitated by ultralarge von Willebrand factor and the presence of platelet aggregating plasma proteins of the family of cysteine proteinases—evidence to support an autoimmune response.[54] TTP is clinically related to other thrombotic microangiopathic conditions, including hemolytic uremic syndrome; malignant hypertension; and preeclampsia, or the pregnancy-induced HELLP (hemolysis, elevated liver enzymes, low platelet count) syndrome.

There are two types of TTP: chronic relapsing and acute idiopathic. **Chronic relapsing TTP** is the more rare type and is usually seen in children. When recognized early enough and successfully treated, the child will experience recurring episodes at approximately 3-week intervals that are usually predictable and responsive to treatment.

Acute idiopathic TTP is much more common and more severe. Early diagnosis and treatment is important because if left untreated it may prove to be fatal within 90 days of onset. Individuals with acute idiopathic TTP have extreme thrombocytopenia, intravascular hemolytic anemia from red cell fragmentation (schistocytosis, an elevated LDL level from tissue injury), and ischemic signs and symptoms most frequently involving the central nervous system.[55] Central nervous system symptoms may include memory disturbances, behavioral irregularities, headaches, or coma.

Plasma exchange (PE) with fresh frozen plasma is the treatment of choice for acute idiopathic TTP, achieving a response rate of 70% to 85%. In addition to PE, steroids (glucocorticoids) are administered. Individuals who do not respond to conventional treatment may be candidates for splenectomy; however, postoperative hemorrhage remains a dangerous complication. Some individuals have responded to immunosuppressive (azothioprine) therapy.[55]

Thrombocythemia

Essential (primary) thrombycythemia (ET) is a clonal myeloproliferative disorder of a multipotent stem cell in which platelets are produced in greater numbers than normal, resulting in platelet counts in excess of 600,000/mm^3. The bone marrow of affected individuals is characterized by hyperplasia of megakaryocytes. Additional manifestations include splenomegaly and periodic episodes of hemorrhage or thrombosis or both.[56]

The exact incidence of essential thrombocythemia is unknown because extensive epidemiologic studies are not available; however, investigators in Denmark estimated the incidence to be 0.59 per 100,000.[57] It is more common in middle-age individuals, with the majority of cases occurring between ages 50 and 60 years. There is no known gender preference, although some reports indicate a greater female prevalence. Evidence also suggests a possible familial connection, with or without other types of myeloproliferative disorders.[58]

Precise mechanisms causing essential thrombocythemia are unknown. It is important to differentiate between reactive (physiologic) thrombocythemia, noted after exercise, postpartum, and as a result of epinephrine, and the essential form, which is associated with additional complications and requires treatment.[56] Platelet increases can also result after splenectomy or an infectious or inflammatory condition.

The platelets of affected individuals appear to have a normal survival time, and evidence suggests that the disorder is caused by increased megakaryocyte production originating at the pluripotential hematopoietic stem cell. Essential thrombocythemia has not been associated with erythrocytosis, which is the hallmark of polycythemia vera; however, recent evidence suggests that, along with an increase in platelets, there may be a concomitant increase in red cells reflecting a close association with myeloproliferative disorders.[59] The presence and degree of erythrocytosis appears to correlate with altered stem cell commitment and development.

Clinical manifestations of essential thrombocythemia vary significantly among individuals. As many as two thirds of affected individuals are diagnosed from a routine CBC. After diagnosis, these individuals may recall events related to thrombosis or hemorrhage.

Microvasculature thrombosis (erythromyalgia), the most common presenting symptom, is frequently manifested in the fingers and toes. It is characterized by warm, congested, red extremities with painful burning sensations, particularly in the forefoot sole and one or more toes. The lower extremities are more frequently affected, and it may be asymmetric. The pain is initiated by standing, exercise, or warmth and relieved by elevation and cooling. In extreme situations, erythromyalgia may lead to acrocyanosis and gangrene.[58]

Arterial thrombosis is more common than venous thrombosis and may involve the coronary and renal arteries. Also reported is involvement of the carotid, mesenteric, and subclavian arteries. Myocardial ischemia and myocardial infarction, without clear evidence of coronary artery disease, have also been observed in individuals with essential thrombocythemia.

Other manifestations related to microvascular thrombosis include neurologic symptoms, of which headache and dizziness are the most common. Other reported symptoms include paresthesias, transient ischemic attacks, strokes, visual disturbances, and seizures.[60] Major thrombotic events that are not directly related to the platelet count are estimated to occur in 20% to 30% of individuals with ET. Other risk factors (e.g., prior history of thrombotic events, advanced age, and duration of thrombocytosis) are identified as better predictors of future thrombotic complications.[61]

In contrast to thrombosis, hemorrhagic manifestations can include bleeding in the gastrointestinal tract; the bleeding may be mistaken for a duodenal ulcer. Other bleeding sites include skin, eyes, urinary tract, gums, tooth sockets (after extraction), joints, and the brain. Hemorrhage is most often not severe, occurring more frequently in individuals with very high platelet counts,[60] and occasionally requires transfusion. Important is recognition that bleeding and clotting may exist simultaneously and individuals will not necessarily be "bleeders" or "clotters."[62]

Since 1980, hydroxyurea (HU), a nonalkylating myelosuppressive agent, has been the drug of choice. HU is relatively effective in causing platelet production suppression; however, long-term use may cause ET to progress to other myelodysplastic syndromes, particularly acute myeloid leukemia.[63]

Other drugs used to treat ET include aspirin and interferon; however, interferon may not work for everyone, and aspirin, as a blood thinner, may contribute to hemorrhagic complications. A newer drug, Anagrelide, is now considered to be the drug of choice. Anagrelide appears to be platelet specific, interfering with platelet maturation rather than production, and as such does not affect red cell and white cell growth and development.[64]

Alterations of Platelet Function

Qualitative alterations in platelet function occur with an increased bleeding time in the presence of a normal platelet count. Qualitative alterations may be acquired or congenital. Congenital alterations (thrombocytopathies) are rare and may be categorized into four types: disorders of platelet adhesion, disorders of platelet aggregation, disorders of platelet secretion, and disorders of procoagulant activity.[65] Clinical manifestations of platelet alterations include petechiae and purpura, mild to moderate mucosal bleeding (bilateral epistaxis, gastrointestinal, genitourinary, and pulmonary), gingival bleeding, and spontaneous bruising.

Disorders of platelet adhesion result from deficiency of a platelet membrane glycoprotein complex Ib/IX (Bernard-Soulier syndrome) or von Willebrand factor. Lack of these proteins prevents platelets from adhering to collagen, resulting in impaired hemostasis and clinical hemorrhage.[66]

Disorders of platelet aggregation are manifested by failure of platelets to aggregate with adenosine diphosphate (ADP), collagen, epinephrine, or thrombin because of a deficiency in the glycoprotein (IIb/IIIa) that acts as a fibrinogen receptor (Glanzmann thrombasthenia). Lack of this protein results in a failure to build "fibrinogen bridges" between platelets (see Fig. 24-16).

Disorders of platelet secretion are characterized by initial normal platelet aggregation with collagen or ADP; however, there is failure of subsequent processes, specifically secretion of prostaglandins and release of granule-bound ADP (gray platelet syndrome, an α-storage pool disease). Disorders of platelet procoagulant activity are extremely rare and are characterized by lack of procoagulant factors normally present in activated platelets and promote the activation of factor X of the coagulation pathway and prothrombin.

Acquired disorders of platelet function are more common than the congenital disorders and may be categorized into three principal causes: drugs, systemic conditions, and hematologic alterations.

Multiple drugs are known to affect platelet function and are listed in Box 26-4. Of this vast array of drugs, aspirin is the only known drug specifically used for its antithrombotic activity.[51] Drugs interfere with platelet function in three ways: inhibition of platelet membrane receptors, inhibition of prostaglandin pathways, and inhibition of phosphodiesterase activity.[67]

Systemic disorders that affect platelet function are chronic renal disease, cardiopulmonary bypass surgery, and anti-

Box 26-4

COMMON DRUGS OR AGENTS* THAT INHIBIT PLATELET FUNCTION†

Nonsteroidal antiinflammatories
- Acetylsalicylic acid (ASA)
- Ibuprofen
- Naproxen
- Indomethacin

B-Lactam antibiotics
- Penicillin G (all penicillin derivatives ending in "cillin")
- Cephalosporins

Cardiovascular drugs
- Nitroglycerin
- Propranolol
- Nifedipine
- Verapamil
- Quinidine
- Diltiazem

Psychotropic drugs
- Tricyclic antidepressants: imipramine
- Phenothiazines: chlorpromazine, promethazine

Anesthetics
- Local: lidocaine, procaine
- General: halothane

Antihistamines
- Diphenhydramine

Food additives or foods
- Ethanol
- Cumin
- Turmeric
- Clove

*Of these drugs and agents, only ASA causes significantly increased bleeding time. Other drugs affect platelet aggregation or bleeding time.
†Generic drug names used in this box.

platelet antibodies associated with autoimmunity disorders. Hematologic disorders that cause platelet dysfunction are chronic myeloproliferative disorders, leukemias, myelodysplastic syndromes, and dysproteinemias.

Disorders of Coagulation

Disorders of coagulation usually are caused by defects or deficiencies of one or more of the clotting factors. (Normal function of the clotting factors is described in Chapter 24.) Qualitative or quantitative abnormalities of clotting factors prevent the enzymatic reactions by which these factors are normally transformed from circulating plasma proteins to a stable fibrin clot (see Fig. 24-17).

Some clotting factor defects are inherited and usually involve a single factor. Two of the most common inherited disorders, the hemophilias and von Willebrand disease, are caused by deficiencies of clotting factors (see Chapter 27). Other coagulation defects are acquired and tend to result from deficient synthesis of clotting factors by the liver. Liver disease is one cause of acquired coagulation deficiency. Another is a dietary deficiency of vitamin K, which is necessary for normal synthesis of the clotting factors.

Other coagulation disorders not caused by quantitative or qualitative clotting factor defects are attributed to pathologic conditions that trigger coagulation inappropriately, engaging the clotting factors and causing detrimental clotting within blood vessels. For example, any cardiovascular abnormality that alters normal blood flow by speeding it up, slowing it down, or obstructing it can create conditions in which coagulation proceeds within the vessels. This is a cause of thromboembolic disease, in which blood clots obstruct blood vessels. Coagulation is also stimulated by the presence of tissue factor, which is released by damaged or dead tissues. Therefore any condition in which tissue decay or damage releases a great deal of tissue thromboplastin, such as occurs in complications of pregnancy, including death of the fetus and placental decay within the mother, can cause widespread and possibly fatal intravascular coagulation. Another cause of detrimental coagulation processes is vasculitis, or inflammation of the blood vessels. Damage to inflamed vessels causes platelet activation, which in turn activates the coagulation cascade. In extensive or prolonged vasculitis, blood clot formation can overcome mechanisms that normally control clot formation and breakdown, leading to clogging of the vessels. In each of these acquired conditions, normal hemostatic function proves detrimental to the body by consuming coagulation factors excessively or by overwhelming normal control of clot formation and breakdown (fibrinolysis).

Impaired Hemostasis

Impaired hemostasis, or the inability to promote coagulation and the development of a stable fibrin clot, is commonly associated with either the lack of vitamin K or specific liver disorders.

Vitamin K Deficiency

Vitamin K, a fat-soluble vitamin, is necessary for synthesis and regulation of normal prothrombin, the prothrombin factors (II, VII, IX, X), and the anticoagulant factors (proteins C and S). The most common cause of vitamin K deficiency is parenteral nutrition in combination with broad-spectrum antibiotics that destroy normal gut flora. Rarely is a deficiency caused by lack of dietary intake.[68]

Parenteral administration of vitamin K is the treatment of choice and usually results in correction. Improvement of clotting tests is usually within 8 to 12 hours. Fresh frozen plasma (FFP) also may be administered and usually is reserved for individuals with life-threatening hemorrhages or who require emergency surgery. Infusion of prothrombin complex concentrations is not recommended because of their thrombogenic activity.[69]

Liver Disease

Individuals with liver disease have a broad range of hemostasis derangements that may be characterized by defects in the clotting or fibrinolytic systems and by platelet function.[69] The usual sequence of events is an initial reduction in clotting factors, which parallels the degree of hepatic parenchymal cell damage or destruction. Factor VII is the first to decline because of its rapid turnover, followed by declines in factors II and X. Factor IX levels are less affected and do not decline until liver destruction is well advanced. Protein C levels also decline early, similar to levels of factor VII; protein S levels decline in the later stages of liver disease. Factor V reduction is of special importance because its plasma level appears to be a direct reflection of liver cell damage.[69]

Other hemostatic alterations in liver disease include increased fibrinolytic activity, which may be primary in origin or a result of disseminated intravascular coagulation (DIC). Increased fibrinolysis results from increased levels and impaired clearance of fibrinolytic activators and decreased levels of inhibitors, such as α_2-antiplasmin.

Thrombocytopenia and thrombocytopathies also occur with liver disease. Thrombocytopenia is related to splenomegaly, which often accompanies liver disease and is associated with portal hypertension. Splenic pooling of platelets is the major cause of thrombocytopenia. Thrombocytopathies are associated with elevated levels of fibrin split products, ethanol, and drugs.

Treatment of hemostatic alterations in liver disease must be comprehensive to cover all aspects related to platelet, clotting, and fibrinolytic dysfunctions. FFP administration is the treatment of choice, but not all individuals tolerate the volume needed to adequately replace all deficient factors. Alternative modalities include the addition of exchange transfusions and platelet concentration to FFP administration.

Consumptive Thrombohemorrhagic Disorders

Consumptive thrombohemorrhagic disorders are a heterogeneous group of conditions that demonstrate the entire range of hemorrhagic and thrombotic pathologic conditions.[70] Symptoms range from subtle to devastating, and these disorders generally are considered to be intermediary disease processes that complicate many primary disease states. Confusion and controversy also exist regarding diagnosis, treatment, and management of consumptive thrombohemorrhagic disorders. No one definition can cover all possible varieties of these disorders; however, *disseminated intravascular coagulation* is the most common term used in the clinical setting to describe a pathologic condition associated with hemorrhage and thrombosis.

Disseminated Intravascular Coagulation

Disseminated intravascular coagulation (DIC) is a complex and highly variable, acquired clinical syndrome with manifestations that are the result of increased protease activity in the blood caused by unregulated release of thrombin with subsequent fibrin formation and accelerated fibrinolysis. The clinical course of DIC ranges from an acute, severe, life-threatening process that is characterized by massive hemorrhage and thrombosis to a chronic, low-grade condition. The chronic condition is characterized by minor laboratory abnormalities with subacute hemorrhage and diffuse microcirculatory thrombosis. DIC may be localized to one specific organ or generalized, involving multiple organs.[71] The clinical course of DIC is determined largely by the intensity of the stimulus, host response, and comorbid conditions.[72]

Because of the complexity and wide variations in manifestations of DIC, diagnosis has been confusing and difficult. To aid in diagnosis, the following definition, based on minimal acceptable criteria, has been developed: "a systemic thrombohemorrhagic disorder seen in association with well-defined clinical situations and laboratory evidence of (1) procoagulant activation, (2) fibrinolytic activation, (3) inhibitor consumption, and (4) biochemical evidence of end-organ damage or failure."[72]

DIC is an intermediary mechanism of disease that is associated with a wide variety of well-defined clinical conditions, specifically those that activate the clotting cascade. The potential for procoagulant activity exists whenever the following clinical situations are present: (1) arterial hypotension, frequently accompanying shock; (2) hypoxemia; (3) acidemia; and (4) stasis of capillary blood flow.[71] Whatever the precipitating cause, the course of DIC is initiated by mechanisms that are the direct result of endothelial damage, tissue damage, and direct activation of factor X.[71]

With tissue damage, intravascular coagulation is initiated by exposure of circulating blood to tissue factor (TF) found in subendothelial cells (fibroblasts and monocytes) or damaged or activated endothelial cells (ECs), also found in subendothelial connective tissue structures.[73] Endothelial damage exposes the negatively charged basement membrane that becomes a hemostatically active vascular surface, precipitating activation of the Hageman factor (XII).

Sepsis is the most common cause of DIC, with prevalence ranging widely from 7.5% to 49%.[74] Potent gram-negative endotoxins, as well as gram-positive microorganisms, have been implicated as a cause of DIC, along with fungi, protozoa (malaria), and viruses (flu, herpes). Hypoxia and low blood flow states associated with cardiopulmonary arrest also can damage the endothelium and activate the intrinsic clotting cascade, triggering DIC.

During sepsis, multiple cytokines are released that play a significant role in the development and maintenance of DIC. These proinflammatory cytokines (tumor necrosis factor–α [TNF-α], interleukins [IL-1, IL-6, IL-8], and platelet activating factor [PAF]) are largely, possibly completely, responsible for the clinical signs and symptoms associated with sepsis. Their major role is activating epithelial cells, causing release of TF and von Willebrand factor, and they have been shown in vitro to increase plasminogen activator inhibitor–1 (PAI-1) synthesis, increase tissue factor activity, and decrease

WHAT'S NEW? Antithrombin Levels in Disseminated Intravascular Coagulation

Acquired antithrombin (AT) deficiency, most notably with DIC, is being used as a predictor of morbidity and mortality in the presence of sepsis. Normal levels of AT are between 75% and 120%. Levels of AT below 70% in plasma were associated with 90% mortality in trauma patients with sepsis; plasma levels below 60% were associated with 100% mortality. The lowest AT levels were found in individuals with sepsis, and AT levels below 65% predicted mortality.

Data from Mammen EF: Antithrombin: its physiological importance and role in DIC, *Semin Thromb Hemost* 24:19, 1998.

thrombomodulin expression, thereby promoting development of thrombi.

DIC is also precipitated by direct tissue damage that causes release of and exposure to TF. Release of TF occurs when normal structures are broken down, such as occurs in ischemia and necrosis, surgical manipulation, and crushing injury. Tissue damage causes injury to the endothelium, complicating the situation and predisposing to the development of DIC. In addition to crushing tissue damage, TF may be released directly into the bloodstream from circulating white cells (monocyte-endotoxin interaction), immune complexes, or cancer cells. Leukemic cells may spontaneously release TF, and malignant cells can also directly activate the tenase complex,[75] a component of the prothrombin activator complex.

In addition to endothelial or tissue damage, which causes release of TF, DIC may be precipitated by direct proteolytic activation of factor X that has been identified as thrombin mimicry[76] and results in proteases directly converting fibrinogen to fibrin. Proteases may come from snake venom, as well as tumor cells. Enzymes from the pancreas and liver also have a direct proteolytic effect and are released during pancreatitis and various stages of liver disease. It appears that direct proteolytic activity does not depend on any type of damage to either the endothelium or tissue.

Miscellaneous causes of DIC have also been identified, most notably blood transfusion. Transfused blood dilutes the clotting factors, as well as circulating naturally occurring antithrombins. In hemolytic transfusion reactions, the endothelium is damaged as a result of the assembly of the complement membrane attack complex rather than the intravascular destruction of red blood cells.[75] Antibody-antigen reactions are also responsible for the development of DIC after anaphylaxis.

The pathophysiology of DIC is shown in Fig. 26-14. DIC is initiated by one of the previously identified etiologies (Box 26-5), activating either the intrinsic or extrinsic clotting cascade. The extrinsic system appears to be the predominant system that is activated. When damage or injury to either tissue or epithelium occurs, the normal physiologic response is the release of TF, which complexes with factor VIIa and directly generates the enzymatic components of the tenase and prothrombinase complexes that are capable of causing an explosive generation of thrombin.[73,75]

The amount of thrombin entering the systemic circulation during DIC exceeds the ability of the body's naturally occurring anticoagulants (proteins C and S; antithrombin [AT]) to regulate it. These anticoagulants require an intact epithelial surface to be active. Therefore, in the presence of damaged epithelium or tissue characteristic of DIC, the activity of the anticoagulants is severely constrained, allowing uninhibited thrombin activity resulting in unrestricted clot formation. Because of the widespread and diffusing clotting activity, clotting factors are consumed. When the clotting factors are all used up, hemorrhage ensues, resulting in the primary pathophysiologic paradox of DIC—*thrombosis in the presence of hemorrhage.*

Thrombin, initially released at the beginning of the clotting cascade, causes platelet aggregation and consumption of clotting factors. It also cleaves fibrinogen into fibrin monomers that polymerize into fibrin clots that become deposited in the microcirculation. This results in microvascular and macrovascular thrombosis, interfering with blood flow and causing peripheral ischemia and end-organ damage.[72]

Once clotting occurs, the fibrinolytic pathway is activated and begins degrading the formed clot. After the coagulation and fibrinolytic systems are activated, large amounts of circulating prothrombin and plasminogen are converted to thrombin and plasmin. Once thrombin and plasmin are circulating systemically, DIC results.[72]

Plasmin, a potent proteolytic enzyme that digests fibrin and fibrinogen, is present in higher than normal amounts. Plasmin is produced when plasminogen is activated by the tissue activators, which are present in endothelial cells and released during tissue damage. Overstimulation of the clotting cascade is also responsible for an abundance of plasmin.

As fibrin is degraded by plasmin, fibrin degradation products (FDPs) are released into the circulation. High concentrations of FDPs, which are potent anticoagulants, further contribute to the bleeding component of DIC. FDPs normally

Box 26-5

MAJOR ETIOLOGIES IDENTIFIED AS ANTECEDENTS TO THE INITIATION AND DEVELOPMENT OF DISSEMINATED INTRAVASCULAR COAGULATION (DIC)

ACUTE FULMINANT DIC

- Obstetric complications
  - Abruptio placentae
  - Retained fetus syndrome
  - Enclampsia
  - Septic abortion
- Intravascular hemolysis
  - Hemolytic transfusion reactions
  - Massive transfusions
- Infections
  - Sepsis (gram negative or positive)
  - Viremias (HIV, varicella, CMV, hepatitis)
- Malignancies
  - Leukeami (acute promyelocytic)
- Crush injuries/tissue necrosis
  - Burns
  - Trauma
- Acute liver disease
  - Obstructive jaundice
  - Acute hepatic failure
- Prothesis
  - LeVeen/Denver shunts
  - Aortic balloon pump
- Vascular disorders

CHRONIC LOW-GRADE DIC

- Cardiovascular disease
- Autoimmune disease
- Renal vascular disorders
- Hematologic disorders
- Inflammatory disorders
- Malignancies

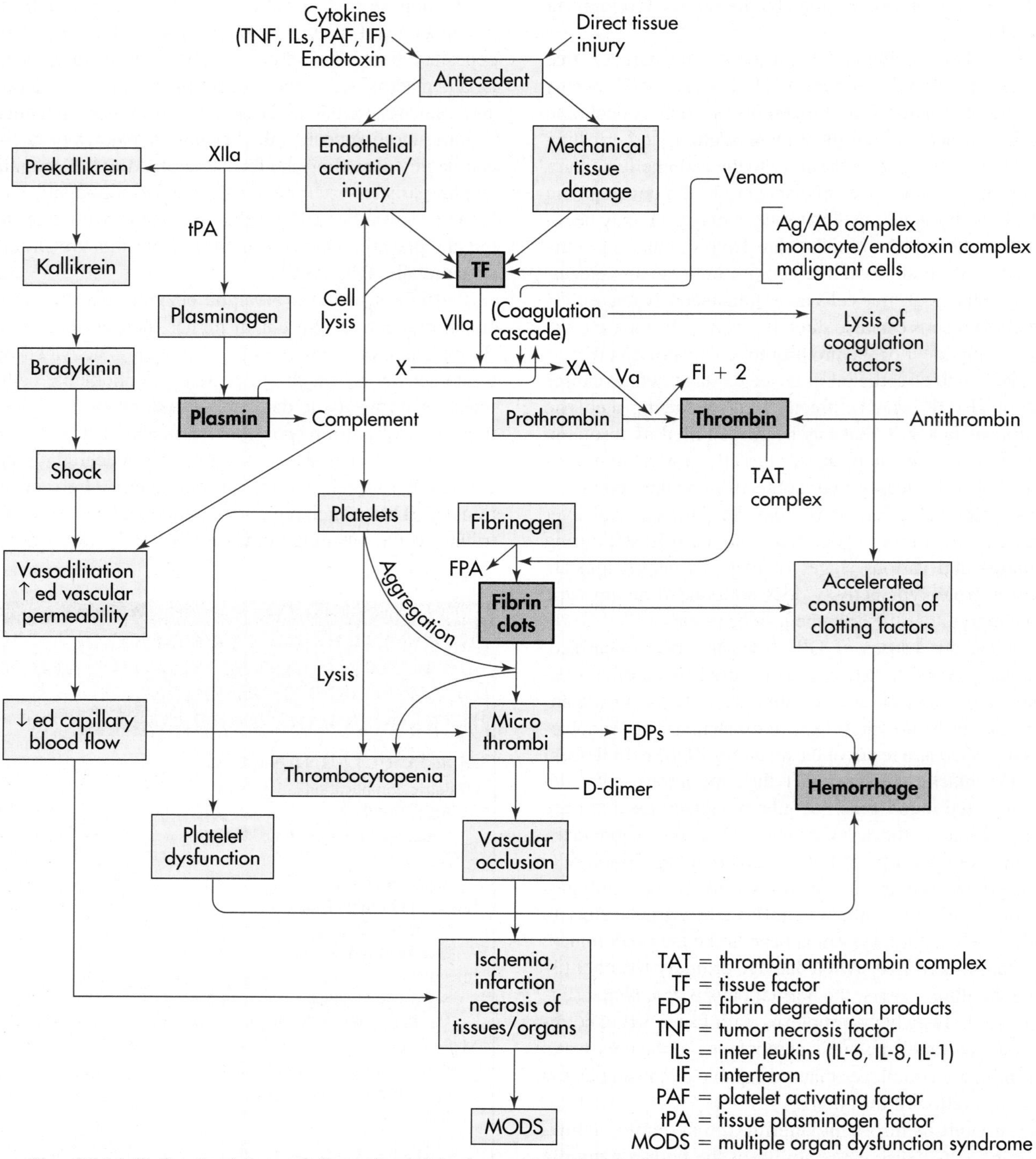

FIG. 26-14 Pathophysiology of disseminated intravascular coagulation (DIC). DIC is initiated by endothelial damage, either directly (tissue damage) or indirectly (activation) causing release of TF. TF initiates the coagulation cascade, which ultimately activates plasmin and thrombin, leading to accelerated use of clotting factors causing clotting and hemorrhage at the same time. TF may also be released by dead tissue. Conversion of X to Xa may also be initiated by venom.

are cleared from the blood by the macrophage system; however, they are not cleared as readily in DIC, which is thought to be caused by a lack of fibronectin. Fibronectin is a glycoprotein with adhesive properties that mediate removal of particulate matter (e.g., fibrin clumps). Low levels of fibronectin in individuals with DIC carry a poor prognosis.[71]

In addition, plasmin activates the kallikrein-kinen and complement systems. Factor XIIa, generated in DIC, acts to convert prekallikrein to kallikrein with later conversion to high-molecular-weight kininogen into circulating kinins.[72] All of these activated systems further contribute to the thrombosis and hemorrhage of DIC.

The obstruction that results from circulatory deposition of thrombin and clot formation interferes with blood flow, causing widespread organ hypoperfusion that can lead to tissue ischemia, infarction, and necrosis. The tissue damage that results from circulatory obstruction further potentiates and complicates the existing DIC process. Because organ perfusion is drastically impaired, manifestations of multisystem organ dysfunction and failure ultimately result.[71] Multisystem organ dysfunction and failure are discussed in Chapter 45.

Platelet interaction with thrombin also plays a significant role in the clotting-bleeding scenario. Thrombin-induced platelet aggregation that occurs early in the clotting cascade initially plays a role in microcirculatory coagulation and obstruction. Eventually the platelets are consumed, causing a thrombocytopenia that increases the hemorrhaging. The positive feedback loop that perpetuates the cycle of thrombosis and hemorrhage persists until the underlying mechanism that precipitated DIC is removed or appropriate therapeutic interventions terminate the process.

Clinical signs and symptoms of DIC present a wide spectrum of possibilities. The initial manifestation depends on whether it manifests as an acute or a chronic condition and what the etiology was that precipitated its onset. Initial signs of acute DIC are rapid development of hemorrhaging, such as oozing from venipuncture sites, arterial lines, and surgical wounds or development of ecchymotic lesions (purpura, petechiae) and hematomas. Other sites of bleeding include the eyes (sclera and conjunctiva), the nose (epistaxis), and the gums. An average individual with DIC demonstrates bleeding at three unrelated sites, and any combination may be observed.[72] Individuals with DIC also manifest a variable level of shock that is out of proportion to the amount of apparent blood loss.[77]

Manifestations of thrombosis are not always as evident, even though thrombosis is often the first pathologic alteration to occur. A large amount of microvascular and macrovascular occlusion may occur that is not clinically obvious. Organ systems that are susceptible to microvascular thrombosis associated with dysfunction include the cardiovascular, pulmonary, central nervous, renal, and hepatic systems. Speedy and accurate clinical interpretations are critical to impede further disruption and destruction. Manifestations of these system dysfunctions include changes in level of consciousness, behavior, and mentation; confusion; seizure activity; oliguria; hematuria; hypoxia; hypotension; hemoptysis; chest pain; and tachycardia. Hemorrhaging into closed compartments of the body, such as the gastrointestinal system, also can occur and may preclude the development of shock.

Cyanosis of the fingers and toes ("blue finger/toe syndrome") and, in some instances, of the nose and breasts may be present. Symmetric parts are often affected and are indicative of microvascular thrombosis that may progress to infarction and gangrene, requiring amputation.[73] Jaundice also may be present and is believed to result from red cell destruction rather than hepatic dysfunction.

Individuals with chronic or low-grade DIC who do not have the overt manifestations of hemorrhaging and thrombosis but instead have subacute bleeding and diffuse thrombosis are described as having a *compensated DIC.*[78] Individuals with this type of DIC demonstrate an increased turnover and decreased survival time of the components of hemostasis. On occasion, an individual may have diffuse or localized thrombosis, but this is not frequently noted.

Diagnosis of DIC is based primarily on clinical manifestations with confirmation provided by laboratory evidence. Because of the complex nature of DIC, laboratory results are highly variable and difficult to interpret without understanding the pathophysiology of DIC.

In general, coagulation tests (prothrombin time [PT], activated partial thromboplastin time [aPTT], reptilase time) provide unreliable data and do not confirm the diagnosis. It would be expected that these tests would be abnormal; however, the results range from shortened times to prolonged times and in many cases are normal. Coagulation factor assay does not contribute further meaningful data to confirm the diagnosis. Coagulation assays done by the standard aPTT- or PT-derived laboratory techniques give uninterpretable results.

FDPs are elevated in 95% to 100% of individuals with DIC; however, presence of FDPs is not necessarily diagnostic for DIC because they may be elevated in other clinical conditions. Presence of FDPs in the blood is diagnostic only for the presence of plasmin and the result of its action on fibrinogen.

The D-dimer test has been used to diagnose DIC. **D-dimer** is a neoantigen produced by plasmin lysis of cross-linked fibrin clots.[79] Monoclonal antibodies are formed against this D-dimer antigen and identified, documenting the activity of thrombin (cross-linking) and plasmin (fibrinolysis). The D-dimer test is the most reliable and specific test for the diagnosis of DIC.

Another laboratory process used in the diagnosis of DIC is performing assays for identifying specific molecular markers associated with thrombin activity. Conversion of prothrombin to thrombin releases an inactive factor, prothrombin fragment 1.2 (F1+2) from the prothrombin molecule, producing an intermediate factor, prethrombin 2. Once generated, prethrombin 2 can be split to produce thrombin that can then proteolyze fibrinogen and thus liberate fibrinopeptide A (FPA) or combine with its major antagonist, antithrombin, and form a stable inactive enzyme inhibitor complex, the thrombin-antithrombin (TAT) complex. Assays of these factors (PF1+2, FPA, TAT) are now generally available to quantify their blood levels, providing evidence of excessive factor Xa (F1+2) and thrombin (FPA) generation.[72]

Antithrombin III (AT III) levels are also assessed for diagnosing and monitoring therapy for DIC. AT III levels are decreased during activation of DIC because of irreversible complexing of thrombin and circulating activated clotting factors with antithrombin, resulting in significant decreases of functional antithrombin. Assays of blood detect this decrease and provide reliable data for diagnosing DIC.

Laboratory diagnosis of DIC is complex and requires evidence of (1) procoagulant activity, (2) fibrinolytic system activation, (3) inhibitor consumption, and (4) end-organ damage. The relationships among these four criteria are summarized in Box 26-6.

Treatment of DIC, like diagnosis, is complex and individualized; it is based on the person's condition, the underlying etiology and the progression of the condition, and changes in the laboratory tests caused by therapy. Specifically it is directed toward (1) eliminating the underlying pathology, (2) restoring hemostasis, and (3) maintaining organ viability.[71] Removal of the underlying pathology is the initial intervention. Once the stimulus for the procoagulant activity is removed, the liver can restore coagulation factors within 24 to 48 hours.[71]

Restoration of hemostasis is more difficult to attain. Heparin has been used frequently; however, its use is controversial and indicated only in certain situations related to DIC. In clinical trials using heparin, results vary widely, therefore there are no standards for its use. Heparin's anticoagulant effect depends on the concentration of functionally active AT III, which is reduced in DIC, and on heparin-neutralizing substances, such as platelet factor 4, that are released from activated platelets in DIC.[80]

Heparin use seems to be effective in DIC caused by a retained dead fetus and acute promyelocytic leukemia. It is indicated also when organ function is compromised by microthrombi or there is a risk of losing an extremity because of vascular occlusion. Heparin's effectiveness in reducing mortality and morbidity in DIC that is precipitated by septic shock has not been established, and its use is contraindicated where there is evidence of postoperative bleeding, peptic ulcer, or central nervous system bleeding.

Replacement therapy (interventions based on restoring the balance of coagulation factors, deficient coagulation factors, platelets, and other coagulation elements) is gaining importance as a treatment modality. Its use is not without controversy, however. A major concern with using replacement therapy is "adding fuel to the fire." No evidence exists to indicate or contraindicate replacement therapy; clinical judgment is apparently the key factor in deciding on its use.

AT III has been available for a number of years and appears to be most useful in DIC related to sepsis. Low levels of AT III correlate with sepsis-initiated DIC; therefore its use in this situation is strongly recommended.[73] AT III is an α_2-globulin that inactivates thrombin, plasmin, and other serine proteases of coagulation, including factors IXa, Xa, XIa, XIIa, and VIIa, thus inhibiting coagulation.[79] AT III augments the activity of heparin; therefore use of AT III with heparin has not been established. Use of AT III is still relatively new, and clinical guidelines for its efficacy in DIC have not been fully established.

Antifibrinolytics are another group of drugs that may be used in the treatment of DIC but should be used only if other treatment modalities have been unsuccessful. No clear evidence exists to justify their use except in instances of life-threatening hemorrhaging that is not controlled by blood component replacement therapy.[73]

Maintenance of organ viability is accomplished primarily by adequate fluid replacement to sustain adequate circulating blood volume and to maintain optimal tissue and organ perfusion. Fluid resuscitation may also be required to restore blood pressure, cardiac output, and urine output to normal parameters.

Thromboembolic Disease

Abnormal clots occur occasionally within the vascular system. A stationary clot that adheres to the vessel wall is called a **thrombus** (Fig. 26-15). Thrombi are composed of fibrin and blood cells. The proportion of each depends on the location of their formation and the hemodynamics of the blood flow in that particular area. **Arterial thrombi** form in the arterial system under conditions of high blood flow and are composed mostly of platelet aggregates held together

Box 26-6

LABORATORY DIAGNOSTIC CRITERIA FOR DISSEMINATED INTRAVASCULAR COAGULATION (DIC)

GROUP I TESTS (INDICATORS OF PROCOAGULANT ACTIVATION)

1. Elevated prothrombin fragment 1+2
2. Elevated fibrinopeptide A
3. Elevated fibrinopeptide B
4. Elevated thrombin-antithrombin (TAT) complex
5. Elevated D-dimer

GROUP II TESTS (INDICATORS OF FIBRINOLYTIC ACTIVITY)

1. Elevated D-dimer
2. Elevated fibrin degradation products (FDPs)
3. Elevated plasmin
4. Elevated plasmin-antiplasmin (PAP) complex

GROUP III TESTS (INDICATORS OF INHIBITOR CONSUMPTION)

1. Decreased antithrombin III
2. Decreased alpha-2 antiplasmin
3. Decreased heparin cofactor II
4. Decreased protein C or S
5. Elevated TAT complex
6. Elevated PAP complex

GROUP IV TESTS (INDICATORS OF END-ORGAN DAMAGE/FAILURE)

1. Elevated lactic dehydrogenase (LDH)
2. Elevated creatinine
3. Decreased pH
4. Decreased Pao_2

Satisfactory criteria for laboratory diagnosis of DIC requires one abnormality in each of groups I through III and at least two abnormalities in group IV.

Data from Bick RL: Disseminated intravascular coagulation: pathophysiological mechanisms and manifestations, *Semin-Thromb Hemost* 24(1):3, 1998.

by fibrin strands. **Venous thrombi** form in conditions of low flow and are composed mostly of red cells with larger amounts of fibrin and very few platelets.[81]

Thrombi may block blood flow within a vessel that supplies nutrients to tissues critical to survival, such as the heart, brain, or lungs. A thrombus has the potential to separate from the vessel wall and travel within the bloodstream to a different location. When this occurs, the thrombus becomes an **embolus.**

The mobile embolus travels within the bloodstream until it comes to a point in a blood vessel that is smaller than itself, causing it to lodge at that location in the vessel. Once it is lodged, blood flow into the distal portions of the circulatory system is blocked; thus tissues and organs that depend on delivery of blood from that particular section of the circulatory system are deprived of blood. Deprivation of an adequate blood supply to these tissues or organs has the potential to cause injury or death.

Prethrombotic conditions predispose an individual to the development of thrombi. The prethrombotic state in general is caused by **hypercoagulability,** or a tendency to coagulate more rapidly than is normal, within the vasculature. Hypercoagulability may be attributable to hereditary or acquired causes. (Congenital hypercoagulability and thrombosis are discussed in Chapter 27.)

Acquired hypercoagulability and thrombosis. The acquired hypercoagulable states are caused mostly by conditions that promote venous stasis. The most common clinical states that predispose to thromboembolic phenomena are major surgery (orthopedic), acute myocardial infarction, congestive heart failure, limb paralysis, spinal injury, malignancy, advanced age, the postpartum period, and bed rest longer than 1 week. Risk of developing thromboemboli is increased by age, previous thrombi development, and hereditary risk factors.[82] During these clinical states, development of thrombi is greatest because of predisposing factors that promote thrombus formation. These factors are referred to as the **triad of Virchow** and are (1) injury to the blood vessel endothelium, (2) abnormalities of blood flow, and (3) hypercoagulability of the blood.

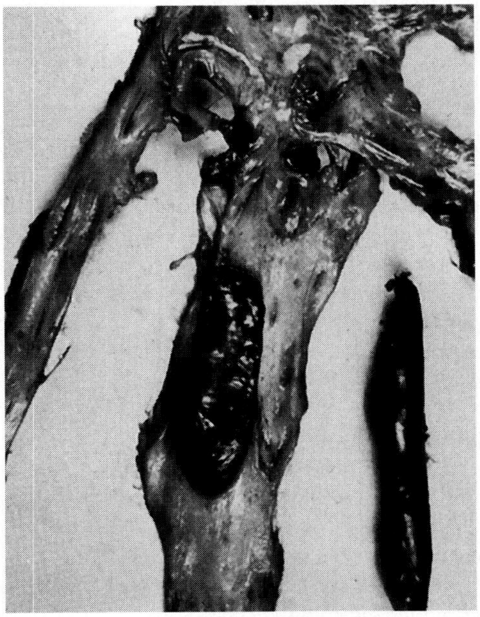

FIG. 26-15 Thrombus. Thrombus arising in valve pocket at upper end of superficial femoral vein. Postmortem clot on the right is shown for comparison. (From McLachlin J, Paterson JC: *Surg Gynecol Obstet* 93:1, 1951.)

Endothelial injury to blood vessels from a variety of sources is the most significant cause of thrombus formation and may, by itself, precipitate the development of thrombi.[13] Initial endothelial injury exposes subendothelial collagen (and other platelet activators) and release of tissue factor. These activities initiate platelet adhesions and aggregation, promoting the individual development of atherosclerotic plaques that progress to further vessel damage and occlusion. Specific causes of vessel endothelial injury are hemodynamic alterations associated with hypertension and turbulent blood flow that occurs in other arterial disorders. Injury may also occur in the presence of radiation injury, exogenous chemical agents (cigarette toxins), endogenous agents (cholesterol), bacterial toxins or endotoxins, or immunologic complex deposits. Whatever the precipitating cause of endothelial injury, it is a potent thrombogenic agent.

Abnormalities of blood flow, specifically turbulence and stasis, contribute to thrombus formation by interfering with laminar flow. Laminar flow is such that the cellular components of blood are located centrally within the vessel, separated from the vascular endothelium by a slower-moving, clear zone of plasma.[13] Interruption of laminar flow by turbulence and stasis promotes thrombus formation by bringing platelets into contact with the endothelium. In addition, clotting factors that may become activated are inhibited from being diluted by fresh-flowing blood, and clotting factor inhibitors are not brought into the area to prevent formation of thrombi. Endothelial cells are also activated by turbulence and stasis, creating an environment for local thrombosis, leukocyte adhesion, and multiple other endothelial cell manifestations.

Clinical conditions in which stasis and turbulence occur include ulcerated atherosclerotic plaques (myocardial infarction), aneurysms, cardiac valve disorders, hyperviscosity conditions (polycythemia vera), and deformed red cells (sickle cell anemia).

Hypercoagulability is the condition in which an individual is at risk for but does not necessarily develop thrombosis.[83] By itself it is a rare cause of thrombosis due to primary or secondary causes. Primary causes include congenital conditions related to protein C, protein S, and AT III deficiencies, abnormal clotting factor V, and fibrinogen variants (see Chapter 27). Secondary causes include a variety of clinical conditions that have been discussed previously. It is not well understood why there is not a greater incidence of thrombosis formation in hypercoagulable states.

Whether episodes of thromboembolism are life threatening depends on the site of vessel occlusion. Therapy consists of removal or breakdown of the clot and supportive measures. Anticoagulant therapy is effective in preventing arterial thrombosis; it is not useful in treating arterial thrombosis. Parenteral heparin is the major anticoagulant used to treat thromboembolism; however, it may contribute to thrombus formation. Oral coumarin drugs also are widely used, particularly for outpatients.

More aggressive therapy may be indicated for such conditions as pulmonary embolism, coronary thrombosis, or deep venous thrombosis. Streptokinase and urokinase activate the fibrinolytic system and are administered to accelerate the lysis of known thrombi. Thrombolytic therapy has limited uses and is prescribed cautiously because it can cause hemorrhagic complications.

It must be pointed out that protein S and C conditions and AT III deficiency also may be acquired and contribute to a hypercoagulable state (see Chapter 27). Conditions associated with an acquired protein deficiency include DIC, liver disease, infection, deep venous thrombosis, adult respiratory distress syndrome, L-asparaginase therapy, hemolytic uremic syndrome, and thrombocytic thrombocytopenic purpura. The postoperative state also predisposes an individual to protein C or S deficiency; however, its role in contributing to deep venous thrombosis remains unclear.[84]

SUMMARY REVIEW

Alterations of Leukocyte Function

1. Quantitative alterations of leukocytes (too many or too few) can be caused by bone marrow dysfunction or premature destruction of cells in the circulation.
2. Leukocytosis (a leukocyte count higher than normal) is usually a response to stress or physiologic response, or both, to invasion of microorganisms.
3. Leukopenia (a leukocyte count lower than normal) is caused by pathologic conditions, such as malignancies and hematologic disorders.
4. Granulocytosis (particularly caused by neutrophilia) occurs in response to infection.
5. When the demand for neutrophils exceeds the supply in the circulation, bone marrow releases immature cells, causing a shift-to-the-left.
6. Eosinophilia results most commonly from parasitic invasion and ingestion or inhalation of toxic foreign particles.
7. Basophilia is seen in hypersensitivity reactions because of the high content of histamine and subsequent release.
8. Monocytosis occurs during the late or recuperative phase of infection when macrophages (mature monocytes) phagocytose surviving microorganisms and debris.
9. Granulocytopenia, a condition resulting in a decrease in neutrophils, can be a life-threatening condition if sepsis occurs; often it is caused by chemotherapeutic agents, severe infection, and radiation.
10. Infectious mononucleosis (IM) is a self-limiting, nonneoplastic, lymphoproliferative syndrome caused by infection of B cells, most commonly the Epstein-Barr virus (EBV), a herpes-type virus.
11. IM most commonly affects young adults between 15 and 35 years of age who have not had previous EBV infection during childhood.
12. Most cases of EBV infectious mononucleosis start with fever and sore throat, a temperature elevation lasting 7 to 10 days, and enlargement and tenderness of the cervical lymph nodes from inflammation at the site of viral entry.
13. The common pathologic feature of all forms of leukemia is an uncontrolled proliferation of leukocytes.
14. All leukemias can be designated as (a) lymphocytic, (b) myelocytic or myelogenous, or (c) monocytic. The acute leukemias are divided into two major types: (a) acute nonlymphoblastic leukemia (ANLL) or acute myelogenous leukemia (AML) and (b) acute lymphoblastic leukemia (ALL).
15. The two principal types of chronic leukemia are (a) chronic granulocytic leukemia (CGL) or chronic myelocytic leukemia (CML) and (b) chronic lymphocytic leukemia (CLL).
16. Although the exact cause of leukemia is unknown, it is considered a clonal disorder. A high incidence of acute leukemias and CLL is reported in certain families, suggesting a genetic predisposition.
17. In leukemia, blasts (precursor cells) "crowd out" the marrow and cause cellular proliferation of the other cell lines to cease.
18. The major clinical manifestations of leukemia include fatigue caused by anemia, bleeding caused by thrombocytopenia, fever secondary to infection, anorexia, and weight loss.
19. Chemotherapy is the treatment of choice for leukemia. Acute leukemias are associated with a 20% to 50% long-term survival rate. Chronic leukemias are associated with a longer life expectancy.
20. Chronic leukemias progress differently from acute leukemias, advancing slowly and without warning.
21. Multiple myeloma is a neoplasm of B cells (immature plasma cells) and mature plasma cells. It is characterized by multiple malignant tumor masses of plasma cells scattered throughout the skeletal system and sometimes in soft tissue.
22. The exact cause of multiple myeloma is unknown, but genetic factors and chronic stimulation of the mononuclear phagocyte system by bacteria, viral agents, and chemicals have been suggested.
23. The major clinical manifestations for multiple myeloma include recurrent infections caused by suppression of the humoral immune response and renal disease as a result of Bence Jones proteinuria.
24. Chemotherapy is the treatment for multiple myeloma. Survival is still only 2 to 3 years with chemotherapy, however.

Alterations of Lymphoid Function

1. The number of lymphocytes is decreased (lymphocytopenia) in most acute infections and in some immune deficiency syndromes.
2. Lymphocytosis occurs in viral infections, infectious mononucleosis, infectious hepatitis, leukemia, lymphomas, and some chronic infections.
3. Lymphomas are tumors of primary lymphoid tissue (thymus and bone marrow) or secondary tissue (lymph nodes, spleen, tonsils, and intestinal lymphoid tissue). The two major types

of malignant lymphomas are Hodgkin disease and non-Hodgkin disease.
4. Distinctive abnormal chromosomes are present in multiple cells of the lymph nodes of an individual with Hodgkin disease. The abnormal cell is called a Reed-Sternberg cell.
5. A virus might be involved in the pathogenesis of Hodgkin disease. Some familial clustering suggests an unknown genetic mechanism.
6. An enlarged, painless mass or swelling, most commonly in the neck, is an initial sign of Hodgkin disease. Local symptoms are produced by lymphadenopathy, usually caused by pressure or obstruction.
7. Treatment of Hodgkin disease includes radiation therapy and chemotherapy. A cure is possible regardless of stage of Hodgkin disease; however, individuals treated with chemotherapy who relapse in less than 2 years have a poor prognosis.
8. The cause of lymph node enlargement and cancerous transformation in non-Hodgkin lymphoma is unknown. Immunosuppressed persons have a greater incidence of non-Hodgkin lymphoma, suggesting an immune mechanism.
9. Generally, with non-Hodgkin lymphoma, the swelling of lymph nodes is painless and the nodes have enlarged and transformed over a period of months or years.
10. Individuals with non-Hodgkin lymphoma can survive for long periods. Treatment is with chemotherapy.
11. Burkitt lymphoma involves the jaw and facial bones and occurs in children from east-central Africa and New Guinea.

Alterations of Splenic Function

1. Splenomegaly (enlargement of the spleen) is not necessarily considered pathologic but may indicate underlying pathology.
2. Splenomegaly results from a wide variety of conditions, most notably those caused by acute inflammatory or infectious processes or those that produce splenic congestion or infiltration.
3. Hypersplenism (overactivity) is associated with splenomegaly and pancytopenia.

Alterations of Platelets and Coagulation

1. Thrombocytopenia is characterized by a platelet count below 100,000 platelets/mm^3 of blood; a count below 50,000/mm^3 increases the potential for hemorrhage associated with minor trauma.
2. Secondary thrombocytopenia commonly is associated with autoimmune diseases and viral infections; bacterial sepsis, which may cause disseminated intravascular coagulation (DIC), also results in thrombocytopenia.
3. Heparin-induced thrombocytopenia develops in approximately 2% to 15% of individuals receiving heparin.
4. Immune thrombocytopenic purpura (ITP) is a major cause of platelet destruction, frequently affecting females, and results in hemorrhaging that ranges from minor development of petechiae to major bleeding from mucosal sites.
5. Thrombotic thrombycytopenic purpura (TTP) causes platelet aggregation leading to microcirculatory occlusion.
6. Thrombocythemia is characterized by a platelet count greater than 600,000/mm^3 of blood and is symptomatic when the count exceeds 1,000,000/mm^3 and when the risk for intravascular clotting (thrombosis) is high.
7. Primary thrombocythemia is caused by accelerated platelet production in the bone marrow characterized by hyperplasia of megakaryocytes.
8. Alterations in normal platelet adherence or aggregation prevent platelet plug formation and may result in prolonged bleeding times.
9. Platelet dysfunction results from changes in the cellular contents (such as proteins and enzymes) and integrity (alterations of platelet membrane).
10. Disorders of coagulation usually are caused by defects or deficiencies of one or more of the clotting factors.
11. Coagulation is impaired when there is a deficiency of vitamin K because of insufficient production of prothrombin and clotting factors II, VII, IX, and X.
12. Liver disease accounts for a pattern of hemostatic derangement caused by a disruption of the synthesis of clotting factors.
13. DIC is a complex syndrome resulting from a variety of clinical conditions that cause release of tissue factor and results in activation and circulation of plasmin and thrombin.
14. DIC is characterized by a cycle of intravascular clotting followed by active bleeding because of accelerated consumption of coagulation factors, platelets, and diffuse fibrinolysis.
15. Thromboembolic disease results from a fixed (thrombus) or moving (embolism) clot that blocks blood flow within a vessel, denying nutrients to tissues distal to the occlusion; death can result when clots are located in the heart, brain, or lungs.
16. Hypercoagulability is the result of deficient anticoagulation proteins. Secondary causes are conditions that promote venous stasis.
17. The term *triad of Virchow* refers to three factors that can cause thrombus formation: (1) loss of integrity of the vessel wall, (2) abnormalities of blood flow, and (3) alterations in the blood constituents.

KEY TERMS

Acute idiopathic TTP, *887*
Acute leukemia, *870*
Agranulocytosis, *867*
Arterial thrombus, *894*
Basopenia, *868*
Basophilia, *868*
Bence Jones protein, *876*
Burkitt lymphoma, *884*
Chronic leukemia, *870*
Chronic relapsing TTP, *887*
Congestive splenomegaly, *885*
Consumptive thrombohemorrhagic disorder, *890*
D-dimer, *893*
Disseminated intravascular coagulation (DIC), *890*
Embolus, *895*
Eosinopenia, *868*
Eosinophilia, *867*
Essential (primary) thrombocythemia (ET), *887*
Granulocytopenia, *867*
Granulocytosis, *867*
Heterophilic antibody, *870*
Hodgkin disease, *879*
Hypercoagulability, *895*
Hypersplenism, *884*
Immune thrombocytopenic purpura (ITP), *886*
Impaired hemostasis, *889*
Infectious mononucleosis (IM), *868*
Infiltrative splenomegaly, *885*
Leukemia, *870*

KEY TERMS—cont'd

REFERENCES

1. Chandrasoma P, Taylor CR: *Concise pathology,* Norwalk, CT, 1995, Lange.
2. Russin SJ, Fillipo BH, Alder AG: Neutropenia in adults: what is its clinical significance? *Postgrad Med* 88:209, 1990.
3. Munshi HG, Montgomery RB: Severe neutropenia: a diagnostic approach, *Western J Med* 172(4):248, 2000.
4. Watts RG: Neutropenia. In Lee GR et al, editors: *Wintrobe's clinical hematology,* Baltimore, 1999, Williams & Wilkins.
5. Bohme A et al: L-tryptophan related eosinophilia-myalgia syndrome possibly associated with a chronic B-lymphocyte leukemia, *Ann Hematol* 77:235, 1998.
6. Barth H et al: Is there any relationship between eosinphilia myalgia syndrome (EMS) and fibromyalgia syndrome (FMS)? An analysis of clinical and immunological data, *Adv Exper Med Biol* 467:487, 1999.
7. Meisel SR et al: Peripheral monocytosis following acute myocardial infarction: incidence and its possible role as a bedside marker of the extent of cardiac injury, *Cardiology* 90:52, 1998.
8. Athens JW: Variations of leukocytes in disease. In Lee GR et al, editors: *Wintrobe's clinical hematology,* ed 9, Philadelphia, 1993, Lea & Febiger.
9. Hickey SM, Strasburger VC: What every pediatrician should know about infectious mononucleosis in adolescents, *Pediatr Clin North Am* 44(6):1541, 1997.
10. Peter J, Ray CG: Infectious mononucleosis, *Pediatr Rev* 19:276, 1998.
11. Willis JL: Mono: tough for teens and twenty-somethings, *FDA Consumer* 32(3):32, 1998.
12. Goodshall SE, Kirchner JT: Infectious mononucleosis: complexities of a common syndrome, *Postgrad Med* 107(7):175, 2000.
13. Cotran RS et al: *Robbins' pathologic basis of disease,* ed 6, Philadelphia, 1999, W.B. Saunders.
14. Omori M: Mononucleosis, 2000. Available at www.emedicine.com.
15. Cozad J: Infectious mononucleosis, *Nurs Pract* 21(3):14, 1996.
16. Auwaerter PG: Infectious mononucleosis in middle age, *JAMA* 281(5):454, 1999.
17. Bailey RE: Diagnosis and treatment of infectious mononucleosis, *Am Fam Physician* 49(4):879, 1994.
18. Haller A et al: Severe respiratory insufficiency complicating Epstein-Barr virus infection: case report and review, *Clin Infect Dis* 21(1):206, 1995.
19. Bates S, Friedman J: Index of suspicion, *Pediatr Rev* 19(4):137, 1998.
20. Gunz FW: The dread leukemias and the lymphomas: their nature and their prospects. In Wintrobe MM, editor: *Blood, pure and eloquent: a story of discovery, of people, and of ideas,* New York, 1980, McGraw-Hill.
21. American Cancer Society: *Cancer facts and figures,* New York, 1999, American Cancer Society.
22. American Cancer Society: Statistics 2000: cancer facts and figures, 2000. Available at www3.cancer.org.
23. Devine SM, Larson RA: Acute leukemia in adults: recent development in diagnosis and treatment, *CA Cancer J Clin* 44:326, 1994.
24. Gorin NC et al: Feasibility and recent improvement of autologous stem cell transplantation for acute myelocytic leukemia in patients over 60 years of age: importance of the source of stem cells, *Br J Haematol* 110(4):887, 2000.
25. Williams M: Gastrointestinal manifestations of graft-versus-host disease: diagnosis and management, *AACN Clin Issues* 10(4):500, 1999.
26. Cancer in focus: the war on cancer: giant leaps at the bench, small steps in the trench, *J NIH Res* 3:41, 1991.
27. Gado K et al: Role of interleukin-6 in the pathogenesis of multiple myeloma, *Cell Biol Int* 24(4):195, 2000.
28. Cotran RS et al: *Robbins' pathologic basis of disease,* ed 4, Philadelphia, 1989, W.B. Saunders.
29. Kelly T et al: Matrix metalloproteinases in multiple myeloma, *Leuk Lymphoma* 37(3-4):273, 2000.
30. Cotran RS et al: *Robbins' pathologic basis of disease,* ed 5, Philadelphia, 1994, W.B. Saunders.
31. Lee GR et al, editors: *Wintrobe's clinical hematology,* ed 9, Philadelphia, 1993, Lea & Febiger.
32. Ullrich S, Zolla-Pazner S: Immunoregulatory circuits in myeloma, *Clin Hematol* 11:87, 1982.
33. Defonzo R et al: Renal function in patients with multiple myeloma, *Medicine (Baltimore)* 57:151, 1978.
34. George ED, Sadovsky R: Multiple myeloma: recognition and management, *Am Fam Physician* 59(7):1885, 1999.
35. Harris NL: A practical approach to the pathology of lymphoid neoplasms: a revised European-American classification from the international Lymphoma Study Group. In Devita VT, Hellman S, Rosenberg SA, editors: *Important advances in oncology 1995,* Philadelphia, 1995, Lippincott.
36. 1993 Revised classification for HIV infections and expanded surveillance case definition for AIDS among adolescents and adults, *MMWR Morb Mortal Wkly Rep* 41:1, 1993.
37. Diehl V et al: The cell origin of Hodgkin disease, *Semin Oncol* 17:660, 1990.
38. Chapman AL, Rickinson AB: Epstein-Barr virus in Hodgkin's disease, *Ann Oncol* 9(suppl 5):S5, 1998.
39. Kadin M et al: Eosinophils are the major source of transforming growth factor beta 1 in nodular sclerosing Hodgkin disease, *Am J Pathol* 142:11, 1993.
40. Wensing B, Farrell PJ: Regulation of cell growth by Epstein-Barr virus, *Microbes Infect* 2(1):77, 2000.
41. Shurin SB: The spleen and its disorders. In Hoffman R et al, editors: *Hematology: basic principles and practice,* New York, 2000, Churchill Livingstone.
42. Chapman WC, Newman M: Disorders of the spleen. In Lee GR et al, editors: *Wintrobe's clinical hematology,* Baltimore, 1999, Williams & Wilkins.
43. Jandl JH: *Blood: textbook of hematology,* ed 2, Boston, 1996, Little, Brown.
44. Rutherford CJ, Frenkel EP: Thrombocytopenia: issues in diagnosis and therapy, *Med Clin North Am* 78(3):555, 1994.

45. Bussel J, Cines D: Immune thrombocytopenia purpura, neonatal alloimmune thrombocytopenia, and post-transfusion purpura. In Hoffman R et al, editors: *Hematology: basic principles and practice,* ed 2, New York, 1995, Churchill Livingstone.
46. Lathan LO, Staggers SL: Ancrod: the use of snake venom in the treatment of patients with heparin-induced thrombocytopenia and thrombosis undergoing coronary artery bypass grafting: nursing management, *Heart Lung* 25(6):451, 1996.
47. Warkentin TE: Heparin-induced thrombocytopenia: a ten-year retrospective, *Annu Rev Med* 50:129, 1999.
48. Karpatkin S: Autoimmune (idiopathic) thrombocytopenic purpura, *Lancet* 349:1531, 1997.
49. McMillan R: The pathogenesis of chronic immune (idiopathic) thrombocytopenic purpura, *Semin Hematol* 37(1 suppl 1):5, 2000.
50. Porcelijn L, von dem Borne AE: Immune-mediated thrombocytopenias: basic and immunological aspects, *Baillieres Clin Haematol* 11(2):331, 1998.
51. George JN, Shatti SJ: Acquired disorders of platelet function. In Hoffman R et al, editors: *Hematology: basic principles and practice,* ed 2, New York, 1995, Churchill Livingstone.
52. George JN et al: Idiopathic thrombocytopenia purpura: a practice guideline developed by explicit methods for the American Society of Hematology, *Blood* 88(1):30, 1996.
53. George JN: Treatment options for chronic idiopathic (immune) thrombocytopenic purpura, *Semin Hematol* 37(1 suppl 1):31, 2000.
54. Rock G et al: Thrombotic thrombocytopenic purpura treatment in the year 2000, *Haematologica* 85(4):410, 2000.
55. Moake JL: Thrombotic thrombocytopenic purpura today, *Hosp Pract* 34(7):53, 1999.
56. Jantumen RE et al: Essential thrombocythemia at diagnosis: causes of diagnostic evaluation and presence of positive diagnostic findings, *Ann Hematol* 77:101, 1998.
57. Jensen MK et al: Incidence, clinical features and outcome of essential thrombocythemia in a well defined geographical area, *Eur J Haematol* 65(2):132, 2000.
58. Levine SP: Thrombocytosis. In Lee GR et al, editors: *Wintrobe's clinical hematology,* Baltimore, 1999, Williams & Wilkins.
59. Jantumen RE: Development of erythrocytosis in the course of essential thrombocythemia, *Ann Hematol* 78:219, 1999.
60. Barbui T, Finazzo G: Clinical parameters for determining when and when not to treat essential thrombocythemia, *Semin Hematol* 36(1 suppl 2):14, 1999.
61. Murphy S: Diagnostic criteria and prognosis in polycythemia vera and essential thrombocythemia, *Semin Hematol* 36(1 suppl 2):9, 1999.
62. Hoffman R, Silverstein MN, Hromas R: Primary thrombocythemia. In Hoffman R et al, editors: *Hematology: basic principles and practice,* ed 2, New York, 1995, Churchill Livingstone.
63. Gilbert HS: Historical perspective on the treatment of essential thrombocythemia and polycythemia vera, *Semin Hematol* 36(1 suppl 2):19, 1999.
64. Silverstein MN, Tefferi A: Treatment of essential thrombocythemia with Anagrelide, *Semin Hematol* 36(1 suppl 2):23, 1999.
65. Bennett JS: Hereditary disorders of platelet function. In Hoffman R et al, editors: *Hematology: basic principles and practice,* ed 2, New York, 1995, Churchill Livingstone.
66. Wyrick-Glatzel J: Quantitative and qualitative vascular and platelet disorders, both congenital and acquired. In Harming DM, editor: *Clinical hematology and fundamentals of hemostasis,* Philadelphia, 1997, Davis.
67. Bick RL: Platelet function defects associated with hemorrhage or thrombosis, *Med Clin North Am* 78(3)577, 1994.
68. Staudinger T et al: Management of acquired coagulation disorders in emergency and intensive care medicine, *Semin Thromb Hemost* 22(1): 93, 1996.
69. Mammen EF: Coagulation defects in liver disease, *Med Clin North Am* 78(3):545, 1994.
70. Marder VJ et al: Consumptive thrombohemorrhagic disorders. In Colman RW et al, editors: *Hemostasis and thrombosis: basic principles and clinical practice,* ed 3, Philadelphia, 1994, Lippincott.
71. Bell TN: Coagulation and disseminated intravascular coagulation. In Secor VH, editor: *Multisystem organ failure: pathophysiology and clinical implications,* ed 2, St Louis, 1996, Mosby.
72. Bick RL et al: Disseminated intravascular coagulation: clinical and pathophysiological mechanisms and manifestations, *Haemostasis* 29:111, 1999.
73. Joist JH: Disseminated intravascular coagulation. In Baue AD, Faist E, Fry DE, editors: *Multiple organ failure,* New York, 2000, Springer.
74. Vervloet MG et al: Derangement of coagulation and fibrinolysis in critically ill patients with sepsis and septic shock, *Semin Thromb Hemost* 24(1):33, 1998.
75. Baglin T: Disseminated intravascular coagulation: diagnosis and treatment, *BMJ* 312:683, 1996.
76. Johnson PC: Disseminated intravascular coagulation. In Fry DE, editor: *Multiple system organ failure,* St Louis, 1996, Mosby.
77. Grosset ABM, Rodgers GM: Acquired coagulation disorders. In Lee GR et al, editors: *Wintrobe's clinical hematology,* Baltimore, 1999, Williams & Wilkins.
78. Bick RL: Dissseminated intravascular coagulation: objective clinical and laboratory diagnosis, treatment and assessment of therapeutic response, *Semin Thromb Hemost* 22(1):69, 1996.
79. Furlong MA, Furlong BR: Disseminated intravascular coagulation, 2000. Available at www.emedicine.com.
80. Riewald M, Reiss H: Treatment options for clinically recognized disseminated intravascular coagulation, *Semin Thromb Hemost* 24(1):53, 1998.
81. Hirsch J et al: Overview of the thrombotic process and its therapy. In Colman RW et al, editors: *Hemostasis and thrombosis: basic principles and clinical practice,* ed 3, Philadelphia, 1994, Lippincott.
82. Toulon P, Perez P: Screening for risk factors for thrombosis using a new generation of assays developed to evaluate the functionality of the protein C anticoagulant pathway, *Hematol Oncol Clin North Am* 14(2): 379, 2000.
83. Whiteman T, Hassouna HI: Hypercoagulable states, *Hematol Oncol Clin North Am* 14(2):355, 2000.
84. Bick RL, Kaplan H: Syndromes of thrombosis and hypercoagulability: congenital and acquired causes of thrombosis, *Med Clin North Am* 82(3):409, 1998.

CHAPTER 27

Alterations of Hematologic Function in Children

NANCY E. KLINE

CHAPTER OUTLINE

This chapter briefly explains fetal and neonatal hematopoiesis and postnatal changes in blood as a foundation for understanding the pathophysiology of specific blood disorders in childhood. Among the diseases that affect erythrocytes are acquired disorders, such as iron deficiency anemia, hemolytic disease of the newborn, and anemia of infectious disease, and inherited disorders, such as glucose-6-phosphate dehydrogenase (G6PD) deficiency, hereditary spherocytosis, sickle cell disease, and the thalassemias. Disorders of coagulation and platelets include inherited hemorrhagic diseases, such as the hemophilias, and antibody-mediated hemorrhagic diseases, which include idiopathic thrombocytopenic purpura, autoimmune neonatal thrombocytopenias, and autoimmune vascular purpuras. Finally, leukocyte disorders, such as leukemia and the lymphomas (both non-Hodgkin lymphoma and Hodgkin disease), are discussed.

FETAL AND NEONATAL HEMATOPOIESIS

As the developing embryo becomes too large for oxygenation of tissues by simple diffusion, the production of erythrocytes begins within the vessels of the yolk sac. Shortly after 2 weeks of gestation, circulating erythrocytes play a major role in delivering oxygen to the tissues. At approximately the eighth week of gestation, the site of erythrocyte production shifts from the vessels to the liver sinusoids and the production of leukocytes and platelets begins in the liver and spleen. Erythropoiesis in the liver and, to a lesser extent, in the spleen and lymph nodes reaches a peak at approximately 4 months. Hepatic blood formation declines steadily thereafter but does not disappear entirely during the remainder of gestation. By the fifth month of gestation, hematopoiesis begins to occur in the bone marrow and increases rapidly until hematopoietic (red) marrow fills the entire bone marrow space. By the time of delivery the marrow is the only significant site of hematopoiesis.

In neonates and young infants, hematopoietic marrow progressively fills the bony cavities of the entire axial skeleton (skull, vertebrae, ribs, sternum), the long bones of the limbs, and many intramembranous bones. (These structures are described in Chapter 42.) Fatty (yellow) marrow gradually replaces hematopoietic marrow in some bones. During childhood, hematopoietic tissue retreats centrally to the vertebrae, ribs, sternum, pelvis, scapulae, skull, and proximal ends of the femur and humerus.

In diseases characterized by hemolysis, erythrocyte production can increase as much as eight times the normal because erythropoietin causes hematopoietic marrow to increase in volume. Initially, hematopoietic marrow expands

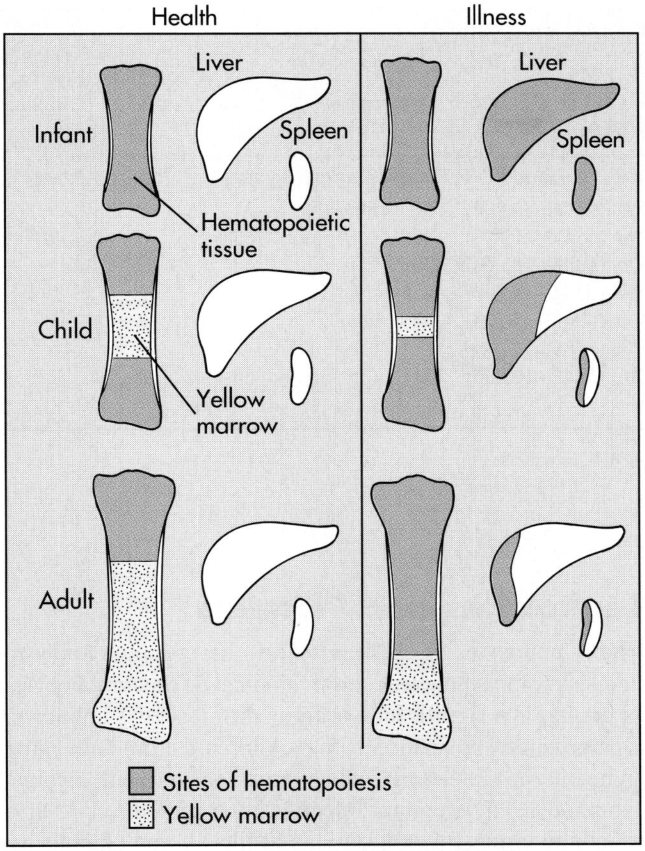

FIG. 27-1 Sites of hematopoiesis in health and illness. With normal maturation, red marrow is partly replaced by yellow marrow in the shafts of the long bones. In adults, red marrow is largely restricted to the proximal ends of the femur and humerus. In response to hemolysis, red marrow replaces yellow marrow in the long bones. In infants, whose long bones already are filled with red marrow, additional hematopoiesis takes place in the liver and spleen. In children and adults, red marrow can replace yellow marrow in response to hemolysis, necessitating less hematopoiesis in the liver and spleen.

from the ends of the long bones toward the middle of the shafts, replacing fatty marrow. Next, blood cell production begins to occur outside the marrow cavities, especially in the liver and spleen. Extramedullary hematopoiesis is more likely to occur in children than in adults because the bony cavities of children already are filled with red marrow (Fig. 27-1). This is why hemolytic disease causes especially pronounced enlargement of the spleen and liver in children.

The erythrocytes undergo striking changes during gestation, particularly during the first two trimesters, during which they nearly double in numbers and in hemoglobin content. A proportionate increase in hematocrit also occurs. By the end of gestation the erythrocyte count has more than tripled but the size of each erythrocyte has decreased.

A biochemically distinct type of hemoglobin is synthesized during fetal life. The three **embryonic hemoglobins (Gower 1, Gower 2, and Portland)** and the **fetal hemoglobin (Hb F)** are composed of two alpha and two gamma chains of polypeptides, whereas the adult hemoglobins (Hb A and Hb A_2) are composed of two alpha and two beta chains. (The structure of an adult hemoglobin molecule is illustrated in Fig. 24-11, and types of hemoglobin are defined in Table 24-5.) Some unknown regulatory mechanism promotes gamma chain synthesis and inhibits beta and delta chain synthesis in utero. This results in production of embryonic or fetal hemoglobin. After birth, gamma chain synthesis is inhibited, whereas beta and delta chain synthesis is facilitated, resulting in production of adult hemoglobins.

Fetal hemoglobin has greater affinity for oxygen than does adult hemoglobin because it interacts less readily with an enzyme (2,3-diphosphoglycerate [2,3-DPG]) that inhibits hemoglobin-oxygen binding. The decreased inhibitory effects of 2,3-DPG enable fetal blood to transport oxygen despite the relative lack of oxygen in the uterine environment. The increased affinity for oxygen enables Hb F to bind with maternal oxygen in the placental circulation.

During the first trimester, nearly all of the hemoglobin in the fetus is embryonic, but some Hb A can be detected. Therefore it is possible to identify as early as 16 to 20 weeks of gestation some disorders of adult hemoglobin, such as sickle cell anemia and thalassemia major. In the 6-month-old fetus, Hb F constitutes 90% of the total. This percentage then begins to decline. At birth, neonatal hemoglobin consists of 70% Hb F, 29% Hb A, and 1% Hb A_2. Between 6 and 12 months of age, normal adult hemoglobin percentages are established (see Chapter 24).

POSTNATAL CHANGES IN THE BLOOD

Blood cell counts tend to rise above adult levels at birth and then decline gradually throughout childhood. Table 27-1 lists normal ranges during infancy and childhood. The immediate rise in values is the result of accelerated hematopoiesis during fetal life, increased numbers of cells that result from the trauma of birth, and cutting of the umbilical cord. These events surrounding the birth also are accompanied by a "shift to the left," that is, the presence of large numbers of immature erythrocytes and leukocytes (particularly granulocytes) in peripheral blood (see Chapter 26). The shift to the left disappears as the infant develops, usually within the first 2 to 3 months of life. Other unique postnatal characteristics, particularly of lymphocytes, may be caused by exogenous factors, such as viral infections.

Average blood volume in the full-term neonate is 85 ml/kg of body weight. The premature infant has a slightly larger blood volume of 90 ml/kg of body weight, with the mean increasing to 150 mg/kg during the first few days after birth. In both full-term and premature infants, blood volume decreases during the first few months. Thereafter the average blood volume is 75 to 77 ml/kg, which is similar to that of older children and adults.

Erythrocytes

The hypoxic intrauterine environment stimulates erythropoietin production in the fetus. This accelerates fetal erythropoiesis, producing polycythemia (excessive proliferation of erythrocyte precursors) of the newborn. After birth the oxy-

Table 27-1 Hematologic Values during Infancy and Childhood

Age	Hemoglobin (g/dl) Mean	Hemoglobin (g/dl) Range	Hematocrit (%) Mean	Hematocrit (%) Range	Reticulocytes (%) Mean	MCV (fl) Lowest	Leukocytes (WBC/mm³) Mean	Leukocytes (WBC/mm³) Range	Neutrophils (%) Mean	Neutrophils (%) Range	Lymphocytes (%) Mean*	Eosinophils (%) Mean	Monocytes (%) Mean
Cord blood	16.8	13.7–20.1	55	45–65	5.0	110	18,000	(9,000–30,000)	61	(40–80)	31	2	6
2 wk	16.5	13.0–20.0	50	42–66	1.0		12,000	(5,000–21,000)	40		63	3	9
3 mo	12.0	9.5–14.5	36	31–41	1.0		12,000	(6,000–18,000)	30		48	2	5
6 mo to 6 yr	12.0	10.5–14.0	37	33–42	1.0	70–74	10,000	(6,000–15,000)	45		48	2	5
7–12 yr	13.0	11.0–16.0	38	34–40	1.0	76–80	8,000	(4,500–13,500)	55		38	2	5
Adult													
Female	14	12.0–16.0	42	37–47	1.6	80	7,500	(5,000–10,000)	55	(35–70)	35	3	7
Male	16	14.0–18.0	47	42–52		80							

From Behrman R et al, editors: *Nelson textbook of pediatrics,* Philadelphia, 1992, W.B. Saunders.
*Relatively wide range.
fl, femtoliters; *MCV,* mean corpuscular volume; *WBC,* white blood cells.

gen from the lungs saturates arterial blood and the amount of oxygen delivered to the tissues increases. In response to the change from a placental to a pulmonary oxygen supply during the first few days of life, levels of erythropoietin and the rate of blood cell formation decrease. The very active rate of fetal erythropoiesis is reflected by the large numbers of immature erythrocytes (reticulocytes) in the peripheral blood of full-term neonates. After birth the number of reticulocytes decreases about 50% every 12 hours so that it is rare to find an elevated reticulocyte count after the first week of life. A decrease in extramedullary hematopoiesis also occurs at this time. In the peripheral blood the erythrocyte count drops for 6 to 8 weeks after birth. During this period of rapid growth the rate of erythrocyte destruction is greater than that in later childhood and adulthood. In full-term infants, normal erythrocyte life span is 60 to 80 days; in premature infants it may be as short as 20 to 30 days; and in children and adolescents it is the same as that in adults—120 days. (Mechanisms of hemolysis are described in Chapter 24.)

In the premature infant the postnatal fall in hemoglobin and hematocrit values is more marked than in the full-term infant. In the preschool and school-age child, there is a gradual rise in hemoglobin, hematocrit, and red blood cell count. Values in males and females first begin to diverge in adolescence. In the female the gradual hemoglobin increase continues into early puberty, at which time it stabilizes. In the male the hemoglobin increase keeps pace with growth and maturation and eventually surpasses that of the female. This higher value in the mature male is related to androgen secretion.

Metabolic processes within the erythrocytes of neonates differ significantly from those of erythrocytes in the normal adult. The relatively young population of erythrocytes in the newborn consumes greater quantities of glucose than do erythrocytes in adults. Several enzymes that regulate glucose consumption are increased in the erythrocytes of neonates, with a subsequent increase in the rate of glycolysis.

Leukocytes and Platelets

The lymphocytes of children tend to have more cytoplasm and less compact nuclear chromatin than do the lymphocytes of adults. The significance of these differences is unknown. One possible explanation is that children tend to have more frequent viral infections, which are associated with atypical lymphocytes. Even minor infections, in which the child fails to exhibit clinical manifestations of illness, and administration of immunizations may result in lymphocyte changes.[1]

The lymphocyte count is high at birth and continues to rise in some healthy infants during the first year of life. Then a steady decline occurs throughout childhood and adolescence until lower adult values are reached. It is unknown whether these developmental variations are physiologic or are a pathologic response to frequent viral infections and immunizations in children.

At birth the neutrophil count is very high and rises during the early days of life.[2] After 2 weeks, neutrophil counts fall to within or below normal adult ranges. By approximately 4 years of age the neutrophil count is the same as that of an adult. White children have slightly higher counts than black children.[3]

Eosinophil count is high in the first year of life and is higher in children than in teenagers or adults.[4] Monocyte counts are high in the first year of life and then decrease to adult levels. No relationship between age and basophil count has been found.

Platelet counts in full-term neonates are comparable to platelet counts in adults and remain so throughout infancy and childhood.[5] Controversy exists as to whether premature infants tend to have thrombocytopenia.

DISORDERS OF ERYTHROCYTES

Anemia is the most common blood disorder in children. Like the anemias of adulthood, the anemias of childhood are caused by ineffective erythropoiesis or premature destruction of erythrocytes. The most common cause of insufficient erythro-

Table 27-2 Anemias of Childhood

Cause	Anemic Condition
DEFICIENT ERYTHROPOIESIS OR HEMOGLOBIN SYNTHESIS	
Decreased stem cell population in marrow (congenital or acquired pure red cell aplasia)	Normocytic-normochromic anemia
Decreased erythropoiesis despite normal stem cell population in marrow (infection, inflammation, cancer, chronic renal disease, congenital dyserythropoiesis)	Normocytic-normochromic anemia
Deficiency of a factor or nutrient needed for erythropoiesis	
Cobalamin (vitamin B_{12}), folate	Megaloblastic anemia
Iron	Microcytic-hypochromic anemia
INCREASED OR PREMATURE HEMOLYSIS	
Alloimmune disease (maternal-fetal Rh, ABO, or minor blood group incompatibility)	Hemolytic disease of the newborn (HDN)
Autoimmune disease (idiopathic autoimmune hemolytic anemia, symptomatic systemic lupus erythematosus, lymphoma, drug-induced autoimmune processes)	Autoimmune hemolytic anemia
Inherited defects of plasma membrane structure (spherocytosis, elliptocytosis, stomatocytosis) or cellular size or both (pyknocytosis)	Hemolytic anemia
Infection (bacterial sepsis, congenital syphilis, malaria, cytomegalovirus infection, rubella, toxoplasmosis, disseminated herpes)	Hemolytic anemia
Intrinsic and inherited enzymatic defects (deficiencies of glucose-6-phosphate dehydrogenase [G6PD], pyruvate kinase, 5′-nucleotidase, glucose phosphate isomerase)	Hemolytic anemia
Inherited defects of hemoglobin synthesis	Sickle cell anemia Thalassemia
Disseminated intravascular coagulation (see Chapter 26)	Hemolytic anemia
Galactosemia	Hemolytic anemia
Prolonged or recurrent respiratory or metabolic acidosis	Hemolytic anemia
Blood vessel disorders (cavernous hemangioma, large vessel thrombus, renal artery stenosis, severe coarctation of the aorta) (see Chapter 30)	Hemolytic anemia

poiesis is iron deficiency, which may result from insufficient dietary intake or chronic loss of iron caused by bleeding. The hemolytic anemias of childhood may be divided into two large categories. The first category consists of disorders that result from premature destruction caused by intrinsic abnormalities of the erythrocytes, and the second category consists of disorders that result from damaging extraerythrocytic factors. The hemolytic anemias are inherited, congenital, or both.

The most dramatic form of acquired congenital hemolytic anemia is **hemolytic disease of the newborn (HDN)**, also termed **erythroblastosis fetalis.** HDN is an alloimmune disease in which maternal blood and fetal blood are antigenically incompatible, causing the mother's immune system to produce antibodies against fetal erythrocytes. Fetal erythrocytes that have been attacked by (i.e., bound to) maternal antibodies are recognized as foreign or defective by the fetal mononuclear phagocyte system and are removed from the circulation by phagocytosis, usually in the fetal spleen. (For a complete discussion of HDN, see p. 904.) Other acquired hemolytic anemias—some of which begin in utero—include those caused by infections or the presence of toxic chemicals.

The inherited forms of hemolytic anemia result from intrinsic defects of the child's erythrocytes, any of which can lead to erythrocyte removal by the mononuclear phagocyte system. Structural defects include abnormal cellular size and abnormalities of plasma membrane structure (spherocytosis). Intracellular defects include enzyme deficiencies, the most common of which is G6PD deficiency, and defects of hemoglobin synthesis, which manifest as sickle cell disease or thalassemia, depending on which component of hemoglobin is defective. These and other causes of childhood anemia, some more common than others, are listed in Table 27-2.

Acquired Disorders

Iron Deficiency Anemia

Iron deficiency anemia is the most frequent blood disorder of infancy and childhood, with the highest incidence occurring between 6 months and 2 years of age. Incidence is not related to gender or race, but socioeconomic factors are important because they affect nutrition. Recent studies document the risk of iron deficiency anemia in children of single, homeless women.[6] Iron deficiency anemia is a common disorder in children because of their extremely high need for iron for normal growth to occur.

Between 4 years of age and the onset of puberty, dietary iron deficiency is uncommon. During adolescence, however, it is relatively common, especially in menstruating females. Rapid growth, together with the average teenager's dietary habits, causes iron depletion. (Mechanisms of iron depletion are described in Chapter 24.)

Pathophysiology

Although inadequate intake of iron is the most common cause of iron deficiency anemia during the first few years of life and during adolescence, blood loss is the most frequent cause in childhood. Chronic iron deficiency anemia from occult (hidden) blood loss may be caused by a gastrointestinal lesion, parasitic infestation, or hemorrhagic disease. As many as one third of infants with severe iron deficiency anemia have chronic intestinal blood loss induced by exposure to a heat-labile protein in cow's milk. Such exposure causes an inflammatory gastrointestinal reaction that damages the mucosa and results in diffuse hemorrhage.

The amount of iron available for hemoglobin synthesis in the infant depends on iron stores present at birth, rate of growth, the amount of dietary iron absorbed, and physiologic or pathologic loss of iron. During the period of inactive erythropoiesis immediately after birth, iron from erythrocytes that die at the end of their normal life span is stored, as hemosiderin, in bone marrow and liver tissue. This creates an iron reserve that can be used in lieu of dietary intake. The greatest stores are present 4 to 8 weeks after birth. Until erythropoiesis resumes, these iron stores are mobilized. In the premature infant, resumption of erythropoiesis depletes iron stores within 6 to 12 weeks; in the full-term infant, depletion takes longer—about 16 to 20 weeks. Once iron stores have been used, the infant depends on dietary iron.

The amount of dietary iron available for erythropoiesis depends on which foods are consumed. Iron-fortified cereals, green and yellow vegetables, fruits, and milk are common in the average 6-month-old infant's diet and provide iron in the amount of 0.9 to 1.5 mg/kg/day, amounts that satisfy the normal average daily requirement. Iron-fortified formulas are available commercially and are being used with increasing frequency.

Clinical Manifestations

The symptoms of mild anemia—lethargy and lassitude—usually are not present or detectable in infants and young children, who are unable to describe these symptoms. Therefore parents usually do not notice any change in the child's behavior or appearance until moderate anemia has developed. General irritability, decreased activity tolerance, weakness, and lack of interest in play are nonspecific indications of anemia. In mild to moderate iron deficiency anemia (hemoglobin of 6 to 10 g/dl), compensatory mechanisms of tissue oxygenation, such as increased amounts of 2,3-DPG within erythrocytes and a shift of the oxyhemoglobin dissociation curve, may be so effective that few clinical manifestations are apparent. When the hemoglobin falls below 5 g/dl, however, pallor, anorexia, tachycardia, and systolic murmurs may occur.

Splenomegaly is evident in 10% to 15% of children with iron deficiency anemia, and, if the condition is long-standing, the sutures of the skull may be widened. Chronic anemia also may result in decreased physical growth and developmental delays. Some children exhibit pica, a behavior in which nonfood substances are eaten. Because children with iron deficiency anemia may be obese, underweight, or of normal weight, other manifestations of undernutrition must be identified.

Iron deficiency anemia may affect neurologic and intellectual function. Some research findings indicate that low iron in the blood affects attention span, alertness, and learning ability, even when anemia is not severe.[7]

Evaluation and Treatment

The most definitive test for differentiating iron deficiency from other microcytic states is the absence of iron stores in the bone marrow. However, measurement of serum ferritin iron concentration, transferrin saturation, iron-binding capacity, and, more recently, serum transferring receptors may prevent proceeding to actual bone marrow evaluation.[8] Evaluation and treatment of iron deficiency anemia in children are similar to evaluation and treatment in adults (see Chapter 25). Oral administration of simple ferrous salts usually is satisfactory, but additional vitamin C may be needed to promote absorption. Administration of supplementary trace metals or other vitamins is not necessary. If malabsorption is the cause of the anemia (or if oral administration has not been successful), iron dextran (Imferon) is given intravenously. Iron therapy is continued for at least 2 months after erythrocyte indexes have returned to normal in order to replenish iron stores.[9,10]

Dietary modification is required to prevent recurrences of iron deficiency anemia, The child's intake of iron-rich foods is increased, and the intake of cow's milk may be restricted, with the exact amount depending on the child's age (from 16 to 32 ounces). Limiting milk intake makes the child hungrier for other iron-rich foods and prevents gastrointestinal blood loss in children whose anemia is aggravated or caused by inflammatory reactions to proteins in cow's milk.

Hemolytic Disease of the Newborn

HDN can occur only if antigens on fetal erythrocytes differ from antigens on maternal erythrocytes. The antigenic properties of erythrocytes are determined genetically: they may be type A, B, or O and may or may not include Rh antigen D. Erythrocytes that express Rh antigen D are Rh positive; those that do not are Rh negative. Maternal-fetal incompatibility exists if mother and fetus differ in ABO blood type or if the fetus is Rh positive and the mother is Rh negative. (The antigenic properties of erythrocytes are described in Chapter 6.)

ABO incompatibility occurs in about 20% to 25% of all pregnancies, but only 1 in 10 cases of ABO incompatibility results in HDN. Rh incompatibility occurs in fewer than 10% of pregnancies and rarely causes HDN in the first incompatible fetus. Even after five or more pregnancies, only 5% of women have babies with hemolytic disease. Usually erythrocytes from the first incompatible fetus cause the mother's immune system to produce antibodies that affect the fetuses of subsequent incompatible pregnancies. Only one in three cases of HDN is caused by Rh incompatibility; most cases are caused by ABO incompatibility.

Pathophysiology

If the mother and fetus have antigenically incompatible erythrocytes, HDN will result (1) if the mother's blood contains preformed antibodies against fetal erythrocytes or produces them on exposure to fetal erythrocytes, (2) if sufficient amounts of antibody (usually immunoglobulin G [IgG]) cross the placenta and enter fetal blood, and (3) if IgG binds with sufficient numbers of fetal erythrocytes to cause widespread antibody-mediated hemolysis or splenic removal. (Antibody-mediated cellular destruction is discussed in Chapter 6.)

Maternal antibodies may be formed against type B erythrocytes if the mother is type A or against type A if the mother is type B. Usually, however, the mother is type O and the fetus is A or B. ABO incompatibility can cause HDN even if fetal erythrocytes do not escape into the maternal circulation during pregnancy. This occurs because the blood of most adults already contains anti-A or anti-B antibodies, which are produced on exposure to certain foods or infection by gram-negative bacteria. (Anti-O antibodies do not exist because type O erythrocytes are not antigenic.) Therefore IgG against type A or B erythrocytes usually is preformed in maternal blood and can enter the fetal circulation throughout the first incompatible pregnancy.

Anti-Rh antibodies, on the other hand, are formed *only* in response to the presence of incompatible (Rh-positive) erythrocytes in the blood of an Rh-negative mother. Sources of exposure include fetal blood that is mixed with the mother's blood at the time of delivery, transfused blood, and, rarely, previous sensitization of the mother by her own mother's incompatible blood.

The first Rh-incompatible pregnancy usually presents no difficulties because very few fetal erythrocytes cross the placental barrier during gestation. When the placenta detaches at birth, however, large numbers of fetal erythrocytes usually enter the mother's bloodstream. If the mother is Rh negative and the fetus is Rh positive, the mother produces anti-Rh antibodies. The capacity of the mother's immune system to produce anti-Rh antibodies depends on many factors, including her genetic capacity to make antibodies against the Rh antigen D, the amount of fetal-to-maternal bleeding, and the occurrence of any bleeding earlier in the pregnancy. Anti-Rh antibodies persist in the bloodstream for a very long time, and if the next offspring is Rh positive, the mother's anti-Rh antibodies can enter the fetus's bloodstream and destroy the erythrocytes. Antibodies against Rh antigen D are of the IgG class and easily cross the placenta.

IgG-coated fetal erythrocytes are destroyed extravascularly, primarily by mononuclear phagocytes in the spleen. As hemolysis proceeds, the fetus becomes anemic. Erythropoiesis accelerates, particularly in the liver and spleen, and immature nucleated cells (erythroblasts) are released into the bloodstream (hence the name *erythroblastosis fetalis*) (Fig. 27-2). The degree of anemia depends on the length of time the antibody has been in the fetal circulation, antibody concentration, and the ability of the fetus to compensate for increased hemolysis. Unconjugated (indirect) bilirubin, which is formed during breakdown of hemoglobin, is transported across the placental barrier into the maternal circulation and is excreted by the mother. **Hyperbilirubinemia** occurs in the neonate after birth because excretion of lipid-soluble unconjugated bilirubin through the placenta no longer is possible.

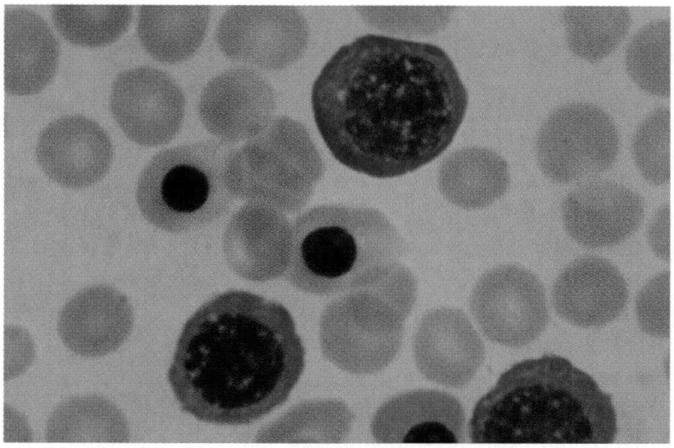

FIG. 27-2 Rh incompatibility in hemolytic disease of the newborn. Shows immature red blood cells not normally found in blood. Large purple cells are erythroblasts; nucleated red blood cells are normoblasts. Normal red blood cells also shown (×500). (Copyright © Ed Reschke.)

The pathophysiologic effects of HDN are more severe in Rh incompatibility than in ABO incompatibility. ABO incompatibility may resolve after birth without life-threatening complications. Maternal-fetal incompatibility in which a mother with type O blood has a child with type A or B blood usually is so mild that it does not require treatment.

Rh incompatibility is more likely than ABO incompatibility to cause severe or even life-threatening anemia, death in utero, or damage to the central nervous system (CNS). Severe anemia alone can cause death as a result of cardiovascular complications (see Chapter 25). Extensive hemolysis also results in increased levels of unconjugated bilirubin in the neonate's circulation. If bilirubin levels exceed the liver's ability to conjugate and excrete bilirubin, some of it is deposited in the brain, causing cellular damage and eventually, if the neonate does not receive exchange transfusions, death.

Fetuses that do not survive anemia in utero usually are stillborn, with gross edema in the entire body, a condition called **hydrops fetalis.** Death can occur as early as 17 weeks of gestation and results in spontaneous abortion.

Clinical Manifestations

Neonates with mild HDN may appear healthy or slightly pale, with slight enlargement of the liver and spleen. Pronounced pallor, splenomegaly, and hepatomegaly indicate severe anemia, which predisposes the neonate to cardiovascular failure and shock. Life-threatening Rh incompatibility is rare today, largely because of the routine use of Rh immune globulin.

Because the maternal antibodies remain in the neonate's circulatory system after birth, erythrocyte destruction can continue. This causes hyperbilirubinemia and **icterus neonatorum (neonatal jaundice)** shortly after birth. Without replacement transfusions, in which the child receives Rh-negative erythrocytes, the bilirubin is deposited in the brain, a condition termed **kernicterus.** Kernicterus produces cerebral damage and usually causes death **(icterus gravis neonatorum).**

Infants who do not die may have mental retardation, cerebral palsy, or high-frequency deafness.

Evaluation and Treatment

Routine evaluation of fetuses at risk for HDN (i.e., fetuses resulting from Rh- or ABO-incompatible matings) include the Coombs test. The indirect Coombs test measures antibody in the mother's circulation and indicates if the fetus is at risk for HDN. The direct Coombs test measures antibody already bound to the surfaces of fetal erythrocytes and is used primarily to confirm the diagnosis of antibody-mediated HDN. Determining prior history of fetal hemolytic disease, as well as diagnostic tests, may help predict the severity of the disorder. Diagnostic measures include maternal antibody titers, fetal blood sampling, amniotic fluid spectrophotometry, and ultrasound fetal assessment.[11]

The key to treatment of HDN resulting from Rh incompatibility lies in prevention (immunoprophylaxis). One of the success stories of immunology has been the spectacular results obtained through the use of Rh immune globulin (RhoGAM), a preparation of antibody against Rh antigen D. If an Rh-negative woman is given Rh immune globulin within 72 hours of exposure to Rh-positive erythrocytes, she will not produce antibody against the D antigen and the next Rh-positive baby will be protected (Fig. 27-3). The injected antibodies remain in the mother's bloodstream long enough to prevent her immune system from producing its own anti-Rh antibodies but not long enough to affect subsequent off-

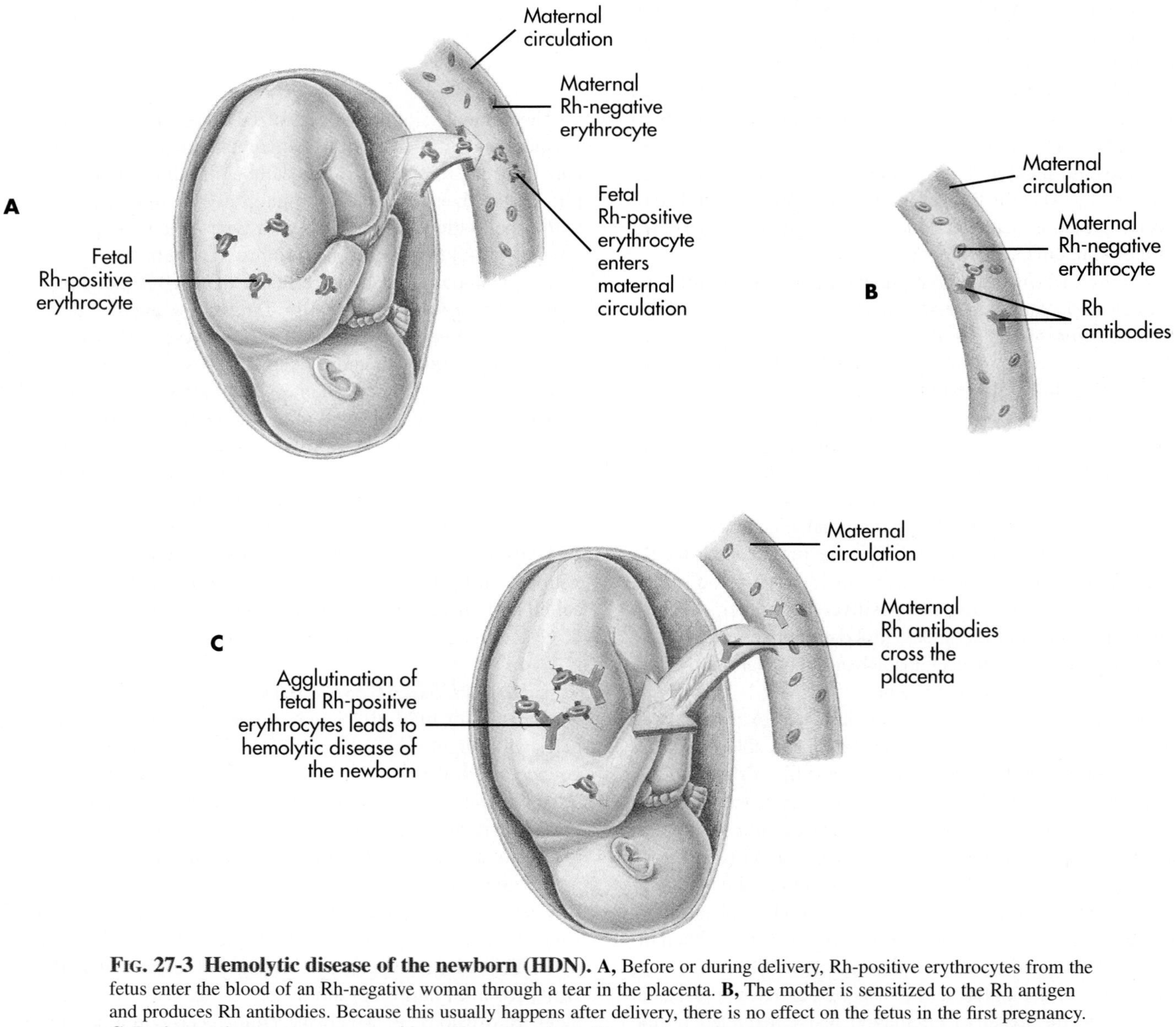

FIG. 27-3 Hemolytic disease of the newborn (HDN). A, Before or during delivery, Rh-positive erythrocytes from the fetus enter the blood of an Rh-negative woman through a tear in the placenta. **B,** The mother is sensitized to the Rh antigen and produces Rh antibodies. Because this usually happens after delivery, there is no effect on the fetus in the first pregnancy. **C,** During a subsequent pregnancy with an Rh-positive fetus, Rh-positive erythrocytes cross the placenta, enter the maternal circulation, and stimulate the mother to produce antibodies against the Rh antigen. The Rh antibodies from the mother cross the placenta, using agglutination and hemolysis of fetal erythrocytes, and HDN develops. (Modified from Seeley RR, Stephens TD, Tate P: *Anatomy and physiology,* ed 3, St Louis, 1995, Mosby.)

spring. The mother must be given Rh immune globulin injections after the birth of each Rh-positive baby and after an abortion. Also, the mother must be especially careful not to receive a transfusion containing Rh-positive blood, because this also would stimulate production of anti-Rh antibodies. In many hospitals, Rh immune globulin is given prophylactically at 28 weeks to all pregnant Rh-negative women with Rh-positive partners. Immunoprophylaxis with Rh immune globulin, unfortunately, appears to be underutilized in the United States. Failure to use immunoprophylaxis, such as in cases of unrecognized abortion, has led to a small increase in mothers who will require comprehensive treatment during subsequent pregnancies.[11,12]

If antigenic incompatibility of the mother's erythrocytes is not discovered in time to administer prophylactic immune globulin (RhoGAM) and a child is born with HDN, treatment consists of exchange transfusions in which the neonate's blood is replaced with new Rh-positive blood that is not contaminated with anti-Rh antibodies. This treatment is instituted during the first 24 hours of extrauterine life to prevent kernicterus. Phototherapy also is used to reduce the toxic effects of unconjugated bilirubin.

Jaundice and indirect hyperbilirubinemia are reduced when the infant is exposed to a high intensity of light in the visible spectrum, the most effective being the blue range (from 420 to 470 nm). Bilirubin in the skin absorbs light energy, which, by photoisomerization, converts the toxic unconjugated bilirubin into conjugated isomers that are excreted in the bile. Phototherapy also causes autosensitization that results in oxidation reactions. Breakdown products from the oxidation reactions are excreted by the liver and kidney without need for conjugation. The therapeutic effect of phototherapy depends on the light energy emitted in the effective wavelengths, the distance between the infant and the light source, and the amount of skin exposed; the rate of hemolysis and the infant's ability to excrete bilirubin also are factors in determining the effectiveness of phototherapy in lowering serum bilirubin levels.

Anemia of Infectious Disease

Infections of the newborn, often initially acquired by the mother and transmitted to the fetus, may result in a hemolytic anemia with clinical manifestations similar to those of HDN. Congenital syphilis, toxoplasmosis, cytomegalic inclusion disease, rubella, coxsackievirus B infection, herpesvirus infection, and bacterial sepsis can all cause hemolytic anemia in the neonate.

The exact mechanism of anemia caused by congenital infections is unclear. In some instances it is related to direct injury of erythrocyte membranes or erythrocyte precursors by the infectious organism. In other instances it results from traumatic destruction of erythrocytes during their passage through inflamed capillaries.

Inherited Disorders

A number of inherited and intrinsic erythrocyte defects are known to cause increased hemolysis (see Table 27-2). These defects may be associated with enzymatic abnormalities that disrupt metabolic processes and prevent normal biochemical balance within the cell, with alterations of hemoglobin structure or synthesis, or with plasma membrane defects accompanied by changes in erythrocyte size or shape.

Glucose-6-Phosphate Dehydrogenase Deficiency

Glucose-6-phosphate dehydrogenase (G6PD) deficiency is an inherited, X-linked, recessive disorder, most fully expressed in homozygous males, although partial expression and a carrier state are possible in heterozygous females. (X-linked inheritance is discussed in Chapter 4.) The deficiency is present in 10% of black Americans and also tends to occur in Sephardic Jews, Greeks, Iranians, Chinese, Filipinos, and Indonesians, with a frequency ranging from 5% to 40%.

Pathophysiology

G6PD is an enzyme that normally enables erythrocytes to maintain metabolic processes despite injurious conditions, such as the presence of certain drugs (sulfonamides, antimalarial agents, salicylates, or naphthaquinolones); ingestion of fava beans (a dietary staple in some Mediterranean areas); hypoxemia; infection; fever; or acidosis. Therefore G6PD deficiency is usually asymptomatic unless one of these stressors is present. Erythrocyte damage in affected children begins after intense or prolonged exposure to one of these substances or conditions, and it ceases when they are removed. In black American males the G6PD defect becomes more pronounced as the erythrocyte ages; in other populations the defect is profound even in young erythrocytes. By ingesting a substance with oxidant properties, such as a salicylate (aspirin), a pregnant woman may precipitate an episode of hemolysis in a fetus with G6PD deficiency.

In the absence of G6PD, oxidative stressors damage hemoglobin and the plasma membranes of erythrocytes and they possibly interfere with the activities of other enzymes within the cell. Hemoglobin is oxidized progressively to methemoglobin, sulfmethemoglobin, and denatured globin-glutathione complexes. Eventually, exposure to oxidating substances results in the precipitation of insoluble hemoglobin inclusions, called *Heinz bodies,* within the cell. Plasma damage and the presence of Heinz bodies cause hemolysis, chiefly in the spleen.

Clinical Manifestations

In Asian and Mediterranean infants, G6PD deficiency is likely to be associated with icterus neonatorum. The most common clinical manifestation of G6PD deficiency is acute hemolytic anemia, usually after infections or the ingestion of certain oxidative drugs. The fava bean produces a severe hemolytic reaction called *favism* in infants with G6PD deficiency.[13]

Hemolytic episodes are characterized by pallor, icterus, dark urine, back pain, and, in severe cases, shock, cardiovascular collapse, and death. Between hemolytic episodes, anemia is absent and erythrocyte survival is normal.

Evaluation and Treatment

Direct or indirect demonstration of reduced G6PD activity in erythrocytes is required for evaluation. Satisfactory screening test results are based on discoloration of methylene blue and reduction of methemoglobin. Immediately after a hemolytic episode, reticulocytes and young erythrocytes predominate. Because young erythrocytes have significantly higher enzyme activity than do older cells, testing should be performed a few weeks after a crisis so that a low level of enzyme activity can be demonstrated. G6PD activity that is within the low normal range in the presence of a high reticulocyte count suggests G6PD deficiency. G6PD deficiency also can be detected by electrophoretic analysis.

Prevention of hemolysis is the most important therapeutic measure. Males belonging to high-risk groups (Greeks, Southern Italians, Sephardic Jews, Filipinos, Chinese, Africans, Thais) should be tested for the defect before being given drugs known to be oxidant. When hemolysis has occurred, supportive treatment may include blood transfusions and oral iron therapy. Spontaneous recovery generally follows treatment.

Hereditary Spherocytosis

Hereditary spherocytosis, also known as *congenital hemolytic anemia* or *congenital acholuric jaundice,* is the most common of the hemolytic disorders in which there is no abnormality of hemoglobin.

Pathophysiology

Transmitted as an autosomal dominant trait, hereditary spherocytosis is presumed to represent new mutations in about 25% of cases. The defect is believed to be caused by an undefined abnormality of proteins or spectrins of the erythrocyte membrane. Affected cells are unduly permeable to sodium and acquire a particular characteristic structure (Fig. 27-4). An increased concentration of intracellular sodium is believed to lead to increased use of adenosine triphosphate (ATP) to drive the so-called cation pump. Early aging and destruction of erythrocytes are believed to result from metabolic overwork and loss of erythrocyte membrane.[14]

Circulation of blood to the spleen creates a metabolic environment that is stressful to spherocyte cells, and repeated passages through this stressful environment result in their sequestration and destruction. The spherocyte is relatively rigid and passes with difficulty through the small openings between the splenic cords and sinuses. Thus the spleen is intimately involved in the hemolytic process.

Clinical Manifestations

With onset in the neonatal period or in early infancy, anemia and hyperbilirubinemia are severe enough to require phototherapy or exchange transfusions. During infancy and childhood, severity of the anemia varies widely but tends to be similar within families. Slight jaundice usually is present. Moderate expansion of the marrow cavity of the skull may occur because of compensatory mechanisms to overproduce cells. After infancy the spleen almost always is enlarged. Although gallstones have been reported to occur as early as 4 to 5 years of age, they usually do not develop until late childhood or early adolescence. If the spleen is not surgically removed, gallstones will form in approximately one half of cases. Aplastic crises are the most serious complications during childhood.[15]

Evaluation and Treatment

It is important to evaluate the family history, blood smear, and studies of osmotic fragility and autohemolysis. As yet, however, no single test is specific for the diagnosis of hereditary spherocytosis.[14] Surgical removal of the spleen invariably produces a clinical cure and should be performed when the child is 5 years of age or older.

Sickle Cell Disease

Sickle cell disease is a group of disorders characterized by the presence of an abnormal form of hemoglobin—**hemoglobin S (Hb S)**—within the erythrocytes. Hb S is formed by a genetic mutation in which one amino acid (valine) replaces another (glutamic acid) (Fig. 27-5, *A*). Hb S, the so-called sickle hemoglobin, reacts to deoxygenation and dehydration by solidifying and stretching the erythrocyte into an elongated

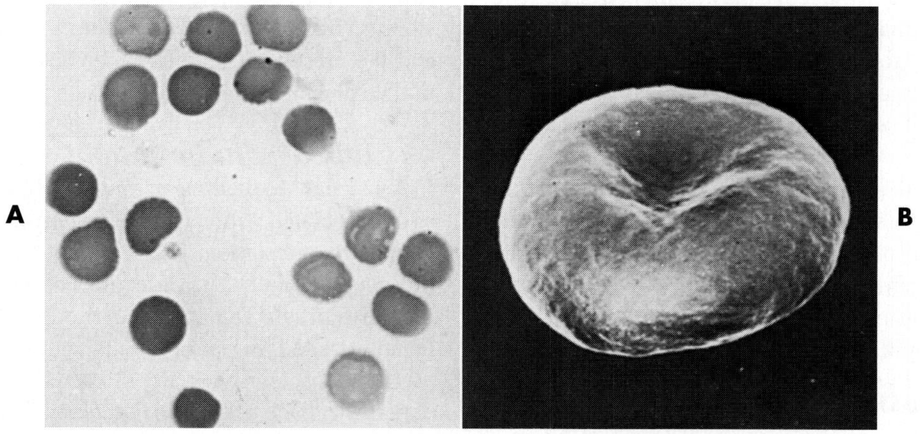

FIG. 27-4 The microspherocyte. A, Blood smear from patient with hereditary spherocytosis (Wright stain). **B,** Scanning electron micrograph. (Courtesy Dr. M Bessis. From Miale JB: *Laboratory medicine: hematology,* ed 6, St Louis, 1982, Mosby.)

sickle shape. This change has a variety of pathologic consequences, including hemolytic anemia.

Sickle cell disease is an inherited, autosomal recessive disorder that is expressed as sickle cell anemia, sickle cell–thalassemia disease, or sickle cell–hemoglobin C disease, depending on mode of inheritance (Table 27-3). (See Chapter 4 for a discussion of genetic inheritance of disease.) **Sickle-cell anemia,** a homozygous form, is the most severe. **Sickle cell–thalassemia** and **sickle cell–Hb C disease** are heterozygous forms in which the child simultaneously inherits another type of abnormal hemoglobin from one parent. **Sickle cell trait,** in which the child inherits Hb S from one parent and normal hemoglobin (Hb A) from the other, is a heterozygous carrier state that rarely has clinical manifestations. All forms of sickle cell disease are lifelong conditions and have no known cure.

Sickle cell disease tends to occur in persons with origins in equatorial countries, particularly central Africa, the Near East, the Mediterranean area, and parts of India. In the United States, sickle cell disease is most common in blacks, with a reported incidence ranging from 1 in 400 to 1 in 500 live births. In the general population the risk of two black American parents having a child with sickle cell anemia is 0.7%. Sickle cell hemoglobin C disease is less common (1 in 800 births), and sickle cell–thalassemia occurs in 1 in 1700 births.

Sickle cell trait occurs in 7% to 13% of black Americans, whereas its incidence among East Africans may be as high as 45%. The sickle cell trait may provide protection against lethal forms of malaria, a genetic advantage to carriers who reside in endemic regions for malaria (Mediterranean and African zones) but no advantage to carriers living in the United States.

Pathophysiology

Deoxygenation is probably the most important variable in determining the occurrence of sickling.[16] The degree of deoxygenation required to produce sickling varies with the percentage of Hb S in the cells. Sickle trait cells will sickle at oxygen tensions of about 15 mm Hg, whereas those from an individual with sickle cell disease will begin to sickle at about 40 mm Hg. Hb S that is not bound with oxygen forms aggregates of semisolid gel that become stacked within the erythrocyte, stretching it into an elongated crescent (Figs. 27-5, *C,* and 27-6). Sickled erythrocytes are stiff and cannot change shape as easily as normal cells when they pass through the microcirculation. (The reversible deformability of erythrocytes is described in Chapter 24.) As a result, sickled erythrocytes tend to plug the blood vessels, causing vascular occlusion, pain, and organ infarction. Sickled cells undergo hemolysis in the spleen or become sequestered there, causing blood pooling and infarction of splenic vessels. The anemia that follows triggers erythropoiesis in the marrow and, in extreme cases, in the liver.

Sickling usually is not permanent; most sickled erythrocytes regain a normal shape after reoxygenation and

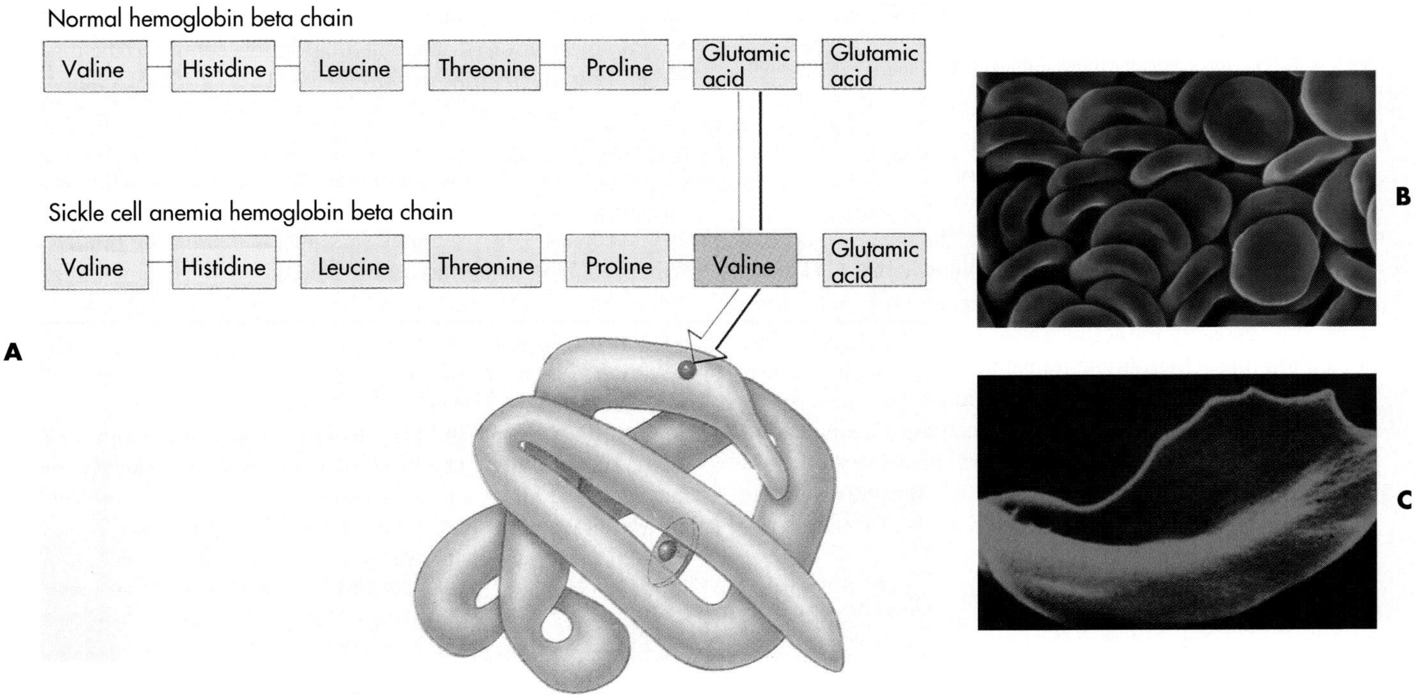

FIG. 27-5 Sickle cell hemoglobin. A, Sickle cell hemoglobin is produced by a recessive allele of the gene encoding the beta chain of the protein hemoglobin. It represents a single amino acid change—from glutamic acid to valine at the sixth position on the chain. In this model of a hemoglobin molecule, the position of the mutation can be seen near the end of the upper arm. **B,** Color-enhanced electron micrograph shows normal erythrocytes. **C,** Illustration of the characteristic shape of a red cell containing the abnormal hemoglobin. (**A,** From Raven PH, Johnson GB: *Biology,* ed 3, Boston, 1993, Times Mirror Higher Education Group. By permission of McGraw-Hill Companies. **B,** Copyright © 1995 Dennis Kunkel Microscopy, Inc. **C,** Courtesy Miale JB: *Laboratory medicine: hematology,* ed 6, St Louis, 1982, Mosby.)

Table 27-3 Inheritance of Sickle Cell Disease

Hemoglobin Inherited From First Parent	Hemoglobin Inherited From Second Parent	Form of Sickle Cell Disease in Child
Hb S (an abnormal hemoglobin)	Hb S	Sickle cell anemia: homozygous inheritance in which the child's hemoglobin is mostly Hb S, with the remainder Hb F (fetal hemoglobin)
Hb S	Defective or insufficient alpha or beta chains of Hb A (alpha- or beta-thalassemia)	Sickle cell: thalassemia disease (heterozygous inheritance of Hb S and alpha- or beta-thalassemia)
Hb S	Hb C or D (both abnormal hemoglobins)	Sickle cell: hemoglobin C (or D) disease (heterozygous inheritance of hemoglobin S and either C or D)
Hb S	Normal hemoglobins (mostly Hb A)	Sickle cell trait, the carrier state (heterozygous inheritance of Hb S and normal hemoglobin)

NOTE: See Chapter 24 for a description of normal fetal and adult hemoglobins.

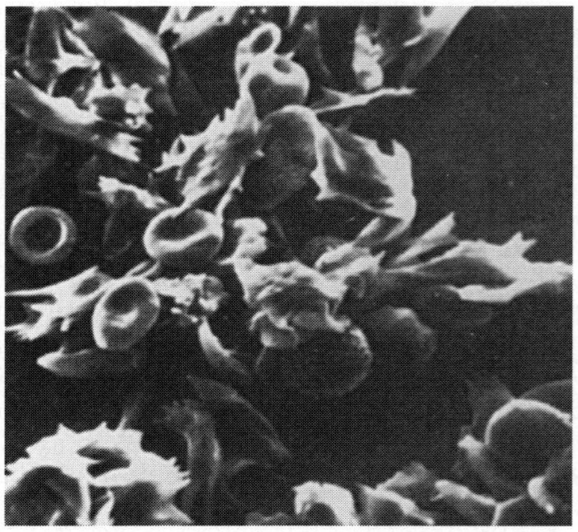

FIG. 27-6 Normal and sickle-shaped blood cells. Scanning electron micrograph of normal and sickle-shaped red blood cells. The irregularly shaped cells are the sickle cells; the circular cells are the normal blood cells. (From Raven PH, Johnson GB: *Biology,* ed 3, Boston, 1993, Times Mirror Higher Education Group. By permission of McGraw-Hill Companies.)

rehydration. Irreversible sickling is not caused by irreversible hemoglobin changes but rather by irreversible plasma membrane damage caused by sickling. The precise nature of the permanent membrane injury is not known, but it is known that, while in the sickled state, the plasma membrane loses some of its capacity for active transport, permitting an influx of calcium ions. (Membrane transport and the effects of calcium influx are described in Unit I.) In persons with sickle cell anemia, in which the erythrocytes contain a high percentage of Hb S (75% to 95%), up to 30% of the erythrocytes can become irreversibly sickled. Occasionally, irreversible sickling occurs in sickle cell disease but never in the carrier state (sickle cell trait).

Sickling is an occasional, intermittent phenomenon that can be triggered or sustained by one or more of the following stressors: decreased oxygen tension (Po_2) of the blood (i.e., hypoxemia), increased hydrogen ion concentration in the blood (decreased pH), increased plasma osmolality, decreased plasma volume, and low temperature (Fig. 27-7). The same decrease in Po_2 will cause the most sickling in persons with sickle cell anemia (high concentrations of Hb S), the second most in children with sickle cell–thalassemia, the third most in those with sickle cell–hemoglobin C disease, and the least or none in those with sickle cell trait. The duration of the Po_2 decrease also is important, because sickling tends to occur only after the inciting stimulus has been present for some time.

The level of Po_2 in the microcirculation also affects sickling because hemoglobin releases whatever oxygen it is carrying to tissues. The Po_2 normally is lower in the microcirculation. The added reduction in Po_2 caused by persistent hypoxemia—induced by stressors—eventually results in sickling in the microcirculation of all cells that contain Hb S in that site (not throughout the body). Sickling within the microcirculation decreases blood flow as sickled cells clog the vessels. Slow blood flow promotes hypoxemia and perpetuates sickling. Finally, decreased blood pH decreases hemoglobin's affinity for oxygen. As less oxygen is taken up by hemoglobin in the lungs, Po_2 drops, promoting sickling further.

Polymerization of sickle hemoglobin is central to the disorder. **Polymerization** stiffens the sickle erythrocyte, changing it from a flexible, nourishing cell to an inflexible obstacle that starves and damages tissues.

Increased osmolality of the plasma (increased concentration of solutes; see Chapters 1 and 3) draws water out of the erythrocytes. This promotes sickling by raising the relative Hb S content in erythrocytes. Decreased plasma volume, which occurs in states of dehydration, causes the blood to become viscous (thick and sticky). Increased viscosity of the blood is the final common pathway leading to many pathologic effects of sickle cell disease. Viscous blood flows slowly and promotes vascular obstruction by increasing opportunities for sickling while decreasing opportunities for reoxygenation in the lungs. This is an example of positive feedback in a vicious cycle of events. Low temperatures precipitate sickle crisis, presumably because of vasoconstriction.[16]

Once sickling begins, it tends to perpetuate itself until Po_2 returns to normal; then it ceases spontaneously. The extent, severity, and clinical manifestations of sickling depend to a great extent on the percentage of hemoglobin that is Hb S. That is why homozygous inheritance of Hb S produces the severest form of sickle cell disease—sickle cell anemia. Heterozygous inheritance of sickle cell disease results in less sickling because the individual's erythrocytes contain other forms of abnormal hemoglobin that, although

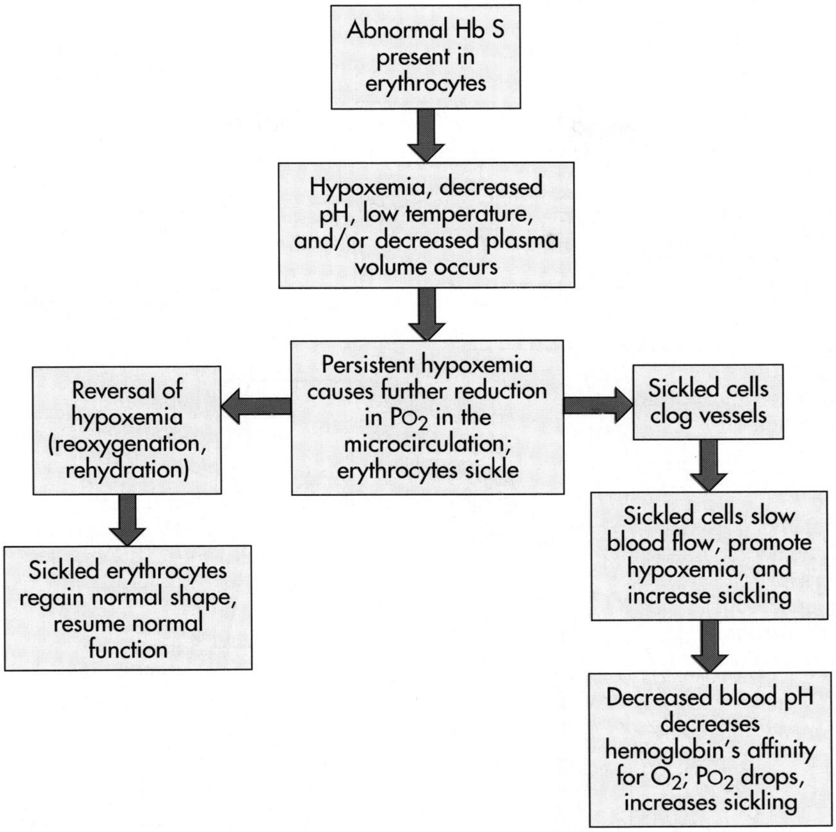

FIG. 27-7 Sickling of erythrocytes.

defective, do not participate in sickling to any great degree. Heterozygous inheritance (sickle cell trait), in which abnormal hemoglobin is inherited from one parent and normal hemoglobin from the other, rarely results in sickling because normal fetal hemoglobin (Hb F) and adult hemoglobin (Hb A) do not participate in sickling at all. Anemia persists because Hb F does not live 120 days.

Clinical Manifestations

When sickling occurs, the general manifestations of hemolytic anemia—pallor, fatigue, jaundice, and irritability—sometimes are accompanied by acute manifestations called *crises.* Extensive sickling can precipitate four types of crises: (1) vasoocclusive (or thrombotic) crisis, (2) aplastic crisis, (3) sequestration crisis, or rarely (4) hyperhemolytic crisis. Sites of specific dysfunction are shown in Fig. 27-8.

Vasoocclusive crisis (thrombotic crisis) begins with sickling in the microcirculation. As blood flow is obstructed by tangled masses of rigid, sickled cells, vasospasm occurs and a "logjam" effect brings all blood flow through the vessel to a halt. Unless the process is reversed, thrombosis and infarction (death caused by lack of oxygen) of local tissue follow. Vasoocclusive crisis is extremely painful and may last for days or even weeks, with an average duration of 4 to 6 days. The frequency of this type of crisis is variable and unpredictable.

Vasoocclusive crises may develop spontaneously or be precipitated by infection, exposure to cold, dehydration, low Po_2, acidosis (low pH), or localized hypoxemia. Symmetric, painful swelling of the hands and feet (hand-foot syndrome) caused by infarction in the small vessels of the extremities often is the initial manifestation of sickle cell disease in infancy. In older children and adults the large joints and surrounding tissue become painful and swollen. Priapism (persistent erection of the penis) may occur if penile veins become obstructed. Severe abdominal pains often are caused by infarction in abdominal structures. Strokes resulting from cerebral occlusion may leave the child with paralysis (usually hemiplegia) or other CNS deficits.

WHAT'S NEW? New Understandings of Acute Chest Syndrome

Acute chest syndrome is the presence of a new pulmonary infiltrate (involving at least one complete lung segment—not atelectasis) with chest pain, a temperature of more than 38.5° C, increased respiratory rate (tachypnea), wheezing, or cough in an individual with sickle cell disease. An injured, underventilated, and inflamed lung becomes "spleenlike" as sickle red cells attach to its endothelium, fails to be reoxygenated, and eventually undergoes more inflammation and lung infarction. The prognosis is poor, and infarction is a leading cause of morbidity. The incidence is about 12.8 cases per 1000 patient-years and is the most common condition at the time of death.

Data from Platt OS: The acute chest syndrome of sickle cell disease, *N Engl J Med* 342(25):1904, 2000 (editorial).

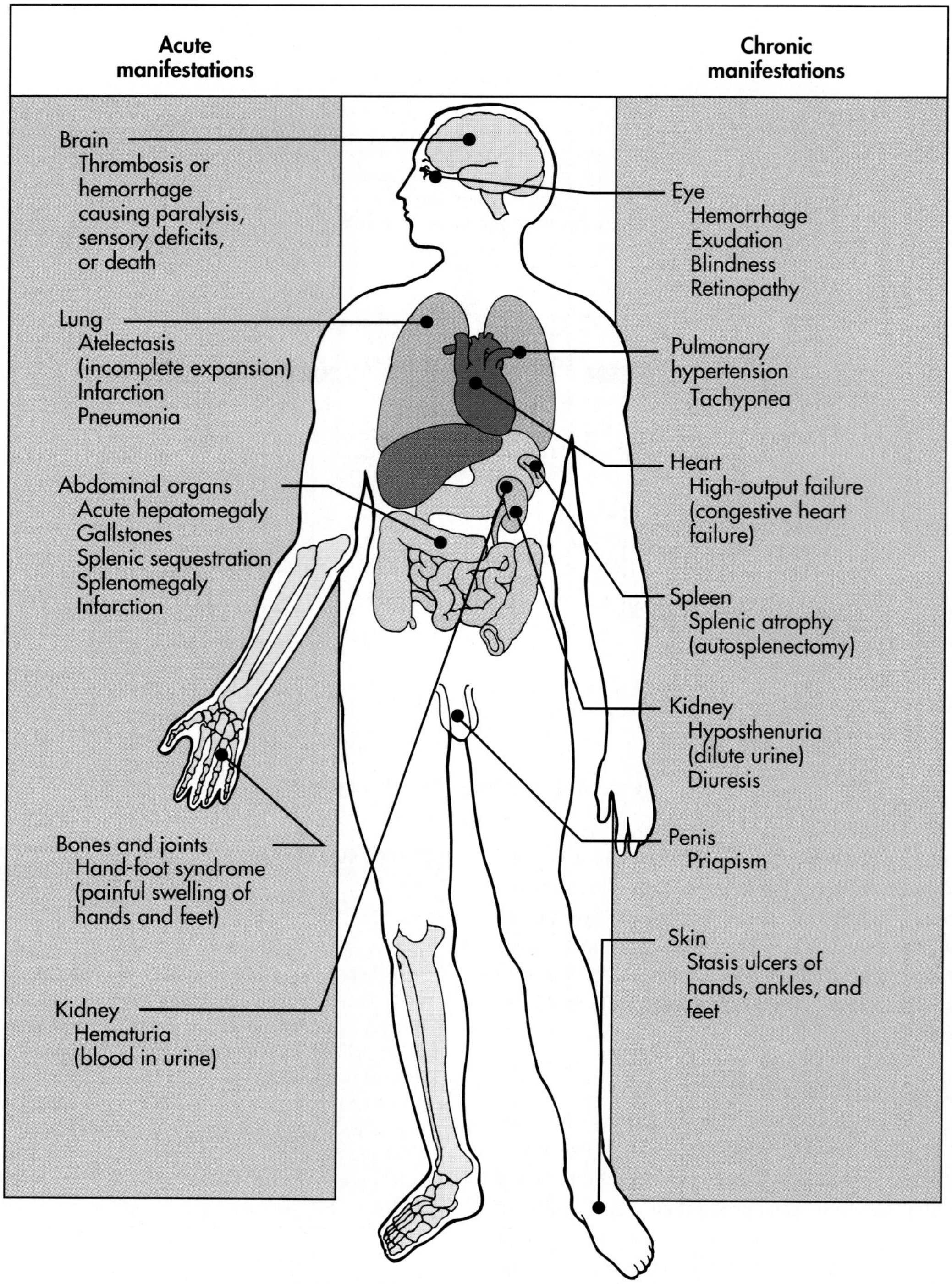

FIG. 27-8 Clinical manifestations of sickle cell disease.

Aplastic crisis consists of profound anemia caused by diminished erythropoiesis despite increased need for new erythrocytes. In sickle cell anemia, erythrocyte survival is only 10 to 20 days. Normally a compensatory increase in erythropoiesis (five to eight times normal) replaces the cells lost through premature hemolysis. If this compensatory response is compromised, aplastic crisis develops in a very short time.

In **sequestration crisis,** large amounts of blood become acutely pooled in the liver and spleen. This type of crisis is seen only in the young child. Because the spleen can hold as much as one fifth of the body's blood supply at one time, mortality rates up to 50% have been reported, with death caused by cardiovascular collapse. If blood volume and pressure are maintained by hydration and blood transfusion, much of the sequestered blood eventually is remobilized. Removal of the spleen is the treatment for recurrent sequestration crises and may be performed after the child reaches 5 years of age.[17]

Hyperhemolytic crisis is unusual but may occur in association with certain drugs or infections. The concomitant presence of G6PD deficiency (see p. 907) contributes to hyperhemolytic episodes, especially when combined with infections.

Although intravascular sickling and hemolysis can begin by 6 to 8 weeks of age, clinical manifestations are not yet present. Clinical manifestations of sickle cell disease usually do not appear until the infant is at least 6 months old, at which time the postnatal decrease in Hb F causes concentrations of Hb S to rise.

Infection is the most frequent cause of death because of sickle cell disease. Sepsis and meningitis develop in as many as 10% of children with sickle cell anemia during the first 5 years of life, with a mortality rate of 25%. Survival time is unpredictable, and many young adults die in their twenties.

Glomerular disease and renal failure cause substantial morbidity.[18] Proteinuria is an early manifestations of sickle nephrology.

Sickle cell–Hb C disease is usually milder than sickle cell anemia. The peripheral blood smear reveals many target cells resulting from the presence of Hb C. The main clinical problems are related to vasoocclusive crises and are believed to result from higher hematocrit values and viscosity. In older children, sickle cell retinopathy, renal necrosis, and aseptic necrosis of the femoral heads occur along with obstructive crises.

Sickle cell–thalassemia has the mildest clinical manifestations of all the sickle cell diseases. Even though most of the child's hemoglobin is Hb S (60% to 90%), normal hemoglobins (Hb A and Hb F) also are present. The normal hemoglobins, particularly Hb F, inhibit sickling. In addition, the erythrocytes tend to be small (microcytic) and to contain relatively little hemoglobin (hypochromic). Their small size makes them less likely than normal-size cells to clog the microcirculation, even when in a sickled state.

The sickle cell trait does not affect life expectancy or interfere with daily activities. However, on rare occasions, severe hypoxia caused by shock, vigorous exercising at high altitudes, flying at high altitudes in unpressurized aircraft, or undergoing anesthesia is associated with vasoocclusive episodes in persons with sickle cell trait. These cells form an ivy shape instead of a sickle shape.

Evaluation and Treatment

The parents' hematologic history and clinical manifestations may suggest that a child has sickle cell disease, but hematologic tests are necessary for diagnosis. If the sickle solubility test confirms the presence of Hb S in peripheral blood, hemoglobin electrophoresis provides information about the amount of Hb S in erythrocytes. Prenatal diagnosis can be made after chorionic villus sampling as early as 8 to 10 weeks of gestation or amniotic fluid analysis at 15 weeks of gestation. Newborn screening for sickle cell disease should be performed according to state law.

Treatment advances over the past 25 years have significantly decreased morbidity and mortality in children with sickle cell disease.[19] Aggressive management of fever, early diagnosis of *acute chest syndrome* (hypoxia, decreased hemoglobin, progressive multilobar pneumonia, fat emboli), judicious use of transfusions, and proper treatment of pain can improve quality of life and prognosis for these children.[20,21] Treatment of sickle cell disease consists of supportive care aimed at preventing consequences of anemia and avoiding crises. Crises can be prevented by avoiding fever, infection, acidosis, dehydration, constricting clothes, and exposure to cold. Immediate correction of acidosis and dehydration with appropriate intravenous fluids is imperative. Infections require aggressive antibiotic therapy. Oxygen is not needed unless the child becomes hypoxic.[22] Pain associated with sickle cell disease is very complex, requiring continuous adjustment of analgesics.[23] Therapeutic use of antisickling agents (urea, cyanate, carbamoyl phosphate) currently is regarded as unsafe and ineffective. The most definitive approach to the treatment of sickle cell disease involves a permanent alteration in the hemoglobin phenotype. Bone marrow transplantation has been successful in persons with homozygous sickle cell disease. Recently, a transplant of blood cells from the umbilical cord of a newborn was done. To avoid increased acidosis, acetaminophen is preferable to salicylates for antipyretic therapy. Immunization against influenza and pneumococcal organisms should be seriously considered. Blood transfusion, including hypertransfusion therapy (e.g., packed red blood cells to raise the hematocrit to a level of 35% for a period of time), can be effective but must be weighed against the risks of hepatitis, human immunodeficiency virus (HIV), hemosiderosis, and iron and splenic overload. Oral maintenance therapy with folic acid is needed to meet the increased demands of chronic hemolytic anemia. Splenectomy may be performed if sequestration crises recur.

Genetic counseling and psychologic support are important for the child and family. Recently, a genetic technique called **preimplantation genetic diagnosis** has been performed on

WHAT'S NEW? The Use of Hydroxyurea in Children with Sickle Cell Anemia

Hydroxyurea increases hemoglobin F synthesis in individuals with sickle cell anemia. Well-organized adult clinical trials have shown that hydroxyurea was able to significantly deter the clinical severity of this disease. However, until recently the safety and efficacy of hydroxyurea in children with sickle cell anemia had not been determined. Fifty-two children with sickle cell disease were treated at the maximum tolerated dose of hydroxyurea for 1 year. Hemoglobin concentration, mean corpuscular volume, and fetal hemoglobin increased significantly. Decreases in white blood cell, neutrophil, platelet, and reticulocyte counts also occurred, but these were mild and reversed upon temporary discontinuation of the drug. Phase III trials are needed to determine if hydroxyurea can prevent chronic organ damage in children with sickle cell anemia.

Data from Carache S: Mechanism of hydroxyurea in the management of sickle cell anemia in adults, *Semin Hematol* 34(2 suppl 3):15, 1997; Kinney TR et al: Safety of hydroxyurea in children with sickle cell anemia: results of the HUG-KIDS study, a phase I/II trial. Pediatric Hydryoxyurea Group, *Blood* 94(5):1550, 1999; Ware RE, Zimmerman SA, Schultz WH: Hydroxyurea as an alternative to blood transfusions for the prevention of recurrent stroke in children with sickle cell disease, *Blood* 94(9):3022, 1999.

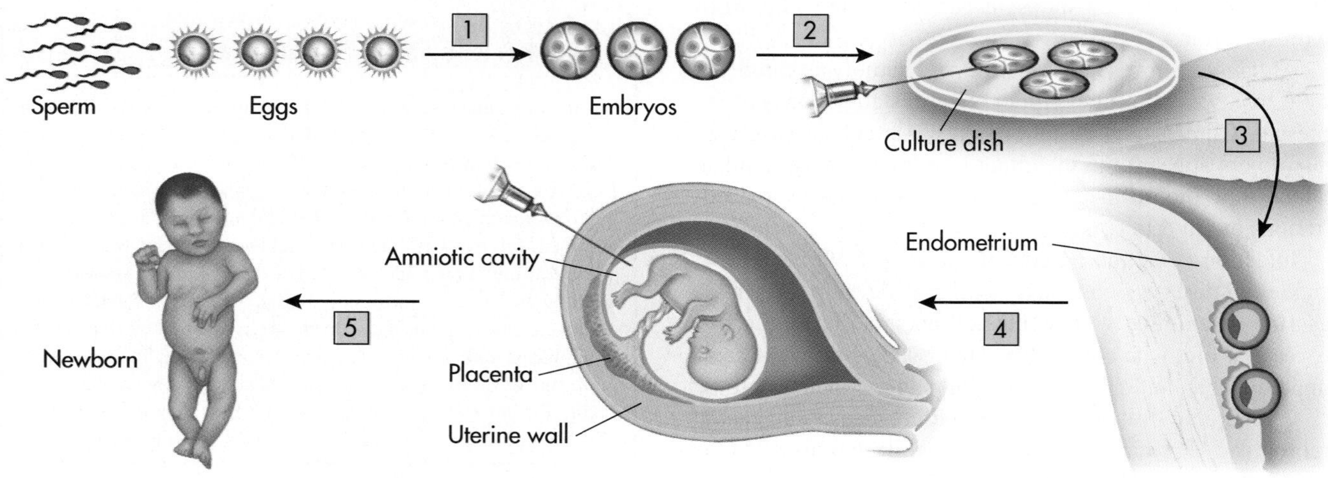

FIG. 27-9 Prepregnancy sickle cell test. (This technique has potential for other inherited diseases.) *1,* Fertilization produces several embryos. *2,* The embryos are tested for the presence of the gene. *3,* The embryo(s) without the gene are implanted. *4,* Amniocentesis confirms whether the fetus or fetuses does not have the sickle cell gene. *5,* Woman has a normal child.

parents to diagnose whether their offspring will or will not carry the gene for sickle cell disease. Fig. 27-9 summarizes this prepregnancy sickle cell test. Genetic counseling enables persons with sickle cell disease or trait to make informed decisions about transmitting this genetic disorder to their offspring, because there is a 25% chance with each pregnancy that a child born to two parents with sickle cell trait will have sickle cell disease.

Thalassemias

The alpha- and beta-thalassemias are inherited autosomal recessive disorders that cause an impaired rate of synthesis of one of the two chains—alpha or beta—of adult hemoglobin (Hb A). The disorder was named **thalassemia,** which is derived from the Greek word for *sea,* because it was defined initially in persons with origins near the Mediterranean Sea. Beta-thalassemia, in which synthesis of the beta globin chain is slowed or defective, is prevalent among Greeks, Italians, and some Arabs and Sephardic Jews. Alpha-thalassemia, in which the alpha chain is affected, is most common among Chinese, Vietnamese, Cambodians, and Laotians. Both alpha-thalassemia and beta-thalassemia are common among black Americans.

Alpha- and beta-thalassemia can be major or minor, depending on how many of the genes that control alpha or beta chain synthesis are defective and whether the defects are inherited homozygously (thalassemia major) or heterozygously (thalassemia minor). Pathophysiologic effects range from mild microcytosis to death in utero, depending on the number of defective genes and mode of inheritance. The anemic manifestation of thalassemia is microcytic-hypochromic hemolytic anemia.

◆ *Pathophysiology*

Normally two genes control beta chain synthesis and four genes control alpha chain synthesis. The number of genetic defects in the controlling genes determines the severity of the disorder. As in sickle cell disease the hemoglobin abnormality usually consists of the substitution of a single amino acid for another amino acid. Other molecular abnormalities that cause thalassemia are two amino acid substitutions, amino acid deletions or fusions, and synthesis of elongated chains.

The fundamental defect in beta-thalassemia is the uncoupling of alpha and beta chain synthesis. Beta chain production is depressed—moderately in the heterozygous form, **beta-thalassemia minor,** and severely in the homozygous form, **beta-thalassemia major** (also called **Cooley anemia**). Depression of beta chain synthesis results in erythrocytes having a reduced amount of hemoglobin and accumulations of free alpha chains. The free alpha chains are unstable and easily precipitate in the cell. Most erythroblasts that contain precipitates are destroyed by mononuclear phagocytes in the marrow, resulting in ineffective erythropoiesis and anemia. Some of the precipitate-carrying cells do mature and enter the bloodstream, but they are destroyed prematurely in the spleen, resulting in mild hemolytic anemia.

There are four forms of alpha-thalassemia:

1. **Alpha trait** (the carrier state), in which a single alpha chain–forming gene is defective
2. **Alpha-thalassemia minor,** in which two genes are defective
3. **Hemoglobin H disease,** in which three genes are defective
4. **Alpha-thalassemia major,** a fatal condition in which all four alpha-forming genes are defective

Death is inevitable because alpha chains are absent and oxygen cannot be released to the tissues.

Beta-thalassemia occurs more commonly than does alpha-thalassemia. Occasionally synthesis of gamma or delta polypeptide chains is defective, resulting in gamma- or delta-thalassemia. (Hemoglobin chains are described in Chapter 24.)

Clinical Manifestations

Beta-thalassemia minor causes mild to moderate microcytic-hypochromic anemia, mild splenomegaly, bronze coloring of the skin, and hyperplasia of the bone marrow. The degree of reticulocytosis depends on the severity of the anemia, resulting in skeletal changes. Hemolysis of immature (and therefore fragile) erythrocytes may cause a slight elevation in serum iron and indirect bilirubin levels. Persons with beta-thalassemia minor usually are asymptomatic.

Persons with beta-thalassemia major may become quite ill. Anemia is severe and results in a significant cardiovascular burden, with high-output congestive heart failure. In the past, death resulted from cardiac failure. Today, blood transfusions can increase life span by one to two decades, and death usually is caused by hemochromatosis (from transfusions). (Hemosiderosis and hematochromatosis are described in Chapter 25.) Liver enlargement occurs as a result of progressive hemosiderosis, whereas enlargement of the spleen is caused by extramedullary hematopoiesis and increased destruction of red blood cells. Spinal impairment that starts in infancy retards linear growth.[24] Bone marrow hyperplasia causes a characteristic deformity of the facial bones, as the nasal bridge, mandible, and maxilla widen.

Persons who inherit the mildest form of alpha-thalassemia, the alpha trait, usually are symptom free, having, at most, mild microcytosis. Alpha-thalassemia minor has clinical manifestations that are virtually identical to those of beta-thalassemia minor: mild microcytic-hypochromic reticulocytosis, bone marrow hyperplasia, increased serum iron concentrations, and moderate splenomegaly.

Signs and symptoms of alpha-thalassemia are similar to those of beta-thalassemia major but milder. Moderate microcytic-hypochromic anemia, enlargement of the liver and spleen, and bone marrow hyperplasia are evident.

Alpha-thalassemia major causes hydrops fetalis and fulminant intrauterine congestive heart failure. In addition to edema and massive ascites, the fetus has a grossly enlarged heart and liver. Diagnosis usually is made postmortem. Prenatal screening for this disorder can be performed by use of chorionic villus sampling. These cells can be analyzed, and a deoxyribonucleic acid (DNA) genetic map can be constructed and evaluated for the abnormalities characteristic of hydrops fetalis.

Both alpha-thalassemia major and beta-thalassemia major are life threatening. Children with thalassemia major generally are weak, fail to thrive, show poor development, and experience cardiovascular compromise with high-output failure secondary to anemia. Untreated, they will die by 5 to 6 years of age.

Evaluation and Treatment

Evaluation of thalassemia is based on familial disease history, clinical manifestations, and blood tests. Peripheral blood smears that show microcytosis and hemoglobin electrophoresis that demonstrates diminished amounts of alpha or beta chains are used to make the diagnosis. Analysis of fetal DNA from withdrawn amniotic fluid is used as a screening test to detect hydrops fetalis (alpha-thalassemia major). Newborn screening for thalassemia should be done according to state law.

Persons who are "silent" carriers or have thalassemia minor generally have few if any symptoms and require no specific treatment. Therapies to support and prolong life are necessary, however, for thalassemia major. There is no cure for either condition. Prenatal diagnosis and genetic counseling may be the most important therapeutic measures offered.

At present, thalassemia major is treated with the following therapies:

1. Blood transfusions, which can return hemoglobin and hematocrit levels to normal, thus alleviating the anemia-induced cardiac failure. Iron overload and hemochromatosis are complications of transfusion therapy.
2. Iron chelation therapy in combination with hypertransfusion (transfusion to a hematocrit of 35 ml/dl).
3. Splenectomy, which can reduce the need for transfusions by eliminating the site of hemolysis, thus prolonging erythrocyte survival.

DISORDERS OF COAGULATION AND PLATELETS

Inherited Hemorrhagic Disease

Hemophilias

Awareness of a serious bleeding disorder in males was documented nearly 2000 years ago in the Babylonian Talmud, which exempted from the rite of circumcision those boys having male relatives prone to excessive bleeding. In 1803 the first description of this disorder appeared in the medical literature, where it was noted to be X linked in nature and associated with joint bleeding and crippling.

Table 27-4 lists the coagulation factors. Until 1952 the term *hemophilia* was reserved for deficiency of factor VIII (antihemophilic factor). Since that time two additional coagulation proteins, factor IX (plasma thromboplastin component [PTC]) and factor XI (plasma thromboplastin antecedent [PTA]), have been identified and their deficiency associated with similar clinical manifestations. Congenital deficiencies of these three plasma clotting factors—VIII, IX, XI—account for 90% to 95% of the hemorrhagic bleeding disorders collectively called hemophilia.

Types of Hemophilia

Hemophilia A (classic hemophilia) is caused by factor VIII deficiency. It is the most common of the hemophilias. Hemophilia A is inherited as an X-linked recessive disorder that affects males and is transmitted by females; its estimated incidence is 1 per 10,000 male births.

Hemophilia B (Christmas disease), caused by factor IX deficiency, also is transmitted as an X-linked recessive trait and is clinically indistinguishable from factor VIII deficiency. Approximately 15% of cases, or 1 in every 25,000 to 30,000 males born with hemophilia, are caused by factor IX.[25]

Hemophilia A and hemophilia B occur with varying degrees of clinical severity, depending on concentrations of

Table 27-4 The Coagulation Factors

International Numbers	Synonyms	Comment
I	Fibrinogen	Number rarely used—congenital deficiency known (afibrinogenemia)
II	Prothrombin	Number rarely used—congenital deficiency known
III	Thromboplastin	No specific factor identified
IV	Calcium	Number rarely used
V	Labile factor, proaccelerin	Congenital deficiency known (parahemophilia, Owren disease)
VI	Activated labile factor, accelerin	No longer differentiated from factor V
VII	Stable factor, SPCA, proconvertin	Congenital deficiency known
VIII	Antihemophilic factor (AHF) or globulin (AHG)	Hemophilia A (classic hemophilia)—results from congenital deficiency
IX	Christmas factor, plasma thromboplastin component (PTC)	Hemophilia B—results from congenital deficiency
X	Stuart-Prower factor	Congenital deficiency known
XI	Plasma thromboplastin antecedent, PTA	Congenital deficiency known
XII	Hageman factor	No clinical symptoms associated with congenital deficiency
XIII	Fibrin-stabilizing factor	Congenital deficiency known

From Behrman R et al, editors: *Nelson textbook of pediatrics,* Philadelphia, 1992, W.B. Saunders.

clotting factor VIII or IX in the blood. Severe hemophilia (concentration of clotting factors less than 1% of normal) is associated with spontaneous bleeding. In moderate hemophilia (1% to 5% of normal), bleeding usually occurs only after trauma; in the mild form (5% to 35% of normal), bleeding occurs only after severe trauma or surgery. The severity of hemophilia is similar in all affected members of a family.

Hemophilia C (factor XI deficiency) occurs as an autosomal recessive disease and occurs equally in males and females. Bleeding usually is less severe than in hemophilia A or B.

Von Willebrand disease results from an inherited autosomal dominant trait with variable clinical manifestations and hematologic findings. The factor VIII deficiency differs from that of hemophilia A in mode of inheritance and response to treatment. In hemophilia A the deficiency is inherited as an X-linked recessive trait, whereas in von Willebrand disease it is inherited as an autosomal dominant trait. The most important difference, however, is in responses to the infusion of plasma. In von Willebrand disease, infusion of plasma causes factor VIII activity to increase for several days because infusion of factor VIII temporarily induces endogenous synthesis of factor VIII.

Pathophysiology

Two types of defects dominate the hereditary defects of hemophilia to date: gene deletions and point mutations. Both types of genetic defects are associated with severe hemophilia A, in which no factor VIII circulates in the blood. To date, about 50 deletion mutations in the gene for factor VIII have been identified at the molecular level and about 34 independent deletion mutations in the factor IX gene have been found to be the cause of hemophilia B.[26,27] The molecular defect that leads to hemophilia is identical among members of a given family; however, the deletional mutation has been unique in each family studied.[26]

Point mutations, in which a single base in the DNA is mutated to another base, represent a second type of mutation that causes hemophilia. When a point mutation gives rise to a de novo stop codon (nonsense mutation), translation of the protein ceases and a shortened version of the protein is synthesized. Usually the protein is destroyed intracellularly and never reaches the plasma. This type of defect is associated with severe hemophilia, that is, with coagulant activity levels below 1%.[26] Point mutations in which one amino acid is substituted for another can cause phenotypes of varying severity. The mutation of an important amino acid can destroy protein function, activation, or folding; inhibit intracellular processing; or cause protein clearance.[26] Unlike deletional mutations, point mutations at the same site have been recorded in different families with hemophilia.

Table 27-4 summarizes the types of coagulation disorders. Not all the disorders are discussed in this chapter because some are extremely rare (congenital dysfibrinogenemias) and others have no clinical significance (e.g., Hageman factor deficiency, a condition in which profound laboratory deficiency of factor XII is associated with absolutely no clinical defects).

Clinical Manifestations

Children with severe hemophilia start to bleed at different ages. In one study 44% of children demonstrated their first bleeding episode before 1 year of age.[28] Although there is no transfer of maternal clotting factor to the fetus, many boys with hemophilia are circumcised without excessive bleeding. Normal hemostasis is achieved in these infants because clotting is activated through the extrinsic coagulation cascade, which does not involve factors VII, IX, or XI.

During the first year, spontaneous bleeding often is minimal, but hematoma formation may result from injections and from firm holding (e.g., under the arms). Easy bruising or hemarthrosis (bleeding into joints) or both occur with ambulation. By 3 to 4 years of age, 90% of children with hemophilia have had episodes of persistent bleeding from relatively minor traumatic lacerations (e.g., to the lip or tongue). This usually is the first clinical manifestation of hemophilia. Hemorrhage into the elbows, knees, and ankles causes pain, limits joint movement, and predisposes the child to degenerative joint changes. Spontaneous hematuria and epistaxis are troublesome but minor complications.

Recurrent bleeding, both spontaneous and after minor trauma, is a lifelong problem. Many affected persons experience phases or cycles of spontaneous bleeding episodes. Mechanisms that cause this phenomenon are unknown. Intracranial hemorrhage and bleeding into the neck or abdomen constitute life-threatening emergencies.

Evaluation and Treatment

Although laboratory tests are of primary value in the evaluation of hemorrhagic disorders, the history and physical assessment also should be given careful consideration. The three phases of coagulation can be assessed individually by simple, reliable tests. In any hemorrhagic condition the adequacy of phase III should be determined first. Unless adequate fibrinogen is present, the blood is incapable of coagulation; thus other laboratory tests that require formation of a visible clot will be invalid. Phase III can be evaluated by the **thrombin time,** the time required for plasma to clot after the addition of bovine thrombin. Fibrinogen can be measured by chemical or immunologic methods.

Phase II is assessed by the **prothrombin time (PT),** the time required for plasma to clot after the addition of thromboplastin and calcium. If phase III is intact, a prolonged prothrombin time indicates a deficiency involving factors II, V, VII, or X, alone or in combination. Specific assays for each of the factors are available.

Phase I, the most complex part of coagulation, can be evaluated by several tests. The **activated partial thromboplastin time (PTT)** is the time required for clotting of plasma that has been activated by incubation with kaolin when calcium and platelets (or partial thromboplastin) are added. PTT assesses the adequacy of factors XII, XI, IX, and VII. The **prothrombin consumption time** is a standard prothrombin test of serum instead of plasma. Because prothrombin is used up during coagulation, the serum normally contains little prothrombin and the serum prothrombin time is prolonged. Deficiencies of the phase I factors are associated with poor use of prothrombin. If the serum and plasma prothrombin times are similar, deficiency of a phase I factor is likely. The **thromboplastin generation** test is the most sensitive of all phase I tests. The test can precisely identify deficiencies of factors VIII and IX. If the PTT, prothrombin consumption, or thromboplastin generation test results are abnormal, the way in which they can be corrected identifies the specific deficiency.

The treatment of hemophilia has advanced during the past 50 years. Plasma first was used in the 1920s, and by the 1940s it was used routinely to treat persons with hemophilia. The disadvantages of fresh frozen plasma (FFP), which is low in factor VIII per volume of plasma, led to the development of cryoprecipitate. In 1964 cryoprecipitate (quick-frozen precipitate), which is rich in factor VIII per volume, was used to treat persons with hemophilia. Although cryoprecipitate advanced the treatment of hemophilia A, it has several disadvantages. The most notable complication is the possibility of transmission of viral diseases. Factor VIII concentrates were first introduced in 1965. In addition to the predictable factor VIII content, other advantages of the early factor VIII concentrates included greater purity than cryoprecipitate and less contamination with other plasma proteins.[29] The recent cloning of the factor VIII gene and the development of recombinant factor VIII have resulted in new factor VIII products that minimize the risk of transmission of viral infection (e.g., HIV and hepatitis)[30] and are potentially less expensive than plasma-derived factor VIII. However, transmission of viral diseases (e.g., hepatitis A, hepatitis C, hepatitis G) continues to occur.[31-34]

Continuous prophylaxis from ages 2 to 18 years reduces the incidence of joint damage and synovitis, which remain the primary causes of disability in people with hemophilia.[35,36]

Congenital Hypercoagulability and Thrombosis

Hereditary bleeding disorders, such as hemophilia, have been recognized and treated for centuries; however, the counterpart of these disorders, **thrombophilia,** has not been recognized until very recently. The inherited thrombophilic conditions generally are caused by defects in the clotting factors that inhibit clot formation; thus the balance between bleeding and clotting is directed toward the clotting aspects of hemostasis. Defects in specific proteins (C and S) and antithrombin (AT), as well as resistance to activated protein C (APC) and hyperhomocystinemia, are the major recognized causes of inherited thrombophilia.[37]

Both proteins C and S are inhibitors of coagulation and depend on vitamin K for synthesis in the hepatocytes of the liver. Decreased levels of either of these proteins interfere with the normal homeostatic balance of procoagulant and anticoagulant activity at the endothelial level. Protein C and S deficiency states predispose affected individuals to thrombosis, especially venous thrombosis of the lower extremities.

Inheritance of **protein C deficiency** is autosomal dominant. Heterozygotes have protein C levels 50% to 60% of normal and may develop superficial thrombophlebitis, deep venous thrombosis, or pulmonary embolism in their late teens and early twenties. The majority of these thrombotic events (75%) occur spontaneously, whereas only 25% are the result of predisposing conditions.[37] Homozygotes have less than 1% of normal levels of protein C and tend to develop thrombosis of the cutaneous vessels with large areas of skin necrosis. It is rare for individuals with protein C deficiency to develop arterial thrombosis.

Protein C deficiency exists in two forms: types I and II. Type I, the most common form, involves a reduction in both biologic and immunologic activity of protein C.[37] Type I is caused by deletion of the entire gene. In type II, the less common form, there is a normal level of protein C antigen but decreased functional levels of activity.[38]

Neonatal purpura fulminans is a fatal syndrome found in infants who are homozygous or double heterozygous for types I and II protein deficiency. Manifestations of this syndrome are ecchymosis that becomes apparent on the first day of life and develops around the head, trunk, and extremities. These cutaneous manifestations often are accompanied by cerebral thrombosis and infarction. The lesions apparent on the skin often coalesce and demonstrate ulceration and necrosis. The infant rarely survives, and the condition is refractory to heparin or antiplatelet therapy.[39]

Treatment for protein C deficiency is heparin for acute episodes of thrombosis. Long-term therapy is required and consists of either oral warfarin sodium (Coumadin) or subcutaneous heparin (2500 to 5000 units) every 12 hours. Protein C concentrates have been developed; however, they have not yet been formally approved for treatment.

Protein S deficiency is similar to protein C deficiency, and the inheritance pattern (autosomal dominant) is also similar. Heterozygotes demonstrate a strong tendency for deep venous thrombosis, with the first incidence often occurring before age 25 years. Other manifestations include superficial thrombophlebitis and pulmonary emboli. There are predisposing conditions for thrombi development in some cases, with evidence of spontaneous thrombi development in most cases.

Protein S deficiency exists in two forms: type I and type II. Type I is identified as a quantitative deficiency and manifests as low levels of protein S antigen and activity, and type II is identified as a qualitative deficiency with low levels of free protein S and normal levels of free and total protein S antigen.[38]

Homozygotes demonstrate severe manifestations of the condition and may develop a form of purpura fulminans in the neonatal period. It also is possible that the homozygous state may lead to uterine death.[37] Treatment with heparin and Coumadin is similar to that of protein C deficiency.

Antithrombin III (AT III) deficiency is inherited as an autosomal dominant condition, with the heterozygote state being the most common. AT III also exists in two forms, type I and type II, with type I being a quantitative deficiency of the AT III antigen. Type II is characterized as a dysfunctional form: normal levels of AT III are present but with reduced activity.

Individuals with AT III deficiency are at risk for early development of venous thrombosis and pulmonary embolism. These events often occur in the middle to late teens, with the potential of occurring as early as 10 years of age. The deep veins of the lower extremities most commonly are involved, with the iliofemoral vein being the most common site of involvement. Other sites include the mesenteric veins, vena cava, renal veins, and retinal veins. Cerebral thromboses also have been described. Arterial thrombotic events are rare. In some cases, thrombosis is precipitated by predisposing conditions, such as surgery, trauma, pregnancy, oral contraceptives, and infection.[39]

The treatment of choice for AT III deficiency is heparin. Antiplatelet agents (e.g., aspirin, dipyridamole) may be used, as well as AT III concentrates.

Antibody-Mediated Hemorrhagic Disease

The antibody-mediated hemorrhagic diseases are a group of disorders caused by the immune response. Antibody-mediated destruction of platelets or antibody-mediated inflammatory reactions to allergens damage blood vessels and cause seepage into tissues. The thrombocytopenic purpuras may be intrinsic or idiopathic, or they may be transient phenomena transmitted from mother to fetus. The inflammatory, or "allergic," purpuras occur in response to allergens in the blood. All these disorders first appear during infancy or childhood.

Idiopathic Thrombocytopenic Purpura

Acute **idiopathic thrombocytopenic purpura (ITP) (autoimmune or primary thrombocytopenic purpura)** is the most common of the thrombocytopenic purpuras of childhood. It is a disorder of platelet consumption in which antiplatelet antibodies bind to the plasma membranes of platelets, causing platelet sequestration and destruction by mononuclear phagocytes in the spleen and other lymphoid tissues at a rate that exceeds the ability of the bone marrow to produce them.

Pathophysiology

Platelets have several tissue-specific antigens on their plasma markers that may be targets for antiplatelet antibody. In approximately 70% of cases of ITP, there is an antecedent viral disease (e.g., cytomegalovirus [CMV], Epstein-Barr virus [EBV], HIV, parvovirus, or viral respiratory infection), thus suggesting that viral sensitization has occurred. The interval between infection and onset of purpura is 1 to 4 weeks. A comparison with purpura seen in adults has identified an immune mechanism as the basis for ITP. High levels of IgG have been found bound to platelets and may represent immune complexes on the platelet surface.[40-43]

Clinical Manifestations

One to four weeks after a viral infection, bruising and a generalized petechial rash often occur with acute onset. Asymmetric bleeding is typical and is found most frequently on the legs and trunk. Hemorrhagic bullae of the gums, lips, and other mucous membranes may be prominent. Epistaxis (nose bleeding) may be severe and difficult to control. Except for the signs of bleeding, the child appears well. The acute phase of the disease associated with spontaneous hemorrhages lasts 1 to 2 weeks, but thrombocytopenia often persists. Although its incidence is less than 1%, intracranial hemorrhage is the most serious complication of ITP. In some cases the onset is more gradual and clinical manifestations consist of moderate bruising and a few petechiae.

Evaluation and Treatment

Laboratory examination reveals a reduced platelet count, and the few platelets observed on a peripheral blood smear are large in size, reflecting increased bone marrow production. The Ivy bleeding time is prolonged. Bone marrow aspiration reveals megakaryocytes in normal or increased numbers and normal erythrocytes and granulocytes.

Even without treatment, the prognosis for children with ITP is excellent. Seventy-five percent recover completely within 3 months. After the initial acute phase, spontaneous clinical manifestations subside. By 6 months after onset, 80% to 90% of affected children have regained normal platelet counts.[44]

Because of the short life span of platelets (10 days), fresh blood or platelets are of no value or of transient benefit; however, their use is indicated when life-threatening hemorrhage occurs. For some children, corticosteroid therapy reduces the severity and shortens the duration of the initial phase by suppressing the immune attack on platelets.[45,46]

Intravenous IgG has been demonstrated to increase the platelet count in some children with ITP, but it is quite costly.[47,48] A newer product, anti-D, is a gamma globulin fraction containing a high proportion of antibodies to the RhO (D) antigen of the red blood cells. Intravenous anti-D is a safe and effective treatment for Rh-positive, nonsplenectomized individuals with ITP, although it is expensive.[49,50]

Parents should be instructed to protect the child from falls or other trauma that might result in bleeding. Splenectomy should be reserved for chronic cases that fail to respond to nonsurgical intervention.[51]

Autoimmune Neonatal Thrombocytopenias

Antibody-mediated thrombocytopenic purpura occurs in neonates in either autoimmune or alloimmune form. Both forms are characterized by the immunologic destruction of platelets by antibodies (IgG) against tissue-specific antigens expressed by the platelets (i.e., platelet-specific antigens).

Autoimmune neonatal thrombocytopenia was first noted in the early 1950s when it was observed that mothers with ITP frequently delivered infants who were transiently thrombocytopenic. Neonatal thrombocytopenia was observed in approximately 50% of infants at risk and lasted an average of 1 month. As platelet counts returned to normal, there was a concomitant drop in the level of maternal antiplatelet antibody on the child's platelets. The antibody is directed against antigens common to maternal and neonatal platelets.[52] The prognosis generally is favorable. Incidence of intracranial hemorrhage in these infants is not well documented, but when it does occur, it is not clear whether it is related to the birth process or not.[53,54]

Neonatal alloimmune thrombocytopenic purpura (NATP) is less common, occurring in approximately 1 in 5000 births. NATP is suspected in thrombocytopenic infants of mothers with normal platelet counts and no history of purpura. The disorder is caused by the production of a maternal antibody against a fetal platelet-specific antigen inherited from the father and not shared by the mother. More than 50% of NATP cases are associated with the presence of the $P1^A1$ antigen on neonatal and paternal platelets but not on maternal platelets.

It is not known why NATP occurs in only half of the neonates genetically at risk for NATP. Because 98% of the population show $P1^A1$ positivity, approximately 1 in 50 pregnancies would be expected to show maternal-fetal incompatibility, but the incidence of NATP is 100 times less. NATP does not develop in neonates born to some mothers with high antiplatelet antibody levels.

The diagnosis of NATP is confirmed by detection in the maternal serum of antibody that reacts with platelets from the infant and father but not with platelets from the mother. In approximately 75% to 85% of cases, NATP recurs in subsequent pregnancies. Purpura usually develops in the affected infant shortly after delivery, and intracranial, renal, and gastrointestinal hemorrhages are possible. The mortality rate from intracranial hemorrhage has been estimated at 10% to 15%.

Most of the life-threatening clinical manifestations of both transient neonatal thrombocytopenia and NATP can be avoided through cesarean delivery. If the mother has antiplatelet disease, however, surgery can result in hemorrhage and serious maternal morbidity. Maternal morbidity resulting from NATP during pregnancy is low (less than 5%): the principal maternal risk is bleeding from surgical incisions during cesarean delivery. This poses a problem for the obstetrician. The incidence of transient thrombocytopenia in infants born to mothers with NATP is about 50%. If all deliveries were cesarean, half the mothers would undergo cesarean delivery unnecessarily. Conversely, if all deliveries were vaginal, half the infants—those with thrombocytopenia—would be at risk for intracranial bleeding. A considerable amount of research has focused on methods of predicting whether the fetus is thrombocytopenic so that the route of delivery can be chosen to minimize the risks for both mother and child. No satisfactory method has been found, despite reports from many laboratories that fetal platelet counts correlate closely with levels of antiplatelet antibody on maternal platelets or in the maternal circulation. Equally unreliable are predictions of neonatal thrombocytopenia based on immunosuppression with corticosteroids. Research continues in such areas as the identification of specific subclasses of antiplatelet antibodies.

Autoimmune Vascular Purpura

Autoimmune vascular purpura (allergic purpura) is caused by antibody-mediated injury of blood vessel walls, typically arterioles and capillaries. The inflammatory reaction is to foreign proteins or chemicals in the blood (microorganisms, drugs, or other chemicals).

Autoimmune vascular purpura usually is seen in children, with the incidence decreasing in adolescents and adults and occurring only rarely in elderly persons. The average age at onset is 5 years, with a slightly higher proportion of males affected. Purpura occurs as vessel integrity is disrupted by inflammatory processes, causing effusion of serosanguineous exudate to perivascular tissues.

Clinical manifestations vary and include headache, anorexia, fever, abdominal pain, arthralgias, and skin lesions (urticaria and erythema). The lesions usually are located symmetrically on the proximal portions of the extremities, particularly on the legs and buttocks, and may be accompanied by itching or paresthesias.[55] Abdominal pain results from hemorrhage into the bowel, which may lead to colic, nausea, and vomiting. These symptoms may precede the appearance of skin lesions. The pain usually is midabdominal but may radiate to other parts of the abdomen. Constipation may occur.

Some forms of autoimmune vascular purpura may produce joint pain and tenderness. Periarticular swelling and edema of the hands and feet are common, but hemarthrosis does not occur. These symptoms may precede the onset of symptoms associated with abdominal pain and purpura. Subacute glomerulonephritis occurs in some cases but usually is reversible.

The characteristic skin lesions (purpura and cutaneous manifestations of allergy), accompanied by a history of joint and abdominal pain, are clues for diagnosis. Laboratory test results often reveal no major abnormalities. Attacks may last several weeks and may recur at odd intervals and with changing manifestations with each episode. Treatment, if necessary, consists of the alleviation of symptoms.

LEUKEMIA AND LYMPHOMA

Leukemia, the most common malignancy of childhood, represents approximately 33% of all childhood cancers. Childhood lymphoma is the third most common malignant neoplasm of children in the United States, representing approximately 11% of all childhood cancers. (See Chapter 26 for a discussion of leukemia in adults.)

Leukemia

Of the varieties of childhood leukemia, 80% to 85% of leukemias in children are acute lymphoblastic leukemia (ALL) or acute undifferentiated leukemia (AUL). The remaining 15% to 20% are acute nonlymphocytic leukemias (ANLLs) (which include myeloblastic, promyelocytic, monocytic, and myelomonoblastic leukemias) and the very rare red blood cell leukemia, erythroleukemia. Because the vast majority of ANLLs involve the myeloblastic cell, many experts refer to the disease as acute myelogenous leukemia (AML). Leukemia accounts for 25% of cases of cancer in black children and 34% of cases of cancer in white children. Approximately 2200 new cases are diagnosed each year in the United States.[56,57] Of those 2200 children, 1700 are diagnosed with ALL. Both a juvenile form and an adult form of chronic granulocytic leukemia (CGL) can develop in children, but CGL is uncommon and accounts for only 2% of all leukemias in childhood. Chronic lymphocytic leukemia (CLL) is virtually nonexistent in children.

The peak incidence for childhood ALL is between 2 and 6 years of age. Although this peak is very evident in white children in the United States, it is not observed in black children. The reason for this difference is unknown, but it may be related to genetic susceptibility or to exposure to the environmental influences that might play a role in leukemia. Further, acute leukemia is nearly twice as common in white children as in nonwhite children (4.2 : 100,000 versus 2.4 : 100,000, respectively). For a white child the risk of acute leukemia developing before age 10 years is 1 : 2800.[57] Childhood ALL also is more common in boys than in girls (1.3 : 1.0).

Types of Leukemia

A number of different classifications are used for the leukemias. First, acute leukemia is differentiated from chronic leukemia. Second, the cell line determines whether lymphoid cells or myeloid cells are involved. In acute leukemia this difference separates ALL from ANLL and vice versa. Then, within each of these categories, further subdivisions have been developed. (See Chapter 26 for a discussion of leukemias in adults.)

Cytogenic studies of leukemic cells are performed routinely at most major treatment centers during the diagnostic process. Abnormal morphologic characteristics, as well as abnormalities in the number of copies of chromosomes, are found in leukemic cells. Hyperdiploidy (increased number of chromosome copies) is associated with a good prognosis. Other genetic abnormalities include chromosome translocations and fragility (break sites). Translocations are more common in children with a poor prognosis. Some oncogenes have been associated with various types of childhood leukemia, including *src, abl,* N-*ras*, and *c-myb*.[58-60]

Two additional classifications of ALL (morphologic and immunologic) have proved clinically useful because they have prognostic value. Although a number of different morphologic classifications have been developed, the accepted system was developed by a cooperative effort of French, American, and British scientists and is known as the French-American-British Cooperative Group (FAB) classification.[61,62] This system divides lymphoblasts into three categories—L1, L2, and L3—on the basis of histologic appearance of the abnormal lymphoblast. Approximately 85% of cases of ALL are of the L1 subtype; less than 15% are L2, a subtype more common in adults with ALL; and the L3 subtype, which is rare, occurs in fewer than 1% of children with ALL.

The immunologic classification of ALL is evolving as advances are made in immunologic techniques.[63] Because of the new techniques, distinguishing between lymphoblastic and nonlymphoblastic leukemia is much easier than in the past, when the degree of immaturity of the cell sometimes made such distinction difficult. In addition, immunologic classifications have assisted clinicians in determining the degree of aggressive therapy needed.

Immunologic classification has been used on identification of various surface markers. Five categories of ALL have been identified on the basis of their presumed origin from thymic cells (T cells) and bursa-equivalent cells (B cells) of normal lymphocytes:

1. T cell ALL, characterized by the presence of abnormal T lymphocytes and found more commonly in older boys whose diagnosis includes mediastinal masses, high white blood cell counts, and hepatosplenomegaly (20% of ALL)
2. B cell ALL, characterized by the presence of abnormal B lymphoblasts and associated with a poor prognosis (5% of ALL)
3. Pre–B cell ALL, characterized by the presence of pre-B lymphoblasts (20% of ALL)

4. Unclassified ALL, also known as *null cell* (meaning neither T nor B lymphoblasts), and now classified as early B cell lineage (15% of ALL)
5. Common ALL, characterized by the presence of a specific antigen known as *common ALL antigen*, or common lymphocytic leukemia antigen (CALLA), recently designated cellular differentiation 10 or CD-10, in which the actual cell usually is considered to be of the B lineage (39% of ALL)

The identification of CALLA is important because this type of ALL has a more favorable prognosis.

Subtypes of ANLL also have been classified by the FAB system according to the morphologic and cytochemical characteristics of the leukemic cell. Seven categories have been established:

1. M1 involves cells that are myeloblastic without differentiation.
2. M2 involves cells that are myeloblastic with differentiation.
3. M3 involves the promyelocyte.
4. M4 involves the myeloblastic and monoblastic cell lines.
5. M5 involves monoblasts.
6. M6 involves precursors of erythrocytes.
7. M7 involves precursors of megakaryocytes.

Nearly half of all childhood ANLL is M1 or M2. Another one third is categorized as M4 or M5. ANLL subtypes M3, M6, and M7 are quite rare.[64]

Pathogenesis

The exact cause of childhood leukemia is unclear. Investigations have focused on genetic susceptibility, environmental factors, and viral infections (see Chapter 12). Observations of a familial tendency and links with a number of inherited disorders have implicated genetic factors in the origin of leukemia. For example, if ALL develops in one identical twin, the risk for disease in the other twin is estimated at 25%,[65] particularly during the first year after diagnosis of the leukemic twin. After approximately 7 years the risk to the unaffected twin returns to the same risk as that of the general population. Some evidence suggests that multiple cases of leukemia occur in families. The incidence of leukemia in siblings of leukemic children is reported to be between 1 : 720 and 1 : 1000, which represents a fourfold risk over that of the general population.[66,67]

Inherited diseases that predispose a child to leukemia (both ALL and ANLL) include Down syndrome (1 : 74 before age 10 years), Fanconi anemia (1:12 before age 21 years), Bloom syndrome (1 : 8 before age 26 years), and ataxia-telangiectasia (1 : 8 before age 25 years).[57] Leukemia also has been associated with known genetic diseases, such as congenital agammaglobulinemia. ANLL in children sometimes is associated with loss or deletion of chromosome 7.[64] ANLL can develop from preexisting myeloproliferative disorders that also are preleukemia syndromes. When these disorders progress to ANLL, an insidious pattern of leukemic dysfunction usually is revealed.

Most research on environmental factors as etiologic agents has centered on exposure to ionizing radiation. Atomic bomb survivors have an increased risk for leukemia. The degree of risk depends on the distance from the epicenter. The peak incidence period is 4 to 8 years after exposure to the radiation.[68] Whereas ANLL most often develops in adults who are exposed to radiation, ALL is more likely to develop in children. The therapeutic use of x-rays for thymic enlargement in children also has been linked to subsequent development of ALL in children.[69] In a more recent study, no increased risk of childhood leukemia was found in children who had received small doses of radiation from diagnostic x-rays.[70] Some doubt remains concerning the relative risk of prenatal exposure to radiation. Although it is likely that in utero radiation presents a cancer risk to the fetus, the magnitude of the risk is uncertain.[71] Although most studies of radiation exposure have focused on artificial radiation sources, there is considerable interest in natural background radiation, particularly the possible role of radon exposure in subsequent childhood and adult cancers.[72]

Electromagnetic field (EMF) exposure from power poles and small appliances has been studied as a causative factor in acute leukemias. Some studies suggest an increased risk in malignant diseases with exposure to electromagnetic fields.[73-75] Other studies, however, have not supported these findings, and further investigation is ongoing.[76-78]

Although chemicals such as benzene have been associated with the development of ANLL in adults, no evidence suggests a similar chemical or drug association in childhood leukemia. Leukemia (primarily ANLL) has been reported as a secondary malignancy (development of a second cancer after the first) in children treated for Hodgkin disease and Wilms tumor, although such cases are rare. In most cases the children received both chemotherapy (alkylating agents or dactinomycin) and radiation therapy for the primary cancer, perhaps accounting for the subsequent development of another cancer.

Leukemic "clusters" that represent a greater number of leukemia cases occurring in a particular geographic location have raised speculation about environmental factors or infectious patterns of transmission. Careful follow-up, however, has failed to document the abnormal clustering.[79] Explanations for this phenomenon therefore are statistical artifact and coincidence. However, one reported leukemic cluster in the town of Woburn, Massachusetts, has been linked to possible water supply contamination by chemicals from factory waste.[80]

Another area of interest has been the role of viruses in the development of leukemia. Viruses clearly have been shown to cause leukemia in a number of animals, including cats, fowl, and mice. Scientists have linked retroviruses with several adult cancers, including (1) human T cell leukemia/lymphoma virus (HTLV-I) with an unusual form of adult T cell leukemia, (2) HTLV-II with hairy cell leukemia, and (3) HIV with Kaposi sarcoma.[27] However, retroviruses have not been linked with childhood leukemia.

Clinical Manifestations

Few variations appear in the presenting symptoms of the various cell types of acute leukemias. The onset may be abrupt or insidious, but the most common symptoms reflect the consequence of bone marrow failure, which results in decreased red blood cells and platelets and changes in white blood cells. Pallor, fatigue, petechiae, purpura, bleeding, and fever generally are present. Approximately 45% of children have a hemoglobin level below 7 g/dl; in contrast to adults, children seem to demonstrate fewer symptoms. If acute blood loss occurs, however, characteristic symptoms of tachycardia, air hunger, restlessness, and thirst may be present. Epistaxis, excessive bruising, and hematuria frequently occur in children with severe thrombocytopenia. Three fourths of children with ALL have platelet counts below 100,000/mm^3 at diagnosis, and 28% have platelet counts below 20,000/mm^3. Half of all children newly diagnosed with ANLL have platelet counts below 50,000/mm^3. Disseminated intravascular coagulation occurs more commonly with ANLL, particularly with promyelocytic leukemia. The granules in the leukemic promyelocytes may then indicate thromboplastin activity.

Fever usually is present as a result of two causes: (1) infection associated with the decrease in functional neutrophils and (2) hypermetabolism associated with the ongoing rapid growth and destruction of leukemic cells. In most children with ALL, the total white blood count is less than 10,000/mm^3, and with ANLL most have white cell counts below 50,000/mm^3. In a few children, however, the peripheral white blood count can go well above 100,000/mm^3. White blood cell counts greater than 200,000/mm^3 can cause leukostasis, an intravascular clumping of cells that results in infarction and hemorrhage, usually in the brain and lung. An excessive leukocyte count at diagnosis is the most important predictor of prognosis in ALL.[56]

Renal failure as a result of hyperuremia (high uric acid levels) can be associated with ALL, particularly at diagnosis. Cell breakdown results as a natural process in the presence of a high white blood cell count or as a result of cellular breakdown caused by chemotherapy. Uric acid levels rise as an end product of purine metabolism from cellular destruction. Because the major excretory pathway is through the kidney, urates can precipitate in renal tubules or ureters and can lead to oliguria and acute renal failure. Renal failure is preventable if uric acid levels are monitored and treatment is aimed at optimal hydration, alkalinization of urine to assist with the excretion of soluble urates, and blockage of further uric acid formation by administration of the drug allopurinol.

Extramedullary invasion with leukemic cells can occur in nearly all body tissue. Most children with ALL have some extramedullary involvement at diagnosis. Leukemic invasion of tissue other than bone marrow is believed to represent metastatic infiltration. Hepatosplenomegaly and lymphadenopathy, resulting from extramedullary hematopoiesis, occur in nearly one half of children with ALL, but they are less common in children with ANLL.

The CNS is a common site of infiltration of extramedullary leukemias, although fewer than 10% of children with ALL have CNS involvement at diagnosis. CNS infiltration manifests later in the course of the disease. Because successful chemotherapy prolongs the time of remission, the incidence of CNS involvement has increased. The most common symptoms of CNS involvement relate to increased intracranial pressure, causing early-morning headaches, nausea, vomiting, irritability, and lethargy. Prophylactic CNS treatment therefore is necessary, because systemic treatment with chemotherapy does not cross the blood-brain barrier.

Gonadal involvement, with testicular and ovarian infiltration, has been demonstrated in postmortem examination in 57% and 35% of children, respectively. Clinical detection of gonadal involvement is much less frequent. The incidence of testicular involvement, like CNS involvement, has increased with lengthened duration of remission. Prophylactic treatment has not been successful and currently is not recommended.

Leukemic infiltration into bones and joints is frequent in children. Reports of bone or joint pain actually lead to the diagnosis of leukemia in some children. In most children, bone pain is characterized as migratory, vague, and without areas of swelling or inflammation. If joint pain is the primary symptom and some swelling is associated with the pain, however, misdiagnoses of rheumatoid arthritis and rheumatic fever may occur.

Other organs reported to be sites of leukemic invasion include the kidneys, heart, lungs, thymus, eyes, skin, and gastrointestinal tract. Of these, the kidneys, lungs, and gastrointestinal tract are the most frequently reported sites. Skin involvement is more common in ANLL than in ALL.

Children with leukemia usually have had symptoms for only 1 week before diagnosis. In 1990 a nationwide study was begun to document the symptom profile of children with cancer, including leukemia. The 5-year study investigated the relationship of demographic and socioeconomic factors.

Evaluation and Treatment

Although blood test results can raise the clinician's suspicion of leukemia, a bone marrow aspiration is required to establish the diagnosis. The **blast cell** is the hallmark of acute leukemia (Fig. 27-10). The blast cell is a relatively undifferentiated cell characterized by diffusely distributed nuclear chromatin, with one or more nucleoli and basophilic cytoplasm (Fig. 27-11).

Healthy children have fewer than 5% blast cells in the bone marrow and none in the peripheral blood. The bone marrow is categorized on the basis of blast percentage. Normal bone marrow is called M1 marrow; M2 and M3 represent an increased percentage of blasts in the sample. This categorization system should not be confused with the similar terminology used to denote subtypes of ANLL. In ALL the bone marrow often is replaced by 80% to 100% blast cells, with a reduction in normally developing red blood cells and granulocytes. The marrow, which is considered hypercellular, is composed of a homogeneous population of cells. Occasionally, however, the marrow appears hypocellular, making the diagnosis difficult to differentiate from aplastic anemia. When this occurs, bone marrow biopsy or biopsy of extramedullary sites is necessary to confirm the diagnosis (Fig. 27-12).

Combination chemotherapy, with or without radiation therapy to localized sites, such as the CNS, is the treatment

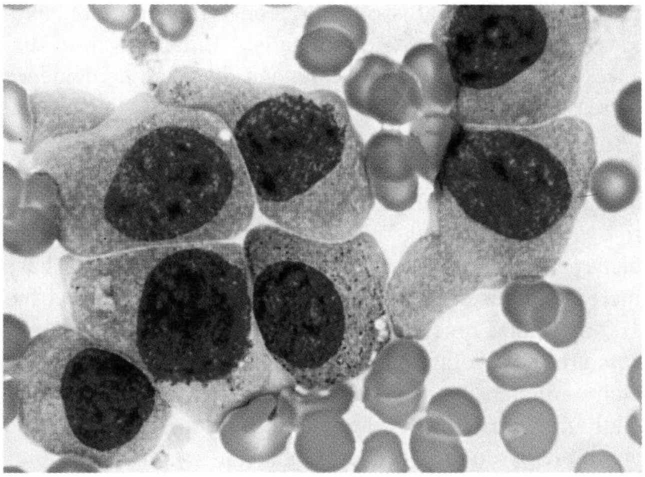

FIG. 27-10 Monoblasts from acute monoblastic leukemia. Monoblasts in a marrow smear from a patient with acute monoblastic leukemia (M5A). The monoblasts are larger than myeloblasts and usually have abundant cytoplasm, frequently with delicate scattered azurophilic granules. (From Damjanov I, Linder J, editors: *Anderson's pathology,* ed 10, St Louis, 1996, Mosby.)

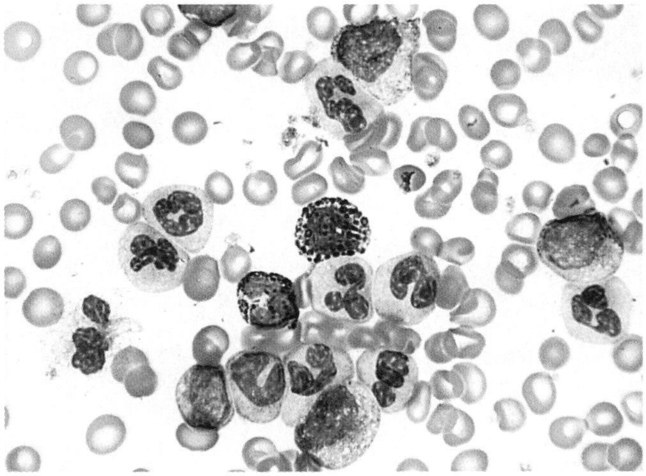

FIG. 27-11 Leukocytosis and basophilia in chronic myeloid leukemia. Blood smear from child with chronic myeloid leukemia showing marked leukocytosis and basophilia. Karyotype analysis identified a Philadelphia chromosome (Wright-Giemsa stain). (From Damjanov I, Linder J, editors: *Anderson's pathology,* ed 10, St Louis, 1996, Mosby.)

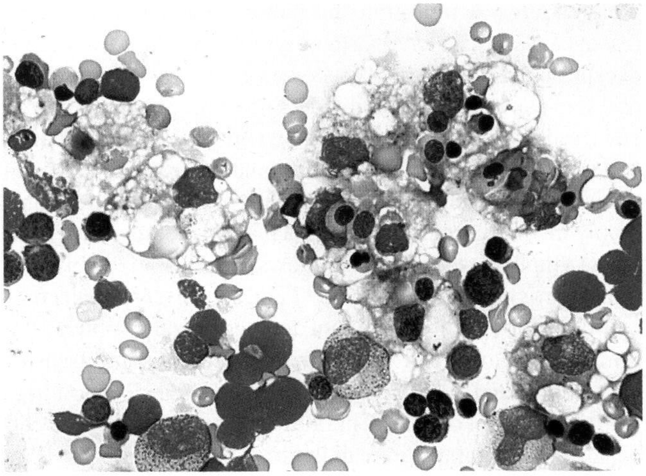

FIG. 27-12 Bone marrow aspirate from a child with T cell lymphoma in a lymph node biopsy. There is marked histiocytic hyperplasia. Two of the histiocytes contain phagocytosed red cells. The histiocytic hyperplasia regressed with disease remission and recurred with relapse of the lymphoma (Wright-Giemsa stain). (From Damjanov I, Linder J, editors: *Anderson's pathology,* ed 10, St Louis, 1996, Mosby.)

of choice for acute leukemia. In ALL, identification of various risk groups has led to the development of different intensities of drug protocols. Thus treatment is tailored specifically for a particular risk group. (Table 27-5 outlines the various prognostic factors for ALL that are considered in determining the degree of risk.)

Most ALL treatment programs have four distinct phases: (1) induction of remission, (2) preventive therapy for the CNS, (3) intensification (also called *consolidation*), and (4) maintenance. In remission induction, the goal is no clinical evidence of disease and a normal bone marrow biopsy result, which is achieved in 95% of children with ALL. Children with persistent leukemia at the end of 1 month of induction therapy have a dismal prognosis.[81] Prophylactic CNS treatment has included both chemotherapy and radiation in the past, but evidence increasingly has shown that this therapy, although effective in preventing CNS leukemia, adversely affects neurologic and intellectual function. A marked incidence of learning disabilities has been identified in children previously treated to prevent CNS disease.[82] New, less toxic treatment protocols are now being studied to deal with this problem.[83] Once remission is achieved, an intensification phase of treatment begins. This treatment is necessary because leukemic cells will continue to be present despite successful remission. Thus the goal of the intensification phase is to further decrease and eliminate the remaining leukemic cells. Intensification therapy often overlaps prophylactic CNS treatment. The final phase of initial treatment is called *maintenance therapy*. The goal of this phase is to maintain disease control. The optimal duration of maintenance therapy is not well defined, but it usually continues for 2.5 to 3 years. During maintenance therapy, intermittent "pulses" of new drugs may be given. Periods of intensified therapy are believed to minimize development of drug-resistant leukemic cells.

ALL is a curable disease. This prognosis is a dramatic reversal of the outlook for a child diagnosed with this disease 30 years ago, when ALL was uniformly fatal and the average survival time was only 2 to 3 months. Today, with prompt and appropriate treatment, 70% to 80% of children with ALL are cured. Those children with the more favorable early pre–B cell or CALLA-positive ALL have a survival rate of 90%.[84]

Prognostic factors in ANLL are not as well defined as they are for ALL because of the small number of affected children and their overall poor prognosis.[85] The goal of treatment for ANLL is similar to that of ALL except that much more aggressive chemotherapy is administered. With intensive chemotherapy, significant bone marrow suppression is necessary

Table 27-5 Prognostic Factors in Acute Lymphoblastic Leukemia (ALL)

Prognostic Factor	Better Prognosis	Worse Prognosis
*Age		
<2 yr or >10 yr		X
2–7 yr	X	
*Gender		
Male		X
Female	X	
*Initial white blood count		
>50,000/mm³		X
<10,000/mm³	X	
Race		
Black		X
White	X	
Morphology		
L_2 or L_3		X
L_1	X	
*Immunology		
T or B cell ALL		X
Early pre–B cell or common lymphocytic leukemia antigen (CALLA)	X	
Leukemic involvement		
Mediastinal mass		X
Central nervous system involvement at diagnosis		X
Splenic enlargement		X

*The four most reliable prognostic factors. Initial prognostic factors become less effective predictors with increasing length of remission. Age and gender are not significant after 15 months of continuous remission, and white blood count is not significant after 24 months of continuous remission.

but predisposes children to infection, bleeding, and anemia. The use of colony-stimulating factor (CSF), which stimulates the rapid proliferation of specific blood cell lines, is a recent advance that now shortens this period of bone marrow aplasia (CSFs are discussed in Chapter 24). Although initial remission is achieved relatively easily in all cases of ALL, successful and lasting remission can be achieved in only 70% to 80% of children with ANLL.[86] If remission is achieved, further treatment, called *continuation therapy*, is required. The specific intensity, timing, and length of continuation therapy are controversial. The use of either a stem cell or bone marrow transplantation (BMT) is an important treatment consideration in ANLL. Because long-term remission and cure of ANLL are difficult to achieve with chemotherapy alone, transplant often is recommended after the first remission is achieved. Transplant is the treatment of choice after relapse of ANLL. The long-term survival rate for children with ANLL, whether treated with chemotherapy or chemotherapy and BMT, is approximately 40%.[87]

Lymphomas

Non-Hodgkin lymphoma (NHL) and Hodgkin disease make up approximately 11% of all childhood cancer. Approximately 750 cases of childhood lymphoma are diagnosed in the United States annually.[57] Either group of diseases is rare before age 5 years, and the relative incidence increases throughout childhood. NHL is 1.5 times more common than Hodgkin disease in children. Boys are more likely to be diagnosed with a malignant lymphoma than are girls, and the high-risk groups have been identified. At particular risk are children with inherited or acquired immune deficiency syndromes. These children have been found to have increased rates of lymphoreticular cancers that range from 100 to 10,000 times the rate of normal children. The cancers are most commonly NHLs.[88] Children who are artificially immunosuppressed after organ transplantation, especially if cyclosporine is the immunosuppressive agent, also are at increased risk for lymphomas.

Non-Hodgkin Lymphoma

The classification of NHL has been confusing because of the heterogeneity of this group of diseases. Generally, most classification systems divide NHL into two categories, nodular or diffuse, on the basis of cellular pattern. Whereas one half of all adults with NHL have a nodular form of the disease, children rarely demonstrate this pattern. Nodular disease represents a less aggressive form of lymphoma. Almost without exception, childhood NHL becomes evident as a diffuse disease and can be further subdivided into three groups: (1) large cell (histiocytic), (2) lymphoblastic, and (3) small noncleaved cell (Burkitt or non-Burkitt lymphoma). Large cell NHL often involves chromosomal translocations. Disease sites commonly involve extranodal sites, such as brain, lung, bone, and skin. Lymphoblastic NHL also shows chromosomal translocations, particularly chromosome 7 and 14. Disease sites commonly include the mediastinum and peripheral lymph nodes. Small noncleaved cell NHL involves chromosome translocations of 8 and 14. It is believed that this translocation triggers the *c-myc* oncogene. Children with small noncleaved cell NHL commonly have intraabdominal disease at diagnosis.

An area of intensive study concerns the apparent biologic similarities of NHL and ALL in children. These two diseases are cytologically identical, and the histologic distinction between them is indicated by the degree of infiltration in the blood and bone marrow. The more bone marrow involvement and the less nodal and organ infiltration that are present, the more likely the disease is to be classified as ALL. Childhood NHL also is much more like ALL in its clinical manifestations and much less like Hodgkin disease or adult NHL.

As in ALL, immunophenotyping is an important part of the classification of childhood NHL. Almost 45% of the disease in children originates from T cells; an equal number originates from B cells. The remaining group, which represents 10% of childhood NHLs, is classified as non-T, non-B.

Pathogenesis

The origin of NHL in childhood is still elusive. Although defective host immunity is implicated in most children in whom NHL develops, an immune deficit cannot be identified. Viral etiology is suggested, but the role in development of human lymphoma is still unclear. The strongest correlation exists between EBV and African Burkitt lymphoma. This form of NHL is associated with a break point on chromosome 8 that is located near the *c-myc* oncogene.[89] The relationship between EBV infection and Burkitt lymphoma outside Africa is weak, however, even though the tumor is histopathologically and clinically indistinguishable. Chronic immunostimulation also has been suggested as a factor in the development of lymphomas because these diseases are seen more frequently when chronic persistent antigenic stimulation occurs from infection, such as malaria or intestinal parasites. Genetic susceptibility also may play a role in the process of malignant transformation. There is increased evidence of NHL in children with congenital immune deficiency syndromes, such as Wiskott-Aldrich syndrome, ataxia-telangiectasia, and Bloom syndrome. Children with acquired immunodeficiency syndrome (AIDS) also are at greater risk for NHL.[88,90] HIV-infected children who develop NHL may have already had a lymphoproliferative disorder such as lymphoid interstitial pneumonitis (LIP) or pulmonary lymphoid hyperplasia (PLH).

Clinical Manifestations

In children, NHL has been found to arise from any lymphoid tissue. Signs and symptoms therefore are specific for the site involved. Some children have such widespread involvement that no original site can be determined. Because childhood NHL is a rapidly progressive disease, symptoms generally are present only a few weeks before diagnosis is made. Rapidly enlarging lymphoid tissue and painless lymphadenopathy are common in about one third of children with abdominal sites of involvement, usually representing a gastrointestinal origin for the disease. Symptoms often include abdominal pain and vomiting, but a palpable mass is not always present. Most children with abdominal symptoms have diffuse, small noncleaved cell NHL (Burkitt or non-Burkitt) of B cell origin. If the tumor recurs, it appears again in the abdomen before distant spread.

The other frequent site of childhood NHL is the chest region. An anterior mediastinal mass, with or without pleural effusion, often is present. If the mass is large enough, respiratory compromise, tracheal compression, and superior vena cava syndrome may arise, which constitute a medical emergency. Children with anterior mediastinal involvement often are male adolescents and usually have diffuse lymphoblastic lymphoma of T cell origin. This form of diffuse lymphoblastic lymphoma often evolves into extensive bone marrow involvement and is considered to be an overt leukemic phase; therefore it is referred to as *leukemic transformation.* CNS involvement and testicular infiltration often then occur. CNS involvement occurs in about 30% of individuals with NHL, usually causing multiple deep-seated lesions within the brain parenchyma. In children with AIDS, NHL is the most common mass lesion found in the brain.[90]

Bone marrow involvement is less common than other primary sites, whereas CNS involvement is common. Relatively few children (10% to 20%) with NHL have lymphoid tissue involvement of the head and neck (Waldeyer ring, nasopharynx, sinuses). Signs and symptoms include tonsillitis, sinusitis, and a painless nasopharyngeal mass. In African Burkitt lymphoma, involvement of facial bones, particularly the jaw, is common, although this occurs infrequently in non-African cases.

Evaluation and Treatment

Diagnosis is made by biopsy of disease sites, usually the involved lymph nodes. Other sites of biopsy include the tonsils, bone marrow, spleen, liver, bowel, or skin. Advances in understanding the disease and progress in treatment strategies have meant that most children with NHL are cured of the disease. Optimal treatment is still being developed, but combination chemotherapy, with or without radiation therapy for prevention of CNS involvement, is being used successfully.[91] Treatment programs are based on the same four phases used in ALL. Radiation therapy may be combined with chemotherapy because lymphoma cells are easily destroyed by radiation. Because of the delay in diagnosis, CNS lymphomas are difficult to treat successfully. Intrathecal chemotherapy is needed in addition to systemic chemotherapy to induce remission.

Children with advanced small noncleaved cell lymphoma of the abdomen have the poorest prognosis. Although remission occurs in more than 90% of these children, most experience subsequent relapses. Even in the presence of advanced lymphoblastic lymphoma, however, 60% to 80% of children can be cured. Children with localized disease in more easily treated sites are likely to be cured with prompt and appropriate treatment. Overall, children with localized diseases have a 90% survival rate and those with advanced disease have a 70% to 80% survival rate.[91]

Hodgkin Disease

Although the etiologic agent for **Hodgkin disease,** a lymphoma, has not been identified in children, an infectious mode of transmission has been implicated. Major interest currently concerns viral activity, particularly in light of the association between the Epstein-Barr virus and African Burkitt lymphoma.[92] Many persons with Hodgkin disease have high EBV titers. At this time, however, the evidence is not sufficient to link EBV infection to Hodgkin disease.

The interest in a viral cause of Hodgkin disease has been supported by epidemiologic studies.[93-95] Childhood factors that might influence the time of exposure to an infectious agent were studied. A striking similarity between the epidemiology of Hodgkin disease in children and the prevaccine era of poliomyelitis supports the theory that Hodgkin disease may be the rare consequence of a common infection. Gutensohn[96] suggested that the pathogenesis of Hodgkin disease in children may differ from that of adults.

Clustering of cases within families may suggest a genetic predisposition to the disease or common exposure to a causative agent. In families where twins are concordant, elevated risk of Hodgkin disease ranges from threefold among first-degree relatives to sevenfold in siblings.[97]

Hodgkin disease is rare in childhood. It occurs infrequently in children younger than 2 years, and few cases are observed before age 5 years. A gradual rise in incidence occurs through age 11 years, with a marked increase through adolescence that continues into the thirties. The annual incidence of Hodgkin disease in the United States is 4 : 1,000,000 in children younger than 15 years.

Individuals typically have painless supraclavicular or cervical adenopathy. These nodes are firm and rubbery and may be sensitive to palpation if they have grown rapidly. At least two thirds of individuals have mediastinal involvement that may cause symptoms ranging from a nonproductive cough to trachael or bronchial compression leading to airway obstruction. Systemic symptoms may include fatigue, anorexia, weight loss, fever, drenching night sweats, and pruritis.

The Ann Arbor staging system considers extent and location of disease, as well as substage classifications that consider systemic symptoms (presence of fever of 38° C for three consecutive days, drenching night sweats, or unexplained loss of 10% or more of body weight in the six months preceding diagnosis). Combination chemotherapy used in conjunction with involved field low-dose radiation has been shown to be an effective treatment, with long-term cure rates reported from 70% to 90%.[98-100]

SUMMARY REVIEW

Fetal and Neonatal Hematopoiesis

1. After 2 weeks of gestation, circulating erythrocytes play a major role in delivering oxygen to the tissues.
2. Erythropoiesis in the liver and, to a lesser extent, in the spleen and lymph nodes reaches a peak at about 4 months.
3. By the fifth month of gestation, hematopoiesis begins to occur in the bone marrow, and by the time of delivery it is the only significant site of hematopoiesis.
4. A biochemically distinct type of hemoglobin is synthesized during fetal life, including Gower 1, Gower 2, and Portland.

Postnatal Changes in the Blood

1. Blood cells tend to rise above adult levels at birth and then decline gradually throughout childhood.
2. The immediate rise in blood cell counts is the result of increased hematopoiesis during fetal life, trauma of birth, and cutting of the umbilical cord.

Disorders of Erythrocytes

1. Iron deficiency anemia is the most frequent blood disorder of infancy and childhood; the highest incidence occurs between 6 months and 2 years of age.
2. Hemolytic disease of the newborn (HDN) results from incompatibility between the maternal and the fetal blood, which may involve differences in Rh factors or blood type (ABO). Maternal antibodies enter the fetal circulation and cause hemolysis of fetal erythrocytes. Because the immature liver is unable to conjugate and excrete the excess bilirubin that results from the hemolysis, icterus neonatorum or kernicterus or both can develop. Kernicterus, which also may result from other causes, causes increased breakdown of red blood cells or decreased liver output of enzymes.
3. Infections of the newborn, often acquired by the mother and transmitted to the infant, may result in hemolytic anemia.
4. Glucose-6-phosphate dehydrogenase (G6PD) deficiency is an inherited enzyme deficiency in erythrocytes that results in a disruption of a common pathway of glycolysis, shortening erythrocyte life span.
5. Hereditary spherocytosis is the most common of the hereditary hemolytic states in which there is no abnormality of hemoglobin. The basic defect is an undefined abnormality of the proteins or spectrins of the erythrocyte membrane in which affected cells are unduly permeable to sodium and acquire a characteristic structure.
6. Sickle cell disease is a genetically determined defect of hemoglobin synthesis, inherited by an autosomal recessive transmission and causing a change in the shape of a red blood cell that results in decreased oxygen or hydration. It is most common among Africans, black Americans, and those of Mediterranean descent.
7. The thalassemias are a heterogeneous group of hereditary hypochromic anemias of varying severity. Basic genetic defects include abnormalities of messenger ribonucleic acid (RNA) processing or deletion of genetic materials, resulting in a decrease in the chains for hemoglobin.

Disorders of Coagulation and Platelets

1. Hemophilia is a condition characterized by impairment of the coagulation of blood and subsequent tendency to bleed. The classic disease is hereditary and limited to males, being transmitted through the female to the second generation. Many similar conditions attributable to the absence of various clotting factors are now recognized.
2. Von Willebrand disease is a dominantly inherited disease characterized by a vascular abnormality that produces a prolongation of bleeding time and by decreased levels of clotting factor VIII. The platelets in von Willebrand disease have decreased adhesiveness because the plasma factor is absent.
3. Disorders of congenital hypercoagulability and thrombosis include protein C deficiency, protein S deficiency, neonatal purpura fulminans, and antithrombin III deficiency.
4. The acquired antibody-mediated hemorrhagic diseases include idiopathic thrombocytopenic purpura (ITP), autoimmune neonatal thrombocytopenia, and autoimmune vascular purpura.
5. ITP, the most common of the childhood thrombocytopenic purpuras, is a disorder of platelet consumption in which antiplatelet antibodies bind to the plasma membranes of platelets. This results in platelet sequestration and destruction by mononuclear phagocytes at a rate that exceeds the ability of the bone marrow to produce them.
6. Autoimmune neonatal thrombocytopenia is an antibody-mediated disorder that occurs in either autoimmune or alloimmune form.
7. The autoimmune vascular purpuras (allergic purpuras) are caused by the body's responses to allergens in the blood.

Leukemia and Lymphoma

1. The childhood leukemias include, in order of their rate of incidence, acute lymphoblastic, acute nonlymphoblastic, and the very rare chronic granulocytic leukemia.
2. Although the cause of childhood leukemia is not known, it is probably the result of multiple interactions between hereditary or genetic predisposition and environmental influences.
3. Acute lymphoblastic leukemia is a potentially curable disease, with more than 70% to 80% of cases cured.
4. The lymphomas of childhood are non-Hodgkin lymphoma and Hodgkin disease.
5. The origin of non-Hodgkin lymphoma is unknown. Factors that have been implicated include defective host immunity, a viral agent, chronic immunostimulation, and genetic predisposition.
6. Non-Hodgkin lymphoma has a favorable prognosis, with a 70% to 80% cure rate.
7. Hodgkin disease is thought to be caused by a yet unidentified etiologic agent.
8. Hodgkin disease is a readily curable disease with survival statistics similar to those of adults.

KEY TERMS

Activated partial thromboplastin time (PTT), *917*
Alpha-thalassemia major, *914*
Alpha-thalassemia minor, *914*
Alpha trait, *914*
Antithrombin III (AT III) deficiency, *918*
Aplastic crisis, *912*
Autoimmune neonatal thrombocytopenia, *919*
Autoimmune vascular purpura (allergic purpura), *919*
Beta-thalassemia major (Cooley anemia), *914*
Beta-thalassemia minor, *914*
Blast cell, *922*
Embryonic hemoglobin (Gower 1, Gower 2, and Portland), *901*
Fetal hemoglobin (Hb F), *901*
Glucose-6-phosphate dehydrogenase (G6PD) deficiency, *907*
Hemoglobin H disease, *914*
Hemoglobin S (Hb S), *908*
Hemolytic disease of the newborn (HDN) (erythroblastosis fetalis), *903*
Hemophilia A (classic hemophilia), *915*
Hemophilia B (Christmas disease), *915*
Hemophilia C (factor XI deficiency), *916*
Hereditary spherocytosis, *908*
Hodgkin disease, *925*
Hydrops fetalis, *905*
Hyperbilirubinemia, *905*
Hyperhemolytic crisis, *912*
Icterus gravis neonatorum, *905*
Icterus neonatorum (neonatal jaundice), *905*
Idiopathic thrombocytopenic purpura (ITP) (autoimmune or primary thrombocytopenic purpura), *918*
Kernicterus, *905*
Neonatal alloimmune thrombocytopenic purpura (NATP), *919*
Neonatal purpura fulminans, *918*
Non-Hodgkin lymphoma (NHL), *924*
Polymerization, *910*
Preimplantation genetic diagnosis, *913*
Protein C deficiency, *917*
Protein S deficiency, *918*
Prothrombin consumption time, *917*
Prothrombin time (PT), *917*
Sequestration crisis, *912*
Sickle cell anemia, *909*
Sickle cell disease, *908*
Sickle cell trait, *909*
Sickle cell–Hb C disease, *909*
Sickle cell–thalassemia, *909*
Thalassemia, *914*
Thrombin time, *917*
Thrombophilia, *917*
Thromboplastin generation, *917*
Vasoocclusive crisis (thrombotic crisis), *911*
von Willebrand disease, *916*

REFERENCES

1. Graham BS: Pathogenesis of respiratory syncytial virus vaccine-augmented pathology, *Am J Respir Crit Care Med* 152:563, 1995.
2. Schelonka RL et al: Differentiation of segmented and band neutrophils during the early newborn period, *J Pediatr* 127:298, 1995.
3. Caramihai E et al: Leukocyte count differences in healthy white and black children, *J Pediatr* 86:252, 1975.
4. Cunningham AS: Eosinophil counts—age and sex differences, *J Pediatr* 87:426, 1975.
5. Kuhne T, Imbach P: Neonatal platelet physiology and pathophysiology, *Eur J Pediatr* 157(2):97, 1998.
6. Looker AC et al: Prevalence of iron deficiency in the United States, *JAMA* 277(12):973, 1997.
7. Prasad AN, Prasad C: Iron deficiency: non-hematological manifestations, *Prog Food Nutr Sci* 15(4):255, 1991.
8. Farhi DC, Leubbers EL, Rosenthal NS: Bone marrow findings in childhood anemia: prevalence of transient erythroblastopenia of childhood, *Arch Pathol Lab Med* 122(7):638, 1998.
9. Lukens JN: Iron metabolism and iron deficiency. In Miller DR, Baehner RL, Miller LP, editors: *Blood diseases of infancy and childhood,* ed 7, St Louis, 1995, Mosby.
10. Nickerson HJ: Treatment of iron deficiency anemia and associated protein-losing enteropathy in children, *J Pediatr Hematol Oncol* 22(1): 50, 2000.
11. Bowman J: The management of hemolytic disease in the fetus and newborn, *Semin Perinatol* 21(1):39, 1997.
12. Urbaniak SJ: The scientific basis of antenatal prophylaxis, *Br J Obstet Gynaecol* 105(suppl 18):11, 1998.
13. Hampl JS et al: Acute hemolysis related to consumption of fava beans: a case study and medical nutrition therapy approach, *J Am Diet Assoc* 97(2):182, 1997.
14. Iolascon A et al: Hereditary spherocytosis: from clinical to molecular defects, *Haematologica* 83(3):240, 1998.
15. Delhommeau F et al: Natural history of hereditary spherocytosis during the first year of life, *Blood* 95(2):393, 2000.
16. Mankad VN: Sickle cell disease and other disorders of abnormal hemoglobin. In Miller DR, Baehner RL, Miller LP, editors: *Blood diseases of infancy and childhood,* ed 7, St Louis, 1995, Mosby.
17. Gill FM et al: Clinical events in the first decade of a cohort of infants with sickle cell disease: cooperative study of sickle cell disease, *Blood* 86:776, 1995.
18. Wigfall DR: Prevalence and clinical correlates of glomerulopathy in children with sickle cell disease, *J Pediatr* 136(6):749, 2000.

19. Wethers DL: Sickle cell disease in childhood: part I. Laboratory diagnosis, pathophysiology and health maintenance, *Am Fam Physician* 62(5):1013, 2000.
20. Platt OS: The acute chest syndrome of sickle cell disease, *N Engl J Med* 342(25):1904, 2000.
21. Wethers DL: Sickle cell disease in childhood: part II. Diagnosis and treatment of major complications and recent advances in treatment, *Am Fam Physician* 62(6):1309, 2000.
22. Beyer JE: Judging the effectiveness of analgesia for children and adolescents during vaso-occlusive events of sickle cell disease, *J Pain Symptom Manage* 19(1):63, 2000.
23. Okpala I: The management of crisis sickle cell disease, *Eur J Haematol* 60(1):1, 1998.
24. Caruso-Nicoletti M et al: Short stature and body proportion in thalassaemia, *J Pediatr Endocrinol Metab* 11(suppl 3):811, 1998.
25. Guy GP et al: An unusual complication in a gravida with factor IX deficiency: case report with review of the literature, *Obstet Gynecol* 80(3, pt 2):502, 1992.
26. Furie B, Furie BC: Molecular and cellular biology of blood coagulation, *N Engl J Med* 326(12):800, 1992.
27. Reitz M Jr et al: A retrovirus associated with human adult T-cell leukemia-lymphoma. In Magrath I, O'Conor G, Ramot B, editors: *Pathogenesis of leukemia and lymphomas: environmental influences,* New York, 1984, Raven Press.
28. Poolman H et al: When are children diagnosed as having severe haemophilia and when do they start to bleed? A 10-year single-centre PUP study, *Eur J Pediatr* 158(suppl 3):S166, 1999.
29. Roberts HR: Factor VIII replacement therapy: issues and future prospects, *Ann N Y Acad Sci* 614:106, 1991.
30. Ludlam CA: Viral safety of plasma-derived factor VIII and IX concentrates, *Blood Coagul Fibrinolysis* 8(suppl 1):S19, 1997.
31. Centers for Disease Control and Prevention: Transmission of hepatitis C virus infection associated with home infusion therapy for hemophilia, *Morb Mortal Wkly Rep* 46(26):597, 1997.
32. Chudy M: A new cluster of hepatitis A infection in hemophiliacs traced to a contaminated plasma pool, *J Med Virol* 57(2):91, 1999.
33. Soucie JM et al: Hepatitis A virus infections associated with clotting factor concentrate in the United States, *Transfusion* 38(6):573, 1998.
34. Woefel J: GB virus C/hepatitis G virus infection in HIV infected patients with haemophilia despite treatment with inactivated clotting factor concentrates, *Arch Dis Child* 80(5):429, 1999.
35. Astermark J et al: Primary prophylaxis in severe haemophilia should be started at an early age but can be individualized, *Br J Haematol* 105(4):1109, 1999.
36. Liesner RJ: Prophylaxis in haemophilic children, *Blood Coagul Fibrinolysis* 8(suppl 1):S7, 1997.
37. Spencer FA: Protein C, protein S and antithrombin deficiencies, *J Thromb Thrombolysis* 9(1):127, 2000.
38. Nizzi FA, Kaplan HS: Protein C and S deficiency, *Semin Thromb Hemostasis* 25(3):265, 1999.
39. Bick RL: Hypercoagulability and thrombosis, *Med Clin North Am* 78(3):635, 1994.
40. George JN, Raskob GE: Idiopathic thrombocytopenic purpura: a concise summary of the pathophysiology and diagnosis in children and adults, *Semin Hematol* 35(1):5, 1998.
41. Karpatkin S: Autoimmune thrombocytopenic purpura, *Blood* 56:329, 1981.
42. Lightsey AL, Koenig HM: Platelet associated immunoglobulin G in childhood idiopathic thrombocytopenic purpura, *J Pediatr* 94:20, 1979.
43. Winiarski J: Mechanisms in childhood idiopathic thrombocytopenic purpura (ITP), *Acta Paediatr Suppl* 424:54, 1998.
44. Bussel JB, Corrigan JJ: Platelet and vascular disorders. In Miller DR, Baehner RL, Miller LP, editors: *Blood diseases of infancy and childhood,* ed 7, St Louis, 1995, Mosby.
45. Carcao MD: Short-course oral prednisone therapy in children presenting with acute immune thrombocytopenia (ITP), *Acta Paediatr Suppl* 424:71, 1998.
46. Vesely S: Self-reported diagnostic and management strategies in childhood idiopathic thrombocytopenic purpura: results of a survey of practicing pediatric hematology/oncology specialists, *J Pediatr Hematol Oncol* 22(1):55, 2000.
47. Blancette V, Freeman J, Garvey B: Management of chronic immune thrombocytopenia purpura in children and adults, *Semin Hematol* 35(suppl 1):36, 1998.
48. Laosombat V: Intravenous gamma globulin for treatment of chronic idiopathic thrombycotopenic purpura in children, *J Med Assoc Thai* 83(2):160, 2000.
49. Frieberg A, Mauger D: Efficacy, safety, and dose response of intravenous anti-D immune globulin (WinRho SDF) for the treatment of idiopathic thrombocytopenic purpura in children, *Semin Hematol* 35(suppl 1):23, 1998.
50. Scaradavou A, Bussel JB: Clinical experience with anti-D in the treatment of idiopathic thrombocytopenic purpura, *Semin Hematol* 35(suppl 1):52, 1998.
51. Taratino MD: Treatment options for chronic immune (idiopathic) thrombocytopenia purpura in children, *Semin Hematol* 37(suppl 1): 35, 2000.
52. Dixon RH, Rosse WF: Platelet antibody in autoimmune thrombocytopenia, *Br J Haematol* 31:129, 1975.
53. Payne SD et al: Maternal characteristics and risk of severe neonatal thrombocytopenia and intracranial hemorrhage in pregnancies complicated by autoimmune thrombocytopenia, *Am J Obstet Gynecol* 177(1): 149, 1997.
54. Valat AS et al: Relationships between severe neonatal thrombocytopenia and maternal characteristics of pregnancies associated with autoimmune thrombocytopenia, *Br J Haematol* 103(2):397, 1998.
55. Hilgartner MW, Corrigan JJ Jr: Coagulation disorders. In Miller DR, Baehner RL, Miller LP, editors: *Blood diseases of infancy and childhood,* ed 6, St Louis, 1995, Mosby.
56. Margolin JF, Poplack DG: Acute lymphocytic leukemia. In Pizzo PA, Poplack DG, editors: *Principles and practices of pediatric oncology,* ed 3, Philadelphia, 1997, Lippincott-Raven.
57. Wingo PA et al: Annual report to the nation on the status of cancer, 1973-1996, with a special section on lung cancer and tobacco smoking, *J Natl Cancer Inst* 91(8):675, 1999.
58. Biondi A, Masera G: Molecular pathogenesis of childhood acute lymphoblastic leukemia, *Haematologica* 83(7):651, 1998.
59. Ma SK, Wan TS, Chan LC: Cytogenetics and molecular genetics of childhood leukemia, *Hematol Oncol* 17(3):91, 1999.
60. Strout MP, Caligiuri MA: Developments in cytogenetics and oncogenes in acute leukemia, *Curr Opin Oncol* 9(1):8, 1997.
61. Bennett J et al: French-American-British (FAB) Cooperative Group: the morphological classification of acute lymphoblastic leukaemia—concordance among observers and clinical correlations, *Br J Haematol* 47:553, 1981.
62. Khalidi HS et al: Acute lymphoblastic leukemia. Survey of immunophenotype, French-American-British classification, frequency of myeloid antigen expression, and karyotypic abnormalities in 210 pediatric and adult cases, *Am J Clin Pathol* 111(4):467, 1999.
63. Orafo A: Clinically useful information provided by the flow cytometric immunophenotyping of hematological malignancies: current status and future directions, *Clin Chem* 45(10):1708, 1999.
64. Golub TR, Weinstein HJ, Grier HE: Acute myelogenous leukemia. In Pizzo PA, Poplack DG, editors: *Principles and practices of pediatric oncology,* ed 3, Philadelphia, 1997, Lippincott-Raven.
65. McMahon B, Levy M: Prenatal origin of childhood leukemia: evidence from twins, *N Engl J Med* 270:1082, 1964.
66. Draper GJ, Heaf MM, Kennier-Wilson LM: Occurrence of childhood cancers among sibs and estimation of familial risks, *J Med Genet* 14: 81, 1977.
67. Miller RW: Persons with exceptionally high risk of leukemia, *Cancer Res* 27:2420, 1967.
68. Alexander FE, Greaves MF: Ionising radiation and leukaemia potential risks: review based on the workshop held during the 10th Symposium on Molecular Biology of Hematopoesis and Treatment of Leuke-

mia and Lymphomas at Hamburg Germany on 5 July 1998, *Leukemia* 12(8):1319, 1998.
69. Murray R, Heckel P, Hempelmann L: Leukemia in children exposed to ionizing radiation, *N Engl J Med* 261:585, 1959.
70. Doll R, Wakeford R: Risk of childhood cancer from fetal irradiation, *Br J Radiol* 70:130, 1997.
71. Boice JD, Miller RW: Childhood and adult cancer after intrauterine exposure to ionizing radiation, *Teratology* 59(4):227, 1999.
72. Axelson O: Cancer risk from exposure to radon in homes, *Environ Health Perspect* 103(S2):37, 1995.
73. Hardell L et al: Exposure to extremely low frequency electromagnetic fields and the risk of malignant diseases: an evaluation of epidemiological and experimental findings, *Eur J Cancer Prev* 4:3, 1995.
74. Levallois P: Do power frequency magnetic fields cause leukemia in children? *Am J Prev Med* 11:263, 1995.
75. Thomas DC et al: Residential magnetic fields predicted from wiring configurations: relationships to childhood leukemia, *Bioelectromagnetics* 20(7):414, 1999.
76. Petridou E: Electrical power lines and childhood leukemia: a study from Greece, *Int J Cancer* 73(3):345, 1997.
77. Pool R: Is there an EMF-cancer connection? *Science* 249:1096, 1990.
78. Savitz DA, John EM, Kleckner RC: Magnetic field exposure from electrical appliances and childhood cancer, *Am J Epidemiol* 131:763, 1990.
79. Waller LA et al: Detection and assessment of clusters of disease: an application to nuclear power plant facilities and childhood leukemia in Sweden, *Stat Med* 14:3, 1995.
80. Lagakos SW, Wessen BJ, Zelen M: An analysis of contaminated well water and health effects in Woburn, Massachusetts, *J Am Stat Assoc* 81: 583, 1986.
81. Siverman LB et al: Induction failure in acute lymphoblastic leukemia of childhood, *Cancer* 85(6):1395, 1999.
82. Koh S et al: Anterior lumbosacral radiculopathy after intrathecal methotrexate treatment, *Pediatr Neurol* 21(2):576, 1999.
83. Hodgson PS: The neurotoxicity of drugs given intrathecally (spinal), *Anesth Analg* 88(4):797, 1999.
84. Crist W et al: Clinical and biological features predict poor prognosis, *Med Pediatr Oncol* 13:135, 1986.
85. Grier HE et al: Prognostic factors in childhood acute myelogenous leukemia, *J Clin Oncol* 5:1026, 1987.
86. Buckley JD et al: Remission induction in children with acute nonlymphocyte leukemia using cytosine arabinoside and doxorubicin or daunorubicin: a report from the Children's Cancer Study Group, *Med Pediatr Oncol* 17:382, 1989.
87. Krischer JP et al: Long-term results in the treatment of acute nonlymphocytic leukemia: a pediatric oncology group study, *Med Pediatr Oncol* 17:401, 1989.
88. Granovsky MO: Cancer in human immunodeficiency virus–infected children: a case series from the Children's Cancer Group and the National Cancer Institute, *J Clin Oncol* 16(5):1729, 1998.
89. Magrath IT: Malignant non-Hodgkin's lymphoma in children, *Hematol Oncol Clin North Am* 1:577, 1987.
90. Mueller BU, Pizzo PA: Cancer in children with primary or secondary immunodeficiencies, *J Pediatr* 126:1, 1995.
91. Shad A, Mcgrath I: Malignant non-Hodgkin's lymphomas in children. In Pizzo PA, Poplack DG, editors: *Principles and practices of pediatric oncology,* ed 3, Philadelphia, 1997, Lippincott-Raven.
92. Hudson MM, Donaldson SS: Hodgin's disease. In Pizzo PA, Poplack DG, editors: *Principles and practices of pediatric oncology,* ed 3, Philadelphia, 1997, Lippincott-Raven.
93. Gutensohn N, Cole P: Childhood social environment and Hodgkin's disease, *N Engl J Med* 304:135, 1981
94. Gutensohn N, Shapiro D: Social class risk factors among children with Hodgkin's disease, *Int J Cancer* 30:433, 1982.
95. Michels KB: The origins of Hodgkin's disease, *Eur J Cancer Prev* 4: 379, 1995.
96. Gutensohn N: Social class and age at diagnosis of Hodgkin's disease: new epidemiologic evidence for the "two-disease hypothesis," *Cancer Treat Resp* 66:689, 1982.
97. Mack TM et al: Concordance for Hodgkin's disease in identical twins suggesting genetic susceptibility to the young-adult form of the disease, *N Engl J Med* 332:413, 1995.
98. Fryer CJ et al: Efficacy and toxicity of 12 courses of ABVD followed by low-dose regional radiation in advanced Hodgkin's disease in children: a report from the Children's Cancer Study Group, *J Clin Oncol* 8:1971, 1990.
99. Hudson MM et al: Efficacy and toxicity of multi-agent chemotherapy and low-dose involved-field radiotherapy in children and adolescents with Hodgkin's disease, *J Clin Oncol* 11:100, 1993.
100. Schellong G, Bramswig JH, Hornig-Franz I: Treatment of children with Hodgkin's disease: results of the German Pediatric Oncology Group, *Ann Oncol* 3:1591, 1992.

CHAPTER 28

Structure and Function of the Cardiovascular and Lymphatic Systems

KATHRYN L. McCANCE

CHAPTER OUTLINE

The function of the circulatory system is simple: to deliver oxygen, nutrients, and other substances to all the body's cells and to remove the waste products of cellular metabolism. Delivery and removal are achieved by a wonderfully complex array of tubing—the blood vessels—connected to a pump—the heart. The heart pumps blood continuously through the blood vessels with cooperation from other systems, particularly the nervous and endocrine systems, which are intrinsic regulators of the heart and blood vessels. Nutrients and oxygen are supplied by the digestive and respiratory systems; gaseous wastes of cellular metabolism are blown off by the lungs; and other wastes are removed by the kidneys.

New and evolving is the role of the vascular endothelium. It is a multifunctional organ whose health is essential to normal vascular physiology and whose dysfunction is a critical factor in the pathogenesis of vascular disease.

CIRCULATORY SYSTEM

The heart pumps blood through two separate circulatory systems, one to the lungs and one to all other parts of the body.

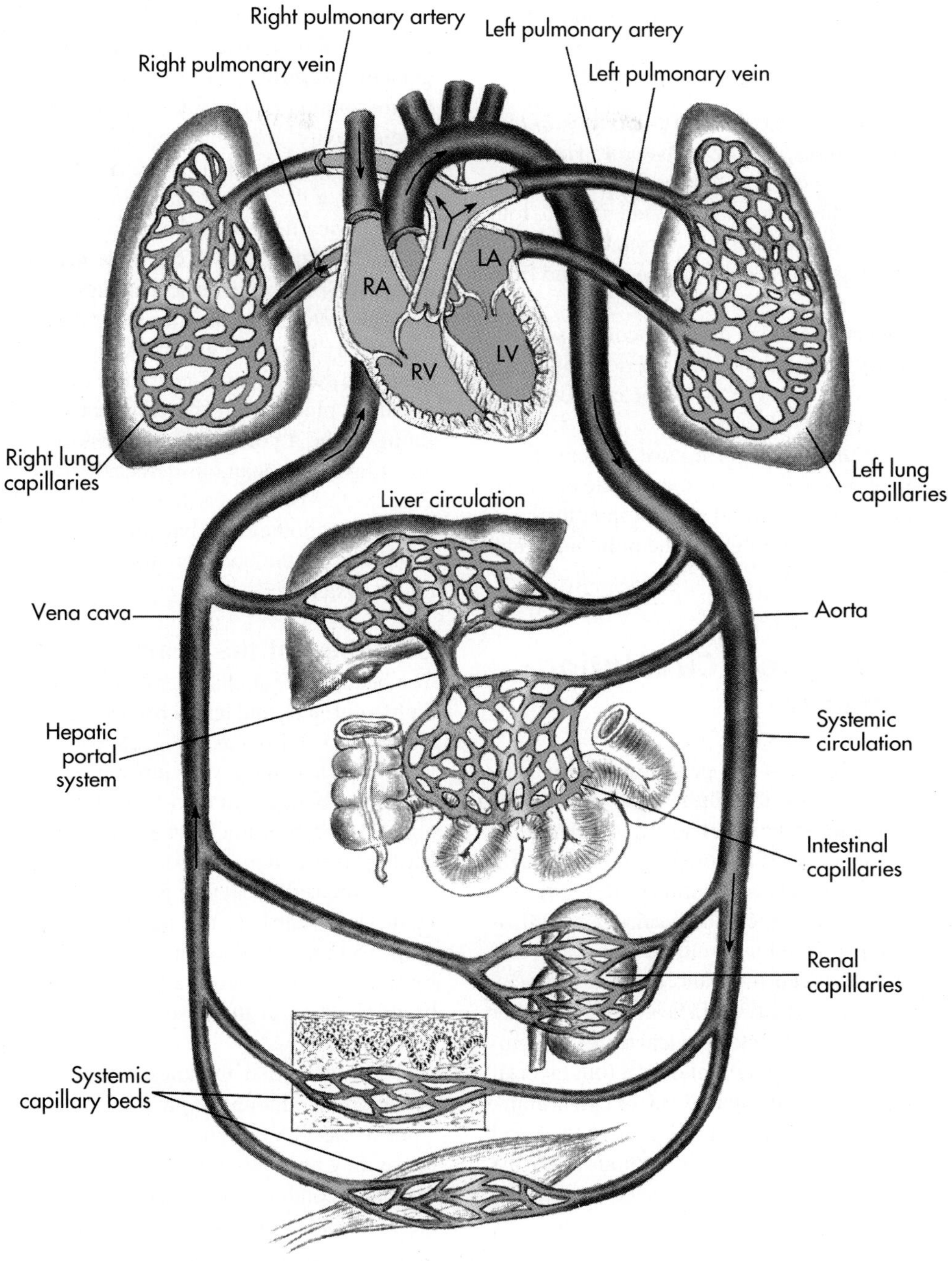

FIG. 28-1 Diagram showing serially connected pulmonary and systemic circulatory systems. Right heart chambers propel unoxygenated blood through pulmonary circulation, while left heart propels oxygenated blood through systemic circulation.

Structures on the right side of the heart, or **right heart,** pump blood through the lungs. (This system, termed the **pulmonary circulation,** is described in Chapter 31.) The left side of the heart, or **left heart,** sends blood throughout the **systemic circulation,** which supplies all of the body except the lungs (Fig. 28-1). These two systems are serially connected; thus the output of one becomes the input of the other.

Arteries carry blood from the heart to all parts of the body, where they branch into even smaller vessels until they become a fine meshwork of capillaries. Capillaries allow the closest contact and exchange between the blood and the interstitial space, or interstitium—the environment in which the cells live. Veins channel blood from capillaries in all parts of the body back to the heart. The plasma passes through the walls of the capillaries into the interstitial space. This fluid eventually is returned to the cardiovascular system by vessels of the lymphatic system.

THE HEART

The adult heart weighs less than 1 pound and is about the size of a fist. It lies obliquely (diagonally) in the **mediastinum,** an area above the diaphragm and between the lungs. The heart of a normal woman is smaller and lighter than that of a normal man.

Heart structures can be categorized by function:

1. *Structural support of heart tissues and circulation of pulmonary and systemic blood through the heart.* This category includes the heart wall and fibrous skeleton, which enclose and support the heart and divide it into four chambers; the valves that direct flow through the chambers; and the great vessels that conduct blood to and from the heart.
2. *Maintenance of heart cells.* This category comprises vessels of the coronary circulation—the arteries and veins that serve the metabolic needs of all the heart cells—and the lymphatic vessels of the heart.
3. *Stimulation and control of heart action.* Among these structures are the nerves and specialized muscle cells that direct the rhythmic contraction and relaxation of the heart muscles, propelling blood throughout the pulmonary and systemic circulatory system.

Structures That Direct Circulation through the Heart

Heart Wall

The heart wall has three layers—the pericardium, myocardium, and endocardium. The **pericardium** is a double-walled membranous sac that encloses the heart (Fig. 28-2). The pericardium has several functions. It (1) prevents displacement of the heart during gravitational acceleration or deceleration, (2) is a physical barrier that protects the heart against infection and inflammation from the lungs and pleural space, and (3) contains pain receptors and mechanoreceptors that can elicit reflex changes in blood pressure and heart rate. The outer layer of the pericardium, the **parietal pericardium,** is composed of a surface layer of mesothelium over a thin layer of connective tissue. The **visceral pericardium,** or epicardium, is the inner layer of the pericardium. At one point the visceral pericardium folds back and becomes continuous with the parietal pericardium, allowing the large vessels to enter and leave the heart without breaching the pericardial layers.

The visceral and parietal pericardia are separated by a fluid-containing space called the **pericardial cavity.** The **pericardial fluid** (10 to 30 ml), which is secreted by cells of the mesothelium, lubricates the membranes that line the pericardial cavity, enabling them to slide over one another with a minimum of friction as the heart beats. The amount and character of the pericardial fluid are altered by inflammation of the pericardium (see Chapter 29).

The thickest layer of the heart wall, the **myocardium,** is composed of cardiac muscle and is anchored to the heart's fibrous skeleton. The thickness of the myocardium varies tremendously from one heart chamber to another. Thickness is related to the amount of resistance the muscle must overcome to pump blood from the different chambers. The internal lining of the myocardium is composed of connective tissue and a layer of squamous cells called the **endocardium** (see Fig. 28-2). The endocardial lining of the heart is continuous with the endothelium that lines all the arteries, veins, and capillaries of the body, creating a continuous, closed circulatory system.

Chambers of the Heart

The heart has four chambers: the **right atrium, left atrium, right ventricle,** and **left ventricle.** (Blood flow through these chambers is illustrated in Fig. 28-3.) The atria are smaller than the ventricles and have thinner walls. The wall of the right atrium is about 2 mm thick, and the wall of the left atrium is about 3 to 5 mm thick. The ventricles have a thicker myocardial layer and make up much of the bulk of the heart. The wall of the right ventricle is about 3 to 5 mm thick, and that of the left ventricle, the most muscular chamber, is about 13 to 15 mm. It is now known that the ventricles are formed by a continuum of muscle fibers that take origin from the fibrous skeleton at the base of the heart (chiefly around the aortic orifice).[1]

The myocardial thickness of each cardiac chamber depends on the amount of pressure or resistance it must overcome to eject blood. The two atria have the thinnest walls because they are low-pressure chambers that serve as storage units and conduits for blood that is emptied into the ventricles. Normally, there is little resistance to flow from the atria

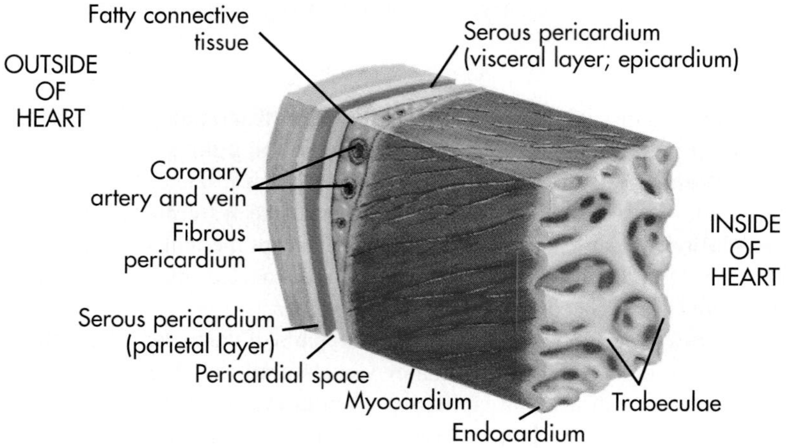

FIG. 28-2 Wall of the heart. This section of the heart wall shows the fibrous pericardium, the parietal and visceral layers of the serous pericardium (with the pericardial space between them), the myocardium, and the endocardium. Note the fatty connective tissue between the visceral layer of the serous pericardium (epicardium) and the myocardium. Note also that the endocardium covers beamlike projections of myocardial muscle tissue, called *trabeculae.* (From Thibodeau GA, Patton KI: *Anatomy and physiology,* ed 4, St Louis, 1999, Mosby.)

to the ventricles. The ventricles, on the other hand, must propel blood all the way through the pulmonary or systemic circulation. The ventricular myocardium must also be strong enough to pump against pressures in the pulmonary or systemic vessels. The mean pulmonary capillary pressure, which is the major force favoring movement of fluid out of the pulmonary capillaries into the interstitium, is only 15 mm Hg. By comparison, the mean arterial pressure is about 92 mm Hg. Pressure is greatest in the systemic circulation, driven by the left ventricle; the left ventricle's myocardium is several times thicker than that of the right ventricle.

The right ventricle is shaped like a crescent, or triangle, enabling it to function like a bellows and efficiently eject large volumes of blood through a very small valve into the low-pressure pulmonary system. The left ventricle is larger and bullet shaped, helping it to eject blood through a relatively large valve opening into the high-pressure systemic circulation.

The ventricles are structurally more complex than the atria. Each ventricle contains muscle fibers that divide it roughly into an **inflow tract,** which receives blood from the atrium, and an **outflow tract,** which sends blood to the circulation (see Fig. 28-3).

Normally, blood does not flow between the chambers of the right side of the heart and the chambers of the left side of the heart. The adult right and left sides of the heart are separated by an intact septal membrane. The atria are separated by the interatrial septum, and the ventricles by the interventricular septum. The interventricular septum is an extension of the fibrous skeleton of the heart. Indentations of the endocardium form valves that separate the atria from the ventricles and the ventricles from the aorta and pulmonary arteries.

Fibrous Skeleton of the Heart

Four rings of dense fibrous connective tissue provide a firm anchorage for the attachments of the atrial and ventricular musculature, as well as the valvular tissue. The fibrous rings are adjacent and form a central, fibrous supporting structure collectively termed the *anuli fibrosi cordis.*

Valves of the Heart

One-way blood flow through the heart is ensured by the four heart valves. During ventricular relaxation the two **atrioventricular valves** open and blood flows from the higher-pressure atria to the relaxed ventricles. With increasing ventricular pressure these valves close and prevent backflow into the atria as the ventricles contract. The **semilunar valves** of the heart open when intraventricular pressure exceeds aortic and pulmonary pressures and blood flows out of the ventricles and into the pulmonary and systemic circulations. After ventricular contraction and ejection, intraventricular pressure falls and the **pulmonic** and **aortic semilunar valves** close, preventing backflow into the right and left ventricles (Fig. 28-4; see also Fig. 28-3).

The heart valve openings are guarded by flaps of tissue called *leaflets* or *cusps* that are attached to the papillary muscles by the **chordae tendineae** (see Fig. 28-3). The **papillary muscles** are extensions of the myocardium that pull the cusps

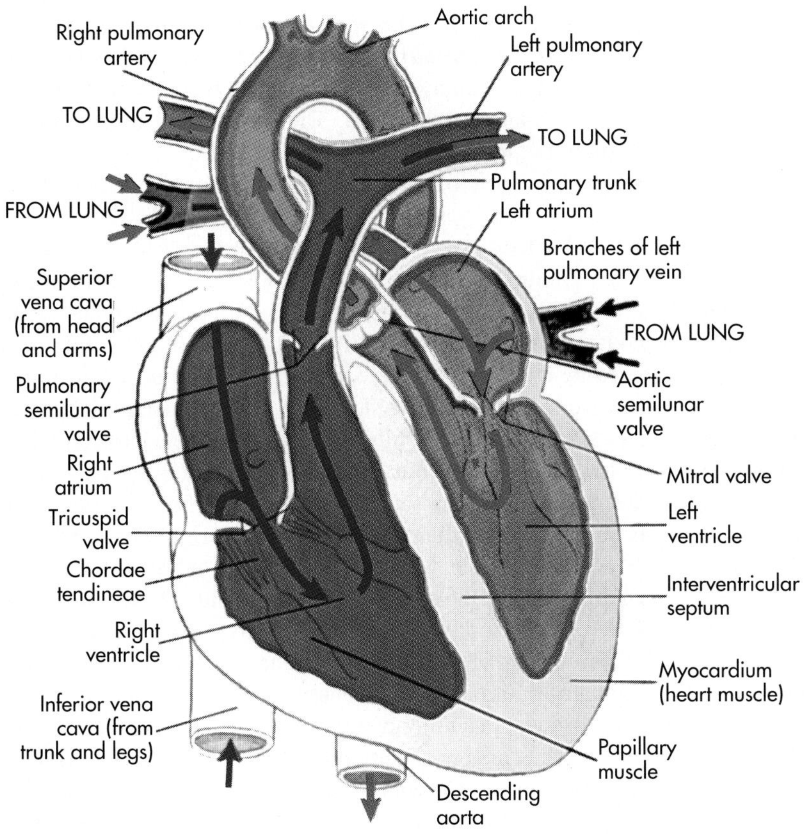

FIG. 28-3 Structures that direct blood flow through the heart. *Arrows* indicate path of blood flow through chambers, valves, and major vessels. (Modified from Thibodeau GA: *Anatomy and physiology,* St Louis, 1987, Mosby.)

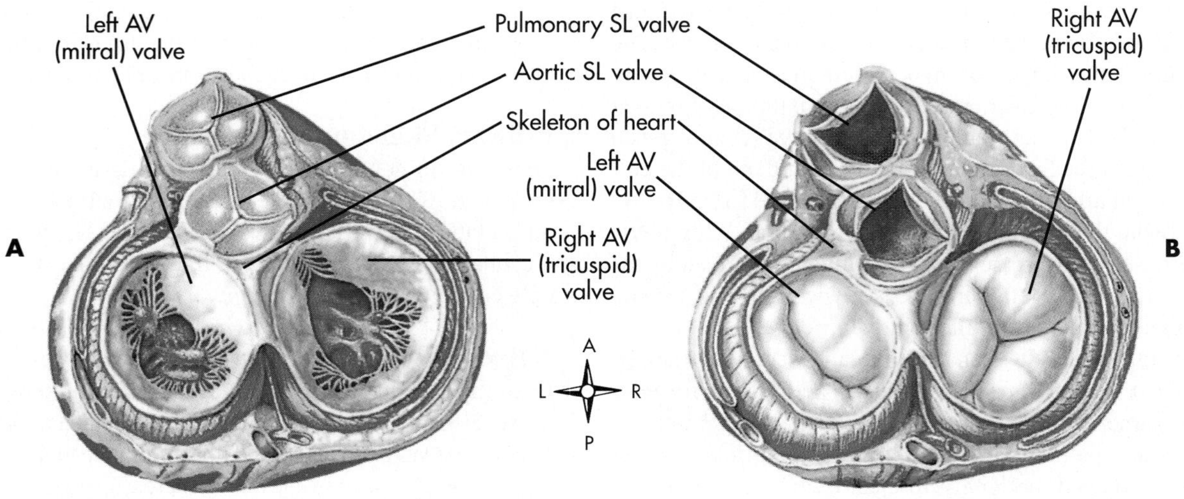

FIG. 28-4 Structure of the heart valves. A, The heart valves in this drawing are depicted as viewed from above (looking down into the heart). Note that the semilunar *(SL)* valves are closed and the atrioventricular *(AV)* valves are open, as when the atria are contracting. **B,** Similar to **A** except that the semilunar valves are closed and the atrioventricular valves are open, as when the ventricles are contracting. (From Thibodeau GA, Patton KI: *Anatomy and physiology,* ed 4, St Louis, 1999, Mosby.)

together and downward at the onset of ventricular contraction, thus preventing their backward expulsion into the atria. (See p. 935 for a description of pressure changes and valvular function.)

The right atrioventricular valve is called the **tricuspid valve** because it has three cusps. The tricuspid opening (orifice) has the largest diameter of all the heart valves. The left atrioventricular valve is a bicuspid (two-cusp) valve called the **mitral valve.** The mitral valve resembles a cone-shaped funnel that extends into the cusps, which are connected by a fibrous tissue called the *commissure.* The anterior cusp of the mitral valve is continuous with supporting tissues of the aortic semilunar valve cusps and the left coronary valve cusps. (The coronary circulation is described on p. 936.) Thus damage to this continuous tissue can alter function of both the aortic and mitral valves.

The tricuspid and mitral valves function as a unit because the atrium, fibrous rings, valvular tissue, chordae tendineae, papillary muscles, and ventricular walls are connected. Collectively, these six structures are known as the **mitral and tricuspid complex.** Damage to any one of the complex's six components can alter function significantly.

Blood leaves the right ventricle through the pulmonic semilunar valve, and it leaves the left ventricle through the aortic semilunar valve (see Figs. 28-3 and 28-4). Both the pulmonic and aortic semilunar valves have three cup-shaped cusps that arise from the fibrous skeleton. The pulmonic cusps are slightly thinner than the aortic cusps. The lower edges of each cusp are suspended from the root of the pulmonary artery or aorta, with the upper valve edges freely projecting into the vessel lumen. When the ventricles contract, the cusps behave like one-way swinging doors. The force of the blood propels the cusps outward against the vessel wall. When the ventricles relax, blood fills the cusps and causes their free edges to meet in the middle of the vessel, closing the valve and preventing any backflow.

Great Vessels

Blood moves in and out of the heart through several large vessels (see Fig. 28-3). The right heart receives venous blood from the systemic circulation through the **superior** and **inferior venae cavae,** which enter the right atrium. Blood leaves the right ventricle and enters the pulmonary circulation through the **pulmonary artery.** The pulmonary artery divides into **right** and **left pulmonary arteries** to transport unoxygenated blood from the right heart to the right and left lungs. The pulmonary arteries branch further into the pulmonary capillary bed, where oxygen and carbon dioxide exchange occurs.

The four **pulmonary veins,** two from the right lung and two from the left lung, carry oxygenated blood from the lungs to the left side of the heart. The oxygenated blood moves through the left atrium and ventricle and out into the **aorta,** which delivers it to systemic vessels that supply the body.

Blood Flow during the Cardiac Cycle

The pumping action of the heart consists of contraction and relaxation of the myocardial layer of the heart wall. Each contraction and the relaxation that follows it constitute one **cardiac cycle.** (Blood flow through the heart during a single cardiac cycle is illustrated in Fig. 28-5.) During relaxation, termed **diastole,** blood fills the ventricles. The contraction that follows, termed **systole,** propels the blood out of the ventricles and into the circulation. Contraction of the left ventricle is slightly earlier than contraction of the right ventricle.

During diastole, blood from the veins of the systemic circulation enters the thin-walled right atrium from the superior vena cava and the inferior vena cava (see Figs. 28-3 and 28-5). Venous blood from the coronary circulation enters the right atrium through the coronary sinus. The right atrium fills and distends, pushing open the right atrioventricular (tricuspid) valve. This permits blood to fill the right ventricle. The same sequence of events occurs a split second earlier in the left heart. The four pulmonary veins, two from the right lung

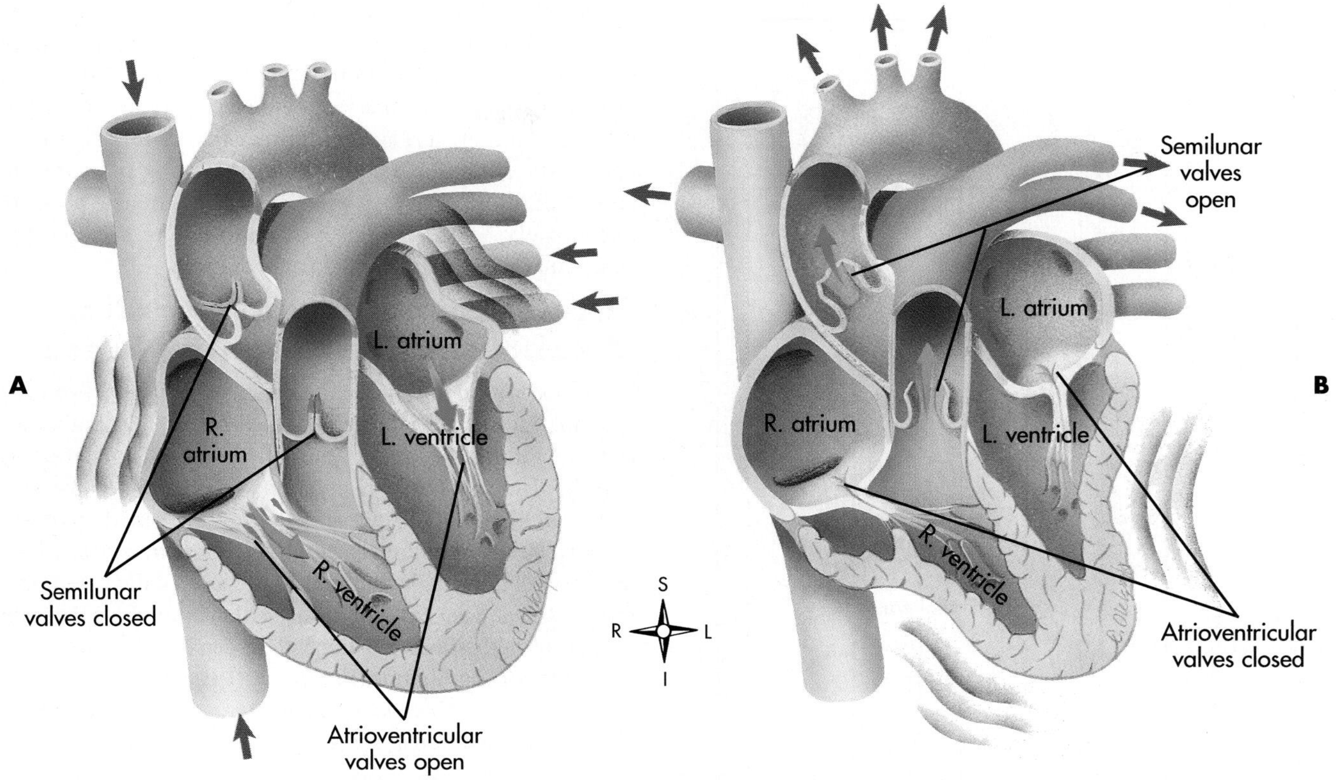

FIG. 28-5 Chambers and valves of the heart. These illustrations depict the action of the heart chambers and valves when the atria contract **(A)** and when the ventricles contract **(B).** (From Thibodeau GA, Patton KI: *Anatomy and physiology,* ed 4, St Louis, 1999, Mosby.)

and two from the left lung, carry blood from the pulmonary circulation to the left atrium. As the left atrium fills, it pushes the cusps of the mitral valve open and blood flows into the left ventricle. Left atrial contraction, "atrial kick," provides a significant increase of blood to the left ventricle. Filling of the right and left sides of the heart occurs during one period of diastole.

Four phases of the cardiac cycle can be identified on initiation of ventricular myocardial contraction (Fig. 28-6):

Phase 1: Systole begins with "isovolumic contraction," so-called because ventricular volume is constant; that is, the lengths of the muscle fibers remain relatively constant. Isovolumic contraction is the first detectable rise in left ventricular pressure. Contraction pushes the atrioventricular valves shut. Their cusps bulge backward but are prevented from opening back into the atria by their anchors, the chordae tendineae (see Fig. 28-3).

Phase 2: When left ventricular pressure reaches that of the aorta, the aortic valve opens and ventricular ejection occurs. Intraventricular pressure and ventricular volume decrease rapidly.

Phase 3: With left ventricular relaxation and decreased ventricular pressure, the aortic valve closes and "isovolumic relaxation" occurs.

Phase 4: When sufficient decreases exist in left ventricular pressure, the mitral valve opens and ventricular filling from the atrium occurs.

Table 28-1 Normal Intracardiac Pressures

	Mean (mm Hg)	Range (mm Hg)
Right atrium	4	0-8
Right ventricle		
Systolic	24	15-28
End-diastolic	4	0-8
Left atrium	7	4-12
Left ventricle		
Systolic	130	90-140
End-diastolic	7	4-12

The ventricle fills rapidly in early diastole and again in late diastole when the atrium contracts. As blood is pushed through the inflow and outflow tracts of the ventricles, it flows around the **crista supraventricularis**—the muscle that separates the inflow from the outflow tracts—and is mixed by passing through the strands of the **trabeculae carneae.** Expulsion of blood from the ventricles marks the end of one cardiac cycle.

Normal Intracardiac Pressures

Normal intracardiac pressures are shown in Table 28-1 and Figs. 28-6 and 28-7. Atrial pressure curves are composed of the **a wave,** which is generated by atrial contraction, and the **v wave,** which is an early diastolic peak caused by filling of the atrium from the peripheral veins. The **x descent** follows the a wave and is produced because of descent of the tricuspid valve ring and by the ejection of blood from both ventricles.

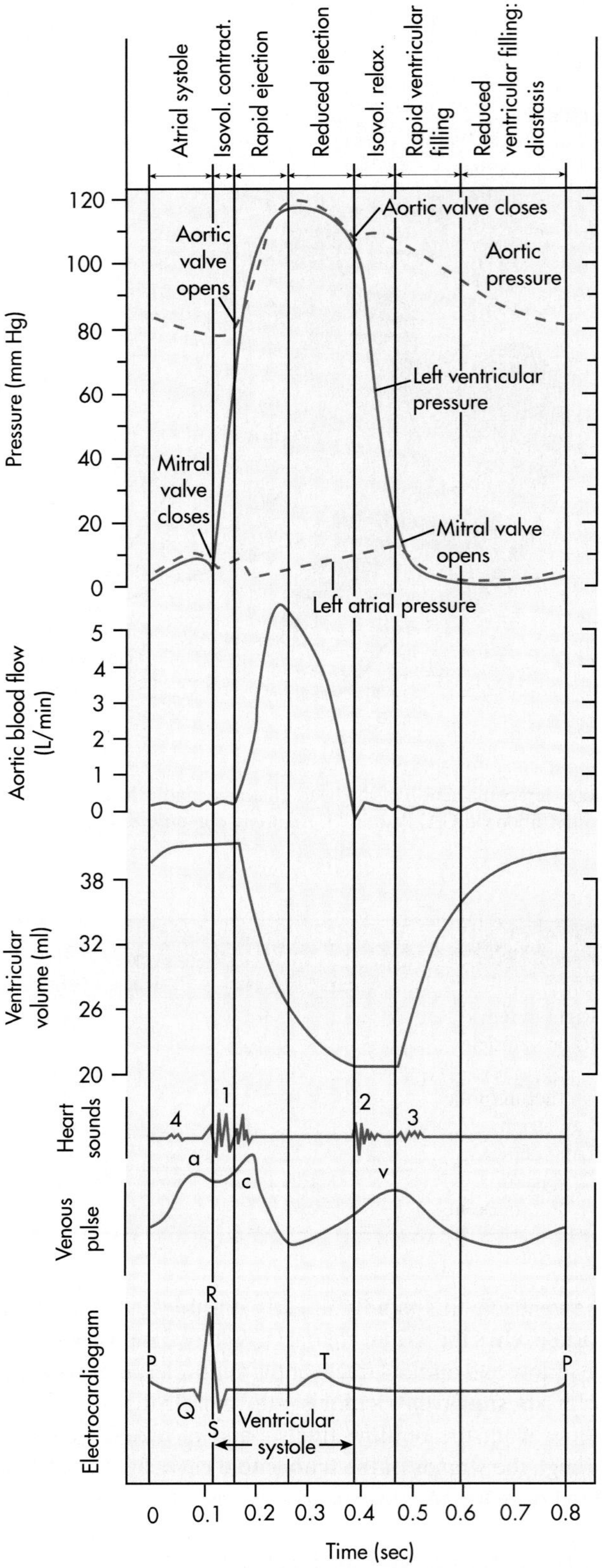

FIG. 28-6 Major phases of cardiac cycle. Schematic at top shows four major phases of cardiac cycle. Left atrial, aortic, and left ventricular pressure pulses correlated in time with aortic flow, ventricular volume, heart sounds, venous pulse, and electrocardiogram for a complete cardiac cycle in the dog. (From Berne RM, Levy MN: *Principles of physiology,* ed 3, St Louis, 2000, Mosby.)

The **y descent** follows the v wave and reflects the rapid flow of blood from the great veins and right atrium into the right ventricle. A small deflection, the **c wave,** occurs after the a wave in early systole and may represent bulging of the mitral valve into the left atrium during early systole. Ventricular pressures are illustrated by a peak systolic pressure and an end-diastolic pressure, which is the ventricular pressure immediately before the onset of systole. The minimal left ventricular pressure occurs in early diastole.

Structures That Support Cardiac Metabolism: The Coronary Vessels

The blood within the heart chambers does not supply oxygen and other nutrients to the cells of the heart. Like all other organs, including the lungs, heart structures are nourished by vessels of the systemic circulation. The branch of the systemic circulation that supplies the heart is termed the **coronary circulation** and consists of **coronary arteries,** which receive blood through openings in the aorta called the **coronary ostia,** and the **cardiac veins,** which empty into the right atrium through another ostium, the opening of a large vein called the **coronary sinus** (Fig. 28-8). (Regulation of the coronary circulation, which is similar to regulation of flow through systemic and pulmonary vessels, is described elsewhere.)

Coronary Arteries

The major coronary arteries are the **right coronary artery** and the **left coronary artery** (see Fig. 28-8). These arteries traverse the epicardium and branch several times. The pattern of branching through the visceral pericardium differs from heart to heart. The branches enter the myocardium and endocardium and branch further to become arterioles and then capillaries. Although the coronary arteries are smaller in women than men, this is attributable to differences in heart weight.

The left coronary artery arises from a single ostium (opening) behind the left cusp of the aortic semilunar valve. This artery ranges from a few millimeters to a few centimeters in length. It passes between the left atrial appendage and the pulmonary artery and generally divides into two branches—the left anterior descending artery and the circumflex artery. Other branches of the left main coronary artery are distributed diagonally across the free wall of the left ventricle.

The **left anterior descending artery,** also called the *anterior interventricular artery,* delivers blood to portions of the left and right ventricles and much of the interventricular septum. The left anterior descending artery travels down the anterior surface of the interventricular septum toward the apex of the heart.

The **circumflex artery** travels in a groove called the **coronary sulcus,** which separates the left atrium from the left ventricle, to the left border of the heart (see Fig. 28-8). It supplies blood to the left atrium and the lateral wall of the left ventricle. The circumflex artery often branches to the posterior surfaces of the left atrium and left ventricle (see Fig. 28-8).

The right coronary artery originates from an ostium behind the right aortic cusp, travels behind the pulmonary artery, and extends around the right heart to the heart's posterior surface,

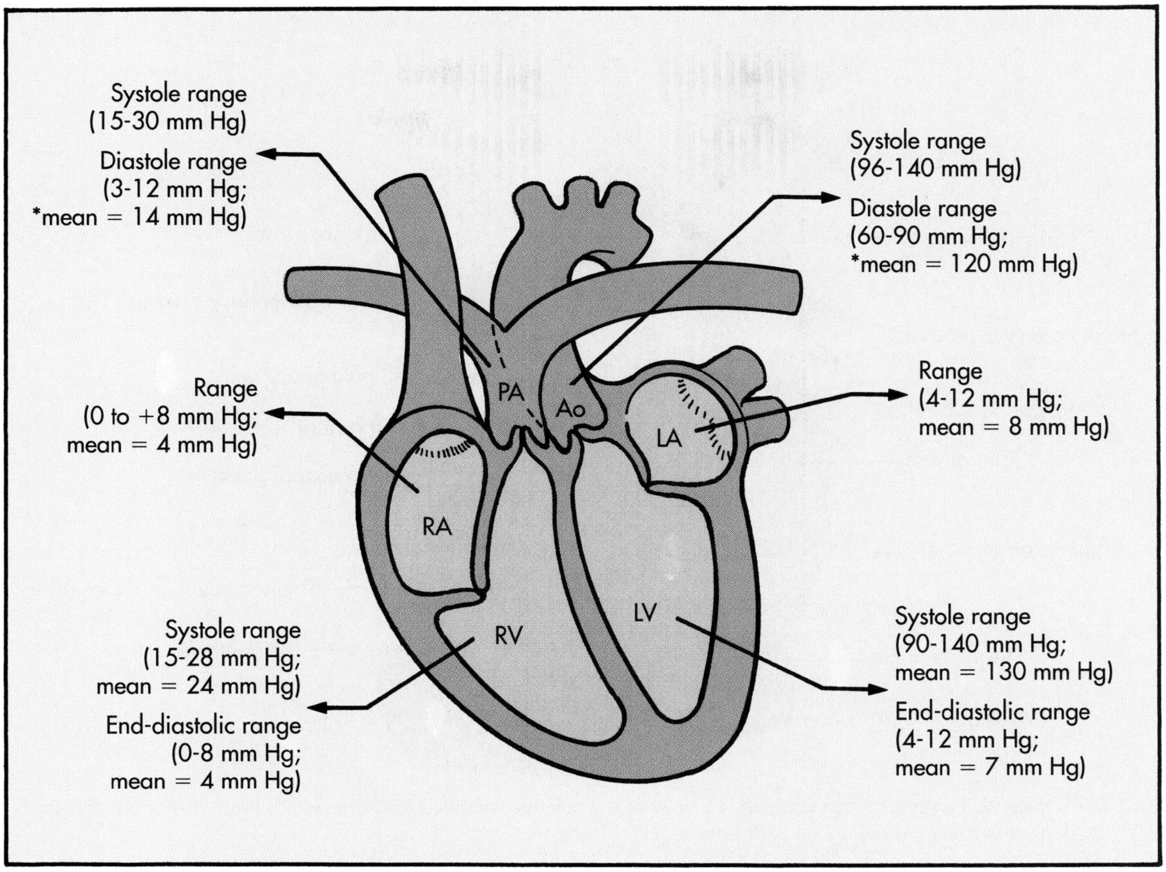

FIG. 28-7 Normal intracardiac pressures. *RA,* Right atrium; *LA,* left atrium; *RV,* right ventricle; *LV,* left ventricle; *PA,* pulmonary artery; *Ao,* aorta; *, main mean pressure.

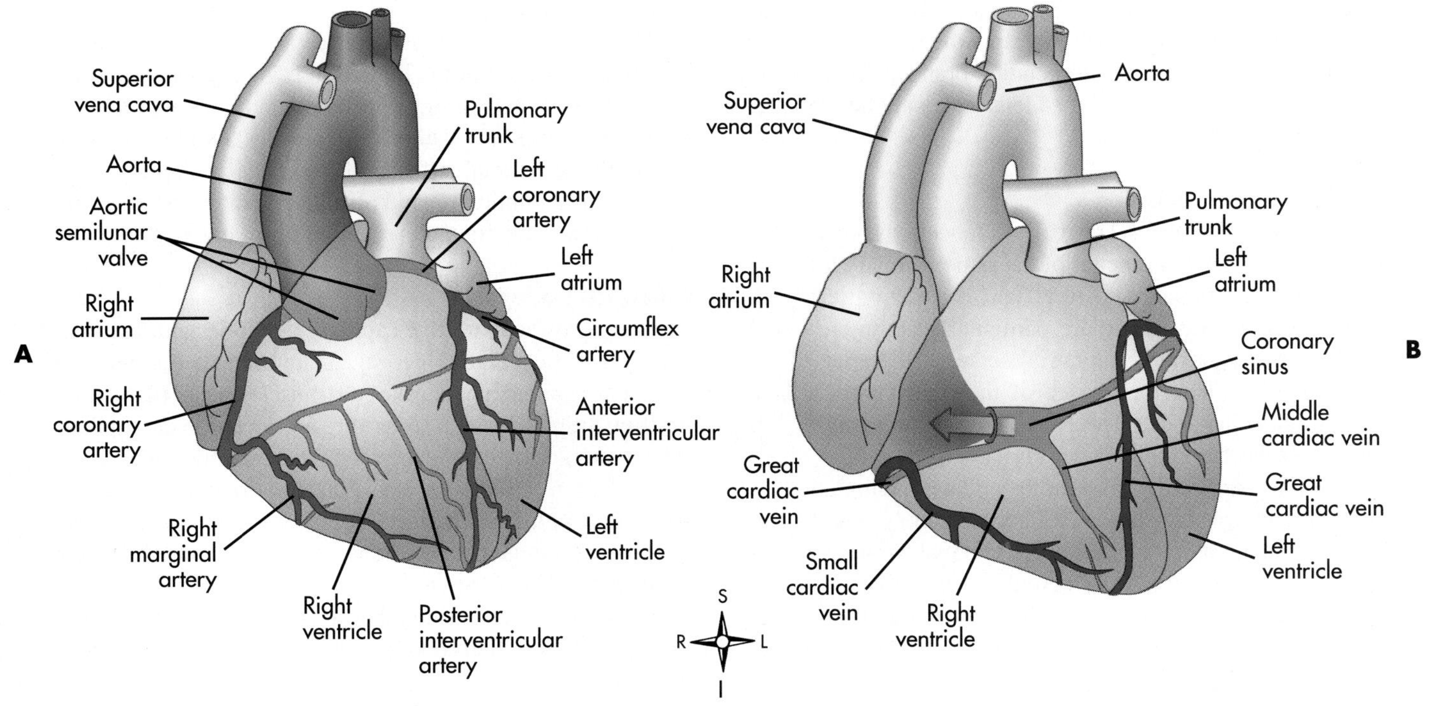

FIG. 28-8 Coronary circulation. A, Arteries. **B,** Veins. Both **A** and **B** are anterior views of the heart. Vessels near the anterior surface are more darkly colored than vessels of the posterior surface seen through the heart. (**A, B,** Modified from Thibodeau GA, Patton KI: *Anatomy and physiology,* ed 4, St Louis, 1999, Mosby.)

Continued

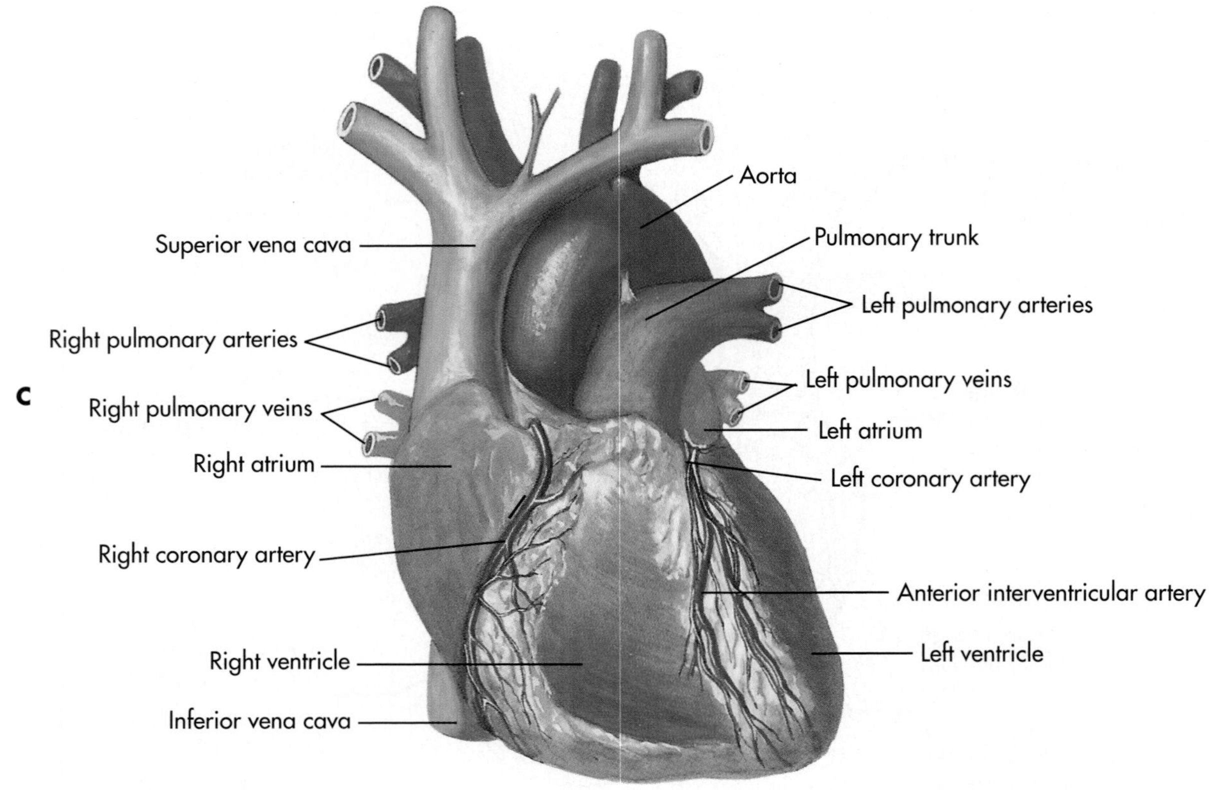

FIG. 28-8, cont'd Coronary circulation. C, View of the anterior (sternocostal) surface. (**C,** From Seeley RR, Stephens TD, Tate P: *Anatomy and physiology,* ed 3, St Louis, 1995, Mosby.)

where it branches to the atrium and the ventricle. The three major branches of the right coronary artery include the conus, which supplies blood to the upper right ventricle; the right marginal branch, which traverses the right ventricle to the apex; and the posterior descending branch, which lies in the posterior interventricular sulcus and supplies smaller branches to both ventricles.

Collateral Arteries

The **collateral arteries** are really connections, or anastomoses, between two branches of the same coronary artery or connections of branches of the right coronary artery with branches of the left. They are particularly common within the interventricular and interatrial septa, at the apex of the heart, over the anterior surface of the right ventricle, and around the sinus node.[2] The epicardium contains more collateral vessels than the endocardium.

The functional importance of the collateral circulation recently has returned to earlier 1960 ideas, namely, that the collateral circulation protects the heart. Gradual coronary occlusion results in the growth of coronary collaterals. Recently, nitric oxide and vascular endothelial growth factor increased coronary collateral growth.[3] Several observations support this protective view:

1. The degree of deterioration of left ventricular function is *inversely* related to the presence of collateral circulation (as seen angiographically).
2. The incidence of aneurysm formation after myocardial infarction is reduced in individuals with significant collateral circulation.
3. The risk for severe consequences of dysrhythmias developing after myocardial infarction is greatly reduced in individuals with well-developed collateral circulations.
4. The presence of collaterals extends the "window of time" for the beneficial effects of reperfusion therapy after myocardial infarction and results in greater improvement in cardiac function and reduction in infarct size.[2]

Coronary Capillaries

The heart has an extensive capillary network, with approximately 3300 capillaries per square millimeter (ca/mm^2) or about one capillary per muscle cell (muscle fiber).[4] Blood travels from the arteries to the arterioles and then into the capillaries, where exchange of oxygen and other nutrients takes place.

Alterations of the cardiac muscles dramatically affect blood flow in the capillaries. For example, in ventricular hypertrophy (enlargement of the ventricular myocardium), the capillary network does not expand along with muscle fiber size. Therefore the same number of capillaries must now perfuse a larger area. This results in decreased exchange of oxygen and nutrients.

Coronary Veins and Lymphatic Vessels

After passing through the extensive capillary network, blood from the coronary arteries drains into the cardiac veins,

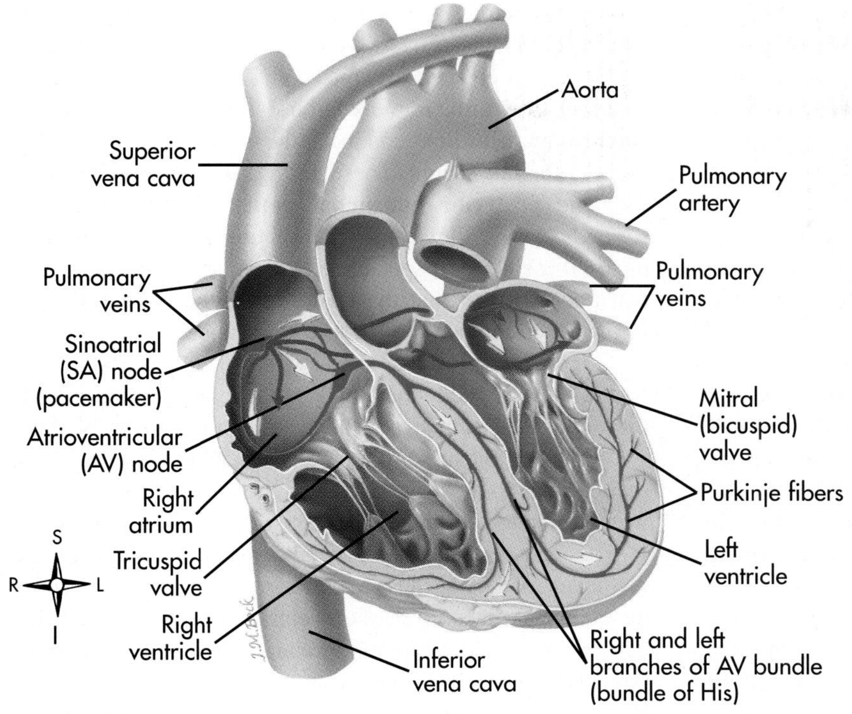

FIG. 28-9 Conduction system of heart. Specialized cardiac muscle cells in the wall of the heart rapidly conduct an electrical impulse throughout the myocardium. The signal is initiated by the SA node (pacemaker) and spreads to the rest of the atrial myocardium and to the atrioventricular (AV) node. The AV node then initiates a signal that is conducted through the ventricular myocardium by way of the atrioventricular bundle (of His) and Purkinje fibers. (Modified from Thibodeau GA, Patton KI: *Anatomy and physiology,* ed 4, St Louis, 1999, Mosby.)

which travel alongside the arteries. Most of the venous drainage of the heart occurs through veins in the visceral pericardium. The veins then feed into the **great cardiac vein** (see Fig. 28-8) and coronary sinus on the posterior surface of the heart, between the atria and ventricles, in the coronary sulcus. Venous coronary blood empties into the right atrium from the coronary sinus. Blood from the left ventricular walls generally is drained through the coronary sinus and its tributaries, which together form the largest system of coronary veins. The great cardiac vein primarily drains the anterior surface of the heart. The **posterior vein of the left ventricle,** the largest on the posterior surface of the heart, branches from the coronary sinus and accompanies the circumflex artery.

The myocardium has an extensive system of lymphatic vessels. With cardiac contraction the lymphatic vessels drain fluid to lymph nodes in the anterior mediastinum that eventually empty into the superior vena cava. The lymphatics are important for protecting the myocardium against injury. (The lymphatic vessels are described on p. 966.)

Structures That Control Heart Action

The continuous, rhythmic repetition of the cardiac cycle (systole and diastole) depends on the transmission of electrical impulses, termed **cardiac action potentials,** through the myocardium. (Action potentials are described in Chapters 1 and 3.) As an electrical impulse passes from cell to cell (fiber to fiber) in the myocardium, it stimulates the fibers to shorten. Shortening causes muscular contraction, or systole. After the action potential passes, the fibers relax and return to their resting length, causing diastole. The muscle fibers of the myocardium are uniquely joined so that action potentials pass from cell to cell very rapidly and efficiently. Therefore an action potential generated in one part of the myocardium passes almost simultaneously through all its contiguous fibers, causing rapid contraction.

The myocardium differs from other muscle tissues in that it contains its own **conduction system**—specialized cells that enable it to generate and transmit action potentials without stimulation from the nervous system. These cells are concentrated at certain sites in the myocardium called **nodes.** Although the heart is innervated by the autonomic nervous system (both sympathetic and parasympathetic fibers), neural impulses are not needed to maintain the cardiac cycle. Thus the heart will beat in the absence of any nervous connection. The cardiac cycle is stimulated by the nodes of specialized cells and "fine-tuned" as needed by the autonomic fibers. The sympathetic and parasympathetic nerves affect the speed of the cardiac cycle (**heart rate,** or beats per minute) and the diameter of the coronary vessels (see Fig. 28-12).

Heart action is influenced also by substances delivered to the myocardium in coronary blood. Nutrients and oxygen are needed for cellular survival and normal function, and hormones and biochemicals affect the strength and duration of myocardial contraction and the degree and duration of myocardial relaxation. Normal or appropriate function depends on the availability of these substances, which is why coronary artery disease can seriously disrupt heart function.

Conduction System

Normally electrical impulses arise in the **sinoatrial node** (SA node, sinus node), which is often called the *pacemaker of the heart.* The SA node is located at the junction of the right atrium and superior vena cava, just above the tricuspid valve (Fig. 28-9). The SA node lies only 1 mm or less beneath the visceral pericardium, making it vulnerable to injury and disease, especially pericardial inflammation.[5] The SA node is nourished by the sinus node artery, which passes through the center of the node. Numerous autonomic nerve endings are within the node. The SA node's **P cells,** so-called because they are pale and primitive appearing, are assumed to be the site of impulse formation.

In the resting adult the SA node generates about 75 action potentials per minute. Each one travels rapidly from cell to cell and through special pathways in the atrial myocardium, causing both atria to contract, beginning systole. Ventricular contraction is delayed because the fibrous skeleton of the heart interrupts cell-to-cell transmission of the electrical impulses. The action potential is transmitted from the atrial to the ventricular myocardium through fibers of the conduction system, traveling first to the **atrioventricular node** (AV node), then to the **bundle of His** (atrioventricular bundle, common bundle), and finally through the **bundle branches** of the interventricular septum to Purkinje fibers in the heart wall (see Fig. 28-9).

The AV node is well situated for mediating conduction between the atria and ventricles. It is located in the right atrial wall above the tricuspid valve and anterior to the ostium of the coronary sinus. There is much variation from one heart to another in the size and length of the AV node fibers. Generally the AV node is thicker and shorter and has fewer P cells than the SA node. Behind the AV node are numerous autonomic ganglia, presumably vagal (parasympathetic).[6] (The nervous systems are described in Chapter 13.) These ganglia may serve as receptors for the vagus nerve and cause slowing of the cardiac cycle.

Conducting fibers from the AV node converge to form the bundle of His. The bundle of His, which is triangular in shape, lies within the posterior border of the interventricular septum. The two lower ends of the triangle give rise to the right and left bundle branches. The **right bundle branch (RBB)** is thin and travels without much branching to the right ventricular apex. Because of its thinness and relative lack of branches, the RBB is susceptible to interruption by damage to the endocardium.

The **left bundle branch (LBB)** arises perpendicularly from the bundle of His and, in some hearts, divides into two branches, or fascicles. The left anterior bundle branch (LABB) passes the left anterior papillary muscle and the base of the left ventricle and crosses the aortic outflow tract. Damage to the aortic valve or the left ventricle can interrupt this branch. The left posterior bundle branch (LPBB) travels posteriorly, crossing the left ventricular inflow tract to the base of the left posterior papillary muscle. This branch spreads diffusely through the posterior inferior left ventricular wall. Blood flow through this portion of the left ventricle is relatively nonturbulent, so the LPBB is somewhat protected from injury caused by wear and tear.

The **Purkinje fibers** are the terminal branches of the right and left bundle branches. They extend from the ventricular apices to the fibrous rings and penetrate the heart wall to the outer myocardium. P cells are found also among the Purkinje fibers.

Because impulses from the SA node arrive at the AV node extremely quickly, investigators have proposed that these nodes are connected by internodal pathways. A special pathway, the **anterior interatrial myocardial band** (or **Bachmann bundle**), conducts the impulse from the SA node to the left atrium. These pathways, the **anterior, middle,** and **posterior internodal pathways,** have been described. These pathways apparently consist of ordinary myocardial cells and specialized conducting fibers. Some researchers assert that these routes are the main pathways for conduction from the SA to the AV node.

Cardiac Excitation

From the SA node the impulse that begins systole spreads throughout the right atrium at a conduction velocity of about 1 m/sec. The Bachmann bundle conducts the impulse from the SA node to the left atrium, and the three internodal pathways conduct the impulse from the SA node to the AV node.

The action potential is delayed in the region of the AV node, possibly because of electrophysiologic differences in the cells that make up the atrioventricular region.[1] The delay between atrial and ventricular excitation permits an additional boost to ventricular filling by atrial contraction (atrial kick). From the AV node the impulse travels from the atrioventricular bundle and through the bundle branches to the Purkinje fibers. Conduction velocities in the atrioventricular and Purkinje fibers are 2 to 4 m/sec, the most rapid in the heart.

Ventricular activation occurs sequentially in three phases: (1) septal activation, (2) apical activation, and (3) basal (upper) and posterior activation. The first areas of the ventricles to be excited are portions of the interventricular septum. The septum is activated from both the RBB and the LBB, although the impulse travels from left to right. The extensive network of Purkinje fibers promotes the rapid spread of the impulse to the ventricular apices. Activation traverses the heart wall from the inside outward (from the endocardium to the epicardium; see Fig. 28-2). The basal and posterior portions of the ventricles are the last to be activated. Deactivation, which begins diastole, occurs in the opposite direction, spreading from the outside inward (epicardium to endocardium). All areas of the ventricle recover at about the same time.

Propagation of Cardiac Action Potentials

Electrical activation of the muscle cells, termed **depolarization,** is caused by the movement of electrically charged solutes (ions) across cardiac cell membranes. Deactivation, called **repolarization,** occurs the same way. (Movement of ions across cell membranes is described in Chapter 1; electrical activation of muscle cells is described in Chapter 40.)

Movement of ions into and out of the cell creates an electrical (voltage) difference across the cell membrane called the *membrane potential.* The resting membrane potential of myocardial cells is -80 to -90 millivolts (mV), and that of SA and AV node cells is -60 mV. During depolarization the inside of the cell becomes less negatively charged. In cardiac cells the difference between resting membrane potential (in millivolts) and the decreased negative charge caused by depolarization is the cardiac action potential. Table 28-2 summarizes the intracellular and extracellular ionic concentrations of cardiac muscle. The various phases of the cardiac action potential are related to changes in the permeability of the cell membrane, primarily to sodium and potassium. *Threshold* is the point at which the cell membrane's selective permeability to sodium and potassium is temporarily disrupted, leading to depolarization.

Normal myocardial cell depolarization and repolarization occur in five phases (Fig. 28-10). Phase 0 consists of depolarization. This phase lasts 1 to 2 milliseconds (ms) and represents rapid sodium entry into the cell. Phase 1 is early repolarization, in which calcium slowly enters the cell. Phase 2, also called the **plateau,** is a continuation of repolarization, with slow entry of calcium and sodium into the cell. Potassium is moved out of the cell during phase 3, with a return to resting membrane potential in phase 4. This time between action potentials corresponds to diastole. If the resting membrane potential becomes more negative, for example with a decrease in extracellular potassium concentration (hypokalemia), it is termed **hyperpolarization.**

The phases of depolarization and repolarization occur somewhat differently in the SA and AV node cells, a difference that enables these cells to generate cardiac action potentials independently. Although the cells of the Purkinje fibers, atria, and ventricles begin with a negative resting membrane potential and proceed to a rapid upstroke, or depolarization (phase 0), a rapid early repolarization (phase 1), a plateau (phase 2), and a rapid later repolarization (phase 3), cells of the SA and AV nodes begin with a less negative resting membrane potential, proceed to a slow upstroke (phase 0), and usually lack a plateau (phase 2) (see Fig. 28-10, *B*). The fast inward current, mediated by sodium ions flowing through "fast channels" in the cell membrane, causes the rapid upstroke of the action potential in Purkinje fibers, atria, and ventricles (see Fig. 28-10, *A*). The slow inward current, mediated by calcium (transient and long-lasting channels) and sodium ions flowing through "slow channels" of the cell membrane, is responsible for the action potential of the SA node and the AV node. Hence, drugs that block calcium have profound effects on the slow inward current and can alter heart rate. Slow channel-blocking drugs, such as verapamil, are used to treat a variety of cardiovascular disorders.

A **refractory period,** during which no new cardiac action potential can be initiated by a stimulus, follows depolarization. This effective or absolute refractory period corresponds to the time needed for the reopening of channels that permit sodium and calcium influx (phase 0 through half of phase 3). A relative refractory period occurs near the end of repolarization, following the effective refractory period. During this time the membrane can be depolarized again but only by a greater-than-normal stimulus. Abnormal refractory periods as a result of disease can cause abnormal heart rhythms, or dysrhythmias, including ventricular fibrillation and cardiac arrest (see Chapter 29).

Normal electrocardiogram. The genesis of the normal electrocardiogram is from electrical activity recorded by skin electrodes, that is, the sum of all cardiac action potentials (Fig. 28-11). The **P wave** represents atrial depolarization. The **PR interval** is a measure of time from the onset of atrial activation to the onset of ventricular activation; it normally ranges from 0.12 to 0.20 second. The PR interval represents the time necessary to travel from the sinus node through the atrium, AV node, and His-Purkinje system to activate ventricular myocardial cells. The **QRS complex** represents the sum of all ventricular muscle cell depolarizations. The configuration and amplitude of the QRS complex vary considerably among individuals. The duration is normally between 0.06 and 0.10 second. During the **ST interval** the entire ventricular myocardium is depolarized. The **QT interval** is sometimes

Table 28-2 Intracellular and Extracellular Ion Concentrations in the Myocardium

Ion	Intracellular Concentration	Extracellular Concentration
Sodium (Na^+)	15 mM	145mM
Potassium (K^+)	150 mM	4mM
Chloride (Cl^-)	5 mM	120 mM
Calcium (Ca^{++})	10^{-7} M	2 mM

mM, Millimoles per kilogram; *M,* moles.

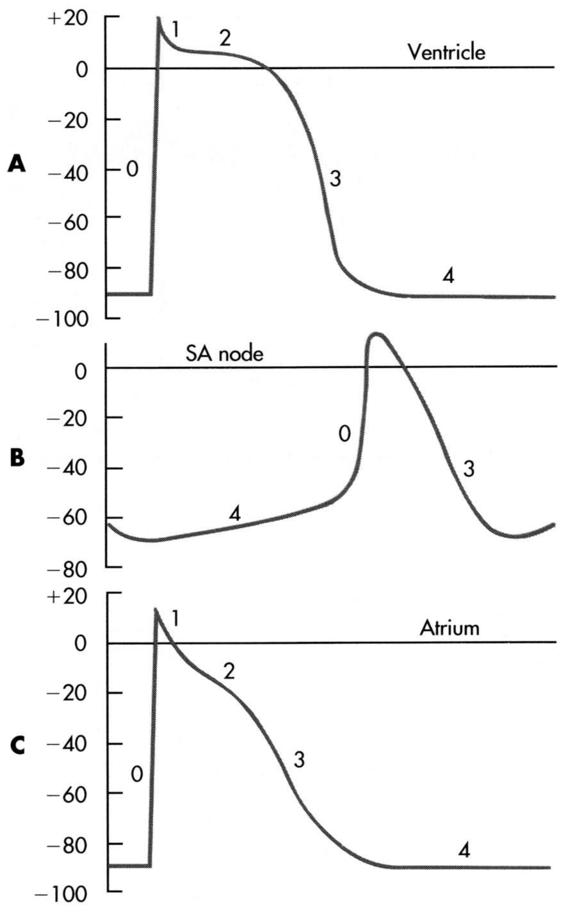

FIG. 28-10 Cardiac action potentials. A, Ventricle. **B,** Sinoatrial (SA) node. **C,** Atrium. Sweep velocity in **B** is one half that in **A** or **C.** (Modified from Berne RM, Levy MN: *Cardiovascular physiology,* ed 8, St Louis, 2001, Mosby.)

called the "electrical systole" of the ventricles. It lasts about 0.4 second, but it varies inversely with the heart rate.

Automaticity. **Automaticity,** or the property of generating spontaneous depolarization to threshold, enables the SA and AV nodes to generate cardiac action potentials without any stimulus. Cells capable of spontaneous depolarization are called **automatic cells.** The automatic cells of the cardiac conduction system can stimulate the heart to beat even when the heart is removed from the body. Spontaneous depolarization is possible in automatic cells because the membrane potential does not "rest" during phase 4. Instead, it slowly creeps toward threshold during the diastolic phase of the cardiac cycle. Because threshold is approached during diastole, phase 4 in automatic cells is called **diastolic depolarization.** The electrical impulse normally begins in the SA node because its cells depolarize more rapidly than other automatic cells.

Rhythmicity. **Rhythmicity** is the regular generation of an action potential by the heart's conduction system. The SA node sets the pace because normally it has the fastest rate, which is why it is called the natural pacemaker of the heart. The SA node depolarizes spontaneously 60 to 100 times per minute. If the SA node is damaged, the AV node will become the heart's pacemaker at a rate of about 40 to 60 spontaneous depolarizations per minute. Eventually, however, conduction cells in the atria usually take over from the AV node. Purkinje fibers are capable of spontaneous depolarization but at a rate of only 30 to 40 beats/min.

Cardiac Innervation

Although the heart's nodes and conduction system generate cardiac action potentials independently, the autonomic nervous system influences the *rate* of impulse generation (firing), depolarization, and repolarization of the myocardium and the strength of atrial and ventricular contraction. Autonomic neural transmission produces changes in the heart and circulatory system faster than metabolic or humoral agents (Fig. 28-12). Speed is important, for example, in stimulating the heart to increase its pumping action during times of stress

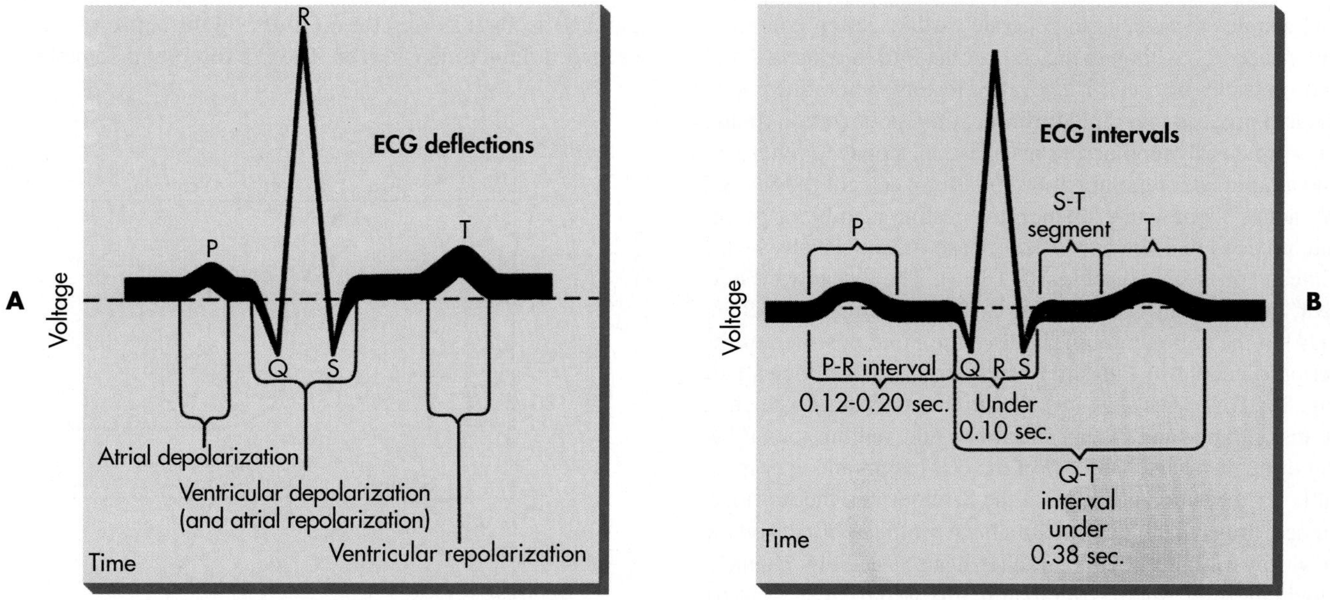

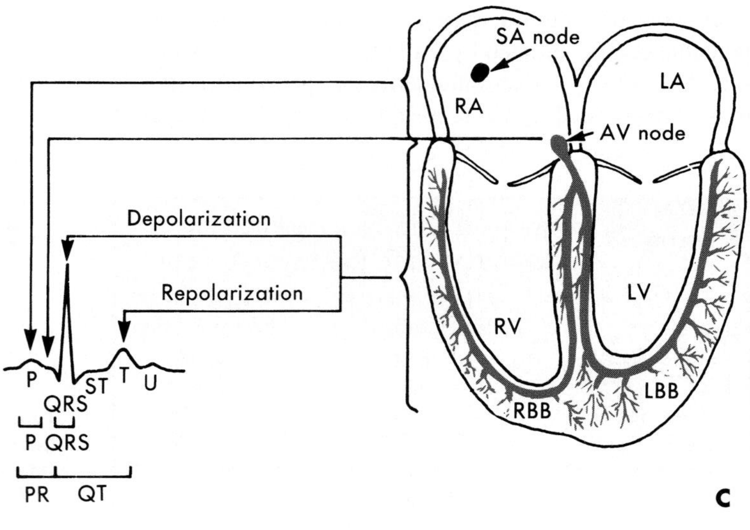

FIG. 28-11 Electrocardiogram (ECG) and cardiac electrical activity. A, Ideal ECG deflections represent depolarization and repolarization of cardiac muscle tissue. **B,** Principal ECG interval among P, QRS, and T waves. Note that the PR wave is measured from the start of the P wave to the end of the Q wave. **C,** Schematic representation of ECG and its relationship to cardiac electrical activity. *SA,* Sinoatrial; *LA,* left atrium; *AV,* atrioventricular; *LV,* left ventricle; *LBB,* left bundle branch; *RBB,* right bundle branch; *RV,* right ventricle; *RA,* right atrium. (**A, B,** From Thibodeau GA, Patton KI: *Anatomy and physiology,* ed 4, St Louis, 1999, Mosby. **C,** From Thibodeau GA: *Anatomy and physiology,* St Louis, 1987, Mosby.

or fear, the so-called *fight or flight response.* Although increased delivery of oxygen, glucose, hormones, and other blood-borne factors sustains increased cardiac activity, the rapid initiation of increased activity depends on the sympathetic and parasympathetic fibers of the autonomic nervous system. (The autonomic nervous sytstem is described and illustrated in Chapter 13.)

Sympathetic and Parasympathetic Nerves

Sympathetic nerve fibers innervate all parts of the atria and ventricles. Parasympathetic fibers from the vagus nerve innervate these structures plus the SA and AV nodes. Strong vagal stimulation can block cardiac action potentials transmitted from the atria. Sympathetic nerves can also shorten the conduction time through the AV node and increase the rhythmicity of the atrioventricular pacemaker fibers.

Efferent sympathetic fibers originate in the thoracic spinal cord and branch into the superior middle and inferior cardiac nerves. The efferent parasympathetic fibers originate in the medulla oblongata and travel by way of the vagus nerves to join the sympathetic nerves in the **cardiac plexus,** a neural junction located at the root of the aorta, in front of the trachea.

Sympathetic nervous activity enhances myocardial performance. Neurally released norepinephrine or circulating catecholamines interact with β-adrenergic receptors on the cardiac cell membranes. The overall effect is an increased influx of Ca^{++} during the action potential plateau. The increased calcium increases the contractile strength of the heart. In addition, sympathetic nervous activity increases heart rate, whereas parasympathetic (vagal) activity decreases heart rate. The vagus nerve releases acetylcholine. In the heart, receptors for these neurotransmitters are found in the myocardium and in the coronary vessels. When the autonomic nervous system is active, the vagal effects usually dominate.

Adrenergic Receptor Function

Sympathetic neural stimulation of the myocardium and coronary vessels depends on the presence of adrenergic receptors, which bind specifically with neurotransmitters of the sympathetic nervous system. (Receptor physiology is discussed in Chapter 1.) The effects of sympathetic stimulation depend on whether (1) α- or β-adrenergic receptors are most plentiful on cells of the effector tissue and (2) the neurotransmitter is norepinephrine or epinephrine.

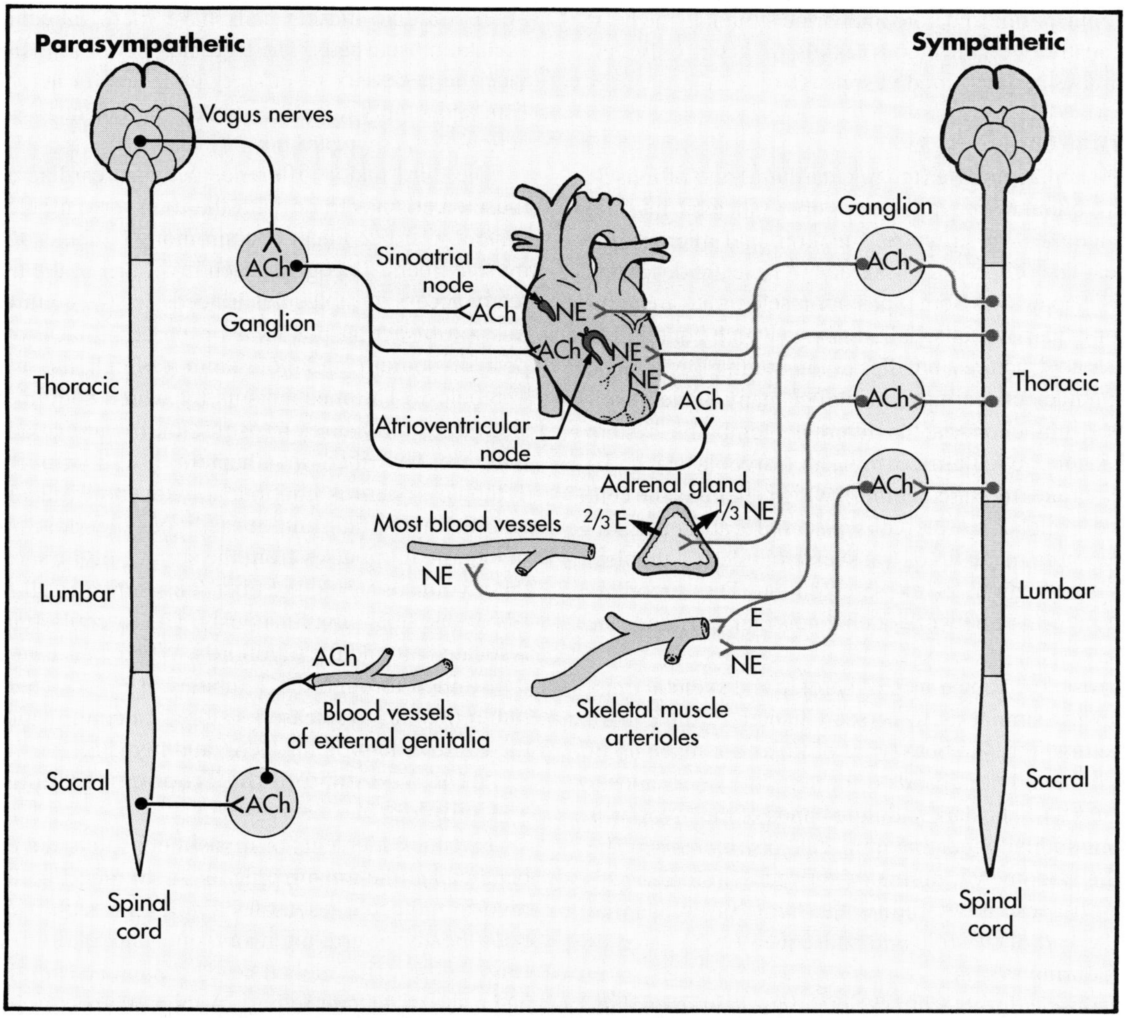

FIG. 28-12 Autonomic innervation of cardiovascular system. *ACh,* Acetylcholine; *NE,* norepinephrine; *E,* epinephrine; *AV,* atrioventricular node.

Overall, cardiovascular structures have more β than α receptors; therefore effects mediated by the β receptors predominate. The β_1 receptors are found mostly in the heart, specifically the conduction system (AV and SA nodes, Purkinje fibers) and the atrial and ventricular myocardium. Norepinephrine binding with β_1 receptors increases the rate of impulse generation (firing) and conduction and also the strength of myocardial contraction during systole. These effects enable the heart to pump more blood. At the same time, epinephrine binds with β_2 receptors, which are most plentiful in the coronary arterioles. This causes the coronary arterioles to dilate, supplying the hard-working myocardium with more oxygen and nutrients (see Table 13-7).

α-Adrenergic receptors are also present in the coronary vessels but in fewer numbers than the β receptors. Norepinephrine binding with $_{\alpha 1}$ receptors in the coronary arteries causes vasoconstriction. The α_2 receptors are located mostly on the sympathetic ganglia and nerve terminals. The effect of norepinephrine on the α_2 receptors is to inhibit release of more norepinephrine, which promotes vasodilation.

Epinephrine stimulates all four types of receptors (β_1, β_2, α_1, α_2) strongly, whereas norepinephrine stimulates α_1, α_2, and β_1 receptors and certain β_2 receptors weakly or not at all. Thus both epinephrine and norepinephrine stimulate the heart (β_1) and constrict certain blood vessels (α_1), but only epinephrine dilates certain blood vessels (β_2).

Myocardial Cells

The cells of cardiac muscle (the myocardium) and of muscle that makes voluntary movement possible (skeletal muscle) are nearly identical in structure, function, and microscopic appearance. (The properties of skeletal muscle are described in detail in Chapter 40.) Both types of muscle tissue are composed of long, narrow cells, called *fibers,* which contain basically the same structures: bundles of longitudinally arranged myofibrils; a nucleus (cardiac muscle) or many nuclei (skeletal muscle); mitochondria; an internal membrane system (the sarcoplasmic reticulum); cytoplasm (sarcoplasm); and a plasma membrane (the sarcolemma), which encloses the cell. Cardiac and skeletal muscle cells also have an "external" membrane system made up of transverse tubules (T tubules) formed by invaginations of the sarcolemma. The sarcoplasmic reticulum forms a network of channels that surrounds the muscle fiber.

The microscopic appearance of cardiac and skeletal muscle is somewhat similar as well (see Chapter 1, Table 1-8). Because the myofibrils in both types of fibers are made up of alternating light and dark bands of protein, the fibers appear striped, or striated. The dark and light bands of the myofibrils make up longitudinal repeating units called *sarcomeres.* The length of the sarcomeres, normally between 1.6 to 2.2 μm, is important because it determines the limits of myocardial stretch at the end of diastole and subsequently the force of contraction during systole.

Cardiac muscle differs from skeletal muscle in several respects that reflect heart function. Cardiac cells are arranged in branching networks throughout the myocardium, whereas skeletal muscle cells tend to be arranged in parallel throughout the length of the muscle. Cardiac fibers have only one nucleus, whereas skeletal muscle cells have many nuclei. Other differences enable cardiac fibers to (1) transmit action potentials quickly from cell to cell, (2) maintain high levels of energy synthesis, and (3) gain access to more ions, particularly sodium and potassium, in the extracellular environment.

Rapid transmission of electrical impulses from cardiac fiber to cardiac fiber is possible because the network of fibers is connected at specialized intercellular junctions called *intercalated disks.* **Intercalated disks** are thickened portions of the sarcolemma that enable electrical impulses to spread quickly in a continuous cell-to-cell (syncytial) fashion. The intercalated disks contain two junctions: desmosomes, which attach one cell to another; and gap junctions, which allow the electrical impulse to spread from cell to cell (see Chapter 1). Together, these junctions provide a low-resistance pathway for impulse propagation.

Unlike skeletal muscle, the heart cannot rest and is in constant need of energy compounds, such as adenosine triphosphate (ATP). Therefore the cytoplasm surrounding the bundles of myofibrils in each cardiac muscle cell contains a superabundance of mitochondria (25% of the cellular volume). Cardiac muscle cells have more mitochondria than skeletal muscle cells. The large number of mitochondria provide the necessary respiratory enzymes for aerobic metabolism and supply quantities of ATP sufficient for the constant action of the myocardium.

The third major difference between cardiac and skeletal muscle cells has to do with the transverse tubule (T tubule) system. Cardiac fibers contain more T tubules than skeletal muscle fibers. This gives each myofibril in the myocardium ready access to molecules it needs for the continuous transmission of action potentials, a process that involves transport of sodium and potassium through the walls of the T tubules. (The mechanisms by which sodium and potassium transport causes transmission of cardiac action potentials are described in Chapters 1 and 40.) Because the T tubule system is continuous with the extracellular space and the interstitial fluid, it facilitates the rapid transmission of electrical impulses from the surface of the sarcolemma to the myofibrils inside the fiber. This activates all the myofibrils of one fiber simultaneously. The sarcoplasmic reticulum is located around the myofibrils. When an action potential is transmitted through the T tubules, it induces the sarcoplasmic reticulum to release its stored calcium, which activates the contractile proteins, actin and myosin.

Actin, Myosin, and the Troponin-Tropomyosin Complex

The thick filaments of **myosin** constitute the central dark band called the **anisotropic,** or **A, bands** (Fig. 28-13). The myosin molecule resembles a golf club with two large bulbous heads protruding from one end of a straight shaft (Fig. 28-14). The bilobed heads contain an actin-binding site and a site of ATPase activity. A thick filament is composed of about 200 myosin molecules bundled together with the heads of the molecules (called cross bridges) facing outward

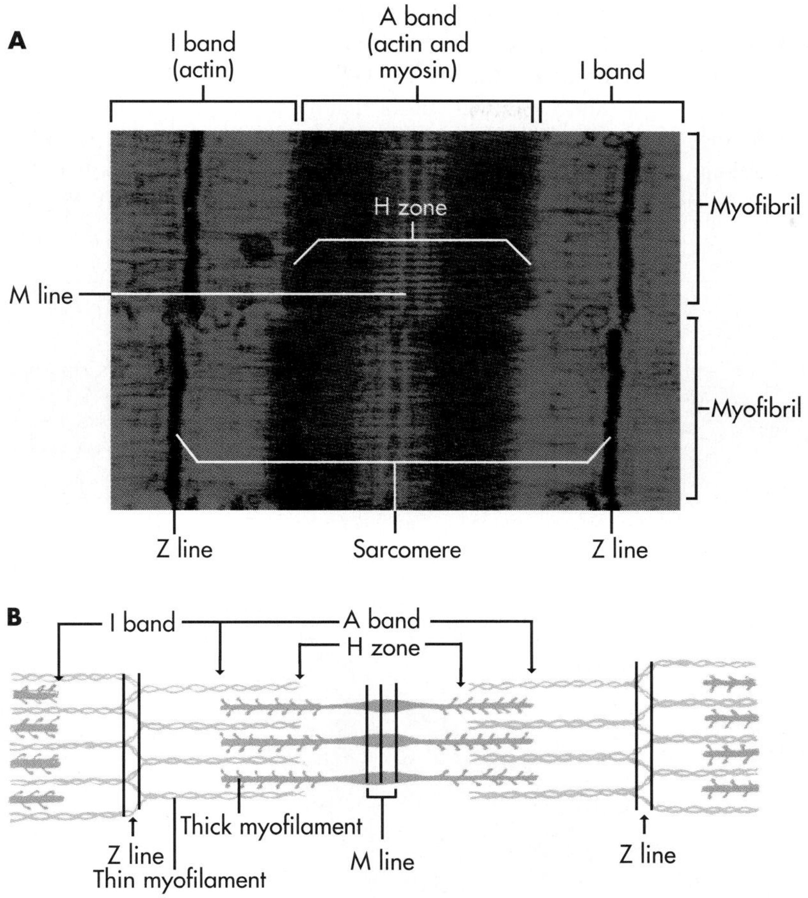

FIG. 28-13 Sarcomere. A, Electron photomicrograph of sarcomere. **B,** Schematic of location and interaction of actin and myosin. (Modified from Thibodeau GA, Patton KT: *Anatomy and physiology,* ed 3, St Louis, 1996, Mosby.)

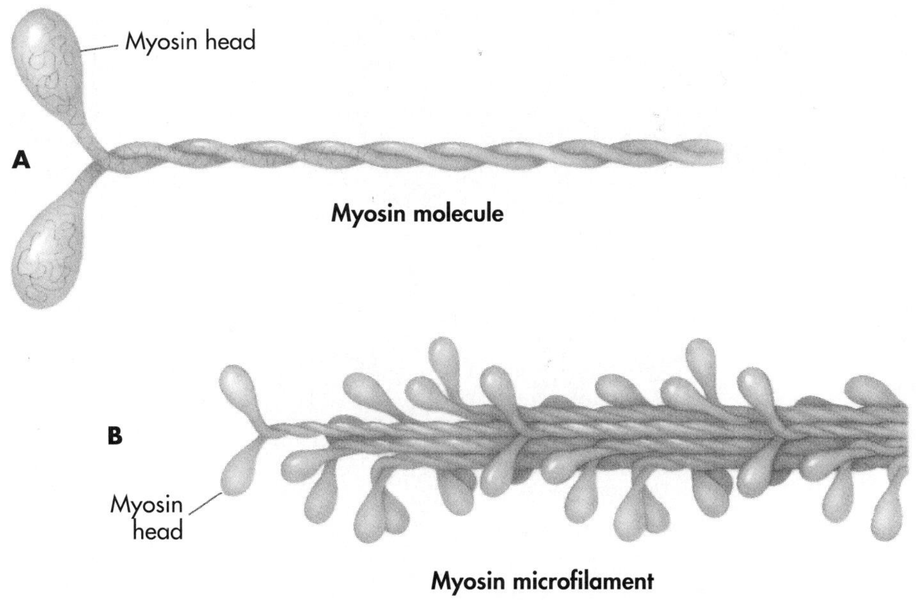

FIG. 28-14 Structure of myosin. A, Each myosin molecule is a coil of two chains wrapped around one another. At the end of each chain is a globular region, much like a golf club, called the *head.* **B,** Myosin molecules usually are combined into filaments, which are stalks of myosin from which the heads protrude at regular intervals. (From Raven RH, Johnson GB: *Understanding biology,* ed 3, Dubuque, Iowa, 1995, Brown.)

(see Fig. 28-14). The actin molecules are part of the thin filaments (Fig. 28-15). The light bands are called **isotropic,** or **I, bands** (see Fig. 28-13). The thin filaments of actin appear light and extend from the **Z line,** a dense fibrous line that crosses the center of each I band. A sarcomere is the area from one dark Z line to an adjacent Z line with a length that varies from 1.6 to 2.2 μm. In the center of a sarcomere is the H zone, a somewhat less dense region. A thin, dark **M line** travels the center of the H zone. A single tropomyosin molecule (a relaxing protein) lies alongside seven actin molecules.

Troponin, another relaxing protein, associates with the tropomyosin molecule, forming the **troponin-tropomyosin complex** (Fig. 28-16). The troponin complex itself has three components. **Troponin T** aids in binding of the troponin complex to actin and tropomyosin; **troponin I** inhibits the ATPase of actomyosin; and **troponin C** contains binding sites for the calcium ions involved in contraction.

Myocardial Metabolism

Cardiac muscle, like other muscle tissue, depends on the constant production of ATP for energy. ATP is produced within the mitochondria mainly from glucose, fatty acids, and lactate. If the myocardium is inadequately perfused because of coronary artery disease, anaerobic metabolism becomes an essential source of energy (see Chapter 1). The en-

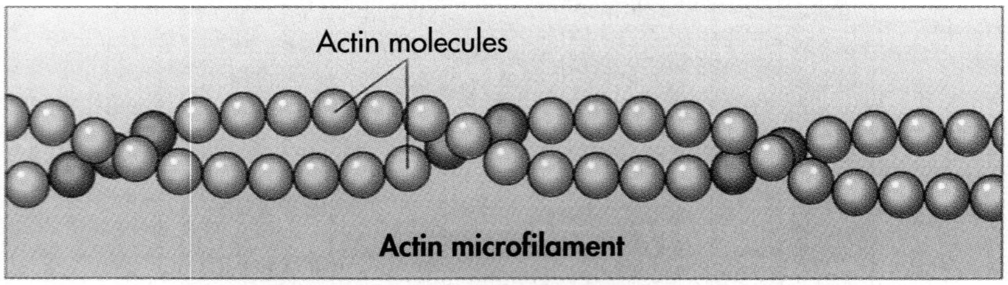

FIG. 28-15 Actin microfilament. (From Raven RH, Johnson GB: *Understanding biology,* ed 3, Dubuque, Iowa, 1995, Brown.)

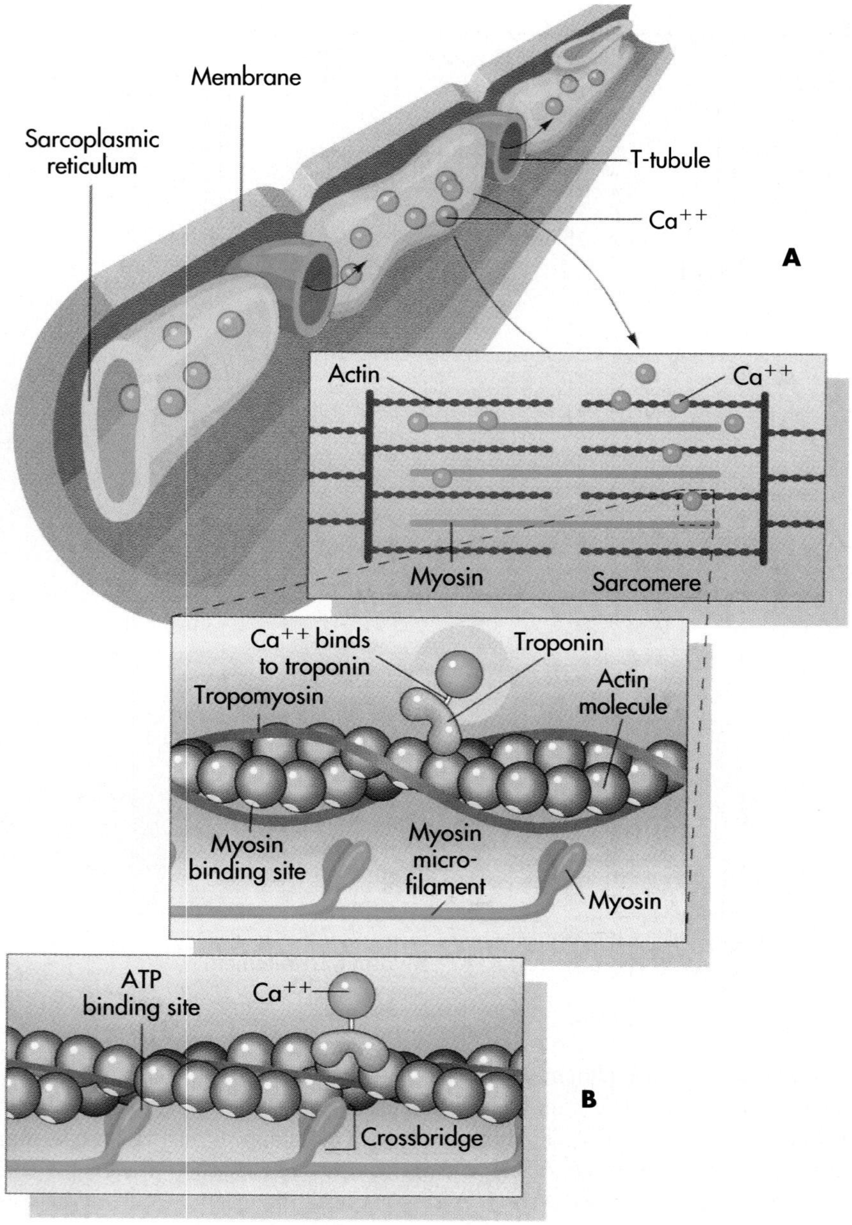

FIG. 28-16 Myofilaments and mechanisms of muscle contraction. A, Thin and thick myofilaments. In resting muscle, calcium ions are stored in the sarcoplasmic reticulum. When an action potential reaches the muscle cell, the T tubules carry the action potential deep into the sarcoplasm. The action potential causes the sarcoplasmic reticulum to release the store of calcium ions. **B,** In resting muscle the myosin binding sites are covered by troponin and tropomyosin. The calcium ions released into the sarcoplasm as a result of action potential bind to the troponin. This binding causes the tropomyosin and troponin to move out of the way of the myosin binding sites, leaving the myosin heads free to bind to the actin microfilament. (From Raven PH, Johnson GB: *Understanding biology,* ed 3, Dubuque, Iowa, 1995, Brown.)

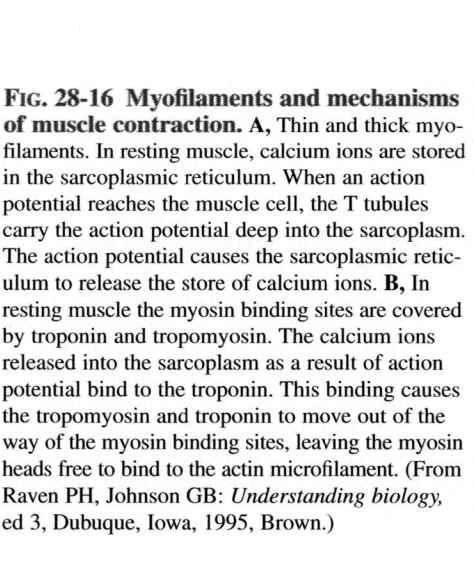

ergy produced by metabolic processes is used for muscle contraction and relaxation, electrical excitation, membrane transport, and synthesis of large molecules. Normally, the amount of ATP produced supplies sufficient energy to pump blood systemically.

Cardiac work often is expressed in terms of **myocardial oxygen consumption** ($M\dot{V}O_2$). Because oxidative metabolism is the main process of cardiac energy generation, the rate of $M\dot{V}O_2$ correlates closely with total cardiac energy requirements. $M\dot{V}O_2$ is determined by three major factors: (1) the amount of wall stress during systole, which can be estimated by measuring the systolic blood pressure; (2) the duration of systolic wall tension, which is measured indirectly by the heart rate; and (3) the contractile state of the myocardium, for which no clinical measurement exists.

The oxygen supply to the myocardium is delivered exclusively by the coronary arteries. From 70% to 75% of the oxygen from the coronary arteries is used immediately by cardiac muscle, leaving little oxygen in reserve. Therefore increased energy needs can be met only by increasing coronary blood flow. When oxygen content decreases, the local concentration of local metabolic factors increases. One of these, adenosine, dilates coronary arterioles, increasing coronary blood flow. Oxygen content of the blood cannot be increased under normal atmospheric conditions, nor can the amount of O_2 extracted from the blood be appreciably increased from the resting level (see Chapter 31). Myocardial O_2 consumption can increase severalfold with exercise and decrease moderately under conditions such as hypotension and hypothermia.[1]

Myocardial Contraction and Relaxation

Myocardial contractility is a change in developed tension at a given resting fiber length. In functional terms, contractility is the ability of the heart muscle to shorten. On a molecular basis, thin filaments of actin slide over thick filaments of myosin, called the **cross-bridge theory of muscle contraction.** Anatomically, contraction occurs when the sarcomere shortens with adjacent Z lines moving closer together (Fig. 28-17). The width of the **A band,** which contains the thick myosin filaments, is unchanged. The movement comes from the long sets of filaments. The degree of shortening of the muscle fibers depends on how much the thin filaments overlap the thick filaments. Maximal contraction occurs when the sarcomere length is 2.2 μm. At 2.2 μm the number of cross-bridge attachments between actin and myosin is maximal.

Cross-Bridge Theory

The globular head-end of the myosin contains a binding site for actin and a separate enzymatic site that catalyzes the breakdown of ATP to adenosine diphosphate (ADP) and inorganic phosphate (see Fig. 28-17). This reaction releases the chemical energy stored in ATP. Magnesium is required for the binding of ATP to the myosin site. The splitting of ATP occurs on the myosin molecule before it attaches to actin, but the ADP and inorganic phosphate (P_i) released remain bound to the active site on myosin. The chemical energy released is transferred to myosin (m), producing a high-energy form of myosin (M):

$$M \cdot ATP \rightarrow M \cdot ADP + P_i$$

The binding of this high-energy form of myosin to actin through a cross bridge releases the energy stored in myosin (e.g., ADP and P_i), producing the force necessary for movement of the cross bridge. With the attachment of actin to myosin at the cross bridge, the myosin head molecule undergoes a position change, exerting traction on the rest of the myosin bridge, causing the thin filaments to slide past the thick filaments (see Fig. 28-17). During contraction each cross bridge undergoes cycles of attachment, movement, and dissociation from the thin filaments.

Calcium and Excitation-Contraction Coupling

Excitation-contraction coupling is the process by which an action potential in the plasma membrane of the muscle fiber triggers the cycle of events leading to cross-bridge activity and contraction. Activation of this cycle depends on the availability of calcium.

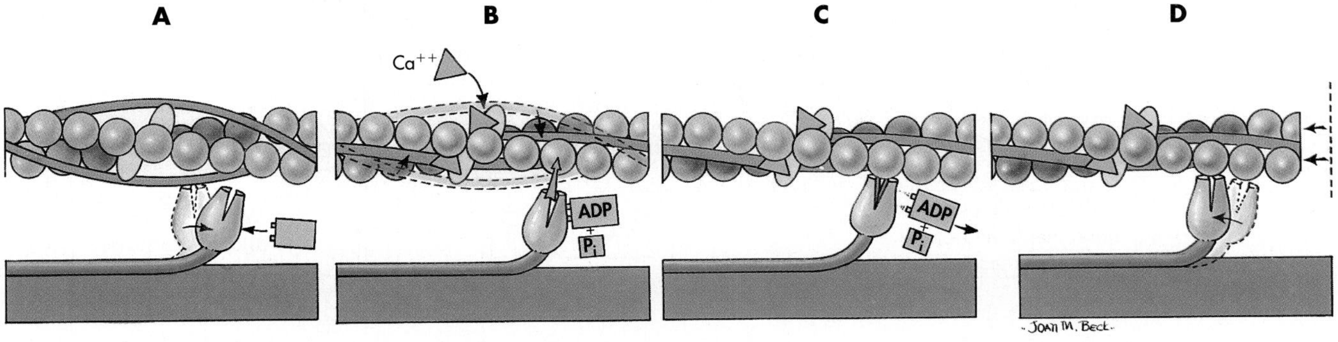

FIG. 28-17 Cross-bridge theory of muscle contraction. A, Each myosin cross bridge in the thick filament moves into a resting position after an adenosine triphosphate (ATP) molecule binds and transfers its energy. **B,** Calcium ions released from the sarcoplasmic reticulum bind to troponin in the thin filament, allowing tropomyosin to shift from its position blocking the active sites of actin molecules. **C,** Each myosin cross bridge then binds to an active site on a thin filament, displacing the remnants of ATP hydrolysis—adenosine diphosphate (ADP) and inorganic phosphate (P_i). **D,** The release of stored energy from step A provides the force needed for each cross bridge to move back to its original position, pulling actin along with it. Each cross bridge will remain bound to actin until another ATP molecule binds to it and pulls it back into its resting position, **A.** (From Thibodeau GA, Patton KI: *Anatomy and physiology,* ed 4, St Louis, 1999, Mosby.)

Calcium is stored in the tubule system and the sarcoplasmic reticulum. It enters the myocardial cell from the interstitial fluid after electrical excitation, which increases the membrane permeability to calcium. Two types of calcium channels (L-type and T-type) are identified in cardiac tissues. The L-type, or long-lasting, channels are the predominant type of calcium channels and are the channels blocked by **calcium channel–blocking drugs** (verapamil, nifedipine, diltiazem). Their major effect is to decrease the strength of cardiac contraction. The T-type, or transient, channels are much less abundant in the heart and are not blocked by calcium channel–blocking drugs.[1] Calcium that enters the cell from the interstitial fluid triggers release of calcium from the storage sites. The storage sites most important for contraction are from the sarcoplasmic reticulum. Calcium from these sites diffuses toward the myofibrils, where it binds with troponin.

The calcium-troponin complex facilitates the contraction process. In the resting state, troponin I is bound to actin and the configuration of the tropomyosin molecule is such that it covers the sites where the myosin heads bind to actin. Thus interaction between actin and myosin is prevented. Calcium binding to troponin inhibits troponin C (which enhances troponin I–actin binding). This in turn causes tropomyosin to move away, thus uncovering the binding sites on the myosin heads. Myosin and actin can now form cross bridges, and ATP can be dephosphorylated to ADP. Sliding of the thick and thin filaments can now occur, and the muscle contracts.

Myocardial Relaxation

Adequate relaxation is just as vital to optimal cardiac function as contraction, and calcium, troponin, and tropomyosin also facilitate relaxation. After contraction, free calcium ions are actively pumped out of the cell back into the interstitial fluid or reaccumulated in the sarcoplasmic reticulum and stored. Troponin releases its bound calcium. The tropomyosin complex blocks the active sites on the actin molecule, preventing cross bridges with the myosin heads. Each tropomyosin molecule is held in this blocking position by a molecule of troponin. Troponin is bound to both tropomyosin and actin (see Figs. 28-16, *A,* and 28-17).

Factors Affecting Cardiac Performance

Four factors affect cardiac performance directly: preload, afterload, heart rate, and myocardial contractility. **Preload** (pressure generated at the end of diastole) and **afterload** (resistance to ejection during systole) depend on both the heart and the vascular system. Heart rate and contractility are characteristics of the cardiac tissue per se and are influenced by neural and humoral mechanisms (Fig. 28-18). To understand the role of these factors in cardiac performance, it is first necessary to understand two physical laws that explain the mechanisms of heart action: the Frank-Starling law of the heart and Laplace's law.

Frank-Starling Law of the Heart

Cardiac muscle, like other muscle, increases its strength of contraction when it is stretched. This relationship was described in 1914 by a British physiologist, Ernest Starling, who based his studies on the earlier work of a German physiologist, Otto Frank. In 1914 Starling wrote that "the output of any heart can be varied within wide limits by alterations

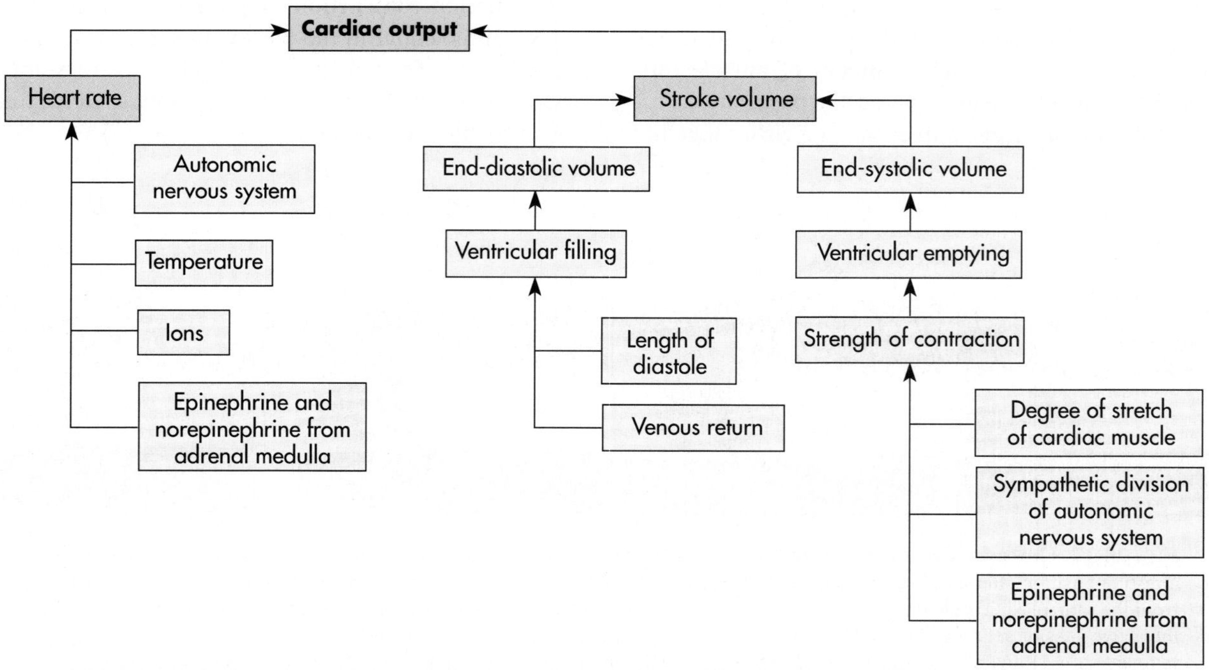

FIG. 28-18 Factors affecting cardiac performance. Cardiac output, which is amount of blood (in liters) ejected by the heart per minute, depends on heart rate (beats per minute) and stroke volume (milliliters of blood ejected during ventricular systole).

of the venous inflow, and that within these limits it varie rectly as the venous inflow. So long as the functional co tion of the heart remains constant, the amount put ou each beat depends directly on the diastolic filling."

The **Frank-Starling law of the heart,** or the len tension relationship of cardiac muscle, relates resting sa mere length, expressed as the volume of blood in the h at the end of diastole, or **end-diastolic volume,** to ten generation, described as development of left ventricular p sure. Thus the volume of blood in the heart at the end o astole (the length of its muscle fibers) is directly relate the force of contraction during the next systole. Altho the change in pressure is related to volume of the ventr and, consequently, to the length of the ventricular mu fibers, it is common to use preload (i.e., filling pressure an index of ventricular volume. The length-tension mec nism is the major mechanism by which the normal right left ventricles maintain equal minute outputs even tho their stroke outputs may vary considerably during normal piration. For example, changes in volume occur wher individual assumes a reclining position after being i standing position; the volume of blood returning to the h temporarily increases. The right ventricle stretches to accommodate this increase in volume and thereby increases its force of contraction. A larger stroke volume (i.e., the amount of blood ejected per beat) is pumped to the lungs, generating higher pressures. Pulmonary vascular pressure increases, causing a rise in the left ventricular filling pressure or preload. Left ventricular volume and pressure increase. The left ventricle pumps a larger stroke volume, and arterial vascular pressure rises.

The mechanical function of the heart is characterized by a number of length-tension curves (Fig. 28-19). Factors that increase contractility (i.e., positive inotropic), such as sympathetic nerve stimulation, cause the heart to operate on a higher length-tension curve (curve A in Fig. 28-19). A higher tension or increase in ventricular stroke volume is generated without a necessary change in left ventricular end-diastolic volume or fiber length. Heart failure (curve C in Fig. 28-19) is characterized by a lower length-tension curve (see Chapter 29). The failing or dilated heart may not be able to use the Frank-Starling law of the heart because its fibers are lengthened maximally already. The failing heart is unable to respond sig-

Laplace's Law

In **Laplace's law,** wall tension is related directly to the product of intraventricular pressure and internal radius and inversely to the wall thickness. This relationship can be calculated by Laplace's equation:

$$T = (p \times \nu)/\mu\text{m}$$

where T = wall tension, p = intraventricular pressure, ν = internal radius of the sphere, and μm = wall thickness. In other words, the amount of tension generated in the wall of the ventricle (or any chamber or vessel) to produce a given intraventricular pressure depends on the size (radius and wall thickness) of the ventricle.

The law of Laplace is useful for understanding aneurysm formation, distensibility in blood vessels, and the effects of ventricular dilation on myocardial contraction. Dilation is an important factor in heart failure (see Chapter 29). With a dilated ventricle, myocardial fibers in the wall must develop greater tension to produce a given pressure within the ventricle. The disadvantage of dilation is that the increased force,

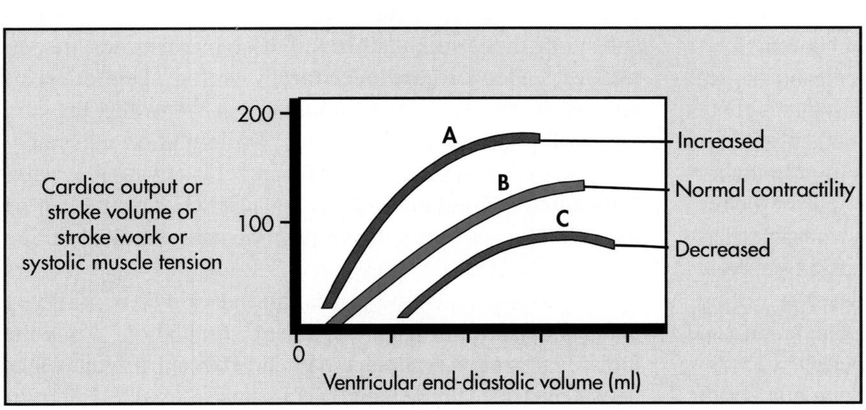

FIG. 28-19 Frank-Starling law of the heart. Relationship between length and tension in heart. End-diastolic volume determines end-diastolic length of ventricular muscle fibers and is proportional to tension generated during systole, as well as to cardiac output, stroke volume, and stroke work. A change in myocardial contractility causes the heart to perform on a different length-tension curve. *A,* Increased contractility; *B,* normal contractility; *C,* heart failure or decreased contractility. (See text.)

[redacted] velop a [redacted] decrease [redacted] g the ability [redacted] sure generated in the left [redacted] e, or left ventricular **end-** [redacted] ermined by end-diastolic vol- [redacted] ank-Starling law, which stretches [redacted] rs, which in turn develop tension, or [redacted] n. Within a physiologic range of muscle [redacted] m to 2.4 μm), increased preload increases [redacted] t (volume of blood pumped per minute; see [redacted]). In monitoring preload the clinician measures in- [redacted] f left ventricular end-diastolic pressure. Pressure [redacted] ges are important because increased left ventricular fill- [redacted] g pressures "back up" into the pulmonary circulation, where they force plasma out through vessel walls, causing fluid to accumulate in lung tissues (pulmonary edema; see Chapter 32). Treatment goals are to maintain an end-diastolic volume that will maintain or increase cardiac output.

Afterload

Left ventricular afterload is the resistance or impedance to ejection of blood from the left ventricle. It is the load the muscle must move after it starts to contract. Aortic systolic pressure is a good index of afterload. Low aortic pressures (decreased afterload) enable the heart to contract more rapidly, whereas high aortic pressures (increased afterload) slow contraction and cause higher workloads against which the heart must function so it can eject less blood. Pressure in the ventricle must exceed aortic pressure before blood can be pumped out during systole. Afterload involves a force-velocity relationship; that is, the lighter the afterload, the faster the contraction, and the heavier the afterload, the slower the contraction.

In addition to influencing the speed of shortening, afterload is related to extent of shortening. Increases in aortic pressure, with a constant preload, result in decreased blood pumped by the left ventricle. Decreased aortic pressure allows the left ventricle to pump a larger volume.

Heart Rate

The average heart rate in normal adults is about 70 beats/min. The average heart rate is significantly greater in children. Heart rate diminishes by 10 to 20 beats/min during sleep and can accelerate to more than 100 beats/min during muscular activity or emotional excitement. In well-conditioned athletes at rest the heart rate is normally about 50 to 60 beats/min. In highly trained or elite athletes the resting heart rate can be below 50 beats/min. Highly trained athletes have a lower resting heart rate, greater stroke volume, and lower peripheral resistance in active muscles than they had before training. The low resting heart rate is the result of an increased vagal stimulation and lower sympathetic stimulation.[1] The lowered peripheral resistance is thought to be caused by an increase in the number of arterioles in skeletal muscle. The decrease in peripheral resistance increases the venous return, causing the cardiac output to increase.[1] As the resting heart rate falls in individuals during physical training, the end-diastolic fiber length of the ventricles increases; this occurs because the longer duration of diastole results in greater filling. The increased end-diastolic fiber length increases stroke volume, which helps compensate for the decreased heart rate.

Neural factors, including neural reflexes, and hormonal and chemical factors influence the heart rate. Neural control is exerted by both the central and autonomic nervous systems. Hormonal factors include the catecholamines (norepinephrine and epinephrine), thyroid hormones, growth hormones, and pancreatic hormones. (Hormonal function is described in Unit VI.) Stimulation by the sympathetic nervous system increases the rhythmicity of the cardiac pacemaker (SA node), whereas the parasympathetic stimulation has an inhibiting effect.

Cardiovascular Control Centers in the Brain

The major **cardiovascular control center** is in the brain stem in the medulla with secondary areas in the hypothalamus, the cerebral cortex, the thalamus, and complex networks of exciting or inhibiting interneurons (connecting neurons) throughout the brain. The hypothalamic centers regulate cardiovascular responses to changes in temperature; the cerebral cortex centers adjust cardiac reaction to a variety of emotional states; and the medullary control center regulates heart rate and blood pressure (see p. 962 for blood pressure regulation). The medullary neurons often are classified as cardiac and vasomotor (vasoconstrictor or vasodilator) centers; however, because these centers are not discrete anatomic areas and actually constitute diffuse networks of interneurons, it is preferable to call the entire area the *cardiovascular control center.*

The nerve fibers from the cardiovascular control center synapse with the autonomic neurons (see Chapter 13 and Table 13-7). When the parasympathetic nerves to the heart are stimulated, the sympathetic nerves to the heart, arterioles, and veins usually are inhibited. The opposite also is true: when the sympathetic nerves are stimulated, the parasympathetic nerves usually are inhibited. Because parasympathetic excitation and simultaneous sympathetic inhibition generally depress cardiac function (e.g., decrease the heart rate), these interneurons often are referred to as the **cardioinhibitory center.** Excitation occurs with parasympathetic inhibition and sympathetic stimulation, and these interneurons are collectively called the **cardioexcitatory center.** Therefore heart rate can be slowed by two simultaneous events that begin in the cardiovascular control center: (1) inhibition of sympathetic stimulation of the SA node and (2) activation of parasympathetic stimulation of the SA node. Heart rate can be increased by activation of sympathetic nerves and inhibition of parasympathetic nerves.

The resting heart rate in healthy individuals is primarily under the control of parasympathetic stimulation. While the individual is at rest, parasympathetic effects from the vagus nerves override sympathetic effects in the SA node. Interruption of the vagus nerves causes significant tachycardia (abnormally fast heart rate) because the inhibitory parasympathetic influence is lost.

Neural Reflexes

Two important neural reflexes that affect heart rate and rhythm are the Bainbridge reflex and the baroreceptor reflex. The **Bainbridge reflex** causes the heart rate to increase after intravenous infusions of blood or other fluid. The increased rate is thought to be caused by a reflex mediated by volume receptors in the atria that are innervated by the vagus nerves. (Volume receptors are thought to respond to increased plasma volume.) The magnitude of the change in heart rate depends on the initial heart rate. If the initial rate is slow, intravenous infusion usually accelerates it, but if the initial rate is rapid, infusions usually will slow it down.[1] Contractility usually is not affected by the Bainbridge reflex.

The **baroreceptor reflex** facilitates blood pressure changes and heart rate changes. The baroreceptor reflex is mediated by tissue pressure receptors (pressoreceptors) in the aortic arch and carotid arteries. (Because the receptors respond to mechanical factors, they are also called *aortic* and *carotid mechanoreceptors.*) The pressoreceptors increase their rate of discharge when stretched by blood pressure elevations. Neural impulses are then transmitted over the glossopharyngeal nerve (ninth cranial nerve) from the carotid artery and through the vagus nerve from the aorta to the cardiovascular control centers in the medulla. These centers initiate an increase in parasympathetic activity and a decrease in sympathetic activity, causing blood vessels to dilate and heart rate to decrease. In the heart the initial response is caused by a decrease in sympathetic stimulation, but most of the decrease in heart rate is probably the result of increased parasympathetic activity. Responses to the baroreceptor reflex return the blood pressure to its previous level, which may or may not be normal. The higher the blood pressure, the greater the reflexive decrease in heart rate.

If blood pressure is decreased, the baroreceptor reflex accelerates heart rate and causes vessels to constrict. These responses raise blood pressure back toward normal. The pressoreceptors are more effective in compensating for a decrease in arterial blood pressure than a rise in pressure.[7]

Neural receptors in the lungs cause heart rate to increase during inspiration and decrease during expiration. The increase in heart rate during inspiration is caused by the stretching (activation) of vagal fibers in the lungs that cause heart rate to speed up by inhibiting the cardioinhibitory center of the medulla. Inhibition of this center allows unopposed sympathetic acceleration of heart rate.

Hormones and Biochemicals

Hormones and biochemicals affect the arteries, arterioles, venules, capillaries, and contractility of the myocardium. Norepinephrine increases heart rate, enhances myocardial contractility, and constricts blood vessels. Epinephrine dilates vessels of the liver and skeletal muscle and also causes an increase in myocardial contractility. Some adrenocortical hormones, such as hydrocortisone, potentiate the effects of the catecholamines.

Thyroid hormones enhance sympathetic activity, promoting an increase in cardiac output. The exact mechanism by which this occurs is not known. A decrease in growth hormone, as well as thyroid and adrenal hormones, results in bradycardia (heart rate below 60 beats/min), reduced cardiac output, and low blood pressure.

Myocardial Contractility

Stroke volume, or the volume of blood ejected during systole, depends on the *force* of contraction, which depends on myocardial contractility, or the degree of myocardial fiber shortening. Two major factors determine the force of contraction: (1) changes in the stretching of the ventricular myocardium caused by changes in ventricular volume (preload) and (2) alterations in the sympathetic activation of the ventricles. Increased flow of blood from the veins into the heart distends the ventricle by increasing preload. Greater preload increases the stroke volume and, subsequently, cardiac output. Increased output then causes increased venous return, atrial volume and pressure, and eventually end-diastolic volume and stroke volume.

Myocardial contractility is difficult to measure because measurement requires keeping preload, afterload, and heart rate constant. Only when these factors are held constant can changes in cardiac performance be attributed to changes in the inotropic (contractile) state of the myocardium itself.

Factors affecting contractility are called **inotropic agents.** Positive inotropic agents increase the velocity of myocardial contraction (phase 0) and stroke volume. The positive inotropic agents are excess thyroid hormone, epinephrine, norepinephrine, dopamine or isoproterenol infusion, and calcium salt infusion. The negative inotropic agents decrease the velocity of myocardial contraction and the stroke volume. These agents include alcohol, procainamide, quinidine, and propranolol.

Myocardial contractility is affected also by oxygen and carbon dioxide levels (tensions) in the coronary blood. (Blood gases are discussed in Chapters 3 and 31.) Different degrees of arterial oxygen deficiency—termed *hypoxemia*—affect contractility differently. With severe hypoxemia (arterial oxygen saturation less than 50%), contractility is decreased. With less severe hypoxemia (saturation more than 50%), contractility is stimulated. Moderate degrees of hypoxemia may increase contractility by enhancing the myocardial response to circulating catecholamines.[1]

Factors Determining Cardiac Output

Cardiac output is the volume of blood flowing through either the systemic or the pulmonary circuit per minute and is expressed in liters per minute. Heart rate and stroke volume determine cardiac output. The volume to which the ventricle fills is determined by the ventricular filling pressure and the compliance of the ventricle. The filling pressure of the right ventricle is the **right atrial pressure,** and the filling pressure of the left ventricle is the **left atrial pressure.** The cardiac output is determined by multiplying the heart rate and the stroke volume. Normal cardiac output is about 5 L/min for a

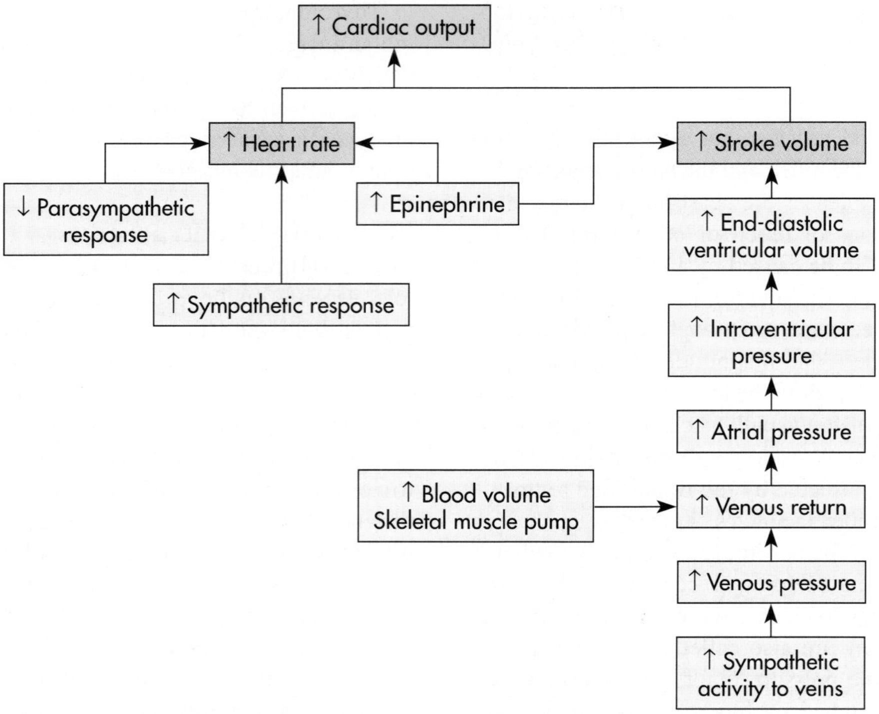

FIG. 28-20 Major factors determining increased cardiac output.

resting adult. A summary of the major factors that determine cardiac output is presented in Fig. 28-20. (Also see discussion of heart rate and myocardial contractility [stroke volume], pp. 950 and 951.)

The ventricle does not eject all of the blood it contains; the amount ejected is called the **ejection fraction,** or the stroke volume divided by the end-diastolic volume. The end-diastolic volume of the normal ventricle is about 70 to 80 ml/m^2; the normal ejection fraction of the resting heart is about 60% to 75%. The ejection fraction is increased by factors that increase contractility (e.g., sympathetic nervous system activity), and a decrease in ejection fraction is a hallmark of ventricular failure.

SYSTEMIC CIRCULATION

The arteries and veins of the systemic circulation are illustrated in Fig. 28-21. Blood from the left side of the heart flows through the aorta and into the systemic arteries. The **arteries** branch into small **arterioles** that branch further into the smallest vessels, the **capillaries,** where nutrient exchange between the blood and tissues occurs. Blood from the capillaries then enters tiny **venules** that join together to form the larger **veins,** which return venous blood to the right heart. **Peripheral vascular system** is an imprecise term used to describe the part of the systemic circulation that supplies the skin and the extremities, particularly the legs and feet.

Structure of Blood Vessels

Blood vessel walls are composed of three layers: the tunica intima (innermost or intimal layer), the tunica media (middle or medial layer), and the tunica externa or adventitia (outermost or external layer). These structures are illustrated in Figs. 28-22 and 28-23. The **tunica intima** is composed of a layer of squamous epithelium or endothelium, a layer of connective tissue, and a basement membrane. (These cellular structures are described in Chapter 1.) The **tunica media** is composed of smooth muscle fibers mixed with elastic fibers. The **tunica externa,** or adventitia, has a thin layer of connective tissue containing elastic and collagenous fibers that run lengthwise in the vessel. Blood vessel walls vary in thickness depending on the thickness or absence of one or more of these three layers. Cells of the larger vessels are nourished by the **vasa vasorum,** small vessels located in the tunica externa. The vasa vasorum arise from the blood vessel itself or from other vessels nearby.

Arterial Vessels

Arterial walls are composed of elastic connective tissue, fibrous connective tissue, and smooth muscle. The two types of arteries are elastic and muscular. The **elastic arteries** have a very thick tunica media that contains more elastic fibers than smooth muscle fibers. Elastic arteries include the aorta and its major branches and the pulmonary trunk. Elasticity enables the vessel to stretch as blood is ejected from the heart during systole. During diastole, elasticity promotes recoil of the arteries, which is important for maintaining blood pressure within the vessels.

The **muscular arteries** are the medium-size and small arteries farther from the heart than the elastic arteries. They contain fewer elastic fibers and more muscle fibers than the elastic arteries because, being farther from the heart, they have less need of the properties of stretch and recoil. The function of the muscular arteries is to distribute blood to arterioles throughout the body. They also play a role in con-

A

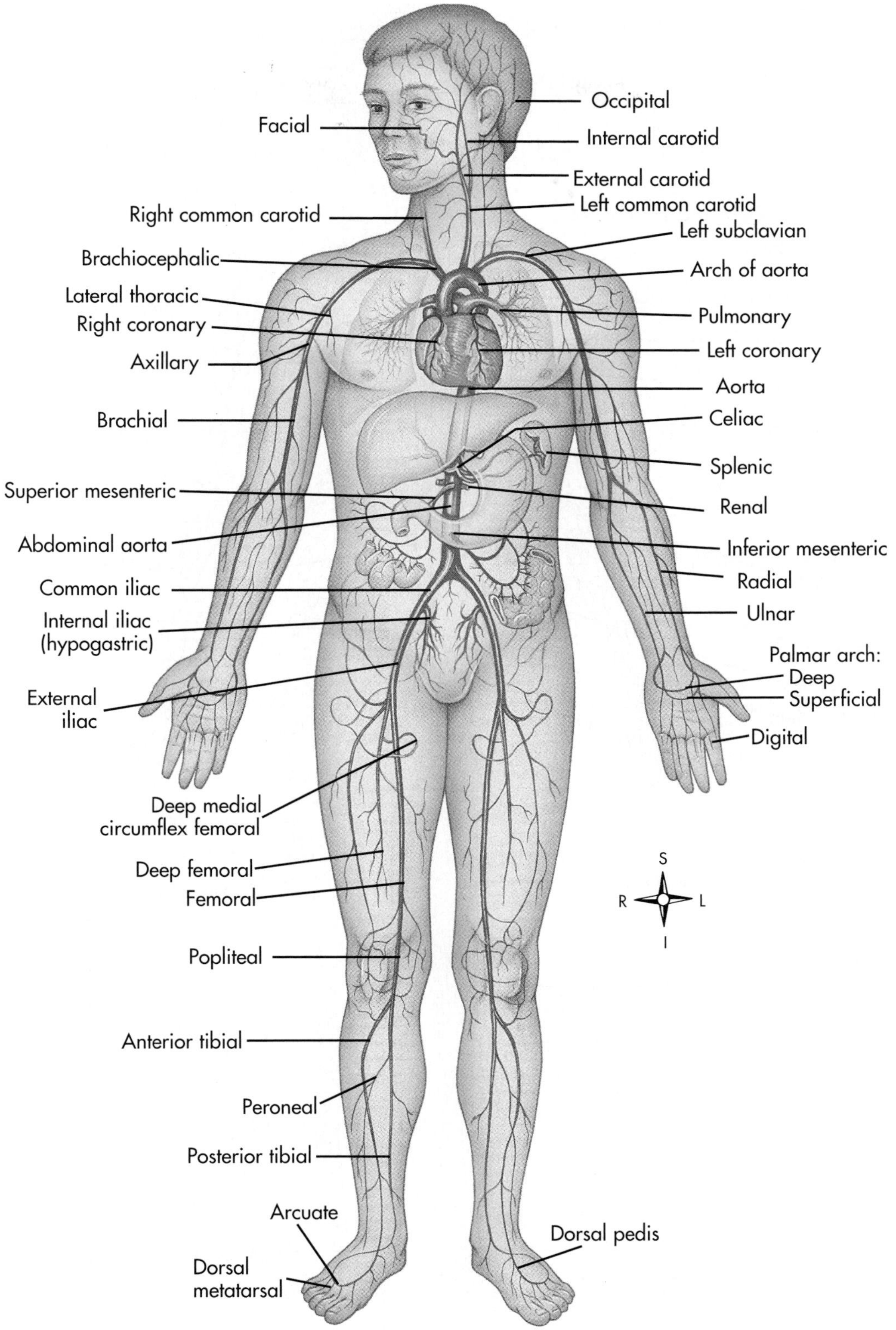

FIG. 28-21 Circulatory system. A, Principal arteries of the body. (From Thibodeau GA, Patton KI: *Anatomy and physiology*, ed 4, St Louis, 1999, Mosby.)

Continued

trolling blood flow because their smooth muscle can be stimulated to contract or relax. Contraction narrows the vessel **lumen** (the internal cavity of the vessel), which diminishes flow through the vessel. This condition is termed **vasoconstriction.** The smooth muscle layer also can be stimulated to relax, which permits more blood to flow through the vessel lumen. This state is called **vasodilation.**

An artery becomes an arteriole where the diameter of its lumen narrows to less than 0.5 mm. The arterioles are composed almost exclusively of smooth muscle, with little elastic

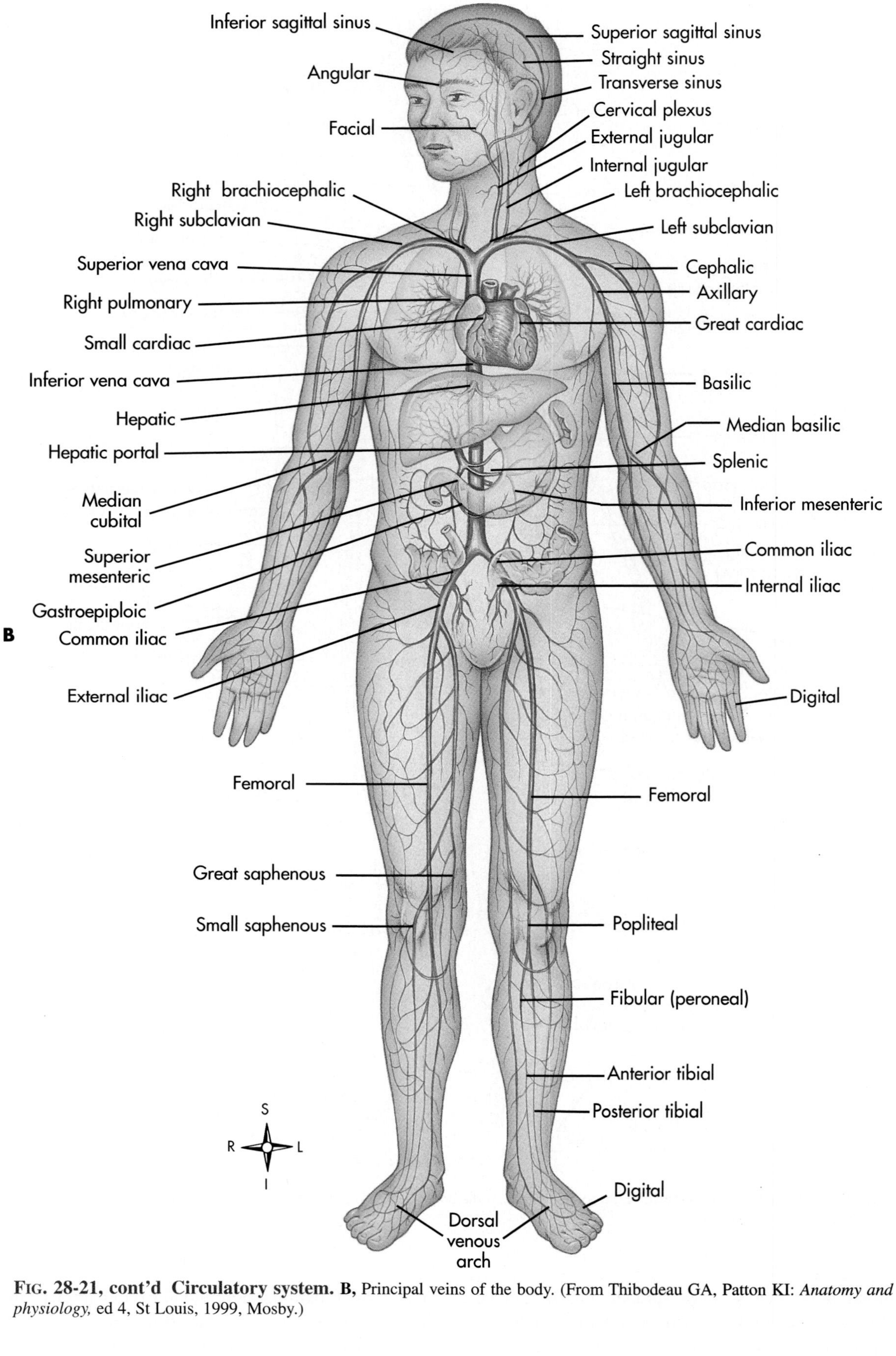

FIG. 28-21, cont'd Circulatory system. B, Principal veins of the body. (From Thibodeau GA, Patton KI: *Anatomy and physiology,* ed 4, St Louis, 1999, Mosby.)

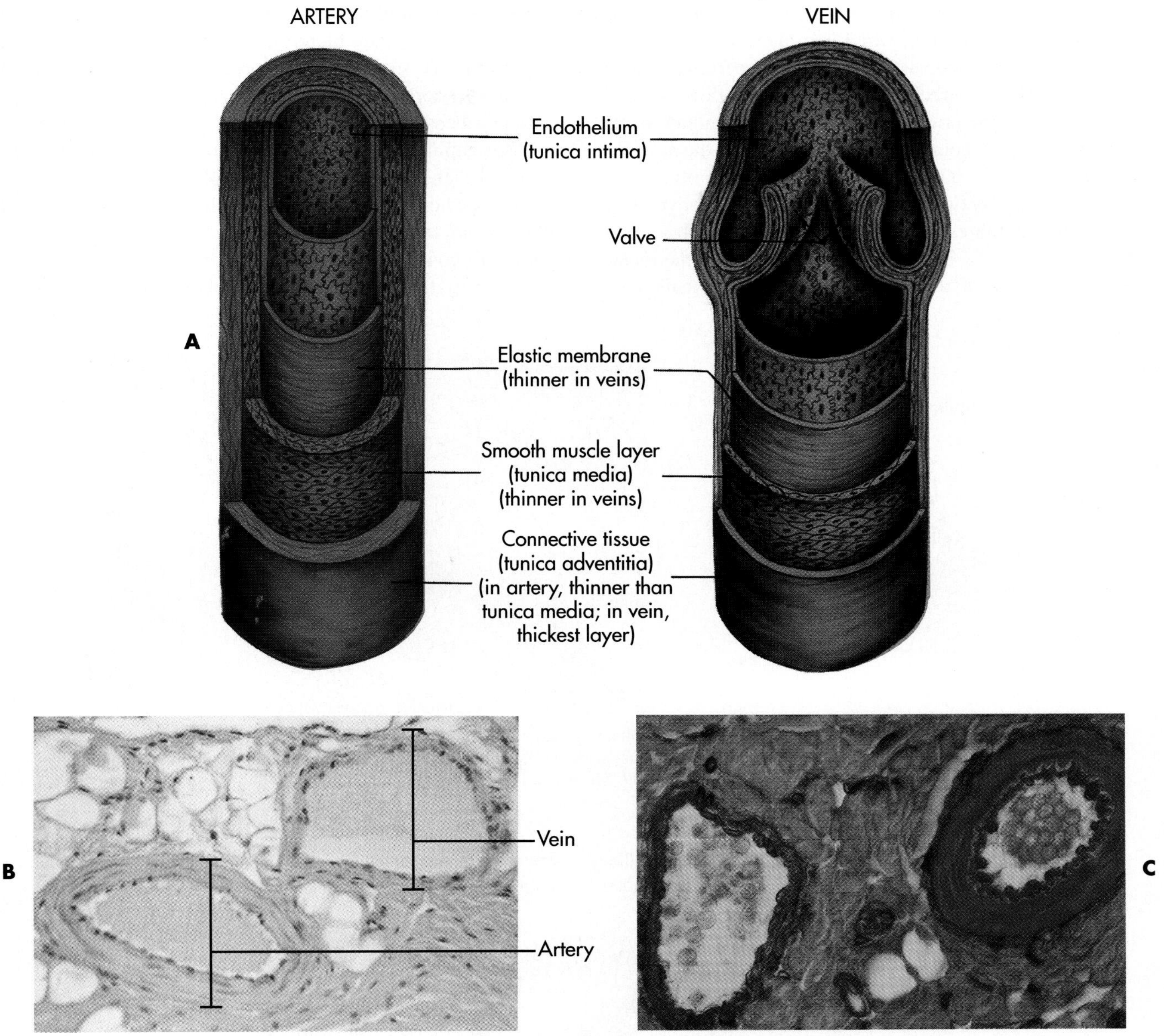

FIG. 28-22 Schematic drawings and micrograph of artery and vein. A, Shown are the comparative thickness of three coats: outer coat (tunica adventitia), muscle coat (tunica media), and lining of endothelium (tunica intima). Note that muscle and outer coats are much thinner in veins than in arteries and that veins have valves. **B,** Micrograph (250×) of a cross section of tissue containing both an artery *(left)* and a vein *(right)*. Note the thickness of the smooth muscle (tunica media) in the artery compared with the vein. **C,** Micrograph showing both an artery and vein. The tunica media is much thicker in the artery. (**A,** Modified from Thompson JM et al: *Mosby's clinical nursing,* ed 4, St Louis, 1997, Mosby. **B,** From Thibodeau GA, Patton KT: *Anatomy and physiology,* ed 3, St Louis, 1996, Mosby. **C,** Copyright © Ed Reschke.)

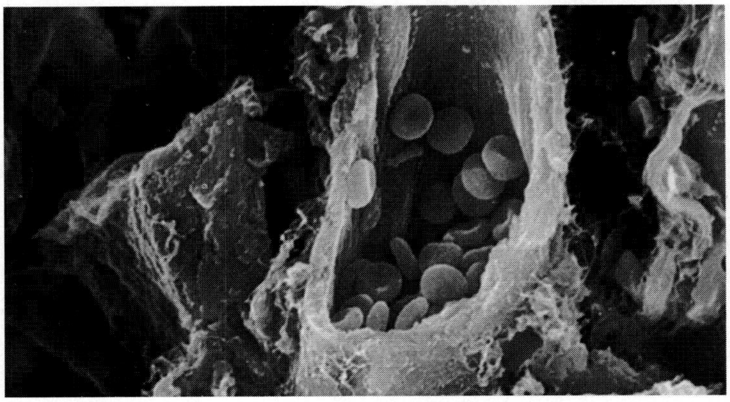

FIG. 28-23 This ruptured tube is a blood vessel. It is full of red blood cells, which move through these blood vessels transporting oxygen and carbon dioxide from one place to another in the body. (From Raven RH, Johnson GB: *Biology,* ed 3, St Louis, 1992, Mosby).

tissue. Arterioles regulate the flow of blood into the capillaries by vasoconstriction, which retards the flow of blood into the capillaries, and vasodilation, which permits blood to enter the capillaries freely (Fig. 28-24). The thick, smooth muscle layer of the arterioles is a major determinant of the resistance blood encounters as it flows through the systemic circulation.

The capillary network is composed of connective channels, or thoroughfares, called **metarterioles,** and "true" capillaries (Fig. 28-25). The capillaries branch from the metarterioles, meeting at a ring of smooth muscle called the **precapillary sphincter.** As the sphincters contract and relax, they regulate blood flow through the capillaries. Appropriately stimulated, the precapillary sphincters help maintain arterial pressure and regulate selective flow to vascular beds.

The capillary walls are very thin, making possible the rapid exchange of substrates, metabolites, and special products (e.g., hormones) between the blood and the interstitial fluid, from which they are taken up by the cells. The capillary wall consists of a single layer of endothelial cells surrounded by the thin basement membrane of the tunica in-

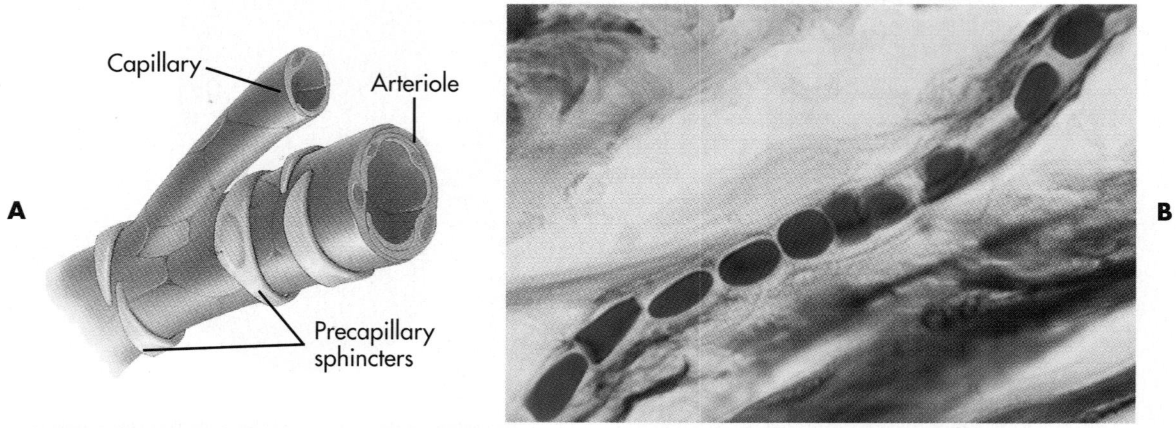

FIG. 28-24 Capillary wall. A, Capillaries have a wall composed of only a single layer of flattened cells, whereas the walls of the larger vessels also have smooth muscle. **B,** Capillary with red blood cells in single file (500×). (**A,** From Thibodeau GA, Patton KI: *Anatomy and physiology,* ed 4, St Louis, 1999, Mosby. **B,** Copyright © Ed Reschke.)

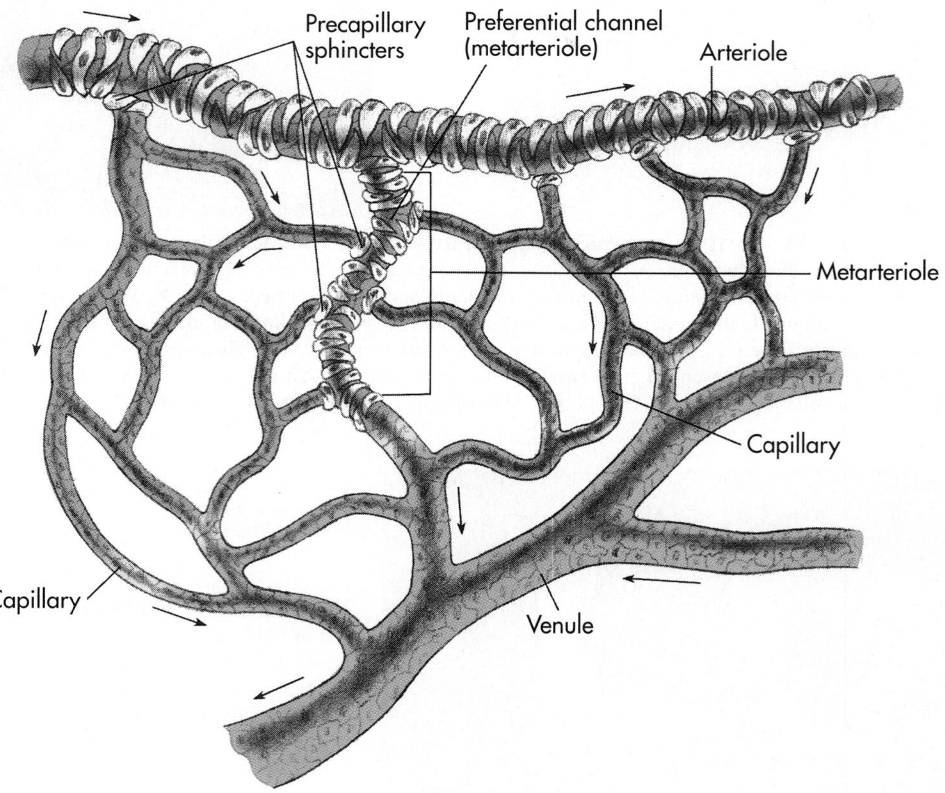

FIG. 28-25 Capillary network. Blood enters network as arterial blood and exits as venous blood.

tima. A single endothelial cell may form the entire vessel wall if the capillary has no tunica media or tunica externa. In some capillaries the endothelial cells contain oval windows or pores termed **fenestrations.** Fenestrations generally are covered by a thin diaphragm.

Substances pass between the capillary lumen and the interstitial fluid in several ways: (1) through junctions between endothelial cells, (2) through fenestrations in endothelial cells, (3) in vesicles moved by active transport across the endothelial cell membrane, or (4) by diffusion through the endothelial cell membrane. (Movement across cell membranes is described in Chapter 1.) A single capillary may be only 0.5 to 1 mm in length and 0.01 mm in diameter, but the capillaries are so numerous that their total surface area may be more than 600 m^2, or larger than 100 football fields.

Control of Vessel Contraction or Relaxation: Vasomotion

The **endothelium** functions as a semipermeable membrane separating the blood from the body and allowing the transport of macromolecules from the blood to the interstitial space. It is known that the endothelium performs other vital functions, including regulation of smooth muscle tone, cell proliferation, synthesis and release of vasoactive chemicals, unimpeded blood flow because of its nonadhesive surface, antithrombogenesis, and fibrinolysis. Box 28-1 summarizes some of the more important functions. It secretes substances that promote contraction or relaxation, or **vasomotion,** of the vascular smooth muscle.

Veins

The smallest venules closest to the capillaries have an inner lining, composed of the endothelium of the tunica intima and surrounded by fibrous tissue. The largest venules, those farthest from the capillaries, are surrounded by a few smooth muscle fibers comprising a thin tunica media.

Compared with arteries, veins are thin walled and fibrous with a larger diameter (see Fig. 28-22). A given vein is larger than the artery that lies within the same sheath. Veins are more numerous than arteries. In veins the tunica externa has less elastic tissue than in arteries, so veins do not recoil after distention as quickly as arteries. Like arteries, veins receive

Box 28-1

ENDOTHELIUM FUNCTIONS AND VASOACTIVE SUBSTANCES

DILATORS

Prostacyclin: A prostaglandin formed from arachidonic acid that can relax vascular smooth muscle through increases in cAMP. The primary function is to inhibit platelet adherence to the endothelium.

Nitric oxide (NO): Also known as endothelial-derived relaxing factor (EDRF). Bradykinin prompts the endothelium to synthesize and release nitric oxide (NO), a potent vasodilator. Continuous small amounts of NO overcome the vessel's natural tendency to constrict.

CONSTRICTORS

Endothelin: Also known as endothelium-derived contracting factor, a potent constrictor. Overproduction can cause hypertension.

Angiotensin II: Angiotensin converting enzyme converts the peptide angiotensin I to angiotensin II. Angiotensin II, another potent vasoconstrictor, can block the release of nitric oxide and prostacyclin. Angiotensin II has multiple functions beyond its hemodynamic effects and plays a key role in the inflammatory response. It (1) increases vascular permeability (through prostaglandins and vascular endothelial growth factor [VEGF]); (2) participates in the recruitment of infiltrating cells; (3) participates in the regulation of the expression of adhesion molecules by resident cells; and (4) contributes to tissue repair by regulation of cell growth and matrix synthesis. Thus angiotension II is involved in both antiinflammatory and proinflammatory reactions. Binding of angiotensin I to angiotensin II type 1 receptor is responsible for most of its physiologic reactions.

PLATELET AND MONOCYTE ADHESION

Monocytes and macrophages: The endothelium helps regulate the number of inflammatory cells (monocytes and macrophages) that bind to the vessel wall. Monocytes increase plaque deposition. A reduction in NO causes an increase in the oxidation of low-density lipoprotein.

CELL GROWTH AND INHIBITION

Nitric oxide, prostacyclin: Inhibits cellular growth.

Angiotensin II: Stimulates growth.

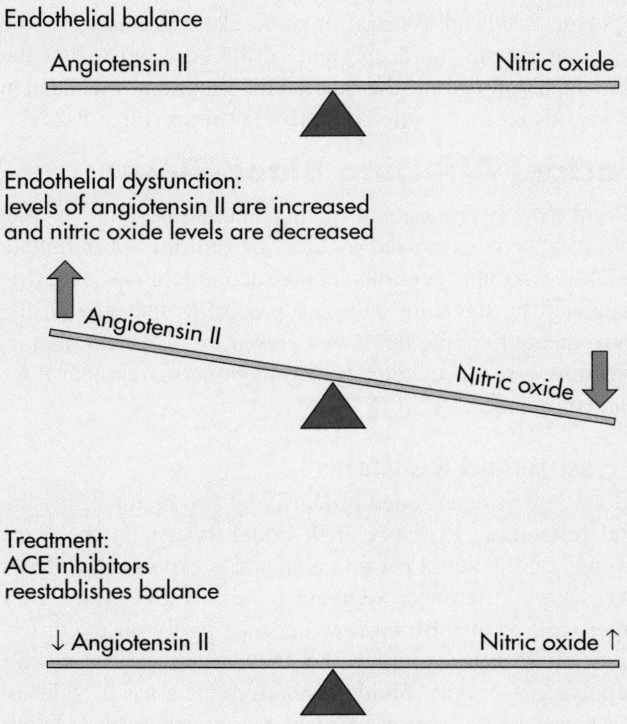

Data from Haendeler J, Berk BC: Angiotensin II mediated signal transduction: important role of tyrosine kinases, *Regul Pept* 95(1-3): 1, 2000; Suzuki Y, Ruiz-Ortega M, Egido J: Angiotensin II: a double-edged sword in inflammation, *J Nephrol* 13(suppl 3):S101, 2000. Figure adapted from Rockett JL: Endothelial dysfunction and the promise of ACE inhibitors, *Am J Nurs* 99(10):44, 1999.

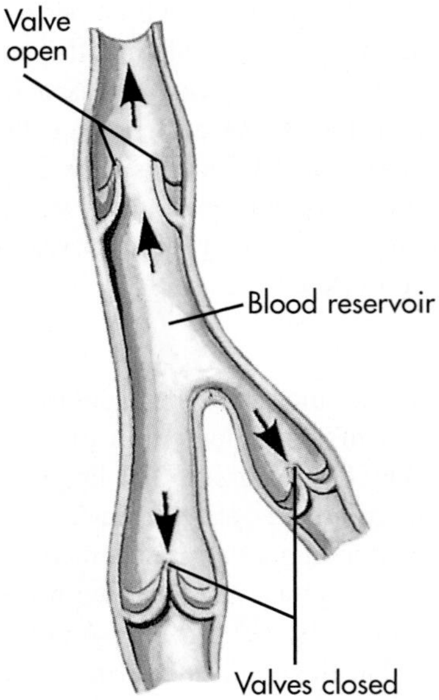

FIG. 28-26 Valves of vein. Pooled blood is moved toward heart as valves are forced open by pressure from volume of blood downstream. (From Thibodeau GA, Patton KT: *Anatomy and physiology,* ed 3, St Louis, 1996, Mosby.)

nourishment from the tiny vasa vasorum. Some veins, most commonly in the lower limbs, contain valves that regulate the one-way flow of blood toward the heart (Fig. 28-26). These valves are folds of the tunica intima and resemble the semilunar valves of the heart. Backflow in veins of the legs is stopped as the flaps of the valves fill with blood and block the vessel. The position of the valves also facilitates blood flow in the proper direction during venous compression. When a person stands up, contraction of the skeletal muscles of the legs compresses the deep veins of the legs and assists the flow of blood toward the heart. This important mechanism of venous return is called the **muscle pump** (Fig. 28-27).

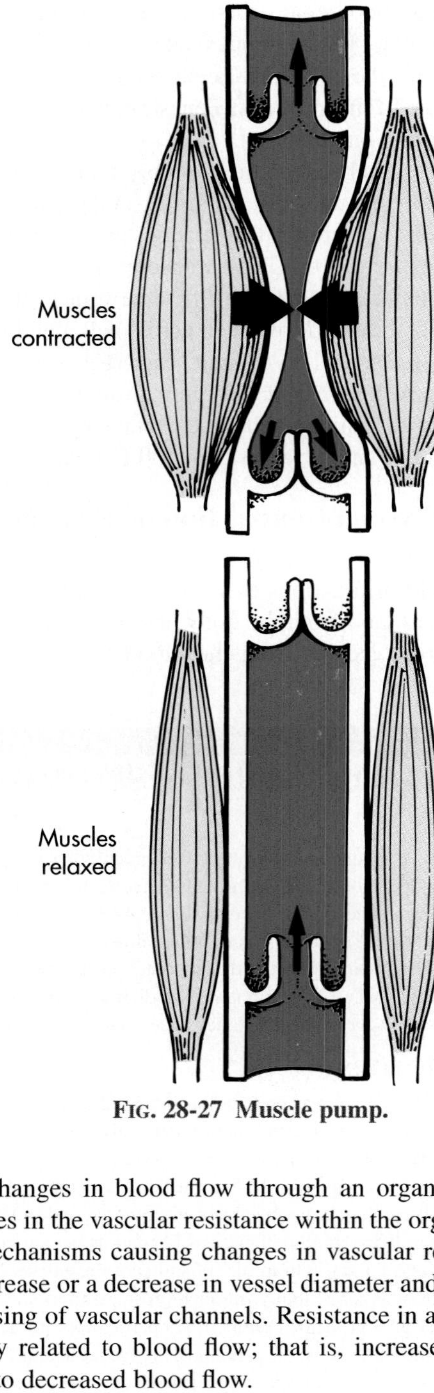

FIG. 28-27 Muscle pump.

Factors Affecting Blood Flow

Blood flow is the amount of fluid moved per unit of time and usually is expressed as liters or milliliters per minute (ml/min) or cubic centimeters per second (cm^3/sec). Flow is regulated by the same physical properties that govern the movement of simple fluids in a closed, rigid system, that is, pressure, resistance, velocity, turbulent versus laminar flow, and compliance.

Pressure and Resistance

Blood flow is determined primarily by two factors: pressure and resistance. **Pressure** in a liquid system is the force exerted on the liquid per unit area and is expressed as dynes per square centimeter (dyn/cm^2), millimeters of mercury (mm Hg), or torr. Blood flow depends partly on the difference between pressures in the arterial and venous vessels supplying the organ. Fluid moves from the arterial "side" of the capillaries, a region of greater pressure, to the venous side, a region of lesser pressure.

Resistance is the opposition to force. In the cardiovascular system most opposition to blood flow is provided by the diameter and length of the blood vessels themselves. Therefore changes in blood flow through an organ result from changes in the vascular resistance within the organ. The major mechanisms causing changes in vascular resistance are an increase or a decrease in vessel diameter and the opening or closing of vascular channels. Resistance in a vessel is inversely related to blood flow; that is, increased resistance leads to decreased blood flow.

Blood flow *(Q)* through a vessel can be calculated from measurements of pressure at the inflow end of the vessel (P_1), pressure at the outflow end of the vessel (P_2), and resistance *(R)*. The difference between P_1 and P_2 often is referred to as the change in pressure and is expressed as δP. The following formula, which expresses **Poiseuille's law,** shows the relationship among blood flow, pressure, and resistance:

$$Q = \delta P/R$$

where Q = blood flow, δP = the pressure difference ($P_1 - P_2$), and R = resistance.

Resistance to flow cannot be measured directly, but it can be calculated if the pressure difference and flow volumes are

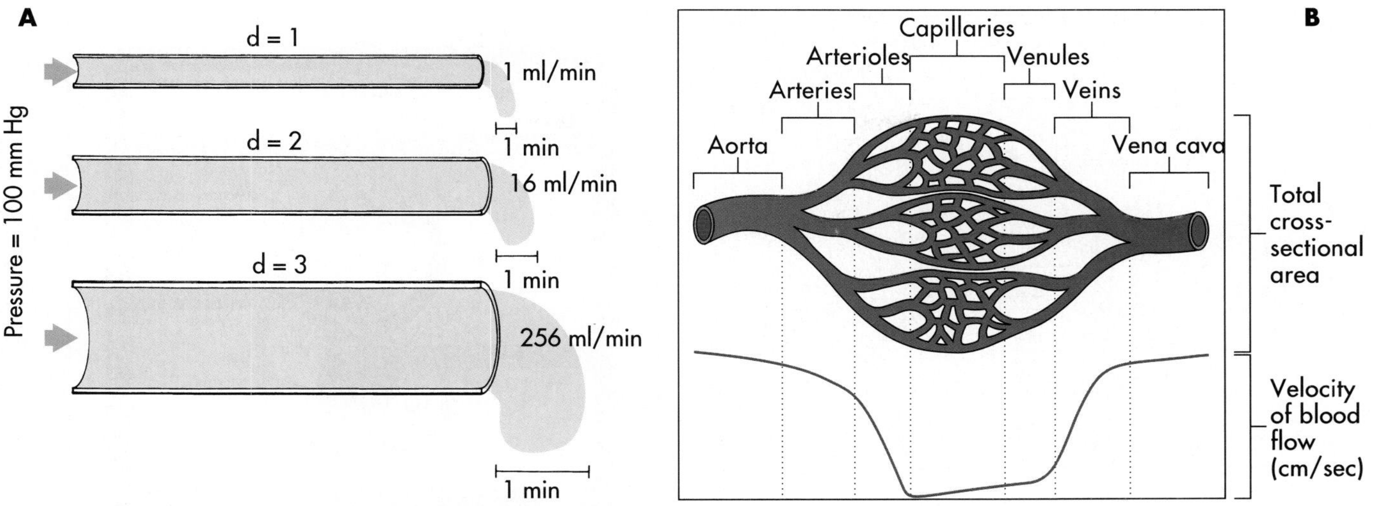

FIG. 28-28 Lumen diameter, blood flow, and resistance. A, Effect of lumen diameter on flow through vessel. *d,* Diameter. **B,** Blood flows with great speed in the large arteries. However, branching of arterial vessels increases the total cross-sectional area of the arterioles and capillaries, reducing the flow rate. When capillaries merge into venules and venules merge into veins, the total cross-sectional area decreases, causing the flow rate to increase. (**B,** From Thibodeau GA, Patton KI: *Anatomy and physiology,* ed 4, St Louis, 1999, Mosby.)

known. To determine resistance, the equation for flow is rearranged as follows:

$$R = \delta P/Q$$

Flow varies inversely with the viscosity of the fluid. Thick fluids move more slowly and cause greater resistance to flow than thin fluids. The viscosity of blood depends on its red cell content. The greater the percentage of red cells in the blood, the more viscous the blood. This relationship is expressed as the hematocrit—the ratio of the volume of red blood cells to the volume of whole blood (see Chapter 24). A high hematocrit reduces flow through the blood vessels, particularly the microcirculation (arterioles, capillaries, venules). Conditions in which the hematocrit is elevated, such as dehydration, cyanotic congenital heart disease (see Chapter 30), or polycythemia (see Chapter 25), can lead to increased cardiac work as a result of increased vascular resistance.

The viscosity of blood also increases if blood flow becomes very slow or stagnates **(anomalous viscosity).** Anomalous viscosity is generally not significant unless cardiac output is low. (Shock is described in Chapter 45.)

Poiseuille's formula for resistance to fluid flow through a tube takes into account the length of the tube, the viscosity of the fluid, and the radius of the tube's lumen. Resistance *(R)* is proportional to a constant $8/\pi$, the viscosity of the blood (η), and the length of the vessel *(l),* and it is inversely proportional to the fourth power of the lumen's radius (ν^4).[1] Thus

$$R = \frac{8\eta l}{\pi\nu 4}$$

Because this equation was derived using straight, rigid tubes with steady, streamlined flow, it cannot be applied directly to the vascular system. Nevertheless, it is a useful model of vascular resistance.

The most important factor determining resistance *in a single vessel* is the caliber of the vessel's lumen, expressed in Poiseuille's formula as its radius and in Fig. 28-28 as its diameter. Small changes in the lumen's radius lead to large changes in vascular resistance. Because vessel length is relatively constant, length is not as important as lumen size in determining flow through a single vessel.

Generally, resistance to flow is greater in longer tubes because resistance increases with length. That resistance increases with increased length is demonstrated by comparing flow of the same amount of blood under the same pressure through vessels arranged in different configurations. Blood flowing through the distributing arteries, beginning with branches off the aorta and ending at arterioles in the capillary bed, encounters more resistance than blood flowing through the capillary bed itself, where flow is distributed among many short, tiny branches arranged in parallel. This is because the distributing arteries comprise a long system of tubes connected in series (end to end), whereas the arterioles and capillaries comprise a short system of many vessels arranged in parallel (side by side) (Fig. 28-29). Although the arterioles are arranged in series with the distributing arteries and the capillaries, they are arranged in parallel with other arterioles. Similarly, the capillaries are in series with the metarterioles, but they are in parallel with other capillaries.

Resistance to flow through a system of vessels, or **total resistance,** depends not only on characteristics of individual vessels but also on whether the vessels are arranged in series or in parallel (see Fig. 28-29). For vessels arranged in series, total resistance equals the sum obtained by adding all the individual resistances calculated using Poiseuille's formula. For vessels arranged in parallel, total resistance equals the sum of the reciprocals *(I/R)* of the individual resistances.

Total resistance is related to the total cross-sectional area of a system of vessels in parallel and to the number of vessels in parallel that make up the total cross-sectional area. The larger the total cross-sectional area, as in the capillary system, the lower the resistance. However, if a cross-sectional

A
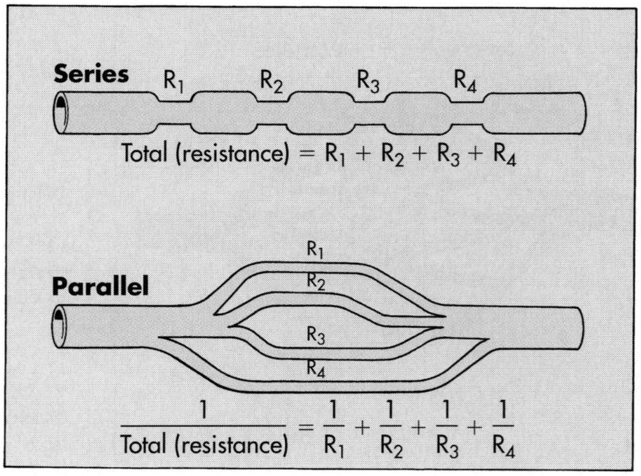

B
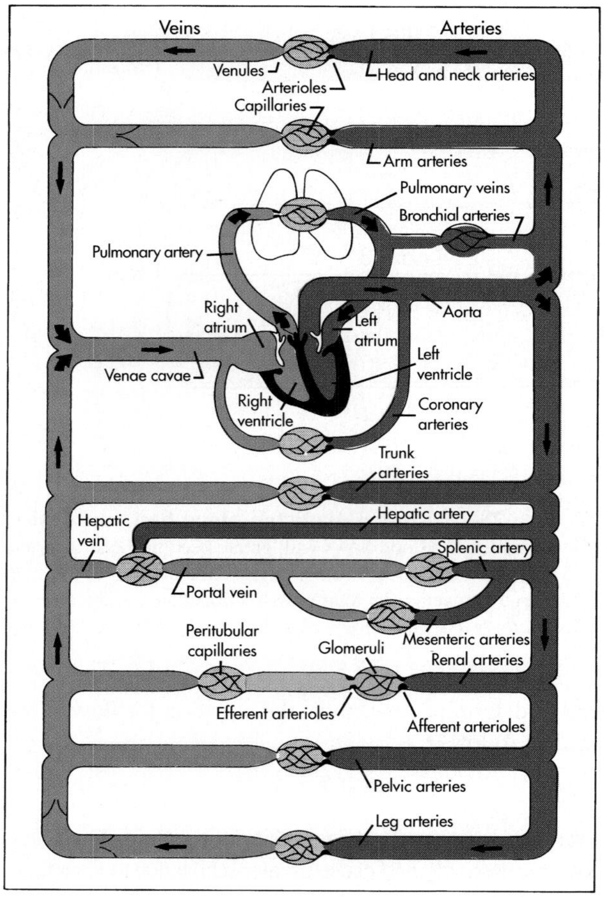

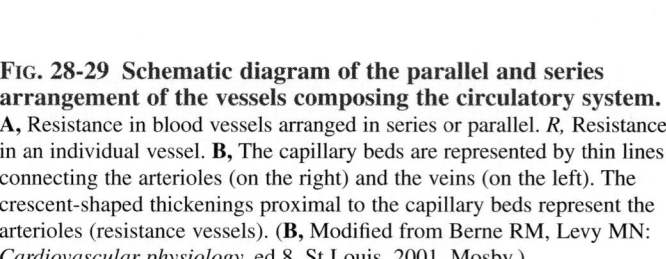

FIG. 28-29 Schematic diagram of the parallel and series arrangement of the vessels composing the circulatory system. **A,** Resistance in blood vessels arranged in series or parallel. *R,* Resistance in an individual vessel. **B,** The capillary beds are represented by thin lines connecting the arterioles (on the right) and the veins (on the left). The crescent-shaped thickenings proximal to the capillary beds represent the arterioles (resistance vessels). (**B,** Modified from Berne RM, Levy MN: *Cardiovascular physiology,* ed 8, St Louis, 2001, Mosby.)

area is made up of a very large number of parallel vessels, the overall resistance will be greater than it would be if the cross-sectional area were made up of only two or three parallel vessels. Therefore resistance is greater in smaller vessels than in larger vessels. The total cross-sectional area of the arteriolar system is greater than that of the arterial system (see Fig. 28-28); the greater number of arterioles arranged in parallel, however, leads to great resistance to flow in the arteriolar system. Because resistance reaches a maximal level in the arteries, they are sometimes called the "stopcocks" of the vascular system. The pressure drop is greatest across the arterioles. Many capillaries arise from each arteriole so that the total cross-sectional area of the capillary bed is very large and resistance is low, despite the fact that the cross-sectional area of each capillary is less (which normally increases resistance) than that of each arteriole. As a result, blood flow becomes quite slow in the capillaries, analogous to water flow in a river. A narrow river whose bed widens flows more slowly through the wide section than through the narrow section. The slow velocity of flow in each vessel promotes optimal capillary-tissue exchange.

Neural Control of Total Peripheral Resistance

Total resistance in the systemic circulation, sometimes called *total peripheral resistance,* is determined primarily by change in the diameter of the arterioles. Reflex control of total cardiac output and peripheral resistance includes (1) sympathetic stimulation of heart, arterioles, and veins and (2) parasympathetic stimulation of the heart only.

The autonomic nervous system is monitored by the cardiovascular control center in the brain (see p. 950). The hypothalamic centers regulate vascular (and cardiac) responses to changes in temperature. When the body's core temperature exceeds normal, the hypothalamus reflex initiates dilation of arterioles and veins in the skin. This causes shunting of blood to the skin, where heat is lost from sweating, radiation, conduction, or convection. When body core temperature decreases below normal, surface vessels constrict, shunting blood to the vital organs. Vasoconstriction is regulated by an area of the brain stem that maintains a constant (tonic) output of norepinephrine from sympathetic fibers in the peripheral arterioles. This tonic activity is essential for maintenance of blood pressure.

During exercise and stress, the sympathetic fibers that stimulate vasodilation of skeletal muscle arterioles are thought to be under the direct control of the cerebral cortex and hypothalamus and *not* the medullary centers.[8] Information about pressure and resistance is sensed by neural receptors (baroreceptors and chemoreceptors) in arterial walls and delivered to the medullary centers.

Baroreceptors

Major stretch receptors are located in the aorta and in the carotid sinus (Fig. 28-30). These baroreceptors respond to changes in smooth muscle fiber length by altering their rate

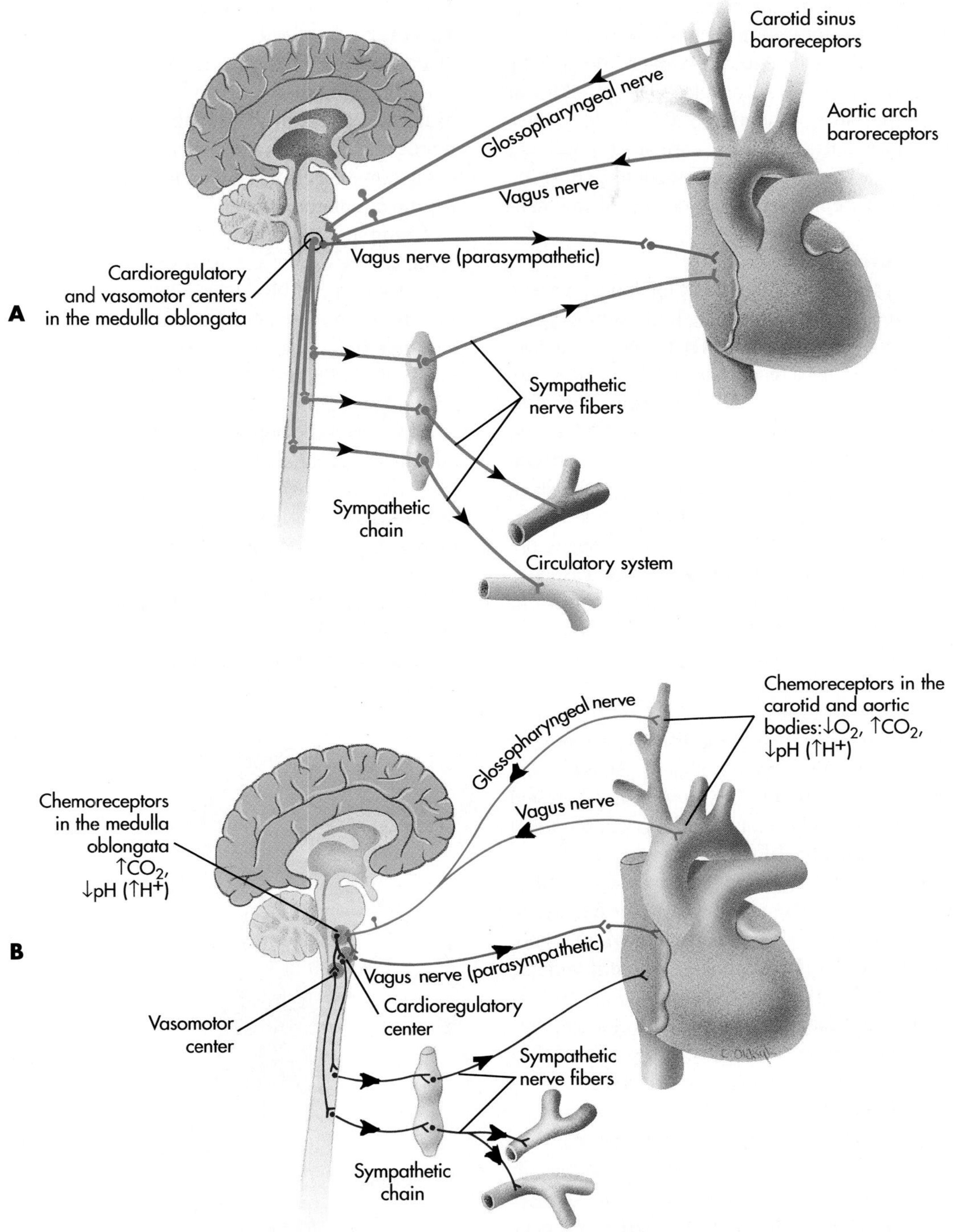

FIG. 28-30 Baroreceptor and chemoreceptor reflex control of blood pressure. A, Baroreceptor reflexes. Baroreceptors located in the carotid sinuses and aortic arch detect changes in blood pressure. Action potentials are conducted to the cardioregulatory and vasomotor centers. The heart rate can be decreased by the parasympathetic system; the heart rate and stroke volume can be increased by the sympathetic system. The sympathetic system also can constrict or dilate blood vessels. **B,** Chemoreceptor reflexes. Chemoreceptors located in the medulla oblongata and in the carotid and aortic bodies detect changes in blood oxygen, carbon dioxide, or pH. Action potentials are conducted to the medulla oblongata. In response, the vasomotor center can cause vasoconstriction or dilation of blood vessels by the sympathetic system, and the cardioregulatory center can cause changes in the pumping activity of the heart through the parasympathetic and sympathetic systems. (From Seeley RR, Stephens TD, Tate P: *Anatomy and physiology,* ed 3, St Louis, 1995, Mosby.)

of discharge, and they supply sensory information to the cardiovascular center that regulates blood pressure. (Technically they are *mechanoreceptors,* but they usually are called *baroreceptors* or *pressoreceptors.*) The rate of firing of the baroreceptors increases and decreases with changes in blood pressure. An increase in arterial pressure increases the rate of firing of both the carotid sinus and aortic arch baroreceptors. These impulses travel up the afferent nerves to the medulla (e.g., the cardiac control center) and (1) slow heart rate by decreasing sympathetic discharge and increasing parasympathetic discharge (vagus nerve), (2) decrease myocardial contractility by inhibiting sympathetic discharge, and (3) increase arteriolar and venous dilation by decreasing sympathetic discharge to smooth muscle. The net effect of this major blood pressure–regulating reflex is to reduce blood pressure to normal by decreasing cardiac output (heart rate and stroke volume) and peripheral resistance. (Postural changes and the baroreceptor reflex are discussed in Chapter 29.)

Arterial Chemoreceptors

Specialized areas within the medulla oblongata and aortic and carotid arteries are sensitive to concentrations of oxygen, carbon dioxide, and hydrogen ions (pH) in the blood (see Fig. 28-30, *B*). Although these receptors, called *chemoreceptors,* are more important for the control of respiration, they also transmit impulses to the medullary cardiovascular centers that regulate blood pressure. A decrease in arterial oxygen concentration or pH causes a reflexive increase in blood pressure, whereas an increase in carbon dioxide causes an increase in blood pressure. Blood pressure changes are carried out by smooth muscle layers in the vessels. Vasoconstriction raises blood pressure, and vasodilation lowers it. The major chemoreceptive reflex is caused by alterations in arterial oxygen concentration. The effects of altered pH or carbon dioxide levels are minor.

Velocity

Blood velocity is the *distance* blood travels in a unit of time, usually centimeters per second (cm/sec). Blood velocity is directly related to blood flow (*amount* of blood moved per unit of time) and inversely related to the cross-sectional area of the vessel in which the blood is flowing.

The relationship between velocity and flow can be understood by thinking of a river. The volume of water flowing in a river is the same whether the river is narrow or wide. Where the river narrows, the water flows quickly; where it widens, the water flows slowly. The volume of water moving between the river banks does not change. In the body, as blood moves from the aorta to the capillaries, the total cross-sectional area of the vessels increases and velocity of flow decreases.

Laminar Versus Turbulent Flow

Flow through any tubular system is either laminar or turbulent. Normally, blood flow through the vessels is laminar. In **laminar flow,** concentric layers of molecules move "straight ahead." Each concentric layer flows at a different velocity (Fig. 28-31). The cohesive attraction between the fluid and the vessel wall prevents the molecules of blood that are in contact with the wall from moving. The next thin layer of blood is able to slide slowly past the stationary layer and so on until, at the center, the blood velocity is greatest. The centermost concentric layer of fluid is not slowed by friction against the vessel wall. Large vessels have room for a large center layer; therefore they have less resistance to flow and greater flow and velocity than smaller vessels.

Where flow is obstructed, the vessel turns, or blood flows over rough surfaces, it becomes **turbulent** with whorls or eddy currents that produce noise, causing a murmur to be heard on auscultation. Resistance increases with turbulence.

Vascular Compliance

Vascular compliance is the increase in volume a vessel is able to accommodate for a given increase in pressure (e.g., $C = VP$). Compliance depends on the ratio of elastic fibers to muscle fibers in the vessel wall. The elastic arteries are more compliant than the muscular arteries; the veins are more compliant than either type of artery and serve as storage areas for the circulatory system.

Compliance determines a vessel's response to pressure changes. For example, with a very small increase in pressure, a large volume of blood can be accommodated by the venous system. In the less compliant arterial system, where smaller volumes and higher pressures are normal, small variations in pressure cause little or no change in the volume of blood within the arterial vessels.

Stiffness is the opposite of compliance. Several conditions and disorders can cause stiffness, with the most common being arteriosclerosis (see Chapter 29). Arteriosclerosis increases the rigidity or stiffness of arterial walls, which in turn increases peak arterial pressure at a given volume of blood.

Regulation of Blood Pressure

Arterial Pressure

Arterial pressure is constantly regulated to maintain tissue **perfusion,** or blood supply to the capillary beds, during a

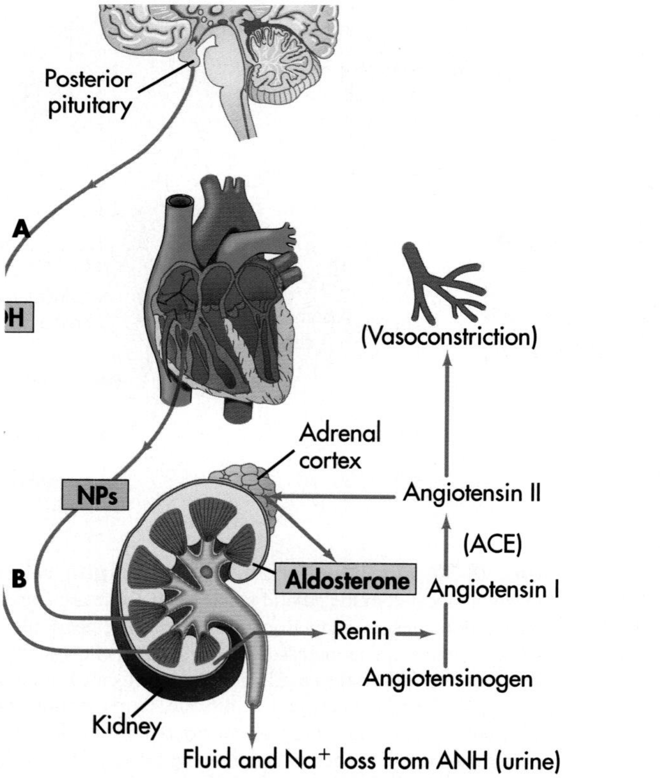

FIG. 28-31 **Laminar and turbulent flow. A,** Laminar flow. Fluid flows in long, smooth-walled tubes as if it is composed of a large number of concentric layers. **B,** Turbulent flow. Turbulent flow is caused by numerous small currents flowing crosswise or oblique to the long axis of the vessel, resulting in flowing whorls and eddy currents. (From Seeley RR, Stephens TD, Tate P: *Anatomy and physiology,* ed 3, St Louis, 1995, Mosby.)

wide range of physiologic conditions, including changes in body position, muscular activity, and circulating blood volume. The **mean arterial pressure (MAP),** which is the average pressure in the arteries throughout the cardiac cycle, depends on the elastic properties of the arterial walls and the *mean* volume of blood in the arterial system. MAP can be approximated from the measured values of the systolic *(Ps)* and diastolic *(Pd)* pressures by means of the following formula: $MAP = Pd + 1/3(Ps - Pd$, or pulse pressure). The major factors and relationships that regulate arterial blood pressure are summarized in Fig. 28-32.

Effects of Cardiac Output

The cardiac output (minute volume) of the heart can be changed by alterations in heart rate, stroke volume (volume of blood ejected during each ventricular contraction), or both. An increase in cardiac output without a decrease in peripheral resistance will cause both arterial volume and mean blood pressure to increase. The higher arterial pressure increases blood flow through the arterioles. On the other hand, a decrease in the cardiac output causes an immediate drop in mean arterial blood pressure and arteriolar flow (Table 28-3).

Effects of Total Peripheral Resistance

Total peripheral resistance is determined primarily by a change in the diameter of the arterioles: arteriolar constriction raises mean arterial pressure by preventing the free flow of blood into the capillaries. Dilation has the opposite effect. Reflex control of vasoconstriction and vasodilation is mediated by the sympathetic nervous system.

Effect of Hyperemia

When metabolic activity is increased in the heart, skeletal muscle, and other muscular organs, it causes an increase

Table 28-3 Factors That Affect Mean Arterial Pressure and Capillary Flow

	Mean Arterial Pressure	Capillary Flow
PERIPHERAL RESISTANCE*		
Increased	Increased	Decreased
Decreased	Decreased	Increased
HEART RATE†		
Increased	Increased	Increased
Decreased	Decreased	Decreased
STROKE VOLUME‡		
Increased	Increased	Increased
Decreased	Decreased	Decreased

From Little RC: *Physiology of the heart and circulation,* ed 3, St Louis, 1985, Mosby.
*Cardiac output maintained constant.
†Peripheral resistance and stroke volume constant.
‡Peripheral resistance and heart rate constant.

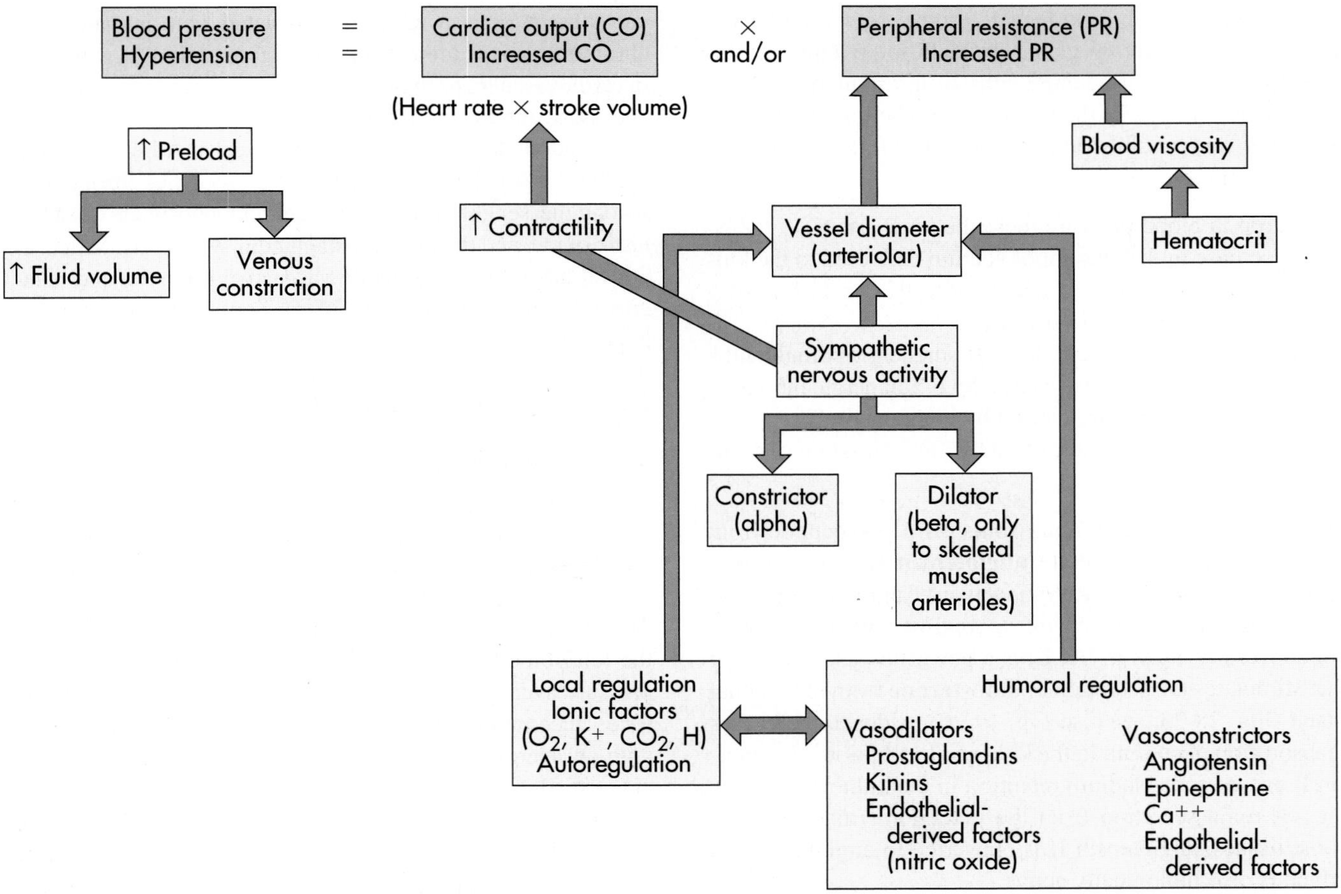

FIG. 28-32 Factors regulating blood flow.

in blood flow termed **hyperemia.** For example, the blood flow to exercising skeletal muscle increases in proportion to the activity of the muscle. This condition, known as *active (exercise) hyperemia,* is the result of arteriolar dilation and autoregulation of blood flow within the active organ.

Effects of Hormones

Many hormones cause contraction or relaxation of arteriolar smooth muscle. By constricting or dilating arterioles in specific vascular beds, hormones can (1) increase the blood supply to vital organs requiring more flow in times of stress, (2) redistribute blood volume during hemorrhage or shock, and (3) regulate heat loss.

Epinephrine, the hormone released from the adrenal medulla, causes vasoconstriction in most vascular beds (exceptions are the liver and skeletal muscles). However, the effects of norepinephrine (from the sympathetic nervous system and adrenal medulla) are quantitatively more vasoconstrictive than the effects of epinephrine.

Antidiuretic hormone, renin-angiotensin system, natriuretic peptides, and adrenomedullin. Blood pressure can be influenced by factors that change the total volume of blood in the circulatory system. Antidiuretic hormone (ADH) is released by the posterior pituitary and causes reabsorption of water by the kidney. With reabsorption the blood plasma volume will increase, increasing blood pressure (see Chapters 3 and 19 and Fig. 19-19).

Renin is an enzyme synthesized and secreted by the juxtaglomerular cells of the kidney. It also has been found in the adrenal cortex, salivary gland, prolactin-producing and luteinizing hormone–producing cells of the pituitary, arterial smooth muscle cells in the vascular endothelium, brain, myocardium, and possibly other tissues.[9] The following factors control renin release:

1. A drop in blood pressure (e.g., the renal artery)
2. A decrease in the amount of sodium delivered to the kidney (although recent evidence indicates a role for chloride in regulating renin secretion)[9]
3. Stimulation of renin release by β-adrenergic stimuli and a decrease in renin release caused by β-adrenergic inhibitors
4. Reduced renin release caused by angiotensin II
5. Increased renin release caused by low potassium concentrations in plasma

Once in the circulation, renin splits off a polypeptide from angiotensinogen to generate **angiotensin I.** Angiotensin I appears to by physiologically inactive.[9] Angiotensin I, however, is converted by an enzyme to **angiotensin II.** Angiotensin converting enzyme (ACE) is a powerful vasoconstrictor that stimulates the secretion of **aldosterone** from the adrenal gland (Fig. 28-33; see also Fig. 19-20). Aldosterone causes reabsorption of sodium in the kidneys. In addition, angiotensin II causes some sodium retention in the kidneys and suppresses renin secretion from the juxtaglomerular cells.[9] In some tissues, angiotensin II is converted to angiotensin III, which is also biologically active.

This kidney-based renin-angiotensin system serves as an important regulatory loop. For example, decreases in blood pressure or sodium delivery to the kidneys (macula densa), as might occur after hemorrhage or extracellular volume deficits (dehydration), stimulate secretion of renin, which forms angiotensin I, which is converted to angiotensin II and restores blood pressure. Sodium retention also results from increased secretion of aldosterone. Overall, the renin-angiotensin system is activated after volume depletion or hypotension or both, and it is suppressed after volume repletion and hypertension.

Angiotensin II is now considered a growth promoter in cardiovascular tissues, and the resultant vascular hypertrophy is a significant factor in the pathogenesis of hypertension. Angiotensin II plays a role in the kidney, not only as a regulator of blood flow but also in the development of structural changes (i.e., hypertrophy). A central role for the renin-angiotensin system is experimental vascular hypertension in the renal system. Angiotensin II has been implicated in the progression of heart failure (see Chapter 29).

Another mechanism that can change blood plasma volume and therefore blood pressure is the **natriuretic peptides (NPs)** (see Fig. 28-33).

Adrenomedullin

Adrenomedullin (ADM) is a recently discovered, widely dispersed peptide present in numerous tissues with powerful vasodilatory activity. Originally isolated from human pheochromocytoma (tumor of the adrenal medulla), it is present in cardiovascular, pulmonary, renal, gastrointestinal, cerebral, and endocrine tissues. It is synthesized and secreted from vascular endothelial and smooth muscle cells. Adrenomedullin mediates vasodilatory and natriuretic properties through the second messenger cyclic adenosine monophosphate (cAMP), nitric oxide, and the renal prostaglandin system. ADM acts as a local autocrine or paracrine vasoactive hormone and is increased in the plasma in various cardiorenal diseases such as hypertension, chronic renal failure, and congestive heart failure. Overall, ADM appears to play an important role in fluid and electrolyte balance and cardiorenal regulation.[10-12]

Venous Pressure

The main determinants of venous blood pressure are (1) the volume of fluid within the veins and (2) the compliance (distensibility) of the vessel walls. Veins have much thinner walls than arteries and are more distensible than arteries. The venous system accommodates approximately 60% of the total blood volume at any given moment, with venous pressure averaging less than 10 mm Hg. Conversely, the arteries accommodate about 15% of the total blood volume, with an average arterial pressure (blood pressure) of about 100 mm Hg.

The sympathetic nervous system controls compliance. The walls of the veins are highly innervated by sympathetic fibers that, when stimulated, cause venous smooth muscle to con-

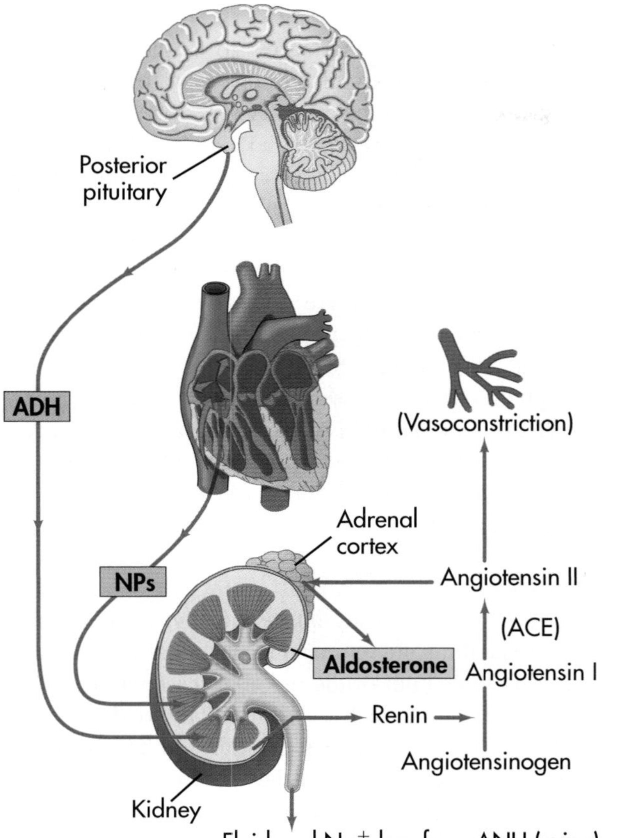

FIG. 28-33 Three mechanisms that influence total plasma volume. The antidiuretic hormone (ADH) mechanism and renin-angiotensin and aldosterone mechanisms tend to increase water retention and thus increase total plasma volume. The natriuretic peptides antagonize these mechanisms by promoting water loss and sodium loss, thus promoting a decrease in total plasma volume. *ACE,* Angiotensin converting enzyme. (Modified from Thibodeau GA, Patton KI: *Anatomy and physiology,* ed 4, St Louis, 1999, Mosby.)

tract. This increases muscle tone (i.e., prevents distention) rather than causing vasoconstriction, as occurs in arterial vessels. The effect of increased muscle tone is to stiffen the wall of the vein, which reduces distensibility and increases blood pressure, forcing more blood through the veins and into the right heart.

Two other mechanisms that increase venous pressure and venous return to the heart are (1) the skeletal muscle pump and (2) the respiratory pump. During skeletal muscle contraction the veins within the muscles are partially compressed, causing a decrease in venous capacity and increased return to the heart. The respiratory pump acts during inspiration, when the veins of the abdomen are partially compressed by the downward movement of the diaphragm. Increased abdominal pressure moves blood toward the heart.

Regulation of Coronary Circulation

Flow of blood *(F)* in the coronary circulation, as in vascular beds, is directly proportional to the perfusion pressure *(P)* and inversely proportional to the vascular resistance *(R)* of the bed ($F = P/R$). **Coronary perfusion pressure** is the difference between pressure in the aorta and pressure in the coronary vessels of the right atrium. Aortic pressure is the driving pressure that perfuses vessels of the myocardium. Mechanisms of vasodilation and vasoconstriction normally maintain coronary blood flow despite stresses imposed by the constant contraction and relaxation of the heart muscle and despite shifts (within a physiologic range) of coronary perfusion pressure.

Several anatomic factors influence coronary blood flow. Because of their location, the aortic valve cusps obstruct coronary blood flow by pushing against the openings of the coronary arteries during systole. Also during systole, the coronary arteries are compressed by ventricular contraction. These anatomic factors have a **systolic compressive effect,** which is particularly evident in the subendocardial layers of the left ventricular wall and can greatly decrease coronary blood flow. Therefore most coronary blood flow in the left ventricle occurs during diastole. During the period of systolic compression, when flow is slowed or stopped, oxygen is supplied by **myoglobin,** a protein that is present in heart muscle that binds oxygen during diastole

WHAT'S NEW?

The Natriuretic Peptides: Atrial Natriuretic Peptide (ANP), Brain Natriuretic Peptide (BNP), C-type Natriuretic Peptide (CNP), and Urodilation

These peptides help regulate sodium excretion (natriuresis), diuresis, vasodilation, and antagonism of the renin-angiotensin system. **Atrial natriuretic peptide (ANP)** or factor is primarily synthesized and stored in right atrial monocytes. In addition, under pathologic conditions, the left ventricle may secrete ANP. **Brain natriuretic peptide (BNP)** was originally isolated from paracrine brain and named *brain natriuretic peptide.* The name is misleading, however, because BNP is mostly synthesized, stored, and secreted from cardiac cells (i.e., atria). BNP is proposed to be a biochemical marker that may provide a screening test for left-ventricle dysfunction. **Natriuretic peptide (NP)** secretion is stimulated by monocyte stretch (for example, increased intravascular volume and blood pressure) and changes in body posture that increase central venous pressure. In addition to stretch, certain neurohormones increase NP secretion, including angiotensin II, endothelin, and norepinephrine. The NPs promote sodium (natriuretic) loss and water (diuretic) loss from the kidneys. They also cause vasodilation of the afferent arterioles. Because of their principal physiologic effects (natriuresis, diuresis, vasodilation) investigators suggest the NP system as an important counterregulatory system to the effects of angiotensin II, endothelin, and norepinephrine.

Data from Colderone A et al: Nitric oxide, atrial natriuretic peptide, and cyclic GMP inhibit the growth-promoting effects of norepinephrine in cardiac monocytes and fibroblasts, *J Clin Invest* 101:812, 1998; Kim SD, Piano MR: The natriuretic peptides: physiology and role in left-ventricle dysfunction, *Biol Res Nurs* 2(1):15, 2000.

and then releases it when blood levels of oxygen fall during systole.

Autoregulation

Autoregulation (automatic self-regulation) enables individual vessels to regulate blood flow by altering their own arteriolar resistances. Autoregulation in the coronary circulation maintains constant blood flow at perfusion pressures (mean arterial pressure) between 60 and 180 mm Hg when other influencing factors are held constant. Thus autoregulation ensures constant coronary blood flow despite shifts in the perfusion pressure within the stated range.

The mechanism of autoregulation is not known, but two explanations have been proposed: the myogenic hypothesis and the metabolic hypothesis. The myogenic hypothesis proposes that autoregulation originates in vascular smooth muscle, presumably of the arterioles, as a response to an increase in arterial pressure. Smooth muscle stretches in response to an increase in perfusion pressure. The stretching eventually stimulates contraction of the smooth muscles, which increases vascular resistance. Initially, coronary blood flow increases with the abrupt distention of the blood vessels. The return of more normal flow follows constriction of the arterioles. This mechanism also works in the opposite direction; that is, vasodilation is stimulated by decreased arterial pressure.

The myogenic hypothesis illustrates the law of Laplace (tension equals pressure times radius). Increased coronary perfusion pressure increases the pressure against the vessel wall, and the stretch increases the vessel's radius, resulting in an increase in wall tension. The increase in tension stimulates constriction of the vessel to a radius less than the original radius, so that the product of pressure (increased) times radius (decreased) is restored to normal.

The metabolic hypothesis of autoregulation, which is better documented, proposes that autoregulation of coronary vessels originates in the myocardium. The stimulus is a drop in coronary perfusion pressure or an increase in the metabolic needs of the myocardium (e.g., because of strenuous exercise). With an increased myocardial oxygen requirement, myocardial cells release substances that promote vasodilation. Substances implicated include CO_2, O_2 (reduced O_2 tension), hydrogen ions (lactic acid), potassium ions, and adenosine. The best known of these substances is adenosine, a potent vasodilator released in response to a decrease in myocardial oxygenation. Little evidence supports the concept that CO_2 hydrogen ions or O_2 plays a significant *direct* role in regulating coronary flow.[1] Low coronary blood flow, hypoxemia, and increased metabolic activity of the heart can all increase the heart muscle's need for oxygen.[1] An increased concentration of adenosine in the interstitial fluid decreases the resistance of the coronary arterioles and increases blood flow. Perfusion strongly correlates with the amount of adenosine released. When coronary perfusion pressure is increased, the increased flow washes out the vasodilatory substances. As the dilators are washed out, vasoconstriction occurs and returns flow toward normal.

Autonomic Regulation

Stimulation of the sympathetic nerves to the heart causes a marked increase in coronary blood flow, even though it also causes vasoconstriction of the coronary vessels. Why? The increased coronary flow is caused by acceleration of heart rate and enhancement of myocardial contractility (more forceful systole). Although the longer, forceful myocardial contraction and the tachycardia (heart rate greater than 100 beats/min) tend to restrict coronary flow, the increase in myocardial metabolism tends to counteract these factors by dilating the coronary arterioles.[1] Therefore the net effect of sympathetic stimulation is to increase coronary blood flow.

Although the coronary vessels themselves contain sympathetic (α- and β-adrenergic) and parasympathetic neural receptors, coronary blood flow is regulated locally through metabolic autoregulation. Metabolic autoregulation overrides neurogenic influences.[1]

LYMPHATIC SYSTEM

The lymphatic system is a special vascular system that picks up excess tissue fluid and returns it to the bloodstream. Normally, fluid is forced out of the blood at the arterial end of the capillary bed and is reabsorbed into the bloodstream at the venous end (Fig. 28-34), yet capillary outflow exceeds venous reabsorption by about 3 L/day so some fluid lags behind in the interstitium. To maintain sufficient blood volume in the cardiovascular system, this fluid must eventually rejoin the bloodstream, which is the function of the lymphatic system.

The lymphatic system consists of lymphatic vessels and the lymph nodes (Fig. 28-35). (Lymph nodes and lymphoid tissues are described in Chapters 6 and 24.) In this pumpless system a series of valves ensures one-way flow of the excess interstitial fluid (now called *lymph*) toward the heart. The lymphatic capillaries are closed at the ends (Fig. 28-36).

Lymph consists primarily of water and small amounts of dissolved proteins, mostly albumin, that are too large to be reabsorbed into the less permeable blood capillaries. Once within the lymphatic system, lymph travels successively through larger and larger vessels called **lymphatic venules** and **lymphatic veins.** The lymphatic vessels run in the same sheaths with the arteries and veins and eventually drain into one of two large ducts in the thorax—the right lymphatic duct and the thoracic duct. The **right lymphatic duct** drains lymph from the right arm and the right side of the head and thorax, whereas the larger **thoracic duct** receives lymph from the rest of the body (see Fig. 28-35). The right lymphatic duct and the thoracic duct drain lymph into the right and left subclavian veins, respectively.

The lymphatic veins are thin walled, like the veins of the cardiovascular system. In the larger lymphatic veins, endothelial flaps form valves similar to those in the circulatory veins (see Fig. 28-26). The valves permit lymph to flow in only one direction because lymphatic vessels are compressed intermittently by contraction of skeletal muscles, pulsatile expansion of an artery in the same sheath, and contraction of the smooth muscles in the walls of the lymphatic vessel.

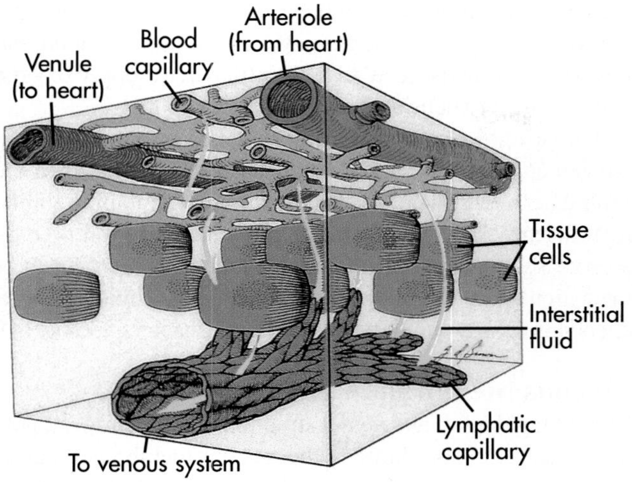

FIG. 28-34 Role of the lymphatic system in fluid balance. Fluid from plasma flowing through the capillaries moves into interstitial spaces. Although much of this interstitial fluid is either absorbed by tissue cells or reabsorbed by capillaries, some of the fluid tends to accumulate in the interstitial spaces. As this fluid builds up, it tends to drain into lymphatic vessels that eventually return the fluid to the venous blood. (From Thibodeau GA, Patton KI: *Anatomy and physiology,* ed 4, St Louis, 1999, Mosby.)

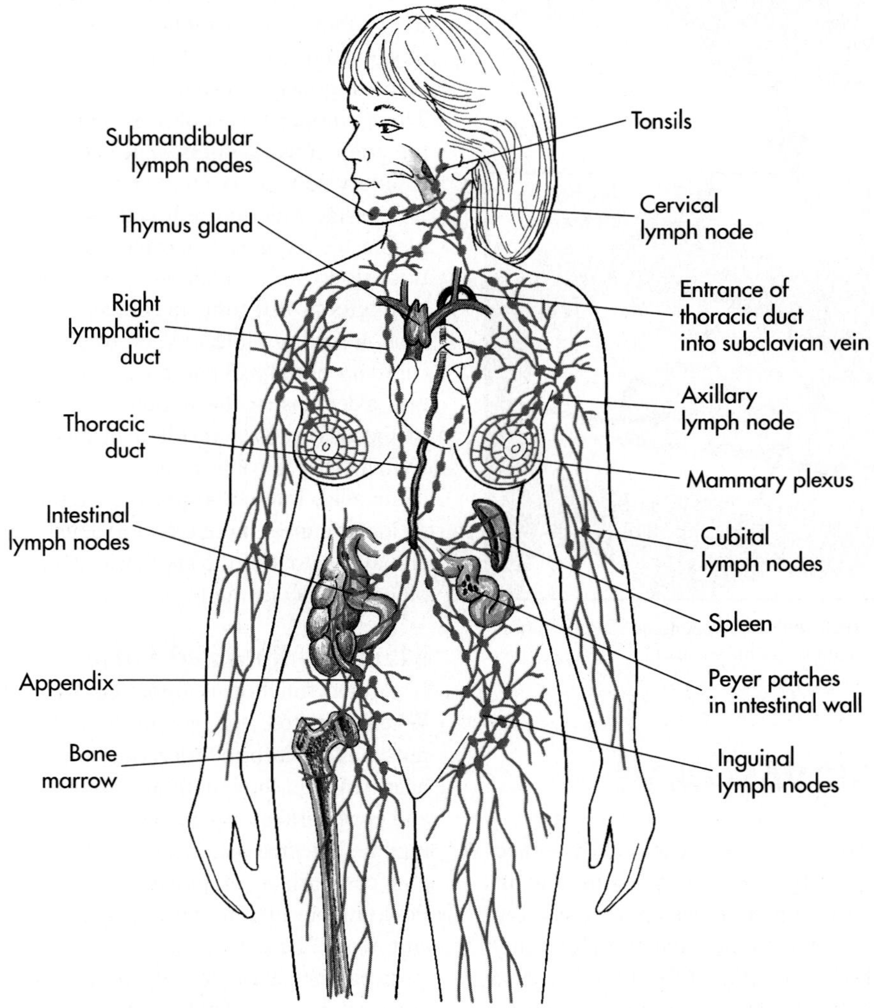

FIG. 28-35 Schematic representation of lymphatic vessels, larger lymphatic trunks, and lymph nodes. (Modified from Seeley RR, Stephens TD, Tate PT: *Anatomy and physiology,* ed 3, St Louis, 1995, Mosby.)

As lymph is transported toward the heart, it is filtered through thousands of bean-shaped lymph nodes clustered along the lymphatic vessels (see Fig. 28-35). Lymph enters the node through several **afferent lymphatic vessels,** filters through the sinuses in the node, and leaves by way of **efferent lymphatic vessels.** Lymph flows slowly through the node, which facilitates the phagocytosis of foreign substances within the node and prevents them from reentering the bloodstream. (Phagocytosis is described in Chapter 7.)

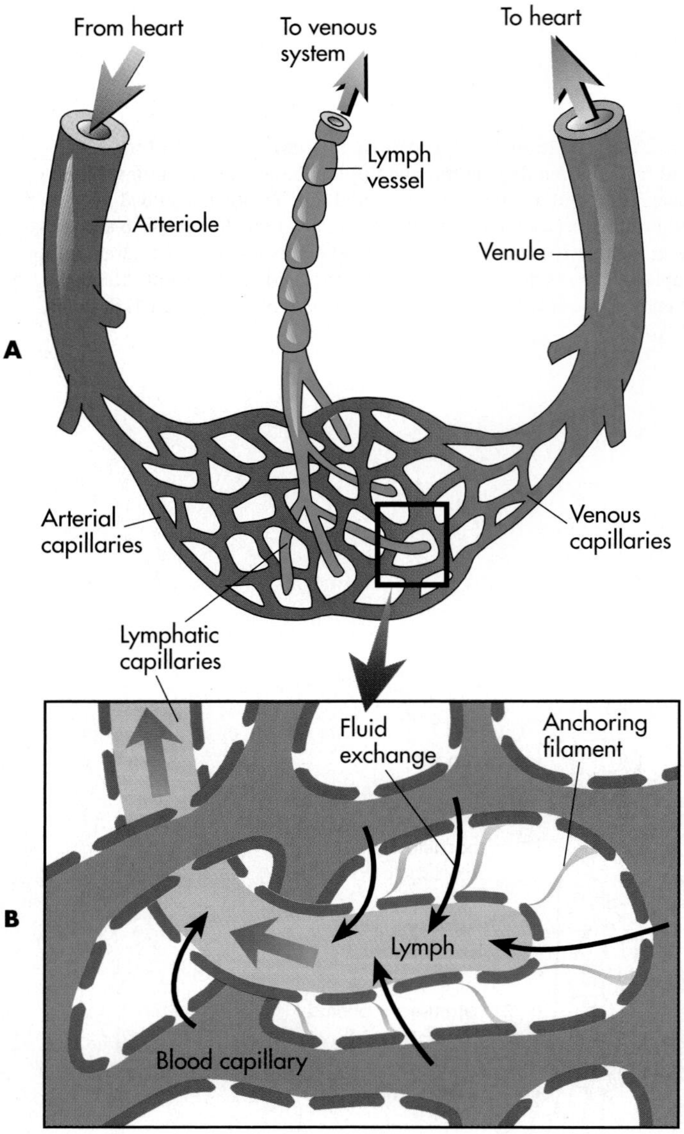

FIG. 28-36 Lymphatic capillaries. A, Schematic representation of lymphatic capillaries. **B,** Anatomic components of microcirculation.

TESTS OF CARDIOVASCULAR FUNCTION

Historically, cardiac function was first measured by subjective means and by simple objective observations that included the individual's sensorium, mucous membrane color, and a manually palpated pulse. Currently, many sophisticated methods measure heart function, ranging from no-risk, noninvasive electrocardiography to relatively high-risk, invasive cardiac catheterization.

Noninvasive Assessment of Function

Sensorium of the Individual

Often, the first observation indicating an impairment of cardiac function is a decreased level of consciousness. Should the pumping ability of the heart decrease for any reason, the amount and pressure of blood ejected from the heart will decrease. Consequently, the amount and pressure of blood that reaches all body tissues will be insufficient to supply oxygen and nutrients to cells and remove waste products.

Perhaps no other system is more sensitive to a decrease in oxygen and nutrient supply, particularly of glucose, than the central nervous system. A decrease in cardiac pumping ability, if sufficiently severe, will almost immediately be followed by a decrease in neural efficiency, which includes impairment of mentation and such simple motor functions as conjugate gaze, enunciation, and pupillary reflexes (see Chapters 13 and 14).

Mucous Membrane Color

When lung, blood, and vessel structure and function are normal, a darkening or bluing of the mucous membranes, called *cyanosis,* signifies decreased cardiac function. Mucous membrane color is a reflection of hemoglobin saturation in the capillary blood (see Chapters 24 and 29). Hemoglobin that is well oxygenated and well saturated takes on a bright red color, whereas poorly oxygenated hemoglobin is dark red or purple. These colors are best observed in the mucous membranes of the conjunctivae, gums, nail beds, and genitalia, where the capillary network is dense and the epithelium is thin.

Cardiac function indirectly affects the affinity of hemoglobin for oxygen. If cardiac function decreases and blood flow slows in the capillary beds, two changes occur. First, hemoglobin will come in contact with tissues for an extended time, allowing more oxygen to diffuse into the tissues. The capillary blood will darken, as will mucous membranes. Second, a decrease in the amount of oxygen delivered per minute to the tissues will result in a metabolic acidosis, as cells switch from aerobic to anaerobic metabolism and produce lactic acid. Interstitial pH and capillary blood pH will drop. Acidosis causes more oxygen to dissociate from hemoglobin and diffuse out of the capillaries (see Chapter 31). Capillary blood in mucous membranes will darken further.

Manually Palpated Pulse

If cardiac function is impaired, the pulse will be affected. When palpated, changes in the radial, femoral, and carotid pulses offer information regarding heart rate, regularity of heart rhythm, the length and strength of ventricular systole, and peripheral artery patency. A decrease in cardiac function may be detected as a decrease in pulsatile strength. A bilateral comparison of pulses may reveal decreased pulsatile flow unilaterally, in which case arterial narrowing or occlusion would be suspected.

Irregular heartbeats (dysrhythmias) may be reflected in changes in pulse rhythmicity and pulse pressure per beat. Turbulent blood flow caused by valve or septal disease may be reflected in the carotid pulses and felt as a "thrill." A pulsatile thrill elsewhere may indicate a fistula, or an opening, between an artery and a nearby vein.

Auscultation of Heart Sounds

Auscultation (auditory examination) of the heart is done with a stethoscope placed over the valve, chamber, or great vessel being examined. Different sounds are normally heard over

Table 28-4 Normal Heart Sounds

Sound	Event in Cardiac Style	Cause of Sound	Comments
First sound (S_1)	Beginning of ventricular systole	Closure of atrioventricular valves, particularly mitral valve	With S_2, the loudest heart sound normally heard
Second sound (S_2)	End of ventricular systole	Closure of semilunar valves, particularly aortic valves	With S_1, the loudest heart sound normally heard
Third sound (S_3)	Early ventricular diastole (filling)	Vibration of ventricular walls as blood rushes in	Normally heard only in children and young adults
Fourth sound (S_4)	Atrial systole during late ventricular diastole (filling)	Uncertain, but thought to be the result of a sudden change in filling rate (i.e., shudder of the left ventricle)	Rarely heard in the normal heart

different heart structures during systole and diastole. The dominant sounds are made by the four heart valves as they close. The first sound, S_1, is made by atrioventricular valve closure. The second, S_2, is made by closure of the aortic and pulmonic semilunar valves. The first two heart sounds provide information about heart rate, heart rhythm, and the length of ventricular systole.

Abnormal heart sounds indicate abnormalities of the heart valves or chamber walls. In healthy adults, only S_1 and S_2 can be heard. Abnormalities of these sounds or detection of the third and fourth heart sounds (S_3 and S_4) indicates disease. The mechanisms causing the normal heart sounds are listed in Table 28-4. Causes of abnormal heart sounds, or **adventitious sounds,** are listed in Table 28-5.

Cardiography

Electrocardiography, typically the 12-lead electrocardiogram (ECG), gives information about heart rate and rhythm, the effects of electrolytes or drugs on the heart, and the electrical orientation of the cardiac muscle. An ECG gives no direct information about the contractile state or mechanical performance of the heart.

Einthoven's triangle places the heart in the center of a triangle, with angles placed at the right shoulder, the left shoulder, and the pubic area. Body fluids conduct electrical potential differences that can be detected by bipolar or unipolar electrical leads placed on the skin. Einthoven's triangle gives a triaxial (three-axis) reference for the detection of cardiac electrical potentials.

Serial 12-lead ECGs are of primary importance in establishing the presence of myocardial infarction. This examination has become part of the routine hospital admission assessment, even when the admitting diagnosis is not cardiac in nature, because it establishes baseline information about the electrical function of the heart. Also, recent ECGs can be compared with ECGs obtained from the same individual in the past. Changes in the ECG over time assist in determining the cause, amount, or nature of changes in cardiac anatomy and physiology. (Fig. 28-11 depicts a normal ECG.)

In conjunction with a 12-lead ECG, a vectorcardiogram can assist one to (1) precisely locate the site of a myocardial infarction, (2) diagnose conduction defects, and (3) diagnose chamber hypertrophy. Commonly, five electrodes are placed over the precordium, one electrode is placed on the left leg, and one is placed on the back of the neck. Recorded in conjunction with the ECG, the electrodes of the vectorcardiogram provide a series of dots over time that represent the vector of the heart in microseconds.

Pulse Tracing

The pulsation described by the flow of blood through an artery during the cardiac cycle can be drawn as a waveform plotting pressure against time (Fig. 28-37). The waveform can be obtained noninvasively by placing a transducer on the skin over the carotid artery while the individual's head is turned slightly away from the transducer. In conjunction with phonocardiography and an ECG, the arterial pulse tracing gives a reference for the phonocardiograph and assists in the timing of the events of the cardiac cycle.

Like an arterial pulse tracing, a venous pulse tracing gives a reference for the phonocardiograph and assists in the timing of the cardiac cycle. A venous pulse tracing is obtained by placing a transducer over the jugular vein at the supraclavicular area near the manubrium. A waveform is produced that reflects pressures in the vein over time during the cardiac cycle.

Vibrations at the apex of the heart during the cardiac cycle are recorded by placing a transducer at the point of maximal impulse. An apexcardiogram is used to assist in the timing of the cardiac cycle and is made along with a phonocardiogram and an ECG.

A **phonocardiogram** is made by placing microphones over the precordium. An ECG is recorded simultaneously as a reference point. By recording the sounds made during the cardiac cycle, the phonocardiogram can assist one to time the events and length of diastole and systole. Abnormal sounds can also be examined more closely for timing, characteristics, and sources of those sounds.

An **echocardiogram** is an ultrasonic examination. The skin is first prepared by applying a lubricating agent (usually cooking oil), and a piezoelectric crystal is placed against the chest. Ultrasonic sound waves are then generated and directed into the cardiac structures, which reflect the waves at different angles and lengths according to structure and density. The crystal picks up these deflected waves and passes them through a transducer, which transforms the waves into electrical impulses. The impulses are displayed on an oscilloscope and are viewed with a simultaneously recorded ECG.

Like an ECG, an echocardiogram is recorded continuously over time so that changes in the heart during the cardiac cycle

Table 28-5 Abnormal Heart Sounds

Sound	Cause of Sound	Typical Underlying Abnormality
Accentuated S_1	Forceful closure of mitral valve	Rapid heart rate resulting from exercise, anemia, or hyperthyroidism
		Mitral valve stenosis (narrowing)
Diminished S_1	Premature partial closure of the mitral valve before systole, so that systole causes only the completion of closure	Prolonged diastole resulting from blockage in conduction system that slows impulse conduction to or within the atrioventricular node
	Failure of the mitral valve to close completely	Mitral valve incompetence (regurgitation)
Accentuated S_2	Forceful closure of the aortic or pulmonic semilunar valve, which closes late and must close quickly	Prolonged systole resulting from high blood pressure in the systemic or pulmonary circulation; systole is slightly prolonged so as to force all the blood out against high pressure
	Valvular stiffness, which increases the impact of closure	Aortic valve syphilis
Diminished S_2	Gentle closure of aortic semilunar valve	Low blood pressure in the systemic arteries, which reduces pressure that pushes valve leaflets shut
	Gentle closure of aortic semilunar valve caused by incomplete opening	Aortic stenosis
Split heart sounds (S_1 and S_2)	Delayed closure of various heart valves, usually caused by late right ventricular systole	Normal increase in venous return to the right heart with inspiration
		Conduction defects involving the right or left bundle branches
		Defect of the interatrial septum that raises pressures in the right heart
		Pulmonic semilunar valve stenosis, which causes delayed closure
Gallop sounds		
S_3 (in adults)	Possibly the "thud" of blood hitting noncompliant ventricular walls at the start of ventricular filling	Myocardial damage that stiffens muscle and prevents relaxation during systole
S_4 (in children)	Ejection of blood into overfilled ventricle during atrial systole	Incomplete emptying of ventricle during systole of preceding cardiac cycle, causing overfilling and overdistention during next cycle; causes include myocardial damage or disease, aortic stenosis, high blood pressure, fluid overload (see Chapter 3)
Murmurs	Turbulent blood flow at high blood pressure	Irregularity, constriction, or dilation of any structure that blood flows through, such as valvular stenosis or incompetence, perforation of interatrial or interventricular septum
		Increased rate of flow (blood flow) through normal structures (e.g., during pregnancy)
Rub	Friction within the pericardium, usually caused by disruption of the pericardial fluid; loss of fluid causes the visceral and parietal pericardium to rub against one another	Surgery, infection, inflammation, or adhesion that damages the parietal or visceral pericardium
Click	Sudden, abnormal movement of an aortic or pulmonic semilunar valve leaflet	Valve prolapse, in which valve leaflets open backward as well as forward; usually resulting from increase in valve opening (anulus)
Snap	Opening of stenotic (stiff) atrioventricular valve (mitral or tricuspid)	Atrioventricular valve stenosis
Hum	Vibration of heart walls or vessel walls caused usually by movement during turbulent blood flow at low pressure	Irregularity of any structure that blood flows through; normal in jugular veins of children

(e.g., valve position, chamber size, myocardial wall position) can be examined. Information about cardiac anatomy and function, including stroke volume and cardiac output, is gained.

Magnetic Resonance Imaging

Magnetic resonance imaging (MRI) is based on the principle that the frequency of energy (resonant frequency) given up by a nucleus is exactly proportional to the surrounding magnetic field (see Chapter 13). Hydrogen nuclei present in high concentrations in body water and fat tend to align parallel to a magnetic field (the individual is placed on a magnet). This orientation can be disturbed by energy at the proper frequency, and the recovery of nuclear orientation releases energy that can be detected. If the magnetic field is different in one part of the body compared with another, the hydrogen

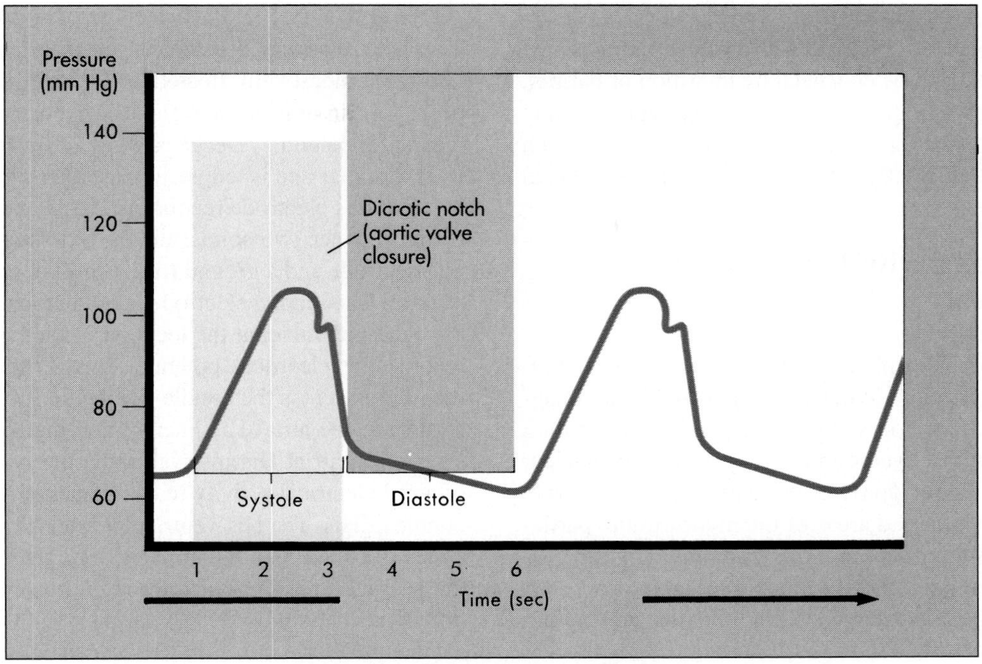

FIG. 28-37 Arterial pulse waveforms.

nuclei will release energy at slightly different frequencies. Thus spatial information (e.g., different body sections) can be encoded in the nuclear frequency.[13]

Anatomy and physiology of the great blood vessels and myocardium are depicted in three dimensions with excellent resolution. Ventricular function can be evaluated using indices of ventricular function, such as ejection fraction. Rapidly moving sequences (MRI) can determine regional wall motion and myocardial deformation. Also, flow direction and velocity can be quantitatively determined. The clinical application of MRI for coronary artery angiography is unclear because of interference from cardiac and respiratory motion.

Doppler Studies

A Doppler study is made by using a handheld microphone placed on the skin over a lubricating gel. The microphone amplifies and can record sounds made by blood flowing in peripheral vessels. The Doppler microphone is placed over the vessel to be studied, and sounds related to obstructions to flow, vessel wall mobility, and heart murmurs are transmitted through the gel to the microphone. The microphone amplifies sound waves so that they are audible to the human ear.

Stress Testing

Cardiac activity during exercise is examined during a stress test. Stress testing elicits signs and symptoms of heart disease and coronary artery disease that may not appear at rest. A 12-lead ECG, blood pressure measurement, and bipolar ECG strip recording are done before the study and at regular intervals during and after the study. Cardiac stress from exercise is induced by having the individual walk on a treadmill. Other, less frequently used forms of exercise include stair climbing (the Stairmaster's double two-step) and bicycle ergometry. The individual exercises until the maximal heart rate for gender and age is reached or until other subjective or objective indicators of cardiac dysfunction or distress appear. Subjective indicators include chest pain, extreme fatigue, extreme dyspnea, leg pain, or the individual's request to stop the test. Objective criteria are ST segment elevation or depression, SA node or atrial dysrhythmias, AV node dysrhythmias, ventricular dysrhythmias, elevated or decreased blood pressure, signs of cerebral hypoxia, and signs of circulatory insufficiency.

A stress test is useful also in determining the rate or progress of recovery from a myocardial infarction or cardiac surgery. Recently, graded exercise in individuals with low-to-moderate-risk chest pain evaluated in an emergency department was shown to be a prognostic indicator of adverse cardiac events.[14] When a differential diagnosis for chest pain has been difficult to determine, stress testing may help distinguish coronary artery insufficiency from other causes of pain. There is some risk associated with stress testing. The mortality rate is about 1 per 10,000, and the morbidity rate is approximately 24 per 10,000.[15] The risk is greater when the test is performed soon after an acute ischemic event.

Chest X-ray Examinations

In a chest x-ray examination the size and contour of the heart and related structures are visualized. A chest x-ray examination is a routine part of a cardiac examination. The most commonly obtained views are anteroposterior and lateral, with the individual upright and the lungs fully expanded.

Invasive Assessment of Function

Invasive studies generally carry a greater risk to the individual than noninvasive studies, with the possible exception of stress testing. Ingestion of substances is considered invasive.

X-ray Films with Barium

The cardiac silhouette obtained with routine radiographic studies of the chest can be enhanced by ingestion of barium. The contrast medium causes the esophagus to appear white on the x-ray film, creating a bright background against which the heart is more distinctly outlined. X-ray films are taken using four different axes.

Nuclear Imaging with Radiolabeled Pharmaceuticals

Hot Spot Imaging

Technetium pyrophosphate (^{99m}TcPYP) is injected intravenously into a resting individual during a "hot spot" imaging examination. Two hours after injection, the distribution pattern of the radioactive solution is recorded by nuclear scan. During the 2-hour delay, the injected material will have been taken up by infarcted areas of the myocardium, particularly 1 to 3 days after the onset of symptoms. This study is not definitive during the first 12 hours after an infarct.

Hot spot imaging is used when (1) there is a conflicting history for myocardial infarction, (2) there are equivocal ECG abnormalities, or (3) an individual's cardiac enzymes have been elevated because of surgery or trauma. Such small amounts of the injected material are used in this examination that the risks associated with radioactive substances are not an issue.

Cold Spot Imaging

Thallium is the radioactive substance injected intravenously during a perfusion imaging examination. During stress testing and at the peak of exercise, thallium is injected intravenously. After a 1- or 2-minute delay the distribution of thallium within the myocardium is determined by nuclear scan, and it is again determined after a period of rest. Thallium typically is not taken up by areas of ischemic or infarcted myocardium, creating "cold spots." Cold spots disappear at rest if the ischemia is reversible and remain at rest if infarction has occurred. Perfusion imaging is useful to differentiate a myocardial infarction from reversible angina (cardiac pain) in the presence of conflicting or equivocal enzymatic and historical data. Risks associated with perfusion imaging are the same as for stress testing. No risk attributable to the small quantity of injected material has been documented.

Tomographic Studies

In the past 10 years, **single photon emission computed tomography (SPECT)** has been used increasingly in cardiac imaging. A series of planar images are obtained from an individual around 180 or 360 degrees. A computer creates a set of transaxial images from these planar images, allowing the radioisotope distribution to be displayed in three dimensions. SPECT, along with many other tomographic modalities (e.g., positron emission tomography [PET], x-ray computed tomography [CT]), uses a computer-based algorithm during reconstruction of the planar images, called *filtered back projection.* PET is believed to be more accurate than SPECT (see Chapter 13). The main disadvantages of the PET technology are its limited availability and high costs.

Atrioventricular Bundle Electrocardiography

Two electrode-tipped catheters are inserted percutaneously into the femoral vein, floated up the inferior vena cava, and positioned in or near the right atrium during atrioventricular bundle (His bundle) electrocardiography. The first electrode is quadripolar and is lodged against the right atrial wall. Two poles of this electrode record the difference in electrical potential between two points, and the other two poles are a pacing electrode and a ground (that allow for pacing of the right atrium). The second electrode is bipolar and is placed across the tricuspid valve, at the location of the bundle of His, and records the electrical potentials across the bundle. These recordings across the bundle divide the PR interval into two segments: the atrial-His interval and the His-ventricular interval. The atrial-His interval is the interval from the onset of atrial electrical activity to the arrival of the impulse at the bundle of His. The His-ventricular interval is the interval between the passage of the impulse through the His bundle and the passage of the impulse through the ventricular conduction system and muscle.

His bundle electrocardiography can detect secondary sites of impulse generation (ectopic foci), as well as accessory pathways of conduction. Other conduction defects and the effects of drugs on conduction also can be illuminated. Risks related to this procedure can be grave and include dysrhythmias, death, vessel or heart perforation, clot or plaque embolization, and kidney failure.

Cardiac Catheterization

One or both sides of the heart can be examined using cardiac catheterization. This procedure requires the use of fluoroscopy and strict sterile techniques and takes place in a specially equipped catheterization laboratory. Local anesthesia is given, and a catheter is introduced percutaneously into the vasculature and passed caudally into the atrium and ventricle. For a right-heart catheterization, the catheter is placed in the brachial or femoral vein. The femoral artery is commonly used for a left-heart study. Once the catheter has been guided into the atrium, pressures are recorded, blood samples are obtained to examine oxygen content, and a contrast medium is injected to visualize chamber function and valve patency. The catheter is then passed into the ventricles and the sequence repeated.

Cardiac catheterization provides a means to visualize the chambers of the heart continuously, although for a short time. A great deal of information can be obtained about heart structure and function. Pressures in each chamber and across heart valves can be precisely measured, along with timing of events in the cardiac cycle. Of particular value is the ability to compare the oxygen content of blood in each heart chamber.

Risks for this procedure have decreased over time, and mortality rates range from 0.1% to 0.3%.[16] Morbidity rates, including serious and relatively minor complications, ranged from 3.1% to 10.1% in 1968,[17] but the morbidity rate currently is less than 0.5%.[18] One of the most serious complications of cardiac catheterization is the development of dysrhythmias and the possible sequelae of inflammation. Death usually is caused by cardiac arrest after ventricular fibrillation.

Coronary Angiography

Fluoroscopic visualization of the coronary arteries and left heart structures using contrast dye (e.g., iodine) is called **coronary angiography** or arteriography. Like cardiac catheterization, this study takes place in a catheterization laboratory using local anesthesia and a sterile field. A catheter is threaded into the left ventricle through the femoral artery. A ventriculogram generally is performed first. Contrast dye is injected into the apex of the ventricle, and the next few cardiac cycles are visualized and filmed. The contrast dye used is 66% diatrizoate meglumine and 10% diatrizoate sodium, an iodine preparation that is not tolerated by individuals who are allergic to iodine. Like cardiac catheterization, coronary angiography is used to gain information about the structure and function of the ventricles and related valves.

After the ventriculogram, catheters are introduced individually into the ostia of the coronary arteries. When the catheter is in position, 5 to 10 ml of contrast dye is mechanically and rapidly injected into the artery and the results are visualized and filmed. Dye injection is repeated with the individual tilted at various angles to afford views of the artery other than the anteroposterior view. The catheter is then either moved to the next artery to be studied or withdrawn to conclude the study. Pressures in the left side of the heart are usually obtained, but blood samples are not. The right side of the heart is not studied.

The risks of this procedure are similar to those of cardiac catheterization, with exceptions. Because the blood supply to the cardiac muscle is briefly interrupted when dye is introduced into the coronary arteries, angina (chest pain) caused by ischemia (lack of oxygen) is much more common. Coronary artery spasms also can occur. Interrupted flow also causes decreased heart rate (bradycardia), as well as some tachydysrhythmias, hypotension, and ST segment depression.

The administration of nitroglycerin sublingually or directly into the coronary artery can dilate the artery sufficiently to alleviate ischemic complications. Persistent bradycardia is corrected by having the individual cough to stimulate the heart rate or, in severe cases, by the administration of atropine. Bradycardia is such a common complication that a temporary pacer often is introduced into the right ventricle through the femoral vein at the beginning of coronary angiography. Heparin is given to avoid thrombus formation. The effects of heparin may be reversed after the procedure by using protamine.

Combined Indicators of Cardiac Function

Cardiac function can be evaluated using indicators calculated from pressures and flow rates in the heart and vessels. Table 28-6 defines the indicators most frequently used in the clinical setting.

Aging and the Cardiovascular System

Cardiovascular disease is the most common cause of hospitalization and death in the elderly population in Western society. The most common cardiovascular pathologic condition is coronary atherosclerosis. It is difficult to describe normal physiologic changes in cardiac function with aging because many pathologic changes are usually present as well. Studies of the effect of age on cardiovascular function must be rigorous in their distinction between persons who are free of disease and those who have disease that may be evident only during stress testing. A consistent finding is the large variation in the older population for nearly every cardiovascular variable. These variations are in part the result of a sharp increase in the prevalence of coronary disease with advancing age and in part the result of major age-associated changes in life-style (e.g., fitness status).[19]

Arterial stiffening occurs with aging even in the absence of clinical hypertension (Fig. 28-38).[19] These changes apparently result from alterations within the vascular media, including age-associated changes in cross linking of collagen, an increase in the amount of collagen, and changes in the nature of elastin.[19] Systolic arterial pressure increases (even in the absence of clinical hypertension) within the clinically "normal" range are considered to result from the age-associated increase in arterial stiffness (see Fig. 28-38). The increased arterial stiffness may not be related strictly to an age-associated change in vascular structure but also may be caused by changes in baroreceptor activity. Baroreceptor activity may decrease with age, slowing physiologic adjustment to changes in blood pressure because of vasodilation or vasoconstriction. In addition, plasma catecholamines increase with aging, which may be a result of exaggerated central nervous system adrenergic flow, possibly associated with blunting of baroreceptor sensitivity,[19] yet elevated plasma catecholamine levels in older individuals are associated with a decreased postsynaptic β-adrenergic response of the heart vasculature. In addition, plasma catecholamine levels are not correlated or are inversely correlated with arterial pressure in elderly persons with normotension or hypertension. In populations in whom the increase in arterial stiffness with age is blunted, the arterial pressure increase with age is also blunted.[19] Recent observations indicate that arterial stiffening is reduced in older individuals who regularly engage in vigorous exercise.[20]

Stress testing is used to uncover changes in functional capacity that are not apparent at rest. In contrast to the subtle age effects on resting cardiac tests, more dramatic changes occur during exercise. Table 28-7 summarizes age-associated changes at rest and during exercise. Overall, long-term exercise conditioning in older individuals increases aerobic capacity and decreases arterial stiffness and left ventricular function.

In summary, age does not appear to significantly alter left ventricular performance except in the presence of a superimposed stress such as severe exercise or disease, particularly dysrhythmia or hypertension. In these instances, impaired diastolic relaxation and systolic emptying may occur. Recent research is focused on decreased endothelial vasoreactivity and prolonged diastolic relaxation. Impaired nitric oxide signaling may contribute to slowed ventricular relaxation.[21] Impaired systolic emptying may be related to a decreased responsiveness to catecholamine β-adrenoreceptor stimulation.[19,20]

Table 28-6 Indicators of Cardiac Function

Indicator	Definition*	Common Cause of Abnormality
Heart rate (HR)	Number of heartbeats (cardiac cycles) per min Normal adult value: 70 beats/min	Ischemia, electrolyte disturbances, drug toxicity
Cardiac output (CO)	Amount of blood (in liters) moved by the heart in 1 min Normal range: 4-8 L/min	Decrease indicates heart failure Increase indicates decreased systemic vascular resistance, common in sepsis
Cardiac index (CI)	Relationship between cardiac output and body surface area (BSA, in square meters) Normal range: 2.8-4.2 L/min/m^2	Decrease indicates heart failure Increase indicates decreased systemic vascular resistance, common in sepsis
Stroke volume (SV)	Amount of blood (in milliliters) ejected by the left ventricle during systole, i.e., per beat Normal range: 60-100 ml/beat	Decrease indicates heart failure Increase indicates decreased systemic vascular resistance, common in sepsis
Stroke volume index (SVI)	Relationship between stroke volume and body surface area Normal range: 33-47 ml/beat/m^2	Decrease indicates heart failure Increase indicates decreased systemic vascular resistance, common in sepsis
Oxygen consumption index (VO_2I)	Amount of oxygen (VO_2 in milliliters) consumed per minute in relation to BSA	Decrease: sedation, anesthesia, hypothermia Increase: elevated temperature, sepsis, seizures
Stroke work index (SWI)	Amount of work (expressed as done) by the left or right ventricle per systole per square meter of BSA Normal value: 35 g/m^2	Decreases within specific ranges indicate cardiogenic or hypovolemic shock (see Chapter 45) Increase: elevated systemic vascular resistance
Systemic mean arterial pressure (MAP)	Mean blood pressure (in millimeters of mercury) in the systemic arteries Normal range: 70-100 mm Hg	Elevated: epinephrine release, diseases of arteries, primary hypertension Decreased: cardiac failure, decreased vascular resistance of sepsis
Pulmonary vascular resistance (PVR)	Relationship among cardiac output, preload, and afterload, expressed as units of force of resistance per second per centimeter of water Normal value: less than 250 dyn/sec/cm^{-5}	Increased: acute respiratory distress syndrome (ARDS), pneumonia, primary pulmonary hypertension, congestive heart failure Decreased: late shock
Systemic vascular resistance (SVR)	Same definition as for PVR Normal range: 770-1500 dyn/sec/cm^{-5}	Increased: epinephrine release Decreased: inflammatory response

*Values given are for adults at rest.

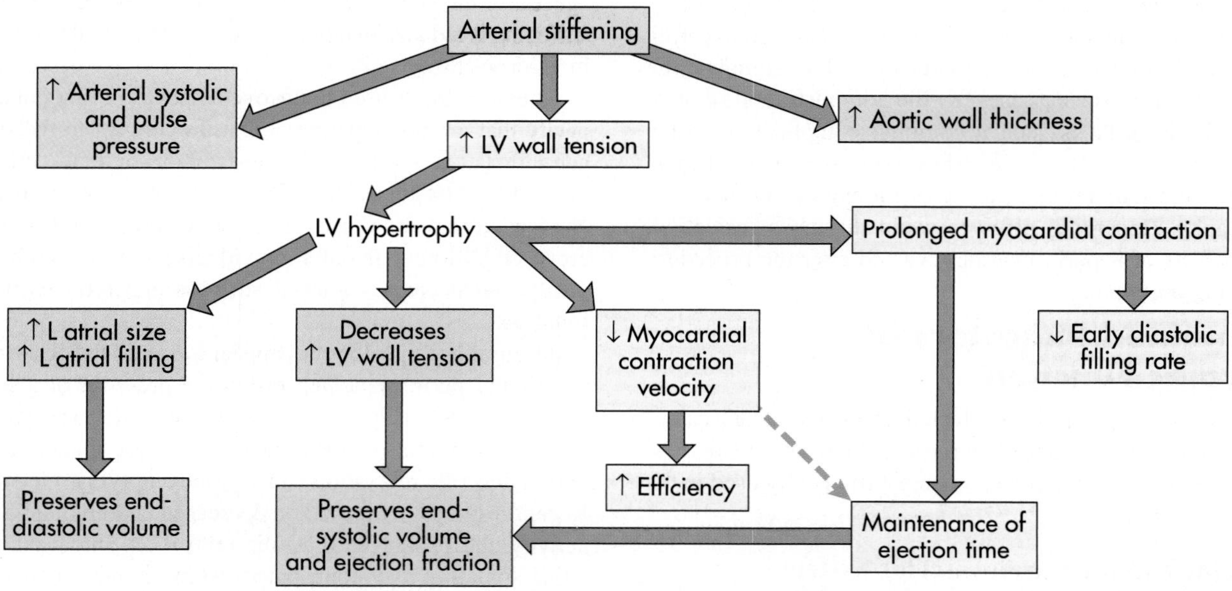

Fig. 28-38 Cardiac consequences of age-associated increase in arterial (central) stiffness. *LV*, left ventricular; *L*, left.

Table 28-7 Cardiovascular Function in Elderly Persons

Determinant	Resting Cardiac Performance	Exercise Cardiac Performance
Cardiac output	Unchanged or slightly decreased in women only	Declines because of a decrease in heart rate and stroke volume
Heart rate	Slight decrease	Increases less than in younger people, possibly because of decreased cardiovascular response to catecholamines; overall slight decrease
Stroke volume	Slight increase	Slight increase
Ejection fraction	Unchanged	Increases more from rest to exercise in younger people than in older people
Afterload	Increased	Uncertain
End-diastolic volume	Unchanged	Smaller for women
End-systolic volume	Unchanged	Lesser increase
Contraction	Increased because of prolonged relaxation	Decreases with vigorous exercise*
Cardiac dilation	No change	Increases at end-diastole and end-systole
$\dot{V}O_2$ max	Not applicable	Declines because of a decline in skeletal muscle mass

Data from Gerstenblith G, Lakatta EG: Aging and the cardiovascular system. In Willerson JT, Cohn JN, editors: *Cardiovascular medicine,* New York, 1995, Churchill Livingstone.
*As measured by end-systolic volume/systolic blood pressure (ESV/SBP), an index of contractility.

SUMMARY REVIEW

Circulatory System

1. The circulatory system is the body's transport system. It delivers oxygen, nutrients, metabolites, hormones, neurochemicals, proteins, and blood cells through the body and carries metabolic wastes to the kidneys and lungs for excretion.
2. The circulatory system consists of the heart and blood vessels and is made up of two separate, serially connected systems: the pulmonary circulation and the systemic circulation.
3. The pulmonary circulation is driven by the right side of the heart. The function of the pulmonary circulation is to deliver blood to the lungs for oxygenation.
4. The systemic circulation is driven by the left side of the heart, and its function is to move oxygenated blood throughout the body.
5. The lymphatic vessels collect fluids from the interstitium and return the fluids to the circulatory system.

The Heart

1. The heart consists of four chambers (two atria and two ventricles), four valves (two atrioventricular valves and two semilunar valves), a muscular wall, a fibrous skeleton, a conduction system, nerve fibers, systemic vessels (the coronary circulation), and openings where the great vessels enter the atria and ventricles.
2. The heart wall, which encloses the heart and divides it into chambers, is made up of three layers: the pericardium (outer layer), the myocardium (muscular layer), and the endocardium (inner lining).
3. The myocardial layer of the two atria, which receive blood entering the heart, is thinner than the myocardial layer of the ventricles, which must be stronger to squeeze blood out of the heart.
4. The right and left sides of the heart are separated by portions of the heart wall called the *interatrial septum* and the *interventricular septum.*
5. Unoxygenated (venous) blood from the systemic circulation enters the right atrium through the superior and inferior venae cavae. From the atrium the blood passes through the right atrioventricular (tricuspid) valve into the right ventricle. In the ventricle the blood flows from the inflow tract to the outflow tract and then through the pulmonic semilunar valve (pulmonary valve) into the pulmonary artery, which delivers it to the lungs for oxygenation.
6. Oxygenated blood from the lungs enters the left atrium through the four pulmonary veins (two from the left lung and two from the right lung). From the left atrium the blood passes through the left atrioventricular valve (mitral valve) into the left ventricle. In the ventricle the blood flows from the inflow tract to the outflow tract and then through the aortic semilunar valve (aortic valve) into the aorta, which delivers it to systemic arteries of the entire body.
7. The heart valves ensure the one-way flow of blood from atrium to ventricle and from ventricle to artery.
8. Oxygenated blood enters the coronary arteries through an opening in the aorta, and unoxygenated blood from the coronary veins enters the right atrium through the coronary sinus.
9. The pumping action of the heart consists of two phases: diastole, during which the myocardium relaxes and the chambers fill with blood, and systole, during which the myocardium contracts, forcing blood out of the ventricles. A cardiac cycle consists of one systolic contraction and the diastolic relaxation that follows it. Each cardiac cycle makes up one *heartbeat.*
10. The conduction system of the heart generates and transmits electrical impulses (cardiac action potentials) that stimulate systolic contractions. The autonomic nerves (sympathetic and parasympathetic fibers) can adjust heart rate and systolic force, but they do not stimulate the heart to beat.
11. The normal electrocardiogram is the sum of all action potentials. The P wave represents atrial depolarization; the QRS complex is the sum of all ventricular cell depolarizations. The ST interval occurs when the entire ventricular myocardium is depolarized.

12. Cardiac action potentials are generated by the sinoatrial node at the rate of about 75 impulses per minute. The impulses can travel through the conduction system of the heart, stimulating myocardial contraction as they go.
13. Cells of the cardiac conduction system possess the properties of automaticity and rhythmicity. Automatic cells return to threshold and depolarize rhythmically without outside stimulus. The cells of the sinoatrial node depolarize faster than other automatic cells, making it the natural pacemaker of the heart. If the sinoatrial node is disabled, the next fastest pacemaker, the atrioventricular node, takes over.
14. Each cardiac action potential travels from the sinoatrial (SA) node to the atrioventricular (AV) node to the bundle of His (atrioventricular bundle), through the bundle branches, and finally to the Purkinje fibers. There the impulse is stopped. It is prevented from reversing its path by the refractory period of cells that have just been polarized. The refractory period ensures that diastole (relaxation) will occur, thereby completing the cardiac cycle.
15. Adrenergic receptor number, type, and function govern autonomic (sympathetic) regulation of heart rate, contractile force, and dilation or constriction of coronary arteries. The presence of specific receptors (α_1, α_2, β_1, β_2) in the myocardium and coronary vessels determines the effects of the neurotransmitters norepinephrine and epinephrine.
16. Unique features that distinguish myocardial cells from skeletal cells enable myocardial cells to transmit action potentials faster (through intercalated disks), synthesize more adenosine triphosphate (ATP) (because of a large number of mitochondria), and have readier access to ions in the interstitium (because of an abundance of transverse tubules). These combined differences enable the myocardium to work constantly, which skeletal muscle is not required to do.
17. Cross bridges between actin and myosin enable contraction to occur. Calcium and its interaction with the troponin complex facilitate the contraction process. With troponin release of calcium, myocardial relaxation begins.
18. Cardiac performance is affected by preload, afterload, heart rate, and myocardial contractility.
19. Preload, or pressure generated in the ventricles at the end of diastole, depends on the amount of blood in the ventricle. Afterload is the resistance to ejection of the blood from the ventricle. Afterload depends on pressure in the aorta.
20. Heart rate is determined by the SA node and by components of the autonomic nervous system, including cardiovascular control centers in the brain, neuroreceptors in the atria and aorta, hormones, and catecholamines (epinephrine and norepinephrine).
21. Contractility is the potential for myocardial fiber shortening during systole. It is determined by the amount of stretch during diastole (i.e., preload) and by sympathetic stimulation of the ventricles.
22. The Frank-Starling law of the heart states that the myocardial stretch determines the force of myocardial contraction (the greater the stretch, the stronger the contraction).
23. Laplace's law states that the amount of contractile force generated within a chamber depends on the radius of the chamber and the thickness of its wall (the smaller the radius and the thicker the wall, the greater the force of contraction).

Systemic Circulation

1. Blood flows from the left ventricle into the aorta and from the aorta into arteries that eventually branch into arterioles and capillaries, the smallest of the arterial vessels. Oxygen, nutrients, and other substances needed for cellular metabolism pass from the capillaries into the interstitium, where they are available for uptake by the cells. Capillaries also absorb products of cellular metabolism from the interstitium.
2. Venules, the smallest veins, receive capillary blood. From the venules the venous blood flows into larger and larger veins until it reaches the venae cavae, through which it enters the right atrium.
3. Vessel walls consist of three layers: the tunica intima (inner layer), the tunica media (middle layer), and the tunica externa (outer layer).
4. Layers of the vessel wall differ in thickness and composition from vessel to vessel, depending on the vessel's size and location within the circulatory system. In general, the tunica media of arteries close to the heart contains a greater proportion of elastic fibers because these arteries must be able to distend during systole and recoil during diastole. Distributing arteries farther from the heart contain a greater proportion of smooth muscle fibers because these arteries must be able to constrict and dilate to control blood pressure and volume within specific capillary beds.
5. Blood flow into the capillary beds is controlled by the contraction and relaxation of smooth muscle bands (precapillary sphincters) at junctions between metarterioles and capillaries. The endothelium is probably a source of prostaglandins that control vasomotion.
6. Blood flow through the veins is assisted by the contraction of skeletal muscles (the muscle pump), and backflow in the lower body is prevented by one-way valves, particularly in the deep veins of the legs.
7. Blood flow is affected by blood pressure; resistance to flow within the vessels; blood consistency (which affects velocity); anatomic features that may cause turbulent or laminar flow; and compliance (distensibility) of the vessels.
8. Poiseuille's law describes the relationship of blood flow, pressure, and resistance as the difference between pressure at the inflow end of the vessel and pressure at the outflow end divided by resistance within the vessel.
9. According to Poiseuille's formula, resistance depends on the vessel's length and radius and on the viscosity of the blood. The greater the vessel's length and the blood's viscosity and the narrower the radius of the vessel's lumen, the greater the resistance within the vessel.
10. Total peripheral resistance, or the resistance to flow within the entire systemic circulatory system, depends on the combined lengths and radii of all the vessels within the system and on whether the vessels are arranged in series (greater resistance) or in parallel (lesser resistance).
11. Poiseuille's law and Poiseuille's formula are based on physical laws governing the behavior of fluids in a straight tube. In the body, blood flow is influenced also by neural stimulation (of vasoconstriction or vasodilation) and by autonomic features that cause turbulence within the vascular lumen (e.g., protrusions from the vessel wall, twists and turns, bifurcations).
12. Arterial blood pressure is influenced and regulated by factors that affect cardiac output (heart rate and stroke volume), total resistance within the system, and blood volume.

13. Venous blood pressure is influenced by blood volume within the venous system and compliance of the venous walls.
14. Blood flow through the coronary circulation is governed not only by the same principles as flow through other vascular beds but also by adaptations dictated by cardiac dynamics. First, blood flows into the coronary arteries during diastole rather than systole because, during systole, the cusps of the aortic semilunar valve block the openings of the coronary arteries. Second, systolic contraction inhibits coronary artery flow by compressing the coronary arteries.
15. Autoregulation enables the coronary vessels to maintain optimal perfusion pressure despite systolic effects, and myoglobin in heart muscle stores oxygen for use during the systolic phase of the cardiac cycle.

Lymphatic System

1. The vessels of the lymphatic system run in the same sheaths with the arteries and veins.
2. Lymph (interstitial fluid) is absorbed by lymphatic venules in the capillary beds and travels through ever larger lymphatic veins until it is emptied through the right or left thoracic duct into the right or left subclavian vein.
3. As lymph travels toward the thoracic ducts, it is filtered by thousands of lymph nodes clustered around the lymphatic veins. The lymph nodes are sites of immune function.

Tests of Cardiovascular Function

1. Observable signs of cardiovascular disease include a decreased level of consciousness (caused by insufficient perfusion of brain tissue) and cyanosis, particularly mucous membrane color (caused by insufficient perfusion of vascular beds of the skin).
2. Palpable signs of cardiovascular disease include abnormal pulses of the radial, femoral, and carotid arteries.
3. Abnormal heart sounds, which are detected by auscultation with a stethoscope or by phonocardiography, are auditory signs of cardiovascular disease.
4. Stress tests elicit clinical manifestations of cardiovascular disease that might not be present at rest.
5. Noninvasive diagnostic tests include electrocardiography (ECG) and Holter monitoring, which detect disturbances of impulse generation or conduction; pulse tracings and Doppler studies, which detect abnormalities of blood flow; phonocardiography; ultrasound (echocardiography), which detects structural and functional abnormalities over time; and chest x-ray films, which detect cardiac enlargement and structural abnormalities. Recently, magnetic resonance imaging has been used to study the anatomy and physiology of the great vessels, flow, direction and velocity, and myocardial deformation.
6. Invasive diagnostic tests involve intravenous injection of radiolabeled substances (barium x-rays, nuclear imaging) or the introduction of a catheter that is threaded through the vascular system to the heart (atrioventricular bundle ECG, cardiac catheterization, coronary angiography).
7. Cardiac catheterization is used to measure the oxygen content and pressure of blood in the heart's chambers and to inject contrast media for x-ray examination of the size and shape of the chambers and valves. Injection of contrast medium in the coronary arteries (coronary angiography), on the other hand, permits visualization of the coronary circulation and every tissue perfused by the coronary arteries.

Aging and the Cardiovascular System

1. Much controversy exists regarding the effects of normal aging on the cardiovascular system. Separating the physiologic from the pathologic alterations is difficult because of the presence of arteriosclerosis in a majority of the elderly population.
2. Recent studies have documented no change in cardiac output, a slight decrease in heart rate, and a slight increase in stroke volume in healthy (lack of ischemic heart disease) elderly persons at rest. No changes were noted at rest in ejection fraction. A slight increase in afterload (e.g., as systolic blood pressure) and prolonged left ventricular relaxation were noted.
3. With exercise the healthy elderly subjects demonstrated a decrease in maximum oxygen consumption and no age-related changes in cardiac output but did demonstrate significant decreases in heart rate and increases in stroke volume. Thus the healthy elderly subjects maintained a normal cardiac output during exercise by dilating the ventricle and using the Frank-Starling mechanism to increase stroke volume.
4. Contrary to previous studies, recent studies have found no age-related increase with exercise for systolic blood pressure and systemic vascular resistance.

KEY TERMS

A band, *947*
a wave, *935*
Adrenomedullin (ADM), *964*
Adventitious sound, *969*
Afferent lymphatic vessel, *967*
Afterload, *948*
Aldosterone, *964*
Angiotensin I, *964*
Angiotensin II, *964*
Anisotropic band, *944*
Anomalous viscosity, *959*
Anterior interatrial myocardial band (Bachmann bundle), *940*
Anterior internodal pathway, *940*
Aorta, *934*
Aortic semilunar valve (aortic valve), *933*
Arteriole, *952*
Artery, *952*
Atrioventricular node (AV node), *940*
Atrioventricular valve, *933*
Automatic cell, *942*
Automaticity, *942*
Autoregulation, *966*
Bachmann bundle, *940*
Bainbridge reflex, *951*
Baroreceptor reflex, *951*
Blood flow, *958*
Blood velocity, *962*
Bundle branch, *940*
Bundle of His (atrioventricular bundle, common bundle), *940*
c wave, *936*
Calcium channel–blocking drug, *948*
Capillary, *952*
Cardiac action potential, *939*
Cardiac cycle, *934*
Cardiac output, *951*
Cardiac plexus, *941*
Cardiac vein, *936*
Cardioexcitatory center, *950*
Cardioinhibitory center, *950*
Cardiovascular control center, *950*

KEY TERMS—cont'd

REFERENCES

1. Berne RM, Levy MN, editors: *Physiology,* ed 4, St Louis, 1998, Mosby.
2. Werner GS et al: Immediate changes of collateral function after successful recanalization of chronic total coronary occlusion, *Circulation* 102(24):2959, 2000.
3. Matsunaga T et al: Ischemia-induced coronary collateral growth is dependent on vascular endothelial growth factor and nitric oxide, *Circulation* 102(25):3098, 2000.
4. Underhill SL et al, editors: *Cardiac nursing,* Philadelphia, 1982, Lippincott.
5. James TN: Pericarditis and the sinus nodes, *Arch Intern Med* 110:305, 1962.
6. James TN: The coronary circulation and conduction system in acute myocardial infarction, *Prog Cardiovasc Dis* 10:410, 1968.
7. Kirchheim HR: Systemic arterial baroreceptor reflexes, *Physiol Rev* 56(1):110, 1976.

8. Vander AJ, Sherman JH, Luciano DS: *Human physiology: the mechanisms of body function,* ed 6, New York, 1994, McGraw-Hill.
9. Kim SD: Measurement of the renin-angiotensin system in heart failure, *Biol Res Nurs* 1(3):210, 2000.
10. Jougasaki M, Burnett JC: Adrenomedullin: potential in physiology and pathophysiology, *Life Sci* 66(10):855, 2000.
11. Hinson JP, Kapas S, Smith DM: Adrenomedullin, a multifunctional regulatory peptide, *Endocr Rev* 21(2):138, 2000.
12. Ueta Y et al: A physiological role for adrenomedullin in rats; a potent hypotensive peptide in the hypothalamo-neurohypophysial system, *Exp Physiol* 85(spec):163S, 2000.
13. Duerinckx AJ: Imaging of coronary artery disease—MR, *J Thorac Imaging* 16(1):25-34, 2001.
14. Diercks DB et al: Identification of patients at risk by graded exercise testing in an emergency department chest pain center, *Am J Cardiol* 86(3):289, 2000.
15. Rochmis P, Blackburn H: Exercise tests: a survey of procedures, safety, and litigation experience in approximately 170,000 tests, *JAMA* 217: 1061, 1971.
16. Abrams HL: Complications of coronary arteriography. In Abrams HL, editor: *Angiography: vascular and interventional radiology,* ed 3, Boston, 1983, Little, Brown.
17. Braunwald E: Cooperative study on cardiac catheterization, *Circulation* 37(suppl 3), 1968.
18. Silverman BD, Neeld JB Jr: Evaluation of the cardiac patient for noncardiac surgery, *J Med Assoc Ga* 73(5):315, 1984.
19. Gerstenblith G: Consequences of vascular aging: concepts for the clinician, *Ital Heart J* 1(suppl 3):S103, 2000.
20. Vaitkevicius PV, Fleg JL: An abnormal exercise treadmill test in an asymptomatic older patient, *J Am Geriatr Soc* 44(1):83, 1996.
21. Zieman SJ et al: Upregulation of the nitric oxide–cGMP pathway in aged myocardium: physiological response to l-arginine, *Circ Res* 88(1):97, 2001.

CHAPTER 29

Alterations of Cardiovascular Function

VALENTINA L. BRASHERS

CHAPTER OUTLINE

The pathophysiology of heart disease is now known to be much more complicated than just structural and hemodynamic changes. Today the focus is on the genetic, neurohumoral, and inflammatory mechanisms that underlie tissue and cellular processes, such as endothelial injury, remodeling, stunning, reperfusion injury, and autoimmune disease.

DISEASES OF THE ARTERIES AND VEINS

Arteriosclerosis

Arteriosclerosis is a chronic disease of the arterial system characterized by abnormal thickening and hardening of the vessel walls. In arteriosclerosis the tunica intima undergoes a series of changes that decrease the artery's ability to change lumen size. Smooth muscle cells and collagen fibers migrate into the tunica intima, causing it to stiffen and thicken. This process gradually narrows the arterial lumen (Fig. 29-1). Changes in lipid, cholesterol, and phospholipid metabolism within the tunica intima also contribute to arteriosclerosis. Although these structural changes may be part of the normal aging process, they can cause or worsen pathophysiologic conditions such as high blood pressure, insufficient perfusion of tissues, or weakening and outpouching of arterial walls.

Atherosclerosis

Atherosclerosis is a form of arteriosclerosis in which the thickening and hardening of the vessel walls are caused by soft deposits of intraarterial fat and fibrin that harden over time. Atherosclerosis is not a single disease entity. It can take several forms, depending on the anatomic location, the individual's age and genetic and physiologic status, and the risk factors to which each individual may have been exposed. It is the leading contributor to coronary artery and cerebrovascular disease. (Atherosclerosis of the coronary arteries is described on p. 1000; atherosclerosis of the cerebral arteries is discussed in Chapter 16.)

Pathophysiology

Atherosclerosis is an inflammatory disease.[1,2,3,4] Pathologically, the lesions progress from endothelial injury and

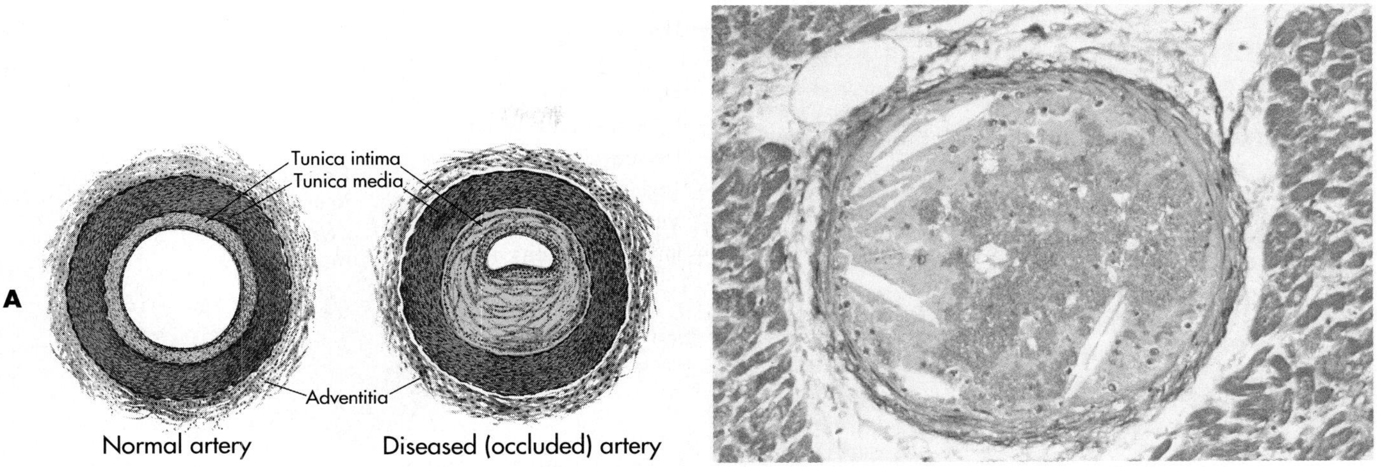

FIG. 29-1 Arteriosclerosis. A, Cross section of a normal artery and an artery altered by disease. **B,** A small artery in the myocardium is occluded by a mass of blue-staining platelets, yellow-staining red cells, and cholesterol bodies. (B from Damjanov I, Linder J, editors: *Anderson's pathology,* ed 10, St Louis, 1996, Mosby.)

dysfunction to fatty streak to fibrotic plaque to complicated lesion (Fig. 29-2). Atherosclerosis begins with injury to the endothelial cells that line artery walls. Possible causes of **endothelial injury** include smoking, hypertension, diabetes (insulin resistance), hyperhomocystinemia, dyslipidemia, autoimmune phenomena, vessel shear wall stress, and increased C-reactive protein and fibrinogen.[5,6,7,8] There is increasing evidence that infection may be a cause of endothelial injury. Other risk factors include endotoxemia and peridontal disease.[9,10] Microorganisms that have been implicated include cytomegalovirus, *Chlamydia pneumoniae*, and *Helicobacter pylori*.[11,12,13,14,15] Once injury has occurred, endothelial dysfunction and inflammation lead to the following pathophysiologic events:

1. Injured endothelial cells become inflamed and cannot make normal amounts of antithrombotic and vasodilating cytokines (Figs. 29-3 and 29-4).[16,17]
2. Numerous inflammatory cytokines are released, including tumor necrosis factor–α (TNF-α), interferon-γ, interleukin-1, and heat shock proteins.[3]
3. Growth factors are also released, including angiotensin II, fibroblast growth factor, and platelet-derived growth factor, which stimulate smooth muscle cell proliferation in the affected vessel.[2,18]
4. Macrophages adhere to the injured endothelium via adhesion molecules (intracellular adhesion molecule-1, P selectin, CD18).[3]
5. These macrophages release enzymes and toxic oxygen radicals that further injure the vessel wall and result in oxidation of low-density lipoprotein (LDL).

The oxidation of LDL is an important step in atherogenesis. Hypertension with increased levels of angiotensin II has been linked to increased LDL oxidation via stimulation of the angiotensin receptor AT_1.[19,20,21] Smoking and diabetes also increase LDL oxidation. Oxidized LDL is toxic to endothelial cells and causes smooth muscle proliferation and abnormal vasoconstriction.[22,23] Oxidized LDL is engulfed by the macrophages, which then penetrate into the intima of the vessel. Macrophages filled with oxidized LDL are called **foam cells**. Currently, investigators are studying antioxidant vitamins and whether they prevent LDL oxidation including beta-carotene and vitamin E.[24,25]

Once these lipid-laden foam cells accumulate in significant amounts, they form a lesion called a **fatty streak** (see Fig. 29-2). These lesions can be found in the walls of arteries of most people, even young children. Once formed, fatty streaks produce more toxic oxygen radicals and cause immunologic and inflammatory changes, resulting in progressive damage to the vessel wall. Decreasing levels of LDL can cause regression of atherosclerotic lesions and can improve endothelial function.[22] Increasing attention is being given to the evaluation of children for dyslipidemia so that early dietary intervention to prevent atherosclerosis can be initiated.[26,27,28]

At this point, smooth muscle cells proliferate, produce collagen, and migrate over the fatty streak, forming a **fibrous plaque** (see Fig. 29-2). This results in further endothelial cell dysfunction, necrosis of underlying vessel tissue, and narrowing of the vessel lumen as the lesion protrudes out from the wall. Vessel obstruction can become significant enough to reduce blood flow to distal tissues, especially during exercise. Although some permanent scarring has occurred by this step in atherogenesis, aggressive reversal of risk factors such as dyslipidemia can result in lesion regression and improved tissue perfusion.[29,30]

As the plaque continues to develop, it can ulcerate or rupture, resulting in platelet adherence to the lesion. Fibrous plaques can become "unstable" and rupture even before they occlude the vessel significantly through a process of apoptosis of cells at the margins of the lesions or through the release

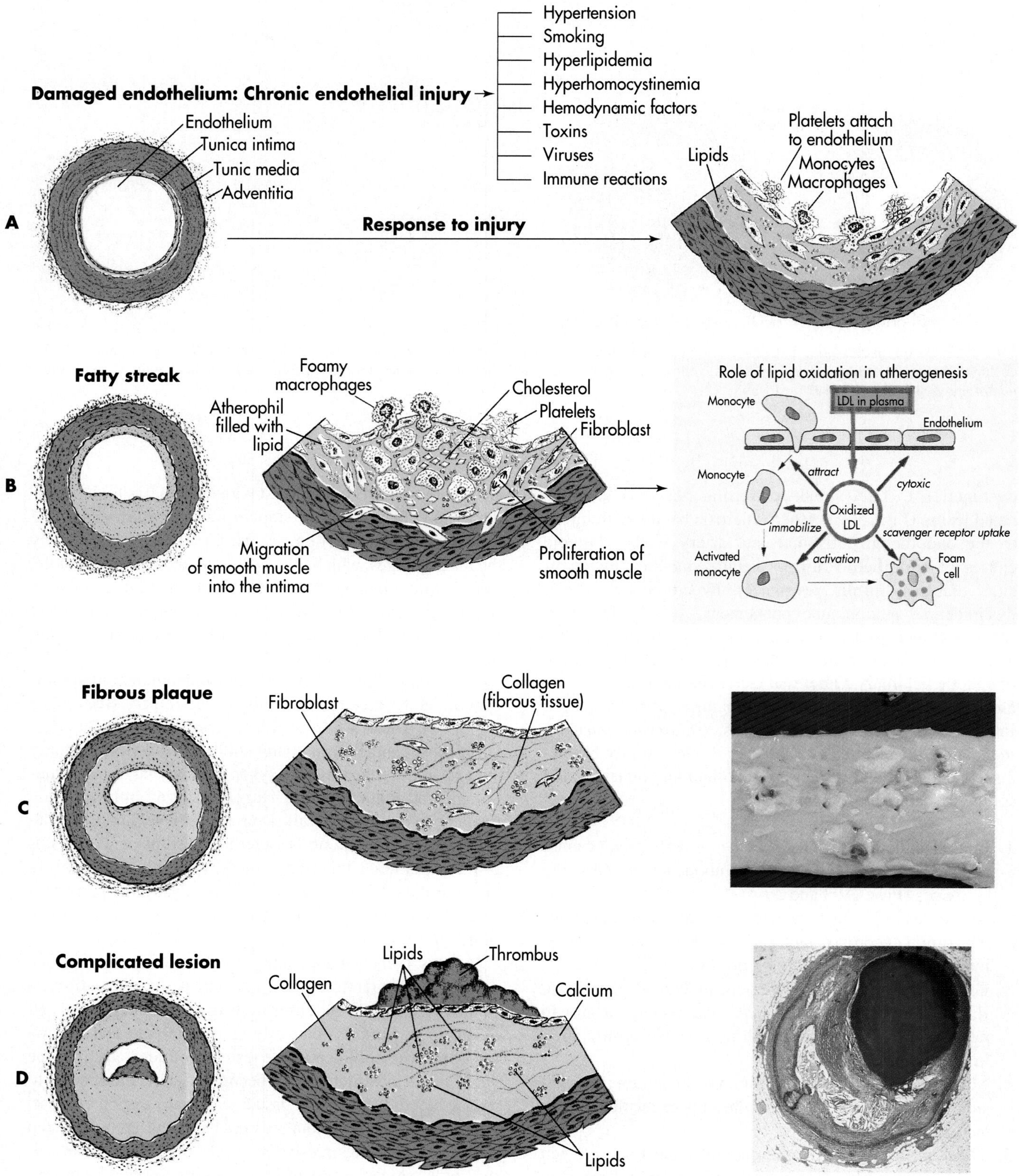

FIG. 29-2 Progression of atherosclerosis. A, Damaged endothelium. **B,** Diagrams of fatty streak and lipid core formation; diagram of oxidized LDL (i.e., combining of oxygen free radicals with LDL). (Micrographs and diagrams of lipid formation and foam cell formation from Damjanov I, Linder J, editors: *Anderson's pathology,* ed 10, St Louis, 1996, Mosby.) **C,** Diagram of fibrous plaque; micrograph of fibrous plaques (fibrolipid) in human aorta. Raised plaques are visible: some are yellow, others are white. One plaque is complicated by red thrombus deposition. **D,** Diagram of complicated lesion; micrograph of coronary thrombus: thrombus is red, collagen is blue. *LDL,* Low-density lipoprotein. (Micrographs and diagrams of lipid formation and foam cell formation from Damjanov I, Linder J, editors: *Anderson's pathology,* ed 10, St Louis, 1996, Mosby.)

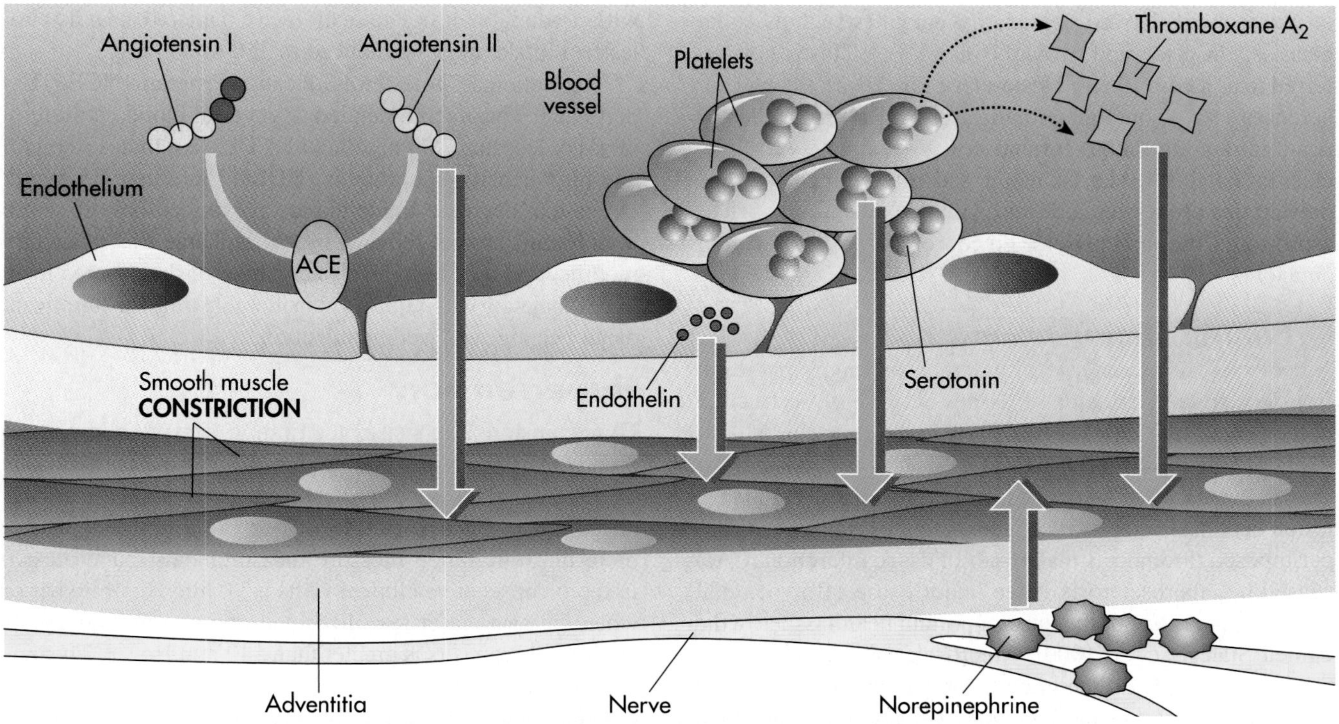

FIG. 29-3 The endothelium regulates vasomotion (constriction and dilation) and platelet aggregation by releasing a variety of constricting and dilating substances. Constricting factors include arachidonic and metabolites, such as thromboxane A_2 (which aspirin inhibits), and a potent amino acid peptide called *endothelin*. The endothelium also converts angiotensin I into angiotensin II by the menbrane-bound angiotensin-converting enzyme that aso metabolizes the endogenous endothelium-dependent vasodilator, bradykinin. (Modified from Stern S, editor: *Silent myocardial ischemia*, St Louis, 1998, Mosby.)

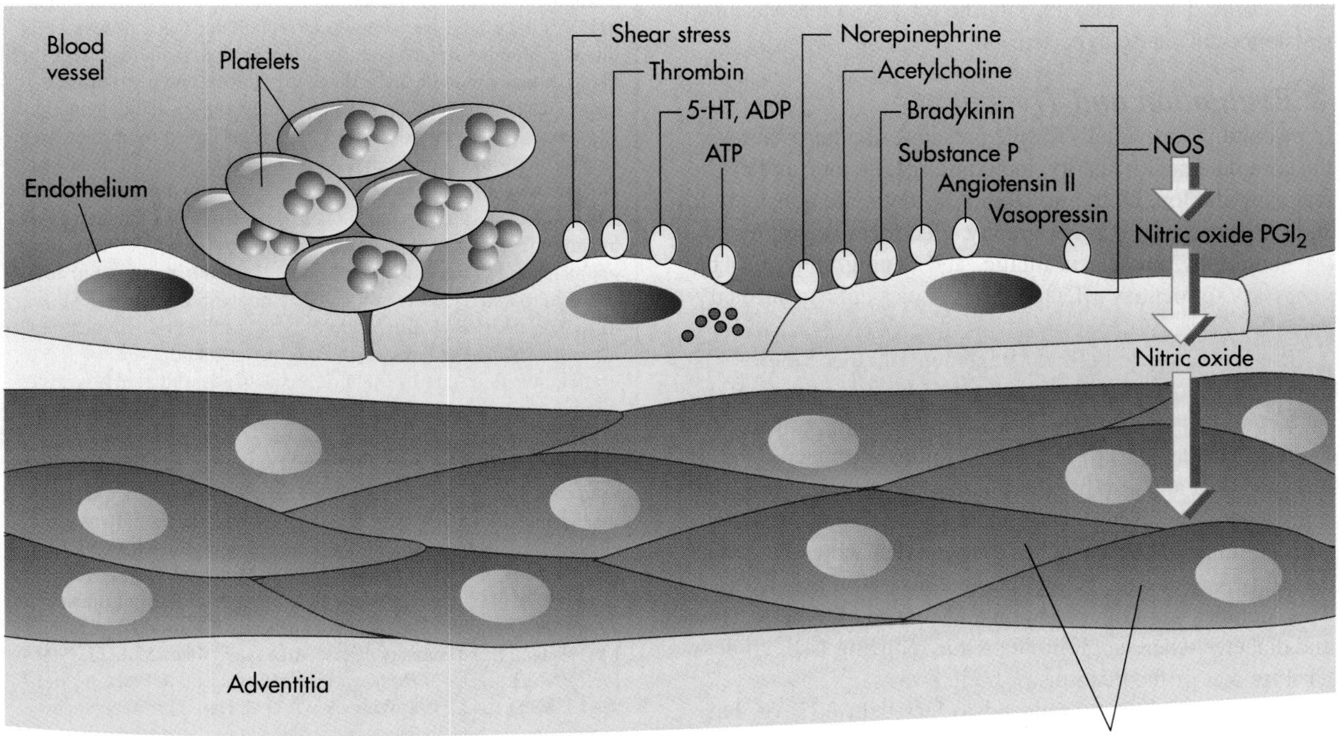

FIG. 29-4 Factors causing endothelium-dependent vasodilation. A variety of exogenous pharmacologic substances, platelet-derived factors, and shear stress can promote release of nitric oxide by stimulating nitric oxide synthase (NOS). Prostacyclin (PGI_2) causes relaxation of vascular smooth muscle cells by cyclic adenosine monophosphate (cAMP)-dependent mechanism, and both nitric oxide and PGI_2 inhibit platelet aggregation. *5-HT*, Serotonin; *ADP*, adenosine diphosphate; *ATP*, adenosine triphosphate. (Modified from Stern S, editor: *Silent myocardial ischemia*, St Louis, 1998, Mosby.)

of macrophage-derived degradative enzymes such as collagenases, elastases, and stromolysins.[2,3,31,32,33] This is now referred to as a **complicated lesion** (see Fig. 29-2). Platelet adherence to the plaque can initiate the coagulation cascade and result in rapid thrombus formation with complete vessel occlusion causing tissue ischemia and infarction. Efforts to prevent this process include antiplatelet medications such as aspirin and the new platelet glycoprotein IIb/IIIa receptor antagonists.[34]

Clinical Manifestations

Atherosclerosis presents with symptoms and signs that result from inadequate perfusion of tissues because of obstruction of the vessels that supply them. Early in the course of the disease, partial vessel obstruction may lead to transient ischemic events, often associated with exercise or stress. As the lesion becomes complicated, increasing obstruction with superimposed thrombosis may result in tissue infarction. CAD caused by atherosclerosis is the major cause of myocardial ischemia and is one of the most important health issues in the United States (see p. 1000). Atherosclerotic obstruction of the vessels supplying the brain is the major cause of stroke. Similarly, any part of the body may become ischemic when its blood supply is compromised by atherosclerotic lesions. Often, more than one vessel will become involved with this disease process so that an individual may present with symptoms from several ischemic tissues at the same time, and disease in one area may indicate that the individual is at risk for other ischemic complications elsewhere. Finally, diffuse atherosclerotic disease may elevate the total systemic vascular resistance and cause hypertension.

Evaluation and Treatment

In evaluating individuals for the presence of atherosclerosis, the complete health history, including risk factors, and physical examination, including laboratory data, are considered. Judicious use of roentgenography, electrocardiography, ultrasonography, nuclear scanning, and angiography may be necessary to identify affected vessels, particularly coronary vessels.

The primary goal in the management of atherosclerosis is to restore adequate blood flow to the affected tissues. If an individual has presented with acute ischemia (e.g., myocardial infarction [MI], stroke), interventions are specific to the diseased area and are discussed under those topics. In situations where the disease process does not require immediate intervention, management focuses on removing the initial causes of vessel damage and preventing lesion progression. This includes smoking cessation and control of hypertension and diabetes where appropriate, while reducing LDL cholesterol by diet or medications or both.

Fat intake should be reduced to less than 30% of daily calorie consumption, with no more than 10% saturated fats, no more than 10% polyunsaturated fats, and 10% to 15% monounsaturated fats. Monounsaturated fats reduce atherogenesis while avoiding the problems of polyunsaturated fats with production of free radicals (see Chapter 10). Daily cholesterol intake must be reduced to 250 to 300 mg.

The National Cholesterol Education Program (NCEP) Expert Panel[35] has recommended target total blood cholesterol levels of less than 200 mg/dl, with LDLs less than 130 mg/dl and high-density lipoproteins (HDLs) more than 35 mg/dl. Drugs that decrease lipidemia are prescribed only if serum lipoproteins are not reduced by a reasonable trial of dietary modification or if lipid levels are dangerously elevated in an individual who will require a considerable time for significant dietary change and weight reduction.

Hypertension

Hypertension is consistent elevation of systemic arterial blood pressure. Approximately 50 million Americans 6 years of age and older have hypertension. Individuals are diagnosed as having hypertension when the average of two or more diastolic blood pressure measurements made on two or more consecutive clinical visits is 90 mm Hg or higher or when the average of systolic blood pressure measurements made on three visits is greater than 140 mm Hg.[36,37] The new classification presented in Table 29-1 describes the stages of blood pressure.[36] "Optimal" blood pressure is associated with the lowest cardiovascular risk, whereas those who fall

WHAT'S NEW? Vitamins and Heart Disease

Folate (lowers serum homocysteine levels) and vitamin E (an antioxidant) have both been shown to reduce the risk cardiovascular disease. Homocysteine is an amino acid that is increased in the blood of many individuals with atherosclerosis and heart disease. It has been shown to participate in endothelial injury and dysfunction. Elevated levels of homocysteine have been linked to an increased risk for both myocardial infarction and stroke, even in those people with few other risk factors for atherosclerotic disease. Although a few individuals have a specific enzyme deficiency that can cause hyperhomocysteinemia (methylenetetrahydrofolate reductase), most people can reduce their levels of homocysteine by taking in additional amounts of folate and B_{12}. Vitamin E has also been shown to reduce the risk of atherosclerotic disease in both smokers and nonsmokers, and reduces cardiovascular risk at dosages of 100 to 400 IU per day. Interestingly, a recent study showed it was not helpful in reducing the risk of myocardial infarction or stroke in a group of high-risk individuals.

Data from Giles SH et al: Association between total homocysteine and the likelihood for a history of acute myocardial infarction by race and ethnicity: results from the Third National Health and Nutrition Examination Survey, *Am Heart J* 139:446, 2000; Neunteufl T et al: Effects of vitamin E on chronic and acute endothelial dysfunction in smokers, *J Am Coll Cardiol* 35(2):277, 2000; Spencer AP, Carson DS, Crouch MA: Vitamin E and coronary disease, *Arch Intern Med* 159:1313, 1999; Welch GN, Loscalzo J: Homocysteine and atherothrombosis, *N Engl J Med* 338(15):1042, 1998; Willinek WA et al: High-normal serum homocysteine concentrations are associated with an increased risk of early atherosclerotic carotid artery wall lesions in healthy subjects, *J Hypertens* 18(4):425, 2000; Yusuf S et al: Vitamin E supplementation and cardiovascular events in high-risk patients: the Heart Outcomes Prevention Study Investigators, *N Engl J Med* 342:154, 2000.

into the "high normal" category are at risk for developing hypertension unless life-style modification is instituted. All stages of hypertension are associated with increased risk of cardiovascular disease events. Stage 1, previously termed "mild," is the most common form of high blood pressure in the adult population. All stages of hypertension need effective long-term therapy.[36] The World Health Organization (WHO) developed a new classification scheme in 1999; it is similar to the Joint National Committee (JNC) Report VI, described in Table 29-1, except that WHO calls the stages of hypertension "Grade" 1 through 3 and includes a separate category called "Isolated Systolic Hypertension." This new category includes those individuals with a systolic pressure greater than or equal to 140 and a diastolic pressure less than 90.[37] Isolated systolic blood pressure is now recognized as an important indicator of cardiovascular risk and should be treated aggressively.[38,39,40,41]

Hypertension is caused by increases in cardiac output, total peripheral resistance, or both. (The many factors affecting cardiac output and peripheral resistance are described in Chapter 28. See Figs. 28-18 and 28-28.) Cardiac output is increased by any condition that increases heart rate or stroke volume, whereas peripheral resistance is increased by any factor that increases blood viscosity or reduces vessel diameter, particularly arteriolar diameter.

Individuals with hypertensive disease may have combined systolic and diastolic hypertension or isolated systolic hypertension. Most cases of combined systolic and diastolic hypertension have no known cause and therefore are diagnosed as **primary hypertension.** Primary hypertension, also called *essential* or *idiopathic hypertension,* affects 90% to 95% of hypertensive individuals.[42] **Secondary hypertension** is caused by altered hemodynamics associated with a primary disease, such as arteriosclerosis. Although many diseases can cause secondary hypertension, this form of hypertension accounts for only 5% to 8% of cases. **Isolated systolic hypertension** is elevated systolic blood pressure accompanied by normal diastolic blood pressure (below 90 mm Hg). Isolated systolic hypertension is a manifestation of increased cardiac output or rigidity of the aorta or both.

Table 29-1 Classification of Blood Pressure for Adults Age 18 Years or Older

Category	Systolic (mm Hg)	Diastolic (mm Hg)
Optimal	<120	<80
Normal	<130	<85
High normal	130-139	85-89
Hypertension		
Stage 1 (mild)	140-159	90-99
Stage 2 (moderate)	160-179	100-109
Stage 3 (severe)	≥180	≥110

From Anonymous. (1997). The sixth report of the Joint National Committee on Prevention, Detection, Evaluation, and Treatment of High Blood Pressure. *Archives of Internal Medicine* 157:2413, 1977.

The National Health and Nutrition Examination Survey III (Phase 2) reported a significant reduction in morbidity and mortality from hypertension. This decline is believed to be from improved hypertension awareness, management, and control. Of concern, however, are more recent observations that the rate of these improvements is leveling off, especially in minority populations.[36]

Factors Associated with Primary Hypertension

A specific cause for primary hypertension has not been identified, and a combination of genetic and environmental factors is thought to be responsible for its development. Genetic predisposition to hypertension is thought to be polygenic. The inherited defects are associated with renal sodium excretion, cell membrane sodium or calcium transport, and sympathetic response to neurogenic hormones (see "What's New? Genetics of Primary Hypertension"). Factors associated with primary hypertension include (1) family history of hypertension; (2) advancing age; (3) gender (men younger than 55 years and women older than 74 years); (4) black race; (5) high dietary sodium intake; (6) glucose intolerance (diabetes mellitus); (7) cigarette smoking; (8) obesity; (9) heavy alcohol consumption; and (10) low dietary intake of potassium, calcium, and magnesium. Many of these factors are also risk factors for other cardiovascular disorders. In fact, hypertension, dyslipidemia, and glucose intolerance often are found together.[43,44,45]

Although populations with high dietary sodium intake have long been shown to have a high incidence of hypertension, recent studies indicate that low dietary potassium, calcium, and magnesium intakes are also risk factors (see "Nutrition and Disease: Diet Modification Can Lower

WHAT'S NEW? Genetics of Primary Hypertension

It is estimated that heritability accounts for about 30% to 40% of primary hypertension. By studying families and by using special genetic markers, scientists have identified several candidate genes likely to be playing a role in the pathogenesis of hypertension. Most of these genes are related to the renin-angiotensin-aldosterone (RAA) system and include those for the angiotensin II receptor, angiotensinogen, and renin. Other genes that have been implicated include those involved with other modulators of vascular tone, such as endothelial nitric oxide synthase, G protein receptor kinase, adrenergic receptors, and the calcium transport system. Several genes are being studied that influence renal salt and water transport (in addition to the RAA) such as a sodium-hydrogen antiporter gene and other genes that affect salt sensitivity. Finally, the genetics of insulin resistance, obesity, dyslipidemia, and hypertension as a cluster of traits is being elucidated.

Data from An P, Rice T, Rao DC: A review of recent genetic epidemiological studies of blood pressure, *CVR&R* 21:85, 2000; Farfel Z, Henry R, Iiri T: Mechanisms of disease: the expanding spectrum of G protein diseases, *N Engl J Med* 340(1):12, 1999; Giner V et al: Renin-angiotensin system genetic polymorphisms and salt sensitivity in essential hypertension, *Hypertension* 35:512, 2000.

Cholesterol").[46,47,48,49] The nicotine in cigarette smoke is a vasoconstrictor that can elevate both systolic and diastolic blood pressure acutely. In habitual smokers an individual cigarette may not raise blood pressure, yet habitual smoking is associated with a high incidence of severe hypertension, myocardial hypertrophy, and death resulting from CAD.[36,50] The incidence of hypertension is higher among heavy drinkers of alcohol (more than three drinks per day) than among abstainers, but moderate drinkers (two to four drinks per week) appear to have lower blood pressures, as well as lower cardiovascular mortality, than either abstainers or heavy drinkers.[36,51]

NUTRITION & DISEASE

Diet Modifications Can Lower Cholesterol*

Although many nutrition recommendations remain controversial, there is consensus among health and nutrition professionals that most Americans should lower their intake of dietary fat and alter its composition. The National Cholesterol Education Program (NCEP) encourages people with high total cholesterol and LDL cholesterol to start with a step I diet that has less than 30% of the total calories coming from fat, 8% to 10% of calories from saturated fat, and less than 300 mg of cholesterol per day. If lipid levels do not decrease after 3 months, a step II diet is tried in which less than 30% of calories come from total fat, less than 7% from saturated fat, and less than 200 mg from cholesterol. Drug therapy may need to be initiated if a lipid-lowering response does not occur after 3 months on a step II diet. People with high-fat baseline diets who lose weight can decrease their cholesterol by 25% with good compliance. Suggestions for lowering fat and saturated fat include (1) avoiding fats as spreads or for flavoring, (2) avoiding or reducing consumption of meat, (3) using specially manufactured low-fat foods (e.g., fat-free salad dressings), (4) modifying common foods to be lower in fat (e.g., remove skin from chicken), and (5) replacing a high-fat food with its low-fat equivalent (e.g., skim milk instead of whole milk).

Other persons may choose to count fat grams (20% of a 2000-kcal diet would be about 45 grams of fat per day) and stay within that limit per day. Labels on food products and nutritional information at fast food restaurants make counting fat grams much easier.

More aggressive diets are also an option for those with high lipid values. These diets contain 10% of total calories from fat, less than 3% from saturated fatty acids (SFAs) and less than 5 mg of cholesterol per day with a minimal amount of animal fat. When decreasing fat, what choices are left for meals? Nuts have been shown to lower serum cholesterol levels. Walnuts lowered low-density lipoprotein (LDL) cholesterol by about 16%, and almonds or hazelnuts reduced serum cholesterol by 8% to 10%. Walnuts have a very low ratio of saturated fatty acids to polyunsaturated fatty acids, as well as a high percentage of fat from α-linolenic acid. Including a 1-oz portion of nuts in a low-fat diet should pose no problem while keeping calories under control.

Changing the source of protein may be a method to further lower cholesterol. A meta-analysis found that consuming 31 to 47 g of soy protein per day significantly decreases serum cholesterol and LDL cholesterol. Evidence suggests that soy protein enhances secretion of bile acids and upregulates LDL-receptor activity. Soy protein may be especially helpful in the diets of children diagnosed with familial hypercholesterolemia.

Fat can be replaced with soluble fibers that are known to lower cholesterol levels. Fibers that have been shown to lower cholesterol and LDL levels include pectins (found in many fruits), gums, mucilages, legumes, oats, and carrots. The amount of reduction varies with the source of fiber. Psyllium has been shown to lower LDL levels by 14% in persons with hypercholesterolemia. Two mechanisms have been proposed for the cholesterol-lowering effect: (1) fiber binds the bile acids, which lowers cholesterol to replete the bile acid pool, and (2) bacteria in the colon ferment fiber to compounds (acetate, propionate, butyrate) that inhibit cholesterol synthesis.

Adding garlic to the diet also may lower cholesterol. Researchers have found that 900 mg of powdered garlic (equivalent of 1½ cloves of garlic) reduced both total cholesterol and LDL cholesterol by about 12%. Taking garlic pills might be an alternative; however, a consumer advocacy group recently analyzed commercial garlic supplements and found enormous variations in the amount of active compounds they contain. Fortunately, cooking does not destroy the allicin (the cardioprotective chemical formed when garlic is crushed) and so the recommendation is simply to include cooked or raw garlic frequently in meals.

Trans-fatty acids are found in many foods, and new data indicate that they may increase a person's risk of a heart attack. The amount of trans-fatty acids in typical margarine ranges from 10% to 30% of total fat and often exceeds 25% in cookies, crackers, pastries, and deep-fried foods, such as French fries and doughnuts. Researchers have found that trans-fatty acids raise LDL cholesterol; lower the good (high-density lipoprotein [HDL]) cholesterol; and may negatively affect levels of lipoprotein (a), a hereditary risk factor for heart disease.

What should a person do? Be wary of products that list "partially hydrogenated oil" on the ingredient list, minimize use of both butter and margarine (choose a fat-free or more liquid version in a tub), cook or bake with olive oil or canola oil, avoid deep fat–fried items, and choose commercially baked items that are either fat free or made with canola or olive oil. What we do not eat may make a difference in our cardiovascular health also. Rapidly accumulating data indicate that serum homocysteine concentration is a risk factor for coronary artery disease. Acquired homocysteinemia may be the result of vitamin B_6, folic acid, or vitamin B_{12} deficiency. It is possible that a vitamin B_6 deficiency could be a possible risk factor for atherosclerotic disease. Certainly, including foods high in vitamin B_6, such as bananas, broccoli, chicken, dried beans, lean pork, peanut butter, potatoes, tuna fish, and whole wheat bread, can be helpful. Epidemiologic evidence that eating no fish at all may be detrimental for the heart is remarkably consistent; however, increasing fish intake beyond one or two servings per week is unlikely to reduce coronary risk substantially in healthy men free of coronary disease.

Many recommendations for lowering fat in the diet are directed to the adult population. However, some parents have felt the need to severely restrict the fat intake in their children's diet, resulting in children failing to thrive. At this time the recommendation is that children younger than 2 years should not be placed on a fat-restricted diet. Children older than 2 years with high cholesterol levels can follow the NCEP step diet guidelines.

*Data from Anderson TJ et al: Systemic nature of endothelial dysfunction in atherosclerosis, *Am J Cardiol* 75:71B, 1995; Glore SR et al: Soluble fiber and serum lipids: a literature review, *J Am Diet Assoc* 94:425, 1994; Huff MW: Research horizons in hyperlipidemia and atherosclerosis, *Can J Cardiol* 5(7):VIII, 1989; Kristal AR et al: Long-term maintenance of a low-fat diet: durability of fat-related habits in the women's health trial, *J Am Diet Assoc* 92:553, 1992; Lovati MR et al: Soybean protein diet increases low density lipoprotein receptor activity in mononuclear cells from hypercholesterolemic patients, *J Clin Invest* 80(5):1498, 1987.

Pathophysiology

Chronic hypertension damages the walls of systemic blood vessels. Prolonged vasoconstriction and high pressures within these vessels, particularly the arteries and arterioles, stimulate the vessels to thicken and strengthen to withstand the stress. Arterial smooth muscle undergoes hypertrophy (cellular enlargement) and hyperplasia (cellular proliferation). Eventually the tunica intima and tunica media undergo fibromuscular thickening sufficient to narrow their lumina. At this point, regardless of stimuli that cause vasoconstriction, the vessels are permanently narrowed.

Hypertensive injury of vessel walls also stimulates the biochemical mediators of inflammation (histamine, leukotrienes, prostaglandins) to increase the permeability of the vascular endothelium. As permeability increases, sodium, calcium, water, plasma proteins, and other blood-borne (humoral) substances enter vessel walls, causing further thickening and, in the case of calcium, increasing responsiveness to stimuli that cause smooth muscle contraction (i.e., vasoconstriction) (Fig. 29-5). (Inflammation is discussed in Chapter 7.)

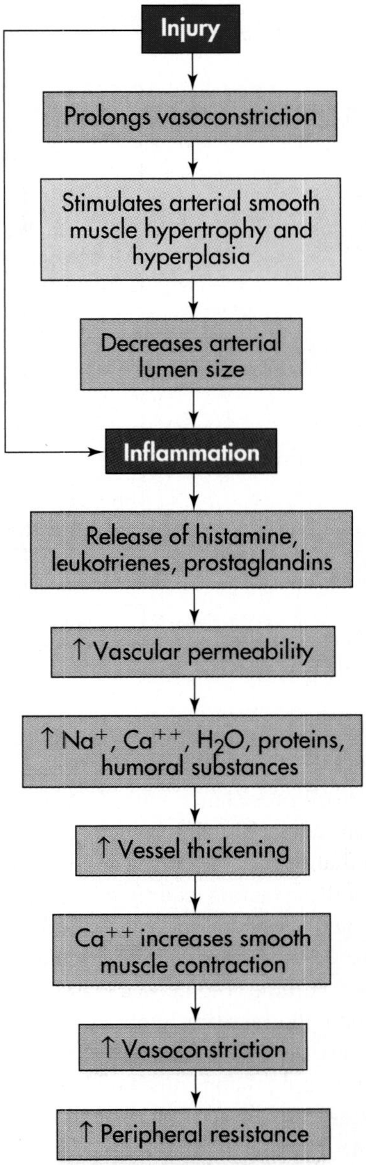

FIG. 29-5 Summary of pathophysiology of hypertension.

In the coronary vessels, hypertension causes or aggravates other conditions, such as atherosclerosis, that diminish vessel caliber (Fig. 29-6). Therefore hypertension combined with CAD increases the risk of coronary artery occlusion and infarction of myocardial tissue.

Primary hypertension. Despite research by numerous investigators, the exact pathogenesis of primary hypertension has not been established. In view of the multiple, interdependent factors involved in normal blood pressure regulation, is seems likely that no single cause or defect will be identified.

Primary hypertension is the result of an extremely complicated interaction of genetics and the environment mediated by a host of neurohumoral effects. The genetic contribution to essential hypertension is discussed in the "What's New? Genetics of Primary Hypertension" box on p. 985.[52,53,54] These genes interact with diet, smoking, age, and the other risk factors to cause chronic changes in vasomotor tone and blood volume. There are many theories to explain these complex interactions. Currently the most frequently cited theories include (1) overactivity of the sympathetic nervous system; (2) overactivity of the renin-angiotensin-aldosterone system; (3) alterations in other neurohumoral mediators of blood volume and vasomotor tone, such as atrial natriuretic peptide, brain natriuretic peptide, and adrenomedullin (a vasodilating and natriuretic peptide); and (4) a complex interaction involving insulin resistance and endothelial function.

The sympathetic nervous system has been implicated in both the development and the maintenance of high blood pressure and plays a role in hypertensive end-organ damage.[55,56] In addition, there is increasing evidence for genetic changes in adrenergic receptors leading to maladaptive responses of the cardiovascular system to sympathetic stimulation.[57] Overstimulation of the α-adrenergic and β-adrenergic receptors results in vasoconstriction and increased cardiac output, thus raising the blood pressure.

The renin-angiotensin-aldosterone system plays an important role in blood pressure regulation by modulating vascular tone and influencing salt and water retention by the kidneys.[58]

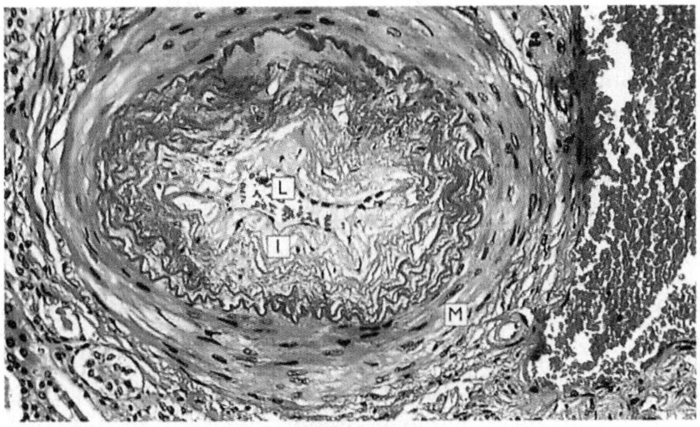

FIG. 29-6 Dramatic hypertension change in small arterioles. Fibrous intimal proliferation *(I)* with reduction in lumen vessel caliber (radius) *(L)* and normal media *(M)*. (From Stevens A, Lowe J: *Pathology,* St Louis, 1995, Mosby.)

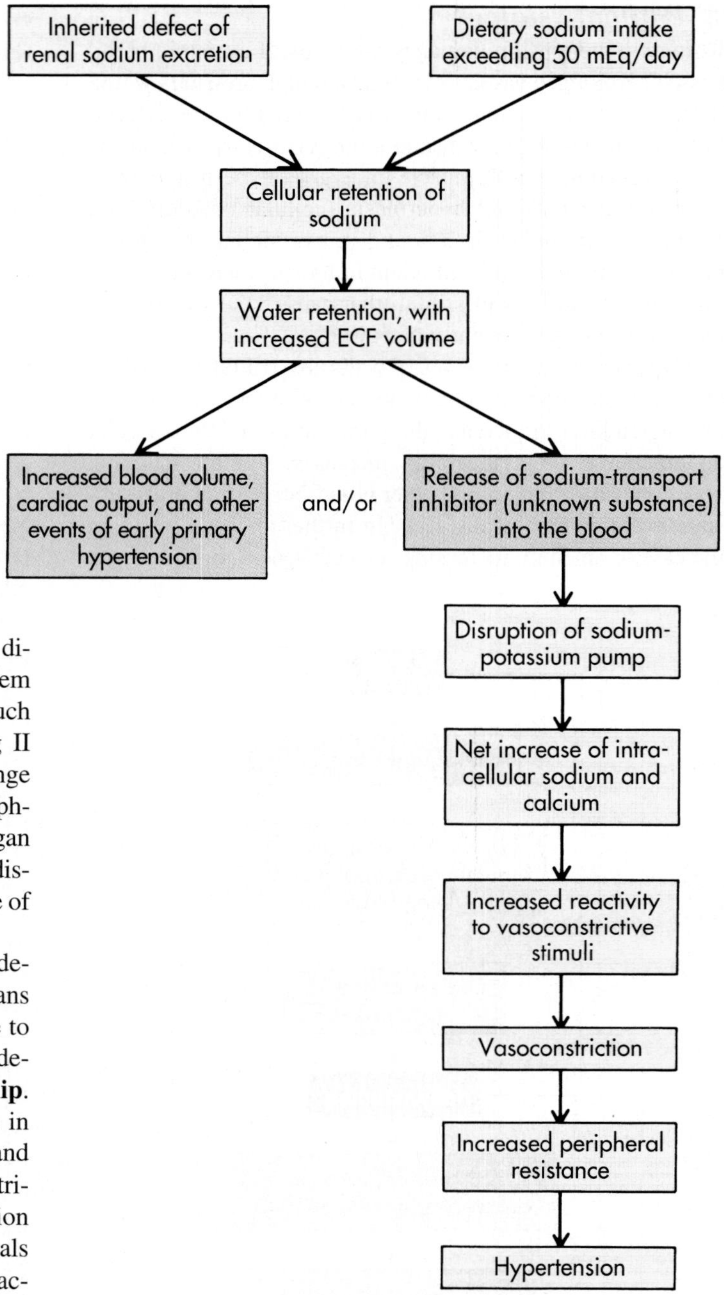

FIG. 29-7 Two related mechanisms of sodium-induced primary hypertension. *ECF,* Extracellular fluid.

Angiotensin II (Ang II) not only causes vasoconstriction directly, but indirectly increases sympathetic nervous system activity and can affect the release of normal vasodilators, such as prostaglandins and nitric oxide.[59,60] Furthermore, Ang II mediates **arteriolar remodeling,** which is structural change in the vessel wall resulting in permanent increases in peripheral resistance. Finally, Ang II is associated with end-organ effects of hypertension, including atherosclerosis, renal disease, and cardiac hypertrophy (see "What's New? The Role of Angiotensin II in Cardiovascular Disease.").[61,62]

One probable contributor to primary hypertension is a defect in sodium excretion by the kidneys. This defect means that the kidney requires a higher level of arterial pressure to stimulate it to excrete sodium and water and has been described as a shift in the **pressure-natriuresis relationship**. Catecholamines and angiotensin II play significant roles in affecting the pressure-natriuresis relationship (pp. 957 and 989).[53,63,64] In addition, atrial natriuretic peptide, brain natriuretic peptide, and adrenomedullin affect renal salt excretion and blood pressure.[65,66] Finally, poor intake of other minerals such as calcium, magnesium, and potassium can alter the activity of the renal sodium-potassium pump, leading to sodium retention (i.e., if these cations are low, sodium, a cation, is retained) and changes in intracellular calcium with resultant vascular reactivity.[46,47,49] The defect in renal sodium excretion is aggravated by dietary sodium intake of more than 50 mEq per day (Fig. 29-7).

Insulin resistance and associated endothelial dysfunction have been implicated as a primary cause of primary hypertension even in the absence of clinical diabetes.[67] A significant portion of people with primary hypertension are insulin resistant. Insulin resistance is associated with decreased endothelial release of nitric oxide and other endogenous vasodilators, and with alterations in renal function.[68,69] Furthermore, sympathetic nervous system activity is increased in insulin resistance,[70] and Ang II activity is increased by high levels of insulin as noted in type 2 diabetes.[71] Interestingly, treatment of hypertension with ACE inhibitors or Ang II receptor blockers can improve insulin sensitivity, whereas treatment of insulin resistance with diabetic drugs in many individuals can reduce blood pressure.[72,73]

It is likely that primary hypertension is an interaction between many of these factors leading to sustained increases in blood volume and peripheral resistance. Early primary hypertension consists of a series of cardiovascular adjustments to increased blood volume (Fig. 29-8). First, cardiac output increases to handle the increased volume of blood circulating through the heart. As the systemic arteries sense the volume increase, their autoregulatory mechanisms try to slow things down by causing vasoconstriction. Because blood volume remains high, the increase in total peripheral resistance caused

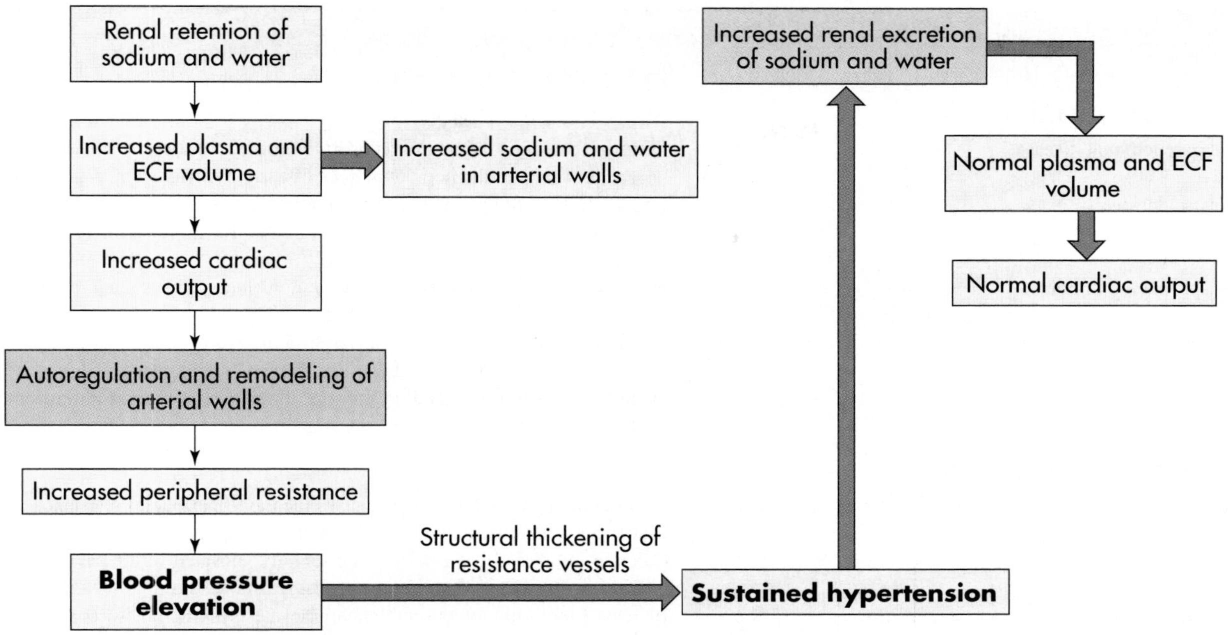

FIG. 29-8 Primary hypertension. Hemodynamic events of early primary hypertension *(thin arrows)* and established primary hypertension *(thick arrows). ECF,* Extracellular fluid volume.

WHAT'S NEW? The Role of Angiotensin II in Cardiovascular Disease

Angiotensin II (Ang II) plays a role in essential hypertension, atherosclerosis, myocardial hypertrophy, ischemic heart disease, and renal disease. It is both a circulating hormone (through the renin-angiotensin-aldosterone system) and a local mediator that is produced in many tissues; in each case it has its effect via stimulation of several tissue receptors (for example, AT_1 receptor). Ang II increases vasomotor tone by direct stimulation of vascular smooth muscle contraction and through the inhibition of endothelial nitric oxide and prostaglandin release. It increases intravascular volume through the stimulation of renal salt and water retention (with aldosterone), shifts the pressure-natriuresis relationship, and alters glomerular hemodynamics. In addition to these physiologic roles for Ang II, it can also be considered a toxin produced in response tissue injury. In blood vessels, Ang II stimulates smooth muscle cell and fibroblast proliferation with thickening of the vessel wall (remodeling). This is important in causing sustained increases in peripheral vascular resistance in chronic hypertension and glomerular scarring in hypertensive and diabetic renal disease, and it may contribute to the atherosclerotic process. It also inhibits the endothelium's ability to resist monocyte and platelet adhesion and thus promotes intravascular inflammation and clotting. In the heart, Ang II also causes remodeling, resulting in hypertrophy and fibrosis of myocardial tissue after ischemic injury or in response to persistent increases in afterload, as seen in hypertension. Ang II is seen as an important mediator of congestive heart failure. Angiotensin-converting enzyme (ACE) inhibitors and Ang II receptor blockers have been demonstrated to be effective drugs in the treatment of hypertension, in preventing diabetic and hypertensive renal disease, in preventing or reducing vascular and myocardial remodeling, and in improving survival in individuals who have had a myocardial infarction or who have congestive heart failure.

Data from du Cailar G et al: Left ventricular adaptation to hypertension and plasma renin activity, *J Hum Hypertens* 14(3):181, 2000; Gibbons GH: The pathophysiology of hypertension. The importance of angiotensin II in cardiovascular remodeling, *Am J Hypertens* 11:177S, 1998; Hansson L et al: Effect of angiotensin-converting-enzyme inhibition compared with conventional therapy on cardiovascular morbidity and mortality in hypertension: the Captopril Prevention Project (CAPPP) randomised trial, *Lancet* 353(9153): 611, 1999; Moser M: In the management of hypertension is it blood pressure lowering alone or specific effects of specific medications that reduce cardiovascular events? *J Clin Hypertens* 2:10, 2000; Rockett J: Endothelial dysfunction and the promise of ACE inhibitors, *Am J Nurs* 99:44, 1999; Schmermund A et al: Cardiac production of Ang II and its pharmacologic inhibition: effects on the coronary circulation, *Mayo Clinic Proc* 74:503, 1999.

by vasoconstriction leads to hypertension. As the hypertension progresses, the increase in peripheral resistance becomes the primary pathophysiologic cause of the increase in blood pressure, even as blood volume returns toward normal.

Secondary hypertension. Secondary hypertension is caused by a systemic disease process that raises peripheral vascular resistance or cardiac output. If the cause is identified and removed before permanent structural changes occur, blood pressure returns to normal. Table 29-2 summarizes the pathogenesis of major forms of secondary hypertension.

Isolated systolic hypertension. Rigidity of the aorta is the chief vascular cause of isolated systolic hypertension and is common in the elderly population. Elevations of systolic pressure alone usually are caused by increases in cardiac

Table 29-2 Pathogenesis of Major Forms of Secondary Hypertension by Cause

Primary Disease	Pathogenesis of Hypertension
RENAL DISORDERS	
Renal parenchymal disease	Disturbances in filtration and reabsorption of serum sodium, potassium, and calcium initiate the hemodynamics of early hypertension
Renovascular disease	Impaired blood flow and renal ischemia invoke the compensatory renin-angiotensin-aldosterone mechanism in an effort to raise the renal perfusion pressure
Renin-producing tumors	Elevated blood renin levels invoke elevations in angiotensin and aldosterone, which cause blood pressure to rise
Renal failure	Disturbances in filtration and reabsorption of serum sodium, potassium, and calcium initiate the hemodynamics of early hypertension
Primary sodium retention	Disturbance in filtration and/or reabsorption of serum sodium initiates the hemodynamics of early hypertension
ENDOCRINE DISORDERS	
Acromegaly	Excess human growth hormone causes increased peripheral resistance
Hypothyroidism	Mucopolysaccharide deposits in vascular tissue increase resistance
Hypercalcemia	Calcium ion directly affects vascular tonicity; elevated serum calcium levels increase vascular tone and peripheral resistance
Hyperthyroidism	Increased inotropic effect on the heart elevates systolic pressure; diastolic pressure decreases as a result of decreased peripheral resistance
Adrenal disorders Cortical disturbances Cushing syndrome	Glucocorticoids facilitate sodium and water retention, initiating the hemodynamics of early hypertension
Primary aldosteronism	Excess aldosterone promotes sodium retention and initiation of the hemodynamics of early hypertension
Congenital adrenal hyperplasia	Excess production of adrenocortical hormones promotes sodium and water retention
Medullary disturbance: pheochromocytoma	Excess catecholamines raise vascular tone and increase peripheral resistance
Extraadrenal chromaffin tumors	Excess catecholamines raise vascular tone and increase peripheral resistance
VASCULAR DISORDERS	
Coarctation of the aorta	Decreased blood flow in distal areas initiates maximum peripheral resistance as an autoregulatory effort to adjust perfusion pressure
Arteriosclerosis	Loss of elasticity in vessel walls results in increased peripheral resistance
PREGNANCY-INDUCED HYPERTENSION	Pathogenesis unclear
NEUROLOGIC DISORDERS	
Elevated intracranial pressure (brain tumor, encephalitis, respiratory acidosis of pulmonary or central nervous system [CNS] origin)	Higher systemic blood pressure required to maintain adequate cerebral perfusion
Quadriplegia, acute porphyria, familial dysautonomia, lead poisoning, Guillain-Barré syndrome	Interface with neural control of blood pressure initiates increased systemic blood pressure
ACUTE STRESS	
Surgery, psychogenic hyperventilation, hypoglycemia, burns, pancreatitis, alcohol withdrawal, sickle cell crisis, resuscitation, increased intravascular volume	Acute stress precipitates release of catecholamines and glucocorticoids
DRUGS AND OTHER SUBSTANCES	
Oral contraceptives and estrogen	Unknown; possibly caused by sodium retention, plasma retention, weight gain, changes in levels and actions of renin, angiotensin, and aldosterone
Corticosteroids	Same as for Cushing disease
Sympathetic stimulants, appetite suppressants, antihistamines	Raises vascular tone and increases vascular resistance
Licorice	Contains glycerrhizic acid, a mineralocorticoid causing salt and water retention
Monoamine oxidase inhibitors	Hypertension may develop in an individual who routinely takes a monoamine oxidase (MAO) inhibitor with ingestion of a food containing tyramine, such as aged cheese

From Kaplan NM: *Clinical hypertension,* ed 5, Baltimore, 1990, Williams & Wilkins.

Table 29-3 Pathologic Effects of Sustained, Complicated Primary Hypertension

Site of Injury	Mechanism of Injury	Potential Pathologic Effect
Heart		
Myocardium	Increased workload combined with diminished blood flow through coronary arteries	Left ventricular hypertrophy, myocardial ischemia, left heart failure
Coronary arteries	Accelerated atherosclerosis (coronary artery disease)	Myocardial ischemia, myocardial infarction, sudden death
Kidneys	Renin and aldosterone secretion stimulated by reduced blood flow	Retention of sodium and water, leading to increased blood volume and perpetuation of hypertension
	Reduced oxygen supply	Tissue damage that compromises filtration
	High pressures in renal arterioles	Nephrosclerosis leading to renal failure
Brain	Reduced blood flow and oxygen supply; weakened vessel walls, accelerated atherosclerosis	Transient ischemic attacks, cerebral thrombosis, aneurysm, hemorrhage, acute brain infarction
Eyes (retinas)	Reduced blood flow	Retinal vascular sclerosis
	High arteriolar pressure	Exudation, hemorrhage
Aorta	Weakened vessel wall	Dissecting aneurysm (see p. 994)
Arterial vessels of lower extremities	Reduced blood flow and high pressures in arterioles, accelerated atherosclerosis	Intermittent claudication, gangrene

output or total peripheral vascular resistance or both. Isolated systolic hypertension caused by increased cardiac output can be secondary to dysfunction of the aortic semilunar valve (aortic valve insufficiency), any abnormal opening between heart chambers (arterioventricular fistula, patent ductus arteriosus; see Chapter 30), thyrotoxic crisis (thyroid storm), Paget disease of the bone, and beriberi.

Rigidity of the aorta is caused by arteriosclerosis, which increases total peripheral vascular resistance. Changes associated with aging alter the aortic valve so that increased cardiac output is needed to maintain blood flow into the systemic circulation. Isolated systolic hypertension is now recognized as an important risk factor for cardiovascular disease and stroke, and it should be treated aggressively.[38,39,40,41]

Complicated hypertension. **Complicated hypertension** is sustained primary hypertension that has pathologic effects besides hemodynamic alterations and fluid and electrolyte imbalances. Complicated hypertension commonly compromises the structure and function of the vessels themselves—namely, the heart, aorta, kidneys, eyes, brain, and lower extremities. The two major mechanisms of tissue damage are ischemia and edema. Ischemia deprives tissues of the oxygen and nutrients they need for survival and function. Leakage of fluids into the interstitial space, and even hemorrhage, are caused by high pressures in the vessels. The heart is particularly susceptible to injury because although high cardiac output is stimulating myocardial hypertrophy, vasoconstriction is diminishing blood flow through the coronary arteries. The pathophysiology of complicated hypertension is summarized in Table 29-3.

Cardiovascular complications include left ventricular hypertrophy, angina pectoris, congestive heart failure (left heart failure), coronary artery disease, myocardial infarction, and sudden death. Myocardial hypertrophy in response to hypertension is mediated by several neurohormonal substances, especially Ang II (see "What's New? The Role of Angiotensin II in Cardiovascular Disease," p. 989). This results in changes in the myocyte proteins, apoptosis of myocytes, and deposition of collagen into the heart muscle. In addition, the increased size of the heart muscle increases demand for coronary perfusion, such that, over time, contractility of the heart is impaired and the individual is at increased risk for heart failure.[74,75] Vascular complications include the formation, dissection, and rupture of aneurysms (outpouchings in vessel walls); intermittent claudication; and gangrene resulting from vessel occlusion. Possible renal complications are parenchymal damage, nephrosclerosis, renal arteriosclerosis, and renal insufficiency or failure. Microalbuminuria (small amounts of protein in the urine) occurs in 10% to 25% of individuals with essential hypertension and is now recognized as an early sign of impending renal dysfunction and significantly increased risk for cardiovascular events.[76,77,78]

Changes in the vascular beds can be estimated by viewing the arterioles of the retina. Complications specific to the retina include retinal vascular sclerosis, exudation, and hemorrhage. Cerebrovascular complications are similar to those of other arterial beds and include transient ischemia, stroke, cerebral thrombosis, aneurysm, and hemorrhage.

Malignant hypertension (rapidly progressive hypertension in which diastolic pressure is usually above 140 mm Hg) can cause encephalopathy, a profound cerebral edema that disrupts cerebral function and causes loss of consciousness. Encephalopathy occurs because high arterial pressure renders the cerebral arterioles incapable of regulating blood flow to the cerebral capillary beds. Capillary permeability is increased by high hydrostatic pressures in the capillaries, and vascular fluid exudes into the interstitial space. If blood pressure is not reduced, cerebral edema and cerebral dysfunction increase until death occurs. Organ damage resulting from malignant hypertension is life threatening. Besides encephalopathy, malignant hypertension can cause papilledema, cardiac failure, uremia, retinopathy, and cerebrovascular accident. This should be considered a hypertensive emergency and managed with rapid administration of parenteral vasodilators with the goal of lowering the blood pressure by 25% within minutes to 2 hours.[36]

Clinical Manifestations

The early stages of hypertension have no clinical manifestations other than elevated blood pressure. Most important, no signs and symptoms cause the individual to seek health care; thus hypertension is called a **lanthanic (silent) disease**. Some hypertensive individuals never have signs, symptoms, or complications, whereas others become very ill, in which case hypertension can cause death. Still others have anatomic and physiologic damage caused by past hypertensive disease despite current blood pressures within normal ranges.

The chance of developing primary hypertension increases with age, over and above the natural rise in blood pressure associated with aging. In individuals at risk for primary hypertension, the factors leading to development of hypertension accumulate during the first 2 or 3 decades of life. Although hypertension usually is thought to be an adult health problem, it is important to remember that hypertension does occur in children and is being diagnosed with increasing frequency.[36] Usually, however, increased peripheral resistance and early hypertension develop in the second, third, and fourth decades of life. If elevated blood pressure is not detected and treated, it becomes established and may begin to accelerate atherosclerosis when the individual is 30 to 50 years of age. This sets the stage for the complications of hypertension that begin to appear during the fourth, fifth, and sixth decades of life.

Most clinical manifestations of hypertensive disease are caused by complications that damage organs and tissues outside the vascular system. Besides elevated blood pressure, the signs and symptoms therefore tend to be specific for the organs or tissues affected. Evidence of heart disease, renal insufficiency, central nervous system dysfunction, impaired vision, impaired mobility, vascular occlusion, or edema can all be caused by sustained hypertension. (See appropriate chapters for specific clinical manifestations of organ dysfunction.)

Evaluation and Treatment

A single elevated blood pressure reading does not mean that a person has hypertension; the diagnosis requires documenting increased blood pressure on at least three different occasions. Some people tend to have high readings whenever they come into a health care setting (sometimes called "white coat syndrome") or if they have had recent caffeine intake or have been smoking. Many clinicians use 24-hour ambulatory blood pressure monitoring in selected individuals to document the blood pressure during their daily activities and to determine if a management modality is working throughout the day. Twenty-four-hour blood pressure measurement is better correlated than clinic measurements with the risk of target organ damage and is indicated in individuals who are suspected of white coat hypertension, hypotensive episodes, drug resistance, or autonomic dysfunction.[36,79] Further routine diagnostic tests for the evaluation of hypertension include complete blood count, urinalysis, biochemical blood profile (fasting glucose, sodium, potassium, creatinine, total cholesterol, high-density cholesterol, triglycerides), and an electrocardiogram (ECG). Individuals who have elevated blood pressure are assumed to have primary hypertension unless their history, physical examination, or initial diagnostic screening indicates secondary hypertension.

Hypertension usually is managed with both pharmacologic and nonpharmacologic methods. An overview of the current recommendations for the management of hypotension is illustrated in Fig. 29-9. Treatment begins with reducing or eliminating risk factors. Life-style modification can prevent hypertension from developing in those individuals who fall into the "high normal" category, can control the blood pressure in mild hypertension, and can enhance the effects of drug treatment for those with more significant blood pressure elevation. The usual dietary recommendations are to restrict sodium intake to 2 g per day, to increase potassium intake, to restrict saturated fat intake, and to adjust calorie intake as required to maintain optimum weight. Increasing calcium and protein intake also has been suggested (see "Nutrition and Disease: Diet and Hypertension"). An exercise program that promotes endurance and relaxation usually is recommended. Physical training increases stroke volume, which has

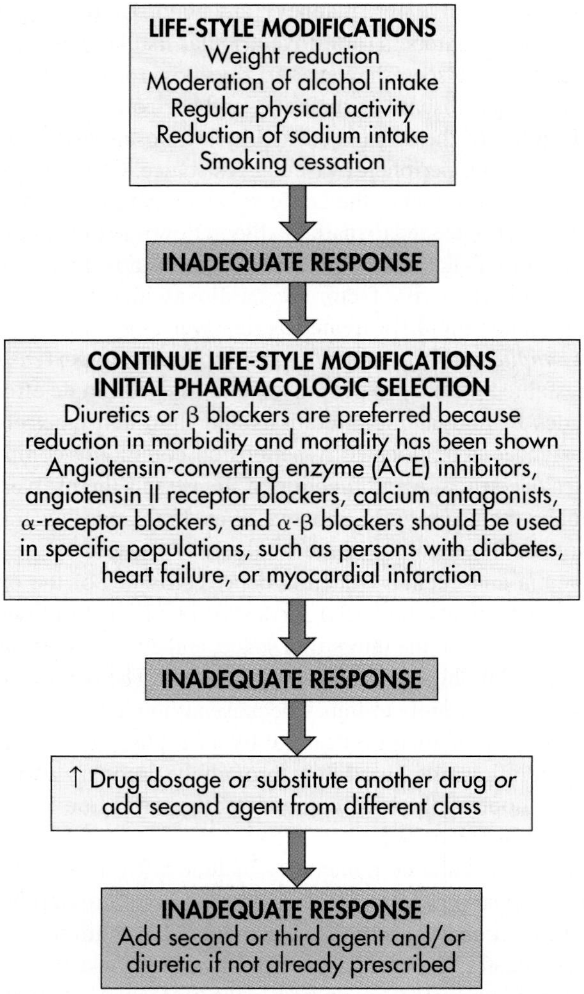

FIG. 29-9 Summary treatment recommendations for hypertension. (From The sixth report of the Joint National Committee on Prevention, Detection, Evaluation, and Treatment of High Blood Pressure, *Arch Int Med* 157:2430,1997.)

the effect of lowering heart rate and hence systolic blood pressure. Relaxation is expected to reduce levels of circulating catecholamines, which has the effect of reducing vascular tone and blood pressure. Individuals are counseled to stop smoking to eliminate vasoconstrictor effects of nicotine.

Pharmacologic treatment of hypertension reduces the risk of end-organ damage and prevents major diseases, such as myocardial ischemia and stroke.[80] The two classes of drugs that have been shown unequivocally to significantly reduce the risk of these sequelae are diuretics and adrenergic blockers (especially beta-blockers). Recently, calcium channel blockers, angiotensin-converting enzyme (ACE) inhibitors, and angiotensin II receptor blockers are being used as first-line treatments.[37,81] Because of the various side effects and special mechanisms of action of these medications, the initial choice of antihypertensive therapy should be tailored to meet the needs of the individual. If blood pressure control cannot be achieved with a single pharmacologic agent, additional drugs may need to be added to the regimen. Diuretics reduce blood pressure initially by facilitating renal excretion of sodium and water, thereby reducing blood volume and cardiac output. Subsequently, the cardiovascular system adjusts to restore cardiac output, but reduced blood pressure is maintained because peripheral resistance is lower. Adrenergic blockers interfere with the transmission of the neurohumoral facilitators (e.g., norepinephrine) of vasoconstriction and cardiac stimulation. These agents bind with adrenergic receptors, preventing receptor binding with neurohumoral stimulators of increased cardiac output and vasoconstriction. Calcium channel blockers lower blood pressure by blocking calcium influx to smooth muscle cells. This decreases vascular reactivity and promotes vasodilation. Angiotensin inhibitors reduce blood pressure by preventing the renin-angiotensin mechanism from acting on the vascular smooth muscle, adrenal cortex, kidney, and brain stem. Captopril, for example, acts by inhibiting the enzyme that converts inactive angiotensin I to the active form, angiotensin II. With less active angiotensin II in the blood, blood pressure decreases and the risk of renal and cardiac complications diminish.

NUTRITION & DISEASE

Diet and Hypertension

Sodium intake has long been linked to hypertension. Recently, studies suggest that low potassium, calcium, and magnesium intake can affect the pressure-natriuresis relationship, cause vasoconstriction, and alter the sodium/potassium pump and thus contribute to the development of hypertension. Restricting sodium intake is most effective in lowering blood pressure for certain groups, primarily blacks, the elderly, and those with diabetes. The average sodium intake in the United States is approximately 6 grams per day. Sodium restriction to less than 2 grams per day is safe for everyone and is recommended for all individuals with hypertension (but is not currently recommended for normotensive individuals). High dietary potassium intake is useful in both preventing hypertension and improving blood pressure control in those with established primary hypertension. Adequate dietary intake of potassium is about 90 mmol per day and ideally should come from foods high in potassium, such as fresh fruits and vegetables. Potassium supplements are indicated for those with hypokalemia due to diuretics. Although dietary supplements of calcium and magnesium are not currently recommended, the Dietary Approaches to Stop Hypertension (DASH) studies suggest that increased intake of foods rich in calcium and magnesium can significantly lower the blood pressure. High protein diets have been correlated with lowering the blood pressure, but this remains controversial. Other general recommendations for individuals with hypertension include lowering dietary fats, increasing omega-3 fatty acids, and weight loss for obese patients.

Data from Griffith LE et al: The influence of dietary and nondietary calcium supplementation on blood pressure: an updated metaanalysis of randomized controlled trials, *Amer J Hypertens* 12(1 part 1):84, 1999; Katz A et al: Effect of a mineral salt diet on 24-h blood pressure monitoring in elderly hypertensive patients, *J Hum Hypertens* 13(11): 777, 1999; Kawamo Y et al: Effects of potassium supplementation on office, home and 24 hour blood pressure in patients with essential hypertension, *Amer J Hypertens* 11:1141, 1999; Moore TJ et al: Effect of dietary patterns on ambulatory blood pressure results from the Dietary Approaches to Stop Hypertension (DASH) Trial. DASH Collaborative Research Group, *Hypertension* 34(3):472, 1999.

Orthostatic (Postural) Hypotension

The term **orthostatic (postural) hypotension** means a decrease in both systolic and diastolic arterial blood pressure on standing. When a normal individual stands up, the resultant gravitational changes on the circulation are compensated for by several mechanisms that include reflex arteriolar and venous constriction, increased heart rate, and mechanical factors, such as the closure of valves in the venous system, pumping of the leg muscles, and a decrease in intrathoracic pressure. The normally increased sympathetic activity during upright posture is mediated through stretch receptors (baroreceptors) in the carotid sinus and the aortic arch (see Chapter 28). Their reflex response to shifts in volume caused by postural changes leads to a prompt increase in heart rate and constriction of the systemic arterioles. Thus, despite a marked decrease in cardiac output, arterial blood pressure is maintained.

Orthostatic hypotension often is accompanied by dizziness, blurring or loss of vision, and syncope or fainting. Fainting is caused by insufficient vasomotor compensation and reduction of blood flow through the brain. The normal or compensatory vasoconstrictor response to standing is thus replaced by a marked vasodilation and blood pooling in the muscle vasculature, as well as in the splanchnic and renal beds.

Orthostatic hypotension may be acute and temporary or chronic. **Acute orthostatic hypotension,** or temporary type, is caused when the normal regulatory mechanisms are sluggish. This delay may be the result of (1) anatomic variation, (2) altered body chemistry, (3) drug action (e.g., antihypertensives or antidepressants), (4) prolonged immobility caused by illness, (5) starvation, (6) physical exhaustion, (7) any condition that produces volume depletion (e.g., massive diuresis, potassium or sodium depletion), and (8) venous pooling (e.g., pregnancy, extensive varicosities of the lower extremities). Elderly persons are susceptible to this type of orthostatic hypotension, in which postural reflexes apparently are slowed as part of the aging process. This is not a universal finding in the elderly population, however.

The two forms of **chronic orthostatic hypotension** are (1) secondary to a specific disease and (2) idiopathic or primary. The diseases that cause secondary orthostatic hypotension are endocrine disorders (e.g., adrenal insufficiency, diabetes mellitus), metabolic disorders (e.g., porphyria), or diseases of the central or peripheral nervous system (e.g., intracranial tumors, cerebral infarcts, Wernicke encephalopathy, peripheral neuropathies). Cardiovascular autonomic neuropathy is a frequent cause of orthostatic hypotension in diabetes and is a serious and often overlooked complication.[82]

Idiopathic, or primary, orthostatic hypotension is the term for hypotension in which there is no known initial cause. It affects men more often than women and usually occurs between the ages of 40 and 70 years. Up to 30% to 49% of the elderly population may be affected by orthostatic hypotension; it is a significant risk factor for falls and associated injuries.[83,84] In addition to cardiovascular symptoms, impotence and bowel and bladder dysfunction often are found in this type. Orthostatic hypotension is also a feature of multiple system atrophy (MSA), in which there are multiple central nervous system degenerative changes.

No curative treatment is available for idiopathic orthostatic hypertension. In the secondary form, syncope ceases when the underlying disorder is corrected. Several treatments can help acute and chronic orthostatic hypotension, including liberalization of salt intake, raising the head of the bed, thigh-high stockings, and volume expansion with mineralocorticoids.

Aneurysm

An **aneurysm** is a localized dilation or outpouching of a vessel wall or cardiac chamber. The law of Laplace can provide an understanding of the hemodynamics of an aneurysm (Fig. 29-10). (The law of Laplace is discussed in detail in Chapter 28.) Presumably, formation of a ventricular wall aneurysm occurs when intraventricular tension stretches the noncontracting infarcted muscle (Fig. 29-11, *B*). The stretching produces infarct expansion, a weak and thin layer of necrotic muscle, and fibrous tissue that bulges with each systole. With time, the aneurysm becomes more fibrotic but continues to bulge with each systole, thus acting as a "reservoir" for some of the stroke volume.

The aorta is particularly susceptible to aneurysm formation because of constant stress on the vessel wall and the absence of penetrating vasa vasorum in the adventitial layer (see Fig. 29-11, *A*). Atherosclerosis may be the most common cause of aneurysms because plaque formation erodes the vessel wall. Arteriosclerosis and hypertension are found in more than half of all individuals with aneurysms. Syphilis and other infections also can cause aortic aneurysms. A review of the literature suggests that for those aortic aneurysms not clearly related to atherosclerosis, contributing factors may include (1) the presence of a genetic marker, (2) deficiencies in wall collagen or collagen-elastin connections, (3) elastin failure from excessive protease activity or the production of nonfunctional elastin with aging, or (4) an increased turnover of aortic collagen. These changes can be inflammatory and involve the processes of aortic vessel wall remodeling and apoptosis.[85] Another important cause of aortic aneurysms of the thoracic aorta is Marfan syndrome. This inherited collagen-vascular disease carries a high mortality rate due to rupture of the ascending thoracic aorta unless surgical repair with graft placement is done.[86]

True aneurysms involve all three layers of the arterial wall and are best described as a weakening of the vessel wall. Most are fusiform and circumferential (Fig. 29-12). **False**

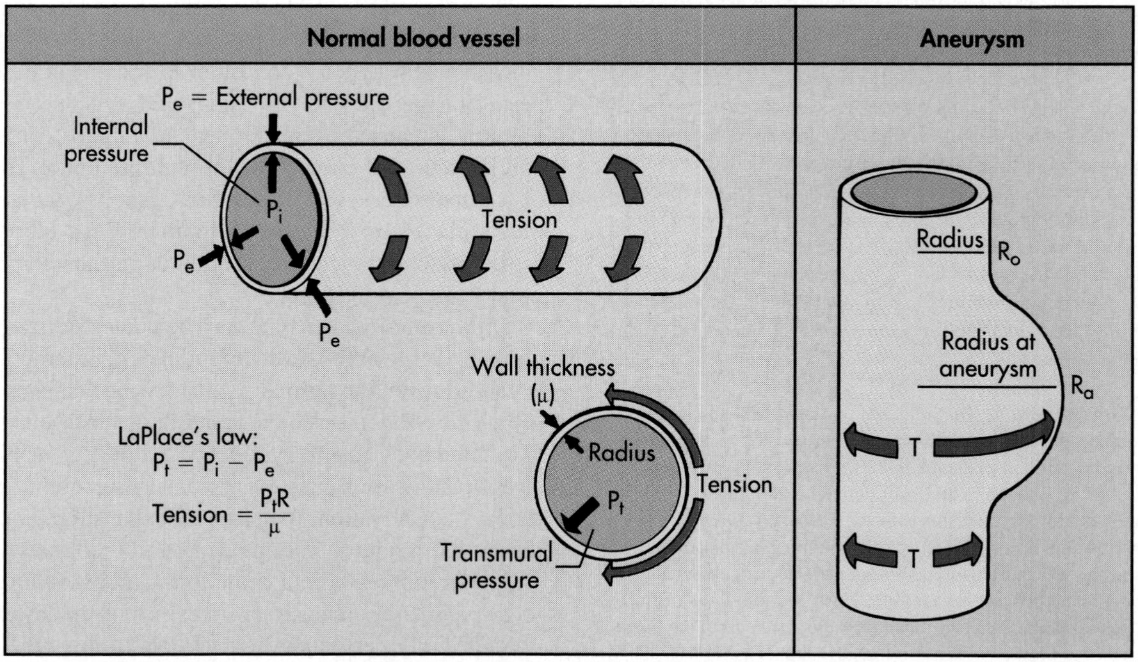

FIG. 29-10 Pressure-tension and wall thickness relations in blood vessels or cardiac chambers (Laplace's law). (From Kissane JM, editor: *Anderson's pathology,* ed 9, St Louis, 1990, Mosby.)

aneurysms and **saccular aneurysms** are usually the result of trauma. These aneurysms are caused by a dissection of the layers of the arterial wall, so that blood is contained at the point of aneurysm by the adventitial layer (dissecting saccular aneurysm) or by a clot (false aneurysm).

Clinical manifestations of aneurysm include a variety of symptoms. Aortic aneurysms can be very painful. Symptoms of dysphagia (difficulty in swallowing) and dyspnea (breathlessness) are caused by the pressure of a thoracic aneurysm on surrounding organs. An abdominal aneurysm can impair flow to an extremity and cause symptoms of ischemia. Cerebral aneurysms, which frequently occur in the circle of Willis, are associated with signs and symptoms of increased intracranial pressure. Signs and symptoms of stroke occur when cerebral aneurysms leak. (Cerebral aneurysms are described in Chapter 16.)

A

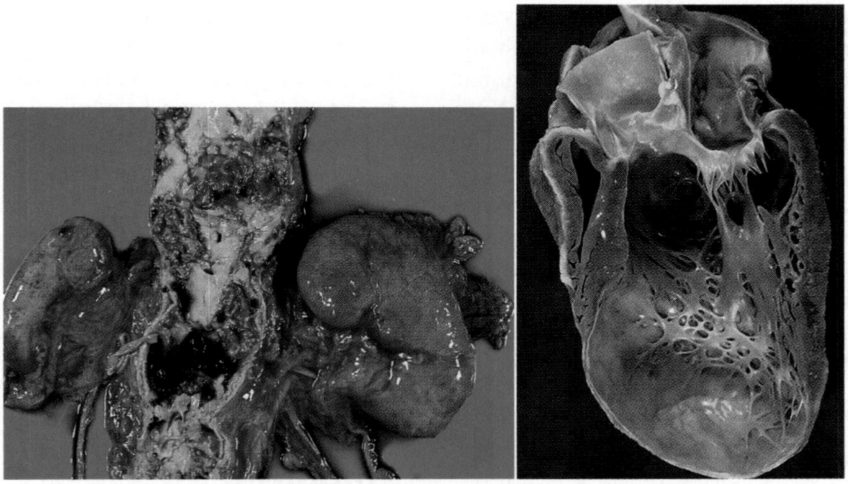

B

FIG 29-11 Aneurysms. A, Abdominal aortic atherosclerotic aneurysm. **B,** In a long-axis view of the left ventricle there is a large, thin-walled apical aneurysm that does not contain thrombus. (From Damjanov I, Linder J, editors: *Anderson's pathology,* ed 10, St Louis, 1996, Mosby.)

A

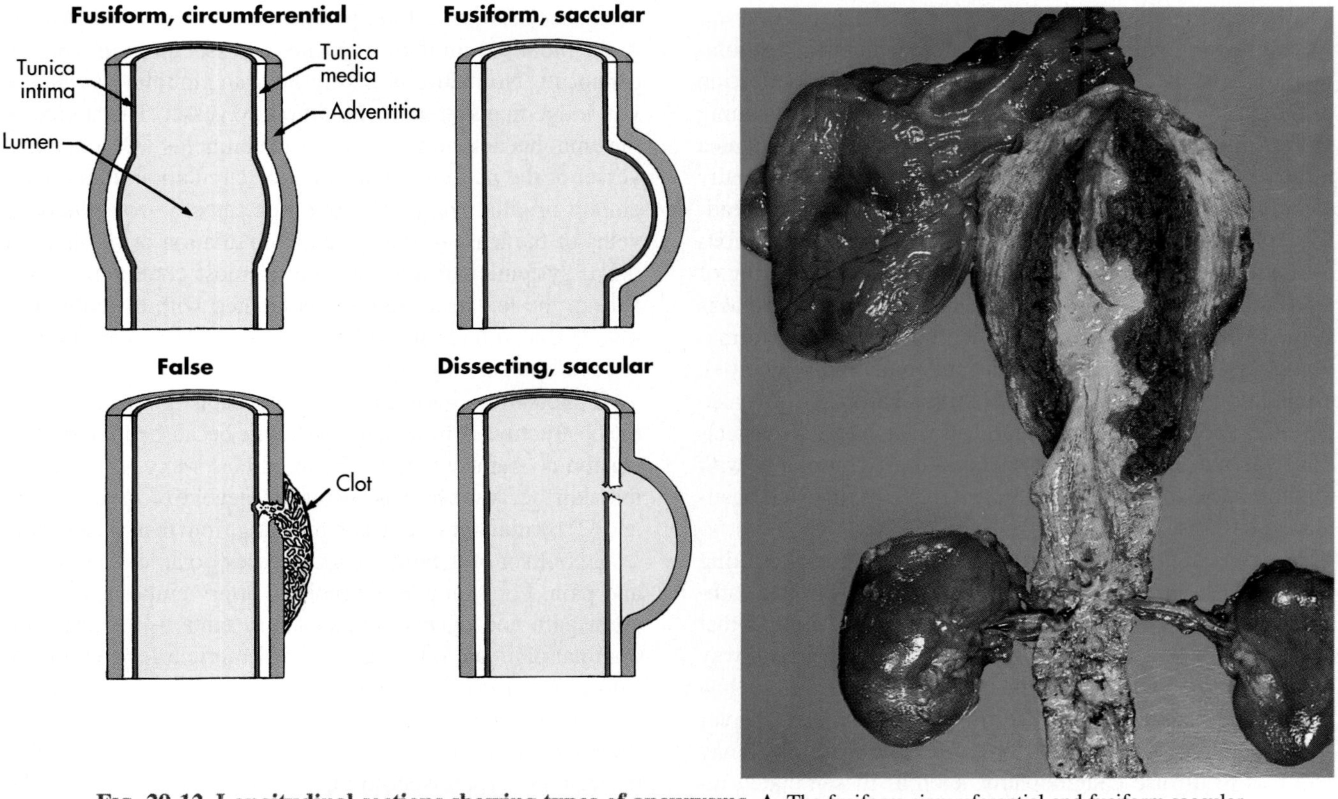

B

FIG. 29-12 Longitudinal sections showing types of aneurysms. A, The fusiform circumferential and fusiform saccular aneurysms are true aneurysms, caused by weakening of the vessel wall. False and saccular aneurysms involve a break in the vessel wall, usually caused by trauma. **B,** Dissecting aneurysm of thoracic aorta. (B from Damjanov I, Linder J, editors: *Anderson's pathology,* ed 10, St Louis, 1996, Mosby.)

Medical treatment of aneurysms depends on the location of the aneurysm and includes maintaining a low blood volume and low blood pressure to decrease mechanical forces thought to contribute to vessel wall dilation. Medical treatment is indicated for slow-growing aortic aneurysms, particularly in early stages, and includes smoking cessation, reducing blood pressure and blood volume, and beta-adrenergic blockage.[87,88] For those aneurysms that are dilating rapidly, surgical treatment frequently is indicated. Cerebral aneurysms must be treated immediately to prevent the possiblity of rupture. Saccular aneurysms are repaired more easily than fusiform and circumferential aneurysms.[89] Surgery should be done when aortic aneurysms reach 5 cm in diameter and usually includes replacement with a prosthetic graft.[90] If the weakness or separation of vascular layers spreads, the aneurysm becomes a **dissecting aneurysm** (Fig. 29-12, *B*). Dissecting aneurysms and leaking aneurysms require emergency treatment. Leaking cerebral aneurysms, especially those associated with vascular spasms as a compensatory mechanism, are treated with clot-stabilizing drugs and a number of clinical measures designed to reduce intracranial pressure and induce hemodynamic stability before surgical intervention.

Thrombus Formation

A **thrombus** is a blood clot that remains attached to a vessel wall (see Fig. 29-13). A detached thrombus is called a **thromboembolus.** Thrombi tend to develop wherever intravascular conditions promote activation of the coagulation, or clotting, cascade. These conditions include intimal irritation, roughening, inflammation, traumatic injury, infection, and low blood pressures or obstructions that cause blood stasis and pooling within the vessels. (Mechanisms of coagulation are described in Chapter 24.) In the arteries, activation of the coagulation cascade usually is caused by roughening of the tunica intima by atherosclerosis. Invasion of the tunica intima by an infectious agent also roughens the normally smooth lining of the artery, causing platelets to adhere readily. Anatomic changes of an artery can stimulate thrombus formation, particularly if the change results in a pooling of arterial blood. This can occur, for example, in blood that is pooled within an aneurysm. In the veins, thrombus formation is associated more often with inflammation (phlebitis), a condition termed **thrombophlebitis.** Thrombi form also on heart valves altered by calcification or bacterial vegetation. Valvular thrombi are associated most commonly with inflammation of the endocardium (endocarditis) and rheumatic heart disease.

Shock (circulatory failure), particularly shock resulting from septicemia, can activate the intrinsic and extrinsic pathways of coagulation. The impaired cellular metabolism that occurs with all types of shock activates the extrinsic pathway of coagulation, whereas blood stasis caused by very low blood pressures activates the intrinsic pathway (see Chapter 24). Thrombus formation may be confined to one area or may progress to diffuse coagulopathy, such as disseminated intravascular coagulation (see Chapter 26).

A thrombus poses two potential threats to the circulation. First, the thrombus may grow large enough to occlude the artery, causing ischemia in tissue supplied by the artery. Second, the thrombus may dislodge, becoming a thromboembolus that travels through the vascular system until it occludes flow into a distal systemic vascular bed. Venous thrombi can make it more difficult for blood to drain from distant venous beds (especially the legs), resulting in edema. Venous thrombi can also embolize and travel to the pulmonic vascular bed (see Chapter 32).

Pharmacologic treatment includes the administration of heparin and warfarin derivatives. These derivatives interfere with the clotting cascade by accelerating the activity of antithrombin III, thereby slowing or stopping thrombus growth. Pharmacologic treatment also includes the intravenous or intraarterial administration of streptokinase, which dissolves the thrombus.

A balloon-tipped catheter can be used to remove or compress a thrombus. This type of catheter is inserted into the vessel containing the thrombus at a point proximal to the thrombus and is threaded past the thrombus until the tip of the catheter is past the thrombus. The balloon on the tip of the catheter is then inflated and drawn backward out of the vessel, pulling out the clot by a dredging action. Various combinations of drug and catheter therapies are sometimes used concurrently.

Embolism

Embolism is the obstruction of a vessel by an **embolus**—a bolus of matter that is circulating in the bloodstream. The embolus may consist of a dislodged thrombus; an air bubble; an aggregate of amniotic fluid; an aggregate of fat, bacteria, or cancer cells; or a foreign substance. An embolus travels in the bloodstream until it reaches a vessel through which it cannot fit. No matter how tiny it is, an embolus eventually will lodge in a systemic or pulmonary vessel. The source of the embolus determines whether the embolus will lodge in a vessel of the pulmonary or systemic circulation. Pulmonary emboli originate on the venous side (mostly from the deep veins of the legs) of the systemic circulation or in the right heart; systemic (or arterial) emboli most commonly originate in the left heart and are associated with thrombi after myocardial infarction, valvular disease, left heart failure, endocarditis, and dysrhythmias.

Embolism causes ischemia or infarction in tissues distal to the obstruction. A limb that is ischemic because of arterial occlusion is characterized (1) by an almost waxy whiteness of the skin because the vasculature is devoid of erythrocytes, and (2) by numbness and pain resulting from neural ischemia.

Embolism of a central organ causes organic dysfunction and pain. For example, pulmonary artery embolism causes chest pain and dyspnea; renal artery embolism causes abdominal pain and oliguria; and mesenteric artery embolism causes abdominal pain and a paralytic, ischemic bowel. Infarction and subsequent necrosis of a central organ are life threatening, not only because of organ dysfunction but also because of sepsis. Necrotic tissue is a rich medium for the growth of bacteria from the lungs; bowel; and, occasionally, bladder. Necrosis of the bladder, in particular, can quickly lead to peritonitis or septicemia.

Embolism of a coronary or cerebral artery is an immediate threat to life if the embolus severely obstructs a major vessel. Occlusion of a coronary artery will cause a myocardial infarction (see p. 1011), whereas occlusion of a cerebral artery causes a stroke (see Chapter 16).

Thromboembolism

Thromboembolism is a vascular obstruction by a dislodged thrombus. The most common source of arterial thromboemboli to the systemic circulation is the heart. Mitral or aortic valvular disease, especially that associated with abnormal heart rhythms (atrial fibrillation and flutter), causes thrombus formation on roughened vascular surfaces and in atrial blood as a result of stasis. More than half of these thromboemboli lodge in the lower extremities (in the femoral and popliteal arteries). Others lodge in the coronary arteries and the cerebral vasculature.

Heart failure is associated with an increased risk of thrombotic complications, although the mechanism for this increased risk is unclear. There is evidence that abnormalities of prothrombotic markers are associated with ischemic heart disease, independent of the presence of systolic or diastolic dysfunction.

Air Embolism

Room air that enters the circulation through intravenous lines is probably the most common cause of air embolism. Room air is about 70% nitrogen. Although nitrogen dissolves quickly in blood, large amounts of air cannot be dissolved rapidly enough to prevent the displacement of blood in the arterioles and capillary beds. Ischemia and necrosis occur when air totally blocks a vessel.

Air also can be introduced into the bloodstream if trauma to the chest causes air from the lungs to enter the vascular space. For example, gunshot wounds and puncture wounds of the thorax sometimes introduce air emboli. Treatment for air embolism is supportive, including bed rest and supplemental oxygen, once the connection between the source of air and the vascular system is eliminated.

Amniotic Fluid Embolism

The great intraabdominal pressures generated during labor and delivery may force amniotic fluid into the bloodstream of the mother through the highly vascular uterine wall. Amniotic fluid not only displaces blood, reducing oxygen, nutrient, and waste exchange, but also introduces antigens, cells, and protein aggregates that trigger inflammation, coagulation, and the immune response within the bloodstream. Capillary beds usually are affected by amniotic fluid emboli, especially the capillary beds of the lungs and kidneys. Treatment is supportive and may include dialysis, particularly after a cesarean delivery or hysterectomy.

Bacterial Embolism

Isolated bacteria in the bloodstream do not cause embolism, but aggregates of bacteria may be large enough to do so. The most common cause of bacterial embolism is subacute bacterial endocarditis, during which clumps of vegetation are dislodged from infected cardiac valves and ejected into the pulmonary or systemic circulation. A less common cause is erosion of an artery or vein by bacteria at a source of infection, such as an abscess. Treatment for bacterial embolism includes bed rest, supplemental oxygen, and antibiotics to eradicate the source of infection.

Fat Embolism

Trauma to the long bones is associated with fat embolism, particularly in the lungs. Two mechanisms have been proposed to account for the generation of fat emboli after skeletal trauma. The first is that trauma to the bones initiates defective fat metabolism, causing globules of fat to form in the blood. Platelets adhere to these globules until the conglomerate is large enough to lodge in a capillary bed. The second possible explanation is that globules of fat are released from fatty bone marrow exposed by fracture. Again, platelets adhere to the fat globules and embolism occurs.

Treatment for fat embolism consists of prompt immobilization of fractures and supportive measures that include administration of supplemental oxygen, steroids, and glucose. Steroid administration may decrease the inflammation that occurs with vascular occlusion. Inflammation in the pulmonary bed is especially dangerous because it can cause adult respiratory distress syndrome (ARDS) (see Chapter 32). Intravenous administration of glucose is thought to prevent inappropriate fat metabolism.

Foreign Matter

Foreign matter can enter the bloodstream during trauma or through an intravenous or intraarterial line. If the bolus of foreign matter is relatively large, it usually is removed surgically. Small particles, such as drug precipitates, small glass shards, or fibers from linen, are sometimes introduced unintentionally into a vessel through intravenous injections or manipulation of monitoring lines. Once in the blood, these small particles initiate the coagulation cascade. The thromboemboli that form around the particles are large enough to occlude a vessel and result in ischemia. Treatment is aimed at preventing thrombus formation around the particle, dissolution of the particle, and supportive measures to alleviate ischemia.

Peripheral Arterial Disease

Thromboangiitis Obliterans (Buerger Disease)

Thromboangiitis obliterans (Buerger disease), which tends to occur in young men who are heavy cigarette smokers, is an inflammatory disease of the peripheral arteries. The inflammatory lesions are accompanied by thrombi and sometimes by vasospasm of arterial segments. Inflammation, thrombus formation, and vasospasm eventually can occlude and obliterate (render physiologically useless) portions of small and medium-size arteries in the feet and sometimes in the hands.[91,92] Typically affected are the digital, tibial, and plantar arteries of the feet and the digital, palmar, and ulnar arteries of the hands. The disease sometimes is associated with inflammation of adjacent veins and nerves. The pathogenesis of thromboangiitis obliterans is not known.

The chief symptoms of thromboangiitis obliterans are pain and tenderness of the affected part. Clinical manifestations are caused by sluggish blood flow and include rubor (redness of the skin), which is caused by dilated capillaries under the skin, and cyanosis, which is caused by blood that remains in the capillaries after its oxygen has diffused into the interstitium. Chronic ischemia causes the skin to thin and become shiny and the nails to become thickened and malformed. In advanced disease, ischemia resulting from vessel obliteration can cause gangrene.[92]

The most important part of treatment is cessation of cigarette smoking. All other measures are aimed at improving circulation to the foot or hand. Vasodilators are prescribed to alleviate vasospasm, and exercises are taught that use gravity to improve blood flow. If vasospasm persists, sympathectomy may be performed. Gangrene necessitates amputation.[93]

Raynaud Phenomenon and Disease

Raynaud phenomenon and **Raynaud disease** are both characterized by attacks of vasospasm in the small arteries and arterioles of the fingers and, less commonly, the toes. Although the clinical manifestations of the phenomenon and the disease are the same, their causes differ. Raynaud phenomenon is secondary to systemic diseases, particularly collagen vascular disease (scleroderma), pulmonary hypertension, thoracic outlet syndrome, myxedema trauma, serum sickness (see Chapter 8), or long-term exposure to environmental conditions, such as cold or vibrating machinery in the workplace. (The effects of segmental vibration are described in Chapter 2.) Raynaud disease, however, is a primary vasospastic disorder of unknown origin. Raynaud disease tends to affect young women and to consist of vasospastic attacks triggered by brief exposure to cold or by emotional stress. Blood vessels in these individuals demonstrate endothelial dysfunction with decreased nitric oxide production.[94] Genetic predisposition may play a role in its development.[95] There is some evidence that Raynaud phenomenon may be the presenting feature of an underlying malignancy. In these cases the vascular disease is characterized by sudden onset and rapid progression of severe digital ischemia.

The clinical manifestations of the vasospastic attacks of either disorder are changes in skin color and sensation caused by ischemia. Vasospasm occurs with varying frequency and severity and causes pallor, numbness, and the sensation of cold in the digits. Attacks tend to be bilateral, and manifestations usually begin at the tips of the digits and progress to the proximal phalanges. Sluggish blood flow resulting from ischemia may cause the skin to appear cyanotic. Rubor follows as vasospasm ends and the capillaries become engorged with oxygenated blood. Rubor often is accompanied by throbbing and paresthesias. Skin color returns to normal after the attack, but frequent, prolonged attacks interfere with cellular metabolism, causing the skin of the fingertips to thicken and the nails to become brittle. In severe, chronic Raynaud phenomenon or disease, ischemia eventually can cause ulceration and gangrene. This outcome is rare, however.

Treatment for Raynaud phenomenon consists of removing the stimulus or treating the primary disease process. Attacks of vasospasm sometimes can be alleviated at their onset by an exercise in which the arms are swung forward and backward. This maneuver increases hydrostatic pressure (and perfusion pressure) in the arteries by means of centrifugal force.

Treatment of Raynaud disease is limited to prevention or alleviation of vasospasm itself, because no underlying disorder has been identified. The exception to this tenet is found in cases where Raynaud phenomenon is associated with a malignancy. Surgical removal of the malignancy or administration of nifedipine may resolve the ischemia. For Raynaud phenomenon not associated with malignancy, treatment is limited to amelioration of symptoms. Stimuli that trigger attacks (e.g., emotional stress, cold) are avoided, and cigarette smoking is stopped to eliminate the vasoconstricting effects of nicotine. Exercises that build centrifugal force in the extremities also are helpful in the early stages of vasospasm. If attacks of vasospasm become frequent or prolonged, vasodilators such as dibenzylchlorethamine, reserpine, or calcium channel blockers may be helpful. Ang II receptor blockers have also been found to relieve the vasospasm.[96] A topical paste made of KY jelly and sodium nitrate (increases nitric oxide) can also help vasodilate.[97] Sympathectomy, which is not always effective, is the next line of treatment. If ischemia leads to ulceration and gangrene, amputation is necessary.

Diseases of the Veins

Varicose Veins and Chronic Venous Insufficiency

A **varicose vein** is a vein in which blood has pooled. Varicose veins—typically the saphenous veins of the legs—are distended, tortuous, and palpable. Varicose veins are caused by (1) trauma to the saphenous veins that damages one or more valves; or (2) gradual venous distention caused by a combination of standing for long periods, which diminishes the action of the muscle pump, and the action of gravity on blood within the legs.

Veins are thin-walled, highly distensible vessels. Normally, valves prevent backflow and pooling of blood. If a valve is damaged, permitting backflow, a section of the vein is subjected to the pressure exerted by a larger volume of blood under the influence of gravity. The vein swells as it becomes engorged and surrounding tissue becomes edematous because increased hydrostatic pressure pushes plasma through the stretched vessel wall.

Valvular incompetence also is caused by venous distention that develops over time in individuals who habitually stand for long periods, wear constricting garments, or cross the legs at the knees. Distention progresses until the pressure in the vein damages venous valves, rendering the valves incompetent. Damaged valves cannot maintain normal venous pressure, which causes hydrostatic pressure in the vein to increase. As the vein distends further, it becomes tortuous, and edema develops in the extremity.

Varicose veins and valvular incompetence can progress to **chronic venous insufficiency (CVI).** CVI is inadequate venous return over a long period. It causes pathologic changes as a result of ischemia in the vasculature, skin, and supporting tissues. CVI is marked by chronic pooling of blood in the veins of the lower extremities and leads to hyperpigmentation of the skin over the feet and ankles. Edema of the feet and ankles becomes marked and may progress proximally to the knees.

Circulation to the extremities becomes so sluggish that the metabolic demands of the cells for oxygen, nutrients, and waste removal are barely met. Any trauma or pressure can therefore lower the oxygen supply to injurious levels by further reducing blood flow into the area. Cell death occurs, and necrotic tissue develops into **venous stasis ulcers.** Persistent ulceration develops because the high metabolic demands of healing tissue—particularly an increased need for oxygen—cannot be met by the existing circulation. Venous stasis ulcers are susceptible to infection because poor circulation impairs the delivery of the cells and biochemicals of the immune and inflammatory responses. (The role of inflammation in processes of healing is described in Chapter 7.)

Treatment of varicose veins and CVI begins conservatively. The individual wears antiembolism stockings and avoids standing and other factors, such as constrictive clothing, that contribute to venous stasis. If conservative treatment is ineffective, saphenous vein stripping is performed.[98]

Thrombus Formation in Veins

Deep venous thrombosis (DVT) is a common and important complication of hospitalization, especially in those individuals who undergo orthopedic or obstetric procedures. The likelihood of DVT is related to the number of clinical risk factors, such as cancer, paralysis, bedridden condition, or inherited hypercoagulable condition.[99,100] The process of thrombus formation in the veins is the same as that of thrombus formation in the arteries. Venous thrombi are more common than arterial thrombi, however, because flow and pressure are lower in the veins than in the arteries (Fig. 29-13). Three factors promote venous thrombosis: (1) venous stasis caused by immobility, age, and left heart failure; (2) vessel damage caused by trauma or intravenous medications; and (3) hypercoagulability such as that seen in pregnancy, oral contraceptive use, coagulation disorders, and some cancers.

The inflammatory response triggered by the clotting cascade causes extreme tenderness, swelling, and redness in the area of thrombus formation. The major danger associated with deep venous thrombosis is that a portion of the thrombus will embolize to the lungs, causing a pulmonary embolus (see Chapter 32).[101] Thrombi that form in superficial veins almost always are caused by trauma to the venous intima and rarely embolize.

The clinical manifestations of deep venous occlusion differ markedly from those of arterial occlusion. Venous thrombosis is most often asymptomatic, so evaluation of risk factors is vital to diagnosis. With venous occlusion the skin is discolored rather than pale (ranging from an angry red to deep blue-purple), edema is prominent, and pain is most marked at the site of occlusion, although extreme edema can render

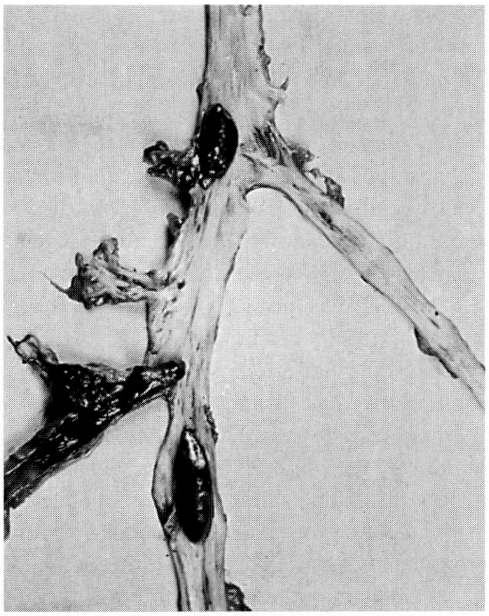

FIG. 29-13 Multiple venous thrombi. (From Rosai J: *Ackerman's surgical pathology,* ed 8, vol 2, St Louis, 1996, Mosby.)

all the skin of the limb quite tender. Neuralgia develops if the edema causes soft tissues to compress local nerves.

Diagnosis is made with Doppler ultrasonography, venous plethysmography, or a venogram. Management requires anticoagulation with heparin. A new subfraction of heparin, called *low-molecular-weight heparin,* is as effective as and safer than unfractionated heparin in the management of venous thrombosis.[102,103,104] Catheter-directed administration of thrombolytics is indicated in some individuals and can reduce the risk of complications, such as venous stasis ulcers.[105] Prevention of DVT is the best form of management and includes the prophylactic use of heparin, low-molecular-weight heparin, warfarin, caval fiter, or compression stockings.[42,102,103,104,105,106,107] Close follow-up is crucial because recurrence of DVT is common.[106]

Superior Vena Cava Syndrome

Superior vena cava syndrome (SVCS) is a progressive occlusion of the superior vena cava (SVC) that leads to venous distention in the upper extremities and head. The leading cause of SVCS is bronchogenic cancer (75% of cases), followed by lymphomas (15%) and metastasis of other cancers (7%). If these conditions are not treated by antibiotics, syphilitic aortic aneurysms, tuberculosis, and mediastinal fibrosis can cause SVCS. Benign causes of SVCS include histoplasmosis and benign tumors such as retrosternal goiter. Invasive therapies, including pacemaker wires, central venous catheters, and pulmonary artery catheters, can lead to acute and chronic SVCS in about 0.3% to 4% of individuals undergoing these therapies and an important cause of SVCS. The right main stem bronchus abuts the SVC so that cancers occurring in this bronchus may press on the SVC. The SVC is also a relatively low-pressure vessel that lies in the closed thoracic compartment; therefore tissue expansion within the thoracic compartment can easily compress the SVC. Finally, the SVC is surrounded by lymph nodes and lymph chains that commonly become involved in thoracic cancers and compress the SVC during tumor growth. In individuals with small cell lung cancers, the presence of SVCS is a favorable prognostic sign, possibly because mediastinal metastases to lymph nodes near the SVCS occur early in the disease. When these enlarged nodes lead to SVCS, the malignancy may be detected earlier than in those individuals without SVCS. When onset of SVCS is slow, collateral venous drainage to the azygous vein usually has time to develop. Chronic SVCS can also be caused by arteriovenous shunts and by lymphadenopathy in cystic fibrosis and goiter.

Clinical manifestations of SVCS include edema and venous distention in the upper extremities and face, including the ocular beds. Individuals may complain of a feeling of fullness in the head, or tightness of shirt collars, necklaces, and rings. Cerebral and central nervous system edema may cause headache, visual disturbance, and impaired consciousness. The skin of the face and arms is purple and taut, and capillary refill time is prolonged. Respiratory distress may be present because of edema of bronchial structures or compression of the bronchus by a carcinoma. Diagnosis is made by chest roentgenogram, Doppler studies, computed tomography (CT), magnetic resonance imaging (MRI), and ultrasound.

Treatment of SVCS may be delayed for 24 hours to determine its cause. With slow onset and the development of collateral venous drainage, SVCS is generally not a vascular emergency but, rather, an oncologic emergency. Treatment includes radiation therapy and the administration of diuretics, steroids, and anticoagulants, as necessary.[108] Treatment also may include bypass surgery using various grafts; thrombolysis, both locally and systemically; balloon angioplasty; and placement of intravascular stents.[109] Stents, particularly Gianturco self-expandable stents, are most effective when the obstruction is not totally enveloped by tumor.[110]

Coronary Artery Disease, Myocardial Ischemia, and Myocardial Infarction

Coronary artery disease (CAD), myocardial ischemia, and myocardial infarction form a pathophysiologic continuum that impairs the pumping ability of the heart by depriving the heart muscle of blood-borne oxygen and nutrients. The earliest lesions of the continuum are those of **coronary artery disease**—virtually any vascular disorder that narrows or occludes the coronary arteries By far the most common cause of coronary artery obstruction is atherosclerosis (Fig. 29-14). CAD can diminish the myocardial blood supply until deprivation impairs myocardial metabolism enough to cause **ischemia,** a local state in which the cells are temporarily deprived of blood supply. They remain alive but cannot function normally. Persistent ischemia or the complete occlusion of a coronary artery causes **infarction,** or death, of the deprived myocardial tissue. Infarction constitutes the often-fatal event known as the "heart attack."

Development of Coronary Artery Disease

CAD is the single largest killer of American males and females, resulting in 466,101 deaths in the United States in 1997—about 1 of every 5 deaths. Two Americans suffer a heart attack every minute from coronary disease, and one of these will die. From 1987 to 1997, the death rate from CAD declined approximately 25% but the actual number of deaths declined only 0.9%.[111] Lifetime risk of death from CAD for a man aged 40 years is 49%; lifetime risk for women is 32%.[112] In the 1960s, researchers began to identify risk factors that contribute to the onset and escalation of CAD. Because CAD usually is caused by atherosclerotic obstruction of the vessels, those conditions that promote plaque formation are important risk factors for myocardial ischemia. The factors were classified as either modifiable or nonmodifiable. The nonmodifiable risk factors refer to variables that cannot be altered by persons wishing to decrease their risk of cardiovascular disease. These include advanced age, male gender (until 60 years of age), black or Asian race, genetic predisposition (which many consider modifiable if genetic risk includes hypertension and dyslipidemia, which are treatable), and diabetes mellitus type 1. The modifiable risk factors include dys-

A

B

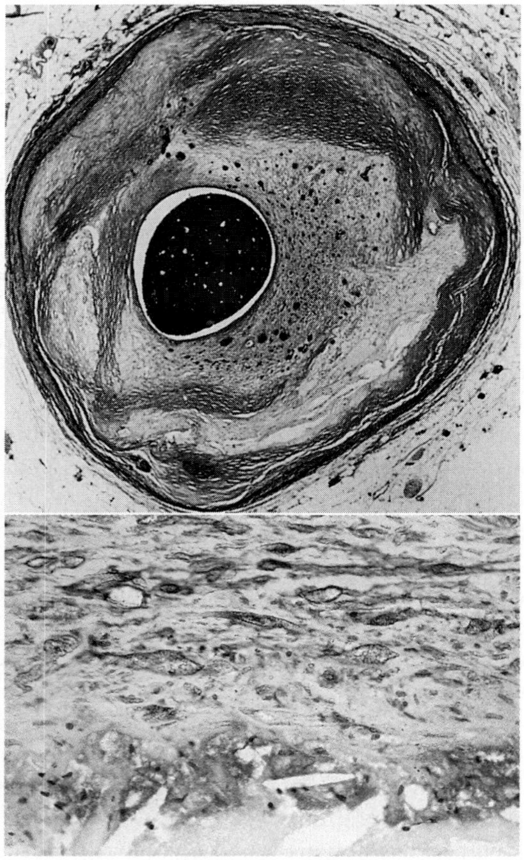

FIG. 29-14 Atherosclerosis. A, Concentric coronary plaque. The lumen is central. There are multiple, new small blood vessels within the plaque, the late result of disruption. **B,** Cell types in a fibrolipid plaque. The plaque cap (brownish) contains numerous elongated smooth muscle cells; some contain lipid. Macrophages are clustered on the edge of the core. (From Damjanov I, Linder J, editors: *Anderson's pathology,* ed 10, St Louis, 1996, Mosby.)

lipidemia (high levels of circulating lipoproteins), lipoprotein (a) (Lp[a]), hyperhomocysteinemia, hypertension, cigarette smoking, diabetes mellitus type 2, obesity, sedentary life-style, psychosocial factors (e.g., stress), estrogen deficiency (?), and heavy alcohol consumption. The role that some of the modifiable risk factors play in precipitating or exacerbating cardiovascular disease is controversial. Dyslipidemia (e.g., hypercholesterolemia), hypertension, and cigarette smoking have, however, been identified objectively as most predictive of CAD. Newly identified risk factors for coronary disease include fibrinogen, serum amyloid, C-reactive protein, uric acid, and infectious agents.[113,114]

Dyslipidemia

The strong link between CAD and elevated plasma lipoprotein concentrations is well documented.[35] The term **lipoprotein** refers to lipids, phospholipids, cholesterol, and triglycerides bound to carrier proteins. Lipids (cholesterol in particular) are required by most cells for the manufacture and repair of plasma membranes. Cholesterol is also a necessary component for the manufacture of such essential substances as bile acids and steroid hormones. Although cholesterol can easily be obtained from dietary fat intake, most body cells also can manufacture cholesterol.

The cycle of lipid metabolism is complex. Dietary fat is packaged into particles known as **chylomicrons** in the small intestine. Chylomicrons are required for absorption of fat; they function by transporting exogenous lipid from the intestine to the liver and peripheral cells. Chylomicrons are the least dense of the lipoproteins and primarily contain triglyceride. Some of the triglyceride may be removed and either stored by adipose tissue or used by muscle as an energy source. The chylomicron remnants, composed mainly of cholesterol, are taken up by the liver. A series of chemical reactions in the liver results in the production of several lipoproteins that vary in density and function. These include **very-low-density lipoproteins (VLDLs),** primarily triglyceride and protein; **low-density lipoproteins (LDLs),** mostly cholesterol and protein; and **high-density lipoproteins (HDLs),** mainly phospholipids and protein.

Increased VLDL (triglyceride) is a risk factor for coronary disease, primarily in middle-aged men and in individuals who have other lipoprotein abnormalities or diabetes.[115] A high level of LDL is a strong indicator of coronary risk. Increased LDL has been shown to result in endothelial dysfunction and increased oxidation by macrophages with incorporation of the oxidized LDL into the coronary vessel wall, a key step in atherogenesis (see p. 980 and Fig. 29-2, *B*). There are several subtypes of LDL; smaller LDL particles are more atherogenic.[116,117] **Lipoprotein (a) (Lp[a])** is a genetically determined molecular complex between LDL and a serum glycoprotein called *apolipoprotein A* that also has been shown to be a risk factor for atherosclerosis.[118,119,120]

HDLs, however, are thought to prevent or delay atherogenesis and thus are thought to be protective. They bring excess cholesterol back from the tissues to the liver where it can be metabolized (reverse cholesterol transport), inhibit smooth muscle proliferation, stimulate endothelial repair, stimulate vasodilator prostaglandins, and facilitate fibrinolysis.[121] These functions of HDL are so important in preventing atherosclerosis that low levels of HDL have been shown to be as much or more of a risk for coronary disease as high levels of total cholesterol or LDL, and low levels of HDL may even be a risk if total cholesterol levels are normal.[116,122]

Most individuals with a lipoprotein abnormality have a combination of environmental and genetic predisposing factors. A high dietary intake of saturated fats is the single most important modifiable risk factor for hypercholesterolemia; because smoking and alcohol consumption may also contribute, dietary and life-style modifications are the primary management tools. Other causes of dyslipidemia include a high intake of trans–fatty acids or underlying systemic diseases. The most common systemic disease associated with dyslipidemia is diabetes mellitus. Other causes include hypothyroidism, pancreatitis, and nephrosis. Unfortunately, for many individuals with moderate or severe increases in serum cholesterol, management also must include one or more medications to achieve adequate reductions in serum lipoproteins. These medications include those that reduce cholesterol production by the liver or enhance cholesterol secretion. The most effective medications inhibit the activity of 3-hydroxy-3-methylglutaryl-coenzyme A (HMG-CoA) reductase, an important enzyme in the synthesis of LDL by the liver. Commonly called "statins," this group of drugs is known to reduce the risk of atherosclerotic

WHAT'S NEW? Novel Coronary Risk Factors

Although the conventional risk factors for coronary artery disease have been well established over the years, several new markers have been associated with an increased risk for atherosclerosis and cardiovascular disease. Among these are indicators of inflammation such as C-reactive protein and soluble intercellular adhesion molecule-1. In addition, antibodies to infectious agents such as *Chlamydia pneumoniae* and serum endotoxin have been associated with an increased risk for cardiovascular events. Evidence for increased thrombogenic activity also has been found to be an indicator of coronary disease; relevant factors include fibrinogen, fibrinolytic activity, platelet activity, and antiphospholipid antibodies. Increased serum uric acid is associated with obesity, dyslipidemia, and hypertension, and has been found to be an independent risk factor for cardiovascular mortality. The clinical utility of these novel risk factors is still being explored.

Data from Danesh J: Coronary heart disease, *Helicobacter pylori,* dental disease, *Chlamydia pneumoniae,* and cytomegalovirus: meta-analyses of prospective studies, *Am Heart J* 138(5 part 2):S434, 1999; Danesh J et al: Risk factors for coronary heart disease and acute-phase proteins. A population-based study, *Euro Heart J* 20(13):954, 1999; Fang J, Alderman MH: Serum uric acid and cardiovascular mortality, *JAMA j1003*283:2404, 2000; Kullo IF, Gau GT, Tajik AJ: Novel risk factors for atherosclerosis, *Mayo Clin Proc* 75:369, 2000; Libby P, Ridker P: Novel inflammatory markers of coronary risk: theory versus practice, *Circulation* 100:1148, 1999; Ridker PM et al: C-reactive protein and other markers of inflammation in the prediction of cardiovascular disease in women, *N Engl J Med* 342(12):836, 2000.

cardiovascular disease.[116,123,124,125] Low levels of HDL do not respond well to diet changes but do respond to exercise and some medications.[126,127]

In people with a genetic defect (familial dyslipoproteinemia), very high levels of VLDL and LDL and/or low levels of HDL can result in symptomatic coronary disease as early as childhood. These genetic defects cause abnormalities in lipid-metabolizing enzymes and abnormal cellular lipid receptors (Table 29-4). In some cases, treatment must begin in childhood.[128]

Table 29-4 Familial Dyslipoproteinemias

Name	Laboratory Findings[a]	Clinical Features	Therapy
Type I; exogenous hyperlipidemia; fat-induced hypertriglyceridemia	Cholesterol normal Triglycerides increased 3 times Chylomicrons increased	Abdominal pain Hepatosplenomegaly Skin and retinal lipid deposits Usual onset: childhood	Low-fat diet
Type IIa; hypercholesterolemia	Triglycerides normal LDL increased Cholesterol increased	Premature vascular disease Xanthomas of tendons and bony prominences Common Onset: all ages	Low–saturated fat and low-cholesterol diet Cholestyramine[b] Colestipol[c] Lovastatin[d] Nicotinic acid[e] Neomycin[f] Intestinal bypass
Type IIb; combined hyperlipidemia; carbohydrate-induced hypertriglyceridemia	LDL, VLDL increased Cholesterol increased Triglycerides increased	Same as IIa	Same as IIa; *plus* carbohydrate restriction Clofibrate[g] Gemfibrozil[h] Lovastatin
Type III; dysbetalipoproteinemia	IDL or chylomicron remnants increased Cholesterol increased Triglycerides increased	Premature vascular disease Xanthomas of tendons and bony prominences Uncommon Onset: adulthood	Weight control Low-carbohydrate, low–saturated fat, and low-cholesterol diet Alcohol restriction Clofibrate Gemfibrozil Lovastatin Nicotinic acid Estrogens[i] Intestinal bypass
Type IV; endogenous hyperlipidemia; carbohydrate-induced hypertriglyceridemia	Glucose intolerance Hyperuricemia Cholesterol normal or increased VLDL increased Triglycerides increased	Premature vascular disease Skin lipid deposits Obesity Hepatomegaly Common onset: adulthood	Weight control Low-carbohydrate diet Alcohol restriction Clofibrate Nicotinic acid Intestinal bypass
Type V; mixed hyperlipidemia; carbohydrate and fat-induced hypertriglyceridemia	Glucose intolerance Hyperuricemia Chylomicrons increased VLDL increased LDL increased Cholesterol increased Triglycerides increased 3 times	Abdominal pain Hepatosplenomegaly Skin lipid deposits Retinal lipid deposits Onset: childhood	Weight control Low-carbohydrate and low-fat diet Clofibrate Lovastatin Nicotinic acid Progesterone[j] Intestinal bypass

[a] *LDL,* Low-density lipoprotein; *VLDL,* very-low-density lipoprotein; *IDL,* intermediate-density lipoprotein.
[b] *Cholestyramine* (Questran), anion exchange resin; binds bile acids; enhances cholesterol excretion.
[c] *Colestipol* (Colestid), same as cholestyramine.
[d] *Lovastatin,* 3-hydroxy-3-methylglutaryl-coenzyme A (HMG-CoA) reductase inhibitor; decreases cholesterol synthesis in the liver.
[e] *Nicotinic acid* (niacin), decreases release of free fatty acids from adipose tissue; increases lipogenesis in liver; decreases glucagon release; most effective for type V disorder.
[f] *Neomycin,* experimental medication; questionable mode of action; decreases LDLs.
[g] *Clofibrate* (Atromid-S), decreases release of free fatty acids from adipose tissue; decreases hepatic secretion of VLDL and increases catabolism of VLDL.
[h] *Gemfibrozil* (Lopid), similar to clofibrate but increases HDLs more.
[i] *Estrogens,* decrease IDL levels in type III disorders; experimental.
[j] *Progesterone,* decreases plasma triglycerides in type V disorders; experimental.

Hyperhomocysteinemia

Hyperhomocysteinemia occurs because of a genetic lack of the enzyme that breaks down homocysteine (an amino acid) and/or a nutritional deficiency of folate, cobalamin (vitamin B_{12}), or pyridoxine (vitamin B_6). It increases risk of coronary artery disease to the same degree as does smoking or hypercholesterolemia. Mechanisms by which it contributes to coronary disease and resultant myocardial ischemia include associated increases in LDL, decreases in endogenous vasodilators, and an increased tendency for thrombosis. Serum levels can be measured randomly, or after a methionine "load" that can help identify individuals at risk, although routine testing of all individuals is not currently recommended. Prevention and management are focused on increasing the dietary intake of folate and B vitamins.

Hypertension

Hypertension is responsible for a twofold to threefold increased risk of atherosclerotic cardiovascular disease, and about 35% of atherosclerotic cardiovascular events may be attributable to this risk factor alone. A reduction in systolic blood pressure of only 12 to 13 mm Hg can reduce the risk of CAD by as much as 21%.[20] It contributes to endothelial injury, a key step in atherogenesis (see p. 980), and causes myocardial hypertrophy, which increases myocardial demand for coronary flow.

Cigarette Smoking

Studies indicate that 30% of the annual mortality from CAD is traceable to cigarette smoking.[129,130] Passive (environmental) smoking increases the risk of coronary artery disease by 25%.[131] The mechanism by which smoking increases atherosclerosis is uncertain. Nicotine stimulates the release of catecholamines (epinephrine and norepinephrine), which increase heart rate and peripheral vascular constriction. As a result, blood pressure increases, as do cardiac workload and oxygen demand. Elevated catecholamines also stimulate release of free fatty acids. In one study, men and women who smoked more than 15 cigarettes per day were found to have lower HDL levels and higher LDL, cholesterol, and triglyceride levels. Cigarette smoking causes endothelial dysfunction and increases in vessel wall thickness; it also increases platelet adhesiveness, thereby increasing the risk of clot formation within the arteries.[132] Further, the carbon monoxide in cigarette smoke reduces the oxygen content of arterial blood. Hypoxemia (insufficient oxygen in arterial blood) may promote atherosclerosis by decreasing the availability of oxygen to the vessel walls and increasing vessel wall permeability. The cadmium in cigarette smoke may be related to elevations in blood pressure. The risk of CAD increases with heavy smoking and decreases when smoking is stopped. After smoking is discontinued, the risks associated with CAD may decrease as much as 50% in 1 year.

Diabetes Mellitus

Diabetes mellitus is an important risk factor for CAD. The 7-year risk for myocardial infarction in individuals with type 2 diabetes mellitus is 45%, or about 2.5 times the rate in the nondiabetic population.[116,133] Diabetic dyslipoproteinemia includes increased LDL and triglycerides, as well as decreased HDL. Glycation of LDL protein decreases LDL uptake by the liver, increases hepatic synthesis of LDL, and increases LDL oxidation. Close control of the blood sugar may help prevent these abnormalities and reduce cardiovascular events.[134] Glucose intolerance, hyperinsulinemia, dyslipidemia, and obesity probably share a genetic etiology and have been grouped into a syndrome classification called **syndrome X,** which requires multiple therapeutic interventions to lower the risk of atherosclerotic coronary disease.[43] The precise role of insulin resistance (even in the absence of clinical diabetes) in atherogenesis and coronary artery disease is still being defined, but it is clearly an important risk factor for heart disease.

Genetic Predisposition

A complete discussion of genetic predisposition, including familial hypercholesterolemia, is in Chapter 5. Men and women with a family history of CAD have an overall increased risk of death from coronary heart disease (irrespective of other risk factors) that has been estimated to be as much as 1.5 to 2.0 times as high as those without a family history.[135]

Obesity

Abdominal obesity has been shown to be a risk factor for CAD.[136,137] Obesity also affects the risk profile by predisposing individuals to hypertension, dyslipidemias, and impaired glucose tolerance; weight loss is associated with an improvement in these risk factors.[138] Studies consistently have reported a decrease in HDL levels associated with obesity. As obesity progresses, the heart increases in size, resulting in increased oxygen consumption and increased workload.

Sedentary Life-Style

Investigations of physical exercise and coronary heart disease have shown that a sedentary life-style predisposes to CAD and that physical exercise may delay or prevent its development.[139,140] Physical exercise may reduce blood pressure, decrease the urge to smoke and eat, improve carbohydrate metabolism, and improve psychologic outlook.[141] (Increased fibrinolysis with decreased blood clotting has been noted in individuals who exercise regularly.) In addition, persons who are habitually physically active tend to have higher plasma HDL levels than do sedentary individuals. There is no evidence that exercise increases development of coronary collateral vessels or results in regression of atheromatous plaques. Physical activity does increase heart volume and mass, increase cardiac capillary vascularity, and decrease heart rate, however—all of which may protect from the effects of ischemic damage.

Alcohol

Moderate alcohol intake (2 to 10 drinks per week) is associated with as much as a 25% reduction in coronary disease and a 50% decrease in sudden cardiac death.[142,143,144] Alcohol reduces coronary risk by increasing HDL and improving hemostatic factors, such as fibrinogen.[145] Red wine offers additional benefits probably because it contains antioxidants and flavenoids.[146,147] Heavier use of alcohol is known to increase body weight, triglyceride levels, and systolic blood pressure and may impair left ventricular function. Some studies have demonstrated a direct cardiotoxic effect of excessive alcohol on myocardial tissue, resulting in collagen accumulation, diminished nucleic acid pools, and loss of membrane transport systems. Further research is needed to clarify this issue.

Women and Coronary Artery Disease

The incidence of CAD is lower in premenopausal women than in age-matched men. In postmenopausal women the incidence of CAD increases rapidly and by 70 years of age approaches the same rate as that for men.

The postmenopausal state is one of estrogen and progesterone deficiency and is characterized by an increase in LDL and total cholesterol,[148] an increase in some women of Lp(a),[149] increased insulin resistance, and worsening hemostatic profiles.[150] The same association is reported between early surgical menopause (bilateral oophorectomy) and risk for CAD. Hysterectomy with the retention of one ovary is associated with little or no increased risk of CAD. Retrospective and observational studies have suggested that synthetic estrogen therapy (i.e., ERT and HRT) reduces the risk of coronary events by 35% to 50% in postmenopausal women.[151] These data showed estrogen's ability to lower LDL and raise HDL; however, for some, estrogen also raised triglycerides. Investigators today, however, report that these studies may have been confounded by the self-selection of the women using HRT. That is, women who chose to take HRT were healthier to begin with. The newest studies are randomized, controlled trials and are prospective. The Heart and Estrogen/Progestin Replacement Study (HERS) trial enrolled 2763 women with documented coronary heart disease. Overall, 172 women in the synthetic HRT group and 176 women in the placebo group had a myocardial infarction or died from heart disease during the study. HERS, like earlier studies, found that women taking hormones were more likely to have blood clots in their legs and lungs. The increased risk of coronary events among HRT users was most pronounced in the first year. Presumably, HRT initially increases the tendency to produce blood clots. In the HERS study, this trend was reversed by the third year of treatment; by the fourth year, the end of the study, there was no difference in heart attacks between the groups. In April, 2000, preliminary results of the unpublished Women's Health Initiative were released. This is a 9-year, randomized, prospective study—the largest to date (final results expected in 2005)—designed to help define synthetic HRT's place in *preventing* CHD. Despite the fact that the participants had no history of CHD, those who received hormones experienced more cardiac problems, including heart attacks, during the first 2 years of the study. From the HERS study, it is clear that if a woman already has cardiovacular problems, she should not start taking HRT. Until more data are available from the Women's Health Initiative and other prospective studies, the decision to take HRT to *prevent* heart attacks is very controversial. The development of new synthetic estrogen receptor modulators (SERMS) may provide drugs that maximize the benefits of postmenopausal estrogen replacement without the risks of breast cancer and vascular thrombosis. In addition, undocumented from prospective longitudinal studies is the effect of a healthy life-style without hormone replacement (i.e, diet, exercise, supplements, stress reduction, etc.) on preventing heart disease.

It is interesting to note that estrogens do not reduce the incidence of CAD in men. The reason for the difference between male and female susceptibility to CAD is not understood. Recent research that examined endogenous estrogens and androgens and cardiovascular mortality in older women found no support for a causal or preventive role for these hormones and cardiovascular mortality.

Smoking is an important risk factor for the development of CAD, especially in young females. Younger females now constitute the greatest risk group for adopting the smoking habit. The decline in smoking over the past 25 years has been greater among males than females. Smoking cessation improves survival rates for both healthy women and women who have had an MI.

Women with diabetes have a greater risk of CAD than men with diabetes, and thus diabetes eliminates any female advantage in the development of CAD. Even an abnormal glucose tolerance *alone* is a risk factor for CAD because of poorer glucose control (as assessed by higher levels of hemoglobin A_{1c} [Hb A_{1c}]). This effect is thought to exist for some time before there is evidence of diabetic levels of glycemia and the onset of non-insulin-dependent diabetes.

A portion of the gender difference in CAD susceptibility is likely related to plasma lipids. In North America, women 20 to 40 years of age tend to have lower LDL levels and VLDL levels and higher plasma levels of HDLs. This female advantage, especially the ratio of LDL to HDL, diminishes gradually after menopause, with increasing levels of LDL and decreasing levels of HDL. Triglycerides also may be independently associated with increasing risk of CAD in women but not in men. Lp(a) is strongly associated with the development of CAD, especially in women. In fact, one of the possible effects of estrogen replacement therapy for reducing risk of CAD is its ability to lower Lp(a).[149]

Type A Personality

Beginning in the 1950s, Friedman and Rosenman[152] and other investigators argued compellingly that persons with type A personality are at higher risk for the development of coronary disease. Individuals with type A personality are described as hard driving, aggressive, compulsive, domineering, and deadline conscious.[153]

As a result of these studies, a review panel recognized type A behavior as a risk factor for CAD in 1981.[154] Since the early 1980s, however, a large number of contradictory findings have been reported regarding the risk status of type A behavior.[154] Several studies have failed to demonstrate an association between type A behavior and the extent of CAD. However, recent reports discuss life-style interventions that include a reduction in stress and type A behavior (especially suppressed hostility) as resulting in improvement in many other risk factors and better overall cardiovascular outcomes.[141,155] Perhaps the relationship between emotions and CAD is mediated through already implicated physiologic mechanisms regulated by the central nervous system, such as increased blood pressure, plasma lipids, and hemostasis. Acute stress has certainly been shown to increase catecholamines and is associated with precipitating myocardial infarction and sudden death in individuals with coronary disease.

Myocardial Ischemia

Pathophysiology

The coronary arteries normally supply blood flow sufficient to meet the demands of the myocardium as it labors under varying workloads. Oxygen extraction from these vessels occurs with maximal efficiency. If efficient exchange does not meet myocardial oxygen needs, healthy coronary arteries are able to dilate to increase the flow of oxygenated blood to the myocardium. A variety of pathologic mechanisms can interfere with blood flow through the coronary arteries, giving rise to myocardial ischemia. Narrowing of a major coronary artery by more than 50% impairs blood flow sufficiently to hamper cellular metabolism under conditions of increased myocardial demand (see Fig. 29-14).

The most common cause of myocardial ischemia is atherosclerosis. Plaque formation within the arterial system often results in occlusion of vessel lumina, depriving the myocardium of oxygen and nutrients. Thrombus formation in the coronary arteries may result from ulceration of atherosclerotic plaques. The growing mass of plaque, platelets, fibrin, and cellular debris eventually can narrow the lumen enough to impede blood flow (see Fig. 29-2). Platelet aggregations are known to release the prostaglandin thromboxane A_2, a potent vasoconstrictor capable of causing spasm of the coronary arteries. Thromboxane A_2 also promotes platelet aggregation, resulting in a vicious positive-feedback cycle of vasoconstriction and platelet buildup in the vessel walls.

Myocardial ischemia develops if coronary blood flow or the oxygen content of coronary blood is not sufficient to meet the metabolic demands of myocardial cells. Imbalances between blood supply and myocardial demand can result from a number of conditions. Supply is reduced by the following factors:

1. Hemodynamic factors, such as increased resistance in coronary vessels, hypotension, or decreased blood volume (e.g., from hemorrhage)
2. Cardiac factors, such as decreases of diastolic filling time, increases in heart rate, or valvular incompetence
3. Hematologic factors, such as the oxygen content of the blood
4. Systemic disorders that reduce blood flow or the availability of oxygen (e.g., shock)

Myocardial ischemia usually is caused by increased resistance in coronary vessels, but because the myocardium has little tolerance for hypoxia, it is particularly vulnerable (along with brain tissue) to the hypoxemia caused by respiratory disease (e.g., chronic obstructive pulmonary disease [COPD]), anemia, or erythrocyte disorders that interfere with oxygen binding (see Chapters 25 and 32). Demand is increased by the following factors:

1. High systolic blood pressure
2. Increased ventricular volume
3. Increased thickness of the myocardium (e.g., left ventricular hypertrophy caused by increased systemic resistance, such as occurs with aortic valve stenosis and hypertension)
4. Increased heart rate resulting from exercise, stress, hyperthyroidism, anemia, or hyperviscosity of the blood (e.g., polycythemia)
5. Conditions that heighten the myocardium's contractile response (such as exercise)

Ischemia occurs if demand exceeds supply. For example, in an individual with CAD, supply may be adequate for myocardial function while the individual is at rest if respiratory and erythrocyte functions are normal. Any factor that increases demand, such as strenuous exercise, or decreases supply, such as the development of anemia or respiratory disease, places the individual at risk for an episode of myocardial ischemia.

Myocardial cells become ischemic within 10 seconds of coronary occlusion. After several minutes the heart cells lose the ability to contract, thus hampering pump function and depriving the myocardium of a glucose source necessary for aerobic metabolism. Anaerobic processes take over, and lactic acid accumulates. Cardiac cells remain viable for approximately 20 minutes under ischemic conditions. If blood flow is restored, aerobic metabolism resumes, contractility is restored, and cellular repair begins. If the coronary arteries cannot compensate for lack of oxygen, myocardial infarction occurs (Fig. 29-15).

Clinical Manifestations

Individuals with reversible myocardial ischemia present clinically in several ways. Chronic coronary obstruction results in recurrent predictable chest pain called **stable angina**. Abnormal vasospasm of coronary vessels results in unpredictable chest pain called **Prinzmetal angina**. Myocardial ischemia that does not cause detectable symptoms is called **silent ischemia**.

Stable angina. Angina pectoris is chest pain caused by myocardial ischemia. The discomfort is usually transient, lasting approximately 3 to 5 minutes. If blood flow is restored, no permanent change or damage results. **Angina pectoris** is typically experienced as substernal chest discomfort, ranging from a sensation of heaviness or pressure to moderately severe pain. Individuals often describe the sensation by clenching a fist over the left sternal border. Discomfort may radiate to the neck, lower jaw, left arm, and left shoulder, or, occasionally, to the back or down the right arm. Discomfort is commonly mistaken for indigestion. The pain is presumably caused by the buildup of lactic acid or abnormal stretching of the ischemic myocardium that irritates myocardial nerve fibers. These afferent sympathetic fibers enter the spinal cord from levels C3 to T4, accounting for the variety of locations and radiation patterns of anginal pain. Pallor, diaphoresis, and dyspnea may be associated with the pain. Stable angina is caused by gradual luminal narrowing and hardening of the arterial walls, so that affected vessels cannot dilate in response to

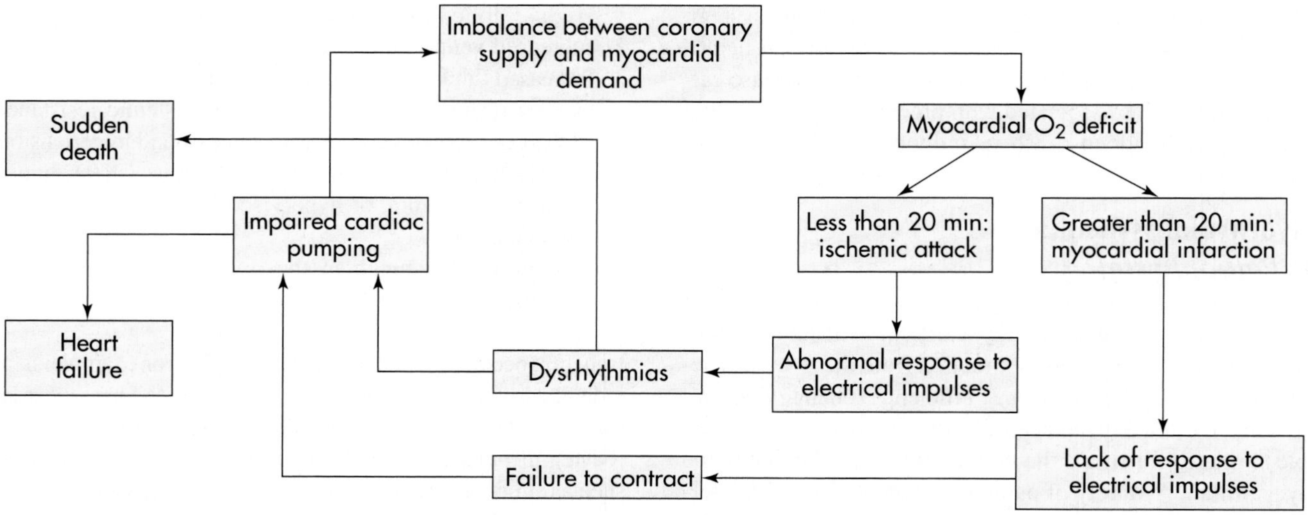

FIG. 29-15 Cycle of ischemic events.

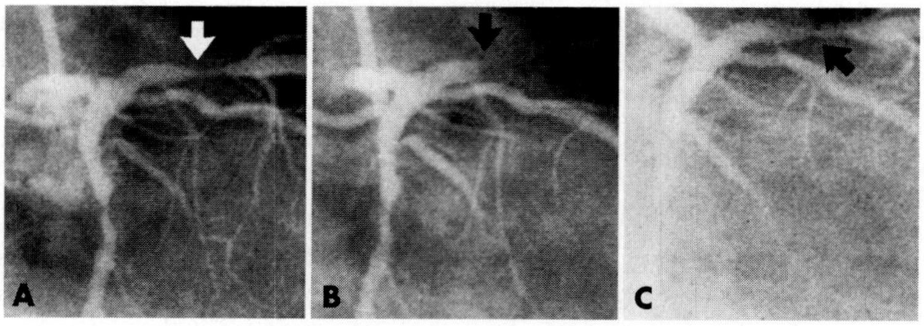

FIG. 29-16 Angiogram. A, Baseline. **B,** Transient total occlusion of left anterior descending branch of the left coronary artery after mental stress. **C,** After nitrates and nifedipine, artery reopened to same diameter as baseline. (From Stern S, editor: *Silent myocardial ischemia,* St Louis, 1998, Mosby.)

increased myocardial demand associated with physical exertion or emotional stress. The pain is usually relieved by rest and nitrates; lack of relief indicates an individual may be developing infarction.

Prinzmetal angina. Prinzmetal angina is chest pain attributable to transient ischemia of the myocardium that occurs unpredictably and almost exclusively at rest. Pain is caused by vasospasm of one or more major coronary arteries with or without associated atherosclerosis. The pain frequently occurs at night during rapid eye movement sleep and may have a cyclic pattern of occurrence. The angina may result from hyperactivity of the sympathetic nervous system, increased calcium reflux in arterial smooth muscle, or impaired production or release of prostaglandin or thromboxane.

Silent ischemia and mental stress (induced ischemia). Myocardial ischemia often does not cause detectable symptoms such as angina. Ischemia can be totally asymptomatic and referred to as silent ischemia. In addition, myocardial ischemia can be silent in the majority of episodes in individuals who also experience angina. Recent studies have addressed the pathophysiologic differences between silent and symptomatic ischemia. One proposed mechanism for the absence of angina in silent myocardial ischemia is the presence of a global or regional abnormality in left ventricular symptomatic afferent innervation. Such abnormality might occur as part of a metabolic dysfunction in diabetes mellitus, following surgical denervation during coronary artery bypass grafting (CABG) or cardiac transplantation, or following ischemic local nerve injury by myocardial infarction.[156]

Another area that is receiving renewed interest is the lack of angina, even though an artery is occluded, in some individuals during mental stress (see Figs. 29-16, 29-17, and 29-18).[157] Rozansky and colleagues documented myocardial ischemia by radionuclide angiography (RNA) during mental stress; the majority of these cases (83%) were silent ischemias.[158] They also noted a smaller increase in heart rate during mental stress than during exercise, although the systolic blood response was comparable and the diastolic blood pressure response is even greater with mental stress. These observations confirmed in similar studies that the increases in blood pressure induced by mental stress and increases in myocardial oxygen demand may play a role in the pathophysiology of myocardial ischemia induced by mental stress.[156]

Silent myocardial ischemia is very prevalent in individuals with a variety of acute and chronic coronary syndromes. Silent ischemia is detected with greater sensitivity and specificity using stress radionucleotide imaging than by exercise electrocardiogram testing alone.[156]

Evaluation and Treatment

Physical examination may disclose extra, rapid heart sounds (left ventricular gallop or S_3), indicating impaired left ventricular function during the ischemic attack. The presence of **xanthelasmas** (small fat deposits) around the eyelids or **arcus**

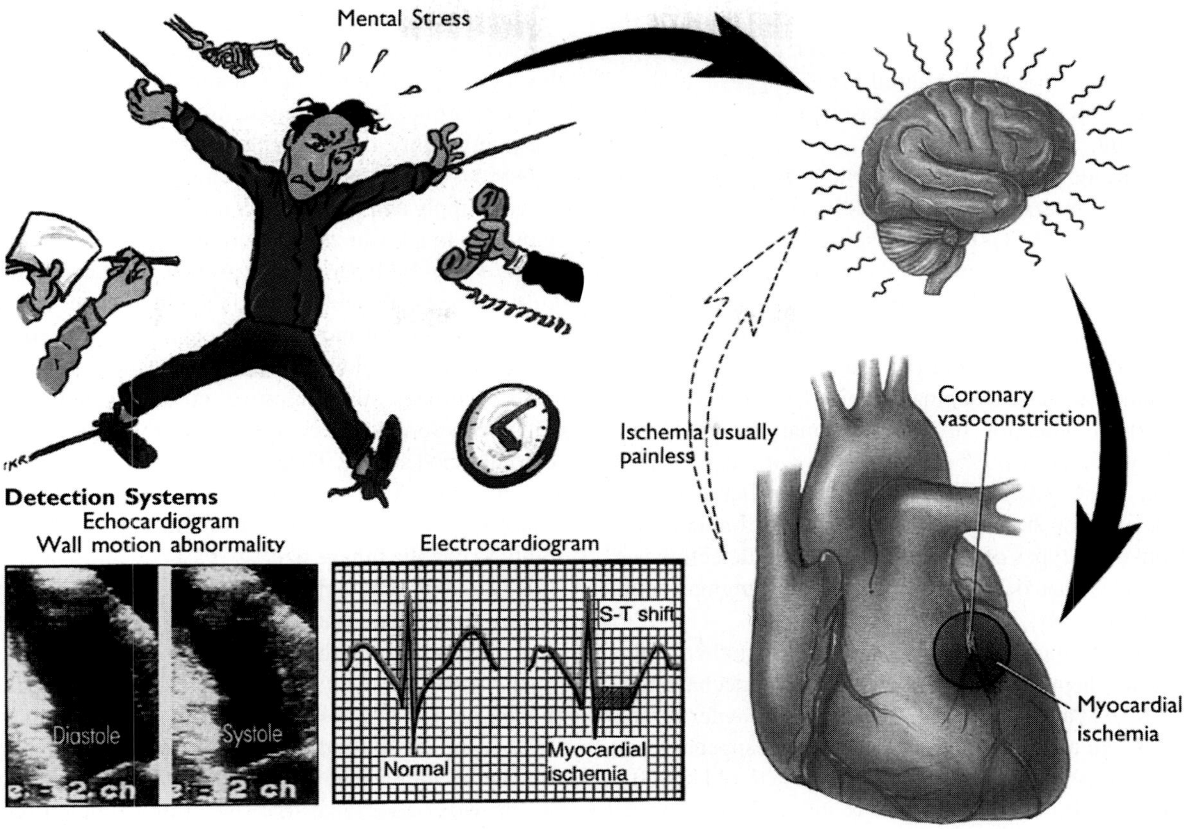

FIG. 29-17 The ischemic cost of aggravation. Linkages among daily mental and emotional stimuli, brain activity, and coronary and myocardial physiology. (From Papodemetrion V et al: Transient coronary occlusion with mental stress, *Am Heart J* 132:1299, 1996.)

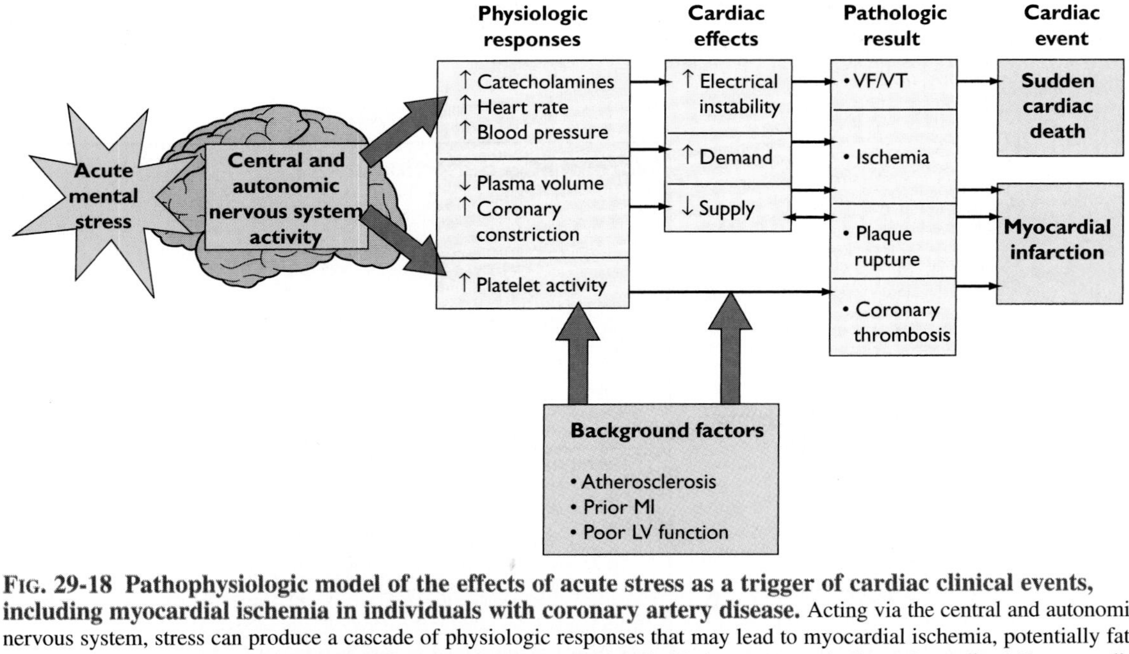

FIG. 29-18 Pathophysiologic model of the effects of acute stress as a trigger of cardiac clinical events, including myocardial ischemia in individuals with coronary artery disease. Acting via the central and autonomic nervous system, stress can produce a cascade of physiologic responses that may lead to myocardial ischemia, potentially fatal dysrhythmia, plaque rupture, or coronary thrombosis. *VF,* Ventricular fibrillation; *VT,* ventricular tachycardia; *MI,* myocardial infarction; *LV,* left ventricular. (From Kranz DS et al: Mental stress as a trigger of myocardial ischemia and infarction. In Deedwania PC, Tofler GH, editors: *Triggers and timing of cardiac events*, ed 2, London, 1996, W.B. Saunders.)

senilis of the eyes (a yellow lipid ring around the cornea) suggests dyslipidemia and possible atherosclerosis. The presence of peripheral or carotid arterial bruits suggests probable atherosclerotic disease and increases the likelihood that CAD is present.

Electrocardiography is a critical tool for the diagnosis of myocardial ischemia. Because many individuals have normal electrocardiograms (ECGs) in the absence of pain, diagnosis requires that electrocardiography be performed during an attack of angina. Transient ST segment depression and T wave inversion are characteristic signs of subendocardial ischemia. ST elevation, indicative of transmural ischemia, is seen in individuals with variant angina (Fig. 29-19). The ECG can also give some indication of which coronary artery is involved. Approximately 30% of individuals with angina will have nondiagnostic ECG tracings and require other diagnostic studies. Exercise stress testing is useful in differentiating angina from other types of chest pain, as well as detecting ischemic changes that occur in the absence of anginal pain (silent ischemia).

Radioisotope imaging with thallium-201 is another technique used to diagnose CAD. Active transport mechanisms (the Na^+, K^+ATPase system) cause thallium to enter myocardial cells. An area of myocardial infarction appears as a region of diminished activity or no activity (a "cold spot"). Defects that are absent at rest but can be induced by exercise represent ischemia. A newer test called **SPECT (single-photon emission computed tomography)** is even more effective at identifying ischemia and estimating coronary risk.

Coronary angiography is useful in determining the anatomic extent of CAD. The procedure is expensive and carries some risk; thus it is used primarily to evaluate for possible percutaneous transluminal angioplasty (PTCA) or coronary artery bypass graft (CABG) surgery for individuals whose noninvasive studies suggest severe disease.

The primary aim of therapy for myocardial ischemia and angina is to reduce myocardial oxygen consumption by favorably altering its various determinants. The factors most amenable to pharmacologic manipulation are blood pressure, heart rate, contractility, and left ventricular volume.

Nitrates are often the drug of choice because they increase oxygen supply and reduce demand. Nitrates cause peripheral veins and, to a lesser extent, peripheral arteries to dilate. Dilation reduces both peripheral vascular resistance and venous return to the heart (preload) and thereby reduces left ventricular filling pressure and left ventricular volume. Reduced filling pressure and volume decrease workload (myocardial demand). Nitrates also improve coronary blood flow by reducing coronary artery spasm and thereby increase myocardial blood supply. These drugs cannot enhance vasodilation in coronary vessels altered by atherosclerosis or arteriosclerosis because these disorders impair the vessels' ability to change lumen size.

β-Adrenergic blocking agents have had great impact on therapy for ischemic heart disease in the past 20 years. By blocking β receptors, these medications can increase oxygen supply and reduce myocardial demand. Beta-blockers diminish catecholamine-induced elevations of heart rate, myocardial contractility, and blood pressure. Coronary blood flow also can be augmented by beta-blockade. Reduction in heart rate provides additional diastolic filling time for coronary perfusion, leading to enhanced oxygen delivery to the heart.

Calcium plays a key role in the electrical excitation of cardiac cells and in mechanical contraction of the myocardial and vascular smooth muscle cells (see Chapter 28). By blocking the influx of calcium into myocardial cells and vascular smooth muscle cells, the pacemaker activity of the sinoatrial (SA) node and conduction properties of the atrioventricular (AV) node can be modified. Combinations of nitrates, beta-blockers, and calcium antagonists may provide

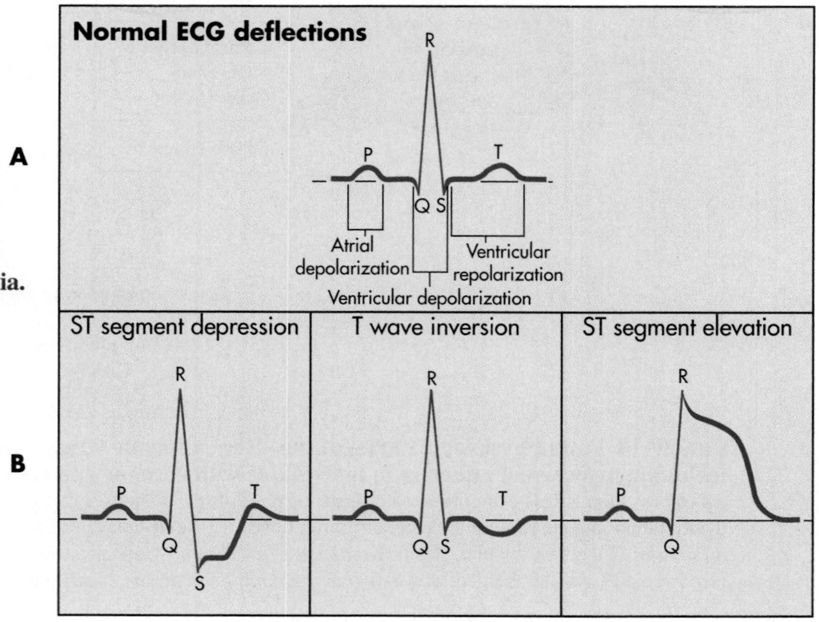

FIG. 29-19 Electrocardiogram (ECG) and ischemia. **A,** Normal ECG. **B,** Electrocardiographic alterations associated with ischemia.

dramatic relief from clinical manifestations of ischemic heart disease and make more invasive interventions unnecessary. The effects of these drugs are summarized in Table 29-5.

Experimental evidence linking platelet aggregation with decreased coronary blood flow has led to the use of antiplatelet agents for individuals with ischemic heart disease. Effective antiplatelet agents include aspirin, sulfinpyrazone, dipyridamole, or the new platelet glycoprotein IIb/IIIa receptor antagonists.[15] Aggressive reversal of risk factors, especially lipid lowering therapy, can reverse disease progression and improve outcomes. This type of secondary prevention reduces the risk of subsequent myocardial infarction.[29,116,123,159]

Percutaneous transluminal coronary angioplasty (PTCA) is a procedure whereby stenotic (narrowed) coronary vessels are dilated with a balloon dilation catheter. The lesion most suitable for angioplasty is one that is discrete, concentric, located in a proximal portion of the vessel, noncalcified, and less than 10 mm in length.[150] PTCA is generally used to treat single-vessel disease, but it can be effective with multiple-vessel disease or restenosis of a coronary artery bypass graft. Restenosis of the artery is the major complication of the procedure; however, placement of a coronary stent can reduce this risk.[160]

Ischemic heart disease can be surgically treated by a **coronary artery bypass graft.** A saphenous vein from the thigh is most commonly used to bypass the obstructed coronary artery. A technique using the left internal mammary artery (LIMA) rather than the saphenous vein has shown significant improvement in long-term graft patency. In selected individuals a procedure called **minimally invasive direct coronary artery bypass (MIDCAB)** can allow for effective bypass grafting of the heart, but with minimal disruption of the chest wall and without cardiopulmonary bypass or cardioplegia; thus, recovery times are much shorter.[161] One of the most common indications for bypass surgery is incapacitating angina in an individual who has good left ventricular function and technically operable coronary arteries but who has not responded to medical therapy. Although surgery has been shown to relieve angina, it does not halt the progress of atherosclerosis or prolong life except when multiple coronary vessels are obstructed or when the left main coronary artery is blocked. A successful coronary artery bypass graft can, however, diminish the probability of lethal insult to the coronary tissues and can markedly improve quality of life. Newer therapies for refractory angina include transmyocardial laser revascularization (TMR) and gene therapy for myocardial angiogenesis.[162,163,164]

Acute Coronary Syndromes

The process of atherosclerotic plaque progression is usually gradual. However, when there is sudden coronary obstruction due to thrombus formation over an atherosclerotic plaque, the acute coronary syndromes result. **Unstable angina** causes reversible myocardial ischemia and is a harbinger of impending infarction (pp. 1011). **Myocardial infarction** results when there is prolonged ischemia causing irreversible damage to the heart muscle. Sudden cardiac death can occur in any of the acute coronary syndromes.

The American Heart Association Committee on Vascular Lesions provided criteria for subdividing coronary atherosclerotic plaque progression into five phases, with different lesion types corresponding to each phase.[30] The main point of this system is that some atherosclerotic lesions are "stable" and progress by gradually occluding the vessel lumen, whereas other lesions are "unstable" or complicated lesions and (even before there is any significant coronary occlusion) are prone to sudden plaque rupture and thrombus formation, resulting in the acute coronary syndromes of unstable angina, myocardial infarction, and even sudden death. Figure 29-20 provides an overview of the steps in the development of the acute coronary syndromes. Plaques that are unstable and prone to rupture are those with a core that is especially rich in deposited oxidized LDL and those with thin fibrous caps.[31,165,166,167] Plaque disruption (erosions, fissuring, or rupture) occurs

Table 29-5 Effects of Antianginal Agents on Myocardial Supply and Demand

	Nitrates	β Blockers	Calcium Antagonists
DEMAND			
Wall tension	Decrease	Increase	Increase or no apparent effect
Systolic blood pressure	Decrease	Decrease	Decrease
Ventricular volume	Decrease	Increase	Decrease or no apparent effect
Heart rate	Increase	Decrease	Increase, decrease, or no apparent effect
Contractility	No apparent effect	Decrease	Decrease
SUPPLY			
Coronary blood flow	Increase	Increase or no apparent effect	Increase
Coronary vascular resistance	Decrease	Increase or no apparent effect	Decrease
Coronary spasm	Decrease	Increase or no apparent effect	Decrease
Diastolic perfusion time	Decrease	Increase	Decrease, increase, or no apparent effect
Collateral blood flow	Increase	No apparent effect	Decrease

From Kafka KR, Meltzer AH, Frishman WH: *Hosp Formulary* 20(1):1144, 1985.

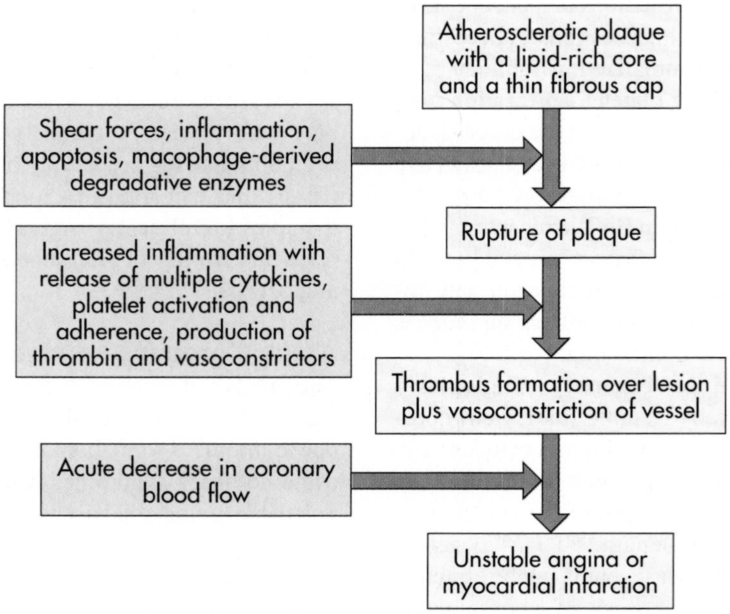

FIG. 29-20 Pathogenesis of the acute coronary syndromes.

due to shear forces, inflammation with release of multiple inflammatory mediators, secretion of macrophage-derived degradative enzymes, and apoptosis of cells at the edges of the lesions.[31,168] Exposure of the plaque substrate activates the clotting cascade.[164] In addition, platelet activation results in the release of coagulants and exposure of platelet glycoprotein IIb/IIIa surface receptors, resulting in further platelet aggregation and adherence.[166] The resulting thrombus can form very quickly. Vessel obstruction is further exacerbated by the release of vasoconstrictors such as thromboxane A_2.[165,166] The thrombus may break up before permanent myocyte damage has occurred (unstable angina) or it may cause prolonged ischemia with infarction of the heart muscle (myocardial infarction). Some individuals have sudden cardiac death without underlying histologic evidence of infarction.[169]

Box 29-1

CLASSIFICATION OF UNSTABLE ANGINA

National Heart Lung and Blood Institute Criteria

1. Angina at rest (usually lasting more than 20 minutes)
2. Exertional angina of new onset (within 2 months) of at least class III severity by the criteria of the Canadian Cardiovascular Society Classification (CCSC)
3. Recent (within 2 months) worsening of angina as reflected by an increase in severity of at least one CCSC class to at least CCSC class III

From Braunwald E, Jones RJ, Mark DB: Diagnosing and managing unstable angina. Agency for Health Policy and Research, *Circulation* 90:613, 1994.

Unstable Angina

Unstable angina is a form of acute coronary syndrome that results in reversible myocardial ischemia. Important, however, is that it signals that the atherosclerotic plaque has become complicated, and infarction may soon follow.

Pathophysiology

A fairly small fissuring or superficial erosion of the plaque leads to transient episodes of thrombotic vessel occlusion and vasoconstriction at the site of plaque damage. This thrombus is labile and occludes the vessel for no more than 10 to 20 minutes, with return of perfusion before significant myocardial necrosis occurs. Careful pathologic examination frequently reveals some myocyte damage, presumably due to distal embolization of the thrombus fragments.[170]

Clinical Manifestations

Unstable angina presents as new onset angina, angina that is occurring at rest, or angina that is increasing in severity or frequency (Box 29-1). Individuals may experience increased dyspnea, diaphoresis, and anxiety as the angina worsens. Those with unstable angina at rest have the greatest risk of subsequent infarction or death.[170]

Evaluation and Management

Physical examination may reveal evidence of ischemic myocardial dysfunction such as tachycardia, S_3 gallop, or pulmonary congestion. The ECG most commonly reveals ST segment depression and T wave inversion during pain that resolves as the pain is relieved. The ECG may be inconclusive in up to one third of individuals with unstable angina, for whom further evaluation is necessary. The cardiac isoenzymes (CPK-MB, LDH_1) remain normal. Sensitive markers of myocyte damage such as the troponins may increase transiently in up to 40% of individuals diagnosed with unstable angina.[170,171,172] Emergency echocardiography may reveal abnormal cardiac contraction. Approximately 20% of individuals with unstable angina will progress to

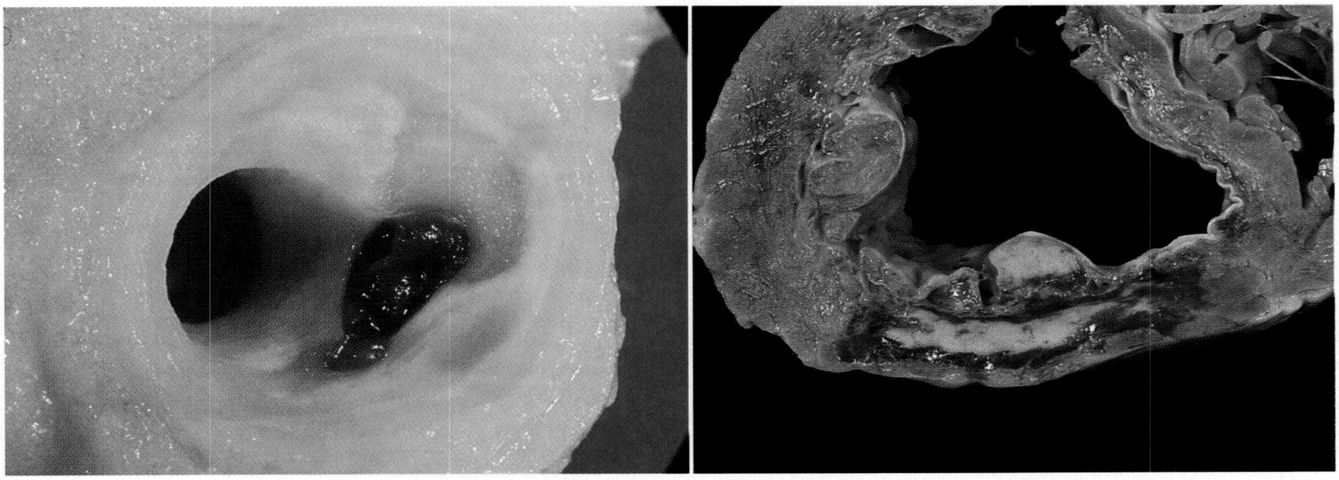

FIG. 29-21 Plaque disruption and myocardial infarction. A, Plaque disruption. The cap of the lipid-rich plaque has become torn with the formation of a thrombus, mostly inside the plaque. **B,** Myocardial infarction. This infarct is 6 days old. The center is yellow and necrotic with a hemorrhagic red rim. The responsible coronary artery occlusion is probably in the right coronary artery. The infarct is on the posterior wall. (From Damjanov I, Linder J, editors: *Anderson's pathology,* ed 10, St Louis, 1996, Mosby.)

myocardial infarction or death within 30 days; unfortunately, up to 4% of individuals with unstable angina are inadvertently discharged from the emergency room, resulting in considerable risk for subsequent infarction and death.[173] Management of unstable angina requires some form of antithrombotic therapy. In most cases, individuals are given aspirin, ticlopidine, or clopidogrel, followed by intravenous unfractionated heparin.[174] Many patients are now being treated with low-molecular-weight heparin, IIb/IIIa platelet receptor antagonists, direct thrombin inhibitors (e.g., Hirudin), thrombolytics, or immediate intervention with percutaneous transluminal angioplasty (PTCA) or coronary artery bypass grafting (CABG).[100,172,175,176]

Myocardial Infarction

When coronary blood flow is interrupted for an extended period of time, myocyte necrosis occurs. This results in myocardial infarction (MI). There are two major types of myocardial infarction, non–Q wave (subendocardial) infarction and Q wave (transmural) infarction.

Pathophysiology

Plaque progression, disruption, and subsequent clot formation is the same for myocardial infarction as it is for the other acute coronary syndromes (see Fig. 29-21, *A*; see also Fig. 29-20). In this case, however, the thrombus is less labile and occludes the vessel for a prolonged period, such that myocardial ischemia progresses to myocyte necrosis and death. If the thrombus breaks up before complete distal tissue necrosis has occurred, the infarction will involve only the myocardium directly beneath the endocardium and will not be associated with the classic Q wave tracing on the ECG (subendocardial or non–Q wave MI). It is especially important to recognize this form of acute coronary syndrome because recurrent clot formation on the disrupted atherosclerotic plaque is likely unless some intervention is undertaken as soon as possible. If the thrombus lodges permanently in the vessel, the infarction will extend through the myocardium all the way from endocardium to epicardium, resulting in severe cardiac dysfunction and the characteristic Q wave on ECG (transmural or Q wave MI).

Cellular injury. Cardiac cells can withstand ischemic conditions for about 20 minutes before cellular death takes place. After only 30 to 60 seconds of hypoxia, ECG changes are visible. Yet even if cells are metabolically altered and nonfunctional, they can remain viable if blood flow returns within 20 minutes. Recent reports suggest that previous recurrent episodes of myocardial ischemia can result in myocyte adaptation to oxygen deprivation and preservation of myocardium. This process, termed **ischemic preconditioning,** is being studied to determine if it has potential prophylactic or therapeutic uses.[177,178,179]

After 8 to 10 seconds of decreased blood flow, the affected myocardium becomes cyanotic and cooler. Myocardial oxygen reserves are used very quickly (within about 8 seconds) after complete cessation of coronary flow. Glycogen stores decrease as anaerobic metabolism begins. Unfortunately, glycolysis can supply only 65% to 70% of the total myocardial energy requirement and produces much less ATP than aerobic processes. Hydrogen ions and lactic acid accumulate. Because myocardial tissues have poor buffering capabilities and myocardial cells are very sensitive to low cellular pH, accumulation of these products further compromises the myocardium. Acidosis may make the myocardium more vulnerable to the damaging effects of lysosomal enzymes and may suppress impulse conduction and contractile function, thereby leading to heart failure.

Oxygen deprivation also is accompanied by electrolyte disturbances—specifically, loss of potassium, calcium, and magnesium from cells. Myocardial cells deprived of necessary oxygen and nutrients lose contractility, thereby diminishing the pumping ability of the heart. Normally, the myocardium takes up varying quantities of catecholamines (epinephrine and norepinephrine). Significant arterial occlusion causes the myocardial cells to release catecholamines, predisposing the individual to serious imbalances of sympathetic and parasympathetic function, irregular heartbeats (dysrhythmia), and heart failure. Catecholamines mediate the release of glycogen, glucose, and stored fat from body cells. Therefore plasma concentrations of free fatty acids and glycerol rise within 1 hour after onset of acute myocardial infarction. Excessive levels of free fatty acids can have a harmful detergent effect on cell membranes. Norepinephrine elevates blood sugar levels through stimulation of liver and skeletal muscle cells. It also suppresses pancreatic B cell activity, which reduces insulin secretion and elevates blood glucose further. Not surprisingly, hyperglycemia is noted approximately 72 hours after an acute myocardial infarction.

Angiotensin II is released during myocardial ischemia and contributes to the pathogenesis of myocardial infarction in several ways. First, it results in the systemic effects of peripheral vasoconstriction and fluid retention. These homeostatic responses are counterproductive in that they increase myocardial work and thus exacerbate the effects of the loss of myocyte contractility. Angiotensin II is also released locally, where it is a growth factor for vascular smooth muscle cells, myocytes, and cardiac fibroblasts; promotes catecholamine release; and causes coronary artery spasm (see "What's New? The Role of Angiotensin II in Cardiovascular Disease," p. 989).[180,181,182]

Cellular death. After about 20 minutes of myocardial ischemia, irreversible hypoxic injury causes cellular death and tissue necrosis. (Types of necrosis are described in Chapter 2.) Necrosis of myocardial tissue results in the release of certain intracellular enzymes through the damaged cell membranes into the interstitial spaces. The lymphatics pick up the enzymes and transport them into the bloodstream, where they can be detected by serologic tests.

Structural and functional changes. Myocardial infarction results in both structural and functional changes of cardiac tissues (Fig. 29-22). Table 29-6 outlines the tissue changes that may follow myocardial infarction. Gross tissue

Table 29-6 Tissue Changes After Myocardial Infarction

Time After Myocardial Infarction	Tissue Changes	Stage of Healing Process
6-12 hours	No gross changes; subcellular cyanosis with decreased temperature	Not begun
18-24 hours	Pale to gray-brown; slight pallor	Inflammatory response; intercellular enzyme release
2-4 days	Visible necrosis: yellow-brown in center and hyperemic around edges	Proteolytic enzymes remove debris; catecholamines, lipolysis, and glycogenolysis elevate plasma glucose and increase free fatty acids to assist depleted myocardium recovery from anaerobic state
4-10 days	Area soft, with fatty changes in center, regions of hemorrhage in infarcted area	Debris cleared; collagen matrix laid down
10-14 days	Weak, fibrotic scar tissue with beginning revascularization	Healing continues but area very mushy, vulnerable to stress
6 wks	Scarring usually complete	Tough inelastic scar replaces necrotic myocardium

NOTE: Processes of tissue healing are described and illustrated in Chapter 7.

A 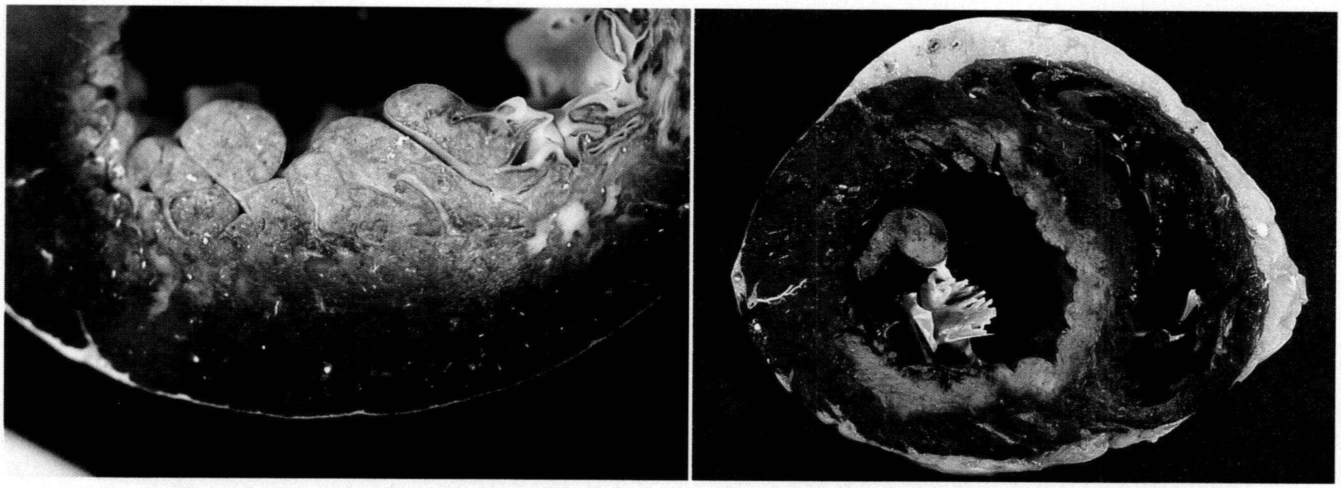 B

FIG. 29-22 Myocardial infarction. A, Local infarct confined to one region. **B,** Massive large infarct caused by occlusion of three coronary arteries. (From Damjanov I, Linder J, editors: *Anderson's pathology,* ed 10, St Louis, 1996, Mosby.)

changes in the area of infarction may not become apparent for several hours, despite almost immediate onset (within 30 to 60 seconds) of electrocardiographic changes. Cardiac tissue surrounding the area of infarction also undergoes changes that can be categorized into (1) **myocardial stunning,** a temporary loss of contractile function that persists for hours to days after perfusion has been restored; (2) **hibernating myocardium,** tissue that is persistently ischemic and undergoes metabolic adaptation to prolong myocyte survival until perfusion can be restored; and (3) **myocardial remodeling,** a process mediated by angiotensin II that causes myocyte hypertrophy and loss of contractile function in the areas of the heart distant from the site of infarction. All these changes can be limited through rapid restoration of coronary flow and the use of angiotensin-converting enzyme (ACE) inhibitors.

The severity of functional impairment depends on the size of the lesion and the site of infarction. Functional changes can include (1) decreased cardiac contractility with abnormal wall motion, (2) altered left ventricular compliance, (3) decreased stroke volume, (4) decreased ejection fraction, (5) increased left ventricular end-diastolic pressure, and (6) SA node malfunction. Life-threatening dysrhythmias and heart failure often follow myocardial infarction.

Repair. Myocardial infarction causes a severe inflammatory response that ends with wound repair (see Chapter 7). Repair consists of degradation of damaged cells, proliferation of fibroblasts, and synthesis of scar tissue. Many cell types, hormones, and nutrient substrates must be available for optimal healing to proceed. Within 24 hours, leukocytes infiltrate the necrotic area and proteolytic enzymes from scavenger neutrophils degrade necrotic tissue. A pseudodiabetic state often develops as catecholamines released from damaged cells stimulate release of glucose and free fatty acids. By the second week, insulin secretion increases to mobilize glucose from the repair processes. The collagen matrix that is deposited is initially weak, mushy, and vulnerable to reinjury. Unfortunately, it is at this time in the recovery period (10 to 14 days after infarction) that individuals feel more capable of increasing activities and may stress the newly formed scar tissue. After 6 weeks the necrotic area is completely replaced by scar tissue, which is strong but unable to contract and relax like healthy myocardial tissue.

Clinical Manifestations

The first symptom of acute myocardial infarction is usually sudden, severe chest pain. The pain is similar to that in angina pectoris but is more severe and persistent and is not relieved by nitrates. It may be described as heavy and crushing, such as a "truck sitting on my chest." Radiation to the neck, jaw, back, shoulder, or left arm is common. Some individuals (especially those who are elderly or diabetic) experience no pain, thereby having a "silent" infarction. Infarction often stimulates a sensation of unrelenting indigestion. Nausea and vomiting may occur because of reflex stimulation of vomiting centers by pain fibers. Vasovagal reflexes from the area of the infarcted myocardium also may affect the gastrointestinal tract. Catecholamine release results in sympathetic stimulation, producing diaphoresis and peripheral vasoconstriction that cause the skin to become cool and clammy. Fever may develop in the first 24 hours and persist for 1 week because of inflammatory activity within the myocardium.

A variety of cardiovascular changes may be found on physical examination. With an acute myocardial infarction, blood pressure may initially decrease. The drop in blood pressure reflexively activates the sympathetic nervous system to compensate and then causes a temporary increase in heart rate and blood pressure. Abnormal extra heart sounds (S_3, S_4) reflect left ventricular dysfunction. Inflammation can cause pericardial friction rub, along with a variety of cardiac murmurs.

Laboratory data reveal leukocytosis and elevated sedimentation rate, both of which indicate inflammation. The individual's blood sugar usually is elevated, and the glucose tolerance level may remain abnormal for several weeks.

A transient rise in plasma enzyme levels can confirm the occurrence of myocardial infarction and indicate its severity. The enzymes released by myocardial cells include creatine kinase (CK) and lactic dehydrogenase (LDH). These enzymes exist in several different active molecular forms called *isoenzymes,* which are present in different amounts within particular tissues. If serologic tests show abnormally high levels of isoenzymes associated with cardiac tissue (CK-MB, LDH_1), acute myocardial infarction probably has occurred. Of the isoenzymes, CK-MB is most specific for myocardial infarction, although its level may also increase in individuals with certain other conditions (e.g., muscular dystrophy, hypothermia, COPD associated with left heart failure and pulmonary embolism, extensive third-degree burns, small bowel infarction). Elevation of CK-MB and LDH_1 may be noted at characteristic times, and laboratory confirmation that an infarction has occurred may be delayed up to 12 hours. The cardiac troponins (troponin I and troponin T) are more specific markers for myocardial injury (see "What's New? Cardiac Troponins in the Diagnosis of Myocardial Infarction"). The amount of troponin and CK elevation may be correlated with severity of infarction. The higher the serum concentration of CK-MB and troponin is, the more extensive the tissue damage that has occurred. Blood is drawn for enzyme determinations as soon as possible after the onset of symptoms, and serial enzyme levels are assessed for several days. Three consecutive days of negative enzyme elevations rule out myocardial infarction.

Myocardial infarction can occur in various regions of the heart wall and may be described as anterior, inferior, posterior, or lateral depending on the anatomic location (Fig. 29-23). Twelve-lead ECGs help to localize the affected area through identification of Q waves and changes in ST segments and T waves (Fig. 29-24). The infarcted myocardium is surrounded by a zone of hypoxic injury, which may progress to necrosis, undergo remodeling, or return to normal. Infarcted tissue is electrically silent and does not contribute to the ECG. Transmural infarcts are large enough to create inscription of a Q wave on the ECG (Q wave infarction). Small infarcts are usually subendocardial and do not create

WHAT'S NEW? **Cardiac Troponins in the Diagnosis of Myocardial Infarction**

The diagnosis of myocardial infarction is most often made on the basis of ECG changes and the measurement of elevated levels of cardiac isoenzymes (CK-MB, LDH_1) in the blood. The cardiac isoenzymes, however, can take several hours to become positive and are relatively nonspecific in that they can also be elevated in muscle diseases, heart failure, pulmonary emboli, COPD, and other unrelated conditions. In recent years, highly sensitive enzyme immunoassays have been developed for troponin I and troponin T, which are protein subunits released from tropomyosin during myocyte injury. Unfortunately, the sensitivity of these markers for use in the diagnosis of acute MI is no better than CPK-MB. Troponin T, however, has been found to be a valuable prognostic indicator of post-MI outcome, as has Troponin I. Troponin I is more sensitive in detecting slight myocyte injury in unstable angina and is also more specific than CPK-MB for the diagnosis of acute myocardial infarction. Measurement of Troponin I is currently indicated in the initial evaluation of all individuals with chest pain suspected of myocardial ischemia.

Data from Dhond MR: Cardiac troponins, *CVR&R* 21:20, 2000; Johnson PA et al: Cardiac troponin T as a marker for myocardial ischemia in patients seen at the emergency department for acute chest pain, *Am Heart J* 137(6):1137, 1999; Rice MS, MacDonald DC: Appropriate roles of cardiac troponins in evaluating patients with chest pain, *J Amer Board Fam Practice* 12(3):214, 1999; Schuchert A et al: Prehospital testing for troponin T in patients with suspected acute myocardial infarction, *Am Heart J* 138(1 part 1):45, 1999.

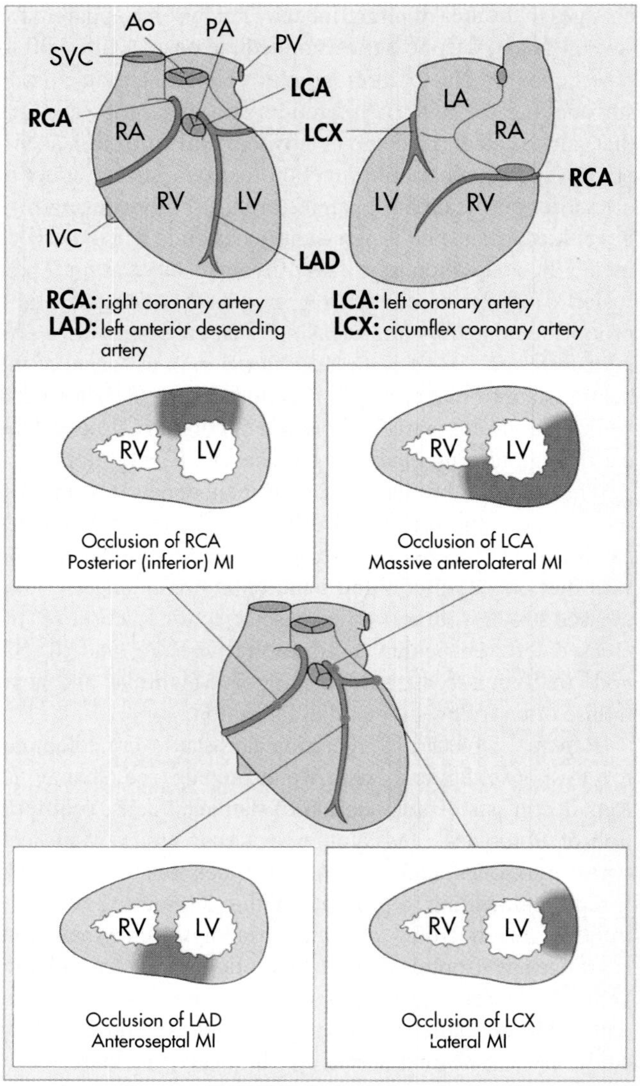

Fig. 29-23 Site of myocardial infarction *(MI)* and vessel involvement. *Ao,* Aorta; *PA,* pulmonary artery; *PV,* pulmonary vein; *LV,* left ventricle; *RV,* right ventricle; *IVC,* inferior vena cava; *RA,* right atrium; *SVC,* superior vena cava; *LA,* left atrium. (Modified from Stevens A, Lowe J: *Pathology,* St Louis, 1995, Mosby.)

a Q wave (non–Q wave infarction). Adjacent to the zone of hypoxic injury is a zone of reversible ischemia. Ischemic and injured myocardial tissue causes ST and T wave changes. As the myocardium heals, the ST segment and T waves gradually return to normal but abnormal Q waves generally persist.

Radionucleotide imaging with thallium-201 can provide a diagnostic picture in individuals with acute or healed myocardial infarction. Technetium-99m pyrophosphate is also taken up by areas of myocardial infarction, which appear as "hot spots." Unfortunately, the area of infarction must be large enough to visualize the hot spot, and the scan may remain positive for many months after infarction.

Evaluation and Treatment

The diagnosis of acute myocardial infarction is made on the basis of ECG, serial enzyme alterations, troponins, radionucleotide imaging, and physical examination (see Clinical Manifestations). Acute myocardial infarction requires immediate admission to a hospital with a coronary care unit, if possible. Aspirin should be administered to all individuals immediately on recognition of myocardial infarction (ticlopidine or clopidrogel if allergic to aspirin). Pain relief is of utmost importance and involves the use of sublingual or topical nitroglycerine and morphine sulfate. Continuous close monitoring of cardiac rhythms and enzymatic changes is especially important. The first 24 hours after onset of symptoms is the time of highest risk for sudden death. In complicated cases, invasive monitoring techniques (e.g., arterial, central venous pressure, and Swan-Ganz lines) may be required. If the infarction is diagnosed within a few hours of the onset of pain and the individual has no contraindications, thrombolytic therapy with tissue plasminogen activator (t-PA) or the newest thrombolytic, called **TNK-t-PA,** should be administered.[183,184,185] Alternatively, emergent PTCA has been shown to be as or more effective than thrombolytics, especially in those suffering from shock. PTCA with stent placement (often with the use of platelet glycoprotein IIb/IIIa receptor antagonists) is becoming the treatment of choice for many individuals with acute myocardial infarction.[15,160,186,87,188]

Bed rest, followed by gradual return to activities of daily living, reduces the myocardial oxygen demands of the compromised heart. Pain relief is of utmost importance. If sublingual nitroglycerin is ineffective, small, carefully titrated doses of morphine sulfate (4 to 6 mg) may be given for anal-

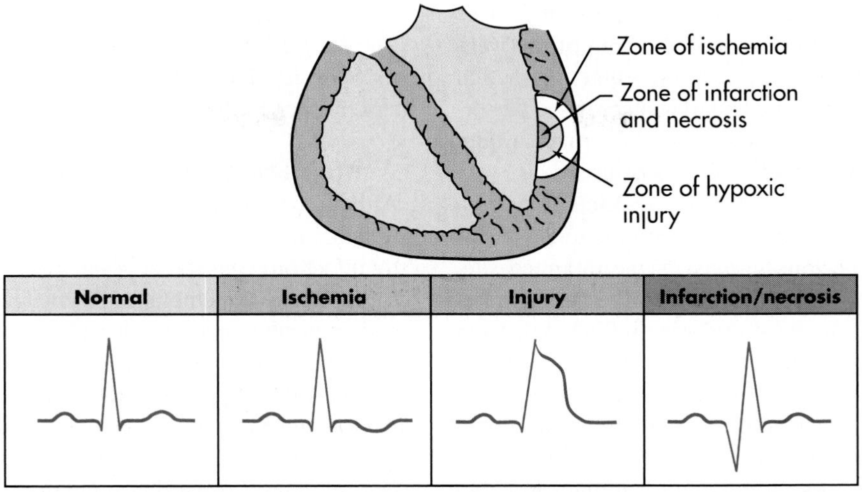

FIG. 29-24 **Electrocardiographic alterations associated with the three zones of myocardial infarction.**

gesia, sedation, and vasodilation. Supplemental oxygen (2 to 4 L/min) is administered to increase arterial oxygen content and deliver more oxygen to the ischemic myocardium. Dietary measures are aimed at preventing nausea and vomiting, and consumption of sodium, saturated fats, sugar, and caffeine is limited. Stool softeners are given to eliminate the need for straining, which can precipitate bradycardia (i.e., vasovagal response) and can be followed by increased venous return to the heart, causing possible cardiac overload.

Additional therapies that should be used in the management of acute myocardial infarction include ACE inhibitors and beta-blockers, which have been shown to improve survival and cardiac function after MI.[183,189] Risk reduction, especially lipid-lowering therapy, is important to reduce the risk of future acute coronary events.[127]

Complications

The number and severity of postinfarction complications depend on the location and extent of necrosis, the individual's physiologic condition before the infarction, and the availability of swift therapeutic intervention.

Dysrhythmias (arrhythmias), which are disturbances of cardiac rhythm, are the most common complication of acute myocardial infarction, affecting more than 90% of individuals. Dysrhythmias can be caused by ischemia, hypoxia, autonomic nervous system imbalances, lactic acidosis, electrolyte abnormalities, alterations of impulse conduction pathways or conduction defects, drug toxicity, or hemodynamic abnormalities. Dysrhythmias may originate from the atria, ventricles, nodal regions, or conduction tissues. The seriousness of dysrhythmias depends on the hemodynamic consequences. There is no ventricular contraction in ventricular fibrillation; consequently, there is no cardiac output. Atrial fibriilation, however, does not affect ventricular contraction and thus can be tolerated by most individuals. (Dysrhythmias are described on p. 1035.) Prophylactic use of antiarrhythmics, such as lidocaine and amiodarone, do not improve mortality; however, individuals at high risk should be considered for implantable cardioverter-defibrillators (ICDs).[190,191,192]

Acute myocardial infarction usually is accompanied by some degree of left ventricular failure (congestive heart failure), which is characterized by pulmonary congestion, reduced myocardial contractility, and abnormal heart wall motion (see p. 1029). Anterior infarction is associated with more severe left heart failure than is inferior infarction. Mortality from acute myocardial infarction is directly related to the reduction in stroke volume caused by the infarcted ventricle. If cardiac output is insufficient to maintain normal arterial pressure and to perfuse the kidneys and other organs adequately, cardiogenic shock develops. Cardiogenic shock characteristically develops if 40% or more of the left ventricular myocardium is infarcted. (Cardiogenic shock is discussed in Chapter 45.)

Inflammation of the pericardium (pericarditis) is a frequent complication of acute myocardial infarction. Pericardial friction rubs often are noted 2 to 3 days later, associated with anterior chest pain that worsens with respiratory effort. Specific treatment is not required; however, corticosteroids dramatically relieve symptoms.

Dressler postinfarction syndrome, which is essentially a delayed form of acute pericarditis, can occur from 1 week to several months after acute myocardial infarction. Although poorly understood, the syndrome is thought to be an immunologic (antigen-antibody) response to the necrotic myocardium. Pain, fever, friction rub, pleural effusion, and arthralgias may accompany this syndrome. Steroids may alleviate symptoms.

Organic brain syndrome may occur in acute or chronic form if blood flow to the brain is impaired secondary to myocardial infarction. Transient ischemic attacks or an outright cerebrovascular accident may result from thromboemboli that have broken loose from coronary arteries or cardiac valves.

Cardiac complications of myocardial infarction include rupture of heart structures. Necrosis of tissue in or around the papillary muscles can cause rupture of these muscles or of the chordae tendineae. Factors that lead to rupture of the free wall of the infarcted ventricle include thinning of the wall, poor collateral flow, shearing effect of muscular contraction against the stiffened necrotic area, marked necrosis at the terminal end of the blood supply, and aging of the myocardium with laceration of the myocardial microstructure.

Rupture of the wall of the infarcted ventricle may be a consequence of aneurysm formation. According to the law of Laplace, with decreased muscle mass at the infarcted site, the wall is weakened and tension stretches the noncontracting infarcted heart muscle, thus producing infarct expansion or aneurysm formation (see discussion of aneurysm, p. 994). Decreased muscle mass causes an increase in the radius of the ventricle, and because the radius is directly proportional to pressure and tension, both increase with time. The wall of the aneurysm becomes more fibrotic but continues to bulge with systole. The bulge results in impaired pump function. Although rare, rupture may occur when the tension becomes too great. Death in individuals with a left ventricular aneurysm is usually related to ventricular tachydysrhythmias and not to ventricular rupture. Left ventricular aneurysm is a late complication of myocardial infarction, occurring months or years after the acute event.

Infarctions around septal structures that separate the heart chambers can lead to septal rupture. Ruptures are associated with audible, harsh cardiac murmurs, increased left ventricular end-diastolic pressure, and decreased systemic blood pressure.

Systemic thromboembolism is commonly found during postmortem examinations of individuals who have died of myocardial infarction. Thromboemboli may disseminate from debris and clots that collect inside dilated aneurysmal sacs or from the infarcted endocardium. Pulmonary emboli are especially common, as are deep venous thrombi of the legs. Early mobilization and prophylactic anticoagulation therapy should reduce the incidence of this complication.

Sudden death resulting from cardiac arrest is often caused by dysrhythmias, particularly ventricular fibrillation. Other dysrhythmias may be equally lethal. Widespread knowledge of cardiopulmonary resuscitation has increased the probability of survival during the first few hours after cardiac insult. Immediate intervention and careful monitoring have also reduced mortality and have improved chances for long-term survival. Several factors, however, contribute to the risk of death during acute infarction or reduce the chances of long-term survival, despite the best possible treatment. They are (1) degree of left ventricular dysfunction, (2) degree of left ventricular ischemia, (3) potential for ventricular dysrhythmias, and (4) age of the individual.

DISORDERS OF THE HEART WALL

Disorders of the Pericardium

Pericardial disease is often a localized manifestation of another disorder, such as infection (bacterial, viral, fungal, rickettsial, parasitic); trauma or surgery; neoplasm; or a metabolic, immunologic, or vascular disorder (uremia, rheumatoid arthritis, systemic lupus erythematosus, periarteritis nodosa). The pericardial response to injury from these diverse causes may consist of acute pericarditis, pericardial effusion, or constrictive pericarditis.

Acute Pericarditis

Although frequently idiopathic, **acute pericarditis** (acute inflammation of the pericardium) is also commonly caused by infection, connective tissue disease, or radiation therapy. The pericardial membranes become inflamed and roughened, and an exudate may develop (Fig. 29-25).

Symptoms include sudden onset of severe chest pain that worsens with respiratory movements and with lying down. Although the pain may radiate to the back, it is generally felt in the anterior chest and may be confused initially with the pain of acute myocardial infarction. Individuals with acute pericarditis may also report dysphagia, restlessness, irritability, anxiety, weakness, and malaise.

Physical examination often discloses low-grade fever and sinus tachycardia. Friction rub—a short, scratchy, grating sensation similar to the sound of sandpaper—may be heard at the cardiac apex and left sternal border and is pathognomonic for pericarditis. The rub is caused by the roughened pericardial membranes rubbing against each other. Friction rubs are not always present and may be intermittently heard. ECG changes may reflect inflammatory processes through diffuse ST segment elevation without Q waves. The ECG may remain abnormal for days or even weeks.[193] Echocardiography may reveal a small pericardial effusion.[194]

Treatment for uncomplicated acute pericarditis consists of relieving symptoms. Analgesics are given to relieve pain, but doses are limited to avoid excessive respiratory depression in individuals who are already limiting respiratory effort because of pain. Salicylates and nonsteroidal antiinflammatory drugs reduce inflammation. Corticosteroids may diminish symptoms, but rebound pain may occur after the steroids are

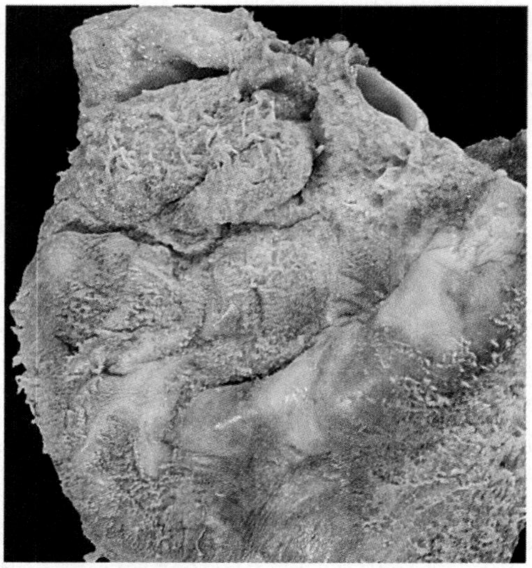

FIG. 29-25 Acute pericarditis. Note shaggy coat of fibers covering surface of heart. (From Damjanov I, Linder J: *Pathology: a color atlas,* St Louis, 2000, Mosby.)

discontinued. Rest is helpful during episodes of acute pain. Exploration of the underlying cause is important. If pericardial effusion develops, aspiration of the excessive fluid may be necessary. Acute pericarditis is usually self-limiting but occasionally may progress to chronic constrictive pericarditis.

Pericardial Effusion

Pericardial effusion—the accumulation of fluid in the pericardial cavity—can occur in all forms of pericarditis. The fluid may be a transudate, such as the serous effusion that develops with left heart failure, overhydration, or hypoproteinemia. More often, however, the fluid is an exudate, which reflects pericardial injury and inflammation (Fig. 29-26). (Types of exudate are described in Chapter 7.) If the fluid is serosanguineous, the underlying cause is likely to be tuberculosis, neoplasm, uremia, or radiation. Idiopathic serosanguineous (cause unknown) effusion is possible, however. Effusions of frank blood are generally related to aneurysms, trauma, or coagulation defects. If chyle leaks from the thoracic duct, it may enter the pericardium and lead to cholesterol pericarditis.

Pericardial effusion, even in large amounts, is not necessarily clinically significant, except that it indicates an underlying disorder. The important consideration is whether the fluid creates sufficient pressure to cause cardiac compression, which is a serious condition known as **tamponade.** If an effusion develops gradually, the pericardium can stretch to accommodate large quantities of fluid without compressing the heart. If the fluid accumulates rapidly, however, even a small amount (50 to 100 ml) may cause serious tamponade. The danger is that pressure exerted by the pericardial fluid eventually will equal diastolic pressure within the heart chambers. The first structures to be affected by tamponade are the right atrium and ventricle, where diastolic pressures are normally lowest. Compression by pericardial fluid interferes with right atrial filling during diastole, resulting in increased venous pressure, systemic venous congestion, and signs and symptoms of right heart failure (distention of the jugular veins, edema, hepatomegaly). Decreased atrial filling leads to decreased ventricular filling, decreased stroke volume, and reduced cardiac output. Life-threatening circulatory collapse may occur.

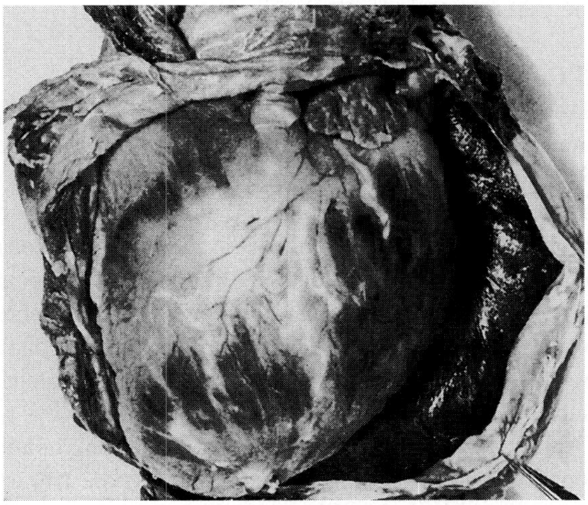

FIG. 29-26 Exudate of blood in the pericardial sac from rupture of aneurysm. (From Anderson WAD, Scotti TM: *Synopsis of pathology,* ed 10, St Louis, 1980, Mosby.)

The most significant clinical finding is pulsus paradoxus, in which arterial blood pressure during expiration exceeds arterial pressure during inspiration by more than 10 mm Hg. Pulsus paradoxus indicates tamponade. This clinical finding reflects impairment of diastolic filling of the left ventricle plus reduction of blood volume within all four cardiac chambers. Presence of a large pericardial effusion or tamponade magnifies the normally insignificant effect of inspiration on intracardiac flow and volume.

Other clinical manifestations of pericardial effusion are distant or muffled heart sounds, poorly palpable apical pulse, dyspnea on exertion, and dull chest pain. A chest roentgenogram may disclose a "water-bottle" configuration of the cardiac silhouette. An echocardiogram can detect an effusion as small as 20 ml and is considered the most accurate and reliable method of diagnosis.

Treatment of pericardial effusion or tamponade generally consists of pericardiocentesis (aspiration of excessive pericardial fluid). Pericardiocentesis is both diagnostic and therapeutic: the fluid is analyzed to identify the cause of the effusion, and its removal alone may bring dramatic relief from symptoms. Persistent pain may be treated with analgesics, antiinflammatory medications, or steroids. Surgery may be required if the underlying cause of tamponade is trauma or aneurysm.

Individuals with acute pericarditis secondary to certain underlying conditions may have pericardial effusion. This manifestation is common in (1) individuals with uremia who are in need of dialysis and have fluid overload and left ventricular failure; (2) individuals who have lymphoma or breast cancer or who are receiving radiation therapy; (3) individuals who are taking drugs such as procainamide and minoxidil; and (4) individuals who have undergone surgery that involved an incision of the heart wall. If an effusion is neoplasm induced, chemotherapeutic agents may be injected into the pericardial space. Triamcinolone also may be injected into the pericardium to induce pericardial sclerosis and prevent further fluid accumulation.[195]

Constrictive Pericarditis

Constrictive pericarditis or **restrictive pericarditis** (chronic pericarditis) was synonymous with tuberculosis years ago (Fig. 29-27). Currently in the United States, this form of pericardial disease is more often idiopathic or associated with radiation exposure, rheumatoid arthritis, uremia, or coronary artery bypass graft. In constrictive pericarditis, fibrous scarring with occasional calcification of the pericardium causes the visceral and parietal pericardial layers to adhere, obliterating the pericardial cavity. The fibrotic lesions encase the heart in a rigid shell. Like tamponade, constrictive pericarditis compresses the heart and eventually reduces cardiac output. Unlike tamponade, however, constrictive pericarditis never develops suddenly.

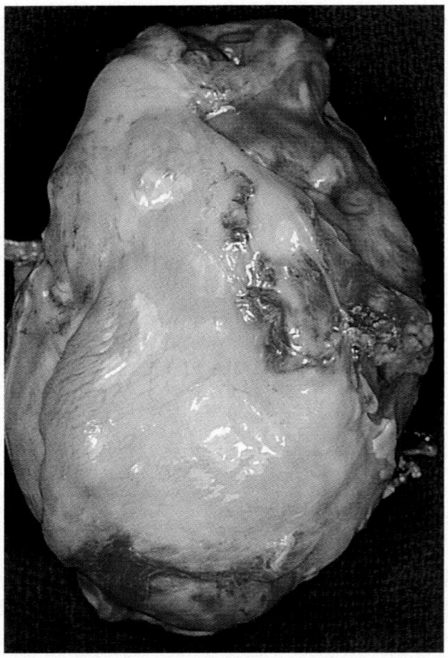

Fig. 29-27 Constrictive pericarditis. The fibrotic pericardium encases the heart in a rigid shell. (From Damjanov I, Linder J: *Pathology: a color atlas,* St Louis, 2000, Mosby.)

Because the onset of constrictive pericarditis is gradual, clinical manifestations seldom include pulsus paradoxus. Symptoms tend to be exercise intolerance, dyspnea on exertion, fatigue, and anorexia. Clinical assessment shows weight loss, edema, distention of the jugular vein, and hepatic congestion. Restricted ventricular filling may cause a pericardial knock (early diastolic sound).

ECG findings include T wave inversions and atrial fibrillation. An echocardiogram may suggest evidence of nonspecific pericardial thickening. CT is best able to detect constrictive processes. Chest roentgenograms frequently disclose prominent pulmonary vessels and calcification of the pericardium. Some individuals require diagnostic thoracotomy in order to make the diagnosis, especially in cases of postoperative restrictive pericarditis.[196]

Initial treatment for constrictive pericarditis is pharmacologic and dietary. Digitalis glycosides, diuretics, and sodium restriction are often prescribed. If these modalities are not successful, surgical excision of the restrictive pericardium is indicated. After surgery, most individuals exhibit significant improvement. For individuals with severe restrictive disease, pericardiectomy may prevent untimely death from heart failure.

Disorders of the Myocardium: The Cardiomyopathies

The **cardiomyopathies** are a diverse group of diseases that primarily affect the myocardium itself. Most are the result of underlying cardiovascular disorders, such as ischemic heart disease or hypertension. Cardiomyopathies can also be secondary to infectious disease, exposure to toxins, systemic connective tissue disease, infiltrative and proliferative disorders, or nutritional deficiencies. Despite this large number of possible causes, most cases of cardiomyopathy are idiopathic; that is, their cause is unknown. The cardiomyopathies are categorized as dilated, hypertrophic, restrictive, or obliterative, depending on their hemodynamic effects (Fig. 29-28 and Table 29-7). An individual may display characteristics of more than one type.

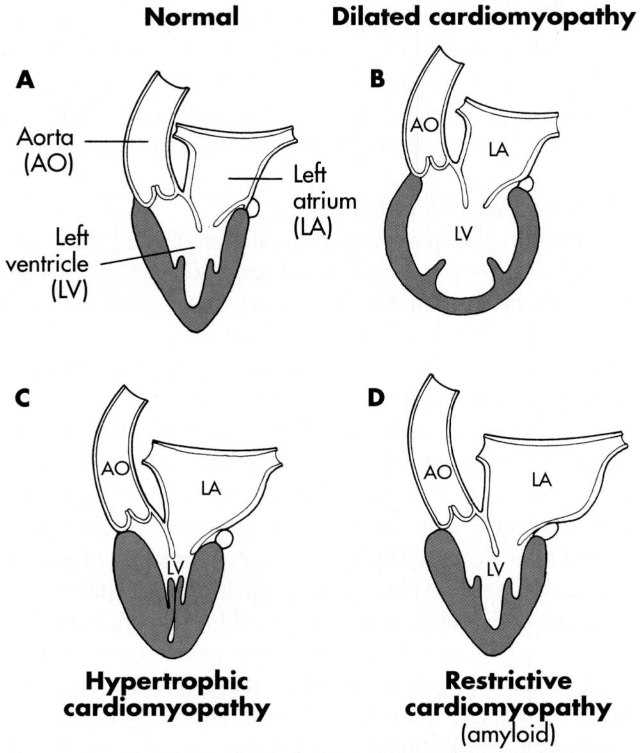

Fig. 29-28 Diagram showing major distinguishing pathophysiologic features of the types of cardiomyopathy. A, The normal heart. **B,** In the dilated type of cardiomyopathy, the heart has a globular shape and the largest circumference of the left ventricle is not at its base but midway between apex and base. **C,** In the hypertrophic type the wall of the left ventricle is greatly thickened; the left ventricular cavity is small, but the left atrium may be dilated because of poor diastolic relaxation of the ventricle. **D,** In the restrictive type the left ventricular cavity is of normal size but, again, the left atrium is dilated because of the reduced diastolic compliance of the ventricle. (From Kissane JM, editor: *Anderson's pathology,* ed 9, St Louis, 1990, Mosby.)

Dilated Cardiomyopathy

Dilated cardiomyopathy (congestive cardiomyopathy) is characterized by ventricular dilation and grossly impaired systolic function, leading to dilated heart failure (Fig. 29-29). The most common causes are ischemic heart disease or valvular heart disease. The basic problem is diminished myocardial contractility, which is reflected in diminished systolic performance of the heart. Dilated cardiomyopathy causes decreased ejection fractions, increased end-diastolic and residual volumes, decreased ventricular stroke volume, and biventricular failure.

About one half of the cases of dilated cardiomyopathy are idiopathic, and the remainder result from some known disease process. Idiopathic dilated cardiomyopathy has a familial origin in 20% to 30% of cases, although the specific genes are yet to be identified.[197,198] Autoimmune processes also have

Table 29-7 Effects of Cardiomyopathies on Circulation Through the Heart

	Type of Cardiomyopathy		
Effect	**Dilated**	**Hypertrophic**	**Restrictive**
HEMODYNAMIC			
Cardiac output	Decreased	Normal	Normal or decreased
Stroke volume	Decreased	Normal or increased	Decreased
Ventricular filling pressure	Increased	Normal or increased	Increased
Ejection fraction	Decreased	Increased	Normal or decreased
Inflow resistance	Normal	Increased	Increased
Outflow tract obstruction	None	Increased	None
Formation of intracardiac thrombi	Increased	None	Increased
STRUCTURAL OR FUNCTIONAL			
Chamber size	Increased	Normal or decreased	Decreased or normal
Myocardial mass	Increased	Increased	Normal or increased
Endocardial thickness	Normal or increased	Increased	Increased
Contractility	Decreased	Increased or decreased	Normal or decreased
Mitral valve competence	Decreased	Decreased	Decreased

Data from DeSanctis RW: *Sci Am Med* 1(1-XIV):1, 1990; Wenger NK, Ablemann WH, Roberts WC. In Hurst JW et al, editors: *The heart, arteries, and veins,* ed 7, New York, 1990, McGraw-Hill.

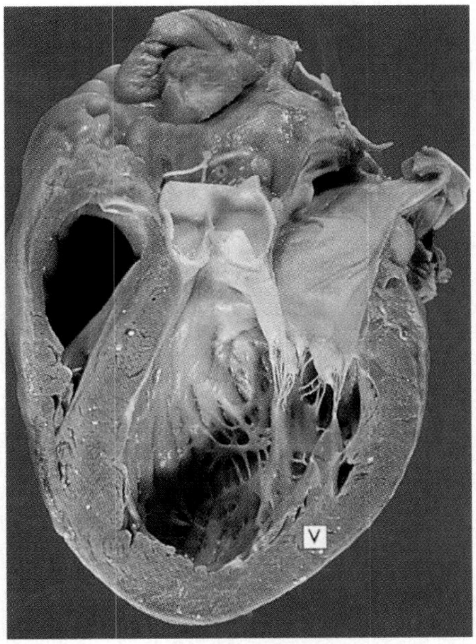

FIG. 29-29 Dilated cardiomyopathy. The dilated left ventricle has a thin wall *(V).* (From Stevens A, Lowe J: *Pathology,* St Louis, 1995, Mosby.)

been implicated.[199] Serious myocardial damage can result from certain drugs used in cancer chemotherapy, especially doxorubicin and daunorubicin. Cardiotoxicity increases with dosage, and the severity of the toxic reaction is directly related to the cumulative dose. Recurrent ischemia without infarction has been implicated as a cause of dilated cardiomyopathy, but the most common cause is heart failure resulting from extensive or recurrent myocardial infarction.

A disproportionate number of individuals with idiopathic dilated cardiomyopathy are alcoholics. Heavy consumption of alcohol is thought to cause cardiomyopathy through three mechanisms: (1) a direct toxic effect of alcohol or of its metabolites; (2) effects of nutritional deficits, especially thiamine deficiency; and (3) toxic effects of beverage additives such as cobalt. In addition, chronic alcoholic cardiomyopathy may be related to underlying viral infection.[200] In contrast to other forms of cardiomyopathy, the progression of myocardial dysfunction may be stopped or reversed if alcohol consumption is reduced or stopped early in the course of the disease.

Peripartum cardiomyopathy is another idiopathic form of dilated cardiomyopathy. The cardiomyopathy usually develops in the first 3 to 4 months after completion of a pregnancy, after the period of maximum physiologic stress is thought to have ended.[201] A few cases have resulted from acute myocardial inflammation (myocarditis).

A third group of dilated cardiomyopathies may be the late consequences of previous viral, bacterial, or parasitic infections or an autoimmune process. Endocardial biopsies have shown that a significant number of these cases also involve active myocarditis. The implications of these findings remain unclear. (Pathophysiologic effects of the cardiomyopathies are summarized in Table 29-8.)

The most common symptoms of dilated cardiomyopathy are dyspnea and fatigue. Pulmonary congestion is expected, but acute pulmonary edema is not. Palpitations are common, and associated dysrhythmias may cause dizziness (syncope). Systemic and pulmonary emboli are common complications. Chest pain may be present, but it is unlike anginal pain.

In the presence of dilated heart failure, blood pressure is often elevated. Extra heart sounds and cardiac murmurs may be present as well. Dilated cardiomyopathy may be difficult to distinguish from acute myocarditis, valvular heart disease, CAD, and hypertensive heart disease.

Treatment for dilated cardiomyopathy consists of salt restriction and the prescription of digitalis glycosides, vasodilators, and diuretics. Anticoagulants are given to prevent

Table 29-8 Pathophysiologic Effects of the Cardiomyopathies

	Type of Cardiomyopathy		
Pathophysiology	**Dilated**	**Hypertrophic**	**Restrictive**
Major symptoms	Fatigue, weakness, palpitations	Dyspnea, angina pectoris, fatigue, dizziness (syncope), palpitations	Dyspnea, fatigue
Cardiomegaly	Moderate to marked	Mild to moderate	Mild
Hypertrophy	Left ventricular myocardium	Left ventricular myocardium and interventricular septum	Left ventricular myocardium
Alterations of chamber volume	Volume increased	Volume decreased, particularly in left ventricle	Volume normal to decreased
Alterations of chamber compliance	Compliance increased	Compliance decreased, particularly in left ventricle	Compliance decreased, particularly in left ventricle
Alterations of systolic function (myocardial contractility)	Contractility decreased in left ventricle	Contractility increased or vigorous	None
Valvular incompetence	Atrioventricular valves, particularly mitral	Mitral valve	Atrioventricular valve
Conduction defects	Intraventricular	Nonspecific	Atrioventricular
Dysrhythmias	Sinoatrial tachycardia; atrial and ventricular dysrhythmias	Atrial and ventricular dysrhythmias	Tachydysrhythmias
Thromboembolism	Systemic or pulmonary	Systemic or pulmonary	Systemic or pulmonary
Associated conditions	Alcoholism, pregnancy, infection, nutritional deficiency, exposure to toxins	Possible inherited defect of muscle growth and development	Infiltrative disease
Eventual cardiovascular event	Left heart failure	Left heart failure	Right heart failure

pulmonary and systemic embolism. Bed rest for extended periods can be used to reduce the workload of the weakened heart. Corticosteroids and immunosuppressants can benefit individuals with documented inflammatory disease, and vasodilators are administered to combat congestion. Venous dilation reduces preload by promoting peripheral venous pooling, thereby decreasing central blood volume and alleviating pulmonary congestion. Arterial dilation reduces afterload and aortic impedance, making it easier for the failing left ventricle to eject blood. Combinations of these drugs have been effective in improving symptoms, although there is no indication that they prolong life. Myocardial pacemakers (pacing) can improve cardiac output in many individuals.[202]

The prognosis is variable and depends on the degree of ventricular dysfunction. Left heart failure is the cause of death in 75% of individuals. Sudden death caused by dysrhythmias also occurs. The majority of deaths occur within 5 years.

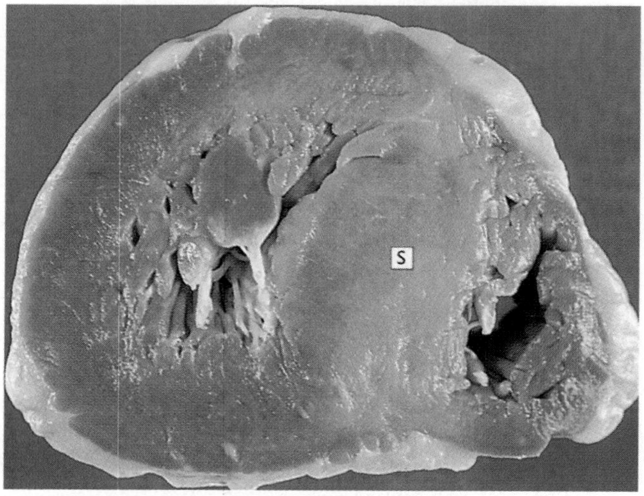

FIG. 29-30 Hypertrophic cardiomyopathy. There is marked left ventricular hypertrophy. This often affects the septum *(S)*. (From Stevens A, Lowe J: *Pathology,* St Louis, 1995, Mosby.)

Hypertrophic Cardiomyopathy

Hypertrophic cardiomyopathy is most commonly the result of hypertension or valvular heart disease and is mediated by Ang II (see p. 988, and "What's New? Role of Angiotensin II in Cardiovascular Disease," on p. 989). Asymmetric septal hypertrophy, muscular subaortic stenosis, and idiopathic hypertrophic subaortic stenosis are all names for another form of hypertrophic cardiomyopathy that causes asymmetric thickening of the myocardium. An autosomal dominant inheritance has been linked to this disorder. Although its origin is unknown, the basic abnormality appears to reside in the contractile elements of the heart muscle. The hallmark of hypertrophic cardiomyopathy is disproportionate thickening of the interventricular septum (Fig. 29-30). There is disorganization of the septal muscle cells and greater hypertrophy of the ventricular septum than of the ventricular chambers. Thus, externally the heart may appear to be of normal size. Additional pathologic changes include abnormalities of collagen deposition and altered contractile proteins in the myocytes.[203,204]

Thickening of the septum results in a hyperdynamic state, with subsequent increased myocardial contractility and ejection fraction. In some individuals, contractility is actually decreased.[205] Diastolic relaxation is impaired and ventricular compliance is decreased (increased stiffness). If the septum is asymmetrically enlarged, it actually may obstruct left ventricular outflow and result in decreased cardiac output. Under these circumstances, any condition or medication that increases contractility also increases the degree of obstruction. For example, nitroglycerin aggravates obstruction by increasing the heart rate, decreasing chamber size, and decreasing blood pressure (afterload). Hypertrophic cardiomyopathy is associated with sudden onset of ventricular tachycardia or fibrillation and sudden death.

Major clinical manifestations of hypertrophic cardiomyopathy are angina, syncope, palpitations, and left heart failure. Myocardial infarction can occur if the hypertrophied myocardium outgrows its blood supply. Dysrhythmias are common, and extra heart sounds and murmurs are not unusual. Electrocardiography discloses left ventricular hypertrophy and dysrhythmias if any are present. Echocardiograms and cardiac catheterization are used to confirm the diagnosis.

Beta-blockers, such as propranolol, are favored for initial therapy because they may decrease left ventricular stiffness and reduce the heart rate enough to permit a longer time for ventricular filling. Verapamil has proved effective, but the other calcium antagonists have not been consistently shown to be beneficial. Surgical resection of the hypertrophic tissue may be done to relieve symptoms in individuals who do not respond to pharmacologic therapy. The prophylactic placement of an implantable cardioverter-defibrillator can reduce the incidence of sudden death in high-risk individuals.[206] Although the course and prognosis of hypertrophic cardiomyopathy vary, long-term survival is expected.

Restrictive Cardiomyopathies

Restrictive cardiomyopathy usually is caused by an infiltrative disease of the myocardium, such as amyloidosis, hemochromatosis, or glycogen storage disease. The myocardium becomes rigid and noncompliant, impeding ventricular filling and raising filling pressures during diastole. The overall clinical and hemodynamic picture mimics and may be confused with that of constrictive pericarditis.

The most common clinical manifestation of restrictive cardiomyopathy is congestive heart failure, particularly right heart failure. Cardiomegaly and dysrhythmias are common. In most cases there is no therapy for restrictive cardiomyopathy other than treating the underlying disease process. Death occurs as a result of congestive failure or dysrhythmias.

Disorders of the Endocardium

Valvular Dysfunction

Disorders of the endocardium, the innermost lining of the heart wall, all damage the heart valves, which are made up of endocardial tissue. Endocardial damage can be either congenital or acquired. The acquired forms cause inflammatory, ischemic, traumatic, degenerative, or infectious alterations of valvular structure and function.

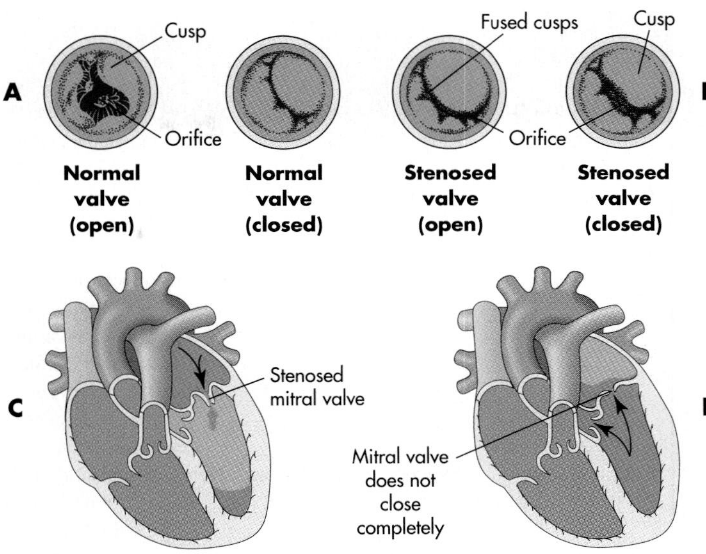

FIG. 29-31 Valvular stenosis and regurgitation. A, Normal position of the valve leaflets, or cusps, when the valve is open and closed. **B,** Open position of a stenosed valve *(left)* and open position of a closed regurgitant valve *(right)*. **C,** Hemodynamic effect of mitral stenosis. The stenosed valve is unable to open sufficiently during left atrial systole, inhibiting left ventricular filling. **D,** Hemodynamic effect of mitral regurgitation. The mitral valve does not close completely during left ventricular systole, permitting blood to reenter the left atrium.

The usual cause of acquired valvular dysfunction is inflammation of the endocardium secondary to acute rheumatic fever or infective endocarditis (see p. 1027). Structural alterations of the heart valves lead to stenosis, incompetence, or both.

In **valvular stenosis** the valve orifice is constricted and narrowed, impeding the forward flow of blood and increasing the workload of the cardiac chamber "behind" the diseased valve (Fig. 29-31). Intraventricular or atrial pressure increases in the chamber to overcome resistance to flow through the valve. Increased pressure causes the myocardium to work harder, causing myocardial hypertrophy. In **valvular regurgitation** (also called insufficiency or incompetence) the valve leaflets, or cusps, fail to shut completely, permitting blood flow to continue even when the valve is supposed to be closed (see Fig. 29-31). During systole some blood leaks back into the atrial chamber "upstream." Valvular regurgitation increases the volume of blood the heart must pump and increases the workload of both atrium and ventricle. Valvular incompetence causes cardiomegaly. Increased volume leads to chamber dilation, and increased workload leads to hypertrophy. Although all four heart valves may be affected, those of the left heart (mitral and aortic semilunar valves) are far more commonly affected than those of the right heart (tricuspid and pulmonic semilunar valves).

Valvular dysfunction stimulates chamber dilation and myocardial hypertrophy, both of which are compensatory mechanisms intended to increase the pumping capability of the heart. Eventually, myocardial contractility is diminished, the ejection fraction is reduced, diastolic pressure increases, and the ventricles fail from overwork. Depending on the severity of the valvular dysfunction and the capacity of the

Table 29-9 Clinical Manifestations of Valvular Stenosis and Regurgitation

Manifestation	Aortic Stenosis	Mitral Stenosis	Aortic Regurgitation	Mitral Regurgitation	Tricuspid Regurgitation
Cardiovascular outcome*	Left ventricular failure	Right ventricular failure	Left heart failure	Left heart failure	Right heart failure
General symptoms	Fatigue	Fatigue, weakness		Fatigue, weakness	Peripheral edema (with heart failure)
Respiratory effects	Dyspnea on exertion	Dyspnea on exertion, orthopnea, paroxysmal nocturnal dyspnea, predisposition to respiratory infections, hemoptysis, pulmonary hypertension, edema	Dyspnea with effort	Dyspnea; occasional hemoptysis	Dyspnea
Central nervous system effects	Syncope, especially on exertion	Neural deficits only associated with emboli (e.g., hemiparesis)	Syncope	None	None
Gastrointestinal effects	None	Ascites; hepatic angina with hepatomegaly	None	None	Ascites, hepatomegaly (with heart failure)
Pain	Angina pectoris	Chest pain	Chest pain (anginal)	None	Palpitations
Heart rate, rhythm	Bradycardia, dysrhythmias (with heart failure)	Palpitations (atrial fibrillation)	Palpitations, water-hammer pulse	Palpitations	Atrial fibrillations
Heart sounds	Systolic murmur	Diastolic murmur, accentuated first heart sound, opening snap	Diastolic and systolic murmurs	Murmur throughout systole	Murmur throughout systole
Most common cause	Congenital, rheumatic fever	Rheumatic fever	Bacterial endocarditis; aortic root disease	Floppy valve; coronary artery disease	Congenital

Data from Braunwald E, editor: *Heart disease: a textbook of cardiovascular medicine,* ed 4, Philadelphia, 1992, W.B. Saunders; Hancock EW: *Sci Am Med* 1(1-XIII):1, 1996.

*Untreated disease.

heart to compensate, valvular alterations cause a range of symptoms and some degree of incapacitation (Table 29-9). The effects of valvular dysfunction are treated with cardiac glycosides, diuretics, dietary salt restriction, and antibiotics until prosthetic valve replacement becomes necessary.

Stenosis

Aortic stenosis. **Aortic stenosis** has three common causes: (1) inflammatory damage caused by rheumatic heart disease, (2) congenital malformation (see Chapter 3), and (3) degeneration thickening and calcification (see Chapter 2). The orifice of the aortic semilunar valve narrows, causing diminished blood flow from the left ventricle into the aorta (Figs. 29-31 and 29-32). Outflow obstruction increases pressure within the left ventricle as it tries to eject blood through the narrowed opening.

Aortic stenosis tends to develop gradually. Clinical manifestations include decreased stroke volume, reduced systolic blood pressure, and narrowed pulse pressure (difference between systolic and diastolic pressure). Heart rate is often slow, and pulses are faint. Resistance to flow gives rise to a crescendo-decrescendo systolic heart murmur. Left ventricular hypertrophy develops to compensate for the increased workload. Eventually, hypertrophy increases myocardial oxygen demand, which the coronary arteries may not be able to supply. If this occurs, ischemia may cause attacks of angina. Untreated aortic stenosis can lead to dysrhythmias, myocardial infarction, and heart failure. Most symptoms of aortic stenosis are attributable to diminished stroke volume, which results in diminished tissue perfusion.

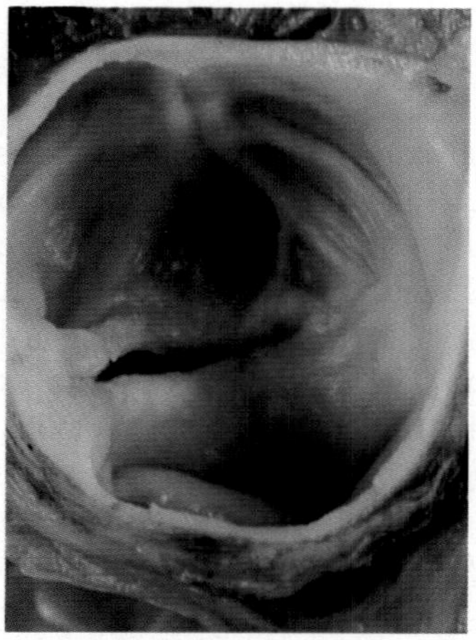

FIG. 29-32 Aortic stenosis. Mild stenosis in valve leaflets of a young adult. (From Damjanov I, Linder J: *Pathology: a color atlas,* St Louis, 2000, Mosby.)

Mitral stenosis. **Mitral stenosis** impairs the flow of blood from the left atrium to the left ventricle. Mitral stenosis is caused most commonly by acute rheumatic fever or bacterial endocarditis, although uncommonly it can be congenital. Narrowing of the orifice occurs as inflammatory lesions in the valvular leaflets heal (Fig. 29-33). Scarring causes the leaflets to become fibrous and fused and the chordae tendineae to become shortened.

Clinical manifestations depend on the size of the valvular orifice. As in aortic stenosis, impedance to blood flow results in incomplete emptying of the left atrium and elevated atrial pressure, as the chamber tries to force blood through the stenotic valve. Continued increases in left atrial volume and pressure cause chamber dilation and hypertrophy. The risk of developing atrial dysrhythmias (especially fibrillation) and dysrhythmia-induced thrombi is high. As mitral stenosis progresses, symptoms of decreased cardiac output occur, especially during exertion. Continued elevation of left atrial pressure and volume causes pressure to rise in the pulmonary circulation. The outcomes of untreated chronic mitral stenosis are pulmonary hypertension, edema, and right ventricular failure.

Atrial enlargement is demonstrated by chest roentgenograms and electrocardiography. Blood flow through the stenotic valve gives rise to a rumbling decrescendo diastolic murmur. The first heart sound (S_1) is often accentuated and somewhat delayed because of increased left atrial pressure. Other signs and symptoms are generally those of pulmonary congestion and right heart failure.

Regurgitation

Aortic regurgitation. **Aortic regurgitation** is caused by a variety of disorders that affect the valve cusps and aortic root, such as rheumatic fever, bacterial endocarditis, syphilis, hypertension, connective tissue disorders (e.g., Marfan syndrome), and atherosclerosis. The hemodynamic repercussions depend on the size of the "leak." During systole, blood is ejected from the left ventricle into the aorta. If the aortic semilunar valve fails to close completely, some of the ejected blood flows back into the left ventricle. Volume overload occurs in the ventricle because it receives blood from the left atrium during diastole and blood from the aorta during systole. Over time, the end-diastolic volume of the left ventricle increases and myocardial fibers stretch to accommodate the extra fluid. Compensatory dilation permits the left ventricle to increase its stroke volume and maintain cardiac output. Ventricular dilation and hypertrophy eventually cease to compensate for aortic incompetence, and heart failure develops.

Clinical manifestations include widened pulse pressure resulting from increased stroke volume and backflow. Turbulence across the aortic valve during diastole produces a characteristic murmur. Large stroke volume and rapid runoff of blood from the aorta result in prominent carotid pulsations and throbbing peripheral pulses (water-hammer pulse). Other symptoms are usually associated with heart failure that occurs when the ventricle can no longer enlarge. Dysrhythmias and endocarditis are common complications of aortic regurgitation.

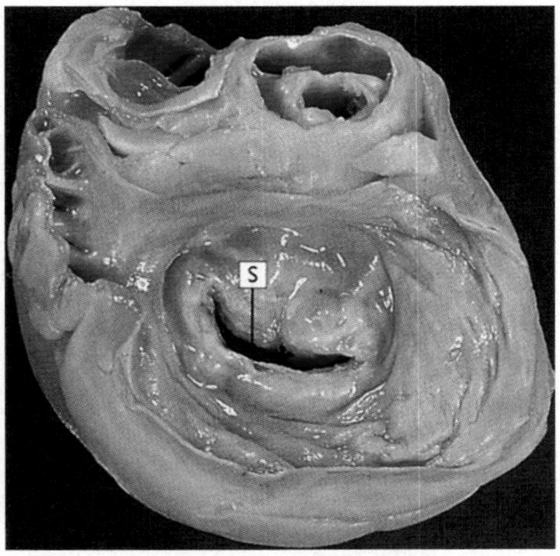

FIG. 29-33 Mitral stenosis with classic "fish mouth" orifice. (From Stevens A, Lowe J: *Pathology,* ed 2, London, 2000, Mosby.)

Mitral regurgitation. **Mitral regurgitation,** unlike mitral stenosis, has a variety of causes. It is common in the general population, occurring in up to 19% of healthy men and women.[207] The most common are mitral valve prolapse and rheumatic heart disease. Other causes include infective endocarditis, CAD, connective tissue diseases (Marfan syndrome), and congestive cardiomyopathy. Mitral regurgitation permits backflow of blood from the left ventricle into the left atrium during ventricular systole, giving rise to a loud pansystolic (throughout systole) murmur that radiates into the back and axilla. The left ventricle becomes dilated and hypertrophied to maintain adequate cardiac output, despite increased volume from the left atrium. The volume of backflow reentering the left atrium gradually increases, causing atrial dilation. As the left atrium enlarges, the valve structures stretch and become deformed, leading to further backflow. As mitral valve regurgitation progresses, left ventricular function may become impaired to the point of failure. Eventually, increased atrial pressure also causes pulmonary hypertension and failure of the right ventricle. Mitral incompetence is usually well tolerated—often for years—until ventricular failure occurs. Most clinical manifestations are caused by heart failure.

Tricuspid regurgitation. **Tricuspid regurgitation** is more common than tricuspid stenosis and usually is associated with cardiac failure and dilation of the right ventricle secondary to high blood pressure in the pulmonary circulation or right ventricle. Rheumatic heart disease and infective endocarditis are less common causes. Tricuspid valve incompetence leads to volume overload in the right ventricle, increased systemic venous blood pressure, and right heart failure. Pulmonic semilunar valve dysfunction can have the same consequences as tricuspid valve dysfunction.

Mitral Valve Prolapse Syndrome

Mitral valve prolapse syndrome is a condition in which the anterior and posterior cusps of the mitral valve billow upward (prolapse) into the atrium during systole (Fig. 29-34). The cusps are enlarged, thickened, and scalloped, possibly secondary to collagenous abnormalities, and the chordae tendineae may be elongated, permitting the valve cusps to stretch

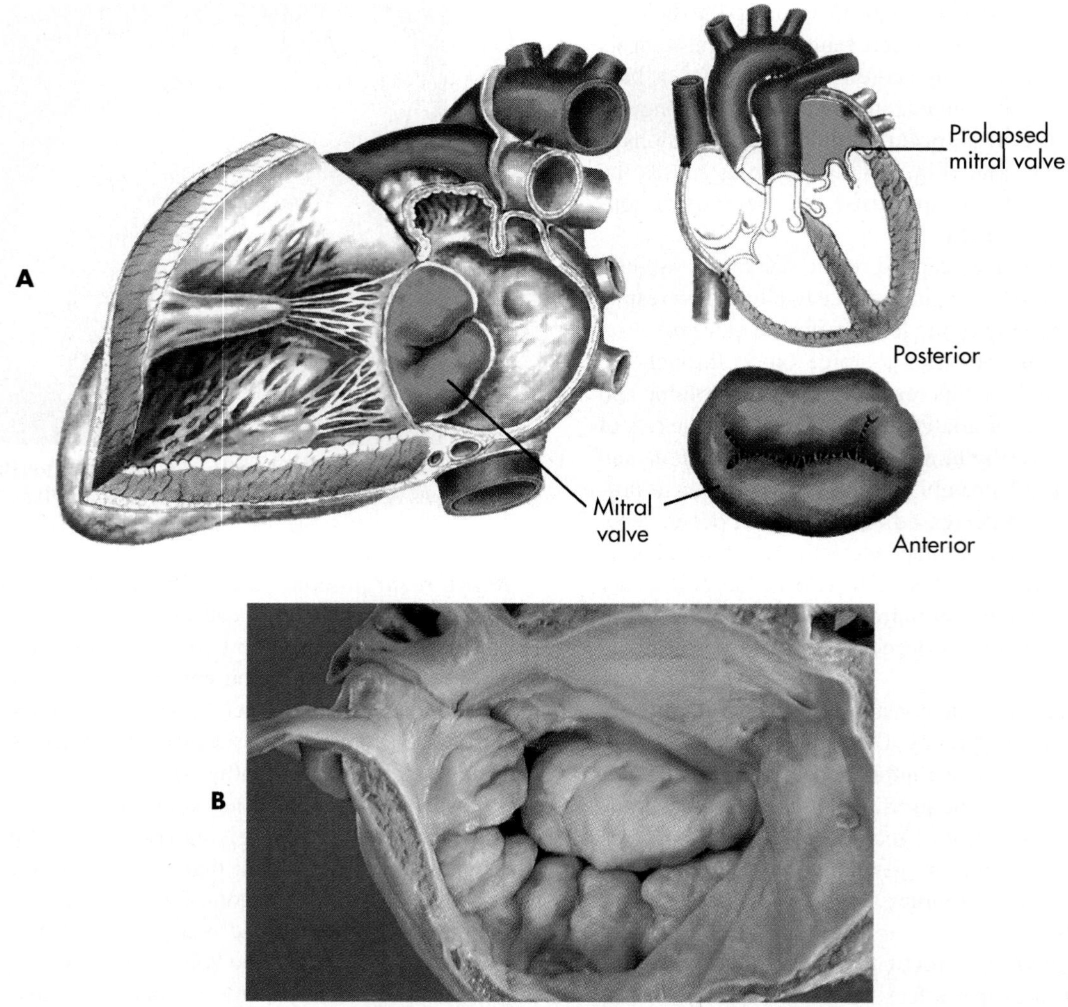

FIG 29-34 Mitral valve prolapse. A, Normal mitral valve *(lower right)* and prolapsed mitral valve *(left)*. Prolapse permits the valve leaflets to billow back into the atrium during left ventricular systole. The billowing causes the leaflets to part slightly, permitting regurgitation into the atrium. **B,** Looking down on the mitral valve, the ballooning of the leaflets is seen. (B from Stevens A, Lowe J: *Pathology,* St Louis, 1995, Mosby.)

upward. Mitral regurgitation occurs if the ballooning valve permits blood to leak into the atrium.

Although previous studies have suggested that the prevalence of mitral valve prolapse may be as high as 5% to 35%, a recent study suggests it is much less common (less than 3%).[208] Mitral valve prolapse tends to be most prevalent in young women. Studies suggest an autosomal dominant inheritance pattern. Because mitral valve prolapse often is associated with other inherited connective tissue disorders (Marfan syndrome, Ehlers-Danlos syndrome, osteogenesis imperfecta), it may result from a genetic or environmental disruption of valvular development during the fifth or sixth week of gestation. There may be a relationship between symptomatic mitral valve prolapse and hyperthyroidism. Other neuroendocrine abnormalities have been suggested, including polymorphisms of the Ang II type 1 (AT_1) receptor.[209]

Many cases of mitral valve prolapse are completely asymptomatic. Cardiac auscultation on routine physical examination may disclose a regurgitant murmur or midsystolic click in an otherwise healthy individual, or echocardiography may demonstrate the condition in the absence of auscultatory findings. Symptomatic mitral valve prolapse can cause palpitations related to dysrhythmias, tachycardia, light-headedness, syncope, fatigue (especially in the morning), lethargy, weakness, dyspnea, chest tightness, hyperventilation, anxiety, depression, panic attacks, and atypical chest pain. Many symptoms are vague and puzzling and are unrelated to the degree of prolapse. Mitral valve prolapse was once considered a psychiatric malady. Research has suggested that individuals with mitral valve prolapse have an autonomic dysfunction in which inordinate quantities of catecholamines are produced, with or without adrenergic stimulation. This finding could explain why mitral valve prolapse causes such a variety of subjective complaints.

Its high incidence rate suggests that mitral valve prolapse may be a normal variant rather than a pathologic entity. Although severe sequelae—such as chorda rupture, ventricular failure, systemic emboli, and sudden death—are possible, the disorder is actually associated with minimal mortality and morbidity. Most individuals experience no physical limitations. In fact, the psychologic effects of chest pain and knowledge of the diagnosis may be more disabling than the disease itself.

Evaluation of mitral valve prolapse includes physical assessment and laboratory evaluation. Echocardiography is the procedure of choice for diagnosing the disorder. Cardiac angiography is rarely necessary to confirm the diagnosis.

The majority of individuals with mitral valve prolapse have very few complications and require no treatment.[208,210] Management is matched to the degree of mitral regurgitation. If regurgitation is present, antibiotic prophylaxis for infective endocarditis is given before invasive procedures but physical activities are not restricted. Occasionally, beta-blockers are required to alleviate syncope, severe chest pain, or palpitations. Hypovolemia (resulting from diuretics or donating blood) is avoided because it can decrease ventricular volume, thereby increasing stress on the prolapsed mitral valve. Surgical repair or valve replacement may be required and is often successful, with few complications.[211]

Acute Rheumatic Fever and Rheumatic Heart Disease

Rheumatic fever is a diffuse, inflammatory disease caused by a delayed immune response to infection by the group A β-hemolytic streptococcus. In its acute form, rheumatic fever is a febrile illness characterized by inflammation of the joints, skin, nervous system, and heart. If untreated, rheumatic fever can cause scarring and deformity of cardiac structures, resulting in **rheumatic heart disease.**

The incidence of acute rheumatic fever declined in the United States during the 1960s, 1970s, and early 1980s because of medical and socioeconomic improvements, as well as changes in the virulence of group A streptococci. Recent outbreaks in the United States and abroad corresponded to the reappearance of highly virulent strains.[212] These virulent microorganisms have different M protein serotypes than the less pathogenic strains and can be identified as nephritogenic or rheumatogenic.[213] Because crowding and poor hygiene are environmental risk factors for acute rheumatic fever, the disease continues to be a major cause of death and disability for underprivileged populations.

The acute disease occurs most frequently in children between 5 and 15 years of age. Only 3% of those in whom pharyngeal streptococcal infection develops acquire acute rheumatic fever. Because the β-hemolytic streptococcus infection must persist for some time to cause acute rheumatic fever, appropriate antibiotic therapy given within the first 9 days of infection usually prevents rheumatic fever. Initiation of antibiotic therapy 2 weeks after the start of streptococcal infection does not prevent rheumatic fever in susceptible individuals.

The incidence of rheumatic fever tends to run in families, lending support to the concept of genetic predisposition, perhaps involving an abnormal immune response to antigens expressed by the bacterial membrane. Individuals who have experienced one attack of acute rheumatic fever are more susceptible than the general population to recurrent attacks.

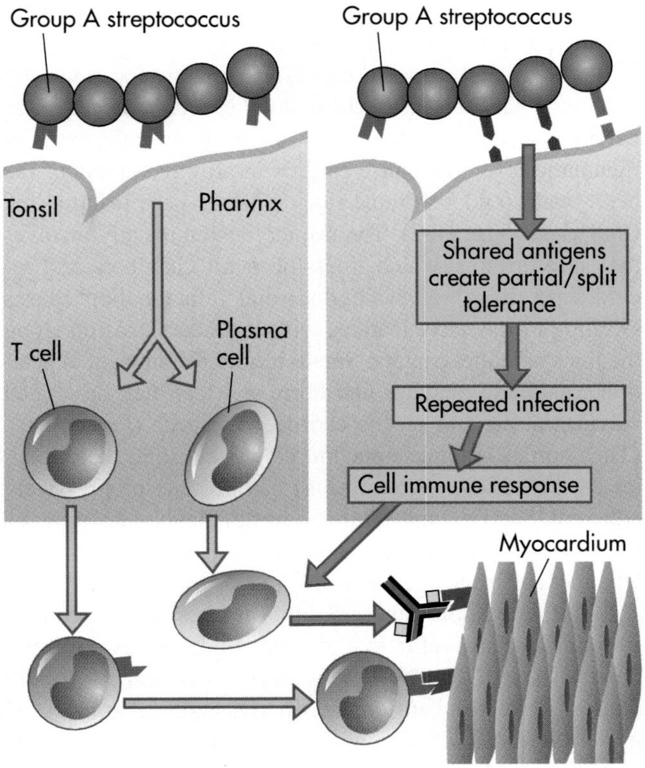

FIG. 29-35 Possible mechanisms whereby molecular mimicry could help induce rheumatic fever. *Left,* Group A streptococci infecting the pharynx and sensitizing both B cells primed for humoral antibody response and T cells capable of cell-mediated immune response against streptococcal cross-reacting epitopes within autologous tissues, such as the heart. *Right,* An alternative pathologic mechanism whereby sharing of antigens between the streptococcus and various autologous human tissues allows a state of partial tolerance to exist. This in turn downregulates an effective eliminative immune response by the host and sets the stage for a series of indolent repetitive group A streptococcal infections, eventually producing rheumatic heart disease through the direct cross-reactive mechanisms shown.

Pathophysiology

Acute rheumatic fever can develop *only* as a sequel to pharyngeal infection by group A β-hemolytic streptococcus. Streptococcal skin infections do not progress to acute rheumatic fever, although both skin and pharyngeal infections can cause acute glomerulonephritis. Acute rheumatic fever probably affects the heart, joints, central nervous system, and skin through an abnormal humoral and cell-mediated immune response to the M proteins on the microorgamisms that cross react with normal tissues (Fig. 29-35).[213] These antigens can bind to receptors on heart, muscle, and brain cells. They also have an affinity for membrane receptors within synovial joints, where they trigger an autoimmune response.

Diffuse, proliferative, and exudative inflammatory lesions develop in the connective tissues, especially in the heart, joints, and skin. The inflammation may subside before treatment, leaving behind damage to the heart valves and increasing the individual's susceptibility to recurrent acute rheumatic fever after any subsequent streptococcal infections. Repeated attacks of acute rheumatic fever cause chronic proliferative changes in the previously mentioned organs as a result of scarring, granulomas, and thromboses.

Approximately 10% of cases of rheumatic fever develop rheumatic heart disease. Rheumatic heart disease begins as **carditis,** or inflammation of the heart. Even mild cases of rheumatic fever can cause carditis in all three layers of the heart wall (endocardium, myocardium, pericardium; see Chapter 28, Fig. 28-2). The primary lesion usually involves the endocardium, which lines the heart chambers and includes the heart valves. Endocardial inflammation causes swelling of the valve leaflets, with secondary erosion along the lines of leaflet contact. Small, beadlike clumps of vegetation containing platelets and fibrin are deposited on eroded valvular tissue and on the chordae tendineae (Fig. 29-36). (The chordae tendineae anchor the valve leaflets; see Chapter 28, Fig. 28-3). These lesions can become progressively adherent. Scarring and shortening of the involved structures occur over time. The valves lose their elasticity, and the leaflets may adhere to each other.

If inflammation penetrates the myocardium, localized fibrin deposits develop that are surrounded by areas of necrosis. These fibrinoid necrotic deposits are called *Aschoff bodies.* Pericardial inflammation is usually characterized by serofibrinous effusion within the pericardial cavity. Cardiomegaly and left heart failure may occur during episodes of untreated acute or recurrent rheumatic fever. Conduction defects and atrial fibrillation are frequently associated with rheumatic heart disease.

Clinical Manifestations

Many common clinical manifestations of acute rheumatic fever—fever, lymphadenopathy, arthralgia, nausea, vomiting, epistaxis, abdominal pain, and tachycardia—are associated with other disorders as well and are by no means diagnostic of the disease. The major specific manifestations of acute rheumatic fever are carditis, acute migratory polyarthritis, chorea, and erythema marginatum, which may occur singly or in combination after a latent period of 1 to 5 weeks after streptococcal infection of the pharynx.

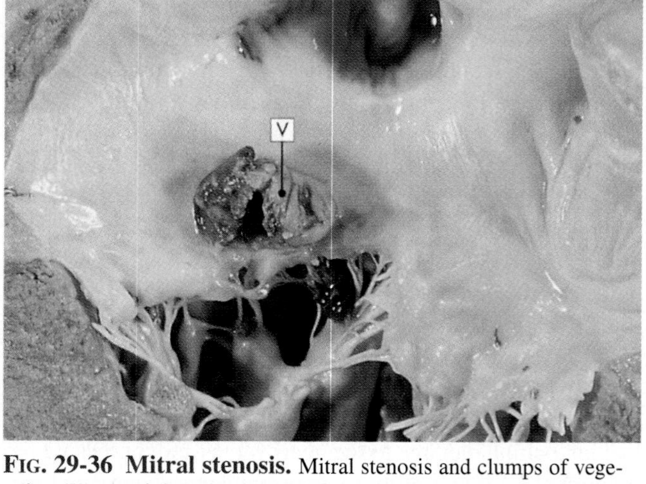

FIG. 29-36 Mitral stenosis. Mitral stenosis and clumps of vegetation *(V)* containing platelets and fibrin. Mitral leaflets are thickened and fused and have clumps of vegetation containing platelets and fibrin. (From Stevens A, Lowe J: *Pathology,* St Louis, 1995, Mosby.)

Carditis. The earliest cardiac manifestation of acute rheumatic fever may be a previously undetected murmur caused by mitral or aortic semilunar valve dysfunction. Chest pain is caused by pericardial inflammation. Pericardial effusion produces an audible friction rub. Extra heart sounds, heart block (see p. 1035), atrial fibrillation, and a prolonged PR interval are frequently associated with chronic rheumatic heart disease.

Polyarthritis. The classic presenting manifestation of acute rheumatic fever is acute migratory polyarthritis (inflammation of more than one joint). Although all of the synovial joints may be involved, the large joints of the extremities are most frequently affected. Two or more joints are usually involved simultaneously or in succession. Exudative synovitis causes heat, redness, swelling, severe pain, and tenderness but no permanent disability. Palpable subcutaneous nodes often develop over bony prominences and along extensor tendons. They do not interfere with joint function and often go unnoticed.

Chorea. **Sydenham chorea**, or **St. Vitus dance**, is a disorder of the central nervous system characterized by sudden, aimless, irregular, involuntary movements. (Chorea is described in Chapter 15.) It is the most definitive sign of rheumatic fever; patients should receive immediate antibiotic treatment if they have not yet received it.[213] It is more common in girls than in boys and may occur several months after the streptococcal infection. The chorea is self-limiting. It runs its course within weeks or months and has no permanent neural sequelae.

Erythema marginatum. **Erythema marginatum** is a distinctive truncal rash that often accompanies acute rheumatic fever. It consists of nonpruritic, pink, erythematous macules that never occur on the face or hands. The rash is transitory and may change in appearance within minutes or hours. Heat (e.g., bathing) darkens the rash. The macules may fade in the center and be mistaken for ringworm.

Evaluation and Treatment

When correlated with findings from physical assessment, laboratory values lend significant support to the diagnosis of acute rheumatic fever. A throat culture positive for group A β-hemolytic streptococci can be an important finding when associated with certain physical signs. Cultures may be negative when the rheumatic attack begins, however. Documented recent scarlet fever is another potentially strong diagnostic aid to acute rheumatic fever, but diagnosis of scarlet fever also depends on a positive throat culture and may be difficult to distinguish from other disorders associated with a similar rash. A high or rising antistreptolysin O (ASO) antibody titer is a more accurate means of diagnosing the presence of a streptococcal infection. Most strains of group A β-hemolytic streptococcus produce a hemolytic factor called *streptolysin O.* Antibodies against this hemolytic factor increase as the individual's immune system fights the disease. ASO antibody titers higher than 250 Todd units in adults and 333 Todd units in children are considered elevated. Several other antibody tests are sensitive prognosticators of streptococcal infection. These include antideoxyribonucleotidase (anti-DNase B), antihyaluronidase, and antistreptozyme (ASTZ).

Elevated white blood cell count, erythrocyte sedimentation rate, and C-reactive protein indicate inflammation. All three are usually increased at the time cardiac or joint symptoms begin to appear. They are more useful in identifying an acute inflammatory process and suggesting prognosis than in diagnosing acute rheumatic fever. The levels of these tests decrease as the inflammatory process resolves.

In 1944 the Jones criteria (Table 29-10) were established to assist in the diagnosis of acute rheumatic fever. The criteria have been modified several times by the American Heart Association, most recently in 1992.[214] No single laboratory test, sign, or symptom is pathognomonic of acute rheumatic fever, but certain combinations of criteria indicate that acute disease is probably present.

Therapy for acute rheumatic fever is aimed at eradicating the streptococcal infection. This is accomplished by a 10-day regimen of oral penicillin or erythromycin administration. Salicylates are used as antiinflammatory agents for both rheumatic carditis and arthritis. Serious carditis may require that cardiac glycosides, corticosteroids, diuretics, and bed rest be added to the regimen.[213] Surgical repair of damaged valves may be necessary in cases of chronic recurrent rheumatic fever or carditis. Active disease is considered resolved when (1) the murmur has disappeared or cardiac status becomes stable, (2) major manifestations are no longer present, (3) the individual is afebrile, and (4) the erythrocyte sedimentation rate is normal or stabilized. This may take 1 to 6 months.

Research suggests that a rheumatic recurrence will develop in 50% to 65% of children with known rheumatic fever if they have another group A streptococcal infection. Recurrence rates decline with the length of time elapsed since the last infection. To prevent recurrence of acute rheumatic fever, continuous prophylactic antibiotic therapy is necessary for as long as 5 years.[213]

Table 29-10 Jones Criteria (Revised) for Diagnosis of Rheumatic Fever

Criteria	Description
Major manifestations	Carditis, polyarthritis, chorea, erythema marginatum, subcutaneous nodes
Minor manifestations	Clinical: previous rheumatic fever or rheumatic heart disease, arthralgia, fever
	Laboratory: elevated appearance of C-reactive protein, leukocytosis
	Electrocardiographic: prolonged PR interval
Supporting evidence of streptococcal infection	Increased titer of streptococcal antibodies: antistreptolysin O (ASO)
	Other: positive throat culture for group A *Streptococcus;* recent scarlet fever

From Dajani AS et al: *JAMA* 264(22):2919, 1990.

Infective Endocarditis

Infective endocarditis is a general term used to describe inflammation of the endocardium—especially the cardiac valves. Causal agents include bacteria, viruses, fungi, rickettsiae, and parasites, but bacterial infection, particularly by streptococci or staphylococci, is most common.[215] Infective endocarditis was once a lethal disease, but morbidity and mortality diminished significantly with the advent of antibiotics and improved diagnostic techniques.

Risk factors for infective endocarditis include acquired valvular heart disease (especially mitral valve prolapse) and implantation of prosthetic heart valves.[216,217] Congenital lesions associated with highly turbulent flow, such as ventricular septal defect, are also risk factors. (Congenital lesions are discussed in Chapter 30.) Other risk factors include a previous attack of infective endocarditis, male gender, intravenous drug abuse, long-term indwelling catheterization (e.g., for pressure monitoring, hyperalimentation, or hemodialysis), and recent cardiac surgery.

Pathophysiology

The pathogenesis of infective endocarditis is a complex process that requires at least three critical elements (Fig. 29-37). First, the endocardium (e.g., heart valve) must be "prepared," usually by endothelial damage, for microorganism colonization. Second, blood-borne microorganisms must adhere to the damaged endocardial surface. Third, the adherent microorganisms must proliferate and promote the propagation of infective endocardial vegetation.

The first critical element, endocardial damage, exposes the endothelial basement membrane. The basement membrane contains a type of collagen that attracts platelets and thereby stimulates thrombus formation on the membrane. Platelet activation and thrombus formation can cause an inflammatory reaction termed **nonbacterial thrombotic endocarditis.** Infective endocarditis cannot develop unless microorganisms gain access to the bloodstream. Microorganisms may enter the bloodstream as a result of minor procedures, such as dental cleaning or bladder catheterization, or they may spread from uncomplicated upper respiratory or skin infections. Any time pathogens gain access to the bloodstream, the potential for endocardial infection exists. Bacteremia and adherence constitute the second critical element. Adherence of microorganisms to the endocardial surface is facilitated by the coexistence of nonbacterial thrombotic endocarditis. It should be noted, however, that highly invasive organisms can cause infective endocarditis even on the healthy, intact endocardium. The third critical element, bacterial proliferation and vegetation formation, is also promoted by coexistent nonbacterial thrombotic endocarditis.

Not all microorganisms are capable of colonization. This capability, which determines the microorganism's pathogenicity, depends on the organism's ability to survive interactions with circulating serum complement, antibodies, and platelets aggregated on the endocardial surface. Complement, antibodies, and platelets may serve as effective inhibitors to bacterial colonization.

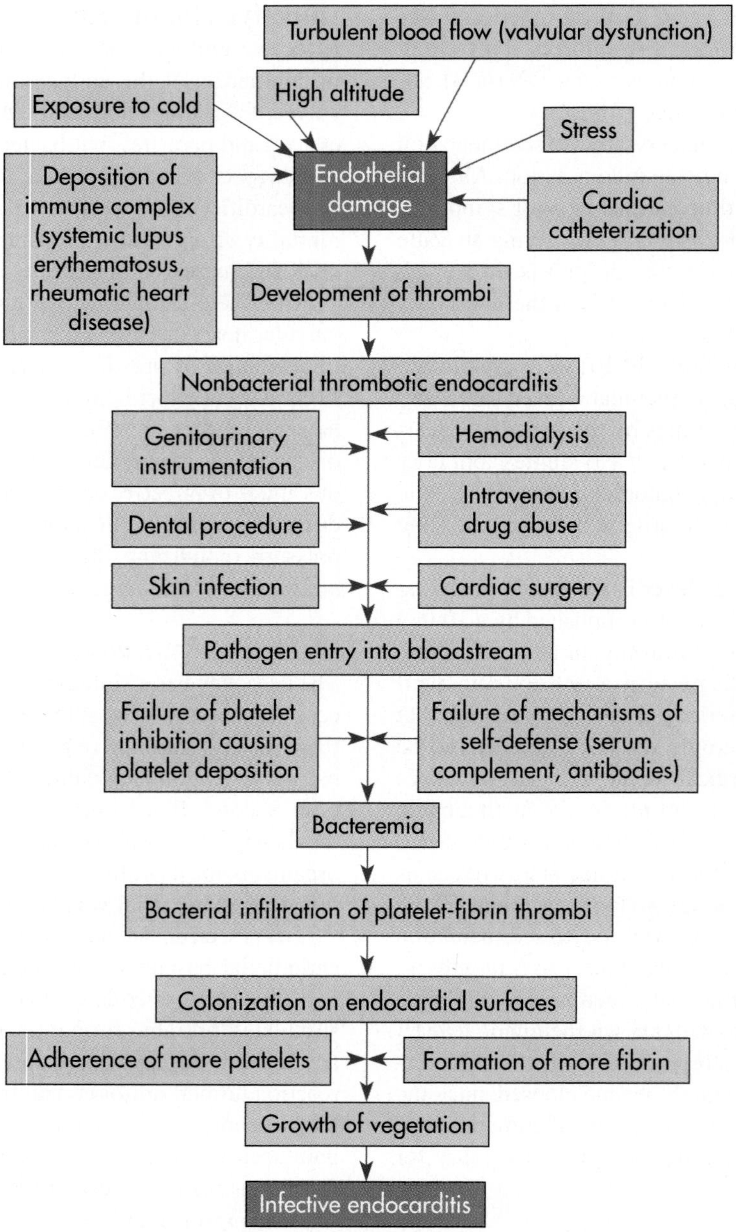

FIG. 29-37 Pathogenesis of infective endocarditis.

In addition to circumventing the host's defense mechanisms, the circulating microorganisms must adhere to the endocardial surface to initiate endocardial infection. Studies suggest that bacteria are able to synthesize extracellular polysaccharides, such as dextran or fibronectin, which promote stickiness on endocardial surfaces.

Once the endocardial surface is colonized, formation of infected vegetation proceeds by a series of complex steps (Fig. 29-38). Within 3 to 6 hours after infection, microbial replication occurs and bacterial colonies form within aggregates of fibrin and platelets. Within 24 hours, infected vegetation has increased in size, with colonies of microorganisms sandwiched between layers of fibrin and platelets. Bacteria may accelerate fibrin formation by activating the clotting cascade in some as yet undetermined manner. As the growing bacterial colonies become progressively enmeshed in the tight fibrin network, which contains few phagocytic cells, they become less and less susceptible to the host's mechanisms of self-defense. Although endocardial tissue is constantly bathed in antibody-containing blood and is surrounded by scavenging monocytes and polymorphonuclear leukocytes, bacterial colonies are inaccessible to host defenses because they are embedded in the protective fibrin clots. The lesions can form anywhere on the endocardium but usually occur on the endocardial surfaces of heart valves and surrounding structures (see Fig. 29-38).

◆ *Clinical Manifestations*

Infective endocarditis may be acute, subacute, or chronic. It causes varying degrees of valvular dysfunction and may be

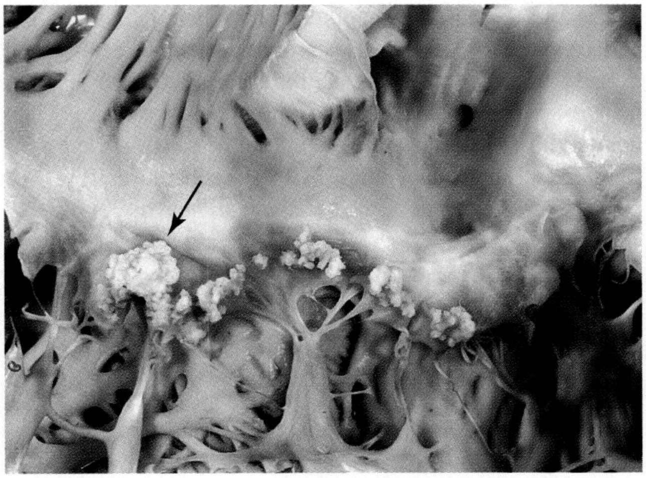

FIG. 29-38 Bacterial endocarditis of mitral valve. Lesion in combination with old rheumatic valvulitis. (From Damjanov I, Linder J: *Pathology: a color atlas,* St Louis, 2000, Mosby.)

associated with manifestations involving any number of organ systems (lungs, eyes, kidneys, bones, joints, central nervous system), making diagnosis exceedingly difficult. The "classic" findings of fever; cardiac murmur; and petechial lesions of the skin, conjunctiva, and oral mucosa are not always present.

Signs and symptoms of infective endocarditis are caused by infection and inflammation, systemic spread of microemboli, and immune complex deposition in various organs. A history of fever, anorexia, weight loss, back pain, and night sweats; a new or significantly changed cardiac murmur; petechiae; positive blood cultures; an elevated erythrocyte sedimentation rate; and urine abnormalities make the diagnosis quite clear. Sudden onset of severely debilitating symptoms indicates acute disease.

If infective endocarditis extends farther into the heart wall and invades the conduction system, electrocardiography may show a prolonged PR interval, left bundle branch block, or complete heart block (see p. 1035). Emboli may travel to the coronary arteries and cause an acute myocardial infarction.

Evaluation and Treatment

Diagnostic evaluation includes blood cultures to identify microorganisms.[65] Criteria for the diagnosis of infective endocarditis include persistent bacteremia, new regurgitant murmurs, vascular complications, and appropriate echocardiographic findings.[218] Echocardiography is used to identify the anatomic location of the infection and any intracardiac complications. If peripheral emboli are suggested, organ scans can be performed to confirm their presence. Antimicrobial therapy generally is given for 4 to 6 weeks, beginning with intravenous administration and ending with oral administration. In some cases, two different antibiotics are given simultaneously to eliminate the offending microorganism and prevent the development of drug resistance. Penicillin and streptomycin commonly are used to treat infective endocarditis. Other drugs may be necessary to treat left heart failure secondary to valvular dysfunction.[65,219]

Recurrent infective endocarditis or severe impairment of the heart valves may require implantation of prosthetic valves. Unfortunately, the presence of an artificial valve is itself a significant risk factor for infective endocarditis. Valve failure and valve-induced embolization are known sequelae of prosthetic valve placement.

Individuals who are known to be at risk for infective endocarditis can avoid the disease by taking antibiotics before and after any procedure that carries the risk of transient bacteremia. Such procedures include dental cleaning, genitourinary instrumentation, and open cardiovascular surgery. The American Heart Association recently published new recommendations concerning the prevention of infective endocarditis.[215]

Cardiac Complications in Acquired Immunodeficiency Syndrome (AIDS)

There is growing evidence that up to 20% of individuals infected with the human immunodeficiency virus (HIV) have cardiac involvement consisting of myocarditis, endocarditis, pericarditis, or cardiomyopathy.[220] Cardiac involvement can result from the HIV itself, inflammation, other infections, malignancy, or drugs. In addition to HIV infection, the cardiac involvement may be induced by the accompanying inflammatory response. Infection also may be caused by a variety of bacterial, viral, protozoan, mycobacterial, and fungal pathogens. Malignancies, such as lymphoma and Kaposi sarcoma, frequently are seen in individuals with AIDS and can affect the heart. Anti-HIV drugs or drugs used to combat opportunistic infections may produce toxic lesions. Myocarditis is the most common pathologic finding, followed by infective endocarditis and dilated cardiomyopathy.[220]

Clinical manifestations of cardiac disease are seen in about 10% of those with HIV. Left heart failure is the most common cardiac manifestation and is related to left ventricular dilation and dysfunction. Pericardial effusion, ventricular dysrhythmias, ECG changes, and right ventricular dilation and hypertrophy are other less common findings. Treatment includes antibiotic therapy when appropriate and relief of symptoms.

MANIFESTATIONS OF HEART DISEASE

Heart Failure

Types

Heart failure is a general term used to describe several types of cardiac dysfunction that result in inadequate perfusion of tissues with vital blood-borne nutrients. Most causes of heart failure result from dysfunction of the left ventricle (systolic and diastolic heart failure). The right ventricle also may be dysfunctional, especially in pulmonary disease (right ventricular failure). Finally, some conditions cause inadequate perfusion despite normal or elevated cardiac output (high-output failure).

Left Heart Failure (Congestive Heart Failure)

Left heart failure is commonly called *congestive heart failure* and can be further categorized as systolic heart failure or diastolic heart failure. Synonyms for these terms are systolic ventricular dysfunction and diastolic ventricular dysfunction. These two types of heart failure can occur together in one individual or singly.

Systolic heart failure is defined as an inability of the heart to generate an adequate cardiac output to perfuse vital tissues. Cardiac output depends on the heart rate and stroke volume. Stroke volume is influenced by three major factors: contractility, preload, and afterload (see Chapter 28).

Contractility is reduced by diseases that disrupt myocyte activity. Myocardial infarction is the most common cause of decreased contractility; other causes include myocarditis and cardiomyopathies. Myocardial ischemia results in a process called **ventricular remodeling,** which causes progressive myocyte contractile dysfunction over time. When contractility is decreased, stroke volume falls and left ventricular end-diastolic volume (LVEDV) increases. This increase causes dilation of the heart and an increase in preload (Fig. 29-39).

Preload, or LVEDV, increases with decreased contractility (see above) or an excess of plasma volume (intravenous fluid administration, renal failure, mitral valvular disease). Increases in LVEDV can actually improve cardiac output to a certain point, but as preload continues to rise, it causes a stretching of the myocardium that eventually can lead to

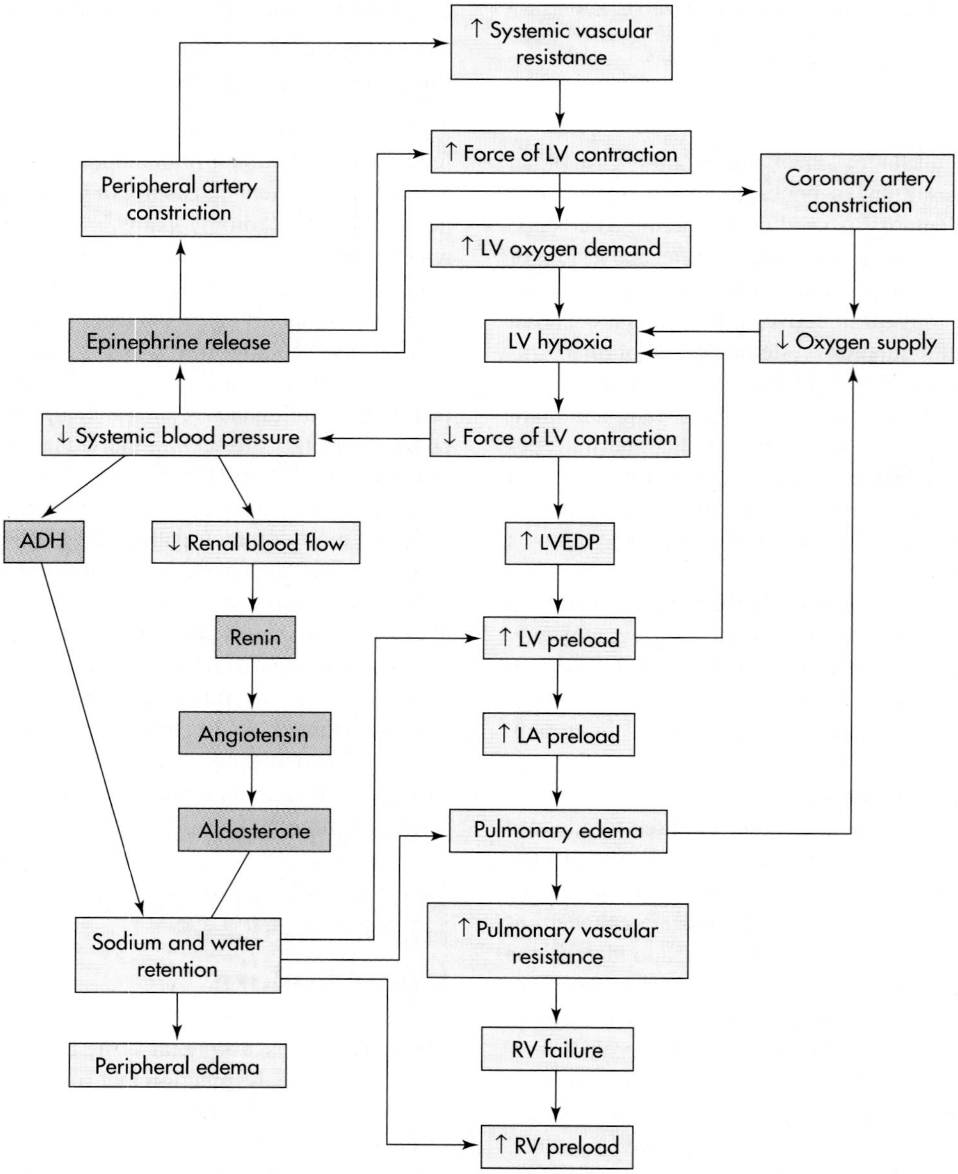

FIG. 29-39 Left heart failure (congestive heart failure) from elevated systemic vascular resistance. Left heart failure leads to right heart failure. Systemic vascular resistance and preload are exacerbated by renal and adrenal mechanisms. *LV,* Left ventricular; *LVEDP,* left ventricular end-diastolic pressure; *LA,* left atrial; *ADH,* antidiuretic hormone; *RV,* right ventricular.

dysfunction of the sarcomeres and decreased contractility (Fig. 29-40).

Increased afterload is most commonly a result of increased peripheral vascular resistance (PVR), such as that seen with hypertension (Fig. 29-41); it can also be the result of aortic valvular disease. With increased PVR, there is resistance to ventricular emptying and more workload for the left ventricle, which responds with hypertrophy of the myocardium. Hypertrophy results in an increase in oxygen demand by the thickened myocardium and leads to changes in the myocytes themselves, also called *ventricular remodeling*. In addition, hypertrophy results in the deposition of collagen between the myocytes; this can disrupt the integrity of the muscle, decrease contractility, and make the ventricle more likely to dilate and fail.

As cardiac output falls, renal perfusion diminishes with activation of the renin-angiotensin-aldosterone system, which acts to increase PVR and plasma volume, thus increasing afterload and preload further. In addition, baroreceptors in the central circulation detect the decrease in perfusion and stimulate the sympathetic nervous system to cause yet more vasoconstriction and the hypothalamus to produce antidiuretic hormone. This vicious cycle of decreasing contractility, increasing preload, and increasing afterload causes progressive worsening of left heart failure (Fig. 29-42).

In addition to these hemodynamic interactions, systolic congestive heart failure is characterized by a complex constellation of neurohumoral and inflammatory processes. These processes involve a large number of important mediators:

1. *Catecholamines.* Sympathetic nervous system activation initially compensates for a decrease in cardiac output by increasing heart rate and peripheral vascular resistance. However, catecholamines cause numerous deleterious effects on the myocardium, including direct toxicity to myocytes, induction of myocyte apoptosis, myocardial remodeling, down-regulation of adrenergic receptors, facilitation of arrhythmias, and potentiation of autoimmune effects on the heart muscle.[221,222,223]
2. *Angiotensin II.* Activation of the renin-angiotensin-aldosterone system not only causes increases in preload and afterload, but also causes direct toxicity to the myocardium. Ang II mediates remodeling of the ventricular wall, with associated loss of contractility (see "What's New? The Role of Angiotensin II in Cardiovascular Disease" p. 989).[223] High circulating levels of Ang II are associated with an increased mortality in individuals with congestive heart failure (CHF).[224]
3. *Arginine vasopressin.* Arginine vasopressin is also known as antidiuretic hormone and causes both peripheral vasoconstriction and renal fluid retention. These actions exacerbate hyponatremia and edema in CHF.[222,223,225]
4. *Natriuretic peptides.* Atrial and brain natriuretic peptides are increased in CHF and may have some protective effect by decreasing preload.[223,226]
5. *Endothelial hormones.* Endothelin is a potent vasoconstrictor and is associated with a poor prognosis in individuals with CHF.[222,223]
6. *Endotoxin.* Increased serum levels of endotoxin have been found in many individuals with CHF, especially those with significant peripheral edema, and has been linked to myocyte apoptosis and release of tumor necrosis factor and interleukins.[227,228]
7. *Tumor necrosis factor–α (TNF-α) and interleukin-6 (IL-6)*: TNF-α is elevated in CHF and contributes to myocardial remodeling, downregulates the synthesis of the vasodilator nitric oxide, induces myocyte apoptosis, and may contribute to weight loss and weakness in individuals with CHF (cardiac cachexia).[226,229,230] IL-6 is also high in individuals with severe CHF and cardiogenic shock and may contribute to further deleterious immune activation.[227]

The interaction of these neurohumoral and inflammatory processes results in a gradual decline in myocardial function. Pathologically, the heart muscle exhibits progressive changes in myocyte myofilaments, decreased contractility, myocyte apoptosis and necrosis, abnormal fibrin deposition in the ventricle wall, myocardial hypertrophy, and changes

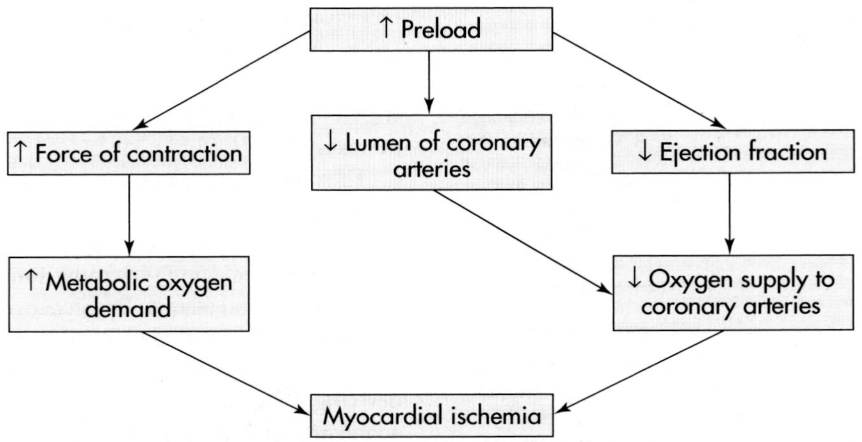

FIG. 29-40 The effect of elevated preload on myocardial oxygen supply and demand.

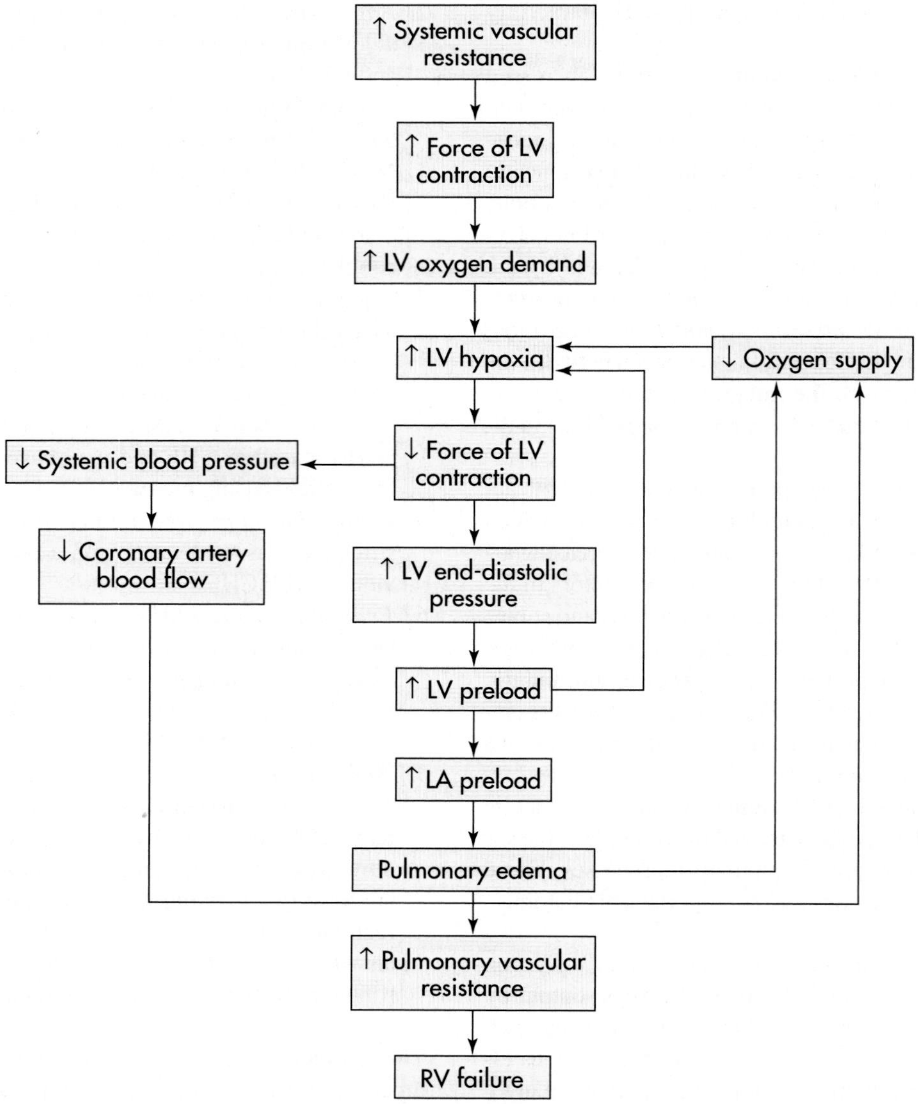

FIG. 29-41 Left heart failure resulting from systemic hypertension. Left heart failure leads to right heart failure. *LV,* Left ventricular; *LA,* left atrial; *RV,* right ventricular.

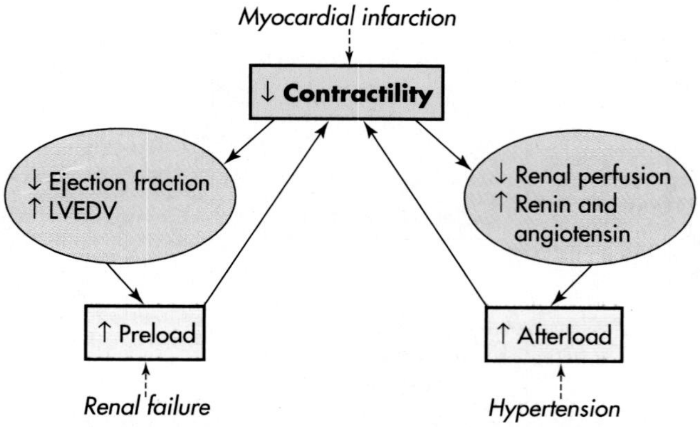

FIG. 29-42 The vicious cycle of systolic heart failure. Although the initial insult may be one of primary decreased contractility (e.g., myocardial infarction), increased preload (e.g., renal failure), or increased afterload (e.g., hypertension), all three factors play a role in the progression of left heart failure (LHF). *LVEDV,* Left ventricular end-diastolic volume.

in the ventricular chamber geometry.[221] These changes reduce myocardial function and cardiac output and lead to increased morbidity and mortality. These discoveries have led to the routine use of ACE inhibitors or Ang II receptor blockers plus beta-blockers in the management of CHF, which has resulted in significant decreases in morbidity and mortality.[65,231,232,233,234]

The clinical manifestations of left heart failure are the result of pulmonary vascular congestion and inadequate perfusion of the systemic circulation. Individuals experience dyspnea, orthopnea, cough of frothy sputum, fatigue, decreased urine output, and edema. Physical examination often reveals pulmonary edema (cyanosis, rales, pleural effusions), hypotension or hypertension, an S_3 gallop, and evidence of underlying CAD or hypertension. The diagnosis is made with echocardiography, revealing decreased cardiac output and cardiomegaly; some people may require invasive catheterization to document underlying coronary disease.

Management of systolic left heart failure is aimed at interrupting the worsening cycle of decreasing contractility, increasing preload, and increasing afterload, as well as blocking the neurohormonal mediators of myocardial toxicity. The **acute onset of left (congestive) heart failure** is most often the result of acute myocardial ischemia and must be managed in conjunction with managing the underlying coronary disease (see p. 1000). Oxygen, nitrate, and morphine administration improve myocardial oxygenation and help relieve coronary spasm while lowering preload through systemic venodilation. Intravenous inotropic drugs, such as dopamine or dobutamine, increase contractility and can help raise the blood pressure in hypotensive individuals. Diuretics reduce preload, and ACE inhibitors reduce both preload and afterload by decreasing aldosterone levels and reducing PVR. Short-acting intravenous beta-blockers also have been found to reduce mortality. Finally, individuals with severe systolic failure may benefit from acute coronary bypass or percutaneous transluminal coronary angioplasty (PTCA). These people are frequently supported with the intraaortic balloon pump (IABP) until they can be taken safely to the operating room; the IABP is positioned in the aorta just distal to the aortic valve and is inflated during diastole to improve coronary perfusion and deflated during systole to reduce afterload.

Management of **chronic left heart failure** also relies on increasing contractility and reducing preload and afterload. Salt restriction, avoidance of nonsteroidal antiinflammatory medications, and institution of exercise training can improve symptoms.[235,236] The inotropic drug of choice in chronic systolic heart failure is digoxin. Although digoxin was found to be safe in the treatment of chronic CHF in one large study,[237] researchers have more recently raised questions about a possible increase in mortality in some individuals.[238,239,240] Salt restriction and diuretics are effective in reducing preload, and spironolactone has been shown to significantly reduce mortality when added to standard therapy.[241] ACE inhibitors reduce preload and afterload and have been shown to reduce mortality in left heart failure by as much as 30%.[231,234,238] Beta-blockers improve symptoms and increase survival but must be used carefully to avoid hypotension.[232,233,242] Although many individuals with left heart failure die suddenly from dysrhythmias, prophylactic administration of antidysrhythmics has not been consistently shown to improve survival. In indivdiuals with sustained ventricular tachycardia, amiodarone or implantable cardioverter-defibrillators should be considered.[243] Coronary bypass surgery or PTCA may improve perfusion to ischemic myocardium ("hibernating" myocardium) and improve cardiac output. Finally, heart transplant may need to be considered.

Diastolic heart failure can occur singly or along with systolic heart failure. Isolated diastolic heart failure is defined as pulmonary congestion despite a normal stroke volume and cardiac output. It is the cause of 25% to 40% of all cases of left heart failure and is more common in women.[244] It results from decreased compliance of the left ventricle and

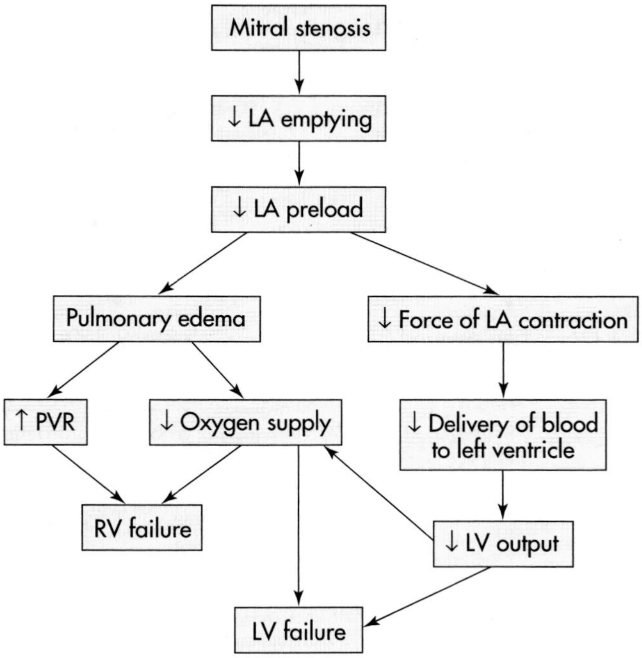

FIG. 29-43 Left atrial failure caused by mitral stenosis. *LA,* Left atrial; *PVR,* pulmonary vascular resistance; *LV,* left ventricular.

abnormal diastolic relaxation such that a normal LVEDV results in an increased left ventricular end-diastolic pressure (LVEDP). This pressure is reflected back into the pulmonary circulation and results in pulmonary edema. The major causes of diastolic dysfunction include hypertension-induced myocardial hypertrophy and myocardial ischemia with resultant ventricular remodeling (see What's New? The Role of Angiotensin II in Cardioascular Disease, p. 989). Other causes include aortic valvular disease, mitral valve disease (Fig. 29-43), and cardiomyopathies.

Individuals with diastolic dysfunction present with dyspnea on exertion; fatigue; evidence of pulmonary edema (rales on auscultation, pleural effusions); and evidence of underlying coronary disease, hypertension, or valvular disease. Diagnosis is made initially by echocardiography, which demonstrates poor ventricular filling with normal ejection fractions. Precise measurements of pressures require catheterization. Management is aimed at improving ventricular relaxation and prolonging diastolic filling times to reduce diastolic pressure. Calcium channel blockers, beta-blockers, and ACE inhibitors have been used with varying success. Inotropic drugs are not indicated in isolated diastolic heart failure because contractility and ejection fraction are not affected. An innovative surgical technique that involves the transplantation of a portion of the latissimus dorsi muscle into the wall of the noncompliant left ventricle (dynamic cardiomyoplasty) is being tried, with some early success. Mortality is lower with diastolic failure than with systolic; however, risk of death is four times that of the population without heart failure.[245]

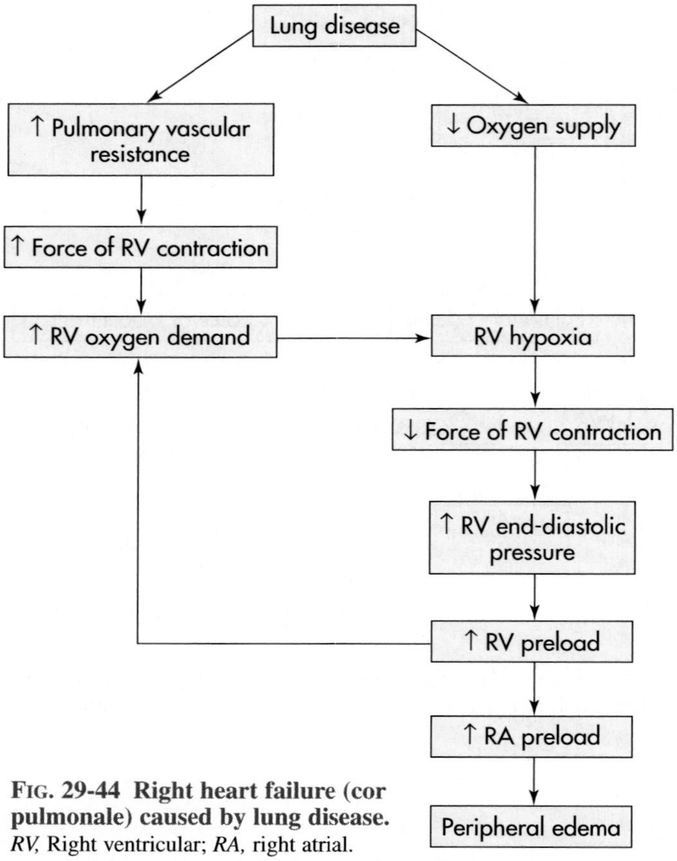

FIG. 29-44 Right heart failure (cor pulmonale) caused by lung disease. *RV,* Right ventricular; *RA,* right atrial.

Right Heart Failure

Right heart failure can result from left heart failure caused by an increase in left ventricular filling pressure that is reflected back into the pulmonary circulation. As pressure in the pulmonary circulation rises, the resistance to right ventricular emptying increases (Fig. 29-44). The right ventricle is poorly prepared to compensate for this increased workload and will dilate and fail. When this happens, pressure will rise in the systemic venous circulation, resulting in peripheral edema and hepatosplenomegaly. Treatment relies on management of the left ventricular dysfunction as just outlined. When right heart failure occurs in the absence of left heart failure, it is caused most commonly by diffuse hypoxic pulmonary disease such as COPD, cystic fibrosis, and ARDS. The mechanisms for this type of right ventricular dysfunction *(cor pulmonale)* are discussed in Chapter 32.

High-Output Failure

High-output failure is the inability of the heart to adequately supply the body with blood-borne nutrients, despite adequate blood volume and normal or elevated myocardial contractility. In high-output failure the heart increases its output but the body's metabolic needs are still not met. Common causes of high-output failure are anemia, septicemia, hyperthyroidism, and beriberi (Fig. 29-45).

Anemia decreases the oxygen-carrying capacity of the blood (see Chapter 25). Metabolic acidosis occurs as the

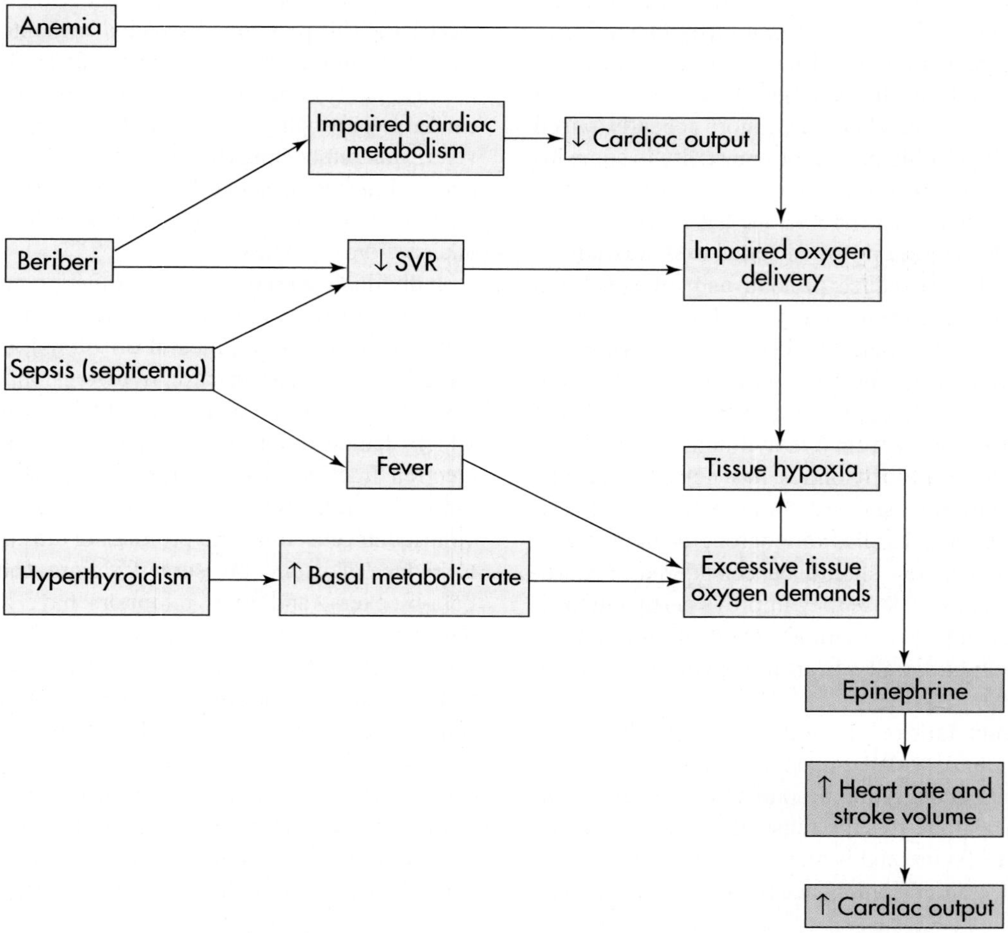

FIG. 29-45 High-output failure. *SVR,* Systemic vascular resistance.

body's cells switch to anaerobic metabolism (see Chapter 3). In response to metabolic acidosis, heart rate and stroke volume increase in an attempt to circulate blood faster. If anemia is severe, however, even maximum cardiac output does not supply the cells with enough oxygen for metabolism.

In septicemia, disturbed metabolism, bacterial toxins, and the inflammatory process cause systemic vasodilation and fever. Faced with a lowered systemic vascular resistance (SVR) and an elevated metabolic rate, cardiac output increases to maintain blood pressure and prevent metabolic acidosis. In overwhelming septicemia, however, the heart may not be able to raise its output enough to compensate for vasodilation. Body tissues show signs of inadequate blood supply despite a very high cardiac output.

Hyperthyroidism accelerates cellular metabolism through the actions of elevated levels of thyroxine from the thyroid gland. This may occur chronically (thyrotoxicosis) or acutely (thyroid storm). Because the body's demand for oxygen threatens to cause metabolic acidosis, cardiac output increases. If blood levels of thyroxine are high and the metabolic response to thyroxine is quite vigorous, even an abnormally elevated cardiac output may be inadequate.

In the United States, beriberi (thiamine deficiency) usually is caused by malnutrition secondary to chronic alcoholism. Beriberi actually causes a mixed type of heart failure. Thiamine deficiency impairs cellular metabolism in all tissues, including the myocardium. In the heart, impaired cardiac metabolism leads to insufficient contractile strength. In blood vessels, thiamine deficiency leads mainly to peripheral vasodilation, which decreases SVR. Heart failure ensues as decreased SVR triggers increased cardiac output, which the impaired myocardium is unable to deliver. The strain of demands for increased output in the face of impaired metabolism may deplete cardiac reserves until low-output failure begins.

Dysrhythmias

A dysrhythmia, or arrhythmia, is a disturbance of heart rhythm. Normal heart rhythms are generated by the SA node and travel through the heart's conduction system, causing the atrial and ventricular myocardium to contract and relax at a regular rate that is appropriate to maintain circulation at various levels of physical activity (see Chapter 28). Dysrhythmias range in severity from occasional "missed" or rapid beats to serious disturbances that impair the pumping ability of the heart, contributing to heart failure and death. Dysrhythmias can be caused by either an abnormal rate of impulse generation (Table 29-11) by the SA node or other pacemaker or the abnormal conduction of impulses (Table 29-12) through the heart's conduction system, including the myocardial cells themselves.

Table 29-11 Disorders of Impulse Formation

Type	Electrocardiogram	Effect	Pathophysiology	Treatment
Sinus bradycardia	P rate 60 or less PR interval normal QRS for each P	Increased preload Decreased mean arterial pressure	Hyperkalemia: slows depolarization Vagal hyperactivity: unknown Digoxin toxicity common Late hypoxia: lack of adenosine triphosphate (ATP)	If hypotensive, treat cause and support Follow with sympathomimetics, cardiotonics, and pacer Vagolytics
Simple sinus tachycardia	P rate 100-150 PR interval normal QRS for each P	Decreased filling times Decreased mean arterial pressure Increased myocardial demand	Catecholamines: rise in resting potential, calcium influx Fever: unknown Early failure and lung disease: hypoxic cell metabolism Hypercalcemia	Oxygen, bed rest Calcium blockers
Premature atrial contractions (PACs) or beats*	Early P waves that may have changed morphology PR interval normal QRS for each P	Occasional decreased filling time and mean arterial pressure	Electrolyte disturbances: decrease all phases Hypoxia and elevated preload: cell membrane disturbances Hypercalcemia	Treat underlying cause Digoxin
Sinus dysrhythmia	Rate varies P-P regularly irregular, short with inspiration, long with exhalation PR interval normal QRS for each P	Variable filling times Variable mean arterial pressures Variable oxygen demand	Unknown Common in young children and young adults	None

*Most common in adults.
†Life threatening in adults.

Continued

Table 29-11 Disorders of Impulse Formation—cont'd

Type	Electrocardiogram	Effect	Pathophysiology	Treatment
Atrial tachycardia (includes premature atrial tachycardia if onset is abrupt)	P rate 151-250 P morphology may differ from sinus P PR interval normal P/QRS ratio variable	Decreased filling time Decreased mean arterial pressure Increased myocardial demand	Same as PACs: leads to increased atrial automaticity, atrial reentry Digoxin toxicity: common	Control ventricular rate Digoxin, calcium blockers, vagus stimulation Pace to override
Atrial flutter*	P rate 251-300, morphology may vary from sinus P PR interval usually not observable P/QRS ratio variable	Decreased filling time Decreased mean arterial pressure	Same as atrial tachycardia Aging	Same as atrial tachycardia Synchronous cardioversion
Atrial fibrillation*	P rate >300 and usually not observable No PR interval QRS rate variable and rhythm irregular	Same as atrial flutter	Same as atrial tachycardia Aging	Same as atrial tachycardia
Idiojunctional rhythm	P absent or independent QRS normal, rate 41-59, regular	Decreased cardiac output from loss of atrial contribution to ventricular preload Decreased mean atrial pressure as a result of bradycardia	Atrial and sinus bradycardia, standstill, or block	Same as sinus bradycardia
Junctional bradycardia	P absent or independent QRS normal, rate 40 or less	Same as idiojunctional rhythm	Same as idiojunctional rhythm Vagal hyperactivity	Same as sinus bradycardia
Premature junctional contractions (PJCs) or beats	Early beats without P waves QRS morphology normal	Decreased cardiac output from loss of atrial contribution to ventricular preload for that beat	Hyperkalemia (6-5.4 mEq/L) Hypercalcemia, hypoxia, and elevated preload (see PACs)	Same as PAC
Accelerated junctional rhythm	P absent or independent QRS morphology normal, rate 60-99	Decreased cardiac output from loss of atrial contribution to ventricular preload	Same as PJCs	Same as PAC
Junctional tachycardia	P absent or independent QRS morphology normal, rate 100 or more	Decreased cardiac output from loss of atrial contribution to ventricular preload Increased myocardial demand because of tachycardia	Same as PJCs	Same as PAC
Idioventricular rhythm†	P absent or independent QRS >0.11 and rate 20-39	Same as idiojunctional rhythm	Sinus, atrial, and junctional bradycardia, standstill, or block	Same as sinus bradycardia
Ventricular bradycardia†	P absent or independent QRS >0.11 and rate 60-21	Same as idiojunctional rhythm	Same as idiojunctional rhythm	Same as sinus bradycardia
Agonal rhythm/ electromechanical dissociation†	P absent or independent QRS >0.11 and rate 20 or less	Absent or barely present cardiac output and pulse Not compatible with life	Depolarization and contraction not coupled: electrical activity present with little or no mechanical activity Usually caused by profound hypoxia	Vigorous pharmacology aimed at restoring rate and force Usually ineffective May attempt to pace
Ventricular standstill or asystole†	P absent or independent QRS absent	No cardiac output Not compatible with life	Profound ischemia, hyperkalemia, acidosis	Same as agonal rhythm, including electrical defibrillation

*Most common in adults.
†Life threatening in adults.

Table 29-11 Disorders of Impulse Formation—cont'd

Type	Electrocardiogram	Effect	Pathophysiology	Treatment
Premature ventricular contractions (PVCs) or depolarizations*	Early beats with P waves QRS occasionally opposite in deflection from usual QRS	Same as premature junctional contractions	Same as PJCs, including aging and induction of anesthesia Impulse originates in cell outside normal conduction system and spreads through intercalated disks	Pharmacology to change thresholds, refractory periods; reduce myocardial demand, increase supply Removal of cause
Accelerated ventricular rhythm	P absent or independent QRS >0.11 and rate 41-99	Same as accelerated junctional rhythm	Same as PVCs	Same as PVCs
Ventricular tachycardia†	P absent or independent QRS >0.11 and rate 100 or more	Same as junctional tachycardia	Same as PVCs	Same as PVCs, including electrical cardioversion
Ventricular fibrillation†	P absent QRS >300 and usually not observable	Same as ventricular standstill	Same as PVCs Rapid infusion of potassium	Same as PVCs including electrical defibrillation

*Most common in adults.
†Life threatening in adults.

Table 29-12 Disorders of Impulse Conduction

Type	Electrocardiogram	Effect	Pathophysiology	Treatment
Sinus block	Occasionally absent P, with loss of QRS for that beat	Occasional decrease in cardiac output Increase in preload for the following beat	Local hypoxia, scarring of intraatrial conduction pathways, electrolyte imbalances Increased atrial preload	Conservative Usually do not progress in severity Pharmacologic treatment includes vagolytics, sympathomimetics, pacing
First-degree block*	PR interval >0.2	None	Same as sinus block Hyperkalemia (>7 mEq/L) Hypokalemia (<3.5 mEq/L) Formation of myocardial abscesses in endocarditis	Conservative Discovery and correction of cause
Second-degree block, Mobitz I, or Wenckebach*	Progressive prolongation of PR interval until one QRS is dropped Pattern of prolongation resumes	Same as sinus block	Hypokalemia (<3.5 mEq/L) Faulty cell metabolism in atrioventricular (AV) node Severity increases as heart rate increases Supports theory that AV node is fatiguing Digoxin toxicity, β blockade Coronary artery disease (CAD), myocardial infarction (MI), hypoxia, increased preload, valvular surgery and disease, diabetes	Same as sinus block

*Most common in adults.
†Life threatening in adults.

Continued

Table 29-12 Disorders of Impulse Conduction—cont'd

Type	Electrocardiogram	Effect	Pathophysiology	Treatment
Second-degree block or Mobitz II	Same as sinus block	Same as sinus block	Hypokalemia (<3.5 mEq/L) Faulty cell metabolism below AV node Antidysrrhythmics, cyclic antidepressants CAD, MI, hypoxia, increased preload, valvular surgery and disease, diabetes	More aggressively than Mobitz I, since can progress to type III Pacemaker after pharmacologic treatment
Third-degree block†	P waves present and independent of QRS No observed relationship between P and QRS Always atrioventricular (AV) dissociation	Same as idiojunctional rhythm	Hypokalemia (<3.5 mEq/L) Faulty cell metabolism low in bundle of His MI, especially inferior wall, as nodal artery interrupted; results in ischemia of AV node	Pharmacologic until pacemaker inserted Temporary pacing if caused by inferior MI, since ischemia usually resolves
Atrioventricular dissociation	P waves present and independent of QRS, but not always because of block (e.g., ventricular tachycardia) AV dissociation not always third-degree block	Decreased cardiac output from loss of atrial contribution to ventricular preload Variable effect on myocardial demand, depending on ventricular rate	May result from third-degree block or accelerated junctional or ventricular rhythm, or be caused by sinus, atrial, and junctional bradycardias	Treat according to cause Pacemaker or reducing rate of AV or ventricular discharge, or increasing rate of sinus or AV node discharge
Ventricular block	QRS >0.11 R-S-R′ in V_1, V_2, V_5, V_6	None	Faulty cell metabolism in right and left bundle branches	Isolated right bundle branch block (RBBB) or left bundle branch block (LBBB) or hemiblock not treated
			RBBB more common than LBBB because of dual blood supply to left bundle branch Congestive heart failure, mitral regurgitation, especially anterior MI, because of infarct of fascicles Left anterior hemiblock more common than left posterior hemiblock, since posterior fascicles have dual blood supply	If acute and/or associated with acute anterior MI, treated with permanent pacer and vigorous pharmacology
Aberrant conduction	QRS >0.11	None unless ventricular rate abnormalities present	Conduction of impulse through intercalated disks, since conduction system transiently blocked because of hypoxia, electrolyte imbalances, digoxin toxicity, excessively rapid rates of discharge	Correct underlying cause

*Most common in adults.
†Life threatening in adults.

Table 29-12 Disorders of Impulse Conduction—cont'd

Type	Electrocardiogram	Effect	Pathophysiology	Treatment
Preexcitation syndromes (Wolff-Parkinson-White and Lown-Ganong-Levine)	P present with QRS for each P PR interval >0.12 and QRS >0.11 because of presence of delta wave in PR interval	None	Congenital presence of accessory pathways (bundle of Kent and fiber of Mahaim) that conduct very rapidly and bypass the AV node, causing early ventricular depolarization in relation to atrial depolarization Prone (reason unknown) to tachycardias and atrial fibrillation that can result in very rapid ventricular rates	Aimed at lining up refractory periods of accessory pathway and AV node to prevent reentry May slow rate with pharmacology May surgically cut pathways

*Most common in adults.
†Life threatening in adults.

SUMMARY REVIEW

Diseases of the Arteries and Veins

1. Atherosclerosis is a form of arteriosclerosis and is the leading contributor to coronary artery and cerebrovascular disease.
2. Atherosclerosis is an inflammatory disease that begins with endothelial injury (smoking, hypertension, diabetes [insulin resistance], hyperhomocystinemia, dyslipidemia, etc.) and progresses through several stages to become a fibrotic plaque.
3. Once a plaque has formed, it can rupture, resulting in thrombosis and vasoconstriction leading to obstruction of the lumen and inadequate perfusion of distal tissues.
4. Hypertension is a sustained elevation of the system arterial blood pressure resulting from increases in cardiac output or total peripheral resistance or both. Hypertension can be primary (without known cause) or secondary (caused by disease or drugs).
5. The risk factors for hypertension include a positive family history; male gender; advanced age; black race; obesity; high sodium intake; low potassium, calcium, and magnesium intake; diabetes mellitus; labile blood pressure; cigarette smoking; and heavy alcohol consumption.
6. Primary hypertension is the result of extremely complicated interactions of genetics and the environment mediated by a host of neurohumoral effects. These genes interact with diet, smoking, age, and the other risk factors to cause chronic changes in vasomotor tone and blood volume.
7. The most frequently cited theories of the pathogenesis of primary hypertension include (1) overactivity of the sympathetic nervous system; (2) overactivity of the renin-angiotensin-aldosterone system; (3) alterations in other neurohumoral mediators of blood volume and vasomotor tone such as atrial natriuretic peptide, brain natriuretic peptide, and adrenomedullin; and (4) a complex interaction involving insulin resistance and endothelial function.
8. Clinical manifestations of hypertension result from damage of organs and tissues outside the vascular system. These include heart disease, renal disease, central nervous system problems, and musculoskeletal dysfunction.
9. Hypertension is managed pharmacologically, using diuretics, adrenergic blockers, calcium channel blockers, angiotensin-converting enzyme (ACE) inhibitors, and angiotensin II receptor blockers (losartan). Nonpharmacologic methods include cessation of smoking, dietary modifications, and exercise.
10. Orthostatic hypotension is a drop in blood pressure that occurs on standing. The compensatory vasoconstriction response to standing is altered by a marked vasodilation and blood pooling in the muscle vasculature.
11. Orthostatic hypotension may be acute or chronic. The acute form is caused by a delay in the normal regulatory mechanisms. The chronic forms are secondary to a specific disease or are idiopathic in nature.
12. The clinical manifestations of orthostatic hypotension include fainting and may involve cardiovascular symptoms, as well as impotence and bowel and bladder dysfunction.
13. An aneurysm is a localized dilation of a vessel wall, to which the aorta is particularly susceptible.
14. A thrombus is a clot that remains attached to a vascular wall. Arteriosclerosis can generate thrombus formation through roughening of the intima that activates the clotting cascade. Thrombus formation may be discrete or diffuse.
15. An embolus is a mobile aggregate of a variety of substances that occludes the vasculature. Sources of emboli include clots, air, amniotic fluid, bacteria, fat, and foreign matter.
16. The most common cause of arterial thrombotic emboli is the heart, as a result of mitral and aortic valvular disease and atrial fibrillation, followed by myxomas. Tissues affected include the lower extremities, the brain, and the heart.
17. Emboli to the central organs cause tissue death in lungs, kidneys, and mesentery.

18. The generation of air emboli requires a connection between the vascular compartment and a source of air. These emboli cause ischemia and necrosis when a vessel is totally blocked.
19. Amniotic fluid may be forced into the bloodstream and generate an embolus during the labor and delivery of pregnancy.
20. Aggregates of bacteria in the vasculature may be large enough to form an embolus.
21. Fat emboli are caused mainly by trauma to the long bones, either through defective fat metabolism after trauma or through the release of fat globules from bone marrow exposed by fracture.
22. The introduction of foreign matter into the vasculature can occur with trauma and also can occur in a hospital setting in which intravenous and intraarterial lines are being used.
23. Vasospastic disorders include Raynaud disease, involving arterioles of the extremities; variant angina, involving coronary arteries; and Buerger disease, involving arteries of the hands and feet.
24. Diabetic lesions of the arteries may be caused by a defect in glycoprotein metabolism that involves the capillary basement membranes in kidneys, retinas, and extremities.
25. Varicosities are areas of veins in which blood has pooled, usually in the saphenous veins. Varicosities may be caused by damaged valves as a result of trauma to the valve or by chronic venous distention involving gravity and venous constriction.
26. Chronic venous insufficiency is inadequate venous return over a long period that causes pathologic ischemic changes in the vasculature, skin, and supporting tissues.
27. Venous stasis ulcers follow the development of chronic venous insufficiency and probably develop as a result of the borderline metabolic state of the cells in the affected extremities.
28. Deep venous thrombosis occurs in individuals who have venous stasis (immobility, age, left heart failure), vein wall damage (trauma, intravenous medications), or hypercoagulable states (pregnancy, oral contraceptives, malignancy, genetic coagulopathies).
29. Deep venous thrombsis is often asymptomatic but may lead to potentially fatal pulmonary emboli; thus prevention and careful assessment in individuals at risk is crucial.
30. Coronary artery disease (CAD) is spasm or occlusion of the coronary arteries and is most often the result of atherosclerotic lesions that limit the flow of blood to the heart.
31. Many risk factors contribute to the onset and escalation of CAD, including advanced age, male gender (under the age of 60), hypertension, dyslipidemia (including elevated Lp[a]), hyperhomocysteinemia, diabetes mellitis, smoking, obesity, sedentary life-style, psychosocial factors, estrogen deficiency, elevated fibrinogen, serum amyloid, C-reactive protein, and possibly infectious agents.
32. Coronary artery disease results in an imbalance between coronary supply of blood and myocardial demand for oxygen and nutients such that reversible myocardial ischemia or irreversible infarction may result.
33. Reversible myocardial ischemia presents clinically in several ways. Chronic coronary obstruction results in recurrent predictable chest pain called stable angina. Abnormal vasospasm of coronary vessels results in unpredictable chest pain called Prinzmetal angina. Myocardial ischemia that does not cause detectable symptoms is called silent ischemia.
34. Stable angina is evaluated by noninvasive techniques of assessing coronary flow with or without exercise (stress electrocardiogram [ECG], thallium, or single-photon emission computed tomography [SPECT]). Management may include life-style changes, vasodilators, percutaneous transluminal angioplasty (PTCA), or coronary bypass surgery.
35. When there is sudden coronary obstruction because of thrombosis formation over a ruptured atherosclerotic plaque, the acute coronary syndromes result. Unstable angina causes reversible myocardial ischemia and is a harbinger of impending infarction. Myocardial infarction results when there is prolonged ischemia causing irreversible damage to the heart muscle. Sudden cardiac death can occur in any of the acute coronary syndromes.
36. Unstable angina occurs due to transient episodes of thrombotic vessel occlusion and vasoconstriction at the site of plaque damage, with return of perfusion before significant myocardial necrosis occurs. This must be managed aggressively with antithrombotic agents to prevent myocardial infarction.
37. When coronary blood flow is interrupted for an extended period of time, myocyte necrosis occurs; this is called myocardial infarction (MI). There are two major types of myocardial infarction: non–Q wave (subendocardial) infarction and Q wave (transmural) infarction. In addition to myocyte necrosis, other changes in the heart with MI include hibernating, stunning, and remodeling of the myocardium.
38. Acute coronary syndromes are assessed by measuring serum enzymes, such as creatinine kinase and troponins, as well as looking for characteristic changes in the ECG. Management may include thrombolytic drugs, antithrombotic drugs, vasodilators, PTCA, or immediate surgery.
39. Dysrhythmias, congestive heart failure, and sudden death are the most common complications of the acute coronary syndromes.

Disorders of the Heart Wall

1. Inflammation of the pericardium (pericarditis) may result from innumerable sources (infection, drug therapy, tumors). Pericarditis presents with symptoms that are physically troublesome, but in and of themselves they are not life threatening.
2. Fluid may collect within the pericardial sac (pericardial effusion). Cardiac function may be severely impaired if a large volume of fluid accumulates rapidly.
3. Cardiomyopathies are a diverse group of primary myocardial disorders that are poorly understood. The cardiomyopathies are categorized as dilated (congestive), restrictive (rigid and noncompliant), and hypertrophic (asymmetric). Size of the cardiac muscle walls and chambers may increase or decrease, depending on the type of cardiomyopathy, thereby altering contractile activity.
4. Hemodynamic integrity of the cardiovascular system depends to a great extent on properly functioning cardiac valves. Congenital or acquired disorders that result in stenosis or incompetence or both can structurally alter the valves.
5. Characteristic heart sounds, cardiac murmurs, and systemic complaints assist in determination of which valve is abnormal. If severely compromised function exists, a prosthetic heart valve may be surgically implanted to replace the faulty one.
6. Mitral valve prolapse (MVP) is a common finding, especially in young women. Although not grossly abnormal, the mitral valve leaflets do not position themselves properly during systole. MVP may be a completely asymptomatic condition, or it may result in severe subjective symptoms. Af-

flicted valves may be at greater risk for developing infective endocarditis.
7. Rheumatic fever is an inflammatory disease that results from a delayed autoimmune response to a streptococcal infection. The disorder usually resolves without sequelae if treated early.
8. Severe or untreated cases of rheumatic fever may progress to rheumatic heart disease, a potentially disabling cardiovascular disorder.
9. Infective endocarditis is a general term for inflammation of the endocardium, especially the cardiac valves. A wide range of conditions predisposes to the development of this disorder. In the mildest cases, valvular function may be slightly impaired by vegetations that collect on the valve leaflets. If infective endocarditis is left unchecked, severe valve abnormalities, chronic bacteremia, and systemic emboli may occur as vegetations break off the valve surface and travel through the bloodstream. Antibiotic therapy can limit the extent of this disease.
10. Human immunodeficiency virus is associated with cardiac abnormalities, including myocarditis, endocarditis, pericarditis, and cardiomyopathy. Left heart failure is the most frequent clinical manifestation.

Manifestations of Heart Disease

1. Heart failure is an inability of the heart to supply the metabolism with adequate circulatory volume and pressure.
2. Left heart failure is commonly called congestive heart failure and can be categorized as systolic heart failure or diastolic heart failure.
3. Systolic heart failure is defined as an inability of the heart to generate an adequate cardiac output to perfuse vital tissue.
4. Cardiac output depends on the heart rate and stroke volume. Stroke volume is influenced by contractility, preload, and afterload. Myocardial infarction is the most common cause of decreased contractility. Myocardial ischemia results in ventricular remodeling that causes progressive myocyte contractile dysfunction over time.
5. Preload (left ventricular end-diastolic volume [LVEDV]) is increased when there is decreased contractility or an excess of plasma volume.
6. Increased afterload is most commonly the result of increased peripheral vascular resistance. This increase in resistance decreases ventricular emptying and makes more workload for the left ventricle, resulting in hypertrophy and ventricular remodeling. The vicious cycle of decreasing contractility, increasing preload, and increasing afterload causes progressive worsening.
7. Neurohumoral mechanisms of CHF include abnormalities in the sympathetic nervous system, the renin-angiotensin-aldosterone system, arginine vasopressin, natriuretic peptides, endothelial hormones, endotoxin, and inflammatory cytokines.
8. The clinical manifestations of left heart failure are the result of pulmonary vascular congestion and inadequate systemic perfusion.
9. Management of left heart failure relies on increasing contractility and reducing preload and afterload.
10. Diastolic heart failure can occur singly or together with systolic heart failure. The major causes of diastolic dysfunction include hypertension-induced myocardial hypertrophy and ischemia with resultant ventricular remodeling.
11. Right heart failure can result from left heart failure and/or diffuse hypoxic pulmonary disease, such as chronic obstructive pulmonary disease (COPD), cystic fibrosis, and adult respiratory distress syndrome (ARDS). These mechanisms are discussed in Chapter 32.
12. High output failure is the inability of the heart to adequately supply the body with blood-borne nutrients despite adequate volume and normal or elevated myocardial contractility. Common causes are anemia, sepsis, hyperthyroidism, and beriberi.
13. A dysrhythmia (arrhythmia) is a disturbance of heart rhythm. Dysrhythmias range in severity from occasional missed beats or rapid beats to disturbances that impair myocardial contractility and are life threatening.
14. Dysrhythmias can occur because of an abnormal rate of impulse generation or the abnormal conduction of impulses.

KEY TERMS

KEY TERMS—cont'd

REFERENCES

1. Danesh J: Smoldering arteries? Low-grade inflammation and coronary heart disease, *JAMA* 82(22):2169, 1999.
2. Libby P: Changing concepts of atherogenesis, *J Intern Med* 247(3): 349, 2000.
3. Ross R: Mechanisms of disease: atherosclerosis—an inflammatory disease, *N Engl J Med* 340(2):115, 1999.
4. Sinisalo J et al: Relation of inflammation to vascular function in patients with coronary heart disease, *Atherosclerosis* 149(2):403, 2000.
5. Danesh J et al: Risk factors for coronary heart disease and acute-phase proteins. A population-based study, *Euro Heart J* 20(13):954, 1999.
6. Malek AM, Alper SI, Izumo S: Hemodynamic shear stress and its role in atherosclerosis, *JAMA* 282(21) 2035, 1999.
7. Welch GN, Loscalzo J: Homocysteine and atherothrombosis, *N Engl J Med* 338(15):1042, 1998.
8. Willinek WA et al: High-normal serum homocysteine concentrations are associated with an increased risk of early atherosclerotic carotid artery wall lesions in healthy subjects, *J Hypertens* 18(4):425, 2000.
9. Wiedermann CJ et al: Association of endotoxemia with carotid atherosclerosis and cardiovascular disease: prospective results from the Bruneck Study, *J Am Coll Cardiol* 34(7):1975, 1999.
10. Wu T et al: Examination of the relation between periodontal health status and cardiovascular risk factors: serum total and high density lipoprotein cholesterol, C-reactive protein, and plasma fibrinogen, *Am J Epidemiol* 151(3):273, 2000.
11. Epstein S, Zhou YF, Zhu J: Potential role of cytomegalovirus in the pathogenesis of restenosis atherosclerosis, *Am Heart J* 138(5, part 2 suppl):S476, 1999.
12. Gupta S: *Chlamydia pneumoniae,* monocyte activation, and azithromycin in coronary heart disease. *Am Heart J* 138(5, part 2):S539, 1999.
13. Haider AW, Wilson PWF, Larson MG: *Chlamydia, H. pylori,* and cytomegalovirus seropositivity and risk of cardiovascular disease: the Framingham Heart Study, *J Am Coll Cardiol* 33:314A, 1999.
14. Kusters J, Kuipers E: *Helicobacter* and atherosclerosis, *Am Heart J* 138(5, part 2 suppl):S523, 1999.
15. Vorchheimer DA, Badimon JJ, Fuster VL: Platelet glycoprotein IIb/IIIa receptor antagonists in cardiovascular disease, *JAMA* 281(15): 1407, 1999.
16. Britten MB, Zeiher AM, Schachinger V: Clinical importance of coronary endothelial vasodilator dysfunction and therapeutic options, *J Intern Med* 245(4):315, 1999.
17. John S, Schmieder RE: Impaired endothelial function in arterial hypertension and hypercholesterolemia: potential mechanisms and differences, *J Hypertens* 18(4):363, 2000.
18. Frohlich ED: Current pathophysiologic considerations in essential hypertension, *Med Clin No Amer* 81:1113, 1997.
19. Adams MR et al: Atherogenic lipids and endothelial dysfunction: mechanisms in the genesis of ischemic syndromes, *Ann Rev Med* 51: 149, 2000.
20. He J, Whelton PK: Elevated systolic blood pressure as a risk factor for cardiovascular and renal disease, *J Hypertens* 17(2):S7, 1999.
21. Kita T: LOX-1, a possible clue to the missing link between hypertension and atherogenesis, *Circulation Res* 84:1113, 1999.
22. Dupuis J et al: Cholesterol reduction rapidly improves endothelial function after acute coronary syndromes. The RECIFE (reduction of cholesterol in ischemia and function of the endothelium) trial, *Circulation* 99(25):3227,1999.
23. Schachinger V et al: A positive family history of premature coronary artery disease is associated with impaired endothelium-dependent coronary blood flow regulation, *Circulation* 100(14):1502, 1999.
24. Kinlay S. Fang JC, Hikita H: Plasma alpha tocopherol and coronary endothelium-dependent vasodilator function, *Circulation* 100:219, 1999.
25. Neunteufl T et al: Effects of vitamin E on chronic and acute endothelial dysfunction in smokers, *J Am Coll Cardiol* 35(2):277, 2000.
26. Berenson GS et al: Association between multiple cardiovascular risk factors and atherosclerosis in children and young adults. The Bogalusa Heart Study, *N Engl J Med* 338(23), 1650, 1998.
27. Sparling PB, Snow TK, Beavers BD: Serum cholesterol levels in college students: opportunities for education and intervention, *J Am Coll Health* 48(3):123, 1999.

28. Stewart KJ et al: Dietary fat and cholesterol intake in young children compared with recommended levels, *J Cardiopulmon Rehab* 9(2): 112, 1999.
29. Eisenberg DA: Cholesterol lowering in the management of coronary artery disease: the clinical implications of recent trials, *Am J Med* 104(2A):2S, 1998.
30. Steinberg D, Gotto AM: Preventing coronary artery disease by lowering cholesterol levels. Fifty years from bench to bedside, *JAMA* 282(21): 2043, 1999.
31. Ravn HB, Falk E: Histopathology of plaque rupture, *Cardiol Clin* 17(2):263, 1999.
32. Rothwell PM et al: Evidence of a chronic systemic cause of instability of atherosclerotic plaques, *Lancet* 335:19, 2000.
33. Zaman AG et al: The role of plaque rupture and thrombosis in coronary artery disease, *Atherosclerosis* 149(2):251, 2000.
34. Gonzalez ER: Antiplatelet therapy in atherosclerotic cardiovascular disease, *Clin Therapeutics* 20(suppl B):B18, 1998.
35. National Cholesterol Education Program (NCEP) Expert Panel: Summary of the second report of the National Cholesterol Expert Panel on detection, evaluation, and treatment of high blood cholesterol in adults (adult treatment panel II), *JAMA* 269(3):3015, 1993.
36. Anonymous: 1999 World Health Organization–International Society of Hypertension guidelines for the management of hypertension. Guidelines subcommittee, *J Hypertens* 17(2), 151, 1999.
37. Anonymous: The Sixth Report of the Joint National Committee on Prevention, Detection, Evaluation, and Treatment of High Blood Pressure, *Arch Intern Med* 157:2413, 1997.
38. Hall WD: Risk reduction associated with lowering systolic blood pressure: review of clinical trial data, *Am Heart J* 138(3):225, 1999.
39. Kannel WB: Historical perspectives on the relative contributions of diastolic and systolic blood pressure elevation to cardiovascular risk profile, *Am Heart J* 138(3):S2205, 1999.
40. Port S et al: Systolic blood pressure and mortality, *Lancet* 355(9199): 175, 2000.
41. Swales J: Current clinical practice in hypertension: the EISBERG (evaluation and interventions for systolic blood pressure elevation-regional and global) project, *Am Heart J* 138(suppl 3 part 2):S231, 1999.
42. Agnelli G, Sonaglia F: Prevention of venous thromboembolism, *Thrombosis Res* 97(1):V49, 2000.
43. Fagan T, Deedwania PC: The cardiovascular dysmetabolic syndrome, *Am J Med* 105 (1A):77S, 1998.
44. Hsueh WA, Law RE: Cardiovascular risk continuum: implications of insulin resistance and diabetes, *Am J Med* 105 (1A):4S, 1998.
45. Mikhail N, Golub MS, Tuck ML. Obesity and hypertension, *Prog Cardiovas Dis* 42(1):39, 1999.
46. Griffith LE et al: The influence of dietary and nondietary calcium supplementation on blood pressure: an updated meta-analysis of randomized controlled trials, *Am J Hypertens* 12(1 part 1):84, 1999.
47. Katz A et al: Effect of a mineral salt diet on 24-h blood pressure monitoring in elderly hypertensive patients, *J Hum Hypertens* 13(11):777, 1999.
48. Kawamo Y et al: Effects of potassium supplementation on office, home and 24 hour blood pressure in patients with essential hypertension, *Am J Hypertens* 11:1141, 1999.
49. Moore TJ et al: Effect of dietary patterns on ambulatory blood pressure: results from the Dietary Approaches to Stop Hypertension (DASH) Trial. DASH Collaborative Research Group, *Hypertension* 34(3):472, 1999.
50. Verdecchia P et al: Cigarette smoking, ambulatory blood pressure and cardiac hypertrophy in essential hypertension, *J Hypertens* 13:1209, 1995.
51. Vriz O et al: The effects of alcohol consumption on ambulatory blood pressure and target organs in subjects with borderline to mild hypertension. HARVEST Study Group, *Am J Hypertens* 11:230, 1998.
52. An P, Rice T, Rao DC: A review of recent genetic epidemiological studies of blood pressure, *CVR&R* 21:85, 2000.
53. Giner V et al: Renin-angiotensin system genetic polymorphisms and salt sensitivity in essential hypertension, *Hypertension* 35(1 part 2): 512, 2000.
54. Farfel Z, Henry R, Iiri T: Mechanisms of disease: the expanding spectrum of G protein diseases, *N Engl J Med* 340(1):12, 1999.
55. Mancia G et al: Sympathetic activation in the pathogenesis of hypertension and progression of organ damage, *Hypertension* 34(4 part 2): 724, 1999.
56. Morimoto S et al: Sympathetic activation and contribution of genetic factors in hypertension with neurovascular compression of the rostral ventrolateral medulla, *J Hypertens* 17(11):1577, 1999.
57. Supiano MA et al: Sympathetic nervous system activity and alpha-adrenergic responsiveness in older hypertensive humans, *Am J Physiol* 276(3 part 1):E519, 1999.
58. Stroth U, Unger T: The renin-angiotensin system and its receptors, *J Cardiovasc Pharmacol* 33(suppl 1):S21, 1999.
59. Brooks DP, Ruffolo RR Jr: Pharmacological mechanism of angiotensin II receptor antagonists: implications for the treatment of elevated systolic blood pressure, *J Hypertens* 17(suppl 2):S27, 1999.
60. Romero JC, Reckelhoff JF: State-of-the-art lecture. Role of angiotensin and oxidative stress in essential hypertension, *Hypertension* 34(4 part 2):943, 1999.
61. Gibbons GH: The pathophysiology of hypertension. The importance of angiotensin II in cardiovascular remodeling, *Am J Hypertens* 11: 177S, 1998.
62. Klingbeil AU et al: Hyper-responsiveness to angiotensin II is related to cardiac structural adaptation in hypertensive subjects, *J Hypertens* 17(6):825, 1999.
63. Hall JE, Brands MW, Henegar JR: Angiotensin II and long-term arterial pressure regulation: the overriding dominance of the kidney, *J Am Soc Nephrol* 10(suppl 12):S258, 1999.
64. Okuguchi T et al: Significance of sympathetic nervous system in sodium-induced nocturnal hypertension, *J Hypertens* 17(7):947, 1999.
65. Bayer AS et al: Diagnosis and management of infective endocarditis and its complications, *Circulation* 98(25):2936, 1998.
66. Bettencourt P et al: Brain natriuretic peptide as a marker of cardiac involvement in hypertension, *Int J Cardiol* 69(2):169, 1999.
67. Osei K: Insulin resistance and systemic hypertension, *Am J Cardiol* 84(1A):33J, 1999.
68. Cleland SJ et al: Insulin action is associated with endothelial function in hypertension and type 2 diabetes, *Hypertension* 35(1 part 2):507, 2000.
69. Raij L: Nitric oxide, salt sensitivity, and cardiorenal injury in hypertension, *Semin Nephrol* 19(3):296, 1999.
70. Watanabe K et al: Relationship between insulin resistance and cardiac sympathetic nervous function in essential hypertension, *J Hypertens* 17(8):1161, 1999.
71. Nickeng G, Bohm, M: Interaction between insulin and AT_1 receptor. Relevance for hypertension and arteriosclerosis, *Basic Res Cardiol* 93(suppl 2):135, 1998.
72. Higashiura K et al: Effect of an angiotensin II receptor antagonist, candesartan, on insulin resistance and pressor mechanisms in essential hypertension, *J Hum Hypertens* 13(suppl 1):S71, 1999.
73. Lender D et al: A double blind comparison of the effects of amlodipine and enalapril on insulin sensitivity in hypertensive patients, *Am J Hypertens* 12(3):298, 1999.
74. du Cailar G et al: Left ventricular adaptation to hypertension and plasma renin activity, *J Hum Hypertens* 14(3):181, 2000.
75. Yamamoto S et al: On the nature of cell death during remodeling of hypertrophied human myocardium, *J Molecul Cell Cardiol* 32(1): 161, 2000.
76. Bianchi S, Bigazzi R, Campese VM: Microalbuminuria in essential hypertension: significance, pathophysiology, and therapeutic implications, *Am J Kidney Dis* 34(6):973, 1999.
77. Campese VM, Bianchi S, Bigazzi R: Association between hyperlipidemia and microalbuminuria in essential hypertension, *Kidney Int* 71(suppl):S10, 1999.
78. Mimran A, Ribstein J, Du Cailar G: Microalbuminuria in essential hypertension, *Curr Opin Nephrol Hypertens* 8(3):359, 1999.
79. Staessen JA et al: Predicting cardiovascular risk using conventional vs ambulatory blood pressure in older patients with systolic hypertension, *JAMA* 282:539, 1999.

80. Hansson L: The Hypertension Optimal Treatment study and the importance of lowering blood pressure, *J Hypertens* 17(suppl):S9, 1999.
81. Pickering, T: Advances in the treatment of hypertension, *JAMA* 281(2):114 1999.
82. Maser RE, Lenhard MJ, DeCherney GS: Cardiovascular autonomic neuropathy: the clinical significance of its determination, *Endocrinologist* 10(1):27, 2000.
83. Ooi WL, Hossain M, Lipsitz LA: The association between orthostatic hypotension and recurrent falls in nursing home residents, *Am J Med* 108(2):106, 2000.
84. Owens PE, Lyons SP, O'Brien ET: Arterial hypotension: prevalence of low blood pressure in the general population using ambulatory blood pressure monitoring, *J Hum Hypertens* 14(4):243, 2000.
85. Grange JJ, Davis V, Baxter BT: Pathogenesis of abdominal aortic aneurysm: an update and look toward the future, *Cardiovasc Surg* 5(3): 256, 1997.
86. Devereux R, Roman M: Aortic disease in Marfan's syndrome, *N Engl J Med* 340:1358, 1999.
87. Chen K et al: Acute thoracic aortic dissection: the basics, *J Emerg Med* 15, 859, 1997.
88. Englund R: Expansion rates of small abdominal aortic aneurysms, *Aust & New Zea J Surg* 68(1):25, 1998.
89. Taylor BV, Kalman PG: Saccular aortic aneurysms, *Ann Vasc Surg* 13(6):555, 1999.
90. Zarins CK, Harris EJ: Operative repair for aortic aneurysms: the gold standard, *J Endovasc Surg* 4(3), 232, 1997.
91. Kurata A et al: Thromboangiitis obliterans: classic and new morphological features, *Virchows Arch* 436(1):59, 2000.
92. Wysokinski WE et al: Sustained classic clinical spectrum of thromboangiitis obliterans (Buerger's disease), *Angiology* 51(2):141, 2000.
93. Shegematsu H, Shigematsu, K: Factors affecting the long-term outcome of Buerger's disease (thromboangiitis obliterans), *Int Angiol* 18: 58, 1999.
94. Freedman RR, Girgis R, Mayes MD: Endothelial and adrenergic dysfunction in Raynaud's phenomenon and scleroderma, *J Rheumatol* 26(11):2386, 1999.
95. Smyth AE et al: A case-control study of candidate vasoactive mediator genes in primary Raynaud's phenomenon, *Rheumatology* (Oxford) 38(11):1094, 1999.
96. Dziadzio M et al: Losartan therapy for Raynaud's phenomenon and scleroderma: clinical and biochemical findings in a fifteen-week, randomized, parallel-group, controlled trial, *Arthritis & Rheum* 42(12): 2646, 1999.
97. Tucker AT, Pearson RM, Cooke ED, Benjamin N: Effect of nitric-oxide-generating system on microcirculatory blood flow in skin of patients with severe Raynaud's syndrome: a randomized trial, *Lancet* 354(9191):1670, 1999.
98. Lees TA et al: A survey of the current management of varicose veins by members of the Vascular Surgical Society, *Ann Royal Coll Surg Eng* 1(6):407, 1999.
99. Anderson DR et al: Thrombosis in the emergency department, *Arch Intern Med* 159:477, 1999.
100. Antman EM, Cohen M: Newer antithrombin agents in acute coronary syndromes, *Am Heart J* 138(suppl):S563, 1999.
101. Meignan M et al: Systematic lung scans reveal a high frequency of silent pulmonary embolism in patients with proximal deep venous thrombosis, *Arch Intern Med* 160(2):159, 2000.
102. Ageno W: Treatment of venous thromboembolism, *Thrombosis Res* 97(1):V63, 2000.
103. Hull RD et al: Low-molecular-weight heparin vs heparin in the treatment of patients with pulmonary embolism. American-Canadian Thrombosis Study Group, *Arch Intern Med* 160(2):229, 2000.
104. Hyers TM: Venous thromboembolism, *Am J Respir Care Med* 159:1, 1999.
105. Horne MK, Chang R: Thrombolytic therapy for deep venous thrombosis? *JAMA* 282, 2164, 1999.
106. Heit JA et al: Predictors of recurrence after deep vein thrombosis and pulmonary embolism, *Arch Intern Med* 160:761, 2000.
107. Stratton MA et al: Prevention of venous thromboembolism, *Arch Intern Med* 160:334, 2000.
108. Haapoja IS, Blendowski C: Superior vena cava syndrome, *Semin Oncol Nurs* 15(3):183, 1999.
109. Kee ST: Superior vena cava syndrome L treatment with catheter-directed thrombolysis and endovascular shunt placement, *Radiology* 206:187, 1998.
110. Schindler N, Vogelzang RL: Superior vena cava syndrome. Experience with endovascular stents and surgical therapy, *Surg Clin North Am* 79(3):683, 1999.
111. American Heart Association: *2000 heart and stroke statistical update*. Dallas, Tex, 1999, American Heart Association.
112. Lloyd-Jones DM, Larson MG, Beiser A, Levy D: Lifetime risk of developing coronary heart disease, *Lancet* 353, 89, 1999.
113. Libby P, Ridker, P: Novel inflammatory markers of coronary risk: theory versus practice, *Circulation* 100:1148, 1999.
114. Ridker PM et al: C-reactive protein and other markers of inflammation in the prediction of cardiovascular disease in women, *N Engl J Med*. 342(12):836, 2000.
115. Gotto AM Jr: Triglyceride as a risk factor for coronary artery disease, *Am J Cardiol* 82(9A):22Q, 1998.
116. Ansell BJ, Watson KE, Fogelman AM: An evidence-based assessment of the NCEP Adult Treatment Panel II guidelines. National Cholesterol Education Program, *JAMA* 282(21):2051, 1999.
117. Gotto AM Jr et al: Relation between baseline and on-treatment lipid parameters and first acute major coronary events in the Air Force/Texas Coronary Atherosclerosis Prevention Study (AFCAPS/TexCAPS), *Circulation* 101(5):477, 2000.
118. Linde R: Apo B and Lp(a): a clinician's perspective, *Endocrinologist* 10(2):83, 2000.
119. Miwa K et al: Lipoprotein (a) is a risk factor for occurrence of acute myocardial infarction in patients with coronary vasospasm, *J Am Coll Cardiol* 35(5):1200, 2000.
120. Seman LJ et al: Lipoprotein (a)-cholesterol and coronary heart disease in the Framingham Heart Study, *Clin Chem* 45(7):1039, 1999.
121. Kwiterovich PO Jr: The antiatherogenic role of high-density lipoprotein cholesterol, *Am J Cardiol* 82(9A):13Q, 1998.
122. Ballantyne CM et al: Influence of low HDL on progression of coronary artery disease and response to fluvastatin therapy, *Circulation* 99(6):736, 1999.
123. Blumenthal RS: Statins: effective antiatherosclerotic therapy, *Am Heart J* 139(4):577, 2000.
124. LaRosa JC, He J, Vupputuri S: Effect of statins on risk of coronary disease: a meta-analysis of randomized controlled trials, *JAMA* 282(24): 2340, 1999.
125. Pitt B et al: Aggressive lipid-lowering therapy compared with angioplasty in stable coronary artery disease *N Engl J Med* 341:70, 1999.
126. Harper CR, Jacobson TA: New perspectives on the management of low levels of high-density lipoprotein cholesterol, *Arch Intern Med* 159(10):1049, 1999.
127. Rubins HB et al: Gemfibrozil for the secondary prevention of coronary heart disease in men with low levels of high-density lipoprotein cholesterol, *N Eng J Med* 341:410, 1999.
128. Rifkind BM, Schucker B, Gorder DJ: When should patients with heterozygous familial hypercholesterolemia be treated? *JAMA* 281:180, 1999.
129. Ockene IS, Miller NH: Cigarette smoking, cardiovascular disease, and stroke: a statement for healthcare professionals from the American Heart Association: American Heart Association Task Force on Risk Reduction, *Circulation* 96:3243, 1997.
130. Villablanca AC, McDonald JM, Rutledge JC: Smoking and cardiovascular disease, *Clin Chest Med* 21(1):159, 2000.
131. He J et al: Passive smoking and the risk of coronary heart disease—a meta-analysis of epidemiologic studies, *N Engl J Med* 340(12):920, 1999.
132. Poredos P, Orehek M, Tratnik E: Smoking is associated with dose-related increase of intima-media thickness and endothelial dysfunction, *Angiology* 50(3):201,1999.

133. Yuan S, Liu Y, Zhu L: Vascular complications of diabetes mellitus, *Clin Exp Pharmacol Physiol* 26(12):977, 1999.
134. Herman WH: Clinical evidence: glycaemic control in diabetes, *Brit Med J* 319(7202):104, 1999.
135. Boer JM et al: The joint impact of family history of myocardial infarction and other risk factors on 12-year coronary heart disease mortality, *Epidemiology* 10(6):767, 1999.
136. He J et al: Dietary sodium intake and subsequent risk of cardiovascular disease in overweight adults, *JAMA* 282:2027, 1999.
137. Morricone L et al: The role of central fat distribution in coronary artery disease in obesity: comparison of nondiabetic obese, diabetic obese, and normal weight subjects, *Internat J Obesity Related Metabol Dis* 23(11):1129, 1999.
138. Grundy SM: Primary prevention of coronary heart disease: integrating risk assessment with intervention, *Circulation* 100(9):988, 1999.
139. Hakim AA et al: Effects of walking on coronary heart disease in elderly men: the Honolulu Heart Program, *Circulation* 100(1):9, 1999.
140. Ornish D et al: Intensive lifestyle changes for reversal of coronary heart disease, *JAMA* 280:2001, 1998.
141. Lisspers J et al: Multifactorial evaluation of a program for lifestyle behavior change in rehabilitation and secondary prevention of coronary artery disease, *Scand Cardiovasc J* 33(1):9, 1999.
142. Albert CM et al: Moderate alcohol consumption and the risk of sudden cardiac death among US male physicians, *Circulation* 100(9): 944, 1999.
143. Gaziano JM et al: Light-to-moderate alcohol consumption and mortality in the Physicians' Health Study enrollment cohort. *J Am Coll Cardiol* 35(1):96, 2000.
144. Wannamethee SG, Shaper AG: Type of alcoholic drink and risk of major coronary heart disease events and all-cause mortality, *Am J Public Health* 89(5):685, 1999.
145. Rimm EB et al: Moderate alcohol intake and lower risk of coronary hart disease: meta-analysis of effects on lipids and haemostatic factors, *Brit Med J* 319:1523, 1999.
146. Bell JR et al: Catechin in human plasma after ingestion of a single serving of reconstituted red wine, *Am J Clin Nutrition* 71(1):103, 2000.
147. Caccetta RA et al: Ingestion of red wine significantly increases plasma phenolic acid concentrations but does not acutely affect ex vivo lipoprotein oxidizability *Am J Clin Nutrition* 71(1):67, 2000.
148. de Aloysio D et al: The effect of menopause on blood lipid and lipoprotein levels. The Icarus Study Group, *Atherosclerosis* 147(1):147, 1999.
149. Shlipak MG et al: Estrogen and progestin, lipoprotein (a), and the risk of recurrent coronary heart disease events after menopause, *JAMA* 283: 1845, 2000.
150. Greendale GA, Lee MP, Arriola ER: The menopause, *Lancet* 353: 571, 1999.
151. Sites CK: Hormones, women, and cardiovascular disease: primary vs. secondary prevention after menopause, *Endocrinologist* 10(2):113, 2000.
152. Friedman M, Rodenman RH: *Type A behavior and your heart*, New York, 1974, Knopf.
153. Rose MI: Type A behavior pattern: a concept revisited, *Can Med Assoc J* 136:345, 1987.
154. Review Panel on Coronary-Prone Behavior and Coronary Heart Disease: Coronary-prone behavior and coronary heart disease a critical review, *Circulation* 63:1199, 1981.
155. Twisk JW et al: Changes in daily hassles and life events and the relationship with coronary heart disease risk factors: a 2-year longitudinal study in 27-29-year-old males and females, *J Psychosom Res* 46(3): 229, 1999.
156. Calnon EA, Beller GA: Observations of silent myocardial ischemia by nuclear cardiology techniques. In Stern S, editor: *Silent myocardial ischemia,* St Louis, 1998, Mosby.
157. Gottdiener JS, Kop WJ, Krantz DS: Mental stress and silent myocardial ischemia: evidence, mechanisms and clinical implications. In Stern S, editor: *Silent myocardial ischemia,* St Louis, 1998, Mosby.
158. Rozansky A: Mental stress and the induction of silent myocardial ischemia in patients with coronary artery disease, *N Engl J Med* 318: 1005, 1988.
159. Waters D: Comparison of aggressive lipid lowering with atorvastatin vs revascularization treatments (AVERT) and conventional care for the reduction of ischemic events in patients with stable coronary artery disease, *CVR&R* 21:36, 2000.
160. Antoniucci D et al: Primary coronary infarct artery stenting in acute myocardial infarction, *Am J Cardiol* 84(5):505, 1999.
161. Edgar WF, Eibersole N, Mayfield MG: MIDCAB, *Am J Nursing* 99(7):40, 1999.
162. Allen KB et al: Comparison of transmyocardial revascularization with medical therapy in patients with refractory angina, *N Engl J Med* 341(14):1029, 1999.
163. Burkhoff D et al: Transmyocardial laser revascularisation compared with continued medical therapy for treatment of refractory angina pectoris: a prospective randomised trial. ATLANTIC Investigators: Angina Treatments-Lasers and Normal Therapies in Comparison, *Lancet* 354(9182):885, 1999.
164. Losordo DW, Vale PR, Isner JM: Gene therapy for myocardial angiogenesis, *Am Heart J* 138(2 part 2):132, 1999.
165. Fuster V, Fayad Z, Badimon JJ. Acute coronary syndromes: biology, *Lancet* 353(suppl 2):5, 1999.
166. Patel VB, Topol EJ: The pathogenesis and spectrum of acute coronary syndromes: from plaque formation to thrombosis, *Cleve Clin J Med* 66(9):561, 1999.
167. Yamagishi M et al: Morphology of vulnerable coronary plaque: insights from follow-up of patients examined by intravascular ultrasound before an acute coronary syndrome, *J Am Coll Cardiol* 35(1):106, 2000.
168. Shah P: Plaque disruption and thrombosis. Potential role of inflammation and infection, *Cardiol Clin* 17(2):271, 1999.
169. Burke AP et al: Plaque rupture and sudden death related to exertion in men with coronary artery disease, *JAMA* 281: 921, 1999.
170. Koenig W et al: C-Reactive protein, a sensitive marker of inflammation, predicts future risk of coronary heart disease in initially healthy middle-aged men: results from the MONICA (Monitoring Trends and Determinants in Cardiovascular Disease) Augsburg Cohort Study, 1984 to 1992, *Circulation* 99(2):237, 1999.
171. Jurlander B et al: Coronary angiographic findings and troponin T in patients with unstable angina pectoris, *Am J Cardiol* 85(7):810, 2000.
172. White HD: Optimal treatment of patients with acute coronary syndromes and non-ST-elevation myocardial infarction, *Am Heart J* 138(suppl):S105, 1999.
173. Pope JH et al: Missed diagnoses of acute cardiac ischemia in the emergency department, *N Engl J Med* 342(16):1163, 2000.
174. Tan WA, Moliterno DJ: Aspirin, ticlopidine, and clopidogrel in acute coronary syndromes: underused treatments could save thousands of lives, *Cleve Clin J Med* 66:615, 1999.
175. Harrington, RA: Overview of clinical trials of glycoprotein IIb-IIIa inhibitors in acute coronary syndromes, *Am Heart J* 138(suppl):S276, 1999.
176. Verheugt FW: Acute coronary syndromes: interventions, *Lancet* 353(suppl 11):16, 1999.
177. Ferrari R et al: Ischemic preconditioning, myocardial stunning, and hibernation: basic aspects, *Am Heart J* 138(2, part 2 suppl):S61, 1999.
178. Gerber BL et al: Myocardial perfusion and oxygen consumption in reperfused noninfarcted dysfunctional myocardium after unstable angina—direct evidence for myocardial stunning in humans, *J Am Coll Cardiol* 34(7):1939, 1999.
179. Noda T et al: Evidence for the delayed effect in human ischemic preconditioning: prospective multicenter study for preconditioning in acute myocardial infarction, *J Am Coll Cardiol* 34(7):1966, 1999.
180. Sanchis J et al: Predictors of early and late ventricular remodeling after acute myocardial infarction, *Clin Cardiol* 22(9):581, 1999.
181. Schmermund A et al: Cardiac production of Ang II and its pharmacologic inhibition: effects on the coronary circulation, *Mayo Clin Proc* 74: 503, 1999.

182. Yousef ZR, Redwood SR, Marber MS: Postinfarction left ventricular remodeling: where are the theories and trials leading us? *Heart* 83:76, 2000.
183. Gersh BJ: Optimal management of acute myocardial infarction at the dawn of the next millennium, *Am Heart J* 138(2 part 2):188, 1999.
184. Todd S et al: Dietary antioxidant vitamins and fiber in the etiology of cardiovascular disease and all-causes mortality: results from the Scottish Heart Health Study, *Am J Epidem* 150(10):1073, 1999.
185. Van de Werf F et al: Safety assessment of single-bolus administration of TNK tissue-plasminogen activator in acute myocardial infarction: the ASSENT-1 trial. The ASSENT-1 investigators, *Am Heart J* 137(5): 786, 1999.
186. Ferguson JJ, Taqi K: IIb/IIIa receptor blockade in acute myocardial infarction, *Am Heart J* 138(2 part 2):164, 1999.
187. Gibson CM: Primary angioplasty compared with thrombolysis: new issues in the era of glycoprotein IIb/IIIa inhibition and intracoronary stenting, *Ann Intern Med* 130(10):841, 1999.
188. Roe MT, Moliterno DJ: Emerging treatment of acute coronary syndromes with platelet glycoprotein IIB/IIIA inhibitors, *J Thromb Thrombolysis* 7(3):247, 1999.
189. Maggioni AP, Latini R: How to use ACE-inhibitors, beta-blockers, and newer therapies in AMI, *Am Heart J* 138(2 part 2):183, 1999.
190. Buxton AE et al: A randomized study of the prevention of sudden death in patients with coronary artery disease. Multicenter Unsustained Tachycardia Trial Investigators, *N Engl J Med* 341(25):1882, 1999.
191. Naccarelli GV et al: Amiodarone: clinical trials, *Curr Opin Cardiol* 15(1):64, 2000.
192. Sadowski ZP et al: Multicenter randomized trial and a systematic overview of lidocaine in acute myocardial infarction, *Am Heart J* 137(5):792, 1999.
193. Chan TC, Brady WJ, Pollack M: Electrocardiographic manifestations: acute myopericarditis, *J Emerg Med* 17(5):865, 1999.
194. Colletti C: Emergency: pericarditis, *Am J Nurs* 99(10):35, 1999.
195. Maisch B et al: Intrapericardial treatment of inflammatory and neoplastic pericarditis guided by pericardioscopy and epicardial biopsy—results from a pilot study, *Clin Cardiol* 22(suppl):I17, 1999.
196. Henein MY et al: Restrictive pericarditis, *Heart* 82(3):389, 1999.
197. Graham RM, Owens W: Pathogenesis of inherited forms of dilated cardiomyopathy, *N Engl J Med* 341(23):1759, 1999.
198. Tiret L et al: Lack of association between polymorphisms of eight candidate genes and idiopathic dilated cardiomyopathy: the CARDIGENE study, *J Am Coll Cardiol* 35(1):29, 2000.
199. Muller J et al: Immunoglobulin adsorption in patients with idiopathic dilated cardiomyopathy, *Circulation* 101(4):385, 2000.
200. Constant J: The alcoholic cardiomyopathies—genuine and pseudo, *Cardiology* 91(2):92, 1999.
201. Chan F, Ngan Kee WD: Idiopathic dilated cardiomyopathy presenting in pregnancy, *Can J Anaesthesia* 46(12):1146, 1999.
202. Watanabe T et al: Evaluation of appropriate pacing with myocardial perfusion and cardiac function as a treatment of end-stage idiopathic dilated cardiomyopathy, *Pacing Clin Electrophysiol* 22(12):1844, 1999.
203. Redwood CS, Moolman-Smook JC, Watkins H: Properties of mutant contractile proteins that cause hypertrophic cardiomyopathy, *Cardio Res* 44(1):20, 1999.
204. Shirani J, Pick R, Roberts WC, Maron B: Morphology and significance of the left ventricular collagen network in young patients with hypertrophic cardiomyopathy and sudden cardiac death, *J Am Coll Cardiol* 35(1):36, 2000.
205. Marian AJ: Pathogenesis of diverse clinical and pathological phenotypes in hypertrophic cardiomyopathy, *Lancet* 355(9197):58, 2000.
206. Maron BJ et al: Efficacy of implantable cardioverter-defibrillators for the prevention of sudden death in patients with hypertrophic cardiomyopathy, *N Engl J Med* 42(6):365, 2000.
207. Singh JP et al: Prevalence and clinical determinants of mitral, tricuspid, and aortic regurgitation (the Framingham Heart Study), *Am J Cardiol* 83(6):897, 1999.
208. Freed LA et al: Prevalence and clinical outcome of mitral-valve prolapse, *N Engl J Med* 341(1):1, 1999.
209. Szombathy T et al: Angiotension II type 1 receptor gene polymorphism and mitral valve prolapse syndrome, *Am Heart J* 139(1 part 1): 101, 2000.
210. Gilon D et al: Lack of evidence of an association between mitral-valve prolapse and stroke in young patients, *N Engl J Med* 341(1):8, 1999.
211. Phillips MR et al: Repair of anterior leaflet mitral valve prolapse: chordal replacement versus chordal shortening, *Ann Thorac Surg* 69(1): 25, 2000.
212. Markowitz M: Pioneers and modern ideas. Rheumatic fever—a half-century perspective, *Pediatrics* 102(1 part 3):272, 1998.
213. Stollerman GH: Rheumatic fever, *Lancet* 349(9056):935, 1997.
214. Djani AS et al: Guidelines for the diagnosis of rheumatic fever: Jones criteria, updated 1993, *Circulation* 87:302, 1993.
215. Dajani AS et al: Prevention of bacterial endocarditis. Recommendations by the American Heart Association, *JAMA* 277:1794, 1997.
216. Dyson C, Barnes RA, Harrison GA: Infective endocarditis: an epidemiological review of 128 episodes, *J Infect* 38(2):87, 1999.
217. Strom BL et al: Dental and cardiac risk factors for infective endocarditis. A population-based, case-control study, *Ann Intern Med* 129: 761, 1998.
218. Durack DT, Lukes AS, Bright DK: New criteria for diagnosis of infective endocarditis: utilization of specific echocardiographic findings: Duke Endocarditis Service, *Am J Med* 96:200, 1994.
219. Thatai D, Turi ZG: Current guidelines for the treatment of patients with rheumatic fever, *Drugs* 57(4):545, 1999.
220. Barbaro G et al: Cardiac involvement in the acquired immunodeficiency syndrome: a multicenter clinical-pathologicalstudy. Gruppo Italiano per lo Studio Cardiologico dei pazienti affetti da AIDS Investigators, *AIDS Res Human Retroviruses* 14(12):1071, 1998.
221. Mann DL: Mechanisms and models in heart failure: a combinatorial approach, *Circulation* 100(9):999, 1999.
222. Pepper GS, Lee RW: Sympathetic activation in heart failure and its treatment with beta-blockade, *Arch Intern Med* 159(3):225, 1999.
223. Schrier RW, Abraham WT: Hormones and hemodynamics in heart failure, *N Engl J Med* 341(8):577, 1999.
224. Roig E et al: Clinical implications of increased plasma angiotensin II despite ACE inhibitor therapy in patients with congestive heart failure, *Euro Heart J* 21(1):53, 2000.
225. Stark J: The interrelation between renal and cardiac function: physiology and pathophysiology with a focus on congestive heart failure, *Crit Care Clin No Amer* 10(4):411, 1998.
226. Albert NM: Advanced systolic heart failure: emerging pathophysiology and current management *Prog Cardiovasc Nurs* 13(3):14, 1998.
227. Brunkhorst FM et al: Pyrexia, procalcitonin, immune activation and survival in cardiogenic shock: the potential importance of bacterial translocation, *Int J Cardiol* 72(1):3, 1999.
228. Niebauer J et al: Endotoxin and immune activation in chronic heart failure: a prospective cohort study, *Lancet* 353:1838, 1999.
229. Agnoletti L et al: Serum from patients with severe heart failure downregulates eNOS and is proapoptotic: role of tumor necrosis factor-alpha *Circulation* 100(19):1983, 1999.
230. Baig MK et al: The pathophysiology of advanced heart failure, *Heart & Lung* 28(2):87, 1999.
231. Califf RM, Cohn JN: Cardiac protection: evolving role of angiotensin receptor blockers, *Am Heart J* (1 part 2):S15, 2000.
232. Hjalmarson A et al: Effects of controlled-release metoprolol on total mortality, hospitalizations, and well-being in patients with heart failure: the Metoprolol CR/XL Randomized Intervention Trial in congestive heart failure (MERIT-HF). MERIT-HF Study Group, *JAMA* 283(10): 1295, 2000.
233. Parmley WW: Surviving heart failure: Robert L. Frye lecture, *Mayo Clin Proc* 75(1):111, 2000.
234. St. John Sutton M et al: Cardiovascular death and left ventricular remodeling two years after myocardial infarction: baseline predictors

and impact of long-term use of captopril: information from the Survival and Ventricular Enlargement (SAVE) trial, *Circulation* 96(10): 3294, 1997.

235. Belardinelli R et al: Randomized, controlled trial of long-term moderate exercise training in chronic heart failure: effects on functional capacity, quality of life, and clinical outcome, *Circulation* 99(9):1173, 1999.
236. Page J, Henry D: Consumption of NSAIDs and the development of congestive heart failure in elderly patients—an underrecognized public health problem, *Arch Intern Med* 160(6):777, 2000.
237. Anonymous: The effect of digoxin on mortality and morbidity in patients with heart failure. The Digitalis Investigation Group, *N Engl J Med* 336(8):525, 1997.
238. Gambassi G et al: Effects of angiotensin-converting enzyme inhibitors and digoxin on health outcomes of very old patients with heart failure. SAGE Study Group: Systematic Assessment of Geriatric drug use via Epidemiology, *Arch Intern Med* 160(1):53, 2000.
239. Lindsay SJ et al: Digoxin and mortality in chronic heart failure. UK heart investigation, *Lancet* 354(9183):1003, 1999.
240. Spargias KS, Hall AS, Ball SG: Safety concerns about digoxin after acute myocardial infarction, *Lancet*. 354(9176):391, 1999.
241. Pitt B et al: The effect of spironolactone on morbidity and mortality in patients with severe heart failure. Randomized Aldactone Evaluation Study Investigators, *N Engl J Med* 341(10):709, 1999.
242. Bonet S et al: Beta-adrenergic blocking agents in heart failure—benefits of vasodilating and nonvasodilating agents according to patients' characteristics: a meta-analyis of clinical trials, *Arch Intern Med* 160(5):621, 2000.
243. Bello D, Massie BM: The current role of amiodarone in patients with congestive heart failure, *Cleve Clin J Med* 65(9):479, 1998.
244. Diller PM et al: Congestive heart failure due to diastolic or systolic dysfunction. Frequency and patient characteristics in an ambulatory setting, *Arch Fam Med* 8(5):414, 1999.
245. Vasan RS et al: Congestive heart failure in subjects with normal versus reduced left ventricular ejection fraction: prevalence and mortality in a population-based cohort, *J Am Coll Cardiol* 33(7):1948, 1999.

CHAPTER 30

Alterations of Cardiovascular Function in Children

JEAN ANNE CONNOR

CHAPTER OUTLINE

Cardiovascular disease in children can be classified as congenital or acquired heart disease. Congenital heart disease is the most common. The diagnosis and management of congenital heart defects continue to improve with the use of fetal echocardiography, early interventional catheterization, or surgical repair. Acquired heart defects in children continue to present challenges to the practitioner; although guidelines for diagnosing acquired defects are available, work is needed in developing standards of treatment and long-term follow-up.

DEVELOPMENT OF THE CARDIOVASCULAR SYSTEM

Developmental Anatomy

Embryology

Cardiogenesis begins at approximately 3 weeks' gestation; however, most cardiovascular development occurs between the fourth and seventh weeks.[1] The heart arises from the mesenchyme and begins in development as an enlarged blood vessel with a large lumen and a muscular wall (Fig. 30-1, *A*). Initially, two lateral endocardial heart tubes fuse to form a single structure (Fig. 30-1, *B*). During the fifth week of gestation, the midsection of this tube begins to grow faster than it ends. This single heart tube elongates and rotates to the right (D-loop formation), creating a bulboventricular loop by approximately the twenty-eighth day[1] (Fig. 30-1, *C*). Also at this time the first fetal heart contractions occur. At this stage the primitive heart structures include a common atrium; common ventricle; the sinus venosus, which eventually evolves into the superior and inferior venae cavae; the bulbus cordis, which eventually evolves into the ventricular outflow tracts; and the truncus arteriosus, which eventually yields the main pulmonary artery and aorta (Fig. 30-1, *D*). By the fourth week of gestation, cardiovascular septation, ventricular development, aortic arch evolution, and circulation begin.

Cardiac Septation

Separation first begins when collections of mesenchymal cells cause the endocardial lining of the heart to bulge into the internal lumen. These changes, known as **endocardial cushions**, are instrumental in closing the atrial septum, dividing the atrioventricular (AV) canals into the right and left AV orifices, and closing the interventricular septum. Altered formation of the endocardial cushions can result in ostium primum atrial septal defects, ventricular septal defects (VSDs), malformation of the AV valves, or a complete AV defect.

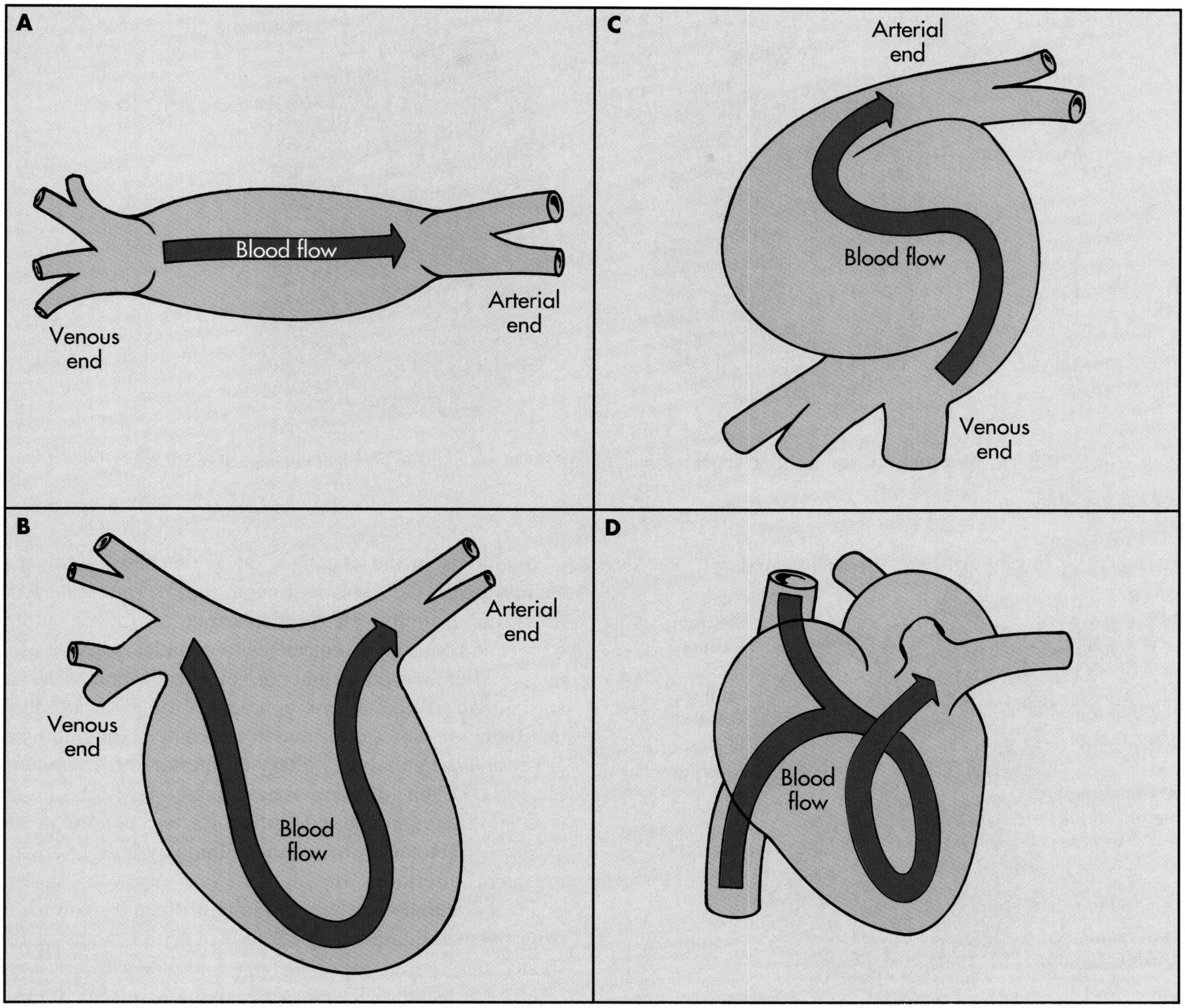

FIG. 30-1 Embryologic development of the heart. A, The earliest heart structure consists of a muscular tube with a large lumen. About the fifth week of gestation, the tube, **B,** bulges and, **C,** twists until, **D,** the ends come together and fuse.

Atrial separation begins when two thin membranelike structures, known as the **septum primum** and the **septum secundum**, grow toward the area of the endocardial cushions (Fig. 30-2). The septum primum forms along the posterior wall of the common atrium and grows downward toward the center portion of the heart. The gap between the two structures, known as the **ostium primum**, normally closes by extensions from the endocardial cushions. At the time of closure, fenestrations or openings develop in the superior portion of the septum primum, creating the **ostium secundum**. Failure of the septum primum to fuse with the endocardial cushions results in an ostium primum defect in the atrial septum near the atrioventricular valve area.

The septum secundum is also a fenestrated, membranelike structure located anteriorly that grows toward the endocardial cushions. During fetal development this structure does not completely fuse with the endocardial cushions to achieve complete atrial septal closure. The nonfused septum secundum and ostium secundum result in the formation of a flapped orifice known as the **foramen ovale**, which allows the right-to-left shunting necessary for fetal circulation. Altered development in any of these structures can lead to an atrial septal defect.

Ventricular septation develops when the muscular ridge located at the apex, the endocardial tissue, and the bulbar ridges in the bulbus cordis fuse (Fig. 30-3). Closure of the interventricular septum ensures communication between the right ventricle (RV) and the pulmonary artery and between the left ventricle (LV) and the aorta. Further evolution of the endocardial tissue gives rise to the membranous ventricular septum and the AV valves. The conal portion of the ventricular septum that separates the aorta from the pulmonary artery forms from the **bulbus cordis**.

When the single primitive heart tube begins to form the D-loop, the venous and arterial poles of the heart are fixed, resulting in torsion within the anterosuperior region of the

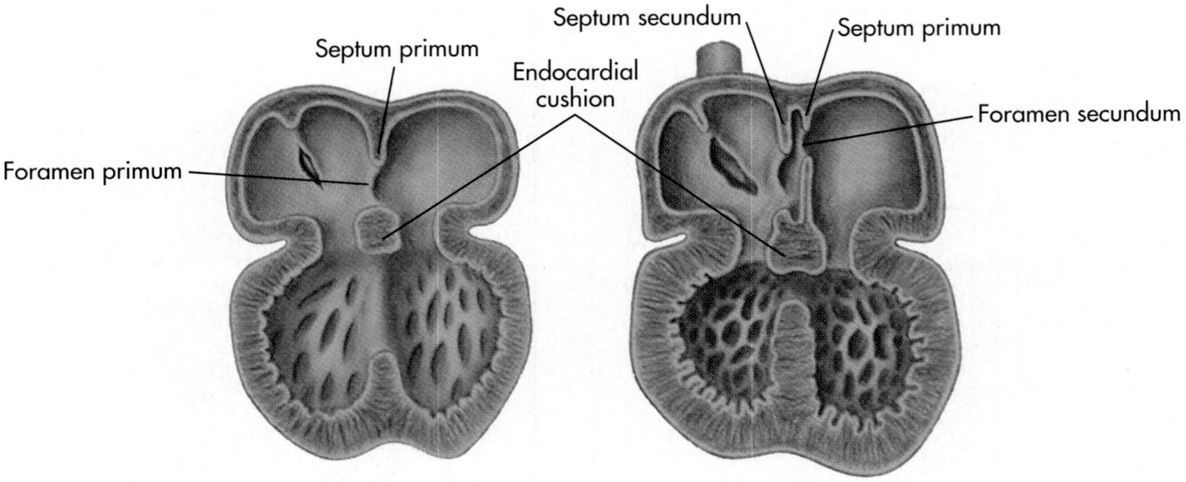

FIG. 30-2 Development of the cardiac septa. (From Thompson JM et al: *Mosby's clinical nursing*, ed 4, St Louis, 1997, Mosby.)

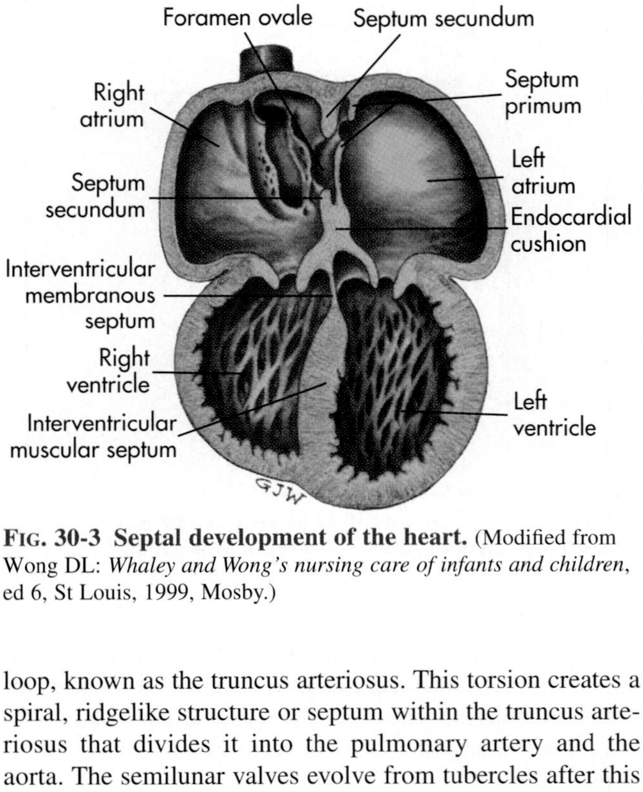

FIG. 30-3 Septal development of the heart. (Modified from Wong DL: *Whaley and Wong's nursing care of infants and children*, ed 6, St Louis, 1999, Mosby.)

loop, known as the truncus arteriosus. This torsion creates a spiral, ridgelike structure or septum within the truncus arteriosus that divides it into the pulmonary artery and the aorta. The semilunar valves evolve from tubercles after this division is complete.

Before this division occurs, however, two large arteries form at the distal end of the truncus arteriosus. They give rise to the six aortic arches. By the fifth week of gestation, the first two pairs disappear and the third eventually evolves into the common carotid artery, the external carotid artery, and part of the internal carotid artery. The fourth pair of aortic arches will form part of the true aortic arch and the proximal segment of the right subclavian artery. The fifth pair disappears; however, the sixth pair yields the proximal and branch pulmonary arteries with lung parenchyma and the **ductus arteriosus.**

Swellings in the conal region at the base of the main trunk separate the right ventricular outflow (pulmonary outflow) tract from the left ventricular outflow (aortic outflow) tract. The conus also contributes to complete closure of the interventricular septum, and normal reabsorption of the subaortic conal region ensures rotation of the great arteries so that the aorta is posterior and to the right of the pulmonary artery and the pulmonary artery is anterior and to the left of the aorta. Despite division of the truncus arteriosus and separation of the right and left outflow tracts, a communication exists between the aorta and the pulmonary artery known as the ductus arteriosus.

Fetal circulation differs physiologically and anatomically from postnatal circulation because of the presence of fetal shunts and altered metabolic needs of the various organs (Fig. 30-4). Fetal oxygenation occurs in the placenta instead of the fetal lungs because they are deflated and therefore nonfunctional. In addition, the fetal liver is only partially functional; therefore the majority of blood is diverted away from these areas through fetal shunts. Because the fetal brain requires maximum concentrations of oxygen and nutrients for growth, fetal circulation is streamlined to ensure optimal perfusion to the brain.

In utero the fetus receives blood carrying oxygen and nutrients from the placenta through the umbilical vein. Fetal arterial oxygen tension is much lower than in the postnatal period—approximately 20 to 30 torr. Yet, despite this hypoxemic state, tissue hypoxia does not occur, because of high fetal cardiac output of approximately 400 ml/kg/min.[2] The blood travels to the liver, where a portion enters the portal and hepatic circulation; approximately half the flow is diverted away from the liver through the ductus venosus and into the inferior vena cava. Because the blood received from the inferior vena cava yields a higher pressure, blood entering the right atrium (RA) from the inferior vena cava is shunted through the foramen ovale and into the left atrium (LA) and is then pumped through the left ventricle (LV) and into the

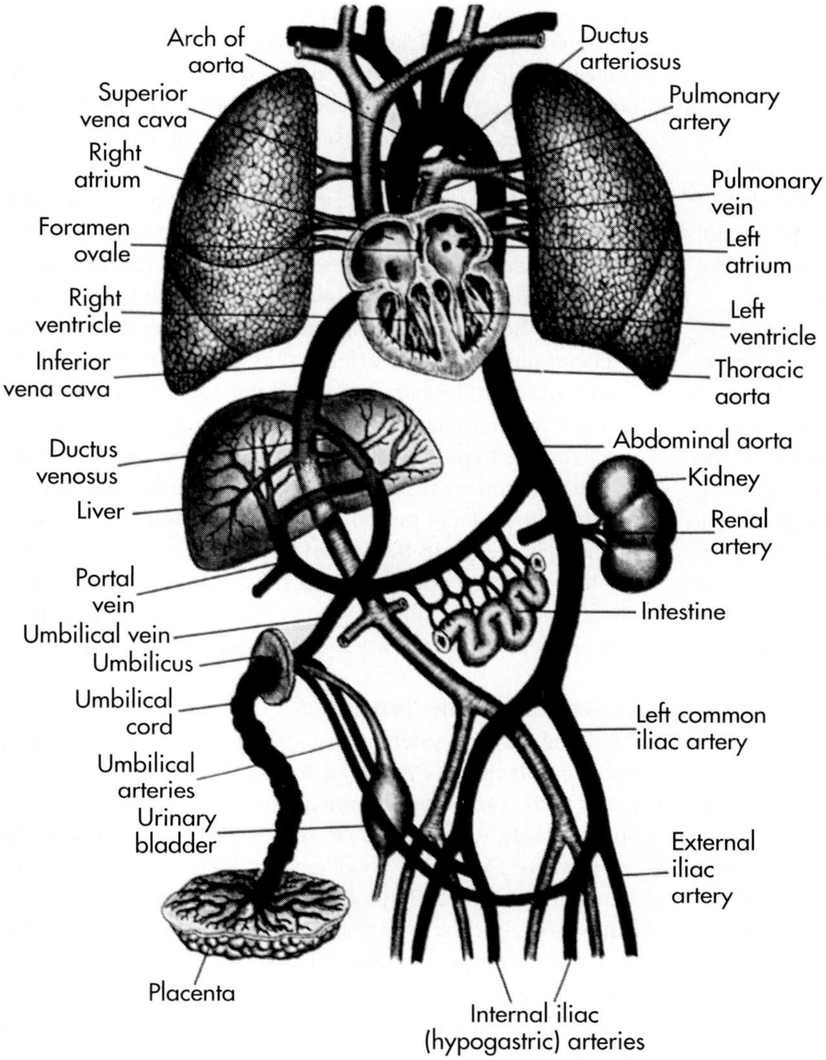

FIG. 30-4 Fetal circulation. Circulation of the fetus reflects the fact that oxygenation of fetal blood does not take place in the lungs, but rather in the placenta. Therefore the pulmonary circulatory system is essentially "bypassed." Instead of traveling from the right heart to the lungs, as occurs after birth, most blood entering the right heart passes through the ductus arteriosus and into the systemic circulation.

aorta. Approximately two thirds of the blood flows to the head and upper extremities. Because this blood is mainly from the placenta, the brain and coronary arteries receive the blood with the highest oxygen concentration. The remaining blood flows into the descending aorta.

Less-saturated blood, with an oxygen tension of 15 to 19 torr, returns from the upper body, head, neck, and arms and travels from the superior vena cava (SVC) into the RA. A small portion of this blood flows into the right ventricle (RV) and out the pulmonary artery (PA) and enters the nonfunctioning lungs. Most of the blood, however, bypasses the lungs by flowing through the ductus arteriosus and into the descending aorta. Blood from the descending aorta returns to the placenta through two umbilical arteries.[1]

The collapsed lungs and low oxygen tension induce vasoconstriction, creating high pulmonary vascular resistance. This is transmitted to the right side of the heart and the pulmonary arteries. Conversely, fetal systemic resistance is low because of the large-volume placenta and ductus arteriosus. Therefore, because blood flow follows the path of least resistance, high pulmonary resistance diverts most of the blood flow into the pulmonary artery, through the ductus arteriosus, and into the aorta. From there it travels into the low-resistance placenta.

Transitional Circulation

At birth a series of circulatory changes occur that affect blood flow, vascular resistance, and oxygen tension. The most important change that takes place in the circulation is the shift of gas exchange from the placenta to the lungs. In addition, alterations in pressure and volume of blood flowing through the heart chambers functionally close the ductus arteriosus, ductus venosus, and foramen ovale. A decrease of pulmonary vascular resistance and an increase of systemic vascular resistance lead to changes in the size and shape of the heart chambers.

Clamping of the umbilical cord and expansion of the lungs at birth shift gas exchange from the placenta to the lungs. Removal of the low-resistance placenta from circulation also causes an immediate increase in systemic vascular resistance to about twice that before birth. Conversely, pulmonary vascular resistance decreases because of expansion of the lungs with the infant's respirations and exposure to more oxygen-rich blood.

Closure of Fetal Shunts

Once the umbilical cord is tied, the umbilical arteries and vein, which comprise the cord, vasoconstrict and undergo fibrous changes. Therefore blood flow through the ductus venosus falls instantly and absence of fetal shunting through this vessel usually occurs within the first 7 days of life. The ductus venosus evolves into the **ligamentum venosum**.

Increased pulmonary venous return and decreased inferior vena cava return cause functional closure of the foramen ovale within the first month of life. In the fetus the foramen ovale is held open by the blood flow from the high-pressure right side, reflecting pulmonary vascular resistance, to the lower-pressure area on the left side of the heart, reflecting systemic vascular resistance. At birth the pressure gradients reverse, causing the valve flaps of the foramen ovale to close. Functional closure occurs by the adherence of these flaps to the atrial septum. Anatomic closure occurs within the first month of life after deposition of fibrin tissue and cell products permanently seals the flaps closed. Until this occurs, any condition that stimulates an increase in the right-sided pressures or causes dilation of the right atrium can reopen the foramen ovale. Conditions in which a patent foramen ovale may continue past the first month of life include pulmonary hypertension, RV failure, and tricuspid atresia.

The ductus arteriosus closes more gradually. Increased oxygen saturation in the systemic arterial blood is thought to be the major stimulus causing vasoconstriction of the ductus arteriosus. In addition, a decrease in the amount of endogenous prostaglandins promoting dilation and the release of vasoactive substances stimulate further ductal closure. Vasoconstriction of the ductal medial smooth muscle shortens and thickens the intima of the ductal wall within 15 to 18 hours after birth. Permanent closure is complete 10 to 21 days after birth. Fibrous tissue adheres to the remaining structure, and the ductus arteriosus eventually evolves into the ligamentum arteriosum. Conditions that involve low arterial oxygen saturations, such as cyanotic heart disease, decreased medial muscle layer within the ductus, or increased levels of circulating vasodilating substances in the blood, may delay or prevent ductal closure.[3]

Postnatal Development

The infant's cardiopulmonary system is proportionally larger in relation to body surface area than the adult's. The infant's heart points at a transverse angle, but as the lungs and heart mature, the heart shifts lower in the chest and is rotated at a more oblique angle. Unlike the adult heart, the newborn heart has RV dominance with a thickened RV wall. This is because of the high pulmonary vascular resistance in the fetal circulation that subjects the right ventricle to high afterload, which in turn causes the right ventricular myocardium to become as thick and strong as the left.

After birth the right ventricular myocardium begins to thin out as the pulmonary vascular resistance drops. As systemic vascular resistance increases, the left ventricular myocardium becomes thicker. By 1 month of age, the newborn's ventricles are approximately equal in weight. As the child grows, the heart size increases accordingly. The weight of the heart doubles during the first year of life and increases six times that by 9 years of age.[4]

Postnatal changes involve a rise in arterial oxygen tension and an increase in alveolar oxygenation that stimulates vasodilation, resulting in a decrease in pulmonary vascular resistance. During the first 2 to 9 weeks of life, the inner medial linings of the small pulmonary arterioles thin out in response to decreased pulmonary arterial pressure. This increased diameter of the pulmonary vessels, along with further development of the pulmonary bed in response to lung growth, results in a decrease in pulmonary vascular resistance. By 2 months of age, pulmonary resistance may approximate adult levels. During the neonatal period, however, care must be taken to maintain homeostasis because of hyperactivity of the pulmonary bed. Adverse conditions, such as alveolar hypoxia, acidosis, and hypothermia, may trigger pulmonary vasoconstriction and lead to pulmonary hypertension.

Postnatal Hemodynamics

As stated earlier, systemic vascular resistance begins to rise once the placenta is removed from the circulation. Normal levels in the infant range from approximately 10 to 15 Wood units × body surface area (in square meters) and gradually increase to 15 to 30 Wood units × body surface area (in square meters) by childhood.[5] Likewise, the systolic pressure is low in the full-term newborn (approximately 39 to 59 mm Hg), reflecting the decreased LV strength. As the left ventricle becomes more developed, the systolic pressure rises steadily until it equals adult levels once the child reaches puberty.

The heart rate of the newborn ranges from 100 to 180 beats/min, which gradually decreases as the child grows. Similarly, the newborn's cardiac output is high, which is a reflection of the fetal circulation described earlier. Oxygen consumption doubles at birth; to maintain adequate oxygen delivery, the cardiac output also remains high. These changes, however, cause minimal cardiac reserve in the newborn. Additional stressors could increase oxygen demands and result in acute deterioration. By 2 months of age, oxygen consumption decreases by half. As the newborn grows, stroke volume steadily increases while the heart rate decreases.[3]

Postnatal Circulation

Postnatal circulation allows the lungs to oxygenate the venous blood and allows saturated blood to be delivered to the systemic circulation. Desaturated blood returning from the superior vena cava, inferior vena cava, and coronary veins enters the right atrium and is pumped to the right ventricle through the tricuspid valve. The right ventricle then pumps the blood through the pulmonic valve to the pulmonary artery; the blood flows to the lungs, where it is oxygenated. The oxygenated blood returns from the lungs through the pulmonary veins and enters the left atrium. The left atrium pumps blood to the left ventricle through the mitral valve. The left ventricle then pumps blood through the aortic valve and into the aorta. The coronary arteries receive the saturated blood along with delivery to the systemic circulation.

CONGENITAL HEART DEFECTS

Congenital heart disease is the leading cause of death, excluding prematurity, during the first year of life (Table 30-1).[6] It is estimated that as many as 35% of deaths caused by congenital heart defects occur in the first year of life and that one third of children born with congenital heart disease will die as a result of their cardiac disease.[7] Currently there are more than 35 documented types of congenital heart defects and the frequency of occurrence in the United States is on the rise. Although researchers have not determined the reason for this increase, one explanation is that it may be the result of improved methods of detection.

The underlying cause of congenital heart disease is known in only 10% of cases. Several factors place the fetus at risk for developing congenital heart disease, including prenatal, environmental, and genetic factors. Among the prenatal factors are maternal rubella, maternal insulin-dependent diabetes, maternal alcoholism, maternal age (older than 40 years), maternal phenylketonuria, and maternal hypercalcemia (Table 30-2). The use of some drugs during pregnancy is associated with an above-average incidence of congenital heart disease. Examples of these drugs include thalidomide, lithium, phenytoin (Dilantin), warfarin, and dextroamphetamine sulfate. The incidence of heart defects has also been found to be higher in stillbirths, spontaneous abortions, and low-birth-weight or small-for-gestational-age infants.[3]

Genetic factors also have been implicated in the development of congenital heart disease, although the mechanism of causation is often multifactorial. In general, the likelihood of unaffected parents having a child with congenital heart disease ranges from 2% to 6%.[6]

Table 30-1 Critical Times in Fetal Heart Development Related to Specific Defects

Defect	Critical Time in Gestation
Transposition of the great vessels	Third to fourth week
Patent ductus arteriosus	Third to eighth week
Anomalous pulmonary venous connection	Third to eighth week
Tricuspid or mitral atresia	Third to sixth week
Ventricular septal defect (muscular)	Fourth to sixth week
Coarctation of the aorta	Fourth week on
Truncus arteriosus	Sixth to seventh week
Ventricular septal defect (membranous)	Sixth to seventh week
Persistent foramen ovale	Eighth week on

Keith JD, Rowe RD, Vlad P, editors: *Heart disease in infancy and childhood,* ed 3, New York, 1978, Macmillan.

Etiology

The etiology of congenital heart disease is unknown. Early epidemiologic studies report a multifactorial influence to be the cause of up to 90% of cardiac anomalies, with a recurrence rate of 2% to 6%.[6] Associated risk factors include maternal, gestational, and familial conditions. Maternal risk factors are discussed in the previous section. Exposure to teratogens in utero may also be a risk factor. Likewise, fetal exposure to

Table 30-2 Environmental Factors and Associated Congenital Heart Defects

Cause	Type of Congenital Heart Defect
INFECTION	
Intrauterine	Patent ductus arteriosus (PDA), pulmonary stenosis, coarctation of aorta
Systemic viral	PDA, pulmonary stenosis, coarctation of aorta
Rubella	PDA, pulmonary stenosis, coarctation of aorta
Coxsackie B5	Endocardial fibroelastosis
RADIATION	Specific cardiovascular effect not known
METABOLIC DISORDERS	
Diabetes	Ventricular septal defect (VSD), cardiomegaly, transposition of the great vessels
Phenylketonuria (PKU)	Coarctation of aorta, PDA
Hypercalcemia	Supravalvular aortic stenosis, pulmonic stenosis; aortic hyperplasia
DRUGS	
Thalidomide	No specific lesion
Dextroamphetamine	One case of reported transposition
Alcohol	Tetralogy of Fallot, atrial septal defect, VSD
PERIPHERAL CONDITIONS	
Increased maternal age	VSD, tetralogy of Fallot (relationship unclear)
Antepartal bleeding	Various defects (relationship unclear)
Prematurity	PDA, VSD
High altitude	PDA, atrial septal defect (increased incidence)

active maternal infections, such as rubella, herpesvirus, coxsackievirus B5, and cytomegalovirus, may be a risk.

Chromosomal aberrations account for about 6% of all congenital heart defects (Table 30-3). Many genetic and hereditary diseases are associated with congenital heart defects, although the mechanism of causation is unknown (Table 30-4). As many as 50% of infants with trisomy 21 have a congenital heart defect, either an AV canal defect or a VSD. Extracardiac defects are noted in as many as 35% of infants with cardiac lesions. Recently, prospective studies utilizing chromosomal analysis have suggested that congenital cardiac malformations may be the result of a single gene defect.[5]

Because of improved screening methods, surgical interventions, and management, children with congenital heart defects are now surviving into adulthood and bearing children of their own. Studies report a 5% to 15% incidence of congenital heart disease in offspring of a parent having a congenital heart lesion. If two siblings have a congenital cardiac anomaly, the recurrence risk is 9%, and if three siblings have a congenital cardiac anomaly, the rate jumps to a 50% chance that the next child also will have a cardiovascular malformation. If one of the lesions is a left-sided obstructive lesion, the incidence is documented to be even higher.

Classification and Clinical Manifestations

There are more than 35 different types of congenital anomalies that can be classified into four categories based on blood flow pattern: (1) lesions increasing pulmonary blood flow; (2) lesions decreasing pulmonary blood flow; (3) obstructive lesions, where right- or left-sided outflow tract obstructions curtail or prohibit blood flow out of the heart; and (4) mixed lesions, where desaturated blood and saturated blood mix

Table 30-3 Genetic Factors and Congenital Heart Defects

Chromosomal Aberrations or Syndrome	Incidence of Defects	Type of Defect
Trisomy 13	80%	Ventricular septal defect (VSD), atrial septal defect (ASD), patent ductus arteriosus (PDA), anomalous pulmonary venous connection, bicuspid aorta, overriding aorta
Trisomy 18	90%	VSD, PDA, patent foramen ovale, bicuspid aortic valve, dextrocardia
Down syndrome	12%–44%	Endocardial cushion defects, VSD, PDA, ASD, transposition of great vessels, tetralogy of Fallot, persistent truncus arteriosus, coarctation of aorta, endocardial fibroelastosis
Cri du chat syndrome	20%	PDA, mixed defects
Turner syndrome	20%–40%	Coarctation of aorta, pulmonary stenosis, subaortic and aortic stenosis, PDA, septal defects

Data from Doyle EF, Rutkowski M: Etiology of congenital heart disease, *Cardiovasc Clin* 2:1, 1970.

Table 30-4 Disorders Coexistent with Congenital Heart Defects

Disorder	Associated Cardiovascular Defect
CONNECTIVE TISSUE DISORDERS	
Marfan syndrome	Aortic or mitral regurgitation, aortic aneurysm
Hurler syndrome	Pseudoatherosclerosis
Hunter syndrome	Pseudoatherosclerosis, hypertension
Osteogenesis imperfecta	Incompetent aortic valve
COMPLEX SYNDROMES	
Kartagener syndrome	Dextrocardia
Holt-Oram syndrome	Atrial septal defect (ASD), ventricular septal defect (VSD)
Ellis–van Creveld syndrome	Defect or absence of atrial septum
Laurence-Moon-Biedl syndrome	Tetralogy of Fallot, single ventricle, transposition of aorta
INBORN ERRORS OF METABOLISM	
Pompe disease	Cardiomegaly, left heart failure
Homocuptinuria	Thromboembolic episodes, pulmonic and aortic regurgitation
PHAKOMATOSIS	
Neurofibromatosis (von Recklinghausen disease)	Hypertension, pheochromocytoma
von Hippel–Lindau disease	Hypertension, pheochromocytoma
Sturge-Weber-Dimitri disease	Anomalies of carotid and meningeal arteries
VASCULAR MALFORMATIONS	
Osler-Weber-Rendu disease (hereditary hemorrhagic telangiectasia)	Atrioventricular fistula, telangiectasia
Milroy disease (lymphedema)	Hypoplasia of lymphatic vessels

Data from Doyle EF, Rutkowski M: Etiology of congenital heart disease, *Cardiovasc Clin* 2:1, 1970.

within the chambers or great arteries of the heart (Table 30-5). By classifying lesions in this way, the clinical manifestations, as well as associated sequelae, are more predictable.

Clinical manifestations are lesion dependent. Lesions increasing pulmonary blood flow include defects that allow blood flow to shunt from the high-pressure left side to the lower-pressure right side, resulting in pulmonary congestion and right heart failure. Lesions that cause decreased pulmonary blood flow are generally complex and result in cyanosis. Obstructive lesions limit the amount of blood flow out of the ventricles. The two types of obstructive lesions are right-sided lesions that result in cyanosis and left-sided lesions that result in congestive heart failure. Mixed lesions result in a variable amount of mixing and pulmonary blood flow; the clinical manifestations usually consist of left heart failure and hypoxemia that may be associated with cyanosis.

Congestive Heart Failure

Congestive heart failure (CHF) is a common complication of many congenital heart defects. In addition, it can occur as the result of decreased myocardial function or excessive metabolic demands. The most common causes of CHF in infancy, however, are pressure and volume overloads secondary to congenital disease. (Table 30-6 lists the congenital heart defects that cause CHF by age.) Ninety percent of children who develop CHF do so within 12 months of age, often by the age of 6 months.

Pathophysiology

In general, the pathophysiologic mechanisms of CHF in infants and children are very similar to those in adults. The same compensatory mechanisms are activated in the face of inadequate cardiac output. A decrease in blood pressure stimulates stretch receptors and baroreceptors in the aorta and carotid arteries, which in turn stimulate the sympathetic

Table 30-5 Classification of Congenital Heart Defects

Classification	Shunt Direction	Newborn Presentation	Specific Defects
Lesions increasing pulmonary blood flow	Left to right	Acyanotic congestive heart failure	Patent ductus arteriosus, atrial septal defect, ventricular septal defect, complete atrioventricular canal defect
Lesions decreasing pulmonary blood flow	Right to left	Cyanotic	Tetralogy of Fallot, tricuspid atresia
Obstructive lesions*	None	Low cardiac output Shock	Coarctation of the aorta, hypoplastic left heart syndrome, aortic stenosis, pulmonary stenosis
Mixed lesions†	Variable	Variable	Transposition of the great arteries, total anomalous pulmonary venous connection, truncus arteriosus

*If patent ductus arteriosus closes, newborns with hypoplastic left heart syndrome, coarctation of the aorta, or critical aortic stenosis will present with shock. Newborns with aortic stenosis or pulmonary stenosis may have only mild symptoms depending on severity of stenosis.

†Transposition of the great arteries and truncus arteriosus will present with cyanosis as patent ductus arteriosus closes. Total anomalous pulmonary venous connection usually presents with congestive heart failure.

Table 30-6 Congenital Heart Defects Causing Congestive Heart Failure

Age	Congenital Heart Defect
Time of birth	Hypoplastic left heart syndrome
	Volume overload caused by tricuspid regurgitation
	Arterial venous fistula
Birth to 1 wk	Hypoplastic left heart syndrome
	Aortic atresia
	Transposition of the great vessels
	Coarctation of the aorta
	Total anomalous pulmonary venous connection (TAPVC) with obstruction
	Patent ductus arteriosus (PDA) in premature infants
First 4 wk	Coarctation of the aorta
	TAPVC
	Large left-to-right shunt caused by ventricular septal defect (VSD), PDA in premature infants
	Tricuspid atresia
	All previously mentioned defects
4–6 wk	Transposition of the great vessels
	Large left-to-right shunt caused by endocardial cushion defect
6 wk to 6 mo	VSD
6 mo	Endocardial fibroelastosis
	Persistent truncus arteriosus with large left-to-right shunt

nervous system. With the release of catecholamines and the stimulation of β receptors, heart rate and the force of myocardial contraction increase. Venous smooth muscle tone also increases, which increases return of venous blood to the heart. Sympathetic stimulation also decreases blood flow to the kidneys, skin, spleen, and extremities so that maximum flow to the brain, heart, and lungs can be maintained. Decreased blood flow to the kidneys causes the release of renin, angiotensin, and aldosterone. This cycle results in retention of sodium and fluid by the kidneys, which in turn increases volume in the circulatory system.

The myocardium hypertrophies in CHF, which increases ventricular pressure. The myocardial fibers also stretch to accommodate the increased volume. This increases contractility and hence the force of ventricular contraction. Both hypertrophy and increased stretch eventually fail to maintain cardiac output as CHF progresses. A review of the Frank-Starling law of the heart (see Chapter 28) is useful for an understanding of the cycle of compensation and decompensation that occurs in CHF.

WHAT'S NEW? Endocarditis Risk

Children with congenital heart disease are at risk for developing endocarditis. Although the risk is low, transient bacteria have been identified in patients following dental and surgical procedures and instrumentation involving mucosal surfaces. A blood-borne pathogen can settle in areas of the heart where there is high turbulence, an abnormal valve or vessel, or an artificial material such as a valve or homograft. *Streptococcus viridans* (α-hemolytic streptocci) is the most common pathogen following dental or oral procedures. *Enterococcus faecalis* (enterococci) is the most common bacterium following genitourinary and gastrointestinal tract surgery or instrumentation. The American Heart Association has provided updated guidelines for the prevention of bacterial endocarditis. The type and dose of antibiotic prophylaxis recommended depend on the procedure and the cardiac classification of risk for endocarditis.

Clinical Manifestations

Although CHF in children has many causes, it is often difficult to determine right or left ventricular failure. When assessing a child with CHF, a combination of symptoms generally is present. Usually, both ventricles are involved by the time signs and symptoms are apparent.[4]

Left heart failure in infants is manifested as poor feeding and sucking, often leading to failure to thrive. In left heart failure, dyspnea, tachypena, and diaphoresis may be accompanied by retractions, grunting, and nasal flaring, wheezing, coughing, and rales.[3] Common skin changes, such as pallor or mottling, are often present.

Hepatomagaly (enlargement of the liver) is atypically attributable to systemic venous congestion caused by right ventricular failure. In infants the normal liver is sharp-edged and palpable 1 to 2 cm below the costal margin. However, the absence of hepatomegaly does not rule out CHF.

Puffy eyelids, periorbital edema, and weight gain without caloric increase are common manifestations of right ventricular failure in infants. Peripheral edema, which is a common finding in adults, is usually more difficult to detect in infants and young children.[3] The clinical manifestations of CHF are given in Box 30-1.

Evaluation and Treatment

A thorough physical examination with emphasis on cardiac and pulmonary findings will often reveal the degree of CHF. Plotting the child's growth (height, weight, head circumference) is an important method of assessing failure to thrive. An electrocardiogram (ECG) should be performed to determine the presence of dysrhythmias or hypertrophy. A chest roentgenogram is useful in assessing the presence of cardiomegaly and signs of increased pulmonary circulation.

Treatment is aimed at decreasing cardiac workload and increasing the efficiency of the heart. Medical management initially consists of diuretics, such as furosemide. Depending on the degree of CHF, other diuretics can be used in combination with furosemide to counteract potassium losses. Medi-

Box 30-1

CLINICAL MANIFESTATIONS OF CONGESTIVE HEART FAILURE

IMPAIRED MYOCARDIAL FUNCTION	PULMONARY CONGESTION	SYSTEMIC VENOUS CONGESTION
Tachycardia	Tachypnea	Weight gain
Sweating (inappropriate)	Dyspnea	Hepatomegaly
Decreased urinary output	Retractions (infants)	Peripheral edema, especially periorbital
Fatigue	Flaring nares	Ascites
Weakness	Exercise intolerance	Neck vein distention (children)
Restlessness	Orthopnea	
Anorexia	Cough, hoarseness	
Pale, cool extremities	Cyanosis	
Weak peripheral pulses	Wheezing	
Decreased blood pressure	Grunting	
Gallop rhythm		
Cardiomegaly		

From Wong DL et al: *Whaley and Wong's nursing care of infants and children,* ed 6, St Louis, 1999, Mosby.

cations, such as digoxin (Lanoxin), an inotropic agent, are also used to increase myocardial contractility. Afterload reducers have recently been employed to further manage severe CHF.[3,4]

Hypoxemia

Heart defects that allow desaturated blood to enter the systemic system without passing through the lungs result in hypoxemia and cyanosis. Hypoxemia occurs when arterial oxygen tension is below normal and results in low oxygen arterial saturations and cellular function alteration. **Cyanosis**, a blue discoloration of the mucous membranes and nail beds, results from deoxygenated hemoglobin in a concentration of at least 5 g/dl of blood or from arterial saturations less than 85%.[3,5] Anemia may mask the signs of hypoxemia, whereas children who are polycythemic with a normal arterial saturation may appear cyanotic. Older children who have an unrepaired septal defect with a left-to-right shunt may become cyanotic because of pulmonary vascular changes secondary to increased pulmonary blood flow. Because of these progressive pulmonary vascular changes, pulmonary vascular resistance increases to exceed or equal vascular resistance, resulting in a reversal of shunting known as **Eisenmenger syndrome**. Three types of defects cause hypoxemia and cyanosis:

1. Lesions that cause right ventricular outflow tract obstruction and shunting from the right side of the heart to the left side, as in tetralogy of Fallot (see p. 1062)
2. Defects involving the mixing of saturated and unsaturated blood within the heart chambers, as in a univentricular heart
3. Defects in children with transposition of the great arteries (see p. 1070), in which two parallel circulations exist and survival depends on the existence of a patent ductus arteriosus or septal shunt

◆ *Clinical Manifestations*

Infants with mild hypoxemia may only occasionally show signs of cyanosis when stressed and otherwise may exhibit near-normal age-projected growth and development. Infants with severe hypoxemia may display signs of feeding intolerance, poor weight gain, tachypnea, and dyspnea. Children with chronic hypoxemia are small for age, display cognitive and motor skill delays, experience shortness of breath with exertion, fatigue easily, and have exercise intolerance. Severe hypoxemia will lead to tissue hypoxia, metabolic acidosis, hyperventilation, poor perfusion, and eventually shock.

In response to chronic hypoxemia, polycythemia occurs as the body generates additional red blood cells to increase the oxygen-carrying capacity of the blood. However, anemia may result because of limited stores of iron, and the increased velocity of the blood limits the amount of circulating platelets and other coagulation factors. Polycythemia also places children at risk for thromboembolic events, especially infants with severe cyanosis and iron deficiency anemia. In addition to the 2% risk of cerebrovascular accidents, there is a 2% chance that children with right-to-left shunting will develop a brain abscess.[5] Clubbing of the nailbeds occurs because of chronic tissue hypoxemia and polycythemia.

Defects Increasing Pulmonary Blood Flow

Cardiac lesions that increase pulmonary blood flow include defects that involve septal abnormalities or communications between the great arteries. These allow the shunting of blood from the high-pressure left side to the lower-pressure right side. Infants with left-to-right shunts are acyanotic and, depending on the degree of shunting, will often develop signs and symptoms of congestive heart failure. Children with signifiant left-to-right shunts left untreated are at risk for the developing of irreversible pulmonary hypertension.

Patent Ductus Arteriosus

The **patent ductus arteriosus (PDA)** is a vessel located between the junction of the main and left pulmonary artery and the lesser curvature of the descending aorta just distal to the left subclavian artery. During fetal circulation the PDA allows blood to shunt from the pulmonary artery to the aorta. At birth, once the placenta is removed and the lungs are expanded, the PDA will start to constrict within the first hours of life. Closure of the PDA in full-term infants is usually noted between 15 hours of life and 2 weeks of age.[8] As an isolated defect, PDA occurs in 5% to 10% of all congenital cardiac defects.[3] In premature infants, studies have shown that the incidence of PDA is as high as 20% in newborns less than 1750 g.[9]

◆ *Pathophysiology*

Failure of the PDA to close results in persistent patency of the ductus arteriosus. The hemodynamic effects of PDA depend on the size of the lumen and the resistance in the pulmonary and systemic circulations.[6] At birth the pulmonary and systemic vascular resistances are almost equal and are reflected in the pulmonary artery and aorta, respectively. Therefore shunting is minimal. However, as pulmonary vascular resistance falls, a reversal of fetal shunting occurs. Blood now begins to shunt left to right, from the aorta to the pulmonary artery. The hemodynamic effect is increased pulmonary blood flow, resulting in an increased workload on the left side of the heart. The increased workload is caused by increased pulmonary venous return to the left atrium and, potentially, an increase in right ventricular pressure if pulmonary vascular changes occur in response to the increased blood flow, leading to an increase in pulmonary vascular pressure (see Fig. 30-5, *C*).

◆ *Clinical Manifestations*

Once pulmonary vascular resistance has fallen, infants with PDA will characteristically have a continuous-machinery type murmur heard best at the left upper sternal border throughout systole and diastole. If the PDA is significant, the infant will also have bounding pulses, an active precordium, a thrill upon palpation, and signs and symptoms of CHF. Infants with a small PDA will usually remain asymtpomatic.

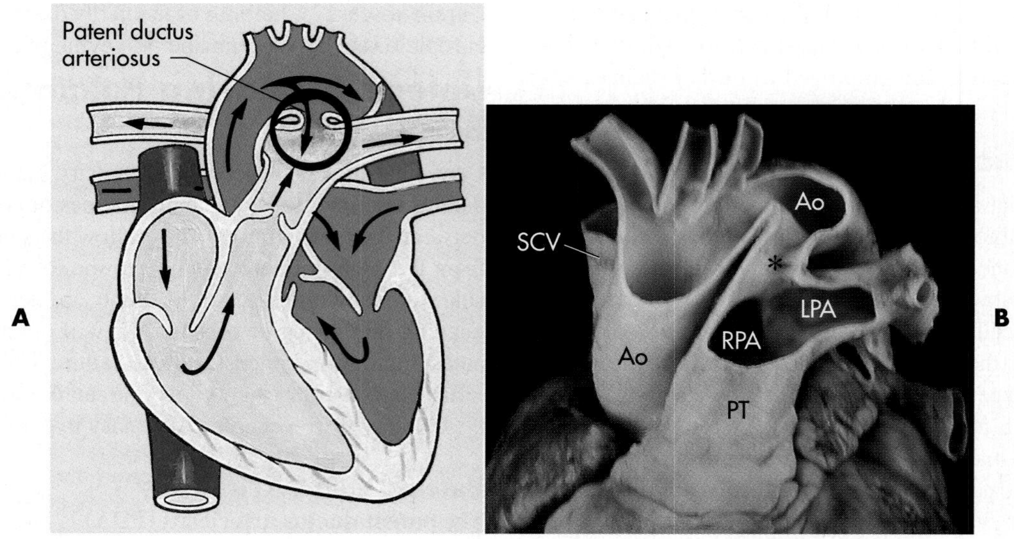

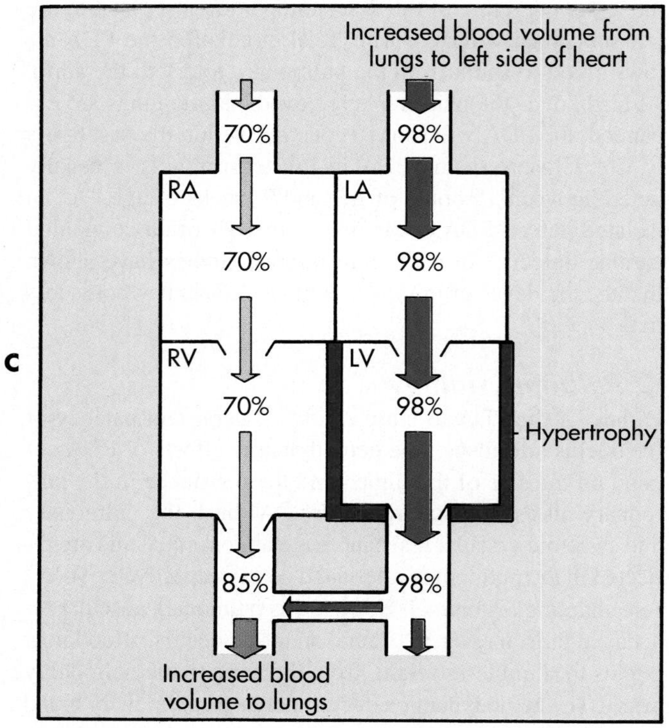

Fig. 30-5 Patent ductus arteriosus (PDA). A, PDA with left-to-right shunt. **B,** PDA (*) in an adult with pulmonary hypertension. **C,** Changes in oxygen saturation, left ventricular volume, and the myocardium caused by left-to-right shunt through a PDA. *SCV,* Subclavian vein; *Ao,* aorta; *LPA,* left pulmonary artery; *RPA,* right pulmonary artery; *PT,* pulmonary trunk; *RA,* right atrium; *RV,* right ventricle; *LA,* left atrium; *LV,* left ventricle. (A from Wong DL: *Whaley and Wong's nursing care of infants and children,* ed 6, St Louis, 1999, Mosby; B from Damjanov I, Linder J, editors: *Anderson's pathology,* ed 10, St Louis, 1996, Mosby; C from Whaley LF, Wong DL: *Nursing care of infants and children,* ed 4, St Louis, 1991, Mosby.)

Evaluation and Treatment

Chest roentgenogram will reveal left atrial and ventricular enlargement and increased pulmonary vascular markings. An ECG may demonstrate ventricular enlargement, particularly on the left, but in most cases it is within normal ranges. Echocardiography and auscultation can confirm the diagnosis based on the characteristic continuous-machinery type of murmur. Cardiac catheterization is not warranted if the results of all noninvasive studies are consistent with the diagnosis.

PDA closure in asymptomatic children is recommended by 2 years of age because of the risk of subacute bacterial endocarditis. Premature infants who develop respiratory distress are initially given indomethacin, a prostaglandin inhibitor, to close the duct.[9] If this is unsuccessful, more invasive measures are taken to close the duct.

Currently the most widely used method for PDA closure is surgical closure involving ligation and division of the ductus. Cardiopulmonary bypass is not needed because of the extracardiac location of the lesion. The rate of successful closure is 100%. Mortality associated with surgical intervention nears 0%; however, there continues to be some morbidity caused by the approach through a left thoracotomy incision.[10,22,12,13,14]

Several other options for PDA closure are available depending on the size of the child and the PDA. Many specialists perform coil embolization of the PDA during catheterization. The catheter is advanced into the ductal opening and

A 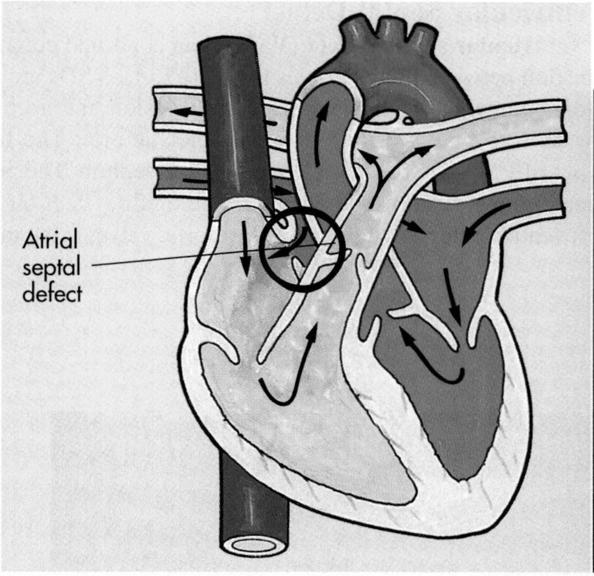

B 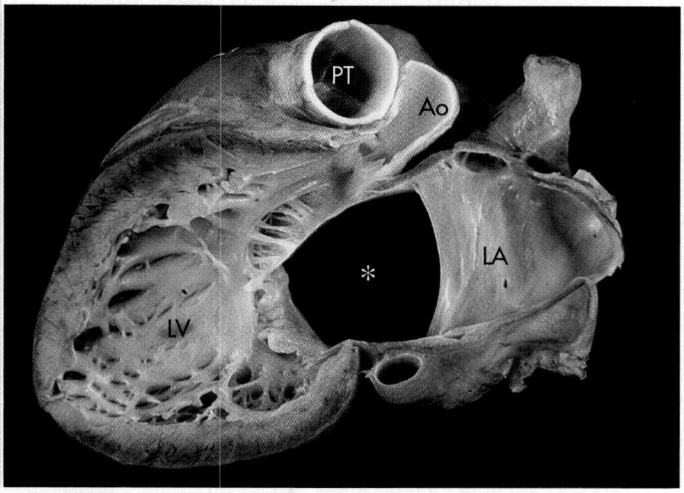

FIG. 30-6 Atrial septal defect (ASD). A, Abnormal opening between the atria causing blood from the higher-pressure left atrium to flow into the lower-pressure right atrium. **B,** Complete ASD (*) form in children. *PT,* Pulmonary artery trunk; *Ao,* aorta; *LA,* left atrium; *LV,* left ventricle. (A from Wong DL: *Whaley and Wong's nursing care of infants and children*, ed 6, St Louis, 1999, Mosby; B from Damjanov I, Linder J, editors: *Anderson's pathology*, ed 10, St Louis, 1996, Mosby.)

ejecting multiple coils into the lumen that embolize and prohibit flow through the duct. The greatest advantages to this procedure are the avoidance of a surgical procedure and thoracotomy pain and a brief observation stay in the hospital.[11,12,13,15]

Another option is closure through video-assisted thoracoscopic surgery. This procedure involves making three small incisions in the left lateral wall, through which a probe is inserted. A clip is then placed around the vessel to occlude it. An advantage of this procedure is that there is less associated morbidity because of the avoidance of a thoracotomy incision.[16,17,18,19]

Atrial Septal Defect

An **atrial septal defect (ASD)** is an abnormal communication between the atria (Fig. 30-6, *A* and *B*). As an isolated lesion, it is the fourth most common congenital heart defect, occurring in 5% to 10% of all congenital cardiac defects. The three major types are an ostium primum defect, an opening found low in the septum that may be associated with atrioventricular valve abnormalities, especially mitral insufficiency; an ostium secundum defect, an opening in the center of the septum (this is the most common type of atrial defect); and a sinus venosus defect, an opening that occurs high up in the atrial septum near the SVC and RA junction. This defect is often associated with partial anomalous pulmonary venous connection.

Pathophysiology

Although the pressure difference between the two atria is minimal, the ASD allows blood to be shunted from left to right because of the slightly higher pressure of the left atrial chamber. Right atrial and ventricular enlargement develops as a result of left-to-right shunting. Children with ASD are generally asymptomatic and rarely display signs of cardiac failure. Moderate to large ASDs allow an increase in pulmonary blood flow, and, over time, pulmonary vascular changes can occur, eventually resulting in pulmonary hypertension.

Clinical Manifestations

Because most children with ASD are asymptomatic, diagnosis usually is made during a routine physical examination by the auscultation of a crescendo-decrescendo systolic ejection murmur that reflects increased blood flow through the pulmonary valve. The location of the murmur is between the second and third intercostal spaces along the left sternal border. A wide fixed splitting of the second heart sound is also characteristic of ASD, reflecting volume overload to the right ventricle causing prolonged ejection time and delay of pulmonic valve closure.

Evaluation and Treatment

In most cases an echocardiogram is sufficient to confirm the diagnosis of an ASD. A chest roentgenogram may reveal cardiomegaly and increased pulmonary vascular markings in an asymptomatic child, although this is rare. An ECG often reflects right axis deviation and diastolic overload of the right ventricle.[3]

ASD closure generally is recommended before the child reaches school age, because if left unrepaired, pulmonary hypertension and right ventricular hypertrophy occurs, placing the child at risk for the development of CHF, atrial dysrhythmias, or embolic events by 20 years of age. Surgical closure is the corrective method of choice and involves a pericardial patch or suture closure of the defect, depending on the size of the opening. Repair is done through a midsternal approach with the use of cardiopulmonary bypass.

Sinus venosus defects require a slightly different approach that consists of a synthetic patch to close the opening and baffle the anomalous right pulmonary venous drainage to the left atrium.

Operative mortality associated with ASD closure is near 0%, with minimal morbidity.[18,20,21] Device closure done in the catheterization laboratory and video-assisted thoracoscopic surgery are currently being investigated.[17,22,23,24,25]

Ventricular Septal Defect

A **ventricular septal defect (VSD)** is an abnormal communication between the ventricles (Fig. 30-7, *A*). VSDs are the most common type of congenital heart lesion and account for 25% to 33% of all congenital heart defects. The four types of VSDs are based on location in the septum. The perimembranous type, which occurs in the outflow tract on the left ventricle immediately below the aortic valve, is the most

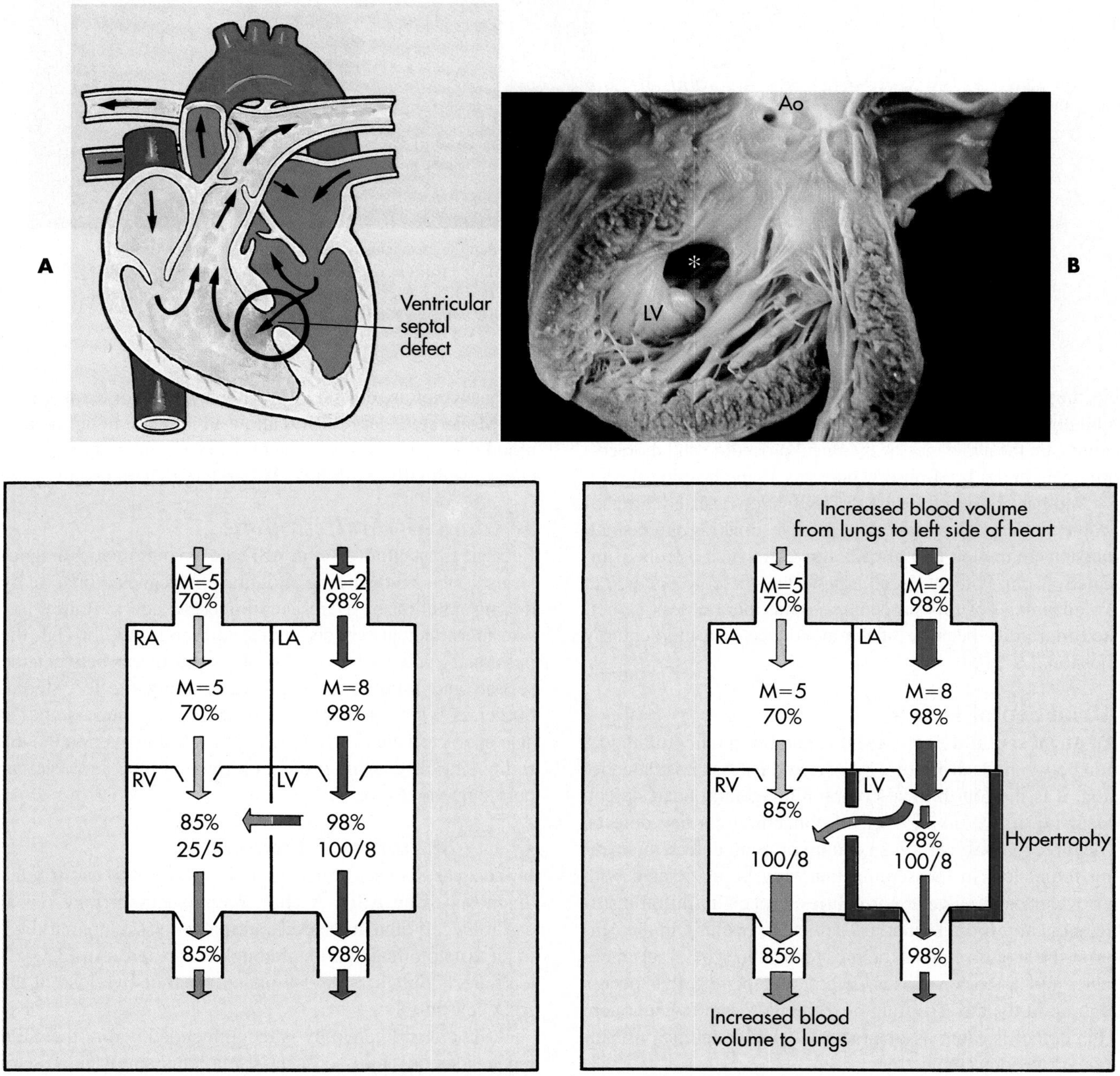

FIG. 30-7 Ventricular septal defects (VSDS). A, VSD with left-to-right shunt. **B,** Muscular (*) defect (opened left ventricles). **C,** Hemodynamics of a small VSD with left-to-right shunt. Mean (M) indicates mean of pressure; systolic/diastolic pressures are in mm Hg; and percentages indicate oxygen saturation. **D,** Hemodynamics of a large VSD with left-to-right shunt. Like the shunting that occurs in preductal coarctation of the aorta, the shunting pictured here causes left ventricular overload and hypertrophy. *Ao,* Aorta; *LV,* left ventricle; *RA,* right atrium; *RV,* right ventricle; *LA,* left atrium. (A from Wong DL: *Whaley and Wong's nursing care of infants and children*, ed 6, St Louis, 1999, Mosby; B from Damjanov I, Linder J, editors: *Anderson's pathology*, ed 10, St Louis, 1996, Mosby; C and D from Whaley LF, Wong DL: *Nursing care of infants and children*, ed 4, St Louis, 1991, Mosby.)

common type, accounting for up to 80% of all VSDs. Muscular VSDs, which occur low in the ventricular septum between the trabeculae, are most likely to close spontaneously and are difficult to reach because of their location low in the apex. Supracristal VSDs occur in the infundibulum, below the pulmonary valve. AV canal VSDs occur posterior and inferior to the membranous system, beneath the septal cusp of the tricuspid valve and inferior to the papillary muscles of the conus.

Pathophysiology

The direction of shunting in a child with a VSD is from the high-pressure left side to the lower-pressure right side. The amount of shunting depends on the size of the defect and the degree of pulmonary vascular resistance. Small VSDs present increased resistance to shunting and limit blood flow through the defect; thus the degree of pulmonary vascular congestion and ventricular chamber enlargement is minimal (Fig. 30-7, *C*).

After about 12 weeks of life, when pulmonary vascular resistance has decreased, moderate-size to large VSDs allow a large amount of shunting from left to right. However, it is the LV rather than the RV that is under pressure and volume overload because most of the shunting occurs during systole when the RV contracts. The shunted blood goes directly out the right ventricle and into the pulmonary artery rather than remaining in the RV cavity (Fig. 30-7, *D*). Therefore there is enlargement of the main pulmonary artery, LA, and LV. LV hypertrophy occurs to effectively pump the additional volume. Eventually the heart is unable to handle the increased volume and CHF develops.

Over time the pulmonary bed also undergoes changes because of increased pulmonary blood flow caused by the left-to-right shunting. In an attempt to maintain normal blood volume, vessels undergo changes that increase their resistance to flow. The smooth muscle layer in the arteriolar walls enlarges, and proliferation of the intimal layer occurs. The effect of these changes is a decrease in the diameter of the pulmonary vessels, which increases the resistance to blood flow and produces a decrease in the amount of blood volume going to the lungs. These changes eventually become irreversible, and pulmonary vascular resistance continues to rise. In some cases it exceeds systemic vascular resistance, causing the shunt through the VSD to reverse direction. Deoxygenated blood now flows into the systemic circulation, and cyanosis occurs, a phenomenon known as *Eisenmenger syndrome.*

Clinical Manifestations

Clinical manifestations in children with VSDs depend on the age of the child, size of the defect, and level of pulmonary vascular resistance. Newborns with small VSDs are relatively asymptomatic. Initially no murmur is present because the newborn's high pulmonary vascular resistance causes equalization of the pressures between both ventricles. Once PVR has dropped, left-to-right shunting occurs, creating a murmur. Infants with large VSDs display symptoms of CHF and poor weight gain. Adults who develop pulmonary vascular obstructive disease as a result of unrepaired VSD will be cyanotic and have clubbing.

On physical examination a loud, harsh, holosystolic murmur and systolic thrill can be detected at the left lower sternal border that radiate to the neck. The intensity of the murmur reflects the pressure gradient across the VSD. An apical diastolic rumble may be present with a moderate to large defect, reflecting mitral regurgitation.

Evaluation and Treatment

ECG and chest roentgenograms show the size of shunting through the defect. The ECG of an individual with a small VSD may be normal, whereas an ECG of an individual with a large VSD may reveal biventricular hypertrophy and LA enlargement. Chest roentgenographic findings are significant for cardiomegaly and increased pulmonary vascular markings; again, the severity is directly related to the magnitude of shunting. An echocardiogram identifies the position, size, degree of shunting, and dimensions of the LA, LV, and RV chambers. It can also provide an estimate of pulmonary artery and RV pressures and pulmonary vascular resistance. Cardiac catheterization may be performed to determine hemodynamics and, in some instances, the location of other VSDs.

Many VSDs spontaneously close during the first year of life.[3] Infants with symptoms of CHF and poor weight gain despite medical management should have their VSD corrected as soon as possible. Left-to-right shunting with a pulmonary flow–systemic flow (Qp:Qs) ratio of greater than 2:1 or evidence of elevated pulmonary vascular resistance is an indication for early surgical closure. Closure of the VSD at this time is to prevent the development of pulmonary vascular obstructive disease.

Placement of a pulmonary artery band to decrease the amount of pulmonary blood flow was initially used as a palliative procedure but is now rarely used unless the presence of an additional lesion makes complete repair impossible. Patch closure, using a synthetic material such as Dacron, is accomplished through a sternotomy and with the use of cardiopulmonary bypass. A transatrial approach is preferable to a right ventriculotomy because of the increased incidence of conduction disturbances.[18,26,27] Contraindications for VSD closure include evidence of pulmonary vascular obstructive disease or Eisenmenger syndrome. Occlusion devices for VSD closure that are performed in the cardiac catherization lab are now under investigation.[28,29]

Atrioventricular Canal Defect

An **atrioventricular canal (AVC) defect** results from nonfusion of the endocardial cushions during fetal life, yielding abnormalities in both the atrial and ventricular septa and atrioventricular valves (Fig. 30-8). This defect accounts for as many as 5% of all congenital heart defects, and approximately 30% of AVC defects occur in children with Down syndrome.[3,30,31] The three types of AVC defects are based on the cardiac components involved. **Complete AVC (CAVC) defects** consist of an inlet VSD, a primum type of ASD, and clefts in both the mitral and tricuspid valves. **Partial AVC**

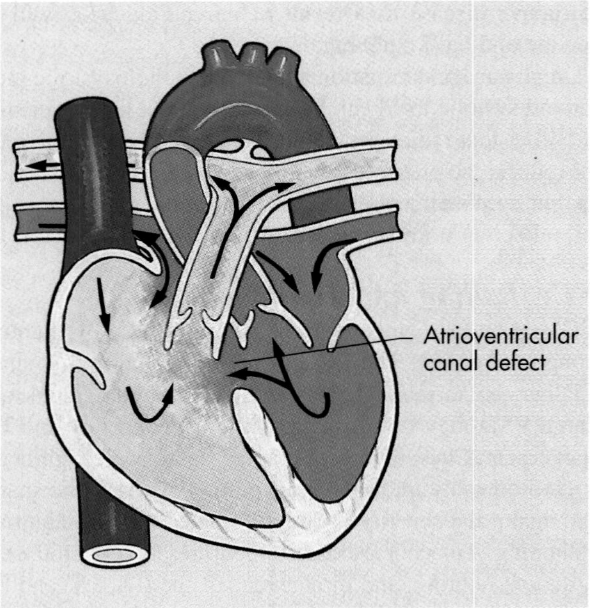

FIG. 30-8 Atrioventricular canal defect. (From Wong DL: *Whaley and Wong's nursing care of infants and children*, ed 6, St Louis, 1999, Mosby.)

(PAVC) defects consist of a primum type of atrial septal defect (ASD) and a cleft in the septal or anterior leaflet of the mitral valve. **Transitional AVC (TAVC) defects** involve partial fusion of the endocardial cushions, resulting in variable atrioventricular valve abnormalities.

Pathophysiology

Hemodynamic abnormalities seen in AVC defects depend on the components of the lesion and the level of pulmonary vascular resistance. Shunting is minimal during the neonatal period when pulmonary vascular resistance is high. However, once pulmonary vascular resistance drops, left-to-right shunting occurs through the septal defects, resulting in increased pulmonary blood flow and CHF.

PAVC defects mimic the hemodynamics of secundum ASD in which the left-to-right shunting through the primum ASD causes RA and RV dilation and increased pulmonary blood flow. The mitral regurgitation that occurs caused by the cleft mitral valve is not hemodynamically significant because blood that flows back into the LA from the LV is immediately shunted into the RA through the primum ASD, resulting in decompression of the LA.

CAVC defects reflect the hemodynamics of both an ASD and a VSD, resulting in biatrial and biventricular enlargement. RA and RV volume overload occurs because of shunting through the primum ASD and tricuspid regurgitation. Likewise, LA and LV volume overload occurs because of shunting through the VSD and mitral regurgitation.

Clinical Manifestations

Children with PAVC defects are generally asymptomatic. Findings on physical examination are similar to those of secundum ASD except for the systolic regurgitant murmur of mitral regurgitation at the apex. At 4 to 12 weeks of age, when pulmonary vascular resistance drops, children with CAVC defects begin to show symptoms of CHF. Physical findings are similar to those found in individuals with VSDs in addition to the systolic murmur radiating to the back and apex, reflecting mitral regurgitation; a middiastolic rumble at the left lower sternal border or apex reflects stenosis of the mitral or tricuspid valve; and signs of CHF, especially frequent respiratory infections.

Evaluation and Treatment

The ECG generally demonstrates a superior left axis deviation, first-degree AV block, and RV hypertrophy or right bundle branch block. The ECG of CAVC defects may also have LV hypertrophy. Chest roentgenogram shows cardiomegaly of all four chambers in the presence of mitral regurgitation, increased pulmonary vascular changes, and a prominent main pulmonary artery. Echocardiography allows visualization of the components of the defect, including continuity between the AV valves, their sizes, and chordal attachments. Cardiac catheterization confirms the location of septal defects, AV valve abnormalities, degree of left-to-right shunting, and presence of pulmonary hypertension.

Timing of surgical repair depends on the severity of symptoms, degree of shunting, and level of pulmonary vascular resistance. The current trend is to perform complete repair between 6 and 12 months of life[18] to avoid the development of pulmonary vascular changes. Surgical repair is performed through a midsternotomy implementing a one- or two-patch repair to close the septal defects and repair the involved AV valves. Mortality has declined below 10% unless the child is a newborn, has severe AV valve incompetence, or has a small LV. Postoperative complications include heart block, dysrhythmias, or mitral regurgitation requiring further surgical intervention or valve replacement.[30,31]

Defects Decreasing Pulmonary Blood Flow

Defects decreasing pulmonary blood flow involve obstruction to pulmonary blood flow and septal communications. Because of RV outflow tract obstruction, right-sided pressures exceed left-sided pressures, resulting in right-to-left shunting. Children with these defects have hypoxemia and cyanosis.

Tetralogy of Fallot

Tetralogy of Fallot consists of four defects: a VSD that is high in the septum and usually large, an overriding aorta that straddles the VSD, pulmonary stenosis, and RV hypertrophy (Fig. 30-9, *A*). It is the most common cyanotic congenital heart defect and accounts for 10% of all defects.[3]

Pathophysiology

Tetralogy of Fallot develops during two phases of embryologic growth: (1) during the division of the truncus arteriosus by the spiral septum in the third or fourth week of gestation and (2) during the division of the ventricles between the fourth

A
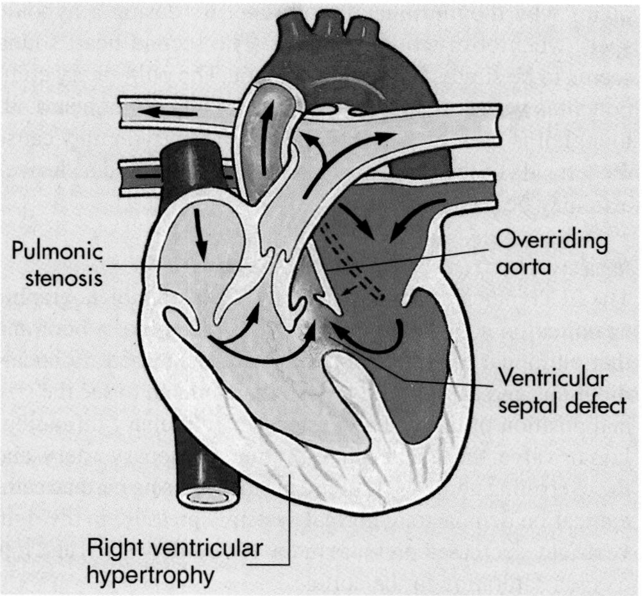

B
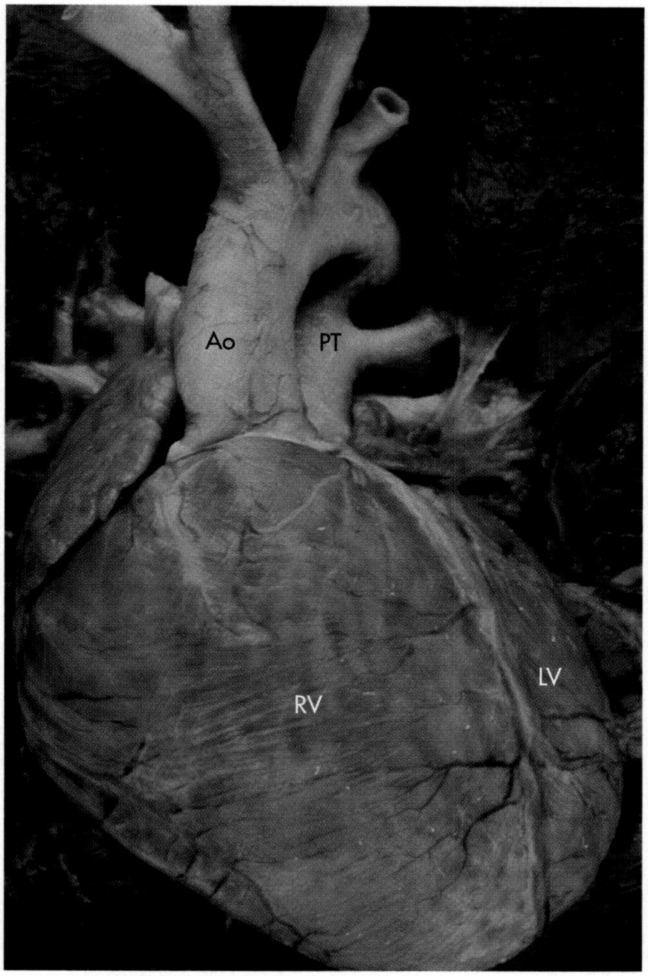

C
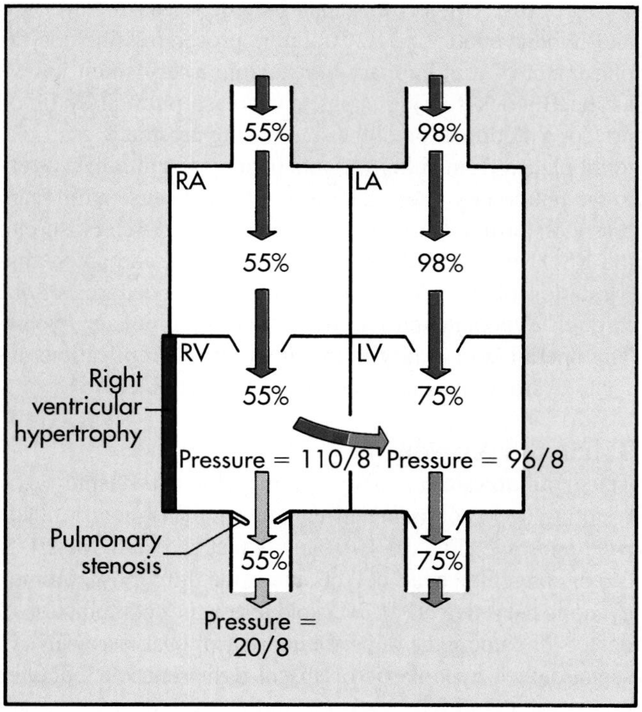

FIG. 30-9 Tetralogy of Fallot. A, Anatomic defects in tetralogy of Fallot. **B,** Complete transposition of the aorta and pulmonary artery. **C,** Hemodynamics of tetralogy of Fallot with right-to-left shunt. *Ao,* aorta; *PT,* pulmonary trunk; *RV,* right ventricle; *LV,* left ventricle; *RA,* right atrium; *LA,* left atrium. (A from Wong DL: *Whaley and Wong's nursing care of infants and children*, ed 6, St Louis, 1999, Mosby; B from Damjanov I, Linder J, editors: *Anderson's pathology*, ed 10, St Louis, 1996, Mosby; C from Whaley LF, Wong DL: *Nursing care of infants and children*, ed 4, St Louis, 1991, Mosby.)

and eighth weeks of gestation. Normally, as these events progress, the truncal septum fuses with the bulbar ridges and, in turn, with the endocardial cushions. The membranous portion of the interventricular septum grows upward to meet the endocardial cushions, and ultimately all of these tissues come together to complete the interventricular septum.

The embryologic error that causes tetralogy of Fallot is not known for certain, but two theories have been proposed.[1] The first is that the truncus arteriosus divides unevenly, resulting in great vessels of unequal size. Because of this asymmetry, the part of the spiral septum that normally fuses with the AV septa is not where it should be, causing a VSD. Concomitantly, pulmonary stenosis develops because there is a larger than normal amount of tissue in the infundibulum of the right ventricle. (This infundibulum is on the ventricular side of the pulmonic valve.) The second theory proposes that infundibular overgrowth in the right ventricle is the major developmental anomaly. The extra tissue restricts the blood flow through the pulmonary artery, causing the artery to be smaller than normal at birth. Concomitantly, the aorta is subjected to greater than normal blood flow during fetal life, causing it to be larger than normal at birth. In addition, infundibular overgrowth in the right ventricle prevents normal closure of the ventricular septum, causing the VSD.

The pathophysiology associated with tetralogy of Fallot varies widely, depending primarily on the degree of pulmonary stenosis but also on the size of the VSD and the pulmonary and systemic resistance to flow. Because the VSD is usually large, pressures may be equal in the right and left ventricles. Therefore the major determinant of shunt direction through the VSD is the difference between pulmonary and systemic vascular resistance (see Fig. 30-9, *C*). Infants who have little or no shunting are acyanotic and are known as "pink tets." If pulmonary vascular resistance is higher than systemic resistance, the shunt is from right to left. If systemic resistance is higher than pulmonary resistance, the shunt is from left to right. Because many factors can alter the balance between pulmonary and systemic resistance, shunt direction is not necessarily constant.

Pulmonary stenosis decreases blood flow to the lungs and, consequently, the amount of oxygenated blood that returns to the left heart. If blood also shunts from right to left through the VSD, deoxygenated blood mixes with the small amount of relatively oxygenated blood returning from the lungs. The result is low O_2 saturation (hypoxemia) in the systemic circulation. The body attempts to compensate for hypoxemia by producing more red cells (thereby causing polycythemia) and by increasing blood flow to the lungs through collateral bronchial vessels.

Clinical Manifestations

As long as the ductus arteriosus remains open, the newborn's pulmonary blood flow may be adequate. As the ductus closes, however, cyanosis becomes apparent. Chronic hypoxemia causes clubbing of the fingers and toes (see Chapter 32).

A common manifestation of tetralogy of Fallot is the sudden onset of dyspnea, cyanosis, and restlessness, sometimes called a hypoxic spell or a "tet spell," that generally occurs with crying and exertion. The cause of these episodes is unknown, but it is theorized that the RV outflow tract goes into spasm or the systemic resistance drops suddenly.[7,18] In either case the relative or actual increase in pulmonary vascular resistance increases the right-to-left shunt and the cyanosis. Infants often have difficulty with feeding because the exertion required increases hypoxia, and therefore they experience slow growth and failure to thrive.

Squatting is a spontaneous compensatory mechanism used by older children to alleviate hypoxic spells. Squatting and its variants increase systemic resistance while decreasing venous return to the heart from the inferior vena cava. The decrease of systemic return makes relatively more oxygenated blood available to the body. The increase of systemic resistance also reverses the shunt through the VSD to a left-to-right shunt, which has the effect of increasing pulmonary blood flow. Through both of these mechanisms, squatting decreases the degree of hypoxemia temporarily.

The typical heart murmur of tetralogy is a pulmonary systolic ejection murmur caused by the obstruction in the outflow tract, which creates turbulence during systole. The smaller the obstruction, the louder the murmur is. This explains why the murmur often disappears during a hypoxic spell, when obstruction increases. The second heart sound seems to be single, but in fact it is not. The pulmonary component is very soft and delayed and usually is not heard, although it is present. The enlarged right ventricle may cause the left side of the chest to be more prominent, and a "heave" also may be palpated.

Evaluation and Treatment

The ECG indicates RV hypertrophy. Chest roentgenographic examination shows that the heart is shaped like a boot and that pulmonary vascular markings are decreased. Echocardiograms and angiograms enable the clinician to see the size and position of the VSD, the stenotic pulmonary infundibulum or valve, the smaller-than-normal pulmonary artery, and the overriding aorta. Measurements made during cardiac catheterization demonstrate normal systemic pressure in the right ventricle, decreased pressure in the RV outflow tract, and low oxygen saturation in the aorta.

The current trend is to repair tetralogy of Fallot before 1 year of life. Triggers for repair include increasing cyanosis and hypercyanotic spells. Palliative procedures include the placement of a pulmonary-to-systemic artery shunt known as the Blalock-Taussig shunt to increase pulmonary blood flow or a modification of the shunt using prosthetic graft material placed from either the subclavian or innominate artery to the pulmonary artery. These shunts may cause pulmonary artery distortion. Corrective repair involves patch closure of the VSD, resection of infundibular stenosis, and patch augmentation of the RV outflow tract. The procedure is done through a median sternotomy on cardiopulmonary bypass. The operative mortality is less than 5%. Complications include dysrhythmias and occasionally heart block.[18,26]

Tricuspid Atresia

Tricuspid atresia consists of an imperforate tricuspid valve, resulting in no communication between the right atrium and right ventricle (Fig. 30-10). This defect accounts for 2% to 3% of congenital heart defects and is the third most common cyanotic heart defect.[3,18] Tricuspid atresia is a combination of defects, including the imperforate tricuspid valve as well as a septal defect, hypoplastic or absent right ventricle, enlarged mitral valve and left ventricle, and varying degrees of pulmonic stenosis.[26] Tricuspid atresia may also be associated with transposition of the great vessels. The most common type of tricuspid atresia involves a hypoplastic right atrium with decreased pulmonary blood flow and a VSD and is not associated with transposition.[3]

Pathophysiology

Systemic blood returns through the superior and inferior venae cavae to the right atrium. Because there is no opening between the right atrium and right ventricle, blood flows through the ASD into the left atrium, mixing with blood returning from the pulmonary circulation. The blood then enters the left ventricle. Most of this blood goes out into the systemic circulation through the aorta, but varying amounts

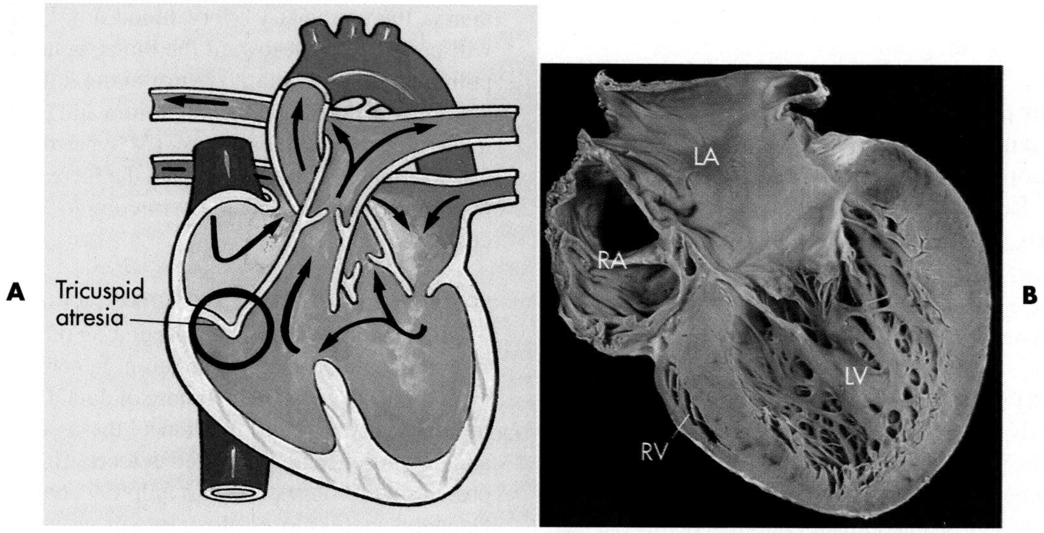

FIG. 30-10 Tricuspid atresia. A, No communication from the right atrium to right ventricle. **B,** Tricuspid atresia with absent right atrioventricular connection with a hypoplastic right ventricle (four-chamber view). *LA,* Left atrium; *RA,* right atrium; *LV,* left ventricle; *RV,* right ventricle. (A from Wong DL: *Whaley and Wong's nursing care of infants and children,* ed 6, St Louis, 1999, Mosby; B from Damjanov I, Linder J, editors: *Anderson's pathology,* ed 10, St Louis, 1996, Mosby.)

pass through the VSD into the hypoplastic right ventricle and then out through the pulmonary valve to the lungs. Pulmonary circulation depends on the presence of a VSD and the presence of a functioning right ventricle of reasonable capacity. If the right ventricle is absent, the pulmonary valve is usually imperforate as well. If this is the case, a PDA is necessary to ensure that some blood flows into the pulmonary circulation.[32]

Pulmonary circulation also depends on the relationship between pulmonary and systemic vascular resistance. As long as pulmonary resistance is lower than systemic resistance, blood flows through the VSD from left to right, feeding the pulmonary circulation. If pulmonary resistance rises above systemic resistance, blood will not reach the pulmonary circulation through the VSD.

◆ *Clinical Manifestations*

Some degree of central cyanosis is common in tricuspid atresia, depending on the amount of pulmonary blood flow. Growth failure also is common. Children experience exertional dyspnea, tachypnea, and hypoxemia. Long-term effects of hypoxia are polycythemia and clubbing. These children also may display hypercyanotic spells. Hepatomegaly may be present if the ASD is restrictive or congestive heart failure occurs as a result of increased pulmonary blood flow.

The murmur heard with tricuspid atresia may have several components. The VSD causes a systolic regurgitant murmur; the larger the VSD, the softer and shorter the murmur is likely to be. A narrowly split second heart sound caused by decreased pulmonary blood flow may be present, or the pulmonic component may be absent when no VSD is involved.

◆ *Evaluation and Treatment*

Chest roentgenographic examination shows a heart size that is normal or slightly increased. ECG shows RA, LA, and LV hypertrophy. Echocardiography and cardiac catheterization depict left-to-right shunting at the ventricular level, inability of blood flow to enter the right ventricle, and the presence of associated defects.

Newborns who are ductal dependent are immediately given prostaglandins to maintain adequate pulmonary blood flow. Initial surgical intervention involves the placement of a Blalock-Taussig shunt (or its modifications). If the ASD is restrictive, a Rashkind procedure may be performed during catheterization. Children who experience increased pulmonary blood flow may require the placement of a pulmonary artery band. Corrective repair involves closing the septal defects, taking down the previous shunts or band, and connecting the superior and inferior venae cavae to the pulmonary artery to separate the pulmonary systemic circulation (Fontan-Kreutzer procedure and its modifications). Postoperative complications include pleural effusions, elevated pulmonary vascular resistance, LV dysfunction, and dysrhythmias.[17,18,33]

Obstructive Defects

Obstructive defects are conditions in which anatomic stenosis (narrowing) in either the right or left outflow tract causes obstruction to blood flow and results in a pressure load on the ventricles and decreased output. The difference between the obstruction is the gradient that reflects the severity of the narrowing; the higher the gradient is, the more obstruction to flow and increased afterload on the ventricle, with resultant decreased cardiac output. The location is classified according to the location of the narrowing in relation to the valve. Valvular stenosis refers to stenosis of the valve itself; subvalvular indicates that the stenotic area is below the valve or in the ventricular outflow tract; and supravalvular is the area above the valve in the great artery. The obstructive defects include coarctation of the aorta, aortic stenosis, pulmonary stenosis, and hypoplastic left heart syndrome.

Symptoms associated with the defect depend on the site of stenosis.

Coarctation of the Aorta

Coarctation of the aorta (COA) is a narrowing of the lumen of the aorta that impedes blood flow. This defect accounts for 8% to 10% of all congenital heart defects.[54] COA is almost always in a juxtaductal position, although it can occur anywhere between the origin of the aortic arch and the bifurcation of the aorta in the lower abdomen. As many as 85% of individuals with COA have a bicuspid aortic valve (Fig. 30-11).

Pathophysiology

COA commonly develops because of an abnormal contractile ductal tissue that constricts at the time of ductal closure.[3] COA causes a condition in which there are higher pressures above the site of stenosis and lower pressures below the site. In preductal COA the right ventricle acts as a systemic pump, sending unoxygenated blood through the ductus into the descending aorta below the coarctation (Fig. 30-12). In postductal COA the right ventricle cannot pump enough blood through the ductus to the descending aorta because of pressure caused by the narrowed aorta. Systolic pressures increase in the ascending aorta and left ventricle and decrease in the descending aorta beyond the COA (Fig. 30-13). To bypass the COA, collateral circulation, which involves small arteries arising from the subclavian arteries, joins intercostal arteries that flow into the descending aorta. This bypasses the COA and supplies more oxygenated blood to the lower extremities. The direction of shunting through the ductus depends on the pressure difference between the pulmonary artery and aorta. When blood pressure is greater in the aorta than in the pulmonary artery, blood flow through the ductus will be left to right toward the lungs, resulting in increased pulmonary blood volume return to the left side of the heart. This places a strain on the left atrium and left ventricle, leading to congestive heart failure. LV hypertrophy develops because of increased afterload from the increased volume of the pulmonary circulation and obstruction to flow caused by the coarctation.

Clinical Manifestations

Clinical manifestations vary depending on the severity of the coarctation and age of presentation. In newborns the onset of symptoms depends on the timing of ductal closure after a fall in pulmonary vascular resistance, the location of the COA, and the presence of associated defects. The newborn usually presents with congestive heart failure secondary to LV failure. Once the ductus closes, these infants will deteriorate rapidly from the development of hypotension, acidosis, and shock. Older children may not be diagnosed until hypertension is noted. Hypertension is noted in the upper extremities with decreased or absent pulses in the lower extremities, accompanied by cool mottled skin and, occasionally, leg cramps during exercise caused by tissue anoxia. Hypertension may cause dizziness, headache, fainting, or epistaxis. A systolic ejection murmur, heard best on the left interscapular area, is caused by rapid blood flow through the narrowed area.

Evaluation and Treatment

A chest roentgenogram shows an enlarged heart with congested lung fields in newborns. Rib notching between the fourth and eighth ribs may be seen in children older than 5 years, reflecting erosion of the ribs from enlarged collat-

A

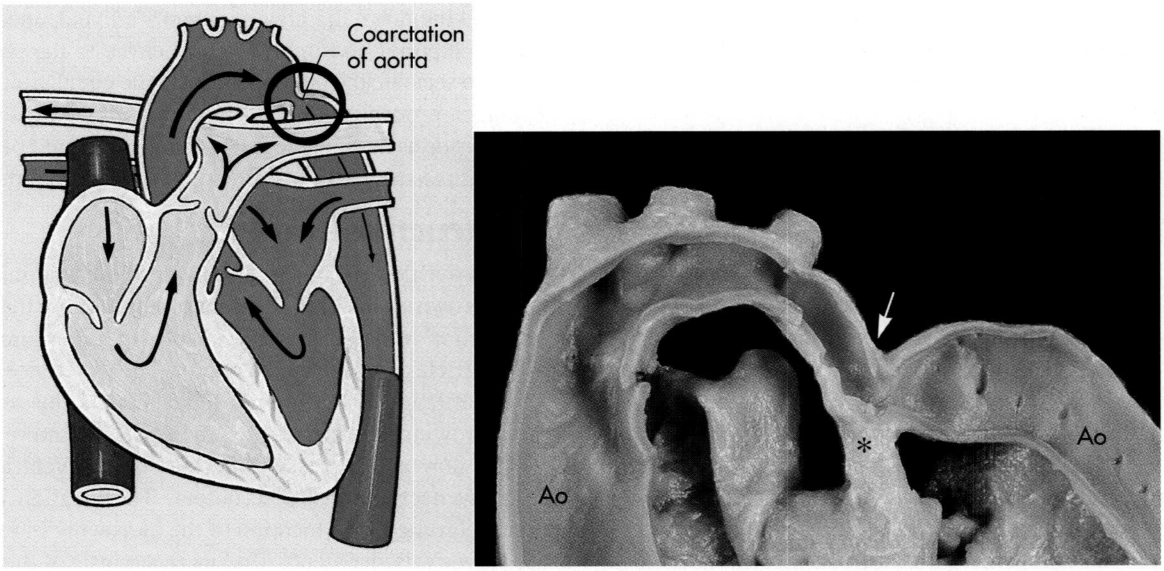

B

FIG. 30-11 Postductal and preductal coarctation of the aorta. A, Postductal coarctation occurs distal to ("after") the insertion of the closed ductus arteriosus into the aortic arch. Preductal coarctation occurs proximal to ("before") insertion of the patent ductus arteriosus. The coarctation consists of a flap of tissue that protrudes from the tunica media of the aortic wall. **B,** Coarctation of the aorta with typical indentation of the aortic wall (arrow) opposite the ductal arterial ligament (*). *Ao,* Aorta. (A from Wong DL: *Whaley and Wong's nursing care of infants and children*, ed 6, St Louis, 1999, Mosby; B from Damjanov I, Linder J, editors: *Anderson's pathology*, ed 10, St Louis, 1996, Mosby.)

eral vessels from the ascending aorta to the descending aorta, bypassing the coarctation. An ECG may be normal or reveal LV hypertrophy. An echocardiogram will confirm the diagnosis and rule out other intracardiac defects. Cardiac catheterization and/or MRI is performed only if the echocardiogram is inconclusive.

The first step in treatment of the symptomatic infant is stabilization, which may require prostaglandin administration, mechanical ventilation, and inotropic support to maintain adequate cardiac output. Once this is achieved, surgical intervention is indicated. Surgical repair for infants younger than 1 year consists of either a subclavian flap aortoplasty technique to enlarge the constricted area or resection with end-to-end anastomosis of the arch segments. Depending on the arch morphology, a modification of this procedure enlarges the aorta beyond the area of constriction. For children older than 1 year, surgical repair consists of either resection with end-to-end anastomosis or prosthetic patch enlargement of the area of constriction.[18,34] Cardiopulmonary bypass is not required because of the extracardiac nature of the lesion, and the approach is through a left thoracotomy.

Postoperative complications include recoarctation and paradoxical postoperative hypertension. Residual permanent hypertension requiring continued medical therapy is related to age at repair; therefore surgical intervention is recommended at the time of diagnosis. Operative mortality for infants is less than 5%, and for children older than 1 year, it is less than 1%.[18] Balloon dilation angioplasty in newborns has been successfully performed. However, aortic aneurysm formation and a high rate of restenosis have been noted;[35,36,37,38] therefore surgical repair remains the correction of choice for the newborn.[39,40,41]

Aortic Stenosis

Aortic stenosis is a narrowing of the aortic outflow tract (Fig. 30-14). The lesion accounts for 5% of all congenital heart defects.[3] Valvular stenosis is caused by malformation or fusion of the cusps. It is the most common type of aortic stenosis, tends to be progressive, and can lead to sudden death as a result of low cardiac output or myocardial infarction. For children with mild to moderate aortic stenosos, exercise restrictions are advised.[32] Less common forms of aortic stenosis are subvalvular stenosis caused by a constricting fibrous ring below the valve and supravalvular stenosis that occurs above the valve.

Pathophysiology

Obstruction to blood flow out the aorta causes an increased workload on the left ventricle, resulting in left ventricle hypertrophy (LVH). LV failure may develop, leading to an

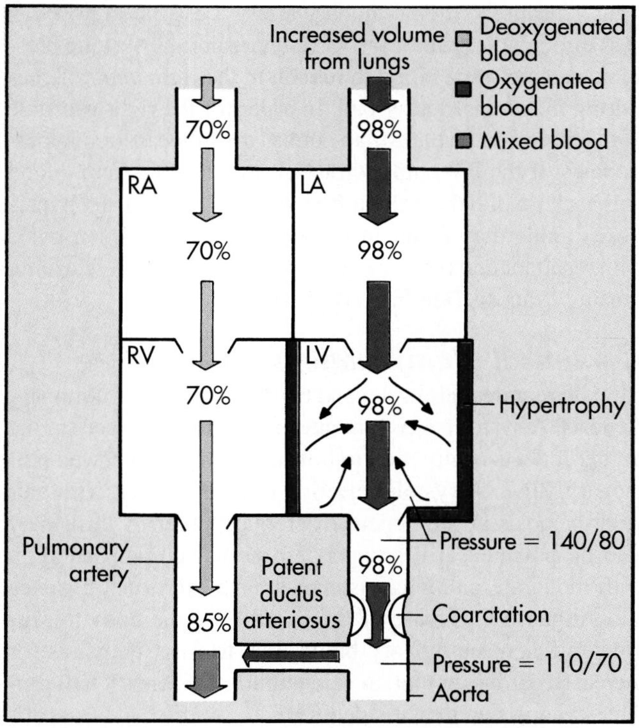

FIG. 30-12 Hemodynamics of preductal coartation of the aorta with a patent ductus arteriosus. The left-to-right shunt through the ductus arteriosus increases the volume of blood in the pulmonary circulation. Afterload (dashed arrows) is increased in the left heart by (1) increased return from the lungs and (2) decreased ventricular outflow caused by the coarctation. The outcome is left heart failure (congestive heart failure). *RA,* right atrium; *LA,* left atrium; *RV,* right ventricle; *LV,* left ventricle.

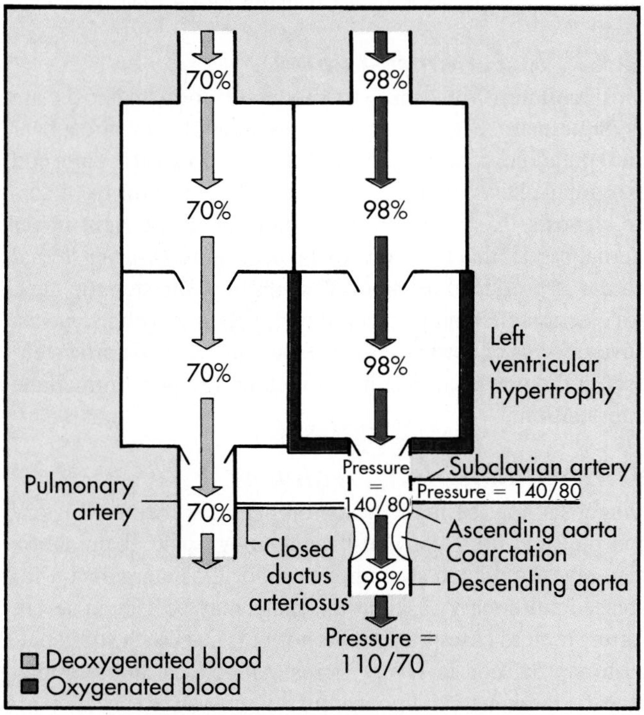

FIG. 30-13 Hemodynamics of postductal coarctation of the aorta. Blood pressure increases in the ascending aorta and subclavian artery and decreases in the descending aorta. These pressure changes eventually occur in the parts of the systemic circulation served by arteries that branch from the aorta before and after the coarctation.

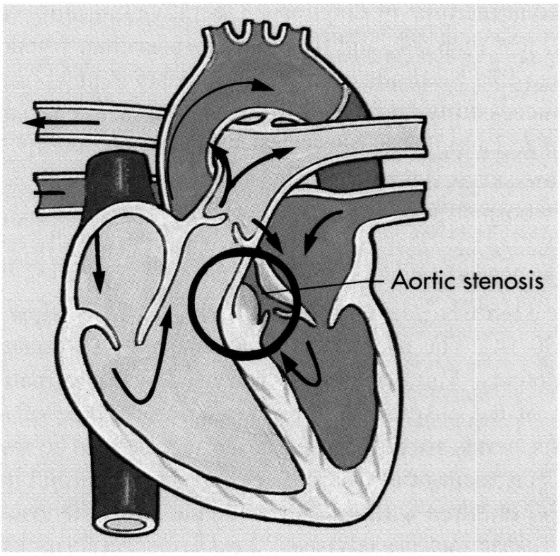

FIG. 30-14 Aortic stenosis. Narrowing of the aortic valve causing resistance to blood flow in the left ventricle, decreased cardiac output, left ventricular hypertrophy, and pulmonary congestion. (From Wong DL: *Whaley and Wong's nursing care of infants and children,* ed 6, St Louis, 1999, Mosby.)

increase in LA pressure and a backup in the system, eventually resulting in pulmonary vascular congestion and pulmonary arterial hypertension. LVH can decrease coronary artery perfusion, resulting in myocardial infarction, or it can alter the LV papillary muscle, causing mitral insufficiency.

Clinical Manifestations

Most children with mild to moderate aortic stenosis are asymptomatic. Signs of exercise intolerance may not appear until preadolescence. Syncopal episodes, epigastric pain, and exertional chest pain may occur in more severe forms of aortic stenosis. A systolic ejection murmur at the right upper sternal border that transmits to the neck and left lower sternal border is produced by blood flow through the stenotic area. An ejection click may be heard with valvular aortic stenosis. Severe forms of aortic stenosis, especially critical aortic stenosis in the newborn, result in shock and require immediate intervention.

Evaluation and Treatment

Diagnosis may be made based on previous medical history and physical findings. Chest roentgenographic examination may reveal a dilated ascending aorta or LV enlargement. Increased pulmonary vascular markings may be seen in severe forms. In mild cases the ECG is normal. LVH with strain pattern may be seen in severe forms. An echocardiogram may reveal a thickened and poorly fucntioning left ventricle with abnormal closure of the aortic valve. Cardiac catheterization will determine the location, cause, and severity of obstruction.

The presence of ST segment changes on ECG, severe congestive heart failure, and evidence of discrete stenosis at the aortic outflow tract are indications for intervention. Balloon aortic valvuloplasty is a palliative procedure that is performed for valvular aortic stenosis; however, it is associated with complications, including aortic insufficiency and dysrhythmia.[42] Aortic valvotomy, under inflow occlusion or cardiopulmonary bypass, is currently performed for valvular aortic stenosis. Operative mortality remains high in infants (up to 20%), although older children have a mortality close to 0%.[33] As many as 25% of individuals require a second surgery within 10 years for restenosis, at which time valve replacement may be the procedure of choice.

Subvalvular aortic stenosis and supravalvular aortic stenosis require surgical repair involving excision of the area causing the constriction. For subvalvular aortic stenosis involving a small LV outflow tract and aortic annulus, a Konno procedure may be done to enlarge the LV outflow tract and aortic annulus with a patch.

Pulmonary Stenosis

Pulmonary stenosis is the narrowing of the pulmonary outflow tract. This may be in the form of abnormal thickening of the valve leaflets or narrowing of the arterial (supravalvular) or ventricular (subvalvular) side of the valve (Fig. 30-15, *A*). **Pulmonary atresia** is the severe form of pulmonary stenosis and involves complete fusion of the commissures, allowing no blood flow out of the pulmonary artery. Pulmonary stenosis accounts for 5% to 8% of all congenital heart defects.[3]

Pathophysiology

Pulmonary stenosis creates resistance to blood flow from the right ventricle to the pulmonary artery. Less blood flow can pass through the pulmonary valve under normal systolic pressure, causing some blood to remain in the right ventricle, resulting in increased afterload. In order for the right ventricle to maintain adequate cardiac output, the myocardium hypertrophies. If the RV outflow tract obstruction is severe, blood will back up into the right atrium, causing dilation and hypertrophy. This may result in reopening of the foramen ovale with resultant unoxygenated blood shunting to the left atrium, causing cyanosis (see Fig. 30-15, *B*).

Clinical Manifestations

Clinical manifestations depend on the severity of pulmonary stenosis. A systolic ejection murmur at the left upper sternal border reflects obstruction to flow through the narrowed pulmonary valve. A systolic ejection click is present with valvular stenosis at the upper left sternal border. A thrill may also be palpated at the upper left sternal border. Children with moderate pulmonary stenosis have exertional dyspnea and fatigability because of the inability of the body to provide sufficient pulmonary blood flow to meet demands for increased cardiac output. Severe pulmonary stenosis will produce cyanosis and right-sided CHF.

Evaluation and Treatment

A chest roentgenogram shows a normal-size heart with a prominent main pulmonary artery caused by poststenotic dilation. An ECG is normal but may reveal right axis deviation and RV hypertrophy with moderate pulmonary stenosis. Echocardiography confirms the diagnosis and detects asso-

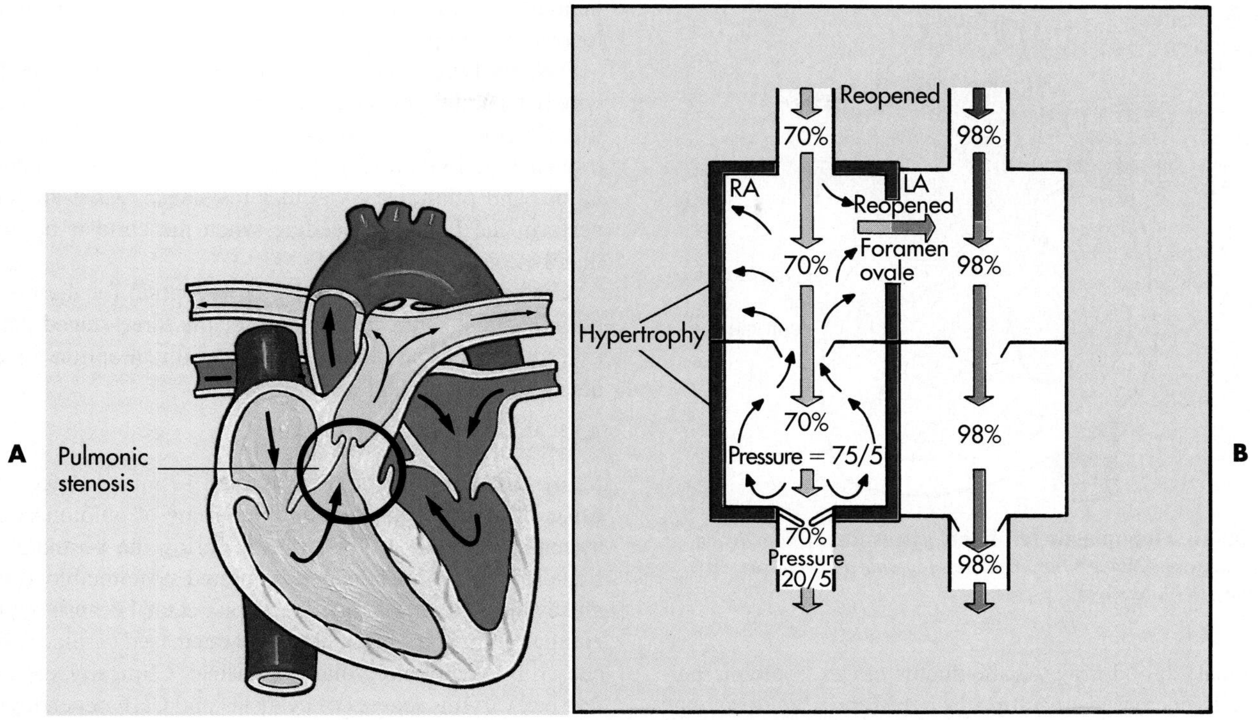

FIG. 30-15 Pulmonary stenosis. A, Obstruction of right ventricular outflow caused by pulmonary stenosis. Pressure on the ventricular side of the pulmonic semilunar valve (pulmonary valve) is much greater than that on the pulmonary arterial side. This difference disrupts the normal pressure gradient across the valve. Pulmonary stenosis increases ventricular afterload by decreasing blood flow through the valve, which causes ventricular hypertrophy. **B,** The backup of ventricular afterload into the right atrium reopens the foramen ovale. Venous blood then flows from the area of higher pressure (the right atrium) to the area of lower pressure (the left atrium), causing a left-to-right shunt. Cyanosis occurs if enough venous blood shunts from right to left to reduce oxygen saturation in the systemic circulation by 3% to 5%. *RA,* Right atrium; *LA,* left atrium. (A from Wong DL: *Whaley and Wong's nursing care of infants and children*, ed 6, St Louis, 1999, Mosby; B from Whaley LF, Wong DL: *Nursing care of infants and children*, ed 4, St Louis, 1991, Mosby.)

ciated defects. Cardiac catheterization further demonstrates pulmonary artery anatomy.

Mild pulmonary stenosis may not require intervention but will be observed closely with prophylaxis for subacute bacterial endocarditis. Treatment is indicated when a significant pressure gradient is detected across the RV outflow tract.

Critical pulmonary stenosis must be addressed immediately. The treatment of choice is balloon angioplasty. This procedure is considered highly effective in decreasing the pressure gradient across the pulmonic valve and is noted to have few associated complications.[43] Surgical correction involves a pulmonary valvotomy incising the fused commissures. Operative mortality is less than 1%.[3] Both valvotomy and balloon angioplasty may result in some pulmonary valve incompetence, and long-term follow-up may reveal the need for further intervention.

Hypoplastic Left Heart Syndrome

Hypoplastic left heart syndrome (HLHS) refers to the abnormal development of the left-sided cardiac structures, resulting in obstruction to blood flow from the LV outflow tract. HLHS involves underdevelopment of the left ventricle, aorta, and aortic arch, as well as mitral atresia or stenosis (Fig. 30-16). Therefore infants with HLHS depend on a well-functioning right ventricle and the presence of a PDA or atrial septal communication for survival. HLHS accounts for 1% of all congenital heart defects and is considered the most complex congenital defect.

Pathophysiology

Because of the high pressures caused by LV outflow tract obstruction, saturated blood enters the left atrium and mixes with desaturated blood in the right atrium through an atrial septal communication. Blood flow follows the normal pathways through the right side of the heart. Exiting the pulmonary artery, the mixed-saturation blood flows through the ductus and to the descending aorta. The amount of blood flow that travels to the pulmonary and systemic circulations depends on vascular resistance in the respective systems. Retrograde blood flow through the hypoplastic ascending aorta provides coronary and cerebral blood flow.

Clinical Manifestations

Newborn infants with HLHS generally are born full term and initially appear healthy. Mild cyanosis, tachypnea, poor feeding, and dyspnea usually manifest during the first week of life. Congestive heart failure develops because of increased

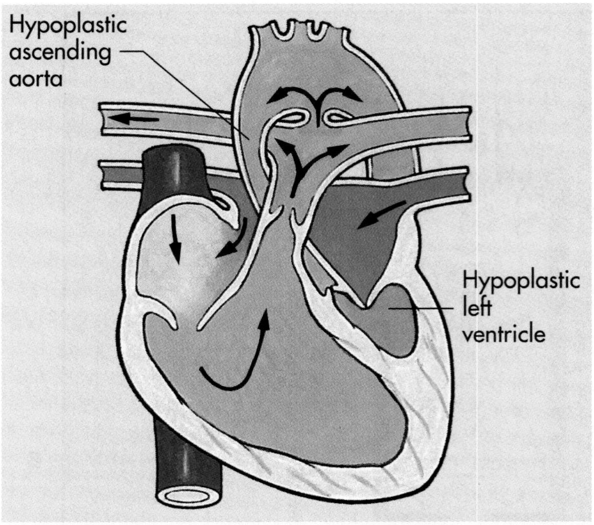

FIG. 30-16 Hypoplastic left heart syndrome. (From Wong DL: *Whaley and Wong's nursing care of infants and children*, ed 6, St Louis, 1999, Mosby.)

pulmonary blood flow. As the ductus closes, systemic perfusion is decreased, resulting in hypoxemia, acidosis, and shock. Usually no heart murmur is detected. The second heart sound is loud and single because of aortic atresia.

Evaluation and Treatment

A chest roentgenogram shows cardiomegaly and increased pulmonary venous congestion. ECG shows RV hypertrophy and diminished left-sided forces. Echocardiography reveals the components of the defect with a diminutive LV cavity, hypoplastic aortic valve and arch, and hypoplastic or absent mitral valve with a dilated RV cavity. This study makes cardiac catheterization unnecessary.

Prostaglandin infusion to maintain patency of the ductus arteriosus is essential for newborn infant survival. Immediate correction of acidosis, inotropic support for adequate cardiac output, and ventilatory manipulation to balance systemic and pulmonary blood flow prevent further deterioration and achieve stabilization.

Surgical intervention includes a three-stage approach that begins with a Norwood procedure. The Norwood procedure consists of an atrial septectomy, placement of a pulmonary-to-systemic artery shunt to maintain adequate pulmonary blood flow, creation of a permanent communication between the right ventricle and aorta, and patch augmentation of the aorta. Postoperative complications include imbalance of systemic and pulmonary blood flow, leading to inadequate cardiac output and persistent heart failure. In most centers, survival after the Norwood procedure is now averaging greater than 50%.[44,45,46,47,48,49]

The second stage is the bidirectional Glenn procedure, which is performed between 6 and 12 months of age, depending on the child's clinical status, pulmonary vascular resistance, and ventricular function. This involves joining the superior vena cava to the pulmonary artery. Complications include superior vena cava syndrome, pleural effusion, and low cardiac output.

The third stage is the Fontan procedure, described earlier, which separates the systemic from the pulmonary circulation. Timing for surgical repair depends on the child's ventricular function, presence of atrioventricular valve regurgitation, and pulmonary vascular resistance. Most surgeons perform the Fontan procedure when the child is approximately 2 years of age.[44,45,46]

Cardiac transplant may also be an option for these newborns.[50] Most surgical centers offer the three-staged palliative surgeries as an initial approach, with an option for cardiac transplantation later in life.[44,48,51]

Mixed Defects

Many complex defects are classified as mixed defects because of their dependence on the mixing of pulmonary and systemic circulations for survival during the postnatal period. This mixing results in desaturated systemic blood flow and cyanosis. Pulmonary congestion occurs because of preferential pulmonary blood flow and decreased cardiac output caused by ventricular volume overload. Clinically, each defect has varying degrees of cyanosis and CHF depending on the various components of the lesion.

Transposition of the Great Arteries

Transposition of the great arteries (TGA) refers to a condition in which the aorta arises from the RV and the pulmonary artery from the LV (Fig. 30-17, *A*). The result is two separate, parallel circuits in which unoxygenated blood circulates continuously through the systemic circulation and oxygenated blood circulates repeatedly through the pulmonary circulation. This condition is incompatible with extrauterine life unless a communication exists between the two circuits to provide the necessary oxygen to the body. Communication is accomplished through mixing of pulmonary and systemic circulations through a PDA, ASD, or VSD (see Fig. 30-17, *B*). Dextro–transposition of the great arteries (D-TGA) is the most common cyanotic congenital heart defect and accounts for 10% of all congenital heart defects; "dextro" refers to the aorta remaining to the right of the pulmonary artery.

Two factors allow newborns with complete transposition to survive long enough to be treated. First, blood from the two closed systems can mix through the ductus arteriosus for a short time after birth if pulmonary vascular resistance remains high. Some mixing also may occur through the foramen ovale. If the child has a VSD, mixing occurs through that opening as well.

Pathophysiology

It is not known precisely which embryologic events lead to transposition, but researchers have proposed that the fault lies in the development of conal tissue in the fibrous skeleton of the heart.[7] The conus is a segment of muscle that separates the atrioventricular (tricuspid and mitral) valves from the semilunar (aortic and pulmonic) valves. (The fibrous skel-

A

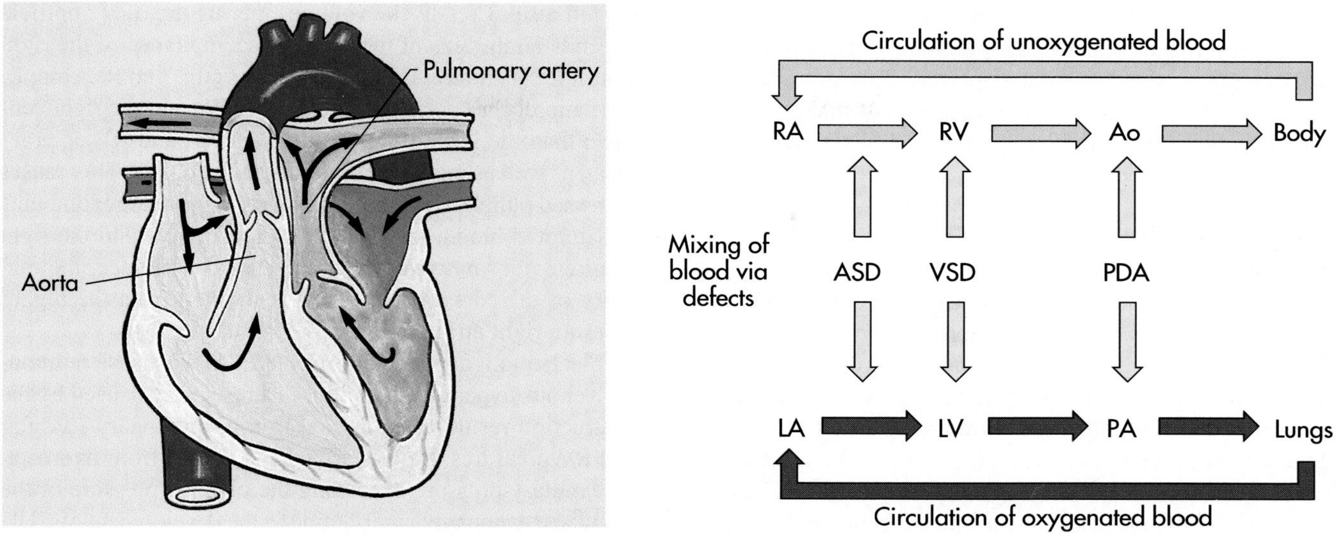

B

FIG. 30-17 Hemodynamics in transposition of the great vessels (TGV). A, Complete transposition of the great vessels with an intact interventricular septum. The aorta arises from the right ventricle and the pulmonary artery from the left. **B,** Oxygen saturation in the two parallel circuits. *RA,* Right atrium; *RV,* right ventricle; *Ao,* aorta; *ASD,* atrial septal defect; *VSD,* ventricular septal defect; *PDA,* patent ductus arteriosus; *LA,* left atrium; *LV,* left ventricle; *PA,* pulmonary artery. (A from Wong DL: *Whaley and Wong's nursing care of infants and children,* ed 6, St Louis, 1999, Mosby; B from Whaley LF, Wong DL: *Nursing care of infants and children,* ed 4, St Louis, 1991, Mosby.)

eton and heart valves are described and illustrated in Chapter 28; see Fig. 28-4.) Normally, the conus grows more on the left side, under the pulmonic valve. This pushes the pulmonic valve anteriorly and to the left of the aortic valve. Some researchers believe that in transposition of the great vessels, nearly the opposite occurs; that is, the conus beneath the aortic valve grows more, pushing the aortic valve until it is anterior (forward) and superior to the pulmonic valve. This causes the aorta to rise anteriorly and to the right of the pulmonary artery.[1] The interventricular septum is intact in about 60% of cases of transposition; a VSD is present in the remaining 40%. Pulmonary stenosis is associated with the transposition in about 4% to 6% of children with intact septums and in 28% to 31% of children with VSDs.[1] The discussion that follows is limited to the pathophysiology of complete transposition with an intact interventricular septum.

Clinical Manifestations

The degree of mixing permitted by fetal structures determines the type and severity of clinical manifestations. Cyanosis may be mild shortly after birth and worsen during the first day because of functional closure of the ductus arteriosus. Low oxygen levels in the blood (hypoxemia) cause metabolic acidosis, tachycardia, and tachypnea. The presence of a PDA or large septal defect allows for more mixing and results in only mild cyanosis, but the infant may develop congestive heart failure.

The first heart sound is normal, and the second sound may be heard as a single sound even though both the aortic and pulmonic valves are functioning. The single S_2 may occur because transposition places the aortic valve closer to the chest wall than the pulmonic valve. No murmur is noted with transposition of the great arteries with an intact ventricular septum.

Evaluation and Treatment

On chest roentgenogram the heart has a characteristic shape—like an egg on its side—and pulmonary vascular markings are increased. The heart may be enlarged if the infant is a few weeks old and has a VSD. ECG findings reveal a right-axis deviation and some RV hypertrophy. Echocardiography confirms the diagnosis of transposition of the great arteries. Cardiac catheterization is necessary to determine the coronary anatomy; measure ventricular ratios; and, if need be, perform a balloon septostomy.

Surgical repair during the newborn period involves the Jatene (arterial switch) operation that transposes the great arteries. The coronary arteries are removed from the aorta before the arterial switch is performed and reimplanted without torsion or kinking into the aorta. This establishes normal blood flow with the left ventricle as the systemic pump. Complications include narrowing at the sites of the great artery anastomoses and coronary insufficiency.[18,33]

Mustard and Senning operations (the creation of an intra-atrial tunnel to baffle the systemic venous blood flow to the mitral valve and the pulmonary venous blood flow to the tricuspid valve) are no longer the procedures of choice because the right ventricle must perform as the systemic pump. Long-term follow-up of children with Mustard and Senning operations revealed significant rates of RV failure and dysrhythmias.

The Rastelli procedure is used with children with transposition, VSD, and severe pulmonary stenosis. This procedure involves closing the VSD with a baffle by rerouting LV blood through the VSD to the aorta. The pulmonary valve is closed, and a right ventricle–to–pulmonary artery prosthetic or homograft valved conduit is placed. This procedure requires prosthetic conduit replacement as the child grows and is associated with ventricular failure and dysrhythmias in the postoperative period.

Total Anomalous Pulmonary Venous Connection

Total anomalous pulmonary venous connection (TAPVC), or total anomalous pulmonary venous return, occurs when the pulmonary veins abnormally connect to the right side of the heart either directly or through one or more systemic veins that drain into the right atrium (Fig. 30-18). An ASD generally is present also. This defect is extremely rare, accounting for only 1% of all congenital heart defects. The four types of TAPVC are based on the site of drainage. Supracardiac TAPVCs are the most common form (50%) and drain to the SVC through the vertical or innominate vein. Cardiac TAPVCs (20%) drain directly into the right atrium or through the coronary sinus. Infracardiac TAPVCs (20%) traverse the diaphragm and drain into the portal or hepatic vein or the IVC. Mixed TAPVCs (10%) are a combination of the various types. Partial anomalous venous connection is a condition in which only one or a few of the pulmonary veins, usually the right-sided veins, drain to the right atrium or one of its tributaries.[3]

Pathophysiology

Physiologically, TAPVC can be differentiated into two groups: nonobstructive and obstructive, depending on the absence or presence of obstruction to pulmonary venous drainage. The hemodynamics of the nonobstructive group involves the right atrium receiving the oxygenated blood that would normally flow into the left atrium. The amount of blood shunted into the left atrium versus the volume entering the right ventricle depends on the size of the ASD and compliance of the right ventricle. Therefore, if the ASD is restrictive and RV compliance approaches normal, more blood will enter the right ventricle than the left atrium, resulting in RA and RV enlargement, as well as increased pulmonary blood flow. This causes increased pulmonary venous blood return and larger amounts of saturated blood. If the ASD is unrestrictive and the right ventricle does not thin out to increase compliance, the majority of mixed saturated blood is shunted from the higher pressure right atrium to the left atrium.

The hemodynamics of obstructed TAPVC cause pulmonary venous hypertension because of resistance caused by the obstruction resulting in an elevation in pulmonary vascular and RV pressures. Pulmonary edema occurs from hydrostatic capillary pressure exceeding the osmotic pressure of the blood and eventually contributing to the development of CHF. This group has a strong association with the infracardiac type of TAPVC and is a surgical emergency.

Clinical Manifestations

The predominant clinical manifestation in infants with TAPVC is cyanosis caused by mixture of oxygenated and deoxygenated blood entering the systemic circulation. The degree of cyanosis is inversely related to the amount of pulmonary blood flow. Children with unobstructed TAPVC may be asymptomatic until pulmonary vascular resistance drops, at which time pulmonary blood flow will increase, resulting in signs of CHF, particularly growth retardation and frequent pulmonary infections, in addition to mild cyanosis. Obstructed TAPVC results in cyanosis and rapid deterioration necessitating immediate surgical correction, or death will occur.

The physical examination also may reveal a systolic murmur at the left upper sternal border and a middiastolic murmur

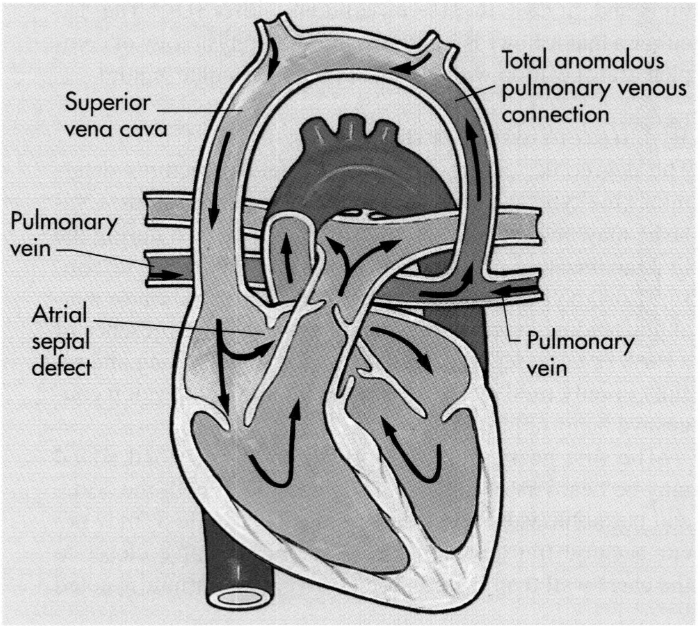

FIG. 30-18 Hemodynamics of total anomalous pulmonary venous connection (TAPVC). In the form of TAPVC represented here, the pulmonary veins enter the left anomalous vertical vein instead of the left atrium. From the left anomalous vertical vein, the mixed blood from the lungs flows into the superior vena cava through an innominate vein (literally, a "vein without a name"). Oxygen saturation within the four heart chambers, the pulmonary artery, and the aorta is the same. Blood pressure in the right heart exceeds that in the left heart because the right heart is receiving blood from both the pulmonary and systemic circulatory systems. (Abnormal vessels are shaded.) (From Wong DL: *Whaley and Wong's nursing care of infants and children*, ed 6, St Louis, 1999, Mosby.)

at the left lower sternal border. Occasionally a venous hum may be detected. A murmur may be absent in obstructed TAPVC. A characteristic quadruple rhythm, consisting of S_1, widely split S_2, and S_3 or S_4, or a gallop rhythm is also present.

Evaluation and Treatment

The ECG shows a right-axis defect (RAD); RV hypertrophy; and, occasionally, RA hypertrophy. The chest roentgenogram of unobstructed TAPVC reveals cardiomegaly, increased pulmonary vascular markings, and a snowman or figure-8 appearance in the supracardiac type. A chest roentgenogram of obstructed TAPVC shows a normal-size heart and a ground-glass appearance of the lung fields, reflecting pulmonary venous congestion or edema. The echocardiogram reveals the abnormal pulmonary venous connections. Cardiac catheterization confirms the site of anomalous connection, the degree of pulmonary blood flow, and the oxygen saturations in the various chambers. The aorta and pulmonary artery have nearly identical oxygen saturations caused by complete mixing of the pulmonary and systemic venous returns to the right atrium.

Surgical repair varies with the type of TAPVC and whether the defect is obstructed or unobstructed. Obstructed lesions are repaired at the time of diagnosis, whereas the unobstructed type generally is repaired during infancy. The procedure is performed on cardiopulmonary bypass and involves anastomosis of the common pulmonary vein to the left atrium; ligating the common pulmonary vein; and closing the ASD, as in the supracardiac and infracardiac types. Repair of the supracardiac type involves baffling the pulmonary venous drainage to the LA. This repair has the highest success rate because of the low technical difficulty, whereas infracardiac repair is associated with a high mortality (up to 25%) and morbidity. Potential complications include reobstruction; atrial dysrhythmias, including sick sinus syndrome; pulmonary artery hypertension; and LV dysfunction.[18,33]

Truncus Arteriosus

Truncus arteriosus is the failure of the large embryonic artery and the truncus arteriosus to divide into the pulmonary artery and the aorta. This results in a single vessel arising from both ventricles, providing blood flow to both the pulmonary and systemic circulations (Fig. 30-19, *A*). This common trunk straddles the VSD (always present) and has a single valve with three or four leaflets, which may result in stenosis or regurgitation. The incidence is 2% of all congenital heart defects, and a right aortic arch is present 50% of the time. There are four types of truncus arteriosus. Type I is the most common (60%) and involves the main pulmonary artery arising from the truncus and then dividing into the right and left pulmonary arteries. Type II is less common (20%) and involves the pulmonary arteries arising from the posterior aspect of the truncus. Type III is the least common (10%) and involves the pulmonary arteries arising from the

A

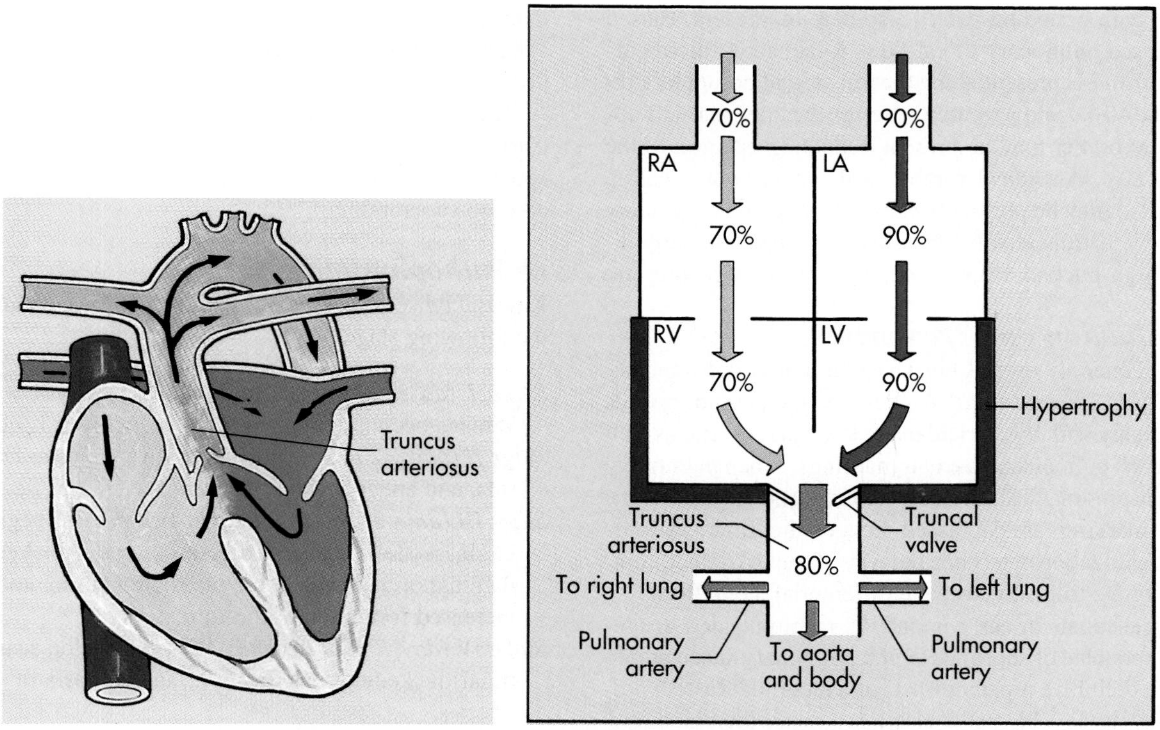

B

FIG. 30-19 Truncus arteriosus. A, Persistent truncus arteriosus. The truncus arteriosus fails to divide into the pulmonary artery and aorta, and the interventricular septum fails to close at the top. Blood from both ventricles mixes in the truncus arteriosus and then enters the pulmonary and systemic circuits. **B,** Alterations of hemodynamics and oxygen saturation by persistent truncus arteriosus. *RA,* Right atrium; *LA,* left atrium; *RV,* right ventricle; *LV,* left ventricle. (A from Wong DL: *Whaley and Wong's nursing care of infants and children,* ed 6, St Louis, 1999, Mosby; B from Whaley LF, Wong DL: *Nursing care of infants and children,* ed 4, St Louis, 1991, Mosby.)

lateral aspect of the truncus. Type IV, also known as pseudotruncus, is now considered a severe form of tetralogy of Fallot with the bronchial arteries arising from the descending aorta to supply the lungs.[3]

Pathophysiology

Blood flow from both the right and left ventricles is pumped into the main truncus, resulting in mixing of the pulmonary and systemic circulations (see Fig. 30-19, *B*). The differential flow out to either the pulmonary bed or the systemic circulation depends on the pulmonary and systemic vascular resistances. Generally the pulmonary vascular resistance is less than the systemic vascular resistance, resulting in the majority of blood flow traveling to the lungs. This may be altered, however, because of pulmonary stenosis, small pulmonary arteries, or increased pulmonary vascular resistance. Pulmonary vascular disease develops early with this defect because of increased pulmonary blood flow.

Clinical Manifestations

Physical findings depend on the amount of pulmonary blood flow and the presence of other cardiac anomalies. If pulmonary stenosis is present, the newborn will present with cyanosis, caused by already elevated pulmonary vascular resistance, but no CHF. Conversely, if pulmonary stenosis is not present, the newborn initially will have mild to moderate cyanosis that worsens with activity. Once pulmonary vascular resistance drops, the pulmonary bed will receive preferential flow and the infant will have signs of CHF. A wide pulse pressure with bounding pulses also may be present, caused by increased pulmonary blood flow. A harsh systolic regurgitant murmur is present along the left sternal border as a result of the VSD, and a systolic click at the apex and left upper sternal border may be present, reflecting opening of the truncal valve. An apical rumble with or without a gallop rhythm also may be present because of increased pulmonary blood flow. If truncal valve insufficiency exists, an early diastolic, high-pitched, decrescendo murmur may be present.

Evaluation and Treatment

An ECG generally reveals biventricular hypertrophy and occasionally LA hypertrophy. A chest roentgenogram reveals cardiomegaly with biventricular and LA enlargement, as well as increased pulmonary vascular markings. When pulmonary stenosis is present, the heart size is normal and the pulmonary vascular markings are decreased. Echocardiography and cardiac catheterization determine the type of truncal defect, competency of the truncal valve, and differential blood flow.

Surgical repair in early infancy is recommended to prevent the sequelae of severe CHF and pulmonary vascular disease. The definitive repair consists of a modified Rastelli procedure involving VSD patch closure to divert the blood flow from the LV outflow tract into the truncus. The pulmonary arteries are excised from the aorta and connected to the right ventricle through a valved homograft—namely, aortic and pulmonary artery segments or cadaver tissue that is specially preserved. Synthetic conduits may be used but tend to calcify and develop narrowing within the lumen, leading to obstruction and the need for early replacement. Mortality varies depending on the type of truncal anomaly (20% to 50%).[26] Postoperative complications include heart failure, residual VSD, dysrhythmias, and pulmonary hypertension. The right ventricle to pulmonary artery homograft requires replacement because it becomes inadequate for somatic growth.

ACQUIRED CARDIOVASCULAR DISORDERS

Acquired heart diseases are those disease processes or abnormalities that occur after birth. They result from various causes, such as infection, genetic disorders, autoimmune processes in response to infection, environment factors, or autoimmune diseases. Examples of acquired heart diseases include Kawasaki disease, myocarditis, rheumatic heart disease, cardiomyopathy, and systemic hypertension. This chapter discusses Kawasaki disease and systemic hypertension. Myocarditis, rheumatic heart disease, and cardiomyopathy are discussed in Chapter 29.

Kawasaki Disease

Kawasaki disease, otherwise known as mucocutaneous lymph node syndrome, is an acute, self-limiting systemic vasculitis that may result in cardiac sequelae. It was first described in 1967 by Dr. Thomisakyu Kawasaki. Although Kawasaki disease occurs throughout the world, the greatest number of cases are reported in Japan.[52]

Kawasaki disease is primarily a condition of young children. Eighty percent of cases are seen in children younger than 5 years of age, with the incidence peaking in the toddler age group. Males are affected slightly more than females. Its peak incidence is in winter and spring.[3,53]

The etiology of Kawasaki disease remains unknown. Current etiologic theories center on an immunologic response to an infectious, toxic, or antigenic substance (including superantigen).[3,53]

Pathophysiology

Kawasaki disease progresses pathologically and clinically in the following stages:

Stage I (days 0 to 12). Small capillaries, arterioles, and venules become inflamed, as does the heart itself.

Stage II (days 12 to 25). Inflammation spreads to larger vessels, and aneurysms of the coronary arteries develop.

Stage III (days 26 to 40). Medium-size arteries begin granulation process, causing coronary artery thickening; inflammation resolves in the microcirculation; and there is increased formation of thrombi.

Stage IV (day 40 and beyond). Vessels develop scarring, intimal thickening, calcification, and stenosis of coronary arteries.

Clinical Manifestations

The clinical course of the disease progresses in three stages: acute, subacute, and convalescent. In the acute phase the child has fever, conjunctivitis, oral changes ("strawberry" tongue), rash, and lymphadenopathy and is often irritable.

During this phase, myocarditis may develop. The subacute phase begins when the fever ends and continues until the clinical signs have resolved. It is at this time that the child is most at risk for coronary artery aneurysm development. Desquamation of the palms and soles occurs at this time, as well as marked thrombocytosis. The convalescent phase is marked by the continued elevation of the erythrocyte sedimentation rate and platelet count.[3,53] Arthritis still may be present. This phase continues until all laboratory values return to normal—usually about 6 to 8 weeks after onset.[3,4]

Evaluation and Treatment

The diagnosis is based on the diagnosis criteria for Kawasaki disease, which state that the child must exhibit five of six criteria, including fever (Box 30-2). These children usually have leukocytosis, increased erythrocyte sedimentation rates, marked thrombocytosis, and elevated liver enzymes. An echocardiogram is obtained at the time of diagnosis as a baseline to assess for coronary aneurysms or inflammation. Serial echocardiograms are obtained after treatment to assess for future development of coronary aneurysms.

The use of high-dose aspirin and intravenous immunoglobulin during the acute phase has decreased the mortality of Kawasaki disease and has reduced the incidence of coronary abnormalities from approximately 65% to less than 25% at 6 to 8 weeks after initiation of therapy.[53] Most children recover completely from Kawasaki disease, including the regression of aneurysms. The most common cardiovascular sequela is coronary thrombosis. Current studies are investigating long-term results of the disease.[54]

Systemic Hypertension

Hypertension (HTN) in children differs from adult hypertension in etiology and presentation. Children diagnosed with HTN are often found to have some underlying disease, such as renal disease or coarctation of the aorta (Box 30-3). In recent years an increased prevalence of primary HTN in older children has been noted. Researchers are now focusing on primary HTN in older children in relation to morbidity and mortality and the presence of early atherosclerotic disease.[3,32]

Box 30-2

DIAGNOSTIC CRITERIA FOR KAWASAKI DISEASE

The child must exhibit five of the following six criteria, including fever:

1. Fever for 5 or more days (often diagnosed with shorter duration of fever if other symptoms are present)
2. Bilateral conjunctival infection without exudation
3. Changes in the oral mucous membranes, such as erythema, dryness, and fissuring of the lips; oropharyngeal reddening; or "strawberry tongue"
4. Changes in the extremities, such as peripheral edema, peripheral erythema, and desquamation of palms and soles, particularly periungual peeling
5. Polymorphous rash, often accentuated in the perineal area
6. Cervical lymphadenopathy

Modified from Wong DL et al: *Whaley and Wong's nursing care of infants and children,* ed 6, St Louis, 1999, Mosby.

Box 30-3

CONDITIONS ASSOCIATED WITH SECONDARY HYPERTENSION IN CHILDREN

RENAL DISORDERS

Congenital defects
- Polycystic kidney, ectopic kidney, horseshoe kidney, etc.
- Obstructive anomalies
- Hydronephrosis

Renal tumor
- Wilms tumor
- Retrovascular

Abnormalities of renal arteries
Renal vein thrombosis
Acquired disorders
- Glomerulonephritis—acute or chronic
- Pyelonephritis
- Nephritis associated with collagen disease

CARDIOVASCULAR DISEASE

Coarctation of the aorta
Arteriovenous fistulae
Patent ductus arteriosus
Aortic or mitral insufficiency

METABOLIC AND ENDOCRINE DISEASES

Adrenal tumors
- Adenoma
- Phenochromocytoma
- Neuroblastoma
- Cushing syndrome
- Adrenogenital syndrome
- Hyperthyroidism
- Aldosteronism
- Hypercalcemia
- Diabetes mellitus

NEUROLOGIC DISORDERS

Space-occupying lesions of cranium (increased intracranial pressure)
- Tumors, cysts, hematoma
- Cerebral edema
- Encephalitis (including Guillain-Barré and Reye syndromes)

MISCELLANEOUS CAUSES

Drugs (corticosteroids, oral contraceptives, pressor agents, amphetamines)
Burns
Genitourinary surgery
Trauma (e.g., stretching of femoral nerve with leg traction)
Insect bites (e.g., scorpion)
Intravascular overload (blood, fluid)
Hypernatremia
Toxemia of pregnancy
Heavy metal poisoning

From Wong DL et al: *Whaley and Wong's nursing care of infants and children,* ed 6, St Louis, 1999, Mosby.

Systemic hypertension in children is defined as systolic and diastolic blood pressure levels greater than the ninety-fifth percentile for age and gender on at least three occasions.[3,32] The Second Task Force on Blood Pressure Control in Children has added height as an additional criterion to the blood pressure guide.[55,56]

Pathophysiology

Hypertension is classified as (1) primary (or essential) hypertension, in which a specific cause cannot be identified; or (2) secondary hypertension, in which a cause is secondary to another alteration (see Box 30-3).[3] In infants and children a cause of HTN is almost always found. In general, the younger the child with significant hypertension, the more likely that a correctable cause can be found. Therefore a thorough evaluation needs to be done.[44,57,58]

The pathophysiology of primary HTN in children is not clearly understood but may result from a complex interaction of a strong disposing genetic component with disturbances in sympathetic vascular smooth muscle tone, humoral agents (angiotensin, catecholamines), renal sodium excretion, and cardiac output (Fig. 30-20). Ultimately these factors impair the ability of the peripheral vascular bed to adjust its own resistance to meet tissue perfusion needs.

Clinical Manifestations

Most children with systemic HTN are asymptomatic. It is necessary that a thorough history and physical examination be obtained. The examination should include an accurate blood pressure measurement on three separate occasions using a cuff of appropriate size (Tables 30-7 and 30-8).[3,55,56]

Certain factors influence blood pressure in children. Children who are overweight are often hypertensive.[59] Smoking is also associated with an increased risk for HTN. The gender or race of the child has not been an associated risk factor for primary HTN.[55]

Evaluation and Treatment

In children the history and physical examination should be directed at determining the etiology of HTN, such as coarctation of the aorta or renal disease (Table 30-9). If coarctation of the aorta is found, surgical or interventional correction is initiated. A complete blood count, serum chemistry levels, urinalysis, urine culture, lipid profile, and renal ultrasound are part of the routine evaluation for renal disease (Box 30-4). If HTN is found to be essential, or primary, in nature, nonpharmacologic therapy is used initially. Moderate weight loss can decrease systolic and diastolic pressures in many children. Appropriate diet, regular physical activity, and avoidance of smoking have been shown to be effective in reducing blood pressure.[3,56]

Drug therapy is controversial in children with primary hypertension; however, when nonpharmacologic therapy fails, a staged approach with the use of diuretics and/or beta-blockers and vasodilators is indicated.[3,60] The current emphasis on preventive cardiology, especially for children, is significant because many investigators believe signs of atherosclerosis are present from childhood.[59]

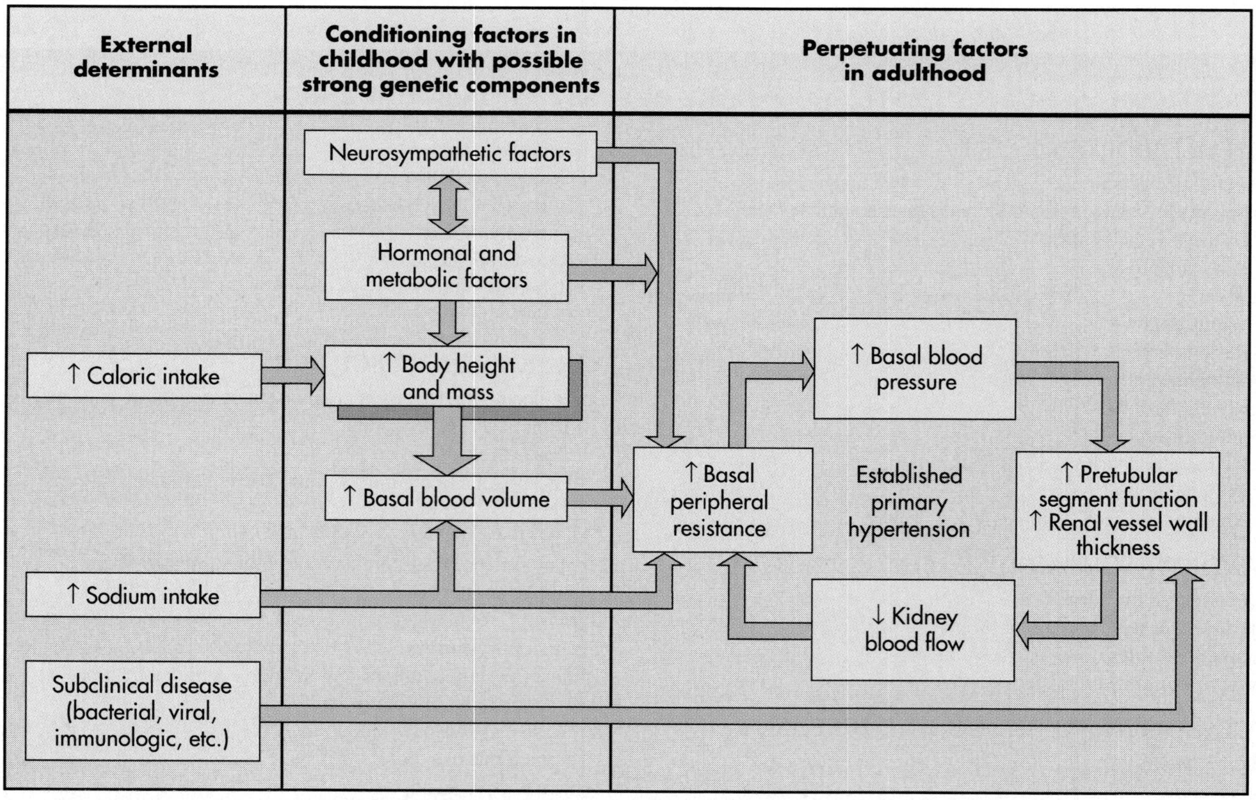

FIG. 30-20 Mechanisms believed to influence blood pressure in children. According to this model, a critical factor in the development of hypertension is obesity during childhood. Increased body mass, coupled with excessive sodium intake, can cause primary hypertension in children or set the stage for its development later in life.

Table 30-7 Suggested Normal BP Values (mm Hg) by Ausculatory Method (Systolic/Diastolic K5)

Age (yrs)	Mean BP Levels	90th Percentile	95th Percentile
6-7	104/55	114/73	117/78
8-9	106/58	117/76	120/82
10-11*	108/60	120/77	124/82
12-13*	112/62	124/78	128/83
14-15			
Boys	116/66	132/80	138/86
Girls	112/68	126/80	130/83
16-18			
Boys	121/70	136/82	140/86
Girls	110/68	125/81	127/84

From Park MK: *Pediatric cardiology for practitioners,* ed 3, St Louis, 1996, Mosby; modified from Goldring D et al: *Journal of Pediatrics* 91:884, 1977; Prineas RJ et al: *Hypertension* 1 (suppl):18, 1980.
BP, Blood pressure; *K5,* the phase V of Korotkoff sound.
*Values for ages 10-13 yr have been extrapolated from these two studies using age-related increments from other studies.

Table 30-8 Normative BP Levels (Systolic/Diastolic [Mean]) by Dinamap Monitor in Children 5 Yr Old and Younger

Age	Mean BP Levels (in mm Hg)	90th Percentile	95th Percentile
1-3 days	64/41 (50)	75/49 (50)	78/52 (62)
1 mo-2 yr	95/58 (72)	106/68 (83)	110/71 (86)
2-5 yr	101/57 (74)	112/66 (82)	115/68 (85)

From Park MK: *Pediatric cardiology for practitioners,* ed 3, St Louis, 1996, Mosby; modified from Park MK, Menard SM: *American Journal of Diseases in Children* 143:860, 1989.
BP, Blood pressure.

Table 30-9 Most Common Causes of Chronic Sustained Hypertension

Age-Group	Causes
Newborn	Renal artery thrombosis, renal artery stenosis, congenital renal malformation, COA, bronchopulmonary dysplasia
<6 yr	Renal parenchymal disease, COA, renal artery stenosis
6-10 yr	Renal artery stenosis, renal parenchymal disease, primary hypertension
>10 yr	Primary hypertension, renal parenchymal disease

From Park MK: *Pediatric cardiology for practitioners,* ed 3, St Louis, 1996, Mosby; modified from Report of the Second Task Force on Blood Pressure Control in Children. *Pediatrics* 79:1, 1987.
COA, Coarctation of the aorta.

Box 30-4

ROUTINE AND SPECIAL LABORATORY TESTS FOR HYPERTENSION

LABORATORY TESTS	SIGNIFICANCE OF ABNORMAL RESULTS
Urinalysis, urine culture, blood urea nitrogen, and creatinine levels	Renal parenchymal disease
Serum electrolyte levels (hypokalemia)	Hyperaldosteronism, primary or secondary Adrenogenital syndrome Renin-producing tumors
ECG, chest roentgenogram	Cardiac cause of hypertension, also baseline function
Intravenous pyelography (or ultrasonography, radionuclide studies, computed tomography of the kidneys)	Renal parenchymal diseases Renovascular hypertension Tumors (neuroblastoma, Wilms tumor)
Plasma renin activity, peripheral	High-renin hypertension Renovascular hypertension Renin-producing tumors Some caused by Cushing syndrome Some caused by essential hypertension

From Park MK: *Pediatric cardiology for practitioners,* ed 3, St Louis, 1996, Mosby.
ECG, Electrocardiogram; *COA,* coarctation of the aorta.

Continued

Box 30-4

ROUTINE AND SPECIAL LABORATORY TESTS FOR HYPERTENSION—cont'd

LABORATORY TESTS	SIGNIFICANCE OF ABNORMAL RESULTS
Plasma renin activity, peripheral—cont'd	Low-renin hypertension Adrenogenital syndrome Primary hyperaldosteronism
24-hr urine collection for 17-ketosteroids and 17-hydroxycorticosteroids	Cushing syndrome Adrenogenital syndrome
24-hr urine collection for catecholamine levels and vanillylmandelic acid	Pheochromocytoma Neuroblastoma
Aldosterone	Hyperaldosteronism, primary or secondary Renovascular hypertension Renin-producing tumors
Renal vein plasma renin activity	Unilateral renal parenchymal disease Renovascular hypertension
Abdominal aortogram	Renovascular hypertension Abdominal COA Unilateral renal parenchymal diseases Pheochromocytoma

From Park MK: *Pediatric cardiology for practitioners,* ed 3, St Louis, 1996, Mosby.
ECG, Electrocardiogram; *COA,* coarctation of the aorta.

SUMMARY REVIEW

Development of the Cardiovascular System

1. The heart arises from the mesenchyme and begins as an enlarged blood vessel with a large lumen and a muscular wall. By approximately the eighth week of gestation, all structures of the fetal heart and vascular system are present.
2. The endocardial cushions are instrumental in closing the atrial septum, dividing the atrioventricular canals into the right and left atrioventricular orifices, and closing the septum.
3. In the fetus the pulmonary and systemic circulatory systems are connected by the foramen ovale, an opening between the atria; by the ductus arteriosus, a fetal vessel that joins the pulmonary artery to the aorta; and by the ductus venosus, a fetal vessel that connects the inferior vena cava to the umbilical vein.
4. Fetal circulation is different from postnatal circulation because of the presence of fetal shunts and altered metabolic needs of the various organs.
5. Fetal blood flow depends on resistance for its distribution through the body. Resistance in the pulmonary circulation is higher than resistance in the systemic circulation, so myocardial thickness is about the same in the right heart and the left heart.
6. After birth, systemic resistance increases and pulmonary resistance decreases.
7. Pulmonary vascular resistance drops suddenly at birth because the lungs expand and the pulmonary vessels dilate. It continues to decrease gradually during the first 6 to 8 weeks after birth. Decreased resistance causes the right myocardium to thin out.
8. Systemic vascular resistance increases markedly at birth because severance of the umbilical cord removes the low-resistance placenta from the systemic circulation. Increased systemic resistance causes the left myocardium to thicken.
9. Changes in resistance cause the fetal connections between the pulmonary and systemic circulatory systems to disappear. The foramen ovale closes functionally at birth and anatomically several months later; the ductus arteriosus closes functionally 15 to 18 hours after birth and anatomically within 10 to 21 days; and the ductus venosus closes within 1 week after birth.
10. At birth a series of circulatory changes occur that affect blood flow, vascular resistance, and oxygen tension. The most important change is the shift of gas exchange from the placenta to the lungs.
11. After birth, significant postnatal changes occur, including thinning of the right ventricular myocardium as the pulmonary vascular resistance drops. As the systemic vascular resistance increases, the left ventricular myocardium becomes thicker.

Congenital Heart Defects

1. Most congenital cardiovascular defects have begun to develop by the eighth week of gestation, and most have many causes, both environmental and genetic.
2. Environmental risk factors associated with the incidence of congenital heart defects typically are maternal conditions. Among these are viral infections, diabetes, drug intake, alcohol intake, metabolic disorders, and advanced maternal age.
3. Genetic factors associated with congenital heart defects include but are not limited to Down syndrome, trisomy 13, trisomy 18, cri du chat syndrome, and Turner syndrome. It now appears, however, that most genetic mechanisms of causation are multifactorial.
4. Classification of congenital heart defects is based on whether they (a) cause blood flow to the lungs to increase or decrease, (b) obstruct ventricular blood flow patterns, or (c) cause mixing of unoxygenated and oxygenated blood.
5. Congestive heart failure is usually the result of congenital heart defects that increase blood volume and pressure in the pulmonary circulation. Clinical manifestations are almost the same as the manifestations of congestive heart failure in

adults. Unique manifestations in children include failure to thrive and periorbital edema.

6. Cyanosis, a bluish discoloration of the skin, indicates that the tissues are not receiving adequate oxygenated blood. Cyanosis can be caused by defects that (a) restrict blood flow into the pulmonary circulation; (b) overload the pulmonary circulation, causing pulmonary hypertension, pulmonary edema, and respiratory difficulty; and (c) cause large amounts of unoxygenated blood to shunt from the pulmonary to the systemic circulation.
7. Congenital defects that maintain or create direct communication between the pulmonary and systemic circulatory systems cause blood to shunt from one system to another, mixing oxygenated and unoxygenated blood and increasing blood volume and pressure on the receiving side of the shunt.
8. The direction of shunting through an abnormal communication depends on differences in pressure and resistance between the two systems. Flow is always from an area of high pressure to an area of low pressure.
9. Acyanotic congenital defects that increase pulmonary blood flow consist of abnormal openings (patent ductus arteriosus, atrial septal defect, ventricular septal defect, atrioventricular canal defect, or truncus arteriosus) that permit blood to shunt from left (systemic circulation) to right (pulmonary circulation). Cyanosis does not occur because the left-to-right shunt does not interfere with the flow of oxygenated blood through the systemic circulation.
10. If the abnormal communication between the left and right circuits is large, volume and pressure overload in the pulmonary circulation leads to congestive heart failure.
11. In truncus arteriosus the main trunk fails to divide longitudinally into the aorta and pulmonary artery. All blood from both ventricles enters the truncus, so that mixed blood is delivered by both circulatory systems, causing cyanosis and CHF.
12. In heart defects that decrease pulmonary blood flow (tetralogy of Fallot, tricuspid atresia), myocardial hypertrophy cannot compensate for restricted right ventricular outflow. Flow to the lungs decreases, and cyanosis is caused by an insufficient volume of oxygenated blood.
13. Obstruction of ventricular outflow commonly is caused by pulmonary stenosis, aortic stenosis, coarctation of the aorta, interrupted aortic arch, or hypoplastic left heart syndrome.
14. Despite obstruction, ventricular outflow remains normal because of compensatory ventricular hypertrophy stimulated by increased afterload and, in postductal coarctation of the aorta, development of collateral circulation around the coarctation.
15. Left heart failure can develop as a result of right ventricular obstruction if afterload backs up into the pulmonary circulation. Congestive heart failure can result from left ventricular obstruction in preductal coarctation of the aorta, in which left-to-right shunting through the patent ductus arteriosus greatly increases blood flow into the pulmonary circulation.
16. Complex congenital defects that depend on mixing of the pulmonary and systemic circulations for survival during the postnatal period include complete transposition of the great arteries, total anomalous pulmonary venous connection, and double-outlet right ventricle. This mixing results in desaturated systemic blood flow and cyanosis.
17. In complete transposition of the great vessels, the circulatory systems are not connected serially or through a shunt, so that oxygenated blood remains permanently in the pulmonary circulation and unoxygenated blood remains permanently in the systemic circulation. Survival depends on patency of the ductus arteriosus; after that, surgical intervention is mandatory.
18. Total anomalous pulmonary venous connection is caused by the persistance of the fetal common pulmonary artery and the lack of pulmonary venous return to the left atrium. All blood from the pulmonary and systemic circulations enters the right atrium. Mixed blood enters the left atrium through an atrial septal defect; it then flows into the systemic circulation and causes cyanosis. Obstruction in the common pulmonary vein causes pressure to back up into the lungs, leading to congestive heart failure.
19. Treatment for all congenital defects is surgical correction of the anomaly and management of cyanosis and left heart failure.

Acquired Cardiovascular Disorders

1. The most common acquired cardiovascular disorders of childhood are Kawasaki disease, rheumatic heart disease, and hypertension.
2. Kawasaki disease is an acute systemic vasculitis that also may result in the development of coronary artery aneurysms and thrombosis.
3. Primary hypertension in children is the same as that in adults, except that it is more likely to be in an early, asymptomatic stage.

KEY TERMS

Aortic stenosis, *1067*
Atrial septal defect (ASD), *1059*
Atrioventricular canal (AVC) defect, *1061*
Bulbus cordis, *1049*
Coarctation of the aorta (COA), *1066*
Complete AVC (CAVC) defect, *1061*
Cyanosis, *1057*
Ductus arteriosus, *1050*
Eisenmenger syndrome, *1057*
Endocardial cushion, *1048*
Foramen ovale, *1049*
Hypoplastic left heart syndrome (HLHS), *1069*
Kawasaki disease, *1074*
Ligamentum venosum, *1052*
Ostium primum, *1049*
Ostium secundum, *1049*
Partial AVC (PAVC) defect, *1061*
Patent ductus arteriosus (PDA), *1057*
Pulmonary atresia, *1068*
Pulmonary stenosis, *1068*
Septum primum, *1049*
Septum secundum, *1049*
Systemic hypertension, *1076*
Tetralogy of Fallot, *1062*
Total anomalous pulmonary venous connection (TAPVC), *1072*
Transitional AVC (TAVC) defect, *1062*
Transposition of the great arteries (TGA), *1070*
Tricuspid atresia, *1064*
Truncus arteriosus, *1073*
Ventricular septal defect (VSD), *1060*

REFERENCES

1. Ban Praagh R, Takoo A: *Etiology and morphogenesis of congenital heart disease*, Mount Kisco, NY, 1980, Future Publishing Company.
2. Teitel DF et al: Effects of birth related events in central flow pattern, *Pediatr Res* 22(5): 577, 1987.
3. Park MK: *Pediatric cardiology for the practitioner*, St Louis, 1996, Mosby.
4. Wong, DL: *Whaley and Wong's nursing care of infants and children*, St Louis, 1999, Mosby.
5. Hazinski MF: *Nursing care of the critically ill child*, St Louis, 1992, Mosby.
6. Edwards WD: *Congenital heart disease*, St Louis, 1996, Mosby.
7. Moller JH, Neal WA: *Fetal, neonatal, and infant cardiac disease*, Norwalk, Conn, 1990, Appleton & Lange.
8. Garson A et al: *The science and practice of pediatric cardiology*, ed 2, Baltimore, 1998, Williams & Wilkins.
9. Gersony W et al: Effects of indomethacin in premature infants with patent ductus arteriosus: results of a national collaborative study, *J Pediatr* 102:895, 1983.
10. Ambalavanan SK: The optimal elective management of patent ductus arteriosus (PDA) in older children [letter; comment], *J Pediatr Surg* 32(4):661, 1997.
11. Galal O et al: The role of surgical ligation of patent ductus arteriosus in the era of the Rashkind device, *Ann Thorac Surg* 63(2):434, 1997.
12. Gray DT, Weinstein MC: Decision and cost-utility analyses of surgical versus transcatheter closure of patent ductus arteriosus: should you let a smile be your umbrella? *Med Decis Making* 18(2):187, 1998.
13. LeBlanc JG et al: The evolution of ductus arteriosus treatment, *Int Surg* 85(1):1, 2000.
14. Sullivan ID: Patent arterial duct: when should it be closed? *Arch Dis Child* 78(3):285, 1998.
15. Hijazi ZM, Geggel RL: Transcatheter closure of patent ductus arteriosus using coils, *Am J Cardiol* 79(9):1279, 1997.
16. Burke RP et al: Video assisted throacoscopic surgery for patent ductus arteriosus in low birth weight neonates and infants, *Pediatrics* 104(2 part 1):227, 1999.
17. Burke RP et al: Video assisted thorascopic surgery for congenital heart disese, *J Thorac Cardiovasc Surg* 109:499, 1995.
18. Chang AC et al: *Pediatric cardiac intensive care*, Baltimore, 1998, Williams & Wilkins.
19. Oto O et al: Ligation of patent ductus arterious by the method of video-assisted thoracoscopic surgery and our other VATS experiences, *J Cardiovasc Surg (Torino)* 39(3):379, 1998.
20. Bitchell DP et al: Minimal access approach for the repair of atrial septal defect: the initial 135 patients, *Ann Thorac Surg* 70(1):115, 2000.
21. Moodie DS, Sterba R: Long-term outcomes excellent for atrial septal defect repair in adults, *Cleve Clin J Med* 67(8):591, 2000.
22. Berger FM et al: Comparison of results and complications of surgical and Amplatzer device closure of atrial septal defects, *J Thorac Cardiovasc Surg* 118(4):674, 1999.
23. Cao Q et al: Transcatheter closure of multiple atrial septal defects. Initial results and value for two- and three-dimensional transoesophageal echocardiography, *Eur Heart J* 21(11);941, 2000.
24. Hausdorf GR et al: Transcatheter closure of atrial septal defect with a new flexible, self-centering device (the STARFlex Occluder), *Am J Cardiol* 84(9):1113, 1999.
25. Pedra CA et al: Transcatheter closure of atrial septal defects using the Cardio-Seal implant, *Heart* 84(3):320, 2000.
26. Mavroudis C, Backer CL: *Pediatric cardiac surgery*, St Louis, 1994, Mosby.
27. Nygren A et al: Preoperative evaluation and surgery in isolated ventricular septal defects: a 21 year perspective, *Heart* 83(2):198, 2000.
28. Hijazi ZM et al: Transcatheter closure of single muscular ventricular septal defects using the amplatzer muscular VSD occluder: initial results and technical considerations, *Catheter Cardiovasc Interv* 49(2): 167, 2000.
29. Ruiz CE et al: First FDA approval under humanitarian device exemption of a septal occluder for fenestrated fontan and muscular ventricular septal defects [editorial], *Catheter Cardiovasc Interv* 50(2):159, 2000.
30. El-Najdawi EK et al: Operation for partial atrioventricular septal defect: a forty-year review, *J Thorac Cardiovasc Surg* 119(5):880, 2000.
31. Fukuda T et al: Complete atrioventricular septal defect and Ebstein's anomaly, *Pediatr Cardiol* 20(3);232, 1999.
32. Emmanouilides GC et al: *Heart disease in infants, children and adolescents*, Baltimore, 1995, Williams & Wilkins.
33. Castenada AR et al: *Cardiac surgery of the neonate and infant*, Philadelphia, 1994, W.B. Saunders.
34. Suzuki T et al: Modified end-to-end anastomosis combined with subclavian flap aortoplasty for repair of coarctation of the aorta with extended hypoplasia of the aortic isthmus, *J Card Surg* 14(5):359, 1999.
35. Koerselman J et al: Balloon angioplasty of coarctation of the aorta: a safe alternative for surgery in adults: immediate and mid-term results, *Catheter Cardiovasc Interv* 50(1):28, 2000.
36. Maheshwari S et al: Balloon angioplasty of postsurgical recoarctation in infants: the risk of restenosis and long-term follow-up, *J Am Coll Cardiol* 35(1):209, 2000.
37. Saba SE et al: Balloon coarctation angioplasty: follow-up of 103 patients [see comments], *J Invasive Cardiol* 12(8):402, 2000.
38. Weber HD, Cyran SE: Initial results and clinical follow-up after balloon angioplasty for native coarctation, *Am J Cardiol* 84(1):113, 1999.
39. Gibbs JL: Treatment options for coarctation of the aorta [editorial], *Heart* 84(1):11, 2000.
40. Jenkins NP, Ward C: Coarctation of the aorta: natural history and outcome after surgical treatment, *QJM* 92(7):365, 1999.
41. Seirafi PA et al: Repair of coarctation of the aorta during infancy minimizes the risk of late hypertension, *Ann Thorac Surg* 66(4):1378, 1998.
42. Egito ES et al: Transvascular balloon dilation for neonatal critical aortic stenosis: early and midterm results, *J Am Coll Cardiol* 29(2):442, 1997.
43. Radtke W, Lock J: Balloon dilation catheters, *Pediatr Clin North Am* 37(1):193, 1990.
44. Bove EL: Current status of staged reconstruction for hypoplastic left heart syndrome, *Pediatr Cardiol* 19(4):308, 1998.
45. Bove EL: Surgical treatment for hypoplastic left heart syndrome, *Jpn J Thorac Cardiovasc Surg* 47(2):47, 1999.
46. Cohen DM, Allen HD: New developments in the treatment of hypoplastic left heart syndrome [see comments], *Curr Opin Cardiol* 12(1): 44, 1997.
47. Daebritz SH et al: Results of Norwood stage I operation: comparison of hypoplastic left heart syndrome with other malformations, *J Thorac Cardiovasc Surg* 119(2):358, 2000.
48. Gutgesell HP, Massaro TA: Management of hypoplastic left heart syndrome in a consortium of university hospitals, *Am J Cardiol* 76:809, 1995.
49. Kern JH et al: Survival and risk factor analysis for the Norwood procedure for hypoplastic left heart syndrome, *Am J Cardiol* 80(2):170, 1997.
50. Razzouk AJ et al: Transplantation as a primary treatment for hypoplastic left heart syndrome: intermediate-term results, *Ann Thorac Surg* 62: 1, 1996.
51. Dajani AS et al: Prevention of bacterial endocarditis. Recommendations by the American Heart Associatin [see comments], *Circulation* 96(1):358, 1997.
52. Seymour JJ, Dickinson ET: Delayed cardiovascular sequelae from Kawasaki syndrome, *Am J Emerg Med* 16(6):579, 1998.
53. Park AH et al: Patterns of Kawasaki syndrome presentation, *Int J Pediatr Otorhinolaryngol* 40(1):41, 1997.
54. Nakamura Y et al: Mortality rates for patients with a history of Kawasaki disease in Japan, *J Pediatr* 128(1):75, 1996.
55. Sinaiko AR: Hypertension in children, *N Engl J Med* 335(26):1968, 1996.

56. Task Force: Update on the task force on high blood pressure in children and adolescents: a working group from the national blood pressure education program, *Pediatrics* 98:649, 1987.
57. Bartram U et al: Causes of death after the modified Norwood procedures: a study of 122 postmortem cases, *Ann Thorac Surg* 64(6):1795, 1997.
58. Rudolph AM et al: *Rudolph's pediatrics*, Stamford, Conn, 1996, Appleton & Lange.
59. Feinstein JA, Quivers ES: Pediatric preventive oncology: healthy habits now, healthy hearts later [see comments], *Curr Opin Cardiol* 12(1):70, 1997.
60. Hoekelman RA et al: *Primary Pediatric Care*, St Louis, 1997, Mosby.

CHAPTER 31

Structure and Function of the Pulmonary System

VALENTINA L. BRASHERS

CHAPTER OUTLINE

The pulmonary system consists of the lungs, airways, chest wall, and pulmonary circulation. Its primary function is the exchange of gases between the environmental air and the blood. There are three steps in this process: (1) *ventilation,* the movement of air into and out of the lungs; (2) *diffusion,* the movement of gases between air spaces in the lungs and the bloodstream; and (3) *perfusion,* the movement of blood into and out of the capillary beds of the lungs to body organs and tissues. The first two functions are carried out by the pulmonary system and the third by the cardiovascular system (see Chapter 28). Normally the pulmonary system functions efficiently under a variety of conditions and with little energy expenditure.

STRUCTURES OF THE PULMONARY SYSTEM

The pulmonary system is made up of two lungs, their airways, and the blood vessels that serve them (Fig. 31-1) and the chest wall, or thoracic cage. The lungs are divided into lobes, three in the right lung (upper, middle, lower) and two in the left lung (upper, lower). Each lobe is further divided into segments and lobules. The space between the lungs, which contains the heart, great vessels, and esophagus, is called the *mediastinum.* A set of tubes, or conducting airways, delivers air to each section of the lung. The lung tissue that surrounds the airways supports them, preventing their distortion or collapse as gas moves in and out during ventilation.

The lungs are protected from a variety of exogenous contaminants by a series of mechanical barriers (Table 31-1). These defense mechanisms are so effective that contamination of the lung tissue itself, particularly by infectious agents, is rare. (Other mechanisms of self-defense are discussed in Chapters 6 and 7.)

Conducting Airways

The conducting airways are the portion of the pulmonary system that provides a passage for the movement of air into and out of the gas-exchange portions of the lung. They consist of upper and lower airways. The **nasopharynx, oropharynx,** and related structures often are called the *upper airway* (Fig. 31-2). These structures are lined with a ciliated mucosa with a very rich vascular supply. The mucosal lining warms and humidifies inspired air and removes foreign particles from it as it passes into the lungs. During quiet breathing, gas usually flows through the nose, nasopharynx, and oropharynx to the lower airways. The mouth and oropharynx also are used for ventilation when the nose is obstructed or when increased flow is required, such as during exercise. Filtering and humidifying are not, however, as efficient with mouth breathing.

The **larynx** connects the upper and lower airways. The structure of the larynx consists of the endolarynx and its surrounding triangular-shaped bony and cartilaginous structures. The endolarynx is formed by two pairs of folds that form the false vocal cords (supraglottis) and the true vocal cords. The slit-shaped space between the true cords forms the glottis (see Fig. 31-2). The vestibule is the space above the false vocal cords. The laryngeal box is formed of three large cartilages—

the epiglottis, thyroid, and cricoid—and three smaller catilages—the arytenoid, corniculate, and cuneiform—that are connected by ligaments. The supporting cartilages prevent collapse of the larynx during inspiration and swallowing. The internal laryngeal muscles control vocal cord length and tension, and the external laryngeal muscles move the larynx as a whole. Both sets of muscles are important to swallowing, respiration, and vocalization. The internal muscles contract during swallowing to prevent aspiration into the trachea and also contribute to voice pitch.

The **trachea,** which is supported by U-shaped cartilage, connects the larynx to the **bronchi,** the conducting airways of the lungs. The trachea divides into the two main airways, or bronchi, at the **carina** (see Fig. 31-1). This area is very sensitive and when stimulated can cause coughing and airway narrowing. The right main bronchus extends from the trachea more vertically than the left main bronchus, so that aspirated fluids or foreign particles tend to enter the right lung rather than the left. The right and left main bronchi enter the lungs at the **hili,** or "roots" of the lungs, along with the pulmonary blood and lymphatic vessels. From the hili the main bronchi branch into lobar bronchi, then to segmental and subsegmental bronchi, and finally end at the sixteenth division in the smallest of the conducting airways, the terminal **bronchioles** (Fig. 31-3). With these multiple divisions, the cross-sectional area of the airways increases to 20 times that of the trachea. This results in decreased velocity or airflow into the gas-exchange portion of the lung and allows for optimal gas diffusion.[1]

The bronchial walls have three layers: an epithelial lining, a smooth muscle layer, and a connective tissue layer. In the large bronchi (to approximately the tenth division), the connective tissue layer contains cartilage. The epithelial lining of the bronchi contains single-celled exocrine glands—the mucus-secreting **goblet cells**—and ciliated cells. High columnar pseudostratified epithelium lines the larger airways, changing to columnar cuboidal epithelium in the bronchioles (types of epithelium are illustrated in Chapter 1). The submucosal glands of the bronchial lining also produce mucus, contributing to the mucous blanket that covers the bronchial epithelium. The ciliated epithelial cells rhythmically beat this mucous blanket toward the trachea and pharynx, where it can be swallowed or expectorated by coughing. Foreign particles and microorganisms that are not expelled by mucociliary clearance and coughing are attacked by cellular components of the inflammatory response and antibodies of the secretory immune system (see Unit III). The biochemical mediators released early in inflammation also play a part in antibody-mediated hypersensitivity reactions, such as asthma, because they stimulate bronchial smooth muscles to constrict.

With branching, the layers of epithelium that line the bronchi become thinner (Fig. 31-4). Ciliated cells and goblet

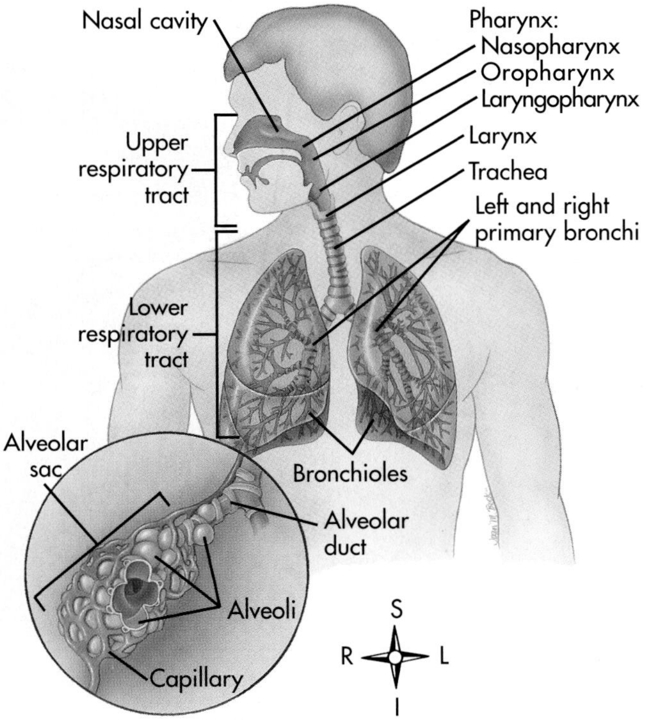

FIG. 31-1 Structural plan of the respiratory system. *Inset* shows alveolar sacs where the interchange of oxygen and carbon dioxide takes place through the walls of the grapelike alveoli. Capillaries surround the alveoli. (From Thibodeau GA, Patton KI: *Anatomy and physiology,* ed 4, St Louis, 1999, Mosby.)

Table 31-1 Pulmonary Defense Mechanisms

Structure or Substance	Mechanism of Defense
Upper respiratory tract mucosa	Maintains constant temperature and humdification of gas entering the lungs; traps and removes foreign particles, some bacteria, and noxious gases from inspired air
Nasal hairs and turbinates	Trap and remove foreign particles, some bacteria, and noxious gases from inspired air
Mucous blanket	Protects trachea and bronchi from injury; traps most foreign particles and bacteria that reach the lower airways
Cilia	Propel mucous blanket and entrapped particles toward the oropharynx, where they can be swallowed or expectorated
Alveolar macrophages	Ingest and remove bacteria and other foreign material from alveoli by phagocytosis (see Chapters 6 and 7)
Irritant receptors in nares (nostrils)	Stimulation by chemical or mechanical irritants triggers sneeze reflex, which results in rapid removal of irritants from nasal passages
Irritant receptors in trachea and large airways	Stimulation by chemical or mechanical irritants triggers cough reflex, which results in removal of irritants from the trachea and large airways

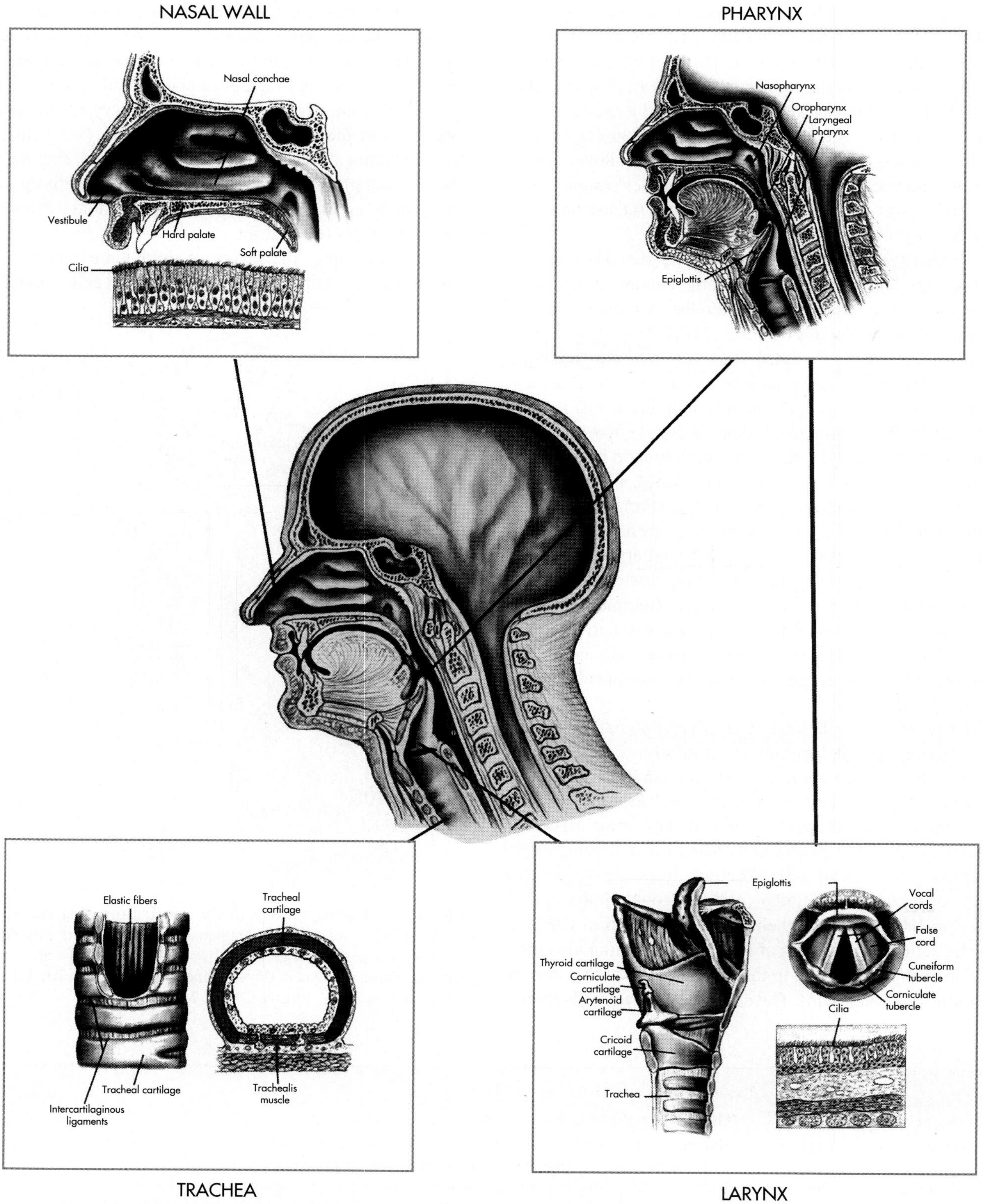

FIG. 31-2 Structures of the upper airway. (Modified from Thompson JM et al: *Mosby's clinical nursing,* ed 4, St Louis, 1997, Mosby.)

cells become more sparse, and smooth muscle and connective tissue layers thin toward the terminal bronchioles.[2]

Gas-Exchange Airways

The conducting airways terminate in gas-exchange airways, where oxygen (O_2) enters the blood and carbon dioxide (CO_2) is removed from it. The gas-exchange airways are made up of **respiratory bronchioles, alveolar ducts,** and **alveoli.** These structures together are sometimes called the **acinus** (see Fig. 31-3), and all of them participate in gas exchange.

The bronchioles from the sixteenth through the twenty-third divisions contain increasing numbers of alveoli and are

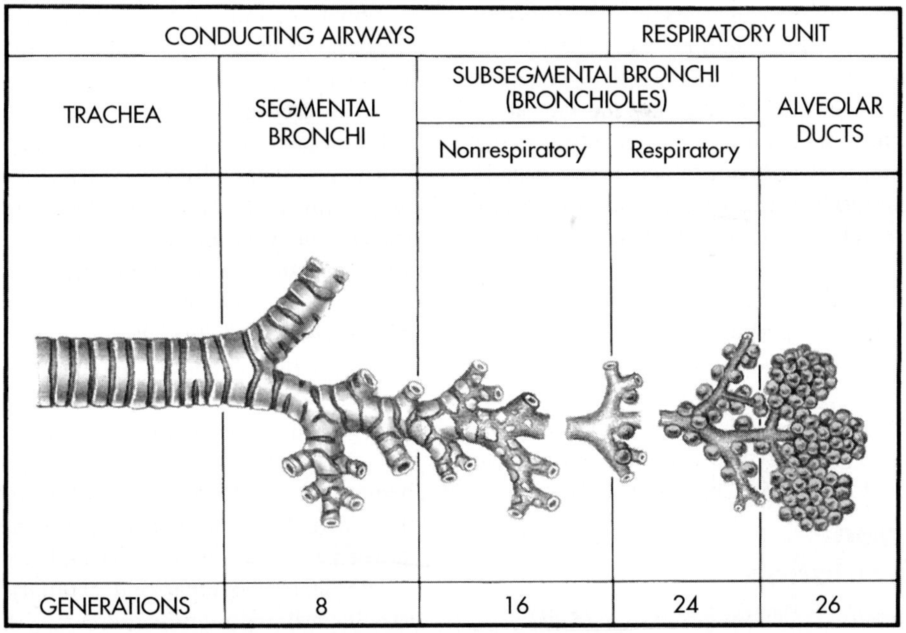

FIG. 31-3 Structures of the lower airway. (From Thompson JM et al: *Mosby's clinical nursing,* ed 4, St Louis, 1997, Mosby.)

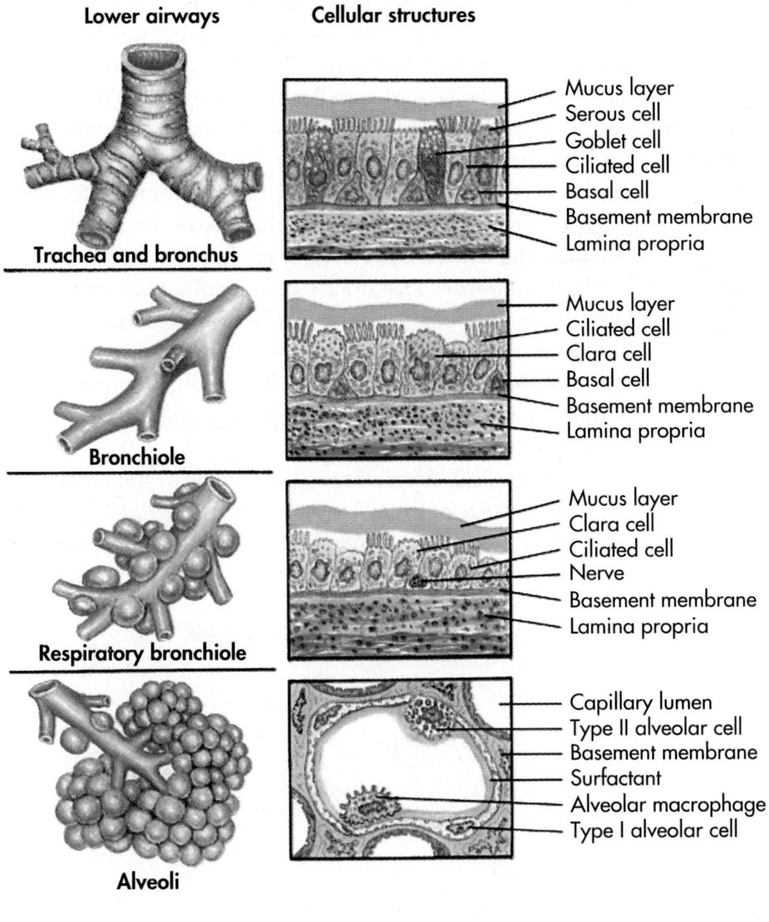

FIG. 31-4 Changes in the bronchial wall with progressive branching. (From Wilson SF, Thompson JM: *Respiratory disorders,* St Louis, 1990, Mosby.)

called *respiratory bronchioles.* The walls of the respiratory bronchioles are very thin, consisting of an epithelial layer devoid of cilia and goblet cells, very little smooth muscle fiber, and a very thin and elastic connective tissue layer. These bronchioles end in alveolar ducts, which lead to alveolar sacs made up of numerous alveoli.

The alveoli are the primary gas-exchange units of the lung, where oxygen enters the blood and carbon dioxide is removed (Fig. 31-5). Tiny passages called *pores of Kohn* permit some air to pass through the septa from alveolus to alveolus, promoting collateral ventilation and even distribution of air among the alveoli. In cross sections, alveoli appear similar to common sponges. The lungs contain approximately 25 million alveoli at birth and 300 million by adulthood.

The alveolar septa consist of an epithelial layer and a thin, elastic basement membrane but no muscle layer (Fig. 31-6). Two major types of epithelial cells appear in the alveolus. Type I alveolar cells provide structure, and type II alveolar cells secrete **surfactant,** a lipoprotein that coats the inner surface of the alveolus and facilitates its expansion during inspiration.

Like the bronchi, alveoli contain cellular components of inflammation and immunity, particularly the mononuclear phagocytes. The mononuclear phagocytes of the lungs are called *alveolar macrophages.* These cells ingest foreign material that reaches the alveolus and prepare it for removal through the lymphatics. (Phagocytosis and the mononuclear phagocyte system are described in Chapters 6 and 7.)

Pulmonary and Bronchial Circulation

The pulmonary circulation facilitates gas exchange, delivers nutrients to lung tissues, acts as a reservoir for the left ventricle, and serves as a filtering system that removes clots, air, and other debris from the circulation (Fig. 31-7).

Despite the fact that the entire cardiac output from the right ventricle goes into the lungs, the pulmonary circulation has a lower pressure and resistance than the systemic circulation. Pulmonary arteries are exposed to about one fifth the pressure of the systemic circulation and have a much thinner muscle layer. (Systemic vessels are described in Chapter 28.) Mean pulmonary artery pressure is 18 mm Hg; mean aortic pressure is 90 mm Hg.

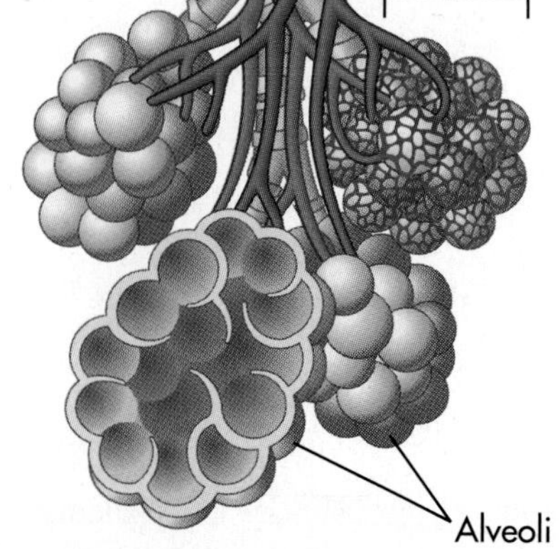

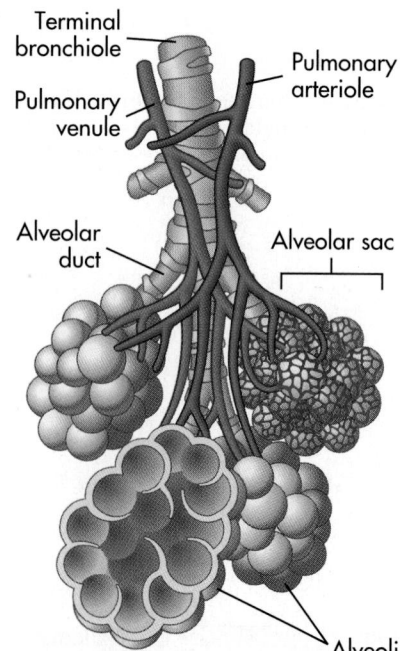

FIG. 31-5 Alveoli. Bronchioles subdivide to form tiny tubes called alveolar ducts, which end in clusters of alveoli called alveolar sacs. (From Thibodeau GA, Patton KI: *Anatomy and physiology,* ed 4, St Louis, 1999, Mosby.)

About one third of the pulmonary vessels are filled with blood (perfused) at any given time. More vessels become perfused when right ventricular cardiac output increases. Therefore increased delivery of blood to the lungs does not normally increase mean pulmonary artery pressure.

The pulmonary artery divides and enters the lung at the hilus with each main bronchus and branches with the bronchus at every division, so that every bronchus and bronchiole has an accompanying artery or arteriole. The arterioles, less than 1 mm in diameter, regulate blood flow through their respective capillary beds.

The arterioles divide at the terminal bronchiole to form a network of pulmonary capillaries around the acinus. The capillaries are an integral part of the alveolar septa. Capillary walls consist of an endothelial layer and a thin basement membrane, which often fuses with the basement membrane of the alveolar septum. This results in very little separation between blood in the capillary and gas in the alveolus.

The shared alveolar and capillary walls compose the **alveolocapillary membrane,** a very thin membrane made up of the alveolar epithelium, the alveolar basement membrane, an interstitial space, the capillary basement membrane, and the capillary endothelium (Fig. 31-8). These extremely thin alveolar walls are easily damaged and can leak plasma and blood into the alveolar space. Gas exchange occurs across the alveolocapillary membrane. With normal perfusion, approximately 100 ml of blood in the pulmonary capillary bed is spread very thinly over 70 to 100 m^2 of alveolar surface area. The alveolocapillary membrane efficiently exposes large quantities of blood to gas in the alveoli. Any disorder that thickens the membrane impairs gas exchange.

Each pulmonary vein drains several pulmonary capillaries. Unlike the pulmonary arteries, which follow the branching bronchi, pulmonary veins are dispersed randomly throughout the lung and then leave the lung at the hili and enter the left atrium. They are similar to veins in the systemic circulation, but they have no valves.

The bronchial circulation is part of the systemic circulation. It supplies nutrients to the conducting airways, large pulmonary vessels, and membranes (pleurae) that surround

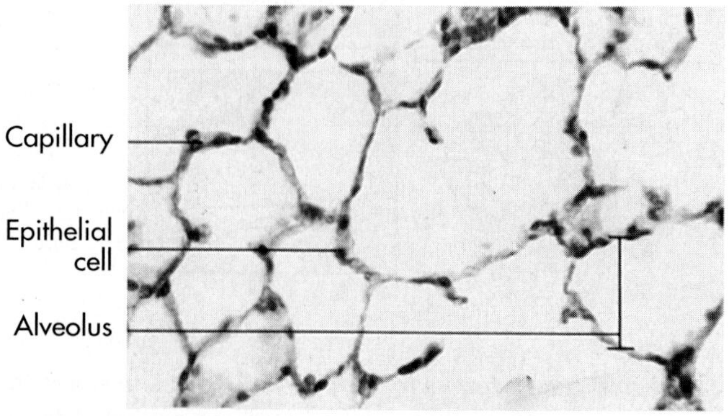

FIG. 31-6 Photomicrograph of lung, showing several alveoli. Note the proximity of the capillary to the alveolar wall. (From Thibodeau GA: *Anatomy and physiology,* St Louis, 1987, Mosby.)

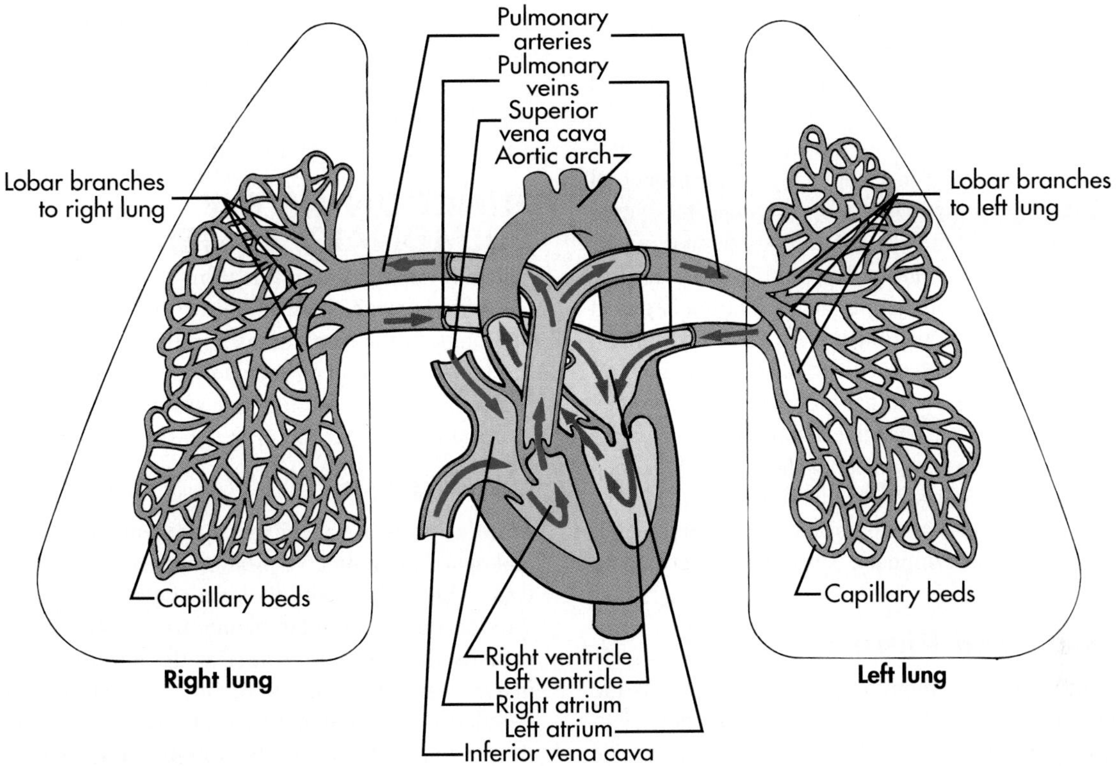

FIG. 31-7 The pulmonary circulation. The right and left pulmonary veins and arteries and the branching capillaries are illustrated.

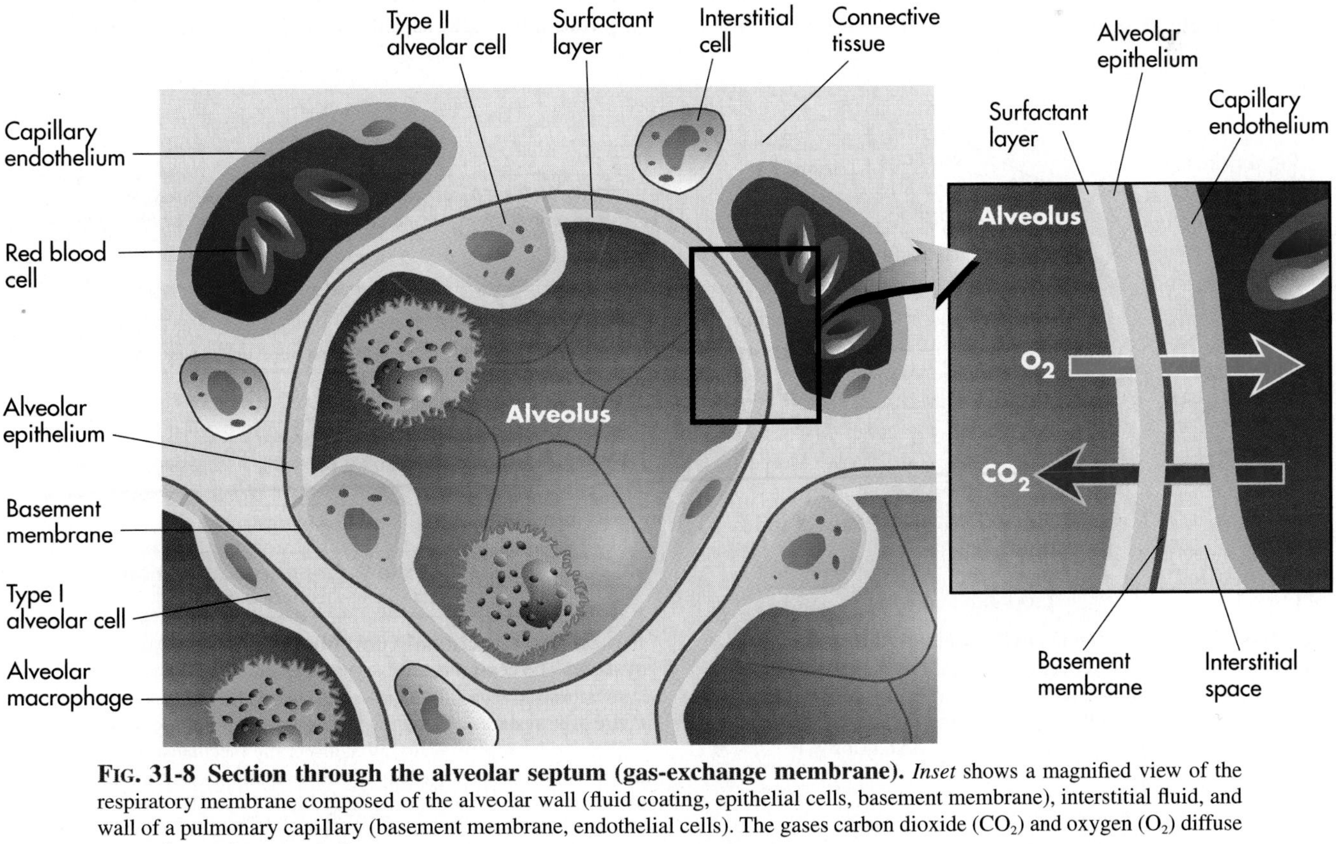

FIG. 31-8 Section through the alveolar septum (gas-exchange membrane). *Inset* shows a magnified view of the respiratory membrane composed of the alveolar wall (fluid coating, epithelial cells, basement membrane), interstitial fluid, and wall of a pulmonary capillary (basement membrane, endothelial cells). The gases carbon dioxide (CO_2) and oxygen (O_2) diffuse across the respiratory membrane.

the lungs. The bronchial circulation is unique in that not all of its capillaries drain into its own venous system. Some of the bronchial capillaries empty into the pulmonary vein and contribute to the normal venous admixture (mixing of oxygenated and deoxygenated blood) or right-to-left shunt (right-to-left shunts are described in Chapter 32). The bronchial circulation does not participate in gas exchange but warms and moistens inspired air and provides airway nourishment.[3]

Lung vasculature also includes deep and superficial lymphatic capillaries. The deep lymphatic capillaries begin at the level of the terminal bronchioles; there are no lymphatic structures in the acinus. Fluid and alveolar macrophages migrate from the alveoli to the terminal bronchioles, where they enter the lymphatic system. The superficial lymphatic capillaries drain the membrane that surrounds the lungs. Both deep and superficial lymphatic vessels leave the lung at the hilus. The lymphatic system plays an important role in keeping the lung free of fluid. (The lymphatic system is described in Chapter 28.)

Chest Wall and Pleura

The chest wall (skin, ribs, intercostal muscles) protects the lungs from injury, and its muscles, in conjunction with the diaphragm, perform the muscular work of breathing. The **thoracic cavity** is contained by the chest wall and encases the lungs (Fig. 31-9). A serous membrane called the **pleura** adheres firmly to the lungs. It then folds over itself and attaches firmly to the chest wall. The membrane covering the lungs is the visceral pleura; that lining the thoracic cavity is the parietal pleura. The area between the two pleurae is called the **pleural space,** or pleural cavity. Normally only a thin layer of fluid secreted by the pleura (pleural fluid) fills the pleural space. This lubricates the pleural surfaces, allowing the two layers to slide over each other without separating. Pressure in the pleural space is usually negative or subatmospheric (-4 to -10 mm Hg).

FUNCTION OF THE PULMONARY SYSTEM

The pulmonary system functions to (1) ventilate the alveoli, (2) diffuse gases into and out of the blood, and (3) perfuse the lungs so that the organs and tissues of the body receive blood that is rich in oxygen and low in carbon dioxide. Each component of the pulmonary system contributes to one or more of these functions (Fig. 31-10).

Ventilation

Ventilation is the mechanical movement of gas or air into and out of the lungs. Ventilation often is misnamed **respiration,** which is actually the exchange of oxygen and carbon dioxide during cellular metabolism. "Respiratory rate" is actually the ventilatory rate, or the number of times gas is inspired and expired per minute. The amount of effective ventilation is calculated by multiplying the ventilatory rate (breaths per minute) by the volume of air per breath (liters per breath, tidal volume). This is called the **minute volume** and expressed in liters per minute.

Carbon dioxide (CO_2), the gaseous form of carbonic acid (H_2CO_3), is a product of cellular metabolism. The lung eliminates about 10,000 milliequivalents (mEq) of carbonic acid per day in the form of CO_2, which is produced at the rate of approximately 200 ml/min. CO_2 elimination is necessary to

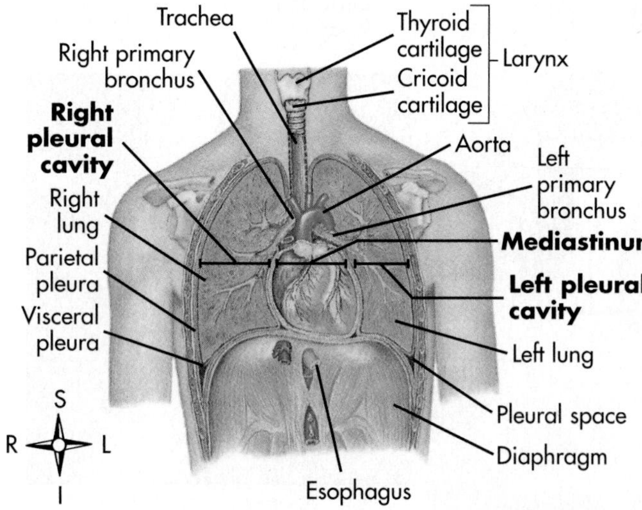

FIG. 31-9 Thoracic (chest) cavity and related structures. The thoracic ("chest") cavity is divided into three subdivisions (left and right pleural divisions and mediastinum) by a partition formed by a serous membrane called the pleura. (From Thibodeau GA, Patton KI: *Anatomy and physiology,* ed 3, St Louis, 1996, Mosby.)

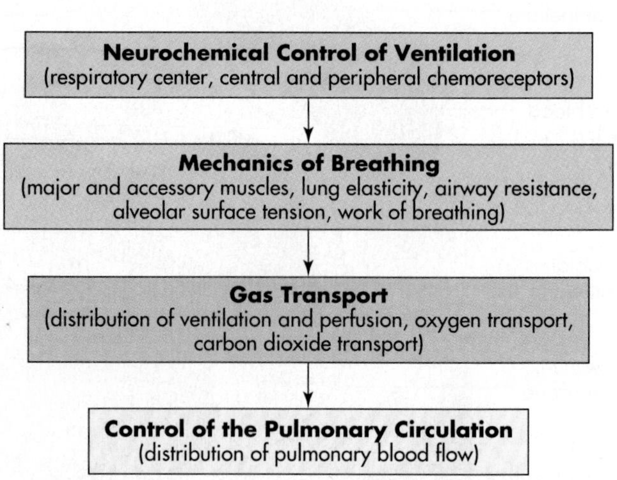

FIG. 31-10 Functional components of the respiratory system. The central nervous system responds to neurochemical stimulation of ventilation and sends signals to the chest wall musculature. The response of the respiratory system to these impulses is influenced by several factors that affect the mechanisms of breathing and therefore affect the adequacy of ventilation. Gas transport between the alveoli and pulmonary capillary blood depends on a variety of physical and chemical activities. The control of the pulmonary circulation plays a role in the appropriate distribution of blood flow.

maintain a normal arterial CO_2 ($Paco_2$) of 40 mm Hg and normal acid-base balance (see Chapter 3 for a discussion of acid-base regulation).

The adequacy of **alveolar ventilation** *cannot* be accurately determined by observation of ventilatory rate, pattern, or effort. If a health care professional needs to determine the adequacy of ventilation, an arterial blood gas analysis must be performed to measure $Paco_2$.

Neurochemical Control of Ventilation

Although breathing is usually involuntary, voluntary breathing is necessary for talking, singing, laughing, and deliberately holding one's breath, because homeostatic changes in ventilatory rate and volume are adjusted automatically by the nervous system to maintain normal gas exchange. The mechanisms that control respiration are very complex.

The **respiratory center** in the brain stem controls respiration by transmitting impulses to the respiratory muscles, causing them to contract and relax (Fig. 31-11). The respiratory center is composed of several groups of neurons located bilaterally in the brain stem: the dorsal respiratory group (DRG), the ventral respiratory group (VRG), the pneumotaxic center, and the apneustic center.[4] The basic automatic rhythm of respiration is set by the DRG, a cluster of inspiratory nerve cells located in the medulla that sends efferent impulses to the diaphragm and inspiratory intercostal muscles. The DRG also receives afferent impulses from **peripheral chemoreceptors** in the carotid and aortic bodies and from several different types of receptors in the lungs. The VRG, also located in the medulla, contains both inspiratory and expiratory neurons. It is almost inactive during normal, quiet respiration, becoming active when increased ventilatory

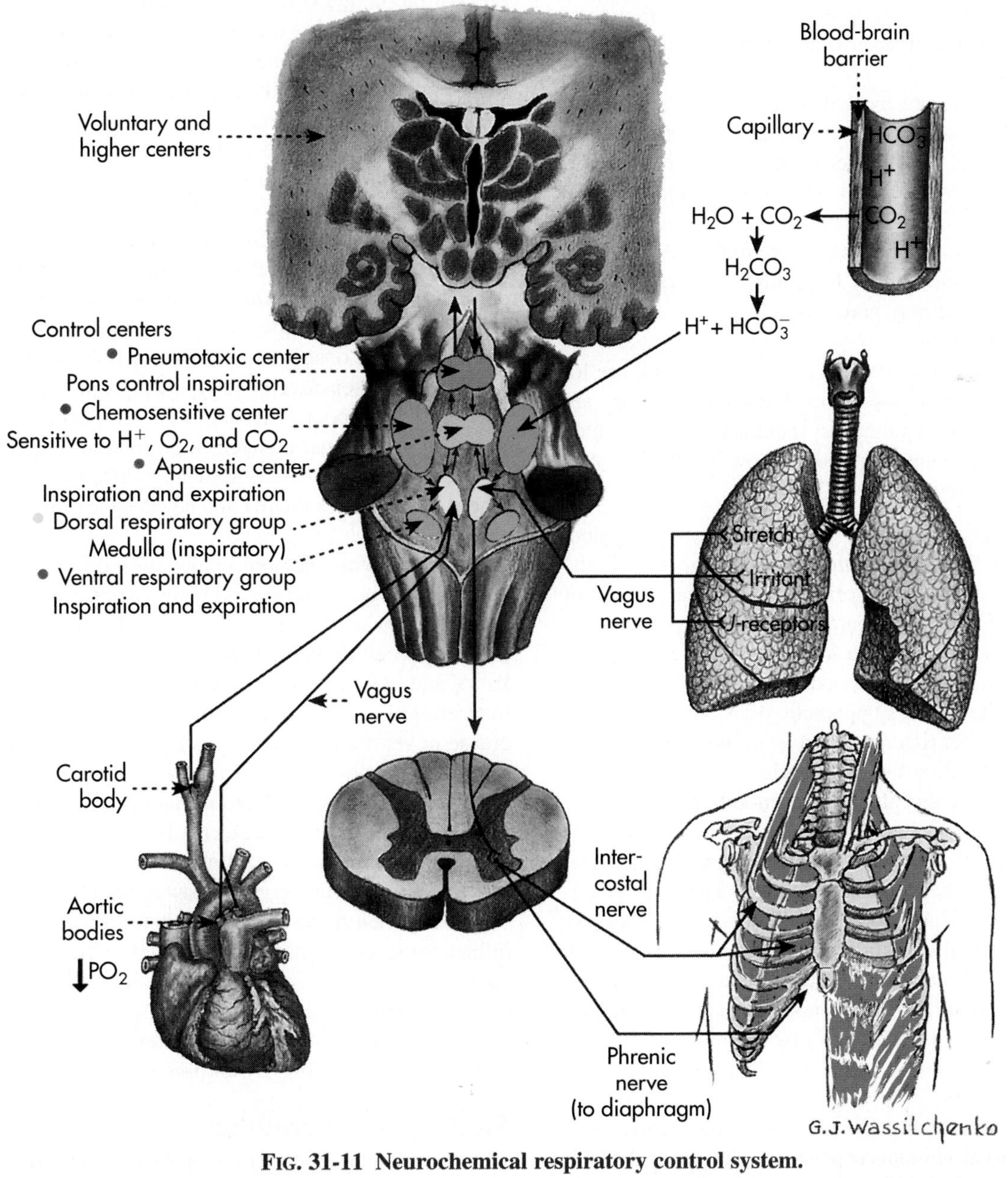

FIG. 31-11 Neurochemical respiratory control system.

effort is required. The pneumotaxic center and apneustic center, situated in the pons, do not generate primary rhythm but rather act as modifiers of the inspiratory depth and rate established by the medullary centers.[4] Breathing can be modified by input from the cortex, the limbic system, and the hypothalamus, and the pattern of breathing can be influenced by emotion and by disease.

Lung Receptors

Three types of lung receptors send impulses from the lungs to the dorsal respiratory group:

1. **Irritant receptors** are found in the epithelium of the conducting airways. They are sensitive to noxious aerosols (vapors), gases, and particulate matter (e.g., inhaled dusts), which cause them to initiate the cough reflex. When stimulated, irritant receptors also cause bronchoconstriction and increased ventilatory rate. These receptors are located primarily in the proximal larger airways and are nearly absent in the distal airways; thus it is possible for secretions to accumulate in the distal respiratory tree without initiating cough.[5]
2. **Stretch receptors** are located in the smooth muscles of airways and are sensitive to increases in the size or volume of the lungs. They decrease ventilatory rate and volume when stimulated, an occurrence sometimes referred to as the *Hering-Breuer expiratory reflex.* This reflex is active in newborns and assists with ventilation.[6] In adults, this reflex is active only at high tidal volumes (such as with exercise) and may play a role in protecting against excess lung inflation.[7]
3. ***J*-receptors** (juxtapulmonary capillary receptors) are located near the capillaries in the alveolar septa. They are sensitive to increased pulmonary capillary pressure, which stimulates them to initiate rapid, shallow breathing; hypotension; and bradycardia.[4]

The lung is innervated by the autonomic nervous system (ANS). Fibers of the sympathetic division of the ANS in the lung branch from the upper thoracic and cervical ganglia of the spinal cord. Fibers of the parasympathetic division of the ANS travel in the vagus nerve to the lung. (Structures and function of the ANS are discussed in detail in Chapter 13.) The parasympathetic and sympathetic divisions of the ANS control airway caliber (interior diameter of the airway lumen) by stimulating bronchial smooth muscle to contract or relax. The parasympathetic receptors cause smooth muscle to contract, whereas sympathetic receptors cause it to relax. Bronchial smooth muscle tone depends on equilibrium, that is, equal stimulation of contraction and relaxation. The parasympathetic division of the ANS is the main controller of airway caliber under normal conditions. Constriction occurs if the irritant receptors in the airway epithelium are stimulated by irritants in inspired air, by endogenous substances (e.g., histamine, serotonin, prostaglandins), by many drugs, and by humoral substances.

Chemoreceptors

Chemoreceptors monitor the pH, $Paco_2$, and Pao_2 of arterial blood. **Central chemoreceptors** monitor arterial blood indirectly by sensing changes in the pH of cerebrospinal fluid (CSF). They are located near the respiratory center and are sensitive to hydrogen ion concentration in the CSF. (Chapter 3 describes the relationship between ions and the pH, or acid-base status, of body fluids.) The pH, or concentration of hydrogen ions in the CSF, reflects $Paco_2$ because, unlike H^+ ions, carbon dioxide in arterial blood diffuses across the blood-brain barrier (the capillary wall separating blood from cells of the central nervous system) into the CSF until the partial pressure of carbon dioxide (Pco_2) is equal on both sides. Carbon dioxide that has entered the CSF combines with H_2O to form carbonic acid, which subsequently dissociates into hydrogen ions that are capable of stimulating the central chemoreceptors. In this way $Paco_2$ regulates ventilation through its impact on the pH (hydrogen ion content) of the CSF.[6]

If alveolar ventilation is inadequate, $Paco_2$ increases. Carbon dioxide diffuses across the blood-brain barrier until Pco_2 in blood and CSF reaches equilibrium. As the central chemoreceptors sense the resulting decrease in pH (increase in hydrogen ion concentration), they stimulate the respiratory center to increase the depth and rate of ventilation. Increased ventilation causes the Pco_2 of arterial blood to decrease below that of the CSF, and carbon dioxide diffuses back out of the CSF, returning its pH to normal.

The central chemoreceptors are sensitive to very small changes in the pH of CSF (equivalent to a 1 to 2 mm Hg change in Pco_2) and are able to maintain a normal $Paco_2$ under many different conditions, including strenuous exercise. If inadequate ventilation, or hypoventilation, is long term (e.g., in chronic obstructive pulmonary disease), these receptors become insensitive to small changes in $Paco_2$ and regulate ventilation poorly. In addition, prolonged increases in $Paco_2$ result in renal compensation through bicarbonate retention. This bicarbonate gradually diffuses into the CSF where it normalizes the pH and negates the effect on ventilatory drive.[7]

The peripheral chemoreceptors are located in aortic bodies, the aortic arch, and carotid bodies at the bifurcation of the carotids, near the baroreceptors (see Chapter 28). Although the peripheral chemoreceptors are sensitive to changes in $Paco_2$ and pH, they are primarily sensitive to oxygen levels in arterial blood (Pao_2) and are responsible for all of the increase in ventilation that occurs in response to arterial hypoxemia.[4] As Pao_2 and pH decrease, peripheral chemoreceptors, particularly in the carotid bodies, send signals to the respiratory center to increase ventilation. The peripheral chemoreceptors are not as sensitive as the central chemoreceptors. The Pao_2 must drop well below normal (to approximately 60 mm Hg) before the peripheral chemoreceptors have much influence on ventilation. If $Paco_2$ is elevated as well, however, ventilation increases much more than it would in response to either abnormality alone. The peripheral chemoreceptors become the major stimulus to ventilation when the central chemoreceptors are "reset" by chronic hypoventilation.

Mechanics of Breathing

The mechanical aspects of inspiration and expiration are known collectively as the *mechanics of breathing* and involve

(1) major and accessory muscles of inspiration and expiration, (2) elastic properties of the lungs and chest wall, and (3) resistance to airflow through the conducting airways. Alterations in any of these properties increase the work of breathing, or the metabolic energy that must be expected to achieve adequate ventilation and oxygenation of the blood.

Major and Accessory Muscles

The major muscles of inspiration are the diaphragm and the external intercostal muscles (muscles between the ribs) (Fig. 31-12). The diaphragm is a dome-shaped muscle that separates the abdominal and thoracic cavities. When the diaphragm contracts, it flattens downward, increasing the volume of the thoracic cavity, and creates a negative pressure that draws gas into the lungs. Contraction of external intercostal muscles elevates the anterior portion of the ribs. This increases the volume of thoracic cavity by increasing its front-to-back (anteroposterior [AP]) diameter. Although the external intercostal muscles may contract during quiet breathing, inspiration at rest usually is assisted by the diaphragm only.

The accessory muscles of inspiration are the sternocleidomastoid and scalene muscles. Like the external intercostal muscles, these muscles enlarge the thorax by increasing its AP diameter. The accessory muscles of inspiration assist inspiration when minute volume (volume of air inspired and expired per minute) is very high, such as during strenuous exercise, or when the work of breathing is increased because of disease. The accessory muscles do not increase the volume of the thorax as efficiently as the diaphragm does.

There are no major muscles of expiration because normal, relaxed expiration is passive and requires no muscular effort. The accessory muscles of expiration, the abdominal and internal intercostal muscles, assist expiration when minute volume is high, during coughing, or when airway obstruction is present. When the abdominal muscles contract, intraabdominal pressure increases, pushing up the diaphragm and decreasing the volume of the thorax. The internal intercostal muscles pull down the anterior ribs, decreasing the AP diameter of the thorax.

Alveolar Surface Tension

Surface tension occurs at any gas-liquid interface and refers to the tendency for liquid molecules that are exposed to air to adhere to one another. This phenomenon can be seen, for example, in a glass of liquid that is about to overflow or in the way liquids "bead" when splashed on a waterproof surface. In both examples this phenomenon decreases the surface area exposed to the air.

Within a sphere, such as an alveolus, surface tension tends to make expansion difficult. According to the law of Laplace, the pressure *(P)* required to inflate a sphere is equal to two times the surface tension ($2T$) divided by the radius *(r)* of the sphere, or $P = (2T/r)$. As the radius of the sphere (or alveolus) becomes smaller, more and more pressure is required to inflate it. If the alveoli were lined with a waterlike fluid, taking breaths would be extremely difficult.

Alveolar ventilation, or distention, is made possible by surfactant, which lowers the surface tension by coating the air-liquid interface in the alveoli. Surfactant, a lipoprotein produced by type II alveolar cells, has a detergent-like effect that separates the liquid molecules, thereby decreasing alveolar surface tension.

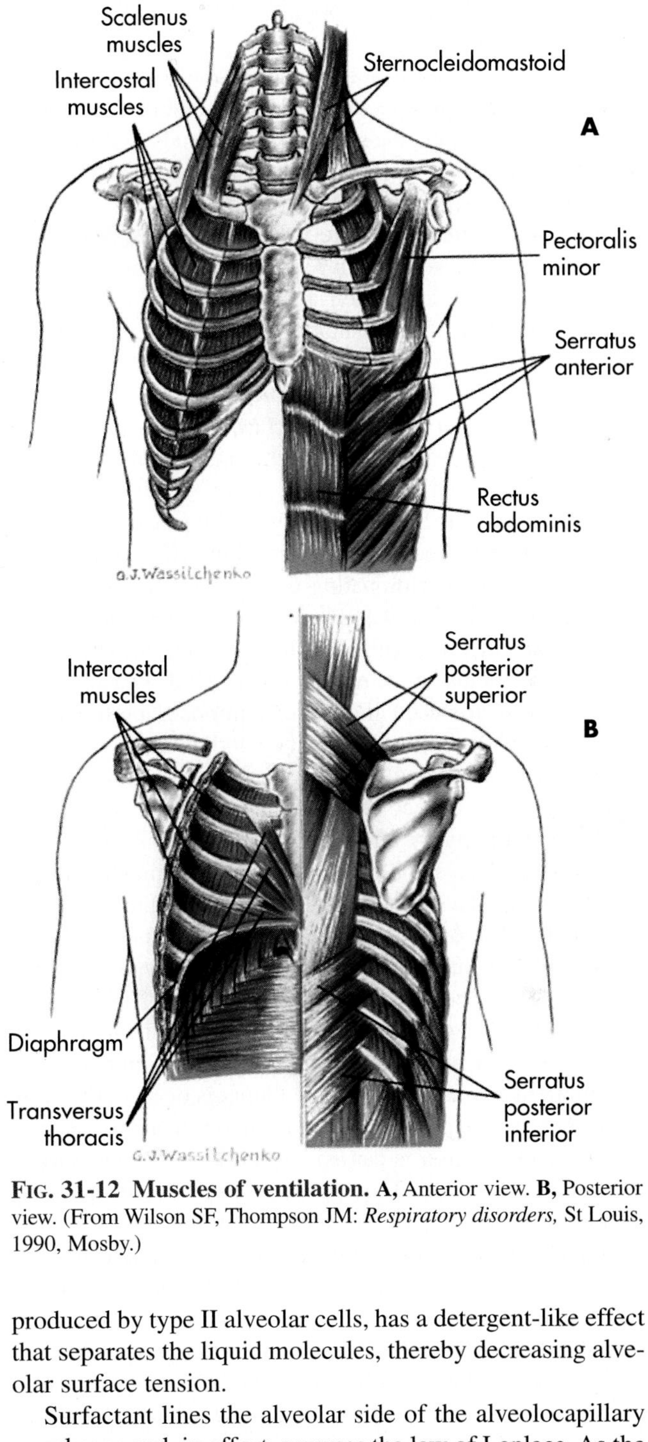

FIG. 31-12 Muscles of ventilation. A, Anterior view. **B,** Posterior view. (From Wilson SF, Thompson JM: *Respiratory disorders,* St Louis, 1990, Mosby.)

Surfactant lines the alveolar side of the alveolocapillary membrane and, in effect, reverses the law of Laplace. As the radius of a surfactant-lined sphere (alveolus) grows smaller, the surface tension *decreases,* and as the radius grows larger, the surface tension *increases.* This occurs because the surfactant molecules have much weaker intermolecular attraction compared with the liquid molecules. The surfactant molecules occupy most of the air-fluid interface and disrupt the intermolecular forces that tend to collapse the alveoli.[3] Therefore the alveoli are much easier to inflate at low lung volumes (i.e., after expiration) than at high volumes (i.e., after inspiration). If surfactant production is disrupted or surfactant is not produced in adequate quantities, alveolar surface tension increases and results in alveolar collapse, decreased lung expansion, increased work of breathing, and severe gas-exchange abnormalities.

The decrease in surface tension caused by surfactant is also responsible for keeping the alveoli free of fluid. In the absence of surfactant, the surface tension tends to attract fluid into the alveoli. In addition, surfactant participates in host defense against respiratory pathogens.[8]

Elastic Properties of the Lung and Chest Wall

The lung and chest wall have elastic properties that permit expansion during inspiration and return to resting volume during expiration. The elasticity of the lungs is caused both by elastin fibers in the alveolar walls and surrounding the small airways and pulmonary capillaries and by surface tension at the alveolar air-liquid interface. The elasticity of the chest wall is the result of the configuration of its bones and musculature.

Elastic recoil is the tendency of the lungs to return to the resting state after inspiration. Normal elastic recoil permits passive expiration, eliminating the need for major muscles of expiration. Passive elastic recoil may be insufficient during labored breathing (high minute volume), in which case the accessory muscles of expiration are used. The accessory muscles also are used if disease comprises elastic recoil (e.g., in emphysema) or blocks the conducting airways.

Normal elastic recoil depends on an equilibrium between opposing forces of recoil in the lungs and chest wall. Under normal conditions the chest wall tends to recoil by expanding outward. This can be observed readily during open heart surgery. When the sternum is split to open the thoracic cavity, the chest wall moves outward laterally. The tendency of the chest wall to recoil by expanding is balanced by the tendency of the lungs to recoil or collapse around the hili. The tendency of the lungs to collapse can be demonstrated if the chest is opened without mechanically ventilating the lungs (e.g., at postmortem examination). As the thorax is opened, the lungs immediately collapse, like inflated balloons that have been released. This reaction is caused by elastic recoil and surface tension in the alveoli. The opposing forces of the chest wall and lungs create, in part, the negative intrapleural pressure.

Balance between the outward recoil of the chest wall and inward recoil of the lungs occurs at the resting level, at the end of expiration. During inspiration, the diaphragm and intercostal muscles contract, air flows into the lungs, and the chest wall expands. Muscular effort is needed to overcome the resistance of the lungs to expansion. During expiration the muscles relax and the elastic recoil of the lungs causes the thorax to decrease in volume until, once again, balance between the chest wall and lung recoil forces is reached[9] (Fig. 31-13).

Compliance is the measure of lung and chest wall distensibility. It represents the relative ease with which these structures can be stretched. Compliance is therefore the reciprocal of elasticity. Compliance is determined by alveolar surface tension and the elastic recoil of the lung and chest wall. It can be measured with the following formula:

$$C = \frac{\Delta V}{\Delta P}$$

where C = compliance in liters per centimeter of water, ΔV = volume change (usually tidal volume), and ΔP = pressure change (airway or pleural pressure) in centimeters of water.[10]

Increased compliance indicates that the lungs or chest wall is abnormally easy to inflate and has lost some elastic recoil. A decrease indicates that the lungs or chest wall is abnormally stiff or difficult to inflate. Compliance is increased in emphysema and decreased in adult respiratory distress syndrome, pneumonia, pulmonary edema, and fibrosis. (These disorders are described in Chapter 32.)

Airway Resistance

Airway resistance, which is similar to resistance to blood flow (described in Chapter 28), is determined by the length, radius, and cross-sectional area of the airways and density, viscosity, and velocity of the gas (Poiseuille's law). Resistance is computed by dividing change in pressure *(P)* by rate of flow *(F)*, or $R = P/F$ (Ohm's law) and can easily be measured in the pulmonary function laboratory.[4] Airway resistance is normally very low. One half to two thirds of total airway resistance occurs in the nose. The next highest resistance is in the oropharynx and larynx. There is very little resistance in the conducting airways of the lungs because of their large cross-sectional area. The most common causes of increased airway resistance are swelling (edema), obstruction (i.e., mucous plugging), and spasm of bronchial smooth muscle (bronchospasm), all of which decrease the radius of the airways. Resistance increases as the diameter of the airways (total cross-sectional area) decreases.

Work of Breathing

The work of breathing is determined by the muscular effort (and therefore oxygen and energy) required for ventilation. The work of breathing is normally very low but may increase considerably in diseases that disrupt the equilibrium between forces exerted by the lung and chest wall. More muscular effort is required when lung compliance is decreased (e.g., in pulmonary edema), chest wall compliance is decreased (e.g., in spinal deformity or obesity), or airways are obstructed by bronchospasm or mucous plugging (e.g., in asthma or bronchitis). An increase in the work of breathing can result in a marked increase in oxygen consumption and metabolic demand, which can cause significant morbidity in individuals with severe lung disease.

Measurement of Gas Pressure

A gas is made up of millions of molecules moving randomly. As they move, they collide with each other and the wall of the space in which they are contained. These collisions exert pressure. If more molecules are present in the space, the pressure, or number of collisions, increases (Fig. 31-14). If the same number of gas molecules is contained in a small and a large container, the pressure is greater in the small container because more collisions occur in the smaller space. Heat increases the speed of the molecules, which increases the number of collisions. Therefore pressure also increases at higher temperatures.

Barometric pressure (P_B) (atmospheric pressure) is the pressure exerted by gas molecules in air at specific altitudes.

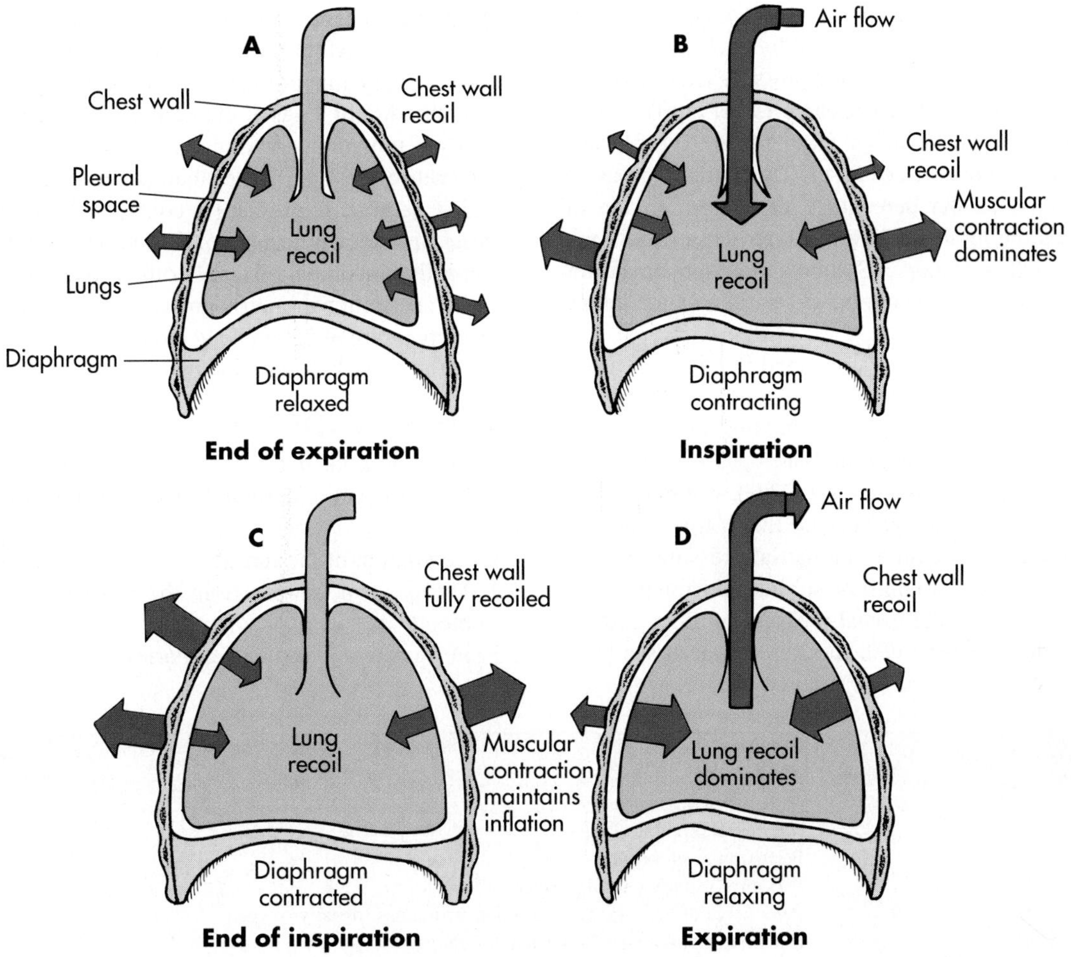

FIG. 31-13 Interaction of forces during inspiration and expiration. A, Outward recoil of the chest wall equals inward recoil of the lungs at the end of expiration. **B,** During inspiration, contraction of respiratory muscles, assisted by chest wall recoil, overcomes tendency of lungs to recoil. **C,** At the end of inspiration, respiratory muscle contraction maintains lung expansion. **D,** During expiration, respiratory muscles relax, allowing elastic recoil of the lungs to deflate the lungs.

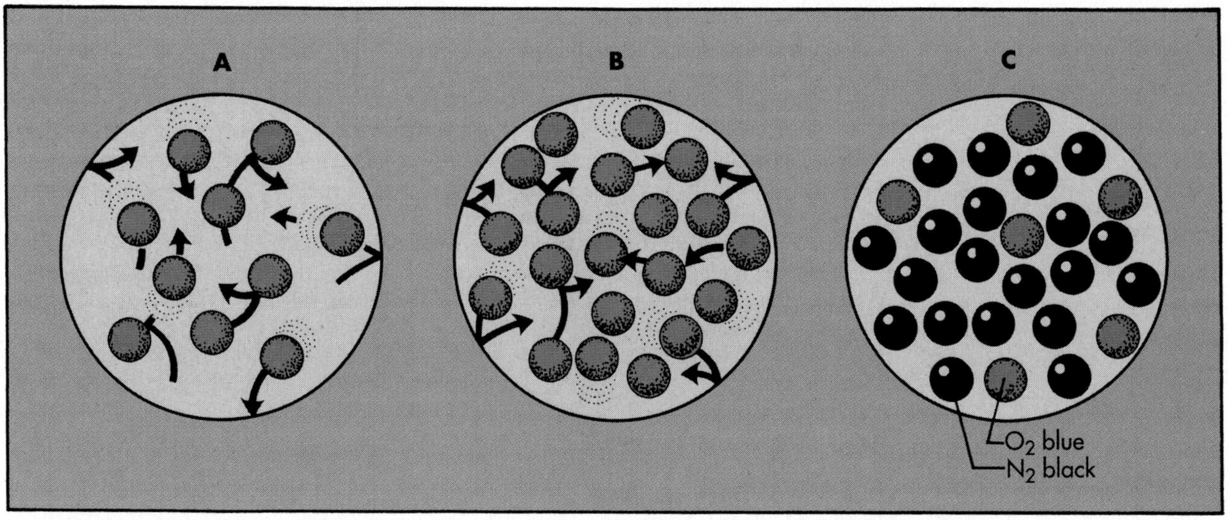

FIG. 31-14 Relationship between number of gas molecules and pressure exerted by the gas in an enclosed space. A, Theoretically, 10 molecules of the same gas exert a total pressure of 10 within the space. **B,** If the number of molecules is increased to 20, total pressure is 20. **C,** If there are different gases in the space, each gas exerts a partial pressure: here the partial pressure of nitrogen (N_2) is 18, that of oxygen (O_2) is 6, and total pressure is 24.

At sea level, barometric pressure is 760 mm Hg. This number is the sum of the pressure exerted by each gas in the air at sea level. The portion of the total pressure exerted by any individual gas is its **partial pressure** (see Fig. 31-14). At sea level the air is made up of oxygen (20.9%), nitrogen (78.1%), and a few other trace gases. The partial pressure of oxygen is equal to the percentage of oxygen in the air (20.9%) times the total pressure (760 mm Hg), or 159 mm Hg ($760 \times 0.209 = 158.84$). (Symbols used in the measurement of gas pressures and pulmonary ventilation are defined in Table 31-2.)

The amount of water vapor contained in a gas mixture is determined by the temperature of the gas and is unrelated to barometric pressure. Gas that enters the lungs becomes saturated with water vapor (humidified) as it passes through the upper airway. At body temperature (37° C), water vapor exerts a pressure of 47 mm Hg. Because this is true regardless of total (barometric) pressure, the partial pressure of water vapor (always 47 mm Hg) must be subtracted from the barometric pressure before the partial pressure of other gases in the mixture can be determined. In saturated air at sea level, the partial pressure of oxygen is therefore $(760 - 47) \times 0.209 = 149$. All pressure and volume measurements made in pulmonary function laboratories specify the temperature and humidity of a gas at the time of measurement.

Many pressure measurements are stated as variations from barometric pressure, rather than percentages of it. On such scales, barometric pressure is considered zero, and pressure varies up or down from zero. Physiologic pressure measurements that involve fluids, rather than gases, are measured as variations from barometric pressure. For example, a systolic blood pressure of 120 mm Hg indicates that systolic pressure is 120 mm Hg above barometric pressure.

Gas Transport

Gas transport, the delivery of oxygen to the cells of the body and the removal of carbon dioxide, has four steps:

1. Ventilation of the lungs
2. Diffusion of oxygen from the alveoli into the capillary blood
3. Perfusion of systemic capillaries with oxygenated blood

Table 31-2 Common Pulmonary Abbreviations

Symbol	Definition
V	Volume or amount of gas
Q	Perfusion or blood flow
P	Pressure (usually partial pressure) of a gas
S	Percentage of hemoglobin saturation with a gas (usually oxygen)
F	Fraction of gas, or gas flow (in a laboratory test)
C	Content or amount of gas
C_T	Thoracic compliance
E	Expired gas
i	Inspired gas
A	Alveolar gas
a	Arterial blood
$\bar{v}$	Mixed venous or pulmonary artery blood
D	Dead space
Pa_{O_2}	Partial pressure of oxygen in arterial blood
P_{AO_2}	Partial pressure of oxygen in alveolar gas
Pa_{CO_2}	Partial pressure of carbon dioxide in arterial blood
$P\bar{v}_{O_2}$	Partial pressure of oxygen in mixed venous or pulmonary artery blood
$P(A - a)_{O_2}$	Difference between alveolar and arterial partial pressure of oxygen (A − a [gradient])
P_B	Barometric or atmospheric pressure
Sa_{O_2}	Saturation of hemoglobin (in arterial blood) with oxygen
$S\bar{v}_{O_2}$	Saturation of hemoglobin (in mixed venous blood) with oxygen
Ca_{O_2}	Content or amount (volume) of oxygen in arterial blood
$C\bar{v}_{O_2}$	Content of oxygen in mixed venous blood
$C(a - \bar{v})_{O_2}$	Oxygen content difference between arterial and mixed venous blood
$\dot{V}_A$	Alveolar ventilation
$\dot{V}_D$	Dead-space ventilation
$\dot{V}_E$	Minute volume
VC	Vital capacity
V_T	Tidal volume or average breath
$\dot{Q}T$	Total perfusion or blood flow (cardiac output)
$\dot{V}/\dot{Q}$	Ratio of ventilation to perfusion
Fi_{O_2}	Fraction of inspired oxygen
FRC	Functional residual capacity
IC	Inspiratory capacity

NOTE: Subscripts identify the particular gas, volume, or pressure being discussed. A dot ($\dot{}$) means measurement over time, usually 1 minute.

4. Diffusion of oxygen from systemic capillaries into the cells

Steps in the transport of carbon dioxide occur in reverse order:

1. Diffusion of carbon dioxide from the cells into the systemic capillaries
2. Perfusion of the pulmonary capillary bed by venous blood
3. Diffusion of carbon dioxide into the alveoli
4. Removal of carbon dioxide from the lung by ventilation

If any step in gas transport is impaired by a respiratory or cardiovascular disorder, gas exchange at the cellular level is compromised.

Distribution of Ventilation and Perfusion

Effective gas exchange depends on an approximately even distribution of gas (ventilation) and blood (perfusion) in all portions of the lungs. The lungs are suspended from the hili in the thoracic cavity. When the individual is in an upright position (sitting or standing), gravity pulls the lungs down toward the diaphragm and compresses their lower portions or bases. The alveoli in the upper portions, or apices, of the lungs contain a greater residual volume of gas and are larger and less numerous than those in the lower portions. Because surface tension increases as the alveoli become larger, the larger alveoli in the upper portions of the lung are more difficult to inflate (less compliant) than the smaller alveoli in the lower portions of the lung. Therefore during ventilation most of the tidal volume is distributed to the bases of the lungs, where compliance is greater.

The heart pumps against gravity to perfuse the pulmonary circulation. As blood is pumped into the lung apices of a sitting or standing individual, some blood pressure is dissipated in overcoming gravity. As a result, blood pressure at the apices is lower than that at the bases. Because greater pressure causes greater perfusion, the bases of the lungs are better perfused than the apices (Fig. 31-15). Thus ventilation and perfusion are greatest in the same lung portions: the lower lobes. Ventilation and perfusion depend on body position. If a standing individual assumes a supine or side-lying position, the areas of the lungs that are then most dependent become the best ventilated and perfused.

Distribution of perfusion in the pulmonary circulation also is affected by alveolar pressure (gas pressure in the alveoli). The pulmonary capillary bed differs from the systemic capillary bed in that it is surrounded by gas-containing alveoli. If the gas pressure in the alveoli exceeds the blood pressure in the capillary, the capillary collapses and flow ceases. This

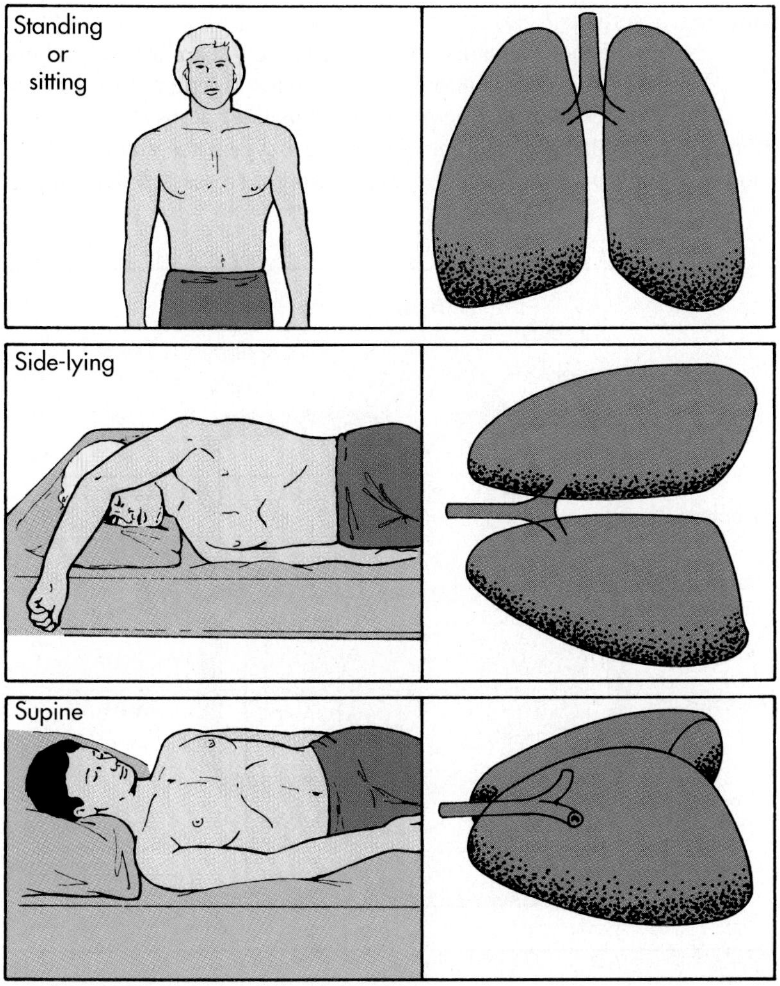

FIG. 31-15 Pulmonary blood flow and gravity. The greatest volume of pulmonary blood flow will normally occur in the gravity-dependent areas of the lungs. Body position has a significant effect on the distribution of pulmonary blood flow.

is most likely to occur in portions of the lung where blood pressure is lowest and alveolar gas volume and therefore pressure are greatest, that is, the apex of the lung.

The lungs are divided into three zones on the basis of the relationships among all the factors affecting pulmonary blood flow. Alveolar pressure plus the forces of gravity, arterial blood pressure, and venous blood pressure affect the distribution of perfusion (Fig. 31-16).

Zone I is where alveolar pressure exceeds pulmonary arterial and venous pressures. The capillary bed collapses, and normal blood flow ceases. Normally zone I is a very small part of the lung at the apex. Zone II is the portion where alveolar pressure is greater than venous pressure but not arterial pressure. Blood flows through zone II, but it is impeded to a certain extent by alveolar pressure. Zone II is normally above the level of the left atrium. In zone III both arterial and venous pressures are greater than alveolar pressure and blood flow is not affected by alveolar pressure. Zone III is in the base of the lung. Blood flow through the pulmonary capillary bed increases in regular increments from the apex to the base.

Although both blood flow and ventilation are greater at the base of the lungs than at the apices, they are not perfectly matched in any of the zones. Perfusion exceeds ventilation in the bases of the lungs, and ventilation exceeds perfusion in the apices of the lung. The relationship between ventilation and perfusion is expressed as a ratio called the **ventilation-perfusion ratio,** or $\dot{V}/\dot{Q}$. The normal $\dot{V}/\dot{Q}$ ratio is 0.8. This is the amount by which perfusion exceeds ventilation under normal conditions.

Oxygen Transport

Approximately 1000 ml (1 L) of oxygen is transported to the cells each minute. Oxygen is transported in the blood in two forms. A small amount dissolves in plasma, and the remainder binds to hemoglobin molecules. Without hemoglobin, oxygen would not reach the cells in amounts sufficient to maintain normal metabolic function. (Hemoglobin is discussed in detail in Chapter 24; cellular metabolism is discussed in Chapter 1.)

Diffusion Across the Alveolocapillary Membrane

The alveolocapillary membrane is the ideal medium for oxygen diffusion because it has a large total surface area (70 to 100 m^2) and is very thin (0.5 μm). In addition, the partial pressure of oxygen molecules (PO_2) is much greater in alveolar gas than in capillary blood, a condition that promotes rapid diffusion down the concentration gradient from the alveolus into the capillary.

The amount of oxygen in the alveoli (PAO_2) depends on the amount of oxygen in the inspired air (see p. 1094) and on the amount of air that remains in the alveoli and tracheobronchial tree between breaths **(physiologic dead space).** This can be estimated by using the alveolar gas equation:

$$PAO_2 = 149 - PaCO_2/0.8 \text{ (the respiratory quotient)}$$

This value is approximately 104 with relaxed breathing; therefore a pressure gradient of approximately 60 mm Hg facilitates the diffusion of oxygen from the alveolus into the capillary (Fig. 31-17). Different values for PAO_2 can be calculated if there are changes in the inspired oxygen content or the $PaCO_2$, which are common occurrences in clinical settings.[4]

Blood remains in the pulmonary capillary for about 0.75 seconds, but only 0.25 seconds is required for oxygen concentration to equilibrate (equalize) across the alveolocapillary membrane. Therefore oxygen has ample time to diffuse into the blood, even during increased cardiac output,

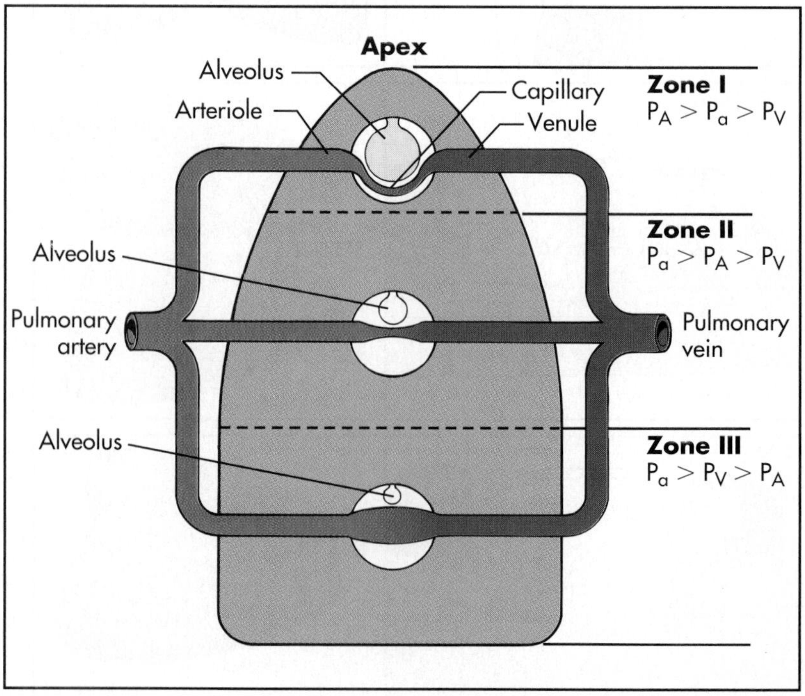

FIG. 31-16 Gravity and alveolar pressure. Effects of gravity and alveolar pressure on pulmonary blood flow in the three lung zones. In zone I, alveolar pressure *(P_A)* is greater than arterial and venous pressure, and no blood flow occurs. In zone II, arterial pressure *(P_a)* exceeds alveolar pressure, but alveolar pressure exceeds venous pressure *(P_V)*. Blood flow occurs in this zone, but alveolar pressure compresses the venules (venous ends of the capillaries). In zone III, both arterial and venous pressures are greater than alveolar pressure and blood flow fluctuates, depending on the difference between arterial and venous pressures.

which speeds blood flow, shortening the time the blood remains in the capillary.

Determinants of Arterial Oxygenation

As oxygen diffuses across the alveolocapillary membrane, it dissolves in the plasma, where it exerts pressure (the partial pressure of oxygen in arterial blood, or PaO_2). As the PaO_2 increases, oxygen moves from the plasma into the red blood cells (erythrocytes) and binds with hemoglobin molecules. Oxygen continues to bind with hemoglobin until the hemoglobin binding sites are filled or saturated. Oxygen then continues to diffuse across the alveolocapillary membrane until the PaO_2 (oxygen dissolved in plasma) and P_AO_2 equilibrate, eliminating the pressure gradient across the alveolocapillary membrane. At this point diffusion ceases (see Fig. 31-17).

Normally approximately 20 ml of oxygen is transported per 100 ml of blood. Because oxygen is not very soluble in plasma, most of the oxygen molecules bind with hemoglobin. Plasma carries only about 0.3 ml of oxygen per 100 ml of blood (at sea level). Although the remaining 19.7 ml is carried by hemoglobin, it is the small amount of oxygen dissolved in plasma that is responsible for oxygen's partial pressure (PaO_2) in the blood.

Although PaO_2 is important in that it provides the driving pressure that loads the hemoglobin with oxygen, it gives little information about the *amount* of oxygen carried in the blood. This amount, which is measured in milliliters per deciliter (100 ml) of blood, is the **oxygen content** of the blood. The total oxygen content of the blood depends on the amount of oxygen chemically combined with hemoglobin, as well as that dissolved in the blood. To calculate the total arterial oxygen content, we must know (1) hemoglobin concentration, or the amount of hemoglobin that is available to bind with oxygen (hemoglobin [Hb] in grams per deciliter); (2) the oxygen saturation or percentage of available hemoglobin that is bound to oxygen (SaO_2); and (3) the partial pressure of oxygen (PaO_2). The maximum amount of oxygen that can be transported by hemoglobin is 1.34 ml/g. The amount of oxygen that can be physically dissolved in blood is 0.003 ml/dl per mm Hg PO_2. If these specific values are known, the oxygen content of arterial blood can be calculated.[11]

$$O_2 \text{ content} = (Hb \times SaO_2 \times 1.34) + (PaO_2 \times 0.003)$$

To calculate the oxygen content of venous blood, the partial pressure of mixed venous blood ($P\bar{v}O_2$) and venous oxygen saturation ($S\bar{v}O_2$) are substituted for the arterial values in the basic formula. Normal venous oxygen content is 15 to 16 ml/dl.

Because hemoglobin transports all but a small fraction of the oxygen carried in arterial blood, increases in hemoglobin concentration affect the oxygen content of the blood. Decreases in hemoglobin concentration below the normal value of 15 ml/dl of blood reduce oxygen content, and increases in

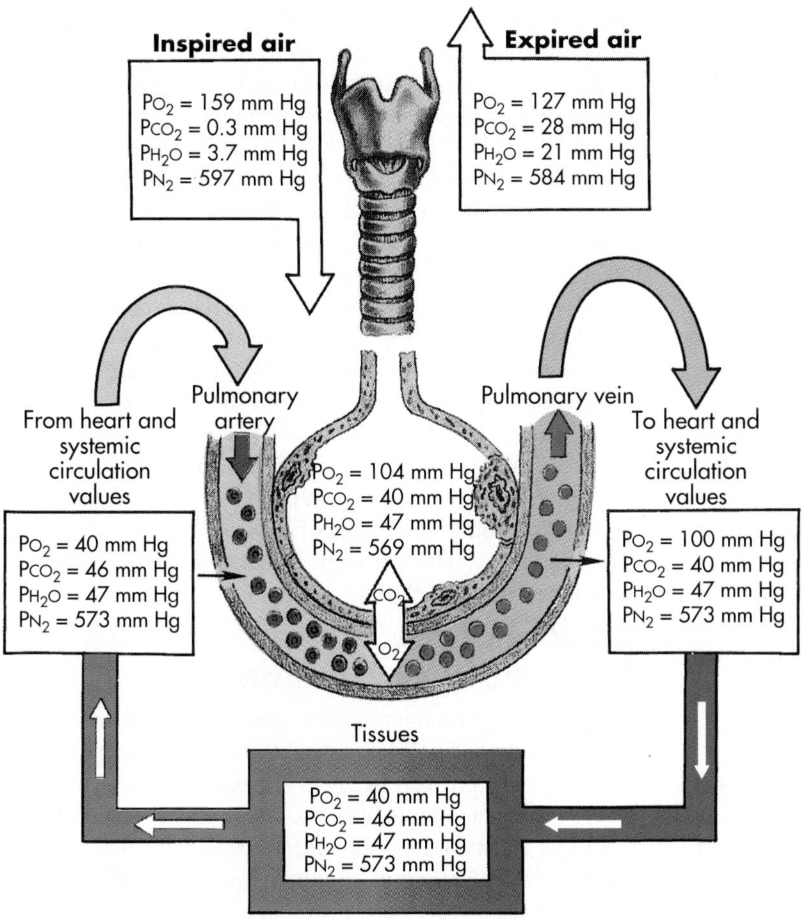

FIG. 31-17 Partial pressure of respiratory gases in normal respiration. These are average values. The values of PO_2, PCO_2, and PN_2 fluctuate from breath to breath.

hemoglobin concentration may minimize the impact of impaired gas exchange. In fact, an increase in hemoglobin concentration is a major compensatory mechanism in pulmonary diseases that impair gas exchange. For this reason, measurement of hemoglobin concentration is important in the assessment of individuals with pulmonary disease. If cardiovascular function is normal, the body's initial response to low oxygen content is to speed up cardiac output. In individuals who also have cardiovascular disease, this compensatory mechanism does not work, making increased hemoglobin concentration an even more important compensatory mechanism. (Hemoglobin structure and function are described in Chapter 24.)

Oxyhemoglobin Association and Dissociation

When hemoglobin molecules bind with oxygen, **oxyhemoglobin (HbO_2)** is formed. Binding occurs in the lungs and is called *oxyhemoglobin association* or *hemoglobin saturation with oxygen* (Sao_2). The reverse process, where oxygen is released from hemoglobin, occurs in the body tissues at the cellular level and is called *hemoglobin desaturation.* When hemoglobin saturation and desaturation are plotted on a graph, the result is a distinctive S-shaped curve known as the **oxyhemoglobin dissociation curve** (Fig. 31-18).

Several factors can change the relationship between Po_2 and So_2, causing the oxyhemoglobin dissociation curve to shift to the right or left (see Fig. 31-18). A shift to the right depicts hemoglobin's decreased affinity for oxygen or an increase in the ease with which oxyhemoglobin dissociates and oxygen moves into the cells. A shift to the left depicts hemoglobin's increased affinity for oxygen, which promotes association in the lungs and inhibits dissociation in the tissues.

The oxyhemoglobin dissociation curve is shifted to the right by acidosis (low pH) and hypercapnia (increased $Paco_2$). In the tissues the increased levels of carbon dioxide and hydrogen ions produced by metabolic activity decrease the affinity of hemoglobin for oxygen. The curve is shifted to the left by alkalosis (high pH) and hypocapnia (decreased $Paco_2$). In the lungs, as carbon dioxide diffuses from the blood into the alveoli, the blood carbon dioxide level is reduced and the affinity of hemoglobin for oxygen is increased. The shift in the oxyhemoglobin dissociation curve by changes in carbon dioxide and hydrogen ion concentration in the blood is called the **Bohr effect.**[12]

The oxyhemoglobin curve is shifted also by changes in body temperature and increased or decreased levels of 2,3-diphosphoglycerate (2,3-DPG), a substance normally present in erythrocytes. Hyperthermia and increased 2,3-DPG levels shift the curve to the right. Hypothermia and decreased 2,3-DPG levels shift the curve to the left.

Carbon Dioxide Transport

Approximately 200 ml of CO_2 is produced by the tissues per minute as a by-product of cellular metabolism. This CO_2 equilibrates with carbonic acid ($H_2O + CO_2 \leftrightharpoons H_2CO_3 \leftrightharpoons H + HCO_3^-$) and must be eliminated continuously to prevent acidosis. The elimination of carbon dioxide by the lungs plays an important role in the regulation of acid-base balance (see Chapter 3).

CO_2 is carried in the blood in three ways: (1) dissolved in plasma (Pco_2), (2) as bicarbonate, and (3) as carbamino compounds. As CO_2 diffuses out of the cells into the blood, it dissolves in the plasma. Approximately 10% of the total CO_2 in venous blood and 5% of the CO_2 in arterial blood is carried dissolved in the plasma (Pco_2). As CO_2 moves into the blood, it diffuses into the red blood cells. Within the red blood cells, carbon dioxide, with the help of the enzyme carbonic anhydrase, combines with water to form carbonic acid and then quickly dissociates into H^+ and HCO_3^-. As carbonic acid dissociates, the H^+ binds to hemoglobin, where it is buffered, and the HCO_3^- moves out of the red blood cell into the plasma. Approximately 60% of the CO_2 in venous blood and 90% of the CO_2 in arterial blood are carried in the form of bicarbonate. The remainder combines with blood proteins, hemoglobin in particular, to form carbamino compounds. Approximately 30% of the CO_2 in venous blood and 5% of the CO_2 in arterial blood are carried as carbamino compounds (see Fig. 3-9).

CO_2 is 20 times more soluble than O_2 and diffuses quickly from the tissue cells into the blood. The amount of CO_2 that is able to enter the blood is enhanced by diffusion of oxygen out of the blood and into the cells. Reduced hemoglobin (hemoglobin that is dissociated from oxygen) is able to carry more CO_2 than hemoglobin that is saturated with O_2. Therefore the drop in So_2 at the tissue level increases the ability of hemoglobin to carry CO_2 back to the lung.

The diffusion gradient for CO_2 in the lung is only approximately 6 mm Hg (venous Pco_2 = 46 mm Hg; alveolar Pco_2 = 40 mm Hg), yet CO_2 is so soluble in the alveolocapillary membrane that the CO_2 in the blood quickly diffuses into the alveoli, where it is removed from the lung with each expiration. Diffusion of CO_2 in the lung is so efficient that diffusion defects that cause hypoxemia (low oxygen content of the blood) do not cause hypercapnia (excessive carbon dioxide in the blood).

The diffusion of CO_2 out of the blood also is enhanced by oxygen binding with hemoglobin in the lung. As hemoglobin binds with O_2, the amount of CO_2 carried by the blood is decreased. Thus, in the tissue capillaries, O_2 dissociation from hemoglobin facilitates the pickup of CO_2, and the binding of O_2 to hemoglobin in the lungs facilitates the release of CO_2 from the blood. This effect of oxygen on CO_2 transport is called the **Haldane effect.**[13]

Control of the Pulmonary Circulation

The caliber of pulmonary artery lumina decreases as smooth muscle in arterial walls contracts. Contraction increases pulmonary artery pressure. Caliber increases as these muscles relax, decreasing blood pressure. Contraction (vasoconstriction) and relaxation (vasodilation) apparently occur in response to local humoral conditions, even though the pul-

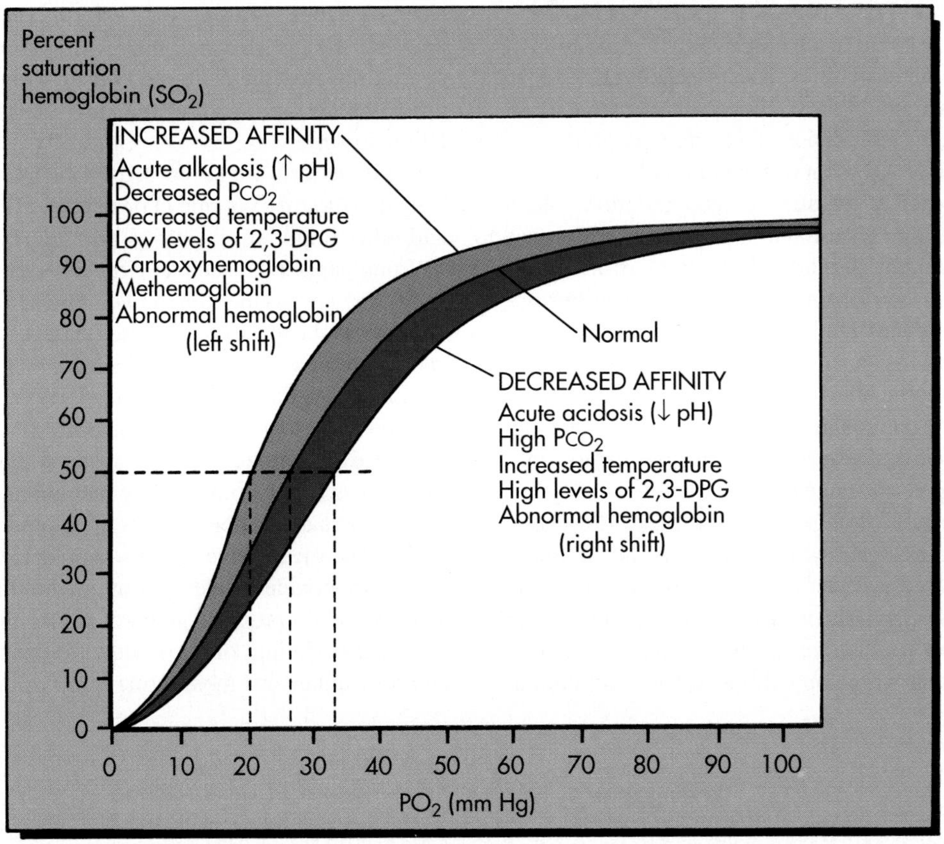

FIG. 31-18 Oxyhemoglobin dissociation curve. The horizontal or flat segment of the curve at the top of the graph is sometimes called the *arterial portion,* or that part of the curve where oxygen is bound to hemoglobin. This portion of the curve is flat because partial pressure changes of oxygen between 60 and 100 mm Hg do not significantly alter the percent saturation of hemoglobin with oxygen. The wide range of partial pressures of oxygen (Pao_2)—60 to 100 mm Hg, represented by the flat part of the curve—allows adequate hemoglobin saturation at a variety of altitudes. For example, a Pao_2 of 100 mm Hg at sea level results in a hemoglobin saturation with oxygen of 98%. At an altitude of 5000 feet the Pao_2 is about 70 mm Hg and hemoglobin saturation is 94%, only 4% less than at sea level. If the relationship between Sao_2 and Pao_2 were linear (in a downward-sloping straight line) instead of flat between 60 and 100 mm Hg, there would be inadequate saturation of hemoglobin with oxygen. For example, with a Pao_2 of 70 mm Hg the saturation would be only 70%, which is equivalent to normal venous oxygen saturation, and life could not be sustained at altitudes much above sea level. The steep part of the oxyhemoglobin dissociation curve occurs after the Pao_2 drops below 60 mm Hg and represents the rapid dissociation of oxygen from hemoglobin. During this phase there is rapid diffusion of oxygen from the blood into tissue cells. Conditions associated with altered affinity of hemoglobin for O_2 are listed. P_{50} is the Pao_2 at which hemoglobin is 50% saturated, normally 26.6 mm Hg. A lower than normal P_{50} represents increased affinity of hemoglobin for O_2; a high P_{50} is seen with decreased affinity. Note that variation from the normal is associated with decreased (low P_{50}) or increased (high P_{50}) availability of O_2 to tissues *(dotted lines).* The *shaded area* shows the entire oxyhemoglobin dissociation curve under the same circumstances. *2,3-DPG,* 2,3-diphosphatidylglycerate. (From Lane EE, Walker JF: *Clinical arterial blood gas analysis,* St Louis, 1987, Mosby.)

monary circulation is innervated by the ANS in the same manner as the systemic circulation.

The most important cause of pulmonary artery constriction is a low alveolar Po_2 (PAO_2). Vasoconstriction caused by alveolar hypoxia, often termed **hypoxic vasoconstriction,** can affect only one portion of the lung (i.e., one lobe that is obstructed, decreasing the PAO_2) or the entire lung. If only one segment of the lung is involved, the arterioles to that segment constrict, shunting blood to other, well-ventilated portions of the lung. This reflex improves the lung's efficiency by better matching ventilation and perfusion. If alveolar hypoxia affects all segments of the lung, however, pulmonary hypertension (elevated pulmonary artery pressure) can result. The pulmonary vasoconstriction caused by low alveolar Po_2 is reversible if the alveolar Po_2 is corrected. Chronic alveolar hypoxia can result in permanent pulmonary artery hypertension, which eventually leads to cor pulmonale and heart failure.

Acidemia also causes pulmonary artery constriction. If the acidemia is corrected, the vasoconstriction is reversed. (Respiratory acidosis and metabolic acidosis are described in Chapter 3.) It is important to note that an elevated $Paco_2$ without a drop in pH does not cause pulmonary artery constriction. Other biochemical factors that affect the caliber of vessels in pulmonary circulation are histamine, prostaglandins, serotonin, nitric oxide, and bradykinin.[14]

TESTS OF PULMONARY FUNCTION

Several laboratory tests aid in the diagnosis and evaluation of pulmonary system abnormalities. Most of them are easy to perform at hospitals and clinics. They provide valuable information as to the possible cause of a respiratory abnormality and evaluate the progression or resolution of disease.

Spirometry is used to measure forced expiration, which frequently is affected by diffuse pulmonary disease. Because the pulmonary system has remarkable reserves, disease may become well established before clinical manifestations appear. Spirometry enables clinicians to detect restrictive or obstructive deficits early in the course of disease. Restrictive lung diseases restrict the lung's volume: the lungs are unable to expand normally, diminishing the amount of gas that can be inspired. Obstructive diseases affect gas flow: airflow into and out of the lungs is obstructed.

Spirometry measures both volume and flow. The test is performed with a spirometer, which is a water-filled cylinder into which an inverted cylinder or bell has been inserted. A length of tubing runs from the inverted bell to a mouthpiece through which a person breathes during testing. The bell is attached to a pen that writes on calibrated paper rotating at a constant speed. As a person performs various breathing maneuvers, the inverted bell moves up and down, causing the pen to move on the calibrated paper. This produces a spirogram, which is a record of the individual's ventilation in relation to time (Fig. 31-19). Clinically, the most important spirometric tests are the forced vital capacity (FVC) and the forced expiratory volume in one second (FEV_1). (These tests and other important measures are described in Table 31-3.)

Lung capacities, such as vital capacity and total lung capacity, are always the sum of two or more volumes. Norms for volumes and capacities are based on age, gender, and height and are referred to as *predicted values.* Changes from predicted or baseline values are taken into account in diagnosing and assessing respiratory disorders.

Diffusing capacity is a measure of the rate of gas diffusion across the alveolocapillary membrane. Oxygen, or more commonly carbon monoxide, is used to measure diffusing capacity. The measurement is made by determining how much carbon monoxide is taken up by the blood and dividing this amount by the pressure gradient across the alveolocapillary membrane. Helium often is added to the gas mixture to obtain a simultaneous measurement of **residual volume (RV),**

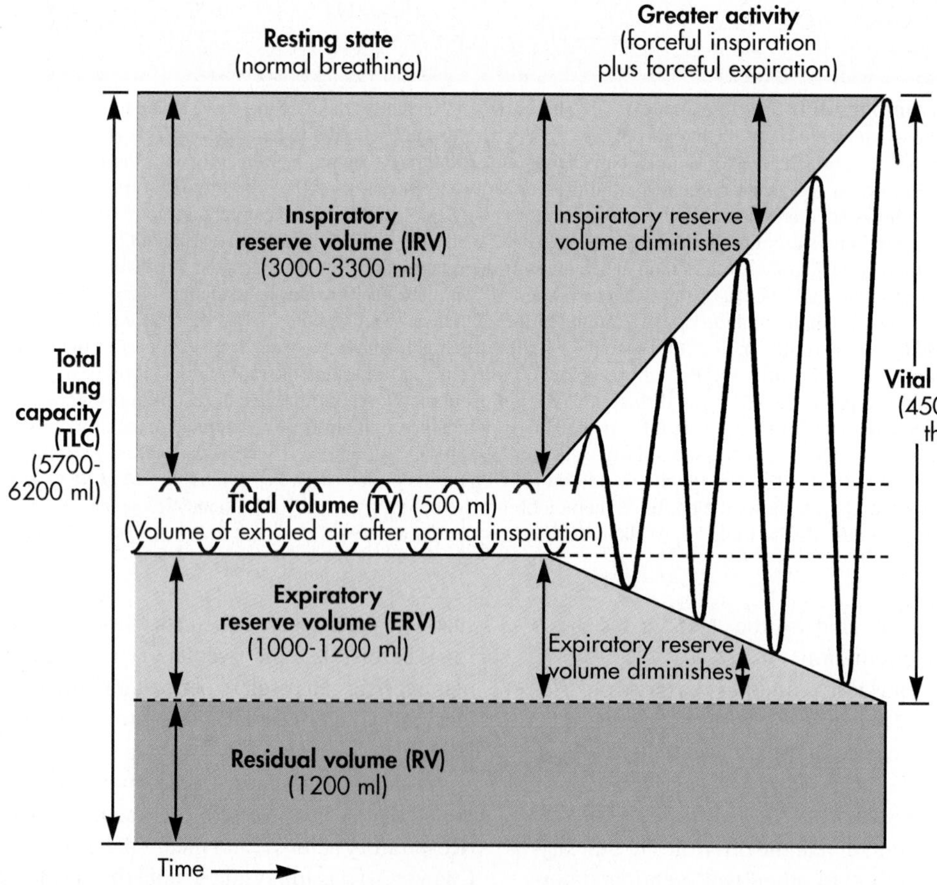

FIG. 31-19 Spirogram. During normal, quiet respirations the atmosphere and lungs exchange about 500 ml of air *(TV).* With a forcible inspiration, about 3300 ml more air can be inhaled *(IRV).* After a normal inspiration and normal expiration, approximately 1000 ml more air can be forcibly expired *(ERV).* Vital capacity is the amount of air that can be forcibly expired after a maximal inspiration and indicates, therefore, the largest amount of air that can enter and leave the lungs during respiration. Residual volume is the air that remains trapped in the alveoli. (From Thibodeau GA, Patton KI: *Anatomy and physiology,* ed 4, St Louis, 1999, Mosby.)

functional reserve capacity (FRC), and **total lung capacity (TLC).** Individuals are asked to perform ventilatory maneuvers similar to those of spirometry. A decreased diffusing capacity can be the result of an abnormal ventilation-perfusion ratio or an actual diffusion defect. Diffusing capacity is decreased in individuals with emphysema.

Arterial blood gas analysis commonly is performed for individuals with suggested or diagnosed pulmonary disease. Direct analysis of the pH and gas concentrations in arterial blood provides valuable information about an individual's gas exchange and acid-base status. Acidosis (low pH), alkalosis (high pH), ventilatory alterations, and decreased $Pa{O_2}$ can be diagnosed accurately only by arterial blood gas analysis. A blood gas report may be divided into an acid-base/ventilation portion and an oxygenation portion. (Normal values for arterial blood gases are given in Table 31-4.) (Acid-base alterations are described in Chapter 3.) Oximetry can be used to monitor oxygen saturation once the arterial blood gas analysis has accurately measured the $Pa{O_2}$, but it does not measure $Pa{CO_2}$ or pH.

Signs and symptoms of most respiratory abnormalities first appear when the system is stressed during exercise. Therefore, if pulmonary disease is suspected, the individual is evaluated at rest and during exercise. During exercise the usual procedures are spirometry and withdrawal of arterial blood for gas analysis. The exercise usually consists of riding a stationary bicycle or walking on a treadmill. Exercise testing enables clinicians to detect early changes in respiratory function and begin treatment. Exercise tests also are used in planning and evaluating exercise and rehabilitation programs.

Chest radiographs are among the most common examinations of the pulmonary system. A few of the abnormalities detected in chest radiographs are air trapping in the alveoli and airways (e.g., in asthma or emphysema), consolidation of lung tissue (in pneumonia or pulmonary edema), cavities (abscesses or tuberculosis), and nodules (lung cancer). Often pulmonary abnormalities are detected in routine chest radiographs of asymptomatic individuals. Various radiographic techniques are available for the diagnosis and evaluation of respiratory disorders.

Aging and the Pulmonary System

Most knowledge about pulmonary structure and function is based on norms for the middle years. Less is known about structure and function in very young (see Chapter 33) and elderly persons, but a few normal physiologic (developmental and degenerative) changes are known to occur from birth to old age. An understanding of these changes is needed to provide appropriate care and to differentiate between normal alterations and disease. Normal alterations include (1) loss of

Table 31-3 Values Measured by Spirometry

Symbol	Ventilatory Property Measured
FVC	Forced vital capacity: maximum amount of gas that can be displaced from the lung during a forced expiration
FEV_1	Forced expiratory volume in 1 sec: maximum amount of air that can be expired from the lung in 1 sec
FEV_1/FVC	Percentage of maximum inspiration that is expired in 1 sec, usually 80% of FVC
FEV_3	Forced expiratory volume in 3 sec; maximum amount of gas that can be expired in 3 sec
FEV_3/FVC	Percentage of FVC that is expired in 3 sec; usually 95% of FVC
$FEF_{25\%-75\%}$	Forced expiratory flow rate during the middle 50% of expiration; sometimes reported as maximum midexpiratory flow rate (MMFR)

Table 31-4 Normal Ranges for Arterial and Mixed Venous Blood Gases

Measurement	Arterial Blood	Mixed Venous Blood*	Clinical Notes
Acid-base status (pH)	7.35–7.45	7.33–7.43	Most important acid-base value; detects acidosis or alkalosis
Partial pressure of carbon dioxide ($P{CO_2}$)	35–45 mm Hg	41–57 mm Hg	Measures adequacy of ventilation and respiratory contribution of acid-base abnormality (respiratory acidosis)
Bicarbonate (HCO_3^-)	22–26 mEq/L	24–28 mEq/L	Measures metabolic contribution to acid-base abnormality (metabolic acidosis); calculated from pH and $P{CO_2}$
Base excess (BE)	− 2 to + 2	0 to + 4	Reflects deviation of bicarbonate concentration from normal
Partial pressure of oxygen ($P{O_2}$) (sea level)	80–100 mm Hg	35–40 mm Hg	Indicates driving pressure that causes oxygen-hemoglobin binding; varies with age and barometric pressure
Saturation of hemoglobin with oxygen ($S{O_2}$)	96%–98%	70%–75%	Indicates abnormalities of oxyhemoglobin association and dissociation; may be measured directly or calculated from $P{O_2}$, pH, and body temperature
Concentration of hemoglobin in the blood	15 g/dl	15 g/dl	Detects alterations of gas transport caused by anemia

*Mixed venous (pulmonary artery) blood is analyzed for critically ill individuals and those undergoing cardiac catheterization (it is not practical to withdraw samples except from a pulmonary artery catheter). Mixed venous blood gas analysis, in conjunction with arterial analysis, provides important information about the adequacy of cardiac output and tissue oxygenation.

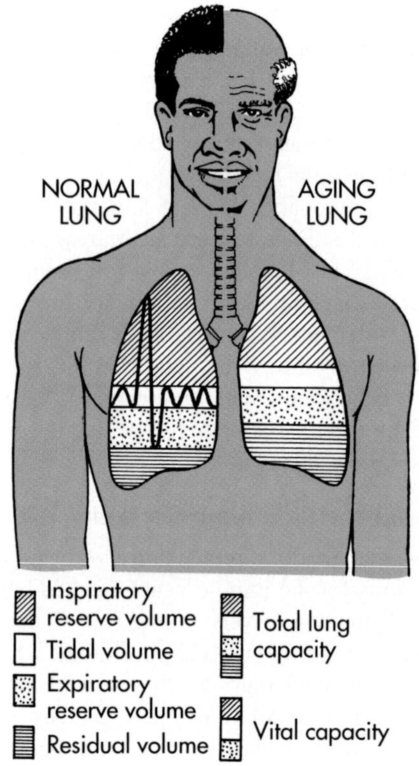

FIG. 31-20 Changes in lung volumes with aging. With aging, note particularly the decrease in vital capacity and the increase in residual volume.

elastic recoil, (2) stiffening of the chest wall, (3) alterations in gas exchange, and (4) increases in flow resistance (Fig. 31-20). These changes are influenced by environmental factors, respiratory disease, body size, and race.[15]

During adulthood and as age advances, the alveoli tend to lose alveoli wall tissue and capillaries. This process diminishes alveolar surface area available for gas diffusion and decreases airway support provided by normal lung tissues. Mechanical changes involve elastic properties of the lungs and chest wall. Chest wall compliance decreases with age because the ribs become ossified (less flexible) and joints become stiffer. As a result the chest wall loses some of its ability to expand. In addition, respiratory muscle strength and endurance decrease by up to 20% by age 70.[16] These mechanical changes in the lung and chest wall, along with structural changes in the alveoli, reduce ventilatory capacity in old age. Vital capacity decreases and residual volume increases; however, total lung capacity remains unchanged. These changes decrease ventilatory reserves and lead to decreased ventilation-perfusion ratios.[17] With advancing age, there is also increased immune dysregulation, asymptomatic low-grade inflammation, and increased risk of infection.[18]

Alterations in gas exchange are reflected by blood gas analysis. With advancing age, pH and Pco_2 do not change much, even though it has been documented that the chemoreceptors become less sensitive to gas partial pressures with age. The elderly have a decreased compensatory response to hypercapnia and hypoxemia; however, the perception of dyspnea remains intact and is even enhanced.[16] Po_2 declines with age as a result of structural and mechanical changes, such as loss of alveolar surface area and increased ventilation-perfusion mismatch. The maximum Pao_2 in an elderly individual at sea level can be estimated by multiplying the person's age by 0.3 and subtracting the product from 100. For example, an 80-year-old individual would have an estimated maximum Po_2 of 76 mm Hg ($0.3 \times 80 = 24$; $100 - 24 = 76$). There is also a decrease in the capillary network.

The decrease in Pao_2 and diminished ventilatory reserve in the elderly person lead to a decrease in exercise tolerance. Furthermore, the elderly are at greater risk for respiratory depression caused by medications. Changes in respiratory function can vary considerably from person to person, however. Changes also are affected by activity and fitness earlier in life. A very active, physically fit individual will, all else being equal, have fewer changes in function at any age than one who has been sedentary. Respiratory muscle strength and endurance decrease with age but can be enhanced with exercise.[19]

SUMMARY REVIEW

Structures of the Pulmonary System

1. The pulmonary system consists of the lungs, airways, chest wall, and pulmonary and bronchial circulation.
2. Air is inspired and expired through the conducting airways, which include the nasopharynx, oropharynx, trachea, bronchi, and bronchioles to the sixteenth division.
3. Gas exchange occurs in structures beyond the sixteenth division: the respiratory bronchioles, alveolar ducts, and alveoli. Together these structures compose the acinus.
4. The chief gas-exchange units of the lungs are the alveoli. The membrane that surrounds each alveolus and contains the pulmonary capillaries is called the alveolocapillary membrane.
5. The gas-exchange airways are served by the pulmonary circulation, a separate division of the circulatory system. The bronchi and other lung structures are served by a branch of the systemic circulation called the bronchial circulation.
6. The chest wall, which contains and protects the contents of the thoracic cavity, consists of the skin, ribs, and intercostal muscles, which lie between the ribs.
7. The chest wall is lined by a serous membrane called the parietal pleura; the lungs are encased in a separate membrane called the visceral pleura. The area where these two pleurae come into contact and slide over one another is called the pleural space.

Function of the Pulmonary System

1. The pulmonary system enables oxygen to diffuse into the blood and carbon dioxide to diffuse out of the blood.
2. Ventilation is the process by which air flows into and out of the gas-exchange airways.

3. Successful ventilation involves the mechanics of breathing: the interaction of forces and counterforces involving the muscles of inspiration and expiration, alveolar surface tension, elastic properties of the lungs and chest wall, and resistance to airflow.
4. The major muscle of inspiration is the diaphragm. When the diaphragm contracts, it moves downward in the thoracic cavity, creating a vacuum that causes air to flow into the lungs.
5. The alveoli produce surfactant, a lipoprotein that lines the alveoli. Surfactant reduces alveolar surface tension and permits the alveoli to expand more easily as air flows in.
6. Compliance is the ability of the lungs and chest wall to expand during inspiration. Lung compliance is ensured by adequate production of surfactant; chest wall expansion depends on flexibility.
7. Elastic recoil is the tendency of the lungs and chest wall to return to their resting state after inspiration. The elastic recoil forces of the lungs and chest wall are in opposition and pull on each other, creating the normally negative pressure of the pleural space.
8. Most of the time ventilation is involuntary. It is controlled by the sympathetic and parasympathetic divisions of the autonomic nervous system, which adjust airway caliber (by causing bronchial smooth muscle to contract or relax) and control the rate and depth of ventilation.
9. Neuroreceptors in the lungs (lung receptors) monitor the mechanical aspects of ventilation. Irritant receptors sense the need to expel unwanted substances, stretch receptors sense lung volume (lung expansion), and *J*-receptors sense alveolar size.
10. Chemoreceptors in the circulatory system and brain stem sense the effectiveness of ventilation by monitoring the pH status of cerebrospinal fluid and the oxygen content (Po_2) of arterial blood.
11. The pulmonary circulation is innervated by the autonomic nervous system, but vasodilation and vasoconstriction are controlled mainly by local and humoral factors, particularly arterial oxygenation and acid-base status.
12. Gas transport depends on ventilation of the alveoli, diffusion across the alveolocapillary membrane, perfusion of the pulmonary and systemic capillaries, and diffusion between systemic capillaries and tissue cells.
13. Efficient gas exchange depends on an even distribution of ventilation and perfusion within the lungs. Both ventilation and perfusion are greatest in the bases of the lungs because the alveoli in the bases are more compliant (their resting volume is low) and perfusion is greater in the bases as a result of gravity.
14. Almost all of the oxygen that diffuses into pulmonary capillary blood is transported by hemoglobin, a protein contained within red blood cells. The remainder of the oxygen is transported dissolved in plasma.
15. Oxygen enters the body by diffusing down the concentration gradient, from high concentrations in the alveoli to lower concentrations in the capillaries. Diffusion ceases when alveolar and capillary oxygen pressures equilibrate.
16. Oxygen is loaded onto hemoglobin by the driving pressure exerted by Pao_2 in the plasma. As pressure decreases at tissue level, oxygen dissociates from hemoglobin and enters tissue cells by diffusion, again down the concentration gradient.
17. Carbon dioxide is more soluble in plasma than oxygen is and diffuses readily from tissue cells into plasma. Carbon dioxide returns to the lungs dissolved in plasma, as bicarbonate, or in carbamino compounds (e.g., bound to hemoglobin).
18. Vasoconstriction of the pulmonary arterial system is caused by alveolar hypoxia, acidemia, and inflammatory mediators—histamine, serotonin, prostaglandins, and bradykinin.

Tests of Pulmonary Function

1. Spirometry measures both volume and flow rate during forced expiration.
2. The alveolar-arterial oxygen gradient is used to evaluate the cause of hypoxia.
3. Diffusing capacity is a measure of the gas diffusion rate at the alveolocapillary membrane.
4. Arterial blood gas analysis can be used to determine pH and oxygen and carbon dioxide concentrations.
5. Radiographic examination of the chest evaluates air trapping, consolidation, cavity formation, or presence of tumors.

Aging and the Pulmonary System

1. Aging affects the mechanical aspects of ventilation by decreasing chest wall compliance and elastic recoil of the lungs. Changes in these elastic properties reduce ventilatory reserve.
2. Aging causes the Pao_2 to decrease but does not affect the $Paco_2$.

KEY TERMS

Acinus, *1084*
Alveolar duct, *1084*
Alveolar ventilation, *1089*
Alveolocapillary membrane, *1086*
Alveolus (pl., alveoli), *1084*
Arterial blood gas analysis, *1101*
Bohr effect, *1098*
Bronchiole, *1083*
Bronchus (pl., bronchi), *1083*
Carina, *1083*
Central chemoreceptor, *1090*
Chest radiograph, *1101*
Compliance, *1092*
Diffusing capacity, *1100*
Elastic recoil, *1092*
Functional reserve capacity (FRC), *1101*
Goblet cell, *1083*
Haldane effect, *1098*
Hilus (pl., hili), *1083*
Hypoxic vasoconstriction, *1099*
Irritant receptor, *1090*
J-receptors, *1090*
Larynx, *1082*
Minute volume, *1088*
Nasopharynx, *1082*
Oropharynx, *1082*
Oxygen content, *1097*
Oxyhemoglobin (HbO_2), *1098*
Oxyhemoglobin dissociation curve, *1098*
Partial pressure (tension) of a gas, *1094*
Peripheral chemoreceptor, *1089*
Physiologic dead space, *1096*
Pleura (pl., pleurae), *1088*
Pleural space (pleural cavity), *1088*
Residual volume (RV), *1100*
Respiration, *1088*
Respiratory bronchiole, *1084*
Respiratory center, *1089*
Spirometry, *1100*

KEY TERMS—cont'd

Stretch receptor, *1090*
Surface tension, *1091*
Surfactant, *1086*
Thoracic cavity, *1088*
Total lung capacity (TLC), *1101*
Trachea, *1083*
Ventilation, *1088*
Ventilation-perfusion ratio (mismatch) ($\dot{V}/\dot{Q}$), *1096*

REFERENCES

1. Ruppel G: The respiratory system. In Egan DF, Scanlan CL, Wilkins RL, editors: *Egan's fundamentals of respiratory care,* ed 7, St Louis, 1999, Mosby.
2. Corrin B: *Pathology of the lungs,* London, 2000, Churchill Livingstone.
3. Mercer RR, Crapo JD: Normal anatomy and defense mechanisms of the lung. In Baum GL et al, editors: *Textbook of pulmonary diseases,* ed 6, London, 1998, Lippincott-Raven.
4. West JB: *Respiratory physiology: the essentials,* ed 6, Philadelphia, 2000, Lippincott Williams & Wilkins.
5. Wideicombe JG: Sensory neurophysiology of the cough reflex, *J Allergy Clin Immunol* 98(5):S84, 1996.
6. Beachey W, Scanlan CL: Acid-base balance and the regulation of respiration. In Egan DF, Scanlan CL, Wilkins RL, editors: *Egan's fundamentals of respiratory care,* ed 7, St Louis, 1999, Mosby.
7. Caruana-Montaldo B, Gleeson K, Zwillich C: The control of breathing in clinical practice, *Chest* 117(1):205, 2000.
8. McCormack F: The structure and function of surfactant protein-A, *Chest* 111(6):114S, 1997.
9. Guyton AC, Hall JE: *Textbook of medical physiology,* ed 10, Philadelphia, 2000, W.B. Saunders.
10. Ward ME, Roussos C, Macklem PT: Respiratory mechanics. In Murray JF, Nadel JA, editors: *Textbook of respiratory medicine,* ed 3, Philadelphia, 2000, W.B. Saunders.
11. Gross GW, Scanlan CL: Gas exchange and transport. In Egan DF, Scanlan CL, Wilkins RL, editors: *Egan's fundamentals of respiratory care,* ed 7, St Louis, 1999, Mosby.
12. Piantadosi CA, Yuh-Chi TH: Respiratory function of the lung. In Baum GL et al, editors: *Textbook of pulmonary diseases,* ed 6, London, 1998, Lippincott-Raven.
13. Giovannini I et al: Quantitative effect of changes in blood CO_2 tension mediated by the Haldane effect, *J Appl Physiol* 87:862, 1999.
14. Dumas JP et al: Hypoxic pulmonary vasoconstriction, *Gen Pharmacol* 33(4):289, 1999.
15. Crapo RO: The aging lung. In Mahler DA, editor: *Pulmonary disease in the elderly patient,* New York, 1993, Marcel Dekker.
16. Oskvig R: Special problems in the elderly, *Chest* 115(5):158S, 1999.
17. Mahler DA, editor: *Pulmonary disease in the elderly patient,* New York, 1993, Marcel Dekker.
18. Meyer KC et al: Immune dysregulation in the aging human lung, *Am J Respir Crit Care Med* 153(3):1072, 1996.
19. Chen HI, Kuo CS: Relationship between respiratory muscle function and age, sex, and other factors, *J Appl Physiol* 66:943, 1989.

CHAPTER 32

Alterations of Pulmonary Function

VALENTINA L. BRASHERS

CHAPTER OUTLINE

Pulmonary disease is often classified as acute or chronic, obstructive or restrictive, and infectious or noninfectious; it is caused by lung or heart failure. Because skillful and knowledgeable clinical care plays a major role in decreasing respiratory mortality and morbidity, the clinician with a clear understanding of the pathophysiology of common respiratory problems can greatly affect the outcome for each individual.

CLINICAL MANIFESTATIONS OF PULMONARY ALTERATIONS

Signs and Symptoms of Pulmonary Disease

Pulmonary disease is associated with many signs and symptoms. The most common of these are cough and dyspnea. Other manifestations include chest pain, abnormal sputum, hemoptysis, altered breathing patterns, cyanosis, and fever. The signs and symptoms present and their specific characteristics often help in identifying the underlying disorder.

Dyspnea

Dyspnea is the subjective sensation of uncomfortable breathing, the feeling of being unable to get enough air. It is often described as breathlessness, air hunger, shortness of breath, labored breathing, and preoccupation with breathing. Dyspnea is a common symptom of respiratory disease.

Dyspnea is usually caused by diffuse and extensive pulmonary disease but can be caused by focal pulmonary disorders as well. Disturbances of ventilation, gas exchange, or ventilation-perfusion relationships can cause dyspnea, as can increased work of breathing or diseases that damage lung tissue (lung parenchyma).

Many mechanisms have been proposed to explain the complex sensation of dyspnea, but no single mechanism has been found to be responsible in all situations. The most commonly accepted explanation is the *length/tension inappropriateness theory,* which involves stimulation of receptors in respiratory muscles. According to this theory, the perception of dyspnea develops when muscle spindles in intercostal muscles are stimulated by a disparity between the tension generated by the muscles and the tidal volume (change in muscle fiber length) that results. This can occur if increased airway resistance or decreased compliance results in respiratory effort that is greater than appropriate for the ventilation achieved. A second explanation involves the stimulation of central and peripheral chemoreceptors. It has long been known that decreased pH, hypercapnia, and hypoxemia can cause dyspnea. Stimulation of chemoreceptors causes dyspnea in many lung diseases in which oxygenation and gas exchange are impaired. A third explanation is stimulation of the afferent receptors in the lung (the stretch receptors, irritant receptors, and *J*-receptors), which send impulses to the central nervous system through the vagus nerve. *J*-receptors, for example, trigger dyspnea in individuals with pulmonary edema and pulmonary microemboli. (The neurochemical control of ventilation is described in Chapter 31.) Other receptors in the face, upper airway, and chest wall can contribute to the sensation of dyspnea. Other factors contributing to the sensation of dyspnea include increased work of breathing, respiratory muscle fatigue, decreased breathing reserve, and strong emotions, particularly anxiety and anger. There is general agreement that neurologic control and function of respiratory muscles are the common elements in most clinical experiences of dyspnea and that the sensation perceived is that of increased respiratory effort.[1]

The signs of dyspnea include flaring of the nostrils, use of accessory muscles of respiration, and retraction (pulling back) of the intercostal spaces. In dyspnea caused by parenchymal disease (e.g., pneumonia), retractions of tissue between the ribs (subcostal and intercostal retractions) are observed more frequently than supercostal retractions (retractions of tissues above the ribs), which predominate in upper airway obstruction.

Dyspnea can occur frequently or in specific circumstances. The first episode commonly occurs with exercise and is called *dyspnea on exertion.* Pulmonary congestion tends to cause dyspnea when the individual is lying down. This type is called **orthopnea.** Orthopnea is caused by the horizontal position, which redistributes body water, causes the abdominal contents to exert pressure on the diaphragm, and decreases the efficiency of the respiratory muscles. Orthopnea is generally relieved by sitting up in a forward-leaning posture or supporting the upper body on several pillows. Some individuals with left ventricular failure wake up at night gasping for air and must sit up or stand to relieve the dyspnea. This type of positional dyspnea is termed **paroxysmal nocturnal dyspnea (PND).** PND results from fluid in the lungs caused by the redistribution of body water while the individual is recumbent.

Abnormal Breathing Patterns

Normal breathing (eupnea) is rhythmic and effortless. Ventilatory rate is 8 to 16 breaths per minute, and tidal volume ranges from 400 to 800 ml. A short expiratory pause occurs with each breath, and the individual takes an occasional deeper breath or sigh. Sigh breaths, which help maintain normal lung function, are usually 1.5 to 2 times the normal tidal volume and occur approximately 10 to 12 times per hour.

The rate, depth, regularity, and effort of breathing undergo characteristic alterations in response to physiologic and pathophysiologic conditions. Patterns of breathing automatically adjust to minimize the work of respiratory muscles. Strenuous exercise or metabolic acidosis induces **Kussmaul respiration (hyperpnea).** Kussmaul respiration is characterized by a slightly increased ventilatory rate, very large tidal volume, and no expiratory pause.

Labored, or obstructed, breathing occurs if the airways are obstructed, as in chronic obstructive pulmonary disease (COPD). Obstructed breathing consists of slow ventilatory rate, large tidal volume, increased effort, and prolonged inspiration or expiration, depending on the site of obstruction. Audible wheezing (whistling sounds) or stridor (high-pitched sounds made during inspiration) is often present.

Restricted breathing is commonly caused by disorders, such as pulmonary fibrosis, that stiffen the lungs or chest wall and decrease compliance. Restricted breathing is characterized by small tidal volumes and rapid ventilatory rate (tachypnea).

Panting occurs with exercise. Shock and severe cerebral hypoxia (insufficient oxygen in the brain) contribute to gasping respirations that consist of irregular, quick inspirations with an expiratory pause. Sighing respirations consist of irregular breathing characterized by frequent, deep sighing inspirations. Sighing respirations are caused by anxiety.

Cheyne-Stokes respirations are characterized by alternating periods of deep and shallow breathing. Apnea lasting 15 to 60 seconds is followed by ventilations that increase in volume until a peak is reached, after which ventilation (tidal volume) decreases again to apnea. Cheyne-Stokes respirations result from any condition that slows the blood flow to the brain stem, which in turn slows impulses sending information to the respiratory centers of the brain stem. Neurologic impairment above the brain stem is also a contributing factor.

Hypoventilation and Hyperventilation

Hypoventilation is inadequate alveolar ventilation in relation to metabolic demands. It is caused by alterations in pulmonary mechanics or in the neurologic control of breathing. When alveolar ventilation is normal, CO_2 is removed from the lungs at the same rate at which it is produced by cellular metabolism. This maintains arterial and alveolar P_{CO_2} at normal levels (40 mm Hg). With hypoventilation, CO_2 removal does not keep up with CO_2 production and Pa_{CO_2} increases, causing hypercapnia (Pa_{CO_2} greater than 44 mm Hg). (Table 31-2 contains the definition of gas partial pressure and other pulmonary abbreviations.) This results in respiratory acidosis, which can affect the function of many tissues throughout the body. Hypoventilation and hypercapnia occur when minute volume (tidal volume times respiratory rate) is reduced.

Hypoventilation is often overlooked until it is severe because breathing pattern and ventilatory rate may appear normal. Blood gas analysis (i.e., measurement of the Pa_{CO_2} of arterial bood) reveals the hypercapnia. Pronounced hypoventilation can cause somnolence or disorientation. In addition, hypoventilation with hypercapnia results in secondary hypoxemia.

Hyperventilation is alveolar ventilation that exceeds metabolic demands. The lungs remove CO_2 at a faster rate than it is produced by cellular metabolism, resulting in decreased $Paco_2$ or **hypocapnia** ($Paco_2$ less than 36 mm Hg). Like hypoventilation, hyperventilation can be determined only by arterial blood gas analysis. Hyperventilation commonly occurs with severe anxiety, acute head injury, and conditions that cause insufficient oxygenation of the blood. Recent evidence suggests that significant hypocapnia can contribute to lung injury in some disorders.[2]

Cough

Cough is important to clear the airways of large amounts of inhaled material, excessive secretions, or abnormal substances, such as edema or pus. Most coughs are initiated in the larynx and in the tracheobronchial tree by both mechanical and chemical "irritant" receptor stimulation. There are few such receptors in the most distal bronchi and the alveoli; thus it is possible for significant amounts of secretions to accumulate in the distal respiratory tree without initiating cough. Other cough receptors are located in the external auditory canal, diaphragm, pericardium, pleura, and stomach. Stimulation of cough receptors is transmitted centrally through the vagus nerve, and central modulation of the cough reflex can be influenced by opiates and serotoninergic agents.

Acute cough is cough that resolves within 2 to 3 weeks of the onset of illness or resolves with treatment of the underlying condition. It is most commonly the result of upper respiratory infections, allergic rhinitis, acute bronchitis, pneumonia, congestive heart failure, pulmonary embolus, or aspiration. **Chronic cough** is defined as cough that has persisted for more than 3 weeks, although some authors have suggested that 7 or 8 weeks is a more appropriate timeframe because acute cough and bronchial hyperreactivity can be prolonged in some cases of viral infection. In nonsmokers, chronic cough is almost always due to postnasal drainage syndrome, asthma, or gastroesophageal reflux disease. In smokers, chronic bronchitis is the most common cause of chronic cough, although lung cancer must always be considered. Up to 33% of individuals taking angiotensin-converting enzyme inhibitors for cardiovascular disease develop chronic cough that resolves with discontinuation of the drug.[3]

Hemoptysis

Hemoptysis is the coughing up of blood or bloody secretions. Hemoptysis is sometimes confused with hematemesis, which is the vomiting of blood. Blood that is coughed up is usually bright red, has an alkaline pH, and is mixed with frothy sputum, whereas blood that is vomited is dark, has an acidic pH, and is mixed with food particles.

The most common causes of hemoptysis are bronchiectasis, lung cancer, bronchitis, and pneumonia.[4] Tuberculosis remains an important cause of hemoptysis but is less common in the United States than in many other parts of the world. Hemoptysis results from damage to the lung parenchyma with rupture of pulmonary vessels or from inflammation, injury, or cancer of the bronchial tree. The amount and duration of bleeding (i.e., a sudden large amount versus a persistent slight amount) provide important clues about the source of the bleeding. Bronchoscopy combined with chest computed tomography (CT) can identify the cause in up to 93% of cases of hemoptysis.[4]

Cyanosis

Cyanosis is a bluish discoloration of the skin and mucous membranes caused by increasing amounts of desaturated or reduced hemoglobin (which is bluish) in the blood. Cyanosis generally develops when 5 g of hemoglobin is desaturated, regardless of hemoglobin concentration. For example, if total hemoglobin concentration is 15 g/dl of blood, 5 g/dl must be desaturated to cause cyanosis. If total hemoglobin (Hb) is 11 g/dl, 5 g/dl must still be desaturated for cyanosis to occur.

Cyanosis can be caused by decreased arterial oxygenation (low Pao_2), pulmonary or cardiac right-to-left shunts, decreased cardiac output, cold environments, or anxiety. In adults, cyanosis is not evident until severe hypoxemia is present and therefore is an insensitive indicator of respiratory distress. Lack of cyanosis does not necessarily indicate that oxygenation is normal. For example, severe anemia (inadequate hemoglobin concentration) and carbon monoxide poisoning (in which hemoglobin binds to carbon monoxide instead of to oxygen) can cause inadequate oxygenation of tissues without causing cyanosis. Individuals with polycythemia (an abnormal increase in numbers of red blood cells), however, may have cyanosis when oxygenation is adequate. Because polycythemia causes hemoglobin concentration to be greater than normal, 5 g/dl can be desaturated, causing cyanosis, without having much effect on oxygenation. Therefore the significance of cyanosis as a clinical finding must be interpreted in relation to the underlying pathophysiology. If cyanosis is suggested, the Pao_2 should be measured. Central cyanosis (decreased oxygen saturation of hemoglobin in arterial blood) is best seen in buccal mucous membranes and lips. Peripheral cyanosis (slow blood circulation in fingers and toes) is best seen in nail beds.

Pain

Pain caused by pulmonary disorders originates in the pleurae, airways, or chest wall. Pleural pain is the most common pain caused by pulmonary disease and is usually sharp or stabbing in character. Infection and inflammation of the parietal pleura cause pain when the pleura stretches during inspiration. The pain is usually localized to a portion of the chest wall, where a unique breath sound called a *pleural friction rub* may be heard over the painful area. Laughing or coughing makes pleural pain worse. Pleural pain is also common with pulmonary infarction (tissue death) caused by pulmonary embolism. In the case of infarction the pain emanates from the area around the infarction.

Pulmonary pain is central chest pain that is pronounced after coughing and occurs in individuals with infection and inflammation of the trachea or bronchi (tracheitis or tracheobronchitis). Central chest pain must be differentiated

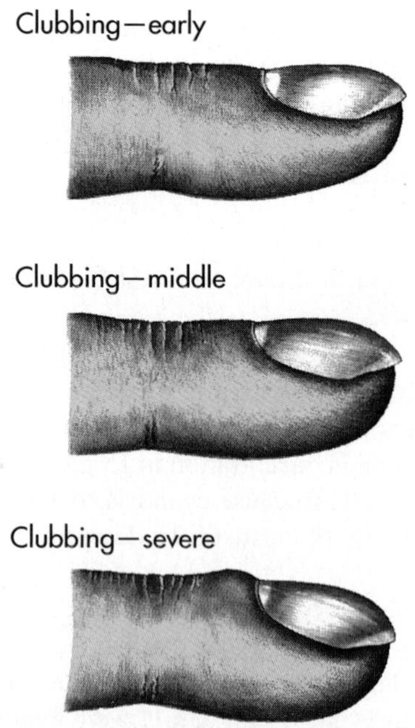

FIG. 32-1 Clubbing of fingers caused by chronic hypoxemia. (From Seidel HM et al: *Mosby's guide to physical examination,* ed 4, St Louis, 1999, Mosby.)

from cardiac pain (see Chapter 29). High blood pressure in the pulmonary circulation (pulmonary hypertension) can cause pain during exercise that is often mistaken for cardiac pain (angina pectoris).

Pain in the chest wall is muscle pain or rib pain (costochondritis). The common causes of chest wall pain are excessive coughing, which makes the muscles sore, and rib fractures. Chest wall pain often mimics pleural pain.

Clubbing

Clubbing is the selective bulbous enlargement of the end (distal segment) of a digit (finger or toe) (Fig. 32-1) whose severity can be graded from 1 to 5 based on the extent of nail bed hypertrophy and the amount of changes in the nails themselves. Usually it is painless. Clubbing is commonly associated with diseases that interfere with oxygenation, such as bronchiectasis, cystic fibrosis, pulmonary fibrosis, lung abscess, and congenital heart disease. Lung cancer, especially of the small cell type, is sometimes associated with clubbing even in the absence of significant hypoxemia.[5] Its pathogenesis is unknown.

Abnormal Sputum

The color, consistency, odor, and amount of sputum vary with different pulmonary disorders. A distinctive color or odor may indicate infection by a specific microorganism. Changes in the amount and consistency of sputum provide information about progression of disease and effectiveness of therapy. The gross and microscopic appearances of sputum enable the clinician to identify cellular debris or microorganisms that aid in diagnosis and choice of therapy.

Conditions Caused by Pulmonary Disease or Injury

Hypercapnia

Hypercapnia, or increased carbon dioxide in the arterial blood (increased Pa_{CO_2}), is caused by hypoventilation of the alveoli. As discussed in Chapter 31, carbon dioxide is easily diffused from the blood into the alveolar space; thus minute volume (respiratory rate times tidal volume) determines not only alveolar ventilation but also Pa_{CO_2}. Hypoventilation is often overlooked because breathing pattern and ventilatory rate may appear normal; it is important to obtain blood gas analysis to determine the severity of hypercapnia and resultant respiratory acidosis (acid-base balance is described in Chapter 3).

There are many causes of hypercapnia. Most are a result of decreased drive to breathe or an inadequate ability to respond to ventilatory stimulation. Causes include (1) depression of the respiratory center by drugs; (2) diseases of the medulla, including infections of the central nervous system or trauma; (3) abnormalities of the spinal conducting pathways, as in spinal cord disruption or poliomyelitis; (4) diseases of the neuromuscular junction or of the respiratory muscles themselves, as in myasthenia gravis or muscular dystrophy; (5) thoracic cage abnormalities, as in chest injury or congenital deformity; (6) large airway obstruction, as in tumors or sleep apnea; and (7) increased work of breathing or physiologic dead space, as in emphysema.

Hypercapnia and the associated respiratory acidosis can result in several important clinical manifestations. Of greatest concern are electrolyte abnormalities that occur in response to the low pH that may cause dysrhythmias. Individuals also may have somnolence and even be in coma because of changes in intracranial pressure associated with high levels of arterial carbon dioxide, which causes cerebral vasodilation. Alveolar hyperventilation with increased alveolar carbon dioxide limits the amount of oxygen available for diffusion into the blood, leading to hypoxemia.

Hypoxemia

Hypoxemia, or reduced oxygenation of arterial blood (reduced Pa_{O_2}), is caused by respiratory alterations, whereas **hypoxia,** or reduced oxygenation of cells in tissues, may be caused by alterations of other systems as well. (Hypoxia can occur anywhere in the body; if it occurs in arterial blood, it is correctly called hypoxemia.) Although hypoxemia can lead to tissue hypoxia, tissue hypoxia can result from other abnormalities, such as low cardiac output or cyanide poisoning, that have no relation to alterations of pulmonary function.

The five causes of hypoxemia are (1) decreased oxygen content (P_{O_2}) of inspired gas, (2) hypoventilation, (3) diffusion abnormalities, (4) abnormal ventilation-perfusion ratios, and (5) pulmonary right-to-left shunt (Table 32-1). The physiologic mechanisms for each cause of hypoxemia are different, and each requires different clinical management.

The P_{O_2} of arterial blood depends on the P_{O_2} of inspired gas (P_{IO_2}). If the P_{O_2} of inspired gas is below normal, less

Table 32-1 Causes of Hypoxemia

Mechanism	Common Clinical Cause
Decrease in inspired oxygen	High altitude Low oxygen content of gas mixture Enclosed breathing spaces (suffocation)
Hypoventilation	Lack of neurologic stimulation of the respiratory center (oversedation, drug overdose, neurologic damage) Chronic obstructive pulmonary disease
Alveolocapillary diffusion abnormality	Emphysema Fibrosis Edema
Ventilation-perfusion mismatch	Asthma Chronic bronchitis Pneumonia
Shunting	Adult respiratory distress syndrome Respiratory distress syndrome of the newborn (hyaline membrane disease) Atelectasis

oxygen is available to diffuse into the blood. The most common cause of a decrease in inspired oxygen is the drop in atmospheric pressure that occurs at high altitudes. PIO_2 drops proportionately with atmospheric pressure, resulting in a decrease in PaO_2. Hypoxemia caused by high altitude is prevented by the use of supplemental oxygen.

Hypoventilation of the alveoli causes elevated $PaCO_2$ (hypercapnia). If oxygen-rich gas is not delivered to the alveoli, the oxygen content of alveolar gas (PAO_2) decreases as $PaCO_2$ increases. As PAO_2 decreases, less oxygen diffuses into the blood, causing hypoxemia. This type of hypoxemia can be completely corrected if alveolar ventilation is improved by increases in the rate and depth of breathing. Hypoventilation is a common cause of hypoxemia in unconscious persons, individuals receiving extensive sedation, and individuals who have COPD.

Diffusion of oxygen through the alveolocapillary membrane is impaired if the alveolocapillary membrane is thickened or the surface area available for diffusion is decreased. Abnormal thickness, as occurs with edema (tissue swelling) and fibrosis (formation of fibrous lesions), increases the time required for diffusion across the alveolocapillary membrane. If diffusion is slowed enough, the PO_2 of alveolar gas and capillary blood does not have time to equilibrate during the fraction of a second that blood remains in the capillary. Destruction of alveoli, such as that which occurs in emphysema, decreases the surface area available for diffusion. Hypercapnia is rarely produced by impaired diffusion because carbon dioxide diffuses so easily from capillary to alveolus that the individual with impaired diffusion would die from hypoxemia before hypercapnia could occur.

An abnormal ventilation-perfusion ratio ($\dot{V}/\dot{Q}$) is the most common cause of hypoxemia (Fig. 32-2). Normally, alveolocapillary lung units receive almost equal amounts of ventilation and perfusion. The normal $\dot{V}/\dot{Q}$ is 0.8 to 0.9 because perfusion is somewhat greater than ventilation in the lung bases. $\dot{V}/\dot{Q}$ mismatch refers to an abnormal distribution of ventilation and perfusion. Hypoxemia can be caused by inadequate ventilation of well-perfused areas of the lung (low $\dot{V}/\dot{Q}$). Blood passing through pulmonary capillaries is exposed to less oxygen than normal. Mismatching of this type is called *shunting* and occurs in asthma as a result of bronchoconstriction and in pulmonary edema and pneumonia when alveoli are filled with fluid. A pulmonary right-to-left shunt exists when blood passes through portions of the pulmonary capillary bed that receive no ventilation, either because the airway leading to the alveoli is completely obstructed or because the alveoli are collapsed or filled with fluid and cellular debris. Blood flows through the pulmonary circulation without being oxygenated. This results in decreased systemic PaO_2 and hypoxemia. $PaCO_2$ is usually not affected except by

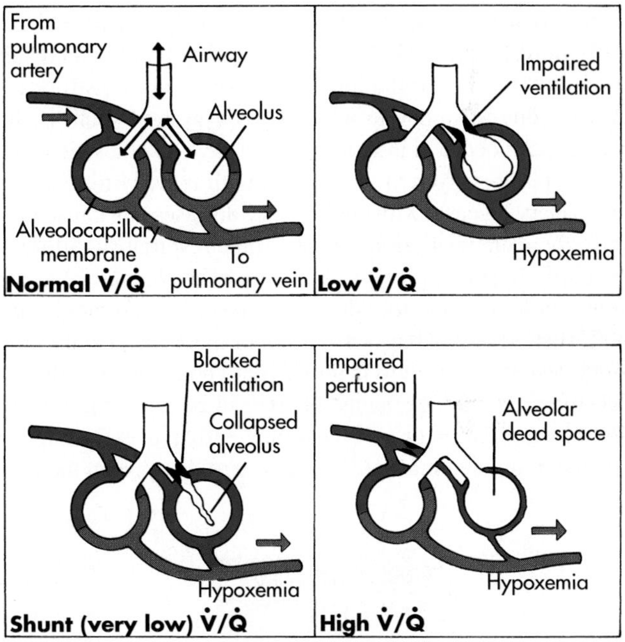

FIG. 32-2 Ventilation-perfusion abnormalities.

severe shunting. Hypoxemia resulting from shunting does not respond to increases in supplemental inspired oxygen concentration because a portion of the pulmonary capillary bed is never exposed to the oxygen-rich gas. This makes hypoxemia produced by shunting very difficult to treat. Shunting is the cause of hypoxemia in adult respiratory distress syndrome (ARDS) and respiratory distress syndrome of the newborn.

Hypoxemia also can be caused by poor perfusion of well-ventilated portions of the lung (high $\dot{V}/\dot{Q}$), resulting in wasted ventilation. In this case, oxygen in the alveoli is not exposed to circulating blood. The result is a decrease in Pa_{O_2}. The most common cause of high $\dot{V}/\dot{Q}$ is a pulmonary embolus that impairs blood flow to a segment of the lung. An area where alveoli are ventilated but not perfused is termed *alveolar dead space.*

Acute Respiratory Failure

Respiratory failure is defined as inadequate gas exchange, that is, hypoxemia, where $Pa_{O_2} \leq 50$ mm Hg or where $Pa_{CO_2} \geq 50$ mm Hg with pH ≤ 7.25. Respiratory failure can result from direct injury to the lungs, airways, or chest wall or indirectly due to injury to another body system such as the brain. It can occur in individuals who have an otherwise normal respiratory system or in those with underlying chronic pulmonary disease. Most pulmonary diseases can cause episodes of acute respiratory failure. If the respiratory failure is primarily hypercapnic, it is the result of inadequate alveolar ventilation and the individual must receive ventilatory support, such as with a bag-valve mask or mechanical ventilator. If the respiratory failure is primarily hypoxemic, it is the result of inadequate exchange of oxygen between the alveoli and the capillaries (see Hypoxemia, earlier in this chapter) and the individual must receive supplemental oxygen therapy. Many patients have a combined hypercapnic and hypoxemic respiratory failure and require both kinds of support.

Pulmonary Edema

Pulmonary edema is excess water in the lung. The normal lung contains very little water or fluid. It is kept dry by lymphatic drainage and a balance among capillary hydrostatic pressure, capillary oncotic pressure, and capillary permeability. In addition, surfactant lining the alveoli repels water, keeping fluid from entering the alveoli. Predisposing factors for pulmonary edema include heart disease, ARDS, and inhalation of toxic gases. The pathogenesis of pulmonary edema is shown in Fig. 32-3.

The most common cause of pulmonary edema is heart disease (see Chapter 29). When the left ventricle fails, filling pressures on the left side of the heart increase and cause a concomitant increase in pulmonary capillary hydrostatic pressure. When the hydrostatic pressure push exceeds oncotic pressure, which holds fluid in the capillary, fluid moves out into the interstitium, or interstitial space (the space within the alveolar septum between alveolus and capillary). Initially fluid is picked up by lymphatic vessels and removed from the lung. When the flow of fluid out of the capillaries exceeds the lymphatic system's ability to remove it, pulmonary edema develops.

Pulmonary edema usually begins to develop at a pulmonary capillary wedge pressure or left atrial pressure of 20 mm Hg. If the capillary oncotic pressure is decreased for any reason (e.g., anemia or decreased plasma proteins), pulmonary edema develops at a lower hydrostatic pressure. Individuals with chronically elevated hydrostatic pressure tend to develop pulmonary edema at higher left atrial pressures.

Another cause of pulmonary edema is capillary injury that increases capillary permeability. Capillary injury causes

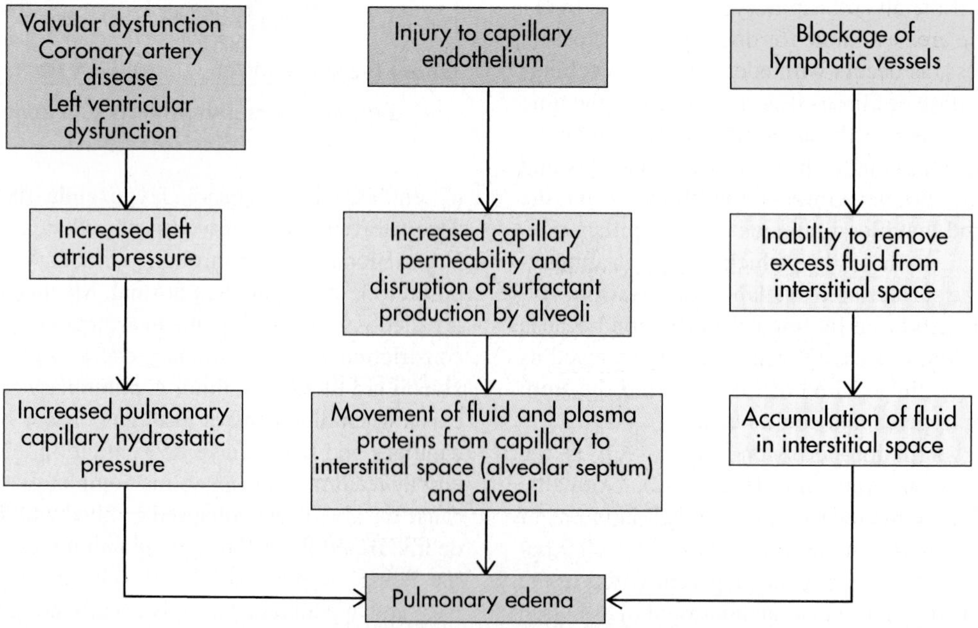

FIG. 32-3 Pathogenesis of pulmonary edema.

edema in cases of ARDS or inhalation of toxic gases, such as ammonia. Capillary injury causes water and plasma proteins to leak out of the capillary and move into the interstitium. When plasma proteins move into the lung interstitium, they increase the interstitial oncotic pressure, which is usually very low. As the interstitial oncotic pressure begins to equal capillary oncotic pressure, water moves out of the capillary and into the lung. (This phenomenon is discussed in Chapter 3, Fig. 3-1.)

Pulmonary edema also can result from obstruction of the lymphatic system. Drainage can be blocked by compression of lymphatic vessels, edema, tumors and fibrotic tissue, and increased systemic venous pressure that elevates hydrostatic pressure of the large pulmonary veins into which the pulmonary lymphatic system drains. This can happen in left-sided heart failure.

Clinical manifestations of pulmonary edema include dyspnea, orthopnea, hypoxemia, and increased work of breathing. Physical examination may reveal inspiratory crackles (rales), dullness to percussion over the lung bases, and evidence of ventricular dilatation (S_3 gallop and cardiomegaly). In severe edema, pink, frothy sputum is expectorated and P_{CO_2} increases.

The treatment of pulmonary edema depends on its cause. If the edema is caused by increased hydrostatic pressure, therapy is geared toward reducing blood pressure with diuretics, vasodilators, and drugs that improve the contraction of the heart muscle. If edema is the result of increased capillary permeability resulting from injury, the treatment is focused on removing the offending agent and supportive therapy to maintain adequate ventilation and circulation. Individuals with either type of pulmonary edema require supplemental oxygen. Mechanical ventilation also is used if edema significantly impairs ventilation and oxygenation.

Aspiration

Aspiration is the passage of fluid and solid particles into the lung. It tends to occur in individuals whose normal swallowing mechanism and cough reflex are impaired by a decreased level of consciousness or central nervous system abnormalities. Predisposing factors include altered level of consciousness caused by substance abuse, sedation, or anesthesia; seizure disorders; cerebrovascular accident; myasthenia gravis (a neuromuscular disorder); and Guillain-Barré syndrome (inflammation of the nerves). Aspiration is also common in children with tracheoesophageal fistula (a congenital abnormality in which the trachea and esophagus communicate; see Chapter 39). The right lung, particularly the right lower lobe, is more susceptible to aspiration than the left lung because the branching angle of the right main stem bronchus is straighter than the branching angle of the left main stem bronchus.

The effects of aspiration depend on the material aspirated. The aspiration of large food particles or gastric fluid with pH of less than 2.5 has serious consequences. Solid food particles can obstruct a bronchus, resulting in bronchial inflammation and collapse of airways distal to the obstruction. If the aspirated solid is not identified and removed by bronchoscopy, a chronic, local inflammation develops that may lead to recurrent infection and bronchiectasis (permanent dilation of the bronchus). Once the pathologic process has progressed to bronchiectasis, surgical resection of the affected area is usually required.

Aspiration of acidic gastric fluid may cause severe pneumonitis (localized lung inflammation). Bronchial damage includes inflammation, loss of ciliary function, and bronchospasm. In the alveoli, acidic fluid damages the alveolocapillary membrane. This allows plasma and blood cells to move from capillaries into the alveoli, resulting in hemorrhagic pneumonitis. The lung becomes stiff and noncompliant as surfactant production is disrupted, leading to further edema and collapse. Hypoventilation may develop as this progresses, and systematic complications, such as hypotension, may occur.

The clinical manifestations of aspiration include the sudden onset of choking and intractable cough with or without vomiting, fever, dyspnea, and wheezing. Some individuals have no symptoms acutely; instead they have recurrent lung infections, chronic cough, or persistent wheezing over months and even years.[6]

Preventive measures for individuals at risk are more effective than treatment of known aspiration. Individuals undergoing surgery do not receive food or fluid for several hours before surgery. Antacids are sometimes given to persons at risk to keep gastric pH above 2.5. Individuals who have difficulty swallowing are fed with extreme caution and positioned to minimize the likelihood of aspiration. Nasogastric tubes, which often are used to remove stomach contents, also can cause aspiration if fluid and particulate matter are regurgitated.

The rate of deaths resulting from aspiration-caused pneumonitis is greater than 50%. Treatment includes supplemental oxygen and mechanical ventilation with positive end-expiratory pressure (PEEP). Fluids are restricted to decrease blood volume and minimize pulmonary edema. Steroids often are administered during the first 72 hours after aspiration, although their effectiveness is not well documented. Bacterial pneumonia may develop as a complication of aspiration pneumonitis. If bacterial pneumonia occurs, it is treated with organism-specific antibiotics.

Atelectasis

Atelectasis is the collapse of lung tissue. The two types of atelectasis are compression and absorption:

1. **Compression atelectasis** is caused by the external pressure exerted by a tumor, fluid, or air in the pleural space or by an abdominal distention pressing on a portion of the lung, causing the alveoli to collapse.
2. **Absorption atelectasis** results from removal of air from obstructed or hypoventilated alveoli or from inhalation of concentrated oxygen or anesthetic agents.

Clinical manifestations of atelectasis are similar to those of pulmonary infection: dyspnea, cough, fever, and leukocytosis.

Atelectasis tends to occur after surgery. Intraoperative high-dose supplemental oxygen in combination with general anesthesia increases the likelihood of postoperative atelectasis.[7] In addition, individuals are often in pain, breathe shallowly, are reluctant to change position, and produce viscous secretions that tend to pool in dependent portions of the lung after surgical procedures, especially those involving the thorax or upper abdomen. Prevention and treatment of postoperative atelectasis usually include deep breathing (often with the aid of an incentive spirometer), frequent position changes, and early ambulation. Deep breathing is beneficial because it (1) promotes the ciliary clearance of secretions, (2) stabilizes the alveoli by redistributing surfactant, and (3) permits collateral ventilation of the alveoli through pores of Kohn in the alveolar septa. The pores of Kohn, which open only during deep breathing, allow air to pass from well-ventilated alveoli to obstructed alveoli, minimizing their tendency to collapse and facilitating obstruction removal (Fig. 32-4).

Bronchiectasis

Bronchiectasis is persistent abnormal dilation of the bronchi. It usually occurs in conjunction with other respiratory conditions and can be caused by obstruction of an airway with mucous plugs, atelectasis, aspiration of a foreign body, infection, cystic fibrosis, tuberculosis, congenital weakness of the bronchial wall, or impaired defense mechanisms. Bronchiectasis is also associated with a number or systemic disorders such as rheumatologic disease, inflammatory bowel disease, and acquired immunodeficiency syndrome (AIDS). The underlying cause of bronchiectasis is found in less than 40% of cases.[8] Bronchiectasis is frequently associated with inflammation of the bronchi **(bronchitis)** and has similar symptoms (see p. 1131).

Bronchial dilation (Fig. 32-5) may be **cylindrical,** with symmetrically dilated airways as is commonly seen after pneumonia and is reversible; **saccular,** in which the bronchi become large and balloonlike; or **varicose,** in which constrictions and dilations deform the bronchi. In both varicose and saccular bronchiectasis, the smaller bronchial divisions are plugged with secretions or obliterated by fibrosis. Large anastomoses (connections) develop between the bronchial and pulmonary blood vessels, increasing blood flow through the bronchial circulation. These anastomoses are thought to cause the hemoptysis experienced by individuals with bronchiectasis. Airway damage leads to bronchospasm and copious production of purulent mucus. Ventilation-perfusion abnormalities develop and result in hypoxemia. In severe cases, $Paco_2$ also may be elevated.

The symptoms of bronchiectasis may date back to a childhood illness or infection. The disease is commonly associated with recurrent lower respiratory tract infections and expectoration of voluminous amounts of purulent sputum (measured in cupfuls). If the individual is not receiving antibiotics, the sputum has a foul odor. Hemoptysis and clubbing of the fingers are common. Pulmonary function studies show decreases in vital capacity (VC) and expiratory flow rates. Bronchiectasis is often associated with bronchitis and atelectasis. Hypoxemia eventually leads to cor pulmonale (see p. 1134). The goals of treatment for bronchiectasis are removal of secretions and prevention of infection.

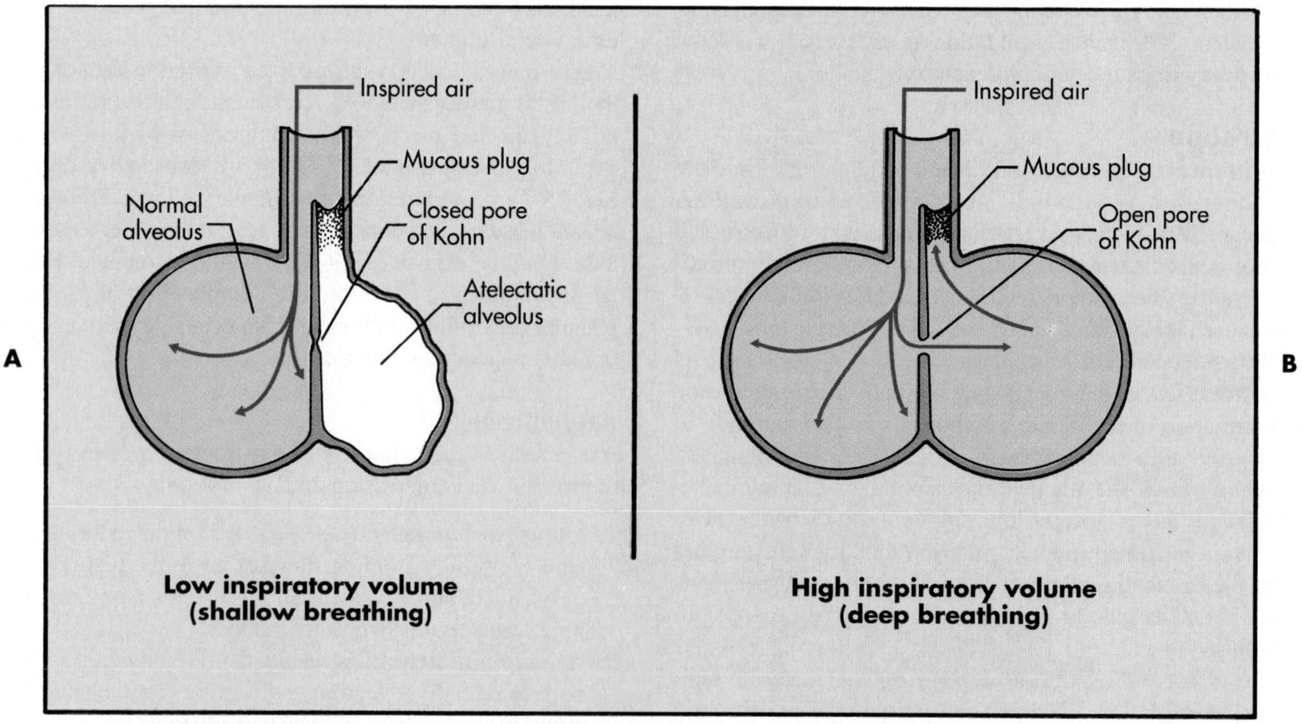

FIG. 32-4 Pores of Kohn. A, Absorption atelectasis caused by lack of collateral ventilation through pores of Kohn. **B,** Restoration of collateral ventilation during deep breathing.

Bronchiolitis

Bronchiolitis is an inflammatory obstruction of the small airways or bronchioles. It is most common in children (see Chapter 33). In adults it usually occurs with chronic bronchitis but can occur in otherwise healthy individuals in association with an infection or inhalation of toxic gases. Atelectasis or emphysematous destruction of the alveoli may develop distal to the inflammatory lesion. Bronchiolitis is usually diffuse. A decrease in the ventilation-perfusion ratio results in hypoxemia and carbon dioxide retention.

Bronchiolitis is often preceded by an upper respiratory infection. Manifestations include a rapid ventilatory rate; marked use of accessory muscles; low-grade fever; dry, nonproductive cough; and hyperinflated chest. If bronchiolitis is caused by an inhalation injury, pulmonary edema occurs rapidly and then quickly clears. One to two weeks later, respiratory distress develops, and infiltrates are seen on chest radiographs. Bronchiolitis is treated with appropriate antibiotics, steroids, and chest physical therapy (humidified air, coughing and deep breathing, postural drainage).

Bronchiolitis obliterans is a late-stage fibrotic process that occludes the airways and causes permanent scarring of the lungs. This process can occur in all causes of bronchiolitis but is most common after lung transplantation, where it affects almost 50% of recipients. Diagnosis is made by spirometry and bronchoscopy with biopsy. Treatment includes corticosteroids and other immunosuppressive agents.[9]

Pleural Abnormalities

Pneumothorax

Pneumothorax is the presence of air or gas in the pleural space caused by a rupture in the visceral pleura (which surrounds the lungs) or the parietal pleura and chest wall (see Chapter 31). As air separates the visceral and parietal pleurae, it destroys the negative pressure of the pleural space. This disrupts the state of equilibrium that normally exists between elastic recoil forces of the lung and chest wall. No longer held in check by the recoil forces of the chest wall, the lung fulfills its tendency to recoil by collapsing toward the hilus (Fig. 32-6).

In **open pneumothorax (communicating pneumothorax),** air pressure in the pleural space equals barometric pressure because air that is drawn into the pleural space during inspiration (through the damaged chest wall and parietal pleura or through the lungs and damaged visceral pleura) is forced back out during expiration. In **tension pneumothorax,** however, the site of pleural rupture acts as a one-way valve, permitting air to enter on inspiration but preventing its escape by closing up during expiration. As more and more air enters the pleural space, air pressure in the pneumothorax begins to exceed barometric pressure. The pathophysiologic effects of tension pneumothorax are life threatening. Air pressure in the pleural space pushes against the already recoiled lung, causing compression atelectasis, and against the mediastinum, compressing and displacing the heart and great vessels.

Spontaneous pneumothorax, which occurs unexpectedly in healthy individuals (usually men) between ages 20 and 40 years, is caused by the spontaneous rupture of blebs (blisterlike formations) on the visceral pleura. Bleb rupture can occur during sleep, rest, or exercise. The ruptured bleb or blebs are usually located in the apexes of the lungs. The cause of bleb formation is not known, although more than 80% of these individuals have been found to have emphysema-like changes in their lungs even if they have never smoked or have no known genetic disorder. Tension pneumothorax can develop with bleb rupture.

Clinical manifestations of spontaneous pneumothorax begin with sudden pleural pain, tachypnea, and possibly mild dyspnea. The manifestations depend on the size of the pneumothorax. If the pneumothorax is large or if there is a tension

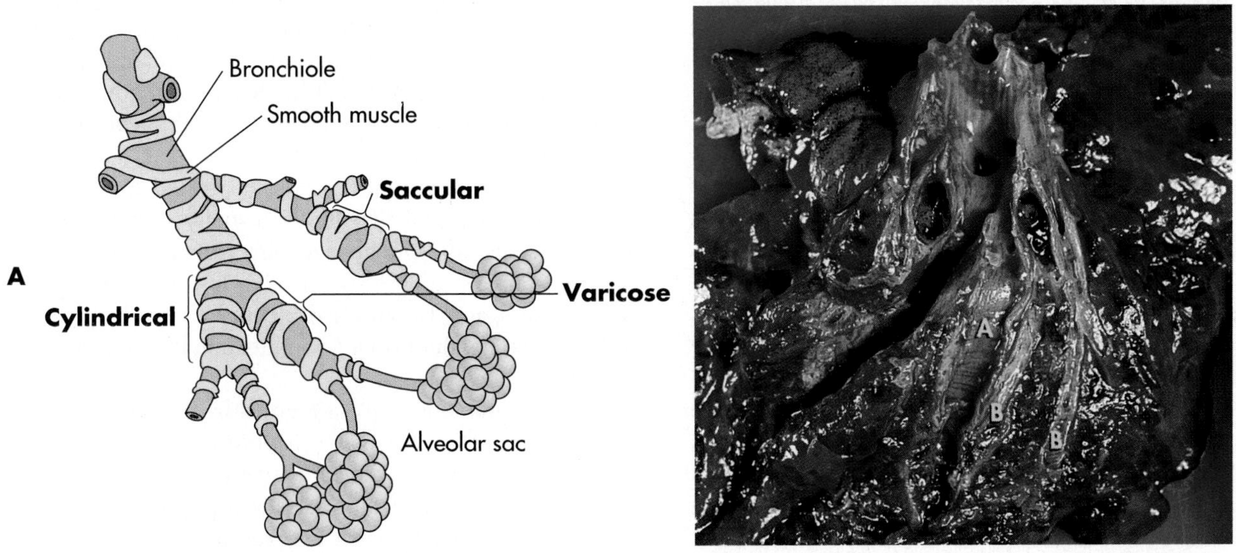

FIG. 32-5 Bronchiectasis. A, Types of bronchiectasis. **B,** Cylindrical bronchiectasis. The dilated bronchi **(A)** and bronchioles **(B)** can be dissected almost to the pleural surface. (**B,** From Damjanov I, Linder J, editors: *Anderson's pathology,* ed 10, St Louis, 1996, Mosby.)

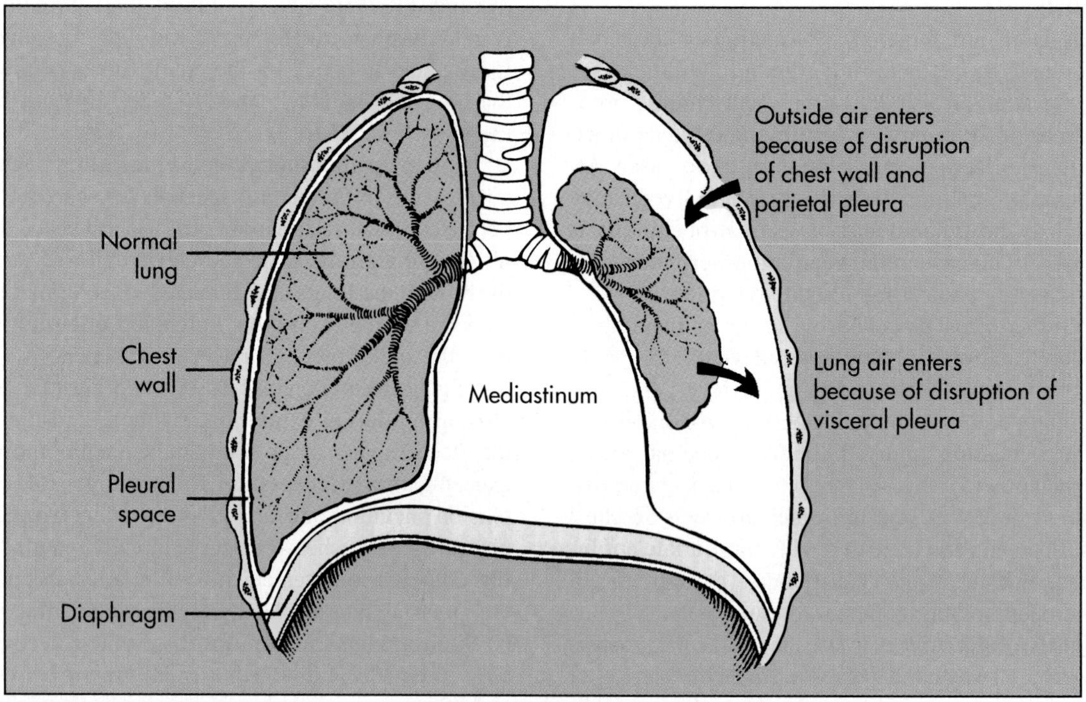

FIG. 32-6 Pneumothorax. Air in the pleural space causes the lung to collapse around the hilus and may push mediastinal contents (heart and great vessels) toward the other lung.

pneumothorax, it may push the mediastinum toward the unaffected lung, causing the chest to appear asymmetric. Hypoxemia may develop. Lung collapse causes diminished breath sounds over the affected lung. Diagnosis is made with chest radiographs. CT scanning is used after the individual is stabilized to determine the risk of recurrence. Small open pneumothorax can be managed with observation and supplemental oxygen or with simple aspiration using a small catheter.[10]

A **secondary pneumothorax** can be caused by chest trauma, such as a rib fracture or stab and bullet wounds that tear the pleura; rupture of a bleb or bulla (larger vesicle), as occurs in COPD; or mechanical ventilation, particularly if it includes PEEP.

The pathophysiology and clinical manifestations of secondary pneumothorax are similar to those of spontaneous pneumothorax. Occasionally air enters the mediastinum. Secondary pneumothorax (and other open pneumothoraces if large enough) is treated with a chest tube that is attached to a water-seal drainage system with suction. After the pneumothorax is evacuated and the pleural rupture is healed, the chest tube is removed.

Tension pneumothorax, in which air in the pleural space cannot escape through the rupture, is a life-threatening emergency. As increasing positive pressure in the pleural space compresses lung tissue and thoracic blood vessels, venous return and cardiac output decrease. Clinical manifestations of tension pneumothorax include severe hypoxemia, dyspnea, and hypotension (low blood pressure), as well as other signs and symptoms of pneumothorax. Deterioration occurs rapidly, and shock and bradycardia (reduced heart rate) may develop.

Tension pneumothorax requires immediate treatment. A chest tube is placed quickly, usually after physical examination alone. If a chest tube is not readily available, a large-bore needle is inserted into the pleural space to decompress it until a chest tube can be placed. An outward gush of air as the needle or chest tube is inserted confirms the presence of tension pneumothorax. The chest tube is connected to a water-seal drainage and suction until the damaged pleura is healed.

In some situations, the pleural tear does not heal spontaneously and it is necessary to prevent recurrence of the pneumothorax by a process called *pleurodesis.* This procedure uses the chest tube to instill a caustic substance, such as talc, into the pleural space. The resultant inflammation and scarring as the pleura heals result in closure of the pleural tear. Some individuals require thoracotomy with pleurectomy.

Pleural Effusion

Pleural effusion is the presence of fluid in the pleural space. The source of the fluid is usually blood vessels or lymphatic vessels lying beneath either pleura, but occasionally the source is an abscess or other lesion that drains into the pleural space. Because the pleura is a relatively permeable membrane, fluids that accumulate in the lung can cross into the pleural space.

Like pneumothorax, pleural effusion can cause compression atelectasis and displace mediastinal contents. Unlike pneumothorax, however, pleural effusion does not cause the lung to collapse as a result of elastic recoil. Because there is no communication between the pleural space and environmental air, pressure in the pleural space remains negative and atelectasis is caused solely by pressure exerted by the effusion.

Table 32-2 Mechanisms of Pleural Effusion

Type of Fluid/Effusion	Source of Accumulation	Primary or Associated Disorder
Transudate (hydrothorax)	Watery fluid that diffuses out of capillaries beneath the pleurae (i.e., capillaries in lung or chest wall)	Cardiovascular disease that causes high blood pressure; liver or kidney disease that disrupts plasma protein production, causing hypoproteinemia (decreased oncotic pressure in the blood vessels)
Exudate	Fluid rich in proteins (leukocytes, plasma proteins of all kinds; see Chapter 7) that migrates out of the capillaries	Infection, inflammation, or malignancy of the pleurae that stimulates mast cells to release biochemical mediators that increase capillary permeability
Empyema (pus)	Detritus of infection (microorganisms, leukocytes, cellular debris) dumped into the pleural space by blocked lymphatic vessels	Pulmonary infections, such as pneumonia; lung abscesses; infected wounds
Hemothorax (blood)	Hemorrhage into the pleural space	Traumatic injury, surgery, rupture, or malignancy that damages blood vessels
Chylothorax (chyle)	Chyle (milky fluid containing lymph and fat droplets) that is dumped by lymphatic vessels into the pleural space instead of passing from the gastrointestinal tract to the thoracic duct	Traumatic injury, infection, or disorder that disrupts lymphatic transport

NOTE: The principles of diffusion are discussed in Chapter 1; mechanisms that increase capillary permeability and cause exudation of cells and proteins are discussed in Chapter 7.

The most common mechanism of pleural effusion is migration of fluids and other blood components through the walls of intact capillaries bordering the pleura. Pleural effusions that enter the pleural space from the intact blood vessels can be transudative or exudative. In **transudative effusion,** the fluid, or transudate, is watery and diffuses out of the capillaries as a result of disorders that increase blood pressure or decrease capillary oncotic pressure. Examples are congestive heart failure, in which venous and left atrial pressures are increased, and liver or kidney disorders that cause hypoproteinemia. Hypoproteinemia decreases capillary oncotic pressure, which promotes diffusion of water out of the capillaries. (This mechanism is discussed in Chapter 3.)

Exudative effusion is less watery and contains high concentrations of white blood cells and plasma proteins. Exudative effusion occurs in response to inflammation, infection, or malignancy and involves inflammatory processes that increase capillary permeability (see Chapter 7). When stimulated by biochemical mediators of inflammation, junctions in the capillary endothelium separate slightly, enabling leukocytes and plasma proteins to migrate out into affected tissues. Mechanisms of pleural effusion are summarized in Table 32-2.

Small collections of fluid normally can be drained away by the lymphatics. Large effusions cause clinical manifestations related to their volume and the rate at which they accumulate in the pleural space. Dyspnea, compression atelectasis with impaired ventilation, and mediastinal shift occur with large effusions. Pleural pain is present if the pleura is inflamed, and cardiovascular manifestations occur in a large, rapidly developing **hemothorax** (hemorrhage into the pleural space). A pleural friction rub can be heard over areas of extensive effusion.

If the effusion is causing considerable impairment of pulmonary function, thoracentesis (needle aspiration) may be performed to drain the fluid from the pleural space. A pleural effusion can contain several liters of fluid.

Empyema

Empyema (infected pleural effusion), or the presence of pus in the pleural space, is a complication of respiratory infection, usually pneumonia caused by *Staphylococcus aureus, Escherichia coli,* anaerobic bacteria, or *Klebsiella pneumoniae* (*Staphylococcus* is responsible for more than 90% of empyemas in children). Empyema is thought to develop when the pulmonary lymphatics become blocked, leading to an outpouring of contaminated lymphatic fluid into the pleural space. They often occur adjacent to a pneumonia (parapneumonic) when the effusion becomes infected. Empyemas can occur also after thoracic surgery or in association with intraabdominal infection.

Individuals with empyema have clinical manifestations of toxicity, including cyanosis, fever, tachycardia (rapid heart rate), cough, and pleural pain. Breath sounds are decreased directly over the empyema. Diagnosis is made by chest radiographs and thoracentesis, although positive cultures from fluids are obtained only about 50% of the time. Therefore the offending microorganism is usually identified by its preponderance in a sputum culture.

The treatment for empyema is similar to that for pneumonia (see p. 1127). Antibiotics are given, and thoracentesis is performed to drain the pleural space. Chest tube placement with continuous drainage is often required.[11] In severe cases, surgical debridement of the pleural space is performed to prevent reaccumulation.

Pleurisy

Pleurisy (pleuritis) is inflammation of the pleura. Pleurisy causes the pleura to become reddened and covered with an exudate of lymph, fibrin, and cellular elements and may lead to pleural effusion. The most common signs and symptoms of pleurisy are chills, fever, and pain on inspiration. Often a pleural friction rub can be heard over the affected area. Pleurisy is frequently preceded by an upper respiratory infection.

Abscess Formation and Cavitation

An **abscess** is a circumscribed area of suppuration and destruction of lung parenchyma. Abscess formation follows **consolidation** of lung tissue, in which inflammation causes alveoli to fill with fluid, pus, and microorganisms. Necrosis (death and decay) of consolidated tissue may progress proximally until it communicates with a bronchus. If this occurs, the abscess empties into the bronchus, leaving a cavity that has a radiographic appearance similar to that of a lesion of tuberculosis. **Cavitation** is the process of abscess emptying and cavity formation. The diagnosis is made by radiography.

Pneumonia caused by aspiration, *Klebsiella,* or *Staphylococcus* is the most common cause of abscess formation. Aspiration abscess is usually associated with alcohol abuse, seizure disorders, general anesthesia, and swallowing disorders. The clinical manifestations of abscess formation are similar to those of pneumonitis: fever, cough, chills, sputum production, and pleural pain. Abscess communication with a bronchus causes a severe cough, copious amounts of often foul-smelling sputum, and occasionally hemoptysis.

Treatment includes the administration of appropriate antibiotics and chest physical therapy, including chest percussion and postural drainage. Sometimes bronchoscopy is performed to drain the abscess. Mortality rates are influenced by the severity of the primary disease that initially caused consolidation and by the virulence of the causative microorganism. Overall, the mortality rate for lung abscess remains at about 20% but can be as high as 50% when *Staphylococcus aureus* is the causative microorganism.[12]

Pulmonary Fibrosis

Pulmonary fibrosis is an excessive amount of fibrous or connective tissue in the lung. It can be caused by healing (formation of scar tissue) after active disease (e.g., ARDS, tuberculosis) or by inhalation of harmful substances (e.g., coal dust, asbestos). When no cause for the development of fibrosis is known, it is called *idiopathic pulmonary fibrosis.*

Fibrosis causes a marked loss of lung compliance. The lung becomes stiff and difficult to ventilate, and the diffusing capacity of the alveolocapillary membrane may decrease, causing hypoxemia. Diffuse pulmonary fibrosis has a poor prognosis, with a median survival of less than 5 years despite treatment with corticosteroids.[13]

Chest Wall Restriction

If the chest wall is deformed, immobilized, or made heavy by fat, the work of breathing is increased and ventilation may be compromised due to a decrease in tidal volume. The degree of ventilatory impairment depends on the severity of the chest wall abnormality. Grossly obese individuals are often dyspneic on exertion or when recumbent. Individuals with severe kyphoscoliosis (lateral bending and rotation of the spinal column, with distortion of the thoracic cage) often have dyspnea on exertion that can progress to respiratory failure. Such individuals are also susceptible to lower respiratory tract infections. Both obesity and kyphoscoliosis are risk factors for respiratory disease in individuals admitted to a hospital for other problems, particularly those who require surgery. Other musculoskeletal abnormalities that can impair ventilation are ankylosing spondylitis (rheumatoid arthritis of the spine; see Chapters 41 and 42) and pectus excavatum, or funnel chest (a deformity characterized by depression of the sternum).

Impairment of respiratory muscle function caused by neuromuscular disease also can restrict the chest wall or impair pulmonary function. Muscle weakness can result in hypoventilation, inability to remove secretions, and hypoxemia. The most common cause of hospital admission for individuals with neuromuscular diseases such as poliomyelitis, muscular dystrophy, myasthenia gravis, and Guillain-Barré syndrome is respiratory difficulty. (See Unit V for a more complete discussion of these disorders.)

Flail Chest

Flail chest results from the fracture of several consecutive ribs in more than one place, or the fracture of the sternum plus several consecutive ribs. These multiple fractures result in instability of a portion of the chest wall, causing paradoxic movement of the chest with breathing. During inspiration the unstable portion of the chest wall moves inward, and during expiration it moves outward, impairing movement of gas in and out of the lungs (Fig. 32-7).

The clinical manifestations of flail chest are pain, dyspnea, unequal chest expansion, hypoventilation, and hypoxemia. Treatment is internal fixation by controlled mechanical ventilation until the chest wall has stabilized.

Inhalation Disorders

Exposure to Toxic Gases

Inhalation of gaseous irritants can cause significant respiratory dysfunction. Commonly encountered toxic gases include smoke, ammonia, hydrogen chloride, sulfur dioxide,

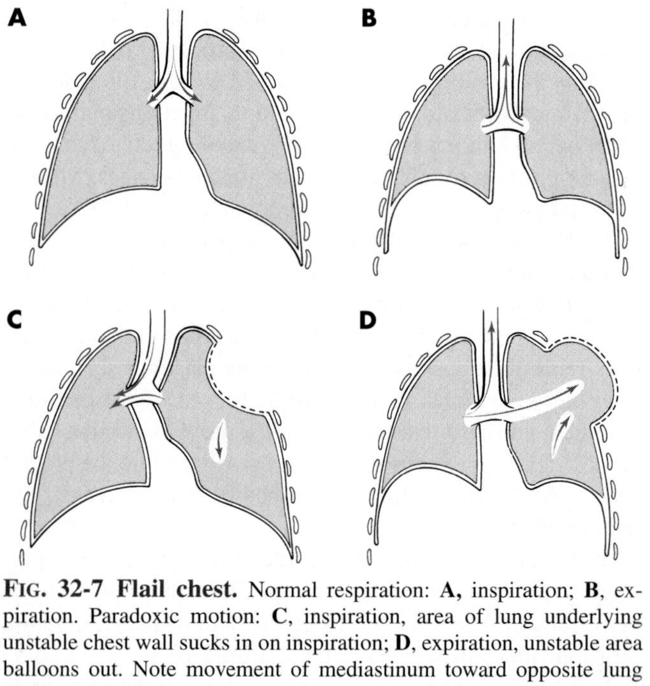

FIG. 32-7 Flail chest. Normal respiration: **A,** inspiration; **B,** expiration. Paradoxic motion: **C,** inspiration, area of lung underlying unstable chest wall sucks in on inspiration; **D,** expiration, unstable area balloons out. Note movement of mediastinum toward opposite lung during inspiration.

chlorine, phosgene, and nitrogen dioxide. Inhalation of a toxic gas results in severe inflammation of the airways, alveolar and capillary damage, and pulmonary edema. (The cellular effects of toxic gases are described in Chapter 2.) Initial symptoms include burning of the eyes, nose, and throat; coughing; chest tightness; and dyspnea. Hypoxemia is common. Treatment includes supplemental oxygen, mechanical ventilation with PEEP, and support of the cardiovascular system. Steroids sometimes are used, although their effectiveness has not been well documented. Most individuals respond quickly to therapy. Some, however, may improve initially and then deteriorate as a result of bronchiectasis or bronchiolitis (inflammation of the bronchioles).

Prolonged exposure to high concentrations of supplemental oxygen can result in a relatively rare iatrogenic condition known as **oxygen toxicity.** Although there is great individual variation in susceptibility to oxygen toxicity, generally the higher the concentration and longer the exposure, the more likely the occurrence of toxicity. Oxygen concentrations of 50% to 75% for greater than 24 to 48 hours have been associated with injury to cells of the lungs. The basic underlying mechanism of injury is a severe inflammatory response mediated primarily by oxygen radicals. The result is damage to alveolocapillary membranes, disruption of surfactant production, interstitial and alveolar edema, and decrease in compliance. Toxicity is often undetected because it occurs in individuals who are already in acute respiratory failure. Clinical manifestations are indistinguishable from those of ARDS. Treatment involves ventilatory support and reduction of inspired oxygen concentration to less than 60% as soon as tolerated by the individual. Other treatments being studied include the administration of antioxidants and surfactant.[14]

Pneumoconiosis

Pneumoconiosis represents any change in the lung caused by inhalation of inorganic dust particles, usually in the workplace. As in all cases of environmentally acquired lung disease, the individual's history of exposure is important in determining the diagnosis. Pneumoconiosis often occurs after years of exposure to the offending dust, and manifestations are often difficult to differentiate from those resulting from smoking.

The dusts of silica, asbestos, and coal are the most common causes of pneumoconiosis. Others include talc, fiberglass, clays, mica, slate, cement, cadmium, beryllium, tungsten, cobalt, aluminum, and iron. No matter what the substance, the dust deposits are permanent. Treatment therefore is palliative and focuses on preventing further exposure and improving working conditions.

Silicosis is a type of pneumoconiosis resulting from the inhalation of free silica (silicon dioxide) and silica-containing compounds. Silica exposure causes acute inflammation and chronic fibrosis of the lung tissue and has been shown to result in apoptosis of lung cells.[15] The silica produces fibrous nodules within the lung. Exposed individuals usually remain asymptomatic long after the nodules are visible on chest radiography. When clinical manifestations do appear, they include cough and dyspnea. Silicosis is also a predisposing factor for lower respiratory tract infection. There is no specific treatment for the disease, although corticosteroids may produce some improvement. Silica exposure occurs in mining and other industries involved with the extraction and processing of ores; preparation and use of sand; and manufacture of pipe, building, and roofing materials.

Coal worker pneumoconiosis (coal miner lung, black lung) is caused by coal dust deposits in the lung. Its mild form is asymptomatic, except for possible chronic bronchitis. Its advanced form consists of severe pulmonary fibrosis. Individuals usually are seen with a productive cough and wheezing. Symptoms are more severe with advanced disease and mimic those of chronic bronchitis (see p. 1124). Diagnosis is made by history of exposure and characteristic chest radiographs. There is no specific treatment for coal worker pneumoconiosis. Individuals with the mild form of the disease usually do well. Those with more complicated forms often develop marked cardiopulmonary dysfunction.

Asbestos exposure affects not only factory workers but also individuals who live in areas of asbestos emission. Asbestos exposure can result in a type of pulmonary fibrosis called **asbestosis** or in tumor formation, depending on the amount of exposure. It is caused by inhalation of hydrous silicates of various metals in fibrous form. Asbestos fibers cause inflammation, release of toxic oxygen radicals, and cellular apoptosis leading to both fibrosis and cancers such as mesothelioma.[16] The most prominent clinical manifestations of fibrosis are dyspnea on exertion, a nonproductive cough, hypoxemia, and decreased lung volume. Progressive disease may lead to respiratory failure and cardiac complications. Asbestos workers who smoke have a marked increase in risk for developing bronchogenic cancer (see p. 1136).

Allergic Alveolitis

Inhalation of organic dusts can result in an allergic inflammatory response called **extrinsic allergic alveolitis (hypersensitivity pneumonitis).** Many allergens can cause this disorder, including grains, silage, bird droppings or feathers, wood dust (particularly redwood and maple), cork dust, animal pelts, coffee beans, fish meal, mushroom compost, and molds that grow on sugar cane, barley, and straw. The lung inflammation, or pneumonitis, occurs after repeated, prolonged exposure to the allergen.

Allergic alveolitis can be acute, subacute, or chronic. The acute form causes a fever, cough, dyspnea, and chills a few hours after exposure that resolve without treatment in 1 to 3 days. With continued exposure, the disease becomes chronic and pulmonary fibrosis develops. (The mechanisms of hypersensitivity reactions are discussed in Chapter 8.) Chronic allergic alveolitis causes weight loss, fever, fatigue, and gradually progressive respiratory failure. Diagnosis is made by serum antibody testing, chest x-ray, bronchoscopy, and CT.[17]

Systemic Disorders

Several systemic diseases affect the airways, pleurae, or lung parenchyma, causing fibrosis, vasculitis, pulmonary hemorrhage, or granuloma formation. Clinical manifestations of lung involvement are usually nonspecific, and the diagnosis is based on involvement of other organs. There is usually no specific treatment, although corticosteroids frequently are used. Some of the systemic diseases affecting the lung are granulomatous disorders such as sarcoidosis, Wegener granulomatosis, lymphomatoid granulomatosis, and eosinophilic granuloma; connective tissue diseases such as rheumatoid disease, systemic lupus erythematosus, scleroderma, polymyositis or dermatomyositis, Sjögren syndrome, and polyarteritis nodosa; angioimmunoblastic or immunoblastic lymphadenopathy, a disease of the lymph nodes; cystic fibrosis (see Chapter 33); and Goodpasture syndrome, a renal disorder.

PULMONARY DISORDERS

Adult Respiratory Distress Syndrome

Adult respiratory distress syndrome (ARDS) is a fulminant form of respiratory failure characterized by acute lung inflammation and diffuse alveolocapillary injury. Identified within the past 25 years, the syndrome affects an estimated 200,000 to 250,000 people per year in the United States. Advances in therapy have decreased the overall mortality rate to

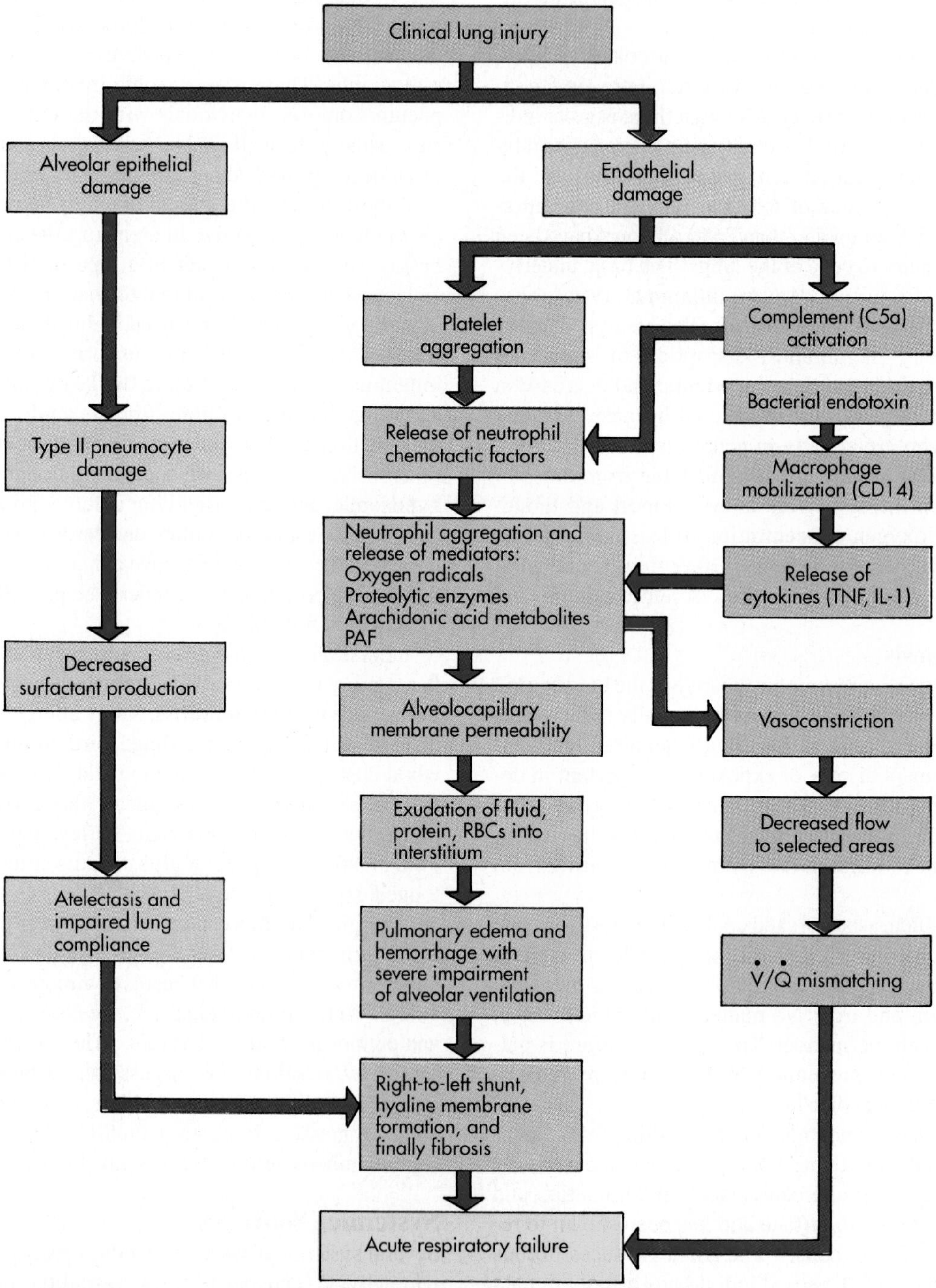

FIG. 32-8 Pathogenesis of adult respiratory distress syndrome (ARDS). *TNF,* Tumor necrosis factor; *IL-1,* interleukin-1; *PAF,* platelet-activating factor; *RBCs,* red blood cells.

less than 40%, although older people and those with severe infections continue to have a much higher mortality rate.[18] Most survivors, however, have almost normal lung function 1 year after the acute illness. ARDS is the result of injury to the lung by numerous unrelated causes. The most common predisposing factors are sepsis and multiple trauma (especially when multiple transfusions are received); however, there are many other causes, including pneumonia, burns, aspiration, cardiopulmonary bypass surgery, pancreatitis, drug overdose, smoke or noxious gas inhalation, oxygen toxicity, radiation therapy, and disseminated intravascular coagulation.[18]

Pathophysiology

All disorders that result in ARDS acutely injure the alveolocapillary membrane and cause severe pulmonary edema (Fig. 32-8). The alveolocapillary damage can occur directly, as with the aspiration of highly acidic gastric contents or inhalation of toxic gases, or indirectly from chemical mediators released in response to systemic disorders, as with sepsis and trauma. Whether the damage is direct or indirect, the common pathway for alveolocapillary membrane injury is a massive inflammatory response by the lungs. Several cell types and inflammatory mediators play key roles in the lung injury. The most important of these are neutrophils, macrophages, complement, endotoxin, interleukin-1 (IL-1), and tumor necrosis factor (TNF).[19,20]

The initial injury to the lungs damages the pulmonary capillary endothelium, activating complement and stimulating platelet aggregation, and intravascular thrombus formation. Platelets release substances that attract and activate neutrophils. In ARDS caused by sepsis, endotoxin (lipopolysaccharide [LPS]) is recognized by the CD14 receptor on macrophages and results in chemotaxis of large numbers of neutrophils to the lungs. A cascade of inflammatory mediators is released by the macrophages, including TNF, IL-1, alpha and beta chemokines, and other interleukins.[20]

The role of neutrophils is central to the development of ARDS. Activated neutrophils release a battery of inflammatory mediators, among them proteolytic enzymes, oxygen free radicals (superoxide radicals, hydrogen peroxide, hydroxyl radicals), arachidonic acid metabolites (prostaglandins, thromboxanes, leukotrienes), and platelet-activating factor. These mediators cause extensive damage of the alveolocapillary membrane and greatly increase capillary membrane permeability.

Increased capillary permeability, a hallmark of ARDS, allows fluids, proteins, and blood cells to leak from the capillary bed into the pulmonary interstitium and alveoli. The resulting pulmonary edema and hemorrhage severely reduce lung compliance and impair alveolar ventilation (Fig. 32-9).

Mediators released by neutrophils, and to a certain extent by macrophages, also cause pulmonary vasoconstriction. Pulmonary hypertension occurs early in the course of the disease secondary to vasoconstriction and to vascular occlusion by aggregated neutrophils, macrophages, and platelets. Because vasoconstriction occurs more in some vascular beds than others, there is decreased blood flow to selected areas of the lungs resulting in $\dot{V}/\dot{Q}$ mismatching.

The initial lung injury damages the alveolar epithelium and the vascular endothelium. Surfactant is inactivated, and its production by type II alveolar cells is impaired as alveoli and respiratory bronchioles fill with fluid or collapse. The lungs become less compliant, resulting in decreased ventilation of alveoli, right-to-left shunting of pulmonary blood flow, and increased work of breathing.

Twenty-four to forty-eight hours after the acute, hemorrhagic phase of ARDS, hyaline membranes form, and after approximately 7 days, fibrosis progressively obliterates the alveoli, respiratory bronchioles, and interstitium. This leads to a decrease in functional residual capacity (FRC) and even more severe right-to-left shunting. The result of this overwhelming inflammatory response by the lungs is acute respiratory failure.

The chemical mediators responsible for the alveolocapillary damage of ARDS often cause widespread inflammation, endothelial damage, and capillary permeability throughout the body resulting in the systemic inflammatory response syndrome (SIRS), which then leads to multiple organ dysfunction syndrome (MODS). In fact, death may not be caused by respiratory failure alone but by MODS associated with ARDS. (MODS is discussed in Chapter 45.)

Clinical Manifestations

The classic signs and symptoms of ARDS are rapid, shallow breathing; respiratory alkalosis; marked dyspnea; decreased lung compliance; hypoxemia unresponsive to oxygen therapy (refractory hypoxemia); and diffuse alveolar infiltrates seen on chest radiographs, without evidence of cardiac disease. Symptoms develop as the disease progresses. Initially individuals hyperventilate, causing respiratory alkalosis. As the work of breathing increases because of the decrease in compliance caused by alveolar filling and collapse, the individual

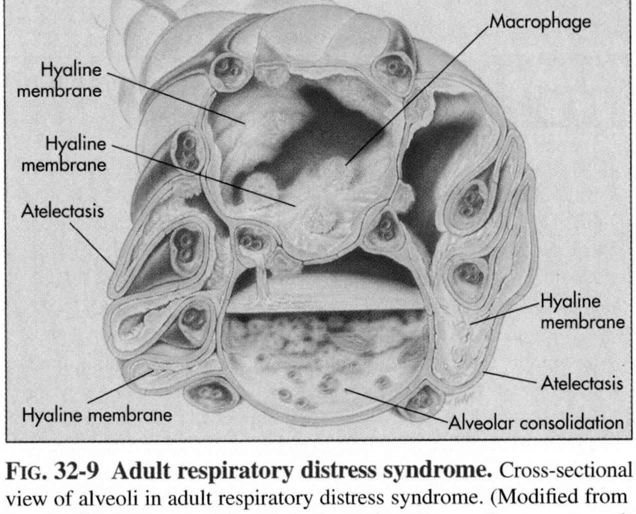

FIG. 32-9 Adult respiratory distress syndrome. Cross-sectional view of alveoli in adult respiratory distress syndrome. (Modified from Des Jardins T, Burton GG: *Clinical manifestations and assessment of respiratory disease*, ed 3, St Louis, 1995, Mosby.)

experiences dyspnea and hypoxemia. Hypoxemia worsens despite oxygen therapy, and diffuse crackles can be heard on auscultation. Eventually metabolic acidosis develops because of the increased work of breathing and cellular hypoxia, and fluffy infiltrates appear on chest radiograhs. If ARDS is not reversed, respiratory acidosis develops and further hypoxemia results in hypotension, decreased cardiac output, and death. The clinical course of progressive ARDS can be summarized as follows: hyperventilation → respiratory alkalosis → dyspnea and hypoxemia → metabolic acidosis → respiratory acidosis → further hypoxemia → hypotension, decreased cardiac output → death.

Evaluation and Treatment

Diagnosis is made on the basis of physical examination, analysis of blood gases, and radiologic examination. Initial physical examination may show fine crackles, and the chest film may be clear or show a few scattered infiltrates. With progressive respiratory involvement, crackles are heard throughout the lungs and radiographs show extensive bilateral infiltrates. The criteria for diagnosis of ARDS were established in 1994 and include refractory hypoxemia, a chest x-ray with bilateral infiltrates, and the exclusion of cardiogenic pulmonary edema.[21] Further diagnostic testing may include CT of the chest and bronchoscopy.[22]

Treatment is based on early detection, supportive therapy, and prevention of complications. Traditional therapy involves mechanical ventilation with PEEP and high oxygen concentrations. Numerous alternative modalities of ventilation are being tested, including noninvasive positive pressure ventilation, permissive hypercapnia, prone positioning, extracorporeal gas exchange, and partial liquid ventilation; some of these methods have shown apparent reductions in mortality rates.[23,24] Sedation may be employed to decrease oxygen consumption. If necessary, drugs are given to increase cardiac output. Steroid administration remains controversial because it has not been demonstrated to alter the outcome of ARDS.

Many studies are underway investigating new ways to prevent or treat ARDS. Prophylactic immunotherapy, antibodies against endotoxin, antioxidants, surfactant replacement, nitric oxide inhalation, and inhibition of various inflammatory mediators are among the possibilities being tested.[22,25]

WHAT'S NEW? The Role of Nitric Oxide in Adult Lung Disease

Nitric oxide (NO) is a gaseous molecule that has many effects in the normal lung, including vasodilation and bronchodilation. Changes in NO production have been implicated in many lung disease processes. Decreased production of NO by the pulmonary vascular endothelium results in vasoconstriction in both primary and secondary forms of pulmonary hypertension (e.g., individuals with COPD and cor pulmonale produce only 50% of the normal amount of NO). Although its role is less clear in the pathogenesis of asthma, it has been suggested that NO may potentiate bronchoconstriction and airway remodeling. NO also has been implicated in inflammatory lung injury such as that seen in acute respiratory distress syndrome. Nitric oxide inhalation as therapy is being studied in all of these diseases.

Data from Hart HC: Nitric oxide in adult lung disease, *Chest* 115(5): 1407, 1999.

Postoperative Respiratory Failure

Although usually not as severe as ARDS, postoperative respiratory failure can result in the same pathophysiology and clinical manifestations as ARDS. Smokers are at risk, particularly if they have preexisting lung disease. Limited cardiac reserve, chronic renal failure, chronic hepatic disease, and infection also increase the tendency to develop postoperative respiratory failure. Surgical procedures involving the thorax or abdomen carry the greatest risk.

The most common postoperative pulmonary problems are atelectasis, pneumonia, pulmonary edema, and pulmonary emboli. These problems usually result in reduced FRC, decreased compliance, and ventilation-perfusion mismatch. Individuals in whom respiratory failure develops usually have had a period of hypotension during surgery, and many have sepsis.

Prevention of postoperative respiratory failure includes frequent turning, deep breathing, and early ambulation to prevent atelectasis and accumulation of secretions. Humidification of inspired air can help loosen secretions. Incentive spirometry gives individuals immediate feedback about tidal volumes, which encourages them to breathe deeply. Supplemental oxygen is given for hypoxemia, and antibiotics are given as appropriate to treat infection. If respiratory failure develops, the individual may require mechanical ventilation for a time. Treatment is then similar to that for ARDS.

Obstructive Pulmonary Disease

Obstructive pulmonary disease is characterized by airway obstruction that is worse with expiration. Either more force (i.e., use of accessory muscles of expiration) is required to expire a given volume of air or emptying of the lungs is slowed or both. The unifying symptom of obstructive pulmonary disease is dyspnea; the unifying sign is wheezing. Individuals have an increased work of breathing, ventilation-perfusion mismatching, and a decreased forced expiratory volume in one second (FEV_1). The most common obstructive diseases are asthma, chronic bronchitis, and emphysema. Because many individuals have both chronic bronchitis and emphysema, these diseases together are often called chronic obstructive pulmonary disease (COPD). Asthma is more acute and intermittent than COPD, even though it can be chronic (Fig. 32-10).

Asthma

Asthma is defined as

> a chronic inflammatory disorder of the airways in which many cells and cellular elements play a role, in particular, mast cells, eosinophils, T lymphocytes, macrophages, neutrophils, and epithelial cells. In susceptible individuals, this inflammation causes recurrent episodes of wheezing, breathlessness, chest tightness, and coughing, particularly at night

or in the early morning. These episodes are usually associated with widespread but variable airflow obstruction that is often reversible, either spontaneously or with treatment. The inflammation also causes an associated increase in the existing bronchial hyperresponsiveness to a variety of stimuli. Subbasement membrane fibrosis may occur in some patients with asthma and these changes contribute to persistent abnormalities of lung function (reference 26, p. 8).

Most attacks of asthmatic bronchospasm are short lived, with freedom from symptoms between episodes. However, airway inflammation is present even in asymptomatic individuals.

Asthma occurs at all ages, with approximately half of all cases developing during childhood and another third before age 40. It has been estimated that approximately 5% of adults and 7% to 10% of children in the United States have asthma.[27] Despite the recent increased numbers and availability of antiasthma drugs, asthma morbidity and mortality have risen in the past 20 years. Asthma is a familial disorder, and there is increasing evidence that genetics play an important and complex role in the etiology of the disease. It is likely that genes are inherited for increased interleukin 4 (IL-4) and immunoglobulin E (IgE) responses to allergens, and for bronchial hyperresponisveness.[28] Apparently, environmental factors interact with inherited factors to increase the risk of asthma and to cause attacks of bronchospasm. For example, childhood exposure to high levels of allergens in the environment, cigarette smoke, air pollution, or respiratory viruses is associated with an increased likelihood of

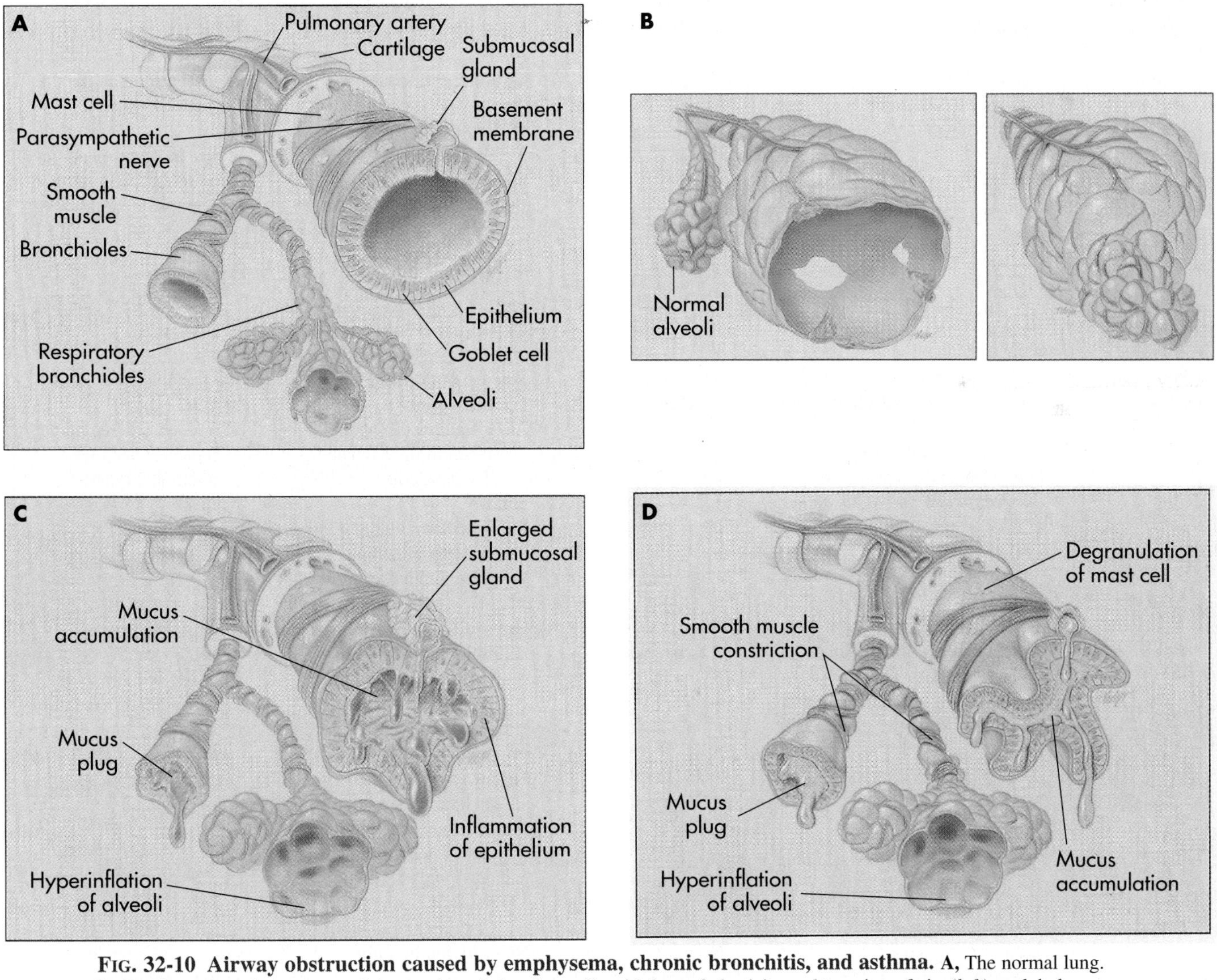

FIG. 32-10 Airway obstruction caused by emphysema, chronic bronchitis, and asthma. A, The normal lung. **B,** Emphysema: enlargement and destruction of alveolar walls with loss of elasticity and trapping of air; *(left)* panlobular emphysema showing abnormal weakening and enlargement of all air spaces distal to the terminal bronchioles (normal alveoli shown for comparison only); *(right)* centrilobular emphysema showing abnormal weakening and enlargement of the respiratory bronchioles in the proximal portion of the acinus. **C,** Chronic bronchitis: inflammation and thickening of mucous membrane with accumulation of mucus and pus leading to obstruction; characterized by cough. **D,** Bronchial asthma: thick mucus, mucosal edema, and smooth muscle spasm causing obstruction of small airways; breathing becomes labored and expiration is difficult. (Modified from Des Jardins T, Burton GG: *Clinical manifestations and assessment of respiratory disease,* ed 3, St Louis, 1995, Mosby.)

developing asthma, especially in those children with a family history of asthma.[29-31] The severity of acute asthma attacks varies among individuals, over time, and with the degree of exposure to inciting factors.

Types of Asthma

Asthma classification has changed in recent years. Many references still refer to extrinsic and intrinsic asthma based on whether the inflammation and airway hyperresponsiveness are mediated by IgE (atopic). Recently, a consensus was reached for a system of asthma classification based on clinical severity rather than on underlying pathophysiologic differences (Table 32-3); this scheme correlates better with management choices and clinical outcomes.[26]

Pathophysiology

Inflammation resulting in hyperresponsiveness of the airways is the major pathologic feature of asthma. IgE and irritant-mediated mast cell degranulation (see Chapter 8) causes the release of a large number of inflammatory mediators, such as histamine, prostaglandins, and leukotrienes.[32] In addition, chemotactic factors are produced that result in bronchial infiltration by neutrophils, eosinophils, and lymphocytes. The resulting inflammatory process produces bronchial smooth muscle spasm, vascular congestion, increased vascular permeability, edema formation, production of thick tenacious mucus, impaired mucociliary function (see Fig. 32-10), thickening of airway walls, and increased contractile response of

Table 32-3 Asthma Classification Based on Severity

Disease Category	Symptoms	Nocturnal Symptoms	Daily Medication for Long-Term Control	Medication for Quick Relief
Step 4: Severe persistent	Continual symptoms Limited physical activity Frequent exacerbations	Frequent	**Two daily medications:** Antiinflammatory agent (high-dose) inhaled glucocorticoid **and** Long-acting bronchodilator (inhaled or oral beta$_2$-agonist or theophylline) **and** Oral glucocorticoid	Short-acting, inhaled beta$_2$-agonist Daily use or increasing use indicates need for additional long-term therapy
Step 3: Moderate persistent	Daily symptoms Daily use of inhaled, short-acting beta$_2$-agonist Exacerbations affect activity Exacerbations at least twice weekly and may last for days	More frequent than once weekly	**One or two daily medications:** Antiinflammatory agent (medium-dose inhaled glucocorticoid) **and/or** Medium-dose inhaled glucocorticoid plus long-acting bronchodilator	Short-acting, inhaled beta$_2$-agonist Daily use or increased use indicates need for additional long-term therapy
Step 2: Mild persistent	Symptoms more frequent than twice weekly but less than once per day Exacerbations may affect activity	More frequent than twice monthly	**One-daily medication:** Antiinflammatory agent (low-dose inhaled glucocorticoid, cromolyn, or nedocromil) **or** Sustained-release theophylline NOTE: Leukotriene modifiers may be considered for individuals at least 12 yr old	Short-acting, inhaled beta$_2$-agonist Daily use or increasing use indicates need for additional long-term therapy
Step 1: Mild intermittent	Symptoms no more frequent than twice weekly Asymptomatic and with normal PEFR between exacerbations Exacerbations brief (hours to days) Intensity of exacerbations varies	No more frequent than twice monthly	**No daily medication**	Short-acting, inhaled beta$_2$-agonist Use more than twice weekly may indicate need to initiate long-term therapy

PEFR, Peak expiratory flow rate.

bronchial smooth muscle. Other inflammatory cytokines, such as TNF and IL-1, have been found to alter muscarinic receptor function leading to increased levels of acetylcholine, which causes bronchial smooth muscle contraction and mucus secretion. These changes, combined with the epithelial cell damage caused by eosinophil infiltration, produce acute airway hyperreponsiveness and obstruction. In cases of significant allergen exposure, symptoms can recur 4 to 12 hours after the initial attack due to persistent eosinophil and lymphocyte activation. This is called the *late asthma response,* and it can be even more severe than the initial attack. Recent studies have identified important roles for nitric oxide and reduced airway pH in the pathogenesis of asthma and airway inflammation.[33-35] Untreated inflammation can lead to long-term airway damage that is irreversible (airway remodeling).[32,36]

Airway obstruction increases resistance to airflow and decreases flow rates, including expiratory flow. Impaired expiration causes hyperinflation distal to obstructions, altered pulmonary mechanics, and increased work of breathing. Changes in resistance to airflow are not uniform throughout the lungs. Because of regional differences in airway resistance, the distribution of inspired air is uneven, with more air flowing to the less resistant portions.

Hyperventilation is eventually triggered by lung receptors responding to increased lung volume and obstruction. Continued air trapping increases intrapleural and alveolar gas pressures and causes decreased perfusion of the alveoli. Increased alveolar gas pressure, decreased ventilation, and decreased perfusion lead to variable and uneven ventilation-perfusion relationships within different lung segments. The result is early hypoxemia without CO_2 retention. Hypoxemia further increases hyperventilation through stimulation of the respiratory center, causing $Paco_2$ to decrease and pH to increase (respiratory alkalosis). As the obstruction becomes more severe, however, the number of alveoli being inadequately ventilated and perfused increases, a point at which CO_2 retention and respiratory acidosis develop. Respiratory acidosis signals respiratory failure.[37]

Clinical Manifestations

During full remission, individuals are asymptomatic and pulmonary function tests are normal. During partial remission, there are no clinical symptoms but pulmonary function tests are abnormal. During attacks, individuals are dyspneic and respiratory effort is marked. Breath sounds are decreased except for considerable wheezing. Because the severity of alterations in blood gases is difficult to evaluate by clinical signs alone, arterial blood gas tensions should be measured. Similarly, a peak flow measurement should be obtained early in an acute attack because it is common for the clinical examination to underestimate the degree of airway obstruction, often leading to inadequate intervention.

A sensation of chest constriction, inspiratory and expiratory wheezing, dyspnea, nonproductive coughing, prolonged expiration, tachycardia, and tachypnea occur at the beginning of an attack. With severe attacks the accessory muscles of respiration are prominent. As the episode resolves, coughing produces a thick, stringy mucus with casts of the small airways that can be seen microscopically.

Evaluation and Treatment

Spirometry shows decreases in expiratory flow rate, forced expiratory volume (FEV), and forced vital capacity (FVC) (see Chapter 31). FRC and total lung capacity (TLC) are increased. Blood gas analysis shows hypoxemia with early respiratory alkalosis or late respiratory acidosis.

The most successful treatment of asthma is elimination of the causative agents. Acute episodes are treated with drugs that are geared toward reversing bronchospasm and airway inflammation.

Over the years, powerful β-adrenergic agonists have been relied on to control asthma, but these drugs do not treat the underlying inflammation. Antiinflammatory agents should be used in significant asthma to reduce the frequency and severity of asthma attacks and to prevent long-term damage to the airways. Despite some controversy about the safety of β-adrenergic agonists and their proper use, most recent studies indicate that they are safe and effective adjuncts to long-term antiinflammatory treatment. Other bronchodilators, such as ipratropium (an inhaled anticholinergic drug), also have been shown to safely supplement antiinflammatories. Recommended antiinflammatory drugs include cromolyn sodium, which stabilizes mast cells and suppresses activation of other inflammatory cells, and low-dose, inhaled corticosteroids, which decrease the inflammatory response and bronchial reactivity in the airways.[26,38,39] In recent years a new class of drugs has been introduced that blocks the production and activity of leukotrienes. Although their role in the management of chronic asthma continues to be elucidated, these drugs have been found to be safe and effective for individuals who fail to respond adequately to inhaled corticosteroids.[38,40]

If bronchospasm is not reversed by usual measures, the individual is considered to have severe bronchospasm, or **status asthmaticus.** With severe bronchospasm the work of breathing can be 5 to 10 times that of normal. When air

WHAT'S NEW? Treatment of Asthma with Leukotriene Antagonists

The recognition that asthma is an inflammatory disease has led to increased interest in antiinflammatory agents that are less toxic and easier to administer than the inhaled or oral corticosteroids. A new class of agents has been approved for treatment of asthma that acts through the blocking of leukotrienes (inflammatory mediators of bronchoconstriction and airway inflammation in asthma). Although not yet approved for small children, these drugs, including zafirlukast and montelukast, have been found to be a safe and effective addition to the management of asthma. Their long-term efficacy in preventing airway remodeling is still not proven. Inhaled corticosteroids remain the first line of antiinflammatory therapy, but the antileukotriene drugs are likely to play an increasingly important role in the management of asthma.

Data from Drazen JM, Israel E, O'Bryne PM: Drug therapy: treatment of asthma with drugs modifying the leukotriene, *N Engl J Med* 340(3): 197, 1999.

NUTRITION & DISEASE

Chronic Obstructive Pulmonary Disease (COPD)

Malnutrition is a major concern for individuals with COPD because they have increased energy expenditure, decreased energy intake, and impaired oxygenation. Malnutrition (1) adversely affects exercise tolerance by limiting skeletal and respiratory muscle strength and aerobic capacity, (2) limits surfactant production, (3) reduces cell-mediated immune responses, (4) reduces protein synthesis, and (5) increases morbidity and mortality. The medical nutrition therapy goal is to maintain an acceptable and stable weight for the person. This can be accomplished by including foods of high energy density, frequent snacking, soft foods and beverages, assistance with shopping and meal preparation, simplified meal preparation, participation in home-delivered meal programs, and sharing meals with others. Protein intake should be maintained at 1.0 to 1.5 g/kg of body weight, and a daily vitamin C supplement should be added to the diet if the individual is still smoking.

Data from Pouw EM et al: Early non-elective readmission for chronic obstructive pulmonary disease is associated with weight loss, *Clin Nutr* 19(2):95, 2000; Schols AM: Nutrition in chronic obstructive pulmonary disease, *Curr Opin Pulm Med* 6(2):110, 2000.

trapping is severe, paradoxic pulse (a systolic blood pressure decrease of more than 10 mm Hg during inspiration) and pneumothorax are common. If status asthmaticus continues, hypoxemia worsens, expiratory flows and volumes decrease further, and the individual begins to tire. Acidosis develops as arterial PCO_2 begins to rise. Asthma becomes life threatening at this point if treatment does not reverse this process quickly. A silent chest (no audible air movement) and a PCO_2 of more than 70 mm Hg are ominous signs.

Chronic Obstructive Pulmonary Disease

Chronic obstructive pulmonary disease (COPD) is defined as pathologic lung changes consistent with emphysema or chronic bronchitis. It is a syndrome characterized by abnormal tests of expiratory airflow that do not change markedly over time, and without a reversible response to pharmacological agents. It is the fourth leading cause of death and affects more than 14 million people in the United States, and unlike most diseases, it has had a significant increase in prevalence and mortality over the past 30 years.[41] COPD is primarily caused by cigarette smoke; both active and passive smoking have been implicated. Other risks include genetics, occupational exposures, and air pollution.[42]

Chronic Bronchitis

Chronic bronchitis is defined as hypersecretion of mucus and chronic productive cough that continues for at least 3 months of the year (usually the winter months) for at least 2 consecutive years. Incidence is increased in smokers (up to twentyfold) and even more so in workers exposed to air pollution. It is a major health problem for the elderly population. Repeated infections are common.

Pathophysiology

Inspired irritants not only increase mucus production but also increase the size and number of mucous glands and goblet cells in airway epithelium. The mucus produced is thicker and more tenacious than normal. This sticky mucus coating makes it much more likely that bacteria, such as *Haemophilus influenzae* and *Streptococcus pneumoniae,* will become embedded in the airway secretions, where they reproduce rapidly. Ciliary function is impaired, reducing mucus clearance further. The lung's defense mechanisms are therefore compromised, increasing susceptibility to pulmonary infection and injury. As infection and injury increase mucus production further, the bronchial walls become inflamed and thickened from edema and accumulation of inflammatory cells. (The pathogenesis of chronic bronchitis is shown in Fig. 32-11.)

Initially chronic bronchitis affects only the larger bronchi, but eventually all airways are involved. The thick mucus and hypertrophied bronchial smooth muscle obstruct the airways and lead to closure, particularly during expiration, when the airways are narrowed (Fig. 32-12). The airways collapse early in expiration, trapping gas in the distal portions of the lung. Obstruction eventually leads to ventilation-perfusion mismatch, hypoventilation (increased $PaCO_2$), and hypoxemia.

Clinical Manifestations

The symptoms that lead individuals with chronic bronchitis to seek medical care include decreased exercise tolerance, wheezing, and shortness of breath. Individuals usually have a productive cough ("smoker's cough"), and evidence of airway obstruction (decreased FEV_1) is shown by spirometry. Hypoxemia may occur with exercise. As the disease progresses, copious amounts of sputum are produced, accompanied by frequent pulmonary infections. FVC and FEV_1 become markedly reduced, and FRC and residual volume (RV) are increased as airway obstruction and air trapping become more pronounced.

Airway obstruction results in decreased alveolar ventilation and increased $PaCO_2$. Marked hypoxemia leads to polycythemia (overproduction of erythrocytes) and cyanosis. If not reversed, hypoxemia leads to pulmonary hypertension and eventually results in cor pulmonale (see Chapter 31) and can lead to severe disability or death. (Table 32-4 lists the common clinical manifestations of chronic bronchitis.)

Evaluation and Treatment

Diagnosis is made on the basis of physical examination, chest radiograph, pulmonary function tests, and blood gas analyses; these tests reflect the progressive nature of the disease. The best "treatment" for chronic bronchitis is prevention, because pathologic changes are not reversible. By the time an individual seeks medical care for symptoms, considerable airway damage is present. If the individual stops smoking, disease progression can be halted. If smoking is stopped before symptoms occur, the risk of chronic bronchitis decreases considerably and eventually reaches that of nonsmokers.

Bronchodilators and expectorants are prescribed to increase airway caliber, improve secretion removal, and maximize gas exchange. Chest physical therapy, including deep breathing, postural drainage when 30 ml or more of sputum

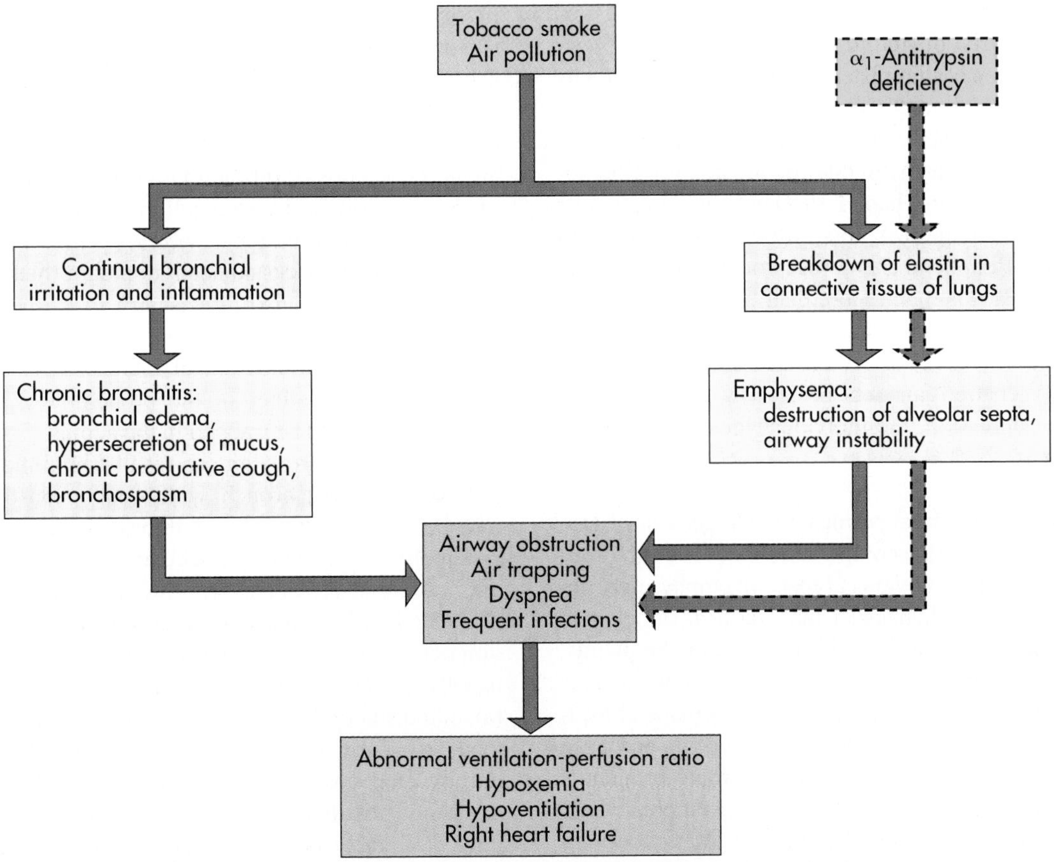

FIG. 32-11 Pathogenesis of chronic bronchitis and emphysema (chronic obstructive pulmonary disease [COPD]). (*Dashed arrows* indicate role of α_1-antitrypsin deficiency, if present.)

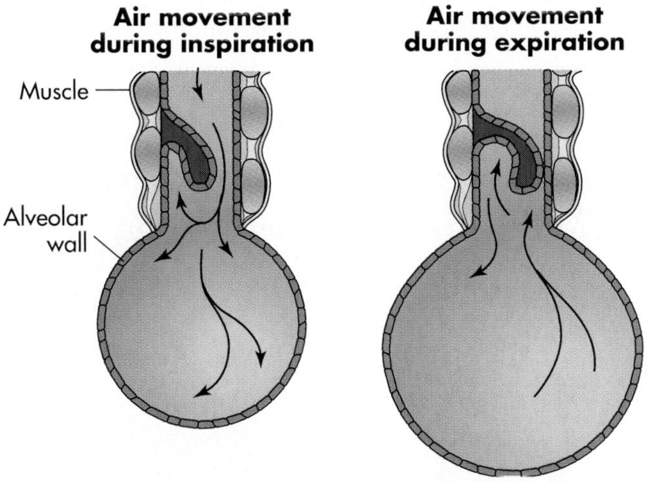

FIG. 32-12 Mechanisms of air trapping in chronic obstructive pulmonary disease (COPD). Mucous plugs and narrowed airways cause air trapping and hyperinflation on expiration. During inspiration the airways enlarge, allowing gas to flow past the obstruction. During expiration the airways narrow and prevent gas flow. This mechanism of air trapping, known as ball valving, occurs in asthma and chronic bronchitis.

Table 32-4 Clinical Manifestations of Chronic Obstructive Lung Disease

Clinical Manifestations	Bronchitis	Emphysema
Productive cough	Classic sign	Late in course with infection
Dyspnea	Late in course	Common
Wheezing	Intermittent	Minimal
History of smoking	Common	Common
Barrel chest	Occasionally	Classic
Prolonged expiration	Always present	Always present
Cyanosis	Common	Uncommon
Chronic hypoventilation	Common	Late in course
Polycythemia	Common	Late in course
Cor pulmonale	Common	Late in course

is produced per day, and percussion, also is used to remove secretions and open airways. Teaching of individuals includes nutritional counseling, respiratory hygiene, recognition of the early signs of infection, and techniques that relieve dyspnea, such as pursed-lip breathing. The role of antibiotics in the management of acute exacertations of chronic bronchitis has been controversial. Recent reports support the use of antibiotics in all persons with increased sputum production or other indications of worsening bronchitis.[43,44] Steroids sometimes are used late in the course of the disease but should be reserved only for those people in whom less toxic therapies are inadequate and who demonstrate some improvement after a trial of steroid therapy.

Low-flow oxygen is administered with care to individuals with severe hypoxemia and CO_2 retention. Because of the chronic elevation of $Paco_2$, the central chemoreceptors no longer act as the primary stimulus for breathing. (Chemoreceptors are described in Chapter 31.) This role is taken over by the peripheral chemoreceptors, which are sensitive to changes in Pao_2. Peripheral chemoreceptors do not stimulate breathing if the Pao_2 is much more than 60 mm Hg. Therefore, if oxygen therapy causes Pao_2 to exceed 60 mm Hg, the stimulus to breathe is lost, $Paco_2$ increases, and apnea results. If adequate oxygenation cannot be achieved without resulting in respiratory depression, the individual must be mechanically ventilated.[45]

Emphysema

Emphysema is abnormal permanent enlargement of gas-exchange airways (acini) accompanied by destruction of alveolar walls and without obvious fibrosis. In emphysema, obstruction results from changes in lung tissues, rather than mucus production and inflammation, as in chronic bronchitis. The major mechanism of airflow limitation in emphysema is loss of elastic recoil. Some degree of emphysema is considered normal in elderly individuals. When it occurs earlier in life, however, it is usually secondary to chronic bronchitis and cigarette smoking, but it may be primary emphysema.

Primary emphysema, which accounts for 1% to 2% of all cases of emphysema, is commonly linked to an inherited deficiency of the enzyme α_1-antitrypsin. α_1-Antitrypsin is a major component of α_1-globulin, a plasma protein. Normally α_1-antitrypsin inhibits the action of many proteolytic enzymes (enzymes that break down proteins). Individuals who have α_1-antitrypsin deficiency (an autosomal recessive trait) have an increased likelihood of developing emphysema because proteolysis in lung tissues is not inhibited. Homozygous individuals have a 70% to 80% likelihood of developing lung disease. (Mechanisms of genetic inheritance are described in Chapter 4.) Persons with α_1-antitrypsin deficiency who smoke are even more susceptible to emphysema than those with the deficiency alone.[46] α_1-Antitrypsin deficiency is suggested in individuals who develop emphysema before age 40 years (or in their early forties) and in nonsmokers who develop emphysema. (The principles of risk factor analysis are discussed in Chapter 5.)

Secondary emphysema also is caused by an inability of the body to inhibit proteolytic enzymes in the lung. It results from an insult to the lungs from inhaled toxins, such as cigarette smoke and air pollution. Not all smokers develop emphysema, but approximately 20% are especially susceptible and develop significant lung damage if they continue to smoke.

Pathophysiology

Emphysema begins with destruction of alveolar septa, probably because of elastin breakdown within the septa. It is postulated that inhaled oxidants, such as those in cigarette smoke and air pollution, tip the normal balance of elastases (proteolytic enzymes) and antielastases (such as α_1-antitrypsin) such that elastin is destroyed at an increased rate. This is the same mechanism by which the genetic loss of α_1-antitrypsin causes emphysema.[44] Septal destruction eliminates portions of the pulmonary capillary bed and increases the volume of air in the acinus. Expiration becomes difficult because loss of elastic recoil reduces the volume of air that can be expired passively. Hyperinflation of alveoli causes large air spaces (bullae) and air spaces adjacent to pleura (blebs) to develop. Septal destruction also affects airway caliber because the force that normal alveoli exert on bronchiolar walls is diminished. The combination of increased RV in the alveoli and diminished caliber of the bronchioles causes part of each inspiration to be trapped in the acinus (Fig. 32-13). Additional airway narrowing can result from inflammatory hyperreactivity of the bronchi with bronchoconstriction, which may be partially reversible with bronchodilators.

Emphysema can be centriacinar (centrilobular) or panacinar (panlobular), depending on the site of involvement (Fig. 32-14). In **centriacinar emphysema,** septal destruction occurs in the respiratory bronchioles and alveolar ducts, usually in the upper lobes of the lung. The alveolar sac (alveoli distal to the respiratory bronchiole) remains intact. It tends to occur in smokers with chronic bronchitis. **Panacinar emphysema** involves the entire acinus with damage more randomly distributed and involving the lower lobes of the lung. It tends to occur in elderly persons and in those with α_1-antitrypsin deficiency.

Clinical Manifestations

Individuals with emphysema usually have dyspnea on exertion that later progresses to marked dyspnea, even at rest (see

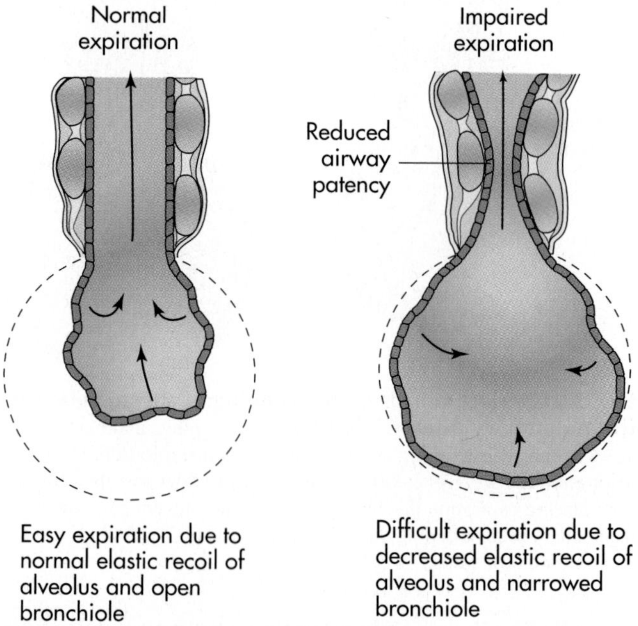

FIG. 32-13 Mechanisms of air trapping in emphysema. Damaged or destroyed alveolar walls no longer support and hold open the airways, and alveoli lose their property of passive elastic recoil. Both of these factors contribute to collapse during expiration.

Table 32-4). There is little cough and very little sputum production. The individual often is thin, has tachypnea with prolonged expiration, and must use accessory muscles for ventilation. The anteroposterior diameter of the chest is increased, and the chest has a hyperresonant sound with percussion. To increase lung capacity, the individual often leans forward with arms extended and braced on knees when sitting.

Evaluation and Treatment

The most definitive evidence for the presence of emphysema is obtained from pulmonary function measurements. Pulmonary function tests indicate obstruction to gas flow during expiration. Airway collapse and air trapping in distal portions of the lung lead to a decrease in FVC and FEV_1 and an increase in FRC, RV, and TLC. TLC can increase to twice the normal value. Diffusing capacity is decreased because of destruction of the alveolocapillary membrane. On radiographs the diaphragm appears flattened and the lung fields appear translucent. Marked and persistent overdistention of the lungs is suggestive of emphysema. Arterial blood gas measurements are usually normal until late in the disease. The disease course is usually prolonged, with increasing dyspnea and intermittent bouts of infection that culminate in failure of the right side of the heart (cor pulmonale) and death.

Treatment for emphysema has changed little in recent decades, although new therapies are being evaluated for the future.[47] Smoking cessation is the most important intervention and must occur early before irreversible damage becomes extensive. Inhaled anticholinergic agents (e.g., ipratropium) are now considered first-line therapy for emphysema.[42,48] A stepwise approach of adding β_2-adrenergic agonists and, frequently, other bronchodilators is suggested. Oral corticosteroids are beneficial only in a small percentage of individuals and should be used only as a last resort for individuals found to be steroid responsive.[49] Low-flow oxygen can improve symptoms and prevent cor pulmonale in selected individuals.[41] Dyspnea can be improved by relaxation exercises, reconditioning, and breathing retraining.[50] Lung volume reduction surgery and lung transplant can be considered.[51,52]

Respiratory Tract Infections

Respiratory tract infections are the most common cause of short-term disability in the United States. Most of these infections—the common cold, pharyngitis (sore throat), and laryngitis—involve only the upper airways. Although the lungs have direct contact with the atmosphere, they remain sterile under most circumstances. Infections of the lower respiratory tract occur most frequently in the young, the very old, or individuals with impaired immunity or underlying disease. In all cases the body's normal defense mechanisms are impaired.

Pneumonia

Pneumonia is infection of the lower respiratory tract caused by bacteria, viruses, fungi, protozoa, or parasites. It is the sixth leading cause of death in the United States. The incidence and mortality of pneumonia are highest in the elderly. Risk factors for pneumonia include advanced age, immunocompromise, underlying lung disease, alcoholism, altered

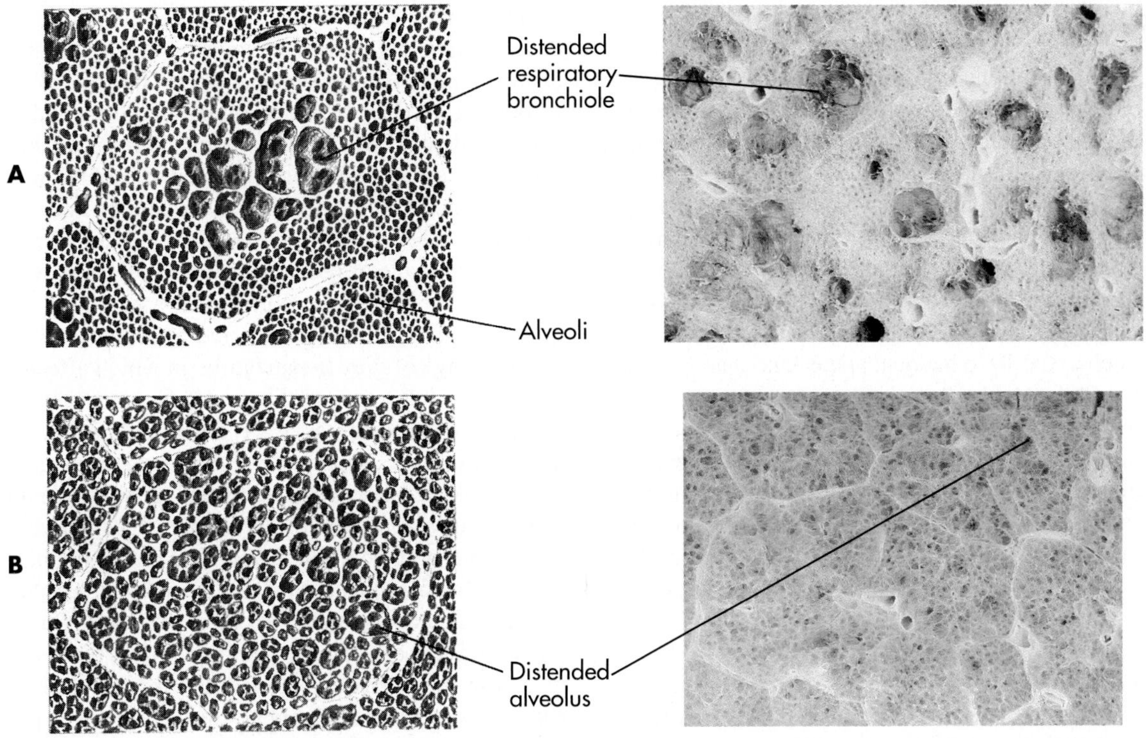

FIG. 32-14 Types of emphysema. **A**, Centriacinar emphysema. **B**, Panacinar emphysema. (Micrographs from Damjanov I, Linder J, editors: *Anderson's pathology,* ed 10, St Louis, 1996, Mosby.)

consciousness, smoking, endotracheal intubation, malnutrition, and immobilization. The causative microorganism influences the symptoms and signs with which the patient presents, how the pneumonia should be treated, and the prognosis. Community-acquired pneumonia tends to be caused by different microorganisms than those infections acquired in the hospital (nosocomial). In addition, the characteristics of the individual are important in determining which etiologic microorganism is likely; for example immunocompromised persons tend to be susceptible to opportunistic infections that are uncommon in normal adults. In general, nosocomial infections and those affecting immunocompromised individuals have a higher mortality rate than community-acquired pneumonias. Some of the most common causal microorganisms include the following:[53,54]

COMMUNITY ACQUIRED	NOSOCOMIAL PNEUMONIA	IMMUNO-COMPROMISED INDIVIDUALS
Streptococcus pneumoniae	*Pseudomonas aeruginosa*	*Pneumocystis carinii*
Mycoplasma pneumoniae	*Staphylococcus aureus*	*Mycobacterium tuberculosis*
Haemophilus influenzae	*Klebsiella pneumoniae*	Atypical mycobacteria
Oral anaerobic bacteria	*Escherichia coli*	Fungi
Influenza virus		Respiratory viruses
Legionella pneumophila		Protozoa
Chlamydia pneumoniae		Parasites
Moraxella catarrhalis		

The most common community-acquired pneumonia is caused by *Streptococcus pneumoniae* (also known as the pneumococcus), which has a relatively low overall mortality rate, although it is higher in the elderly.[53] *Mycoplasma pneumoniae* is a common cause of pneumonia in young people, especially those living in group housing such as dormitories and army barracks. Influenza is the most common viral community-acquired pneumonia in adults. *Legionella* species can contaminate cooling systems and water supplies leading to outbreaks of disease, such as the 1976 incident at the American Legion Convention in Philadelphia. *Pseudomonas aeruginosa,* other gram-negative organisms, and *Staphylococcus aureus* are the most common etiologic agents in nosocomial pneumonia.[55] Immunocompromised (human immunodeficiency virus, transplant) individuals are especially susceptible to *Pneumocystis carinii,* mycobacterial infections, and fungal infections of the respiratory tract. These infections can be difficult to treat and have a high mortality rate.

Pathophysiology

Aspiration of oropharyngeal secretions is the most common route of lower respiratory tract infection; thus the nasopharynx and oropharynx constitute the first line of defense for most infectious agents.[56] Another route of infection is through the inhalation of microorganisms that have been released into the air when an infected individual coughs, sneezes, or talks, or from aerosolized water, such as that from contaminated respiratory therapy equipment. This route of infection is most important in viral and mycobacterial pneumonias and in *Legionella* outbreaks. Pneumonia can also occur when bacteria are spread to the lungs in the blood from bacteremia that can result from infection elsewhere in the body or from intravenous drug abuse.

In healthy individuals, pathogens that reach the lungs are expelled or held in check by mechanisms of self-defense (see Chapters 6, 7, and 31). If a microorganism gets past the upper airway defense mechanisms, such as the cough reflex and mucociliary clearance, the next line of defense is the alveolar macrophage. This phagocyte is capable of removing most infectious agents without setting off significant inflammatory or immune responses. However, if the microorganism is virulent or present in large enough numbers, it can overwhelm the alveolar macrophage and result in a full-scale activation of the body's defense mechanisms, including the release of multiple inflammatory mediators, cellular infiltration, and immune activation.[56] These inflammatory mediators and immune complexes can damage bronchial mucous membranes and alveolocapillary membranes, causing the acini and terminal bronchioles to fill with infectious debris and exudate. In addition, some microorganisms release toxins from their cell walls that can cause further lung damage. The accumulation of exudate in the acinus leads to dyspnea and to $\dot{V}/\dot{Q}$ mismatching and hypoxemia.

Pneumococcal Pneumonia

The pathogenesis of pneumococcal pneumonia *(Streptococcus pneumoniae)* is best understood (Fig. 32-15). *Streptococcus pneumoniae* organisms initiate the inflammatory response (see Chapter 7), and inflammatory exudate causes aveolar edema. Edema creates a medium for the multiplication of bacteria and aids in the spread of infection into adjacent portions of the lung. The involved lobe undergoes consolidation (solidification of the tissue caused by filling with exudate). A stage of red hepatization follows in which alveoli fill with blood cells, fibrin, edematous fluid, and pneumococci, giving lung tissue a red appearance. This passes into the stage of gray hepatization, in which affected tissues become gray because of fibrin deposition over the pleural surfaces and the presence of fibrin and leukocytes (neutrophils) in the consolidated alveoli, where phagocytosis is rapidly taking place. With resolution, increasing numbers of macrophages appear in the alveolar spaces, the neutrophils degenerate, and the fibrin threads and remaining bacteria are digested by macrophages and removed by lymphatic vessels. Usually infection is limited to one or two lobes. Rapid lysis of pneumococcal bacteria (as occurs with antibiotic treatment) results in the release of intracellular bacterial proteins that can be toxic. The best known of these proteins is pneumolysin, which is cytotoxic to virtually every cell in the lung and

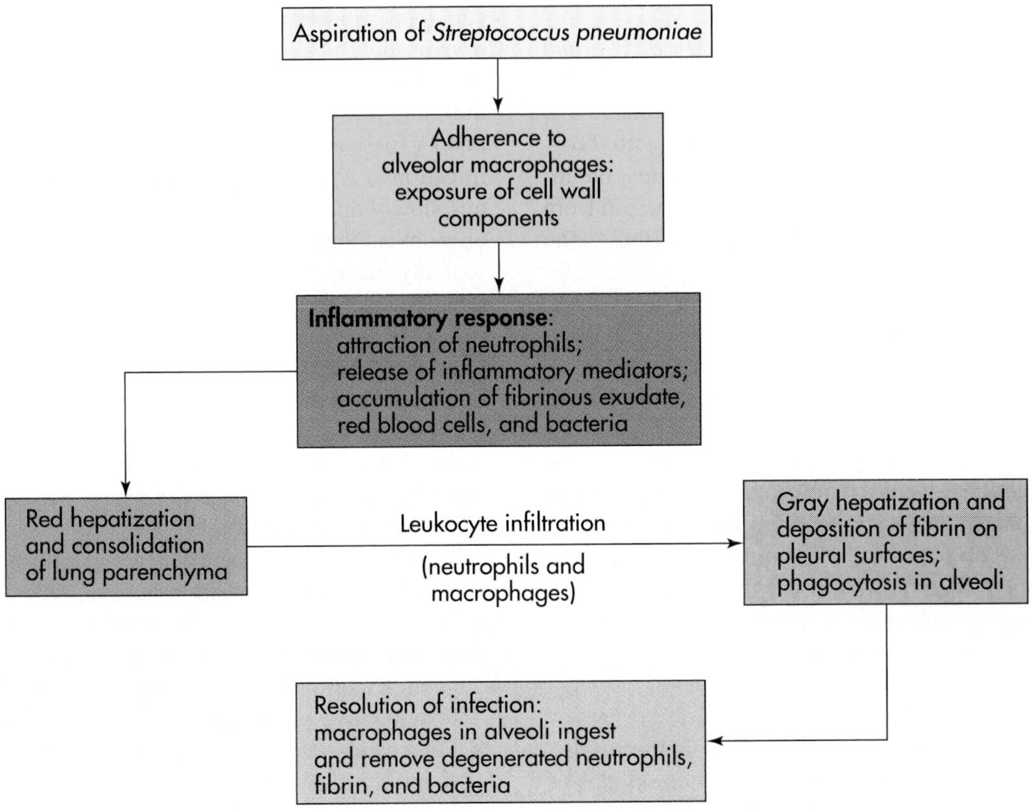

FIG. 32-15 Pathophysiologic course of pneumococcal pneumonia.

is partially responsible for the worsening in clinical symptoms sometimes seen in individuals immediately after they begin antibiotic treatment.[57]

Viral Pneumonia

Viral pneumonia is usually mild and self-limiting, but it can set the stage for a secondary bacterial infection by providing an ideal environment for bacterial growth and by damaging ciliated epithelial cells, which normally prevent pathogens from reaching the lower airways. Viral pneumonia can be a primary infection (e.g., influenza pneumonia) or a complication of another viral illness (e.g., chickenpox, measles). The virus not only destroys the ciliated epithelial cells but also invades the goblet cells and bronchial mucous glands. Sloughing of destroyed bronchial epithelium occurs throughout the respiratory tract, preventing mucociliary clearance. Bronchial walls become edematous and infiltrated with leukocytes.

Clinical Manifestations

Most cases of pneumonia are preceded by an upper respiratory infection, which is usually viral. This is then followed by the onset of cough, dyspnea, and fever. The cough is often productive but may be nonproductive, especially in viral pneumonia. Other symptoms include chills, malaise, and pleuritic chest pain. Physical examination may reveal signs of pulmonary consolidation, such as inspiratory crackles, increased tactile fremitus, egophony, and whispered pectoriloquy. Individuals may also demonstrate symptoms and signs of underlying systemic disease or sepsis.

Evaluation and Treatment

The diagnosis of pneumonia is confirmed by finding infiltrates on chest x-ray. These infiltrates may be patchy, lobar, or diffuse. The white blood cell count is usually elevated and, in the case of bacterial pneumonia, displays a preponderance of polymorphonucleocytes on differential. Sputum Gram stain is indicated in all patients with pneumonia, and sputum and blood cultures should be done in all hospitalized persons.[53,54] In immunocompromised or severely ill individuals, further diagnostic testing, such as transtracheal aspiration, bronchoscopy, or lung biopsy, may be necessary to identify the etiologic organism.[58]

The first step in the management of pneumonia is establishing adequate ventilation and oxygenation. Most individuals have hypoxemia and a respiratory alkalosis, although persons with underlying lung disease may require ventilation. Adequate hydration and good pulmonary hygiene (e.g., deep breathing, coughing, chest physical therapy) are also important.

Antibiotics are used to treat bacterial infections and should be chosen based on the likely causative microorganism (community acquired versus nosocomial) and the underlying condition of the individual. The sputum Gram stain and culture can also guide the choice of treatment. Viral pneumonia is usually treated with supportive therapy, although antivirals may be indicated in severe infection. Infections with opportunistic organisms may be polymicrobial and require multiple drugs, including antifungals.

Tuberculosis

Tuberculosis (TB) is an infection caused by *Mycobacterium tuberculosis,* an acid-fast bacillus that usually affects the lungs but may invade other body systems. It is estimated that approximately 1.86 billion people are infected with TB—32% of the world population.[59] In the United States, the incidence of TB decreased from 1950 to 1980, increased from 1985 to 1992, and has decreased once again since 1992.[60] The largest increases have occurred in men age 25 to 44 years; in children younger than age 15 years; and in Hispanic, black, and Asian populations. The major reason for this trend is the epidemic of acquired immunodeficiency syndrome (AIDS). Individuals with AIDS are highly susceptible to respiratory infections, including multidrug-resistant TB. These highly resistant microorganisms have developed because a large number of individuals do not consistently take their medications, allowing resistant strains to be selected and spread.[61] Emigration of infected individuals from high-prevalence countries, transmission in crowded institutional settings, homelessness, substance abuse, and lack of access to medical care also have contributed to the spread of TB.

◆ *Pathophysiology*

Like some types of pneumonia, tuberculosis is transmitted from person to person in airborne droplets. Microorganisms lodge in the lung periphery, usually in the upper lobe. Once the bacilli are inspired into the lung, they multiply and cause nonspecific pneumonitis (lung inflammation). Some bacilli migrate through the lymphatics and become lodged in the lymph nodes, where they encounter lymphocytes and initiate the immune response.

Inflammation in the lung causes neutrophils and then alveolar macrophages to migrate to the area. These cells are phagocytes that engulf the bacilli and begin the process by which the body's defense mechanisms isolate the bacilli, preventing their spread. The neutrophils and macrophages seal off the colonies of bacilli, forming a granulomatous lesion called a *tubercle* (see Chapter 7). Infected tissues within the tubercle die, forming cheeselike material called *caseation necrosis.* (Necrosis is described in Chapter 2.) Collagenous scar tissue then grows around the tubercle, completing isolation of the bacilli. The immune response is complete after 10 days or so, preventing further multiplication of the bacilli.

Once the bacilli are isolated in tubercles and immunity develops, tuberculosis may remain dormant for life. If the immune system is impaired, however, or if live bacilli escape into the bronchi, active disease occurs and may spread through the blood and lymphatics to other organs. Endogenous reactivation of dormant bacilli in elderly persons may be caused by poor nutritional status, insulin-dependent diabetes, long-term corticosteroid therapy, and other debilitating diseases.

◆ *Clinical Manifestations*

In many infected individuals, tuberculosis is asymptomatic. In others, symptoms develop so gradually that they are not noticed until the disease is advanced. However, symptoms can appear in immunosuppressed individuals within weeks of exposure to the bacillus. Common clinical manifestations include fatigue, weight loss, lethargy, anorexia (loss of appetite), and a low-grade fever that usually occurs in the afternoon. (These are common signs and symptoms of all chronic infections.) A cough that produces purulent sputum develops slowly and becomes more frequent over several weeks or months. Night sweats and general anxiety are often present. Dyspnea, chest pain, and hemoptysis may also occur as the disease progresses.

◆ *Evaluation and Treatment*

Tuberculosis is diagnosed by a positive tuberculin skin test (purified protein derivative [PPD]), sputum culture, and chest radiographs. A positive tuberculin skin test indicates that an individual has been infected and has produced antibodies against the bacillus. By itself the positive skin test does not indicate the presence of active disease. It is important that the material used for skin testing be standardized to minimize the number of false-positive and false-negative results. Those who have received the tuberculosis vaccine with bacille Calmette-Guérin (BCG) will also have a positive PPD.

When active pulmonary disease is present, the tubercle bacillus can be cultured from the sputum and may be seen with an acid-fast stain. Chest radiographs of individuals with current or previous active disease demonstrate characteristic changes. Nodules, calcifications, cavities, and hilar enlargement (enlarged mediastinal lymph nodes) commonly are seen in the upper lobes. A positive skin test indicates the need for yearly chest radiographs to detect active disease.

Tuberculosis is graded as follows to aid in evaluation and determination of appropriate therapy:[62]

0—no tuberculosis, no exposure, no infection
1—exposure to tuberculosis, no infection
2—tuberculosis infection, no disease
3—tuberculosis, active disease
4—tuberculosis, no active disease
5—tuberculosis suspected

Treatment consists of antibiotic therapy to control active or dormant tuberculosis and prevent transmission. The choice of drugs and the duration of treatment depend on the individual's health history, the likelihood of bacterial resistance to certain drugs, and the presence of active disease. The waxy coat of *M. tuberculosis* renders it impermeable to many common drugs. Before the increase in tuberculosis incidence during the past decade, treatment with two effective drugs generally was sufficient. Isoniazid with either rifampin or ethambutol usually was used for 6 to 9 months. Today, with the increased numbers of immunosuppressed and susceptible individuals and drug-resistant bacilli, the recommended treatment for those at high risk is a combination of four drugs: isoniazid, rifampin, pyrazinamide, and ethambutol or streptomycin.[63] Newer drugs being tested include rifapentine and immune amplifiers.[64,65]

In the past, individuals with active tuberculosis were isolated from the community and their families in sanitariums.

Today individuals remain at home or, rarely, in the hospital, until sputum cultures show that the active bacilli have been eliminated. This usually takes a few weeks to 2 months if the antibiotics are taken conscientiously. If the individual's cooperation is in question, it is advisable for the administration of the drugs to be supervised by health care workers.

Acute Bronchitis

Acute bronchitis is acute infection or inflammation of the airways or bronchi. Acute bronchitis commonly follows a viral illness and is usually self-limiting. Many of the clinical manifestations are similar to those of pneumonia (i.e., fever, cough, chills, malaise), but physical examination does not reveal signs of pulmonary consolidation and chest radiographs show no infiltrates. Individuals with viral bronchitis have a nonproductive cough that frequently occurs in paroxyms and is aggravated by cold, dry, or dusty air. Purulent sputum may be produced. Chest pain often develops from the effort of coughing. Treatment consists of rest, aspirin, humidity, and a cough suppressant, such as codeine.

Individuals with bacterial bronchitis have a productive cough, fever, and pain behind the sternum (breast bone) that is aggravated by coughing. It is rare in previously healthy adults except after viral infection but is common in those with COPD. Bacterial bronchitis is treated with rest, aspirin, humidity, and antibiotics (usually a pencillinase-resistant penicillin). If the cough is nonproductive, a cough suppressant is given, because a dry cough can cause bronchial irritation and damage. Acute bronchitis may progress to pneumonia.

Pulmonary Vascular Disease

Blood flow through the lungs can be disrupted by a number of disorders that result in occlusion of the vessels, an increase in pulmonary vascular resistance, or destruction of the vascular bed. The consequences of altered pulmonary blood flow may be of no functional significance or can result in severe and life-threatening changes in ventilation-perfusion ratios. Major disorders include pulmonary embolism, pulmonary hypertension, and cor pulmonale.

Pulmonary Embolism

Pulmonary embolism is occlusion of a portion of the pulmonary vascular bed by an embolus: a thrombus (blood clot), a tissue fragment, lipids (fats), or an air bubble (Fig. 32-16). The most common emboli are thrombi dislodged from deep veins in the thigh. They also can originate in the pelvis, particularly in pregnant women. Symptomatic pulmonary embolism occurs in approximately 30% of cases of untreated deep venous thrombosis.[66]

Risk factors for **pulmonary thromboembolism,** the obstruction of a pulmonary vessel by a thrombus, include many conditions and disorders that promote blood clotting (see Chapter 24). Clotting within the vessels is promoted by venous stasis (slowing or stagnation of blood flow through the veins), hypercoagulability (increased tendency of the blood to form clots), and injuries to the endothelial cells that line the vessels. Venous stasis is usually caused by immobility associated with prolonged bed rest or sitting, obesity, neurologic disease, or old age, but it also can be caused by pregnancy, congestive heart failure, sickle cell disease, and systemic lupus erythematosus. Hypercoagulability can result from coagulation disorders of the blood, malignancy, or oral contraceptive use. Clot formation also proceeds if vessel damage occurs, as in traumatic injury, surgery, or spontaneous rupture (e.g., cerebrovascular accident). Deep venous thrombosis and pulmonary embolism are frequent complications of hospitalization, especially in individuals who undergo obstetric or orthopedic procedures.[67] No matter what its source, a blood clot becomes an embolus when all or part of it breaks away from the site of formation and begins to travel in the bloodstream. (Thromboembolism is described further in Chapter 24.)

Although the overall incidence of pulmonary embolism has declined in recent years, it remains an important cause of death, especially in elderly and hospitalized persons.[68] One half of the deaths occur within 2 hours of embolization, which often is undetected and therefore untreated.

Pathophysiology

The impact or effect of the embolus depends on the extent of pulmonary blood flow obstruction, the size of the affected vessels, the nature of the embolus, and the secondary effects. Pulmonary emboli can occur as any of the following:

1. Massive occlusion: an embolus that occludes a major portion of the pulmonary circulation (i.e., main pulmonary artery embolus)
2. Embolus with infarction: an embolus that is large enough to cause infarction (death) of a portion of lung tissue
3. Embolus without infarction: an embolus that is not severe enough to cause permanent lung injury
4. Multiple pulmonary emboli, which may be chronic or recurrent

Depending on its pattern of occurrence and severity, pulmonary embolism causes varying degrees of hypoxic vasoconstriction,

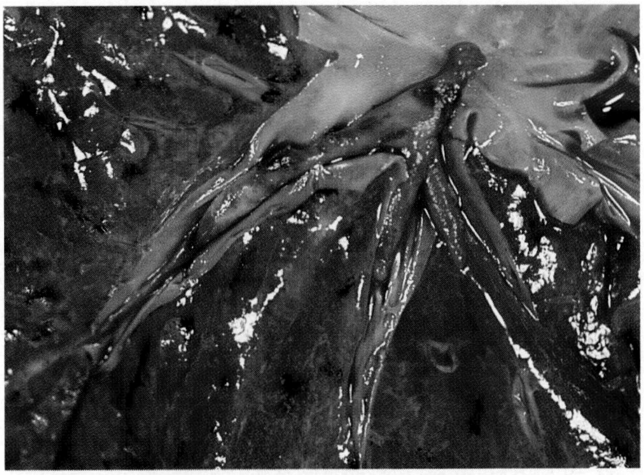

FIG. 32-16 Pulmonary embolus. The embolus extends into major branches of the pulmonary artery. (From Damjanov I, Linder J, editors: *Anderson's pathology,* ed 10, St Louis, 1996, Mosby.)

decrease in surfactant, atelectasis, and release of neurohumoral substances such as histamine, serotonin, and thromboxane. The embolus also may cause systemic hypotension, decreased cardiac output, and pulmonary hypertension, which, when severe, results in acute right ventricular failure and death. The pathogenesis of pulmonary embolism caused by a thrombus is summarized in Fig. 32-17.

If the embolus does not cause infarction, the clot is dissolved by the fibrinolytic system (see Chapter 24) and pulmonary function returns to normal. If pulmonary infarction occurs, shrinking and scarring develop in the affected area of the lung. (Infarction, or cellular death caused by lack of blood supply, is described in detail in Chapter 2.)

Clinical Manifestations

In most cases the clinical manifestations of pulmonary embolism are nonspecific; therefore evaluation of risk factors and predisposing factors is an important aspect of diagnosis. More than 90% of pulmonary emboli are the consequence of clots that were initially formed in the veins of the legs and pelvis. The characteristic symptoms and signs of deep vein thrombosis are leg pain and leg swelling. Sometimes the thrombus is palpable, but often the legs appear normal or signs are masked by superficial thrombophlebitis. Calf asymmetry, when documented with a tape measure, is one of the most important findings in deep venous thrombosis. This clinical finding is often overlooked in the assessment of individuals with suspected deep vein thrombosis; calf asymmetry of more than 1 cm increases the likelihood of a deep vein thrombosis from 27% to 56% in an at-risk individual.

Massive occlusion causes profound shock, hypotension, tachypnea, tachycardia, severe pulmonary hypertension, and chest pain. Diagnosis can be difficult because the signs mimic those of other cardiopulmonary problems.[66] Once these manifestations occur, death is imminent. Manifestations of emboli that cause infarction are pleural pain, dyspnea, pleural friction rub, pleural effusion, hemoptysis, fever, and leukocytosis. On chest radiographs the infarcted portion of the lung shows up as a nonspecific infiltrate in a classic wedge shape bordering the pleura. Pulmonary infarction is most likely in individuals with underlying pulmonary disease.

Pulmonary embolism without infarction is the most common type and is the most difficult to evaluate. The individual usually has sudden onset of tachypnea, tachycardia, dyspnea, and unexplained anxiety. Occasionally syncope (fainting) or pleural pain occurs. Recurrent pulmonary emboli occur in individuals who have had a history of previous emboli. Recurrent emboli may not be detected until progressive incapacitation, precordial pain, anxiety, dyspnea, and right ventricular enlargement are exhibited.

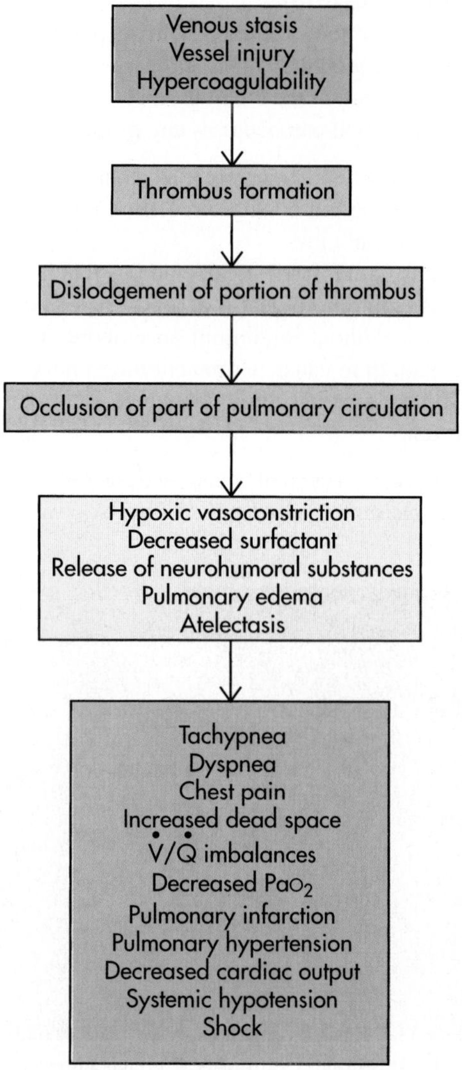

FIG. 32-17 Pathogenesis of massive pulmonary embolism caused by a thrombus (pulmonary thromboembolism).

Evaluation and Treatment

Routine chest radiographs and pulmonary function tests are not definitive tests for pulmonary embolism. Pulmonary embolism is suggested if arterial blood gas analyses demonstrate unexplained hypoxemia and hyperventilation. A blood test called a D-dimer is a sensitive but nonspecific test for pulmonary embolism that can help with diagnosis.[69] A ventilation-perfusion scan is used to detect areas of the lung that demonstrate normal ventilation but an absence of perfusion. If this scan is inconclusive, a pulmonary angiogram may be indicated. Newer tests being evaluated include spiral volumetric CT and magnetic resonance imaging.[70,71]

The ideal treatment for pulmonary embolism is prevention through risk factor analysis and elimination of predisposing factors for individuals at risk. (Risk factor analysis is described in Chapter 5.) Venous stasis in hospitalized individuals is minimized by leg elevation, bed exercises, position changes, early postoperative ambulation, and pneumatic calf compression. Clot formation is also prevented by prophylactic low-dose anticoagulant therapy; unfortunately, many individuals do not receive adequate prophylactic treatment.[72]

Anticoagulant therapy is the primary treatment for pulmonary embolism. Intravenous administration of heparin is begun immediately and is followed by oral doses of coumarin. Recent studies indicate that low-molecular-weight heparin is as safe and effective as standard heparin but is easier to administer.[73,74] If massive life-threatening embolism occurs, a fibrinolytic agent, such as streptokinase, is sometimes used.

Pulmonary Hypertension

Pulmonary hypertension is high blood pressure in the pulmonary arteries. Normally, pulmonary artery pressure is lower than systemic artery pressure. *Pulmonary hypertension* is defined as a rise in pulmonary artery pressure of 5 to 10 mm Hg above normal (pressure is normally 15 to 18 mm Hg).

Primary pulmonary hypertension is very rare. It has no known cause, usually occurs in women between ages 20 and 40 years, and may be hereditary. Primary pulmonary hypertension has a poor prognosis: most individuals die within 5 years of diagnosis.

Secondary pulmonary hypertension is more common. It can be secondary to any respiratory or cardiovascular disorder that (1) increases the volume or pressure of blood entering the pulmonary arteries or (2) narrows or obstructs the pulmonary arteries. The first cause overloads the pulmonary circulation from without; the second elevates blood pressure by increasing resistance to flow within the lungs.

Pathophysiology

In primary hypertension the small pulmonary arteries (arterioles) become narrow or obliterated as a result of hypertrophy (enlargement) of smooth muscle in the vessel walls and formation of fibrous lesions around the vessels. The mechanisms that cause these changes are not known but may be related to endothelial dysfunction.[75] Vessel narrowing or obliteration increases resistance and causes the pulmonary hypertension. Pressures in the left ventricle, which receives blood from the lungs, remain normal, but high pressures generated in the lungs are transmitted to the right ventricle, which supplies the pulmonary arteries. Eventually the right ventricle fails. Right ventricular disease resulting from pulmonary hypertension is termed **cor pulmonale.** Oxygenation is not severely affected, although mild hypoxia and cyanosis do occur. Death eventually results from cor pulmonale. (Mechanisms of heart failure are described in Chapter 29.)

There are four causes of secondary pulmonary hypertension:

1. Elevated left ventricular filling pressures, as occur in coronary artery disease and mitral valve disease
2. Increased blood flow through the pulmonary circulation (left-to-right shunts), as occurs with a ventricular septal defect or patent ductus arteriosus
3. Obliteration or obstruction of the pulmonary vascular bed by a pulmonary embolus or by chronic destruction of an alveolar wall (i.e., emphysema)
4. Vasoconstriction of the vascular bed, as occurs with hypoxemia, acidosis, or their combination

Secondary pulmonary hypertension can be reversed if the primary disorder is resolved. If hypertension persists, hypertrophy occurs in the medial smooth muscle layer of the arterioles. The larger arteries stiffen, and hypertension progresses until pulmonary artery pressure equals systemic blood pressure. The result is right ventricular hypertrophy and eventual cor pulmonale. The pathogenesis of heart failure caused by secondary pulmonary hypertension is shown in Fig. 32-18.

Clinical Manifestations

Pulmonary hypertension may not be detected until pulmonary artery pressure is equal to systemic blood pressure. The symptoms are often masked by primary pulmonary or cardiovascular disease. The first indication of pulmonary hypertension is often an abnormality seen on a chest radiograph (enlarged right heart border) or an electrocardiogram that shows right ventricular hypertrophy. Manifestations of fatigue, chest discomfort, tachypnea, and dyspnea, particularly with exercise, are common.

Evaluation and Treatment

Diagnosis of pulmonary hypertension can be made only with right-sided heart catheterization. The diagnosis of primary pulmonary hypertension is made when all other causes of hypertension, such as mitral stenosis (see Chapter 29), COPD, and pulmonary embolus, have been ruled out.

There is no effective treatment for primary pulmonary hypertension except lung transplantation, but supplemental oxygen, digitalis, and diuretics are used as palliative measures. α-adrenergic blockers, β-adrenergic agonists, and inhaled nitric oxide (NO) are being evaluated, but only epoprostenol (prostacyclin) has been found to improve hemodynamics and prolong survival.[76,77]

The most effective treatment for secondary pulmonary hypertension is treatment of the primary disorder. If the underlying cause is removed, pulmonary hypertension disappears.

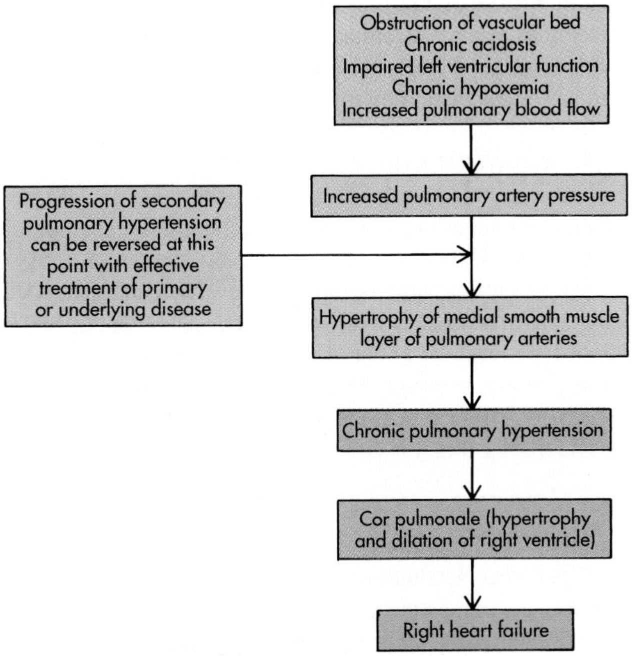

FIG. 32-18 Pathogenesis of pulmonary hypertension and cor pulmonale.

Once pulmonary hypertension has persisted long enough for hypertrophy of the medial smooth muscle layer to develop, however, as it does with chronic hypoxemia, it is no longer reversible. Treatment often includes supplemental oxygen to reverse hypoxic vasoconstriction. Diuretics and digitalis are used judiciously to treat right ventricular failure.

Cor Pulmonale

Cor pulmonale, also called *pulmonary heart disease,* consists of right ventricular enlargement (hypertrophy, dilation, or both). It is secondary to pulmonary hypertension caused by disorders of the lungs or chest wall.

Pathophysiology

Cor pulmonale develops as pulmonary hypertension creates chronic pressure overload in the right ventricle similar to that created in the left ventricle by systemic hypertension. (Systemic hypertension is discussed in Chapter 29.) Pressure overload increases the work of the right ventricle and causes hypertrophy of the normally thin-walled heart muscle. Acute hypoxemia, such as might occur with pneumonia, can exaggerate pulmonary hypertension and dilate the ventricle as well. Right ventricular filling pressures are normal until failure occurs. The right ventricle usually fails when pulmonary artery pressure equals systemic blood pressure.

Clinical Manifestations

The clinical manifestations of cor pulmonale may be obscured by primary respiratory disease and appear only during exercise testing. The heart appears normal at rest, but with exercise, cardiac output falls. The electrocardiogram shows right ventricular hypertrophy. Chest pain is common. The pulmonary component of the second heart sound, which represents closure of the pulmonic valve, may be accentuated, and a pulmonic valve murmur also may be present. Tricuspid valve murmur may accompany the development of right ventricular failure. Peripheral edema, hepatic congestion, and jugular venous distention often may be detected.

Evaluation and Treatment

Diagnosis is made on the basis of physical examination, radiologic examination, and electrocardiogram or echocardiogram or both. Physical examination findings are often similar to those of chronic lung disease with dyspnea and distended neck veins. The goal of treatment for cor pulmonale is to decrease the workload of the right ventricle by lowering pulmonary artery pressure. Treatment is the same as for pulmonary hypertension, and its success depends on reversal of the underlying lung disease.

Lip Cancer

Cancer of the lip is more prevalent in men, with 3100 new cases per year accounting for about 1% of all cancers in men.[78] Long-term exposure to sun, wind, and cold over a period of years results in dryness, chapping, hyperkeratosis, and predisposition to malignancy. The lower lip is the most common site.

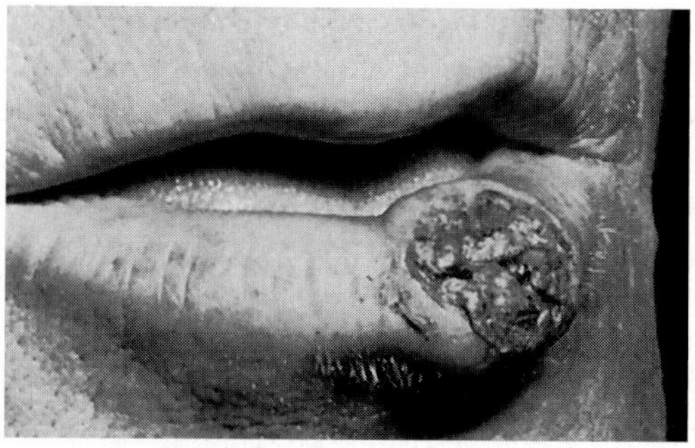

FIG. 32-19 Lip cancer. Carcinoma of the lower lip with central ulceration and raised, rolled borders. (From del Regato JA, Spjut HJ, Cox JD: *Ackerman and del Regato's cancer,* ed 2, St Louis, 1985, Mosby.)

Box 32-1

STAGING OF LIP CANCER

STAGE I

Primary tumor less than 2 cm; no palpable nodes

STAGE II

Primary tumor 2 to 4 cm; no palpable nodes

STAGE III

Primary tumor larger than 4 cm; metastatic lymph nodes

STAGE IV

Large primary tumors; nodes fixed to mandible or distant metastases

Pathophysiology

The most common form of lower lip cancer is termed *exophytic.* The lesion usually develops in the outer part of the lip along the vermilion border. The lesion becomes thickened and evolves to an ulcerated center with a raised border (Fig. 32-19). Verrucous-type lesions are less common. They have an irregular surface, follow cracks in the lip, and tend to extend toward the inner surface. Squamous cell carcinoma is the most common cell type. Basal cell carinoma does not develop unless there is extension beyond the mucous membrane or vermilion border of the lip.

Clinical Manifestations

Malignant lesions often are preceded by the development of a blister that evolves into a superficial ulceration. In some cases there is a history of recurrent scales that precede development of a bleeding ulceration. Metastases to the cervical lymph nodes have a low rate of occurrence (2% to 8%) and are more likely when the primary lesion is thicker and exists for a longer period.[79]

Evaluation and Treatment

Diagnosis is commonly made by clinical history and presentation of the lesion. Biopsy confirms the presence of malignant cells. The staging for lip cancer is summarized in Box 32-1. Surgical excision is effective for smaller lesions. Larger lesions that require extensive resection may need

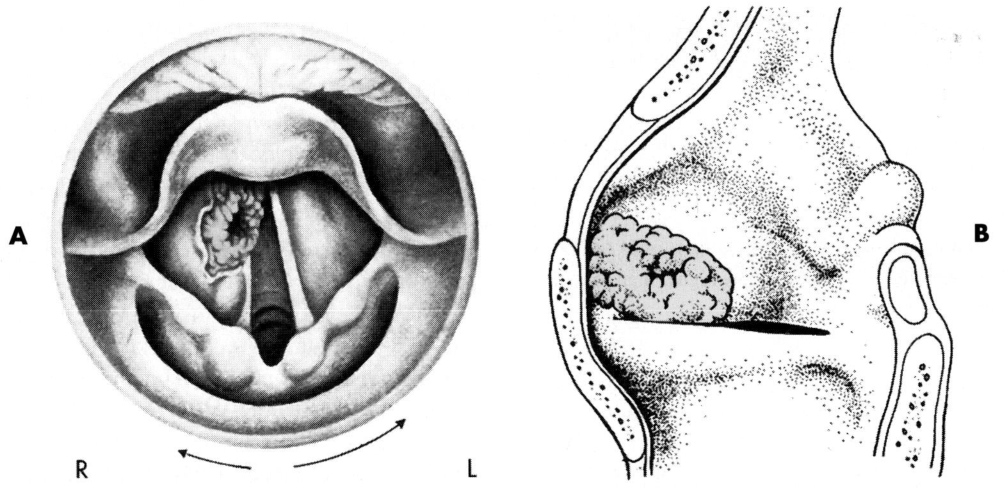

FIG. 32-20 Laryngeal cancer. A, Mirror view of carcinoma of right false cord partially hiding true cord. **B,** Lateral view. (From del Regato JA, Spjut HJ, Cox JD: *Ackerman and del Regato's cancer,* ed 2, St Louis, 1985, Mosby.)

subsequent cosmetic surgeries. Interstitial irradiation and radioactive implants have proved effective for control of primary lesions.[80] The prognosis for recovery is excellent, and deaths are usually the result of inadequate treatment.

Laryngeal Cancer

Cancer of the larynx represents approximately 2% to 3% of all cancers in the United States. There are approximately 10,600 new cases per year, 8600 of them in men.[78] The risk of laryngeal cancer is increased by the amount of tobacco smoked; risk is further heightened with the combination of smoking and alcohol consumption.[81] The highest incidence is in men between 50 and 75 years of age.

Pathophysiology

Carcinoma of the true vocal cords (glottis) is more common than that of the supraglottic structures (epiglottis, aryepiglottic folds, arytenoids, and false cords). Tumors of the subglottic area are rare. Squamous cell carcinoma is the most frequent cell type, although small cell carcinomas also occur (Fig. 32-20). Metastasis develops by spread to the draining lymph nodes, and distant metastasis, usually to the lung, is rare.

Clinical Manifestations

The presenting symptoms of laryngeal cancer include hoarseness, dyspnea, and cough. Progressive hoarseness is the most significant symptom and can result in voice loss. Dyspnea is rare in the case of supraglottic tumors but can be severe in subglottic tumors. Cough occurs less commonly and may follow swallowing. Laryngeal pain or a sore throat is likely to be present with supraglottic lesions.[82]

Evaluation and Treatment

Evaluation of the larynx includes external inspection and palpation of the larynx and the lymph nodes in the neck. Indirect laryngoscopy provides a stereoscopic view of the structure and movement of the larynx. A biopsy also can be obtained during this procedure. Direct laryngoscopy provides specific visualization of the tumor. Plain films of the larynx and CT facilitate the identification of tumor boundaries and the degree of extension to surrounding tissue.

Radiation therapy has shown good results for early carcinoma of the vocal cords. Chemotherapy may be useful as an adjunct to surgery.[83] Partial laryngectomies are the preferred treatment for small supraglottic and subglottic malignancies. Total laryngectomy is required when lesions are extensive and involve the cartilage.

WHAT'S NEW? Carcinogens in Tobacco Smoke and Lung Cancer

Tobacco smoke causes 90% of male lung cancer and 80% of female lung cancer in the United States. There are 55 carcinogens in tobacco smoke, 20 of which have been linked definitively with lung cancer. The carcinogens that are thought to play the largest role in lung cancer are the polycyclic aromatic hydrocarbons and the tobacco-specific nitrosamines. Although the precise mechanism by which these carcinogens cause cancer has yet to be elucidated, they have been directly linked to oncogene activation and tumor-suppressor gene inhibition. Some people have an abnormality in the enzyme glutathione S-transferase, which is important in the detoxification of tobacco smoke carcinogens. These individuals have an increased risk for lung cancer.

Data from Hecht SS: Tobacco smoke carcinogens and lung cancer, *J Natl Cancer Inst* 91(14):1194, 1999.

Lung Cancer

Lung cancers (bronchogenic carcinomas) arise from the epithelium of the respiratory tract. As such, the term *lung cancer* excludes other pulmonary tumors, including sarcomas, lymphomas, blastomas, hematomas, and mesotheliomas. Lung cancer is an epidemic in the United States, with an estimated 164,000 new cases in 2000. It accounts for 13% of all cancers in both men and women but is responsible for 31% of all cancer deaths in men and 25% of all cancer

Box 32-2

IMPORTANT TRENDS FOR LUNG CANCER

INCIDENCE

An estimated 164,000 new cases in 2000: 89,500 in males and 71,600 in females.

MORTALITY

An estimated 156,900 deaths in 2000: 89,300 in males and 66,000 in females. The death rate for women is now higher than that of any other cancer.

RISK FACTORS

Heavy cigarette smoking (more than 20 cigarettes/day) is the number one risk factor. Passive smoking (exposure to someone else's cigarette smoke) increases the risk of lung cancer. Occupational risk factors include exposure to asbestos dust, arsenic, chromium, nickel, ionizing radiation, chloromethyl ethers, coal products, mustard gas, and vinyl chloride. Cigarette smoking and exposure to asbestos may have a synergistic effect on the production of lung cancer.

WARNING SIGNS

A persistent cough, sputum streaked with blood, chest pain, recurring attacks of pneumonia or bronchitis.

EARLY DETECTION AND PREVENTION

Lung cancer is very difficult to detect early. If a smoker quits at the time of early cellular changes, altered bronchial lining often returns to normal. Periodic chest x-ray films, sputum cytologic analysis, and low-dose computed tomography can detect presymptomatic, early-stage lung cancers, particularly of the squamous cell type; however, no conclusive evidence of reduction in lung cancer mortality as a consequence of screening has been found.

TREATMENT

Surgery, radiation therapy, and chemotherapy are all used. Surgery is usually the treatment of choice, and with improved ventilation machinery and antibiotics, surgical complications are infrequent. Tumor spread requiring chemotherapy or radiation therapy is evident in about one third of all surgical lung cancer patients.

SURVIVAL

Only 14% of white and 11% of black patients live 5 or more years after diagnosis. Non–small cell carcinomas are considered separately from small cell carcinomas (see text). Rates have improved only slightly over a recent 10-year period.

From Greenlee RT et al: Cancer statistics 2000, *CA Cancer J Clin* 50(1): 7, 2000.

deaths in women[78] (Box 32-2). Although the mortality rate for lung cancer has leveled off in men, it is still rising in women. The lung cancer death rate for women is higher than that of any other cancer, including breast cancer, because of increased cigarette smoking by women.[84] Deaths from lung cancer appear at 35 to 44 years of age; a sharp increase occurs between ages 45 and 55 years; and the incidence continues to increase through ages 65 to 74 years, after which it levels off and decreases among the very old.

The most common cause of lung cancer is cigarette smoking. Heavy smokers have about a 25 times greater chance of developing lung cancer than nonsmokers. Passive smoking at home and in the workplace is associated with as much as a 30% increase in the risk for lung cancer.[85] Cigarette smoke contains several organ-specific carcinogens, and smoking has been causally related to carcinogenesis at several sites, including the larynx, oral cavity, esophagus, and urinary bladder. Genetic predisposition to developing lung cancer, which is evident in analysis of pedigrees, also plays a role in its pathophysiology (see Chapter 5).

The cancer death rates for pipe and cigar users are about equal to those of cigarette smokers for cancer of the larynx, oral cavity, and esophagus. The incidence of lung cancer decreases among people who stop smoking, and it reaches a level almost as low as that of nonsmokers 15 years after smoking has stopped. Theories of carcinogenesis are discussed in Chapter 11.

Environmental or occupational risk factors associated with lung cancer include benzopyrene and radon particles associated with uranium mining, radiation, and nuclear bombs. Others are polycyclic aromatic hydrocarbons and arsenicals, asbestos fibers, diesel exhaust, nitrogen mustard gases, nickel, silica, vinyl chloride, and chlormethyl methyl ether. Air pollution, coal, and iron mining are also considered risk factors.

Types

At least 12 different cell types of tumors are included under the broad heading of lung cancer. The four major histologic types are squamous cell carcinoma, small cell carcinoma, large cell carcinoma, and adenocarcinoma (including bronchioalveolar cell carcinoma). For clinical and therapeutic reasons, however, lung cancers are frequently classified as small cell lung cancer (SCLC; 25% of all lung cancers) and non-SCLC (NSCLC; 75% of all lung cancers). Characteristics of these tumors, including evaluation and treatment, are listed in Table 32-5. Some controversy exists as to the most frequently encountered cell type of bronchogenic carcinoma. In the past, squamous cell carcinoma was considered the most common type, but the incidence of adenocarcinoma is currently greater. Common sites of involvement for all four types of bronchogenic carcinoma are shown in Fig. 32-21. (Tumor biology is the subject of Chapter 10.)

Primary carcinomas of the lung and large metastatic tumors receive their blood supply from the bronchial arteries. The advancing tumor edge and small metastatic lesions receive their blood supply from the pulmonary circulation. Regional chemotherapeutic perfusion has not provided successful palliation for lung cancer.

Non–Small Cell Lung Cancer

Squamous cell carcinoma. Squamous cell carcinoma accounts for about 30% of bronchogenic carcinomas, representing a sharp decline in incidence in the past two decades. These tumors are typically located near the hilus and project into bronchi.

Because of the location in the central bronchi, obstructive manifestations are nonspecific and include nonproductive cough or hemoptysis. Pneumonia and atelectasis are often associated with squamous cell carcinoma (Fig. 32-22, *A*). Chest

Table 32-5 Characteristics of Lung Cancers

Tumor Type	Growth Rate	Metastasis	Means of Diagnosis	Clinical Manifestations and Treatment
Squamous cell carcinoma	Slow	Late; mostly to hilar lymph nodes	Biopsy, sputum analysis, bronchoscopy, electron microscopy, immunohistochemistry	Cough, sputum production, airway obstruction; treated surgically
Adenocarcinoma	Moderate	Early	Radiography, fiber-optic bronchoscopy, electron microscopy	Pleural effusion; treated surgically
Large cell carcinoma	Rapid	Early and widespread	Sputum analysis, bronchoscopy, electron microscopy (by exclusion of other cell types)	Chest wall pain, pleural effusion, cough, sputum production, hemoptysis, airway obstruction resulting in pneumonia (if airways involved); treated surgically
Small cell (oat cell) carcinoma	Very rapid	Very early; to mediastinum or distally in lung	Radiography, sputum analysis, bronchoscopy, electron microscopy, immunohistochemistry, and clinical manifestations (cough, chest pain, dyspnea, hemoptysis, localized wheezing)	Airway obstruction, signs and symptoms of excessive hormone secretion; treated by chemotherapy and ionizing radiation to thorax and central nervous system

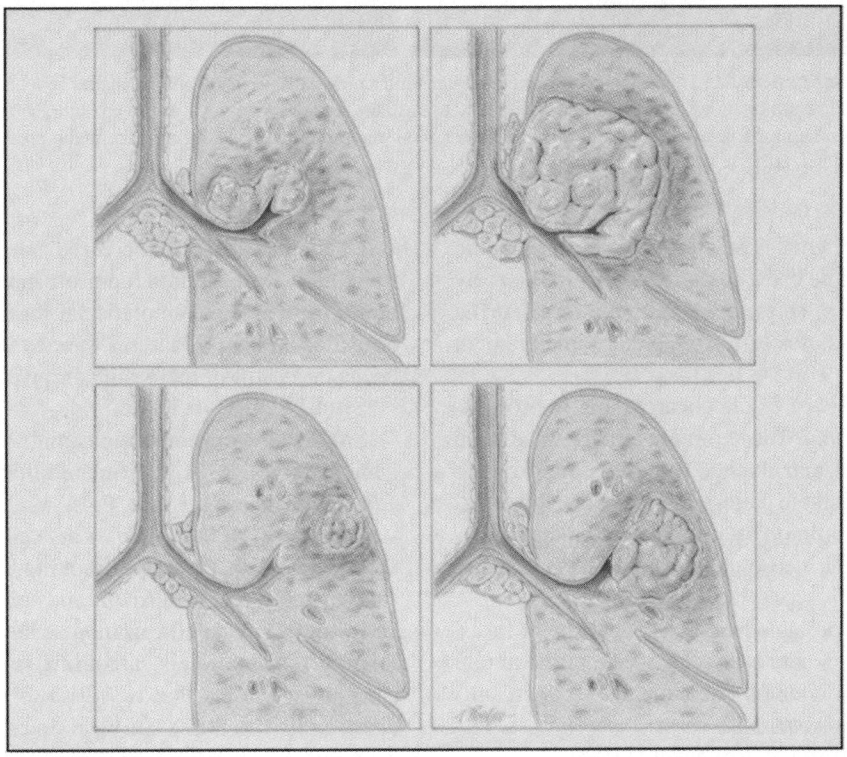

FIG. 32-21 **Cancer of the lung. A,** Squamous (epidermoid) cell carcinoma. **B,** Small cell (oat cell) carcinoma. **C,** Adenocarcinoma. **D,** Large cell carcinoma. (Tumor characteristics are summarized in Table 32-5.) (From Des Jardins T, Burton GG: *Clinical manifestations and assessment of respiratory disease,* ed 3, St Louis, 1995, Mosby.)

pain is a late symptom associated with large tumors. These tumors can remain fairly well localized and tend not to metastasize until late in the course of the disease. The preferred treatment is surgical resection, although once metastasis has taken place, total surgical resection is difficult and survival rates dramatically decrease. Although chemotherapy has limited effectiveness, adjuvant treatment with newer agents has been shown to improve survival and quality of life.[86]

Adenocarcinoma. **Adenocarcinoma** (tumor arising from glands) of the lung constitutes 35% to 40% of all bronchogenic carcinomas (Fig. 32-22, *B*). The recent increase in incidence of adenocarcinoma has been ascribed to the increasing frequency of lung cancer in women, environmental and occupational carcinogens, and changes in the histologic criteria for diagnosis. These tumors, which are usually smaller than 4 cm, more commonly arise in the peripheral regions of

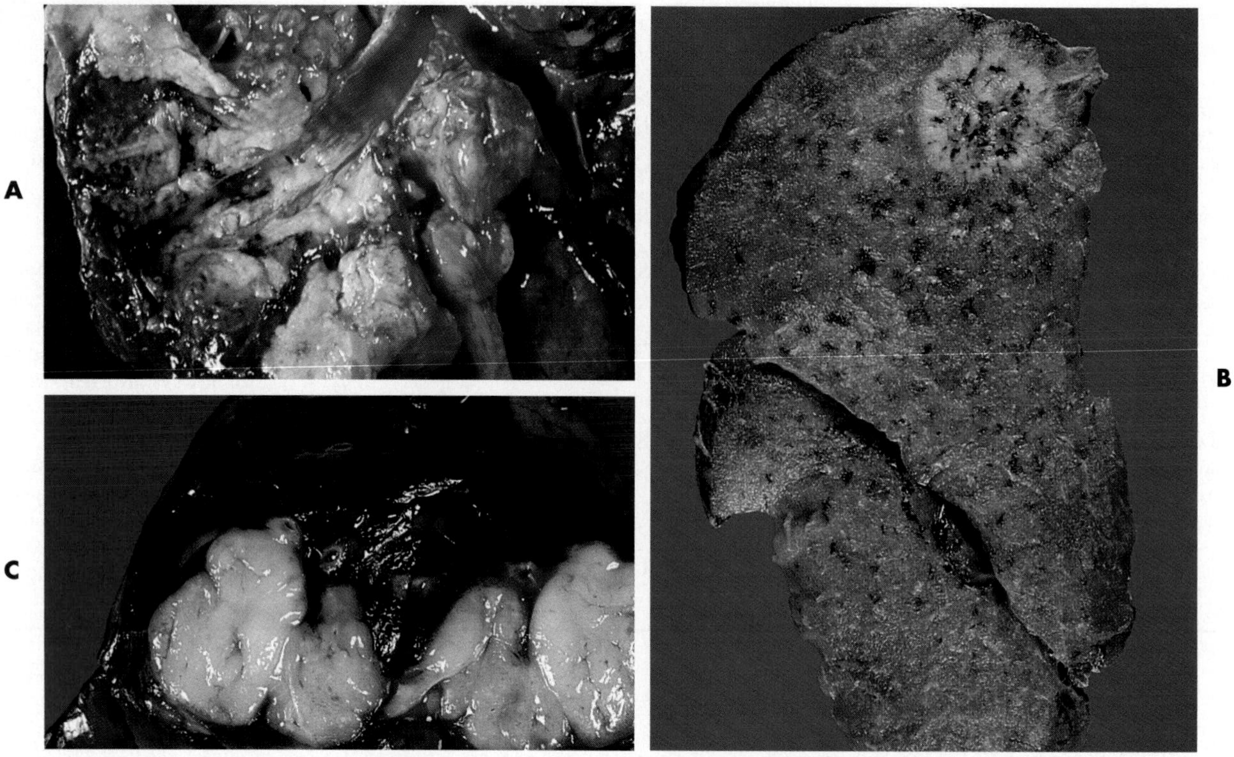

FIG. 32-22 Lung cancer. **A,** Squamous cell carcinoma. This hilar tumor originates from the main bronchus. **B,** Peripheral adenocarcinoma. The tumor shows prominent black pigmentation, suggestive of having evolved in an anthracotic scar. **C,** Small cell carcinoma. The tumor forms confluent nodules. On cross sectioning, the nodules have an encephalid appearance. (From Damjanov I, Linder J, editors: *Anderson's pathology,* ed 10, St Louis, 1996, Mosby.)

the pulmonary parenchyma. They may be asymptomatic and discovered by routine chest roentgenogram in the early stages, or the individual may seek treatment for pleuritic chest pain and shortness of breath from pleural involvement by the tumor.

Included in the category of adenocarcinoma is bronchioloalveolar cell carcinoma. These tumors tend to arise from the terminal bronchioles and alveoli. They are slow-growing tumors with an unpredictable pattern of metastasis. Metastasis occurs through the pulmonary arterial system and mediastinal lymph nodes. This cell type has the weakest association with smoking.

Surgical resection is possible in a high proportion of cases, but because metastasis occurs early, the 5-year survival rate is less than 10%. Newer chemotherapeutic agents are resulting in increased survival rates.[86]

Large Cell Carcinoma (Undifferentiated)

Undifferentiated large cell carcinomas constitute 10% to 15% of bronchogenic carcinomas. This cell type has lost all evidence of differentiation and is therefore commonly referred to as **undifferentiated large cell anaplastic cancer.** Because large cell carcinomas show none of the histologic findings of squamous cell carcinoma or adenocarcinoma, they are diagnosed by a process of exclusion. The cells are generally larger than leukocytes and contain large, darkly stained nuclei. These tumors commonly arise peripherally but are found centrally and can grow to distort the trachea and cause widening of the carina.

Once metastasis has occurred, surgical therapy is limited to palliative procedures (comfort measures) designed to relieve obstructive pneumonitis or prevent recurrence of pleural effusion. Neither radiation therapy nor chemotherapy has been successful in increasing survival.

Small Cell Carcinoma

Small cell carcinomas constitute 20% to 25% of bronchogenic carcinomas. It is estimated that most of these tumors are central in origin (see Figs. 32-21 and 32-22, *C*). Cell sizes range from 6 to 8 μm. This cell type has the strongest correlation with cigarette smoking. Because these tumors show a rapid rate of growth and tend to metastasize early and widely, small cell carcinomas have the worst prognosis. Staging for small cell carcinoma is divided into only two categories: limited disease (20% to 30%) versus extensive disease (70% to 80%). Survival time for untreated small cell carcinoma is usually 1 to 3 months; with treatment, however, approximately 10% of individuals are alive at 2 years.[87]

Small cell carcinoma is most often associated with ectopic hormone production, production of hormones by tumors of nonendocrine origin, or production of an inappropriate hormone by an endocrine gland. Neuroendocrine cells containing neurosecretory granules exist throughout the tracheobronchial tree. Ectopic hormone production is important to the clinician because resulting signs and symptoms (called *paraneoplastic syndromes*) may be the first manifestation of the underlying cancer. The most common paraneoplastic syndrome associated with small cell lung cancer is the syndrome of inappropriate antidiuretic hormone secretion, which occurs in up to 40% of individuals.[87] Small cell carcinomas also commonly produce gastrin-releasing peptide, calcitonin, arginine vasopressin, and adrenocorticotropic hormone (ACTH). As a result of ACTH secretion, individuals with lung cancer secrete large quantities of 17-hydroxysteroids and 17-ketosteroids, leading to the development of an atypical Cushing syndrome. Signs and symptoms related to this condition include muscular weakness, facial edema, hypokalemia, alkalosis, hyperglycemia, hypertension, and increased pigmentation. They are treated primarily with chemotherapy and radiation therapy, with temporary remission.

◆ *Pathogenesis*

Tobacco smoke contains as many as 20 documented lung carcinogens and is responsible for causing 80% to 90% of lung cancers.[88] These carcinogens, along with probable inherited genetic predisposition to cancers, result in multiple genetic abnormalities in bronchial cells, including deletions of chromosomes, activation of oncogenes, and inactivation of tumor-suppressor genes. Further, cellular damage is caused by smoke-induced toxic oxygen radical production. The most common genetic abnormality associated with lung cancer is loss of the tumor-suppressor gene p53; mutations in this gene have been found in 50% to 60% of non–small cell lung cancers and 90% of small cell cancers.[89] Once lung cancer is initiated by these carcinogen-induced mutations, further tumor development is promoted by growth factors, such as epidermal growth factor.

The bronchial mucosa suffers multiple carcinogenic "hits" due to repetitive exposure to cigarette smoke, and eventually epithelial cell changes begin to be visible on biopsy. These changes progress from metaplasia to carcinoma in situ, and finally to invasive carcinoma. Further, tumor progression includes invasion of surrounding tissues and, finally, metastasis to distant sites, including the brain, bone marrow, and liver.

◆ *Clinical Manifestations*

Symptoms of early-stage, localized disease are nonspecific and are likely to be attributed by the individual to the effects of smoking. The clinical manifestations are ambiguous and insidious; they include coughing, sputum production, hemoptysis, pneumonia, airway obstruction, and pleural effusions. Table 32-5 summarizes the clinical manifestations according to tumor type. By the time manifestations are severe enough to motivate the individual to seek medical advice, the disease is usually advanced.

◆ *Evaluation and Treatment*

Diagnosis and treatment for each cell type of lung cancer are summarized in Table 32-5. Smoking cessation is the only proven way to reduce the risk of lung cancer. Trials with other measures, such as dietary modification, are underway.[90,91]

Other Lung Cancers

Bronchial carcinoid tumors represent about 1% of all lung tumors. The tumor cells have dense granules containing neuroendocrine-like hormones, but they rarely produce endocrine symptoms (carcinoid syndrome).

WHAT'S NEW? Early Detection of Lung Cancer—An Enhanced Role for Screening

Until recently, the American Cancer Society and other oncology groups have recommended against routine screening for lung cancer. Even though treatment is far more effective in early-stage cancers, older studies had failed to demonstrate a clear survival benefit for screening. Recently, it has been noted that radiographic screening for lung cancer can be greatly improved using a technique called low-dose computed tomography. This technique uses much less radiation than conventional computed tomography and, when compared with routine chest x-ray, can detect four times as many early lung cancers. The role of low-dose computed tomography in screening for lung cancer continues to be evaluated, but it is likely to become an important tool.

Data from Henschke CI et al: Early Lung Cancer Action Project: overall design and findings from baseline screening, *Lancet* 354(9143):99, 1999; Smith RA et al: American Cancer Society guidelines for the early detection of cancer, *Cancer J Clin* 50:34, 2000.

Carcinoid tumors tend to occur earlier in life than bronchogenic carcinoma, although they can occur through the seventh decade of life.[92] The average age at diagnosis is about 45 years, and carcinoid tumors are not related to smoking. The tumors arise more commonly in the main or segmental bronchi, are easily visualized bronchoscopically, and are found on routine chest radiographs. Cells are not recovered from bronchial washings because the tumor is covered with normal mucosa. These tumors are slow-growing cancers, and 50% of individuals with bronchial carcinoid tumors are asymptomatic. Local surgical resection is curative if metastasis has not occurred; this can often be done by bronchoscopic laser electrocautery.[93]

Adenocystic tumors (cylindromas) and **mucoepidermoid carcinomas** are rare bronchial gland tumors. They arise predominantly in the trachea or large airways and cause obstruction. They can be malignant and metastasize early, although distal pulmonary metastases are usually slow growing. Thus it is not unusual for an individual to survive 10 to 15 years after diagnosis.

Mesotheliomas arise from the pleura and are often aggressive malignant tumors. Most arise from the pleural surface (80%). Benign pleural mesotheliomas have a slow clinical onset and are usually asymptomatic, but over a period of years they can cause dyspnea and mild pleuritic pain. These tumors can grow to be very large and fill the entire pleural cavity. Mesotheliomas are more likely to be malignant than benign. Current management of malignant mesothelioma includes a combination of pleuropneumonectomy, chemotherapy, radiation, and hyperthermia.[94]

There is a clear association between asbestos exposure and malignant mesothelioma, especially in asbestos workers, although the minimum amount of exposure that constitutes risk has not been determined. Some individuals develop mesothelioma after minimal asbestos exposure. A long latent interval between exposure to asbestos and appearance of mesothelioma usually occurs, and onset of symptoms may take 20 to 30 years.[95]

Staging

The histologic cell type and the stage of the disease are the major factors that influence choice of therapy for individuals. The currently accepted system for the staging of lung cancer is the **TNM classification** (Table 32-6). This system is a code in which T denotes the extent of the primary tumor, N indicates the nodal involvement, and M describes the extent of metastasis. Staging of lung cancer is illustrated in Fig. 32-23.

Table 32-6 1997 Revised International System for Staging Lung Cancer

Symbol	Definition
Primary Tumor (T)	
T0	No evidence of tumor
Tx	Tumor that cannot be assessed or is not apparently radiologically or bronchoscopically (malignant cells in bronchopulmonary secretions)
Tis	Carcinoma in situ
T1	Tumor with the following characteristics:
a	Size: ≤3 cm
b	Airway location: in lobar bronchus or distal airways
c	Local invasion: none, surrounded by lung or visceral pleura
T2	Tumor with any of the following characteristics:
a	Size: >3 cm
b	Airway location: involvement of the main bronchus (distance to the carina is 2 cm or more) or presence of atelectasis or obstructive pneumonitis that extends to hilar region but does not involve the entire lung
c	Local invasion: involvement of the visceral pleura
T3	Tumor with the following location or invasion:
a	Size: any
b	Airway location: tumor in the main bronchus (within 2 cm of the carina) or tumor with atelectasis or obstructive pneumonitis of the entire lung
c	Local invasion: invasion of chest wall (including superior sulcus tumors), diaphragm, mediastinal pleura, or parietal pericardium
T4	Tumor with the following location or invasion:
a	Size: any
b	Airway location: satellite tumor nodule(s) within the ipsilateral primary-tumor lobe of the lung
c	Local invasion: invasion of the mediastinum, heart, great vessels, trachea, esophagus, vertebral body, or carina; or presence of malignant pleural/pericardial effusion
Lymph Nodes (N)	
Nx	Regional lymph nodes cannot be assessed
N0	Absence of regional lymph node involvement
N1	Presence of metastasis to ipsilateral peribronchial or ipsilateral hilar lymph nodes or both (including direct extension to intrapulmonary nodes)
N2	Presence of metastasis to ipsilateral mediastinal or subcarinal lymph nodes or both
N3	Presence of metastasis to any of the following lymph node groups: contralateral mediastinal, contralateral hilar, ipsilateral or contralateral scalene, or supraclavicular
Distant Metastasis (M)	
Mx	Metastasis cannot be assessed
M0	Absence of distant metastasis
M1	Presence of distant metastasis (separate metastatic tumor nodule[s] in the ipsilateral nonprimary-tumor lobe[s] of the lung also are grouped as M1)
Stage Grouping—TNM Subsets	
Stage 0	TisN0M0
Stage 1A	T1N0M0
Stage 1B	T2N0M0
Stage IIA	T1N1M0
Stage IIB	T2N1N0;T3N0M0
Stage IIIA	T3N1M0;T(1-3)N2M0
Stage IIIB	T4, any N, M0; any T, N3M0
Stage IV	Any T; any N; M1

From Mountain CF: Revisions in the international system for staging lung cancer, *Chest* 111(6):1710, 1997.

NOTE: The uncommon superficial tumor of any size with its invasive component limited to bronchial wall is classified T1 even in the case of extension to main bronchus.

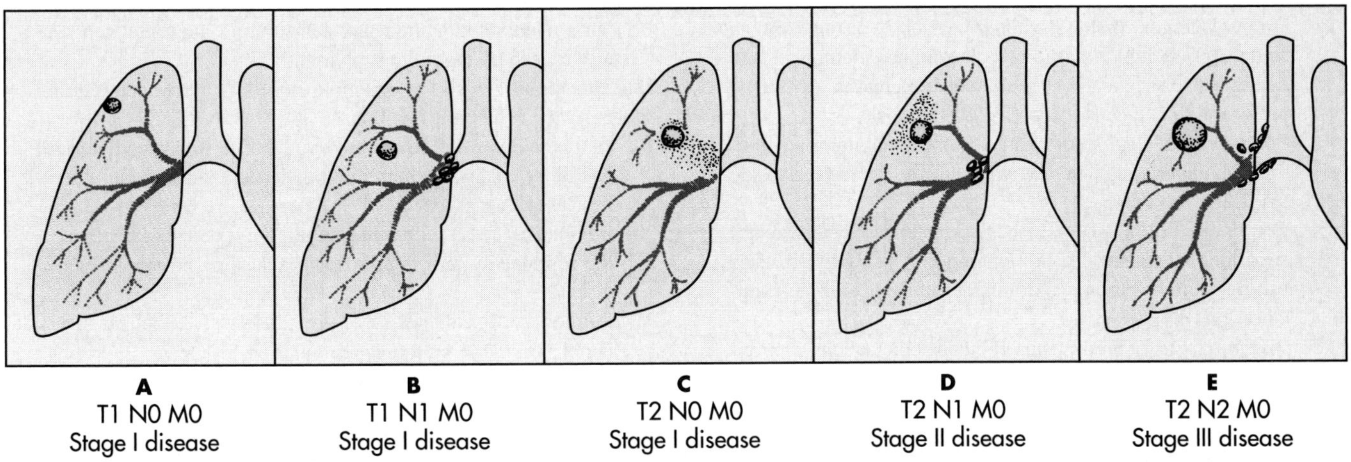

FIG. 32-23 Staging of lung cancer by the TNM classification system. A, B, Stage I disease includes tumors classified as T1, with or without metastasis to the lymph nodes in the ipsilateral hilar region. **C,** Also included in stage I are tumors classified as T2 but having no nodal or distant metastases. **D,** Stage II disease includes those tumors classified as T2, with metastasis only to the ipsilateral hilar lymph nodes. **E,** Stage III includes all tumors more extensive than T2 or any tumor with metastasis to the lymph nodes in the mediastinum or with distant metastasis.

SUMMARY REVIEW

Clinical Manifestations of Pulmonary Alterations

1. Dyspnea is a feeling of breathlessness and increased respiratory effort.
2. Abnormal breathing patterns are adjustments made by the body to minimize the work of respiratory muscles. They include Kussmaul, obstructed, restricted, gasping, and Cheyne-Stokes respirations, and sighing.
3. Hypoventilation is decreased alveolar ventilation caused by airway obstruction, chest wall restriction, or altered neurologic control of breathing. Hypoventilation causes increased $Paco_2$.
4. Hyperventilation is increased alveolar ventilation produced by anxiety, head injury, or severe hypoxemia. Hyperventilation causes decreased $Paco_2$.
5. Coughing is a protective reflex that expels secretions and irritants from the lower airways.
6. Hemoptysis is expectoration of bloody mucus, which can be caused by bronchitis, tuberculosis, abscess, neoplasms, and other conditions that cause hemorrhage from damaged vessels.
7. Cyanosis is a bluish discoloration of the skin caused by desaturation of hemoglobin, polycythemia, or peripheral vasoconstriction.
8. Chest pain can result from inflamed pleurae, trachea, bronchi, or respiratory muscles.
9. Clubbing of the fingertips is associated with diseases that interfere with oxygenation of the tissues.
10. Hypoxemia is a reduced Pao_2 caused by (a) decreased oxygen content of inspired gas, (b) hypoventilation, (c) diffusion abnormality, (d) ventilation-perfusion mismatch, or (e) shunting.
11. Pulmonary edema is excess water in the lung caused by disturbances of capillary hydrostatic pressure, capillary oncotic pressure, or capillary permeability. A common cause is left-sided heart failure that increases the hydrostatic pressure in the pulmonary circulation.
12. Atelectasis is the collapse of alveoli resulting from compression of the lung tissue or absorption of gas from obstructed alveoli.
13. Bronchiectasis is abnormal dilation of the bronchi secondary to another pulmonary disorder, usually infection or inflammation.
14. Pneumothorax is the accumulation of air in the pleural space. It can be caused by spontaneous rupture of weakened areas of a pleura or secondary to pleural damage caused by disease, trauma, or mechanical ventilation.
15. Pleural effusion is the accumulation of fluid in the pleural space, usually resulting from disorders that promote transudation or exudation from capillaries underlying the pleura but occasionally resulting from blockage or injury that causes lymphatic vessels to drain into the pleural space.
16. Empyema is the presence of pus in the pleural space (infected pleural effusion). The source of the pus is usually lymphatic drainage from sites of bacterial pneumonia.
17. Pleurisy is inflammation of the pleura.
18. Pulmonary fibrosis is an excessive amount of connective tissue in the lung. It diminishes lung compliance and may be idiopathic or caused by disease.
19. Chest wall compliance is diminished by obesity and kyphoscoliosis, which compress the lungs, and by neuromuscular diseases that impair chest wall muscle function.
20. Flail chest results from rib or sternal fractures that disrupt the mechanics of breathing.
21. Inhalation of noxious gases or prolonged exposure to high concentrations of oxygen can damage the bronchial mucosa or alveolocapillary membrane and cause inflammation or acute respiratory failure.
22. Pneumoconiosis, which is caused by inhalation of dust particles in the workplace, including coal dust, can cause pulmonary fibrosis, susceptibility to lower airway infection, and tumor formation.
23. Silicosis is a type of pneumoconiosis caused by inhalation of silica.
24. Allergic alveolitis is an allergic or hypersensitivity reaction to many allergens.
25. Bronchiolitis is the inflammatory obstruction of small airways. It is most common in children.

Pulmonary Disorders

1. Acute respiratory failure is caused by inadequate gas exchange or ventilation ($Pao_2 \leq 50$ mm Hg or $Paco_2 \geq 50$ mm Hg and $pH \leq 7.25$).

2. Adult respiratory distress syndrome (ARDS) results from an acute, diffuse injury to the alveolocapillary membrane and decreased surfactant production, which increases membrane permeability and causes edema and atelectasis.
3. Postoperative respiratory failure is most common in individuals undergoing surgery who smoke or have chronic disease.
4. Obstructive pulmonary disease is characterized by airway obstruction that causes difficult expiration. Obstructive disease can be acute or chronic and includes asthma, chronic bronchitis, and emphysema.
5. In asthma, obstruction is caused by episodic attacks of bronchospasm, bronchial inflammation, mucosal edema, and increased mucus production.
6. Extrinsic asthma is caused by an immune response to allergens or other irritants.
7. Intrinsic asthma is not caused by allergens and occurs in adults older than 35 years.
8. A local imbalance between the parasympathetic and sympathetic divisions of the autonomic nervous system is thought to facilitate bronchospasm in individuals with intrinsic asthma.
9. Chronic bronchitis causes airway obstruction resulting from bronchial smooth muscle hypertrophy and production of thick, tenacious mucus.
10. In emphysema, destruction of the alveolar septa and loss of passive elastic recoil lead to airway collapse and obstruct gas flow during expiration.
11. Emphysema in which septal deterioration is caused by α_1-antitrypsin deficiency or old age tends to be panacinar.
12. Emphysema in which septal deterioration results from smoking tends to be centriacinar.
13. Chronic obstructive pulmonary disease (COPD) is the coexistence of chronic bronchitis and emphysema.
14. Upper respiratory tract infections, which are the most common cause of short-term disability in the United States, include rhinitis (the common cold), pharyngitis, and laryngitis.
15. Serious lower respiratory tract infections, which occur most frequently in very old persons and individuals with impaired immunity or underlying disease, include pneumonia and tuberculosis.
16. Pneumococcal pneumonia is an acute lung infection resulting in an inflammatory response with four phases: (a) consolidation, (b) red hepatization, (c) gray hepatization, and (d) resolution.
17. Viral pneumonia is an acute, self-limiting lung infection usually caused by the influenza virus.
18. Tuberculosis is a lung infection caused by *Mycobacterium tuberculosis* (tubercle bacillus).
19. In tuberculosis the inflammatory response isolates colonies of bacilli by enclosing them in tubercles and surrounding the tubercles with scar tissue.
20. Bacilli may remain dormant within the tubercles for life or, if the immune system breaks down, cause recurrence of active disease.
21. Pulmonary vascular diseases are caused by embolism or hypertension in the pulmonary circulation.
22. Pulmonary embolism is occlusion of a portion of the pulmonary vascular bed by a thrombus (most common), a tissue fragment, or an air bubble. Depending on its size and location, the embolus can cause hypoxic vasoconstriction, pulmonary edema, atelectasis, pulmonary hypertension, shock, and even death.
23. Pulmonary hypertension (pulmonary artery pressure 5 to 10 mm Hg above normal) is caused by (a) elevated left ventricular pressure, (b) increased blood flow through the pulmonary circulation, (c) obliteration or obstruction of the vascular bed, or (d) active constriction of the vascular bed produced by hypoxemia or acidosis.
24. Cor pulmonale is right ventricular enlargement caused by chronic pulmonary hypertension. Cor pulmonale progresses to right ventricular failure if the pulmonary hypertension is not reversed.
25. Lip cancer is most common in men and represents about 1% of all cancers. In the most common cell type, squamous cell, metastasis is rare when lesions are diagnosed and treated early.
26. Laryngeal cancer occurs primarily in men and represents 2% to 3% of all cancers. Squamous cell carcinoma of the true vocal cords is most common and manifests with a clinical symptom of progressive hoarseness.
27. Lung cancer, the most frequent cause of cancer death in the United States, is commonly caused by cigarette smoking.
28. Cancer cell types include squamous cell carcinoma, small cell (oat cell) carcinoma, adenocarcinoma, large cell carcinoma, bronchial adenoma, and mesothelioma. Each type arises in a characteristic site or type of tissue, causes distinctive clinical manifestations, and differs in likelihood of metastasis and prognosis.
29. Bronchial carcinoid and adenocystic tumors are rare tumors of the bronchial airways.

KEY TERMS

Abscess, *1116*
Absorption atelectasis, *1111*
Acute cough, *1107*
Adenocarcinoma, *1137*
Adenocystic tumor (cylindroma), *1139*
Adult respiratory distress syndrome (ARDS), *1118*
Asbestosis, *1117*
Aspiration, *1111*
Asthma, *1120*
Atelectasis, *1111*
Bronchial carcinoid tumor, *1139*
Bronchiectasis, *1112*
Bronchiolitis, *1113*
Bronchiolitis obliterans, *1113*
Bronchitis, *1112*
Cavitation, *1116*
Centriacinar emphysema, *1126*
Cheyne-Stokes respirations, *1106*
Chronic bronchitis, *1124*
Chronic cough, *1107*
Chronic obstructive pulmonary disease (COPD), *1124*
Clubbing, *1108*
Coal worker pneumoconiosis (coal miner lung, black lung), *1117*
Compression atelectasis, *1111*
Consolidation, *1116*
Cor pulmonale, *1133*
Cough, *1107*
Cyanosis, *1107*
Cylindrical bronchiectasis, *1112*
Dyspnea, *1105*
Emphysema, *1126*
Empyema (infected pleural effusion), *1115*
Extrinsic allergic alveolitis (hypersensitivity pneumonitis), *1117*
Exudative effusion, *1115*

KEY TERMS—cont'd

Flail chest, *1116*
Hemoptysis, *1107*
Hemothorax, *1115*
Hypercapnia, *1106*
Hyperventilation, *1107*
Hypocapnia, *1107*
Hypoventilation, *1106*
Hypoxemia, *1108*
Hypoxia, *1108*
Kussmaul respiration (hyperpnea), *1106*
Mesothelioma, *1139*
Mucoepidermoid carcinoma, *1139*
Open pneumothorax (communicating pneumothorax), *1113*
Orthopnea (positional dyspnea), *1106*
Oxygen toxicity, *1117*
Panacinar emphysema, *1126*
Paroxysmal nocturnal dyspnea (PND), *1106*
Pleural effusion, *1114*
Pleurisy (pleuritis), *1115*
Pneumoconiosis, *1117*
Pneumonia, *1127*
Pneumothorax, *1113*
Pulmonary edema, *1110*
Pulmonary embolism, *1131*
Pulmonary fibrosis, *1116*
Pulmonary thromboembolism, *1131*
Saccular bronchiectasis, *1112*
Secondary pneumothorax, *1114*
Silicosis, *1117*
Small cell carcinoma, *1138*
Spontaneous pneumothorax, *1113*
Squamous cell carcinoma, *1136*
Status asthmaticus, *1123*
Tension pneumothorax, *1113*
TNM classification, *1140*
Transudative effusion, *1115*
Tuberculosis, *1130*
Undifferentiated large cell carcinoma (undifferentiated large cell anaplastic cancer), *1138*
Varicose bronchiectasis, *1112*

REFERENCES

1. Manning HL, Schwartzstein RM: Mechanisms of disease pathophysiology of dyspnea, *N Engl J Med* 333(23):1547, 1995.
2. Laffey JG, Kavanagh BP: Carbon dioxide and the critically ill—too little of a good thing? *Lancet* 354(9186):1283, 1999.
3. Irwin RS et al: Managing cough as a defense mechanism and as a symptom: a consensus panel report of the American College of Chest Physicians, *Chest* 115(2 suppl):133s, 1998.
4. Hirshberg B et al: Hemoptysis: etiology, evaluation, and outcome in a tertiary referral hospital, *Chest* 112(2):440, 1997.
5. Sridhar KS, Lobo CF, Altman RD: Digital clubbing and lung cancer, *Chest* 114(6):1535, 1998.
6. Baharloo F et al: Tracheobronchial foreign bodies: presentation and management in children and adults, *Chest* 115(5):1357, 1999.
7. Rothen HU et al: Prevention of atelectasis during general anaesthesia, *Lancet* 345:1387, 1995.
8. Cohen M, Sahn SA: Bronchietasis in systemic diseases, *Chest* 116(4): 1063, 1999.
9. Boehler A et al: Bronchiolitis obliterans after lung transplantation: a review, *Chest* 114(5):1411, 1998.
10. Miller AC: Treatment of spontaneous pneumothorax: the clinician's perspective on pneumothorax management, *Chest* 113(5):1423, 1998.
11. Lim TK: Management of pleural empyema, *Chest* 116(3):845, 1999.
12. Hirshberg B et al: Factors predicting mortality of patients with lung abscess, *Chest* 115(3):746, 1999.
13. Ziesche R et al: A preliminary study of long-term treatment with interferon gamma-1b and low-dose prednisone in patients with idiopathic pulmonary fibrosis, *N Engl J Med* 341(17):1254, 1999.
14. Capellier G et al: Oxygen toxicity and tolerance, *Minerva Anestegiolica* 65(6):388, 1999.
15. Lim Y et al: Silica-induced apoptosis in vitro and in vivo, *Toxicol Lett* 108(2-3):335, 1999.
16. Kinnula VL: Oxidant and antioxidant mechanisms of lung disease caused by asbestos fibres, *Eur Respir J* 14(3):706, 1999.
17. Schuyler M, Cormier Y: The diagnosis of hypersensitivity pneumonitis, *Chest* 111(3):534, 1997.
18. Hudson LD, Steinberg KP: Epidemiology of acute lung injury and ARDS, *Chest* 115(1 suppl):74s, 1999.
19. Kollef MH, Schuster DP: The acute respiratory distress syndrome, *N Engl J Med* 332:27, 1995.
20. Martin TR: Lung cytokines and ARDS: Roger S Mitchell lecture, *Chest* 116(1 suppl):2s, 1999.
21. Bernard GR et al: The American European Consensus Conference on ARDS: definitions, mechanisms, relevant outcomes and clinical trial coordination, *Am J Respir Crit Care Med* 149:818, 1994.
22. Wyncoll DLA, Evans TW: Acute respiratory distress syndrome, *Lancet* 354(9177):497, 1999.
23. Rocker GM et al: Noninvasive positive pressure ventilation: successful outcome in patients with acute lung injury ARDS, *Chest* 115(1):173, 1999.
24. Vollman KM, Aulbach RK: Acute respiratory distress syndrome. In Kinney MR et al, editors: *AACN clinical reference for critical care nursing,* ed 4, St Louis, 1998, Mosby.
25. Sachdeva RC, Guntapalli KK: Acute respiratory distress syndrome, *Crit Care Clin* 13(3):503, 1997.
26. Second Expert Panel on the Management of Asthma, National Heart, Lung, and Blood Institute: *Highlights of the Expert Panel Report 2: guidelines for the diagnosis and management of asthma,* pub no NIH 97-4051A, Bethesda, Md, 1997, National Institutes of Health.
27. Mannino DM et al: Surveillance for asthma—United States, 1960-1995, *MMWR CDC Surveil Summ* 47(1):1, 1998.
28. Borrish L: Genetics of allergy and asthma, *Ann Allergy Asthma Immunol* 82:413, 1999.
29. Martinez FD: Role of respiratory infections in onset of asthma and chronic pulmonary disease, *Clin Exp Allergy* 29(suppl 2):53, 1999.
30. Charpin D, Dutau H: Role of allergens in the natural history of childhood asthma, *Pediatr Pulmonol* 18:34, 1999.
31. Nicolai T: Air pollution and respiratory disease in children: what is the clinically relevant impact? *Pediatr Pulmonol* 18:9, 1999.
32. Fahy JV, Corry DB, Boushey HA: Airway inflammation and remodeling in asthma, *Curr Opin Pulmon Med* 5(1):15, 2000.
33. Ashutosh K: Nitric oxide and asthma: a review, *Curr Opin Pulmon Med* 6(1):21, 2000.
34. Hart CM: Nitric oxide in adult lung disease, *Chest* 115(5):1407, 1999.
35. Hunt JF et al: Endogenous airway acidification—implications for asthma pathophysiology, *Am J Respir Crit Care Med* 161(3):694, 2000.
36. Reed CE: The natural history of asthma in adults: the problem of irreversibility, *J Allergy Clin Immunol* 103:539, 1999.
37. Chernjack RM: Physiologic diagnosis and function in asthma, *Clin Chest Med* 16:567, 1995.
38. Lipworth BJ: Leukotriene-receptor antagonists, *Lancet* 353(9146):67, 1999.
39. Owen CL: New directions in asthma management, *Am J Nurs* 99(3):26, 1999.
40. Drazen JM, Israel E, O'Byrne PM: Drug therapy: treatment of asthma with drugs modifying the leukotriene, *N Engl J Med* 340(3):197, 1999.
41. Kerstjens HAM: Clinical evidence: stable chronic obstructive pulmonary disease, *BMJ* 319(7208):495, 1999.

42. Strategies in preserving lung health and preventing COPD and associated diseases. The National Lung Health Education Program (NLHEP), *Chest* 113(2 suppl):123S, 1998.
43. Grossman RF: The value of antibiotics and the outcomes of antibiotic therapy in exacerbations of COPD, *Chest* 113:2495, 1998.
44. Senior RM, Anthonisen NR: Chronic obstructive pulmonary disease (COPD), *Am J Respir Crit Care Med* 157:s139, 1998.
45. Hoo GW, Hakimian M, Santiago SM: Hypercapnic respiratory failure in COPD patients: response to therapy, *Chest* 117(1):169, 2000.
46. Crystal RG: Alpha-1 antitrypsin deficiency. In Fishman AP, editor: *Update: pulmonary diseases and disorders,* New York, 1992, McGraw-Hill.
47. Barnes PJ: New therapies for chronic obstructive pulmonary disease, *Thorax* 53:137, 1998.
48. Celli BR: Standards for the optimal management of COPD, *Chest* 113(4 suppl):283s, 1998.
49. Boushey HA: Glucocorticoid therapy for chronic obstructive pulmonary disease, *N Engl J Med* 340(25):1990, 1999.
50. Griffiths TL et al: Results at 1 year of outpatient multidisciplinary pulmonary rehabilitation: a randomized controlled trial, *Lancet* 355 (9201):362, 2000.
51. O'Brien GM et al: Improvements in lung function, exercise and quality of life in hypercapnic patients after lung volume reduction surgery, *Chest* 115:75, 1999.
52. Trulock EP: Lung transplantation for COPD, *Chest* 113(4 suppl):269s, 1998.
53. Bernstein JM: Treatment of community-acquired pneumonia—IDSA guidelines, *Chest* 315(3 suppl):9S, 1999.
54. Brown PD, Lerner SA: Community acquired pneumonia, *Lancet* 352(9136):1295, 1999.
55. Khurana S, Litaker D: The dilemma of nosocomial pneumonia: what primary care physicians should know, *Cleveland Clin J Med* 67(1):25, 2000.
56. Nelson S et al: Pathophysiology of pneumonia, *Clin Chest Med* 16:1, 1995.
57. Toumanen EI, Austrian R, Masure HR: Pathogenesis of pneumococcal infection, *N Engl J Med* 332:1280, 1995.
58. Liebler JM, Markin CJ: Fiberoptic bronchoscopy for diagnosis and treatment, *Crit Care Clin* 16(1):82, 2000.
59. Dye C et al: Global burden of tuberculosis: estimated incidence, prevalence, and mortality by country, *JAMA* 282(7):677, 1999.
60. McCray E: The epidemiology of tuberculosis in the United States, *Clin Chest Med* 18:99, 1997.
61. Mitchison DA: How drug resistance emerges as a result of poor compliance during short-course chemotherapy for tuberculosis, *Int J Tuberculosis Lung Dis* 2:10, 1998.
62. American Thoracic Society: Diagnostic standards and classification of tuberculosis, *Am Rev Respir Dis* 142(3):725, 1990.
63. Basso LA, Blanchard JS: Resistance to antitubercular drugs, *Adv Exp Med Biol* 456:115, 1998.
64. Schraufnagel DE: Tuberculosis treatment for the beginning of the next century, *Int J Tuberculosis Lung Dis* 3(8):651, 1999.
65. Temple ME, Nahata MC: Rifapentine: its role in the treatment of tuberculosis, *Ann Pharmacother* 33(11):1203, 1999.
66. Hyers TM: Venous thromboembolism, *Am J Respir Care Med* 159:1, 1999.
67. Heit JA et al: Risk factors for deep vein thrombosis and pulmonary embolism, *Arch Intern Med* 160:809, 2000.
68. Silverstein MD et al: Trends in the incidence of deep vein thrombosis and pulmonary embolism, *Arch Intern Med* 158:585, 1998.
69. Indik JH, Alpert JS: Detection of pulmonary embolism by D-dimer assay, spiral computed tomography and magnetic resonance imaging, *Prog Cardiovasc Dis* 42(4):261, 2000.
70. Kline JA et al: New diagnostic tests for pulmonary embolism, *Ann Emerg Med* 35(2):168, 2000.
71. Mullins MD et al: The role of spiral volumetric computed tomography in the diagnosis of pulmonary embolism, *Arch Intern Med* 160:293, 2000.
72. Stratton MA et al: Prevention of venous thromboembolism, *Arch Intern Med* 160:334, 2000.
73. Hull RD et al: Low molecular-weight heparin vs heparin in the treatment of patients with pulmonary embolism: American-Canadian thrombosis study group, *Arch Intern Med* 160(2):229, 2000.
74. Litin SC, Heit JA, Mees KA: Use of low-molecular-weight heparin in the treatment of venous thromboembolic disease: answers to frequently asked questions, *Mayo Clin Proc* 73:545, 1998.
75. Galie N et al: Primary pulmonary hypertension: insights into pathogenesis from epidemiology, *Chest* 114(3 suppl):184S, 1998.
76. Gaine SP, Rubin LJ: Primary pulmonary hypertension, *Lancet* 352 (9129):719, 1998.
77. Hoeper MM et al: A comparison of the acute hemodynamic effects of inhaled nitric oxide and aerosolized iloprost in primary pulmonary hypertension, *J Am Coll Cardiol* 35(1):176, 2000.
78. Greenlee RT et al: Cancer statistics, 2000, *CA Cancer J Clin* 50(1):7, 2000.
79. Onercl M, Yilmaz T, Gedikoghi G: Tumor thickness as a predictor of cervical lymph node metastasis in squamous cell carcinoma of the lower lip, *Otolaryngol Head Neck Surg* 122(1):139, 2000.
80. De Visscher JG et al: A comparison of results after radiotherapy and surgery for stage 1 squamous cell carcinoma of the lower lip, *Head Neck* 21(6):526, 2000.
81. Szyfter K et al: Molecular and cellular alterations in tobacco smoke-associated larynx cancer, *Mutation Res* 445(2):259, 1999.
82. Sessions RB, Harrison LB, Hong WK: Laryngeal cancer. In Devita VT Jr, Hellman S, Rosenberg S, editors: *Cancer: principles and practice of oncology,* Philadelphia, 1993, Lippincott.
83. Laccourreye O et al: Chemotherapy combined with conservation surgery in the treatment of early larynx cancer, *Curr Opin Oncol* 119(3):200, 1999.
84. Wingo PA et al: Annual report to the nation on the status of cancer, 1973-1996, with a special section on lung cancer and tobacco smoking, *J Natl Cancer Inst* 91(8):675, 1999.
85. Brown KG: Lung cancer and environmental tobacco smoke: occupational risk to non-smokers, *Environ Health Perspect* 107(suppl 6):885, 1999.
86. Bunn PA, Kelly K: New chemotherapeutic agents prolong survival and improve quality of life in non–small cell lung cancer: a review of the literature and future directions, *Clin Cancer Res* 4(5):1087, 1998.
87. Adjel AA, Marks RS, Bonner JA: Current guidelines for the management of small cell lung cancer, *Mayo Clin Proc* 74:809, 1999.
88. Hecht SS: Tobacco smoke carcinogens and lung cancer, *J Natl Cancer Inst* 91(14):1194, 1999.
89. Schreiber G et al: Molecular genetic analysis of primary lung cancer and cancer metastatic to the lung, *Anticancer Res* 19:1109, 1999.
90. Biesalski HK et al: European Consensus Statement on Lung Cancer: risk factors and prevention. Lung Cancer Panel, *CA Cancer J Clin* 48: 167, 1998.
91. Le Marchand L et al: Intake of flavonoids and lung cancer, *J Natl Cancer Inst* 92(2):154, 2000.
92. Rosado de Christensen ML et al: Thoracic carcinoids radiologic-pathologic correlation, *Radiographics* 19(3):707, 1999.
93. Van Boxem TJ et al: High-resolution CT in patients with intraluminal typical bronchial carcinoid tumors treated with bronchoscopic therapy, *Chest* 117(1):125, 2000.
94. Butchart EG: Contemporary management of malignant pleural mesothelioma, *Oncologist* 4(6):488, 1999.
95. DeKlerk N: Environmental mesothelioma. In Jaurand ML, Bignon J, editors: *The mesothelial cell and mesothelioma,* New York, 1994, Marcel Dekker.

CHAPTER 33

Alterations of Pulmonary Function in Children

DEBORAH K. FROH

CHAPTER OUTLINE

Alterations of respiratory function in children are influenced by age, development, gender, race, genetic dominance, and environmental conditions. Newborns are especially vulnerable to a variety of upper and lower airway infections caused by immunologic immaturity. Structural differences in infants and children also render them less competent to tolerate conditions causing increased work of breathing. Access to medical care and timeliness of immunizations influence the incidence and severity of pulmonary disorders.

STRUCTURE AND FUNCTION

A number of structural characteristics of the pulmonary system influence the way in which infants and children respond to respiratory disturbances. These include structural characteristics of the upper and lower airways, chest wall and lung dynamics, metabolic requirements, immunologic immaturity, and physiologic control of respiration.

Upper Airway

All conducting airways (the portions of airway that do not conduct gas exchange) are present at birth and change only in size throughout childhood. Branching of the bronchial tree is, in fact, complete by the sixteenth week of fetal life.

Because infants and children naturally have smaller-diameter airways than do adults, they suffer exponentially more obstruction for a given degree of mucosal edema or secretion accumulation. The relative sizes of tonsils, adenoids, and epiglottis, likewise, are proportionately greater in the young child and, with swelling, can impose a significant site of obstruction. Infants up to 2 to 3 months of age are "obligatory nose breathers" and are unable to breathe *in* through their mouths. Nasal congestion is therefore a serious threat to the young infant.

Lower Airway

Although the tracheobronchial tree is complete at birth, there are fewer alveoli in the neonate than in the older child or adult. Further, there is a reduced number or size (or both) of pores of Kohn that allow collateral ventilation. The quantity of alveoli increases until 8 years of age, after which the alveoli increase in size and complexity.

The structural changes that occur during the last trimester transform the lungs, with widening of airspaces at the expense of interstitial tissue. Capillaries grow into the distal respiratory units, which keep subdividing to maximize surface area. Specialized cell types, such as type II cells, become manifest (Fig. 33-1).

Surfactant is a lipid-protein mix that is produced by type II cells and is critical for maintaining alveolar expansion (and thus allowing normal gas exchange). It lines alveoli and reduces surface tension, preventing alveolar collapse at the end of each exhalation. Without surfactant the alveoli tend to stay closed, demanding greater inspiratory force and work of breathing to reexpand the alveoli on the next breath. Deficiency of surfactant is often seen in premature infants and causes respiratory distress syndrome (RDS) or hyaline membrane disease. This surfactant deficiency reflects developmental immaturity. Surfactant lipid is produced by 20 to 24 weeks of gestation and is secreted into the fetal airways

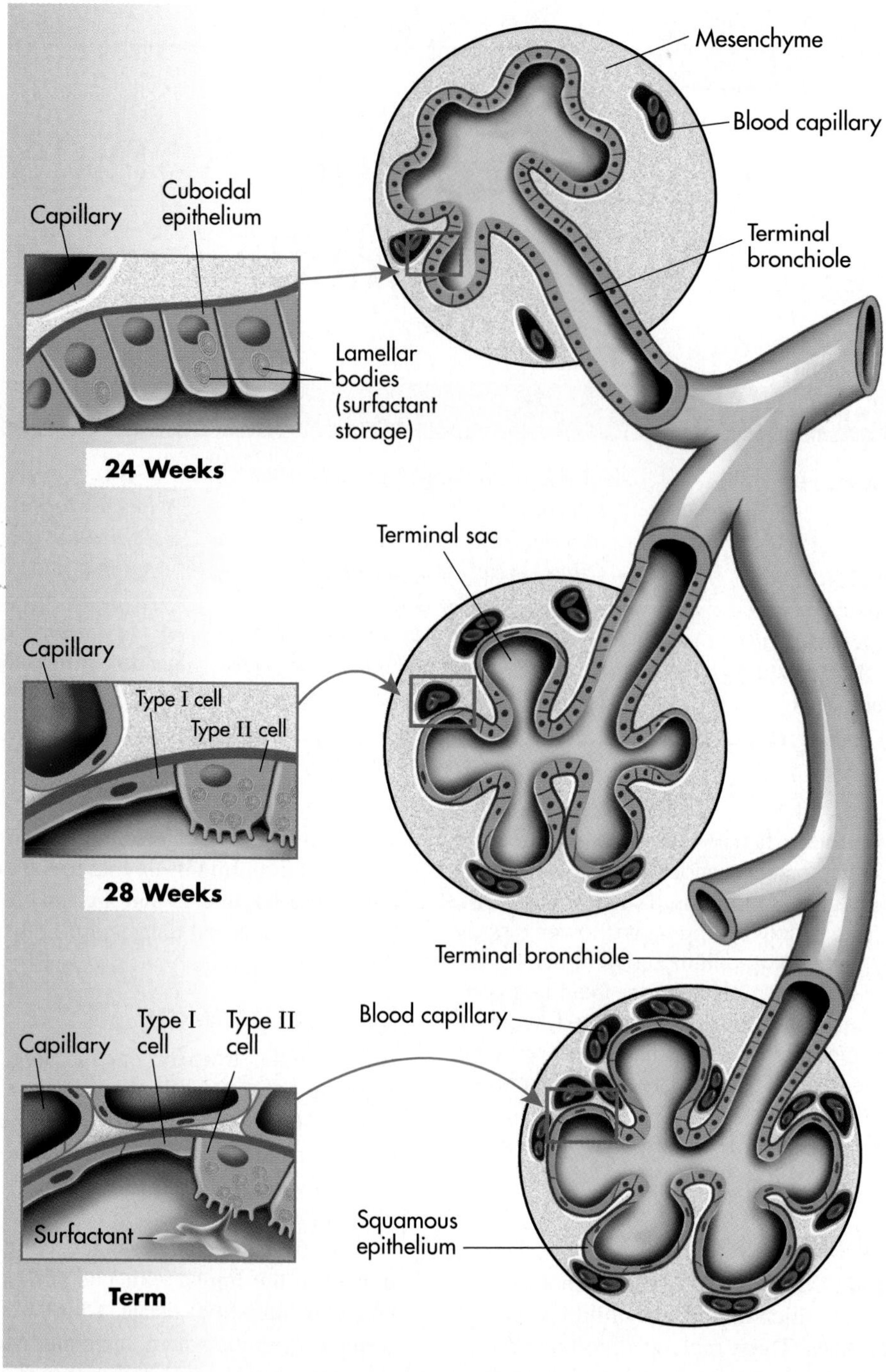

FIG. 33-1 Prenatal development of the alveolar unit. Epithelial cells differentiate into type II and type I cells. Mature type II tests are cuboidal, have apical microvilli, and contain lamellar bodies for surfactant storage and secretion. Type I cells are derived from type II cells and consist of flattened epithelium overlying capillaries, thus forming part of the desired thin air-blood barrier. During fetal development the pulmonary capillaries initially are randomly distributed in mesenchyme. They progressively arrange around the epithelial tubes and establish close contacts to the lining epithelium. Overall, the volume of mesenchyme decreases and that of the potential airspace increases.

by 30 weeks. The more premature the infant, the higher the risk of RDS.

Chest Wall Dynamics

Chest wall compliance is high in infants, particularly premature infants. The cartilaginous structures of the thoracic cage are not yet well ossified (ossification continues to occur throughout childhood), and the chest wall is easily collapsible. During inspiration in the young child, air is drawn in by the downward movement of the diaphragm, but the resulting negative pressure causes the "soft" chest wall to be drawn *inward* (Fig. 33-2); this produces so-called *paradoxic breath-*

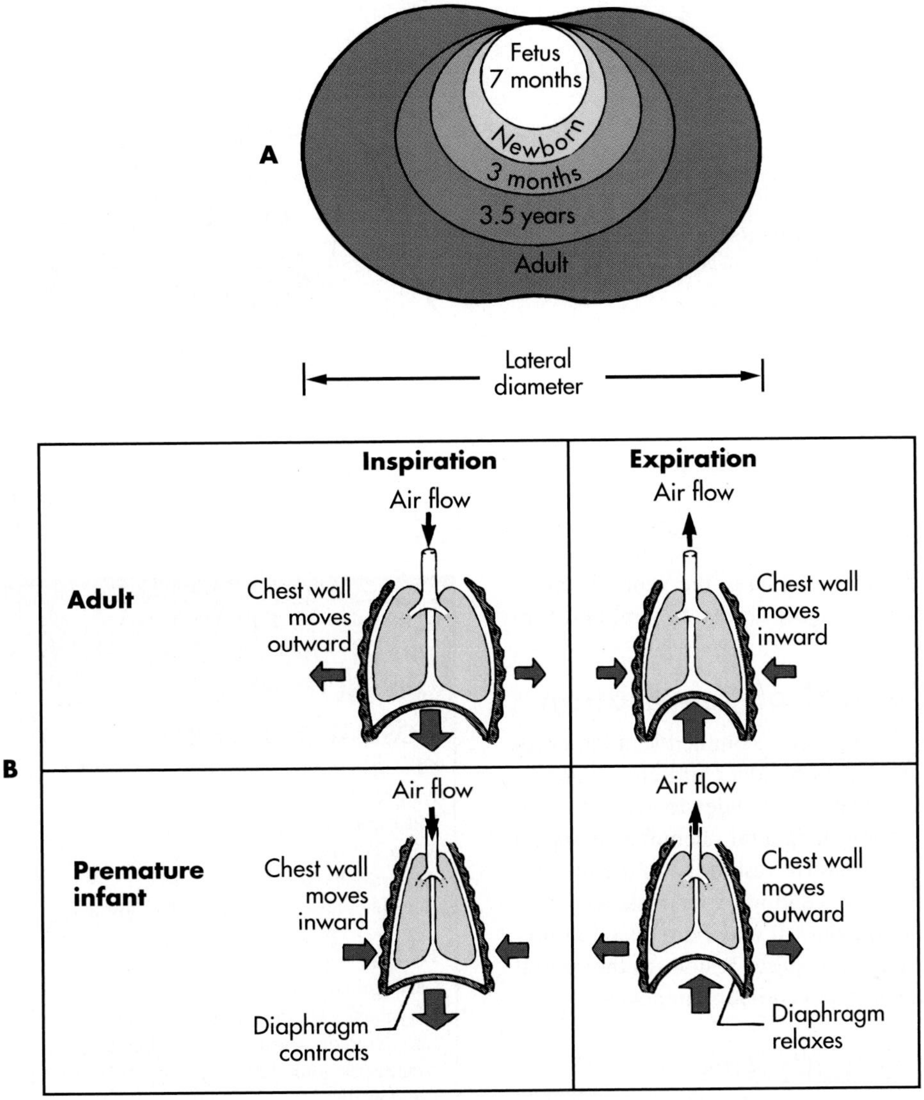

FIG. 33-2 Developmental differences in the chest wall and lung mechanics. A, Changes in chest wall shape with age. **B,** Differences in lung mechanics caused by differences in chest wall compliance (degree of rigidity) in premature infants and adults. (*Arrows* indicate direction of airflow, chest wall movement, and diaphragm movement.)

ing, or *diaphragmatic breathing.* Paradoxic breathing is especially seen during rapid eye movement (REM) sleep of premature infants. With pulmonary compromise the accessory muscles also are drawn inward, creating retraction of the intercostal and supraclavicular spaces (Fig. 33-3).

Resting lung volume, or **functional residual capacity (FRC),** represents the balance point between the natural elastic recoil of the lungs (to collapse) and the elastic recoil of the chest wall (to expand). In the face of an overly compliant chest wall, infants up to about 1 year of age are thought to maintain their FRC and avoid atelectasis by muscular "braking" of their expiration. This may occur either by active glottic narrowing or by increased activity of the inspiratory intercostal muscles.

Metabolic Characteristics

The basal metabolic rate of a child is greater than that of an adult, and thus oxygen consumption ($\dot{V}O_2$) is greater per unit of body weight. The $\dot{V}O_2$ of the child's normal pulmonary state accounts for up to 25% of the total $\dot{V}O_2$. The work of breathing increases $\dot{V}O_2$ exponentially with respiratory distress. Less muscle glycogen reserve limits the efficiency of accessory muscles, and consequently fatigue, with lactic acidosis, occurs quickly. Children also have a high proportion of extracellular fluid; they more quickly lose fluid from fever, from environmental heat, or in association with tachypnea (causing evaporation from the respiratory tract) and become dehydrated.

Immunologic Incompetence

Passive immunity with immunoglobulin G (IgG) is normally conveyed transplacentally from the mother to the fetus beginning at 20 weeks of gestation; thus levels are lower in preterm than term infants. Breastfeeding allows further transfer after birth. Because IgG has a half-life of approximately 21 days, the placentally transferred antibodies will be gone after a few months. Babies are able to make IgG, IgM, and IgA, and levels increase slowly with age. Cell-mediated

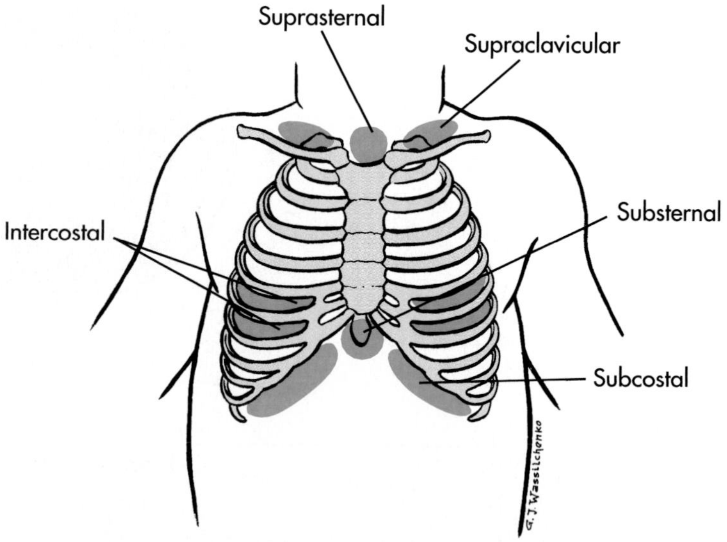

FIG. 33-3 Areas of chest muscle retraction. (From Wong DL: *Whaley and Wong's nursing care of infants and children,* ed 6, St Louis, 1999, Mosby.)

immunity is also not fully developed in the neonate, creating a situation of enhanced susceptibility to viral and fungal infections.

Physiologic Control of Respiration

The newborn, for up to 3 weeks, has a blunted ventilatory response to hypoxia compared with older children and adults. The mechanisms for this are not well understood but may reflect reduced activity of the peripheral chemoreceptors (in the carotid body) and nonadaptive responses in the respiratory center (in the brain stem). Ventilatory response to hypercarbia is normal in term infants but may be reduced in premature infants. Congenital or acquired lesions of the central nervous system may cause hypoventilation or apnea.

PULMONARY DISORDERS

Pulmonary dysfunction can be categorized into disorders of either the upper airway or lower airway. Signs of acute respiratory failure, however, remain the same regardless of etiology. These include the following:

- Increased respiratory effort with retractions (see Fig. 33-3) or gasping; apnea in some conditions
- Cyanosis or pallor
- Agitation
- Decreased level of consciousness
- Cardiovascular signs: tachycardia, mottled color, or bradycardia
- Physiologic compromise reflected by hemoglobin desaturation, hypoxemia, hypercarbia, and acidosis

Disorders of the Upper Airways

The crucial issue in the upper airways is patency. The most common causes of *acute-onset* **upper airway obstruction (UAO)** in children are infections, **foreign body aspiration**, angioedema, and trauma. *Chronic* UAO has many etiologies, including congenital malformations affecting the airway, cartilaginous weakness, vocal cord paralysis, and subglottic stenosis. Chronic upper airway symptoms should prompt referral to a pediatric pulmonologist or an otolaryngologist because specialized diagnostic studies may be needed. A list of causes of pediatric UAO can be found in Box 33-1.

Box 33-1

CAUSES OF UPPER AIRWAY OBSTRUCTION IN CHILDREN ACCORDING TO SITE OF OBSTRUCTION

NOSE AND PHARYNX

Choanal atresia
Lingual thyroid or thyroglossal cyst
Macroglossia
Micrognathia
Hypertrophic tonsils/adenoids
Retropharyngeal or peritonsillar abscess

LARYNX

Laryngomalacia
Laryngeal web, cyst or laryngocele
Laryngotracheobronchitis (viral croup)
Acute spasmodic laryngitis (spasmodic croup)
Epiglottitis
Vocal cord paralysis
Laryngotracheal stenosis
Intubation
Foreign body
Cystic hygroma
Subglottic hemangioma
Laryngeal papilloma
Angioneurotic edema
Laryngospasm (hypocalcemic tetany)
Psychogenic stridor

TRACHEA

Tracheomalacia
Bacterial tracheitis
External compression

From Leung AKC, Cho H: Diagnosis of stridor in children, *Am Fam Physician* 60(8):2289, 1999.

The site and nature of the obstruction are often discernible by assessing the noise associated with breathing, the

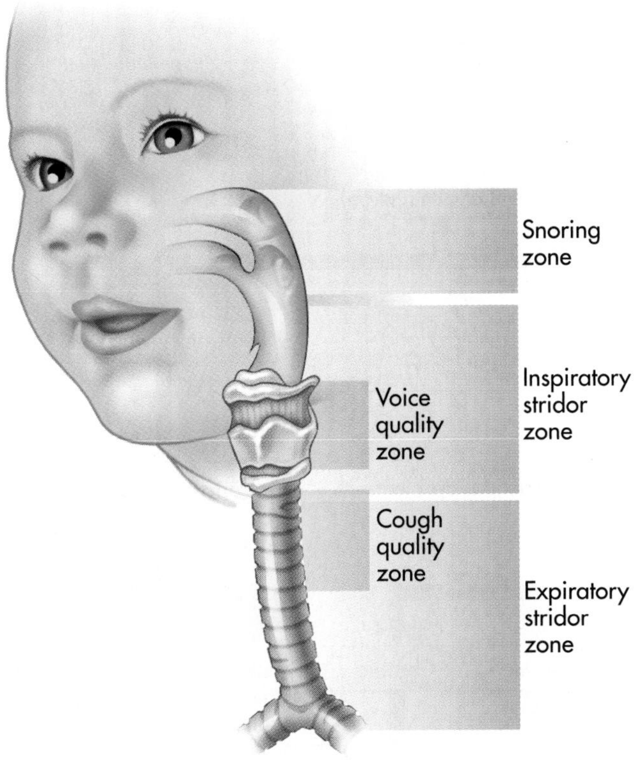

FIG. 33-4 Listening can help locate the site of airway obstruction. A loud, gasping snore suggests enlarged tonsils or adenoids. In inspiratory stridor, the airway is compromised at the level of the supraglottic larynx, vocal cords, subglottic region, or upper trachea. Expiratory stridor or central wheeze results from narrowing or collapse of the lower trachea or bronchi. Airway noise during both inspiration and expiration often represents a fixed obstruction of the vocal cords or subglottic space. Hoarseness or a weak cry is a by-product of obstruction at the vocal cords. If a cough is croupy or low pitched, suspect tracheal pathology. (Redrawn from Eavey RD: A sound workup for evaluating airway obstructions, *Contemp Pediatr* 3(6):78, 1986; used with permission; original illustration by Paul Singh-Roy.)

quality of the voice or cry, and presence of feeding difficulties.[1,2] This assessment can often be made by observation. Likewise, the severity of the problem can to a great extent be judged by simple visual observation of signs, including retractions, nasal flaring, gasping or obstructed breaths, anxiety, restlessness, or need to maintain a specific head or body position. Agitation should be regarded as a likely sign of hypoxemia or obstruction. In acute UAO, increasing the child's anxiety, as by excessive examination, can worsen the condition further. The child should be kept as calm as possible. The clinician should never attempt a pharyngeal examination if there is any suspicion of epiglottitis or retropharyngeal abscess, because this maneuver may precipitate acute obstruction of the airway.

The sounds of the child's breathing can provide key clues (Fig. 33-4). A sonorous, snoring noise is typical for nasopharyngeal obstruction, such as adenotonsillar hypertrophy. A common sign of pediatric UAO is **stridor,** a harsh, vibratory sound of variable pitch due to turbulent flow through the partially obstructed airway. A diagnostic approach to stridor is outlined in Fig. 33-5. Whether it is present in inspiration or expiration, or both, reflects the site of the problem. In general, *inspiratory* stridor is generated with obstruction of the *extrathoracic* airway (above the thoracic inlet), which includes the supraglottic structures, the larynx, the subglottic space, and the upper trachea. *Expiratory* stridor or a monophonic wheeze may be generated by an obstruction in the *intrathoracic* airway (the mid to lower trachea and central bronchi). *Biphasic* stridor typically reflects obstruction at the glottis (e.g., vocal cord paralysis) itself or a *fixed* rather than a *dynamic* lesion in the subglottic space (e.g., hemangioma or subglottic stenosis). Biphasic noise may sometimes mean abnormalities of both extrathoracic and intrathoracic trachea (long-segment stenosis or malacia).

Abnormalities of voice or cry (weak or hoarse) suggest problems at the larynx, such as vocal cord paralysis. Muffling of the voice, especially in an acute setting, suggests supralaryngeal obstruction, such as epiglottitis or retropharyngeal abscess. Pronounced cough may be an irritative symptom, such as due to aspirated foreign body, or may be a sign of tracheal obstruction. The cough associated with croup or trachael foreign body is usually harsh and barking.

Airway obstruction occurs more early in infants than in older children. Obviously, airway luminal size is smaller along with body size, but any decrease in luminal diameter will be much more significant. This is because airway resistance is proportional to the inverse of the *fourth* power of the radius; thus a decrease to half the original diameter increases resistance sixteenfold. Furthermore, an infant's cartilaginous structures are more collapsible and thus are prone to creating or contributing to a situation of upper airway obstruction.

Infections

Infections of the upper airway (Table 33-1) are common in children, and some have the potential to cause life-threatening emergencies. Recognition and rapid evaluation of these problems are crucial pediatric care skills.

Croup

Classic **croup** is an acute **laryngotracheobronchitis** and is common among young children from 6 months to 5 years,

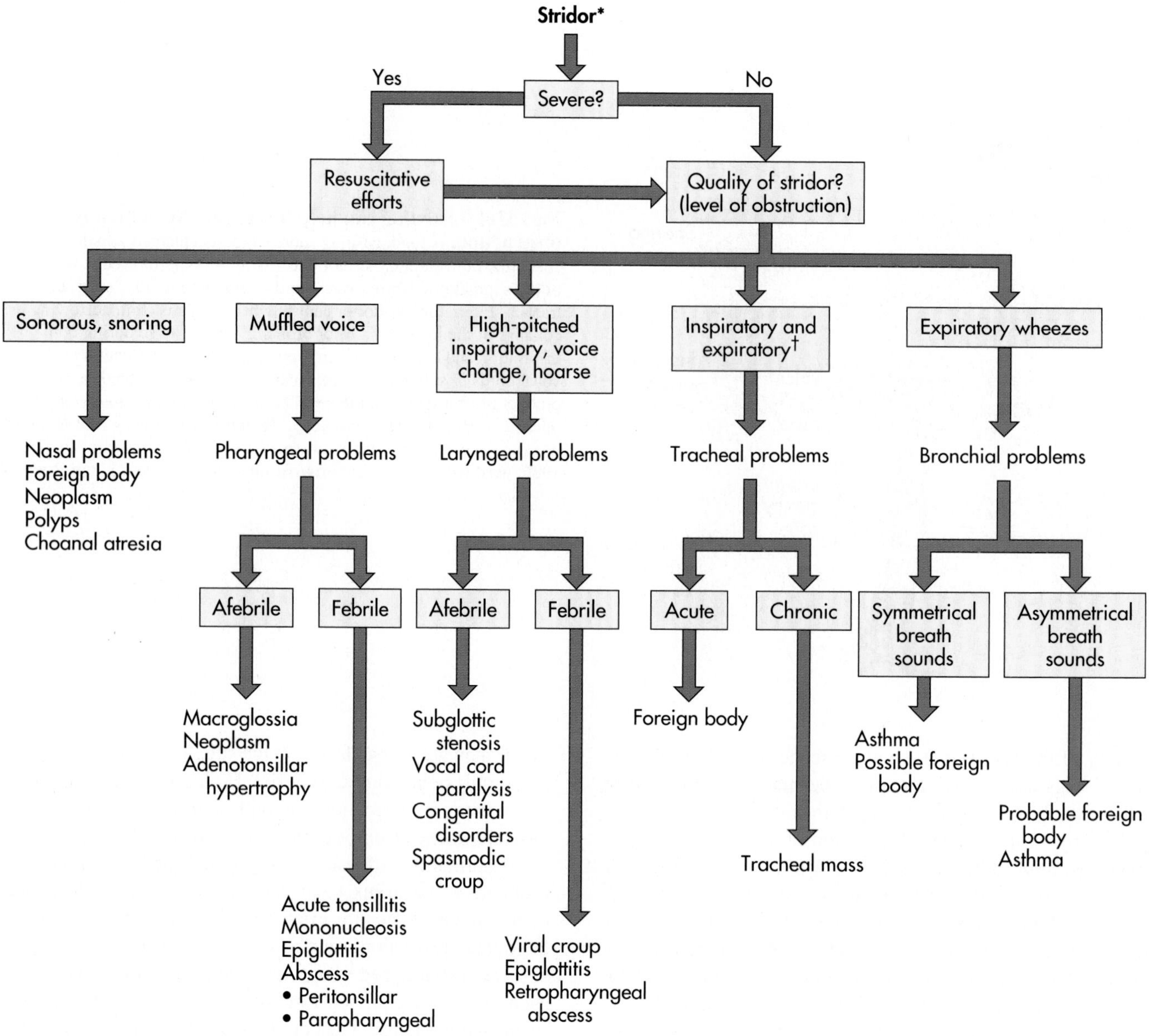

* The age of the patient must be considered in making a specific diagnosis
† Laryngeal problems are frequently associated with inspiratory and expiratory stridor

FIG. 33-5 Diagnostic approach to stridor. (Adapted from Handler SD: Stridor. In Fleisher GR, Ludwig S, editors: *Textbook of pediatric emergency medicine,* Baltimore, 1993, Williams & Wilkins.)

with peak incidence at age 1 to 2 years.[3,4] In 85% of cases, croup is caused by a virus, most commonly parainfluenza but sometimes others such as influenza A or respiratory syncytial virus. The incidence of croup is highest in late autumn and winter, corresponding to parainfluenza season. Croup is more common in boys than girls. In a significant portion of affected children, croup is a recurrent problem during childhood, and in about 15% of cases there is a family history of croup.

Pathophysiology

The pathophysiology of viral croup is due primarily to subglottic edema from the infection. The mucous membranes of the larynx are tightly adherent to the underlying cartilage, whereas those of the subglottic space are looser and thus allow accumulation of mucosal and submucosal edema. Furthermore, the cricoid cartilage is structurally the narrowest point of the airway, making edema in this area critical. As depicted in Fig. 33-6, increased resistance to airflow leads to increased work of breathing, which generates more negative intrathoracic pressure, which, in turn, may exacerbate dynamic collapse of the upper airway.

Clinical Manifestations

Typically there is a prodrome of rhinorrhea, sore throat, and low-grade fever for a few days. The child then develops the characteristic seal-like barking cough and, in severe cases, inspiratory stridor. Most cases are mild and resolve sponta-

Table 33-1 Comparison of Upper Airway Infections

Condition	Age	Onset	Etiology	Pathophysiology	Symptoms
Acute laryngotracheobronchitis	6 mo–3 yr	Usually gradual	Viral	Inflammation from vocal cords to bronchial lumina	Harsh cough; stridor; low-grade fever; may have nasal discharge, conjunctivitis
Acute tracheitis	1–12 yr	Abrupt or following viral illness	*Staphylococcus aureus*	Inflammation of upper trachea	High fever; toxic appearance; thick harsh cough; purulent secretions; may prefer head elevation
Epiglottitis	2–6 yr	Abrupt	*Haemophilus influenzae* Group A streptococcus	Inflammation of supraglottic structures	Severe sore throat; high fever; toxic appearance; muffled voice; may drool; sits erect and quietly
Retropharyngeal abscess	>6 yr	Gradual, 2–5 days	*Staphylococcus aureus* Group B hemolytic streptococcus	Abscess in posterior pharyngeal wall	Similar to epiglottitis
Peritonsillar abscess	>9 yr	May be abrupt	Group B hemolytic streptococcus, *Staphylococcus aureus*	Abscess within or around tonsil	Similar to epiglottitis; may have trismus

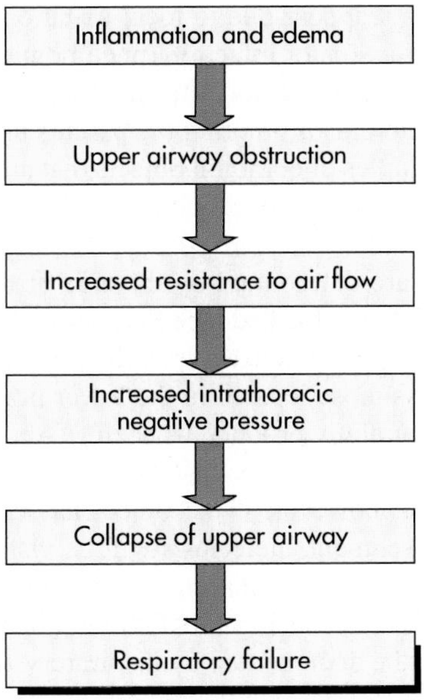

FIG. 33-6 Upper airway obstruction with croup.

neously after several more days. Occasionally, however, upper airway obstruction becomes severe and requires urgent management.[4]

Spasmodic croup is another clinical entity that is characterized by similar hoarseness, barking cough, and stridor but of sudden onset, usually at night and without viral prodrome. It often resolves as quickly as it develops. The etiology is unknown.

Evaluation and Treatment

The degree of symptoms determines the level of treatment. Most children have just a barking cough and viral symptoms and may need no specific treatment. However, the presence of stridor (especially at rest), retractions, or agitation suggests a sicker child.

Croup therapy has been the subject of debate for years, particularly the role of glucocorticoids. The consensus from numerous controlled studies is that there is a demonstrable benefit by 6 hours after a single dose of either dexamethasone (0.15 to 0.6 mg/kg) or nebulized budesonide (2 mg).[5,6] Dexamethasone has a biologic half-life of 36 to 72 hours, long enough to carry the child through the acute phase of the illness before it naturally subsides. The use of steroids in outpatient management of croup is expected to have a huge impact on related hospitalizations and health care costs.

Traditional therapy for croup has included mist. However, scientific studies have neither supported nor refuted its benefit. Acute use of nebulized epinephrine is extremely helpful when significant respiratory distress is present. Epinephrine is usually given as either 5 ml of a 1:1000 solution of L-epinephrine or as 0.5 ml of racemic epinephrine (2.25%) mixed with 2.5 ml of normal saline. It stimulates α- and β-adrenergic receptors and is thought to decrease airway secretions and mucosal edema. However, its effect lasts only 2 hours and should be considered a temporizing measure until concomitantly given steroids begin to take effect. Thus children who are given nebulized epinephrine should be observed for 2 to 3 hours to ensure that they will remain stable if released, and close follow-up is mandatory.

Acute Epiglottitis

Acute epiglottitis is a severe, life-threatening, rapidly progressive infection of the epiglottis and surrounding area. Historically, cases were nearly always due to *Haemophilus influenzae* type b. However, since the advent of *H. influenzae* immunization, acute epiglottitis incidence has decreased to only 10% to 20% of previous levels and has become an adult as well as a pediatric disease.[7-10] Current pediatric cases usually represent vaccine failures or are caused by alternative pathogens such as group A streptococci.[11]

Clinical Manifestations

In the classic form of the disease, a child between 2 and 6 years of age suddenly develops high fever, sore throat, inspiratory stridor, and severe respiratory distress. The child appears ill and anxious and has a voice that sounds muffled.

Drooling and dysphagia (inability to swallow) are common. Death may occur in a few hours. Nasotracheal intubation or tracheotomy is mandatory in instances of rapidly increasing obstruction. Examination of the throat may trigger laryngospasm and cause respiratory collapse. Pneumonia, cervical lymph node inflammation, otitis, and, rarely, meningitis or septic arthritis may occur during the course of epiglottitis.

Evaluation and Treatment

Despite its decreasing incidence, all pediatric practitioners must be familiar with epiglottitis as a life-threatening emergency. The essentials are recognition, avoiding disturbing the child (which could worsen the obstruction), securing the airway by the most experienced personnel (usually an anesthesiologist and otolaryngologist), and intravenous antibiotics. Despite the severe presentation of epiglottitis, resolution with treatment is usually rapid, with intubation rarely needed for more than a few days.

Other Acute Upper Airway Infections

Bacterial tracheitis. **Bacterial tracheitis** can cause rapidly fatal airway obstruction. It is most often caused by *S. aureus* or *H. influenzae*. Onset may be sudden and mimic epiglottitis, or it may complicate a preexisting viral upper respiratory infection or croup. The presence of airway edema and copious purulent secretions leads to obstruction; sometimes there is even formation of a tracheal pseudomembrane or mucosal sloughing. Management is similar to epiglottitis with placement of an artificial airway and intravenous antibiotics.

Retropharyngeal abscess. Retropharyngeal abscess usually occurs in children under 2 years of age in the setting of either nasopharyngeal infection or penetrating local injury. Clinical signs include fever, dysphagia, drooling, stridor, respiratory distress, and stiff neck. This condition requires intravenous antibiotics and, sometimes, incision and drainage.

Tonsillar infections. Tonsillar infections occasionally are severe enough to cause UAO.[12] A classic example, now rare due to immunization, is **diphtheria,** which causes sore throat and dysphagia along with fever, malaise, headache, and nausea. There is significant swelling of the tonsils and pharynx, and there may be a tenacious membrane covering the mucosa.

Peritonsillar abscess is usually unilateral and a complication of acute tonsillitis.[12] Children have fever, sore throat, dysphagia, trismus, pooling of saliva, and muffled voice. Peritonsillar bulging (Fig. 33-7) and cervical adenopathy on the same side are usually visible. The abscess must be drained and the child given antibiotics. The most common causative microorganism is group A β-hemolytic streptococcus.

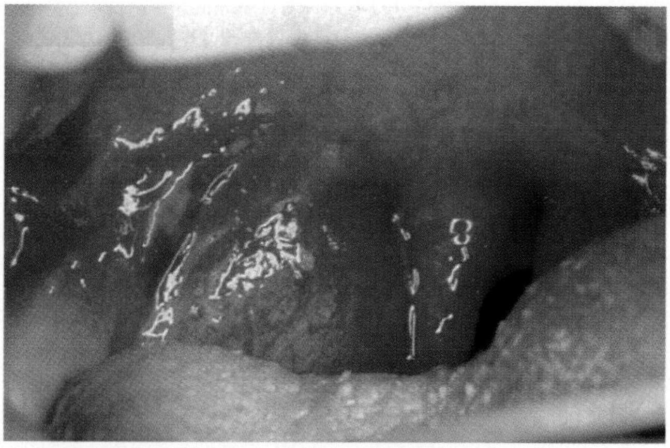

FIG. 33-7 Peritonsillar abscess. Suppuration is evident within the areolar tissue between the tonsil and the superior pharyngeal constrictor muscle, as well as between the anterior and posterior tonsillar pillars. (From Whiting JL, Chow AW: Life-threatening infections of the mouth and throat, *J Crit Illness* 2(7):36, 1987.)

Foreign Body Aspiration

Most children who aspirate a foreign object are between 1 and 3 years of age. Often the aspiration either is not witnessed or does not seem significant to the parent, so fewer than one third of children who aspirate an object seek medical care during the first 24 hours.[13,14] At the time of the aspiration event, the child may cough, choke, gag, or wheeze; occasionally stridor or cyanosis occurs. There may then be a quiescent interval of minutes to even weeks or months before symptoms reappear due to local irritation, granulation, bronchial obstruction, or infection (pneumonia or bronchiectasis). Pronounced inspiratory stridor, cough, and wheezing are typical symptoms prompting the parents to seek medical attention. Examples of common objects that are aspirated include nuts, sunflower seeds, hot dog chunks, popcorn, coins, and small toys.[13-15]

Symptoms are determined by the size of the object and the site in which it is located (see Fig. 33-4). Foreign bodies lodged in the upper trachea typically produce inspiratory stridor, whereas those located in the lower intrathoracic airways more commonly produce wheezing. About 75% of aspirated foreign bodies lodge in a bronchus. Many objects are not radiopaque; however, if the object has completely occluded a lung segment, atelectasis will be visible on a chest x-ray examination or air will accumulate distal to the obstruction if the object is causing a ball-valve effect. This effect can sometimes be documented by inspiratory and expiratory chest films (Fig. 33-8). In a younger child, bilateral decubitus films may show failure to compress the obstructed lung when in the "down" postion.

Most foreign bodies can be removed by bronchoscopy; rarely is a pulmonary lobectomy required. Food particles, which are soft, must be removed, as well as hard objects, because infection will otherwise occur. Objects lodged in the laryngeal or subglottic regions are particularly dangerous because of their potential for complete or near-complete airway occlusion.[16]

Other Causes of Upper Airway Compromise

Angioedema

Angioedema is a localized edema involving the deep, subcutaneous layers of skin or mucous membranes. It may occur with deficiency of C1 esterase inhibitor (hereditary angioedema), IgE-mediated allergies, anaphylaxis, or other systemic allergic reactions. Generally, angioedema causes facial swelling first, particularly of the eyes and lips, and

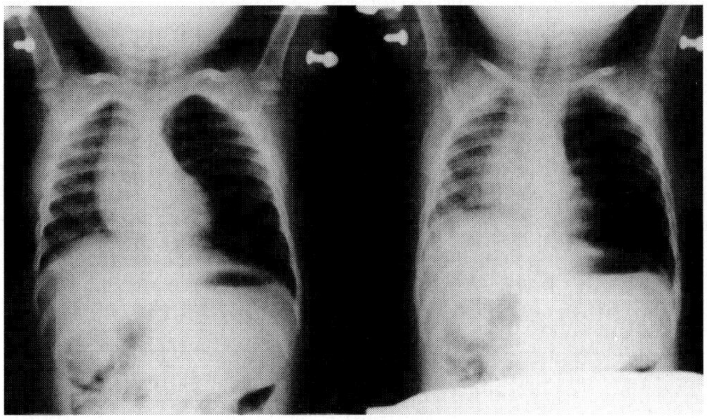

FIG. 33-8 Foreign body aspiration. Inspiratory *(left)* and expiratory *(right)* chest radiographs of a child who aspirated a portion of a potato into the left main stem bronchus. Left lung field is hyperaerated and the mediastinum is shifted to the right on expiration due to left-sided obstructive emphysema. (From Kenna MA, Bluestone CD: Foreign bodies in the air and food passages, *Pediatr Rev* 10(1):25, 1988.)

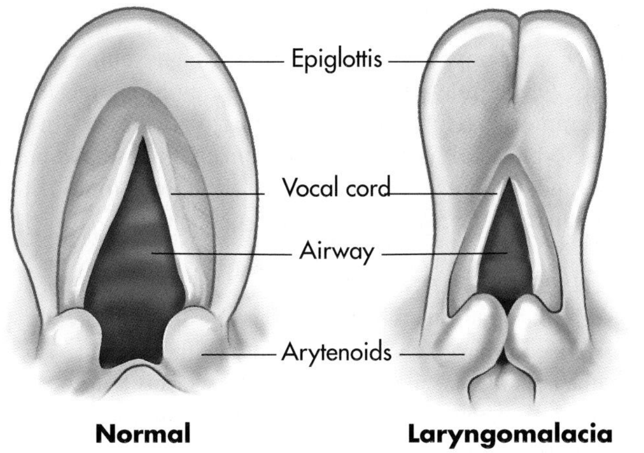

FIG. 33-9 Laryngomalacia. In the normal larynx *(left)*, supralaryngeal structures maintain their upright orientation during inspiration. In contrast, in infants with laryngomalacia (*right*), there is inward prolapse of the arytenoid masses, which include the prominent cuneiform tubercles and the arytenoid cartilages. The glottis becomes partially covered, and airflow is impeded. Sometimes the edges of the epiglottis curl inward, further exacerbating the obstruction. In expiration, these structures are "blown" aside passively.

then progresses to airway swelling.[17] Prompt recognition and treatment with epinephrine will usually prevent progression to complete airway obstruction.[18]

Subglottic Stenosis

Traumatic injury to the upper airway with development of **subglottic stenosis** is a well-described complication of endotracheal intubation.[19] Factors that contribute to subglottic stenosis include long-term assisted ventilation, use of an endotracheal tube that is too large, excessive movement of the tube, and individual susceptibility.[20] The occurrence of subglottic stenosis can be minimized by ensuring that the tube size allows a small air leak during inspiration (at a peak inspiratory force of approximately 25 mm Hg) and that the tube is securely taped. Sedation is generally required to reduce head movement for children who are intubated. For significant subglottic stenosis, tracheostomy or tracheal reconstructive surgery may be needed.[21,22]

Laryngomalacia and Tracheomalacia

Laryngomalacia is the most common cause of chronic stridor in babies, but it is usually mild and improves spontaneously over the first year of life as the supralaryngeal cartilage structures stiffen. In laryngomalacia, the epiglottis or arytenoids or both fold inward with inspiration, partially covering the glottis (Fig. 33-9). Typical signs of laryngomalacia include inspiratory stridor beginning in the first days or weeks of life, accentuated with activity, and sometimes positional (worse supine or head flexed). There may be feeding difficulties, but they are usually mild. Cry is normal.

In **tracheomalacia,** the tracheal cartilages tend to collapse during the respiratory cycle. Symptoms are more subtle than in laryngomalacia. There may be low-pitched inspiratory stridor for malacia of the upper trachea or centrally located, single-pitch (monophonic) wheeze for malacia of the mid to distal trachea. Both laryngomalacia and tracheomalacia can be suspected clinically and confirmed by bronchoscopy.

Vocal Cord Paralysis

In the normal situation, the vocal cords move apart to facilitate inspiration and move together to vocalize. Paralysis of one or both vocal cords may affect both breathing and speech. In infants and children, vocal cord dysfunction is usually a consequence of other problems, such as surgical trauma to the recurrent laryngeal nerve during cardiac surgery or Arnold-Chiari malformation of the brain stem, where the nucleus ambiguus acts as the "relay station" for laryngeal function. **Vocal cord paralysis** sometimes resolves spontaneously or with correction of the underlying problem, such as decompression of hydrocephalus. However, tracheostomy is sometimes required for bilateral vocal cord paralysis as a temporary or permanent measure.[23]

Congenital Malformations

Congenital malformations of the trachea and bronchial tree cause airway obstruction. Affected infants develop obvious airway symptoms or feeding difficulties or both. Many children are first thought to have gastroesophageal reflux as the principal problem. Lesions include laryngeal webs, cysts, clefts, subglottic hemangiomas, and abnormalities involving the great vessels that result in tracheal compression (vascular rings).[24] Surgical management is usually required in these conditions.[25,26]

Obstructive Sleep Apnea

Obstructive sleep apnea syndrome (OSAS) is defined by partial or complete UAO during sleep, with disruption of normal ventilation and normal sleep patterns. Childhood OSAS is common, with an estimated prevalence of 2% to 3%.[27,28] In children, unlike adults, OSAS occurs equally among males and females.

Pathophysiology

The pathophysiology of childhood OSAS may be multifactorial in origin. In otherwise healthy children, the most common predisposing factor is adenotonsillar hypertrophy, which causes physical impingement on the nasopharyngeal airway. OSAS may also occur in obese children and those with craniofacial anomalies or neurologic disorders. In addition to physical narrowing, other mechanisms have been suggested, such as abnormalities in the motor tone of the upper airways or abnormal arousal mechanisms.

Clinical Manifestations

Usually there is a history of snoring and labored breathing during sleep that may be continuous or intermittent. There may be episodes of increased respiratory effort but no audible airflow, often terminated by snorting, gasping, repositioning, or arousal. Sleep is often described as restless. Occasionally, daytime sleepiness is reported.

Disorders of the Lower Airways

Lower airway disease is one of the leading causes of morbidity in the first year of life and continues to be an important component of other illnesses. Pulmonary conditions commonly observed include perinatal conditions, such as newborn respiratory distress syndrome; congenital malformations; asthma; cystic fibrosis; infections; aspiration syndrome; and acute respiratory distress syndrome.

Respiratory Distress Syndrome

Respiratory distress syndrome (RDS) of the newborn, also known as **hyaline membrane disease (HMD),** is the leading cause of death in the newborn, accounting for 20% to 30% of deaths in premature newborns. Hyaline membrane disease is outlined in Box 33-2. The major predispos-

Box 33-2

HYALINE MEMBRANE DISEASE

EPIDEMIOLOGY
- Worldwide
- Prematurity predisposes
- Cesarean section without labor predisposes
- Perinatal asphyxia predisposes
- Male > female
- White > black
- Second-born twin at greater risk
- PROM spares
- IUGR spares
- Maternal stress spares
- Maternal diabetes predisposes if <37 weeks
- Maternal hemorrhage predisposes

CLINICAL SIGNS
- Onset near the time of birth
- Retractions and tachypnea
- Expiratory grunt
- Cyanosis
- Systemic hypotension
- Characteristic chest film
- Course to death or improvement 3–5 days
- Fine inspiratory rales
- Hypothermia
- Peripheral edema
- Pulmonary edema

PATHOPHYSIOLOGY
- Reduced lung compliance
- Reduced FRC
- Poor lung distensibility
- Poor alveolar stability
- Right-to-left shunts
- Reduced effective pulmonary blood flow
- If hypotensive and hypoxic, poor peripheral perfusion, poor renal perfusion, myocardial malfunction
- Patent ductus arteriosus contributes

PATHOBIOCHEMISTRY
- Respiratory acidosis
- Decreased saturated phospholipids
- Low AF L/S ratio
- Low surfactant-associated proteins
- Decreased total serum proteins
- Decreased fibrinolysis
- Low thyroxine levels

PATHOLOGY
- Atelectasis
- Injury to epithelial cells, edema
- Membrane contains fibrin and cellular products
- No tubular myelin
- Osmiophilic lamellar bodies decreased early, increased later

ETIOLOGY
- Surfactant deficiency during disease
- Probable inadequate hormonal (corticoid) stimulus in utero
- DPL synthesis impaired or destruction increased or both
- Autonomic dysfunction

PREVENTION
- Prenatal glucocorticoids for >24 hours
- Surfactant replacement before 1–2 hours

From Hansen T, Corbet A: Disorders of the transition. In Taeusch HW, Ballard RA, editors: *Avery's diseases of the newborn,* ed 7, Philadelphia, 1998, W.B. Saunders.

PROM, prolonged rupture of membranes (>16 hours); *IUGR,* intrauterine growth retardation; *FRC,* functional residual capacity; *AF,* amniotic fluid; *L/S,* lecithin/sphingomyelin; *DPL,* dipalmitoyl lecithin.

ing factor is prematurity, but occasionally RDS is seen in other situations, most notably infants of diabetic mothers. Additional factors increasing risk include cesarean delivery. It is more common in boys than girls and in whites than nonwhites. The incidence of RDS (in the absence of preventive treatment) is approximately 50% to 60% at 29 weeks of gestation and decreases significantly by 36 weeks. Antenatal stress on the fetus may accelerate lung maturation and decrease RDS risk. In special circumstances, such as elective early delivery (e.g., for maternal health reasons), RDS risk is assessed by sampling amniotic fluid for quantitation of secreted surfactant lipids, the basis of the lethicin/sphingomyelin (L/S) ratio (value of 2.0 or greater predicts low risk). Another common test looks for presence of the lipid phosphatidylglycerol, which also reflects lung maturity.

Pathophysiology

RDS is caused by surfactant deficiency and, secondarily, a deficiency in alveolar surface area for gas exchange. Premature infants are born with many underdeveloped and small alveoli that are difficult to inflate. Those that are available for gas exchange do not have adequate surfactant to maintain alveolar distention at end expiration. The chest wall is weak and highly compliant.[29] The net effect is *atelectasis* (Fig. 33-10), which is difficult for the neonate to overcome because it requires a significant negative inspiratory pressure to open the alveoli with each breath. The infant uses more oxygen to sustain the work of breathing and becomes hypoxemic and hypercapnic. Hypoxia and atelectasis cause pulmonary vasoconstriction and increase intrapulmonary resistance and shunting (Fig. 33-11). This results in hypoperfusion of the lung and a decrease in effective pulmonary blood flow. Increased pulmonary vascular resistance causes a partial return to fetal circulation, with right-to-left shunting of blood through the ductus arteriosus and foramen ovale.

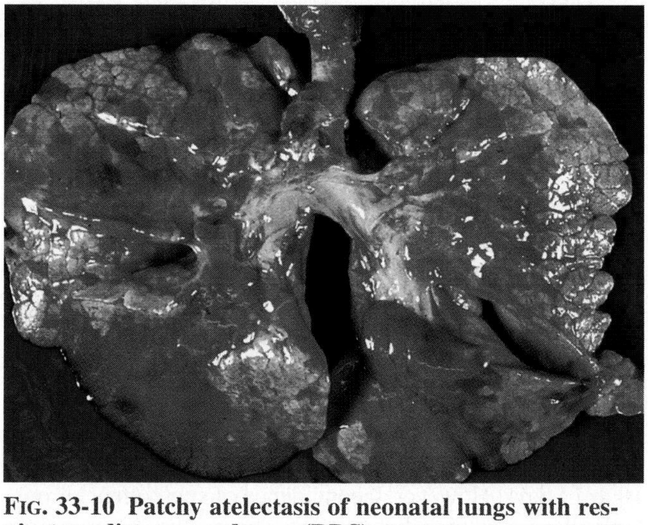

FIG. 33-10 Patchy atelectasis of neonatal lungs with respiratory distress syndrome (RDS). (From Damjanov I, Linder J, editors: *Anderson's pathology,* ed 10, St Louis, 1996, Mosby.)

Capillary permeability increases and epithelium may be damaged because of ventilation-induced injury, together resulting in the leakage of plasma proteins. Fibrin deposits in the airspaces create the appearance of "hyaline membranes" for which the disorder is named. The plasma proteins leaked into the airspace have the additional adverse effect of interfering with the function of surfactant that may be present.

To make the situation more complex, prolonged hypoxemia activates anaerobic glycolysis, which produces increased amounts of lactic acid and promotes metabolic acidosis. Because the collapsed alveoli are unable to get rid of excess carbon dioxide, respiratory acidosis also develops. Lowered pH causes further vasoconstriction. With inadequate pulmonary circulation and alveolar perfusion, the oxygen content of the blood continues to decrease, pH decreases, and materials needed for surfactant production are not circulated to the alveoli. The pathogenesis of RDS is summarized in Fig. 33-11.

Clinical Manifestations

Signs of RDS appear within minutes of birth. Some neonates require resuscitation at birth because of asphyxia or initial severe respiratory distress. Tachypnea (respiratory rate over 60 breaths per minute), expiratory grunting or whining, intercostal and subcostal retractions, nasal flaring, and poor color are the most striking clinical manifestations of RDS. The natural course is characterized by progressive hypoxemia and dyspnea. Apnea and irregular respirations occur as the infant tires. The typical chest radiograph shows diffuse, fine granular densities within the first 6 hours of life. RDS can progress to death in severe cases, but in most cases the clinical manifestations reach a peak within 3 days, after which there is gradual improvement.

Evaluation and Treatment

Diagnosis is made on the basis of clinical manifestations, chest radiographs, and, occasionally, confirmatory analysis (e.g., L/S ratio) of amniotic fluid or tracheal aspirates. The ultimate treatment for RDS would be prevention of premature birth, but in the meantime there have been significant advances.

The first is antenatal treatment with glucocorticoids for women in preterm labor. Glucocorticoids induce a significant and rapid acceleration of lung maturation, and there is extensive evidence that maternal steroid therapy significantly reduces the incidence of RDS, intraventricular hemorrhage, and death.[30,31] This treatment is currently recommended in the setting of preterm labor at 24 to 34 weeks of gestation unless delivery is imminent; ideally, dosing continues for 48 hours while attempts are made to halt labor.

The second major advance in RDS treatment has been exogenous surfactant, either synthetic or purified from animal sources and instilled down an endotracheal tube.[32] Current protocols recommend prophylactic administration to infants weighing less than 1000 g beginning within 15 to 30 minutes of birth, after the infant is stabilized. Repeat dos-

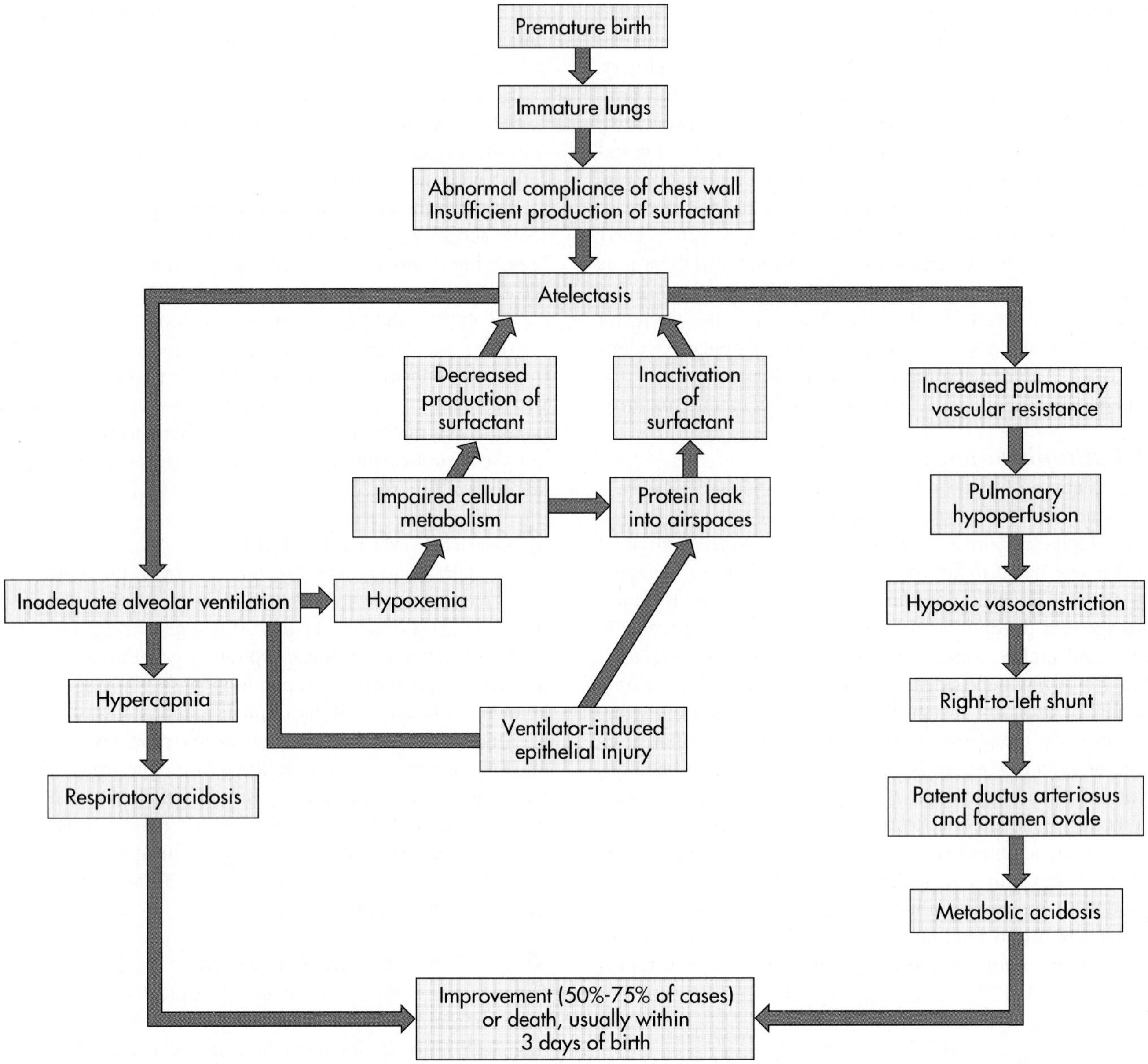

FIG. 33-11 Pathogenesis of respiratory distress syndrome (RDS) of the newborn. RDS is also known as hyaline membrane disease.

ing is usually given every 12 hours during the first few days. There is usually a dramatic improvement in oxygenation. For infants weighing more than 1000 g, surfactant replacement is based on clinical need. Therapy with surfactant should be considered complementary to antenatal glucocorticoids, which promote not only accelerated surfactant synthesis but also enhanced structural development of the lung and beneficial effects on mechanisms of fluid clearance from the lung.

The third advance in RDS treatment has been in supportive care. Newborns with RDS need oxygen and often support, such as continuous positive airway pressure or mechanical ventilation. There is a great deal of current interest in establishing which strategies, such as choice of tidal volume or use of high-frequency oscillation, will produce the least amount of ventilator-induced lung injury.[33] The extremely preterm infant is particularly vulnerable. Ventilation may interfere with alveolarization and surfactant metabolism and may aggravate the proinflammatory state that is believed to accompany premature birth and RDS, as reflected by abnormal cytokine profiles in the lung. A combination of factors may lead to subsequent development of chronic lung disease or bronchopulmonary dysplasia.

Approximately 50% to 70% of infants with RDS survive with treatment. In many cases, recovery is complete within 10 to 14 days. However, the incidence of subsequent chronic lung disease is significant among very low–birth weight infants.

WHAT'S NEW? Nitric Oxide Improves Oxygenation

Nitric oxide (NO) is a potent vasodilator and reduces pulmonary vascular resistance. Inhaled NO in low doses (2 to 20 parts per million) improves oxygenation in cases of neonatal pulmonary hypertension by decreasing extrapulmonary shunting through a patent ductus arteriosus or a patent foramen ovale or both. In parenchymal lung disease (such as respiratory distress syndrome, meconium aspiration, or pneumonia), NO may reverse intrapulmonary shunting by redistribution of pulmonary blood flow, enhancing ventilation-perfusion matching. Because of its short half-life, it is metabolized in the pulmonary circulation before it can cause systemic side effects. NO has been used primarily in term or near-term infants with hypoxic respiratory failure. Despite enthusiasm about NO, further study is needed to assess its benefits, especially in other groups, such as preterm infants and older children with acute respiratory distress syndrome.

Data from American Academy of Pediatrics Committee on Fetus and Newborn: Use of inhaled nitric oxide, *Pediatrics* 106(2 pt 1):344, 2000; Day RN et al: Acute response to inhaled nitric oxide in newborns with respiratory failure and pulmonary hypertension, *Pediatrics* 98:698, 1996; Smyth R: Inhaled nitric oxide treatment for preterm infants with hypoxic respiratory failure, *Thorax* 55(suppl 1):51, 2000.

Bronchopulmonary Dysplasia

Bronchopulmonary dysplasia (BPD) is a chronic disease usually resulting from acute respiratory disease in the neonatal period. There is a wide spectrum of clinical severity.[34] Risk factors for development of BPD include prematurity; lung immaturity in the neonate less than 28 weeks of age or less than 1500 g; RDS in the neonatal period; high inspired O_2 concentrations; positive-pressure ventilation, especially if prolonged and associated with sustained alveolar distention ("volutrauma"); patent ductus arteriosus; and vitamin A deficiency.[35,36]

The reported incidence of BPD varies because of differences in diagnostic criteria. Criteria are based on abnormalities visible on x-ray films and clinical criteria, such as persistent oxygen requirement. It is estimated that 10% to 35% of very low–birth weight infants develop BPD.[37,38]

Pathophysiology

The evolution of classic BPD occurs over several weeks and includes an early exudative inflammatory phase, followed by a fibroproliferative phase. There usually are both bronchiolar and interstitial changes. Early findings are hyaline membranes, bronchial necrosis, inflammatory debris, and obliterative bronchiolitis. There is inhomogeneous aeration and development of cysts. Extensive remodeling occurs in alveolar units, which have thickened walls and poor septation; there may be marked interstitial fibrosis. Fig. 33-12 illustrates the pathophysiology of BPD. To a significant extent, cytokines may be responsible for the abnormal alveolarization and injury response that lead to BPD.[39]

Pulmonary alterations of BPD include scarring and emphysema. Alveoli fail to multiply, and alveolar walls or capillaries become inflamed and may be destroyed. The pulmonary arteries have smaller lumina and thicker walls than are normal for the infant's age, causing pulmonary hypertension. Ciliated epithelium is lost, and mucous plugs and debris clog the airways. Ventilation-perfusion mismatch is severe, and the infant may develop an infection, cor pulmonale, and right-sided heart failure.[40,41]

Clinical Manifestations

Clinically, the severely affected infant exhibits hypoxemia and hypercapnia caused by ventilation-perfusion mismatch and diffusion defects. Intermittent bronchospasm, mucous plugging, and pulmonary hypertension characterize the clinical course. A heterogeneous lung parenchyma is caused by atelectasis, cysts, and air trapping, creating frequent alterations in clinical appearance. The infant seems stable or improving and then suddenly deteriorates, becoming dusky and agitated ("BPD spell"). These episodes also may be caused by a sudden increase in pulmonary vascular resistance or, occasionally, by the development of an extrapleural air leak.

Infants with severe BPD require prolonged, assisted ventilation with cautious weaning. Diuretics are used to control pulmonary edema. Bronchodilators are employed to reduce airway resistance. Early antiinflammatory therapies, such as steroids, may facilitate weaning but introduce other risks.[42] Nutritional needs are high and must be met to promote growth and healing; the infant usually can be fed enterally. Early supplemental vitamin A, which plays a role in normal lung development, may be required in low–birth weight infants.[34,35,43] Infection is a constant threat because of invasive lines, the endotracheal tube, and a compromised immune system.

Mortality rates have been reported to be as high as 40% in hospitalized infants. Death is usually caused by infection or respiratory failure. Most infants who survive are discharged with home oxygen therapy (some on ventilators) and experience frequent respiratory infections and growth retardation. Gradual improvement is usually noted in the first 2 years, but pulmonary function may remain abnormal for many years.[34,44] Home mortality is usually caused by other complications, such as infection or cor pulmonale.

Cystic Fibrosis

Cystic fibrosis (CF) is an autosomal recessive inherited disorder that results from defective epithelial ion transport. On a simplistic level, CF is associated with abnormal secretions that may cause obstructive problems within the respiratory, digestive, and reproductive tracts. However, research suggests that there may be additional issues, such as an intrinsic proinflammatory state and weaknesses in local immune defenses.

The CF gene has been located on chromosome 7. Its mutation results in the abnormal expression of the protein **cystic fibrosis transmembrane regulator (CFTR),** which is a chloride channel present on the surface of many types of epithelial cells, including those lining airways, bile ducts, pancreas, sweat ducts, and vas deferens. CF affects primarily

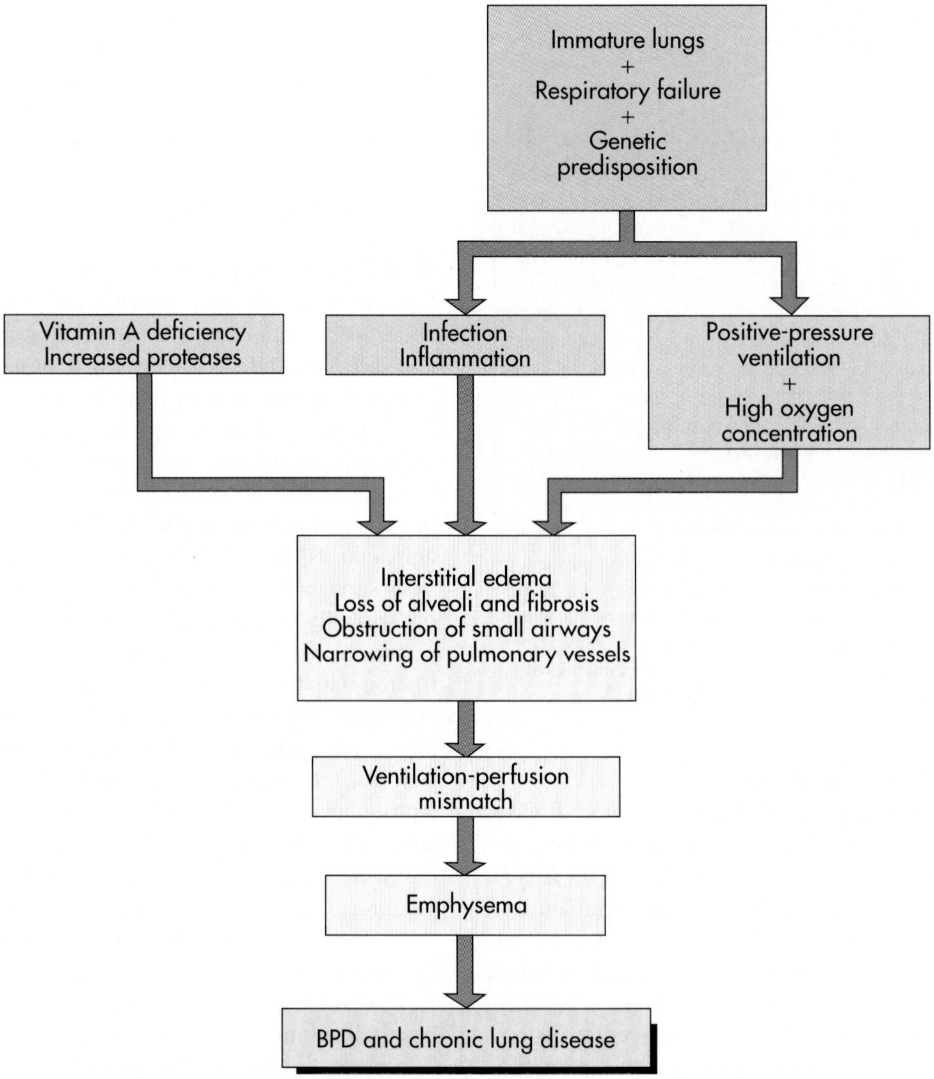

FIG. 33-12 Pathophysiology of bronchopulmonary dysplasia (BPD).

whites (approximately 1 in 3500) but is occasionally seen in other groups as well.[45] Estimated carrier frequency is high (1 in 29 whites in the United States). Carriers are healthy.

Pathophysiology

Although CF is a multiorgan disease, respiratory failure is almost always the cause of death. The typical features of CF lung disease are mucus plugging, chronic inflammation, and infection. These lead to microabscess formation, bronchiectasis, patchy consolidation and pneumonia, peribronchial fibrosis, and cyst formation (Fig. 33-13). There is a progressive decrease in the amount of available and functional lung tissue. The pathophysiology for these changes is outlined in Fig. 33-14. Peripheral bullae may develop because of obstruction and airway wall weakening, and pneumothorax may occur. Hemoptysis, sometimes life threatening, may occur because of erosion of enlarged bronchial arteries that develop in response to the inflammation associated with bronchiectasis. Over a long period of time, pulmonary vascular remodeling occurs because of localized hypoxia and arteriolar vasoconstriction; pulmonary hypertension and cor pulmonale may develop.

The mucus plugging seen in CF probably results from both increased production of mucus and altered physicochemical properties of the mucus. Mucus-secreting airway cells (goblet cells and submucosal glands) are increased in number and size. CF mucus is dehydrated and viscous because of abnormal chloride secretion and sodium absorption. Mucin glycoproteins in CF are also highly sulfated, which may make the mucus layer more rigid.[46,47] Finally, after secretion, CF mucus is made more viscous by DNA and filamentous (F) actin from degraded neutrophils.[48,49]

Chronic inflammation contributes to long-term lung damage, and there is evidence that this process may even begin in infancy.[50] Abnormal cytokine profiles, such as deficient interleukin-10 (IL-10), may promote inflammation.[51] Neutrophils are present in great excess in CF airways, and one of their products, neutrophil elastase, has the following detrimental effects: (1) direct damage to lung structural proteins, such as elastin; (2) induction of airway cells to produce IL-8,

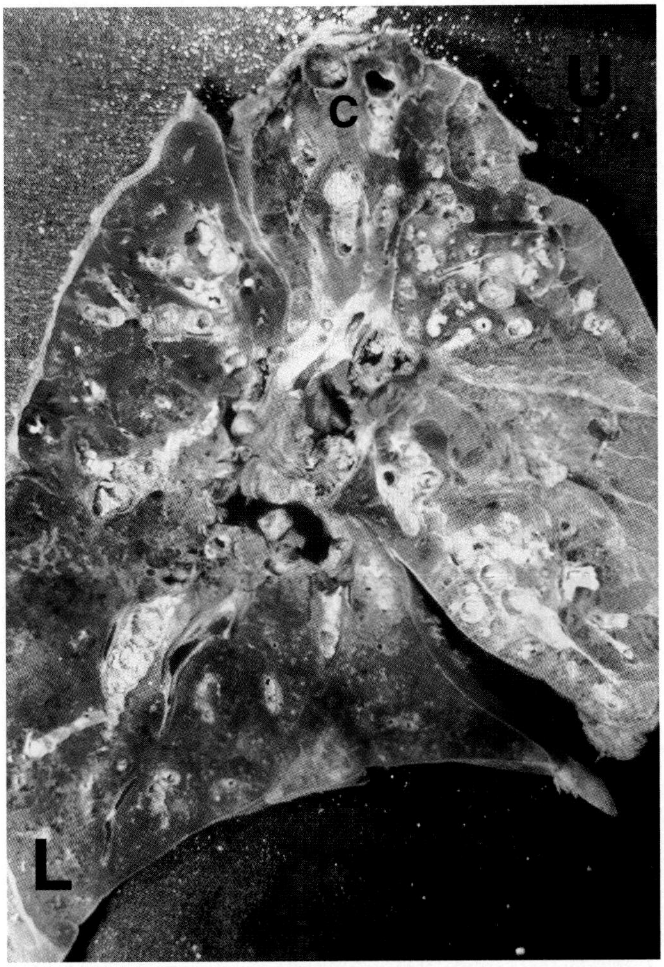

FIG. 33-13 Pathology of the lung in end-stage cystic fibrosis. Key features are widespread mucus impaction of airways and bronchiectasis (especially in upper lobe, *U*), with hemorrhagic pneumonia in the lower lobe *(L)*. Small cysts *(C)* are present at the apex of the lung. (From Kleinerman J, Vauthy P: *Pathology of the lung in cystic fibrosis,* Atlanta, 1976, Cystic Fibrosis Foundation.)

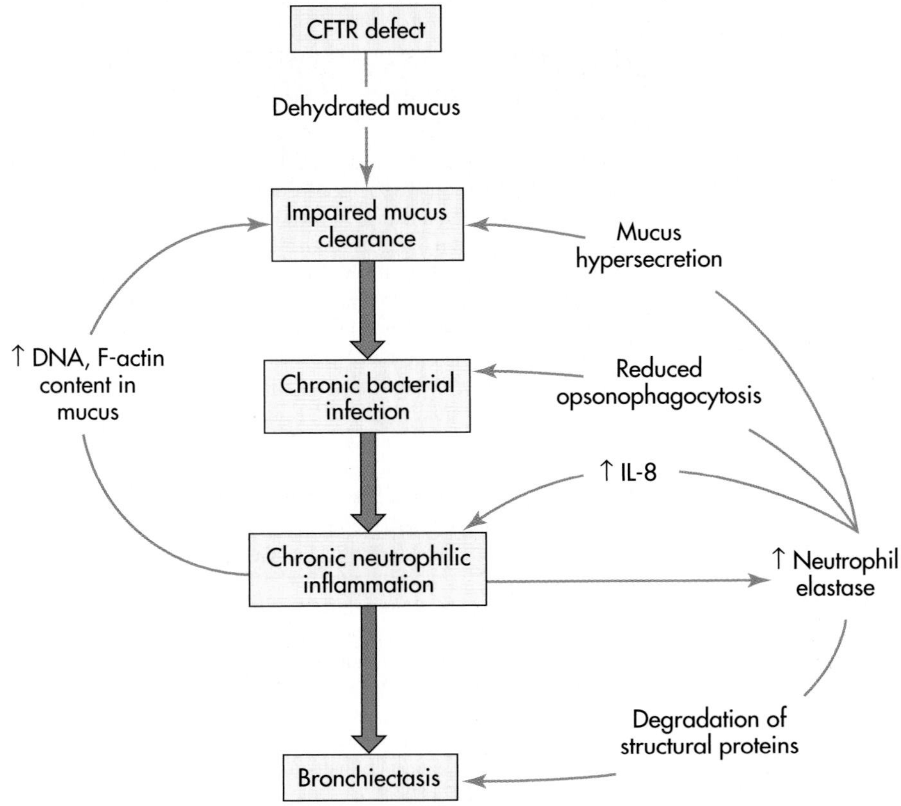

FIG. 33-14 Pathogenesis of cystic fibrosis lung disease.

a strong attractant for neutrophils and thus a means for augmenting a local "vicious cycle" of inflammation; (3) cleavage of IgG and complement components important for opsonization and phagocytosis of pathogens; and (4) direct stimulation of mucus secretion by mucus-producing cells.

Children with CF have a propensity for chronic endobronchial infection that remains poorly understood. It is likely that local factors in the CF airway microenvironment favor bacterial colonization, because there is no systemic immune defect. *Staphylococcus aureus* is common, and *Pseudomonas aeruginosa* ultimately colonizes airways in 75% of children with CF. *Pseudomonas* acquisition has been linked with more rapid decline in pulmonary function.[52] Persistence of this microorganism incites chronic local inflammation, airway damage, bronchiectasis, microabscess formation, and foci of hemorrhagic pneumonia.

Clinical Manifestations

The median age at diagnosis is 6 months; nearly 75% of cases are diagnosed by 1 year. Approximately 10% of cases are not diagnosed until after age 10, however, and usually have milder symptoms. The most common manifestations are respiratory and gastrointestinal. Respiratory symptoms include persistent cough or wheeze and recurrent or severe pneumonia. Physical signs developing over time include barrel chest and digital clubbing. Classic gastrointestinal manifestations include meconium ileus at birth, failure to thrive, and malabsorptive symptoms, such as frequent loose and oily stools. About 10% of CF patients do not experience gastrointestinal problems and are termed "pancreatic sufficient". A handful of specific CFTR mutations are predictive of this milder digestive and nutritional phenotype. More subtle manifestations of CF include chronic sinusitis, nasal polyps, and rectal prolapse. Males with CF are typically infertile (98%). Complications of CF may include liver disease (approximately 5%) and diabetes mellitus (10% to 25%). Overall severity of CF lung disease is highly variable and has not proven predictable on the basis of genotype; even affected siblings may have disparate courses.

Evaluation and Treatment

The standard method of diagnosis is the sweat test, which will reveal sweat chloride concentration in excess of 60 mEq/L. Genotyping for CFTR mutations is also available as an alternative or supplemental method but may fail to confirm up to 10% of cases because of a lack of ability to screen for every described CF-associated mutation. There are more than 800 mutations, but most standard laboratory panels include fewer than 100 mutations.

Treatment is primarily focused on pulmonary health and on nutrition, which seem to be related. Common pulmonary therapies include techniques to promote mucus clearance, such as chest physical therapy and related mechanical devices; bronchodilators; and aerosolized DNase, which acts to liquefy mucus.[48] Antibiotic practices vary, with both prophylactic and treatment strategies being used. *Pseudomonas aeruginosa* suppression using inhaled maintenance antibiotics (tobramycin) has been shown to have a beneficial clinical impact.[53] Intravenous antibiotics are used to treat major flare-ups of pulmonary infection, which may be either subacute or acute. Individuals with end-stage lung disease may consider lung transplantation.

Approximately 90% of children with CF have pancreatic insufficiency, of variable extent, and need to take pancreatic enzymes (for absorption of nutrients) before meals and snacks for their entire lifetime. Fat-soluble vitamins (A, D, E, and K) must be supplemented. Caloric needs are high, especially with advancing lung disease, and high-calorie supplements or even gastrostomy feeding may be warranted.

Despite the often high maintenance requirements of individuals with CF, most should be expected to live high-quality lives for a long time. Most will survive to adulthood, and the situation will improve with new approaches to treatment and, possibly, even cure.

Respiratory Infections

Infections may be localized to the bronchioles and bronchi, alveoli, interstitium, or pleura. The cause and site of infections are related to the age of the child, seasonal variables, and environmental exposures. Infants and young children tend to have more viral infections, especially during late autumn to early spring. Environmental factors may include presence of siblings, day-care exposure, and other variables.

Bronchiolitis

Bronchiolitis has a peak incidence during winter and spring and is a major reason for hospital admission for children younger than 1 year, particularly children of lower socioeconomic status.[54] Bronchiolitis causes obstruction of the

WHAT'S NEW? A Cure for Cystic Fibrosis?

After sequencing the CF gene in 1989, hopes were voiced for a gene therapy "cure" within 5 years. Ideally, the normal CFTR gene could be inhaled or sprayed into the lungs and disease progression halted. The task has proven more formidable than expected. Different methods, such as viral vectors or lipid-DNA complexes, have demonstrated problems of low efficiency of gene transfer, lack of persistence of gene transfer, or significant host immune responses. Nevertheless, increasingly promising results have been obtained. Since 1993, a number of limited gene transfer experiments have been completed in individuals with CF. Some of these have provided "proof of concept" in that normal CFTR mRNA (transcribed from the transferred DNA) was seen in at least a small portion of epithelial cells, and local chloride transport could be at least partially corrected. New and modified strategies continue to be developed to make the process efficient, practical, and safe.

Data from Albelda SM, Wiewrodt R, Zuckerman JB: Gene therapy for lung disease: hype or hope? *Ann Intern Med* 132(8):649, 2000; Hyde SC et al: Repeat administration of DNA/liposomes to the nasal epithelium of patients with cystic fibrosis, *Gene Ther* 7(13):1156, 2000; Zuckerman JB et al: A phase I study of adenovirus-mediated transfer of the human cystic fibrosis transmembrane conductance regulator gene to a lung segment of individuals with cystic fibrosis, *Hum Gene Ther* 10(18):2973, 1999.

bronchioles by submucosal edema, increased secretions, and bronchospasm. It is often more severe in the first year of life and in children with underlying lung or heart disease. Bronchiolitis can be caused by respiratory syncytial virus (RSV) (more than 50% of cases), adenoviruses, influenza, parainfluenza, and mycoplasma in older children.

Pathophysiology

Viral infection causes necrosis of the bronchial epithelium and destruction of ciliated epithelial cells. There is infiltration with lymphocytes around the bronchioles and a cell-mediated hypersensitivity to viral antigens with release of lymphokines causing inflammation, as well as activation of eosinophils, neutrophils, and monocytes.[55] The submucosa becomes edematous, and cellular debris and fibrin form plugs within the bronchioles.

Edema of the bronchiolar wall, accumulation of mucus and cellular debris, and possibly bronchospasm narrow many peripheral airways. Other airways become partially or completely occluded. Atelectasis occurs in some areas of the lung and hyperinflation in others.

The mechanics of breathing are disrupted by bronchiolitis. There is air trapping, and FRC is approximately twice normal. Compliance is decreased because the lungs are already highly inflated and because airway resistance within the lung is uneven and increased. The decrease in compliance and the increase in airway resistance result in a substantial increase in the work of breathing.

Serious alterations in gas exchange occur because of airway obstruction and patchy atelectasis. Hypoxemia develops because of ventilation-perfusion mismatch, and hypercapnia may occur in severe cases.

Clinical Manifestations

Children with bronchiolitis have tachypnea, expiratory wheezing, cough, rhinorrhea, mild fever, and varying grades of respiratory distress. Chest radiographs often reveal hyperexpanded lungs, patchy or peribronchial infiltrates, and, sometimes, atalectasis of the right upper lobe. Severely affected infants appear anxious and distressed because of dyspnea or hypoxemia. The thoracic cage is overexpanded, particularly in its anteroposterior diameter. The infant takes rapid, short breaths, and wheezing and rales are often heard on auscultation. With overexpansion of the lungs, the diaphragm is flattened, causing downward displacement of the liver and spleen. Abdominal distention results from air swallowing. The tidal volume decreases. Some individuals have persistent high airway resistance and airway hyperresponsiveness long after resolution of the viral process.[56-58]

Evaluation and Treatment

Diagnosis is made by physical examination (e.g., rhinitis, cough, wheezing, chest retractions, tachypnea) and radiologic examination. Nasal washings may be tested for specific viral agents, such as RSV. Treatment is determined by the severity of the disease and age of the child. Infants younger than 1 year are most at risk for acute respiratory failure and may require assisted ventilation. Supplemental oxygen is given as needed, and adequate hydration should be maintained. Bronchodilators have not been scientifically validated as consistently providing significant benefit but are widely tried on an empiric basis. Likewise, steroids are not of proven benefit. Antiviral agents (ribavirin) for RSV may be considered for severe cases, but therapy is costly and efficacy unclear. Prophylactic treatment with RSV-specific monoclonal antibody is recommended for high-risk infants under 2 years old.

Pneumonia

Pneumonia involves inflammation and infection in the terminal airways and alveoli. It is a major cause of morbidity and mortality, particularly in developing countries. The most common agents are viral, followed by bacteria and mycoplasma. In children, fungal pneumonia is rare. Opportunistic infections occur only in the immunocompromised child and are not discussed further in this chapter.

Bacterial pneumonia usually results from inhalation of microbes dispersed in ambient air or in secretion droplets (person-to-person spread) or by aspiration of one's own nasopharyngeal bacteria. Once in the alveolar region, bacteria encounter local host defenses, such as opsonins and IgG, which prepare bacteria for ingestion by alveolar macrophages. If these mechanisms fail, neutrophils will be recruited and an intense, cytokine-mediated inflammation will ensue. Vascular engorgement, edema, and a fibrinopurulent exudate occur. Alveolar filling precludes gas exchange and, if extensive, could lead to respiratory failure.[59] If sepsis occurs at the same time, shock and end-organ hypoperfusion will cause metabolic acidosis. A spreading viral infection of the lower respiratory tract sometimes sets the stage for bacterial infection by causing epithelial damage and reduced mucociliary clearance.

The most common bacterial pathogens for young children beyond the neonatal period are listed in Table 33-2. Pneumococcal pneumonia is the most common and manifests acutely and with variable severity. It is usually lobar in pattern. Staphylococcal and group A streptococcal pneumonia can be particularly fulminant and necrotizing, with a high incidence of accompanying empyema, pneumatoceles, and sepsis. *Haemophilus influenzae* pneumonia has become rare because of widespread immunization. It is hoped that the recent release of a new pneumococcal vaccine that is immunogenic for infants, the most susceptible group, will lead to a similar dramatic reduction in pneumococcal disease.

Viral pneumonia is acquired by direct contact, droplet transmission, or aerosol. There is initial destruction of ciliated epithelium of the distal airway, with sloughing of cellular material. A mononuclear-predominant inflammatory response occurs, in the interstitium initially, and may later involve the alveoli as well.

The most common cause of viral pneumonia in infants is RSV, usually in the winter to early spring. A number of other viruses are important, including parainfluenza, influenza, and adenoviruses. Certain serotypes of adenovirus can cause necrotizing disease, sometimes leading to obliterative bronchiolitis and significant lung disability.

Table 33-2 Common Causes of Bacterial Pneumonia

Causal Agent	Age	Onset	Signs and Symptoms
Streptococcus pneumoniae (pneumococcus)	1–4 years	Acute, often follows an upper respiratory infection, winter and early spring	High fever, productive cough, pleuritic pain, increased respiratory rate, decreased breath sounds in area of consolidation; lobar pattern or "round pneumonia" on radiograph
Staphylococcus aureus	1 wk–2 yr	Acute, winter months; may be primary or secondary	High fever, cough, respiratory distress; sepsis frequent; pleural effusion and pneumatoceles common
Group A streptococci	All ages	Acute, any season	High fever, chills, respiratory distress, sepsis or shock; empyema and pneumatoceles common

Atypical pneumonia *(Mycoplasma pneumoniae, Chlamydia pneumoniae)* is the most common cause of community-acquired pneumonia for school-age children and young adults. *Chlamydia pneumoniae* is clinically indistinguishable from and is typically grouped with *Mycoplasma pneumoniae* as "atypical" pneumonia. Transmission is person to person, with a 2- to 3-week incubation period. There is usually only upper respiratory tract involvement.

Mycoplasma microorganisms lack cell walls but have a limiting membrane and a specialized tip for attaching to ciliated respiratory epithelial cells. Local sloughing of cells occurs. Peribronchial lymphocytic infiltration develops, along with neutrophil recruitment to the airway lumen. The pattern resembles bronchitis or bronchopneumonia.

Onset is usually gradual, resembling a typical upper respiratory infection with low-grade fever and prominent cough. Cases are not usually clinically severe, and full recovery should be expected.

Evaluation and Treatment

Diagnosis of pneumonia is based on clinical findings and chest radiograph confirmation. A bacterial pneumonia will initially produce a patchy infiltration and later cause a segmental or lobar disease. A unilateral lobar consolidation on a chest x-ray film is frequently associated with *Streptococcus pneumoniae.* A consolidation associated with a pleural effusion is almost always caused by *H. influenzae* type b or, if the patient is younger than 1 year, *S. aureus.* Aspiration pneumonia characteristically produces perihilar or lower lobe infiltrates.

Some pneumonias may be treated on an outpatient basis; however, many children require oxygen supplementation and, occasionally, assisted ventilation. This is particularly true with infants who have a viral interstitial pneumonia, such as RSV. In addition, adequate hydration, nutrition, and supportive pulmonary therapy are required to reduce the duration and severity of illness. Many hospitalized infants are markedly tachypneic and unable to coordinate their breathing with swallowing; they may require enteral feeding. Aspiration is always a risk with infants in respiratory distress.

Appropriate antibiotic administration for bacterial pneumonias is usually instituted for a minimum of 10 days, and longer for *S. aureus* or group A streptococci. The decision to discontinue an antibiotic should be determined by clinical criteria and improvement of x-ray abnormalities.

Aspiration Pneumonitis

Aspiration pneumonitis is caused by a foreign substance, such as food, secretions, or environmental compounds, entering the lung and causing inflammation. The aspiration of meconium from amniotic fluid can occur at birth. Meconium contains bile salts from the fetal intestinal tract that cause inflammation. Neurologically compromised children or children undergoing sedation or anesthesia may aspirate oral secretions (containing anaerobic bacteria) or stomach contents. The severity of lung injury after an aspiration incident is determined by the amount of material aspirated, the pH of the aspirated material, and the presence of pathogenic bacteria. Very low pH or very high pH will cause a significant inflammatory response. With hydrocarbon ingestions, lung injury is determined by the volatility and viscosity of the aspirated substance. A low-viscosity substance, such as gasoline or lighter fluid, is the most toxic; high-viscosity hydrocarbons, such as petroleum jelly or mineral oil, are much less likely to cause a pneumonitis. Treatment for aspiration pneumonitis depends on the material aspirated. Strategies for prevention of aspiration are an important part of the therapeutic plan for every person and are important at every well-child visit. Children at highest risk are toddlers, children with poor airway reflexes or gastroesophageal reflux, or both.

Asthma

Asthma is an obstructive airway disease characterized by reversible airflow obstruction, bronchial hyperreactivity, and inflammation. It is the most prevalent chronic disease in childhood, affecting 5% to 10% of all children, and has become more prevalent in the past two decades. In the prepubertal years, more boys than girls are affected. Inner-city black and Hispanic children have higher morbidity and mortality rates than white children.[60] The mortality rate rose among children with asthma from 1980 to 1993[61] but may be leveling off.[62] Asthma-related deaths almost always occur outside the hospital setting.

There are currently many theories regarding the mechanisms of disease in childhood asthma. The wide spectrum of clinical disease probably reflects a complex interaction between *genetic* susceptibility and *environmental* factors, including allergens and infections, particularly viral respiratory infections.[63-67] A number of experts postulate that a key determinant of asthma is the T-lymphocyte phenotype being tipped toward a "Th_2 response" in which CD4 T-helper (Th) cells produce specific cytokines, such as IL-4, IL-5, and IL-13, that promote an atopic/allergic response in the airways as opposed to a "Th_1 response" characteristic of delayed-type hypersensitivity and phagocyte-mediated host defense.[68,69] IL-4 and IL-13 are particularly important for B cell switching to favor IgE production; IL-5 is crucial for local differentiation and enhanced survival of eosinophils within the airways.

It is possible that certain early childhood respiratory viral infections could favor the Th_2-predominant phenotype and contribute to inducing asthma in susceptible individuals. It has also been suggested that *lack* of sufficient early exposure to viruses and aeroallergens could favor the Th_2 phenotype in the airways and permit induction of asthma. This so-called "hygiene hypothesis" has been offered as an explanation for the higher prevalence of asthma in Westernized countries than in less developed countries, for example, and for the inverse relationship between number of siblings and incidence of atopy. These theories about the origins of asthma are interesting although not solidly proven, and the only link between viruses and asthma that is universally accepted is that viruses frequently precipitate acute exacerbations of asthma.

There is significant evidence that asthma has a strong genetic component, but asthma clearly involves a number of genes.[70] Population genomic screening has led to the proposal of a number of candidate genes or chromosomal regions that are associated with asthma, as well as with associated phenotypes, such as bronchial hyperresponsiveness, high levels of serum IgE, and sensitization to allergens.

Pathophysiology

Examination of postmortem lung specimens of individuals who died from asthma reveals abnormalities consistent with both acute and chronic changes in the airways. There is extensive mucous plugging, mucosal edema, and denudation of bronchial and bronchiolar epithelium. Eosinophilia is present in the submucosa, and a multicellular inflammatory infiltrate accumulates in the airways. Thickening of the basement membrane, airway smooth muscle hypertrophy, and mucous gland hypertrophy are often noted, sometimes even in pathology specimens from mild asthmatics, providing evidence that there may be long-term airway structural changes associated with asthma.

In a full-blown asthma attack **(status asthmaticus),** there are components of bronchospasm, as well as acute airway inflammation directed by a number of cells and the mediators they secrete. Mucous plugging, edema, and cellular infiltration lead to further airway narrowing. There is partial obstruction creating a "ball-valve" effect leading to segmental hyperinflation, which may become extreme and compromise effective tidal volume. Measures of expiratory flow rates, such as FEV_1 and peak flow, are markedly reduced.

For acute allergen-induced asthma, the paradigm of the "early asthmatic response" remains useful (Fig. 33-15, *A*). This begins immediately after exposure and lasts up to 2 hours. The allergen binds to preformed IgE on the surface of mucosal mast cells, and crosslinking of these IgE molecules triggers degranulation of the mast cell, releasing mediators such as histamine, leukotrienes, prostaglandin D_2, platelet-activating factor, and certain cytokines. These mediators cause airway smooth muscle constriction (bronchospasm), increased vascular permeability (mucosal edema), and mucus secretion. The "late asthmatic response" starts 4 to 8 hours after exposure and may persist up to 24 hours (Fig. 33-15, *B*). The response is characterized by inflammatory cell recruitment (neutrophils, eosinophils, basophils, lymphocytes) that was triggered earlier by chemotactic factors and upregulation of endothelial adhesion molecules. Another wave of mediator release occurs, again inciting bronchospasm, edema, and mucus secretion. Epithelial damage and impaired mucociliary function may be seen because of direct toxic effects of products such as major basic protein from eosinophils. This local injury stimulates local nerve endings, which may aggravate bronchoconstriction and mucus secretion through autonomic pathways. In chronic asthma, some of these mechanisms may be operational on an ongoing basis. Chronically increased numbers of inflammatory cells may lead to long-term changes, such as goblet cell hyperplasia and airway wall remodeling (subepithelial fibrosis, smooth muscle hypertrophy).

The typical arterial blood gas abnormalities in acute asthma are hypoxemia, hypocarbia, and respiratory alkalosis. Because bronchial obstruction is nonuniform, ventilation is likewise uneven, causing ventilation mismatch and hypoxemia. The degree of hypoxemia is usually mild, however, and arterial saturations of less than 90% indicate severe airway obstruction. Pulmonary circulation may be altered by regional hypoxic vasoconstriction, as well as the effect of increased intra-alveolar pressure (caused by hyperinflation) to decrease perfusion of alveolar capillaries. Typically, respiratory rate is elevated to compensate for hypoxemia, with reduced minute ventilation because of increased airway resistance and lung hyperinflation. Thus arterial P_{CO_2} is low (30 to 35 mm Hg), and even a normal value should be of concern. Retention of CO_2 is a late finding, usually occurring only if FEV_1 falls to around 15% to 20% of predicted values, and reflects inadequate alveolar ventilation and increased functional dead space. Alterations of pH homeostasis usually start with respiratory alkalosis caused by hyperventilation. With severe airway obstruction, the end result of the pathophysiologic processes may be respiratory failure with acute CO_2 retention and respiratory acidosis. Metabolic acidosis may accompany life-threatening asthma, especially when left ventricular filling and thus cardiac output become compromised because of severe hyperinflation.

Clinical Manifestations

In a typical acute asthma attack, the major complaints are cough, wheeze, and shortness of breath. There may or may not have been signs of a preceding upper respiratory infection, such as rhinorrhea or low-grade fever. In children, 70% to 80% of acute wheezing episodes are associated with viral

A

B

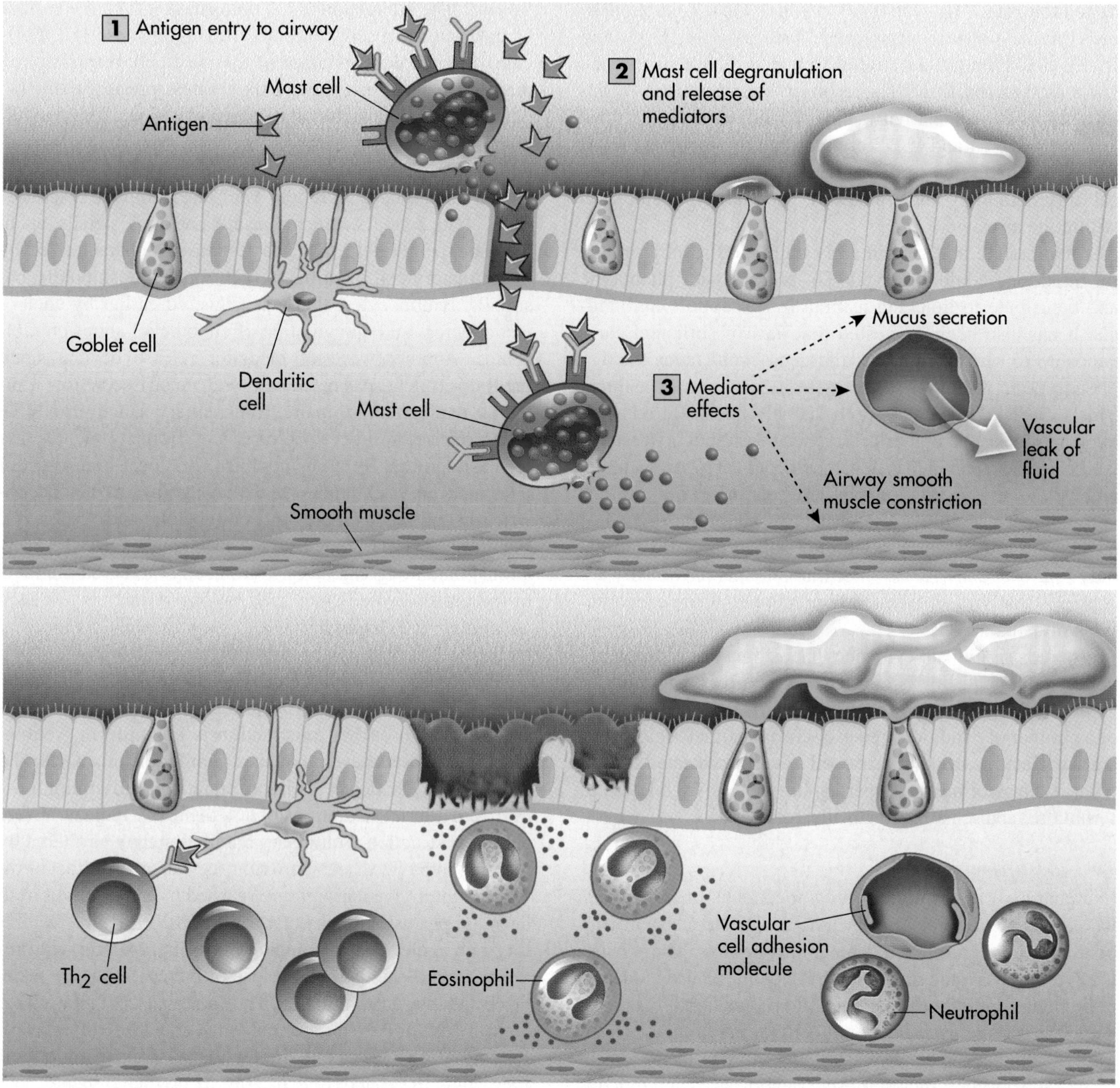

FIG 33-15 Asthmatic responses. A, In the early asthmatic response, inhaled antigen *(1)* binds to preformed IgE on mast cells. Mast cells degranulate *(2)* and release mediators such as histamine, leukotrienes, prostaglandin D_2, platelet-activating factor, and others. Acute inflammation opens intercellular tight junctions, allowing antigen to penetrate and activate submucosal mast cells. Secreted mediators *(3)* induce active bronchospasm, edema, and mucus secretion. Inflammatory responses are set in motion by chemotactic factors and upregulation of adhesion molecules *(not shown)*. At the same time, as shown on the left, antigen may be received by dendritic cells that process and later present it, either in regional lymph nodes to naive (Th_0) T lymphocytes or locally to memory Th_2 cells in the airway mucosa (see **B**). **B,** In the late asthmatic response, there are areas of epithelial damage caused at least in part by toxicity of eosinophil products (major basic protein, eosinophilic cationic protein, eosinophil-derived neurotoxin, and eosinophil peroxidase). Many inflammatory cells have been recruited by chemokines and upregulation of vascular cell adhesion molecules. Local T lymphocytes display a predominant Th_2 cytokine profile. They produce IL-4 and IL-13, which promote switching of B cells to favor IgE production, and IL-3, IL-5, and granulocyte-macrophage colony–stimulating factor, which encourage eosinophil differentiation and survival.

respiratory infections. In infants and toddlers under 2 years old, the most common of these is RSV. In older children and adults, the major viral trigger is rhinovirus.

On physical examination, there is expiratory wheezing that is often described as high pitched and musical and there is prolongation of the expiratory phase of the respiratory cycle. Sometimes hyperinflation is visible. Respiratory rate is elevated, as is heart rate. Nasal flaring and accessory muscle use are evident, with retractions in the substernal, subcostal, intercostal, suprasternal, or sternocleidomastoid areas. Infants may appear to be "head bobbing" because of sternocleidomastoid muscle use. Pulsus paradoxus may be present. The child may appear anxious or diaphoretic, important signs of respiratory compromise.

Findings in chronic asthma may include hyperinflation of the thorax (barrel chest) or pectus excavatum. Clubbing should not be seen in asthma and, if present, should trigger evaluation for other conditions, such as cystic fibrosis.

Evaluation and Treatment

For objective evaluation of asthma, the best indicators are measures of pulmonary function typically obtained through spirometry. The child takes a maximal inspiration followed by a maximal, fast exhalation; expiratory flow rates are calculated from volume exhaled over time. The forced expiratory volume in 1 second (FEV_1) and the midexpiratory flow rate ($FEF_{25\%-75\%}$, or forced expiratory flow rate between 25% and 75% of total exhaled volume) are reduced in acute asthma and sometimes at baseline in chronic asthma. During acute asthma, however, individuals may be too dyspneic to perform this maneuver or it may precipitate coughing. In following chronic asthma, these measures are useful in guiding management. In addition, reduced flow rates may be supportive evidence in making a diagnosis of asthma, as may documentation of bronchial hyperreactivity (in response to challenge, such as exercise or inhaling methacholine) or response to an inhaled bronchodilator. For home management of asthma, peak flow meters are often used. Peak flow measures are less reliable and less reproducible than those obtained by spirometry but can be helpful once a baseline value has been established on the basis of repeated measurements over a period of time. Decreases in peak flow can then be interpreted meaningfully, especially by families, to help modify treatment in the face of increased symptoms or intercurrent illness.

Rapid-acting bronchodilators, such as albuterol (a β_2-adrenergic agonist), for management of acute asthma are typically used, as well as systemic steroids for moderate to severe attacks to decrease inflammatory responses in the lung. Inhaled ipratropium bromide is an anticholinergic agent that contributes to bronchodilation by inhibiting vagal tone; it is sometimes used together with albuterol for acute treatment for additive effect or sometimes as an alternative, though less effective, for those who cannot tolerate β_2-adrenergic agonists because of side effects.

There is a growing number of options for management of chronic asthma depending on chronicity and severity of symptoms, as well as individual compliance issues. Guidelines have been outlined and widely distributed by a National Institutes of Health (NIH) expert panel.[71] For individuals with persistent symptoms, daily "controller" medication is recommended. This category includes inhaled cromolyn or nedocromil, inhaled steroids, oral leukotriene modifiers (see "What's New? Treatment of Asthma with Leukotriene Antagonists" in Chapter 32), and inhaled long-acting β_2-adrenergic agonists, such as salmeterol.

Acute Respiratory Distress Syndrome

Acute respiratory distress syndrome (ARDS) is a condition resulting from a direct pulmonary insult (such as pneumonia, aspiration, near-drowning, or smoke inhalation) or a systemic insult (such as sepsis or multiple trauma), either of which activates an inflammatory response that causes alveolocapillary injury. *Adult respiratory distress syndrome* is the historical term for this condition, but its recognition in children has led to renaming it *acute respiratory distress syndrome.* Clinically, ARDS is characterized by severe hypoxemia, decreased pulmonary compliance, and diffuse densities on chest radiograph. ARDS accounts for approximately 10% of total patient days and one third of all deaths in pediatric intensive care units.[72] The mortality rate in pediatric ARDS remains high, at approximately 50%.[73,74]

Pathophysiology

The hallmark of ARDS is lung inflammation. There is activation of a number of systems and mediators (Fig. 33-16), including complement, cytokines, arachidonic acid metabolites, platelet-activating factor, reactive oxygen species, and others. Sources of these mediators include neutrophils, activated platelets, macrophages, and injured endothelium. In early ARDS, there is pulmonary neutrophil influx along with intraluminal fibrin and platelet aggregation. Injury to the endothelial and endothelial barriers results in capillary leak and noncardiogenic pulmonary edema. Edema fluid contains plasma proteins that can inactivate surfactant, contributing further to alveolar collapse. This fluid also has procoagulant activity, leading to fibrin clotting within airspaces. During the acute phase, the pulmonary microcirculation is compromised by the formation of thrombi composed of fibrin, platelets, and leukocytes.

The early accumulation of edema fluid in the airspaces results in decreased lung compliance, decreased functional residual volume, and increased dead space. There is ventilation-perfusion mismatching, intrapulmonary shunting, and hypoxemia. Diffuse pulmonary thrombosis contributes further to the formation of pulmonary edema by increasing capillary hydrostatic pressure and may lead to pulmonary hypertension.

In the fibroproliferative phase, type II alveolar cells proliferate and there is alveolar septal thickening and collagen deposition. Interstitial fibrosis can be evident as early as 10 days after the initial insult. Similarly, vascular changes may occur, including obliteration of the microcirculation and thickening of the walls of pulmonary arterioles and arteries, which can lead to chronic pulmonary hypertension in survivors.

Clinical Manifestations

ARDS develops acutely after the initial insult, usually within 24 hours (although occasionally it is delayed up to a few days). There is progressive respiratory distress and severe hypoxemia with poor response to oxygen supplementation. Initially, hyperventilation occurs, but CO_2 retention may ultimately occur because of inadequate functional airspace and respiratory muscle fatigue. Severity of the overall picture is modified by comorbid factors, such as the presence of sepsis or multiorgan failure and whether there are complications, such as nosocomial pneumonia.

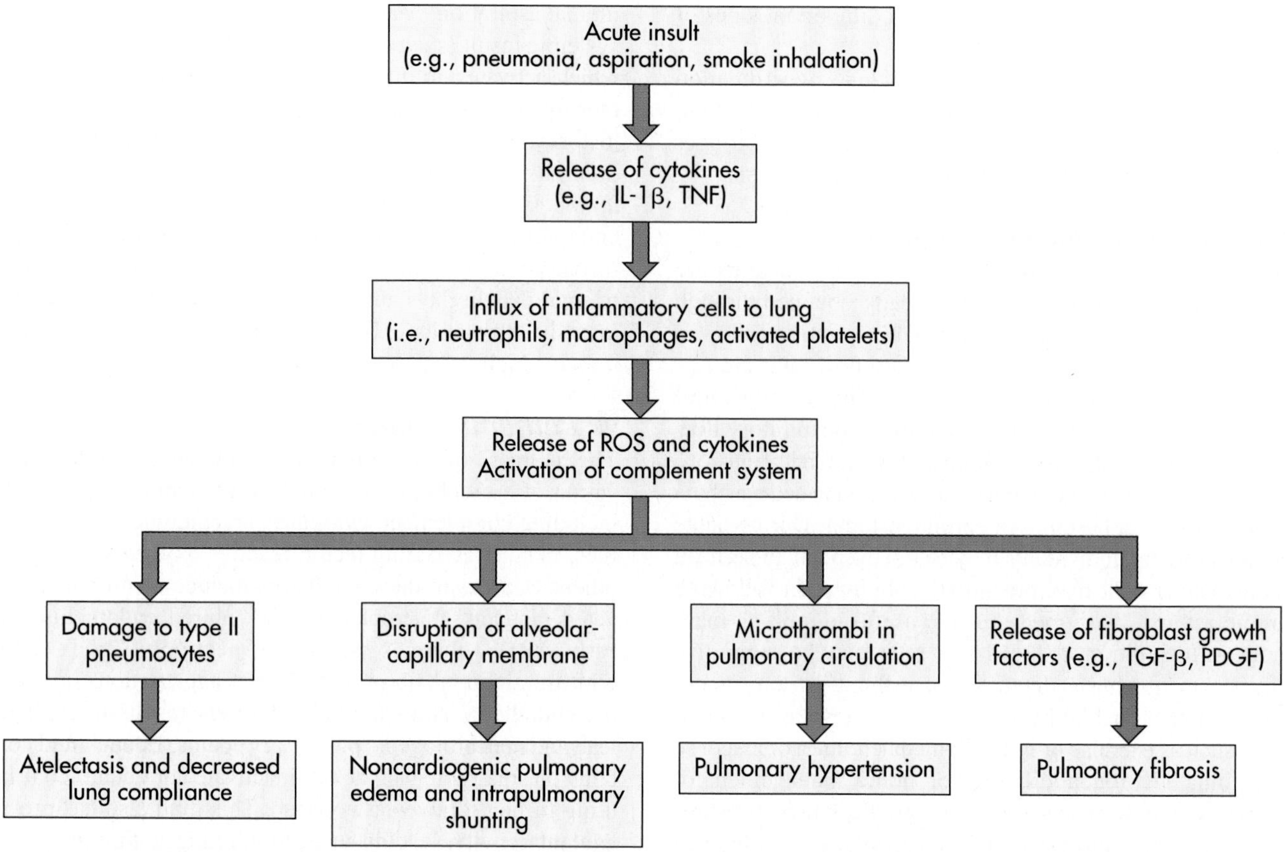

FIG. 33-16 Proposed mechanisms for the pathogenesis of acute respiratory distress syndrome (ARDS). *IL-1β,* Interleukin-1β; *TNF,* tumor necrosis factor; *ROS,* reactive oxygen species; *TGF-β,* transforming growth factor–β; *PDGF,* platelet-derived growth factor. (From Soubani AO, Pieroni R: Acute respiratory distress syndrome: a clinical update, *South Med J* 92(5):452, 1999.)

Evaluation and Treatment

Treatment of ARDS remains supportive in nature. Of course, any underlying condition, such as sepsis, must be treated. Beyond that, the goals are maintaining adequate tissue oxygenation, minimizing acute lung injury, and avoiding iatrogenic pulmonary complications. Most individuals with ARDS require mechanical ventilation and often relatively high levels of positive end-expiratory pressure to promote alveolar recruitment and stabilization and redistribution of alveolar edema fluid into the interstitium. Various ventilation strategies have been described for ARDS, such as low tidal volumes, permissive hypercapnia, prone positioning, inverse inspiratory/expiratory ratio, and high-frequency oscillator ventilation. Liquid ventilation through perfluorocarbons instilled in the lungs is being investigated. These fluids have low surface tension and are efficient carriers of oxygen and carbon dioxide. Other therapies, such as surfactant and nitric oxide, offer theoretic promise, but their efficacy in pediatric ARDS has not yet been validated.

SUDDEN INFANT DEATH SYNDROME

Sudden infant death syndrome (SIDS) remains a disease of unknown cause. It is defined as "sudden death of an infant under 1 year of age which remains unexplained after a thorough case investigation, including performance of a complete autopsy, examination of the death scene, and review of the clinical history".[75] SIDS is the leading cause of infant death beyond the neonatal period in the United States.

The incidence of SIDS is low during the first month of life but sharply increases in the second month of life, peaks at 3 to 4 months old, and is unusual after 6 months of age. It is more common in male (60%) than female (40%) infants. It almost always occurs during nighttime sleep, when infants are least likely to be observed. A seasonal variation has been noted, with higher frequencies during the winter months. This has been related to a higher rate of respiratory tract infection during those months, and such infections are often reported to have preceded the death.

Clinical risk groups include babies who were preterm or low birth weight, multiple births, and siblings of prior SIDS victims (fourfold to sixfold increased risk). The occurrence of an apparent life-threatening event seems to predict increased SIDS risk. Nevertheless, about three quarters of all SIDS victims have no known predisposing clinical risk factor.

Additional risk factors fall into the categories of socioeconomic or maternal factors and factors in the baby's sleeping situation.[76-80] Maternal factors that predict increased SIDS risk are maternal smoking,[76] young maternal age (under 20 years), unmarried mother, less prenatal care, poverty, and illicit drug use. Risk factors that relate to the baby's sleeping situation are prone positioning (and to a lesser extent, side sleeping), sleeping on soft bedding, and overheating. Prone sleeping was concluded to be a major and modifiable risk factor. Epidemiologic studies have shown that SIDS rates decreased by 40% to 70% in countries, including the United States, where massive public campaigns warned against prone sleeping for infants.[75,81] Infants should sleep on their backs. Other avoidable risk factors include loose bedding materials and sleeping on top of any soft surface (such as sheepskins, quilts, comforters, pillows, adult-type mattresses, or waterbeds). Bed sharing with parents increases risk in some situations.[79,80] Overwrapping the infant or overheating the room also appear to increase risk, particularly if the infant is sleeping prone.

The etiology of SIDS remains unknown. A leading hypothesis is that there may be developmental immaturity of ventilatory and arousal responses to hypoxemia or hypercarbia. Alternative theories involve increased vagal tone; sudden intrapulmonary shunting because of abnormalities of surfactant or pulmonary vessels; or exaggerated inflammation, eosinophil degranulation, and massive cytokine release causing pulmonary edema in response to either bacterial pathogens from the nasopharynx or viral respiratory tract infections.

Currently, the best strategy to reduce SIDS is thought to be avoidance of all the controllable risk factors, particularly unsafe sleeping practices and maternal smoking. Parents of infants with clinical risk should be taught cardiopulmonary resuscitation as a precaution. Although home monitoring has not been proven to decrease the incidence of SIDS, some at-risk infants may warrant cardiorespiratory monitoring after careful consideration of the individual situation.

SUMMARY REVIEW

Structure and Function

1. The airways of infants and children are narrower from the trachea through the terminal bronchioles, thus making them more prone to obstruction than the airways of adults.
2. Infants and young children continue to form new alveoli until approximately age 8, after which they simply increase in size as the body grows.
3. Surfactant production is an important marker of developmental maturity of the fetal lung.
4. The immature chest wall is soft and compliant, contributing to inefficient mechanisms of breathing.
5. Children have greater oxygen consumption than adults.
6. Immune mechanisms are not fully developed at birth, making young infants more susceptible to infection.
7. Physiologic control of breathing may be impaired during the first few weeks of life.

Pulmonary Disorders

1. Physical examination can provide important clues in assessing the location and nature of upper airway obstruction.
2. Viral croup (laryngotracheobronchitis) is the most common cause of acute upper airway obstruction in children and usually affects children ages 6 months to 5 years. Subglottic edema may be mild to severe. Parainfluenza is the most common cause.
3. Acute epiglottitis is a life-threatening emergency that is now rarely seen because of vaccination against *Haemophilus influenzae,* the primary causative microorganism. Other bacteria, such as group A streptococci, can also cause epiglottitis.
4. Other bacterial infections of the airway can pose serious threats, including bacterial tracheitis, retropharyngeal abscess, and peritonsillar infections.
5. Aspiration of a foreign body should be considered whenever there is a sudden onset of stridor, coughing, wheezing, or hoarseness. This usually occurs in 1- to 3-year-olds. Occasionally, diagnosis is delayed and symptoms may be attributed to asthma, bronchitis, or pneumonia without recognition of the underlying cause.
6. Chronic upper airway obstruction may be manifested by stridor, abnormal cry, wheezing, or dyspnea. The most common cause of stridor in infants is laryngomalacia. Other causes include subglottic stenosis, vocal cord paralysis, and vascular rings.
7. Obstructive sleep apnea usually occurs in older children rather than infants and is underdiagnosed. Typical symptoms are snoring, gasping, and restless sleep. The most common cause in children is adenotonsillar hypertrophy.
8. Respiratory distress syndrome (RDS) of the newborn usually occurs in premature infants who are born before surfactant production and alveolocapillary development are complete. Atelectasis and hypoventilation cause shunting, hypoxemia, and hypercapnia.
9. Bronchopulmonary dysplasia is a chronic lung disease of infancy and early childhood that is usually the consequence of acute respiratory disease in the newborn period. Most often this occurs in infants who were premature and required ventilatory support. Contributing factors include structural immaturity, inflammation, and disordered lung repair processes.
10. Cystic fibrosis (CF) is an autosomal recessive disease characterized by thick, tenacious mucus, plugging of airways, chronic pulmonary infection, and bronchiectasis. The other major manifestations are digestive and nutritional, related to pancreatic insufficiency. Median survival is currently 32 years, with mortality primarily related to lung disease.
11. Bronchiolitis occurs in infants and toddlers, usually in the winter and early spring. It is caused by viruses, most commonly respiratory syncytial virus (RSV). There is extensive edema, inflammation, and damage to the bronchiolar epithelium. Infants with underlying lung disease or heart disease experience more severe illness and should be given injections of monoclonal antibody against RSV as a preventive measure.
12. Childhood pneumonia can be caused by viruses, bacteria, or *Mycoplasma.* Lobar pneumonia is usually bacterial (especially

pneumococcal). Certain bacteria, such as *Staphylococcus aureus* and group A streptococci, can cause particularly fulminant disease, as well as abscesses and empyema.

13. Aspiration pneumonitis can occur because of lung inflammation from entry of toxins (e.g., accidental ingestion) or irritants. Aspiration of oropharyngeal bacteria can occur because of an impaired airway, because of loss of protective reflexes in neurologically impaired children, or during anesthesia.
14. Asthma is an obstructive airway disease with episodes of acute respiratory symptoms (cough, wheeze, dyspnea) and intermittent or chronic subacute symptoms. It is the most common chronic condition in children. It is a disease of local airway inflammation, with exacerbation in response to triggers, such as infections or allergens. Inflammatory cell infiltration, mucosal edema, mucous plugging of airways, and epithelial damage are seen, and there is evidence of long-term remodeling of airways.

Sudden Infant Death Syndrome

1. Sudden infant death syndrome (SIDS) usually occurs in children under 6 months of age during sleep in the prone position. The cause is unknown. However, some known risk factors are avoidable, such as maternal smoking, prone sleeping, soft bedding surfaces, and overheating.

KEY TERMS

Acute epiglottitis, *1151*
Acute respiratory distress syndrome (ARDS), *1165*
Angioedema, *1152*
Aspiration pneumonitis, *1162*
Asthma, *1162*
Atypical pneumonia *(Mycoplasma pneumoniae, Chlamydia pneumoniae), 1162*
Bacterial pneumonia, *1161*
Bacterial tracheitis, *1152*
Bronchiolitis, *1160*
Bronchopulmonary dysplasia (BPD), *1157*
Croup syndrome, *1149*
Cystic fibrosis (CF), *1157*
Cystic fibrosis transmembrane regulator (CFTR), *1157*
Diphtheria, *1152*
Foreign body aspiration, *1148*
Functional residual capacity (FRC), *1147*
Laryngomalacia, *1153*
Laryngotracheobronchitis, *1149*
Obstructive sleep apnea syndrome (OSAS), *1153*
Peritonsillar abscess, *1152*
Pneumonia, *1161*
Respiratory distress syndrome (RDS) of the newborn (hyaline membrane disease), *1154*
Spasmodic croup, *1151*
Status asthmaticus, *1163*
Stridor, *1149*
Subglottic stenosis, *1153*
Sudden infant death syndrome (SIDS), *1166*
Surfactant, *1145*
Tracheomalacia, *1153*
Upper airway obstruction, *1148*
Vocal cord paralysis, *1153*

REFERENCES

1. Eavey RD: A sound workup for evaluating airway obstruction, *Contemp Pediatr* 3(6):78, 1986.
2. Leung AKC, Cho H: Diagnosis of stridor in children, *Am Fam Physician* 60(8):2289, 1999.
3. Kaditis AG, Wald ER: Viral croup: current diagnosis and treatment, *Pediatr Infect Dis J* 17(9):827, 1998.
4. Klassen TP: Croup, a current perspective, *Pediatr Clin North Am* 46(6): 1167, 1999.
5. Ausejo M et al: The effectiveness of glucocorticoids in treating croup: meta-analysis, *BMJ* 319:595, 1999.
6. Geelhoed GC: Croup, *Pediatr Pulmonol* 23:370, 1997.
7. Hickerson SL et al: Epiglottitis: a 9-year case review, *South Med J* 89(5):487, 1996.
8. Carey MJ: Epiglottitis in adults, *Am J Emerg Med* 14(4):421, 1996.
9. Gonzalez-Valdapena H et al: Epiglottitis and *Haemophilus influenzae* immunization: the Pittsburgh experience—a five-year review, *Pediatrics* 96(3 pt 1):424, 1995.
10. Midwinter KI, Hodgson D, Yardley M: Paediatric epiglottis: the influence of the *Haemophilus influenzae* b vaccine, a ten-year review in the Sheffield region, *Clin Otolaryngol Allied Sci* 24(5):447, 1999.
11. Wenger JK: Supraglottitis and group A streptococcus, *Pediatr Infect Dis J* 16(10):1005, 1997.
12. Whiting JL, Chow AW: Life-threatening infections of the mouth and throat, *J Crit Illness* 2(7):36, 1987.
13. Blazer S, Naveh Y, Friedman A: Foreign body in the airway, a review of 200 cases, *Am J Dis Child* 134:68, 1980.
14. Kenna MA, Bluestone CD: Foreign bodies in the air and food passages, *Pediatr Rev* 10(1):25, 1988.
15. Fitzpatrick PC, Guarisco JL: Pediatric airway foreign bodies, *J La State Med Soc* 150(4):138, 1998.
16. Halvorson DJ et al: Management of subglottic foreign bodies, *Ann Otol Rhinol Laryngol* 105(7):541, 1996.
17. Nielsen EW et al: C1 inhibitor and diagnosis of hereditary angioedema in newborns, *Pediatr Res* 35(2):184, 1994.
18. Ewan PW: Clinical study of peanut and nut allergy in 62 consecutive patients: new features and associations, *BMJ* 312(7038):1074, 1996.
19. Shinkwin CA, Gibbin KP: Tracheostomy in children, *J R Soc Med* 89(4):188, 1996.
20. Othersen HB Jr: Subglottic tracheal stenosis, *Semin Thorac Cardiovasc Surg* 6(4):200, 1994.
21. Brodner DC, Guarisco JL: Subglottic stenosis: evaluation and management, *J La State Med Soc* 151(4):159, 1999.
22. Cotton RT: Management of subglottic stenosis, *Otolaryngol Clin North Am* 33(1):111, 2000.
23. deJong AL et al: Vocal cord paralysis in infants and children, *Otolaryngol Clin North Am* 33(1):131, 2000.
24. Gormley PK et al: Congenital vascular anomalies and persistent respiratory symptoms in children, *Int J Pediatr Otorhinolaryngol* 51(1):23, 1999.
25. Dennie CJ, Coblentz CL: The trachea: pathologic conditions and trauma, *Can Assoc Radiol* 44(3):157, 1993.
26. Dunham ME et al: Management of severe congenital tracheal stenosis, *Ann Otol Rhinol Laryngol* 103(5, pt 1):351, 1994.
27. Marcus CL: Sleep-disordered breathing in children, *Curr Opin Pediatr* 12:208, 2000.
28. Redline S et al: Risk factors for sleep-disordered breathing in children: associations with obesity, race, and respiratory problems, *Am J Respir Crit Care Med* 159:1527, 1999.

29. Verma RP: Respiratory distress syndrome of the newborn infant, *Obstet Gynecol Surv* 50(7):542, 1995.
30. Crowley P, Chalmers I, Keirse MJNC: The effects of corticosteroid administration before preterm delivery: an overview of the evidence from controlled trials, *Br J Obstet Gynaecol* 97:11, 1990.
31. NIH Consensus Development Conference Statement: Effect of corticosteroids for fetal maturation on perinatal outcomes, *Am J Obstet Gynecol* 173:246, 1995.
32. Rodriguez RJ, Martin RJ: Exogenous surfactant therapy in newborns, *Respir Care Clin North Am* 5(4):595, 1999.
33. Jobe AH, Ikegami M: Lung development and function in preterm infants in the surfactant treatment era, *Annu Rev Physiol* 62:825, 2000.
34. Eber E, Zach MS: Long term sequelae of bronchopulmonary dysplasia (chronic lung diseases of infancy), *Thorax* 56(4):317, 2001.
35. Robbins ST, Fletcher AB: Early vs delayed vitamin A supplementation in very-low-birth-weight infants, *JPEN J Parenter Enteral Nutr* 17(3): 220, 1993.
36. Inder TE et al: Plasma vitamin A levels in the very low birthweight infant—relationship to respiratory outcome, *Early Hum Dev* 52(2): 155, 1998.
37. Parker RA, Lindstrom DP, Cotton RB: Improved survival accounts for most, but not all, of the increase in bronchopulmonary dysplasia, *Pediatrics* 90(5):663, 1992.
38. Vanhatalo AM et al: Incidence of bronchopulmonary dysplasia during an 11-year period in infants weighing less than 1500 g at birth, *Ann Chir Gynaecol Suppl* 208:113, 1994.
39. Jobe AH, Ikegami M: Mechanisms initiating lung injury in the preterm, *Early Hum Dev* 53(1):81, 1998.
40. Behrman RE, Kliegman RM, Arvin AM: *Nelson textbook of pediatrics,* ed 16, Philadelphia, 2000, W.B. Saunders.
41. Carey BE, Trotter C: Bronchopulmonary dysplasia, *Neonatal Net* 15(4):73, 1996.
42. Bancalari E: Corticosteroids and neonatal chronic lung disease, *Eur J Pediatr* 157(suppl 1):S31, 1998.
43. Shenai JP, Mellen BG, Chytil F: Vitamin A status and postnatal dexamethasone treatment in bronchopulmonary dysplasia, *Pediatrics* 106(3):547, 2000.
44. Speer CP, Silverman M: Issues relating to children born prematurely, *Eur Respir J* 27(suppl):13S, 1998.
45. Kosorok MR, Wei WH, Farrell PM: The incidence of cystic fibrosis, *Stat Med* 15(5):449, 1996.
46. Cheng P et al: Increased sulfation of glycoconjugates by cultured nasal epithelial cells from patients with cystic fibrosis, *J Clin Invest* 84(1):68, 1989.
47. Sangadala S, Bhat UR, Mendicino J: Structures of sulfated oligosaccharides in human trachea mucin glycoproteins, *Mol Cell Biochem* 126(1): 37, 1993.
48. Shak S et al: Recombinant human DNase I reduces the viscosity of cystic fibrosis sputum, *Proc Natl Acad Sci USA* 87(23):9188, 1990.
49. Vasconcellos CA et al: Reduction in viscosity of cystic fibrosis sputum by gelsolin, *Science* 263(5149):969, 1994.
50. Khan TZ et al: Early pulmonary inflammation in infants with cystic fibrosis, *Am J Respir Crit Care Med* 151:1075, 1995.
51. Bonfield TL, Konstan MW, Berger M: Altered respiratory epithelial cell cytokine production in cystic fibrosis, *J Allergy Clin Immunol* 104(1): 72, 1999.
52. Henry RL, Mellis CM, Petrovic L: Mucoid *Pseudomonas aeruginosa* is a marker of poor survival in cystic fibrosis, *Pediatr Pulmonol* 12:158, 1992.
53. Burns JL et al: Effect of chronic intermittent administration of inhaled tobramycin on respiratory microbial flora in patients with cystic fibrosis, *J Infect Dis* 179(5):1190, 1999.
54. Spencer N et al: Deprivation and bronchiolitis, *Arch Dis Child* 74(1): 50, 1996.
55. Stark JM et al: Respiratory syncytial virus infection enhances neutrophil and eosinophil adhesion to cultured respiratory epithelial cells: roles of CD18 and intercellular adhesion molecule-1, *J Immunol* 156(12): 4474, 1996.
56. Castleman WL et al: Viral bronchiolitis during early life induces increased number of bronchiolar mast cells and airway hyperresponsiveness, *Am J Pathol* 137(4):821, 1990.
57. Sigurs N et al: Respiratory syncytial virus bronchiolitis in infancy is an important risk factor for asthma and allergy at age 7, *Am J Respir Crit Care Med* 161(5):1501, 2000.
58. Stein RT et al: Respiratory syncytial virus in early life and risk of wheeze and allergy by age 13 years, *Lancet* 354(9178):541, 1999.
59. Light RB: Pulmonary pathophysiology of pneumococcal pneumonia, *Semin Respir Infect* 14(3):218, 1999.
60. Weiss KB, Gergen PJ, Crain EE: Inner-city asthma: the epidemiology of an emerging US public health concern, *Chest* 101(6, suppl):362S, 1992.
61. Asthma mortality and hospitalization among children and young adults—United States, 1980-1993, *MMWR Morb Mortal Wkly Rep* 45(17):350, 1996.
62. Sly RM: Decreases in asthma mortality in the United States, *Ann Allergy Asthma Immunol* 85(2):121, 2000.
63. Gern JE: Viral and bacterial infections in the development and progression of asthma, *J Allergy Clin Immunol* 105(2 Pt 2):S497, 2000.
64. Nafstad P, Magnus P, Jaakkola JJK: Early respiratory infections and childhood asthma, *Pediatrics* 106(3):E38, 2000.
65. Holt PG et al: Microbial stimulation as an aetiologic factor in atopic disease, *Allergy* 54:12, 1999.
66. Martinez FD et al: Asthma and wheezing in the first six years of life, *N Engl J Med* 332:133, 1995.
67. Platts-Mills TAE, Rakes G, Heymann PW: The relevance of allergen exposure to the development of asthma in childhood, *J Allergy Clin Immunol* 105:S503, 2000.
68. Colavita AM, Reinach AJ, Peters SP: Contributing factors to the pathobiology of asthma: the Th_1/Th_2 paradigm, *Clin Chest Med* 21(2):263, 2000.
69. Fahy JV: Reducing IgE levels as a strategy for the treatment of asthma, *Clin Exp Allergy* 30(suppl 1): 16, 2000.
70. Howard TD, Meyers DA, Bleecker ER: Mapping susceptibility genes for asthma and allergy, *J Allergy Clin Immunol* 105:S477, 2000.
71. National Institutes of Health, National Heart, Lung, and Blood Institute: *Expert panel report 2: guidelines for the diagnosis and management of asthma*, NIH Pub. No. 97-4051A, 1997.
72. Schears GJ, Costarino AT: Complexity of inflammatory mediators in acute respiratory distress syndrome (ARDS), *J Pediatr* 135:144, 1999.
73. Soubani AO, Pieroni R: Acute respiratory distress syndrome: a clinical update, *South Med J* 92(5):450, 1999.
74. Moloney-Harmon PA: When the lung fails. Acute respiratory distress syndrome in children, *Crit Care Nursing Clin North Am* 11(4):519, 1999.
75. American Academy of Pediatrics Task Force on Infant Sleep Position and Sudden Infant Death Syndrome: Changing concepts of sudden infant death syndrome: implications for infant sleeping environment and sleep position, *Pediatrics* 105(3):650, 2000.
76. Alm B et al: A case-control study of smoking and sudden infant death syndrome in the Scandinavian countries, 1992 to 1995. The Nordic Epidemiological SIDS Study, *Arch Dis Child* 78(4):329, 1998.
77. Daltveit AK et al: Sociodemographic risk factors for sudden infant death syndrome: associations with other risk factors. The Nordic Epidemiological SIDS Study, *Acta Paediatr* 87(3):284, 1998.
78. Leach CE et al: Epidemiology of SIDS and explained sudden infant deaths. CESDI SUDI Research Group, *Pediatrics* 104(4):e43, 1999.
79. Mitchell EA et al: Risk factors for sudden infant death syndrome following the prevention campaign in New Zealand: a prospective study, *Pediatrics* 100(5):835, 1997.
80. Kemp JS et al: Unsafe sleep practices and an analysis of bedsharing among infants dying suddenly and unexpectedly: results of a four-year, population-based, death-scene investigation study of sudden infant death syndrome and related deaths, *Pediatrics* 106(3):E41, 2000.
81. DeJonge GA et al: Sleeping position for infants and cot death in the Netherlands 1985-1991, *Arch Dis Child* 69:660, 1993.

CHAPTER 34

Structure and Function of the Renal and Urologic Systems

SUE E. HUETHER

CHAPTER OUTLINE

The primary function of the kidney is to maintain a stable internal environment for optimal cell and tissue metabolism. The kidneys accomplish these life-sustaining tasks by balancing solute and water transport, excreting metabolic waste products, conserving nutrients, and regulating acids and bases. The kidney also has an endocrine function, secreting the hormones renin, erythropoietin, and 1,25-dihydroxyvitamin D_3 for regulation of blood pressure, erythrocyte production, and calcium metabolism, respectively. In times of severe fasting the kidney also can synthesize glucose from amino acids, performing the process of gluconeogenesis. The formation of urine is achieved through the processes of filtration, reabsorption, and secretion by the glomeruli and tubules within the kidney. The bladder stores the urine that it receives from the kidney by way of the ureters. Urine is then removed from the body through the urethra.

STRUCTURES OF THE RENAL SYSTEM

Structures of the Kidney

The **kidneys** are paired organs located on the posterior abdominal wall outside the peritoneal cavity. They lie on either side of the vertebral column with their upper and lower poles extending from the twelfth thoracic to the third lumbar vertebrae (Fig. 34-1). Each kidney is approximately 11 cm long, 5 to 6 cm wide, and 3 to 4 cm thick. A tightly adhering capsule (the **renal capsule**) surrounds each kidney, and the kidney then is embedded in a mass of fat. The capsule and fatty layer are covered with a double layer of **renal fascia,** fibrous tissue that attaches the kidney to the posterior abdominal wall.

The cushion of fat and the position of the kidney between the abdominal organs and muscles of the back protect it from trauma. The right kidney is slightly lower than the left; it is displaced downward by the overlying liver. A medial indentation (the **hilum**) contains the entry and exit for the renal blood vessels, nerves, lymphatic vessels, and ureter.

The gross structure of the kidney can be identified when it is divided from top to bottom in a coronal plane (Fig. 34-2). The major components are the outer **renal cortex** and the inner **renal medulla.** The cortex contains all the glomeruli and portions of the tubules. The medulla is formed by the straight segments of the proximal and distal tubules and the collecting ducts. It consists of a series of wedges, called **renal pyramids,** with an outer zone close to the cortex and an inner zone. **Renal columns** extend from the cortex down between the renal pyramids. The apexes of the pyramids project into a **minor calyx** (a cup-shaped cavity), which joins

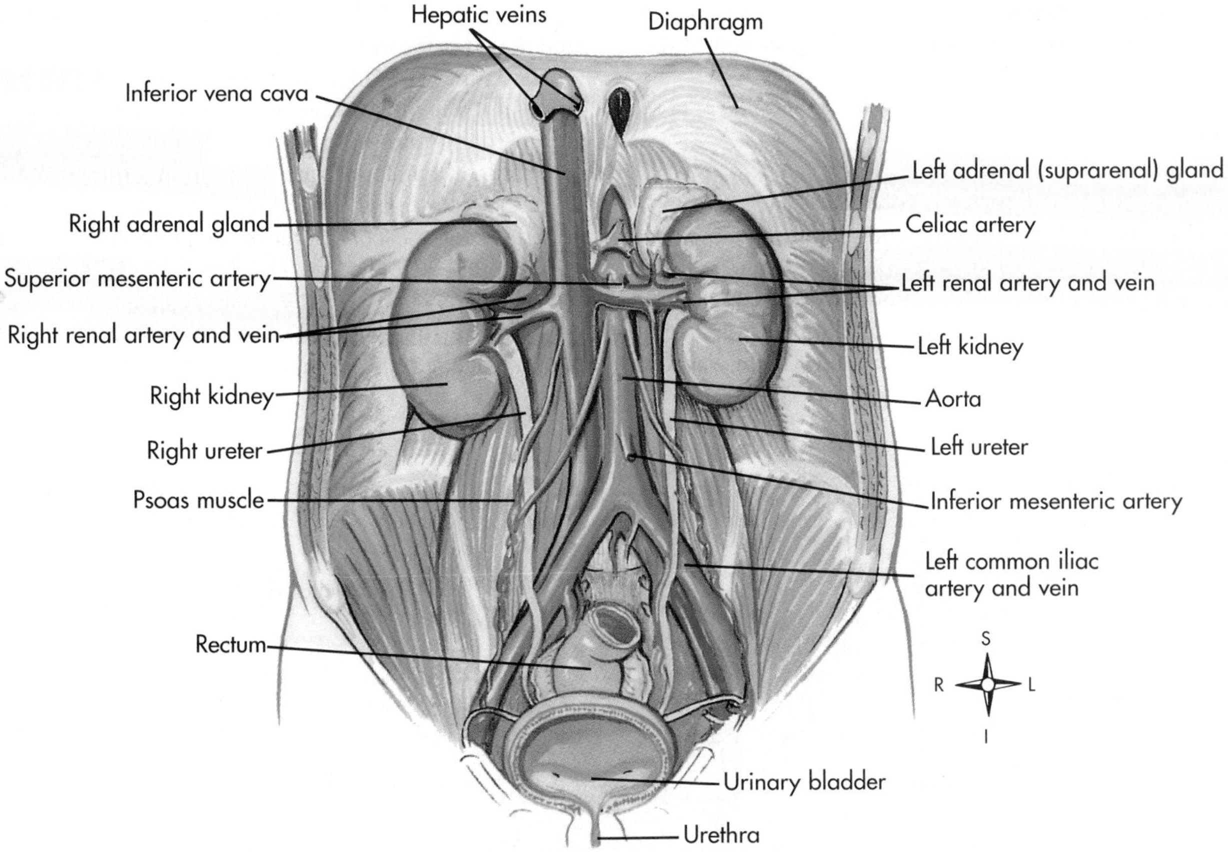

FIG. 34-1 Organs of the urinary system. (From Thibodeau GA, Patton KI: *Anatomy and physiology,* ed 4, St Louis, 1999, Mosby.)

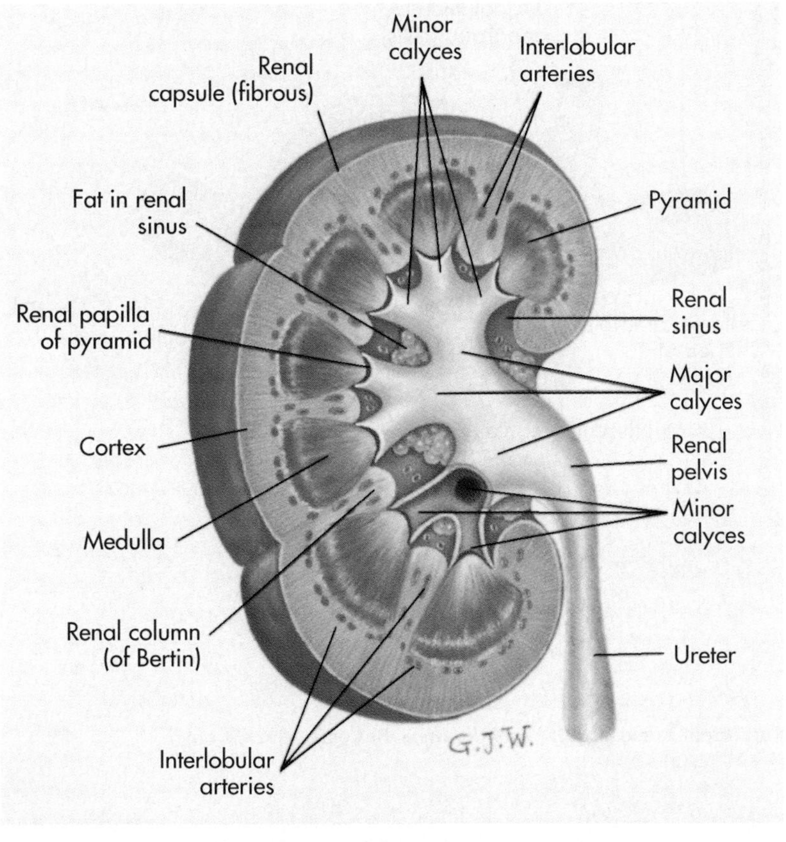

FIG. 34-2 Kidney structure. (From Brundage DJ: *Renal disorders,* St Louis, 1992, Mosby.)

together to form a **major calyx.** The major calyces join to form the **renal pelvis,** an extension of the upper end of the ureter.

Nephron

The **nephron** is the functional unit of the kidney. Approximately 1.2 million nephrons are contained in each kidney. The nephron is a tubular structure with subunits that include the renal corpuscle, proximal convoluted tubule, loop of Henle, distal convoluted tubule, and collecting duct, all of which contribute to the formation of final urine (Fig. 34-3). The different structures of the epithelial cells lining various segments of the tubule facilitate the special functions of secretion and reabsorption (Fig. 34-4).

The kidney has three kinds of nephrons: (1) **superficial cortical nephrons** (85% of all nephrons), which extend only partially into the medulla; (2) **midcortical nephrons** with short or long loops; and (3) **juxtamedullary nephrons,** which lie close to and extend deep into the medulla and are important for the concentration of urine (Fig. 34-5). The **glomerulus** (Fig. 34-6; see also Fig. 34-3) is a tuft of capillaries, the glomerular capillaries, that loop into a circular capsule, the **Bowman capsule,** like fingers pushed into bread dough. Together, the glomerulus and Bowman capsule are

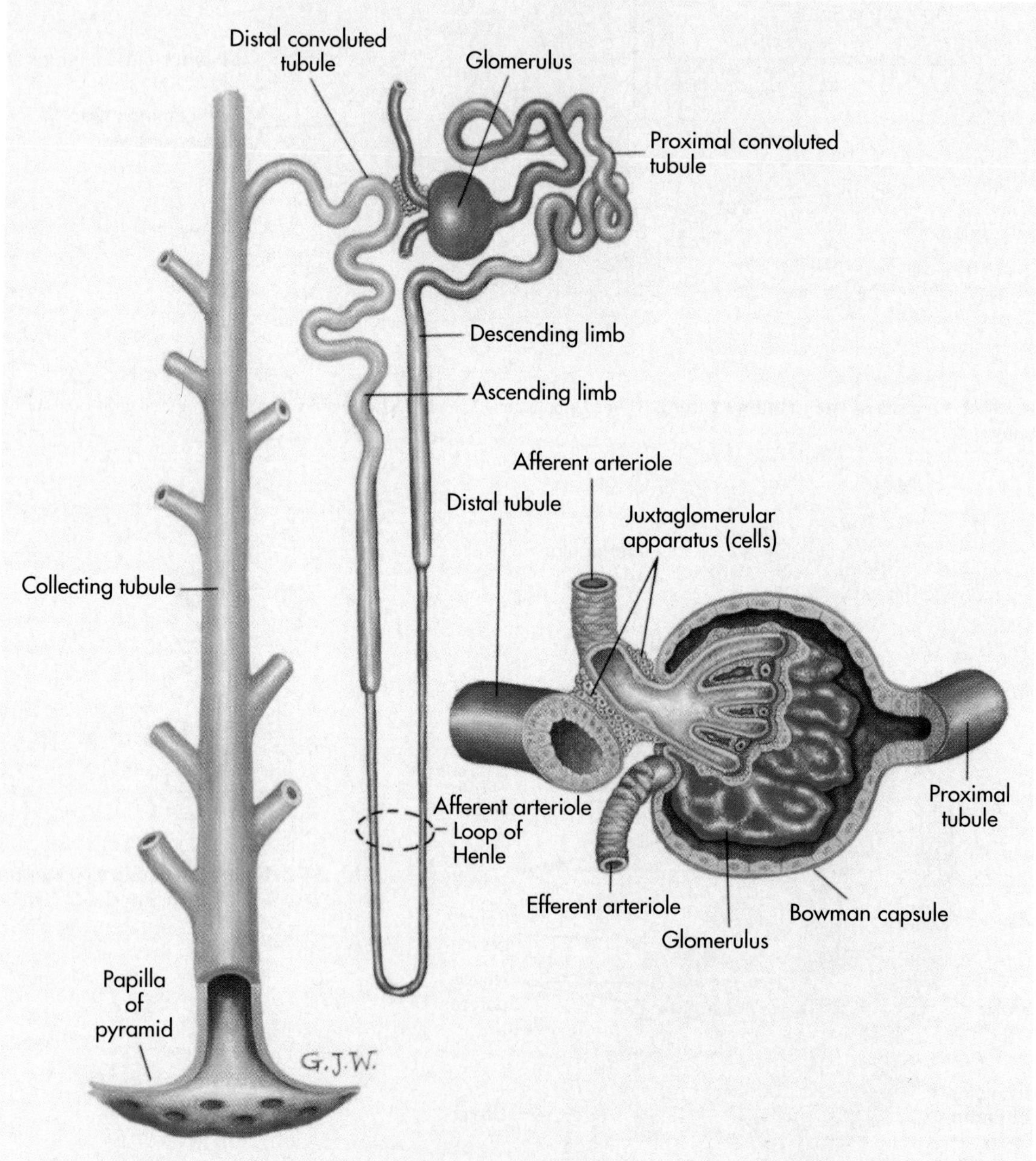

FIG. 34-3 Components of the nephron. (From Brundage DJ: *Renal disorders,* St Louis, 1992, Mosby.)

called the **renal corpuscle. Mesangial cells** (shaped like smooth muscle cells) and the mesangial matrix lie between and support the glomerular capillaries.[1] They have contractile and phagocytic properties, similar to monocytes, and produce vasoactive substances that may influence the glomerular filtration rate (GFR) by regulating glomerular capillary blood flow. The space inside the Bowman capsule is called the **Bowman space.**

The wall of the glomerular capillary serves as a filtration membrane (the **glomerular filtration membrane**) and has three layers: (1) an inner capillary endothelium, (2) a middle basement membrane, and (3) an outer layer of capillary epithelium (also called *podocytes* or *visceral epithelium*). Each layer has unique structural properties that allow all components of the blood to filter through, with the exception of blood cells and plasma proteins with a molecular weight greater than 70,000 (Fig. 34-7; see also Fig. 34-6). The **glomerular endothelium** is composed of cells in continuous contact with the basement membrane. It is perforated by many small openings or windows, called *fenestrae.* The middle basement membrane is a negatively charged, selectively permeable network of glycoproteins and mucopolysaccharides and may be secreted by the epithelial cells.[2] The **glomerular epithelium** has specialized cells called **podocytes.** Footlike processes radiate from the podocytes and adhere to the basement membrane. The foot processes of one podocyte interlock with the foot processes of adjacent podocytes, forming an elaborate network of intercellular clefts. These clefts are called **filtration slits** or slit membranes and modulate filtration.[3]

The glomerular filtration membrane separates the blood of the glomerular capillaries from the fluid in the Bowman space. The glomerular filtrate passes through the three layers of the glomerular membrane and forms the primary urine. The endothelial cells and basement membrane of the filtration membrane express negatively charged glycoproteins and form a filtration barrier to anionic proteins.

The glomerulus is supplied by the afferent arteriole and drained by the efferent arteriole. A group of specialized cells known as **juxtaglomerular cells** are located around the afferent arteriole where it enters the renal corpuscle (see Fig. 34-3). Between the afferent and efferent arterioles is a portion of the distal convoluted tubule with specialized cells known as **macula densa** (see Fig. 34-6). Together the juxtaglomerular cells and macula densa cells form the **juxtaglomerular apparatus (JGA)** (see Fig. 34-3). Control of renal blood flow, glomerular filtration, and renin secretion occurs at this site.

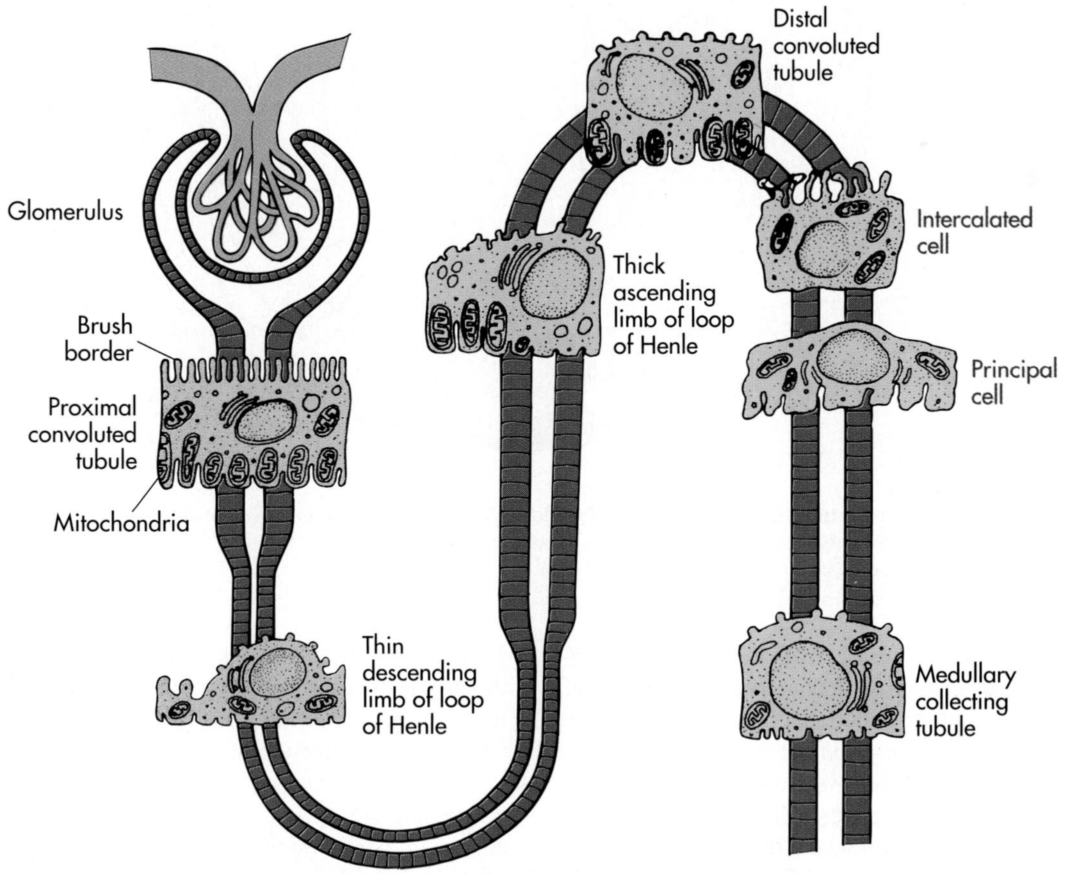

FIG. 34-4 Epithelial cells of the various segments of nephron tubules. The brush border and high number of mitochondria in the cells of the proximal convoluted tubule permit reabsorption of 60% of the glomerular filtrate. *Intercalated cells* (blue) secrete either H^+ (reabsorb HCO_3^-) or HCO_3^- and reabsorb K^+. *Principle cells* (blue) reabsorb Na^+ and water and secrete K^+. (Modified from Berne RM, Levy MN, editors: *Principles of physiology,* St Louis, 1993, Mosby.)

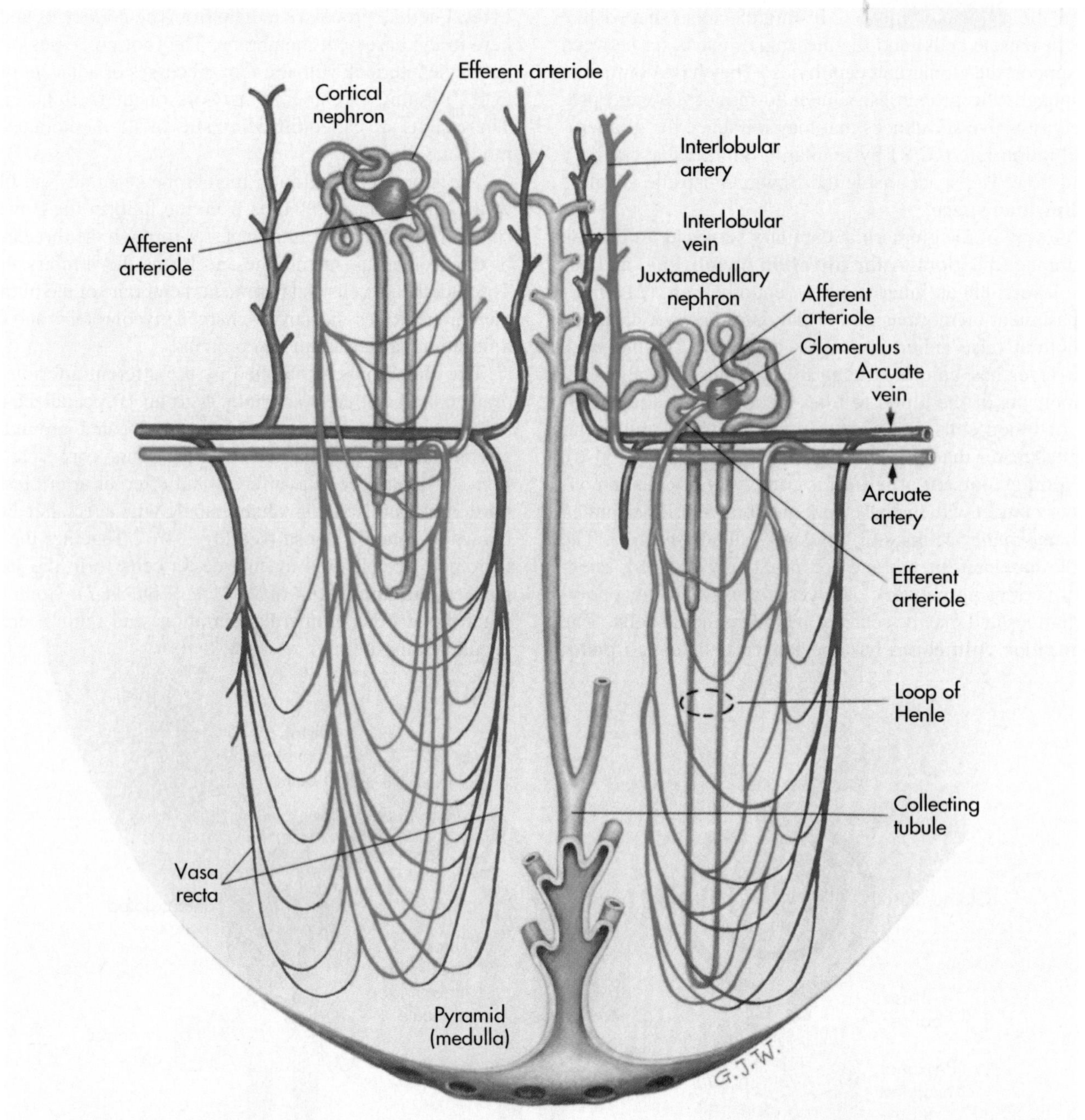

FIG. 34-5 The nephron unit with its blood vessels. Blood flows through nephron vessels as follows: interlobular artery, afferent arteriole, glomerulus, efferent arteriole, peritubular capillaries (around the tubules), venules, interlobular vein. (From Brundage DJ: *Renal disorders,* St Louis, 1992, Mosby.)

The **proximal tubule** continues from the Bowman space and has an initial convoluted segment (pars convoluta) and then a straight segment (pars recta) that descends toward the medulla (see Fig. 34-3). The proximal tubular lumen consists of one layer of cuboidal cells with a surface layer of microvilli that increases reabsorptive surface area. This is the only surface inside the nephron where the cells are covered with microvilli (a brush border) (see Fig. 34-4). The proximal tubule joins the **loop of Henle,** a hairpin loop composed of thick and thin portions of a descending segment that goes into the medulla. The tube then loops and becomes the thickening ascending segment that extends toward the cortex. The thin segment is composed of thin squamous cells with no active transport function. The cells of the thick segment are cuboidal and actively transport several solutes.

The more numerous cortical nephrons have glomeruli originating close to the surface of the cortex or in the midcortex, unlike the juxtamedullary nephrons, whose glomeruli are located deep in the cortex close to the medulla. The major structural difference between the glomeruli in the two types of nephrons is the length of the loop of Henle. In cortical nephrons the loop is short and may not extend into the

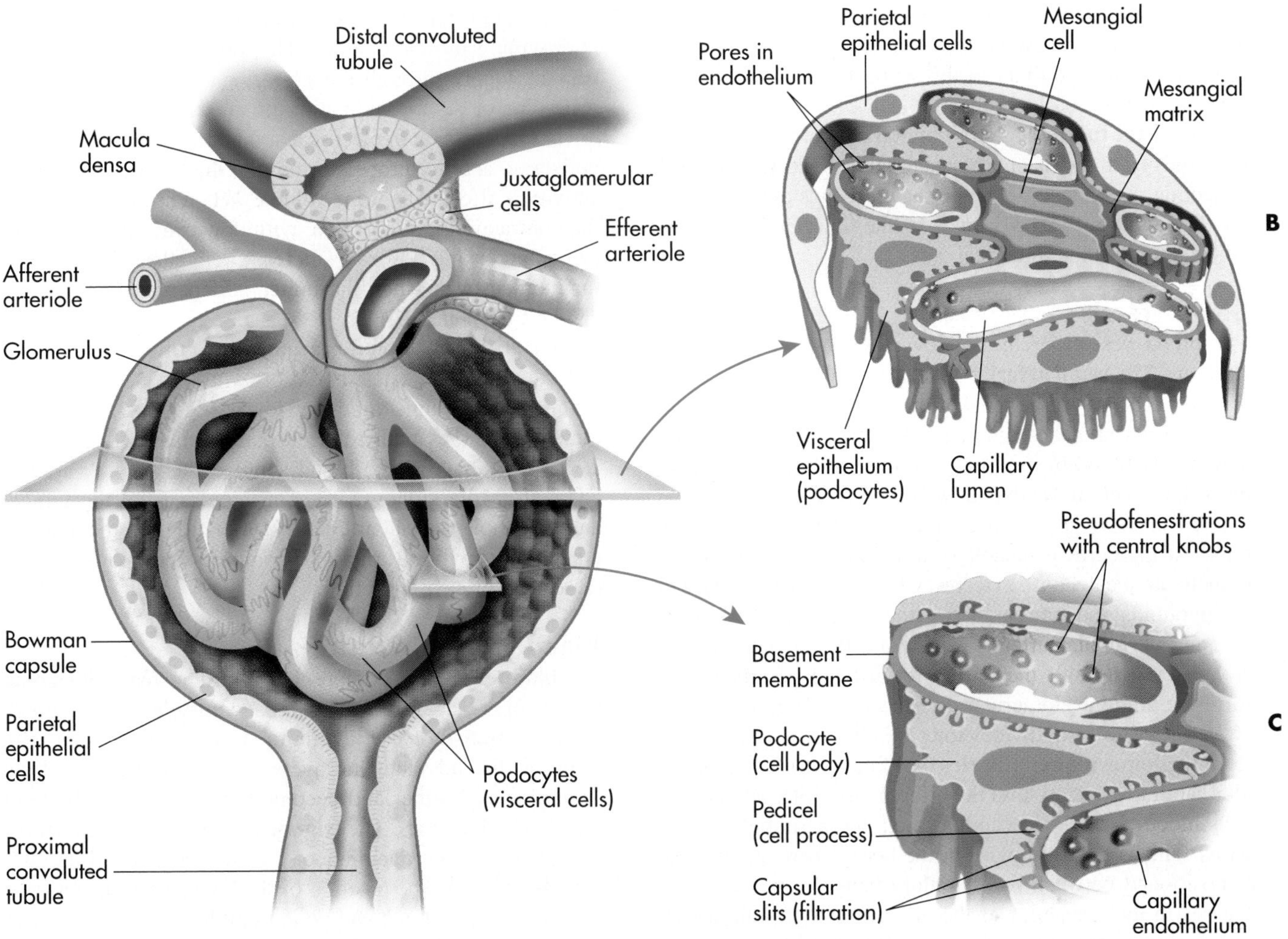

FIG. 34-6 Anatomy of the glomerulus and juxtaglomerular apparatus. **A,** Longitudinal cross section of glomerulus and juxtaglomerular apparatus. **B,** Enlargement of glomerular capillary filtration membrane. **C,** Horizontal cross section of glomerulus.

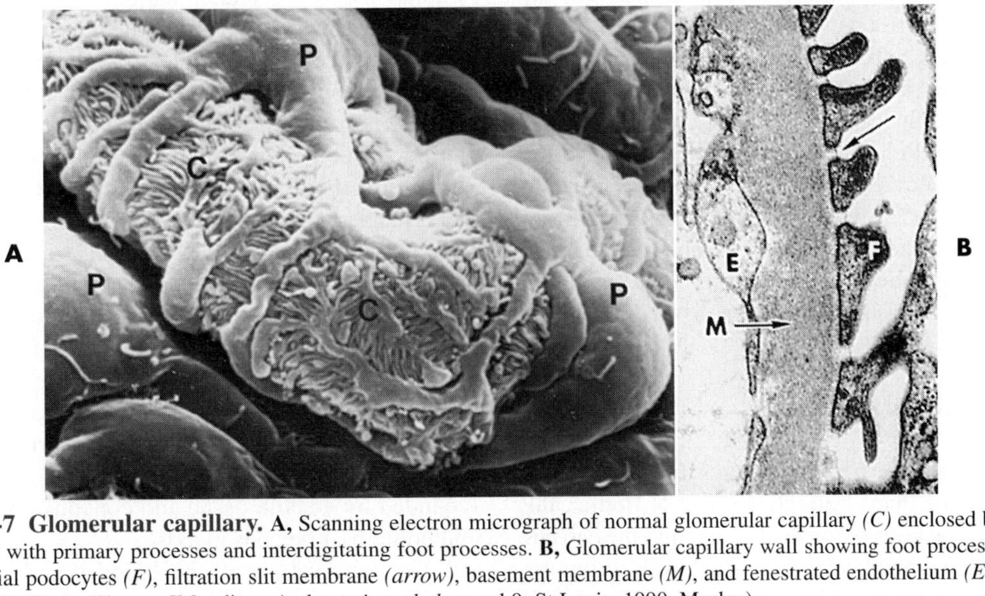

FIG. 34-7 Glomerular capillary. **A,** Scanning electron micrograph of normal glomerular capillary *(C)* enclosed by podocytes *(P)* with primary processes and interdigitating foot processes. **B,** Glomerular capillary wall showing foot processes of endothelial podocytes *(F)*, filtration slit membrane *(arrow)*, basement membrane *(M)*, and fenestrated endothelium *(E)*. (×40,000.) (From Kissane JM, editor: *Anderson's pathology,* ed 9, St Louis, 1990, Mosby.)

medulla. The loops of Henle for the juxtamedullary nephrons, however, may extend the whole length of the medulla (40 mm). Juxtamedullary nephrons represent about 12% of the total number of nephrons.

The **distal tubule** has straight and convoluted segments. It extends from the macula densa to the **collecting duct.** The collecting duct is a large tubule that descends down the cortex, through the renal pyramids of the inner and outer medullae, and into the minor calyx.

Blood Vessels

The blood vessels of the kidney closely parallel nephron structure. The **renal arteries** arise as the fifth branches of the abdominal aorta. At the renal hilum they divide into anterior and posterior branches and then subdivide into lobar arteries that supply blood to the lower, middle, and upper thirds of the kidney. The **interlobar arteries** are further subdivisions that travel down the renal columns and between the pyramids. At the cortical medullary junction, interlobar arteries branch into the **arcuate arteries,** which arch over the base of the pyramids and run parallel to the surface of the kidney.

The interlobular arteries arise from the arcuate arteries and extend through the cortex toward the periphery and form the afferent glomerular arterioles (see Fig. 34-5). The afferent arteriole subdivides into a fistlike structure of four to eight **glomerular capillaries** (see Fig. 34-6). The glomerular capillaries empty into the efferent arteriole, which conveys blood to a second capillary bed, the peritubular capillaries. This is the only place in the body where an arteriole is positioned between two capillary beds. Increases or decreases in the resistance of the afferent and efferent arterioles increase or decrease glomerular filtration.

The **peritubular capillaries** surround the convoluted portions of the proximal and distal tubules and the loop of Henle (see Fig. 34-5). The peritubular capillaries are adapted differently for the cortical and juxtamedullary nephrons. The peritubular capillaries surrounding the tubules of the cortical nephrons are similar to capillaries in other tissues. For the juxtamedullary nephrons a network of capillaries called the **vasa recta** forms loops and closely follows the loops of Henle. The capillaries of the vasa recta are the only blood supply to the medulla. They influence the osmolar concentration of the medullary extracellular fluid, which is important to the formation of a concentrated urine. All capillaries then drain into the venous system. The renal veins follow the arterial path in a reverse direction and have the same names as the arteries. The renal vein empties into the inferior vena cava. The lymphatic vessels tend also to follow the distribution of the blood vessels.

Urinary Structures

Ureters

The urine formed by the nephrons flows from the distal tubules and collecting ducts through the duct of Bellini, the **renal papillae** (projections of the ducts), and into the calyces and is collected in the renal pelvis (see Fig. 34-2). From the renal pelvis, urine is funneled into the **ureters.** Each adult ureter is approximately 30 cm long and is composed of long, intertwining muscle bundles. The lower ends of the ureters pass obliquely through the posterior aspect of the bladder wall. The close approximation of muscle cells permits the direct transmission of electrical stimulation, and the resulting peristaltic activity propels urine into the bladder. Peristaltic activity is affected by urine volume. When urine flow is slow, the contraction is segmented, with downward propulsion of urine. Increasing flow rates increase peristalsis. Peristalsis is maintained even when the ureter is denervated, so ureters can be transplanted.

Sensory innervation for the upper part of the ureter arises from the tenth thoracic nerve roots, with referred pain to the umbilicus. The innervation of lower segments arises from the sacral nerves with referred pain to the vulva or penis. The ureters have a rich blood supply. The primary arteries come from the kidney with contributions from the lumbar and superior vesical arteries. Contraction of the bladder during **micturition** (urination) compresses the lower end of the ureter, preventing reflux.

Bladder and Urethra

The **bladder** is a bag composed of a basket weave of smooth muscle fibers that forms the **detrusor muscle** and its smooth lining of transitional epithelium. As the bladder fills with urine, it distends and the layers of transitional epithelium slide past each other and become thinner as the volume of the bladder increases. The **trigone** is a smooth triangular area lying between the openings of the two ureters and the urethra (Fig. 34-8). The position of the bladder varies with age and gender. In infants and young children the bladder rises above the symphysis pubis, providing easy access for percutaneous aspiration. In adults it lies in the true pelvis, in front of the rectum and in front of the uterus in women. Inferiorly, the bladder sits on the prostate in men and on the anterior vagina in women. The bladder has a profuse blood supply, accounting for the bleeding that readily occurs with trauma, surgery, or inflammation.

The **urethra** extends from the inferior side of the bladder to the outside of the body. Two muscles called *sphincters* control excretion of urine from the bladder through the urethra. A ring of smooth muscle forms the **internal urethral sphincter** at the junction of the urethra and bladder. The **external urethral sphincter** is composed of striated muscles and is under voluntary control. The entire urethra is lined with mucus-secreting glands. The female urethra is short (3 to 4 cm). The male urethra is long (18 to 20 cm) and has three segments: prostatic, membranous, and cavernous. The prostatic urethra is closest to the bladder. It passes through the prostate gland and contains the openings of the ejaculatory ducts. The membranous urethra is the segment that passes through the floor of the pelvis. The cavernous segment forms the remainder of the tube. The cavernous segment is surrounded by erectile tissue and contains the openings of the bulbourethral mucous glands.

The innervation of the bladder and internal urethral sphincter is supplied by parasympathetic fibers of the au-

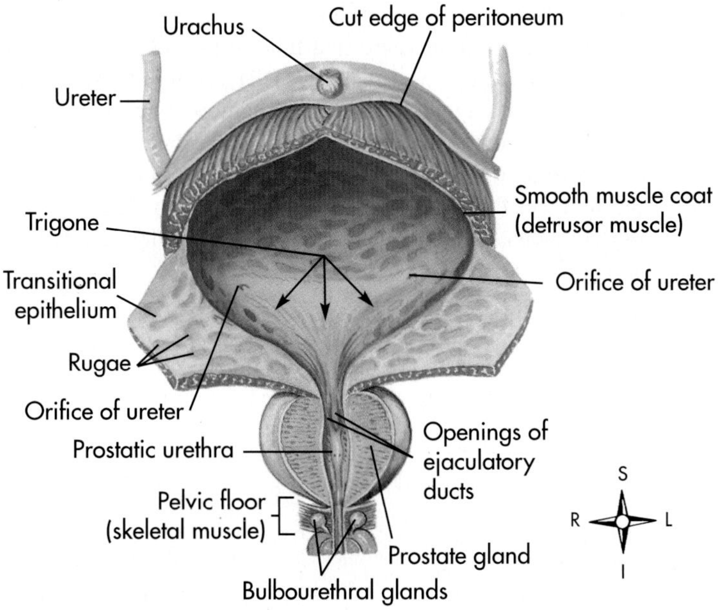

FIG. 34-8 Structure and location of the urinary bladder. Frontal view of a dissected urinary bladder (male) in a fully distended position. (From Thibodeau GA, Patton KI: *Anatomy and physiology,* ed 4, St Louis, 1999, Mosby.)

tonomic nervous system. They primarily pass with the arteries to and from the sacral levels of the spinal cord. Sensory fibers may extend as high as the T6 portion of the spinal cord. Motor fibers from the pudendal nerve supply the external urethral sphincter. The reflex arc required for micturition is stimulated by mechanoreceptors, which respond to stretching of tissue. The mechanoreceptors sense bladder fullness and send impulses to the sacral level of the cord with bladder filling. When the bladder accumulates 250 to 300 ml of urine, the bladder contracts and the internal urethral sphincter relaxes through activation of the spinal reflex arc (known as the *micturition reflex*). At this time a person feels the urge to void. In older children and adults, the reflex can be inhibited or facilitated by impulses coming from the brain, resulting in voluntary control of micturition.

RENAL BLOOD FLOW

The kidneys are highly vascular organs and usually receive 1000 to 1200 ml of blood per minute, or about 20% to 25% of the cardiac output. With a normal hematocrit of 45%, about 600 to 700 ml of blood flowing through the kidney per minute is plasma. From the renal plasma flow (RPF), 20% (approximately 120 to 140 ml/min) is filtered at the glomerulus and passes into the Bowman capsule. The filtration of the plasma per unit of time is known as the **glomerular filtration rate (GFR),** and the GFR is directly related to the perfusion pressure in the glomerular capillaries.

The remaining 80% (about 480 ml) of plasma flows through the efferent arterioles to the peritubular capillaries. The ratio of glomerular filtrate to RPF per minute (120/600 = 0.20) is called the *filtration fraction.* Normally all but 1 to 2 ml of the glomerular filtrate is reabsorbed and returned to the circulation by the peritubular capillaries.

The GFR is directly related to renal blood flow (RBF), which is regulated by intrinsic autoregulatory mechanisms,

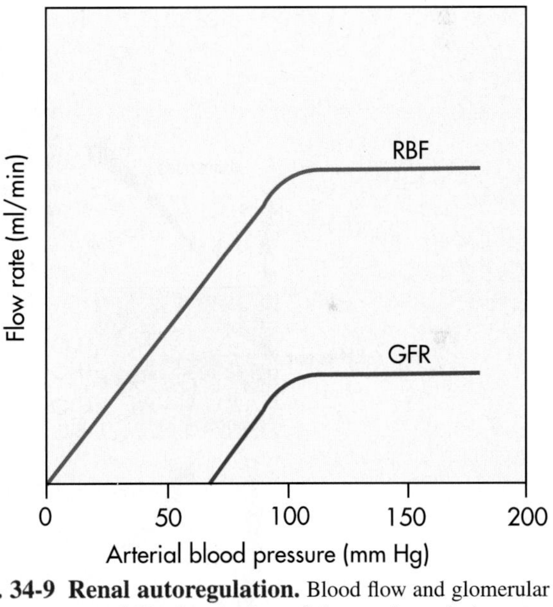

FIG. 34-9 Renal autoregulation. Blood flow and glomerular filtration rate are stabilized in the face of changes in perfusion pressure. (From Berne RM, Levy MN, editors: *Principles of physiology,* ed 3, St Louis, 2000, Mosby.)

neural regulation, and hormonal regulation. In general, blood flow to any organ is determined by the arteriovenous pressure differences across the vascular bed. If mean arterial pressure decreases or vascular resistance increases, RBF decreases.

Autoregulation

In the kidney a local mechanism tends to keep the rate of blood flow and therefore the GFR fairly constant over a range of arterial pressures between 80 and 180 mm Hg (Fig. 34-9). This means that changes in afferent arteriolar resistance and arteriolar pressure occur in the same direction. For example, as systemic blood pressure increases, the afferent arterioles constrict, preventing an increase in glomerular blood flow and filtration pressure. Opposite processes occur with a decrease in systemic blood pressure. Therefore RBF and GFR are relatively constant. This "constant" state is maintained by some intrinsic autoregulatory mechanism mediating the arteriolar resistance changes. The purpose of renal autoregulation is to prevent wide fluctuations in systemic arterial pressure from being transmitted to the glomerular capillaries. In this way, large fluctuations in GFR are prevented and solute and water excretion is constantly maintained when arterial pressure changes.

One mechanism responsible for the autoregulatory response in the kidney is probably a **myogenic mechanism.** As arterial pressure declines, the stretch on the afferent arteriolar wall decreases and the arteriole relaxes, with an increase in RBF; an increase in arteriolar pressure causes the arteriole to contract and decreases RBF. **Tubuloglomerular feedback** is a second mechanism for autoregulation of RBF and GFR. The macula densa of the distal tubule in the JGA senses changes in flow rate and sodium chloride content of the lumenal fluid. This information initiates a signal causing compensatory changes in afferent arteriolar resistance and GFR.[4]

Neural Regulation

The blood vessels of the kidney are innervated by the sympathetic noradrenergic fibers that cause arteriolar vasocon-

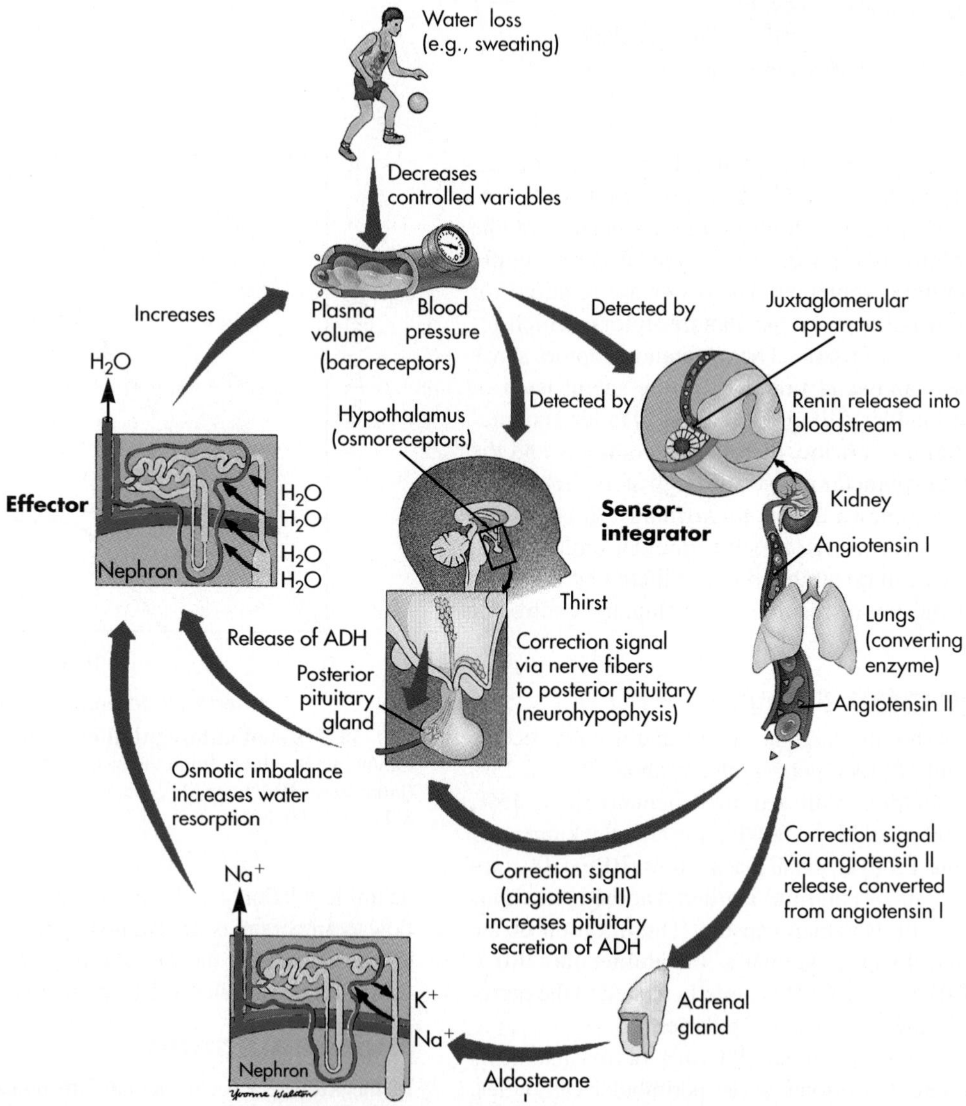

FIG. 34-10 Cooperative roles of antidiuretic hormone (ADH) and aldosterone in regulating urine and plasma volume. The drop in blood pressure that accompanies loss of fluid from the internal environment triggers the hypothalamus to rapidly release ADH from the posterior pituitary gland. ADH increases water reabsorption by the kidney by increasing water permeability of the distal tubules and collecting ducts. The drop in blood pressure is also detected by each nephron's juxtaglomerular apparatus, which responds by secreting renin. Renin triggers the formation of angiotensin II, which stimulates release of aldosterone from the adrenal cortex. Aldosterone then slowly boosts water reabsorption by the kidneys by increasing reabsorption of NaCl. Because angiotensin II also stimulates secretion of ADH, it serves as an additional link between the ADH and aldosterone mechanisms. (From Thibodeau GA, Patton KI: *Anatomy and physiology*, ed 4, St Louis, 1999, Mosby.)

striction. The innervation of the kidney comes primarily from the celiac ganglion and greater splanchnic nerve (see Fig. 13-25). The afferent and efferent arterioles are richly innervated, but nerves have not been observed in the glomerular capillaries.

The RBF is reflexly related to the systemic arterial pressure. When systemic arterial pressure decreases, increased renal sympathetic nerve activity is mediated reflexively through the carotid sinus and the baroreceptors of the aortic arch. This stimulates renal arteriolar vasoconstriction and decreases both RBF and GFR. Thus RBF still changes when systemic arterial pressure is significantly reduced, although autoregulatory processes dampen the response. The decreased RBF decreases the GFR and diminishes excretion of sodium and water, promoting an increase in blood volume and thus an increase in systemic pressure. The afferent and efferent arterioles are innervated by sympathetic nerves. The nerves are stimulated by decreased blood volume and cause vasoconstriction and decreased glomerular filtration.

Exercise, body position, and hypoxia also influence RBF. Exercise and change of body position activate renal sympathetic neurons and cause mild vasoconstriction. Severe hypoxia stimulates the chemoreceptors of the carotid and aortic bodies and decreases RBF by means of sympathetic stimulation. Hemorrhage induces intense sympathetic stimulation and vasoconstriction, and both GFR and blood flow are reduced.

Hormones and Other Factors

Hormonal factors and many mediators can alter the resistance of the renal vasculature by stimulating vasodilation or vasoconstriction. A major hormonal regulator of RBF is the **renin-angiotensin system,** which can increase systemic arterial pressure and change RBF. Renin is an enzyme formed and stored in the cells of the arterioles of the JGA (see Fig. 34-3). Several complex physiologic mechanisms stimulate the release of renin. These mechanisms are principally decreased blood pressure in the afferent arterioles, which reduces stretch of the juxtaglomerular cells; decreased sodium chloride concentration in the distal convoluted tubule; and sympathetic nerve stimulation of β-adrenergic receptors on the juxtaglomerular cells.[5]

When renin is released, it cleaves an α-globulin (angiotensinogen) in the plasma to form angiotensin I, which is physiologically inactive. In the presence of a converting enzyme, angiotensin I is converted to angiotensin II and angiotensin III. Angiotensin II stimulates secretion of aldosterone by the adrenal cortex (see Chapter 19), is also a potent vasopressor, and inhibits renin release. Angiotensin III has less of an effect than angiotensin II. Numerous physiologic effects of the renin-angiotensin system serve the purpose of stabilizing systemic blood pressure and preserving the extracellular fluid volume during hypotension or hypovolemia, including sodium reabsorption, systemic vasoconstriction, sympathetic nerve stimulation, thirst stimulation, and drinking. (The combined effects of the renin-angiotensin system and antidiuretic hormone [ADH] are summarized in Fig. 34-10.) Angiotensin II is also produced within the kidney.

Natriuretic peptides are a group of peptide hormones with **atrial natriuretic peptide (ANP)** secreted from cells in the right atrium.[6] When right atrial pressure rises, ANP inhibits secretion of renin, inhibits angiotensin-induced secretion of aldosterone, relaxes vascular smooth muscle, and inhibits sodium and water absorption by kidney tubules. The result is decreased blood volume and blood pressure.[7] Other hormones and mediators that influence renal blood flow are summarized in Table 34-1.

Table 34-1 Hormones, Mediators, and Renal Blood Flow

Hormone or Mediator	Effect on Renal Blood Flow
Adenosine	Produced within kidney; causes vasoconstriction of afferent arteriole; decreases RBF and GFR
Angiotensin II	Produced systemically and within kidneys; constricts afferent and efferent arterioles; decreases RBF and GFR
Atrial natriuretic peptide	Produced by atria of the heart with hypertension and increased blood volume; causes vasodilation of afferent arteriole and vasoconstriction of efferent arteriole; modest increase in GFR with little change in RBF
Bradykinin	Produced in kidney from kininogen and causes vasodilation by release of nitric oxide and prostaglandins; increases RBF and GFR
Dopamine	Produced by the proximal tubule; increases RBF; inhibits renin secretion
Endothelin	Produced by renal vessel endothelial cells, mesangial cells, and distal tubule cells in response to bradykinin, angiotensin II, epinephrine, and stretch; most active with renal disease; profound vasoconstriction of afferent and efferent arterioles; decreases RBF and GFR
Histamine	Produced locally within the kidney; modulates RBF in basal state and during inflammation; increases RBF by decreasing afferent and efferent arteriolar resistance and does not decrease GFR
Nitric oxide	Produced by renal vessel endothelial cells with increased stretch and by stimulation of acetylcholine, histamine, bradykinin, ATP; increases vasodilation of afferent and efferent arterioles
Prostaglandins PGI_2, PGE_2	Produced locally within kidney with decreased RBF; dampen vasoconstriction caused by sympathetic nerves and angiotensin II; prevent harmful vasoconstriction and renal ischemia
Urodilatin	Produced by distal tubule and collecting duct when there is increased circulating volume and increased blood pressure; inhibits sodium and water reabsorption from medullary part of collecting duct producing diuresis

RBF, Renal blood flow; *GFR,* glomerular filtration rate.

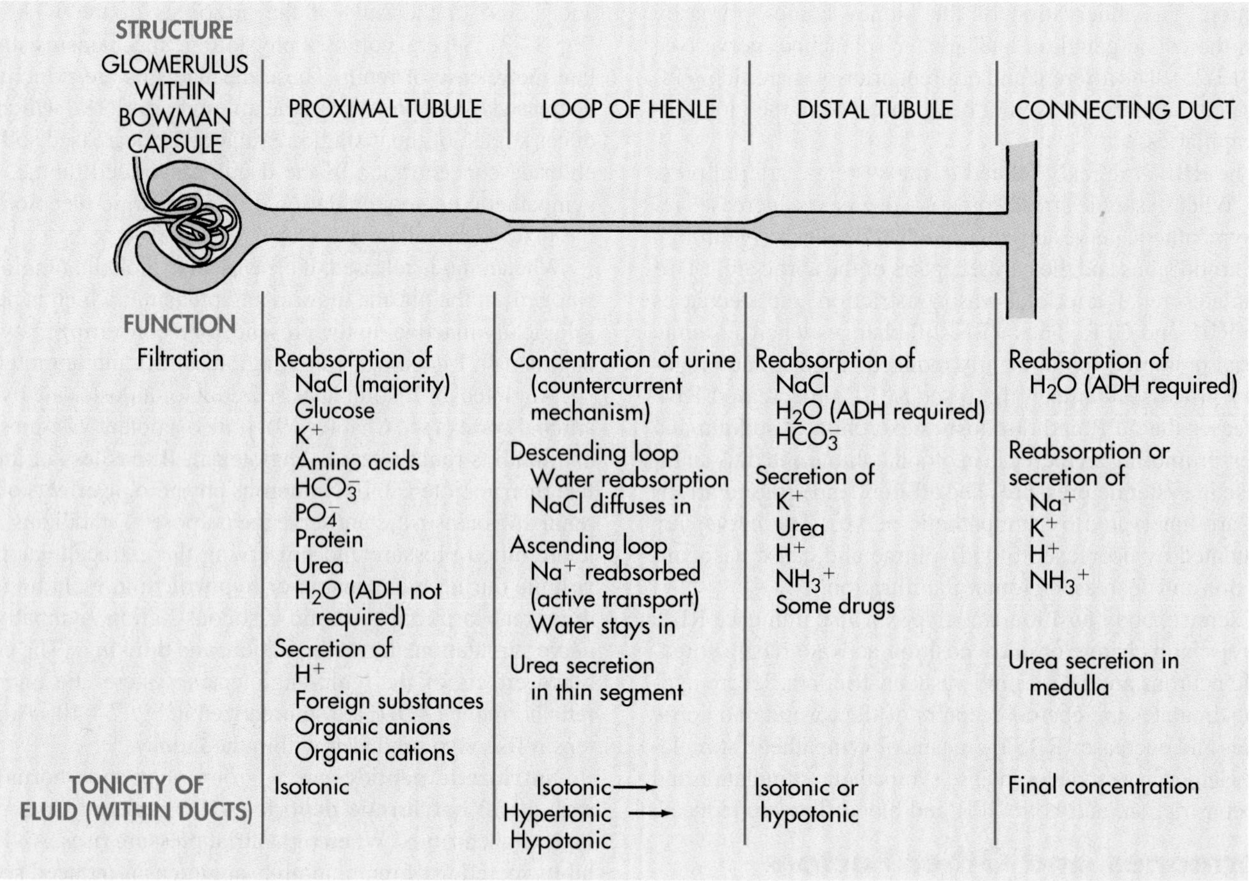
STRUCTURE
GLOMERULUS WITHIN BOWMAN CAPSULE
PROXIMAL TUBULE
LOOP OF HENLE
DISTAL TUBULE
CONNECTING DUCT
FUNCTION
Filtration
Reabsorption of
NaCl (majority)
Glucose
K^+
Amino acids
HCO_3^-
PO_4^-
Protein
Urea
H_2O (ADH not required)
Secretion of
H^+
Foreign substances
Organic anions
Organic cations
Concentration of urine (countercurrent mechanism)
Descending loop
Water reabsorption
NaCl diffuses in
Ascending loop
Na^+ reabsorbed (active transport)
Water stays in
Urea secretion in thin segment
Reabsorption of
NaCl
H_2O (ADH required)
HCO_3^-
Secretion of
K^+
Urea
H^+
NH_3^+
Some drugs
Reabsorption of
H_2O (ADH required)
Reabsorption or secretion of
Na^+
K^+
H^+
NH_3^+
Urea secretion in medulla
TONICITY OF FLUID (WITHIN DUCTS)
Isotonic
Isotonic→
Hypertonic →
Hypotonic
Isotonic or hypotonic
Final concentration

FIG. 34-11 Major functions of nephron segments. *ADH,* Antidiuretic hormone. (Modified from Wong DL : *Whaley and Wong's nursing care of infants and children,* ed 6, St Louis, 1999, Mosby.)

KIDNEY FUNCTION

Nephron Function

The nephron can perform many functions simultaneously. It filters the plasma at the glomerulus and reabsorbs and secretes different substances at various parts of its tubular structure (Fig. 34-11). The function of the nephron is to form a filtrate of protein-free plasma. This process, known as **ultrafiltration,** occurs across the glomerular capillaries. The nephron then regulates the filtrate to maintain body fluid volume, electrolyte composition, and pH within narrow limits.

Regulation of the filtrate occurs through two processes: tubular reabsorption and tubular secretion. **Tubular reabsorption** is the movement of fluids and solutes from the tubular lumen to the peritubular capillary plasma. Transfer of substances from the plasma of the peritubular capillary to the tubular lumen is **tubular secretion.** The transport mechanisms are both active and passive (processes defined in Chapter 1). The elimination of a substance in the final urine is known as **excretion** (Fig. 34-12).

Glomerular Filtration

The fluid filtered by the glomerular capillary filtration membrane is protein free but contains electrolytes such as sodium, chloride, and potassium and organic molecules such as creatinine, urea, and glucose in the same concentrations as in plasma. Like other capillary membranes, the glomerulus is freely permeable to water and relatively impermeable to large colloids such as plasma proteins. The size of the molecules and their electrical charge are important factors affecting the permeability of substances crossing the glomerulus. The small size of the filtration slits or pores in the membrane restricts the passage of proteins and other macromolecules. The negative charge along the filtration membrane further impedes the passage of negatively charged macromolecules (because like forces repel each other). Positively charged macromolecules therefore permeate the membrane more readily than neutrally charged particles.

Capillary pressure, as well as electrical charge, has an effect on glomerular filtration. The hydrostatic pressure within the capillary is the major force for inducing water and solutes across the filtration membrane and into the Bowman capsule. This pressure is determined indirectly by the efficiency of cardiac contraction and directly by the systemic arterial pressure and the resistances to blood flow in the afferent and efferent arterioles. Two forces oppose the filtration effects of the glomerular capillary hydrostatic pressure (P_{GC}): (1) the hydrostatic pressure in the Bowman space (P_{BC}) and (2) the effective oncotic pressure of the glomerular capillary blood

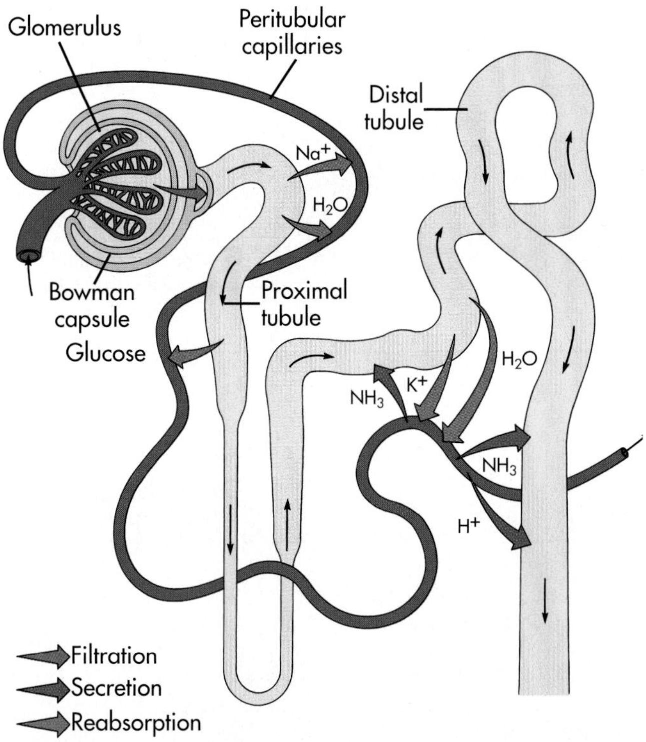

FIG. 34-12 Glomerular filtration, tubular reabsorption, and tubular secretion. The three processes by which the kidneys excrete urine. From proximal convoluted tubules, sodium and glucose are reabsorbed into peritubular capillaries by active transport. Water reabsorption by osmosis follows. From distal convoluted tubules, sodium is reabsorbed by active transport. Osmotic reabsorption of water from them occurs when ADH is present. Secretion of ammonia and hydrogen occurs from peritubular capillaries into distal tubules by active transport. (From Thibodeau GA, Patton KI: *Anatomy and physiology,* ed 4, St Louis, 1999, Mosby.)

(π_{GC}). (As explained in Chapter 3, hydrostatic pressure is a pushing force in relation to water and oncotic pressure is a pulling force.) Because the fluid in the Bowman space normally contains only minute amounts of protein, it normally does not have an oncotic influence on the plasma of the glomerular capillary (Fig. 34-13).

The combined effect of forces favoring and forces opposing filtration determines the filtration pressure. The **net filtration pressure (NFP)** is the sum of forces favoring and opposing filtration and is expressed by the following equation:

$$\text{NFP} = (P_{GC} + \pi_{BC}) \text{ (forces favoring filtration)} - (P_{BC} + \pi_{GC}) \text{ (forces opposing filtration)}$$

The estimated values contributing to the forces of net filtration are presented in Table 34-2.

As the protein-free fluid is filtered into the Bowman capsule, the plasma oncotic pressure increases and the hydrostatic pressure decreases. The increase in glomerular capillary oncotic pressure is great enough to reduce the net filtration pressure to zero at the efferent end of the capillary and to stop the filtration process effectively. The low hydrostatic pressure and increased oncotic pressure in the efferent arteriole then are transferred to the peritubular capillaries and facilitate reabsorption of fluid from the proximal tubules.

Filtration Rate

The total volume of fluid filtered by the glomeruli averages 180 L/day, or approximately 120 ml/min, a phenomenal amount considering the size of the kidneys. Because only 1 to 2 L of urine is excreted per day, 99% of the filtrate is reabsorbed into the peritubular capillaries and returned to the blood. The factors determining the GFR are directly related to the pressures that favor or oppose filtration. Any changes in afferent or efferent arteriolar resistance will alter glomerular capillary hydrostatic pressure and GFR. Vasoconstriction of one or the other of these two arterioles produces opposite effects on glomerular pressure. For example, if the afferent arteriole constricts, blood flow decreases, with a corresponding drop in glomerular pressure. The GFR then decreases, and body fluids are conserved. Conversely, constriction of the efferent arteriole increases the net filtration pressure and the GFR increases. When both afferent and efferent arterioles constrict, little change occurs in filtration pressure, but RBF is reduced and so is the GFR.

Obstruction to the outflow of urine (caused by strictures, stones, or tumors along the urinary tract) can cause a retrograde increase in pressure at the Bowman capsule and a decrease in GFR. Excessive loss of protein-free fluid from vomiting, diarrhea, use of diuretics, or excessive sweating can increase glomerular capillary oncotic pressure and decrease the GFR. Renal disease can also cause changes in pressure relationships by altering capillary permeability and the surface area available for filtration (see Chapter 35).

Tubular Transport

By the end of the proximal tubule, approximately 60% to 70% of filtered sodium and water and about 50% of urea have been reabsorbed, along with 90% or more of potassium, glucose, bicarbonate, calcium, phosphate, amino acids, and uric acid. All this occurs by active transport. Chloride, water, and urea are reabsorbed passively but are linked to the active transport of sodium (cotransport). Active transport in the renal tubules can be limited as the carrier molecules become saturated, a phenomenon known as **transport maximum (T_m).** Transport maximums exist for most substances actively transported by the tubular epithelium. The reabsorption of glucose is a significant example. Glucose is coupled to sodium transport and is almost completely reabsorbed in the proximal tubule. Like other actively transported substances, glucose has a maximal transport capacity, or renal threshold. This means that when the carrier molecules for glucose become saturated, the excess will be excreted in the urine. Normally, the plasma level and filtered glucose load are not high enough to saturate the carrier mechanism. When the plasma glucose reaches 180 mg/dl, however, as occurs in the individual with uncontrolled diabetes mellitus, the threshold for glucose is achieved. Any further increase in the plasma level causes loss of glucose in the urine.

Proximal tubule. Active reabsorption of sodium is the primary function of the proximal tubule. Water, most electrolytes, and organic substances are cotransported with sodium.

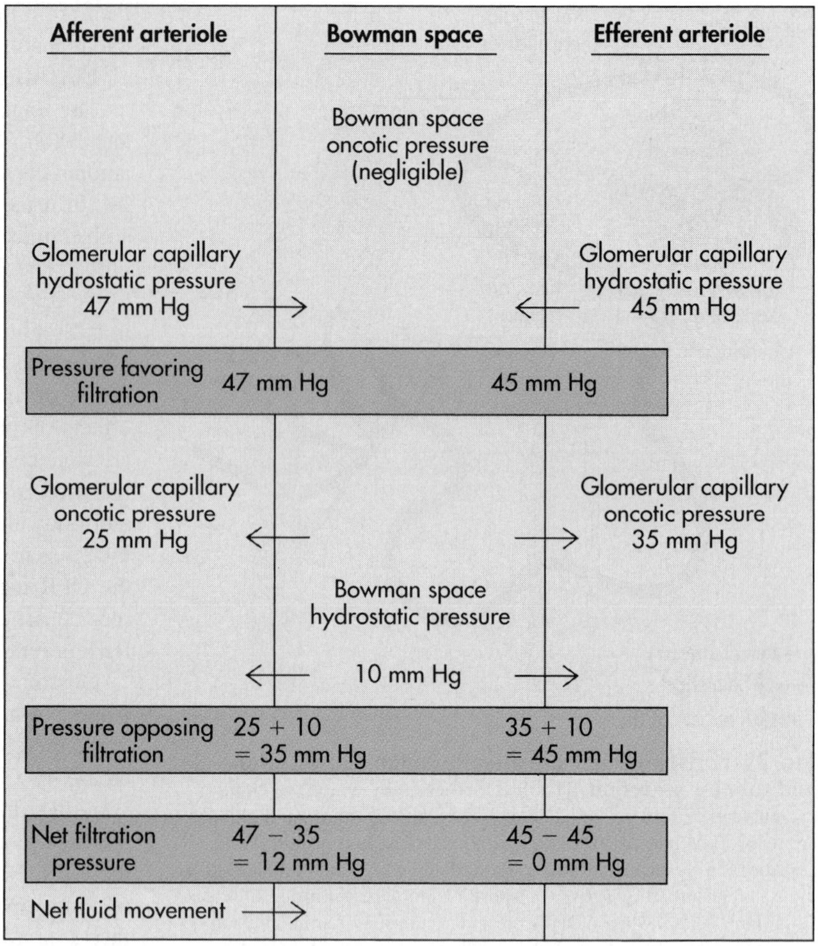

FIG. 34-13 Glomerular filtration pressures.

Table 34-2 Glomerular Filtration Pressures

Forces	Pressures	Beginning of Capillary (Pressures, mm Hg)	End of Capillary (Pressures, mm Hg)
PROMOTING FILTRATION			
Glomerular capillary hydrostatic pressure	P_{GC}	47	45
Bowman capsule oncotic pressure	π_{BC}	Negligible effect	
OPPOSING FILTRATION			
Bowman capsule hydrostatic pressure	P_{BC}	10	10
Glomerular capillary oncotic pressure	π_{GC}	25	35
NET FILTRATION PRESSURE		12	0

The osmotic force generated by active sodium transport promotes the passive diffusion of water out of the tubular lumen and into the peritubular capillaries. Passive transport of water is further enhanced by the elevated oncotic pressure of the blood in the peritubular capillaries. The reabsorption of water leaves an increased concentration of urea within the tubular lumen, creating a gradient for its passive diffusion to the peritubular plasma.

As the positively charged sodium ions leave the tubular lumen, negatively charged chloride ions passively follow to maintain electroneutrality. Because the luminal membrane (the inside of the tubule) of the proximal tubular cell has a limited permeability to chloride, however, chloride reabsorption lags behind sodium.

Hydrogen ions are actively exchanged for sodium ions. The hydrogen ions (H^+) then combine with bicarbonate (HCO_3^-). Bicarbonate is completely filtered at the glomerulus, and approximately 90% is reabsorbed in the proximal tubule. This process also occurs to a lesser extent in the ascending loop of Henle and the distal tubule.

In the tubular lumen, hydrogen and bicarbonate ions form carbonic acid (H_2CO_3). The carbonic acid rapidly breaks down, or dissociates, to carbon dioxide (CO_2) and water (H_2O) in the presence of the enzyme carbonic anhydrase, which is in the luminal membrane. The CO_2 and H_2O then diffuse into

Table 34-3 Substances Transported by Renal Tubules

Reabsorption	Secretion
Albumin	Choline
Ascorbate	Creatinine
Fructose	Histamine
Galactose	Methyl guanidine
Glucose	Para-aminohippurate
Glutamate	Penicillin
Phosphate	Steroid glucuronides
Sulfate	Thiamine
Xylose	

the tubular cell, where carbonic anhydrase again catalyzes the CO_2 and H_2O to form HCO_3^- and H^+. The H_2CO_3 thus produces H^+ and HCO_3^-. The H^+ is secreted again, and HCO_3^- combines with sodium and is transported to the peritubular capillary blood.

Thus, because bicarbonate is not highly permeable at the peritubular capillary membrane, it is reabsorbed as CO_2 and H_2O, which are readily diffusible. One of the unusual aspects of this process is that the bicarbonate molecule filtered at the glomerulus is not the same molecule that is reabsorbed (because it dissociates) and the hydrogen ion secreted by the proximal tubule is not excreted in the urine. Bicarbonate is thus conserved, and the hydrogen is reabsorbed as water. Therefore these ions normally do not contribute to the urinary excretion of acid or the addition of acid to the blood (Fig. 34-14).

In addition to the proximal tubular secretion of hydrogen ions, secretory transport mechanisms exist for creatinine, other organic bases, and endogenous and exogenous organic acids, including para-aminohippurate and penicillin (Table 34-3). These secretory mechanisms are important for eliminating drugs and other exogenous chemical products from the body. Frequently, exogenous substances are conjugated with sulfate and glucuronic acid by the liver and then actively secreted by the renal tubules. This has important clinical implications because many drugs and their metabolites are eliminated from the body in this way. When the renal tubules are damaged, metabolic by-products and drugs may accumulate, causing toxic levels in the body.

Loop of Henle and distal tubule. The filtrate entering and leaving the proximal tubule is essentially isoosmotic with the plasma and has a concentration of about 285 mOsm. Although approximately 65% of salt and water is reabsorbed along the proximal tubule, they are reabsorbed in equal amounts, causing only minor changes in the osmotic and electrolyte concentrations of the fluid flowing into the loop of Henle. Therefore any concentration or dilution of urine occurs at more distal sites of the nephron, principally in the loop of Henle and collecting ducts. Near the top of the renal pyramids, the interstitial osmolality reaches 1200 mOsm/L.

These quantitative changes taking place in the loop of Henle are related to the length of the loop and its depth of penetration into the medulla. The structural features of the medullary hairpin loops provide the kidney with the ability

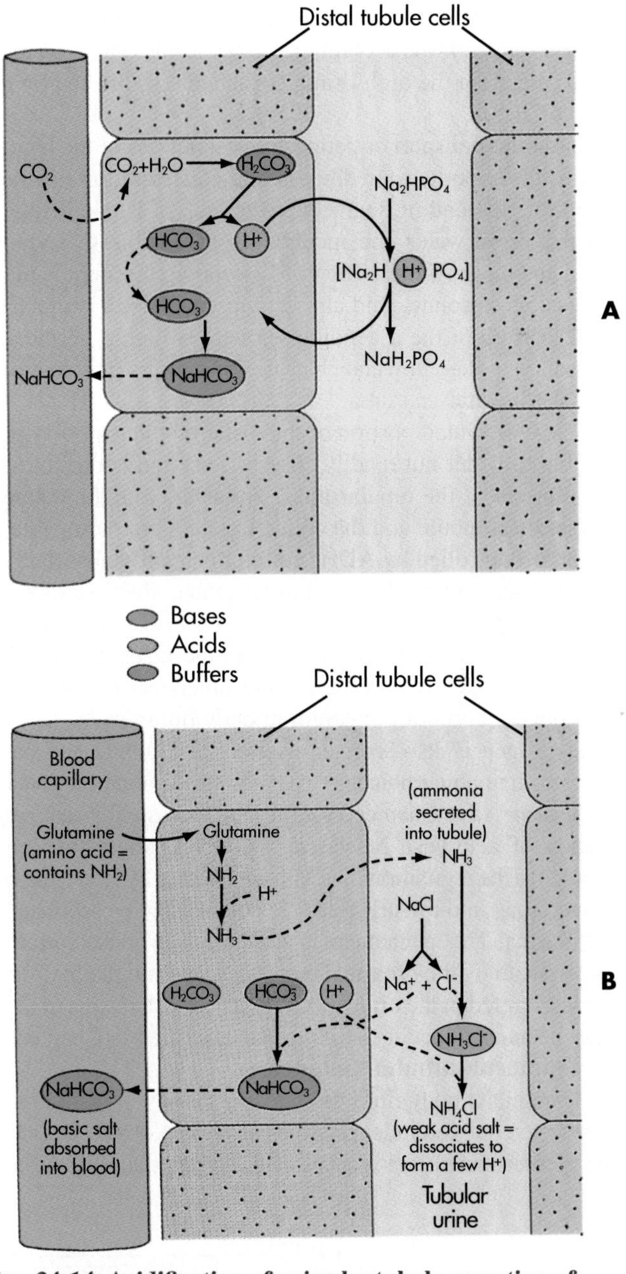

FIG. 34-14 Acidification of urine by tubule excretion of ammonia (NH_3). A, Acidification of urine and conservation of base by distal renal tubule excretion of H^+. **B,** An amino acid (glutamine) moves into tubule cell and loses an amino group (NH_2) to form ammonia, which is secreted into the urine. In exchange, the tubule cell absorbs a basic salt (mainly $NaHCO_3$) into blood from urine. (From Thibodeau GA, Patton KI: *Anatomy and physiology,* ed 3, St Louis, 1996, Mosby.)

to concentrate urine and conserve water for the body. The transition of the filtrate into urine is a function of the concentrating ability of the loops and final adjustments in urine composition made by the distal tubule and collecting duct.

The primary function of the loop of Henle is to establish a hyperosmotic state within the medullary interstitial fluid. This is achieved by reabsorbing more solute than water into the interstitium. The fluid leaving the ascending limb of the loop is therefore hypoosmotic, or more dilute than the fluid that entered. This dilution allows the distal tubule and collecting duct to make final adjustments in the concentration or dilution of the excreted urine according to body needs. The vasa recta act to maintain the high osmotic gradient established by the loop of Henle.

Different transport or permeability functions of the loop of Henle are important for dilution and concentration of urine. The thin, descending segment of the loop of Henle is highly permeable to water and moderately permeable to sodium, urea, and other solutes. The thin, ascending segment is more permeable to solutes and almost impermeable to water. The thick portion of the ascending segment is highly permeable to sodium, potassium, and chloride and significantly less permeable to water and urea.

The convoluted portion of the distal tubule is poorly permeable to water but readily absorbs ions and contributes to the dilution of the tubular fluid. The later, straight segment of the distal tubule and the collecting duct are permeable to water as controlled by ADH. Sodium is readily absorbed by the later segment of the distal tubule and collecting duct under the regulation of the hormone aldosterone (see Chapter 19). Potassium is actively secreted in these segments and is also controlled by aldosterone and other factors related to the concentration of potassium in body fluids.[8]

Hydrogen is also secreted by the distal tubule and combines with nonbicarbonate buffers for the elimination of acids in the urine. (See Chapter 3 for further discussion of renal regulation of acid-base balance.) The distal tubule thus contributes to the regulation of acid-base balance by excreting hydrogen ions into the urine and by adding new bicarbonate to the plasma. The mechanism is similar to the conservation of bicarbonate by the proximal tubule, except that the hydrogen ion is excreted in the urine. (The specific mechanisms of acid-base balance and acid excretion are described in Chapter 3.)

Glomerulotubular Balance

To regulate body fluid balance, the kidney must not reabsorb or excrete too much sodium or water. Normally, 99% of the glomerular filtrate is reabsorbed. When the GFR spontaneously decreases or increases, the renal tubules, primarily the proximal tubules, automatically adjust their rate of reabsorption of sodium and water to balance the change in GFR. This prevents wide fluctuations in sodium and water excretion into the urine and maintains sodium and water balance.[9]

Concentration and Dilution of Urine

The production of a concentrated urine involves a **countercurrent exchange system,** in which fluid flows in opposite directions through parallel tubes. A concentration gradient causes fluid to be exchanged across the parallel pathways. In the nephron the fluid moves up and down the parallel sides of the hairpin loop of Henle in the medulla. The longer the loop, the greater the concentration gradient because the concentration gradient increases from the cortex to the tip of the medulla. The loops of Henle serve as multipliers of the concentration gradient, and the vasa recta act as a countercurrent exchanger for maintaining the gradient.[10]

Water, Sodium, and Chloride

The process is initiated in the thick ascending limb of the loop of Henle with the active transport of chloride and sodium out of the tubular lumen and into the medullary interstitium (Fig. 34-15). Because the lumen of the ascending limb is impermeable to water, water cannot follow the sodium/chloride transport. This lack of luminal permeability causes the ascending tubular fluid to become hypoosmotic and the medullary interstitium to become hyperosmotic. The descending limb of the loop, which receives fluid from the proximal tubule, is highly permeable to water, but it is the only place in the nephron that does not actively transport either sodium or chloride. Sodium and chloride may, however, diffuse into the descending tubule from the interstitium. The hyperosmotic interstitium causes water to move out of the descending limb, and the remaining fluid in the descending tubule becomes increasingly concentrated as it flows toward the tip of the medulla. As the tubular fluid rounds the loop and enters

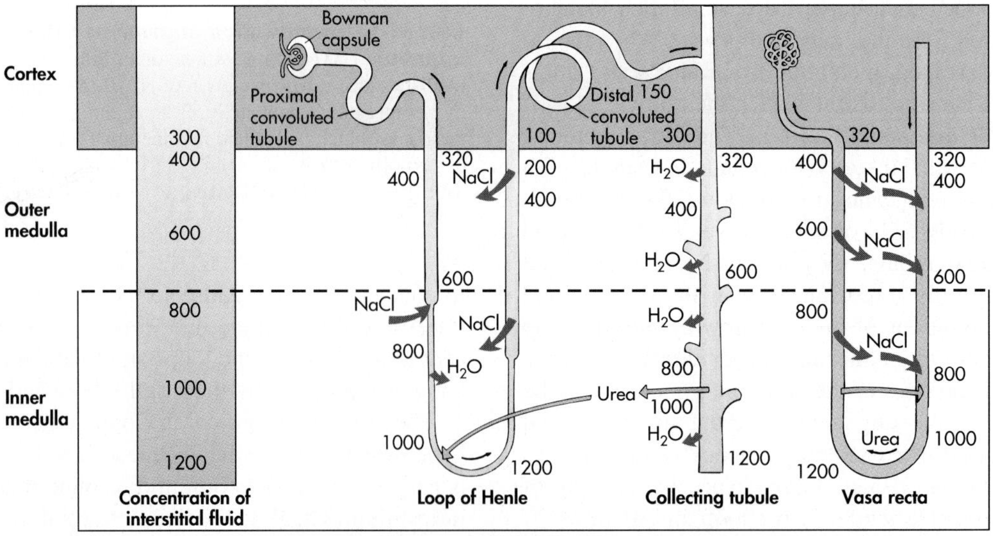

FIG. 34-15 Countercurrent mechanism for concentrating and diluting urine. (NOTE: numbers on illustration represent milliosmoles [mOsm].)

the ascending limb, sodium and chloride are removed and water is retained. The fluid then becomes more and more dilute as it encounters the distal tubule.

The slow rate of blood flow and the hairpin structure of the vasa recta allow blood to flow through the medullary tissue without disturbing the osmotic gradient. As blood flows into the descending limb of the vasa recta, it encounters the increasing osmotic concentration gradient of the medullary interstitium. Water moves out, and sodium and chloride diffuse into the descending vasa recta. The plasma becomes increasingly concentrated as it flows toward the tip of the medulla.

As the blood flow passes into the ascending limb and back toward the cortex, the surrounding interstitial fluid becomes comparatively more dilute. Water then moves back into the vasa recta, and sodium and chloride diffuse out. The net result is a preservation of the medullary osmotic gradient. If blood were to flow rapidly through the vasa recta, as occurs in some renal diseases, the medullary concentration gradient would be washed away and the ability to concentrate urine and conserve water would be lost. The efficiency of water conservation is related to the length of the loops: the longer the loops, the greater the ability to concentrate the urine. Many desert animals have very long loops and can reabsorb water so efficiently that they rarely need to drink.

Urea

Urea is an end product of protein metabolism and is the major constituent of urine along with water. The glomerulus freely filters urea, and tubular reabsorption of urea depends on urine flow rate with less reabsorption at higher flow rates. Approximately 50% of urea is excreted in the urine, and 50% is recycled within the kidney. The recycling of urea from the tubules and collecting ducts contributes to the osmotic gradient within the medulla and is necessary for the concentration and dilution of urine. Because urea is an end product of protein metabolism, individuals with protein deprivation cannot maximally concentrate their urine.

Catecholamines

With hemorrhage or extracellular fluid depletion, there is activation of sympathetic nerves to release norepinephrine and the adrenal medulla to release epinephrine. Sodium and water are reabsorbed by the proximal tubule, the thick ascending limb of the loop of Henle, the distal tubule, and the collecting duct.[9]

Antidiuretic Hormone

The distal tubule in the cortex receives the hypoosmotic urine from the ascending limb of the loop of Henle. The concentration of the final urine is controlled by ADH, which is secreted from the posterior pituitary, or neurohypophysis. ADH increases water permeability in the last segment of the distal tubule and along the entire length of the collecting ducts, which pass through the inner and outer zones of the medulla.

In the presence of ADH, water reabsorption is high. Most of the water is reabsorbed in the medullary collecting ducts because of the high osmotic gradient in the medullary interstitium. The water diffuses into the ascending limb of the vasa recta and returns to the systemic circulation. The excreted urine can have a high osmotic concentration, up to 1400 mOsm. The volume is normally reduced to about 1% of what was filtered at the glomerulus.

ADH secretion is therefore one cause of **oliguria,** or diminished excretion of urine, that is, less than 400 ml/day or 30 ml/hr. Fluid imbalance may be related to the syndrome of inappropriate secretion of ADH, which is a cause of water excess (see Chapter 3). Inadequate secretion of ADH results in diabetes insipidus, the excretion of a large volume of dilute urine.

In the absence of ADH, **water diuresis,** an increase in excretion of a highly dilute urine, takes place. The distal tubules and collecting ducts become impermeable to water. Water remains in the tubular lumen and is excreted as a dilute and large volume of urine. Because ADH has no effect on sodium reabsorption, it continues to be actively transported from the distal tubule. (The mechanism for the regulation of ADH and plasma osmolality is described in Chapter 3.)

Urodilantin and Atrial Natriuretic Peptide

Urodilantin and ANP are encoded by the same gene and have a similar structure. ANP is secreted by the cardiac atria, and **urodilantin** is secreted by the distal tubules and functions only in the kidney. Both are stimulated by a rise in blood pressure and an increase in extracellular fluid volume. ANP inhibits ADH secretion, and ADH regulates water reabsorption and promotes water excretion. Urodilantin inhibits NaCl and water reabsorption in the medullary part of the collecting duct.

Diuretics as a Factor in Urine Flow

A **diuretic** is any agent that enhances the flow of urine. Clinically, diuretics interfere with renal sodium reabsorption and reduce extracellular fluid volume. Diuretics are commonly used to treat hypertension and edema caused by heart failure, cirrhosis, and nephrotic syndrome.

Different diuretics affect different sites of tubular function and may produce side effects that alter acid-base and electrolyte balance. Therefore health professionals need to understand their indications for use, mechanisms of action, and toxic side effects. Diuretics are divided into four general categories: (1) osmotic diuretics, (2) carbonic anhydrase inhibitors (inhibitors of urinary acidification), (3) inhibitors of loop sodium or chloride transport, and (4) aldosterone antagonists. (The physiologic mechanism related to each category is summarized in Table 34-4).

Renal Hormones

Certain hormones are either activated or synthesized by the kidney. These hormones have significant systemic effects and include the active form of vitamin D, erythropoietin, and natriuretic hormone (see p. 1179).

Vitamin D

Vitamin D is a hormone that can be obtained in the diet or synthesized by the action of ultraviolet radiation on cholesterol in the skin. These forms of vitamin D_3 (cholecalciferol) are inactive and require two hydroxylations to establish a

Table 34-4 Action of Diuretics

Diuretic	Site of Action	Action	Side Effects
OSMOTIC DIURETIC			
Mannitol Glycerol Urea	Proximal tubule	Freely filtered but not reabsorbed; osmotically attracts water and diminishes sodium reabsorption	Hypokalemia, dehydration
CARBONIC ANHYDRASE INHIBITORS			
Acetazolamide	Proximal tubule	Inhibits carbonic anhydrase; blocks hydrogen ion secretion and reabsorption of sodium and bicarbonate	Hypokalemia, systemic acidosis, alkaline urine
INHIBITORS OF SODIUM/CHLORIDE REABSORPTION			
Thiazides	Between end of ascending loop and beginning of distal tubule	Blocks sodium and chloride reabsorption; mildly suppresses carbonic anhydrase	Hypokalemia, metabolic alkalosis
Furosemide Ethacrynic acid Torsemide	Thick ascending limb of Henle loop	Blocks active transport of chloride, sodium, and potassium	Hypokalemia, uric acid retention
Bumetanide	Cortical vasodilation	Increased rate of urine formation	Hypokalemia, uric acid retention
POTASSIUM SPARING			
Spironolactone	Distal tubule	Inhibits aldosterone, blocks sodium reabsorption, and results in potassium retention	Hyperkalemia, nausea, confusion, gynecomastia
Triamterene and amiloride	Distal tubule	Blocks sodium reabsorption and inhibits potassium excretion	Nausea, vomiting, headache, granulocytopenia, skin rash

metabolically active form. The first step occurs in the liver with hydroxylation at the twenty-fifth carbon, and the second hydroxylation occurs at the first carbon position in the kidneys. The end product is 1,25-dihydroxycholecalciferol, or 1,25-dihydroxyvitamin D_3 (1,25-OH_2D_3).

Vitamin D is necessary for the absorption of calcium and phosphate by the small intestine. The renal hydroxylation step is stimulated by parathyroid hormone. A decreased plasma calcium level (less than 10 mg/dl) stimulates the secretion of parathyroid hormone. Parathyroid hormone then stimulates a sequence of events that help restore plasma calcium back toward normal:

Calcium mobilization from bone

Synthesis of 1,25-dihydroxyvitamin D_3

↓

Absorption of calcium from the intestine

↓

Increased renal calcium reabsorption

↓

Decreased renal phosphate reabsorption

Serum phosphate fluctuations also influence the renal hydroxylation of vitamin D. Decreased levels stimulate active 1,25-OH_2D_3 formation, and increased levels inhibit formation. This results in compensatory changes in phosphate absorption from bone and the intestine. The clinical significance of the role of the kidney in calcium and phosphate metabolism is evident in renal disease. Patients with renal disease have a deficiency of 1,25-OH_2D_3 and manifest symptoms of disturbed calcium and phosphate balance (see Chapter 3).

Erythropoietin

Erythropoietin stimulates the bone marrow to produce red blood cells in response to tissue hypoxia. (Erythrocyte production is discussed in Chapter 24.) The stimulus for erythropoietin release is decreased oxygen delivery in the kidneys. The anemia of chronic renal failure, in which kidney cells have become nonfunctional, may be related to the lack of this hormone.

TESTS OF RENAL FUNCTION

The Concept of Clearance

A number of specific renal functions can be measured by renal clearance. Renal clearance techniques determine how much of a substance can be cleared from the blood by the kidneys per given unit of time. The application of this principle permits an indirect measure of GFR, tubular secretion, tubular reabsorption, and renal blood flow.

Clearance and Glomerular Filtration Rate

The GFR provides the best estimate of functioning renal tissue. Loss or damage to nephrons leads to a corresponding decrease in GFR. The measurement of GFR requires use of a substance that has a stable plasma concentration; is freely filtered at the glomerulus; and is not secreted, reabsorbed, or metabolized by the tubules. Inulin (a fructose polysaccharide) is one substance that meets the criteria for measurement of GFR.

The kidney "clears" inulin from the plasma by filtering it at the glomerulus, reabsorbing nearly all of the fluid, and excreting the inulin left behind in the urine. The amount of inulin filtered is equal to the volume of plasma filtered (GFR) multiplied by the plasma concentration of inulin (P_{IN}). The amount of inulin in the urine is equal to a volume of urine per unit of time ($\dot{V}$) (usually 24 hours) multiplied by the inulin concentration of urine (U_{IN}). Because all the inulin filtered is excreted in the urine,

$$GFR \times P_{IN} = U_{IN} = \dot{V}$$

GFR can be calculated by rearranging the formula:

$$GFR\ (ml/min) = \frac{(U_{IN} \times \dot{V})}{P_{IN}}$$

The accurate determination of inulin clearance requires constant infusion to maintain a stable plasma level. This is time consuming and inconvenient. Therefore the clearance of creatinine, a natural substance produced by muscle and released into the blood at a relatively constant rate, is commonly used clinically. It is freely filtered at the glomerulus, but a small amount is secreted by the renal tubules. Therefore creatinine clearance overestimates the GFR but within tolerable limits. Creatinine clearance provides a good measure of GFR because only one blood sample is required in addition to a 24-hour volume of urine. The GFR estimated by creatinine clearance is calculated as follows:

$$GFR = \frac{(U_{CR} \times \dot{V})}{P_{CR}}$$

Similar calculations can be made for all solutes excreted in the urine per unit of time. Substances freely filtered at the glomerulus but with a clearance less than inulin or creatinine have been reabsorbed along the tubules. For example, glucose is completely reabsorbed and has a clearance rate of nearly zero. Conversely, substances secreted by the tubules have a clearance rate greater than inulin or creatinine (i.e., greater than 1.0).

Clearance and Renal Blood Flow

The standard clearance formula also can be used to estimate RPF and RBF. The substance used for this evaluation is para-aminohippurate (PAH). Some PAH is filtered at the glomerulus, and most of the remainder is secreted into the tubules in one circulation through the kidney. If all the PAH were removed from the plasma during a single pass through the kidney, total RPF could be determined. Because the supporting and nonsecreting structures of the kidney receive 10% to 15% of effective renal blood flow (ERBF), clearance of PAH measures only what is known as the **effective renal plasma flow (ERPF),** which is 85% to 90% of the true renal plasma flow:

$$ERBF = ERPF$$
$$1 - Hematocrit$$
$$(1.0 - 0.45)$$

The estimation of ERBF can then be calculated by considering the hematocrit in the following formula:

$$ERPF = C_{PAH} = \frac{U_{PAH}\dot{V}}{P_{PAH}}$$

where C_{PAH} = renal clearance of PAH, U_{PAH} = PAH in urine, and P_{PAH} = PAH in plasma.

Blood Tests

Plasma Creatinine Concentration

A long-term decline in GFR over weeks or months is reflected in the **plasma creatinine (P_{CR}) concentration** (normal value = 0.7 to 1.2 mg/dl). The P_{CR} concentration has a stable value when the GFR is stable because creatinine has a constant rate of production as a product of muscle metabolism. The amount filtered is approximately equal to the amount excreted, and a small amount is secreted by kidney tubules. When the GFR declines, the P_{CR} increases proportionately. Thus the GFR and P_{CR} are inversely related. If the GFR were to decrease by 50%, the filtration and excretion of creatinine would be reduced by 50% and creatinine would accumulate in plasma to twice the normal value. Therefore elevated P_{CR} values represent decreasing GFR. In the new steady state, however, the total amount of creatinine excreted in the urine would remain the same because of the proportionate decrease in GFR and increase in P_{CR}.

The application of this principle is simple and useful for monitoring progressive changes in renal function. The test is most valuable for monitoring the progress of chronic rather than acute renal disease because it takes 7 to 10 days for the plasma creatinine level to stabilize when GFR declines. Serial measures can be obtained over a long time and plotted as a curve of glomerular function. The P_{CR} also becomes elevated during trauma or breakdown of muscle tissue. In such instances the value is then not useful for estimating GFR.

Blood Urea Nitrogen

The concentration of urea nitrogen in the blood reflects glomerular filtration and urine-concentrating capacity. Because urea is filtered at the glomerulus, blood urea nitrogen (BUN) levels increase as glomerular filtration drops. Because urea is reabsorbed by the blood through the permeable tubules, the BUN rises in states of dehydration and acute and chronic renal failure when passage of fluid through the tubules is slowed. BUN also varies as a result of altered protein intake and protein catabolism and therefore is a poor measure of GFR. The normal range for BUN in the adult is 10 to 20 mg/dl of blood.

Urinalysis

Urinalysis is a noninvasive and relatively inexpensive diagnostic procedure. The best results are obtained from a fresh, cleanly voided specimen, because decay permits changes in the composition of urine. Urinalysis includes evaluation of color, turbidity, protein, pH, specific gravity, sediment, and supernatant.

Urine normally has a clear, light yellow color because of urochrome and other pigments. When formed substances (crystals, blood cells, or casts) are in the urine, it appears turbid. Protein in the urine creates marked foaming when shaken, and the foam is yellow or orange when the urine contains bile pigments. Urine does not normally contain protein or bile.

Urine pH normally ranges between 5.0 and 6.5, but it may vary from 4.5 to 8.0. Urine is more alkaline after eating and then declines before the next meal. Because sleep is accompanied by intermittent hypoventilation, a person produces more acidic urine after awakening.

Specific Gravity

Specific gravity is an estimated measure of the solute concentration of the urine. Specific gravity of any solution is measured by comparing the weight of the solution with an equal volume of distilled water. Hence, specific gravity is not a true measure of the number or concentration of particles, but it correlates well with osmolality and is a useful clinical tool. Specific gravity usually is measured with a hydrometer in a cylinder of urine; the normal value is 1.016 to 1.022. Dipstick evaluations may be falsely high when urine pH is less than 6 and falsely low when the pH is more than 7.

The final urine osmolality is primarily a function of ADH, which controls water reabsorption in the collecting ducts. If the kidney is unable to concentrate or dilute urine, given a stimulus, the cause is usually a malfunction of the renal tubules or inappropriate ADH secretion by the posterior pituitary gland. The state of hydration also affects the urine specific gravity, so hydration status should be evaluated before making a diagnosis. This determination is helpful for differentiating oliguria caused by intrinsic renal disease from hypovolemia as a result of dehydration.

Urine Sediment

The urine sediment is examined microscopically and may contain cells, casts, crystals, and bacteria. Epithelial cells may be seen in the microscopic field because they are shed naturally throughout the urinary tract.

Red Blood Cells

Normal urine contains few or no red blood cells. If a large number of red cells are present, this is known as **hematuria** and the sediment may be red. An alkaline or hypotonic urine causes lysis of red cells, however, so that the cells will not be seen. Urine then will be positive for hemoglobin, and the specific gravity will be elevated. Hematuria can occur with the administration of anticoagulants and with several renal diseases.

Casts

Casts (accumulations of cellular precipitates) originate in the renal tubules, from which they take their shape. They are cylindric with distinct borders. All casts have a precipitated microprotein matrix and arise primarily from the ascending limb of the distal tubule. Red cell casts indicate bleeding into the tubules; white cell casts are associated with an inflammatory process. Epithelial cell casts indicate degeneration of the tubular lumen or necrosis of the renal tubules. The type of cast identified suggests the disease process occurring in the kidney.

Crystals

Numerous kinds of **crystals** can be observed in the urine. They may be composed of cystine, uric acid, calcium oxalate, or phosphate. They may not be initially observable, but as the urine cools, crystals will form. Crystals tend to form in a concentrated acidic or alkaline urine. Generally, they are not clinically significant. Crystal formation is diagnostically significant, usually indicating inflammation, infection, or a metabolic disorder.

White Blood Cells

White blood cells (WBCs) in the urine (a condition termed **pyuria**) are primarily indicative of urinary tract infection, particularly when bacteria are present. Glomerulonephritis and nephrotic syndrome also may demonstrate pyuria, but usually in combination with proteinuria, red cells, and casts. The finding of WBC casts reflects a kidney infection, because these casts are not formed in the bladder or prostate. If WBCs are present in the urine, a culture should be done for specific identification of bacteria and sensitivity of bacteria to antibiotics.

Other Measures

Dipsticks and reagent strips are available for other substances in the urine, including glucose, bilirubin, urobilinogen, leukocyte esterase and nitrates, ketones, proteins, hemoglobin, and myoglobin.[2]

Aging and Renal Function

Throughout life the kidney responds to an increased workload by compensatory hypertrophy. This hypertrophy is marked in individuals who have donated a kidney for transplant or have lost functioning nephrons from trauma or disease. The glomeruli increase in diameter, and the tubules enlarge effectively to maintain the regulatory functions of the kidney. Hypertrophy occurs more rapidly and with a larger size increase in younger individuals and in those with high protein intake.

Changes in the kidneys occur throughout life, with a linear decrease in renal blood flow and GFR.[11] With aging the number of nephrons decreases. The primary mechanism appears to be a change in the renal vasculature and perfusion pattern, which leads to a reduction in numbers of nephrons. The rate of nephron loss accelerates between 40 and 80 years of age. By 75 years of age the nephron population is reduced by 30% to 50%, with loss of renal mass occurring primarily in the cortex.[2] Degenerative changes within nephrons also occur with aging. The glomerular capillaries atrophy, with a reduction in the branching vessels. The glomeruli then may disappear completely. The arcuate and interlobular arteries become tortuous, contributing to ischemia. The loss of the glomerular tuft may cause a shunt between the afferent and efferent arterioles. Although loss of juxtaglomerular nephrons still allows the vasa recta to be perfused, the combination of events contributes to a decreasing ability to excrete a concentrated urine. Thus the specific gravity of the urine in older individuals tends to be on the low side of normal.

Tubular transport changes with aging. Glucose, bicarbonate, and sodium are not as efficiently reabsorbed, and hyperkalemia is more common because of decreased secretion. Response to acid or base loads is delayed and prolonged. Sudden or large changes in pH or fluid load may lead to serious imbalances with increased risk of hypervolemia or hypovolemia. Acute losses or chronic fluid deficits can lead to renal insufficiency in the elderly person. Administration of drugs eliminated by renal processes may require dose modifications and more astute observations for toxic side effects. The T_m for glucose reabsorption decreases with age, contributing to a greater amount of glucose in the urine. This is an important consideration when glycosuria is used for screening or monitoring the process of diabetes mellitus in elderly persons. These changes occur independently of disease, however, indicating a normal process of aging. An age-related decline in renal activation of vitamin D decreases intestinal absorption of calcium. Previous or concurrent renal disease or urinary tract obstruction may amplify age-related changes in function.

SUMMARY REVIEW

Structures of the Renal System

1. The kidneys are paired structures lying bilaterally between the twelfth thoracic and third lumbar vertebrae.
2. The kidney is composed of an outer cortex and an inner medulla.
3. The calyces join to form the renal pelvis, which is continuous with the upper end of the ureter.
4. The nephron is the urine-forming unit of the kidney and is composed of the glomerulus, proximal tubule, hairpin loops of Henle, distal tubule, and collecting duct.
5. The glomerulus contains loops of capillaries. The capillary walls serve as a filtration membrane for the formation of the primary urine.
6. The proximal tubule is lined with microvilli to increase surface area and enhance reabsorption.
7. The hairpin loops of Henle transport solutes and water, contributing to the hypertonic state of the medulla.
8. The distal tubule adjusts acid-base balance by excreting acid into the urine and forming new bicarbonate ions.
9. The ureters extend from the renal pelvis to the posterior wall of the bladder. Urine flows through the ureters by means of peristaltic contraction of the ureteral muscles.
10. The bladder is a bag composed of the detrusor and trigone muscles and innervated by parasympathetic fibers. When accumulation of urine reaches 250 to 300 ml, mechanoreceptors, which respond to stretching of tissue, stimulate the micturition reflex.

Renal Blood Flow

1. Renal blood flows at about 1000 to 1200 ml/min, or 20% to 25% of the cardiac output.
2. Blood flow through the glomerular capillaries is maintained at a constant rate in spite of a wide range of arterial pressures (autoregulation).
3. The glomerular filtration rate (GFR) is the filtration of plasma per unit of time and is directly related to the perfusion pressure of renal blood flow.
4. Autoregulation of renal blood flow and sympathetic neural regulation of vasoconstriction maintain a constant GFR.
5. Renin is an enzyme secreted from the juxtaglomerular apparatus; it causes the generation of angiotensin, a potent vasoconstrictor. The renin-angiotensin system is thus a regulator of renal blood flow.
6. Natriuretic hormone from the right atrium of the heart promotes sodium and water loss by inhibiting aldosterone.

Kidney Function

1. The major function of the nephron is urine formation, which involves the processes of glomerular filtration, tubular reabsorption, and tubular secretion and excretion.
2. Glomerular filtration is favored by capillary hydrostatic pressure and opposed by oncotic pressure in the capillary and hydrostatic pressure in the Bowman capsule. The balance of favoring and opposing filtration forces is known as net filtration pressure (NFP).
3. The GFR is approximately 120 ml/min, and 99% of the filtrate is reabsorbed.
4. The proximal tubule reabsorbs about 60% to 70% of the filtered sodium and water and 90% of other electrolytes.
5. Because most molecules are reabsorbed by active transport, the carrier mechanism can become saturated at a point known as the transport maximum (T_m). Molecules not reabsorbed are excreted with the urine.
6. The distal tubules actively reabsorb sodium and secrete potassium and hydrogen for the regulation of electrolyte and acid-base balance.
7. The concentration of the final urine is a function of the level of antidiuretic hormone (ADH) that stimulates the distal tubules and collecting ducts to reabsorb water. The countercurrent exchange system of the long loops of Henle and their accompanying capillaries establishes a concentration gradient within the renal medulla to facilitate the reabsorption of water from the collecting duct.
8. The distal nephron regulates acid-base balance by excreting hydrogen ions and forming new bicarbonate.
9. The kidney secretes or activates a number of hormones that have systemic effects, including 1,25-OH_2D_3 and erythropoietin.

Tests of Renal Function

1. Tests that measure renal clearance indicate how much of a substance can be cleared from the blood by the kidneys per given amount of time.

2. Creatinine, a substance produced by muscle, is measured in both plasma and urine to calculate a commonly used clinical measurement of GFR.
3. Both the plasma creatinine concentration and the blood urea nitrogen (BUN) levels indicate glomerular function. Plasma creatinine is measured to monitor progressive renal dysfunction; BUN is an indicator of hydration status.
4. Urinalysis involves evaluation of color, turbidity, protein, pH, specific gravity, sediment, and supernatant.
5. Presence of bacteria, red blood cells, white blood cells, casts, or crystals in the urine sediment may indicate a renal disorder.

Aging and Renal Function

1. As a person grows older, a decrease occurs in the number of nephrons. Both renal blood flow and glomerular filtration rate decline.
2. Tubular transport and reabsorption decrease with age. Response to acid-base changes and reabsorption of glucose are delayed. Drugs eliminated by the kidney can accumulate in the plasma, causing toxic reactions.

KEY TERMS

Arcuate artery, *1176*
Atrial natriuretic peptide (ANP), *1179*
Bladder, *1176*
Bowman capsule, *1172*
Bowman space, *1173*
Cast, *1188*
Collecting duct, *1176*
Countercurrent exchange system, *1184*
Crystal, *1188*
Detrusor muscle, *1176*
Distal tubule, *1176*
Diuretic, *1185*
Effective renal plasma flow (ERPF), *1187*
Excretion, *1180*
External urethral sphincter, *1176*
Filtration slit, *1173*
Glomerular capillary, *1176*
Glomerular endothelium, *1173*
Glomerular epithelium, *1173*
Glomerular filtration membrane, *1173*
Glomerular filtration rate (GFR), *1177*
Glomerulus, *1172*
Hematuria, *1188*
Hilum, *1170*
Interlobar artery, *1176*
Internal urethral sphincter, *1176*
Juxtaglomerular apparatus (JGA), *1173*
Juxtaglomerular cell, *1173*
Juxtamedullary nephron, *1172*
Kidney, *1170*
Loop of Henle, *1174*
Macula densa, *1173*
Major calyx, *1172*
Mesangial cell, *1173*
Micturition, *1176*
Midcortical nephron, *1172*
Minor calyx, *1170*
Myogenic mechanism, *1178*
Natriuretic peptide, *1179*
Nephron, *1172*
Net filtration pressure (NFP), *1181*
Oliguria, *1185*
Peritubular capillary, *1176*
Plasma creatinine (P_{CR}) concentration, *1187*
Podocyte, *1173*
Proximal tubule, *1174*
Pyuria, *1188*
Renal artery, *1176*
Renal capsule, *1170*
Renal column, *1170*
Renal corpuscle, *1173*
Renal cortex, *1170*
Renal fascia, *1170*
Renal medulla, *1170*
Renal papilla, *1176*
Renal pelvis, *1172*
Renal pyramid, *1170*
Renin-angiotensin system, *1179*
Specific gravity, *1188*
Superficial cortical nephron, *1172*
Transport maximum (T_m), *1182*
Trigone, *1176*
Tubular reabsorption, *1180*
Tubular secretion, *1180*
Tubuloglomerular feedback, *1178*
Ultrafiltration, *1180*
Urea, *1185*
Ureter, *1176*
Urethra, *1176*
Urinalysis, *1188*
Urine pH, *1188*
Urodilantin, *1185*
Vasa recta, *1176*
Water diuresis, *1185*

REFERENCES

1. Haas CS et al: Regulatory mechanism in glomerular mesangial cell proliferation, *J Nephrol* 12(6):405, 1999.
2. Brenner BM: *Brenner and Rector's the kidney,* vol 1, ed 6, Philadelphia, 2000, W.B. Saunders.
3. Pavenstadt H: Roles of the podocyte in glomerular function, *Am J Physiol Renal Physiol* 278(2):F173, 2000.
4. Welch WJ, Wilcox CS, Thomson SC: Nitric oxide and tubuloglomerular feedback, *Semin Nephrol* 19(3):251, 1999.
5. Valtin H, Schafer JA: *Renal function,* ed 3, Boston, 1995, Little, Brown.
6. Kramer HS: Atrial natriuretic peptides and the natriuretic hormone(s): regulatory roles and therapeutic applications. In Gronick HC, editor: *Concepts of nephrology,* vol 19, St Louis, 1996, Mosby.
7. Thibault G, Amiri F, Garcia R: Regulation of natriuretic peptide secretion by the adult heart, *Am J Physiol* 276(6 pt 2):1977, 1999.
8. Palmer LG: Potassium secretion and the regulation of distal nephron K channels, *Am J Physiol* 277(6 pt 2):821, 1999.
9. Koeppen BM, Stanton BA: *Renal physiology,* ed 3, St Louis, 2001, Mosby.
10. Knepper MA, Chou CL, Layton HB: How is urine concentrated by the renal inner medulla? In Bourke E, Mallick NP, Pollak VE, editors: *Moving points in nephrology,* vol 12, Basel, 1993, Karger.
11. Beck LH: The aging kidney. Defending a delicate balance of fluid and electrolytes, *Geriatrics* 55(4):26, 2000.

CHAPTER 35

Alterations of Renal and Urinary Tract Function

SUE E. HUETHER

CHAPTER OUTLINE

Renal and urinary function can be affected by a variety of disorders. The most common type of urinary dysfunction is infection of the bladder. The urinary tract also can be obstructed by stones or tumors. Renal function can be impaired by disorders of the kidney itself or by many systemic diseases. Because the kidney filters the blood, it is directly linked to every other organ system. Renal failure, whether acute or chronic, is therefore a life-threatening condition.

URINARY TRACT OBSTRUCTION

Urinary tract obstruction, or obstructive uropathy, is an interference with the flow of urine at any site along the urinary tract (Fig. 35-1). The obstruction causes urine accumulation behind the obstruction, leading to infection or damage to involved organs. Obstruction can be congenital or acquired. Among the numerous causes are tumors, stones (calculi), trauma, edema, pregnancy, benign prostatic hyperplasia or carcinoma, inflammation of the gastrointestinal tract, or loss of ureteral peristaltic activity or bladder muscle function. Urinary tract obstructions can develop acutely or evolve insidiously over weeks or months.

Consequences

The pathophysiologic consequences of urinary tract obstruction are related to (1) location within or outside the urinary tract, (2) unilateral or bilateral involvement, (3) partial or complete obstruction, (4) short-term or long-term duration, and (5) the underlying cause. Obstruction of urine flow increases hydrostatic pressure and dilation of structures behind the site of occlusion. Pressure increases are less severe in the lower urinary tract because more surface area is available for dilation.

Obstruction of the ureter causes **hydroureter** (accumulation of urine in the ureter). Retrograde increases in hydrostatic pressure involving the renal pelvis and calyces produce **hydronephrosis** (accumulation of urine in the renal collecting system). Acute, complete obstructions cause an increase in pressure that is transmitted to the proximal tubule and decreases glomerular filtration. If the obstruction is complete, the glomerular filtration rate (GFR) will decline to zero, with resulting renal failure. Complete unilateral obstruction reduces renal blood flow and GFR and is reflected by an increased plasma creatinine level.[1]

Chronic partial obstruction causes compression of the kidney structures from accumulation of urine, with ischemic atrophy of the papilla and medulla. Although the kidneys initially increase in size, progressive atrophy follows, with eventual loss of renal mass and smaller kidneys. The accompanying tubular damage decreases renal ability to conserve sodium and water and to excrete hydrogen ion and potassium. The resulting failure to concentrate the urine may produce excessive urine volumes even though the GFR has declined. Sodium and bicarbonate are wasted, with an increased risk of dehydration and metabolic acidosis.

Relief of urinary tract obstruction is usually followed by a variable period of diuresis (commonly called *postobstructive diuresis*) with losses of large amounts of urine. The diuresis is related to salt and water retention during the period

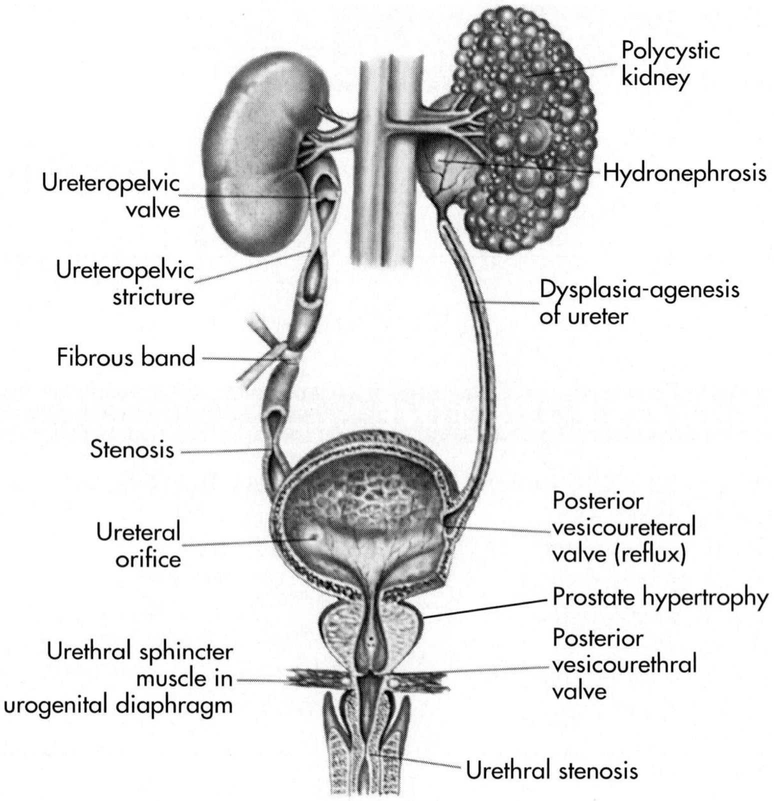

FIG. 35-1 Major sites of urinary tract obstruction. (Modified from Wong DL: *Whaley and Wong's nursing care of infants and children,* ed 6, St Louis, 1999, Mosby.)

of obstruction and a return to a normal GFR. The diuresis lasts for a few days, usually without symptoms of volume depletion such as postural hypotension or elevated blood urea nitrogen (BUN) and plasma creatinine levels.

An uncommon result of obstruction relief is an excessive loss of sodium and water (greater than 10 L/day). In some cases of chronic obstruction, diuresis may not be significant after relief of obstruction because the GFR returns to normal slowly or not at all.

Complications of urinary tract obstruction include infection and renal failure. The type of complication depends on the site of obstruction. Obstructions below the bladder cause infection because the accumulated urine is an excellent medium for bacterial growth. Acute or chronic renal failure occurs with prolonged bilateral obstruction (see p. 1206). Acute renal failure can be prevented if the obstruction is relieved within 1 week. Chronic renal failure may be insidious.

Obstructive Disorders

Kidney Stones

Calculi, or **renal stones** (nephrolithiasis), are masses of crystals and protein and are a common cause of urinary tract obstruction in adults. The incidence of renal stones at autopsy is approximately 5%. Approximately 1% of the U.S. population will have a renal stone at some time.[2] Caucasians are at highest risk.

The three major kinds of renal stones are (1) calcium oxylate (75% to 80%), (2) struvite (magnesium, ammonium, phosphate) (15%), and (3) uric acid (7%). Cystine stones account for less than 1% of all renal stones.

Pathophysiology

The formation of stones is complicated and not entirely understood. Contributing factors include high urinary concentration of stone-forming substances, urine pH that affects solubility, low urine output, tubular defects, facilitators and inhibitors of crystal growth, various diseases, drugs, and diet. Inhibitors of crystal aggregation (nephrocalcin) are normally present in the urine. One theory of stone formation is a reduced excretion of these inhibitors in the urine.[3]

The stone begins with a nucleus, or **nidus,** that evolves in the presence of stone-forming substances such as calcium oxalate, calcium phosphate, or struvite. It may become trapped within the urinary tract and attract other crystals, forming a stone. A high urinary saturation of stone-forming substances enhances crystal formation and stone growth (Fig. 35-2).

Some types of stones are aggregates of different substances. For example, people with high concentrations of uric acid attract calcium oxalate crystals onto a uric acid nidus even though urinary calcium and oxalate levels are normal. The pH of the urine affects the solubility of many stone-forming substances. For instance, an alkaline urine decreases the solubility and enhances the crystallization of calcium carbonate and calcium phosphate. Keeping the urine more acidic increases the solubility of these substances and helps prevent supersaturation and stone formation. Uric acid tends to crystallize in an acidic urine, particularly when the pH remains below 5.5 and urine volume is low. Calcium oxalate and cystine stones form independently of the urine pH.

Stones usually grow on the papillae or in the renal tubules, calyces, or renal pelvis. Stones also may form in the ureter or

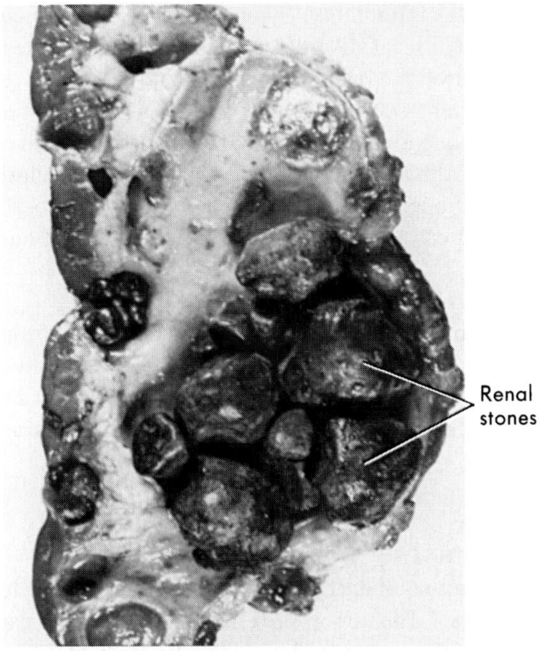

FIG. 35-2 Hydronephrosis. Hydronephrosis with renal stones in renal pelvis and calyces. (From Kissane JM, editor: *Anderson's pathology,* ed 9, St Louis, 1990, Mosby.)

bladder. Many stones are less than 5 mm in diameter and are readily passed with the urine. Large stones are sometimes called **staghorn calculi,** because they grow in the pelvis and extend into the calyces to form branching stones. Renal failure may be a consequence unless the stones are surgically removed.

Calcium stones are the smallest and most common stones. They occur most commonly in middle-age men with a familial history of stone formation. Most are formed of calcium oxalate or an aggregate of calcium oxalate and calcium phosphate. Approximately 80% of them are idiopathic, although they frequently are associated with hypercalciuria and hyperuricosuria (a high level of uric acid in urine). Prolonged immobilization resulting in bone demineralization or hyperparathyroidism can precipitate hypercalciuria and stone formation. Struvite stones (magnesium, ammonium, phosphate) are precipitated by infection with urea-splitting microorganisms[4] (e.g., *Pseudomonas* and *Proteus*) and are more common in women. With such infections, an alkaline urine is produced and large stones tend to form in the kidney or bladder.

Uric acid stones are caused by gout, an increase in uric acid production and hyperuricosuria. High-purine diets (consisting of meat, fish, and poultry) also can contribute to elevated levels of uric acid. Formation of uric acid stones is enhanced by a concentrated and acidic urine. Thus regional enteritis and ulcerative colitis can precipitate the formation of uric acid stones. These diseases may cause fluid loss and a metabolic acidosis that develops from loss of bicarbonate (see Chapter 3). Individuals with the rare hereditary disorder cystinuria develop cystine stones. In cystinuria an error in cystine metabolism causes decreased tubular reabsorption of cystine with an increased amount of this relatively insoluble substance in the urine.

WHAT'S NEW? Kidney Stone Inhibitors

Adhesion of urinary crystals to the apical surface of renal tubular cells is a critical step in stone formation. Several specific anions are inhibitors of calcium oxalate (CaOx) nucleation and aggregation, including nephrocalcin, uroponin, and glycosaminoglycans. These inhibitors work by preventing crystal adhesion to renal cells and crystal aggregation. Tamm-Horsfall protein inhibits CaOx aggregation in urine with high pH, and other proteins inhibit stone formation in acidic urine. Renal lithostathine inhibits growth of calcium carbonate crystals. Crystal retention and calculus formation may be caused by alterations in these urinary anions.

Data from Selvan R, Kalaiselvi P: A novel basic protein from human kidney which inhibits calcium oxalate crystal growth, *BJU Int* 86(1):7, 2000; Shirane Y et al: Study of inhibition mechanisms of glycosaminoglycans on calcium oxalate monohydrate crystals by atomic force microscopy, *Urol Res* 27(6):426, 1999.

Clinical Manifestations

Pain is the hallmark symptom of a renal stone. The location and severity vary with the site of occurrence. The presence of stones above the ureters is usually asymptomatic unless an infection or obstruction occurs. A stone obstructing the ureter causes a colicky pain as the rhythmic contractions of the ureter attempt to advance the stone. Distention and spasm of the ureter follow from the accumulation of urine behind the stone. The pain may be in the flank or at the costovertebral angle (between the last rib and the lumbar vertebrae), or it may radiate into the groin if the stone is lower in the ureter. The pain can be exquisitely severe, requiring narcotic analgesia for relief, and is frequently accompanied by nausea and vomiting. Gross or microscopic hematuria (blood in the urine) may be present.

Evaluation and Treatment

The diagnosis of renal stones requires a thorough medical and family history, diet history, previous history of urinary tract disease, and use of medications. Both blood and urine tests should be performed to evaluate the presence of stone-forming substances. Urine pH and the presence of red or white blood cells should be evaluated. The GFR can be estimated by assessing the BUN and plasma creatinine (see Chapter 34). A plain (flat plate) film of the abdomen and an intravenous pyelogram will identify the presence of radiopaque stones and confirm the anatomic location.

The purpose of treatment is to prevent new stone formation and reduce the size of stones that have already formed.[5] Calcium stones reduce with difficulty, but struvite, uric acid, and cystine stones may dissolve with appropriate therapy. The principal components of treatment are (1) reducing the concentration of stone-forming substances by increasing the flow of urine with a high fluid intake and (2) decreasing the amount of the substance in the urine by decreasing dietary intake or endogenous production. The solubility of stone-forming substances often can be enhanced by altering the pH of the urine. Calcium stones are often treated with thiazide diuretics and allopurinol; cystine stones are treated with D-penicillamine, captopril, and alpha-mercaptopropionylglycine. Surgical removal may be required for large stones, obstruction, recurrent infections, or intractable pain. Smaller stones may pass spontaneously, or they can be extracted by instrumentation. Extracorporeal ultrasonic or laser lithotripsy is a relatively noninvasive procedure that uses high-frequency sound waves to fragment stones for excretion in the urine.[6,7]

Neurogenic Bladder

Neurogenic bladder is a functional urinary tract obstruction caused by an interruption of the nerve supply to the bladder. The neurologic disruption can occur in the central nervous system or at the level of the spinal cord.

Pathophysiology

Bladder paralysis interferes with the normal flow of urine and is related to the level of the neural lesion. Upper motor neuron lesions in (or below) the cortex but above the sacral level of the spinal cord cause loss of voluntary control of voiding. Lower motor neuron lesions (sacral level of the spinal cord) disrupt the sacral reflex arc and cause loss of both voluntary and involuntary control of urination. Some disease states or trauma may affect only the sensory or motor innervation of the bladder. (The types of neurogenic bladder are reviewed in Table 35-1.)

Clinical Manifestations

Infection with a neurogenic bladder may be associated with bladder distention and urine retention, placement of catheters, or the development of stones caused by bone resorption from physical immobility. Symptoms are often difficult to interpret because of disordered sensation and the presence of other neurologic disturbances. The individual may experience a burning sensation but not pain. The development of fever is frequently accompanied by chills and shivering, which aid in differentiating fever caused by other neurologic lesions. Neurogenic bladder must be properly diagnosed and treated, or it can lead to deterioration of renal function.[8]

Evaluation and Treatment

Sterile sampling of urine for bacterial analysis confirms the presence of bacteriuria. Antibiotic treatment for specific microorganisms is required. Urodynamic evaluations are required for diagnosis and treatment selection for neurogenic bladder.[9]

Tumors

Renal Tumors

Renal adenomas (benign tumors) are solid, rarely detected small tumors.[10] The tumors are encapsulated and are usually located near the cortex of the kidney. Because they can become malignant, they are usually surgically removed. **Renal cell carcinoma** is the most common renal neoplasm (85% of all renal neoplasms) and represents about 2% of cancer deaths.[11] Renal cell carcinoma occurs in men (18,700 new cases in 2001) more often than in women (12,100 new cases in 2001).[12] The 5-year survival rate is about 60%.[12]

Pathogenesis

An association has been identified between tobacco use, obesity, analgesic use, and the incidence of renal cell carcinoma.[13-15] Renal cell carcinomas are adenocarcinomas and are classified according to cell type and extent of metastasis. Clear cell tumors are the most common and have a better prognosis than granular cell or spindle tumors. Confinement

Table 35-1 Classification of Neurogenic Bladder

Type of Neurogenic Bladder	Cause	Neural Lesion	Clinical Manifestations	Treatment
Uninhibited (loss of cortical inhibition)	Lack of voluntary control in infancy, multiple sclerosis	Upper motor neuron	Smaller urine volume, frequency, urgency, incontinence, enuresis	Anticholinergic medication Intermittent catheterization
Reflex or automatic (reflex arc maintained below lesion with spontaneous voiding)	Spinal cord transection, cord tumors, multiple sclerosis above level T12 of cord	Upper motor neuron	Involuntary voiding that may include incomplete emptying with retention and infection	Catheter or condom drainage; stimulation of reflex arc by stroking perineum, abdomen, or rectum
Autonomous (loss of cortical inhibition and interruption of spinal reflex arc)	Sacral cord trauma, tumors, herniated disk, abdominal surgery with transection of pelvic parasympathetic nerves	Lower motor neuron	Overflow incontinence in which bladder does not empty spontaneously with stretch-fullness	Catheter, urinary diversion surgery
Motor paralysis (sensory functions intact)	Lesions at levels S2, S3, S4; poliomyelitis; trauma; tumors	Lower motor neuron	Overflow incontinence caused by loss of bladder contraction	Manual compression (Credé maneuver)
Sensory paralysis (motor functions intact)	Posterior lumbar nerve roots, diabetes mellitus, tabes dorsalis	Lower motor neuron	Dribbling, overflow incontinence; loss of sensation of bladder fullness	Bladder training to empty at regular intervals (e.g., every 3 hr)

within the renal capsule, together with treatment, is associated with a better survival rate. The tumors usually occur unilaterally and spread through the lymph nodes and blood vessels to the lungs, liver, lymph nodes, and bone (Fig. 35-3).[16]

Clinical Manifestations

The classic clinical manifestations of renal cell carcinoma are hematuria, flank pain, palpable flank mass, and weight loss, but these symptoms occur in fewer than 10% of cases. Such signs and symptoms represent an advanced stage of disease, whereas earlier stages are often silent. Hematuria is the most common presenting symptom.[17] The flank pain is usually dull and aching. Tumor palpation is generally difficult but easier in thin people. Systemic manifestations include weight loss and fatigue; intermittent fever from tumor toxins; anemia from hematuria and lack of erythropoietin or polycythemia from secretion of erythropoietic factor; altered liver function with elevated serum alkaline phosphatase, prothrombin, and bilirubin; and hypertension from elevated renin levels. The most common sites of distant metastasis are the lung, lymph nodes, liver, bone, thyroid, and central nervous system.[18]

Evaluation and Treatment

Diagnosis is based on the clinical symptoms, plain x-ray films of the abdomen, intravenous pyelography, renal angiography, and computed tomography. (Staging of renal cell carcinoma is presented in Table 35-2.) Treatment is usually surgical removal of the affected kidney (radical nephrectomy) with combined use of chemotherapeutic agents and biologic response modifiers (i.e., interferon-alpha and interleukins).[19] Hormonal agents (antiestrogen drugs) are less effective. Radiation therapy may also be used. Immediate relief of obstruction caused by invading tumors can be obtained by placing ureteral catheters past the obstruction or by inserting a nephrostomy tube percutaneously into the renal pelvis. If the obstruction is not treatable, urinary diversion procedures may be required to prevent chronic infection. Survival is related to tumor grade, tumor cell type, and extent of metastasis.

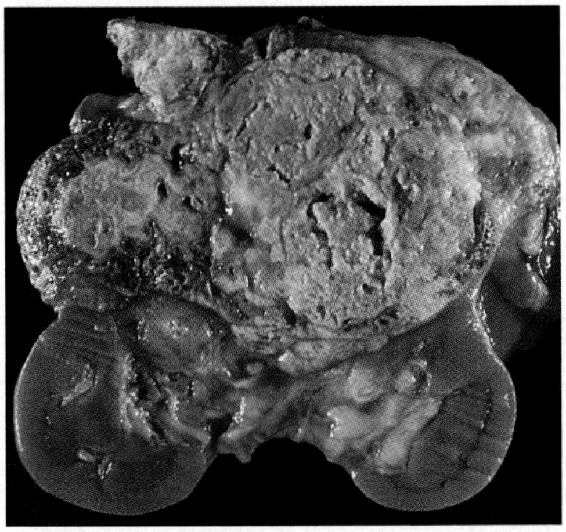

FIG. 35-3 Renal cell carcinoma. Renal cell carcinomas usually are spheroidal masses composed of yellow tissue mottled with hemorrhage, necrosis, and fibrosis. (From Damjanov I, Linder J, editors: *Anderson's pathology,* ed 10, St Louis, 1996, Mosby.)

Bladder Tumors

Bladder tumors represent about 3% of all malignant tumors and are the fifth most common malignancy.[11] Approximately 54,500 people develop bladder cancer each year, and 11,700 die of it.[11] The development of bladder cancer is highest in men older than age 60 years.

Pathogenesis

The risk of bladder cancer is greater for men who smoke[20] or work in the chemical, rubber, and textile industries. Bladder cancer is diagnosed at a higher stage in women.[21] Bladder cancer is associated with mutations in the tumor-suppressor gene *p53* with overexpression of the *p53* protein product; other genes are under study.[22] The tumor is usually composed of transitional cells (the cells lining the bladder) and may have a papillary growth pattern (a tuftlike lesion attached to a stalk) (Fig. 35-4). Nonpapillary tumors (representing 10% of bladder tumors) are not as common as papillary tumors, but they tend to be more invasive and have a poorer prognosis. Metastasis is usually to lymph nodes, liver, bones, and lungs. Staging for bladder carcinoma is presented in Table 35-3. Secondary bladder cancer develops by invasion of cancer from bordering organs, such as cervical carcinoma in women or prostatic carcinoma in men.

Clinical Manifestations

Bladder tumors may be asymptomatic or accompanied by hematuria. Advanced cancers are associated with pelvic pain and frequent urination.

Evaluation and Treatment

Diagnosis is made by cystoscopy (visual examination of the urinary tract through a cystoscope), cell studies, biologic markers,[23] urograms (x-ray examinations), and transurethral biopsy. Treatment is related to the type and size of the lesion. Transurethral resection is the treatment of choice for superficial tumors because of the high propensity for bladder tumors to recur. Endoscopic treatment with the neodymium: yttrium-aluminum-garnet (Nd:YAG) laser has also proven effective.[24] Carcinoma in situ is treated with intravesicular (inside the bladder) bacille Calmette-Guérin (BCG) or interferon, which induces a local immune response.[25] Chemotherapeutic agents also have been used with some success to

Table 35-2 Staging of Renal Cell Carcinoma

Stage	Metastasis
I	Tumor confined within kidney capsule
II	Invasion through renal capsule and renal vein but within surrounding fascia
III	Involvement of regional lymph nodes and vena cava
IV	Distant metastases

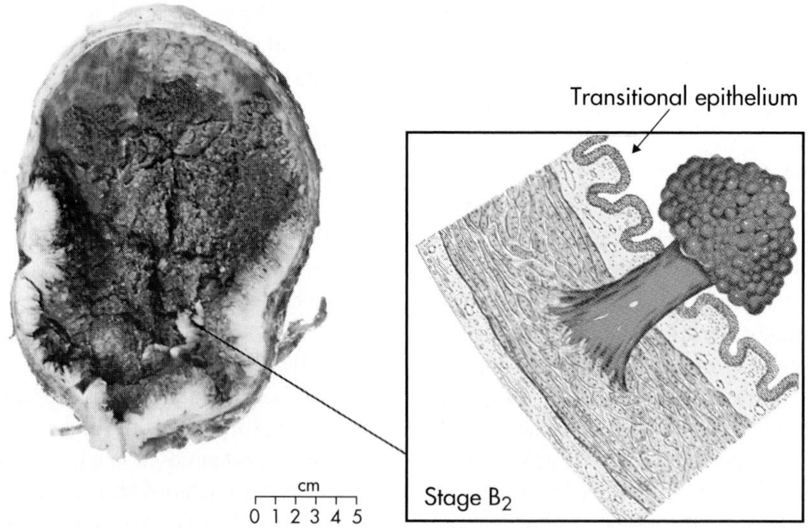

FIG. 35-4 Cystectomy specimen. Multiple papillary tumors cover greater part of bladder wall. (From Kissane JM, editor: *Anderson's pathology,* ed 9, St Louis, 1990, Mosby.)

Table 35-3 Staging of Bladder Carcinoma

Stages	Metastasis
0	Limited to mucosal involvement
A	Submucosal involvement
B	Involvement of the muscularis layer
C	Invasion of the perivesical fat
D_1	Spread to regional lymph nodes
D_2	Spread to distant sites, bone, and visceral organs

prevent recurrence. Radiation therapy is not as effective, and candidates for radiation must be carefully selected based on tumor type. Chemotherapy may be combined with radiation and surgical resection. Cystectomy is standard for invasive bladder cancer.[26] Because of the risk of recurrence, cystoscopic evaluations are performed every 3 to 6 months after initial treatment.

URINARY TRACT INFECTION

Causes

Urinary tract infections (UTIs) are usually caused by bacteria. At risk are premature newborns; prepubertal children; sexually active and pregnant women; women treated with antibiotics that disrupt vaginal flora; spermicide users; estrogen-deficient postmenopausal women; individuals with indwelling catheters; and persons with diabetes mellitus, neurogenic bladder, or urinary tract obstruction. Cystitis is more common in women because of the shorter urethra and the closeness of the urethra to the anus (increasing the possibility of bacterial contamination). Up to 30% of women may have a lower UTI at some time in their life.[27] Infections are diagnosed by culture of specific microorganisms with counts of 10,000 bacteria/ml of freshly voided urine. Bacterial contamination of the normally sterile urine usually occurs by retrograde movement of gram-negative bacilli into the urethra and bladder and then to the ureter and kidney. Gram-positive microorganisms, fungi, or tubercular bacilli are less common causes of infection. A UTI can occur anywhere along the urinary tract, including the urethra, prostate, bladder, ureter, and kidney.

Several factors normally combine to protect against UTIs. Most bacteria are washed out of the urethra during micturition. The low pH and high osmalality of urea and secretions from the uroepithelium provide a bactericidal effect. The ureterovesical junction closes during bladder contraction, preventing reflux of urine to the ureters and kidneys. Both the longer urethra and prostatic secretions decrease the risk of infection in men.[28]

Types

Cystitis

Cystitis is an inflammation of the bladder, the most common site of UTI. The morphologic appearance of the bladder through cystoscopy describes different types of cystitis. With mild inflammation the mucosa is hyperemic (red). More advanced cases may show diffuse hemorrhage (called *hemorrhagic cystitis*), pus formation, or suppurative exudate (called *suppurative cystitis*) on the epithelial surface of the bladder. Prolonged infection may lead to sloughing of the bladder mucosa with ulcer formation (termed *ulcerative cystitis*). The most severe infections may cause necrosis of the bladder wall (termed *gangrenous cystitis*). Generally, the infections are uncomplicated.[29]

◆ *Pathophysiology*

The most common infecting microorganisms are *Escherichia coli, Klebsiella, Proteus, Pseudomonas,* and *Staphylococcus.* The disease may occur alone or in association with pyelonephritis or prostatitis. Expression of type 1 fibriae by *E. coli* with attachment to the uroepithelium is thought to be the initial step of infection. Some women may be genetically susceptible to certain strains of *E. coli* attachment.[30] Infection initiates an inflammatory response and the symptoms of cystitis. The inflammatory edema in the bladder wall stimulates discharge of stretch receptors with small

WHAT'S NEW? Pregnancy and Urinary Tract Infection

Urinary tract infection (UTI) during pregnancy is common beginning at week 6 and peaking at 22 to 24 weeks and can result in preterm delivery if not treated. The infection is related to ascending infection from ureteral dilation, increased bladder volume, decreased bladder and ureteral tone, urinary stasis, and ureterovesical reflux. Decreased urine concentration is related to physiologic increases in plasma volume. Increased urine progestin and estrogens may affect bacterial resistance of the lower urinary tract. Glucosuria is common during pregnancy and may promote bacterial growth. The causative microorganisms are the same as those that cause UTI in nonpregnant women: *Escherichia coli, Proteus mirabilis,* and *Klebsiella pneumoniae.*

Data from Connolly A, Thorp JM Jr: Urinary tract infections in pregnancy, *Urol Clin North Am* 25(4):779, 1999; Delzell JE, Lefevre ML: Urinary tract infections during pregnancy, *Am Fam Physician* 61(3): 713, 2000.

volumes of urine, producing the urgency and frequency of urination associated with cystitis.

Clinical Manifestations

Many individuals with bacteriuria are asymptomatic. The clinical manifestations of cystitis, however, usually include frequency, urgency, dysuria (painful urination), and suprapubic and low back pain. Hematuria, cloudy urine, and flank pain are more serious symptoms. Approximately 10% of individuals with bacteriuria have no symptoms, and 30% of individuals with symptoms are abacteriuric.[31] Elderly persons with cystitis may be asymptomatic, and elderly women may have a higher risk of mortality.[32,33]

Evaluation and Treatment

Evaluation of the urine for bacteria is the most important diagnostic procedure. Risk factors, such as urinary tract obstruction, should be identified and treated. Evidence of bacteria from urine culture and sensitivity warrants treatment with a microorganism-specific antibiotic. A single large dose of antibiotic or a 3-day course may be effective when symptoms are of short duration and there are no complications.[34] Three to five days of treatment is most common. Elderly people with obstructive disorders may require 7 to 14 days of treatment.[35] From 20% to 25% of women have relapsing infection within 7 to 10 days, requiring prolonged antibiotic therapy.[36] Follow-up urine cultures should be obtained 1 week after initiation of treatment and again at monthly intervals for 3 months. Clinical symptoms frequently are relieved, but bacteriuria may still be present. Repeat cultures should be obtained every 3 to 4 months until 1 year after treatment for evaluation of recurrent infection.

"Nonbacterial" Cystitis

A significant number of women have symptoms of cystitis, such as frequency, urgency, and dysuria, but with negative urine cultures. It is more common in women age 20 to 30 years and is called **urethral syndrome.**[37] The cause has been obscure, but now there is evidence that inflamed or infected microscopic paraurethral glands connected to the distal third of the urethra in the prevaginal space are the anatomic location of this syndrome. These glands are homologous to the prostate and stain histologically for prostate-specific antigen. The glands are evaluated by palpation of the sides of the urethra through the anterior vaginal wall. Treatment with antibiotics is usually effective, although symptoms may recur.[38]

A persistent and chronic form of "nonbacterial" cystitis occurring primarily in women is **interstitial cystitis.** The cause is not known, but an autoimmune reaction may be responsible for the inflammatory response, which includes mast cell activation, altered epithelial permeability, and sensory nerve sensitivity.[39] The inflammation is associated with a derangement of the bladder mucosa that makes it more susceptible to penetration by bacteria. Inflammation and fibrosis of the bladder wall are accompanied by the presence of hemorrhagic ulcers (Hunner ulcers). Characteristic symptoms include bladder fullness, frequency, small urine volume, and lower abdominal pain. No single treatment is effective, and different approaches are used for symptom relief.[40]

Table 35-4 Common Causes of Pyelonephritis

Predisposing Factors	Pathologic Mechanisms
Kidney stones	Obstruction and stasis of urine contributing to bacteriuria and hydronephrosis; irritation of epithelial lining with entrapment of bacteria
Vesicoureteral reflux	Chronic reflux of urine up the ureter and into kidney during micturition contributing to bacterial infection
Pregnancy	Dilation and relaxation of ureter with hydroureter and hydronephrosis; partly caused by obstruction from enlarged uterus and partly from ureteral relaxation caused by higher progesterone levels
Neurogenic bladder	Neurologic impairment interfering with normal bladder contraction with residual urine and ascending infection
Instrumentation	Introduction of organisms into urethra and bladder by catheters and endoscopes introduced into the urinary tract for diagnostic purposes
Female sexual trauma	Movement of organisms from the urethra into the bladder with infection and retrograde spread to kidney

Acute Pyelonephritis

Pyelonephritis is an infection of the renal pelvis and interstitium. The causative microorganism is usually bacterial *(E. coli)* but can be a fungus or virus. (Common causes of pyelonephritis are summarized in Table 35-4.) Urinary obstruction and reflux of urine from the bladder (vesicoureteral reflux) are the most common underlying risk factors. (See Chapter 36 for a discussion of vesicoureteral reflux in children.) One or both kidneys may be involved. Most cases occur in women. The responsible microorganism is usually *E. coli, Proteus,* or *Pseudomonas.* The latter two microorganisms are more commonly associated with infections after urethral instrumentation or urinary tract surgery. These microorganisms also split urea to ammonia, making an alkaline urine that increases the risk of stone formation. Seeding from the kidney from bacteremia is less common.

Pathophysiology

The infection probably is spread by ascending microorganisms along the ureters, but spread may occur also by way of the bloodstream. The inflammatory process is usually focal and irregular, affecting primarily the pelvis, calyces, and medulla. The infection causes medullary infiltration of white blood cells with renal inflammation, renal edema, and purulent urine. The release of phagocytic lysozymes and oxygen radicals and the presence of other inflammatory mediators may damage tubular cells.[41] In severe infections, localized abscesses may form in the medulla and extend to the cortex. The tubules are primarily affected, but the glomeruli are usually spared. Necrosis of renal papillae can develop (Fig. 35-5). After the acute phase, healing occurs with deposition of scar tissue and atrophy of affected tubules. The number of bacteria decreases until the urine again becomes sterile. Acute pyelonephritis rarely causes renal failure.[42,43]

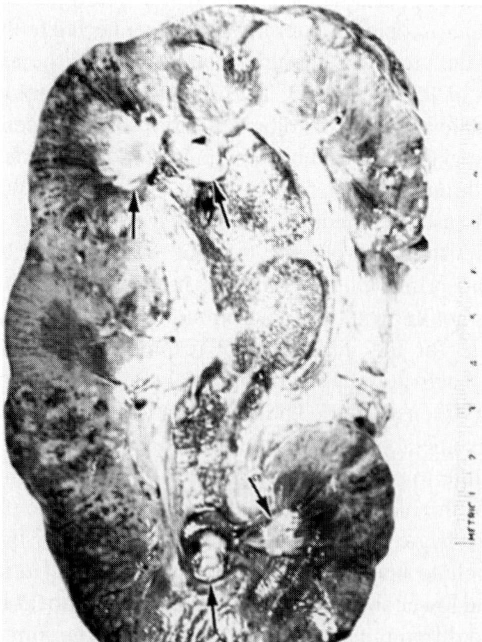

FIG. 35-5 Acute pyelonephritis. Papillary necrosis resulting from acute pyelonephritis and obstruction. Note necrotic papillae *(arrows);* mottled patchy cortical infiltrate of acute pyelonephritis; and congested, dilated renal pelvis. (From Kissane JM, editor: *Anderson's pathology,* ed 9, St Louis, 1990, Mosby.)

Clinical Manifestations

The onset of symptoms is usually acute, with fever, chills, flank or groin pain, frequency, dysuria, and costovertebral tenderness. Children and older adults may have nonspecific symptoms such as fever and malaise.

Evaluation and Treatment

Differentiating cystitis from pyelonephritis by clinical symptoms alone is difficult. The specific diagnosis is established by urine culture. The presence of antibody-coated bacteria is associated more closely with pyelonephritis.[44] White blood cell casts indicate pyelonephritis, but they are not always present in the urine.

Uncomplicated acute pyelonephritis responds well to 2 weeks of microorganism-specific antibiotic therapy. Follow-up urine cultures are obtained at 1 and 4 weeks after treatment if symptoms recur.[45] Antibiotic-resistant microorganisms or reinfection may occur in cases of urinary tract obstruction or reflux. Intravenous pyelography and voiding cystourethrography identify surgically correctable lesions.

Chronic Pyelonephritis

Chronic pyelonephritis is a persistent or recurrent autoimmune infection of the kidney with inflammation and scarring of the kidney. One or both kidneys may be involved. Recurrent infections from acute pyelonephritis may be associated with chronic pyelonephritis. The urine in chronic pyelonephritis may, however, contain only a few white cells and bacteria.[46] Generally, chronic pyelonephritis is more likely to occur in patients who have renal infections associated with some type of obstructive pathologic condition. This includes renal stones and vesicoureteral reflux.

Pathophysiology

Chronic urinary tract obstruction prevents elimination of bacteria in the normal flow of urine, resulting in progressive inflammation that causes fibrosis and scarring. The renal pelvis and calyces become dilated and blunted. Gradual destruction of the tubules occurs, with areas of atrophy or dilation and diffuse scarring. Impairment of function may affect urine-concentrating ability, with the excretion of a dilute urine, and can lead to chronic renal failure.

The lesions of chronic pyelonephritis are sometimes termed *chronic interstitial nephritis* because the inflammation and fibrosis are located in the interstitial spaces between the tubules. Chronic interstitial nephritis occurs from causes other than chronic pyelonephritis, including drug toxicity from analgesics such as phenacetin, aspirin, and acetaminophen; ischemia; irradiation; and immune complex diseases.

Clinical Manifestations

The early symptoms of chronic pyelonephritis are often minimal and may include hypertension. They may be similar to acute pyelonephritis, with frequency, dysuria, and flank pain, although milder and more vague. Progression leads to renal failure.

Evaluation and Treatment

The urinalysis usually shows white blood cells and less commonly white blood cell casts. Bacteriuria may be associated with the presenting symptoms. Intravenous pyelogram and ultrasound reveal a small kidney with a characteristic "clubbing" of the affected calyces. Treatment is related to the underlying cause. When obstruction occurs, it must be relieved. Antibiotics may be given, and recurrent infection requires prolonged antibiotic therapy.

GLOMERULAR DISORDERS

Immunologic mechanisms are primarily responsible for glomerular disease, with the exception of hereditary disorders, nephritis associated with systemic diseases, and vascular pathologic conditions. The onset of glomerular disease may be sudden or insidious, with hypertension, edema, and an elevated BUN. Low levels of serum complement are associated with acute poststreptococcal glomerulonephritis (APSGN) and normal levels with immunoglobulin A (IgA) nephropathy and idiopathic rapidly progressive glomerulonephritis (RPGN).[47] Some individuals are asymptomatic, and the disease is detected through the presence of microscopic hematuria from a routine urinalysis. The most definitive indication of glomerular disease is microscopic evaluation of tissue obtained by renal biopsy. The presence of clinical symptoms such as edema, hypertension, urinary changes, or systemic diseases associated with glomerular injury provides supporting evidence for the diagnosis.

Different types of glomerular disease may be associated with patterns of urinary sediment. Urine in diseases associated with a **nephrotic sediment** has massive proteinuria, lipiduria, and microscopic or no hematuria. Urine in diseases associated with a **nephritic sediment** is characterized by hematuria with red cell casts, white cell casts, and varying degrees of proteinuria, which is usually not severe. The sediment of chronic glomerular disease has waxy casts, granular casts, and less proteinuria and hematuria than nephrotic or nephritic sediment. Severe glomerular disease is usually associated with diffuse lesions and may demonstrate oliguria, hypertension, and renal failure. Focal lesions tend to produce less severe clinical symptoms. In some instances, hematuria may occur with excessive amounts of urine protein (e.g., in renal symptoms of lupus erythematosus and membranous proliferative glomerulonephritis).

Reduced GFR during glomerular disease is evidenced by the plasma creatinine concentration or creatinine clearance (see Chapter 34). Glomerular damage causes a decrease in glomerular membrane surface area, glomerular capillary blood flow, and driving hydrostatic pressure. In the presence of hypoalbuminemia, plasma fluid tends to move to the interstitial spaces, contributing to decreased blood volume, decreased renal blood flow, and decreased glomerular capillary hydrostatic pressure with a decline in GFR.

Edema is commonly associated with nephrotic syndrome (see p. 1204) or may be caused by salt and water retention from reduced GFR. Excessive fluid retention may cause systemic and pulmonary edema, requiring the use of diuretics or dialysis. The volume expansion that accompanies salt and water retention leads to hypertension. Excessive renin production is usually not a cause of hypertension in glomerular diseases unless it is associated with ischemia, as in uremia (see p. 1205), or with profound hypovolemia.

Death occurs in 2% to 5% of all persons during acute glomerular disease. During the first few weeks, the major life-threatening problems are acute renal insufficiency with fluid, electrolyte, and acid-base imbalances; acute hypertension that may cause hypertensive encephalopathy; circulatory failure; and pulmonary edema.

Glomerulonephritis

Glomerulonephritis is an inflammation of the glomerulus that can be caused by a variety of factors, including immunologic abnormalities, effects of drugs or toxins, vascular disorders, and systemic diseases. In most cases the exact cause of glomerular injury may be unknown. Immunologic alterations are most frequently responsible for glomerular injury (Fig. 35-6).[48,49] Glomerular disease is the most common cause of chronic and end-stage renal failure.

Types

The classification of glomerulonephritis is arbitrary and can be described according to cause, pathologic lesions, disease progression, or clinical presentation.[50] (Types of glomerular lesions are reviewed in Table 35-5, and features of types of glomerulonephritis are summarized in Table 35-6.)

Acute Glomerulonephritis

Acute glomerulonephritis is frequently associated with a group A (nephritogenic strain) poststreptococcal infection (acute poststreptococcal glomerulonephritis). The disease has an abrupt onset and usually occurs 7 to 10 days after a streptococcal infection of the throat (5% to 10% incidence) or skin (25% incidence), commonly in children (see Chapter 36).

Table 35-5 Types of Glomerular Lesions

Lesion	Characteristics
Diffuse	Relatively uniform involvement of most (>50%) or all glomeruli; most common form of glomerulonephritis
Focal	Changes in only some glomeruli (<50%), whereas others are normal
Segmental-local	Changes in one part of the glomerulus with other parts unaffected
Mesangial	Deposits of immunoglobulins in the mesangial matrix
Membranous	Thickening of the glomerular capillary wall
Proliferative	Increase in the number of glomerular cells
Sclerotic	Glomerular scarring from previous glomerular injury
Crescentic	Accumulation of proliferating cells within the Bowman space making the appearance of a crescent

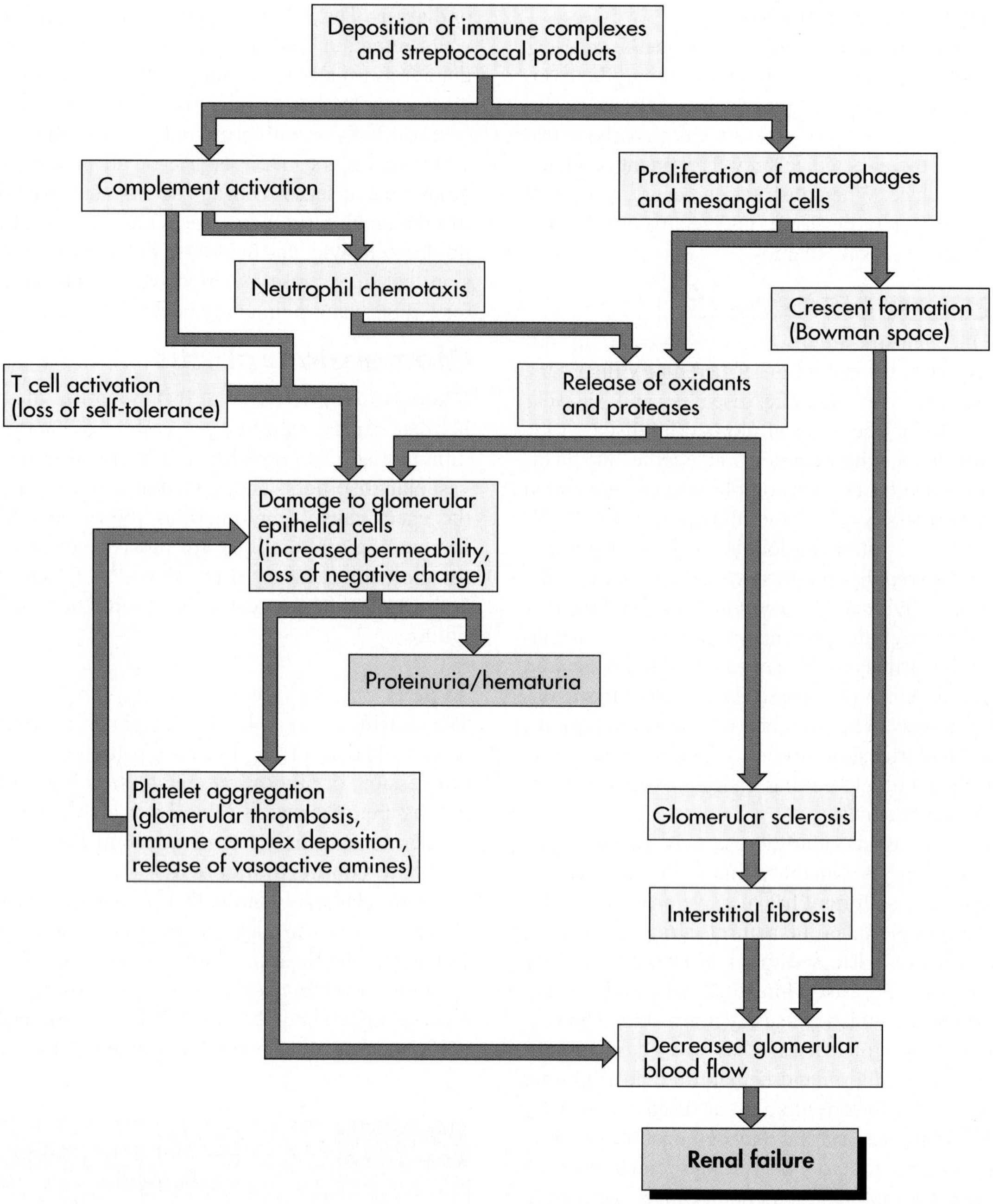

FIG. 35-6 Mechanisms of glomerular injury. (Adapted from Couser WG: rapidly progressive glomerulonephritis: classification, pathogenetic mechanisms, and therapy, *Am J Kidney Dis* 11(6):449, 1988.)

Sporadic occurrences have been observed after bacterial endocarditis, which may be associated with streptococcal or staphylococcal microorganisms, or after viral diseases such as varicella, hepatitis B, and hepatitis C.

Symptoms usually occur 10 to 21 days after infection and include hematuria, red blood cell casts, proteinuria, decreased GFR, oliguria, edema, and hypertension. The edema of acute glomerulonephritis tends to be around the eyes but may involve dependent areas such as the feet and ankles. Occasionally, ascites or pleural effusions develop. Serum complement levels are usually low because they are consumed by the initial infection. Immunofluorescent findings from renal biopsy indicate the presence of immune complex deposits in the glomerulus (complement C3 and IgG) and neutrophil and macrophage recruitment and activation, with diffuse mesangial cell and capillary endothelial cell proliferation of the entire glomeruli (Fig. 35-7).[51,52] The thickening of the glomerular membrane contributes to the decreased GFR. Activated complement inflammatory cytokines and growth factors attack epithelial cells, altering membrane permeability and leading to proteinuria. More severe renal disease is observed after a prolonged infection before antibiotic therapy, but there is no specific treatment for the glomerulonephritis. Most individuals, especially children, recover without significant loss of renal function or recurrence of the disease.

Table 35-6 Features of the Common Types of Glomerulonephritis

Type and Cause	Pathophysiology
Poststreptococcal Group A β-hemolytic streptococcus	Usually diffuse lesions; subepithelial deposits of IgG and complement complexes; infiltration of neutrophils and monocytes; proliferation of mesangial and epithelial cells; with occlusion of glomerular capillary blood flow and decreased glomerular filtration
Rapidly progressive or crescentic Nonspecific response to glomerular injury; can occur in any severe glomerular disease	Diffuse lesions; accumulation of fibrin, macrophages, and epithelial cell proliferation into the Bowman space forms crescents and occludes glomerular capillary blood flow decreasing glomerular filtration; anti–glomerular basement membrane antibodies lead to necrotizing, proliferative glomerulonephritis and renal failure
Membranoproliferative Usually idiopathic; associated with hypocomplementemia Type I: activation of classical complement pathway with nephrotic syndrome Type II: activation of alternate complement pathway with hematuria	Diffuse lesions; mesangial cell proliferation; thickening of basement membrane; subendothelial deposits of immune complex occlude glomerular capillary blood flow and decrease glomerular filtration
IgA nephropathy (Berger disease) Usually idiopathic; elevated IgA plasma levels	Usually focal, some diffuse lesions; mesangial cell proliferation with IgA deposits; release of inflammatory mediators with crescent formation, sclerosis, interstitial fibrosis, and decreased GFR
Minimal change disease (lipoid nephrosis) Usually idiopathic	Diffuse fusion of epithelial foot processes; loss of negative charge in basement membrane and increased permeability lead to severe proteinuria and nephrotic syndrome
Focal glomerulosclerosis Usually idiopathic	Similar to minimal change disease with focal glomerulosclerosis from hyaline deposits in the glomerular membrane resulting in proteinuria and nephrotic syndrome
Membranous nephropathy Usually idiopathic; can be associated with systemic diseases, i.e., hepatitis B virus, systemic lupus erythematosus, solid malignant tumors	Diffuse thickening of glomerular basement membrane and capillary wall from deposits of antibody and complement; increased permeability with proteinuria and nephrotic syndrome

IgG, Immunoglobulin G; *IgA,* immunoglobulin A; *GFR,* glomerular filtration rate.

A B C

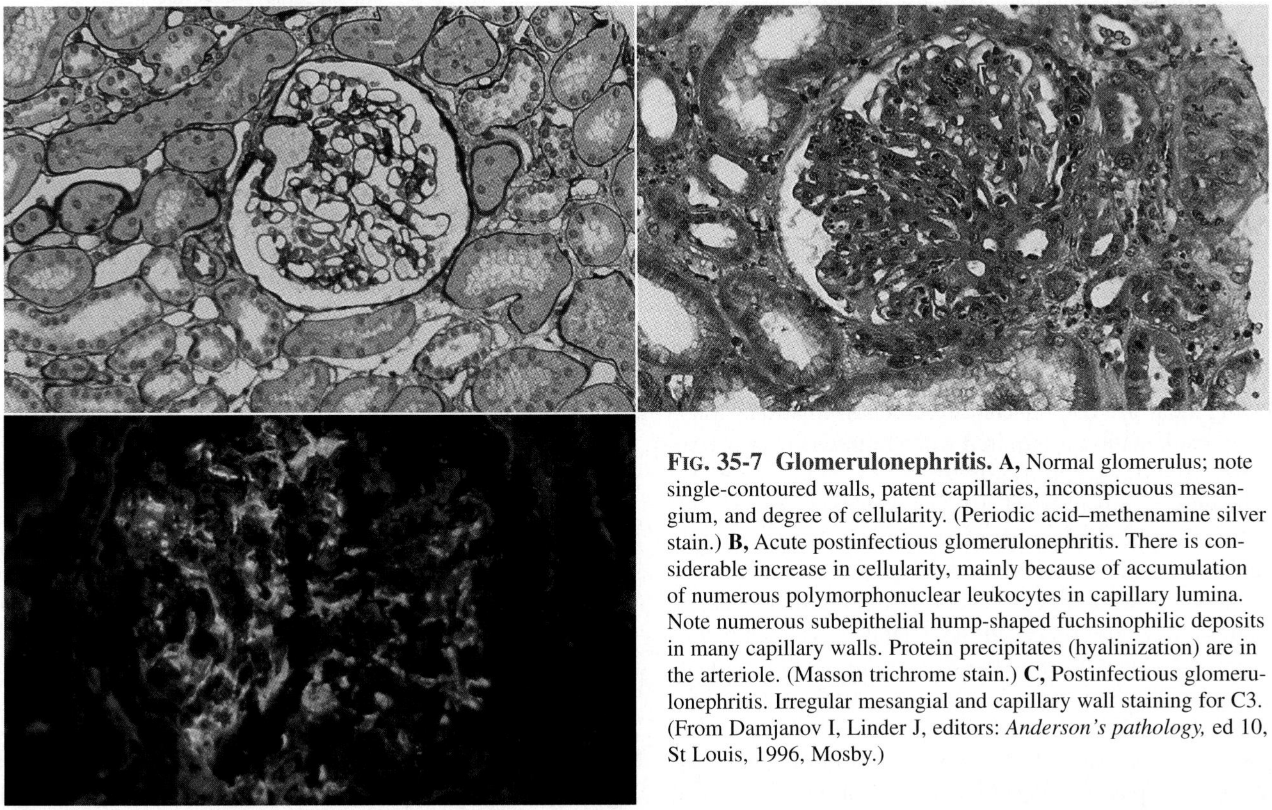

FIG. 35-7 Glomerulonephritis. A, Normal glomerulus; note single-contoured walls, patent capillaries, inconspicuous mesangium, and degree of cellularity. (Periodic acid–methenamine silver stain.) **B,** Acute postinfectious glomerulonephritis. There is considerable increase in cellularity, mainly because of accumulation of numerous polymorphonuclear leukocytes in capillary lumina. Note numerous subepithelial hump-shaped fuchsinophilic deposits in many capillary walls. Protein precipitates (hyalinization) are in the arteriole. (Masson trichrome stain.) **C,** Postinfectious glomerulonephritis. Irregular mesangial and capillary wall staining for C3. (From Damjanov I, Linder J, editors: *Anderson's pathology,* ed 10, St Louis, 1996, Mosby.)

IgA Nephropathy

IgA nephropathy is the most common form of glomerulonephritis in developed countries, especially Asia. The cause is unknown. The disease manifests with gross or microscopic (30% to 40%) hematuria 24 to 48 hours after an upper respiratory or gastrointestinal viral infection. Proteinuria, edema, and hypertension are less common. Abnormal glycosylated IgA, produced by the bone marrow, and complement molecules are trapped in the glomerular mesangium. Mesangial cells respond with proliferation from autocrine growth factors and release oxidants and proteases, contributing to glomerular injury and glomerulosclerosis. Treatment is symptomatic and prognosis is variable, with 50% progressing to renal failure.[53]

Rapidly Progressive Glomerulonephritis

Rapidly progressive glomerulonephritis (RPGN) is also known as subacute, crescentic, or extracapillary glomerulonephritis.[54] The disease affects primarily adults in their fifties and sixties and may be idiopathic or associated with a number of proliferative glomerular diseases (with diffuse proliferation of extracapillary cells), such as poststreptococcal glomerulonephritis and Goodpasture syndrome. Antineutrophil cytoplasmic antibodies with associated vasculitis are common in this disease.[55]

Anti–glomerular basement membrane disease (Goodpasture syndrome) is an example of RPGN. The disease is associated with antibody formation against both pulmonary capillary and glomerular basement membranes with pulmonary hemorrhage and glomerulonephritis. The disease is rare but occurs most commonly in men 20 to 30 years of age (lung hemorrhage) and older adults (renal disease).

By the time RPGN is diagnosed, renal insufficiency is apparent. There is extensive proliferation of cells into Bowman space. The cells become mixed with fibrin and form crescent-shaped deposits (Fig. 35-8). Typically, the glomerular injury is accompanied by a rapid decline in glomerular function progressing to renal failure in a few weeks or months. Hematuria is common and may be accompanied by proteinuria, edema, or hypertension.

RPGN has a relatively poor prognosis if not diagnosed and treated early. Plasma exchange combined with immunosuppression improves renal function.[51,56] Antiviral therapy reduces severity related to hepatitis C virus.[51,56] Anticoagulants, such as heparin or warfarin, may be of some benefit in reducing the fibrin component of crescent formation. Dialysis or transplantation is required when failure is irreversible.

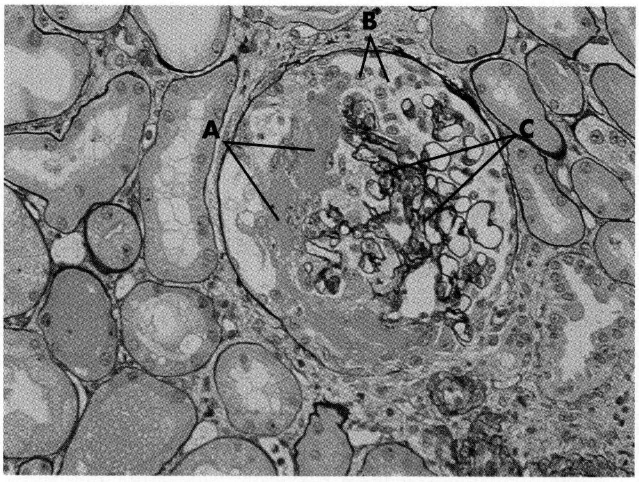

FIG. 35-8 Anti–glomerular basement membrane nephritis. Glomerulus with a fresh crescent consisting of fibrin and cells in the urinary space *(A)*. There is disruption of the basement membrane of the Bowman capsule, with migration of cells from the interstitium into the urinary space *(B)*. The capillary tufts *(C)* are distorted and compressed because of the crescent. Note the free erythrocytes in tubular lumina. The interstitium is mildly edematous. (Periodic acid–methenamine silver stain.) (Modified from Damjanov I, Linder J, editors: *Anderson's pathology,* ed 10, St Louis, 1996, Mosby.)

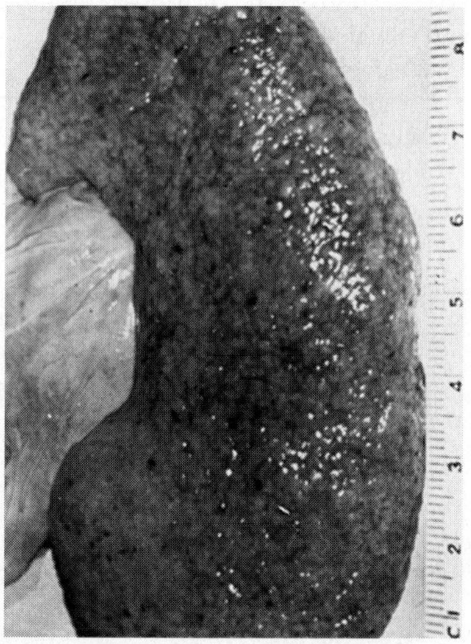

FIG. 35-9 End-stage chronic glomerulonephritis. Pebbly surface corresponds to surviving hypertrophied nephrons amid atrophy. (From Kissane JM, editor: *Anderson's pathology,* ed 9, St Louis, 1990, Mosby.)

Chronic Glomerulonephritis

Chronic glomerulonephritis encompasses several glomerular diseases with a progressive course leading to chronic renal failure. There may be no history of renal disease before the diagnosis, although several years of proteinuria and hematuria may have preceded the diagnosis. Various pathologic changes are evident in the glomerulus. Proliferation of mesangial cells (cells in connective tissue supporting the glomerular capillaries) may be focal or diffuse with segmental fibrosis and glomerular deterioration. Secondary tubular dilation and atrophy may develop. Hypercholesterolemia also has been associated with progressive glomerular injury. The proposed mechanism is related to glomerulosclerosis. The primary cause may be difficult to establish because advanced pathologic changes may obscure specific disease characteristics (Fig. 35-9). Insulin-dependent diabetes mellitus and lupus erythematosus are secondary causes of chronic glomerular injury.[57]

◆ *Pathophysiology*

Patterns of antigen-antibody complex deposition within the glomerular capillary filtration membrane have been estab-

Table 35-7 Immunologic Pathogenesis of Glomerulonephritis

Glomerular Injury	Mechanism
Soluble immune-complex glomerulonephritis (90%)	Formation of antibodies stimulated by the presence of endogenous or exogenous antigens results in circulating soluble antigen-antibody complexes, which are deposited in glomerular capillaries; glomerular injury occurring with complement activation and release of immunologic substances that lyse cells and increase membrane permeability; immune deposits with a microscopic appearance that fluoresce in a *granular pattern* when stained with fluorescein and viewed under ultraviolet light; severity of glomerular injury related to the number of complexes formed; a type III hypersensitivity
Anti–glomerular basement membrane glomerulonephritis (5%)	Antibodies are formed and act directly against the glomerular basement membrane; immune response that causes crescent formation and a *linear pattern* of immunofluorescence; generally associated with rapidly progressive renal failure such as Goodpasture syndrome
Alternative complement pathway	A relatively obscure mechanism associated with low levels of complement and membranoproliferative glomerulonephritis
Cell-mediated immunity	A delayed hypersensitivity response that damages the glomerulus; actual cellular mechanism not clearly understood

lished using light, electron, and immunofluorescent microscopy for different disease processes (Table 35-7). Electron microscopy differentiates morphologic changes within the glomerular capillary wall. Staining with fluorescein identifies different antibodies (i.e., IgG or IgA) and their configurations when viewed under ultraviolet light with a microscope (see Fig. 35-7, *C*).

Three types of immune mechanisms contribute to acute glomerular injury: (1) deposition of circulating soluble antigen-antibody complexes, (2) formation of antibodies specific against the glomerular basement membrane, and (3) streptococcal release of neuramidase, which alters IgG with binding of anti-IgG to the glomerulus.[58] The response of glomerular cells to inflammatory mediators leads to cell proliferation, sclerosis, and chronic impaired renal function. The severity of glomerular damage and renal insufficiency is related to the size, number, location (focal or diffuse), duration of exposure, and type of antigen-antibody complexes.

Glomerular damage generally occurs from activation of biochemical mediators of inflammation (complement, leukocytes, fibrin), which begins after the antibody or antigen-antibody complexes have localized in the glomerular capillary wall. Complement is deposited with the antibodies, followed by a sequence of metabolic events that initiate an attack on the glomerular membrane. Complement activation can serve as a chemotactic stimulus for attraction of neutrophils and monocytes. The neutrophils and monocytes further the inflammatory reaction by releasing lysosomal enzymes and reactive oxygen species, which damage glomerular cell walls.[52]

These processes alter membrane permeability and may cause loss of the negative electrical charge across the glomerular filtration membrane. Membrane damage can lead to platelet aggregation and degranulation, whereby platelets release vasoactive amines such as serotonin or histamine. These substances then increase glomerular permeability. Changes in membrane permeability and electrical charge permit the passage of protein molecules or red blood cells into the urine, causing proteinuria or hematuria or both. The coagulation system also may be activated and lead to fibrin deposition in the Bowman space, contributing to crescent formation (deposition of substances in the Bowman space). (Coagulation is discussed in Chapter 24.) Membrane proliferation, deposits in the membrane, mesangial proliferation, and swelling reduce renal blood flow and depress glomerular filtration.

Clinical Manifestations

Two major changes in the urine distinguish glomerulonephritis: (1) hematuria with red blood cell casts and (2) proteinuria exceeding 3 to 5 g/day, with albumin as the major protein. Several disorders may produce hematuria because bleeding can occur anywhere along the urinary tract. The characteristics of hematuria from red blood cells escaping through the glomerular membrane include a smoky brown-tinged urine, red blood cell casts, and an accompanying proteinuria. Bleeding from sites lower in the urinary tract may produce a pink- or red-colored urine. Glomerular bleeding provides prolonged contact with the acidic urine and transforms hemoglobin to methemoglobin, which has a brownish color and no blood clots. The immune-mediated inflammatory response with cellular infiltration decreases GFR, which leads to fluid retention. Salt and water are reabsorbed, contributing to fluid volume expansion and hypertension. The history and physical examination may disclose findings that differentiate glomerular disease from another source of urinary tract bleeding. Gross proteinuria is associated with nephrotic syndrome; a decrease in urine output accompanies a decreased GFR.

Mild proteinuria and hematuria may occur during the early years of the disease. Blood pressure may be normal. After 10 or 20 years, renal insufficiency begins to develop, followed by nephrotic syndrome and an accelerated progression to end-stage renal failure. Symptom patterns vary depending on the underlying cause. Steroids usually do not change the course of the disease, and dialysis or kidney transplantation ultimately may be necessary.

Evaluation and Treatment

The diagnosis of glomerular disease is confirmed by the progressive development of clinical manifestations and laboratory findings of abnormal urinalysis with proteinuria, red blood cells, white blood cells, and casts. In APSGN the streptococcal exoenzymes are elevated, such as antistreptolysin O and antistreptokinase. Serum complement is decreased, and serum creatinine concentration is elevated. Creatinine clearance evaluates the extent of glomerular damage. Microscopic evaluation from renal biopsy provides a specific determination of renal injury and type of pathology.

Management principles for treating glomerulonephritis are related to treating the primary disease, preventing or minimizing immune responses, and correcting accompanying problems such as edema, hypertension, hyperkalemia, and hyperlipidemia. Specific treatment regimens are necessary for particular types of glomerulonephritis.

Nephrotic Syndrome

Nephrotic syndrome is the excretion of 3.5 g or more of protein in the urine per day. The large amount of urine protein is characteristic of glomerular injury. Other findings include hypoalbuminemia, edema, hyperlipidemia, and lipiduria (Table 35-8). Lipoid nephrosis (minimal change disease), membranous glomerulonephritis, and focal glomerulosclerosis are directly related to nephrotic syndrome, although these conditions can occur with other types of glomerular disease.[59]

Secondary forms of nephrotic syndrome occur as a result of other organic pathologic processes. Systemic diseases often implicated in secondary nephrotic syndrome include diabetes mellitus, amyloidosis, systemic lupus erythematosus, and Henoch-Schönlein purpura. Nephrotic syndrome also is seen in association with certain drugs, infections, malignancies, and vascular disorders. When present as a secondary complication with renal diseases, nephrotic syndrome often signifies a more serious prognosis.

Pathophysiology

Loss of plasma proteins, particularly albumin and some immunoglobulins, occurs across the injured glomerular filtration membrane (Fig. 35-10). Disturbances in the glomerular basement membrane, which may be metabolic, biochemical, or physiochemical, lead to increased permeability to protein. Hypoalbuminemia results from urinary loss of albumin combined with a diminished synthesis of replacement albumin by the liver. Albumin is lost in the greatest quantity because of its high plasma concentration and low molecular weight.

Increased synthesis of plasma proteins may be insufficient to compensate for losses. Factors such as decreased dietary intake of protein from anorexia or malnutrition, or accompanying liver disease, may contribute to lower levels of plasma albumin. Loss of immunoglobulins may increase susceptibility to infections.

Clinical Manifestations

Proteinuria is an excessive amount of protein in the urine (up to 10 g/24 hr).[60] Many of the clinical manifestations of nephrotic syndrome are related to loss of serum proteins (see Table 35-8).[61]

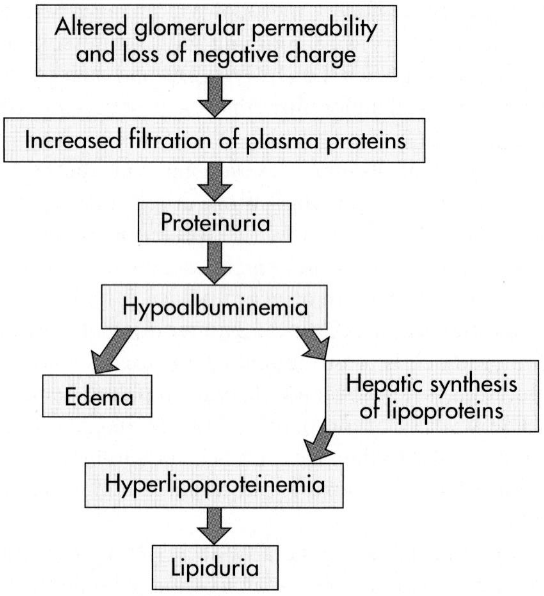

FIG. 35-10 Pathophysiology of nephrotic syndrome.

Table 35-8 Clinical Manifestations of Nephrotic Syndrome

Manifestation	Contributing Factors	Result
Proteinuria	Increased glomerular permeability, decreased proximal tubule reabsorption	Edema, increased susceptibility to infection from loss of immunoglobulins
Hypoalbuminemia	Increased urinary losses of protein	Edema
Edema	Hypoalbuminemia (decreased oncotic pressure, sodium and water retention, increased aldosterone and antidiuretic hormone [ADH] secretion), unresponsiveness to atrial natriuretic peptides	Soft, pitting, generalized edema
Hyperlipidemia	Decreased serum albumin; increased hepatic synthesis of very-low-density lipoproteins; increased cholesterol, phospholipids, triglycerides	Increases atherogenesis
Lipiduria	Sloughing of tubular cells containing fat (oval fat bodies); free fat from hyperlipidemia	Fat droplets that may float in urine
Decreased vitamin D	The globulin to which 1,25-vitamin D is attached for transport passes through the glomerulus and is lost in the urine	Decreased absorption of calcium from gut

Edema may be the first symptom (see Chapter 3). Renal edema is associated with hypoalbuminemia and is soft, pitting, and in areas of low tissue pressure, such as the periorbital regions. According to Starling's law, hydrostatic pressure acts to force fluid into the interstitial space at the arterial end of the capillaries. The hydrostatic pressure is balanced by the oncotic pressure of the plasma proteins, which tends to draw the fluid back into the capillaries at the venous end (see Chapter 3). Plasma albumin concentration in nephrotic syndrome is often reduced to 20% of normal, with a considerable decrease in the plasma oncotic pressure. The threat of decreased plasma volume from the accumulation of fluid in the tissues stimulates compensatory mechanisms. Among these mechanisms are activation of the renin-angiotensin-aldosterone system and antidiuretic hormone (ADH), which together lead to excessive sodium and water retention. The nephrotic kidney is also unresponsive to atrial natriuretic peptide with increased sodium and water retention.[62] Increased lymph flow may allow some compensation. Edema in the interstitial space may facilitate lymph flow by elevating tissue pressure, facilitating the return of interstitial fluid into the plasma compartment.

Levels of all the plasma lipids (triglycerides, phospholipids, cholesterol) are elevated, producing a hyperlipidemia. Hyperlipidemia is primarily related to increased synthesis by the liver, decreased lipoprotein catabolism,[63] reduced plasma oncotic pressure from hypoalbuminemia, and increased hepatic delivery of cholesterol precursors.[64] **Lipiduria** is manifested by lipid casts or free fat droplets that leak across the glomerular capillary walls and into the urine. Tubular epithelial cells that reabsorb lipoprotein also may be shed and appear in the urine as "oval fat bodies."

The hormone 25-hydroxycholecalciferol (vitamin D_3) is normally bound to a circulating globulin. If this is lost in the urine, there will be decreased absorption of intestinal calcium and hypocalcemia (see Chapter 3). Symptoms of vitamin D deficiency will develop, including low plasma levels of ionized calcium, secondary hyperparathyroidism, and osteomalacia.

Evaluation and Treatment

Nephrotic syndrome is diagnosed when the protein level in a 24-hour urine collection is greater than 3.5 g. Serum albumin decreases (to less than 3 g/dl), and serum cholesterol, phospholipids, and triglycerides increase. Fat bodies may be present in the urine. The specific pathology is identified by renal biopsy.

Nephrotic syndrome is commonly treated with a normal-protein, low-fat diet; salt restriction; diuretics; steroids; and occasionally albumin replacement.[65] Because the nephrotic state is caused primarily by protein depletion, dietary protein supplements (up to 100 g) are essential, unless renal failure has occurred. Diuretics may be used, particularly loop diuretics such as furosemide or ethacrynic acid, to control edema or hypertension. Care must be taken to observe for hypovolemia and hypokalemia or potassium toxicity in the presence of renal insufficiency. Aldactone may be combined with loop diuretics to suppress aldosterone activity and conserve potassium.

Because hyperlipidemia is associated with hypoalbuminemia, correction occurs when normal plasma albumin levels are reestablished. A low–saturated fat diet may be helpful in chronic nephrosis as a way of slowing down atherogenic processes. Drugs such as clofibrate are not safe to use when renal insufficiency exists. The underlying cause of nephrotic syndrome should be treated specifically if it is known.

RENAL FAILURE

Classification of Renal Dysfunction

The terms *renal insufficiency, renal failure, azotemia,* and *uremia* are all associated with decreasing renal function. Often, they are used synonymously, although with some distinctions. Generally, **renal insufficiency** refers to a decline in renal function to about 25% of normal or a GFR of 25 to 30 ml/min. Levels of serum creatinine and urea are mildly elevated. **Renal failure** often refers to significant loss of renal function. When less than 10% of renal function remains, this is termed **end-stage renal failure (ESRF).**

Renal failure may be acute and rapidly progressive (within hours), although the process may be reversible. Renal failure also can be chronic, progressing to ESRF over a period of months or years.[66] **Uremia** is a syndrome of renal failure and includes elevated blood urea and creatinine levels accompanied by fatigue, anorexia, nausea, vomiting, pruritus, and neurologic changes. The terms *azotemia* and *uremia* are sometimes incorrectly used interchangeably. **Azotemia** means increased serum urea levels and frequently increased creatinine levels as well. Renal insufficiency or renal failure causes azotemia. *Uremia* represents the numerous consequences related to renal failure, including retention of toxic wastes, deficiency states, and electrolyte disorders. Both azotemia and uremia indicate an accumulation of nitrogenous waste products in the blood, a common characteristic that explains the overlap in definitions of terms.

Types

Acute Renal Failure

Acute renal failure (ARF) is an abrupt reduction in renal function. Acute renal failure is usually associated with oliguria (urine output of less than 30 ml/hr or less than 400 ml/day), although urine output may be normal or increased. BUN and creatinine values are elevated. Most types of acute renal failure are reversible if diagnosed and treated early.[67] Acute renal failure can be caused by different clinical conditions, including severe hypotension, vascular obstruction, severe glomerular disease, or it can occur following administration of radiocontrast media. Acute renal failure is commonly classified as prerenal, intrarenal, or postrenal (Table 35-9). A combination of ischemic or hepatotoxic factors may produce acute renal failure.[68]

Pathophysiology

Prerenal acute renal failure is the most common cause of ARF and is caused by impaired renal blood flow. The GFR declines because of the decrease in filtration pressure. Poor

Table 35-9 Classification of Acute Renal Failure

Area of Dysfunction	Possible Causes
Prerenal	Hypovolemia Hemorrhagic blood loss (trauma, gastrointestinal bleeding, complications of childbirth) Loss of plasma volume (burns, peritonitis) Water and electrolyte losses (severe vomiting or diarrhea, intestinal obstruction, uncontrolled diabetes mellitus, inappropriate use of diuretics) Hypotension or hypoperfusion Septic shock Cardiac failure or shock Massive pulmonary embolism Stenosis or clamping of renal artery
Intrarenal	Acute tubular necrosis (postischemic or nephrotoxic) Glomerulopathies Malignant hypertension Coagulation defects
Postrenal	Obstructive uropathies (usually bilateral) Ureteral obstruction (edema, tumors, stones, clots) Bladder neck obstruction (enlarged prostate)

perfusion can result from renal vasoconstriction, hypotension, hypovolemia, hemorrhage, or inadequate cardiac output. Acute prerenal failure may occur when chronic renal failure exists if a sudden stress is imposed on already marginally functioning kidneys. Failure to restore blood volume or blood pressure may cause acute tubular necrosis or acute cortical necrosis.[69]

Intrarenal acute renal failure may result from acute tubular necrosis, cortical necrosis, acute glomerulonephritis, vascular disease (malignant hypertension, disseminated intravascular coagulation, and renal vasculitis), or interstitial disease (drug allergy). **Acute tubular necrosis (ATN)** is the most common cause of acute renal failure.[70] The terms *acute tubular necrosis* and *acute renal failure* are sometimes used interchangeably, but the conditions are not the same because acute renal failure can occur without ATN. ATN is generally described as postischemic or nephrotoxic.

ATN caused by ischemia occurs most frequently after surgery (40% to 50% of cases), but ATN is also associated with sepsis, obstetric complications, severe burns, or trauma. A severe episode of hypotension often associated with hypovolemia is a significant contributing event. The ischemia generates toxic oxygen free radicals and inflammatory mediators that cause cell swelling, injury, and necrosis, a form of reperfusion injury, particularly in the outer medulla.[71,72] Nephrotoxic ATN can be produced by numerous antibiotics, but the aminoglycosides (neomycin, gentamicin, tobramycin) are the major culprits. The drugs tend to accumulate in the renal cortex and may not cause renal failure until after treatment is complete. Radiocontrast media (x-ray media) and cisplatin also may be nephrotoxic. Dehydration, advanced age, concurrent renal insufficiency, and diabetes mellitus tend to enhance nephrotoxicity from either aminoglycosides or radiocontrast media. Other substances such as excessive myoglobin (oxygen-transporting substance in muscles), carbon tetrachloride, heavy metals (mercury, arsenic), methoxyflurane anesthesia, or bacterial toxins may promote renal failure. Necrosis caused by nephrotoxins is usually uniform and limited to the proximal tubules. Ischemic necrosis tends to be patchy and may be distributed along any part of the nephron.

Three pathophysiologic explanations have been proposed to account for the oliguria of ATN.[73] All three mechanisms probably contribute to oliguria in varying degrees throughout the course of the disease (Fig. 35-11). The classic explanation is the *tubular obstruction theory.* This theory suggests that ischemia of the tubules causes sloughing of cells, cast formation (composed of granular and epithelial cells), or ischemic edema, resulting in tubular obstruction. Obstruction then causes a retrograde increase in pressure and reduces the GFR. Renal failure can occur within 24 hours.

The *back leak theory* suggests that glomerular filtration remains normal but that tubular reabsorption of filtrate is accelerated because of changes in permeability caused by ischemia. Most studies of renal function in ATN, however, indicate a decrease in glomerular filtration, and back leak may be only a minor aspect of acute failure (Fig. 35-12).

Alterations in renal blood flow are considered by some authorities to be a major cause of decreased glomerular filtration and decreased intrarenal blood flow. The exact mechanism is unknown, although afferent arteriolar constriction may be produced by an intrarenal release of angiotensin II. Specific vasoactive agents released from endothelial cells may contribute to regional hypoxia. Ischemia also may contribute to changes in glomerular permeability and decreased GFR.

Postrenal acute renal failure is rare and occurs with urinary tract obstruction that affects the kidneys bilaterally (e.g., bladder outlet obstruction, prostatic hypertrophy, or bilateral ureteral obstruction). A pattern of several hours of anuria with flank pain followed by polyuria is a characteristic finding. This type of renal failure can occur after diagnostic catheterization of the ureters, a procedure that may cause edema of the tubular lumen.

◆ *Clinical Manifestations*

The clinical progression of acute renal failure with recovery of renal function occurs in three phases: oliguria, diuresis, and recovery. Oliguria begins within 1 day after a hypotensive event and lasts for 1 to 3 weeks, but it may regress in several hours or extend for several weeks, depending on the duration of ischemia and severity of toxic injury. Anuria (urine output less than 50 ml/day) is uncommon in ATN, but 10% to 20% of cases have nonoliguric failure. Anuria suggests bilateral renal artery occlusion, obstructive uropathy, or acute cortical necrosis. Nonoliguric failure usually represents less severe injury. The urine output may vary in volume, but the BUN and plasma creatinine concentrations increase (plasma creatinine is inversely proportional to the GFR).

Other early manifestations depend on the underlying cause of renal failure. Individuals who have experienced trauma or surgery or persons in a catabolic state may have more rapid

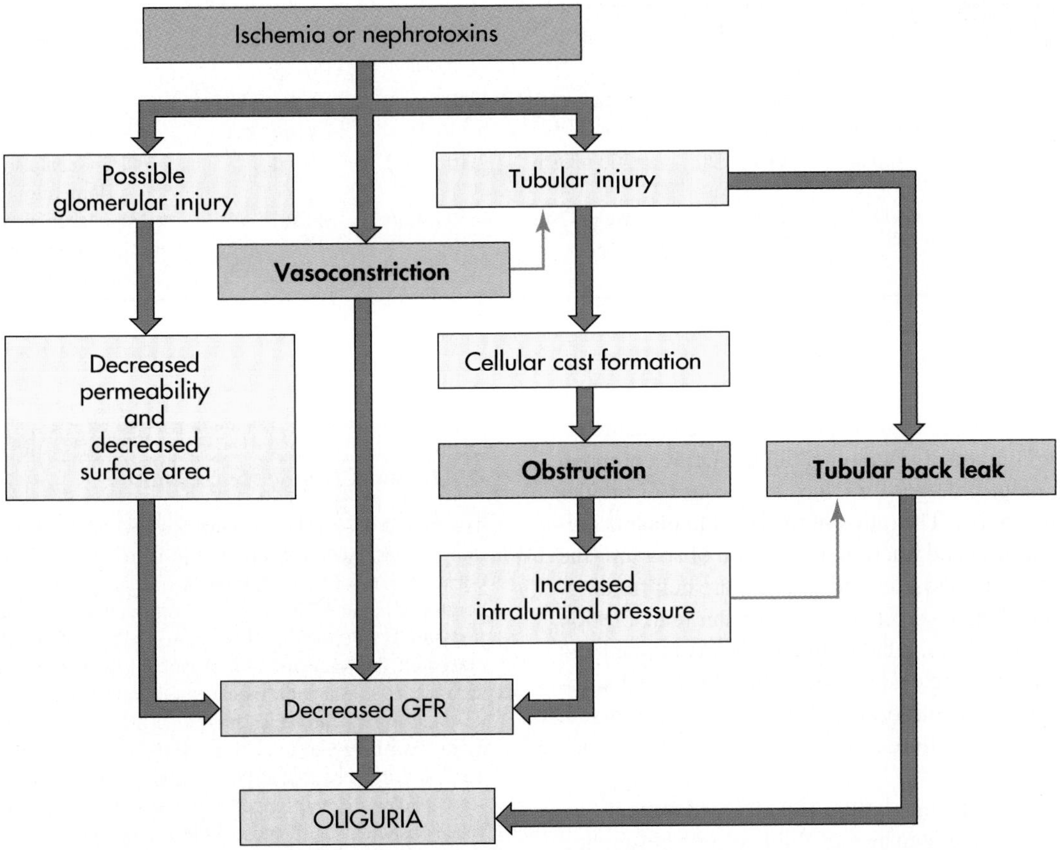

FIG. 35-11 Mechanisms of oliguria in acute renal failure. *GFR,* Glomerular filtration rate.

elevations in BUN. They are prone to hyperkalemia and hyperphosphatemia from cellular breakdown. Fluid retention may cause edema. Symptoms of congestive heart failure develop in persons with cardiac disease. Nausea, vomiting, and fatigue accompany uremia and electrolyte imbalances. Wound healing is delayed, and the risk of infection, particularly pneumonia, is greater. Nonoliguric renal failure generally has a better prognosis because of fewer complications. Oliguric patients may require maintenance dialysis to attenuate symptoms of renal failure.

As renal function improves, increase in urine volume (diuresis) is progressive. During the early diuretic phase the tubules are still damaged. Sodium and potassium are lost in the urine, and there is a greater risk for hypokalemia. Volume depletion may ensue, with fluid losses of 3 to 4 L/day. Fluid and electrolyte balance must be carefully monitored and excessive urinary losses replaced.

Serial measurements of plasma creatinine provide an index of renal function during the recovery phase. Return to normal status may take 3 to 12 months, and approximately 30% of individuals do not have full recovery of a normal GFR or tubular function.

◆ *Evaluation and Treatment*

The diagnosis of ATN is related to the cause of the disease. A history of surgery, trauma, or cardiovascular disorders is common. Exposure to nephrotoxins also must be considered.

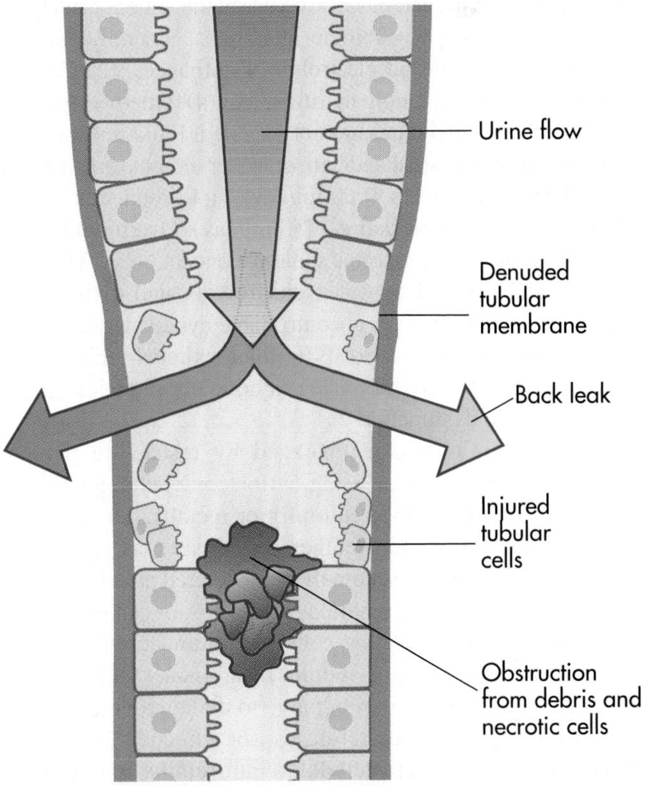

FIG. 35-12 Theories of oliguria. Diagram representing the back leak and obstruction theories of oliguria in acute renal failure.

Table 35-10 Differentiation of Acute Oliguric Renal Failure

	Urine Volume	Urine Specific Gravity	Urine Osmolality	Urine Sodium	BUN/Plasma Creatinine	FE_{Na}*
Prerenal failure	<400ml	1.016-1.020	>500 mOsm	<10 mEq/L	>15:1	<1% (seen also in acute glomerulonephritis)
Acute tubular necrosis	<400ml	1.010-1.012	<400 mOsm	>30 mEq/L	<15:1	>1% (seen also in urinary tract obstruction and renal parenchymal disease)

$$^*FE_{Na} = \frac{\text{Urine Na/plasma Na}}{\text{Urine creatinine/plasma creatine}} \times 100.$$

The diagnostic challenge is to differentiate prerenal acute renal failure from intrarenal acute renal failure. Urine composition provides helpful diagnostic clues to changes in tubular function (Table 35-10). The ratios of the BUN to plasma creatinine concentration and fractional excretion of sodium (the ratio of filtered sodium to excreted sodium) are helpful diagnostic indicators. The tests reflect renal tubular reabsorption ability. In prerenal failure, tubular function is maintained and salt, water, and urea are reabsorbed. With ATN, reabsorption and urinary concentration abilities are compromised. Other causes of renal failure also may exhibit similar clinical findings.

Prevention of acute renal failure is a major treatment factor and involves (1) maintenance of fluid volume before and after surgery or diagnostic procedures and (2) use of mannitol. Mannitol causes renal vasodilation with increased renal blood flow and GFR.

The primary goal of therapy is to maintain the individual's life until renal function has recovered. Management principles directly related to physiologic alterations generally include (1) correcting fluid and electrolyte disturbances, (2) treating infections, (3) maintaining nutrition, and (4) remembering that drugs or their metabolites are not excreted. Fluid replacement must be carefully calculated with consideration of urine losses, insensible losses (up to 1000 ml/day), and production of endogenous water by oxidation (450 ml/day). Overhydration of patients dilutes their plasma sodium concentration. **Dialysis** (mechanical removal of water, electrolytes, and toxins from the blood) is indicated for uncontrollable hyperkalemia or acidosis or severe fluid overload. Continuous renal replacement therapy is particularly promising in critically ill patients with multiple organ dysfunction.[74]

Hyperkalemia can be managed by restricting dietary sources of potassium or using cation-ion exchange resins, which may be administered orally or rectally. These resins exchange potassium for another cation, such as sodium in the bowel, and the potassium then is excreted attached to the resin. Dialysis may be required, or potassium can temporarily be driven back into the cells by administering glucose and insulin or by infusing sodium bicarbonate. Glucose metabolism causes potassium to move to the intracellular fluid, and insulin infusions therefore can be effective in shifting potassium from the extracellular to intracellular space, along with the transport of glucose, within 30 minutes. (Glucose metabolism is discussed in Chapter 20.) Causing alkalemia with sodium bicarbonate also shifts potassium into cells in exchange for hydrogen ions.

NUTRITION & DISEASE
Acute and Chronic Renal Failure

Traditional approaches to nutrition and azotemic control rely on renal replacement therapy and protein and fluid restriction. The consequences of these approaches have been episodic and partial control of azotemia; inadequate nitrogenous and caloric therapy, particularly in critically ill patients; and loss of amino acids during dialysis. Continuous renal replacement therapy has permitted new approaches to nutrition management with adaptation to individual needs. Calories can be given to meet daily energy expenditure, nitrogen can be given to achieve neutral nitrogen balance, and vitamins and trace elements can be given to meet expected demands. Adequate nutritional support promotes renal recovery and may prevent consequences of muscle weakness and immune dysfunction.

Indices of malnutrition have also been established for individuals with end-stage renal disease; 20% to 50% are estimated to be malnourished, with morbidity and mortality significantly affected. Catabolism and nutrient loss during dialysis are well documented. Effects of dietary restriction must be closely monitored, and appropriate enteral supplementation must be provided. A supplemented very-low-protein diet can be safely used in patients with chronic renal failure without adverse effects on the clinical and nutritional status of the individual and may delay the onset of end-stage renal failure. Intradialytic parenteral nutrition and use of amino acid dialysate are promising options.

Data from Aparicio M et al: *Journal of the American Society of Nephrology* 11:708-716, 2000; Bellomo R, Ronco C: *Am J Kidney Dis* 28(5, suppl 3):S58, 1996; Ikizler TA, Hakim RM: *Kidney Int* 50(2):343, 1996; Kierdorf HP: *New Horiz* 3(4):699, 1995.

Careful monitoring of the electrocardiogram for peaking T waves is essential for patients with hyperkalemia. Intravenous infusion of calcium is the most rapid method of treating cardiac effects of hyperkalemia. Calcium decreases the threshold potential and reduces the membrane excitability caused by hyperkalemia (see Chapter 3). Calcium should be used only in emergencies, however, because hypercalcemia also may cause cardiac arrest.

Azotemia is generally controlled and nutrition maintained with a low-protein, high-carbohydrate diet. Essential amino acid replacement can be given orally or parenterally. Adequate carbohydrate intake slows protein catabolism and helps pre-

WHAT'S NEW? Continuous Renal Replacement Therapy

Continuous renal replacement therapy (CRRT) is a treatment that provides a form of continuous dialysis for acute renal failure. It is replacing intermittent hemodialysis (IHD) or peritoneal dialysis, particularly for critically ill individuals. Generally, there are two forms of CRRT, hemofiltration and hemodiafiltration. Each may be further subdivided into arteriovenous or venovenous, depending on the site of vascular access. Hemofiltration removes excess fluid and solutes (urea, creatinine, sodium, potassium) by pumping blood through the semipermeable membranes of a hemofilter in a compartment of ultrafiltrate. Individuals must be carefully monitored for either volume excess or deficit and electrolyte imbalance. Hemodiafiltration is a combination of hemofiltration and hemodialysis with the removal of solutes by diffusion gradients from the blood across semipermeable membranes to a dialysis solution. In clinical trials comparing CRRT and IHD in critically ill patients, CRRT proved to be a better treatment and resulted in better outcomes. Fluids, wastes, and inflammatory mediators are removed in a controlled manner, and there are better metabolic control, hemodynamic stability, and tissue oxygenation. There are opportunities for early and aggressive nutritional support, decreased duration of acute renal failure, and prevention of multiple organ failure.

Data from Druml W: Metabolic aspects of continuous renal replacement therapies, *Kidney Int Suppl* 72:S56, 1999; Meyer MM: Renal replacement therapies, *Crit Care Clin* 16(1):29, 2000; van Bommell E et al: *Am J Nephrol* 15(3):192, 1995.

vent hyperkalemia. Because sepsis is a common serious or fatal complication of renal failure, observation for signs of infection and early treatment with antibiotics are necessary. Drug dosage levels may require adjustment if they are metabolized or excreted by the kidneys. Recovery may take up to 1 year.

Chronic Renal Failure

The kidney has many important regulatory functions, including body fluid volume, solute concentration and dilution, acid-base balance, excretion of waste products, and secretion of hormones that regulate red blood cell production, blood pressure, and calcium metabolism. Progressive and irreversible loss of renal function **(chronic renal failure),** regardless of the cause, affects these vital processes with changes manifest throughout all organ systems. The kidneys, however, exhibit remarkable adaptive abilities, and symptomatic changes resulting from increased creatinine, urea, and potassium and alterations in salt and water balance usually do not become apparent until the renal function declines to less than 25% of normal.

Pathophysiology

Different theories have been proposed to account for the adaptation to loss of renal function. One view suggests that the adaptive response depends on the particular location of kidney damage. For example, tubular interstitial diseases damage primarily the tubular or medullary parts of the nephron, producing problems such as renal tubular acidosis, salt wasting, and difficulty diluting or concentrating the urine. When there is primarily vascular or glomerular damage, proteinuria, hematuria, and nephrotic syndrome are more prominent. This theory is useful for planning treatment in early stages of renal failure when symptomatic differences in renal disease may be distinct.

A second theory, the *intact nephron hypothesis,* proposes that loss of nephron mass with progressive kidney damage causes the remaining nephrons to sustain normal or increased function. These nephrons are capable of a compensatory expansion in their rates of filtration, reabsorption, and secretion. They also can maintain a constant rate of excretion in the presence of a declining GFR. The increased workload is achieved primarily by hypertrophy and hyperfunction of the remaining nephrons.

The intact nephron hypothesis explains adaptive changes in solute and water regulation that occur with advancing renal failure. Although the urine of an individual with chronic renal failure may contain abnormal amounts of protein and red and white blood cells or casts, the major end products of excretion will be similar to normally functioning kidneys until advanced stages of renal failure, when there is a significant reduction of functioning nephrons.[75]

The *hyperfiltration hypothesis* provides an explanation for progressive failure of intact nephrons. Continued long-term exposure to increased capillary pressure and flow leads to glomerulosclerosis and loss of GFR.[76,77] This pathology is common to diabetic and hypertensive nephropathy. Use of angiotensin-converting enzyme inhibitors combined with other drugs (calcium channel blockers or beta blockers) slows this process.[78,79] Table 35-11 summarizes factors contributing to the pathophysiology of chronic renal failure.

Creatinine and Urea Clearance

Creatinine is constantly released from muscle and excreted primarily by glomerular filtration with relatively no reabsorption and some secretion. In a steady state, the amount produced approximates the amount filtered and excreted. If either the rate of production or the GFR changes, the plasma concentration of creatinine changes until the amount excreted again equals the amount produced. Therefore, if the GFR falls, as in chronic renal failure, the plasma creatinine level increases by a reciprocal amount to maintain a constant rate of excretion. Because no significant tubular adjustment occurs for creatinine (i.e., tubular secretion), the plasma levels continue to increase as the GFR decreases. This relationship allows the plasma creatinine concentration to serve as an estimate of changing glomerular function.[80] (This relationship is represented in Fig. 35-13.)

The clearance of urea is similar, although urea is both filtered and reabsorbed and varies with the state of hydration and diet. Urea clearance therefore is less than the GFR. If protein intake and metabolism are constant, however, plasma levels increase as the GFR declines. Thus no tubular adaptation modifies urea levels because urea is excreted primarily by glomerular filtration.

Sodium and Water Balance

Levels of sodium must be regulated within narrow limits, because sodium is the major extracellular solute. In chronic

Table 35-11 Factors Contributing to Pathophysiology of Renal Failure

Factor	Characteristics
Creatinine and urea clearance	In chronic renal failure, the GFR falls and the plasma creatinine concentration increases by a reciprocal amount; because there is no regulatory adjustment for creatinine, plasma levels continue to rise and serve as an index of changing glomerular function. As GFR declines, urea clearance increases. (NOTE: Urea is both filtered and reabsorbed and varies with the state of hydration.)
Sodium and water balance	In chronic renal failure, sodium load delivered to nephrons exceeds normal, so excretion must increase; thus less is reabsorbed. Obligatory loss occurs, leading to sodium deficits and volume depletion. As GFR is reduced, ability to concentrate and dilute urine diminishes.
Phosphate and calcium balance	Changes in acid-base balance affect phosphate and calcium balance. The major disorders associated with chronic renal failure are reduced renal phosphate excretion, decreased renal synthesis of 1,25-$(OH)_2$ vitamin D_3, and hypocalcemia. Hypocalcemia leads to secondary hyperparathyroidism, GFR falls, and progressive hyperphosphatemia, hypocalcemia, and dissolution of bone result.
Hematocrit	Because of anemia that accompanies chronic renal failure, lethargy, dizziness, and low hematocrit are common.
Potassium balance	In chronic renal failure, tubular secretion of potassium increases until oliguria develops. Use of potassium-sparing diuretics also may precipitate elevated serum potassium levels. As disease progresses, total body potassium levels can rise to life-threatening levels and dialysis is required.
Acid-base balance	In early renal insufficiency, acid excretion and bicarbonate reabsorption are increased to maintain normal pH. When GFR reaches 30% to 40%, metabolic acidosis begins. When end-stage renal failure develops, the metabolic acidosis may be severe enough to require dialysis.

GFR, Glomerular filtration rate.

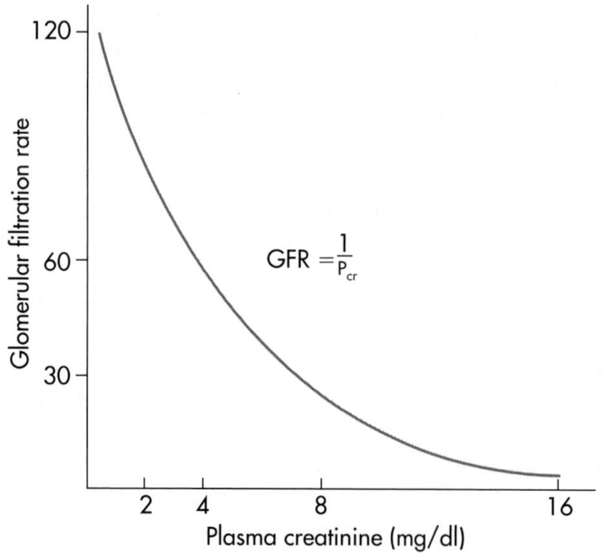

FIG. 35-13 Plasma creatinine (P_{CR}) and glomerular filtration rate (GFR).

renal failure the sodium load delivered to each remaining nephron is greater than normal, so the fractional excretion of sodium (the ratio of excreted to filtered sodium) must increase to maintain normal sodium balance. Increased excretion of sodium is accomplished by a decrease in the fractional reabsorption of sodium (ratio of reabsorbed to filtered sodium). Although the tubules exhibit a compensatory increased reabsorption, a large obligatory loss remains.[81]

Although the nephron is highly efficient at excreting sodium, it has difficulty conserving sodium when GFR decreases to 25% (approximately 25 ml/min) of normal. At this GFR an obligatory loss of 20 to 40 mEq of sodium per day occurs. If dietary intake is less than this amount, sodium deficits and volume depletion occur. These may be caused by osmotic diuresis from loss of urea or by an inability to inhibit natriuretic hormone after a sudden decrease in sodium intake.

The regulation of water balance and osmolality is normally achieved by urinary concentration mediated by ADH. As GFR is reduced, ability to concentrate and dilute the urine diminishes. In earlier stages of renal failure, this may be caused by osmotic diuresis produced by increased fractional excretion of solutes by the remaining nephrons or by a decreased tubular response to ADH. Individual nephrons can maintain water balance until severe renal failure occurs and GFR declines to 15% to 20% of normal with extensive loss of nephron and tubular function. At this stage the urinary concentration becomes fixed and approaches that of the plasma at 285 mOsm/L with a specific gravity of about 1.010.

Potassium Balance

Urinary excretion of potassium is related primarily to distal tubular secretion mediated by aldosterone and sodium-potassium adenosine triphosphatase (see Chapter 3). In renal failure there is increased tubular secretion that provides effective regulation until the onset of oliguria. Larger amounts of potassium are also lost through the bowel.[82] Although nonoliguric patients can maintain potassium excretion with normal dietary intake, they are more prone to develop hyperkalemia with increased loading (i.e., use of salt substitutes). Use of potassium-sparing diuretics, such as spironolactone (Aldactone), volume depletion, acute infection, severe acidosis, or marked hyperglycemia also may precipitate elevated levels of serum potassium. With progression of disease to end-stage renal failure, total body potassium can increase to life-threatening levels and must be controlled by dialysis.[83]

Table 35-12 Calcium and Phosphate Metabolism in Chronic Renal Failure

Kidney	Plasma	Bone
Decreased renal production of vitamin D_3	Decreased source of calcium from gut	Decreased calcium deposition
	Increased PTH secretion	
Decreased phosphate excretion	Elevated phosphate	
	Formation of $CaHPO_4$	
	Decreased ionized calcium	
Increased phosphate excretion (phosphaturia)	Increased PTH secretion (secondary hyperparathyroidism)	Release of calcium and phosphate
Increased calcium reabsorption and increased vitamin D formation (increased intestinal absorption of calcium)	Increased calcium	Osteitis fibrosa, osteomalacia, calcium deposits in soft tissue (occurs when kidney fails to respond to PTH secretion because of loss of renal mass and calcium and phosphate continue to be absorbed from bone)

PTH, Parathyroid hormone.

Acid-Base Balance

The intake of a normal diet produces 50 to 100 mEq of hydrogen per day. These ions are secreted from the renal tubules and excreted in the urine combined with phosphate and ammonia buffers (buffering is described in Chapter 3). During early stages of renal insufficiency, normal pH is maintained by an increased rate of acid excretion and bicarbonate reabsorption by individual nephrons. Metabolic acidosis begins to develop when the GFR decreases by 30% to 40%, primarily because of decreased ammonia synthesis and decreased bicarbonate reabsorption. Phosphate buffers remain effective until late stages of chronic renal failure. When end-stage renal failure develops, serum bicarbonate levels stabilize at 15 to 20 mEq/L, partly because the excess hydrogen is buffered by anions in bone. Individuals with end-stage renal failure develop metabolic acidosis, which may be severe enough to require dialysis.

Phosphate and Calcium Balance

The metabolism of calcium and phosphate is mediated by parathyroid hormone (PTH) and vitamin D. Changes in acid-base balance also influence the status of calcium and phosphate (see Chapter 3). The major calcium and phosphate disorders associated with chronic renal failure are reduced renal phosphate excretion, decreased renal synthesis of 1,25-$(OH)_2$ vitamin D_3 (the active form of vitamin D), and hypocalcemia (Table 35-12).

In early chronic renal failure, excreted phosphate levels decrease and the plasma phosphate concentration increases because of the decrease in GFR. The elevated plasma phosphate binds calcium ($CaHPO_4$), causing hypocalcemia. The decreased calcium stimulates the secretion of PTH. The PTH causes release of calcium from bone and enhanced urinary excretion of phosphate. The adaptive effect is a secondary hyperparathyroidism with return of phosphate and calcium levels toward normal (see Chapter 20). With each incremental loss of GFR, however, the effectiveness of PTH in maintaining phosphate balance diminishes. Reducing the dietary intake of phosphate and providing calcium supplementation are helpful at this early stage of failure. When the GFR declines to 25% of normal, however, PTH is no longer effective in maintaining serum phosphate levels. The persistent decreased GFR and hyperparathyroidism cause progressive hyperphosphatemia, hypocalcemia, and dissolution of bone (e.g., osteitis fibrosa, osteomalacia).[84]

Hypocalcemia and bone disease are accelerated by impaired synthesis of 1,25-vitamin D_3 when loss of functioning nephrons is significant and GFR is less than 25% of normal. Lack of the active form of vitamin D reduces intestinal absorption of calcium and impairs the effectiveness of calcium and phosphate resorption from bone by PTH. The toxicity of uremia also may suppress vitamin D action in the gut. This depletion can be treated with vitamin D supplements, but larger than normal doses are required. A negative calcium balance also occurs when acidosis is present, which is common in chronic renal failure. Generally, patients with advanced chronic renal failure have high phosphate and low serum calcium concentrations. The secondary hyperparathyroidism, however, may cause calcium levels to approach normal, and in a small percentage of cases they may be elevated.

Hematocrit

Normochromic-normocytic anemia accompanies chronic renal failure because of inadequate production of erythropoietin, decreased red blood cell life span, and blood loss related to diseased kidneys and the uremic state. Lethargy, dizziness, and low hematocrit are common findings.[85]

Lipids

Hypertriglyceridemia occurs in 30% to 70% of individuals with chronic renal failure. There is a high ratio of high-density lipoprotein (HDL) to low-density lipoprotein (LDL) with accelerated atherosclerosis.[86] Uremia produces a deficiency of lipoprotein lipase in capillary endothelium of muscle and fat tissue and decreased hepatic triglyceride lipase. Decreased lipolytic activity results in a reduction of HDL. Apolipoprotein B is also elevated, accelerating atherogenesis.

Proteins

Proteinuria and a catabolic state contribute to the negative nitrogen balance of chronic renal failure. Muscle protein diminishes, and serum levels of albumin, complement, and transferrin are frequently low. Proteinuria may independently cause renal damage by promoting inflammation and fibrosis.[87] The amount of proteinuria is also related to the extent of renal injury and predicts disease progression.[88] Restricting dietary protein intake slows the decline in GFR in chronic renal failure, particularly in the case of diabetic nephropathy.[89]

Table 35-13 Systemic Effects of Uremia

System	Manifestations	Mechanisms	Treatment
Skeletal	Osteitis fibrosa (bone inflammation with fibrous degeneration); bone demineralization (principally subperiosteal loss of cortical bone in the fibers, lateral ends of the clavicles, and lamina dura of the teeth); spontaneous fractures, bone pain; osteomalacia (rickets) with end-stage renal failure	Bone resorption associated with hyperparathyroidism, vitamin D deficiency, and demineralization; lowered calcium and raised phosphate levels	Control of hyperphosphatemia to reduce hyperparathyroidism; administration of calcium and aluminum hydroxide antacids, which bind phosphate in the gut, together with a phosphate-restricted diet; vitamin D replacement; avoidance of magnesium antacids because of impaired magnesium excretion
Cardiopulmonary	Hypertension, pericarditis with fever, chest pain, and pericardial friction rub, pulmonary edema, Kussmaul respirations	Extracellular volume expansion as cause of hypertension; hypersecretion of renin also associated with hypertension; fluid overload associated with pulmonary edema and acidosis leading to Kussmaul respirations	Volume reduction with diuretics that are not potassium sparing (to avoid hyperkalemia); angiotensin-converting enzyme (ACE) inhibitors; combination of propranolol, hydralazine, and minoxidil for those with high levels of renin; bilateral nephrectomy with dialysis or transplantation
Neurologic	Encephalopathy (fatigue, loss of attention, difficulty problem solving); peripheral neuropathy (pain and burning in the legs and feet, loss of vibration sense and deep tendon reflexes); loss of motor coordination, twitching, fasciculations, stupor, and coma with advanced uremia	Uremic toxins associated with end-stage renal disease	Dialysis
Endocrine	Retarded growth in children	Decreased growth hormone	Exogenous recombinant human growth hormone
	Osteomalacia	Elevated parathyroid hormone levels	Same as for Skeletal above
	Higher incidence of goiter	Decreased thyroid hormone	Replacement when indicated
Hematologic	Anemia, usually normochromic normocytic; platelet disorders with prolonged bleeding times	Reduced erythropoietin secretion associated with loss of renal mass, leading to reduced red cell production in the bone marrow; uremic toxins associated with shortened red cell survival	Dialysis; recombinant human erythropoietin and iron supplementation; conjugated estrogens; DDAVP (1-desamino-8-D-arginine vasopressin); transfusion
Gastrointestinal	Anorexia, nausea, vomiting; mouth ulcers, stomatitis, urinous breath (uremic fetor), hiccups, peptic ulcers, gastrointestinal bleeding, and pancreatitis associated with end-stage renal failure	Retention of urea, metabolic acids, and other metabolic waste products, including methylguanidine	Protein-restricted diet for relief of nausea and vomiting
Integumentary	Abnormal pigmentation and pruritus	Retention of urochromes, contributing to sallow, yellow color; high plasma calcium levels associated with pruritus	Dialysis with control of serum calcium levels
Immunologic	Increased risk of infection that can cause death	Suppression of cell-mediated immunity; reduction in number and function of lymphocytes, diminished phagocytosis	Routine dialysis
Reproductive	Sexual dysfunction: menorrhagia, amenorrhea, infertility, and decreased libido in women; decreased testosterone levels, infertility, and decreased libido in men	Elevated hormones: luteinizing hormone (LH), follicle-stimulating hormone (FSH), prolactin, and LH-releasing hormone; decreased testosterone, estrogen, and progesterone	No specific treatment

Carbohydrates

Glucose intolerance because of insulin resistance is common in chronic renal failure. A protein molecule found in uremic serum may interfere with insulin action at a postreceptor site. Secondary parahyperthyroidism and vitamin D deficiency may be contributing factors.[90]

Clinical Manifestations

The clinical manifestations of chronic renal failure are often described using the term *uremia.* Uremia refers to a number of symptoms caused by a decline in renal function with the accumulation of toxins in the plasma. The specific mechanisms contributing to toxic symptoms are unknown, although studies have shown that urea and creatinine are only minimally responsible. A combination of other end products of metabolism is associated with toxic symptoms and accompanies accumulations of urea and creatinine. Generally, the symptoms include anorexia, nausea, vomiting, diarrhea, weight loss, pruritus, edema, and neurologic changes (Table 35-13).

Evaluation and Treatment

Evaluation of chronic renal failure is based on the history and presenting signs and symptoms. Elevated serum creatinine concentrations and urea nitrogen are consistent with chronic renal failure. Ultrasound, intravenous pyelogram, or plain x-ray films show small kidney size. Renal biopsy confirms the diagnosis.

Dietary Management

The management of nutrition is essential for the person with chronic renal failure. Generally, nutritional management requires limiting the intake of some nutrients. Loss of renal function causes retention of end products of protein metabolism and alterations in the ability to maintain fluid and electrolyte balance. Regulation of food and fluid intake may delay the need for dialysis. Diet therapy is planned according to individual needs by considering the type and severity of renal disease. The major objective is to maintain adequate nutrition while preventing the accumulation of metabolic waste products.[91]

Sodium and Fluids

Sodium requirements for individuals with renal failure vary widely depending on the type of renal disease and use of diuretics. Glomerular disease tends to cause sodium retention, whereas tubulointerstitial diseases lead to sodium wasting. Sodium requirements can be evaluated by determining 24-hour urinary sodium levels. Usually sodium and fluids are restricted in patients with renal failure.

Fluid intake is usually limited to the amount of urine output, plus an additional amount for insensible water losses (500 to 1000 ml). Higher insensible losses occur with fever, excessive sweating, and elevations greater than 5000 feet.

Potassium

Potassium is usually retained in chronic renal failure and requires dietary restriction. In the presence of anuria or oliguria, potassium is restricted to 0.5 mEq/kg of body weight per day (i.e., 50 mEq/day, or about 2 g/day). Many individuals with renal failure can control serum potassium levels if foods high in potassium are avoided.

Caloric Intake

Adequate caloric intake is necessary to maintain ideal body weight. Calories are usually supplied in the form of fats and carbohydrates when protein intake is restricted. Individuals with chronic renal failure often have anorexia as a result of nausea, altered taste sensation, or psychologic depression, making it difficult to maintain an adequate caloric intake. A caloric intake of 35 kcal/kg of body weight per day usually spares tissue protein as a source of calories. Activity levels and metabolic rate also should be considered when calculating caloric intake.

During dialysis, most water-soluble vitamins are lost into the dialysis bath, requiring replacement to maintain normal body requirements. Minerals, such as zinc and magnesium, also may be lost and must be replaced.[92] Zinc replacement improves taste sensation and appetite.

When conservative management of chronic renal failure with diet, diuretics, and fluid restriction is no longer effective, dialysis or transplantation becomes a necessary form of treatment. Indications for initiating dialysis include uncontrollable hypertension, hyperkalemia, and signs of uremia, particularly neuropathies. When signs of neuropathy develop, dialysis should be initiated as soon as possible to prevent permanent damage.

Erythropoietin

Anemia of renal failure can be successfully treated with recombinant human erythropoietin. Individuals are significantly less lethargic and experience an increased sense of well-being, increased appetite, and improved sleeping patterns. Supplemental iron and vitamin B_{12} are also given.[93]

SUMMARY REVIEW

Urinary Tract Obstruction

1. Obstruction can occur anywhere in the urinary tract and is usually caused by renal stones or tumors. The most serious complications are hydronephrosis, hydroureter, and infection caused by accumulation of urine behind the obstruction.
2. The most common kidney stone is formed from calcium and most often causes obstruction by lodging in the ureter.
3. Obstruction can be caused by a neural lesion that interrupts innervation of the bladder. The dysfunction is called a neurogenic bladder.
4. Renal cell carcinoma is the most common renal neoplasm. The larger neoplasms tend to metastasize to the lung, liver, and bone.
5. Bladder tumors are commonly composed of transitional cells with a papillary appearance and a high rate of recurrence.

Urinary Tract Infection

1. Urinary tract infections (UTIs) are usually caused by bacteria, commonly from the retrograde movement of bacteria into the urethra and bladder.
2. Cystitis is an inflammation of the bladder commonly caused by bacteria, although types of "nonbacterial" cystitis may be caused by other conditions or by an autoimmune reaction.
3. Pyelonephritis is an acute or a chronic inflammation of the renal pelvis that may cause abscess formation and scarring with an alteration in renal function. Pyelonephritis may be acute or chronic.

Glomerular Disorders

1. Glomerulonephritis is a group of related diseases of the glomerulus that can be caused by immune responses, toxins or drugs, vascular disorders, and other systemic diseases.
2. Acute glomerulonephritis commonly results from inflammatory damage to the glomerulus as a consequence of immune reactions after a streptococcal infection.
3. IgA nephropathy is a common cause of glomerulonephritis with deposition of abnormal serum IgA and complement, which causes glomerular injury and sclerosis.
4. Rapidly progressive glomerulonephritis (RPGN) is associated with injury that results in proliferation of glomerular capillary endothelial cells and rapid loss of renal function.
5. Chronic glomerulonephritis is related to a variety of diseases that cause deterioration of the glomerulus and progressive loss of renal function.
6. Immune mechanisms in glomerulonephritis are the deposition of antigen-antibody complexes and the formation of antibodies specific for the glomerular basement membrane.
7. Nephrotic syndrome is the excretion of at least 3.5 g of protein in the urine per day. Its principal symptoms are hypoproteinuria, hyperlipidemia, and edema.
8. Nephrotic syndrome is caused by a loss of plasma proteins, principally albumin and some immunoglobulins, across the injured glomerular filtration membrane.

Renal Failure

1. Acute renal failure is classified as prerenal, intrarenal, or postrenal and is usually accompanied by oliguria with elevated plasma blood urea nitrogen (BUN) and plasma creatinine levels.
2. Prerenal acute failure is caused by decreased renal perfusion with a decreased glomerular filtration rate (GFR), ischemia, and tubular necrosis.
3. Intrarenal acute renal failure is associated with several systemic diseases but is commonly related to acute tubular necrosis (ATN).
4. Postrenal failure is associated with diseases that obstruct the flow of urine from the kidneys.
5. Chronic renal failure represents a progressive loss of renal function. Plasma creatinine levels gradually become elevated as GFR declines, sodium is lost in the urine, potassium is retained, acidosis develops, calcium and phosphate metabolism are altered, hematocrit drops, and serum lipids increase.

KEY TERMS

REFERENCES

1. Milam DF: Causes of upper urinary tract obstruction. In Jacobson HR, Striker GE, Klahr S: *The principles and practice of nephrology,* St Louis, 1995, Mosby.
2. Krane JR, Siroky MB, Fitzpatrick JM: *Clinical urology,* Philadelphia, 1994, Lippincott.
3. Coe FL et al: *Kidney stones: medical and surgical management,* Philadelphia, 1996, Lippincott-Raven.
4. Kramer G, Klingler HC, Steiner GE: Role of bacteria in the development of kidney stones, *Curr Opin Urol* 10(1):35, 2000.
5. Goldfarb DS, Coe FL: Prevention of recurrent nephrolithiasis, *Am Fam Physician* 8:2269, 1999.
6. Weir MJ, Tariq N, Honey RJ: Shockwave frequency affects fragmentation in a kidney stone model, *J Endourol* 14(7):547, 2000.
7. Taari K, Lehtoranta K, Rannikko S: Holmium:YAG laser for urinary stones, *Scand J Urol Nephrol* 33(5):295, 1999.
8. Madersbacher HG: Neurogenic bladder dysfunction, *Curr Opin Urol* 9(4):303, 1999.
9. Fowler CJ: Neurological disorders of micronutrition and their treatment, *Brain* 122(pt 7):1213, 1999.
10. Licht MR: Renal adenoma and oncocytoma, *Semin Urol Oncol* 13(4): 262, 1995.
11. American Cancer Society: *Cancer facts and figures*, 2000. Available at www3.cancer.org/cancerinfo.

12. Bahnson RR: Renal and urinary tract neoplasia. In *National Kidney Foundation: primer on kidney diseases,* San Diego, 1994, Academic Press.
13. Sweeney C, Farrow DC: Differential survival related to smoking among patients with renal cell carcinoma, *Epidemiology* 11(3):344, 2000.
14. Van Poppel H et al: Precancerous lesions in the kidney, *Scand J Urol Nephrol Suppl* (205):136, 2000.
15. Gago-Dominguez et al: Regular use of analgesics is a risk factor for renal cell carcinoma, *Br J Cancer* 81(3):354, 1999.
16. Bichler KH, Wechsel HW: The problematic nature of metastasized renal cell carcinoma, *Anticancer Res* 19(2C):1463, 1999.
17. Smith JA: Genitourinary tumors. In Jacobson HR, Striker GE, Klahr S, editors: *The principles and practice of nephrology,* St Louis, 1995, Mosby.
18. Vetter JM: Metastasis of renal-cell carcinoma: a pathologist's theoretical view. In Bollack CG, Jacqmin D, editors: *Basic research and treatment of renal cell carcinoma metastasis,* New York, 1990, Wiley-Liss.
19. Figlin RA: Renal cell carcinoma: management of advanced disease, *J Urol* 161(2):381, 1999.
20. Brennan P et al: Cigarette smoking and bladder cancer in men: a pooled analysis of 11 case-control studies, *Int J Cancer* 86(2):289, 2000.
21. van der Poel HG, Mungan NA, Witjes JA: Bladder cancer in women, *Int Urogynecol J Pelvic Floor Dysfunct* 10(3):207, 1999.
22. Rabbani F, Cordon-Cardo C: Mutation of cell cycle regulators and their impact on superficial bladder cancer, *Urol Clin North Am* 27(1):83, 2000.
23. Zlotta AR, Schulman CC: Biological markers in superficial bladder tumors and their prognostic significance, *Urol Clin North Am* 27(1):179, 2000.
24. Frimberger D, Zaak D, Hofstetter A: Endoscopic fluorescence diagnosis and laser treatment of transitional cell carcinoma of the bladder, *Semin Urol Oncol* 18(4):264, 2000.
25. Brown DH, Wagner TT, Bahnson RR: Interferons and bladder cancer, *Urol Clin North Am* 27(1):178, 2000.
26. Hassen W, Droller MJ: Current concepts in assessment and treatment of bladder cancer, *Curr Opin Urol* 10(4):291, 2000.
27. Kurowski D: The women with dysuria, *Am Fam Physician* 57(9):2155, 1998.
28. Roberts JA: Pathophysiology of bacterial cystitis, *Adv Exp Med Biol* 462:325, 1999.
29. Orenstein R, Wong ES: Urinary tract infection in adults, *Am Fam Physician* 59(5):1125, 1999.
30. Sussman M, Gally DL: The biology of cystitis: host and bacterial factors, *Annu Rev Med* 50:149, 1999.
31. Sanford JP: Urinary tract symptoms and infection, *Annu Rev Med* 26: 485, 1975.
32. Childs SJ, Egan RJ: Bacteriuria and urinary infections in the elderly, *Urol Clin North Am* 23(1):43, 1996.
33. Molander U et al: A longitudinal cohort study of elderly women with urinary tract infections, *Maturitas* 34(2):127, 2000.
34. Naber KG: Short-term therapy of acute uncomplicated cystitis, *Curr Opin Urol* 9(1):57, 1999.
35. Nygaard IE, Johnson JM: Urinary tract infections in elderly women, *Am Fam Physician* 53(1):175, 1996.
36. Madersbacher HG, Thalhammer F, Marberger M: Pathogenesis and management of recurrent urinary tract infection in women, *Curr Opin Urol* 10(1):29, 2000.
37. O'Dowd TC et al: Urethral syndrome: a self-limiting illness, *BMJ* 288: 1349, 1984.
38. Gittes RF, Nakamura RM: Female urethral syndrome: a female prostatis? *West J Med* 164(5):435, 1996.
39. Sant GR, Theoharides TC: Interstitial cystitis, *Curr Opin Urol* 9(4): 297, 1999.
40. Erickson DR: Interstitial cystitis: update on etiologies and therapeutic options, *J Womens Health Gend Based Med* 8(6):745, 1999.
41. Roberts JA: Management of pyelonephritis and upper urinary tract infections, *Urol Clin North Am* 26(4):753, 1999.
42. Kooman JP et al: Acute pyelonephritis: a cause of acute renal failure? *Neth J Med* 57(5):185, 2000.
43. Talner LB et al: Acute pyelonephritis: can we agree on terminology? *Radiology* 192(2):297, 1994.
44. Ratner JJ et al: Bacteria-specific antibody in the urine of patients with acute pyelonephritis and cystitis, *J Infect Dis* 143:404, 1981.
45. Korman TM, Grayson ML: Treatment of urinary tract infections, *Aust Fam Physician* 24(12):2205, 1995.
46. Rubin RH, Cotran RS, Tolkoff-Rubin NE: Urinary tract infection, pyelonephritis, and reflux nephropathy. In Brenner BM, Rector RC, editors: *The kidney,* ed 5, Philadelphia, 1996, W.B. Saunders.
47. Couser WG: Glomerulonephritis, *Lancet* 353:1509, 1999.
48. Yoshizawa N: Acute glomerulonephritis, *Intern Med* 39(9):687, 2000.
49. Hricik DE, Chung-Park M, Sedor UR: Glomerulonephritis, *N Engl J Med* 339(13):888, 1998.
50. Glassock RJ, Cohen AH: The primary glomerulopathies, *Dis Mon* 42(6):329, 1996.
51. Kluth DC, Rees AJ: New approaches to modify glomerular inflammation, *J Nephrol* 12(2):66, 1999.
52. Nordstrand A, Horgren M, Holm SE: Pathogenic mechanism of acute post-streptococcal glomerulonephritis, *Scand J Infect Dis* 31(6):523, 1999.
53. Wardle EN: Rationales for treating IgA nephropathies, *Ren Fail* 22(1): 1, 2000.
54. Erwig LP, Rees AJ: Rapidly progressive glomerulonephritis, *J Nephrol* 112(suppl 2):S111, 1999.
55. Hagen EC et al: Diagnostic value of standardized assays for anti-neutrophil cytoplasmic antibodies in idiopathic systemic vasculitis. EC/BCR Project for ANCA Assay Standardization, *Kidney Int* 53(3): 743, 1998.
56. Stegmayr BC et al: Plasma exchange or immunoadsorption in patients with rapidly progressive crescentic glomerulonephritis. A Swedish multi-center study, *Int J Artif Organs* 22(2):81, 1999.
57. Gonick HG: *Current nephrology,* vol 11, St Louis, 1994, Mosby.
58. Madaio MP: Postinfectious glomerulonephritis. In Jacobson HR, Striker GE, Klahr S: *The principles and practice of nephrology,* St Louis, 1995, Mosby.
59. Schena FP: Primary glomerulonephritides with nephrotic syndrome. Limitations of therapy in adult patients, *J Nephrol* 12(suppl 2):S125, 1999.
60. Bergstein JM: A practical approach to proteinuria, *Pediatr Nephrol* 13(8):697, 1999.
61. Kaysen GA: Nonrenal complications of nephrotic syndrome, *Annu Rev Med* 45:201, 1994.
62. Coe FL et al, editors: *The yearbook of nephrology,* St Louis, 1992, Mosby.
63. de Sain–van der Velden MG: Increased VLDL in nephrotic patients results from a decreased catabolism while increased LDL results from increased synthesis, *Kidney Int* 53(4):994, 1998.
64. Kaysen GA, de Sain–van der Velden MG: New insights into lipid metabolism in the nephrotic syndrome, *Kidney Int* 71:S18, 1999.
65. Kuhn K et al: Treatment of severe nephrotic syndrome, *Kidney Int* 64: S50, 1998.
66. Schrierer RW: *Diseases of the kidney,* New York, 1997, Little, Brown.
67. Alkhunaizi AM, Schrier RW: Management of acute renal failure: new perspectives, *Am J Kidney Dis* 28(3):315, 1996.
68. Agmon Y, Brezis M: Acute renal failure: a multifactorial syndrome. In Bourke E, Mallick NP, Pollak BE, editors: *Moving points in nephrology,* Basel, 1993, Karger.
69. Nissenson AR: Acute renal failure: definition and pathogenesis, *Kidney Int* 66:S7, 1998.
70. Mandal AK, Lightfoot BO, Treat RC: Mechanisms of protection in acute renal failure, *Circ Shock* 11(3):245, 1983.
71. Nath KA, Norby SM: Reactive oxygen species and acute renal failure, *Am J Med* 109(8):665, 2000.
72. Johnson KS, Weinberg JM: Postischemic renal injury due to oxygen radicals, *Curr Opin Nephrol Hypertens* 2(4):625, 1993.
73. Agrawal M, Swartz R: Acute renal failure, *Am Fam Physician* 61(7):2077, 2000.

74. Ronco C et al: Future technology for continuous renal replacement therapies, *Am J Kidney Dis* 28(5, suppl 3):S121, 1996.
75. Bricker NS, Morrin PA, Kime SW Jr: The pathologic physiology of chronic Bright's disease. An exposition of the "intact nephron hypothesis," *J Am Soc Nephrol* 8(9):1470, 1997.
76. Sackman H et al: Contrasting renal functional reserve in very long-term type I diabetic patients with and without nephropathy, *Diabetologia* 43(2):177, 2000.
77. Schmieder RE et al: Glomerular hyperfiltration during sympathetic nervous system activation in early essential hypertension, *J Am Soc Nephrol* 8(6):893, 1997.
78. Bakis GL et al: Preserving renal function in adults with hypertension and diabetes: a consensus approach. National Kidney Foundation Hypertension and Diabetes Executive Committees Working Group, *Am J Kidney Dis* 36(3):646, 2000.
79. Chantrel F, Moulin B, Hannedouche T: Blood pressure, diabetes and diabetic nephropathy, *Diabetes Metab* 26(suppl 4):37, 2000.
80. Walser M: Assessing renal function from creatinine measurements in adults with chronic renal failure, *Am J Kidney Dis* 32(1):23, 1998.
81. Andreucci M et al: Diuretics in renal failure, *Miner Electrolyte Metab* 25(1-2):32, 1999.
82. Kupin WL, Narins RG: The hyperkalemia of renal failure: pathophysiology, diagnosis, and therapy. In Bourke E, Mallick NP, Pollak BE, editors: *Moving points in nephrology,* Basel, 1993, Karger.
83. Giovannetti S, Cupisti A, Barsotti G: The metabolic acidosis of chronic renal failure: pathophysiology and treatment. In Berlyn GM, editor: *The kidney today,* Basel, 1992, Karger.
84. Hoyland JA, Picton ML: Cellular mechanisms of renal osteodystrophy, *Kidney Int Suppl* 73:S8, 1999.
85. Eckhardt KY: Pathophysiology of renal anemia, *Clin Nephrol* 53 (1 suppl):S2, 2000.
86. Kaysen GA, de Sain-van der Velden MG: New insights into lipid metabolism in the nephrotic syndrome, *Kidney Int Suppl* 71:S18, 1999.
87. Burton C, Harris KP: The role of proteinuria in the progression of chronic renal failure, *Am J Kidney Dis* 27(6):765, 1996.
88. Klahr S: Mechanisms of progression of chronic renal damage, *J Nephrol* 12(suppl 1):S53, 1999.
89. Fouque D et al: Low protein diets delay end-stage renal disease in non-diabetic adults with chronic renal failure, *Cochrane Database Syst Rev* (2):CD001892, 2000.
90. Mak RH: 1,25-Dihydroxyvitamin D_3 corrects insulin and lipid abnormalities in uremia, *Kidney Int* 53(5):1353, 1998.
91. Mitch WE, Maroni BJ: Factors causing malnutrition in patients with chronic uremia, *Am J Kidney Dis* 33(1):176, 1999.
92. Zima T et al: Trace elements in end-stage renal disease. 2. Clinical implication of trace elements, *Blood Purif* 17(4):187, 1999.
93. Macdougall IC: Strategies for iron supplementation: oral versus intravenous, *Kidney Int Suppl* 69:S61, 1999.

CHAPTER 36

Alterations of Renal and Urinary Tract Function in Children

SUE E. HUETHER

CHAPTER OUTLINE

Some renal and urinary disorders occur in children as well as adults. In childhood, however, the kidney and genitourinary structures continue to develop, so that renal dysfunction may be associated with mechanisms and manifestations different from those in adults. In addition, some renal and urinary disorders are congenital. Many of these involve structural anomalies of the renal system.

STRUCTURE AND FUNCTION OF THE RENAL SYSTEM IN CHILDREN

Development of the Renal System

The embryonic kidneys develop as three sets of sequentially replaced organs (Fig. 36-1). First, the pronephros arise at the level of the cervical and upper thoracic regions during the third fetal week. The mesonephros begin development more caudally about the fourth fetal week and begin excretory function in the sixth week. Metanephros, the permanent kidneys, arise distal to the bifurcation of the aorta. The metanephros have two parts—the metanephric duct that buds off the mesonephric duct and metanephrogenic tissue. The ureteric bud (metanephric duct) grows dorsocranially and starts subdividing to become the collecting system for the kidneys. By the fifth fetal month, it will have progressively branched into the collecting ducts. The metanephrogenic tissue atop the terminal branches of the collecting ducts develops into primitive glomeruli and uriniferous tubules. Establishing the connection between the uriniferous tubules and the collecting ducts is a vital part of kidney development; errors in this stage can result in polycystic kidneys.

After glomeruli and tubules form, the tissues organize and progressively differentiate over approximately 30 days. Initial glomerular development is staggered, so there are glomeruli in various stages. In fact, a few of the first glomeruli formed degenerate and disappear during the later stages of pregnancy. Progressive development continues into the ninth fetal month, when all metanephrogenic tissue disappears.

As the embryo develops and the vertebral column straightens, the kidneys appear to ascend to the sacral area at about 6 weeks, to the third lumbar area by the third month, and to the first lumbar area at term. The kidneys rotate 90 degrees as they ascend so that renal tissue is lateral and the collecting system is medial.

While the kidneys mature, the cloaca becomes the urogenital sinus. It then differentiates into the vesicourethral canal, which forms the bladder and the upper urethra, and the urogenital sinus, which forms the main part of the urethra.

At birth the kidneys occupy a large portion of the posterior abdominal wall, and the ureters are proportionately shorter than those of an adult. All the nephrons are present at birth, and their number does not increase as the kidney grows and matures. The kidney reaches adult size by adolescence and, because of maturation of the tubular system, increases in weight tenfold from birth.

Urine formation and excretion begin by the third month of gestation, contributing to the amniotic fluid. In infancy the bladder lies close to the abdominal wall, making urinary bladder aspiration for diagnostic purposes a relatively simple

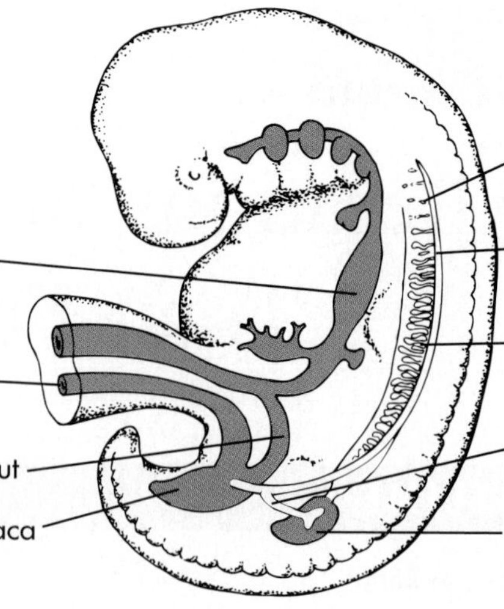

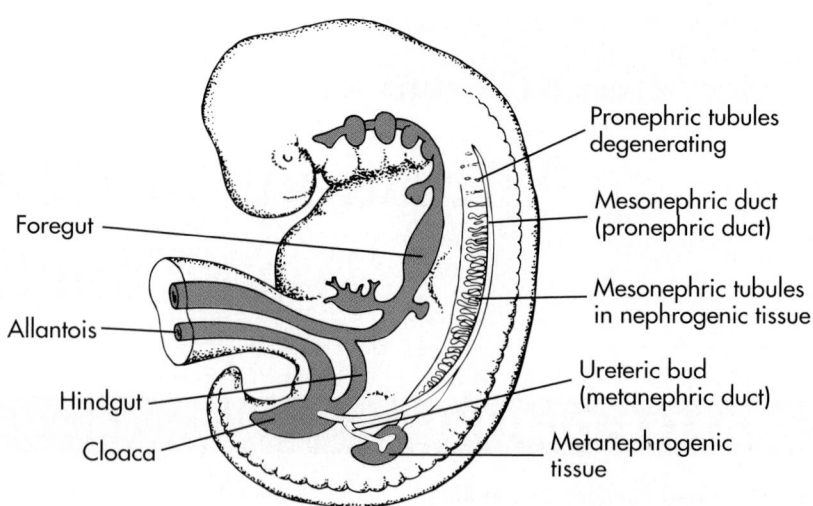

FIG. 36-1 Topography of the pronephros, mesonephros, and metanephric primordium. (From Netter F, Shapter R, Yonkman F, editors: *The ciba collection of medical illustrations*, vol 6. Kidneys, ureters, and urinary bladder, Summit, NJ, 1973, Ciba Pharmaceutical Corporation.)

Table 36-1 Average Daily Urine Output in Children

Age	Output (ml/day)
1 and 2 days	15-50
3-10 days	50-300
10 days–2 mo	250-400
2 mo–1 yr	400-500
1-3 yr	500-600
5-8 yr	700-1000
8-14 yr	700-1500

From Kempe CH, Silver KH, O'Brien D: *Current pediatric diagnosis and treatment,* Los Altos, Calif, 1982, Lange Medical Publishers.

procedure. The bladder descends into the pelvis with growth, changing from a cylindric organ to the adult pyramidal shape. Although small amounts of urine are found in the bladder at birth, the newborn may not void for 12 to 24 hours. (The average daily urine output is shown in Table 36-1.)

Immediately at birth the renal blood flow and glomerular filtration rate (GFR) increase because of a decrease in vascular resistance and the need to perform excretory functions no longer performed by the placenta. Renal vascular resistance remains higher in newborns and infants, however, which may be attributed to increased levels of circulating renin. The resistance progressively declines during the first year of development, with an increasing fraction of the cardiac output going to the kidney. The GFR continues to increase, becoming stable at 1 or 2 years but retaining 30% to 50% of adult levels until the end of the first year. Although glomerular filtration is important in removing nitrogenous and other wastes, the amount of urea to be removed is small.

Fluid and Electrolyte Balance in Children

Because the kidney develops from the center toward the periphery, renal distribution of blood flow during the newborn period is primarily to the renal medulla. The result is a preferential flow to the medullary nephrons, which have comparatively short loops at this stage of development. The combination of higher blood flow and shorter loops produces a more dilute urine—approximately 600 to 700 mOsm. The dilute urine is accentuated by a low rate of urea excretion because urea is necessary to establish the concentration gradient in the medulla. Urea excretion is low primarily because infants are in a high anabolic state and use their protein for growth.

Because of a high hydrogen ion concentration, limited ability to regulate the internal environment, and lowered osmotic pressure, the infant's renal system has a narrow chemical safety margin. The immaturity and smaller surface area of the tubules also may diminish the water reabsorption response to antidiuretic hormone (ADH). An immature tubular transport capacity means that the ability to excrete a potassium load, reabsorb bicarbonate, or buffer hydrogen with ammonia does not become efficient until approximately 2 years of age. Consequently, any disturbance, such as diarrhea, infection, fasting for diagnostic tests, or improper feeding, can rapidly lead to severe acidosis and fluid imbalance because the infant can rapidly develop overhydration, or edema.

After birth the proportion of total body water to body weight does not change markedly. Considerable change occurs, however, in the location of that body water as the child matures (see Chapter 3). The percentage of extracellular fluid volume of the newborn infant is nearly double that of the adult. Decrease in extracellular fluid volume occurs in two different periods of rapid growth—infancy and adolescence.

Not only does the infant have a greater content of extracellular fluid, but also the fluid exchange rate is greater. The adult takes in and excretes approximately 2000 ml of water daily, representing 5% of the total body fluid and 14% of the extracellular fluid. In contrast, the infant's daily exchange of 600 to 700 ml represents 290% of the total or nearly 50% of the extracellular volume, making control of dehydration and overhydration more difficult.

The composition of body fluids differs slightly with age. The total electrolyte concentration in extracellular fluids is greater in the newborn than in the adult. The concentration of sodium, chloride, phosphates, and organic acids is also greater. The concentration of bicarbonate ions is lower in the infant than in the older child, with a mild acidosis evidenced by a lowered pH. These variations, combined with a lowered plasma protein level, cause a reduced oncotic pressure of the vascular compartment and favor accumulation of fluid in the tissue spaces and an increased GFR. In the healthy child, these differences remain for a few weeks or months. The premature infant and the normal newborn infant are usually in a state of well-compensated acidosis and potential edema.

ALTERATIONS IN RENAL FUNCTION IN CHILDREN

Structural Abnormalities

Variations from the normal anatomic structure of the urinary tract occur in 10% to 15% of the total population. The structural abnormalities range from minor, nonpathologic, or easily correctable anomalies to those that are incompatible with life. For example, the kidneys may fail to ascend from the pelvis to the abdomen, causing ectopic kidneys—which usually function normally. The kidneys also may fuse as they ascend, causing a single U-shaped **horseshoe kidney**. Approximately one third of individuals with horseshoe kidneys are asymptomatic, and the most common problems are hydronephrosis, infection, and stone formation.[1] Collectively, structural anomalies of the renal system account for approximately 45% of cases of renal failure in children.

Some anomalies are obvious at birth, whereas others remain latent. The following structural anomalies are commonly associated with urinary tract malformations:[2]

Low-set, malformed ears
Chromosomal disorders, especially trisomy 13 (Patau syndrome) and trisomy 18
Absent abdominal muscles (prune-belly syndrome)
Anomalies of the spinal cord and lower extremities
Imperforate anus or genital deviation
Wilms tumor
Congenital ascites
Cystic disease of the liver
Positive family history of renal disease (hereditary nephritis or cystic disease)

Hypospadias

Hypospadias is a congenital condition in which the urethral meatus is located on the ventral side or undersurface of the penis. The meatus can be located anywhere on the glans, the penile shaft, the base of the penis, the penoscrotal junction, or the perineum (Fig. 36-2). This is the most common anomaly of the penis and occurs in about 1 in 300 infant boys. The etiology is multifactoral and related to disruptions in male hormones, including testerone biosynthesis defects, 5α-reductase mutations, hormones administered for in vitro fertilization, and other environmental factors.[3] **Chordee**, or penile torsion, may accompany hypospadias. In chordee a shortage of skin on the ventral surface causes the penis to bend or to "bow" ventrally (Fig. 36-3).[4] Penile torsion is a counterclockwise twist of the penile shaft. Partial absence of the foreskin and cryptorchidism (undescended testes, see Chapter 22) are associated with the anomaly.[5]

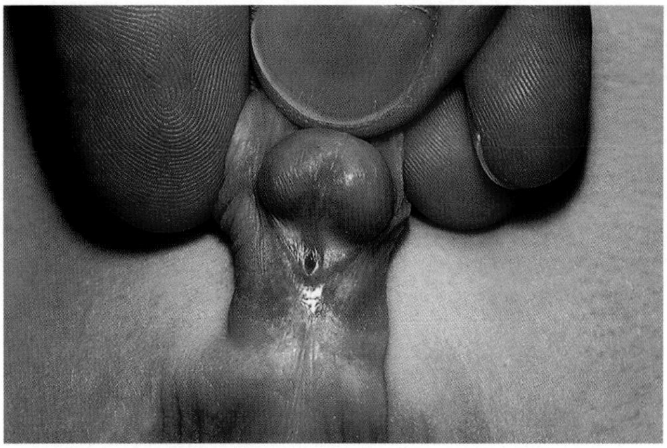

FIG. 36-2 Hypospadias. (Courtesy MC Gleason, MD, San Diego; from Wong DL: *Whaley and Wong's nursing care of infants and children*, ed 6, St Louis, 1999, Mosby.)

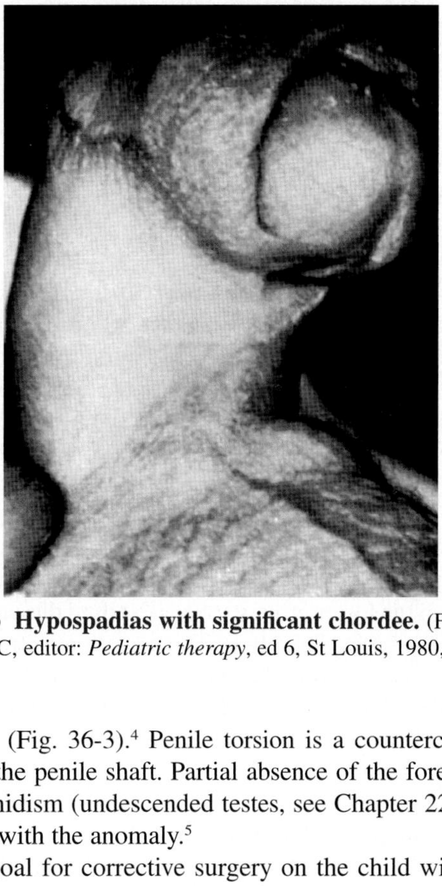

FIG. 36-3 Hypospadias with significant chordee. (From Shirkey HC, editor: *Pediatric therapy*, ed 6, St Louis, 1980, Mosby.)

The goal for corrective surgery on the child with hypospadias is a cosmetically acceptable, straight penis with the urinary meatus at the tip. Formerly performed in two or more stages, hypospadias repairs are now done in one stage. Improvements in microsurgical techniques have improved outcomes and decreased complications.[6] Surgery is usually performed between 6 and 12 months of age.

Surgery is most effective between 18 and 30 months of age, when the penis has reached sufficient size. Psychologically, the preferred time to perform the correction is before the child enters school and before he develops castration and mutilation anxiety.

WHAT'S NEW? Improved Techniques for Hypospadias Repair

Lack of sufficient penile skin to correct hypospadias deformities lead surgeons to try many different options: meatal flaps, free skin grafts, and bladder mucosa grafts. Use of buccal mucosa to reconstruct the urethra has been successful. Buccal mucosa is elastic, of an ideal thickness, and easy to obtain from a donor site that heals quickly. Techniques have also been developed to preserve the neurovascular bundle. Lasers and tissue solder are also being evaluated.

Data from Brock JW: Autologous buccal mucosal graft for urethral reconstruction, *Urology* 44(5):753; Dean GE, Burno DK, Zaontz MR: Chordee repair utilizing a novel technique ensuring neurovascular bundle preservation, *Tech Urol* 6(1):5, 2000; King, LR: Bladder mucosal grafts for severe hypospadias: a successful technique, *J Urol* 152:2338, 1994; Snodgrass W: Changing concepts in hypospadias repair, *Curr Opin Urol* 9(6):513, 1999.

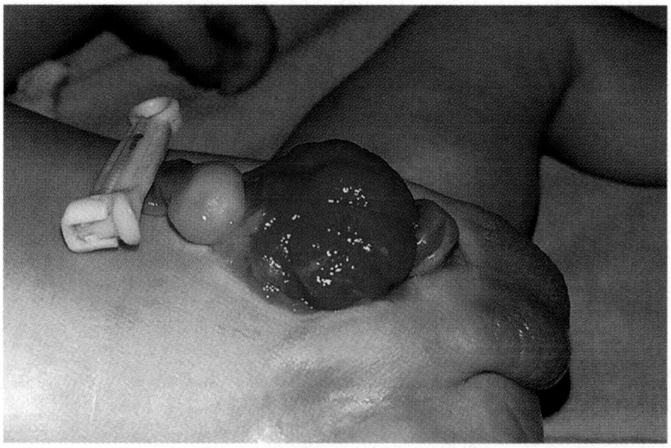

FIG. 36-4 Exstrophy of bladder. (Courtesy H. Gil Rushton, MD, Children's National Medical Center, Washington, DC; from Wong DL: *Whaley and Wong's nursing care of infants and children*, ed 6, St Louis, 1999, Mosby.)

Epispadias

Epispadias and exstrophy of the bladder are the same congenital defect but expressed to a different degree. In male epispadias the urethral opening is on the dorsal surface of the penis. In females a cleft along the ventral urethra usually extends to the bladder neck. The incidence of epispadias is about 1 in 40,000 to 118,000 births. Twice as many boys as girls present with this defect.

In boys the urethral opening may be small and situated behind the glans (anterior epispadias) or a fissure may extend the entire length of the penis and into the bladder neck (posterior epispadias). Children with anterior epispadias can be continent with perhaps only stress incontinence, but those with posterior epispadias will experience constant dribbling of urine.

Exstrophy of the Bladder

Exstrophy of the bladder is an extensive congenital anomaly in which the lower urinary tract is exposed directly to the surface of the body (Fig. 36-4). The posterior portion of the bladder mucosa is exposed and appears bright red through a fissure in the adbominal wall. The incidence of exstrophy of the bladder is about 1 in 400,000 live births. Boys are predominant by a ratio of 3:1.[7]

Exstrophy of the bladder is caused by intrauterine failure of the abdominal wall and the mesoderm of the anterior bladder to fuse. The rectus muscles below the umbilicus are separated, and the pubic rami (bony projections of the pubic bone) are not joined. In addition, the posterior aspect of the pelvis is externally rotated, which retroverts the acetabula and causes external rotation of the feet.[8] This causes a waddling gait when the child first learns to walk, but most children quickly learn to compensate. Urine seeps onto the abdominal wall from the ureters, causing a constant odor of urine and excoriation of the surrounding skin. Because the exposed bladder mucosa becomes hyperemic and edematous, it bleeds easily and is painful. It should be covered with Silastic or a plastic dressing (Glad Wrap or Saran Wrap) for protection from diaper irritation while permitting urine drainage.

The unrepaired exstrophic bladder is cosmetically unacceptable and prone to cancerous changes as soon as 1 year after birth. Ideally, the bladder and pubic defect should be closed before the infant is 48 hours old. Reconstruction of the internal and external genitalia can be done when girls reach their late teens. Epispadias repair in boys is better done at 2 to 3 years of age as are bladder neck reconstruction, ureteral implantation, and bladder augmentation. Objectives of management include preservation of renal function, attainment of urinary control, prevention of infection, reconstructive repair of the defect, and improvement of sexual function and quality of life.

Hypoplastic or Dysplastic Kidneys

During embryologic development the ureteric duct grows into the metanephric tissue, triggering the formation of the kidneys. If this growth does not occur, the kidney is absent—a condition called **renal aplasia**. Occasionally a **hypoplastic kidney**, a very small normal kidney, may develop. These aberrations may be unilateral or bilateral; the occurrence may be incidental or familial. Bilateral hypoplastic kidneys are a common cause of chronic renal failure in children. Segmental hypoplasia (the Ask-Upmark kidney) is not the result of developmental abnormalities but a deformity acquired secondary to intrarenal reflux.[9]

Renal dysplasia usually results from abnormal differentiation of the renal tissues; for example, primitive glomeruli and tubules, cysts, and nonrenal tissue (such as cartilage) are found in the dysplastic kidney. Dysplasia usually is associated also with a functional or organic obstruction of the collecting system. The obstruction may begin before birth, as in prune-belly syndrome, posterior urethral valves, or ureteroceles.

Renal Agenesis

Renal agenesis (failure of a kidney to grow or develop) may be unilateral or bilateral, and it may occur randomly or be

WHAT'S NEW? Prenatal Diagnosis of Congenital Genitourinary Anomalies

Prenatal ultrasound can detect an infant's gender (important in diagnosing gender-linked hereditary disorders) and possibly genital epispadias, unilateral renal agenesis, pelvic kidney, and double collecting system. In addition, color Doppler ultrasound can detect the lack of renal arteries and renal agenesis. Advances are being made in fetal therapy for obstructive uropathy.

Data from Freedman, AL, Johnson, MP, Gonzalez R: Fetal therapy for obstructive uropathy: past, present, future? *Pediatr Nephrol* 14(2):167, 2000; Isaksen CV et al: Fetuses and infants with congenital urinary system anomalies: correlation between prenatal ultrasound and postmortem findings, *Ultrasound Obstet Gynecol* 15(3):177, 2000.

Table 36-2 Corticosteroid Treatment in Children with Nephrotic Syndrome

Response to corticosteroid	Incidence (%)	Outcomes
Steroid responsive	93	Single course of therapy, low recurrence rate
Steroid dependent (frequently relapsing)	7	Intermittent exacerbations with remissions for several years
Steroid resistant	Rare	Resistance to steroids, eventual development of chronic renal failure

clearly hereditary. The kidney is usually polycystic and dysplastic. The condition may occur as an isolated entity or as a problem associated with other unrelated disorders.[10]

Unilateral renal agenesis occurs in approximately 1 of 1000 live births. Males are more often affected, and it is usually the left kidney that is absent. The single kidney is often completely normal so that the child can expect a normal, healthy life. The normal solitary kidney grows because of compensatory hypertrophy before and after birth, and by the time the child is several years older, the volume of this kidney may approach twice the normal size.[11a]

In some instances, however, the single kidney is abnormally formed and associated with abnormalities of its collecting system.[11b] Extrarenal congenital abnormalities are relatively more common with unilateral renal agenesis.

Bilateral renal agenesis (also called **Potter syndrome**) occurs in about 1 in 3000 live births, and 75% of affected infants are male. Bilateral renal agenesis results from either an abnormal development of the normal progression from pronephros to mesonephros to metanephros or an isolated bilateral failure of development of the ureteral buds. The term *Potter syndrome* refers to the association with a specific group of facial anomalies (wide-set eyes, parrot-beak nose, low-set ears, and receding chin). Affected infants rarely live more than a few hours. Most die of respiratory distress caused by associated pulmonary hypoplasia rather than from renal failure. Approximately 40% of affected infants are stillborn.

Glomerular Disorders

Glomerulonephritis

Glomerulonephritis includes a number of renal disorders in which proliferation and inflammation of the glomeruli are secondary to an immune mechanism (Table 36-2). (The major glomerulopathies are described in Chapter 35.) Chronic glomerulonephritis accounts for 53% of renal failure in children and is responsible for most school-age and teenage children requiring dialysis and kidney transplantation.

Poststreptococcal Glomerulonephritis

Acute poststreptococcal glomerulonephritis (PSGN) is one of the most common noninfectious renal diseases in children. It occurs after a throat or skin infection with certain strains of group A β-hemolytic streptococci and is characterized by a sudden onset of gross hematuria, edema, hypertension, and renal insufficiency.

Pharyngeal infections are most common during cold weather; skin infections from impetigo, infected insect bites, or varicella sores usually occur during warm weather. The pathophysiology of PSGN in children is similar to that occurring in adults (see Chapter 35). Antigen-antibody complexes with deposits of IgG, IgA, and C_3 complement in the glomerulus initiates glomerular injury and inflammation. Increased vascular permeability and loss of negative charge, along the glomerular vascular membrane, leads to hematuria and proteinuria. The most severely affected children develop acute renal failure with oliguria.

Typically a child is in good health until the onset of an upper respiratory or skin infection. One to two weeks later, mild proteinuria (less than 2 g per 4 hr), hematuria, and periorbital edema appear. The urine is usually smoky brown or cola colored because of the presence of red blood cells, and the volume is reduced. The onset of symptoms in the child is abrupt and consists of flank or midabdominal pain, irritability, general malaise, and fever. Acute hypertension may cause headache; vomiting; somnolence; and other central nervous system (CNS) manifestations, including seizures. Cardiovascular symptoms are related to circulatory overload and are compounded by hypertension. These include dyspnea; tachypnea; and an enlarged, tender liver. As many as half the children affected are asymptomatic.

The disease usually runs its course in 1 month, but urine abnormalities may be found up to 1 year after the onset. Some children become oliguric and develop rapidly progressive glomerulonephritis, whereas others slowly progress to chronic glomerulonephritis. Prolonged proteinuria and abnormal GFR indicate an unfavorable prognosis. More than 95% recover completely.

Treatment is symptom specific. Because oliguria and hypertension are common, fluid, sodium, and potassium intakes are restricted. Bed rest, antihypertensive medication, and diuretic agents are indicated during the acute phase.

Acute glomerulonephritis (AGN) may be accompanied by a positive throat or skin culture for *Streptococcus*. The urine usually contains red blood cells and proteins. As a precautionary measure, penicillin is given in therapeutic doses for

10 to 14 days to eradicate residual streptococci. Early treatment of streptococcal infections with antibiotics does not preclude the development of the disease. Family members of the affected child should have throat or skin cultures and be treated with penicillin if a culture is positive.[12]

Immunoglobulin A Nephropathy

Immunoglobulin A (IgA) nephropathy is one of the many types of glomerulonephritis and occurs almost twice as frequently in males as in females. It is characterized by deposition mainly of IgA, but also some immunoglobulin M (IgM) and complement proteins,[13] in the mesangium of the glomerular capillaries, even though there is no evidence of systemic immunologic disease such as systemic lupus erythematosus or anaphylactoid purpura. The damage to the glomerulus can progress to glomerulosclerosis and tubular interstitial involvement, which is usually reversible.[14]

Children with the disease have recurrent gross hematuria, often after a respiratory infection. Most continue to have microscopic hematuria between the attacks of gross hematuria. Many also have a mild proteinuria in spite of otherwise normal renal function. Treatment is supportive. Long-term follow-up should consist of checking blood pressure, urinalysis, proteinuria levels, and renal function every 6 to 12 months.[15] Approximately 20% of affected children develop the progressive form of the disease, however, with hypertension and decreasing renal function. Hypertriglyceridemia and hyperuricemia are predictors of poor outcome.[16] These children eventually require dialysis and transplantation.

Henoch-Schonlein Nephritis—IgA Nephropathy

Henoch-Schonlein nephritis is an IgA nephropathy that affects the glomerular blood vessels. The most typical lesion is segmental focal glomerulonephritis with IgA deposits in the mesangium. Transient hematuria without functional impairment is more common in children. However, the development of interstitial fibrosis and crescent formation from subepithelial immune deposits along with the glomeruli with crescent formation increases the risk of chronic renal failure.[17]

Hemolytic-Uremic Syndrome

Hemolytic-uremic syndrome is an acute disorder characterized by hemolytic anemia originating in the microcirculation and thrombocytopenia. It is the most common cause of acute renal failure in young children.[18] The cause remains unknown, although an association between hemolytic-uremic syndrome and both bacterial and viral agents has been established. Hemolytic-uremic syndrome is the most frequent cause of acute renal failure in children. *Escherichia coli* is the most common associated organism in the United States.[19] The disease occurs in infants and children younger than 4 years. When it occurs in adults, it is often associated with pregnancy or use of oral contraceptives. The prognosis has improved dramatically in recent years, with more than 90% of children surviving and most regaining normal renal function.

Pathophysiology

In hemolytic-uremic syndrome, verotoxin from *E. coli* damages red blood cells and endothelial cells. The endothelial lining of the glomerular arterioles becomes swollen and occluded with platelets and fibrin clots. Narrowed vessels damage erythrocytes as they pass through. These damaged burr cells, helmet cells, and fragmented red blood cells are removed by the spleen, causing acute hemolytic anemia. Fibrinolysis, the process of dissolution of a clot, acts on precipitated fibrin, causing the fibrin split products to appear in serum and urine. The platelet clustering within damaged vessels, combined with the damage and removal of platelets, produces thrombocytopenia. Other tissues, including the brain, liver, heart, and intestines, are often involved.

Clinical Manifestations

A prodromal gastrointestinal illness (fever, vomiting, diarrhea) or, less frequently, an upper respiratory infection often precedes the onset of hemolytic-uremic syndrome by 1 to 2 weeks. After a symptom-free 1- to 5-day period, the sudden onset of pallor, bruising or purpura, irritability, and oliguria heralds the onset of the disease. Slight fever, anorexia, vomiting, diarrhea (with the stool characteristically watery and blood stained), abdominal pain, mild jaundice, and circulatory overload are accompanying symptoms. Seizures and lethargy indicate CNS involvement. Renal failure is apparent within the first days of onset. The renal failure causes metabolic acidosis, azotemia, hyperkalemia, and often hypertension.

Evaluation and Treatment

Clinical evaluation includes history of preexisting illness, presenting symptoms, and urine and blood analysis. Management consists of maintaining nutrition and fluid and electrolyte balance and controlling hypertension and seizures.[18] When renal failure occurs, early and frequent peritoneal dialysis is indicated. Blood transfusions with packed red cells are needed to maintain reasonable hemoglobin levels.

Nephrotic Syndrome

In children with nephrotic syndrome the kidney is usually the only or principal organ involved. This condition is termed **primary nephrotic syndrome**. If it results from a systemic disease or other causes (e.g., drugs, toxins), it is called **secondary nephrotic syndrome** (see Chapter 35).

Approximately 95% of cases of nephrotic syndrome in children occur in the absence of systemic or preexisting renal disease. Primary nephrotic syndrome is found predominantly in preschool children, with a peak incidence of onset between 2 and 3 years of age. It is rare after 8 years of age. Boys are affected more frequently than girls. No prevalent racial or geographic distributions are evident. The incidence is approximately 3 per 100,000 children per year.

Pathophysiology

Nephrotic syndrome is a term used to describe a symptom complex characterized by proteinuria, hypoproteinemia, hyperlipidemia, and edema. Transient hematuria or hypertension may occur. Nephrotic syndrome is a clinical and biochemical state that may develop during the course of several different renal or systemic diseases. (The pathophysiology and common clinical manifestations of nephrotic syndrome in adults are described in Chapter 35.) **Minimal change nephrotic syndrome** is found in 85% of children with idiopathic nephrosis. The mechanism of increased glomerular permeability is unknown but is related, in part, to loss of negative charge within the glomerular capillary wall. The glomeruli appear normal, and immunoglobulin deposition is usually absent. The only change is fusion of epithelial cell podocytes.[12,20] The hyperlipidemia results from both increased hepatic synthesis and decreased plasma catabolism.[21] In nephrotic syndrome not due to minimal change disease, the distal tubules are unable to excrete salt. This may be related to vascular hyperpermeability in primary nephrotic syndrome. The severe edema may lead to hypovolemia.[22,23] Focal segmental glomerulosclerosis is present in approximately 20% of children with nephrotic syndrome and is more common in blacks. The more severe the proteinuria, the more likely that end stage renal disease will occur.[24a]

Clinical Manifestations

Onset of nephrotic syndrome is insidious, with periorbital edema as the first sign. The edema is most noticeable in the morning but subsides during the day as fluid shifts to the abdomen and lower extremities (Fig. 36-5). Because toddlers have picky eating habits, parents are often pleased with the weight gain associated with edema. Parents become alerted to an abnormality when they notice diminished, "frothy," or "foamy" urine and when edema becomes pronounced with ascites, respiratory difficulty from pleural effusion, and labial or scrotal swelling.

Edema of the intestinal mucosa may cause diarrhea, anorexia, and poor absorption. Edema often masks the malnutrition caused by malabsorption and protein loss. Because of protein deficiency, changes in the quality of hair indicate a malnourished state. Pallor, with shiny skin and prominent veins, is also common. Blood pressure is usually normal or slightly decreased. The child has an increased susceptibility to infection, especially pneumonia, peritonitis, cellulitis, and septicemia. Irritability, fatigue, and lethargy are common. Infants born with congenital nephrotic syndrome have large fontanelles, have separated cranial sutures, and may show gingival hyperplasia.[24b]

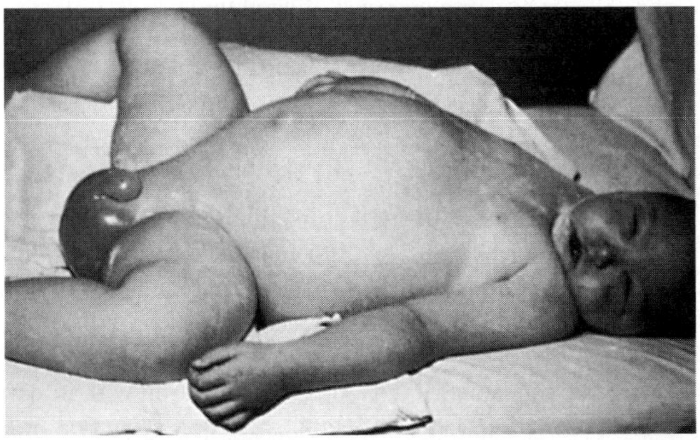

FIG. 36-5 Child with nephrotic syndrome. (From Shirkey HC, editor: *Pediatric therapy*, ed 6, St Louis, 1980, Mosby.)

Evaluation and Treatment

The diagnosis of nephrotic syndrome is evident from the finding of proteinuria, hyperlipidemia, and lipiduria. Several diagnostic tests, including kidney biopsy, may be required to determine whether the cause is an intrinsic renal disease or a consequence of systemic disease.

The goals of treatment are to reduce the excretion of protein and to maintain a protein-free urine. Prevention or treatment of infection, control of edema, establishment of a balanced nutritional state, and restoration of normal metabolic processes are also important in managing the disorder. Corticosteroids are the primary therapeutic agents, and outcomes in children are often described according to their response to steroid therapy (Table 36-3). Basic management of nephrotic syndrome includes activity as tolerated; a low-sodium, well-balanced diet; glucocorticosteroids (prednisone), diuretics (furosemide [Lasix]), and immunosuppressive agents (cyclophosphamide [Cytoxan], azathioprine [Imuran]); paracentesis (for ascites); and skin care.

Adults and children respond differently to management. Most children have complete remission; few adults do. Most children have minimal or no pathologic renal changes. The prognosis for ultimate recovery is quite good. Although relapses are common, usually after respiratory infections or live-virus immunizations, most children can look forward to a healthy future. Even those with frequent relapses usually have a spontaneous resolution before 30 years of age.[25] Renal transplant is performed for those children who progress to renal failure.[26]

Obstructive Disorders

Urinary Tract Infections

Urinary tract infections (UTIs) are rare in newborns and are usually caused by bacteria from the bloodstream settling in the urinary tract. UTIs are most common in 7- to 11-year-old girls as a result of bacteria, usually a pathogenic strain

Table 36-3 Primary Glomerulonephritis in Children

Classification	Findings
Cause	Poststreptococcal infection Related to other bacterial or viral infection Unknown
Immunologic mechanism	Antigen-antibody complex Anti–glomerular basement membrane disease No immunologic cause established
Histopathology	No lesion Diffuse, focal, or segmented Membranous, proliferative, or combination of types Lobular, exudative, necrotizing, and other types Chronic with glomerular proliferation
Clinical manifestations of disease	Acute glomerulonephritis Persistent (chronic) glomerulonephritis Idiopathic nephrotic syndrome

WHAT'S NEW? Allergy and Minimal Change Nephropathy

Minimal change nephropathy (MCN) in children has been associated with allergy to cow's milk, eggs, pork, inhaled pollen, and house dust. Children with MCN have increased type Th-2 lymphocytes and increased type II immunoglobulin E (IgE) receptors on B cells. The Th-2 subset of lymphocytes produces interleukins (IL-4, IL-5, and IL-6) with long-lasting production of IgE and immunoglobulin G (IgG). Children with MCN who go into remission with steroid therapy have decreased IL-4-induced type II IgE receptors. Although the cause of this disease remains unknown, abnormal T cell function is probably implicated and further research is clarifying the relationship among allergy, immune cytokines, and MCN.

Data from Cho BS et al: Up-regulation of interleukin-4 and CD23/FcepsilonRII in minimal change syndrome, *Pediatr Nephrol* 13(3): 199, 1999; Neuhaus TJ et al: *Clin Exp Immunol* 100:475, 1995; Wardle EN: *Nephron* 74(2):422, 1996.

of *E. coli*, ascending the urethra. Individual susceptibility, bacterial virulence, and the host's anatomy (presence of reflux, obstruction, stasis, or stones) affect the severity of the disease. The recurrence rate is approximately 30% to 40%.[27]

Cystitis, or infection of the bladder, results in mucosal inflammation and congestion. This causes detrusor muscle hyperactivity and a resulting decrease in the bladder capacity. It also can lead to reflux of urine up the ureters. Transient reflux caused by the cystitis, or chronic vesicoureteral reflux, can send bacteria all the way to the kidney, causing acute or chronic pyelonephritis. Either of these can cause renal abscesses or scarring.

Differentiating whether an infection is in the bladder or the kidneys is difficult based on symptoms alone. Infants usually develop nausea, vomiting, diarrhea, or jaundice. Children may present with fever of undetermined origin, frequency, urgency, enuresis or incontinence in a previously dry child, abdominal pain, foul-smelling urine, and sometimes hematuria. Acute pyelonephritis usually causes chills, fever, and flank or abdominal pain along with enlarged kidney(s) caused by edema. Chronic pyelonephritis may be asymptomatic.

Diagnosis of UTIs is by urine culture. An accompanying urinalysis can show pyuria and microscopic hematuria. Dipstick analysis for nitrite and/or leukocyte esterase is also sensitive.[28] The presence of casts in the urine can indicate pyelonephritis. Ultrasound, cortical scintigraphy, or computed tomography (CT) scan may be necessary to rule out obstructions or abscesses.

With treatment, UTI symptoms are usually relieved in 1 to 2 days and the urine becomes sterile. Sulfonamides are the drug of choice, with the usual treatment lasting 7 to 10 days. More potent medications may be required if the child has been previously treated for a UTI or has congenital abnormalities of the urinary tract. About 3 to 6 weeks after treatment is completed, all children with a first UTI should have a voiding cystourethrogram done to rule out reflux.[29] It is important not to rush this test because the UTI can cause mild to severe reflux. If reflux is found, an intravenous pyelogram may be done to check for renal damage or scarring. Follow-up urine cultures should be done 2 to 3 weeks after the medication is completed and every 3 months for the next 1 to 2 years to monitor for recurrence and for normal renal development and function, even if the child is asymptomatic.

Surgical correction of reflux or obstruction is necessary before the urinary tract can be sterilized. Children who develop frequent recurrences and who do not have surgically correctable anomalies may need prophylactic antibiotic therapy. These children also require regular cultures to rule out asymptomatic infections with resistant microorganisms.

Vesicoureteral Reflux

Vesicoureteral reflux (VUR) is the retrograde flow of bladder urine into the ureters. Reflux allows infected urine from the bladder to be repeatedly swept up into the kidneys. The reflux perpetuates infection by preventing complete emptying of the bladder, because infected, refluxed urine drains back into the bladder at the end of each voiding. In addition, the reflux allows the maximal intravesical pressure to be transmitted to the renal calyces and pyramids. The combination of reflux and infection is an important cause of pyelonephritis, especially in children younger than 5 years.

Vesicoureteral reflux occurs more frequently in girls by a ratio of 10:1 and is uncommon in blacks. Its incidence is approximately 1 in 1000 children, and siblings of those affected have a 25% chance of developing reflux. Although reflux is considered abnormal at any age, the shortness of the submucosal segment of the ureter during infancy and childhood renders the antireflux mechanism relatively inefficient and delicate. Thus reflux is seen commonly in association with infections during early childhood but rarely in older children and adults. (Among adults with UTIs, the incidence of reflux is approximately 5%.)

Reflux may be unilateral or bilateral, and it can be classified or graded (Fig. 36-6) for comparative purposes:

Grade I—reflux into a nondilated distal ureter
Grade II—reflux into the upper collecting system without dilation
Grade III—reflux into dilated ureter or blunting of calyceal fornices
Grade IV—reflux into a grossly dilated ureter
Grade V—massive reflux with ureteral dilation and tortuosity and effacement of the calyceal details; occurs almost exclusively in male infants[30]

Pathophysiology

Primary reflux results from a congenitally abnormal or ectopic insertion of the ureter into the bladder. In some infants, VUR may be related to inadequate relaxation of the external urethral sphincter.[31] Occasionally the condition is hereditary. Secondary reflux is more serious and may be transient or persistent. It develops in association with infection, malformations of the ureterovesical (UV) junction, increased intravesical pressures, and surgery on the UV junc-

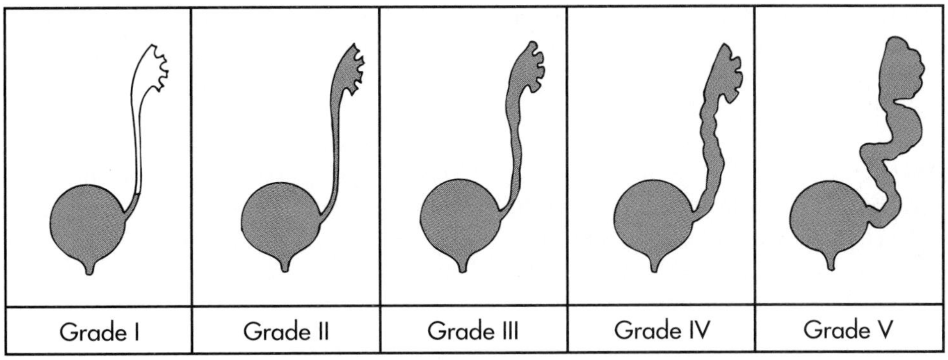

FIG. 36-6 Grades of reflux. (From Retik A, Cukier J, editors: *Pediatric urology*, Baltimore, 1987, Williams & Wilkins.)

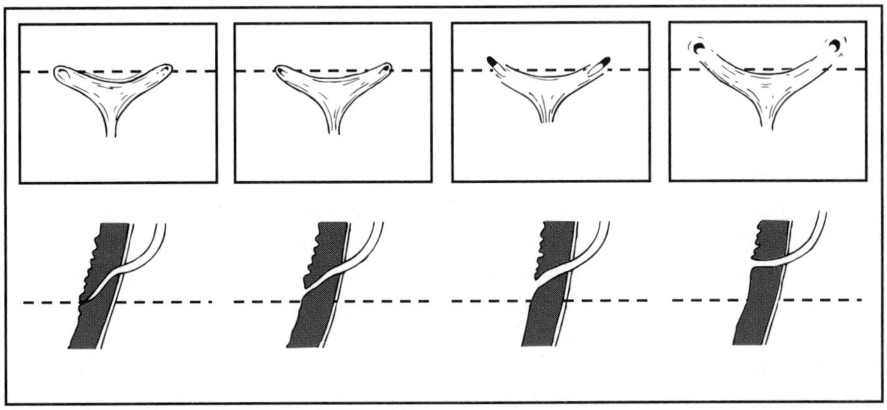

FIG. 36-7 Normal and abnormal configuration of the ureteral orifices. *Left to right*, Progressive lateral displacement of the ureteral orifices and shortening of the intramural tunnels. *Top row*, Endoscopic appearance. *Bottom row*, Sagittal view through the intramural ureter. (From Behrman R et al, editors: *Nelson textbook of pediatrics*, Philadelphia, 1992, W.B. Saunders.)

tion (Fig. 36-7). Urinary tract infection associated with VUR may lead to renal scarring, particularly when there is pyelonephritis.[32]

Clinical Manifestations

Children with reflux have recurrent UTIs or unexplained fever, poor growth and development, irritability, and feeding problems. Both children and adults may have a family history of reflux or UTI, pain with voiding, and signs of urinary obstruction or neuropathy.

Evaluation and Treatment

In addition to the history of recurrent UTIs and other symptoms, a voiding cystourethrogram (VCUG) and an intravenous pyelogram may be required for diagnosis. Most children with vesicoureteral reflux respond to nonoperative management aimed at prevention and treatment of infection. Spontaneous remission of grades I and II reflux may occur in 30% to 60% of children younger than 5 years. Children with grades III and IV reflux need long-term monitoring and prophylactic antibiotics.[33] Recurrent infection may require surgical intervention. In cases of grade V reflux, early surgical intervention is indicated to prevent renal scarring, although spontaneous resolution can occur during the first year.[30] Siblings of children with vesicoureteral reflux should have a screening VCUG performed. Up to 46% have been found to have asymptomatic vesicoureteral reflux.[34]

Wilms Tumor

Wilms tumor is an embryonal tumor of the kidney. The tumor was first described in 1814 and was named after Max Wilms, a German surgeon who wrote a detailed explanation of it in 1899. At that time Wilms proposed that the tumor was of embryonic origin and arose from undifferentiated mesoderm. Because it is an embryonal tumor of the kidney, Wilms tumor is also known by the histologic name of *nephroblastoma.*

The incidence of Wilms tumor remains constant in the United States, with 7.8 cases per 1 million persons ages 1 to 14 years. This means that approximately 400 children are diagnosed each year in the United States, or 1 in every 10,000 children will develop a Wilms tumor. Most children are between 1 and 5 years of age when they are diagnosed. The peak incidence occurs between 2 and 3 years of age. Wilms tumor is the most common childhood cancer of the urinary tract. There are no associations between frequency and gender; however, Wilms tumor is slightly more common in females and in black children than in white children.[35]

Microscopically, Wilms tumor is composed of three cellular components: stromal, epithelial, and blastemic. This occurs because blastemic cells, which are primitive and undifferentiated, may have partially developed into epithelial or stromal tissue. With each of these three cellular components, varying stages of differentiation may be evident.

Pathogenesis

Wilms tumor has both sporadic and inherited origins. The sporadic form occurs in children with no known genetic predisposition. Inherited cases, which are relatively rare, are transmitted in an autosomal dominant fashion.

In both cases, Wilms tumor has been linked to the deletion or inactivation of genes on the short arm of chromosome 11.[36] The deletion or inactivation of these genes demonstrated that the mechanism for development of Wilms tumor involved tumor-suppressor genes. Three tumor-suppressor genes have now been identified.[37] *WT1* and *WT2* have been localized to chromosome 11, 17, and 19. A third gene, *WT3*, may be located on chromosome 16q. It has been associated with the familial form of Wilms tumor.[38]

The pathogenesis of both the sporadic and inherited forms of Wilms tumor is similar to retinoblastoma. In the inherited form of the disease, the child inherits the loss of one copy of the Wilms tumor–suppressor gene (*WT3*) in all of the primitive metanephric blastemic (fetal renal) cells that normally differentiate into the renal tubules and glomeruli. All that is needed is the loss of the other copy of the gene for a Wilms tumor to develop. Because many cells are vulnerable to the loss of this second copy of the gene, bilateral presentation of Wilms tumor (tumor in both kidneys) occurs occasionally in the inherited form of the disease. In the sporadic form of Wilms tumor, both copies of the gene are lost during fetal development. Because normal renal development occurs during the eighth to the thirty-fourth week of gestation, gene loss likely occurs during this time.[39]

Eighteen percent of children who have Wilms tumor also have a number of congenital anomalies. Children with these abnormalities are usually found to have large deletions of the short arm of chromosome 11. Besides loss of the Wilms tumor–suppressor genes, several other important genes are lost, resulting in the anomalies. The anomalies associated with Wilms tumor are aniridia (lack of an iris in the eye), hemihypertrophy (an asymmetry of the body), and genitourinary malformations (i.e., horseshoe kidneys, hypospadias, ureteral duplication, polycystic kidneys, uterine abnormalities).[40,41] Children with both congenital anomalies and Wilms tumor are more likely to have the inherited bilateral form of the disease.

Clinical Manifestations

Most Wilms tumors (90%) are enlarging asymptomatic upper abdominal masses at the time of diagnosis. Many tumors are actually discovered by the child's parent, who feels or notices an abdominal swelling, usually while dressing or bathing the child. The child appears healthy and thriving. Other presenting complaints include vague abdominal pain (37%), hematuria (21%), and fever (23%).[42] Hypertension also may be present. The reported frequency is quite variable, from 25% to as high as 63% in one report.[43] Hypertension is probably caused by either encroachment by the tumor on the blood supply or secretion of renin by the tumor.

Wilms tumor may occur in any part of the kidney and varies greatly in size at the time of diagnosis. The tumor generally appears as a solitary mass surrounded by a smooth, fibrous external capsule and may contain cystic or hemorrhagic areas. A pseudocapsule generally separates the tumor from the renal parenchyma.

Evaluation and Treatment

On physical examination the tumor feels firm, nontender, and smooth. The mass is generally confined to one side of the abdomen. Should the tumor be palpable past the midline of the abdomen, it may be very large or may be arising from a horseshoe or ectopic kidney. Once an abdominal mass is detected, an abdominal ultrasound may be the initial study and may demonstrate a solid intrarenal mass. Abdominal CT scan or magnetic resonance imaging also may be obtained before biopsy and surgical removal of the tumor.

Diagnosis is based on surgical biopsy. Additional laboratory and radiologic studies are used to evaluate the presence or absence of metastasis. The most common sites of metastasis are regional lymph nodes and the lungs. Metastases also occur in the liver, brain, and bone.

Several staging systems for Wilms tumor have been developed. The most widely accepted system was developed by the National Wilms Tumor Study Group (Table 36-4). The system is based on surgical findings and the extent of disease at diagnosis.[40]

Surgical exploration and resection begin the treatment of Wilms tumor. The abdomen is explored to determine the extent of disease. In the case of bilateral disease, surgical intervention may include heminephrectomy of the less involved kidney and nephrectomy of the other. Wilms tumor is considered radiosensitive, and radiation therapy has been found to be most effective if begun 1 to 3 days after surgery. Radiation is not needed for stages I or II disease; it may be used in stages III and IV disease. Radiation therapy also is used for lung, nonresectable liver, brain, bone, and lymph node metastases should they be present. The optimal protocol for chemotherapy is still under study for each stage of Wilms tumor. Further studies are needed to determine the ultimate value of each approach.[35]

Table 36-4 Staging of Wilms Tumor

Stage	Tumor Characteristics
Stage I	Tumor limited to the kidney, completely resected
Stage II	Tumor ascending beyond the kidney but appearing to be totally resected
Stage III	Residual nonhematogenous tumor confined to the abdomen
Stage IV	Hematogenous metastases
Stage V	Bilateral disease either at diagnosis or later

NOTE: Staging system of the Third National Wilms Tumor Study Group (NWTS-3).

Tremendous advances have been made in the treatment and cure of Wilms tumor. Before the 1930s, 90% of children died of Wilms tumor. Today, with modern treatment, the overall cure rate is as high as 95% for children with stage I through stage III disease. Prognosis is generally poor for children with metastases, although this is one of the few tumors for which lung metastases have been cured.

Various factors affect the child's prognosis. These include tumor weight at diagnosis, the age of the child, lymph node invasion, and histologic category. The most important prognostic factors, however, appear to be the histologic category and regional lymph node involvement (Table 36-5). Children with a favorable history and no metastatic sites have a 90% survival rate. Even those children with less favorable results do very well, with up to an 80% survival rate.[44]

Enuresis

Enuresis refers to the involuntary passage of urine by a child who is beyond the age when voluntary bladder control should have been acquired. Bladder control is accomplished by most children before the age of 4 years. Five years of age is more accurate and widely accepted, however, and is determined largely by cultural beliefs and practices of parents regarding toilet training. In 80% of children, enuresis occurs at night only and is then called **nocturnal enuresis**.

Types

Primary enuresis refers to a condition in which the child has never been continent. Secondary enuresis, or acquired enuresis, occurs when a child who has experienced a period of dryness of at least 3 to 6 months after toilet training becomes incontinent again. **Secondary enuresis** may be diurnal (daytime), nocturnal, or a combination of both. (Types of incontinence are defined in Table 36-6.)

The incidence of enuresis is difficult to determine because it is not a problem that parents readily share with others and because definitions vary according to cultural norms and family practices. Some families start toilet training before 1 year of age and expect continence by the age of 1 to 1½ years, whereas other families do not expect dryness earlier than 5 years. According to research data, the incidence of enuresis in children older than 5 years ranges from 15% to 26%. Boys are more enuretic than girls by a ratio of 3 : 2. Teenage enuresis is usually a continuation of childhood bed-wetting.

Theories

Theories about the cause of enuresis abound. A combination of factors is likely to be responsible for enuresis. All or part of each one might be operating in a given child. A reasonable approach is to eliminate organic or physiologic causes for enuresis before exploring the psychologic ones.

Organic causes of enuresis account for 2% to 10% of cases. The causes include urinary tract infections; neurologic disturbances; congenital defects of the meatus, urethra, and bladder neck; allergies; or alteration in renal tubular ion and water transport related to prostaglandin secretion.[45] Disorders that increase the normal output of urine, such as diabetes mellitus and diabetes insipidus, or disorders that impair the concentrating ability of the kidney, such as chronic renal failure or sickle cell disease, must be considered in the evaluation of enuresis.

Enuresis in children is possibly caused by a maturational lag. Studies have demonstrated that the child with enuresis has a smaller functional bladder capacity than a nonenuretic child.[46] A number of children show a general developmental delay along with elevated intravesical pressure and spikelike detrusor contractions during bladder filling. Enuresis may spontaneously disappear in these children as they get older. Other studies have shown that children with enuresis completely fill and empty their bladder several times each night because of a constant urine output and a stable level of antidiuretic hormone (ADH). Children who remain dry usually have elevated levels of ADH and thus a decreased urine output

Table 36-5 National Wilms Tumor Study-3 Survival Rates

	Relapse-free survival, 4 years (percent)	Four-year survival (percent)
Stage I/FH	89	95.6
Stage II/FH	87.4	91.1
Stage III/FH	82.0	90.9
Stage IV/FH	70.0	80.9

From Green DM et al: *CA Cancer J Clin* 46(1):56, 1996.
FH, Favorable histology.

Table 36-6 Classification of Incontinence

Types of Incontinence	Definition
Total incontinence	Inability to store any urine; indicates an anatomic or functional absence of urinary sphincters (e.g., epispadias, myelomeningocele) or a bypassing of urinary sphincters (e.g., vesicovaginal fistula)
Overflow incontinence	Frequent dribbling that relieves a constantly full bladder; occurs when urinary outlet is obstructed
Urge incontinence	Sudden and uncontrollable need to void that cannot be suppressed; suggests bladder irritation
Precipitate voiding	Voiding without a preceding urge to void; suggests neurologic origin
Stress incontinence	Uncontrollable voiding that occurs when intravesical pressure momentarily exceeds intravesical resistance, as in "giggle incontinence"
Paradoxic incontinence	Incontinence in spite of normal voiding; suggests an ectopic ureteral orifice outside the urinary sphincter mechanism (e.g., a girl who is constantly wet, yet voids normally)

at night.[47] Still other studies indicated loss of diurnal variation in ADH.[48]

Genetic factors as a cause of enuresis are being investigated. Linkages have been proposed between nocturnal enuresis and chromosomes 8, 12, 13, and 22.[49] Bed-wetting does occur with high frequency among parents, siblings, and other near relatives of symptomatic children. These observations are further supported by a high concordance rate in enuretic monozygotic twins.

Recent research studying sleep and nocturnal enuresis indicate that enuresis may be related to non–rapid eye movement (non-REM) sleep, and that enuretics may spend more time in stage 3 sleep with a greater depth of sleep.[50,51] This is in contrast to earlier reports that proposed that enuresis occurs as the child moves from the deeper stages of non-REM to the REM stage.

A variety of psychosocial theories also have been postulated as explanations of enuresis. Enuresis has been associated with temper tantrums, fear reactions, excitability, low birth weight, and minimal brain dysfunction.[52]

Behavioral interventions—such as self-awakening techniques, enuresis alarms, and motivational therapy—have the best results in treating enuresis. Desmopressin acetate nasal spray, a synthetic ADH, is best used when other treatments have not worked and a "quick fix" is required for social reasons, such as sleepovers.[47,53,54,55] Psychotherapy and behavior modification are recommended when enuresis is associated with psychologic stress.

SUMMARY REVIEW

Structure and Function of the Renal System in Children

1. Because of high hydrogen ion concentration, limited ability to regulate the internal environment, and lowered osmotic pressure, infants have a narrow chemical safety margin.
2. Any disturbance, such as diarrhea, infection, fasting, or feeding alterations, can lead rapidly to severe acidosis and fluid imbalance in infants.
3. The composition of body fluids differs with age, thus making children more vulnerable to pathophysiologic changes.
4. Because the kidney develops from the medulla to the cortex, blood flow to the medullary nephrons is limited in infancy and infants thus have limited urine-concentrating capacity.

Alterations in Renal Function in Children

1. Congenital renal disorders affect 10% to 15% of the population. These disorders range in severity from minor, easily correctable anomalies to those incompatible with life.
2. Hypospadias is a congenital condition in which the urethral meatus is located on the undersurface of the penis; epispadias is a congenital condition in which the urethral opening is located on the dorsal surface of the penis.
3. Epispadias is a mild form of exstrophy—a congenital condition that affects the urethra and bladder neck. The urethral opening in boys is on the dorsal surface of the penis.
4. Exstrophy of the bladder is a congenital malformation in which the pubic bones are separated, the lower portion of the abdominal wall and anterior wall of the bladder are missing, and the back wall of the bladder is everted through the opening.
5. A dysplastic kidney is the result of abnormal differentiation of renal tissues. The hypoplastic kidney is a very small but otherwise normal kidney.
6. Renal agenesis is the failure of a kidney to grow or develop. The condition may be unilateral or bilateral and may occur as an isolated entity or in association with other disorders.
7. Glomerulonephritis is an inflammation of the glomeruli characterized by hematuria, edema, and hypertension. The cause is unknown, but poststreptococcal glomerulonephritis may follow infections, especially those of the upper respiratory tract. Deposition of IgA immunoglobulins in the mesangium of the glomerular capillaries leads to immunoglobulin A nephropathy.
8. Henoch-Schonlein nephritis is an IgA nephropathy that affects glomerular blood vessels.
9. Hemolytic-uremic syndrome is an acute disorder characterized by hemolytic anemia, acute renal failure, and thrombocytopenia.
10. Nephrotic syndrome is a term used to describe a symptom complex characterized by proteinuria, hypoproteinemia, hyperlipidemia, and edema. Metabolic, biochemical, or physiochemical disturbance in the glomerular basement membrane may lead to increased permeability to protein.
11. Urinary tract infections can result from general sepsis in the newborn but are caused by bacteria ascending the urethra in older children. The bladder alone is infected in cystitis. The infection ascends to the kidney or kidneys in pyelonephritis. Urinary tract anomalies must be surgically corrected to prevent frequent recurrent infections.
12. Vesicoureteral reflux, which refers to the retrograde flow of bladder urine into the ureters, provides mechanisms for bladder infection in children, whose ureters are shorter than those of adults.
13. Wilms tumor is an embryonal tumor of the kidney that usually presents between birth and 5 years of age. The tumor can be successfully treated by surgery, with a combination of drugs and, sometimes, radiation therapy.
14. Enuresis refers to the involuntary passage of urine.
15. Enuresis may occur during the day (diurnally) or night (nocturnally). The disorder tends to occur during non–rapid eye movement (non-REM) sleep and can have a variety of organic and psychologic causes.

KEY TERMS

Chordee, *1219*
Cystitis, *1224*
Enuresis, *1227*
Epispadias, *1220*
Exstrophy of the bladder, *1220*
Glomerulonephritis, *1221*
Hemolytic-uremic syndrome, *1222*
Henoch-Schonlein nephritis, *1222*
Horseshoe kidney, *1219*
Hypoplastic kidney, *1220*
Hypospadias, *1219*
Minimal change nephrotic syndrome, *1223*
Nephrotic syndrome, *1222*
Nocturnal enuresis, *1227*
Potter syndrome, *1221*
Primary enuresis, *1227*
Primary nephrotic syndrome, *1222*
Renal agenesis, *1220*
Renal aplasia, *1220*
Renal dysplasia, *1220*
Secondary enuresis, *1227*
Secondary nephrotic syndrome, *1222*
Urinary tract infection (UTI), *1223*
Vesicoureteral reflux, *1224*
Wilms tumor (nephroblastoma), *1225*

REFERENCES

1. McAninch JW: Disorders of the kidneys. In Taragho EA, McAninch JW, editors: *Smith's general urology*, Norwalk, Conn, 1995, Appleton & Lange.
2. Kelalis PP, Lowell RK, Bellmam BA: *Clinical pediatric oncology*, ed 3, Philadelphia, 1992, W.B. Saunders.
3. Silver RI: What is the etiology of hypospadias? A review of recent research, *Del Med J* 72(8):343, 2000.
4. Caesar RE, Caldamone AA: The use of free grafts for correcting penile chordee, *J Urol* 164(5):1691, 2000.
5. Speakman MJ, Azmy AF: Skin chordee without hypospadias—an underrecognized entity, *Br J Urol* 69(4):428, 1992.
6. Borer JG, Retik AB: Current trends in hypospadias repair, *Urol Clin North Am* 26(1):15, 1999.
7. Ben-Chaim J et al: Bladder exstrophy from childhood to adult life, *J R Soc Med* 89(1):39P, 1996.
8. Sponseller PD et al: The anatomy of the pelvis in the exstrophy complex, *J Bone Joint Surg Am* 77(2):177, 1995.
9. Holliday MA, Barratt TM, Avner ED: *Pediatric nephrology*, ed 2, Baltimore, 1994, Williams & Wilkins.
10. Hitchcock T, Burge DM: Renal agenesis: an acquired condition? *J Pediatr Surg* 29(3):454, 1994.
11a. Glazebrook KN, McGrath FP, Steele BT: Prenatal compensatory renal growth: documentation with US, *Radiology* 189(3):733, 1993.
11b. Cascio S, Paran S, Puri P: Associated urological anomalies in children with unilateral renal agenesis, *J Urol* 162(3 Pt 2):1081, 1999.
12. Behrman R, Kliegman R, Jenson H, editors: *Nelson textbook of pediatrics*, ed 16, Philadelphia, 2000, W.B. Saunders.
13. Nakagawa H et al: Significance of glomerular deposition of C3c and C3d in IgA nephropathy, *Am J Nephrol* 20(2):122, 2000.
14. Lai FM et al: Characterization of early IgA nephropathy, *Am J Kidney Dis* 36(4):703, 2000.
15. Andreoli SP: Chronic glomerulonephritis in childhood, *Pediatr Clin North Am* 42(6):1487, 1995.
16. Syrhanen J, Mustonen J, Pasternack A: Hypertriglyceridaemia and hyperuricaemia are risk factors for progression of IgA nephropathy, *Nephrol Dial Transplant* 15(1):34, 2000.
17. Rieu P, Noel LH: Henoch-Schonlein nephritis in children and adults. Morphological features and clinicopathological correlations, *Ann Med Interne* (Paris) 150(2):151, 1999.
18. Trachtman H, Christen E: Pathogenesis, treatment, and therapeutic trials in hemolytic uremic syndrome, *Curr Opin Pediatr* 11(2):162, 1999.
19. Green DA, Murphy WG, Uttley WS: Haemolytic uraemic synrome: prognostic factors, *Clin Lab Haematol* 22(1):11, 2000.
20. Travis LB: Nephrotic syndrome. In Rudolph AM, Hoffman JIE, Rudolph CD: *Rudolph's pediatrics*, Norwalk, Conn, 1996, Appleton & Lange.
21. Chesney RW: The idiopathic nephrotic syndromes, *Curr Opin Pediatr* 11(2):158, 1999.
22. Rostoker G, Behar A, Lagrue G: Vascular permeability in nephrotic edema, *Nephron* 85(3):194, 2000.
23. Vande Walle JG, Donckerwolcke RA, Koomans HA: Pathophysiology of edema formation in children with nephrotic syndrome not due to minimal change disease, *J Am Soc Nephrol* 10(2):323, 1999.
24a. Korbet SM: Clinical picture and outcome of primary focal segmental glomerulosclerosis, *Nephrol Dial Transplant* 14(suppl 3):68, 1999.
24b. Mattoo TK: Gingival hyperplasia in congenital and infantile nephrotic syndrome, *Pediatr Nephrol* 11(3):388, 1997.
25. Warshaw BL: Nephrotic syndrome in children, *Pediatr Ann* 23(9):495, 1994.
26. Wyhl E et al: Impact of recurrent nephrotic syndrome after renal transplantation in young patients, *Pediatr Nephrol* 12(7):529, 1998.
27. Le Saux N, Pham B., Moher D: Evaluating the benefits of antimicrobial prophylaxis to prevent urinary tract infections in children: a systemic review, *CMAJ* 163(5):523, 2000.
28. Gorelick MH, Shaw KN: Screening tests for urinary tract infection in children: a meta-analysis, *Pediatrics* 104(5):e54, 1999.
29. Kass EJ, Kernen KM, Carey JM: Paediatric urinary tract infection and the necessity of complete urological imaging, *BJU Int* 86(1):94, 2000.
30. Sillen U: Viscoureteral reflux in infants, *Pediatr Nephrol* 13(4):355, 1999.
31. Chandra M, Maddix H: Urodynamic dysfunction in infants with vesicoureteral reflux, *J Pediatr* 136(6):754, 2000.
32. Jakobsson G, Jacobson SH, Hjalmas K: Vesico-ureteric reflux and other risk factors for renal damage: identification of high- and low-risk children, *Acta Pediatr Suppl* 88(431):31, 1999.
33. Wan J et al: An analysis of social and economic factors associated with follow-up of patients with vesicoureteral reflux, *J Urol* 156(2 pt 2):668, 1996.
34. Peeden JN, Noe HN: Is it practical to screen for familial vesicoureteral reflux within a private pediatric practice? *Pediatrics* 89(4):758, 1992.
35. Julian JC, Merguerian PA, Shortliffe L: Pediatric genitourinary tumors, *Curr Opin Oncol* 7:265, 1995.
36. Lee SB, Haber DA: Wilms tumor and the WT1 gene, *Exp Cell Res* 264(1):74, 2001.
37. Rapley EA et al: Evidence of susceptibility genes to familial Wilms tumor in addition to WT1, FWT1 and FWT2, *Br J Cancer* 83(2):177, 2000.
38. Tay JS: Molecular genetics of Wilms' tumor, *J Paediatr Child Health* 31(5):379, 1995.
39. Belasco J, Chatten J, D'Angio G: Wilms tumor. In Sutow W, Fernbach D, Vietti T, editors: *Clinical pediatric oncology*, ed 3, St Louis, 1984, Mosby.
40. Neville HL, Ritchey ML: Wilms' tumor: overview of National Wilms' Tumor Study Group results, *Urol Clin North Am* 27(3):435, 2000.
41. Nicholson HS et al: Uterine anomalies in Wilms' tumor survivors, *Cancer* 78(4):887, 1996.

42. Green DM: The diagnosis and management of Wilms' tumor, *Pediatr Clin North Am* 32:735, 1985.
43. Sukarochana K, Tolentino W, Kiesewetter WB: Wilms' tumor and hypertension, *J Pediatr Surg* 7:573, 1972.
44. Mitchell C et al: The treatment of Wilm's tumor: results of the United Kingdom Children's Cancer Study Group (UKCCSG) second Wilm's tumour study, *Br J Cancer* 83(5):602, 2000.
45. Kuznetsova AA et al: Possible role of prostaglandins in pathogenesis of nocturnal enuresis in children, *Scand J Urol Nephrol* 34(1):27, 2000.
46. Troup CW, Hodgson NB: Nocturnal functional bladder capacity in enuretic children, *J Urol* 105:129, 1971.
47. Stark M: Assessment and management of the care of children with nocturnal enuresis: guidelines for primary care, *Nurs Practit Forum* 5(3): 170, 1994.
48. Uygur MC, Ergen A, Remzi D: Enuresis nocturna: new concepts in pathophysiology, *Int Urol Nephrol* 27(4):439, 1995.
49. Gontard A et al: Molecular genetics of nocturnal enuresis: linkage to a locus on chromosome 22, *Scand J. Urol Nephrol Suppl* 202:76, 1999.
50. Hunsballe J: Sleep studies based on electroencephalogram energy analysis, *Scand J Urol Nephrol Suppl* 202:28, 1999.
51. Neveus T et al: Sleep of children with enuresis: a polysomnographic study, *Pediatrics* 103(6 part 1):1193, 1999.
52. Retik A, Cukier J, editors: *Pediatric urology*, Baltimore, 1987, Williams & Wilkins.
53. Glazener CM, Evans JH: Desmopressin for nocturnal enuresis in children, *Cochrane Database Syst Rev* (2):CD002112, 2000.
54. Harari MD, Moulden A: Noctural enuresis: what is happening? *J Paediatr Child Health* 36(1):78, 2000.
55. Natochin YV, Kuznetsova AA: Nocturnal enuresis: correction of renal function by desmopressin and diclofenac, *Pediatr Nephrol* 14(1):42, 2000.

CHAPTER 37

Structure and Function of the Digestive System

SUE E. HUETHER

CHAPTER OUTLINE

The digestive system breaks down ingested food, prepares it for uptake by the body's cells, provides body water, and eliminates wastes. This system consists of the gastrointestinal tract and accessory organs of digestion: the liver, gallbladder, and exocrine pancreas.

Food breakdown begins in the mouth with chewing and continues in the stomach, where food is churned and mixed with acid, mucus, enzymes, and other secretions. From the stomach, the fluid and partially digested food pass into the small intestine, where biochemicals and enzymes secreted by the liver and exocrine pancreas break the food down into absorbable components of proteins, carbohydrates, and fats. These nutrients pass through the walls of the small intestine into blood vessels and lymphatics that carry them to the liver for storage or further processing.

Ingested substances and secretions that are not absorbed in the small intestine pass into the large intestine, where fluid continues to be absorbed. Fluid wastes travel to the kidneys and are eliminated in the urine. Solid wastes pass into the rectum and are eliminated from the body through the anus.

Except for chewing, swallowing, and defecation of solid wastes, the movements of the digestive system (gastrointestinal motility) are all controlled by hormones and the autonomic nervous system. As ingested substances move through the gastrointestinal tract, they trigger the release of hormones that stimulate or inhibit (1) the muscular contractions that mix and propel food from the esophagus to the anus and (2) the timely secretion of substances that aid in digestion. The autonomic innervation, both sympathetic and parasympathetic, is controlled by centers in the brain and by local stimuli that are mediated at plexuses (networks of nerve fibers) within the gastrointestinal walls.

THE GASTROINTESTINAL TRACT

The **gastrointestinal tract (alimentary canal)** consists of the mouth, esophagus, stomach, small intestine, large intestine, rectum, and anus (Fig. 37-1). It carries out the following digestive processes:

1. Ingestion of food
2. Propulsion of food and wastes from the mouth to the anus
3. Secretion of mucus, water, and enzymes
4. Mechanical digestion of food particles
5. Chemical digestion of food particles
6. Absorption of digested food
7. Elimination of waste products by defecation

Histologically, the gastrointestinal tract consists of four layers. From the inside out they are the mucosa, submucosa, muscularis, and serosa or adventitia. These concentric layers vary in thickness, and each layer has sublayers (Fig. 37-2). Intrinsic nerves are located solely within the gastrointestinal tract and are controlled by local and autonomic nervous system stimuli through the **enteric plexus,** which comprises three nerve plexuses located in different layers of the

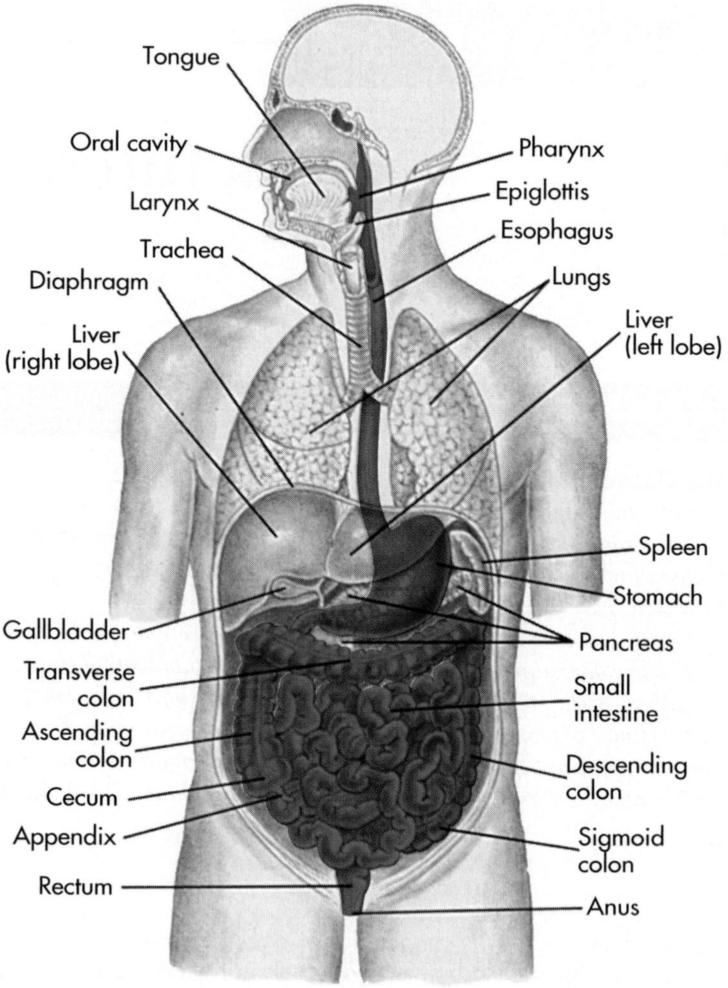

FIG. 37-1 Structure and function of the digestive system. Digestion begins in the mouth with chewing, which breaks down food mechanically and mixes it with saliva. Swallowing propels chewed food through the esophagus to the stomach, where acids and stomach motility liquefy it further. Next the liquefied food enters the small intestine, where secretions of the intestinal walls, liver, gallbladder, and pancreas digest it into absorbable nutrients. Nutrients are absorbed through intestinal walls, and unabsorbed wastes enter the large intestine (colon), where fluids are removed. Solid wastes then enter the rectum and leave the body through the anus. (From Thompson JM et al: *Mosby's clinical nursing*, ed 4, St Louis, 1997, Mosby.)

gastrointestinal walls. The **submucosal plexus (Meissner plexus)** is located in the muscularis mucosae, the **myenteric plexus (Auerbach plexus)** in the muscle layers (tunica muscularis), and the **subserosal plexus** just beneath the serosa. These enteric nerve circuits regulate motility, blood flow, and secretions.[1]

Mouth and Esophagus

The **mouth** is a reservoir for the chewing and mixing of food with saliva. As food particles become smaller and move around in the mouth, the taste buds and olfactory nerves are continuously stimulated, adding to the satisfaction of eating. The tongue's surface contains thousands of chemoreceptors, or taste buds, that can distinguish salty, sour, bitter, and sweet tastes. Tastes and food odors help to initiate salivation and the secretion of gastric juice in the stomach. There are 32 permanent teeth in the adult mouth, and they are important for speech and mastication.

Salivation

The three pairs of **salivary glands** (the submandibular, sublingual, and parotid glands) (Fig. 37-3) secrete about 1 L of saliva per day. **Saliva** consists mostly of water that contains varying amounts of mucus; sodium; bicarbonate; chloride; potassium; and **salivary α-amylase (ptyalin),** an enzyme that initiates carbohydrate digestion in the mouth and stomach.

Both sympathetic and parasympathetic divisions of the autonomic nervous system control salivation. Because cholinergic parasympathetic fibers stimulate the salivary glands, atropine (an anticholinergic agent) inhibits salivation and makes the mouth dry. β-Adrenergic stimulation from sympathetic fibers also increases salivary secretion. The salivary glands are not regulated by hormones.

The composition of saliva depends on the rate of secretion (Fig. 37-4). Aldosterone can increase an exchange of sodium for potassium, increasing sodium conservation and potassium excretion. The bicarbonate concentration of saliva sustains a pH of about 7.4, which neutralizes bacterial acids and prevents tooth decay. Saliva also contains immunoglobulin A (IgA), which helps to prevent infection. Exogenous fluoride (e.g., fluoride in drinking water) is absorbed and then secreted in the saliva, providing additional protection against tooth decay.

Swallowing

The **esophagus** is a hollow muscular tube approximately 25 cm long that conducts substances from the oropharynx to the stomach (see Fig. 37-1). Swallowed food is moved to the

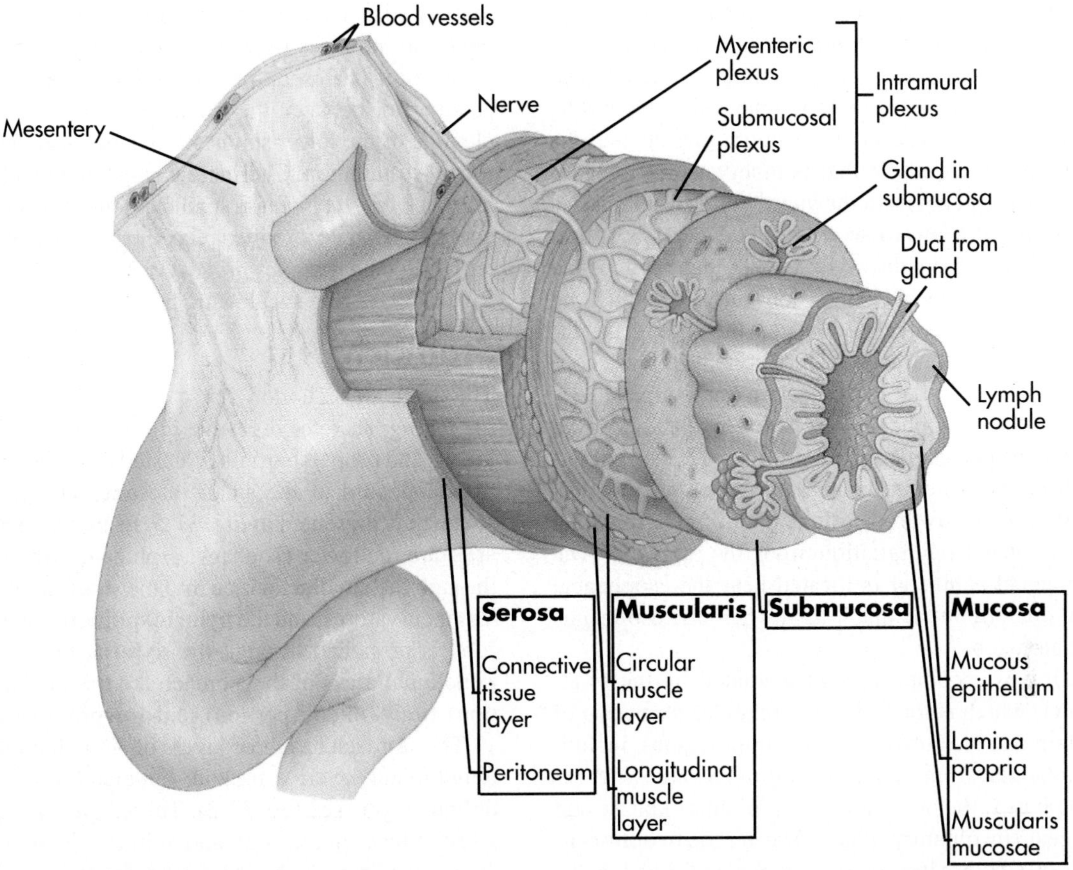

FIG. 37-2 Wall of the gastrointestinal (GI) tract. The wall of the GI tract is made up of four layers with a network of nerves between the layers. Shown here in a generalized diagram of a segment of the GI tract. Note that the serosa is continuous with a fold of serous membrane called a *mesentery*. Note also that digestive glands may empty their products into the lumen of the GI tract by way of ducts. (From Thibodeau GA, Patton KI: *Anatomy & physiology*, ed 4, St Louis, 1999, Mosby.)

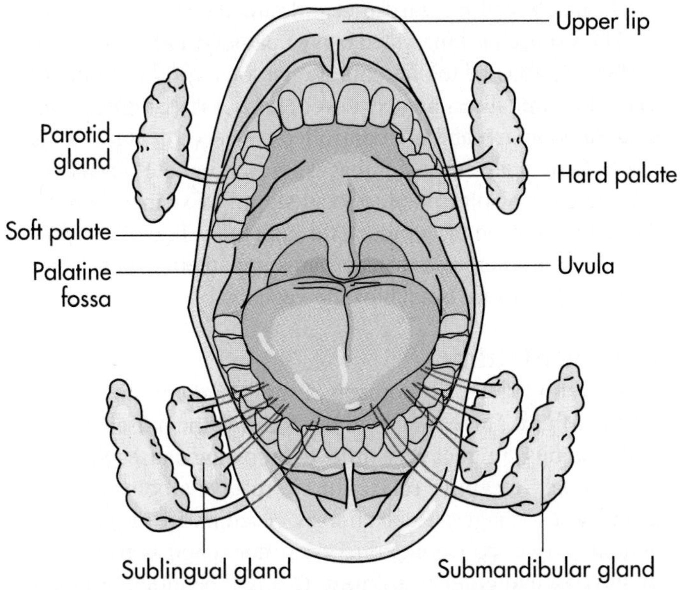

FIG. 37-3 Structures of the mouth. (From Phipps WJ et al: *Medical-surgical nursing: concepts and clinical practice*, ed 6, St Louis, 1999, Mosby.)

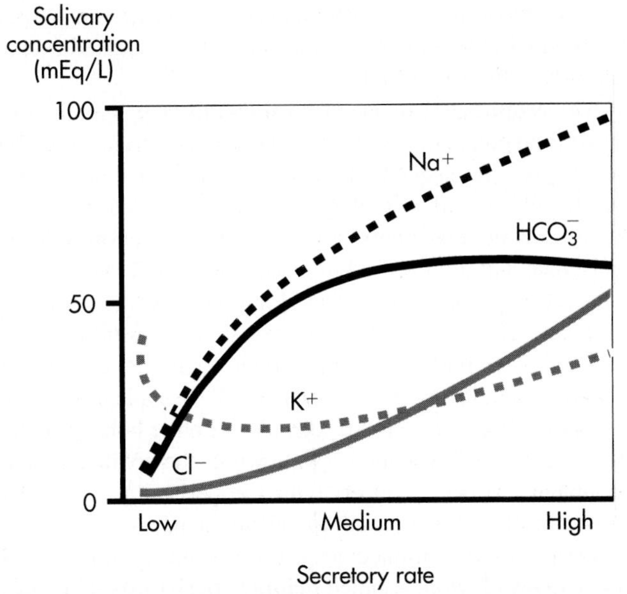

FIG. 37-4 Salivary electrolyte concentrations and flow rate. Changes in concentration of sodium (Na^+), potassium (K^+), chloride (Cl^-), and bicarbonate (HCO_3^-) with increases in flow rate of saliva. *Black dotted line*, Sodium; *solid black line*, bicarbonate; *solid red line*, chloride; *dotted red line*, potassium.

stomach by **peristalsis,** the sequential contraction and relaxation of outer longitudinal and inner circular layers of muscles. The upper third of the esophagus contains striated muscle that is directly innervated by motor neurons. The middle third contains a mix of striated and smooth muscle, and the lower third is smooth muscle that is innervated by preganglionic cholinergic fibers from the vagus nerve. The muscles are activated in a downward sequence. Peristalsis is stimulated when afferent fibers distributed along the length of the esophagus sense changes in wall tension caused by stretching as food passes. The greater the tension, the greater the intensity of esophageal contraction. Occasionally, intense contractions cause pain similar to "heartburn" or angina.

Each end of the esophagus is opened and closed by a sphincter. The **upper esophageal sphincter (cricopharyngeal muscle)** prevents entry of air into the esophagus during respiration.[2] The **lower esophageal sphincter (cardiac sphincter)** prevents regurgitation from the stomach. The lower esophageal sphincter is located near the esophageal hiatus—the opening in the diaphragm where the esophagus ends at the stomach.

Swallowing is a complex event mediated by the swallowing center, which is located in the reticular formation of the brain stem and also involves other brain regions, including the insula/claustrum and cerebellum.[3] Swallowing occurs in two phases: the oropharyngeal (voluntary) phase and the esophageal (involuntary) phase. During the **oropharyngeal phase of swallowing**, food is segmented into a bolus by the tongue and forced posteriorly toward the pharynx as the tongue pushes upward against the hard palate. The superior constrictor muscle of the pharynx contracts, preventing movement of food into the nasopharynx. At the same time, respiration is inhibited and the epiglottis slides downward to prevent the bolus from entering the larynx and trachea. The movements of the tongue and pharyngeal constrictors propel the food into the esophagus in a series of coordinated events taking less than 1 second.[4]

The **esophageal phase of swallowing** begins as the bolus of food enters the esophagus. The bolus is transported by peristalsis—the sequential waves of muscular contractions that travel down the esophagus and are preceded by receptive waves of relaxations.[5] The wave of relaxation reduces resistance and allows food to pass, after which the wave of contraction pushes food farther along. The lower esophageal sphincter relaxes just before the arrival of a peristaltic wave. The sphincter muscles return to their resting tone after the bolus of food passes into the stomach. The esophageal phase of swallowing takes 5 to 10 seconds, with the bolus moving 2 to 6 cm/sec. Throughout swallowing, the sphincters and esophagus work in concert with the peristaltic wave that moves food from the mouth to the stomach.

Peristalsis that immediately follows the oropharyngeal phase of swallowing is called **primary peristalsis**. If a bolus of food becomes stuck in the esophageal lumen, the distention of the esophageal wall stimulates **secondary peristalsis**, a wave of contraction and relaxation that is independent of voluntary swallowing. This is in response to stretch receptors that are stimulated by increased wall tension, causing an increase in impulses from the swallowing center of the brain.

When it is closed, the lower esophageal sphincter serves as a barrier between the stomach and esophagus. The muscle tone of the lower sphincter changes with neural and hormonal stimulation. Cholinergic vagal input and the digestive hormone *gastrin* increase sphincter tone. Nonadrenergic, noncholinergic vagal impulses relax the lower esophageal sphincter, as do the hormones *progesterone, secretin,* and *glucagon*. Relaxation during swallowing is mediated by the vagus.[6]

Stomach

The **stomach** is a hollow, muscular organ that stores food during eating, secretes digestive juices; mixes food with these juices; and propels partially digested food, called **chyme**, into the duodenum of the small intestine. The anatomy of the stomach is presented in Fig. 37-5. Its major anatomic boundaries are the lower esophageal sphincter, where food passes through the **cardiac orifice** into the stomach; the greater and lesser curvatures; and the **pyloric sphincter**, which relaxes as food is propelled through the **pylorus** into the duodenum. Functional areas of the stomach are the **fundus** (upper portion), **body** (middle portion), and **antrum** (lower portion).

The stomach has three layers of smooth muscle: an outer, longitudinal layer; a middle, circular layer; and an inner, oblique layer (see Fig. 37-5). These layers become progressively thicker in the body and antrum, where food is mixed, churned, and pushed out into the duodenum. The glandular epithelium is discussed in the section about secretory functions of the stomach (see p. 1236).

Blood is supplied to the stomach by a branch of the celiac artery. The blood supply is so abundant that nearly all arterial vessels must be occluded before ischemic changes occur in the stomach wall. The splenic vein drains the right side of the stomach, and the gastric vein drains the left side.

The stomach is innervated by sympathetic and parasympathetic divisions of the autonomic nervous system. Some of the autonomic fibers are extrinsic; that is, they originate outside the stomach and are controlled by nerve centers in the brain. Others are intrinsic; that is, they originate within the stomach and also respond to local stimuli. Extrinsic sympathetic fibers reach the stomach through the celiac plexus (solar plexus), whereas extrinsic parasympathetic fibers enter through the gastric branch of the vagus nerve.

Gastric Motility

In its resting state the stomach is small and contains about 50 ml of fluid. There is no wall tension, and the muscle layers in the fundus contract very little. Swallowing causes the fundus to relax (receptive relaxation) to receive a bolus of food from the esophagus. Relaxation is coordinated by efferent, nonadrenergic, noncholinergic vagal fibers and is facilitated by **gastrin** and **cholecystokinin**, two polypeptide hormones secreted by the gastrointestinal mucosa. (The actions of digestive hormones are summarized in Table 37-1.) Food is stored in vertical or oblique layers as it arrives in the fundus, whereas fluids flow relatively quickly down to the antrum.

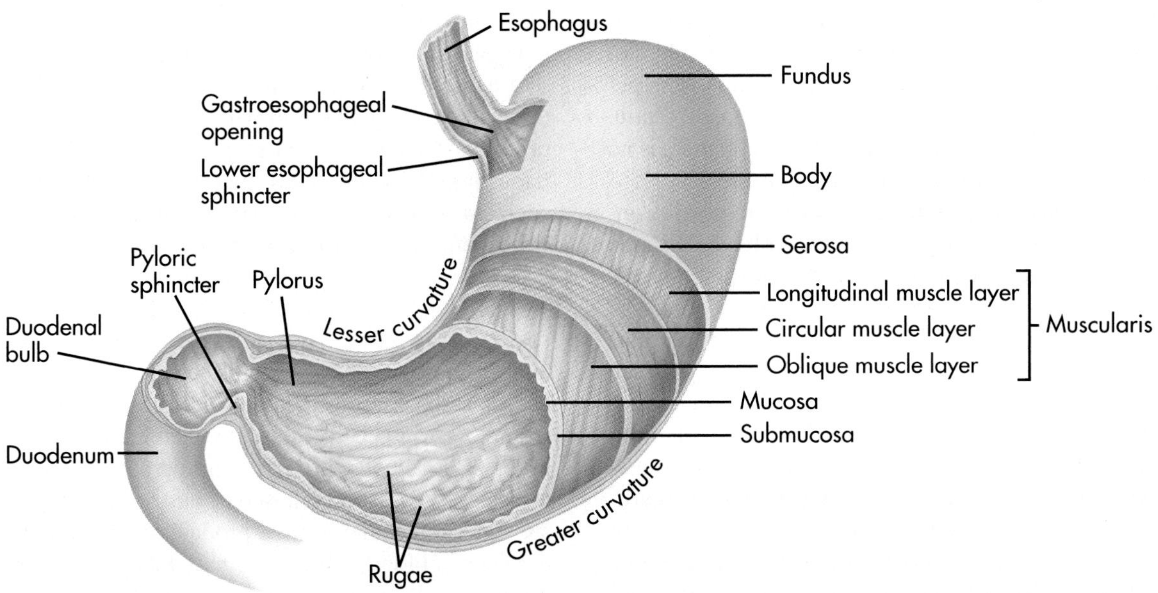

FIG. 37-5 Stomach. A portion of the anterior wall has been cut away to reveal the muscle layers of the stomach wall. Note that the mucosa lining the stomach forms folds called *rugae*. (From Thibodeau GA, Patton KI: *Anatomy & physiology*, ed 4, St Louis, 1999, Mosby.)

Table 37-1 Selected Hormones and Neurotransmitters of the Digestive System

Source	Hormone	Stimulus for Secretion	Action
Mucosa of the stomach	Gastrin	Presence of partially digested proteins in the stomach	Stimulates gastric glands to secrete hydrochloric acid and pepsinogen
Mucosa of the small intestine	Motilin	Presence of acid and fat in the duodenum	Increases gastrointestinal motility
	Secretin	Presence of chyme (acid, partially digested proteins, fats) in the duodenum	Stimulates pancreas to secrete alkaline pancreatic juice and liver to secrete bile; decreases gastrointestinal motility
	Cholecystokinin	Same as for secretin	Stimulates gallbladder to eject bile and pancreas to secrete alkaline fluid; decreases gastric motility
	Enteroglucagon	Intraluminal fats and carbohydrates	Weakly inhibits gastric and pancreatic secretion and enhances insulin release, lipolysis, ketogenesis, and glycogenolysis
	Peptide YY	Intraluminal fat and bile acids	Inhibits postprandial gastric acid and pancreatic secretion and delays gastric and small bowel emptying

Modified from Thibodeau, GA, Patton KT: *Structure and function of the body,* ed 11, St Louis, 1999, Mosby.
NOTE: The digestive hormones are not secreted into the gastrointestinal lumen but rather into the bloodstream, in which they travel to target tissues. There are more than 30 peptide hormone genes expressed in the gastrointestinal tract and more than 100 hormonally active peptides. (From Rehfield JF: The new biology of gastrointestinal hormones, *Physiol Rev* 70(4):1087, 1990.)

Gastric (stomach) motility increases with the initiation of peristaltic waves, which sweep over the body of the stomach toward the antrum. The rate of peristaltic contractions is approximately three per minute and is influenced by neural and hormonal activity. Gastrin, **motilin** (an intestinal hormone), and the vagus nerve increase contraction by lowering the threshold potential of muscle fibers. (The neural and biochemical mechanisms of muscle contraction are described in Chapter 40.) Sympathetic activity and **secretin** (another intestinal hormone) are inhibitory and raise the threshold potential. The rate of peristalsis is mediated by pacemaker cells that initiate a wave of depolarization (basic electrical rhythm), which moves from the upper part of the stomach to the pylorus.

The mixing and emptying of food (chyme) from the stomach take several hours. Mixing occurs as food is propelled toward the antrum. As food approaches the pylorus, the velocity of the peristaltic wave increases, forcing the contents back toward the body of the stomach. This **retropulsion** effectively mixes food with digestive juices, and the oscillating motion breaks down large food particles. With each peristaltic wave a small portion of the gastric contents (chyme) passes through the pylorus and into the duodenum. The pylorus is about 1.5 cm long and is always open about 2.0 mm. It opens wider during antral contraction. Normally there is no regurgitation from the duodenum into the antrum.

The rate of **gastric emptying** (movement of gastric contents into the duodenum) depends on the volume, osmotic pressure, and chemical composition of the gastric contents. Larger volumes of food increase gastric pressure, peristalsis, and rate of emptying. Solids, fats, and nonisotonic solutions delay gastric emptying. (Osmotic pressure and tonicity are described in Chapters 1 and 3.) Products of fat digestion, which are formed in the duodenum by the action of bile from the liver and enzymes from the pancreas, stimulate the secretion of cholecystokinin. This hormone inhibits gastric motility and decreases gastric emptying so that fats are not emptied into the duodenum at a rate that exceeds the rate of bile and enzyme secretion. Osmoreceptors in the wall of the duodenum are sensitive to the osmotic pressure of duodenal contents. The arrival of hypertonic or hypotonic gastric contents activates the osmoreceptors, which delay gastric emptying to facilitate formation of an isoosmotic duodenal environment. The rate at which acid enters the duodenum also influences gastric emptying. Secretions from the pancreas, liver, and duodenal mucosa neutralize gastric acid in the duodenum. The rate of emptying is adjusted to the duodenum's ability to neutralize the incoming acidity.[7]

Gastric Secretion

Stimulated by eating, the stomach secretes large volumes of gastric juices or gastric secretions. Specialized cells located throughout the gastric mucosa produce mucus, acid, enzymes, hormones, and intrinsic factor. (Intrinsic factor is necessary for the intestinal absorption of vitamin B_{12}.) The hormones are secreted into the blood and travel to target tissues in the bloodstream. The other gastric secretions are released directly into the stomach lumen. Mucus covers the entire mucosa, forming a protective barrier against acid and proteolytic enzymes, which otherwise would damage the gastric lining.[8]

In the fundus and body of the stomach the **gastric glands** of the mucosa are the primary secretory units (Fig. 37-6). Several of these glands (three to seven) empty into a common duct known as the **gastric pit**. The **parietal cells (oxyntic cells)** within the glands secrete hydrochloric acid and intrinsic factor. The **chief cells** within the glands secrete **pepsinogen**, an enzyme precursor that is readily converted to **pepsin** (a proteolytic enzyme) in the gastric juice. The pyloric gland mucosa in the antrum synthesizes and releases the hormone *gastrin*.

The composition of gastric juice depends on volume and flow rate (Fig. 37-7). Potassium remains relatively constant, but its concentration is greater in gastric juice than in plasma. The rate of secretion varies with the time of day. Generally the rate and volume of secretion are lowest in the morning and highest in the afternoon and evening. Loss of gastric juices through vomiting, drainage, or suction may decrease body stores of sodium and potassium.

Gastric secretion is inhibited by unpleasant odors and tastes and by rage, fear, or pain. These sensations and emotions cause a discharge of sympathetic impulses and inhibit parasympathetic impulses. Increased secretions may be associated with feelings of aggression or hostility and may contribute to some forms of gastric pathology.

Acid

The major functions of gastric acid are to dissolve food fibers, act as bactericide against swallowed organisms, and convert pepsinogen to pepsin. The production of acid by the parietal cells requires the transport of hydrogen and chloride from the parietal cells to the stomach lumen. Acid is formed in the parietal cells, primarily through the hydrolysis of water (Fig. 37-8). At a high rate of gastric secretion, bicarbonate moves into the plasma, producing an "alkaline tide" in the venous blood, which also may result in a more alkaline urine.[9]

Acid secretion by parietal cells is stimulated by acetylcholine (a neurotransmitter), gastrin (a hormone), and histamine (a biochemical mediator) and is inhibited by somatostatin (a hormone). The vagus nerve also releases acetylcholine and stimulates the secretion of histamine. Histamine secretion is also stimulated by gastrin. Histamine is stored in enterochro-

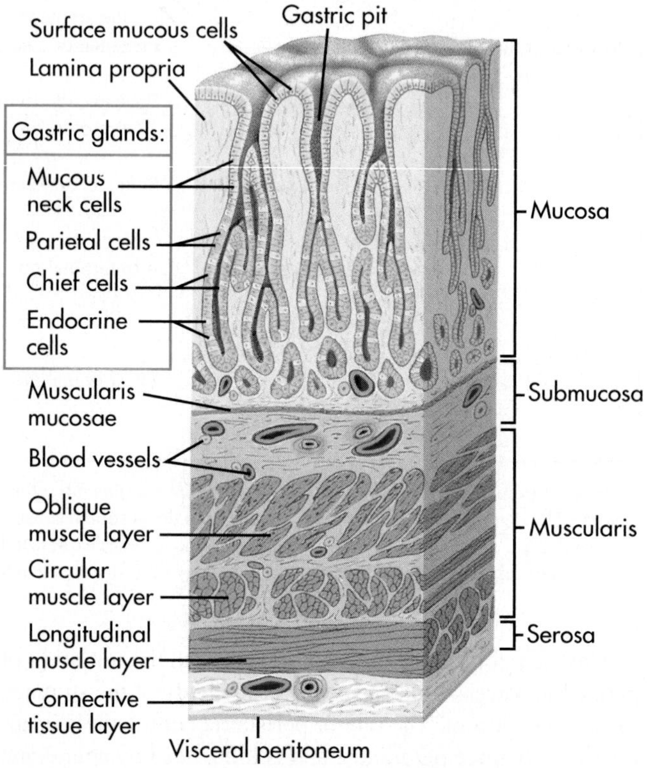

FIG. 37-6 Gastric pits and gastric glands. Gastric pits are depressions in the epithelial lining of the stomach. At the bottom of each pit is one or more tubular *gastric glands*. Chief cells produce the enzymes of gastric juice, and parietal cells produce stomach acid. (From Thibodeau GA, Patton KI: *Anatomy & physiology*, ed 4, St Louis, 1999, Mosby.)

maffin cells (mast cells; see Chapter 7) in the gastric mucosa. Histamine receptors in the gastric mucosa are H2 receptors (unlike those in the bronchial mucosa, which are H1 receptors). The drug *cimetidine* is an H2 antagonist and is therefore effective in suppressing acid secretion in persons with ulcers. Prostaglandins inhibit the secretion of acid.[10] Enterogastrones, such as gastric inhibitory peptide, and secretin inhibit acid secretion.

Pepsin

Acetylcholine, gastrin, and secretin stimulate the chief cells to release pepsinogen during eating. Gastrin indirectly stimulates pepsinogen secretion through a cholinergic reflex that it causes while stimulating acid secretion. Pepsinogen is quickly converted to pepsin at any pH below 5.0, but the optimum pH for pepsin activation is 2.0. Pepsin is a proteolytic enzyme that breaks down protein-forming polypeptides in the stomach. Once chyme has entered the duodenum, the alkaline environment of the duodenum inactivates pepsin.

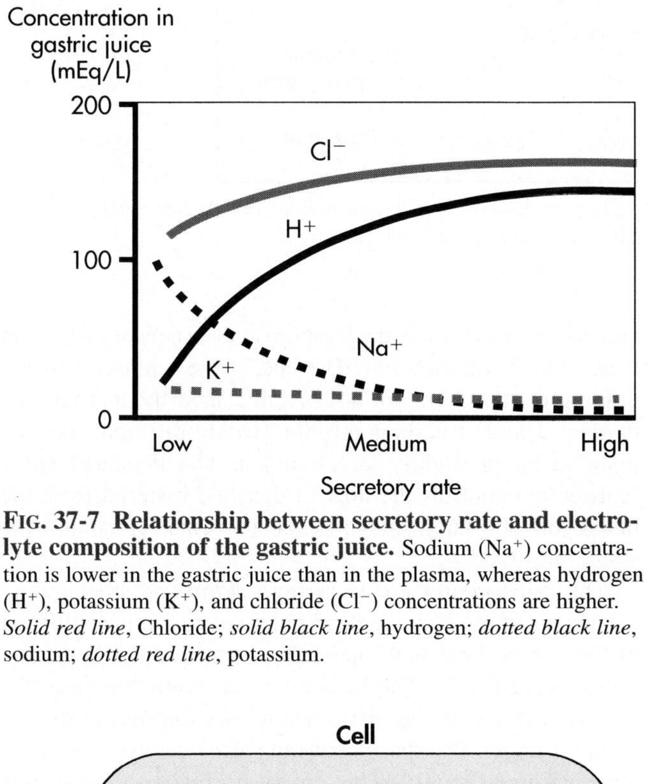

FIG. 37-7 Relationship between secretory rate and electrolyte composition of the gastric juice. Sodium (Na^+) concentration is lower in the gastric juice than in the plasma, whereas hydrogen (H^+), potassium (K^+), and chloride (Cl^-) concentrations are higher. *Solid red line*, Chloride; *solid black line*, hydrogen; *dotted black line*, sodium; *dotted red line*, potassium.

Mucus

The gastric mucosa is protected from the digestive actions of acid and pepsin by a coating of mucus called the **mucosal barrier**. Gastric mucosal blood flow is important to maintaining mucosal barrier function.[11] The quality and quantity of mucus and the tight junctions between epithelial cells make gastric mucosa relatively impermeable to acid. Prostaglandins and nitric oxide protect the mucosal barrier by stimulating the secretion of mucus and bicarbonate and by inhibiting secretion of acid. A break in the protective barrier may occur because of exposure to aspirin, *Helicobacter pylori*, ethanol, regurgitated bile, or ischemia. Breaks cause inflammation and ulceration.

Phases

The secretion of gastric juice is influenced by numerous stimuli that together facilitate the process of digestion. The phases of gastric secretion are the cephalic phase, the gastric phase, and the intestinal phase (Fig. 37-9).

Cephalic phase. The anticipatory and sensory experiences of smelling, seeing, tasting, chewing, and swallowing food contribute to the **cephalic phase** of secretion.[12] The cephalic phase of gastric secretion is mediated by the vagus nerve through the myenteric plexus. Acetylcholine (ACh) is liberated and stimulates the parietal and chief cells to secrete acid and pepsinogen, respectively. The G cells in the antrum release gastrin into the bloodstream, through which it travels to the gastric glands and stimulates acid secretion.

Insulin secretion by the endocrine pancreas, which is stimulated by hyperglycemia, is also a strong stimulus for gastric secretion and is mediated by the vagus through sensors located in the hypothalamus. Maintenance of steady serum glucose levels suppresses the gastric response to insulin.

Gastric phase. The **gastric phase of secretion** begins with the arrival of food in the stomach. Two major stimuli have a secretory effect: (1) distention of the stomach and (2) the presence of digested protein. The vagus and enteric nerve plexuses are stimulated by distention and contribute

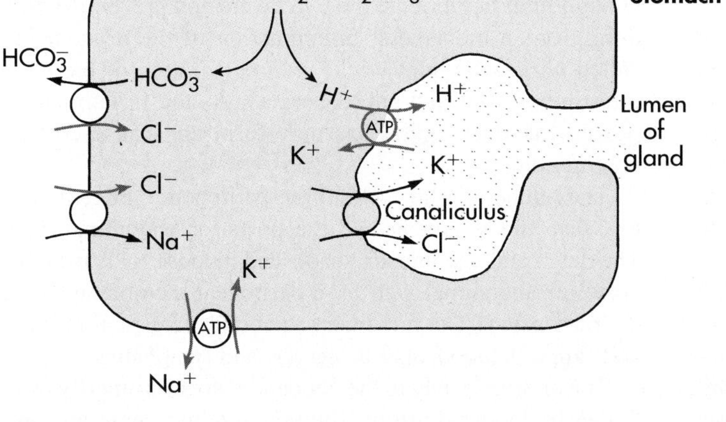

FIG. 37-8 One mechanism for secretion of hydrochloric acid. *ATP*, Adenosine triphosphate. (From Berne RM, Levy MN, editors: *Principles of physiology*, ed 2, St Louis, 1996, Mosby.)

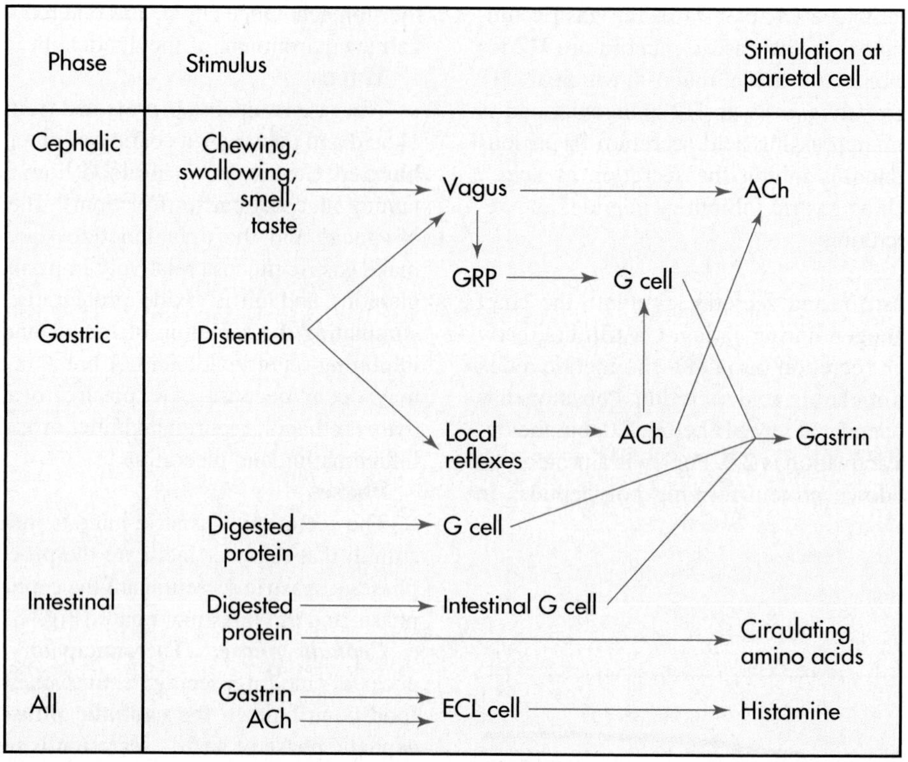

FIG. 37-9 Mechanisms for stimulating acid secretion. *ACh*, Acetylcholine; *GRP*, gastrin-releasing peptide; *ECL*, enterochromaffin-like cell. (From Johnson LR: *Gastrointestinal physiology*, ed 5, St Louis, 1997, Mosby.)

to gastric secretion through a local reflex. Both neural reflexes are mediated by acetylcholine and can be blocked by atropine. As digestion proceeds, products of protein breakdown, stimulating the release of gastrin from **G cells** in the antrum. Proteins in the stomach buffer the acid gastric juice and increase the gastric pH. Caffeine stimulates acid secretion, as does calcium.

Intestinal phase. The movement of chyme from the stomach into the duodenum initiates the **intestinal phase of secretion.** This phase represents a slowdown of the gastric secretory response and appears to be hormonally mediated by a hormone called *entero-oxyntin*. Gastric inhibitory peptide decreases gastric motility and the secretion of acid and pepsin when chyme enters the duodenum. The intestinal absorption of some amino acids (products of protein breakdown) also stimulates gastric secretion. The intestinal phase of gastric secretion is limited by the fact that acidic chyme in the duodenum tends to inhibit both gastric acid secretion and gastric motility. Acid in the duodenum stimulates the release of hormones that inhibit acid secretion while stimulating pepsinogen secretion. One of these hormones, cholecystokinin-pancreozymin, inhibits gastrin-stimulated acid production. Other intestinal hormones probably also act synergistically to regulate gastric secretion.

Small Intestine

The **small intestine** is about 5 meters long and is functionally divided into three segments: the **duodenum, jejunum,** and **ileum** (Fig. 37-10). The duodenum begins at the pylorus and ends where it joins the jejunum at a suspensory ligament called the *Treitz ligament*. The end of the jejunum and beginning of the ileum are not distinguished by an anatomic marker. These structures are not grossly different, but the jejunum has a slightly larger lumen. The **ileocecal valve (sphincter)** controls the flow of digested material from the ileum into the large intestine and prevents reflux into the small intestine.[13]

The **peritoneum** is the serous membrane surrounding the organs of the abdomen and pelvic cavity. It is analogous to the pericardium and pleura that surround the heart and lungs, respectively. The visceral peritoneum lies over the organs, and the parietal peritoneum lines the wall of the abdominal cavity. The space between these two layers is called the **peritoneal cavity**. This cavity normally contains just enough fluid to lubricate the two layers and prevent friction during organ movement. Inflammation of the peritoneum, called *peritonitis*, may occur with perforation of the large intestine or after abdominal surgery. As the inflammatory process resolves, adhesions may form and cause colonic obstruction.

The duodenum lies behind the peritoneum, or retroperitoneally, and is attached to the posterior abdominal wall. The ileum and jejunum are suspended in loose folds from the posterior abdominal wall by a peritoneal membrane called the **mesentery**. The mesentery facilitates intestinal motility and supports blood vessels, nerves, and lymphatics.

The arterial supply to the duodenum arises primarily from the gastroduodenal artery. The jejunum and ileum are sup-

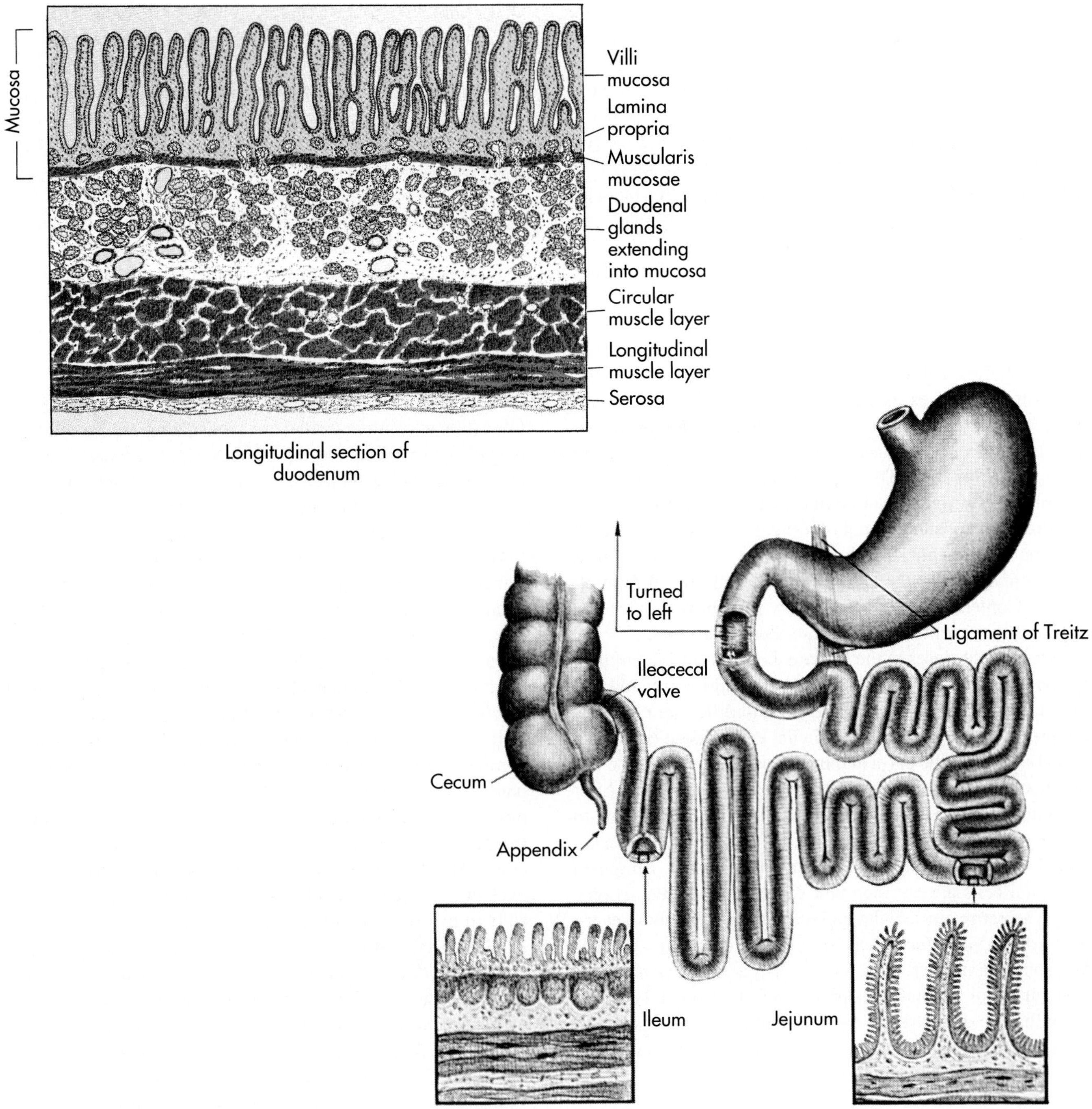

FIG. 37-10 The small intestine. (Modified from Thompson JM et al: *Mosby's clinical nursing*, ed 4, St Louis, 1997, Mosby.)

plied by branches of the superior mesenteric artery. The superior mesenteric vein joins the splenic vein and empties into the portal circulation to the liver. The regional lymph nodes and lymphatics drain into the thoracic duct. Both divisions of the autonomic nervous system innervate the small intestine. Secretion, motility, pain sensation, and intestinal reflexes (e.g., relaxation of the lower esophageal sphincter) are mediated by parasympathetic nerves. Sympathetic activity inhibits motility and produces vasoconstriction. Intrinsic motor innervation is mediated by the myenteric plexus (Auerbach plexus) and the submucosal plexus (Meissner plexus).

The smooth muscles of the small intestine are arranged in two layers: a longitudinal, outer layer; and a thicker, inner circular layer (see Fig. 37-10). Mucosal folds (plica) within the small intestine slow the passage of food, thereby providing more time for digestion and absorption. The folds are most numerous and prominent in the jejunum and upper ileum (see Fig. 37-10).

Absorption occurs through **villi,** which cover the mucosal folds and are the functional units of the intestine. (Villi are illustrated in Fig. 37-10). Each villus secretes some of the enzymes necessary for digestion and absorbs nutrients. A villus is composed of absorptive columnar cells and mucus-secreting goblet cells of the mucosal epithelium. Near the surface, columnar cells closely adhere to each other at sites called *tight junctions*. Water and electrolytes are absorbed through these intercellular spaces. The surface of each columnar epithelial cell contains tiny projections called **microvilli** (see Fig. 37-10). Together the microvilli create a mucosal surface known as the **brush border**. The villi and microvilli greatly increase the surface area available for absorption. Coating the brush border is an "unstirred" layer of fluid that is important for the absorption of substances other than water and electrolytes. The **lamina propria** (a connective tissue layer of the mucous membrane) lies beneath the epithelial cells of the villi and contains lymphocytes; plasma cells, which produce immunoglobulins; and macrophages.

Central arterioles ascend within each villus and branch into a capillary array that extends around the base of the columnar cells and cascades down to the venules that lead to the portal circulation. The opposing ascending and descending blood flow provide a countercurrent exchange system for absorbed substances and blood gases. A central **lacteal**, or lymphatic channel, is also contained within each villus and is important for the absorption and transport of fat molecules. Contents of the lacteals flow to regional nodes and channels that eventually drain into the thoracic duct.[14]

Between the bases of the villi are the crypts of Lieberkühn, which extend to the submucosal layer. Undifferentiated and secretory cells are located here. The undifferentiated cells are precursors of columnar epithelial cells. These cells arise from the base of the crypt and move toward the tip of the villus, maturing in shape and function as they progress. After becoming columnar cells and completing their migration to the tip of the villus, they function for a few days and then are sloughed into the intestinal lumen and digested. Sloughed epithelial cells are an important source of endogenous protein. The entire epithelial population is replaced about every 4 to 7 days. Many factors can influence this process of cellular proliferation. Starvation, vitamin B_{12} deficiency, and cytotoxic drugs or irradiation suppress cell division and shorten the villi. The decreased absorption that results can cause diarrhea and malnutrition. Nutrient intake and intestinal resection stimulate cell production.

Intestinal Digestion and Absorption

The process of digestion is initiated in the stomach by the actions of hydrochloric acid and pepsin, which break down food fibers and proteins. The chyme that passes into the duodenum is a liquid that contains small particles of undigested food. Digestion is continued in the proximal portion of the small intestine by the action of pancreatic enzymes, intestinal enzymes, and bile salts. Here carbohydrates are broken down to monosaccharides and disaccharides; proteins are degraded further to amino acids and peptides; and fats are emulsified and reduced to fatty acids and monoglycerides (Fig. 37-11). These nutrients, along with water, vitamins, and electrolytes, are absorbed across the intestinal mucosa by active transport, diffusion, or facilitated diffusion. Products of carbohydrate and protein breakdown move into villus capillaries and then to the liver through the portal vein. Digested fats move into the lacteals and eventually reach the liver through the systemic circulation. Intestinal motility exposes nutrients to a large mucosal surface area by mixing chyme and moving it through the lumen. Different segments of the gastrointestinal tract absorb different nutrients. Sites of absorption are shown in Fig. 37-12.

Water and Electrolytes

The epithelial cell membranes of the small intestine are formed of lipids and therefore are hydrophobic, or tend to repel water. (The properties of cell membranes are described in Chapter 1.) Therefore water and electrolytes are transported in both directions (toward the capillary blood or toward the intestinal lumen) through the tight junctions and intercellular spaces rather than across cell membranes. Water diffuses passively according to hydrostatic pressure and in relation to osmotic gradients established by the active transport of sodium and other substances. Approximately 85% to 90% of the water that enters the gastrointestinal tract each day is absorbed in the small intestine. The remaining water and electrolytes are absorbed at a constant rate in the colon.[15] Sodium passes through the tight junctions and is actively transported across cell membranes. The proximal part of the small intestine is more permeable to sodium than the distal part. Sodium is transported into the intestinal cells in exchange for hydrogen at the brush border, and chloride actively enters the cell in exchange for bicarbonate to maintain electroneutrality in the ileum. There is also a sodium pump at the basolateral membrane. Sodium and glucose share a common carrier mechanism, so that sodium absorption is enhanced by glucose transport (Fig. 37-13). Potassium moves passively across the tight junctions with changes in the electrochemical gradient. Net potassium secretion occurs in the colon. Because of potassium secretion in the colon and the exchange of chloride for bicarbonate, prolonged diarrhea results in hypokalemic metabolic acidosis.

Carbohydrates

Carbohydrate (starch, table sugar, milk, sugar, maltose) accounts for at least 50% of the American diet. Because only monosaccharides (galactose, glucose, fructose) are absorbed by the intestinal mucosa, the complex carbohydrates (polysaccharides and oligosaccharides) must be hydrolyzed to their simplest form (see Fig. 37-10). Ribose, a 5-carbon sugar that forms part of ribonucleic acid (RNA), adenosine triphosphate (ATP), and deoxyribonucleic acid (DNA), is an important part of the diet. Salivary and pancreatic amylases break down starches to oligosaccharides by splitting α-1,4-glucosidic linkages of long-chain molecules. The major oligosaccharides are sucrose (glucose-fructose), maltose (glucose-glucose), and lactose (glucose-galactose). Approximately half of starch hydrolysis occurs in the stomach and about half in the duodenum. In the small intestine the oligosaccharides are hydrolyzed by brush-border enzymes, mainly sucrase, maltase, and lactase, to their respective monosaccharides (fructose, glucose, galactose). The sugars then pass through the unstirred layer by diffusion. At the cell membrane, glucose and galactose are actively transported with a sodium carrier and fructose is absorbed passively. Consequently glucose and galactose are

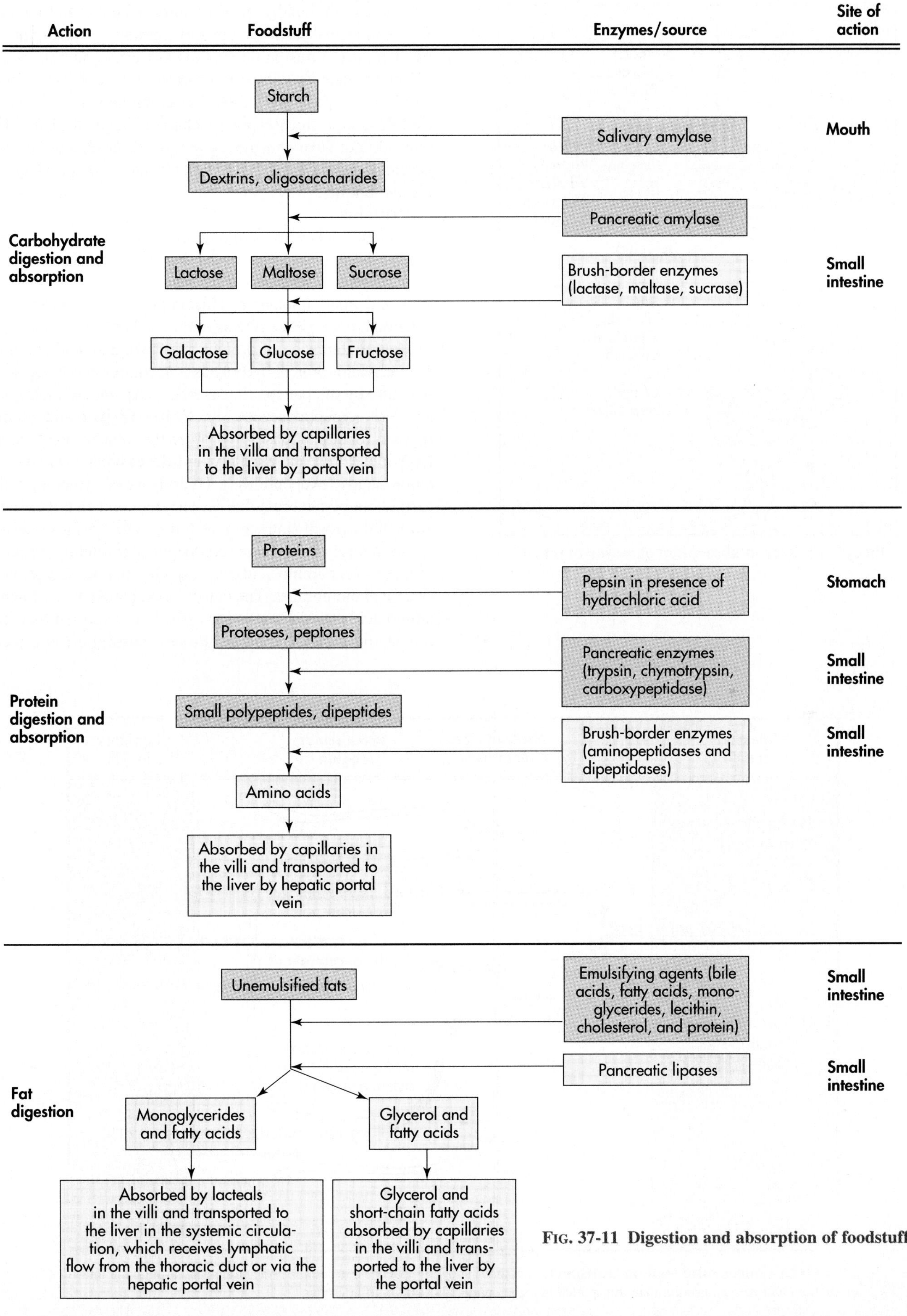

FIG. 37-11 Digestion and absorption of foodstuffs.

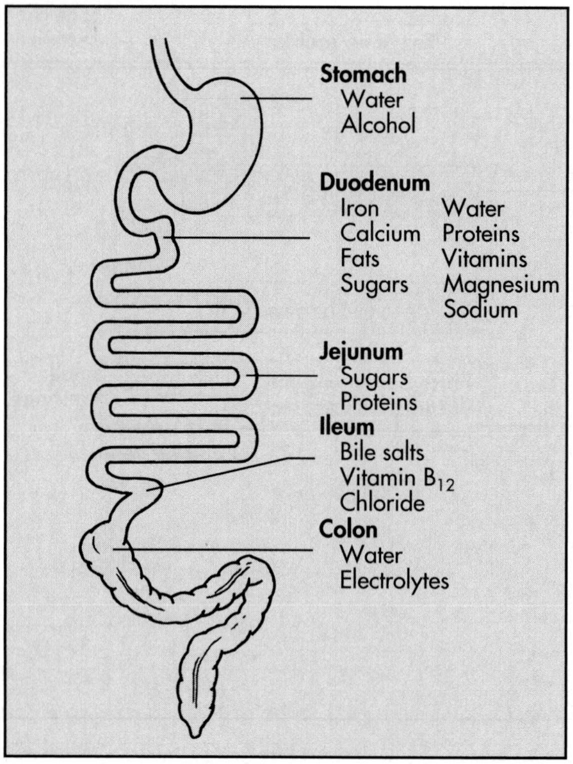

FIG. 37-12 Sites of absorption of major nutrients.

absorbed more rapidly than fructose. Insulin is not required for the intestinal absorption of carbohydrates. Fructose passes by facilitated diffusion into the bloodstream, and glucose and galactose enter by diffusion or active transport. The sugars are absorbed primarily in the duodenum and upper jejunum. Cellulose is a glucose polysaccharide found in plants. Humans do not have enzymes to digest cellulose, but the undigested material contributes to volume and stimulates large intestine motility.

Proteins

Protein intake varies among different populations. Adults require 44 to 56 g of protein per day. Approximately 20 to 30 g of protein is derived endogenously from shed epithelial cells and small amounts of plasma proteins. Most protein is absorbed; only 5% to 10% is eliminated in the stool.

Gastric digestion of protein by pepsin and acid is not essential. Major protein hydrolysis is accomplished in the small intestine by the pancreatic enzymes: trypsin, chymotrypsin, and carboxypeptidase (see Fig. 37-10). **Trypsin** and **chymotrypsin** (endopeptidase) hydrolyze the interior bonds of the large molecules, and **carboxypeptidases** break away the end amino acids (exopeptidase). Hydrolysis of proteins is also carried out by the brush-border enzymes and enzymes in the epithelial cytosol (intracellular fluid). The brush-border enzymes hydrolyze the large oligopeptides (proteins composed of three to six amino acids) into smaller peptides, which can cross cell membranes. The cytosol then breaks them down to amino acids. Amino acids are actively transported by a carrier at the basal membrane. Protein absorption is directly

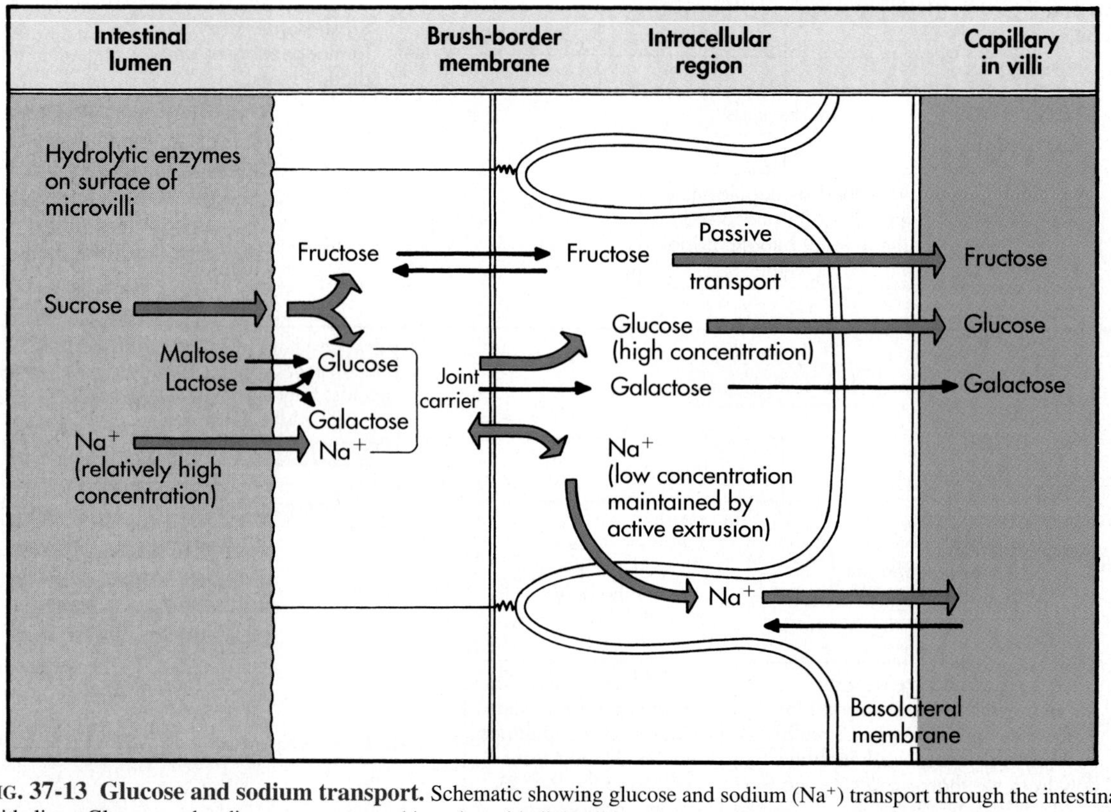

FIG. 37-13 Glucose and sodium transport. Schematic showing glucose and sodium (Na^+) transport through the intestinal epithelium. Glucose and sodium are transported into the epithelial cell by a joint carrier.

linked to the active transport of sodium. There are three groups of free amino acids:

1. Neutral amino acids (methionine, glycine, phenylalanine, tryptophan)
2. Basic amino acids (arginine, ornithine, lysine, cystine)
3. Proline and hydroxyproline

Each group enters the circulation through a specific mechanism of transport. A small amount of protein may be taken into the cells by pinocytosis (see Chapter 1).

Like the sugars, proteins are absorbed primarily in the proximal area of the small intestine. Protein absorption is impaired if inadequate amounts of proteolytic enzymes are secreted from the pancreas, as occurs with cystic fibrosis.

Fats

Approximately 90 to 100 g of fat is consumed daily by the average American. Fat is an important source of calories and is a primary structural component of cell membranes and organelles. Sources of dietary fat are reviewed in Box 37-1. Although triglycerides are the major dietary lipids, cholesterol, phospholipids, and fat-soluble vitamins also have nutritional importance. The digestion and absorption of fat occur in four phases: (1) emulsification and lipolysis, (2) micelle formation, (3) fat absorption, and (4) resynthesis of triglycerides and phospholipids.

The mechanical action of the stomach and small intestine disperses the triglyceride droplets into small particles. **Emulsification** is the process by which emulsifying agents (fatty acids, monoglycerides, lecithin, cholesterol, protein, bile salts) in the intestinal lumen cover the small fat particles and prevent them from re-forming into fat droplets (decrease their surface tension). Emulsified fat is then ready for **lipolysis** (lipid hydrolysis) by pancreatic lipase, phospholipase, and hydrolase. **Lipase** breaks down triglycerides to diglycerides, monoglycerides, free fatty acids, and glycerol (see Fig. 37-11). The action of lipase requires the presence of colipase, a pancreatic enzyme that allows lipase to penetrate the triglyceride molecule. **Phospholipase** cleaves fatty acids from phospholipids, and **hydrolase** breaks cholesterol esters into fatty acids and cholesterol.

The products of lipid hydrolysis must be made water soluble if they are to be absorbed efficiently from the intestinal lumen. This is accomplished by the formation of water-soluble molecules known as **micelles** (Fig. 37-14). Micelles are formed of bile salts, the products of fat hydrolysis, fat-soluble vitamins, and cholesterol. The fats form the core of the micelle, and the polar bile salts form an outer shell, with the hydrophobic ("water-hating") side facing the interior and the hydrophilic ("water-loving") side facing the aqueous (water-like) content of the intestinal lumen. Because the unstirred layer of the brush border is aqueous, the micelles readily diffuse through it. The micelles maintain the fat molecules in the dissolved or solubilized form, which allows them to move more rapidly from the micelle toward the absorbing surface of

Box 37-1

DIETARY FAT

SATURATED FATTY ACID (PALMITIC ACID [$C_{16}H_{32}O_2$])

Each carbon atom in the chain is linked by single bonds to adjacent carbon and hydrogen atoms; atoms are solid at room temperature and found in animal fat and tropical oils (coconut and palm oil); they increase low-density lipoprotein (LDL) cholesterol ("bad" cholesterol) blood levels and increase the risk of coronary artery disease

UNSATURATED FATTY ACID

Unsaturated fatty acids are soft or liquid at room temperature; omega 6 fatty acids are found in plants and vegetables (olive, canola, and peanut oils), and omega 3 fatty acids are found in fish and shellfish

1. Monounsaturated fatty acids (oleic acid [$C_{18}H_{34}O_2$])
   Contain one double bond in the carbon chain and are found in both plants and animals; may be beneficial in reducing blood cholesterol, glucose levels, and systolic blood pressure; do not lower high-density lipoprotein (HDL) cholesterol ("good" cholesterol) level; low HDL levels have been associated with coronary heart disease
2. Polyunsaturated fatty acids (linoleic acid [$C_{18}H_{32}O_2$])
   Contain two or more double bonds in the carbon chain and are found in plants and fish oils; omega 6 fatty acids lower total and LDL cholesterol blood levels; high levels of polyunsaturated fatty acids may lower LDL; omega 3 fatty acids lower blood triglyceride levels and reduce platelet aggregation and reduce blood clotting tendency; are necessary for growth and development and may prevent coronary artery disease, hypertension, cancer, inflammatory and immune disorders

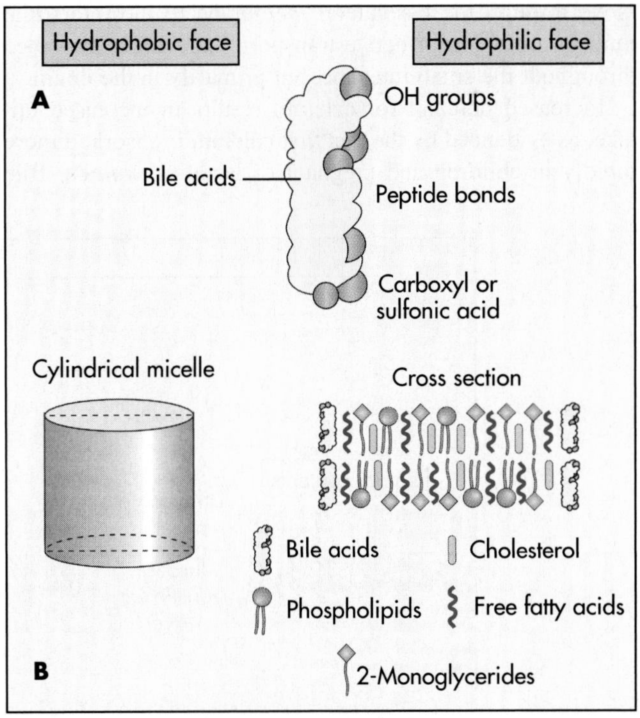

FIG. 37-14 Structure of bile acid and micelle. A, A bile acid molecule in solution. The molecule is amphipathic in that it has a hydrophilic face and a hydrophobic face. The amphipathic structure is key in the ability of the bile acids to emulsify lipids and form micelles. **B,** A model of the structure of a bile acid–lipid mixed micelle, an emulsified fat. (From Berne RM, Levy MN, editors: *Principles of physiology*, ed 3, St Louis, 2000, Mosby.)

the intestinal epithelium. The fat products of the micelle then readily diffuse through the epithelial cell membrane, while the bile salts remain in the lumen and proceed to the ileum, where they are absorbed into the circulation and returned to the liver (Fig. 37-15). Almost all of the bile salts are recycled in this way.

When the fat products reach the inside of the epithelial cell, they are resynthesized into triglycerides and phospholipids. The triglycerides are covered with phospholipids, lipoproteins, and cholesterol to become particles called **chylomicrons**. The chylomicrons travel to the basolateral membrane of the columnar epithelial cells, where they are extruded into the intercellular spaces of the villus. From here they enter the lacteals and lymphatic channels and, eventually, the systemic circulation.

Minerals and Vitamins

The recommended intake of calcium ranges from 1000 to 1500 mg/day. Between 500 and 600 mg is secreted or shed into the lumen with desquamated epithelial cells. Not all this calcium is absorbed. Daily absorption of calcium is approximately 600 mg. This amount increases with increased intake. When its concentration in the lumen is greater than 5 mmol/L, calcium is absorbed by passive diffusion. At concentrations less than 5 mmol/L, calcium is transported actively across cell membranes, bound to a carrier protein. The carrier formation requires the presence of the active form of vitamin D (1,25-dihydroxyvitamin D). The calcium-protein complex moves into the epithelial cell, where the calcium binds to proteins or other substances. Then these complexes move through the basolateral membrane to the interstitial fluid by diffusion or active transport. Calcium is absorbed throughout the small intestine, but primarily in the ileum.

Increased demand for calcium results in increased uptake, as evidenced by the fact that calcium is absorbed more rapidly in children and pregnant or lactating women. Bile salts enhance calcium absorption indirectly by facilitating the absorption of vitamin D. In addition, bile salts promote the absorption of free fatty acids, which, at high concentrations, bind calcium and form soaps in the intestinal lumen. In older individuals, calcium is absorbed less readily because of inadequate amounts of the active form of vitamin D.

The recommended intake of **magnesium** for adults is 300 to 350 mg/day. Approximately 50% of it is absorbed by active transport or passive diffusion in the jejunum and ileum. Phosphate is also absorbed in the small intestine by passive diffusion and active transport.

The levels of **iron** in the body are regulated primarily by intestinal absorption and secretion. The average intake ranges from 15 to 30 mg/day. Of this amount, menstruating women absorb 1.0 to 1.5 mg and men absorb 0.15 to 1.0 mg. Generally the amount of iron absorbed is equal to the amount required. Iron is absorbed more rapidly if a deficiency exists. The primary sources of iron are heme from hemoglobin and myoglobin from animal protein. This iron is rapidly absorbed by the epithelial cells of the duodenum and jejunum. Inorganic iron (e.g., iron in fruits, cereals, eggs, vegetables) is also readily absorbed. The presence of vitamin C reduces ferric iron to ferrous iron, which is the form more easily absorbed. Calcium phosphate and phosphoproteins (milk and antacids) in the intestinal lumen bind iron and reduce absorption. Tea also binds iron by forming iron tannate complexes.

Iron is bound to intestinal transferrin in the small bowel and is absorbed and bound to the protein ferritin and to amino acid chelates in the cytosol of epithelial cells. Transport of iron across the basolateral membrane is determined by the amount of iron in the circulation. It is transported in the blood by plasma transferrin and is carried to body tissues. During hemorrhage, pregnancy, or growth, iron is actively transported from the epithelial cell to the plasma, where it is carried by the globulin protein transferrin (see Chapter 24).

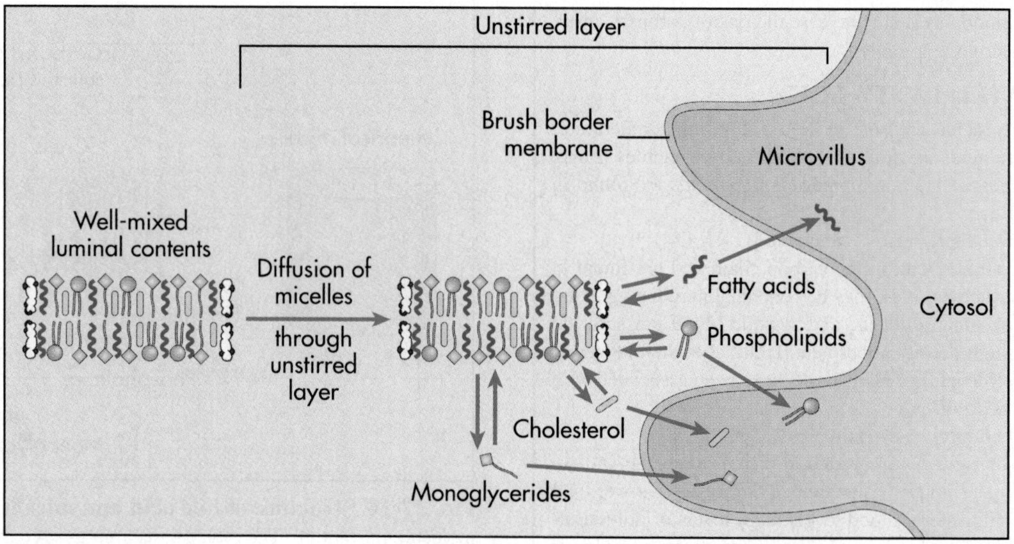

FIG. 37-15 Lipid absorption in the small intestine. Micelles of bile salts and products of lipid digestion diffuse through the unstirred layer and among the microvilli. As digestive products are absorbed from free solution by epithelial cells of the villi, more digestive products dissociate from the micelles. (From Berne RM, Levy MN, editors: *Principles of physiology*, ed 3, St Louis, 2000, Mosby.)

When there is less need for iron, it remains in the cell and is carried into the lumen when the cell is sloughed from the end of the villus. The intestinal cells require 3 days to increase their rate of iron absorption after hemorrhage. This is because the need for iron is perceived by the precursor cells in the crypts of Lieberkühn, and they take 3 days to mature and migrate to the tips of the villi, where they absorb more iron.

The absorption of **vitamins** is summarized in Table 37-2. Most of the water-soluble vitamins are absorbed passively or by sodium-dependent active transport. Most vitamin B_{12} (cobalamin) is bound to intrinsic factor (making it resistant to digestion) and absorbed in the terminal ileum, although a small amount of the vitamin is absorbed in its free (unbound) form. Because intrinsic factor is secreted by gastric cells of the stomach, gastric resection and gastric atrophy with achlorhydria diminish the secretion of intrinsic factor and hence the absorption of vitamin B_{12}. Lack of vitamin B_{12} prevents normal erythrocyte maturation and causes pernicious (macrocytic) anemia. (Anemias are discussed in Chapter 25.)

Vitamin B_{12} is present in animal protein and is particularly abundant in liver and kidney. Gastric and pancreatic enzymes release vitamin B_{12} from food, after which the vitamin binds to intrinsic factor through an intermediary transport protein. The intrinsic factor–vitamin B_{12} complex then attaches to specific receptor sites on epithelial cells of the terminal ileum, where it is absorbed. After several hours the vitamin enters the plasma, attaches to the carrier protein transcobalamin, and is transported to tissues.

Intestinal Motility

The movements of the small intestine facilitate both digestion and absorption. Chyme coming from the stomach stimulates intestinal movements that mix in secretions from the liver, pancreas, and intestinal glands. A churning motion brings the luminal content into contact with the absorbing cells of the villi. Propulsive movements then advance the chyme toward the large intestine.

Intestinal motility is affected by two movements: haustral segmentation and peristalsis. **Haustral segmentation**, which occurs more frequently than peristalsis, consists of localized rhythmic contractions of the circular smooth muscles.[16] The contractions occur at different rates in different parts of the small intestine. Frequency is greatest (12 per minute) in the upper small intestine and least (8 per minute) in the distal part of the ileum. Haustral segmentation divides and mixes the chyme, bringing it into contact with the absorbent mucosal surface. It also helps to propel the chyme toward the large intestine. The frequency of the haustral segmentation is regulated intrinsically by the frequency of the basic electrical rhythm (BER), which arises in the myenteric plexus of longitudinal smooth muscle. Although the basic rate of contraction is controlled intrinsically, the force of contraction can be enhanced by vagal stimulation (i.e., extrinsically).

Peristaltic movements involve short segments (about 10 cm) of longitudinal smooth muscle. The wave of contraction moves slowly (1 to 2 cm/sec) to allow time for digestion and absorption.

The intestinal villi move with contractions of the muscularis mucosae, a very thin layer of muscle that separates the mucosa and submucosa. Absorption is promoted by the swaying of villi in the luminal contents. Contractile activity also helps to empty the central lacteals, which contain products of fat digestion.

Neural reflexes along the length of the small intestine facilitate motility, digestion, and absorption. Through reflex action, receptors in one part of the intestine transmit signals that influence the function of another part. The **ileogastric reflex** inhibits gastric motility when the ileum becomes distended. This prevents the continued movement of chyme into an already distended intestine. The **intestinointestinal reflex** inhibits intestinal motility when one part of the intestine is overdistended. Both of these reflexes require extrinsic innervation. The **gastroileal reflex**, which is activated by an increase in gastric motility and secretion, stimulates an increase in ileal motility. This empties the ileum and prepares

Table 37-2 Intestinal Absorption of Vitamins

Vitamin	Mechanisms of Absorption	State of Absorption
FAT-SOLUBLE VITAMINS		
A (retinol)	Micelle formation with bile salts	Upper small intestine
D (1,25 dihydroxycalciferol)		
E (tocopherol)		
K		
WATER-SOLUBLE VITAMINS		
B_1 (thiamine)	Active transport (sodium dependent)	Duodenum and jejunum
B_2 (riboflavin)	Unknown	Duodenum and jejunum
Niacin (nicotinic acid)	Passive diffusion	Jejunum
C (ascorbic acid)	Active transport (sodium dependent)	Ileum
Folic acid	Active transport (sodium dependent)	Jejunum
B_{12} (cobalamin)	Active transport (intrinsic factor dependent)	Terminal ileum
B_6 (pyridoxine, pyridoxamine, pyridoxal)	Passive diffusion	Jejunum
Pantothenic acid	Passive diffusion	Duodenum and jejunum
Biotin	Unknown	Unknown

it to receive more chyme. The gastroileal reflex is probably regulated by the hormone gastrin or through the autonomic nerves.

During prolonged fasting or between meals, particularly overnight, slow waves sweep along the entire length of the intestinal tract from the stomach to the terminal ileum. This is known as the *interdigestive myoelectric complex*, and it appears to propel residual gastric and intestinal contents into the colon.

The ileocecal valve (sphincter) marks the junction between the terminal ileum and the large intestine. This valve is intrinsically regulated and is normally closed. The arrival of peristaltic waves from the last few centimeters of the ileum causes the ileocecal valve to open, allowing a small amount of chyme to pass through. Distention of the upper large intestine causes the sphincter to constrict, preventing further distention or retrograde flow of intestinal contents.

Large Intestine

The **large intestine** is approximately 1.5 m long and consists of the cecum, appendix, colon (ascending, transverse, descending, and sigmoid), rectum, and anal canal (Fig. 37-16). The **cecum** is a pouch that receives chyme from the ileum. Attached to the cecum is the **vermiform appendix**, an appendage having little or no physiologic function. From the cecum, chyme enters the **colon,** a four-part length of intestine that loops upward, traverses the abdominal cavity, and descends to the anal canal. The four parts of the colon are the **ascending colon, transverse colon, descending colon,** and **sigmoid colon**. Two sphincters control the flow of intestinal contents through the cecum and colon: the ileocecal valve, which admits chyme from the ileum to the cecum, and the **O'Beirne sphincter**, which controls the movement of wastes from the sigmoid colon into the rectum. A thick (2.5 to 3 cm) portion of smooth muscle surrounds the anal canal, forming the **internal anal sphincter**. Overlapping it distally is the striated muscle of the **external anal sphincter**.

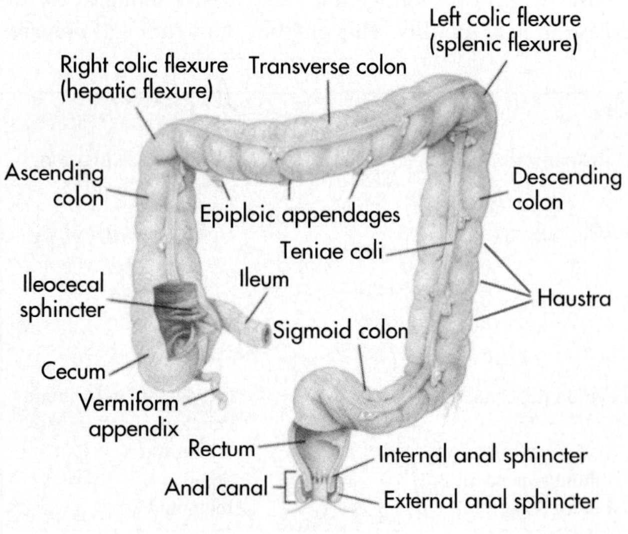

FIG. 37-16 Large intestine (i.e., cecum, colon, and rectum) and anal canal. The teniae coli and epiploic appendages are along the length of the colon. (From Seeley RR, Stephens TD, Tate PP: *Anatomy & physiology*, ed 3, St Louis, 1995, Mosby.)

In the cecum and colon the longitudinal muscle layer consists of three longitudinal bands called **teniae coli** (see Fig. 37-16). The teniae coli are shorter than the colon, giving the colon its "gathered" appearance. The circular muscles of the colon separate the gathers into outpouchings called **haustra**. The haustra become more or less prominent with the contractions and relaxations of the circular muscles. The mucosal surface of the colon has rugae (folds), particularly between the haustra, and **Lieberkühn crypts** but no villi. Columnar epithelial cells and mucus-secreting goblet cells form the mucosa throughout the large intestine. The columnar epithelium absorbs fluid and electrolytes, and the mucus-secreting cells lubricate the mucosa.

The myenteric plexus regulates motor and secretory activity independently of the extrinsic system. Extrinsic parasympathetic innervation occurs through the vagus and extends from the cecum up to the first part of the transverse colon. Vagal stimulation increases rhythmic contraction of the proximal colon. Extrinsic parasympathetic fibers reach the distal colon through the pelvic nerves and can increase motility throughout the colon. The internal anal sphincter is usually in a state of contraction, and its reflex response is to relax when the rectum is distended. The intrinsic nerve plexuses provide the major innervation of the internal anal sphincter, which also receives sympathetic innervation to maintain contraction and parasympathetic innervation that facilitates relaxation when the rectum is full. The external anal sphincter is innervated by branches of the sacral division of the spinal cord. Sympathetic innervation of this sphincter arises from the celiac and superior mesenteric ganglia and the sphincter nerve. The external anal sphincter is paralyzed after destruction of the lower spinal cord, but the internal sphincter is not. Sympathetic activity in the entire large intestine modulates intestinal reflexes, conveys somatic sensations of fullness and pain, participates in the defecation reflex, and constricts blood vessels. The blood supply of the large intestine and rectum is derived primarily from branches of the superior and inferior mesenteric artery.[17]

The primary type of colonic movement is segmental. The circular muscles contract and relax at different sites, shuttling the intestinal contents back and forth between the contracting and relaxing haustra, most commonly during fasting. The movements massage the intestinal contents, now called the **fecal mass**, and facilitate the absorption of water. Propulsive movement occurs with the proximal-to-distal contraction of several haustral units. Peristaltic movements also occur and promote the emptying of the colon. The **gastrocolic reflex** initiates propulsion in the entire colon, usually during or immediately after eating, when chyme enters from the ileum. The gastrocolic reflex causes the fecal mass to pass rapidly into the sigmoid colon and rectum, stimulating defecation. Gastrin and cholecystokinin participate in stimulating this reflex. Epinephrine inhibits contractile activity.

Approximately 500 to 700 ml of chyme flows from the ileum to the cecum per day. Most of the water is absorbed in the colon by diffusion and active transport. The electrochemical gradient established by sodium movement enhances the diffusion of serum potassium from the capillaries in the lumen. Aldosterone increases membrane permeability to sodium, thereby increasing both the diffusion of sodium into the cell and its active transport across the basolateral membrane to the interstitial fluid. (See Chapter 19 for a discussion of aldosterone secretion.) This increases the cell-to-lumen diffusion gradient for potassium. Potassium moves outward, and chloride is absorbed with sodium as the complementary anion. Chloride also enters the cell in exchange for bicarbonate.

Absorption and epithelial transport occur in the cecum, ascending colon, transverse colon, and descending colon. By the time the fecal mass enters the sigmoid colon, the mass consists entirely of wastes and is called the feces. **Feces**, or excrement, consists of food residue, unabsorbed gastrointestinal secretions, shed epithelial cells, and bacteria.

The movement of feces into the sigmoid colon and rectum stimulates the **defecation reflex (rectal reflex)**. The rectal wall stretches and the tonically constricted internal anal sphincter (smooth muscle with autonomic nervous system control) relaxes, creating the urge to defecate. The defecation reflex can be overridden voluntarily by contraction of the external anal sphincter and muscles of the pelvic floor. The rectal wall gradually relaxes, reducing tension, and the urge to defecate passes. Retrograde contraction of the rectum may displace the feces out of the rectal vault until a more convenient time for evacuation. Pain or fear of pain associated with defecation (e.g., rectal fissures or hemorrhoids) can inhibit the defecation reflex. The defecation reflex is regulated by parasympathetic and cholinergic fibers. Voluntary inhibition or facilitation of defecation is mediated from cortical projections onto the medulla and down to sacral segments of the cord.

Defecation is facilitated by squatting or sitting because these positions straighten the angle between the rectum and anal canal and increase the efficiency of straining (increasing intraabdominal pressure). Intraabdominal pressure is increased by initiating the Valsalva maneuver. This maneuver consists of inhaling and forcing the diaphragm and chest muscles against the closed glottis. This increases both intrathoracic and intraabdominal pressure, which is transmitted to the rectum.

Intestinal Bacteria

The type and number of bacteria vary greatly throughout the normal gastrointestinal tract, with an increasing number of bacteria from the stomach to the distal colon. The stomach is relatively sterile because of the secretion of acid that kills ingested pathogens or inhibits bacterial growth. Bile acid secretion, intestinal motility, and antibody production suppress bacterial growth in the duodenum, and in the duodenum and jejunum there is a low concentration of aerobes (10^{-1} per ml to 10^{-4} per ml), primarily streptococci, lactobacilli, staphylococci, enterobacteria, and *Bacteroides*.[18] There are no anaerobes proximal to the ileum. Anaerobes are found distal to the ileocecal valve. They constitute about 95% of the fecal flora in the colon and contribute one third of the solid bulk of feces. *Bacteroides*, clostridia, anaerobic lactobacilli, and coliforms are the most common microorganisms from the ileum to the cecum.

The intestinal tract is sterile at birth but becomes colonized with *Escherichia coli, Clostridium welchii*, and *Streptococcus* within a few hours. Within 3 to 4 weeks after birth, the normal flora is established. The intestinal bacteria do not have major digestive or absorptive functions. They do play a role in the metabolism of bile salts (contributing to the intestinal reabsorption of bile and the elimination of toxic bile metabolites); the metabolism of estrogens, androgens, and lipids and conversion of unabsorbed carbohydrates to absorbable organic acids; metabolism of various nitrogenous substances and drugs; and protection against exogenous infection.[19]

ACCESSORY ORGANS OF DIGESTION

The liver, gallbladder, and exocrine pancreas all secrete substances necessary for the digestion of chyme. These secretions are delivered to the duodenum through ducts (Fig. 37-17). The liver produces bile, which contains salts necessary for fat digestion and absorption. Between meals, bile is stored in the gallbladder. The exocrine pancreas produces enzymes needed for the complete digestion of carbohydrates, proteins, and fats. The exocrine pancreas also produces an alkaline fluid that neutralizes chyme, creating a duodenal pH that supports enzymatic action. The liver receives nutrients absorbed by the small intestine and metabolizes or synthesizes these nutrients into forms that can be absorbed by the body's cells. It then releases the nutrients into the bloodstream or stores them for later use.

Liver

The **liver**, which weighs 1200 to 1600 g, is the largest organ in the body. It is located under the right diaphragm and is divided into right and left lobes. The larger, right lobe is divided further into the caudate and quadrate lobes (Fig. 37-18). The falciform ligament separates the right and left lobes and attaches the liver to the anterior abdominal wall. A fibrous cord called the *round ligament (ligamentum teres)* extends along the free edge of the falciform ligament. The round ligament is the remnant of the umbilical vein and extends from the umbilicus to the inferior surface of the liver. The coronary ligament branches from the falciform ligament and extends over the superior surface of the right and left lobes, adhering the liver to the inferior surface of the diaphragm. The liver is covered by a fibroelastic capsule called the Glisson capsule. The **Glisson capsule** contains blood vessels, lymphatics, and nerves. When the liver is diseased or swollen, distention of the capsule causes pain and the lymphatics may ooze fluid into the peritoneal space.

The metabolic functions of the liver require a large amount of blood. The liver receives blood from both arterial and venous sources. The hepatic artery branches from the

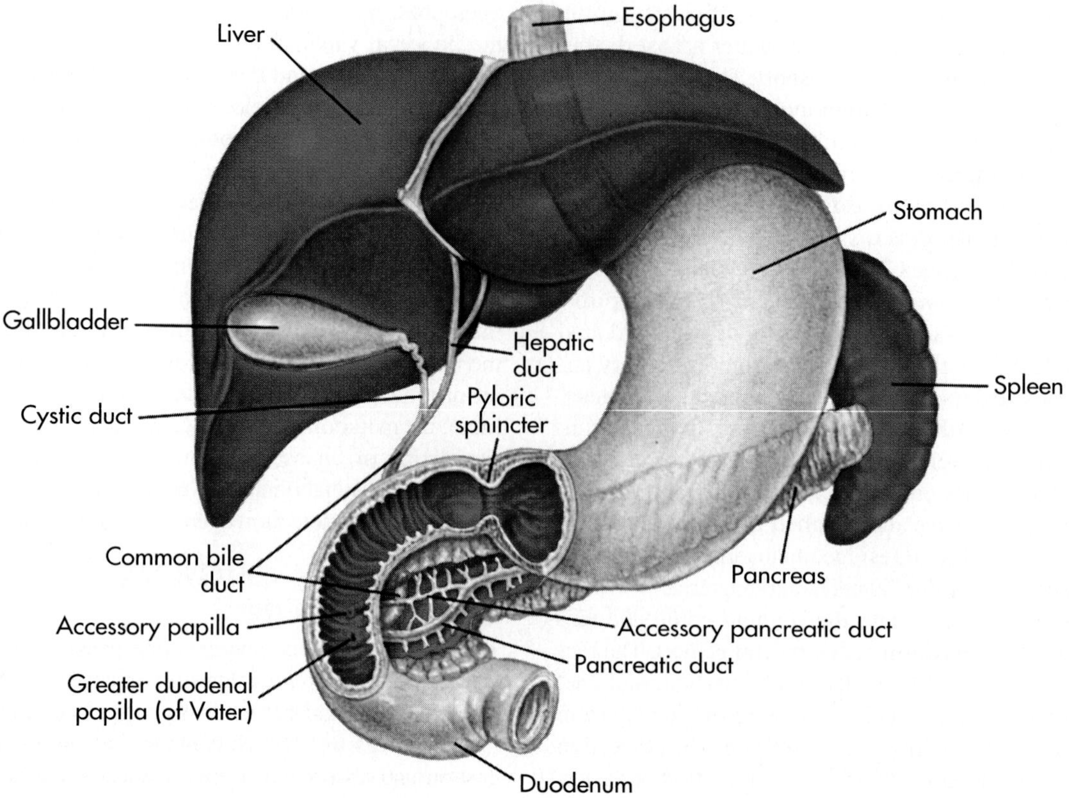

FIG. 37-17 Location of the liver, gallbladder, and exocrine pancreas, which are the accessory organs of digestion. (From Thompson JM et al: *Mosby's clinical nursing*, ed 4, St Louis, 1997, Mosby.)

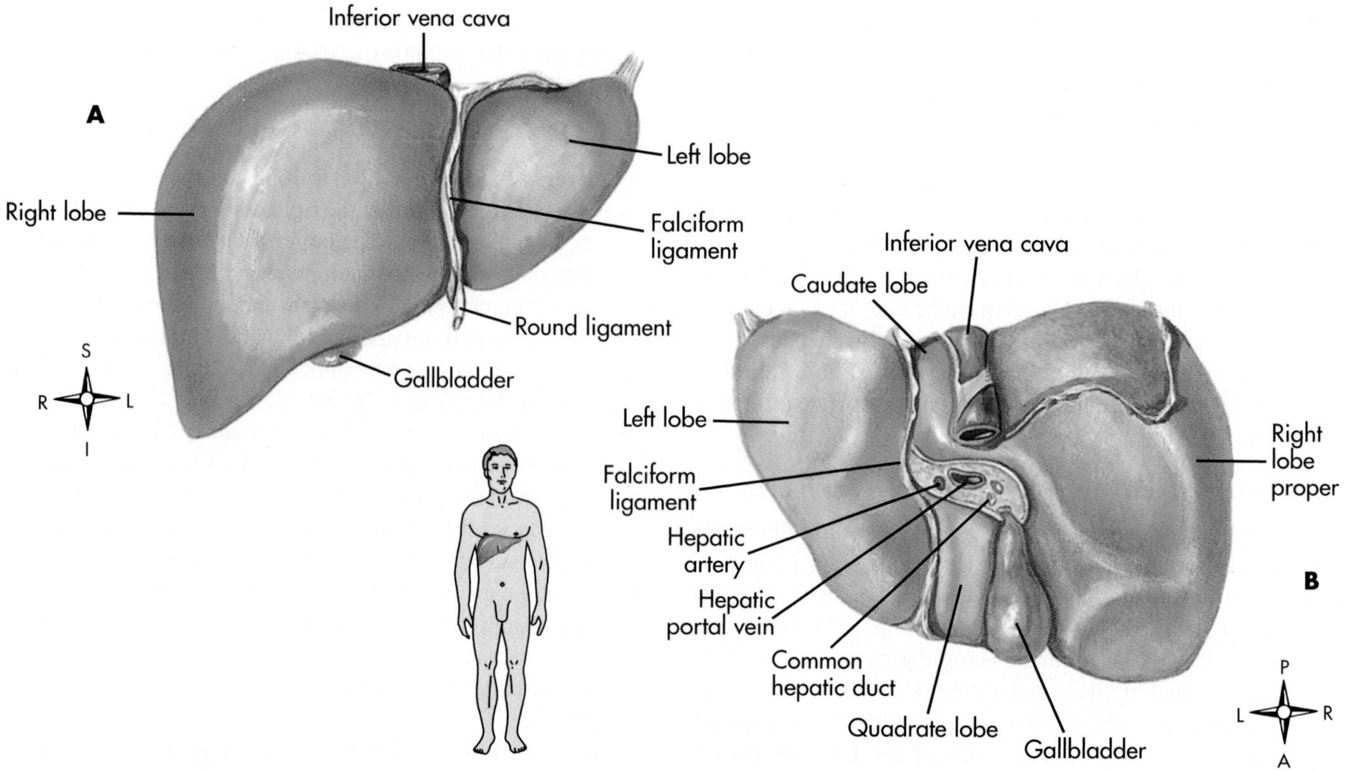

FIG. 37-18 Gross structure of the liver. A, Anterior view. **B,** Inferior view. (From Thibodeau GA, Patton KI: *Anatomy & physiology*, ed 4, St Louis, 1999, Mosby.)

abdominal aorta and provides oxygenated blood at the rate of 400 to 500 ml/min (about 25% of the cardiac output). The hepatic portal vein, which receives deoxygenated blood from the inferior and superior mesenteric veins and the splenic vein, delivers about 1000 to 1200 ml/min to the liver. Portal venous blood constitutes 70% of the blood supply to the liver. This blood carries some oxygen and is rich in nutrients that have been absorbed from the digestive tract.

Within the liver lobes are multiple, smaller anatomic units called **liver lobules** (Fig. 37-19). The lobules are formed of cords or plates of **hepatocytes,** which are the functional cells of the liver. These cells are capable of regeneration; therefore damaged or resected liver tissue can regrow. Lipocytes are star-shaped cells that store lipids, including vitamin A. Small capillaries, or **sinusoids**, are located between the plates of hepatocytes. The sinusoids receive a mixture of venous and arterial blood from branches of the hepatic artery and portal vein. Blood from the sinusoids drains to a central vein in the middle of each liver lobule. Venous blood from all the lobules then flows into the hepatic vein, which empties into the inferior vena cava. Small channels known as **bile canaliculi** are adjacent to hepatocytes and conduct bile, which is produced by the hepatocytes, outward to bile ducts and eventually drain into the **common bile duct** (see Fig. 37-19). The common bile duct empties bile into the duodenum through an opening called the **major duodenal papilla** (sphincter of Oddi).[20]

The sinusoids of the liver lobules are lined with highly permeable endothelium. This permeability enhances the transport of nutrients from the sinusoids into the hepatocytes, where they are metabolized. The sinusoids are also lined with phagocytic cells known as **Kupffer cells**. Kupffer cells are part of the mononuclear phagocyte system (see Chapter 24). **Stellate cells** contain retinoids (vitamin A) and are contractile and may regulate sinusoidal blood flow. They remove foreign substances from the blood and trap bacteria. **Pit cells** are natural killer cells found in the sinusoidal lumen; they are important in tumor defense.[21] Between the endothelial lining of the sinusoid and the hepatocyte is the **Disse space**, which drains interstitial fluid into the hepatic lymph system.

Secretion of Bile

The liver assists intestinal digestion by secreting 700 to 1200 ml of bile per day. **Bile** is an alkaline, bitter-tasting, yellowish green fluid that contains bile salts (conjugated bile acids), cholesterol, bilirubin (a pigment), electrolytes, and water. It is formed by hepatocytes and secreted into the canaliculi. **Bile salts,** which are conjugated bile acids, are required for the intestinal emulsification and absorption of fats. Having facilitated fat emulsification and absorption, most bile salts are actively absorbed in the terminal ileum and returned to the liver through the portal circulation for resecretion.[22] The recycling of bile salts is termed the **enterohepatic circulation** (Fig. 37-20).

Bile has two fractional components: the acid-dependent fraction and the acid-independent fraction. Hepatocytes secrete the **bile acid–dependent fraction** of the bile. This fraction consists of bile acids, cholesterol, lecithin (a phospholipid), and bilirubin (a bile pigment). The **bile acid–independent fraction** of the bile, which is secreted by the hepatocytes and epithelial cells of the bile canaliculi, is a bicarbonate-rich aqueous fluid that gives bile its alkaline pH.

Bile salts are conjugated in the liver from primary and secondary bile acids. The **primary bile acids** are cholic acid and chenodeoxycholic (chenic) acid. These acids are synthesized from cholesterol by the hepatocytes. The **secondary bile acids** are deoxycholic acid and lithocholic acid. These acids are formed in the small intestine by the action of intestinal bacteria, after which they are absorbed and flow to the liver (see Fig. 37-20). Both forms of bile acids are conjugated with amino acids (glycine or taurine) in the liver to form bile salts. Conjugation makes the bile acids more water soluble, thus restricting their diffusion from the duodenum and ileum. The primary and secondary bile acids together form the **bile acid pool**. Other components of bile include phospholipids and cholesterol.

Bile salts are planar molecules; that is, they are hydrophobic on one end and hydrophilic on the other. When the concentration of bile salts is adequate or has reached the **critical micelle concentration**, the molecules form micelles with their hydrophilic side toward the watery chyme of the intestine and their hydrophobic side surrounding fat molecules such as cholesterol, free fatty acids, and phospholipids (see Fig. 37-14). Micelle formation facilitates the absorption of fat by the intestinal mucosa.

Bile secretion is called **choleresis**. A **choleretic agent** is a substance that stimulates the liver to secrete bile. One strong

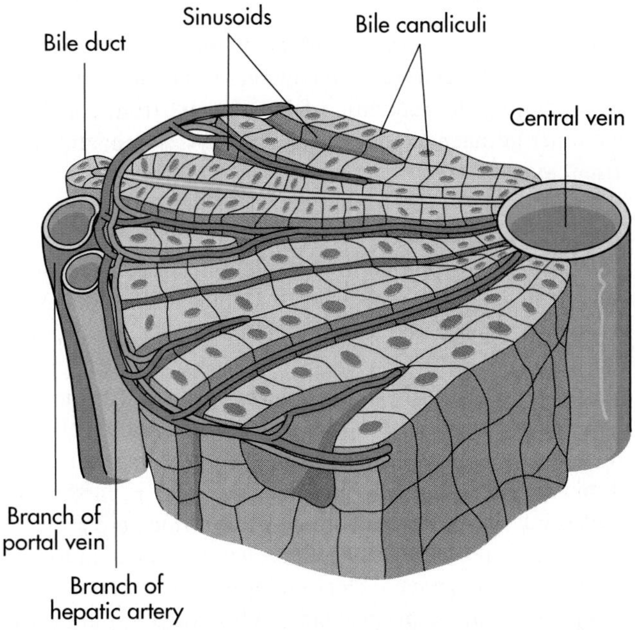

FIG. 37-19 Diagrammatic representation of a liver lobule. A central vein is located in the center of the lobule with plates of hepatic cells disposed radially. Branches of the portal vein and hepatic artery are located on the periphery of the lobule, and blood from both perfuses the sinusoids. Peripherally located bile ducts drain the bile canaliculi that run between the hepatocytes.

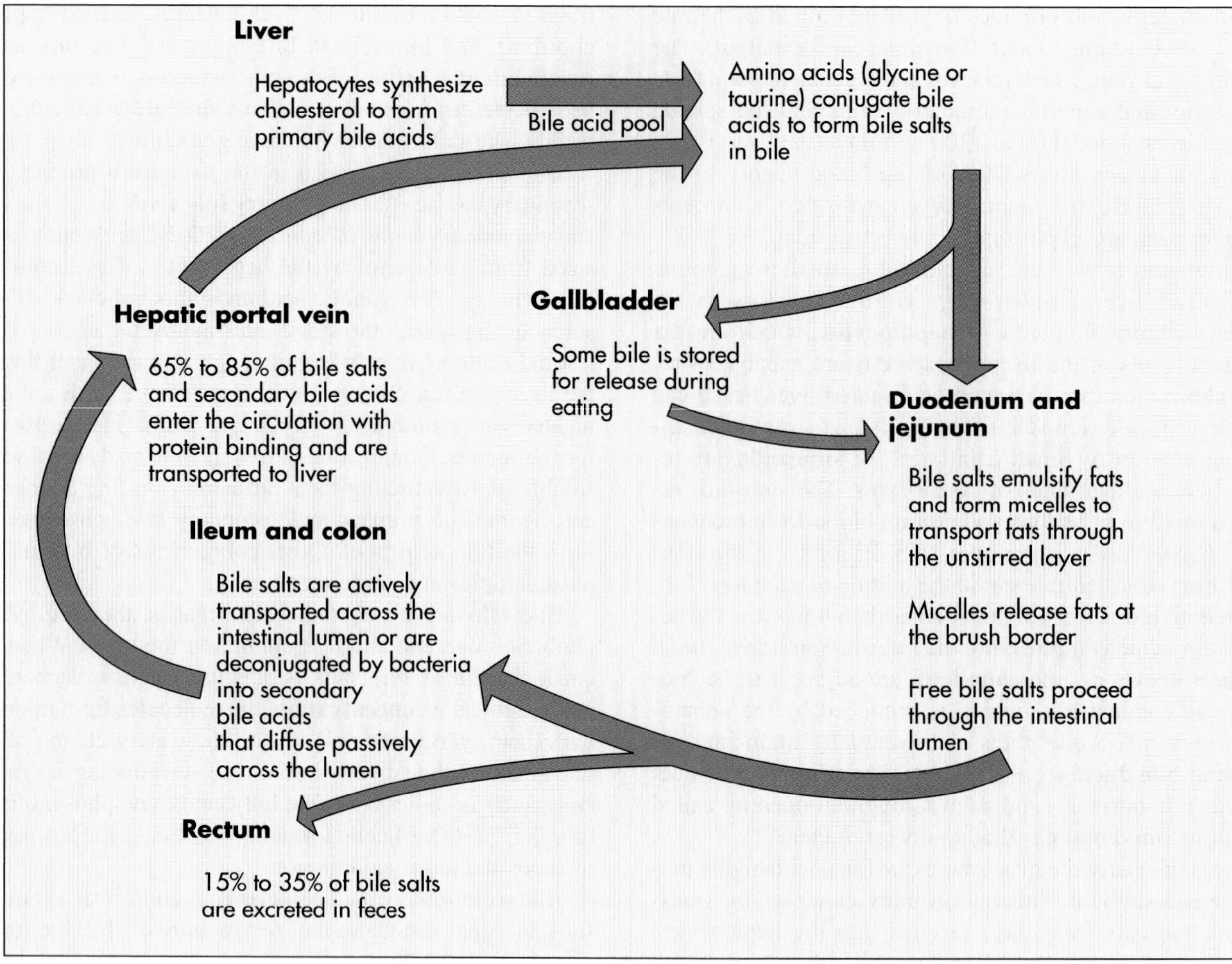
Liver
Hepatocytes synthesize cholesterol to form primary bile acids
Bile acid pool
Amino acids (glycine or taurine) conjugate bile acids to form bile salts in bile
Gallbladder
Some bile is stored for release during eating
Hepatic portal vein
65% to 85% of bile salts and secondary bile acids enter the circulation with protein binding and are transported to liver
Duodenum and jejunum
Bile salts emulsify fats and form micelles to transport fats through the unstirred layer
Micelles release fats at the brush border
Free bile salts proceed through the intestinal lumen
Ileum and colon
Bile salts are actively transported across the intestinal lumen or are deconjugated by bacteria into secondary bile acids that diffuse passively across the lumen
Rectum
15% to 35% of bile salts are excreted in feces

FIG. 37-20 The enterohepatic circulation of bile salts.

stimulus is a high concentration of bile salts. Other choleretics include secretin, which increases the rate of bile flow by promoting the secretion of bicarbonate from canaliculi and other intrahepatic bile ducts; cholecystokinin; and vagal stimulation.

Metabolism of Bilirubin

Bilirubin is a byproduct of destruction of aged red blood cells. It gives bile a greenish black color and produces the yellow tinge of jaundice. Aged red blood cells are taken up and destroyed by macrophages of the mononuclear phagocyte system, primarily in the spleen and liver. (In the liver these macrophages are Kupffer cells.) Within these cells, hemoglobin is separated into its component parts—heme and globin (Fig. 37-21). The globin component is further degraded into its constituent amino acids, which are recycled to form new protein. The heme moiety is converted to biliverdin by the enzymatic cleavage of iron. The iron attaches to transferrin in the plasma and can be stored in the liver or used by the bone marrow to make new red blood cells. The biliverdin is enzymatically converted to bilirubin in the macrophage of the mononuclear phagocytic system and then is released into the plasma. In the plasma, bilirubin binds to albumin and is known as **unconjugated bilirubin**, or free bilirubin, which is lipid soluble.

In the liver, unconjugated bilirubin moves from plasma in the sinusoids into the hepatocyte. Within hepatocytes it joins with glucuronic acid to form **conjugated bilirubin,** which is water soluble. Conjugation transforms bilirubin from a lipid-soluble substance that can cross biologic membranes to a water-soluble substance that can be excreted in the bile. When conjugated bilirubin reaches the distal ileum and colon, it is deconjugated by bacteria and converted to **urobilinogen.** Most of the urobilinogen is then excreted in the urine, and a small amount is eliminated in feces.

Vascular and Hematologic Functions

Because of its extensive vascular network, the liver can store a large volume of blood. The amount stored at any one time depends on pressure relationships in the arteries and veins. The liver can also release blood to maintain systemic circulatory volume in the event of hemorrhage.

Kupffer cells in the sinusoids of the liver remove bacteria and foreign particles from the portal blood. Because the liver receives all of the venous blood from the gut and pancreas, the Kupffer cells play an important role in destroying intestinal bacteria and preventing infections.

The liver also has hemostatic functions. It synthesizes prothrombin; fibrinogen; and factors I, II, VII, IX, and X, all of which are necessary for effective clotting (see Chapter 24).

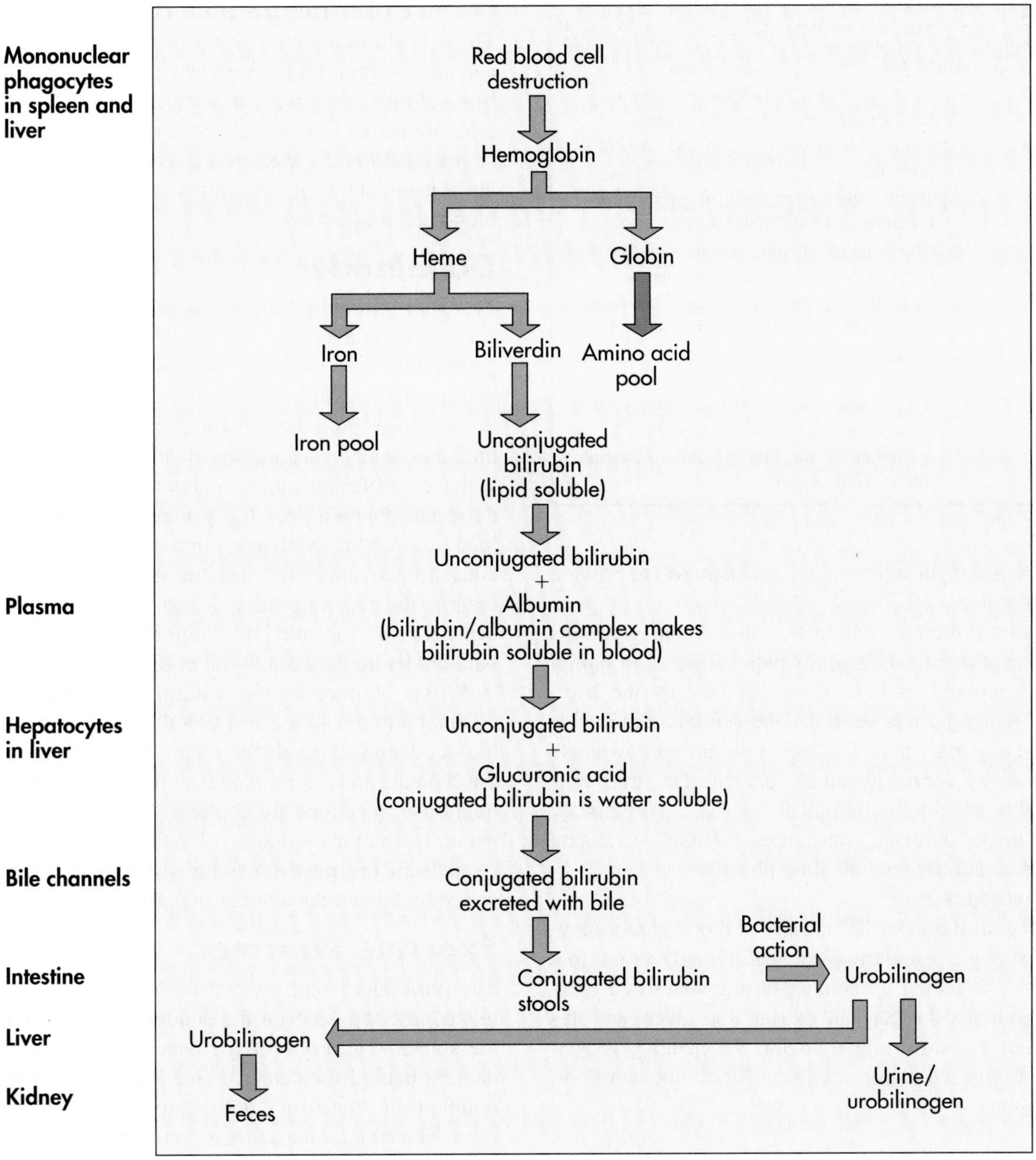

FIG. 37-21 Bilirubin metabolism.

Vitamin K, a fat-soluble vitamin, is essential for the synthesis of other clotting factors. Because bile salts are needed for reabsorption of fats, vitamin K absorption depends on adequate bile production in the liver. Impairment of vitamin K absorption diminishes production of clotting factors and increases risk of bleeding.

Metabolism of Nutrients

Fats

Fat is synthesized from carbohydrate and protein, primarily in the liver. Fat absorbed by lacteals in the intestinal villi enters the liver through the lymphatics, primarily as triglycerides. In the liver the triglycerides can be hydrolyzed to glycerol and free fatty acids and used to produce metabolic energy (adenosine triphosphate [ATP]), or they can be released into the bloodstream as lipoproteins (lipids bound to proteins). The lipoproteins are carried by the blood to adipose cells for storage. The liver also synthesizes phospholipids and cholesterol, which are needed for the hepatic production of bile salts, steroid hormones, components of plasma membranes, and other special molecules.

Proteins

Protein synthesis requires the presence of all the essential amino acids (obtained only from food), as well as nonessential amino acids. Proteins perform many important roles in the body and are summarized in Table 37-3.

Within hepatocytes, amino acids are converted to carbohydrates by the removal of ammonia (NH_3), a process known as **deamination**. The ammonia is converted to urea by the liver and passes into the blood to be excreted by the kidneys. Depending on need, the ketoacids are converted to fatty acids for fat synthesis and storage or are oxidized by

Table 37-3 Proteins in the Body

Role	Example
Contraction	Actin and myosin enable muscle contraction
Energy	Proteins can be metabolized for energy
Fluid balance	Albumin, a major source of plasma oncotic pressure
Protection	Antibodies and complement protect against infection and foreign substances
Regulation	Enzymes control chemical reactions; hormones regulate many physiologic processes
Structure	Collagen fibers provide structural support to many parts of the body; keratin strengthens skin, hair, and nails
Transport	Hemoglobin transports oxygen and carbon dioxide in the blood; plasma proteins serve as transport molecules; proteins in cell membranes control movement of materials into and out of cells

the Krebs tricarboxylic acid cycle (see Chapter 1) to provide energy for the liver cells.

The plasma proteins, including albumins and globulins (with the exception of γ-globulin, which is formed in lymph nodes and lymphoid tissue), are synthesized by the liver. The liver also synthesizes several nonessential amino acids and serum enzymes, including aspartate aminotransferase (AST; previously serum glutamate oxaloacetate transaminase [SGOT]), alanine aminotransferase (ALT; previously serum glutamate pyruvate transaminase [SGPT]), lactate dehydrogenase (LDH), and alkaline phosphatase.

Carbohydrates

The liver contributes to the stability of blood glucose levels by releasing glucose during states of hypoglycemia (low blood sugar) and taking up glucose during states of hyperglycemia (high blood sugar) and storing it as glycogen (glyconeogenesis) or converting it to fat. When all glycogen stores have been used, the liver can convert amino acids and glycerol to glucose.

Metabolic Detoxification

The liver alters exogenous and endogenous chemicals (e.g., drugs), foreign molecules, and hormones to make them less toxic or less biologically active. This process, called **metabolic detoxification (biotransformation),** diminishes intestinal or renal tubular reabsorption of potentially toxic substances and facilitates their intestinal and renal excretion. In this way alcohol, barbiturates, amphetamines, steroids, and hormones (including estrogens, aldosterone, antidiuretic hormone, and testosterone) are metabolized or detoxified, preventing excessive accumulation and adverse effects.

Although metabolic detoxification is usually protective, sometimes the end products of metabolic detoxification become toxins. Those of alcohol metabolism, for example, are acetaldehyde and hydrogen. Excessive intake of alcohol over a prolonged period causes these end products to damage hepatocytes. Acetaldehyde damages cellular mitochondria, and the excess hydrogen promotes fat accumulation. This is how alcohol impairs the liver's ability to function.

Storage of Minerals and Vitamins

The liver stores certain vitamins and minerals, including iron and copper, in times of excessive intake and releases them in times of need. The liver can store vitamins B_{12} and D for several months and vitamin A for several years. The liver also stores vitamins E and K. Iron is stored in the liver as ferritin, an iron-protein complex, and is released as needed for red blood cell production.

Gallbladder

The **gallbladder** is a saclike organ that lies on the inferior surface of the liver (Fig. 37-22). The primary function of the gallbladder is to store and concentrate bile between meals. During the interdigestive period, bile flows from the liver through the right or left hepatic duct into the common hepatic duct and meets resistance at the closed **sphincter of Oddi**, which controls flow into the duodenum and prevents reflux of duodenal contents into the pancreatobiliary system.[23] Bile then flows to the **cystic duct** into the gallbladder, where it is concentrated and stored. The mucosa of the gallbladder wall readily absorbs water and electrolytes, leaving a high concentration of bile salts, bile pigments, and cholesterol. The gallbladder holds about 90 ml of bile.

Within 30 minutes after eating, the gallbladder begins to contract and the sphincter of Oddi relaxes, forcing bile into the duodenum through the major duodenal papilla. During the cephalic and gastric phases of digestion, gallbladder contraction is mediated by cholinergic branches of the vagus nerve. Hormonal regulation of gallbladder contraction is derived from the release of cholecystokinin and motilin secreted by the duodenal mucosa in the presence of fat.

Exocrine Pancreas

The **pancreas** is approximately 20 cm long, with its head tucked into the curve of the duodenum and its tail touching the spleen. The body of the pancreas lies deep in the abdomen, behind the stomach (see Fig. 37-22). The pancreas is unique in that it has both endocrine and exocrine functions. The endocrine pancreas secretes insulin, glucagon, somatostatin, and pancreatic polypeptide.[7]

The **exocrine pancreas** is composed of acini and networks of ducts that secrete enzymes and alkaline fluids with important digestive functions. The acinar cells are organized into spherical lobules around small secretory ducts (see Fig. 37-22). Secretions drain into a system of ducts that leads to the **pancreatic duct (Wirsung duct),** which empties into the common bile duct at the **ampulla of Vater**. In some individuals an accessory duct (the duct of Santorini) branches off the pancreatic duct and drains directly into the duodenum at an opening called the *minor duodenal papilla.*

Arterial blood is supplied to the pancreas by branches of the celiac and superior mesenteric arteries. Venous blood leaves the head of the pancreas through the portal vein, with the body and tail being drained through the splenic vein. All hormonal pancreatic secretions also pass through the portal vein into the liver.

Pancreatic innervation arises from preganglionic parasympathetic fibers of the vagus nerve. These fibers activate

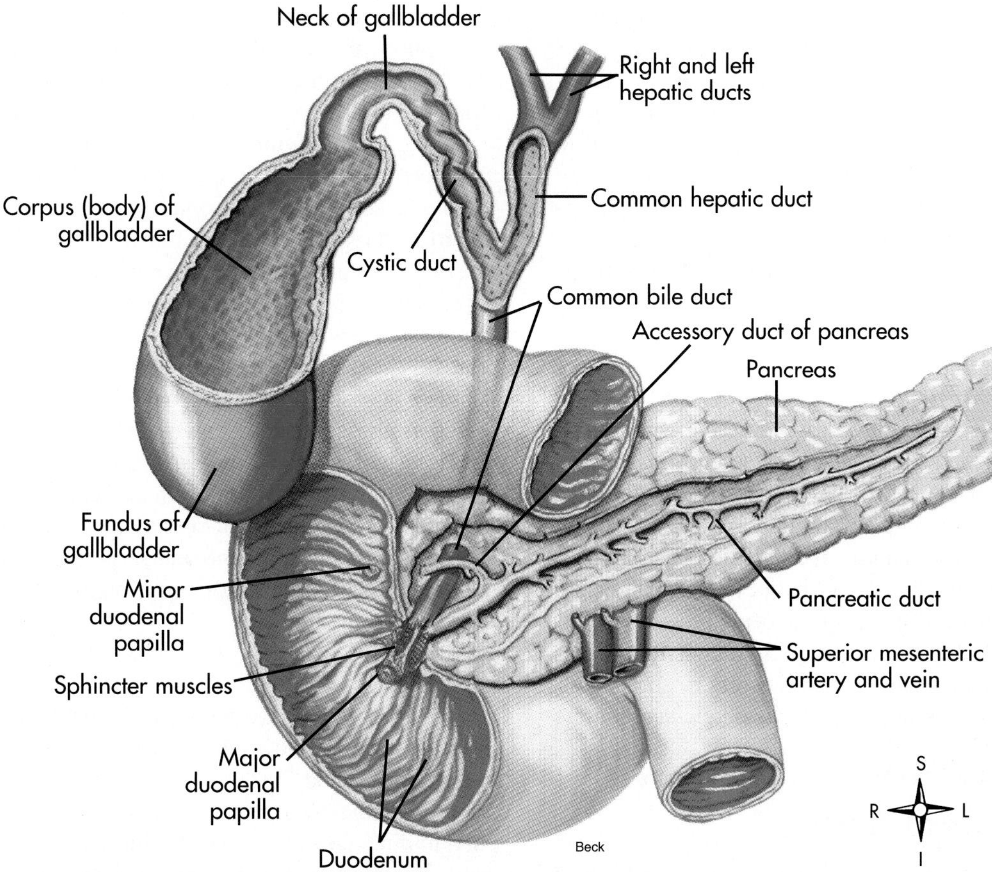

FIG. 37-22 Common bile duct and its tributaries. Obstruction of either the hepatic or the common bile duct by stone or spasm prevents bile from being ejected into the duodenum. (From Thibodeau GA, Patton KI: *Anatomy & physiology*, ed 4, St Louis, 1999, Mosby.)

postganglionic fibers, which stimulate enzymatic and hormonal secretion. Sympathetic postganglionic fibers from the celiac and superior mesenteric plexuses innervate the blood vessels and cause vasoconstriction and inhibit pancreatic secretion.

The aqueous secretions of the exocrine pancreas are isotonic and contain potassium, sodium, bicarbonate, and chloride. Sodium and potassium concentrations are about equal to those in the plasma. The concentration of bicarbonate in pancreatic juice varies directly with the secretory flow rate. As bicarbonate secretion increases, chloride secretion decreases to maintain a constant anionic concentration. The highly alkaline pancreatic juice neutralizes the acidic chyme that enters the duodenum from the stomach and provides the alkaline medium needed for the actions of digestive enzymes.

In the pancreas, transport of water and electrolytes through the ductal epithelium involves both active and passive mechanisms. The secretory cells of the acini actively transport hydrogen into the blood and bicarbonate into the duct lumen. Potassium and chloride are secreted by diffusion according to changes in electrochemical potential gradients. As the secretion flows down the duct, water is osmotically transported into the juice until it becomes isoosmotic. At low flow rates, bicarbonate is exchanged passively for chloride, but at higher flow rates there is less time for this exchange and bicarbonate concentration increases. Because eating stimulates the flow of pancreatic juice, the juice is most alkaline when it needs to be—during digestion.

The pancreatic enzymes hydrolyze proteins, carbohydrates, and fats. The proteolytic (protein-digesting) enzymes include trypsin, chymotrypsin, and carboxypeptidase. These enzymes are secreted in their inactive forms—that is, as trypsinogen, chymotrypsinogen, and procarboxypeptidase—to protect the pancreas from the digestive effects of its own enzymes. For further protection the pancreas produces **trypsin inhibitor**, which prevents the activation of proteolytic enzymes while they are in the pancreas. Once in the duodenum, the inactive forms (proenzymes) are activated by **enterokinase**, an enzyme secreted by the duodenal mucosa. Trypsinogen is the first proenzyme to be activated. Its conversion to trypsin stimulates the conversion of chymotrypsinogen to chymotrypsin and procarboxypeptidase to carboxypeptidase. Each of these enzymes cleaves specific peptide bonds to reduce polypeptides to smaller peptides.

Pancreatic α-amylase is secreted in active form and digests carbohydrate by cleaving interior α-1,4-glucosidic bonds at an optimum pH of approximately 6.9. **Pancreatic lipases** hydrolyze triglyceride, cholesterol, and phospholipids to free fatty acids and uronoglycerides.

Secretion of the aqueous and enzymatic components of pancreatic juice is controlled by hormonal and vagal stimuli. Secretin stimulates the acinar and duct cells to secrete the bicarbonate-rich fluid that neutralizes chyme and prepares it for enzymatic digestion. As chyme enters the duodenum, its acidity (pH of 4.5 or less) stimulates the **S cells** (secretin-producing cells) of the duodenum to release secretin, which is absorbed by the intestine and delivered to the pancreas in the bloodstream. In the pancreas, secretin causes ductal and acinar cells to release alkaline fluid. Secretin also inhibits the actions of gastrin, thereby decreasing gastric acid secretion and motility. The overall effect is to neutralize contents of the duodenum.

Enzymatic secretion follows, stimulated by cholecystokinin and acetylcholine. Cholecystokinin is released in the duodenum in response to the essential amino acids and fatty acids already present in chyme. Cholecystokinin and acetylcholine both act on the acinar cells, causing enzyme release. Once in the small intestine, activated pancreatic enzymes inhibit the release of more cholecystokinin and acetylcholine. This feedback mechanism inhibits the secretion of more pancreatic enzymes. Acetylcholine is liberated from pancreatic branches of the vagus nerve during the cephalic phase of digestion. Pancreatic polypeptide is released after eating and inhibits postprandial pancreatic exocrine secretion. (Table 37-1 summarizes hormonal stimulation of pancreatic secretions.)

TESTS OF DIGESTIVE FUNCTION

Gastrointestinal Tract

Although important diagnostic information can be obtained from the patient's medical history and presenting symptoms, numerous disease-specific tests must be performed to evaluate the structure and function of the gastrointestinal tract. A description of selected studies is presented in Tables 37-4 and 37-5. Radiography and imaging techniques, including ultrasound and radionuclide and computed tomography (CT) scanning, are common procedures for evaluating structure and function. Plain roentgenograms using contrast media such as barium- or iodine-containing compounds can be used to outline the gastrointestinal lumen, biliary tree and pancreatic ducts, fistulae, and arteriovenous systems. CT scanning is particularly useful for diagnosis of pancreatic or hepatic tumors or cysts. Ultrasonic scanning is a safe, simple, and relatively inexpensive technique used to detect liver-related jaundice and intraabdominal masses, particularly abscesses.

Fiberoptic endoscopy, using flexible endoscopes, allows direct visualization of the gastrointestinal tract. A biopsy channel allows tissue sampling, and suction can be applied to remove gastrointestinal secretions or blood. Analysis of stool, gastric secretions, and plasma provides important clues to infection, malabsorption syndromes, ulcerative lesions, and tumor growth.

Liver

A variety of diagnostic tests can be performed to evaluate liver function (Table 37-6).[24,25] Imaging techniques similar to those described for the gastrointestinal tract are also useful to evaluate liver structure and function. Plasma chemistry findings are also altered with many liver diseases because of release of cytoplasmic enzymes into the circulation when there is damage to the hepatocyte. Of particular importance are elevations of aminotransferases and LDH. Ob-

Table 37-4 Selected Studies of Gastrointestinal Structure

Test	Description	Application
Plain roentgenograms	Use of high-energy electromagnetic radiation to evaluate tissue structure by radiopacity or radiolucency	Visualization of the position, size, and structure of abdominal contents
Air or barium contrast roentgenograms	Introduction of radiopaque substances into the upper or lower gastrointestinal tract	Enhanced visualization of the contours, position, and size of the gastrointestinal tract to detect umbilical hernia, ulcers, diverticula, congenital anomalies, polyps, tumors, strictures, obstructions
Endoscopy Esophagoscopy (esophagus) Gastroscopy (stomach) Duodenoscopy (duodenum) Colonoscopy (large intestine) Sigmoidoscopy (sigmoid colon)	Passage of rigid or flexible (fiberoptic) endoscope into the gastrointestinal tract for visualization or biopsy	Visualization or biopsy of inflamed hernias, polyps, ulcers, strictures, varices, tumors, sites of bleeding, mucosal or neoplastic lesions and for culture of *Helicobacter pylori* from stomach
Ultrasound	Use of piezoelectric crystal to generate sound waves that are reflected from tissue interfaces to provide an image	Imaging of abdominal organs (gallbladder, liver, pancreas, spleen), masses, stones, abscesses, structural abnormalities
Computed tomography (CT)	Use of a computer to integrate differences in absorption of a large number of x-rays to produce a cross-sectional image; may be done with contrast agents	Imaging of gallbladder, liver, pancreas, spleen, cysts, hematomas, abscesses, stones, extrahepatic bile ducts, and portal vein
Magnetic resonance imaging (MRI)	Projection of differences in magnetic properties of molecules within different cells and tissues, using the field of a large magnet	Same applications as CT scan; can also detect blood flow and vessel patency

struction of bile canaliculi or ducts results in regurgitation of bile back into the hepatic sinusoids and into the circulation, with elevation of bilirubin levels. Prothrombin times are often prolonged with both hepatitis and chronic liver disease. In severe disease, other plasma proteins, such as albumin and globulins, may be diminished as a result of hepatocyte damage. Liver biopsies are often performed to evaluate the extent of liver involvement or degeneration with cirrhosis or hepatitis.

Gallbladder

Evaluation of structural alterations in the gallbladder may be achieved by the use of various imaging techniques. Table 37-7 summarizes these techniques. Obstruction of the common ducts from stones, tumors, or inflammation prevents the flow of bile from the liver and gallbladder from reaching the gastrointestinal tract. Both the conjugated and total serum bilirubin values are elevated, urine urobilinogen is increased, stools are clay colored, and jaundice develops. Fat absorption can be impaired and the prothrombin time prolonged if vitamin K is not absorbed. With inflammation of the gallbladder, the white cell count is elevated.

Exocrine Pancreas

Tests of pancreatic function are summarized in Table 37-8. Evaluation of plasma and urinary amylase provides particularly significant measures of pancreatic function. Inflammation or obstruction of the pancreas results in an increase in serum amylase levels. Decreased renal absorption of amylase results in increased urine amylase levels. Increased stool fat can reflect pancreatic insufficiency caused by decreased lipase secretion when biliary function is normal.

Aging and the Gastrointestinal System

Age-related changes in gastrointestinal function begin to occur before 50 years of age. Tooth enamel and dentin wear down, making the teeth vulnerable to cavities. Teeth are lost, frequently as a result of periodontal (gum) disease or recession of the gums. Taste buds decline in number, and the sense of smell diminishes. Together these losses decrease the sense of taste. Salivary secretion decreases and contributes to dry mouth. In very old persons, these oral and sensory changes make eating less pleasurable and reduce appetite. Food may not be chewed or lubricated sufficiently, making swallowing difficult. The esophagus develops decreased motility.

Age also diminishes gastric motility and volume, including secretion of bicarbonate and gastic mucus.[26] Acid content of gastric juice is related to gastric atrophy, which results in hypochlorhydria (insufficient hydrochloric acid) and delayed gastric emptying, best managed with frequent and

Table 37-5 Selected Tests of Gastrointestinal Function

Test	Normal Findings	Clinical Significance of Abnormal Findings
Stool studies	Resident microorganisms: clostridia, enterococci, *Pseudomonas,* a few yeasts	Detection of *Salmonella typhi* (typhoid fever), *Shigella* (dysentery), *Vibrio cholerae* (cholera), *Yersinia* (enterocolitis), *Escherichia coli* (gastroenteritis), *Staphylococcus aureus* (food poisoning), *Clostridium botulinum* (food poisoning), *Clostridium perfringens* (food poisoning), *Aeromonas* (gastroenteritis)
	Fat: 2-6 g/24 hr	Steatorrhea (increased values) can result from intestinal malabsorption or pancreatic insufficiency
	Pus: none	Large amounts of pus are associated with chronic ulcerative colitis, abscesses, and anal-rectal fistula
	Occult blood: none (OrthoTolidin or guaiac test)	Positive tests associated with bleeding
	Ova and parasites: none	Detection of *Entamoeba histolytica* (amebiasis), *Giardia lamblia* (giardiasis), and worms
D-Xylose absorption	5-Hr urinary excretion: 4.5 g/L Peak blood level: >30 mg/dl	Differentiation of pancreatic steatorrhea (normal D-xylose absorption) from intestinal steatorrhea (impaired D-xylose absorption)
Gastric acid stimulation	11-20 mEq/hr after stimulation	Detection of duodenal ulcers, Zollinger-Ellison syndrome (increased values), gastric atrophy, gastric carcinoma (decreased values)
Manometry (use of water-filled catheters connected to pressure transducers passed into the esophagus, stomach, colon, or rectum to evaluate contractility)	Values vary at different levels of the intestine	Inadequate swallowing, motility, sphincter function
Culture and sensitivity of duodenal contents	No pathogens	Detection of *Salmonella typhi* (typhoid fever)
Breath tests		
Glucose breath test or D-xylose	Negative for hydrogen or CO_2	May indicate intestinal bacterial overgrowth
Urea breath test	Negative for isotopically labeled CO_2	Presence of *Helicobacter pylori* infection

Table 37-6 Common Liver Function Tests

Test	Normal Value	Interpretation
SERUM ENZYMES		
Alkaline phosphatase	13-39 U/L	Increases with biliary obstruction and cholestatic hepatitis
γ Glutanyltransferase	Male 12-38 U/L Female 9-31 U/L	Increases with biliary obstruction and cholestatic hepatitis
Aspartate amino transferase (AST; previously serum glutamate oxaloacetate transaminase [SGOT])	5-40 U/L	Increases with hepatocellular injury
Alanine amino transferase (ALT; previously serum glutamate pyruvate transaminase [SGPT])	5-35 U/L	Increases with hepatocellular injury
LDH (lactate dehydrogenase)	90-220 U/L	Isoenzyme LD_5 is elevated with hypoxic and primary liver injury
5′-Nucleotidase	2-11 U/L	Increases with increase in alkaline phosphatase and cholestatic disorders
BILIRUBIN METABOLISM		
Serum bilirubin		
Indirect (unconjugated)	<0.8 mg/dl	Increases with hemolysis (lysis of red blood cells)
Direct (conjugated)	0.2-0.4 mg/dl	Increases with hepatocellular injury or obstruction
Total	<1.0 mg/dl	Increases with biliary obstruction
Urine bilirubin	0	Decreases with biliary obstruction
Urine urobilinogen	0-4 mg/24 hr	Increases with hemolysis or shunting of portal blood flow
SERUM PROTEINS		
Albumin	3.5-5.5 g/dl	Reduced with hepatocellular injury
Globulin	2.5-3.5 g/dl	Increases with hepatitis
Total	6-7 g/dl	
Albumin/globulin (A/G) ratio	1.5:1 to 2.5:1	Ratio reverses with chronic hepatitis or other chronic liver disease
Transferrin	250-300 μg/dl	Liver damage with decreased values, iron deficiency with increased values
α-Fetoprotein	6-20 ng/ml	Elevated values in primary hepatocellular carcinoma
BLOOD CLOTTING FUNCTIONS		
Prothrombin time (PT)	11.5-14 sec or 90%-100% of control	Increases with chronic liver disease (cirrhosis) or vitamin K deficiency
Partial thromboplastin time (PTT)	25-40 sec	Increases with severe liver disease or heparin therapy
BSP (bromsulphalein) excretion	<6% retention in 45 min	Increased retention with hepatocellular injury

Table 37-7 Diagnostic Evaluation of the Gallbladder

Test	Application
Plain roentgenogram of the abdomen	Visualization of calcified gallstones
Oral cholecystogram (use of an oral contrast medium such as iodopanoic acid, which is excreted with bile and concentrated in the gallbladder for visualization by radiography; may be administered as a double dose)	Visualization of gallstones; evaluation of filling and emptying of gallbladder
Intravenous cholangiography (use of intravenous contrast agents for visualization of gallbladder and bile ducts)	Diagnosis of acute gallbladder inflammation (cholecystitis) or disease of bile ducts
Cholecystosonography (ultrasound imaging of gallbladder and bile ducts)	Preferred method for detecting gallstones; differentiation of hepatic disease from biliary obstruction; diagnosis of chronic cholecystitis
Cholescintigraphy (radioisotope imaging of gallbladder)	Diagnosis of cholecystitis in individuals allergic to iodine-containing contrast agents; diagnosis of cystic duct obstruction
Endoscopic retrograde cholangiography (instillation of contrast medium through cannulation of ampulla of Vater with a duodenoscope)	Differentiation of intrahepatic or extrahepatic obstructive jaundice
Computed tomography (CT)	Diagnosis of biliary obstruction or malignancy when ultrasound is not successful

small meals. Decreased production of intrinsic factor leads to pernicious anemia. The villi of the small intestine become broader and shorter, perhaps because of a decrease in cell turnover. Intestinal absorption, motility, and blood flow decrease, impairing nutrient absorption. Proteins, fats, minerals (including iron and calcium), and vitamins are absorbed more slowly and in lesser amounts, and absorption of carbohydrates, particularly lactose, is decreased.[27,28] Although constipation is often described as a condition of old age, it is probably caused by life-style factors rather than physiologic decline. Lifelong bowel habits, current diet, lack of fluid intake, and immobility are likely causes of constipation in elderly persons.[29]

The liver decreases in size and weight with advancing age. Cell numbers and their regeneration decrease. However, liver function test results often remain within relatively normal ranges. Alterations in liver function in older individuals are usually a sign of a pathologic condition. Liver blood flow decreases with age and can influence efficiency of drug metabolism. Oxidative metabolism of drugs may be decreased.[30] The pancreas undergoes structural changes, such as fibrosis, fatty acid deposits, and atrophy. Pancreatic secretion decreases, but there is usually no observable dysfunction.[28,31] Aging does not cause apparent changes in the structure and function of the gallbladder and bile ducts, but incidence of gallstones increases.

Table 37-8 Selected Tests of Pancreatic Function

Test	Normal Value	Clinical Significance
Serum amylase	60-180 Somogyi units/ml	Elevated levels with pancreatic inflammation
Serum lipase	1.5 Somogyi units/ml	Elevated levels with pancreatic inflammation (may be elevated with other conditions; differentiates with amylase isoenzyme study)
Urine amylase	35-260 Somogyi units/hr	Elevated levels with pancreatic inflammation
Secretin test	Volume 1.8 ml/kg/hr Bicarbonate concentration: >80 mEq/L Bicarbonate output: >10 mEq/L/30 sec	Decreased volume with pancreatic disease as secretin stimulates pancreatic secretion
Stool fat	2-5 g/24 hr	Measures fatty acids; decreased pancreatic lipase increases stool fat

SUMMARY REVIEW

The Gastrointestinal Tract

1. The major functions of the gastrointestinal tract are the mechanical and chemical breakdown of food and the absorption of digested nutrients.
2. The gastrointestinal tract is a hollow tube that extends from the mouth to the anus.
3. The walls of the gastrointestinal tract have several layers: mucosa, muscularis mucosae, submucosa, tunica muscularis (circular muscle and longitudinal muscle), and serosa.
4. The peritoneum is a double layer of membranous tissue. The visceral layer covers the abdominal organs, and the parietal layer extends along the abdominal wall.
5. Except for swallowing and defecation, which are controlled voluntarily, the functions of the gastrointestinal tract are controlled by extrinsic and intrinsic autonomic nerves and intestinal hormones.
6. Digestion begins in the mouth, with chewing and salivation. The digestive component of saliva is α-amylase, which initiates carbohydrate digestion.
7. The esophagus is a muscular tube that transports food from the mouth to the stomach. The tunica muscularis in the upper part of the esophagus is striated muscle, and that in the lower part is smooth muscle.
8. Swallowing is controlled by the swallowing center in the reticular formation of the brain. The two phases of swallowing are the oropharyngeal phase (voluntary swallowing) and the esophageal phase (involuntary swallowing).
9. Food is propelled through the gastrointestinal tract by peristalsis: waves of sequential relaxations and contractions of the tunica muscularis.
10. The lower esophageal sphincter opens to admit swallowed food into the stomach and then closes to prevent regurgitation of food back into the esophagus.
11. The stomach is a baglike structure that secretes digestive juices, mixes and stores food, and propels partially digested food (chyme) into the duodenum.
12. The vagus nerve stimulates gastric (stomach) secretion and motility.
13. The hormones *gastrin* and *motilin* stimulate gastric emptying; the hormones *secretin* and *cholecystokinin* delay gastric emptying.
14. Mucus is secreted throughout the stomach and protects the stomach wall from acid and digestive enzymes.
15. Gastric glands in the fundus and body of the stomach secrete intrinsic factor, which is needed for vitamin B_{12} absorption, and hydrochloric acid, which dissolves food fibers, kills microorganisms, and activates the enzyme *pepsin*.
16. Chief cells in the stomach secrete pepsinogen, which is converted to pepsin in the acid environment created by hydrochloric acid.
17. Acid secretion is stimulated by the vagus nerve, gastrin, and histamine and inhibited by sympathetic stimulation and cholecystokinin.
18. The three phases of acid secretion by the stomach are the cephalic phase (anticipation and swallowing), the gastric phase (food in the stomach), and the intestinal phase (chyme in the intestine).
19. The small intestine is 5 m long and has three segments: the duodenum, jejunum, and ileum.

20. The duodenum receives chyme from the stomach through the pyloric valve. The presence of chyme stimulates the liver and gallbladder to deliver bile and the pancreas to deliver digestive enzymes. Bile and enzymes flow through an opening guarded by the sphincter of Oddi.
21. Bile is produced by the liver and is necessary for fat digestion and absorption. Bile's alkalinity helps to neutralize chyme, thereby creating a pH that enables the pancreatic enzymes to digest proteins, carbohydrates, and sugars.
22. Enzymes secreted by the small intestine (maltase, sucrose, lactase), pancreatic enzymes, and bile salts act in the small intestine to digest proteins, carbohydrates, and fats.
23. Digested substances are absorbed across the intestinal wall and then transported to the liver, where they are metabolized further.
24. The ileocecal valve connects the small and large intestines and prevents reflux into the small intestine.
25. Villi are small fingerlike projections that extend from the small intestinal mucosa and increase its absorptive surface area.
26. Sugars, amino acids, and fats are absorbed primarily by the duodenum and jejunum; bile salts and vitamin B_{12} are absorbed by the ileum. Vitamin B_{12} absorption requires the presence of intrinsic factor.
27. Bile salts emulsify and hydrolyze fats and incorporate them into water-soluble micelles, which transport them through the unstirred layer to the brush border of the intestinal mucosa. The fat content of the micelles readily diffuses through the epithelium into lacteals (lymphatic ducts) in the villi. From there fats flow into lymphatics and into the systemic circulation, which delivers them to the liver.
28. Minerals and water-soluble vitamins are absorbed by both active and passive transport throughout the small intestine.
29. Peristaltic movements created by longitudinal muscles propel the chyme along the intestinal tract, while contractions of the circular muscles (haustral segmentation) mix the chyme.
30. The ileogastric reflex inhibits gastric motility when the ileum is distended.
31. The intestinointestinal reflex inhibits intestinal motility when one intestinal segment is overdistended.
32. The gastroileal reflex increases intestinal motility when gastric motility increases.
33. The large intestine consists of the cecum, appendix, colon (ascending, transverse, descending, and sigmoid), rectum, and anal canal.
34. The teniae coli are three bands of longitudinal muscle that extend the length of the colon.
35. Haustra are pouches of colon that are formed with alternating contraction and relaxation of the circular muscles.
36. The mucosa of the large intestine contains mucus-secreting cells and mucosal folds, but no villi.
37. The large intestine massages the fecal mass and absorbs water and electrolytes.
38. Distention of the ileum with chyme causes the gastrocolic reflex, or the mass propulsion of feces to the rectum.
39. Defecation is stimulated when the rectum is distended with feces. The conically contracted internal anal sphincter relaxes, and if the voluntarily regulated external sphincter relaxes, defecation occurs.
40. The largest number of intestinal bacteria are in the colon. They are anaerobes consisting of *Bacteroides*, clostridia, coliforms, and lactobacilli.
41. The intestinal tract is sterile at birth and becomes totally colonized within 3 to 4 weeks.
42. Endogenous infections of the gastrointestinal tract occur by excessive proliferation of bacteria, perforation of the intestine, or contamination from neighboring structures.

Accessory Organs of Digestion

1. The liver is the largest organ in the body. It has digestive, metabolic, hematologic, vascular, and immunologic functions.
2. The liver is divided into the right and left lobes and is supported by the falciform, round, and coronary ligaments.
3. Liver lobules consist of plates of hepatocytes, which are the functional cells of the liver.
4. The hepatocytes synthesize 700 to 1200 ml of bile per day and secrete it into the bile canaliculi, which are small channels between the hepatocytes. The bile canaliculi drain bile into the common bile duct and then into the duodenum through an opening called the *major duodenal papilla (sphincter of Oddi).*
5. Sinusoids are capillaries located between the plates of hepatocytes. Blood from the portal vein and hepatic artery flows through the sinusoids to a central vein in each lobule and then to the hepatic vein and inferior vena cava.
6. Kupffer cells, which are part of the mononuclear phagocyte system, line the sinusoids and destroy microorganisms in sinusoidal blood.
7. The primary bile acids are synthesized from cholesterol by the hepatocytes. The primary acids are then conjugated to form bile salts. The secondary bile acids are the product of bile salt deconjugation by bacteria in the intestinal lumen.
8. Most bile salts and acids are recycled. The absorption of bile salts and acids from the terminal ileum and their return to the liver are known as the *enterohepatic circulation of bile.*
9. Bilirubin is a pigment liberated by the lysis of aged red blood cells in the liver and spleen. Unconjugated bilirubin is fat soluble and can cross cell membranes. Unconjugated bilirubin is converted to water-soluble, conjugated bilirubin by hepatocytes and is secreted with bile.
10. The gallbladder is a saclike organ located in the inferior surface of the liver. The gallbladder stores bile between meals and ejects it when chyme enters the duodenum.
11. Stimulated by cholecystokinin, the gallbladder contracts and forces bile through the cystic duct and into the common bile duct. The sphincter of Oddi relaxes, enabling bile to flow through the major duodenal papilla into the duodenum.
12. The pancreas is a gland located behind the stomach. The endocrine pancreas produces hormones (glucagon and insulin) that facilitate the formation and cellular uptake of glucose. The exocrine pancreas secretes an alkaline solution and the enzymes (trypsin, chymotrypsin, carboxypeptidase, α-amylase, lipase) that digest proteins, carbohydrates, and fats.
13. Secretin stimulates pancreatic secretion of alkaline fluid, and cholecystokinin and acetylcholine stimulate secretion of enzymes. Pancreatic secretions originate in acini and ducts of the pancreas and empty into the duodenum through the common bile duct or an accessory duct that opens directly into the duodenum.

Tests of Digestive Function

1. Numerous diagnostic tests are performed to evaluate structure and function (digestion, secretion, absorption) of the gastrointestinal tract. Roentgenograms and scans are most commonly used to evaluate structure, in addition to direct

observation by endoscopy. Gastric and stool analysis and blood studies provide important information about digestion, absorption, and secretion.
2. Plasma chemistry levels and imaging procedures are commonly used to diagnose alterations in liver function. Of particular importance are the enzymes lactate dehydrogenase (LDH), aspartate aminotransferase (AST), and alanine aminotransferase (ALT). Plasma bilirubin levels reflect alterations in bilirubin and bile metabolism, and prothrombin times are prolonged in hepatitis and chronic liver disease.
3. Obstructive diseases of the gallbladder are evident by elevated serum bilirubin, elevated urine urobilinogen, and increased stool fat. The serum leukocytes become elevated with inflammation of the gallbladder.
4. The most significant indicators of pancreatic dysfunction are serum amylase and stool fat. Both values are increased with diseases of the pancreas.

Aging and the Gastrointestinal System

1. Advancing age is often associated with the loss or wearing down of teeth, diminished senses of taste and smell, and diminished salivary secretions, all of which may make eating difficult and reduce appetite.
2. Aging reduces gastric motility and secretions, particularly of hydrochloric acid. These changes slow gastric digestion and emptying.
3. Intestinal motility and absorption of carbohydrates, proteins, fats, and minerals decrease with age.

KEY TERMS

Ampulla of Vater, *1252*
Antrum of stomach, *1234*
Ascending colon, *1246*
Bile, *1249*
Bile acid pool, *1249*
Bile acid–dependent fraction, *1249*
Bile acid–independent fraction, *1249*
Bile canaliculi, *1247*
Bile salts, *1249*
Bilirubin, *1250*
Body of stomach, *1234*
Brush border, *1240*
Carboxypeptidase, *1242*
Cardiac orifice, *1234*
Cecum, *1246*
Cephalic phase of secretion, *1237*
Chief cell, *1236*
Cholecystokinin, *1234*
Choleresis, *1249*
Choleretic agent, *1249*
Chylomicron, *1244*
Chyme, *1234*
Chymotrypsin, *1240*
Colon, *1246*
Common bile duct, *1247*
Conjugated bilirubin, *1250*
Critical micelle concentration, *1249*
Cystic duct, *1252*
Deamination, *1251*
Defecation reflex (rectal reflex), *1247*
Descending colon, *1246*
Disse space, *1249*
Duodenum, *1238*
Emulsification, *1243*
Enteric plexus, *1231*
Enterohepatic circulation, *1249*
Enterokinase, *1253*
Esophageal phase of swallowing, *1234*
Esophagus, *1232*
Exocrine pancreas, *1252*
External anal sphincter, *1246*
Fecal mass, *1246*
Feces, *1247*
Fundus of stomach, *1234*
G cell, *1238*
Gallbladder, *1252*
Gastric emptying, *1236*
Gastric gland, *1236*
Gastric phase of secretion, *1237*
Gastric pit, *1236*
Gastrin, *1234*
Gastrocolic reflex, *1246*
Gastroileal reflex, *1245*
Gastrointestinal tract (alimentary canal), *1231*
Glisson capsule, *1247*
Haustral segmentation, *1245*
Haustrum (pl., haustra), *1246*
Hepatocyte, *1249*
Hydrolase, *1243*
Ileocecal valve (sphincter), *1238*
Ileogastric reflex, *1245*
Ileum, *1238*
Internal anal sphincter, *1246*
Intestinal phase of secretion, *1238*
Intestinointestinal reflex, *1245*
Iron, *1244*
Jejunum, *1238*
Kupffer cell, *1249*
Lacteal, *1240*
Lamina propria, *1240*
Large intestine, *1246*
Lieberkühn crypts, *1246*
Lipase, *1243*
Lipolysis, *1243*
Liver, *1247*
Liver lobule, *1249*
Lower esophageal sphincter (cardiac sphincter), *1234*
Magnesium, *1244*
Major duodenal papilla, *1249*
Mesentery, *1238*
Metabolic detoxification (biotransformation), *1252*
Micelle, *1243*
Microvillus, *1240*
Motilin, *1235*
Mouth, *1232*
Mucosal barrier, *1237*
Myenteric plexus (Auerbach plexus), *1232*
O'Beirne sphincter, *1246*
Oropharyngeal phase of swallowing, *1234*
Pancreas, *1252*
Pancreatic α-amylase, *1253*
Pancreatic duct (Wirsung duct), *1252*
Pancreatic lipase, *1253*
Parietal cell (oxyntic cell), *1236*
Pepsin, *1236*
Pepsinogen, *1236*
Peristalsis, *1234*
Peristaltic movement, *1245*
Peritoneal cavity, *1238*
Peritoneum, *1238*
Phospholipase, *1243*
Pit cell, *1249*
Primary bile acid, *1249*
Primary peristalsis, *1234*
Pyloric sphincter, *1234*
Pylorus, *1234*
Retropulsion, *1235*
S cell, *1254*
Saliva, *1232*
Salivary α-amylase (ptyalin), *1232*
Salivary gland, *1232*
Secondary bile acid, *1249*
Secondary peristalsis, *1234*
Secretin, *1235*
Sigmoid colon, *1246*
Sinusoid, *1247*
Small intestine, *1238*
Sphincter of Oddi, *1250*
Stellate cell, *1249*
Stomach, *1234*
Submucosal plexus (Meissner plexus), *1232*
Subserosal plexus, *1232*

KEY TERMS—cont'd

Swallowing, *1234*
Teniae coli, *1246*
Transverse colon, *1246*
Trypsin, *1242*
Trypsin inhibitor, *1253*
Unconjugated bilirubin, *1250*
Upper esophageal sphincter (cricopharyngeal muscle), *1234*
Urobilinogen, *1250*
Vermiform appendix, *1246*
Villus (pl., villi), *1239*
Vitamin, *1245*

REFERENCES

1. Furness JB: types of neurons in the enteric nervous system, *J Auton Nerv Syst* 81(1):87, 2000.
2. Lang IM, Shaker R: An overview of the upper esophageal sphincter, *Curr Gastroenterol Rep* 2(3):185, 2000.
3. Zald DH, Pardo JV: The functional neuroanatomy of voluntary swallowing, *Ann Neurol* 46(3):281, 1999.
4. Aly YA, Abdel-Aty H: Normal oesophageal transit time on digital radiography, *Clin Radiol* 54(8):545, 1999.
5. Sifrim D, Janssens J: Secondary peristaltic contractions, like primary peristalsis, are preceded by inhibition in the human esophageal body, *Digestion* 57(1):73, 1996.
6. Diamant NE: Neuromuscular mechanisms of primary perstalsis, *Am J Med* 103(5A):40S, 1997.
7. Johnson LR: *Gastrointestinal physiology*, ed 6, St Louis, 2000, Mosby.
8. Pabst MA, Wachter C, Holzer P: Morphologic basis of the functional gastric acid barrier, *Lab Invest* 74(1):78, 1996.
9. Helander HF, Keeling DJ: Cell biology of gastric acid secretion, *Baillieres Clin Gastroenterol* 7(1):1, 1993.
10. Wolf MM, Soll AH: The physiology of gastric acid secretion, *N Engl J Med* 319(26):1707, 1988.
11. Kawano S, Tsuji S: Role of mucosal blood flow: a conceptional review in gastric mucosal injury and protection, *J Gastroenterol Hepatol* 15(suppl): D1, 2000.
12. Nederkoorn C, Smulders FT, Jansen A: Cephalic phase responses, craving, and food intake in normal subjects, *Appetite* 35(1):45, 2000.
13. Thompson AB et al: Small bowel review: part 1, *Can-S-Gastroentrol* 12(7):487, 1998.
14. Kvietys PR, Barrowman JA, Granger ND: *Pathophysiology of the splanchnic circulation*, Boca Raton, Fla, 1987, CRC Press.
15. Ashton KA et al: Basal and meal-stimulated colonic absorption, *Dis Colon Rectum* 39(8):865, 1996.
16. Husebye E: The patterns of small bowel motility: physiology and implications in organic disease and functional disorders, *Neurogastroenterol Motil* 11(3):141, 1999.
17. Rosenblum JD, Boyle CM, Schwartz LB: The mesenteric circulation. Anatomy and physiology, *Surg Clin North Am* 77(2):289, 1997.
18. Mims CA et al: *Medical microbiology*, ed 2, St Louis, 1998, Mosby.
19. Marshall JC: Gastrointestinal flora and its alterations in critical illness, *Curr Opin Clin Nutr Metab Care* 2(5):405, 1999.
20. Zakim D, Bayer TD: *Hepatology: a textbook of liver disease*, ed 3, Philadelphia, 1996, W.B. Saunders.
21. Luxon BA: Anatomy and physiology of the liver and biliary tree. In Bacon BR, DiBisceglie AM, editors: *Liver disease: diagnosis and management,* Philadelphia, 2000, Churchill Livingston.
22. Agellon LB, Torchia EC: Intracellular transport of bile acids, *Biochim Biophys Acta* 1486(1):198, 2000.
23. Toouli J, Craig A: Sphincter of Oddi function and dysfunction, *Can J Gastroenterol* 14(5):411, 2000.
24. Johnson DE: Special considerations in interpreting liver function tests, *Am Fam Physician* 59(8):2223, 1999.
25. Aranda-Michel J, Sherman KE: Tests of the liver: use and misuse, *Gastroenterologist* 6(1):34, 1998.
26. Guslandi M, Pellegrini A, Sorghi M: Gastric mucosal defences in the elderly, *Gerontology* 45(4):206, 1999.
27. Timiras PS: *Physiological basis of aging and geriatrics*, ed 2, Boca Raton, Fla, 1994, CRC Press.
28. Saltzman JR, Russell RM: The aging gut. Nutritional issues, *Gastroenterol Clin North Am* 27(2):309, 1998.
29. Wilson JA: Constipation in the elderly, *Clin Geriatr Med* 15(3):499, 1999.
30. Schmucker DL: Aging and the liver: an update, *J Gerontol A Biol Sci Med Sci* 53(5):B315, 1998.
31. Glaser J, Stienecker K: Pancreas and aging: a study using ultrasonography, *Gerontology* 46(2):93, 2000.

CHAPTER 38

Alterations of Digestive Function

SUE E. HUETHER

CHAPTER OUTLINE

The gastrointestinal tract is a continuous, hollow organ that extends from the mouth to the anus. It includes the esophagus, stomach, small intestine (duodenum, jejunum, ileum), large intestine (ascending, transverse, descending, and sigmoid colon), and rectum.

Disorders of the gastrointestinal tract disrupt one or more of its functions. Structural and neural abnormalities can slow, obstruct, or accelerate the movement of chyme at any level of the gastrointestinal tract. Inflammatory and ulcerative conditions of the gastrointestinal wall disrupt secretion, motility, and absorption. Many clinical manifestations of gastrointestinal tract disorders are nonspecific: that is, they can be caused by a variety of impairments. These manifestations are described in the next section.

DISORDERS OF THE GASTROINTESTINAL TRACT

Clinical Manifestations of Gastrointestinal Dysfunction

Anorexia

Anorexia is lack of a desire to eat despite physiologic stimuli that would normally produce hunger. Anorexia is a nonspecific symptom that is often associated with nausea, abdominal pain, and diarrhea. Disorders of other organ systems, including cancer, heart disease, and renal disease, are often accompanied by anorexia. (See p. 1284 for a discussion of anorexia nervosa.)

Vomiting

Vomiting is the forceful emptying of stomach and intestinal contents (chyme) through the mouth. Several types of stimuli initiate the vomiting reflex, including the presence of ipecac or copper salts in the duodenum; severe pain; distention of the stomach or duodenum; torsion or trauma affecting the ovaries, testes, uterus, bladder, or kidney; and activation of the chemoreceptor trigger zone in the medulla. 5-Hydroxytryptamine (5-HT, i.e., serotonin) stimulates the emetic center and appears to be released from enterochromaffin cells in the intestinal wall and possibly from neurons in the brain stem.[1,2,3]

Nausea and retching usually precede vomiting. **Nausea** is a subjective experience that is associated with many different conditions. Specific neural pathways have not been identified with nausea. Hypersalivation and tachycardia are common associated symptoms. **Retching** begins with deep inspiration. The glottis closes, intrathoracic pressure falls, and the esophagus becomes distended. Simultaneously the abdominal muscles contract, creating a pressure gradient from abdomen to thorax. The lower esophageal sphincter and body of the stomach relax, but the duodenum and antrum of the stomach go into spasm. The reverse peristalsis and pressure gradient force chyme from the stomach and duodenum up into the esophagus. Because the upper esophageal sphincter is closed, chyme does not enter the mouth. As the abdominal muscles relax, the contents of the esophagus drop back into the stomach. This process may be repeated several times before vomiting occurs. A diffuse sympathetic discharge causes the tachycardia, tachypnea, and sweating that accompany retching and vomiting. The parasympathetic system mediates copious salivation, increased gastric motility, and relaxation of the upper and lower esophageal sphincters.

Vomiting usually follows retching. The duodenum and antrum of the stomach produce retrograde peristalsis while the body of the stomach and esophagus relax. When the stomach is full of gastric contents, the diaphragm is forced high into the thoracic cavity by strong contractions of the abdominal muscles. The higher intrathoracic pressure forces the upper esophageal sphincter to open, and chyme is expelled from the mouth. Then the stomach relaxes and the upper part of the esophagus contracts, forcing the remaining chyme back into the stomach. The lower esophageal sphincter then closes. The cycle is repeated if there is a volume of chyme remaining in the stomach.

Spontaneous vomiting that is not preceded by nausea or retching is called **projectile vomiting**. Projectile vomiting is caused by direct stimulation of the vomiting center by neurologic lesions (e.g., tumors, aneurysms) involving the brain stem. The metabolic consequences of vomiting are fluid, electrolyte, and acid-base disturbances (see Chapter 3).

Constipation

Constipation is difficult or infrequent defecation and may affect up to 14% of the population.[4] Because patterns of bowel evacuation differ greatly among individuals, constipation must be individually defined. It usually means a decrease in the number of bowel movements per week, hard stools, and difficult evacuation. Normal bowel habits range from two or three evacuations per day to one per week.

Pathophysiology

Constipation can be caused by neurogenic disorders of the large intestine in which neurotransmitters are altered or neural pathways are absent or degenerated.[5] An example is Hirschsprung disease (congenital megacolon)—the absence of ganglion cells in the myenteric plexus of the large intestine. Constipation is usually evident from birth, because the colon is incapable of the propulsive movements that move feces into the rectum (see Chapter 39). Other disorders associated with constipation include acquired megacolon (enlarged or dilated colon), pelvic hiatal hernia, multiple sclerosis, spinal cord trauma, and cerebrovascular disease (Box 38-1).

Many functional or mechanical conditions can slow intestinal transit time. Muscle weakness or pain caused by abdominal surgery can impair or inhibit defecation. Normally the abdominal muscles are used to create the intraabdominal pressure required to evacuate the rectum. Weakness or pain can interfere with the generation of adequate intraabdominal pressure. Lesions of the anus, such as inflamed hemorrhoids, fissures, or fistulae, make defecation painful because of stretching. With the urge to defecate, the sphincter becomes hypertonic, and the stool is not eliminated.

A low-residue diet (the habitual consumption of highly refined foods) decreases the volume and number of stools and causes constipation. Increased consumption of cereals, fruits, and vegetables adds nonabsorbable fiber to the feces and is conducive to regular and easy evacuations.

A sedentary life-style and lack of regular exercise are frequent causes of constipation. Lack of access to toilet facilities and consistent suppression of the urge to empty the bowel are other causes. Depression often impairs bowel evacuation, partly because depressed individuals tend to be sedentary and lack the motivation to eat a healthy diet. The problem is made worse if antidepressant drugs (e.g., anticholinergics) are used to treat the depression. Anticholinergics block parasympathetic impulses in the gastrointestinal tract, thereby impairing motility.

Box 38-1

CAUSES OF CONSTIPATION

- Megacolon (enlarged or dilated colon)
- Abdominal muscle weakness
- Painful anal lesions
- Low-residue diet
- Sedentary life-style
- Delayed spontaneous defecation
- Emotional depression
- Selected drugs
  - Opiates
  - Anticholinergics
  - Antacids (calcium carbonate, aluminum hydroxide)
- Systemic diseases
  - Hypothyroidism
  - Diabetic neuropathy

Excessive use of antacids containing calcium carbonate or aluminum hydroxide often results in constipation. Opiates, particularly codeine, tend to inhibit bowel motility.

Clinical Manifestations

Changes in bowel evacuation patterns—such as less frequent defecation, smaller stool volume, difficulty in evacuating the rectum, or a feeling of bowel fullness and discomfort—require investigation.

Evaluation and Treatment

The patient's medical history, physical examination, and stool diaries provide precise clues regarding the nature of constipation. Functional constipation (i.e., constipation resulting from life-style or bowel habits) usually has a long history. Dysfunctional constipation is more likely to be sudden. Sudden-onset constipation can accompany the development of organic lesions and requires careful evaluation.

The individual's description of frequency, stool consistency, associated pain, and presence of blood is significant. Blood may be present as a result of bleeding hemorrhoids or a neoplastic lesion of the colon. Cramping abdominal pain may be symptomatic of partial bowel obstruction. In assessing frequency, it is important to discover whether evacuation was stimulated by enemas or cathartics (laxatives). Palpation discloses colonic distention, masses, and tenderness. Stool transit time is evaluated. Digital examination of the rectum is performed to assess sphincter tone and detect anal lesions. Proctosigmoidoscopy is used to visualize the lumen directly. A barium enema may be required if no lesions are directly visualized and symptoms continue after simple treatment.

The treatment for dysfunctional constipation is to manage the underlying lesion or disease. Management of functional constipation likewise depends on its cause. Treatment usually consists of bowel retraining, in which the individual establishes a satisfactory bowel evacuation routine without becoming preoccupied with bowel movements. Moderate exercise, increased fluid and fiber intake, bulk supplements (e.g., Metamucil, Konsyl), stool softeners, and laxative agents are useful for some individuals. Enemas can be used to establish bowel routine, but they should not be used habitually.

Diarrhea

Diarrhea is an increase in the frequency of defecation and the fluidity and volume of feces. Many factors determine stool volume and consistency, including water content of the colon and the presence of unabsorbed food, unabsorbable material, and intestinal secretions. Stool volume in the normal adult averages less than 200 g/day. Stool volume in children depends on age and size. An infant may pass up to 100 g/day. The adult intestine processes approximately 9 L of luminal content per day; 2 L is ingested, and the remaining 7 L consists of intestinal secretions. Of this volume, 99% of the fluid is absorbed—90% (7 to 8 L) in the small intestine and 9% (1 to 2 L) in the colon. Normally, approximately 150 ml of water is excreted daily in the stool.

Pathophysiology

Diarrhea in which the volume of feces is increased is called large-volume diarrhea. Large-volume diarrhea generally is caused by excessive amounts of water or secretions or both in the intestines. Small-volume diarrhea, in which the volume of feces is not increased, usually results from excessive intestinal motility. The three major mechanisms of diarrhea are osmotic, secretory, and motile.[6] (Specific mechanisms of diarrhea in children are described in Chapter 39.)

In **osmotic diarrhea** a nonabsorbable substance in the intestine draws water into the lumen by osmosis. The excess water and the nonabsorbable substance cause large-volume diarrhea. Lactase deficiency is the most common cause of osmotic diarrhea. Loss of pancreatic enzymes can be a contributing factor. In this condition the nonabsorbable substance is milk sugar, or lactose. Lactose remains in the intestinal lumen because it is not digested and absorbed (see p. 1278). Excessive ingestion of synthetic, nonabsorbable sugars (e.g., sorbitol) has a similar effect.

Secretory diarrhea is a form of large-volume diarrhea caused by excessive mucosal secretion of fluid and electrolytes or inhibition of sodium chloride absorption. Primary causes are bacterial enterotoxins (particularly those released by cholera or strains of *Escherichia coli*) and neoplasms (such as gastrinoma or thyroid carcinoma). These tumors produce hormones that stimulate intestinal secretion.

Large-volume diarrhea also can result from excessive motility of the intestine. The cause is usually a lesion that impairs autonomic control of motility, such as diabetic neuropathy. Excessive motility decreases transit time, mucosal surface contact, and opportunities for fluid absorption. Therefore a larger volume of stool reaches the rectum, producing urgency and frequency of elimination.

Small-volume diarrhea usually is caused by an inflammatory disorder of the intestine, such as ulcerative colitis or Crohn disease. Inflammation of the colon causes cramping pain, urgency, and frequency. Small-volume diarrhea also can be caused by fecal impaction, a severe form of constipation. In this case the diarrhea consists of secretions (mucus and fluid) produced by the colon to lubricate the impacted feces and move it toward the anal canal. These secretions flow around the impaction and cause low-volume, secretory diarrhea.

Motility diarrhea is caused by resection of the small intestine, surgical bypass of an area of the intestine, or fistula formation between loops of intestine. Food is not mixed properly, and there is impaired digestion and increased motility.

Clinical Manifestations

Diarrhea can be acute or chronic, depending on its cause. Systemic effects of prolonged diarrhea are dehydration, electrolyte imbalance, metabolic acidosis, and weight loss. Manifestations of acute bacterial or viral infection include fever, with or without cramping pain. Fever, cramping pain, and bloody stools accompany diarrhea caused by inflammatory bowel disease. Steatorrhea (fat in the stools) and diarrhea are common signs of malabsorption syndromes.

Evaluation and Treatment

A thorough history is taken to document the onset and frequency of diarrhea. Exposure to contaminated food or water is indicated if the individual has traveled in foreign countries or areas where drinking water might be contaminated. Iatrogenic diarrhea is suggested if the individual has undergone abdominal radiation therapy, intestinal resection, or treatment with selected drugs (e.g., antibiotics, diuretics, antihypertensives, laxatives).[7] Physical examination helps the clinician to identify underlying systemic disease. Stool culture, examination of stool specimens for blood, abdominal roentgenograms, and intestinal biopsies provide more specific data.

Treatment for diarrhea includes restoration of fluid and electrolyte balance, management of distressing symptoms, and treatment of causal factors. In older adults and children, dehydration and electrolyte imbalance may be severe and require intravenous fluid therapy. Nutritional deficiencies need to be corrected in cases of chronic diarrhea or malabsorption. Substances that solidify stools decrease frequency and water content. Natural bran and commercial preparations of psyllium, such as Konsyl and Metamucil, are inexpensive and effective treatments for mild diarrhea. Opium alkaloids such as Lomotil suppress motility, relieve cramping, and reduce stool volume and frequency.

Abdominal Pain

Abdominal pain is the presenting symptom of a number of gastrointestinal diseases. (The physiology of pain is described in Chapter 14.) The causal mechanisms of abdominal pain are mechanical, inflammatory, or ischemic. Generally the abdominal organs are not sensitive to mechanical stimuli, such as cutting, tearing, or crushing. These organs are, however, sensitive to stretching and distention, which activate nerve endings in both hollow and solid structures. The onset of pain is associated with rapid distention; gradual distention causes little pain. Traction on the peritoneum caused by adhesions, distention of the common bile duct, or forceful peristalsis resulting from intestinal obstruction causes pain because of increased tension. Capsules that surround solid organs, such as the liver and gallbladder, contain pain fibers that are stimulated by stretching if these organs swell.

Biochemical mediators of the inflammatory response, such as histamine, bradykinin, and serotonin, stimulate organic nerve endings and produce abdominal pain. The edema and vascular congestion that accompany chemical, bacterial, or viral inflammation also cause painful stretching. Obstruction of blood flow from the distention of bowel obstruction or mesenteric vessel thrombosis produces the pain of ischemia, and increased concentrations of tissue metabolites stimulate pain receptors.

Abdominal pain can be parietal (somatic), visceral, or referred. **Parietal pain** arises from the parietal peritoneum. This pain is more localized and intense than visceral pain, which arises from the organs themselves. Nerve fibers from the parietal peritoneum travel with peripheral nerves to the spinal cord, and the sensation of pain corresponds to skin dermatomes T6 and L1. Parietal pain lateralizes because, at any particular point, the parietal peritoneum is innervated from only one side of the nervous system.

Visceral pain arises from a stimulus acting on an abdominal organ. It is usually felt near the midline in the epigastrium (upper midabdomen), midabdomen, or lower abdomen. The pain is poorly localized and is dull rather than sharp. Its location is generally related to the corresponding skin dermatomes of the affected organ. Visceral pain is diffuse and vague because nerve endings in abdominal organs are sparse and multisegmented. Pain arising from the stomach, for example, is experienced as a sensation of fullness, cramping, or gnawing in the midepigastric area.

Referred pain is visceral pain felt at some distance from a diseased or an affected organ. Referred pain is usually well localized and is felt in skin or deeper tissues that share a central afferent pathway with the affected organ. Generally, referred pain develops as the intensity of a visceral pain stimulus increases. Intense gallbladder pain is, for example, referred to the back between the scapulae (shoulder blades). The pain may begin as a vague discomfort in the right epigastric region and then, as inflammation worsens, progress to a sharp, localized, referred pain between the shoulder blades.

Gastrointestinal Bleeding

Numerous disorders cause bleeding in the gastrointestinal tract. Upper **gastrointestinal bleeding**, which is defined as bleeding in the esophagus, stomach, or duodenum, is commonly caused by bleeding ulcers. Other causes include esophageal or gastric varices, a Mallory-Weiss tear at the esophageal gastric junction from severe retching, or cancer. Lower gastrointestinal bleeding—or bleeding from the jejunum, ileum, colon, or rectum—can be caused by polyps, inflammatory disease, cancer, or hemorrhoids. Acute, severe gastrointestinal bleeding is life threatening. Mortality depends on the volume and rate of blood loss, associated disease, age, and effectiveness of treatment.[8,9]

The signs of gastrointestinal bleeding are defined in Table 38-1. Acute blood loss is usually characterized by **hematemesis** (the presence of blood in the vomitus),

Table 38-1 Presentations of Gastrointestinal Bleeding

Presentation	Definition
Acute bleeding	
Hematemesis	Bloody vomitus; either fresh, bright red blood or dark, grainy, digested blood with "coffee grounds" appearance
Melena	Black, sticky, tarry, foul-smelling stools caused by digestion of blood in the gastrointestinal tract
Hematochezia	Fresh, bright red blood passed from the rectum
Occult bleeding	Trace amounts of blood in normal-appearing stools or gastric secretions; detectable only with a guaiac test

hematochezia (bright red or burgundy blood from the rectum), or **melena** (dark, tarry stools). **Occult bleeding** is usually caused by slow, chronic blood loss that results in iron deficiency anemia as iron stores in the bone marrow are slowly depleted. Physiologic response to gastrointestinal bleeding depends on the amount and rate of the loss (Fig. 38-1). Changes in blood pressure and heart rate are the best indicators of massive blood loss in the gastrointestinal tract. Blood losses of 1000 ml or more over a short time cause a decrease in cardiac output, a decrease in systolic and diastolic blood pressure, and an increase in pulse rate. With losses of 1000 ml or more, the heart rate is greater than 100 beats/min and systolic blood pressure is less than 100 mm Hg. During the early stages of blood volume depletion, the peripheral vascular

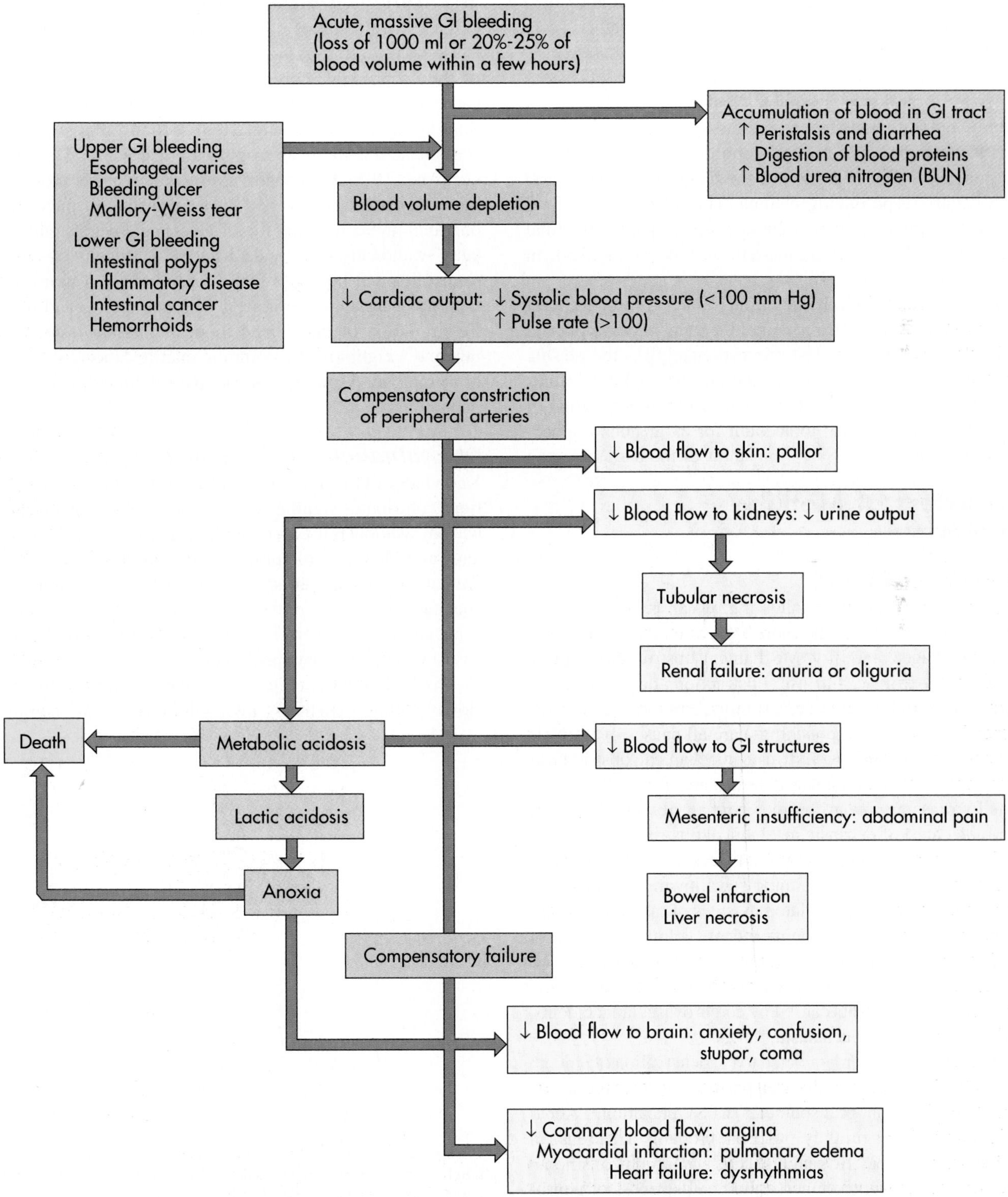

FIG. 38-1 Pathophysiology of gastrointestinal (GI) bleeding.

compartment constricts to shunt blood to vital organs, including the brain (see Chapter 28). Signs that this is happening are postural hypotension (a drop in blood pressure that occurs with a change from the recumbent position to a sitting or upright position), light-headedness, and loss of vision. If blood loss continues, hypovolemic shock progresses. Diminished blood flow to the kidneys causes decreased urine output and may lead to oliguria (low urine output), tubular necrosis, and renal failure. Ultimately, insufficient cerebral and coronary blood flow causes irreversible anoxia and death.

The accumulation of blood in the gastrointestinal tract is irritating and increases peristalsis, causing diarrhea. If bleeding is from the lower gastrointestinal tract, the diarrhea is frankly bloody. Bleeding from the upper gastrointestinal tract also can be rapid enough to produce bright red stools, but generally some digestion of the blood components will have occurred, producing melena. The digestion of blood proteins originating from massive upper gastrointestinal bleeding is reflected by an increase in blood urea nitrogen (BUN) levels (see Fig. 38-1).

The hematocrit and hemoglobin values are not the best indicators of acute gastrointestinal bleeding because plasma and red cell volume are lost proportionately. As the plasma volume is replaced, the hematocrit and hemoglobin values begin to reflect the extent of blood loss. The interpretation of these values is modified to account for exogenous replacement of fluids and the hydration status of the tissues.

Disorders of Motility

Dysphagia

Pathophysiology

Dysphagia is difficulty swallowing. It can result from mechanical obstruction of the esophagus or a disorder that impairs esophageal motility. Mechanical obstructions can be intrinsic or extrinsic. Intrinsic obstructions originate in the wall of the esophageal lumen. Tumors, strictures, and diverticular herniations (outpouchings) are all causes of intrinsic mechanical obstruction. Extrinsic mechanical obstructions originate outside the esophageal lumen and narrow the esophagus by pressing inward on the esophageal wall. The most common cause of extrinsic mechanical obstruction is tumor.

Functional dysphagia is caused by neural or muscular disorders that interfere with voluntary swallowing or peristalsis. Disorders that affect the striated muscles of the upper esophagus interfere with the oropharyngeal (voluntary) phase of swallowing. Typical causes of functional dysphagia in the upper esophagus are dermatomyositis (a muscle disease) and neurologic impairments caused by cerebrovascular accidents, Parkinson disease, or achalasia.[10]

Achalasia is a disorder related to (1) denervation of smooth muscle in the middle and lower portions of the esophagus, and (2) lower esophageal sphincter (LES) relaxation.[11] Achalasia results from neural dysfunction, probably a decrease in the number of myenteric ganglion cells and atrophy of smooth muscle cells. Disrupted innervation results in loss of neuromuscular coordination and muscle tone at the lower end of the esophagus. The three mechanisms that impair swallowing are decreased peristalsis of the middle esophagus, loss of tone in the LES, and decreased relaxation of the LES after swallowing. Food accumulates above the obstruction and distends the esophagus (Fig. 38-2). As hydrostatic pressure increases, food is slowly forced past the obstruction into the stomach.

Clinical Manifestations

Clinical manifestations of dysphagia vary according to the cause and location of the obstruction. Distention and spasm of the esophageal muscles during eating or drinking may cause a mild or severe stabbing pain at the level of obstruction. Discomfort occurring 2 to 4 seconds after swallowing is associated with upper esophageal obstruction. Discomfort occurring 10 to 15 seconds after swallowing is more common in obstructions of the lower esophagus. If the cause of obstruction is a growing tumor, dysphagia begins with difficulty swallowing solids and advances to difficulty swallowing semisolids and liquids.[12] If the cause is loss of motor function, dysphagia is experienced with both solids and liquids. Regurgitation of undigested food, unpleasant taste, vomiting, and weight loss are common manifestations of all types of dysphagia. Aspiration of esophageal contents can lead to pneumonia.

Evaluation and Treatment

Knowledge of the individual's history and clinical manifestations contributes significantly to a diagnosis of dysphagia. A barium swallow is used to visualize the contours of the esophagus and identify structural defects. Manometry documents the duration and amplitude of abnormal pressure changes associated with obstruction or loss of neural regulation. Esophageal endoscopy is performed to examine the esophageal mucosa and obtain biopsy specimens.

The individual is taught to manage symptoms by eating slowly, eating small meals, taking fluid with meals, and sleep-

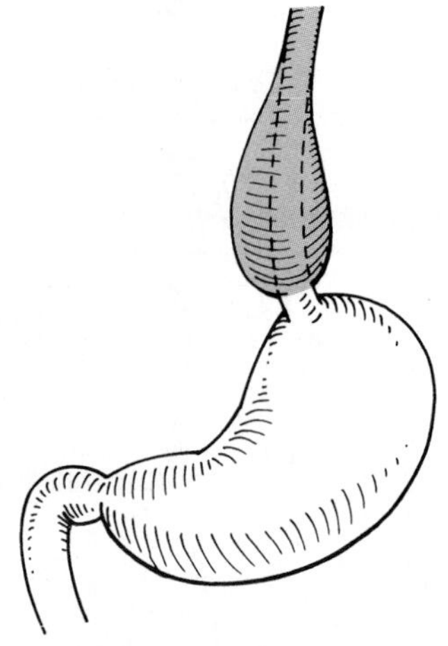

FIG. 38-2 Achalasia. Decreased muscle tone and peristaltic function prevent food from entering the stomach, causing esophageal distention. (From Phipps WP et al: *Medical-surgical nursing: concepts and clinical practice*, ed 4, St Louis, 1991, Mosby.)

ing with the head elevated to prevent regurgitation and aspiration. Anticholinergic drugs, such as dicyclomine (Bentyl), or botulinum toxin (inhibits acetylcholine) may alleviate achalasia.[13] Definitive treatments include mechanical dilation of the esophageal sphincter and surgical separation of the lower esophageal muscles with a longitudinal incision (myotomy). Myotomy widens the passage into the stomach.

Gastroesophageal Reflux Disease (GERD)

Gastroesophageal reflux is the reflux of chyme from the stomach to the esophagus. The LES may relax spontaneously and transiently 1 to 2 hours after eating, permitting gastric contents to regurgitate into the esophagus. The acid is usually neutralized and cleared from the esophagus by peristaltic action within 1 to 3 minutes, and sphincter tone is restored. Gastroesophageal reflux that does not cause symptoms is known as *physiologic reflux*. In some individuals, however, a combination of factors causes an inflammatory response to reflux called **reflux esophagitis**.

Pathophysiology

Normally the resting tone of the LES maintains a zone of high pressure that prevents gastroesophageal reflux. In individuals who develop reflux esophagitis, this pressure tends to be lower than normal. Vomiting, coughing, lifting, or bending that increases abdominal pressure can contribute to the development of reflux esophagitis. The severity of the esophagitis depends on the composition of the gastric contents, the length of time they are in contact with the esophageal mucosa, and epithelial resistance to acid.[14] If the chyme is highly acidic or contains bile salts and pancreatic enzymes, reflux esophagitis can be severe. In individuals with weak esophageal peristalsis, refluxed chyme remains in the esophagus longer than usual. This increases the amount of time the esophageal mucosa is exposed to acids, bile, and enzymes. The presence of hiatal hernia contributes to reflux. Finally, delayed gastric emptying contributes to reflux esophagitis by (1) lengthening the period during which reflux is possible, and (2) increasing the acid content of chyme. Disorders that delay emptying include gastric or duodenal ulcers, which can cause pyloric edema; strictures that narrow the pylorus; and hiatal hernia, which can weaken the LES.[15]

Reflux esophagitis causes inflammatory responses in the esophageal wall, such as hyperemia, increased capillary permeability, edema, tissue fragility, erosion, and ulcerations (Fig. 38-3). Fibrosis, basal cell hyperplasia, and elongation of papillae are common.[16] Precancerous lesions (Barrett esophagus) can be a long-term consequence.[17]

Clinical Manifestations

The clinical manifestations of reflux esophagitis are heartburn, regurgitation of acidic chyme, and upper abdominal pain within 1 hour of eating. The symptoms worsen if the individual lies down or if intraabdominal pressure increases (e.g., as a result of coughing, vomiting, or straining at stool). Symptoms may be present when no acid is in the esophagus.[16] Edema, fibrosis (strictures), esophageal spasm, or decreased esophageal motility may result in dysphagia. Alcohol or acid-containing foods, such as citrus fruits, can cause discomfort during swallowing. There also is an association between acid reflux, asthma, and chronic cough.[18]

Evaluation and Treatment

Diagnosis of reflux esophagitis is based on clinical manifestations. Esophageal endoscopy shows edema and erosion, and allows for evaluation of dysplastic changes (Barrett esophagus) and the development of esophageal carcinoma. A barium swallow is used to identify associated conditions, such as hiatal hernia, gastric ulcers, and abnormal contours of the esophageal lumen. Ambulatory pH monitoring evaluates acidity near the LES.

Antacids relieve symptoms by neutralizing gastric contents. Elevation of the head of the bed 6 inches prevents reflux. Weight reduction and cessation of smoking also help to alleviate symptoms. Proton pump inhibitors are more effective than H_2 receptor antagonists or prokinetics for severe disease.[19] Laparoscopic fundoplication is the most common surgical treatment.[20]

Hiatal Hernia

Pathophysiology

Hiatal hernia, a type of diaphragmatic hernia, is the protrusion (herniation) of the upper part of the stomach through the diaphragm and into the thorax. The two types of hiatal hernia are (1) sliding (direct) hiatal hernia, and (2) paraesophageal (rolling) hiatal hernia (Fig. 38-4). In **sliding hiatal hernia** (the most common type, 90%) the stomach slides or moves into the thoracic cavity through the esophageal hiatus, an opening in the diaphragm for the esophagus and vagus nerves. A congenitally short esophagus, trauma, or weakening of the

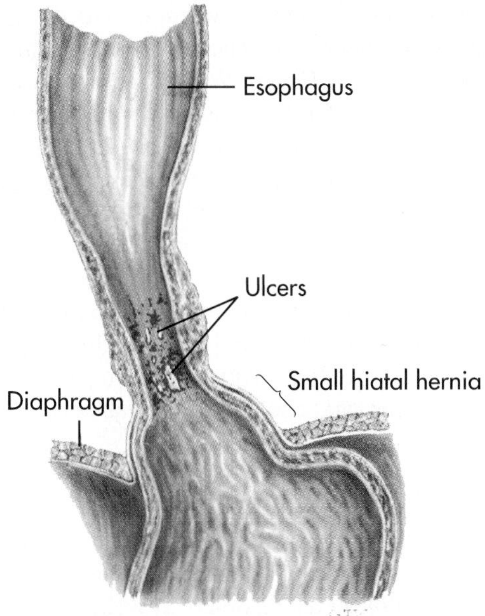

FIG. 38-3 Esophagitis with esophageal ulcerations. (From Doughty DB, Jackson DB: *Gastrointestinal disorders*, St Louis, 1993, Mosby.)

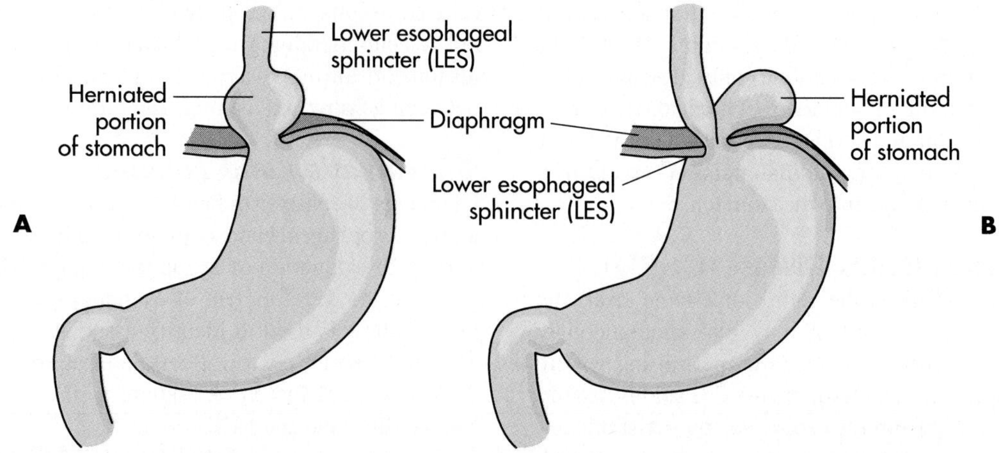

FIG. 38-4 Types of hiatal hernia. A, In sliding hiatal hernia the visceral peritoneum remains intact and restrains the size of the hernia. **B,** In paraesophageal hernia the membrane becomes thinned out or defective, allowing a true peritoneal sac to protrude into the posterior mediastinum, where negative intrathoracic pressure causes it to enlarge. (From Phipps WP et al: *Medical-surgical nursing: concepts and clinical practice*, ed 6, St Louis, 1999, Mosby.)

diaphragmatic muscles at the gastroesophageal junction contributes to the hernia. While the individual is in the supine position, the lower esophagus and stomach are pulled into the thorax. Standing causes the stomach to "slide" back into the abdomen. Sliding hiatal hernia is exacerbated by factors that increase intraabdominal pressure. Therefore coughing, bending, tight clothing, ascites, obesity, or pregnancy accentuates the hernia. This type of hernia is associated with gastroesophageal reflux and esophagitis because the hernia diminishes the resting pressure of the LES. In pregnant women with sliding hiatal hernia, progesterone and estrogen may lower the resting pressure of the LES further.

Paraesophageal hiatal hernia (rolling hiatal hernia) is herniation of the greater curvature of the stomach through a secondary opening in the diaphragm (see Fig. 38-4). As the stomach protrudes through the opening into the thorax, it lies alongside the esophagus. The gastroesophageal junction remains below the diaphragm. With paraesophageal hernia, reflux is uncommon. The position of a portion of the stomach above the diaphragm, however, causes congestion of mucosal blood flow and can lead to gastritis and ulcer formation. A mechanical strangulation of the hernia is a major complication, and surgical correction is required. Strangulation occludes blood vessels and causes vascular engorgement, edema, ischemia, and hemorrhage. Hiatal hernias of both types tend to occur in conjunction with several other diseases, including reflux, peptic ulcer, cholecystitis (gallbladder inflammation), cholelithiasis (gallstones), chronic pancreatitis, and diverticulosis.

◆ *Clinical Manifestations*

Hiatal hernias are often asymptomatic. Generally a wide variety of symptoms develop later in life and are associated with other gastrointestinal disorders as well. Manifestations of the various types of hiatal hernia are difficult to distinguish and include gastroesophageal reflux, dysphagia, heartburn, and epigastric pain.[21] Regurgitation and substernal discomfort after eating are common.

◆ *Evaluation and Treatment*

Diagnostic procedures include barium roentgenogram and endoscopy. A chest roentgenogram often will show the protrusion of the stomach into the thorax, indicating paraesophageal hiatal hernia.

Treatment for sliding hiatal hernia is usually conservative. The individual can diminish reflux by eating small, frequent meals and avoiding the recumbent position after eating. Abdominal supports and tight clothing are avoided, and weight control is recommended for obese individuals. Antacids alleviate reflux esophagitis. Anticholinergic drugs are contraindicated because they relax the LES and delay gastric emptying. Individuals who are uncomfortable at night benefit from sleeping in a semi-Fowler position. Surgery (fundoplication) may be performed if medical management fails to control symptoms.[22]

Pyloric Obstruction

◆ *Pathophysiology*

Pyloric obstruction is the narrowing or blocking of the opening between the stomach and the duodenum. This condition can be congenital (see Chapter 39) or acquired. Acquired obstruction is caused by peptic ulcer disease or carcinoma near the pylorus. Duodenal ulcers are more likely than gastric ulcers to obstruct the pylorus. Ulceration causes obstruction resulting from inflammation, edema, spasm, fibrosis, or scarring. Tumors cause obstruction by growing into the pylorus.

◆ *Clinical Manifestations*

Early in the course of pyloric obstruction, the individual experiences vague epigastric fullness, which becomes more distressing after eating and later in the day. Nausea and epigastric pain may occur as the muscles of the stomach contract in attempts to force chyme past the obstruction. These symptoms disappear when the chyme finally moves into the duodenum. As obstruction progresses, anorexia develops, sometimes accompanied by weight loss. Severe obstruction causes

Table 38-2 Common Causes of Intestinal Obstruction

Cause	Pathophysiology
Herniation	Protrusion of the intestine through a weakness in the abdominal muscles or through the inguinal ring
Intussusception	Telescoping of one part of the intestine into another; this usually causes strangulation of the blood supply; more common in the ileocecal area in infants 10-15 months of age than in adults
Torsion (volvulus)	Twisting of the intestine on its mesenteric pedicle, with occlusion of the blood supply; often associated with fibrous adhesions in the small intestine; occurs most frequently in the large intestine in the elderly
Diverticulosis	Inflamed saccular herniations (diverticuli) of the mucosa and submucosa through the tunica muscularis of the colon; diverticuli are interspersed between thick, circular, fibrous bands; most common in obese individuals older than 60 years
Tumor	Tumor growth into the intestinal lumen; adenocarcinoma of the colon and rectum is the most common tumoral obstruction; most common in individuals older than 60 years
Paralytic (adynamic) ileus	Loss of peristaltic motor activity in the intestine; associated with abdominal surgery, pertonitis, hypokalemia, ischemic bowel, spinal trauma, or pneumonia; affects both small and large intestine
Fibrous adhesions	Peritoneal irritation from surgery or trauma leads to formation of fibrin and adhesions that attach to intestine, omentum, or peritoneum and can cause obstruction; most common in small intestine

gastric distention and atony (lack of muscle tone and gastric motility). Gastric distention stimulates gastric secretion, which increases the feeling of fullness. Rolling or jarring of the abdomen produces a sloshing sound called the *succussion splash*. At this stage, vomiting is a cardinal sign of obstruction. It is usually copious and occurs several hours after eating. The vomitus contains undigested food but no bile. Prolonged vomiting leads to dehydration, which is accompanied by a hypokalemic and hypochloremic metabolic alkalosis caused by loss of potassium and gastric acid. Because food does not enter the intestine, stools are infrequent and small. Prolonged pyloric obstruction causes malnutrition, dehydration, and extreme debilitation.

Evaluation and Treatment

Diagnosis is based on clinical manifestations, a history of ulcer disease, and examination of residual gastric contents. Endoscopy is performed if gastric carcinoma is the suggested cause of pyloric obstruction. Barium studies are contraindicated because the barium may harden and be retained in the stomach.

Obstructions resulting from ulceration often resolve with conservative management. Gastric drainage is used to decompress the stomach and restore normal motility. Gastric secretions that contribute to inflammation and edema can be suppressed with omeprazole or cimetidine. Fluids and electrolytes (saline and potassium) are given intravenously to effect rehydration and correct hypokalemia and alkalosis (see Chapter 3). Severely malnourished individuals may require parenteral hyperalimentation (intravenous nutrition). Surgery may be required to treat gastric carcinoma or persistent obstruction caused by fibrosis and scarring.[23]

Intestinal Obstruction

Intestinal obstruction can be caused by any condition that prevents the normal flow of chyme through the intestinal lumen (Tables 38-2 and 38-3). Criteria for classifying intestinal obstruction are summarized in Table 38-4. Intestinal obstruction is classified by cause as simple or functional. Simple obstruction is mechanical blockage of the lumen by a lesion; functional obstruction is a failure of motility (paralytic ileus). Simple obstruction of the small intestine from fibrous adhesions is the most common type of intestinal obstruction. Acute obstructions usually have mechanical causes, such as adhesions or hernias. Chronic or partial obstructions are more often associated with tumors or inflammatory disorders, particularly of the large intestine. Common causes of intestinal obstruction in children are presented in Chapter 39.

Table 38-3 Large and Small Bowel Obstruction

Cause	Pathophysiology
Small bowel obstruction	Adhesions: secondary to previous abdominal surgeries—50%-70% Hernia: inguinal, ventral, or femoral—20%-25% Tumors: may be associated with intussception—10%
Large bowel obstruction	Colon/rectal cancer—90% Volvulus—4%-5% Diverticular disease—3% Other causes (inflammatory bowel disease, adhesions, hernia)

From Feldman M et al: *Sleisenger & Fordtran's gastrointestinal liver disease*, Philadelphia, 1998, W.B. Saunders; Moses BV: Surgical corrections of the small intestine. In Ratnaike RN, editor: *Small bowel disorders*, London, 2000, Arnold Press.

Pathophysiology

The consequences of intestinal obstruction are related to its onset and location and the length of intestinal tract proximal to the obstruction. The major pathophysiologic alterations are presented in Fig. 38-5. Obstruction leads to intestinal distention and the loss of fluids and electrolytes. Distention begins almost immediately, as gases and fluids accumulate proximal to the obstruction. The major source of gas is swallowed air, but some is contributed by bacterial fermentation. Distention decreases the intestine's ability to absorb water and electrolytes and increases the net secretion of these substances into the lumen. Within 24 hours, up to 8 L of fluid

Table 38-4 Classification of Intestinal Obstruction

Criteria for Classification	Definition
ONSET	
Acute	Sudden onset; often caused by torsion, intussusception, or herniation
Chronic	Protracted onset; more commonly from tumor growth or progressive formation of strictures
EXTENT OF OBSTRUCTION	
Partial	Incomplete obstruction of intestinal lumen
Complete	Complete obstruction of intestinal lumen
LOCATION OF OBSTRUCTING LESION	
Intrinsic	Obstruction develops within intestinal wall; examples: luminal edema or hemorrhage, foreign bodies (gallstones), tumors, or intraluminal fibrosis causing obstruction
Extrinsic	Obstruction originates outside the intestine; examples: tumors, torsion, fibrosis, hernia, intussusception
EFFECTS ON INTESTINAL WALL	
Simple	Luminal obstruction without impairment of blood supply
Strangulated	Luminal obstruction with occlusion of blood supply
Closed loop	Obstruction at each end of a segment of the intestine
CAUSAL FACTORS	
Mechanical	Blockage of the intestinal lumen by intrinsic or extrinsic lesions; usually treated surgically
Functional (paralytic ileus)	Paralysis of the intestinal musculature as a result of trauma, peritonitis, electrolyte imbalances, or spasmolytic agents; usually treated surgically

and electrolytes enters the lumen in the form of saliva, gastric juice, bile, pancreatic juice, and intestinal secretions. Copious vomiting or sequestration of fluids in the intestinal lumen prevents their reabsorption and produces severe fluid and electrolyte disturbances. Extracellular fluid volume and plasma volume decrease, causing dehydration. Hemoconcentration (decreased plasma volume) elevates hematocrit, decreases central venous pressure, and causes tachycardia. Severe dehydration leads to hypovolemic shock.

If the obstruction is at the pylorus or high in the small intestine, metabolic alkalosis develops initially as a result of excessive loss of hydrogen ions that normally would be reabsorbed from the gastric juice. With prolonged obstruction or obstruction lower in the intestine, metabolic acidosis is more likely to occur because bicarbonate from pancreatic secretions and bile cannot be reabsorbed. Hypokalemia can be extreme, promoting acidosis and atony of the intestinal wall. Metabolic acidosis also may be accentuated by ketosis, the result of declining carbohydrate stores caused by starvation. If pressure from the distention is severe enough, it occludes the arterial circulation and causes ischemia, necrosis, perforation, and peritonitis. Fever and leukocytosis are often associated with strangulation. Lack of circulation permits the buildup of significant amounts of lactic acid, which worsen the metabolic acidosis. Bacterial proliferation and translocation across the mucosa causes peritonitis or sepsis.

Clinical Manifestations

Signs and symptoms of intestinal obstruction are consistent with the pathophysiology. Colicky pains followed by vomiting are the cardinal symptoms. Typically the pain occurs intermittently. Sweating, nausea, and hypotension occur as an autonomic response. Pain intensifies for seconds or minutes as a peristaltic wave of muscle contraction meets the obstruction. The passing of the wave is followed by a pain-free interval. With severe distention the pain may diminish in intensity. If strangulation occurs, the pain loses its colicky character, becoming more constant and severe as ischemia progresses to necrosis or perforation.

Vomiting and distention vary, depending on the level of the obstruction. Obstruction at the pylorus causes early, profuse vomiting of clear gastric fluid. Obstruction in the proximal small intestine causes mild distention and vomiting of bile-stained fluid. Obstruction lower in the intestine causes more pronounced distention because a greater length of intestine is proximal to the obstruction. In this case, vomiting may not occur or may occur later and contain fecal material. Partial obstruction can cause diarrhea or constipation, but complete obstruction usually causes constipation only. Complete obstruction increases the number of bowel sounds, which may be tinkly and accompanied by peristaltic rushes and crampy, abdominal pain. Signs of dehydration, hypovolemia, and metabolic acidosis may be observed as early as 24 hours after the occurrence of complete obstruction. Distention may be severe enough to push against the diaphragm and decrease lung volume. This can lead to atelectasis and pneumonia, particularly in debilitated individuals.

Evaluation and Treatment

Evaluation is based on clinical manifestations and includes ultrasound and radiography.[24] Successful management requires early identification of the site and type of obstruction. Replacement of fluid and electrolytes and decompression of the lumen with gastric or intestinal suction are essential forms

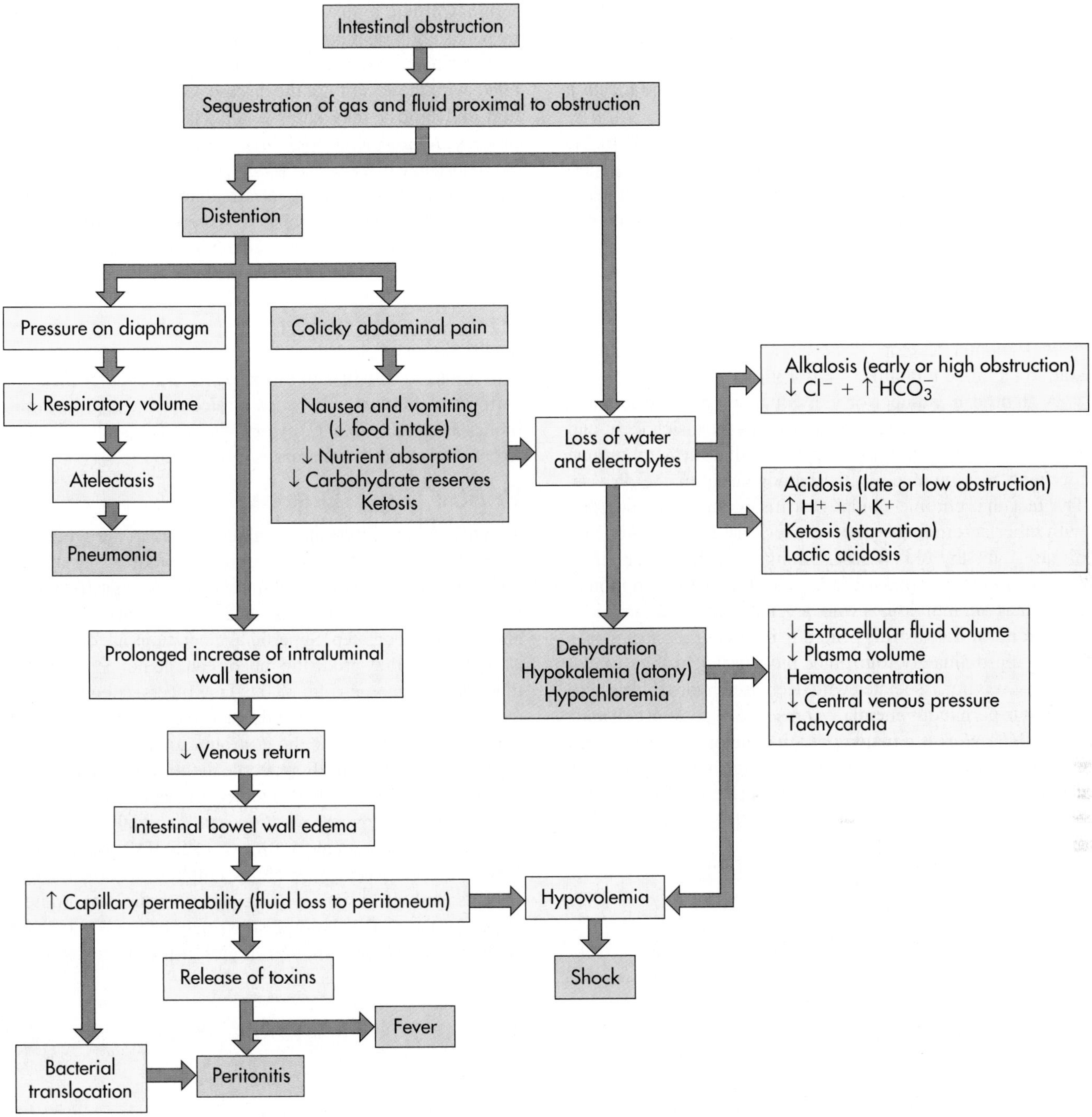

FIG. 38-5 Pathophysiology of intestinal obstruction.

of therapy. Immediate surgical intervention is required for strangulation and complete obstruction.

Gastritis

Gastritis is an inflammatory disorder of the gastric mucosa. It can be acute or chronic and can affect the fundus or antrum or both. **Acute gastritis** erodes the surface epithelium in a diffuse or localized pattern. The erosions are usually superficial.

Acute gastritis is usually injury of the protective mucosal barrier by drugs, chemicals, or *Helicobacter pylori*. Nonsteroidal antiinflammatory drugs, such as aspirin, ibuprofen, naproxen, and indomethacin, are known to cause gastritis, perhaps because they inhibit prostaglandins, which normally stimulate the secretion of mucus (Fig. 38-6).[25] Alcohol, histamine, digitalis, and metabolic disorders such as uremia are contributing factors. *H. pylori* infection causes inflammation, pain, nausea, and vomiting.[26] The clinical manifestations of acute gastritis can include vague abdominal discomfort, epigastric tenderness, and bleeding. Healing usually occurs spontaneously within a few days. Discontinuing injurious drugs, using antacids, or decreasing acid secretion with cimetidine facilitates healing.

Chronic gastritis tends to occur in elderly individuals and causes thinning and degeneration of the stomach wall. Chronic gastritis usually is classified as type A (fundal) or type B (antral), depending on the pathogenesis and location of the lesions.

Chronic fundal gastritis, also called *atrophic gastritis*, is the most rare and severe type. The gastric mucosa degenerates extensively in the body and fundus of the stomach, leading to gastric atrophy. Loss of chief cells and parietal cells diminishes secretion of pepsinogen, hydrochloric acid, and intrinsic factor. Because acid secretion is insufficient, the feedback mechanism that normally inhibits gastrin secretion is impaired, causing elevated plasma levels of gastrin. Pernicious anemia develops because intrinsic factor is unavailable to facilitate vitamin B_{12} absorption.

A significant number of individuals with chronic fundal gastritis have antibodies to parietal cells, intrinsic factor, and gastric cells in their sera, suggesting that an autoimmune mechanism is involved in the pathogenesis of the disease. The fact that chronic fundal gastritis occurs in association with other autoimmune diseases, such as diabetes, Addison disease, and thyroid disease, strengthens this association. Chronic fundal gastritis is a risk factor for gastric carcinoma, particularly in individuals who develop pernicious anemia.

Chronic antral gastritis generally involves the antrum only and is approximately four times more frequent than fundal gastritis. It is not associated with decreased hydrochloric acid secretion, pernicious anemia, or presence of parietal cell antibodies. *H. pylori* is a major causative factor associated with chronic atrophic antral gastritis.[27] In approximately 10% of cases, antibodies to gastrin-secreting cells are found in the serum. Chronic reflux of bile may contribute to the gastritis by persistently disrupting the mucosal barrier.

Signs and symptoms of chronic gastritis often do not correlate with the severity of the disease. Gastroscopic examination and biopsy may show a long-standing inflammatory process and gastric atrophy in an individual with no history of abdominal distress. *H. pylori* infection is evidence for *H. pylori* gastritis. Failure to stimulate acid secretion confirms achlorhydria (diminished secretion of hydrochloric acid). The gastric secretions also can be evaluated for the presence of intrinsic factor. Individuals may report vague symptoms, including anorexia, fullness, nausea, vomiting, and epigastric pain. Gastric bleeding may be the only clinical manifestation of gastritis.

Symptoms usually can be managed with smaller meals; a soft, bland diet; and avoidance of alcohol and aspirin. Antibiotics are used to treat *H. pylori*. Vitamin B_{12} is administered to correct pernicious anemia.

Peptic Ulcer Disease

A **peptic ulcer** is a break, or an ulceration, in the protective mucosal lining of the lower esophagus, stomach, or duodenum. Such breaks expose submucosal areas to gastric secretions and autodigestion. Peptic ulcers can be acute or chronic, and superficial or deep. Superficial ulcerations are called *erosions* because they erode the mucosa but do not penetrate the muscularis mucosae (Fig. 38-7). True ulcers extend through the muscularis mucosae and damage blood vessels, causing hemorrhage, or perforate the gastrointestinal wall.

Approximately 5 million people in the United States have peptic ulcer disease.[28] Risk factors for peptic ulcer disease are smoking, *H. pylori* infection, and habitual use of nonsteroidal antiinflammatory drugs (NSAIDs) or alcohol. Some chronic diseases, such as emphysema, rheumatoid arthritis, and cirrhosis, are associated with the development of peptic ulcers. Psychologic stress may be a risk factor for peptic ulcer disease, although studies of life stress and ulcer

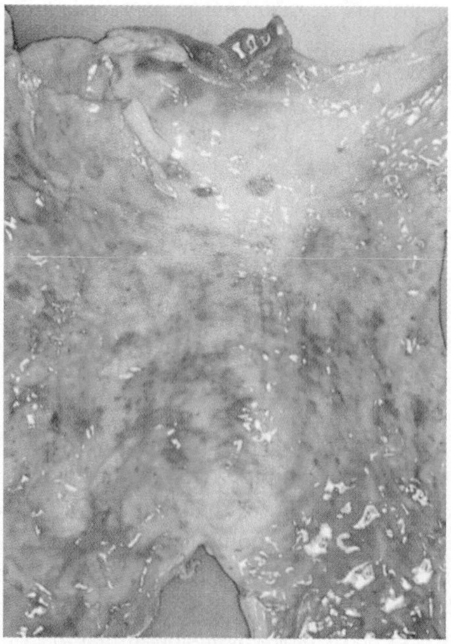

FIG. 38-6 Acute erosive gastritis. Acute erosive gastritis is shown in the opened stomach. The mucosa appears hyperemic, and the foci of superficial ulceration are manifest as scattered, small, red areas termed *erosions*. (From Stevens A, Lowe J: *Pathology*, London, 1995, Mosby.)

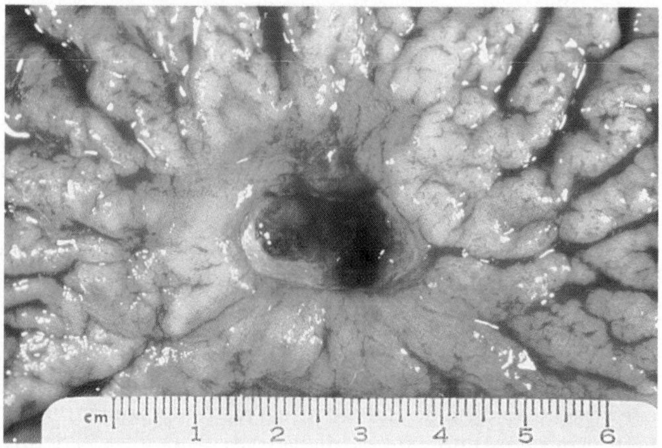

FIG. 38-7 Chronic peptic ulcer. Gross photograph of a chronic peptic ulcer located in the lesser curvature, straddling the antrum and corpus of the stomach. (From Damjanov I, Linder J, editors: *Anderson's pathology*, ed 10, vol 2, St Louis, 1996, Mosby.)

disease are inconclusive.[29] Individuals with multiple stressors, poor coping skills, and persistent anxiety and depression in the presence of recurrent peptic ulcers may require psychiatric management.[30] The exact mechanism of causation is not known.

Duodenal Ulcers

Duodenal ulcers occur with greater frequency than other types of peptic ulcers and affect 10% to 15% of the population.[31] The incidence of duodenal ulcers is approximately the same among men and women in the United States.[32] Duodenal ulcers tend to develop in younger persons and in individuals with type O blood.

Pathophysiology

Infection with *H. pylori* is a major cause of duodenal ulcers.[33] Hypersecretion of acid and pepsin is a contributing cause, and inadequate secretion of bicarbonate by the duodenal mucosa also may be a factor. Other factors that contribute to ulcer formation are as follows:

1. A greater than usual number of parietal (acid-secreting) cells in the gastric mucosa
2. High serum gastrin levels that remain high longer than normal after eating and continue to stimulate secretion of acid and pepsin (may be caused by *H. pylori*)
3. Failure of the feedback mechanism whereby acid in the gastric antrum inhibits gastrin release
4. Rapid gastric emptying, which overwhelms the buffering capacity of the bicarbonate-rich pancreatic secretions
5. Association of *H. pylori* with death of mucosal epithelial cells and elevated levels of gastrin and pepsinogen
6. *H. pylori* release of toxins and enzymes that promote inflammation and ulceration
7. Use of NSAIDs, which inhibit prostaglandins
8. Acid production stimulated by cigarette smoking
9. Decreased mucosal bicarbonate secretion

All these factors, singly or in combination, cause acid and pepsin concentrations in the duodenum to penetrate the mucosal barrier and cause ulceration (Fig. 38-8).[34,35]

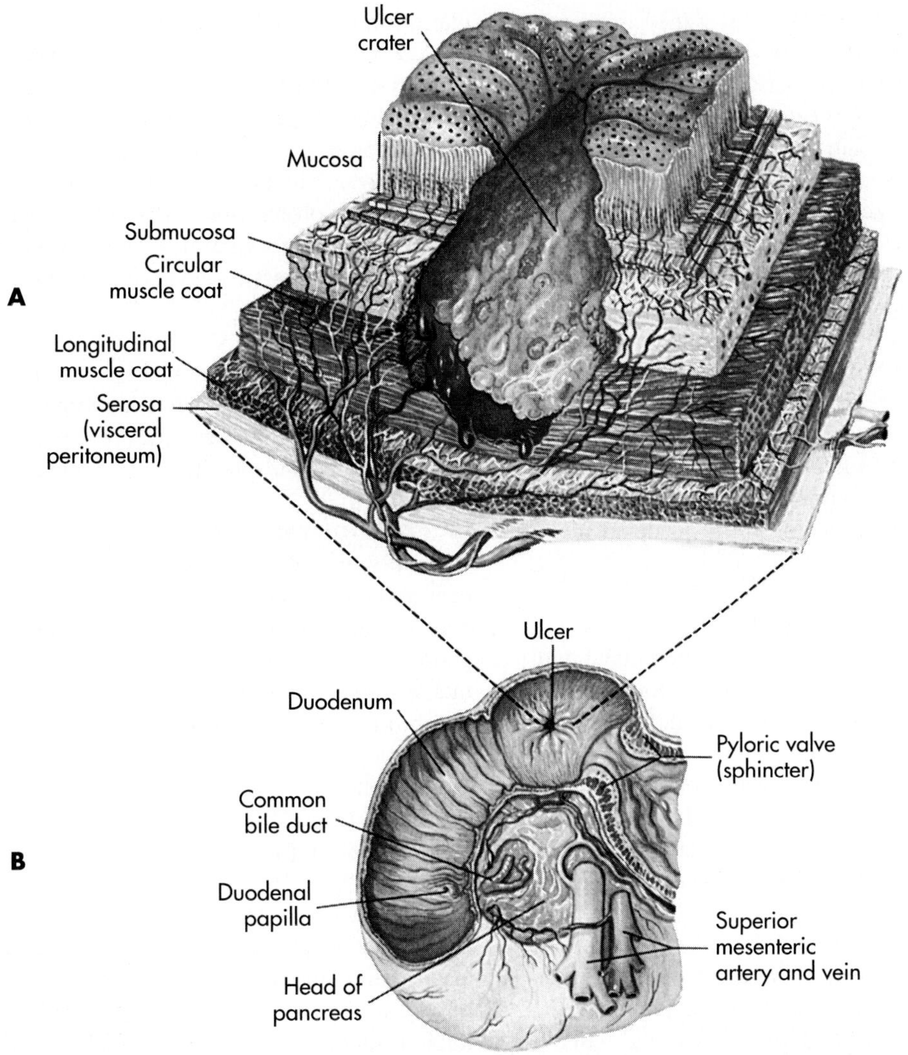

FIG. 38-8 Duodenal ulcer. A, A deep ulceration in the duodenal wall extending as a crater through the entire mucosa and into the muscle layers. **B,** Duodenal ulcer.

Continued

C

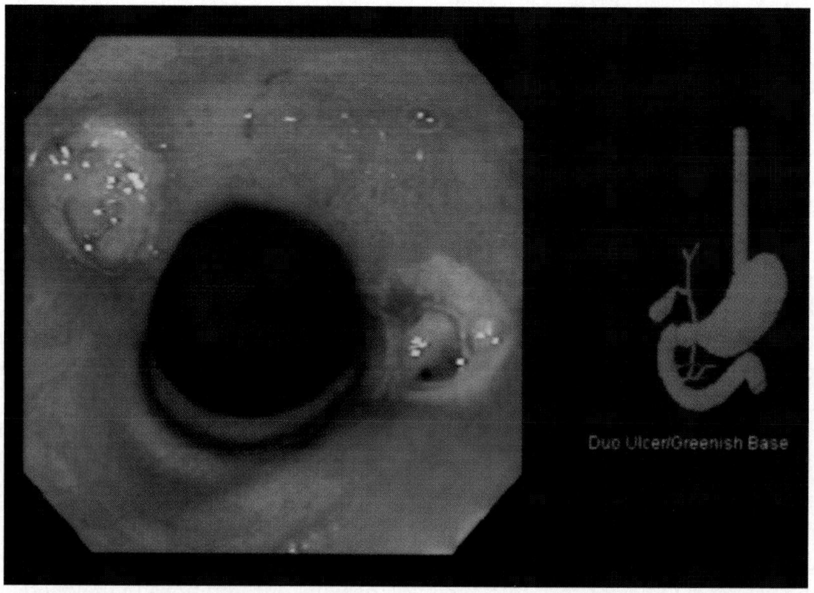

Fig. 38-8, cont'd Duodenal ulcer. C, Bilateral (kissing) duodenal ulcers in a person using nonsteroidal antiinflammatory drugs (NSAIDs). (C, courtesy David Bjorkman, M.D., University of Utah School of Medicine, Department of Gastroenterology.)

Clinical Manifestations

The characteristic manifestation of a duodenal ulcer is chronic intermittent pain in the epigastric area. The pain begins 30 minutes to 2 hours after eating, when the stomach is empty. It is not unusual for pain to occur in the middle of the night and disappear by morning. The pain results from sensorineural stimulation by acid, muscle spasm, or both. Pain is relieved rapidly by ingestion of food or antacids, creating a typical "pain-food-relief" pattern. Some individuals with duodenal ulcer have no symptoms, particularly elderly persons; the first manifestation may be hemorrhage or perforation, particularly with a history of NSAID or anticoagulant use.

Duodenal ulcers often heal spontaneously but recur within months. Exacerbations tend to develop in the spring and fall. Healing is accompanied by relief of pain. Constant, unremitting pain may be caused by complications, such as intestinal obstruction or perforation. Bleeding from duodenal ulcers causes hematemesis or melena.

Evaluation and Treatment

Several diagnostic approaches are used to differentiate duodenal ulcers from gastric ulcers or gastric carcinoma. Barium roentgenograms may show an anatomic deformity created by the ulcer crater. If the roentgenographic examination is inconclusive, flexible endoscopic evaluations may be performed. Radioimmune assays of gastrin levels are evaluated to identify ulcers associated with gastric carcinomas. The urea breath test and positive findings from gastric biopsy detect *H. pylori* infection.[36]

Management of duodenal ulcers is aimed at relieving the causes and effects of hyperacidity. Antacids neutralize gastric contents, elevate pH, inactivate pepsin, and relieve pain. Acid secretion can be suppressed with drugs (e.g., cimetidine) that block histamine (H2) receptors and inhibit the secretion of acid. Proton pump inhibitors (Omeprazole) inhibit acid production. Therapy with bismuth, metronidazole or clarithromycin, and either amoxicillin or tetracycline for *H. pylori* usually prevents relapse.[37,38] Ulcer-coating agents, such as sucralfate and colloidal bismuth, promote healing. Anticholinergic drugs may be used to inhibit gastric secretion, suppress gastric motility, and delay gastric emptying. Surgical resection may be required for bleeding or perforating ulcers or obstruction.[39] Risk of duodenal ulcer may be reduced with a diet high in vitamin A and fiber.[40a] Clinical trials are in progress for a vaccine against *H. pylori*.[40b]

Gastric Ulcers

Gastric ulcers are ulcers of the stomach. They occur with about equal frequency in males and females, usually between the ages of 55 and 65 years, and are about one fourth as common as duodenal ulcers (Table 38-5 and Fig. 38-9).

Pathophysiology

Generally gastric ulcers develop in the antral region, adjacent to the acid-secreting mucosa of the body. The primary defect is an abnormality that increases the mucosal barrier's permeability to hydrogen ions. Gastric secretion may be normal or less than normal.

Chronic gastritis is often associated with development of gastric ulcers and may precipitate ulcer formation by limiting the mucosa's ability to secrete a protective layer of mucus (Fig. 38-10). Decreased mucosal synthesis of prostaglandin may be one factor causing decreased mucus secretion.[41]

Other factors associated with gastric ulcer development include duodenal reflux of bile and use of ulcerogenic drugs (aspirin and indomethacin). Reflux of bile is caused by loss of tone at the pyloric sphincter. The pyloric sphincter may fail to respond to stimuli that normally increase resting tone, such as entry of acid, protein, and fat into the duodenum.

An increased concentration of bile salts disrupts the gastric mucosa; this disruption may decrease the electrical po-

Table 38-5 Characteristics of Gastric and Duodenal Ulcers

Characteristics	Gastric Ulcer	Duodenal Ulcer
INCIDENCE		
Age at onset	50-70 years	20-50 years
Family history	Usually negative	Positive
Gender (prevalence)	Equal in women and men	Equal in women and men
Stress factors	Increased	Average
Ulcerogenic drugs	Normal use	Increased use
Cancer risk	Increased	Not increased
PATHOPHYSIOLOGY		
Abnormal mucus	May be present	May be present
Parietal cell mass	Normal or decreased	Increased
Acid production	Normal or decreased	Increased
Serum gastrin	Increased	Normal
Serum pepsinogen	Normal	Increased
Associated gastritis	More common	Usually not present
Helicobacter pylori	May be present (60%-80%)	Often present (95%-100%)
CLINICAL MANIFESTATIONS		
Pain	Located in upper abdomen Intermittent Pain-antacid-relief pattern Food-pain pattern	Located in upper abdomen Intermittent Pain-antacid or food-relief pattern Nocturnal pain common
Clinical course	Chronic ulcer without pattern of remission and exacerbation	Pattern of remissions and exacerbations for years

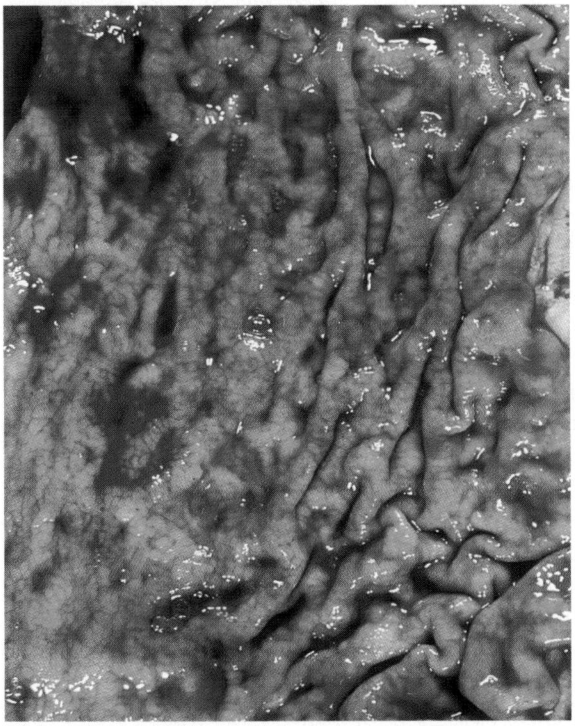

FIG. 38-9 Macroscopic appearance of benign gastric ulcers. (From Damjanov I, Linder J, editors: *Anderson's pathology,* vol 2, ed 10, St Louis, 1996, Mosby.)

tential across the gastric mucosal membrane. The break damages the mucosal barrier by permitting hydrogen ions to diffuse into the mucosa, where they disrupt permeability and cellular structure. A vicious cycle can be established as the damaged mucosa liberates histamine, which stimulates the increase of acid and pepsinogen production, blood flow, and capillary permeability. The disrupted mucosa becomes edematous and loses plasma proteins. Destruction of small vessels causes bleeding.

Clinical Manifestations

The clinical manifestations of gastric ulcers are similar to those of duodenal ulcers (see Table 38-5). The pattern of pain, food, and relief is common, but the pain of gastric ulcers also may occur immediately after eating. Another difference is that gastric ulcers tend to be chronic rather than alternate between periods of remission and exacerbation. Gastric ulcers also cause more anorexia, vomiting, and weight loss than duodenal ulcers. The evaluation and treatment of gastric ulcers are similar to the evaluation and treatment of duodenal ulcers.

Stress Ulcers

A **stress ulcer** is an acute form of peptic ulcer that tends to accompany severe illness, systemic trauma, or neural injury. Emotional stress may be associated with stress ulcer.[42] Usually, multiple sites of ulceration are distributed within the stomach or duodenum. Decreased mucosal blood flow is an important contributing event in stress ulcer formation.[43] Stress ulcers may be classified as ischemic ulcers or Cushing ulcers.

Ischemic ulcers develop within hours of an event—such as hemorrhage, multisystem trauma, severe burns, heart failure, or sepsis—that causes ischemia of the stomach and duodenal mucosa. Stress ulcers that develop as a result of burn injury are frequently called **Curling ulcer**.

The shock, anoxia, and sympathetic responses produced by the precipitating event decrease mucosal blood flow, leading

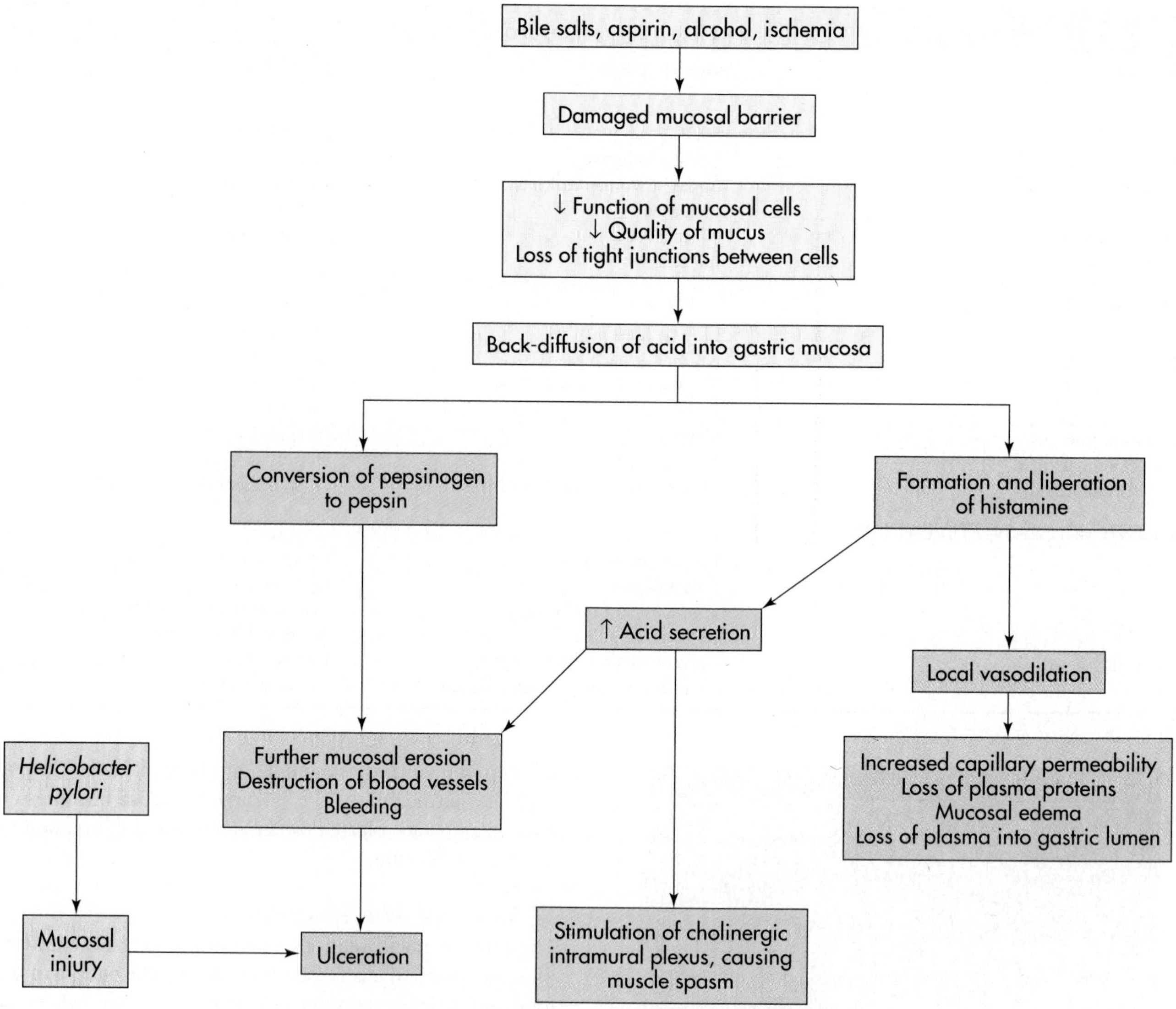

FIG. 38-10 Pathophysiology of gastric ulcer formation.

to ischemia. Because the metabolism of the mucosal cells declines as a result of lack of arterial blood, the mucosal lining degenerates. Acid diffuses back into the mucosa, causing inflammation, ulceration, hemorrhage, and necrosis. The ulcerative process is accelerated if bile or pancreatic enzymes are regurgitated from the duodenum.

Cushing ulcer is a stress ulcer associated with severe head trauma or brain surgery. This ulcer results from decreased mucosal blood flow and hypersecretion of acid caused by overstimulation of the vagal nuclei. Excessive acid damages the mucosal barrier, initiating the processes summarized in Fig. 38-10.

The primary clinical manifestation of stress ulcers is bleeding. Other symptoms may not be present. The bleeding may be slight or, if a small vessel is perforated, amount to hundreds of milliliters. Use of prophylactic antacids and H_2 receptor blockers and suppression of vagal stimulation with anticholinergic drugs are effective forms of therapy. Stress ulcers seldom become chronic.

Surgical Treatment of Ulcer

Advances in the medical treatment of peptic ulcer disease have reduced the number of cases requiring surgery to 10% to 15%. Despite this small percentage, clinicians care for a significant number of individuals who undergo upper gastrointestinal surgery and experience long-term complications. The most common indications for ulcer surgery are recurrent or uncontrolled bleeding and perforation of the stomach or duodenum.[44] The primary objectives of surgical treatment are to reduce stimuli for acid secretion, decrease the number of acid-secreting cells in the stomach, and correct complications of ulcer disease (Table 38-6).

Acute complications of gastrectomy or anastomosis, such as poor wound healing, abscess formation, or suture failure, are relatively uncommon except in the debilitated person. Chronic complications, however, occur more often and are likely to develop if a large portion of the stomach has been removed. These complications and their pathophysiologic mechanisms are described in the next section.

Table 38-6 Surgical Management of Peptic Ulcer Disease

Procedure	Definition	Purpose
Neural surgery		
Vagotomy	Severance of the vagus nerve	Eliminate neural stimulus of acid secretion
Selective vagotomy	Severance of vagal branches supplying acid-secreting (parietal) cells	Eliminate neural stimulus of acid secretion
Gastric surgery		
Pyloroplasty	Surgical widening or removal of obstruction of the pylorus	Facilitate gastric emptying
Antrectomy (partial gastrectomy)	Removal of the antrum	Eliminate hormonal stimulus of acid secretion—that is, the gastrin-secreting cells of the antral mucosa
Subtotal gastrectomy	Removal of most of the body and all of the antrum of the stomach	Remove acid-secreting and gastrin-secreting mucosa
Anastomosis (Billroth operation)	Reattachment of stomach to duodenum (Billroth I) or jejunum (Billroth II)	Restore continuity of the gastrointestinal tract after resection

Postgastrectomy Syndromes

Postgastrectomy syndromes are a group of signs and symptoms that occur after gastric resection. They are caused by changes in motor and control functions of the stomach and upper small intestine.[45]

Dumping Syndrome

Dumping syndrome is the rapid emptying of hypertonic chyme from the surgically created, residual stomach into the small intestine 10 to 20 minutes after eating. It occurs with varying severity in 5% to 10% of individuals who have undergone partial gastrectomy or pyloroplasty. It is not common in individuals who have undergone a Billroth II anastomosis accompanied by vagotomy. Factors that promote dumping syndrome include (1) loss of gastric capacity, (2) loss of emptying control when the pylorus is removed, and (3) loss of feedback control by the duodenum when it is removed. Rapid gastric emptying and creation of a high osmotic gradient within the small intestine cause a sudden shift of fluid from the vascular compartment to the intestinal lumen. Plasma volume decreases, causing vasomotor responses, such as increased pulse rate, hypotension, weakness, pallor, sweating, and dizziness. Rapid distention of the intestine produces a feeling of epigastric fullness, cramping, nausea, vomiting, and diarrhea.[46]

A less common form of dumping syndrome, termed *late dumping syndrome*, occurs 1 to 2 hours after eating. The symptoms include weakness, diaphoresis, and confusion, but they cannot be explained by rapid gastric emptying. After a high-carbohydrate meal, individuals who have undergone gastrectomy may develop hypoglycemia, which causes the symptoms. The hypoglycemia is caused by an increase in insulin secretion stimulated by the hyperglycemia that follows eating. Other hormonal responses may also participate in the development of hypoglycemia.

Most cases of dumping syndrome respond well to dietary management.[47] Frequent small meals that are high in protein and low in carbohydrates relieve symptoms. Other measures include drinking fluids between meals instead of at mealtime and reclining on the left side after eating. Some cases require surgical intervention, including reconstruction of the pylorus or a gastrojejunostomy.[45] Octreotide reduces abdominal and vasomotor symptoms of dumping syndrome by unknown mechanisms.[48]

Alkaline Reflux Gastritis

Alkaline reflux gastritis is a stomach inflammation caused by reflux of bile and alkaline pancreatic secretions that contain proteolytic enzymes and disrupt the mucosal barrier. This form of gastritis occurs in 5% to 20% of individuals who have undergone gastrectomy or pyloroplasty. Clinical manifestations include nausea, bilious vomiting (vomiting in which the vomitus contains bile), and sustained epigastric pain that worsens after eating and is not relieved by antacids.[49] Endoscopy shows a hemorrhagic and friable gastric mucosa. Conservative management is often difficult because antacids do not consistently improve symptoms. Avoidance of aspirin and alcohol may decrease gastric irritation, and a low-fat diet may limit bile secretion. Surgical correction may ultimately be required.

Afferent Loop Obstruction

Afferent loop obstruction is an unusual problem that may occur after gastrojejunostomy (Billroth II; see Table 38-6). The problem is caused by volvulus, hernia, adhesion, or stenosis in the duodenal stump on the proximal side of the gastrojejunostomy. Partial obstruction causes bile and pancreatic secretions to accumulate and distend the loop. Obstruction also causes delayed emptying. The symptoms of afferent loop obstruction include intermittent severe pain and epigastric fullness after eating. Vomiting usually relieves symptoms. Conservative management consists of a low-fat diet. Surgical correction is required for complete obstruction.

Diarrhea

Diarrhea is one of the most common long-term alterations caused by gastric surgery. Diarrhea can accompany dumping syndrome or occur as a solitary symptom. Diarrhea can occur as frequent, persistent elimination of liquid stool or as intermittent, precipitous, and unpredictable elimination of a large volume of stool. Both types can be either mild or severe. Postgastrectomy diarrhea appears to be related to rapid gastric emptying, particularly after intake of large amounts of high-carbohydrate liquids, which increase the osmotic gradient and attract water into the intestinal lumen. Small, dry meals and anticholinergic drugs are effective control measures.

Weight Loss

Weight loss frequently follows gastric resection. Inadequate food intake is a common cause, because many individuals cannot tolerate carbohydrates or a normal-size meal. Foods may be poorly absorbed because the stomach is less able to mix, churn, and break down food particles. Vomiting, diarrhea, and malabsorption of fats also contribute to weight loss.

Anemia

Anemia after gastrectomy results from iron, vitamin B_{12}, or folate deficiency. Iron malabsorption may be caused by decreased acid secretion. Acid changes iron from a trivalent to a divalent molecule, making it easier to absorb. Iron absorption is also compromised in individuals who have undergone a Billroth II procedure because the duodenum is no longer available to absorb iron.

Vitamin B_{12} deficiency may occur several years after gastrectomy. Contributing factors include loss of parietal cells, which secrete intrinsic factor. (Intrinsic factor facilitates absorption of vitamin B_{12}; see Chapter 37.) Vitamin B_{12} absorption is also compromised if gastric contents are not mixed adequately with pancreatic enzymes, such as may occur after a Billroth II anastomosis.

Folate deficiency is related to poor intake or malabsorption. Management of deficiencies consists of replacement of iron and folate with supplements. Vitamin B_{12} can be administered monthly by injection.

Malabsorption Syndromes

Malabsorption syndromes interfere with nutrient absorption in the small intestine. Historically malabsorption disorders have been classified as maldigestion or malabsorption. **Maldigestion** is failure of the chemical processes of digestion that take place in the intestinal lumen or at the brush border of the intestinal mucosa. **Malabsorption** is the failure of the intestinal mucosa to absorb (transport) the digested nutrients. Frequently maldigestion and malabsorption are interrelated or occur together, making classification difficult. Generally, however, maldigestion is caused by deficiencies of enzymes, such as pancreatic lipase or intestinal lactase, that are necessary for digestion. Inadequate secretion of bile salts and inadequate reabsorption of bile in the ileum also contribute to maldigestion. Malabsorption is the result of mucosal disruption caused by gastric or intestinal resection, vascular disorders, or intestinal disease.

Pancreatic Insufficiency

The pancreatic enzymes (lipase, amylase, trypsin, chymotrypsin) are required for the digestion of proteins, carbohydrates, and fats. **Pancreatic insufficiency** is the deficient production of these enzymes by the pancreas. Causes of pancreatic insufficiency include chronic pancreatitis, pancreatic carcinoma, pancreatic resection, and cystic fibrosis. Significant damage to or loss of pancreatic tissue must occur before enzyme levels decrease sufficiently to cause maldigestion. Although pancreatic insufficiency causes poor digestion of all nutrients, fat maldigestion is the chief problem. Salivary amylase and enzymes secreted by the intestinal brush border assist in carbohydrate and protein digestion, but these enzymes do not digest fats. Absence of pancreatic bicarbonate in the duodenum and jejunum causes an acidic pH that worsens maldigestion by preventing activation of pancreatic enzymes that are present. Maldigestion, a large amount of fat in the stool (steatorrhea), and weight loss are the most common signs of pancreatic insufficiency.[50]

Lactase Deficiency

Deficiency of disaccharidase at the brush border of the small intestine is caused by a congenital defect in which a single enzyme, usually lactase, is lacking. **Lactase deficiency** inhibits the breakdown of lactose (milk sugar) into monosaccharides and therefore prevents lactose digestion and absorption across the intestinal wall. Lactase deficiency is most common in blacks. The deficiency usually does not develop until adulthood. Secondary (acquired) lactase deficiency can be caused by several diseases of the intestine, including gluten-sensitive enteropathy (see Chapter 39), enteritis, and bacterial overgrowth.

The undigested lactose remains in the intestine, where bacterial fermentation causes gases to form. Undigested lactose also increases the osmotic gradient in the intestine, causing irritation and osmotic diarrhea. Clinical manifestations of lactase deficiency are bloating, crampy pain, diarrhea, and flatulence. The disorder is diagnosed by a lactose-tolerance test.[51] Avoiding milk products and adhering to a lactose-free diet relieve symptoms.

Bile Salt Deficiency

Conjugated bile acids (bile salts) are necessary for the digestion and absorption of fats. Bile salts are conjugated in the bile that is secreted from the liver. When bile enters the duodenum, the bile salts aggregate with fatty acids and monoglycerides to form micelles. Micelle formation solubilizes fat molecules and allows them to pass through the unstirred layer at the brush border (see Chapter 37). A minimum concentration of bile salts, termed the *critical micelle concentration*, is required to allow micelles to form. Therefore conditions that decrease the production or secretion of bile result in decreased micelle formation and fat malabsorption. These conditions include advanced liver disease, which decreases production of bile salts; obstruction of the common bile duct, which decreases flow of bile into the duodenum; intestinal stasis (lack of motility), which permits overgrowth of intestinal bacteria that deconjugate bile salts; and diseases of the ileum, which prevent the reabsorption and recycling of bile salts (enterohepatic circulation).

Clinical manifestations of bile salt deficiency are related to poor intestinal absorption of fat and fat-soluble vitamins (A, D, E, K). Increased fat in the stools (steatorrhea) leads to diarrhea and decreased plasma proteins. The losses of fat-soluble vitamins and their effects include the following:

1. Vitamin A deficiency results in night blindness.
2. Vitamin D deficiency results in decreased calcium absorption with bone demineralization (osteoporosis), bone pain, and fractures.
3. Vitamin K deficiency prolongs prothrombin time, leading to spontaneous development of purpura (bruising) and petechiae.
4. Vitamin E deficiency has uncertain effects but may cause testicular atrophy and neurologic defects in children.

The most effective treatment for fat-soluble vitamin deficiency is to increase medium-chain triglycerides in the diet, for example, by using coconut oil for cooking. Vitamins A, D, and K are given parenterally.

Inflammatory Bowel Disease

Ulcerative Colitis

Ulcerative colitis is a chronic inflammatory disease that causes ulceration of the colonic mucosa, usually in the rectum and sigmoid colon. The lesions appear in susceptible individuals between 20 and 40 years of age. Risk factors include family history of disease and Jewish descent, and the disease is more prevalent among white populations.

Although the cause of ulcerative colitis is unknown, dietary, infectious, genetic, and immunologic factors are all suggested causes.[52,53] The hypothesis that inflammation is caused by infectious agents is not supported by consistent identification of specific viruses or bacteria in affected individuals. The familial tendency to develop ulcerative colitis and the occurrence of disease in identical twins support a genetic theory of causation. Perhaps most significant are immunologic factors associated with the disease. Anticolon antibodies have been identified in the sera of individuals with ulcerative colitis. Lymphocytes (T cells) in individuals with ulcerative colitis may have cytotoxic effects on the epithelial cells of the colon, as well as damage caused by inflammatory cytokines (interleukins [IL-1, IL-2, IL-6, IL-8] and tumor necrosis factor [TNF-α]), toxic oxygen radicals, interferon-γ (IFN-γ), and IL-10.[54] Furthermore, autoimmune disorders, such as systemic lupus erythematosus and erythema nodosum, may accompany ulcerative colitis.

Pathophysiology

The primary lesion of ulcerative colitis begins with inflammation at the base of the crypt of Lieberkühn in the large intestine, primarily the left colon, with neutrophil infiltration. The disease is most severe in the rectum and sigmoid colon. The mucous layer is thinner than normal. The mucosa is hyperemic and may appear dark red and velvety (Fig. 38-11). Inflammatory cytokines released from leukocytes, macrophages, and neutrophils cause tissue damage.[54] Small erosions form and coalesce into ulcers. Abscess formation occurs in the crypts. Necrosis and ragged ulceration of the mucosa ensue. Edema and thickening of the muscularis mucosae may narrow the lumen of the involved colon. Mucosal destruction causes bleeding, cramping pain, and an urge to defecate.[55] Frequent diarrhea, with passage of small amounts of blood and purulent mucus, is common. Loss of the absorptive mucosal surface and decreased colonic transit time cause large volumes of watery diarrhea.

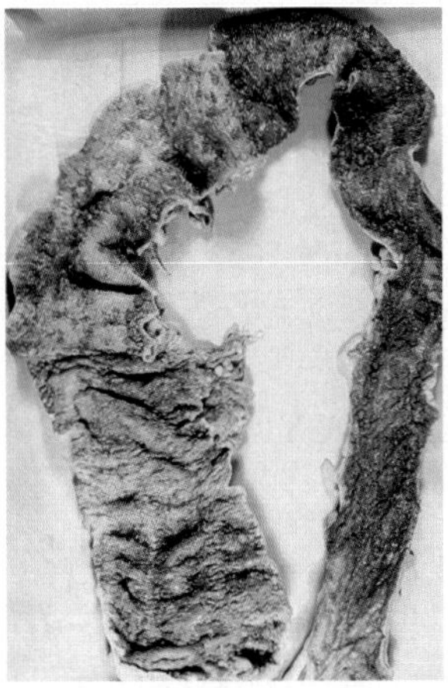

FIG. 38-11 Acute ulcerative colitis. Colitis with extensive mucosal ulceration involving the entire colon. (From Damjanov I, Linder J, editors: *Anderson's pathology*, ed 10, St Louis, 1996, Mosby.)

Clinical Manifestations

The course of ulcerative colitis consists of intermittent periods of remission and exacerbation. Clinical manifestations vary with the severity and extent of disease. Mild ulcerative colitis involves less mucosa, so that frequency of bowel movements, bleeding, and pain are minimal. Severe forms may involve the entire colon and are characterized by fever; elevated pulse rate; frequent diarrhea (10 to 20 movements per day); urgency; obviously bloody stools; and continuous, crampy pain. Dehydration, weight loss, anemia, and fever result from fluid loss, bleeding, and inflammation. Complications include toxic megacolon, anal fissures, hemorrhoids, and perirectal abscess. Severe hemorrhage is rare, but chronic blood loss may precipitate hypotension and shock. Edema, strictures, or fibrosis can obstruct the colon. Perforation is an unusual but possible complication. The risk of left-sided colon cancer increases significantly after many years of ulcerative colitis.[56]

Evaluation and Treatment

Diagnosis of ulcerative colitis is based on the medical history and clinical manifestations. Sigmoidoscopy shows an inflamed and hemorrhagic mucosa. A barium enema and roentgenograms may show loss of haustra, ulceration, and irregular mucosa. The laboratory data include low hemoglobin values, hypoalbuminemia, and low serum potassium levels. Infectious causes are ruled out by stool culture. The symptoms of ulcerative colitis are very similar to those of Crohn disease, making differential diagnosis difficult.[57]

Treatment depends on the severity of symptoms and the extent of mucosal involvement. The disease is often treated with sulfasalazine (a combination of a sulfa drug and aminosalicylates). Steroids and salicylates suppress the inflammatory response and help to alleviate the cramping pain.[57]

Table 38-7 Features of Ulcerative Colitis and Crohn Disease

Feature	Ulcerative Colitis	Crohn Disease
INCIDENCE		
Age at onset	Any age; 10-40 years most common	Any age; 10-30 years most common
Family history	Less common	More common
Gender (prevalence)	Equal in women and men	About equal in women and men
Cancer risk	Increased	Is increasing
PATHOPHYSIOLOGY		
Location of lesions	Colon & rectum, no "skip" lesions	All of GI tract: mouth to anus, "skip" lesions common
Inflammation and ulceration	Mucosal layer involved	Entire intestinal wall involved
Granulomas	Rare	Common
Friable mucosa	Common	Less common
Anal and perianal fistuale and abscesses	Rare	Common
Narrowed lumen and possible obstruction	Rare	Common
CLINICAL MANIFESTATIONS		
Abdominal pain	Occasional	Common
Diarrhea	Common	Common
Bloody stools	Common	Less common
Abdominal mass	Rare	Common
Small intestinal malabsorption	Rare	Common
Steatorrhea	Rare	Common
Clinical course	Remissions and exacerbations	Remissions and exacerbations

Broad-spectrum antibiotics may be prescribed if bacterial infection is suggested. For unknown reasons, nicotine may have a protective effect in ulcerative colitis but not in Crohn disease.[58] Severe, unremitting disease can require hospital admission and administration of intravenous fluids. Extreme malnutrition may require intravenous hyperalimentation. Surgical resection of the colon or a colostomy may be performed if other forms of therapy are unsuccessful.[59]

Crohn Disease

Crohn disease (granulomatous colitis or regional enteritis) is an idiopathic inflammatory disorder that affects any part of the gastrointestinal track from the mouth to the anus. In a small percentage of cases, Crohn disease is difficult to differentiate from ulcerative colitis (Table 38-7). Risk factors and theories of causation are the same as those for ulcerative colitis. Like ulcerative colitis, Crohn disease tends to run in families. Ten to twenty percent of affected individuals have a positive family history. Increased suppressor T cell activity with cytokine-mediated damage and alterations in immunoglobulin A (IgA) production are the immunologic factors associated with Crohn disease. Smoking, dietary substances, and bacteria not part of the normal flora also may be causal factors.

Pathophysiology

The inflammatory process of Crohn disease begins in the intestinal submucosa and spreads across the intestinal wall to involve the mucosa and serosa. The most common site of the disease is the ileocolon, but both the large and small intestines may be involved. The inflammation can affect some haustral segments but not others, creating a pattern called *skip lesions*. One side of the intestinal wall may be affected but not the other.

The ulcerations of Crohn disease produce longitudinal and transverse fissures that extend inflammation into lymphoid tissue. The typical lesion is a granuloma having cobblestone projections of inflamed tissue surrounded by areas of ulceration (Fig. 38-12). (Granulomas are described in Chapter 7.) Fistulae may form in the perianal area between loops of intestine or extend into the bladder.

Clinical Manifestations

Individuals with Crohn disease may have no specific symptoms other than an "irritable bowel" for several years. Diarrhea is the most common sign, with passage of blood and mucus. Diarrhea can result from decreased colonic absorption, bypass fistulae, bacterial overgrowth, and the presence of bile in the colon that inhibits water absorption.[60] Other manifestations are related to the location and extent of intestinal involvement. Inflammation of the ileum, for example, causes tenderness in the lower right side of the abdomen. Weight loss and lower abdominal pain accompany Crohn disease. If the ileum is involved, the individual may be anemic as a result of malabsorption of vitamin B_{12}. There also may be deficiencies in folic acid, vitamin D absorption, and calcium. Proteins may be lost, leading to hypoalbuminemia. Anal manifestations occur in about 30% of cases, including anal fissure, perianal abscess, and fistula.[52] Individuals with Crohn disease of long duration are also at risk for intestinal adenocarcinoma, particularly in the small intestine.[61] Complications include obstruction, fistulae, abscess formation, and chronic blood loss.

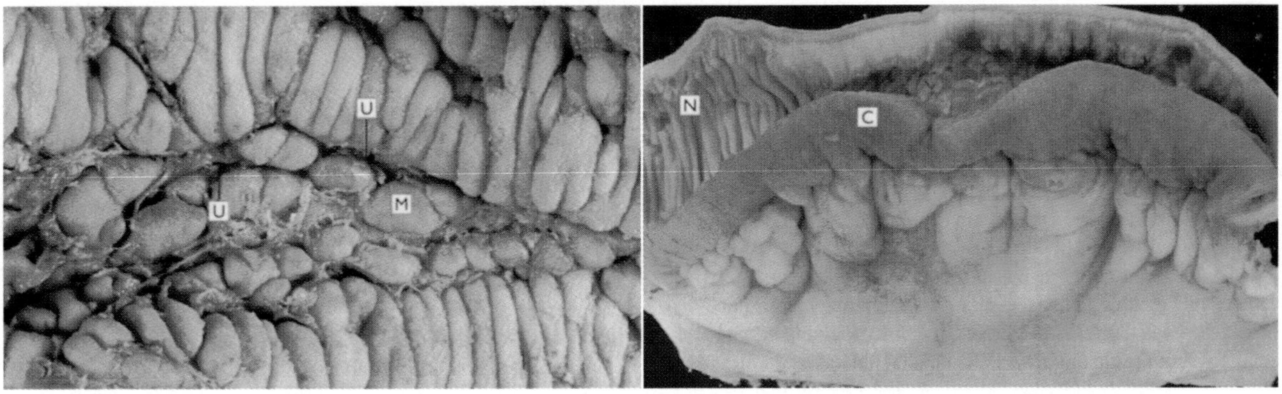

FIG. 38-12 Crohn disease. A, The mucosa in Crohn disease demonstrates a cobblestone pattern as a result of fissured ulcers *(U)* with intervening areas of edematous mucosa *(M).* **B,** Compared with normal small bowel wall *(N),* the Crohn segment *(C)* shows wall thickening that has caused a stenosis. (From Stevens A, Lowe J: *Pathology*, London, 1995, Mosby.)

Evaluation and Treatment

The diagnosis and treatment of Crohn disease are similar to the diagnosis and treatment of ulcerative colitis. Treatment with immunomodulatory agents can be effective. Surgery is generally performed to manage complications such as strictures, fistula, abscess, and perforation, or to relieve obstruction.[62]

Diverticular Disease

Diverticula are herniations or saclike outpouchings of mucosa through the muscle layers of the colon wall. **Diverticulosis** is asymptomatic diverticular disease. **Diverticulitis** represents inflammation. Diverticular disease is most common in individuals over 60 years of age, particularly those who live in developed countries where much of the diet consists of refined foods.

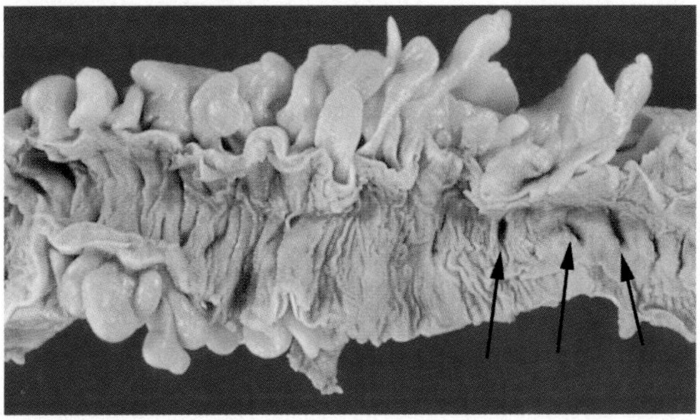

FIG. 38-13 Diverticular disease. In diverticular disease, the outpouches (arrows) of mucosa seen in the sigmoid colon appear as slitlike openings from the mucosal surface of the opened bowel. (Modified from Stevens A, Lowe J: *Pathology*, London, 1995, Mosby.)

Pathophysiology

Although diverticula can occur anywhere in the gastrointestinal tract, the most frequent site is the sigmoid colon. The diverticula form at weak points in the colon wall, usually where arteries penetrate the tunica muscularis to nourish the mucosal layer. The colonic mucosa herniates through the smooth muscle layers (Fig. 38-13). A common associated finding is thickening of the circular and longitudinal (teniae coli) muscles surrounding the diverticula. Hypertrophy and contraction of these muscles increase intraluminal pressure and degree of herniation. Habitual consumption of a low-residue diet reduces fecal bulk, thus reducing the diameter of the colon. According to the law of Laplace (see Chapter 28), wall pressure increases as the diameter of a cylindrical structure decreases. Therefore pressure within the narrow lumen can increase enough to rupture the diverticula. Diverticulitis can cause abscess formation or peritonitis.[63]

Clinical Manifestations

Symptoms of diverticular disease are usually vague or absent. Cramping pain of the lower abdomen can accompany constriction of the hypertrophied colonic muscles. Diarrhea, constipation, distention, or flatulence may occur. Diverticula with an obstructed opening become inflamed or abscesses form, and the individual develops fever, leukocytosis (increased white blood cell count), and tenderness of the lower left quadrant. Right lower quadrant pain and severe complications, such as hemorrhage, peritonitis, bowel obstruction, and fistula formation, are rare.

Evaluation and Treatment

Diverticula are often discovered during diagnostic procedures performed for other problems. Ultrasound, sigmoidoscopy, or barium enema are used for diagnosis of uncomplicated diverticuli. Abdominal computed tomography (CT) is used for complicated cases.

An increase of dietary fiber intake frequently relieves symptoms. Uncomplicated diverticulitis is treated with antibiotics. Surgical resection may be required if there are severe complications.[64]

Appendicitis

Appendicitis is an inflammation of the vermiform appendix, which is a projection from the apex of the cecum. It is the most common surgical emergency of the abdomen and affects

NUTRITION & DISEASE
Diverticulitis and Diet

Daily consumption of fiber-enriched foods is recommended for the prevention of diverticula. A high-fiber diet increases fecal bulk, decreases transit time, lowers intracolonic pressures, and eases stool elimination. The recommendation for fiber is 20 to 35 g/day. Some examples of high-fiber choices are whole wheat bread and other grain products, baked potato with skin, fresh fruit with skins, raw vegetables, beans, peas, legumes, wheat bran, and brown rice. Side effects may include flatulence, intestinal rumbling, cramps, and diarrhea. A gradual increase in dietary fiber over a month or two helps to avoid these problems. Other potential problems with an excessively high fiber diet (greater than 40 to 45 g) might include a decrease in nutrient absorption because of the increased volume of intestinal contents, which in turn decreases the ability of the digestive enzymes to come in contact with the food. An increase of water (eight 8-oz glasses) is important so intestinal blockage will not occur. For small children and elderly persons a high-fiber diet increases the volume of food needed to meet energy requirements, and that increase may be difficult to obtain. Although some doctors recommend restricting nuts; seeds; and foods containing seeds such as berries, kiwi, and tomatoes that might lodge in the pouches, there is no evidence that this happens. If the diverticula become inflamed, a low-fiber, low-residue (no milk products), or elemental diet, or in complicated cases TPN, is required to prevent continued irritation of the inflamed tissue.

Data from Bennett WG, Cerda JJ: *Postgrad Med* 99(2):153, 1996; Ozick LA, Salazar CO, Donelson SS: *Gastroenterologist* 2(4):299, 1994.

7% to 12% of the population. The most common occurrence is between 20 and 30 years of age, although it may develop at any age.

Pathophysiology

The exact cause of appendicitis is controversial. Obstruction of the lumen with stool, tumors, or foreign bodies with consequent bacterial infection and inflammation[65] is a common theory. The obstructed lumen does not allow drainage of the appendix, and as mucosal secretion continues, intraluminal pressure increases. The resultant increased pressure decreases mucosal blood flow, and the appendix becomes hypoxic. The mucosa ulcerates, promoting bacterial or other microbial invasion with further inflammation and edema. Inflammation may involve the distal or entire appendix. Gangrene develops from thrombosis of the luminal blood vessels, followed by perforation.

Clinical Manifestations

Epigastric or periumbilical pain is the typical symptom of an inflamed appendix. The pain may be vague at first, increasing in intensity over 3 to 4 hours. It may subside and then recur with a shift of location to the right lower quadrant. Right lower quadrant pain is associated with extension of the inflammation to the surrounding tissues. Nausea, vomiting, and anorexia follow the onset of pain, and fever is common. Diarrhea occurs in some individuals, particularly children; others have a sensation of constipation. Perforation, peritonitis, and abscess formation are the most serious complications of appendicitis.

Evaluation and Treatment

In addition to clinical manifestations, the clinician can usually locate the painful site with one finger. Rebound tenderness is usually referred to the right lower quadrant. The white blood cell count ranges from 10,000 to 16,000 cells/mm^3, with increased neutrophils. C-reactive protein is elevated.[66] Roentgenograms of the abdomen, CT scans, and ultrasound assist diagnostic accuracy.

Antibiotics and appendectomy is the treatment for simple or perforated appendicitis. Surgery provides quick recovery for simple appendicitis. Recovery is more complicated in cases of perforation or abscess formation.[67]

Vascular Insufficiency

The stomach and intestines are supplied by three branches of the abdominal aorta: the celiac axis and the superior and inferior mesenteric arteries. Because of the rich collateral circulation, at least two of the supplying vessels must be compromised to cause ischemia.[68] Atherosclerotic lesions, thrombi, and emboli can develop in these vessels, occluding blood flow and causing ischemia or necrosis in the gastrointestinal tract.

Chronic mesenteric insufficiency can develop secondary to congestive heart failure, acute myocardial infarction, dysrhythmias, hemorrhage, stenosis, thrombus formation, aortic aneurysm, or any condition that decreases arterial blood flow. Elderly individuals with arteriosclerosis are particularly susceptible. Chronic occlusion is often accompanied by formation of collateral circulation that may be able to nourish the resting intestine. After eating, however, when the intestine requires more blood, the arterial supply may be insufficient. Ischemia develops, causing a cramping abdominal pain, called *abdominal angina*, after meals. Progressive vascular obstruction eventually causes continuous abdominal pain and necrosis of the intestinal tissue.

Colicky abdominal pain after eating is a cardinal symptom of chronic mesenteric insufficiency. Some individuals suffer significant weight loss because they stop eating to control the pain. Chronic segmental ischemia may lead to strictures and destruction.

Acute occlusion of mesenteric blood flow results from dissecting aortic aneurysms or emboli. Embolic obstruction is associated with atrial fibrillation, mitral valve disease, and heart valve prostheses. The superior mesenteric artery has a more direct line of flow from the aorta; therefore emboli enter it more readily than the inferior branch, causing ischemia and necrosis of the small intestine. Ischemia and necrosis alter membrane permeability. There is initially increased motility, which is followed by absence of motility from the ischemia. The damaged intestinal mucosa cannot produce enough mucus to protect itself from digestive enzymes.[69] Mucosal alteration causes fluid to move from the blood vessels into the bowel wall and peritoneum. Fluid loss causes hypovolemia and further decreases in intestinal blood flow. As intestinal infarction progresses, shock, fever, bloody diarrhea, leukocytosis, and abdominal distention develop. Abdominal pain may be severe. Bacteria invade the necrotic intestinal wall, causing gangrene and peritonitis.

Diagnosis of mesenteric artery occlusion is based on clinical manifestations, mesenteric artery angiography, and abdominal radiography. Bruit can frequently be heard over the occluded artery. After angiography a vasodilating agent may be injected into the vessels to improve the circulation. Surgery is required to remove necrotic tissue or repair sclerosed vessels. Mortality is high for individuals with acute occlusion and compromised cardiac output.

Disorders of Nutrition

Obesity

Obesity is defined as body mass index that corresponds to greater than 120% of ideal body weight. Obesity is a major nutritional problem in the United States and is associated with the three leading causes of death: cardiovascular disease, cancer, and diabetes mellitus.

Obesity is an imbalance between energy intake and expenditure, usually associated with excessive caloric intake. It can be classified as either exogenous (resulting from an excess of ingested calories) or endogenous (resulting from inherent metabolic problems).[70] Physiologically, obesity can be classified according to the structure and distribution of the adipose tissue itself. Child-onset obesity is both hyperplastic (caused by a greater than normal *number* of fat cells) and hypertrophic (caused by a greater than normal *size* of fat cells). In children the adipose tissue is dispersed over the entire body and few metabolic abnormalities exist. Adult-onset obesity is hypertrophic, the adipose tissue is centrally located, and metabolic abnormalities are more common. Increased visceral fat is associated with ischemic heart disease, hyperlipidemia, hypertension, and glucose intolerance.[71] Genotype is an important predisposing factor.

Several theories have been postulated to explain the physiology of obesity, and multiple environmental and genetic factors explain its development:

1. *Genetic theory*—the obese (ob) gene product *leptin* is expressed predominantly in adipose tissue and may function to control body fat stores by regulating food intake (satiety) and energy expenditure.[72,73] Alterations in the expression of the ob gene and the B_2 adrenoceptor gene may result in excessive body fat stores.[74] The B_2 adrenoceptor gene, located primarily in adipose tissue, regulates resting metabolic rate and fat oxidation. Insulin may be an important regulatory hormone.
2. *Fat-cell theory*—individuals with hyperplastic fat (adipose) cells are overweight because they have an excessive number of fat cells, and the number increases whenever a positive energy balance occurs.
3. *Lipoprotein-lipase (LPL) theory*—LPL promotes fat storage, and obese individuals may have elevated levels of LPL in their fat cells, which rise even higher after weight reduction; the LPL works against the maintenance of reduced body weight and stimulates the fat cells to return to their hypertrophic size.
4. *Lipostatic theory*—obese individuals may have a higher hypothalamic set-point, which makes it difficult for them to maintain weight loss.
5. *Thermogenetic theory*—obese people are believed to have very few brown fat cells, which are the mitochondria-rich fat cells responsible for heat production, so they cannot burn off excess energy but, rather, store it as fat.[75]
6. *Sodium-potassium-adenosine triphosphatase (ATPase) pump theory*—this enzyme pump (which transports sodium out of the cell and potassium into the cell and splits adenosine triphosphate, releasing energy) is lacking in obese individuals, leading to a lack of energy release and obesity.
7. *Diabetes-associated theory*—excessive food intake stimulates hyperinsulinemia and promotes high blood levels of glucose, which is stored as glycogen in the liver or as triglycerides in the adipose cells, thereby enhancing hypertrophy and hyperplasia of fat cells in the already obese person.
8. *Psychologic causation theory*—obese people are directed more by external cues, such as the sight, smell, and taste of food, than by internal cues, such as hunger and satiety; another psychologic theory postulates that eating creates the desire to eat more.

Pathophysiology

Obese individuals are at risk for coronary artery disease resulting from hypercholesterolemia and hypertension. Abnormal obesity increases risks for diabetes, hypertension, and cardiovascular disease.[76] Obesity is also a risk factor for breast, cervical, endometrial, and liver cancer in women. Obese men are at greater risk for prostatic, colon, and rectal cancer.[77] Pulmonary function can be compromised by a large amount of adipose tissue overlying the chest cage. Gas exchange, vital capacity, and expiratory volume all decrease, causing low arterial oxygen tension and high carbon dioxide tension. Sleep apnea can occur. Exercise intolerance and pain in the fingers and weight-bearing joints, particularly the knees, are common. Joint pain may be caused by premature erosion of cartilage.[78]

Evaluation and Treatment

Obesity is evaluated by a number of methods, including use of height and weight tables, body mass index (ratio of weight to height), skinfold thickness, hydrostatic weighing, measurement of oxygen intake, and bioelectric impedance analysis. If excess fat interferes with physiologic or psychologic functioning, treatment may be initiated.

Obesity is a chronic disease with various approaches to treatment.[79] The treatment for obesity caused by excessive nutrient intake is a regimen of reduced nutrient intake and increased energy expenditure. Age at onset, laboratory data about metabolic function (e.g., glucose tolerance tests, serum triglyceride, and cholesterol analyses), and distribution of adipose tissue determine the weight-reduction goal. Individuals with adult-onset obesity can reduce the size of their adipose cells and achieve a standard weight. Those with child-onset obesity may never achieve a standard weight.

The goal of weight reduction is to return the adipose cells to normal size and correct any associated metabolic abnormalities. The diet and exercise regimen is tailored to the unique problems of each obese individual. Self-motivation and a support system are critical aspects of treatment. Additional treatments, such as psychotherapy, behavioral modification, medications, and surgery, are prescribed as needed.[80]

Anorexia Nervosa and Bulimia Nervosa

Many young adults and adolescents—as many as 1% of women and adolescent girls in the United States—are affected by two complex and related eating disorders: anorexia nervosa and bulimia. They occur rarely in black women, and only 5% to 10% of cases are men.[81] Risk factors include genetic, familial, biologic, psychologic, and social factors. There is an association between sexual assault history and eating disorders.[82] An increasing number of children, young men, and elderly women are experiencing eating disorders, often with an associated depression, anxiety, or personality disorder.[83] **Anorexia nervosa** is a psychologic and physiologic syndrome characterized by the following:[84]

1. A fear of becoming obese despite progressive weight loss
2. A distorted body image: the perception that the body is fat when it is actually underweight
3. Body weight 15% less than normal for age and height because of refusal to eat
4. In women and girls, absence of three consecutive menstrual periods

Persons with anorexia nervosa frequently deny they have any eating problem. As the disease progresses, muscle and fat depletion give the individual a skeleton-like appearance. Iron deficiency anemia promotes fatigue, and low white blood cell count increases risk of infection. Reproductive functioning is affected, including ovarian function, menstruation, fertility, and pregnancy. Postural hypotension, edema, bradycardia, hypothermia, low total body potassium, constipation, and sleep disturbances may ensue. The loss of 25% to 30% of ideal body weight can eventually lead to death caused by starvation-induced cardiac failure.[85] Most organ systems are affected by progressive starvation. Diagnosis of anorexia nervosa involves a thorough medical history, physical and psychologic examination, and ruling out other causes of anorexia and malnutrition.[86]

There are no universally accepted treatments. Treatment objectives for anorexia nervosa include reversing the compromised physical state, promoting insights and knowledge about the disorder, mutual goals, interaction with family members, restoring development growth, and modifying food habits. Correction of nutritional status may require intensive treatment, including total parenteral nutrition. When the individual demonstrates the willingness to eat food for nourishment, dietary protein, carbohydrate, and fat are introduced in tolerable amounts. Psychotherapy begins as soon as the physical symptoms are stabilized and may continue for several years.

Bulimia nervosa is more common than anorexia and typically begins as an attempt to lose weight. The group at risk is the same as that for anorexia nervosa, except that bulimia tends to occur in slightly older, less affluent women. Diagnosis of bulimia is based on these findings:[87]

1. Recurrent episodes of binge eating during which the individual fears not being able to stop
2. Self-induced vomiting, use of laxatives, fasting to oppose the effect of binge eating, or excessive exercise
3. Two binge-eating episodes per week for at least 3 months

Because of negative connotations associated with self-stimulated vomiting and purging, individuals who have bulimia binge and purge secretly. Bulimic individuals may binge and purge as often as 20 times each day. Weight will fluctuate about 10 pounds. Continual vomiting of acidic chyme can cause pitted teeth, pharyngeal and esophageal inflammation, and tracheoesophageal fistulae. Overuse of laxatives can cause rectal bleeding. Secret binging isolates the bulimic individual and leads to depression and anger that is turned inward. A vicious cycle of depression, overeating to try to feel better, vomiting and purging to maintain a normal weight, and returning depression perpetuates this eating disorder. Mood symptoms are often worse in the winter.[88]

Because persons with bulimia are usually older than individuals with anorexia nervosa and usually have separated from a family core, individual or group counseling is the treatment focus. Individuals with bulimia rarely have physical problems requiring hospital care.

Bulimorexia combines the major components of anorexia nervosa and bulimia. Individuals with bulimorexia binge and gorge with food, vomit and purge with laxatives, and starve themselves intermittently. Risk factors and treatment objectives for bulimorexia are the same as for anorexia nervosa.

Starvation

Starvation is a reduction in energy intake leading to weight loss. Short-term starvation and long-term starvation have different effects. Therapeutic short-term starvation is part of many weight-reduction programs because it causes an initial rapid weight loss that reinforces the individual's motivation to diet. Therapeutic long-term starvation is used in medically controlled environments to facilitate rapid weight loss in morbidly obese individuals. Pathologic long-term starvation can be caused by poverty; chronic diseases of the cardiovascular, pulmonary, hepatic, and digestive systems; malabsorption syndromes; HIV infection; and cancer. In-hospital starvation primarily affects individuals with functional and cognitive deficits and inadequate caloric intake.[89]

Short-term starvation, or extended fasting, consists of several days of total dietary abstinence or deprivation. The body responds with protective mechanisms. For 4 to 6 hours after the last meal, the body is in a well-fed state and its energy requirements are supplied by glucose from recently ingested carbohydrates. Once all available energy has been absorbed from the intestine, glycogen in the liver is converted to glucose through **glycogenolysis**, the splitting of glycogen into glucose. This process peaks within 4 to 8 hours, and gluconeogenesis begins. **Gluconeogenesis** is the formation of glucose from noncarbohydrate molecules: lactate, pyruvate, amino acids, and the glycerol portion of fats. Like glycogenolysis, gluconeogenesis takes place within the liver. Both of these processes deplete stored nutrients and thus cannot meet the body's energy needs indefinitely. Proteins continue to be catabolized to a minimal degree, providing carbon for the synthesis of glucose.

Long-term starvation begins after several days of dietary abstinence and eventually causes death. Absolute deprivation of food causes **marasmus** or protein energy malnutrition. Protein deprivation in the presence of carbohydrate intake is called **kwashiokor**. Marasmic kwashiokor is a combination of chronic energy deficiency and chronic or acute protein deficiency.[90,91] The major characteristic of long-term starvation is a decreased dependence on gluconeogenesis and an increased use of ketone bodies (products of lipid and pyruvate metabolism) as a cellular energy source. During long-term starvation, depressed insulin levels and increased glucagon, cortisone, epinephrine, and growth hormones promote lipolysis in adipose tissue. Lipolysis liberates fatty acids, which supply energy to cardiac and skeletal muscle cells, and ketone bodies, which sustain brain tissue. Fatty acid or ketone body oxidation meets most of the energy needs of the cells. (Some glucose is still needed as fuel for brain tissue.) Once the supply of adipose tissue is depleted, proteolysis begins. The breakdown of muscle and visceral protein is the last process to supply energy for life. Death results from severe alterations in electrolyte balance and loss of renal, pulmonary, and cardiac function.

Adequate ingestion of appropriate nutrients is the obvious treatment for starvation. In medically induced starvation the body is maintained in a ketotic state until the desired amount of adipose tissue has been lysed. Starvation imposed by chronic disease, long-term illness, or malabsorption is treated with enteral or parenteral nutrition.

DISORDERS OF THE ACCESSORY ORGANS OF DIGESTION

The accessory organs of digestion (liver, gallbladder, pancreas) secrete substances necessary for digestion and, in the case of the liver, carry out metabolic functions needed to maintain life. Inflammatory disease is a common cause of accessory organ dysfunction. Inflammation disrupts secretory function and prevents secretions from flowing into the duodenum. Lack of accessory organ secretions is a major cause of maldigestion and malabsorption in the small intestine. Other causes of accessory organ dysfunction are obstruction of ducts by aggregates in the secretions themselves (e.g., obstruction of bile flow by gallstones) or by tumors. (Cancers of the digestive tract are described at the end of this chapter.)

Clinical Manifestations of Liver Disorders

Of all the accessory organ disorders, acute or chronic liver disease leads to the most systemic, life-threatening complications. These complications include portal hypertension, ascites, hepatic encephalopathy, jaundice, and hepatorenal syndrome.

Portal Hypertension

Portal hypertension is abnormally high blood pressure in the portal venous system. Pressure in this system is normally 3 mm Hg; portal hypertension is an increase to at least 10 mm Hg. The portal veins carry blood from the gastrointestinal tract, pancreas, and spleen to the liver. In the liver the blood flows through the sinusoids and empties into the hepatic veins, which carry it into the inferior vena cava. The inferior vena cava delivers blood to the right atrium. The portal veins, sinusoids, and hepatic veins compose the portal venous system.

Pathophysiology

Portal hypertension is caused by disorders that obstruct or impede blood flow through any component of the portal venous system or vena cava. The obstruction can occur in the liver as a result of thrombosis, inflammation, or fibrosis of the sinusoids, as occurs in cirrhosis of the liver, viral hepatitis, or schistosomiasis (a parasitic infection). Portal outflow to the vena cava can be impeded by hepatic vein thrombosis or cardiac disorders—such as failure of the right side of the heart or constrictive pericarditis—that impair the pumping ability of the right heart. This causes blood to back up and increase pressure in the portal system. The most common cause of portal hypertension is obstruction caused by cirrhosis of the liver (see p. 1294), and increased portal blood flow from anterior splanchnic vasodilation.[92]

High pressure in the portal veins causes collateral vessels to open between the portal veins and the systemic veins, in which blood pressure is considerably lower (Fig. 38-14). This enables blood to bypass the obstructed portal vessels. The collateral veins develop in the esophagus, anterior abdominal wall, and rectum. High pressure and increased flow volume are transmitted through these veins from the portal to the systemic venous circulation.

Long-term portal hypertension causes several problems that are difficult to treat and can be fatal:[93]

1. **Varices** (distended, tortuous, collateral veins): prolonged elevation of pressure in collateral veins causes their transformation into varices, particularly in the lower esophagus and stomach but also in the rectum.
2. **Splenomegaly** (enlargement of the spleen): caused by increased pressure in the splenic vein, which branches from the portal vein.
3. **Ascites** (the accumulation of fluid in the peritoneal cavity, which is the space between the visceral peritoneum and the parietal peritoneum): caused in part by increased

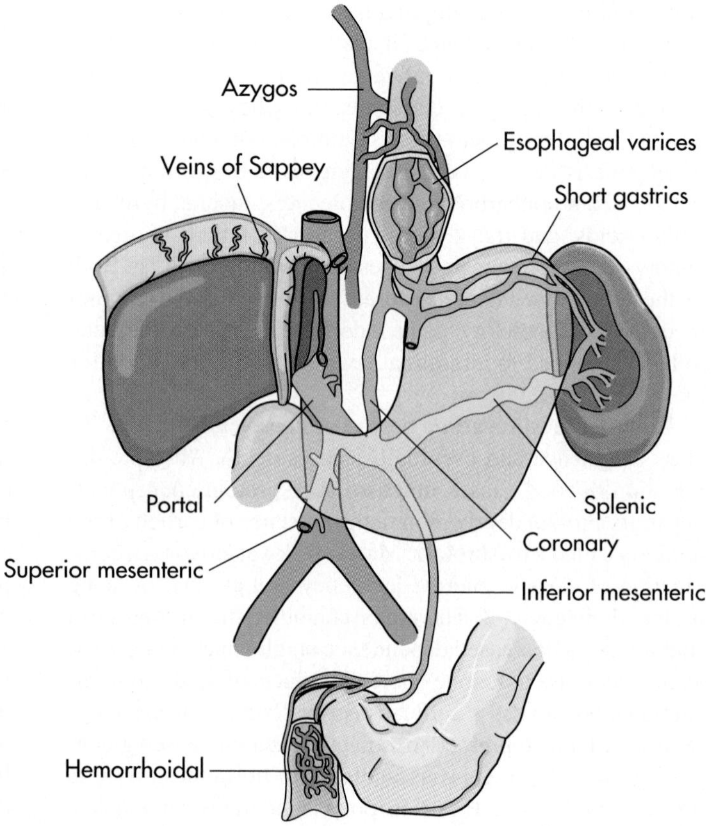

FIG. 38-14 Varices related to portal hypertension. Portal vein, its major tributaries, and the most important shunts (collateral veins) between the portal and caval systems. (From Phipps WP et al: *Medical-surgical nursing: concepts and clinical practice*, ed 6, St Louis, 1999, Mosby.)

pressure in the mesenteric tributaries of the portal vein. Hydrostatic pressure forces water out of these vessels and into the peritoneal cavity. (This process, termed *transudative effusion*, is described in Chapter 32.)

4. **Hepatic encephalopathy** (also called portosystemic encephalopathy): characterized by central nervous system disturbances with astrocyte changes that lead to alterations of consciousness.

Blood that is shunted through collateral vessels to the systemic veins bypasses the liver, where toxins, hormones, and other harmful substances normally are removed. Hepatic encephalopathy results from the presence of these substances, particularly ammonia, in blood that reaches the brain.[94]

Clinical Manifestations

The vomiting of blood from bleeding **esophageal varices** is the most common clinical manifestation of portal hypertension.[95] Slow, chronic bleeding from varices causes anemia or melena. Usually the bleeding is from varices that have developed slowly over a period of years.

Rupture of esophageal varices causes hemorrhage and voluminous vomiting of dark-colored blood. The ruptured varices are usually painless. Rupture is caused by a combination of erosion by gastric acid and elevated venous pressure. Mortality from ruptured esophageal varices ranges from 30% to 60%. Recurrent bleeding of esophageal varices indicates a poor prognosis. Most individuals die within 1 year.

Evaluation and Treatment

Diagnosis of portal hypertension is often made at the time of variceal bleeding and confirmed by endoscopy and evaluation of portal venous pressure. Distended collateral veins may radiate over the abdomen, giving rise to caput medusae (Medusa's head). The individual usually has a history of jaundice, hepatitis, or alcoholism.

Beta-blockers can be effective in preventing variceal bleeding. Emergency management of bleeding varices includes compression of the varices with an inflatable tube or balloon, band ligation, and injection of a sclerosing agent.[95] Surgical construction of a portacaval shunt (anastomosis of the portal vein to the inferior vena cava) may decompress the varices, but this treatment can precipitate encephalopathy or liver failure resulting from reduced hepatic blood flow. There is no effective, definitive treatment for portal hypertension. Liver transplant is an option for liver failure.

Ascites

Ascites is the accumulation of fluid in the peritoneal cavity. Ascites traps body fluid in a "third space" from which it cannot escape. The effect is to reduce the amount of fluid available for normal physiologic functions. Cirrhosis is the most common cause of ascites. Other diseases associated with ascites include heart failure, constrictive pericarditis, abdominal malignancies, nephrotic syndrome, and malnutrition. Twenty-five percent of individuals who develop ascites caused by cirrhosis die within 1 year. Continued heavy drinking is associated with this mortality rate.

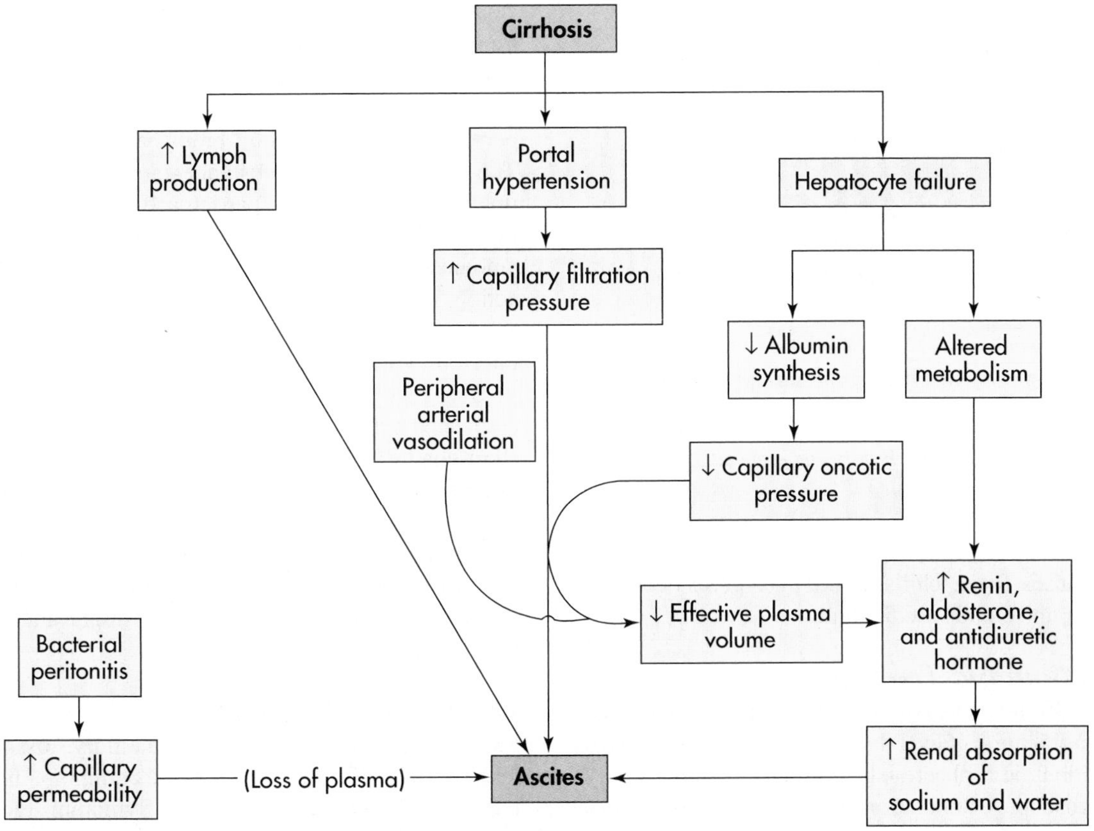

FIG. 38-15 Mechanisms of ascites caused by cirrhosis.

Pathophysiology

Several factors contribute to the development of ascites. Impaired excretion of sodium by the kidneys promotes water retention, but the initiating event is not clear. The *overflow theory* proposes that renal sodium retention is stimulated by portal hypertension with intravascular hypervolemia and overflow into the peritoneal cavity. This imbalance tends to push water into the peritoneal cavity. Portal hypertension also increases the production of hepatic lymph, which "weeps" into the peritoneal cavity. The *underfill theory* proposes an increase in hepatic sinusoidal hydrostatic pressure and decreased oncotic pressure with weeping of lymph fluid from the surface of the liver. There is a decrease in effective circulating plasma volume, stimulating the kidney to retain more sodium and water, leading to intravascular volume overload. The *arterial vasodilation theory* proposes that circulating nitric oxide triggers peripheral vasodilation early in the course of cirrhosis and stimulates renal sodium retention through renin-angiotensin-aldosterone, increased sympathetic tone, and changes in the intrarenal blood flow.[96]

In cases of cirrhosis, both portal hypertension and decreased production of albumin by hepatocytes contribute to the ascites. Besides reducing albumin synthesis, deranged liver metabolism permits the accumulation of hormones that regulate sodium and water balance. Excessive amounts of aldosterone and antidiuretic hormone remain in the blood, stimulating the kidneys to retain sodium and water. High aldosterone levels can be attributed also to increased secretion mediated by excessive plasma renin activity. The increased plasma renin activity may develop because of decreased metabolic function of the liver, increased renal secretion stimulated by low blood flow, or both.

As ascites sequesters more and more body fluid, the kidneys respond by retaining sodium and water in amounts exceeding intake. Retention of sodium and water expands plasma volume, thereby accelerating portal hypertension and ascites formation.

Ascites can be complicated by bacterial peritonitis. Peritonitis involves an inflammatory response that worsens ascites by increasing mesenteric capillary permeability. As plasma seeps out of the permeable mesenteric capillaries, it adds to the volume of ascitic fluid. Fig. 38-15 summarizes the mechanisms by which cirrhosis of the liver causes ascites.

Clinical Manifestations

The accumulation of ascitic fluid causes weight gain, abdominal distention, and increased abdominal girth (Fig. 38-16). Large volumes of fluid (10 to 20 L) displace the diaphragm and cause dyspnea by decreasing lung capacity. Respiratory rate increases, and the individual assumes a semi-Fowler position to relieve the dyspnea. Some peripheral edema is usually present. Approximately 10% of individuals with ascites develop bacterial peritonitis, either spontaneously or as a result of paracentesis (needle aspiration of ascitic fluid).

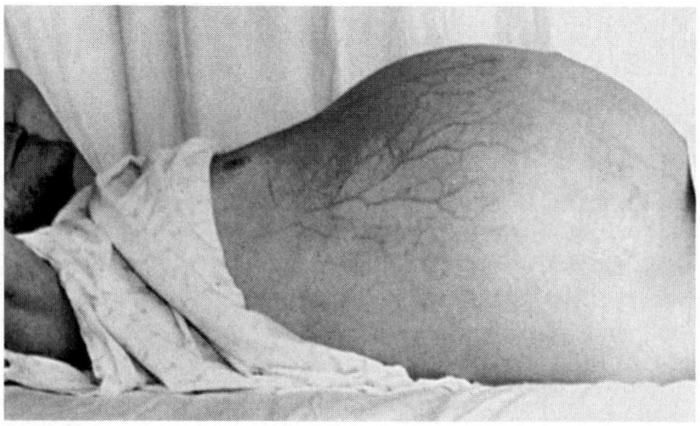

FIG. 38-16 Massive ascites in an individual with cirrhosis. Distended abdomen, dilated upper abdominal veins, and inverted umbilicus are classic manifestations. (From Prior JA, Silberstein JS, Stang JM: *Physical diagnosis: the history and examination of the patient*, ed 6, St Louis, 1981, Mosby.)

Peritonitis causes fever, chills, abdominal pain, decreased bowel sounds, and cloudy ascitic fluid.

Evaluation and Treatment

Diagnosis of ascites is usually based on clinical manifestations and identification of liver disease. Paracentesis is used to aspirate ascitic fluid for bacterial culture, biochemical analysis, and microscopic examination. The goal of treatment is to relieve discomfort. If the restoration of liver function is possible (e.g., in ascites caused by viral hepatitis), the ascites diminishes spontaneously. In the meantime, dietary salt restriction and potassium-sparing diuretics can reduce ascites. Strong diuretics, such as furosemide or ethacrynic acid, may be used. Albumin may be given.[97] Serum electrolytes are monitored carefully because the individual is at risk for hyponatremia and hypokalemia.

Palliative measures include paracentesis to remove 1 or 2 L of ascitic fluid and relieve respiratory distress. This procedure can have serious complications, however. The removal of too much fluid relieves pressure on blood vessels and carries the risk of hypotension, shock, or death. Despite repeated paracenteses, ascitic fluid reaccumulates in individuals with irreversible disease, drawing more albumin and electrolytes out of the vascular compartment. Paracentesis is also likely to cause peritonitis. Individuals with ascites and portal hypertension have a poor prognosis.

Hepatic Encephalopathy

Hepatic encephalopathy (portosystemic encephalopathy) is a complex neurologic syndrome characterized by impaired cerebral function, flapping tremor (asterixis), and electroencephalogram (EEG) changes. The syndrome may develop rapidly during acute fulminant hepatitis or slowly during the course of chronic liver disease. Risk factors in the presence of advanced liver disease include gastrointestinal bleeding, increased dietary protein, electrolyte imbalance, and hypoxia.

Pathophysiology

Hepatic encephalopathy probably results from a combination of biochemical alterations that affect neurotransmission. The astrocyte is the most vulnerable.[98] Liver dysfunction and collateral vessels that shunt blood around the liver to the systemic circulation both permit toxins absorbed from the gastrointestinal tract to circulate freely to the brain. Also, permeability of the blood-brain barrier may be increased. The most hazardous substances are end products of intestinal protein digestion, particularly ammonia.[99] The digestion of blood from leaking or ruptured varices adds to the amount of ammonia present in systemic blood, as does the action of ammonia-forming bacteria in the colon. Ammonia that reaches the brain may alter cerebral energy metabolism, interfere with neurotransmitters, or cause edema.[100]

Blood levels of ammonia do not account for all symptoms associated with hepatic encephalopathy. The accumulation of short-chain fatty acids, serotonin, tryptophan, and false neurotransmitters probably contributes to neural derangement.[101] Excessive γ-aminobutyric acid (GABA), an inhibitory neurotransmitter, may contribute to reduced levels of consciousness. Infection, hemorrhage, electrolyte imbalance, sedatives, and analgesics can also precipitate stupor and coma in the presence of liver disease.

Clinical Manifestations

Subtle changes in personality, memory loss, irritability, lethargy, and sleep disturbances are common initial manifestations of hepatic encephalopathy. Symptoms then can progress to confusion, flapping tremor of the hands, stupor, convulsions, and coma. Coma is usually a sign of liver failure and ultimately results in death.

Evaluation and Treatment

Diagnosis of hepatic encephalopathy is based on a history of liver disease and clinical manifestations. Electroencephalography and blood chemistry tests, including blood ammonia levels, provide supportive data. There is no specific diagnostic test.

Correction of fluid and electrolyte imbalances and withdrawal of depressant drugs metabolized by the liver are the first steps in the treatment of hepatic encephalopathy. Reduction of blood ammonia levels is a major objective. This is accomplished by restricting dietary protein intake and eliminating intestinal bacteria. Neomycin is effective in sterilizing the bowel, but it can be nephrotoxic. Lactulose may be administered to prevent ammonia absorption in the colon. Lactulose passes unabsorbed into the large intestine, where bacteria hydrolyze it to a watery acid. The acid (1) converts ammonia to nonabsorbable ammonium and (2) produces diarrhea, which limits the amount of time feces are available for ammonia production by intestinal bacteria.

Jaundice

Jaundice (icterus) is a yellow or greenish pigmentation of the skin caused by **hyperbilirubinemia** (plasma bilirubin concentrations above 1.2 mg/dl). Hyperbilirubinemia and jaundice can result from excessive hemolysis of red blood cells or disorders of the bile ducts or liver cells (Fig. 38-17). Jaundice in newborns is caused by impaired bilirubin uptake and conjugation (see Chapter 39).

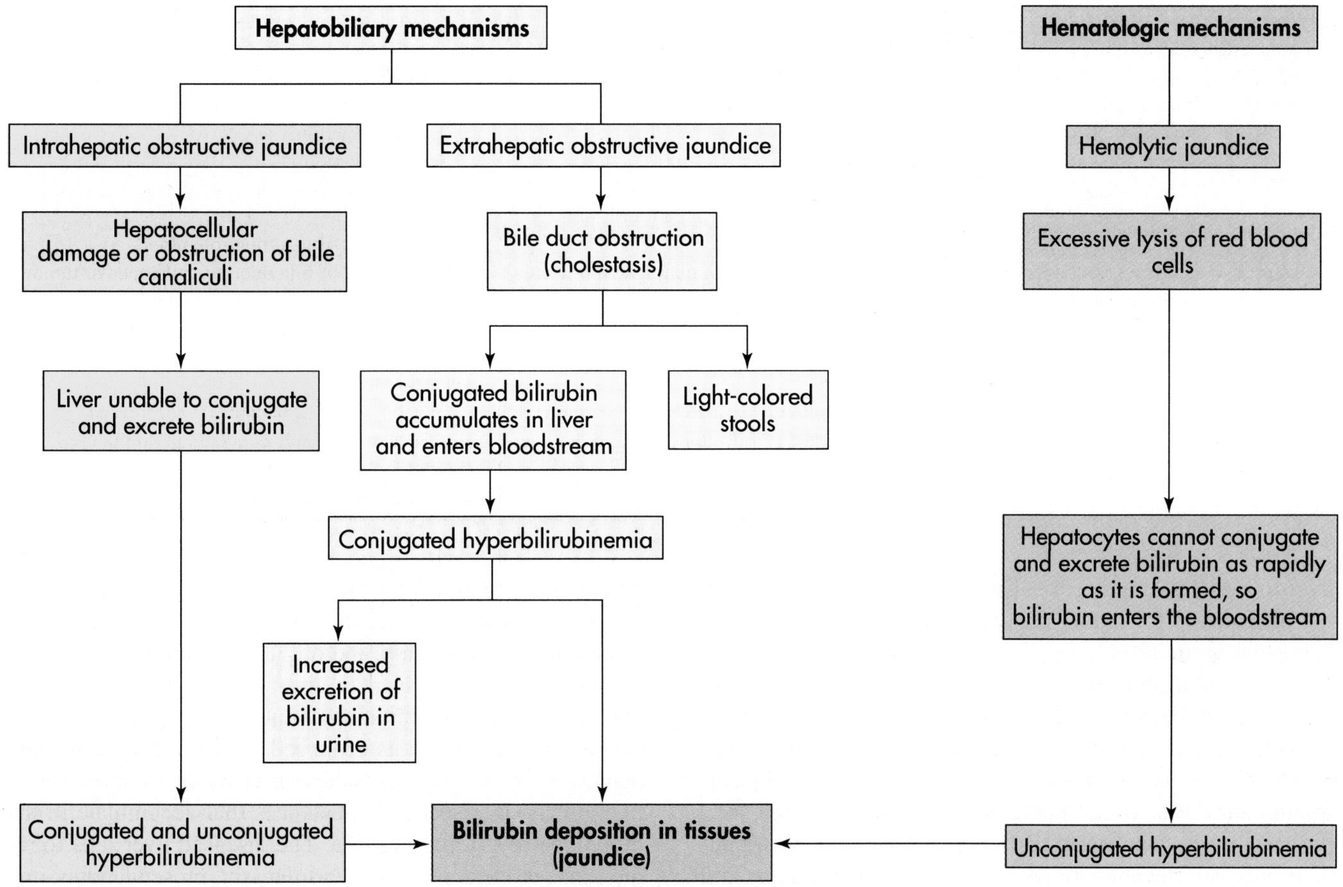

FIG. 38-17 Mechanisms of jaundice.

Pathophysiology

Obstructive jaundice can result from extrahepatic or intrahepatic obstruction.[102] *Extrahepatic obstructive jaundice* develops if the common bile duct is occluded by a gallstone or tumor. Because the bile duct is obstructed, bilirubin is conjugated by the hepatocytes but cannot flow into the duodenum. Therefore it accumulates in the liver and enters the bloodstream, causing hyperbilirubinemia. Because conjugated bilirubin is water soluble, it appears in the urine. The stools may be light colored or clay colored because they lack bile pigments. The stools also lack urobilinogen because bile is not available for conversion to urobilinogen.

Intrahepatic obstructive jaundice involves disturbances in hepatocyte function and obstruction of bile canaliculi. The uptake, conjugation, and excretion of bilirubin are affected because of elevated levels of both conjugated and unconjugated bilirubin. Hepatocellular damage increases plasma concentrations of unconjugated bilirubin. The major disorder, however, is obstruction of bile canaliculi, which diminishes flow of conjugated bilirubin into the common bile duct. In mild cases, some of the bile canaliculi open. Consequently the amount of bilirubin in the intestinal tract may be only slightly decreased. The stools may appear normal or light colored.

Excessive hemolysis (breakdown) of red blood cells can cause **hemolytic jaundice**. An increased amount of unconjugated bilirubin is formed through metabolism of the heme component of destroyed red blood cells. The extra amount of unconjugated bilirubin exceeds the conjugation ability of the liver, causing blood levels of unconjugated bilirubin to rise. Unconjugated bilirubinemia is the major cause of hemolytic jaundice. Because unconjugated bilirubin is not water soluble, it is not excreted in the urine. The reserve conjugation ability of the liver usually prevents long-term unconjugated hyperbilirubinemia greater than 4 to 5 mg/dl. Severe hemolytic crisis, as occurs with sickle cell disease (see Chapter 27), is a cause of hemolytic jaundice. Hemolytic drugs also can cause jaundice. If unconjugated hyperbilirubinemia exceeds 5 mg/dl, both hemolytic and liver disorders are indicated.

Hyperbilirubinemia and jaundice can be caused also by metabolic defects that impair the uptake or conjugation of unconjugated bilirubin in the liver. Gilbert disease, for example, causes an elevation of unconjugated bilirubin in the plasma but no other symptoms of liver disease. Gilbert disease is probably caused by an inherited deficiency of glucuronyl transferase enzyme, which is required for the hepatic uptake of unconjugated bilirubin. The causes of jaundice are summarized in Table 38-8.

Clinical Manifestations

The clinical manifestations of jaundice vary and are related to the underlying pathology. Conjugated hyperbilirubinemia may cause the urine to darken several days before the onset of jaundice. The complete obstruction of bile flow from the

Table 38-8 Three Common Types of Jaundice

Type	Mechanism	Causes
Hemolytic jaundice (predominately unconjugated bilirubin)	Destruction of erythrocytes	Membrane defect of erythrocytes Immune reaction Severe infection Toxic substances in the circulation (e.g., snake venom) Transfusion of incompatible blood
Obstructive jaundice (predominately conjugated bilirubin)	Obstruction of passage of conjugated bilirubin from liver to intestine	Obstruction of bile duct by gallstones or tumor (extrahepatic obstructive jaundice) Obstruction of bile flow through the liver (intrahepatic obstructive jaundice) Drugs
Hepatocellular jaundice	Failure of liver cells (hepatocytes) to conjugate bilirubin and of bilirubin to pass from liver to intestine	Genetic defect of hepatocyte (decreased enzymes), such as occurs in premature infants (see Chapter 39) Severe infections

liver to the duodenum causes light-colored stools. With partial obstruction the stools are normal in color and bilirubin is present in the urine.

Fever, chills, and pain often accompany jaundice resulting from viral or bacterial inflammation of the liver (e.g., viral hepatitis). Manifestations of liver injury from any cause commonly include anorexia, malaise, and fatigue. Yellow discoloration may first occur in the sclera of the eye and then progress to the skin. Pruritus frequently accompanies jaundice with an elevation of serum alkaline phosphatase and bilirubin accumulation in the skin.[103]

Evaluation and Treatment

Laboratory evaluation of serum establishes whether elevated plasma bilirubin is conjugated or unconjugated or both. Unconjugated bilirubinemia results from hemolysis or hereditary disorders of bilirubin metabolism. Elevations of conjugated bilirubin indicate liver injury or extrahepatic obstruction. The history and physical examination identify underlying disorders, such as alcoholism, exposure to hepatitis virus, or gallbladder disease. The treatment for jaundice consists of correcting the cause.

Hepatorenal Syndrome

Hepatorenal syndrome consists of advanced liver disease and functional renal failure with oliguria, sodium and water retention (with or without ascites and peripheral edema), hypotension, and peripheral vasodilation. Renal disorders associated with liver disease can have numerous causes, but hepatorenal syndrome is usually associated with alcoholic cirrhosis and fulminant hepatitis. The renal failure is not caused by primary renal disease or other extrinsic factors, but rather by systemic arterial vasodilation and vasoconstriction of the renal circulation.[104]

Pathophysiology

Oliguric hepatic failure generally accompanies a sudden decrease in blood volume secondary to massive gastrointestinal bleeding or hypotension caused by failing liver function. Hypotension also can be caused by the excessive use of diuretics to treat ascites with decreased renal blood flow, glomerular filtration rate, and oliguria. A significant number of individuals with advanced liver disease develop oliguria unrelated to any precipitating event. Inappropriate constriction of renal arterioles is proposed as the causative mechanism. Intrarenal vasoconstriction may result from the selective effects of vasoactive substances that accumulate in the blood because of liver failure. The diseased liver fails to remove excessive angiotensin, vasopressin, prostaglandins, and catecholamines from the blood. These substances travel to the kidneys and cause vasoconstriction. Vasoconstriction also may be a compensatory response to portal hypotension and the pooling of blood in the splanchnic circulation. The exact reason for the vasoconstriction is unknown[105] but is related to vasoconstrictive mediators[106] and sympathetic nerve stimulation. Systemic vasodilation caused by increases in nitric oxide and other substances may also contribute to vascular alterations and renal failure in advanced liver disease.[107]

Clinical Manifestations

The onset of hepatorenal manifestations may be gradual or acute. Oliguria and complications of advanced liver disease, including jaundice, ascites, and gastrointestinal bleeding, are usually present. Systolic blood pressure is usually below 100 mm Hg. Nonspecific symptoms of hepatorenal syndrome include anorexia, weakness, and fatigue.

Evaluation and Treatment

Despite oliguria, serum potassium levels do not become dangerously elevated until the terminal stages of the hepatorenal syndrome. Blood urea increases, followed by an increase in creatinine concentration. Urine osmolality is increased, but urine sodium concentrations are below normal. Urine specific gravity is above 1.015. Treatment may include systemic vasoconstrictors, transjugular intrahepatic portosystemic shunt, or simultaneous administration of plasma volume expansion and vasoconstrictors.[108] Liver transplant reverses symptoms.

Table 38-9 Characteristics of Viral Hepatitis

Characteristic	Hepatitis A	Hepatitis B	Hepatitis D	Hepatitis C	Hepatitis E	Hepatitis G
Size of virus	27 nm RNA virus	47 nm DNA virus	36 nm RNA virus, defective virus with HBsAg coat	30-60 nm RNA virus	32 nm RNA virus	30-60 nm RNA virus
Incubation period	30 days	60-180 days	30-180 days	35-60 days	15-60 days	Unknown
Route of transmission	Fecal-oral, parenteral, sexual	Parenteral, sexual	Parenteral, ? fecal-oral, sexual	Parenteral	Fecal-oral	Parenteral, sexual
Onset	Acute with fever	Insidious	Insidious	Insidious	Acute	Unknown
Carrier state	Negative	Positive	Positive	Positive	Negative	Positive
Severity	Mild	Severe; may be prolonged or chronic	Severe	Mild to severe	Severe in pregnant women	Unknown
Chronic hepatitis	No	Yes	Yes	Yes	No	Unknown
Age-group affected	Children and young adults	Any	Any	Any	Children and young adults	Any
Prophylaxis	Hygiene, immune serum globulin	Hygiene, HBV vaccine	Hygiene, HBV vaccine	Hygiene, screening blood, interferon-alpha	Hygiene, safe water	

RNA, Ribonucleic acid; *DNA,* deoxyribonucleic acid; *HBsAg,* hepatitis B surface antigen; *HBV,* hepatitis B virus.

The prognosis for hepatorenal syndrome is usually poor and is related to liver function. Secondary problems, including fluid and electrolyte disorders, bleeding, infections, and encephalopathy, are vigorously treated.

Disorders of the Liver

Viral Hepatitis

Viral hepatitis is a relatively common systemic disease that affects primarily the liver. Six strains of viruses cause various types of hepatitis: hepatitis A virus (HAV), hepatitis B virus (HBV), hepatitis D virus (HDV), hepatitis C virus (HCV), and hepatitis E virus (HEV). Hepatitis A used to be known as infectious hepatitis, and hepatitis B as serum hepatitis. Hepatitis G virus is usually not a significant cause of liver disease but it may be associated with fulminant hepatitis.[109] Characteristics of the various types are presented in Table 38-9.

Types

Hepatitis A. The hepatitis A virus can be recovered from the feces, bile, and sera of infected individuals. The usual mode of transmission is the fecal-oral route (contaminated food or water), but the virus can be spread also by the transfusion of infected blood. Approximately 45% of adults in urban areas have HAV antibodies in their blood. The disease spreads readily in crowded, unsanitary conditions, usually through contaminated food or water. Person-to-person spread is more likely to occur in settings such as day care centers or institutions for the mentally retarded, where there is close contact between clients and caregivers.[110]

The incubation period (the time between exposure and onset of symptoms) for hepatitis A is 4 to 6 weeks (Fig. 38-18). Fecal shedding of the virus is greatest for 10 to 14 days before the onset of symptoms and during the first week of symptoms and up to 3 months after onset of symptoms.[111] The disease is most contagious during this time. Antibodies to HAV (anti-HAV) develop about 4 weeks after infection. The serum immunoglobulin M (IgM) concentration increases initially and is followed by an increase of serum immunoglobulin G (IgG). IgG levels remain elevated for several years after infection, creating immunity to the disease. (See Chapter 6 for a description of immune functions.)

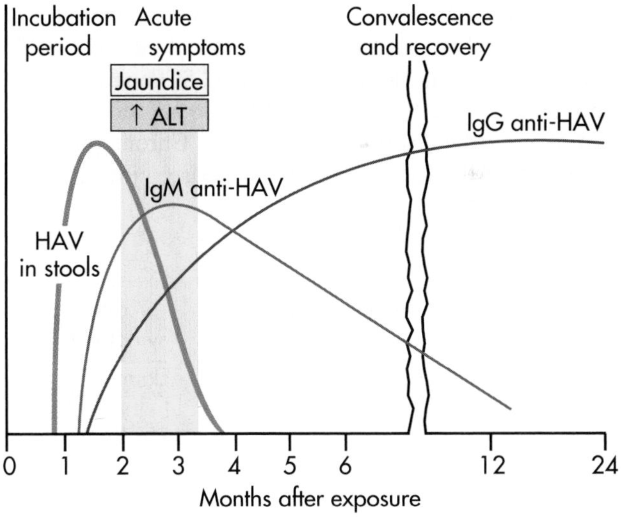

FIG. 38-18 Course of infection with the hepatitis A virus (HAV). *IgM,* Immunoglobulin M; *IgG,* immunoglobulin G.

Hepatitis B. Hepatitis B is transmitted through contact with infected blood, body fluids, or contaminated needles.

Hepatitis B is also a sexually transmitted disease (see Chapter 23). Transmission among homosexual men may be by oral or genital contact with bleeding lesions in the rectal mucosa. People receiving hemodialysis, multiple blood transfusions, or immunosuppressive drugs have a greater risk of exposure or less resistance to HBV. Mother-infant transmission occurs if the mother becomes infected during the third trimester of pregnancy. Approximately 0.3% of adults in the United States carry the hepatitis B surface antigen (HBsAg) marker for active HBV.[112]

Three types of viral particles are involved in HBV infection. The larger (47 nm) Dane particle probably represents the intact HBV. The Dane particle has a double-layered outer coat and carries the hepatitis B surface antigen (HBsAg), which was originally called the *Australia antigen*. HBsAg can be identified in the serum by radioimmunoassay. Hepatitis B core antigen (HBcAg) usually is not detected in the serum. The HBeAg is a derivative of HBcAg and is a marker of HBV replication. The HBV has an incubation period of 6 to 8 weeks. The initial serologic change is a transient increase in IgM. Levels of IgG antibodies to HBsAg rise more slowly and remain elevated for years (Fig. 38-19).

Hepatitis C. Hepatitis C virus (non-A, non-B hepatitis) causes most cases of posttransfusion hepatitis. Hepatitis C antibody is present in 1.8% of the United States population with new infections from intravenous drug use.[113] The risk for developing hepatitis C is greater with large volumes of blood replacement and among intravenous drug users. HCV is a ribonucleic acid (RNA) virus; the U.S. Food and Drug Administration (FDA) has approved an assay for screening hepatitis C antibodies in blood products. Chronic hepatitis C is a risk factor for chronic liver disease, cirrhosis, and carcinoma.[114]

Hepatitis D. The hepatitis D virus (HDV) occurs in individuals with hepatitis B. The delta virus depends on the hepatitis B virus for its replication because the coat of the delta virus consists of HBsAg molecules that are on the surface of the HBV virus. Parenteral drug users have a high incidence of HDV infection. Hepatitis D has been shown to suppress replication of hepatitis B virus.[115] The clinical course of HDV is similar to that of hepatitis A and B, although it is sometimes more severe.

Hepatitis E. Hepatitis E is most common in developing countries and is transmitted by the fecal-oral route,[116] usually

WHAT'S NEW? New Hepatitis Viruses

Five hepatitis viruses are currently recognized: A, B, C, D, and E. Two new viruses have provisionally been designated as hepatitis F virus and hepatitis G virus. Hepatitis F is an enteric virus isolated from human stool and transmitted experimentally to primates. Hepatitis G virus (HGV) is associated with acute and chronic non-ABCDE hepatitis and has worldwide distribution. It is transmitted parenterally but does not seem to cause classic hepatitis in most cases. Whether HGV causes chronic hepatitis is still unknown. The hepatitis GB agents are non-ABCDE viruses and consist of two flavivirus-like viruses: GBV-A and GBV-B. GBV-C and HGV appear to be different strains of the same virus and will require genetic coding for differentiation. It is likely that there is at least one blood-borne hepatitis virus to be discovered to explain hepatitis syndromes.

Data from Linnen J et al: *Science* 271:505, 1996; Fry DE: The ABCs of hepatitis, *Adv Surg* 33:413, 1999; Robaczewska M et al: Hepatitis G virus: molecular organization, methods of detection, prevalence, and disease association, *Int J Infect Dis* 3(4):220, 1999.

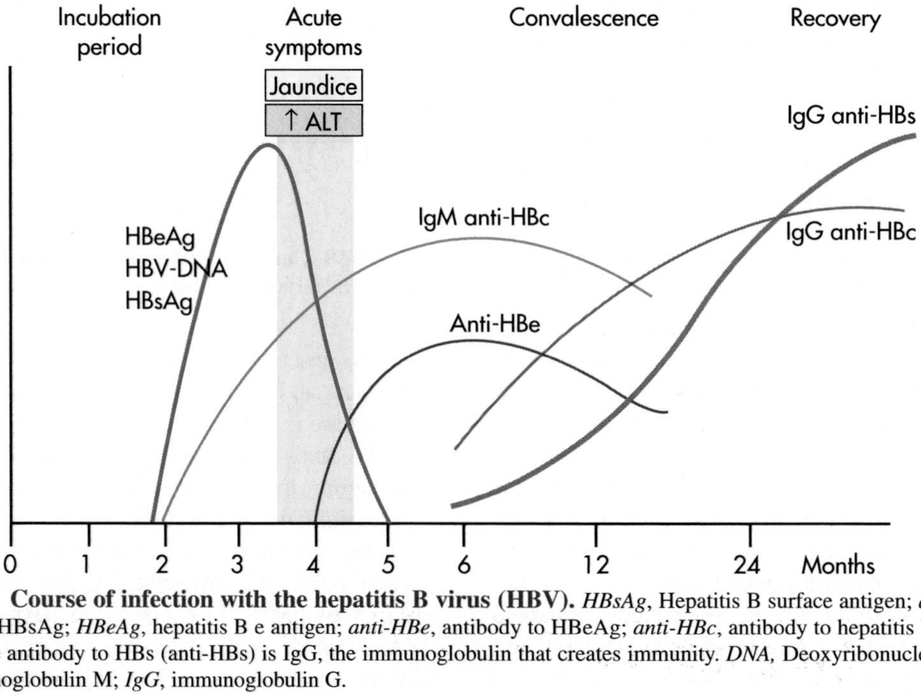

FIG. 38-19 Course of infection with the hepatitis B virus (HBV). *HBsAg*, Hepatitis B surface antigen; *anti-HBs*, antibody to HBsAg; *HBeAg*, hepatitis B e antigen; *anti-HBe*, antibody to HBeAg; *anti-HBc*, antibody to hepatitis B core antigen. The antibody to HBs (anti-HBs) is IgG, the immunoglobulin that creates immunity. *DNA*, Deoxyribonucleic acid; *IgM*, immunoglobulin M; *IgG*, immunoglobulin G.

by contaminated water. It is more prevalent among adults and has the highest mortality in pregnant women. Clinically, it resembles HAV.

Hepatitis G. Hepatitis G virus is a recently discovered parenterally and sexually transmitted virus. Currently there is still much unknown about this virus. No association with hepatocellular carcinoma is reported.[117,118]

Pathophysiology

The pathologic lesions of hepatitis are similar to those caused by other viral infection. Hepatic cell necrosis, scarring, Kupffer cell hyperplasia, and infiltration by mononuclear phagocytes occur with varying severity. Cellular injury is promoted by cell-mediated immune mechanisms (i.e., cytotoxic T cells and natural killer cells). Regeneration of hepatic cells begins within 48 hours of injury. The inflammatory process can damage and obstruct bile canaliculi, leading to cholestasis and obstructive jaundice. In milder cases the liver parenchyma is not damaged. Damage tends to be most severe in cases of hepatitis B and hepatitis C. Hepatitis B is also associated with acute fulminating hepatitis, a rare form of the disease that is characterized by massive hepatic necrosis. Acute fulminating hepatitis causes severe encephalopathy, which is manifested as confusion, stupor, and coma. Liver failure can occur, leading to intestinal bleeding, cardiorespiratory insufficiency, and renal failure. Mortality is high, but recovery can be complete.

Clinical Manifestations

The clinical manifestations of the various types of hepatitis are very similar. The spectrum of manifestations ranges from absence of symptoms to fulminating hepatitis, with rapid onset of liver failure and coma. Acute viral hepatitis causes abnormal liver function test results. The serum aminotransferase values, aspartate transaminase (AST) and alanine transaminase (ALT), are elevated, but their elevation may not be consistent with the extent of cellular damage. The clinical course of hepatitis usually consists of three phases: the prodromal, icteric, and recovery phases.

Prodromal phase. The **prodromal phase** of hepatitis begins about 2 weeks after exposure and ends with the appearance of jaundice. Fatigue, anorexia, malaise, nausea, vomiting, headache, hyperalgia, cough, and low-grade fever are prodromal symptoms that precede the onset of jaundice. Food odors often cause nausea, and changes in taste suppress the desire to smoke and drink alcohol. Right upper abdominal pain is common, and a weight loss of 2 to 4 kg is not unusual. The infection is highly transmissible during this phase.

Icteric phase (jaundice). The **icteric phase** begins about 1 to 2 weeks after the prodromal phase and lasts 2 to 6 weeks. Hepatocellular destruction and intrahepatic bile stasis cause jaundice (icterus). The urine may be dark and the stools clay colored before the onset of jaundice. The icteric phase is the actual phase of illness. The liver is enlarged, smooth, and tender, and percussion over the liver causes pain. During the icteric phase, gastrointestinal and respiratory symptoms subside but fatigue and abdominal pain may persist or become more severe. Serum bilirubin levels range from 5 to 10 mg/dl, with both conjugated and unconjugated fractions increasing. The jaundice may last 2 to 6 weeks or longer. Mild and transient itching often accompanies jaundice. The prothrombin time may be prolonged in individuals with more serious forms of the disease.

Recovery phase. The posticteric or **recovery phase** begins with resolution of jaundice, about 6 to 8 weeks after exposure. Although the liver may still be enlarged and tender, symptoms diminish. In most cases, liver function test results return to normal within 2 to 12 weeks after the onset of jaundice.

Chronic hepatitis may begin at this point and is associated with HBV infection. **Chronic active hepatitis** is the persistence of clinical manifestations and liver inflammation after acute hepatitis B, hepatitis C, and hepatitis D. Liver function tests remain abnormal for longer than 6 months, and HBsAg persists. Chronic, active hepatitis B is a predisposition to cirrhosis and primary hepatocellular carcinoma. Hepatitis C can be transmitted from mothers to infants.[119]

Evaluation and Treatment

The most specific diagnostic test for viral hepatitis is serologic analysis for HBsAg, which is the marker for HBV. Diagnosis of type A hepatitis is based on the presence of anti-HAV, as is the diagnosis of HCV. The assay for HDV is the total antibody to hepatitis D and antigen (anti-HDV). A test for HEV has not been developed. Liver function tests also can indicate other viral liver diseases, drug toxicity, or alcoholic hepatitis.

There is no specific treatment for acute viral hepatitis. Physical activity may be restricted. A low-fat, high-carbohydrate diet is beneficial if bile flow is obstructed. Interferon can be useful in the treatment of chronic hepatitis B and hepatitis C.[120]

To prevent transmission of hepatitis A, hand washing and use of gloves for disposing of bedpans and fecal matter are imperative. There should be no direct contact with blood or body fluids of patients with hepatitis B or hepatitis C. The administration of immune globulin before exposure or early in the incubation period can prevent hepatitis A. A vaccine for HAV and HBV is now available.[121] Interferon-α is effectively used for the treatment of chronic hepatitis B. Prophylactic immune globulin administered before exposure can also prevent hepatitis B, as can lamivudine for selected individuals.[122] Prophylaxis is recommended for health care workers and others who are at risk for contact with infected body fluids.[123]

Fulminant Hepatitis

Fulminant hepatitis is a clinical syndrome resulting in severe impairment or necrosis of liver cells and potential liver failure. The disorder may occur as a complication of hepatitis C or hepatitis B, particularly HBV infection compounded by infection with the delta virus. Toxic reactions to drugs and congenital metabolic disorders also can cause fulminant hepatitis.

Causative mechanisms of fulminant hepatic failure are poorly understood. Hepatocytes become edematous, and patchy areas of necrosis and inflammatory cell infiltrates disrupt the parenchyma. The death of hepatocytes may be caused by viral or immunologic damage.

Fulminant hepatitis usually develops 6 to 8 weeks after the initial symptoms of viral hepatitis or a metabolic liver disorder. Anorexia, vomiting, abdominal pain, and progressive jaundice are initial signs, followed by ascites and gastrointestinal bleeding. Hepatic encephalopathy is manifested as lethargy, altered motor functions, and coma. Liver function tests show elevations of both direct and indirect serum bilirubin, serum transaminases, and blood ammonia. Prothrombin time is prolonged.

Treatment of fulminant hepatitis is supportive. The hepatic necrosis is irreversible, and 60% to 90% of affected children die. Liver transplantation may be life saving.[124] Survivors usually do not develop cirrhosis or chronic liver disease. A bioartificial liver is being tested as a bridge to transplant.[125]

Cirrhosis

Cirrhosis is an irreversible inflammatory disease that disrupts liver structure and function and is a leading cause of death in the United States. Disorganization of hepatic tissues is caused by diffuse fibrosis and nodular regeneration. Nodules of regenerated tissue form between fibrous bands, giving the liver a cobbly appearance. The liver may be larger or smaller than normal, and usually it is firm or hard when palpated. A variety of disorders can cause cirrhosis. Therefore it is often classified by cause (Table 38-10).

The precise process of cellular injury depends on the cause of cirrhosis, and the causes are not all clearly understood. Structural changes result from fibrosis, which is a consequence of inflammation. The parenchyma of the liver becomes distorted, and biliary channels may be altered or obstructed, producing jaundice. Obstruction caused by cirrhosis can cause portal hypertension (see p. 1285). New vascular channels can form shunts, and blood from the portal vein bypasses the liver. These vascular changes compromise liver function further, and the process of regeneration is replaced by hypoxia; necrosis; atrophy; and, ultimately, liver failure.

Cirrhosis develops slowly over a period of years. Its severity and rate of progression depend on the cause. If toxins, such as alcohol, are involved, the rate of cell death and the severity of inflammation depend on the amount of toxin present.[126]

Alcoholic Cirrhosis

Alcoholic hepatitis is a precursor of cirrhosis characterized by inflammation, degeneration, and necrosis of hepatocytes, infiltration of polymorphonuclear leukocytes and lymphocytes, immunologic alterations, and lipid peroxidation. The injured hepatocytes contain Mallory bodies (hyaline endoplasmic reticulum). The presence of Mallory bodies indicates the onset of fibrosis. The mechanism of hepatocyte injury is not clearly understood, but immunologic factors are suggested. Serum IgA is often elevated in individuals with alcoholic hepatitis, and liver antigens and antibodies have been identified in persons with progressive alcoholic liver disease. The inflammation and necrosis caused by alcoholic hepatitis stimulate the fibrosis characteristic of the cirrhotic stage of disease.[127]

Deaths from alcohol-related liver disease have increased over the past decade. The incidence of alcoholic cirrhosis is greatest in middle-age men. In the United States, mortality resulting from cirrhosis is highest among nonwhites. Although alcoholic cirrhosis is the most prevalent of the various types of cirrhosis, the occurrence of cirrhosis among persons with alcoholism is relatively low (approximately 25%). The amount and duration of alcohol consumption are positively related to the extent of liver damage. Abuse of any type of alcoholic beverage can cause cirrhosis. Malnutrition may add to the risk of cirrhosis in alcohol abusers.

Pathophysiology

Alcoholic cirrhosis is caused by the toxic effects of alcohol on the liver, immunologic alterations, and lipid peroxidation.[128] Alcoholic cirrhosis is also associated with HCV.[129] The oxidative metabolism of alcohol occurs primarily in the liver (see Chapter 2). Alcohol is transformed to acetalde-

Table 38-10 Cirrhosis of the Liver

Type and Disease Name	Causal Mechanisms	Pathophysiology
Alcoholic cirrhosis, Laennec cirrhosis, portal cirrhosis, fatty cirrhosis	Toxic effects of chronic, excessive alcohol intake; acetylaldehyde formed by alcohol metabolism damages hepatocytes	Fatty liver, inflammation (alcoholic hepatitis), and derangement of the lobular architecture by necrosis and fibrosis (cirrhosis)
Biliary cirrhosis (intrahepatic or extrahepatic obstruction of bile flow)		
Primary biliary cirrhosis	Unknown; possibly an autoimmune mechanism	Inflammation and scarring of lobular bile ducts
Secondary biliary cirrhosis	Obstruction by neoplasms, strictures, or gallstones	Inflammation and scarring of bile ducts proximal to the obstruction
Postnecrotic cirrhosis	Viral hepatitis caused by hepatitis C; drugs or other toxins; autoimmune destruction	Replacement of necrotic tissue with cirrhotic tissue, particularly fibrous, nodular scar tissue
Metabolic cirrhosis	Metabolic defects and storage disease, such as α1-antitrypsin deficiency, glycogen storage disease, hemochromatosis, Wilson disease, galactosemia	Inflammation and scarring with specific morphologic changes related to cause

hyde. Excessive amounts of acetaldehyde significantly alter hepatocyte function. Mitochondrial function is impaired, decreasing oxidation of fatty acid. Enzyme and protein synthesis may be depressed or altered, and hormone and ammonia degradation is diminished. Acetaldehyde inhibits export of proteins from the liver, alters metabolism of vitamins and minerals, promotes liver fibrosis, and induces malnutrition.[130] Reactive oxygen species formed from metabolism of ethanol can injure liver cells by lipid peroxidation. Alcohol may also stimulate the formation of autoantibodies specific to hepatic cells. Cellular damage initiates an inflammatory response. Inflammation and necrosis result in excessive collagen formation. Dense bands of fibrosis surround regenerative hepatocellular nodules. Fibrosis and scarring alter the structure of the liver and obstruct biliary and vascular channels.[131] Examples of liver damage are shown in Fig. 38-20.

Alcoholic cirrhosis begins with fatty infiltration and cirrhosis. The relationship among these stages of alcoholic liver disease is not clear. Fatty infiltration can occur without subsequent hepatitis or cirrhosis. Fat deposition (deposition of triglycerides) within the liver is caused primarily by increased lipogenesis and decreased fatty acid oxidation by hepatocytes. Lipids mobilized from adipose tissue or dietary fat intake may contribute to fat accumulation. Cessation of alcohol intake reverses the fatty accumulation.

Clinical Manifestations

Fatty infiltration causes no specific symptoms or abnormal liver function test results. The liver is usually enlarged, however, and the individual has a history of continuous alcohol intake during the previous weeks or months. Anorexia, nausea, jaundice, and edema develop with advanced fatty infiltration or the onset of alcoholic hepatitis (Fig. 38-21).

The clinical manifestations of alcoholic hepatitis can be mild or severe. Nonspecific symptoms include fatigue, weight loss, and anorexia.[132] Toxic effects of alcohol also can cause testicular atrophy, reduced libido, azoospermia, and decreased testosterone in men.[133] Manifestations of acute illness include nausea, anorexia, fever, abdominal pain, and jaundice. Cirrhosis is a multiple-system disease and causes hepatomegaly, splenomegaly, ascites, gastrointestinal hemorrhage, portal hypertension, hepatic encephalopathy, and esophageal varices. Anemia results from blood loss, poor nutrition, and hypersplenism. Risk for infection is greater, in part because of altered macrophage function.[134] The presence of numerous and severe manifestations increases the risk of death. The clinical features of alcoholic cirrhosis depend on the duration of the disease and the severity of liver damage.

Evaluation and Treatment

The diagnosis of alcoholic hepatitis is based on the individual's history and clinical manifestations. The results of liver function tests are abnormal, and serologic studies show elevated serum enzymes and bilirubin, decreased serum albumin, and prolonged prothrombin time.

Liver biopsy can confirm the diagnosis of cirrhosis, but biopsy is not necessary if clinical manifestations of cirrhosis are evident. Liver function test results are usually abnormal and reflect the severity of liver damage. In severe disease with a poor prognosis, the serum albumin concentration is very low, prolonged prothrombin times cannot easily be corrected with vitamin K therapy, and serum bilirubin levels are high.

There is no specific treatment for alcoholic cirrhosis, but many of the complications are treatable. Rest; a nutritious diet; and management of complications, such as ascites, gastrointestinal bleeding, and encephalopathy, are essential. Cessation of alcohol consumption slows the progression of liver damage, improves clinical symptoms, and prolongs life. Although the liver damage is irreversible, measures that halt the inflammation and destruction of liver cells prolong life.

Biliary Cirrhosis

Biliary cirrhosis differs from alcoholic cirrhosis in that the damage and inflammation leading to cirrhosis begin in bile canaliculi and bile ducts, rather than in the hepatocytes. The two types of biliary cirrhosis are *primary* and *secondary*. Although both involve bile duct pathology, they differ with respect to cause, risk factors, and mechanisms of obstruction and inflammation.

Primary biliary cirrhosis. **Primary biliary cirrhosis** is an autoimmune disease related to mitochondrial autoantibodies.[135] The disease is characterized by inflammation and destruction of small intrahepatic bile ducts with portal inflammation and, ultimately, fibrosis. Women are affected more commonly than men. Symptoms rarely develop before the

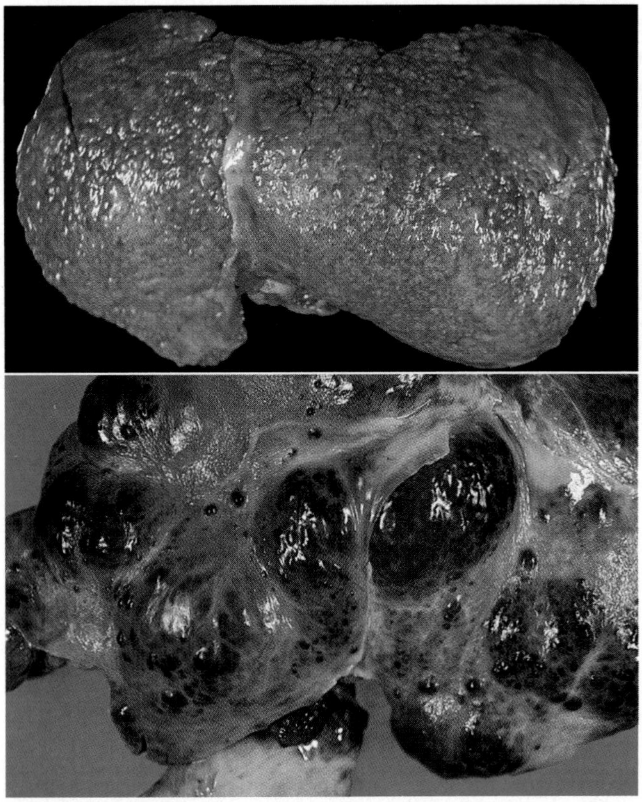

A

B

FIG. 38-20 Cirrhosis. **A,** Micronodular cirrhosis. **B,** Macronodular cirrhosis. (From Damjanov I, Linder J, editors: *Anderson's pathology*, ed 10, St Louis, 1996, Mosby.)

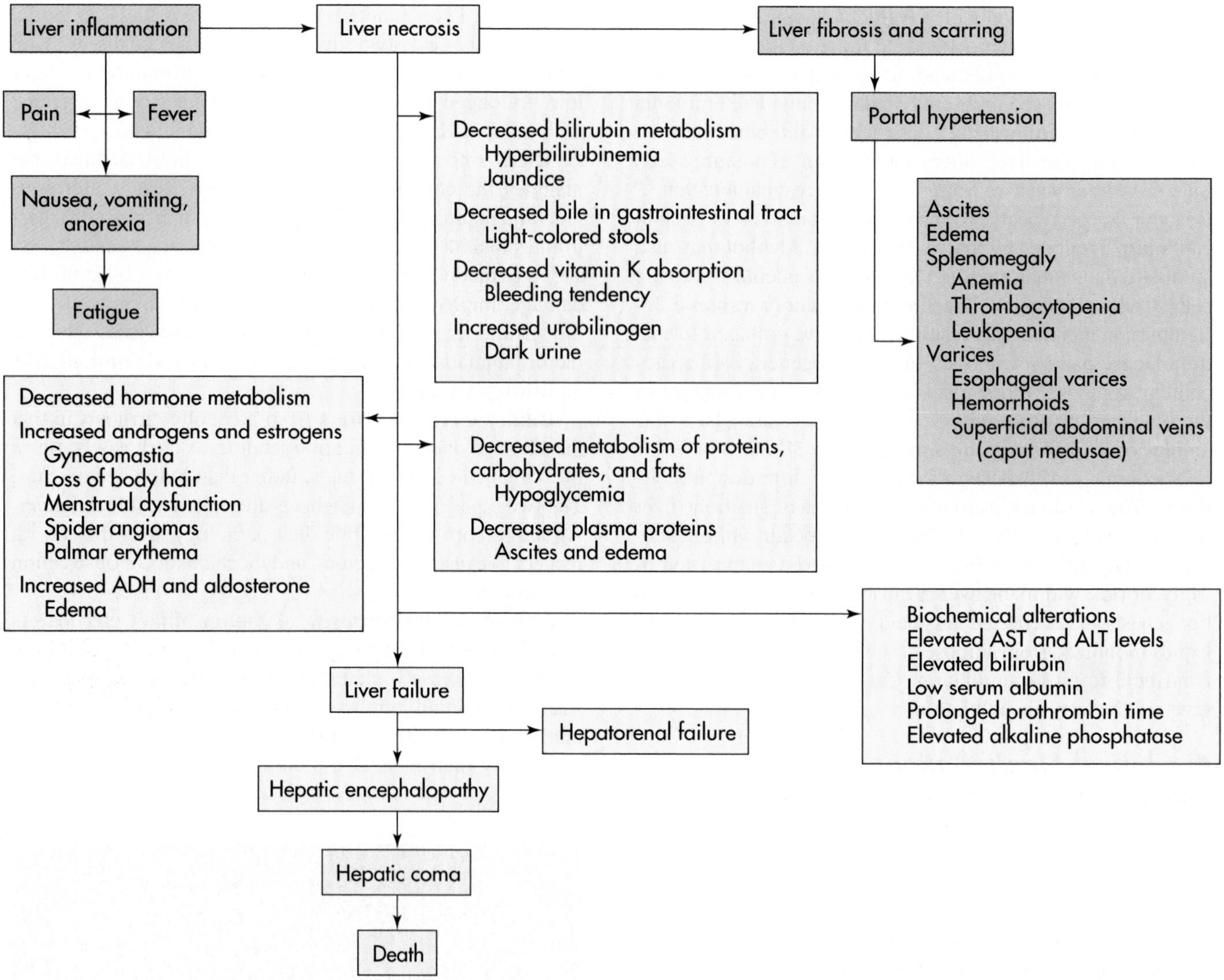

FIG. 38-21 Clinical manifestations of cirrhosis. *ADH*, Antidiuretic hormone; *AST*, aspartate transaminase; *ALT*, alanine transaminase.

age of 30 years. Primary biliary cirrhosis frequently accompanies collagen diseases.[136]

Primary biliary cirrhosis develops insidiously. It begins with inflammation, destruction, fibrosis, and obstruction of the intrahepatic bile ducts. Nodular regeneration and cirrhosis follow. Portal hypertension develops during the later stages of the disease.[137]

A significant number of individuals with primary biliary cirrhosis are asymptomatic. The earliest manifestations are pruritus, hyperbilirubinemia, jaundice, and light-colored stools. These symptoms are caused by intrahepatic obstruction of bile flow. Steatorrhea and fat-soluble vitamin deficiencies are present in some cases. Cirrhosis, symptoms of portal hypertension and encephalopathy, and ultimately liver failure develop. Life expectancy is approximately 5 to 10 years after onset of symptoms.

Serologic tests show elevated alkaline phosphatase levels and hyperlipidemia, with or without other clinical manifestations. Most individuals have a circulating IgG antimitochondrial antibody that is not found in other types of liver disease. Evaluation involves ruling out biliary obstruction caused by gallstones, tumor, or inflammation of the common bile duct (i.e., secondary biliary cirrhosis). Liver biopsy usually confirms the diagnosis of primary biliary cirrhosis.

Corticosteroids or azathioprine or both are used to suppress the immune response. No specific treatment is available. The distressing pruritus may be relieved by cholestyramine, which binds bile salts in the intestine. Intramuscular injections of vitamins D and K alleviate the vitamin deficiency. The other symptoms of cirrhosis are managed as they develop. Long-term treatment with ursodiol slows progression and decreases the need for liver transplant.[138]

Secondary biliary cirrhosis. **Secondary biliary cirrhosis** develops when there is prolonged partial or complete obstruction of the common bile duct or its branches. The obstruction may be caused by gallstones, tumors, fibrotic strictures, or chronic pancreatitis. Biliary atresia and cystic fibrosis cause secondary biliary cirrhosis in children.

Chronic obstruction to bile flow increases pressure in the hepatic bile duct and results in the accumulation of bile in the centrilobular spaces. Necrotic areas develop and are followed by proliferation and inflammation of the portal ducts that result in edema and fibrosis. Pools of bile form when the portal ducts rupture into surrounding necrotic areas. Injury is accompanied by regeneration of hepatic cells with the development of finely nodular cirrhosis.

Clinical manifestations are similar to those of primary biliary cirrhosis, with jaundice and pruritus the most distressing symptoms. Right upper quadrant pain is common, and a low-grade fever may be present from bile duct inflammation (cholangitis).

Cholangiography provides the most definitive diagnosis. Laboratory tests usually show elevated conjugated bilirubin and alkaline phosphatase levels. Aminotransferase increases if there is an accompanying cholangitis. Surgery or endoscopy relieves obstruction, prolongs survival, and diminishes or resolves symptoms. Continued obstruction leads to advanced cirrhosis and liver failure.

Postnecrotic Cirrhosis

Postnecrotic cirrhosis is a consequence of many types of chronic, severe liver disease. Of individuals with hepatitis C, 25% develop postnecrotic cirrhosis. Liver injury results from drugs or toxins; inherited metabolic disorders, such as Wilson disease; α_1-antitrypsin deficiency; advanced alcoholic cirrhosis; or primary biliary cirrhosis that progresses to postnecrotic cirrhosis.

Clinical manifestations represent a progression of symptoms associated with an earlier stage of liver disease. Portal hypertension with ascites, bleeding varices, hypersplenism, and encephalopathy are the most prominent symptoms. As a consequence of progressive liver injury, broad and dense bands of fibrosis separate islands of liver cells, giving the liver a nodular appearance. The liver is small in size and distorted in shape.

Diagnosis is confirmed by needle biopsy, and treatment is directed toward relief of symptoms. Death usually occurs as a result of bleeding or encephalopathy.

Disorders of the Gallbladder

Obstruction and inflammation are the most common disorders of the gallbladder. Obstruction is caused by **gallstones,** which are aggregates of substances in the bile. The gallstones may remain in the gallbladder or be ejected, with bile, into the cystic duct. Gallstones that become lodged in the cystic duct obstruct the flow of bile into and out of the gallbladder and cause inflammation. Gallstone formation is termed cholelithiasis. Inflammation of the gallbladder or cystic duct is known as cholecystitis.

Cholelithiasis

Cholelithiasis is a prevalent disorder in developed countries, where incidence is 10% to 20%. The actual incidence is unknown because many individuals who have gallstones are asymptomatic. Gallstones are of two types: cholesterol and pigmented.[139] Cholesterol stones are the most common (Fig. 38-22). Risk factors include obesity; middle age; female gender; American Indian ancestry; and gallbladder, pancreatic, or ileal disease. Pigmented stones, which are common, occur later in life and are associated with cirrhosis.

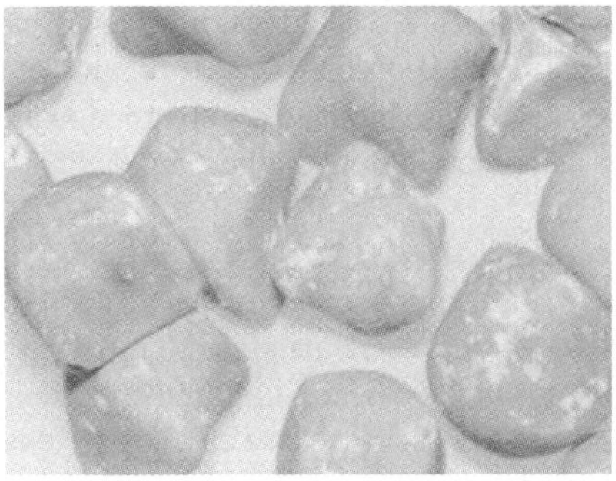

FIG. 38-22 Cholesterol stones. Stones are round and faceted; they can be 0.5 to 3 cm in size but are typically large. Biochemical analysis reveals over 50% cholesterol composition with lesser amounts of calcium salts so, strictly, most such stones are of mixed composition. (From Stevens A, Lowe J: *Pathology*, London, 1995, Mosby.)

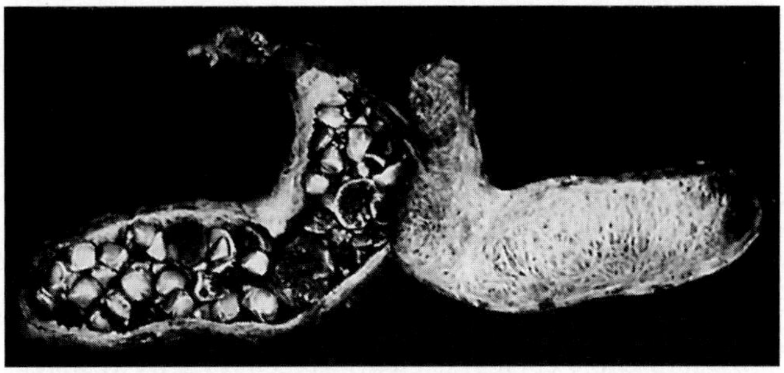

FIG. 38-23 Resected gallbladder containing mixed gallstones. (From Kissane JM, editor: *Anderson's pathology*, ed 9, St Louis, 1990, Mosby.)

Pathophysiology

Cholesterol gallstones form in bile that is supersaturated with cholesterol produced by the liver. Supersaturation sets the stage for cholesterol crystal formation, or the formation of "microstones." More crystals then aggregate on the microstones, which grow to form "macrostones." This process usually occurs in the gallbladder, which may have decreased motility. The stones may lie "silent" or become lodged in the cystic or common duct, causing pain and cholecystitis. Gallstone formation may be such that the stones accumulate and fill the entire gallbladder (Fig. 38-23).

It is not known why the hepatocytes secrete bile that is supersaturated with cholesterol. Proposed mechanisms include (1) an enzymatic defect that affects the hepatocytes' synthesis of cholesterol; (2) diminished secretion of bile acids, which normally promote cholesterol solubility; (3) decreased resorption of bile salts from the ileum, which decrease the bile acid pool; and (4) some combination of these mechanisms. In obese individuals the mechanism appears to involve cholesterol synthesis, whereas in nonobese individuals, it appears to involve decreased secretion of bile acids.

Pigmented stones are created by cholesterol, calcium bilirubinate, or pigmented polymers. The formation of pigmented stones is associated with biliary tract obstruction and bacterial degradation and precipitation of biliary lipids.[140]

Clinical Manifestations

Epigastric and right hypocondrium pain and intolerance to fatty foods are the cardinal manifestations of cholelithiasis. Vague symptoms include heartburn; flatulence; epigastric discomfort; and food intolerances, particularly to fats and cabbage. The pain, frequently called *biliary colic* is most characteristic and is caused by the lodging of one or more gallstones in the cystic or common duct.[141] The pain can be intermittent or steady. It usually is located in the right upper quadrant and radiates to the mid-upper back. Jaundice indicates that the stone is located in the common bile duct. Abdominal tenderness and fever indicate cholecystitis.

Evaluation and Treatment

Diagnosis is based on the patient's medical history, physical examination, and radiographic evaluation. An oral cholecystogram usually outlines the stones. Intravenous cholangiography is used to differentiate cholelithiasis from other causes of extrahepatic biliary obstruction if the cholecystogram is negative. Endoscopic or percutaneous cholangiography is also a diagnostic option.

Laparoscopic cholecystectomy is the preferred treatment for gallstones that cause obstruction or inflammation. An alternative treatment is the administration of drugs that dissolve the stones. For example, the bile acid chenodeoxycholic acid (CDCA) can completely or partially dissolve cholesterol gallstones. Ursodeoxycholic acid (UDCA), which is structurally similar to CDCA, is also effective; is less toxic to hepatocytes; and does not cause fatty diarrhea, as does CDCA.

Cholecystitis

Cholecystitis can be acute or chronic. Both forms are almost always caused by the lodging of a gallstone in the cystic duct. Obstruction causes the gallbladder to become distended and inflamed. The pain is similar to that caused by gallstones. Pressure against the distended wall of the gallbladder decreases blood flow. Ischemia, necrosis, and perforation of the gallbladder are possible. Fever, leukocytosis, rebound tenderness, and abdominal muscle guarding are common findings. Serum bilirubin and alkaline phosphatase levels may be elevated. Nevertheless, the acute abdominal pain of cholecystitis must be differentiated from the pain caused by other disorders, such as pancreatitis, myocardial infarction, and acute pyelonephritis of the right kidney. Cholangiography or radioactive scan can confirm a diagnosis of cholecystitis.

Narcotics may be required to control pain, and antibiotics (e.g., gentamicin and clindamycin) are often prescribed to manage bacterial infection in severe cases. Persistent symptoms or development of chronic cholecystitis punctuated by recurrent acute attacks usually requires gallbladder resection (cholecystectomy). If pancreatic abscesses develop, they usually are resected.[142]

Disorders of the Pancreas

Pancreatitis, or inflammation of the pancreas, is a relatively rare and potentially serious disorder. Incidence is about equal in men and women and is more common between 50 and 60 years of age. Pancreatitis can be acute or chronic. It is associated with several other clinical conditions, including alcoholism, obstructive biliary tract disease (particularly cholelithiasis), peptic ulcers, trauma, and hyperlipidemia; and with certain drugs.[143] The risk of mortality increases with the development of infection or pulmonary, cardiac, and renal complications.

Acute Pancreatitis

Pathophysiology

Acute pancreatitis (acute hemorrhagic pancreatitis) is usually a mild disease, but about 20% of those afflicted develop a severe pancreatic inflammation requiring hospital care. Although the precise pathogenic mechanism or sequence of events often is unknown, alcoholism and biliary tract obstruction are commonly associated. The most common theory is that pancreatitis develops because of an injury or disruption of the pancreatic ducts or acini, which permits leakage of pancreatic enzymes (trypsin, chymotrypsin, and elastase) into pancreatic tissue. The leaked enzymes become activated in the tissue, initiating autodigestion and acute pancreatitis (Fig. 38-24). Bile reflux into the pancreas occurs if gallstones obstruct the common bile duct and bile contributes to attacks of acute pancreatitis.[144] The activated proteolases (trypsin and elastase) and lipases break down tissue and cell membranes, causing edema, vascular damage, hemorrhage, and necrosis.[145] (Fatty necrosis is described in Chapter 2.) Toxic enzymes and inflammatory mediators (TNF-α, IL-1β, IL-6, IL-8, IL-10, C5a, ICAM, and substance P) are released into the bloodstream and cause injury to vessels and other organs, such as the lungs and kidneys.[146] Myocardial depression and shock can develop secondary to release of vasoactive peptides. These systemic effects are major causes of multiple-organ failure and mortality.

Clinical Manifestations

Epigastric or midabdominal pain is the cardinal symptom of acute pancreatitis. The pain may radiate to the back because

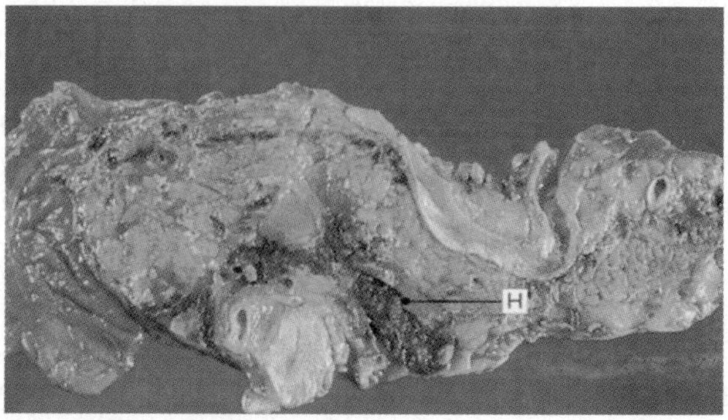

FIG. 38-24 Acute pancreatitis. The pancreas appears edematous and is commonly hemorrhagic. (From Stevens A, Lowe J: *Pathology*, London, 1995, Mosby.)

of the retroperitoneal location of the pancreas. The pain is caused by edema, which distends the pancreatic ducts and capsule; chemical irritation and inflammation of the peritoneum; and irritation or obstruction of the biliary tract. Fever and leukocytosis accompany the inflammatory response. Nausea and vomiting are caused by hypermotility or paralytic ileus secondary to the pancreatitis or peritonitis.

Abdominal distention accompanies bowel hypermotility and the accumulation of fluids in the peritoneal cavity. Hypotension and shock occur frequently because plasma volume is lost as enzymes and kinins released into the circulation increase vascular permeability and dilate vessels. Hypovolemia, hypotension, and myocardial insufficiency result. A small percentage of individuals develop tachypnea and hypoxemia secondary to pulmonary edema, atelectasis, or pleural effusions caused by circulating pancreatic enzymes. In severe cases, hypovolemia decreases renal blood flow sufficiently to impair renal function. Tetany may develop as a result of deposition of calcium in areas of fat necrosis or as a decreased response to parathormone. Transient hyperglycemia also can occur if glucagon is released from damaged A cells in the pancreatic islets. Multiple organ failure accounts for most deaths with severe pancreatitis. In hemorrhagic pancreatitis, some individuals develop flank or periumbilical ecchymosis, a sign of poor prognosis.

Evaluation and Treatment

Diagnosis of pancreatitis is based on clinical findings, identification of associated disorders, and laboratory studies. Elevated serum amylase is a characteristic diagnostic feature. The amylase level usually rises within 12 hours after the onset of symptoms and returns to normal within 3 to 5 days in most cases. Urine amylase and serum lipase also are elevated. Elevated C-reactive protein is a marker of severity.[147] The ratio of amylase clearance to creatinine clearance by the kidney can be diagnostic because, in cases of pancreatitis, amylase clearance increases significantly compared with creatinine clearance. Acute pancreatitis is difficult to diagnose because several other disorders can cause similar clinical and laboratory findings. These disorders include perforating duodenal ulcer, acute cholecystitis, small-bowel obstruction, and kidney stones. Ultrasound and computed tomography (CT) scan are used in more severe cases to evaluate extent of involvement and complications.

The goal of treatment for acute pancreatitis is to stop the process of autodigestion and prevent systemic complications. Narcotic medications may be needed to relieve pain. Meperidine hydrochloride (Demerol) is used instead of morphine because it causes less spasm of the sphincter of Oddi than morphine. To decrease pancreatic secretions and "rest the gland," oral food and fluids are withheld and continuous gastric suction is instituted. Nasogastric suction may not be necessary with mild pancreatitis but may help relieve pain and prevent paralytic ileus in individuals who are nauseated and vomiting. Enteral nutrition with use of jejunal tube feedings is often effective. Parenteral fluids are essential to restore blood volume and prevent hypotension and shock. Parenteral hyperalimentation should be initiated when enteral feeding is not tolerated.[148] Drugs that decrease gastric acid production (e.g., cimetidine) can decrease stimulation of the pancreas by secretin. Antibiotics may control infection. The risk of mortality increases significantly with the development of pulmonary, cardiac, and renal complications.

Chronic Pancreatitis

Structural or functional impairment of the pancreas leads to **chronic pancreatitis**. Chronic alcohol abuse is the most common cause.[149] Chronic pancreatitis causes continuous or intermittent abdominal pain, which usually intensifies after a meal. Pain is associated with increased intraductal pressure, increased tissue pressure, ischemia, neuritis, or ongoing injury.[150] Occasionally manifestations of pancreatic enzyme deficiency, such as steatorrhea or a malabsorption syndrome, are present. To correct enzyme deficiencies and prevent malabsorption, oral enzyme replacements are taken before and during meals. Loss of islet cell function can cause insulin-dependent diabetes. Cessation of alcohol intake is essential for the management of chronic pancreatitis.

Fibrosis, strictures, continued inflammation, and pancreatic cysts are common lesions of chronic pancreatitis. The cysts are walled-off areas or pockets of pancreatic juice, necrotic debris, or blood within or adjacent to the pancreas. Surgical drainage or partial resection of the pancreas may be required to relieve pain and prevent cystic rupture.[151] Chronic pancreatitis is a risk factor for pancreatic cancer.

CANCER OF THE DIGESTIVE SYSTEM

Cancer of the Gastrointestinal Tract

Cancer of the Esophagus

Carcinoma of the esophagus is a rare disease.[152] The incidence in the United States and Europe is less than 1% of new cancers per year.[153] The incidence in the United States is higher in blacks than in whites and peaks at about 60 years of age.

Dietary factors, particularly deficiencies of trace elements and vitamins, possibly influence carcinogenesis. Esophageal cancer is strongly associated with malnutrition caused by poor economic conditions, special dietary habits, or alcoholism.[154] Alcohol use and tobacco use have long been established as risk factors for esophageal cancer. The risk of esophageal cancer increases with the amount of alcohol consumed. Alcohol abuse, in combination with dietary zinc deficiency, renders the esophageal mucosa susceptible to carcinogens. Although heavy cigarette smoking is known to increase the risk of esophageal cancer, esophageal cancer is found more frequently in pipe and cigar smokers than cigarette smokers.

Reflux esophagitis is associated with carcinomas of the esophagus, as is sliding hiatal hernia. Both of these conditions can cause erosive esophagitis and ulceration that can eventually lead to metaplasia and neoplastic changes.

Pathogenesis

Carcinoma of the esophagus is usually squamous cell carcinoma or, less commonly, adenocarcinoma. Adenocarcinomas of the esophagus are frequently secondary to infiltration by a gastric carcinoma or to the presence of Barrett (dysplastic) epithelium (columnar rather than squamous epithelium in the lower esophagus), which is associated with chronic gastroesophageal reflux. Carcinomas can occur at any level of the esophageal tract but are most common where the esophagus joins the stomach (the gastroesophageal junction).[155,156]

The pathogenesis of esophageal carcinoma is facilitated by (1) alterations of esophageal structure and function that permit food and drink to remain in the esophagus for prolonged periods; (2) ulceration and metaplasia caused by esophageal reflux; and (3) long-term exposure to irritants, such as alcohol and tobacco, that cause neoplastic transformation (see Chapter 11). Chronic inadequate nutrition can impair both structure and function of the esophagus. Nutritional deprivation, particularly deficiencies of vitamin A and zinc, results in mucosal changes that make the esophageal mucosa vulnerable to neoplastic changes. Mutation of the TP53 gene is an early event in Barrett adenocarcinoma.[157]

Clinical Manifestations

The two main manifestations of esophageal carcinoma are chest pain and dysphagia. The most common type of pain is heartburn (pyrosis). It is initiated by eating spicy or highly seasoned foods and by lying down. Dysphagia (pain on swallowing), another common symptom, is usually pressurelike and may radiate posteriorly between the scapulae. Odynophagia may be initiated by the swallowing of cold liquids. Spontaneous chest pain is more difficult to diagnose positively. Some individuals with esophageal cancer complain of a constant retrosternal pain that radiates to the back. Dysphagia usually progresses rapidly. It is mostly painless during the early stages of esophageal carcinoma.

Evaluation and Treatment

Individuals who present with dysphagia undergo endoscopy so that specimens can be obtained and examined for neoplastic change. CT studies of the thorax also are used for diagnosis. Untreated esophageal cancer metastasizes rapidly and therefore has a poor prognosis. The lymphatic vessels of the esophagus are continuous with vital mediastinal structures and drain to the lymph nodes from the neck of the celiac axis, making it impossible to remove all the lymph nodes with the tumor. Removal of the primary lesion and the local lymph nodes, however, can benefit the individual with esophageal cancer. If the malignancy has not spread beyond these sites, cure is likely. If spread has occurred, however, an incomplete resection is of little benefit.

Cancer of the Stomach

Although the incidence of gastric cancer has declined in the United States, it still represents about 2% (21,500 cases) of all new cancer cases annually.[153] In countries such as Japan, the British Isles, and Iceland, the incidence of stomach cancer has remained high consistently. The incidence rate in Japan is one of the highest in the world. Studies of Japanese immigrants to the United States show that offspring who are born and raised in the United States have an incidence rate comparable to that of other Americans. These data illustrate the importance of environmental factors, such as diet, to carcinogenesis.

The most important risk factors in causing gastric cancer are (1) infection with *Helicobacter Pylori*; (2) salt added to food; (3) food additives (e.g., nitrates) in pickled or salted foods (e.g., bacon); and (4) low intake of fruits and vegetables. Vitamin C and carotenoids are possible protective factors. Dietary salt enhances the conversion of nitrates to carcinogenic nitrosamines in the stomach. Salt is also caustic to the stomach and can cause chronic atrophic gastritis. Finally, hypertonic salt solutions delay gastric emptying. Delayed emptying increases the time during which carcinogenic nitrosamines can exert their effects on the stomach mucosa. Infection with *H. pylori* and severe chronic gastritis change the mucosal cell proliferation pattern, increasing the risk for gastric and duodenal carcinoma.[158,159,160]

The metabolism of nitrates and nitrites is very complex. Nitrates interact with amino acids in the stomach to form nitrosamines. The conversion of these carcinogenic nitrosamines is enhanced at a low pH by iodides and thiocyanates. Nitrates are thought to be active only when converted to nitrites and to cause stomach cancer once atrophic gastritis has occurred.

The incidence of gastric cancer is greater in males than in females. Other nonenvironmental risk factors are a family history of gastric adenocarcinoma; blood type (blood group A); and pernicious anemia, which causes atrophy of the gastric mucosa in the same locations where gastric tumors arise.

Pathogenesis

Gastric cancer usually begins in the glands of the stomach mucosa. Approximately 50% of all gastric cancers develop in the prepyloric antrum (Fig. 38-25). Atrophic gastritis and intestinal metaplasia are strongly linked to the development of gastric cancer.[161] Insufficient acid secretion by the atrophic mucosa creates a relatively alkaline environment that permits bacteria to multiply and act on nitrates. The resulting increase

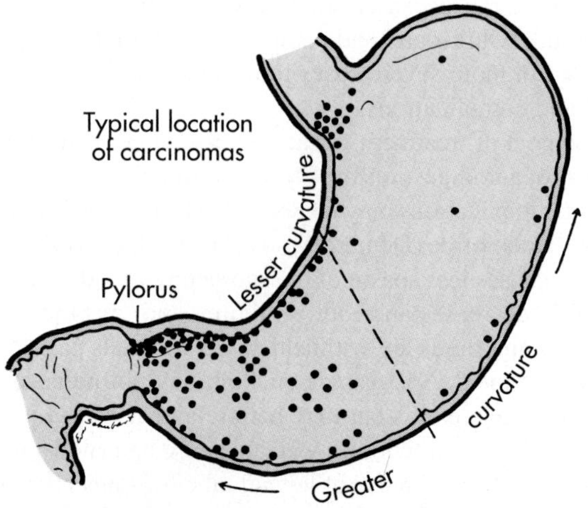

FIG. 38-25 Typical sites of stomach cancer. (From del Regato JA, Spjut HJ, Cox JD: *Cancer: diagnosis, treatment, and prognosis*, ed 2, St Louis, 1985, Mosby.)

in nitrosoamines damages the deoxyribonucleic acid (DNA) of mucosal cells further, promoting metaplasia and neoplasia. Duodenal reflux may also contribute to intestinal metaplasia. The reflux contains caustic bile salts that destroy the mucosal barrier that normally protects the stomach.

◆ *Clinical Manifestations*

The early stages of gastric cancer are generally asymptomatic or produce vague symptoms such as loss of appetite (especially for meat), malaise, and "indigestion." Later manifestations of gastric cancer include unexplained weight loss, upper abdominal pain, vomiting, change in bowel habits, and anemia caused by persistent occult bleeding. The prognosis is poor because symptoms do not occur until the tumor has penetrated the muscle layers of the stomach; spread to surrounding tissues; and entered the draining lymph nodes and veins, causing distant metastases. Generally the first manifestations of carcinoma are caused by distant metastases.

◆ *Evaluation and Treatment*

The choice of diagnostic tests depends on the clinical manifestations at the time of presentation. Most symptoms suggest a problem in the upper gastrointestinal tract, and the lesion is shown by a barium roentgenogram. Direct endoscopic visualization and biopsy usually establish the diagnosis. Another definitive technique is microscopic examination of exfoliated cells obtained by lavage during endoscopy.

Surgery is the treatment for gastric cancer. Staging is determined by pathologic findings after resection. Radiation therapy is generally unsuccessful, and immunotherapy is still experimental. Chemotherapy sometimes reduces the tumor. Individuals who respond well to chemotherapy generally live longer than those who do not.

Cancer of the Colon and Rectum

Cancer of the lower intestinal tract (colorectal cancer) is the second most frequent cause of cancer death in the United States for both men and women. Colorectal cancer accounts for 10% to 15% of all cancer deaths.[153] Cancer of the colon tends to occur in individuals older than 50 years. It is rare in children. Worldwide, the prevalence of colorectal cancer is highest in populations with high socioeconomic standards, possibly because of dietary and lifestyle habits.[162,163] Cancer of the small intestine is rare and represents less than 1% of gastrointestinal cancers.

◆ *Pathogenesis*

Genetic events are associated with the development of colonic cancer (Fig. 38-26). Alterations in the p53 gene are present in 85% of colorectal cancers.[164,165] Allelic deletion on chromosomes 5, 17, and 18 appears to promote transition from normal to malignant colon mucosa. Dietary factors, including high fat, low fiber, and low calcium, may promote somatic mutations. Promoting mechanisms are related to prolonged contact of the fecal mass with colon mucosa[166] and substances produced by microflora of the sigmoid colon.[167,168] Lower risk for colon cancer is associated with diets high in cereal grains, vegetables, folic acid, and calcium and/or vitamin D; hormone replacement therapy; physical activity; and use of nonsteroidal antiinflammatory drugs.[169,170,171]

Many colorectal cancers develop from adenomatous polyps (chromosome 5 mutation). A polyp, or papilloma, is a fingerlike projection arising from the mucosal epithelium. Most polyps are benign. The adenomatous polyposis coli (APC) gene was first identified as the gene mutated in an inherited syndrome of colon cancer known as familial adenomatous polyposis coli (FAP).[172] The two major types of neoplastic polyps are pedunculated (stalk) adenomatous polyps

WHAT'S NEW? Prevention of Colon Cancer

Cancer of the colon is a major cause of cancer death. Nonsteroidal antiinflammatory drugs (NSAIDs) including aspirin decrease the incidence and mortality from colon cancer in humans by 45% to 50%. It has been observed that NSAIDs inhibit the proliferation rate, alter the cell cycle distribution, and induce apoptosis in colon cancer cell lines. In addition, dietary supplements of calcium; vitamins A, C, and E; carotenoids; and omega-3 fatty acids reduce cancers and abnormal epithelial proliferation in animals. The lipid fraction of wheat bran has demonstrated colon tumor inhibitor properties.

Data from DuBois RN et al: *Cancer Res* 56(4):733, 1996; Eastwood GL: *Dig Dis* 14(2):119, 1996; Dubois RN: Review article: cyclooxygenase—a target for colon cancer prevention, *Aliment Pharmacol Ther* 14(sppl 1):64, 2000; Reddy BS et al: Prevention potential of wheat bran fractions against experimental colon carcinogenesis: implications for human colon cancer prevention, *Cancer Res* 60(17):4792, 2000.

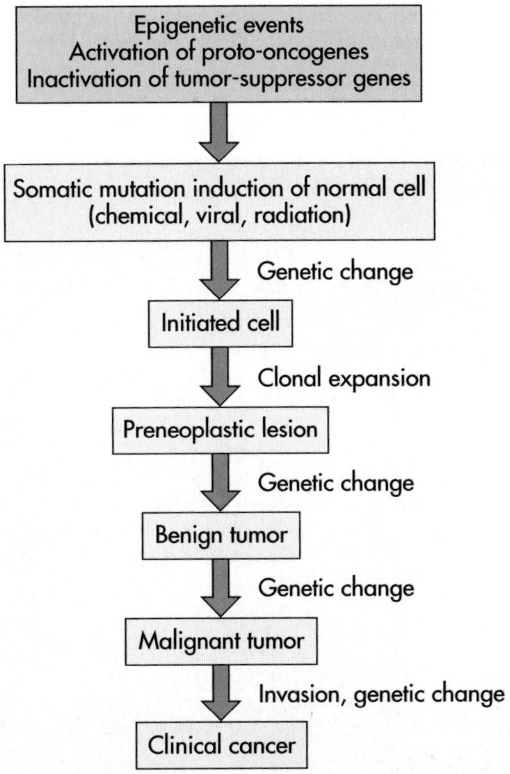

FIG. 38-26 Multistage development of colonic cancer.

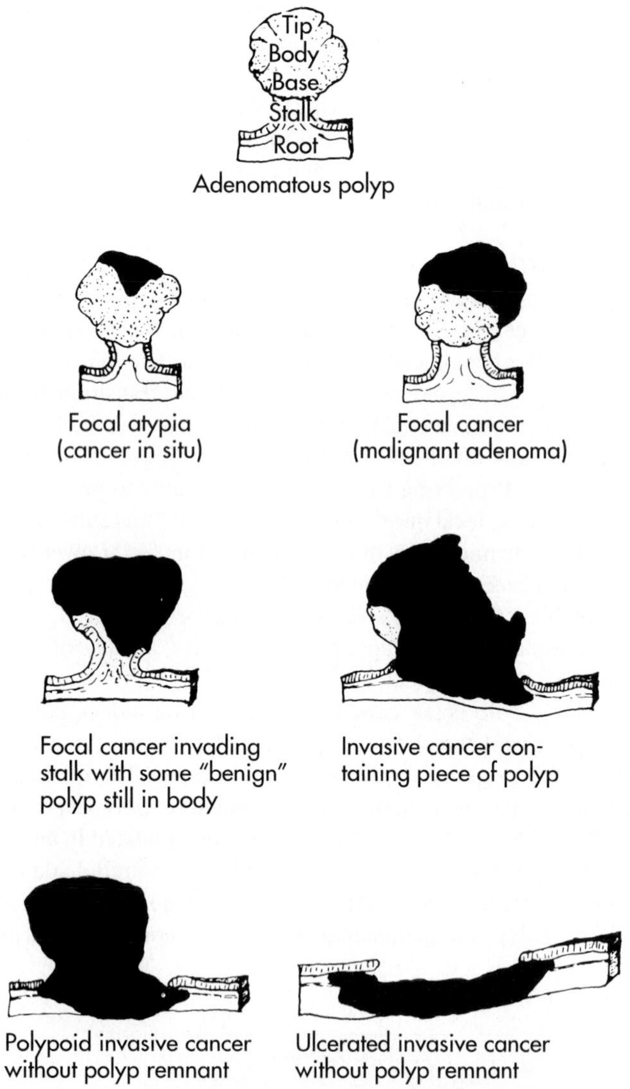

and sessile (papillary or villous) adenomas (Fig. 38-27). Once the adenoma traverses the muscularis mucosae, it becomes invasive and highly malignant. Adenomas can be detected early, however, and the submucosa may not be penetrated for several years. The larger the polyp is, the greater the risk of colorectal cancer. Although lesions larger than 1.5 cm occur less frequently, they are more likely to be malignant than those smaller than 1.0 cm. The adenomatous polyp forms in an area of epithelial cell hyperproliferation and crypt dysplasia. Table 38-11 gives other conditions commonly confused with colorectal cancer.

Most colorectal cancers are moderately differentiated adenocarcinomas. Progression to cancer is a multistep process and involves several suppressor genes that result in cell regulation abnormalities.[173] These tumors have a long preinvasive phase, and when they invade they tend to grow slowly. Because the lymphatic channels are located underneath the muscularis mucosae, the lesions must traverse this layer before metastasis can occur.

◆ *Clinical Manifestations*

Tumors of the right (ascending) and left (descending) colon evolve into two distinct tumor types. On the right side the lesions are polypoid and extend along one wall of the cecum and ascending colon. Clinical manifestations include pain, a palpable mass in the lower right quadrant, anemia, and dark red or mahogany-colored blood mixed with the stool (Fig. 38-28). These large, bulky tumors become necrotic and ulcerated, contributing to persistent blood loss and anemia. Obstruction is unusual because the feces are more liquid.

Tumors of the left, or descending, colon start as small, elevated, buttonlike masses. This type grows circumferentially and spreads along the entire bowel wall, eventually ulcerat-

B

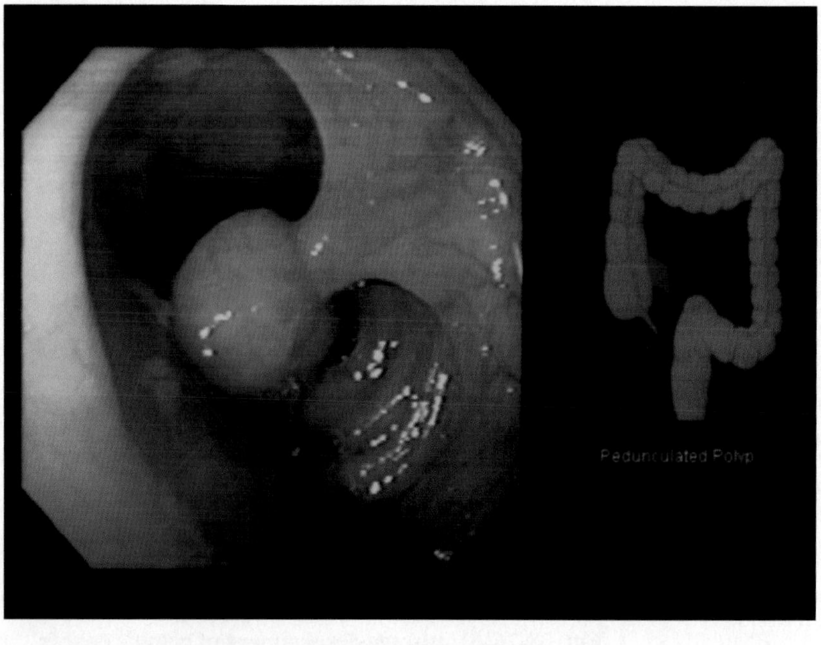

FIG. 38-27 Development of cancer of the colon from adenomatous polyps. A, The tumor becomes invasive if it penetrates the muscularis mucosae and enters the submucosal layer. **B,** Endoscopic image of pedunculated polyp in descending colon. (A from del Regato JA, Spjut HJ, Cox JD: *Cancer: diagnosis, treatment, and prognosis*, ed 2, St Louis, 1985, Mosby; B courtesy David Bjorkman, M.D., University of Utah School of Medicine, Department of Gastroenterology.

ing in the middle as the tumor penetrates the blood supply. Obstruction is frequent but occurs slowly. Manifestations include progressive abdominal distention, pain, vomiting, constipation, need for laxatives, cramps, and bright red blood on the surface of the stool.

Systemic lymphatic spread occurs along the aorta to the mesenteric and pancreatic lymph nodes. Liver metastasis follows invasion of the mesenteric veins (left colon) or superior veins (right colon), which drain into the portal circulation.

Rectal carcinomas are defined as tumors occurring up to 15 cm from the anal opening. Tumors of the rectum can spread through the rectal wall to nearby structures: the prostate in men and the vagina in women. Penetration occurs more readily in the lower third of the rectum because it has

Table 38-11 Conditions Commonly Confused with Colorectal Cancer

Condition	Significant Characteristics
Diverticulitis	Left-sided pain similar to that of appendicitis; tender lower left quadrant. Associated findings: nausea, vomiting, fever, obstruction, anorexia, and leukocytosis; mucosa is intact, and perforation, peritonitis, and abscesses occur more frequently than in cancer; proctosigmoidoscopy or barium enema used to distinguish from cancer:
Chronic ulcerative colitis	Younger people with chronic attacks of bloody diarrhea, crampy abdominal pain, fever, malnutrition, and dehydration; usually involves the left colon and rectum; endoscopy, barium enema, and biopsy performed for definitive diagnosis
Crohn disease (granulomatous colitis)	Generally involves the right colon; chronic diarrhea with abdominal cramps, fever, weight loss, and often a palpable abdominal mass; difficult at times to distinguish Crohn disease from ulcerative colitis; endoscopic examination and barium enema used to distinguish from cancer
Appendicitis	Vague abdominal symptoms, often with a tender or nontender mass in the lower right quadrant; associated symptoms: mild fever and leukycytosis; barium enema used to distinguish cancer of the cecum from appendiceal abscess
Thrombosed hemorrhoids	Examination shows a tender, swollen, bluish painful mass in the anus; patient will have a history of hemorrhoids

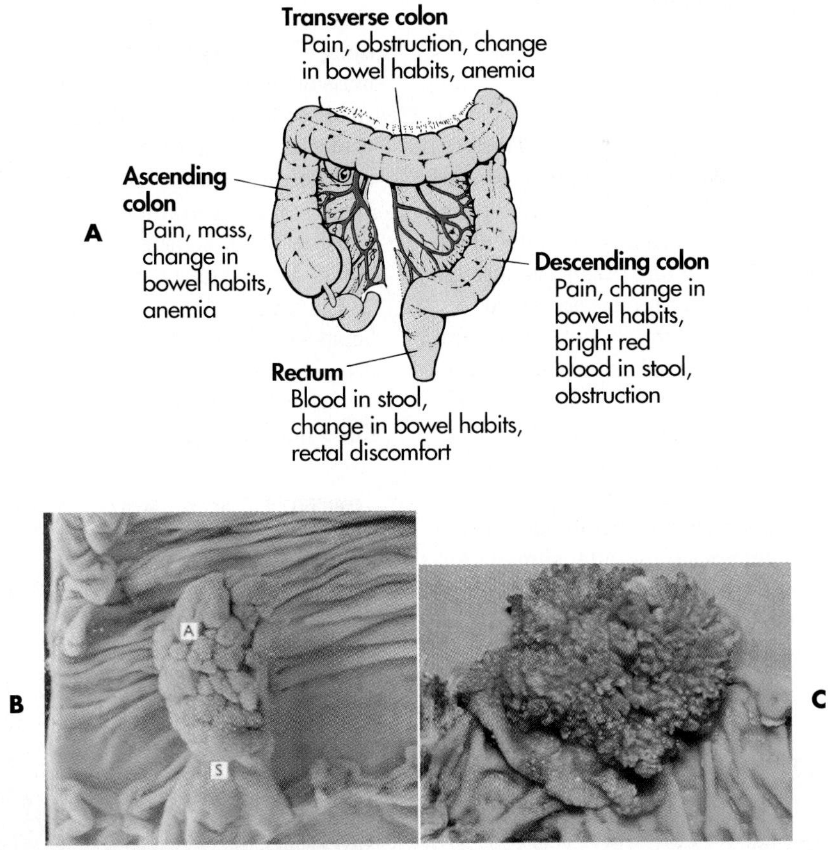

FIG. 38-28 Signs and symptoms of colorectal cancer by location of primary lesion. A, Clinical manifestations are listed in order of frequency for each region (lymphatics of colon also shown). **B,** Tubular adenomata *(A)* are rounded lesions 0.5 to 2 cm in size that are generally red and sit on a stalk *(S)* of normal mucosa that has been dragged up by traction of the polyp in the bowel lumen. C, Villous adenomata are frondlike lesions about 0.6 cm thick that occupy a broad area of mucosa generally 1 to 5 cm in diameter. (B and C from Stevens A, Lowe J: *Pathology*, London, 1995, Mosby.)

no serosal covering. Systemic and pulmonary metastases occur through the hemorrhoidal plexus, which drains into the vena cava.

Evaluation and Treatment

Individuals with a family history of polyps should be screened using colonoscopy, with removal of polyps when polyps are found. Screening asymptomatic at-risk individuals over age 50 includes fecal occult blood tests and sigmoidoscopy or colonoscopy.[174] A diet rich in vegetables, grains, fruit, and calcium and low in fat can modify cancer risk.[175,176] Genetic markers have been developed to identify inherited forms of colorectal cancer.[177,178]

The staging of colorectal cancer involves preoperative testing and operative exploration. Preoperative testing begins with physical examination of the abdomen to detect liver enlargement and ascites and palpate appropriate lymph nodes. Elevations of carcinoembryonic antigen (CEA) are often detected in the sera of individuals with colorectal carcinoma. The amount of CEA in the serum is a function of the stage of the disease and the type of tumor. Operative staging consists of careful exploration during surgery and biopsy of possible metastases. The Dukes classification for staging of colorectal cancer is as follows:

Stage A: cancer limited to the bowel wall
Stage B: cancer extending through the bowel wall
Stage C: nodal metastases regardless of extension into bowel wall
Stage D: distant metastases regardless of primary size

Treatment for cancer of the colon is always surgical. The location and amount of colon resected depend on the site of the cancer. Resection and anastomosis can be performed for cancer of the ascending, transverse, descending, or sigmoid colon and upper rectum. These surgeries are performed through abdominal incisions, and natural defecation is preserved.

Growths in the lower portion of the rectum require removal of the entire rectum. The proximal end of the descending colon is brought out through a small incision in the abdominal wall and becomes a permanent colostomy. Prognosis after surgery depends on the stage and location of the tumor.

Radiation therapy is often given before surgery in the hope that it will shrink the tumor, alter the malignant cells, or do both, so that these cells will not survive after surgery. Adjuvant chemotherapy is used to treat metastatic disease and cases with a high risk of recurrence. Immunotherapy can boost the immune response. Recombinant vaccines for colon cancer are in clinical trials.[179,180]

Cancer of the Accessory Organs of Digestion

Cancer of the Liver

Cancer in the liver is usually caused by metastatic spread from a primary site elsewhere in the body. Primary liver cancer is relatively rare in the United States but is common in densely populated parts of the Far East, southern Africa, China, and Greece. In the United States the number of deaths from liver cancer is greatest among Asians and Pacific Islanders (third leading cause of cancer deaths). For reasons not understood, incidence is higher in males than in females. Primary liver cancer is rare before the age of 40 years and most common during the sixth decade. Together, primary and secondary liver cancer accounts for less than 2% of all cancer deaths in the United States.[153]

Risk factors for primary liver cancer include the following:

1. Infection with hepatitis B virus (HBV), hepatitis C virus (HCV), and hepatitis D virus (HDV), particularly in conjunction with cirrhosis, acts either as a carcinogen or as a cocarcinogen in chronically infected hepatocytes.[181]
2. Chronic liver disease, especially cirrhosis.
3. Exposure to mycotoxins. The most significant mycotoxins are the aflatoxins, particularly those produced by *Aspergillus flavus,* a mold found on spoiled corn, peanuts, and grain. Aflatoxins cause mutation of the p53 suppressor gene.[182]
4. Heavy smoking and heavy drinking of alcohol.[183]

Pathogenesis

Primary carcinomas of the liver are hepatocellular or cholangiocellular. **Hepatocellular carcinoma (hepatocarcinoma)** develops in the hepatocytes, whereas **cholangiocellular carcinoma (cholangiocarcinoma)** develops in the bile ducts. Hepatocellular carcinoma can be nodular (consisting of multiple, discrete nodules), massive (consisting of a large tumor mass having satellite nodules), or diffuse (consisting of very small nodules distributed throughout most of the liver). Hepatocellular carcinoma is the type of primary liver cancer that is closely associated with cirrhosis (Fig. 38-29). Because carcinoma of the liver invades the hepatic and portal veins, it often spreads to the heart and lungs. Other sites of metastases are the brain, kidney, and spleen.

Cholangiocellular carcinomas occur less frequently than hepatocellular carcinomas. This type of primary liver cancer is most common in areas where liver fluke infestation is prevalent, such as southeast China. The mechanism by which fluke infestation causes cholangiocellular carcinoma is un-

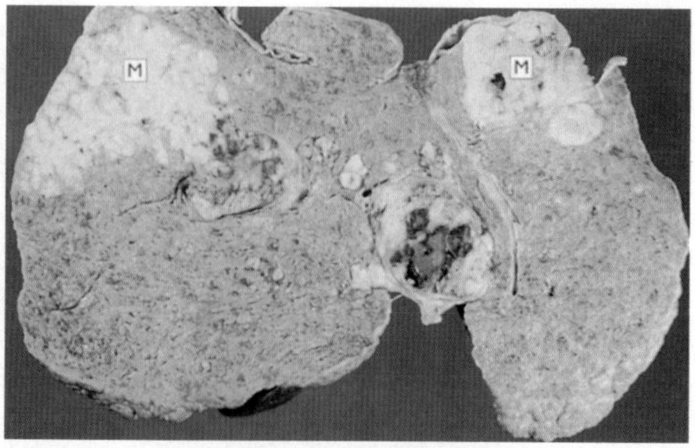

FIG. 38-29 Hepatocellular carcinoma. Macroscopically, hepatocellular carcinomas may be single or multifocal. They usually develop in a liver already affected by cirrhosis. Tumor appears as an abnormal mass *(M)* within the liver. (From Stevens A, Lowe J: *Pathology,* London, 1995, Mosby.)

known. Cholangiocellular carcinoma can occur anywhere along the bile duct and extend directly into the liver, usually as a solitary lesion. It is difficult to distinguish an invasion of cholangiocellular carcinoma from a metastatic adenocarcinoma except by neoplastic changes found in nearby ducts.

Clinical Manifestations

The clinical presentation of liver cancer in adults is characterized by vague abdominal symptoms, such as nausea and vomiting, fullness, pressure, and dull ache in the right hypochondrium. Manifestations of hepatocellular carcinoma can occur slowly or abruptly. In individuals with cirrhosis, deepening jaundice or abrupt lack of appetite is a sign of hepatocellular carcinoma. Obstruction by the tumor can cause sudden worsening of portal hypertension and development of ascites. As the tumor enlarges, it causes pain. Cholangiocellular carcinoma more commonly presents insidiously as pain, loss of appetite, weight loss, and gradual onset of jaundice. Some carcinomas of the liver rupture spontaneously, causing hemorrhage. Others are discovered accidentally during evaluation of a bone fracture or surgical exploration.

Evaluation and Treatment

There is no specific test for the diagnosis of liver cancer. The diagnosis is based on biopsy findings, laboratory findings, radiologic examination, and exploratory laparotomy.

Levels of alkaline phosphatase, serum glutamic oxaloacetic transaminase (AST), and serum glutamic pyruvic transaminase (ALT) are commonly elevated in individuals with hepatocellular carcinoma. α-Fetoprotein is elevated (in excess of 400 ng/ml) in individuals with advanced hepatocellular carcinoma. Excessive levels of α-fetoprotein have been correlated with hepatitis B antigen, rapid tumor growth, and poor tumor differentiation. Erythrocytosis is secondary to erythropoietin production.

In individuals without cirrhosis, liver scans can document filling defects. CT or ultrasonography is used to detect solid tumors, but neither can distinguish benign from malignant tumors. A liver biopsy can be diagnostic unless scattered nodules are missed by the examiner.

Surgical resection is possible only if the tumor is localized to a removable lobe of the liver. Tumors of the posterior segment of the right lobe are not resectable, because this segment contains the right hepatic vein. Chemotherapeutic agents are administered systemically or locally. Radiation is not part of the treatment regimen, because the dosages needed for effectiveness exceed the tolerance of liver tissue. Liver transplant and alcohol injection are alternatives for small tumors.[184]

The overall median survival rate for those with symptomatic liver cancer is only 3 to 4 months. Surgery is hazardous and usually not undertaken if the individual has cirrhosis. Most individuals develop metastases after surgical resection, but long-term survival is possible.

Cancer of the Gallbladder

Cancer of the gallbladder is more common in women than in men by a ratio of about 4 to 3.[153] It occurs rarely before the age of 40 years and is most common between the ages of 50 and 60 years. Obesity is a risk factor. Native populations in North and South America have greater risk.[185] Most gallbladder cancer is caused by metastasis. Primary carcinoma of the gallbladder is rare and is usually associated with chronic cholecystitis and cholelithiasis.

Pathogenesis

Most primary carcinomas of the gallbladder are adenocarcinomas. A few are squamous cell carcinomas. p53 gene mutation and overexpression and K-ras gene mutation occur.[186] Invasion of the liver occurs early. Spreading occurs to the cystic and periportal lymph nodes with invasion of the pancreas and retroperitoneal lymph nodes. Direct invasion of the stomach and the duodenum can cause pyloric obstruction. Infection often accompanies cancer of the gallbladder. Generalized peritonitis, gangrene, perforation, and liver abscesses are potential complications of infection.

Clinical Manifestations

A typical presentation of carcinoma of the gallbladder is steady, upper-right-quadrant pain for about 2 months. Other manifestations include diarrhea, belching, weakness, loss of appetite, weight loss, and vomiting. Obstructive jaundice can occur if an enlarging tumor presses on the extrahepatic ducts.

Evaluation and Treatment

Early diagnosis of cancer of the gallbladder is not possible. Therefore individuals with gallstones, especially older women, are evaluated carefully. Inflammatory disorders, such as cholangitis (bile duct inflammation) and peritonitis, often obscure an underlying malignancy. The most specific diagnostic procedures include ultrasonography, CT, and (magnetic resonance imaging) MRI.

Complete surgical resection of the gallbladder is the only effective treatment. Because advanced malignancies cannot be resected, gallbladders containing stones are removed as a preventive measure. The prognosis of gallbladder cancer is extremely poor; most individuals die within 1 year after surgery.[187]

Cancer of the Pancreas

Pancreatic cancer now ranks fourth in men and fifth in women as a cause of cancer deaths in the United States. The incidence of pancreatic cancer rises steadily with age. Males are affected slightly more often than females and blacks more often than whites. Pancreatic cancer accounts for about 28,200 deaths annually in the United States.[153] Mortality is nearly 100%. The cause of pancreatic cancer is not known, and with the exception of an association of risk with cigarette smoking, no external risk factors have been identified.[153] Pancreatitis is associated with 50% of pancreatic cancers.[188]

Pathogenesis

Cancer of the pancreas can arise from exocrine or endocrine cells. Most pancreatic tumors arise from exocrine cells in the ducts and are called *ductal adenocarcinomas*. Tumors arising in small ducts invade nearby glandular tissue, penetrate the covering of the pancreas, and extend into

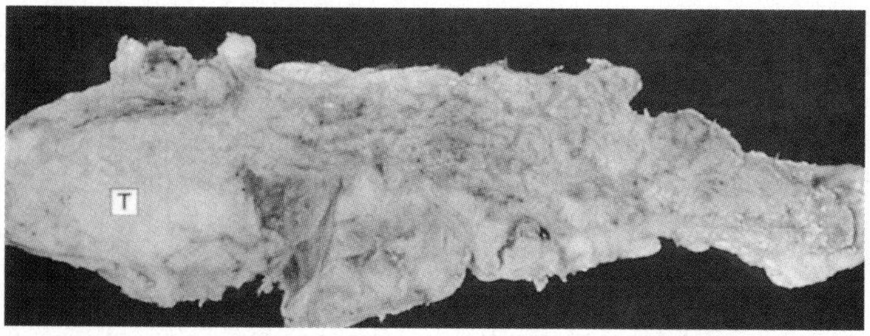

FIG. 38-30 Hepatocellular carcinoma. Tumors appear as gritty, gray, hard nodules *(T)* irregularly invading the adjacent gland and local structures. (From Stevens A, Lowe J: *Pathology*, London, 1995, Mosby.)

Table 38-12 Cancer of the Gut, Liver, and Pancreas

Organ	Percentage of Deaths of All Cancers	Risks	Cell Type	Common Manifestations
Esophagus	2%	Malnutrition Alcohol Tobacco Chronic reflux	Squamous cell Adenocarcinoma	Chest pain Dysphagia
Stomach	2%	Salty food Nitrates and nitrosamines Gastric atrophy	Adenocarcinoma Squamous cell	Anorexia Malaise Weight loss Upper abdominal pain Vomiting Occult blood
Colorectal	10%	Polyps Ulcerative colitis Diverticulitis High–refined carbohydrate, low-fiber, high-fat diet	Adenocarcinoma (left colon grows in ring; right colon grows as mass)	Pain Mass Anemia Bloody stool Obstruction Distention
Liver	2%	Hepatitis B, C, and D viruses Cirrhosis Intestinal parasite Aflatoxin from moldy peanuts	Hepatomas Cholangiomas	Pain Anorexia Bloating Weight loss Portal hypertension Ascites ± jaundice
Pancreas	5%	Chronic pancreatitis Cigarette smoking Alcohol (?) Diabetic women	Adenocarcinoma (exocrine part of gland, ductal epithelium)	Weight loss Weakness Nausea Vomiting Abdominal pain Depression ± jaundice May have insulin-secreting tumors with symptoms of hypoglycemia

From American Cancer Society: *CA Cancer J Clin* 44(1), 1997.
All the above cancers are within the top 10 causes of death from cancer.

surrounding tissues.[189] A K-ras mutation is the most common genetic alteration and there are also tumor suppressor gene alterations, including p53, p16, and DCC. Growth factors may be overexpressed.[190]

Ductal adenocarcinomas can occur in the head, body, or tail of the pancreas. Tumors of the head quickly spread to obstruct the common bile duct and portal vein (Fig. 38-30). These tumors can then infiltrate the superior mesenteric artery, the vena cava, and the aorta. Cancer cells that enter the blood vessels can form emboli. Tumors of the body and tail infiltrate the posterior abdominal wall. Lymphatic invasion occurs early and rapidly and involves local and regional lymph nodes. Venous invasion causes metastases to the liver. Tumor implants on the peritoneal surface can obstruct veins and promote development of ascites.

Ductal adenocarcinomas arising in the head of the pancreas cause biliary obstruction somewhat early in the disease. Individuals with such tumors survive slightly longer than those with cancer of the body and tail, presumably because they seek medical attention earlier.

Tumors of the endocrine pancreas are rare neoplasms of the islets of Langerhans known as *apudomas*. The first four letters in *apudoma* derive from *amine precursor uptake* and *decarboxylation*. The apudomas are so named because they contain neurosecretory granules. Endocrine neoplasms are fatal because they secrete abnormal amounts of hormones, such as insulin.

Clinical Manifestations

Cancer of the body and tail of the pancreas is generally asymptomatic until there is intraductal obstruction or the tumor invades adjacent tissue. Frequently vague back pain is an initial symptom. Jaundice develops in most cases, usually caused by obstruction of the bile duct.[191] Because obstruction impairs enzyme secretion and flow to the duodenum, pancreatic cancer causes fat and protein malabsorption, resulting in weight loss. Distant metastases are found in the neck nodes, the lungs, and the brain. Most individuals die of hepatic failure, malnutrition, or systemic diseases.

Evaluation and Treatment

A laparotomy is often performed, particularly if jaundice is present. Ultrasonography and CT may be needed to confirm the need for a laparotomy, especially in individuals without jaundice. Laparotomy is used to establish a definitive diagnosis, evaluate the extent of disease, and determine whether palliative bypass surgery (i.e., cholecystojejunostomy and gastrojejunostomy) is needed. Most individuals require palliative double bypass of the blocked bile ducts, as well as gastrojejunostomy to prevent duodenal obstruction.

Many surgeons recommend a total pancreatectomy because cancer of the pancreas seldom consists of a single lesion. Chemotherapy and radiation therapy are seldom beneficial except as palliative measures. Because almost all pancreatic cancers are advanced at the time of diagnosis, staging has little relevance in determining treatment. Cancers of the gastrointestinal tract are summarized in Table 38-12.

SUMMARY REVIEW

Disorders of the Gastrointestinal Tract

1. Anorexia (loss of appetite), vomiting, constipation, diarrhea, abdominal pain, and evidence of gastrointestinal bleeding are clinical manifestations of many disorders of the gastrointestinal tract.
2. Vomiting is the forceful emptying of the stomach effected by gastrointestinal contraction and reverse peristalsis of the esophagus. It is usually preceded by nausea and retching, with the exception of projectile vomiting, which is associated with direct stimulation of the vomiting center in the brain.
3. Constipation is frequently caused by unhealthy dietary and bowel habits combined with lack of exercise. Constipation also can result from a disorder that impairs intestinal motility or obstructs the intestinal lumen.
4. Diarrhea can be caused by excessive fluid drawn into the intestinal lumen by osmosis (osmotic diarrhea), excessive secretion of fluids by the intestinal mucosa (secretory diarrhea), or excessive gastrointestinal motility.
5. Abdominal pain is caused by stretching, inflammation, or ischemia (insufficient blood supply). Abdominal pain originates in the organs themselves (visceral pain) or in the peritoneum (parietal pain). Visceral pain is frequently referred to the back.
6. Obvious manifestations of gastrointestinal bleeding are hematemesis (vomiting of blood), melena (dark, tarry stools), and hematochezia (frank bleeding from the rectum). Occult bleeding can be detected only by testing stools or vomitus for the presence of blood.
7. Dysphagia is difficulty in swallowing. It can be caused by a mechanical or functional obstruction of the esophagus. Functional obstruction is an impairment of esophageal motility.
8. Achalasia is a form of functional dysphagia caused by loss of esophageal innervation.
9. Gastroesophageal reflux is the regurgitation of chyme from the stomach into the esophagus. An inflammatory response (reflux esophagitis) ensues if the esophageal mucosa is repeatedly exposed to acids and enzymes in the regurgitated chyme.
10. Hiatal hernia is the protrusion of the upper part of the stomach through the hiatus (esophageal opening in the diaphragm) at the gastroesophageal junction. Hiatal hernia can be sliding or paraesophageal.
11. Pyloric obstruction is the narrowing or blockage of the pylorus, which is the opening between the stomach and the duodenum. It can be caused by a congenital defect, inflammation and scarring secondary to a gastric ulcer, or tumor growth.
12. Intestinal obstruction prevents the normal movement of chyme through the intestinal tract. It is usually mechanical—that is, caused by torsion, herniation, or tumor.
13. The most severe consequences of intestinal obstruction are fluid and electrolyte losses, hypovolemia, shock, intestinal necrosis, and perforation of the intestinal wall.
14. Gastritis is an acute or a chronic inflammation of the gastric mucosa.
15. Regurgitation of bile, use of antiinflammatory drugs or alcohol, and some systemic diseases are associated with gastritis.
16. Chronic gastritis of the fundus and body is the most severe form of gastritis. It can result in gastric atrophy and decreased secretion of hydrochloric acid, pepsinogen, and intrinsic factor.
17. Chronic gastritis of the antrum, the most common type, is not usually associated with impaired secretion or gastric atrophy.
18. Appendicitis is the most common surgical emergency of the abdomen. Obstruction of the lumen leads to increased pressure, ischemia, and inflammation of the appendix. Without surgical resection, inflammation may progress to gangrene, perforation, and peritonitis.
19. A peptic ulcer is a circumscribed area of mucosal inflammation and ulceration caused by excessive secretion of gastric acid, disruption of the protective mucosal barrier, or both.
20. The three types of peptic ulcers are duodenal, gastric, and stress ulcers.
21. Duodenal ulcers, the most common peptic ulcers, are associated with increased numbers of parietal (acid-secreting) cells

in the stomach, elevated gastrin levels, and rapid gastric emptying. Pain occurs when the stomach is empty, and pain is relieved with food or antacids. Duodenal ulcers tend to heal spontaneously and recur frequently.
22. Gastric ulcers develop near parietal cells, generally in the antrum, and tend to become chronic. Gastric secretions may be normal or decreased, and pain may occur after eating.
23. Ischemic stress ulcers develop suddenly after severe illness, systemic trauma, or neural injury. Ulceration follows mucosal damage caused by ischemia (decreased blood flow to the gastric mucosa).
24. Cushing ulcer is a stress ulcer caused by head trauma. Ulceration follows hypersecretion of hydrochloric acid caused by overstimulation of the vagal nuclei.
25. Postgastrectomy syndromes are long-term complications that follow gastrectomy—the resection of all or part of the stomach. The postgastrectomy syndromes include dumping syndrome, alkaline reflux gastritis, afferent loop obstruction, diarrhea, weight loss, and anemia.
26. Dumping syndrome is the rapid emptying of chyme into the small intestine. It causes an osmotic shift of fluid from the vascular compartment to the intestinal lumen, which decreases plasma volume.
27. Alkaline reflux gastritis is stomach inflammation caused by the reflux of bile and pancreatic secretions from the duodenum into the stomach. These substances disrupt the mucosal barrier and cause inflammation.
28. Afferent loop obstruction is an obstruction of the duodenal stump on the proximal side of a gastrojejunostomy. Biliary and pancreatic secretions accumulate in the stump, causing distention, intermittent pain, and vomiting.
29. Malabsorption syndromes result in impaired digestion or absorption of nutrients.
30. Pancreatic insufficiency causes malabsorption associated with impaired digestion. The pancreas does not produce sufficient amounts of the enzymes that digest protein, carbohydrates, and fats into components that can be absorbed by the intestine.
31. Deficient lactase production in the brush border of the small intestine inhibits the breakdown of lactose. This prevents lactose absorption and causes osmotic diarrhea.
32. Bile salt deficiency causes fat malabsorption and steatorrhea (fatty stools). Bile salt deficiency can result from inadequate secretion of bile, excessive bacterial deconjugation of bile, or impaired reabsorption of bile salts caused by ileal disease.
33. Ulcerative colitis is an inflammatory disease that causes ulceration, abscess formation, and necrosis of the colonic and rectal mucosa. Cramping pain, bleeding, frequent diarrhea, dehydration, and weight loss accompany severe forms of the disease. A course of frequent remissions and exacerbations is common.
34. Crohn disease is similar to ulcerative colitis, but it affects both the large and small intestines, and ulceration tends to involve all the layers of the lumen. "Skip lesion" fissures and granulomas are characteristic of Crohn disease. Abdominal tenderness, nonbloody diarrhea, and weight loss are the usual symptoms.
35. Diverticula are outpouchings of colonic mucosa through the muscle layers of the colon wall. Diverticulosis is the presence of these outpouchings; diverticulitis is inflammation of the diverticula.
36. Vascular insufficiency in the intestine is associated most often with occlusion or obstruction of the mesenteric vessels or insufficient arterial blood flow. The resulting ischemia and necrosis produce abdominal pain, fever, bloody diarrhea, hypovolemia, and shock.
37. Obesity can be classified as exogenous or endogenous, and adipose (fat) cells as hyperplastic or hypertrophic.
38. Susceptibility to obesity may involve an excessive number of fat cells, increased amounts of lipoprotein in fat cells, high biologic set-point controlled by the hypothalamus, presence of relatively few brown (thermoregulating) fat cells, high blood glucose levels associated with type 2 diabetes, or decreased action of the adenosine triphosphatase (ATPase) pump.
39. Obesity increases the risk of developing coronary artery disease, cancer, and pulmonary disorders.
40. Anorexia nervosa, or self-imposed starvation, is a psychogenic disorder primarily of adolescent and young women. It causes significant weight loss and developmental delays and can be fatal.
41. Bulimia (binging and purging) involves eating normal or large amounts of food and then purging by inducing vomiting or abusing laxatives. Severe weight loss is rare, but frequent vomiting causes tooth decay, pharyngitis, and esophagitis.
42. Short-term starvation, or lack of dietary intake for 3 or 4 days, stimulates mobilization of stored glucose by two metabolic processes: glycogenolysis (splitting of glycogen into glucose) and gluconeogenesis (formation of glucose from noncarbohydrate molecules).
43. Long-term starvation triggers the breakdown of ketone bodies and fatty acids. Eventually proteolysis (protein breakdown) begins, and death ensues if nutrition is not restored.

Disorders of the Accessory Organs of Digestion

1. Portal hypertension, ascites, hepatic encephalopathy, jaundice, and hepatorenal syndrome are complications of many liver disorders.
2. Portal hypertension is an elevation of portal venous pressure to at least 10 mm Hg. It is caused by increased resistance to venous flow in the portal vein and its tributaries, including the sinusoids and hepatic vein.
3. Portal hypertension is the most serious complication of liver disease because it can cause potentially fatal complications, such as bleeding varices, ascites, and hepatic encephalopathy.
4. Ascites is the accumulation and sequestration of fluid in the peritoneal cavity, often as a result of portal hypertension and decreased concentrations of plasma proteins.
5. Hepatic encephalopathy (portal systemic encephalopathy) is impaired cerebral function caused by blood-borne toxins (particularly ammonia) not metabolized by the liver. Toxin-bearing blood may bypass the liver in collateral vessels opened as a result of portal hypertension, or diseased hepatocytes may be unable to carry out their metabolic functions.
6. Manifestations of hepatic encephalopathy range from confusion and asterixis (flapping tremor of the hands) to loss of consciousness, coma, and death.
7. Jaundice (icterus) is a yellow or greenish pigmentation of the skin or sclera of the eyes caused by increases in plasma bilirubin concentration (hyperbilirubinemia).
8. Obstructive jaundice is caused by obstructed bile canaliculi (intrahepatic obstructive jaundice) or obstructed bile ducts

outside the liver (extrahepatic obstructive jaundice). Bilirubin accumulates proximal to sites of obstruction, enters the bloodstream, and is carried to the skin and deposited.
9. Hemolytic jaundice is caused by destruction of red blood cells at a rate that exceeds the liver's ability to metabolize unconjugated bilirubin.
10. Hepatorenal syndrome is functional kidney failure caused by advanced liver disease, particularly cirrhosis with portal hypertension. Renal failure is caused by a sudden decrease in blood flow to the kidneys, usually as a result of massive gastrointestinal hemorrhage or liver failure. Its chief clinical manifestation is oliguria.
11. Viral hepatitis is an infection of the liver caused by a strain of the hepatitis virus: hepatitis A virus (HAV); hepatitis B virus (HBV); or non-A, non-B hepatitis. Although they differ with respect to modes of transmission and severity of acute illness, all types cause hepatic cell necrosis, Kupffer cell hyperplasia, and infiltration of liver tissue by mononuclear phagocytes. These changes obstruct bile flow and impair hepatocyte function.
12. The clinical manifestations of viral hepatitis depend on the stage of infection. Fever, malaise, anorexia, and liver enlargement and tenderness characterize the prodromal phase (stage 1). Jaundice and hyperbilirubinemia mark the icteric phase (stage 2). During the recovery phase (stage 3), symptoms resolve. Recovery takes several weeks.
13. Fulminant hepatitis is a complication of hepatitis B (with or without hepatitis D infection) or non-A, non-B hepatitis. It causes widespread hepatic necrosis and is often fatal.
14. Cirrhosis is an inflammatory disease of the liver that causes disorganization of lobular structure, fibrosis, and nodular regeneration. Cirrhosis can result from hepatitis or exposure to toxins, such as acetaldehyde (a product of alcohol metabolism). The disease causes progressive irreversible liver damage, usually over a period of years.
15. Alcoholic cirrhosis impairs the hepatocytes' ability to oxidize fatty acids, synthesize enzymes and proteins, degrade hormones, and clear portal blood of ammonia and toxins. The inflammatory response includes excessive collagen formation, fibrosis, and scarring, which obstruct bile canaliculi and sinusoids. Bile obstruction causes jaundice. Vascular obstruction causes portal hypertension, shunting, and varices.
16. Primary biliary cirrhosis is the inflammatory destruction of intrahepatic bile ducts. Its cause is unknown.
17. Secondary biliary cirrhosis develops from prolonged obstruction of bile flow with increased pressure in the hepatic bile ducts that causes pooling of bile and necrosis of tissue. Relief of obstruction relieves symptoms of jaundice and pruritus. Continued obstruction causes cirrhosis and liver failure.
18. Postnecrotic cirrhosis is the consequence of many severe, chronic liver diseases. Fibrosis, atrophy, and nodular regeneration are characteristic of liver structure with severely altered liver function and manifestations, including portal hypertension, ascites, bleeding varices, and encephalopathy.
19. Cholelithiasis (the formation of gallstones) is a common disorder of the gallbladder. Gallstones form in the bile as a result of the aggregation of cholesterol crystals (cholesterol stones) or precipitates of unconjugated bilirubin (pigmented stones). Gallstones that fill the gallbladder or obstruct the cystic or common bile duct cause abdominal pain and jaundice.
20. Cholecystitis is an inflammation of the gallbladder. It is usually associated with obstruction of the cystic duct by gallstones.
21. Acute pancreatitis (pancreatic inflammation) is a serious but relatively rare disorder. Some unknown factor injures the pancreatic ducts or acini. Injury permits leakage of digestive enzymes into pancreatic tissue, where they become activated and begin the process of autodigestion, inflammation, and destruction of tissues. Release of pancreatic enzymes into the bloodstream or abdominal cavity causes damage to other organs.
22. Chronic pancreatitis results from structural or functional impairment of the pancreas. It causes recurrent abdominal pain and digestive disorders.

Cancer of the Digestive System

1. Cancer of the esophagus is rare and tends to occur in people older than 60 years. Alcohol and tobacco use, reflux esophagitis, and nutritional deficiencies are associated with esophageal carcinoma.
2. Dysphagia and chest pain are the primary manifestations of esophageal cancer. Early treatment of tumors that have not spread into the mediastinum or lymph nodes results in a good prognosis.
3. Gastric carcinoma is associated with high salt intake, food preservatives (nitrates and nitrites), and atrophic gastritis.
4. Approximately 50% of all gastric cancers are located in the prepyloric antrum. Clinical manifestations (weight loss, upper abdominal pain, vomiting, hematemesis, anemia) develop only after the tumor has penetrated the wall of the stomach.
5. Cancer of the colon and rectum (colorectal cancer) is the second most common cancer death in the United States. Preexisting polyps are highly associated with adenocarcinoma of the colon.
6. Tumors of the right (ascending) colon are usually large and bulky; tumors of the left (descending, sigmoid) colon develop as small, buttonlike masses. Manifestations of colon tumors include pain, bloody stools, and change in bowel habits.
7. Rectal carcinoma is located up to 15 cm from the opening of the anus. The tumor spreads transmurally to the vagina in women or to the prostate in men.
8. Metastatic invasion of the liver is more common than primary cancer of the liver.
9. Primary liver cancers are associated with chronic liver disease (cirrhosis and hepatitis B). Hepatocellular carcinomas arise from the hepatocytes, whereas cholangiocellular carcinomas arise from the bile ducts. Primary liver cancer spreads to the heart, lungs, brain, kidney, and spleen through the circulation.
10. Cancer of the gallbladder is relatively rare and tends to occur in women older than 50 years. Adenocarcinoma is most common. Because clinical manifestations occur late in the disease, metastases to lymph channels have usually occurred by the time of diagnosis, and the prognosis is poor.
11. Cancer of the pancreas now ranks fifth as a cause of cancer deaths. The one known risk factor is heavy cigarette smoking. Most tumors are adenocarcinomas that arise in the exocrine cells of ducts in the head, body, or tail of the pancreas. Symptoms may not be evident until the tumor has spread to surrounding tissues. Treatment is palliative, and mortality is nearly 100%.

KEY TERMS

Achalasia, *1266*
Acute gastritis, *1271*
Acute pancreatitis (acute hemorrhagic pancreatitis), *1298*
Afferent loop obstruction, *1277*
Alcoholic cirrhosis, *1294*
Alcoholic hepatitis, *1294*
Alkaline reflux gastritis, *1277*
Anorexia, *1261*
Anorexia nervosa, *1284*
Appendicitis, *1281*
Ascites, *1285*
Biliary cirrhosis, *1295*
Bulimia nervosa, *1284*
Bulimorexia, *1284*
Cholangiocellular carcinoma (cholangiocarcinoma), *1304*
Cholecystitis, *1298*
Cholelithiasis (gallstone), *1297*
Chronic active hepatitis, *1293*
Chronic gastritis, *1272*
Chronic pancreatitis, *1299*
Cirrhosis, *1294*
Constipation, *1262*
Crohn disease, *1280*
Curling ulcer, *1275*
Cushing ulcer, *1276*
Diarrhea, *1263*
Diverticula, *1281*
Diverticulitis, *1281*
Diverticulosis, *1281*
Dumping syndrome, *1277*
Duodenal ulcer, *1273*
Dysphagia, *1266*
Esophageal varices, *1286*
Fulminant hepatitis, *1293*
Gallstone, *1297*
Gastric ulcer, *1274*
Gastritis, *1271*
Gastroesophageal reflux, *1267*
Gastrointestinal bleeding, *1264*
Gluconeogenesis, *1285*
Glycogenolysis, *1285*
Hematemesis, *1264*
Hematochezia, *1265*
Hemolytic jaundice, *1289*
Hepatic encephalopathy, *1286*
Hepatocellular carcinoma (hepatocarcinoma), *1304*
Hepatorenal syndrome, *1290*
Hiatal hernia, *1267*
Hyperbilirubinemia, *1288*
Icteric phase of hepatitis, *1293*
Intestinal obstruction, *1269*
Ischemic ulcer, *1275*
Jaundice (icterus), *1288*
Kwashiorkor, *1285*
Lactase deficiency, *1278*
Long-term starvation, *1285*
Malabsorption, *1278*
Maldigestion, *1278*
Marasmus, *1285*
Melena, *1265*
Motility diarrhea, *1263*
Nausea, *1262*
Obesity, *1283*
Obstructive jaundice, *1289*
Occult bleeding, *1265*
Osmotic diarrhea, *1263*
Pancreatic insufficiency, *1278*
Pancreatitis, *1298*
Paraesophageal hiatal hernia, *1268*
Parietal pain, *1264*
Peptic ulcer, *1272*
Portal hypertension, *1285*
Postnecrotic cirrhosis, *1297*
Primary biliary cirrhosis, *1295*
Prodromal phase, *1293*
Projectile vomiting, *1262*
Pyloric obstruction, *1268*
Recovery (posticteric) phase of hepatitis, *1293*
Referred pain, *1264*
Reflux esophagitis, *1267*
Retching, *1262*
Secondary biliary cirrhosis, *1296*
Secretory diarrhea, *1263*
Short-term starvation, *1284*
Sliding hiatal hernia, *1267*
Splenomegaly, *1285*
Starvation, *1284*
Stress ulcer, *1275*
Ulcerative colitis, *1279*
Varices, *1285*
Viral hepatitis, *1291*
Visceral pain, *1264*
Vomiting, *1262*

REFERENCES

1. Bountra C et al: Towards understanding the aetiology and pathophysiology of the emetic reflex: novel approaches to antiemetic drugs, *Oncology* 53(suppl 1):102, 1996.
2. Gale JD: Serotonergic mediation of vomiting, *J Pediatr Gastroenterol Nutr* 21(suppl 1):S22, 1995.
3. Meadows N: The central control of vomiting, *J Pediatr Gastroenterol Nutr* 21(suppl 1):S20, 1995.
4. Stewart WF et al: Epidemiology of constipation (EPOC) study in the United States: relation of clinical subtypes to sociodemographic features, *Am J Gastroenterol* 94(12):3530, 1999.
5. Mitolo-Chieppa D et al: Cholinergic stimulation and nonadrenergic, noncholinergic relaxation of human colonic circular muscle in idiopathic chronic constipation, *Dig Dis Sci* 43(12):2716, 1998.
6. Haubrich WS, Schaffrer F, Berk JE: *Bockus gastroenterology*, vol 1, ed 5, Philadelphia, 1995, W.B. Saunders.
7. Ratnaike RN, Jones TE: Mechanisms of drug-induced diarrhoea in the elderly, *Drugs Aging* 13(3):245053, 1998.
8. Gostout CJ: Acute gastrointestinal bleeding: what are the issues the new millennium will resolve? *Gastrointest Endosc Clin N Am* 10(1): 89, 2000.
9. Ruigomez A et al: Overall mortality among patients surviving an episode of peptic ulcer bleeding, *J Epidemiol Community Health* 54(2): 130, 2000.
10. Mujica VR, Conklin J: When it's hard to swallow. What to look for in dysphagia, *Postgrad Med* 105(7):131, 1999.
11. Podas T et al: Achalasia: a critical review of epidemiological studies, *Am J Gastroenterol* 93(12):2345, 1998.
12. Nellemann H, et al: Bread and barium. Diagnostic value in patients with suspected primary esophageal motility disorders, *Acta Radiol* 41(2):145, 2000.
13. Bittinger M, Wienbeck M: Pneumatic dilation in achalasia, *Can J Gastroenterol* 15(3):195, 2001.
14. Orlando RC: Mechanisms of reflux-induced epithelial injuries in the esophagus, *Am J Med* 108(suppl 4a):104S, 2000.
15. Johanson JF: Epidemiology of esophageal and supraesophageal reflux injuries, *Am J Med* 108(suppl 41):99S, 2000.
16. Haggitt RC: Histopathology of reflux-induced esophageal and supraesophageal injuries, *Am J Med* 108(suppl 4a):109S, 2000.
17. Koop H: Reflux disease and Barrett's esophagus, *Endoscopy* 32(2): 101, 2000.
18. Richter JE: Gastroesophageal reflux disease and asthma: the two are directly related, *Am J Med* 108(suppl 4a):153S, 2000.
19. DeVault KR: Overview of medical therapy for gastroesophageal reflux disease, *Gastroenterol Clin N Am* 28(4):831, 1999.
20. Hogan WJ, Shaker R: Life after antireflux surgery, *Am J Med* 108 (suppl 4a):181S, 2000.
21. Hashemi M, Sillin LF, Peters JH: Current concepts in the management of paraesophageal hiatal hernia, *J Clin Gasterol* 29(1):8, 1999.
22. Spivak H, Lelcuk S, Hunter JG: Laparoscopic surgery of the gastroesophageal junction, *World J Surgery* 23(4):356, 1999.

23. Khandekar S, Chandler ST, Trewby PN: Successful medical treatment of peptic pyloric stenosis: Dr Sippy revisited, *J R Coll Physicians Lond* 32(4):3540, 1998.
24. Cerro P et al: Sonographic diagnosis of intussusceptions in adults, *Abdom Imaging* 25(1):45, 2000.
25. Tytgat GN: Ulcers and gastritis, *Endoscopy* 32(2):108, 2000.
26. Yardley JH, Hendrix TR: Gastritis and gastropathy. In Yamada T, Alpers DH, Laine L, editors: *Atlas of gastroenterology*, ed 3, p 221, Philadelphia, 1999, Lippincott Williams & Wilkins.
27. Oksanen A et al: Atrophic gastritis and *Helicobacter pylori* infection in outpatients referred for gastroscopy, *Gut* 46(4):460, 2000.
28. Vakil N, Fennerty B: The economics of eradicating *Helicobacter pylori* infection in duodenal ulcer disease, *Am J Med* 100(5A):605, 1996.
29. Shigemi J, Mino Y, Tsuda T: The role of perceived job stress in the relationship between smoking and the development of peptic ulcers, *J Epidemiol* 9(5):320, 1999.
30. Levenstein S: The very model of a modern etiology: a biopsychosocial view of peptic ulcer [review], *Psychosom Med* 62(2):176, 2000.
31. Kurata JH: Epidemiology of peptic ulcer disease. In Swabb EA, Szabo S, editors: *Investigation and basis for therapy*, New York, 1991, Marcel Dekker.
32. Schineller BA, Ramchandani D: Psychologic factors associated with peptic ulcer disease, *Med Clin North Am* 75(4):865, 1991.
33. Qureshi WA, Graham DY: Diagnosis and management of *Helicobacter pylori* infection, *Clin Cornerstone* 1(5):18, 1999.
34. Gisbert JP et al: *H. pylori*-negative duodenal ulcer prevalence and causes in 774 patients, *Dig Dis Sci* 44(11):2295, 1999.
35. Tovey FI, Hobsley M: Is *Helicobacter pylori* the primary cause of duodenal ulceration? *J Gastroenterol Hepatol* 14(11):1053, 1999.
36. Freston JW: Management of peptic ulcers: emerging issues, *World J Surg* 24(3):250, 2000.
37. Frazer AG et al: An audit of low dose triple therapy for eradication of *Helicobacter pylori, NZ Med J* 109(1027):290, 1996.
38. Megraud F, Marshall BJ: How to treat *Helicobacter pylori*: first-line, second-line, and future therapies, *Gastroenterol Clin North Am* 29(4): 759, 2000.
39. Dubois F: New surgical strategy for gastroduodenal ulcer: laparoscopic approach, *World J Surg* 24(3):270, 2000.
40a. Aldoori WH et al: Prospective study of diet and the risk of duodenal ulcer in men, *Am J Epidemiol* 145{1}:42, 1997.
40b. Lee CK: Vaccination against *Helicobacter pylori* in non-human primate models and humans, *Scand J Immunol* 53(5):437, 2001.
41. Tatsuguchi A et al: Localisation of cyclooxygenase 1 and cyclooxygenase 2 in *Helicobacter pylori*–related gastritis and gastric ulcer tissues in humans, *Gut* 46(6):782, 2000.
42. Aoyma N et al: Peptic ulcer after the Hanshin-Awaji earthquake: increased incidence of bleeding gastric ulcer, *Am J Gastroenterol* 93(3): 311, 1998.
43. van der Voort PH, Zandstra DF: Pathogenesis, risk factors, and incidence of upper gastrointestinal bleeding after cardiac surgery: is specific prophylaxis in routine bypass procedures needed? *J Cardiothorac Vasc Anesth* 14(3):293, 2000.
44. Jamieson GG: Current status of indications for surgery in peptic ulcer disease, *World J Surg* 24(3):256, 2000.
45. Mehagnoul-Schipper DJ et al: Sympathoadrenal activation and the dumping syndrome after gastric surgery, *Clin Auton Res* 10(5):301, 2000.
46. Carvajal SH, Mulvihill SJ: Postgastrectomy syndromes: dumping and diarrhea, *Gastroenterol Clin North Am* 23(2):261, 1994.
47. Khoshoo V et al: Nutritional management of dumping syndrome associated with antireflux surgery, *J Pediatr Surg* 29(11):1452, 1994.
48. Hasler WL, Soudah HC, Owyang C: Mechanisms by which octreotide ameliorates symptoms in the dumping syndrome, *J Pharmacol Exp Ther* 277(3):1359, 1996.
49. Klingler PJ et al: Indications, technical modalities and results of the duodenal switch operation for pathologic duodenogastric reflux, *Hepatogastroenterology* 46(25):97, 1999.
50. Bruno MJ et al: Maldigestion associated with exocrine pancreatic insufficiency: implications of gastrointestinal physiology and properties of enzyme preparations for a cause-related and patient-tailored treatment, *Am J Gastroenterol* 90(9):1383, 1995.
51. Shaw AD, Davies GJ: Lactose intolerance: problems in diagnosis and treatment, *J Clin Gastroenterol* 28(3):208, 1999.
52. Allison MC et al: *Inflammatory bowel disease*. St Louis, 1998, Mosby.
53. Geerling BJ et al: Diet as a risk factor for the development of ulcerative colitis, *Am J Gastroenterol* 95(4):1108, 2000.
54. Murata Y et al: The role of proinflammatory and immunoregulatory cytokines in the pathogenesis of ulcerative colitis, *J Gastroenterol* 30 (suppl 8):56, 1995.
55. Kirsner JB: *Inflammatory bowel disease*, ed 5, Philadelphia, 2000, W.B. Saunders.
56. Gasche C: Complications of inflammatory bowel disease, *Hepatogastroenterology* 47(31):49, 2000.
57. Karlinger K et al: The epidemiology and the pathogenesis of inflammatory bowel disease, *Eur J Radiol* 35(3):154, 2000.
58. Thomas GA et al: Role of smoking in inflammatory bowel disease: implications for therapy, *Postgrad Med J* 76(895):273, 2000.
59. Hanover SB: Ulcerative colitis. In Lichtenstein LM, Fauci AS, editors: *Current therapy in allergy, immunology, and rheumatology*, ed 5, St Louis, 1996, Mosby.
60. Winar SJ, editor: *Management of gastrointestinal diseases*, vol 2, New York, 1992, Gower Medical Publishing.
61. Mellemkjaer L et al: Crohn's disease and cancer risk (Denmark), *Cancer Causes Control* 11(2):145, 2000.
62. Krupnick AS, Morris JB: The long-term results of resection and multiple resections in Crohn's disease, *Sem Gastrointest Dis* 11(1):41, 2000.
63. Stollman NH, Raskin JB: Diverticular disease of the colon, *J Clin Gastroenterol* 29(3):241, 1999.
64. Wolff BG, Devine RM: Surgical management of diverticulitis, *Am Surg* 66(2):153, 2000.
65. Carr NJ: The pathology of acute appendicitis, *Ann Diagn Pathol* 4(1): 46, 2000.
66. Andersson RE et al: Repeated clinical and laboratory examinations in patients with an equivocal diagnosis of appendicitis, *World J Surg* 24(4):479, 2000.
67. Hardin DM Jr: Acute appendicitis: review and update, *Am Fam Physician* 60(7):2027, 1999.
68. Patel A, Kaleya RN, Sammartano JR: Pathophysiology of mesenteric ischemia, *Surg Clin North Am* 72(1):31, 1992.
69. Kvietys PR, Barrowmand A, Granger ND: *Pathophysiology of the splanchnic circulation*, vol 1, Boca Raton, Fla, 1987, CRC Press.
70. Ravussin E, Swinburg GA: Pathophysiology of obesity, *Lancet* 340: 404, 1992.
71. Matsuzawa Y et al: Pathophysiology and pathogenesis of visceral fat obesity, *Obes Res* 3(suppl 2):187S, 1995.
72. Considine RV: Weight regulation, leptin and growth hormone, *Horm Res* 48(suppl 5):116, 1997.
73. Houseknecht et al: The biology of leptin: a review, *J Anim Sci* 75(5): 1405, 1998.
74. Leroy P et al: Expression of the ob gene in adipose cells: regulation by insulin, *J Biol Chem* 271(5):2365, 1996.
75. Hamann A, Flier JL, Lowell BB: Decreased brown fat markedly enhances susceptibility to diet-induced obesity, diabetes, and hyperlipidemia, *Endocrinology* 137(1):21, 1996.
76. Alexander JK: Obesity and coronary heart disease, *Am J Med Sci* 321(4):215, 2001.
77. Khaodhiar L, McCowen KC, Blackburn GL: Obesity and its comorbid conditions, *Clin Cornerstone* 2(3):17, 1999.
78. Bray GA: The obese patient. In Smith LH, editor: *Major problems in internal medicine*, vol 9, Philadelphia, 1985, W.B. Saunders.
79. Stunkard AJ: Current views on obesity, *Am J Med* 100(2):230, 1996.
80. Becker DE, Freudenberg N: Developing comprehensive approaches to prevention and control of obesity among low-income, urban, African-American women, *J Am Med Womens Assoc* 56(2):59, 2001.

81. National Institute of Mental Health: *Eating disorders*, NIH Pub 93-3477, Washington, DC, 1993, US Government Printing Office.
82. Law SA, Golding JM: Sexual assault history and eating disorder among White, Hispanic, and African-American women and men, *Am J Public Health* 86(14):579, 1996.
83. Emous SJ: Eating disorders in adolescent girls, *Pediatr Int* 42(1):107, 2000.
84. American Psychiatric Association: *Diagnostic and statistical manual of mental disorders*, ed 4, Washington, DC, 1994, Academic Press.
85. Hartman D: Anorexia nervosa: diagnosis, aetiology, and treatment, *Postgrad Med* 71(842):712, 1995.
86. Kohn M, Golden NH: Eating disorders in children and adolescents: epidemiology, diagnosis, and treatment, *Paediatr Drugs* 3(2):91, 2001.
87. Mehler PA: Eating disorders: bulimia nervosa, *Hosp Pract (Off Ed)* 31(2):107, 1996.
88. Lam RW, Golder EM, Gerwal A: Seasonality of symptoms in anorexia and bulimia nervosa, *Int J Eat Disord* 19(1):35, 1996.
89. Incalzi RA et al: Energy intake and in-hospital starvation, *Arch Intern Med* 156(4):425, 1996.
90. Mahan LK, Escott-Stump S, editors: *Krause's food, nutrition and diet therapy*, ed 10, Philadelphia, 2000, W.B. Saunders.
91. Stipanuk MH: *Biochemical and physiological aspects of human nutrition*, Philadelphia, 2000, W.B. Saunders.
92. Bosch J, Garcia-Pagan JC: Complications of cirrhosis. I. Portal hypertension, *J Hepatol* 32(suppl 2):141, 2000.
93. Bosch J: The sixth Carlos E. Rubio memorial lecture. Prevention and treatment of variceal hemorrhage, *P R Health Sci J* 19(1):57, 2000.
94. Butterworth KF, Borsatto R: Complications of cirrhosis III. Hepatic encephalopathy, *J Hepatol* 32(suppl 1):171, 2000.
95. Binmoeller KF, Borsatto R: Variceal bleeding and portal hypertension, *Endoscopy* 32(3):189, 2000.
96. Palmer BF: Pathogenesis of ascites and renal salt retention in cirrhosis, *J Investig Med* 47(5):183, 1999.
97. Gentilini P et al: Albumin improves the response to diuretics in patients with cirrhosis and ascites: results of a randomized, controlled trial, *J Hepatol* 30(4):639, 1999.
98. Hazell AS, Butterworth RF: Hepatic encephalopathy: an update of pathophysiologic mechanisms, *Proc Soc Exp Bio Med* 222(2):99, 1999.
99. Shimamoto C, Hirata I, Katsu K: Breath and blood ammonia in liver cirrhosis, *Hepatogastroenterology* 47(32):443, 2000.
100. Clemmeson JO et al: Cerebral herniation in patients with acute liver failure is correlated with arterial ammonia concentration, *Hepatology* 29(3):648, 1999.
101. Schafer DF, Jones EA: Hepatic encephalopathy. In Zakim D, Boyer TD, editors: *Hepatology: a textbook of liver disease,* vol 1, ed 2, Philadelphia, 1990, W.B. Saunders.
102. Rossi RL, Traverso LW, Pimentel F: Malignant obstructive jaundice: evaluation and management, *Surg Clin North Am* 76(1):63, 1996.
103. Raiford DS: Pruritus of chronic cholestasis, *QJM* 88(9):603, 1995.
104. Wong F, Blendis L: Pathophysiology and treatment of hepatorenal syndrome, *Gastroenterologist* 6(2):133, 1998.
105. Bataller R et al: Hepatorenal syndrome, *Forum (Genova)* 8(1):62, 1998.
106. Moore K: Renal failure is acute liver failure, *Eur J Gastroenterol Hepatol* 11(9):967, 1999.
107. Gines P, Arroyo V, Rodes J: Ascites and hepatorenal syndrome: Pathogenesis and treatment strategies. In Schrier RW et al, editors: *Advances in internal medicine*, vol 3, p 99, St Louis, 1998, Mosby.
108. Arroyo V, Jimemez W: Complications of cirrhosis. II. Renal and circulatory dysfunction. Lights and shadows in an important clinical problem, *J Hepatol* 32(suppl 1):157, 2000.
109. Sheng L et al: Hepatitis G virus infection in acute fulminant hepatitis: prevalence of HGV infection and sequence analysis of a specific viral strain, *J Viral Hepat* 5(5):301, 1998.
110. Ciocca M: Clinical course and consequences of hepatitis A infection, *Vaccine* 18(suppl 1):S71, 2000.
111. Yotsuyanagi H et al: Prolonged fecal excretion of hepatitis A virus in adult patients with hepatitis A is determined by polymerase chain reaction, *Hepatology* 24:10, 1996.
112. Gerety RJ: *Hepatitis B*, Orlando, Fla, 1985, Academic Press.
113. Lawence SP: Advances in the treatment of hepatitis C. In Schrier RW, editor: *Advances in internal medicine*, vol 45, St Louis, 2000, Mosby.
114. Boyer N, Marcellin P: Natural history of hepatitis C and the impact of anti-viral therapy, *Forum (Genova)* 10(1):4, 2000.
115. Tong MJ, Terrault NA, Klintmalm G: Hepatitis B transplantation: special conditions, *Semin Liver Dis* 20(suppl 1):25, 2000.
116. Nanda SK et al: Protracted viremia during acute sporadic hepatitis E virus infection, *Gastroenterology* 108:225, 1995.
117. Karayiannis P et al: Natural history and molecular biology of hepatitis G virus/GB virus C, *Clin Diagn Virol* 10(2-3):103, 1998.
118. Mandell GL, Bennett JE, Dolin R: *Principles and practice of infectious diseases*, vol 2, Philadelphia, 2000, Churchill Livingstone.
119. Ohto H et al: Transmission of hepatitic C from mothers to infants, *N Engl J Med* 330:744, 1994.
120. Lin OS, Keeffe EB: Current treatment strategies for chronic hepatitis B and C, *Annu Rev Med* 52:29, 2001.
121. Shouval D: Vaccines for prevention of viral hepatitis, *Haemophilia* 4(4):587, 1998.
122. Malik AH, Lee WM: Chornic hepatitis B virus infection: treatment strategies for the next millennium, *Ann Intern Med* 132(9):723, 2000.
123. Maddrey WC: Chronic viral hepatitis: diagnosis and management, *Hosp Pract*, February 15, 1994.
124. Shakil AO, Mazariegos GV, Kramer DJ: Fulminant hepatic failure, *Surg Clin North Am* 79(1):77, 1999.
125. Kaptanoglu L, Blei AT: Current status of liver support systems, *Clin Liver Dis* 4(3):711, 2000.
126. Hill DB, Kugelmas M: Alcoholic liver disease. Treatment strategies for the potentially reversible stages, *Postgrad Med* 103(4):261, 1998.
127. Savolainen V et al: Early perivenular fibrosis—precirrhotic lesions among moderate alcohol consumers and chronic alcoholics, *J Hepatol* 23(5):524, 1995.
128. Zetterman RZ: Alcoholic liver disease. In Gitnick G, editor: *Current hepatology*, vol 16, St Louis, 1996, Mosby.
129. Lieber CS: Alcoholic liver disease: new insights in pathogenesis lead to new treatments, *J Hepatol* 32(suppl 1):113, 2000.
130. Greenwel P: Acetaldehyde-mediated collagen regulation in hepatic stellate cells, *Alcohol Clin Exp Res* 23(5):930, 1999.
131. Walsh K, Alexander G: Alcoholic liver disease, *Postgrad Med* 76(895): 280, 2000.
132. Walsh K, Alexander G: Alcoholic liver disease, *Postgrad Med* 76(895): 280, 2000.
133. Gavaler JS, van Thiel DH: Ethanol: its adverse effects upon the hypothalamic pituitary-gonadal axis, *J Lab Clin Med* 101:21, 1983.
134. Gomez F, Ruiz P, Schreiber AD: Impaired function of macrophage Fcg receptors and bacterial infection in alcoholic cirrhosis, *N Engl J Med* 331:1122, 1994.
135. Mackay IR: Autoimmunity and primary biliary cirrhosis, *Baillieres Best Pract Res Clin Gastroenterol* 14(04):519, 2000.
136. Heathcote EJ: Management of primary biliary cirrhosis. The American Association of the Study of Liver Disease practice guidelines, *Hepatology* 31(4):1005, 2000.
137. Heathcote EJ: Management of primary biliary cirrhosis. The American Association of the Study of Liver Disease practice guidelines, *Hepatology* 31(4):1005, 2000.
138. Heathcote J: Update on primary biliary cirrhosis, *CanJ Gastroenterol* 14(1):43, 2000.
139. Carey MC: Pathogenesis of gallstones, *Am J Surg* 165(4):410, 1993.
140. Donovan JM: Physical and metabolic factors in gallstone pathogenesis, *Gastroenterol Clin North Am* 28(1):75, 1999.
141. Berger MY et al: Abdominal symptoms: do they predict gallstones? A systemic review, *Scand J Gastroenterol* 35(1):70, 2000.
142. Venu RP et al: Endoscopic transpapillary drainage of pancreatic abscess: technique and results, *Gastrointest Endosc* 51(4 Pt 1):391, 2000.
143. Sakorafas GH, Tsiotou AG: Etiology and pathogenesis of acute pancreatitis: current concepts, *J Clin Gastroenterol* 30(4):343, 2000.

144. Arendt T et al: Gallstones, the choledochoduodenal junction and initiation of acute pancreatitis: are two stones the culprit rather than one stone? *Med Hypothesis* 54(4):570, 2000.
145. Dugernier T, Laterre PF, Reynaert MS: Ascites fluid in severe acute pancreatitis: from pathophysiology to therapy, *Acta Gastroenterol Belg* 63(3):264, 2000.
146. Bhatia M et al: Inflammatory mediators in acute pancreatitis, *J Pathol* 190(2):117, 2000.
147. Kemppainen EA et al: Advances in the laboratory diagnostics of acute pancreatitis, *Ann Med* 30(2):169, 1998.
148. Erstad BL: Enteral nutrition support in acute pancreatitis, *Ann Pharmacother* 34(4):514, 2000.
149. Layer P, DiMagno EP: Early and late onset in idiopathic and alcoholic chronic pancreatitis. Different clinical courses, *Surg Clin North Am* 79 (4):847, 1999.
150. Owyang C: Chronic pancreatitis. In Yamada T, Alpers DH, Laine L, editors: *Atlas of gastroenterology*, ed 3, p 433, Phialdelphia, 1999, Lippincott Williams & Wilkins.
151. Pitchumoni CS: Chronic pancreatitis: pathogenesis and management of pain, *J Clin Gastroenterol* 27(2):101, 1998.
152. O'Reilly MA, O'Reilly PM, Glees J: The radiological features of primary small-cell carcinoma of the esophagus, *Dysphagia* 11(3):191, 1996.
153. American Cancer Society: *Estimated new cancer cases and deaths by sex for all sites, United States, 2000*, 2000, American Cancer Society. [www3.cancer.org/cancerinfo/sitecenter]
154. Heath EI et al: Adenocarcinoma of the esophagus: risk factors and prevention, *Oncology (Huntingt)* 14(4):507, 2000.
155. Blot WJ, McLaughlin JK: The changing epidemiology of esophageal cancer, *Semin Oncol* 33(3):71, 2000.
156. Lam AK: Molecular biology of esophageal squamous cell carcinoma, *Crit Rev Oncol Hematol* 33(2):71, 2000.
157. Audrezet MP et al: Molecular analysis of the TP52 gene in Barrett's adenocarcinoma, *Hum Mutat* 7(2):109, 1996.
158. Alexander GA, Brawley OW: Association of *Helicobacter pylori* infection with gastric cancer, *Mil Med* 165(1):21, 2000.
159. Bechi P et al: *Helicobacter pylori* and cell proliferation of the gastric mucosa: possible implications for gastric carcinoma, *Am J Gastroenterol* 91(2):271, 1996.
160. Kuipers EJ: Review article: relationship between *Helicobacter pylori*, atrophic gastritis, and gastric cancer, *Alimen Pharmacol Ther* 12(suppl 1):25, 1998.
161. Houben GM, Stockbrugger RW: Bacteria in the aetio-pathogenesis of gastric cancer: a review, *Scand J Gastroenterol* 212(suppl):13, 1995.
162. Lipkin M et al: Dietary factors in human colorectal cancer, *Ann Rev Nutr* 19:545, 1999.
163. Slattery ML et al: Lifestyle and colon cancer: an assessment of factors associated with risk, *Am J Epidemiol* 150(8):869, 1999.
164. Ahen JD: The genetic basis of colorectal cancer risk, *Adv Intern Med* 41:531, 1996.
165. Jen J et al: Allelic loss of chromosome 18q and prognosis in colorectal cancer, *N Engl J Med* 331:213, 1994.
166. Ahnen DJ: Genetics of cancer, *West J Med* 154(6):700, 1991.
167. Kanazawa K et al: Factors influencing the development of sigmoid colon cancer: bacteriologic and biochemical studies, *Cancer* 77(suppl 8):1701, 1996.
168. Potter JD: Colorectal cancer: molecules and populations, *J Natl Cancer Inst* 91(11):916, 1999.
169. Baron JA et al: Calcium supplements for the prevention of colorectal adenomas. Calcium polyp prevention study, *N Engl J Med* 340:101, 1999.
170. Holt PR: Studies of calicum in food supplements in humans, *Ann N Y Acad Sci* 889:128, 1999.
171. Willett WC: Goals for nutrition in the year 2000, *CA Cancer J Clin* 49(6):331, 1999.
172. Goss KH, Groden J: Biology of the adenomatous polyposis coli tumor suppressor, *J Clin Oncol* 18(9):1967, 2000.
173. Winawer SJ: Natural history of colorectal cancer, *Am J Med* 106(1A): 3S, 1999.
174. Lieberman D: How to screen for colon cancer, *Ann Rev Med* 49:163, 1998.
175. Hill MJ: Mechanisms of diet and colon carcinogenesis, *Eur J Cancer Prev* 8(suppl 1):S95, 1999.
176. Vargas PA, Alberts DS: Primary prevention of colorectal cancer through dietary modification, *Cancer* 70(suppl 5):1229, 1992.
177. Chung-Faye GA et al: Gene therapy strategies for colon cancer, *Mol Med Today*, 6(2):8207, 2000.
178. Petersen GM et al: Genetic testing and counseling for hereditary forms of colorectal cancer, *Cancer* 86(suppl 11):2540, 1999.
179. Schlom J et al: Strategies in the development of recombinant vaccines for colon cancer, *Semin Oncol* 26(6):672, 1999.
180. Sobrero A et al: New directions in the treatment of colon cancer: a look to the future, *Eur J Cancer* 36(5):559, 2000.
181. Weimann A, Oldhafer KJ, Pichlmayr R: Primary liver cancers, *Curr Opin Oncol* 7(4):387, 1995.
182. Okuda K: Hepatocellular carcinoma, *J Hepatol* 32(suppl 1):225, 2000.
183. Kuper H et al: Tobacco smoking, alcohol consumption and their interaction in the causation of hepatocellular carcinoma, *Int J Cancer*, 85(4):498, 2000.
184. Bismuth H, Majno PE, Adam R: Liver transplantation for hepatocellular carcinoma, *Semin Liver Disease* 19(3):311, 1999.
185. Lowenfels AB et al: Epidemiology of gallbladder cancer, *Hepatogastroenterology* 46(27):1529, 1999.
186. Levin B: Gallbladder carcinoma, *Ann Oncol* 4:129, 1999.
187. Sheth S, Bedford A, Chopra S: Primary gallbladder cancer: recognition of risk factors and the role of prophylactic cholecystectomy, *Am J Gastroenterol* 95(6):1402, 2000.
188. Lowenfels AB, Maisonneuve P, Lankisch PG: Chronic pancreatitis and other risk factors for pancreatic cancer, *Gastroenterol Clin North Am* 28(3):673, 1999.
189. Poston GJ, Gillespie J, Guillou PJ: Biology of pancreatic cancer, *Gut* 32(7):800, 1991.
190. Sakorafas GH, Tsiotou AG, Tsiotos GG: Molecular biology of pancreatic cancer; oncogenes, tumour suppressor genes, growth factors, and their recpetors from a clinical perspective, *Cancer Treat Rev* 26(1):29, 2000.
191. Krech RL, Walsh D: Symptoms of pancreatic cancer, *J Pain Symptom Manage* 6(6):360, 1991.

CHAPTER 39

Alterations of Digestive Function in Children

DEBORAH B. EVERS

CHAPTER OUTLINE

Disorders of the gastrointestinal tract in children include anomalies with structural and functional alterations, as well as enzyme deficiencies. Structural alterations can occur throughout the gastrointestinal tract and include cleft lip and palate, esophageal atresia, tracheoesophageal fistula, pyloric stenosis, aganglionic megacolon, and imperforate anus. Gastroesophageal reflux, hepatic and pancreatic enzyme deficiencies, and bacterial or viral invasions of the gastrointestinal tract also contribute to the diseases and gastrointestinal clinical manifestations in children.

DISORDERS OF THE GASTROINTESTINAL TRACT

Congenital Impairment of Motility

Cleft Lip and Cleft Palate

Cleft lip (harelip) and **cleft palate,** developmental anomalies of the first branchial arch, are the fourth most common congenital disability in the United States (Fig. 39-1).[1] In whites the incidence of cleft lip or cleft palate ranges from 1 in 600 to 1 in 1250 births. The incidence of cleft lip, with or without cleft palate, is 1 in 600 births, whereas the incidence of cleft palate alone is about 1 in 1000 births. Incidence is lower in black populations and higher in Japanese populations. Cleft lip, with or without cleft palate, is more frequent in females. Both anomalies can be unilateral or bilateral, and both anomalies can be partial or complete.

In most cases, cleft lip and cleft palate are caused by multiple gene-environment interactions, including maternal tobacco and alcohol use and genetic variations of the transforming growth factor–alpha gene.[2-4] Preliminary data offer evidence that maternal hyperhomocysteinemia may also be a factor associated with having offspring with nonsyndromic orofacial clefts.[5] (This phenomenon, called *multifactorial inheritance,* is discussed in Chapter 4.) Together, these factors reduce the amount of neural crest mesenchyme that migrates into the area that will develop into the face of the embryo. If the amount is sufficiently reduced, clefting occurs.[6] The cleft can be part of a syndrome determined by single mutant genes or part of a chromosomal defect, usually trisomy 13. Rarely, the cleft is caused by a teratogenic agent, such as an anticonvulsant drug.

Pathophysiology

Cleft lip

Cleft lip is caused by the incomplete fusion of the nasomedial or intermaxillary process during the second month of embryonic development. The deformity develops during a period of very rapid fetal growth. The cleft causes structures of the face and mouth to develop without the normal restraints of encircling lip muscles. A characteristic depression or flattening of the infant's midfacial contour may occur because normal antagonistic forces across the midline are absent, and growth of the involved facial segments is disturbed. The facial cleft may affect not only the lip but also the external nose, the nasal cartilages, the nasal septum, and the alveolar processes.

The cleft is usually just beneath the center of one nostril. The defect may occur bilaterally and may be symmetric or asymmetric. The cleft can range in severity from a slight indentation of the lip to a fissure that extends to the nostril, causing a sagging and flattening of the nose. The failure of lip fusion by 35 days of gestation may impair closure of the palatal shelves. The more complete the cleft lip, the greater the chance that teeth in the line of the cleft will be missing or malformed.

Cleft Palate

Cleft palate is often associated with cleft lip but may occur without it. Cleft palate results from the failure of the primary palatal shelves, or processes, to fuse during the third month of gestation. The fissure may affect only the uvula and soft palate, or it may extend forward to the nostril and involve the hard palate and the maxillary alveolar ridge. It may be unilateral or bilateral, with the cleft occupying the midline posteriorly and as far forward as the alveolar process, where it deviates to the involved side. Clefts involving the palate only are usually but not necessarily in the midline. In some cases the vomer and nasal septum are partly or completely undeveloped. When these facial bones are involved, the nasal cavity may freely communicate with the oral cavity.

Clinical Manifestations

Feeding the infant with cleft lip usually presents no difficulty if the cleft lip is simple and the palate intact. Nursing at breast or bottle depends on suction developed by pressing the nipple against the hard palate with the tongue. Closure of the lips is not necessary, but the tongue must work harder if the infant cannot purse his or her lips. A baby with cleft palate usually requires large, soft nipples with cross-cut openings. Although

WHAT'S NEW? Folic Acid Helps Decrease the Risk of Orofacial Clefts

Folic acid supplementation during pregnancy has been shown to be effective in decreasing the incidence of neural tube defects. The benefits of folic acid supplementation for women who are planning a pregnancy are supported by a study of 891 mothers and infants. Results showed that women who took multivitamins with folic acid surrounding the time of conception had a 25% to 50% lower risk of producing children with orofacial clefts.

Data from Shaw GM et al: Risks of orofacial clefts in children born to women using multivitamins containing folic acid periconceptually, *Lancet* 346:393, 1995.

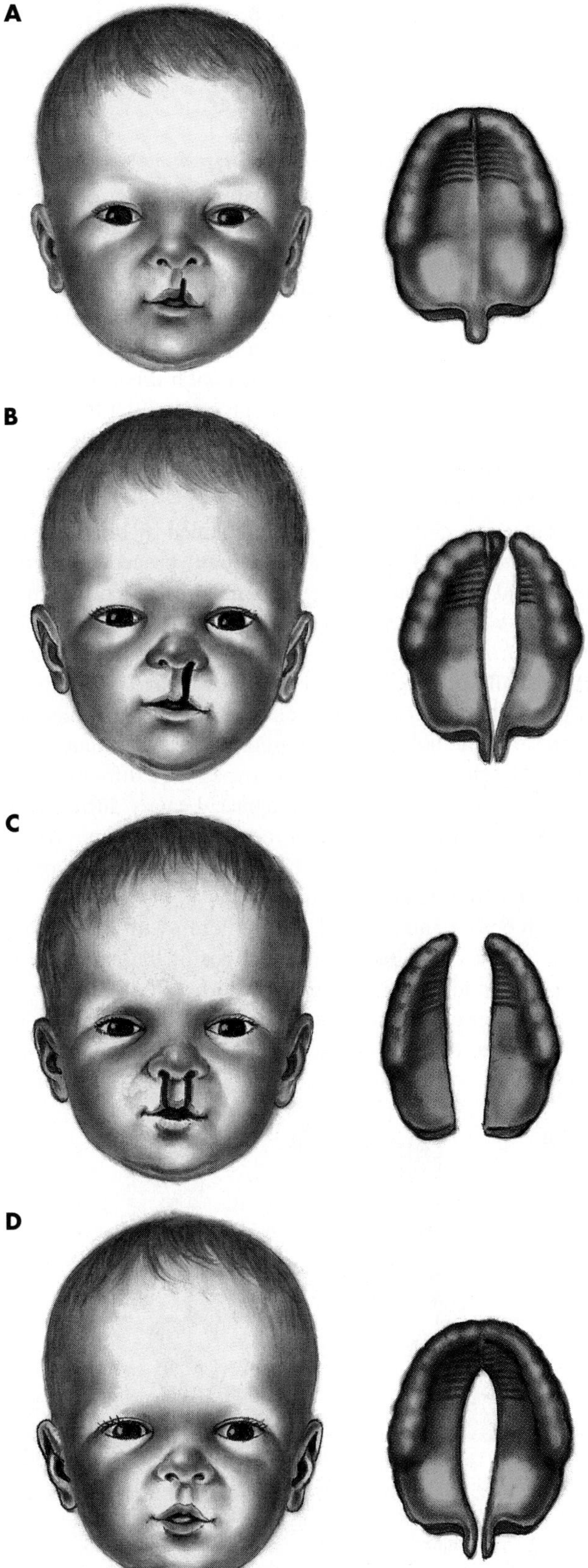

FIG. 39-1 Variations in clefts of the lip and palate. **A,** Notch in vermilion border. **B,** Unilateral cleft lip and palate. **C,** Bilateral cleft lip and cleft palate. **D,** Cleft palate. (From Wong DL: *Whaley and Wong's nursing care of infants and children,* ed 6, St Louis, 1999, Mosby.)

most infants with cleft palate can be successfully breast-fed, it may be impossible for some because of an unproductive suck.[7] An orthodontic prosthesis for the roof of the mouth may facilitate sucking for some infants.

Evaluation and Treatment

Facial x-ray films confirm the extent of bone deformity. Soft tissue alterations are evaluated by history and physical examination.

The nature and extent of the cleft, the infant's condition, and the method of surgical correction proposed determine the course of treatment. Surgical correction is often planned in stages. The lip is united first. Although this can be done within a few weeks of birth, most surgeons prefer to wait until the infant is 2 to 3 months old to allow sufficient growth to occur. The initial repair may be revised when the child is 4 to 5 years old.

Repair of a cleft lip that is accompanied by bilateral cleft palate is technically more difficult, so the procedure is often performed in two steps. The lip is repaired when the infant is a few weeks old. The palate is closed after the child is weaned from the nipple but before he or she has begun to talk, usually at about 12 to 18 months of age.[8] The aim of surgery is to obtain an airtight closure of the palatal cleft and to preserve the mobility and length of the soft palate. Even with early closure, the child may experience difficulty sealing off the nasopharynx from the buccal cavity during swallowing and while pronouncing certain consonants. Speech training and special attention by a prosthodontist and orthodontist are almost always required.

Both before and after surgery, children with cleft lip and palate tend to have recurrent infections of the paranasal sinuses and middle ear. Parents should be alerted to this increased risk so that otitis media can be detected and treated earlier to decrease the chance of long-term scarring and subsequent hearing loss.[9,10] Breast-milk feedings have been found to be associated with a lower incidence of otitis media in these infants.[11] Hypertrophy of the tonsils and adenoids is common. Children with an orofacial cleft are at an increased risk of being infected by *Streptococcus mutans* and *Lactobacillus* at a very early age. Such colonization indicates a high risk for caries in the primary dentition.[12] Displacement of the maxillary arches and malposition of the teeth usually require orthodontic correction.

Esophageal Malformations

Congenital malformations of the esophagus occur in 1 of 3000 to 4500 live births. Esophageal atresia is a condition in which the esophagus ends in a blind pouch. **Esophageal atresia** is usually accompanied by a fistula between the esophagus and the trachea. This connection is called a **tracheoesophageal fistula (TEF).** Either defect can occur alone, however (Fig. 39-2).

Pathophysiology

The esophageal abnormalities are thought to arise from defective differentiation as the trachea separates from the esophagus during the fourth to sixth weeks of embryonic development. Defective growth of endodermal cells leads to atresia. Incomplete fusion of the lateral walls of the foregut leads to incomplete closure of the laryngotracheal tube and fistula formation.

Clinical Manifestations

Polyhydramnios is reported to occur in 14% to 90% of mothers of affected infants.[13] The blind end of the proximal esophagus has a capacity of only a few milliliters. As the infant with esophageal atresia swallows oral secretions, the pouch fills and overflows into the pharynx, resulting in drooling and occasionally in aspiration (see Fig. 39-2, *A* and *C*).

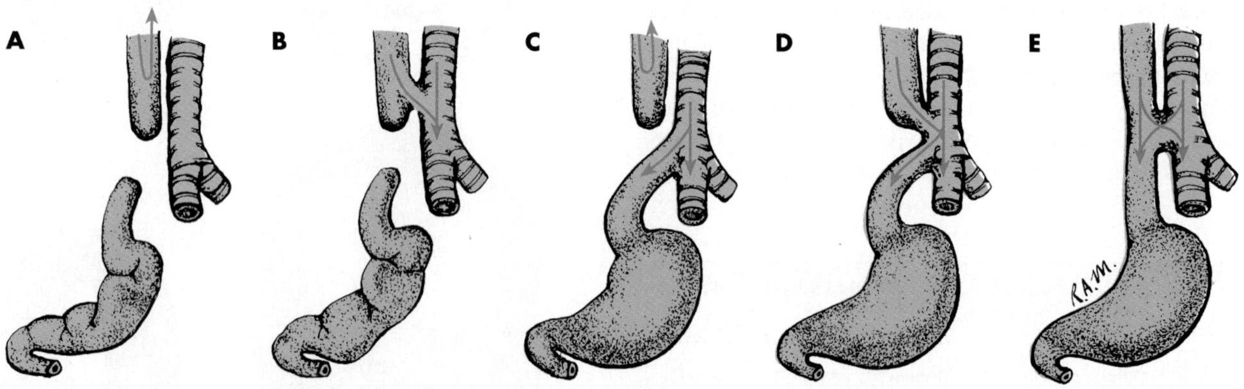

FIG. 39-2 Five types of esophageal atresia and tracheoesophageal fistula. A, Simple esophageal atresia. Proximal esophagus and distal esophagus end in blind pouches, and there is no tracheal communication. Nothing enters the stomach; regurgitated food and fluid may enter the lungs. **B,** Proximal and distal esophageal segments end in blind pouches, and a fistula connects the proximal esophagus to the trachea. Nothing enters the stomach; food and fluid enter the lungs. **C,** Proximal esophagus ends in a blind pouch, and a fistula connects the trachea to the distal esophagus. Air enters the stomach; regurgitated gastric secretions enter the lungs through the fistula. **D,** Fistula connects both proximal and distal esophageal segments to the trachea. Air, food, and fluid enter the stomach and the lungs. **E,** Simple tracheoesophageal fistula between otherwise normal esophagus and trachea. Air, food, and fluid enter the stomach and the lungs. Between 85% and 90% of esophageal anomalies are type C; 6% to 8% are type A; 3% to 5% are type E; and fewer than 1% are type B or D. (From Wong DL: *Whaley and Wong's nursing care of infants and children,* ed 6, St Louis, 1999, Mosby.)

If a fistula connects the trachea with the distal esophagus, the abdomen fills with air and becomes distended. The distention may be great enough to interfere with breathing (see Fig. 39-2, *C* to *E*). If the fistula connects the proximal esophagus to the trachea, the first feeding after birth will be problematic (see Fig. 39-2, *B, D,* and *E*). As the infant drinks, the blind end of the esophagus and the mouth fill with fluid. When the infant tries to take a breath, the fluid is aspirated into the lungs, which triggers protective cough and choke reflexes. Intermittent cyanosis may result. Plain water or glucose is recommended for the initial feeding to minimize the dangers associated with aspiration. If an abnormality of the esophagus is indicated, oral feedings are withheld until a diagnosis is confirmed.

Pulmonary complications are compounded by reflux of air and gastric secretions into the tracheobronchial tree through the fistula (see Fig. 39-2, *D* and *E*), causing severe chemical irritation. The upper lobe of the right lung is most commonly involved because of its proximity to the tracheoesophageal fistula. Infants with esophageal atresia but no fistula have a scaphoid (boat-shaped), gasless abdomen. In fistula without atresia (Fig. 39-2, *E*), the usual symptoms are recurrent aspiration, pneumonia, and atelectasis that remains "silent" for days or even months.

In at least 50% of infants with esophageal defects, other congenital anomalies are present as well. Cardiovascular anomalies are the most common, but other digestive tract, urinary, vertebral, and central nervous system defects can accompany esophageal atresia and tracheoesophageal fistula.

Evaluation and Treatment

Esophageal atresia is usually diagnosed at birth, when attempts to pass a small-bore orogastric or nasogastric tube into the stomach fail. X-ray films show the catheter coiled in the upper esophageal pouch. Barium x-ray examinations are used by some investigators.[14]

Treatment is surgical. Esophageal continuity is restored, and the fistula is eliminated. Surgery is usually undertaken after birth, sometimes in stages. The child may continue to have problems with aspiration, gastroesophageal reflux, and esophagitis after surgical repair.[15,16] The overall survival rate for infants with esophageal defects is approximately 75%.[17]

Pyloric Stenosis

Pyloric stenosis is an obstruction of the pyloric sphincter caused by hypertrophy of the sphincter muscle. It is one of the most common disorders of early infancy and affects infants between the ages of either 1 and 2 weeks or 3 and 4 months.[18] The incidence of pyloric stenosis among males is approximately 5 in 1000, whereas among females it is only 1 in 1000. Whites are affected more frequently than blacks or Asians, and full-term infants are affected more frequently than premature infants.[19] Increased gastrin secretion by the mother in the last trimester of pregnancy increases the likelihood of pyloric stenosis in the infant. The overproduction of gastric secretions in the infant may be caused by stress-related factors in the mother. Exogenous administration of prostaglandin E is associated with an increased incidence of pyloric stenosis. There is an increased incidence of pyloric stenosis in children with Down syndrome; 6.9% of children have a parent who had pyloric stenosis, and 4.9% have a close relative affected.[20,21] Pyloric stenosis occurs in approximately 20% of male and 10% of female descendants of mothers who had pyloric stenosis.[22]

Pathophysiology

The circular muscle of the pylorus is grossly enlarged because of an increase in cell size (hypertrophy) and an increase in cell number (hyperplasia).[23] Research has shown that transforming growth factor–alpha plays a role in stimulating this increase in muscle mass.[24] The mucosal lining of the pyloric opening is folded and the lumen is narrowed by the encroaching muscle. Because of the extra peristaltic effort necessary to force the gastric contents through the narrow pylorus, the muscle layers of the stomach may become hypertrophied as well.

Clinical Manifestations

Between 2 and 3 weeks after birth, an infant who has fed well and gained weight begins to vomit without apparent reason. The vomiting gradually becomes more forceful. In some cases, stomach contents may shoot out 3 or 4 feet. Food is often regurgitated through the nose. The forceful, or projectile, vomiting usually occurs immediately after eating, and the vomitus consists of the bulk of the feeding plus some food retained from previous feedings but is almost always free of bile. Infants frequently are hungry and want to eat again after vomiting.[25]

Prolonged retention of food in the stomach is a characteristic feature of pyloric stenosis. In infants with pyloric stenosis, food is present after 4 hours unless vomiting has occurred. Constipation is the rule because not much food reaches the intestine.

In severe untreated cases, increased gastric peristalsis and vomiting lead to severe fluid and electrolyte imbalances (hypochloremic metabolic alkalosis), chronic malnutrition, and weight loss that can be fatal within 4 to 6 weeks. Infants with pyloric stenosis are irritable because of hunger, and they may have esophageal discomfort caused by repeated vomiting and esophagitis. The vomitus may be blood streaked because of rupture of gastric and esophageal vessels.

Evaluation and Treatment

Diagnosis is based on the history of clinical manifestations. Occasionally, gastric peristalsis is observable over the abdomen. A firm, small, movable mass, approximately the size of an olive, is felt in the right upper quadrant in 70% to 90% of infants with pyloric stenosis. Sonography is routinely done because this clearly shows the hypertrophied pyloric muscles and narrowed pyloric channel. This technique is replacing contrast x-ray examinations.[26,27]

Pyloric stenosis is now recognized earlier than in previous decades; the "classic" metabolic derangements (water and electrolyte imbalances) traditionally associated with this condition have been highly uncommon for the past three decades.[28] The standard treatment for hypertrophic pyloric stenosis is a pyloromyotomy, in which the muscles of the pylorus are split and separated. The mortality rate associated with surgical correction is less than 0.5%.

Some infants respond to medical and nutritional management, which is based on the theory that the pylorus will open spontaneously by 6 to 8 months of age if nutrition can be maintained. To maintain nutrition, antispasmodic drugs are given to relax the pylorospasm and the infant is refed after vomiting. Medical management is associated with slow improvement and a higher mortality rate. Endoscopic balloon dilation and treatment with oral or intravenous atropine sulfate have been successful, but studies reporting this are few.[29]

Malrotation

During the tenth week of embryonic development, the emerging ileum and cecum normally rotate, so that the cecum moves into the lower right quadrant of the abdomen and is fixed there by the mesentery. **Malrotation** is a condition in which rotation does not occur and the colon remains in the upper right quadrant, where an abnormal membrane may press on and obstruct the duodenum. The obstructing band over the duodenum, called a **periduodenal band,** is one of the most significant findings in malrotation. Associated abnormalities are seen in 30% to 62% of children in a reported series; 50% of children with duodenal atresia and 33% of those with jejunal atresia have associated malrotation.[30]

Pathophysiology

The small intestine lacks a normal posterior fixation in malrotation because it has only a rudimentary attachment near the origin of the superior mesenteric artery. Therefore the entire mass can twist when the mobile loops of intestine from the duodenojejunal junction to the middle of the transverse colon twist on themselves. The twisting is termed *volvulus.* Intestinal twisting around the rudimentary mesentery angulates and obstructs the intestinal lumen and partly or completely occludes the superior mesenteric artery, causing infarction and necrosis of the entire midgut.

Clinical Manifestations

Although most cases of malrotation-associated volvulus and infarction develop during the neonatal period (50%) or infancy (85% are younger than 1 year), some develop during childhood or even adulthood.[31] In infants the obstruction causes intermittent or persistent bile-stained vomiting after feedings. Abdominal distention is limited initially to the epigastrium because only the stomach and duodenum are dilated. The degree of distention depends on the pressure of swallowed air and the degree of obstruction caused by the volvulus. Dehydration and electrolyte imbalance may occur rapidly because large amounts of pancreatic juice, bile, and gastric secretions are lost through vomiting. Fever usually ensues. Pain, scanty stools, diarrhea, and bloody stools are associated with progressive volvulus, vascular compression, and infarction of the intestine in infants. Intermittent or partial volvulus may be seen in older children and adults. This may be asymptomatic (25% to 50% of the time) and discovered during unrelated abdominal surgery, or it may cause minor abdominal complaints, such as nausea after meals, recurrent episodes of vomiting, or abdominal pain.[18]

Evaluation and Treatment

Diagnosis of malrotation with volvulus and infarction is based on a review of the clinical manifestations. X-ray films of the abdomen show gas bubbles and distention proximal to the site of obstruction.

Treatment consists of opening the abdomen and reducing the volvulus manually. The surgeon takes the entire intestinal mass in hand and rotates it counterclockwise. Necrotic bowel may be resected and a primary anastomosis performed. When there is gangrene and question of viability of the bowel ends, an enterostomy may be performed. Second-look operations may be done to avoid resection of viable bowel. In cases of malrotation without duodenal obstruction, the operative survival rate is 80%. The operative survival rate is 40% to 50% in cases of malrotation complicated by obstruction caused by periduodenal bands or other intraabdominal anomalies. Resection of large segments of the small intestine results in short-bowel syndrome and its long-term sequelae. Persistence of symptoms after surgical correction suggests pseudo-obstructive motility disorders as the underlying problem.

Meconium Ileus

Meconium is a substance that fills the entire intestine before birth. It consists of intestinal gland secretions and some amniotic fluid. Normally, meconium is passed from the rectum during the first 12 to 72 hours after birth.

Meconium ileus is intestinal obstruction caused by meconium formed in utero that is abnormally sticky and adheres firmly to the mucosa of the small intestine, resisting passage beyond the terminal ileum. The cause is usually a lack of digestive enzymes during fetal life. This meconium is also found to contain albumin, which is not normally found in meconium. The detection of albumin in meconium has been used as a screening test for cystic fibrosis.[32] Neonatal meconium ileus occurs in 10% to 15% of newborns with cystic fibrosis.[33] Partial aplasia of the pancreas is an associated factor, however, and one fifth of infants with meconium ileus are premature or have a history of maternal hydramnios (excessive amniotic fluid). After intestinal atresia and malrotation with volvulus, meconium ileus is the most common cause of small intestinal obstruction in newborns.

Pathophysiology

The terminal ileum is plugged with thick, viscous meconium resulting from the formation of an insoluble, calcium-glycoprotein compound in abnormal mucus. The segment of the ileum proximal to the obstruction is distended with liquid contents, and its walls may be hypertrophied. The segment distal to the obstruction is collapsed and filled with small pellets of pale-colored stool. Meconium in the obstructed segment has the consistency of thick syrup or glue. Peristalsis fails to propel this viscous material through the ileum, so it becomes impacted. Volvulus, atresia, or perforation of the bowel sometimes accompanies meconium ileus.

Clinical Manifestations

Abdominal distention usually develops during the first few days after birth. The infant does not pass meconium and begins to vomit within hours or days of birth. Infants with cystic fibrosis may have signs of pulmonary involvement, such as tachypnea, intercostal retractions, and grunting respirations. The distended abdomen shows patterns of dilated intestinal loops that feel doughlike when palpated. Some of the loops contain scattered, firm, movable masses. Despite hyperactive peristalsis, the rectal ampulla is empty.

Evaluation and Treatment

Radiologic examination is used to confirm the presence of meconium ileus.[34] The sweat test, which is accurate in 90% of infants, is performed to detect or rule out cystic fibrosis. The treatment of choice for cases not complicated by volvulus or perforation is a hyperosmolar enema done using fluoroscopy to evacuate the meconium. Although the success of this technique has not correlated with osmolality of the enema, the overall success rate is higher when meglumine diatrizoate (Gastrografin) is used than when it is not used. Also, the success rate is better when additives, such as polysorbate 80 (Tween 80) and acetylcysteine (Mucomyst), are used.[35] Enterotomy and irrigation are reserved for complicated cases and enema failures.

Survival of infants with meconium ileus is improving, with a 97% to 98% survival rate at 1 year.[36] The mortality rate increases to 70% if obstruction is complicated by peritonitis. After recovery from neonatal meconium ileus, the long-term outlook depends on the severity and progression of pulmonary disease. Recent research demonstrates a clear association of meconium ileus with poor long-term nutritional outcomes in children with cystic fibrosis related to surgical treatment for the ileus and poor essential fatty-acid status.[37]

Distal Intestinal Obstruction Syndrome

Distal intestinal obstruction syndrome (DIOS), formerly called *meconium ileus equivalent,* affects approximately 15% of children and adults with cystic fibrosis.[38] Intestinal contents may become abnormally thick and impact the intestinal lumen, particularly after episodes of dehydration or lack of pancreatic enzymes. Use of high-strength pancreatic enzymes has been implicated in formation of strictures of the ascending colon in children with cystic fibrosis and resultant chronic DIOS.[39,40] The child displays signs and symptoms of intestinal obstruction. In most cases the obstruction is relieved by hypertonic enemas. Meconium ileus and DIOS have been shown to be risk factors for the development of liver disease in those with cystic fibrosis.[38,41]

Obstructions of the Duodenum, Jejunum, and Ileum

Congenital obstruction of the duodenum can be caused by intrinsic malformations or external pressure. Intrinsic obstruction is caused by failure of the duodenum to become patent. The obstruction may be partial or complete and usually is located at or near the major duodenal papilla. Extrinsic obstructions can be caused by peritoneal bands that constrict the duodenum. The duodenum can be obstructed by an annular pancreas—a defect in which the head of the pancreas surrounds part of the duodenum. Congenital obstructions of the jejunum and ileum can be attributable to atresia, stenosis, meconium ileus, megacolon (Hirschsprung disease), intussusception, Meckel diverticulum, intestinal duplication, or strangulated hernia.

In **ileal atresia** or **jejunal atresia,** the intestine ends blindly proximal and distal to an interruption in its continuity, with or without a gap in the mesentery. Stenosis (narrowing of the lumen) causes dilation proximal to the obstruction and luminal collapse distal to it.

Congenital Aganglionic Megacolon

Congenital aganglionic megacolon (Hirschsprung disease) is a functional obstruction of the colon caused by inadequate motility. The exact cause is unknown but appears to involve multiple interacting factors and a complex inheritance pattern that involves the *RET* proto-oncogene.[42] There is an increased incidence in males (3.9 : 1) and increased incidence in the siblings of children with Hirschsprung disease (4%) as compared with the general population incidence of 0.02% (1 : 5000).[43] There is an increased incidence in children with Down syndrome.[20,44] The inheritance pattern seems to change with extension of the aganglionic portion of the colon. Aganglionosis beyond the sigmoid colon appears to be more compatible with a dominant gene pattern with incomplete penetrance. With short-segment Hirschsprung disease (involving the rectum up to the sigmoid colon), the inheritance patterns appear multifactorial with the recessive gene pattern of low penetrance.[45] Interaction of endothelin-3 with endothelin-B receptors has been found to be essential for the development of epidermal melanocytes and enteric neurons. Disruption of the endothelin-B receptor gene has been found to cause aganglionic megacolon in mice, and defects in this receptor gene have been mapped to human chromosome 13. It is postulated that this defect may be the cause of hereditary Hirschsprung disease.[46]

Pathophysiology

Congenital aganglionic megacolon is caused by a malformation of the parasympathetic nervous system. It is characterized by abnormalities of the basement membrane and extracellular matrix and absence of the intramural ganglion cells in the enteric nerve plexuses (Meissner and Auerbach plexuses) along variable lengths of the colon.[43] Lacking neural stimulation, the muscle layers of the colon wall fail to propel feces through the colon, leading to obstruction. In 80%

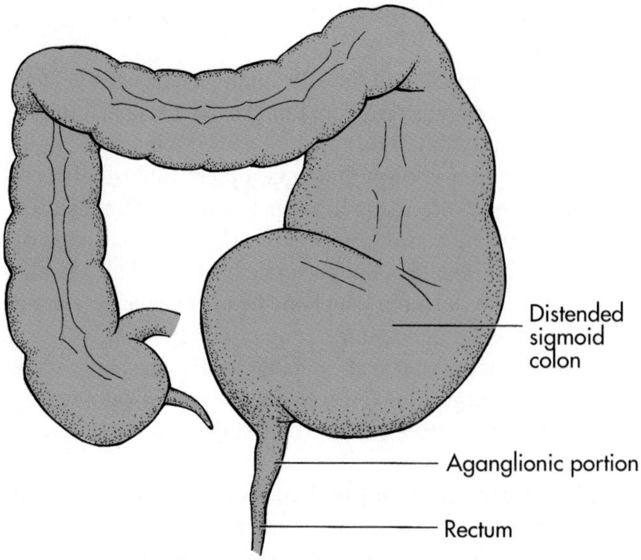

Fig. 39-3 Congenital aganglionic megacolon (Hirschsprung disease). (From Wong DL: *Whaley and Wong's nursing care of infants and children,* ed 6, St Louis, 1999, Mosby.)

of cases the aganglionic segment is limited to the rectal end of the sigmoid colon. In 3% of cases the entire colon lacks ganglion cells. The abnormally innervated colon obstructs fecal movements, causing the proximal colon to become distended; hence the term *megacolon* (Fig. 39-3).

The ganglia normally develop from an advancing neural crest between the muscle layers (tunica muscularis) in the submucosal area (muscularis mucosae) of the intestinal wall. In cases of congenital megacolon, neurologic development is blocked and large, nonmyelinated fibers develop in place of these ganglion cells.[47] The segment of colon that lacks ganglion cells has a relatively normal lumen caliber and wall thickness. In the segment of the colon proximal to it, the lumen is dilated and the muscle hypertrophied. Therefore the abnormal portion of the colon appears to be normal and the normal portion appears to be diseased.

Clinical Manifestations

The extent of the aganglionic portion of the colon determines the severity of the symptoms of congenital aganglionic megacolon. The most distal part of the rectum is always involved. This is the extent of the aganglionic portion in some children, and the child is said to have "ultrashort-segment" Hirschsprung disease and generally has only mild constipation as a symptom. These individuals may not be diagnosed until adulthood. Symptoms of constipation increase in severity as the aganglionic portion extends proximally. Diarrhea may be the first sign, however, because only water can travel around the impacted feces.

The most serious complication in the neonatal period is enterocolitis related to fecal impaction. Bowel dilation stretches and partly occludes the encircling blood and lymphatic vessels, causing edema, ischemia, infarction of the mucosa, and significant outflow of fluid into the bowel lumen. Copious, liquid stools result. Infarction and destruction of the mucosa enable enteric microorganisms to penetrate the bowel wall. Frequently, gram-negative sepsis occurs, accompanied by fever and vomiting. Severe and rapid electrolyte changes may take place, causing collapse and rapid death.

Evaluation and Treatment

Anorectal manometry is a reliable screening tool for the diagnosis of Hirschsprung disease.[48] Serial manometry measurements may be required in neonates.[49] This test has uncovered ultrashort-segment Hirschsprung disease in older children with a history of constipation.[50] The definitive diagnosis is made by rectal biopsy showing an absence of ganglion cells in the submucosa of the colon. X-ray films show dilated loops of colon, and contrast films show aganglionic areas. The infant usually cannot expel the barium.

The involved segment is resected within the first few months of life. For children with short-segment Hirschsprung disease, enemas are given to relieve impaction and laxatives with a dietary and bowel training program are used in preference to surgical intervention.[50] The child is *not* treated for diarrhea.

After surgery, enterocolitis sometimes recurs. If the postoperative enterocolitis is allowed to persist, pseudopolyps may appear. Because these are essentially identical to the lesions of ulcerative colitis, they have malignant potential. Therefore a colectomy is indicated if pseudopolyps develop.

In general, the prognosis of congenital megacolon is satisfactory for children who undergo surgical treatment. Bowel training may be prolonged, but most children achieve bowel continence before puberty.[51]

Anorectal Malformations

Several congenital malformations of anorectal structures can obstruct the passage of feces. The incidence of minor abnormalities is approximately 1 in 500, and that of major anomalies is approximately 1 in 5000.

Congenital anorectal malformations range from mild anal stenosis, which is corrected by simple dilation, to complex deformities, such as anal or rectal agenesis, atresia, and fistula (Fig. 39-4). Deformities that cause complete obstruction are known collectively as **imperforate anus.**

Approximately 40% of infants with anorectal malformations have other developmental anomalies as well. The most commonly associated major anomalies are Down syndrome, congenital heart disease, renal abnormalities, cryptorchidism, esophageal atresia, and malformations of the spine.[20,52-54]

Imperforate anus may not be obvious. It can be detected by gentle insertion of a rectal tube. X-ray films show dilations throughout the intestinal tract. Anal stenosis can be treated by dilations, but all other anorectal malformations require surgical correction. The overall mortality rate is approximately 10%. More than 90% of children with a low (anal) anomaly achieve bowel continence; however, fewer than 30% of those with very high anomalies or anomalies associated with genitourinary fistulae achieve continence.[55-57]

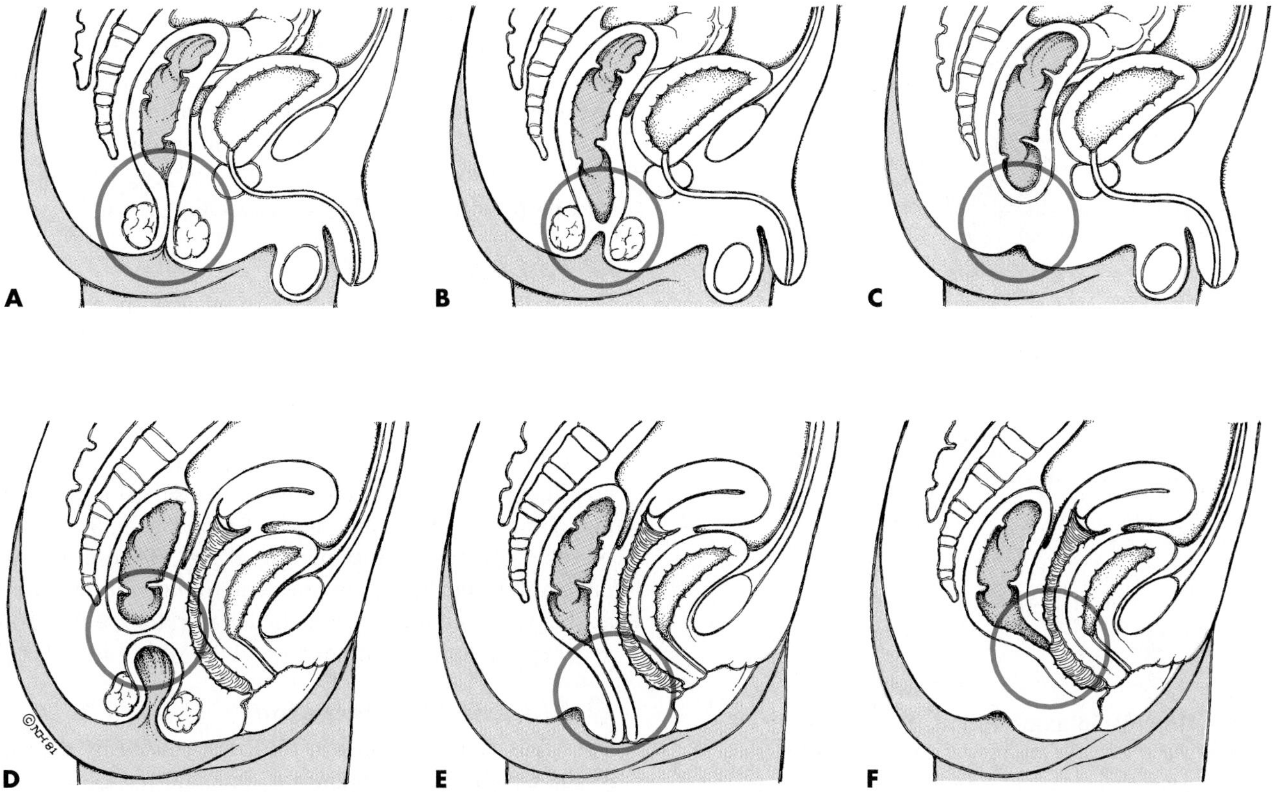

FIG. 39-4 Anorectal stenosis and imperforate anus. A, Congenital anal stenosis. **B,** Anal membrane atresia. **C,** Anal agenesis. **D,** Rectal atresia. **E,** Rectoperineal fistula. **F,** Rectovaginal fistula. (From Wong DL: *Whaley and Wong's nursing care of infants and children,* ed 5, St Louis, 1995, Mosby.)

Acquired Impairment of Motility

Intussusception

The most frequent cause of acquired intestinal obstruction in infants is intussusception. **Intussusception** is the telescoping or invagination of one portion of the intestine into another. Usually, the ileum invaginates the cecum and part of the ascending colon by collapsing through the ileocecal valve. Intussusception involving the ileum and colon (ileocolic intussusception) accounts for 80% to 90% of intestinal obstructions in infants and is two to three times more frequent in males than in females.[58] Nearly 75% of intussusceptions occur before age 2 years; 70% occur before age 1 year. Intussusception is rare in infants younger than 3 months and is infrequent after 36 months. Intussusception has occurred in children of all ages recovering from abdominal surgery; intussusception has been found in children with cystic fibrosis and symptoms of bowel obstruction that were initially misdiagnosed as distal intestinal obstruction syndrome (meconium ileus equivalent).[59,60]

Pathophysiology

Most commonly, the proximal portion of the intestine, the intussusceptum, collapses into the distal portion, the intussuscipiens, in the direction of peristaltic flow (Fig. 39-5). As it does so, the intussusceptum drags its mesentery into the enveloping lumen. Initially, the mesentery is constricted, obstructing venous return. Compression of the mesenteric vessels between the two layers of intestinal wall and at the U-shaped angle at either end of the intussusceptum leads within hours to venous stasis, engorgement, edema, exudation, and further vascular compression. Unless the intussusception is treated, bleeding and gangrene ensue. The tension of the mesentery on the intussusceptum tends to arch the bowel in a curve with its center at the mesenteric root. Edema and compression obstruct the flow of chyme through the intestine.

Clinical Manifestations

The affected infant suddenly develops abdominal pain, becomes irritable (colicky), and draws up the knees. Vomiting occurs soon afterward. A single normal stool may be passed, evacuating the colon distal to the apex of the intussusception. After that, 60% of infants pass "currant jelly" stools, which appear dark and gelatinous because of their blood and mucus content. In one study, less than one third of children had this clinical triad of vomiting, colicky abdominal pain, and bloody stools.[61] Most infants have a tender, sausage-shaped abdominal mass. Abdominal tenderness and distention develop as intestinal obstruction becomes more acute.[62]

Evaluation and Treatment

Diagnosis is based on clinical manifestations, onset of symptoms, and ultrasonography. Ultrasound of the abdomen facilitates establishing a diagnosis; more than 82% of children

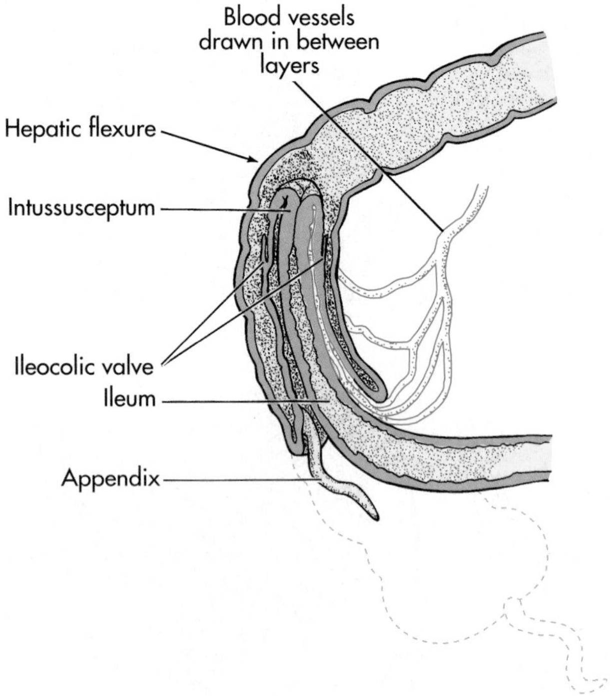

Fig. 39-5 Ileocolic intussusception. (From Wong DL: *Whaley and Wong's nursing care of infants and children,* ed 6, St Louis, 1999, Mosby.)

have positive ultrasound results in both ileocolic and jejuno-intestinal intussusception. Reduction is an emergency procedure involving hydrostatic pressure generated by an air or a barium enema given using fluoroscopic guidance.[63] This technique is successful 45% to 70% of the time. A potential complication of enema reduction is bowel perforation, and for this reason the use of air rather than barium is favored.[64] Surgical reduction is done on children who fail or are not candidates for hydrostatic reduction. Untreated intussusception in infants is nearly always fatal. Most infants recover if the intussusception is reduced within 24 hours.[65] Spontaneous reduction of intussusception may occur in symptomatic or asymptomatic children and occurs more commonly than previously reported. These intussusceptions are usually short-segment, small-bowel intussusceptions with no recognizable lead point.[66] Recurrent intussusception is more frequent after nonsurgical reduction than after surgical reduction. Risk of recurrence cannot be predicted by initial features or symptoms, and children with recurrent intussusception may exhibit fewer symptoms with a shorter interval to bowel necrosis and perforation.[67]

Gastroesophageal Reflux

Gastroesophageal reflux (GER) involves dilation of the esophagus and intrusion of acid contents into it; GER is believed to be related to relaxation or incompetence of the lower esophageal sphincter (see Chapter 38). In newborns, reflux is normal because neuromuscular control of the gastroesophageal sphincter is not fully developed. The frequency of reflux is highest in premature infants and decreases during the first 6 to 12 months of life.

There is an increased incidence of symptomatic reflux in children with neurologic impairment and cerebral palsy.[68] It is thought to be a factor in the stimulation of apnea and reactive airway disease in some children.[69] Reflux is thought to be a contributing cause in infant deaths and sudden infant death syndrome.[70] Increasingly, GER has been recognized as a significant problem for children with cystic fibrosis.[71]

Pathophysiology

Delayed maturation of the lower esophageal sphincter or impaired hormonal or neurotransmitter response mechanisms (i.e., vasoactive intestinal peptide and nitric oxide) are possible causes of inappropriate sphincter relaxation. Factors that maintain lower esophageal sphincter integrity in children include location of the gastroesophageal junction in a high-pressure zone within the abdomen, mucosal gathering within the sphincter, and the angle at which the esophagus is inserted into the stomach. Reflux persists if any of these pressure-maintaining factors is altered. Irritation of the mucosa by acidic gastric contents results in deterioration of the esophageal epithelium and stimulation of the vomiting reflex.[25,72]

Clinical Manifestations

The signs and symptoms of GER are caused by exposure of the esophageal epithelium to refluxed gastric contents. Eighty-five percent of affected infants vomit excessively during the first week of life and usually have other symptoms by 6 weeks.

Vomiting may be forceful and must be differentiated from pyloric stenosis. Aspiration pneumonia develops in one third of infants with GER. In cases that persist into childhood, chronic cough, wheezing, and recurrent pneumonia are common.[73] Repeated vomiting leads to inadequate retention of nutrients, adversely affecting growth and weight gain. Esophagitis from exposure of the esophageal mucosa to acidic gastric contents is manifested by pain, bleeding, and eventually stricture formation and abnormal motility. Approximately 25% of children with GER also have iron deficiency anemia caused by frank or occult blood loss.

Evaluation and Treatment

The clinical manifestations are often adequate to confirm a diagnosis of GER. A barium swallow and esophageal pH monitoring with a probe are useful diagnostic procedures in complex cases.[72]

Mild GER resolves without treatment. Maintaining infants in a flat prone or a left lateral position, particularly during and for the first hour after a feeding, results in fewer or shorter episodes of GER.[74] Infants with GER are excepted from the Academy of Pediatrics' recommended sleep position for healthy infants to decrease the risk of SIDS.[75] Older infants and children achieve better results in an upright (sitting or standing) position while awake, with prone positioning used for sleeping.[74] Thickened feedings may help some infants; however, this has not been shown to be consistently helpful. For some infants, thickened feedings may actually worsen reflux by causing a delay in gastric emptying time.

WHAT'S NEW? An Infant Is Vomiting: Could It be Pyloric Stenosis or Gastroesophageal Reflux?

Recent research has shown that serum bicarbonate levels of 29 mmol/L or greater and serum chloride levels of 98 mmol/L or less have high positive predictive values and are specific in identifying infants with pyloric stenosis. Evaluation of these values help discriminate between pyloric stenosis and gastroesophageal reflux when the history and physical examination fail to do so. Therefore incorporating this additional diagnostic tool when evaluating infants with vomiting of uncertain etiology may prove helpful.

Data from Smith GA, Mihalov L, Shields BJ: Diagnostic aids in the differentiation of pyloric stenosis from severe gastroesophageal reflux during early infancy: the utility of serum bicarbonate and serum chloride, *Am J Emerg Med* 17(1):28, 1999.

Small, frequent feedings and frequent burping are generally universally accepted strategies for managing reflux.[76] Medications to increase motility, increase lower esophageal sphincter pressure, or decrease gastric acid production have been used to treat GER. If no improvement is seen with medical management or the child has life-threatening events with reflux, an antireflux surgical procedure, including gastropexy and fundoplication, is performed. A fundoplication re-creates a valve by wrapping the fundus of the stomach around the lower esophagus.[77]

Impairment of Digestion, Absorption, and Nutrition

Cystic Fibrosis

Cystic fibrosis (CF) of the pancreas, which is also called *mucoviscidosis* or *fibrocystic disease* of the pancreas, is a genetically transmitted disease (mutation of the long arm of chromosome 7) that involves many organs and systems and usually causes death in childhood or young adulthood. It is the most frequent cause of chronic suppurative lung disease in children and is the most common life-threatening inherited disease in the white population. This section focuses on the deficiency of pancreatic enzymes. (Chapter 33 discusses the pulmonary consequences of cystic fibrosis.)

Pathophysiology

The pathophysiologic triad that is the hallmark of CF includes (1) pancreatic enzyme deficiency, which causes maldigestion; (2) overproduction of mucus in the respiratory tract and inability to clear secretions, which cause progressive chronic obstructive pulmonary disease; and (3) abnormally elevated sodium and chloride concentrations in sweat. Exocrine secretions tend to be abnormally thick and to precipitate in the glandular ducts, obstructing flow. Almost all clinical manifestations of CF are a result of overproduction of extremely viscous mucus and pancreatic enzyme deficiency. The full spectrum of involvement is evident from Table 39-1.

Pancreatic function may range from normal to completely ablated. Approximately 85% of patients have pancreatic insufficiency. Obstruction of the pancreatic ducts with thick mucus blocks the flow of pancreatic enzymes and causes degenerative and fibrotic changes in the pancreas. Pancreatic damage eventually can affect the beta cells, resulting in diabetes mellitus in some children. The incidence of diabetes mellitus and cirrhosis in this population has increased as larger numbers of people with cystic fibrosis have moved into young and middle adulthood. Severe problems with maldigestion of proteins, carbohydrates, and fats occur because of insufficient secretion of pancreatic enzymes.[78]

Clinical Manifestations

Clinical manifestations are presented in Table 39-1.

Evaluation and Treatment

Seventy-two-hour stool fat measurements are used to determine the extent of pancreatic function. Stools also may be examined for absence of pancreatic enzymes, particularly trypsin and chymotrypsin. To optimize treatment, the 13Carbon-mixed triglyceride breath test offers a simple, noninvasive way of assessing the need for pancreatic enzyme supplementation in children with cystic fibrosis.[79] Pancreatic replacement enzymes are administered before or with meals. However, even with enzyme replacement, the improvement in digestion is not complete or consistent.[80] High-calorie, high-protein diets with frequent snacks and vitamin supplements are used to treat the malnutrition; however, anorexia is not uncommon in this group secondary to pulmonary disease and frequently large sputum output. To combat the worsening problem of growth failure in children with cystic fibrosis, an increasing number of persons are using nasogastric or gastrostomy tube feedings to supplement oral intake.[81]

Gluten-Sensitive Enteropathy

Gluten-sensitive enteropathy, formerly called *celiac sprue* or *celiac disease,* is the loss of mature villous epithelium caused by ingestion of gluten, the protein component of cereal grains. The gluten in wheat, rye, barley, and oats is toxic to the intestinal epithelial cells of genetically susceptible individuals.[82] The disease occurs largely in whites and has been documented in Asians from India and Pakistan, but it is almost nonexistent in native Africans, Japanese, and Chinese. Prevalence rates in Europe range from 1 in 1000 to 1 in 3000. Recent data suggest that gluten-sensitive enteropathy, traditionally considered rare in the United States, may be as common as in Europe.[83]

The pathogenesis appears to require interaction between a number of intrinsic factors (genetic susceptibility, activation of the immune system) and extrinsic factors (gluten and possibly other environmental factors). Both cellular immunity and humoral immunity are implicated. There are increases in the percentages of T cells, immunoglobulin, and complement in the mucosa of active celiac disease. Immunoglobulin A (IgA) and immunoglobulin M (IgM) antigliadin antibodies have been found in jejunal fluid of persons with untreated disease.[84] Although gluten-sensitive enteropathy is widely perceived as a malabsorption syndrome of childhood, the

Table 39-1 Pathophysiology, Clinical Manifestations, and Complications of Cystic Fibrosis

Organ Involved	Secretory Dysfunction	Clinical Manifestations	Complications
Sweat glands	Elevated concentration of sodium and chloride in sweat	Hyponatremia; hypochloremia	Heat prostration; shock
Intestine			
Newborn	Viscid meconium	Meconium ileus with intestinal obstruction	Meconium peritonitis
Older child and adult	Inspissated (dried out) mucofecal masses (intestinal sludging)	Partial intestinal obstruction with severe cramping pains	Volvulus (obstruction), intussusception (prolapse)
Pancreas (enzyme deficiency)	Inspissation and precipitation of pancreatic secretions, causing obstruction of pancreatic ducts	Absence of pancreatic enzymes, causing malabsorption of food and fatty, bulky stools	Hypoproteinemia; iron deficiency anemia; malnutrition
		Decreased vitamins A, D, E, and K absorption	Vitamins A, D, E, and K deficiency and rectal prolapse
	Insulin deficiency	Glucose intolerance	Diabetes mellitus
Liver	Inspissation and precipitation of bile in biliary system	Focal biliary cirrhosis; shrunken, "hob-nail" liver	Portal hypertension with esophageal varices and hematemesis
Salivary glands	Inspissation and precipitation of secretions in small ducts of submaxillary and sublingual salivary glands	Mild patchy fibrosis of salivary glands	None
Paranasal structures	Viscid mucus	Retention of mucus; clouding seen on sinus roentgenograms	Mucopyoceles (pus accumulations) with nasal deformity or orbital cavity extension
Nose	Nasal polyps	Obstruction of nasal air flow	None
Lungs	Viscid mucus in bronchioles and bronchi	Obstruction of bronchioles causing bronchiolectasis, bronchiectasis, and chronic lung infection	Hemoptysis; pneumothorax; cor pulmonale; respiratory failure
Reproductive tract			
Male	Viscid genital tract secretions during embryologic development, causing failure of formation of normal vas deferens	Sterility	None
Female	Distention of endocervical epithelial cells with cytoplasmic mucin	Decreased fertility	Polypoid cervicitis (cervical inflammation) while taking oral contraceptives

From Rudolph AM, Hoffman JIE: *Pediatrics,* Norwalk, Conn, 1982, Appleton-Century-Crofts.

diagnosis is increasingly being made for the first time in adult life.[85]

◆ *Pathophysiology*

The mucosa of the upper small intestine appears shiny, cobble stoned, and thin in children with gluten-sensitive enteropathy. The major pathophysiologic characteristics of the disease are atrophy of villi in the upper small intestine and malabsorption of most nutrients in the presence of cereal gluten (Fig. 39-6). The atrophy is caused by accelerated shedding of epithelial cells from the villi. To compensate for this loss, epithelial cell production increases, causing hypertrophy of the crypts of Lieberkühn. Increased cell production is not sufficient to keep pace with cell loss, however. Inflammation and edema develop around the enlarged cysts. The villi shorten and atrophy, and their surface cells are not mature enough to sustain absorptive functions. The microvilli and brush border disappear, leaving patches of bald mucosa. The loss of mucosal surface area and brush-border enzymes leads to severe malabsorption. The pathologic process is most pronounced in the duodenum and jejunum. The ileum may be spared. The severity of disease correlates with the length of the small intestinal mucosa involved.

Damage to the mucosa of the duodenum and jejunum has secondary effects that exacerbate malabsorption. The secretion of intestinal hormones, such as secretin and cholecystokinin-pancreozymin, may be diminished. Because these chemical messengers are scarce, secretion of pancreatic enzymes and expulsion of bile from the gallbladder decrease.

Destruction of mucosal cells causes inflammation, and water and electrolytes are secreted, leading to watery diarrhea. In addition, absorption that normally occurs by sodium-dependent active transport or facilitated diffusion is impaired. Carbohydrates, amino acids, dipeptides, water-soluble vita-

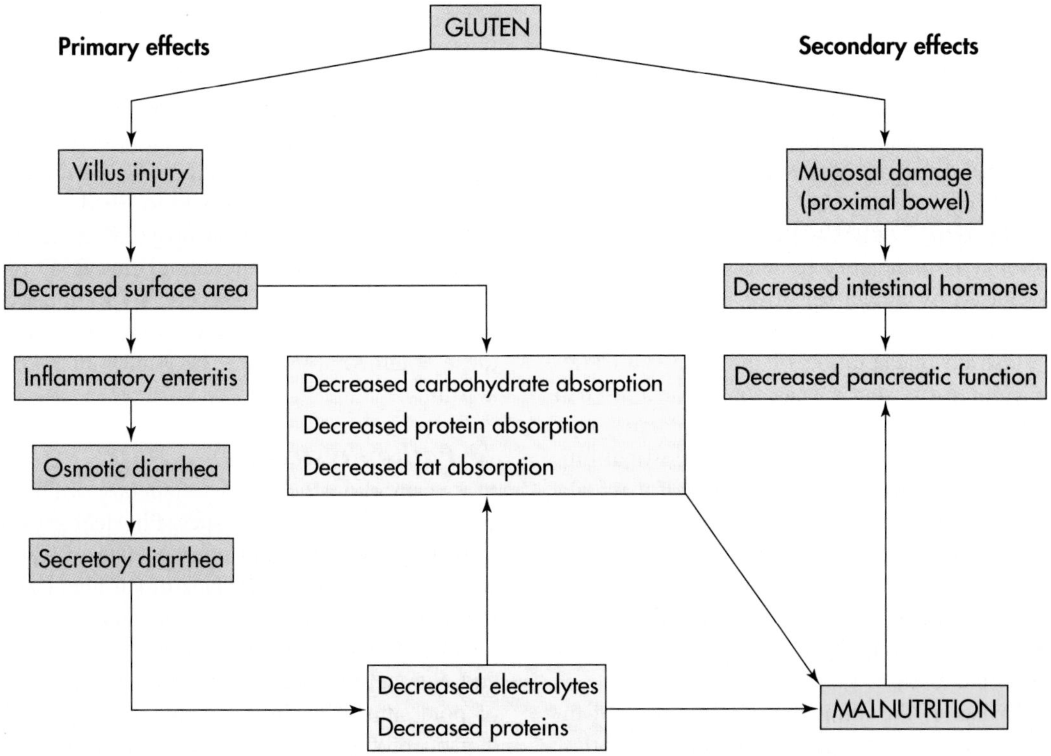

FIG. 39-6 Pathophysiology of gluten-sensitive enteropathy.

mins, bile salts, and cations are not absorbed from the intestinal lumen. Potassium loss, which is more severe than sodium loss, leads to muscle weakness. Magnesium and calcium malabsorption can cause seizures or tetany. Unabsorbed fatty acids combine with calcium, and secondary hyperparathyroidism increases phosphorus excretion, resulting in bone reabsorption. Calcium is no longer available to bind oxalate in the intestine and is absorbed, which causes hyperoxaluria. Gallbladder function may be abnormal, and bile salt conjugation may be decreased.

Fat malabsorption in the jejunum is the major cause of steatorrhea (fatty stools). Malabsorption may be mild early in the disease. Fecal nitrogen is elevated because peptidase deficiencies impair protein absorption. Pancreatic function is decreased, not only because of decreased hormonal levels but also because of malnutrition.

Deficiencies of fat-soluble vitamins are common in children with gluten-sensitive enteropathy. Vitamin K malabsorption leads to hypoprothrombinemia. In one third of cases, iron and folic acid malabsorption are manifested as cheilosis; anemia; and a smooth, red tongue. Vitamin B_{12} absorption is impaired in those with extensive ileal disease. Because the absorption of folate and iron is greatest in the proximal small intestine, deficiencies of these substances are common.

Clinical Manifestations

The onset of clinical manifestations of gluten-sensitive enteropathy depends on the age of the infant when gluten-containing substances are added to the diet. In 50% of affected children, onset occurs by 18 months of age, with latent intervals varying from months to years. Severity of symptoms can vary tremendously.

Diarrhea is an early sign in most infants. The stools are pale, bulky, greasy, and foul smelling, and they may contain oil droplets. Three to five such movements occur daily. As early as 3 or 4 months of age, growth failure, anorexia, and constipation can begin. In older children, constipation is occasionally seen despite steatorrhea. Vomiting and abdominal pain are prominent in infants but unusual in older children. Anorexia is prevalent. The classic physical manifestations of organic failure to thrive, such as abdominal protuberance, wasted buttocks and limbs, and hypotonia, occur in fewer than 50% of infants with gluten-sensitive enteropathy. Growth is usually diminished.[86]

Manifestations of malabsorption, such as rickets, tetany, frank or occult bleeding, or anemia, may be obvious.[87] Some children urinate more at night. The tongue is smooth and red, and the child may bruise and bleed easily. Hypomagnesemia and hypocalcemia cause irritability, tremor, convulsions, tetany, bone pain, osteomalacia, and dental abnormalities. If vitamin D deficiency is prolonged, rickets and clubbing of the terminal phalanges are likely. Eighty-six percent of older children have fingerprint changes (ridge atrophy). In older children, delayed puberty and infertility may be a manifestation of otherwise subtle gluten-sensitive enteropathy. Osteomalacia may be severe; skeletal symptoms were the most prominent finding in 30% of adults with atypical forms of gluten-sensitive enteropathy.[88] Small intestinal lymphoma is also associated with gluten-sensitive enteropathy.[89]

An unusual complication of gluten-sensitive enteropathy in infancy is celiac crisis. Celiac crisis is characterized by severe diarrhea, dehydration, and hypoproteinemia as a result of malabsorption and protein loss.

Evaluation and Treatment

An intestinal biopsy is mandatory to detect the classic mucosal changes caused by gluten-sensitive enteropathy. The initial biopsy generally is followed by a second intestinal biopsy to demonstrate regeneration of intestinal villi after treatment with a gluten-free diet. Occasionally, the child will be rechallenged with gluten at a later point and a biopsy performed a third time to demonstrate return of intestinal mucosal damage. A wide variety of screening tests for malabsorption also may be useful. Serum IgA and immunoglobulin G (IgG) antigliadin (from gluten) antibodies also are measured. Urinary assay to determine the ratio of lactose to mannitol has been successfully used to differentiate children with active gluten-sensitive enteropathy from healthy children or children with inactive disease.[90]

Treatment consists of the immediate and permanent institution of a diet free of cereal grains (wheat, rye, barley, oats, malt). Lactose intolerance is presumed; therefore lactose (milk sugar) also is excluded from the diet. Tolerance to lactose improves with removal of gluten and healing of the mucosa and may be reintroduced at a later point. Infants are routinely given vitamin D, iron, and folic acid supplements to treat deficiencies.

Approximately 25% of children experience recurrent relapses that interfere with growth. For most children, however, the long-term prognosis is excellent. There is an increased incidence of malignant disease, particularly lymphoma, in individuals who fail to respond to gluten-free diets.

Protein Energy Malnutrition

Kwashiorkor and marasmus are the two most common types of malnutrition in children. These disorders are known collectively as **protein energy malnutrition (PEM).** Both are states of long-term starvation (see Chapter 38). **Kwashiorkor** is a severe protein deficiency, and **marasmus** is a severe deficiency of all nutrients. Kwashiorkor is a widespread nutritional problem among children in developing countries and economically destitute populations. The disease usually occurs in infants or children from 1 to 4 years of age who have been weaned from breast milk to a high-starch, protein-deficient diet.

Marasmus can occur at any age, but it is common in children younger than 1 year. In marasmus, starvation is attributable to lack of protein and carbohydrates. One third of the world's children suffer from PEM, with the highest concentrations in Latin America, Asia, and Africa.[91] The mortality risk for children in developing countries has been found to be inversely related to anthropometric indicators (height, weight, head circumference, skinfold thickness, midarm muscle circumference). There is elevated risk even in the mild to moderate range of malnutrition.[92] Poor sanitation and early weaning of breast-fed infants to overdiluted commercial formulas are major risk factors for PEM.

PEM is a complication of some diseases, such as chronic fever, tuberculosis, malignancy, digestive and malabsorptive disorders, and psychogenic illness. Radiation therapy and chemotherapy can also contribute to PEM. Acute and chronic malnutrition is common in hospitalized individuals in the United States. One study found that 25% of hospitalized children had PEM (5.1% severe, 7.7% moderate, and 14.5% mild). Although these results were significantly less than those obtained at the same institution in 1976, they are still alarming.[93]

Pathophysiology

In kwashiorkor, the deficit of dietary amino acids reduces protein synthesis in all tissues. Physical growth and mental growth are stunted, and maintenance of minimal life processes is in jeopardy. The lack of sufficient plasma proteins, particularly albumin, causes systemic pressure changes that result in generalized edema. The volume of total body water and extracellular fluid increases, causing a substantial loss of potassium. The liver swells with stored fat because no hepatic proteins are synthesized to form and release lipoproteins. Pancreatic atrophy and fibrosis may be present. Kwashiorkor also causes malabsorption, reduced bone density, and impaired renal function. If the condition is not reversed, the prognosis is very poor.

Because the intake of all dietary nutrients is reduced to a minimum in marasmus, metabolic processes, including liver function, are preserved but growth is severely retarded. Caloric intake is too low to support protein synthesis for growth or the storage of fat. If more protein is needed than is ingested, muscle wasting occurs. Fat wasting and anemia are common and can be severe. The volume of total body water is high. Serum triglyceride and phospholipid levels increase with increasing severity of malnutrition, but other serum values, such as cholesterol, are normal or slightly reduced. High fasting phospholipid and triglyceride concentrations are predictive of a poor prognosis for these children.[94] Severe vitamin A deficiency commonly results in blindness.[95]

Clinical Manifestations

Retarded physical, mental, and psychologic development; muscle wasting; diarrhea; dermatosis; and infection characterize marasmus. The presence of subcutaneous fat, hepatomegaly, and fatty liver distinguishes kwashiorkor from marasmus. These manifestations are missing in marasmus because caloric intake is not sufficient to support fat synthesis and storage.[96]

Evaluation and Treatment

Evaluation of PEM is based on nutritional history and clinical manifestations. The provision of deficient nutrients will resolve clinical symptoms in 4 to 6 weeks. Physical and mental retardation may not be reversible, however. Nutritional rehabilitation with appropriate environmental stimulation for infants and young children has been shown to resolve or improve cerebral shrinkage, physical growth, and psychomotor development.[97,98]

Failure to Thrive

Failure to thrive (FTT) is the inadequate physical development of an infant or a child. It is manifested as a deceleration in weight gain, a low weight/height ratio, or a low weight/height/head circumference ratio. In the United States, FTT usually affects infants and young children. FTT is a nutritional disorder having organic or nonorganic causes. Nonorganic FTT is most common among psychosocially and economically deprived populations, whereas organic FTT occurs equally in all populations. The incidence of nonorganic FTT is greater than that of organic FTT.[99]

Pathophysiology

Organic FTT has a pathophysiologic cause, such as gastroesophageal reflux, pyloric stenosis, gastroenteritis, infection by intestinal parasites, or congenital anomalies or chronic diseases of major body systems. All these factors reduce the availability of nutrients for maintenance and growth. Psychosocial problems can develop as a result of organic FTT.[100] A chronic disease or congenital anomaly that causes weakness or reduced stature can create developmental, psychosocial, and emotional problems for the child.

Nonorganic FTT occurs in the absence of any gastrointestinal, endocrine, or other chronic diseases. It is usually associated with psychosocial deprivation, although behavior problems may also contribute to its occurrence in the absence of maternal pathologic findings. Behavioral and psychosocial problems may be compounded by inadequate economic resources and lack of knowledge. Generally, the problem in nonorganic FTT is ineffective nurturing by primary caregivers. Infants and children are at risk for nonorganic FTT if their parents or primary caregivers are unable to provide nurturance. A variety of parental stressors may be involved and include the following:

Lack of nurturance in the parents' own childhood
Unwanted pregnancy
Inability to bond with the infant because of health or other problems
Postpartum depression
Family crisis, such as a death or marital problems
Stress caused by single parenthood or social isolation
Mental, emotional, or physical illness

The first few postnatal months appear to be a sensitive period in the relationship between growth and mental development, suggesting a critical need for early diagnosis and aggressive interventions.[101,102]

Clinical Manifestations

Clinical manifestations of organic FTT are retarded growth accompanied by manifestations of the underlying disease. Manifestations of nonorganic FTT are retarded growth plus reduced energy level, reduced responsiveness and interaction with the environment, social isolation, spasticity or rigidity when held or touched, inability to make eye contact or smile, refusal to eat, and rejection of foods. Weight loss and decelerated growth are accompanied by developmental retardation in many areas. Nonorganic FTT is a complex syndrome involving psychosocial, emotional, and parent-child problems that compound the pathophysiologic abnormalities.[103,104] Children with primarily organic FTT have been found to have lower developmental skills, and their parents have been found to have higher emotional distress. Infant stress, vomiting, and feeding disorders have been noted in children with both organic and inorganic FTT.[105,106]

Evaluation and Treatment

Failure to thrive is suggested if a child falls below the third percentile on the growth curve or is falling off a previously established growth curve. Organic FTT is manifested in infancy by weight, height, and head circumference growth that may be parallel to but below the normal ranges. If no genetic, endocrine, or other systemic disorder is identified and if the physical and laboratory examinations show no abnormalities other than delayed growth, an environmental cause is indicated.

Hospital admission is recommended if the diagnosis is unclear or the child is in nutritional or emotional jeopardy. Eating patterns, food preferences, caloric intake, and family interactions can be assessed during the hospital stay. If the cause is environmental, the hospitalized child with FTT usually begins to gain weight.

If an organic problem has been identified, management of FTT consists of treating the cause. Management of nonorganic FTT involves the immediate total care of the child and measures to address (1) the psychosocial and emotional problems of the caregivers and (2) parent-child interactions. Counseling, parental modeling, and long-term family support are sometimes required.[107] Clinical manifestations of organic FTT have inorganic components in the majority of children, and the most successful interventions not only treat the underlying organic cause but also address the psychosocial symptoms.

Necrotizing Enterocolitis

Necrotizing enterocolitis (NEC) is the most common gastrointestinal emergency in the newborn. If left untreated, NEC can result in bowel necrosis, perforation, and death. The overall mortality rate is between 20% and 40%.[108] The exact etiology is unclear. The incidence of NEC is increasing, causing 1500 to 2000 infant deaths every year in the United States.[109] Premature babies are the most likely victims, but it also occurs in full-term infants.[110] Affected infants have a mean gestational age of 31 weeks and weigh about 1500 g.[111] The risk of NEC decreases as the gastrointestinal tract matures.

Pathophysiology

Factors contributing to the development of NEC include infections, immature immunity, maternal age greater than 35 years, perinatal stress, and the effects of medications and feeding practices. Reduced mucosal blood flow leading to hypoxic injury to intestinal mucosa is thought to be a cause. This injury allows bacterial invasion of the bowel wall. Accumulation of gas in the mucosa and submucosa leads to ischemia and necrosis of intestinal segments. The terminal ileum and proximal colon are most often involved.[112] Premature infants have decreased secretory IgA and decreased intestinal T cells. The intestinal mucosal barrier is scanty and motility is slower, increasing the risk for infection.

Clinical Manifestations

Manifestations of NEC usually appear within 2 weeks of birth, with earlier symptoms in full-term infants (5.3 days compared with 15.3 days in premature infants).[113] They range from mild abdominal distention to bowel perforation, sepsis, and death. Abdominal pain, unstable temperature, bradycardia, and apnea are nonspecific signs. Affected infants have abdominal distention, occult or grossly bloody stools, retained gastric contents, and septicemia with elevated white blood cell and falling platelet counts. The more premature the infant, the greater the incidence of NEC and related diseases of prematurity, such as respiratory distress syndrome and immune compromise.

Evaluation and Treatment

Diagnosis is based on clinical manifestations, laboratory results, and plain films of the abdomen that show gas accumulation in the intestine. Treatments include cessation of feeding, gastric suction to decompress the intestines, fluid and electrolyte maintenance, and administration of antibiotics to control sepsis. Surgical resection is the treatment of choice for intestinal perforation; however, for very ill infants weighing less than 1000 g, peritoneal drainage without laparotomy may improve survival.[114] Following treatment of NEC, infants treated by both medical and surgical management are at risk for intestinal obstruction related to the development of strictures.[115] Infants who have extensive resection of necrotic bowel may develop short-bowel syndrome, requiring chronic total parenteral nutrition. Intestinal transplantation is available as a lifesaving option for these children.[116] Low-birth-weight infants are at greatest risk of death from NEC. Prophylaxis with antibiotics, feeding with human milk, and stopping the inflammatory response are helpful treatments.[117,118]

Diarrhea

Diarrhea is a common gastrointestinal problem during infancy and early childhood. Severe diarrhea occurs one to three times during the first 3 years of life. Most episodes are self-limiting and resolve within 72 hours.

The pathophysiologic mechanisms of diarrhea in children are similar to those for adults described in Chapter 38. Prolonged diarrhea is more dangerous in children, however, because they have much smaller fluid reserves than adults. Therefore dehydration can develop rapidly if any disturbance increases fluid secretion into the gastrointestinal lumen (secretory diarrhea), draws fluid into the lumen by osmosis (osmotic diarrhea), or prevents fluid absorption in the intestine.

Infant diarrhea is of special concern because its cause may be a congenital or metabolic anomaly. Infants have low fluid reserves and relatively rapid peristalsis and metabolism. Therefore the danger of dehydration is great.

Common causes of acute diarrhea in infants include congenital aganglionic megacolon, infections, milk-protein allergies, and NEC. Less common causes are adrenogenital syndrome, impaired chloride-bicarbonate exchange, congenital lactase deficiency, glucose-galactose malabsorption, and sucrase-isomaltase deficiency.

Infectious diarrhea in newborns is usually associated with nursery epidemics involving such pathogens as *Escherichia coli, Klebsiella,* staphylococci, *Salmonella,* and *Shigella.* Diarrhea caused by these agents has a rapid onset, and acidosis and shock can occur quickly. *Clostridium difficile,* often associated with previous antibiotic therapy, can cause acute, profuse, watery diarrhea and symptoms of colitis.[119] True milk-protein allergy, which is uncommon, causes bloody, explosive stools after the introduction of milk into the diet.

Acute Diarrhea in Children

Acute diarrhea in children is almost synonymous with acute viral or bacterial gastroenteritis. Viral gastroenteritis tends to be self-limiting. Bacterial gastroenteritis is treated with antibiotics if the causal pathogen can be identified. Other causes of acute diarrhea in the older child include antibiotic therapy, appendicitis, chemotherapy, inflammatory bowel disease, parasitic infestation, parenteral infections, and ingestion of toxic substances.

Rotavirus, the leading cause of severe diarrhea in infants and young children, invades the cells of the intestinal mucosa and, by its presence (even without replicating), damages these cells. Damage decreases viable absorptive surface, causing an imbalance of secretion and absorption that results in diarrhea. This is consistent with a viral toxin–like effect that can take several weeks for recovery of mucosal damage.

Chronic Diarrhea in Children

Children with acute gastroenteritis frequently remain mildly symptomatic for up to 4 weeks; therefore diarrhea that persists longer than 4 weeks is considered to be chronic. Children with chronic diarrhea can be divided into two groups: (1) otherwise well children whose growth is normal and (2) ill children whose growth is retarded. Causes of chronic diar-

WHAT'S NEW? Rotavirus Vaccine and Intussusception: Is There a Link?

Recent research has identified an increased risk of intussusception in infants during the first few weeks after receipt of the licensed trivalent rotavirus vaccine (RotaShield). This situation has resulted in the American Academy of Pediatrics revising their recommendations for the rotavirus vaccine and the manufacturer voluntarily removing the product from the market.

Data from Centers for Disease Control and Prevention: Withdrawal of rotavirus recommendations, *MMWR* 48(43):1007, 1999.

rhea in the first group include abnormal colonic motility, lactose intolerance, encopresis, parasitic infestation, and antibiotic use.[120] Chronic diarrhea in the second group is usually caused by a disease that impairs absorption.

Chronic Nonspecific Diarrhea

Chronic nonspecific diarrhea is a condition in which uncoordinated colonic motility causes forceful expulsion of feces. It affects children between 1 and 5 years of age. Apparently, the lower sigmoid colon remains in a tonically contracted state. Defecation occurs when pressure in the upper sigmoid colon and distal descending colon becomes great enough to force feces through the nonmotile, contracted segment. Prostaglandin synthesis is increased in the jejunum, and there are bile salts in the stools that may act as secretagogues.[120]

In some instances, there is a family history of bowel complaints. As an infant, the child is likely to have experienced colic and diarrhea associated with teething and immunizations. In more than 90% of cases, chronic nonspecific diarrhea resolves by 40 to 50 months of age. The cure frequently accompanies toilet training. Many children with chronic nonspecific diarrhea develop irritable bowel syndrome (which is also called *mucous colitis*) as adults.[121] Children with chronic nonspecific diarrhea usually do well with normal food and fluid intake with a balance of fluid, fiber, fat, and fruit juices.

Primary Lactose Intolerance

Lactose intolerance is the inability to digest milk sugar. It is caused by inadequate production of lactase and is a common cause of diarrhea in children, particularly nonwhite children, under 7 years of age. The malabsorption of lactose results in osmotic diarrhea, in which fluids move by osmosis from the vascular compartment into the intestinal lumen. The undigested sugar is acted on by the colonic bacteria, and intestinal gas is produced. The diarrhea is accompanied by abdominal pain, bloating, and flatulence. Treatment consists of reducing milk consumption. Some children can tolerate lactose in fermented forms, such as cheese and yogurt. Complete restriction of lactose-containing foods is rarely necessary in young infants.[122]

DISORDERS OF THE LIVER

Disorders of Biliary Metabolism and Transport

Physiologic Jaundice of the Newborn

Physiologic jaundice of the newborn is usually a transient, benign icterus that occurs during the first week of life in otherwise healthy, full-term infants; 6.8% of all newborns have physiologic jaundice, with an increased frequency in breast-fed infants. In one study, 49% of full-term breast-fed infants had jaundice with a total bilirubin greater than 10 mg/dl by the third day of life.[123] Physiologic jaundice is caused by mild unconjugated (indirect-reacting) hyperbilirubinemia. A high level of indirect hyperbilirubinemia (greater than 15 mg/dl) is considered pathologic. There is a risk of brain damage (kernicterus) with persistent high indirect hyperbilirubinemia. The mechanism by which bilirubin crosses the blood-brain barrier and precipitates into brain cells is unknown.

Pathophysiology

Physiologic jaundice results from the complex interaction of factors that cause (1) increased bilirubin production, (2) impaired hepatic uptake and excretion of bilirubin, and (3) reabsorption of bilirubin in the small intestine. Serum bilirubin values increase to 5 to 6 mg/dl by the second to fourth day after birth in full-term infants and 10 to 15 mg/dl by the fifth to seventh day in premature infants.

Clinical Manifestations

Physiologic jaundice develops during the second or third day after birth and usually subsides in 1 to 2 weeks in full-term infants and 2 to 4 weeks in premature infants. After this, increasing bilirubin values and persistent jaundice indicate pathologic hyperbilirubinemia. A late rising bilirubin level may also be a manifestation of glucose-6-phosphate dehydrogenase deficiency.[124,125] Bilirubin encephalopathy (kernicterus), which is caused by the deposition of toxic, unconjugated bilirubin in brain cells, usually does not occur in healthy, full-term infants. Premature infants with respiratory distress, acidosis, or sepsis are at greater risk for encephalopathy.

Evaluation and Treatment

Both total and direct (conjugated) bilirubin levels are measured; the direct bilirubin should not exceed 1 mg/dl.[22] Other causes of jaundice must be eliminated to confirm physiologic jaundice. Treatment depends on the degree of hyperbilirubinemia. Physiologic jaundice is usually treated by phototherapy (ultraviolet light).[125] Pathologic jaundice requires an exchange transfusion.

Biliary Atresia

Biliary atresia is a congenital malformation characterized by the absence or obstruction of intrahepatic or extrahepatic bile ducts. Extrahepatic ducts may end in a blind pouch. The cause of the intrauterine injury to the ducts is not clear but is thought to be related to a chromosomal abnormality or active agents, such as infection or drugs.[126] The disease expression is a continuum in which the principal process is one of bile duct destruction. The points of destruction are influenced by the stage of intrauterine development in which injury occurs.[22]

The atresia or obstruction of the bile ducts leads to plugging, inflammation, and fibrosis of the bile canaliculi. Progressive obstruction may lead to biliary cirrhosis (see Chapter 38), portal hypertension, or liver failure.[21]

Jaundice is the primary clinical manifestation of biliary atresia. Other signs are hepatomegaly and acholic (clay-colored) stools. Fat absorption is impaired for lack of bile salts, and the infant may fail to gain weight. Cirrhosis and liver failure lead to death within 2 years if untreated.

Diagnosis of biliary atresia is based on clinical manifestations and liver biopsy. Liver function test results are abnormal. Serum transaminase and alkaline phosphatase values are elevated, and conjugated (direct) serum bilirubin levels rise progressively.

Extrahepatic atresia can be relieved by surgical drainage and correction in approximately 10% of cases. Some infants benefit from the Kasai procedure, in which a hepatic duct remnant is anastomosed to the jejunum or a jejunal segment is anastomosed to the porta hepatis if the patent hepatic duct remnant is not available (Fig. 39-7). Even with initial restoration of bile flow, however, obliteration of intrahepatic bile ducts continues and cirrhosis results. Liver transplantation is the long-term therapy for biliary atresia. Approximately 40% of children with biliary atresia are immediate candidates for transplantation. Approximately 80% of children transplanted for biliary atresia will become long-term survivors with good physical and mental development.[127] The use of reduced and split livers from living, related donors has increased the number of children who survive after receiving transplantation.[128]

Inflammatory Disorders

Hepatitis

The pathophysiology of viral and fulminant hepatitis is described in Chapter 38.

Hepatitis A

Approximately one third of the reported cases of hepatitis A occur in children.[129] Incidence is highest among young children of preschool age. Outbreaks tend to occur in day care centers with large numbers of children who are not toilet trained and staff members who practice poor hand-washing techniques.[130] Hepatitis A in children is usually mild and asymptomatic. Clinical manifestations, however, may include nausea, vomiting, and diarrhea. Because jaundice is absent, infected children appear to have the "flu." Almost all children recover from hepatitis A without residual liver damage.[131]

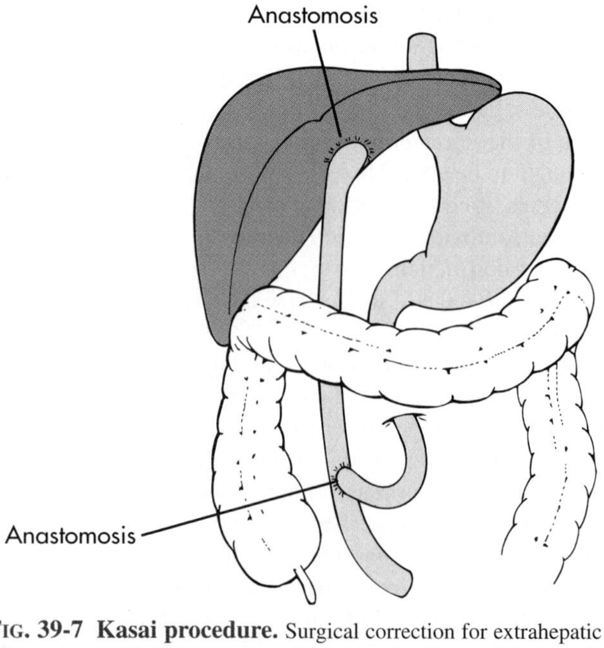

Fig. 39-7 Kasai procedure. Surgical correction for extrahepatic biliary atresia. The jejunal segment between the liver and the bowel may be externalized, creating a double-barrel portoenterostomy.

Hepatitis B

Infants of mothers who are chronic hepatitis B surface antigen (HBsAg) carriers, hemophiliacs who receive frequent blood transfusions, children who abuse parenteral drugs, and children who live in institutions for the mentally retarded are all at risk for hepatitis B virus (HBV) infection. Of newborns infected by their mothers, 90% develop chronic hepatitis and become carriers. The risk of chronic hepatitis is more than 30% for children younger than 6 years who contract hepatitis B; hepatitis B leads to chronic hepatitis in only 5% of cases among populations of all ages.[132] Chronic hepatitis may develop more frequently in young children because of immaturity of the immune system. Infected infants and children are at risk for cirrhosis and hepatocellular carcinoma. The most serious consequence of HBV infection is fulminant hepatitis, which occurs in 1% of cases. Hepatitis D infection (HDV) depends on active infection with HBV. There is evidence that the risk of fulminant hepatitis is higher in individuals with combined infection of HBV and HDV than in those with HBV infection alone.[133] The most effective approach to the treatment of hepatitis B is prevention. The American Academy of Pediatrics has added immunization for hepatitis B to those immunizations recommended for infants. Efforts are underway to immunize children and adolescents who did not receive this series as infants.

Hepatitis C

Hepatitis C in children is associated primarily with blood transfusions. Children who receive frequent transfusions are at highest risk. Between 10% and 50% of affected children develop chronic liver disease. Interferon-α is effective in the treatment of both hepatitis B and hepatitis C.[134]

Chronic Hepatitis

The cause of chronic hepatitis is unknown in most cases, but an autoimmune mechanism is suggested because inflammatory findings are commonly seen in biopsy specimens of the liver. Manifestations of chronic hepatitis include malaise, anorexia, fever, gastrointestinal bleeding, hepatomegaly, edema, and transient joint pain. Serum transaminase and bilirubin levels are elevated. There may be evidence of impairment of synthetic functions of the liver: prolonged prothrombin time and hypoalbuminemia. Diagnosis is based on the clinical manifestations and liver biopsy.

Treatment has variable efficacy and differs by the causative pathogen. Treatment with zidovudine (AZT) and interferon-α has been effective in managing persons coinfected with chronic hepatitis and human immunodeficiency virus (HIV).[135] Interferon-α has been most effective in young children with chronic hepatitis following hepatitis B and C.[136] Young children may respond to alternate-day treatment with steroids.[22]

Cirrhosis

Cirrhosis is the excessive formation of fibrous tissue in response to inflammation and tissue damage (see Chapter 38). Most forms of chronic liver diseases in children can progress to cirrhosis, but they seldom do so. The complications of cirrhosis in children are the same as those in adults: portal hypertension, the opening of collateral vessels between the portal and systemic veins, and varices. In addition, children with cirrhosis experience growth failure caused by nutritional deficits and developmental delay, particularly in gross motor function because of ascites and weakness. The cause of cirrhosis may influence its severity and course. Some types of cirrhosis can be stabilized if the cause is identified and treated early.

Portal Hypertension

The two basic causes of portal hypertension in children are (1) increased resistance to blood flow within the portal system and (2) increased volume of portal blood flow. Increased resistance to flow can occur anywhere in the portal circulatory system. Portal hypertension can accompany cirrhosis, intraabdominal infections, portal vein thrombosis, congenital anomalies of the portal vein, and congenital hepatic fibrosis.

Types

Extrahepatic Portal Hypertension

Extrahepatic (prehepatic) portal venous obstruction causes 50% to 70% of extrahepatic portal hypertension in children. For at least half of these children, no specific cause can be found. Obstruction is almost always in the portal vein and is usually caused by thrombosis. Umbilical infection with or without a history of catheterization of the umbilical vein may be a cause in neonates. Portal vein thrombosis can occur as a complication of intraabdominal infections, pancreatitis, and blunt abdominal trauma. It also has been associated with neonatal dehydration, inflammatory bowel disease, and hypercoagulable states, such as protein C and protein S deficiencies.[22] The liver is usually normal in cases of extrahepatic portal hypertension.

Intrahepatic Portal Hypertension

Cirrhosis is the primary cause of intrahepatic portal hypertension. The most common finding is fibrosis, which increases resistance to portal blood flow by constricting and reducing the compliance of the hepatic sinusoids.

Course of the Disease

The important consequence of portal hypertension in children is the development of collateral circulation, with portosystemic shunting, hypersplenism, and ascites.

Clinical Manifestations

The clinical manifestations of portal hypertension are splenomegaly, upper gastrointestinal bleeding, ascites, and hepatic encephalopathy. Splenomegaly is the most frequent sign of portal hypertension in children. The spleen may be firm or hard, depending on the duration of portal hypertension. Hematemesis, possibly associated with abdominal pain, often accompanies sudden pallor. Melena is observed, either at the time of hematemesis or soon afterward. In children, most episodes of gastrointestinal bleeding are caused by rupture of esophageal varices. Clotting abnormalities caused by altered liver function promote the bleeding. If plasma volume is increased, esophageal varices readily rupture during activities, such as coughing, that increase blood pressure. Acetylsalicylic acid (aspirin), which should not be administered to children, can trigger bleeding, but its exact mechanisms of action are not known. Severe bleeding episodes can cause hypovolemic shock and death. Symptoms of ascites include weight gain, protruding abdomen, and reduced tidal volumes if the ascites is severe. Severe liver disease is characterized by hypoalbuminemia, prolonged prothrombin times, hyperbilirubinemia, electrolyte imbalance, and hypoglycemia.

Hepatic encephalopathy in children can be acute or chronic. Acute encephalopathy is characterized by major disorders of consciousness, which may progress to coma. This may follow an acute episode of variceal bleeding as the impaired liver attempts to metabolize the large protein (nitrogenous) load from the blood. Chronic, or minimal, encephalopathy is characterized by emotional or psychiatric disorders, decreased intellectual functioning, personality disorders caused by minimal brain dysfunction, and spatial disorientation.

Evaluation and Treatment

Assessment of portal hypertension in children must be thorough because the cause dictates the management. The objectives of the clinical investigation are to locate the site of the venous block and identify the disease responsible for the portal hypertension. Thorough physical examination, laboratory tests of liver function, imaging procedures, and biopsy may be included in the diagnostic evaluation (see Chapter 37). Sclerotherapy is the initial treatment of choice for severe esophageal varices in children.[137]

The indications for surgical shunting include gastrointestinal hemorrhage not responsive to sclerotherapy. Surgical venous shunts rarely have been performed on small children because of the high failure rate secondary to vessel occlusion, but they may be an alternative in older children, with some success.[22,138] Surgical shunts had been a contraindication for subsequent liver transplantation but are no longer considered a contraindication, although the shunt does make the transplantation technically more difficult. The transjugular intrahepatic portosystemic shunt (TIPS) procedure is performed for some children. This is a therapeutic option in which a stent is placed between the right hepatic vein and the right or left portal vein to allow shunting of blood without surgical intervention.[139]

The outcome of portal hypertension depends almost entirely on its cause. Children with extrahepatic disease are expected to recover with little morbidity. For children with intrahepatic disease, the prognosis varies.

Metabolic Disorders

More than 5000 genetically determined metabolic pathways have been identified in liver tissue. The earliest possible identification of metabolic disorders is essential because (1) early treatment may prevent permanent damage to vital organs, such as the liver or brain; (2) precise genetic counseling may be possible with prenatal diagnosis; and (3) complications can be minimized, even if cure is not possible. Galactosemia, fructosemia, and Wilson disease are treatable metabolic disorders that have hepatic clinical manifestations. These disorders are presented in Table 39-2.

Wilson Disease

Wilson disease (hepatolenticular degeneration) is an autosomal recessive defect of copper metabolism that causes toxic amounts of copper to accumulate in the liver, brain, kidneys, and corneas. The gene has been mapped to chromosome 13 and is a putative copper-transporting P-type adenosine triphosphatase (ATPase) membrane-spanning protein. It is highly expressed in the liver, kidney, and placenta and is expressed in lower levels in the brain, heart, muscle, and pancreas.[140] This defect in the uptake and excretion of copper by hepatocytes is an important cause of progressive liver disease in children and young adults. Wilson disease is very rare, with an incidence of 1 in 30,000 live births.[141] Between 1 in 200 and 1 in 500 persons are carriers.[22]

Pathophysiology

Two major abnormalities in copper metabolism have been identified: (1) diminished biliary excretion of copper and (2) failure to insert copper into ceruloplasmin (a glycoprotein that transports copper in the blood). A positive copper balance is present from birth in children with Wilson disease, despite increased excretion of copper in the urine. Copper toxicity with accumulation in the liver and brain is the major abnormality. Excesses of copper generate free radicals that disrupt cellular organelles, deoxyribonucleic acids (DNA), microtubules, enzymes, and proteins. Copper overload is related to impaired biliary excretion of copper and may be related to failure of hepatocyte lysosomes to eliminate copper by exocytosis.[142]

Early in the disease, intestinal absorption of copper is normal, as is hepatic clearance of albumin-bound, absorbed copper. As copper-binding proteins in the liver become saturated, hepatic uptake of copper diminishes, with elevated serum copper levels and biochemical and clinical evidence of liver damage caused by copper accumulation. In later stages of the disease, copper accumulates in extrahepatic tissues, including the eyes, brain, and kidneys.

When cerebral copper-binding proteins become saturated, a characteristic pattern of brain damage develops, particularly in the basal ganglia. Neural effects include intention tremor, unsteady gait, dystonia, and behavioral changes. Manifestations of renal tubular injury usually appear simultaneously. The uptake of copper by red blood cells is thought to cause hemolytic anemia, a condition sometimes seen early in the clinical course of Wilson disease.

Clinical Manifestations

The clinical manifestations of Wilson disease may begin as young as 4 years of age, when control mechanisms responsible for copper homeostasis and biliary excretion should have matured. The mean age at diagnosis in one large study was 15.5 years.[143]

The classic clinical presentation of Wilson disease is a triad of neuromuscular abnormalities, intention tremors, dysarthria (indistinct speech), and dystonia (disordered muscu-

Table 39-2 Galactosemia, Fructosemia, and Wilson Disease

	Galactosemia	Fructosemia	Wilson Disease
Mechanism of disease	Deficiency of galactase and phosphate, uridyl transferase An autosomal recessive trait Cannot convert galactose to glucose Toxic accumulation of galactose in body tissues, liver, and brain	Deficiency of fructose-1-phosphate aldolase An autosomal recessive trait Cannot metabolize fructose, sucrose, or honey; occurs when breast milk is replaced with cow's milk Toxic accumulation of fructose in body tissues	Probably autosomal recessive: defect on chromosome 13 Defect in copper excretion by liver Impaired transport of copper in blood caused by diminished transport protein (ceruloplasmin) Toxic accumulations of copper in liver, brain, kidney, corneas
Clinical manifestations	High levels of blood galactose Vomiting Hypoglycemia May have failure to thrive Symptoms of cirrhosis at 2 to 6 months—jaundice Mental retardation if not treated Cataracts if not treated	High levels of blood fructose Vomiting Hypoglycemia May have failure to thrive Hepatomegaly Jaundice Seizures	Intention tremors Indistinct speech Dystonia Greenish yellow rings in cornea Hepatomegaly Jaundice Anorexia Renal tubular defects
Evaluation	Presence of reducing substances in urine when infant is receiving lactose	Detailed dietary history Liver or intestinal mucosa biopsy	Low plasma ceruloplasmin
Treatment	Galactose-free diet	Fructose-, sucrose-, honey-free diet Vitamin C supplementation	Chelation therapy to remove copper from body Decreased dietary intake of copper Liver transplant

lar tonicity): (1) Kayser-Fleischer rings (accumulation of copper in the limbus of the cornea, causing a greenish yellow ring), (2) cirrhosis associated with elevated serum copper, and (3) low ceruloplasmin levels. Initial symptoms vary from malaise and abdominal pain to jaundice. Changes in mental and motor performance may develop at age 6 years or into adult life. The earliest signs of liver involvement include enlargement of the liver and spleen, jaundice, and anorexia. Edema and ascites may develop suddenly, or gastrointestinal hemorrhage may be the initial sign of the disease. Occasionally, Wilson disease begins with a hemolytic crisis caused by the toxic effects of copper on the red blood cells. Cirrhosis develops in all untreated cases. Copper deposition in the kidneys causes a proximal renal tubular defect that results in losses of glucose, amino acids, phosphate, and uric acid in the urine and renal tubular acidosis. All untreated individuals will develop behavioral or psychiatric disorders.

Evaluation and Treatment

Because Wilson disease is rare, it may not be diagnosed until clinical manifestations develop. Laboratory tests detect a serum ceruloplasmin concentration less than 30 mg/dl. Serum copper values may be normal or high, and urine copper values are elevated. Liver biopsy is used to assess structural changes and measure copper concentrations. Although D-penicillamine has traditionally been the drug of choice for Wilson disease, zinc, which has low toxicity, has demonstrated effectiveness.[144] Copper intake is reduced by eliminating organ meats, nuts, legumes, shellfish, and chocolate from the diet. Physiotherapy may accelerate the recovery of gait and muscular coordination. Liver transplantation is the sole resolutive therapy for Wilson disease and is the treatment of choice for persons who develop fulminant hepatic failure or end-stage cirrhosis.[145] Children with untreated Wilson disease die of neural, hepatic, renal, or hematologic complications.

SUMMARY REVIEW

Disorders of the Gastrointestinal Tract

1. Most alterations of digestive function in children are caused by congenital obstructions of the intestinal tract; disorders of digestion, absorption, or nutrition; or liver disease.
2. Cleft lip (harelip) and cleft palate (failure of the bony palate to fuse in the midline) may occur separately or together. The fissure may affect the uvula, soft palate, hard palate, nostril, and maxillary alveolar ridge.
3. Esophageal atresia, a condition in which the esophagus ends in a blind pouch, may occur with or without tracheoesophageal fistula, a connection between the esophagus and the trachea. As the infant swallows oral secretions or ingests milk, the pouch fills, causing either drooling or aspiration into the lungs.
4. Pyloric stenosis, one of the most common disorders requiring surgery in early infancy, is an obstruction of the pyloric outlet caused by hypertrophy and hyperplasia of circular muscles in the pyloric sphincter.
5. Malrotation of the intestine, with an obstructing band and volvulus (twisting of the bowel on itself), may partly or completely occlude the gastrointestinal tract and its blood vessels.
6. Meconium ileus is a condition in the newborn in which intestinal secretions and amniotic waste products produce a thick, tarry plug that obstructs the intestine. From 10% to 15% of children with cystic fibrosis have meconium ileus as neonates.
7. Duodenal, jejunal, and ileal obstructions can be caused by meconium ileus, atresia, congenital aganglionic megacolon, or acquired obstructive disorders.
8. Congenital aganglionic megacolon (Hirschsprung disease) is caused by a malformation of the parasympathetic nervous system in a segment of the colon. It is characterized by the absence of nerves needed for peristalsis.
9. Malformations of the anus and rectum range from mild congenital stenosis of the anus to complex deformities, all of which are classified as imperforate anus.
10. The most frequent cause of acquired intestinal obstruction in infants is intussusception, a condition in which one portion of the bowel telescopes, or invaginates, into another, most commonly in the area of the ileocecal junction.
11. Gastroesophageal reflux is caused by the relaxation or incompetence of the lower esophageal sphincter. Infants are susceptible to reflux because the sphincter is not fully mature, their diet consists of liquids, and they are seldom in an upright position.
12. The pathophysiologic triad that is the hallmark of cystic fibrosis includes pancreatic enzyme deficiency (which causes maldigestion), overproduction of mucus in the respiratory tract, and abnormally elevated sodium and chloride concentrations in sweat. Older children with cystic fibrosis also may have diabetes mellitus caused by damage to endocrine function of the pancreas and chronic liver disease. Affected individuals seldom survive beyond their thirties.
13. Gluten-sensitive enteropathy is a lifelong disease characterized by the loss of mature villous epithelium in the presence of a gluten-containing diet. It results in malabsorption and growth failure.
14. Protein energy malnutrition is a group of disorders resulting from a severe dietary deficiency of proteins (kwashiorkor), carbohydrates, or both (marasmus). Starvation causes stunted mental and physical development. Kwashiorkor occurs most often in young toddlers who have stopped breast-feeding and subsist on a high-carbohydrate diet.
15. Failure to thrive is inadequate physical growth of a child. Organic failure to thrive is caused by genetic, anatomic, or pathophysiologic factors that retard normal growth and development. Nonorganic failure to thrive is caused by nutritional deficits associated with inadequate nurturing.

16. Necrotizing enterocolitis is a disorder in neonates, particularly premature infants, thought to result from stress and anoxia of the bowel wall. Bacteria invade the mucosa and submucosa, resulting in colitis, necrosis, and even perforation of the intestinal wall.
17. Diarrhea in infants and children can rapidly cause dehydration and electrolyte imbalances because fluid reserves are relatively small.
18. The most common cause of acute diarrhea in children is bacterial or viral enterocolitis (infection of the gastrointestinal tract).
19. Chronic diarrhea (diarrhea persisting longer than 4 weeks) can be caused by a wide variety of underlying conditions and frequently leads to growth failure and slow development.

Disorders of the Liver

1. Physiologic jaundice of the newborn is caused by mild hyperbilirubinemia that subsides in 1 to 2 weeks. Pathologic jaundice is caused by severe hyperbilirubinemia and can cause brain damage.
2. Biliary atresia is a congenital malformation of the bile ducts that obstructs bile flow. Atresia causes jaundice, cirrhosis, and liver failure. Biliary atresia is the most common reason for liver transplantation in children.
3. Acute hepatitis has the same clinical course in children and adults, but children have milder cases of the disease. Hepatitis A is the most common form of childhood hepatitis.
4. Cirrhosis is rare in children, but it can develop from most forms of chronic liver disease.
5. Portal hypertension in children usually is caused by extrahepatic obstruction. Thrombosis of the portal vein is the most common cause of portal hypertension in children, and splenomegaly is the most frequent sign.
6. The three most common metabolic disorders that cause liver damage in children are galactosemia, fructosemia, and Wilson disease. All three are inherited as genetic traits and permit the accumulation of toxins in the liver.
7. Wilson disease causes defective copper uptake and metabolism. Unexcreted copper accumulates in the liver, brain, kidney, and corneal cells. Damage from accumulated copper is gradual; the disease is usually not diagnosed before age 4 or 5 years.

KEY TERMS

Biliary atresia, *1329*
Chronic nonspecific diarrhea, *1329*
Cleft lip (harelip), *1314*
Cleft palate, *1314*
Congenital aganglionic megacolon (Hirschsprung disease), *1319*
Cystic fibrosis (CF), *1323*
Distal intestinal obstruction syndrome (DIOS), *1319*
Esophageal atresia, *1316*
Failure to thrive (FTT), *1327*
Gluten-sensitive enteropathy, *1323*
Ileal atresia, *1319*
Imperforate anus, *1320*
Infant diarrhea, *1328*
Infectious diarrhea, *1328*
Intussusception, *1321*
Jejunal atresia, *1319*
Kwashiorkor, *1326*
Lactose intolerance, *1329*
Malrotation, *1318*
Marasmus, *1326*
Meconium, *1318*
Meconium ileus, *1318*
Necrotizing enterocolitis (NEC), *1327*
Nonorganic FTT, *1327*
Organic FTT, *1327*
Periduodenal band, *1318*
Physiologic jaundice of the newborn, *1329*
Protein energy malnutrition (PEM), *1326*
Pyloric stenosis, *1317*
Tracheoesophageal fistula (TEF), *1316*
Wilson disease, *1332*

REFERENCES

1. Edmundson R, Reinhartsen D: The young child with cleft lip and palate: intervention needs in the first three years, *Infants Young Child* 11(2):12, 1998.
2. Lorente C et al: Tobacco use and alcohol use during pregnancy and risk of oral clefts, *Am J Public Health* 90(3):415, 2000.
3. Shaw GM, Lammer EJ: Maternal periconceptual alcohol consumption and risk for orofacial clefts, *J Pediatr* 134(3):298, 1999.
4. Shaw GM et al: Orofacial clefts, parental cigarette smoking, and transforming growth factor–alpha gene variants, *Am J Hum Genet* 58(3): 551, 1996.
5. Wong WY et al: Nonsyndromic orofacial clefts: association with maternal hyperhomocysteinemia, *Tetralogy* 60(5):253, 1999.
6. Romitti Pa et al: Candidate genes for nonsyndromic cleft lip and palate and maternal cigarette smoking and alcohol consumption: evaluation of genotype-environment interactions from a population-based case-control study of orofacial clefts, *Tetralogy* 59(1):39, 1999.
7. Bianecuzzo M: Clinical focus of clefts: yes! Infants with clefts can be breastfed, *AWHONN Lifelines* 2(4):45, 1998.
8. Rohrich RJ et al: Timing of hard palatal closure: a critical long-term analysis, *Plast Reconstr Surg* 98(2):236, 1996.
9. Broen PA et al: Comparison of the hearing histories of children with and without cleft palate, *Cleft Palate Craniofac J* 33(2):127, 1996.
10. Resnick J, Zarem H: Diseases and injuries in the oral region. In Wald WR, Polin RA, editors: *Gellis and Kagan's current pediatric therapy*, ed 15, Philadelphia, 1996, W.B. Saunders.
11. Paradise JL, Elster BA, Tan L: Evidence in infants with cleft palate that breast milk protects against otitis media, *Pediatrics* 94(6 pt 1):853, 1994.
12. Bokhaut B et al: Prevalence of *Streptococcus mutans* and *Lactobacillus* in 18-month-old children with cleft lip and/or palate, *Cleft Palate Craniofac J* 33(5):424, 1996.
13. Novitt-Schumacher R: Alterations in gastrointestinal function. In Ball J, Bindler R, editors: *Pediatric nursing: caring for children,* ed 2, Connecticut, 1999, Appleton & Lange.
14. Gentry E et al: Congenital tracheoesophageal fistula with esophageal atresia, *Int J Pediatr Otorhinolaryngol* 48(3):231, 1999.
15. Lindahl H, Rintala R: Long-term complications in cases of isolated esophageal atresia treated with esophageal anastomosis, *J Pediatr Surg* 30(8):1222, 1995.
16. Robertson DF et al: Late pulmonary function following repair of tracheoesophageal fistula or esophageal atresia, *Pediatr Pulmonol* 20(1): 21, 1995.

17. Sparey C et al: Esophageal atresia in the Northern Region Congenital Anomaly Survey, *Am J Obstet Gyn* 182(2):427, 2000.
18. Welch KJ: *Pediatric surgery,* ed 4, St Louis, 1986, Mosby.
19. Phillips JD: Abdominal surgical emergencies. In Wyllie R, Hyams J, editors: *Pediatric gastrointestinal diseases,* ed 2, Philadelphia, 1999, W.B. Saunders.
20. Armstrong M: The child with a cognitive deficit. In McKinney ES et al, editors: *Maternal-child nursing,* Philadelphia, 2000, W.B. Saunders.
21. Sams CA: The child with a gastrointestinal alteration. In McKinney ES et al, editors: *Maternal-child nursing,* Philadelphia, 2000, W.B. Saunders.
22. Behrman RE, Kliegman R, Jensen HB: *Nelson textbook of pediatrics,* ed 16, Philadelphia, 1999, W.B. Saunders.
23. Oue T, Puri P: Smooth muscle cell hypertrophy versus hyperplasia in hypertrophic pyloric stenosis, *Pediatr Res* 45(6):853, 1999.
24. Shima H, Puri P: Increased expression of transforming growth factor–alpha in hypertrophic pyloric stenosis, *Pediatr Surg Intern* 15(3-4): 198, 1999.
25. Fleisher DR: Functional vomiting disorders in infancy: innocent vomiting, nervous vomiting, and infant rumination syndrome, *J Pediatr* 125(6 pt 2):S84, 1994.
26. Mendelson KL: Emergency abdominal ultrasound in children: current concepts, *Med Health RI* 82(6):198, 1999.
27. Rohrschneider WK et al: Pyloric muscle in asymptomatic infants: sonographic evaluation and discrimination for idiopathic hypertrophic pyloric stenosis, *Pediatr Radiol* 28(6):429, 1998.
28. Papadakis K et al: The changing presentation of pyloric stenosis, *Am J Emerg Med* 17(1):67, 1999.
29. Yamataka A et al: Pyloromyotomy versus atropine sulfate for idopathic hypertrophic pyloric stenosis, *J Pediatr Surg* 35(2):338, 2000.
30. Bailey PV et al: Congenital duodenal obstruction: a 32 year review, *J Pediatr Surg* 28(1):92, 1993.
31. Shelton BK: Intestinal obstruction, *AACN Clin Issues* 10(4):478, 1999.
32. Wilcken B et al: Neonatal screening for cystic fibrosis: a comparison of two strategies for case detection in 1.2 million babies, *J Pediatr* 127(6):965, 1995.
33. Mushtaq I et al: Meconium ileus secondary to cystic fibrosis: the East London experience, *Pediatr Surg Intern* 13(5-6):365, 1998.
34. McAlister WH, Kronemer KA: Emergency gastrointestinal radiology of the newborn, *Radiol Clin North Am* 34(4):819, 1996.
35. Kao SC, Franken EA Jr: Nonoperative treatment of simple meconium ileus: a survey of the Society for Pediatric Radiology, *Pediatr Radiol* 25(2):97, 1995.
36. Murshed R et al: Meconium ileus: a 10 year review of 36 patients, *Eur J Surg* 7(5):275, 1997.
37. Lai HC et al: Nutritional status of patients with cystic fibrosis with meconium ileus: a comparison with patients without meconium ileus and diagnosed early through neonatal screening, *Pediatrics* 105(1, pt 1):53, 2000.
38. Minkes RK et al: Intestinal obstruction after lung transplantation in children with cystic fibrosis, *J Pediatr Surg* 34(10):1489, 1999.
39. Hasler WL: Pancreatic enzymes and colonic strictures with cystic fibrosis: a case-control study, *Gastroenterology* 114(3):608, 1998.
40. Moss RL, Musemeche CA, Feddersen RM: Progressive pan-colonic fibrosis secondary to oral administration of pancreatic enzymes, *Pediatr Surg Int* 13(2-3):168, 1998.
41. Wyllie R: Gastrointestinal manifestations of cystic fibrosis, *Clin Pediatr* 38(12):738, 1999.
42. Zhan J et al: Expression of RET proto-oncogene and GDNF deficit in Hirschsprung disease, *J Pediatr Surg* 34(11):1606, 1999.
43. Hofstra RM et al: A homozygous mutation in the endothelium-2 gene associated with a combined Waardenburg type 2 Hirschsprung phenotype (Shah-Waardenburg syndrome), *Nat Genet* 12(4):445, 1996.
44. Moore SW, Johnson HG: Hirschsprung disease: genetic and functional associations of Down syndrome and Waardenberg syndrome, *Semin Pediatr Surg* 7(3):156, 1998.
45. Kapur RP: Hirschsprung disease and other enteric dysganglionoses, *Crit Rev Clin Lab Sci* 36(3):225, 1999.
46. Oue T, Puri P: Altered endothelin-3 and endothelin-B receptors on mRNA expression in Hirschsprung disease, *J Pediatr Surg* 34(8): 1257, 1999.
47. Sullivan PB: Hirschsprung's disease, *Arch Dis Child* 74(1):5, 1996.
48. Osatakul S, Patrapinyokul S, Osatakul N: The diagnostic value of anorectal manometry as a screening test for Hirschsprung disease, *J Med Assoc Thai* 82(11):1100, 1999.
49. Emir H et al: Anorectal manometry during the neonatal period: its specificity in the diagnosis of Hirschsprung disease, *Eur J Pediatr Surg* 9(2):101, 1999.
50. Staiano A Tozzi A: Diagnosis and treatment of constipation in children, *Curr Opin Pediatr* 10(5):512, 1998.
51. Fonkalsrud EW: Long-term results after colectomy and ileoanal pull-through procedure in children, *Arch Surg* 131(8):881, 1996.
52. Bouchard S, Yazbeck S, Lallier M: Perineal hemangioma, anorectal malformation, and genital anomaly: a new association, *J Pediatr Surg* 34(7):1133, 1999.
53. Clarke SA, Van der Avoirt A: Imperforate anus, Hirschsprung disease, and trisomy 21: a rare combination, *J Pediatr Surg* 34(12):1874, 1999.
54. DeFilippo RE et al: Neurogenic bladder in infants born with anorectal malformations: comparison with spinal and urologic status, *J Pediatr Surg* 34(5):825, 1999.
55. Chen CJ: The treatment of imperforate anus: experience with 108 patients, *J Pediatr Surg* 34(1):1728, 1999.
56. Heikenen JB et al: Colonic motility in children with repaired imperforate anus, *Digest Dis Sci* 44(7):1288, 1999.
57. Pena A et al: Bowel management for fecal incontinence in patients with anorectal malformations, *J Pediatr Surg* 33(1):133, 1998.
58. Winslow BT, Westfall JM, Nicholas RA: Intussusception, *Am Fam Physician* 54(1):213, 1996.
59. deVories S, Sleeboom C, Aronson DC: Postoperative intussusception in children, *Br J Surg* 86(1):81, 1999.
60. Linke F, Eble F, Berger S: Postoperative intussusception in children, *Pediatr Surg Intern* 14(3):175, 1998.
61. Chung JL et al: Intussusception in infants and children: risk factors leading to surgical reduction, *J Formos Med Assoc* 93(6):481, 1994.
62. Macdonald IA, Beattie TF: Intussusception presenting to a paediatric accident and emergency department, *J Accid Emerg Med* 12(3):182, 1995.
63. Schmit P, Rohrschneider WK, Christmann D: Intestinal intussusception survey about diagnostic and nonsurgical therapeutic procedures, *Pediatr Radiol* 29(10):752, 1999.
64. Hadidi AT, El Shal NJ: Childhood intussusception: a comparative study of nonsurgical management, *J Pediatr Surg* 34(2):304, 1999.
65. Roeyen G: Intussusception in infants: an emergency in diagnosis and treatment, *Eur J Emerg Med* 6(1):73, 1999.
66. Kornecki A et al: Spontaneous reduction of intussusception: clinical spectrum, management, and outcome, *Pediatr Radiol* 30(1):58, 2000.
67. Daneman A et al: Patterns of recurrence of intussusception in children: a 17-year review, *Pediatr Radiol* 28(12):913, 1998.
68. Del Giudice E et al: Gastrointestinal manifestations in children with cerebral palsy, *Brain Dev* 21(5):307, 1999.
69. Richter JE: Gastroesophageal reflux disease and asthma: the two are directly related, *Am J Med* 108(4a suppl):153S, 2000.
70. Thach BT: Sudden infant death syndrome: can gastroesophageal reflux cause sudden infant death? *Am J Med* 108(4a suppl):144S, 2000.
71. Button BM: Postural drainage techniques and gastroesophageal reflux in infants with cystic fibrosis, *Eur Respir J* 14(6):1456, 1999.
72. Hillemeier CA: Gastroesophageal reflux: diagnostic and therapeutic approaches, *Pediatr Clin North Am* 43(1):197, 1996.
73. Bauman N, Sandler AD, Smith RJ: Respiratory manifestations of gastroesophageal reflex disease in pediatric patients, *Ann Otol Rhinol Laryngol* 105(1):23, 1996.
74. Tobin JM, McCloud P, Cameron DJ: Posture and gastroesophageal reflux: a case for left lateral positioning, *Arch Dis Child* 76(3):254, 1997.

75. Orenstein SP: Gastroesophageal reflux. In Wyllie R, Hyams, J, editors: *Pediatric gastrointestinal diseases,* ed 2, Philadelphia, 1999, W.B. Saunders.
76. Vandenplas Y: Dietary regimen for regurgitation: recommendations from a working party, *Acta Paediatrica* 87(4):462, 1998.
77. Heloury Y et al: Laparoscopic Nissen fundoplication with simultaneous percutaneous endoscopic gastrostomy in children, *Surg Endosc* 10(8):837, 1996.
78. Anthony H et al: Pancreatic enzyme replacement therapy in cystic fibrosis, *J Pediatr Child Health* 35(2):125, 1999.
79. Amarri S et al: 13Carbon mixed triglyceride breath test and pancreatic enzyme supplementation in cystic fibrosis, *Arch Dis Child* 76(4): 349, 1997.
80. Benabdeslam H et al: Biochemical assessment of the nutritional status of cystic fibrosis patients with pancreatic enzyme extracts, *Am J Clin Nutr* 67(5):912, 1998.
81. Williams SG et al: Percutaneous endoscopic gastrostomy feedings in patients with cystic fibrosis, *Gut* 44(1):87, 1999.
82. Fasano A, Catassi C: Current approaches to the diagnosis and treatment of celiac disease: an evolving spectrum, *Gastroenterology* 120(3): 636, 2001.
83. Hill I et al: The prevalence of celiac disease in at-risk groups of children in the United States, *J Pediatr* 136(1):86, 2000.
84. Troncone R, Greco L, Auricchio S: Gluten-sensitive enteropathy, *Pediatr Clin North Am* 43(2):355, 1996.
85. Green PHR et al: Characteristics of adult celiac disease in the USA: results of a national survey, *Am J Gastroenterol* 96(1):126, 2001.
86. Gemme G et al: Linear growth and skeletal maturation in subjects with treated celiac disease, *J Pediatr Gastroenterol Nutr* 29(3):339, 1999.
87. Fine KD: The prevalence of occult gastrointestinal bleeding in celiac sprue, *N Engl J Med* 334(18):1163, 1996 (see comments).
88. Lupattelli G et al: Severe osteomalacia due to gluten-sensitive enteropathy, *Ann Ital Med Int* 9(1):40, 1994.
89. Egan S et al: Celiac-associated lymphoma: a single institutional experience of 30 cases in the combination chemotherapy era, *J Clin Gastroenterol* 21(2):123,1995.
90. Celli M et al: Rapid gas-chromatographic assay of lactulose and mannitol for estimating intestinal permeability, *Clin Chem* 42(5):752, 1995.
91. Bern C et al: Assessment of potential indicators for protein-energy malnutrition in the algorithm for integrated management of childhood illness, *Bull WHO* 75(1, suppl):87, 1997.
92. Pelletier DL: The relationship between child anthropometry and mortality in developing countries: implications for policy, programs and future research, *J Nutr* 123(10 suppl):2047S, 1994.
93. Hendricks KM et al: Malnutrition in hospitalized pediatric patients: current prevalence, *Arch Pediatr Adolesc Med* 149(10):1118, 1995.
94. Ogunkeye OO, Ighogboja IS: Increase in total serum triglyceride and phospholipid in kwashiorkor, *Ann Trop Paediatr* 12(4):463, 1992.
95. McLaren DS: Vitamin A deficiency disorders, *J Indian Med Assoc* 97 (8):320, 1999.
96. Latham MC: The dermatosis of kwashiorkor in young children, *Semin Dermatol* 10:270, 1991.
97. Gunston GD et al: Reversible cerebral shrinkage in kwashiorkor: an MRI study, *Arch Dis Child* 67:1030, 1992.
98. Proos LA et al: A longitudinal study on anthropometric and clinical development of Indian children adopted in Sweden: growth, morbidity, and development during two years after arrival in Sweden, *Ups J Med Sci* 97:93, 1992.
99. Lopez RF, Schumann L: Clinical health problems: failure-to-thrive, *J Am Acad Nurse Pract* 9(10):489, 1997.
100. Thomas D: Alterations in psychosocial function. In Ball J, Bindler R, editors: *Pediatric nursing: caring for children,* ed 2, Connecticut, 1999, Appleton & Lange.
101. Mackner LM, Starr RH, Black MM: The cumulative effect of neglect and failure-to-thrive on cognitive functioning, *Child Abuse Neglect* 21(7):691, 1997.
102. Tolia V: Very early onset nonorganic failure to thrive in infants, *J Pediatr Gastroenterol Nutr* 20(1):73, 1995.
103. Lemons PK, Dodge NN: Persistent failure-to-thrive: case study, *J Pediatr Health Care* 12(1):27, 1998.
104. Steward DK, Garvin, BJ: Nonorganic failure-to-thrive: a theoretical approach, *J Pediatr Nurs* 12(6):342, 1997.
105. Gahagan S, Holmes R: A stepwise approach to evaluation of undernutrition and failure-to-thrive, *Pediatr Clin North Am* 45(1):169, 1998.
106. Moore J: Feeding to thrive in babies and small children, *Comm Nurse* 3(11):23, 1997.
107. Chatvon I et al: Attachment and feeding problems: a reexamination of non-organic failure-to-thrive and attachment insecurity, *J Am Acad Child Adolesc Psychiatry* 37(11):1217, 1998.
108. Voss M et al: Fulminating necrotizing enterocolitis: outcome and prognostic factors, *Pediatr Surg Int* 13(8):576, 1998.
109. Neu J, Weiss MD: Necrotizing enterocolitis: pathology and prevention, *J Parenteral Enteral Nutr* 23(5, suppl):S13, 1999.
110. Ng S: Necrotizing enterocolitis in the full-term neonate, *J Paediatr Child Health* 37(1):1, 2001.
111. Caplan MS, Jilling T: New concepts in necrotizing enterocolitis, *Curr Opin Pediatr* 13(2):111, 2001.
112. Neu J: Necrotizing enterocolitis: the search for a unifying pathogenic theory leading to prevention, *Pediatr Clin North Am* 43(2):409, 1996.
113. Kabeer A, Gunnlaugsson S, Coren C: Neonatal necrotizing enterocolitis: a 12-year review at a county hospital, *Dis Colon Rectum* 83(8): 866, 1995.
114. Ahmed T, Ein S, Moore A: The role of peritoneal drains in treatment of perforated necrotizing enterocolitis: recommendations from recent experiences, *J Pediatr Surg* 33(10):1468, 1998.
115. Lessin MS, Schwartz DL, Wesselhoeft CW: Multiple spontaneous small bowel anastomosis in premature infants with multisegmental necrotizing enterocolitis, *J Pediatr Surg* 35(2):170, 2000.
116. Vennarecci G: Intestinal transplantation for short gut syndrome attributable to necrotizing enterocolitis, *Pediatrics* 105(2):E25, 2000.
117. Kamitsuka MD, Horton MK, Williams MA: The incidence of necrotizing enterocolitis after introducing standardized feeding schedules for infants between 1250 and 2500 grams and less than 35 weeks gestation, *Pediatrics* 105(2):379, 2000.
118. Ledbetter DJ, Juul SE: Erythropoietin and the incidence of necrotizing enterocolitis in infants with very low birth weight, *J Pediatr Surg* 35(2):178, 2000.
119. Surawicz CM: *Clostridium difficile* disease: diagnosis and treatment, *Gastroenterologist* 6(1):60, 1998.
120. Kneepkens CMF, Hoekstra JH: Chronic nonspecific diarrhea of childhood, *Pediatr Clin North Am* 43(2):375, 1996.
121. Hyams JS, Hyman PE, Rasquin-Weber A: Childhood recurrent abdominal pain and subsequent adult irritable bowel syndrome, *J Dev Behav Pediatr* 20(5):318, 1999.
122. McBean LD, Miller GD: Allaying fears and fallacies about lactose intolerance, *J Am Diet Assoc* 98(6):671, 1998.
123. Gourley GR et al: Neonatal jaundice and diet, *Arch Pediatr Adolesc Med* 153(2):184, 1999.
124. Kaplan M et al: Predischarge bilirubin screening in glucose-6-phosphate dehydrogenase–deficient neonates, *Pediatrics* 105(3 pt 1):533, 2000.
125. Maisels MJ: Clinical rounds in the well-baby nursery: treating jaundiced newborns, *Pediatr Ann* 25(1):548, 1995.
126. Bates MD et al: Biliary atresia: pathogenesis and treatment, *Semin Liver Dis* 18(3):281, 1998.
127. Migliazzi L et al: Long-term survival expectancy after liver transplantation in children, *J Pediatr Surg* 35(1):5, 2000.
128. Casas A et al: Living donor liver transplantation in critically ill children, *Pediatr Transplant* 3(2):104, 1999.
129. Avery ME, First LR: *Pediatric medicine,* ed 2, Baltimore, 1994, Williams & Wilkins.
130. Sadetzki S, Rostmi N, Modan B: Hepatitis A outbreak in a day care center: a community-case report, *Eur J Epidemiol* 15(6):549, 1999.
131. Debray D: Liver failure in children with hepatitis A, *Hepatology* 26(4):1018, 1997.
132. Hyams KC: Risks of chronicity following acute hepatitis B virus infection: a review, *Clin Infect Dis* 20(4):992, 1995.

133. Marsman WA et al: Fulminant hepatitis B virus: recurrence after liver transplantation in two patients also infected with hepatitis delta virus, *Hepatology* 25(2):434, 1997.
134. Murray JA: Interferon therapy for hepatitis B and C, *Postgrad Med* 104(6):25, 1998.
135. Del Pozo MA et al: Interferon alpha treatment of chronic hepatitis C in HIV infected patients receiving zidovudine: efficacy, tolerance, response-related factors, *Hepatogastroenterology* 45(23)1695, 1998.
136. Hoofnagle JH, diBisceglie AM: Drug therapy: the treatment of chronic viral hepatitis, *N Engl J Med* 336(5):347, 1997.
137. Ganguly S et al: Study of portal hypertension in children with special reference to sclerotherapy, *Trop Gastroenterol* 18(3):1119, 1997.
138. Evans S et al: Selective distal splenorenal shunts for intractable variceal bleeding in pediatric portal hypertension, *J Pediatr Surg* 30(8):1115, 1995.
139. Hackworth CA et al: Transjugular intrahepatice portosystemic shunt creation in children: initial clinical experience, *Radiology* 206(1):109, 1998.
140. Pfeil SA, Lynn DJ: Wilson's disease: copper unfettered, *J Clin Gastroenterol* 29(1):22, 1999.
141. Brewer GJ: Recognition, diagnosis, and management of Wilson's disease, *Proc Soc Exp Biol Med* 233(1):39, 2000.
142. Zucker SD, Gollan, SL: Wilson's disease and hepatic copper toxicosis. In Zakim O, Boyer TD, editors: *Hepatology: a textbook of liver disease,* Philadelphia, 1996, W.B. Saunders.
143. Stremmel W et al: Wilson disease: clinical presentation, treatment, and survival, *Ann Intern Med* 115(9):720, 1991.
144. Brewer GJ et al: Treatment of Wilson's disease with zinc XVI: treatment during the pediatric years, *J Lab Clin Med* 137(3):191, 2001.
145. Stracciari A: Effects of liver transplantation on neural manifestation in Wilson disease, *Arch Neurol* 57(3):384, 2000.

CHAPTER 40

Structure and Function of the Musculoskeletal System

CHRISTY L. CROWTHER • LEONA A. MOURAD

CHAPTER OUTLINE

The way an individual functions in daily life, moves about, or manipulates objects physically depends on the integrity of the musculoskeletal system. The musculoskeletal system is actually composed of two systems: (1) the skeleton proper, which is composed of bones and joints, and (2) skeletal muscles. Each of the systems contributes to mobility. The skeleton supports the body and provides leverage to the skeletal muscles so that movement of various parts of the body is possible. Movement of the various body parts is accomplished by contraction of the skeletal muscles and bending or rotation at the joints.

STRUCTURE AND FUNCTION OF BONES

Bones give form to the body, support tissues, and permit movement by providing points of attachment for muscles. Many bones meet in movable joints that determine the type and extent of movement possible. Bones also protect many of the body's vital organs. For example, the bones of the skull, thorax, and pelvis are hard exterior shields that protect the brain, heart, lungs, and reproductive and urinary organs.

The marrow cavities within certain bones serve as sites of blood cell formation. In adults, blood cells originate exclusively in the marrow cavities of the skull, vertebrae, ribs, sternum, shoulders, and pelvis. Bones also have a crucial role in mineral homeostasis, storing minerals (i.e., calcium, phosphate, carbonate, magnesium) that are essential for the proper working of many delicate cellular mechanisms.

Elements of Bone Tissue

Mature bone is a rigid connective tissue consisting of cells, fibers, a gelatinous material termed **ground substance,** and large amounts of crystallized minerals, mainly calcium, that give bone its rigidity. The structural elements of bone are summarized in Table 40-1.

Bone cells enable bone to grow, repair itself, change shape, and continuously synthesize new bone tissue and resorb (dissolve or digest) old tissue. The fibers in bone are made of collagen, which gives bone its tensile strength (the ability to hold itself together). Ground substance acts as a medium for the diffusion of nutrients, oxygen, metabolic wastes, biochemicals, and minerals between bone tissue and blood vessels.

Bone formation begins during fetal life as mesenchymal cells differentiate into chondrocytes (cartilage) or osteoblasts (bone). In mature bone the formation of new tissue begins with the production of an organic matrix by the bone cells. This **bone matrix** consists of ground substances, collagen, and other proteins (see Table 40-1) that take part in bone formation and maintenance.

The next step in bone formation is **calcification,** when minerals are deposited and crystallize. Minerals bind tightly to

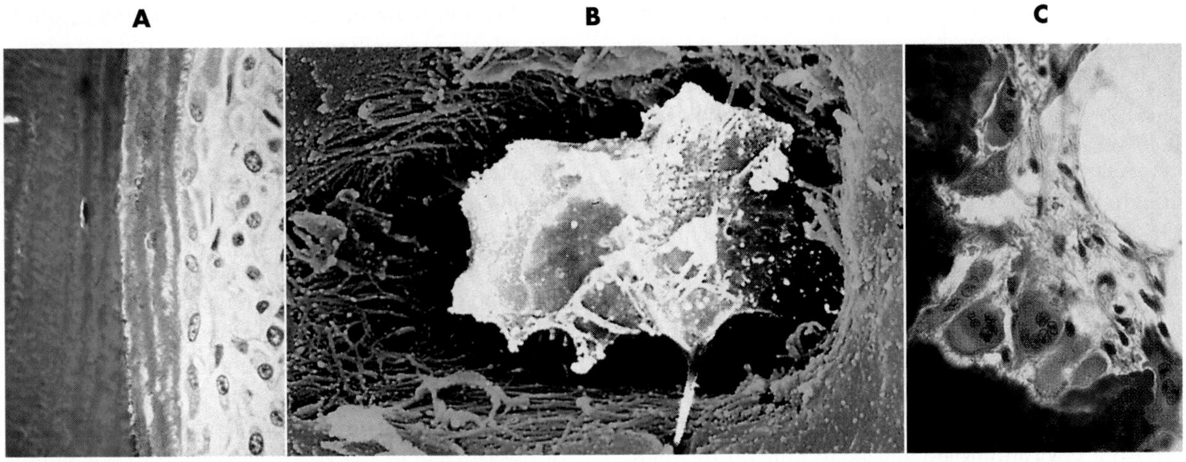

FIG. 40-1 Bone cells. A, Osteoblasts are responsible for the production of collagenous and noncollagenous proteins that compose osteoid. Active osteoblasts are lined up on the osteoid. Note the eccentrically located nuclei. **B,** Osteocyte. Scanning electron micrograph showing an osteocyte within a lacuna. The cell is surrounded by collagen fibers and mineralized bone. **C,** Osteoclasts actively resorb mineralized tissue. The scalloped surface in which the multinucleated osteoclasts rest is termed the *Howship lacuna.* (**A, C,** From Damjanov I, Linder J, editors: *Anderson's pathology,* ed 10, St Louis, 1996, Mosby. **B,** From Erlandsen S, Magney J: *Color atlas of histology,* St Louis, 1992, Mosby.)

Table 40-1 Structural Elements of Bone

Structural Element	Function
BONE CELLS	
Osteoblasts	Synthesize collagen and proteoglycans; stimulate osteoclast resorptive activity
Osteocytes	Maintain bone matrix
Osteoclasts	Resorb bone; assist with mineral homeostasis
BONE MATRIX	
Collagen fibers	Lend support and tensile strength
Proteoglycans	Control transport of ionized materials through matrix
Bone morphogenic proteins	Induce cartilage and bone formation
BMP-1	
BMP-2A	
BMP-3	
BMP-7	
Glycoproteins	
Sialoprotein	Promotes calcification
Osteocalcin	Inhibits calcium-phosphate precipitation; promotes bone resorption
Laminin	Stabilizes basement membranes in bones
Osteonectin	Binds calcium in bones
Albumin	Transports essential elements to matrix; maintains osmotic pressure of bone fluid
α-Glycoprotein	Promotes calcification
Minerals (elements)	
Calcium	Crystallizes to lend rigidity and compressive strength
Phosphate	Regulates vitamin D and thereby promotes mineralization

collagen fibers, producing tensile and compressional strength in bone, and withstand pressure and weight bearing to bone.

Bone Cells

Bone contains three types of cells: osteoblasts, osteocytes, and osteoclasts (Fig. 40-1). **Osteoblasts** are the bone-forming cells. Their primary function is to lay down new bone. Once this function is complete, osteoblasts become osteocytes. **Osteocytes** are osteoblasts that have become imprisoned within the mineralized bone matrix. They help maintain bone by synthesizing new bone matrix molecules.[1] **Osteoclasts** function primarily to resorb (remove) bone during process of growth and repair.

Osteoblasts

An **osteoblast** is a cell that produces type I collagen, is responsive to parathyroid hormone (PTH), and produces osteocalcin when stimulated by 1,25-dihydroxyvitamin D.[2] Osteoblasts are active on the outer surface of bones, where they form a single layer of cells. They bring about the formation of new bone by their synthesis of **osteoid** (nonmineralized bone matrix). The mechanism of osteoblast stimulation is reported to be the production of so-called coupling factors generated during the resorption process. Osteoblasts bring about the formation of new bone and the orderly mineralization of bone matrix by concentrating some of the plasma proteins (growth factors) found in the bone matrix and by facilitating the deposit and exchange of calcium and other ions at the site. As new bone is formed, it is shaped and remodeled through the effects of transforming growth factor–beta (TGF-β), as well as other plasma proteins (growth factors) found in the bone marrow (Table 40-2).

The concept of coupling bone formation with bone resorption has been extensively studied yet is still not entirely clear. Studies have shown that osteoblasts release a factor that induces osteoclastic activity by stimulating osteoclasts to remove nonmineralized organic material from bone surfaces, exposing resorption-inducing bone mineral to osteoclastic contact. In contact with bone mineral, osteoclasts can be further stimulated by colony-stimulating factor and interleukins-1, -3, and -6 produced by macrophage cells in the presence of PTH.[3] Thus the cells of the osteoblastic lineage (osteoblasts and osteocytes) form a network of cells in bone that sense the shape and structure of bone and determine where it is appropriate that bone be formed or resorbed, according to Wolfe's law (bone is shaped according to its function).

Osteoblasts have an active state and a resting state. When active, osteoblasts synthesize and secrete osteoid. When in the resting state, they appear dormant. If appropriately stimulated, however, the resting osteoblasts are capable of resuming activity.

Osteocytes

An osteocyte is a transformed osteoblast that is trapped or surrounded in osteoid as it hardens from minerals that enter during calcification (see Fig. 40-1, B). The osteocyte is within a space in the hardened bone matrix called a **lacuna.** Each osteocyte has a higher nucleus/cytoplasm ratio with a thin layer of nonmineralized osteoid around it, similar to the egg white surrounding an egg yolk.

The function of osteocytes is not fully known, but they do synthesize certain matrix molecules assisting bone calcification. They also help concentrate nutrients in the matrix. Osteocytes obtain nutrients from capillaries in the canaliculi, which contain nutrient-rich fluids. Osteocytes also may help synthesize and replace needed elements of the matrix, thus helping to maintain mineral homeostasis with the help of the PTH and osteoblast cells. Through exchanges between these cells, hormone catalysts, and minerals, optimal levels of calcium, phosphorus, and other minerals are maintained in blood plasma. The osteocyte also aids in modifying bone matrix through release of enzymes to dissolve the mineralized walls of the lacunae to prepare the bone for remodeling. Remodeling is described on p. 1345.

Osteoclasts

Osteoclasts are the major resorptive cells of bone. They are large, multinucleated cells with a short life span. Osteoclasts develop from the hematopoietic stem cell in the bone marrow stroma[4] and adjacent vessels and from mononuclear phagocytic cells. Osteoclasts contain lysosomes (digestive

WHAT'S NEW? Growth Factors: Possible New Management Tools

Bone morphogenic proteins (BMPs), part of the transforming growth factor–beta (TGF-β) cytokines, have been found to be powerful inducers of bone formation. BMPs may be important in future treatment of fractures. Animal and preliminary clinical studies using BMPs have shown promise in improved healing of bone and cartilage defects.

Data from Demers C, Hamdy RC: Bone morphogenic proteins, *Sci Med* 6(6):13, 1999.

Table 40-2 Effects of Selected Cytokines (Growth Factors) on Skeletal Tissues

Cytokine (Growth Factor)	Target Tissue	Formation	Resorption
Transforming growth factor–beta	Bone	+, −	+, −
	Cartilage	+, −	−
Transforming growth factor–alpha or epidermal growth factor	Bone	+, −	+
	Cartilage	+	
Insulin-like growth factor	Bone	−	0
	Cartilage	−	?
Fibroblast growth factor	Bone	+, −	0
	Cartilage		?
Platelet-derived growth factor	Bone	+	0
Colony-stimulating factors	Bone	0	+
	Cartilage	?	?
Interferon-gamma	Bone	−	−
	Cartilage	−	?
Tumor necrosis factor	Bone	−	+
	Cartilage	−	+
Interleukin-1, -3, and -6	Bone	+, −	+
	Cartilage	−	+

+, −: Both stimulatory and inhibitory properties on the specific cell listed; 0: no effects presently known; ?: possible effects on cell listed.

vacuoles) filled with hydrolytic enzymes. Fine projections, or microvilli, fan out from the osteoclast cell's surface and are known as **ruffled borders;** these projections result from extensive infoldings of the cell membrane adjacent to the resorptive surface.[4] Osteoclasts in regions of bone resorption lie in pits called *Howship lacunae,* where the osteoclasts' infolded, ruffled borders greatly increase the surface area of the plasma membrane. The infolds end in numerous channels and vesicles in the cell cytoplasm, permitting them to resorb the bone under their ruffled, infolded borders.

Osteoclasts bind to the bone surface of cell attachment proteins called **integrins.**[4] They bring about resorption of bone by secretion of citric and lactic acids, which help dissolve bone minerals, and collagenase, which aids in digesting collagen, along with the action of cytokines (see Table 40-2). Once resorption is completed, the osteoclast disappears by degeneration, either by reversing to its parent cell or through cell mobility from the site, where the osteoclast becomes an inactive, or "resting," osteoclast.

Bone Matrix

Bone matrix is made of the extracellular elements of bone tissue, composed of about 35% organic and 65% inorganic materials.[2] The major organic components are collagen fibers, and the major inorganic components are the calcium and phosphate minerals. Other parts of the bone matrix are the proteins, carbohydrate-protein complexes, and ground substances. Water makes up 5% to 8% of the matrix.

Collagen Fibers

Collagen fibers make up the major organic component of bone matrix. The fibers are approximately 90% type I collagen, which is synthesized and secreted by osteoblasts. Once secreted, the collagen molecules assemble into thin chains called *alpha chains,* which combine in threes to form **fibrils.** The fibrils form a staggered pattern, overlapping nearby fibrils by approximately one fourth their length. This staggered, overlapping pattern creates regular gaps, called *hole zones,* into which mineral crystals are deposited. After mineral deposition the fibrils link together and twist to form ropelike fibers. Collagen fibers then join to form a framework that gives bone its tensile strength and enables it to bear weight.

Collagen is the most abundant macromolecule in the body, accounting for approximately one third of all protein and providing the structural framework for nearly all tissues. Collagen is one of the extracellular components, along with proteoglycans and noncollagenous matrix proteins, of articular cartilage. To date, 14 different types of collagen have been identified. Cartilage-specific collagens include types II (the principal component), VI, IX, X, and XI. Type IX collagen is thought to be the "glue" that holds together the type II collagen scaffold of articular cartilage, helps maintain the structural integrity of cartilage, and resists tensile forces on the joint cartilage. Degradation of type IX collagen by proteolytic enzymes has been seen in the early stages of osteoarthritis and rheumatoid arthritis. Researchers have proposed that this degradation, or "unplugging," may be the mechanism for the degenerative changes seen in osteoarthritic and rheumatoid cartilage. Table 40-3 gives the musculoskeletal distribution of other types of collagen.

Proteoglycans

Proteoglycans are large complexes of numerous polysaccharides attached to a common protein core. They strengthen bone by forming compression-resistant networks between the collagen fibrils. Proteoglycans also control the transport and distribution of electrically charged particles (ions), particularly calcium, through the bone matrix, thereby playing a role in bone calcium deposition and calcification.

Glycoproteins

Glycoproteins are also carbohydrate-protein complexes of bone. Glycoproteins control the collagen interactions that lead to fibril formation. They also may play a role in calcification.

Some of the glycoproteins in bone matrix include bone sialoprotein, osteocalcin, osteonectin, laminin, albumin, and α-glycoprotein. Other proteins recently found in bone matrix are the compounds currently called **bone morphogenic proteins (BMPs)** (see Table 40-1). **Sialoprotein (osteopontin)** makes up about 8% of the noncollagenous matrix of bone and easily binds with calcium.

Osteocalcin is also a calcium-binding protein that binds preferentially to calcium that has already crystallized. The roles of osteocalcin may be to inhibit calcium phosphate precipitation and play a part in bone resorption by recruiting osteoclasts.

Osteonectin is also thought to bind calcium in bones, and laminin stabilizes basement membranes in bones. **Laminin** is an abundant bone matrix protein in humans that is most effective in neurite and axon growth.[4]

Bone albumin is identical to serum albumin (see Chapter 24). In calcified matrix, bone albumin is permanently fixed to bone mineral crystals and remains so until the bone is resorbed. Researchers believe bone albumin transports essential elements such as hormones, ions, and other metabolites to and from the bone cells and maintains the osmotic pressure of **bone fluid** (fluid surrounding mineral crystals and osteoblasts).

Table 40-3 Types of Collagen in Musculoskeletal Tissues

Type of Collagen*	Distribution in Musculoskeletal Tissues
I	Bone, tendon, ligament, intervertebral disk
II	Cartilage, intervertebral disk
IV	Basement cell membrane
V	Codistributed with type I
VI	Ubiquitous
IX	Codistributed with type II
X	Cartilage growth plate
XI	Cartilage
XII	Codistributed with type I
XIII	Molecule has not been isolated in connective tissues to date
XIV	Codistributed with type I

*To date, 14 different types of collagen have been identified.

α-Glycoprotein is thought to be synthesized in the liver, to be released into blood plasma, and to circulate to bone matrix, where it accumulates. α-Glycoprotein's affinity for calcium is 40 times greater than that of albumin. Therefore it probably plays an important role in the calcification of growing bone. α-Glycoprotein also may facilitate bone resorption by activating osteoclasts.

Bone Minerals

Mineralization is the final step in bone formation, after collagen synthesis and fiber formation. Mineralization has two distinct phases: (1) formation of the initial mineral deposit (initiation), and (2) proliferation or accretion of additional mineral crystals on the initial mineral deposits (growth).[4] The majority of the mineral content in the body is an analog of the naturally occurring mineral *hydroxyapatite.*

Table 40-4 lists the sequence in which calcium and phosphate form amorphous (fluid) calcium phosphate compounds that are converted, in stages, to solid hexagonal crystals of **hydroxyapatite (HAP).** As the calcium and phosphorus concentrations increase in the bone matrix, the first precipitate to form is dicalcium phosphate dihydrate (DCPD). Once DCPD precipitation begins, the remaining phases of bone crystal formation proceed until insoluble HAP is produced, with approximately 80% to 90% of the HAP incorporated into the collagen fibers. Amorphous calcium phosphate is distributed throughout the bone matrix.

Types of Bone Tissue

Bone is made up of two types of bony (osseous) tissue: **compact bone (cortical bone)** and **spongy bone (cancellous bone)** (Fig. 40-2). Compact bone makes up approximately 85% of the skeleton; spongy bone makes up the remaining 15%. Both types of bone tissue contain the same structural elements, and, with a few exceptions, both compact tissue and spongy tissue are present in every bone. The major difference between the two types of tissue is the organization of the elements.

Compact bone is highly organized, solid, and extremely strong. The basic structural unit in compact bone is the haversian system (Fig. 40-3). Each **haversian system** is made up of the following:

1. A central canal called the **haversian canal**
2. Concentric layers of bone matrix called **lamellae**
3. Tiny spaces (lacunae) between the lamellae
4. Bone cells (osteocytes) within the lacunae
5. Small channels or canals called **canaliculi**

Each haversian system is a separate cylindric entity that looks like a set of concentric rings. In the center of the haversian system is the haversian canal. The haversian canal runs through the long axis of bone and contains one or two blood vessels and nerve fibers. The blood vessels in the canal communicate with blood vessels in the periosteum (surface cover) and marrow cavity to transport nutrients and wastes to and from the osteocytes contained within the lacunae. Surrounding each haversian canal are the concentric lamellae. Between the lamellae are the lacunae, each of which contains one osteocyte. The lacunae are connected to each other and to the haversian canal by the canaliculi, which run parallel to the horizontal axis of the bone. Each canaliculus encloses a small extension (cytoplasmic process) from the osteocyte contained in the lacuna.

Table 40-4 Sequence of Calcium and Phosphate Compound Formation and Crystallization

Formula	Name	Abbreviation
$Ca(HPO_4) \cdot 2H_2O$	Dicalcium phosphate dihydrate	DCPD
$Ca_4H(PO_4)_3$	Octacalcium phosphate	OCP
$Ca_9(PO_4)_6$ (var.)	Amorphous calcium phosphate	ACP
$Ca_3(PO_4)_2$	Tricalcium phosphate	TCP
$Ca_5(PO_4)_3OH$	Hydroxyapatite	HAP

NOTE: Compounds are listed in the order in which precipitation and crystal formation occur.

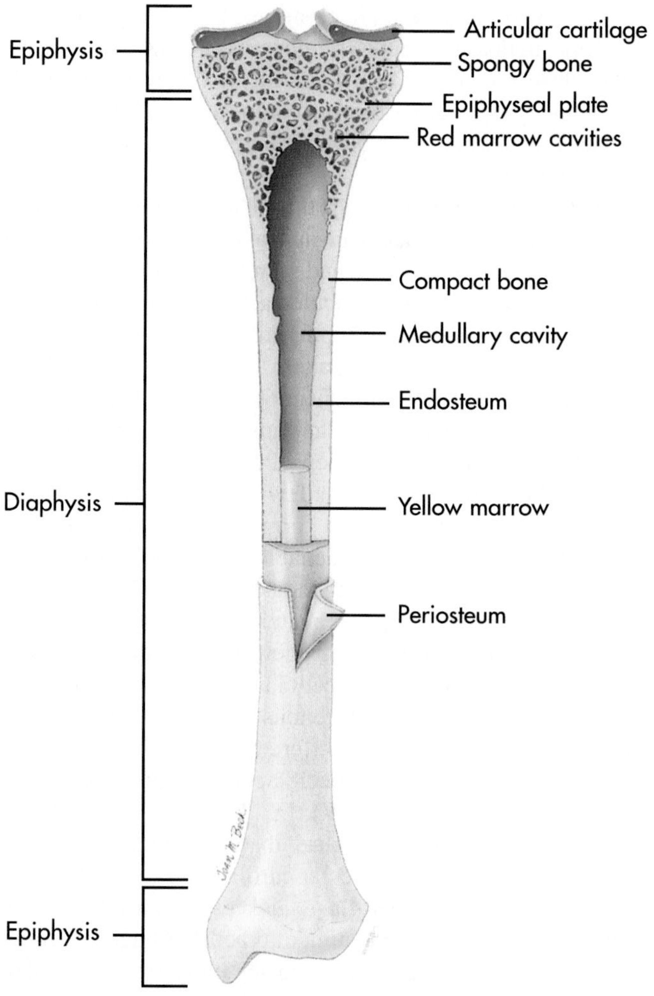

FIG. 40-2 Cross section of bone. Longitudinal section of long bone (tibia) showing cancellous and compact bone. (From Thibodeau GA, Patton KT: *Anatomy and physiology,* ed 4, St Louis, 1999, Mosby.)

Spongy bone is less complex and lacks haversian systems. In spongy bone the lamellae are not arranged in concentric layers but in plates or bars termed **trabeculae** that branch and unite with one another to form an irregular meshwork. The pattern of the meshwork is determined by the direction of stress on the particular bone. The spaces between the trabeculae are filled with red bone marrow. The osteocyte-containing lacunae are distributed between the trabeculae and interconnected by canaliculi. Capillaries pass through the marrow to nourish the osteocytes.

All bones are covered with a double-layered connective tissue called the **periosteum.** The outer layer of the periosteum contains blood vessels and nerves, some of which penetrate to the inner structures of the bone through channels called Volkmann canals (see Fig. 40-3). The inner layer of the periosteum is anchored to the bone by collagenous fibers (Sharpey fibers) that penetrate the bone. Sharpey fibers also help hold or attach tendons and ligaments to the periosteum of bones.[5]

Characteristics of Bone

The human skeleton consists of 206 bones, which constitute the axial skeleton and the appendicular skeleton (Fig. 40-4). The **axial skeleton** consists of 80 bones that make up the skull, vertebral column, and thorax. The **appendicular skeleton** consists of 126 bones that make up the upper and lower extremities, the shoulder girdle (pectoral girdle), and the pelvic girdle. The skeleton contributes about 14% of the weight of the adult body.

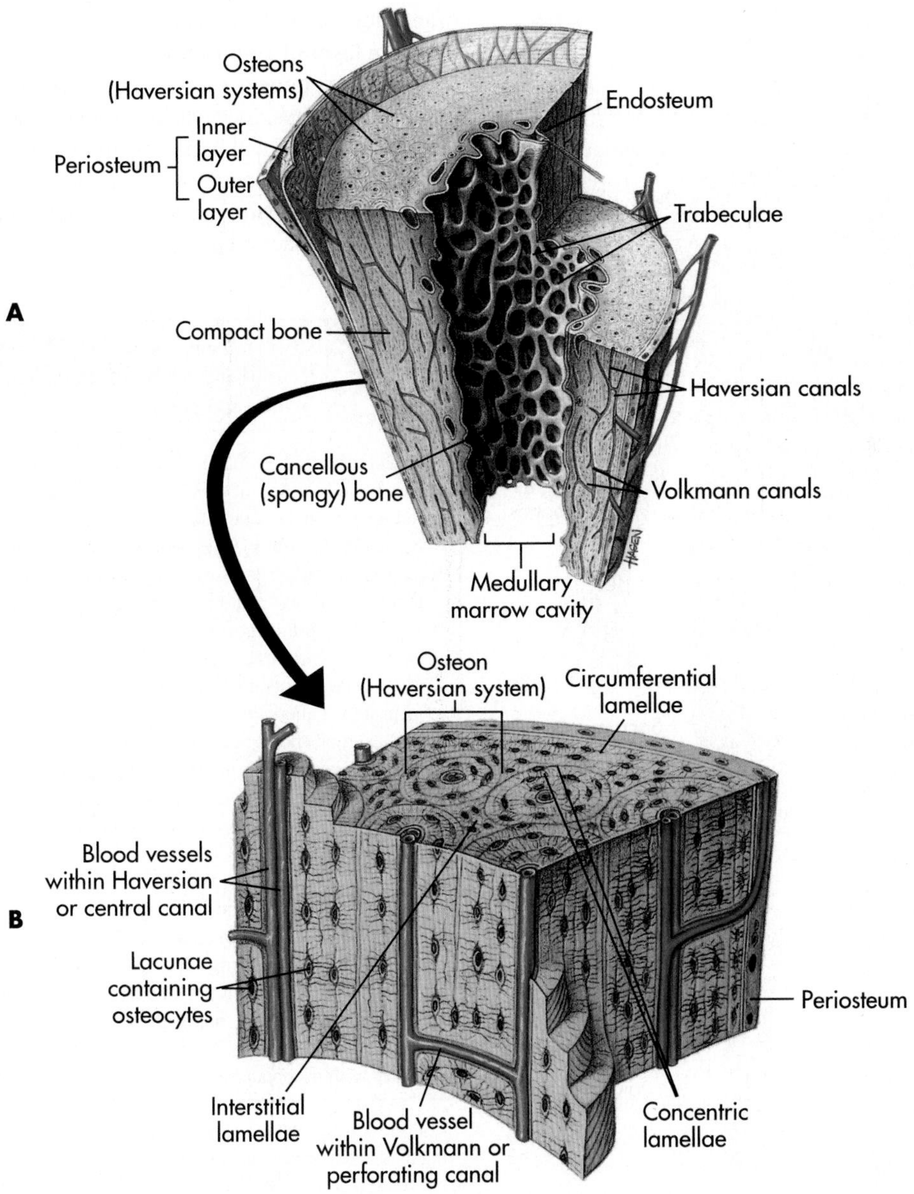

FIG. 40-3 Structure of compact and cancellous bone. A, Longitudinal section of a long bone showing both cancellous and compact bone. **B,** A magnified view of compact bone. (From Thibodeau GA, Patton KT: *Anatomy and physiology,* ed 4, St Louis, 1999, Mosby.)

Bones can be classified by shape as long, flat, short (cuboidal), or irregular. **Long bones** are longer than they are wide and consist of a narrow tubular midportion **(diaphysis)** that merges into a broader neck **(metaphysis)** and a broad end **(epiphysis)** (see Fig. 40-2).

The diaphysis consists of a shaft of thick, rigid compact bone that can tolerate bending forces. Contained within the diaphysis is the elongated marrow (medullary) cavity. The marrow cavity of the diaphysis contains primarily fatty tissue, which is referred to as *yellow marrow.* The yellow marrow assists red bone marrow in hematopoiesis only during times of stress. The yellow marrow cavity of the diaphysis is continuous with marrow cavities in the spongy bone of the metaphysis and diaphysis. The marrow contained within the epiphysis is red because it contains primarily blood-forming tissue (see Chapter 24). A layer of connective tissue, the **endosteum,** lines the outer surfaces of both types of marrow cavity.

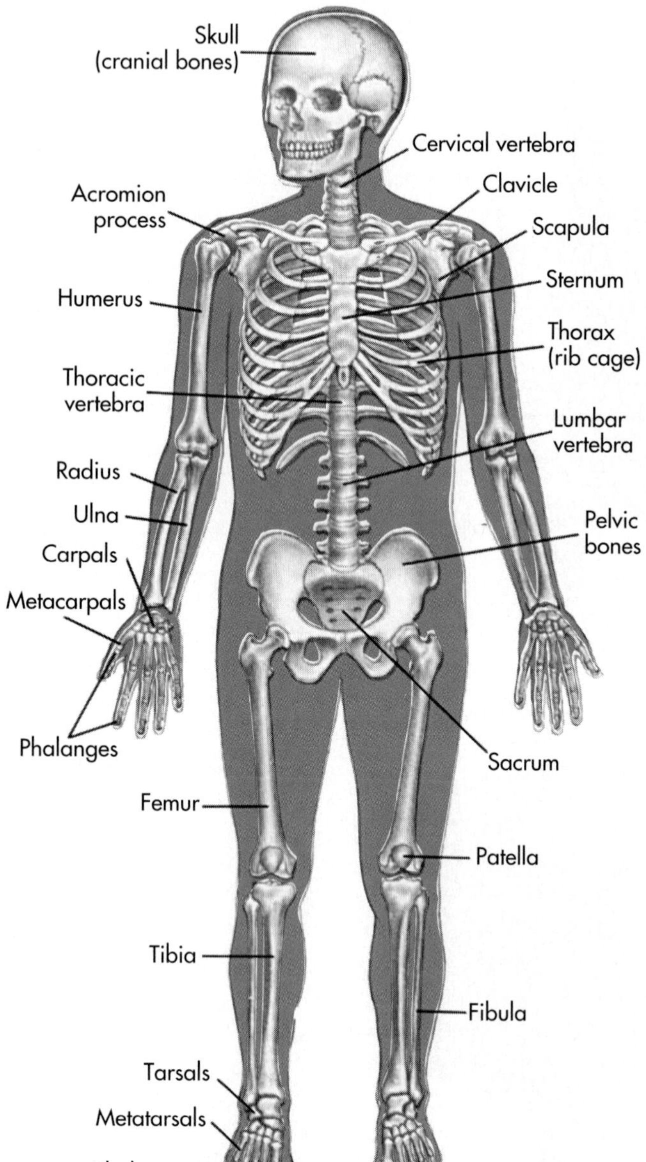

FIG. 40-4 Axial and appendicular skeleton. See text for explanation. (From Thompson JM et al: *Mosby's clinical nursing,* ed 4, St Louis, 1997, Mosby.)

The broadness of the epiphysis allows weight bearing to be distributed over a wide area. The epiphysis is made up of spongy bone covered by a very thin layer of compact bone. In a child the epiphysis is separated from the metaphysis by a cartilaginous **growth plate,** the **epiphyseal plate.** After puberty the epiphyseal plate calcifies and the epiphysis and metaphysis merge. By adulthood the line of demarcation between the epiphysis and metaphysis is undetectable.

In **flat bones,** such as the ribs or scapulae, two plates of compact bone are roughly parallel to each other. Between the compact bone plates is a layer of spongy bone. **Short bones (cuboidal bones),** such as the bones of the wrist or ankle, are often cuboidal in shape. They consist of spongy bone covered by a thin layer of compact bone.

Irregular bones, such as the vertebrae, mandibles, or other facial bones, have various shapes that include thin and thick segments. The thin part of an irregular bone consists of two plates of compact bone with spongy bone between the plates. The thick part consists of spongy bone surrounded by a layer of compact bone.

WHAT'S NEW?

Osteoblasts "Talk" to Osteoclasts, Providing a Mechanism for Stopping Bone Deterioration

If bone builders, osteoblasts, keep ahead of bone destroyers, osteoclasts, bone building occurs. A wide variety of disorders shift this balance and cause bone destruction—resulting in debilitating and even deadly fractures. Investigators have now reported an exciting fundamental mechanism by which osteoblasts communicate with osteoclasts. A new protein—named *osteoprotegrin* (OPG)—turns out to be key in the "conversation" between osteoblasts and osteoclasts. It appears now that osteoblasts and osteoclasts cooperate. This cooperation occurs because of the binding of OPG. OPG binds to a protein called OPG-ligand. This attachment prevents OPG-ligand from promoting osteoclasts into action. Think of OPG-ligand as an automobile's accelerator; stepping on it increases bone loss. OPG, however, is the brake, and when it is activated it promotes bone growth. The balance between the two determines the overall quality of bone. Osteoblasts make both OPG and OPG-ligand. OPG-ligand binds to surface proteins on osteoclasts, triggering proliferation of these cells and increasing their bone destruction. OPG secreted in the bone matrix serves as a decoy (sometimes called decoy receptor), sequestering OPG-ligand and preventing it from triggering bone resorption. OPG-ligand is the essential molecule for osteoclast development. Investigators speculate that by controlling the balance between OPG and OPG-ligand one may be able to treat diseases with associated bone loss.

Data from Kong Y, Penninger JM: Molecular control of bone remodeling and osteoporosis, *Exp Gerontol* 35(8):947, 2000; Travis J: Boning up: turning on cells that build bone and turning off ones that destroy it, *Science News* 257:41, 2000; Wan M et al: Transcriptional mechanisms of BMP-induced osteoprotegrin gene expression, *J Biol Chem* 276(13): 10119, 2001.

Maintenance of Bone Integrity

Remodeling

The internal structure of bone is maintained by **remodeling,** a three-phase process in which existing bone is resorbed and new bone is laid down to replace it. Remodeling is carried out by clusters of bone cells termed **bone-remodeling units.** The bone remodeling units are made up of bone precursor cells that differentiate into osteoclasts and osteoblasts. Precursor cells are located on the free surfaces of bones and along the vascular channels (especially the marrow cavities).

In phase 1 (activation) of the remodeling cycle, a stimulus (e.g., hormone, drug, vitamin, physical stressor) activates the bone cell precursors in a localized area of bone to form osteoclasts. In phase 2 (resorption), the osteoclasts form a "cutting cone," which gradually resorbs bone, leaving behind an elongated cavity termed a *resorption cavity.* The resorption cavity in compact bone follows the longitudinal axis of the haversian system, and the resorption cavity in spongy bone parallels the surface of the trabeculae.

Phase 3 (formation) is the laying down of new bone, termed *secondary bone,* by osteoblasts lining the walls of the resorption cavity. Successive layers (lamellae) in compact bone are laid down until the resorption cavity is reduced to a narrow haversian canal around a blood vessel. In this way, old haversian systems are destroyed and new haversian systems are formed. New trabeculae are formed in spongy bone. The entire process of remodeling takes about 3 to 4 months.

Repair

The remodeling process can repair microscopic bone injuries, but gross injuries, such as fractures and surgical wounds (osteotomies), heal by the same stages as soft tissue injuries, except that new bone, instead of scar tissue, is the final result (see Chapter 7). In bone the stages of wound healing are as follows:

1. *Hematoma formation:* occurs if vessels have been damaged, causing hemorrhage. Fibrin and platelets within the hematoma form a meshwork that is the initial framework for healing with the help of hematopoietic growth factors such as platelet-derived growth factor and TGF-β (see Table 40-2).
2. *Procallus formation:* fibroblasts, capillary buds, and osteoblasts move into the wound to produce granulation tissue called **procallus.** Cartilage is formed as a precursor of bone, and types I, II, and III collagen are formed. Enzymes and growth factors, such as insulin and insulin-like growth factors, plus bone morphogenic protein and osteogenin, aid in this stage of healing.
3. *Callus formation:* osteoblasts in the procallus form membranous or **woven bone (callus).** Enzymes increase the phosphate content and permit the phosphate to join with calcium to be deposited as mineral to harden the callus.
4. *Callus replacement:* osteoblasts continue to replace the callus with lamellar bone or trabecular bone (Fig. 40-5).

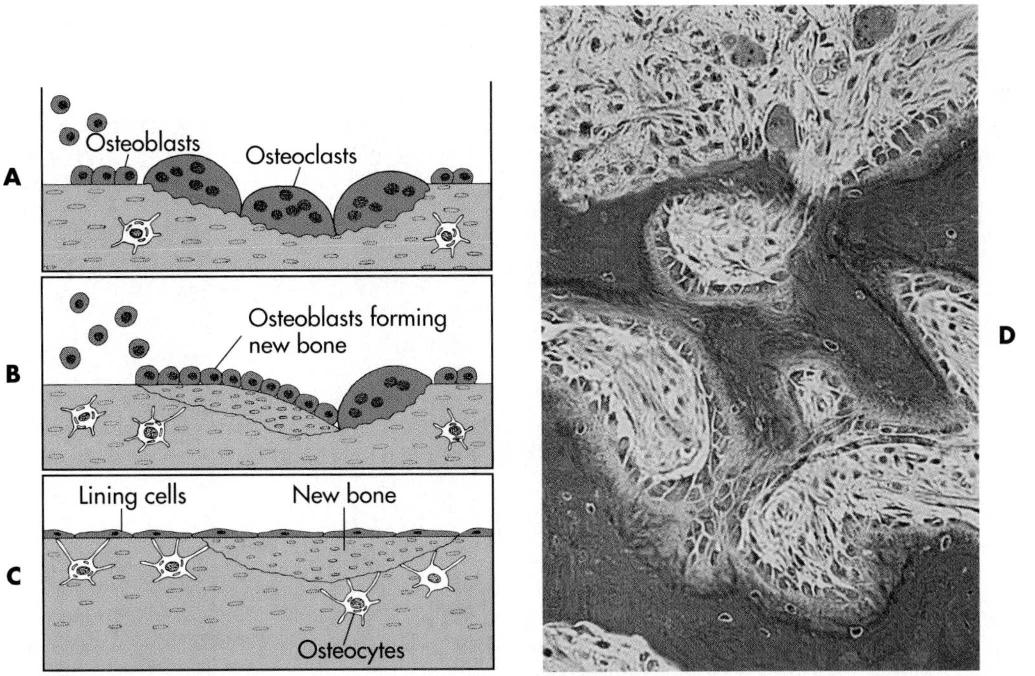

FIG. 40-5 Bone remodeling. In the remodeling sequence, bone sections are removed by the bone-resorbing cells (osteoclasts) and replaced with a new section laid down by bone-forming cells (osteoblasts). The cells work in response to signals generated in that environment. The first phase of remodeling is mediated only by the multinucleated osteoclastic cells. They are activated, scoop out bone **(A),** and resorb it; then the work of the osteoblasts begins **(B).** They form new bone that replaces bone removed by the resorption process **(C).** The sequence takes 4 to 5 months. **D,** Active bone remodeling seen in the settings of primary or secondary hyperparathyroidism. Note the active osteoblasts surmounted on red-stained osteoid. Marrow fibrosis is present. (**A–C,** From Mundy GR: *Bone remodeling and its disorders,* St Louis, 1995, Mosby. **D,** From Damjanov I, Linder J, editors: *Anderson's pathology,* ed 10, St Louis, 1996, Mosby.)

5. *Remodeling:* the periosteal and endosteal surfaces of the bone are remodeled to the size and shape of the bone before injury. Synthesis of other types of collagen recedes in favor of type I, which is the collagen found in bone. This final stage of healing, or remodeling, is vital because bone that has not been remodeled does not have good mechanical properties for weight bearing and mobility.

The speed with which bone heals depends on the severity of the bone disruption; the type and amount of bone tissue that must be replaced (spongy bone heals faster); blood supply and oxygen to the site; presence of growth and thyroid hormones, insulin, vitamins, and other nutrients; presence of systemic disease; effects of aging; and effective treatment, including immobilization and the prevention of complications such as infection. In general, however, hematoma formation occurs within hours of fracture or surgery; formation of procallus by osteoblasts occurs within days; callus formation occurs within weeks; and replacement and contour modeling occur within years—up to 4 years in some cases.

STRUCTURE AND FUNCTION OF JOINTS

The site where two or more bones meet is called a **joint (articulation)** (Fig. 40-6). The primary function of joints is to provide stability and mobility to the skeleton. Whether a joint provides stability or mobility depends on its location and its structure. Generally, joints that stabilize the skeleton have a simpler structure than those that enable the skeleton to move. Most joints provide both stability and mobility to some degree (Fig. 40-7).

Joints are classified based on the degree of movement they permit or on the connecting tissues that hold them together. Based on movement, a joint is classified as a **synarthrosis (immovable joint),** an **amphiarthrosis (slightly movable joint),** or a **diarthrosis (freely movable joint).** On the basis of connective structures, joints are classified broadly as fibrous, cartilaginous, and synovial. Each of these three structural classifications can be subdivided according to the shape and contour of the articulating surfaces (ends) of the bones and the type of motion the joint permits.

Fibrous Joints

A joint in which bone is united directly to bone by fibrous connective tissue is called a **fibrous joint.** Generally, fibrous joints are synarthroses (immovable), but many fibrous joints allow some movement. The degree of movement depends on the distance between the bones and the flexibility of the fibrous connective tissue.

Fibrous joints are further subdivided into three types: sutures, syndesmoses, and gomphoses. A **suture** has a thin layer of dense fibrous tissue that binds together interlocking flat bones in the skulls of young children. Sutures form an extremely tight union that permits no motion. By adulthood the fibrous tissue has been replaced by bone. A **syndesmosis** is a joint in which the two bony surfaces are united by a ligament or membrane. The fibers of ligaments are flexible and stretch, permitting a limited amount of movement. The paired bones of the lower arm (radius and ulna) and the lower leg (tibia and

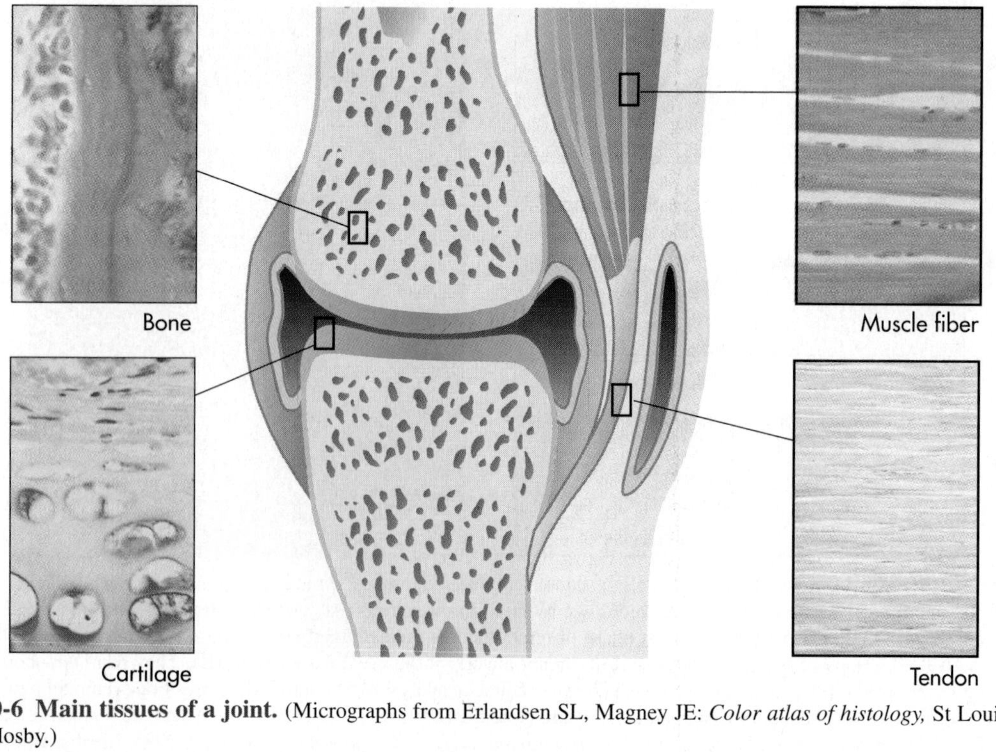

FIG. 40-6 Main tissues of a joint. (Micrographs from Erlandsen SL, Magney JE: *Color atlas of histology,* St Louis, 1992, Mosby.)

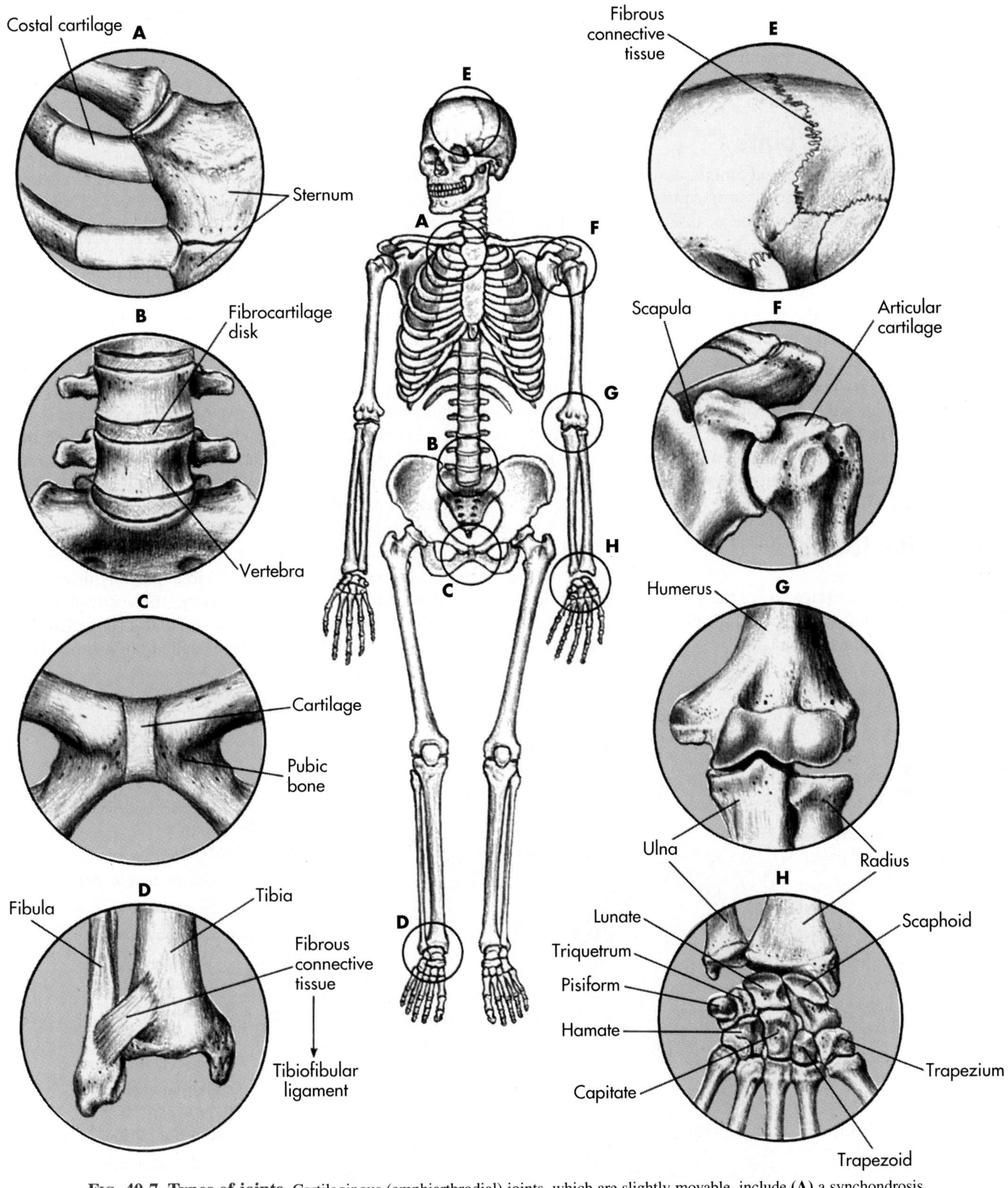

FIG. 40-7 Types of joints. Cartilaginous (amphiarthrodial) joints, which are slightly movable, include **(A)** a synchondrosis that attaches ribs to costal cartilage; **(B)** a symphysis that connects vertebrae; and **(C)** the symphysis that connects the two pubic bones. Fibrous (synarthrodial) joints, which are immovable, include **(D)** the syndesmosis between the tibia and fibula; **(E)** sutures that connect the skull bones; and the gomphosis (not shown), which holds teeth in their sockets. The synovial joints include **(F)** the spheroid type at the shoulder; **(G)** the hinge type at the elbow; and **(H)** the gliding joints of the hand.

fibula) and their ligaments are syndesmotic joints. A **gomphosis** is a special type of fibrous joint in which a conical projection fits into a complementary socket and is held there by a ligament. The teeth held in the maxilla or mandible are gomphosis joints.

Cartilaginous Joints

The two types of cartilaginous joints are symphyses and synchondroses. A **symphysis** is a cartilaginous joint in which bones are united by a pad or disk of fibrocartilage. The articulating surfaces of the two bones are usually covered by a thin layer of hyaline cartilage, and the thick pad of fibrocartilage acts as a shock absorber and stabilizer. Examples of symphyses are the symphysis pubis, which joins the two pubic bones, and the intervertebral disks, which join the bodies of the vertebrae. A **synchondrosis** is a joint in which hyaline cartilage, rather than fibrocartilage, connects the two bones. The joints between the ribs and the sternum are synchondroses. The hyaline cartilage of these joints is called *costal cartilage.* Slight movement at the synchondroses between the ribs and the sternum allows the chest to move outward and upward during breathing.

Synovial Joints

Structure

Synovial joints (diarthroses) are the most movable and the most complex joints in the body (Fig. 40-8). A synovial joint consists of the following parts:

1. A fibrous joint capsule (articular capsule)
2. A synovial membrane that lines the inner surface of the joint capsule
3. A joint cavity (synovial cavity), a space formed by the capsule
4. Synovial fluid, which fills the joint cavity and lubricates the joint surface
5. Articular cartilage, which covers and pads the articulating bony surfaces

Joint Capsule

The fibrous **joint capsule (articular capsule)** is connective tissue that covers the ends of the bones where they meet in the joint. Sharpey fibers firmly attach the proximal and distal capsule to the periosteum and ligaments and tendons, which also reinforce the capsule. The joint capsule is made up of parallel, interlacing bundles of dense, white fibrous tissue. It is richly supplied with nerves, blood vessels, and lymphatic vessels. The nerves in and around the joint capsule are sensitive to the rate and direction of motion, compression, tension, vibration, and pain.

Synovial Membrane

The **synovial membrane (synovium)** is the smooth, delicate inner lining of the joint capsule (Fig. 40-9). It lines the nonarticular portion of the synovial joint and any ligaments or tendons that traverse the joint cavity. The synovial membrane is made up of two layers—a vascular layer called the **subintima** and a thin cellular layer called the **intima.** The

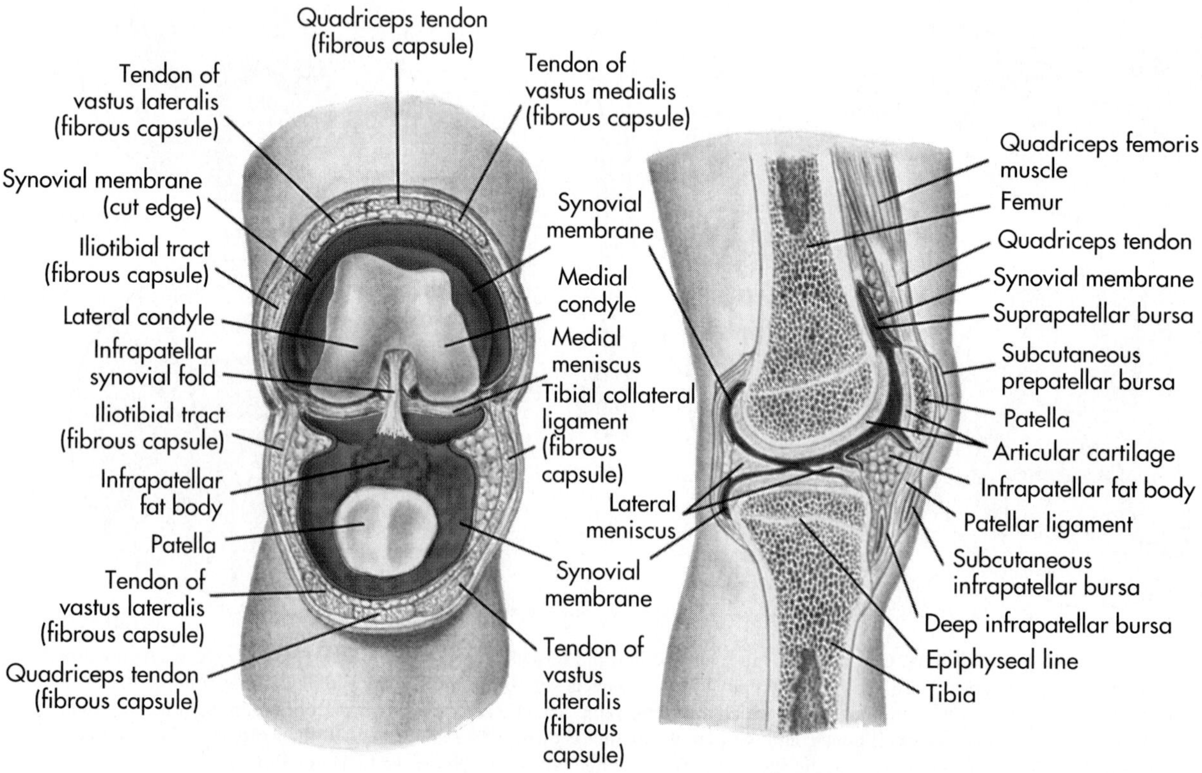

FIG. 40-8 Knee joint (synovial joint). (From Thompson JM et al: *Mosby's manual of clinical nursing,* ed 4, St Louis, 1997, Mosby.)

vascular subintima merges with the fibrous joint capsule and is composed of loose fibrous connective tissue, elastin fibers, fat cells, fibroblasts, macrophages, and mast cells. The intima consists of rows of synovial cells embedded in a fiber-free intercellular matrix. The intima contains two types of synovial cells: type A cells and type B cells. The **type A cells** ingest and remove bacteria and particles of debris by phagocytosis in the joint cavity. (Phagocytosis is described in Chapter 7.) The **type B cells** secrete **hyaluronate**, a binding agent that gives synovial fluid its viscous quality. The synovial membrane is richly supplied with blood and lymphatic vessels; therefore it is capable of rapid repair and regeneration.

Joint Cavity

The **joint cavity (synovial cavity)** is an enclosed, fluid-filled space between the articulating surfaces of the two bones. This small cavity, often called the joint space, enables the two bones to move "against" one another. The synovial cavity is surrounded by the synovial membrane and filled with a clear, viscous, slick fluid called the *synovial fluid.*

Synovial Fluid

Synovial fluid is superfiltrated plasma from blood vessels in the synovial membrane. Synovial fluid lubricates the joint surfaces, nourishes the pad of the articular cartilage that covers the ends of the bones, and contains free-floating synovial cells and various leukocytes that phagocytose joint debris and microorganisms. Loss of synovial fluid leads to rapid deterioration of articular cartilage.

Articular Cartilage

Articular cartilage is a layer of hyaline cartilage that covers the end of each bone (Fig. 40-10). It may be thick or thin, depending on the size of the joint, the fit of the two bone ends, and the amount of weight and shearing force the joint normally withstands. The function of articular cartilage is to reduce friction in the joint and to distribute the forces of weight bearing. Articular cartilage is composed of **chondrocytes** (cartilage cells) (making up about 2% of the tissue) and an intercellular matrix made up of collagen (making up about 10% to 30% of weight), protein polysaccharides

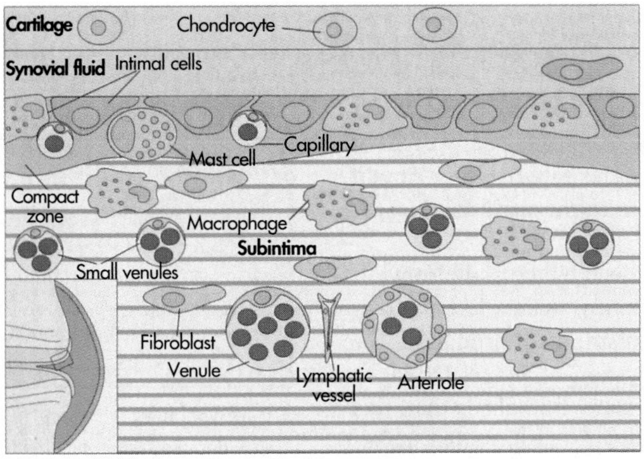

FIG. 40-9 Synovium. Note the delicate synovial lining resting on a fibroadipose subintimal lining rich in capillaries, lymphatics, and nerve endings. (Modified from Klippel JH, Dieppe PA: *Rheumatology,* ed 2, London, 1998, Mosby.)

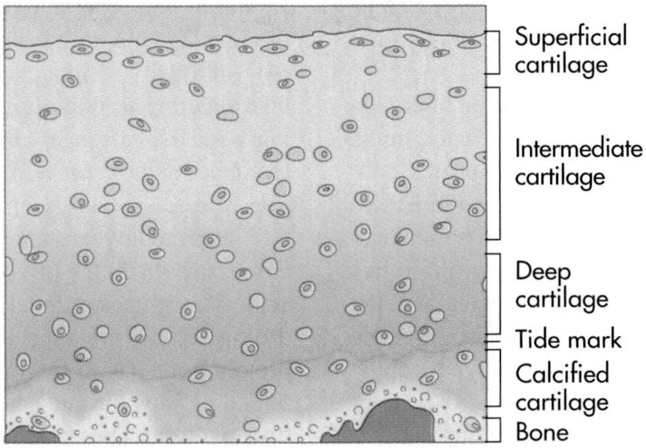

FIG. 40-10 Articular cartilage. Note the different zones within the cartilage. (Modified from Klippel JH, Dieppe PA: *Rheumatology,* ed 2, London, 1998, Mosby.)

Table 40-5 Characteristics of Muscle Fibers

Characteristic	Type I (Red)	Type II (White)
Anatomic location	Deep axial portion of surface muscle	Surface portion of surface muscle
Contraction speed	Slow	Fast
Motor neuron type	Type I, small alpha	Type II, large alpha
Firing frequency	Low, long duration	Rapid, short duration
Resistance to fatigue	High	Low
Myoglobin	High	Low
Capillary supply	Profuse	Intermediate to sparse
Metabolism	Oxidative	Glycolysis
Mitochondria	Many	Few
Enzymes	Lactate dehydrogenase, types 1–3	Lactate dehydrogenase, types 4 and 5
Creatine kinase	Cardiac type	Fast, skeletal
Example (most muscles are mixed)	Greater proportion of slow-contracting fibers in soleus	Greater proportion of fast-contracting fibers in laryngeal and ocular muscles
Glycogen content	Low	High
Intensity of contraction	Low	High
Aerobic metabolic capacity	High	Low
Fiber diameter	Small	Large
Myosin–adenosine triphosphatase (ATPase) activity	Low	High

From Spence AP, Mason EE: *Human anatomy and physiology,* ed 4, St Paul, Minn, 1992, West Publishing Co.

(making up 5% to 10% of weight), and water. The water content ranges from 60% to almost 80% of the net weight of the cartilage, and individual molecules rapidly enter or exit the articular cartilage to contribute to the resiliency of the tissue.[6]

The intercellular matrix is produced by the chondrocytes, which synthesize and extrude collagen, which, like the collagen produced by bone cells, is distributed throughout the cartilage in a highly organized system of fibers. Collagen fibers in cartilage are made up of many fine fibrils that, like bone fibrils, are assembled in an orderly fashion that makes them resistant to physical, metabolic, or chemical breakdown. The main differences between bone collagen and cartilage collagen are the amino acid content of the alpha chains and the composition of the fibrils. Bone collagen fibrils are made up of two type I chains and one type II chain. Approximately 90% of the cartilage collagen fibrils is made up of three identical type II chains, with the remaining 10% made up of types V, VI, IX, X, and XI (Table 40-5).[6]

At the surface of articular cartilage, the collagen fibers run parallel to the joint surface and are closely compacted into a dense, protective mat.[7] (Loss of this dense, compacted configuration at the surface subjects the underlying fibers to splitting and thinning, in which case the cartilage is unable to tolerate weight bearing.) In the middle layer (the proliferative zone) of the cartilage, the fibers are arranged tangential to the surface, which allows them to deform and absorb some of the force of weight bearing. In the bottom layer (the hypertrophic zone) of the cartilage, the fibers are perpendicular to the joint surface, allowing them to resist shear forces, and are embedded in a calcified layer of cartilage called the **tidemark.** The tidemark anchors the collagen fibers to the underlying (subchondral) bone. Collagen fibers are important components of the cartilage matrix because they account for approximately 60% of the dry weight and because they (1) anchor the cartilage securely to underlying bone, (2) provide a taut framework for the cartilage, (3) control the loss of fluid from the cartilage, and (4) prevent the escape of protein polysaccharides (proteoglycans) from the cartilage.

WHAT'S NEW? New Cartilage Repair Treatments

Cartilage repair has always been a disappointing enterprise. Four categories of new treatments are, however, showing promise. They can generally be classified as (1) stimulation of bone marrow to form a repair tissue, (2) transplantation of osteochondral autografts or allografts, (3) implantation of cultured autologous chondrocytes, and (4) use of resorbable collagen scaffold.

Data from Bobic V: Tissue repair techniques of the future: options for articular cartilage injury. Techvest, LLC first annual conference on tissue repair, replacement, and regeneration, Oct 27-28, 1998, New York, NY.

The proteoglycans are macromolecules consisting of proteins, carbohydrates **(glycosaminoglycans),** and hyaluronic acid. The glycosaminoglycans (keratan sulfate and chondroitin sulfate) are attached to the **protein core,** and several protein cores (with their attached glycosaminoglycans) are bound to a hyaluronic acid chain by a special protein called **link protein.** The proteoglycans give articular cartilage its stiff quality and regulate the movement of synovial fluid

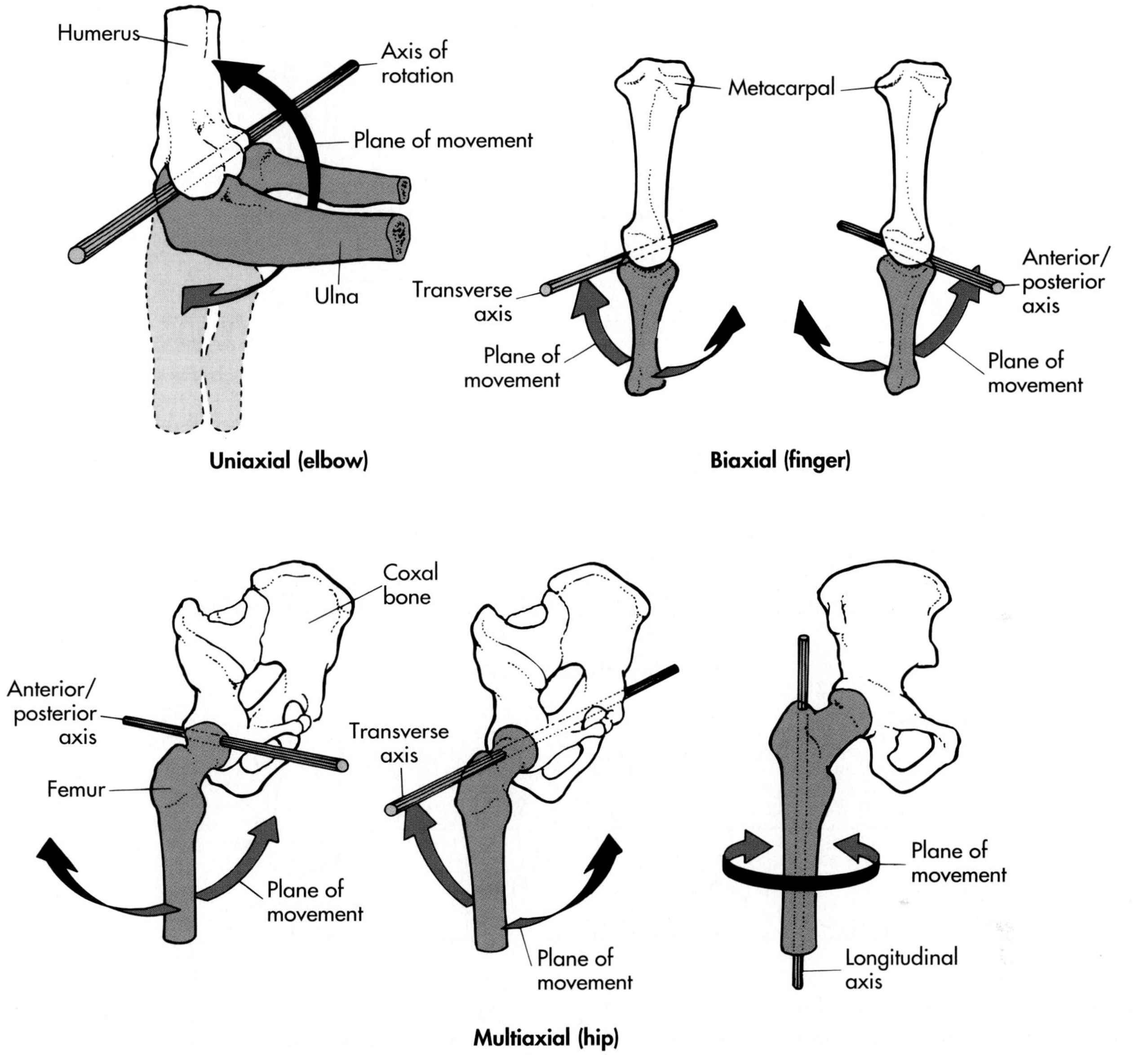

FIG. 40-11 Movements of synovial (diarthrodial) joints.

through the cartilage. Without proteoglycans, normal weight bearing would rapidly and completely press all the synovial fluid out of the cartilage. The proteoglycans act as a pump, permitting enough fluid to be pressed out to ensure that a fluid film is always present on the surface of the cartilage, even after hours of weight bearing. The pumping action of proteoglycans also draws synovial fluid back into the cartilage after a weight-bearing load is released. Mobility and weight bearing are necessary for the pumping action of proteoglycans to occur. Nonuse of a joint quickly reduces the pumping action, which changes the composition of the matrix and interferes with the nutrition of the chondrocytes.

Articular cartilage has no blood vessels, lymph vessels, or nerves. Therefore it is insensitive to pain and regenerates slowly and minimally after injury. Regeneration occurs primarily at sites where the articular cartilage meets the synovial membrane, where blood vessels and nutrients are available.

Movement

Synovial joints are described as uniaxial, biaxial, or multiaxial according to the shapes of the bone ends and the type of movement occurring at the joint (Fig. 40-11). Usually one of the bones is stable and serves as an axis for the motion of the other bone. The body movements made possible by various synovial joints are either circular or angular (Fig. 40-12).

STRUCTURE AND FUNCTION OF SKELETAL MUSCLES

The skeletal muscles are made up of millions of individual fibers that, by the process of contraction and relaxation, do the work necessary to complete movements as varied as a

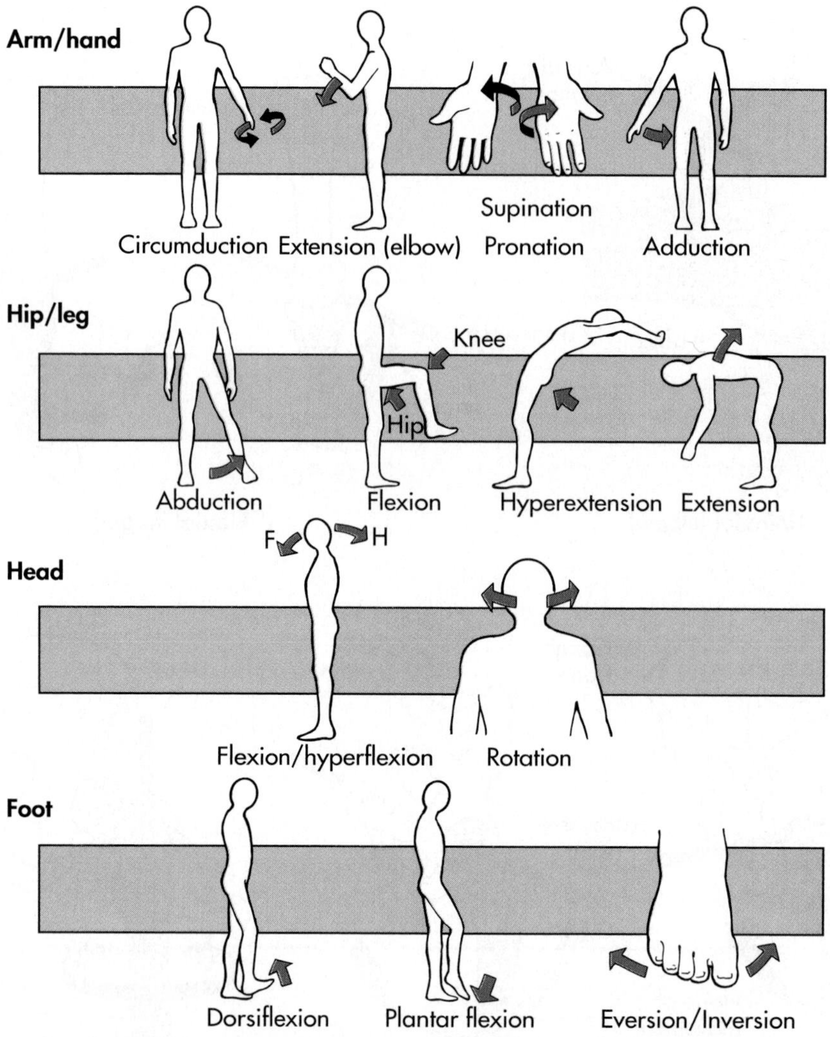

FIG. 40-12 Body movements provided by synovial (diarthrodial) joints.

ballerina's pirouette or an artist's deft stroke (Fig. 40-13). Muscle constitutes 40% of adults' body weight and 50% of children's body weight. Muscle is 75% water, 20% protein, and 5% organic and inorganic compounds. Thirty-two percent of all protein stores for energy and metabolism is contained in muscle.

Whole Muscle

There are more than 350 named muscles; almost all are paired. The body's muscles vary dramatically in size and shape. They range from 2 to 60 cm in length and are shaped according to function. **Fusiform muscles** are elongated muscles shaped like straps and can run from one joint to another. **Pennate muscles** are broad, flat, and slightly fan shaped, with fibers running obliquely to the muscle's long axis. The multipennate deltoid muscle, which flexes and extends the arm, is a good example of a muscle shaped according to its function.

Each skeletal muscle is a separate organ encased in a three-part connective tissue framework called **fascia.** The layers of connective tissue protect the muscle fibers, attach the muscle to bony prominences, and provide a structure for a network of nerve fibers, blood vessels, and lymphatic channels.

The outermost layer, the **epimysium,** is located on the surface of the muscle and tapers at each end to form the **tendon** (Fig. 40-14). Tendons allow a short muscle to exert power on a distant joint where a thick muscle would interfere with joint mobility. The next layer, the **perimysium,** further subdivides the muscle fibers into bundles of connective tissue, or **fascicles.** The **endomysium** surrounds the muscle fascicles, the smallest unit of muscle fibers visible without a microscope. The ligaments, tendons, and fascia are made up of connective tissue that also serves to buffer the limbs from the effects of sudden strains or changes in speed. The rapid recovery necessary for strenuous exercise is supported by the elastic property of muscle and its connective tissue.

Skeletal muscle is described, almost interchangeably, as **voluntary, striated,** or **extrafusal.** "Voluntary" indicates that the muscle is controlled directly by the central nervous system. "Striated" describes the striated, or striped, pattern of skeletal muscle viewed under a light microscope. The striations result from the organization of the muscle fibers into the contractile units called *sarcomeres.* "Extrafusal" distinguishes the skeletal muscle fibers from other contractile fibers located within the sensory organs of the muscle.

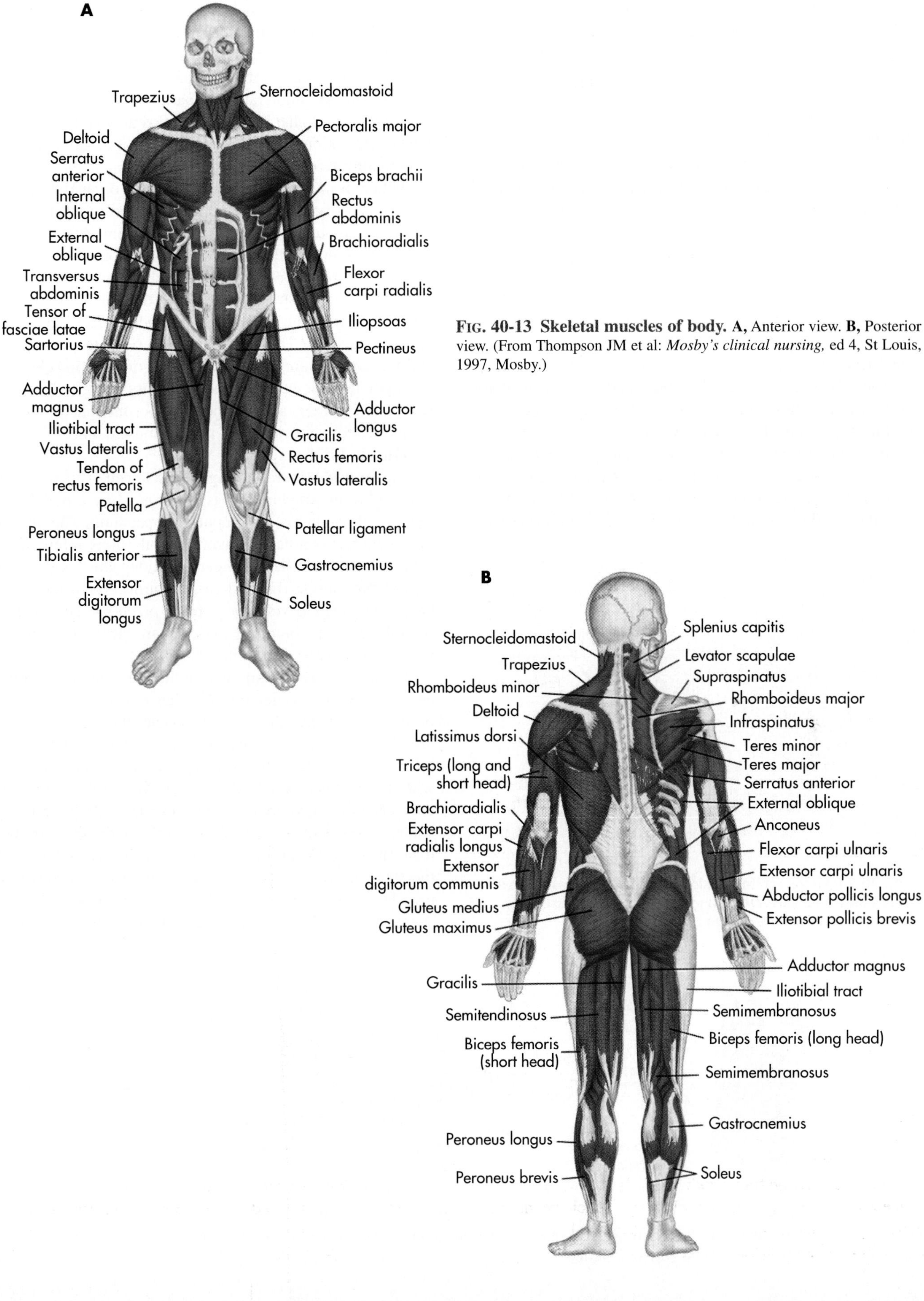

FIG. 40-13 Skeletal muscles of body. A, Anterior view. **B,** Posterior view. (From Thompson JM et al: *Mosby's clinical nursing,* ed 4, St Louis, 1997, Mosby.)

Other components that are visible on gross inspection of the whole muscle include the motor and sensory nerve fibers. These function together with the muscle, innervating portions of it and providing the electrical impulses needed for motor function.

Motor Unit

From the anterior horn cell of the spinal cord, the axons of motor nerves branch out to innervate a specific group of muscle fibers. Each anterior horn cell, its axon (part of a lower motor neuron; see Chapter 13), and the muscle fibers innervated by it are called a **motor unit** (Fig. 40-15). The motor units are composed of lower motor neurons, which extend to skeletal muscles. Often termed the *functional unit* of the neuromuscular system, the motor unit behaves as a single entity and contracts as a whole when it receives an electrical impulse.

The whole muscle may be controlled by several motor nerve axons. These branch to innervate many motor units within the muscle. The whole muscle then may be made up of many motor units. The number of motor units per individual muscle varies greatly. In the calf, for example, one motor axon will innervate approximately 2000 muscle fibers, out of a total of 1,200,000 muscle fibers. This is a high innervation ratio of muscle fibers to axons, and it contrasts markedly with the low innervation ratio in the laryngeal muscles. There, two to three muscle fibers constitute each motor unit, and the innervation ratio can be of great functional significance. The greater the innervation ratio of a particular organ, the greater its endurance. Higher innervation ratios prevent fatigue, and lower innervation ratios allow for precision of movement.

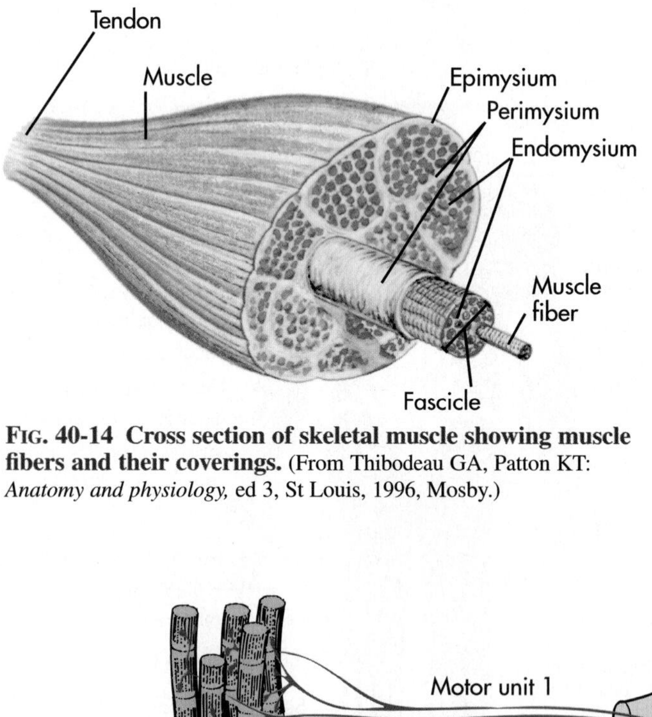

FIG. 40-14 Cross section of skeletal muscle showing muscle fibers and their coverings. (From Thibodeau GA, Patton KT: *Anatomy and physiology,* ed 3, St Louis, 1996, Mosby.)

Sensory Receptors

Although muscles function as effector organs, they also contain sensory receptors and are involved in sending different signals to the central nervous system. Among these are the muscle spindles and Golgi tendon organs. **Spindles** are mechanoreceptors that lie parallel to muscle fibers and respond to muscle stretching. **Golgi tendon organs** are dendrites that terminate and branch to tendons near the neuromuscular junction. The muscle spindles, Golgi tendon organs, and free nerve endings provide a means of reporting changes in length, tension, velocity, and tone in the muscle. This system of afferent signals is responsible for the muscle stretch response and maintenance of normal muscle tone.

Muscle Fibers

Each **muscle fiber** is a single **muscle cell.** This long cell is cylindric in structure and is surrounded by a membrane capable of excitation and impulse propagation. The muscle fiber contains bundles of **myofibrils,** the fiber's functional subunits, in a parallel arrangement along the longitudinal axis of the muscle (Fig. 40-16). At birth the muscle fibers have completed development from precursor cells called **myoblasts.** All voluntary muscles are derived from the mesodermal layer of the embryo.

The type of peripheral nerve influences the muscle fiber and motor unit considerably. Whether motor nerves are fast or slow determines the type of muscle fibers in the motor unit. Type II fibers, also called *white fast-motor fibers,* are innervated by relatively large type II alpha motor neurons with fast conduction velocities. These fibers rely on a short-term anaerobic glycolytic system for rapid energy transfer, whereas type I fibers depend on aerobic oxidative metabolism. Histochemical stains are now routinely used to describe the structure of muscle fibers and contractile elements of muscle biopsy specimens. White muscle **(type II fibers)** stains dark in the enzyme stain adenosine triphosphatase

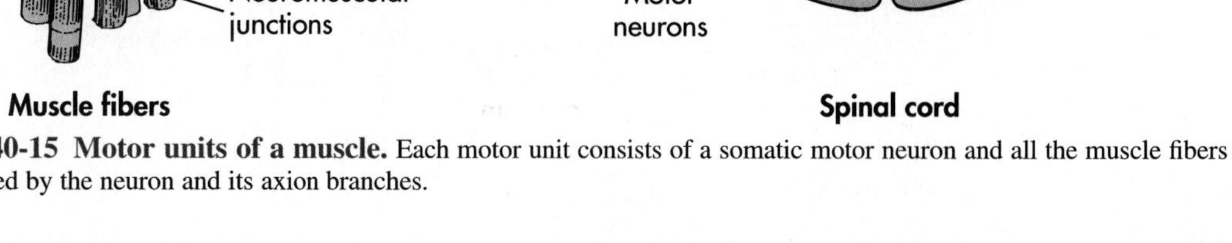

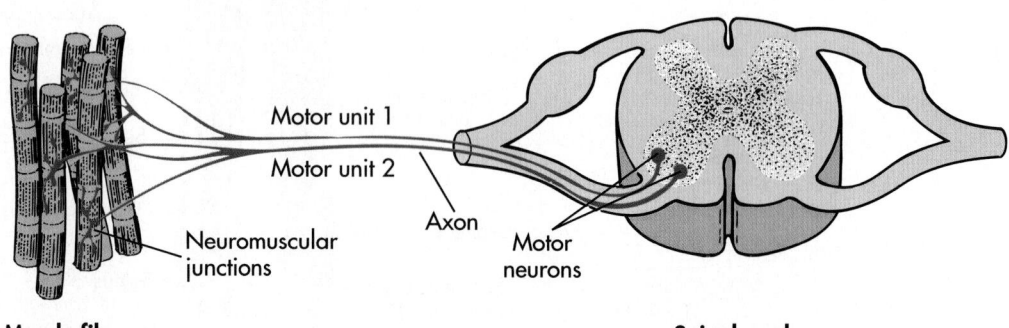

FIG. 40-15 Motor units of a muscle. Each motor unit consists of a somatic motor neuron and all the muscle fibers (cells) supplied by the neuron and its axion branches.

(ATPase) at a pH of 9.4. Red muscle **(type I fibers)** appears lightly stained.

The overlap of muscle fibers that appear with staining gives the checkerboard appearance of muscle biopsy specimens and provides an equal distribution of fiber types throughout the muscle. This overlap also helps compensate for muscle fiber loss and fatigue of individual motor units during activity. In spite of this, some muscles contain proportionally more of one fiber type than another. The postural muscles have more type I fibers, allowing them the high resistance to fatigue that is necessary to maintain the same position for extended periods. The ocular muscles have more type II muscle fibers, allowing them to respond rapidly to visual changes. (Table 40-5 describes the specific characteristics of type I and type II fibers.)

The number of muscle fibers varies according to location. Large muscles, such as the gastrocnemius, have more fibers (1,200,000) than the smaller muscles, such as the lumbrical muscles in the hand (10,000). The diameter of muscle fibers also varies. The closely packed polygons are small (10 to 20 μm) until puberty, when they attain the normal adult diameter of 40 to 80 μm. Women usually have smaller-diameter fibers than men. Small muscles, such as the ocular muscles, are 15 μm in diameter; larger, more proximal muscles are 40 μm. Fiber size can have functional significance. Studies have shown that larger fiber diameter is associated with generation of greater forces. Fiber diameter can be increased by activities that cause hypertrophied muscle, such as exercise or occupational overuse.

The major components of the muscle fiber include the muscle membrane, myofibrils, sarcotubular system, sarcoplasm, and mitochondria (see Fig. 40-16). The **muscle membrane** is a two-part membrane. It includes the **sarcolemma,** which contains the plasma membrane of the muscle cell, and the cell's **basement membrane.** The sarcolemma is 7.5 nm thick and is capable of propagating electrical impulses to initiate contraction. At the motor nerve end-plate, where the nerve impulse is transmitted, the sarcolemma forms the highly convoluted synaptic cleft. The sarcolemma is made up of lipid molecules and protein systems. The protein systems perform special functions, such as transport of nutrients and protein synthesis. They also provide the sodium-potassium pump and include the cell's cholinergic receptor. The basement membrane is 50 nm thick and is composed primarily of proteins and polysaccharides. It serves as the cell's microskeleton and maintains the shape of the muscle cell. The basement membrane also may function in some way to restict further diffusion of electrolytes once they have crossed the sarcolemma.

The **sarcoplasm** is the cytoplasm of the muscle cell and contains the intracellular components that are common to all cells (see Chapter 1). The sarcoplasm is an aqueous substance that provides a matrix that surrounds the myofibrils. It contains numerous enzymes and proteins that are responsible for the cell's energy production, protein synthesis, and oxygen storage. The mitochondria house enzyme systems for energy production, particularly those that regulate such processes as the citric acid cycle and adenosine triphosphate (ATP) formation. Many other structures are present in the sarcoplasm. The ribosomes are composed primarily of ribonucleic acid (RNA) and participate in the process of protein synthesis. The cell nucleus, satellite cells, glycogen granules, and lipid droplets are suspended in the sarcoplasmic matrix. Blood vessels, nerve endings, muscle spindles, and Golgi tendon organs are also directly located within this structure.

Unique to the muscle is the **sarcotubular system,** a network that includes the transverse tubules and the sarcoplasmic reticulum, which crosses the interior of the cell. The **sarcoplasmic reticulum** is made in the same manner as the endoplasmic reticulum in other cells. In the muscle

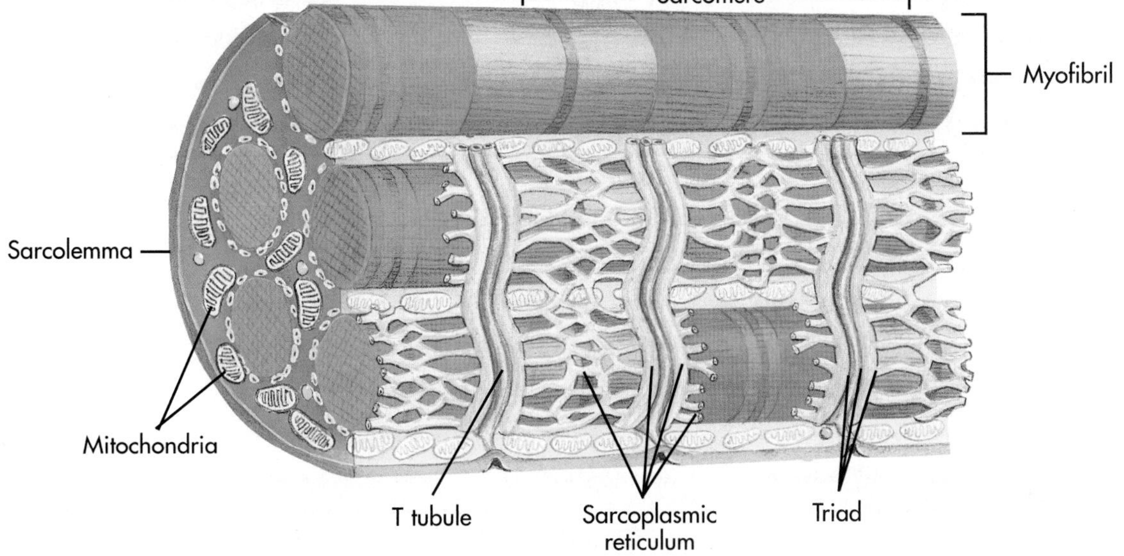

FIG. 40-16 Myofibrils of a skeletal muscle fiber (cell) and overall organization of skeletal muscle. (From Thibodeau GA, Patton KT: *Anatomy and physiology,* ed 4, St Louis, 1999, Mosby.)

cells the sarcoplasmic reticulum is involved in calcium transport, which initiates muscle contraction at the **sarcomere,** a portion of the myofibril. The sarcoplasmic reticulum is composed of tubules that run parallel to the myofibrils. The longitudinal tubules are termed **sarcotubules.** The **transverse tubules,** which are closely associated with the sarcotubules, run across the sarcoplasm and communicate with the extracellular space. Together, the tubules of this membrane system allow for intracellular calcium uptake, regulation, release during muscle contraction, and storage of calcium during muscle relaxation.

Myofibrils. The myofibrils are the functional units of muscle contraction. Each myofibril contains sarcomeres, which appear at intervals (see Fig. 40-16). The sarcomeres are composed of two contractile proteins, **actin** and **myosin.**

The myofibrils are the most abundant subcellular muscle component, equaling 85% to 90% of the total volume. On cross section they are irregular polygons with a mean diameter of less than 1 μm. Each myofibril is composed of serially repeating sarcomeres, separated by Z lines, which give the muscle its striped, cross-striated appearance. Each sarcomere has a dark A band and is flanked by two light I bands (Fig. 40-17). The A band is 1.5 to 1.6 μm long and contains thick myosin filaments. Included in the A band is a lighter zone called the H band, and in the center of the H band is the dark M band, or M line. The I band, which contains actin, is divided at the midpoint of each sarcomere by the Z line. Its length varies with the start of muscle contraction.

Myofibrils are composed of myofilaments. Each myofilament is structured in a closely packed hexagonal arrange-

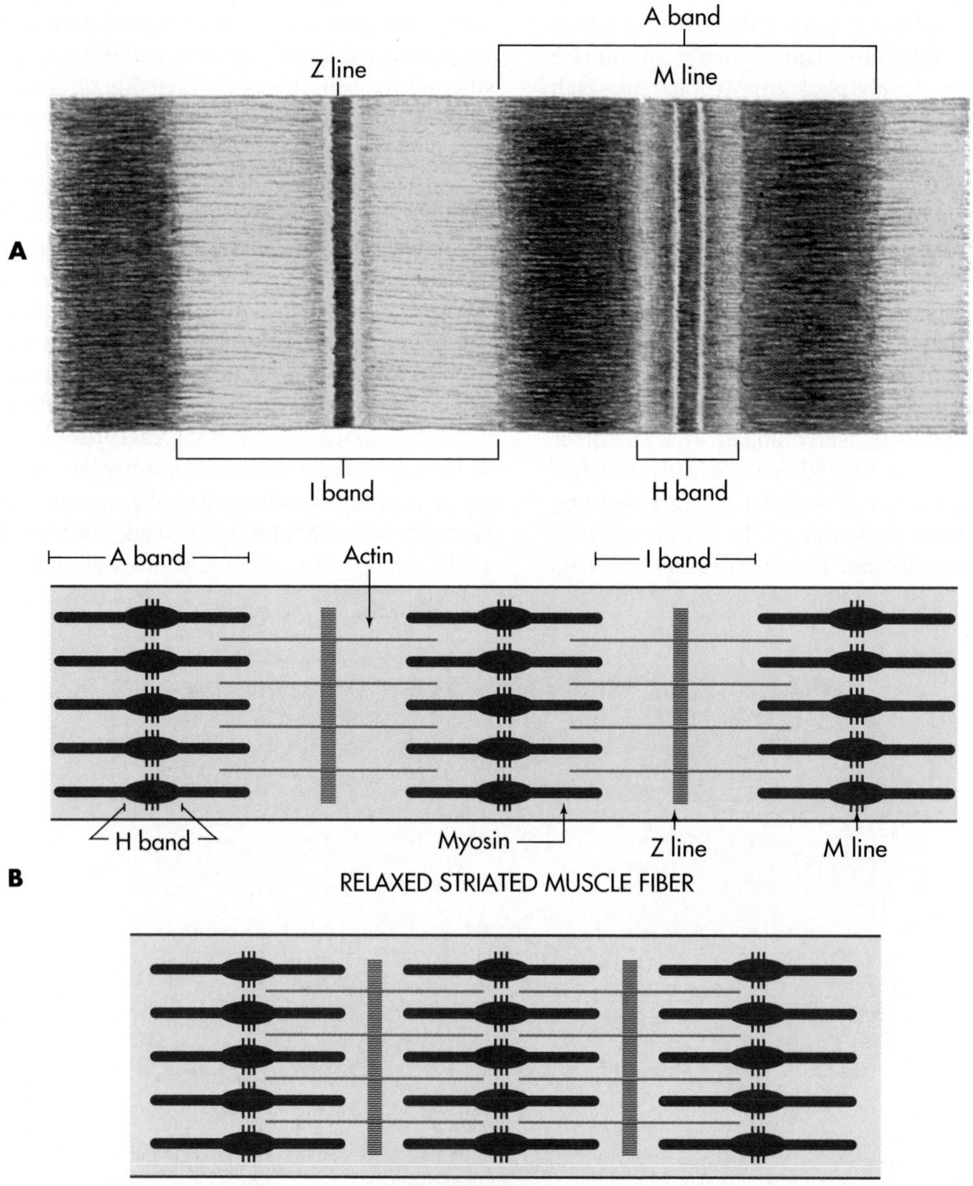

FIG. 40-17 Muscle fibers. A, Lines and bands in striated muscle. **B,** Relationships of bands, actin, myosin, and lines in relaxed and contracted muscle fibers. (Modified from Thompson JM et al: *Mosby's clinical nursing,* ed 3, St Louis, 1993, Mosby.)

ment, with two thin filaments for every thick filament. The thick filament, along with C protein and M line protein, is made up of myosin. Myosin has two subunits, heavy and light meromyosin, which resemble twisted golf club shafts. The thin filaments are twisted double strands made up of actin, troponin, and tropomyosin (see Chapter 28 and Fig. 28-16).

Muscle proteins. At present, 12 proteins have been identified in the muscle fibers.[4] (Table 40-6 outlines their distribution, location, and possible functional significance.) The contractile and regulatory functions of actin, myosin, and the troponin-tropomyosin complex (associated with actin) are the most commonly known. They also account for most of the protein found in the myofibril. The structural and regulatory processes of muscle proteins are less well understood. Alpha actin and beta actin are known to link the filaments. M protein contains the enzyme creatine kinase (CK). Creatine is released when muscle cells are damaged, making serum creatine an important test of pathologic conditions of muscles.

The most abundant proteins, actin and myosin, are also found in other cells, particularly motile cells such as platelets. The complete amino acid sequences of both actin and myosin have been identified. Noteworthy is the presence of the amino 3-methylhistidine, which is found only in the thin filament, actin. Eight-five to ninety percent of 3-methylhistidine is found in skeletal muscle. Because it is excreted unchanged (in the urine) after release from muscle and other tissue, 3-methylhistidine has been used to gauge muscle protein degradation. The amino acids lysine and histidine, in addition to leucine, have been used to study protein synthesis by means of stable isotope infusion and muscle biopsy analysis.

Nonprotein constituents of muscle. Substances such as nitrogen, creatine, creatinine, phosphocreatine, purines, uric acid, and amino acids all serve in the complex process of muscle metabolism. Glycogen and its derivatives are present as energy sources.

Creatine and creatinine metabolism have been used to measure muscle mass. Plasma creatine is taken up by muscle and converted into the high-energy phosphate compound *phosphocreatine* by the enzyme *creatine kinase.* Creatinine is formed in muscle from creatine at a constant rate of 2% per day. (Tests for plasma creatine are discussed in Chapter 34.) Creatine excretion is increased in muscle wasting. This change reflects the reduction in total body creatine stores and loss of muscle mass.

Inorganic compounds, anions (phosphate, chloride), and cations (calcium, magnesium, sodium, potassium) are important in the regulation of protein synthesis, muscle contraction, enzyme systems, and membrane stabilization. Total body potassium (TBK), measured by the K_{40} method, has been used to measure muscle mass, also called *lean body mass.* TBK levels reflect changes in muscle mass seen during growth, malnutrition, and muscle wasting.

Components of Muscle Function

The ultimate function of muscle is to accomplish work. Although variously expressed in such measures as foot-pounds or kilogram-meters, work usually refers to the amount of energy liberated or force exerted over a distance (work = force × distance). Muscles usually contract or tense while doing work. Muscle contraction occurs on the molecular

Table 40-6 Contractile Proteins of Skeletal Muscle Fibrils

Name	Approximate Percentage of Myofibrillar Protein	Location	Function
Myosin	55	A band (thick filament)	Contraction; hydrolyzes ATP and develops tension
Actin	20	I band (thin filament)	Contraction; activates myosin ATPase and interacts with myosin
Troponin	7	Thin filament	Regulatory protein; in presence of Ca^{++}, promotes actin-myosin activation
Tropomyosin	5-7	Thin filament	Regulatory and structural function; links filaments, controls filament length
Alpha (α) actin	10	Z band	Regulatory and structural function; links filaments, controls filament length
Beta (β) actin	2	Z band	Regulatory and structural function; links filaments, controls filament length
M protein	2	M line (center of thick filaments)	Regulatory and structural function; provides enzyme creatine kinase
C protein	2	A band (thick filaments)	Possible structural role
*Titin	Unknown	Z line (thick filament)	Interconnects thin filaments in Z line
Creatine kinase	Unknown	M line	Catalyzes the phosphorylation of ADP to form ATP
*Desmin	Unknown	Z line	Interconnects thin filaments in Z line
*Filamin	Unknown	Z line	Interconnects thin filaments in Z line
*Zeumatin	Unknown	Z line	Interconnects thin filaments in Z line

From Simon SR, editor: *Orthopaedic basic science,* Chicago, 1994, American Academy of Orthopaedic Surgeons.
ATP, Adenosine triphosphate; *ATPase,* adenosine triphosphatase; *ADP,* adenosine diphosphate.

level and leads to the observable phenomenon of muscle movement.

Muscle Contraction at the Molecular Level

Muscle contraction is a four-step process that includes excitation, coupling, contraction, and relaxation. The process involves the electrical properties of all cells and the movement of ions across the plasma membrane (see Chapter 1). The muscle fiber is an excitable tissue. At rest an electric charge of -90 mV is continually maintained across the sarcolemma. This resting potential, generated by the separation of positive and negative charges on either side of the membrane, creates an electrochemical equilibrium caused by the selective permeability of the sarcolemma to electrolytes in the intracellular and extracellular fluids, particularly potassium and sodium.

Excitation, the first step of muscle contraction, begins with the spread of an action potential from the nerve terminal to the neuromuscular junction. The rapid depolarization of the membrane initiates an electrical impulse in the muscle fiber membrane called the **muscle fiber action potential.** As the action potential advances along the sarcolemmal membrane, it spreads to the transverse tubules. (The velocity of conduction is much slower in muscle fibers than in myelinated nerve fibers—only 3 to 5 m/sec compared with 54 to 90 m/sec in nerve fibers.)

The second stage, **coupling,** follows the depolarization of the transverse tubules. This stage consists of the migration of calcium ions, which are stored in the sarcoplasmic reticulum, to the myofilaments. Calcium affects troponin and tropomyosin, muscle proteins that bind with actin when the muscle is at rest. In the presence of calcium, however, both of these proteins are attracted to calcium ions, leaving the actin free to bind with myosin.

Contraction begins as the calcium ions combine with troponin, a reaction that overcomes the inhibitory function of the troponin-tropomyosin system. The thin filament *actin* then slides toward the thick filament, myosin. The two ends of the myofibril shorten after contraction when the myosin heads attach to the actin molecules, forming a cross-bridge that constitutes an actin-myosin complex. ATP, located on the actin-myosin complex, is released when the cross-bridges attach. This is the **sliding filament theory** described by A.F. Huxley in the 1950s, but it is now called the *cross-bridge theory* because of the formation of the actin-myosin cross-bridges, or the process of contraction.[4] The process is so named because the actin actually slides onto the myosin, causing the sarcomere to shorten. The useful distance of contraction of a skeletal muscle is approximately 25% to 35% of the muscle's length.

The last step, **relaxation,** begins as the sarcoplasmic reticulum absorbs the calcium molecules, removing them from interaction with troponin. Calcium is pumped back into the sarcoplasmic reticulum by means of an active transport process. The cross-bridges detach, and the sarcomere lengthens. (The cross-bridge theory of muscle contraction is discussed in Chapter 28.)

Muscle Metabolism

Skeletal muscle requires a constant supply of ATP and phosphocreatine. These substances are necessary to fuel the complex processes of muscle contraction, driving the cross-bridges of actin and myosin together and transporting calcium from the sarcoplasmic reticulum to the myofibril. Other internal processes of the muscular system that require ATP include protein synthesis, which replenishes muscle constituents and accommodates growth and repair. The rate of protein synthesis is related to hormone levels (particularly insulin), amino acid substrates, and overall nutritional status. At rest the rate of ATP formation by oxidation of glucose or acetoacetate is sufficient to maintain internal processes, given normal nutritional status. During activity the need for ATP increases 100-fold. The metabolic pathways for muscle activity in Table 40-7 show reactions to the immediate need for increased ATP caused by contraction. Activity lasting longer than 5 seconds expends the available stored ATP and phosphocreatine.

Stored glycogen and blood glucose are converted anaerobically to sustain brief activity without increasing the demand for oxygen. Anaerobic glycolysis is much less efficient than aerobic glycolysis, using six to eight times more glycogen to produce the same amount of ATP. With increased activity, such as intense exercise, or ischemia, an increase in lactic acid occurs because of the breakdown of glycogen, thus causing a shift in muscle pH (see Table 40-7). This short-term mechanism "buys time" by allowing ATP

Table 40-7 Energy Sources for Muscular Activity

Sources	Reactions
Short-term (anaerobic) sources	Adenosine triphosphate (ATP) $\rightarrow$ Adenosine diphosphate (ADP) + Inorganic phosphate (P_I) + Energy
	Phosphocreatine + ADP $\rightleftharpoons$ Creatine + ATP
	Glycogen/glucose + P_I + ADP $\rightarrow$ Lactate + ATP
Long-term (aerobic) sources	Glycogen/glucose + ADP + P_I + $O_2 \rightarrow H_2O + CO_2$ + ATP
	Free fatty acids + ADP + P_I + $O_2 \rightarrow H_2O + CO_2$ + ATP
	Creatine kinase catalyzes the reversible reaction of ATP to ADP: Creatine phosphate + ADP $\overset{\text{Creatine kinase}}{\rightleftharpoons}$ Creatine + ATP

From Spence AP, Mason EE: *Human anatomy and physiology,* ed 4, St Paul, Minn, 1992, West Publishing Co.

formation in spite of inadequate energy stores or oxygen supply. When the anaerobic threshold is reached and more oxygen is required, physiologic changes occur, including an increase in lactic acid and increases in oxygen consumption, heart rate, respiratory rate, and muscle blood flow.

Strenuous exercise requires oxygen, which activates the aerobic glycogen pathway for ATP formation. During maximal exercise, free fatty acid mobilization and the aerobic glycogen pathways provide ATP over an extended time. These pathways require oxygen both to maintain maximal activity and to return the muscle to the resting state. Maximal exercise increases oxygen uptake 15 to 20 times over the resting state. When this system becomes exhausted or inadequate to respond to the need for ATP, fatigue and weakness finally force the muscle to reduce activity, with a resultant buildup of lactic acid in muscle fibers.

The ability to sustain maximal muscular activity leads to the accumulation of oxygen debt. **Oxygen debt** is the amount of oxygen needed to convert the buildup of lactic acid to glucose and replenish ATP and phosphocreatine stores.[2] For example, after running at maximal speed for 10 seconds, the average person has consumed 1 L of oxygen. At rest, oxygen consumption for the same period is approximately 40 ml. As the person recovers, the measured oxygen debt is 4 L greater than the amount used during activity.

Oxygen consumption is measured to calculate the metabolic cost of activity in normal and diseased muscle. It is an indirect measure of energy expenditure, along with timed tests of activity, heart rate, and respiratory quotient (ratio of carbon dioxide to expired oxygen consumed). Energy expenditure is measured directly by heat production because heat is released whenever work is accomplished.

Another factor that changes energy requirements is muscle fiber type. Type II fibers rely on anaerobic glycolytic metabolism and fatigue readily. Type I fibers can resist fatigue for longer periods because of their capacity for oxidative metabolism.

Muscle Mechanics

Muscle contraction cannot be viewed in isolation. Several factors determine how force is transmitted from the cross-bridges on individual muscle fibers to accomplish whole-muscle contraction. First, when a motor unit responds to a single nerve stimulus, it develops a phasic contraction, also called *twitch.* Because the motor unit contracts in an "all or nothing" manner, the contraction that is generated will be a maximal contraction. The central nervous system smoothly grades the force generated by "recruiting" additional motor units and varying the discharge frequency of each active motor unit. This adding of motor units within the muscle is called **repetitive discharge.**

Recruitment and repetitive discharge of motor units allow the muscle to activate the number of motor units needed to generate the desired force. The total force developed is the sum of the force generated by each motor unit. As the strength, speed, and duration of stimuli increase, the summation of contractions reaches a critical frequency called **tetanus.** When tetanus is reached, no further increase in force can be achieved.

Other variables, such as fiber type, innervation ratio, muscle temperature, and muscle shape, influence the efficiency of muscular contraction. The two muscle fiber types differ in their responses to electrical activity. Tetanus and duration of phasic contractions, which take microseconds to accomplish, are achieved more rapidly in type II than in type I muscle fibers. Low innervation ratios promote control and coordination, whereas high ratios promote strength and endurance. Muscles work best at normal body temperature, 98.6° F (37° C). Finally, muscles with a large cross-sectional area, such as the fan-shaped pennate muscles, develop greater contractile forces than smaller-diameter muscles. The initial length of a muscle and the range of shortening that occurs when the muscle contracts also determine the forces it can generate. The long fusiform muscles have a greater range of shortening and can contract up to 57% of their resting length. A certain amount of elongation is necessary to generate sufficient tension and muscular force. The elongation that occurs during the swing of a golf club or tennis racquet is an example of how stretch improves contractile force.

Types of Muscle Contraction

During **isometric contraction (static or holding contraction),** the muscle maintains constant length as tension is increased. Isometric contraction occurs, for example, when the arm or leg is pushed against an immovable object. The muscle contracts, but the limb does not move.

During **isotonic contraction** the muscle maintains a constant tension as it moves. Isotonic contractions can be **eccentric (lengthening)** or **concentric (shortening).** Positive work is accomplished during concentric contraction, and energy is released to exert force or lift a weight. In contrast, during an eccentric contraction the muscle lengthens and absorbs energy. Negative work is accomplished on the muscle by the load. Eccentric contraction requires less energy to accomplish and has been said to result in the development of pain and stiffness after unaccustomed exercise.

Movement of Muscle Groups

Muscles do not act alone but in groups, often under automatic control. When a muscle contracts and acts as a "prime mover," or **agonist,** its reciprocal muscle, or **antagonist,** relaxes. This is easily tested by holding the right arm in the horizontal position in front of the body and then bending the elbow while feeling the biceps in the front and the triceps in the back with the other hand. The biceps is firm, and the triceps is soft. As the arm is flexed, the muscles change. When the elbow is completely flexed, the biceps is soft and the triceps firm. Completing this movement causes the agonist and antagonist to change automatically; only the movement is commanded, not the alternate contraction and relaxation of the specific muscle groups.

Other associated actions may be seen during walking; as the foot leaves the ground, the paravertebral and gluteal muscles on the opposite sides of the body contract to maintain balance. One notices the loss of the associated muscle's action when paralysis offsets this process and decreases balance. If a person is paralyzed, difficulty in maintaining balance is noticeable.

TESTS OF MUSCULOSKELETAL FUNCTION

Tests of Bone Function

Diagnostic procedures to evaluate bone function include gait analysis, serum calcium and phosphorus, x-ray films, angiography, and bone scanning. Roentgenograms visualize bone structure, because bone absorbs x-ray beams better than soft tissue. Angiography is used to observe bone circulation. Bone scanning is the most frequently used procedure to evaluate bone function and can detect malignancy, trauma, necrosis, infection, metabolic bone disease, and osteoarthritis. Single- or dual-photon absorptiometry is often used to measure density of bones in the extremities (single-photon absorptiometry) and fracture risk of vertebral bodies and the femoral neck (dual-photon absorptiometry). Dual-photon absorptiometry allows the soft tissue component to be subtracted.

Tests of Joint Function

Procedures used to diagnose joint function include arthrography, arthroscopy, magnetic resonance imaging, and synovial fluid analysis. **Arthrography** (the injection of dye into the joint) is particularly useful to diagnose tears in the fibrocartilage of the knee (meniscus) and the rotator cuff of the shoulder. **Arthroscopy** is the direct visualization of a joint through an arthroscope. **Magnetic resonance imaging (MRI)** produces images of body tissues through the use of electromagnetic (radio) waves that alter the atoms (hydrogen ions) in the nuclei of cells being examined. When the radio waves are stopped, the nuclear atoms return to their original positions, emitting energy as signals as they move back. The signals produce visible images for examination and diagnosis. MRI produces excellent contrast of soft tissues for evaluation of musculoskeletal conditions.

Analysis of synovial fluid may reveal inflammatory, septic, and noninflammatory joint diseases, which cause characteristic changes in the color, clarity, viscosity, and cellular elements of the fluid. The presence of blood in the joint fluid (hemarthrosis) usually indicates joint trauma. Normal synovial fluid is sterile, so the presence of bacteria in the fluid always indicates disease. Cell fragments and fibrous tissue in the fluid are the result of inflammation or wear and tear on the articular surfaces.

Tests of Muscular Function

When the individual's history and physical examination disclose abnormalities, such as weakness, atrophy, muscle tenderness, cramps, and stiffness, specific tests of muscle function are in order. One of the most useful tests is the serum CK concentration. CK is found in large quantities in the muscle fibers, and when these are diseased or damaged, CK leaks into the serum. Myoglobin is also detectable in the urine after acute muscle damage caused by crush injury, ischemic disorders, extreme exertion, and some inherited diseases.

Because the muscle membrane tissue is excitable and carries an electrical charge, its capacity to function can be assessed by electromyography. Using sensitive needle electrodes, the **electromyogram (EMG)** records the summation of action potentials of the muscle fibers in each motor unit. The EMG is often compared with the electrocardiogram (ECG), but the activity recorded on the EMG is on a much smaller scale. The amplitude of the ECG is measured in volts, the duration of impulse is recorded in seconds, and both are recorded as the heart rate (e.g., 80 V/60 sec). On the EMG the amplitude is recorded in millivolts and the duration is measured in milliseconds, with a frequency of about 5 to 50 action potentials per second. The motor unit potentials are measured to determine rate of firing, duration, and amplitude. Abnormalities in EMG and nerve conduction velocities help differentiate muscle diseases (myopathy) from peripheral nerve (neuropathy) and neuromuscular junction disorders. The muscle biopsy (using histologic, histochemical, and electron microscopic studies) is used to further define the presence of myopathic and neuropathic disorders, many of which can be diagnosed only by muscle biopsy.

The forearm ischemic exercise test allows the clinician to determine the integrity of the glycolytic pathways and enzyme systems that function during intensive exercise. To perform this test, a catheter is placed in an antecubital vein and venous blood is collected for up to 20 minutes after intensive graded series of workloads at maximal grip strength. Any defects in the glycolytic pathway are expressed by a lack of lactate production, such as is seen in McArdle disease. Mitochondrial disorders are associated with excessive lactate production at two levels of exercise. The absence of ammonia, usually proportional to the rise in lactate, is seen in myoadenylate deaminase deficiency.

Although manual muscle testing of strength and range of motion is still the most common way to detect changes, myometers are becoming increasingly popular. These handheld devices measure strength of contraction in several muscle groups, namely, the neck flexors, shoulder abductors, wrist extensors, hip flexors, knee extensors, and foot dorsiflexors.

A new area of evaluation is genetics. Recent advances in molecular genetics, deoxyribonucleic acid (DNA) libraries, genetic probes, and gene localization techniques have enhanced our knowledge of neuromuscular diseases.

Aging and the Musculoskeletal System

Aging of Bones

Aging is accompanied by the loss of bone tissue. Bones become less stiff, less strong, and more brittle with aging. The bone remodeling cycle takes longer to complete, and the rate of mineralization also slows down. With aging, women experience loss of bone density, accelerated by rapid bone loss during early menopause from increased osteoclastic bone resorption.[8] By age 70, susceptible women have lost an average of 50% of their peripheral cortical bone mass. Bone mass losses to such an extent lead to deformity, pain, stiffness, and a high risk for fractures. Men experience bone loss also but at later ages and much slower rates than women. Also, initial bone masses in men are approximately 30% higher than in women; therefore bone loss in men causes less risk of disability than for women. Men's peak bone mass is related to their race, heredity, hormonal factors (testosterone and estradiol), physical activity, and calcium intake during childhood. Bone loss in both sexes is related to smoking, calcium deficiency, magnesium deficiency, vitamin D deficiency, high protein intake, excess phosphorus intake, overly vigorous exercise, certain prescription and over-the-counter drug use, alcohol intake, and physical inactivity.[9,10] Bone mass can be gained in healthy young women up to the third decade through physical activity, intake of dietary calcium, and magnesium. The use of oral contraceptives and gaining of bone mass is controversial. Height is also lost with aging because of increased spinal curvature.[3,11,12]

Aging of Joints

With aging, cartilage becomes more rigid, fragile, and susceptible to fibrillation because of more cross-linking of collagen and elastin, decreasing water content in the cartilage ground substance, and decreasing concentrations of glycosaminoglycans. Decreased range of motion of the joint is related to the changes in ligaments and muscles. Bones in joints develop evidence of osteoporosis with fewer trabeculae and thinner, less dense bones, making them prone to fractures. Intervertebral disk spaces decrease in height.[3,11]

Aging of Muscles

The function of skeletal muscle depends on many factors that are affected by aging, including the nervous, vascular, and endocrine systems. In the young child the development of muscle tissue is highly dependent on continuing neurodevelopmental maturation. Muscle fiber composition in adults does not change until late in life, but the variation among individuals increases with age.[13] Muscle function remains trainable even into advanced age.[14] Muscle diseases have a definite association with specific age-groups. Muscular dystrophies occur in children, and muscle disabilities related to rheumatic diseases usually occur in advancing age.

Age-related loss in skeletal muscle is referred to as **sarcopenia** and is a direct cause of the age-related decrease in muscle strength. As the body ages, muscle bulk and strength decline slowly; thus strength is maintained into the fifties, with a slow decline in dynamic and isometric strength evident after age 70. Type II fibers also decrease. There is reduced RNA synthesis, loss of mitochondrial volume, and reduction in the size of motor units. The regenerative function of muscle tissue remains normal in aging persons. As much as 30% to 40% of skeletal muscle mass and strength may be lost from the third to ninth decades.[15]

The maximal oxygen intake decreases with age. Reduced basal metabolic rate and decreased lean body mass are also seen in the elderly population. However, strength training can reduce sarcopenia in older women.[15]

SUMMARY REVIEW

Structure and Function of Bones

1. Bones provide support and protection for the body's tissues and organs and are important sources of minerals and blood cells.
2. Bone formation begins with the production of an inorganic matrix by bone cells. Bone minerals crystallize in and around collagen fibers in the matrix, giving bone its characteristic hardness and strength.
3. Bone tissue is continuously being resorbed and synthesized by bone-remodeling units of osteoclasts and osteoblasts.
4. Bones in the body are made up of compact bone tissue and spongy bone tissue. Compact bone is highly organized into haversian systems that consist of concentric layers of crystallized matrix surrounding a central canal that contains blood vessels and nerves. Dispersed throughout the concentric layers of crystallized matrix are small spaces containing osteocytes. Smaller canals, called *canaliculi,* interconnect the osteocyte-containing spaces. The crystallized matrix in spongy bone is arranged in bars or plates. Spaces containing osteocytes are dispersed between the bars or plates and interconnected by canaliculi.
5. There are 206 bones in the body, divided into the axial skeleton and the appendicular skeleton. Bones are classified by shape as long, short, flat, or irregular. Long bones have a broad end (epiphysis), broad neck (metaphysis), and narrow midportion (diaphysis) that contains the medullary cavity.
6. Bone injuries are repaired in stages. Hematoma formation provides the fibrin framework for formation and organization of granulation tissue. The granulation tissue provides a cartilage model for the formation and crystallization of bone matrix. Remodeling restores the original shape and size to the injured bone.

Structure and Function of Joints

1. A joint is the site where two or more bones attach. Joints provide stability and mobility to the skeleton.
2. Joints are classified as synarthroses, amphiarthroses, or diarthroses, depending on the degree of movement they allow. Joints are classified also by the type of connecting tissue holding them together. Fibrous joints are connected by dense fibrous tissue, ligaments, or membranes. Cartilaginous joints are connected by fibrocartilage or hyaline cartilage. Synovial joints are connected by a fibrous joint capsule. Within the capsule is a small, fluid-filled space. The fluid in the space nourishes the articular cartilage that covers the ends of the bones meeting in the synovial joint.

3. Articular cartilage is a highly organized system of collagen fibers and proteoglycans. The fibers firmly anchor the cartilage to the bone, and the proteoglycans control the loss of fluid from the cartilage.
4. Joints help move bones and muscle.

Structure and Function of Skeletal Muscles

1. Skeletal muscle is the largest organ in the body and is made up of millions of individual fibers.
2. Whole muscles vary in size (2 to 60 cm) and shape (fusiform and pennate). They are encased in a three-part connective tissue framework. The fundamental concept of muscle function is the *motor unit,* defined as all muscle fibers innervated by a single motor nerve.
3. Muscle fibers contain bundles of myofibrils arranged in parallel along the longitudinal axis and include the muscle membrane, myofibrils, sarcotubular system, aqueous sarcoplasm, and mitochondria. There are two types of muscle fibers, type I and type II, determined by motor nerve innervation.
4. Myofibrils and myofilaments contain the major muscle proteins, actin and myosin, which interact to form crossbridges during muscle contraction. The nonprotein muscle constituents provide an energy source for contraction and regulate protein synthesis, enzyme systems, and membrane stabilization.
5. Muscle contraction includes excitation, coupling, contraction, and relaxation.
6. Muscle strength is graded by the "all or nothing" phenomenon and recruitment. Speed of contraction is affected by several factors: muscle fiber type, temperature, stretch, and weight of the load.
7. The two types of muscle contraction are isometric and isotonic. Muscle shortening occurs during contraction but can be seen also during pathologic and physiologic contracture.
8. Skeletal muscle requires a constant supply of adenosine triphosphate (ATP) and phosphocreatine to fuel muscle contraction and for growth and repair. ATP and phosphocreatine can be generated aerobically or anaerobically.

Tests of Musculoskeletal Function

1. Various diagnostic procedures are used to evaluate bone function, including gait analysis, serum calcium and phosphorus, x-ray films, angiography, bone scanning, and magnetic resonance imaging.
2. Procedures used to evaluate joint function include arthrography, arthroscopy, magnetic resonance imaging, and synovial fluid analysis.
3. Tests of muscular function include physical examination, serum creatine kinase, myoglobin, electromyogram, muscle biopsy, myometers, and the forearm ischemic exercise test.

Aging and the Musculoskeletal System

1. Muscle bulk and strength slowly decline with aging, although not to a pathologic degree. Age should not be a deterrent to developing an exercise program in older and elderly persons.

KEY TERMS

Actin, *1356*
Agonist, *1359*
Amphiarthrosis (slightly movable joint), *1346*
Antagonist, *1359*
Appendicular skeleton, *1343*
Arthrography, *1360*
Arthroscopy, *1360*
Articular cartilage, *1349*
Axial skeleton, *1343*
Basement membrane, *1355*
Bone albumin, *1341*
Bone fluid, *1341*
Bone matrix, *1338*
Bone morphogenic protein (BMP), *1341*
Bone-remodeling unit, *1345*
Calcification, *1338*
Canaliculus, *1342*
Chondrocyte, *1349*
Collagen fiber, *1341*
Compact bone (cortical bone), *1342*
Concentric (shortening) contraction, *1359*
Contraction, *1358*
Coupling, *1358*
Diaphysis, *1344*
Diarthrosis (freely movable joint), *1346*
Eccentric (lengthening) contraction, *1359*
Electromyogram (EMG), *1360*
Endomysium, *1352*
Endosteum, *1344*
Epimysium, *1352*
Epiphyseal plate (growth plate), *1344*
Epiphysis, *1344*
Excitation, *1358*
Fascia, *1352*
Fascicle, *1352*
Fibril, *1341*
Fibrous joint, *1346*
Flat bone, *1344*
Fusiform muscle, *1352*
Glycoprotein, *1341*
α-Glycoprotein, *1342*
Glycosaminoglycans, *1350*
Golgi tendon organ, *1354*
Gomphosis, *1348*
Ground substance, *1338*
Haversian canal, *1342*
Haversian system, *1342*
Hyaluronate, *1349*
Hydroxyapatite (HAP), *1342*
Integrin, *1341*
Intima, *1348*
Irregular bone, *1344*
Isometric contraction (static or holding contraction), *1359*
Isotonic contraction, *1359*
Joint (articulation), *1346*
Joint capsule (articular capsule), *1348*
Joint cavity (synovial cavity), *1349*
Lacuna, *1340*
Lamella, *1342*
Laminin, *1341*
Link protein, *1350*
Long bone, *1344*
Magnetic resonance imaging (MRI), *1360*
Metaphysis, *1344*
Motor unit, *1354*
Muscle cell, *1354*
Muscle fiber, *1354*
Muscle fiber action potential, *1358*
Muscle membrane, *1355*
Myoblast, *1354*
Myofibril, *1354*
Myosin, *1356*
Osteoblast, *1339*
Osteocalcin, *1341*
Osteoclast, *1339*
Osteocyte, *1339*
Osteoid, *1339*
Osteonectin, *1341*
Oxygen debt, *1359*
Pennate muscle, *1352*
Perimysium, *1352*
Periosteum, *1343*
Procallus, *1345*
Protein core, *1350*
Proteoglycan, *1341*

KEY TERMS—cont'd

Relaxation, *1358*
Remodeling, *1345*
Repetitive discharge, *1359*
Ruffled border, *1341*
Sarcolemma, *1355*
Sarcomere, *1356*
Sarcopenia, *1361*
Sarcoplasm, *1355*
Sarcoplasmic reticulum, *1355*
Sarcotubular system, *1355*
Sarcotubule, *1356*
Short bones (cuboidal bones), *1344*
Sialoprotein (osteopontin), *1341*
Skeletal (voluntary, striated, or extrafusal) muscle, *1352*
Sliding filament theory, *1358*
Spindle, *1354*
Spongy bone (cancellous bone), *1342*
Subintima, *1348*
Suture, *1346*
Symphysis, *1348*
Synarthrosis (immovable joint), *1346*
Synchondrosis, *1348*
Syndesmosis, *1346*
Synovial fluid, *1349*
Synovial joint, *1348*
Synovial membrane (synovium), *1348*
Tendon, *1352*
Tetanus, *1359*
Tidemark, *1350*
Trabecula, *1343*
Transverse tubule, *1356*
Type A synovial cell, *1349*
Type B synovial cell, *1349*
Type I fiber, *1355*
Type II fiber, *1354*
Woven bone (callus), *1345*

REFERENCES

1. Baron R: Anatomy and ultrastructure of bone. In Favus MJ, Christakos S, editors: *Primer on the metabolic bone diseases and disorders of mineral metabolism,* ed 4, Philadelphia, 1999, Lippincott Williams & Wilkins.
2. Seeley RR, Stephens TD, Tate P: *Anatomy and physiology,* ed 3, St Louis, 1995, Mosby.
3. Bouxsein ML, Myers ER, Hayes WC: Biomechanics of age-related fractures. In Marcus R, Feldman D, Kelsey J, editors: *Osteoporosis,* San Diego, 1996, Academic Press.
4. Buckwalter JA, Einhorn TA, Simon SR, editors: *Orthopaedic basic science,* Rosemont, Ill, 1999, American Academy of Orthopaedic Surgeons.
5. Kreamer WJ, Volek JS: Creatinine supplementation: its role in human perforance, *Clin Sports Med* 18(3):651, 1999.
6. Mankin HJ et al: Form and function of articular cartilage. In Simon SR, editor: *Orthopaedic basic science,* Chicago, 1994, American Academy of Orthopaedic Surgeons.
7. Ombregt L et al: Connective tissue. In Ombregt L et al, editors: *A system of orthopaedic medicine,* London, 1995, Saunders.
8. Demers C, Hamdy RC: Bone morphogenic proteins, *Sci Med* 6(6):8, 1999.
9. Greendale GA, Edelston S, Barrett-Conner E: Endogenous sex steroids and bone mass in older men: positive associations with serum estrogens and negative associations with androgens, *J Clin Invest* 100:1755, 1997.
10. Wasnich RD: Vertebral fracture epidemiology, *Bone* 3(suppl):179S, 1996.
11. Carter DR, vander Meulen CH, Beaupre GS: Skeletal development: mechanical consequences of growth, aging, and disease. In Marcus R, Feldman D, Kelsey J, editors: *Osteoporosis,* San Diego, 1996, Academic Press.
12. Reid IR: Menopause. In Favus MJ, Christakos S, editors: *Primer on the metabolic bone diseases and disorders of mineral metabolism,* ed 4, Philadelphia, 1999, Lippincott Williams & Wilkins.
13. Lind M: Growth factors: possible new clinical tools: a review, *Acta Orthop Scand* 67(4):407, 1996.
14. Simkin PA: The musculoskeletal system. In Klippel JH, Dieppe PA, editors: *Rheumatology,* ed 2, St Louis, 1998, Mosby.
15. Curl WW: Aging and exercise: are they compatible in women? *Clin Orthop* 372:156, 2000.

CHAPTER 41

Alterations of Musculoskeletal Function

CHRISTY L. CROWTHER • LEONA A. MOURAD

CHAPTER OUTLINE

Musculoskeletal injuries include fractures, dislocations, sprains, and strains. Fractures are the most serious. Alterations in bones, joints, and muscles may be caused by metabolic disorders, infections, inflammatory or noninflammatory diseases, or tumors.

MUSCULOSKELETAL INJURIES

Skeletal muscles can withstand many penetrating injuries without permanent loss of function. For example, studies of soldiers with severe combat injuries showed that muscle function was preserved after the removal of large portions of muscle tissue. Successful regeneration of skeletal muscle fibers depends primarily on the extent of injury, preservation of vascular supply (and source of nutrition), and the availability of terminal axons for reinnervation.

Skeletal Trauma

Fractures

A **fracture** is a break in the continuity of a bone. A break occurs when force is applied that exceeds the tensile or compressive strength of the bone. The incidence of fractures varies for individual bones according to age and gender. The highest incidence of fractures is in young males (between ages 15 and 24 years) and in adults 65 years of age and older. Fractures of healthy bones, particularly the tibia, clavicle, and lower humerus, tend to occur in young persons and to be the result of trauma. Fractures of the hands and feet are usually caused by accidents in the workplace. The incidence of fractures of the upper femur, upper humerus, vertebrae, and pelvis is highest in older or elderly adults and is often associated with osteoporosis (see p. 1373). There are more than 200,000 fractures of the hip yearly in the United States alone.[1]

Classification

Fractures can be classified as complete or incomplete and open or closed (Fig. 41-1). In a **complete fracture** the bone is broken all the way through, whereas in an **incomplete fracture** the bone is damaged but is still in one piece. Complete or incomplete fractures also can be classified as **open** (formerly referred to as *compound*) if the skin is broken or as **closed** (formerly called *simple*) if it is not. A fracture in which a bone breaks into two or more fragments is termed a **comminuted fracture.** Fractures are classified also according to the direction of the fracture line. A **linear fracture** runs parallel to the long axis of the bone. An **oblique fracture** is a slanted fracture of the shaft of the bone. A **spiral**

fracture encircles the bone, and a **transverse fracture** occurs straight across the bone.

Incomplete fractures tend to occur in the more flexible, growing bones of children. The three main types of incomplete fractures are greenstick, torus, and bowing. A **greenstick fracture** perforates one cortex and splinters the spongy bone. The name is derived from the damage sustained by a young tree branch (a green stick) when it is bent sharply. The outer surface is disrupted, but the inner surface remains intact. Greenstick fractures typically occur in the proximal metaphysis or diaphysis of the tibia, radius, and ulna. In a **torus fracture** the cortex buckles but does not break. **Bowing fractures** usually occur when longitudinal force is applied to bone. This type of fracture is common in children and usually involves the paired radius-ulna or fibula-tibia. A complete diaphyseal fracture occurs in one of the bones of the pair, which disperses the stress sufficiently to prevent a complete fracture of the second bone, which bows. A bowing fracture resists correction (reduction) because the force necessary to reduce it must be equal to the force that bowed it. Treatment of bowing fractures is difficult also because the bowed bone interferes with reduction of the fractured bone. Types of fractures are summarized in Table 41-1.

Fractures may be further classified by cause as pathologic, stress, or transchondral. A **pathologic fracture** is a break at the site of a preexisting abnormality, usually by force that would not fracture a normal bone. Any disease process that weakens a bone (especially the cortex) predisposes the bone to pathologic fracture, commonly associated with tumors, osteoporosis, infections, and metabolic bone disorders.

Stress fractures occur in normal or abnormal bone that is subjected to repeated stress, such as occurs during athletics. The stress is less than the stress that usually causes a fracture. Two types of stress fractures are **fatigue fractures,** caused by abnormal stress or torque applied to a bone with normal ability to deform and recover (e.g., joggers, dancers, military recruits), and **insufficiency fractures,** stress fractures that occur in bones lacking normal ability to deform and recover (i.e., normal weight-bearing or activity fractures the bone).

A **transchondral fracture** consists of fragmentation and separation of a portion of the articular cartilage that covers the end of a bone at a joint. (Joint structures are defined in Chapter 40.) The fragments may consist of cartilage alone or cartilage and bone. Typical sites of transchondral fracture are the distal femur, the ankle, the kneecap, the elbow, and the wrist. Transchondral fractures are most prevalent in adolescents.

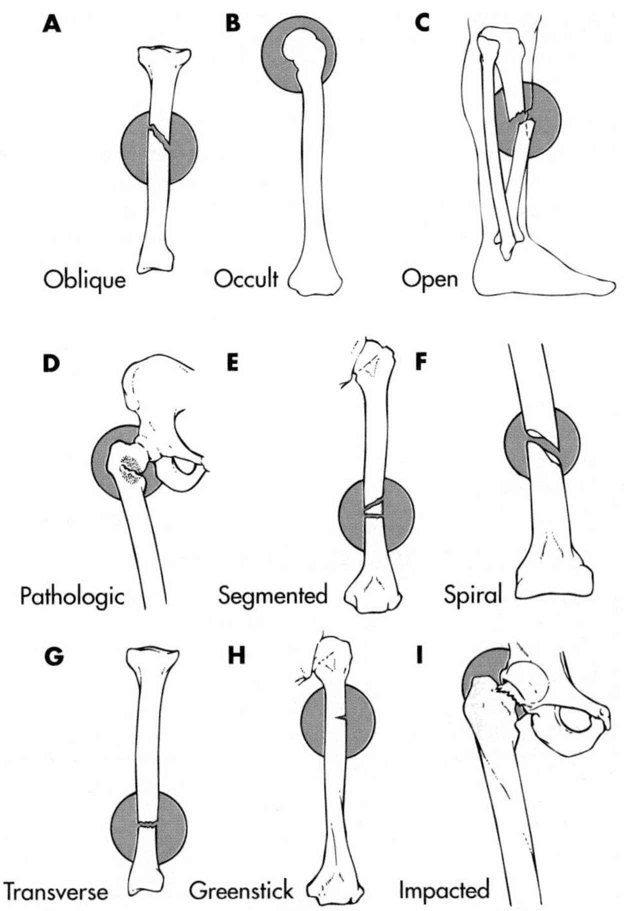

FIG. 41-1 Examples of types of bone fractures. A, Oblique: fracture at oblique angle across both cortices. *Cause:* direct or indirect energy, with angulation and some compression. **B,** Occult: fracture that is hidden or not readily discernible. *Cause:* minor force or energy. **C,** Open: skin broken over fracture; possible soft tissue trauma. *Cause:* moderate to severe energy that is continuous and exceeds tissue tolerances. **D,** Pathologic: transverse, oblique, or spiral fracture of bone weakened by tumor pressure or presence. *Cause:* minor energy or force, which may be direct or indirect. **E,** Segmented: fracture with two or more pieces or segments. *Cause:* direct or indirect moderate to severe force. **F,** Spiral: fracture that curves around cortices and may become displaced by twist. *Cause:* direct or indirect twisting energy or force with distal part held or unable to move. **G,** Transverse: horizontal break through bone. *Cause:* direct or indirect energy toward bone. **H,** Greenstick: break in only one cortex of bone. *Cause:* minor direct or indirect energy. **I,** Impacted: fracture with one end wedged into opposite end of inside fractured fragment. *Cause:* compressive axial energy or force directly to distal fragment. (Redrawn from Mourad L: Musculoskeletal system. In Thompson JM et al, editors: *Mosby's clinical nursing,* ed 6, St Louis, 1997, Mosby.)

Pathophysiology

When a bone is broken, the periosteum and blood vessels in the cortex, marrow, and surrounding soft tissues are disrupted. Bleeding occurs from the damaged ends of the bone and from the neighboring soft tissue. A clot (hematoma) forms within the medullary canal, between the fractured ends of the bone, and beneath the periosteum (Fig. 41-2). Bone tissue immediately adjacent to the fracture dies. This necrotic tissue (along with any debris in the fracture area) stimulates an intense inflammatory response characterized by vasodilation, exudation of plasma and leukocytes, and infiltration by inflammatory leukocytes and mast cells. Within 48 hours after the injury, vascular tissue invades the fracture area from surrounding soft tissue and the marrow cavity, and blood flow to the entire bone is increased. Bone-forming cells in the periosteum, endosteum, and marrow are activated to produce subperiosteal procallus along the outer surface of the shaft and over the broken ends of the bone (Fig. 41-3). Osteoblasts within the procallus synthesize collagen and matrix, which

Table 41-1 Types of Fractures

Type	Definition
TYPICAL COMPLETE FRACTURES	
Closed fracture	Noncommunicating wound between bone and skin
Open fracture	Communicating wound between bone and skin
Comminuted fracture	Multiple bone fragments
Linear fracture	Fracture line parallel to long axis of bone
Oblique fracture	Fracture line at 45-degree angle to long axis of bone
Spiral fracture	Fracture line encircling bone (as a spiral staircase)
Transverse fracture	Fracture line perpendicular to long axis of bone
Impacted	Fracture fragments are pushed into each other
Pathologic	Fracture occurs at a point in the bone weakened by disease, for example, with tumors or osteoporosis
Avulsion	A fragment of bone connected to a ligament or tendon breaks off from the main bone
Compression	Fracture is wedged or squeezed together on one side of bone
Displaced	Fracture with one, both, or all fragments out of normal alignment
Extracapsular	Fragment is close to the joint but remains outside the joint capsule
Intracapsular	Fragment is within the joint capsule
TYPICAL INCOMPLETE FRACTURES	
Greenstick fracture	Break on one cortex of bone with splintering of inner bone surface, commonly occurs in children and elderly persons
Torus fracture	Buckling of cortex
Bowing fracture	Bending of the bone
Stress fracture	Microfracture
Transchondral fracture	Separation of cartilaginous joint surface (articular cartilage) from main shaft of bone

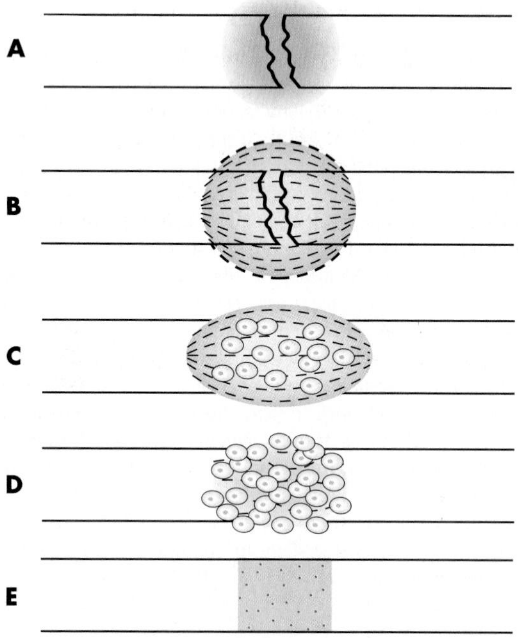

FIG. 41-2 Bone healing (schematic representation). A, Bleeding at broken ends of the bone with subsequent hematoma formation. **B,** Organization of hematoma into fibrous network. **C,** Invasion of osteoblasts, lengthening of collagen strands, and deposition of calcium. **D,** Callus formation; new bone is built up as osteoclasts destroy dead bone. **E,** Remodeling is accomplished as excess callus is resorbed and trabecular bone is laid down. (From Phipps WJ et al: *Medical-surgical nursing: concepts and clinical practice,* ed 6, St Louis, 1999, Mosby.)

becomes mineralized to form callus. As the repair process continues, remodeling occurs, during which unnecessary callus is resorbed and trabeculae are formed along lines of stress. Except for the liver, bone is unique among all body tissues in that it will form new bone, not scar tissue, when it heals after a fracture.

◆ *Clinical Manifestations*

The clinical manifestations of a fracture vary according to the type of fracture, site of the fracture, and associated soft tissue injury. In general, the signs and symptoms of a fracture include impaired function, unnatural alignment (deformity), swelling, muscle spasm, tenderness, pain, and impaired sensation. The position of the bone segments is determined by the pull of attached muscles, gravity, and the direction and magnitude of the force that caused the fracture. One or both segments may be rotated inward or outward on the bone's long axis (rotation), be misaligned at an angle (angulation), slide over the other segment (overriding), or be out of normal position (displaced).

The immediate pain of a fracture is severe and usually caused by the trauma. Subsequent pain may be produced by muscle spasm, overriding of the fracture segments, or damage to adjacent soft tissues. Numbness is common and is caused by swelling, by the pinching or severing of a nerve, by the trauma, or by bone fragments. Pathologic fractures usually cause angular deformity, painless swelling, or generalized bone pain. Pathologic fractures are not usually associated with trauma or trauma-related pain. Stress fractures are painful,

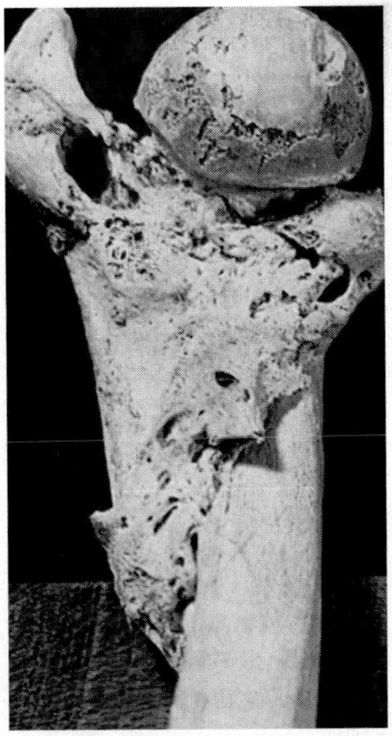

FIG. 41-3 Exuberant callus formation following fracture. (From Rosai J: *Ackerman's surgical pathology,* ed 8, St Louis, 1996, Mosby.)

not because of trauma, but because of accelerated remodeling. The pain occurs during activity and is usually relieved by rest. Stress fractures also cause local tenderness and soft tissue swelling. Transchondral fractures may be entirely asymptomatic or painful during movement. Range of motion in the joint is limited, and movement may evoke audible clicking sounds (crepitus).

Evaluation and Treatment

Treatment of a displaced fracture involves realigning the bone fragments (reduction) close to their normal or anatomic position and holding the fragments in place (immobilization) so that bone union can occur. Several methods are available to reduce a fracture: closed manipulation, traction, and open reduction. Many fractures heal without manipulation—they require only adequate immobilization. A fracture that is malaligned, however, requires more aggressive treatment.

Most fractures can be reduced by closed manipulation: the skin is not opened, and the bone is moved or manipulated into place. Closed manipulation is used when the contour of the bone is in fair alignment and can be maintained well with immobilization.

Traction is used to accomplish or maintain reduction. When bone fragments are displaced (not in their anatomic position), weights are used to apply firm, steady traction (pull) and countertraction to the long axis of the bone. Traction stretches and fatigues muscles that pull the bone fragments out of place, allowing the distal fragment to align with the proximal fragment. Traction can be applied to the skin (skin traction) (Fig. 41-4), directly to the involved bone, or distal to the involved bone (skeletal traction). Skin traction is used when only a few pounds of pulling force are needed to realign the fragments or when the traction will be used for brief times only, such as before surgery or, for children with femoral fractures, for 3 to 7 days before applying a cast. A traction boot is applied to the skin and is closed with self-adhering straps, with weights attached to the foot area of the traction boot. In skeletal traction, a pin or wire is drilled through the bone below the fracture site, and a traction bow, rope, and weights are attached to the pin or wire to apply tension and to provide the pulling force to overcome the muscle spasm and help realign the fracture fragments.

A

B

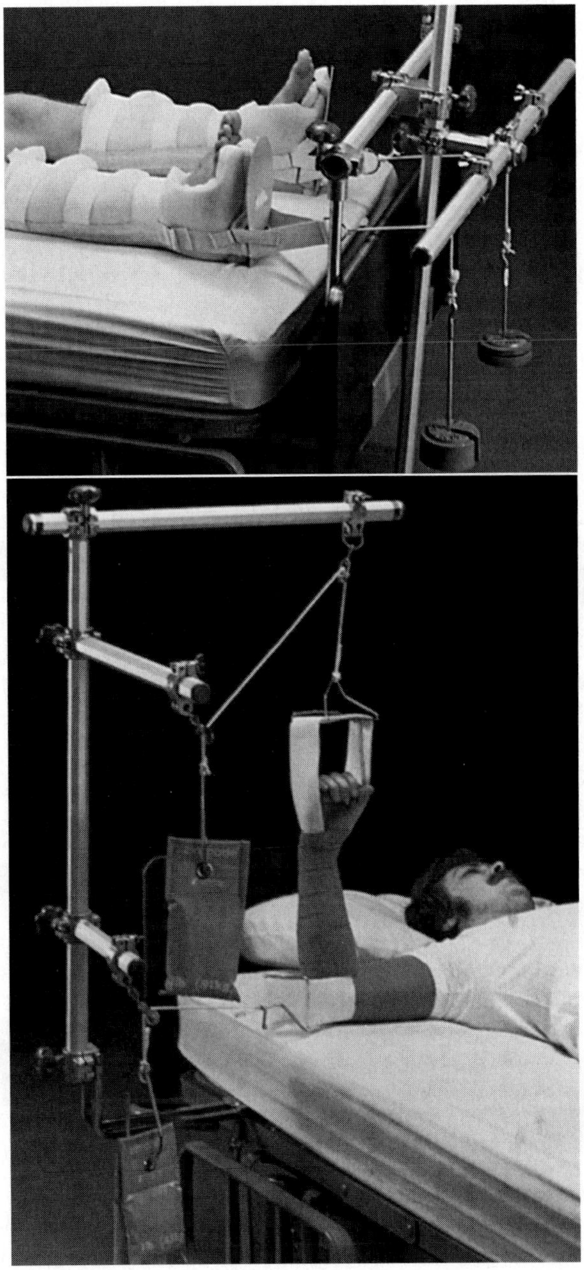

FIG. 41-4 Two types of skin traction. A, Buck extension traction. **B,** Dunlop traction. (From Mourad L: *Orthopedic disorders,* St Louis, 1991, Mosby.)

External fixation is used to reduce and immobilize open fractures. Pins are placed in the bone proximal and distal to

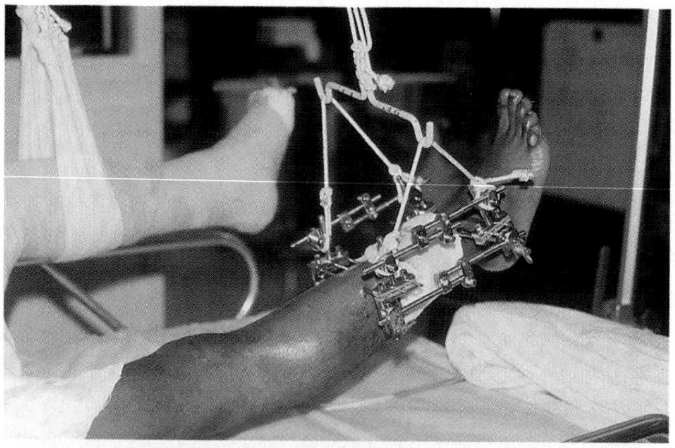

FIG. 41-5 Example of an external fixation device on the right leg. The left leg is in a splint.

the break and then stabilized by an external frame of clamps and rods (Fig. 41-5).

Open reduction is a surgical procedure that exposes the fracture site; the fragments are brought into alignment under direct visualization. Some form of prosthesis, screw, plate, nail, or wire usually is used to maintain the reduction (internal fixation).

Splints and plaster casts are used to immobilize and hold a reduction in place. Improper reduction or immobilization of a fractured bone may result in nonunion, delayed union, or malunion. **Nonunion** is failure of the bone ends to grow together (Fig. 41-6). The gap between the broken ends of the bone fills with dense fibrous and fibrocartilaginous tissue instead of new bone. Occasionally, the fibrous tissue contains a fluid-filled space that resembles a joint and is termed a *false joint,* or *pseudoarthrosis.* **Delayed union** is union that does not occur until approximately 8 to 9 months after a fracture. **Malunion** is the healing of a bone in a nonanatomic position.

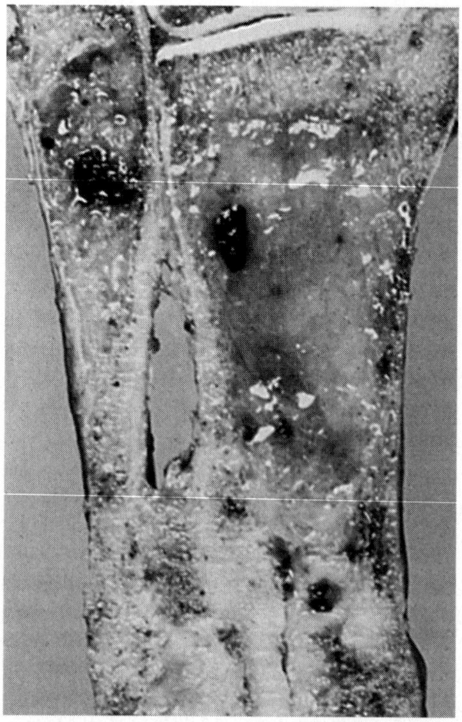

FIG. 41-6 Nonunion of old fracture of tibia and fibula in 53-year-old white man. Multiple fractures had occurred in 2 years previous and necessitated bone grafting. (From Rosai J: *Ackerman's surgical pathology,* ed 8, St Louis, 1996, Mosby.)

Dislocation and Subluxation

Dislocation and subluxation are usually caused by trauma. **Dislocation** is the temporary displacement of two bones in which the two bone surfaces lose contact entirely. If the contact between the two bone surfaces is only partially lost, the injury is called a **subluxation.**

Dislocation and subluxation are most common in persons younger than 20 years and are generally associated with fractures. Dislocation and subluxation, however, may result from congenital or acquired disorders that cause (1) muscular imbalance, as occurs with congenital dislocation of the hip or neurologic disorders; (2) incongruities in the articulating surfaces of the bones, as occurs with rheumatoid arthritis (see p. 1389); or (3) joint instability.

The joints most often dislocated or subluxed are the joints of the shoulder, elbow, wrist, finger, hip, and knee (Fig. 41-7). The shoulder's glenohumeral joint is a relatively unstable joint because the articular surface of the glenoid cavity is only one third as large as the surface of the humeral head. As a result, the glenohumeral joint is frequently injured.

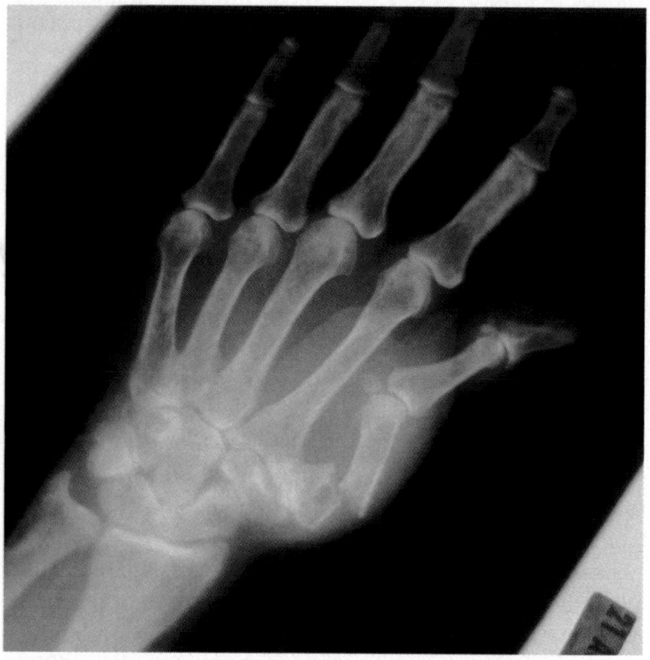

FIG. 41-7 Displaced fracture. X-ray showing a displaced fracture of the base of the first metacarpal, also known as a Bennett fracture.

Physical trauma to the shoulder can cause anterior, posterior, superior, or inferior dislocation. Anterior dislocation is the most common and is usually the result of an indirect force that places the shoulder in extreme external rotation.[2] Posterior dislocations usually occur as a result of trauma. A superior dislocation is rare and usually the result of an extreme forward and upward force on an adducted arm. Inferior displacement is frequently seen in persons with neurologic injuries of the brachial plexus and is believed to be caused by stretching of the supporting muscles or by joint effusion.

Traumatic dislocation of the elbow joint is common in the immature skeleton. In adults an elbow dislocation is usually associated with a fracture of the ulna or head of the radius. Posterior dislocations occur when the individual falls on an outstretched hand with the arm in extension. Anterior dislocations are usually the result of a direct blow to the flexed elbow.

Traumatic dislocation of the wrist usually involves the distal ulna and carpal bones. Any one of the eight carpal bones can be dislocated after an injury. The most common cause is a fall on the hyperextended hand.

Dislocation in the hand usually involves the metacarpophalangeal and interphalangeal joints. Dislocation of the metacarpophalangeal joint is the result of a fall on the outstretched hand that forces the joint into hyperextension. Dislocation of the interphalangeal joint occurs as a result of injury to the fingers in a hyperextended position.

Considerable trauma is needed to dislocate the hip. Anterior hip dislocation is rather rare and is caused by forced abduction, for example, when an individual lands on the feet from a high fall. Posterior dislocation of the hip can occur in an automobile accident in which the flexed knee strikes the dashboard.

The knee is an unstable joint that depends heavily on the soft tissue structures around it for support. Because the knee is an unstable weight-bearing joint exposed to many different types of motion (flexion, extension, rotation), it is one of the most frequently injured joints. A knee dislocation can be anterior, posterior, lateral, medial, or rotary. It is usually the result of a hyperextension injury that occurs during sports activities.

Pathophysiology

Dislocations and subluxations are often accompanied by fracture because stress is placed on areas of bone not normally subjected to stress. In addition, as the bone separates from the joint, it may bruise or tear adjacent nerves, blood vessels, ligaments, supporting structures, and soft tissue. Dislocation of the shoulder may damage the shoulder capsule and the axillary nerve. Damage to the axillary nerve causes anesthesia in the sensory distribution of the nerve and paralysis of the deltoid muscle. Elbow dislocations are accompanied by torn periosteum ligaments and muscle. Bleeding from the damaged periosteum and muscle puts pressure on adjacent arteries that shuts off circulation to and from the forearm and hand. If the pressure is not promptly relieved, ischemic paralysis develops. Dislocations of the hand often result in permanent disability because of damage to the tendons and intricate mechanisms that allow smooth gliding in the joints. Avascular necrosis of the femoral head is a complication seen in hip dislocations. Knee dislocation usually tears both the collateral and cruciate ligaments.

Clinical Manifestations

Signs and symptoms of dislocations or subluxations include pain, swelling, limitation of motion, and joint deformity. Pain may be caused by effusion of inflammatory exudate into the joint or associated tension and ligament injury. Joint deformity is usually caused by muscle contractions that exert pull on the dislocated or subluxated joint. Limitation of motion may be a result of effusion into the joint or the displacement of bones.

Tenderness and deformity are prominent in dislocations of the fingers. Unusual muscle pull and pain often result in abnormal posturing of the fingers; for example, the fingers or thumb may be abnormally flexed. A dislocated elbow is often held in a flexed position, and the joint resists active or passive movement. Pain is the key symptom of shoulder injuries. Attempts to lift the arm aggravate the pain. In most shoulder dislocations, the ability to elevate the arm is minimal and the individual supports the injured arm with the opposite hand. Pain and an abnormal gait or limp or inability to bear full weight usually accompany traumatic dislocation of the hip. The pain is constant and severe and is often felt in the inguinal region or thigh. The thigh and leg may assume a position of inward rotation, adduction, or flexion and appear shortened. In a rare anterior dislocation, the limb is not shortened and the joint is fixed in abduction, outward rotation, and flexion.

Evaluation and Treatment

Evaluation of dislocations and subluxations is based on clinical manifestations and roentgenograms. Treatment consists of reduction and immobilization for 2 to 6 weeks and exercises to maintain normal range of motion in the joint. Depending on the joint, healing is usually complete within months to years.

Support Structures

Sprains and Strains of Tendons and Ligaments

Tendon and ligament injuries can accompany fractures and dislocations. A tendon is fibrous connective tissue that attaches skeletal muscle to bone. A **ligament** is a band of fibrous connective tissue that connects bones where they meet at a joint. Tendons and ligaments support the bones and joints and either facilitate or limit motion. Tendons and ligaments can be torn, ruptured, or completely separated from bone at their points of attachment.

A tear in a tendon is commonly known as a **strain.** Major trauma can tear or rupture a tendon at any site in the body. Most frequently injured are the tendons of the hands and feet, the knee (patellar), the upper arm (biceps and triceps), the thigh (quadriceps), the ankle, and the heel (Achilles). Traumatic rupture of the biceps tendon is often caused by lifting excessive weight with the arms. Rupture of the Achilles tendon occurs when forced dorsiflexion is applied to the foot when it is in plantar flexion.[3] Spontaneous tendon ruptures can occur in individuals receiving local corticosteroid injections and persons with rheumatoid arthritis or systemic lupus erythematosus.

Ligament tears are commonly known as **sprains.** Ligament tears and ruptures can occur at any joint but are most common in the wrist, ankle, elbow, and knee joints. A complete separation of a tendon or ligament from its bony attachment site is known as an **avulsion.** An avulsion is the result of abnormal stress on the ligament or tendon and is commonly seen in young athletes, especially sprinters, hurdlers, and runners.

Strains and sprains are classified as first degree (least severe), second degree, and third degree (most severe).

Pathophysiology

When a tendon or ligament is torn, an inflammatory exudate develops between the torn ends. Later, granulation tissue containing macrophages, fibroblasts, and capillary buds grows inward from the surrounding soft tissue and cartilage to begin the repair process. Within 4 to 5 days after the injury, collagen formation begins. At first, collagen formation is random and disorganized. As the collagen fibers interweave and connect with preexisting tendon fibers, they become organized parallel to the lines of stress. Eventually vascular fibrous tissue fuses the new and surrounding tissues into a single mass. As reorganization takes place, the healing tendon or ligament separates from the surrounding soft tissue. Usually a healing tendon or ligament lacks sufficient strength to withstand strong pull for 4 to 5 weeks after the injury. If strong muscle pull does occur during this time, the tendon or ligament ends may separate again, which causes the tendon or ligament to heal in a lengthened shape with an excessive amount of scar tissue that renders the tendon or ligament functionless. Scar remodeling may take months to years before it is complete.[4]

Clinical Manifestations

Tendon and ligament injuries are painful and are usually accompanied by soft tissue swelling, changes in tendon or ligament contour, and dislocation or subluxation of bones. The pain is generally sharp and localized, and tenderness persists over the distribution of the tendon or ligament. Painful joint swelling can usually be seen in finger and elbow sprains. Flexion deformities of the fingers and thumb occur in injuries to the extensor tendons. Crepitus may accompany tendon injury in the wrist. Pain in the elbow may be accentuated by flexion, supination, and extension of the elbow or by extension of the wrist. Lifting small objects requires extension of the wrist and therefore aggravates the pain. Tendon injuries in the upper arm cause weakness when the individual tries to flex the forearm. Pain is often the key symptom of shoulder injuries. It may be referred to the deltoid muscle or extend down the arm. The pain is usually aggravated by attempts to lift the arms. Depending on the ligament or tendon involved, tendon and ligament injuries in the knee may produce pronounced mobility, lost lateral movement, instability when walking down stairs, semiflexion, crepitus, or an upward shift of the patella.

Evaluation and Treatment

Evaluation is based on clinical manifestations, stress radiography, arthroscopy, or arthrography. When possible, treatment consists of suturing the tendon or ligament ends in close approximation. If this is not possible because of the extent of damage, tendon or ligament grafting may be necessary. Prolonged rehabilitation exercises help ensure that the patient regains nearly normal functions.

Tendinitis and Bursitis

Trauma can also cause painful inflammation of tendons (tendinitis) and bursae (bursitis). Other causes of tendinitis include crystal deposits, postural misalignment, and hypermobility in a joint. Achilles tendinitis is inflammation of the Achilles tendon, one that is frequently inflamed.

Epicondylitis is inflammation of a tendon where it attaches to a bone (at its origin). Epicondylar areas of the humerus, radius, or ulna and the area around the knee are most frequently inflamed. **Lateral epicondylitis,** commonly called **tennis elbow,** is probably the result of irritation of the extensor carpi radialis brevis tendon at its origin.[5] **Medial epicondylitis,** referred to as **golfer's elbow,** is inflammation of the medial humeral epicondyle (Fig. 41-8).

Bursae are small sacs lined with synovial membrane and filled with synovial fluid; they are located between tendons, muscles, and bony prominences. Their primary function is to

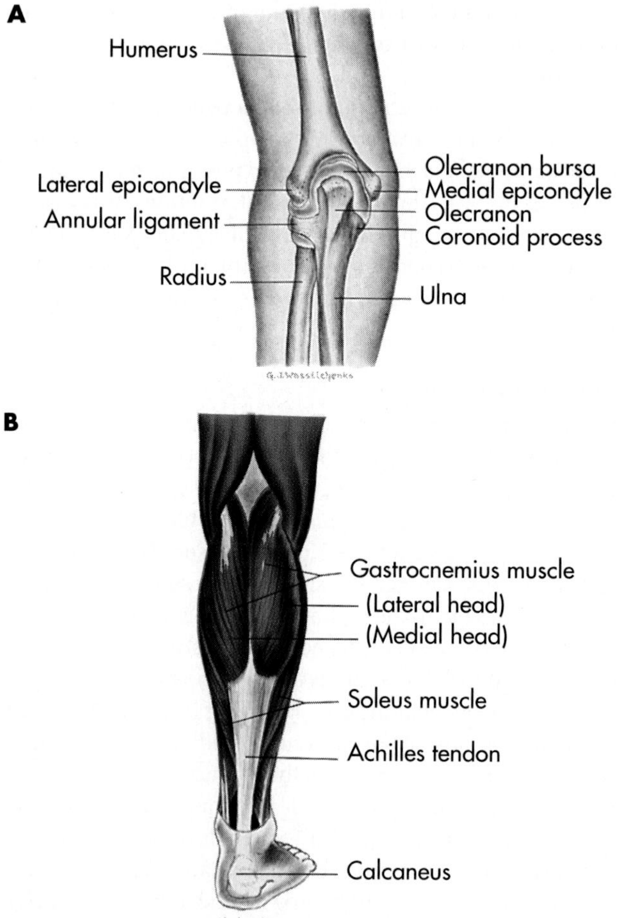

FIG. 41-8 Tendinitis and epicondylitis. A, Medial or lateral epicondyles of humerus, site of epicondylitis. **B,** Achilles tendon, site of frequently occurring tendinitis. (From Mourad L: *Orthopedic disorders,* St Louis, 1991, Mosby.)

separate, lubricate, and cushion these structures. Acute bursitis occurs primarily in the middle years and is caused by trauma. Chronic bursitis can result from repeated trauma.[6] Septic bursitis is caused by wound infection or bacterial infection of the skin overlying the bursae. Bursitis commonly occurs in the shoulder, hip, knee, and elbow.[7]

Pathophysiology

In tendinitis, fluid from inflammation accumulates, causing swelling of the tendon and its enclosing sheath. Inflammatory changes cause thickening of the sheath, which limits movements and causes pain. Microtears cause bleeding, edema, and pain in the involved tendon or tendons. At times, after repeated inflammations, calcium may be deposited in the tendon origin area, causing a calcific tendinitis.

The usual bursitis is an inflammation that is reactive to overuse or excessive pressure. The inflamed bursal sac becomes engorged, and the inflammation can spread to adjacent tissues (Fig. 41-9). The inflammation may decrease with rest, heat, and aspiration of the fluid. (Inflammation is discussed in Chapter 7.)

Clinical Manifestations

Clinical manifestations of tendinitis are usually localized to one side of the joint. Generally there is local pain and more pain with active motion than with passive motion. With tendinitis, the pain is localized over the involved tendon and movement in the affected joint is limited. The onset of pain may be gradual or sudden in bursitis, and movement in the joint is not mechanically limited. Shoulder bursitis impairs arm abduction because of pain. Bursitis in the knee produces pain when climbing stairs, and crossing the legs is painful in bursitis of the hip. Lying on the side of the inflamed trochanteric bursa is also very painful. Signs of infectious bursitis may include the presence of a puncture site, prior corticosteroid injection, severe inflammation, or an adjacent source of infection.[7]

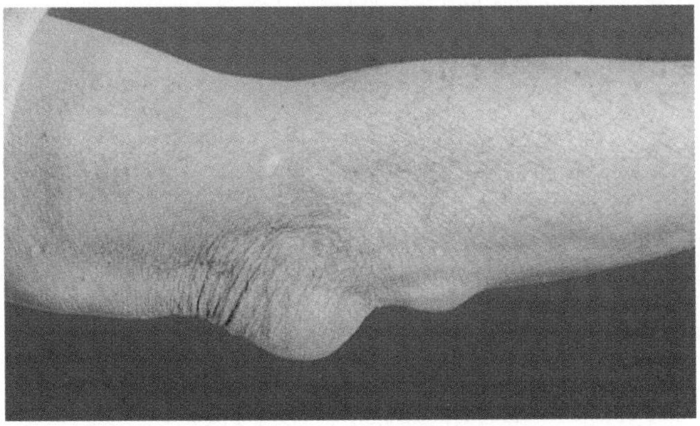

FIG. 41-9 Olecranon bursa. A case of olecranon bursitis in a patient with rheumatoid arthritis. A rheumatoid nodule is also shown. (From Klippel JH, Deippe PA, editors: *Rheumatology,* ed 2, London, 1998, Mosby.)

Evaluation and Treatment

Evaluation of tendinitis, epicondylitis, and bursitis is based on clinical manifestations, physical examination, arthroscopy, arthrography, and possibly magnetic resonance imaging (MRI). Treatment includes immobilization of the joint with a sling, splint, or cast; systemic analgesics; ice or heat applications; or local injection of an anesthetic and a corticosteroid to reduce inflammation. Physical therapy to prevent loss of function begins after acute inflammation subsides.

Muscle Strains

Mild injury such as **muscle strain** is usually seen after traumatic or sports injuries. *Muscle strain* is a general term for local muscle damage. It is often the result of sudden, forced motion causing the muscle to become stretched beyond normal capacity. Knife and gunshot wounds also cause traumatic rupture. Strains often involve the tendon as well. Muscles are ruptured more often than tendons in young people; the opposite is true in the older population. Muscle strain may be chronic when the muscle is repeatedly stretched beyond its usual capacity. There is evidence of tissue disruption with subsequent signs of muscle regeneration and connective tissue repair when a biopsy is performed. Hemorrhage into the surrounding tissue and signs of inflammation also may be present. Regardless of the cause of trauma, muscle cells usually can regenerate. Regeneration may take up to 6 weeks, and the affected muscle should be protected during this time. Types of muscle strain, together with their manifestations and treatment, are summarized in Table 41-2.

A late complication of localized muscle injury is **myositis ossificans.** This condition is thought to be caused by scar tissue calcification and subsequent ossification. Examples include "rider's bone," in which the adductor muscle of the thigh of equestrians becomes calcified, and "drill bone," in which the same complication is seen in the deltoid and

Table 41-2 Muscle Strain

Type	Manifestations	Treatment
First degree (e.g., bench press in untrained athlete)	Muscle overstretched, painful	Ice should be applied 5 or 6 times in the first 24-48 hours; complete rest for up to 2 weeks, followed by weight bearing 3 times per week and range of motion daily
Second degree (e.g., any muscle strain with bruising and pain)	Muscle intact with some tearing pain, mild bruising	Treatment similar to that for first-degree strains, with added mild analgesia; cryokinetics (a treatment system of alternating applications of heat and cold with progressive exercise)
Third degree (e.g., traumatic injury)	Caused by tearing of fascia, muscle rupture palpable, bleeding present	Surgery to approximate ruptured edges; immobilization and rest for 6 weeks, followed by an individualized rehabilitation regimen of strengthening exercises

pectoral muscles of fencers and infantry soldiers, as well as football players after muscle injury to thigh muscles.

Myoglobinuria

Myoglobinuria, also called *rhabdomyolysis,* can be a life-threatening complication of severe muscle trauma. Myoglobinuria is named for the principal manifestation of the condition—an excess of myoglobin (an intracellular muscle protein) in the urine. Muscle cell damage releases the myoglobin. The most severe form is often called *crush syndrome.* Less severe and more localized forms are called **compartment syndromes,** which can lead to **Volkmann ischemic contracture** in the forearm or leg. Crush syndrome first gained notoriety in the reports of injuries seen after the London air raids in World War II. More recently it has been reported in individuals found unresponsive and immobile for long periods, usually after a drug overdose. Myoglobinuria also can be seen after viral infections, administration of certain anesthetic agents, strychnine poisoning, tetanus, heat stroke, electrolyte disturbances, and fractures. Excessive muscular activity also has been implicated in reports of myoglobinuria in athletes, such as long-distance runners, ice skaters, skiers, military recruits, and those subjected to fraternity hazing. Status epilepticus, electroconvulsive therapy, and high-voltage electrical shock are also associated with severe and sometimes fatal myoglobinuria.

If the myoglobinuria is caused by fulminant malignant hyperthermia, severe muscle spasm and rhabdomyolysis can lead to renal failure. Other complications include intraoperative rigidity, tachycardia, cardiac dysrhythmias, metabolic and respiratory acidosis, and temperature elevations up to 43° C, which can occur very rapidly. Cerebral edema, cardiogenic and hypovolemic shock, pulmonary edema, and disseminated intravascular clotting can contribute to the death of an individual with malignant hyperthermia.

Pathophysiology

The weight of a limp extremity can generate enough pressure to produce muscle ischemia (Fig. 41-10). This causes edema, rising compartment pressure, and tamponade that leads to muscle infarction and neural injury and, finally, results in cell loss. Physical interruptions in the sarcolemmal membrane,

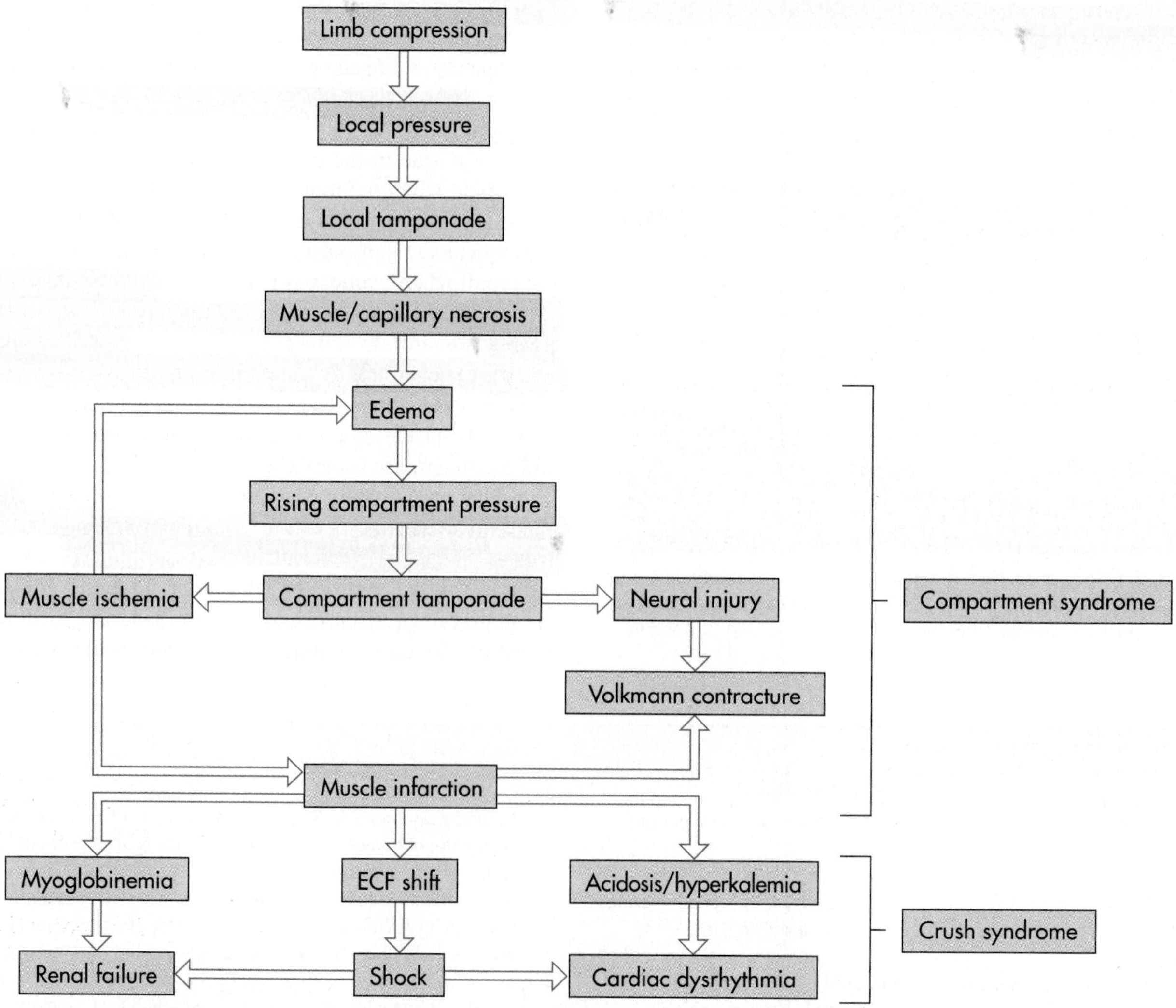

FIG. 41-10 Pathogenesis of compartment syndrome and crush syndrome caused by prolonged muscle compression. *ECF,* Extracellular fluid.

called *holes* or *delta lesions,* suggest that the sarcolemmal membrane may be the route by which muscle constituents are released. (The sarcolemmal membrane, the plasma membrane of the muscle cell, is described in Chapter 40.)

Clinical Manifestations

When myoglobin is released from the muscle cells into the circulation, it can cause a visible, dark reddish brown pigmentation of the urine. The renal threshold for myoglobin is low, approximately 0.5 mg/dl of urine, so that only 200 g of muscle need be damaged to cause visible changes in the urine. Along with the release of myoglobin, creatine kinase (CK) and other serum enzymes are released in massive quantities. The CK level is often 100 times greater than normal (5 to 25 U/ml for women and 5 to 35 U/ml for men). The efflux of proteins and enzymes also includes loss of potassium, phosphate, nucleotides, creatinine, and creatine. Serum hypocalcemia is seen early in the course of myoglobinuria and is followed by late hypercalcemia.

Evaluation and Treatment

Careful and thorough preoperative assessment should alert the anesthesiologist to the possibility of a susceptible individual. A family history of anesthetic problems and previous untoward anesthetic experiences (muscle cramping, unexplained fevers, dark urine) are criteria that require further clarification before administration of a volatile anesthetic.

Priorities in treatment of myoglobinuria include identifying and treating the underlying disorder and preventing life-threatening renal failure. Malignant hyperthermia and myoglobinuria caused by succinylcholine or volatile anesthetic agents can be treated by halting the anesthetic administration and infusing dantrolene sodium (Dantrium). Diluting the pigment using intravenous fluids and administration of mannitol, sodium bicarbonate, and furosemide (Lasix) to "flush" the kidney have been advocated to prevent renal failure. Other secondary problems include electrolyte imbalance, volume depletion, acidosis, hyperuricemia, hyperkalemia, and calcium imbalance. These require specific treatment. Short-term dialysis also may be necessary.

Compartment syndromes may require emergency treatment when blood flow to the affected extremity is compromised because of increased venous pressure, leading to decreased arterial inflow, ischemia, and edema. When clinical evaluation is inconclusive, the rising compartment pressure can be directly measured by inserting a wick catheter, needle, or slit catheter into the muscle. Immediate fasciotomy and debridement have been advocated for pressures of more than 30 mm Hg.[8] Compartments frequently affected are the anterior tibial, deep posterior tibial, volar, hand, and gluteal.

DISORDERS OF BONES

Metabolic Bone Diseases

Metabolic bone disease is characterized by abnormal bone structure that is caused by altered or inadequate biochemical reactions. The altered or inadequate biochemical reactions may be attributable to genetics, diet, or hormones.

Osteoporosis

Osteoporosis is a disease in which the density or mass of bone is reduced. The bone that remains is histologically and biochemically normal, but there is not enough of it to maintain skeletal integrity and mechanical support. Osteoporosis occurs in all populations and at all ages and is a devastating disorder with significant physical, psychosocial, and financial consequences. The disease can be (1) generalized, involving major portions of the axial skeleton, or (2) regional, involving one segment of the appendicular skeleton. Both spongy and compact bone are lost, but spongy bone loss exceeds compact bone loss.

Healthy young women can gain bone mass up to and during the third decade of life through physical activity; dietary calcium, magnesium, and vitamin D intake; adequate body weight; and exposure to sex hormones at puberty.[9] Osteoporosis is the most common metabolic disease. Primary osteoporosis has been subdivided into two types: type I is postmenopausal osteoporosis in the sixth and seventh decades, and type II is also known as *senile osteoporosis*. However, it is uncertain whether these two subgroups are different manifestations of the same disease or two distinct diseases. Secondary osteoporosis occurs as a result of other conditions, as a result of diseases, or from medications.[10]

Because of the decreased bone mass, fractures are major risks for persons with osteoporosis. Wrist fractures in women increase during the sixth decade, and hip fractures increase exponentially from approximately 70 years. The incidence of hip fractures in the United States is expected to rise to 750,000 annually by the year 2050.[11] Vertebral fractures also occur in the latter years of life, mainly in the sixth and seventh decades, with possibly one in three women older than 65 years having a vertebral fracture. The annual direct and indirect costs of osteoporosis are more than 10 to 15 billion dollars.[9] Approximately half the persons with osteoporosis and fractures never walk again.[12] Osteoporosis leads to marked losses of both spongy and trabecular bone, with women losing approximately one half and men approximately one quarter of their spongy bone.

Osteoporosis is most common in white and Asian women. Members of other races, particularly blacks, have denser bones. Whites are therefore more susceptible than other races to osteoporosis caused by loss of bone density with age.

The cause of generalized osteoporosis is multifactorial. Postmenopausal osteoporosis, which occurs in middle-age and older women, is probably caused by a combination of inadequate dietary calcium intake and possibly magnesium, lack of exercise, lack of vitamin D, decreased levels of estrogen, and family history. Excessive phosphorus intake, chiefly through the intake of sodas and junk food, interferes with the calcium/phosphorus balance, resulting in an increased risk of brittle bones. Fluoride has been used for treatment of postmenopausal osteoporosis for years. Although fluoride therapy increased bone formation, at higher doses (150 mg/day) the new bone is structurally abnormal. Newly formed bone shows evidence of mineralization defects, causing spongy and irregular bone.[13-16] Investigators report that, with doses of 25 mg twice daily of sodium fluoride, there was an increase in vertebral bone mass after 3 years without an increase in risk of fracture.[15] Thus fluoride is a controversial issue, and aggressive research must be done to determine if fluoridated water alters the incidence of hip fractures. Before menopause, higher estrogen levels inhibit bone resorption by decreasing the sensitivity of osteoclasts to circulating parathyroid hormone (PTH). Without the inhibitory action of estrogen, PTH overstimulates osteoclasts within the basic multicellular units to initiate the remodeling cycle, which begins with resorption. (Remodeling is described in Chapter 40.) The cause of senile (age-related) osteoporosis remains unclear, but it may be that osteoblasts and osteoclasts shrink, regress to a former state, or undergo alterations that diminish their activity. Reduction in physical activity in older persons may also be a major factor in the bone loss, because preservation of bone mass depends on skeletal stress through muscle contraction and weight bearing.

Insufficient intake or malabsorption of dietary minerals, particularly calcium and possibly magnesium, are factors in the development of osteoporosis. However, among the trace elements in bone and hair, significant differences were found in the contents of zinc, copper, and manganese between unaffected individuals and those with osteoporosis.[17] Calcium absorption from the intestine decreases with age, and studies of individuals with osteoporosis show that their calcium intake is lower than that of age-matched controls. Deficiencies of protein and vitamins, particularly vitamins C and D, also contribute to bone loss. Excessive intakes of caffeine, alcohol, and nicotine along with low body fat have also been considered risk factors.[9,18]

A variety of hormonal imbalances also may contribute to osteoporosis. Skeletal homeostasis depends on a very narrow range of plasma calcium and phosphate concentrations, which are maintained by the endocrine system. Therefore endocrine dysfunction ultimately can cause metabolic bone disease. The hormones most commonly associated with osteoporosis are parathyroid hormone (hyperparathyroidism), cortisol (stress and Cushing syndrome), thyroid hormone (hyperthyroidism), and growth hormone (acromegaly). (Endocrine function is discussed in Unit VI.) Decreased testosterone and estradiol levels contribute to male osteoporosis.[19] Secondary osteoporosis is more common in men (30% to 60% of cases); however, new data reveal that 50% of cases in perimenopausal women are associated with secondary causes.[20]

Secondary osteoporosis is most often due to long-term corticosteroid use. Corticosteroids inhibit osteoblasts and increase bone resorption. Osteoporosis sometimes develops temporarily in individuals receiving large doses of heparin, perhaps because heparin promotes bone resorption by decreasing collagen synthesis or by increasing collagen breakdown. Osteoporosis caused by heparin therapy usually resolves when therapy ceases.

Regional osteoporosis—osteoporosis confined to a region or segment of the appendicular skeleton—usually has a known cause. Classic regional osteoporosis is associated with disuse or immobilization of a limb because of fractures, motor paralysis, or bone or joint inflammation. A negative calcium balance develops early and continues throughout the period of immobilization. After 8 weeks of immobilization, significant osteoporosis is present, although it may develop earlier in persons younger than 20 years or older than 50 years. The pattern of bone loss may be uniform, spotty, or bandlike. Uniform bone loss usually occurs after long immobilization, for example, in persons with quadriplegia or after an amputation. The bone loss initially appears in the appendicular skeleton or pelvis within 2 to 3 months after the paralysis. A uniform distribution of osteoporosis has also been observed in astronauts and in individuals treated with air suspension therapy as a result of weightlessness. A summary of risk factors is given in Table 41-3.

NUTRITION & DISEASE

Trace Elements and Their Effects on Skeletal Tissue*

Flouride accumulates in new bone formation sites and results in a net gain in bone mass; however, at higher doses the new bone may be structurally abnormal.

Magnesium enhances bone turnover by stimulating osteoclastic function and may help with regulation of calcium.

Zinc regulates secretion of calcitonin from the thyroid gland and influences bone turnover; it is essential for enzymes in osteoblasts responsible for collagen synthesis and alkaline phosphatase and also is required for osteoblasts.

Iodine enhances bone turnover, as hormonal forms of thyroxine and triiodothyronine.

Aluminum induces impairment of bone formation by inhibiting osteoblastic function.

Copper induces low bone turnover by suppressing both osteoblastic and osteoclastic function.

Boron may be used by osteoblasts for bone formation and may be related to magnesium in its effect on bone.

Iron functions in mitochondrial oxidative phosphorylation in osteobasts and osteoclasts.

Manganese is required for biosynthesis of mucopolysaccharides in bone matrix formation.

Data from Mahan LK, Escott-Stump S: *Krause's food, nutrition, and diet therapy,* ed 10, Philadelphia, 2000, W.B. Saunders; Okano T: Effects of essential trace elements on bone turnover—in relation to osteoporosis, *Nippon Rinsho* 54(1):148, 1996 (non-English).

*The exact involvement of these trace elements in osteoporosis has not been clarified.

Pathophysiology

Whatever the cause, osteoporosis develops when the remodeling cycle—the process of bone resorption and bone formation—is disrupted, leading to an imbalance in the coupling process. There are two mechanisms of bone loss occurring in two stages: rapid bone loss and slow bone loss. A complete remodeling cycle, consisting of basic multicellular unit activation (see Chapter 40), bone resorption, and bone formation, takes approximately 4 months in a normal, healthy adult. In an individual with osteoporosis, 2 years may be needed to complete one cycle. In normal bone, the frequency of multicellular unit activation, the rate of resorption, and the rate of new bone formation are relatively constant, so that replacement follows resorption immediately and the amount of bone replaced equals the amount of bone resorbed. In bones affected by osteoporosis, this equilibrium can be disrupted by (1) an increase in the number of basic multicellular units activated, (2) an increase in the frequency of basic multicellular unit activation, (3) an increase in the rate of resorption, (4) a delay in the rate of bone formation, or (5) a deficiency of cells in the multicellular unit. Any one of these changes causes a net decrease in total bone mass. Rapid bone loss occurs during early menopause and is osteoclast mediated, whereas slow bone loss is osteoblast mediated, occurring later after early menopause.

If the number of basic multicellular units increases, resorption occurs at more sites, or loci. Loci of resorption become so numerous that new bone is destroyed along with old bone, creating a state of "runaway" resorption. If a normal number of basic multicellular units is activated with abnormal frequency, the result is a net increase in the total amount of bone lost in a given period of time.

Another mechanism causing osteoporosis is an imbalance between the rate of resorption and the rate of new bone formation. Some hormones and drugs are thought to interfere with the relationship between osteoclast activity (bone resorption) and osteoblast activity (bone formation). Anything that causes resorption to speed up or replacement to slow down causes resorption cavities to persist, weakening the bone. Cell communication between osteoblasts and osteoclasts has recently been reported (see What's New? Osteoblasts "Talk" to Osteoclasts, Providing a Mechanism for Stopping Bone Deterioration, Chapter 40, p. 1344). By controlling the ligands and receptors involved in this communication, new therapies will probably emerge.

Osteoporosis also occurs if the basic multicellular units fail to complete the three phases of the remodeling cycle. Failure occurs if the number of osteoclasts and osteoblasts in bone tissue is inadequate. Completion of the remodeling cycle requires delivery of a continuous supply of bone cell precursors from the marrow. Any interruption in the bone's vascular system will interfere with the delivery of osteoclast and osteoblast precursors to bone tissue.

Age-related bone loss occurs when bone formation decreases faster than bone resorption, particularly in the fifth decade. Losses are at the rates of 0.3% to 0.5% yearly in both men and women. Men have greater bone mass than women, which may be a factor in their later involvement with osteoporosis.[21]

Clinical Manifestations

The specific clinical manifestations of osteoporosis depend on the bones involved. The most common manifestations, however, are pain and bone deformity. Fractures are likely to occur because the trabeculae of spongy bone become thin and sparse and compact bone becomes porous. As the bones lose volume, they become brittle and weak and may collapse or become misshapen. Vertebral collapse causes kyphosis (hunchback) and diminished height (Fig. 41-11). Fractures of the long bones (particularly the femur and humerus), distal radius, ribs, and vertebrae are most common. Fracture of the neck of the femur—the so-called broken hip—tends to occur in older or elderly women with osteoporosis. Fatal complications of fractures include fat or pulmonary embolism, hemorrhage, and shock. Approximately 20% of persons may die as a result of surgical complications. Male

Table 41-3 Risk Factors for Osteoporosis

Category	Risk Factors
Genetic	Family history of osteoporotic fracture
	White race
	Increased age
	Female sex
Anthropometric	Small stature
	Fair or pale skinned
	Thin build
Hormonal	Early menopause (normal or surgical)
	Late menarche
	Nulliparity
	Obesity
	Low endogenous hormone levels
Dietary	Low dietary calcium
	Excess protein, sodium intake
	High caffeine intake (controversial)
Lifestyle	Sedentary
	Smoking
	Alcohol (inconsistent)
Concurrent illness and drugs	Hyperparathyroidism
	Rheumatoid arthritis
	Hyperthyroidism
	History of prior fracture
	Neurologic disease, cerebrovascular accident, parkinsonism

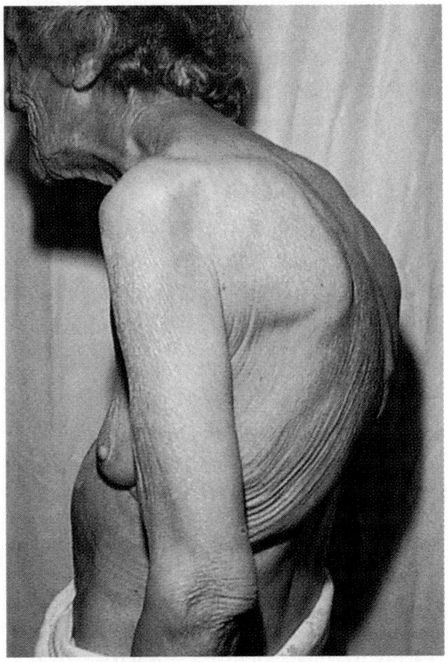

FIG. 41-11 **Kyphosis.** This elderly woman's condition was caused by a combination of spinal osteoporotic vertebral collapse and chronic degenerative changes in the vertebral column. (From Kamal A, Brocklehurst JC: *Color atlas of geriatric medicine,* ed 2, St Louis, 1992, Mosby.)

osteoporosis is usually secondary osteoporosis because of hypogonadism or corticosteroid use.

Evaluation and Treatment

Generally, osteoporosis is detected radiographically as increased radiolucency of bone. By the time abnormalities are detected by x-ray examination, as much as 25% to 30% of bone tissue may have been lost.

Types of radiologic examinations include single- or dual-photon absorptiometry and computed tomography (CT) scans (Fig. 41-12). Other evaluation procedures include tests for levels of serum calcium, phosphorus, and alkaline phosphatase, and protein electrophoresis. Body calcium levels also can be measured by neuron activation analysis, a procedure involving use of radioactive calcium-49, whose gamma activity can be measured with a whole-body counter.

The goals of osteoporosis treatment are to slow down the rate of calcium and bone loss and to stop the disease before it progresses too far. Controversial is the role of calcium intake to both prevent and treat osteoporosis. It is well accepted that oral calcium intake sufficient to maintain normal calcium balance is necessary during adolescence to ensure development of peak bone mass, and that calcium-deficient diets can aggravate bone loss associated with menopause and aging. Although recommendations have been established for young women of 1000 mg of calcium daily and postmenopausal women of 1500 mg daily (with vitamin D) if receiving sex hormone replacement therapy, it has been difficult to translate these recommendations into clear-cut clinical outcomes. A number of investigations lack an association between current calcium intake and bone mineral density. A significant relationship has been observed between an individual's lifetime history of calcium intake and peak bone mineral density. Clinical trials must be done to test the effects of dietary calcium or supplements on bone loss accounting for potential confounding factors, such as menopausal status, estrogen levels, vitamin D levels, magnesium levels, smoking, contraceptive use, usual calcium intake, and level of physical activity.

Magnesium (Mg^{++}), another mineral important for skeletal development, is at risk for being deficient in the diet. It is an essential mineral in many biochemical and physiologic functions, including activation of enzymes, involvement in ATP synthesis, protein synthesis, regulation of membrane channels, and muscle contraction. New evidence suggests that large fluxes of magnesium can cross the cell plasma membrane in either direction following a variety of stimuli, resulting in a modification of activity for several cellular enzymes.[22] Magnesium is important to bone quality by controlling hydroxyapatite crystal growth to prevent formation of brittle bones.[23] It seems reasonable that Mg^{++} is required for normal calcium (Ca^{++}) absorption because severe Mg^{++} deficiency results in hypocalcemia. Elevation of plasma Mg^{++} or Ca^{++} concentration inhibits Mg^{++} and Ca^{++} resorption, leading to hypermagnesiuria and hypercalciuria.[24] An extracellular Ca^{++}/Mg^{++} sensing receptor has been found located on distal tubule cells. Also, recent data have shown a relationship between Mg^{++} and Ca^{++} signaling in pancreatic and other secretory epithelia.[25] Significant extrusion of Mg^{++} from these cells is related to mobilization of intracellular Ca^{++}.[25]

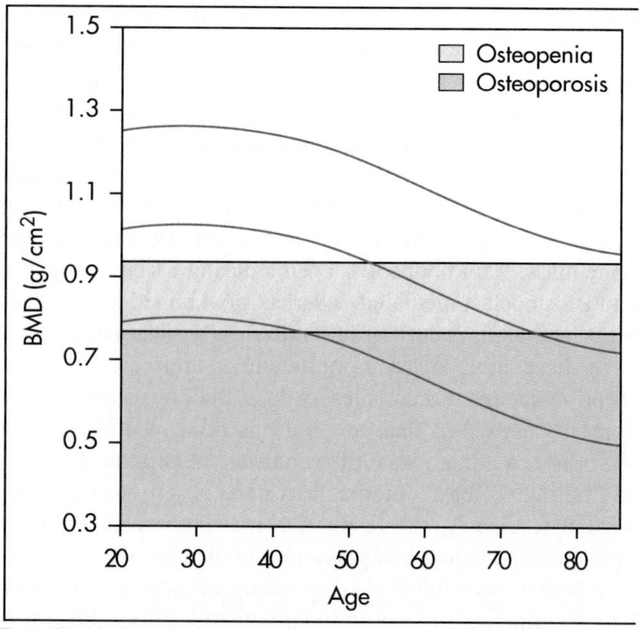

FIG. 41-12 Lumbar spine bone mass density (BMD). The normal female reference curves for lumbar spine BMD are plotted in this graph to include the World Health Organization definitions of osteopenia and osteoporosis. (Redrawn from Collier BD, Fogelman I, Rosenthall L: *Skeletal nuclear medicine,* St Louis, 1996, Mosby.)

Regular, moderate weight-bearing exercise can slow down the bone loss and, in some cases, reverse demineralization because the mechanical stress of exercise stimulates bone formation. Although hormone treatment is controversial, postmenopausal women are given estrogen and progestins in addition to exercise and dietary supplements of calcium and vitamin D. Magnesium may also be recommended. Progesterone alone at higher concentrations may also be effective in postmenopausal women.[26] It is important to reduce the risk of falls and enhance bone quality. Therefore an exercise program to enhance rehabilitation is advised (Fig. 41-13). Important new findings suggest that estrogen may prevent excessive bone loss before and after menopause by limiting osteoclast life span through promotion of apoptosis. This mechanism is mediated by transforming growth factor–beta.[27]

Selective estrogen receptor modulators (SERMs) have been developed to provide the positive effects of estrogen on bone but minimize estrogen's negative effect on breast and endometrial tissues. Raloxifene and tamoxifen are examples of SERMs.

Other treatments include intranasal calcitonin given daily and sodium fluoride given orally. By inhibiting bone resorption, the biphosphates alendronate and risedronate have been effective in reducing hip and vertebral fractures in glucocorticoid-induced osteoporosis and in women with osteoporosis.[28] Men with osteoporosis are treated with biphosphonates and testosterone. Increases in spine bone density are reported after this treatment.[21]

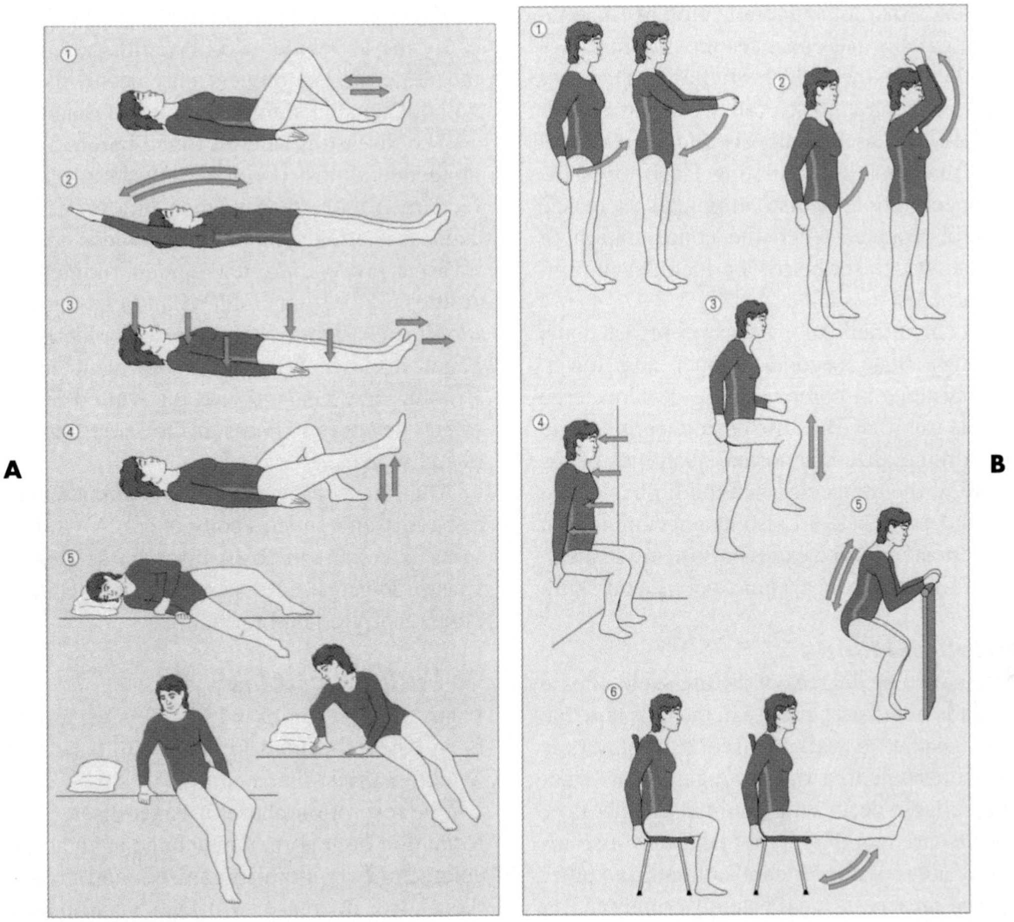

FIG. 41-13 Osteoporosis. A, Exercises for individuals with established osteoporosis of the spine. **B,** Additional exercises for individuals with osteoporosis. (Modified from Klippel JH, Dieppe PA, editors: *Rheumatology,* St Louis, 1994, Mosby.)

Osteomalacia

Osteomalacia is a metabolic disease characterized by inadequate and delayed mineralization of osteoid in mature compact and spongy bone. In osteomalacia the remodeling cycle proceeds normally through osteoid formation, but mineral calcification and deposition do not occur. Bone volume remains unchanged, but the replaced bone consists of soft osteoid instead of rigid bone. Rickets is similar to osteomalacia in pathogenesis, but it occurs in the growing bones of children, whereas osteomalacia occurs in adult bone. (Rickets is described in Chapter 42.)

Both osteomalacia and rickets are rare in the United States and Western Europe but are significant health problems in Great Britain, Ethiopia, Pakistan, Iran, and India. In the United States these diseases occur in elderly persons, in premature infants of very low birth weight, and in individuals adhering to rigid macrobiotic vegetarian diets.

Many factors contribute to the development of osteomalacia, but the most important is a deficiency of vitamin D. The major risk factors in vitamin D deficiency are diets deficient in vitamin D, decreased endogenous production of vitamin D, intestinal malabsorption of vitamin D, renal tubular diseases, and anticonvulsant therapy. Classic vitamin D deficiency is rare in the United States because of the addition of synthetic vitamin D to dairy products and bread.

Disorders of the small bowel, hepatobiliary system, and pancreas are common causes of vitamin D deficiency in the United States, however. In malabsorptive disease of the small bowel, vitamin D and calcium absorption are decreased, so that vitamin D is lost in feces. Liver disease interferes with the metabolism of vitamin D to its more active form, and diseases of the pancreas and biliary system cause a deficiency of bile salts, which are necessary for normal intestinal absorption of vitamin D.

The mechanism by which anticonvulsant drug therapy results in vitamin D deficiency is not completely understood, but researchers think that the anticonvulsants phenobarbital and phenytoin interfere with calcium absorption and increase degradation of vitamin D metabolism in the liver. Renal osteodystrophy is a common cause of osteomalacia.

Pathophysiology

Crystallization of minerals in osteoid requires adequate concentrations of calcium and phosphate. When the concentrations are too low, crystallization (and hence ossification) does not proceed normally.

Vitamin D deficiency disrupts mineralization because vitamin D normally regulates and enhances the absorption of calcium ions from the intestine. A lack of vitamin D causes the plasma calcium concentrations to fall. Low plasma calcium levels stimulate increased synthesis and secretion of PTH. Although the increase in circulating PTH raises the plasma calcium concentration, it also stimulates increased renal clearance of phosphate. When the concentration of phosphate in the bone decreases below a critical level, mineralization cannot proceed normally.

Abnormalities occur in both spongy and compact bone. Trabeculae in spongy bone become thinner and fewer, whereas haversian systems in compact bone develop large channels and become irregular. Because osteoid continues to be produced but not mineralized, abnormal quantities of osteoid build up, coating the trabeculae and the linings of the haversian canals. Excessive osteoid also can accumulate in areas beneath the periosteum. The excess of osteoid leads to gross deformities of the long bones, spine, pelvis, and skull.

Clinical Manifestations

Osteomalacia causes varying degrees of diffuse skeletal pain and tenderness. Pain is noted particularly in the hips, and the individual may be hesitant to walk. Muscular weakness is common and may contribute to a waddling gait. Bone fractures and vertebral collapse occur with minimal trauma. Low back pain may be an early complaint, but pain may also involve ribs, feet, other areas of the vertebral column, and other sites. Uremia may be present in renal osteodystrophy.

Evaluation and Treatment

Laboratory data may include elevated blood urea nitrogen (BUN) and creatinine levels, normal or low serum calcium levels, and a serum inorganic phosphate level that is usually higher than 5.5 mg. Alkaline phosphatase and PTH levels are usually elevated. Radiographic findings show pseudofractures and radiolucent bands perpendicular to the surface of involved bones. A bone biopsy is used to evaluate presence of renal osteodystrophy to determine bone aluminum deposits.

Treatment of osteomalacia includes the following:

1. Adjusting serum calcium and phosphorus levels to normal
2. Suppressing secondary hyperthyroidism
3. Chelating bone aluminum if needed
4. Administering calcium carbonate to decrease hyperphosphatemia
5. Dietary supplements of vitamin D
6. Renal dialysis
7. Renal transplant for renal osteodystrophy

Paget Disease

Paget disease (osteitis deformans) is a state of increased metabolic activity in bone characterized by abnormal and excessive bone remodeling, both resorption and formation. Chronic accelerated remodeling eventually enlarges and softens the affected bones.

Paget disease most often affects the axial skeleton, especially the vertebrae, skull, sacrum, sternum, pelvis, and femur. The disease process may occur in one or more bones without causing significant clinical manifestations.

The disease is seldom found before age 40 years, but its incidence almost doubles each decade from age 50. It affects men more than women in a proportion of 3:2.[29] Because it is often symptomless and can be diagnosed only by invasive procedures, few epidemiologic data are available. Autopsy data from England and Germany indicate that approximately 3% to 4% of persons older than 40 years have Paget disease. It is most prevalent in Australia, Great Britain, New Zealand, and the United States. Paget disease affects several members of the same family in 15% to 30% of individuals.[30]

The cause of Paget disease is unknown, but there appears to be a strong genetic component. A viral connection (slow virus infection) to Paget disease has also been proposed.[30] Classic Paget disease arises as a consequence of disorderly bone resorption and formation.

Pathophysiology

Paget disease begins with excessive resorption of spongy bone. The trabeculae diminish, and bone marrow is replaced by extremely vascular fibrous tissue.

The resorption phase of Paget disease is followed by the formation of abnormal new bone at an accelerated rate. The collagen fibers are disorganized, and glycoprotein levels in the matrix decrease. Mineralization may extend into the bone marrow. Bone formation is excessive around partially resorbed trabeculae, causing them to thicken and enlarge. Eventually, Paget disease progresses to an inactive phase, in which abnormal remodeling is minimal or absent.

Clinical Manifestations

In the skull, abnormal remodeling is first evident in the frontal or occipital regions; then it encroaches on the outer and inner surfaces of the entire skull. The skull thickens and assumes an asymmetric shape. Thickened segments of the skull may compress areas of the brain, producing altered mentality and dementia. Impingement of new bone on cranial nerves causes sensory abnormalities, impaired motor function, deafness, atrophy of the optic nerve, and obstruction of the lacrimal duct. Headache is commonly noted.

Extensive alterations of the facial bones are rare except in the jaw, where sclerosis and thickening of the maxilla and mandible displace teeth and produce malocclusion. In long bones, resorption begins in the subchondral regions of the epiphysis and extends into the metaphysis and diaphysis. Occasionally, Paget disease affects both ends of a tubular bone. In the femur, Paget disease produces an exaggerated lateral curvature. In the tibia, anterior curvature is also exaggerated. Stress fractures are common in the lower extremities.

Clinical manifestations of Paget disease in the vertebral column depend on the level of involvement and are caused by compression of adjacent structures. In the cervical spine, cord compression can lead to spastic quadriplegia. Approximately 1% of persons with Paget disease develop osteogenic sarcoma.

Evaluation and Treatment

Evaluation of Paget disease is made on the basis of radiographic findings of irregular bone trabeculae with a thickened and disorganized pattern. Early disease is detected by bone scanning that shows increased uptake of bone radionuclides. Alkaline phosphatase and urinary hydroxyproline are elevated.

Most individuals require no treatment because the disease is localized and does not cause symptoms. Treatment during active disease is for pain relief, prevention of deformity, or fracture. Biphosphonates and calcitonin (salmon and human) are the mainstays of treatment. Surgery is indicated if there are neurologic complications.[30]

Infectious Bone Disease: Osteomyelitis

Infectious bone disease is expensive and difficult to treat and often culminates in extensive physical disability. Several factors contribute to the difficulty in treating bone infection:

1. Bone contains multiple microscopic channels that are impermeable to the cells and biochemicals of the body's natural defenses. Once bacteria gain access to these channels, they are able to proliferate unimpeded.
2. The microcirculation of bone is highly vulnerable to damage and destruction by bacterial toxins. Vessel damage causes local thrombosis (blockage) of the small vessels, which leads to ischemic necrosis (death) of bone.
3. Bone cells have a limited capacity to replace bone destroyed by infections. Initially, osteoclasts are stimulated by infection to resorb bone, which opens up isolated bone channels so that cells of the inflammatory and immune system can gain access to the infected bone. At the same time, however, resorption weakens the structural integrity of the bone. New bone formation usually lags behind resorption, and the haversian systems in the new bone are incomplete.

Osteomyelitis is a bone infection caused by bacteria; however, fungi, parasites, and viruses also can cause bone infection (Fig. 41-14). It is further categorized according to the pathogen's mode of entry into bone tissue. **Exogenous osteomyelitis** is an infection that enters from outside the body, for example, through open fractures, penetrating wounds, or surgical procedures. In exogenous osteomyelitis, the infection spreads from soft tissues into adjacent bone. **Endogenous (hematogenous) osteomyelitis** is caused by pathogens carried in the blood from sites of infection elsewhere in the body. In hematogenous osteomyelitis, the infection spreads from bone to adjacent soft tissues. Hematogenous osteomyelitis is commonly found in infants, children, and elderly persons. (Osteomyelitis in children is discussed in Chapter 42.) In infants, incidence rates among males and females are approximately equal. In children and older adults, however, males are most commonly affected. Osteomyelitis is a common complication of sickle cell anemia and low oxygen tension.

Staphylococcus aureus is the usual cause of hematogenous osteomyelitis. Other microorganisms include group B streptococci, *Haemophilus influenzae, Salmonella,* and gram-negative bacteria. Group B streptococci and *H. influenzae* tend to infect young children; *Salmonella* infection is associated with sickle cell anemia; and gram-negative infections are most common in older adults and individuals with impaired immunity. Mycobacterial and fungal infections occur in immunocompromised individuals.

Cutaneous, sinus, ear, and dental infections are the primary sources of bacteria in hematogenous bone infections. Soft tissue infections, disorders of the gastrointestinal tract, infections of the genitourinary system, and respiratory infections are also sources of bacterial contamination. In addition, infections after total joint replacements are causes. The vulnerability of specific bone depends on the anatomy of its vascular supply.

In adults, hematogenous osteomyelitis is more common in the spine, pelvis, and small bones. Microorganisms reach the vertebrae through arteries, veins, or lymphatic vessels. The spread of infection from pelvic organs to the vertebrae is well documented. Vaginal, uterine, ovarian, bladder, and intestinal infections can lead to iliac or sacral osteomyelitis.

Exogenous osteomyelitis can be caused by human bites or fist blows to the mouth. Superficial animal or human bites

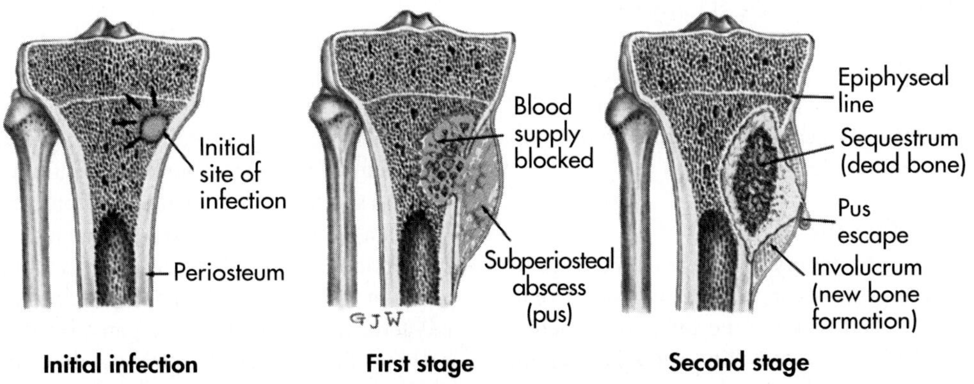

FIG. 41-14 Osteomyelitis showing sequestration and involucrum. (From Mourad L: *Orthopedic disorders,* St Louis, 1991, Mosby.)

inoculate local soft tissue with bacteria that later spread to underlying bone. Deep bites can introduce microorganisms directly onto bone. The most common infecting organism in human bites is *S. aureus.* In animal bites the most common infecting organism is *Pasteurella multocida,* which is part of the normal mouth flora of cats and dogs.

Direct contamination of bones with bacteria can also occur in open fractures or dislocations with an overlying skin wound. Intervertebral disk surgery and operative procedures involving implantation of large foreign objects, such as metallic plates or artificial joints, are associated with exogenous osteomyelitis. Local injections and venous punctures are significant causes of exogenous osteomyelitis. Exogenous osteomyelitis of the arm and hand bones tends to occur in drug abusers. *S. aureus* is the most common pathogen. In general, persons who are chronically ill, have diabetes or alcoholism, or are receiving large doses of steroids or immunosuppressive drugs are particularly susceptible to exogenous osteomyelitis or recurring episodes of this disease.

Pathophysiology

Regardless of the source of the pathogen, the pathologic features of bone infection are similar to those in any other body tissue (see Chapters 6 and 7). First, the invading pathogen provokes an intense inflammatory response. Inflammation in bone is characterized by vascular engorgement, edema, leukocyte activity, and abscess formation. Once inflammation is initiated, the small terminal vessels thrombose and exudate seals the bone's canaliculi. Inflammatory exudate extends into the metaphysis and the marrow cavity and through small metaphyseal openings into the cortex. In children, exudate that reaches the outer surface of the cortex forms abscesses that lift the periosteum off underlying bone. Lifting of the periosteum disrupts blood vessels that enter bone through the periosteum, which deprives underlying bone of its blood supply; this leads to necrosis and death of the area of bone infected, producing **sequestrum,** an area of devitalized bone (see Fig. 41-14). Lifting of the periosteum also stimulates an intense osteoblastic response. Osteoblasts lay down new bone that can partially or completely surround the infected bone. This layer of new bone surrounding the infected bone is called an **involucrum.** Openings in the involucrum allow the exudate to escape into surrounding soft tissue and ultimately through the skin by way of sinus tracts.

In adults, this complication is rare because the periosteum is firmly attached to the cortex and resists displacement. Instead, infection disrupts and weakens the cortex, which predisposes the bone to pathologic fracture.

Clinical Manifestations

Clinical manifestations of osteomyelitis vary with the age of the individual, the site of involvement, the initiating event, the infecting organism, and whether the infection is acute, subacute, or chronic. Acute osteomyelitis causes an abrupt onset of inflammation. If an acute infection is not completely eliminated, the disease may become subacute or chronic. In subacute osteomyelitis, signs and symptoms are usually vague. In the chronic stage, infection is indolent or silent between exacerbations. The microorganisms persist in small abscesses or fragments of necrotic bone and produce occasional flare-ups of acute osteomyelitis. The progression from acute to subacute osteomyelitis may be the result of inadequate or inappropriate therapy or the development of drug-resistant microorganisms.

In the adult, hematogenous osteomyelitis has an insidious onset. The symptoms are usually vague and include fever, malaise, anorexia, and weight loss. Recent infection (urinary, respiratory, skin) or instrumentation (catheterization, cystoscopy, myelography, diskography) usually precedes onset of symptoms.

The primary symptom of acute osteomyelitis in the spine is back pain. The pain may be intermittent or constant, aggravated by motion, and throbbing at rest. It may radiate in a radicular distribution and is commonly accompanied by spinal tenderness and rigidity. Hip contracture occurs in the presence of soft tissue inflammation as a result of irritation of the psoas muscle.

The signs and symptoms of sacroiliac osteomyelitis are generally severe and include local pain, tenderness, and a limp. The pain may radiate to the buttock or the abdomen.

Single or multiple abscesses (Brodie abscesses) characterize subacute or chronic osteomyelitis. Brodie abscesses are circumscribed lesions 1 to 4 cm in diameter, usually in the ends of long bones and surrounded by dense ossified bone matrix. The abscesses are thought to develop when the infectious microorganism has become less virulent or the individual's immune system is resisting the infection somewhat successfully.

In exogenous osteomyelitis, signs and symptoms of soft tissue infection predominate. Inflammatory exudate in the soft tissues disrupts muscles and supporting structures and forms abscesses. Low-grade fever, lymphadenopathy, local pain, and swelling usually occur within days of contamination by a puncture wound. Osteomyelitis in the hand causes exquisite tenderness over the course of tendon sheaths. The fingers are usually in a semiflexed position, and extension usually causes severe pain. Palmar swelling or symmetric swelling of the fingers may be present.

Evaluation and Treatment

Laboratory data show an elevated white cell count. Radiographic studies include radionuclide bone scanning, CT, and MRI. Treatment of osteomyelitis includes antibiotics and debridement with bone biopsy and culture. Initial antibiotic therapy should be intravenous. Chronic conditions may require surgical removal of the inflammatory exudate followed by continuous wound irrigation with antibiotic solutions in addition to systemic treatment with antibiotics. **Hyperbaric oxygen therapy** of 100% oxygen, given at 2 atmospheres of pressure for 2 hours' duration per day for 30 treatments, is also beneficial for chronic refractory osteomyelitis. Implants for total joint replacements may be removed to treat the infected joint more thoroughly.

Bone Tumors

Many different types of tumors involve the skeleton. Bone tumors may originate from bone cells, cartilage, fibrous tissue, marrow, or vascular tissue. Based on the tissue of origin, bone tumors are classified as osteogenic, chondrogenic, collagenic, and myelogenic. Each of the four types arises from one of the four stem cells that are ultimately derived from the primitive mesoderm (Fig. 41-15). In addition, bone tumors may be classified as being of histiocytic, notochordal, lipogenic, and neurogenic origins.

The mesoderm contributes the primitive fibroblast and reticulum cells. The fibroblast is the progenitor of the osteoblast and the chondroblast. Each cell synthesizes a specific type of intercellular ground substance, and the tumor derived from the cell is generally characterized by the type of ground substance produced by the cell. For example, osteogenic tumors usually contain cells that have the appearance of osteoblasts and produce an intercellular substance that can be recognized as osteoid. Chondrogenic tumors contain chondroblasts and produce an intercellular substance similar to chondroid (cartilage). Collagenic tumors contain fibrous tissue cells and produce an intercellular substance similar to the type of collagen found in fibrous connective tissue.

Tumors are also classified as benign or malignant. The differences between malignant and nonmalignant bone tumors are sometimes difficult because the criteria used to differentiate them are vague (see Chapter 10). The criteria used to identify tumor cells as malignant are (1) an increased nuclear/cytoplasmic ratio, (2) an irregular nuclear border, (3) excess chromatin, (4) a prominent nucleolus, and (5) an increase in the number of cells undergoing mitosis. However, many young, rapidly growing, normal cells and cells subjected to inflammation and change in their blood supply also exhibit many of these same characteristics. (Tumor characteristics in general are described in Chapter 10.)

Epidemiology

The incidence of bone tumors varies with age. In children younger than 15 years, the rate of bone tumors is relatively low, constituting approximately 3% of all malignancies. Adolescents have the highest incidence of bone tumors, and adults between 30 and 35 years of age have the lowest incidence. After age 35, the incidence slowly increases until, at age 60, it equals the incidence in adolescents, primarily related to metastatic tumors.

Patterns of Bone Destruction

The general pathologic features of bone tumors include bone destruction, erosion or expansion of the cortex, and periosteal response to changes in underlying bone. The least amount of pathologic damage occurs with benign bone tumors, which push against neighboring tissue. Because they usually have a symmetric, controlled growth pattern, benign bone tumors tend to compress and displace neighboring normal bone tissue, which weakens the bone's structure until it is incapable of withstanding the stress of ordinary use, leading to pathologic fracture. Other tumors invade and destroy adjacent normal bone tissue by producing substances that promote resorption by increasing osteoclast activity or by interfering with a bone's blood supply.

Three patterns of bone destruction by bone tumors have been identified: (1) the geographic pattern, (2) the moth-eaten pattern, and (3) the permeative pattern (Table 41-4).

Tumors that erode the cortex of the bone usually stimulate a periosteal response, that is, new bone formation at the interface between the surface of the bone and the periosteum. Slow erosion of the cortex usually stimulates a uniform periosteal

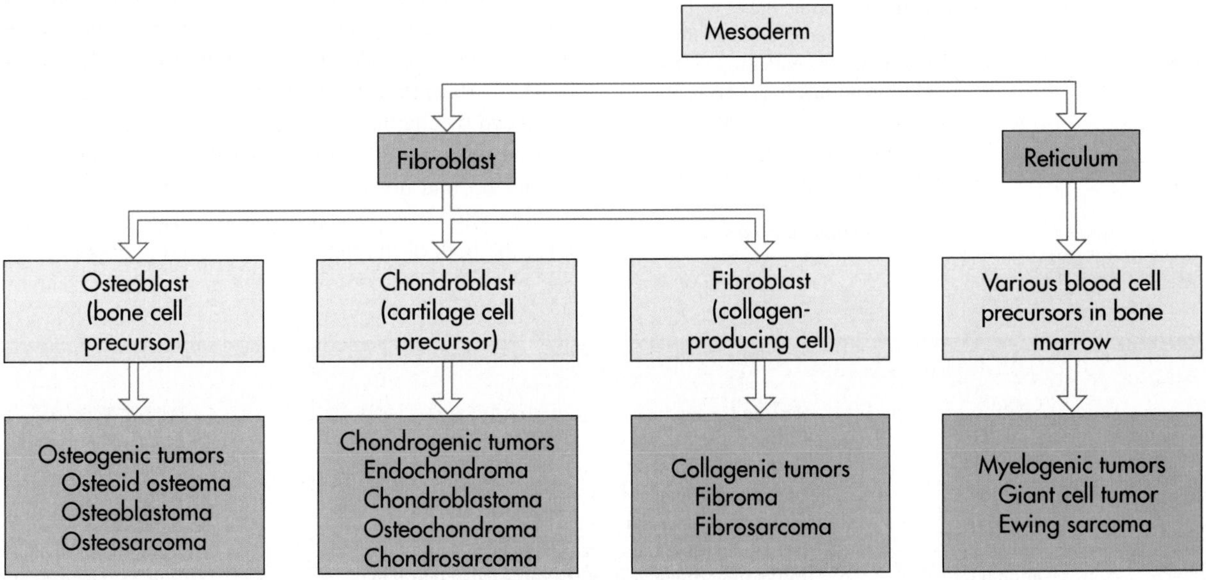

FIG. 41-15 Derivation of bone tumors.

response. Additional layers of bone are added to the exterior surface of the bone to buttress the cortex. Eventually, the additional layers expand the bone's contour. Aggressive penetration of the cortex usually elevates the periosteum and stimulates erratic patterns of new bone formation. Examples of erratic patterns include concentric layers of new bone; a sunburst pattern, in which delicate rays of new bone radiate toward the periosteum from a single focus on the underlying surface; and rays of new bone that grow perpendicularly, creating a brush or bristle pattern.

Diagnosis

A malignant bone tumor must be identified early to allow the survival of the individual and the preservation of the affected limb. However, individuals frequently have only vague symptoms that may be attributed to minor trauma, degenerative changes, or inflammatory conditions. In addition, other conditions may obscure the diagnosis.

Thorough diagnostic studies are needed to determine the exact type and extent of bone tumor present, which also helps determine the optimal treatment regimen. Serum alkaline phosphatase levels are elevated in bone lytic tumors, and they are significantly elevated in osteosarcoma and Ewing sarcoma. Radiologic studies include plain radiologic films, CT scan, and MRI, which has become the examination of choice for the local staging of bone tumors, especially the staging of peripheral osteosarcomas (Table 41-5). MRI is also used to monitor the response of osteosarcomas to radiation or chemotherapy and to detect recurrent disease. A CT scan can evaluate involvement of osteosarcoma in flat bones when the tumor is not well defined on a plain film, can assist in differentiating the tumor, and can locate pulmonary metastases. Radionucleotide bone scans show an increased uptake at the tumor site.

Additional diagnostic studies done for specific bone tumors include a complete blood count and erythrocyte sedimentation rate (to rule out infection, myeloma, or Ewing sarcoma) and serum levels of calcium and phosphorus to detect hypercalcemia. Serum glucose levels may be elevated in chondrosarcoma. Acid phosphatase may show moderate elevations in bone metastases, multiple myeloma, and advanced Paget disease. Serum protein electrophoresis and immunoelectrophoresis are done to rule out multiple myeloma.[31] Fine-needle biopsy is done, usually at the time of surgery, to determine the exact tumor type.

Table 41-4 Patterns of Bone Destruction by Bone Tumors

Type of Destruction	Pattern Seen
Geographic	Well-defined margins separated from surrounding normal bone; well-defined lytic area in affected bone
Moth eaten	Less-defined margin not easily separated from normal bone; areas of partially destroyed bone adjacent to completely lytic areas
Permeative	Poorly demarcated margins; abnormal lytic bone merges imperceptibly with surrounding normal bone

Types

A very large number of lesions are classified as bone tumors. The bone tumors most representative of the four derivative types (see Fig. 41-15)—osteogenic, chondrogenic, collagenic, and myelogenic tumors—are described here.

Osteogenic Tumors: Osteosarcoma

Osteogenic (bone-forming) tumors are characterized by the formation of bone or osteoid tissue with a sarcomatous tissue. The tissue can have the appearance of compact or spongy bone. The most common malignant bone-forming tumor is the osteosarcoma. **Osteosarcomas** account for 38% of bone tumors. The male/female ratio is 3:2, and osteosarcoma occurs predominantly in adolescents and young adults. Sixty percent of osteosarcomas occur in persons younger than 20 years. A secondary peak incidence for osteosarcoma occurs in the 50- to 60-year-old age group, primarily in individuals with a history of radiation therapy several years previously for pelvic or other malignancies (Fig. 41-16).

An osteosarcoma is a malignant bone-forming tumor. It is large, destructive, and most often found in bone marrow; it has a moth-eaten pattern of bone destruction. The borders of the tumor are indistinct and merge into adjacent normal bone. Osteosarcomas always contain osteoid and callus, produced by anaplastic stromal cells, which are atypical, abnormal cells not seen in normal developing bone; they are neither normal nor embryonal. The osteosarcoma may also contain chondroid (cartilage) and fibrinoid tissue that may form the bulk of the tumor. The osteoid is deposited in thick

Table 41-5 Surgical Staging System for Bone Tumors

Stage	Grade	Site (T)	Metastasis (M)
IA	Low (G_1)	Intracompartmental (T_1)	None (M_0)
IB	Low (G_1)	Extracompartmental (T_2)	None (M_0)
IIA	High (G_2)	Intracompartmental (T_1)	None (M_0)
IIB	High (G_2)	Extracompartmental (T_2)	None (M_0)
IIIA	Low (G_1)	Intracompartmental or extracompartmental (T_1 or T_2)	Regional or distant (M_1)
IIIB	High (G_2)	Intracompartmental or extracompartmental (T_1 or T_2)	Regional or distant (M_1)

Data from Simon SR, editor: *Orthopaedic basic science,* Chicago, 1994, American Academy of Orthopaedic Surgeons.

masses or "streamers" between the trabeculae of callus, which infiltrate the normal compact bone, destroy it, and replace it with dense callus and masses of osteoid. Demonstrating the presence of osteoid aids in the diagnosis of osteosarcoma. Bone tissue produced by osteosarcomas never matures to compact bone.

Ninety percent of osteosarcomas are located in the metaphyses of long bones, especially the distal femoral metaphysis, with 50% around the knee area. The tumor typically breaks through the cortex, lifts the periosteum, and forms a soft tissue mass that is *not* covered by a smooth shell of new bone. Lifting of the periosteum stimulates bizarre patterns of new bone formation called a *periosteal reaction.* Distinct osteosarcomas occur on the surface of long bones, called parosteal, periosteal, or high-grade surface osteosarcomas; dedifferentiated parosteal and central osteosarcomas also occur.

The most common initial symptoms are pain and swelling. Initially, the pain is slight and intermittent, but within a short time the pain increases in severity and duration. Pain is usually worse at night and gradually requires medication. Systemic symptoms are uncommon. Usually, a coincidental history of trauma is noted. Occasionally, the individual may have a pathologic fracture.

Surgery is the treatment of choice, with the location of the tumor, its size, malignancy grade, and evidence of metastasis dictating the type and extent of surgery. Preoperative chemotherapy has greatly increased the number of individuals qualifying for limb salvage surgery. Limb salvaging procedures have been made possible by advances in reconstructive techniques and endoprosthetics. Limb salvage ultimately may be successful in as many as 80% of persons. Individuals must have achieved most of their bone growth to be candidates for limb salvage procedures. Skeletally immature individuals may have a limb salvage operation, referred to as a *rotationplasty,* in which the major portions of the thigh, the tumor, and contaminated knee are resected while preserving the nerve supply (sciatic) to the leg and foot. The proximal tibia is internally fixed to the stump of the proximal femur after it has been rotated 180 degrees. The foot is positioned at a desired spot or direction, allowing the ankle joint to function as a knee joint with the foot supplying the traditional role of the tibial stump in a below-knee amputation.

If an amputation is done, individuals are monitored closely with chest roentgenograms and CT. Pulmonary metastases are surgically resected, and chemotherapy is now a common therapy given both before and after operation, using combinations of chemotherapeutic agents.

Chondrogenic Tumors: Chondrosarcoma

Chondrogenic (cartilage-forming) tumors produce cartilage or **chondroid,** a primitive cartilage or cartilage-like substance. The most common chondrogenic tumor is chondrosarcoma, accounting for 20% of bone tumors.

Chondrosarcoma is a tumor of middle-age and older adults. Most cases of primary chondrosarcoma are found in persons between 50 and 70 years of age. Secondary chondrosarcoma (a chondrosarcoma derived from an **endochondroma**) occurs most frequently in young adults between 20 and 30 years of age. The tumor is found more frequently in men than in women.

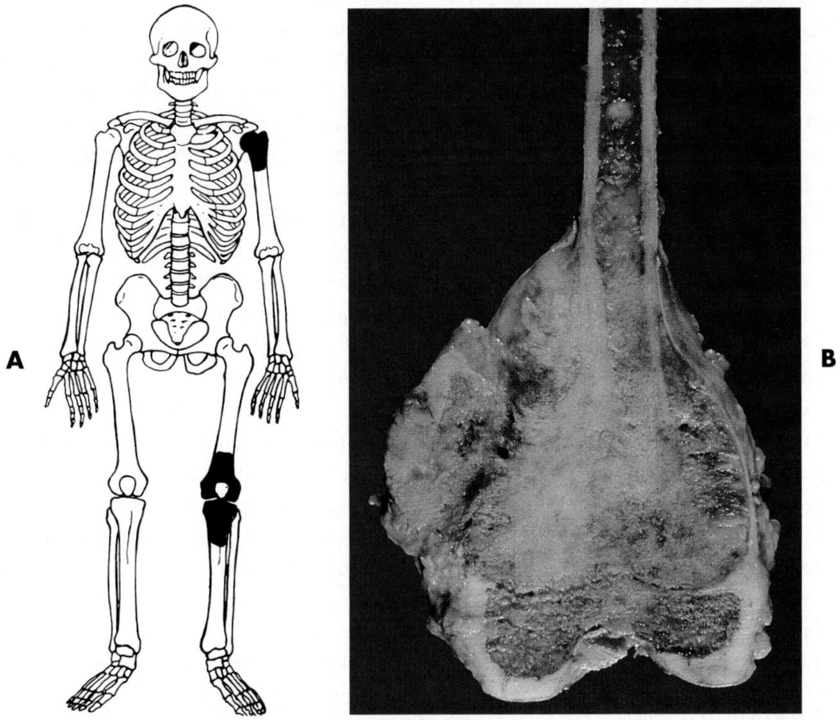

FIG. 41-16 Osteosarcoma. A, Common locations of osteosarcoma. **B,** Femur has a large mass involving the metaphysis of the bone; the tumor has destroyed the cortex, forming a soft tissue component. (From Damjanov I, Linder J, editors: *Anderson's pathology,* ed 10, St Louis, 1996, Mosby.)

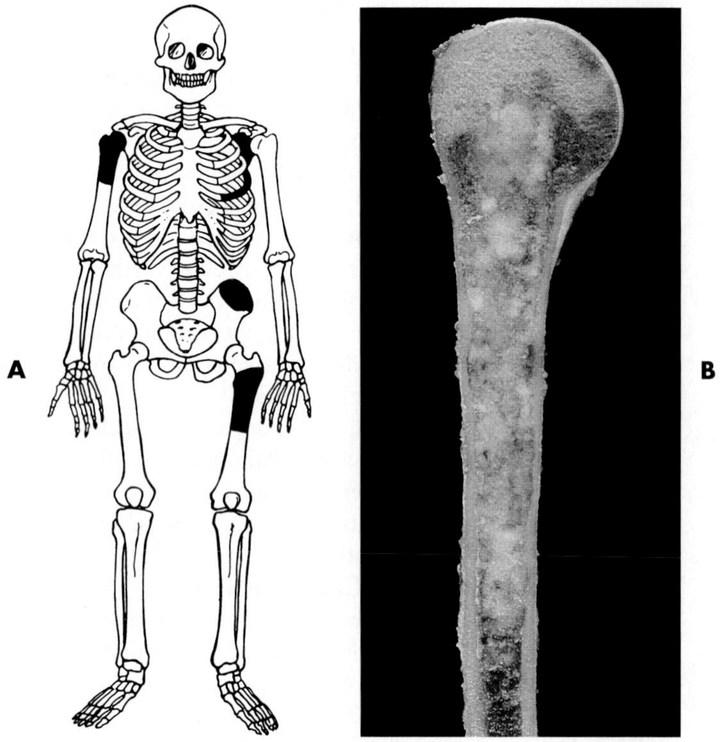

FIG. 41-17 Chondrosarcoma. A, Common locations of chondrosarcoma. **B,** Chondrosarcoma of humerus. (From Damjanov I, Linder J, editors: *Anderson's pathology,* ed 10, St Louis, 1996, Mosby.)

A chondrosarcoma is a large, ill-defined malignant tumor that infiltrates trabeculae in spongy bone. It occurs most often in the metaphysis or diaphysis of long bones, especially the femur, and in the bones of the pelvis (Fig. 41-17). The tumor contains large lobules of hyaline cartilage that are separated by bands of fibrous tissue and anaplastic cells. If located near the end of the bone, the tumor will infiltrate into the joint space. The tumor expands and enlarges the contour of the bone, causes extensive erosion of the cortex, and expands into the soft tissues.

Symptoms associated with the chondrosarcoma have an insidious onset. Local swelling and pain are the usual symptoms that cause the individual to seek treatment. At first the pain is dull and intermittent, and then it gradually intensifies and becomes constant. It may waken the person at night.

Diagnostic studies include radiographs, which must be reviewed carefully for an accurate diagnosis. Biopsy is done at the time of surgery. (If biopsy is done before scheduled surgical incision, seeding of tumor cells could occur.) Sufficient tumor material must be obtained to facilitate an accurate diagnosis.

Surgical excision is generally regarded as the treatment of choice. Many surgically treated individuals demonstrate recurrences, however, so amputation is becoming one treatment of choice. Therefore individuals with tumors located in the limbs have a better prognosis than those with pelvic lesions.

Collagenic Tumors: Fibrosarcoma

Collagenic (collagen-forming) tumors produce fibrous connective tissue. The most typical collagenic tumor is the fibrosarcoma.

Fibrosarcomas represent 4% of the primary malignant bone tumors, with a broad age distribution. They may occur at any age but are most common in adults between 30 and 50 years of age. The incidence is slightly greater in females. Fibrosarcoma may also be a secondary complication of radiation therapy, Paget disease, and long-standing osteomyelitis.

Fibrosarcoma is a solitary tumor that most frequently affects the metaphyseal region of the femur or tibia. The tumor is composed of a firm fibrous mass of tissue that contains collagen, malignant fibroblasts, and occasional osteoclast-like giant cells.

The tumor begins in the marrow cavity of the bone and infiltrates the trabeculae. It demonstrates a permeative growth pattern, destroys the cortex, and extends into the soft tissue. Metastasis to the lung is common.

Symptoms associated with the tumor have an insidious onset, which delays diagnosis. Pain and swelling, the usual symptoms that cause the individual to seek treatment, usually indicate that the tumor has broken through the cortex. Local tenderness, a palpable mass, and limitation of motion also may be present. A pathologic fracture in the affected bone is frequently the reason for seeking medical help. Diagnostic studies include radiographs and MRI.

Radical surgery and amputation are the treatments of choice for fibrosarcoma. Radiation therapy is generally considered ineffective treatment for this tumor.

Myelogenic Tumors

Myelogenic tumors originate from various bone marrow cells. Two types of myelogenic tumors are giant cell tumor and myeloma.

Giant cell tumor. **Giant cell tumor** is the sixth most common of the primary bone tumors, accounting for 4% to 5% of bone tumors. Giant cell tumors have a wide age distribution; however, they are rare in persons younger than 10 years or older than 70 years. Most giant cell tumors are found in persons between 20 and 40 years of age. Unlike most other bone tumors, giant cell tumors affect females more frequently than males.

The giant cell tumor is a solitary, circumscribed tumor that causes extensive bone resorption because of its osteoclastic origin (Fig. 41-18). The tumor is rich in osteoclast-like giant cells and anaplastic stromal cells. It may also contain osteoid, callus, and collagen. The giant cell tumor is located in the center of the epiphysis in the femur, tibia, radius, or humerus. The tumor has a slow, relentless growth rate and is usually contained within the original contour of the affected bone. It may, however, extend into the articular cartilage. When the tumor extends, it is usually covered by periosteum or periosteal bone growth. The tumor also may extend into local soft tissue, but it has a low rate of metastasis to other organs or tissues, although it has a high recurrence rate.

The most common symptoms associated with giant cell tumor are pain, local swelling, and limitation of movement. Diagnostic studies include radiographs, CT, and MRI. Cryosurgery and resection of the tumor with the use of adjuvant polymethylmethacrylate (PMMA) for bone grafts decrease recurrence and are more successful treatments than

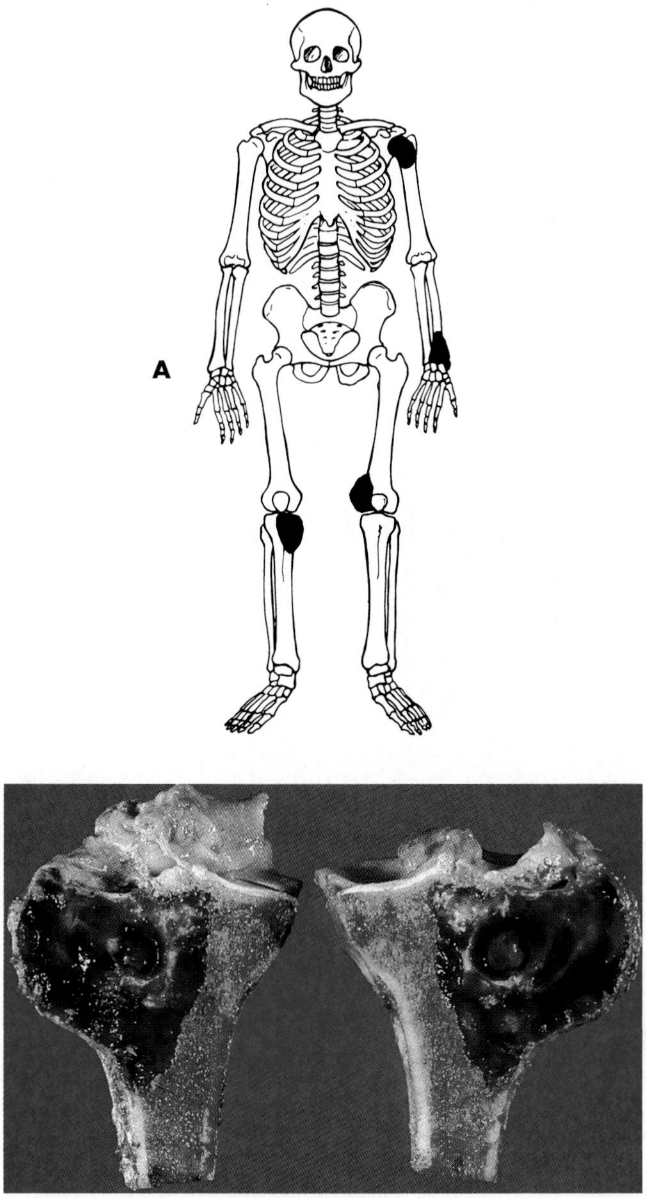

FIG. 41-18 Giant cell tumor of bone. A, Common skeletal locations. **B,** Gross picture of cell tumor of bone (epimetaphysis). (From Damjanov I, Linder J, editors: *Anderson's pathology,* ed 10, St Louis, 1996, Mosby.)

curettage and radiation. Depending on the extent of the tumor and its recurrence, amputation may be necessary.

Myeloma. **Myeloma** is a neoplastic proliferation of immunocytes called *plasma cells.* Myeloma is the most common of the primary malignant tumors of the skeleton and accounts for 27% of bone tumors. The tumor may be solitary or multifocal (known as a *multiple myeloma*). Approximately 15% of the detected myelomas are multiple myelomas (see Chapter 26). Myeloma is common in persons older than 40 years. Males are affected twice as frequently as females, and blacks have a higher incidence than whites.

Myelomas characteristically cause cortical and medullary bone lysis and infiltrate the bone marrow. The most common initial symptom of myeloma is pain, which may be felt in a single bone or the entire skeleton. The usual sites of pain are the lower back, upper spine, pelvis, ribs, and sternum. The pain is initially aching, intermittent, and aggravated by weight bearing. As the disease progresses, pain becomes severe and prolonged. It is common for the individual with myeloma to be treated for a slipped disk or arthritis before the correct diagnosis of myeloma is established. In addition to pain, the individual may complain of weakness, fatigue, weight loss, and anorexia.

Persons with myeloma have a poor prognosis, and the treatment is generally palliative. Pain is relieved with narcotics, and special beds are used to lessen pain and prevent pathologic fractures. Cord decompression may be necessary in persons with spinal myeloma. Radiotherapy and chemotherapy have very limited success.

DISORDERS OF JOINTS

The American College of Rheumatology (ACR) recognizes 13 groups of joint disease (arthropathies). Most of these disorders can be placed into two major categories: noninflammatory joint disease and inflammatory joint disease.

Noninflammatory Joint Disease

Noninflammatory joint disease is differentiated from inflammatory joint disease by (1) the absence of synovial membrane inflammation, (2) the lack of systemic signs and symptoms, and (3) normal synovial fluid. **Degenerative joint disease (osteoarthritis)** is the most prevalent noninflammatory joint disease. Its chief pathologic feature is degeneration and loss of articular cartilage in synovial joints (Fig. 41-19). Degenerative joint disease tends to occur in men and women older than 40 years and becomes more common with increasing age. Although incidence rates are the same in men and women, women are more severely affected.

Medical clinicians are somewhat divided about use of the terms *degenerative joint disease* and *osteoarthritis.* The term *osteoarthrosis* has been used in most recent communications and appears to be the more accepted term in the European literature.

Types of Osteoarthritis

Osteoarthritis (OA) associated with known risk factors, such as joint stress, congenital abnormalities, or joint instability caused by trauma, is referred to as **secondary** (Box 41-1). Idiopathic, formerly **primary,** OA is not associated with known risk factors. Both idiopathic OA and secondary OA have the same pathologic characteristics: (1) erosion of the articular cartilage; (2) sclerosis (thickening and hardening) of bone underneath the cartilage (subchondral sclerosis); and (3) formation of bone spurs, or **osteophytes,** which grossly alter the bony contours and enlarge the joint, possibly even leading to subluxation of the bone from the joint.

Idiopathic OA is the most common type of noninflammatory joint disease, affecting more than 60 million persons in the United States alone. OA is generally distributed throughout the peripheral and central joints of the body and affects adult men more than women until after age 55. The joints most characteristically affected are in the hand, wrist, neck (lower cervical spine), lower back (lumbar spine, sacroiliac),

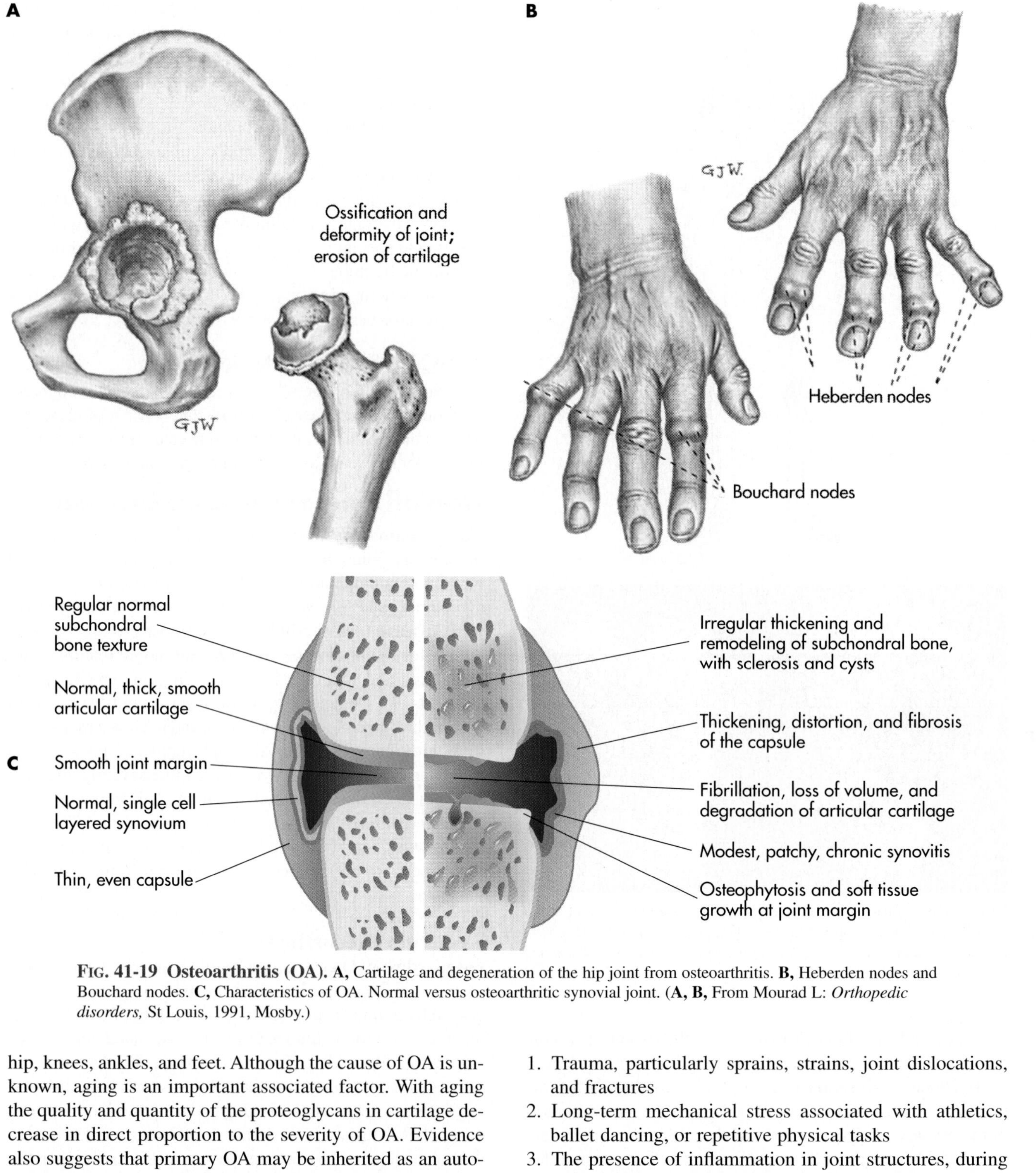

FIG. 41-19 Osteoarthritis (OA). A, Cartilage and degeneration of the hip joint from osteoarthritis. **B,** Heberden nodes and Bouchard nodes. **C,** Characteristics of OA. Normal versus osteoarthritic synovial joint. (**A, B,** From Mourad L: *Orthopedic disorders,* St Louis, 1991, Mosby.)

hip, knees, ankles, and feet. Although the cause of OA is unknown, aging is an important associated factor. With aging the quality and quantity of the proteoglycans in cartilage decrease in direct proportion to the severity of OA. Evidence also suggests that primary OA may be inherited as an autosomal recessive trait, suggesting that defects in one or more of the genes encoding for the structural components of articular cartilage may cause premature cartilage degeneration.

Secondary OA can be caused by any condition that damages cartilage directly; subjects the joint surfaces or underlying bone to chronic, excessive, or abnormal forces; or causes instability in the joint. Specific risk factors include the following:

1. Trauma, particularly sprains, strains, joint dislocations, and fractures
2. Long-term mechanical stress associated with athletics, ballet dancing, or repetitive physical tasks
3. The presence of inflammation in joint structures, during which inflammatory cells release enzymes capable of digesting cartilage cells
4. Joint instability caused by damage to supporting structures, such as the joint capsule, ligaments, or tendons
5. Neurologic disorders (e.g., diabetic neuropathy, Charcot neuropathic joint) in which pain and proprioceptive reflexes are diminished or lost, increasing the tendency for abnormal movement, positioning, or weight bearing

6. Congenital or acquired skeletal deformities
7. Hematologic or endocrine disorders, such as hemophilia, which causes chronic bleeding into the joints, or hyperparathyroidism, which causes bone to lose calcium
8. Drugs (e.g., colchicine, indomethacin, steroids) that stimulate the activity of collagen-digesting enzymes in the synovial membrane

All of these factors alter articular cartilage in some way and accelerate the rate of cartilage loss.

Pathophysiology

The primary defect in primary and secondary OA is loss of articular cartilage. Early in the disease, the articular cartilage loses its glistening appearance, becoming yellow-gray or brownish gray. As the disease progresses, surface areas of the articular cartilage flake off and deeper layers develop longitudinal fissures (fibrillation). The cartilage becomes thin and may be absent over some areas, leaving the underlying bone (subchondral bone) unprotected. Consequently, the unprotected subchondral bone becomes sclerotic (dense and hard). Cysts sometimes develop within the subchondral bone and communicate with the longitudinal fissures in the cartilage. Pressure builds in the cysts until the cystic contents are forced into the synovial cavity, breaking through the articular cartilage on the way. As the articular cartilage erodes, cartilage-coated osteophytes may grow outward from the underlying bone and alter the bone contours and joint anatomy. These spurlike bony projections enlarge until small pieces, called *joint mice,* break off into the synovial cavity. If osteophyte fragments irritate the synovial membrane, synovitis and joint effusion result. The joint capsule also becomes thickened and at times adheres to the deformed underlying bone, which may contribute to the limitation of movement (see Fig. 41-19).

Articular cartilage is probably lost through enzymatic breakdown of the cartilage matrix—the proteoglycans, glycosaminoglycans, and collagen. First, the enzymes break down the macromolecules of proteoglycans, glycosaminoglycans, and collagen into large, diffusible fragments. Then the fragments are taken up by the cartilage cells (chondrocytes) and digested by the cell's own lysosomal enzymes. (Processes of cellular uptake and lysosomal digestion are described in Chapter 1.) The loss of proteoglycans from articular cartilage is a hallmark of the osteoarthritic process.

Enzymatic destruction of articular cartilage begins in the matrix, with destruction of proteoglycans and collagen fibers. Enzymes, particularly stromelysin and acid metalloproteinase, affect proteoglycans by interfering with assembly of the proteoglycan subunit or the proteoglycan aggregate (see Chapter 40); these enzymes are markedly elevated in OA. Changes in the conformation of proteoglycans disrupt the pumping action that regulates movement of water and synovial fluid into and out of the cartilage. Without the regulatory action of the proteoglycan pump, cartilage imbibes too much fluid and becomes less able to withstand the stresses of weight bearing. Also with aging, the proteoglycan content is decreased and water content in cartilage can be increased by as much as 8%, affecting the strength of the cartilage. Persons with OA, even those with fairly extensive cartilage destruction, have elevated levels of proteoglycans or fragments of proteoglycans in their synovial fluid, perhaps indicative of a more pronounced reparative phase. Other studies indicate that cytokines, such as interleukin-1 (see Chapter 40 for discussion of cytokines), may play a major role in cartilage degradation as a result of release and activation of proteolytic

Box 41-1

CLASSIFICATION OF OSTEOARTHRITIS (OA)

CLASSIFICATION BY THE JOINTS INVOLVED

1. Monoarticular, oligoarticular, or polyarticular (generalized)
2. Chief joint site (index joint site) and localization within the joint
   a. Hip (superior pole, medial pole, or concentric)
   b. Knee (medial, lateral, patellofemoral compartments)
   c. Hand (interphalangeal joints or thumb base)
   d. Spine (apophyseal joints or intervertebral disk disease)
   e. Others

CLASSIFICATION INTO PRIMARY AND SECONDARY FORMS OF OA

Primary (idiopathic)

Secondary

1. Indicates that a likely cause can be identified
2. Metabolic causes
   a. Ochronosis
   b. Acromegaly
   c. Hemochromatosis
   d. Calcium crystal deposition
3. Anatomic causes
   a. Slipped femoral epiphysis
   b. Epiphyseal dysplasias
   c. Blount disease
   d. Perthe disease
   e. Congenital dislocation of the hip
   f. Leg length inequality
   g. Hypermobility syndromes
4. Traumatic causes
   a. Major joint trauma
   b. Fracture through a joint or osteonecrosis
   c. Joint surgery (e.g., meniscectomy)
   d. Chronic injury (occupational arthropathies)
5. Inflammatory causes
   a. Any inflammatory arthropathy
   b. Septic arthritis

CLASSIFICATION BY THE PRESENCE OF SPECIFIC FEATURES

1. Inflammatory OA
2. Erosive OA
3. Atrophic or destructive OA
4. OA with chondrocalcinosis
5. Others

Data from Klippel JA, Dieppe PA, editors: *Rheumatology,* ed 2, London, 1998, Mosby.

and collagenolytic enzymes associated with an imbalance of cell responses to growth factor activity.

Enzymes that degrade collagen (i.e., collagenases) probably originate in the chondrocytes or in leukocytes. Collagen breakdown destroys the fibrils that give articular cartilage its tensile strength and exposes the chondrocytes to mechanical stress and enzyme attack. Thus a cycle of destruction begins that involves all the components of articular cartilage—proteoglycans, collagen fibers, and chondrocytes.

Clinical Manifestations

Clinical manifestations of idiopathic or secondary OA typically appear during the fifth or sixth decade of life, although asymptomatic, articular surface changes are common after age 40 years. Pain and stiffness in one or more joints, usually weight bearing or load bearing, are the first symptoms of the disease. Examination usually shows general involvement of both peripheral and central joints. Peripheral joints most often involved are in the hands, wrists, knees, and feet. Central joints most often affected are in the lower cervical spine, lumbosacral spine, shoulders, and hips.

Joint structures are capable of generating a limited number of signs and symptoms. The primary signs and symptoms of joint disease are pain, stiffness, enlargement or swelling, tenderness, limited range of motion, muscle wasting, partial dislocation, and deformity.

Pain and stiffness are the predominant symptoms of OA. They are usually aggravated by weight bearing or use of the joint and relieved by resting the joint. Nocturnal pain is usually not relieved by rest and may be accompanied by paresthesias (numbness, tingling, prickling). Sometimes pain is referred to another part of the body. For example, osteoarthritis of the lumbosacral spine may mimic sciatica, causing severe pain in the back of the thigh along the course of the sciatic nerve. OA in the lower cervical spine may cause brachial neuralgia (pain in the arm) aggravated by movement of the neck. Osteoarthritic conditions in the hip cause pain that may be referred to the lower thigh and knee area.

The actual mechanisms of joint pain are complex and poorly understood, but several explanations are possible. The pain could be caused by articular distention and stretching of the fibrous joint capsule, which has an abundant nerve supply. In addition, inflammation of the joint capsule causes fibrous shrinking, so that movement of the joint in any direction causes painful stretching. Pain also can arise from the subchondral or periarticular bone (Fig. 41-20).

The origin of joint stiffness is unknown. *Joint stiffness* is generally defined as difficulty in initiating joint movement, immobility, or a loss of range of motion. The stiffness usually occurs as joint movement begins, and it dissipates within 30 minutes. Enlargement and bulging of joint contour, commonly described as swelling, may be caused by bone enlargement or the proliferation of osteophytes around the margins of the joint. Swelling also occurs if inflammatory exudate or blood enters the joint cavity, thereby increasing the volume of synovial fluid. This condition, termed **joint effusion,** is caused by (1) the presence of osteophyte fragments in the synovial cavity, (2) drainage of cysts from diseased subchondral bone, or (3) acute trauma to joint structures, resulting in hemorrhage and inflammatory exudation into the synovial cavity.

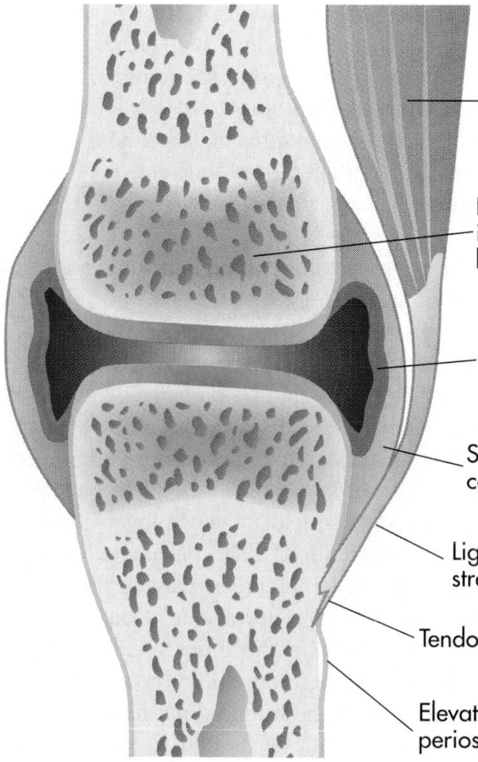

FIG. 41-20 Possible causes of pain in osteoarthritis.

Range of motion is limited to some degree, depending on the extent of cartilage degeneration. Frequently, joint motion is accompanied by sounds of crepitus, creaking, or grating. Hypermobility and subluxation of joints occur in OA secondary to a neurologic disorder.

As OA of the lower extremity progresses, the person may begin to limp noticeably (Fig. 41-21). Having a limp is distressing because it affects the person's independence and ability to do activities of daily living. The affected joint is also more symptomatic after use, such as at the end of the day.[32]

Evaluation and Treatment

Evaluation consists of clinical assessment and radiologic studies, CT scan, arthroscopy, and MRI. Treatment is either conservative or surgical. Conservative treatment includes rest of the involved joint until inflammation, if present, subsides; range of motion to prevent joint capsule contraction; use of a cane, crutches, or walker to decrease weight bearing; weight loss if obesity is present; and analgesic and antiinflammatory drug therapy to reduce swelling and pain. Glucosamine and chondroitin, so-called nutraceuticals, have shown some success in reducing the pain and progression of OA. Intraarticular injection of high-molecular-weight viscosupplements, particularly hyaluronic acid, has also been successful in decreasing knee pain with OA.[33,34] Surgery is used to improve joint movement, correct deformity or malalignment, or create a new joint with artificial implants. There are nearly 250,000 total hip replacements yearly in the United States, most of which are related to OA.

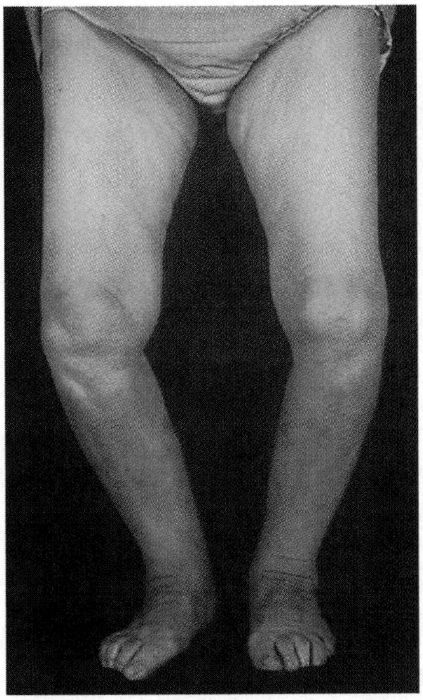

FIG. 41-21 Typical varus deformity of knee osteoarthritis. (From Doherty M: *Color atlas and text of osteoarthritis,* London, 1994, Wolfe.)

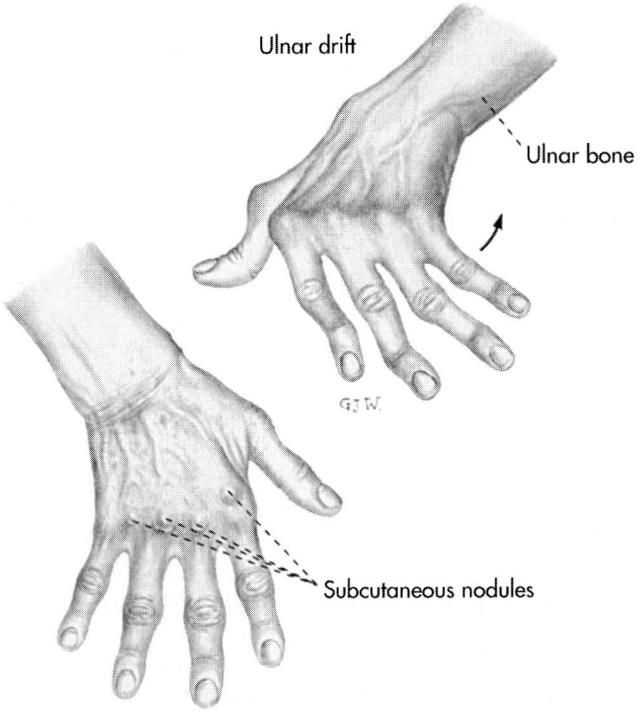

FIG. 41-22 Rheumatoid arthritis of the hand. Note swelling from chronic synovitis of metacarpophalangeal joints, marked ulnar drift, subcutaneous nodules, and subluxation of metacarpophalangeal joints with extension of proximal interphalangeal joints and flexion of distal joints. Note also deformed position of thumb. Hand has wasted appearance. (From Mourad L: *Orthopedic disorders,* St Louis, 1991, Mosby.)

Inflammatory Joint Disease

The second major type of joint disease is **inflammatory joint disease,** commonly termed *arthritis.* Inflammatory joint disease is characterized by inflammatory damage or destruction in the synovial membrane or articular cartilage and by systemic signs of inflammation (fever, leukocytosis, malaise, anorexia, hyperfibrinogenemia).

Inflammatory joint disease can be infectious or noninfectious. In infectious inflammatory joint disease, inflammation is caused by invasion of the joint by bacteria, mycoplasmas, viruses, fungi, or protozoa. These agents can invade the joint through a traumatic wound, surgical incision, or contaminated needle, or they can be delivered by the bloodstream from sites of infection elsewhere in the body, typically bones, heart valves, or blood vessels. In noninfectious inflammatory joint disease, which is the most common form, inflammation is caused by immune reactions or the deposition of crystals of monosodium urate in and around the joint. Rheumatoid arthritis and ankylosing spondylitis are noninfectious inflammatory diseases caused by immune reactions and possibly hypersensitivity reactions;[35] gouty arthritis is a noninfectious inflammatory disease caused by crystal deposition.

Rheumatoid Arthritis

Rheumatoid arthritis (RA) is a systemic autoimmune disease that causes chronic inflammation of connective tissue, primarily in the joints. (Autoimmune disease is described in Chapter 8.) The first joint tissue to be affected is the synovial membrane, which lines the joint cavity (see Chapter 40, Fig. 40-8). Eventually, inflammation may spread to the articular cartilage, fibrous joint capsule, and surrounding ligaments and tendons, causing pain, joint deformity, and loss of function (Fig. 41-22). The joints most commonly affected are in the fingers, feet, wrists, elbows, ankles, and knees, but the shoulders, hips, and cervical spine also may be involved, as well as the tissues of the lungs, heart, kidneys, and skin.

RA affects 1% to 2% of adults and, like most autoimmune diseases, develops most often in women, with a female/male ratio of 3 : 1. The frequency of RA increases from the third decade on, affecting 5% or more of the population ages 70 years and older. Besides inflammation of the joints, RA can cause fever, malaise, rash, lymph node or spleen enlargement, and Raynaud phenomenon (transient lack of circulation to the fingertips and toes).

Despite intensive research, the cause of RA remains obscure. It is probably a combination of genetic, environmental, hormonal, and reproductive factors. RA probably occurs in a genetically susceptible host because of an aberrant immune response to an unidentified antigen. A key genetic element has been localized to the HLA-DR4, HLA-DRB1, and HLA-DP areas of the major histocompatibility complex. Infectious microorganisms that may play a role in the cause of RA include bacteria, mycoplasmas, and viruses (especially Epstein-Barr virus). With long-term or intensive exposure to the antigen, normal antibodies (immunoglobulins [Ig]) become autoantibodies—antibodies that attack host tissues (self-antigens). Because they are usually present in individuals with rheumatoid arthritis, the transformed antibodies are termed **rheumatoid factors (RFs).** The RFs usually consist of two classes of immunoglobulin antibodies (antibodies for IgM and IgG) but occasionally involve antibodies for IgA. Their main antigenic targets are portions of the immunoglobulin molecules. RFs bind with their target self-antigens in blood and synovial membrane, forming immune complexes (antigen-antibody complexes). (See Chapter 6 for a discussion of antigen-antibody binding in the immune response.)

RA has a higher incidence in women, with evidence of hormonal involvement that shows that the disease symptoms lessen during pregnancy and exacerbate in the postpartal period. Evidence for endocrine involvement in RA tissues and cells include (1) presence of androgen and estrogen receptors, (2) high concentrations of biologically active steroids, (3) key enzymes of steroid metabolism, and (4) significant changes of estrogen to androgen ratio. These data strongly suggest that individual immune cells, including synovial macrophages, may behave as steroid-sensitive cells.[36] Most studies on the influence of exogenous hormones and risk of RA have focused on oral contraceptive pills, with inconsistent findings. Fewer studies have been done with hormone replacement; however, new interest has emerged on the role of estrogen and autoimmunity (see What's New? Estradiol-Mediated Alterations of Immune Responses, Chapter 22, p. 769). RA also has seasonal variations, being worse in winter months.

◆ *Pathophysiology*

Cartilage damage in RA is the result of at least three processes:

1. Neutrophils, T cells (particularly CD4 T cells), and other cells in the synovial fluid become activated, degrading the surface layer of articular cartilage.
2. Cytokines, particularly interleukin-1 (IL-1) and tumor necrosis factor–alpha (TNF-α), cause the chondrocytes to attack cartilage.
3. The synovium digests nearby cartilage, releasing inflammatory molecules containing TNF-α and IL-1.

Several types of leukocytes are attracted out of the circulation and to the synovial membrane. The phagocytes of inflammation (neutrophils and macrophages) ingest the immune complexes and, in the process of doing so, release powerful enzymes that degrade synovial tissue and articular cartilage (Fig. 41-23). The immune system's B and T lymphocytes are also activated. The B lymphocytes are stimulated to produce more RFs, and the T lymphocytes produce enzymes that amplify and perpetuate the inflammatory response. Although the precipitating cause is unknown, the newly targeted self-antigens (immunoglobulins) are in relatively constant supply and can thus perpetuate inflammation and the formation of immune complexes indefinitely (Fig. 41-24).

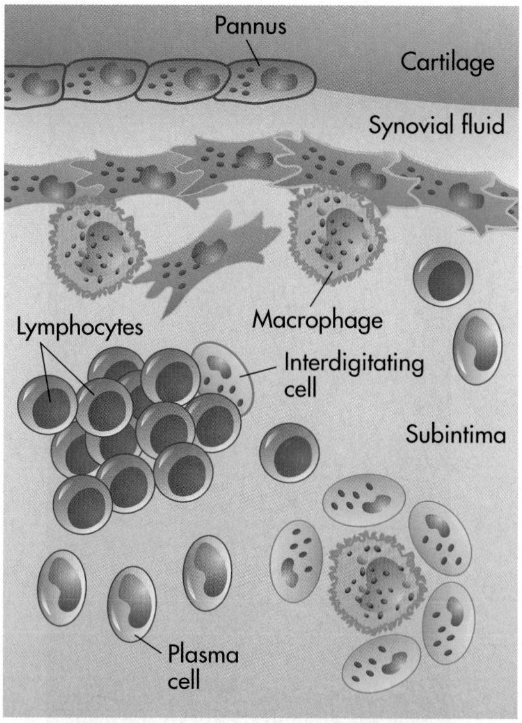

FIG. 41-23 Synovitis. Inflamed synovium showing typical arrangements of macrophages *(red)* and fibroblastic cells.

Inflammatory and immune processes have several damaging effects on the synovial membrane. Along with the swelling caused by leukocyte infiltration, the synovial membrane undergoes hyperplastic thickening as its cells proliferate and enlarge abnormally. As synovial inflammation progresses to involve its blood vessels, small venules become occluded by the hypertrophied endothelial cells, fibrin, platelets, and inflammatory cells, which decrease vascular flow to the synovial tissue. Compromised circulation, coupled with increased metabolic needs because of hypertrophy and hyperplasia, causes hypoxia and metabolic acidosis. Acidosis stimulates the release of hydrolytic enzymes from synovial cells into the surrounding tissue, initiating erosion of the articular cartilage and inflammation in the supporting ligaments and tendons.

Inflammation causes hemorrhage, coagulation, and fibrin deposition on the synovial membrane, in the intracellular matrix, and in the synovial fluid. Over denuded areas of the synovial membrane, fibrin develops into granulation tissue called **pannus.** (Granulation tissue is the tissue produced earliest in the process of healing; see Chapter 7.) Researchers disagree about whether pannus is a cause or an effect of articular cartilage involvement in RA. Some believe that, as RA progresses, pannus extends from the synovial membrane into adjacent articular cartilage and destroys the cartilage. Other researchers think that pannus forms on articular cartilage after the cartilage has been destroyed by inflammation. In any case, pannus formation does not lead to synovial or articular regeneration but rather to formation of scar tissue that immobilizes the joint (Fig. 41-25).

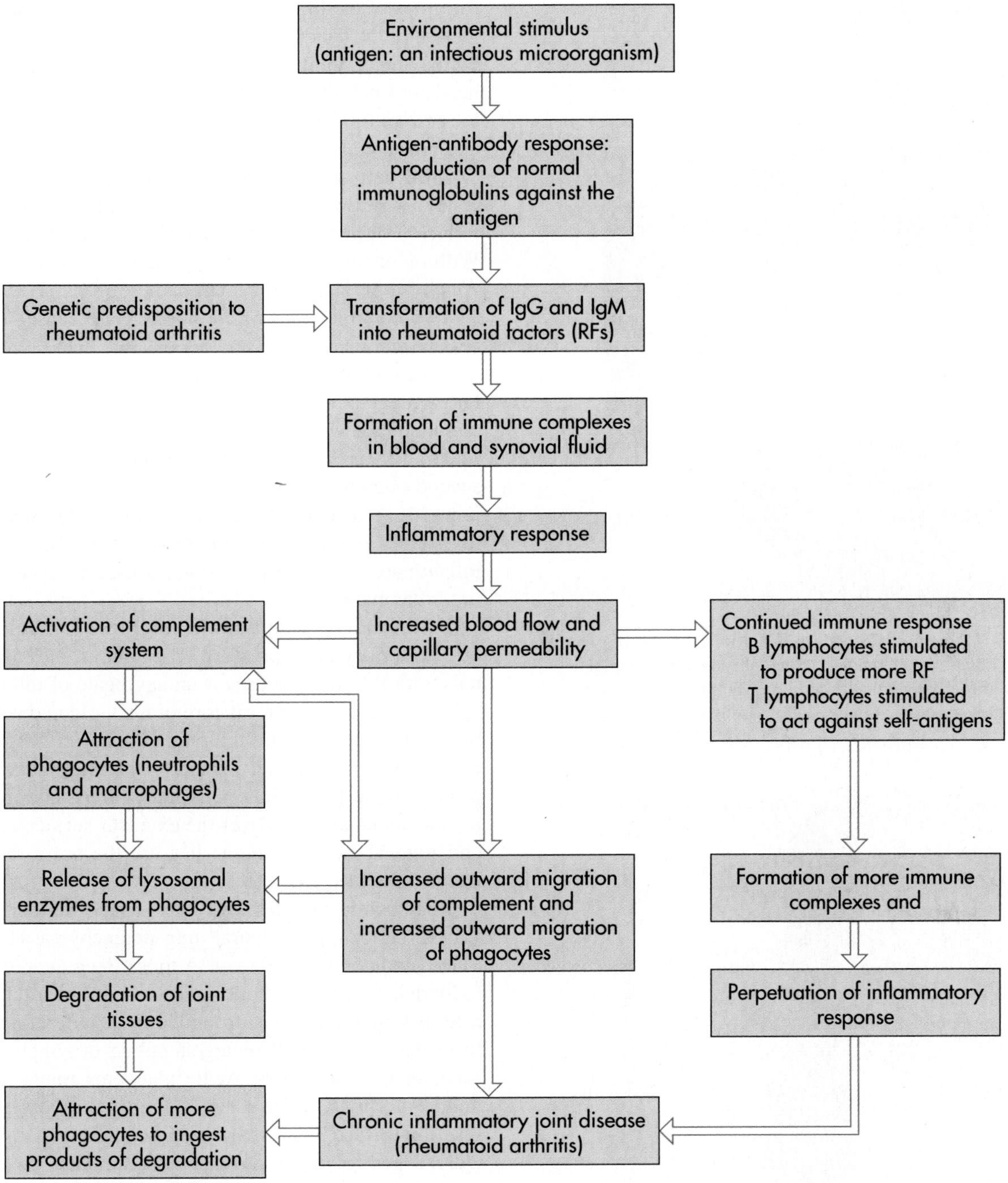

FIG. 41-24 Probable pathogenesis of rheumatoid arthritis. *IgG,* Immunoglobulin G; *IgM,* immunoglobulin M.

Clinical Manifestations

The onset of RA is usually insidious, although as many as 15% of cases have an acute onset. RA begins with general systemic manifestations of inflammation, including fever, fatigue, weakness, anorexia, weight loss, and generalized aching and stiffness. Local manifestations also appear gradually over a period of weeks or months. Typically, the joints become painful, tender, and stiff. Pain early in the disease is caused by pressure from swelling. Later on, the disease pain is caused by sclerosis of subchondral bone and new bone formation. Stiffness usually lasts for about 1 hour after arising in the morning and is thought to be related to synovitis.

Initially the joints most commonly involved are the metacarpophalangeal (MCP) joints, proximal interphalangeal (PIP) joints, and wrists, with later involvement of larger weight-bearing joints.

Joint swelling, which is widespread and symmetric, is caused by increasing amounts of inflammatory exudate (leukocytes, plasma, plasma proteins) in the synovial membrane, hyperplasia of inflamed tissues, and formation of new bone (Fig. 41-26). On palpation, the swollen joint feels warm and the synovial membrane feels "boggy." The skin over the joint may have a ruddy, cyanotic hue and may look thin and shiny.

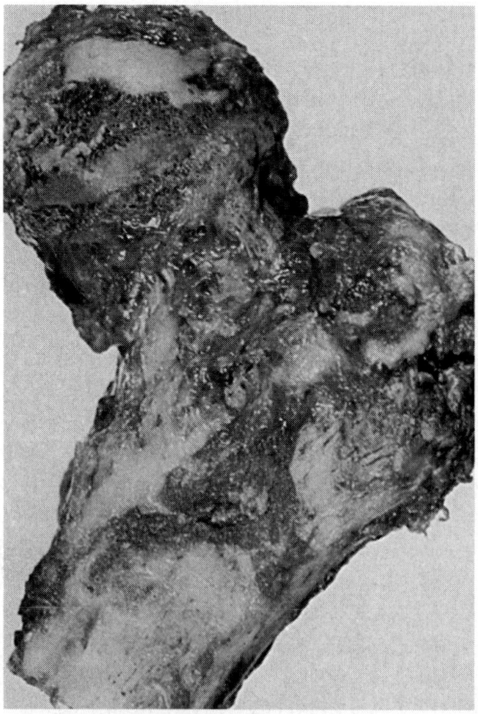

FIG. 41-25 Advanced rheumatoid arthritis involving femur. There is prominent proliferation of synovium and almost complete destruction of overlying articular cartilage. (From Rosai J: *Ackerman's surgical pathology,* ed 8, St Louis, 1996, Mosby.)

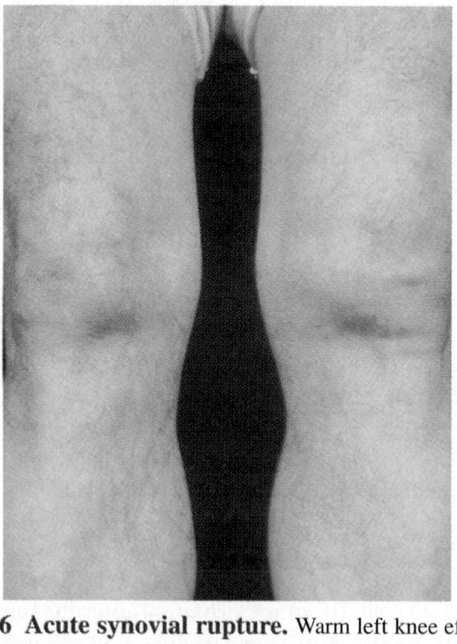

FIG. 41-26 Acute synovial rupture. Warm left knee effusion caused by accompanying synovitis in knee osteoarthritis. Note slight knee swelling. (From Doherty M: *Color atlas and text of osteoarthritis,* London, 1994, Wolfe.)

An inflamed joint may lose some of its mobility. Even mild synovitis can lead to loss of range of motion, which becomes evident after inflammation subsides. Extension becomes limited and is eventually lost if flexion contractures form. Loss of range of motion can progress to permanent deformities of the fingers, toes, and limbs, including ulnar deviation of the hands, boutonnière and swan-neck deformities of the finger joints, plantar subluxation of the metatarsal heads of the foot, and hallux valgus (angulation of the great toe toward the other toes). Flexion contractures of the knees and hips are also common.

Joint deformities cause the physical limitations experienced by persons with RA. Loss of joint motion is quickly followed by secondary atrophy of the surrounding muscles. With secondary muscle atrophy the joint becomes unstable, which further aggravates joint pathology.

Two complications of chronic RA are caused by an excessive amount of inflammatory exudate in the synovial cavity. One complication is the formation of cysts in the articular cartilage or subchondral bone. Occasionally, these cysts communicate with the skin surface (usually the sole of the foot) and can drain through passages called fistulae. The second complication is rupture of a cyst or of the synovial joint itself, usually caused by strenuous physical activity that places excessive pressure on the joint. Rupture releases inflammatory exudate into adjacent tissues, thereby spreading inflammation.

Extrasynovial **rheumatoid nodules,** or swellings, are observed in areas of pressure or trauma in 20% of individuals with RA. Each nodule is an aggregate of inflammatory cells surrounding a central core of fibrinoid and cellular debris. T lymphocytes are the predominant leukocytes in the nodule. B lymphocytes, plasma cells, and phagocytes are found around the periphery. Nodules are found most often in subcutaneous tissue over the extensor surfaces of elbows and fingers. Less common sites are the scalp, back, feet, hands, buttocks, and knees.

Rheumatoid nodules also may invade the skin, cardiac valves, pericardium, pleura, lung parenchyma, and spleen. These nodules are identical to those encountered in some individuals with rheumatic fever and are characterized by central tissue necrosis surrounded by proliferating connective tissue. Also noted are large numbers of lymphocytes and occasional plasma cells. Acute glaucoma may result, with nodules forming on the sclera. Pulmonary involvement may result in diffuse pleuritis or multiple intraparenchymal nodules. Together, the occurrence of pulmonary nodules and pneumoconiosis (chronic inflammation of the lungs from inhalation of dust) creates the syndrome called **Caplan syndrome.** Diffuse pulmonary fibrosis may occur because of immunologically mediated immune complex deposition.

Rheumatoid nodules within the heart may cause valvular deformities, particularly of the aortic valve leaflets Pericardial effusion or other pericardial problems occur in almost 50% of RA patients. Lymphadenopathy of the nodes close to the affected joints may develop. Rheumatoid nodules within the spleen result in splenomegaly. Involvement of blood vessels results in an acute necrotizing vasculitis, characteristic of that noted in other immunologic/inflammatory states. Thromboses of such involved vessels may give rise to myocardial infarctions, cerebrovascular occlusions, mesenteric infarction, kidney damage, and vascular insufficiency in the hands and fingers (Raynaud phenomenon). Vascular changes are noted primarily in individuals receiving steroid therapy; thus there is some concern that the therapy may play a role in initiating these lesions. Changes in skeletal muscle are often noted in the form of nonspecific atrophy secondary to joint dysfunction.

Evaluation and Treatment

Evaluation of RA is by physical examination, roentgenography of the joint, and serologic tests for rheumatoid factor and circulating immune complexes. The American College of Rheumatology lists the following diagnostic criteria for rheumatoid arthritis:

1. Morning stiffness for longer than 1 hour
2. Arthritis of three or more joint areas
3. Arthritis of hand joints
4. Symmetric arthritis
5. Rheumatoid nodules over extensor surfaces or bony prominences
6. Serum rheumatoid factor present in abnormal amounts
7. Radiographic changes

The presence of four or more of the criteria is diagnostic of RA. Criteria 1 through 4 with joint signs or symptoms must be present for 6 weeks.

Treatment is conservative or surgical. Conservative treatment includes rest of the inflamed joint and whole-body rest for several hours daily, use of hot and cold packs, physical therapy, antineoplastic medications, a diet high in calories and vitamins, corticosteroids, antiinflammatory drugs, immunosuppressants, and disease-modifying antirheumatic drugs (DMARDs) taken orally or by injection. Surgical synovectomy may be done early in the disease to decrease inflammatory effusion and remove pannus. Surgery is used to correct deformity or mechanical deficiency in intermediate or late stages of the disease and includes arthrodesis, arthroplasty, or total joint replacement. Recently, there is evidence that total fasting induces a substantial reduction in joint pain, swelling, morning stiffness, and other symptoms in individuals with RA.

WHAT'S NEW? New Therapies for Rheumatoid Arthritis

Treatment for rheumatoid arthritis has rapidly expanded with the introduction of new therapies. Recent pharmaceutical developments are focused on modifying the autoimmune and inflammatory components of RA. Two new agents, leflunomide (Arava) and etanercept (Enbrel), have shown significant promise in relieving RA symptoms. Leflunomide reversibly inhibits an enzyme involved in the autoimmune process, and etanercept competitively inhibits the binding of TNF to TNF receptor sites.

Gene therapy is the latest focus of research. Several preliminary studies have shown success in reducing interleukins and other cytokine levels in synovial fluid. Autologous stem cell transplantation may also be used in the near future.

Some data from Forre O, Haugen M, Hassfeld WG: New treatment possibilities in rheumatoid arthritis, *Scand J Rheumatol* 29(2):73, 2000.

Ankylosing Spondylitis

Ankylosing spondylitis is a chronic, inflammatory joint disease characterized by stiffening and fusion (ankylosis) of the spine and sacroiliac joints. Although inflammation is the primary pathologic process in both RA and ankylosing spondylitis, the two diseases differ in the primary site of inflammation and the end result. In RA the primary site of inflammation is the synovial membrane, resulting in the destruction and instability of synovial joints. In ankylosing spondylitis, the primary pathologic site is the **enthesis** (the point at which ligaments, tendons, and the joint capsule are inserted into bone) and the end results are fibrosis, ossification, and fusion of the joint, primarily the sacroiliac joints and the vertebral column.

The incidence of ankylosing spondylitis is almost equal in men and women, but the disease tends to be more severe in men. In women, ankylosing spondylitis may affect the peripheral joints of the appendicular skeleton rather than the axial skeleton, progress less rapidly, and cause less dramatic spinal changes.

The prevalence of ankylosing spondylitis in the United States is approximately 0.5% to 1% among whites, 3% to 4% among blacks, and 18% to 50% in various nations of American Indians. Worldwide, the disease appears to be most prevalent in whites. The prevalence of ankylosing spondylitis in males is at least 10 times greater than previously considered. It affects men three times as often as women. Many individuals with ankylosing spondylitis remain undiagnosed.

Primary ankylosing spondylitis usually develops in late adolescence or young adulthood, with peak incidence at about 20 years of age. Secondary ankylosing spondylitis affects older age groups and is often associated with other inflammatory diseases (e.g., psoriatic arthropathy, inflammatory bowel disease, Reiter syndrome).

The cause of ankylosing spondylitis is unknown, but the disease is strongly associated with the presence of histocompatibility antigen HLA-B27 on the chromosomes of affected individuals, suggesting a genetic predisposition to the disease. *Klebsiella* infection or other "triggers" may perpetuate the inflammatory response.[37]

Pathophysiology

Ankylosing spondylitis begins with inflammation of fibrocartilage in cartilaginous joints, primarily in the vertebrae. The fibrous tissue of the joint capsule, the cartilage that surrounds intervertebral disks, the entheses, and periosteum are infiltrated by inflammatory cells. As inflammatory cells (chiefly macrophages) and lymphocytes infiltrate and erode bone and fibrocartilage in joint structures, repair begins. Repair of cartilaginous structures begins with the proliferation of fibroblasts. Fibroblasts synthesize and secrete collagen. The collagen becomes organized into fibrous scar tissue that eventually undergoes calcification and ossification. With time, all the cartilaginous structures of the joint are replaced by ossified scar tissue, causing the joint to fuse, or lose flexibility.

Repair of eroded bone begins with osteoblast activation and proliferation. Osteoblasts lay down new bone (callus), which is remodeled and replaced by compact, lamellar bone. Bone repair changes the contour of the bone's surface because the new bone grows outward to form a new enthesis with the end of the eroded ligament. The new enthesis, which forms on top of the old one, is called a **syndesmophyte.** As calcification of the spinal ligaments progresses, the vertebral bodies lose their concave anterior contour and appear square. On radiographs the spine assumes the classic "bamboo spine" appearance of ankylosing spondylitis.

Clinical Manifestations

The most common signs and symptoms of early ankylosing spondylitis are low back pain and stiffness. Typically, the individual with primary disease develops low back pain during the early twenties. The pain is at first insidious but progressively becomes persistent. It is often worse after prolonged rest and is alleviated by physical activity. Early morning stiffness usually accompanies the low back pain, and the individual typically has difficulty sitting up or twisting the spine. Forward flexion, rotation, and lateral flexion of the spine are restricted and painful. Early pain and resultant loss of motion are caused by the underlying inflammation and reflex muscle spasm rather than by soft tissue or bony fusion.

As the disease progresses, the normal convex curve of the lower spine (lumbar lordosis) diminishes and concavity of the upper spine (kyphosis) increases. The individual becomes increasingly stooped. The thoracic spine becomes rounded, the head and neck are held forward on the shoulders, and the hips are flexed (Fig. 41-27).

Inflammation in the tendon insertions of the many costosternal and costovertebral muscles can cause pleuritic chest pain and restricted chest movement. The pain is usually worse on inspiration. Movement in the diaphragm is normal and full. Pressure on the anterior chest wall over the sternum, ribs, and costal cartilages may cause tenderness. Tenderness over the pelvic brim may cause discomfort at night and interfere with sleep because turning onto the iliac crests causes pain. Tenderness over the ischial tuberosities may make sitting on hard seats unbearable. Tenderness in the heels may contribute to a limp or the cautious placement of the feet during walking.

Along with low back pain, many individuals have peripheral joint involvement, uveitis, fibrotic changes in the lungs, cardiomegaly, aortic incompetence, amyloidosis, and Achilles tendinitis. Symptoms may include fatigue, weight loss, low-grade fever, hypochromic anemia, and an increased erythrocyte sedimentation rate.[38]

Evaluation and Treatment

Diagnosis of ankylosing spondylitis is made from the history and physical examination, roentgenograms, and serum analysis for the presence of the histocompatibility antigen HLA-B27. Erythrocyte sedimentation rate is elevated throughout the disease to 10 to 15 mm/hr in males and 10 to 15 mm/hr in females (normal is 0 to 9 mm/hr in males and 0 to 2 mm/hr in females). Alkaline phosphatase levels are frequently elevated. Treatment of individuals with ankylosing spondylitis consists of physical therapy to maintain skeletal mobility and prevent the natural progression of contractures. Prevention of deformity and maintenance of mobility require a continuous program of physical therapy. Exercises are performed several times each day to maintain chest expansion, full extension of the spine, and complete range of motion in the proximal joints.

Nonsteroidal antiinflammatory drugs (NSAIDs) will often provide relief of symptoms within 48 hours.[39] Analgesic medications are prescribed to suppress some of the pain and stiffness and to facilitate exercise. The medications do not prevent disease progression, but they do provide relief from symptoms. Surgical procedures, such as osteotomy, total hip replacement, and cervical spinal fusion, and radiation therapy are sometimes used to provide relief for individuals with end-stage disease or intolerable deformity. Persons should stop smoking to lessen pulmonary problems.

Gout

Gout is a syndrome caused by an inflammatory response to uric acid production or excretion resulting in high levels of uric acid in the blood (hyperuricemia) and in other body flu-

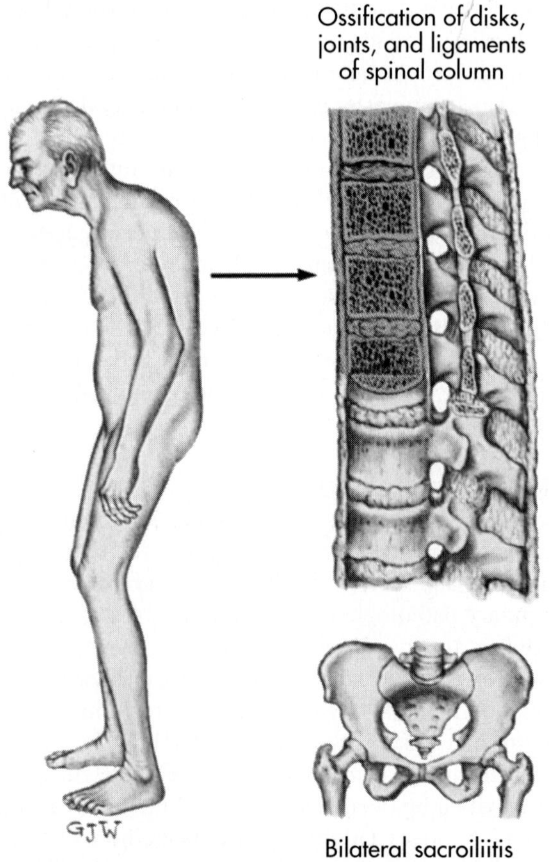

FIG. 41-27 Characteristic posture and sites of ankylosing spondylitis. (From Mourad L: *Orthopedic disorders,* St Louis, 1991, Mosby.)

ids, including synovial fluid. When the uric acid reaches a certain concentration in fluids, it crystallizes, forming insoluble precipitates that are deposited in connective tissues throughout the body. Crystallization in synovial fluid causes acute, painful inflammation of the joint, a condition known as **gouty arthritis.** With time, crystal deposition in subcutaneous tissues causes the formation of small, white nodules, or **tophi,** that are visible through the skin. Crystal aggregates deposited in the kidneys can form urate renal stones and lead to renal failure.

In classic gouty arthritis, monosodium urate crystals form and cause joint inflammation. Pseudogout is caused by the formation of calcium pyrophosphate dihydrate (CPPD) crystals. The effect of either crystal is the same—the onset of an acute inflammatory response (see Chapter 7).

Gout is rare in children and premenopausal women and is uncommon in males younger than 30 years. The peak age of onset in males is between 40 and 50 years, whereas it is somewhat later in females.[40] The risk of developing gouty arthritis is similar in males and females for a particular urate concentration. The plasma urate concentration is an important determinant of the risk of developing gout (Table 41-6).

Uric acid is a weak acid that is ionized at normal body pH and thus occurs in the blood or tissues in the form of urate ion. When ionized, uric acid can form salts with various cations, but 98% of extracellular uric acid is in the form of monosodium urate (uric acid salt). At any time the proportion of uric acid or urate is pH dependent, so the ratio of these two forms varies considerably in urine (Fig. 41-28).

The solubility of urate and uric acid is critical to the development of crystals. Urate is more soluble in plasma, synovial fluid, and urine than in aqueous solutions. The solubility of uric acid in urine rises dramatically as the pH increases above 4. There is little change, however, in the solubility of urate within the normal pH range that exists in the plasma, synovial fluid, and other tissues. Decreasing temperatures cause both urate and uric acid solubility to fall. The pathways of production of uric acid are shown in Fig. 41-29.

Pathophysiology

The pathophysiology of gout is closely linked to purine metabolism (or cellular metabolism of purines) and kidney function. At the cellular level, purines are synthesized to purine nucleotides, which are used in the synthesis of nucleic acids, adenosine triphosphate, cyclic adenosine monophosphate (AMP), and cyclic guanosine monophosphate (GMP). Uric acid is a breakdown product of purine nucleotides (uric acid synthesis and elimination are illustrated in Fig. 41-30). Some individuals with gout have an accelerated rate of purine synthesis accompanied by an overproduction of uric acid. Even with restricted purine consumption, these individuals continue to overproduce uric acid. Other individuals break down purine nucleotides at an accelerated rate that also results in an overproduction of uric acid. Production of uric acid can be the result of an increased turnover of nucleic acids, which is associated with an increased turnover of cells at other body sites. The increased turnover of nucleic acids leads to increased levels of uric acid with a compensatory increase in purine synthesis.

Most uric acid is eliminated from the body through the kidneys. Urate is filtered at the glomerulus and undergoes both reabsorption and excretion within the renal tubules. In primary gout, urate excretion by the kidneys is sluggish. The sluggish excretion may be the result of a decrease in glomerular filtration of urate or an acceleration in urate reabsorption. In addition, monosodium urate crystals are deposited in renal interstitial tissues, causing impaired urine flow. (Kidney function is described in Chapter 34.)

The exact process by which crystals of monosodium urate are deposited in joints and induce gouty arthritis is unknown. However, several mechanisms may be involved, including the following:

Table 41-6 Mean Urate Concentrations by Age and Gender

Characteristic	Mean Urate Levels
Prepuberty	3.5 mg/dl
Males (at puberty)	Steep rise to 5.2 mg/dl
Females (puberty to premenopause)	Slow rise to ≈ 4.0 mg/dl
Females (after menopause)	4.7 mg/dl
Hyperuricemia	
Males	7.0 mg/dl
Females	6.0 mg/dl

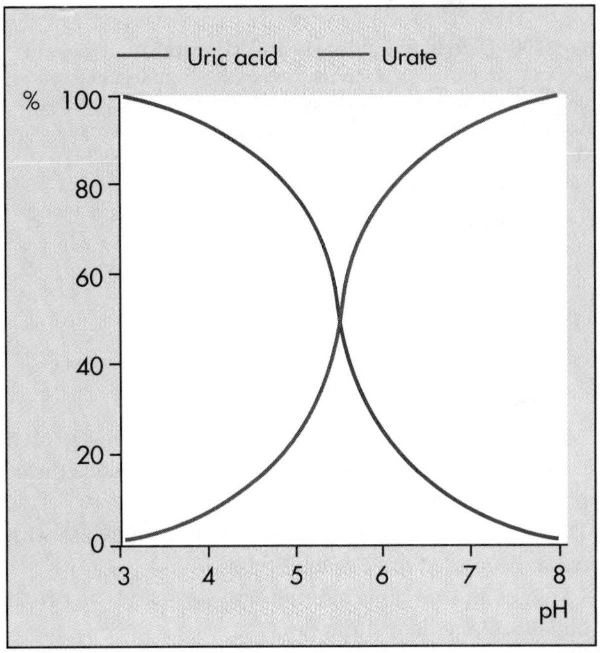

FIG. 41-28 Effect of pH on uric acid and urate equilibrium. At pH 5.7, equal amounts of uric acid and urate are present in the solution. (Redrawn from Klippel JH, Dieppe PA, editors: *Rheumatology,* ed 2, London, 1998, Mosby.)

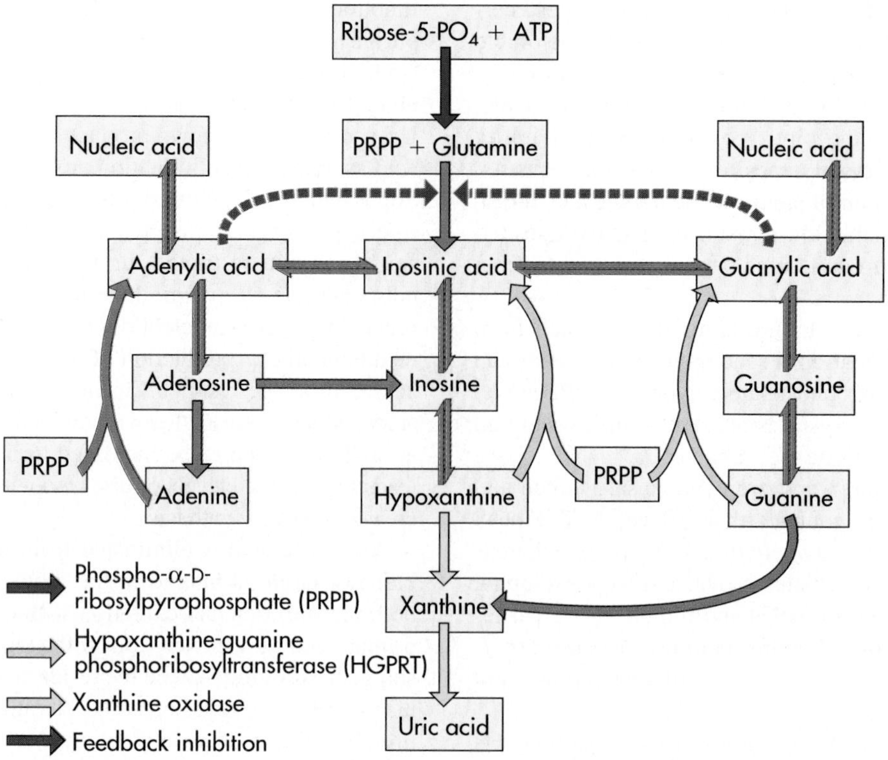

FIG. 41-29 Production of uric acid. The major pathways involved in purine nucleotide synthesis. (Redrawn from Klippel JH, Dieppe PA, editors: *Rheumatology,* ed 2, London, 1998, Mosby.)

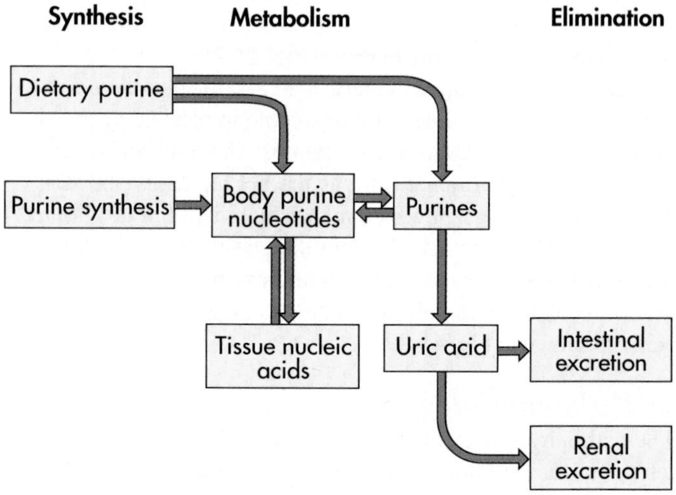

FIG. 41-30 Uric acid synthesis and elimination. Uric acid is derived from purines ingested or synthesized from ingested foods, as well as being recycled following cell breakdown. Uric acid is then eliminated through the kidneys and gastrointestinal tract. (Redrawn from Klippel JH, Dieppe PA, editors: *Rheumatology,* ed 2, London, 1998, Mosby.)

1. Monosodium urate precipitates at the periphery of the body, where lower body temperatures may reduce the solubility of monosodium urate
2. Decreased albumin or glycosaminoglycan levels, which cause decreased urate solubility
3. Changes in ion concentration and decreases of pH that enhance urate deposition
4. Trauma that promotes urate crystal precipitation

The monosodium urate crystals may form in the synovial fluid or in the synovial membrane, cartilage, or other connective tissues in joints and elsewhere, such as in the heart, earlobes, and kidneys. Evidence suggests that an acute attack of gout is the result of the *formation* of crystals rather than the *releasing* of the crystals from connective tissues into the synovial fluid.

Monosodium urate crystals can stimulate and perpetuate the inflammatory response (Fig. 41-31). The presence of the crystals triggers the acute inflammatory response, during which neutrophils are attracted out of the circulation and begin to phagocytize (ingest) the crystals.

Crystals coated with IgG are thought to react with crystallizable fragment (Fc) receptors on the surface of the responding cell (see Fig. 41-31), thereby promoting phagocytosis

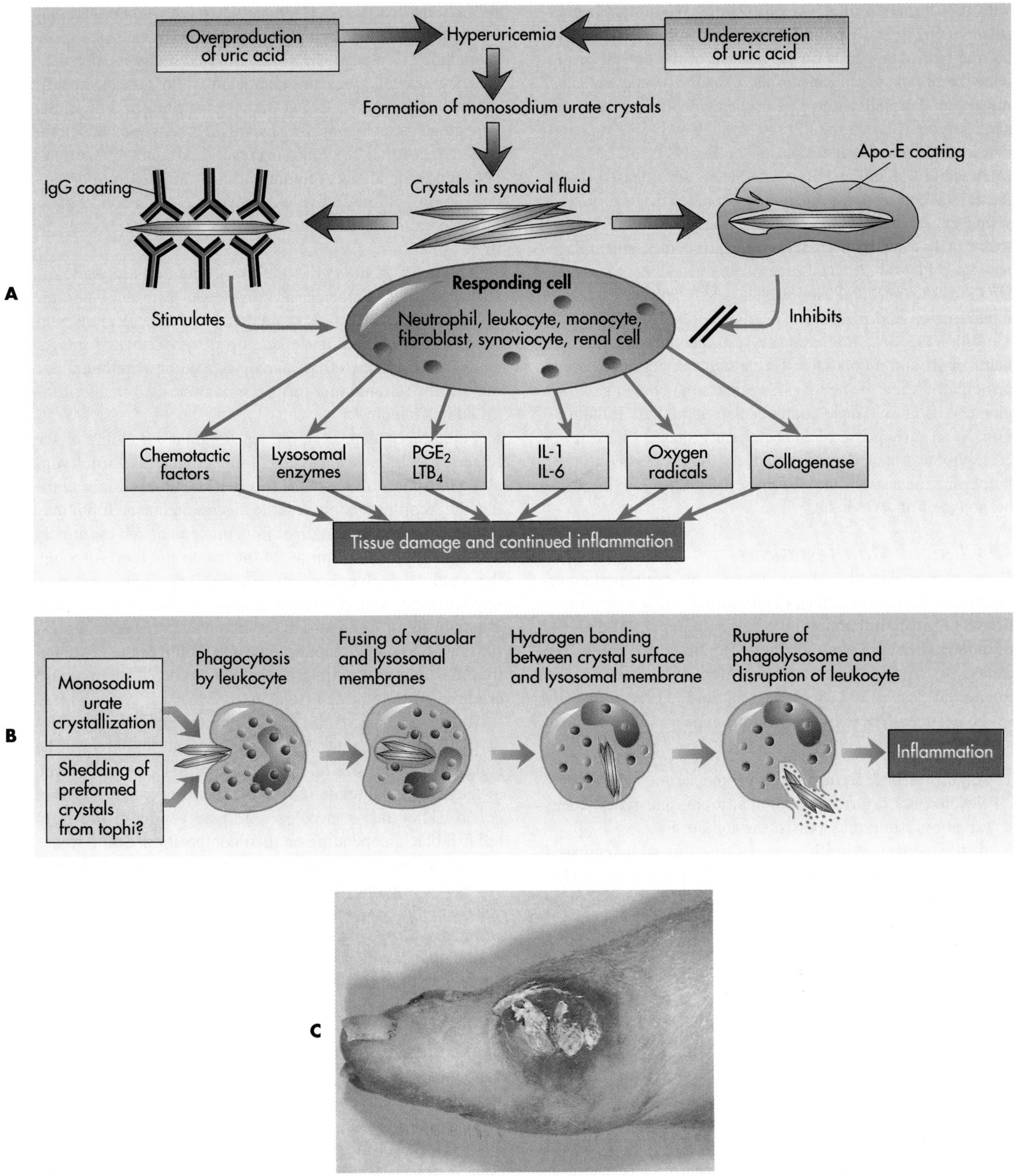

FIG. 41-31 Pathogenesis of acute gouty arthritis. A, Depending on the urate crystal coating, a variety of cells may be stimulated to produce a wide range of inflammatory mediators. **B,** Sequence of events in the production of inflammation response to urate crystals. **C,** Gouty tophus on right foot. (**C,** From Dieppe P et al: *Arthritis and rheumatism in practice,* London, 1991, Gower.)

with the formation of a phagolysosome. When the phagolysosomal enzymes strip the IgG from the surface of the crystal, the hydrogen bands on the surface of the crystal can induce membrane breakdown of the phagolysosome and cause rupture of the cell within.[40] Recent evidence indicates that apolipoprotein-E coating of urate crystals will inhibit phagocytosis and the cellular response (see Fig. 41-31, *A*).

A variety of inflammatory mediators are released during the crystal/cell response, including chemotactic factors, lysosomal enzymes, eicosanoids, prostaglandin E (PGE_2), interleukins (IL-1 and IL-6), reactive oxygen species, and collagenase (see Fig. 41-31, *B*). Some of these mediators stimulate the influx of neutrophils, monocytes, and lymphocytes. (Acute inflammation and phagocytosis are described in Chapter 7.)

Within the joint fluid, urate crystals react particularly with neutrophils and monocytes. Tissue damage begins to occur, principally when the neutrophils release the contents of their phagolysosomes. These contents also perpetuate inflammation. At an early phase of an acute gouty attack, synovial microtophi have been demonstrated. As the process continues, numerous microtophi may be present on the synovial membrane (see Fig. 41-31, *C*).

Clinical Manifestations

Gout is manifested by (1) an increase in serum urate concentration (hyperuricemia), (2) recurrent attacks of monarticular arthritis (inflammation of a single joint), (3) deposits of monosodium urate monohydrate (tophi) in and around the joints, (4) renal disease involving glomerular, tubular, and interstitial tissues and blood vessels, and (5) the formation of renal stones. These manifestations appear in three clinical stages:

1. **Asymptomatic hyperuricemia:** the serum urate level is elevated but arthritic symptoms, tophi, and renal stones are not present; may persist throughout life.
2. **Acute gouty arthritis:** attacks develop with increased serum urate concentrations; tends to occur with sudden or sustained increases of hyperuricemia but can also be triggered by trauma, drugs, and alcohol.
3. **Tophaceous gout:** the third and chronic stage of disease; can begin as early as 3 years or as late as 40 years after the initial attack of gouty arthritis. Progressive inability to excrete uric acid expands the urate pool until urate crystal deposits (tophi) appear in cartilage, synovial membranes, tendons, and soft tissue.

Trauma is the most common aggravating factor. The great toe is subject to chronic strain in walking, and subsequently an acute gout attack may follow long walks. Trauma associated with occupations, such as truck driving, may also precipitate an attack.

Attacks of gouty arthritis occur abruptly, usually in a peripheral joint. The primary symptom is severe pain. Approximately 50% of the initial attacks occur in the metatarsophalangeal joint of the great toe. The other 50% involve the heel, ankle, instep of the foot, knee, wrist, or elbow. The pain is usually noticed at night. Within a few hours the affected joint becomes hot, red, and extremely tender and may be slightly swollen. Lymphangitis and systemic signs of inflammation (leukocytosis, fever, elevated sedimentation rate) are occasionally present. Untreated, mild attacks usually subside in several hours but may persist for 1 or 2 days. Severe attacks may persist for several days or weeks. When the patient recovers, the symptoms resolve completely. Intervals between acute attacks of gouty arthritis are called *intercritical periods.* Some individuals never have a second attack; others experience subsequent attacks 5 to 10 years after the first.

The helix of the ear is the most common site of tophi, which are the characteristic diagnostic lesions of chronic gout. Each tophus consists of a deposit of urate crystals, surrounded by a granuloma made up of mononuclear phagocytes (macrophages) that have developed into epithelial and giant cells. (Granuloma formation is described in and illustrated in Chapter 7.)

Tophaceous deposits produce irregular swellings of the fingers, hands, knees, and feet. Tophi commonly form lumps along the ulnar surface of the forearm, the tibial surface of the leg, the Achilles tendon, and the olecranon bursa. Tophi may produce marked limitation of joint movement and eventually cause grotesque deformities of the hands and feet. Although the tophi themselves are painless, they often cause progressive stiffness and persistent aching of the affected joint. Tophi in the upper extremities may cause nerve compressions such as carpal tunnel syndrome. Tophi in the lower extremities may cause tarsal tunnel syndrome. They may also erode and drain through the skin.

Renal stones are 1000 times more prevalent in individuals with primary gout than in the general population. The stones can be the size of a grain of sand or a piece of gravel, or they can accumulate in massive deposits called *staghorn calculi.* They range in color from pale yellow to brown to reddish black, depending on their composition. Some stones consist of pure monosodium urate; others consist of calcium oxalate or calcium phosphate. Renal stones can form in the collecting tubules, pelvis, or ureters, causing obstruction, dilation, and atrophy of the more proximal tubules and leading eventually to acute renal failure. Stones deposited directly in renal interstitial tissue initiate an inflammatory reaction that leads to chronic renal disease and progressive renal failure.

Treatment

The aims of gout treatment are to terminate the acute gouty attack as promptly as possible, prevent recurring attacks, prevent or reverse complications associated with urate deposits in the joints and kidneys, and prevent formation of kidney stones. Acute gouty arthritis is treated with antiinflammatory drugs. The drugs of choice are nonsteroidal antiinflammatory agents (NSAIDs) and allopurinol. Colchicine is used in individuals unable to tolerate NSAIDs. Hydrocortisone may be injected into the joint to relieve pain. Ice also may relieve some of the inflammation of the joint. Weight bearing on the involved joint is avoided until the acute attack subsides. The individual is put on a low-purine diet, with high fluid intake to increase urinary output. Antihyperuricemic drugs are given to reduce serum urate concentrations.

DISORDERS OF SKELETAL MUSCLE

Muscle weakness and fatigue are common symptoms. In many cases, neural, traumatic, and psychogenic causes provide an adequate explanation for the failure to generate force (weakness) or sustain force (fatigue) seen in myopathies. The pathophysiologic mechanisms in some of the metabolic and inflammatory muscle diseases have been explored, but the cause of many of the myopathies remains obscure. The complex interaction between muscles and nerves affects muscular function as well. Only inherited and acquired disorders of skeletal muscles are discussed here.

Secondary Muscular Dysfunction

Muscular symptoms arise from a variety of causes unrelated to the muscle itself. Secondary muscular phenomena (contracture, stress-related muscle tension, immobility) are common disorders that influence muscular function.

Contractures

Contractures can be pathologic or physiologic. A physiologic muscle contracture occurs in the absence of a muscle action potential in the sarcolemma. Muscle shortening is explained on the basis of failure of the calcium pump in the presence of adenosine triphosphate (ATP). A physiologic contracture is seen in McArdle disease (muscle myophosphorylase deficiency) and malignant hyperthermia. The contracture is usually temporary if the underlying pathology is reversed.

A pathologic contracture is a permanent muscle shortening caused by muscle spasm or weakness. Heel cord (Achilles tendon) contractures are examples of pathologic contractures. They are associated with plentiful ATP and occur in spite of a normal action potential. The most common form of contracture is seen in such conditions as muscular dystrophy (see Chapter 42) and central nervous system (CNS) injury. Contractures also may develop secondary to scar tissue contraction in the flexor tissues of a joint, for example, contracture of burned tissues in the antecubital area of the forearm leading to a flexion contracture.

Stress-Induced Muscle Tension

Abnormally increased muscle tension has been associated with chronic anxiety, as well as a variety of stress-related muscular symptoms, including neck stiffness, back pain, and headache.[41,42] Abnormalities in the CNS, reticular activating system, and autonomic nervous system (ANS) have been implicated. For example, as an individual progressively relaxes, the amplitude of the knee-jerk reflex diminishes. Conversely, individuals with absent reflexes increase tension by such maneuvers as clenching the teeth or hand grip. The underlying pathophysiology may be related to the fact that as a muscle contracts, the muscle spindle is activated. This gamma-feedback system produces a series of impulses that are transmitted to the brain by the sensitive 1A afferent fibers. Unconscious tension is thought to increase the activity of the reticular activating system as well. This influences increasing firing of the efferent loop of the gamma fibers and produces further muscle contraction and increases muscle tension. ANS function that regulates increased blood flow to the muscle during sympathetic activity may be related to increased muscle contraction tension.

Various forms of treatment have been used to reduce the muscle tension associated with stress. Progressive relaxation training, yoga, meditation, and biofeedback are examples of stress reduction therapies. **Biofeedback** uses an integrated electromyogram (EMG) to make recordings from the skin surface. The goal is to teach the individual to control tension that has been functioning maladaptively. It is particularly useful in individuals who have a connection between skeletal muscle tension and pain.[43] **Progressive relaxation training** emphasizes the individual's ability to perceive the difference between tension and relaxation. This technique involves sequential tensing and a relaxing environment. The individual is taught to practice this routine daily, often with the use of audiotaped instructions. By teaching the individual to recognize excessive contraction of skeletal muscle, one hopes to enhance the ability to relax specific muscle groups to relieve tension and thus reduce CNS arousal, as well as ANS arousal.

Fibromyalgia

Fibromyalgia is a chronic musculoskeletal syndrome characterized by diffuse pain, fatigue, and tender points. Increased sensitivity to touch (i.e., tender points), the absence of systemic or localized inflammation, and fatigue and sleep disturbances are common. Because the symptoms are vague, fibromyalgia has often been misdiagnosed or completely dismissed by clinicians. A common misdiagnosis has been chronic fatigue syndrome. From 80% to 90% of individuals affected are women, and the peak age is 30 to 50 years. Although the incidence is unknown, the prevalence is reported to be 2% and increases with age.[44] It is more common than RA, but its cause is still unknown.[45]

The etiology of fibromyalgia has been debated for more than a century. It is unlikely that it is caused by a single factor. The most common precipitating factors include the following:

- Flulike viral illness
- Chronic fatigue syndrome
- Human immunodeficiency virus (HIV) infection
- Lyme disease
- Usually unspecified
- Physical trauma
- Emotional trauma
- Medications, especially steroid withdrawal

Certain rheumatic diseases, such as RA or systemic lupus erythematosus, may coexist if not initially manifest with fibromyalgia. In addition, fibromyalgia may overlap with myofascial pain syndromes (Table 41-7).[44]

Pathophysiology

It is unproved but long suspected that muscle is the end organ responsible for the pain and fatigue. Although studies are small, they have documented more metabolic alterations—lower ATP, lower adenosine diphosphate (ADP), and higher concentrations of AMP—and more alterations in the number of capillaries and fiber area in individuals with fibromyalgia than in study control subjects.[44] Unfortunately, these studies have not proved that these alterations are the result of muscle oxygen problems or reduced physical activity. Most studies have demonstrated that increased muscle tenderness in fibromyalgia is a result of generalized pain intolerance, possibly related to functional abnormalities within the CNS (Fig. 41-32).

It is significant that blood flow in the left and right thalamus is lower in individuals with fibromyalgia than in controls.[46] The thalamus and caudate nucleus are involved in pain perception. A chronic stress response may be involved in producing lower peripheral (e.g., at the muscle site) and central levels of serotonin and involves growth hormone and the classic stress pathway—the hypothalamic-pituitary-adrenal axis (see Chapters 9 and 13). Individuals with fibromyalgia may have an adrenal hyporesponsiveness. Studies of levels of substance P showed a minimal relationship with tenderness on examination.[44]

Table 41-7 Comparison of Fibromyalgia and Myofascial Pain Syndromes

Variable	Fibromyalgia	Myofascial Pain
Location	Generalized	Regional
Examination	Tender points	Trigger points
Response to local therapy	Not sustained	Curative
Gender	Female/male ratio: 10:1	Equal or unknown
Systemic features	Characteristic	Unknown

Clinical Manifestations

The prominent symptom of fibromyalgia is diffuse, chronic pain. The locations of nine pairs of tender points for diagnostic classification of fibromyalgia are shown in Fig. 41-33. The pain often begins in one location, especially the neck and shoulders, but then becomes more generalized. People describe the pain as *burning* or *gnawing*. Fatigue is profound. The effect on everyday life is considerable.[47] Some investigators have found that the majority of women experienced pain and fatigue for more than 90% of their time awake.[47] Fatigue is most notable when arising from sleep and during the midafternoon. Headaches, symptoms of irritable bowel syndrome, and excess sensitivity to cold (Raynaud-like) are reported in 50% of individuals.

Almost 25% of individuals seek psychologic support for depression. Anxiety, particularly in regard to their diagnosis and future, is almost universal.[44] Again, the only reliable finding on examination is the presence of multiple tender points.

Evaluation and Treatment

Because the manifestations of chronic, generalized pain and fatigue are present in many musculoskeletal (e.g., rheumatic) disorders, these disorders should be considered in the diagnosis of fibromyalgia (Tables 41-8 and 41-9).

No one regimen of medication has proved successful for fibromyalgia. Medications that improve sleep may be helpful. Antiinflammatory medications have been used despite the

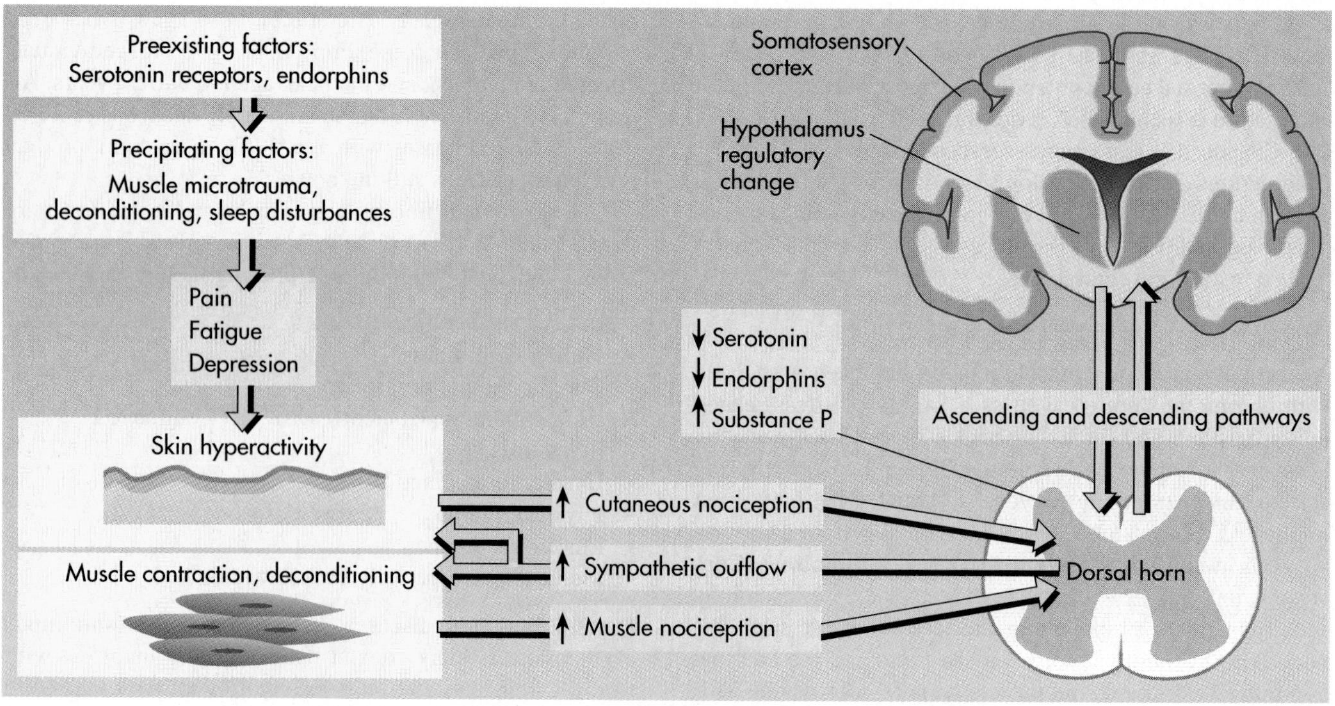

FIG. 41-32 Theoretic pathophysiologic model of fibromyalgia.

fact there is no evidence of tissue inflammation. These medications have not been effective. Certain CNS-active medications, most notably tricyclics, amitriptyline, and cyclobenzaprine, were significantly better than placebos in controlled trials.[44] Amitriptyline significantly improved pain, morning stiffness, and sleep but not tender points. However, these successes occurred in only 25% to 45% of individuals.[44] One of the most important aspects of treatment is education and reassurance (Box 41-2).

Disuse Atrophy

The term **disuse atrophy** describes the pathologic reduction in normal size of muscle fibers after prolonged inactivity from bed rest, trauma (casting), or local nerve damage. The effects of muscular deconditioning associated with lack of physical activity may be apparent in a matter of days. The normal individual on bed rest loses muscle strength from baseline levels at a rate of 3% per day. Bed rest also is associated with cardiovascular, skeletal, and other organ system changes.

Measures to prevent atrophy include frequent forceful isometric muscle contractions and passive lengthening exercises. If reuse is not restored within 1 year, regeneration of muscle fibers becomes impaired.

Table 41-8 Differential Diagnosis of Fibromyalgia

Differential Diagnosis	Helpful Differential Features
Rheumatoid arthritis*	Synovitis, serologic tests, elevated erythrocyte sedimentation rate (ESR)
Systemic lupus erythematosus*	Dermatitis, serositis (renal, central nervous system, etc.)
Polymyalgia rheumatica*	Elevated ESR, elderly persons, response to corticosteroids
Myositis	Increased muscle enzymes, weakness more than pain
Hypothyroidism*	Abnormal thyroid function tests
Neuropathies	Clinical and electrophysiologic evidence of neuropathy

Data from Klippel JH, Dieppe PA, editors: *Rheumatology,* ed 2, London, 1998, Mosby.

*Fibromyalgia may also more commonly coexist with these conditions.

Muscle Membrane Abnormalities

Two defects of the muscle membrane (plasma membrane of the muscle fiber) have been linked to clinical syndromes: the

Table 41-9 Concomitant Conditions with Fibromyalgia

Concomitant Condition	Relationship to Fibromyalgia
Depression	Present in 25%-60% of fibromyalgia cases
Irritable bowel	Present in 50%-80% of fibromyalgia cases
Migraine	Present in 50% of fibromyalgia cases
Chronic fatigue syndrome (CFS)	70% of CFS cases meet criteria for fibromyalgia
Myofascial pain	May be a localized form of fibromyalgia

Data from Klippel JH, Dieppe PA, editors: *Rheumatology,* ed 2, London, 1998, Mosby.

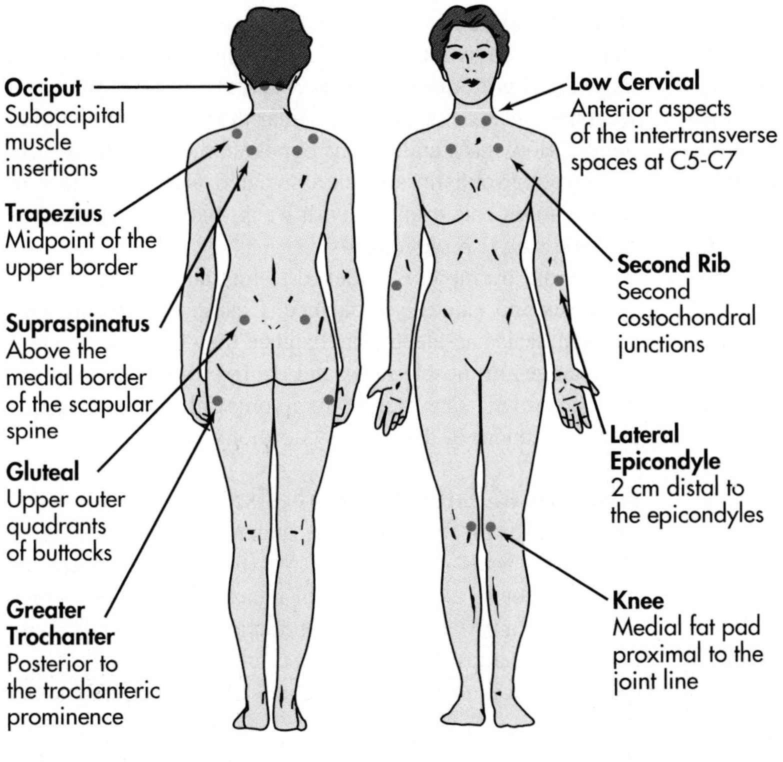

FIG. 41-33 Location of specific tender points for diagnostic classification of fibromyalgia. (Redrawn from Freundlich B, Leventhal L: The fibromyalgia syndrome. In Schumacher HR Jr, Klippel JH, Koopman WJ, editors: *Primer on the rheumatic diseases,* ed 11, Atlanta, 1997, Arthritis Foundation. Copyright © 1997. Reprinted with permission of the Arthritis Foundation, 1330 W. Peachtree St., Atlanta, GA 30309.)

Box 41-2

EDUCATION AND REASSURANCE FOR INDIVIDUALS WITH FIBROMYALGIA

Stress that the illness is real, not imagined.
Explain that fibromyalgia is probably not caused by infection.
Explain that fibromyalgia is not a deforming or deteriorating condition.
Explain that fibromyalgia is neither life-threatening nor markedly debilitating, although it is an irritating presence.
Discuss the role of sleep disturbances and the relationship of neurohormones to pain, fatigue, abnormal sleep, and mood.
Reassure that although the cause is unknown, some information is known about the physiologic changes responsible for the symptoms.
Use muscle "spasms" and, perhaps, low muscle blood flow to lay the groundwork for exercise recommendations.
Assist individual to use aerobic exercise to reduce stress and increase rapid eye movement (REM) sleep.

hyperexcitable membrane seen in the myotonic disorders and the intermittently unresponsive membrane seen in the periodic paralyses. Although these are infrequent disorders, research into the pathologic processes has led to an improved understanding of the cell membrane.

Myotonia

Myotonia is a delayed relaxation after such voluntary muscle contractions as grip, eye closure, or muscle percussion. The distinctive "dive-bomber" noise, audible on needle EMG, is caused by the prolonged depolarization of the muscle membrane. Because the depolarization is not terminated by neuromuscular blocking agents, such as curare, the abnormality has been localized at the muscle membrane; the basic defect is due to ion channel dysfunction.[48] (These structures are described in Chapter 40.)

Myotonia can be reproduced by removing extracellular chloride, thus reducing chloride conductance across the plasma membrane. The delicate balance in which sodium diffuses into the intracellular fluid, potassium diffuses out of the intracellular fluid, and chloride is in flux is thus interrupted. Because the normal diffusion processes (described in Chapter 3) stabilize the membrane, the shift in chloride ions is thought to increase membrane excitability. The chloride abnormality may explain the resting membrane hyperexcitability, but it does not explain the delayed relaxation present in myotonia and has not been detected in human myotonia.

Myotonia is seen in several disorders: myotonia congenita, paramyotonia congenita, myotonic muscular dystrophy, and some forms of periodic paralysis. Most are inherited disorders and are mild in symptomatology, with the exception of myotonic muscular dystrophy (see p. 1424). Myotonia is treated by drugs that reduce muscle fiber excitability, such as procaine, procainamide, phenytoin, and quinine preparations. Recent treatments include acetazolamide, a carbonic anhydrase inhibitor, and verapamil, a calcium channel blocker.

Periodic Paralysis

During an attack of **periodic paralysis,** the muscle membrane is unresponsive to neural stimuli and the resting membrane potential is reduced from -90 to -45 mV. Periodic paralysis is triggered by exercise and any process or medication that increases serum potassium. The disorder is often inherited in an autosomal dominant pattern, although it can be seen in hyperthyroidism.

The paralysis, which leaves the individual flaccid and weak, does not affect the respiratory muscles. Many individuals have myotonia present on examination. In most cases the weakness is accompanied by a change in serum potassium, although in some individuals the change may be negligible. Cardiac dysrhythmias have been present during attacks. Although the biochemical defect remains unknown, changes in the muscle membrane and sarcoplasmic reticulum have been described.

Hypokalemic periodic paralysis is triggered by high-carbohydrate meals, prolonged bed rest, or emotional stress. (The effect of potassium on the resting membrane potential is discussed in Chapter 3.) Glucose and insulin infusions and oral potassium loading are used as provocative tests; oral and intravenous potassium can relieve acute attacks. Treatment includes thiazides, diuretics, and a high-salt diet. Acetazolamide and a low-salt diet are useful for long-term therapy.

Metabolic Muscle Diseases

Disorders in muscle metabolism can be caused by endocrine abnormalities or diseases of energy metabolism, such as glycogen storage disease, enzyme deficiencies, and abnormalities in lipid metabolism and mitochondrial function.

Endocrine Disorders

Often the systemic effects of hormonal imbalance overshadow the individual's muscular symptoms. For example, individuals with thyrotoxicosis may have signs of proximal weakness, paresis of the extraocular muscles (exophthalmic ophthalmoplegia), and, rarely, hypokalemic periodic paralysis. Hypothyroidism is often associated with a decrease in muscle mass and strength, with weak, flabby skeletal muscles and sluggish movements.

Thyroid hormone is believed to regulate muscle protein synthesis and electrolyte balance. Changes in muscle protein synthesis and electrolyte balance may therefore explain the changes in muscle mass and contractility seen in endocrine disorders. The muscle symptoms subside with appropriate treatment of the primary hormonal disorder.

Diseases of Energy Metabolism

Muscle relies on carbohydrates, such as glycogen and lipids (free fatty acids), for energy. When stored glycogen or lipids cannot be used because of a lack of the enzyme necessary to convert energy for contraction, the individual experiences cramps, fatigue, and exercise intolerance. Disorders of muscle metabolism can be self-limiting, such as is

A 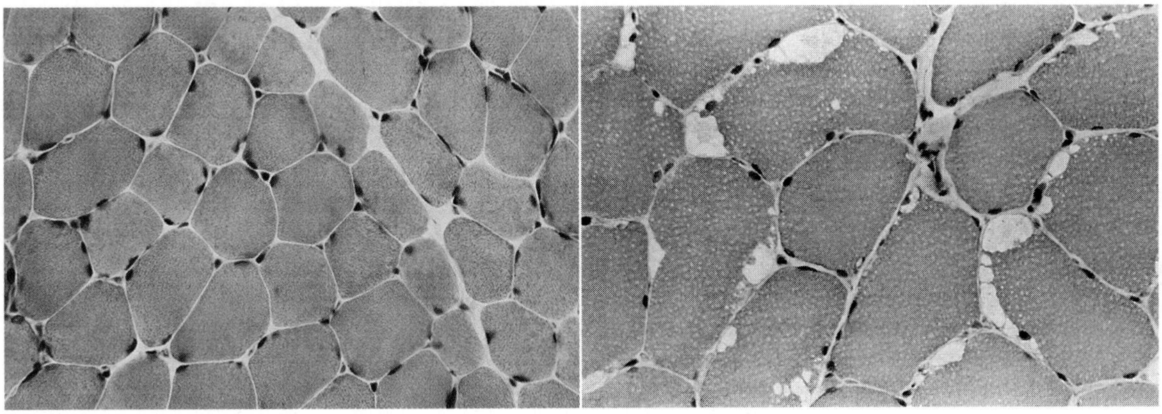 B

FIG. 41-34 McArdle disease. A, Normal muscle fibers. **B,** McArdle disease. Note the (white) peripheral vacuoles. (From Damjanov I, Linder J, editors: *Anderson's pathology,* ed 10, St Louis, 1996, Mosby.)

seen in McArdle disease and some lipid disorders, or cause widespread irreparable muscle destruction, as in acid maltase deficiency.

McArdle Disease

McArdle disease, or myophosphorylase deficiency, was the first myopathy in which a single enzyme defect was identified (Fig. 41-34). Although it is rare, more than 110 cases have been reported from one clinic alone. Individuals with McArdle disease lack muscle phosphorylase, which is responsible for the breakdown of glycogen in muscle. Normally, after the body uses the short-term ATP and phosphocreatine stores, intramuscular lactic acid accumulates as glycogen is used (see Chapter 40). The individual with McArdle disease is not able to break down glycogen or produce lactic acid.

The altered energy production manifests itself in exercise intolerance, fatigue, and painful muscle cramps. When exercise is carried to an extreme, painful muscle contracture and myoglobinuria develop. Some individuals describe a "second wind" phenomenon, in which exercise tolerance increases if they slow their pace once the initial sensation of fatigue commences. This may be caused by the use of free fatty acids as a secondary source of energy. As the disease progresses, some individuals have pronounced muscle weakness and wasting. Other organs are not involved because the absence of phosphorylase is limited to muscle. Generally, individuals with McArdle disease learn to adapt their daily routine to avoid muscle symptoms. Usually the diagnosis of McArdle disease is made by the histochemical evaluation of myophosphorylase activity in frozen sections. There is no staining of myofibrils in affected individuals.

Acid Maltase Deficiency

Acid maltase deficiency is an uncommon glycogen storage disease associated with an accumulation of glycogen in the lysosomes of muscle cells and the cells of other tissues. The usual pathways of glycogen degradation are preserved. The absence of the enzyme acid maltase is responsible for the abnormality in glycogen metabolism, although the exact mechanism is unknown. It is an autosomal recessive disorder, with the gene located on the long arm of chromosome 17.

The infantile form is called **Pompe disease** and is recognized shortly after birth by hypotonia; dysreflexia; and an enlarged heart, tongue, and liver. Hypertrophy of these tissues is thought to be the result of glycogen deposition. Children die of cardiac or respiratory failure within 1 year of diagnosis. The adult variety becomes evident subacutely. The muscular symptoms resemble those of muscular dystrophy or polymyositis (see p. 1423). A distinguishing feature in adults may be the presence of severe respiratory muscle weakness.

Myoadenylate Deaminase Deficiency

An enzyme deficiency that produces changes in skeletal muscle and is associated with exercise intolerance is **myoadenylate deaminase deficiency (MDD).** Because these individuals lack myoadenylate deaminase, they have a poor capacity for sustained energy production. Myoadenylate deaminase is the catalytic enzyme that forms phosphocreatine and ATP during exercise through a metabolic pathway that binds the purine and phosphate molecules that constitute ATP. Persons with MDD differ from those with McArdle disease in that, during the ischemic exercise test, lactate production is normal when ATP and phosphocreatine are synthesized. The enzyme defect has been reported to be common, but in practice it may rarely be recognized as a cause of exercise intolerance.

Lipid Deficiencies

Disorders of lipid metabolism are uncommon but account for severe changes in muscle metabolism. The lipid content of muscle cells consists of the free fatty acids, which are oxidized in the mitochondria. These acids require carnitine and the enzyme carnitine palmityl transferase (CPT) to transport metabolic by-products and energy to the myofibrils. Individuals with CPT deficiency have mild muscular symptoms but can experience bouts of renal failure caused by myoglobinuria. Individuals with a deficiency of carnitine alone have progressive muscle weakness and can experience sudden exacerbations.

Measuring the CPT and carnitine content in muscle aids in the diagnosis. Cells in the muscle biopsy show vacuoles and lipid deposits. Treatments with riboflavin, medium-chain triglycerides, oral carnitine, and prednisone have been suggested.

Inflammatory Muscle Diseases: Myositis

Viral, Bacterial, and Parasitic Myositis

Viral, bacterial, and parasitic infections of varying severity are known to produce inflammatory changes in skeletal muscle, a group of conditions collectively described by the term **myositis.** In tuberculosis and sarcoidosis, chronic inflammatory changes and granulomas are found in muscle, as well as in other affected tissues. In trichinosis, *Trichinella* larvae reside in infected pork and, after ingestion, migrate to the intestinal mucosa and from there to the lymphatics. Symptoms include severe pain, rash, and muscle stiffness. Treatment includes administration of corticosteroids, prednisone, and the antiparasitic agent thiabendazole. Toxoplasmosis, a common parasitic infection, is also associated with a generalized polymyositis that responds rapidly to therapy.

In the tropics, more prevalent disorders include bacterial infections with *Staphylococcus aureus* and parasites such as cysticercus, the larva of the tapeworm *Taenia solium.* Viral infections can be associated with an acute myositis. Muscle pain, tenderness, signs of inflammation, and CK elevation are common manifestations of viral myositis. The self-limiting symptoms of muscle aches and pains during a bout of influenza may actually be a subacute form of viral myopathy.

Polymyositis and Dermatomyositis

Polymyositis (generalized muscle inflammation) and **dermatomyositis** (polymyositis accompanied by skin lesions) are the most common inflammatory muscle diseases requiring long-term care. Prevalence rates may be about 6 per 1,000,000 persons.

Pathophysiology

Polymyositis and dermatomyositis are characterized by inflammation of connective tissue and muscle fibers that presumably causes the extensive necrosis and destruction of muscle fibers. The agent that causes the muscle inflammation has not been identified, but abnormalities in the immune system have been implicated (Fig. 41-35). This family of diseases is now designated as autoimmune because of the presence of autoantibodies in the serum of many individuals. Studies have shown that the inflammatory cells that surround the perimysial and perivascular sites are selectively enriched in B cells and helper T cells in dermatomyositis. There is less vascular involvement in polymyositis, and most of the inflammatory cells, including B cells, T cells, and macrophages, surround the muscle fibers and fascicles.

Clinical Manifestations

The acute symptoms include many of those seen in any inflammatory process: malaise, fever, muscle swelling, pain and tenderness, lethargy, and listlessness. Both illnesses are usually associated with a symmetric proximal muscle weakness and initially can be confused with other myopathies. A thorough evaluation is required to exclude other disorders. Clinical features common in both polymyositis and dermatomyositis are dysphagia, reduced esophageal motility, vasculitis, Raynaud phenomenon, cardiomyopathy, and interstitial pulmonary fibrosis. Some patients have other coexisting collagen vascular disorders, such as rheumatoid arthritis, systemic lupus erythematosus, and progressive systemic sclerosis (formerly called *scleroderma*).

The presence of skin rash, calcinosis, and eyelid edema most often suggests dermatomyositis (Fig. 41-36). The skin rash is a purple (heliotrope) color and involves the eyelids, face, chest, and extensor surfaces of the extremities. Dermatomyositis is slightly more common in children and older adults, with an onset before age 15 years or after age 50 years. The adult with dermatomyositis occasionally has underlying malignancies. Calcinosis, with calcium deposition in the subcutaneous tissue, can be a severe long-term complication of dermatomyositis.

Evaluation and Treatment

The muscle biopsy is striking in dermatomyositis, with most individuals showing inflammatory cells grouped around blood

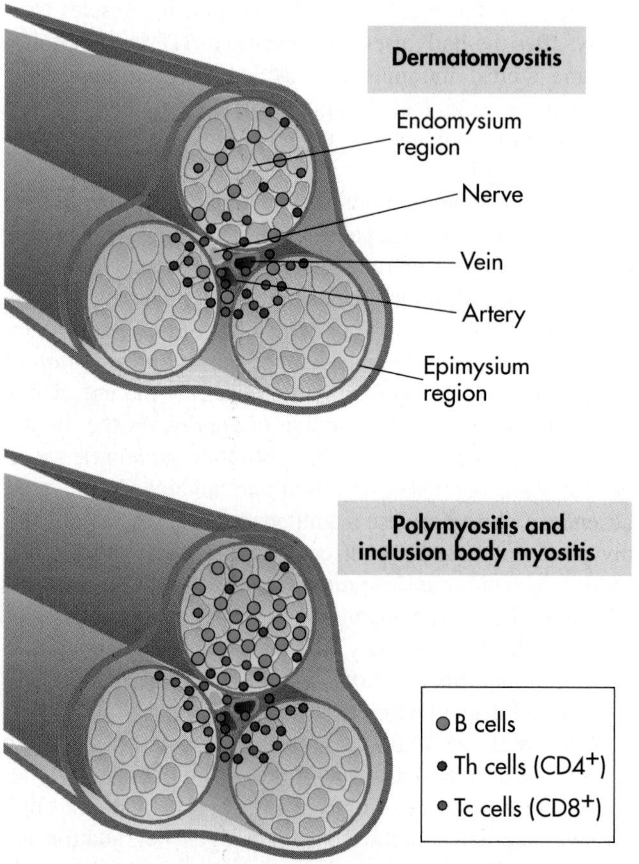

FIG. 41-35 Distribution of CD4 and CD8 lymphocytes in different clinical forms of myositis. Dermatomyositis shows perivascular and CD4 T cells. Polymyositis shows mostly CD8 T cells.

vessels and atrophy of cells in muscle fascicles. This change, perifascicular atrophy, is absent in polymyositis. CK and sedimentation rate are often extremely elevated in both disorders. EMG abnormalities include signs of muscle irritability and myopathic changes—usually large numbers of low-amplitude action potentials of brief duration. The EMG also shows a typical "myopathic" pattern, with short, low-amplitude polyphasic potentials, as well as signs of marked muscle irritability. Muscle biopsy is indispensable for a diagnosis of polymyositis or dermatomyositis as opposed to other myotonic diseases. MRI reveals inflammation and edema of the muscles.

Treatment primarily includes immunosuppressive drugs, although they are not always successful if uniformly applied. Most clinicians choose corticosteroids initially, usually prednisone on a daily or alternating-day schedule, tapering the dosage as the symptoms subside. Successful treatment with azathioprine, methotrexate, and cyclophosphamide has also been reported. Individuals with muscle weakness require careful physiotherapy to design a regular exercise program that prevents contractures and maximizes functional ability.

Toxic Myopathies

The most common cause of **toxic myopathy** is alcohol abuse. Two clinical syndromes are prevalent: (1) an acute attack of muscle weakness, pain, and swelling after a binge or (2) a more chronic, progressive proximal weakness in a drinker of long duration. The incidence of acute alcoholic myopathy has been estimated at up to 20% of individuals admitted with acute alcoholic withdrawal.

The pathologic abnormalities include necrosis of individual muscle fibers; whole segments can be found in the same stage of degeneration. The mechanism by which alcohol affects the muscle fiber is uncertain, but experiments have shown both a direct toxic effect and nutritional deficiency.

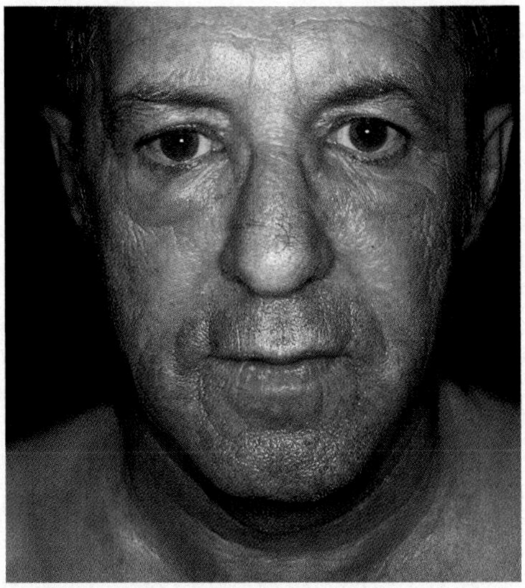

FIG. 41-36 Dermatomyositis. Heliotrope (violaceous) discoloration around the eyes and periorbital edema. (From Habif TP: *Clinical dermatology,* ed 3, St Louis, 1996, Mosby.)

Acute alcoholic myopathy can range from benign cramps and pain resolving in a matter of hours to severe weakness and markedly increased CK associated with myoglobinuria and renal failure. Individuals are prone to repeated attacks following recovery. The only treatment is abstinence from alcohol and improved nutrition. The individual with chronic alcoholic myopathy often has a coexisting peripheral neuropathy that complicates the diagnosis.

Chemical agents have also been implicated in the development of myopathy. The drug chloroquine, an antimalarial and amebicidal agent, in high doses has been associated with the development of generalized muscle weakness, particularly of the proximal muscles. Myopathy has also been caused by emetine (the major constituent of ipecac), vincristine, corticosteroids, and the toxic denatured rapeseed oil.

Rhabdomyolysis and myoglobinuria are often caused by sedatives and narcotics, particularly street heroin, clofibrate (hypolipidemic agent), and the antifibrinolytic aminocaproic acid. Drugs that induce hypokalemia, such as amphotericin B, licorice, and azathioprine, have also been reported to cause myalgia and myopathy.

Repeated intramuscular injections have been associated also with changes in muscle fibers. Local necrosis of muscle fiber and elevated CK have been reported after intramuscular injections of cephalothin, lidocaine, diazepam, and digoxin; these effects were not produced with injections of saline. When drugs are injected over long periods, a chronic focal myopathy develops. Proliferation of connective tissue in both the muscle fiber and overlying skin and subcutaneous tissue has been reported. Over time, segments of the muscles, particularly the deltoid and quadriceps, are converted into fibrotic bands. Pathophysiologic mechanisms for these changes include repeated needle trauma and infection, along with the nonphysiologic acidity and alkalinity of the injected material.

Muscle Tumors

Rhabdomyoma

Rhabdomyoma is an extremely rare benign tumor of muscle that generally occurs in the tongue, neck muscles, larynx, uvula, nasal cavity, axilla, vulva, and heart. These tumors are usually treated by surgical excision and do not recur.

Rhabdomyosarcoma

The malignant tumor of striated muscle is called **rhabdomyosarcoma.** These tumors are highly malignant, with rapid metastasis. They are located in the muscle tissue of the head, neck, and genitourinary tract in 75% of cases. The remainder are in the trunk and extremities.

Three types of rhabdomyosarcoma are differentiated on pathologic section: pleomorphic, embryonal, and alveolar. The pleomorphic, or spindle cell, type is considered to be one of the most highly malignant tumors of the extremities seen in adulthood. Once believed to be a common sarcoma, it is now believed to be very rare.[49] Embryonal tumors are most frequently seen in childhood and appear on biopsy to be shaped like a tadpole or tennis racquet. Alveolar-type tumors appear latticelike and look like lung tissue alveoli.

The diagnosis of rhabdomyosarcoma is made by incisional biopsy and examination of the specimen by a pathologist. On electron microscopy the tissue demonstrates myofilaments and Z-band material; CT scan helps define the tissue borders. Staging is based on pathologic grade of the tumor and is helpful in determining prognosis and treatment.

Treatment consists of a combination of surgical excision, radiation therapy, and systemic chemotherapy. Cure with distant metastasis is unlikely.

Other Tumors

Metastatic deposits of tumors in muscles are rare in spite of the extensive vascular supply of skeletal muscles. It is suggested that local pH or metabolic changes prevent metastatic involvement from other tumors. When adjacent carcinomas do cause muscle damage, it is usually related to the compression of tissue and resultant muscle atrophy.

SUMMARY REVIEW

Musculoskeletal Injuries

1. One of ten persons in the United States experiences an acute musculoskeletal injury each year.
2. The most serious musculoskeletal injury is a fracture. A bone can be completely or incompletely fractured. A closed fracture leaves the skin intact. An open fracture has an overlying skin wound. The direction of the fracture line can be linear, oblique, spiral, or transverse. Greenstick, torus, and bowing fractures are examples of incomplete fractures that occur in children. Stress fractures occur in normal or abnormal bone that is subjected to repeated stress. Fatigue fractures occur in normal bone subjected to abnormal stress. Normal weight bearing can cause an insufficiency fracture in abnormal bone.
3. Dislocation is complete loss of contact between the surfaces of two bones. Subluxation is partial loss of contact between two bones. As a bone separates from a joint, it may damage adjacent nerves, blood vessels, ligaments, tendons, and muscle.
4. Tendon tears are called *strains,* and ligament tears are called *sprains.* A complete separation of a tendon or ligament from its attachment is called an *avulsion.*

Disorders of Bones

1. Metabolic bone diseases are characterized by abnormal bone structure. In osteoporosis the density or mass of bone is reduced because the bone remodeling cycle is disrupted. Osteomalacia is a metabolic bone disease characterized by inadequate bone mineralization. Excessive and abnormal bone remodeling occurs in Paget disease.
2. Osteomyelitis is a bone infection caused *most frequently* by bacteria. Bacteria can enter bone from outside the body (exogenous osteomyelitis) or from infection sites within the body (hematogenous osteomyelitis).
3. Bone tumors originate from bone cells, cartilage cells, fibrous tissue cells, or vascular marrow cells. Each cell produces a specific type of ground substance that is used to classify the tumor as osteogenic (bone cell), chondrogenic (cartilage cell), collagenic (fibrous tissue cell), or myelogenic (vascular marrow cell). Malignant bone tumors are large, aggressively destroy surrounding bone, invade surrounding tissue, and initiate independent growth outside the site of origin. Benign bone tumors are less destructive, limit their growth to the anatomic confines of the bone, and have a well-demarcated border.

Disorders of Joints

1. Noninflammatory joint disease is differentiated from inflammatory joint disease by the absence of synovial membrane inflammation, the absence of systemic signs and symptoms, and the presence of normal synovial fluid.
2. Osteoarthritis is a noninflammatory joint disease characterized by the degeneration and loss of articular cartilage, sclerosis of underlying bone, and formation of bone spurs (osteophytes).
3. Rheumatoid arthritis is an inflammatory joint disease characterized by inflammatory destruction of the synovial membrane, articular cartilage, joint capsule, and surrounding ligaments and tendons. Rheumatoid nodules may also invade the skin, lung, and spleen and involve small and large arteries. Rheumatoid arthritis is a systemic disease that affects the heart, lungs, kidneys, and skin, as well as the joints.
4. Ankylosing spondylitis is a chronic, inflammatory joint disease characterized by stiffening and fusion of the spine and sacroiliac joints.
5. Gout is a metabolic disorder associated with high levels of uric acid in the blood and body fluids. Uric acid crystallizes in the connective tissue of a joint, where it initiates inflammatory destruction of the joint.

Disorders of Skeletal Muscle

1. A pathologic contracture is permanent muscle shortening caused by muscle spasticity, as seen in central nervous system injury or severe muscle weakness.
2. Stress-induced muscle tension is presumably caused by increased activity in the reticular activating system and gamma loop in the muscle fiber. The use of progressive relaxation training and biofeedback has been advocated to reduce muscle tension.
3. Fibromyalgia is a chronic musculoskeletal syndrome characterized by diffuse pain and tender points. Unknown but suspected is that muscle is the end organ responsible for the pain and fatigue. Most cases are in women, and the peak age is 30 to 50 years.
4. Atrophy of muscle fibers and overall diminished size of the muscle are seen after prolonged inactivity. Isometric contractions and passive lengthening exercises decrease atrophy to some degree in immobilized patients.
5. Hyperexcitable membranes cause the physical and electrical phenomenon of myotonia. The disorder is treated with drugs that reduce fiber excitability. Periodic paralysis is caused by

an unresponsive muscle membrane and is accompanied by changes in serum potassium. The biochemical defect is possibly related to changes in the muscle membrane and sarcoplasmic reticulum.
6. Metabolic muscle diseases are caused by endocrine disorders, glycogen storage disease, enzyme deficiencies, and abnormal lipid function. The muscle depends on a complex system of carbohydrates and fats converted by enzymes to produce energy for the muscle cell. Abnormalities in these pathways can inhibit function or cause damage to the muscle fiber. These illnesses are rare, yet they account for significant functional abnormalities.
7. Viral, bacterial, and parasitic infections of muscles produce the characteristic clinical and pathologic changes associated with inflammation. These are usually treatable and self-limiting disorders.
8. Polymyositis (generalized muscle inflammation) and dermatomyositis (polymyositis accompanied with skin rash) are characterized by inflammation of connective tissue and muscle fibers, and muscle fiber necrosis. Cell-mediated and humoral immune factors have been implicated. Treatment with immunosuppressive agents is effective in many cases.
9. The most common toxic myopathy is caused by alcohol abuse. Direct toxic effects of alcohol-producing necrosis of muscle fibers and nutritional deficiency have been suggested. The only treatment is abstinence and improved nutrition. The toxic effects of many drugs on muscle fibers cause local trauma to the muscle fibers from direct effects of the needle, secondary infection, and changes caused by nonphysiologic acidity and alkalinity in the fibers.
10. Sarcomas of muscle tissue are rare. Rhabdomyosarcoma has a uniformly poor prognosis because of an aggressive invasion and early, widespread dissemination. The usual treatment includes surgical excision, radiation therapy, and systemic chemotherapy.

KEY TERMS

Acid maltase deficiency, *1403*
Acute gouty arthritis, *1398*
Ankylosing spondylitis, *1393*
Asymptomatic hyperuricemia, *1398*
Avulsion, *1370*
Biofeedback, *1399*
Bowing fracture, *1365*
Bursae, *1370*
Caplan syndrome, *1392*
Chondrogenic (cartilage-forming) tumor, *1383*
Chondroid, *1383*
Chondrosarcoma, *1383*
Closed (simple) fracture, *1364*
Collagenic (collagen-forming) tumor, *1384*
Comminuted fracture, *1364*
Compartment syndrome, *1372*
Complete fracture, *1364*
Contracture, *1399*
Degenerative joint disease (osteoarthritis), *1385*
Delayed union, *1368*
Dermatomyositis, *1404*
Dislocation, *1368*
Disuse atrophy, *1401*
Endochondroma, *1383*
Endogenous (hematogenous) osteomyelitis, *1379*
Enthesis, *1393*
Epicondylitis, *1370*
Exogenous osteomyelitis, *1379*
Fatigue fracture, *1365*
Fibromyalgia, *1399*
Fibrosarcoma, *1384*
Fracture, *1364*
Giant cell tumor, *1384*
Gout, *1394*
Gouty arthritis, *1395*
Greenstick fracture, *1365*
Hyperbaric oxygen therapy, *1380*
Incomplete fracture, *1364*
Inflammatory joint disease (arthritis), *1389*
Insufficiency fracture, *1365*
Involucrum, *1380*
Joint effusion, *1388*
Lateral epicondylitis (tennis elbow), *1370*
Ligament, *1369*
Linear fracture, *1364*
Malunion, *1368*
McArdle disease, *1403*
Medial epicondylitis (golfer's elbow), *1370*
Muscle strain, *1371*
Myelogenic tumor, *1384*
Myeloma, *1385*
Myoadenylate deaminase deficiency (MDD), *1403*
Myoglobinuria, *1372*
Myositis, *1404*
Myositis ossificans, *1371*
Myotonia, *1402*
Noninflammatory joint disease, *1385*
Nonunion, *1368*
Oblique fracture, *1364*
Open (compound) fracture, *1364*
Osteoarthritis (OA), *1385*
Osteogenic (bone-forming) tumor, *1382*
Osteomalacia, *1377*
Osteomyelitis, *1379*
Osteophyte, *1385*
Osteoporosis, *1373*
Osteosarcoma, *1382*
Paget disease (osteitis deformans), *1378*
Pannus, *1390*
Pathologic fracture, *1365*
Periodic paralysis, *1402*
Polymyositis, *1404*
Pompe disease, *1403*
Primary osteoarthritis, *1385*
Progressive relaxation training, *1399*
Regional osteoporosis, *1374*
Rhabdomyosarcoma, *1405*
Rheumatoid arthritis (RA), *1389*
Rheumatoid factor (RF), *1390*
Rheumatoid nodule, *1392*
Secondary osteoarthritis, *1385*
Sequestrum, *1380*
Spiral fracture, *1364*
Sprain, *1370*
Strain, *1368*
Stress fracture, *1365*
Subluxation, *1368*
Syndesmophyte, *1394*
Tophaceous gout, *1398*
Tophus (pl., tophi), *1395*
Torus fracture, *1365*
Toxic myopathy, *1405*
Transchondral fracture (osteochondritis dissecans), *1365*
Transverse fracture, *1365*
Volkmann ischemic contracture, *1372*

REFERENCES

1. Stevens JA et al: Surveillance for injuries and violence among older adults, *MMWR* 48(SS08):27, 1999.
2. Cole BJ, Warner JJP: Arthroscopic versus open Bankart repair for traumatic anterior shoulder instability, *Clin Sports Med* 19(1):19, 2000.
3. Browner BD et al: *Skeletal trauma: fractures, dislocations, ligamentous injuries,* vol 1, Philadelphia, 1992, W.B. Saunders.
4. Frank CB: Ligament healing: current knowledge and clinical applications, *J Am Acad Orthop Surg* 4(2):74, 1996.
5. Halloran L: Bilateral epicondylitis in a karate instructor, *Orthop Nurs* 17(5):28, 1998.
6. Salzman KL, Lillegard WA, Butcher JD: Upper extremity bursitis, *Am Fam Physician* 56:1797, 1997.
7. Butcher JD, Salzman KL, Lilligard WA: Lower extremity bursitis, *Am Fam Physician* 53:2317, 1996.
8. Blackman PG: A review of chronic exertional compartment syndrome in the leg, *Med Sci Sports Exerc* 32(3 suppl):S4, 2000.
9. Osteoporosis prevention, diagnosis, and therapy: NIH concensus statement online, 17(2):1, March 27-29, 2000. Available at www.odp.od.nih.gov/consensus.
10. Lindsay R, Cosman F: Prevention of osteoporosis. In Favus MJ, editor: *Primer on the metabolic bone diseases and disorders of bone metabolism,* ed 4, Philadelphia, 1999, Lippincott Williams & Wilkins.
11. Moffett JD, Einhorn TA: General orthopedic principles. In Rosen CJ, Glowicki J, Bilezikian JP, editors: *The aging skeleton,* San Diego, 1999, Academic Press.
12. Liscum B: Osteoporosis: the silent disease, *Orthop Nurs* 11(4):21, 1992.
13. Burgener D et al: Fluoride increases typosine kinase activity in osteoblast-like cells: regulatory role for the stimulation of key proliferation and Pi transport across the plasma membranes, *J Bone Miner Res* 10(1):164, 1995.
14. Mundy G, Lance NE: Bone agents. In Klippel JH, Dieppe PA, editors: *Rheumatology,* ed 2, London, 1998, Mosby.
15. Pak YC et al: Treatment of postmenopausal osteoporosis with slow-release sodium fluoride. Final report of randomized controlled clinical trial, *Ann Intern Med* 123:401, 1995.
16. Riggs BL et al: Effect of fluoride treatment on fracture rate in postmenopausal women with osteoporosis, *N Engl J Med* 322:802, 1990.
17. Okano T: Effects of essential trace elements on bone turnover—in relation to osteoporosis, *Nippon Rinsho* 54(1):148, 1996 (non-English).
18. Clark K, Sowers MR: Alcohol dependence, smoking status, reproductive characteristics, and bone mineral density in premenopausal women, *Res Nurs Health* 19(5):399, 1996.
19. Greendale GA, Edelstein S, Barrett-Connor E: Endogenous steroids and bone mineral density in older women and men: the Rancho Bernado study, *J Bone Miner Res* 12:1833, 1997.
20. Marwick C: Consensus panel considers osteoporosis, *JAMA* 283(16):2093, 2000.
21. Orwell, ES: Osteoporosis in men. In Flavus JM, editor: *Primer on the metabolic bone diseases and disorders of bone metabolism,* ed 4, Philadelphia, 1999, Lippincott Williams & Wilkins.
22. Romani AM, Scarpa A: Regulation of cellular magnesium, *Front Biosci* 5:D720, 2000.
23. Weaver CM: Calcium and magnesium requirements of children and adolescents and peak bone mass, *Nutrition* 26(7-8):514, 2000.
24. Quamme GA, de Rouffignac C: Epithelial magnesium transport and regulation by the kidney, *Front Biosci* 5:D694, 2000.
25. Yago MD et al: Intracellular magnesium: transport and regulation in epithelial secretory cells, *Front Biosci* 5:D602, 2000.
26. Eisman JA: Pathogenesis of osteoporosis. In Klippel JA, Dieppe PA, editors: *Rheumatology,* ed 2, London, 1998, Mosby.
27. Hughes DE et al: Estrogen promotes apoptosis of murine osteoclast mediated by TGF-β, *Nat Med* 2(10):1132, 1996.
28. Col NF et al: Individualizing therapy to prevent long-term consequences of estrogen deficiency in postmenopausal women, *Arch Int Med* 159:1458, 1999.
29. de Deuxchaisnes CN, Devogelaer JP: Paget's disease of bone. In Klieppel JH, Dieppe PA, editors: *Rheumatology,* ed 2, London, 1998, Mosby.
30. Siris ES: Paget's disease of bone. In Flavus JM, editor: *Primer on the metabolic bone diseases and disorders of bone metabolism,* ed 4, Philadelphia, 1999, Lippincott Williams & Wilkins.
31. Kastrup JJ, Buseck MS, Lyon JC: Common pitfalls in a bone tumor workup, *Contemp Orthop* 24(5):567, 1992.
32. Norden DK, Boyce EG, Scumacher HR: Stepped-care guide to osteoarthritis therapy, *Orthop Special Edit* 3(3):28, 1994.
33. McAlindon TE et al: Glucosamine and chondroitin for treatment of osteoarthritis: a systemic quality assessment and meta-analysis, *JAMA* 283(11):1469, 2000.
34. Wobig M et al: The role of elastoviscosity in the efficacy of viscosupplementation for osteoarthritis of the knee: a comparison of Hylan G-F 20 and a lower-molecular-weight hyaluronan, *Clin Ther* 21(9):1549, 1999.
35. Behar SM, Porcelli SA: The immunology of inflammatory arthritis, *Sci Med* 3(6):12, 1996.
36. Castagnetta L et al: Endocrine end-points in rheumatoid arthritis, *Ann N Y Acad Sci* 876:180, 1999.
37. Feltcamp TEW, Kahn MW, Lopez de Castro JA: The pathogenetic role of HLS-B27, *Immunol Today* 17(1):5, 1996.
38. Campbell SM: Rheumatoid arthritis: current strategies, *Hosp Med* 34(8):29, 1998.
39. Dougados M: Diagnostic features of ankylosing spndylitis, *Br J Rheumatol* 34(4):301, 1995.
40. Cohen MG, Emmerson BT: Gout. In Klippel JH, Dieppe JA, editors: *Rheumatology,* St Louis, 1994, Mosby.
41. Larsson R, Oberg PA, Larsson SE: Changes of trapezius muscle blood flow and electromyography in chronic neck pain due to trapezius myalgia, *Pain* 79(1):45, 1999.
42. Westgaard RH: Muscle activity as a releasing factor for pain in the shoulder and neck, *Cephaligia* 19(suppl 25):1, 1999.
43. Gandevia SC: Mind, muscles, and motoneurones, *J Sci Med Sport* 2(3):167, 1999.
44. Goldenberg RL: Fibromyalgia, chronic fatigue syndrome, and myofascial pain, *Curr Opin Rheumatol* 8(2):113, 1996.
45. Cunningham ME: Becoming familiar with fibromyalgia, *Orthop Nurs* 15(2):33, 1996.
46. Johansson G et al: Cerebral dysfunction in fibromyalgia: evidence from regional cerebral blood flow measurements to neurological tests and cerebrospinal fluid analysis, *Acta Psychiatr Scand* 91:86, 1995.
47. Buckwalter JA, Lappin DR: The disproportionate impact of chronic arthralgia and arthritis among women, *Clin Orthop* (372):159, 2000.
48. Davies NP, Hanna MG: Neurologic channelopathies: diagnosis and therapy in the new millenium, *Ann Med* 31(6):406, 1999.
49. Miettinen M, Weiss SW: Soft tissue tumors. In Damjanvov I, Linder J, editors: *Anderson's pathology,* ed 10, St Louis, 1996, Mosby.

CHAPTER 42

Alterations of Musculoskeletal Function in Children

KRISTEN LEE CARROLL

CHAPTER OUTLINE

Musculoskeletal alterations in children are very common. They may be congenital, such as clubfoot; hereditary, such as muscular dystrophy; or acquired, such as Legg-Calvé-Perthes disease. Some of these disorders are acute, and the child will recover completely; other disorders are chronic or, in some cases, terminal. An understanding of the pathophysiology of these alterations will aid in providing the best care possible for these children.

MUSCULOSKELETAL DEVELOPMENT IN CHILDREN

Bone Formation

Bone formation, which begins at about the eighth week of gestation, involves two phases: (1) the delivery of bone cell precursors to sites of bone formation and (2) the aggregation of these cells at **primary centers of ossification,** where they mature and begin to secrete osteoid (see Chapter 40). Some of the bone cell precursors are present in fetal connective tissues, whereas others migrate in blood to sites of bone formation after blood vessels have grown into the tissue.

Cellular aggregation and maturation occur in two types of fetal tissue, depending on which bones are being formed. The cranium, facial bones, clavicles, and parts of the jawbone arise from a fetal membrane termed the *mesenchyme*. Bones that develop on or within the mesenchyme grow by the process of **intramembranous formation**. As the mesenchyme becomes vascularized, the immature bone cells aggregate and mature into osteoblasts, which form the centers of ossification. Osteoblasts secrete osteoid, which surrounds them and quickly ossifies, forming the lacunae and canaliculi of compact bone. Spicules of bone radiate from the ossification centers to form the primary trabeculae characteristic of spongy bone. Later, some of the spongy bone is replaced by compact bone.

Endochondral formation is the development of new bone from cartilage. This process, by which the long bones of the appendicular skeleton develop, is more complex than intramembranous formation (Fig. 42-1). First, mesenchymal tissue forms a **cartilage anlage,** which defines the shape of the bone. The cartilage model is subsequently removed and replaced by bone. Endochondral bone formation begins in the outer layer of the cartilage model, which consists of a layer of dense connective tissue called **perichondrium**. The perichondrium contains cells that develop into osteoblasts, forming a collar of bone, termed the **periosteal collar,** around the cartilage model. Cartilage enclosed within the periosteal collar degenerates, and capillaries from outside the perichondrium invade the degenerating cartilage cells, carrying with them osteoblast precursors from the inner layer of the perichondrium and osteoclast precursors from the blood itself.

Endochondral bone formation progresses at the primary center of ossification in the middle of the cartilage model and extends toward either end of the developing bone. At the same time, the periosteal collar thickens and becomes wider toward the epiphyses. By the end of gestation, **secondary centers of ossification** (i.e., the epiphyseal centers) begin to lay down bone at both ends of the cartilage model. Here, too, cartilage within the periosteal collar degenerates, and blood vessels grow inward, delivering bone cell precursors. Once the osteoblasts begin to secrete osteoid, ossification spreads from the secondary centers in all directions until all the cartilage within the model is replaced by bone.

Two regions of cartilage remain at the ends of long bones: (1) articular cartilage over the free ends of the bone and (2) the physeal plate, a layer of cartilage between the metaphysis and epiphysis. (These structures are described and illustrated in Chapter 40; see Fig. 40-2.) The physeal plate retains the ability to form and calcify new cartilage and deposit bone until the skeleton matures roughly 1 year after sexual maturity (11 to 15 years of age in females, 15 to 18 in males).

Bone Growth

Until adult stature is reached, growth in the length of bone occurs at the physeal plate through endochondral ossification. Cartilage cells at the epiphyseal side of the physeal plate multiply and enlarge. As rapidly as new cartilage cells form, cartilage cells at the metaphyseal side of the plate are destroyed and replaced by bone.

In the shaft of new bone, where growth is relatively slow, the bone produced by accretion is compact and dense. The compact bone is thickest where it has to withstand the maximal stresses, which generally occur in the middle of the shaft.

The two physeas of the long bone can have varying strengths. The more active of the two has more power to remodel deformity but can also be more sensitive to injury. The architecture of the physis also dictates its sensitivity to injury. The distal femur, for example, has an undulating pattern increasing its resistance to sheer force; when injured, however, growth disturbance is highly likely.

Growth in the diameter of bone occurs by deposition of new bone on an existing bone surface. Bone matrix is laid down by osteoblasts on the periosteal surface and subsequently becomes calcified. At the same time, bone resorption occurs on the endosteal surface. Endosteal resorption increases the diameter of the medullary cavity, which contains marrow and spongy bone.

Many factors affect the development, physiology, and rate of growth of the epiphyseal plate. Growth hormone must be secreted by the pituitary gland at a constant rate to stimulate the growth plate consistently. Other known factors affecting growth include peptide regulatory factors (e.g., fibroblast growth factor [FGF]); changes in cell-to-cell interactions through cell adhesion molecules (CAMs) and cell junctions; and complex interactions or changes in extracellular matrix (ECM), nutrition, general health, and other hormones (e.g., thyroid hormone, adrenal and gonadal androgens, estrogens). These factors influence both the rate of bone growth and the time of appearance of the secondary ossification centers. When the skeleton is mature, the epiphyseal plate is replaced by bone. This process, termed **physeal closure**, unites the metaphysis and the epiphysis. Physeal closure occurs earlier in females than males because of earlier puberty in females.

Throughout life, bone is constantly being destroyed and re-formed (see Chapter 40), but the process is at its maximum in children approximately 2½ years of age. By young adulthood, bone turnover, or remodeling, occurs at a relatively slow rate.

Skeletal Development

The axial skeleton changes shape with growth. (The axial skeleton and appendicular skeleton are described and illustrated in Chapter 40; see Fig. 40-4). In a newborn the entire spine is concave anteriorly, or **kyphosed**. In the first 3 months

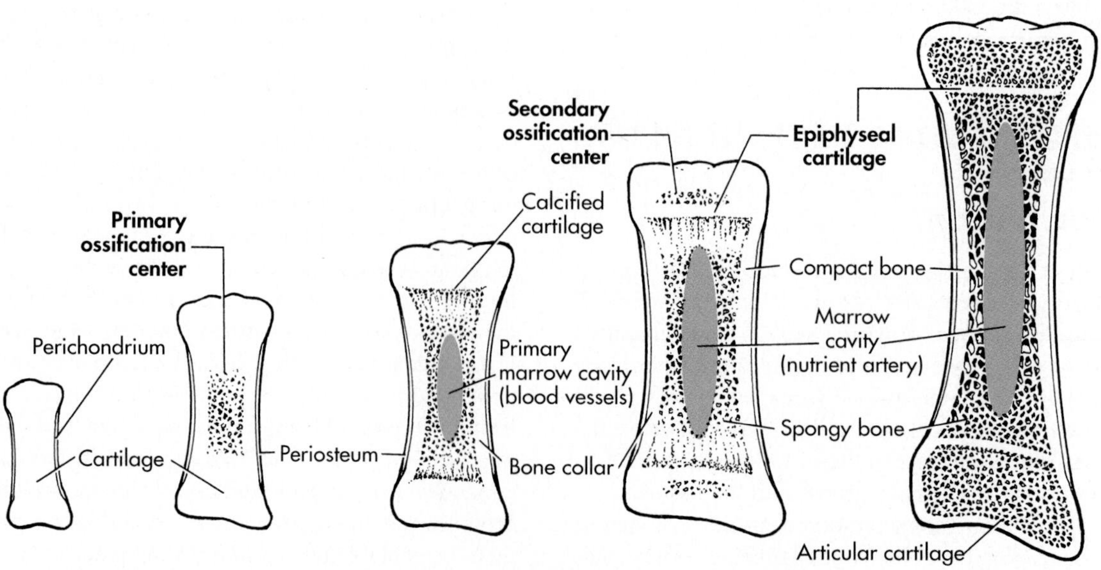

FIG. 42-1 Stages of endochondral bone formation and centers of ossification in long bone.

of life, with the infant's ability to control the head, the upper (cervical) spine begins to arch, or become **lordotic**. The normal lordotic curve of the lower (lumbar) spine begins to develop with sitting.

The appendicular skeleton (the extremities) grows faster during childhood than does the axial skeleton. The newborn has a relatively large head and long spine with disproportionately shorter limbs than an adult. By 1 year of age, 50% of the total growth of the spine has occurred.[1] Therefore failure of the spine to grow (e.g., spinal fusion) does not limit eventual height as much as the premature fusion of the growth plates of the lower extremities. In children with congenital curvature of the spine, growth tends to worsen the deformity rather than to increase the length of the spine.

Besides getting longer, growing bones of the extremities undergo changes in rotation and alignment. In the newborn the proximal femur is rotated forward up to 40 degrees and the tibia is rotated inward. With growth the femur assumes its normal alignment (by 8 years of age) and tibial rotation neutralizes 5 years of age. Bowlegs and knock knees are normal at certain stages of growth. At birth the newborn's legs are bowed because of stresses in utero. **Genu varum (bowleg)** reaches a peak by 2½ years of age, whereas **genu valgum (knock knee)** maximizes by 5 to 6 years of age. If genu varum or genu valgum persists past these ages, a pathologic process rather than a physiologic phase may be present. Pathologic causes of genu varum are Blount disease, rickets, skeletal dysplasias (such as achondroplastic dwarfism), and tramatic injury. Genu valgum may persist also as a result of skeletal dysplasia.

Muscle Growth

The composition and size of muscles vary with age. In the fetus, muscle tissue contains a large amount of water and much intercellular matrix. After birth, both are reduced considerably as the muscle fibers (cells) enlarge by accumulating cytoplasm. Little information is available about the numbers of fibers in a given muscle at various ages, but the total mass of muscle in the body can be estimated from the amount of creatinine excreted in the urine, because the conversion of creatine to creatinine takes place only in muscle (see Chapter 40). Between birth and maturity, the number of muscle nuclei in the body increases 14 times in boys and 10 times in girls. Muscle fibers reach their maximal size in girls at approximately 10 years of age and in boys by 14 years. Growth in length occurs at the ends of muscles, and the increase in length is accompanied by an increase in number of nuclei in the fibers. Muscle fibers increase in diameter as the fibrils become more numerous. The fibrils themselves do not increase in diameter. Connective tissue components of muscle grow where the tendon and muscle meet.

A potent stimulus to the growth of a muscle is the separation of its attachments as the skeleton grows. The length of a muscle fiber is the direct consequence of the range of movement it is called on to perform. The stimulus for the formation of a tendon is probably the pull of the muscle rudiment on undifferentiated connective tissue. The repair of a tendon from which a segment has been removed does not occur if the muscle is prevented from exercising tension on the damaged tendon. Replacement of muscle by tendon (tendinification) sometimes is the result of limitation of movement. If the normal opponents of a muscle are paralyzed, the muscle fails to grow properly, and it may be that the full development of a muscle depends on the progressive rise in the tension exerted on it by its antagonists.

Muscle growth during adolescence is a major factor in weight gain. Gender differences in muscle size and weight are minor in childhood but become considerable with the onset of puberty.

In the infant, muscle accounts for approximately 25% of total body weight, compared with 40% in the adult. In the adult, approximately 55% of muscle weight is in the lower limb muscles, whereas in the infant the majority of the weight is axial musculature. The respiratory and facial muscles are well developed at birth so that the infant can perform the vital functions of breathing and sucking. Other muscle groups, such as the pelvic muscles, take several years to develop fully. Throughout life the weight of the skeletal muscles can be increased by exercise. Less is known about the development of visceral and cardiac muscle. Visceral muscle fibers increase in both number and size, but the increase in fiber size is most important. Fiber enlargement alone can increase the bulk of visceral muscle by as many as eight times. Cardiac muscle also grows mainly by enlargement of existing fibers.

MUSCULOSKELETAL ALTERATIONS IN CHILDREN

Congenital Defects

Syndactyly

The most common congenital defect of the upper extremity is **syndactyly,** or webbing of the fingers (Fig. 42-2). Simple webbing involves the soft-tissue envelope alone and is best released surgically when the child is 1 to 2 years of age. True syndactyly involves fusion of the bones and nails as well as the soft tissues; it may be associated with absence or anomaly of bony or neurovascular units. The primary goal in surgical correction of these defects is to achieve maximal

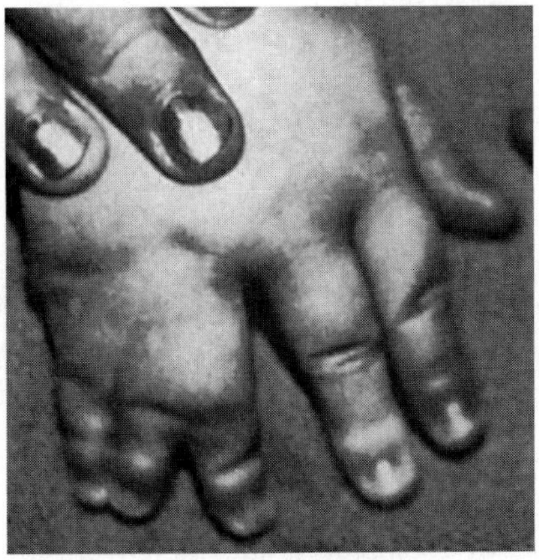

FIG. 42-2 Syndactyly.

function and appearance. Ideally, corrective surgery is deferred until the child is 6 to 12 months of age and completed before the child enters school. **Vestigial tabs,** such as an extra digit, are best removed during the immediate neonatal period, however. Anomalies on the medial or radial aspect of the arm are often associated with abnormalities of blood, heart, or kidneys. Lateral or ulnar-sided defects are less often associated with systemic anomalies and are far more rare.

Developmental Dysplasia of the Hip

Developmental dysplasia of the hip (DDH), formerly known as congenital dislocation of the hip, is an abnormality in the development of the proximal femur, acetabulum, or both. Although most often present at birth, it may occur at any time in the newborn or infant period.

The incidence of true dislocation of the hip or a dislocatable hip is 1 in 1000 live births. Some degree of instability of the hip is present in approximately 10 per 1000 live births. The left hip is affected in 60% of cases with the right hip alone affected only 20% of the time. Bilateral DDH occurs 20% of the time.

Risk factors for DDH include family history, female sex (6:1), metatarsus adductus (20%), torticollis (20%), oligohydramnios, first pregnancy, and breech presentation. First pregnancies and oligohydramnios (deficient volume of amniotic fluid) are thought to limit fetal movement, and breech presentation not only limits movement but places the hips in a position of flexion and adduction. As many as 50% of children with DDH have a history of breech presentation. Maternal hormones that reportedly increase joint laxity also have an effect on DDH, although the exact mechanism is unknown. DDH also is more common in whites and those cultures that swaddle infants with the hips in extension and adduction.

◆ *Pathophysiology*

The hip can be described as subluxated, dislocatable, or dislocated (Fig. 42-3). The subluxated hip maintains contact with the acetabulum but is not well seated within the hip joint. The dislocatable hip is sometimes located but can be dislocated. The dislocated hip has no contact between the femoral head and the acetabulum. Some degree of acetabular dysplasia is present in almost all cases. Typically the acetabulum is shallow or sloping rather than cup shaped.

By approximately 10 weeks of gestation, the femur, acetabulum, and hip joint capsule are well developed. It appears that most dysplasias occur within the second and third trimesters and are often due to positioning factors. Experimentally, DDH can be produced in laboratory animals by placing the developing hip in adduction and extension replicating the breech position. There is, however, a genetic component that is poorly understood. In addition, 2% of DDH are teratologic or due to a systemic syndrome, such as arthrogryposis or spina bifida, where muscle contracture leads to DDH.

If the DDH is left untreated in the growing child, secondary changes occur. As the hip is left subluxated or dislocated, the acetabulum becomes increasingly shallow and the soft tissues shorten about the proximal femur. If the hip is dislocated, the bone acetabulum fills with soft tissue and a false acetabulum forms where the femoral head contacts the iliac crest. An apparent limb length inequity and hip muscle weakness occurs, leading to a waddling gait.

◆ *Clinical Manifestations*

The clinical manifestations vary with the severity of the condition and the age of the child. Signs and symptoms that should be noted include the following:

1. Asymmetry of gluteal or thigh folds
2. Limb length discrepancy (Galeazzi sign)
3. Limitation of hip abduction
4. Positive Ortolani sign (dislocation)
5. Positive Barlow test (reduction)
6. Positive Trendelenburg gait (waddling)
7. Pain (very late)

The child should also be examined for other anomalies, such as torticollis or metatarsus adductus, which can be associated with DDH.

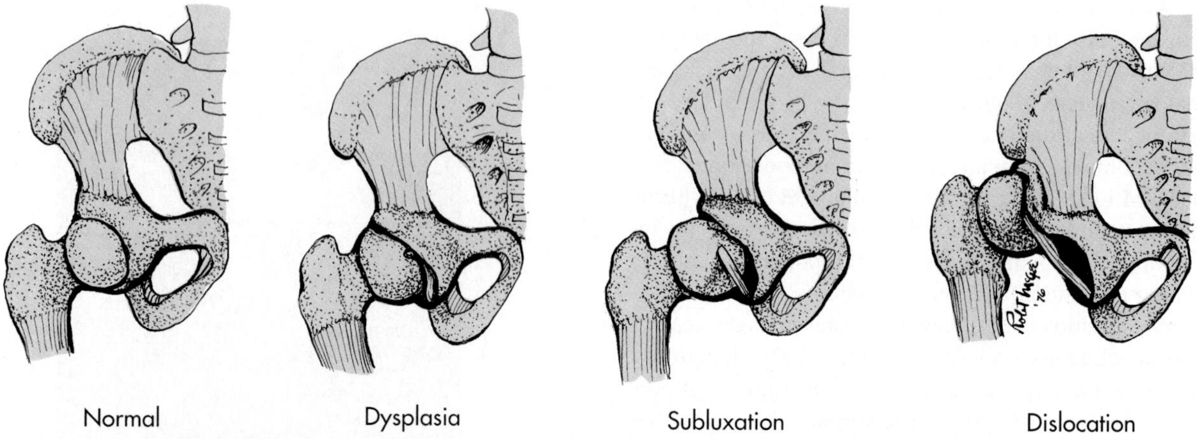

FIG. 42-3 Configuration and relationship of structures in developmental dysplasia of the hip. (From Wong DL: *Whaley and Wong's nursing care of infants and children*, ed 6, St Louis, 1999, Mosby.)

◆ *Evaluation and Treatment*

In the newborn period, clinical examination is the most important diagnostic tool. Real-time ultrasound, in which the hip is examined while the ultrasound is performed, also is extremely valuable in the newborn period, especially in high-risk infants. The use of ultrasound allows visualization of the cartilaginous structures of the hip (the femoral head and the outer lip of the acetabulum), which are not seen on plain roentgenogram. Radiographs are used after age 6 months.[2]

Treatment depends on the age of the child, severity of dysplasia, and duration of dysplasia. The earlier that treatment is begun, the better the result. In children less that 4 months of age, a Pavlik harness can brace the hip in abduction and flexion and the acetabulum will remodel as the femoral head rests centered in the socket. With this treatment, up to 98% of children will have an excellent result. A "closed" reduction (without opening the joint) followed by spica or body casting up to 3 months can be done in children up to 12 months. After 12 months of age, surgical intervention—including opening the joint and cutting and realigning the femur and/or acetabulum—may be required. In teratologic dislocations, bracing often is unsuccessful and surgery is therefore needed.

Deformities of the Foot

Congenital Deformity

Congenital foot deformity is found in roughly 4% of all newborns, and metatarsus adductis accounts for 75% of these (Table 42-1). **Metatarsus adductus** is a forefoot adduction deformity associated with a normal, plantigrade hindfoot and is believed to be secondary to intrauterine positioning. Metatarsus adductus is usually classified by two criteria: flexibility (passively correctable or rigid) and degree of deformity. The degree of deformity (mild, moderate, severe) is ascertained by the heel bisection line. A mild deformity is one in which the heel bisection line passes medial to the third toe; moderate, through the third or fourth toes; and severe, lateral to the fourth toes. It should be emphasized that a majority of children are well served by expectant treatment rather than early surgical intervention. Serial casts during the first 6 months of life are suggested for moderate to severe deformities and those deformities that appear less flexible. Casts may be the below-knee type and are usually undertaken for 6 to 12 weeks. For severe, rigid, and persistent deformities, midfoot capsulotomy and abductor hallucis lengthening can be offered. Unlike tarsometatarsal capsulotomy, this procedure causes less scarring and better overall results. Eighty-seven percent of children usually spontaneously correct by 6 years of age and 95% by 15 years of age. Even in those children with some residual deformity and an oblique medial cuneiform, few sequelae in adult life occur.

Equinovarus Deformity

There are three types of equinovarus (clubfoot): positional equinovarus, idiopathic congenital equinovarus, and teratologic equinovarus (Fig. 42-4). The true positional equinovarus lends itself to rapid correction by application of serial casts. The idiopathic variety is treated by attempting cast correction, followed by surgical intervention of resistant

Table 42-1 Terms Used to Describe Foot Abnormalities

Term	Definition
POSITION	
Abduction	Lateral deviation away from the midline of the body
Adduction	Lateral deviation toward the midline of the body
Eversion	Twisting of the foot outward along its long axis
Inversion	Twisting of the foot inward on its long axis
Dorsiflexion	Bending the foot upward and backward
Plantar flexion	Bending of the foot downward and forward
ABNORMALITY	
Talipes	Congenital abnormality of the foot (clubfoot)
Pes	Acquired deformity of the foot
Varus	Inversion and adduction of the heel and the forefoot
Valgus	Eversion and abduction of the heel and forefoot
Equinus	Plantar flexion of the foot in which the heel is lower than the toes
Calcaneus	Dorsiflexion of the foot in which the heel is lower than the toes
Planus	Flattening of the medial longitudinal arch of the foot (flatfoot)
Cavus	Elevation of the medial longitudinal arch of the foot (high arch)
Equinovarus	Coexistent equinus and varus deformities
Calcaneovarus	Coexistent calcaneus and varus deformities
Equinovalgus	Coexistent equinus and valgus deformities
Calcaneovalgus	Coexistent calcaneus and valgus deformities

NOTE: The positions listed can all be achieved by voluntary movement of the normal foot; an abnormality exists if the foot is fixed in one or more of the positions while at rest.

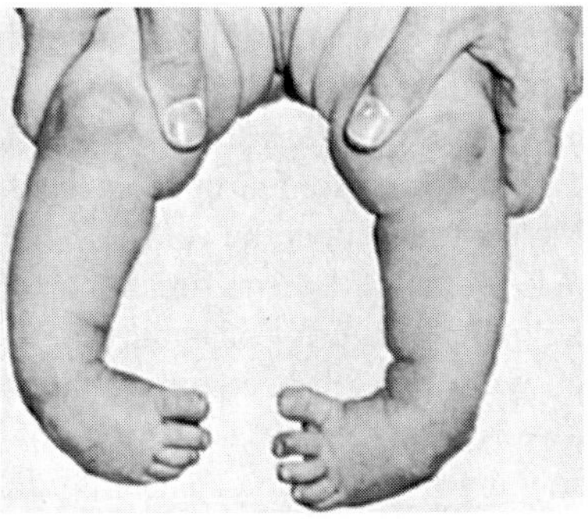

FIG. 42-4 Infant with bilateral congenital talipes equinovarus. (From Brashear HR, Raney RB: *Shand's handbook of orthopedic surgery*, ed 9, St Louis, 1978, Mosby.)

deformities. Teratologic equinovarus nearly always requires surgical correction and/or muscle balancing procedures.

Positional equinovarus. **Positional equinovarus** is one in which the infant's foot is in equinovarus position but does not have a deep posterior or plantar medial crease. It appears to be secondary only to intrauterine position. The foot can be passively brought to a plantigrade position and is amenable to casting. In general, 1 to 3 months of above-knee casting corrects this foot without the need for surgical intervention.

Idiopathic congenital equinovarus. The etiology of idiopathic equinovarus (clubfoot) is unknown. In one human fetal study, all clubfeet were associated with identifiable anterior horn cell changes in L5 and S1. Enterovirus infection, known to potentially cause anterior horn cell damage if present intrauterinely, reaches a peak prevalence in the summer or fall of temperate climates. These two seasons correlate with the peaks of conception in children with clubfeet. Muscle biopsies of both the anterior tibialis long flexors and peroneus brevis muscles in clubfoot reveal that at least 50% show decreased number of muscle fibers and/or abnormal fiber histology. The soleus often has an increase in type 1 fibers, whereas the brevis has a fiber type dispropotion. The more abnormal the histopathology is, the more severe the deformity, and the greater the chance of recurrent deformity following treatment. In addition to neurologic causes, positional abnormalities (e.g., oligohydramnios) have been implicated. The genetic component is unclear and studies are ongoing.

Idiopathic equinovarus occurs in roughly 1 out of every 1000 live births, with males affected twice as often as females. Although these deformities have been historically treated nonoperatively, surgical intervention became much more common after 1950. Initial treatment (birth to 6 months) remains manipulation and casting. Casts are usually changed every 7 to 14 days. If full correction is not attained after casting, a posteromedial surgical release is performed. In all studies the rate of recurrent deformity requiring subsequent operative intervention is repeatedly between 15% and 50%.

Teratologic equinovarus. The most common causes of **teratologic equinovarus** are either neuromuscular (such as spina bifida) or syndromic, as in arthrogryposis or osteochondrodysplasia (such as diastrophic dwarfism). The teratologic clubfoot, unlike the idiopathic type, usually fails casting protocols and requires operative intervention. The surgery is often more extensive than in an idiopathic clubfoot and revision surgery is also more frequent.

Pes planus (flatfoot) deformity. **Pes planus (flatfoot)** is a frequent reason for parental concern. Despite medical evidence to the contrary, it can be very difficult to convince families that a flexible flatfoot is as functional as the one with a "normal" arch. The majority of babies are born with flat (or "fat") feet, with the arch becoming more apparent with age. The relatively benign natural history, however, should not overshadow the importance of accurate diagnosis. Significant ankle valgus, vertical talus, tarsal coalition, and skewfoot must be accurately differentiated from flexible pes planus.

Flexible flatfoot deformity appears to be familial, with occasional association of generalized ligamentous laxity. Careful evaluation of possible occult Achilles contracture is done by holding the hindfoot in varus and dorsiflexing the ankle. Achilles contracture can signify a more severe flatfoot variant. The flexibility of the hindfoot is evaluated by having the child stand on his or her toes or by dorsiflexing the first toe passively with the child in a non-weight-bearing position. This "windlass mechanism" tightens the plantar fascia reconstituting an arch and hindfoot varus if the foot is indeed flexible. If hindfoot flexibility and an "underlying" arch are present, then flexible flatfoot is diagnosed.

By all recent data, the surgical or orthotic treatment of *asymptomatic* flexible pes planus is unnecessary. Custom orthotics, Helfet heel cups, and corrective orthopedic shoes may relieve discomfort but will have no influence over the natural history (clinically or radiographically) of flat feet. Multiple adult studies on army recruits have shown that soldiers with flat feet perform just as well as their counterparts without "fallen" arches.

There is a small subset of children with painful flexible flat feet. For these children, careful attention to a possible Achilles contracture or tarsal coalition (congenital union of the hindfoot bones) must be made. This small group having flexible flat feet with pain are best treated with inexpensive shoe inserts and expectantly watched. If pain continues into adolescence, requiring more aggressive treatment, calcaneal lengthening will correct the pes planus without decreasing hindfoot motion. Arthroereisis has also been studied but the long-term effects of indwelling Silastic within the subtalar joint is still unknown. All surgery carries risk; if a foot is flat but flexible and nonpainful, treatment is not required. The painless flexible flatfoot should be viewed as a variation of normal feet.

Abnormal Density or Modeling of the Skeleton

Osteogenesis Imperfecta

Osteogenesis imperfecta (brittle bone disease) is an inherited disorder of connective tissues that affects primarily bone. The disorder was first described in 1840 as a syndrome in newborns consisting of osteoporosis with fractures and skeletal deformities. Currently, the Sillence classification[3] is replacing the older classification of tarda and congenita. The Sillence system is based on both models of inheritance and clinical findings (Table 42-2). In the more severe forms the child is usually stillborn or dies soon after birth, although some survive into childhood. Osteogenesis imperfecta in its more severe forms is evident at birth because fractures and deformity have occurred in utero. The less severe forms may not become evident until the child begins to walk. Some children with this form experience numerous fractures and can be mistaken for battered children until the diagnosis is made.

The prevalence rate of the most common form is about 1 in 30,000. Inheritance is usually autosomal dominant but can be autosomal recessive. At least four syndromes have been identified that have various clinical manifestations and prognoses (see Table 42-2).

Pathophysiology

The major errors in osteogenesis imperfecta lie in the synthesis of collagen. Genetic studies have shown that the gene responsible for the encoding of collagen easily mutates. These mutations cause osteogenesis imperfecta. The large range of phenotypes includes all mutants of the two collagen structural genes. (Genes are discussed in Chapter 4.) Abnormalities in collagen include (1) an increase in collagen hydroxylysine residue in bones; (2) a decrease in hydroxylysine-norleucine in skin collagen; and (3) absence of α-polypeptide production in cultured skin fibroblasts.[4]

Table 42-2 Sillence Classification of Osteogenesis Imperfecta Syndromes

Type	Genetics	Description
I	Autosomal dominant	Mildest form of osteogenesis imperfecta Mild to moderate bone fragility without deformity Associated with blue sclerae, early hearing loss, easy bruising May have mild to moderate short stature Type 1A: dentinogenesis imperfecta absent Type 1B: dentinogenesis imperfecta present
II	Autosomal dominant or recessive	Perinatal lethal or recessive Extreme fragility of connective tissue, multiple in utero fractures, usually intrauterine growth retardation Soft, large cranium Micromelia, long bones bowed, ribs beaded
III	Autosomal recessive	Progressive deforming phenotype Severe fragility of bones, usually have in utero fractures Severe osteoporosis Relative macrocephaly with triangular facies Fractures heal with deformity and bowing Associated with white sclerae and extreme short stature, scoliosis
IV	Autosomal dominant	Skeletal fragility and osteoporosis more severe than type I Associated with bowing of long bones; light sclerae, ± moderate short stature, ± moderate joint hyperextensibility Type IVA: dentinogenesis imperfecta absent Type IVB: dentinogenesis imperfecta present

From Klippel JH, Dieppe PA, editors: *Rheumatology,* ed 2, London, 1998, Mosby.

A number of metabolic abnormalities have been reported. Some individuals have increased serum thyroxine levels, suggesting hyperthyroidism. This is consistent with the findings of increased sweating, heat intolerance, increased body temperature, a resting tachycardia, and tachypnea. The hyperthyroid findings, however, are not consistent in all individuals with osteogenesis imperfecta. Studies of leukocyte metabolism suggest an uncoupling of oxidative phosphorylation. Reports of alterations of platelet function with defects in adhesion and clot retraction also exist.

Clinical Manifestations

The classic clinical manifestations of osteogenesis imperfecta are osteoporosis and increased rate of fractures, possible bony deformation, triangular facies, possible vascular weakness (i.e., aortic aneurysm), possible blue sclera, and poor dentition. The Sillence classification designated types I through IV based on severity. The most severe, types II and III, are comparable to osteogenesis imperfecta congenita. These two types are characterized by autosomal recessive inheritance and early onset of manifestations. Both can cause stillbirth or severe neonatal deformity and a short life expectancy. Less severe are types I and IV, which are comparable to osteogenesis imperfecta tarda. Type I is slightly more common than types II and III, and type IV is quite rare. Types I and IV are inherited as autosomal dominant traits and vary in age of onset from birth to adulthood. Type IV, especially when the sclera are white, is the least deforming type and is often confused with nonaccidental trauma (child abuse).

Evaluation and Treatment

Evaluation of osteogenesis imperfecta is based on clinical manifestations and serologic tests. Serum alkaline phosphatase is elevated in all forms of the disease. Osteogenesis imperfecta can be diagnosed prenatally by ultrasound or chorionic villi sampling. Quantitative analysis of cultured skin fibroblast collagen by electrophoresis shows a decreased quantity of collagen in the affected individual.

For osteogenesis imperfecta type II, no therapeutic intervention will be effective. For other types of osteogenesis

WHAT'S NEW? Biphosphonate Drug Trial for Osteogenesis Imperfecta

Pamidronate, a biphosphonate compound, was given at 4- to 6-month intervals to children with severe (type III and type IV) osteogenesis imperfecta. Pamidronate inhibits bone resorption by decreasing osteoclastic activity. In the 30 children in the study, bone mineral density increased by 41.9% and fractures decreased by 1.7 per year. Mobility increased in 51% of the children. All children claimed their fatigue and chronic bone pain improved. Despite these findings consistent with decreased bone turnover, fracture healing remained unchanged. A large multicenter study is now trying to refine these treatments for all children with osteogenesis imperfecta.

Data from Francis G et al: Cyclic administration of Pamidronate in children with severe osteogenesis imperfecta, *New Engl J Med* 339:947, 1998.

imperfecta, careful positioning and handling of the newborn may prevent fractures. Beyond the neonatal period, various orthopedic measures are applied, such as prompt splinting of fractures and correction of deformities arising from the progressive bowing or bending of the skeleton by intermedullary rodding of the bones (Fig. 42-5). These are sequentially replaced as the child grows. There presently is a multicenter study of biphosphonate therapy showing promising results in type III, with marked improvements of bone density (up to 30%). Final results are still pending. Genetic counseling for affected families should aim at primary prevention.

Rickets

Rickets is a disorder in which growing bone fails to become mineralized (ossified), resulting in "soft" bones and skeletal deformity. Rickets results from either insufficient vitamin D (rare in industrialized nations), insensitivity to vitamin D, wasting of vitamin D by the kidney, or inability to absorb vitamin D and calcium in the gut. In industrialized nations the most common X-linked dominant form is hypophosphotemic rickets. Vitamin D is the mineral necessary for absorption and metabolism of calcium and phosphate. Rickets in the immature skeleton leads to broad, irregular growth plates as the rows of cells in the growth plate that are to ossify fail to do so as they reach the metaphysis (Fig. 42-6).

Children with rickets are often listless and irritable. They have hypotonia and muscle weakness and may be unable to walk without support. Abnormal parietal flattening and frontal bossing occur in the skull. The calvaria become soft, and the sutures may widen. Cartilaginous attachments of the

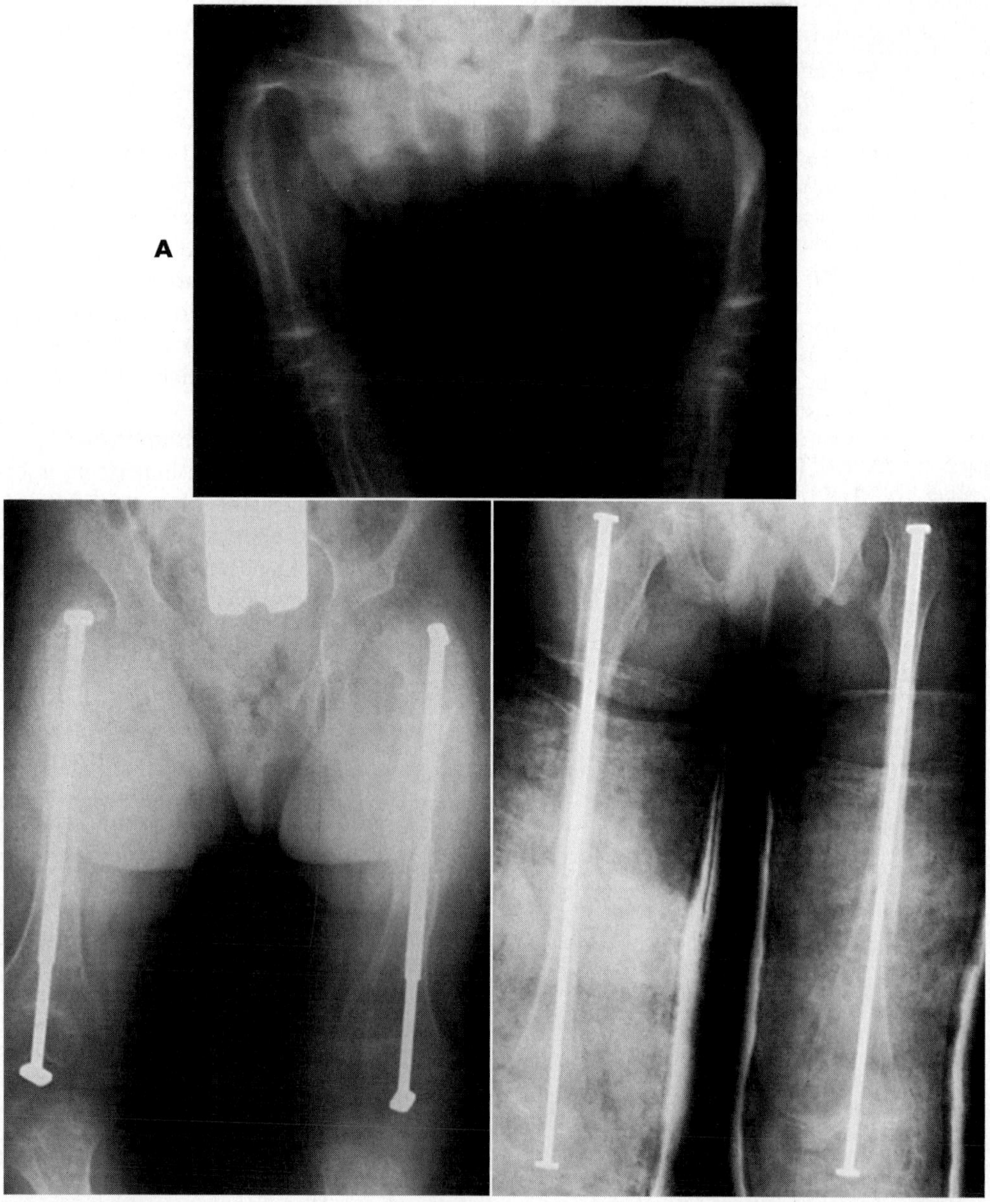

FIG. 42-5 Osteogenesis imperfecta treated with osteotomies and telescoping medullary rods. A, Severe deformity of both femurs. **B,** Same individual after multiple osteotomies with telescoping medullary rod fixation. **C,** Same individual 4 years later demonstrating growth of femurs, no recurrence of deformity, and elongation of rods. (Plaster casts are in place for immobilization of tibial osteotomies.) (From Canale ST, editor: *Campbell's operative orthopaedics,* ed 9, vol 1, St Louis, 1998, Mosby.)

ribs become prominent, and the long bones of the extremities (tibia, femur, radius, ulna) may be bowed. Growth is retarded, and fractures are common.

Like osteogenesis imperfecta, surgical treatment of bony deformity is often required. However, medical management of calcium, phosphorus, and vitamin D levels must be optimized before surgical intervention. Deformity often improves with normalization of bone metabolism.

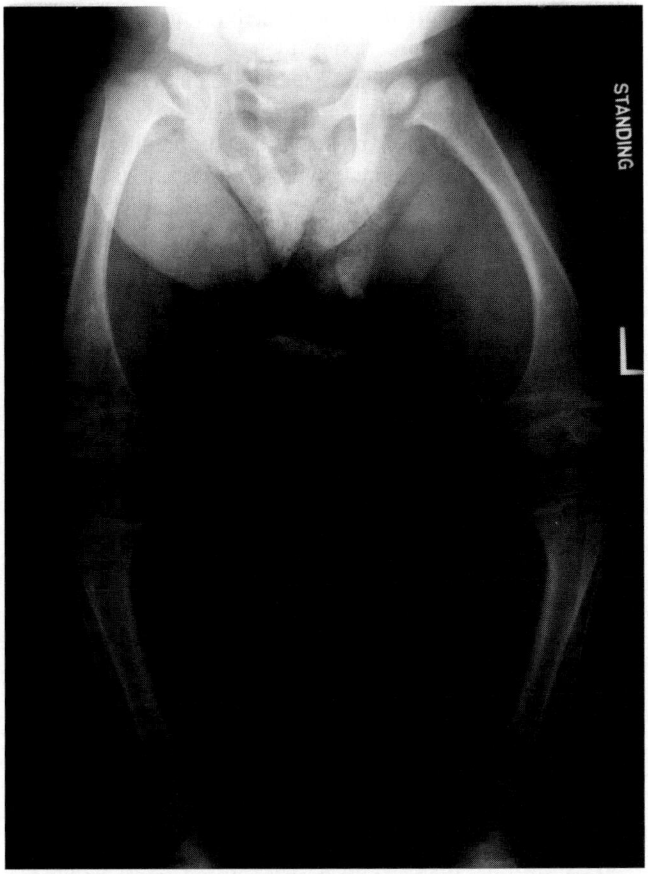

FIG. 42-6 Rickets. This standing radiograph of an 8-year-old female with hypophosphotemic rickets shows cupping and widening of the growth plates throughout the lower extremities. Also note the bowing femoral deformity and hip deformity.

Scoliosis

Scoliosis is a rotational curvature of the spine most obvious in the anterior-posterior plane (Fig. 42-7). It can be classified as nonstructural or structural. **Nonstructural scoliosis** results from a cause other than the spine itself, such as posture, leg length discrepancy, or pain. **Structural scoliosis** is curvature of the spine associated with vertebral rotation. Nonstructural scoliosis can become structural if the underlying cause is not found and treated.

Structural scoliosis can be caused by a great variety of conditions. It can result from congenital skeletal abnormalities (15%), neuromuscular diseases (15%), trauma, extraspinal contractures, bone infections that involve the vertebrae, metabolic bone disorders (e.g., rickets, osteoporosis, osteogenesis imperfecta), joint disease, and tumors. Most cases of structural scoliosis, however, have no known cause, although genetic factors are suggested. Structural scoliosis with no known cause, termed **idiopathic scoliosis**, accounts for at least 65% of cases.

Idiopathic scoliosis is classified as infantile, juvenile, or adolescent, depending on the child's age at the time of onset. In infantile scoliosis, spinal curvature develops during the first 3 years of life; in juvenile scoliosis, curvature develops between the skeletal age of 4 years and the onset of adolescence; and in adolescent scoliosis, it develops after the skeletal age of 10. Adolescent idiopathic scoliosis is the most common. Scoliosis in its milder forms occurs equally in boys and girls once curves measure more than 15 degrees; however, girls are 5 times as likely to have scoliosis than boys.

Pathophysiology

It has been hypothesized that in individuals with adolescent scoliosis, there is an abnormality of the central nervous system involving the balance mechanism in the midbrain. A

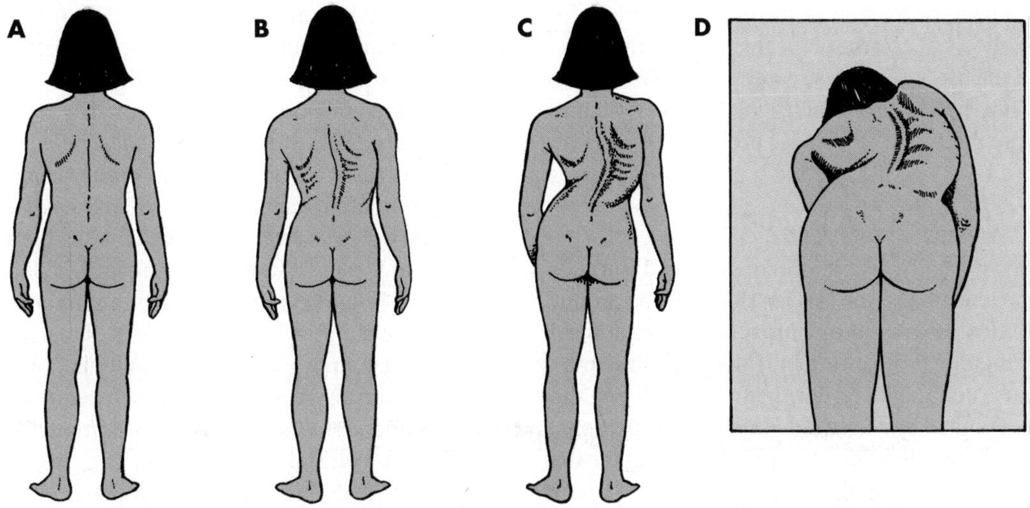

Fig. 42-7 Scoliosis in children. Normal spinal alignment and abnormal spinal curvatures associated with scoliosis. **A,** Normal. **B,** Mild. **C,** Severe. **D,** Rotation and curvature of scoliosis.

genetic component is also suggested because 30% occur within families. Postural and equilibrium dysfunction along with vestibular dysfunction have also been implicated in other studies.

Experimentally, it also has been shown that individuals with adolescent idiopathic scoliosis have an abnormality in the function of the posterior columns of the spinal cord. This results in abnormal proprioception and is not evident clinically except in the presence of scoliosis. The exact cause of scoliosis, however, remains elusive.[5,6]

The earliest pathologic changes, which are probably secondary changes, occur in the soft tissues. The muscles, ligaments, and other soft tissues become shortened on the concave side of the curve. With time, progressive deformities of the vertebral column and ribs develop. In growing children, lateral deviation of the spinal column ceases and one-sided compression of the vertebral bodies on the concave side of the curve begins. Vertebral deformity occurs as asymmetric forces are applied to the epiphyseal center of the ossification by shortened and tight soft tissues on the concave side of the curve. The degree of compression and twisting varies according to the position of the vertebrae in the curve. The compressive force is greatest on the vertebrae in the apex of the concavity, so that the apical vertebrae become most deformed.

The curves increase most rapidly during periods of rapid skeletal growth. If the curve is less than 40 degrees at skeletal maturity, the risk of progression is quite small. In curves greater than 50 degrees, the spine is biomechanically unstable and the curve will in all likelihood continue to progress throughout life. The average rate of progression is 1 degree per year. Curves in the thoracic spine greater than 60 degrees result in decreased pulmonary function, whereas the most common complication of large curves in the lumbar spine is back pain.

Clinical Manifestations

The clinical manifestations of nonstructural scoliosis are mild spinal curvature with prominence of one hip or rounded shoulders. The curvature disappears with forward flexion of the spine, lying down, or traction of the head. Treatment for nonstructural scoliosis is correction of the underlying disorder. The clinical manifestations of structural scoliosis include asymmetry of hip height, asymmetry of shoulder height, shoulder and scapular (shoulder blade) prominence, and rib prominence.

Evaluation and Treatment

Spinal curvature is usually visible or palpable, and muscles on one side of the lower back (the convex side) may be prominent or bulging. Most cases of idiopathic scoliosis are noticed during school screening programs. In girls the deformity may be noticed because clothing does not "hang" properly on the body. Diagnosis is made by roentgenographic examinations.

Treatment of curves between 25 and 35 degrees in the skeletally immature child is with bracing. In most cases the low-profile brace is used. Within the past few years, a brace used only at night, the Charleston bending brace, has been developed. Unfortunately, results with the Charleston brace have shown it to be less effective than the traditional low-profile braces in preventing progression of curves. Occasionally a Milwaukee brace, which has a metal upper structure and neck ring, is needed for curves with an apex higher than midthoracic level. Low-profile and Milwaukee braces are worn for 23 hours daily until skeletal maturity. Bracing will only prevent progression of the curve; it will not correct the curvature. Bracing is not effective in curves greater than 40 degrees or in skeletally mature individuals. Extensive chiropractic manipulations and electrical stimulation have not been shown to change natural history. Surgical treatment with spinal fusion with instrumentation is recommended for curves greater than 40 to 50 degrees. If surgery is indicated, it is better performed during the adolescent years while there is greater flexibility of the curves and less risk of complications.

One dilemma in the treatment of scoliosis is predicting which curves will progress and which will not. Currently, researchers are evaluating platelet calmodulin as a predictor for the severity and progression of adolescent idiopathic scoliosis.[7] Early results have shown a higher platelet calmodulin level in individuals with a progressive curve. If these early results are corroborated in future studies, these levels could be used to avoid unnecessary radiography in individuals with a low risk of progression and more accurately predict which individuals would benefit from brace or surgical treatment.[7]

Bone Infection: Osteomyelitis

Osteomyelitis is an infection of the bone. Occurring twice as often in males as females, acute osteomyelitis may affect infants and children of any age, but it occurs most frequently between 3 and 12 years of age.

Bacteria enter the bone through the bloodstream and lodge in the medullary cavity, where a rich phagocytic mechanism frequently prevents most of the bacteria from establishing an infectious state. In some cases, however, the bacteria may lodge at the end of the venous loops beneath the epiphyseal plate and infection develops because there are no phagocytic cells present to remove the bacteria (Fig. 42-8).[8,9,10]

The microorganism responsible for osteomyelitis varies and is related to the age of the child (Box 42-1). Osteomyelitis in the newborn is caused primarily by *Staphylococcus aureus.* Group B streptococcus and *Escherichia coli* infections are responsible for some cases, especially those of multiple bone involvement and in high-risk infants.[10]

Staphylococcus aureus is the responsible microorganism in 60% to 90% of osteomyelitis cases in older children. *Haemophilus influenzae*, a previously common cause of osteomyelitis in children less than 5 years of age, has now become rare with the improvements in immunization. Gram-negative microorganisms account for an increasing number of infections of the vertebrae,[11,12] whereas *Salmonella* infections are associated with sickle cell disease.

Factors that predispose an individual to the development of osteomyelitis include impetigo, furunculosis, infected lesions of varicella (chickenpox), infected burns, cerebral abscesses, immunization with bacille Calmette-Guérin (BCG) vaccine, prolonged intravenous or central parenteral alimentation, drug addiction, and direct trauma to the area adjacent to the site of osteomyelitis.

Pathophysiology

Osteomyelitis usually begins as a bloody abscess in the metaphysis of the bone. The abscess ruptures under the periosteum and spreads along the bone shaft or into the bone marrow cavity if untreated. Infection rarely spreads down the medullary cavity of the bone but rather first gains entrance to the subperiosteal space in the metaphysis. This is the path of least resistance because the cortex of the bone in this area is porous or mazelike and the inflammatory response blocks spread within the bone.[13] Because of the accumulation of debris caused by the infection, the periosteum may separate and form a shell of new bone around the infected portion of the shaft. Because the periosteum is separated from an adequate blood supply, sections of the bone die with the pieces of dead bone, or **sequestra.** The periosteum that maintains a blood supply generates new bone and is responsible for the appearance of the periosteal new bone, or **involucrum.** The presence of the sequestra and involucrum indicates that the disease has progressed to subperiosteal abscess formation.

In cases where the infection in the metaphysis occurs near the joint, the accumulating pus (bacteria, white blood cells, fluid) creates increasing pressure that may cause a rupture into the joint cavity. If rupture into the joint occurs, the pus causes inflammation and a condition called **secondary septic arthritis.**[10] Although thought uncommon, a recent study shows 40% of children will have adjacent joint involvement with osteomylitis. The most common joint is the knee. Osteomyelitis is most commonly caused by bacteria that reach the metaphysis through the bloodstream but may occur through secondary inoculation of microorganisms caused by trauma or contagious spread of infection from cellulitis in adjacent soft tissue.

Osteomyelitis in infants is frequently associated with septic arthritis because the infant's bone has blood vessels that perforate the growth plate. Because of the unique nature of blood supply to an infant's bones, osteomyelitis and septic arthritis frequently occur together. Normal anatomic variations in infants allow infection to spread directly to the epiphysis, which causes both joint disease and permanent epiphyseal disease. Multiple sites of osteomyelitis are also more common in children younger than 2 years, necessitating bone scan to check other bones when infants are infected. This can then lead to other areas of osteomyelitis and possibly septic arthritis.[14]

Children are susceptible to joint involvement for several reasons (Fig. 42-9). In the immature infant, there is no epiphyseal plate or an ossific nucleus at the end of the bone and the cartilage precursor of bone is penetrated by vascular channels. In these infants the infection begins in the vulnerable

A

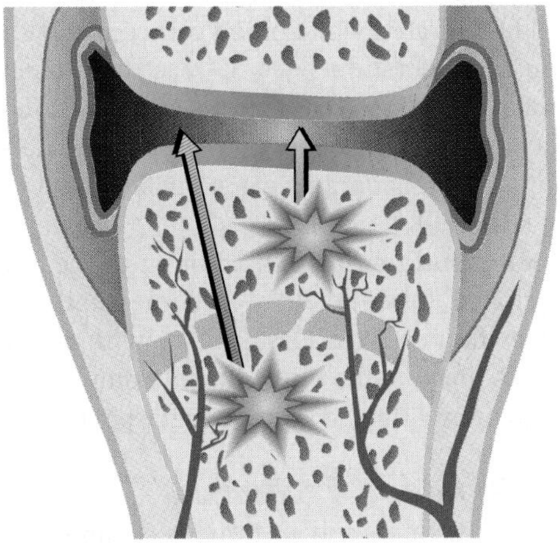

B

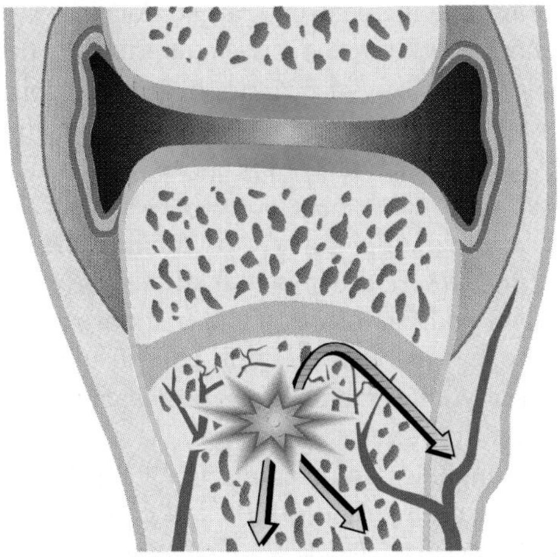

FIG. 42-8 Pathogenesis of acute osteomyelitis differs with age. A, In infants younger than 1 year the epiphysis is nourished by penetrating arteries through the physis, allowing development of the condition within the epiphysis. **B,** In children up to 15 years of age the infection is restricted to below the physis because of interruption of the vessels.

Box 42-1

CAUSATIVE MICROORGANISMS OF OSTEOMYELITIS ACCORDING TO AGE

NEWBORNS

Staphylococcus aureus
Group B streptococcus
Gram-negative enteric rods

INFANTS

Staphylococcus aureus
Haemophilus influenzae

OLDER CHILDREN

Staphylococcus aureus
Pseudomonas
Salmonella
Neisseria gonorrhoeae

ADOLESCENTS AND ADULTS

Pseudomonas
Mycobacterium tuberculosis

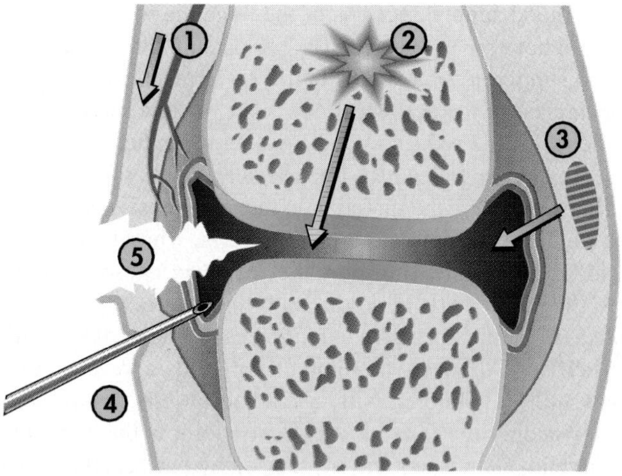

FIG. 42-9 Routes of infection to the joint.

cartilage precursor of the end bone itself and results in rapid destruction of the joint and arrested growth of the bone. For this reason the early detection and treatment of osteomyelitis are crucial if the infant's joint is to be saved from later destruction. As the child matures and the epiphyseal plate forms, a temporary barrier is established against infection because the arterioles end beneath the epiphyseal plate.[13]

In children older than 2 years, the epiphyseal plate prevents the spread of a metaphyseal abscess into the epiphysis and the cortex of the metaphysis is thicker. These anatomic differences increase the likelihood that the metaphyseal abscess will extend into the diaphysis and the blood supply of the bone will be disrupted. The periosteum is also more difficult to perforate in older children; this may lead to a larger subperiosteal abscess that could endanger the periosteal blood supply as well. This process commonly results in extensive sequestrum formation and chronic osteomyelitis.[13]

Osteomyelitis is much less common after the physeal plates are closed, except in the vertebral body. Infection may develop in any part of a bone, and abscesses spread slowly. Destruction of the cortex in a localized area may result in a pathologic fracture.[11,12]

Spread of infection to contiguous joints is related to the child's age. Infection may spread to adjacent joints because the epiphyseal plate of the proximal femur is located within the hip joint capsule; the distal femoral plate is partially located within the knee; and the proximal and distal humeral plates are partially located within the shoulder and elbow joints, respectively. Recent studies have shown, however, that, like infants, older children may demonstrate up to 42% of contiguous joint involvement. Even in areas where the involved osteomylitis was extraarticular, joint involvement occurred; this differs from previous reports in the literature.[14]

Clinical Manifestations

The clinical manifestations of osteomyelitis are age dependent and are related to the differing vascular patterns found in the skeletal system at various ages. Three distinct groups may be identified: (1) infants younger than 1 year, (2) children from 1 year of age to puberty, and (3) adolescents after cessation of bone growth and adults.

Infants. Osteomyelitis may be an acute illness characterized by fever and failure to move the affected limb (pseudoparalysis). Infantile osteomyelitis is characterized by involvement of multiple sites within the same bone or in multiple bones. If untreated, involvement of the adjacent growth plate can result in growth arrest.

Children. Osteomyelitis in children between the ages of 1 year and puberty is characterized by fever and systemic signs of toxicity. The illness is sometimes subacute, with the child complaining of swelling, redness, tenderness, and decreasing ability to bear weight on or move the affected area. Onset can be abrupt. Osteomyelitis during childhood most frequently affects the long bones but also may be found in the pelvis and spine. Clinical manifestations are usually accompanied by elevated white blood cell counts and elevated erythrocyte sedimentation rates. C-reactive protein (CRP), when elevated, is a sensitive sign of osteomyelitis and can rapidly decrease with appropriate treatment. Evidence of infection using roentgenograms can be delayed but bone scan is positive within 48 hours.

Adolescents and adults. In addition to the sites previously mentioned, osteomyelitis in adolescents and adults may involve the vertebrae. Back pain, with a duration of several weeks, may be the only clinical complaint. This age group is less often affected than younger populations.

Evaluation and Treatment

White blood cell counts and erythrocyte sedimentation rates are sometimes elevated, but this is not a consistent finding. Monitoring of erythrocyte sedimentation rates is an indication of response to management but can be delayed. C-reactive protein is more quickly responsive to appropriate treatment. Blood cultures (positive in 30% to 40%) and aspiration of the soft tissue or bone, or both, should be done to identify the causative microorganism. Appropriate antibiotics should be prescribed after culture and sensitivity studies have been completed. A tuberculin test also is administered because *Mycobacterium tuberculosis* is sometimes the responsible microorganism and has recently had a slight resurgence in incidence. Bone scans can be quite helpful with diagnosis and in children younger than 1 year are absolutely required to define if multiple sites are involved.

Treatment includes intravenous (IV) antibiotics or, in highly reliable children and families, a combination of IV and oral antibiotics for 6 weeks. Drainage and margination of bone is required if changes are present on radiographs signifying abscess. Immobilization may help with pain control. If a joint is also infected, this is a *surgical emergency* to avoid damage to the articular cartilage by lysosymes released from the involved neutrophils.

Table 42-3 Incidence of Connective Tissue Diseases in Children

Disease	Annual Rate/10^5	Gender Ratio (Female/Male)	Race Ratio (White/Black)	Peak Age-Group at Risk (yr)	Childhood Onset (%)
Rheumatoid arthritis	40	3:1	Equal	Increases with age (20-50)	5
Systemic lupus erythematosus	6	8:1	1:4	15-45	18
Dermatomyositis	0.8	2:1	1:3	45-65	20
Scleroderma	0.4	3:1	Equal	Increases with age (30-50)	3
Polyarteritis	0.2	1:3	Equal	Midadult	Rare

Data from Hollingworth P. In Klippel JH, Dieppe PA, editors: *Rheumatology,* St Louis, 1994, Mosby.

Death is rare, but serious sequelae may occur. The course of the disease and prognosis depend on the age of the child, the rapidity with which the diagnosis is established, the initiation of early treatment, and maintenance of the treatment for an adequate time. The most serious complications are growth arrest, osseous necrosis, and recurrence. Recurrence with present antibiotic regimens is less than 10%.

Juvenile Rheumatoid Arthritis

The rheumatic diseases are a group of diverse conditions having in common the inflammation of connective tissues. They include rheumatoid arthritis, systemic lupus erythematosus, dermatomyositis, scleroderma, and polyarthritis. Incidence of these disorders in children is estimated in Table 42-3.

Juvenile rheumatoid arthritis (JRA) is the childhood form of rheumatoid arthritis (see Chapter 41). Like adult-onset rheumatoid arthritis, JRA is a syndrome that is often accompanied by systemic manifestations. Approximately 5% of all cases of rheumatoid arthritis begin in childhood. An estimated quarter of a million children in the United States have JRA.

The basic pathophysiology of JRA is the same as that of adult rheumatoid arthritis. The clinical manifestations of JRA may differ, however, beginning with mode of onset. Unlike adult rheumatoid arthritis, which begins insidiously with systemic signs of inflammation and generalized aches, JRA has three distinct modes of onset: arthritis in fewer than five joints (pauciarticular arthritis), arthritis in more than five joints (polyarticular arthritis), and systemic disease. Onset is less gradual in JRA than in adult rheumatoid arthritis. Juvenile rheumatoid arthritis also differs from the adult form in the following respects:[15,16]

1. Predominantly the large joints are affected.
2. Subluxation and ankylosis of the cervical spine are common if the disease progresses.
3. Joint pain is not as severe as in the adult type.
4. Serologic tests often detect antinuclear antibody (ANA).
5. Chronic uveitis is common, especially if ANA positive.
6. Serologic tests seldom detect rheumatoid factor.
7. Rheumatoid nodules are not limited to subcutaneous tissue but are found in the heart, lungs, eyes, and other organs.

Treatment for children with JRA is supportive but not curative. Many children with pauciarticular arthritis who are seronegative for ANA will resolve their symptoms over time. However, with systemic onset (Stills disease) or seropositivity, JRA may progress to true adult RA. The aims of treatment are to control inflammation and other clinical manifestations of the disease and to minimize deformity.

Avascular Diseases of the Bone: Osteochondrosis

The avascular diseases of the bone, collectively termed **osteochondroses,** are caused by insufficient blood supply to growing bones. Disturbances of blood supply to primary and secondary centers of ossification during periods of rapid bone growth result in a variety of skeletal abnormalities.

The cause of the osteochondroses remains obscure. In the past, infection, nutritional deficiencies, and hormonal imbalances were blamed, but these causes have been largely disproven. Currently, vascular impairment and trauma, coupled with an underlying developmental or genetic predisposition, have been identified as probable causes of osteochondroses. The most common osteochondroses are Osgood-Schlatter disease (tibial tubrecle), distal patellar pole (Sindig Larsen-Johansson syndrome), radial head (Panner disease), the navicular bone of the foot (Kohler disese), and calcaneus (Sever disease). All are associated with activity-related pain of the affected region that improves with rest. All are more common in boys than girls and athletes more than nonathletes.

The osteochrondroses involve areas of significant tensile or compressing stress that undergo partial osseous necrosis, progressive bony weakness, and then microfracture. Most of these are associated with trauma and overuse and improve with rest. Antiinflammatories, modification of activities, and even immobilization are used during active disease. Reparative correction by revascularization is the rule, although this may be a lengthy process.

Legg-Calvé-Perthes Disease

Legg-Calvé-Perthes disease, commonly called Perthes disease, is classically thought to be an osteochondroses like those previously described. This self-limited disease of the hip is presumably produced by recurrent interruption of the blood supply to the femoral head. The ossification center first becomes necrotic, collapses, and then is gradually remodeled by live bone.

Legg-Calvé-Perthes disease is relatively common (1 in 5000 children), usually occurring in children between 3 and

10 years of age, with a peak incidence at 6 years. It is more common in boys than in girls by a ratio of about 5:1. The condition is bilateral in approximately 10% of affected children.

The cause of decreased blood supply to the head of the femur is unknown. Several theories have been proposed, including thyroid deficiency; trauma; infection; and protein C and S deficiencies, which cause a hypercoagulable state.[17] A plausible theory is that acute synovitis (infection of the synovial membrane) and increased hydrostatic pressure in the hip joint compress blood vessels that supply the femoral head.

Constitutional factors definitely play a role. Birth weight of children with Legg-Calvé-Perthes disease is much lower than that of unaffected children. Skeletal maturation is delayed an average of 2 years in children with Legg-Calvé-Perthes disease, and affected children are between 2.5 and 7 cm shorter than unaffected children of the same age. Familial occurrence is 30% to 40%. The disease is rare in blacks, and it is frequent in children of Japanese and central European ancestry.

Pathophysiology

Legg-Calvé-Perthes disease runs its natural course in 2 to 5 years. In the incipient stage the soft tissues of the hip (synovial membrane and joint capsule) are swollen, edematous, and hyperemic, often with fluid present in the joint (Fig. 42-10). The joint space widens, and the joint capsule bulges. The first stage lasts only a few weeks. In the second (or active avascular necrotic) stage, the entire epiphysis or the anterior half of the epiphysis of the femoral head is dead and the metaphyseal bone at the junction of the femoral neck and capital epiphyseal plate is softened because of increased blood supply and decalcification. Soon granulation tissue (procallus) and blood vessels invade the dead bone. This stage lasts several months to 1 year.

The third (or regenerative healing) stage ordinarily lasts 2 to 4 years. The dead femoral head is replaced by procallus, and new bone is laid down. Collapse and flattening of the femoral head occur, and the femoral neck becomes short and wide (see Fig. 42-10).

In the fourth (or residual) stage, remodeling takes place and the newly formed bone is organized into a live spongy bone. Children less than 6 years of age at onset have more time to remodel the damage Perthes has caused and have the best outcome.[18] Recent multicenter studies, using the "lateral pillar" classification,[18] have shown that hips younger than 6 years with *no* involvement of the lateral femoral head (type A) do better than those with involvement of the lateral femoral head. Those children with complete collapse of not only the lateral but also the entire femoral head (type C) have the worst prognosis. Long-term studies of type C hips show that without treatment 70% to 90% progress to osteoarthritis by 40 years of age.[19]

Clinical Manifestations

Injury or trauma precedes the onset of clinical manifestations in approximately one third of children with Legg-Calvé-Perthes disease. Onset of symptoms is insidious unless trauma aggravates the disease process. The child frequently complains of a limp or pain for several months. The pain usually is referred to the knee, inner thigh, and groin, following the path of the obturator nerve. In some children, pain may be absent or minimal. If pain is present, it is usually aggravated by activity and relieved by rest.

The typical physical findings include spasm on rotation of the hip in extension, a limitation of internal rotation flexion and adduction. If the child is walking, an abnormal gait, termed a Trendelenberg gait or abductor lurch, is apparent. The child moves his or her trunk toward the affected side with stance to compensate for weak abductor musculature. If the hip pain or limp has been present for a prolonged period, muscles of the hip and thigh atrophy.

Evaluation and Treatment

Diagnosis is confirmed by radiographic examination. Principles of treatment are "containment" (keeping the ball completely in the socket) and motion to maintain the articular cartilage. In the past, children were treated with bed rest and a variety of braces, which have now been shown to be ineffective. Currently, most children can be managed with antiinflammatory medications and bed rest for episodes of synovitis and activity modification (avoidance of jumping activities that place increased stress on the hip). Serial roentgenograms are obtained to monitor the progress of the disease and ensure that the hip remains congruent. Surgery may be necessary if the femoral head becomes subluxated or incongruent with the acetabulum before the reparative process. The ball must be congruent to take on the shape of the socket as remodeling occurs.

Factors affecting the outcome of Legg-Calvé-Perthes disease are the age of the child, the extent of necrosis, and the stage of disease at the time treatment is begun and congruence

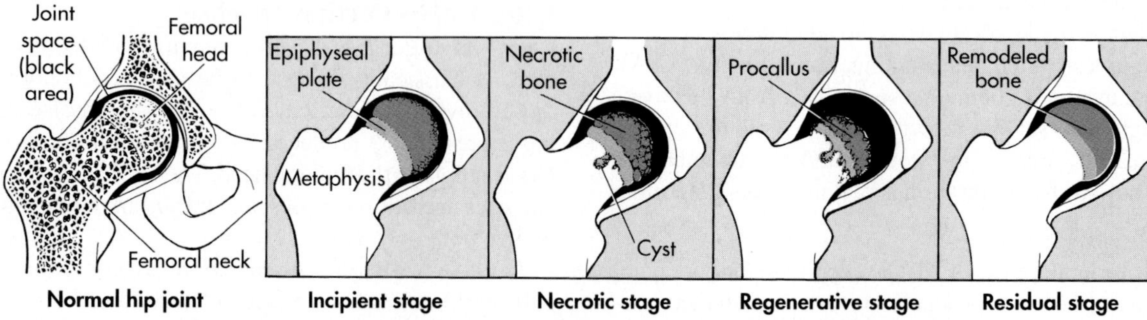

Fig. 42-10 Stages of Legg-Calvé-Perthes disease, a form of osteochondrosis.

of the joint with skeletal maturity. Recent studies have shown that girls, despite earlier skeletal maturity, do as well as boys. Outcome is 70% satisfactory with Herring stage A; for Herring B and C or age greater than 8 years, outcome is guarded. Present prospective studies are evaluating more aggressive early treatment (i.e., osteotomy of the femur or pelvis) on the more involved hips to change long-term outcome.

Osgood-Schlatter Disease

Osgood-Schlatter disease consists of tendinitis of the anterior patellar tendon, within which the patella (kneecap) is embedded, and associated osteochondrosis of the tubercle of the tibia. Osgood-Schlatter disease occurs most frequently in preadolescents and adolescents who participate in sports. The incidence is higher in boys than in girls.

Pathophysiology

The severity of the lesion varies from mild tendinitis to a complete separation of the anterior extension of the tibial epiphysis, which is the part of the epiphysis that contributes to growth of the tibial tubercle. The underlying pathologic alterations also vary. The mildest form of Osgood-Schlatter disease causes ischemic (avascular) necrosis in the region of the bony tibial tubercle, with hypertrophic cartilage formation during the stages of repair. In more severe cases the abnormality involves a true epiphyseal separation of the tibial tubercle, with the characteristics of avascular necrosis described in the section on Legg-Calvé-Perthes disease.

Clinical Manifestations

The child experiences pain and swelling in the region of the patellar tendon and tibial tubercle, which becomes prominent and is tender to direct pressure. The pain is most severe after physical activity that involves vigorous quadriceps contraction or direct local trauma to the tibial tubercle area. Frequently the child experiences sudden acute discomfort referable to the affected region. Sudden onset of pain is caused by a pathologic fracture through an area of ischemic necrosis.

Evaluation and Treatment

Diagnosis is confirmed by roentgenographic examination. The goal of treatment for Osgood-Schlatter disease is to decrease the stress at the tubercle. Often a period of 4 to 8 weeks of restriction from strenuous physical activity, especially activities requiring deep knee bending, is sufficient. If pain relief is not achieved, a cast or brace is required to immobilize the knee, a situation that is particularly difficult if the condition is bilateral.

Gradual resumption of activity is permitted after 8 weeks, but return to unrestricted athletic participation requires an additional 8 weeks to allow for revascularization, healing, and ossification of the tibial tubercle.

Cerebral Palsy

Cerebral palsy (CP) is a static disorder of muscle tone and balance caused by an ischemic insult to the brain, usually perinatally. The incidence is presently 3% to 5% but is increasing with successful resuscitation of premature infants.

Evaluation and Diagnosis

The diagnosis of cerebral palsy can be quite subtle but is often made when gross motor milestones are not met by predicted ages. In some infants, diagnosis can be made as early as 4 months.[20] Cognitive involvement is widely variable and is dependent on the amount of CNS involvement. There are classic patterns: hemiplegia involves one side of the body, diplegia usually involves the lower extremities only, and quadriplegia involves all four extremities. Quadraplegic involvement is most often associated with cognitive involvement, seizure disorder, and aphasia. Many quadriplegics, however, are of normal intelligence and "trapped" within aphasia. When given communication devices, these children are sometimes "discovered," as is their normal intelligence.

Treatment

Treatment of cerebral palsy is multifaceted and undergoing constant evolution. The use of physical and occupational treatments, orthotics, spasticity reduction (by selected dorsal rhizotomy, oral, or intrathecal Baclofen), botulinom-A ("Botox") toxin injections, and surgery are often all used to maximize a child's function. In many centers, a multispecialty approach at "CP clinics" occurs so that a family may, within one clinic visit, see neurology, pediatrics, orthotics, orthopedic surgery, and rehabilitation clinicians.

Children with CP should be carefully followed and given all possible opportunities to flourish. Although CP is a static disorder, progressive deformity for ongoing muscle tone can occur. Monitoring these children as they grow with a multispecialty approach is essential to their best outcome.

Muscular Dystrophy

The **muscular dystrophies** are a group of familial disorders that cause degeneration of skeletal muscle fibers. The muscular dystrophies are the most prevalent of the muscle diseases in childhood and are characterized by progressive, symmetric weakness and wasting of skeletal muscle groups, with increasing disability and deformity.

Classification of the muscular dystrophies is based on age of onset, rate of progression, distribution of muscular involvement, and inheritance patterns. The major clinically and genetically distinct types are the pseudohypertrophic (Duchenne), facioscapulohumeral, limb girdle, and oculopharyngeal dystrophies (Fig. 42-11). Because the clinical findings and genetic inheritance patterns are consistent for each type, some researchers believe that each involves a separate biochemical defect. Genetic research has focused on identifying the site of abnormal gene function for each defect. This will permit more accurate carrier detection and, eventually, description of the biochemical aberration. (Table 42-4 summarizes the types of muscular dystrophy.)

Duchenne Muscular Dystrophy

In 1868 the French neurologist G.B.A. Duchenne described a pseudohypertrophic muscular paralysis associated with large amounts of fat and connective tissue. Today this form of muscular dystrophy, called **Duchenne muscular dystrophy**, is the most common of the muscular dystrophies. Its

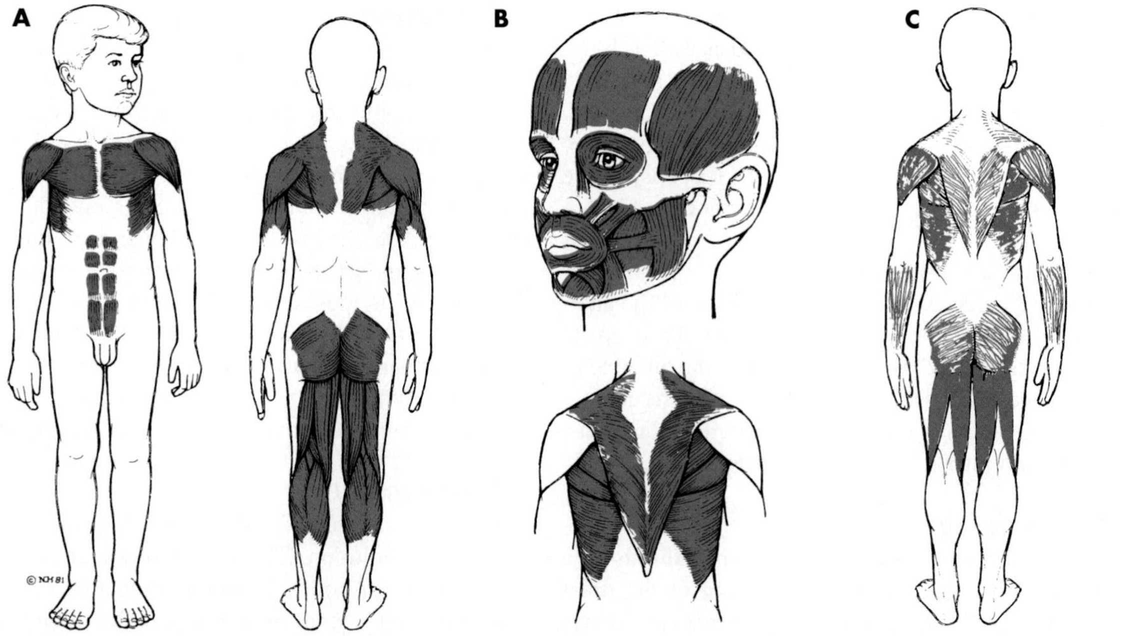

FIG. 42-11 **Initial muscle groups involved in three types of muscular dystrophy. A,** Pseudohypertrophic. **B,** Facioscapulohumeral. **C,** Limb girdle. (From Wong DL: *Whaley and Wong's nursing care of infants and children*, ed 6, St Louis, 1999, Mosby.)

Table 42-4 Major Muscular Dystrophy Syndromes

Disease	Mode of Inheritance	Age at Clinical Onset	Usual Distribution	Rate of Progression	Mental Retardation	Distinguishing Findings
Duchenne muscular dystrophy (DMD)	X-linked recessive	About 3 years	Hips and shoulders, quadriceps femoris, gastrocnemius (pseudohypertrophy)	Rapid	Frequent	Elevated serum enzymes (CPK, LDH, SGOT, aldolase)
Facioscapulohumeral dystrophy	Autodomal dominant	In first or second decade	Shoulder girdle, neck, face, pelvic girdle (late)	Moderate	Occasional	Several distinct muscle pathologic findings
Limb girdle (LG) dystrophy	Poorly defined or recessive	Variable	Pelvic and shoulder girdles	Variable	Variable	Collection of several diseases
Myotonic dystrophy (MyD)	Autosomal dominant	Variable—birth to fifth decade	Distal extensor muscle, eyelids, face, neck, hands, pharynx	Slow, related to age at clinical onset, faster with younger patients	Frequent	Percussion myotonia, cataracts, diabetic GTT despite increased insulin, testicular atropy, decreased IgG

CPK, Creatine phosphokinase; *LDH,* lactate dehydrogenase; *SGOT,* serum glutamic oxaloacetic transaminase; *GTT,* glucose tolerance test; *IgG,* immunoglobulin G.

incidence is approximately 1 in 3500 male births.[21] Classic Duchenne muscular dystrophy occurs only in boys and has a history of X-linked inheritance in half of the cases.

Pathophysiology

The X-linked inherited type of Duchenne muscular dystrophy is thought to be caused by a deletion of a segment of deoxyribonucleic acid (DNA)[21] or a single-gene defect on the short arm of the X chromosome. A protein encoded by the Duchenne muscular dystrophy gene, called **dystrophin**, has been identified.

Dystrophin is present in normal muscle cells and absent in Duchenne muscular dystrophy. Dystrophin mediates anchorage of the actin cytoskeleton of skeletal muscle fibers to the basement membrane through a membrane glycoprotein complex. The complete lack of dystrophin in severe Duchenne dystrophy means that poorly anchored fibers tear themselves apart under the repeated stress of contraction. Free calcium

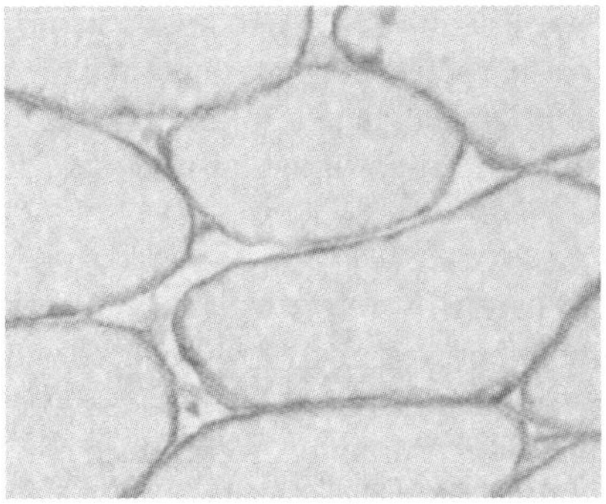

FIG. 42-12 Dystrophin abnormalities. This shows staining of muscle for dystrophin (reddish brown). In Duchenne dystrophy this staining would be absent because no protein is produced. In Becker dystrophy, staining is reduced or patchy. (From Stevens A, Lowe J: *Pathology*, St Louis, 1995, Mosby.)

then enters the muscle cells, causing cell death and fiber necrosis (Fig. 42-12).[22]

There is increased endomysial connective tissue and fat; loss of striations; and concomitant hyaline, granular, and fatty degeneration of fibers. Disorganization of tendinous insertions is associated with fat accumulation in these areas. Although fibers regenerate in the younger child, they are abnormal in many ways and become nonfunctional with time.

Clinical Manifestations

Duchenne muscular dystrophy is usually identified in children approximately 3 years of age, when the parents notice slow motor development with progressive weakness and muscle wasting. Sitting, standing, and walking are delayed, and the child is clumsy, falls frequently, and has difficulty climbing stairs.

Muscular weakness always begins in the pelvic girdle, causing a "waddling" gait. Hypertrophy of the calf muscles is apparent in 80% of cases. The method of rising from the floor by "climbing up the legs" (Gower sign) is characteristic and is caused by weakness of the lumbar and gluteal muscles. The foot assumes an equinovarus position (see Fig. 42-4), and the child tends to walk on the toes because of weakness of the anterior tibial and peroneal muscles. Within 3 to 5 years, muscles of the shoulder girdle become involved. Contractures and wasting of the muscles contribute to muscular atrophy and deformity of the skeleton.

Duchenne muscular dystrophy has serious complications. Pulmonary function is compromised greatly because of marked kyphoscoliosis ("humped" upper spine combined with scoliosis), which usually develops after the child is confined to a wheelchair (Fig. 42-13). The incidence of cardiac involvement in Duchenne muscular dystrophy is as high as 95%. Chronic heart failure may occur in 50% of children. A moderate degree of mental retardation causes these children to have a mean IQ of approximately 80. Smooth muscle dysfunction may cause megacolon, volvulus, cramping pain, and malabsorption in the gastrointestinal tract. The children usually succumb to other pulmonary or cardiac causes and death ensues by the late teens. Only 25% live to age 21.

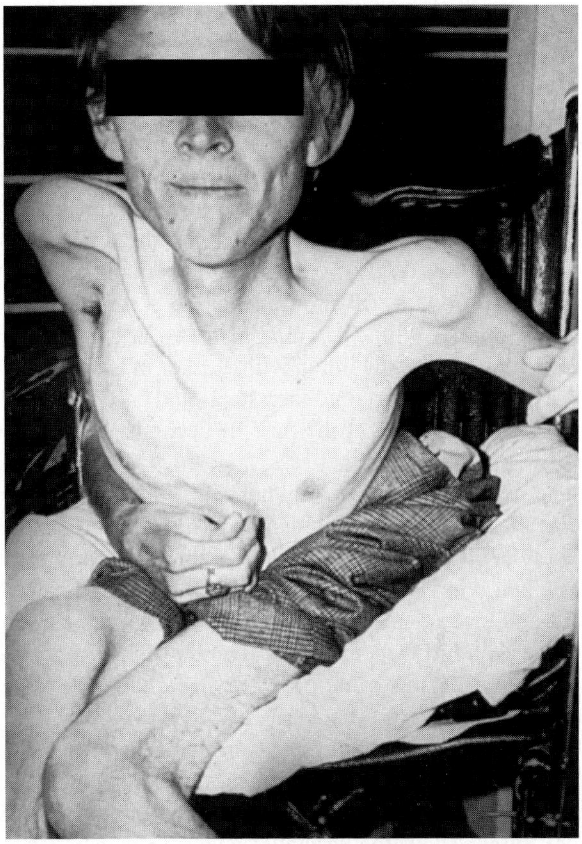

FIG. 42-13 Duchenne muscular dystrophy. An individual with late-stage Duchenne muscular dystrophy, showing severe muscle loss. (From Jorde LB et al: *Medical genetics*, ed 2, St Louis, 1999, Mosby.)

Evaluation and Treatment

Diagnosis is confirmed by measurement of serum enzymes, electromyography (EMG), and muscle biopsy. The serum enzymes, especially creatine phosphokinase (CPK), are increased to more than 10 times normal, even during infancy and before the onset of weakness. Histologic changes in muscle include degeneration of muscle fibers, with variation in fiber size and central nuclei. Fat and connective tissue replace muscle fibers.

Although intrauterine diagnosis is not yet possible, work is being done in this area.[23] Elevated CPK levels at birth are diagnostic indicators of Duchenne muscular dystrophy. Identification of female carriers of the disease cannot be achieved with certainty, but serum CPK is elevated in 60% to 80% of carriers.

There is no effective treatment for Duchenne muscular dystrophy. Maintaining function in unaffected muscle groups for as long as possible is the primary goal. Although activity fosters maintenance of muscle function, strenuous exercise may hasten the breakdown of muscle fibers. Range-of-motion exercises, bracing, and surgical release of contracture deformities are used to maintain normal function as long as possible. Scoliotic surgery is suggested when curves reach greater than 20 degrees to prolong respiratory function or walking ability or both. Genetic counseling is recommended. With X-linked inheritance, male siblings of an affected child have a 50% chance of being affected and female siblings have a 50% chance of being carriers.

Becker Muscular Dystrophy

Becker muscular dystrophy is often called benign Duchenne muscular dystrophy because it shares the X-linked inheritance pattern and similar but milder clinical features. The incidence of Becker dystrophy is one tenth that of Duchenne dystrophy. In Becker dystrophy, mutations in the middle rod region of dystrophin still allow anchorage of muscle to basement membrane. Clinical symptoms often begin between 5 and 15 years of age. Children with Becker muscular dystrophy remain ambulatory into their teens and early 20s; in one study the average age at the time of necessity for a wheelchair was 25 years.

The pattern of muscle weakness for both dystrophies is almost identical, but scoliosis and contractures are rare until the child with Becker muscular dystrophy is permanently wheelchair bound. The changes in creatine kinase levels and EMG and electrocardiogram (ECG) readings are the same as those seen in Duchenne muscular dystrophy. Many individuals live well into middle age. Heart failure is infrequent but can be a cause of premature death and disability.

Maintaining ambulation and careful follow-up for evidence of cardiopulmonary complications are essential measures for long-term care. Children with Becker muscular dystrophy rarely show the mental changes seen in Duchenne dystrophy. The accurate diagnosis of Becker muscular dystrophy is important. If the affected individual marries and has children, all daughters will be carriers of this X-linked recessive disorder. Genetic counseling should be offered to the mother, female siblings, offspring, and any maternal relatives.

Facioscapulohumeral Muscular Dystrophy

Facioscapulohumeral muscular dystrophy is a mild form of progressive, autosomal dominant muscular dystrophy. Age at onset varies from early childhood to adulthood, and the disease affects males and females equally. As the name implies, clinical manifestations begin with weakness and atrophy of facial and shoulder girdle (scapulohumeral) muscles. The illness progresses slowly. Inability to close the eyes completely may be noted from early childhood. The face is expressionless, and pouting of the lips makes whistling impossible. The first symptoms usually include drooping of the shoulders with difficulty in raising the arms above the head. Onset of weakness in the lower limbs often is delayed for 20 to 30 years, and pseudohypertrophy of muscles is rare. Contractures and skeletal deformities develop less frequently and are less prominent than in Duchenne muscular dystrophy.

Treatment includes supportive physiotherapy to prevent contractures and prolong ambulation. Lightweight plastic ankle-foot orthoses (AFOs) for footdrop are extremely helpful. Surgery to stabilize the shoulder is sometimes advised.

Some individuals with facioscapulohumeral muscular dystrophy improve with steroid therapy, particularly if the clinical picture includes rapidly progressive weakness. The disease may be arrested for prolonged periods; however, most individuals remain active and have a normal life expectancy. Vocational training and genetic counseling are important to provide them with the information necessary to plan their future.

Scapuloperoneal Muscular Dystrophy

Scapuloperoneal muscular dystrophy is considered a variant of facioscapulohumeral muscular dystrophy, but distal muscles in the lower extremity are involved early instead of the facial and shoulder muscle weakness that is the early sign in facioscapulohumeral dystrophy. Many individuals seek initial treatment for troublesome footdrop and shoulder weakness. Analysis of inheritance patterns shows that the disease can be inherited either as an autosomal dominant trait or as an X-linked recessive trait.

The initial symptoms may resemble those of several other illnesses, including nemaline myopathy (a congenital muscle disease) and early hypertrophic peripheral neuropathy. A careful diagnostic evaluation therefore is in order. Other clinical findings include hypertrophy of the muscle that extends the toes, brought about by a futile attempt to overcome footdrop, and depressed or absent muscle stretch reflexes. Creatine kinase is elevated 2 to 20 times the normal level; EMG readings show myopathy.

Treatment is directed toward treating symptoms and preserving ambulation and functional ability. Footdrop is easily treated with AFOs. Individuals with scapuloperoneal muscular dystrophy remain ambulatory for 40 or more years. Occasionally, walking may be hampered by paraspinal muscle contractures; in this case a wheelchair may assist the individual to cover long distances. The life span in this disorder is normal. It is important that genetic counseling be available to all persons.

Limb Girdle Muscular Dystrophy

The diagnosis of **limb girdle muscular dystrophy** is considered when acute causes of proximal weakness are eliminated and the clinical findings and genetic pattern exclude Duchenne and facioscapulohumeral muscular dystrophy. The diagnosis is often determined by exclusion because few consistent clinical features make this type of muscular dystrophy unique. In fact, some researchers think that limb girdle dystrophy actually may be several separate diseases awaiting more sophisticated methods of evaluation to give them precise labels. Most individuals have a negative family history, making sporadic disease or an autosomal recessive pattern of inheritance likely. The prevalence rate for limb girdle muscular dystrophy is set at 20 per million.

The initial symptoms include shoulder and pelvic girdle weakness, which are usually noted in the early 20s but can be seen as late as the 40s. The muscle weakness is often asymmetric and progresses at a much slower pace than in Duchenne muscular dystrophy. The biceps and deltoid muscles can be extremely atrophic and weak. Individuals can remain ambulatory for extended periods, often up to 20 years after initial diagnosis. When confined to wheelchairs, they show few of the severe effects of other dystrophies, such as contractures and scoliosis. Heart involvement and mental retardation also are rare.

The individual will have mild elevation in creatine kinase levels and a myopathic pattern on EMG. Muscle biopsy is often more characteristic, with fiber splitting and fibers that appear profusely "moth-eaten" and whorled. Treatment includes supportive measures to maintain ambulation and functional ability and frequent follow-up to eliminate secondary complications such as cardiopulmonary disease.

Musculoskeletal Tumors in Children

Bone Tumors

Bone tumors are uncommon childhood tumors and comprise less than 5% of all childhood malignancies. Of the malignant tumors, osteosarcoma and Ewing sarcoma are the most common. Fortunately, the majority of pediatric tumors are benign, most commonly nonossifying fibroma, chondroma, simple bone cyst, aneurysmal bone cyst, osteoid osteoma, and fibrous dysplasia.

Benign Bone Tumors

Nonossifying fibroma. The **nonossifying fibroma (fibrous cortical deficit)**, which is believed to be a defect in ossification rather than a true tumor, makes up approximately 50% of benign bone tumors. Most fibrous cortical defects resolve spontaneously or are obliterated by reparative ossification or remodeling. In some cases, however, the fibrous cortical defect persists and proliferates, becoming a fibroma. Fibromas are found primarily in children and adolescents. Ninety percent of these tumors occur in persons younger than 20 years.

The nonossifying fibroma is a sharply demarcated, cortical-based tumor surrounded by a dense border of hardened bone. The tumor itself consists of fibrocytes arranged in whorled bundles, fibroblastic tissue, and osteoclast-like giant cells. As the tumor evolves, the fibrocytes imbibe lipids and assume a foamy appearance; thus they are known as *foam cells.* The tumor also contains extensive deposits of hemosiderin pigment. The long axis of the tumor parallels the long axis of the bone.

The nonossifying fibroma is usually asymptomatic and is found incidently on radiographs. In the 1950s, as flouride was added to drinking water, random skeletal surveys were done on hundreds of children. Nonossifying fribromas were discovered in 20% to 30% of all children. The fibroma is generally not treated until it occupies more than 50% of the diameter of the bone or extends more than 3 to 4 cm into the cortex. When the tumor grows to this size, a pathologic fracture may occur and, therefore, curettage and bone grafting of the defect is undertaken.

Simple bone cyst. **Simple bone cysts (SBCs)** are cystic lesions of the central region of the metaphysical region in skeletally mature children. With growth, these lesions may appear within the diaphysis. These children are usually asymptomatic until pathologic fracture or incidental discovery occur. Lesions often heal after a fracture, but large lesions may require treatment. Presently a large prospective, randomized study is comparing steroid injection (the classical treatment for these lesions) versus bone marrow injection for treatment. Very large lesions in weight-bearing areas may require internal fixation and bone grafting.

Aneurysmal bone cyst. **Aneurysmal bone cysts (ABCs)** are typically eccentric, metaphysical lesions that occur in a slightly older population than SBCs. The etiology remains controversial; many consider ABC a lesion secondary to another process, such as giant cell tumor. This lesion must be differentiated from telangestatic sarcoma and, therefore, biopsy is necessary. Once diagnosed, curretage with complete removal of the "pseudolining" must be done with chemical or electrocautery to minimize recurrence. Bone graft is placed in the defect. Even with modern techniques, recurrence can be as high as 21%.[24]

Osteoid osteoma. **Osteoid osteoma,** or the larger counterpart, osteoblastoma, present as painful lesions of the diaphysis or metadiaphysis of long bones. Involvement of the posterior elements of the spine—with resultant "splinting" scoliosis—can occur. Night pain is common, as is relief from symptoms with NSAIDs, as these tumors release prostaglandins. When pain is too extreme to be controlled medually, resection of the "nidus," or central portion, of the lesion is uniformly successful. Computed tomographic (CT) guidance to the lesion is often utilized.

Fibrous dysplasia. **Fibrous dysplasia (FD)** can occur in one bone (monostotic) or in multiple bones (polyostotic). Polyostotic fibrous dysplasia is often a function of the triad Albright syndrome that also includes precocious puberty and cutaneous pigmentation. Although any bone can be affected, the long bones, ribs, and skull are the most common. A radiographic "ground glass" appearance is present primarily in the metaphyseal or metadiaphyseal areas. Deformity can be marked and necessitate operative intervention. When allograft is used to replace fibrous dysplasia bone, it can become involved in the fibrous dysplasia as well. The majority of individuals are observed, however; endocrinology will also be involved if Albright syndrome is present.

Malignant Bone Tumors

Osteosarcoma. **Osteosarcoma**, accounting for 60% of childhood malignant bone tumors, is the most common bone tumor during childhood and originates in bone-producing mesenchymal cells. Between the ages of 10 to 15, osteosarcoma occurs most commonly in the long bones, especially near active physes, such as distal femur and proximal tibia.

Molecular analysis has demonstrated deletion of genetic material on the long arm of chromosome 13, leading to the identification of a tumor suppressor gene as part of the mechanism for tumor development. The oncogene *src* also has been associated with osteosarcoma.

Pathophysiology

Osteosarcoma occurs mainly in the metaphyses of long bones. Most tumors arise in bones involved with the knee joint at the distal end of the femur or proximal end of the tibia. As a tumor of mesenchymal cells, osteosarcoma demonstrates production of osteoid cells.

Osteosarcoma is a bulky tumor that extends beyond the bone into a soft-tissue mass. It may encircle the bone and destroy the trabeculae of the diseased bone. Osteosarcoma disseminates through the bloodstream, usually to the lung. As many as 25% of children diagnosed with osteosarcoma exhibit lung metastases at diagnosis. Other sites of metastatic spread include other bones and visceral organs.

Clinical Manifestations

The most common presenting complaint is pain. There may be swelling, warmth, and redness caused by the vascularity of the tumor. Symptoms may also include cough, dyspnea, and chest pain if lung metastasis is present. If a lower extremity is involved, a limp may be present and a pathologic fracture may result if the disease is extensive.

Initial evaluation includes roentgenographic examination that shows the osteosarcoma's characteristic osteoblastic and osteolytic changes. "Staging" studies to determine not only local extent of the tumor but also possible metastatic spread must be done. These include bone scan (to assess boney spread), magnetic resonance imaging (MRI) of the lesion (to plan surgical resection and to compare to postchemotherapy studies), and chest roentgenograms or CT or both. The chest roentgenogram must be done *before* biopsy because the general anesthetic required for biopsy can give false/positive results on the roentgenogram.

Evaluation and Treatment

Tissue biopsy confirms the diagnosis, although needle biopsy is often sufficient to establish the diagnosis. There are five histologic types of osteosarcoma. The histologic type is determined by the predominant cell type. The tumor is then graded according to degree of malignancy; the higher the number is, the worse the prognosis.

Surgery and chemotherapy are the primary treatments for osteosarcoma. The tumor is resistant to radiation. The 5-year survival rate with most chemotherapy and surgery protocols is 70%.[25]

Chemotherapy is an important component of treatment because as many as 80% of children treated with surgery alone eventually develop metastatic disease. Chemotherapy is used preoperatively to shrink the size of the tumor and minimize metastatic growth. Following chemotherapy, the child is given a short "rest period" to regain strength for surgery. Following adjunctive chemotherapy, the majority of children now undergo "limb salvage" rather than amputation procedures. Using preoperative MRI, the extent of the lesion is mapped and a tumor-free margin is left and reconstructed either with allograft bone or arthoplasty (artificial joint). The long-term survival rates of children treated with limb salvage and chemotherapy is now near equal to amputation in 5 and 10 year survival.[26]

A number of approaches have been used to treat pulmonary metastases. Because pulmonary metastases are generally solitary, thoracotomy with wedge resection has proved the most effective treatment. Investigators have searched for adjuvant treatment to prevent pulmonary metastases, but nothing has proved useful.

Ewing sarcoma. **Ewing sarcoma** is a malignant round cell tumor of bone and soft tissue that has a poor prognosis. It is the second most common and most lethal malignant bone tumor during childhood. This tumor is named after James Ewing, who first identified it as a separate clinical diagnosis in 1921. The most frequent period of diagnosis is between 5 and 15 years of age, and diagnosis is rare after 30 years of age; however, it may be seen in children younger than 3 years. Like osteosarcoma, Ewing sarcoma is slightly more common in males than females and is linked with periods of rapid bone growth. The incidence of Ewing sarcoma is less than 2% in blacks.[27]

Pathophysiology

Ewing sarcoma commonly occurs in the midshaft or diaphysis of long bones or in flat bones. The most frequent sites include the pelvis, femur, and tibia (Fig. 42-14). The femur is involved in most cases, with the pelvis being the second most common site. It can occur in any bone.

Arising from bone marrow, Ewing sarcoma can break through the cortex of the bone to form a soft-tissue mass. It does not form bone, but abundant reactive bone may be present in an attempt to contain this quickly growing lesion. Metastasis occurs early and is usually apparent at diagnosis or within 1 year. The most common sites are the lung, other bones, lymph nodes, bone marrow, liver, spleen, and central nervous system, although any organ is possible.

Clinical Manifestations

Like osteosarcoma, the most common complaint is pain about the diaphysis that increases in severity. A soft-tissue mass is often present. Additional symptoms may include fever, malaise, and anorexia. Known as "the great imitator," Ewing sarcoma can appear radiographically identical to infection or even benign lesions like Langerhan cell granulomatosis. Any pervasive diaphseal lesion must be regarded with a high index of suspicion.

Evaluation and Treatment

In addition to plain roentgenogram, CT and MRI are needed to help establish the diagnosis and extent of the tumor. Bone scan, chest roentgenogram, and chest CT scan are also used to detect metastases. No specific laboratory test is diagnostic; however, the sedimentation rate will be elevated and lactic dehydrogenase (LDH) often is elevated. An elevated LDH level is a poor prognostic sign. Biopsy is used to conclusively establish the diagnosis. The identification of an 11:22 chromosomal translocation within the tumor cells will confirm the diagnosis of Ewing sarcoma.

The use of multidrug chemotherapy has improved survival rates. Recent treatment protocols call for preoperative chemotherapy followed by radiation or surgical resection or both, with continuation of chemotherapy for 12 to 18 months afterwards. Amputation is avoided when possible but may

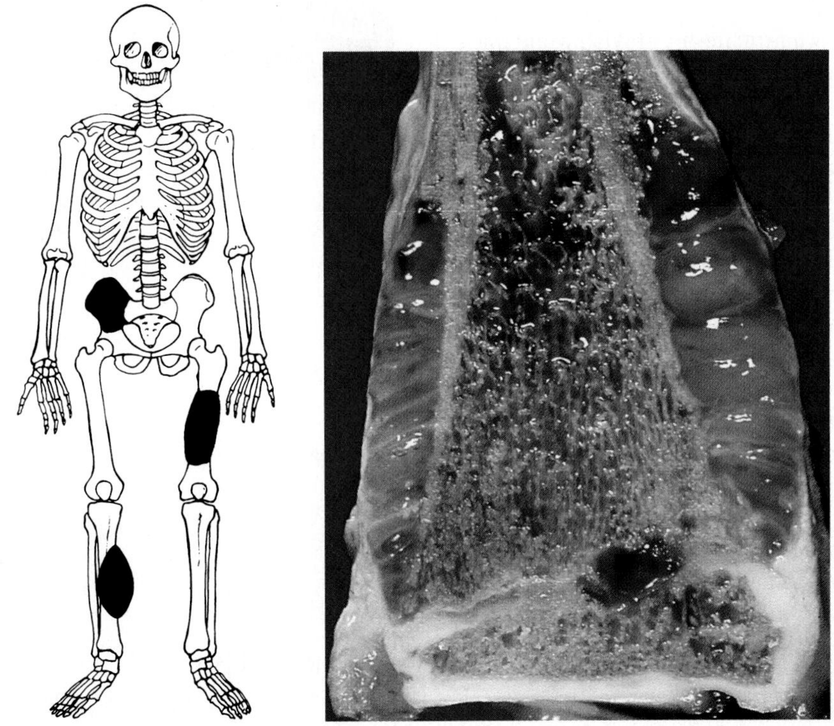

FIG. 42-14 Ewing sarcoma. A, Most common anatomic sites. **B,** Close-up view of Ewing sarcoma of the distal end of the tibia. Tumor extends into the soft tissue. (From Damjanov I, Linder J, editors: *Anderson's pathology*, ed 10, St Louis, 1996, Mosby.)

be considered in lower limb tumors of children younger than 8 years because of the serious discrepancy in bone growth that results if the primary treatment used is radiation, which can damage the physis. Secondary malignancies caused by high dose radiation are also a concern.[28]

Ewing sarcoma has had a dismal prognosis, with 5-year survival rates no better than 5% to 10%. Combinations of aggressive radiation, chemotherapy, and surgical resection have, however, improved the survival rate for localized disease to more than 60%.[29] The major predictor of prognosis appears to be the location of the primary tumor and whether metastases are present at diagnosis. The most favorable sites of involvement are the extremities; the worst prognosis involves tumors of the trunk, particularly the pelvis.

Muscle Tumors

Most soft-tissue tumors in children are benign. Only two malignant soft-tissue tumors occur with any frequency—rhabdomyosarcoma in the younger child and synovial cell sarcoma in the teenager. Both of these occur rarely. The annual incidence is 8.0 per million for white children and 7.7 per million for black children. About 230 children are diagnosed with a soft-tissue tumor each year in the United States. Soft-tissue tumors originate from the primitive mesenchymal cells that normally give rise to muscle, tendons, blood vessels, lymphatic structures, fibrous and connective tissue, and bursa and fascia. Table 42-5 identifies the classification of soft-tissue tumors according to origin. All malignant soft-tissue tumors are characterized as highly aggressive tumors that invade surrounding structures and metastasize early.

Table 42-5 Classification of Tumors by Origin

Tissue	Tumor
Muscle	
Striated	Rhabdomyosarcoma
Smooth	Leiomyosarcoma
Adipose	Liposarcoma
Fibrous	Fibrosarcoma
Synovial mesothelium	Synovial sarcoma
Lymphatic structures	Lymphangiosarcoma
Blood vessels	Hemangiopericytoma
Nerve sheath	Neurogenic sarcoma

Rhabdomyosarcoma (RMS) is the most common soft-tissue sarcoma of childhood and accounts for more than 50% of soft-tissue tumors but less than 3% of all childhood cancers. RMS arises from embryonal rhabdomyoblasts that normally differentiate into mature striated muscle.

RMS can develop anywhere striated muscle is located. The primary locations and percentage range of incidence are the head and neck (including the orbit), 36% to 61%; the trunk, 8% to 33%; the extremities, 14% to 24%; and the genitourinary tract, 10% to 17%. Two age ranges (2 to 6 years and 15 to 19 years) are associated with RMS. More than two thirds of children with RMS are diagnosed by 10 years of age, and RMS is slightly more common in males than females.

Recent studies demonstrate an association between *p53* (a tumor-suppressor gene) mutations and sporadic rhabdomyosarcoma.[30] Three oncogenes (*src,* H/K-*ras,* and *c-myb*) have been associated with this tumor.[31]

Pathophysiology

RMS generally appears as a firm, fleshy, grayish white mass. It sometimes exhibits variations that appear as a cystic polypoid mass. RMS has various appearances, depending on the phase of differentiation of the rhabdomyoblast. The cells may be round, spindle-shaped, tadpole-shaped, or multinucleated giant cells.

At least 20% of children with RMS have metastatic disease at diagnosis. The preferred sites of metastases include the lungs, lymph nodes, bone marrow, liver, brain, and bone. Another 30% have disease that is unresectable, although not widely spread. This also becomes a grave prognosis.

Clinical Manifestations

The signs and symptoms of RMS depend on the anatomic location of the primary tumor and presence of symptomatic metastases. The tumors are usually painless, and early detection of RMS is facilitated by the presence of a palpable or visible mass. Deep-seated tumors may cause functional impairment but can be silent until they are very large. The clinical manifestations of RMS are outlined in Table 42-6.

Evaluation and Treatment

Diagnostic studies during the pretreatment phase are used to determine the extent of the primary tumor and presence or absence of distant metastases. Specific diagnostic studies depend on the primary site, but a combination of radiographic, nuclear, and CT scanning or MRI technology and blood studies is used. A biopsy of the primary tumor is necessary to confirm the diagnosis. Currently, chromosomal abnormalities are being investigated for RMS. Although not widely incorporated into clinical management at this time, identification of the DNA content has value as both a prognostic factor and a determinant of treatment.

RMS is treated by a combination of surgery, radiation, and chemotherapy. Complete surgical resection provides the greatest assurance that cure can be achieved; however, cure occurs in only 16% of children. If surgical resection leads to serious disfigurement or functional disability (e.g., enucleation for orbital tumors or cystectomy for bladder tumors), chemotherapy and radiation serve as the primary treatment and surgery is avoided or minimized. For all tumors except stage I disease, local radiation therapy is given. A variety of combination chemotherapies are used for RMS. Chemotherapy for stage I or II disease is given for 1 year if disease does not recur. For stage III or IV, treatment (combined with radiation therapy) continues an additional year. Intrathecal chemotherapy is given to children whose tumor locations favor central nervous system spread.

The primary prognostic factor in RMS is the degree of residual disease after surgical resection. Children with localized disease (stages I and II) have long-term survival rates of 70% to 80%. If widespread disease is present, long-term survival rates drop to 20%. Orbital tumors have an overall favorable prognosis, probably because of the lack of lymphatics in the area and early physical signs of disease.

Table 42-6 Clinical Manifestations of Rhabdomyosarcoma

Location	Manifestation
HEAD AND NECK	
Orbit	Ptosis Exophthalmos Proptosis
Paranasal sinuses	Nasal obstruction Epistaxis Swelling Chronic sinusitis
Nasopharnx	Hypernasal speech Nasal discharge Visible polypoid mass
Oropharyngeal	Dysphagia Painful mastication
Middle ear	Chronic serous otitis media Discharge from affected ear Facial nerve palsy Conduction hearing loss Visible polypoid mass
EXTREMITIES	
All locations	Deep-seated, fixed palpable mass
RETROPERITONEAL	
All locations	Usually asymptomatic May have vague abdominal pain Bowel or genitourinary obstruction (late) Possible palpable mass
GENITOURINARY	
Vaginal	Abnormal vaginal bleeding Protruding polypoid mass
Prostate	Urinary tract obstruction
Bladder	Urinary retention Straining to void Hematuria
Paratesticular	Mass in scrotum that may be painful

NONACCIDENTAL TRAUMA

Abuse is estimated to occur in over 1.5 million children per year in the United States. The maltreatment may be psychological, sexual, or physical. Of children who suffer physical abuse, 30% are initially seen by an orthopedist. Accurate and appropriate referrals to child protection are not only legally mandated but also essential for the well-being of the child; an abused child who returns unmonitored to an abusive situation has a 15% chance of mortality.

Etiology

Children who are not yet ambulatory and present with a long bone fracture have over a 75% chance of that fracture being caused by **nonaccidental trauma. "Corner" metaphyseal**

fractures, caused by a twisting force, are nearly pathognomonic of abuse but occur only 25% of the time (Fig. 42-15). Fractures at multiple stages of healing are also suggestive, however, osteogenesis imperfecta must be ruled out. The most common presentation is a transverse tibia fracture.[32] After walking age, only 2% of long bone fractures are due to nonaccidental trauma.[33]

Evaluation

If suspected, nonaccidental trauma necessitates early consultation with child protective services. The child should undergo skeletal radiographic survey, especially if less than 2 years of age, and have a complete physical examination to evaluate for patterned bruising, burns, or multiple soft tissue injuries. Ophthalmologic examination should be used to evaluate for retinal hemorrhage caused by shaking. A thorough history must be obtained for all identified injuries. It is important to remember that social isolation can lead to increased likelihood of abuse, but no social strata is immune.

When unclear, bone scan can be helpful in diagnosing subtle injuries, especially rib fractures. Posterior rib fractures are especially likely to be caused by abuse. MRI and CT of the brain can help diagnose injuries caused by shaking.

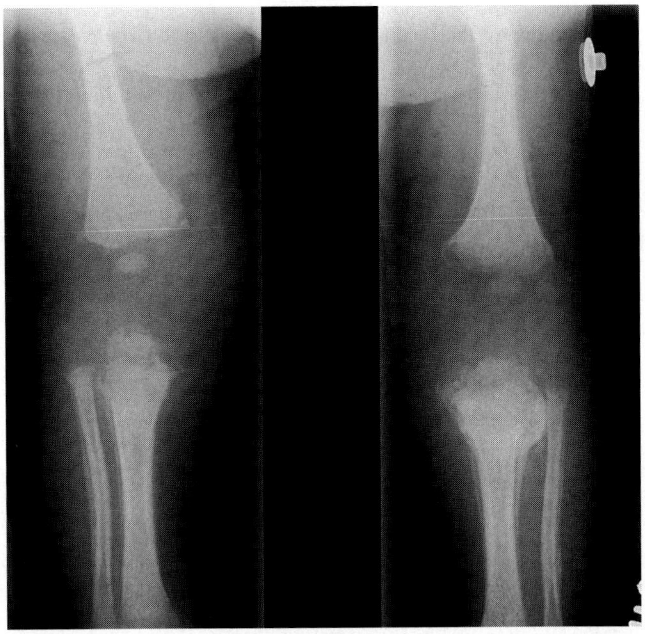

FIG. 42-15 **Corner fracture.** Bilateral knee radiograph showing healing corner fractures of bilateral proximal tibias and distal femurs. Note the varying amount of callus formation signifying fractures at different stages of healing.

Treatment

A nonjudgmental attitude on the part of the treating health care provider is essential. The child and family involved in nonaccidental trauma are delicate and require not only physical but emotional care. Social workers need to be involved early to ensure appropriate medical care to the child. Fortunately, fractures heal quickly in young children; neurologic injury and social disease, however, are much more difficult to cure.

SUMMARY REVIEW

Musculoskeletal Development in Children

1. Skeletal growth and development consist of two concurrent processes in healthy children: (a) the creation of new cells and tissues (growth), and (b) the consolidation of new tissues into a permanent form (maturation).
2. Ossification takes place in two centers in long bones: (a) the primary center, or the diaphysis (the long, central portion of the bone); and (b) the secondary center, or the epiphysis (the end portions of the bone).
3. Until adult stature is reached (17 years for females and 18 years for males), growth in length of bones occurs at the epiphyseal plate through endochondral ossification.
4. Fifty percent of the total growth of the spine has occurred by 1 year of age, and most children have achieved 50% of their adult height by 2 years of age.
5. The appendicular skeleton (extremities) grows faster during childhood than does the axial skeleton.
6. Muscle fibers reach their maximal size in females at 10 years of age and at 14 years of age in males.

Musculoskeletal Alterations in Children

1. The most common congenital defect of the upper extremities is syndactyly (webbing of the fingers).
2. Developmental dysplasia of the hip is a serious and disabling condition in children if not diagnosed and treated.
3. Congenital muscle disorders (myopathies) include absence of muscles, hypoplasia, hyperplasia, and faulty intrinsic development.
4. Osteogenesis imperfecta (brittle bone disease) is an inherited disorder of collagen that affects primarily bones and results in serious fractures of many bones.
5. Rickets is a condition caused by deficiencies in vitamin D, calcium, and usually phosphorus that is characterized by the failure of bones to become mineralized (ossified) and results in skeletal deformity.
6. Scoliosis is a lateral curvature of the spinal column that can be caused by congenital malformations of the spine, poliomyelitis, skeletal dysplasia, spastic paralysis, and unequal leg length but is most often idiopathic.
7. Osteomyelitis is a local or generalized bacterial infection of bone and bone marrow. Bacteria are usually introduced by direct extension from a nearby infection, through the bloodstream, or by trauma.
8. Juvenile rheumatoid arthritis is an inflammatory joint disorder characterized by pain and swelling.
9. Avascular diseases of the bone are collectively referred to as osteochondroses and are caused by an insufficient blood supply to growing bones.
10. Legg-Calvé-Perthes disease is one of the most common osteochondroses. This disorder is characterized by epiphyseal

necrosis or degeneration of the head of the femur followed by regeneration or recalcification.
11. Osgood-Schlatter disease is characterized by inflammation or partial separation of the tibial tubercle caused by chronic irritation, usually as a result of overuse of the quadriceps muscles. The condition is seen primarily in muscular, athletic adolescent males.
12. The muscular dystrophies are a group of genetically transmitted diseases characterized by progressive atrophy of symmetric groups of skeletal muscles without evidence of involvement or degeneration of neural tissue. There is an insidious loss of strength in all forms of the disorder with increasing disability and deformity.
13. Benign bone tumors include nonossifying fibroma, simple bone cysts, aneursysmal bone cysts, osteoid osteoma, and fibrous dysplasia.
14. The two main types of malignant childhood bone tumors are osteosarcoma and Ewing sarcoma.
15. Osteosarcoma, the most common malignant childhood bone tumor, originates in bone-producing mesenchymal cells and is most often located in the distal end of the femur or proximal end of the tibia.
16. Most childhood osteosarcoma cases are diagnosed between 15 and 19 years of age and occur equally in males and females.
17. Ewing sarcoma originates from cells within the bone marrow space and is located most often in the midshaft of long bones or in flat bones.
18. Ewing sarcoma is more common in males and is diagnosed most frequently between the ages of 5 and 15 years.
19. Pain is the usual presenting symptom for either osteosarcoma or Ewing sarcoma.
20. The primary treatments for osteosarcoma are surgery and chemotherapy. The primary treatment for Ewing sarcoma is a combination of chemotherapy, radiation, and surgery.
21. The most common type of childhood soft-tissue tumor is rhabdomyosarcoma.
22. Rhabdomyosarcoma originates from embryonal rhabdomyoblasts that normally differentiate into mature striated muscle.
23. Clinical manifestations of rhabdomyosarcoma depend on the anatomic location; superficial tumors exhibit a painless palpable mass, whereas deep-seated tumors cause functional impairment.
24. Rhabdomyosarcoma is treated with a combination of surgery, radiation, and chemotherapy.

Nonaccidental Trauma

1. Nonaccidental trauma must be considered with any long bone injury in a preambulatory child.
2. Soft tissue injury, corner fractures, and fractures at different stages of healing are extremely helpful in making a diagnosis of nonaccidental trauma.
3. When nonaccidental trauma is suspected, a child must be evaluated radiographically for other fractures, head trauma, and retinal hemorrhage.
4. All social strata are at risk.
5. The health care provider is legally responsible to report suspected nonaccidental trauma.

KEY TERMS

Aneurysmal bone cyst (ABC), *1427*
Becker muscular dystrophy, *1426*
Cartilage anlage, *1409*
Cerebral palsy (CP), *1423*
Corner metaphyseal fracture, *1430*
Developmental dysplasia of the hip (DDH), *1412*
Duchenne muscular dystrophy, *1423*
Dystrophin, *1424*
Endochondral formation of bone, *1409*
Ewing sarcoma, *1428*
Facioscapulohumeral muscular dystrophy, *1426*
Fibrous dysplasia (FD), *1427*
Genu valgum (knock knee), *1411*
Genu varum (bowleg), *1411*
Idiopathic equinovarus, *1414*
Idiopathic scoliosis, *1417*
Intramembranous formation of bone, *1409*
Involucrum, *1419*
Juvenile rheumatoid arthritis (JRA), *1421*
Kyphosed, *1410*
Legg-Calvé-Perthes disease, *1421*
Limb girdle muscular dystrophy, *1426*
Lordotic, *1411*
Metatarsus adductus, *1413*
Muscular dystrophy, *1423*
Nonaccidental trauma, *1430*
Nonossifying fibroma (fibrous cortical deficit), *1427*
Nonstructural scoliosis, *1417*
Osgood-Schlatter disease, *1423*
Osteochondrosis, *1421*
Osteogenesis imperfecta (brittle bone disease), *1414*
Osteoid osteoma, *1427*
Osteomyelitis, *1418*
Osteosarcoma, *1427*
Perichondrium, *1409*
Periosteal collar, *1409*
Pes planus (flatfoot), *1414*
Physeal closure, *1410*
Positional equinovarus, *1414*
Primary center of ossification, *1409*
Rhabdomyosarcoma (RMS), *1429*
Rickets, *1416*
Scapuloperoneal muscular dystrophy, *1426*
Scoliosis, *1417*
Secondary center of ossification, *1410*
Secondary septic arthritis, *1419*
Sequestrum (pl., sequestra), *1419*
Simple bone cyst (SBC), *1427*
Structural scoliosis, *1417*
Syndactyly, *1411*
Teratologic equinovarus, *1414*
Vestigial tab, *1412*

REFERENCES

1. Simkin P: The musculoskeletal system. In Klippel JH, Dieppe PA, editors: *Rheumatology*, ed 2, London, 1998, Mosby.
2. Weintraub S, Grill F: Ultrasonography in developmental dysplasia of the hip, *J Bone Joint Surg Am* 82-A(7):1004, 2000.
3. Sillence D: Osteogenesis imperfecta: an expanding panorama of variants, *Clin Orthop* 159:11, 1981.
4. Zaleske DJ, Doppelt SH, Mankin HJ: Endocrine abnormalities of the immature skeleton. In Lovell WW, Winter RB, editors: *Pediatric orthopedics*, ed 2, Philadelphia, 1986, Lippincott.

5. Barrack R et al: Vibratory hypersensitivity in idiopathic sclerosis, *J Pediatr Orthop* 8(4):389, 1988.
6. Byrd J: Current theories on the etiology of idiopathic scoliosis, *Clin Orthop* 299:114, 1988.
7. Kindsfater K et al: Levels of platelet calmodulin for the prediction of progression and severity of adolescent idiopathic scoliosis, *J Bone Joint Surg Am* 76(8):1186, 1994.
8. Caksen H et al: Septic arthritis in childhood, *Pediatr Int* 42(5):534, 2000.
9. Gillespie WJ et al: Aspects of the microbe: host relationship in staphylococcal hematogenous osteomyelitis, *Orthopedics* 10(3):475, 1987.
10. Hedström SA, Lidgren L: Septic arthritis and osteomyelitis. In Klippel JH, Dieppe PA, editors: *Rheumatology*, ed 2, London, 1998, Mosby.
11. Przybylski GJ, Sharan AD: Single-stage autogenous bone grafting and internal fixation in the surgical management of pyogenic discitis and vertebral osteomyelitis, *J Neurosurg* 94(1 suppl):1, 2001.
12. Ray NJ, Basset RL: Pyogenic vertebral osteomyelitis, *Orthopedics* 8(4):504, 1985.
13. Mader JT et al: The host and skeletal infection: classification and pathogenesis of acute bacterial bone and joint sepsis, *Baillieres Best Pract Res Clin Rheumatol* 13(1):1, 1999.
14. Perlman M et al: The incidence of joint involvement of adjacent osteomyelitis in pediatric patients, *J Pediatr Orthop*, 20(1):40, 2000.
15. Cassidy JT: *Textbook of pediatric rheumatology*, New York, 1982, Wiley & Sons.
16. Hollingworth P: Juvenile chronic arthritis. In Klippel JH, Dieppe PA, editors: *Rheumatology*, ed 2, London, 1998, Mosby.
17. Gluek CS, Crawford A: Association of antithrombotic factor deficiencies and hypofibrinolysis with LCP disease, *J Bone Joint Surg Am* 78:3, 1996.
18. Herring JA et al: The lateral piller classification of L-C-P disease, *J Pediatr Orthop* 12:143, 1992.
19. Schoenecker PL et al: LCP disease in children <6 yr old, *Orthop Rev* 22:201, 1993.
20. Swanson MN et al: Identification of neurodevelopment abnormality at 4 and 8 months by the movement assessment of infants, *Dev Med Child Neuro* 34:321, 1992.
21. Scott MO et al: Duchenne muscular dystrophy gene expression in normal and diseased human muscle, *Science* 239:1418, 1988.
22. Stevens A, Lowe J: *Pathology*, London, 1995, Mosby.
23. Nevo Y et al: Fetal muscle biopsy as a diagnostic tool in Duchenne muscular dystrophy, *Prenat Diag* 19(10):921, 1999.
24. Campanacci M, Capann R, Picci P: Unicameral and aneurysmal bone cysts, *Clin Ortho* 204:25, 1986.
25. Glasser DB et al: Survival, prognosis, and therapeutic response in osteogenic sarcoma: the Memorial Hospital experience, *Cancer* 69:698, 1992.
26. Rougratt BT et al: Limb salvage compared with amputation for osteocarcoma of the distal end of the femur, *J Bone Joint Surg Am* 76A:647, 1994.
27. Ayala AG, Ro JY, Raymond AK: Bone tumors. In Damjanov I, Linder J, editors: *Anderson's pathology*, ed 10, St Louis, 1996, Mosby.
28. Smith LM, Cox RS, Donaldson SS: Second cancers in long term survivors of Ewing's sarcoma, *Clin Orthop* 274:175, 1992.
29. Ruyman FB, Grovas AC: Progress in the diagnosis and treatment of rhabdomyosarcoma and related soft tissue sarcomas, *Cancer Invest* 18(3):223, 2000.
30. Lugo-Vicente H: Molecular biology and genetics affecting pediatric solid tumors, *Bol Asoc Med P R* 92(4-8):72, 2000.
31. Israel MA: Molecular and cellular biology in pediatric malignancies. In Pizzo PA, editor: *Principles and practices of pediatric oncology*, Philadelphia, 1989, Lippincott.
32. King J et al: Analysis of 429 fractures in 189 battered children, *J Pediatr Orthop* 8:585, 1988.
33. Thomas SA et al: Long bone fracture in young children: distinguishing accidental injuries from child abuse, *Pediatrics* 88:471, 1991.

CHAPTER 43

Structure, Function, and Disorders of the Integument

SUE E. HUETHER

CHAPTER OUTLINE

The skin is the largest organ of the body. Combined with the accessory structures of hair, nails, and glands, it forms the integumentary system. The skin covers the entire body and accounts for approximately 20% of the body's weight. The primary function of the skin is to protect the body from the environment by serving as a barrier against microorganisms, ultraviolet radiation, loss of body fluids, and the stress of mechanical forces. The skin also regulates body temperature within a very narrow range and is involved in the production of vitamin D. Touch and pressure receptors provide important protective functions and pleasurable sensations.

STRUCTURE AND FUNCTION OF THE SKIN

Layers of the Skin

The skin is formed of two major layers: a superficial or outer layer of **epidermis** and a deeper layer of **dermis** (the true skin) (Fig. 43-1 and Table 43-1). The subcutaneous tissue, or **hypodermis,** is an underlying layer of connective tissue that contains macrophages, fibroblasts, and fat cells. Each skin layer contains cells that represent progressive stages of skin cell differentiation as the skin grows.

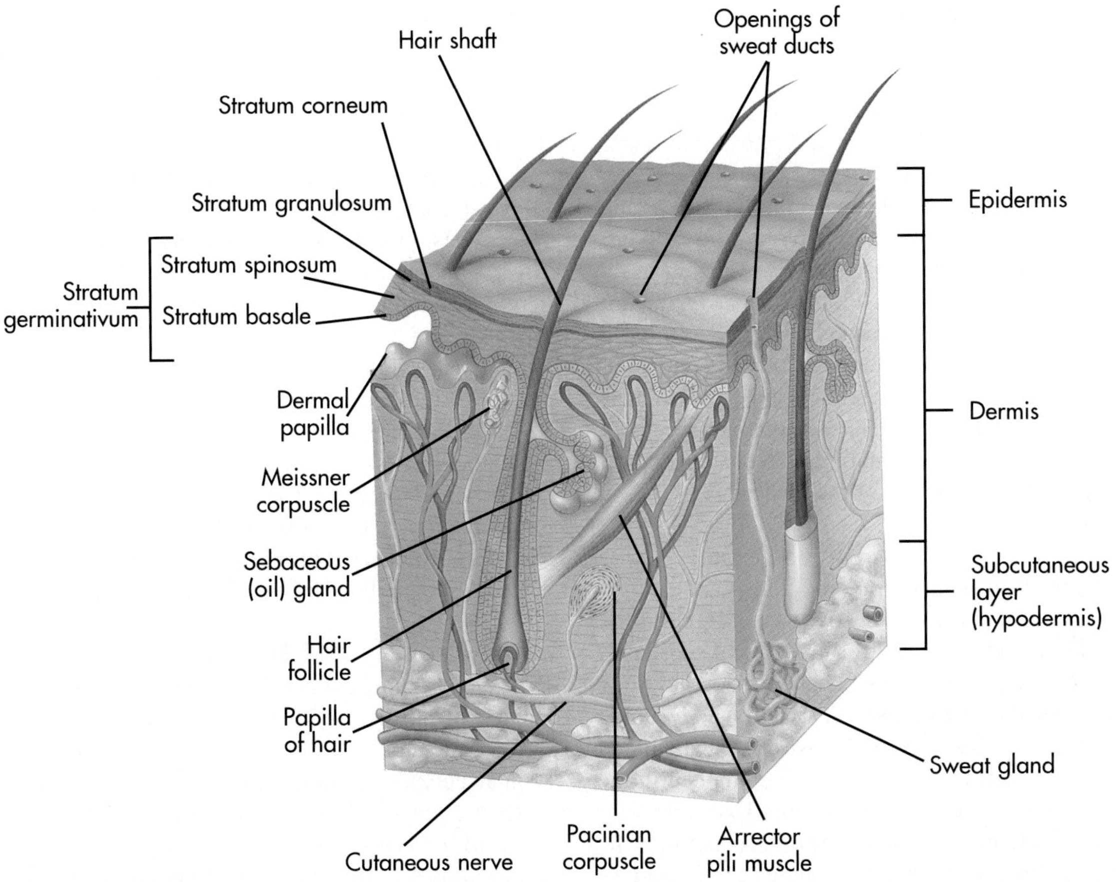

FIG. 43-1 Structure of the skin. (From Thibodeau GA, Patton KT: *Anatomy and physiology*, ed 4, St Louis, 1999, Mosby.)

Table 43-1 Layers of the Skin

Structure	Cell Types	Characteristics
Epidermis	Keratinocytes and melanocytes	Most important layer of skin; normally very thin (0.12 mm) but can thicken and form corns or calluses with constant pressure or friction
	Langerhans cells	Cells with dendrite process and immune functions
Stratum corneum	Keratinocytes and melanocytes	Tough superficial layer covering the body
Stratum lucidum	Keratinocytes and melanocytes	Clear layers of cells containing eleidin, which becomes keratin as cells move up to corneum layer
Stratum granulosum	Keratinocytes and melanocytes	Keratohyalin gives a granular appearance to this layer
Stratum spinosum	New keratinocytes	Polygonal shaped with spinous processes projecting between adjacent keratinocytes
Stratum germinativum	Keratinocytes	Basal layer where keratinocytes divide and move upward to replace cells shed from the surface
Dermis	Collagen, elastin, reticulin, ground substance	Irregular connective tissue layer with rich blood, lymphatic, and nerve supply; contains sensory receptors and special glands
Papillary layer		
Reticular layer		
Hypodermis		Subcutaneous tissue or superficial fascia of varying thickness that connects the overlying dermis to underlying muscle

Epidermis

The epidermis grows continually by shedding the superficial layer of **stratum corneum,** which is formed entirely of keratinocytes and melanocytes. These cells are named for the substances they produce. **Keratinocytes** produce **keratin,** a scleroprotein. Keratin is the main constituent of skin, hair, and nail cells. The thickness of the epidermis varies from 0.3 mm on the eyelids to 1.5 mm on the palms of the hands and soles of the feet. New cells (keratinocytes) formed in the **basal layer (stratum basale)** move upward and differentiate, forming the **spinous layer (stratum spinosum).** Together they form the germinative layer (stratum germinativum). The cells enlarge and then become flattened, stacked, and cornified (stratum corneum) as they ascend to the skin surface.

Cornification, or keratinization, prevents dehydration of deeper skin layers. The average turnover of the epidermis is about 30 days.

The epidermis has three different types of cells that facilitate its functional characteristics: melanocytes, Langerhans cells, and Merkel cells. The **melanocytes** are usually located near the base of the epidermis. They synthesize and secrete the pigment melanin with exposure to sunlight in response to melanocyte-stimulating hormone (MSH). Melanin in the epidermis provides a shield against ultraviolet radiation and determines skin color. **Langerhans cells** migrate to the dermis from the bone marrow. The Langerhans cells initiate an immune response and provide a defense against environmental antigens. **Merkel cells** are associated with touch receptors, and they function as slowly adapting mechanoreceptors when stimulated by deformation of the epidermis.

Dermis

The dermis varies from 1 to 4 mm in thickness and is composed of three types of fibrous connective tissue: (1) collagen, (2) elastin and reticulin, and (3) a gel-like ground substance. The haphazard arrangement of connective tissue allows the skin to be mobile and to stretch and contract with body movement. Hair follicles, sebaceous glands, sweat glands, blood vessels, lymphatic vessels, and nerves are contained in the dermis. The conelike projections of the papillary dermis interface with the epidermis. The papillae provide texture to the surface of the skin by forming what are known as *rete pegs.*

The cells of the dermis include fibroblasts, mast cells, and macrophages. Fibroblasts secrete the connective tissue matrix. Mast cells release histamine and play a role in hypersensitivity reactions in the skin. Macrophages are phagocytic and participate in immune responses.

Hypodermis (Subcutaneous Layer)

The subcutaneous tissue contains the dermal appendages (nails, hair, sebaceous glands, and the eccrine and apocrine sweat glands), the supplying blood vessels of the dermis, and nerves of the autonomic nervous system. A layer of cushioning fat provides a base for the hypodermis.

Dermal Appendages

The **dermal appendages** include the **nails, hair, sebaceous glands,** and the eccrine and apocrine **sweat glands.** The nails are protective keratinized plates that appear at the ends of fingers and toes. Each nail is composed of four structural units: (1) the proximal nail fold, (2) the matrix from which the nail grows, (3) the hyponychium (nail bed), and (4) the nail plate (Fig. 43-2). Nail growth is continuous throughout life at a rate of 1 mm or less per day.

Hair follicles and sebaceous glands are integrated units (see Fig. 43-1). Hair color, density, grain, and pattern of distribution have considerable variability and depend on age, gender, and race. Hair follicles arise from the matrix (or bulb) located deep in the dermis. They extend from the dermis at an angle and have an erector pili muscle attached near the middermis that straightens the follicle when contracted, causing the hair to stand up. Hair growth begins in the bulb, with cellular differentiation of stem cells occurring as the hair progresses up the follicle.[1] Hair is fully hardened, or cornified, by the time it emerges at the skin surface. Hair growth is cyclic, with periods of growth and rest that vary over different body surfaces.

The **sebaceous glands** open onto the surface of the skin through a canal. They are found in greatest numbers on the face, chest, and back with modified glands on the eyelids, lips, nipple, glans penis, and prepuce. Sebaceous glands secrete sebum that is composed primarily of lipids; sebum oils the skin and hair and prevents drying. Growth of sebaceous glands is stimulated by testosterone, and their enlargement is one of the early signs of puberty.

The **eccrine sweat glands** are distributed over the body, with the greatest numbers in the palms of the hands, soles of the feet, and forehead. These secretions are important in thermoregulation and cooling of the body through evaporation. The **apocrine sweat glands** are fewer in number and are located in the axillae, scalp, face, abdomen, and genital area.

Blood Supply and Innervation

The blood supply to the skin is limited to the **papillary capillaries,** or plexus, of the dermis. These capillary loops arise from a subpapillary plexus that is supplied by a deeper horizontal cutaneous arterial plexus. Branches from the deep plexus supply hair follicles and sweat glands. A subpapillary network of veins drains the capillary loops. Arteriovenous anastomoses in the dermis facilitate the regulation of body temperature. Heat loss can be regulated by varying blood flow through the skin by opening and closing the arteriovenous anastomoses in conjunction with evaporative heat loss of sweat. The sympathetic nervous system regulates both vasoconstriction and vasodilation. There are only α-adrenergic receptors in the skin. The lymphatic vessels of the skin arise in the papillary dermis and drain into larger subcutaneous trunks, removing cells, proteins, and immunologic mediators.

Aging and Skin Integrity

Many age-associated changes in the skin are readily observable and appear over the body surface. Both genetic and environmental factors, particularly ultraviolet radiation from

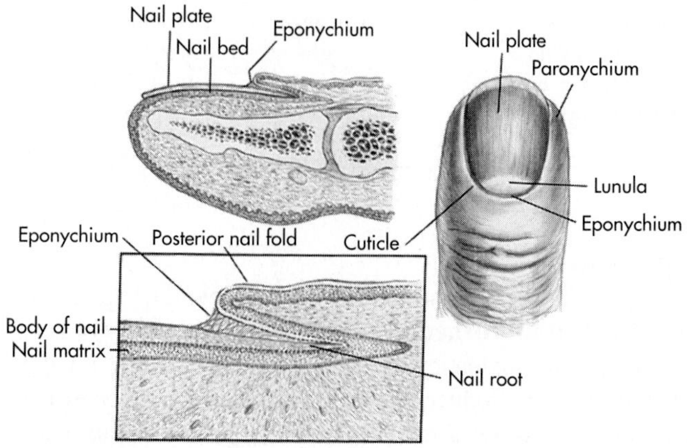

FIG. 43-2 Structures of the nail. (From Thompson JM et al: *Mosby's clinical nursing,* ed 4, St Louis, 1997, Mosby.)

sun exposure, contribute to cutaneous changes with aging.[2] Structurally the skin becomes thinner, drier, and wrinkled with a change in pigmentation.[3] The cellular alterations contributing to the changes include a flattening of the dermoepidermal border with a shortening and decrease in the number of capillary loops. There are fewer melanocytes, with decreased protection against ultraviolet radiation. A significant decrease in the number of Langerhans cells decreases the skin's immune response with aging. The thickness of the dermis also decreases and accounts for the translucent, paper-thin quality of the skin. Loss of the rete pegs gives the skin a smooth, shiny appearance.[4]

The decreased vasculature probably contributes to the atrophy of eccrine, apocrine, and sebaceous glands that causes dry skin. Loss of elastin fibers is associated with wrinkling. The collagen fibers become less flexible and decrease the ability of the skin to stretch and regain shape. Decreased cell proliferation,[5] decreased blood supply, and depressed immune responses also delay wound healing in aging skin. Changes in hair color and distribution also occur. Graying is caused by loss of melanocytes from hair bulbs, and thinning occurs from a gradual decline in the number of hair follicles and growth of finer hair.

The epidermal cells change shape, and the barrier function of the stratum corneum is reduced. There is increased permeability and decreased clearance of substances from the dermis. The accumulation of such substances is related to decreased vascularity and can cause skin irritation. Temperature regulation is compromised in elderly persons, and there is an increased risk for both heat stroke and hypothermia. Loss of cutaneous vasomotion and subcutaneous fat, decreased vascularity, and decreased eccrine sweat production are contributing factors. The pressure and touch receptors and free nerve endings all decrease in number and reduce sensory perception. In summary, many of the protective functions of the skin are decreased with aging.[6]

Tests of Skin Function

Diagnostic evaluations of skin disorders often can be completed by gathering historical information, performing a physical examination, and observing the distribution and characteristics of the presenting lesions. Additional diagnostic studies are summarized in Table 43-2.

Clinical Manifestations of Skin Dysfunction

Lesions

Lesions of the skin are readily observable and easily assessed for distribution and structure. Identification of the morphologic structure and appearance of the skin in combination with a health history is necessary to identify the underlying pathophysiology. Table 43-3 describes and illustrates the basic lesions of the skin. Special skin lesions are described in Table 43-4.

Pressure Ulcers

Pressure ulcers, or pressure sores, are ischemic ulcers resulting from pressure and shearing forces. The term *decubitus ulcer* refers to an ulcer or pressure sore that results when an individual lies in the recumbent position for a long time. The more general terms of pressure sore or ulcer are used here. Factors associated with greatest risk are as follows:[7]

1. Elderly in hospitals and nursing homes
2. Neurologic disorders with loss of mobility and/or sensation (spinal cord injuries, dementia, or cerebrovascular disease)
3. Immobilization
4. Incontinence
5. Debilitation
6. Lying in bed without changing position or relieving pressure over an extended period
7. Lying for hours on hard imaging and operating tables

Text continued on p. 1443

Table 43-2 Summary of Skin Diagnostic Procedures

Test	Purpose
Skin biopsy	Differential diagnosis of cellular structure, i.e., benign growths vs. carcinoma, chronic infections, blistering diseases, and vasculitis
Microscopic immunofluorescence	Identification of antibodies, immunoglobulins, and complement components for diseases such as pemphigus, vasculitis, and discoid lupus erythematosus using fluorescent light on slide-mounted biopsy specimens
Gram stain	Differentiation of gram-positive from gram-negative bacteria according to stain absorption
Culture	Identification of chronic bacterial and fungal infections by incubating skin specimens in culture media
Wood lamp examination	Examination of skin or hair to identify fungus that fluoresces bright yellow-green under ultraviolet light
Patch and scratch tests	Application of suspected allergens to skin patch or scratch for evaluation of immune system responses to known allergens and evaluation of cell-mediated immune function (*Candida albicans,* skin fungus)
Skin scrapings	Application of potassium hydroxide (KOH) and low heat to skin scrapings on a glass slide to identify fungi
Side lighting	Indirect lighting of the skin using light to the side of the lesions to evaluate patterns of depression and elevation of skin lesions
Diascopy	Use of glass or clear plastic pressed on the skin to differentiate erythema caused by dilated capillaries (blanching) from extravasation of blood (no blanching)

Table 43-3 Primary and Secondary Skin Lesions

Primary Skin Lesions	Examples		
MACULE A flat, circumscribed area that is a change in the color of the skin; less than 1 cm in diameter	Freckles, flat moles (nevi), petechiae, measles, scarlet fever	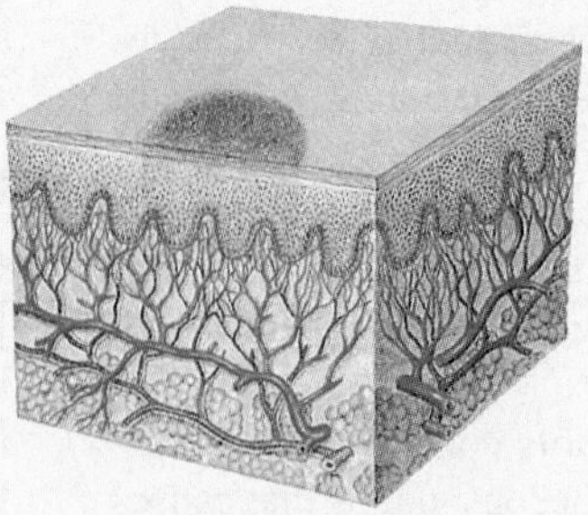	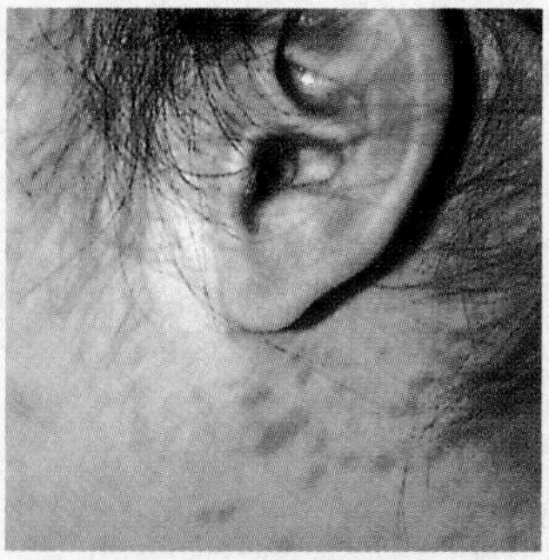 **Macules[c]**
PAPULE An elevated, firm, circumscribed area less than 1 cm in diameter	Wart (verruca), elevated moles, lichen planus	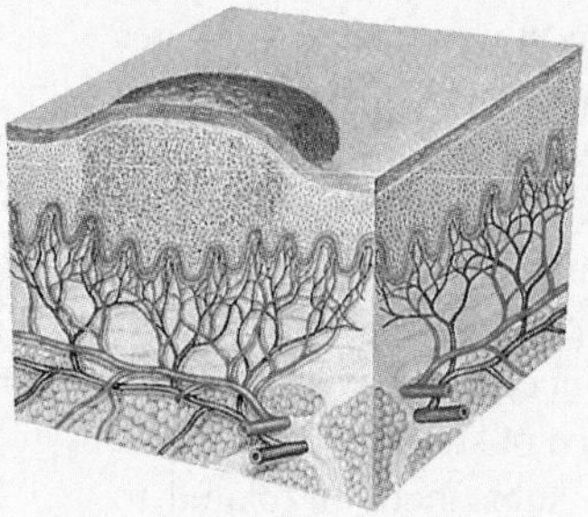	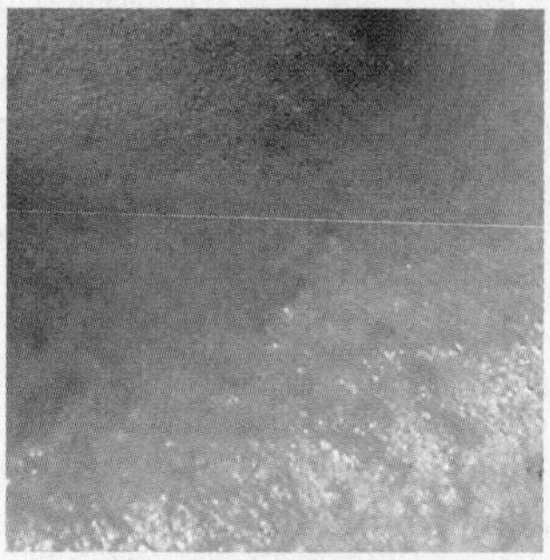 **Flat warts[c] (Courtesy Dr. E Sahn.)**
PATCH A flat, nonpalpable, irregular-shaped macule more than 1 cm in diameter	Vitiligo, port-wine stains, mongolian spots, café au lait spot	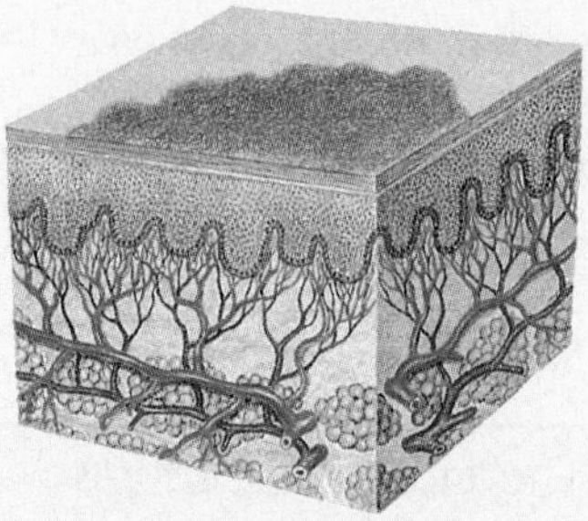	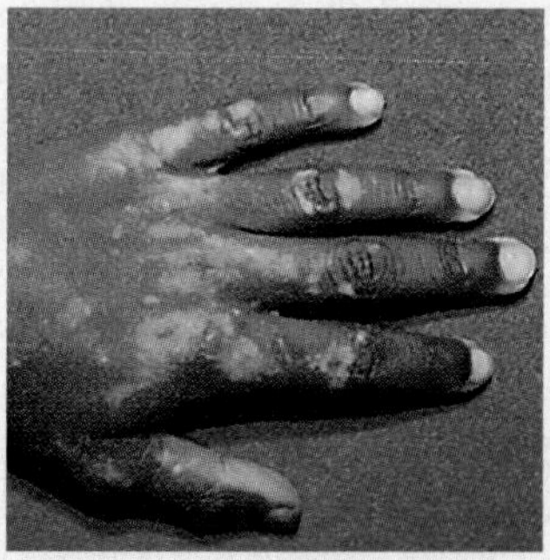 **Vitiligo[h]**
PLAQUE Elevated, firm, and rough lesion with flat top surface greater than 1 cm in diameter	Psoriasis, seborrheic and actinic keratoses	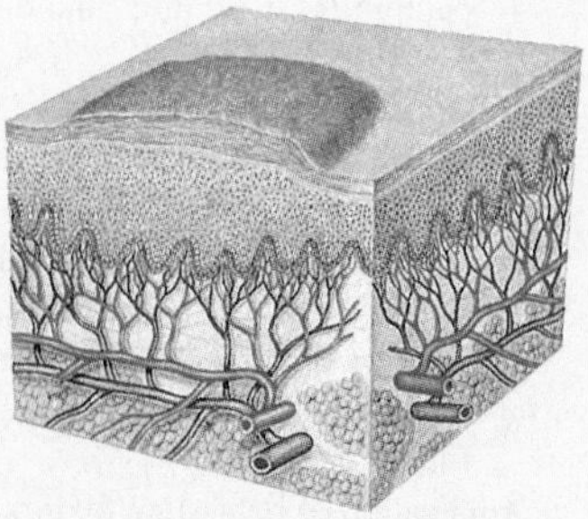	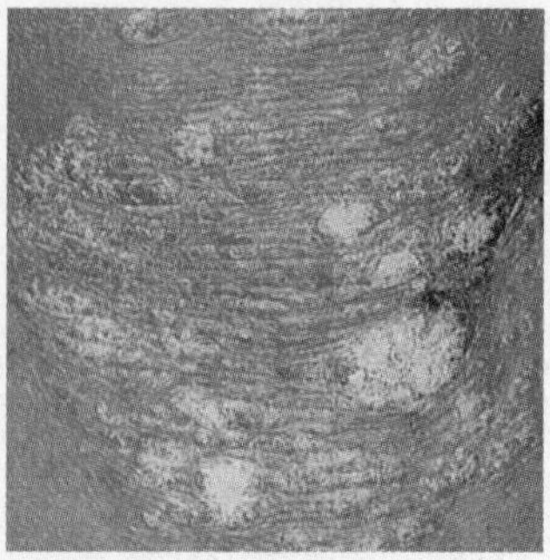 **Plaque[e]**

Table 43-3 Primary and Secondary Skin Lesions—cont'd

Primary Skin Lesions	Examples
WHEAL Elevated, irregular-shaped area of cutaneous edema; solid, transient; variable diameter	Insect bites, urticaria, allergic reaction

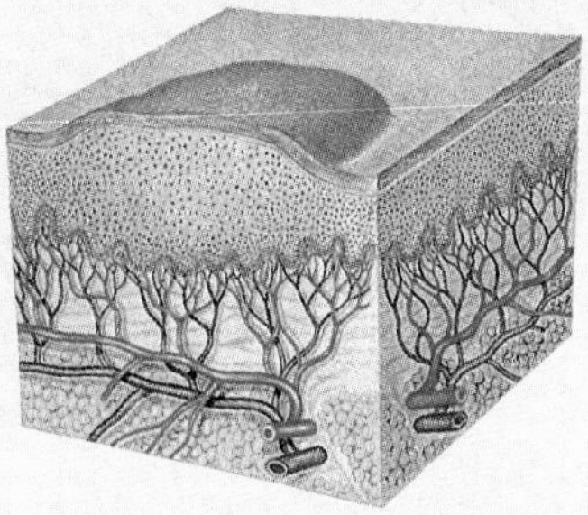
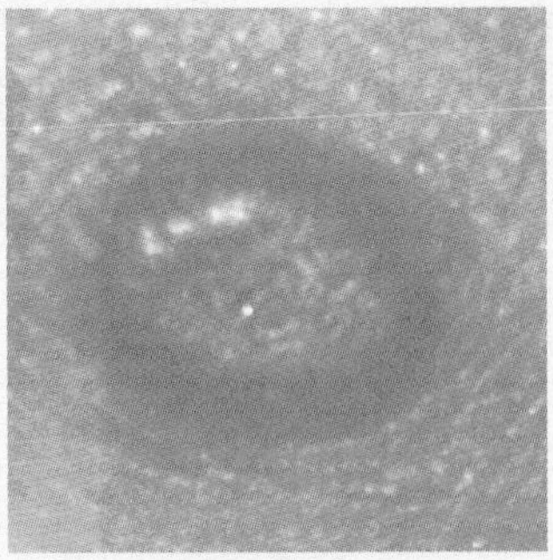

Wheal[c]

Primary Skin Lesions	Examples
NODULE Elevated, firm, circumscribed lesion; deeper in dermis than a papule; 1-2 cm in diameter	Erythema nodosum, lipomas

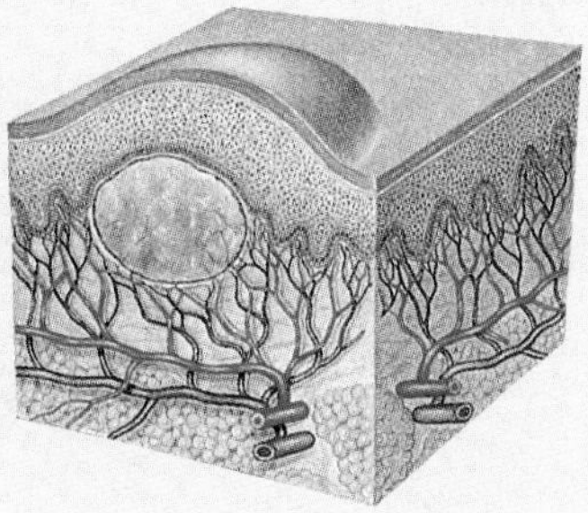
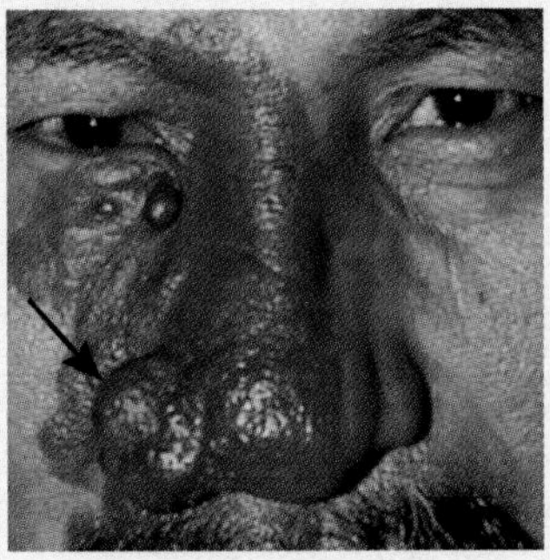

Hypertrophic nodule[d]

Primary Skin Lesions	Examples
TUMOR Elevated, solid lesion; may be clearly demarcated; deeper in dermis; greater than 2 cm in diameter	Neoplasms, benign tumor, lipoma, hemangioma

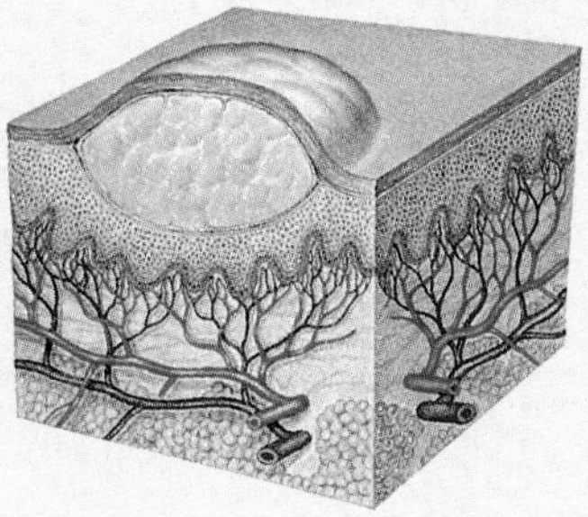
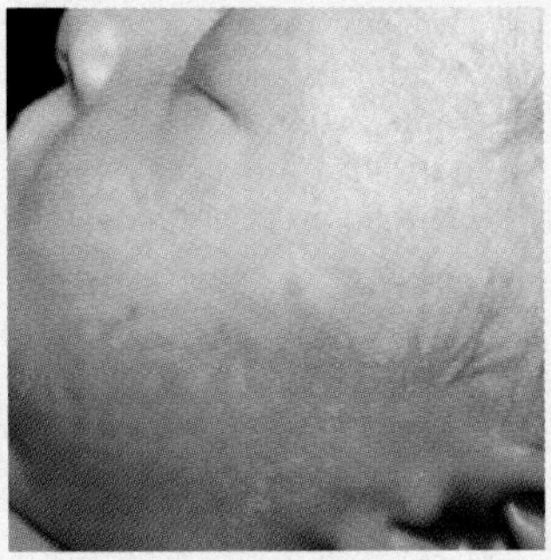

Hemangioma[h]

Primary Skin Lesions	Examples
VESICLE Elevated, circumscribed, superficial, not into dermis; filled with serous fluid; less than 1 cm in diameter	Varicella (chickenpox), herpes zoster (shingles)

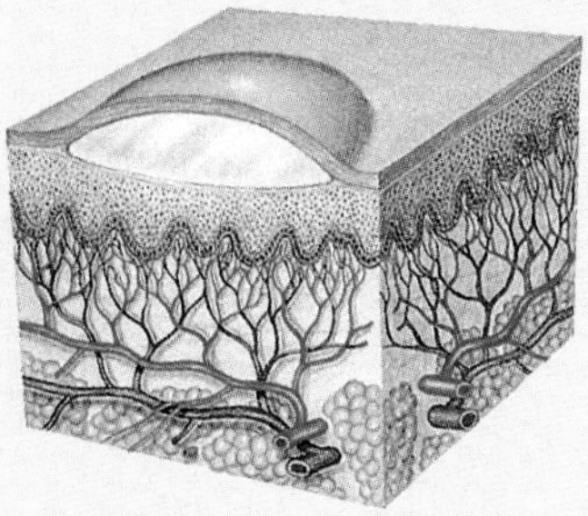
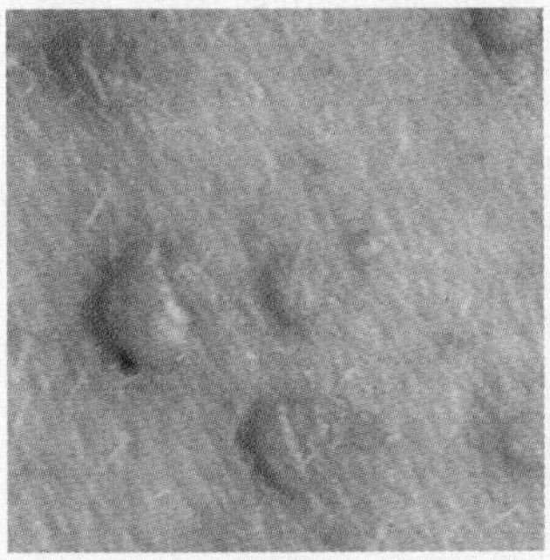

Vesicles[c]

Continued

Table 43-3 Primary and Secondary Skin Lesions—cont'd

Primary Skin Lesions	Examples

BULLA

Vesicle greater than 1 cm in diameter — Blister, pemphigus vulgaris

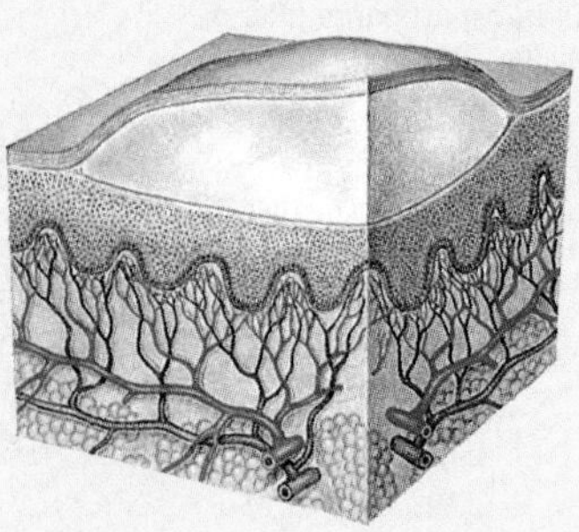

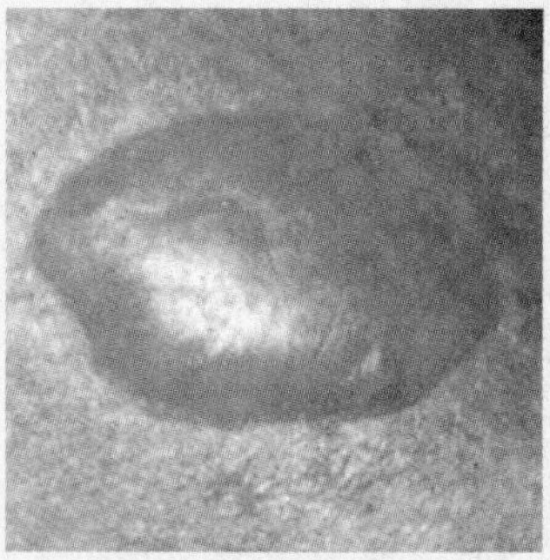

Bulla[c]
(Courtesy Dr. KA Riley.)

PUSTULE

Elevated, superficial lesion; similar to a vesicle but filled with purulent fluid — Impetigo, acne

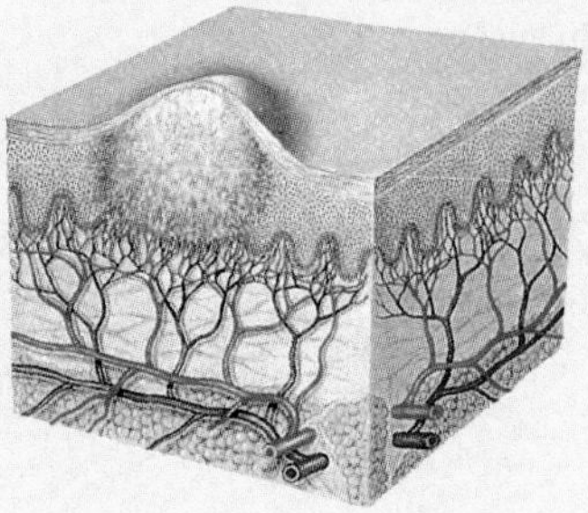

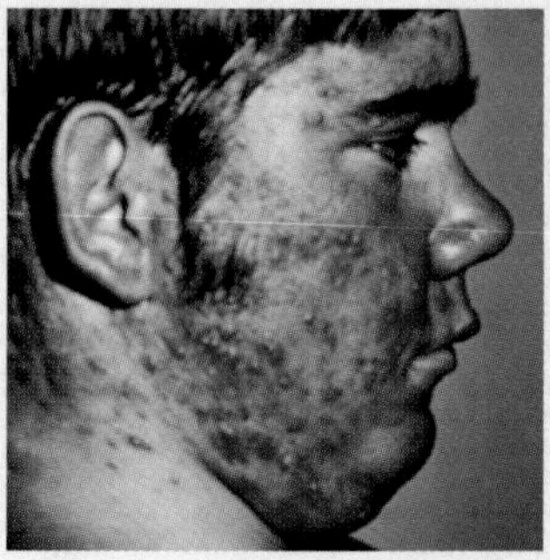

Acne[h]

CYST

Elevated, circumscribed, encapsulated lesion; in dermis or subcutaneous layer; filled with liquid or semisolid material — Sebaceous cyst, cystic acne

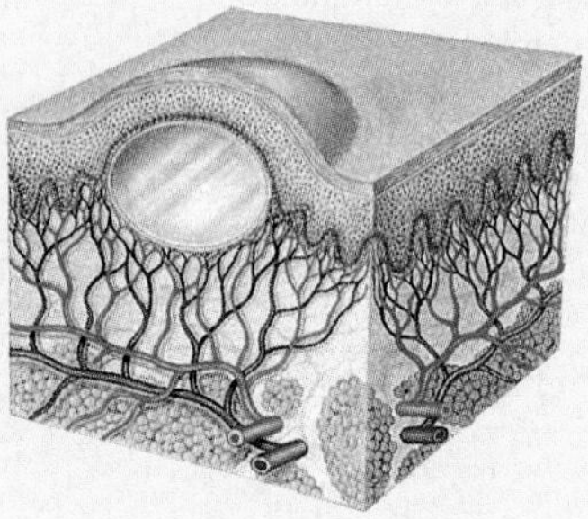

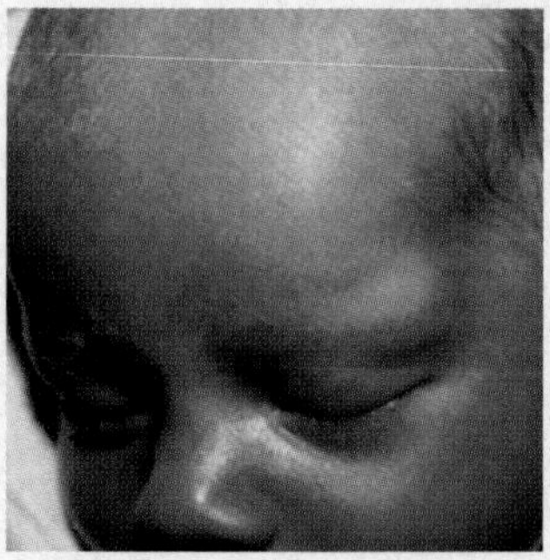

Sebaceous cyst[h]

TELANGIECTASIA

Fine, irregular red lines produced by capillary dilation — Telangiectasia in rosacea

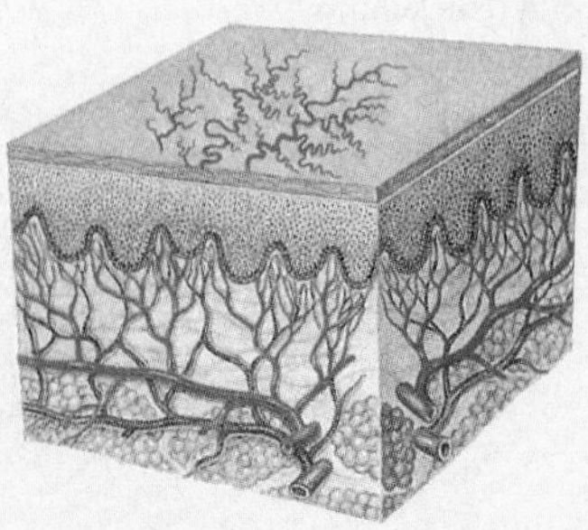

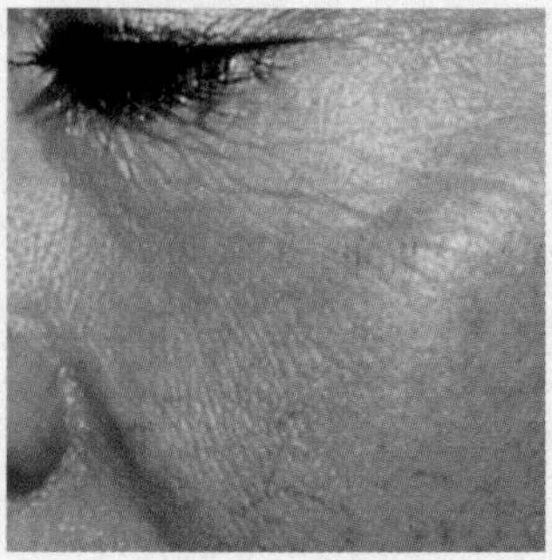

Telangiectasia[d]

Table 43-3 Primary and Secondary Skin Lesions—cont'd

Primary Skin Lesions	Examples		
SCALE Heaped-up, keratinized cells; flaky skin; irregular; thick or thin; dry or oily; variation in size	Flaking of skin with seborrheic dermatitis following scarlet fever, or flaking of skin following a drug reaction; dry skin	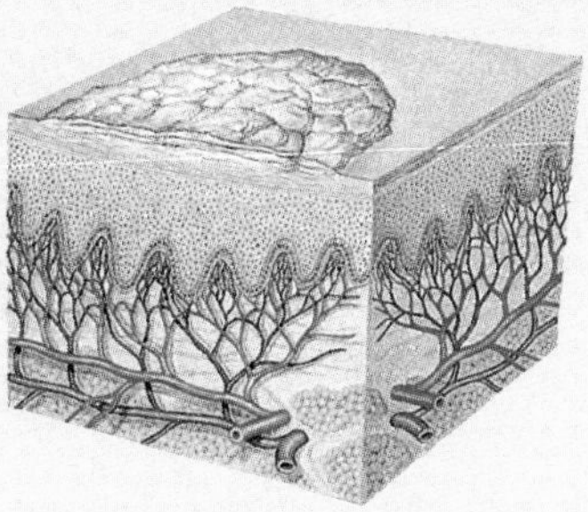	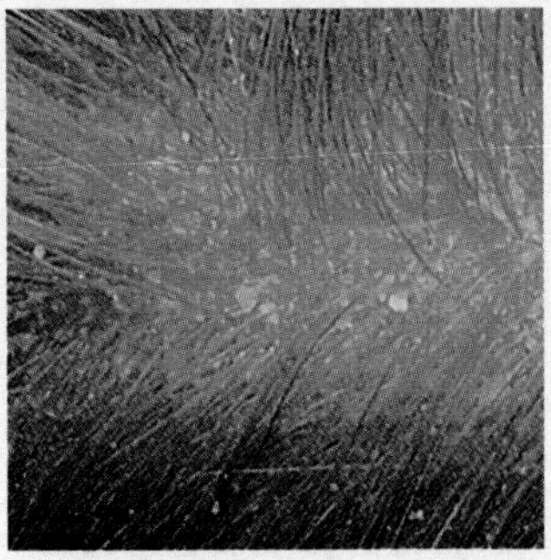 **Fine scaling**[a]
LICHENIFICATION Rough, thickened epidermis secondary to persistent rubbing, itching, or skin irritation; often involves flexor surface of extremity	Chronic dermatitis	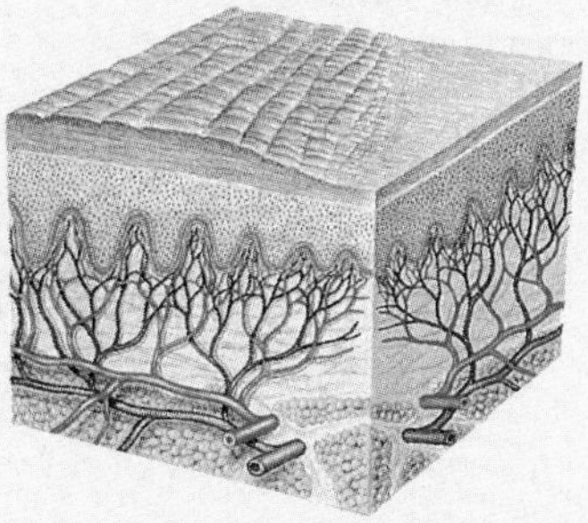	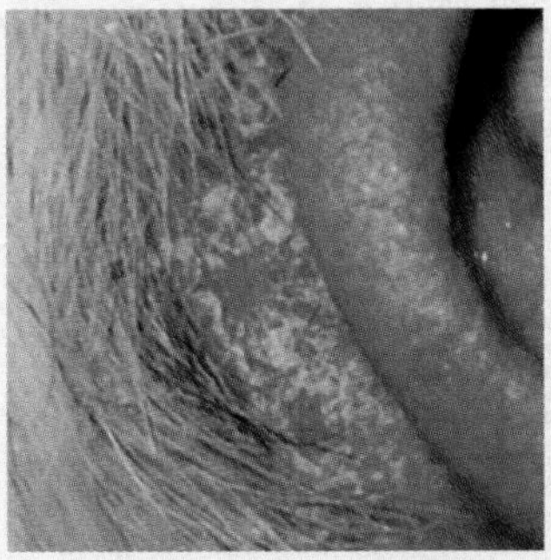 **Stasis dermatitis in early stage**[f]
KELOID Irregular-shaped, elevated, progressively enlarging scar; grows beyond the boundaries of the wound; caused by excessive collagen formation during healing	Keloid formation following surgery	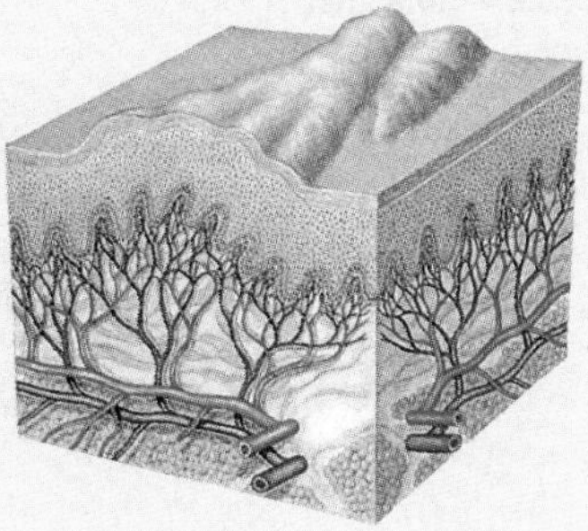	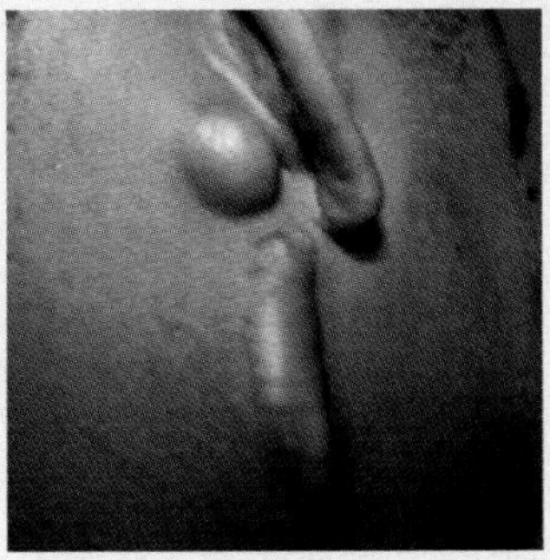 **Keloid**[h]
SCAR Thin to thick fibrous tissue that replaces normal skin following injury or laceration to the dermis	Healed wound or surgical incision	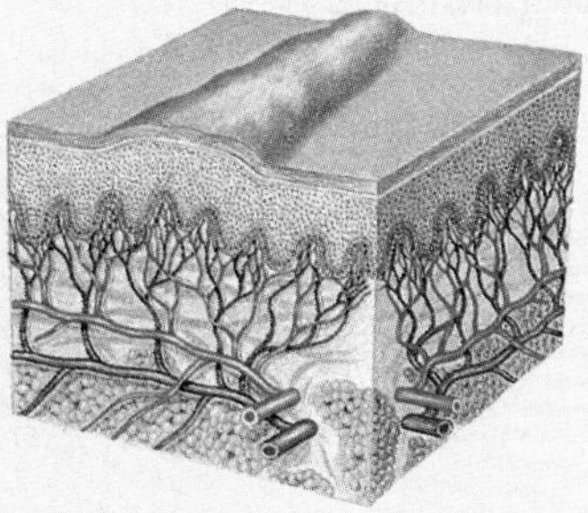	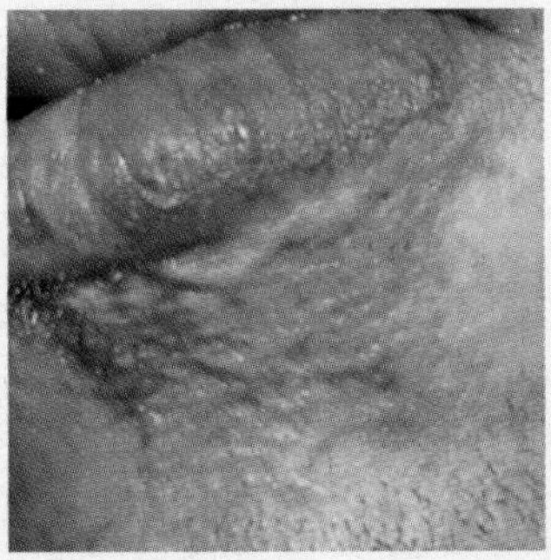 **Hypertrophic scar**[d]

Continued

Table 43-3 Primary and Secondary Skin Lesions—cont'd

Primary Skin Lesions	Examples		
EXCORIATION Loss of the epidermis; linear, hollowed-out, crusted area	Abrasion or scratch, scabies	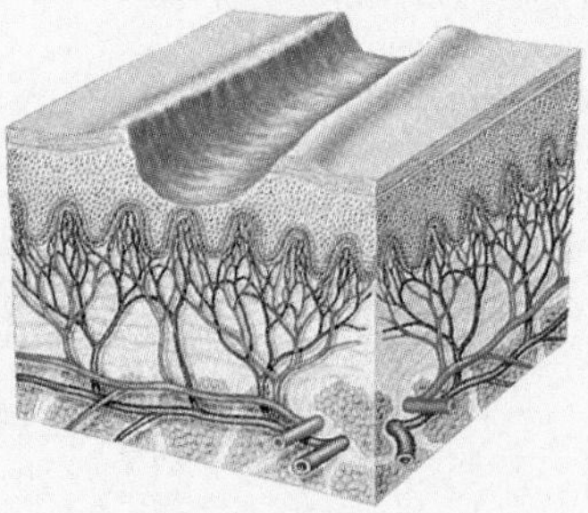	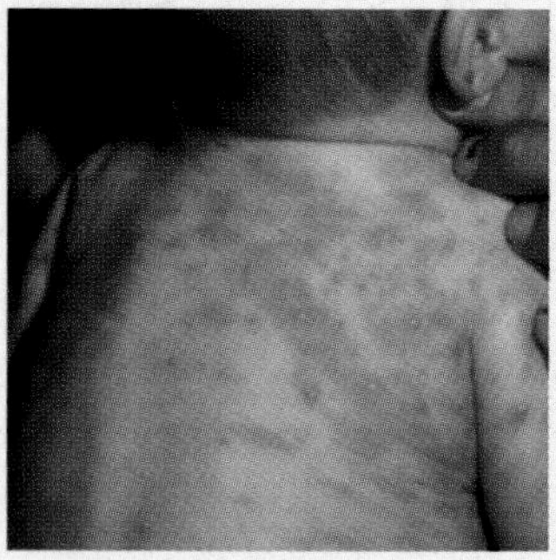 **Scabies[h]**
FISSURE Linear crack or break from the epidermis to the dermis; may be moist or dry	Athlete's foot, cracks at the corner of the mouth	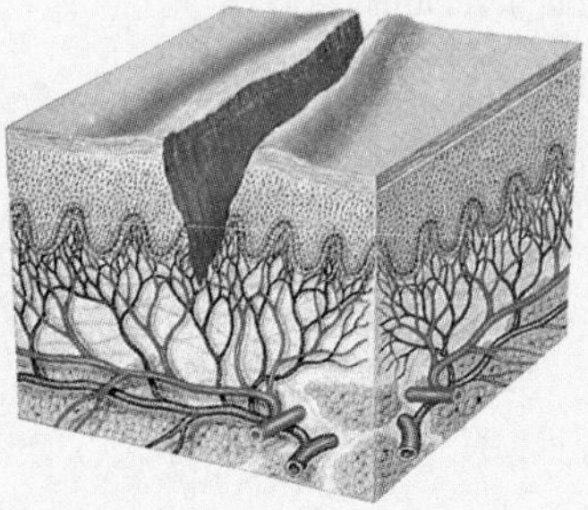	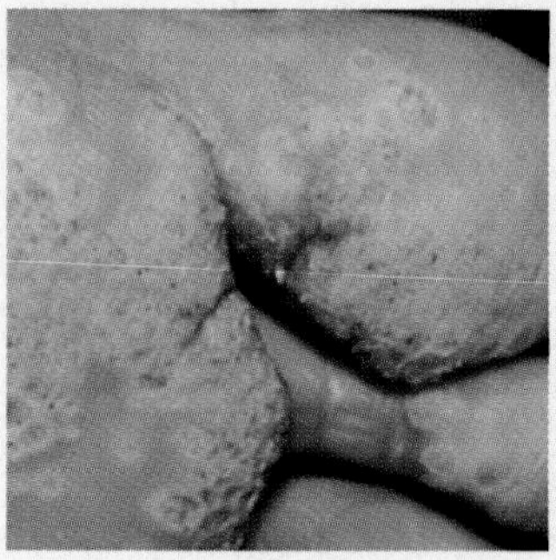 **Fissures[d]**
EROSION Loss of part of the epidermis; depressed, moist, glistening; follows rupture of a vesicle or bulla	Varicella, variola after rupture	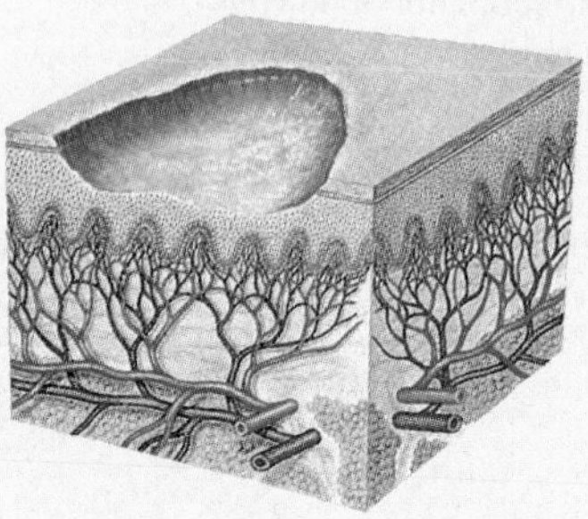	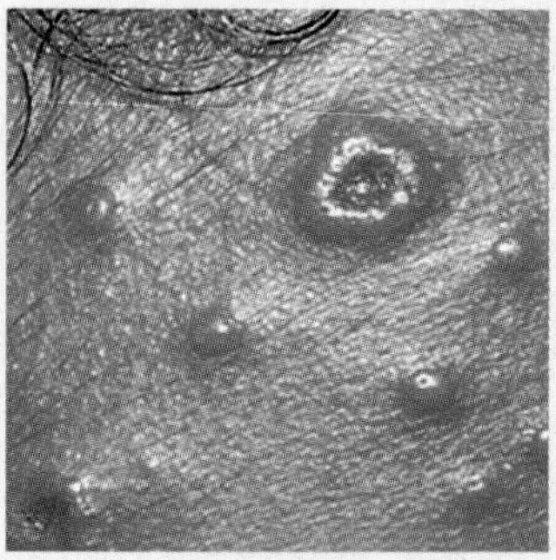 **Erosion[b]**
ULCER Loss of epidermis and dermis; concave; varies in size	Decubiti, stasis ulcers	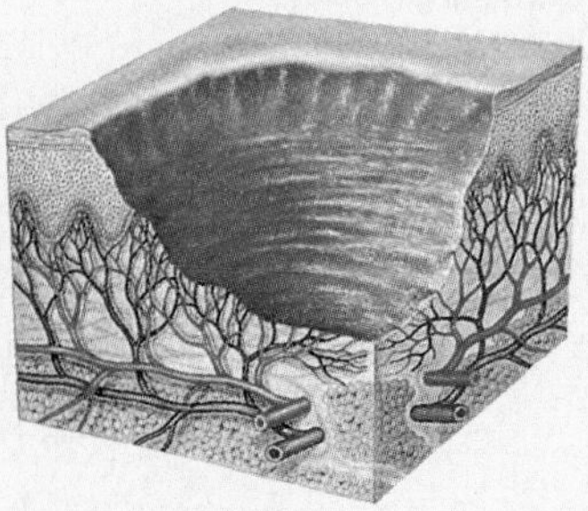	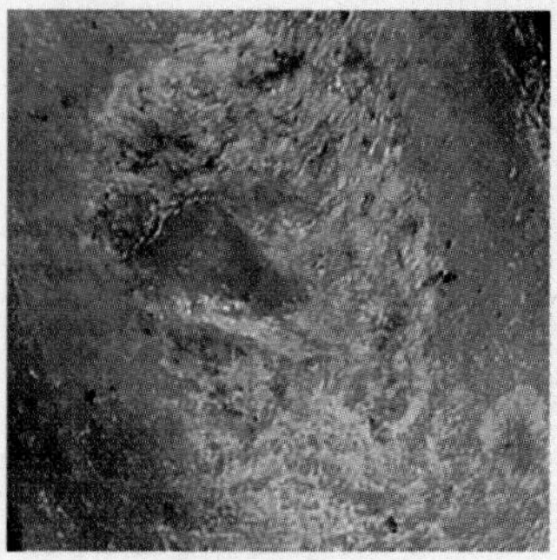 **Stasis ulcer[e]**

Table 43-3 Primary and Secondary Skin Lesions—cont'd

Primary Skin Lesions	Examples
ATROPHY	
Thinning of the skin surface and loss of skin markings; skin appears translucent and paperlike	Aged skin, striae

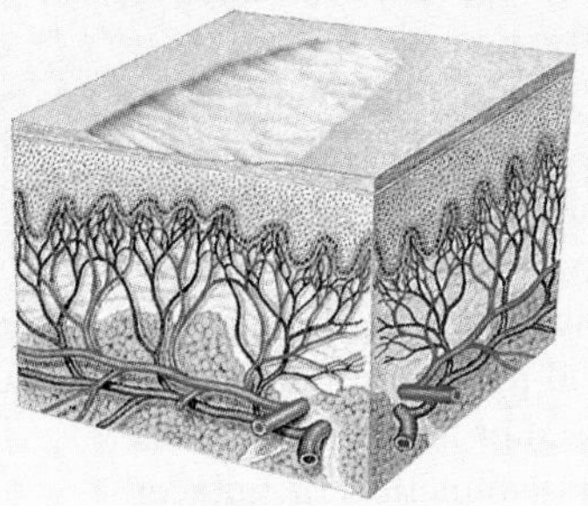

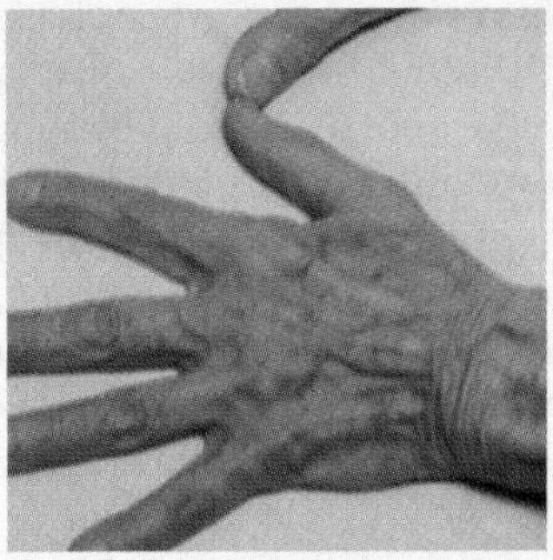

Aged skin[g]

From Thompson JM, Wilson SF: *Health assessment for nursing practice,* St Louis, 1996, Mosby.
[a]Baran R, Dawber RR, Levene GM: *Color atlas of the hair, scalp, and nails,* St Louis, 1991, Mosby.
[b]Cohen BA: *Pediatric dermatology,* London, 1993, Wolfe.
[c]Farrar WE et al: *Infectious diseases,* ed 2, London, 1992, Gower.
[d]Goldman MP, Fitzpatrick RE: *Cutaneous laser surgery: the art and science of selective photo thermolysis,* ed 2, St Louis, 1998, Mosby.
[e]Habif TP: *Clinical dermatology,* ed 3, St Louis, 1996, Mosby.
[f]Marks JG Jr, DeLeo VA: *Contact and occupational dermatitis,* St Louis, 1991, Mosby.
[g]Seidel HM et al: *Mosby's guide to physical examination,* ed 4, St Louis, 1999, Mosby.
[h]Weston WL, Lane AT: *Color textbook of pediatric dermatology,* ed 2, St Louis, 1996, Mosby.

Table 43-4 Special Skin Lesions

Type	Clinical Manifestations
Comedone	A plug of sebaceous and keratin material lodged in the opening of a hair follicle; an open comedone has a dilated orifice (blackhead), and a closed comedone has a narrow opening (whitehead)
Burrow	A narrow, raised, irregular channel caused by a parasite
Petechiae	A circumscribed area of blood less than 0.5 cm in diameter
Purpura	A circumscribed area of blood greater than 0.5 cm in diameter
Telangiectasia	Dilated, superficial blood vessels

8. Chronic diseases accompanied by anemia, edema, renal failure, malnutrition, sepsis, and urinary or fecal incontinence
9. Coarse bed sheets used for turning by dragging, which produces a shearing force

Risk factors for the critically ill include the following:[8]

1. Norepinephrine infusion
2. APACHE II score
3. Fecal incontinence
4. Anemia
5. Length of stay

Pressure sores usually develop over bony prominences. The sacrum, heels, ischia, and greater trochanters are the most common sites. Continuous pressure on tissue between the bony prominence and a resistant outside surface distorts capillaries and occludes the blood flow and oxygen supply. If the pressure is relieved within a few hours, a brief period of reactive hyperemia (redness) occurs with no lasting tissue damage. If the pressure continues unrelieved, the endothelial cells lining the capillaries become disrupted with platelet aggregation, forming microthrombi that block blood flow and cause anoxic necrosis of surrounding tissues. Pressure ulcers can be classified by stages:

I. Nonblanchable erythema of intact skin
II. Partial-thickness skin loss involving epidermis or dermis
III. Full-thickness skin loss involving damage or necrosis of subcutaneous tissue that may extend to, but not through, underlying fascia
IV. Full-thickness skin loss with extensive destruction, tissue necrosis, or damage to muscle, bone, or supporting structures[9]

A layer of dead tissue forms that appears as a blister when there is superficial damage or as a reddish blue discoloration when there is deeper tissue damage. Superficial sores are more common on the sacrum as a result of shearing or friction forces (forces parallel to the skin). Deep sores develop closer to the bone as a result of tissue distortion and vascular occlusion from pressure that is perpendicular to the tissue (over the heels, trochanter, and ischia).

The necrotic tissue initiates an inflammatory response, with pain, fever, and leukocytosis. Although bacteria colonize the dead tissue, the infection is usually localized and self-limiting. Proteolytic enzymes from bacteria and macrophages dissolve necrotic tissues and cause a foul-smelling discharge that resembles, but is not, pus.

Pressure sores are often painful in individuals who do not have loss of sensation from spinal cord trauma or neuropathy. The presence of necrotic tissue produces an inflammatory response with hyperemia, fever, and increased white blood cell count. If the ulceration is large, toxicity and pain lead to loss of appetite, debility, and renal insufficiency. Individuals who are immunosuppressed or have diabetes mellitus may develop infection and inflammation of adjacent tissues (cellulitis) or septicemia.

The primary goal for those at risk for pressure ulcers is prevention.[10] Pressure sores are not prevented by topical agents because they do not relieve the pressure. Frequent turning, use of pressure reduction surfaces, and maintenance of fluid and caloric intake are effective preventive techniques.[11] Nutrition, oxygenation, and fluid balance must be maintained.

Superficial ulcers should be covered with flat, nonbulky dressings that cannot wrinkle and cause increased pressure or friction. Spontaneous healing will occur more quickly when the ulcer is kept moist with an occlusive dressing.[12] Antibiotics are seldom required. Antiseptics, such as hydrogen peroxide or iodine, are damaging to granulation tissue and should not be used.[13] Successful healing requires continued adequate relief of pressure.

Large, deep pressure ulcers may require surgical débridement of necrotic tissue, opening of deep pockets for drainage, and skin grafting for wound closure and successful healing. The myocutaneous flap, a single unit of skin with its underlying muscle and vasculature, has been an effective treatment in large avascular areas over bony prominences. Application of wound tension by range of motion may also promote healing.[14]

Keloids

Keloids are sharply elevated, irregularly shaped, progressively enlarging scars caused by excessive amounts of collagen in the corneum during connective tissue repair. Seemingly inconsequential trauma may result in a keloidal reaction, particularly in blacks and Orientals. Burns incite this reaction more commonly than other types of injury (see Chapter 45).

Excessive or poorly aligned tension on a wound, introduction of foreign material into the skin, and certain types of trauma (e.g., burns) are all provocative factors. Those parts of the body at risk include shoulders, back, chin, ears, and lower legs. Most keloids appear within 1 year of trauma. Individuals 10 to 30 years of age develop lesions much more commonly than do children before puberty or older adults.

Type III collagen is increased with keloids. The increased synthesis of collagen is associated with IL-6 and dermal fibroblasts that have high metabolic and mitotic rates.[15] **Myofibroblasts,** cells with characteristics of both fibroblasts and smooth muscle cells, have been identified as the principal cells in keloids. Collagenase activity in keloids has been found to be normal or increased, but the collagen may be protected from degradation by **proteoglycan,** a glycoprotein present in connective tissue that serves as a binding (cementing) material, and by specific inhibitors of proteolytic enzymes. Genes regulating fibroblast apoptosis may be downregulated in keloid tissue.[16] A familial tendency for keloid formation has been found, with both autosomal recessive and autosomal dominant inheritance patterns reported.

Keloids start as pink or red, firm, well-defined, rubbery plaques that persist for several months after trauma. Later, uncontrolled overgrowth causes extension beyond the site of the original wound and the tumor becomes smoother, irregularly shaped, hyperpigmented, harder, and more symptomatic. The tendency to send out **clawlike prolongations** is typical of keloids (Fig. 43-3).

Preventive measures such as avoiding unnecessary, elective surgeries are of paramount importance. When surgery is necessary for cosmetic reasons, having it done in early childhood is best. Scalpel surgery with strict aseptic technique and avoidance of wound tension is imperative. Treatment of keloids includes multiple approaches including a combination of surgery with intralesional steroids and/or radiotherapy, silicone gel sheeting, pressure, cryotherapy, pulsed dye laser, interferon alfa-2b, and cultured epithelial autografts.[17]

Pruritus

Pruritus, or itching, is a symptom associated with many primary skin disorders, such as eczema, psoriasis, or lice infestations, or it can be a manifestation of systemic disease (e.g., chronic renal failure, cholestatic liver disease, thyroid disorders, iron deficiency) or the use of opiate drugs. Pruritus may be localized or generalized and may move from one location to another.[18] Both central and peripheral nerve pathways are activated.[19]

The actual mechanisms causing pruritus are unknown. Multiple stimuli can produce itching, including histamine, proteases, heat, cold, and chemical and electrical stimulation. Substance P, a neurotransmitter present throughout the nervous system, induces histamine release and wheal formation with itching when injected into the skin. Small c-receptors are sensitive to histamine.[20] Acetylcholine elicits itch but not pain in atopic eczema.[19] Lymphocytes are also present in many

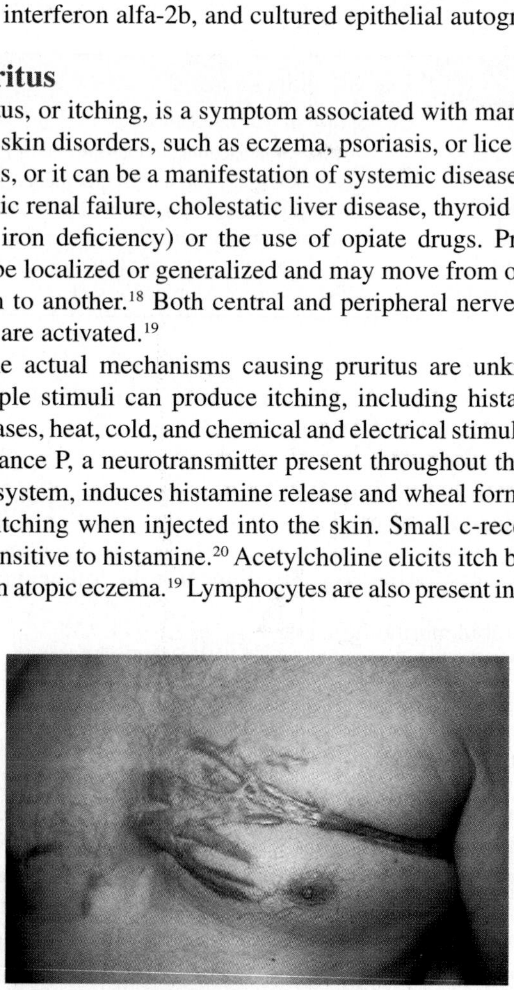

Fig. 43-3 Keloid. (Courtesy Department of Dermatology, School of Medicine, University of Utah.)

itching skin diseases, and lymphokines may be involved in the pathogenesis of itching.[21]

Itching has also been linked to pain, because many stimuli that induce pain produce itching at lower intensities. Central nervous system mechanisms can also modulate itching, and itching is less perceptible when the mind is concentrating on other things. How the central nervous system influences the itch sensation is unclear, but itch and pain may travel in the same neural pathways.[22,23]

Chronic itching is an unpleasant sensation relieved by scratching—often severe enough to cause trauma to the skin, resulting in infection and scarring. Some individuals become so distraught with the constant irritation that they apply heat with enough intensity and duration to produce burns.

Management of localized itching depends on the cause, and the primary condition must be treated. Symptomatic relief may be obtained from antihistamines, which also have a sedative effect. Minor tranquilizers, such as promethazine, may be effective for some causes of pruritus. Itching related to dry, rough skin (xerosis) can be managed with applications of emollients and increased environmental humidity. Topical steroids are immediately effective with some occurrences of pruritus; however, in some instances, pruritus is resistant to any type of therapy.

DISORDERS OF THE SKIN

Disruptions in skin integrity may be precipitated by trauma, abnormal cellular function, infection and inflammation, and systemic diseases. Many skin disorders are benign and self-limiting, whereas others are severe and life threatening.

Inflammatory Disorders

The most common inflammatory disorder of the skin is eczema (eczematous inflammation). **Eczema** is an inflammatory response of the skin caused by endogenous and exogenous agents and is often considered synonymous with dermatitis. Endogenous eczemas include atopic dermatitis and seborrheic dermatitis. Exogenous eczemas include irritant dermatitis and allergic contact dermatitis. Eczematous dermatitis is characterized by erythema, vesicles, scales, and itching. Edema, serous discharge, and crusting occur with continued irritation and scratching. In chronic eczema the skin becomes thickened, leathery, and hyperpigmented from recurrent irritation and scratching. The location of eczema is related to the underlying cause. Eczematous inflammations need to be differentiated from other rashes and dermatoses, particularly psoriasis.

Allergic Contact Dermatitis

Allergic contact dermatitis is a common form of cell-mediated or delayed hypersensitivity. (See Chapter 8 for various types of allergic responses.) Various allergens (e.g., microorganisms, chemicals, foreign proteins, drugs, metals, latex) can form the sensitizing antigen. The response is an interaction of skin barrier function; reaction to irritants; and neuronal response, such as itching.[24] Contact with poison ivy is a common example (Fig. 43-4). As the allergen comes in contact with the skin, the allergen is bound to a carrier protein, forming a sensitizing antigen. The Langerhans cells process the antigen and carry it to T cells that then become sensitized to the antigen. Keratinocytes also may activate lymphocytes and endothelial cells in allergic contact dermatitis.[25] IgE antibodies are recovered in latex allergy and are associated with an immediate allergic response to latex rubber protein.[26]

In delayed hypersensitivity, several hours pass before an immunologic response is apparent. The T cells play an important role because they differentiate and secrete lymphokines that affect macrophage movement and aggregation, coagulation, and other inflammatory responses (see Chapter 2). Sensitization usually develops with first exposure to the antigen, and symptoms of dermatitis occur with reexposure.

The manifestations of allergic contact dermatitis include erythema and swelling with pruritic (itching) vesicular lesions in the areas of allergen contact. The pattern of distribution provides clues to the source of the antigen (e.g., hands exposed to chemical solutions or boundaries from rings and bracelets). Patch tests with specific antigens assist with diagnosis. Removal of the irritant is necessary for resolution of the inflammatory response and tissue repair. Topical or systemic steroids may be required for treatment, depending on the severity of the lesion.

Irritant Contact Dermatitis

Irritant contact dermatitis is a nonimmunologically mediated inflammation of the skin. Chemical irritation from acids

A

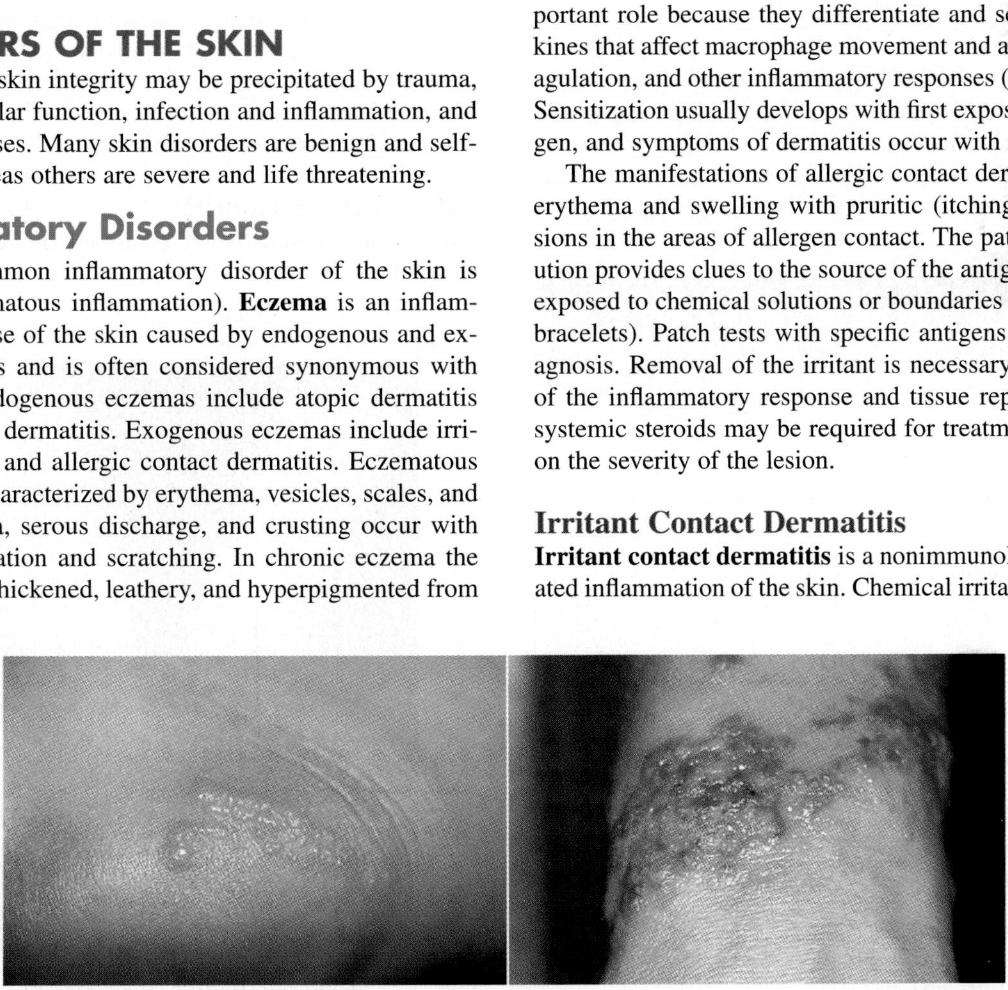

B

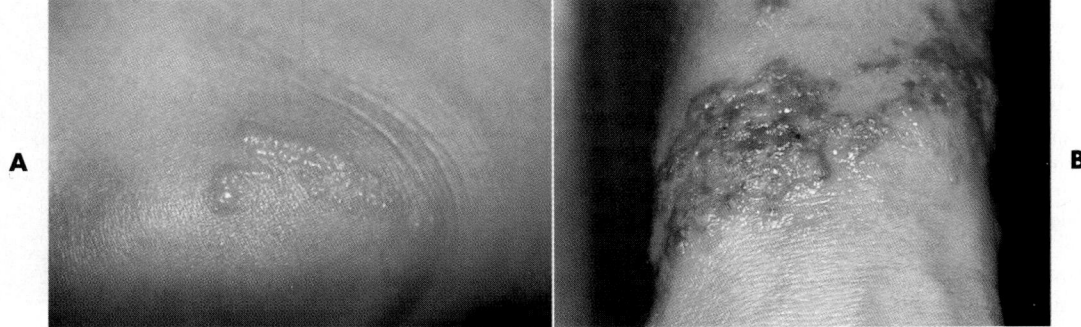

FIG. 43-4 Poison ivy. A, Poison ivy on knee. **B,** Poison ivy dermatitis. (Courtesy Department of Dermatology, School of Medicine, University of Utah.)

and prolonged exposure to soaps and detergents are common causes (Box 43-1). The skin lesions are similar in appearance to allergic contact dermatitis. Removing the source of irritation and use of topical agents constitute effective treatment.

Atopic Dermatitis

Atopic dermatitis affects 9% to 12% of the population[27] and is increasing.[28] It is more common in infancy and childhood; however, some individuals are affected throughout life. Often there is also food allergy.[29] A family history of asthma, allergic rhinitis, dry skin, and eczema accompanies this disorder.

The dermatitis results from the complex activation of mast cells; eosinophils; T lymphocytes; monocytes; and other inflammatory cells that release histamine, lymphokines, interleukins (i.e., IL-4), eosinophil cationic protein,[30] and other inflammatory mediators. Serum immunoglobulin E (IgE) is elevated and IL-8 may be a contributing factor.[31] Eosinophils are elevated and may release major basic protein, which activates mast cells.[32] The interaction of allergen with the immune system results in the chronic inflammation.[33] Inflammation in atopic dermatitis may also be stimulated by *Staphylococcus aureus* antigen and exotoxin activation of T cells.[34]

During adolescence and adulthood the lesions are usually localized to the hands and feet or flexor surfaces (i.e., antecubital fossa, popliteal space) of the arms and legs (Fig. 43-5). The erythema, scaling, and lichenification (thickened and leatherlike skin) are exacerbated by scratching, because the lesions are manifest by itching.[35] The scratching increases susceptibility to infection from *Staphylococcus aureus* and predisposition to cutaneous dissemination of viruses, particularly herpes simplex and vaccinia. Affected individuals also have a higher incidence of cataracts.[36]

Management of atopic dermatitis includes avoidance of known irritants, good lubrication, and preservation of skin moisture. During the acute inflammatory stage, application of open wet compresses, using aluminum acetate solution (Burow solution), soothes itching and cools and moistens the skin. Topical steroids in the lowest possible dosages may be used to treat the lesions. Antibiotics are used to treat staphylococcal infections. Relief of pruritus is difficult, but oral antihistamines occasionally are prescribed, including topical doxepin.[37] Affected individuals should avoid exposure to herpes simplex and vaccination with live virus.

Box 43-1

SUBSTANCES KNOWN TO CAUSE CONTACT DERMATITIS

- Alkalis
  - Soaps
  - Detergents
  - Ammonia preparations
  - Lye
  - Drainpipe cleaners
  - Toilet bowl cleaners
  - Oven cleaners
- Acids
- Metal salts
  - Cyanides of calcium, copper, mercury, nickel, silver, zinc
  - Chlorides of calcium and zinc
- Bromine, chlorine, iodine, fluorine
- Insecticides
- Dusts of lime, zinc, arsenic
- Wood dust from teak, cinchona bark, quinine, pyrethrum
- Tobacco dust from cigars
- Explosive powders
- Hydrocarbons
  - Crude petroleum, lubricating oil, cutting oil
  - Paraffins, mineral oils
  - Asphalt, other tar products
- Soot, peat

Stasis Dermatitis

Stasis dermatitis usually occurs on the legs as a result of venous stasis and edema. The disorder is associated with varicosities, phlebitis, and vascular trauma. First, erythema and pruritus develop and then scaling, petechiae, and hyperpigmentation. Progressive lesions become ulcerated, particularly around the ankles and tibia (Fig. 43-6).

Treatment includes elevating the legs as often as possible, not wearing tight clothes around the legs, and not standing for long periods. Acute inflammations are treated with antibiotics. Chronic lesions with ulceration are treated with wet dressings of Burow solution or silver nitrate. Edema is controlled with external compression.

Seborrheic Dermatitis

Seborrheic dermatitis is a common chronic inflammation of the skin involving the scalp, eyebrows, eyelids, ear canals,

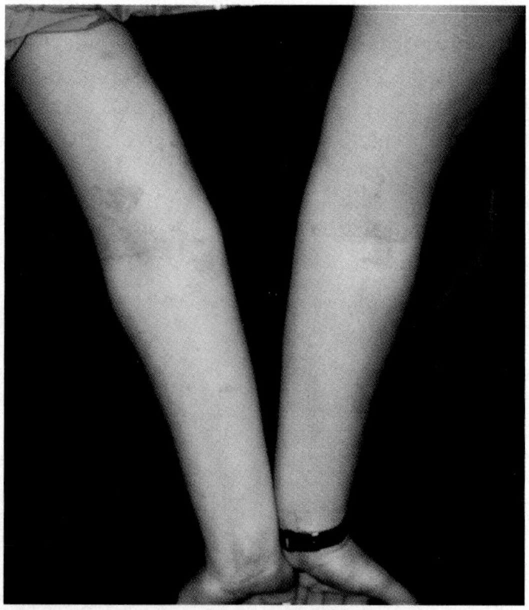

FIG. 43-5 Atopic dermatitis. (Courtesy Department of Dermatology, School of Medicine, University of Utah.)

nasolabial folds, axillae, chest, and back (Fig. 43-7). In infants it is known as *cradle cap.* The cause is unknown, and the lesions appear from infancy to old age, with periods of remission and exacerbation. The lesions appear as scaly, white, or yellowish inflammatory plaques with mild pruritus. Mild cases are treated with shampoos containing sulfur, salicylic acid, or tar. Corticosteroid applications are useful for suppression of severe symptoms but should not be used for maintenance therapy.

Papulosquamous Disorders

Psoriasis, pityriasis rosea, and lichen planus are disorders characterized by inflammatory processes associated with papules, scales, plaques, and erythema. Collectively they are described as **papulosquamous disorders.**

Psoriasis

Psoriasis is a chronic, relapsing, proliferative skin disorder that can occur at any age and affects 1% to 2% of the population.[38] The onset is generally established by 20 years of age. The cause of psoriasis is unknown, but genetic, immunologic, and biochemical alterations have been investigated. T cell activation and consequent cytokine production is a factor in the triggering and maintenance of psoriatic lesions.[39] A family history of psoriasis often is established, and an human leukocyte antigen (HLA)–associated inheritance is likely.[40]

Both the dermis and epidermis are thickened, with cellular hyperproliferation, altered differentiation, and inflammation.[41] The turnover time for shedding the epidermis is decreased from the normal 26 to 30 days to 3 to 4 days. There are increased numbers of germinative cells and an increase in transit time of cells through the dermis. The rapid cellular proliferation does not allow time for cell maturation and keratinization to occur, resulting in a thickened epidermis and plaque formation. The loosely cohesive keratin gives the lesion a silvery appearance. There is frequently capillary dilation and increased vascularization to accommodate the increased cell metabolism. The increased vascularity causes erythema. The types of psoriasis include plaque, guttate, pustular, and erythrodermic. The disease can be mild, moderate, or severe, depending on the size, distribution, and inflammation of the lesions. Early-onset psoriasis is an inflammatory lesion with epidermal hyperproliferation and the presence of activated T lymphocytes.[42] Pustular types of psoriasis show genetic susceptibility and a strong association with major histocompatibility complex (MHC) class 1 and alteration in T cell–mediated cytokines and growth factors.[38] The progress of psoriasis is characterized by remissions and exacerbations. Antimalarial drugs exacerbate existing psoriasis in 18% of individuals.[43] Arthritis develops in approximately 5% of individuals with psoriasis.[44]

The typical psoriatic lesion is a well-demarcated, thick, silvery, scaly, erythematous plaque surrounded by normal skin (Fig. 43-8). Initial lesions usually develop insidiously as small erythematous papules that enlarge and coalesce into larger inflammatory lesions. The lesions are commonly located on the face, scalp, elbows, and knees and at sites of trauma. Lesions that develop in skinfolds are smooth and have a deep red color. The scales are usually loosely adherent and may cause small bleeding points when removed.

In guttate psoriasis, small papules appear suddenly on the trunk and extremities (Fig. 43-9). The lesions may appear a

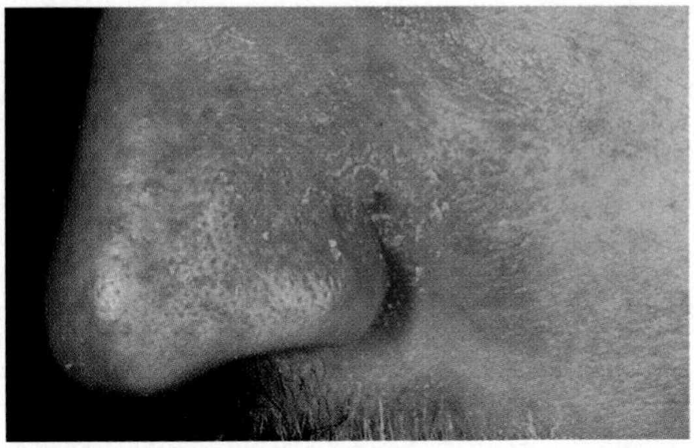

FIG. 43-7 Seborrheic dermatitis. (Courtesy Department of Dermatology, School of Medicine, University of Utah.)

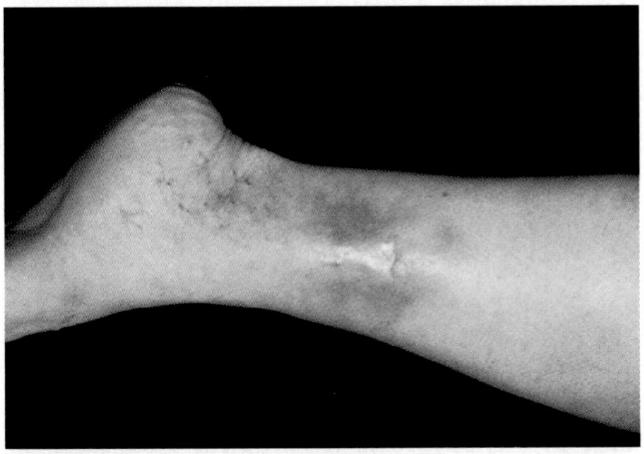

FIG. 43-6 Stasis ulcer. (Courtesy Department of Dermatology, School of Medicine, University of Utah.)

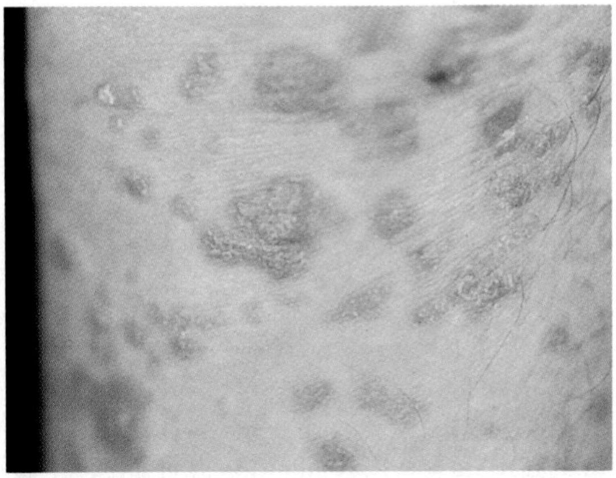

FIG. 43-8 Psoriasis. Typical oval plaque with well-defined borders and silvery scale. (Courtesy Department of Dermatology, School of Medicine, University of Utah.)

few weeks after a streptococcal respiratory infection, and children with psoriasis reflect a tendency to develop guttate psoriasis. Guttate psoriasis may resolve spontaneously in weeks or months.

Treatment is individualized and related to reducing epidermal cell turnover. Mild lesions are usually treated with emollients, keratolytic agents, and corticosteroids. Moderate lesions may respond to ultraviolet light, tar preparations, or a combination of both, and to methotrexate, cyclosporin, and acetretin. Vitamin D_3 (calcitriol) is used to reduce epidermal proliferation.[45,46] Severe disease may require hospitalization with a combination of topical agents and systemic corticosteroids and antimetabolites such as methotrexate. Lesions of the scalp, nails, and genitalia are treated with different lotions and shampoos.

Pityriasis Rosea

Pityriasis rosea is a benign, self-limiting inflammatory disorder that occurs more frequently in young adults, usually during the winter months. The cause is unknown but is thought to be a virus.[47] Pityriasis rosea begins as a single lesion known as a **herald patch** (Fig. 43-10) that is circular, demarcated, salmon-pink, approximately 3 to 4 cm in diameter, and usually located on the trunk. Early lesions are macular and papular. Secondary lesions develop within 14 to 21 days and extend over the trunk and upper part of the extremities. Lesions are rarely located on the face. The lesions emerge as small erythematous papules that expand into characteristic oval lesions. There may be few or hundreds of lesions. The pattern of distribution follows the skin lines around the trunk and resembles a drooping pine tree. As scales flake off from the margin of the lesions, a collarette pattern is formed. Itching is the most common symptom. Occasionally headache, fatigue, or sore throat precedes the development of the lesions.[48]

The diagnosis of pityriasis rosea is made by the clinical appearance of the lesion. It can be confused with secondary syphilis, psoriasis, or seborrheic dermatitis. The disorder is usually self-limiting and resolves in a few months with symptomatic treatment for pruritus. Ultraviolet light, antihistamines, or topical corticosteroids may be used to control itching. Sun exposure facilitates resolution of the lesions.

WHAT'S NEW? Angiogenesis and Skin Disorders

Angiogenesis is the formation of new capillary blood vessels and is a normal component of embryonic development, wound revascularization, inflammation, and malignant growth. The process is regulated by growth factors and proangiogenic cytokines and inhibitors of neovascularization. Defective or uncontrolled angiogenesis is central to the etiology of dermatologic pathologic conditions, including psoriasis, warts, cutaneous melanoma, pyogenic granulomas, hemangiomas, pressure ulcers, and stasis ulcers. An imbalance in the production of angiogenic mediators or deficiency in angiogenic-inhibitory molecules contributes to the development of these disorders.

Data from Arbiser JL: *J Am Acad Dermatol* 34(3):486, 1996; Birch A et al: Expression of basic fibroblast growth factor and vascular endothelial growth factor in primary and metastatic melanoma from the same patients, *Melanoma Res* 9(4):375, 1999; Tomanek RJ, Schatteman GC: Angiogenesis: new insights and therapeutic potential, *Anat Rec* 261(3):126, 2000.

Lichen Planus

Lichen planus is a benign, inflammatory disorder of the skin and mucous membranes. The cause is unknown, but T cells, adhesion molecules, inflammatory cytokines, and antigen-presenting cells are involved.[49] The infiltrate of T cells mediates immunoreactivity against basal layer kerotinocytes, which have altered surface antigens and adhesion molecules.[50] More recently, lichen planus has been linked to hepatitis C virus.[51] Some individuals develop lichenoid lesions after exposure to drugs or film-processing chemicals. The age of onset is usually between 30 and 70 years. The disorder begins with nonscaling, violet-colored pruritic papules, 2 to 10 mm in size, usually located on the wrists, ankles, lower legs, and genitalia (Fig. 43-11). The papules are flat topped and have a polygonal shape, often with a small central depression. New lesions are pale pink and evolve into a dark violet color. Persistent lesions may be thickened and red, forming hypertrophic lichen planus. The lesions often involve the oral mu-

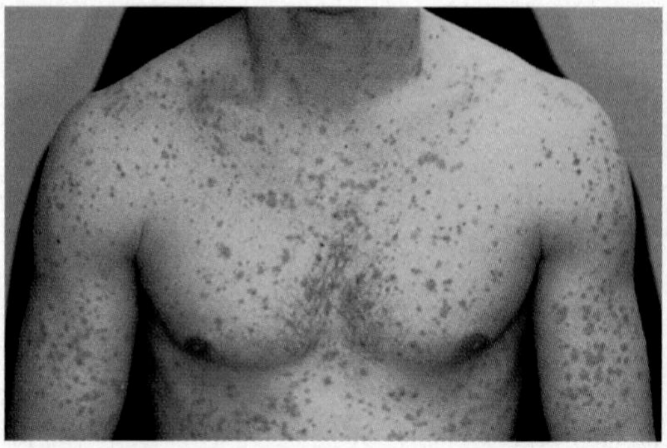

FIG. 43-9 Guttate psoriasis following streptococcal infection. Numerous uniformly small lesions may abruptly occur following streptococcal pharyngitis. (Courtesy Department of Dermatology, School of Medicine, University of Utah.)

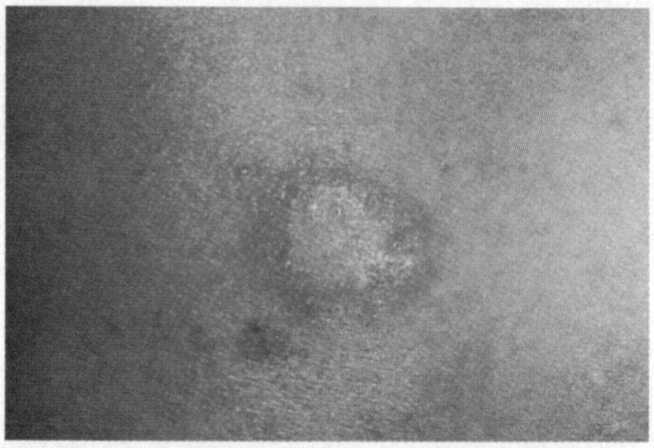

FIG. 43-10 Pityriasis rosea herald patch. A collarette pattern has formed around the margins. (Courtesy Department of Dermatology, School of Medicine, University of Utah.)

cous membranes, appearing as lacy white rings that must be differentiated from leukoplakia or oral candidiasis.[52] Fine white lines can be seen throughout the oral lesions on magnification. Mucous membrane lesions also can develop on the penis and vulvovaginal area. More commonly, oral lesions do not ulcerate, but localized or extensive painful ulcerations can occur. Chronic ulcerated lesions become malignant in 1% of individuals with the disease. Thinning and splitting of nails are common, and part or all of the nail may be shed.

Pruritus is the most distressing symptom. The lesions are self-limiting and may last for months or years, with an average duration of 12 to 18 months. Hyperpigmentation resulting from the inflammation is a common consequence of the lesion. Approximately 20% of individuals have a recurrence. Diagnosis is commonly made by the clinical appearance of the lesion. Treatment is individualized. Antihistamines are given for itching, and topical or systemic corticosteroids may be used to control inflammation. Mucous membrane lesions are treated with topical steroids or with injection into a single lesion.

Acne Vulgaris

Acne vulgaris is an inflammatory disorder of the pilosebaceous follicle (the sebaceous gland contiguous with a hair follicle). It occurs most commonly during adolescence. Details of this disorder are presented in Chapter 44.

Acne Rosacea

Acne rosacea is an inflammation of the skin that develops in middle-age adults. The disease is chronic with episodes of exacerbation.[53] The most common lesions are erythema, papules, pustules, and telangiectasia. They occur in the middle third of the face, including the forehead, nose, cheeks, and chin (Fig. 43-12). The cause is unknown, but the lesions are associated with chronic flushing and sensitivity to the sun. Hypertrophy of the sebaceous glands may be severe enough to produce an irreversible bulbous appearance of the nose, known as *rhinophyma.* Disorders of the eye frequently accompany rosacea, particularly conjunctivitis and, more rarely, keratitis. Facial application of fluorinated topical steroids may precipitate rosacea-like lesions that are difficult to treat.

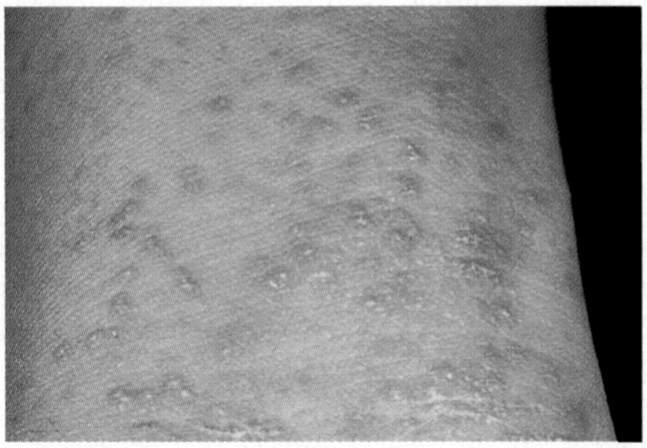

FIG. 43-11 Hypertrophic lichen planus on arms. (Courtesy Department of Dermatology, School of Medicine, University of Utah.)

Hot drinks or alcohol should be taken cautiously because the heat and vasodilation accentuate erythema. Tetracycline is the drug of choice for treatment, and a low maintenance dose may be required after the most severe lesions are controlled. One percent topical metronidazole may be effective.[54] Surgical excision of excessive tissue may be required for rhinophyma. There is controversy regarding the association between gastric *H. pylori* infection and rosacea.[55,56]

Lupus Erythematosus

Lupus erythematosus is an inflammatory disease with cutaneous manifestations. Discoid (or cutaneous) lupus erythematosus (DLE) is limited to the skin and can lead to systemic lupus erythematosus. (Systemic lupus erythematosus [SLE], a diffuse, multisystem disease, is discussed in Chapter 8.)

Discoid Lupus Erythematosus

Discoid lupus erythematosus (DLE) usually occurs in adults, particularly in women in their late 30s or early 40s. The lesions may be single or multiple and of various sizes. Often the lesions are located on light-exposed areas of the skin, and photosensitivity is common. The face is the most common site of lesion involvement, with a characteristic butterfly distribution over the cheeks and bridge of the nose; however, the lesions may occur on any part of the body.

The cause is thought to be an altered immune response to an unknown antigen. DLE may be described as a subset of SLE, with cutaneous manifestations as the only symptom (Fig. 43-13).[57] Skin biopsy with immunofluorescent observation reveals lumpy deposits of immunoglobulins, especially IgM.

The early lesion is asymmetric, with a 1- to 2-cm raised red plaque with a brownish scale. The scale penetrates the hair follicle and leaves a carpet-tack appearance when removed. The lesions persist for months and then resolve spontaneously or atrophy. Healing progresses from the center of the lesion, with a residual telangiectasia and scarring that is usually hypopigmented. Atrophy of the dermis and epidermis that results in a depressed scar can occur. Scalp lesions may lead to hair loss. Other symptoms of cutaneous lupus

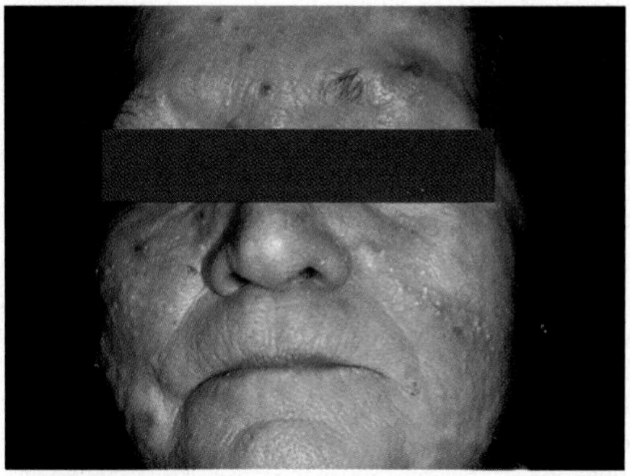

FIG. 43-12 Granulomatous rosacea. Pustules and erythema occur on the forehead, cheeks, and nose. (Courtesy Department of Dermatology, School of Medicine, University of Utah.)

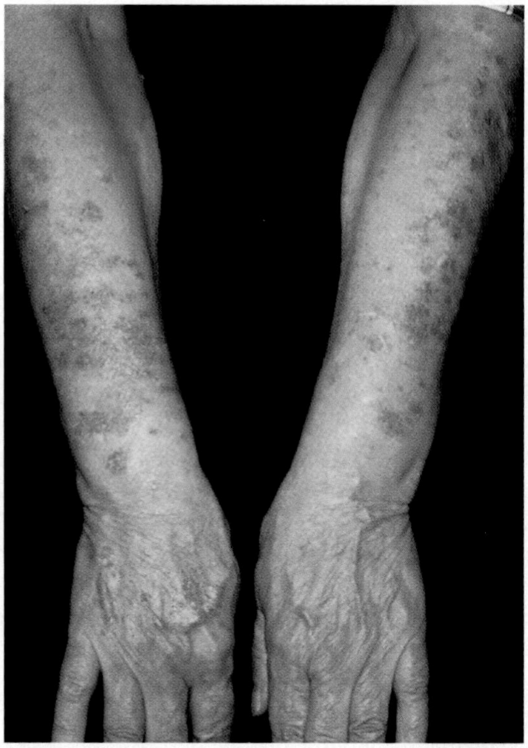

Fig. 43-13 Subacute cutaneous lupus (discoid lupus erythematosus). (Courtesy Department of Dermatology, School of Medicine, University of Utah.)

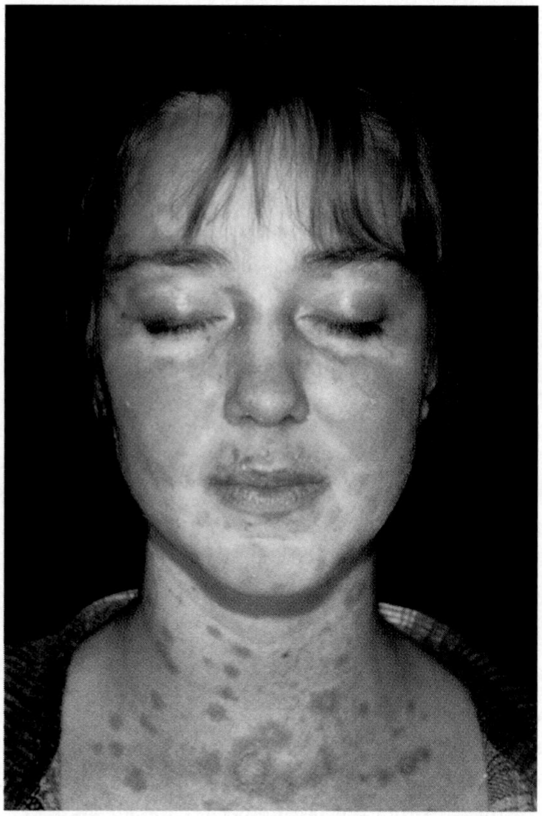

Fig. 43-14 Systemic lupus erythematosus (SLE) flare. Note butterfly-type of rash over cheeks and bridge of nose. (Courtesy Department of Dermatology, School of Medicine, University of Utah.)

erythematosus include alopecia (hair loss), telangiectasias, urticaria, and Raynaud phenomenon. Scarring or atrophic alopecia is a common problem of DLE. Scaling and inflammation lead to destruction of hair follicles, followed by skin that is smooth and white with telangiectasias. Hair loss is random in distribution. Telangiectasias (prominent skin capillaries) are distributed primarily over the palms and fingers in association with erythema. Urticaria of DLE may appear as typical hives, but they usually stay localized, are not pruritic, and last for days. They probably result from immune complex deposition rather than an allergic response. Raynaud phenomenon with a history of episodic vasospasm of the arterioles of the fingers and toes with stress or exposure to cold often precedes the onset of DLE by several years. Raynaud phenomenon is characterized by an initial stage of vasospasm that leads to white, numb, and cold digits followed by cyanosis and then a reactive hyperemia as the vasospasm relaxes.

Diagnosis of DLE is made from the presenting symptoms, biopsy of skin lesions, and Wood tests. Individuals with DLE should use sunscreen or limit direct exposure to the sun because this exacerbates lesions. Initial treatment with topical steroids relieves symptoms. Systemic therapy with antimalarial drugs (e.g., chloroquine sulfate) usually leads to clinical improvement within 1 to 3 months, but these medications must be used with caution to prevent serious side effects.

Systemic Lupus Erythematosus

Systemic lupus erythematosus (SLE) is a chronic inflammatory immune complex disorder that may affect the skin as well as other major body organs. The disease is most common in young women. There is a strong genetic component, with altered cellular immunity and autoantibody production resulting in tissue inflammation and injury. The cause is unknown.[32,58]

The most characteristic clinical manifestations are joint pain, fever, malaise, and diffuse facial erythema, often with a butterfly pattern (Fig. 43-14). Systemic manifestations can include oral ulcers, glomerulonephritis with hypertension and nephrotic syndrome, pleurisy, pericarditis, endocarditis, lymphadenopathy, and splenomegaly. The nervous system may be involved, with polyneuropathy, seizures, and behavioral changes. Anemia and thrombocytopenia are frequently observed in individuals with SLE.[59]

Diagnosis of SLE is based on clinical manifestations and histopathologic findings of low complement levels, the presence of antinuclear antibodies, anti–deoxyribonucleic acid (anti-DNA) antibodies, and deposits of immunoglobulin and complement at the dermoepidermal junction.

Avoidance of sun and ultraviolet light is essential to prevent photosensitivity. Treatment of systemic manifestations depends on the degree and extent of organ system involvement. Antimalarials, salicylates, steroids, and immunosuppressive agents may be used. The disease can be controlled but is not curable.

Vesiculobullous Disorders

Vesiculobullous skin disorders represent a group of diseases that have different causes and clinical courses but share a common characteristic of vesicle, or blister, formation. Two such diseases are pemphigus and erythema multiforme.

Pemphigus

Pemphigus is an autoimmune blistering disease of the skin and oral mucous membranes caused by circulating IgG autoantibodies directed against the cell surface adhesion molecule desmoglein at the desmosomal cell junction in the suprabasal layer of the epidermis. The antibody reaction is thought to cause the intraepidermal blister formation and acantholysis (loss of cohesion between epidermal cells) characteristic of pemphigus.[60] Pemphigus is relatively rare and can occur in all age-groups but is more prevalent between 40 and 50 years of age.

The types of pemphigus are as follows:

1. **Pemphigus vulgaris:** most common form; epidermis separated above the basal layer with blister formation; usually begins with the formation of a blister in the mouth or on the scalp, developing in 6 to 12 months into flaccid bullous lesions that rupture easily, leaving crusty denuded skin; lesions spread to include the face, back, chest, umbilicus, and groin; pressure on the blister may cause it to spread to adjacent skin (Nikolsky sign); complicated by secondary infection of the open lesions.
2. **Pemphigus foliaceus** and **pemphigus erythematosus:** less severe forms of the disease; oral lesions are usually absent; erythema with crusting, scaling, and occasionally bullae develops in more localized areas; blisters in the horizontal plane of the stratum corneum rupture easily, forming crusts; can spread to become more generalized.
3. Rare forms of pemphigus: pemphigus herpetiformis, IgA pemphigus, and paraneoplastic pemphigus.[61]

The diagnosis of pemphigus is made from the clinical manifestations and histologic examination of the skin. Immunofluorescence demonstrates the presence of antibodies at the site of blister formation. The clinical course of the disease may range from rapidly fatal to relatively benign. The primary treatment for pemphigus is systemic corticosteroids, usually in high doses during acute episodes or when there is widespread involvement. Adjuvant immunosuppressive therapy also may be used and decreases the steroid dosage requirement. Newer methods of treatment and a clearer understanding of the pathogenesis have improved the prognosis and decreased the mortality.[62]

Bullous Pemphigoid

Bullous pemphigoid is a more benign disease, with the presence of serum and bound IgG and blistering of the subepidermal skin layer.[63] It occurs more commonly after 60 years of age. The lesions of pemphigoid begin with localized erythema or as pruritic plaques that extend and become edematous. The plaques turn reddish purple by 2 to 3 weeks, with vesicles and bullae emerging on the surface (Fig. 43-15). The bullae do not extend with pressure. The blisters rupture within 1 week and heal rapidly.

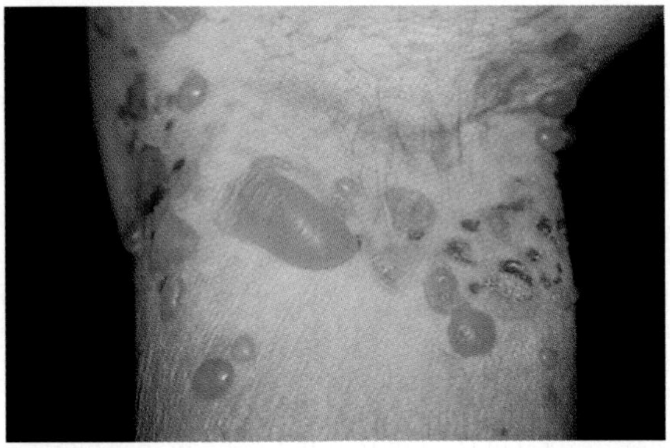

FIG. 43-15 **Bullous pemphigoid.** Generalized eruption with blisters arising from an edematous, erythematous annular base. (Courtesy Department of Dermatology, School of Medicine, University of Utah.)

Diagnosis is by skin biopsy and immunofluorescent examination. The presence of subepidermal blistering and eosinophils distinguishes pemphigoid from pemphigus. Treatment usually includes hydroxyzine (Atarax) for itching and prednisone with an immunosuppressive drug to control blistering. Individuals who respond to treatment with sulfapyridine or dapsone do not require prednisone.

Erythema Multiforme

Erythema multiforme is an acute, recurrent, inflammatory disorder of the skin and mucous membranes, often associated with immunologic or toxic reactions to drugs or microorganisms (e.g., *Mycoplasma pneumoniae,* herpes simplex).[64] It can occur at any age but is more common between 20 and 40 years of age, although it is relatively rare. Immune complex formation and deposition of complement (C3), IgM, and fibrinogen around the superficial dermal blood vessels, basement membrane, and keratinocytes are found in most individuals with erythema multiforme. Edema develops in the superficial dermis, leading to the formation of vesicles and bullae. The lesions vary in clinical presentation and may involve the skin or mucous membranes or both. The characteristic "bull's-eye" or "target" lesions occur on the skin surface with a central dusky region surrounded by concentric rings or alternating edema and inflammation.[65] The lesions usually occur suddenly in groups over 2 to 3 weeks. Urticarial plaques, 1 to 2 cm in diameter, can develop without the target lesion. A vesiculobullous form is characterized by mucous membrane lesions and erythematous plaques over elbows and knees. Single or multiple vesicles or bullae may arise on a part of the plaque, accompanied by pruritus and burning. In the minor form there may be ten to hundreds of lesions.[66] The lesions heal within 3 to 4 weeks (Fig. 43-16).

The most common severe forms in children and young adults are **Stevens-Johnson syndrome** (severe bullous form) and **toxic epidermal necrolysis**, in which there are numerous erythematous bullous lesions on both the skin and mucous membranes. The cause is unknown, but an immune mechanism related to drug administration is involved.[67] Bursts of nitric oxide formation have been proposed as the cause of epidermal apoptosis and necrosis.[68] Prodromal symptoms of fever, headache, malaise, sore throat, and cough develop in approximately one third of the cases. The bullous lesions form erosions and crusts when they rupture. The mouth, air passages, esophagus, urethra, and conjunctiva may be involved. Blindness can result from corneal ulcerations. Difficulty with eating, breathing, and urinating may develop with severe manifestations. The disease can involve the kidneys and extend from the upper respiratory passages into the lungs. Severe forms of the disease can be fatal.

In toxic epidermal necrolysis there is destruction of the epidermis. Both cytotoxic lymphocytes (early) and monocytes-macrophages (late) are involved in this severe blistering disease.[69]

Diagnosis is made by medication history, recognition of the target lesion, or by skin biopsy if the target lesion is absent. Mild acute forms of the disease last 10 to 14 days. Mild forms of the disease, usually self-limiting, require no treatment. Any ongoing drug therapy should be withdrawn or reevaluated and underlying infections treated. Fluid and electrolyte balance should be monitored in severe forms of the disease, and mucous membranes must be carefully managed with a bland diet, warm saline eyewashes, topical anesthetics, or corticosteroids to maintain comfort and prevent infection. High-dose steroids have been used successfully in serious cases.[70] Cutaneous blisters can be treated with wet compresses of Burow solution. Ophthalmic, kidney, and lung involvement require special care. Resolution occurs in 8 to 10 days, usually without scarring. Mucosal lesions may take 6 weeks to heal.

Infections

Cutaneous infections are common forms of skin disease. They generally remain localized; however, serious complications can develop with systemic involvement. The types of skin infection include bacterial, viral, and fungal. Most infections occur superficially; however, systemic signs and symptoms occasionally develop and rarely are life threatening. Aerobes, yeast, and anaerobes comprise the normal flora of the skin and often provide protection against pathogens that cause skin infections, including *Staphylococcus* and *Streptococcus*.[71]

Bacterial Infections

Most bacterial infections of the skin are caused by local invasion of pathogens. Coagulase-positive *S. aureus* and, less frequently, β-hemolytic streptococci are the common causative organisms.[72]

Folliculitis

Folliculitis is a bacterial infection of the hair follicle. *Staphylococcus aureus* is the common causative organism. The infection develops from proliferation of the organism around the opening of the follicle with spread into the follicle. Inflammation is caused by the release of chemotactic factors and enzymes from the bacteria. The lesions appear as pustules with a surrounding area of erythema. They are most prominent on the scalp and extremities and rarely cause systemic symptoms. Prolonged skin moisture, skin trauma, and poor hygiene are associated contributing factors to the development of folliculitis. Cleaning with soap and water and topical application of antibiotics are effective forms of treatment.

Furuncles and Carbuncles

Furuncles, or "boils," are an inflammation of the hair follicles. They may develop from a preceding folliculitis with spread through the follicular wall into the surrounding dermis. The invading organism is usually *S. aureus.* The infecting strain may spread to the skin from the anterior nares. Any skin area with hair can be infected, and one or several lesions may be present. The precipitating events are similar to folliculitis. The initial lesion is a deep, firm, red, painful nodule 1 to 5 cm in diameter (Fig. 43-17). Within a few days the initial erythematous nodules change to a large fluctuant and tender cystic nodule that may be accompanied by cellu-

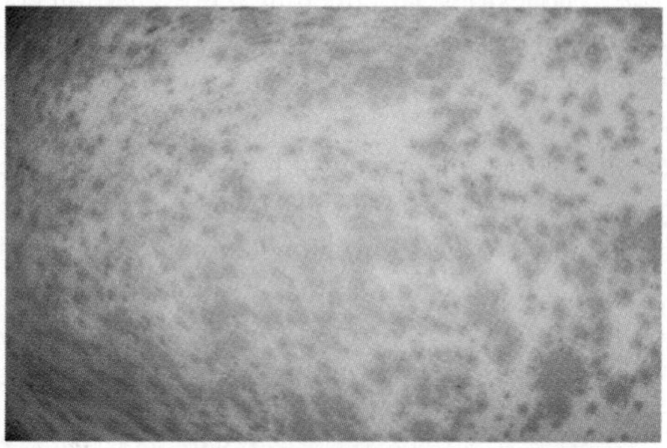

Fig. 43-16 Erythema multiforme caused by doxepin. (Courtesy Department of Dermatology, School of Medicine, University of Utah.)

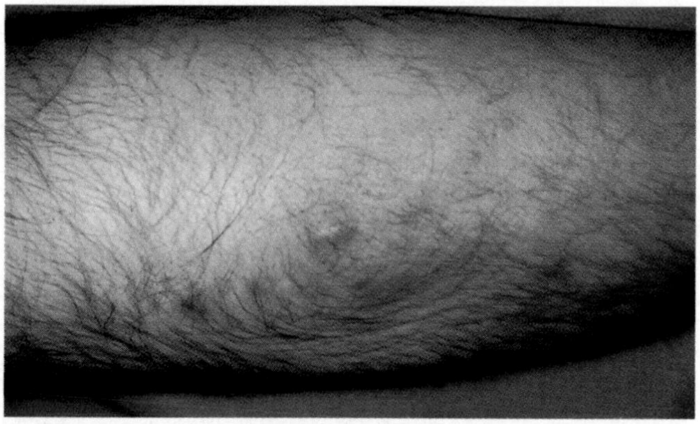

Fig. 43-17 Furuncle of the forearm. (Courtesy Department of Dermatology, School of Medicine, University of Utah.)

litis. No systemic symptoms are present, and the lesion may drain large amounts of pus and necrotic tissue.

Carbuncles are a collection of infected hair follicles. The lesion occurs most frequently on the back of the neck, the upper back, and the lateral thighs. The lesion begins in the subcutaneous tissue and lower dermis as a firm mass that evolves into an erythematous, painful, swollen mass that drains through many openings. Abscesses may develop. Chills, fever, and malaise are systemic symptoms that can occur during the early stages of lesion development.

Furuncles and carbuncles are treated with warm compresses to provide comfort and promote localization and spontaneous drainage. Abscess formation requires incision and drainage, and recurrent infections are treated with systemic antibiotics.

Cellulitis

Cellulitis is an infection of the dermis and subcutaneous tissue usually caused by *Staphylococcus* or group B streptococci.[73] Cellulitis can occur as an extension of a skin wound, an ulcer, or from furuncles or carbuncles. Risk factors include diabetes mellitus, edema, peripheral vascular disease, and tinea pedis.[74] The infected area is erythematous, swollen, and painful. The infection responds to systemic antibiotics, and Burow soaks can be used to relieve pain.

Erysipelas

Erysipelas is an acute superficial infection of the skin (a superficial form of cellulitis) most often caused by group A streptococci. The face, ears, and lower legs are common sites of involvement, and the site of initial infection may not be identified. Chills, fever, and malaise precede the onset of lesions by 4 hours to 20 days. The initial lesions appear as firm, red spots that then enlarge and coalesce to form a clearly circumscribed, advancing, bright red, hot lesion with a raised border. Vesicles may appear over the lesion and at the border, producing a bullous form of the disease.[75] Itching, burning, and tenderness accompany the development of the lesion. Cold compresses provide symptomatic relief, and systemic antibiotics are required to arrest the infection.

Impetigo

Impetigo is a superficial lesion of the skin caused by coagulase-positive *Staphylococcus* or β-hemolytic streptococci. It may complicate atopic dermatitis.[76] The disease occurs in adults but is more common in children (see Chapter 44).

Viral Infections

Herpes Simplex Virus

There are eight types of **herpes simplex virus (HSV),** a group of DNA viruses: HSV-1 (type 1), HSV-2 (type 2), cytomegalovirus (CMV), varicella-zoster virus (type 3), Epstein-Barr virus, and human herpesvirus 6, 7, and 8 (Kaposi sarcoma–associated herpesvirus) cause substantial neurologic morbidity among infants and children.[77,78] A "cold sore" or "fever blister" is a type of HSV-1 infection and is the most common manifestation of the herpes simplex virus.[79] HSV-1 usually occurs in nongenital sites and causes infection of the cornea (herpes keratitis), mouth (gingivostomatitis), and labia (labialis). Individuals receiving cytotoxic therapy for cancer are at risk.

The lesions of HSV-1 appear as a rash or clusters of inflamed and painful vesicles within the mouth, over the tongue, or on the lips and around the nose (Fig. 43-18). Increased sensitivity, paresthesias, and mild burning may occur before onset of the lesion. The vesicles rupture, forming a crust. Lesions may last 2 to 6 weeks. Occasionally, there is an associated upper respiratory infection. Treatment is symptomatic, and the lesions usually resolve within 2 weeks.

Genital infections are more commonly caused by HSV-2. The virus is spread by skin-to-skin mucous membrane contact during viral shedding. Risk of infection is high after sexual contact with infected individuals. After penetrating the skin, HSV is established in the sensory nerve ganglion innervating the primary site. Infection in one area does not protect other areas from subsequent infection. The primary infection is asymptomatic and can be determined only by a rising antibody titer.[80]

The incubation period ranges from 2 to 14 days, and clinical symptoms last 1 to 3 weeks. An individual then continues to shed the virus for 2 to 6 weeks. The virus remains dormant within sensory or autonomic nerve ganglia and can lead to recurrence of the disease. A number of factors stimulate recurrence, including sun exposure, fever, or stress, and lesions are usually located at or near the primary site. Because anti-HSV antibodies develop in response to infection, recurrence is also related to the titer or amount of antibodies present.

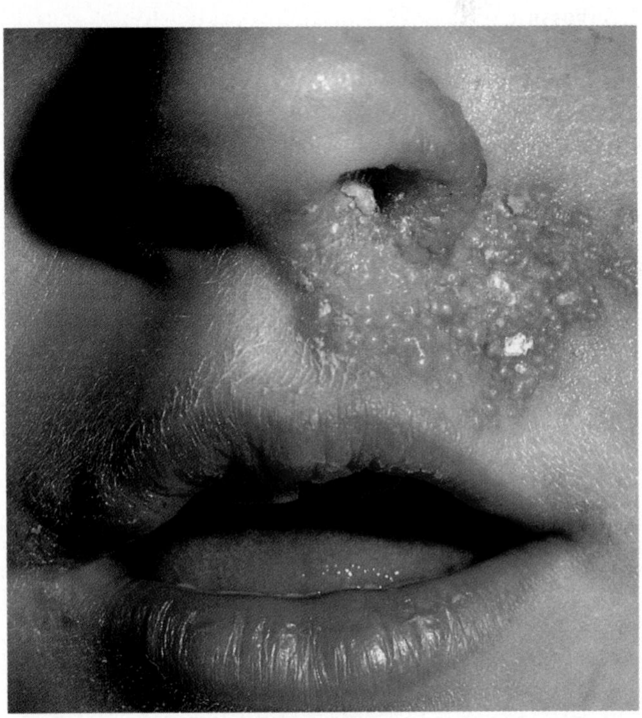

FIG. 43-18 Herpes simplex labialis. Typical presentation with tense vesicles appearing on the lips and extending onto the skin. (From Habif TB: *Clinical dermatology: a color guide to diagnosis and therapy,* ed 3, St Louis, 1996, Mosby.)

Genital herpes (HSV-2) may also occur in primary or recurrent forms, and a large number of infections are sexually transmitted, usually within 3 to 14 days after exposure (see Chapter 23). The lesions begin as small vesicles that progress to ulceration within 3 to 4 days with pain, itching, and weeping. Treatment includes oral or topical administration of an antiviral drug that decreases new lesion formation and promotes healing. A vaccine has been effective in controlling recurrent infection, and progress is being made with prophylactic vaccines.[81]

Herpes Zoster and Varicella

Herpes zoster (shingles) and **varicella** (chickenpox) are caused by the same herpesvirus, varicella-zoster virus (VZV). Varicella occurs as a primary infection followed years later by herpes zoster. Chickenpox usually occurs in children (see Chapter 44).

Herpes zoster, or shingles, has initial symptoms of pain and paresthesia localized to the affected dermatome (the cutaneous area innervated by a single spinal nerve; see Chapter 13), followed by vesicular eruptions along a facial, cervical, or thoracic lumbar dermatome (Fig. 43-19). Some individuals have vesicles scattered outside the area of the dermatoma. Local symptoms are alleviated with compresses, calamine lotion, or baking soda. Persistent pain is a debilitating complication, particularly in the elderly and requires treatment.[82] Antiviral drugs are useful.[83,84] Approximately 20% of individuals experience postherpetic neuralgias.[85] The varicella vaccine is safe and effective and may boost humoral and cellular immunity in the elderly.[86] Treatment includes a topical lidocaine patch, gabapentin, controlled-release oxycodone, and tricyclic antidepressants.[87]

Warts

Warts (verrucae) are benign lesions of the skin caused by the human papillomavirus (HPV). There are many different types of HPV, and specific viruses are associated with specific kinds and locations of lesions. An oncoprotein expressed by HPV is thought to inactivate growth controls regulated by *p53* tumor-suppressor protein.[88] The lesions are round and elevated with a rough, grayish surface; can occur anywhere on the skin;[89] and are transmitted by touch. Common warts (verrucae vulgaris) occur most frequently in children and are usually on the fingers, although they may be located on any skin surface or mucous membrane. Warts vary in shape, size (flat, round, or fusiform), and location (Fig. 43-20). Plantar warts are usually located at pressure points on the bottom of the feet.

Diagnosis of warts is by visualization. Treatment considers age of the individual and size and location of the lesion. Warts can be removed by freezing with liquid nitrogen; electrocautery; vaporization with lasers; application of keratolytics; or application of irritants and corrosives, such as salicylic acid, formaldehyde, interferons, or podophyllum.[90,91] Many warts resolve spontaneously, but there is often recurrence.

Condylomata acuminata (venereal warts) are a highly contagious, sexually transmitted disease. The cauliflower-like lesions occur in moist areas, along the glans of the penis, vulva, and anus (see Chapter 23). HPV is thought to be a primary cause of cervical cancer (see Chapter 22).[92,93,94]

Fungal Infections

The fungi causing superficial skin infections are called *dermatophytes,* and they thrive on keratin (stratum corneum, hair, nails). Fungal disorders are known as *mycoses;* when caused by dermatophytes, the mycoses are termed *tinea* (dermatophytosis or ringworm). **Tinea pedis** is a chronic, superficial fungal infection of the skin of the foot common in adults (Fig. 43-21). In prepubertal children, most scaling disorders of the toes and feet are eczema. **Tinea corporis (ringworm)** and **tinea capitis** (a fungal infection of the scalp) are much more common in children than adults. (See Chapter 44 for a discussion of fungal infections in children.)

Tinea Infections

Tinea infections are fungal infections of the skin and are classified according to their location on the body.[95] The most common sites are summarized in Table 43-5. These infections are common in children (see Chapter 44). Tinea is diagnosed by culture, microscopic examination of skin scrapings

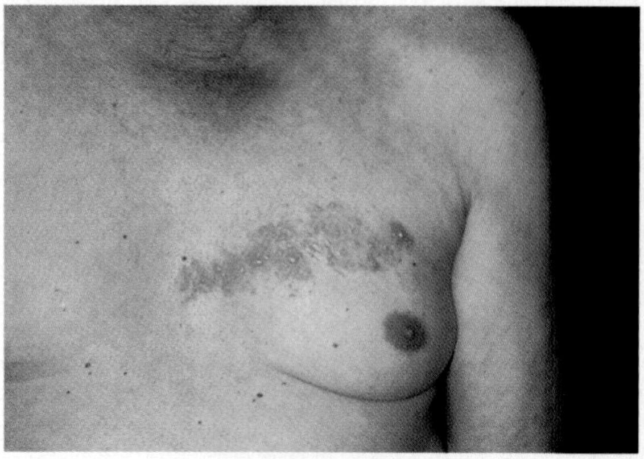

Fig. 43-19 Herpes zoster. Diffuse involvement of a dermatome. (Courtesy Department of Dermatology, School of Medicine, University of Utah.)

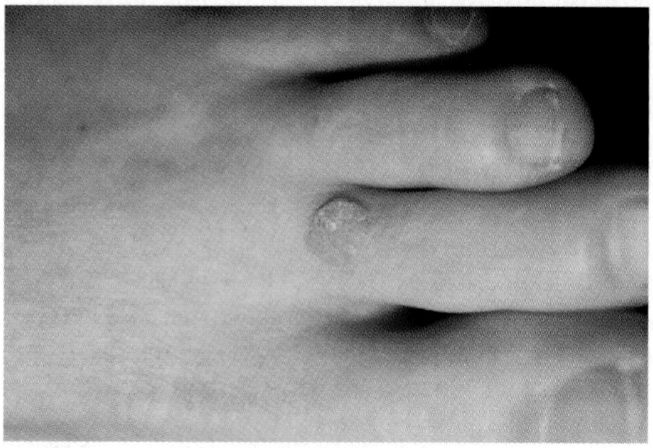

Fig. 43-20 Verruca vulgaris. (Courtesy Department of Dermatology, School of Medicine, University of Utah.)

prepared with potassium hydroxide wet mount, or observation of the skin with an ultraviolet light (Wood lamp). Cultures establish the particular type of fungus and are necessary for hair and nail infections. Fungi have characteristic spores and filaments known as **hyphae** that are more prominent when prepared in potassium hydroxide. The spores fluoresce blue-green when exposed to ultraviolet light. Treatment is related to the type of fungi and includes both topical and systemic antifungal medication.

Candidiasis

Candidiasis is caused by the yeastlike fungus *Candida albicans* and normally can be found on mucous membranes, on the skin, in the gastrointestinal tract, and in the vagina. *C. albicans* can, under certain circumstances, change from a commensal organism to a pathogen, particularly when the immune system is depressed.[96] Factors that predispose to infection include (1) a local environment of moisture, warmth, maceration, or occlusion; (2) the systemic administration of antibiotics; (3) pregnancy; (4) diabetes mellitus; (5) Cushing disease; (6) debilitated states; (7) age younger than 6 months (more likely to get an infection because of decreased immune reactivity); (8) immunosuppression; and (9) certain neoplastic diseases of the blood and monocyte/macrophage system. The resident bacteria on the skin, mainly cocci, inhibit proliferation of *C. albicans.* Cell-mediated immunity plays a major role in the defense against monilial infections. *C. albicans* can activate the complement system by the alternative pathway and can include small abscesses. Candidiasis affects only the outer layers of mucous membranes and skin and occurs in the mouth, vagina, uncircumcised penis, and large skinfolds. Table 43-6 lists the different sites of candidiasis. Depressed phagocytic function has been observed in individuals with extensive lesions.[97]

The initial lesion is a thin-walled pustule that extends under the stratum corneum with an inflammatory base that may burn or itch. The accumulation of inflammatory cells and scale produces a whitish yellow, curdlike substance over the infected area. The lesion ceases to spread when it reaches dry skin.[98]

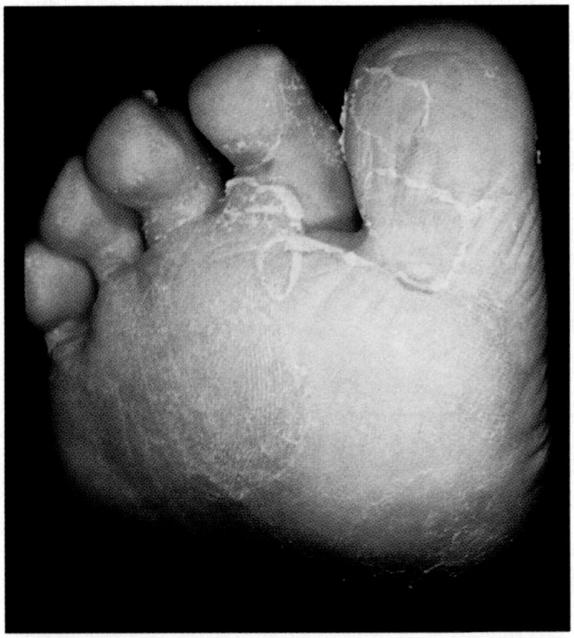

FIG. 43-21 Tinea pedis. Inflammation has extended from the web area onto the dorsum of the foot. (Courtesy Department of Dermatology, School of Medicine, University of Utah.)

Vascular Disorders

Vascular abnormalities are commonly associated with skin diseases, or they may be present as congenital vascular malformations (see Chapter 44) or as vascular responses to local or systemic vasoactive substances. Blood vessels may increase in number, dilate, constrict, or become obliterated by disease processes.

Cutaneous Vasculitis

Vasculitis (angiitis) is an inflammation of the blood vessels. The initiating site of inflammation may be the blood, the vessel wall, or the adjacent tissue. Small vessels are usually affected. Immune complexes, which initiate an uncontrolled inflammatory response, are often the cause of damage, and the lesions are often polymorphic.

Cutaneous vasculitis develops from the deposit of immune complexes in small blood vessels as a toxic response

Table 43-5 Common Sites of Tinea Infections

Site	Clinical Manifestations
Tinea capitis (scalp)	Scaly, pruritic scalp with bald areas; hair breaks easily
Tinea corporis (skin areas, excluding scalp, face, hands, feet, groin)	Circular, clearly circumscribed, mildly erythematous scaly patches with a slightly elevated ringlike border; some forms are dry and macular, and other forms are moist and vesicular
Tinea cruris (groin, also known as "jock itch")	Small erythematous and scaling vesicular patches with a well-defined border that spreads over the inner and upper surfaces of the thighs; occurs with heat and high humidity
Tinea pedis (foot, also known as "athlete's foot")	Occurs between the toes and may spread to the soles of the feet, nails, and skin of toes; slight scaling, macerated painful skin, occasionally with fissures and vesiculation
Tinea manus (hand)	Dry, scaly, erythematous lesions, or moist vesicular lesions that begin with clusters of intensely itching, clear vesicles; often associated with fungal infection of the feet
Tinea unguium or onychomycosis (nails)	A superficial or deep inflammation of the nail that develops yellow-brown accumulations of brittle keratin over all or portions of the nail

to drugs (phenothiazines, barbiturates, sulfonamides) or allergens or as a response to streptococcal or viral infection. The precise mechanism is not known, but the deposit of immune complex activates complement, which is chemotactic for polymorphonuclear leukocytes. The cutaneous form usually resolves in a few weeks and is treated with steroids.

The disorder is also known as *allergic vasculitis* and occurs primarily in adults. A systemic form (cutaneous systemic vasculitis) can involve other organs, including the kidneys, lungs, and gastrointestinal tract.[99] The extremities are the chief sites, primarily the lower legs and feet. The lesions appear as palpable purpuras (from the leakage of blood from damaged vessels) and progress to hemorrhagic bullae with necrosis and ulceration from occlusion of the vessel (Fig. 43-22). Lesions appear in clusters and remain from 1 to 4 weeks. Recurrences are common. Biopsy may disclose the presence of complement or immunoglobulins in the vessel walls.

Identifying and removing the antigen (chemical, drug, or source of infection) is the first step of treatment. Corticosteroids and other drugs may be used when symptoms are severe.[100]

Urticaria

Urticarial lesions are most commonly associated with type I hypersensitivity reactions to drugs (e.g., penicillin, aspirin), certain foods (e.g., strawberries, shellfish), systemic diseases (e.g., intestinal parasites, lupus erythematosus), or physical agents (e.g., heat, cold) (see Chapter 8). The lesions are mediated by IgE-stimulated histamine release, which causes the endothelial cells of skin blood vessels to contract. The leakage of fluid from the vessel appears as wheals, welts, or hives and may be a few leaks or many leaks distributed over the entire body (Fig. 43-23). Most lesions resolve spontaneously within 24 hours, but new lesions may appear. All possible causes should be removed. Antihistamines usually reduce hives and provide relief of itching. Epinephrine or corticosteroids and β-adrenergic agnoists may be required for treatment of severe attacks (i.e., angioderma). Chronic urticaria is probably an autoimmune disease.[101]

Scleroderma

Scleroderma means sclerosis of the skin, and the cause is unknown. The disease is more prominent in women. It may affect the visceral organs or remain localized to the skin. Systemic scleroderma involves the connective tissues of many organs, including the kidney, heart, peripheral nervous system, gastrointestinal tract, and lungs.[102] Only a few organs are involved in some individuals. The cutaneous lesions are most often on the face and hands, neck, and upper chest. The entire skin can be involved, however.

Table 43-6 Sites of Candidiasis

Site	Risk Factors	Clinical Manifestations	Treatment
Vagina (vulvovaginitis)	Heat, moisture, occlusive clothing Pregnancy Systemic antibiotic therapy Diabetes mellitus Sexual intercourse with infected male	Vaginal itching; white, watery, or creamy discharge Red and swollen vaginal and labial membranes with erosions Lesions may spread to anus and groin	Miconazole cream Clotrimazole tablets or cream Nystatin tablets Ketoconazole cream Loose cotton clothing
Penis (balanitis)	Uncircumcised Sexual intercourse with infected female	Pinpoint, red, tender papules and pustules on glans and shaft of penis	Any of creams listed above Topical steroids for severe inflammation
Mouth	Diabetes mellitus Immunosuppressive therapy Inhaled steroids	Red, swollen, painful tongue and oral mucous membranes Localized erosions and plaques appear with chronic infection	Nystatin oral suspension Clotrimazole troches Ketoconazole

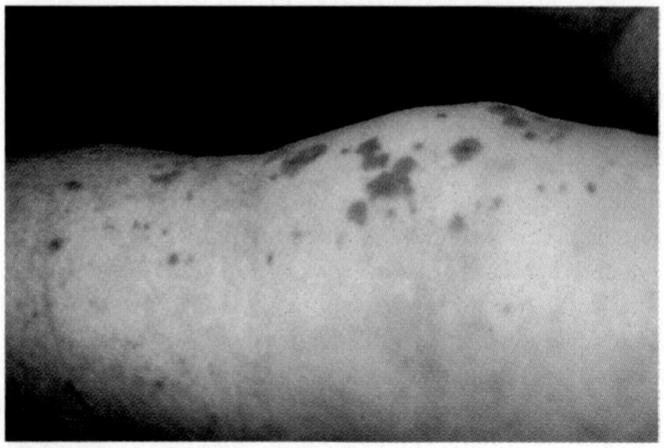

FIG. 43-22 Vasculitis of the leg. (Courtesy Department of Dermatology, School of Medicine, University of Utah.)

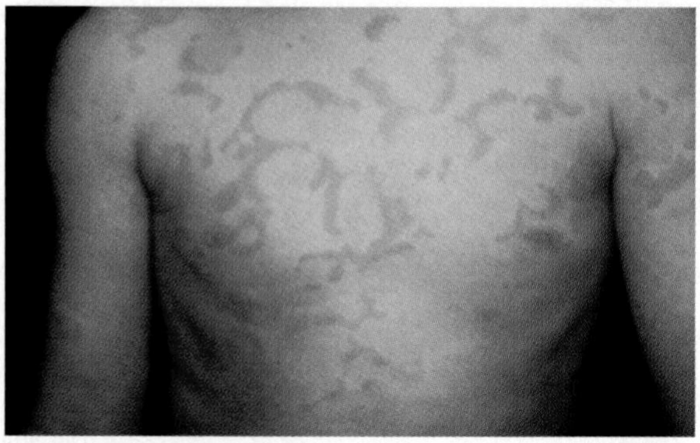

FIG. 43-23 Urticaria. (Courtesy Department of Dermatology, School of Medicine, University of Utah.)

There are massive deposits of collagen with fibrosis, accompanied by inflammatory reactions, vascular changes in the capillary network with a decrease in the number of capillary loops, dilation of the remaining capillaries, enhanced expression of adhesion molecules, and perivascular infiltrates.[103] Fibrosis occurs in the papillary and reticular dermis and in the subcutaneous tissue and deep fascia. Autoimmunity and an immune reaction to a toxic substance are both possible initiating mechanisms of the disease, and autoantibodies are often recovered from the skin and serum of individuals with scleroderma.[104] Impaired regulation of collagen gene expression probably underlies the persistent fibrosis.[105]

The skin is hard, hypopigmented, taut, shiny, and tightly connected to the underlying tissue. The tightness of the facial skin projects an immobile masklike appearance, and the mouth may not open completely. The nose may assume a beaklike appearance. The hands are shiny and sometimes red and edematous (Fig. 43-24). The fingers become tapered and flexed, often with depressed scars and loss of fingertips from atrophy. Raynaud phenomenon with episodic arteriolar vasoconstriction of the fingers contributes to ulcer formation. The nails may be shed. Calcium deposits develop in the subcutaneous tissue and erupt through the skin. Progression to body organs may occur, and death is caused by subsequent respiratory failure, renal failure, cardiac dysrhythmias, or esophageal or intestinal obstruction or perforation. There is no specific treatment, and progression of the disease is variable. Fifty percent of individuals die within 5 years of the onset of scleroderma.

Suitable clothing and a warm environment are essential to protecting the hands. Trauma and smoking should be avoided. Vasodilator drugs or sympathectomy rarely has lasting effects. Symptomatic treatment is required for involved organs (e.g., intestinal resection for obstruction, antibiotics for pneumonitis, regulation of hypertension).[106]

Insect Bites

Ticks

Ticks are significant vectors of transmitted diseases, including Rocky Mountain spotted fever and other rickettsial diseases, tularemia, and Lyme disease. Ticks vary in size from 1 cm to about the size of a comma on this printed page. They embed their heads in the skin to obtain blood. As they gorge themselves on blood, they enlarge to many times their normal size and may release toxins or transmit microorganisms during feeding. In most instances, there is no consequence from a tick bite, with the exception of a papular urticaria at the site of the bite. If mouthparts remain in the skin when the tick is removed, a persistent nodule remains that may require excision; the tick should be removed completely intact. Irritant substances, such as camphor, gasoline, soft wax, or heat from a match, may stimulate the tick to withdraw its head. Applying tick repellant, such as diethyltoluamide (DEET), butopyronoxyl (Indalone), or benzylbenzoate, helps to prevent tick bites.

Lyme disease is a multisystem inflammatory disease caused by the spirochete *Borrelia burgdorferi* transmitted by tick bites and is the most frequently reported vector-borne illness.[107] The highest incidence is among children, and 50% of infected individuals are symptom free. Symptoms of the disease occur in stages. Soon after the bite, there is localized infection (erythema migrans [rash] with or without flulike illness). Within weeks to months after the onset of the illness, there is disseminated infection (secondary erythema migrans, arthralgias, meningitis, neuritis, carditis). Late persistent infection can continue for years (arthritis, encephalopathy, polyneuropathy). An immune response to *B. burgdorferi* may contribute to the pathogenesis of the disease.[108] The microorganism is difficult to culture.

The diagnosis of Lyme disease is based on the clinical presentation and history of tick bite, if known. Serologic tests frequently are used to confirm the diagnosis.[109] Antibiotics are used for treatment.[110] Vaccines are available for prevention in persons 15 to 70 years of age.[111]

Mosquitoes and Flies

There are thousands of species of **mosquitoes** throughout the world. Species from the Culicada family are responsible for malaria, yellow fever, dengue fever, filariasis, and St. Louis encephalitis. Mosquitoes can bite through thin, loose clothing and are attracted by warmth and sweat. The edema, pruritus, and papular lesions of the mosquito bite are caused by the disruption of the skin from the insertion of a blood tube by a female mosquito. Irritating salivary secretions also contain anticoagulants. Reactions vary depending on the sensitivity of the victim.

Several species of flies are blood suckers. The black fly (Simuliidae) is usually found in swarms—near moving bodies of water in the late spring and early summer—and is a vicious biter. The initial bite is painless because the fly injects an anesthetic with the bite. Subsequent lesions are painful and accompanied by significant swelling of surrounding tissues. Systemic reactions, such as fever, headache, and nausea, are common.

Very small flies of the Ceratopogonidae family, also known as "no-see-ums," "midges," "punkies," or sand fleas, are also blood suckers. The bite of the female is particularly

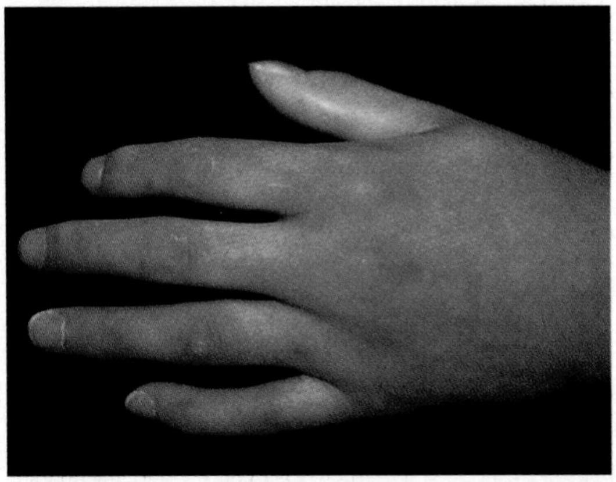

FIG. 43-24 Scleroderma (acrosclerosis). Note inflammation and shiny skin. (Courtesy Department of Dermatology, School of Medicine, University of Utah.)

miserable and produces immediate pain, erythema, and vesicles. Itching and vesicular reactions may persist for weeks.

The fiercest blood-sucking flies are the Tabanidae, or horseflies, deer flies, gadflies, greenheads, and clegs. These flies vary in size from 1 to 5 cm and produce painful, bleeding bites because of their large mouthparts. The bites produce urticaria that may be accompanied by weakness, dizziness, and wheezing.

Wounds produced by biting insects should be cleansed with soap and water, and a local antiseptic should be applied. Local applications of steroid creams or antihistamine will reduce symptoms. Systemic reactions may require more specific medical care.

Benign Tumors

Most benign tumors of the skin are associated with aging. Benign tumors include seborrheic keratosis, keratoacanthoma, actinic keratosis, and moles.

Seborrheic Keratosis

Seborrheic keratosis is a benign proliferation of basal cells that produces smooth or warty elevated lesions. They are usually seen in older people and occur as multiple lesions on the chest, back, and face. The color varies from tan to waxy yellow, flesh colored, or dark brown-black. Lesion size varies from a few millimeters to several centimeters, and they are often oval and greasy appearing with a hyperkeratotic scale (Fig. 43-25). Cryotherapy with liquid nitrogen is effective treatment, and the lesions usually slough 2 to 3 weeks after treatment.

Keratoacanthoma

A **keratoacanthoma** is a benign, self-limiting tumor that arises from hair follicles. It usually occurs on sun-exposed surfaces and develops in individuals between 60 and 65 years of age. The most commonly affected sites are the face, back of the hands, forearms, neck, and legs (Fig. 43-26). The lesion develops in stages with a histologic pattern resembling squamous cell carcinoma:[112]

Proliferative stage. Lesion develops as a rapidly growing, dome-shaped nodule with central crust.

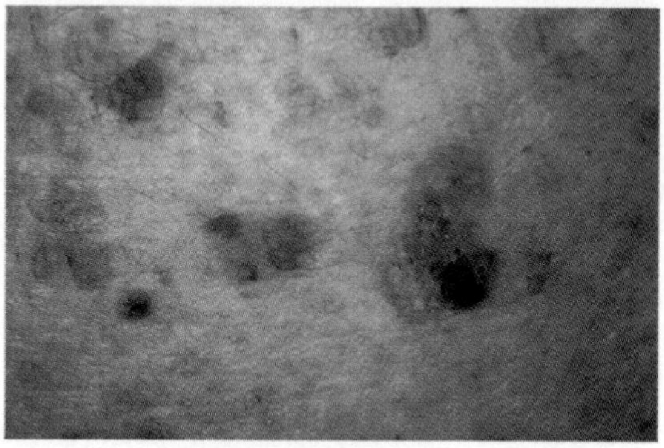

FIG. 43-25 Seborrheic keratosis. Typical lesion that is broad, flat, and comparatively smooth surfaced. (Courtesy Department of Dermatology, School of Medicine, University of Utah.)

Mature stage. Lesion fills with whitish keratin and requires differentiation from squamous cell carcinoma.[113]

Involution stage. This stage occurs over 3- to 4-month period with regression of lesion.

Although the lesions will resolve spontaneously, they can be removed by curettage or excision to improve cosmetic appearance.

Actinic Keratosis

Actinic keratosis is a premalignant lesion found on skin surfaces exposed to the ultraviolet radiation of the sun. The prevalence is highest in individuals with unprotected, light-colored skin. Actinic keratosis is rare in black skin. The lesions appear as pigmented patches of rough, adherent scale (Fig. 43-27). Surrounding areas may have telangiectasias. Freezing with liquid nitrogen provides quick, effective treatment. Excisions also may be performed, providing tissue for cellular analysis. The lesions should continue to be evaluated for progression to squamous cell carcinoma.[114] Protection from the sun with clothing or a sun-blocking agent to prevent lesions from developing elsewhere is advised.

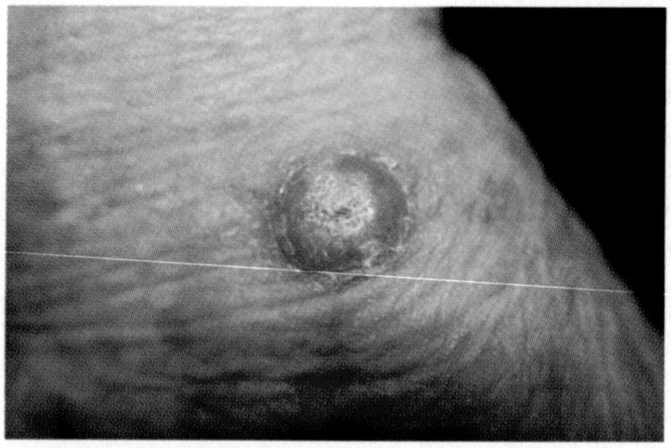

FIG. 43-26 Keratoacanthoma. Classic presentation of a fully developed tumor. Round, smooth, dome-shaped mass with a central keratin-filled crater. (Courtesy Department of Dermatology, School of Medicine, University of Utah.)

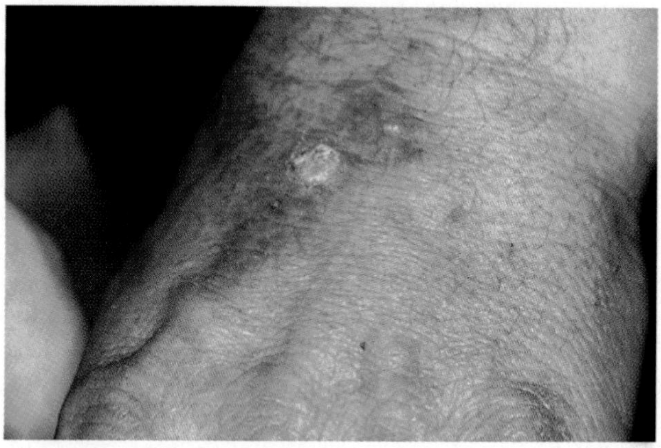

FIG. 43-27 Actinic keratosis. (Courtesy Department of Dermatology, School of Medicine, University of Utah.)

Nevi

Nevi (moles) are pigmented or nonpigmented lesions that form from melanocytes beginning at ages 3 to 5 years. During the early stages of development, the cells accumulate at the junction of the dermis and epidermis and are macular lesions. Over time the cells move down into the dermis and the nevi become nodular and palpable. Nevi may appear on any part of the skin, and they vary in size. They occur singly or in groups and are not disfiguring. Nevi may undergo transition to malignant melanomas (see p. 1460). Nevi irritated by clothing can be excised.

Box 43-2

IMPORTANT TRENDS FOR SKIN CANCER

INCIDENCE*

Approximately 1 million cases per year, with the majority being the highly curable **basal** or **squamous** cell cancers; not as common is the most serious **malignant melanoma** with an estimated 51,400 cases per year

MORTALITY*

Total estimated deaths in 2001 were 9800: 7800 from malignant melanoma, 2000 from other skin cancers

RISK FACTORS

- Excessive exposure to ultraviolet radiation from the sun
- Fair complexion
- Occupational exposure to coal tar, pitch, creosote, arsenic compounds, and radium
- Exposure to human papillomavirus and human immunodeficiency virus
- Skin cancer is negligible in blacks because of heavy skin pigmentation

WARNING SIGNALS*

Any change on the skin, especially a change in the size or color of a mole or other darkly pigmented growth or spot

PREVENTION AND EARLY DETECTION

Avoidance of sun when ultraviolet light is strongest (e.g., 10:00 AM to 3:00 PM); use sunscreen preparations, especially those containing ingredients such as PABA (para-aminobenzoic acid); basal and squamous cell cancers often form a pale, waxlike, pearly nodule or a red, scaly, sharply outlined patch; melanomas are usually dark brown or black pigmentation; they start as small molelike growths that increase in size, change color, become ulcerated, and bleed easily from a slight injury

TREATMENT

There are four methods of treatment: surgery, electrodesiccation (tissue destruction by heat), radiation therapy, or cryosurgery (tissue destruction by freezing); for malignant melanomas, wide and often deep excisions and removal of nearby lymph nodes are required

SURVIVAL*

For basal cell and squamous cell cancers, cure is highly likely with early detection and treatment; malignant melanoma, however, metastasizes quickly; this accounts for a lower 5-year survival rate particularly for white patients with this disease

*Data from American Cancer Society: *Cancer facts and figures 2001*, Atlanta, 2001, The Society.

Cancer

Skin cancers account for about 40% of all cancers, and the incidence in skin cancer is increasing.[115] Basal cell carcinoma and squamous cell carcinoma are the most common skin cancers. Incidence of these carcinomas is greater in men than in women, and incidence increases steadily with age. Malignant melanoma is the most serious skin cancer, affecting 51,400 people per year, and is increasing at a rate of 3% per year.[116] An estimated 10,000 people die of skin cancer each year; 7800 of these deaths are from malignant melanoma.[116] Important trends related to skin cancer are presented in Box 43-2.

Ultraviolet solar radiation causes most skin cancers by inducing mutations in the *p53* tumor-suppressor gene.[117,118] Protection from the sun during the first 10 to 20 years of life significantly reduces the risk of skin cancer.[119] Areas widely exposed to the sun's rays—the face, neck, and hands—are highly vulnerable for such lesions. Outdoor workers (farmers, sailors, fishermen) are high-risk skin cancer populations. Like other cancers, skin cancers progress through stages of initiation, progression, and metastasis.

Basal Cell Carcinoma

Basal cell carcinoma is a surface epithelial tumor of the skin originating from undifferentiated basal or germinative cells. The tumors grow upward and laterally or downward to the dermal epidermal junction (Fig. 43-28). They usually have depressed centers and rolled borders. Early tumors are so small that they are not clinically apparent. Generally these tumors do not invade blood or lymph vessels; thus they do not metastasize beyond the skin. Basal cell carcinoma can cause severe local destruction, however.

Basal cell carcinoma is the most common type of skin cancer in whites and is thought to be caused by sunlight exposure.[120] Lesions are seen most frequently in regions with intense sunlight and on those areas most exposed—namely, the face and neck. Dark-skinned persons and those avoiding sunlight are significantly less likely to develop these malignant tumors. In dark-skinned persons, basal cells contain the

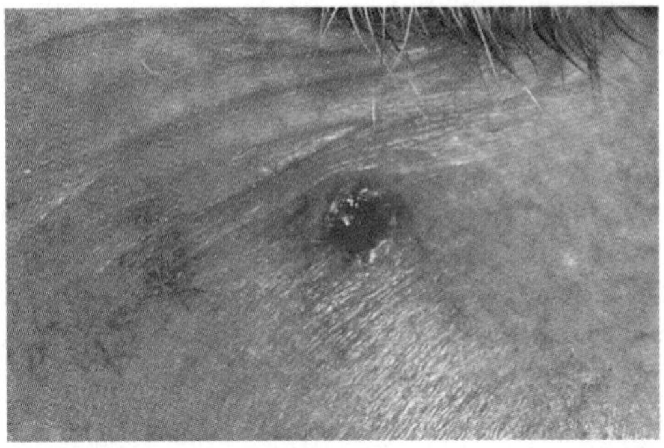

FIG. 43-28 Basal cell carcinoma. Center has ulcerated. (Courtesy Department of Dermatology, School of Medicine, University of Utah.)

pigment melanin, a protective factor against sun exposure. Whereas ultraviolet radiation seems to be the primary causative agent, other factors are implicated: arsenic and genetic factors (i.e., an environmentally induced alteration on chromosome 9 that has tumor-suppressor activity and downregulation of TP53 gene).[121,122] The use of arsenic in insecticides has recently diminished; however, arsenic is found in drinking water from ground wells. Genetic factors are displayed in the less common nevoid basal cell carcinoma syndrome.

These tumors arise in consequence to a defect that prevents the cells from being shed by the normal keratinization process. The maturing process of epidermal cells is called *keratinization;* however, the process of keratinization specifically means the synthesis of fibrous protein or keratin. Basal cell tumors lack the normal keratin proteins, but this may be reversible. Transplantation of basal cell and in vitro cultures shows the property of keratinization can be restored.

The growth rate for these tumors is quite slow. The lesion starts as a nodule (greater than 5 mm across) that is pearly or ivory in appearance and slightly elevated above the skin surface with small blood vessels on the surface. As the lesion grows, it often ulcerates, develops crusting, and is firm to the touch. If left untreated, basal cell lesions invade surrounding tissues and, over months or years, can destroy a nose, an eyelid, or an ear (for treatment, see Box 43-2). Metastatic spread is rare.[123]

Squamous Cell Carcinoma

Squamous cell carcinoma is a tumor of the epidermis characterized by two types: in situ and invasive. Because of the invasive nature of some tumors, squamous cell carcinoma is significantly more malignant if left untreated.[124]

Sunlight causes squamous cell carcinoma.[118] Areas affected are the head and neck (75%) and the hands (15%), with 10% of squamous cell carcinomas occurring elsewhere on the body. In countries where arsenic is higher in drinking water, these tumors are more predominant. Gamma rays and x-rays are also associated with squamous cell carcinoma. In addition, patients who are immunosuppressed experience a greater occurrence.

The exact mechanism for producing squamous cell carcinoma is unknown. Again, the initiator-promoter model can be applied to explain the cancer process (see Chapter 11), particularly with mutation of the *p53* gene.[125] It is unclear whether ultraviolet light produces its harmful effects because of problems in DNA synthesis, repair, or replication.

Invasive squamous cell carcinoma can arise from premalignant lesions of the skin. It rarely arises from normal-appearing skin or "de novo." The premalignant lesions include sun-damaged skin or dysplasias (actinic dermatitis); leukoplasia, or whitish, discolored areas; scars; radiation-induced keratosis; tar and oil keratosis; and chronic ulcers and sinuses. The invasive type grows more rapidly than basal cell carcinomas and can spread to regional lymph nodes. These tumors are firm and increase in both elevation and diameter. The surface may be granular and bleed easily (Fig. 43-29).

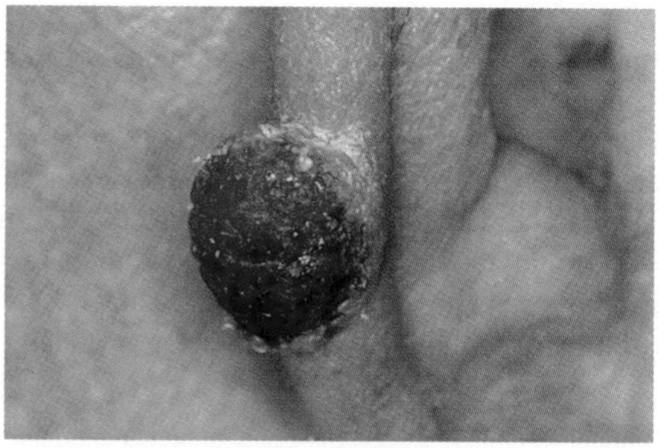

FIG. 43-29 Squamous cell carcinoma. The sun-exposed ear is a common site for squamous cell carcinoma. (Courtesy Department of Dermatology, School of Medicine, University of Utah.)

In situ squamous cell carcinoma is usually confined to the epidermis (intraepidermal) but may extend into the dermis. Common premalignant skin lesions associated with in situ squamous cell carcinomas are actinic (solar) keratosis and Bowen disease. Actinic keratosis is a white, scaly, keratotic (horny) lesion on the exposed areas of the body. Bowen disease is a dysplasia of the basal layer of the dermis or carcinoma in situ. It often is found on unexposed areas of the body and is demonstrated by flat, reddish, scaly patches. These lesions may enlarge to more than 1 cm in diameter, rarely invading surrounding tissue and almost never metastasizing. Other cellular components in the skin (sweat glands, hair follicles, etc.) can give rise to skin cancer, but these cancers are relatively uncommon.

Malignant Melanoma

Melanoma is a malignant tumor of the skin originating from melanocytes, or cells that synthesize the pigment melanin. The incidence of melanoma is increasing, and young to middle-age adults are at highest risk.[126] Early recognition of cutaneous melanomas can have a major impact on surgically curing this disease. The ABCD rule is used as a guide: assymetry, border irregularity, color variation, diameter larger than 6 mm.[127]

Risk factors implicated in melanoma induction include genetic predisposition, exposure to ultraviolet light (solar and artificial), steroid hormone activity, fair hair, light skin with a propensity to sunburn, and freckles.[128,129] Melanomas arise as a result of malignant degeneration of melanocytes located either along the basal layer of the epidermis or in a benign melanocytic nevus. A number of proto-oncogenes have been identified in human malignant melanoma.[130] A nevus, or mole, is an aggregation of melanocytes (Fig. 43-30). These clusters of cells may not be apparent until puberty, when the pigmentation process is initiated by steroid hormones. The relationship between nevi and melanoma makes it important for the clinician to understand the various neval forms (Table 43-7). Most nevi never become suspicious; however, suspicious pigmented nevi should be removed.[131] Indications for biopsy include color change, size change, irregular notched margin, itching, bleeding or oozing, nodularity,

A

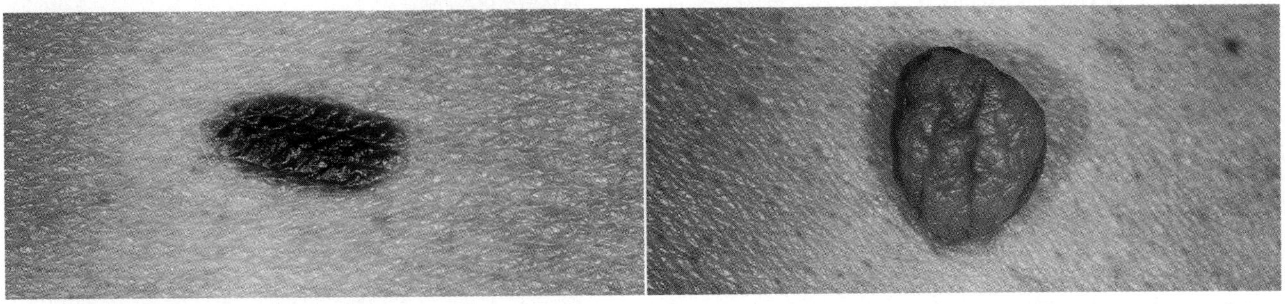

B

FIG. 43-30 Nevi. A, Junction nevus: flat, black, and uniform. **B,** Dermal nevus: pedunculated with a soft, flabby, wrinkled surface. (From Habif TB: *Clinical dermatology: a color guide to diagnosis and therapy,* ed 3, St Louis, 1996, Mosby.)

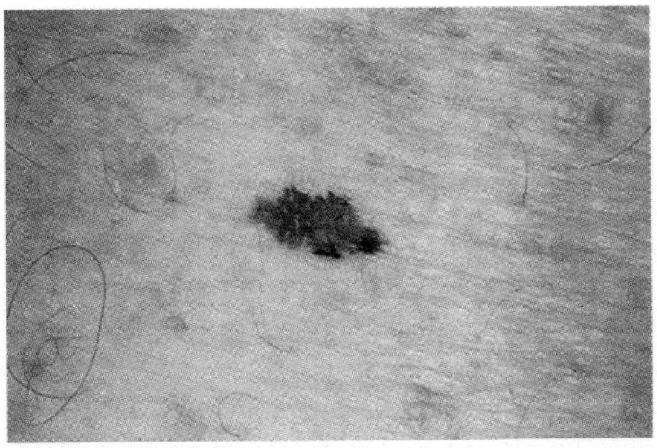

FIG. 43-31 Lentigo malignant melanoma. (Courtesy Department of Dermatology, School of Medicine, University of Utah.)

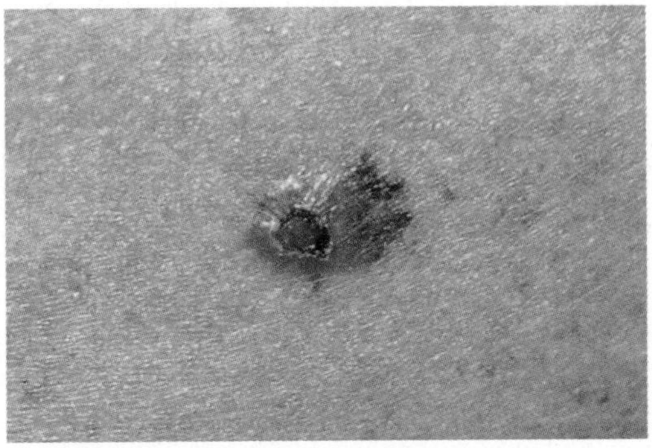

FIG. 43-32 Level 4 melanoma. (Courtesy Department of Dermatology, School of Medicine, University of Utah.)

Table 43-7 Classification of Nevi

Nevi	Common Characteristics
Junctional nevus	Flat, well circumscribed, vary in size up to 2 cm, dark color, hairs may be present; originate in basal layer of epidermis and can eventually reach the cutaneous surface; most likely to develop into a melanoma
Compound nevus	Most common in adolescents; the majority of pigmented lesions in children; rarely does this lesion develop to melanoma; usually 1 cm in size; hairs may be present; surface is elevated and smooth
Intradermal nevus	Small (less than 1 cm) with regular edges and bristlelike hairs; color ranges from skin tone to light brown; has a slight likelihood of developing into a melanoma

scab formation, and ulceration. The clinical varieties of cutaneous melanoma include lentigo malignant melanoma (LMM) (Fig. 43-31), superficial spreading melanoma (SSM) (Fig. 43-32), and primary nodular melanoma (PNM). Clinical characteristics are summarized in Box 43-3.

Treatment of melanoma with no evidence of metastatic disease involves surgical excision to the primary site and regional lymph nodes. The extent of surgery is determined by the staging of disease. Lesions of the extremities have the best prognosis; head and neck lesions and trunk lesions have the poorest prognosis. Only 20% to 40% of patients with regional lymph node involvement are alive and cured at 5 years. Immune response modifiers, vaccines, and gene therapy are under investigation.[132,133,134]

Kaposi Sarcoma

Kaposi sarcoma (KS) is a vascular malignancy with four different presentations:

1. In association with drug-induced immunosuppressions, for example, after kidney transplant
2. An endemic form in equatorial Africa
3. A form presenting on the lower legs of elderly men
4. In association with acquired immunodeficiency syndrome (AIDS)

Kaposi-associated herpesvirus 8 is found in all four forms of KS.[135]

Individuals with AIDS are immunosuppressed, and this allows for opportunistic infections and malignancy. Proliferation of the tumor depends on the presence of platelet-derived growth factors.[136]

The human immunodeficiency virus and cytomegalovirus have been proposed as cofactors in the development of KS.[137] The herpesvirus may be a common etiology for all types of KS.[138] The endothelial cell is thought to be the progenitor of KS. The lesions emerge as purplish brown macules

Box 43-3

CLINICAL CHARACTERISTICS OF VARIETIES OF CUTANEOUS MELANOMA

LENTIGO MALIGNANT MELANOMA	
Frequency	10% to 15% of cutaneous melanomas
Age at diagnosis	50 to 80 years old
Primary location	Head, neck, dorsum of hands
Pigmentation according to thickness	
<1.5 mm (levels I and II)	Tan and brown
>1.5 mm (level III)	Tan, brown, and blue-black
>1.5 mm (levels IV and V)	Nodule formation
SUPERFICIAL SPREADING MELANOMAS	
Frequency	70% of cutaneous melanomas
Age at diagnosis	20 to 60 years old
Primary location	Legs of females; upper back of both genders
Pigmentation according to thickness	
<1.5 mm (levels I and II)	Tan and brown
>1.5 mm (level III)	Tan, brown, and blue-black
>1.5 mm (levels IV and V)	Nodule formation
PRIMARY NODULAR MELANOMA	
Frequency	12% of cutaneous melanomas
Age at diagnosis	20 to 60 years old
Primary location	No specific site preference
Pigmentation according to thickness	
>1.5 mm (level III)	Small nodule (any hue)
>1.5 mm (levels IV and V)	Large nodule (any hue)

and develop into plaques and nodules. They tend to be multifocal rather than spreading by metastasis. The lesions initially appear over the lower extremities in the classic form (Fig. 43-33). The rapidly progressive form associated with AIDS tends to spread symmetrically over the upper body, particularly the face and oral mucosa. The lesions are often pruritic and painful. About 75% of individuals with epidemic KS have involvement of lymph nodes, particularly in the gastrointestinal tract and lungs. Organ involvement is much less common in the classic form. The rapidly progressive form has a poor prognosis and shorter survival rates than the classic form. (See Chapter 23 for a further discussion on AIDS.)

Diagnosis is by skin biopsy, with a high index of suspicion for those with immune deficiency. Local lesions can be excised. Multiple disseminated lesions may be treated with a combination of interferon-α; radiation therapy; and cytotoxic drugs, particularly liposomal doxorubicin.[139] The new retroviral therapies for AIDS treatment is also changing the clinical course of KS. Experimental treatments include angiogenesis inhibitors; hormonal therapies; retinoic acid derivatives; and immune modulators, such as interleukin-12.[140] General response to treatment is poor, but a 2-year survival

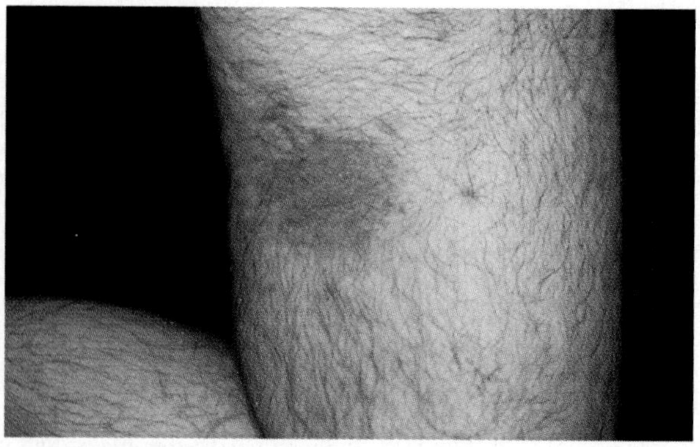

FIG. 43-33 Kaposi sarcoma. The purple lesion commonly seen on the skin. (Courtesy Department of Dermatology, School of Medicine, University of Utah.)

rate is better in individuals with KS alone than in those with KS and an opportunistic infection.

Frostbite

Frostbite is injury to the skin caused by exposure to extreme cold. The areas most commonly affected are fingers, toes, ears, nose, and cheeks. Initially the body responds with alternating cycles of vasoconstriction and vasodilation—"the burning reaction." The mechanism of injury is complex but appears to be related to direct cold injury to cells, indirect injury and cell death from extracellular and intracellular ice crystal formation, and impaired circulation with anoxia because of thrombosis in the exposed area.[141] The inflammatory mediators of frostbite are similar to burns and include prostaglandins, thromboxanes, bradykinin, and histamine. Reperfusion injury is part of the pathophysiology.[142] Frozen skin becomes white or yellowish and is waxy. There is numbness and no sensation of pain.

Skin damage can range from mild to severe. With mild frostbite, redness and discomfort occur during rewarming, followed by a return to normal in a few hours. In more severe cases, cyanosis and mottling develop, followed by redness, swelling, and burning pain on rewarming. Within 24 to 48 hours, vesicles and bullae appear that resolve into crusts that eventually slough off, leaving thin, newly formed skin. The most severe cases result in gangrene with loss of the affected part. Frostbite may be classified by depth of injury after rewarming:[143]

First degree. Superficial, characterized by a numb central white area surrounded by erythema and edema and including partial skin freezing without blistering

Second degree. Full-thickness skin freezing with blistering surrounded by edema and hyperemia

Third degree. Deep, characterized by full-thickness skin and subcutaneous freezing with tissue necrosis and hemorrhagic vesicles

Fourth degree. Deep tissue freezing with full-thickness necrosis and gangrene

Immediate treatment of frostbite is to cover affected areas with other body surfaces and warm clothing. The area should not be rubbed or massaged. Local, dry heat should be avoided. Immersion in a warm water bath (40° to 42° C) until frozen tissue is thawed is the best treatment. Aspirin is used to inhibit prostaglandins, and aloe vera is a topical inhibitor of thromboxane.[144] Pain during the thawing period is severe and should be treated with potent analgesics. Gentle cleansing and no pressure on the skin should be maintained during healing. Amputation of necrotic tissue is delayed until a clear line of demarcation is established.

DISORDERS OF THE HAIR

Alopecia

Male-Pattern Alopecia (Androcentric Alopecia)

Alopecia means loss of hair. Localized hair loss in men is not a disease but a genetically predisposed response to androgens. The mechanism of inheritance is unknown. Within the distribution of hair over the scalp, androgen-sensitive hair follicles are on top and androgen-insensitive follicles are on the sides and back. In genetically predisposed men, the androgen-sensitive follicles are transformed into vellus follicles. The normal hair is shed and replaced by fine, light, short hair. Male-pattern baldness begins with frontotemporal recession and progresses to loss of hair over the top of the scalp. Minoxidil may be used to stimulate hair growth.[145] Affected men may choose to wear wigs, have hair transplants, or have plastic surgery.

Female-Pattern Alopecia

Some women in their 20s and 30s experience progressive thinning and loss of hair over the central part of the scalp.[146] Contrary to male-pattern baldness, no loss of hair occurs along the frontal hairline. Many of these women have elevated levels of serum adrenal androgen dehydroepiandrosterone sulfate (DHEAS).[147] In rare instances a male-pattern baldness develops. Laboratory evaluation of serum androgenic hormones shows elevations, and some women have decreased hair loss when treated with daily doses of spironolactone.

Alopecia Areata

Alopecia areata is a T cell–mediated chronic inflammatory disease directed at hair follicles that results in baldness.[148] Hair loss occurs in multiple areas of the scalp, usually in round patches.[149] The eyebrows, eyelashes, beard, and other areas of the body are rarely involved. The cause is unknown, but stressful events, cell-mediated immune factors (including IL-1),[150] and genetic susceptibility are linked to hair loss. Metabolic disorders, such as Addison disease, thyroid disease, and lupus erythematosus, also are associated with alopecia areata.[151,152,153]

The affected areas of skin are smooth or may have short shafts of hair. The hair shaft is poorly developed and breaks at the surface. Regrowth occurs within 1 to 3 months, but hair loss may recur at the same site. Permanent regrowth of hair usually occurs. Total loss of hair (alopecia totalis) occurs in some young people; the long-term prognosis for total hair regrowth is poor.

Diagnosis is made by observation of the pattern of hair loss. Biopsy may show a lymphocytic infiltrate around the follicle. Intralesional steroids may be used to stimulate hair growth when there are a few small areas of hair loss. Systemic steroids are used for larger areas of alopecia. Topical applications of anthralin also are used to stimulate hair growth. Minoxidil has been tested for use in resistant cases and has been found effective in some cases, and topical immunotherapy is effective for extensive areas.[154,155]

Hirsutism

Hirsutism is the growth and distribution of hair on the face, body, and pubic area in a male pattern. There is also frontotemporal hair recession. These areas of hair growth are androgen sensitive.[156] Variations of hair growth in women are great, and a male pattern can be normal. Women who develop hirsutism may be secreting hormones associated with ovarian or adrenal disease, and such women should be evaluated for polycystic ovaries, adrenal hyperplasia, or adrenal tumors. If no hormonal pathologic conditions exist, treatment may include cosmetic removal of hair, oral contraceptives, glucocorticoids, cimetidine, and finasteride or flutamide.[157,158,159]

DISORDERS OF THE NAIL

Paronychia

Paronychia is an acute or chronic infection of the cuticle. Acute paronychia is manifest by the rapid onset of painful inflammation of the cuticle, usually after minor trauma. An abscess may develop, requiring incision and drainage for relief of pain. The most common causative organisms are staphylococci and streptococci. Occasionally *Candida* will be present.

Chronic paronychia develops slowly, with tenderness and swelling around the proximal or lateral nail folds. One or more fingers or toes may be involved. Individuals whose hands are frequently exposed to moisture are at greatest risk. Manipulation of the cuticle can be predisposing because it opens the space between the proximal nail fold and nail plate, leaving a moist, warm medium for the incubation of pathogenic organisms. The skin around the nail becomes more edematous and painful with progressive infection. Pus may be expressed from the proximal nail fold. The nail plate is usually not affected, although it can become discolored with ridges.

Treatment includes keeping the hands dry. Oral antibiotics are not very effective because they do not penetrate the affected tissues. Topical application of thymol is usually effective.

Onychomycosis

Onychomycosis is a fungal or dermatophyte infection of the nail plate that occurs in 2% to 18% of the population.[160] The most common pattern is a nail plate that turns yellow or white and becomes elevated with the accumulation of hyperkeratotic debris within the plate. Fungal infections of the nail may require culture and microscopy. In psoriasis there is absence of pitting on the nail surface.[161] Treatment is difficult because topical or systemic antifungal agents do not penetrate the nail plate readily. New oral antifungals are effective.[162] Surgical excision of the nail may be required.

SUMMARY REVIEW

Structure and Function of the Skin

1. Skin is the largest organ of the body and equals 20% of body weight.
2. The skin has two layers: the dermis and epidermis.
3. The underlying epidermis contains a basal and a spinous layer with melanocytes, Langerhans cells, and Merkel cells.
4. The dermis is composed of connective tissue elements, hair follicles, sweat glands, sebaceous glands, blood vessels, nerves, and lymphatic vessels.
5. The papillary capillaries provide the major blood supply to the skin, arising from deeper arterial plexuses.
6. Heat loss and heat conservation are regulated by arteriovenous anastomoses that lead to the papillary capillaries.

Aging and Skin Integrity

1. Older skin is thinner and drier and has fewer capillary loops with changes in pigmentation.
2. Loss of melanocytes and hair follicles leads to gray and thinner hair.
3. The skin of older persons is more permeable; there is decreased sweating and loss of thermal regulation with decreased protective functions.
4. Pressure ulcers develop from pressure and shearing forces that occlude capillary blood flow, with resulting ischemia and necrosis. Areas at greatest risk are pressure points over bony prominences, such as the greater trochanter, sacrum, ischia, and heels. Immobilized individuals with fractures and neurologic deficits are most likely to develop pressure ulcers.
5. Pruritus is itching and is associated with many skin disorders. The exact neurologic mechanism is unknown, but pain receptors with low-density stimulation are one theory of irritation. Scratching with skin trauma, potential infection, and scarring are associated with itching.

Disorders of the Skin

1. Contact dermatitis is a form of delayed hypersensitivity that develops with sensitization to allergies, such as metals, chemicals, or poison ivy.
2. Irritant contact dermatitis develops from prolonged exposure to chemicals, such as acids or soaps.
3. Atopic or allergic dermatitis is associated with a family history of allergies, hay fever, elevated immunoglobulin E (IgE) levels, and increased histamine sensitivity. Pruritus and scratching predispose the skin to infection, scaling, and thickening.
4. Stasis dermatitis occurs on the legs and results from venous stasis and edema.
5. Seborrheic dermatitis involves scaly, yellowish, inflammatory plaques of the scalp, eyebrows, eyelids, ear canals, chest, axillae, and back. The cause is unknown.
6. Papulosquamous disorders are characterized by papules, scales, plaques, and erythema.
7. Psoriasis is a chronic autoimmune skin disease with thickening of both the epidermis and dermis, characterized by scaly, erythematous, pruritic plaques.
8. Pityriasis rosea is a self-limiting disease characterized by oval lesions with scales around the edges located along skin lines of the trunk.
9. Lichen planus is a papular, violet-colored inflammatory lesion of unknown origin manifest by severe pruritus.
10. Acne vulgaris is an inflammation of the pilosebaceous follicle.
11. Acne rosacea develops on the middle third of the face with hypertrophy and inflammation of the sebaceous glands.
12. Lupus erythematosus can affect only the skin (discoid) or have a systemic presentation. The inflammatory lesions usually occur in sun-exposed areas, with a butterfly distribution over the nose and cheeks.
13. Pemphigus is a chronic, autoimmune, blistering disease that begins in the mouth or on the scalp and spreads to other parts of the body, often with a fatal outcome. There are two forms: pemphigus vulgaris and bullous pemphigus.
14. Erythema multiforme is an acute inflammation of the skin and mucous membranes with lesions that appear targetlike with alternating rings of edema and inflammation; it is often associated with allergic reactions to drugs. Stevens-Johnson syndrome is a severe form that also involves the mucous membranes.
15. Folliculitis is a bacterial infection of the hair follicle.
16. A furuncle is an infection of the hair follicle that extends to the surrounding tissue.
17. A carbuncle is a collection of infected hair follicles that forms a draining abscess.
18. Cellulitis is a diffuse infection of the dermis and subcutaneous tissue.
19. Erysipelas is a superficial streptococcal infection of the skin commonly affecting the face, ears, and lower legs.
20. Impetigo may have a bullous or an ulcerative form and is caused by *Staphylococcus* or *Streptococcus.*
21. Herpes simplex virus type 1 (HSV-1) causes cold sores but can infect the cornea, mouth, and labia. HSV-2 causes genital lesions and is usually spread by sexual contact.
22. Herpes zoster and varicella are both caused by the same herpesvirus.
23. Warts are benign, rough, elevated lesions caused by papillomavirus. Condylomata acuminata, or venereal warts, are spread by sexual contact.
24. Tinea infections (fungal infections) can occur anywhere on the body and are classified by location (i.e., tinea pedis, tinea corporis, tinea capitis).
25. Candidiasis is a yeastlike fungal infection occurring on skin, on mucous membranes, and in the gastrointestinal tract.
26. Cutaneous vasculitis is an inflammation of skin blood vessels with purpura, ischemia, and necrosis resulting from vessel necrosis.
27. Urticarial lesions are associated with hypersensitivity responses and appear as wheals, welts, or hives.
28. Scleroderma is a sclerosis of the skin that may also affect systemic organs and cause renal failure, bowel obstruction, or cardiac dysrhythmias.
29. Ticks cause a local reaction and can cause systemic disease when mouthparts pierce the skin and remain embedded in the tissue.
30. Lyme disease is a multisystem inflammatory disease caused by *Borrelia burgdorferi* transmitted by tick bites.
31. Mosquitoes can transmit infectious diseases, and the saliva from their bite produces the characteristic itching and wheal formation.
32. Blood-sucking flies are represented by many species, including Ceratopogonidae ("no-see-ums"), Tabanidae (horseflies),

or Simuliidae (black flies). Their bites are usually painful and produce bleeding, and the itching and local reactions may last for days with systemic symptoms of fever and malaise.

33. Seborrheic keratosis is a proliferation of basal cells that produce elevated, smooth, or warty lesions of varying size. They are most common among the elderly population.
34. Keratoacanthoma arises from hair follicles on sun-exposed areas. There are three stages of development, which result in a dome-shaped, crusty lesion filled with keratin that resolves in 3 to 4 months.
35. Actinic keratosis is a pigmented scaly lesion that develops in sun-exposed individuals with fair skin. The lesion may become malignant in the form of squamous cell carcinoma.
36. Nevi arise from melanocytes and may be pigmented or fleshy pink. They occur singly or in groups and may undergo transition to malignant melanoma.
37. Basal cell carcinoma is the most common skin cancer and occurs most frequently on sun-exposed areas.
38. Squamous cell carcinoma is a tumor of the epidermis and can be localized (in situ) or invasive.
39. Malignant melanoma arises from melanocytes; if it is not excised early, metastasis occurs through the lymph nodes.
40. Kaposi sarcoma is a vascular malignancy associated with immune deficiency states.
41. Frostbite usually occurs on cheeks and digits, with direct injury to cells and impaired circulation.

Disorders of the Hair

1. Male-pattern alopecia is an inherited form of irreversible baldness with hair loss in the central scalp and recession of the temporofrontal hairline.
2. Female-pattern alopecia is a thinning of the central hair of the scalp beginning in women at 20 to 30 years of age.
3. Alopecia areata is patchy loss of hair usually associated with stress or metabolic diseases; it is usually reversible.
4. Hirsutism is a male pattern of hair growth in women that may be normal or the result of excessive secretion of androgenic hormones.

Disorders of the Nail

1. Paronychia is an inflammation of the cuticle that can be acute or chronic and is usually caused by staphylococci or streptococci.
2. Onychomycosis is a fungal infection of the nail plate.

KEY TERMS

REFERENCES

1. Jankovic SM, Jankovic SV: The control of hair growth, *Dermatol Online J* 4(1):2, 1998.
2. Hadshiew IM, Eller MS, Gilchrest BA: Skin aging and photoaging: the role of DNA damage and repair, *Am J Contact Dermat* 11(1):19, 2000.
3. Timiras PS: *Physiologic basis of aging and geriatrics,* Boca Raton, Fla, 1994, CRC Press.
4. Gilchrist BA: *Skin and aging processes,* Boca Raton, Fla, 1984, CRC Press.
5. Yaar M: Molecular mechanisms of skin aging, *Adv Dermatol* 10:63, 1996.

6. Gilchrest BA: A review of skin ageing and its medical therapy, *Br J Dermatol* 135(6):867, 1996.
7. Berlowitz DR, Brandeis GH, Anderson J: Predictors of pressure ulcer healing among long-term care residents, *J Amer Geriatric Soc* 45:30, 1997.
8. Theaker C et al: Risk factors for pressure sores in the critically ill, *Anesthesia* 55(3):221, 2000.
9. Clinical guidelines: how to predict and prevent pressure ulcers, *Am J Nurs* 92(7):52, 1992.
10. Xakellis GC, Frantz RA: The cost effectiveness of interventions for preventing pressure ulcers, *J Am Board Fam Pract* 9(2):79, 1996.
11. AGS Clinical Practice Committee: Pressure ulcers in adults: prediction and prevention, *J Am Geriatr Soc* 44(9):1118, 1996.
12. Smith DM: Pressure ulcers in the nursing home, *Ann Intern Med* 123 (6):433, 1995.
13. Fine NA, Mustoe TA: Wound healing. In Greenfield LJ et al, editors: *Surgery: scientific principles and practice,* ed 2, Philadelphia, 1997, Lippincott-Raven.
14. Goldstein B, Saunders JE, Benson B: Pressure ulcers in SCI: does tension stimulate wound healing? *Am J Phys Med Rehabil* 75(2):130, 1996.
15. Xue H, McCauley RL, Zhang W: Elevated interleukin-6 expression in keloid fibroblasts, *J Surg Res* 89(1):74, 2000.
16. Sayah DN et al: Downregulation of apoptosis-related genes in keloid tissues, *J Surg Res* 87(2):209, 1999.
17. English RS, Schenefelt PD: Keloids and hypertrophic scars, *Dermatol Surg* 25(8):631, 1999.
18. Greaves MW, Wall PD: Pathophysiology of itching, *Lancet* 348(9032): 938, 1996.
19. Heyer GR, Hornstein OP: Recent studies of cutaneous nicoception in atopic and non-atopic subjects, *J Dermatol* 26(2):77, 1999.
20. Schmelz M et al: Specific C-receptors for itch in human skin, *J Neurosci* 17(20):8003, 1997.
21. Hagermark O: Itch mediators, *Semin Dermatol* 14(4):271, 1995.
22. Ekblom A: Some neurophysiological aspects of itch, *Semin Dermatol* 14(4):252, 1995.
23. Teofoli P et al: Itch and pain, *Int J Dermatol* 35(3):159, 1996.
24. Mizzuddin N, Marenus KD, Maes DH: Factors defining sensitive skin and its treatment, *Am J Contact Dermat* 9(3):107, 1998.
25. Barker JN: Role of keratinocytes in allergic contact dermatitis, *Contact Dermatol* 26(3):145, 1992.
26. Moussadeh N et al: A new quantitative in vitro for the detection of latex-specific IgE antibodies, *Allerg Immunol* 31(10):343, 1999.
27. Schultz-Larsen F, Hanifin JM: Secular changes in the occurrence of atopic dermatitis, *Acta Dermato Venereol Suppl (Stoch)* 176:7, 1992.
28. Rothe MJ, Grant-Kels JM: Atopic dermatitis: an update, *J Am Acad Dermatol* 35(1):1, 1996.
29. Sicherer SH, Sampson HA: Food hypersensitivity and atopic dermatitis: pathophysiology, epidemiology, diagnosis, and management, *J Allergy Clin Immunol* 104(3 part 2):S114, 1999.
30. Miyasato M et al: Serum levels of eosinophil cationic protein reflect the state of in vitro degranulation of blood hypodense eosinophils in atopic dermatitis, *J Dermatol* 23(6):382, 1996.
31. Kimata H, Lindley I: Detection of plasma interleukin-8 in atopic dermatitis, *Arch Dis Child* 70:119, 1994.
32. Habif TB: *Clinical dermatology: a color guide to diagnosis and therapy,* St Louis, 1996, Mosby.
33. Borish L, Joseph BZ: Inflammation and the allergic response, *Med Clin North Am* 76(4):765, 1992.
34. Kemp AS, Campbell DE: New perspectives on inflammation in atopic dermatitis, *J Paediatr Child Health* 32(1):4, 1996.
35. Wahlgren CF: Itch and atopic dermatitis: an overview, *J Dermatol* 26(11):770, 1999.
36. Nagaki Y, Hayasaka S, Kadoi S: Cataract progression in patients with atopic dermatitis, *J Cataract Refract Surg* 25(1):96, 1999.
37. Drake LA, Fallon JD, Sober A: Relief of pruritus in patients with atopic dermatitis after treatment with topical doxepin cream, *J Am Acad Dermatol* 31:613, 1994.
38. Christophers E: The immunopathology of psoriasis, *Int Arch Allergy Immunol* 110(3):199, 1996.
39. Kreuger JG et al: Successful in vivo blockage of CD25 (high-affinity interleukin-2 receptor) on T cells by administration of humanized anti-Tac antibody to patients with psoriasis, *J Am Acad Dermatol* 43(3): 448, 2000.
40. Asumalahti K et al: A candidate gene for psoriasis near HLS-C, HCR (Pg8) is highly polymorphic with a disease-associated susceptibility allele, *Hum Mol Genet* 9(10):1533, 2000.
41. Peters BP, Weissman FG, Gill MA: Pathophysiology and treatment of psoriasis, *Am J Health Syst Pharm* 57(7):645, 2000.
42. Prinz JC: Which T cells cause psoriasis? *Clin Exp Dermatol* 24(4): 291, 1999.
43. Wolf R, Ruocco V: Triggered psoriasis, *Adv Exp Med Biol* 455:221, 1999.
44. Winchester R: Psoriatic arthritis, *Dermatol Clin* 13(4):779, 1995.
45. Ashcroft DM et al: Systemic review of comparative efficacy and tolerability of calcipotriol in treating chronic plaque psoriasis, *Br Med J* 320(7240):963, 2000.
46. Harrison PV: Topical tacalcitol treatment for psoriasis, *Hosp Med* 61(6):402, 2000.
47. Kempf W, Burg G: Pityriasis rosea—a virus induced skin disease? An update, *Arch Virol* 145(8):1509, 2000.
48. Ginsburg CM: Pityriasis rosea, *Pediatr Infect Dis J* 10(11):858, 1991.
49. Katta R: Lichen planus, *Am Fam Physician* 61(11):3319. 2000.
50. Porter SR et al: Immunologic aspects of dermal and oral lichen planus: a review, *Oral Surg Oral Med Oral Path Oral Radiol Endod* 83:358, 1997.
51. Chuang TY et al: Hepatitis C virus and lichen planus: a case-control study of 340 patients, *J Am Acad Dermatol* 41:787, 1999.
52. Miles DA, Howard MM: Diagnosis and management of oral lichen planus, *Dermatol Clin* 14(2):281, 1996.
53. Wilkin JK: Rosacea: pathophysiology and treatment, *Arch Dermatol* 130(3):359, 1994.
54. Thiboutot DM: Acne and rosacea: new and emerging therapies, *Dermatol Clin* 18(1):63, 2000.
55. Bamford JT et al: Effect of treatment of *Helicobacter pylori* infection on rosacea, *Arch Dermatol* 135(6):659, 1999.
56. Szlachcic A et al: *Helicobacter pylori* and its eradication in rosacea, *J Physiol Pharmacol* 50(5):777, 1999.
57. Yell JA, Mbuagbaw J, Burge SM: Cutaneous manifestations of systemic lupus erythematosus, *Br J Dermatol* 135:355, 1996.
58. Arnett FC: Genetic aspects of human lupus, *Clin Immunol Immunopathol* 63(1):4, 1992.
59. Skaer TL: Medication induced systemic lupus erythematosus, *Clin Ther* 14(4):496, 1992.
60. Amagai M: Pemphigus: autoimmunity to epidermal cell adhesion molecules, *Adv Dermatol* 11:319, 1996.
61. Robinson ND et al: The new pemphigus variants, *J Am Acad Dermatol* 40(5 part 1):649, 1999.
62. Korman NJ: New and emerging therapies in the treatment of blistering diseases, *Dermatol Clin* 18(1):127, 2000.
63. Nousari HC, Anhalt GJ: Pemphigus and bellous pemphigoid, *Lancet* 354(9179):667, 1999.
64. Aurelian L, Kokuba H, Burnett JW: Understanding the pathogenesis of HSV-associated erythema multiforme, *Dermatology* 197(3):219, 1998.
65. Katta R: Taking aim at erythema multiforme. How to spot target lesions and less typical presentations, *Postgrad Med* 107(1):87, 2000.
66. Provost TT, Weston WL: *Bullous diseases,* St Louis, 1993, Mosby.
67. Roujeau JC: Stevens-Johnson syndrome and toxic epidermal necrolysis are severity variants of the same disease which differs from erythema multiforme, *J Dermatol* 24(11):726, 1997.
68. Learner LH et al: Nitric oxide synthase in toxic epidermal necrolysis and Stevens-Johnson syndrome, *J Invest Dermatol* 114(1):196, 2000.
69. LeCleach L et al: Blister fluid T lymphocytes during toxic epidermal necrolysis are functional cytotoxic cells which express human natural killer (NK) inhibitory receptors, *Clin Exp Immunol* 119(1):225, 2000.

70. Cheriyan S et al: The outcome of Stevens-Johnson syndrome treated with corticosteroids, *Allergy Proc* 16(4):151, 1995.
71. Singh G, Marples BM, Klingman AM: Staphylococcus infections in humans, *J Invest Dermatol* 57:149, 1971.
72. Bisno AL, Stevens DL: Streptococcal infections of skin and soft tissues, *N Engl J Med* 334(4):240, 1996.
73. Cox NH, Colver GB, Paterson WD: Management and morbidity of cellulitis of the leg, *J R Soc Med* 91(12):634, 1998.
74. Koutkia P, Mylonakis E, Boyce J: Cellulitis: evaluation of possible predisposing factors in hospitalized patients, *Diagn Microbiol Infect Dis* 34(4):325, 1999.
75. Guberman D et al: Bullous erysipelas: a retrospective study of 26 patients, *J Am Acad Dermatol* 41:733, 1999.
76. Adachi J et al: Increasing incidence of streptococcal impetigo in atopic dermatitis, *J Dermatol Sci* 17(1):45, 1998.
77. Bale JF Jr: Human herpesviruses and neurological disorders of childhood, *Semin Pediatr Neurol* 6(4):278, 1999.
78. Wahren B, Linde A: Virological and clinical characteristics of human herpes virus 6, *Scand J Infect Dis* 80(suppl):105, 1991.
79. Crumpacker CS: Herpes simplex. In Fitzpatrick TB et al, editors: *Dermatology in general medicine,* ed 3, New York, 1987, McGraw-Hill.
80. Stanberry L et al: New developments in epidemiology, natural history and management of genital herpes, *Antiviral Res* 42(1):1, 1999.
81. Krause PR, Straus SE: Herpesvirus vaccines. Development, controversies, and applications, *Infect Dis Clin North Am* 13(1):61, 1999.
82. Whitley RJ, Gnann JW Jr: Therapeutic approaches to the management of herpes zoster, *Adv Exp Med Biol* 458:159, 1999.
83. Alper BS, Lewis PR: Does treatment of acute herpes zoster prevent or shorten postherpetic neuralgia? *J Fam Pract* 49(3):355, 2000.
84. Cohen JI et al: Recent advances in varicella-zoster virus infection, *Ann Intern Med* 130(11):922, 1999.
85. Ragozzino MW et al: Population based study of herpes zoster and its sequelae, *Medicine (Baltimore)* 5(61):310, 1982.
86. Chartrand SA: Varicella vaccine, *Pediatr Clin North Am* 47(2):373, 2000.
87. Kanazi GE, Johnson RW, Dworkin RH: Treatment of postherpetic neuralgia: an update, *Drugs* 59(5):1113, 2000.
88. Lassus J, Ranki A: Simultaneously detected aberrant p53 tumor-suppressor protein and HPV-DNA localized mostly in separate keratinocytes in anogenital and common warts, *Exp Dermatol* 5(2):72, 1996.
89. Prasad CJ: Pathobiology of human papillomavirus, *Clin Lab Med* 15(3):685, 1995.
90. Miller DM, Brodell RT: Human papillomavirus infection: treatment options for warts, *Am Fam Physician* 53(1):135, 1996.
91. Plasencia JM: Cutaneous warts: diagnosis and treatment, *Prim Care* 27(2):423, 2000.
92. Beutner KR et al: Genital warts and their treatment, *Clin Infect Dis* 28(suppl 1):S37, 1999.
93. Myers ER et al: Mathematical model for the natural history of human papillomavirus infection and cervical carcinogenesis, *Am J Epidemiol* 151(12):1158, 2000.
94. Sasieni PD: Human papillomavirus screening and cervical cancer prevention, *J Am Med Womens Assoc* 55(4):216, 2000.
95. Stein DH: Tineas—superficial dermatophyte infections, *Pediatr Rev* 19(11):368, 1998.
96. Rupke SJ: Fungal skin disorders, *Prim Care* 27(2):407, 2000.
97. Di-Silverio A et al: Specific and nonspecific parameters of the host defense system in patients with superficial fungal infections, *Mycoses* 38(11-12):453, 1995.
98. Levitz SM: Overview of host defenses in fungal infections, *Clin Infect Dis* 14(suppl 1):537, 1992.
99. Lotti TM, Comacchi C, Ghersetich I: Cutaneous necrotizing vasculitis. Relation to systemic disease, *Adv Exp Med Biol* 455:115, 1999.
100. Lotti T et al: Cutaneous small-vessel vasculitis, *J Am Acad Dermatol* 39(5 P6 1):667, 1998.
101. Leznoff A: Chronic urticaria, *Can Fam Physician* 44:2170, 1998.
102. Generini S et al: Systemic sclerosis. a clinical review, *Adv Exp Med Biol* 455:73, 1999.
103. Haustein UF, Anderegg U: Pathophysiology of scleroderma: an update, *J Eur Acad Dermatol Venereol* 11(1):1, 1998.
104. Amento EP: Immunologic abnormalities in scleroderma, *Semin Cutan Med Surg* 17(1):18, 1998.
105. Systemic sclerosis: current pathogenetic concepts and future prospects for targeted therapy, *Lancet* 347(9013):1453, 1996 (clinical conference).
106. LeRoy EC: A brief overview of the pathogenesis of scleroderma (systemic sclerosis), *Ann Rheum Dis* 51(2):286, 1992.
107. Orloski KA et al: Surveillance for Lyme disease—United States, 1992-1998, *Mor Mortal Wkly Rep CDC Surveill Summ* 49(3):1, 2000.
108. Filgueira L et al: Human dendritic cells phagocytose and process *Borrelia burgdorferi, J Immunol* 157(7):2998, 1996.
109. Ziska MH, Donta ST, Demarest FC: Physician preferences in the diagnosis and treatment of Lyme disease in the United States, *Infection* 24(2):182, 1996.
110. Wormser GP: Controversies in the use of antimicrobials for the prevention and treatment of Lyme disease, *Infection* 24(2):178, 1996.
111. American Academy of Pediatrics, Committee on Infectious Diseases: Prevention of Lyme disease, *Pediatrics* 105(1 part 1):142, 2000.
112. Beham A et al: Keratoacanthoma: a clinically distinct variant of well differentiated squamous cell carcinoma, *Adv Anat Pathol* 5(5):269, 1998.
113. Cain CT, Niemann TH, Argenyi ZB: Keratoacanthoma versus squamous cell carcinoma: an immunohistochemical reappraisal of p53 protein and proliferating cell nuclear antigen expression in keratoacanthoma-like tumors, *Am J Dermatopathol* 17(4):324, 1995.
114. Moy RL: Clinical presentation of actinic keratoses and squamous cell carcinoma, *J Am Acad Dermatol* 42(1 part 2):8, 2000.
115. American Cancer Society: *Nonmelanoma skin cancer*, Atlanta, 2001. Available at www3.cancer.org/cancerinfo.
116. American Cancer Society: *Estimated new cancer cases and deaths by sex for all sites, United States 2000,* Atlanta, 2000, American Cancer Society. [www3.cancer.org/cancerinfo/sitecenter].
117. Buzzell RA: Carcinogenesis of cutaneous malignancies, *Dermatol Surg* 22(3):209, 1996.
118. Green A et al: Sun exposure, skin cancers and related skin conditions, *J Epidemiol* 9(6 suppl):S7, 1999.
119. Truhan AP: Sun protection in childhood, *Clin Pediatr* 30(12):676, 1991.
120. Rosso S et al: The multicentre south European study 'Helios' II: different sun exposure patterns in the aetiology of basal cell and squamous cell carcinomas of the skin, *Br J Cancer* 73(11):1447, 1996.
121. Boonchai W et al: Expression of p53 in arsenic-related and sporadic basal cell carcinoma, *ArchDermatol* 136(2):195, 2000.
122. Gailani MR et al: Relationship between sunlight exposure and a key genetic alteration in basal cell carcinoma, *J Natl Cancer Inst* 88(6): 349, 1996.
123. Mackie RM: *Skin cancer,* ed 2, St Louis, 1996, Mosby.
124. Goldman GD: Squamous cell cancer: a practical approach, *Semin Cutan Med Surg* 17(2):80, 1998.
125. Leffell DJ: The scientific basis of skin cancer, *J Am Acad Dermatol* 42(1 part 2):18, 2000.
126. Bishop JA: Melanoma, *Hosp Med* 61(2):103, 2000.
127. Koh HK et al: Prevention and early detection strategies for melanoma and skin cancer: current status, *Arch Dermatol* 132:436, 1996.
128. Katsambas A, Nicolaidou E: Cutaneous malignant melanoma and sun exposure: recent developments in epidemiology, *Arch Dermatol* 132 (4):444, 1996.
129. Rodenas JM et al: Sun exposure, pigmentary traits, and risk of cutaneous malignant melanoma: a case-control study in a Mediterranean population, *Cancer Causes Control* 7(2):275, 1996.
130. Dreiling L, Hoffman S, Robinson WA: Melanoma: epidemiology, pathogenesis, and new modes of treatment, *Adv Intern Med* 41:553, 1996.

131. Lober CW: Dysplastic (atypical) nevi: significance and management, *South Med J* 85(9):870, 1992.
132. Klatzmann D: Gene therapy for metastatic malignant melanoma: evaluation of tolerance to intratumoral injection of cells producing recombinant retroviruses carrying the herpes simplex virus type 1 thymidine kinase gene, to be followed by ganciclovir administration, *Hum Gene Ther* 7(2):355, 1996.
133. Nishimura T et al: Application of interleukin 12 to antitumor cytokine and gene therapy, *Cancer Chemother Pharmacol* 38(suppl):S27, 1996.
134. Stingl G et al: Phase I study to the immunotherapy of metastatic malignant melanoma by a cancer vaccine consisting of autologous cancer cells transfected with human IL-2 gene, *Hum Gene Ther* 7(4):552, 1996.
135. Mitsuyasu RT: Update on the pathogenesis and treatment of Kaposi sarcoma, *Curr Opin Oncol* 12(2):174, 2000.
136. Sturzl M et al: Expression of platelet-derived growth factor and its receptor in AIDS-related Kaposi sarcoma in vivo suggests paracrine and autocrine mechanisms of tumor maintenance, *Proc Natl Acad Sci USA* 89(15):7046, 1992.
137. Goopman J: Neoplasms in the acquired immune deficiency syndrome: the multidisciplinary approach, *Semin Oncol* 14(2 suppl 3):1, 1987.
138. Iscovich J et al: Classic kaposi sarcoma: epidemiology and risk factors, *Cancer* 88(3):500, 2000.
139. Yarchoan R: Therapy for Kaposi's sarcoma: recent advances and experimental approaches, *J Acquir Immune Defic Syndr* 1(21 suppl 1): S66, 1999.
140. Gascon P, Schwartz RA: Kaposi's sarcoma. New treatment modalities, *Dermatol Clin* 18(1):169, 2000.
141. Grandberg PO: Freezing cold injury, *Arctic Med Res* 50(suppl 6):76, 1991.
142. Murphy JV et al: Frostbite: pathogenesis and treatment, *J Trauma* 48(1):171, 2000.
143. Greenfield LJ et al: *Surgery: scientific principles and practice,* ed 2, Philadelphia, 1997, Lippincott-Raven.
144. Raine TJ, London MD, Goluch L: Antiprostaglandins and antithromboxanes for treatment of frostbite, *Surg Forum* 31:557, 1980.
145. Savin RC, Atton AV: Minoxidil: update on its clinical role, *Dermatol Clin* 11(1):55, 1993.
146. Norwood OT, Lehr B: Female androgenetic alopecia: a separate entity, *Dermatol Surg* 26(7):679, 2000.
147. Rushton DH: Management of hair loss in women, *Dermatol Clin* 11 (1):47, 1993.
148. Bodemer C et al: Role of cytotoxic T cells in chronic alopecia areata, *J Invest Dermatol* 114(1):112, 2000.
149. Callen JP et al: *Color atlas of dermatology*, Philadelphia, 2000, W.B. Saunders.
150. Hoffmann R, Happle R: Does interleukin-1 induce hair loss? *Dermatology* 191(4):273, 1995.
151. Ghersetich I, Campanile G, Lotti T: Alopecia areata: immunohistochemistry and ultrastructure of infiltrate and identification of adhesion molecule receptors, *Int J Dermatol* 35:28, 1996.
152. Gupta MA, Gupta AK, Watteel GN: Stress and alopecia areata, *Acta Derm Venereol* 77:296, 1997.
153. Sawaya ME, Hordinsky MK: Advances in alopecia areata and androgenic alopecia, *Adv Dermatol* 7:211, 1992.
154. Bertolino AP: Alopecia areata. A clinical overview, *Postgrad Med* 107(7):81, 2000.
155. Madani S, Shapiro J: Alopecia areata update, *J Am Acad Dermatol* 42(4):549, 2000.
156. Bergfeld WF: Hirsutism in women. Effective therapy that is safe for long-term use, *Postgrad Med* 107(7):93, 2000.
157. Tartagni M et al: Comparison of Diane 25 and Diane 35 plus finasteride in the treatment of hirsutism, *Fertil Steril* 73(4):718, 2000.
158. Falsetti L et al: Comparison of finasteride versus flutamide in the treatment of hirsutism, *Eur J Endocrinol* 141(4):361, 1999.
159. Vigersky RA et al: Treatment of hirsute women with cimetidine, *N Engl J Med* 303:1042, 1980.
160. Scher RK: Onychomycosis: therapeutic update, *J Am Acad Dermatol* 40(6 part 2):S21, 1999.
161. Elewski BE: Diagnostic techniques for confirming onychomycosis, *J Am Acad Dermatol* 35(3 part 2):S6, 1996.
162. Gupta AK, Shear NH: A risk-benefit assessment of the new oral antifungal agents used to treat onychomycosis, *Drug Saf* 22(1):33, 2000.

CHAPTER 44

Alterations of the Integument in Children

NOREEN HEER NICOL • SUE E. HUETHER

CHAPTER OUTLINE

Children frequently develop alterations in the skin, which may be minor or severe and localized or generalized. Unfortunately the skin is frequently underrated for its vital roles as a barrier, foundation, and calorie reservoir, as well as its roles in temperature regulation, sensation, grasp, insulation, and individual image. Manifestation of skin diseases in children may differ from those in adults, although the causative mechanisms may be similar. Some diseases resolve spontaneously and require no treatment. Diagnosis is commonly made from the history, appearance, and distribution of the lesion or lesions. Common skin diseases of childhood are presented here.

ACNE VULGARIS

Acne vulgaris is the most common skin disease and affects 85% of the population between the ages of 12 and 25 years. Genetic influences may determine an individual's susceptibility and severity of disease. Severe acne tends to run in families. The incidence of acne is the same in both genders, although severe disease affects males more frequently.

Distinctive pilosebaceous units, known as *sebaceous follicles*, are the sites for development of acne lesions. The follicles are located primarily on the face and upper parts of the chest and back. These follicles have many large sebaceous glands, a small vellus hair, and a dilated follicular canal that is visible as a "pore" on the skin surface. Acne lesions may be divided into inflammatory lesions (pustules, papules, nodules) and noninflammatory lesions (closed and open comedones).[1] In **noninflammatory acne** the comedones are open (blackheads) and closed (whiteheads), with the accumulated material causing distention of the follicle and thinning of follicular canal walls. **Inflammatory acne** develops in closed comedones when the follicular wall ruptures, expelling sebum into the surrounding dermis and initiating inflammation. Pustules form when the inflammation is close to the surface; papules and cystic nodules can develop when the inflammation is deeper, causing mild to severe scarring (Fig. 44-1). Both types of lesions may exist in the same individual.

The exact cause of acne is unknown. The principal factors are follicular hyperkeratinization, excessive sebum production, proliferation of *Propionibacterium acnes* (*P. acnes*), and inflammation secondary to the action of extracellular inflammatory products produced by *P. acnes*. An excessive production and accumulation of sebum appear to be directly related to androgenic hormones and the pathogenesis of acne. Testosterone is converted to dihydrotestosterone in the skin, which increases the size and productivity of the sebaceous glands.[2] Acne begins with sebum accumulation that obstructs the pilosebaceous unit. The mass of accumulated keratinous sebaceous material and bacteria within the pilosebaceous follicle (see Fig. 44-1) causes inflammation when it is exposed to the dermis with rupture of a follicle.

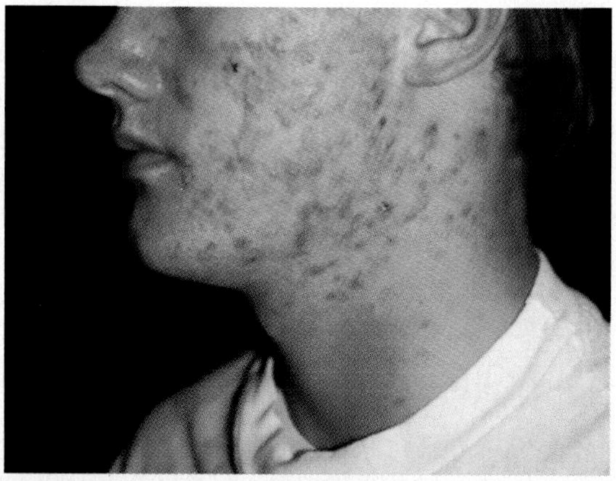

FIG. 44-1 Cystic acne. Multiple pustules (erythematous papules and pustules) are present, and several have become confluent. Note areas of scarring. (Courtesy Department of Dermatology, School of Medicine, University of Utah.)

The *P. acnes* bacteria produce substances that promote inflammation, including chemotactic factors and lipolytic and proteolytic enzymes. The hydrolytic action of the enzymes converts triglycerides into free fatty acids that stimulate inflammation and edema with breakdown of the follicle wall. Chemotactic substance also may be released with mediation of inflammation by attraction of polymorphonuclear leukocytes. Acne conglobata is a highly inflammatory form of acne with the formation of communicating cysts and abscesses beneath the skin. Remissions tend to occur during the summer, perhaps from more exposure to sunlight. External forces—such as cosmetics, use of oral and topical medications, mechanical friction, and occupation—can be etiologic factors. Stress does not cause acne but can make it worse. Self-manipulation of acne must be discouraged because it leads to increased inflammation and potential increased scarring.

Treatment of acne should address these causative factors. Dietary restrictions are not warranted and have no effect on the course of disease. Topical treatment, including topical antibiotics, benzoyl peroxide, salicylic acid, and tretinoin, should be the first line of therapy because it is the least invasive. Use of systemic therapies, including oral antibiotics, sex hormones, corticosteroids, and isotretinoin, should be pursued when first-line therapy fails. Acne surgery, including comedo extraction, intralesional steroids, and cryosurgery, may be useful in selected individuals. Severe scarring may be treated with dermabrasion. With the many successful treatment options for acne which are available, no individual should suffer through severe or disfiguring acne.[3,4]

DERMATITIS

Atopic Dermatitis

Atopic dermatitis (AD) is the most common cause of eczema in children, with a prevalence rate of about 10%. The cause of this chronic relapsing form of pruritic eczema is unknown, but 75% to 80% of individuals with atopic dermatitis have a personal or family history of asthma or allergic rhinitis (hay fever). Onset is usually from 2 to 6 months of age, and 85% of cases occur within the first 5 years of life. There are no specific laboratory features of AD that can be used for diagnostic purposes. An increased serum immunoglobulin E (IgE) level and positive immediate skin tests to a variety of common food and inhalant allergens are seen in approximately 80% of patients. Similarly, blood eosinophilia is a common finding in AD. The basis for the elevated serum IgE levels and eosinophilia in AD is thought to relate to various abnormalities of T cell function, including interleukin-4 production.[5,6]

AD has a constellation of clinical features that include severe pruritus, a long-term course with frequent exacerbations, and characteristic eczematoid appearance and age-dependent distribution of skin lesions. The skin becomes increasingly dry, sensitive, itchy, and easily irritated because the barrier function is impaired. Microscopic epidermal cracks that let water out and irritants and allergens in lead to further drying and cracking, which results in rubbing and scratching. Rubbing and scratching to relieve the itch are actually responsible for many of the clinical changes that are seen (Fig. 44-2). Itching is the hallmark of atopic dermatitis, and the vicious itch-

WHAT'S NEW? Immunologic Treatment Breakthrough in Atopic Dermatitis

Atopic dermatitis is a genetically linked, chronically relapsing, inflammatory skin disease commonly associated with respiratory allergy. This disorder has a complex immunopathogenesis involving both immediate and cellular immune responses. Atopic dermatitis lesions can be clinically classified as acute or chronic; immunopathologic work has been done to determine the difference between the acute and chronic lesion. T cells may be found in uninvolved skin of atopic individuals with dermatitis. These cells are not seen in normal individuals.

Atopic dermatitis has a complex interrelationship with environmental, immunologic, genetic, and pharmacologic factors. Research has been undertaken to clarify the relative contributions of these factors seeking to identify the relevant effector cells and mediators. These factors include the pattern of local cytokine release, the differentiation of helper T cells, multiple roles of IgE, skin-directed cell responses, infectious agents, and superantigens.

This research in immunology and inflammatory skin disease has resulted in the development and approval of a new drug class called *topical immunodulators*. This new class of drugs constitutes the single most important development in the treatment of atopic dermatitis in nearly four decades. Topical tacrolimus (Protopic®), the first medication in this class, was introduced to the United States market in 2001 as a new steroid-free treatment modality. Topical immunomodulators could and likely will, after further testing, be used for other skin-related disease states.

Data from Boguniewicz M et al: A randomized, vehicle-controlled study of tacrolimus ointment for treatment of atopic dermatitis in children. Pediatric Tacrolimus Study Group, *J Allergy Clin Immunol* 102(4 part 1):637, 1998; Leung DYM, Soter NA: Cellular and immunologic mechanisms in atopic dermatitis, *J Am Acad Dermatol* 44(1): S1, 2001. Nicol NH, Boguniewicz M: Understanding and treating atopic dermatitis, *Nurs Pract Forum* 10(2):48, 1999.

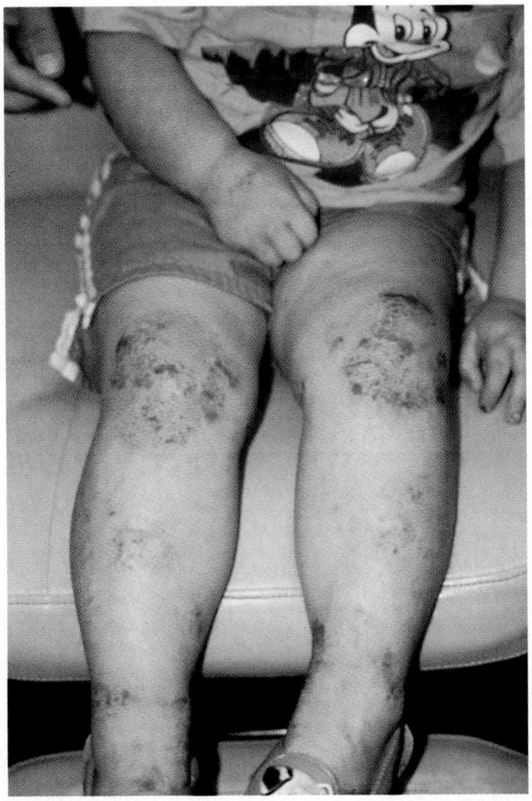

FIG. 44-2 Atopic dermatitis. Characteristic lesions with crusting from irritation and scratching over knees and around ankles. (Courtesy Department of Dermatology, School of Medicine, University of Utah.)

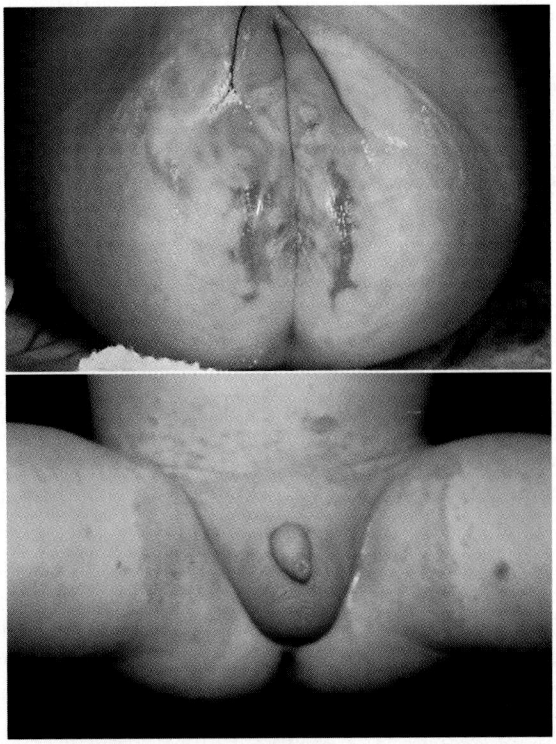

FIG. 44-3 Diaper dermatitis. A, Diaper dermatitis with erosions. **B,** Diaper dermatitis with *Candida albicans* secondary infection. (Courtesy Department of Dermatology, School of Medicine, University of Utah.)

scratch cycle is easily established and difficult to break. The itch continues to be poorly understood. Unlike urticaria, histamine is not considered a major pruritogen in atopic dermatitis.[7] In children the rash appears primarily on the face, scalp, trunk, and extensor surfaces of the arms and legs. In older children and adults the rash tends to be found on the neck, antecubital and popliteal fossae, and hands and feet. Individuals with AD also tend to develop viral, bacterial, and fungal skin infections in the areas with eczema.

Management of patients with AD includes accurate diagnosis and identification and elimination of exacerbating factors, such as irritants, allergens, and emotional stresses. Hydration of the skin is the key to good therapy but is often difficult to achieve. Antiinflammatory agents, such as topical corticosteroids or tar preparations, are necessary during active flares of eczema. In 2001 the first new topical immunomodulator, tacrolimus, was introduced for treatment of moderate to severe eczema. Systemic therapy includes the use of sedating antihistamines and antibiotics. Systemic corticosteroids usually are not warranted in this chronic, non-life-threatening illness.

Diaper Dermatitis

Diaper dermatitis is probably the most common skin disorder of infancy and early childhood. Diaper dermatitis is not a specific disease but rather a variety of inflammatory disorders affecting the lower aspect of the abdomen, genitalia, buttock, and upper portion of the thigh. It is a form of irritant contact dermatitis that is initiated by a combination of factors, including prolonged exposure to and irritation by urine and feces, maceration by wet diapers, airtight plastic diaper covers, and possible increased association with intercurrent illnesses and early introduction of cereals. Disposable diapers do not appear to give any additive protection over cloth.[8] Frequently, diaper dermatitis is secondarily infected with *Candida albicans*.

The lesions vary from mild erythema to erythematous papular lesions. Candidal (monilial) diaper dermatitis is usually very erythematous, with sharp margination and pustulovesicular satellite lesions (Fig. 44-3).

Treatment is changing the diaper frequently to keep the area clean and dry or frequently exposing the perineal area to air. Topical antifungal medication is used to treat *Candida albicans* when present. Short-term use of low-potency topical steroids alternately with antifungals at each diaper change helps to reduce the inflammation. Use of various topical agents to provide a barrier from the irritating agents promotes healing.

INFECTIONS OF THE SKIN

Infectious diseases caused by bacteria, viruses, and fungi constitute the major forms of skin disease. Breaks in the skin integrity, particularly those that inoculate pathogens into the dermis and epidermis, may cause or exacerbate infections.[9,10]

Most infections tend to occur superficially; however, systemic signs and symptoms develop occasionally and rarely are life threatening.

Bacterial Infections

Impetigo Contagiosum

Impetigo is a common bacterial skin infection in infants and children, usually caused by staphylococcus or streptococcus. The disease is more common in midsummer to late summer, with a higher incidence in hot, humid climates. Impetigo is particularly infectious among people living in crowded conditions with poor sanitary facilities. It affects children in good health, but conditions such as anemia and malnutrition are predisposing factors. There are two common types of impetigo: bullous and vesicular. Both start as vesicles with a very thin vesicular roof composed of stratum corneum.

Bullous Impetigo

Bullous impetigo is caused by *Staphylococcus aureus.* The staphylococci produce a bacterial toxin called *exfoliative toxin (ET),* which causes a disruption in cellular adhesion.[11] This form characteristically occurs in newborns and is highly contagious. The source of the infection is usually a staff member in a newborn nursery or a family member with a pustule or who is an asymptomatic carrier. The pathogen is often carried in the anterior nares, perineal region, or fingernails and is transmitted by contact with the individual or contaminated equipment.[12]

The exfoliative toxin stimulates the formation of vesicles, which enlarge or coalesce to form superficial bullae. There may be a few localized lesions or many lesions scattered over the skin. As the bullae rupture, a thin, flat, honey-colored crust appears. The crust is the hallmark of impetigo. A moist, inflamed, serum-weeping base is revealed when the crust is removed. The lesions are often located on the face around the nose and mouth, but the hands and other exposed areas are also frequently involved. Regional lymphadenitis is uncommon.

Vesicular Impetigo

Vesicular impetigo is a contagious, acute, superficial, vesiculopustular form of impetigo caused by group A *Streptococcus pyogenes* (alone or in combination with *Staphylococcus aureus*). The organisms are disseminated by direct physical contact from other infected individuals or through insect bites. The lesions begin as small vesicles with a honey-colored serum. Yellow to white-brown crusts form as the vesicles rupture and extend radially (Fig. 44-4). Untreated lesions may last for weeks and extend to cover a large area. In contrast to bullous impetigo, regional lymphadenitis is common.

The risk of nephritogenic strains of streptococci varies considerably in North America.[13] Aggressive treatment of both patient and patient contacts significantly reduces the chance of acute glomerulonephritis, which is clearly the most significant complication of streptococcal impetigo.

Treatment of choice for both types of impetigo is antibiotics. Antibiotic therapy should be determined by bacterial culture and drug sensitivity. While waiting for these laboratory results, empiric treatment with drugs such as systemic erythromycin or dicloxacillin or topical mupirocin—which give good coverage against staphylococci and streptococci—should be used. Topical mupirocin should be limited to early, small, localized infections. Removal of crusts and scrubbing the lesions with antibacterial soaps have not been shown to be effective.[14] Good hand-washing techniques and isolation of the infected child's washcloth, towels, drinking glass, and linen are important. The highly contagious nature of this disease should be emphasized.

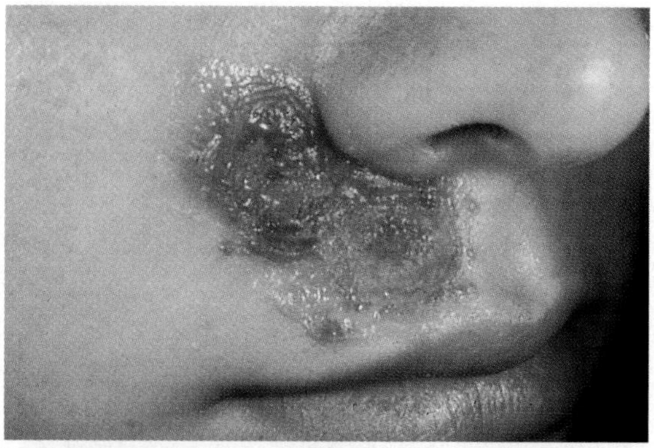

Fig. 44-4 Impetigo and herpes simplex virus (HSV) of upper lip. Note weeping and crusting lesions. (Courtesy Department of Dermatology, School of Medicine, University of Utah.)

Staphylococcal Scalded-Skin Syndrome

Staphylococcal scalded-skin syndrome (SSSS) is the most serious staphylococcal skin infection that affects the skin and usually is seen in infants and children younger than 5 years.[15] SSSS is caused by infection with group II staphylococci, which produce a toxin, an epidermolysin that causes a separation of the skin just below the granular layer of the epidermis. The toxins are usually produced at body sites other than the skin and arrive at the epidermis through the circulatory system. Staphylococci typically are not found in the skin lesions themselves. The syndrome is more common in children younger than 10 years than in adults. Adults have circulating antistaphylococcal antibodies and are better able to metabolize and excrete the toxin. Newborns are at the highest risk because of their lack of immunity (not having prior exposure to the toxin). A case of SSSS in a newborn caused by mother-to-child transmission occurred through breastfeeding when the mother had a breast abscess. Thus breastfeeding should be avoided in cases of breast abscess.[16]

The clinical symptoms begin with fever, malaise, rhinorrhea, and irritability followed by generalized erythema with exquisite tenderness of the skin. There may be an associated impetigo, but the infection often begins in the throat or chest. The erythema spreads from the face and trunk to cover the entire body except the palms, soles, and mucous membranes. Within 48 hours, blisters and bullae may form and the pain is severe (Fig. 44-5). Fluid loss from ruptured blisters and water evaporation from denuded areas may cause dehydration. Perioral and nasolabial crusting and fissures develop. In se-

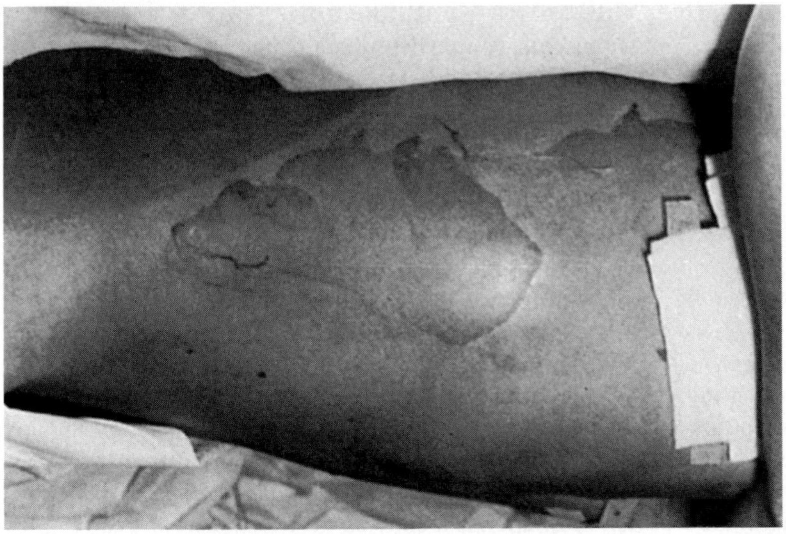

FIG. 44-5 Staphylococcal scalded-skin syndrome (SSSS). The skin lesions, showing desquamation and wrinkling of the skin margins, appeared 1 day after drainage of a staphylococcal abscess. (From Levine G, Norden C: *N Engl J Med* 287:1339, 1972.)

vere cases the skin of the entire body may slough. When secondary infection can be prevented, healing of the involved skin occurs in 10 to 14 days, usually without scarring.

Before medical intervention, culture, histology, or exfoliative cytology must be done to differentiate SSSS from toxic epidermal necrolysis (TEN) (see p. 1480). When the infection is confirmed, treatment with oral or intravenous antibiotics is begun. Topical antibiotics are ineffective. The skin should be treated the same as a severe burn—with meticulous aseptic technique. Special care is required when the lips and eyelids are involved.[17]

Fungal Infections

Fungal disorders are known as *mycoses* and, when caused by dermatophytes (fungi that thrive on keratin), the mycoses are termed *tinea* (dermatophytosis or ringworm).[18] Tinea pedis (a chronic, superficial fungal infection of the skin of the foot) occurs in children but is rare. Most scaling disorders of the toes and feet in prepubertal children are usually eczema (see Chapter 43). Tinea capitis (infection of the scalp) and tinea corporis (infection of the body) are much more common in children than adults. (The different types of tinea are described in Chapter 43.) Dermatophytes may be grouped into three categories based on natural habitat and host preference. Anthropophilic species infect humans, geophilic species are soil-based and may infect both humans and animals, and zoophilic species generally infect nonhuman mammals.[19] These dermatophytes invade the stratum corneum and not the remainder of the epidermis or dermis. The inflammatory response is thought, in part, to be secondary to the toxins released by the dermatophyte. It is important to confirm by culture which microorganism is causing the fungal infection before commencing therapy.

Tinea Capitis

Tinea capitis, a fungal infection of the scalp, is the most common fungal infection of childhood. It rarely affects infants and is seen in children between 2 and 10 years of age.

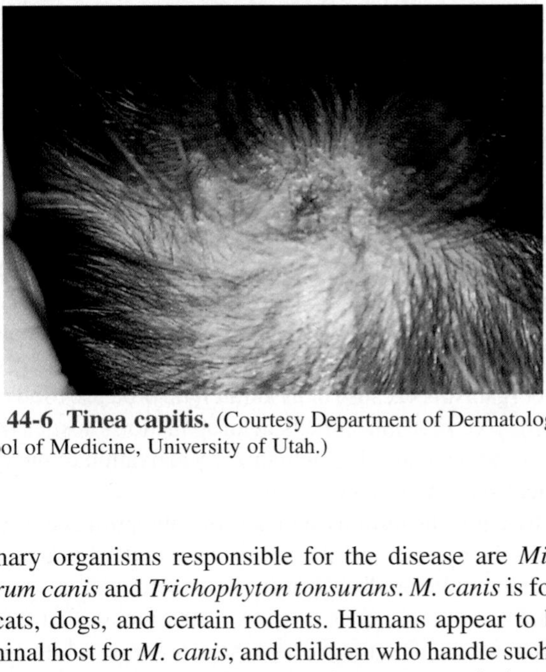

FIG. 44-6 Tinea capitis. (Courtesy Department of Dermatology, School of Medicine, University of Utah.)

Primary organisms responsible for the disease are *Microsporum canis* and *Trichophyton tonsurans*. *M. canis* is found on cats, dogs, and certain rodents. Humans appear to be a terminal host for *M. canis*, and children who handle such animals are possible hosts. Human-to-human transmission does not occur. *T. tonsurans* conversely is transmitted by human-to-human contact. Areas of crowding are the most prevalent environments for this organism, which frequently affects inner-city children. *T. tonsurans* is often the predominant dermatophyte found on inner-city children, and many of these infections are not symptomatic. The prevalence of asymptomatic carriers among household contacts of a child with active *T. tonsurans* disease has been found to be high.[20] Treatment of household contacts with a sporicidal shampoo should be considered and cosleeping and comb sharing must be discouraged. When symptoms are present, the clinical presentations vary, depending on the organism. Frequently the lesions are circular and manifest by broken hairs 1 to 3 mm above the scalp, leaving a partial alopecia 1 to 5 cm in diameter (Fig. 44-6).[21] A slight erythema and scaling with raised borders can be observed.

Diagnosis is best confirmed by performing Wood light examination, potassium hydroxide (KOH) examination, and fungal culture, in that order. *T. tonsurans* does not fluoresce with Wood light examination. Oral griseofulvin is the treatment of choice because topical fungicides do not penetrate to the hair bulb. New agents are currently being tested for resistant strains.[22]

Tinea Corporis

Tinea corporis is a common superficial dermatophyte infection in children. The organisms most commonly responsible for this disease are *M. canis* and *Trichophyton mentagrophytes*. As in tinea capitis, contact with young kittens and puppies is a common source of the disorder. Tinea corporis preferentially affects the nonhairy parts of the face, trunk, and limbs. Lesions are often erythematous, round or oval, scaling patches that spread peripherally with clearing in the center, creating the ring appearance, which is why this disease is commonly referred to as *ringworm*. The lesions are distributed asymmetrically, and multiple lesions (when present) overlap. Potassium hydroxide examination of the scale from the border of the lesions confirms the diagnosis. Most lesions respond well to applications of appropriate topical antifungal medications.[23]

Thrush

Candida albicans infection is a superficial fungal infection that commonly occurs in children. *C. albicans* is part of the normal skin flora in certain individuals and invades susceptible tissue sites if the predisposing factors are not eliminated. *C. albicans* penetrates the epidermal barrier more easily than other organisms because of its keratolytic proteases and other enzymes. *C. albicans* attracts neutrophils to skin sites of invasion and generates inflammation by activation of the complement system within the skin.

Thrush is the term used to describe the presence of *Candida* in the mucous membranes of the mouth of infants and, less commonly, adults. Thrush is characterized by the formation of white plaques or spots in the mouth that lead to shallow ulcers. The tongue may have a dense, white covering. The underlying mucous membrane is red and tender and may bleed when the plaques are removed. The disease is often accompanied by fever and gastrointestinal irritation. The infection commonly spreads to the groin, buttocks, and other parts of the body. Treatment may be difficult and may include oral antifungal washes, such as nystatin oral suspension. Simultaneous treatment of a *Candida* nipple infection or vaginitis in the mother is helpful in reducing the *C. albicans* surface colonization of the infant. Feeding bottles and nipples should be sterilized to prevent reinfection. The diaper area should be kept clean and dry.

Viral Infections

Viral infections of the skin in children are caused by poxvirus, papovavirus, and herpesvirus. The most common infections are described here.

Molluscum Contagiosum

Molluscum contagiosum is a common, highly contagious viral infection of the skin and, occasionally, conjunctiva that affects primarily children. It is transmitted by skin-to-skin contact; autoinnoculation; and fomites, such as clothing, wash devices, and towels. This disease appears to be more common in individuals with atopic dermatitis and a variety of immunodeficient states, including HIV.[24] A poxvirus that induces epidermal cell proliferation causes this disease. The epidermis grows down into the dermis to form saccules containing clusters of virus. The characteristic molluscum body is composed of mature, immature, and incomplete viruses and cellular debris.[25]

The lesions of molluscum are discrete, slightly umbilicated, dome-shaped papules 1 to 5 cm in diameter that appear anywhere on the skin or conjunctiva. The skin distribution in children is mainly on the trunk, face, and extremities (Fig. 44-7). The pubic, genital, and perineal areas are favored in adults (see Chapter 23). Usually, no inflammation surrounds molluscum lesions unless they are traumatized or secondary infection occurs. Scarring occurs with healing.

The best three diagnostic procedures are (1) staining smears of the expressed molluscum body, (2) examining a biopsy, and (3) inoculating a molluscum suspension into cell cultures to demonstrate the cytotoxic reactions. Most lesions are self-limiting and clear in 6 to 9 months if not manipulated. However, because children frequently manipulate these lesions, spontaneous involution may take 2 to 4 years without therapy. The papules can be removed by curette or destroyed with liquid nitrogen. If multiple lesions are present, however, these procedures can be painful to small children and may not be justified. When curettage is used, EMLA® cream used before and after the procedure provides rapid pain relief in children without serious application site reactions.[26] Topical cantharidin can be used to treat these lesions and has been found to be extremely effective and well tolerated with high parental satisfaction.[27] Measures to prevent

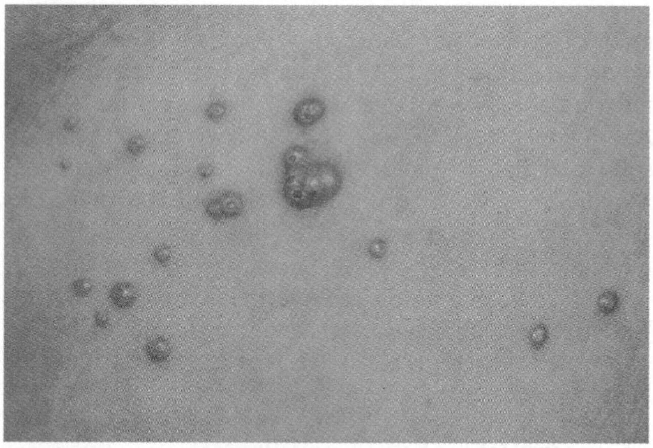

FIG. 44-7 Molluscum contagiosum. Waxy pink globules with umbilicated centers. (From Habif TP: *Clinical dermatology: a color guide to diagnosis and therapy*, ed 3, St Louis, 1996, Mosby.)

spread of infection must be taken. Children must be taught not to manipulate or scratch these lesions. Recurrences are common.

Rubella (German or 3-Day Measles)

Rubella is a common communicable disease of children and young adults caused by a ribonucleic acid (RNA) virus that enters the bloodstream through the respiratory route. This disease is mild in most children. The incubation period ranges from 14 to 21 days. Prodromal symptoms are few but may include enlarged cervical and postauricular lymph nodes, low-grade fever, headache, sore throat, runny nose, and cough. A faint-pink to red, coalescing maculopapular rash develops on the face, with spread to the trunk and extremities 1 to 4 days after the onset of initial symptoms (Fig. 44-8). The rash is thought to be the result of virus dissemination to the skin. The rash subsides after 2 to 3 days, usually without complications. Children are generally not contagious after development of the rash. There is lifelong immunity to rubella—as there is for measles, chickenpox, and roseola—after the disease. Differential presentations of viral diseases producing rashes are given in Table 44-1.

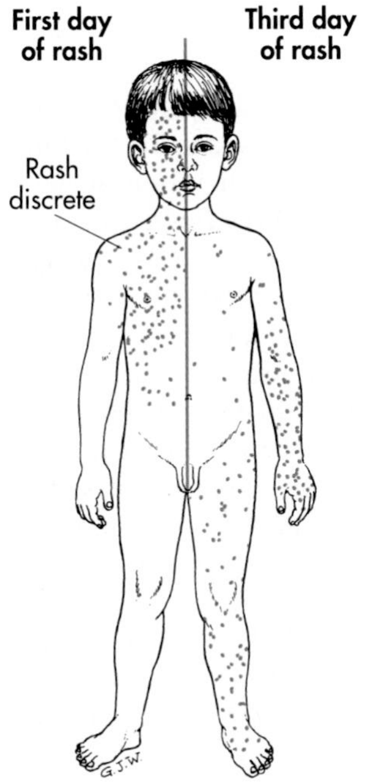

FIG. 44-8 Measles. Full-blown maculopapular rash with tendency to coalesce. (From Wehrle PF, Top FH Sr: *Communicable and infectious diseases*, ed 9, St Louis, 1981, Mosby.)

Vaccination for rubella is usually combined with vaccines for mumps and measles (rubeola) (MMR). Recommendations now state that MMR vaccine should be given at 12 to 15 months of age, so there will not be interference from maternal measles antibody, and again at either 4 to 6 years or 11 to 12 years of age.[28] In the past, parents chose not to give the vaccine because of the misbelief that it would cause the disease. Studies have confirmed that measles or rubella-like illnesses in MMR-vaccinated children are often caused by other viruses.[29] Measles is known to occur in previously immunized children.[30]

Women of childbearing age are immunized if their rubella hemagglutination-inhibition titer is low. Pregnancy should be avoided for 3 months after vaccination because the attenuated virus in the vaccine may remain for this period. Pregnant women who have rubella early in the first trimester may have a fetus that develops congenital defects.

There is no specific treatment for rubella. Recovery is spontaneous, although lymph nodes may remain enlarged for weeks. Supportive therapy includes rest, fluids, and use of a vaporizer. In rare cases a mild encephalitis or peripheral neuritis may follow rubella.

Rubeola (Red Measles)

Rubeola is a highly contagious, acute viral disease of children. It is transmitted by direct contact with droplets from infected persons and is caused by an RNA-containing para-

Table 44-1 Differential Presentation of Viral Diseases Producing Rashes

Viral Disease	Incubation	Prodromal Symptoms	Duration/Characteristics	Clinical Symptoms
Rubella (German measles)	14-21 days	1-2 days Mild fever Malaise Respiratory symptoms	1-3 days Pink-red maculopapular Face and trunk	Enlarged and tender occipital and periauricular nodes
Rubeola (measles)	7-12 days	2-5 days Fever Cough Respiratory symptoms	3-5 days Purple-red to brown maculopapular Face, trunk, extremities	Koplik spots 1-3 days before rash
Roseola (exanthema subitum)	5-15 days	2-5 days High fever	1-3 days Red macular Neck and trunk	Rash develops when fever subsides
Varicella (chickenpox)	11-20 days	1-2 days Low-grade fever Cough May be asymptomatic	7-14 days Red papules, vesicles, pustules in clusters	Eruption of new lesions for 4-5 days Occasional ulcerative lesion in the mouth

myxovirus with an incubation period of 7 to 12 days, during which there are no symptoms. Prodromal symptoms include high fever (up to 40.5° C), malaise, enlarged lymph nodes, runny nose, conjunctivitis, and "barking" cough. Within 3 to 4 days, an erythematous maculopapular rash develops over the head and spreads distally over the trunk, extremities, hands, and feet. Early lesions blanch with pressure, followed by a brownish hue that does not blanch as the rash fades. Characteristic pinpoint white spots surrounded by an erythematous ring develop over the buccal mucosa and are known as *Koplik spots*. These spots precede the rash by 1 to 2 days. The rash then subsides within 3 to 5 days.

Complications associated with measles may be caused by the primary infection or a secondary bacterial infection. Measles encephalitis occurs in about 1 of 800 cases, and most children recover completely. Only a small minority develop permanent brain damage or die. Bacterial complications include otitis media and pneumonia, usually caused by group A hemolytic streptococcus, *Haemophilus influenzae*, or *Staphylococcus aureus* infection.

Measles is prevented by a single vaccination of live attenuated measles virus as previously discussed. There is no specific treatment for measles, and supportive therapy is the same as for rubella. Antibiotic therapy is initiated if secondary bacterial infections develop.

Roseola (Exanthem Subitum)

Roseola is a presumed viral infection of infants between 6 months and 2 years of age, but it can be seen in children as old as 4 years. The incubation period is 5 to 15 days, followed by the sudden onset of fever (38.9° to 40.5° C) that lasts for 3 to 5 days. After the fever an erythematous macular rash that lasts about 24 hours develops primarily over the trunk and neck. Children usually feel well, eat normally, and have few other symptoms. Usually no treatment is required.

Chickenpox and Herpes Zoster

Chickenpox (varicella) and herpes zoster (shingles) are both produced by the varicella-zoster virus (VZV). VZV is a complex herpes group deoxyribonucleic acid (DNA) virus. The incubation period is 10 to 27 days; it averages 14 days. Productive infection occurs within keratinocytes such that the vesicular lesions occur in the epidermis, and an inflammatory infiltrate is often present. Histologically, VZV lesions form intraepidermal vesicles. Infected keratinocytes degenerate, swell, detach from each other, and often contain inclusions surrounded by a clear halo and a circle of darkly staining chromatin. As the vesicle evolves, polymorphonuclear cells enter the vesicle and can lead to a pustular appearance. The vesicle eventually ruptures and is followed by crust formation. On mucous membranes the vesicles rupture and leave superficial, transient ulcers. Varicella occurs in people not previously exposed to VZV, whereas herpes zoster occurs in partially immune individuals who have had varicella.[31]

Chickenpox

Chickenpox is a disease of early childhood, with 90% of children contracting the disease during the first decade of life. It is a highly contagious virus that is spread by close person-to-person contact and by airborne droplets. Introduction of an infected person into a household results in 90% possibility of susceptible persons developing the disease within the incubation period—usually 14 days. Children are contagious for at least 1 day before development of the rash. Transmission of the virus may occur until approximately 5 to 6 days after the onset of the first skin lesions in normal children. In immunocompromised children the virus is recoverable for a longer period, but these children must be considered contagious for at least 7 to 10 days. Chickenpox occurs most commonly in the late winter and early spring. Transmission occurs more readily in temperate climates than in tropical climates.

Healthy children who develop chickenpox have no prodromal symptoms. The first sign of illness may be itching or the appearance of vesicles, usually on the trunk, scalp, or face. The rash later spreads to the extremities. Characteristically, lesions can be seen in various stages of maturation with macules, papules, and vesicles present in a particular area at the same time (Fig. 44-9). The vesicular lesions are superficial and can be easily ruptured. New lesions will erupt for 4 to 5 days, until there are approximately 100 to 300 in different stages of development. The vesicles become crusted, with only the crust remaining, although there may be an occasional vesicle on the palm later in the disease. Although uncommon, ulcerative lesions are sometimes seen in the mouth and, less commonly, on the conjunctiva and pharynx. Fever usually lasts 2 to 3 days and ranges from 38.5° to 40° C.

Complications are rare in children but more common in adults. They can include transient hematuria (from rupture of vesicles in the bladder), epistaxis, laryngeal edema, and varicella pneumonia. One case of chickenpox produces al-

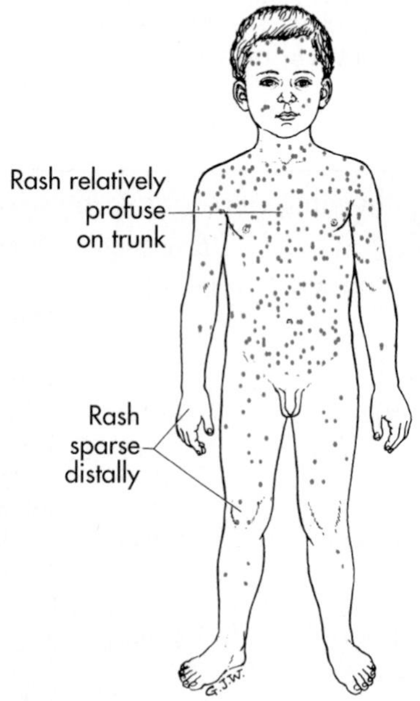

Fig. 44-9 Chickenpox. Generalized, polymorphous eruption. (From Wehrle PF, Top FH Sr: *Communicable and infectious diseases*, ed 9, St Louis, 1981, Mosby.)

most complete immunity against a second attack. The fetus may be malformed (2%) if chickenpox develops in the first trimester of pregnancy.[32] Infants whose mothers have chickenpox at any stage of pregnancy have a higher risk of developing herpes zoster during the first few years of life.

Uncomplicated chickenpox requires no specific therapy. Baths, wet dressings, and oral antihistamines are occasionally helpful to relieve itching and to prevent secondary infection as a result of scratching. Oral antistaphylococcal drugs should be given if secondary bacterial infection is present. Zoster immune globulin may be administered to immunodeficient individuals if given within 72 hours after exposure to chickenpox. Oral antiviral drugs may be valuable in immunosuppressed or other select groups of children.

Chickenpox can now be prevented with a safe and effective vaccine. The American Academy of Pediatrics[33] recommends the chickenpox vaccine for all children between the ages of 12 and 18 months who do not have a history of chickenpox. Healthy children between the ages of 18 months and 13 years also should be immunized with a single dose at the earliest opportunity. Healthy adolescents over 13 years of age and young adults who have no history of chickenpox should receive two doses of the vaccine 4 to 8 weeks apart.

Herpes Zoster

Although herpes zoster (shingles) occurs mainly in adults, approximately 5% of cases are in children younger than 15 years. The course of the disease in children with an immune defect is more complicated and requires intravenous treatment with antiviral agents.[34] The chickenpox virus persists for life in sensory nerve ganglia and reactivates to cause herpes zoster. The eruption of **zoster** consists of groups of vesicles situated on an inflammatory base and following the course of a sensory nerve. Common dermatomal distribution in childhood is thoracic. The base of the lesions frequently appears hemorrhagic, and some of the lesions may become necrotic and ulcerative. In addition to the localized eruption, there are frequently a few scattered lesions resembling chickenpox. Therapy is similar to that for chickenpox unless it is ophthalmic or disseminated zoster, for which systemic antiviral treatment and (when the eye is involved) a referral to an opthalmologist are indicated.

Smallpox

Smallpox (variola) is a highly contagious and deadly but preventable disease. It is caused by poxvirus variolae. Because of worldwide mass immunization, the world is now virtually free of smallpox.[35]

INSECT BITES AND PARASITES

Insect bites and infestations are common causes of skin disorders in children and adults. Skin damage occurs by various mechanisms, including trauma of bites and stings, allergic reactions, transmission of disease, injection of substances that cause local or systemic reactions, and inflammatory reactions from retained mouthparts.

Scabies

Scabies is a contagious disease caused by the itch mite, *Sarcoptes scabiei* (Fig. 44-10, *A*). It is transmitted by close personal contact (see Chapter 23) and by infected clothing and bedding. Scabies is frequently epidemic in areas of overcrowded housing and poor sanitation. Scabies is frequently associated with immunocompromised individuals, such as those with human T-cell leukemia/lymphoma virus I (HTLV-1) and HIV.[36] Infestation is initiated by a female mite that tunnels into the stratum corneum, depositing eggs and creating a burrow several millimeters to 1 centimeter long. Over a 3-week period, the eggs mature into adult mites, which sometimes can be recognized as tiny dots at the end of intact burrows.

Symptoms appear 3 to 5 weeks after infestation. The primary lesions are burrows, papules, and vesicular lesions, with severe itching that worsens at night. Two or three bites, commonly referred to as "breakfast, lunch, and dinner," usually appear in a line on exposed areas of the skin. Itching is

A

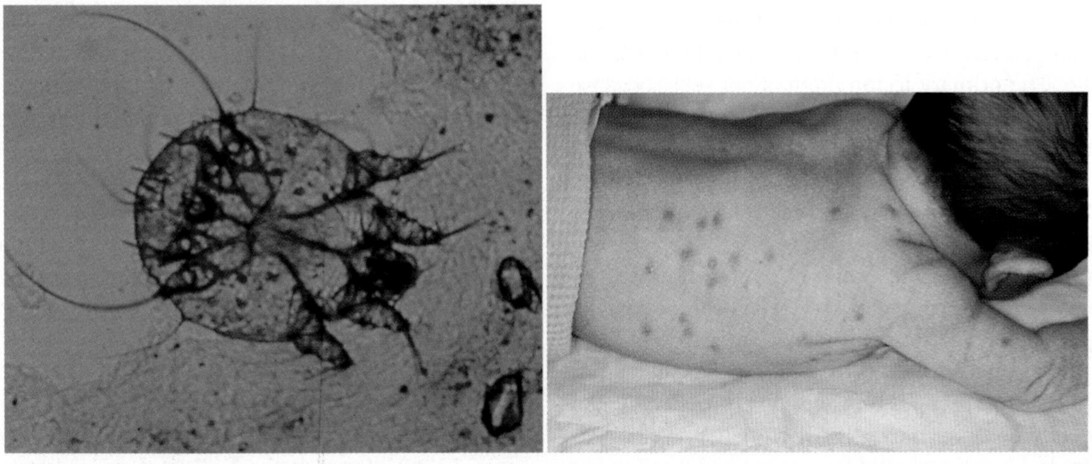

B

FIG. 44-10 Scabies. A, Scabies mite, as seen clinically when removed from its burrow. **B,** Characteristic scabies bites. (Courtesy Department of Dermatology, School of Medicine, University of Utah.)

thought to be related to sensitization to the larval stages of the parasite. In older children and adults the lesions occur in the webs of fingers, axillae, and creases of the arms and wrists; along the belt line; and around the nipples, genitalia, and lower buttocks. Infants and young children have a different pattern of distribution, with involvement of the palms, soles, head, neck, and face (see Fig. 44-10, *B*). Secondary infections and crusting develop from scratching and eczematous changes.

Norwegian scabies is a relatively rare, widespread scabetic infestation with an affinity for severely mentally retarded persons, who are unable to effectively scratch. It is highly contagious and is characterized by heavily crusted lesions on the scalp, elbows, knees, palms, soles, and buttocks.

Diagnosis of scabies is made by observation of the tunnels and burrows and scraping of the skin with microscopic examination of the mite or its eggs or feces. Treatment is the application of a scabicide, such as lindane lotion, cream, or shampoo (Kwell), and is curative. Even with elimination of all viable scabies organisms, itching may persist for 10 days or longer. All clothing and linens should be washed and dried in hot cycles or dry-cleaned.

Pediculosis (Lice Infestation)

The three known types of human lice are (1) the head louse (*Pediculus capitis*), (2) the body louse (*Pediculus corporis*), and (3) the crab or pubic louse (*Phthirus pubis*). They are highly contagious parasites and survive by sucking blood. The female louse reproduces every 2 weeks, producing hundreds of nits as newly hatched lice mate with old. The mouthparts are shaped for piercing and sucking and attach to the skin while feeding. When piercing the skin, the louse secretes a toxic saliva; the mechanical trauma and toxin produce a pruritic dermatitis. Head and body lice are acquired by personal contact, combs, or brushes. Crab lice are spread by body contact, such as contact with an infected adult (see Chapter 23). Sharing clothing is also a common source of transmission.[37]

Itching is the major symptom of lice infestation. In head lice infestation the ova attach to hairs above the ears and in the occipital region. The primary lesion of the body louse is a pinpoint red macule, papule, or wheal with a hemorrhagic puncture site. The primary lesion often is not seen, because it is masked by excoriations, wheals, and crusts. The crab louse is found on pubic hairs but may also involve other body hair such as eyelashes, mustache, beard, and axillae. Young children particularly may become infected with crab lice on their eyebrows or eyelashes.

The live louse, 2 to 3 mm long, is rarely observed, although the ova, or nits, can be observed as oval, yellowish, pinpoint specks fastened to a hair shaft. The ova will fluoresce under an ultraviolet light (Wood lamp) and can be best observed with a microscope. Infestations are easily treated with a pediculicide or scabicide.[38] All clothes, towels, bedding, combs, and brushes should be washed and dried in hot air or boiled, or the clothes should be ironed. Individuals who have close personal contact also should be treated.

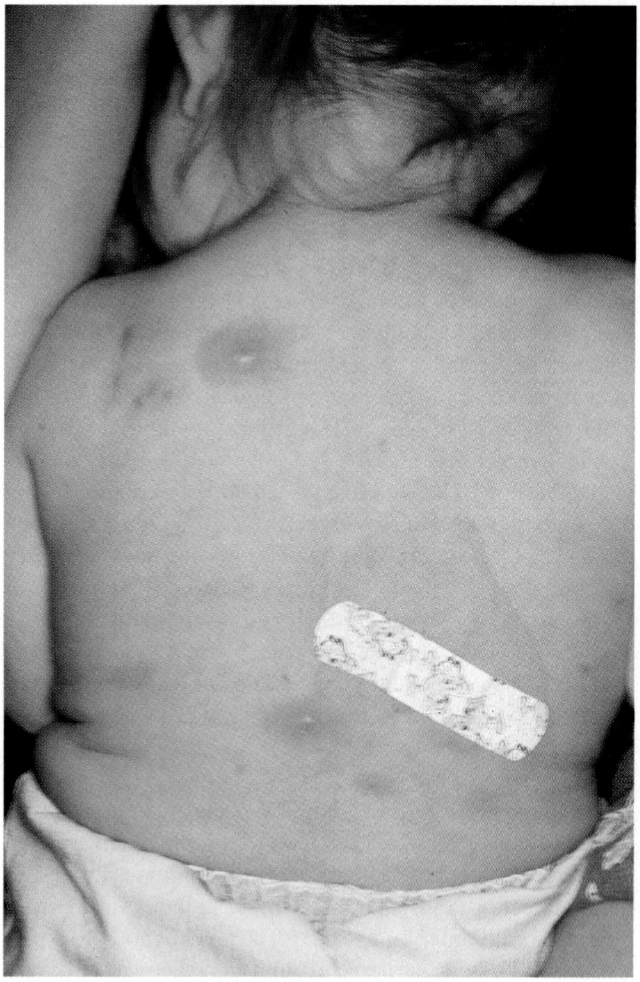

FIG. 44-11 Flea bites. Flea bite producing an urticarial wheal with central puncture.

Fleas

Young children are very susceptible to **flea bites**, and the most common are the bites of cat, dog, and human fleas.[39] Bites occur in clusters along the arms and legs or where clothing fits tightly. The bite produces an urticarial wheal with a central hemorrhagic puncture (Fig. 44-11). Treatment includes spraying carpets, crevices, and furniture with malathion or lindane powder. Infected animals should be treated, and clothes and bedding should be washed in hot water.

Bedbugs

The common bedbug, *Cimex lectularis,* is a blood-sucking, nocturnal parasite of man. Chickens, bats, and some domestic animals are the other hosts for this bug.[40] **Bedbugs** live in the crevices and cracks of floors, walls, and furniture and in bedding or furniture stuffing. They are 3 to 5 mm long and reddish brown. Bedbugs emerge to feed in darkness and attach to the skin to suck blood. Feeding occurs for 5 to 15 minutes, and the bedbug then leaves. It will move long distances to search for food and can travel from house to house.

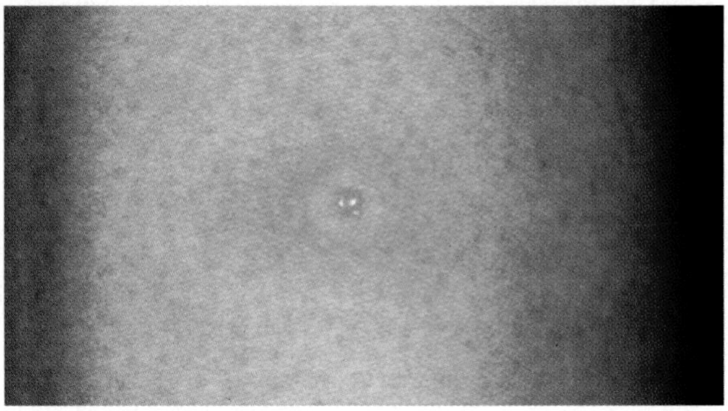

FIG. 44-12 Bullous bedbug bites. (Courtesy Department of Dermatology, School of Medicine, University of Utah.)

If the host has not been previously sensitized, the only symptom is a red macule that develops into a nodule, lasting up to 14 days. In sensitized children and adults, pruritic wheals, papules, and vesicles may form (Fig. 44-12). Secondary infections require treatment. Bedbugs are eliminated by spraying with chlordane or lindane and by cleaning or disposing of bedding, mattresses, and furniture.

VASCULAR DISORDERS

Congenital vascular malformations occur in 10% of all infants.[41] The lesions are developmental in origin, with islands of angioblastic tissue failing to communicate with normal adjacent blood vessels. The most common disorders are strawberry hemangioma, cavernous hemangioma, nevus flammeus, and salmon patches. They are known collectively as *vascular nevi*.[42]

Strawberry Hemangiomas

Strawberry hemangiomas are distinct, raised vascular lesions that may be present at birth but usually emerge 3 to 5 weeks after birth. They proliferate and become bright red and elevated with minute capillary projections that give them a strawberry appearance. Usually only one lesion is present, and it is located on the head and neck area or trunk (Fig. 44-13). After the initial growth, the lesion grows at the same rate as the child and then starts to involute at 12 to 16 months of age. Approximately 90% of strawberry hemangiomas involute by 5 to 6 years of age, usually without scarring.[43]

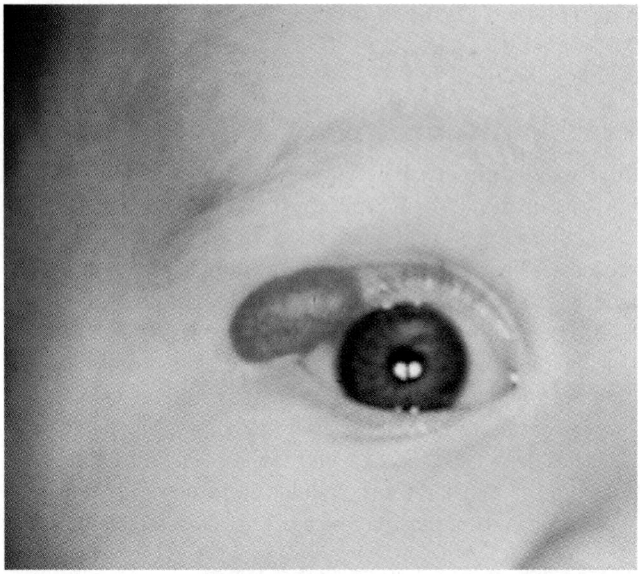

FIG. 44-13 Strawberry hemangioma. (Courtesy Department of Dermatology, School of Medicine, University of Utah.)

Cavernous Hemangiomas

Cavernous hemangiomas are present at birth and have larger and more mature vessels within the lesion than strawberry hemangiomas. Some lesions, however, are composed of a mixture of strawberry and cavernous hemangiomas. They appear primarily on the head and neck area and have a bluish red color with less distinct borders. Cavernous hemangiomas grow rapidly up to 6 months of age and mature by 1 year of age. A period of involution begins and proceeds for 6 to 12 months, with complete involution by 2 to 3 years in 30% of children and by 9 years of age in 90% of children.

Hemangiomas that require treatment are those located near structures such as the eye, nares, auditory canal, or pharynx or those that grow rapidly and are susceptible to trauma or secondary infection (Fig. 44-14). No form of treatment is entirely satisfactory. Surgery, liquid nitrogen, or laser ablation can control bleeding or reduce the size of the lesion, however. The best cosmetic results are obtained when there is spontaneous involution. Ulceration, bleeding, and infection are relatively rare, but cleansing and use of topical antibiotics are effective when they do occur. Open lesions do better when left open to the air, and Telfa dressings are recommended if bandages are required.

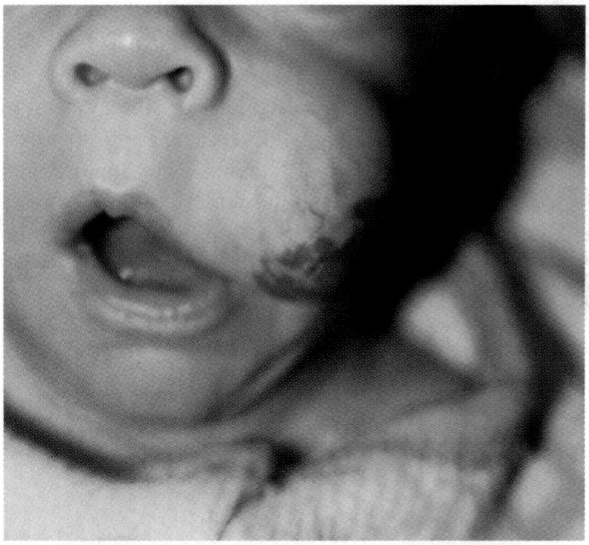

FIG. 44-14 Cavernous hemangioma. (Courtesy Department of Dermatology, School of Medicine, University of Utah.)

Salmon Patches

Salmon patches are macular, pink lesions present at birth and located on the nape of the neck (stork bites), forehead, upper eyelids, or nasolabial fold region. They are one of the most common congenital malformations in the skin. The pink color results from distended dermal capillaries, and 95% fade by 1 year of age. They generally do not present a cosmetic problem.

Port-Wine Stains

Port-wine stains (nevus flammeus) are congenital malformations of the dermal capillaries. The lesions are flat, and their color ranges from pink to dark reddish purple. They are present at birth or within a few days after birth and do not fade with age. Involvement of the face and other body surfaces is common, and the lesions may be large (Fig. 44-15). During adolescence and later adult years, the port-wine stain may become papular and cavernous. Treatments using cryosurgery or tattooing are not very satisfactory. The pulsed dye laser has been used most recently to successfully lighten the color and flatten the more nodular and cavernous lesions.[44] Waterproof cosmetics may be used to cover the lesions.

OTHER SKIN DISORDERS

Miliaria

Miliaria is a dermatosis commonly seen in infants. It is characterized by a vesicular eruption after prolonged exposure to perspiration, with subsequent obstruction of the eccrine ducts. There are two forms of miliaria: miliaria crystallina and miliaria rubra. In **miliaria crystallina**, ductal rupture occurs within the stratum corneum and appears as 1- to 2-mm clear vesicles without erythema. They rupture within 24 to 48 hours and leave a white scale. In **miliari rubra** the ductal rupture occurs in the lower epidermis, with inflammatory cells attracted to the site of the rupture. Miliaria rubra (prickly heat) is characterized by 2- to 4-mm discrete erythematous papules or papulovesicles (Fig. 44-16). Both forms may become secondarily infected, requiring systemic antibiotics. The key to management is avoidance of excessive heat and humidity, which cause sweating. Light clothing, cool baths, and air conditioning assist in keeping the skin surface dry and cool.

Erythema Toxicum Neonatorum

Erythema toxicum neonatorum (toxic erythema of the newborn) is a benign, erythematous accumulation of macules, papules, or pustules that appear at birth or 3 to 4 days after birth. The lesions first appear as a blotchy, macular erythematous rash. The macules vary from 1 mm to 1 cm. When papules or pustules develop, they are light yellow or white and 1 to 3 mm in diameter. There may be few or several hundred lesions, and any body surface can be affected, with the exception of the palms and soles, where there are no pilosebaceous follicles. The cause of the lesion is unknown, and it is self-limiting. No treatment is required.

Toxic Epidermal Necrolysis

Toxic epidermal necrolysis (TEN) is more common in adults but incidence is increasing in children. Hypersensitivity reactions to drugs (sulfonamides, nonsteroidal antiinflammatory agents, anticonvulsants) seem to be the cause of most cases of TEN. The onset of skin eruptions is preceded by malaise; anorexia; fever; and mild inflammation of the eyelids, conjunctiva, mouth, or genitalia. Erythema with tenderness is first described in the axillae and groin, extending over the body surface. Blisters and bullae form, and the entire epidermis may be shed, leaving open, weeping, painful areas of underlying skin. About one third of children have pulmonary complications.[45] TEN must be confirmed by skin biopsy to differentiate from staphylococcal scalded-skin syndrome (see p. 1472) and acute graft-versus-host disease. Skin biopsy shows full-thickness epidermal necrosis and subepidermal blister formation.[46] Treatment requires intensive burn management, preferably in a burn unit. The offending drug must be discontinued.

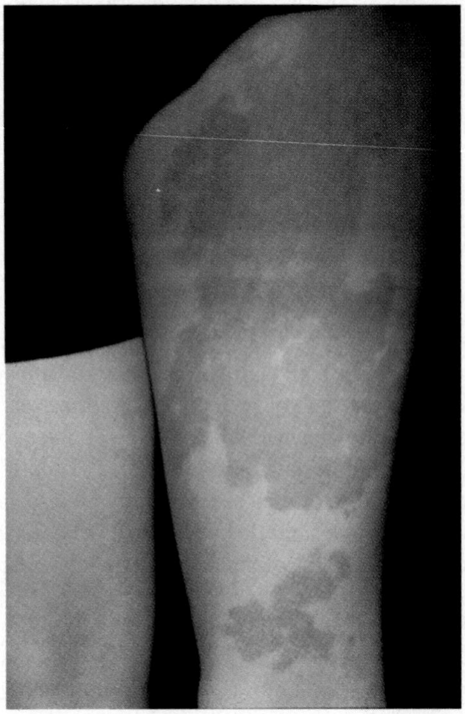

FIG. 44-15 Port-wine hemangioma. Port-wine hemangioma in a child. (Courtesy Department of Dermatology, School of Medicine, University of Utah.)

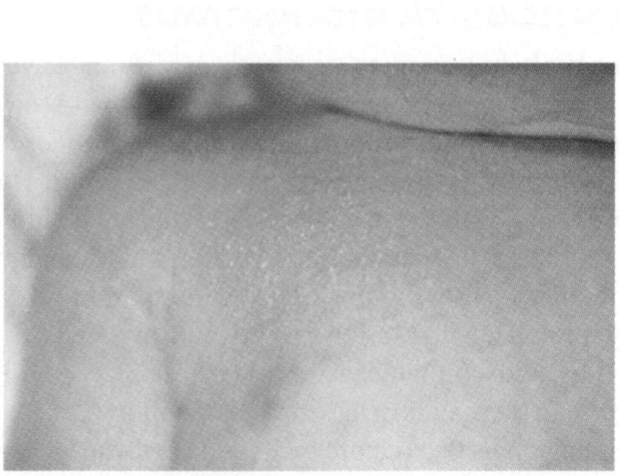

FIG. 44-16 Miliaria rubra. Note discrete erythematous papules or papulovesicles. (Courtesy Department of Dermatology, School of Medicine, University of Utah.)

SUMMARY REVIEW

Acne Vulgaris

1. Acne is a common disorder that affects susceptible pilosebaceous follicles, primarily of the face, neck, and upper trunk. It is characterized by both noninflammatory and inflammatory lesions.

Dermatitis

1. Atopic dermatitis is associated with elevated immunoglobulin E (IgE) levels and a family history of asthma and hay fever. Red, scaly lesions commonly occur on the face, cheeks, and flexor surfaces of the extremities in infants and young children.
2. Diaper dermatitis is a type of irritant contact dermatitis that develops from prolonged exposure to urine and feces and frequently becomes secondarily infected with *Candida albicans*.

Infections of the Skin

1. Impetigo is a contagious bacterial disease occurring in two forms: bullous and vesicular. The toxins from the bacteria produce a weeping lesion with a honey-colored crust.
2. Staphylococcal scalded-skin syndrome (SSSS) is a staphylococcal skin infection that occurs more commonly in young children with low titers of antistaphylococcal antibody. Painful blisters and bullae form over large areas of the skin, requiring systemic antibiotics for treatment.
3. Thrush is a fungal infection of the mouth caused by *Candida albicans*.
4. Tinea capitis and tinea corporis are fungal infections of the scalp and body caused by dermatophytes.
5. Molluscum contagiosum is a poxvirus of the skin that produces pale papular lesions filled with viral and cellular debris.
6. Rubella (3-day measles) is a communicable disease characterized by fever, sore throat, enlarged cervical and postauricular nodes, and a generalized maculopapular rash that lasts 1 to 4 days.
7. Rubeola is a contagious disease with symptoms of high fever; enlarged lymph nodes; conjunctivitis; and a red rash that begins on the head, spreads to the trunk and extremities, and lasts 3 to 5 days. Both bacterial and viral complications may accompany rubeola.
8. Roseola is a benign disease of infants with a sudden onset of fever that lasts 3 to 5 days, followed by a rash that lasts 24 hours.
9. Chickenpox (varicella) is a highly contagious disease caused by the varicella-zoster virus. Vesicular lesions occur on the skin and mucous membranes. Individuals are contagious from 1 day before the development of the rash until about 6 days after the rash develops.
10. Herpes zoster (shingles) is a viral eruption of vesicles on the skin along the distribution of a sensory nerve. Children with immune suppression develop more serious complications.
11. Smallpox (variola) is a highly contagious, deadly disease that has been eradicated worldwide by vaccination.

Insect Bites and Parasites

1. Scabies is an itching lesion caused by the itch mite, which burrows into the skin, forming papules and vesicles. The mite is very contagious and is transmitted by direct contact.
2. Pediculosis (lice infestation) is caused by blood-sucking parasites that secrete a toxic saliva and damage the skin to produce a pruritic dermatitis. Lice are spread by direct contact and are recognized by the ova, or nits, that attach to the shaft of body hairs.
3. Flea bites produce a pruritic wheal with a central puncture site and occur as clusters in areas of tight-fitting clothing.
4. Bedbugs are blood-sucking parasites that live in cracks of floors, furniture, or bedding and feed at night. They produce pruritic wheals and nodules.

Vascular Disorders

1. A strawberry hemangioma is a vascular lesion present at birth that proliferates in size and then grows at the same rate as the child. Most lesions resolve spontaneously by 5 years of age.
2. A cavernous hemangioma is present at birth, has larger vessels than a strawberry hemangioma, and is bluish red. Cavernous hemangiomas usually involute by 9 years of age and may require surgical removal if located near the eyes, nares, or genitalia.
3. Salmon patches are macular pink lesions with dilated capillaries that usually resolve by 1 year of age.
4. Port-wine stains are congenital malformations of dermal capillaries that do not fade with age.

Other Skin Disorders

1. Miliaria is characterized by small pruritic papules or vesicles that result from closure of the sweat duct opening in infants.
2. Erythema toxicum neonatorum is a benign accumulation of macules, papules, and pustules that spontaneously resolves within a few weeks after birth.
3. Toxic epidermal necrolysis (TEN) is similar to SSSS, but the causative agent is usually a drug.

KEY TERMS

REFERENCES

1. Pochi PE et al: Report of the consensus conference on acne classification, *J Amer Acad Dermatol* 24(3):495, 1991.
2. Lucky AW: A review of infantile and pediatric acne, *Dermatology* 196(1):95, 1998.
3. Cargnello JA: Acne: what's new? *Med J Aust* 165(3):153, 1996.
4. Nyguyen QH, Kim YA, Schwartz RA: Management of acne vulgaris, *Am Fam Physician* 50(1):89, 1994.
5. Leung DYM, Soter NA: Cellular and immunologic mechanisms in atopic dermatitis, *J Am Acad Dermatol* 44(1):S1, 2001.
6. Nicol NH, Boguniewicz M: Understanding and treating atopic dermatitis, *Nurse Pract Forum* 10(2):48, 1999.
7. Wahlgren CF: Itch and atopic dermatitis: an overview, *J Dermatol* 26(11):770, 1999.
8. Phillip R, Hughes A, Colding J: Getting to the bottom of nappy rash. ALSPAC survey team. Avon longitudinal study of pregnancy and childhood, *Br J Gen Pract* 47(421):493, 1997.
9. Brook I, Frazier EH, Yeager JK: Microbiology of nonbullous impetigo, *Pediatr Dermatol* 14(3):192, 1997.
10. O'Dell ML: Skin and wound infections: an overview, *Am Fam Physician* 57(10):2424, 1998.
11. 19. Leyden JL: Pathophysiology of certain bacterial diseases. In Soter NA, Baden HP, editors: *Pathophysiology of dermatologic diseases*, ed 2, New York, 1991, McGraw-Hill.
12. Rudy SJ: Superficial fungal infections in children and adolescents, *Nurse Prac Forum* 19(2):56, 1999.
13. Weston WL, Lane AT, Morelli JG: *Color textbook of pediatric dermatology*, ed 2, St Louis, 1996, Mosby.
14. Hacker SM: Common infections of the skin: characteristics, causes, and cures, *Postgrad Med* 96(2):43, 1994.
15. Hoffmann R et al: Staphylococcus scalded skin syndrome (SSSS) and consecutive septicaemia in a preterm infant, *Pathol Res Pract* 190(1): 77, 1994.
16. Raymond J et al: Staphylococcal scalded skin syndrome in a neonate, *Eur J Clin Microbiol Infect Dis* 16(6):453, 1997.
17. Pollack S: Staphylococcal scalded skin syndrome, *Pediatr Rev* 17(1): 18, 1996.
18. Elewski BE: Cutaneous mycoses in children, *Br J Dermatol* 134(suppl 46):7, 1996.
19. Gupta AK et al: An overview of topical antifungal therapy in dermatomycoses. A North American perspective, *Drugs* 55(5):645, 1998
20. Pomeranz AJ et al: Asymptomatic dermatophyte carriers in the households of children with tinea capitis, *Arch Pediatr Adolesc Med* 153(5): 483, 1999.
21. Williams JV et al: Semiquantitative study of tinea capitis and the asymptomatic carrier state in inner-city school children, *Pediatrics* 96(2 part 1):265, 1995.
22. Friedlander SF, Suarez S: Pediatric antifungal therapy, *Dermatol Clin* 16(3):527, 1998.
23. Noble SL, Forbes TC, Stamm PL: Diagnosis and management of common tinea infections, *Am Fam Physician* 58(1):164, 1998.
24. Waugh MA: Molluscum contagiosum, *Dermatol Clin* 16(4):839, 1998.
25. Prasad SM: Molluscum contagiosum, *Pediatr Rev* 17(4):118, 1996.
26. Ronnerfalt L, Fransson J, Wahlgren CF: EMLA cream provides rapid relief for the curettage of molluscum contagiosum in children with atopic dermatitis without causing serious application-site reactions, *Pediatr Dermatol* 15(4):309, 1998.
27. Silverberg NB, Sidbury R, Mancini AJ: Childhood molluscum contagiosum: experience with cautharidin therapy in 300 patients, *J Am Acad Dermatol* 43(3):503, 2000.
28. Watson JC et al: Measles, mumps, and rubella—vaccine use and strategies for elimination of measles, rubella, and congenital rubella syndrome and control of mumps: recommendations of the Advisory Committee on Immunization Practices (ACIP), *MMWR Morb Mortal Wkly Rpt* 47(RR-8):1, 1998.
29. Davidkin I et al: Etiology of measles- and rubella-like illnesses in measles, mumps, and rubella-vaccinated children, *J Infect Dis* 178(6):1567, 1998.
30. Poland GA, Jacobson RM: Failure to reach the goal of measles elimination: apparent paradox of measles infection in immunized persons, *Arch Intern Med* 154(16):1815, 1994.
31. Whitley RJ: Sorivudine: a potent inhibitor of varicella zoster virus replication, *Adv Exp Med Biol* 394:41, 1996.
32. Pastuszak AL et al: Outcome after maternal varicella infection in the first 20 weeks of pregnancy, *N Engl J Med* 330(13):901, 1994.
33. American Academy of Pediatrics, Committee on Infectious Diseases: Recommendations for the use of live attenuated varicella vaccine, *Pediatrics* 95(5):791, 1995.
34. Kakourou T et al: Herpes zoster in children, *J Am Acad Dermatol* 39 (part 1):207, 1998.
35. Ellner PD: Smallpox: gone but not forgotten, *Infection* 26(5):263, 1998.
36. Chosidow O: Scabies and pediculosis, *Lancet* 355(9206):819, 2000.
37. Meinking TL, Taplin D: Infestations: pediculosis, *Curr Probl Dermatol* 24:157, 1996.
38. Bergus GR: Topical treatments for head lice, *J Fam Pract* 42(1):21, 1996.
39. Howard R, Frieden IJ: Papular urticaria in children, *Pediatr Dermatol* 13(3):246, 1996.
40. Huntley AC: Cimex lectularius: what is this insect and how does it affect man? *Dermatol Online J* 5(1):6, 1999.
41. Jacobs AH, Watson RG: The incidence of birthmarks in the neonate, *Pediatrics* 58:218, 1976.
42. Rogers M: The significance of birthmarks, *Med J Aust* 164(10):618, 1996.
43. Low DW: Hemangiomas and vascular malformations, *Semin Pediatr Surg* 3(2):40, 1994.
44. Troilius A, Ljunggren B: Reflectance spectrophotometry in the objective assessment of dye laser-treated port-wine stains, *Br J Dermatol* 132(2):245, 1995.
45. Kim MJ, Lee KY: Bronchiolitis obliterans in children with Stevens-Johnson syndrome: follow-up with high resolution CT, *Pediatr Radiol* 26(1):22, 1996.
46. Rzany B et al: Histopathological and epidemiological characteristics of patients with erythema exudativum multiforme major, Stevens-Johnson syndrome and toxic epidermal necrolysis, *Br J Dermatol* 135(1):6, 1996.

CHAPTER 45

Shock, Multiple Organ Dysfunction Syndrome, and Burns in Adults

KATHLEEN M. BALDWIN • STEPHEN E. MORRIS*

CHAPTER OUTLINE

Shock occurs when the cardiovascular system fails to perfuse tissues adequately, resulting in widespread impairment of cellular metabolism. Because tissue perfusion can be disrupted by any factor that alters heart function, blood volume, or blood pressure, shock has many causes and various clinical manifestations. Ultimately, however, shock from any cause progresses to organ failure and death, unless compensatory mechanisms reverse the process or clinical intervention succeeds. Untreated severe shock overwhelms the body's compensatory mechanisms through positive-feedback loops that initiate and maintain a downward physiologic spiral.

Multiple organ dysfunction syndrome (MODS) is progressive and often the ultimate failure of two or more organ systems following a severe illness or injury. The disease process is initiated and perpetuated by uncontrolled systemic inflammatory and stress responses and is characterized by a hypermetabolic and hyperdynamic state that persists as organ dysfunction develops. For many years the syndrome was referred to as *multiple organ failure* or *multiple systems organ failure*. Gradually it was recognized that the term *organ dysfunction* more accurately describes the syndrome as a process of physiologic deterioration.

Major burns result in extensive immediate tissue injury and thus are a form of trauma with wide-reaching effects on all organ systems. The cause of injury may be thermal contact, flame, chemical agents, or electrical agents; each cause requires a different approach in diagnosis and treatment. Closely associated with thermal burns is smoke inhalation injury, which accounts for about 25% of all burn unit admissions. As a multiorgan problem, thermal injuries can have an overwhelming effect on survival of the burned individual. Regardless of the cause of burns, the result is a final common pathway of physiologic response dependent on the extent of burn surface involvement and depth of tissue destruction.

*Chapter content on "Shock" and "Multiple Organ Dysfunction Syndrome" contributed by Kathleen M. Baldwin; "Burns" contributed by Stephen E. Morris.

SHOCK

Shock can be classified by cause, principal pathophysiologic process, or clinical manifestations. Classification by cause is perhaps the most useful because it suggests the principal pathophysiologic process and focuses on the underlying disorder, which must be treated to prevent the irreversible impairment of cellular metabolism. Shock is classified by cause as cardiogenic (caused by heart failure); neurogenic, or vasogenic (caused by alterations in vascular smooth muscle tone); anaphylactic (e.g., hypersensitivity); septic (caused by infection); or hypovolemic (caused by insufficient intravascular fluid volume). An additional type, traumatic shock, has recently been proposed,[1] which has components of hypovolemic and septic shock.

Cellular Alterations

Because the body is made up of many cells that may function or malfunction at different stages of metabolic impairment, shock causes many diverse signs and symptoms. Subjective complaints are usually nonspecific and may not be particularly helpful to the clinician attempting diagnosis and treatment. The individual may report feeling sick, weak, cold, hot, nauseated, dizzy, confused, afraid, thirsty, and short of breath.

Observable and measurable signs and symptoms often conflict. Blood pressure, cardiac output, and urinary output are usually—but not always—decreased. Respiratory rate is usually increased. Variable indicators of shock include alterations of heart rate, core body temperature, skin temperature, systemic vascular resistance, and skin color. Dyspnea, diaphoresis, and altered sensorium may be obvious.

Impairment of Cellular Metabolism

The final common pathway in all types of shock is impairment of cellular metabolism, which is a complex concept. Fig. 45-1 illustrates the pathophysiology of shock at the cellular level.

Impairment of Oxygen Use

In all types of shock the cell either is not receiving an adequate amount of oxygen or is unable to use oxygen (see Fig. 45-1). In cardiogenic shock, cardiac output is too low to deliver adequate oxygen to the cell. In hypovolemic shock, oxygen delivery is impaired by inadequate numbers of red cells or inadequate volume of intravascular fluid. In neurogenic, anaphylactic, and septic shock, systemic vascular resistance (SVR) is too low and perfusion pressure in the capillaries is inadequate to drive oxygen across cell membranes. In septic shock, hypoxia is made worse by fever, which increases the cell's oxygen consumption rate, and by endotoxic and inflammatory chemical disruption of cell metabolism, which impairs the cells' ability to use oxygen.

Without oxygen the cell shifts from aerobic to anaerobic metabolism. Anaerobic metabolism is a less efficient method of extracting energy from carbon bonds, and the cell begins to use its stores of adenosine triphosphate (ATP) faster than stores can be replaced. Without ATP the cell loses its ability to maintain an electrochemical gradient across its selectively permeable membrane. Specifically, the cell cannot operate the sodium-potassium pump. Sodium and chloride accumulate inside the cell, and potassium exits. Cells of the nervous system and myocardium are profoundly and immediately affected. The resting potentials of these cells are reduced, and action potentials decrease in amplitude. Myocardial depressant factor also decreases the contractility of the heart. A variety of clinical manifestations of impaired central nervous system and myocardial function result.

As sodium moves into the cell, water follows. Throughout the body, the water drawn from the interstitium into the cells is "replaced" by water that is, in turn, drawn out of the vascular space. This decreases circulatory volume. Within the cells, water causes cellular edema that disrupts cellular membranes, releasing lysosomal enzymes that injure the cells internally and leak into the interstitium.

Three positive-feedback loops now begin that further impair oxygen use: (1) activation of the clotting cascade, (2) decreased circulatory volume, and (3) lysosomal enzyme release. First, enzymatic processes are disrupted by the change in the normal ionic and osmotic levels in the cell, as are those processes governed by the physical laws of diffusion. Diffusion of nutrients and wastes into and out of the cell takes longer, and cellular metabolism is further altered. At the same time, diffusion across capillary membranes occurs more slowly as blood flow in the capillary beds becomes sluggish. Sluggish capillary flow decreases tissue perfusion further and activates the clotting cascade (see Chapter 24). The clotting cascade activates the inflammatory response and also accounts for common complications of shock, such as acute tubular necrosis, adult respiratory distress syndrome (ARDS), and disseminated intravascular coagulation (DIC).

Decreased circulatory volume, the second positive-feedback loop, magnifies decreased tissue perfusion in all types of shock. Decreased intravascular volume causes decreased cardiac output in septic shock and further decreases cardiac output in cardiogenic shock. In individuals with anaphylactic, neurogenic, or septic shock and an already dilated vasculature, hypotension worsens as a result of decreased circulatory volume.

The third positive-feedback loop involves the release of lysosomal enzymes. Lysosomal enzymes not only injure the cell that released them, but also injure adjacent cells. By damaging the mechanisms of surrounding cells, lysosomal enzymes extend areas of impaired metabolism and cellular injury.

In addition to decreasing ATP stores, anaerobic metabolism affects the pH of the cell and metabolic acidosis develops. A compensatory mechanism is initiated that enables cardiac and skeletal muscles to use lactic acid as a fuel source, but only for a limited time. The decreasing pH of the cell that is functioning anaerobically has serious consequences. Enzymes necessary for cellular function dissociate under acid conditions. Enzyme dissociation stops cell function, repair, and division. As lactic acid is released systematically, blood pH drops, reducing the oxygen-carrying capacity of the blood (see Chapter 2). Therefore less oxygen is delivered to the cells. Further acidosis triggers the release of more lysosomal enzymes because the low pH disrupts lysosomal membrane integrity.

Impairment of Glucose Use

Impaired glucose use can be caused by either impaired glucose delivery or impaired glucose uptake by the cells (see Fig. 45-1). The reasons for inadequate glucose delivery are the same as those enumerated for inadequate oxygen delivery. In addition, in septic and anaphylactic shock, glucose metabolism may be increased or disrupted because of fever or bacteria, and glucose uptake can be prevented by the presence of vasoactive toxins, endotoxins, histamine, and kinins.

Some of the compensatory mechanisms activated by shock contribute to decreased glucose uptake by the cells. High serum levels of cortisol, growth hormone, and catecholamines account for hyperglycemia and insulin resistance, tachycardia, increased SVR, and increased cardiac contractility. Cells shift to glycogenolysis, gluconeogenesis, and lipolysis to generate

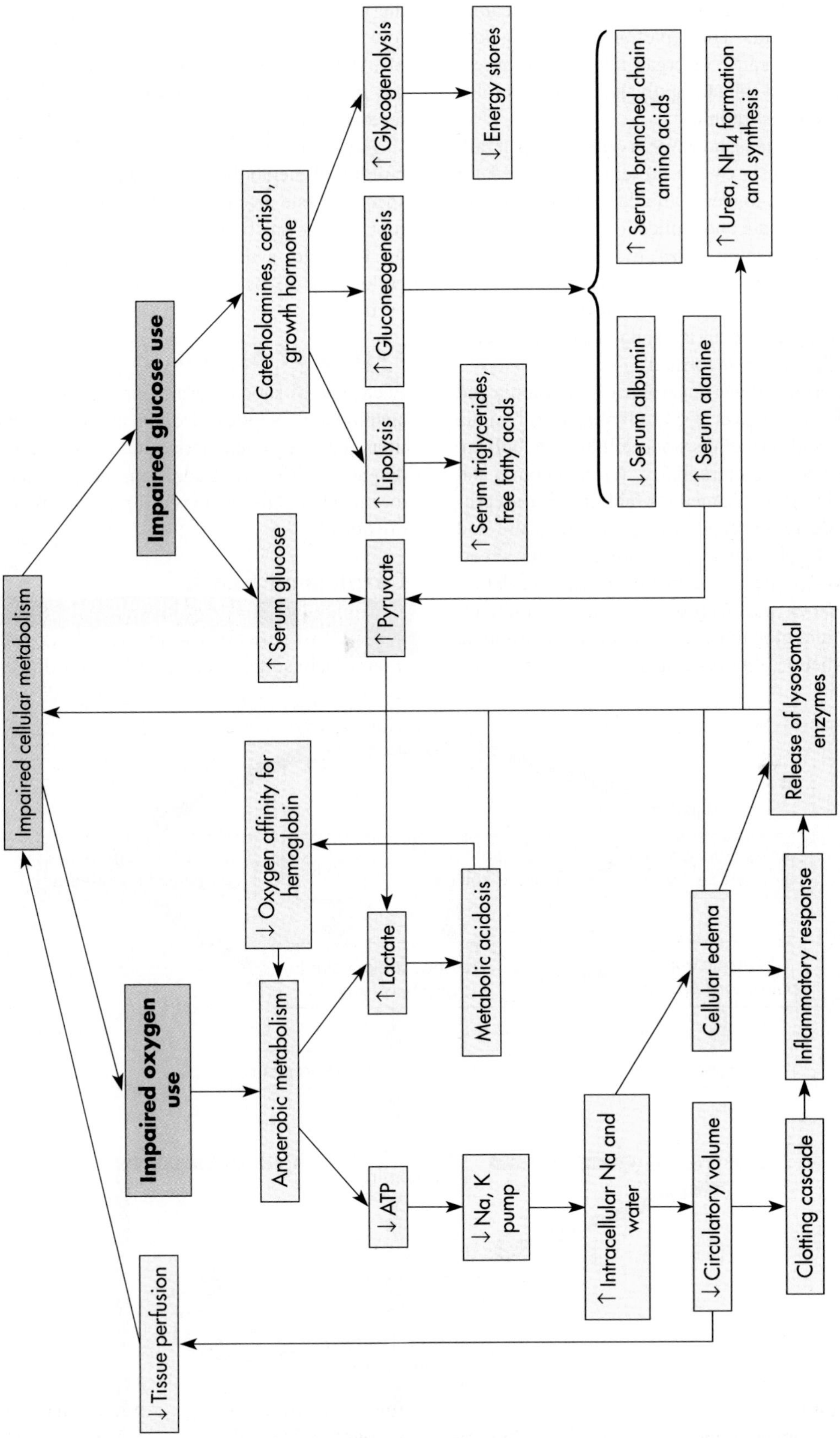

FIG. 45-1 Impairment of cellular metabolism by shock. *ATP,* Adenosine triphosphate.

fuel for survival (see Chapter 1). Except in the liver, kidneys, and muscles, the body's cells have extremely limited stores of glycogen. In fact, total body stores can fuel the metabolism for only about 10 hours. The depletion of fat and glycogen stores is not itself a cause of organ failure, but the energy costs of glycogenolysis and lipolysis are considerable and contribute to the cells' failure.

The depletion of protein is, however, a cause of organ failure. When gluconeogenesis causes proteins to be used for fuel, these proteins are no longer available to maintain cellular structure, function, repair, and replication. The breakdown of protein occurs in starvation states, hyperdynamic metabolic states, and septic shock. Under anaerobic metabolism, protein breakdown liberates alanine, which is converted to pyruvate. In sepsis, pyruvic acid is changed into lactic acid and a positive-feedback loop is formed.

As proteins are broken down anaerobically, ammonia and urea are produced. Ammonia is toxic to living cells. Uremia develops, and uric acid further disrupts cellular metabolism. Proteins are broken down preferentially. Serum albumin and other plasma proteins are consumed for fuel first. Serum protein consumption decreases capillary osmotic pressure and contributes to the development of interstitial edema, creating another positive-feedback loop that decreases circulatory volume. In septic shock, plasma protein breakdown includes breakdown of immunoglobulins, thereby impairing immune system function when it is most needed.

Muscle wasting caused by protein breakdown weakens skeletal and cardiac muscle. Skeletal muscle wasting impairs the muscles that facilitate breathing. Muscle wasting therefore alters the actions of both heart and lungs. The delivery of oxygen and glucose to the cells is directly reduced, as is the removal of waste products, forming another positive-feedback loop.

A final outcome of impaired cellular metabolism is the buildup of metabolic end products in the cell and interstitial spaces. Waste products are toxic to the cells and further disrupt cellular function and membrane integrity. In septic shock, for example, a deficiency in cellular metabolism and the buildup of toxins may precede and cause decreased tissue perfusion.

Types of Shock

Each type of shock (cardiogenic, hypovolemic, neurogenic, anaphylactic, septic) involves numerous clinical manifestations that also characterize many other conditions, making diagnosis difficult. In addition, the body's many compensatory mechanisms can mask, for a time, many definitive signs of shock.

Cardiogenic Shock

Cardiogenic shock results from heart failure from any cause. Most cases of cardiogenic shock follow myocardial infarction or surgery (about 15%) requiring cardiopulmonary

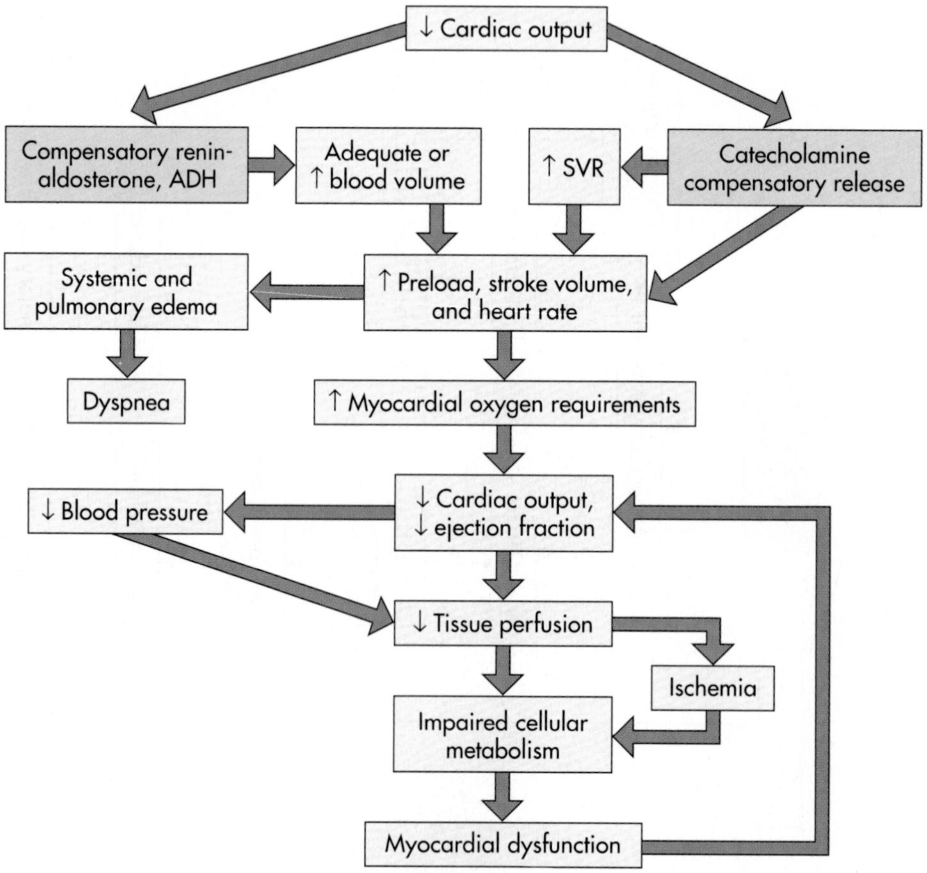

FIG. 45-2 Cardiogenic shock. Shock becomes life threatening when compensatory mechanisms (colored labels) cause increased myocardial oxygen requirements. *ADH,* Antidiuretic hormone; *SVR,* systemic vascular resistance.

bypass.[2] Shock also can follow heart failure from any cause, myocardial stunning, myocardial ischemia, myocardial or pericardial infections, dysrhythmias, tension pneumothorax, and conditions causing excessive right ventricular afterload. Cardiogenic shock is notoriously unresponsive to treatment, with in-hospital mortalities ranging from 50% to 80%.[3] Mortality improves with the use of percutaneous coronary angioplasty and thrombolytic/aspirin therapy following myocardial infarction[4,5] and the use of mechanical assistive devices to improve cardiac function.[2] Age, systolic blood pressure, heart rate, and Killip class have been correlated with increased risk for cardiogenic shock following thrombolytic therapy.[6] The pathophysiology of cardiogenic shock is shown in Fig. 45-2. As cardiac output decreases, renal and hypothalamic adaptive responses maintain or increase blood volume. Blood pressure is maintained through vasoconstriction in response to catecholamine release from the adrenals. Catecholamines also increase contractility and heart rate. Increases in blood volume and vascular resistance succeed in normalizing blood pressure and increasing cardiac performance but at the cost of increasing myocardial demands for oxygen and nutrients. Increasing myocardial requirements further strain the already failing heart, which can no longer pump an adequate volume of blood with sufficient force to perfuse the tissues. The direct effect of decreased tissue perfusion is impaired cellular metabolism. (Normal cellular metabolism is discussed in Chapter 1.)

The clinical manifestations of cardiogenic shock are caused by widespread impairment of cellular metabolism. They include impaired mentation, elevated preload in the systemic and pulmonary vasculature, systemic and pulmonary edema, low cardiac output, dusky skin color, low blood pressure, oliguria, ileus, and dyspnea.

Hypovolemic Shock

Hypovolemic shock is caused by loss of whole blood (hemorrhage), plasma (burns), or interstitial fluid (diaphoresis, diabetes mellitus, diabetes insipidus, emesis, or diuresis) in large amounts. Loss of whole blood or plasma causes hypovolemia directly. Loss of interstitial fluid causes it indirectly by promoting diffusion of plasma from the intravascular to the extravascular space. Hypovolemic shock begins to develop when intravascular volume has decreased by about 15%.

Hypovolemia is offset initially by compensatory mechanisms (Fig. 45-3). Heart rate and SVR increase as a result of catecholamine release by the adrenals. This boosts both cardiac output and tissue perfusion pressures. Compelled by a decrease in capillary hydrostatic pressures, interstitial fluid

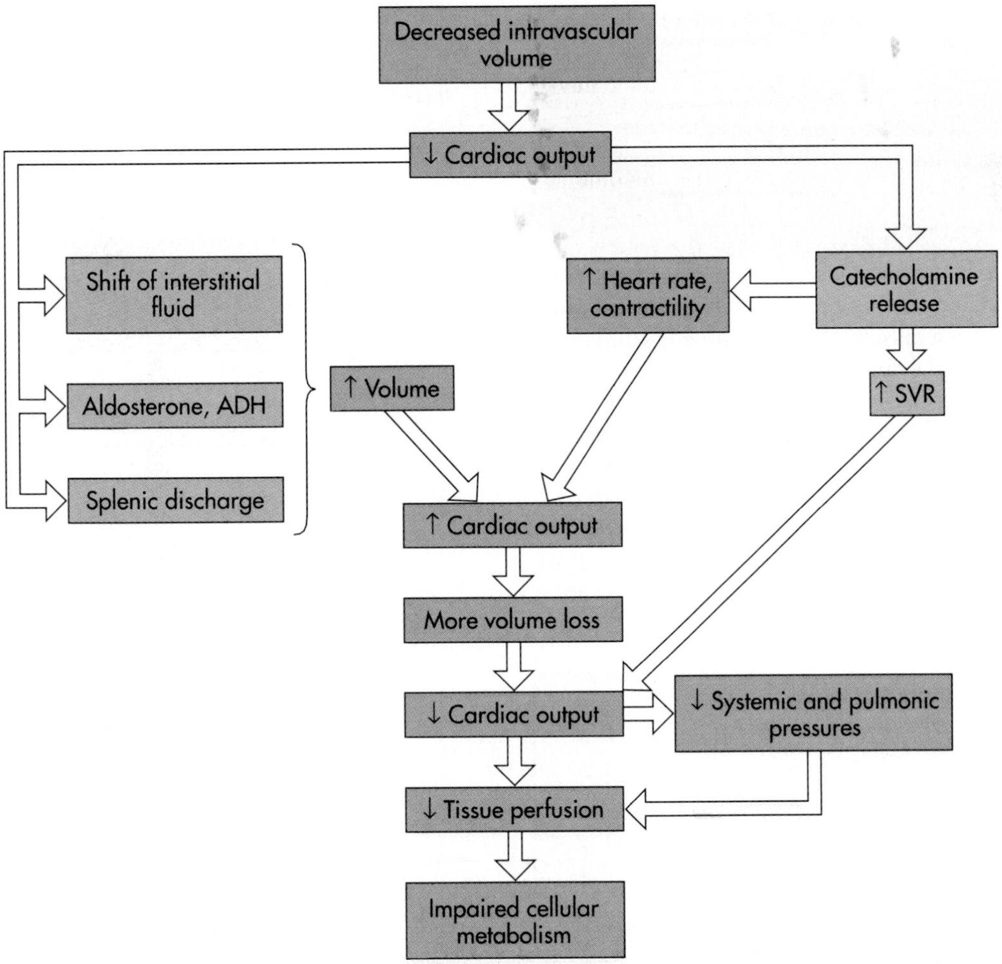

FIG. 45-3 Hypovolemic shock. This type of shock becomes life threatening when compensatory mechanisms *(colored labels)* are overwhelmed by continued loss of intravascular volume. *ADH*, Antidiuretic hormone; *SVR*, systemic vascular resistance.

moves into the vascular compartment. The liver and spleen add to blood volume by disgorging stored red blood cells and plasma. In the kidneys, renin (through several intermediaries) stimulates aldosterone release and the retention of sodium (and hence water), whereas antidiuretic hormone (ADH) from the posterior pituitary gland increases water retention.

These compensatory mechanisms are finite, however. If the initial fluid or blood loss is great or if loss continues, compensation fails, resulting in decreased tissue perfusion. Nutrient delivery to the cells is impaired, and cellular metabolism fails. Mortality for traumatic hemorrhagic shock ranges from 10% to 31%. Prompt control of hemorrhage is the treatment of choice. Fluid replacement is also an important treatment, but the type of fluid used and the rate of replacement are currently controversial.[1] The clinical manifestations of hypovolemic shock include high SVR, poor skin turgor, thirst, oliguria, low systemic and pulmonary preloads, and rapid heart rates.

Neurogenic Shock

Neurogenic shock is sometimes called **vasogenic shock**. Both terms refer to a widespread and massive vasodilation that results from an imbalance between parasympathetic and sympathetic stimulation of vascular smooth muscle (see Chapter 28). Occasionally, parasympathetic overstimulation or sympathetic understimulation persists, causing vasodilation for an extended period. Extreme, persistent vasodilation leads to neurogenic shock (Fig. 45-4). Neurogenic shock creates "relative hypovolemia." Blood volume has not changed, but the amount of space containing the blood has increased, so that SVR decreases drastically; thus pressure in the vessels is inadequate to drive nutrients across capillary membranes, and nutrient delivery to the cells is impaired. As with other types of shock, this leads to impaired cellular metabolism.

Neurogenic shock can be caused by any factor that stimulates parasympathetic activity or inhibits sympathetic activity of vascular smooth muscle. (Parasympathetic stimulation automatically inhibits sympathetic activity and vice versa; see Chapter 28.) Normally, sympathetic stimulation maintains muscle tone. If sympathetic stimulation is interrupted or inhibited, vasodilation occurs. Therefore trauma to the spinal cord or medulla, conditions that interrupt the supply of oxygen to the medulla, or conditions that deprive the medulla of glucose (e.g., insulin reactions) can cause neurogenic shock by interrupting sympathetic activity. Depressive drugs, anesthetic agents, and severe emotional stress and pain are other causes of neurogenic shock.

The clinical hallmark of neurogenic shock is a very low SVR, along with other indicators of excessive parasympathetic activity. Bradycardia is the most obvious manifestation,

WHAT'S NEW? Pyruvate Administration During Hemorrhage

Pyruvate administration during hemorrhage improved cardiovascular and cerebrovascular function, prevented metabolic acidosis, and delayed spontaneous cardiovascular decompensation and death in animal studies.

Data from Morgan PD et al: Intravenous pyruvate prolongs survival during hemorrhagic shock in swine, *Am J Physiol* 277(6 part 2): H2253, 1999.

WHAT'S NEW? Results of Recent Animal Studies on Fluid Resuscitation Following Hemorrhage

1. Resuscitation with whole blood—not packed red blood cells and lactated Ringer solution—restores normal myocardial function.
2. Intrinsic cardiac dysfunction is more closely associated with depth of hypotension than with duration of hypotension.
3. Delayed fluid resuscitation with lactated Ringer solution is equal to and may be superior to convention fluid resuscitation.
4. Controlled fluid resuscitation with lactated Ringer solution or hetastarch increased survival rates when compared to standard fluid resuscitation protocols.
5. A combination of hetastarch and lactated Ringer solution restored mean arterial pressure and prevented early bacterial translocation to mesenteric lymph nodes.

1. Data from Barbee RW, Kline JA, Watts JA: A comparison of resuscitation with packed red blood cells and whole blood following hemorrhagic shock in canines, *Shock* 12(6):449, 1999; *2.* Data from Kline JA et al: Heart function after severe hemorrhagic shock, *Shock* 12(6): 454, 1999; *3.* Data from Novak L et al: Comparison of standard and alternative prehospital resuscitation in uncontrolled hemorrhagic shock and head injury, *J Trauma* 47(5):834, 1999; *4.* Data from Burris D et al: Controlled resuscitation for uncontrolled hemorrhagic shock, *J Trauma* 46(2):216, 1999; *5.* Data from Topaloglu U et al: Hypertonic saline prevents early bacterial translocation in hemorrhagic shock, *Surg Today* 29(1):47, 1999.

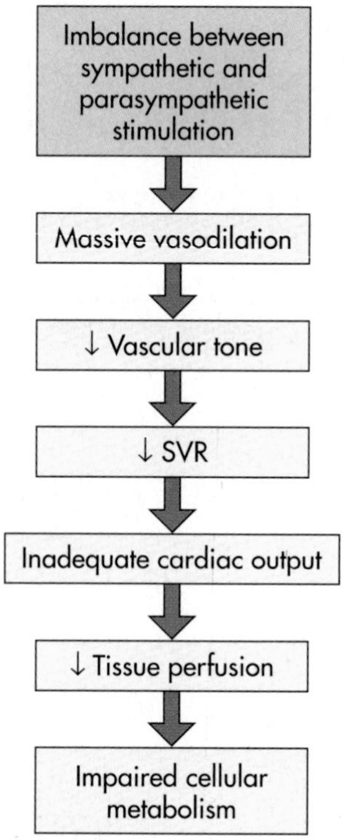

FIG. 45-4 Neurogenic shock. *SVR*, Systemic vascular resistance.

especially in the early stages. Bradycardia may cease when compensatory mechanisms, particularly an increase in sympathetic system activity, have been initiated. The ejection fraction remains high, indicating a healthy myocardium, whereas central venous pressure decreases as the veins dilate. Neurogenic shock causes fainting if blood pressure decreases to the point that cerebral metabolism is not sufficient to support consciousness. Most episodes of fainting are *not* shock, however; for such episodes to progress to shock is rare. By allowing the blood pressure to equalize from head to toe as the individual becomes prone, fainting can actually prevent shock.

Anaphylactic Shock

Anaphylactic shock is the outcome of a widespread hypersensitivity reaction known as *anaphylaxis*. The basic physiologic alteration in anaphylactic shock is the same as that in neurogenic shock—that is, vasodilation, peripheral pooling, and relative hypovolemia leading to decreased tissue perfusion and impaired cellular metabolism (Fig. 45-5). Anaphylactic shock is often more severe than other types of normovolemic shock because the hypersensitivity reaction that triggers vasodilation has other pathophysiologic effects that rapidly involve the entire body.

Anaphylactic shock begins as an allergic reaction—an immune and inflammatory response—to an allergen. (An allergen is an antigen to which an individual is hypersensitive; see Chapters 6, 7, and 8 for discussions of immunity, inflammation, and hypersensitivity.) Some allergens known to cause hypersensitivity reactions are snakebite venom, insect venoms, pollens, shellfish, penicillin, and animal sera. Once in the body, the allergen causes an extensive immune and inflammatory response. The vascular effects of this response include vasodilation and increased vascular permeability, resulting in peripheral pooling and tissue edema. The extravascular effects include constriction of extravascular smooth muscle. Constriction often causes respiratory difficulty because it tends to affect smooth muscle layers in the airway walls (e.g., the larynx and bronchioles; see Chapter 31).

The onset of anaphylactic shock is usually sudden, and progression to death can occur within minutes unless emergency treatment is given. The first manifestations of shock may be anxiety, difficulty in breathing, gastrointestinal cramps, edema, hives (urticaria), and sensations of burning or itching of the skin. A precipitous decrease in blood pressure occurs and is followed by impaired mentation. Other signs include decreased SVR (with high or normal cardiac output)

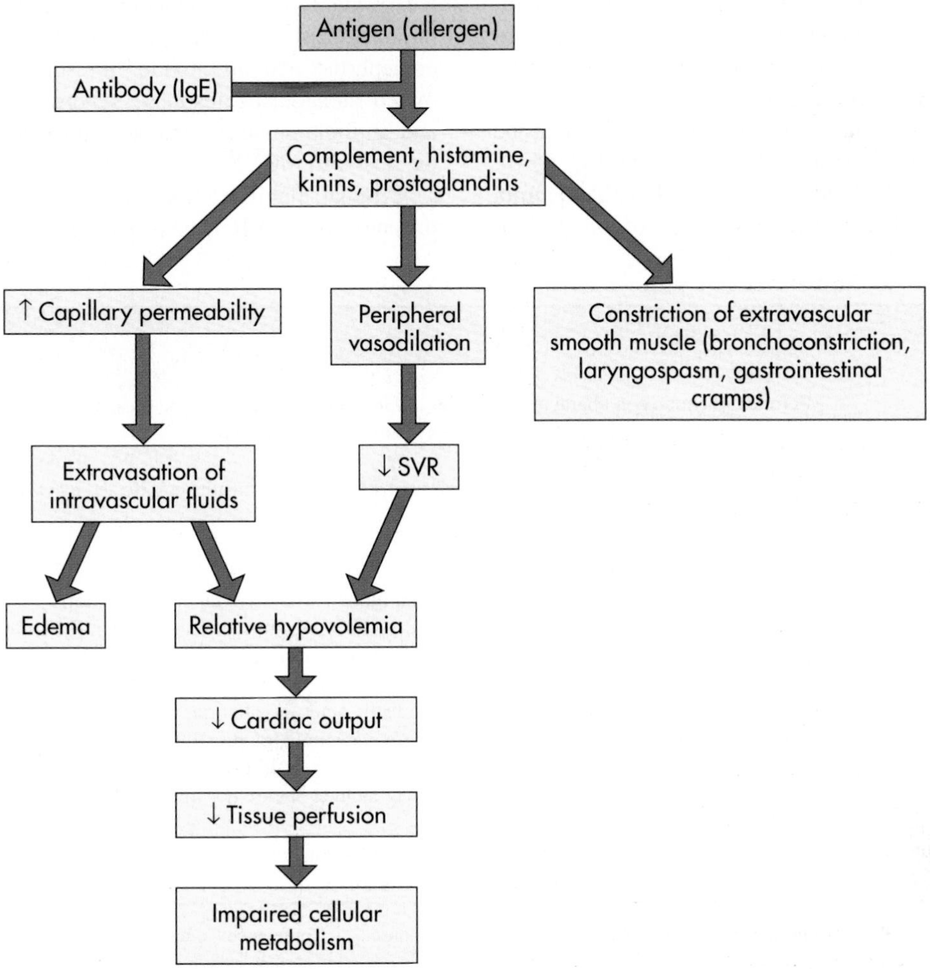

FIG. 45-5 Anaphylactic shock. *IgE*, Immunoglobulin E; *SVR*, systemic vascular resistance.

and oliguria. Treatment begins with removal of the antigen (if possible). Epinephrine is administered to cause vasoconstriction and reverse airway constriction. Volume expanders (e.g., lactated Ringer solution) are given intravenously to reverse the relative hypovolemia, and antihistamines and steroids are given to stop the inflammatory reaction.

Septic Shock

Septic shock is one component of a continuum of progressive dysfunction called the *systemic inflammatory response syndrome (SIRS)*. The syndrome begins with an infection that progresses to bacteremia, then sepsis, then severe sepsis, then septic shock, and then multiple organ dysfunction syndrome (MODS). Consensus on definitions of each component was achieved in 1992,[7] and these definitions are presented in Table 45-1.

Septicemia is the thirteenth most common cause of death in the United States and the leading cause of death of individuals in noncoronary intensive care units.[8] Mortality ranges from 20%[9,10] to 95%.[11] Septic shock is caused most often by gram-negative bacteria, but it can occur from gram-positive bacteria and fungi. Despite advances in antibiotic therapy, gram-negative sepsis has increased dramatically in the past 20 years. Even when properly treated with available therapies, it carries a 35% to 44% crude mortality rate.[8] Prognosis is significantly affected by the source and virulence of the infectious microorganism. Gram-negative sepsis and nosocomial infections result in higher mortality than gram-positive sepsis and community-acquired infections.[12]

Septic shock begins with a nidus of infection that may be readily discernible or extremely difficult to locate (Fig. 45-6). Bacteria then enter the bloodstream to produce bacteremia in one of two ways: (1) directly from the site of infection or (2) from toxic substances released by the bacteria directly into the bloodstream. These toxic substances, which act as triggering molecules in the septic syndrome, include endotoxins released by gram-negative microorganisms,[13] lipoteichoic acids and peptidoglycan released by gram-positive microorganisms, and superantigens.[14,15]

The triggering molecules cause the host to initiate a proinfammatory response. Proinflammatory cells released include polymorphonuclear leukocytes, macrophages, monocytes, and platelets. Proinflammatory mediators released include cytokines (interleukins IL-1, IL-2, IL-6, IL-8, and IL–15; tumor necrosis factor–α; and granulocyte cell–stimulating factor), complement and complement cascade activation, kinins, arachidonic acid metabolites (prostaglandins, prostacyclin, leukotrines, and thromboxane), soluble adhesion molecules, platelet-activating factor, endorphins, vasoactive neuropeptides, histamine, seratonin, monocyte chemoattractant proteins 1 and 2, protolytic enzymes (e.g., elastase and lysosomal enzymes), protein kinase, tyrosine kinase, CD-14, toxic oxygen metabolites (e.g., superoxide, hydroxyl radical, hydrogen peroxide, peroxynitrite), neopterin, and clotting cascade activation.[16] A compensatory antiinflammatory response syndrome is presumed to follow this response.[16,17] Antiinflammatory mediators released include lipopolysaccaride-binding protein; IL-1 receptor antagonist; soluble CD-14; type 2 IL-1 receptor; leukotrine B_4 receptor antagonist; IL-4, IL-10, and -13; soluble tumor necrosis factor receptor; transforming growth factor–β; epinephrine; and nitric oxide.[16] Presumably the end result is a mixed antagonistic response syndrome as proinflammatory and antiinflammatory mediators respond, intensify, and lead the host into MODS.

Clinical manifestations of septic shock are low arterial pressure, low SVR from vasodilation, and an alteration in

Table 45-1 Causes and Definitions of Septic Shock

Cause	Definition
Infection	Microbial phenomenon characterized by an inflammatory response to the presence of microorganisms or the invasion of normally sterile host tissue by those microorganisms
Bacteremia	Presence of viable bacteria in the blood
Systemic inflammatory response syndrome	A systemic inflammatory response to a variety of severe clinical insults manifested by two or more of the following signs: Temperature >38° C or <36° C Heart rate >90 beats/min Respiratory rate >20 breaths/min or arterial blood carbon dioxide level <32 torr White blood cell count >12,000 cells/mm³ <4000 cells/mm³ or containing <10% immature forms (bands)
Sepsis	The systemic response to infections manifested by two or more of the signs listed above
Severe sepsis	Sepsis associated with organ dysfunction, hypoperfusion, or hypotension; hypoperfusion and percussion abnormalities may include but are not limited to lactic acidosis, oliguria, or an acute alteration in mental status
Septic shock	Sepsis with hypotension (systolic blood pressure <90 mm Hg or a reduction >40 mm Hg from baseline) in the absence of other causes for hypotension; this occurs despite adequate fluid resuscitation, along with the presence of perfusion abnormalities that may include but are not limited to lactic acidosis, oliguria, or an active alteration in mental status
Multiple organ dysfunction syndrome	Presence of altered organ function in an acutely ill individual such that homeostasis cannot be maintained without intervention

From American College of Chest Physicians/Society of Critical Care Medicine Consensus Conference Committee: *Crit Care Med* 20(6):864, 1992.

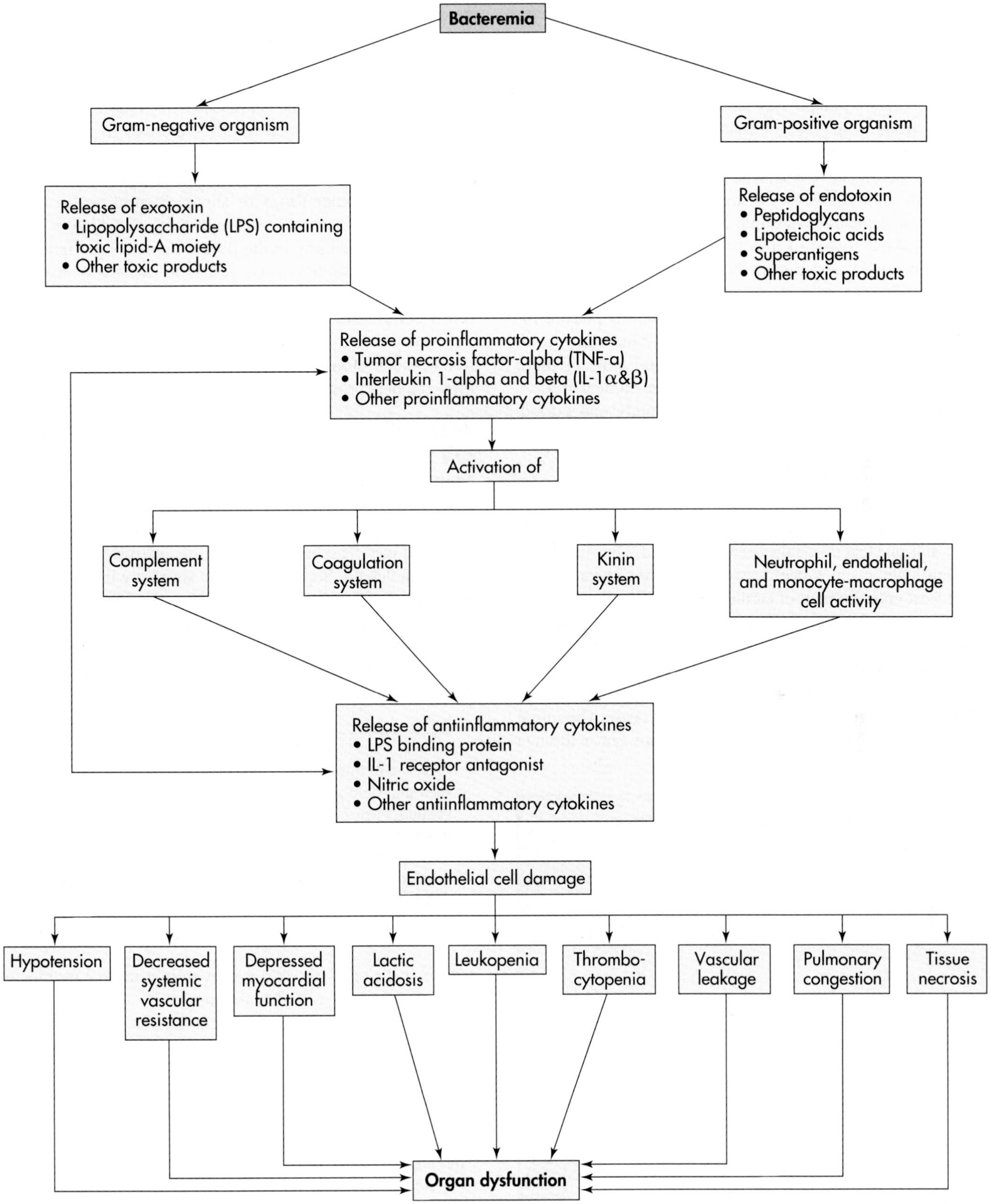

FIG. 45-6 Septic shock cascade. (From Larson V, Barke RA: Gram-negative bacterial sepsis and the sepsis syndrome, *Urol Clin No Amer* 26(4):687, 1999.)

oxygen extraction by all cells. Tachycardia causes cardiac output to remain normal or become elevated, although myocardial contractility is reduced. Temperature instability is present, ranging from hyperthermia to hypothermia. Effects on other organ systems may result in deranged renal function, gastrointestinal mucosa changes that result in release of bacteria from the gut, jaundice, clotting abnormalities, deterioration of mental status, and tachypnea that often progresses to acute respiratory distress syndrome.

Treatment includes multiple drug antimicrobial therapy, removal of the source of infection if one is found, fluid resuscitation, and vasoactive medications to improve hemodynamic performance. Experimental treatment under study includes high-dose corticosteroids; continuous plasma filtration;[18] and immunomodulating therapy,[19] including monoclonal antibodies and vaccines.[20] To date, none of these therapies have proven to be beneficial in clinical trials.[21] Because the septic syndrome is incompletely understood, recommended treatment continues to evolve.

Treatment for Shock

The first treatment for shock is to discover and correct or remove the underlying cause. Although this seems a simple tenet, it is one that is not always remembered. Thus treatment for cardiogenic shock begins with treatment of heart failure or at least enhancement of cardiac output. If hypovolemia is the cause of shock, hemorrhage and other causes of fluid loss must be stopped. In neurogenic shock as a result of spinal cord trauma, stabilization of the spine and surrounding tissue is a beginning, and pain usually can be decreased to a level at which neurally mediated decreases of SVR cease. The initial treatment for anaphylactic shock is to remove or neutralize the antigen. Treatment for septic shock begins with eradication of the infective agent, usually with antimicrobials.

After the underlying cause or condition is corrected as far as possible, treatment is supportive. Intravenous fluid is administered to expand intravascular volume, except in cardiogenic shock, which requires diuresis to reduce preload. Supplemental oxygen is always given. Cardiotonic drugs are given early in cardiogenic shock, and they are given later in other forms of shock. Steroid use in septic shock remains unproven, although there is evidence that a single, high dose early in the illness improves mortality.[22,23] Stress ulcer prophylaxis and gastric tonemetry, to measure splanchnic blood flow, are imperative because the gut is currently believed to be the driver of the septic syndrome.[23]

Once positive-feedback loops are established, intervention in shock is difficult. Prevention and very early treatment offer the best prognosis.

WHAT'S NEW? Current Understanding of Sepsis

1. Despite intensive research in the past 10 years, the incidence and prevalence of sepsis is increasing.
2. The syndrome is quite heterogenous, with many paths leading to septic shock; thus finding a "magic bullet" that will treat all individuals is not likely.
3. Animal models have not proved useful in assessing drug treatments for sepsis; what works in lower-order species doe not work in humans.
4. The microbiology of sepsis is very complex and controlled by multiple microbial mediators.
5. Sepsis has an intricate and dynamic immunopathogenesis.
6. Outcomes for individuals with sepsis hinge on many host-specific factors in addition to the sepsis itself.
7. Definitions for systemic inflammatory response syndrome sepsis and septic shock are not mutually exclusive, making exact diagnosis difficult.
8. Most clinical trials have small samples and are underpowered, making findings questionable.
9. Setting an arbitrary mortality end point of 28 days in clinical trials has been ineffective in adequately assessing interventions.

Data from Opal SM, Cross AS: Clinical trials for severe sepsis past failures, and future hopes, *Inf Dis Clin No Amer* 13(2):285, 1999.

MULTIPLE ORGAN DYSFUNCTION SYNDROME

Multiple organ dysfunction syndrome (MODS) is the progressive dysfunction of two or more organ systems resulting from an uncontrolled inflammatory response to a severe illness or injury. The organ dysfunction can progress to organ failure and death. Sepsis and septic shock are the most common causes of MODS. In 1991 a consensus conference was sponsored by the American College of Chest Physicians and the Society of Critical Care Medicine to develop a set of definitions for sepsis and related disorders (see Table 45-1). At the conference, MODS was defined as follows:[24]

> Presence of altered organ function in an acutely ill person, such that homeostasis cannot be maintained without intervention. Primary MODS is the direct result of a well-defined insult in which organ dysfunction occurs early and can be directly attributable to the insult itself. Secondary MODS develops as a consequence of a host response and is identified within the context of SIRS.

MODS is the end stage of a variety of injuries that terminate in severe, generalized inflammation.

MODS is a relatively new diagnosis, first recognized as a distinct clinical syndrome in the mid-1970s,[25,26] when advances in resuscitation and support technologies allowed many individuals to survive life-threatening illness or trauma only to die of complications of their disease. Today MODS is a leading cause of mortality in surgical intensive care units.[27] Mortality for individuals with MODS is between 45% and 55% for failure of two organ systems; it is higher than 80% when three or more organ systems have failed; and it approaches 100% if the failure of three or more organs persists longer than 4 days.[28] Moreover, mortality has not improved much over the past 15 to 20 years.[8]

Although sepsis and septic shock are the most common causes, MODS can be initiated by any severe injury or disease process that activates a massive systemic inflammatory response by the host. Documented clinical infection is not necessary for its development. Other common triggers are severe trauma, major surgery, burns, circulatory shock, acute pancreatitis, acute renal failure, ARDS, persistent inflammatory foci, and necrotic tissue. MODS is the major cause of death following septic shock, trauma, burn injuries, and ARDS. People at greatest risk for developing MODS are elderly individuals and persons with significant tissue injury or preexisting disease.[29,30] Risk factors for the development of MODS are as follows:

- Age 65 years or older
- Baseline organ dysfunction (e.g., renal insufficiency)
- Bowel infarction
- Coma on admission
- Inadequate, delayed resuscitation
- Malnutrition
- Multiple blood transfusions (more than 6 units per 12 hr)
- Age of packed red blood cells infused during the first 6 hours postinjury[31]
- Persistent infectious focus
- Preexisting chronic disease (e.g., cancer, diabetes)
- Presence of hematoma
- Significant tissue injury
- Steroids

Pathophysiology

In **primary MODS** the organ injury is directly associated with a specific insult, most often ischemia or impaired perfusion from an episode of shock or trauma, thermal injury, soft tissue necrosis, or invasive infection.[27] This decreased perfusion is both local (in the injured organs themselves) and generalized. The generalized hypoperfusion in primary MODS usually cannot be detected clinically. As a result of the insult, a stress response is initiated and stress hormones—in particular, catecholamines—are released. The inflammatory and stress responses are not as evident as in secondary MODS. However, during the inflammatory response in primary MODS it is thought that neutrophils and macrophages are "primed" by cytokines.[27] Any second insult, such as additional tissue injury, infection, or organ ischemia, may then activate the primed cells to produce an exaggerated response of secondary MODS (Fig. 45-7).

The progressive organ dysfunction of **secondary MODS** is the result of an excessive inflammatory reaction, after a latent period following the initial injury, in organs distant from the site of the original injury. It is postulated that the resulting organ trauma is caused by the host response to a second insult rather than being a direct result of the primary injury. Often the second insult is mild but produces a disproportionate response because of the previous priming of leukocytes. The interaction of injured organs then leads to a self-perpetuating inflammation. For example, injured lungs produce large amounts of inflammatory mediators that are released into the circulation and can activate inflammation in virtually all other organs.[32]

Secondary MODS is initiated as primed macrophages release a barrage of mediators, particularly the cytokines tumor necrosis factor (TNF) and IL-1, when stimulated by the delayed postinjury insult. These mediators damage the endothelium throughout the body. If a gram-negative bacterial infection is present, endotoxin released from the bacteria also causes severe damage to endothelial cells. Normal endothelial cells have little interaction with leukocytes, but, when stimulated by TNF, IL-1, or endotoxin, they change to a proinflammatory state and express adhesion molecules that mediate adhesion of neutrophils. The adhered neutrophils then migrate through the endothelium, aggregate in the area of damaged tissue, and amplify the inflammation.[29,30] The activated endothelial cells release nitric oxide (endothelial-derived relaxant factor), a potent vasodilator that is considered an important factor in the blood flow changes and loss of vascular tone seen in systemic inflammation.[33] The injured endothelium also becomes much more permeable, allowing fluid and protein to leak into the interstitial spaces. An important function of normal endothelium is anticoagulation. When damaged, the endothelium loses much of its ability to prevent blood clotting, allowing microvascular thrombi to develop.

The postinjury insult also activates the neuroendocrine system, resulting in a second, more extensive stress response. The normal function of the stress response is to maintain basal and stress-related homeostasis,[34] but in MODS homeostasis cannot be maintained. In fact, the endocrine response becomes excessive and injurious. There is an early increase in circulating catecholamines that contributes to many of the clinical manifestations of MODS, such as tachycardia, hypermetabolism, and increased oxygen consumption. Cortisol, glucagon, insulin, human growth hormone, ADH, and endorphin levels also are increased. Many of these hormones contribute to the extreme catabolic state seen in MODS, and endorphins, which are vasodilators, decrease SVR. The sympathetic nervous system, to compensate for complications resulting from the injury (e.g., fluid loss, hypotension), also is stimulated. The stimulation persists throughout the period of critical illness.[35] The stress response can be amplified by a number of factors, including pain, anxiety, psychosis, and hyperthermia. (Stress response is discussed in detail in Chapter 9.)

Because of endothelial cell damage and the release of mediators, four major plasma cascades are activated: complement, kallikrein-kinin, coagulation, and fibrinolytic. Complement components, particularly the anaphylatoxins C3a and C5a, cause vasodilation by stimulating release of histamine from mast cells. They also have strong chemotactic properties. C5a, especially, causes adhesion and the activation and degranulation of neutrophils. Complement is thought to be a powerful trigger for the exaggerated inflammatory response. Activation of the kinin system results in the production of bradykinin, a very potent vasodilator known to decrease SVR. Coagulation mechanisms also are activated, and because tissue injury and endothelial damage are extensive, microvascular thrombosis occurs throughout the body, resulting in impaired microvascular circulation and organ ischemia.

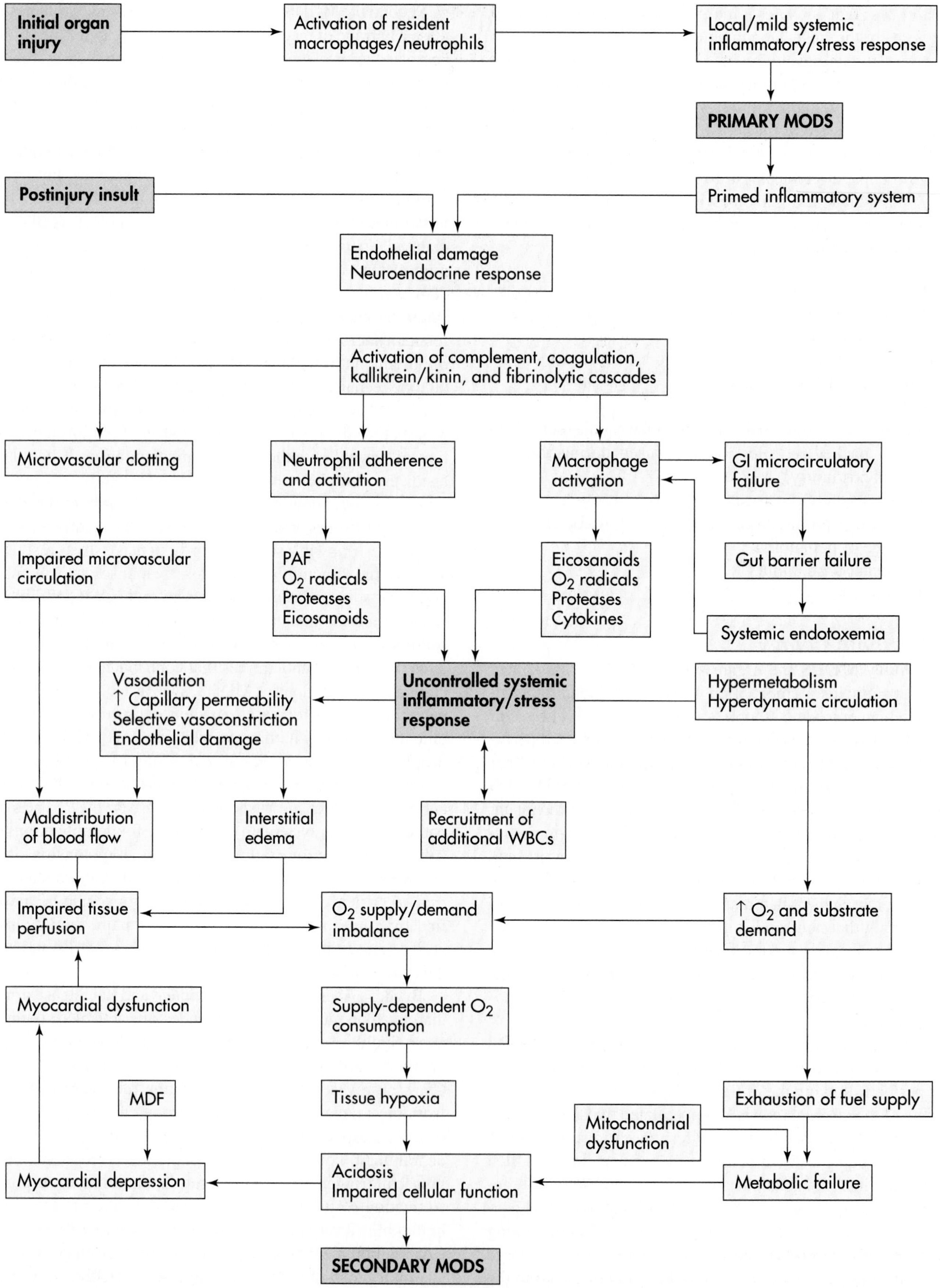

FIG. 45-7 Pathogenesis of multiple organ dysfunction syndrome. *MODS*, Multiple organ dysfunction syndrome; *GI*, gastrointestinal; *PAF*, platelet activating factor; *WBCs*, white blood cells; *MDF*, myocardial depressant factor.

Concurrently, fibrinolytic mechanisms are activated. However, the tendency toward clotting is greater, resulting in a net procoagulant state that can lead to the development of DIC. The overall effect of the activation of the plasma cascades is a hyperinflammatory and hypercoagulant state that contributes to vasodilation, vasopermeability, cardiovascular instability, endothelial damage, and clotting abnormalities.

Once cytokines and other mediators have been released and the plasma enzyme cascades have been activated, a massive systemic inflammatory response develops. It involves several types of inflammatory cells, particularly neutrophils, macrophages, and mast cells. These cells, having been primed by their response to the initial organ injury, now pour large amounts of chemical mediators into tissues and into the systemic circulation. Neutrophils have tremendous inflammatory potential. The accumulation of activated neutrophils in organs is thought to play a key role in the pathogenesis of MODS.[28,36] When neutrophils adhere to the endothelium, they undergo a "respiratory burst" (oxidative burst) and release oxygen radicals. The respiratory burst occurs as the activated neutrophil experiences a sudden increase in oxidative metabolism, producing large quantities of highly toxic oxygen free radicals. These reactive oxygen species are oxygen atoms with an unpaired electron in the outer electron ring. The primary reactive oxygen species produced are superoxide ($O^-{}_2$), hydrogen peroxide (H_2O_2), hydroxyl radical (OH^-), and singlet oxygen (O). Oxygen radicals are extremely damaging to vascular endothelium and tissue cells, attacking deoxyribonucleic acid (DNA), cross linking membrane structures, and inducing membrane peroxidation—reactions that disorganize cell membranes and lead to tissue necrosis.[37]

Other important mediators released by neutrophils are proteases, particularly collagenase and elastase. Proteases directly damage endothelium and neighboring cells, resulting in increased capillary permeability and organ damage. When activated, neutrophils also release platelet activating factor (PAF), a mediator that damages endothelium, stimulates clot formation, and activates increasing numbers of phagocytes. It is important in the propagation of the unregulated inflammation of MODS. Finally, neutrophils release arachidonic acid metabolites (eicosanoids) as a result of lipid peroxidation of their cell membranes. Of the arachidonic acid metabolites (prostaglandins, thromboxanes, leukotrienes), two are particularly important in the pathogenesis of organ hypoperfusion: prostacyclin (PGI_2) and thromboxane A_2 (TXA_2). TXA_2 is a powerful vasoconstrictor, and PGI_2 is a potent vasodilator. When released in varying amounts in different organ beds, they are largely responsible for the maldistribution of blood flow characteristic of MODS. In total, neutrophils produce at least 50 to 60 toxins.[38] Collectively, products released by neutrophils cause endothelial damage, systemic vasodilation, selective vasoconstriction (vasoconstriction of certain organ beds or parts of organ beds), increased vascular permeability, and microvascular coagulation.

Macrophages, present in most tissues, are activated by endotoxin, complement, and monocyte chemotactic substances. Producing more than 30 mediators,[29] macrophages share a key role in the development of the unregulated inflammation of secondary MODS with the neutrophils. Like neutrophils, they produce oxygen radicals, proteases, and arachidonic acid metabolites. In addition, as previously noted, they release TNF and IL-1. It is reported that excessive or prolonged stimulation of macrophages leads to the overproduction of cytokines, which initiates the cycle of harmful effects seen in MODS.[27] TNF and IL-1 share many of the same functions and act synergistically, but TNF appears to be the chief messenger that initiates and perpetuates the inflammatory response.[39] TNF has potent metabolic effects, including fever, anorexia, hyperglycemia, hypermetabolism, and weight loss. It activates neutrophils, damages endothelial cells, and potentiates hypotension and shock. IL-1 also has metabolic effects, inducing fever, hypermetabolism, and muscle wasting. Normally, TNF-α activates cytokines, the coagulation system, fibrinolysis, and neutrophils. With the exception of neutrophil activation, IL-1 causes similar activation in individuals with cancer.[17] In the pathogenesis of MODS, the cytokines are linked to all cellular, hemodynamic, and metabolic alterations.

The gastrointestinal mucosa is particularly vulnerable to inflammatory mediators released by macrophages and neutrophils. Under normal circumstances the gut mucosa serves as a barrier to prevent bacteria from the gastrointestinal tract from entering the systemic circulation. Damage to the mucosa results in microcirculatory failure of the gut and consequent loss of the gut barrier function. The loss of intestinal barrier function leads to the systemic spread of bacteria and/or endotoxin from the gut (systemic endotoxemia). This phenomenon is called *translocation of bacteria.* The idea that the gut acts as a reservoir of bacteria and endotoxin that can initiate or perpetuate the development of MODS is known as the **gut hypothesis.**[39,40] The gut hypothesis provides a possible explanation for the fact that an infectious focus is not always found in individuals with MODS. Although this hypothesis has been substantiated by animal studies and has much support, the evidence from human studies is inconclusive.[25,39,40]

The numerous inflammatory processes operating in MODS cause maldistribution of blood flow and hypermetabolism. **Maldistribution of blood flow** refers to the uneven distribution of flow to various organs and between the large vessels and capillary beds of the body. It is caused by generalized vasodilation, increased capillary permeability, selective vasoconstriction, endothelial damage, and impaired microvascular circulation. It is a major factor in the pathophysiology of MODS. The alterations in blood flow—which can occur at the cellular, organ, or regional level—lead to impaired tissue perfusion and a decreased supply of oxygen to the cells. The organs most severely affected by hypoperfusion are the lungs, splanchnic bed, liver, and kidneys. At the same time, a condition of **hyperdynamic circulation** with increased venous return of blood to the heart exists. This is caused by an increase in cardiac output secondary to the decrease in SVR and to the shunting of blood past closed capillary beds through anatomic precapillary arteriovenous channels. Despite the supernormal systemic blood flow, oxygen delivery to the tissues decreases. Several factors contribute to the problem. First, blood is shunted past selected regional capillary beds. Shunting, caused by loss of autoregulation in some organs, may be an early indicator of progression of sepsis into MODS.[41] This occurs because inflammatory mediators, particularly TXA_2, override the normal vascular control to cause selective vasoconstriction and because injured endothelial cells are unable to respond to normal vasodilator mediators. Second, interstitial edema, resulting from microvascular permeability, contributes to decreased oxygen delivery to cells by increasing the distance oxygen must travel to reach the cells. Third, capillary obstruction occurs because of the formation of microvascular thrombi and the aggregation of leukocytes.

Hypermetabolism, with accompanying alterations in carbohydrate, fat, and lipid metabolism, is initially a compensatory measure to meet the body's increased demands for energy seen in MODS. Over time, however, hypermetabolism becomes detrimental, placing enormous demands on the heart. Hypermetabolism is the result of (1) the neuroendocrine response to stress with the release of catecholamines and cortisol, and (2) the action of TNF and IL-1. With increased metabolism the calorie requirements increase to 1.5 to 2 times normal,[33] and a cardiac output of 1.5 to 2 times normal is usually seen.[42] The alterations in metabolism affect all aspects of substrate utilization. Most important is the catabolism of protein, primarily of skeletal muscle and visceral organs. The extreme catabolism of protein can produce 15 to 20 g of nitrogen per day[29] and rapidly depletes lean body mass. Hyperglycemia occurs as gluconeogenesis by the liver increases and glucose utilization by the cells decreases. Fatty acids are mobilized from adipose tissue. The net result of the hypermetabolism is depletion of oxygen and fuel supplies.

Myocardial depression also accompanies MODS. The cause remains unclear, but possible explanations are the effects of myocardial depressant factor (MDF), TNF, and IL-1 on cardiac contractility; alterations in β-adrenergic receptors in the heart; and hypoxia of the myocardium.[43]

The decreased oxygen delivery to the cells (resulting from the maldistribution of blood flow) and the increased oxygen needs of the cells (resulting from hypermetabolism) combine to create an imbalance in oxygen supply and demand. This imbalance is critical in the pathogenesis of MODS because it results in a pathologic condition known as **supply-dependent oxygen consumption**. Ordinarily the amount of oxygen consumed by the cells depends only on the needs of the cells because there is an adequate reserve of oxygen that can be delivered if required. In MODS, however, the reserve has been exhausted and the amount of oxygen consumed becomes dependent on the amount the circulation is able to deliver. Because the amount is inadequate in MODS, the tissues become hypoxic. Compounding the hypoxic damage to cells is a phenomenon called *reperfusion injury* (see Chapter 2). Much of the organ damage in MODS occurs with the reestablishment of blood flow after a period of ischemia. During the ischemic episode, energy stores and ATP are depleted and the enzyme *xanthine dehydrogenase* is converted to *xanthine oxidase*. With reperfusion of the ischemic tissue, oxygen radicals are formed from oxygen by the action of xanthine oxidase, and they attack the already damaged tissues. Consequently, although reperfusion is necessary to restore oxygen supply to ischemic organs, it can increase the extent of injury. Therefore, because of supply-dependent oxygen consumption and reperfusion injury, tissues become increasingly hypoxic. The result is cellular acidosis, impaired cellular function, and ultimately multiple organ failure.

WHAT'S NEW? Antibiotic-Mediated Release of Lipopolysaccharide (LPS)

Antibiotics, particularly cell wall active antibiotics, have been implicated in increased release of LPS during the sepsis syndrome, increasing proinflammatory cytokines and worsening individual outcomes. The β-lactam antibiotic group is the most potent at LPS release; however, differences in potency between antibiotics within the group have been documented.

Data from Morrison DC et al: Structure-function relationships of bacterial endotoxins contribution to microbial sepsis, *Inf Dis Clin No Amer* 13(2):313, 1999.

Clinical Manifestations

In MODS the organs that show clinical manifestations of failure are not always the organs involved as part of the initial injury, and there is usually a lag time between the initial insult and the development of systemic organ failure. The development of primary MODS is difficult to monitor, but there is a well-established general pattern in the clinical development of secondary MODS.[39] Following the inciting event and aggressive resuscitation of the individual for approximately 24 hours, the individual develops low-grade fever, tachycardia, tachypnea, dyspnea, altered mental status, and a general hyperdynamic and hypermetabolic state (Box 45-1). Following this, the lungs begin to fail and ARDS may appear within 24 to 72 hours (see discussion of ARDS, Chapter 32). Between 7 and 10 days, the hypermetabolic and hyperdynamic state intensifies; bacteremia with enteric organisms is common; and signs of hepatic, intestinal, and renal failure develop. During days 14 to 21, the renal failure and liver failure become more severe. Hematologic failure and myocardial failure are usually later manifestations. Encephalopathy, characterized by mental status changes ranging from confusion to deep coma, may occur at any time. This sequence can evolve rapidly, with death occurring between 14 and 21 days, or it can evolve over a period of weeks. Individuals can recover from either the slowly evolving or the rapidly evolving course.

The clinical manifestations of failure of individual organs in MODS are caused by inflammatory mediator damage, tissue hypoxia, and hypermetabolism. Respiratory failure progresses early to ARDS and is characterized by tachypnea, pulmonary edema with crackles and diminished breath sounds, use of accessory muscles, and hypoxemia. Liver failure, although early in its development, is not clinically detectable until the later stages of MODS, when jaundice, abdominal distention, liver tenderness, muscle wasting, and hepatic encephalopathy appear. All aspects of metabolism, substance detoxification, and immune response are impaired. Albumin and clotting factor synthesis decreases, protein wastes accumulate, and liver tissue macrophages (Kupffer cells) no longer function effectively.

The gastrointestinal system is very sensitive to ischemic and inflammatory injury. Clinical manifestations of bowel involvement are hemorrhage, ileus, stress ulcers, malabsorption, diarrhea or constipation, vomiting, anorexia, abdominal pain, and pancreatitis. Intolerance to enteral feeding may develop. Adding to damage caused by injury to the bowel is bacterial translocation into the bloodstream resulting from the loss of the gut barrier function. The overwhelmed liver is unable to clear the bacteria from the systemic circulation. Thus, regardless of whether infection or some other injury was the precipitating cause of MODS, once intestinal bacteria enter the systemic circulation, it is likely that sepsis will be a problem. Renal failure develops at about the same time and is marked by progressive oliguria, azotemia, and edema. If renal shutdown is severe, anuria, hyperkalemia, and metabolic acidosis occur.

The first manifestations of cardiac failure are similar to those of septic shock: tachycardia, bounding pulse, increased cardiac output, fall in SVR, hypotension, warm skin, and supraventricular dysrhythmias (see Septic Shock, p. 1490). In the terminal stages, profound hypotension and ventricular dysrhythmias may develop. Changes in central nervous system function may be noted. Ischemia and inflammation are responsible for the changes, which include apprehension,

Box 45-1

CLINICAL MANIFESTATIONS OF ORGAN DYSFUNCTION

PULMONARY
- Adult respiratory distress syndrome (ARDS) pattern of respiratory failure (dyspnea, patchy infiltrates, refractory hypoxemia, respiratory acidosis, abnormal O_2 indices)
- Pulmonary hypertension

GASTROINTESTINAL
- Abdominal distention and ascites
- Intolerance to enteral feedings
- Paralytic ileus
- Upper and lower gastrointestinal bleeding (guaiac-positive stools)
- Diarrhea
- Ischemic colitis
- Mucosal ulceration
- Decreased bowel sounds
- Bacterial overgrowth in stool

LIVER
- Increased serum bilirubin level (hyperbilirubinemia)
- Increased liver enzyme levels (serum aspartate transaminase [SAST], serum alanine aminotransferase [SALT], lactic dehydrogenase [LDH], alkaline phosphatase)
- Increased serum ammonia level
- Decreased serum transferrin level
- Jaundice
- Hepatomegaly

GALLBLADDER
- Right upper quadrant tenderness or pain
- Abdominal distention
- Unexplained fever
- Decreased bowel sounds

HYPERMETABOLISM
- Decreased lean body mass
- Muscle wasting
- Severe weight loss
- Negative nitrogen balance
- Hyperglycemia
- Hypertriglyceridemia
- Increased serum lactate levels
- Decreased serum albumin, serum transferrin, prealbumin, retinol-binding protein

RENAL
- Increased serum creatinine level and blood urea nitrogen
- Oliguria, anuria, or polyuria consistent with prerenal azotemia or acute tubular necrosis
- Urinary indices consistent with prerenal azotemia or acute tubular necrosis

CARDIOVASCULAR

Hyperdynamic
- Decreased pulmonary capillary wedge pressure
- Decreased systemic vascular resistance
- Decreased right atrial pressure
- Decreased left ventricular stroke work index
- Increased oxygen consumption
- Increased cardiac output, cardiac index, heart rate

Hypodynamic
- Increased systemic vascular resistance
- Increased right atrial pressure
- Increased left ventricular stroke work index
- Decreased oxygen delivery and consumption
- Decreased cardiac output and cardiac index

CENTRAL NERVOUS SYSTEM
- Lethargy
- Altered level of consciousness
- Fever
- Hepatic encephalopathy

COAGULATION AND HEMATOLOGIC
- Thrombocytopenia
- Disseminated intravascular coagulation

IMMUNE
- Infection
- Decreased lymphocyte count
- Anergy

Modified from Thelan LA et al: *Critical care nursing: diagnosis and management,* ed 3, St Louis, 1998, Mosby.

confusion, disorientation, restlessness, agitation, headache, decreased cognitive ability and memory, and decreased level of consciousness. When ischemia is severe, seizures and coma can occur.

Evaluation and Treatment

Because there is no specific therapy for MODS, early detection is extremely important so that supportive measures can be initiated as soon as possible. Frequent assessment of the clinical status of individuals at known risk is essential. Unfortunately, there is no way to determine with certainty when an organ is failing. One set of criteria for diagnosis of organ dysfunction and failure has been proposed by Deitch[44] (Table 45-2).

Several systems for scoring severity of illness have also been developed. Commonly used systems are the **Acute Physiology and Chronic Health Evaluation II and III (APACHE II and APACHE III)**. The scoring systems use individual variables to describe the relative risks of individuals and to identify where the person is on the continuum of illness progression. However, these scoring systems were developed to assess prognosis in large groups of individuals, not in individuals, and therefore are not well adapted for clinical decision making. They are more useful for research studies.[39] Once organ failure develops, monitoring of laboratory values and hemodynamic parameters is necessary to assess the degree of clinical impairment.

At present the therapeutic management of MODS consists of prevention and support. Prevention of the syndrome is important. First, the initial source of inflammation must be eliminated or controlled if possible. Next, a second insult must be avoided. It is essential to remove any potential site of infection by debriding necrotic tissue, draining abscesses, reducing the numbers of invasive procedures performed, and removing hematomas. Nosocomial infections from contaminated lines and catheters are of concern and must be prevented. Nosocomial infection rates of 15% to 25% have been reported in critically ill individuals.[11] Early reduction of long-bone fractures and surgical repair of injured tissues are also important preventive measures.

The goals of therapy are to control infection, provide adequate tissue oxygenation, restore intravascular volume, and support the function of individual organs. After the initial injury has been aggressively treated and sources of infection have been removed, antibiotics generally are administered. This is important because infection remains a common cause of death.[39] The choice of agents is based on the individual's disease process, but the regimen is usually a combination of antibiotics that covers both gram-negative and gram-positive organisms.

Because oxygen is not stored in the tissues, it must be continuously delivered. Maintaining an arterial oxygen saturation of 88% to 92% is recommended,[45] and hemoglobin levels should be kept above 10 to 12 g/dl.[37,42] Blood transfusions may be necessary to ensure an adequate hemoglobin level. To deliver oxygen to the organs in the face of profound systemic vasodilation, fluid volume must be restored. Therefore aggressive fluid therapy is initiated early in the course of the disease. Usually large volumes of isotonic crystalloid solutions are administered, although colloids (often albumin) also may be added to maintain adequate preload.

Finally, support for individual organ systems must be provided. Respiratory failure is treated with mechanical ventilation with high oxygen concentrations and positive end-expiratory pressures (PEEP). To provide adequate nutrition and metabolic support, the failing gastrointestinal system is supported with enteral feedings. It is now well recognized that enteral feedings help to preserve gut microbial barrier function and are therefore preferred to parenteral feedings. However, if the individual is unable to tolerate the amount of enteral feeding required to meet the enormous metabolic demands, hyperalimentation may be added. Ideally, the feeding formula is carefully calculated to meet the individual's nutritional requirements. Once renal failure is established, dialysis or continuous hemofiltration may be required to maintain fluid and electrolyte balance. To support the failing

Table 45-2 Criteria for Diagnosis of Organ Dysfunction and Failure

Organ or System	Dysfunction	Advanced Failure
Pulmonary	Hypoxia requiring respirator-assisted ventilation for at least 3-5 days	Progressive ARDS requiring PEEP >10 cm H_2O and Fio_2 >0.5
Hepatic	Serum bilirubin ≥2-3 mg/dl or liver function values twice normal or higher	Clinical jaundice with bilirubin ≥8-10 mg/dl
Renal	Oliguria ≤479 ml/24 hr or rising creatinine (≥2-3 mg/dl)	Renal dialysis
Intestinal	Ileus with intolerance to enteral feeding for longer than 5 days	Stress ulcers requiring transfusion; acalculus cholecystitis
Hematologic	PT and PTT ↑ >25% or platelets <50,000-80,000	Disseminated intravascular coagulation
Central nervous system	Confusion, mild disorientation	Progressive coma
Cardiovascular	Decreased ejection fraction or capillary leak syndrome	Hypodynamic response refractory to inotropic support

From Deitch EA: *Ann Surg* 216(2):117, 1992.
ARDS, Adult respiratory distress syndrome; *PEEP,* positive end-expiratory pressure; *Fio_2,* fraction of inspired oxygen in air; *PT,* prothrombin time; *PTT,* partial thromboplastin time.

cardiovascular system, inotropic drugs, such as low-dose dopamine and dobutamine, may be required to maximize cardiac contractility and maintain cardiac output. Vasopressors also are used occasionally to maintain perfusion pressures. Although steroids have antiinflammatory effects, they are controversial because they have not been shown to be effective and may even worsen organ dysfunction.[46]

Recent scientific knowledge about inflammatory mediators has led to many investigational therapies for MODS. Although results from animal studies have been promising, human clinical trials have not confirmed the benefit of any agent. There are still many challenges to be overcome before specific therapies for MODS are used clinically. Whatever therapies prove to be effective, it is likely that they will be used in combination.

BURNS

The total burn incidence in the United States has dropped from 4.2 per 100,000 during 1961 through 1964 to 1.5 per 100,000 during 1993 through 1996.[47] Deaths from fire and burn injuries have decreased 50% to an estimated 5500 burn deaths in 1991, compared with 9000 burn-associated deaths in 1971.[48] This remarkable progress is the result of several factors, including an increased national focus on fire safety and burn prevention, the establishment of regional burn centers, the use of smoke detectors, regulation of consumer product safety, and occupational safety mandates. A decrease in hospitalization reflects a shift to outpatient care and improved prehospital and emergency treatment.

NUTRITION & DISEASE

Immunonutrition

Researchers are currently identifying specific nutrients—in addition to fats, carbohydrates, and proteins—that upregulate the individual's immune system. Enteral formulas containing one or more of the following nutrients may provide additional benefits to some individuals:

Glutamine. Fuels many of the cellular components of the immune system and, in one clinical trial, improved nitrogen balance, reduced infection, lowered microbial colonization, and shortened length of stay.

Arginine. Is a precursor to nitric oxide, a major antiinflammatory cytokine. In research studies, it improved nitrogen balance; promoted wound healing; improved bacteria clearance; enhanced proliferation of leukocytes, the activity of natural killer cells, and production of IL-2; and decreased bacterial translocation from the gut, improving survival from gut-derived sepsis.

Nucleotides. Believed to increase natural killer cell and macrophage activity, improve helper T cell functions, prevent gut atrophy, and decrease gut permeability.

Omega-3 fatty acids. Have increased survival and suppressed autoimmune disease in animal studies.

Diets containing these elements are referred to as "pharmaconutrients" because of their immune-stimulating effects.

Data from DeWitt RC, Kudsk KA: The gut's role in metabolism, mucosal barrier function, and gut immunology, *Inf Dis Clin No Amer* 13(2):465, 1999.

The cause of burns may be **thermal** or **nonthermal**, such as chemical, electrical, or radioactive. Thermal burns are often described as contact, flame, or scald injuries as a result of direct contact with a hot solid object, flames, or heated liquid. Adherent materials (e.g., asphalt, tar, or plastic) may likewise produce a contact burn. Chemical injuries are a result of contact with substances that are directly toxic to skin or the lining of the respiratory or alimentary tract. Such chemicals are often acid, alkali, or organic agents, termed **vesicants**, that cause blistering of the epithelial surfaces. Electrical burns may be the result of the conduction of electrical current through the body with the heating of tissue, or flash over the body surface associated with an electrical discharge.

Burn Wound Depth

The classification of **burn wound depth** is usually based on the physical appearance and the symptoms associated with the affected skin. The definitive diagnosis is determined by the histologic depth of tissue necrosis. Such histologic evaluation, unfortunately, necessitates a skin biopsy. Because of the invasive nature of the biopsy procedure, the clinical depth determination is usually accepted temporarily and the ultimate healing or lack thereof either confirms or alters the assessment. Common burn depth classification describes four types of injury.

First-degree burns are a **partial-thickness injury** involving only the epidermis, without injury to the underlying dermal or subcutaneous tissue (Table 45-3). The skin maintains water vapor and bacterial barrier functions. Many sunburns are first-degree injuries caused by exposure of skin to ultraviolet radiation from the sun. Initially there is local pain and erythema, but no blisters appear for about 24 hours. An extensive first-degree burn may cause systemic responses such as chills, headache, localized edema, and nausea or vomiting. No treatment of extensive first-degree burns is required unless the person is elderly or an infant, in which case severe nausea and vomiting may lead to inadequate fluid intake and dehydration. Therapy consists of intravenous hydration until the nausea and vomiting subside 24 to 72 hours after burn injury. Comfort measures for previously healthy children or adults with extensive first-degree burns consist of aspirin for adults or acetaminophen for children every 4 hours in age-appropriate doses and frequent application of a water-soluble lotion. First-degree burns heal in 3 to 5 days without scarring.

Second-degree burns describe two categories of burn depth with markedly different characteristics. Both of these are partial-thickness injuries, but they evoke vastly different responses. The hallmark of **superficial partial-thickness injury** is the appearance of thin-walled, fluid-filled blisters that develop within just a few minutes after injury. Another dominant characteristic of superficial injury is pain. As blisters break or are removed, nerve endings are exposed to air (Fig. 45-8). Tactile and pain sensors remain intact throughout healing, with each wound care procedure causing extreme pain. Wounds heal in 3 to 4 weeks if the individual is adequately nourished and no complications develop (Fig. 45-9). Scar formation is unusual with this injury. The amount of

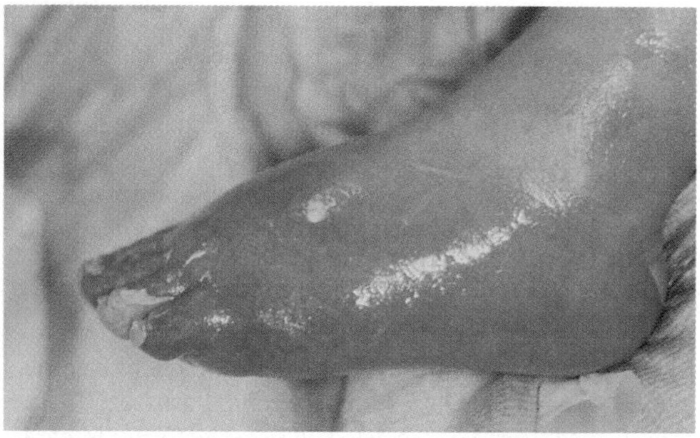

FIG. 45-8 Superficial partial-thickness injury. Scald injury following débridement of overlying blister and nonadherent epithelium. (Courtesy Intermountain Burn Center, University of Utah.)

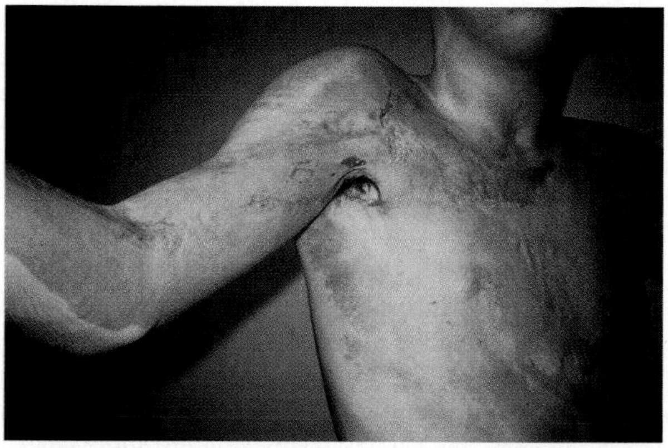

FIG. 45-9 Axillary burn scar contracture. Note the blanching of the anterior axillary fold and small ulceration, both indicating the diminished range of motion. (Courtesy Intermountain Burn Center, University of Utah.)

Table 45-3 Depth of Burn Injury

		Second Degree		Third Degree
Characteristic	**First Degree**	**Superficial Partial Thickness**	**Deep Partial Thickness**	**Full Thickness**
Morphology	Destruction of epidermis only	Destruction of epidermis and some dermis	Destruction of epidermis and dermis, leaving only skin appendages	Destruction of epidermis, dermis, and underlying subcutaneous tissue
Skin function	Intact	Absent	Absent	Absent
Tactile and pain sensors	Intact	Intact	Intact but diminished	Absent
Blisters	Present only after first 24 hr	Present within minutes, thin walled and fluid filled	May appear as fluid-filled blisters; often is layer of flat, dehydrated "tissue paper" that lifts off in sheets	Blisters rare; usually is a layer of flat, dehydrated "tissue paper" that lifts off easily
Appearance of wound after initial debridement	Skin peels at 24-48 hr, normal or slightly red underneath	Red to pale ivory, moist surface	Mottled with areas of waxy white, dry surface	White, cherry red, or black; may contain visible thrombosed veins; dry, hard leathery surface
Healing time	3-5 days	21-28 days	30 days to many months	Will not heal; may close from edges as secondary healing if wound is small
Scarring	None	May be present; low incidence influenced by genetic predisposition	Highest incidence because of slow healing rate promoting scar tissue development; also influenced by genetic predisposition	Skin graft; scarring minimized by early excision and grafting; influenced by genetic predisposition

scarring that develops is a genetically determined trait and is not predictable during the early course of treatment.

Deep partial-thickness burns involve the entire dermis, sparing skin appendages such as hair follicles and sweat glands (see Table 45-3). The burn often looks waxy white and is surrounded by margins of superficial partial-thickness injury. The injury is often clinically indistinguishable from a full-thickness injury (Fig. 45-10), but by 7 to 10 days after burn injury, skin buds and hair will appear from hair follicles, indicating that skin appendages remain. These wounds take weeks to heal, and current therapy consists of surgical removal of the burn wound (excision) followed by application of the person's own unburned skin from another body area (autograft). Wounds that heal slowly produce more scar tissue and continue to be a potential source of infection until closed. In the presence of relative surgical contraindications, such as cardiopulmonary failure, deep partial-thickness wounds are not surgically treated but are allowed to heal primarily. The ultimate healing of deep partial-thickness burns commonly results in hypertrophic scarring with poor functional and cosmetic results.

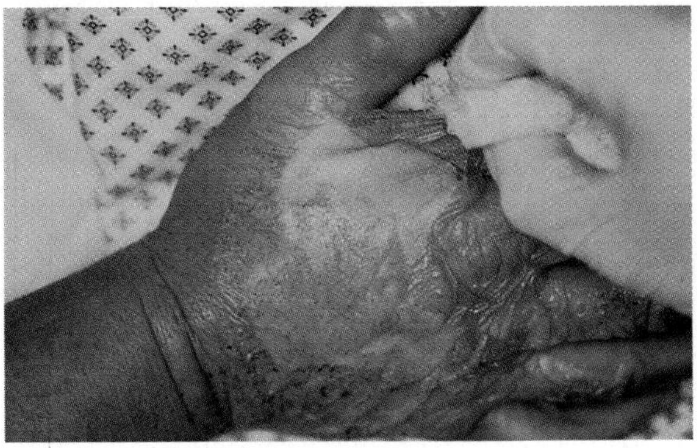

FIG. 45-10 Deep partial-thickness wound. Note pale appearance and minimal exudate. (Courtesy Intermountain Burn Center, University of Utah.)

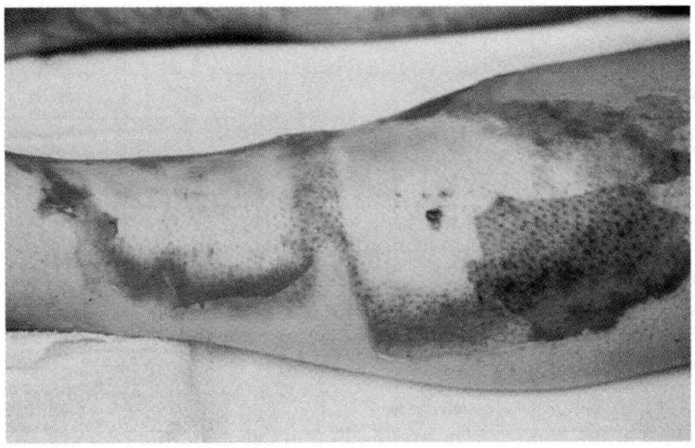

FIG. 45-11 Full-thickness thermal injury. The wound is dry and insensate. (Courtesy Intermountain Burn Center, University of Utah.)

Third-degree burns, or **full-thickness burns**, involve destruction of the entire epidermis; dermis; and, often, underlying subcutaneous tissue (see Table 45-3). On occasion, all underlying subcutaneous tissue is destroyed and muscle or bone may be destroyed. Full-thickness wounds often appear relatively innocuous when their color is white and the delineation between normal and burned skin is not accompanied by a marked color change. Elasticity of the dermis is destroyed, giving the wound a dry, leathery appearance (Fig. 45-11). As marked edema forms, distal circulation may be compromised in areas of circumferential burns. **Escharotomies** (cutting through the burned skin) are performed to release pressure. Full-thickness burns are painless because all nerve endings have been destroyed by the injury.

The extent of the **total body surface area (TBSA)** burn is estimated using either the "rule of nines" (Fig. 45-12) or the Lund and Browder chart (Fig. 45-13). Areas of partial-thickness and full-thickness injury are marked on the diagram in Fig. 45-13. First-degree burns are not included in the TBSA estimate. The surface area of the palm averages 1% of the body surface area over a wide range of ages; thus it can be used to estimate burn areas of irregular size and shape.[49]

Severity of burn injury is a combination of many factors, including age, medical history, extent and depth of injury, and body area involved. The American Burn Association has defined criteria to assist health care professionals in identifying patients who require care at a specialized burn center (Box 45-2). The multidisciplinary burn center is recommended for those persons who are at high risk for morbidity, mortality, or permanent functional loss.

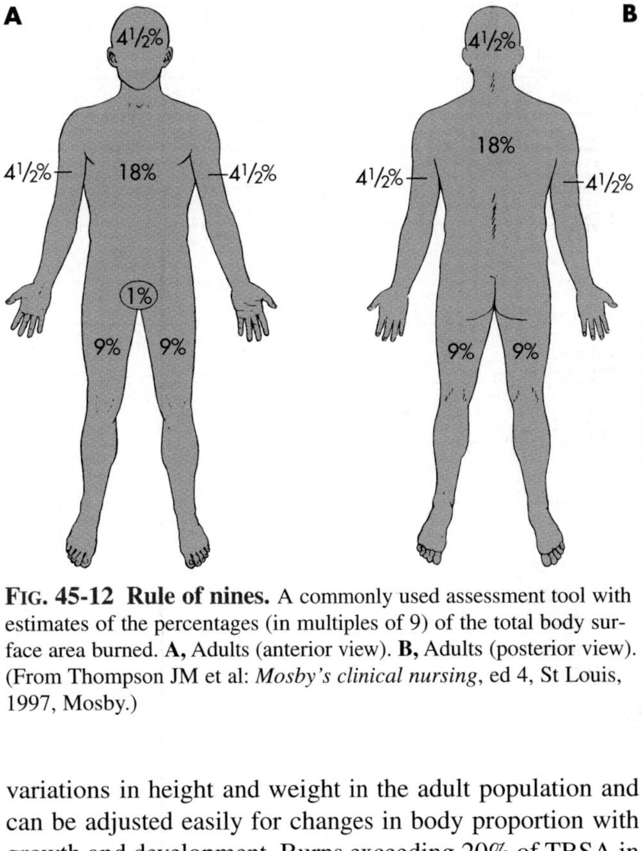

FIG. 45-12 Rule of nines. A commonly used assessment tool with estimates of the percentages (in multiples of 9) of the total body surface area burned. **A,** Adults (anterior view). **B,** Adults (posterior view). (From Thompson JM et al: *Mosby's clinical nursing*, ed 4, St Louis, 1997, Mosby.)

Pathophysiology and Clinical Manifestations

Burn injury results in dramatic changes in most physiologic functions of the body within the first few minutes after the event. The effect of burn depends on two factors—first, the extent of body surface affected and, second, the depth of cutaneous injury. Body surface burn extent is described by the percentage of TBSA injured. This normalizes for the usual variations in height and weight in the adult population and can be adjusted easily for changes in body proportion with growth and development. Burns exceeding 20% of TBSA in most adults are considered to be major burn injuries and are associated with massive evaporative water losses and flux of large amounts of fluid and electrolytes in the body tissues, manifested as generalized edema and circulatory hypovolemia. Depth of cutaneous injury has been categorized in many ways but always depends on the severity of injury of epidermal and dermal elements of the skin and whether the alteration is complete necrosis or a reversible injury.

With a major burn injury, a systemic pathophysiology ensues that requires therapeutic intervention to sustain life. The immediate (acute) physiologic consequences of a major burn injury center around the profound, life-threatening

Area	Birth 1 yr.	1-4 yr.	5-9 yr.	10-14 yr.	15 yr.	Adult	2°	3°	Total	Donor Areas
Head	19	17	13	11	9	7				
Neck	2	2	2	2	2	2				
Ant. Trunk	13	13	13	13	13	13				
Post. Trunk	13	13	13	13	13	13				
R. Buttock	2½	2½	2½	2½	2½	2½				
L. Buttock	2½	2½	2½	2½	2½	2½				
Genitalia	1	1	1	1	1	1				
R. U. Arm	4	4	4	4	4	4				
L. U. Arm	4	4	4	4	4	4				
R. L. Arm	3	3	3	3	3	3				
L. L. Arm	3	3	3	3	3	3				
R. Hand	2½	2½	2½	2½	2½	2½				
L. Hand	2½	2½	2½	2½	2½	2½				
R. Thigh	5½	6½	8	8½	9	9½				
L. Thigh	5½	6½	8	8½	9	9½				
R. Leg	5	5	5½	6	6½	7				
L. Leg	5	5	5½	6	6½	7				
R. Foot	3½	3½	3½	3½	3½	3½				
L. Foot	3½	3½	3½	3½	3½	3½				
						TOTAL				

Cause of Burn ______________________________

Date of Burn ____________

Time of Burn ____________

Age ____________

Sex ____________

Weight ____________

BURN DIAGRAM

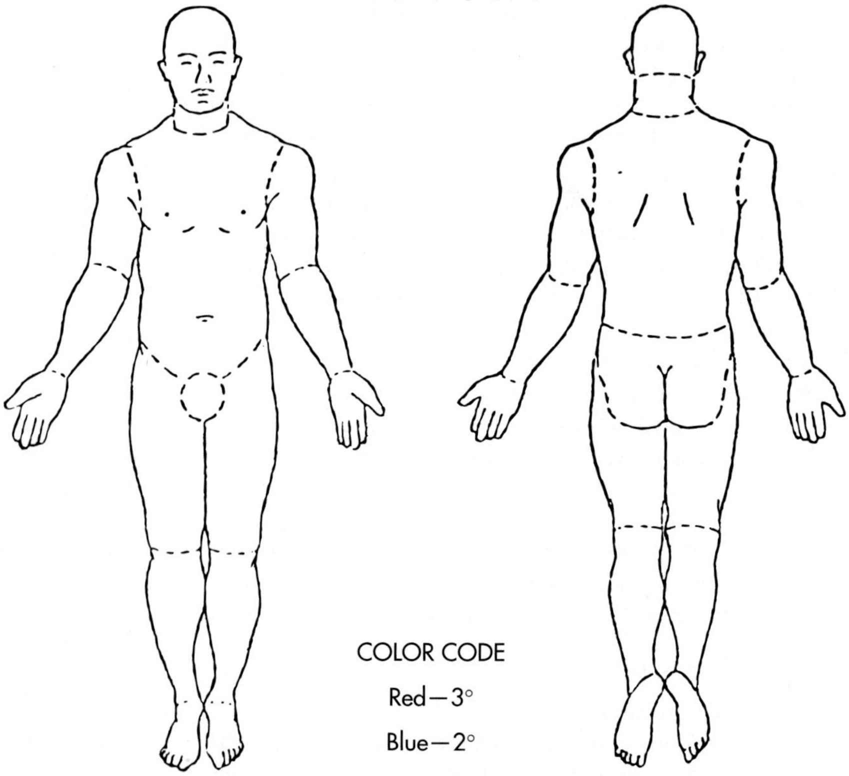

FIG. 45-13 Lund and Browder chart. Regional differences in body surface are calculated based on age. (Courtesy Intermountain Burn Center, University of Utah.)

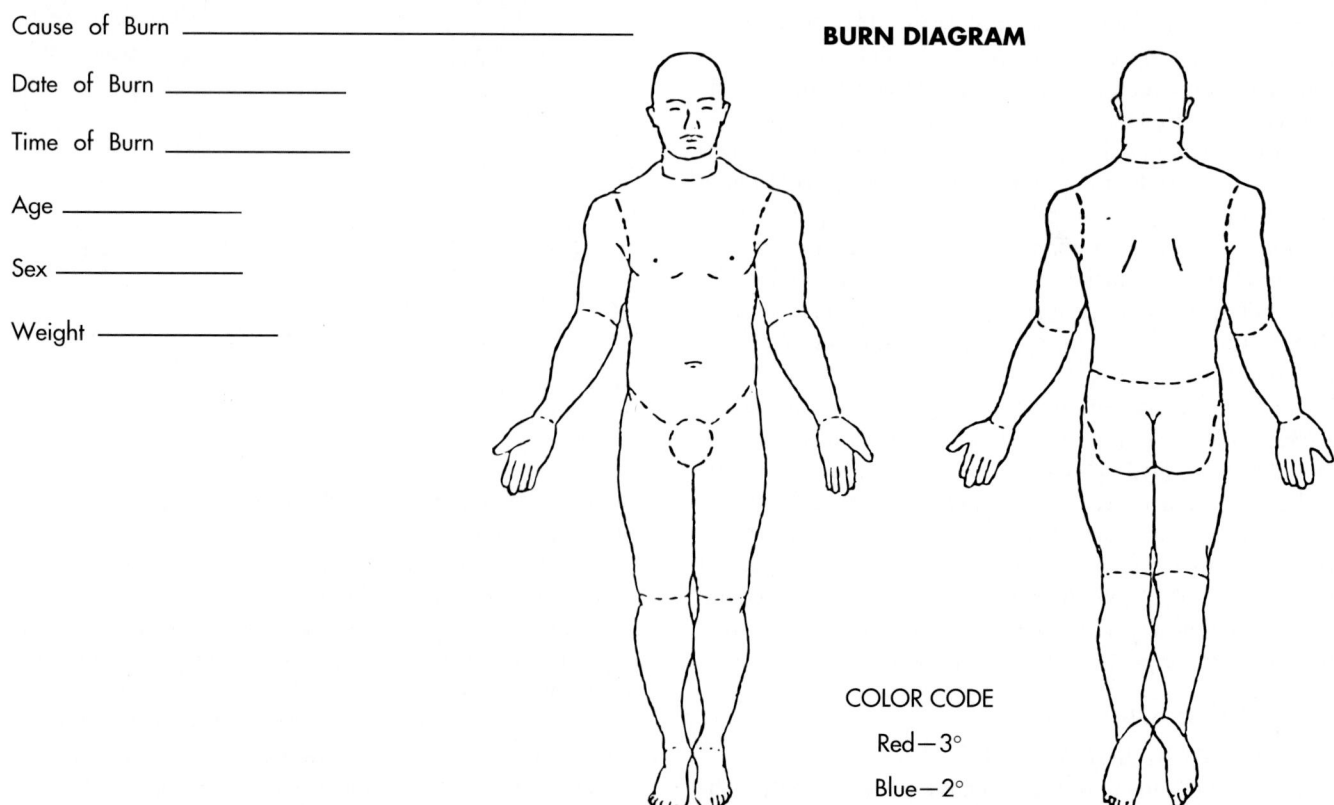

hypovolemic shock that occurs in conjunction with cellular and immunologic disruption within a few minutes of injury (Fig. 45-14). **Burn shock** is a phenomenon consisting of both a hypovolemic cardiovascular component and a cellular component.

Hypovolemia associated with burn shock results from massive fluid losses from the circulating blood volume. The losses are caused by an increase in capillary permeability that persists for approximately 24 hours after burn injury. **Fluid resuscitation** is the administration of intravenous fluids, often lactated Ringer solution, in an effort to restore the circulating blood volume during the period of increasing capillary permeability. In addition to hypovolemia, most other organ systems are affected. Cardiac contractility is diminished during the initial 24-hour resuscitation period with shunting of blood away from the liver, kidney, and gut. This is often termed the *ebb phase* of the response to trauma and can be seen with other severe injuries. Normal blood volume still does not result in restoration of normal cardiac output because of this so-called myocardial depression. Blood flow is shunted away from the kidneys, gut, liver, and other viscera, with an attendant decrease in function of these organs. This may account for the decreased gut barrier function seen in thermal injury.[50]

There is also evidence that cellular metabolism is disrupted with onset of the burn wound, resulting in altered cell membrane permeability and loss of normal electrolyte homeostasis. This cellular defect may be the pathophysiologic process responsible for the genesis of burn shock. Also, the many circulating factors in burn serum may play a role in the generation of cellular abnormalities. Although the cardiovascular and systemic response is intricately interwoven into the cellular response, they are presented here as separate entities for the purpose of describing their components.

Cardiovascular and Systemic Response to Burn Injury

The clinical manifestations of burn shock are the result of more than simple loss of extracellular fluid at the burn wound site. Hypovolemia and numerous local mediators in the burn wound,[51] as well as systemic signals, result in alteration of cellular function throughout the body. The restoration of normal intravascular volume with either saline solutions or colloid materials (e.g., albumin, blood, or dextrans) does not reverse changes such as increases in pulmonary vascular resistance or myocardial contractility.[32,52,53] This is reflected in cardiac output with precipitous decreases that often result in inadequate perfusion of most tissues at the capillary level, which is the hallmark of burn shock. Fluid infusion likewise does not return cardiac output to preburn levels.[54,55] These findings led to the postulation of a specific myocardial depressant factor (MDF).[52,56,57] Other causes also have been suggested, such as reactive oxygen radicals that attack cell membranes and other subcellular organelles as a result of first ischemia and then reperfusion of tissues during burn shock and resuscitation.[58] A third factor

Box 45-2

BURN UNIT REFERRAL CRITERIA

A burn unit may treat adults or children or both.

Burn injuries that should be referred to a burn unit include the following:

1. Partial thickness burns greater than 10% total body surface area (TBSA)
2. Burns that involve the face, hands, feet, genitalia, perineum, or major joints
3. Third-degree burns in any age group
4. Electrical burns, including lightning injury
5. Chemical burns
6. Inhalation injury
7. Burn injury in patients with preexisting medical disorders that could complicate management, prolong recovery, or affect mortality
8. Any patient with burns and concomitant trauma (such as fractures) in which the burn injury poses the greatest risk of morbidity or mortality. In such cases, if the tramua poses the greater immediate risk, the patient may be initally stabilized in a trauma center before being transferred to a burn unit. Physician judgment will be neccessary in such situations and should be in concert with the regional medical control plan triage protocols.
9. Burned children in hospitals without qualified personnel or equipment for the care of children
10. Burn injury in patients who will require special social, emotional, or long-term rehabilitative intervention

From Committee on Trauma: *Resources for optimal care of the injured patient,* Chicago, 1999, American College of Surgeons.

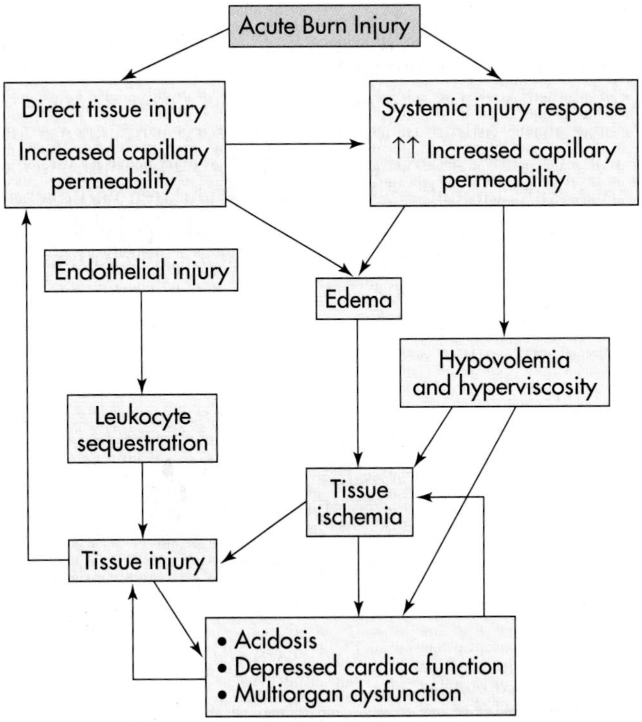

FIG. 45-14 Immediate cellular and immunologic alterations of burn shock.

may be the level of nitric acid after burn injury, which could have a direct myocardial depressant effect.[59,60] The relationship of nitric oxide and myocardial function is not yet totally clear. Gamelli and colleagues[61] found nitric oxide production to be significantly depressed in burned individuals who did not survive their injuries. They postulate that nitric oxide may scavenge reactive oxygen radicals and protect tissues from oxidative injury.

Regardless of the contribution of these mechanisms, fluid resuscitation eventually results in improved outcome of the massively burned person. This resuscitation involves infusion of intravenous fluid at a rate faster than the loss of circulating vascular volume for a period of about 24 hours from the time of burn injury and may require up to 30 L in a major burn. Resuscitation from burn shock can be accomplished using any of a number of infusion protocols. The most frequently used protocol is the Parkland formula.[62] Lactated Ringer solution is employed because it closely approximates extracellular fluid, the repository for fluid lost from the circulatory system during this phase of extensive edema formation (Table 45-4). The use of electrolyte-free fluids, such as D_5W, results in life-threatening hypovolemia and hyponatremia. Resuscitation with hypertonic saline has been used in some medical centers but is reserved for special circumstances; its use can result in adverse outcomes.[63]

The massive edema associated with burn shock is inevitable with fluid resuscitation, and failure to administer resuscitation fluid results in irreversible hypovolemic shock and death. The edema occurs in unburned as well as burned areas (Fig. 45-15). This often leads to mechanical airway obstruction, necessitating tracheal intubation, and increased severity of the interstitial pulmonary edema associated with inhalation injury.

The most reliable criterion for adequate resuscitation of burn shock is urine output. The individual is in hypovolemic shock and will, as a compensatory mechanism, decrease or cease urine output in an effort to preserve circulating volume. The adult receiving sufficient intravenous fluid will excrete urine amounts of 30 to 50 ml/hr; children will excrete 1 ml/kg/hr. If the individual does not have adequate urine output, it often indicates inadequate fluid resuscitation. The massive amount of intravenous fluid required by burned individuals during the shock phase is often intimidating to the person unfamiliar with burns. One common concern is that 30 L of intravenous fluid over 24 hours will result in pulmonary edema. It should be remembered that the individual is in hypovolemic shock and that the fluid is lost almost as fast as it is infused.

Table 45-4 Electrolyte Content of Ringer Lactate Solution and Extracellular Fluid

Electrolyte	Extracellular Fluid* (mEq/L)	Lactated Ringer† (mEq/L)
Sodium	135-145	130
Potassium	3.2-4.5	4
Chloride	95-105	109
Lactate (bicarbonate)	24-28	28

*Normal values may vary slightly between laboratories.
†Plus 80-100 ml free water per liter.

The end point of burn shock is defined as the time when the individual is able to maintain adequate urine output for 2 hours with the hourly fluid administration rate at that individual's maintenance rate (Box 45-3). As burn shock ends, fluid administered remains in the circulating volume and is reflected as increased urine output. The mechanism whereby capillary integrity is restored is unknown but usually occurs about 24 hours after burn injury (Fig. 45-16). After the individual has reached the end point of burn shock, the term used to describe the person's condition is **capillary sealed**. In individuals with large burns, colloid-containing fluids may be given to help maintain oncotic pressure during the resuscitation phase and afterward to enhance the mobilization of interstitial fluids and diuresis.[64]

On completion of resucitation, an infusion (equal to 20% of the calculated blood volume) of type-specific, fresh frozen plasma or commercially available volume expander solution is often administered to maintain intravascular volume.

Cellular Response to Burn Injury

In addition to capillary endothelial permeability changes resulting in vascular fluid losses, transmembrane potential changes occur in cells not directly damaged by heat. The normal potential of −90 mV decreases to nearly −70 mV, with an increase in intracellular sodium and water. Such membrane potential changes may be caused by a circulating shock factor.[65] Other changes can be categorized as (1) a metabolic response to the burn injury or (2) an immunologic response to the burn injury.

Metabolic Response

The metabolic changes after a burn injury were described in 1967 by Welt and associates as "sick cell syndrome."[66] This was considered to be a cell membrane transport defect related to an alteration in the steady state composition characterized by high intracellular concentrations of sodium. Trunkey and

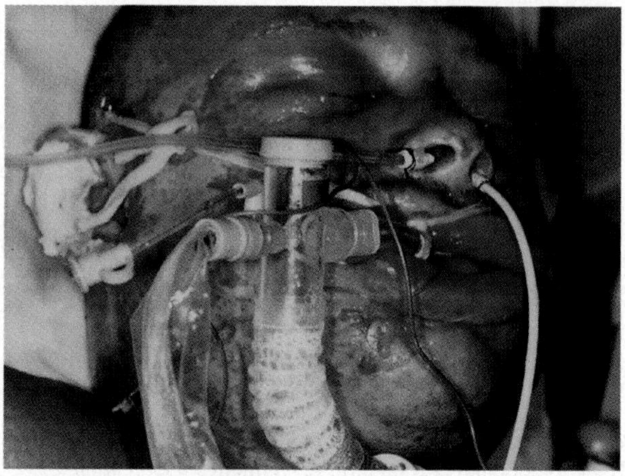

Fig. 45-15 Edema. Superficial facial burns can result in marked swelling, requiring prompt endotracheal intubation to maintain the airway. (Courtesy Intermountain Burn Center, University of Utah.)

colleagues[67] found a marked decrease in primate muscle extracellular water and an increase in both intracellular sodium and water during hypovolemic shock. In addition, other researchers demonstrated an associated decrease in resting membrane potential, a decrease in amplitude of the action potential, and a prolongation of both the repolarization and depolarization times in association with a decreased intracellular potassium concentration.[68,69] The cellular dysfunction of burn injury extends beyond the transmembrane potential disruption and the sodium-potassium pump impairment to include a loss of intracellular magnesium and phosphate[70] and elevated serum lactic dehydrogenase (LDH) levels.[71] Thus impairments of basic cellular function may be the underlying cause of the diminished membrane potentials. The data suggest a decrease in the efficiency of the pump. The failure of rapid intravascular volume repletion to restore membrane potential completely suggests other pathways for cellular metabolic derangement.[72]

Metabolic reactions to the stress of a major burn injury involve the response of the sympathetic nervous system and other homeostatic regulators. Catecholamines are found in elevated amounts in both the serum and urine of burned individuals. Cortisol, glucagon, and insulin levels are elevated, with a corresponding increase in gluconeogenesis, lipolysis, and proteolysis. Changes in lipid metabolism are reflected as an elevation in plasma free fatty acids (FFA) and a decrease in plasma cholesterol and phospholipids.[73] Herndon and colleagues[74] found that the use of propanolol, a nonselective β_1- and β_2-blocker, could attenuate symptoms of the hypermetabolic response, including a decrease in heart rate and lipolysis. Glucose and lactate kinetics are altered after burn injury. Although tissue hypoxia produces lactic acidosis, its persistence in the presence of adequate tissue perfusion suggests an increased rate of glycogenolysis.[75] A small study conducted by Knox and colleagues[76] showed that growth hormone levels are diminished in major burn injuries and appear to improve survival but more clearly affect wound healing.[74]

Burn injury induces an almost immediate hypermetabolic state that persists until wound closure. Wilmore and colleagues[77] described the hypermetabolic state of 20 burned individuals as unrelated to ambient temperatures, with persistent elevation of core body temperatures. The metabolic rate increased with burn size in a curvilinear relationship, with oxygen consumption rarely exceeding two times basal levels. Evaporative water loss and surface cooling are not the primary stimulus for the hypermetabolic state; rather, the hypermetabolism is related to an increase and resetting of the thermal regulatory set-point. A core body temperature of 38.5° C is typical. A reflex arc mobilizes neural or hormonal afferent stimuli to the hypothalamus, producing a catecholamine response clinically manifested as hypermetabolism, hyperthermia, and hyperglycemia.

Evidence also exists that the burn wound itself directly mediates the response to injury at both the local and systemic levels. Cytokines, oxygen radicals, chemotactic substances, and eicosanoids contribute to the systemic inflammatory response and hypermetabolic state. The inflammatory response at the wound level is magnified into a generalized systemic inflammatory response that is often deleterious.[78,79,80] Vasodilation,

Box 45-3

MAINTENANCE FLUID REPLACEMENTS FOLLOWING MAJOR BURN INJURY*

1. *Basal fluid* replacements per day
   1500 ml/day/m² body surface area = 24-hour requirements
2. *Evaporative water loss* from burn wound
   a. Adults: (25 + % total body surface area burn) (m² body surface area) = ml/hr
   b. Children: (35 + % total body surface area burn) (m² body surface area) = ml/hr
3. *Total hourly maintenance fluids*
   Basal fluid requirements per day ÷ 24 hours + evaporative water loss per hour = ml/hr maintenance fluids

Example: A 70-kg adult with a 50% total body surface area burn and a body surface area of 2 m requires the following:
Basal = (1500 ml/day) (2 m² body surface area) = 3000 ml/24 hr, or **125 ml/hr**
Evaporative = (25 + 50% total body surface burn) (2 m² total body surface area) = (75) (2) = **150 ml/hr**
Total maintenance fluids = **125 ml + 150 ml = 275 ml/hr**

*From end of burn shock until wound closure is achieved.

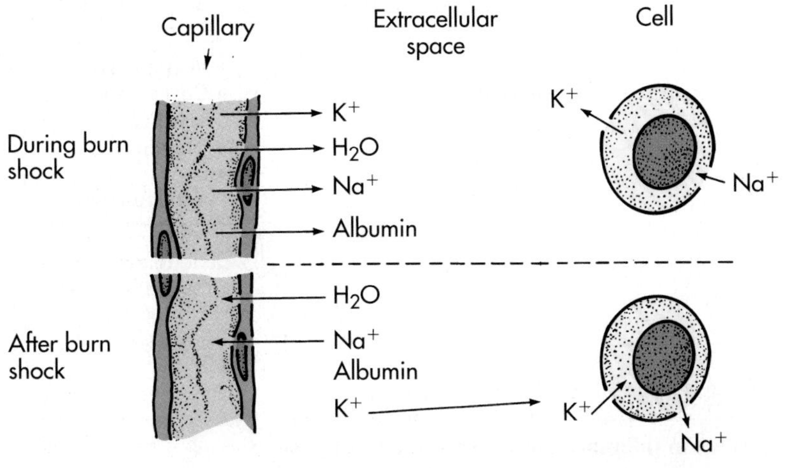

FIG. 45-16 Direction of fluid and electrolyte shifts associated with burn shock. (Courtesy Intermountain Burn Center, University of Utah.)

increased capillary permeability, and edema occur to facilitate healing of the local area. The distribution of the peripheral circulation after burn injury transports both heat and glucose preferentially to the wound. The energy cost of these reparative and transport processes is reflected in the increased metabolism and hyperdynamic circulation.

The extensive evaporative water loss that occurs in burn tissue is a heat-consuming process, and the energy of evaporation is provided by increased visceral heat production. The signal for the response is unknown because individuals whose wounds have been denervated continue to have a **post-traumatic hypermetabolic response**. Hypothalamic function alterations result in the elevation of human growth hormone (hGH) serum levels in the presence of hyperglycemia, a finding opposite that in normal states.[77] Further, the hypermetabolic rate is not decreased during rest, sleep, or warmth.

Evidence of hepatic response to burn injury is characterized by alterations in the clotting factors.[81] A hypercoagulable state develops as manifested by an elevated plasma fibrinogen concentration in the presence of shortened prothrombin time (PT) and activated partial thromboplastin time (PTT).[82]

In summary, extensive burn injury initiates the most marked alterations in body metabolism associated with any illness (Fig. 45-17). Much of the work explaining this response has been conducted by Wilmore,[83,84] who reported that the persistent tachycardia, hyperpnea, hyperpyrexia, and marked body wasting seen in burn injury reflect heightened metabolic activity and accelerated body catabolism. These systemic alterations occur as a result of the cutaneous inflammatory process and are thought to facilitate wound repair. The neural component of this alteration is in response to a sympathetic reaction that releases catecholamines in large amounts.

Immunologic Response

The immunologic response to burn injury is immediate, prolonged, and severe. The result in individuals surviving burn shock is immunosuppression with increased susceptibility to potentially fatal systemic burn wound sepsis.

Several cytokines have been identified in the immediate postburn period. IL-1 is detected in the serum of burned individuals. The level of IL-1 correlates inversely with burn survival; low levels may be associated with a higher mortality.[85] Fatal burn injury has often shown decreased levels of IL-2, which may result in decreased T helper 1 (Th1) lymphocytes. Th1 cells produce IL-2, interferon-γ, and TNF, which help to initiate cellular immunity and immunoglobulin G (IgG) production. IL-4 is elevated after burn injuries and causes a shift in the T helper cell production from Th1 to Th2 lymphocytes. Th2 cells secrete IL-4, which promotes further conversion of nonspecific Th cells to Th2 cells. Th2 cells also produce other cytokines and antibodies.[86] IL-6 levels increase quickly after burn injury and remain elevated for sev-

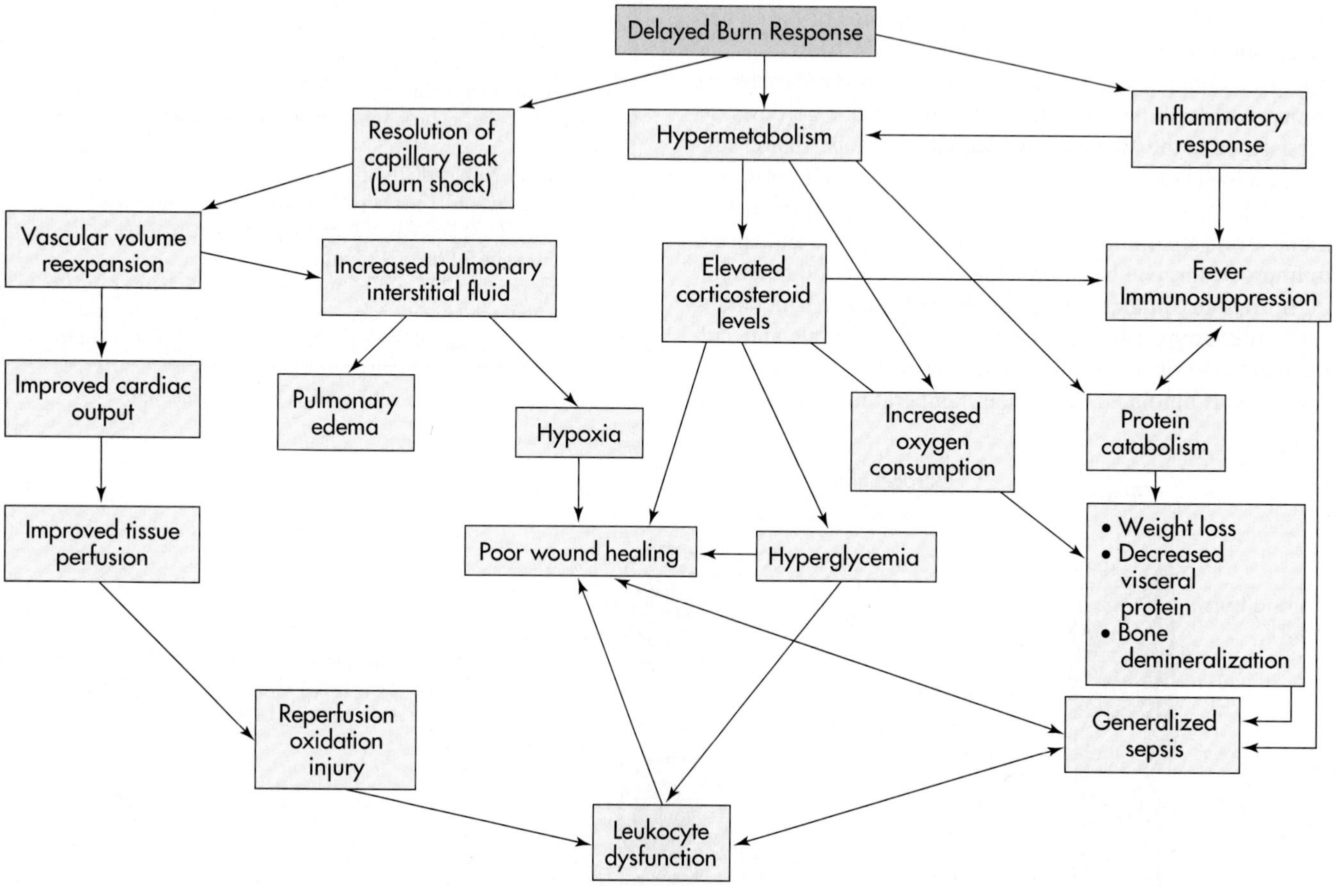

FIG. 45-17 Physiologic alterations in inflammatory burn injury response.

eral weeks. The level of IL-6 correlates with the extent of burn injury.[87] IL-6, together with platelet activating factor, activates polymorphonuclear neutrophils, causing infiltration of neutrophils into burned tissue and adhesion to vascular endothelial surfaces.[88,89] IL-8 levels are elevated after burn injury, with significantly greater elevations seen in individuals with a TBSA burn of 40% or higher. IL-8 activity may play a role in the strong and persistent activation of neutrophils noted in people with large burns.[90] Burn blister fluid contains large amounts of IL-6 and IL-8 in addition to substances such as epidermal growth factor, platelet-derived growth factor, and transforming growth factor.[91]

Macrophages, platelets, neutrophils, and vascular endothelial cells release prostaglandins and leukotrienes, which are the by-products of arachidonic acid metabolism. These chemical mediators cause peripheral vasodilation, pulmonary vasoconstriction, increased capillary permeability, and local tissue ischemia in the burn wound.

A host of chemicals found in burn plasma in altered concentrations also may play a role in burn shock. These include vasoactive amines (histamine, serotonin), products of complement activation (C3a, C5a), prostaglandins, kinins, endotoxin, and metabolic hormones (catecholamines, glucocorticoids). A decrease in complement components C3a and C5a in the circulation after burn injury suggests a nonspecific activation of the complement system.[92] Activation of the complement system in injured tissue results in an inflammatory response caused by release of histamine and serotonin by C3a and C5a, because both histamine and serotonin alter capillary permeability and participate in the mechanism of burn shock along with linin polypeptides and other chemical mediators. Prostaglandins function in the inflammatory process by regulating metabolism of cells of inflammation (see Chapter 7).

Burn shock can induce changes in the integrity of the intestinal wall, facilitating bacterial translocation and endotoxemia.[93] Bacterial translocation from the gut may be a mechanism of infection leading to septic shock after burn injury and other major trauma.[94] Circulating endotoxin is correlated with the development of MODS and death after major burn injury.[95]

White blood cells are also altered at this time, when their need to inhibit sepsis is vital. Natural resistance to infection in burn wounds is a function of the nonspecific immune system; that is, resistance to microorganisms that infect wounds rests almost solely on the ability of phagocytic cells (i.e., granulocytes, macrophages) to leave the bloodstream, migrate to the site of infection, and ingest and kill microorganisms.[96] Normally, opsonins render bacteria susceptible to phagocytosis, but the burn injury triggers a consumptive opsoninopathy. Burn serum contains an inhibitor of C3 conversion that leads to decreased opsonization and polymorphonuclear (PMN) neutrophil dysfunction.[97,98]

Individuals with altered immunocompetence before burn injury are at additional risk for complications. Included in this group are individuals at the extremes of age and those with cardiac disease, malnutrition, immune deficiency disease, and a history of alcohol or drug abuse.[99,100] Additional risk factors include diabetes mellitus and pulmonary or renal dysfunction.

Evaporative Water Loss

One of the major purposes of intact skin is to serve as a barrier to evaporative water loss (EWL) from the body. With major burn injury, this ability of the skin to regulate evaporative water loss is totally disrupted. In a classic study done in 1962, Moncrief and Mason[101] attempted to determine the magnitude of such a loss and determined that daily evaporative water loss was in the range of 20 times normal in the early phase of injury, with gradual decreases as wound closure is achieved. Further studies indicated that insensible water loss through burned skin is not from evaporation of water from sweat glands but rather from water vapor formed within the body and lost through the skin.[102,103]

Calculation of the amount of fluid lost by evaporative water loss includes losses from all sources. Normally the skin is the major source of insensible loss (75%) and the lungs are minor sources (25%), with a total loss of only approximately 600 to 800 ml/day. This changes dramatically with burns, because not only does skin loss increase but also lung loss increases by hypermetabolism and hyperventilation, especially in an intubated individual. Total evaporative losses exceed many liters per day in an adult with large burn wounds. Replacement of the loss is mandatory to prevent volume deficit.

Evaluation and Treatment

Burn recovery is long and stormy, with complications the rule rather than the exception. The goal of burn management is wound closure in a manner that promotes survival. Scar formation with contractures is often a consequence of healing in deep partial-thickness and third-degree burns (Fig. 45-18).

The three essential elements of survival of major burn injury are (1) meticulous wound management, (2) adequate fluids and nutrition, and (3) early surgical excision and grafting. Current therapy for deep-partial and full-thickness burn injury includes surgical removal of the burn tissue (excision) followed by grafting of the person's unburned skin (autograft) to the excised area. Satisfactory wound closure with cultured epithelial autograft (Fig. 45-19) has been inconsistent and

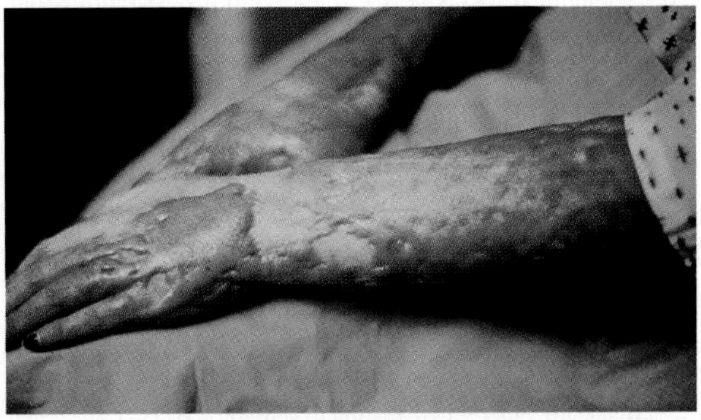

FIG. 45-18 Hypertrophic scarring. Deep partial-thickness thermal injury can result in extensive hypertrophic scarring. (Courtesy Intermountain Burn Center, University of Utah.)

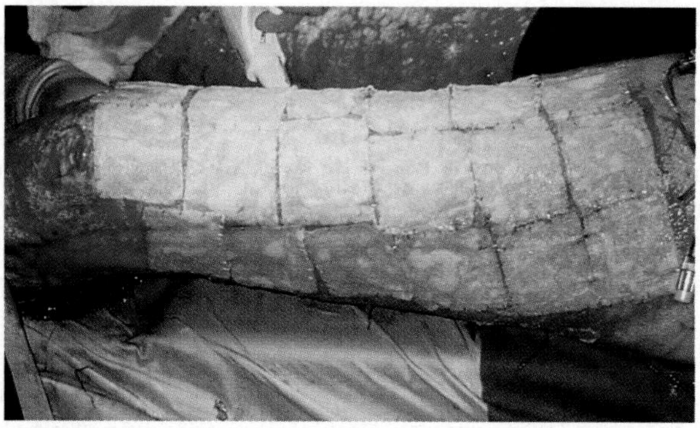

FIG. 45-19 Application of cultured epithelial autografts. The thin sheets of keratinocytes are attached to gauze backing to allow application onto the clean, excised thigh. (Courtesy Intermountain Burn Center, University of Utah.)

costly.[104,105] Advancements in skin replacement technology include sheets of acellular dermal matrix that can be used with thin-meshed autografts or cultured epithelial autografts.[106,107] Current research is also directed at therapies to modulate the hypermetabolic and inflammatory response. Nutritional therapy is focused on early enteral feeding to reduce the potential of gut-mediated sepsis. Ongoing clinical trials using anabolic agents (e.g., recombinant human growth hormone) and pharmacologic agents that modulate inflammatory and endocrine mediators (e.g., ibuprofen, propranolol) show promise in the treatment of severe burn injuries.[64] Burn pain is almost always acute, and treatment strategies usually differ from strategies for chronic pain. In addition to opioid-based agents, new strategies for treatment may include antianxiety agents, hypnosis, and relaxation techniques.[108]

WHAT'S NEW? Burn Care

Immunologic modulation and tissue engineering continue to be areas of significant interest for burn care research. The problem of severe lean body wasting can result in significant debility and even death after burns. Human growth hormone and oxandrolene have been used to mitigate these changes; in the acute setting, human growth hormone was shown to speed donor site healing. In the past the use of oxandrolene in the recovery phase of burn care in conjunction with aggressive nutritional support has been demonstrated to be useful. More recently, a prospective study performed by a group at Brigham and Women's Hospital in Boston was conducted in burned individuals during the postburn period. This study illustrated that these individuals had significantly less weight loss using either recombinant human growth hormone or the anabolic steroid oxandrolene that did those who received the same aggressive nutritional support and physical therapy but did not receive the anabolic substances. Additionally there was a decrease in the loss of nitrogen in these same individuals receiving human growth or oxandrolone, which may indicate better utilization of dietary protein or a decrease in the breakdown of body protein during this early period of burn response.

The technology of burn wound coverage is also changing significantly. A synthetic dermal substitute has been used for some time. However, after the substitute has been applied to the wound, it requires a substantial amount of time for engraftment and then coverage with very thin epithelial autografts. The search for the ideal burn wound covering continues. In an attempt to improve this process, a group from the Karolinska Hospital in Stockholm, Sweden, grafted a cell-free dermis seeded with autologous keratinocytes. The resultant grafts were found to have complete epithelial coverage within 2 weeks of grafting. This and other approaches in development may dramatically change the coverage of burn wounds in the future.

Data from Demling RH, DeSanti L: Oxandrolone, an anabolic steroid, significantly increases the rate of weight gain in the recovery phase of major burns, *J Trauma* 43:47, 1997; Demling RH: Comparison of the anabolic effects and complications of human growth hormone and the testosterone analog, oxandrolone, after severe burn injury, *Burns* 25:215, 1999; Gustafson C-J, Kratz G: Cultured analogous keratinocytes on a cell-free dermis in the treatment of full-thickness wounds, *Burns* 25:330, 1999.

SUMMARY REVIEW

Shock

1. Shock is a widespread impairment of cellular metabolism involving positive-feedback loops that places the individual on a downward physiologic spiral, which, if not reversed, can lead to multiple organ dysfunction syndrome.
2. Types of shock are cardiogenic, hypovolemic, neurogenic, anaphylactic, and septic. A newly identified type of shock, traumatic shock, combines features of hypovolemic shock and septic shock.
3. The final common pathway in all types of shock is impaired cellular metabolism—cells switch from aerobic to anaerobic metabolism. Energy stores drop, and cellular mechanisms relative to membrane permeability, action potentials, and lysozyme release fail.
4. Anaerobic metabolism results in activation of the inflammatory response, decreased circulatory volume, and decreasing pH.
5. Impaired cellular metabolism results in cellular inability to use glucose because of impaired glucose delivery or impaired glucose intake, resulting in a shift of glycogenolysis, gluconeogenesis, and lipolysis for fuel generation.
6. Glycogenolysis is affected for up to 10 hours. Gluconeogenesis results in the use of proteins necessary for structure, function, repair, and replication that leads to more impaired cellular metabolism. Lipolysis is ineffective because of a lack of transport serum proteins and malfunction of the Krebs cycle.
7. Gluconeogenesis contributes to lactic acid, uric acid, and ammonia buildup; interstitial edema; and impairment of the immune system, as well as general muscle weakness leading to decreased respiratory function and cardiac output.
8. Cardiogenic shock is attributable to heart failure and is characterized by a decrease in cardiac output and impaired cellular metabolism.
9. Hypovolemic shock is caused by loss of blood or fluid in large amounts. The use of compensatory mechanisms may be vigorous, but tissue perfusion ultimately decreases and results in impaired cellular metabolism.

10. Neurogenic (vasogenic) shock results from massive vasodilation, causing a relative hypovolemia (even though cardiac output may be high), and results in impaired cellular metabolism.
11. Anaphylactic shock is caused by physiologic recognition of a foreign substance. The inflammatory response is triggered, and a massive vasodilation with fluid shift into the interstitium follows. The relative hypovolemia leads to impaired cellular metabolism.
12. Septic shock begins with impaired cellular metabolism caused by uncontrolled septicemia. The infecting agent triggers the inflammatory and immune responses. It is part of a continuum known as the *systemic inflammatory response syndrome*. Mortality for septic shock is very high.

Multiple Organ Dysfunction Syndrome

1. Multiple organ dysfunction syndrome (MODS) is the progressive failure of two or more organ systems resulting from a systemic inflammatory response after a severe illness or injury. The inflammatory response can be triggered by sepsis, necrotic tissue, trauma, burns, adult respiratory distress syndrome, acute pancreatitis, and other severe injuries.
2. Primary MODS is the immediate local or mild systemic response to the triggering event or illness. It primes the inflammatory system.
3. Secondary MODS is the uncontrollable, excessive systemic inflammatory response that develops after a latent period and results in organ dysfunction.
4. People at greatest risk for developing MODS are elderly individuals, those with significant tissue injury or preexisting disease, and those in whom resuscitation from the initiating illness or injury has been delayed or inadequate.
5. Mortality from MODS is very high: 45% to 55% for failure of two organ systems, 80% for failure of three or more organ systems, and nearly 100% if the failure of three or more organs persists longer than 4 days.
6. Multiple organ dysfunction involves the stress response; release of complement, coagulation, and kinin proteins; changes in the vascular endothelium; and numerous inflammatory processes mediated by substances released by activated neutrophils and macrophages.
7. The consequences of the release of inflammatory mediators in MODS are vasodilation, increased vasopermeability, and selective vasoconstriction resulting in maldistribution of blood flow; hypermetabolism; myocardial depression; and hypoxic injury to cells. Cellular hypoxia and acidosis impair cellular metabolism, leading to organ dysfunction.
8. Clinical manifestations of the development of MODS are general during the first 24 hours: low-grade fever, tachycardia, tachypnea, dyspnea, and altered mental status. Over the next several days, beginning with the lungs, individual organ systems show signs of failure.
9. Because there is no specific therapy for MODS, early detection is extremely important so that supportive measures can be initiated as soon as possible.
10. At present the therapeutic management of MODS consists of prevention or removal of triggering mechanisms and support of individual organs. Recent scientific knowledge about inflammatory mediators has led to many promising future therapies for MODS.

Burns

1. Burns are classified according to depth and extent of injury.
2. First-degree burns involve the superficial skin without loss of protective function.
3. Second-degree burns are superficial (blister formation) or superficial involving partial skin thickness with a waxy white appearance and no involvement of dermal appendages.
4. Third-degree burns involve full skin thickness and often underlying tissues. They are painless and can be life threatening from hypovolemic shock and metabolic and immunologic responses.
5. The total body surface area (TBSA) burned is estimated using either the rule of nines or the Lund and Browder chart. Burns exceeding 20% TBSA are considered major burns.
6. Hypovolemia associated with burn shock is caused by increased capillary permeability with massive fluid losses from blood volume.
7. Altered cell membrane permeability and loss of electrolyte homeostasis contribute to burn shock.
8. Cardiac contractility is decreased during the first 24 hours with shunting of blood away from the liver, kidney, and gut.
9. Fluid resuscitation involves infusion of fluid at a rate faster than the loss of circulating volume for a period of about 24 hours after the burn injury; up to 30 L of fluid may be required for a major burn.
10. The most reliable criterion for adequate resuscitation of burn shock is urine output.
11. Capillary seal is the term used to indicate the end of burn shock.
12. Transmembrane potentials are altered in cells not directly damaged by heat, with impairment of the sodium-potassium pump and loss of magnesium and phosphate.
13. The stress of a major burn activates the sympathetic nervous system with release of catecholamines, cortisol, glucagon, and insulin.
14. Burn injury produces a hypermetabolic state that persists until wound closure and is related to a higher thermal regulatory set-point.
15. The local inflammatory response at the burn site releases cytokines, oxygen radicals, chemotactic factors, and eicosanoids, which leads to a systemic inflammatory response and contributes to hypermetabolism.
16. A posttraumatic hypermetabolic response is associated with increased visceral heat production.
17. Alterations in clotting factors produce a hypercoagulable state following major burns.
18. The immune response following a burn is immediate, prolonged, and severe.
19. Numerous alterations in inflammatory cytokines are evident in the immediate burn period, affecting cellular immunity, antibody production, and attraction of neutrophils and contributing to the vasodilation and increased capillary permeability associated with burn shock.
20. Changes in intestinal wall integrity lead to translocation of bacteria, endotoxemia, and septic shock.
21. White blood cells are altered, and there is decreased opsonization and phagocytosis, contributing to the development of sepsis.
22. Loss of intact skin with a major burn results in significant evaporative water loss contributing to hypovolemia.
23. Treatment of major burns involves meticulous wound management, adequate fluids and nutrition, early surgical excision and grafting, modulation of the hypermetabolic state, and pain management.

KEY TERMS

Acute Physiology and Chronic Health Evaluation II and III (APACHE II and APACHE III), *1498*
Anaphylactic shock, *1489*
Burn shock, *1503*
Burn wound depth, *1499*
Capillary sealed, *1504*
Cardiogenic shock, *1486*
Deep partial-thickness burn, *1500*
Escharotomy, *1501*
First-degree burn, *1499*
Fluid resuscitation, *1503*
Gut hypothesis, *1495*
Hyperdynamic circulation, *1495*
Hypermetabolism, *1496*
Hypovolemic shock, *1487*
Maldistribution of blood flow, *1495*
Multiple organ dysfunction syndrome (MODS), *1492*
Myocardial depression, *1496*
Neurogenic shock (vasogenic shock), *1488*
Nonthermal, *1499*
Partial-thickness injury, *1499*
Posttraumatic hypermetabolic response, *1506*
Primary MODS, *1493*
Secondary MODS, *1493*
Second-degree burn, *1499*
Septic shock, *1490*
Shock, *1483*
Superficial partial-thickness injury, *1499*
Supply-dependent oxygen consumption, *1496*
Thermal, *1499*
Third-degree burn (full-thickness burn), *1501*
Total body surface area (TBSA), *1501*
Vesicant, *1499*

REFERENCES

1. Menezes J et al: A novel nitric oxide scavenger decreases liver injury and improves survival after hemorrhagic shock, *Am J Physiol* 277(1 part 1):G144, 1999.
2. Rippe JM et al: *Intensive care medicine*, ed 3, Boston, 1996, Little, Brown.
3. Hollenberg SM, Kavinsky CJ, Parrillo JE: Cardiogenic shock, *Annals Int Med* 131(1):47, 1999.
4. Hibbard MD et al: Percutaneous transluminal coronary angioplasty in patients with cardiogenic shock, *J Am Coll Cardiol* 19(3):639, 1992.
5. Ranjadayalan K, Umachandran V, Timms A: Clinical impact of introducing thrombolytic and aspirin therapy into the management policy of a coronary care unit, *Am J Med* 93(3):233, 1992.
6. Hasdai D et al: Predictors of cardiogenic shock after thrombolytic therapy for acute myocardial infarction, *J Am Coll Cardiol* 35(1):136, 2000.
7. American College of Chest Physicians/Society of Critical Care Medicine Consensus Conference Committee: Definitions for sepsis and organ failure and guidelines for the use of innovative therapies in sepsis, *Crit Care Med* 20(6):864, 1992.
8. Rangel-Frausto MS: The epidemiology of bacterial sepsis, *Inf Dis Clin No Amer* 13(2):299, 1999.
9. Eidleman LA, Pizov R, Sprung CL: New therapeutic approaches in sepsis: a critical review, *Intensive Care Med* 21:S269, 1995.
10. Parrillo JE: Pathogenetic mechanisms of septic shock, *N Engl J Med* 328(20):1471, 1993.
11. Wiessner WH, Casey LC, Zbilut JP: Treatment of sepsis and septic shock: a review, *Heart Lung* 24:380, 1995.
12. Bone RC: Sepsis and SIRS, *Nephrol Dial Transplant* 9(suppl 4):99, 1994.
13. Morrison DC et al: Structure-function relationships of bacterial endotoxins contribution to microbial sepsis, *Inf Dis Clin No Amer* 13(2):313, 1999.
14. Bernal A et al: Superantigens in human disease, *J Clin Immunol* 19(3):149, 1999.
15. Sriskandan S, Cohen J: Gram-positive sepsis, *Inf Dis Clin No Amer* 13(2):397, 1999.
16. Symeonides S, Balk RA: Nitric oxide in the pathogenesis in sepsis, *Inf Dis Clin No Amer* 13(2):449, 1999.
17. Van der Poll T, van Deventer SJH: Cytokines and anticytokines in the pathogenesis of sepsis, *Inf Dis Clin No Amer* 13(2):413, 1999.
18. Reeves JH et al: Continuous plasma filtration in sepsis syndrome, *Crit Care Med* 27(10):2096, 1999.
19. Pittet D et al: Impact of immunomodulating therapy on morbidity in patients with severe sepsis, *Am J Resp Crit Care Med* 160:852, 1999.
20. Bhattacharjee AK, Cross AS: Vaccines and antibodies in the prevention and treatment of sepsis, *Inf Dis Clin No Amer* 13(2):355,1999.
21. Opal SM, Cross AS: Clinical trials for severe sepsis past failures, and future hopes, *Inf Dis Clin No Amer* 13(2):285, 1999.
22. Briegel J et al: Stress doses of hydrocortisone reverse hyperdynamic septic shock: a prospective, randomized, double-blind, single-center study, *Crit Care Med* 27(4):723, 1999.
23. Dellinger RP: Current therapy for sepsis, *Inf Dis Clin No Amer* 13(2):495, 1999.
24. Bone RC: Why new definitions of sepsis and organ failure are needed, *Am J Med* 95:348, 1993.
25. Baue AE: Multiple, progressive or sequential system failure: a syndrome for the '70s, *Arch Surg* 110(7):779, 1975.
26. Tilney NL, Bailey GL, Morgan AP: Sequential system failure after rupture of abdominal aortic aneurysm: an unsolved problem in postoperative care, *Ann Surg* 178(2):117, 1973.
27. Garrison RN et al: Microvascular changes explain the "two-hit" theory of multiple organ failure, *Annals Surg* 227(6):851, 1998.
28. St. John RC, Dorinsky PM: An overview of multiple organ dysfunction syndrome, *J Lab Clin Med* 124(4):478, 1994.
29. Beal AL, Cerra FB: Multiple organ failure syndrome in the 1990s, *J Am Med Assoc* 271(3):226, 1994.
30. Moore FA, Moore EE: Evolving concepts in the pathogenesis of postinjury multiple organ failure, *Surg Clin North Am* 75(2):257, 1995.
31. Zallen G et al: Age of transfused blood is an independent risk factor for postinjury multiple organ failure, *Am J Surgery* 178(6):570, 1999.
32. Demling RH, Will JA, Belzer FO: Effect of major thermal injury on the pulmonary microcirculation, *Surgery* 83:746, 1978.
33. Demling R et al: Multiple organ dysfunction in the surgical patient: pathophysiology, prevention, and treatment. In Wells SA, editor: *Current problems in surgery*, vol 4, St Louis, 1993, Mosby.
34. Chrousos GP: The hypothalamic-pituitary-adrenal axis and immune-mediated inflammation, *N Engl J Med* 322(20):1351, 1995.
35. Bannan J, Visvanathan K, Zambriskie JB: Structure and function of streptococcal and staphylococcal superantigens in septic shock, *Infect Dis Clin No Am* 13(2):387, 1999.
36. Botha AJ et al: Early neutrophil sequestration after injury: a pathologic mechanism for multiple organ failure, *J Trauma* 39(3):411, 1995.
37. Baker CC, Huynh T: Sepsis in the critically ill patient. In Wells SA et al, editors: *Current problems in surgery*, vol 32, St Louis, 1995, Mosby.
38. Baue AE: The horror autotoxicus and multiple-organ failure, *Arch Surg* 127:1451, 1992.
39. Deitch EA: Multiple organ failure. In Davis JH et al, editors: *Surgery: a problem-solving approach*, ed 2, St Louis, 1995, Mosby.
40. Pope HC et al: Reticuloendothelial system activity and organ failure in patients with multiple injuries, *Arch Surgery* 134:421, 1999.
41. Ince C, Sinaasappel M: Microcirculatory oxygenation and shunting in sepsis and shock, *Crit Care Med* 27(7):1369, 1999.
42. Demling R, LaLonde C, Ikegami K: Physiologic support of the septic patient, *Surg Clin North Am* 74(3):637, 1994.
43. Carpati CM, Astiz ME, Rackow EC: Mechanisms and management of myocardial dysfunction in septic shock, *Crit Care Med* 27(2):231, 1999.
44. Deitch EA: Multiple organ failure: pathophysiology and potential future therapy, *Ann Surg* 216:117, 1992.

45. Wheeler AP, Bernard GR: Treating patients with sepsis, *New Eng J Med* 340(3):207, 1999.
46. Bone RC: Sepsis and controlled clinical trials: the odyssey continues, *Crit Care Med* 23(8):1313, 1995.
47. Clark DE, Dainiak CN, Reeder S: Decreasing incidence of burn injury in a rural state, *Inj Prev* 6(4):259, 2000.
48. Brigham PA, McLoughlin E: Burn incidence and medical care use in the United States: estimates, trends, and data sources, *J Burn Care Rehabil* 17(2):95, 1996.
49. Sheridan RL et al: Planimetry study of the percent of body surface represented by the hand and palm: sizing irregular burns is more accurately done with the palm, *J Burn Care Rehabil* 16(6):605, 1995.
50. Morris SE, Navaratnam N, Herndon DN: A comparison of effects of thermal injury and smoke inhalation on bacterial translocation, *J Trauma* 30(6):639, 1990.
51. Arturson G: Forty years in burns research—the postburn inflammatory response, *Burns* 26:599, 2000.
52. Baxter CR, Cook WA, Shires GT: Serum myocardial depressant factor of burn shock, *Surg Forum* 17:1, 1966.
53. Horton JW et al: Calcium antagonists improve mechanical performance after thermal trauma, *J Surg Res* 87(1):39, 1999.
54. Aikawa N, Martyn JAJ, Burke JF: Pulmonary artery catheterization and thermodilution cardiac output determination in the management of critically burned patients, *Am J Surg* 135:811, 1978.
55. Dobson EL, Warner GF: Factors concerned in the early stages of thermal shock, *Circ Res* 5:69, 1957.
56. Lefer AM, Martin J: Origin of myocardial depressant factor in shock, *Am J Physiol* 218:1423, 1970.
57. Rosenthal SR, Hawley PL, Hakin AA: Purified burn toxic factor and its competition, *Surgery* 71:527, 1972.
58. Horton JW, Burton KP, White DJ: The role of toxic oxygen metabolites in a young model of thermal injury, *J Trauma* 39(3):563, 1995.
59. Onuoha G, Alpar K, Jones I: Vasoactive intestinal peptide and nitric oxide in the acute phase following burns and trauma, *Burns* 27(1):17, 2001.
60. Ungureanu-Longrois D et al: Myocardial contractile dysfunction in the systemic inflammatory response syndrome: role of a cytokine-inducible nitric oxide synthase in cardiac myocytes, *J Mol Cell Cardiol* 27(1):155, 1995.
61. Gamelli RL et al: Burn-induced nitric oxide release in humans, *J Trauma* 39(5):869, 1995.
62. Baxter CR: Fluid volume and electrolyte changes of the early post-burn period, *Clin Plast Surg* 1:693, 1974.
63. Huang PP et al: Hypertonic sodium resuscitation is associated with renal failure and death, *Ann Surg* 221(5):543, 1995.
64. Herndon DN, Spies M: Modern burn care, *Semin Pediatr Surg* 10(1): 28, 2001.
65. Evans JA, Darlington DN, Gann DS: A circulating factor(s) mediates cell depolarization in hemorrhagic shock, *Ann Surg* 312(6):549, 1991.
66. Welt LG et al: Membrane transport defect: the sick cell, *Trans Assoc Am Physicians* 80:217, 1967.
67. Trunkey DD et al: The effect of hemorrhagic shock on intracellular muscle action potentials in the primates, *Surgery* 74:241, 1973.
68. Cunningham JN Jr, Shires GT, Wagner Y: Changes in intracellular sodium and potassium content of red blood cells in trauma and shock, *Am J Surg* 122:650, 1971.
69. Rosenthal SM, Tabor H: Electrolyte changes and chemotherapy in experimental burn and traumatic shock and hemorrhage, *Arch Surg* 51: 244, 1945.
70. Turinsky J, Gonnerman WA, Loose LD: Impaired mineral metabolism in postburn muscle, *J Trauma* 21:417, 1981.
71. Deets DK, Glaviano VV: Plasma and cardiac lactic dehydrogenase activity in burn shock, *Proc Soc Exp Biol Med* 142:412, 1973.
72. Button B et al: Evidence of circulating membrane depolarization factor(s) in hemorrhagic shock, *Shock* 1(suppl):15, 1994.
73. Okamoto R, Glaviano VV, Pindok M: Myocardial lipases and catecholamines in burn shock, *Proc Soc Exp Biol Med* 137:347, 1971.
74. Ikezu T et al: A unique mechanism of desensitization to lipolysis mediated by beta (3)-adrenoreceptor in rats with thermal injury, *Am J Physiol* 277(2 part 1):E316, 1999.
75. Wilmore DW, Aulick HL, Goodwin CW: Glucose metabolism following severe injury, *Acta Chir Scand* 498:3, 1979.
76. Akcay MN et al: The effect of growth hormone on 24-h urinary creatinine levels in burned patients, *Burns* 27(1):42, 2001.
77. Wilmore DW et al: Alterations in hypothalamic function following thermal injury, *J Trauma* 15:697, 1975.
78. Gump FE, Price JB Jr, Kinney JM: Blood flow and oxygen consumption in patients with severe burns, *Surg Gynecol Obstet* 130:23, 1970.
79. Wilmore DW et al: Influence of the burn wound on local and systemic responses to injury, *Ann Surg* 186:444, 1977.
80. Wilmore DW et al: Effect of injury and infection on visceral metabolism and circulation, *Ann Surg* 192:491, 1980.
81. Holder IA, Neely AN: Hageman factor-dependent kinin activation in burns and its theoretical relationship to postburn immunosuppression syndrome and infection, *J Burn Care Rehabil* 11:496, 1990.
82. McManus WF, Eurenius K, Pruitt BA Jr: Disseminated intravascular coagulation in burned patients, *J Trauma* 13:416, 1973.
83. Wilmore DW: *The metabolic management of the critically ill*, ed 2, New York, 1990, Plenum.
84. Wilmore DW, Aulick LH: Metabolic changes in burned patients, *Surg Clin North Am* 58:1173, 1978.
85. Wright K et al: Burn-activated neutrophils and tumor necrosis factor-alpha alter endothelial cell actin cytoskeleton and enhance monolayer permeability, *Surg* 128(2):259, 2000.
86. Goebel A et al: Injury induces deficient interleukin-12 production, but interleukin-12 therapy after injury restores resistance to infection, *Ann Surg* 231(2):253, 2000.
87. Nishiura T et al: Gene expression and cytokine and enzyme activation in the liver after a burn injury, *J Burn Care Rehabil* 21(2):135, 2000.
88. Biffl WL et al: Interleukin-6 delays neutrophil apoptosis via a mechanism involving platelet-activating factor, *J Trauma* 40(4):575, 1996.
89. Choi M et al: Preventing the infiltration of leukocytes by monoclonal antibody blocks the development of progressive ischemia in rat burns, *Plast Reconstr Surg* 96(5):1186, 1995.
90. Iocono JA et al: Interleukin-8 levels and activity in delayed-healing thermal wounds, *Wound Repair Regen* 8(3):216, 2000.
91. Ortega MR, Ganz T, Milner SM: Human beta defensin is absent in burn blister fluid, *Burns* 26(8):724, 2000.
92. Heideman J, Kaijser B, Gelin L: Complement activation and hematologic, hemodynamic, and respiratory reactions early after soft tissue injury, *J Trauma* 18:696, 1978.
93. Grzybowski J et al: Antidietary antigen antibodies in the sera of patients with burns as a potential marker of gut mucosa integrity failure, *J Burn Care Rehabil* 13:194, 1992.
94. Deitch EA, Berg R: Bacterial translocation from the gut: mechanism of infection, *J Burn Care Rehabil* 8:475, 1987.
95. Yao YM et al: The association of circulating endotoxaemia with the development of multiple organ failure in burned patients, *Burns* 21(4): 255, 1995.
96. Benhaim P, Hunt TK: Natural resistance to infection: leukocyte functions, *J Burn Care Rehabil* 13(part 2):287, 1992.
97. Alexander JW et al: Consumptive opsoninopathy: possible pathogenesis in lethal and opportunistic infections, *Ann Surg* 184:672, 1976.
98. Bjornson AB, Altemeier WA, Bjornson HS: Changes in humoral components of host defense following burn trauma, *Ann Surg* 186:96, 1977.
99. Goff DR et al: Cardiac disease and the patient with burns, *J Burn Care Rehabil* 11:305, 1990.
100. McGill V et al: The impact of substance use on mortality and morbidity from thermal injury, *J Trauma* 38(6):931, 1995.
101. Moncrief JA, Mason AD: Water vapor loss in the burned patient, *Surg Forum* 13:38, 1962.
102. Moncrief JA: Burns. In Schwartz SI et al, editors: *Principles of surgery,* ed 2, New York, 1974, McGraw-Hill.
103. Roe CF, Kinney JM: Water and heat exchange in third-degree burns, *Surgery* 56:212, 1964.

104. Ronford V et al: Long-term regeneration of human epidermis on third degree burns transplanted with autologous cultured epithelium grown on a fibrin matrix, *Transplantation* 70(11):1588, 2000.
105. Williamson JS et al: Cultured epithelial autograft: five years of clinical experience with twenty-eight patients, *J Trauma* 39(2):309, 1995.
106. Carsin H et al: Cultured epithelial autografts in extensive burn coverage of severely traumatized patients: a five-year single-center experience with 30 patients, *Burns* 26(4):379, 2000.
107. Wainwright D et al: Clinical evaluation of an acellular allograft dermal matrix in full-thickness burn, *J Burn Care Rehabil* 17(2):124, 1996.
108. Jellish WS et al: Effect of topical local anesthetic application to skin harvest sites for pain management in burn patients undergoing skin-grafting procedures, *Ann Surg* 229(1):115, 1999.

CHAPTER 46

Shock, Multiple Organ Dysfunction Syndrome, and Burns in Children

MARY FRAN HAZINSKI • MARILYN E. JENKINS*

CHAPTER OUTLINE

This chapter reviews shock, multiple organ dysfunction syndrome, and burns in children. It clearly defines the differences between these conditions in children and adults. These differences are noted not only in the pathophysiology section, but also in the epidemiology, clinical manifestations, and treatment and evaluation sections.

SHOCK AND MULTIPLE ORGAN DYSFUNCTION SYNDROME

Shock in children is most often the result of hemorrhage, severe dehydration, progressive heart failure, or sepsis. It may also complicate the care of the child with pulmonary failure (cor pulmonale), drug toxicity, electrolyte or acid-base imbalance, dysrhythmias, or multiple organ failure. (The physiology of shock is discussed in Chapter 45.)

Shock in children is present when there are signs of poor systemic perfusion, regardless of the blood pressure—shock may be present with normal, high, or low blood pressure. When blood pressure is inappropriate for age, the child is in **compensated shock**. If shock is associated with hypotension, the child is in **decompensated shock**.

Multiple organ dysfunction syndrome (MODS) is the failure of at least two organs that results from a single cause and arises 3 to 10 days after the causative event. For example, MODS can develop as a complication of sepsis, cardiopulmonary arrest, or trauma, and typically the signs of organ failure develop within days.

Types of Shock

Shock is categorized as follows:

1. *Hypovolemic shock*: caused by inadequate intravascular volume relative to the vascular space
2. *Cardiogenic shock*: results from impairment of myocardial function
3. *Distributive or vasogenic shock*: associated with inappropriate distribution of blood flow and increased capillary permeability (e.g., septic shock) or central nervous system injury (e.g., neurogenic shock)

Such a classification system is helpful because it indicates the major therapy required (Box 46-1). However, it is inadequate for describing individuals with late or progressive shock, because at that point they are likely to demonstrate widespread cardiovascular dysfunction, including inappropriate intravascular volume relative to the vascular space, severe myocardial dysfunction, and maldistribution of blood flow. In addition, severe shock of any kind, even with successful therapy, may be followed by complications or death. The hypoxic insult can serve to prime cells and may result in reperfusion injury and inflammatory response that further injures cells and produces multiple organ dysfunction. The etiologic classification is also misleading for septic shock,

*Chapter content on "Shock" and "Multiple Organ Dysfunction Syndrome" contributed by Mary Fran Hazinski; "Burns" contributed by Marilyn E. Jenkins.

because sepsis produces elements of hypovolemic and cardiogenic shock in addition to the complications of maldistribution of blood flow. Finally, any individual in shock is likely to develop some myocardial dysfunction and some compromise in organ perfusion and function. Thus all aspects of cardiovascular function and oxygen delivery must be skillfully supported during the treatment of any form of shock.

Hypovolemic Shock

Hypovolemic shock, the most common type of shock in children, is associated with a reduction in the intravascular volume relative to the vascular space. Dehydration and trauma are the most common causes of hypovolemic shock in children. It may also result from a redistribution of blood volume or increased capillary permeability, such as develops following burns or sepsis.

Box 46-1

CLASSIFICATION AND CAUSES OF SHOCK

HYPOVOLEMIC

1. Hemorrhage
   a. External: laceration
   b. Internal: ruptured spleen or liver, vascular injury, fracture (newborn: intracerebral/intraventricular hemorrhage)
   c. Gastrointestinal: bleeding ulcer, ruptured viscus, mesenteric hemorrhage
2. Plasma loss
   a. Burn
   b. Inflammation or sepsis: capillary leak syndrome
   c. Nephrotic syndrome
   d. Third spacing: intestinal obstruction, pancreatitis, peritonitis
3. Fluid and electrolyte loss
   a. Acute gastroenteritis
   b. Excessive evaporative loss (including burns)
   c. Renal pathologic conditions
4. Endocrine
   a. Adrenal insufficiency, adrenogenital syndrome
   b. Diabetes mellitus
   c. Diabetes insipidus
   d. Hypothyroidism (myxedema coma)

CARDIOGENIC

1. Myocardial insufficiency
   a. Dysrhythmia: bradycardia, atrioventricular (AV) block, ventricular tachycardia, supraventricular tachycardia
   b. Cardiomyopathy: myocarditis, ischemia, hypoxia, hypoglycemia, acidosis
   c. Drug intoxication
   d. Hypothermia
   e. Congenital heart disease, including ductal-dependent lesion such as coarctation of the aorta or critical pulmonary stenosis

DISTRIBUTIVE (VASOGENIC)

1. High or normal resistance (increased venous capacitance)
   a. Septic shock
   b. Anaphylaxis
   c. Barbiturate intoxication
2. Low resistance, vasodilation: central nervous system (CNS) injury (i.e., spinal cord transection)

From Hazinski MF: Shock. In Barkin RM, editor: *Pediatric emergency medicine: concepts and clinical practice,* ed 2, St Louis, 1997, Mosby.

When hypovolemia is mild or moderate, such as 5% dehydration or mild hemorrhage, compensatory vasoconstrictive adrenergic responses redistribute blood from the mesenteric, renal, and skin circulation to the heart and brain. Blood pressure is initially maintained as the vasoconstriction reduces the vascular space. Hypotension may not be observed in the child with hypovolemic shock unless intravascular volume loss is rapid or severe.[1] This usually occurs with greater than 10% dehydration in the infant or child or greater than 7% dehydration in the adolescent. A 20% to 25% acute hemorrhage is usually required to produce hypotension in the child with trauma. Thus a normal blood pressure is frequently observed in the child with hypovolemic shock. Hypotension is a sign of severe, decompensated shock.

Hypovolemia may also be caused by an increase in the vascular space relative to intravascular volume. This may be associated with the vasodilation of sepsis or an inflammatory response, following an ischemic insult, or ingestion of β-adrenergic drugs. A relative hypovolemia may also be caused by increased capillary permeability with a redistribution of intravascular volume, such as with burns or increased capillary permeability. The translocation of extravascular fluid to a location that is neither intravascular nor intracellular, as in edema, is termed **"third spacing" of fluids**.

With **distributive (vasogenic) shock**, a normal cardiac output probably is inadequate to maintain blood flow to all tissue beds simultaneously. Although no absolute fluid or blood loss has occurred, volume administration is necessary to ensure that the intravascular volume is adequate relative to the vascular space, and cardiac output must be supported at a level that is higher than normal.

Neurogenic shock is a form of hypovolemic and vasogenic (maldistributive) shock. It is caused by loss of vasomotor tone following severe injury to the spinal cord. Massive vasodilation and loss of sympathomimetic tone result in a larger vascular space and relative hypovolemia.

Compensatory Responses

Adrenergic and renal compensatory mechanisms are stimulated by significant dehydration or hypovolemia. Reduced renal perfusion stimulates the renin-angiotensin-aldosterone system, resulting in renal sodium and water retention. Decreased atrial stretch stimulates the secretion of antidiuretic hormone (ADH, also known as arginine vasopressin [AVP]) and produces free water retention by the kidneys. These mechanisms are similar in adults and children and may help to restore or maintain intravascular volume over time. Neonatal and young infant kidneys, however, are incapable of excreting a concentrated urine, so these compensatory mechanisms are relatively ineffective during the first weeks of life.

Compensatory mechanisms cannot be maintained indefinitely. Systemic vasoconstriction increases left ventricular afterload and myocardial oxygen consumption. Prolonged tachycardia produces impaired subendocardial blood flow and increased myocardial oxygen consumption, which may ultimately contribute to myocardial ischemia. Extreme tachypnea increases oxygen demand and reduces tidal volume. A severe compromise in blood flow and systemic perfusion contributes to cerebral, renal, or hepatic ischemia and possible organ failure (see p. 1522).

Clinical Manifestations

The child with inadequate cardiac output demonstrates signs of inadequate blood flow to some tissue beds and some evidence of organ system failure. When hypovolemic or cardiogenic shock is present, the extremities may feel cool (they cool in a peripheral to proximal fashion). By comparison, excessive skin blood flow may be present in children with sepsis or septic shock. Capillary refill time is often prolonged, despite a warm ambient temperature, and the skin may have a mottled appearance. Urine output decreases if renal perfusion is compromised and is less than 2 ml/kg/hr in infants, less than 1 ml/kg/hr in children, and less than 0.5 ml/kg/hr in adolescents despite adequate fluid intake. Liver enzymes may be elevated if hepatic perfusion is reduced. The development of a metabolic acidosis indicates that blood flow to some tissues is inadequate to support total aerobic metabolism. Hypotension is often *not* present unless or until shock is severe.

The child's level of consciousness and responsiveness may provide valuable information about the severity of illness. The healthy infant should orient to faces, make eye contact, and track bright objects across a visual field. The healthy child is alert and reluctant to be separated from parents or examined by strangers. The critically ill infant or child is often extremely irritable; and lethargy indicates severe deterioration in the child's level of consciousness. A decreased response to painful stimulation is abnormal in the child of any age and usually indicates severe cardiorespiratory or neurologic compromise.[2]

Hypoglycemia may be observed in seriously ill or injured infants and may be associated with cardiovascular or neurologic deterioration. Infants have high glucose needs and low glycogen stores that may be rapidly depleted during stress. However, *hyperglycemia* has been linked with poor survival in some older children with trauma or shock;[3] this high glucose level may result from gluconeogenesis or excessive glucose administration.

Vital signs should be evaluated in light of the child's clinical condition. Normal vital signs are not always appropriate in the seriously ill or injured child (Box 46-2).[2] The clinical manifestations observed in the child with hypovolemic shock are those of inadequate systemic perfusion associated with intravascular volume loss and/or expansion of the vascular space. If compensatory mechanisms are working, adrenergic compensatory mechanisms produce tachycardia and redistribution of blood flow, including signs of peripheral vasoconstriction, cool extremities, delayed capillary refill, and oliguria. Hypotension is often only a late, and preterminal, sign of shock in the child. Table 46-1 contains normal vital signs in children.

The child's heart rate should be appropriate for age and clinical condition. The child in shock is often tachycardic. The **tachycardia** may be primary (dysrhythmia) or secondary to stress (sinus tachycardia). If the heart rate, particularly the ventricular rate, is extremely rapid or if it is present

Box 46-2

ESTIMATING BLOOD PRESSURE IN CHILDREN

The typical "normal" (i.e., median, or fiftieth percentile) systolic blood pressure for a child 1 to 10 years of age may be estimated by adding 90 mm Hg to twice the child's age in years (90 mm Hg + [2 × Age in years]); this corresponds to the fiftieth percentile systolic blood pressure for the child's age. A systolic pressure equal to or less than 70 mm Hg plus twice the child's age in years (70 mm Hg + [2 × Age in years]) is considered hypotensive beyond 1 year of age because this blood pressure corresponds to the fifth percentile systolic blood pressure for age (i.e., only 5% of normal, healthy children will demonstrate a systolic blood pressure lower than that number).

Data from Chameides L, Hazinski MF, editors: *Textbook of pediatric advanced life support,* Dallas, 1997, American Heart Association.

Table 46-1 Normal Pediatric Vital Signs

Age	Awake Heart Rate* (per min)	Sleeping Heart Rate (per min)
Newborn	100-180	80-160
Infant (6 mo)	100-160	75-160
Toddler	80-110	60-90
Preschooler	70-110	60-90
School-age child	65-110	60-90
Adolescent	60-90	50-90
Age		**Respiratory Rate (breaths per min)**
Infant		30-60
Toddler		24-40
Preschooler		22-34
School-age child		18-30
Adolescent		12-16
Age	**Systolic Blood Pressure† (mm Hg)**	**Diastolic Blood Pressure (mm Hg)**
Birth (12 hr, <1000 g)	39-59	16-36
Birth (12 hr, 3-kg weight)	50-70	25-45
Newborn (96 hr)	60-90	20-60
Infant (6 mo)	87-105	53-66
Toddler (2 yr)	95-105	53-66
School-age child (7 yr)	97-112	57-71
Adolescent (15 yr)	112-128	66-80

Modified from Hazinski MF: *Manual of pediatric critical care,* St Louis, 1999, Mosby.

*Heart rate ranges from Gillette PC, Garson A Jr: *Pediatric cardiac dysrhythmias,* New York, 1982, Grune & Stratton.

†Blood pressure ranges taken from the following sources:

Neonate: Versmold H et al: *Pediatrics* 67:107, 1981. 10th-90th percentile ranges used.

Others: Horan MJ, chairman, Task Force on Blood-Pressure Control in Children: *Pediatrics* 79:1, 1987. 50th-90th percentile ranges used.

and: National High Blood Pressure Education Program Working Group in Hypertension Control in Children and Adolescents. Update on the 1987 Task Force Report on High Blood Pressure in Children and Adolescents: a working group report from the National Blood Pressure Education Program. *Pediatrics* 98:649, 1996.

Note: Always consider patient's normal range and clinical condition. Heart and respiratory rates will normally increase with fever or stress.

Table 46-2 Factors Affecting Cardiovascular Performance in Children

Factor	Comments
Heart rate	Normally more rapid in children than in adults. Because the *stroke volume* is smaller than in adults, the *cardiac output* of the child is more closely related to heart rate than stroke volume. *Tachycardia* is expected in the seriously ill or injured child. The most common cause of *bradycardia* in young children is hypoxia and is an ominous sign if present in association with poor perfusion. Urgent treatment is required once bradycardia or supraventricular or ventricular tachycardia produces signs of shock.
Stroke volume	Averages 1.5 ml/kg; affected by conditions altering ventricular preload, compliance, contractility, and afterload.
Ventricular end-diastolic pressure (VEDP)	Optimal pressure for children in shock is unknown. Aggressive fluid administration is linked to improved survival in children with *septic* shock.
Ventricular compliance or distensibility	Can be affected by congenital heart defects such as atrial septal defects (ASDs). If compliance is low, such as in newborns and infants, volume administration may increase VEDP. Hypoplastic ventricles are often noncompliant. Hypertrophied ventricles, noted in children with severe pulmonary stenosis or aortic stenosis, may become fibrotic and noncompliant. Increased compliance may be present in early septic shock.
Contractility	No evidence exists that contractility is significantly lower in newborns, infants, and children than adults. Newborn myocardium does have fewer contractile proteins and higher water content than adult myocardium, but the clinical significance of this is probably minimal.
Afterload	Newborn myocardium *can* adapt to mild, nonacute increases in afterload. Afterload may be increased in children with systemic vasoconstriction or pulmonary hypertension (constrictors include alveolar hypoxia, acidosis, hypothermia, and alveolar distention). Some uncorrected congenital heart defects may increase afterload. Coarctation of the aorta and aortic stenosis increase left ventricular afterload. Pulmonary stenosis increases right ventricular afterload. Afterload may be decreased in septic shock.
Oxygen delivery and consumption	Highest per kilogram body weight during the neonatal period and infancy. Oxygen reserve is smaller in infants and children than in adults, and the young child requires a higher cardiac output and oxygen delivery per kilogram than the adult. Increased oxygen consumption occurs in critically ill newborns exposed to cold because they cannot shiver to generate heat. Other causes of increased oxygen consumption in children and infants include fever, sepsis, pain, and seizures.

in the child with decreased myocardial function, shock may result. In general, if ventricular rate exceeds 200 to 220 beats/min in the infant or 160 to 180 beats/min in the child, ventricular diastolic filling time and coronary artery perfusion time are significantly reduced and stroke volume falls. As a result, cardiac output falls and signs of congestive heart failure or shock develop. Once supraventricular or ventricular tachycardia produces signs of shock, urgent treatment is required.[4]

Bradycardia, an abnormally low heart rate, can cause a fall in cardiac output. In young animal models a fall in heart rate produces a commensurate fall in cardiac output.[4,5] The most common cause of bradycardia in young children is hypoxia. Therefore, if bradycardia is observed, airway patency, oxygenation, and ventilation must be constantly assessed and supported as needed. Bradycardia often indicates impending cardiovascular collapse or cardiac arrest and is the most common terminal cardiac rhythm observed.[4]

The child's stroke volume may be altered by conditions affecting ventricular preload, compliance, contractility, and afterload (Table 46-2). Each of these variables must be evaluated and optimized in the treatment of shock (see Chapter 45).

If the ambient temperature is warm, capillary refill is normally brisk; a prolonged capillary refill time may indicate a compromise in systemic perfusion with some forms of shock. Capillary refill time of less than 1.5 to 2 seconds is normal and may be observed in infants and children with minimal fluid deficit (less than 5% dehydration). If the capillary refill time is 1.5 to 3 seconds in a warm room, a 5% to 10% dehydration is likely to be present, and a refill time over 3 seconds is associated with greater than 10% dehydration.[1,6] Metabolic/lactic acidosis also may be present.

The central venous pressure (CVP) and pulmonary artery wedge pressure (PAWP) (also called *pulmonary artery occlusion pressure* [PAOP]) is 5 to 8 mm Hg or lower, and the cardiac silhouette is typically small (not enlarged) on chest radiograph.

Clinically significant dehydration is associated with weight loss (Table 46-3). Fluid intake and output records (or reports from parents or primary caretakers) reveal a history of inadequate fluid intake or excessive fluid losses. The child with significant dehydration demonstrates dry mucous membranes, a sunken fontanelle (in infants), and poor skin turgor (Table 46-4).[1] The blood urea nitrogen (BUN) and urine specific gravity are usually elevated. The serum sodium concentration and osmolality are affected by the type and severity of dehydration present.

Hemorrhage is another potential cause of hypovolemic shock. To appreciate the significance of any blood lost or drawn for laboratory analysis, the total blood loss should be considered as a percentage of the child's circulating blood volume (Table 46-5).

Acute blood loss (hemorrhage) typically does not compromise peripheral perfusion until 15% to 25% of intravascular volume is lost (an acute intravascular or blood loss of 12 to 16 ml/kg). Tachycardia and peripheral vasoconstriction may be the only early evidence of hemorrhage in the child with trauma (Table 46-6). Once hypotension develops, cardiovascular collapse is imminent and rapid intravascular volume expansion must be provided.

Table 46-3 Dehydration and Hypovolemia

Type of Dehydration	Clinical Indicators
Isotonic dehydration	Fluid output exceeds intake. Loss of free water is proportional to loss of sodium, so serum sodium concentration remains normal. Fluid loss is from intravascular *and* extravascular compartments. Compromises peripheral perfusion when the young child has lost approximately 7%-10% (100 ml/kg) of body weight. Compromises systemic perfusion in the adolescent with acute fluid loss equivalent to 5%-7% of body weight. Produces hypotension (decompensated shock) when the young child has lost 10%-15% (150 ml/kg) of body weight. Produces hypotension in the adolescent with a fluid loss equivalent to 7%-10% of body weight because body water constitutes a smaller percentage of body weight in older children and adults than in young children.
Hypotonic/hyponatremic dehydration	Associated with a proportionally greater loss of sodium than free water; thus the serum sodium falls. Resultant acute fall in serum osmolality produces an acute extravascular fluid shift and further loss of extravascular volume. Fluid loss in hypotonic dehydration primarily from the *intravascular* compartment; thus a compromise in systemic perfusion will be observed following even small quantities of fluid loss. Poor peripheral perfusion occurs in a *child* with a fluid loss equivalent to 5%-7% (50-75 ml/kg) of body weight. Adolescents with hyponatremic dehydration may demonstrate a compromise in peripheral perfusion with a fluid loss equivalent to approximately 3%-5% of body weight. Hypotension will often be observed when fluid loss is equal to approximately 10% (100 ml/kg) of body weight. Hypotension in an adolescent is observed when the fluid loss equals approximately 5%-7% of body weight.
Hypertonic/hypernatremic dehydration	Free water deficit is proportionately greater than the deficit of sodium, so serum sodium concentration rises, increasing serum osmolality and producing an intravascular shift of free water. For this reason the child with hypernatremic dehydration is likely to maintain intravascular volume and systemic perfusion until relatively large quantities of fluid are lost. Compromise in systemic perfusion is not likely to be observed in the *child* with hypernatremic dehydration until *severe* dehydration is present with a fluid loss equivalent to >10% of body weight (or >4% of body weight in the adolescent). Hypotension may not be observed until the fluid loss approximates 15% or more of body weight (>7%-10% of body weight in the adolescent). Hypotension in the child with hypertonic/hypernatremic dehydration indicates a substantial fluid deficit. However, the deficit must be replaced carefully to correct shock and avoid rapid lowering of serum sodium concentrations.

Table 46-4 Assessment of Degree of Dehydration in Isotonic Fluid Losses*

Clinical Parameters	Mild	Moderate	Severe
Body weight loss			
Infant	5% (50 ml/kg)	10% (100 ml/kg)	15% (150 ml/kg)
Adult	3% (30 ml/kg)	6% (60 ml/kg)	9% (90 ml/kg)
Skin turgor	Slightly ↓	↓↓	↓↓↓
Fontanelle	May be flat or depressed	Depressed	Significantly depressed
Mucous membranes	Dry	Very dry	Parched
Skin perfusion	Warm, normal color	Extremities cool Pale color	Extremities cold Mottled or gray color
Heart rate	Mild tachycardia	Moderate tachycardia	Extreme tachycardia
Peripheral pulses	Normal	Diminished	Absent
Blood pressure	Normal	Normal	Reduced
Sensorium	Normal or irritable	Irritable or lethargic	Unresponsive
Urine output	Slightly ↓	Mild oliguria	Marked oliguria or anuria
Azotemia	Absent	Present	Present and severe

From Hazinski MF: Renal disorders. In Hazinski MF, editor: *Manual of pediatric critical care,* St Louis, 1999, Mosby.
*The interpretation of the assessments must be appropriately modified for age and *type* of dehydration (hypotonic or hypertonic).

Redistribution of blood volume associated with systemic vasodilation, high capillary pressure, and transudative fluid losses or capillary leak may produce signs of poor systemic perfusion in the absence of evidence of absolute volume loss. For example, children with end-stage hepatic failure may demonstrate a relative hypovolemia associated with ascites and hepatorenal syndrome. Children demonstrate increased capillary permeability and loss of intravascular volume immediately following a burn. The septic child may also demonstrate systemic edema associated with capillary

Table 46-5 Estimation of Pediatric Circulating Blood Volume

Age of Child	Blood Volume (ml/kg body weight)
Newborn	85-90
Infant	75-80
Child	70-75
Adolescent	65-70

From Hazinski MF. In Hazinski MF, editor: *Manual of pediatric critical care,* St Louis, 1999, Mosby.

Table 46-6 Classification of Pediatric Hemorrhagic Shock in Trauma Patients Based on Clinical Evaluation

System	Very Mild Hemorrhage (<15% Blood Volume Loss)	Mild Hemorrhage (15% to 25% Blood Volume Loss)	Moderate Hemorrhage (25% Blood Volume Loss)	Severe Hemorrhage (40% Blood Volume Loss)
Cardiovascular	Heart rate normal or mildly increased	Tachycardia	Significant tachycardia	Severe tachycardia
	Normal pulses	Peripheral pulses may be diminished	Thready peripheral pulses	Thready central pulses
	Normal blood pressure	Normal blood pressure	Hypotension	Significant hypotension
	Normal pH	Normal pH	Metabolic acidosis	Significant acidosis
Respiratory	Rate normal	Tachypnea	Moderate tachypnea	Severe tachypnea
Central nervous system	Slightly anxious	Irritable, confused	Irritability or lethargy	Lethargy
		Combative	Diminished pain response	Coma
Skin	Warm, pink	Cool extremities, mottling	Cool extremities, mottling or pallor	Cold extremities, pallor or cyanosis
	Capillary refill brisk	Delayed capillary refill	Prolonged capillary refill	
Kidneys	Normal urine output	Oliguria, increased specific gravity	Oliguria, increased blood urea nitrogen (BUN)	Anuria

From Soud T, Pieper P, Hazinski MF. In Hazinski MF, editor: *Nursing care of the critically ill child,* ed 2, St Louis, 1992, Mosby.

leak and further intravascular volume loss. In these children, some evidence of extravascular fluid movement (ascites, systemic edema, or fluid loss to dressings over burns) is usually observed.

Signs of neurogenic shock in the child with recent, severe spinal cord injury include warm skin and hypotension with a low diastolic blood pressure. Signs of poor systemic perfusion also are observed (see Clinical Manifestations below).

Cardiogenic Shock

Cardiogenic shock is present when impaired myocardial function compromises cardiac output. This form of shock is observed most commonly in the following situations:

1. Following cardiovascular surgery or with inflammatory disease of the heart, such as cardiomyopathy and myocarditis
2. With severe forms of obstructive congenital heart disease (hypoplastic left heart, severe aortic stenosis, hypoplastic right ventricle)
3. With drug toxicity or severe electrolyte or acid-base imbalances
4. As a complication of any form of shock and early in septic shock

Compensatory Responses

In the early stages of cardiogenic shock, adrenergic compensatory responses produce tachycardia, peripheral vasoconstriction, and constriction of the splanchnic arteries to divert blood flow from the skin, kidneys, and gut and maintain flow to the heart and brain.[7] If these compensatory mechanisms are sufficient, systemic blood pressure and effective coronary artery and cerebral blood flow may be maintained. However, tachycardia and systemic arterial constriction increase myocardial oxygen consumption. In addition, reduction in gut and kidney blood flow may produce hepatic, mesenteric, or renal ischemia or failure. Decreased renal perfusion stimulates the renin-angiotensin-aldosterone system, as described for hypovolemic shock on p. 1514.

If the mean arterial pressure or pulse pressure falls, stimulation of the baroreceptors in the carotid sinuses and aortic arch is reduced. This reduced baroreceptor activity removes inhibition from the vasomotor center in the medulla, resulting in increased adrenergic stimulation. If myocardial dysfunction progresses, cardiac output and systemic blood pressure ultimately fall. Myocardial ischemia then exacerbates myocardial dysfunction, and multisystem organ failure may result from persistent or severe organ ischemia.

Clinical Manifestations

The child with cardiogenic shock demonstrates signs of inadequate systemic perfusion despite adequate intravascular volume or even relative hypervolemia. This form of shock is generally associated with low cardiac output. The child's extremities are cool to touch (will cool peripherally to proximally), with delayed capillary refill despite a warm, ambient temperature. The skin may be mottled (Fig. 46-1).

Evidence of a high central venous pressure, including hepatomegaly and periorbital edema, is typically present in uncomplicated cardiogenic shock, particularly if right ventricular failure is involved. Evidence of pulmonary edema may be noted on chest radiograph or clinical assessment (including signs of respiratory distress, reduced lung compliance during hand ventilation, or frothy pink sputum suctioned from the endotracheal tube). The cardiac silhouette is usually enlarged on the chest radiograph (unless concurrent hypovolemia is present). If myocardial function is severely compromised, peripheral pulses may be diminished in intensity (dampened) or they may vary in intensity (pulsus alternans).

If a pulmonary artery catheter is in place, the cardiac output may be calculated through thermodilution technique,

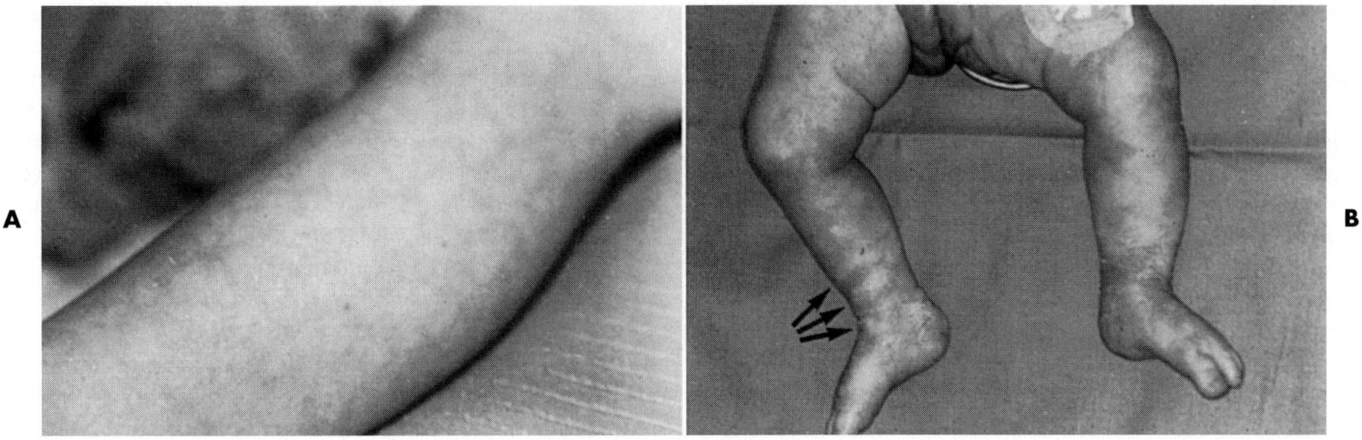

FIG. 46-1 Mottling of skin caused by poor systemic perfusion. A, Mottling of skin color often indicates inadequate tissue oxygenation; this may result from hypoxemia or poor systemic perfusion. This child developed myocardial dysfunction and signs of cardiogenic shock. **B,** Mottled skin color is often associated with other signs of compromise of skin perfusion, including delayed capillary refill. The skin over this infant's right ankle was blanched using three fingers (arrows), and the skin failed to perfuse for more than 5 seconds. This infant suffered from septic shock. (From Hazinski MF: Cardiovascular disorders. In Hazinski MF, editor: *Nursing care of the critically ill child,* ed 2, St Louis, 1992, Mosby.)

continuous monitoring of the mixed venous oxygen saturation, or continuous monitoring of cardiac output. A fall in cardiac output may be detected.

Signs of low cardiac output and cardiogenic shock may be identical to signs of cardiac tamponade. Although some classic signs of tamponade, including muffled heart tones or pulsus paradoxus, may be observed, these signs may be difficult to appreciate if cardiac output and blood pressure are severely compromised. Therefore, if cardiogenic shock is suspected in a child after cardiovascular surgery or any child at risk for the development of pericardial effusion, tamponade should be ruled out through an echocardiogram.

Septic Shock

Sepsis and its complications result from activation of biochemical and physiologic cascades that lead to the formation or activation of cytokines and protein systems that result in vasodilation, increased capillary permeability, maldistribution of blood flow, and cardiovascular dysfunction. Sepsis and its complications may result in organ system dysfunction and death and are a leading cause of death in noncoronary intensive care units.[8] Approximately 25% of all individuals with sepsis develop septic shock, and mean mortality from septic shock is approximately 50%.[9]

Most information about the pathophysiology, clinical progression, and outcome of sepsis has come from adult clinical studies and adult animal models of sepsis. However, it appears that much information gleaned from adult experience is applicable to children. Most sepsis in adults is thought to be initiated by gram-negative infections, although an increasing number of infections are caused by gram-positive microorganisms. Approximately 40% of all nosocomial infections in children are linked to gram-negative infections; 40% to gram-positive infections; and 20% to viruses, fungi, or rickettsial microorganisms.[10]

People at greatest risk for the development of sepsis include those at the extremes of age (infants and children and the elderly); individuals with invasive catheters, surgical incisions, or wounds or burns; immunocompromised persons; and persons receiving long-term antibiotic therapy.[11] Many of these risk factors are present in any seriously ill or injured child or any child with a chronic disease. In fact, more than 50% of children hospitalized in critical care units for longer than 3 weeks are expected to develop nosocomial infections; risk of infection increases with the use of invasive monitoring and support devices.[12] The most common nosocomial infections reported in children include cutaneous infections, bacteremias, and lower respiratory tract infections.[10] Such infections may be prevented with proper hand washing by health care providers before and after patient contact, appropriate sterile and aseptic technique during catheter insertion and tubing changes, and proper sterilization of respiratory therapy equipment. Unfortunately, fewer than 50% of health care providers in pediatric and newborn intensive care units wash their hands before and after every contact.[13,14]

Both proinflammatory and antiinflammatory cytokines serve an essential protective function in fighting infection and modulating the immune response. It is now clear that sepsis remains a disruption in the balance between *proinflammatory* mediators (including tumor necrosis factor–α, interleukins [IL]-1, IL-6, and IL-8; platelet activating factor; arachidonic acid metabolites; leukemia inhibitory factor; nitric oxide; and many kinins) and *antiinflammatory* mediators (IL-4, IL-10, IL-11, and IL-13; transforming growth factor B; colony-stimulating factors; soluble tumor necrosis factor receptor; IL-1 receptor antagonist; and protein C). Extremely high levels of proinflammatory mediators, such as tumor necrosis factor (TNF), nitric oxide, and platelet activating factor can become destructive.[8,15] High proinflammatory cytokine levels have been implicated in the development of sepsis-induced pulmonary injury and microcirculatory disruptions, such as are observed in burns, severe trauma, shock reperfusion syndromes, and multiple organ dysfunction syndrome.[15] Tumor necrosis factor levels are directly related to mortality in newborns and children with meningitis and sepsis.[8,16] Increased nitric oxide concentrations are thought to be responsible for vasodilation, hypotension, and some of the decreased myocardial function that develops during sepsis. Children with sepsis, particularly those with hypotension, have increased total serum nitrite concentrations that probably reflect increased endogenous production of nitric oxide.[17]

During sepsis, endotoxin stimulates the endothelium to become a secretory organ. The endothelium changes from profibrinolytic and anticoagulant to antifibrinolytic and precoagulant, leading to the ultimate development of microthrombin in some areas of the microcirculation, further contributing to maldistribution of blood flow.[18] Mediators (e.g., protein C) that regulate coagulation pathways have been implicated in this process. Low levels of protein C are present in children who develop coagulopathies during sepsis; protein C deficiency is a marker for severe sepsis,[19] although administration of protein C has not consistently improved survival.[20]

There is clear interaction among catecholamines, adrenoreceptors, and glucocorticoids. Endogenous glucocorticoids have an antiinflammatory effect (they decrease activation of proinflammatory mediators), and they modulate vasomotor tone by enhancing cardiovascular and vasomotor response to catecholamines.[21] Septic children may have an actual adrenal insufficiency (caused by adrenal hemorrhage, decreased renal perfusion, inhibition of corticosteroid production by TNF, or actual adrenal disease) or a relative adrenal insufficiency (with inadequate adrenal stress response or decreased response to circulating glucocorticoids). In two recent studies in adults, administered hydrocortisone improved survival;[22,23] however, these results contradict studies performed in the 1980s, so further validation is required. A wide range of plasma cortisol levels have been reported in children with sepsis, and low plasma cortisol levels have been associated with the highest mortality in meningococcemia.[24] For these reasons, when sepsis is present, adrenal insufficiency should be ruled out or treated if present.

Clinical Manifestations

Sepsis and its complications produce a cascade of physical and biochemical changes. The clinical progression of sepsis produced by these changes has been described and defined by a consensus panel of physicians,[25] and these stages have been clinically validated in adults (Table 46-7).[9,26] Application of these consensus terms have also been proposed for children.[11]

Systemic inflammatory response syndrome (SIRS) represents a nonspecific response to a variety of insults, including trauma, burns, pancreatitis, or infection. SIRS is present when the individual demonstrates two or more of the following as an acute change from baseline: fever (greater than 38° C) or hypothermia (less than 36° C), tachycardia, tachypnea, respiratory alkalosis, and alterations in white blood cell count (WBC) (including leukocytes, leukopenia, or an increase in the percentage of immature or band forms of WBCs). These clinical signs may also be altered by age, immune function, and clinical condition. For example, the

Table 46-7 Definitions and Clinical Criteria for Sepsis and Septic Shock, Including Proposed Pediatric Criteria

Clinical Stage	Clinical Criteria
Systemic inflammatory response syndrome (SIRS)	Two or more of the following (as acute change): Fever (>38° C) or hypothermia (<36° C) Tachycardia *Adults:* >90 beats/min *Newborns:* >140 beats/min *Infants:* >120 beats/min *Children:* >90-100 beats/min Tachypnea or hypocarbic respiratory alkalosis ($Paco_2$ <32 mm Hg with spontaneous breathing) *Adults:* rate >20 breaths/min *Infants:* rate >50 to 60 breaths/min *Children:* rate >40 breaths/min Leukocytosis (white blood cell count >12,000/mm³) Leukopenia (white blood cell count <4000/mm³) or >10% band forms
Sepsis	SIRS (two or more of above) plus suspected infection
Severe sepsis	Sepsis plus signs of organ dysfunction, hypoperfusion, or hypotension; signs of organ dysfunction or hypoperfusion may include lactic acidosis, oliguria, or acute alteration in mental status
Septic shock	Severe sepsis plus hypotension despite vigorous volume administration/resuscitation, or normotension maintained with vasopressors *Adults:* fall in systolic blood pressure by 40 mm Hg or more, systolic pressure <90 mm Hg, or diastolic pressure <70 mm Hg *Children* (older than 1 yr): fall in blood pressure from baseline values or systolic pressure <70 mm Hg + (2 × Age in years)

Data from American College of Chest Physicians/Society of Critical Care Medicine Consensus Conference Committee: *Crit Care Med* 20:864, 1992; Hazinski MF et al: *Am J Crit Care* 2:224, 1993.

newborn often develops hypothermia rather than fever as a sign of infection. The child with chronic lung disease and chronic hypercarbia or the child receiving controlled mechanical ventilatory support may not demonstrate a respiratory alkalosis. Because neutrophils are required for the development of fever and many of the local signs of infection, the neutropenic child may demonstrate normothermia despite infection.

Sepsis is a systemic response to infection. It it present when manifestations of SIRS are observed in conjunction with suspected infection; positive blood or other cultures are not necessary for the diagnosis, but suspicion of infection is required. For example, if the child with trauma develops a high fever or pulmonary congestion several days after injury, it is highly likely that an infection is present.

Severe sepsis is present when the individual demonstrates evidence of sepsis (SIRS with suspected infection) and signs of organ dysfunction, hypoperfusion, or hypotension. Altered organ perfusion is signaled by signs of organ system failure. The dysfunctional organ system should be separate from the site of suspected infection. This important distinction will enable separation of signs of severe sepsis from signs of pneumonia and associated respiratory failure.

Septic shock is heralded in the person with severe sepsis by hypotension despite adequate fluid resuscitation or by the necessity for vasopressors to maintain blood pressure. Because children tend to develop hypotension only late in the course of any shock, septic shock should be identified when the child develops more subtle signs of poor perfusion despite adequate fluid resuscitation. If the child with sepsis develops hypotension, decompensated septic shock is present. Mortality from septic shock associated with hypotension may be as high as 46%.[9,27]

Most children with sepsis generate a cardiac output that is higher than normal despite a fall in ventricular ejection fraction. This high cardiac output is associated with ventricular dilation and an increase in ventricular end-diastolic volume, an increase in heart rate, and a fall in systemic vascular resistance. A high cardiac output can usually be maintained if intravascular volume remains adequate. Echocardiography may reveal the reduction in ventricular ejection fraction and left ventricular dilation. If the mixed venous oxygen saturation is monitored continuously (through use of a fiberoptic pulmonary artery catheter), the mixed venous oxygen saturation ($S\bar{v}O_2$) generally rises because cardiac output and oxygen delivery increase while oxygen extraction decreases. Although some tissue beds may be ischemic, overall oxygen extraction does not increase, so the $S\bar{v}O_2$ remains high.[28] When the child with sepsis improves in response to therapy, the $S\bar{v}O_2$ often falls as oxygen extraction increases.

It is now clear that most individuals who develop septic shock have a high cardiac output and a low systemic vascular resistance.[29] Cardiac output usually falls to levels below normal only if the individual has severe underlying cardiovascular dysfunction or if fluid administration is inadequate to maintain intravascular volume. In one clinical study, children who received inadequate volume resuscitation during the first hours of therapy had a significantly higher mortality.[30] With successful and liberal fluid resuscitation, cardiac output is usually high and should return to normal within 24 hours. If cardiac output and heart rate remain high and systemic vascular resistance remains low despite therapy for longer than 24 hours after development of hypotension, resuscitation has not been successful and the septic cascade continues to produce maldistribution of blood flow, with a high mortality.[29]

The terms *warm* versus *cold* septic shock are outdated and imprecise terms and no longer used. Warm shock was thought to be associated with peripheral vasodilation and hyperdynamic cardiovascular function with a high cardiac output. Cold shock was thought to be a preterminal condition associated with a fall in cardiac output and peripheral vasoconstriction. It is now recognized that signs of peripheral vasoconstriction probably indicate inadequate volume resuscitation.

Reperfusion and Inflammatory Injury

Reperfusion (reoxygenation) injury is cellular injury caused by the restoration or reperfusion of physiologic concentrations of oxygen to cells that have been exposed to injurious but nonlethal hypoxic conditions.[31] Reperfusion injury is stimulated by the generation of highly reactive oxygen intermediates (e.g., free oxygen radicals and superoxide) that damage cell membranes, denature proteins, and disrupt chromosomes (see Chapter 2).[32] The amount of free oxygen radical produced is directly related to the severity and duration of the ischemic period. The process is most likely to affect endothelial cells of the microvasculature, causing MODS, and is likely to contribute to the compromise of organ perfusion following shock resuscitation.[32]

An ischemic insult activates white blood cells, priming monocytes and macrophages and contributing to the release of inflammatory mediators or cytokines, including TNF, the interleukins (IL-1, IL-6, and IL-8), and platelet activating factor. These cytokines in turn contribute to vasodilation, increased capillary permeability, and altered platelet function. The ultimate result is a maldistribution of blood flow and a compromise in organ perfusion. The role of these mediators is summarized in Table 6-7.[32] Chapter 45 includes a more comprehensive discussion of MODS.

Signs of organ system failure include but are not limited to lactic acidosis, oliguria, and an acute alteration in mental status (e.g., decrease in Glasgow Coma Scale score of 1 point or more). Box 46-3 lists other potential signs of organ system failure in children.

Evaluation and Treatment

Acidosis may be the most sensitive indicator of inadequate systemic perfusion in children. The development of a metabolic acidosis or a rise in serum lactate concentration indicates the presence of inadequate tissue oxygenation. Hypotension is a late sign of shock in infants and children and often indicates cardiovascular collapse.

Box 46-3

PROPOSED SIGNS OF ORGAN SYSTEM DYSFUNCTION*

CENTRAL NERVOUS SYSTEM

- Acute change in mental status (confusion, agitation, lethargy)
- Glasgow Coma Scale score <15 (previously normal) or decreased by 1

PULMONARY (ARDS)

- Unexplained hypoxemia with suspected sepsis (Pao_2/Fio_2) <175-280 mm Hg)
- Bilateral pulmonary infiltrates with PAOP <18 mm Hg
- Deterioration from baseline†

RENAL (NOT PRERENAL)

- Oliguria (urine output <0.5 ml/kg/hr)
- Increase in serum creatinine from normal with urine sodium <40 mmol/L
- Rise in serum creatinine by 2.0 mg/dl in presence of preexisting renal insufficiency

HEPATOBILIARY

- Elevation in liver function enzymes to twice normal
- Serum bilirubin >2.0 mg/dl

GASTROINTESTINAL

- Paralytic ileus
- Gastrointestinal bleeding†

COAGULATION

- Confirmatory test for DIC (FDP >1 : 40 or D-dimers >2.0)
- Thrombocytopenia or fall in platelet count by 25%
- Elevated prothrombin time and partial thromboplastin time
- Clinical evidence of bleeding

From Hazinski MF et al: *Am J Crit Care* 2(3):224, 1993.

ARDS, Adult respiratory distress syndrome; *PAOP,* pulmonary artery occlusion pressure; *DIC,* disseminated intravascular coagulation; *FDP,* fibrin degradation products.

*Clinical criteria indicating organ system failure. These signs are consistent with organ systm dysfunction or failure in the absence of other attributable causes.

†Indicates criteria that have been added to the lists published in *Bone*[57-59] based on additional references.[60-61]

The child's ventilation and oxygenation should be evaluated whenever shock is present. In addition, evaluation of the child's electrolytes, glucose, BUN, creatinine, liver function, calcium, phosphorus, and cardiac enzyme concentrations may help to determine the cause of the shock or treatment needed.

Hematologic evaluation is necessary if hemorrhage or disseminated intravascular coagulation (DIC) is apparent. Hemoglobin and hematocrit may be artificially normal in the face of an acute hemorrhage; unless volume resuscitation is provided with whole blood, the child's hematocrit ultimately falls. Evaluation for nontraumatic hemorrhage or potential DIC includes a complete blood count, platelets, coagulation tests (prothrombin time [PT], partial thromboplastin time [PTT], bleeding time), and DIC screen (fibrinogen, fibrin split products).

A chest roentgenogram should be taken to evaluate cardiac size and exclude pneumonia, pneumothorax, and pulmonary edema. An arterial blood gas (ABG) measurement monitors progression of acidosis and evidence of oxygenation or ventilation problems associated with respiratory distress. Oximetry enables evaluation of hemoglobin saturation and may indicate the loss of peripheral pulses; however, oximetry should never be used as a "pulse check." Electrocardiogram (ECG) and echocardiogram should be selectively used to evaluate cardiac function and rule out dysrhythmias, effusion, and failure as contributing factors to low cardiac output.

Microbiologic evaluation should be performed as appropriate when infection is suspected. Blood and urine cultures also should be obtained as needed; a Gram stain should be available immediately in these cultures. Evaluation of spinal fluid, stool, and joints may be needed.

Early recognition and therapy are the keys to survival of children in shock. Therefore signs of poor systemic perfusion must be identified as soon as they appear. Supportive therapy then is required to optimize each aspect of cardiovascular and pulmonary function. Throughout therapy it is important to evaluate the child's response to therapy and to monitor for evidence of further deterioration and development of MODS. If signs of MODS develop, organ function must be supported.

The goals of treatment of shock are maximization of oxygen delivery and minimization of oxygen demand. The airway, oxygenation, and ventilation must be supported. Reduction of oxygen demand requires the treatment for fever and pain. In addition, the child should be kept warm, with prevention of shivering. Blood components and, perhaps, intravenous fluids should be warmed before administration to young infants and children with hypothermia. Fear and pain increase oxygen consumption, so care must be taken to reassure the child and treat pain as indicated.

When signs of shock are detected, immediate resuscitation is required. Once systemic perfusion is restored, transfer to a pediatric intensive care unit is advised. During resuscitation, however, continuous evaluation and support of cardiopulmonary function must be provided. Hemodynamic monitoring should be instituted and volume and inotropic support provided as needed. The warmth of the child's extremities, capillary refill, quality of peripheral pulses, level of consciousness and responsiveness, urine output, oxygenation, ventilation, and acid-base status should be assessed throughout shock therapy.

Monitoring of the volume of urine output and specific gravity is useful in determining the child's response to fluid therapy. A urinary catheter should be inserted if shock is present unless the child has sustained pelvic trauma or a urethral tear is suspected. All sources of fluid intake and output should be carefully monitored and recorded hourly, or more frequently if needed.

Initial therapy for any unstable person requires evaluation of airway patency and ventilation. The child should be positioned to support maximal airway patency, and the effectiveness of ventilation should be evaluated constantly. Supplemental oxygen is administered as needed at up to 3 to 6 L/min by nonbreathing mask, head hood, or bag-valve-mask ventilation. Children in shock should be intubated *before* respiratory deterioration or arrest complicates shock management.

The child's heart rate must be adequate to support effective cardiac output and systemic perfusion. The most common pediatric dysrhythmias are listed in Box 46-4. Bradydysrhythmias and extreme tachydysrhythmias should be treated promptly. Pharmacologic therapy, pacing, or synchronized direct current (DC) cardioversion may be required.

The most common ECG findings associated with loss of pulses ("arrest" rhythms) include asystole, electromechanical dissociation (EMD), pulseless ventricular tachycardia, and ventricular fibrillation. Regardless of ECG findings, cardiopulmonary resuscitation—including cardiac compression—must be performed when pulses are lost.

Volume resuscitation is designed to restore intravascular volume relative to the vascular space and optimize ventricular preload. The specific fluid selected and route of administration are determined by the child's clinical condition. In general, however, isotonic **crystalloids** (salt-containing solutions, such as normal saline or lactated Ringer solution) or **colloids** (protein-containing fluids, such as albumin or blood) are administered in boluses of 20 ml/kg. Individuals in septic shock may require a large volume of intravenous fluid to restore and maintain systemic perfusion. More than 40 ml/kg may be administered during the first hour of volume resuscitation, and a total of 100 to 200 ml/kg or more may be required during the first several hours of therapy.[30] In fact, rapid volume administration, particularly during the first hour of therapy, has been linked with improved survival in hypotensive children in septic shock. If intravenous access cannot be achieved in children younger than 6 years, an intraosseous needle should be inserted and intraosseous fluid and drug administration provided through that route.[4]

Unless shock is mild or responds immediately to volume therapy, insertion of a central venous (monitoring) catheter is advisable. Several multilumen catheters are available in pediatric sizes that enable simultaneous monitoring of central venous pressure and administration of fluids.

An intraarterial line should be inserted once initial stabilization has been achieved. This enables reliable, continuous evaluation of arterial pressure. Noninvasive oscillometric blood pressure monitoring devices may not accurately measure low or rapidly falling blood pressures and may *overestimate* the blood pressure.[33] Sphygmomanometry may also yield inaccurate blood pressure measurement; cuff pressure measurement of a person in shock typically *underestimates* the systolic blood pressure (cuff measurements are lower than intraarterial pressure).[34]

Insertion of a pulmonary artery catheter should be considered whenever the child demonstrates shock that is unresponsive to initial volume and vasoactive drug support. A pulmonary artery catheter with thermodilution cardiac output thermistor, a fiberoptic pulmonary artery catheter or both can enable continuous monitoring of mixed venous oxygen saturation or continuous monitoring of cardiac output. Quantification of these variables can be particularly helpful if precise tracking of hemodynamic measurements is desired. This may be necessary in the care of the child with septic shock or MODS.

Box 46-4
MOST COMMON PEDIATRIC DYSRHYTHMIAS

HEART (QRS) RATE TOO SLOW FOR CLINICAL CONDITION

QRS duration (width) normal
- Sinus bradycardia
- Junctional rhythm
- Heart block

QRS duration (width) prolonged
- Supraventricular tachycardia (SVT) with aberrant ventricular conduction
- Ventricular rhythm
- Heart block

HEART (QRS) RATE TOO FAST FOR CLINICAL CONDITION

QRS duration (width) normal
- Sinus tachycardia
- SVT

QRS duration (width) prolonged
- SVT with aberrant ventricular conduction
- Ventricular tachycardia

COLLAPSE (PULSELESS) RHYTHMS

Electromechanical dissociation
Ventricular tachycardia
Ventricular fibrillation
Asystole

From Hazinski MF: Cardiovascular disorders. In Hazinski MF, editor: *Manual of pediatric critical care,* St Louis, 1999, Mosby.

Administration of blood or blood component therapy is necessary to treat hemorrhage or severe coagulopathies. A "normal" hematocrit does not rule out the possibility of hemorrhage; the hematocrit typically falls in a person who has sustained whole blood loss after intravascular fluid shift or replacement of the blood loss with crystalloids or colloids. In general, 10 ml/kg boluses of packed red blood cells are administered.

Transfusion for the child with chronic anemia and shock must be accomplished slowly to prevent hypervolemia and further deterioration in myocardial function. Administration of packed red blood cells at a rate averaging 3 to 5 ml/kg/hr over several hours may be well tolerated, particularly if it is preceded and followed by administration of diuretics. If severe anemia is associated with severe hypervolemia and myocardial dysfunction, an exchange transfusion may be required. If a coagulopathy is present, blood component therapy should be administered to prevent or treat hemorrhage.

Hypoxemia, metabolic acidosis, and electrolyte imbalances depress myocardial function and must be corrected when shock is present. During resuscitation of the child in shock, oxygen is administered and mechanical ventilatory support is usually indicated.

Hypoglycemia may develop rapidly in the critically ill or injured infant because infants have high glucose needs and low glycogen stores. If glucose is needed, however, continuous infusion is preferred to intermittent bolus therapy. In fact, hyperglycemia has been linked to poor outcome in some children with head injury, although it is unclear whether the poor outcome is caused by idiopathic hyperglycemia or excessive glucose administration.[3]

Acute or severe alterations in the serum sodium concentration should be avoided during fluid therapy. Acute changes in serum sodium produce changes in serum osmolality that result in fluid shifts into and out of the vascular spaces. Such fluid shifts can be associated with neurologic complications, including seizures, cerebral edema, and intracranial hemorrhage.[35]

Alterations in serum potassium concentration may affect myocardial contractility and conduction. However, children are far less sensitive than adults to minor changes in serum potassium concentration. Hypokalemia may result from inadequate potassium administration during volume therapy or from excessive potassium losses caused by drug therapy (e.g., furosemide). The serum potassium concentration falls in the presence of alkalosis; this represents an intracellular shift of potassium and is corrected when the pH is normalized. True hypokalemia should be treated with an infusion of potassium chloride at a dose equivalent to 0.5 to 1 mEq/kg administered over several hours.

Hyperkalemia may result from excessive potassium administration or reduced potassium excretion (e.g., in renal failure). Serum potassium concentration also rises when acidosis develops; the rise in serum potassium is caused by a shift of potassium from the intracellular to the vascular space (e.g., exchange with vascular H^+) and falls when the serum pH is corrected.

Both ionized and total calcium concentration should be monitored, and documented hypocalcemia must be treated. Serum ionized calcium concentration is often low (less than 4.5mEq/L) in children with septic shock.[36]

Hypercalcemia may be observed in children with some malignancies, including acute lymphocytic leukemia, lymphomas, and soft tissue sarcomas. Malignant cells often secrete a parathormone-like substance that stimulates bone reabsorption, release of calcium, and rapid cell turnover.[37] Although mild hypercalcemia is not life threatening, extreme hypercalcemia (total serum calcium approaching 19 to 20 mEq/L) may produce renal and cardiovascular complications. Table 46-8 summarizes additional drug therapy for children in shock. If oxygenation, ventilation, heart rate, and intravascular volume are appropriate and myocardial function and systemic perfusion remain poor, vasoactive drug therapy with inotropes is indicated.

Emerging Therapies for Sepsis

A variety of nontraditional therapies for sepsis have intermittently found favor but have failed to produce consistent improvement in survival. Mediator-specific therapies to treat sepsis have improved outcome in laboratory animals and subsets of individuals with sepsis but have failed to improve outcome in large clinical trials. Continuous plasmafiltration has been shown to improve organ function and blood pressure in septic adults and children[38] but also failed to improve survival. Glucocorticoid administration has been successful for infants and children with actual or relative adrenal insufficiency[24] but may not improve survival in all septic individ-

Table 46-8 Drug Therapies for Children in Shock

Type	Indications	Comments
Vasoactive (inotropes)	If oxygenation, ventilation, and intravascular volume are appropriate but myocardial function and systemic perfusion remain poor or heart rate is low	Useful in the treatment of cardiogenic and distributive shock or any shock with impaired myocardial function; goals include increased heart rate, increased cardiac output, redistribution of cardiac output, and increased cardiac contractility
Sympathomimetic	To stimulate particular adrenergic receptors	Receptors targeted will be determined by the child's heart rate, peripheral perfusion, blood pressure, and urine output
Dopamine	To improve renal, coronary artery, mesenteric, and cerebral circulation at low doses and increase heart rate or myocardial function at moderate doses; vasoconstriction may occur at high doses	Popular drug used especially in the presence of oliguria; provides dopaminergic effects (renal, coronary artery, mesenteric, cerebral vasodilation) at low doses; β- and α-adrenergic effects at higher doses
Epinephrine	For resuscitation from cardiopulmonary arrest or cardiovascular collapse; to treat symptomatic bradycardia unresponsive to oxygen therapy and adequate ventilation or in the treatment of hypotension	Effective in increasing mean arterial pressure and improving myocardial function in children with septic shock
Vasodilators	To reduce impedance to ventricular ejection	Because they dilate both arteries and veins, they may reduce ventricular preload and afterload
Antibiotics	For signs of sepsis	Broad spectrum used until a specific causative microorganism is identified
Steroids	For meningitis	Given 20 to 30 min before first dose of antibiotics, steroids may be associated with improvement in auditory function

uals. Although meningococcal sepsis may be an ideal form of sepsis to study because of its consistent presentation and clinical course, a wide variety of therapies have failed to produce improved outcome in this disease.[20]

At this time the best therapies for children with shock include early detection of signs of shock and excellent support of oxygen delivery and organ system function.[15] Prevention of shock is also important. Injury prevention of trauma and treatment of dehydration can eliminate the two leading causes of hypovolemic shock in children. *Haemophilus influenzae* sepsis and meningitis have been virtually eradicated in the United States since the introduction and widespread use of *H. influenzae* vaccine for infants, and immunization against *Neisseria meningitidis* (the causative microoganism of meningococcal sepsis) may similarly reduce the incidence of meningococcal sepsis. Adminstration of colony-stimulating factors to increase white blood cell count in immunosuppressed persons has been shown to decrease infection and sepsis in this high-risk population. Septic shock may also be prevented with good hand-washing technique, early detection of infection, and appropriate antimicrobial therapies for infection and sepsis.

BURNS

Management of pediatric burn injuries requires an understanding of the differences that exist in this population related to etiology of injury, growth and development, physiology, and clinical course. In 1988 the American Burn Association established criteria to guide transfer to a specialized burn center. These recommendations are based on complex management issues related to treatment of acute burns and the long-term rehabilitation needs of children.[39,40]

Burn injuries in children are frequently preventable and are often the result of inadequate supervision, curiosity, inability to escape the burning agent, or intentional abuse. **Scald injuries** are most commonly seen in the very young child and result from exposure to hot water, grease, or other hot liquids. Hot tap water in the bathroom accounts for approximately 21% of scald injuries. Hot water heaters set above 140° F can burn a child in less than 1 second (Table 46-9).

A child's skin is thinner and thus more susceptible to injury than an adult's skin. The extent of injury is determined by the temperature of the burning agent and the duration of exposure. Because very young children may be unable to escape the heat source, the depth of the injury is likely to be greater. The kitchen is also a common site of burn injury for young children and often involves pulling over dishes or appliances containing hot liquids. These types of injuries account for 50% of the burns sustained by children younger than 2 years.[41]

Although **child abuse** can occur at any age, young children are particularly vulnerable to serious injury. Estimates of the incidence of abuse by scalding vary from 4% to 25% of hospital admissions in the pediatric burn population.[41,42,43] Specific characteristics have been identified that raise the index of suspicion of intentional burns. These include a history of previous accidents, a delay in seeking treatment for the injury, inconsistency in the caretaker's report of the accident, a burn pattern that does not coincide with the reported circumstances or the developmental capabilities of the child, and well-demarcated burns of the buttocks or extremities.[44] Forced immersion in hot water typically presents with deep symmetric injuries lacking any evidence of splash wounds (Fig. 46-2). **Contact burns** may also be intentionally inflicted by contact with cigarettes or other hot objects such as curling irons. Young children may inadvertently grasp a hot object. However, the pattern of injury will be confined to the palm. Burns to the dorsum of the hand are viewed with suspicion.[45]

Children 3 to 8 years of age are most frequently injured by flame during fire play. Lighters and matches ignite clothing and cause house fires. Young children may run when clothing ignites and increase the severity of injury. Escape from a burning residence or motor vehicle is often delayed because young children cannot cognitively comprehend the circumstances or physically remove themselves from the danger. **Flame burns** involving flammable liquids, especially gasoline, are more common in older children.

Although flame and scald burns account for the majority of thermal injuries in children, **electrical burns** result from direct contact with high- or low-voltage current. Most

Table 46-9 Time and Temperature Factors in Hot Water Burns

Time (sec)	Temperature (°F)
ADULTS	
31	130
15	135
5	140
1.8	150
YOUNG CHILDREN	
10	130
4	135
1	140
0.5	149

Data from Maley M: *Information Exchange* 4:1, 1991.

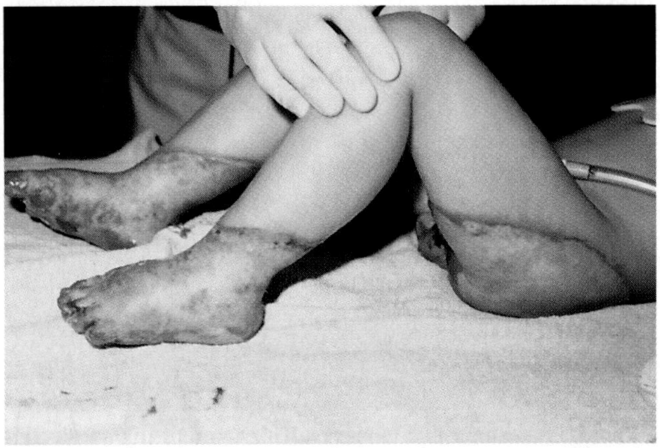

FIG. 46-2 Burn pattern typically seen following forced emersion in hot water.

commonly these injuries occur as a result of risk-taking behavior on the part of young males. Trauma from contact with electrical energy results from the passage of current through vital organs, muscle compartments, and nerve or vascular pathways. Very young children are at risk for injury from chewing on electrical cords or inserting objects into electric outlets (Fig. 46-3). Lightning strikes also account for some electrical burns. **Chemical injuries** are rare in children since they most frequently occur in an industrial setting. The causative agent has important implications for the evaluation, treatment, and prognosis of the child.

Severity of Injury

The severity of burn injury is assessed based on the percentage of the total body surface area (TBSA) involved. Use of the standard rule of nines results in inaccurate calculation of the percentage of TBSA involved in children. Although the infant's trunk and arms are of roughly the same proportion as the adult's, the head and neck make up 18% of TBSA and each lower extremity is 14% of TBSA. A modified rule of nines deducts 1% from the head and adds 0.5% to each leg for each year of life after 2 years.[46] Various charts are available that assign body proportions to children of different ages (Fig. 46-4). These are generally used in pediatric burn facilities and accurately compute the extent of burn injury.

Because thermal trauma represents a three-dimensional wound, the severity of injury is assessed also in relation to the **depth of injury**. The etiology of the burn and the duration of contact with the burning agent are important considerations in determining the depth of injury. In general, the more intense the heat source and the longer the contact, the deeper the resulting injury will be. However, infant skin is extremely fragile and more likely to sustain a deeper burn. This makes the estimation of the depth of burn difficult in very young children, especially following scald injuries (Fig. 46-5). Intentionally inflicted burns tend to be more severe since contact with the burning agent is prolonged. Electrical injuries may also mask the extent of damage on initial assessment. Visible tissue damage may appear minimal despite severe injury to underlying structures.

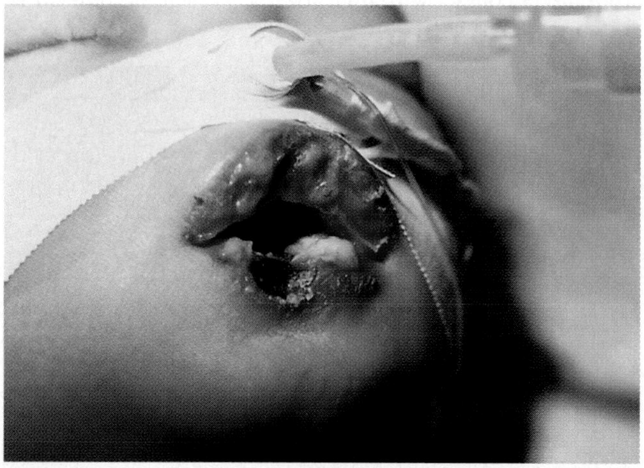

FIG. 46-3 Commissure burn resulting from biting an electrical wire.

Another important factor in assessing the severity of injury is the victim's age. Children younger than 2 years have a significantly higher risk for associated morbidity and mortality following thermal injury. They have not achieved maturity of the immune system and are at increased risk for infection and sepsis. In addition, very young children are intolerant of rapid fluid shifts and demonstrate immature renal function, which negatively affects their ability to retain sodium and water.

The areas of the body injured are another consideration when assessing the severity of the burn. Burns of the hands, feet, and perineum and burns across joints carry the potential for scar formation and contracture that may interfere with function as well as growth and development. Specialized care is required to preserve maximal function. In addition, burns to the face and neck may result in airway compromise as well as deformity from damage to delicate cartilage of the nose and ears.

Concomitant injuries may be suggested by the circumstances of the burn and should always be investigated. Fractures may result from jumping from a window to escape a house fire. Electrical injuries and motor vehicle accidents often result in associated trauma. Any suspicion of intentionally inflicted burns should alert the burn team to assess for other injuries.

Pathophysiology

Major thermal trauma involves all body systems, and the consequences of injury include shock, infection, hypermetabolism, organ failure, and functional limitations. These effects can be magnified in the pediatric population as a result of physiologic immaturity and age-related variation in treatment modalities.

Integument

The local response manifested in the area of trauma includes cellular destruction and damage. Progressive injury caused by **dermal ischemia** may result from ineffective initial management, especially inadequate or delayed resuscitation. An increase in the permeability and hydrostatic pressure of the capillaries results in the loss of fluid, proteins, and electrolytes into the interstitial spaces. A diminishing intravascular oncotic pressure further enhances these losses and results in edema formation. Profound edema can result not only in the area of injury but also in unburned areas. In addition, loss of the protective barrier of the skin increases **evaporative fluid loss** 5 to 10 times more than for unburned skin.[47] Although these losses are maximal in the immediate postburn period, they persist until wound closure.

Circulatory alterations also occur in the area of injury. Reduced blood flow and capillary stasis result from **hemoconcentration,** the release of thromboplastin and clot-activating factors from heat-damaged cells, reduced cardiac output, and edema formation. Circulation in the area of partial-thickness

Burn Estimate and Diagram
Age vs Area

Initial Evaluation

Cause of Burn ____________________

Date of Burn ____________________

Time of Burn ____________________

Age ____________________

Sex ____________________

Weight ____________________

Date of Admission ____________________

Signature ____________________

Date ____________________

Burn Diagram

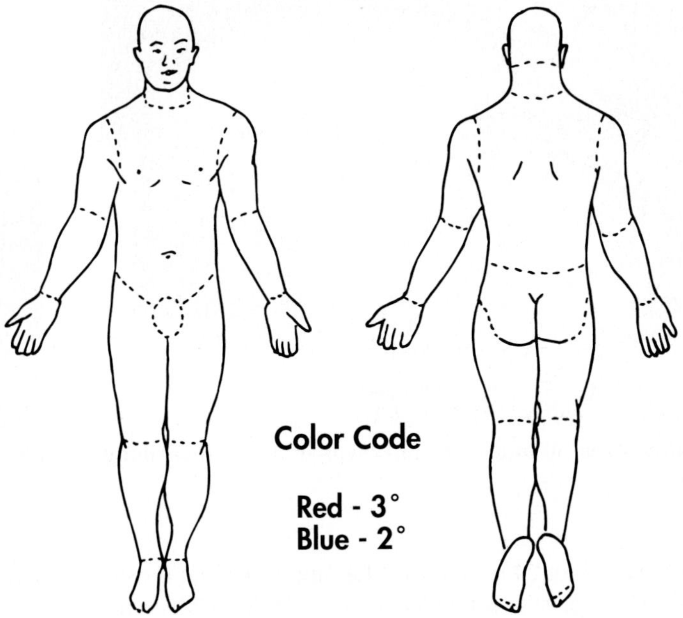

Area	Birth-1 yr	1-4 yr	5-9 yr	10-14 yr	15 yr	Adult	2°	3°	Total	Donor Areas
Head	19	17	13	11	9	7				
Neck	2	2	2	2	2	2				
Ant. Trunk	13	13	13	13	13	13				
Post. Trunk	13	13	13	13	13	13				
R. Buttock	2 1/2	2 1/2	2 1/2	2 1/2	2 1/2	2 1/2				
L. Buttock	2 1/2	2 1/2	2 1/2	2 1/2	2 1/2	2 1/2				
Genitalia	1	1	1	1	1	1				
R. U. Arm	4	4	4	4	4	4				
L. U. Arm	4	4	4	4	4	4				
R. L. Arm	3	3	3	3	3	3				
L. L. Arm	3	3	3	3	3	3				
R. Hand	2 1/2	2 1/2	2 1/2	2 1/2	2 1/2	2 1/2				
L. Hand	2 1/2	2 1/2	2 1/2	2 1/2	2 1/2	2 1/2				
R. Thigh	5 1/2	6 1/2	8	8 1/2	9	9 1/2				
L. Thigh	5 1/2	6 1/2	8	8 1/2	9	9 1/2				
R. Leg	5	5	5 1/2	6	6 1/2	7				
L. Leg	5	5	5 1/2	6	6 1/2	7				
R. Foot	3 1/2	3 1/2	3 1/2	3 1/2	3 1/2	3 1/2				
L. Foot	3 1/2	3 1/2	3 1/2	3 1/2	3 1/2	3 1/2				
						Total				

Shriners Hospitals for Crippled Children Burns Institute **Burn Diagram**

FIG. 46-4 Lund-Browder chart. Modified Lund-Browder chart for estimating body surface area of burn. Burn estimate and diagram by age vs. area: initial evaluation. (Courtesy Shriners Hospitals for Children, Cincinnati Burns Hospital.)

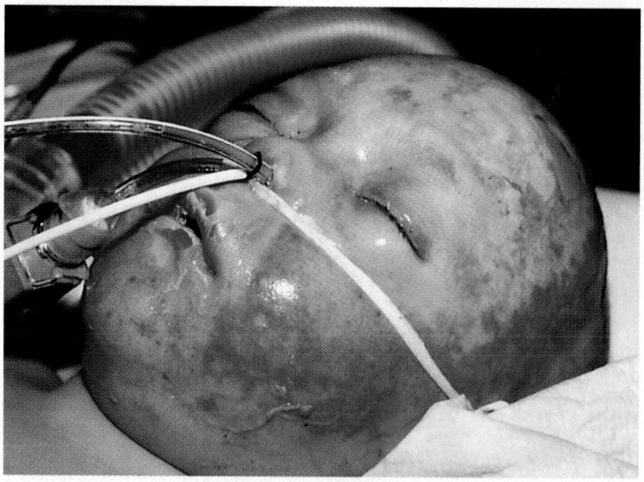

FIG. 46-5 Areas of indeterminant depth of injury in a young child.

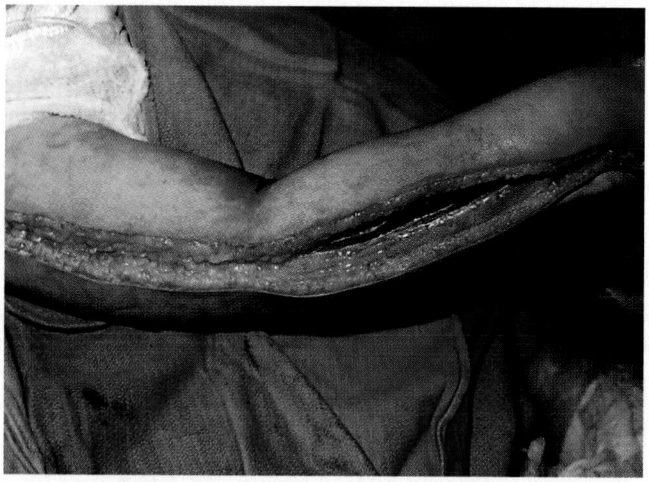

FIG. 46-6 Escharotomy/fasciotomy in a severely burned arm.

wounds ceases for 24 to 48 hours after injury, when it is usually restored. Vascular supply in the area of full-thickness injuries is completely occluded and is not restored until granulation tissue forms or the wound is surgically repaired. The dry, leathery **eschar** provides an ideal environment for bacterial growth. Infection or trauma may convert a partial-thickness injury to a full-thickness one, especially in young children, who have thinner, more delicate skin.

Cardiovascular System

The marked reduction in cardiac output immediately following injury is accompanied by an initial increase in systemic vascular resistance. As fluid is lost into the interstitial spaces, a further reduction in cardiac output occurs, accompanied by vasodilation. Because the infant maintains cardiac output by increasing heart rate preferentially to stroke volume, extremely elevated heart rates result in a decreased filling time and a further reduction in cardiac output.[46] Adequate resuscitation returns cardiac output to normal levels in approximately 24 to 36 hours. Without fluid replacement, cardiac output continues to decrease and results in organ failure and death.

The inefficient and labile peripheral circulation of the infant further complicates management of the burn shock phase of treatment. The rapid fluid shift to the interstitial space and drying of the eschar result in compromised circulation and a resultant tourniquet effect in the extremities. Blood vessels and nerves become entrapped because the fascia cannot expand to accommodate the massive edema. Release of pressure is required to restore blood flow and preserve nerve function (Fig. 46-6).

Constriction of the chest and impairment of respiratory excursion may also result, especially in the very young child because of the increased pliability of the rib cage. Increased **intraabdominal pressure** resulting from massive fluid shifts has been reported in the immediate postburn period. Evaluating 30 children, Greenhalgh and Warden[48,49,50] found that although children with increased intraabdominal pressure readings tended to be younger, larger TBSA injuries and full-thickness components were significantly associated with elevated pressures. Increased intraabdominal pressure has the potential to impair hemodynamics, renal function, and respiratory excursion. Despite maintaining cardiac output with fluid replacement, renal function remains impaired in the presence of increased intraabdominal pressure. Increases in the production and release of the hormones norepinephrine, dopamine, epinephrine, angiotensin, and renin support the clinical finding of profoundly altered renal, pulmonary, and cardiovascular function.

Renal System

Loss of circulating volume into the interstitial spaces results in reduced renal blood flow and decreased glomerular filtration. An important measure of the adequacy of volume replacement is urine excretion. Sufficient volume replacement maintains urine output during resuscitation. Approximately 36 hours after injury, edema fluid begins to mobilize and output increases.

Evidence of pigment in the urine results from the hemolysis of red blood cells. This is especially common following extensive electrical injuries. The release of **myoglobin** may occlude the kidney tubules and result in renal failure.

Children younger than 2 years lack the ability to concentrate urine because of the immaturity of the renal system and are therefore at increased risk for dehydration. In addition, the child has a relatively larger TBSA in relation to weight than the adult. Combined with limited physiologic reserves, increased fluid requirements are necessary for children both during burn shock resuscitation and to compensate for evaporative water losses.[51]

Gastrointestinal System

The gastrointestinal system plays an important role in the pathophysiology of burns. Alterations in blood flow result in decreased perfusion to the gastrointestinal tract. Ischemia may cause erosion and necrosis of gastrointestinal tissue.

Table 46-10 Metabolic Alterations Following Injury

Response	Dominant Factors	Clinical Findings
Ebb response	Loss of plasma volume Shock Low plasma insulin levels	Hyperglycemia Decreased oxygen consumption Depressed resting energy expenditure Decreased blood pressure Cardiac output below normal Decreased body temperature
Flow response		
Acute phase	Elevated catecholamines Elevated glucagon Elevated glucocorticoids Normal or elevated insulin levels High glucagon/insulin ratio	Catabolic Hyperglycemia Increased respiratory rate Increased oxygen consumption Increased body temperature Redistribution of polyvalent cations such as zinc and iron Mobilization of metabolic reserves Increased urinary excretion of nitrogen, sulfur, magnesium, phosphorus, potassium Accelerated gluconeogenesis
Adaptive phase	Stress hormone response subsiding	Anabolic Normoglycemia Energy turnover diminished Convalescence

From Gottschlich M, Alexander JW, Bower RH. In Rombeau JL, Caldwell MD, editors: *Enteral and tube feeding,* Philadelphia, 1990, W.B. Saunders (with permission).

Catecholamine release has been suggested as a factor in the suppression of gastric acid production in the immediate postburn period. Following this initial reduction, gastric acid production exceeds normal levels and increases the risk of erosion. A study of gastrin and cholecystokinin suggests a potential role of these peptides in the neuroendocrine alterations exhibited following burn injury.[52]

Paralytic ileus frequently occurs following major thermal injuries. Although digestion ceases in the stomach and the large bowel, the small intestine maintains motility and absorptive capacity. Intestinal motility returns as fluid losses are replaced unless irreversible necrosis of the bowel has occurred as a result of insufficient perfusion.

Metabolism

Complex metabolic alterations are observed following thermal injury. The extent of metabolic derangement is proportional to the magnitude of TBSA burn sustained. Wilmore[53] demonstrated the linear increase in metabolic rate up to 2½ times normal resting energy expenditure. As burn injury approaches 50% of TBSA, a plateau is reached, limiting further physiologic response to the trauma or other challenges such as infection.

A biphasic pattern of physiologic response is evident in thermally injured children. The initial **ebb phase** occurs during the immediate postburn period and continues for 3 to 5 days. This phase is characterized by reduced oxygen consumption, impaired circulation, and cellular shock. Following the resolution of the shock and the restoration of circulating volume, the metabolic response shifts to a **catabolic** or **(flow) phase** (Table 46-10). A state of **hypermetabolism** ensues, characterized by increased oxygen consumption and elevation of catecholamines, glucocorticoids, and glucagon.

Increased blood flow to the wound supplies additional glucose necessary for tissue repair. Insulin levels are usually normal or even elevated but are inappropriately low in relation to glucagon. Both catecholamines and glucocorticoids act as antagonists to insulin. This effect combined with a tissue resistance to insulin stimulates glycogenolysis and gluconeogenesis, thus increasing glucose flow from the liver.[54]

Metabolic rates slowly return to normal with wound closure. However, a reactivation of the hypermetabolic response may occur with sepsis or organ failure. Limited glucose stores provide additional challenges in the very young child.

Immune Function

Burn trauma–induced immunodepression results in increased susceptibility to infection and sepsis. Although the exact mechanisms responsible for this immunosuppression remain obscure, it is clear that complex interactions of the hypermetabolic response, nutritional support, bacterial translocation, and defects in both specific and nonspecific immune function are involved (Fig. 46-7). In addition, young children are at increased risk for microbial invasion caused by an immature immune system and limited antibody production.

Deitch[55] reported that wound- or gut-derived endotoxemia may be one of the mediators of the hypermetabolic response observed following thermal injury. Endotoxin may increase the permeability of the gut and alter defense mechanisms. Endotoxin is observed in burn serum very early after injury.[56] Indeed some children with burns exhibit immunosuppression for a prolonged period after wound closure is achieved.[57]

Circulating immunoglobulins may be affected by several factors, including age and the severity of injury.[58] Therapeutic interventions such as multiple transfusions, surgical procedures, and antibiotic and anesthetic administration also introduce elements that confound the evaluation of immunosuppressive effects. The alterations in the immune response are complex and result from the interaction of the components of the immune system that are initiated at the time of injury.[59]

Scar Maturation

In normal epidermal healing, minimal disruption in skin color, texture, and thickness occurs. However, burn wounds that extend into the dermis are repaired through **scar formation** and may result in an overgrowth of dermal constituents (Fig. 46-8). Accelerated collagen synthesis most likely begins with high levels of activity in granulation tissue. **Hypertrophic scars** produce a random, nodular orientation of collagen fibers. The red, raised, and rigid appearance of the immature scar is the result of increased vascularity, an increase in the number of fibroblasts, reduced interstitial spaces, and abundant and altered ground substances.[60] As the hypertrophic scar matures, collagen begins to orient in a more parallel fashion and vascularity decreases (Fig. 46-9). Collagen synthesis is very active soon after wound closure, and alteration of the scar can be accomplished before strong cross-linking of the collagen is established.

The length of time required to achieve wound closure is the most reliable predictor of hypertrophic scarring. Deeper burns demonstrate increased scarring caused by the formation of granulation tissue and prolonged healing time. Generally, darker-pigmented races are more susceptible to hypertrophic scarring.[61] Although age has not been found to be a predictor of hypertrophic scar formation, younger individuals are more susceptible to trauma and have greater skin tension and an accelerated rate of collagen synthesis. Increased tension with resultant trauma stimulates inflammation, which in turn results in the formation of additional collagen.

Clinical Manifestations

The clinical manifestations of burn injuries are apparent in all organ systems. Although the cutaneous trauma is the initiator of the chain of responses, it is important to consider all of the likely consequences of the injury. An awareness of the changing patterns of convalescence and the development of complications assists in the identification and early treatment of potential sequelae.

Burn Shock

The pathophysiologic responses result in **hypovolemia** and extracellular sodium depletion in the thermally injured individual. These manifestations are discussed in Chapter 45. Hypotension is a late sign of shock in the child. Heart rate is a more reliable measure. The urine output is a reflection of end-organ perfusion and is therefore the most accurate monitor of the adequacy of fluid resuscitation. Fluid should be delivered at a rate sufficient to maintain urine output at 1 ml/kg/hr in the child. Children weighing more than 50 kg should produce 30 to 50 ml/hr during resuscitation.[51,62] Fluid is titrated to maintain the output within these parameters.

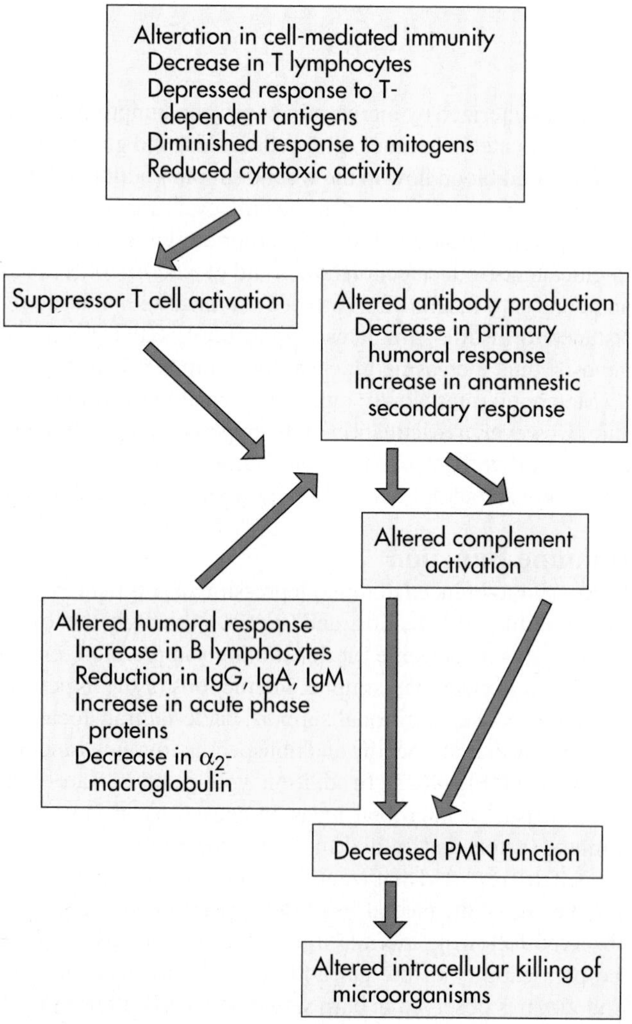

Fig. 46-7 Altered immune function following thermal injury. Cell-mediated immunity, antibody production, humoral response.

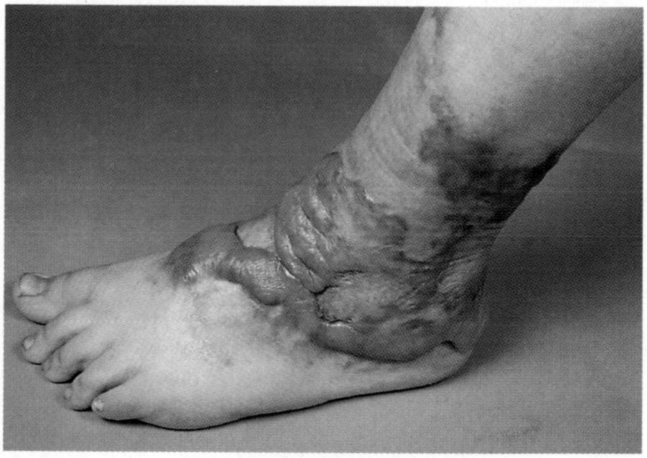

Fig. 46-8 Immature hypertrophic scar.

The fluid of choice for burn shock resuscitation should approximate the fluid lost from the circulating volume—for example, lactated Ringer solution. Children require fluid resuscitation for smaller burns than adults as a result of limited physiologic reserves. The child's relatively greater ratio of body surface area to weight results in increased evaporative water losses and proportionately more fluid during resuscitation. Although **colloid replacement** during burn shock resuscitation remains controversial, replacement may be required in the very young child who fails to respond to fluid replacement.[63] A component for **maintenance fluid** *must* be included in the calculation of fluid needs during resuscitation. Maintenance fluids represent the body requirements in the absence of burn injury. Resuscitation is considered complete when the child is able to maintain urine output for 2 hours with fluid rates at maintenance levels.

Successful resuscitation depends on establishment of intravenous access. Although this is usually accomplished by peripheral or central venous cannulation, circulatory collapse may preclude timely administration of fluid replacement. Cannulation of veins in the pediatric population is further complicated by small vessels and increased subcutaneous fat. Children are good candidates for **intraosseous** cannulation when traditional venous access techniques fail. Blood, drugs, and fluid are readily absorbed by red marrow that drains into medullary venous channels and thus to the systemic circulation. This technique is most effective in children younger than 6 years, because red marrow is replaced by yellow marrow as the child grows. Yellow marrow absorbs fluid less readily than red marrow.[64,65] With proper care and removal as soon as other access is available, complications are minimal.

Pulmonary System

The clinical manifestations of thermal injury related to the pulmonary system include a variety of complications ranging from inhalation injury, pulmonary edema, and respiratory failure to aspiration of gastric contents and pneumonia. Inhalation injury and other pulmonary complications remain the leading cause of death following burn injury in every age-group.[66]

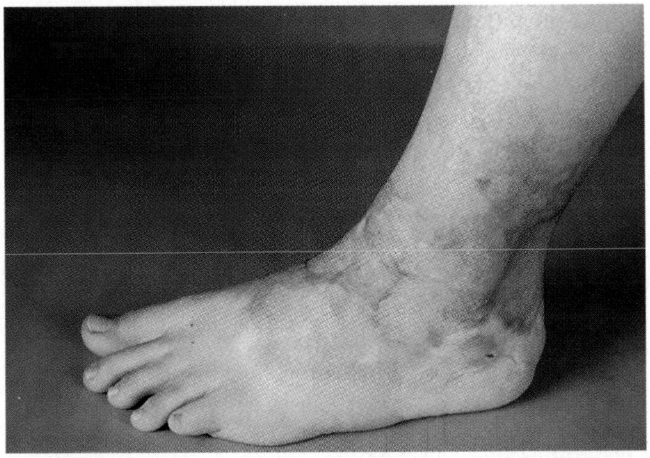

FIG. 46-9 Flat, mature scar after pressure therapy.

Anatomic differences in the pediatric airway affect the response to pulmonary complications as well as therapeutic interventions. The infant airway is positioned anteriorly, making visualization of the cords more difficult. The difficult visualization is further compounded by the relatively large tongue and slanting vocal cords. A small degree of edema results in greatly increased work of breathing in the child (Fig. 46-10). These considerations are particularly important during the resuscitation phase, when progressive edema threatens to obstruct the airway. Significant edema results in impairment of respiratory function unless an artificial airway is inserted (Fig. 46-11). Malposition of an endotracheal tube may result in inadvertent extubation, intubation of the bronchi, and atelectasis. Because of the relatively short length of the infant trachea, alterations of the position of the head and neck can affect tube position despite maintenance of the tube position at the teeth.[67,68,69]

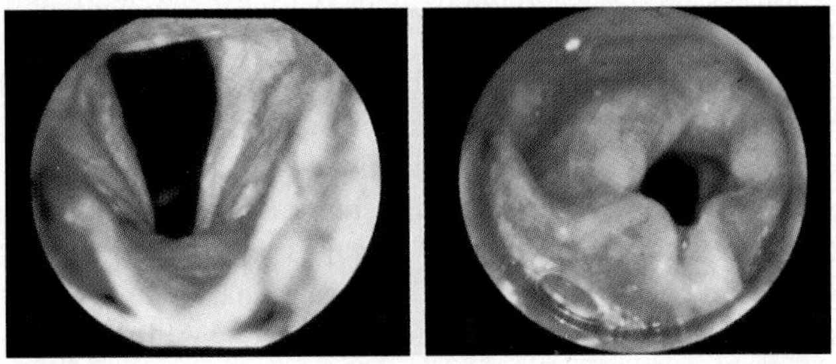

FIG. 46-10 Airways. Adult airway *(left)*; smaller pediatric airway *(right)*.

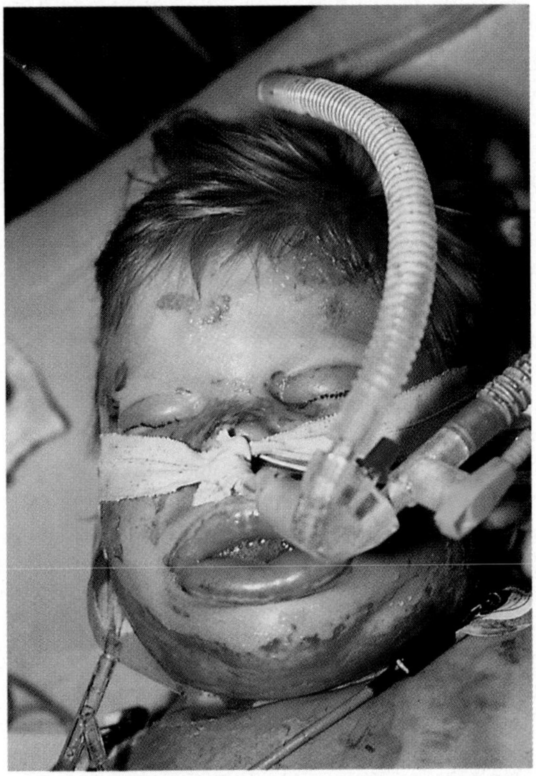

FIG. 46-11 Severe facial edema during burn shock.

Infants compensate for pulmonary compromise by increasing the respiratory rate. However, since the child possesses fewer type I muscle fibers, fatigue related to the increased work of breathing results in more rapid desaturation than in adults. The soft cartilage of the pediatric airway is prone to collapse in the presence of partial obstruction. Children with burns are at increased risk for these events because of underlying respiratory disease or injury.

Therapeutic interventions required for maintenance of pulmonary function have also been implicated in postextubation stridor and barotrauma. A mixture of helium and oxygen has been successfully used to decrease airway resistance and increase the volume of gas exchange following extubation.[70] Recent evidence suggests barotrauma from mechanical ventilation may be minimized by protocols based on permissive hypercapnia. Moderate respiratory acidosis was well tolerated and ventilating pressures maintained below 40 cm.[71] The low incidence of mortality associated with this strategy suggests a reduction in ventilator-induced lung injury.

The consequences of metabolic and physiologic changes occurring during the acute phase of injury remain apparent during convalescence. A predominantly restrictive and obstructive disease pattern has been reported in the child more than 2 years after injury.[72] The rib cage may be physically restricted by scarring in addition to pulmonary damage. Endurance levels may also be affected by the inability to dissipate heat following thermal trauma.[73]

Hypermetabolism

The hypermetabolic response following burn injury profoundly alters the production and utilization of nutrients. As a consequence of these phenomena, caloric requirements increase dramatically. The advent of portable metabolic testing equipment has permitted quantification of individual energy requirements at rest. Mayes and colleagues[74] compared various formulas proposed for the assessment of energy needs with measured energy expenditure. They reported that most existing formulas overestimated the energy needs of the pediatric burn population. This was particularly evident among the infant and toddler age-groups. These investigators recommend an addition of 30% to measured energy expenditure to compensate for stress-related factors such as wound care, pain, and physical activity.

In addition to age, body composition has been found to significantly affect the postburn course. Preexisting obesity has been associated with increased clinical sepsis and associated morbidity.[75] However, the heightened nutrient requirements of the burned child preclude a reduction in nutritional support during the acute phase of recovery. Aggressive nutritional therapy is critical to the recovery of these children, and programs designed to achieve ideal body weight should not be instituted until wound healing is achieved.

The requirements for micronutrients are also increased following thermal injury.[76,77] Hypermetabolism results in a rapid turnover in vitamins and trace minerals important in the wound healing and immune response. A deficiency of specific nutrients interferes with carbohydrate and nucleic acid metabolism, collagen formation, and immune function.

The **thermoregulatory response** following burn injury results in an elevation in core body temperature. Temperature increases to 38° to 39° C to provide maximal comfort and minimal energy expenditure in children with significant burns. Although the mechanism of this metabolic response remains unclear, it is known that failure to maintain body temperature results in more stress and potential circulatory collapse.[78] Therapeutic intervention, such as operative procedures and dressing changes, and transport present situations requiring increased diligence to prevent inadvertent cooling.[79,80] Infants are at increased risk for a precipitous drop in core body temperature caused by an inability to regulate heat loss by shivering. Heat is also lost because of evaporation of water from damaged skin surfaces. Infants and children are especially vulnerable because of the large surface area relative to metabolically active tissue.

Infection

Whereas shock and pulmonary compromise present the most immediate threat after thermal trauma, both local and systemic infections become the primary complication during healing. Initially the burn wound is relatively free of pathogens. However, the dead, avascular tissue and wound exudate provide a fertile environment for bacterial growth. Colonization of the wound is apparent by the fifth postburn day. Gram-positive microorganisms are usually recovered from cultures first, followed by opportunistic gram-negative bacteria. The impaired vascular supply to burned tissue enhances the proliferation of pathogenic microorganisms. Bacterial invasion results in thrombosis and a further impairment of circulation sufficient to convert a partial-thickness injury to a full-thickness wound.

Improvements in treatment have resulted in a reduction in wound infection. Aggressive excision and grafting of the wounds, improved nutritional support, and the development of microorganism-specific topical antimicrobials have contributed to this trend. However, the incidence of septicemia remains relatively constant. This is perhaps explained by the survival of children with burns of increasingly large body surface area. Because the burned child is immune suppressed for many weeks following injury, monitoring and timely identification of infectious processes are essential for optimal management and recovery. Developing resistance to antimicrobial agents underscores the need for diligent environmental control of microorganisms.[81,82]

Functional Limitations

Children require specialized management to ensure optimal functional and cosmetic results. Scar and contracture management is necessary for prolonged periods because of changes in body composition as the child grows and matures. Very young children present unique challenges because the small body size can be difficult to fit with pressure garments and splints, growth is rapid, and cooperation with the rehabilitation program is limited. Children are reluctant to move when doing so causes pain, and they are likely to assume a position of comfort. Unfortunately, this position is often one that results in contracture formation and loss of function. Proper positioning and splint application are necessary to maintain body alignment.

Infant skin is thinner, and the epidermis is more loosely connected to the dermis. This increases the risk of blistering, chafing, and rash formation. The infant also produces less sebum and sweat, which further exacerbates the propensity to skin irritation. Since scar tissue contains no sweat glands, these characteristics of the skin in growing children compound the difficulty in maintaining pressure on maturing scars while cooling the body.

Scar tissue is metabolically active and highly vascular. Collagen is deposited in random patterns, and contraction of the scar can result in disabling deformities. The scar is active as long as it is raised, red, and firm. **Scar maturation** requires 1 to 2 years and depends on individual differences and compliance with the rehabilitation program. The maturation is accompanied by intense itching, which is particularly distressful for infants and toddlers. The delicate skin is easily damaged by scratching or trauma. The mature scar is characterized by increased suppleness, flattening, and pigmented color.

Scar tissue does not grow and expand like normal tissue. Although massage therapy offers some benefit in stretching, functional limitation may develop as the child grows. This is particularly evident over joints. Reconstructive surgery is often necessary to restore anatomic integrity and to promote independent function.

Evaluation and Treatment

The initial assessment conducted on admission to the burn center includes maintenance of an adequate airway, fluid resuscitation to manage burn shock, and the evaluation and treatment of the wound. Other therapies are initiated throughout the course of treatment. Nutritional support is essential to ensure an optimal outcome. Positioning and splinting to prevent contracture formation as well as rehabilitative aspects of therapy are instituted on admission and continue throughout the hospitalization. Psychosocial support is very important for both the child and the family. The information provided should be consistent and honest to allow clarification of concerns.

Fluid Resuscitation

Fluid resuscitation is generally required for children following thermal injuries in excess of 15% to 20% of the TBSA. Fluid is administered to compensate for the fluid and electrolytes extravasating into the interstitial spaces. This replacement restores circulating volume, improves perfusion, and alleviates organ dysfunction associated with impaired circulation.

Various protocols have been proposed as guidelines for fluid administration. It is important to remember that any regimen serves merely as a guideline and will require adjustment based on the individual response of each child. A commonly employed protocol consists of a modification of the Parkland formula (Fig. 46-12). Children require proportionately more fluid during burn shock resuscitation than adults with comparable injuries.[63] Additional fluid loss through an airway damaged by smoke inhalation also increases fluid requirements.[83] The resistance of burn shock to aggressive fluid resuscitation may be managed by an exchange transfusion technique. Banked whole blood is used to replace the circulating volume and remove the circulating inflammatory response factors.[84] This therapeutic modality may benefit children who fail to respond to conventional fluid therapy protocols.

Wound Management

The goals of wound management include prevention of infection, removal of devitalized tissue, and closure of the wound. Burns that are clearly deep dermal or full-thickness injuries are surgically excised as soon as the child is hemodynamically stable following resuscitation. Early excision reduces the incidence of wound infection and systemic sepsis.[85] Coverage of the excised wound is necessary to achieve wound closure. The choice of a coverage technique depends on the availability of donor skin.

Split-thickness sheet grafts are selected for areas of maximal functional and cosmetic results (Fig. 46-13). Children with very large burn injuries often do not have sufficient unburned skin available to use the sheet graft. In these cases the surgeon will employ a meshing technique to expand the available skin and increase the size of the graft. The pattern created heals by migration from the meshed edges. Scar formation is increased, and the mesh pattern will remain clearly visible (Fig. 46-14). The choice of the donor site also affects the final result. Skin obtained below the clavicle is noticeably more yellow than skin above the clavicle. This is an important consideration, especially for grafts to the face.[86] Ongoing research and further refinement of the cultured skin substitutes has produced a source of autologous skin when donor sites are limited.[87,88]

Pulmonary Support

Morbidity and mortality associated with respiratory failure is a consequence of inhalation injury and sepsis-induced multiorgan failure.[89] In order to avoid barotrauma from high ventilating pressures and concentrations of oxygen, current management attempts to support pulmonary function through permissive hypercapnia and high-frequency percussive ventilation.[90] When this therapy fails, improvements in intrapulmonary shunt and pulmonary artery pressures may be realized by the inhalation of nitric oxide. This pulmonary vasodilator has been shown to offer short-term benefit in this population. However, long-term impact on survival remains controversial.[91] Extracorporeal membrane oxygenation (ECMO), another technique available for children resistant to conventional support, allows cardiopulmonary rest by a prolonged bypass. Maximal benefit is associated with a relatively short course of conventional therapy and excision and grafting of burn wounds before the initiation of ECMO.[84,92,93]

Nutritional Support

The heightened metabolic demands following burn injury combined with a poor appetite often necessitate supplementation

Date ____________________

RESUSCITATION CALCULATIONS

I. RESUSCITATION

A. Calculated Resuscitation and Basal Requirement (less than 2 yr—2000 cc/m²)

1. (4 cc × ________ kg × ________ % burn) + (1500 cc × ________ m²) = cc/24 hr

(________________) + (________________) = ________________ cc/24 hr

B. Resuscitation Fluid per 8 hours

1. 1st 8 hours ________________ cc, ________________ cc/hr

2. 2nd 8 hours ________________ cc, ________________ cc/hr

3. 3rd 8 hours ________________ cc, ________________ cc/hr

II. MAINTENANCE FLUIDS

A. Basal fluid requirement—1500 cc/m² (less than 2 yr—2000 cc/m²)

1. Total body surface area ________________ m²

2. 24 hours ________________ cc

3. Hourly ________________ cc/hr

B. Evaporative water loss

1. Adults—(25 + % burn) m² = cc/hr

Children—(35 + % burn) m² = cc/hr

2. Calculated evaporative water loss

a. (________ + ________ % burn) ________ m² = ________ cc/hr; ________ cc/24 hr

C. Total maintenance fluids—basal requirement and evaporative water loss

1. 24 hours ________________ cc

2. Hourly ________________ cc

Shriners Hospitals for Crippled Children Cincinnati Unit

Resuscitation Calculations

FIG. 46-12 Calculation of fluid requirements during burn shock and maintenance needs. (Courtesy Shriners Hospitals for Children, Cincinnati Burns Hospital.)

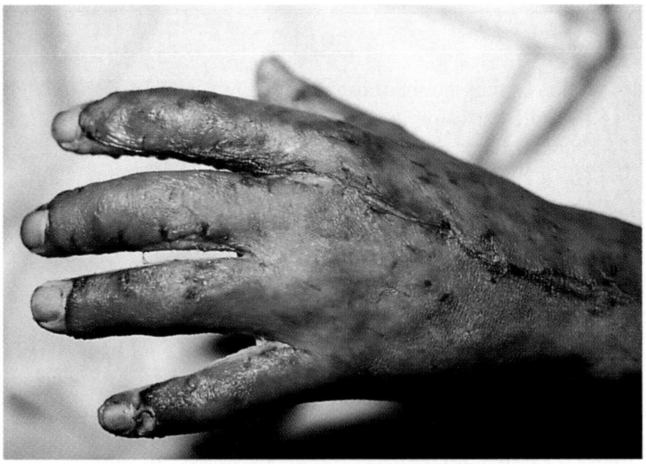

FIG. 46-13 Split-thickness sheet graft.

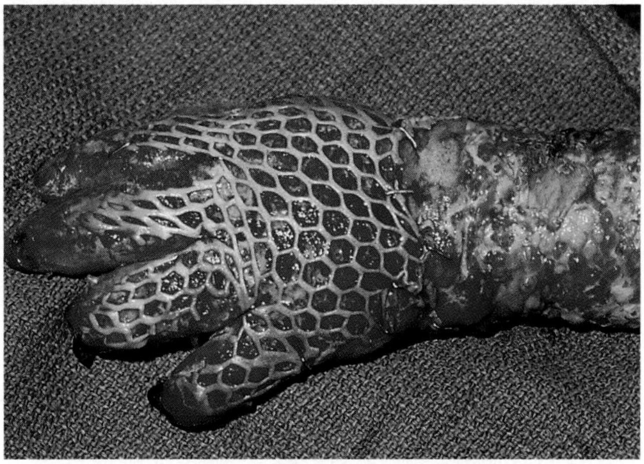

FIG. 46-14 Meshed autograft.

of oral intake. Children with burns in excess of 25% of TBSA frequently require supplementation with tube feeding. Feeding does not need to be delayed pending resolution of paralytic ileus and the resumption of bowel sounds because the small bowel maintains motility and absorptive capability. A small-bore feeding tube placed in the duodenum provides a safe route for the delivery of essential nutrients.[94] Gastric decompression is maintained by a nasogastric tube to prevent aspiration.[95] Parenteral hyperalimentation is reserved for those children who are unable to tolerate enteral support because of attendant risks of catheter sepsis and loss of intestinal integrity.[96] Early initiation of enteral supplementation along with aggressive management of complications permits successful enteral alimentation in most burned children.

Human growth hormone, an anabolic agent, has been administered to blunt the protein catabolism seen following thermal trauma. Investigators have reported sparing of lean body mass and enhanced wound healing following administration of recombinant human growth hormone.[97,98,99] Combined with aggressive nutritional support, this therapy may provide additional benefit to children recovering from burn injuries. Some evidence exists to support ongoing growth delays and weight loss following discharge.[100] Outpatient follow-up should include a nutritional assessment to identify children at risk for further weight loss.

Comfort Management

Pain management presents a significant challenge in the pediatric population. In addition to procedural pain, there is a component of background pain that is present without activity. Pain perception is also affected by the degree of emotional overlay or affective experience.[101] The measurement of pain is particularly challenging in young infants, who lack the language skills to express pain. A variety of tools, from physiologic monitors to behavioral analyses and analog scales, have been developed to measure pediatric pain. Some success has been reported with the use of nonpharmacological intervention to reduce pain and anxiety.[102]

WHAT'S NEW? C-reactive Protein Serum Levels as an Early Indicator of Sepsis

Timely initiation of definitive therapy for sepsis increases the likelihood of a positive outcome. C-reactive protein (CRP), a major acute-phase protein involved in a variety of host-defense processes, was monitored throughout the acute burn phase in 57 children. CRP monitoring predicted the onset of sepsis 2.13 ± 0.5 days before clinical parameters made the diagnosis apparent. This information has the potential to improve the treatment of an individual with a burn injury.

Data from Neely AN, Smith WL, Warden GD: Efficacy of a rise in C-reactive protein serum levels as an early indicator of sepsis in burned children, *J Burn Care Rehabil* 19:102, 1998.

Community Reintegration

Rehabilitation becomes the major focus of care once wound coverage has been achieved and continues until all reconstructive procedures have been completed. This phase may extend over many years in the pediatric population. In addition to the functional aspects of rehabilitation, attention must be directed to psychosocial needs and community reintegration. Children are increasingly surviving massive burn injuries because of advances in care in the past 20 years. However, adaptation to self-image and functional limitations poses serious issues for both the child and the family.[103,104] A method to facilitate the transition from the hospital to the community is the school reentry program offered by many burn centers. These programs provide education for teachers and peers about the injury, appearance, and abilities of the returning child.

A panel of experts have developed and tested a standardized, self-administered questionnaire for children between 5 and 18 years of age. This tool is designed to evaluate the effectiveness of burn management treatments and individual-oriented outcomes. Consistent ongoing measurement of outcomes will provide benchmarks and identify opportunities to continue to improve burn care.[105]

SUMMARY REVIEW

Shock and Multiple Organ Dysfunction Syndrome

1. Shock in children is present when there are signs of poor systemic perfusion, regardless of blood pressure.
2. Hypovolemic shock is the most common type of shock in children. Dehydration and trauma are the most common causes of hypovolemic shock.
3. Hypotension is a sign of severe, decompensated shock.
4. Hypovolemia can be caused by volume loss, an increase in the vascular space relative to the amount of volume, or a redistribution of intravascular volume.
5. Clinical manifestations of hypovolemic shock include inadequate systemic perfusion associated with intravascular fluid loss. Adrenergic compensatory mechanisms include tachycardia, redistribution of blood flow, peripheral vasoconstriction, cool extremities, delayed capillary refill, and oliguria.
6. Neurogenic shock is caused by a loss of vasomotor tone following severe injury to the spinal cord.
7. Clinical manifestations of neurogenic shock include warm skin, hypotension with a low diastolic blood pressure, and poor systemic perfusion.
8. Cardiogenic shock, with decreased cardiac output, is observed most commonly following cardiovascular surgery or with inflammatory diseases of the heart, such as cardiomyopathy and myocarditis. It is also found in children with obstructive congenital heart disease and those with drug toxicity or severe electrolyte or acid-base imbalances.
9. Clinical manifestations of cardiogenic shock include inadequate systemic perfusion despite adequate intravascular volume. Cardiac output is typically low. Adrenergic compensatory mechanisms are similar to those found in hypovolemic shock.
10. Sepsis in children caused by nosocomial infections is linked to gram-negative infections 40% of the time; gram-positive infections 40% of the time; and viruses, fungi, or rickettsial microorganisms 20% of the time. Sepsis can lead to septic shock.
11. Altered cytokine levels are associated with septic shock in children. Tumor necrosis factor (TNF) levels are directly related to mortality in newborns and children with meningitis and sepsis.
12. Sepsis is a systemic response to infection. It is present when manifestations of systemic inflammatory response syndrome (SIRS) are observed. SIRS is present when the individual demonstrates two or more of the following as an acute change from baseline values: fever, hypothermia, tachycardia, tachypnea, respiratory alkalosis, and alterations in the white blood cell count. The newborn often develops hypothermia rather than fever as a sign of infection.
13. Severe sepsis is present when the individual demonstrates evidence of SIRS and signs of organ dysfunction, hypoperfusion, or hypotension.
14. The development of septic shock is heralded when the person with severe sepsis becomes hypotensive despite adequate fluid resuscitation or requires vasopressors to maintain blood pressure.
15. Reperfusion and inflammatory injury stimulate free oxygen radicals that damage cell membranes, denature proteins, and disrupt chromosomes. This process likely affects endothelial cells and the microvasculature, causing multiple organ dysfunction syndrome (MODS).
16. Acidosis may be the most sensitive indicator of inadequate systemic perfusion in children. Hypotension is a late sign of shock in infants and children.
17. The goals of treatment for shock are maximization of oxygen delivery and minimization of oxygen demand. Airway, oxygenation, and ventilation must be supported. The child should be kept warm, and shivering should be prevented. The warmth of the child's extremities, capillary refill, quality of peripheral pulses, level of consciousness and responsiveness, urine output, oxygenation, ventilation, and acid-base status should be assessed throughout shock therapy.
18. Treatment consists of immediate resuscitation, including fluid replacement, ventilation, pharmacologic therapy, electrocardiographic (ECG) analysis, hemodynamic monitoring, administration of blood or blood component therapy, and management of electrolyte and acid-base imbalances.

Burns

1. Burns in children are often the result of inadequate supervision, curiosity, inability to escape the burning agent, or intentional abuse.
2. Scald injuries are commonly seen in the very young child and result from exposure to hot water, grease, or other hot liquids.
3. A child's skin is thinner and thus more susceptible to injury than adult skin. The kitchen and bathroom are common sites of burn injury.
4. It is estimated that from 4% to 25% of hospital admissions for scald injuries are the result of child abuse.
5. Flame burns involving flammable liquids, most notably gasoline, are more common in older children. Risk-taking behaviors in young males can lead to electrical burns. Chemical injuries are rare in children because these injuries are associated with industrial settings.
6. Use of the standard rule of nines results in inaccurate calculation of the percentage of total body surface area (TBSA) involved in children. A modified rule of nines deducts 1% from the head and adds 0.5% to each leg for each year of life after 2 years of age.
7. Major thermal trauma involves all body systems, and the consequences of injury include shock, infection, hypermetabolism, organ failure, and functional limitations. These effects can be magnified in the pediatric population as a result of physiologic immaturity and age-related variation in treatment modalities.
8. Infection or trauma may convert a partial-thickness injury to a full-thickness one, especially in young children, who have thinner, more delicate skin.
9. Marked reduction in cardiac output occurs immediately following injury and is accompanied by an initial increase in systemic vascular resistance. The inefficient and labile peripheral circulation of the infant complicates management of the burn shock phase of treatment. Constriction of the chest and impairment of respiratory excursion may occur in the very young child because of the increased pliability of the rib cage. Younger children are also more susceptible to increased intra-abdominal pressure.
10. Children younger than 2 years lack the ability to concentrate urine because of the immaturity of the renal system and are therefore at increased risk for dehydration. Because children

have a relatively larger body surface area in relation to weight than adults, they require proportionately increased fluid during burn shock resuscitation and to compensate for evaporative water losses.

11. A biphasic pattern of physiologic responses is evident in thermally injured children. The initial ebb phase occurs during the immediate postburn period and continues for 3 to 5 days. This phase is characterized by reduced oxygen consumption, impaired circulation, and cellular shock. Following this phase and the restoration of volume, the metabolic response shifts to a catabolic or flow phase. This phase is characterized by hypermetabolism with an increased oxygen consumption and elevation of catecholamines, glucocorticoids, and glucagon.
12. Some children exhibit immunosuppression for a prolonged period after wound closure is achieved.
13. Although age was not found to be a predictor of hypertrophic scarring, children have greater skin tension and an accelerated rate of collagen synthesis.
14. Children require fluid resuscitation for smaller burns than the adult population as a result of limited physiologic reserves. Colloid replacement may be required in the very young child who fails to respond to fluid replacement. Resuscitation is considered complete when the child is able to maintain urine output for 2 hours with fluid rates at maintenance levels.
15. The leading cause of death in children following burn injury, as in adults, is pulmonary complications.
16. Children require specialized management to ensure optimal functional and cosmetic results. Long-term scar and contracture management is necessary because of changes in body composition as the child grows and matures.

KEY TERMS

Bradycardia, *1516*
Cardiogenic shock, *1518*
Catabolic (flow) phase, *1529*
Chemical injury, *1526*
Child abuse, *1525*
Colloid, *1523*
Colloid replacement, *1531*
Compensated shock, *1513*
Contact burn, *1525*
Crystalloid, *1523*
Decompensated shock, *1513*
Depth of injury, *1526*
Dermal ischemia, *1526*
Distributive (vasogenic) shock, *1514*
Ebb phase, *1529*
Electrical burn, *1525*
Eschar, *1528*
Evaporative fluid loss, *1526*
Flame burn, *1525*
Fluid resuscitation, *1533*
Hemoconcentration, *1526*
Hypermetabolism, *1529*
Hypertrophic scar, *1530*
Hypovolemia, *1530*
Hypovolemic shock, *1514*
Intraabdominal pressure, *1528*
Intraosseous, *1531*
Maintenance fluid, *1531*
Multiple organ dysfunction syndrome (MODS), *1513*
Myoglobin, *1528*
Neurogenic shock, *1514*
Rehabilitation, *1535*
Reperfusion (reoxygenation) injury, *1521*
Scald injury, *1525*
Scar formation, *1530*
Scar maturation, *1533*
Sepsis, *1519*
Shock, *1513*
Split-thickness sheet graft, *1533*
Systemic inflammatory response syndrome (SIRS), *1520*
Tachycardia, *1515*
Thermoregulatory response, *1532*
Third spacing of fluid, *1514*

REFERENCES

1. Gorelick MH, Shaw KN, Murphy KO: Validity and reliability of clinical signs in the diagnosis of dehydration in children, *Pediatrics* 99:E6, 1997.
2. Hazinski MF: Children are different. In Hazinski MF, editor: *Manual of pediatric critical care,* St Louis, 1999, Mosby.
3. Michaud LJ et al: Elevated initial blood glucose levels and poor outcome following severe brain injuries in children, *J Trauma* 31:1356, 1991.
4. Chameides L, Hazinski MF, editors: *Textbook of pediatric advanced life support,* Dallas, 1997, American Heart Association.
5. Rudolph AM: *Congenital diseases of the heart*, Chicago, 1974, Year Book Medical.
6. Sevedra JM et al: Capillary refill (skin turgor) in the assessment of dehydration, *Am J Dis Child* 145:296, 1991.
7. Hazinski MF: Cardiovascular disorders. In Hazinski MF, editor: *Manual of pediatric critical care*, St Louis, 1999, Mosby.
8. Bone RC: Toward a theory regarding the pathogenesis of the systemic inflammatory response syndrome: what we do and do not know about cytokine regulation, *Crit Care Med* 24:63, 1996.
9. Rangel-Frausto MS et al: The natural history of the systemic inflammatory response syndrome (SIRS): a prospective study, *JAMA* 273: 117, 1995.
10. Singh-Naz N et al: Risk factors for nonsocomial infections in critically ill children; a prospective cohort study, *Crit Care Med* 24:875, 1996.
11. Hazinski MF et al: Epidemiology, pathophysiology, and clinical presentation of gram-negative sepsis, *Am J Crit Care* 2:224, 1993.
12. Milliken J et al: Nosocomial infections in a pediatric intensive care unit, *Crit Care Med* 16:233, 1988.
13. Davenport SE: Frequency of handwashing by registered nurses caring for infants on radiant warmers and in incubation, *Neonatal Network* 11:21, 1992.
14. Donowitz LO: Hand-washing technique in a pediatric intensive care unit, *Am J Dis Child* 141:683, 1987.
15. Wheeler AP, Bernard G: Treating patients with severe sepsis, *New Engl J Med* 340:207, 1999.
16. Sullivan JS et al: Correlation of plasma cytokine elevation with mortality rate in children with sepsis, *J Pediatr* 120:510, 1992.
17. Wong HR et al: Nitric oxide production in critically ill patients, *Arch Dis Child* 74:482, 1996.
18. Glauser MP: Pathophysiologic basis of sepsis; considerations for future strategies of intervention, *Crit Care Med* 28(suppl):S4, 2000.
19. Fisher CJ: Protein C levels as a prognostic indicator of outcome in sepsis and related diseases, *Crit Care Med* 28(suppl):S49, 2000.

20. Giroir B: Meningococcemia as a model for testing the hypothesis of antiseptic therapies, *Crit Care Med* (suppl):S57, 2000.
21. Sprung CL: Corticosteroids in septic shock. Resurrection of the last rites? *Crit Care Med* 26:627, 1998.
22. Bollaert PE et al: Reversal of late septic shock with supra-physiologic doses of hydrocortisone, *Crit Care Med* 26:645, 1998.
23. Briegel J et al: Stress doses of hydrocortisone reverse hyperdynamic septic shock; a prospective, randomized, double-blind, single-center study, *Crit Care Med* 27:723, 1999.
24. Riordan et al: Admission cortisol and adrenocorticotrophic hormone levels in children with meningococcal disease: evidence of adrenal insufficiency? *Crit Care Med* 27:2257, 1999.
25. American College of Chest Physicians/Society of Critical Care Medicine Consensus Conference Committee: Definitions for sepsis and organ failure and guidelines for the use of innovative therapies in sepsis, *Crit Care Med* 20:864, 1992.
26. Bone RC: Sepsis and its complications: the clinical problem, *Crit Care Med* 22(suppl):S8, 1994.
27. Barrier SL, Lowry SF: An overview of mortality risk prediction in sepsis, *Crit Care Med* 23:376, 1995.
28. Dantzker D: Oxygen delivery and utilization in sepsis, *Crit Care Med* 5:81, 1989.
29. Parker MM et al: Serial cardiovascular variables in survivors and nonsurvivors of human septic shock: heart rate as an early predictor of prognosis, *Crit Care Med* 15:923, 1987.
30. Carcillo JA, Davis AL, Zaritsky A: Role of early fluid resuscitation in pediatric septic shock, *JAMA* 266:1242, 1991.
31. Damjanov I, Linder J: *Anderson's pathology*, ed 10, St Louis, 1996, Mosby,
32. Waxman D: Shock: ischemia, reperfusion, inflammation, *New Horiz* 4:153, 1996.
33. Hutton P et al: An assessment of the Dinamap 845, *Anesthesiology* 39:261, 1984.
34. Cohn JN: Blood pressure measurement in shock: mechanisms of inaccuracy in auscultatory and palpatory methods, *JAMA* 199:188, 1967.
35. Oh MS, Carroll HJ: Electrolyte and acid-base disorders. In Chernow B, editor: *The pharmacologic approach to the critically ill patient*, ed 3, Baltimore, 1994, Williams & Wilkins.
36. Zaritsky A et al: CPR in children, *Ann Emerg Med* 16:1107, 1987.
37. Whitlock D, Whitlock J, Coates TD: Hematologic and oncologic emergencies requiring critical care. In Hazinski MF, editor: *Nursing care of the critically ill child*, ed 2, St Louis, 1992, Mosby.
38. Reeves JH et al: Continuous plasmafiltration in sepsis syndrome, *Crit Care Med* 27:2096, 1999.
39. Committee on Trauma: *Resource for optimal care of the injured patient* [pamphlet], 1999, American College of Surgeons.
40. Sheridan R et al: Early burn center transfer shortens the length of hospitalization and reduces complications in children with serous burn injuries, *J Burn Care Rehabil* 20:347, 1999.
41. Maley M: Scald in the kitchen, *Info Exchange* 9:1, 1993.
42. Purdue GF, Hunt JL, Prescott PR: Child abuse by burning—an index of suspicion, *J Trauma* 28:221, 1988.
43. Renz BM, Sherman R: Abusive scald burns in infants and children, *Am Surgeon* 59:329, 1993.
44. Warner JE, Hansen DJ: The identification and reporting of physical abuse by physicians: a review and implications for research, *Child Abuse Negl* 18:11, 1994.
45. Devlin BK, Reynolds E: Child abuse: how to recognize it, how to intervene, *Am J Nurs* 94(3):26, 1994.
46. Helvig E: Pediatric burn injuries, *AACN Clin Issues* 4:433, 1993.
47. Gordon MD, Winfree JH: Fluid resuscitation after major burn. In Carrougher GJ, editor: *Burn care and therapy*, St. Louis, 1998, Mosby.
48. Greenhalgh DG, Warden GD: The importance of intra-abdominal pressure measurements in burned children, *J Trauma* 36(5):685, 1994.
49. Mars M, Hadley GP: Raised compartmental pressure in children: a basis for management, *Injury* 29(3):183, 1998.
50. Meldrum DR et al: Prospective characterization and selective management of the abdominal compartment syndrome, *Am J Surgery* 174:667, 1997.
51. Warden GD: Burn shock resuscitation, *World J Surg* 16:16, 1992.
52. Cone JB et al: Alterations in gastrointestinal peptides after thermal injury in humans, *J Burn Care Rehabil* 14(6):663, 1993.
53. Wilmore DW: Nutrition and metabolism following thermal injury, *Clin Plast Surg* 1:603, 1974.
54. Gottschlich MM: Nutrition in the burned pediatric patient. In Samour PQ, Helm KK, Lange C, editors: *Handbook of pediatric nutrition*, Gaithersburg, Md, 1999, Aspen.
55. Deitch EA: Nutritional support of the burn patient, *Crit Care Med* 11(3):735, 1995.
56. Hiki N et al: Endotoxemia and specific antibody behavior against different endotoxins following multiple injuries, *J Trauma* 38(5):794, 1995.
57. Ogle CK et al: A long-term study and correlation of lymphocyte and neutrophil function in the patient with burns, *J Burn Care Rehabil* 11(2):105, 1990.
58. Stratta RJ et al: Immunologic parameters in burned patients: effect of therapeutic interventions, *J Trauma* 26(1):7, 1986.
59. Harris BH, Gelfand JA: The immune response to trauma, *Semin Pediatr Surg* 4(2):77, 1995.
60. Staley MJ, Richard RL: Scar management. In Richard RL, Staley MJ, editors: *Burn care and rehabilitation: principles and practice*, Philadelphia, 1994, Davis.
61. Deitch EA et al: Hypertrophic burn scars: analysis of variables, *J Trauma* 23:895, 1983.
62. Yowler CJ, Fratianne RB: Current status of burn resuscitation, *Clin Plast Surg* 27:1, 2000.
63. Cocks AJ, O'Connell A, Martin H: Crystalloids, colloids, and kids: a review of paediatric burns in intensive care, *Burns* 24:717, 1998.
64. Evans RJ et al: Intraosseous infusion—a technique available for intravascular administration of drugs and fluids in the child with burns, *Burns* 21(7):552, 1995.
65. Hurren JS, Dunn KW: Intraosseous infusion for burn resuscitation, *Burns* 21(4):285, 1995.
66. Carrougher GJ: Inhalation injury, *AACN Clin Issues* 4:367, 1993.
67. Conrardy PA et al: Alteration of endotracheal tube position, *Crit Care Med* 4(2):8, 1976.
68. Scharar SR: Endotracheal tube tip position in an infant with severe burns, *J Burn Care Rehabil* 16:654, 1995.
69. Trout S et al: Influence of head and neck position on endotracheal tube tip position on chest x-ray examination: a potential problem in the infant undergoing intubation, *J Burn Care Rehabil* 15:405, 1994.
70. Rodeberg DA et al: Use of a helium-oxygen mixture in the treatment of postextubation stridor in pediatric patients with burns, *J Burn Care Rehabil* 16:476, 1995.
71. Sheridan RL et al: Permissive hypercapnia as a ventilatory strategy in burned children: effect on barotrauma, pneumonia, and mortality, *J Trauma* 39(5):854, 1995.
72. Mlcak RP et al: Increased physiological dead space/tidal volume ratio during exercise in burned children, *Burns* 21(5):337, 1995.
73. Desai MH et al: Does inhalation injury limit exercise endurance in children convalescing from thermal injury? *J Burn Care Rehabil* 14:16, 1993.
74. Mayes T et al: Evaluation of predicted and measured energy requirements in burned children, *J Am Diet Assoc* 96(1):24, 1996.
75. Gottschlich MM et al: Significance of obesity on nutritional, immunologic, hormonal, and clinical outcome parameters in burns, *J Am Diet Assoc* 93(11):1261, 1993.
76. Gosling P et al: Serum copper and zinc concentrations in patients with burns in relation to burn surface area, *J Burn Care Rehabil* 16:481, 1995.
77. Gottschlich MM, Warden GD: Vitamin supplementation in the burn patient, *J Burn Care Rehabil* 11:275, 1990.
78. Kelemen JJ et al: Effect of ambient temperature on metabolic rate after thermal injury, *Ann Surg* 223:406, 1996.
79. Fiege A, Rutherford WF, Nelson DR: Factors influencing patient thermoregulation in flight, *Air Med J* 15(1):18, 1996.

80. Kagan R, Jenkins M: Transport and management of children with burns and inhalation injuries. In Jaimovich DG, Vidyasagar D, editors: *Handbook of pediatric and neonatal transport medicine*, Philadelphia, 1996, Hanley & Belfus.
81. Neely AN, Holder IA: Antimicrobial resistance, *Burns* 25:17, 1999.
82. Peck MD et al: Surveillance of burn wound infections: a proposal for definitions, *J Burn Care Rehabil* 19:386, 1998.
83. Zak AL et al: Acute respiratory failure that complicates the resuscitation of pediatric patients with scald injuries, *J Burn Care Rehabil* 20:391, 1999.
84. Heink NR: Fluid resuscitation and the role of exchange transfusion in pediatric burn shock, *Crit Care Nurs* 12(7):50, 1992.
85. Peterson SR, Umphred E, Warden GD: The incidence of bacteremia following burn wound excision, *J Trauma* 22:274, 1982.
86. Greenhalgh DG: The healing of burn wounds, *Dermatol Nurs* 8(1):13, 1996.
87. Boyce ST et al: Assessment with the dermal torque meter of skin pliability after treatment of burns in cultured skin substitutes, *J Burn Care Rehabil* 21:55, 2000.
88. Boyce ST et al: The 1999 clinical research award. Cultured skin substitutes combined with Integra Artificial Skin to replace native skin autograft and allograft for the closure of excised full-thickness burns, *J Burn Care Rehabil* 20:453, 1999.
89. Brown DL et al: Inhalation injury severity scoring system: a quantitative method, *J Burn Care Rehabil* 17:552, 1996.
90. Cortiella J, Mlcak R, Herndon D: High frequency percussive ventilation in pediatric patients with inhalation injury, *J Burn Care Rehabil* 20:232, 1999.
91. Sheridan RL et al: Low-dose inhaled nitric oxide in acutely burned children with profound respiratory failure, *Surgery* 126:856, 1999.
92. Goretsky MJ et al: The use of extracorporeal life support in pediatric burn patients with respiratory failure, *J Pediatr Surg* 30:620, 1995.
93. Pierre EJ et al: Extracorporeal membrane oxygenation in the treatment of respiratory failure in pediatric patients with burns, *J. Burn Care Rehabil* 19:131, 1998.
94. Gottschlich MM: Early and perioperative support. In Matarese L, Gottschlich MM, editors: *Contemporary nutrition support practice*, Philadelphia, 1998, W.B. Saunders.
95. Jenkins M, Gottschlich M, Warden G: Enteral support during operative procedures, *J Burn Care Rehabil* 15:199, 1994.
96. Herndon DN et al: Failure of TPN to improve liver function, immunity, and mortality in thermally injured patients, *J Trauma* 27:195, 1987.
97. Gore DC et al: Effect of exogenous growth hormone on whole-body and isolated-limb protein kinetics in burned patients, *Arch Surg* 126:38, 1991.
98. Herndon DN et al: Effects of recombinant human growth hormone on donor-site healing in severely burned children, *Ann Surg* 212(4):424, 1990.
99. Jeevanandam M et al: Decreased growth hormone levels in the catabolic phase of severe injury, *Surgery* 111:495, 1992.
100. Mittendorfer B et al: Younger pediatric patients with burns are at risk for postdischarge weight loss, *J Burn Care Rehabil* 16:589, 1995.
101. Gordon M et al: Use of pain assessment tools: is there a preference? *J Burn Care Rehabil* 19:451, 1998.
102. Turner JG et al: The effect of therapeutic touch on pain and anxiety in burn patients, *J Adv Nurs* 28:10, 1998.
103. Kendall-Grove KJ et al: Rates of dysfunction in parents of pediatric patients with burns, *J Burn Care Rehabil* 19:312, 1998.
104. LeDoux J et al: Relationship between parental emotional states, family environment and the behavioral adjustment of pediatric burn survivors, *Burns* 24:425, 1998.
105. Daltroy LH et al: American Burn Association/Shriners Hospitals for Children burns outcomes questionnaire: construction and psychometric properties, *J Burn Care Rehabil* 21:29, 2000.

INDEX OF SPECIAL FEATURES

ALGORITHMS

LIFESPAN CONTENT

Pediatric

Aging

NUTRITION AND DISEASE BOXES

WHAT'S NEW? BOXES

INDEX

Page numbers followed by f indicate figures; t, tables; b, boxes. Syndromes and disorders appear in **boldface** type.

C

H

O

V

MOST COMMON LABORATORY VALUES

Constituent	Normal Mean Value and Some Ranges	Normal Range in SI Units
ELECTROLYTES	Total <1% of plasma weight	
Na^+	142 mEq/L	136–142 mmol/L
K^+	4 mEq/L	3.8–5.0 mmol/L
Ca^{++}	5 mEq/L	2.1–2.6 mmol/L
Mg^{++}	3 mEq/L	1.25–1.75 mmol/L
Cl^-	103 mEq/L	95–103 mmol/L
HCO_3^-	27 mEq/L	21-28 mmol/L
Phosphate (mostly HPO_4^{2-})	2 mEq/L	0.5–1.25 mmol/L
SO_4^{2-}	1 mEq/L	0.25–0.75 mmol/L
PROTEINS	7.3 g/dl	64–83 g/L
Albumins	4.5 g/dl	33–52 g/L
Gamma globulin	0.5–1.6 g/dl	5–16 g/L
Globulins	2.5 g/dl	23–35 g/L
Fibrinogen	0.3 g/dl	2–4 g/L
BLOOD GASES		
pH	7.4	—
CO_2 content (arterial)	40 mm Hg	4.66–5.32 kPa
O_2 content (arterial)	94 mm Hg	12.64–13.30 kPa
Bicarbonate	21–28 mEq/L	21–28 mmol/L
NUTRIENTS		
Glucose and other carbohydrates	100 mg/dl	3.85–6.05 mmol/L
Total amino acids	40 mg/dl	1.50–2.50 mmol/L
Total lipids	400–800 mg/dl	4.0–8.0 g/L
Cholesterol	150–250 mg/dl	3.9–6.5 mmol/L
Triglycerides	75–165 mg/dl	0.85–1.89 mmol/L
Phospholipids	150–380 mg/dl	1.50–3.80 g/L
Free fatty acids	9.0–15.0 mM/L	—
Individual vitamins	0.0001–2.5 mg/dl	—
Individual trace elements	0.001–0.3 mg/dl	—
WASTE PRODUCTS		
Urea (BUN)	7–18 mg/dl	2.9–8.2 mmol/L
Uric acid	2–6 mg/dl	0.120–0.360
Creatinine	1 mg/dl	53–106 μmol/L
Creatinine clearance	107–139 ml/min	1.78–2.32 mmol/L
Uric acid (from nucleic acids)	5 mg/dl	0.120–0.360 mmol/L
Bilirubin (direct)	Up to 0.3 mg/dl	Up to 5.1 μmol/L
Bilirubin (indirect)	0.1–1.0 mg/dl	1.7–17.1 μmol/L

s, Serum.